DRUG INFORMATION HANDBOOK for ONCOLOGY

A Complete Guide to Combination Chemotherapy Regimens

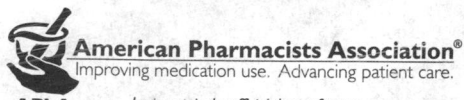

American Pharmacists Association®
Improving medication use. Advancing patient care.

APhA

Lexicomp is the official drug reference for the American Pharmacists Association.

11th Edition

SENI

Diedra
PharmD, MB

Lexicomp®

DRUG INFORMATION HANDBOOK for ONCOLOGY

A Complete Guide to Combination Chemotherapy Regimens

Diedra L. Bragalone, PharmD, MBA, BCOP, BCPS
Senior Editor
Pharmacotherapy Specialist
Lexi-Comp, Inc

Lexicomp®

APhA

NOTICE

This data is intended to serve the user as a handy reference and not as a complete drug information resource. It does not include information on every therapeutic agent available. The publication covers more than 300 commonly used drugs and is specifically designed to present important aspects of drug data in a more concise format than is typically found in medical literature or product material supplied by manufacturers.

The nature of drug information is that it is constantly evolving because of ongoing research and clinical experience and is often subject to interpretation. While great care has been taken to ensure the accuracy of the information and recommendations presented, the reader is advised that the authors, editors, reviewers, contributors, and publishers cannot be responsible for the continued currency of the information or for any errors, omissions, or the application of this information, or for any consequences arising therefrom. Therefore, the author(s) and/or the publisher shall have no liability to any person or entity with regard to claims, loss, or damage caused, or alleged to be caused, directly or indirectly, by the use of information contained herein. Because of the dynamic nature of drug information, readers are advised that decisions regarding drug therapy must be based on the independent judgment of the clinician, changing information about a drug (eg, as reflected in the literature and manufacturer's most current product information), and changing medical practices. Therefore, this data is designed to be used in conjunction with other necessary information and is not designed to be solely relied upon by any user. The user of this data hereby and forever releases the authors and publishers of this data from any and all liability of any kind that might arise out of the use of this data. The editors are not responsible for any inaccuracy of quotation or for any false or misleading implication that may arise due to the text or formulas as used or due to the quotation of revisions no longer official.

Certain contributors have written for this book in their private capacities. No official support or endorsement by any federal or state agency or pharmaceutical company is intended or inferred.

The publishers have made every effort to trace any third party copyright holders, if any, for borrowed material. If they have inadvertently overlooked any, they will be pleased to make the necessary arrangements at the first opportunity.

If you have any suggestions or questions regarding any information presented in this data, please contact our drug information pharmacists at (330) 650-6506. Book revisions are available at our website at http://www.lexi.com/home/revisions/.

This manual was produced using Lexi-Comp's Information Management System™ (LIMS) — A complete publishing service of Lexi-Comp, Inc.

Lexicomp®

1100 Terex Road • Hudson, Ohio • 44236
(330) 650-6506

Wolters Kluwer
Health

ISBN 978-1-59195-317-3

TABLE OF CONTENTS

Oncology Editorial Advisory Panel 2
Editorial Advisory Panel 3
Preface 11
Use of the Drug Information Handbook for Oncology 12
Pregnancy Categories 16
Reducing Oncology Medication Errors 18

ALPHABETICAL LISTING OF DRUGS 25

CHEMOTHERAPY REGIMEN INDEX 1500

ALPHABETICAL LISTING OF CHEMOTHERAPY REGIMENS 1511

SPECIAL TOPICS 1781
- Cancer Treatment-Related Complications 1782
- Cancer-Related Topics 1829
- Stem Cell Transplantation 1887
- Drug Development, Approval, and Distribution 1898
- Hazardous Drugs 1904

APPENDIX 1915
- Abbreviations and Measurements 1916
- Assessment of Renal Function 1924
- Comparative Drug Charts 1934
- Laboratory Values 1940

PHARMACOLOGIC CATEGORY INDEX 1947

ONCOLOGY EDITORIAL ADVISORY PANEL

Diedra L. Bragalone, PharmD, MBA, BCOP, BCPS
Pharmacotherapy Specialist
Lexi-Comp, Inc

Stephanie S. Minich, PharmD, BCOP
Pharmacotherapy Specialist
Lexi-Comp, Inc

Jennifer Fisher Lowe, PharmD, BCOP
Pharmacotherapy Contributor
Lexi-Comp, Inc

William J. Dana, PharmD, FASHP
Pharmacy Quality Assurance
Harris County Hospital District

Michael S. Edwards, PharmD, MBA, BCOP
Chief, Oncology Pharmacy
Director, Oncology Pharmacy Residency Program
Walter Reed Army Medical Center

Tracy Hagemann, PharmD
Associate Professor
College of Pharmacy
The University of Oklahoma

Mark T. Holdsworth, PharmD, BCOP
Associate Professor of Pharmacy & Pediatrics
Pharmacy Practice Area Head
College of Pharmacy
The University of New Mexico

Patrick J. Kiel, PharmD, BCPS, BCOP
Clinical Pharmacy Specialist
Hematology and Stem Cell Transplant
Indiana University Simon Cancer Center

Polly E. Kintzel, PharmD, BCPS, BCOP
Clinical Pharmacy Specialist-Oncology
Spectrum Health

Nicholas A. Link, PharmD, BCOP
Clinical Specialist, Oncology
Hillcrest Hospital

Melissa Makii, PharmD, BCPS
Clinical Pharmacy Specialist
Pediatric Oncology
Rainbow Babies & Children's Hospital

EDITORIAL ADVISORY PANEL

Matthew A. Fuller, PharmD, BCPS, BCPP, FASHP
Clinical Pharmacy Specialist, Psychiatry
Cleveland Department of Veterans Affairs Medical Center
Associate Clinical Professor of Psychiatry and *Clinical Instructor of Psychology*
Case Western Reserve University
Adjunct Associate Professor of Clinical Pharmacy
University of Toledo

Jason C. Gallagher, PharmD, BCPS
Clinical Pharmacy Specialist, Infectious Diseases
and *Clinical Associate Professor*
Temple University Hospital

Jennifer L. Gardner, PharmD
Neonatal Clinical Pharmacy Specialist
Texas Children's Hospital

Meredith D. Girard, MD, FACP
Medical Staff
Department of Internal Medicine
Summa Health Systems
Assistant Professor Internal Medicine
Northeast Ohio Medical University (NEOMED)

Morton P. Goldman, RPh, PharmD, BCPS, FCCP
Senior Editor
Lexi-Comp, Inc

Julie A. Golembiewski, PharmD
Clinical Associate Professor and *Clinical Pharmacist, Anesthesia/Pain*
Colleges of Pharmacy and Medicine
University of Illinois

Jeffrey P. Gonzales, PharmD, BCPS
Critical Care Clinical Pharmacy Specialist
University of Maryland Medical Center

Roland Grad, MDCM, MSc, CCFP, FCFP
Associate Professor
Department of Family Medicine
McGill University

Larry D. Gray, PhD, ABMM
Director, Clinical Microbiology
TriHealth Laboratories
Bethesda and Good Samaritan Hospitals

Tracy Hagemann, PharmD
Associate Professor
College of Pharmacy
The University of Oklahoma

JoEllen L. Hanigosky, PharmD
Clinical Coordinator
Department of Hematology/Oncology/Bone Marrow Transplant
Children's Hospital of Akron

Martin D. Higbee, PharmD
Associate Professor
Department of Pharmacy Practice and Science
The University of Arizona

Jane Hurlburt Hodding, PharmD
Executive Director, Inpatient Pharmacy Services and Clinical Nutrition Services
Long Beach Memorial Medical Center and Miller Children's Hospital

Mark T. Holdsworth, PharmD, BCOP
Associate Professor of Pharmacy & Pediatrics
and *Pharmacy Practice Area Head*
College of Pharmacy
The University of New Mexico

Edward Horn, PharmD, BCPS
Clinical Specialist, Transplant Surgery
Allegheny General Hospital

Collin A. Hovinga, PharmD
Director of Research and Associate Professor
Dell Children's Medical Center
UT Austin School of Pharmacy

Darrell T. Hulisz, PharmD
Associate Professor
Department of Family Medicine
Case Western Reserve University

John J. Lewin III, PharmD, BCPS
Clinical Specialist, Neurosciences Critical Care
The Johns Hopkins Hospital

Jeffrey D. Lewis, PharmD, MACM
Associate Dean and Associate Professor of Pharmacy Practice
Cedarville University School of Pharmacy

John Lindsley, PharmD, BCPS
Cardiology Clinical Pharmacy Specialist
The Johns Hopkins Hospital

Nicholas A. Link, PharmD, BCOP
Clinical Specialist, Oncology
Hillcrest Hospital

Jennifer Fisher Lowe, PharmD, BCOP
Pharmacotherapy Contributor
Lexi-Comp, Inc

Sherry Luedtke, PharmD
Associate Professor
Department of Pharmacy Practice
Texas Tech University HSC School of Pharmacy

Melissa Makii, PharmD, BCPS
Clinical Pharmacy Specialist
Pediatric Oncology
Rainbow Babies & Children's Hospital

Vincent F. Mauro, BS, PharmD, FCCP
Professor of Clinical Pharmacy
and *Adjunct Professor of Medicine*
Colleges of Pharmacy and Medicine
The University of Toledo

Barrie McCombs, MD, FCFP
Medical Information Service Coordinator
The Alberta Rural Physician Action Plan

Christopher McPherson, PharmD
Clinical Pharmacist
Neonatal Intensive Care Unit
St. Louis Children's Hospital

Timothy F. Meiller, DDS, PhD
Professor
Oncology and Diagnostic Sciences
Baltimore College of Dental Surgery
Professor of Oncology
Marlene and Stewart Greenebaum Cancer Center
University of Maryland Medical System

Geralyn M. Meny, MD
Medical Director
American Red Cross, Penn-Jersey Region

Charla E. Miller, RPh, PharmD
Neonatal Clinical Pharmacy Specialist
Wolfson Children's Hospital

Julie Miller, PharmD
Pharmacy Clinical Specialist, Cardiology
Columbus Children's Hospital

Katherine Mills, PharmD
Pharmacotherapy Contributor
Lexi-Comp, Inc

Leah Millstein, MD
Assistant Professor
Division of General Internal Medicine
University of Maryland School of Medicine

Stephanie S. Minich, PharmD, BCOP
Pharmacotherapy Specialist
Lexi-Comp, Inc

Kim Moeller, RN, MSN, OCN, ACNS-BC
Advanced Practice Nurse
Summit Oncology Associates

Kevin M. Mulieri, BS, PharmD
Pediatric Hematology/Oncology Clinical Specialist
Penn State Milton S. Hershey Medical Center
Instructor of Pharmacology
Penn State College of Medicine

Elizabeth A. Neuner, PharmD, BCPS
Infectious Diseases Clinical Specialist
The Cleveland Clinic Foundation

Joni Lombardi Stahura, BS, PharmD, RPh
Pharmacotherapy Specialist
Lexi-Comp, Inc

Kim Stevens, RN
Home Care
Samaritan Regional Health System

Stephen Marc Stout, PharmD, MS, BCPS
Pharmacotherapy Specialist
Lexi-Comp, Inc

Dan Streetman, PharmD, RPh
Pharmacotherapy Specialist
Lexi-Comp, Inc

Darcie-Ann Streetman, PharmD, RPh
Clinical Pharmacist
University of Michigan Health System

Carol K. Taketomo, PharmD
Director of Pharmacy and Nutrition Services
Children's Hospital Los Angeles

Mary Temple Cooper, PharmD
Pediatric Clinical Research Specialist
Hillcrest Hospital

Elizabeth A. Tomsik, PharmD, BCPS
Manager
Adverse Drug Reactions Group
Lexi-Comp, Inc

Dana Travis, RPh
Pharmacotherapy Specialist
Lexi-Comp, Inc

Jennifer Trofe-Clark, PharmD
Clinical Transplant Pharmacist
Hospital of The University of Pennsylvania

John N. van den Anker, MD, PhD, FCP, FAAP
Vice Chair of Pediatrics for Experimental Therapeutics
and *Chief and Professor of Evan and Cindy Jones Pediatric Clinical Pharmacology*
Children's National Medical Center
Professor of Pediatrics, Pharmacology & Physiology
George Washington University School of Medicine and Health Sciences

Heather L. VandenBussche, PharmD
Professor of Pharmacy, Pediatrics
Pharmacy Practice
Ferris State University College of Pharmacy

Amy Van Orman, PharmD, BCPS
Pharmacotherapy Specialist
Lexi-Comp, Inc

Kristin Watson, PharmD, BCPS
Assistant Professor, Cardiology
and *Clinical Pharmacist, Cardiology Service*
Heart Failure Clinic
University of Maryland Medical Center

David M. Weinstein, PhD, RPh
Manager
Metabolism, Interactions, and Genomics Group
Lexi-Comp, Inc

Anne Marie Whelan, PharmD
Associate Professor
College of Pharmacy
Dalhouise University

Sherri J. Willard Argyres, MA, PharmD
Medical Science Pharmacist
Lexi-Comp, Inc

John C. Williamson, PharmD, BCPS
Pharmacy Clinical Coordinator, Infectious Diseases
Wake Forest Baptist Health

Nathan Wirick, PharmD
Infectious Disease and Antibiotic Management Clinical Specialist
Hillcrest Hospital

EDITORIAL ADVISORY PANEL

PREFACE

The *Drug Information Handbook for Oncology* was designed to meet the needs of all oncology professionals involved in prescribing, preparing, and administering therapy. Presented in a concise and uniform format, this book contains monographs with information pertaining to both antineoplastic agents and ancillary or supportive care medications. This handbook serves as a portable quick reference while providing comprehensive oncology-related drug information. Organized like a dictionary for ease-of-use, a drug monograph can be quickly located by generic name.

The Chemotherapy Regimen section provides a comprehensive presentation of cancer chemotherapy regimens. The regimens are listed alphabetically by regimen name (acronym). An index lists regimens by indication. In addition, a special Combination Chemotherapy Regimen field in each drug monograph will link you to the applicable regimens.

A special topics section addresses issues regarding Cancer Treatment-Related Complications (eg, oral mucositis / stomatitis, management of chemotherapy-induced nausea and vomiting, management of infections); Cancer-Related Topics (eg, chemotherapy and cancer treatment during pregnancy, chemotherapy and obesity, principles of anticancer therapy, common toxicity criteria, venous thromboembolism in the cancer patient); and Safe Handling of Hazardous Drugs.

The appendix section includes information related to conversions, renal function, comparative drug charts, and laboratory reference values for adults. A pharmacologic category index provides a practical approach to categorizing drugs by their respective therapeutic classification.

We know you will find this handbook to be a valuable source of information and we welcome comments or suggestions to further improve future editions.

USE OF THE DRUG INFORMATION HANDBOOK FOR ONCOLOGY

The *Drug Information Handbook for Oncology* is divided into six sections.

The first section is a compilation of introductory text pertinent to the use of this book.

The drug information section of the handbook, in which all drugs are listed alphabetically, details information pertinent to each drug. Extensive cross-referencing is provided by U.S. brand names, Canadian brand names, and index terms.

The Chemotherapy Regimen section provides a comprehensive presentation of cancer chemotherapy regimens. The regimens are listed alphabetically by regimen name (acronym). An index at the beginning of this section lists regimens by indications. In addition, a special Combination Chemotherapy Regimen field in each drug monograph will link you to the applicable regimens.

The Special Topics section contains important cancer-related issues (ie, chemotherapy and cancer treatment during pregnancy, chemotherapy and obesity, principles of anticancer therapy, and safe handling of hazardous drugs). These issues are discussed in detail.

The fifth section is an appendix section.

The last section of this handbook is an index listing drugs in their unique pharmacologic category.

Alphabetical Listing of Drugs

Drug information is presented in a consistent format and provides the following:

Generic Name	U.S. adopted name
Pronunciation Guide	Phonetic pronunciation
Related Information	Cross-reference to other pertinent drug information found elsewhere in this handbook
Brand Names: U.S.	Trade names (manufacturer-specific) found in the United States. The symbol [DSC] appears after trade names that have been recently discontinued.
Brand Names: Canada	Trade names found in Canada
Index Terms	Includes names or accepted abbreviations of the generic drug; may include common brand names no longer available; this field is used to create cross-references to monographs
Generic Availability (U.S.)	Indicates availability of generic products in the United States.
Pharmacologic Category	Unique systematic classification of medications
Use	Information pertaining to appropriate FDA-approved indications of the drug.
Unlabeled Use	Information pertaining to non-FDA-approved indications of the drug.

Labeled Contraindications	Information pertaining to inappropriate use of the drug as dictated by approved labeling.
Pregnancy Risk Factor	Five categories established by the FDA to indicate the potential of a systemically absorbed drug for causing risk to fetus.
Lactation	Indicates if the drug listed in the monograph is present in breast milk and the manufacturers' recommendation for use while breast-feeding (where recommendation of American Academy of Pediatrics differs, notation is made).
Warnings/Precautions	Precautionary considerations, hazardous conditions related to use of the drug, and disease states or patient populations in which the drug should be cautiously used. Boxed warnings, when present, are clearly identified and are adapted from the FDA approved labeling. Consult the product labeling for the exact black box warning through the manufacturer's or the FDA website.
Adverse Reactions	Side effects are grouped by percentage of incidence (if known) and/or body system
Drug Interactions	
Metabolism/Transport Effects	If a drug has demonstrated involvement with cytochrome P450 enzymes, or other metabolism or transport proteins, this field will identify the drug as an inhibitor, inducer, or substrate of the specific enzyme(s) (eg, CYP1A2 or UGT1A1). CYP450 isoenzymes are identified as substrates (minor or major), inhibitors (weak, moderate, or strong), and inducers (weak or strong).
Avoid Concomitant Use	Designates drug combinations which should not be used concomitantly, due to an unacceptable risk:benefit assessment. Frequently, the concurrent use of the agents is explicitly prohibited or contraindicated by the product labeling.
Increased Effect/Toxicity	Drug combinations that result in a increased or toxic therapeutic effect between the drug listed in the monograph and other drugs or drug classes.
Decreased Effect	Drug combinations that result in a decreased therapeutic effect between the drug listed in the monograph and other drugs or drug classes.
Ethanol/Nutrition/Herb Interactions	Presents a description of the interaction between the drug listed in the monograph and ethanol, food, or herb/nutraceuticals.
Storage/Stability	Information regarding storage of product. Provides the time and conditions for which a solution or mixture will maintain full potency. For example, some solutions may require refrigeration after reconstitution while stored at room temperature prior to preparation.
Reconstitution	Includes comments on solution choice with time or conditions for the mixture to maintain full potency before administration
Mechanism of Action	How the drug works in the body to elicit a response
Pharmacodynamics/Kinetics	The magnitude of a drug's effect depends on the drug concentration at the site of action. The pharmacodynamics are expressed in terms of onset of action and duration of action. Pharmacokinetics are expressed in terms of absorption, distribution (including appearance in breast milk and crossing of the placenta), protein binding, metabolism, bioavailability, half-life, time to peak serum concentration, and elimination.

Dosing	The amount of drug to be typically given or taken during therapy; may include the following:
Adult	The recommended amount of drug to be given to adult patients
Adult & Geriatric	This combined field is only used to indicate that no specific adjustments for elderly patients were identified. However, other issues should be considered (eg, renal or hepatic impairment). Also refer to Geriatric Considerations for additional information related to the elderly.
Geriatric	A suggested amount of drug to be given to elderly patients; may include adjustments from adult dosing (lack of information in the monograph may imply that the drug is not used in the elderly patient or no specific adjustments could be identified)
Pediatric	Suggested amount of drug to be given to neonates, infants, and children. The following age group definitions are utilized to characterize age-related dosing unless otherwise specified in the monograph: Neonate (0-28 days of age), infant (>28 days to 1 year of age), children (1-12 years of age), and adolescent (13-18 years of age).
Renal Impairment	Suggested dosage adjustments based on compromised renal function; may include dosing instructions for patients on dialysis
Hepatic Impairment	Suggested dosage adjustments based on compromised liver function
Adjustment for Toxicity	Suggested dosage adjustments in the event specific toxicities related to therapy are noted, such as hematologic toxicities related to cancer chemotherapy
Combination Regimens	List of combination chemotherapy regimens in which the drug is a component
Usual Infusion Concentrations	Information describing the usual concentrations of drugs for administration in the pediatric and adult populations as appropriate. Concentrations are derived from the literature, manufacturer recommendation, or organizational recommendations (eg, the Institute for Safe Medication Practices [ISMP]) and are universally established. Institution-specific standard concentrations may differ from those listed.
Administration	Information regarding the recommended final concentrations, rates of administration for parenteral drugs, or other guidelines when giving the medication
Emetic Potential	Likelihood that the drug will cause nausea or vomiting
Vesicant/Extravasation Risk	Indicates whether the drug is considered to be a vesicant and likely to cause significant morbidity if the infusion infiltrates soft tissues
Extemporaneous Preparations	Directions for preparing oral or rectal suppositories or liquid formulations from solid drug products. May include stability information and references.
Monitoring Parameters	Laboratory tests and patient physical parameters that should be monitored for safety and efficacy of drug therapy.
Test Interactions	Listing of assay interferences when relevant; (B) = Blood; (S) = Serum; (U) = Urine
Dietary Considerations	Specific dietary modifications and/or restrictions
Additional Information	Pertinent information about specific brands

Product Availability	Provides availability information on products that have been approved by the FDA, but not yet available for use. Estimates for when a product may be available are included, when this information is known. May also provide any unique or critical drug availability issues.
Prescribing and Access Restrictions	Provides information on any special requirements regarding the prescribing, obtaining or dispensing of drugs, including access restrictions pertaining to drugs with REMS elements and those drugs whose access restrictions are not REMS-related.
Medication Guide Available	Identifies drugs that have an FDA-approved Medication Guide.
Dosage Forms	Information with regard to form, strength, and availability of the drug in the United States. **Note:** Additional formulation information (eg, excipients, preservatives) is included when available. Please consult product labeling for further information.
Dosage Forms: Canada	Information with regard to form, strength, and availability of products that are uniquely available in Canada, but currently not available in the United States.
Controlled Substance	Contains controlled substance schedule information as assigned by the United States Drug Enforcement Administration (DEA) or Canadian Controlled Substance Act (CDSA). CDSA information is only provided for drugs available in Canada and not available in the U.S.
References	Recommended for additional information

Chemotherapy Regimens

The Chemotherapy Regimen section provides a comprehensive presentation of cancer chemotherapy regimens. The regimens are listed alphabetically by regimen name (acronym). An index lists regimens by indications. In addition, a special Combination Chemotherapy Regimen field in each drug monograph will guide you to the applicable regimens.

Special Topics

Important cancer-related issues (ie, managing infections, oral mucositis / stomatitis, chemotherapy and cancer treatment during pregnancy, chemotherapy and obesity, principles of anticancer therapy, chronic pain management [cancer], hospice [end of life] care, palliative care medicine [cancer], hematopoietic stem cell transplantation, safe handling of hazardous drugs, venous thromboembolism in the cancer patient) are discussed in detail.

Appendix

The appendix offers a compilation of tables, guidelines, nomograms, algorithms, and conversion information which can often be helpful when considering patient care.

Pharmacologic Category Index

This index provides a useful listing of drugs by their pharmacologic classification.

PREGNANCY CATEGORIES

Pregnancy Categories (sometimes referred to as pregnancy risk factors) are a letter system currently required under the *Teratogenic Effects* subsection of the product labeling. The system was initiated in 1979. The categories are required to be part of the package insert for prescription drugs that are systemically absorbed.

The categories are defined as follows:

A Adequate and well-controlled studies in pregnant women have not shown that the drug increases the risk of fetal abnormalities.

B Animal reproduction studies show no evidence of impaired fertility or harm to the fetus; however, no adequate and well-controlled studies have been conducted in pregnant women.
or
Animal reproduction studies have shown adverse events; however, studies in pregnant women have not shown that the drug increases the risk of abnormalities.

C Animal reproduction studies have shown an adverse effect on the fetus. There are no adequate and well-controlled studies in humans and the benefits from the use of the drug in pregnant women may be acceptable, despite its potential risks.
or
Animal reproduction studies have not been conducted.

D Based on human data, the drug can cause fetal harm when administered to pregnant women, but the potential benefits from the use of the drug may be acceptable, despite its potential risks.

X Studies in animals or humans have demonstrated fetal abnormalities (or there is positive evidence of fetal risk based on reports and/or marketing experience) and the risk of using the drug in pregnant women clearly outweighs any possible benefit (for example, safer drugs or other forms of therapy are available).

The categories do not take into consideration nonteratogenic effects (that information is currently presented separately). In 2008, the Food and Drug Administration (FDA) proposed new labeling requirements which would eliminate the use of the pregnancy category system and replace it with scientific data and other information specific to the use of the drug in pregnant women. These proposed changes were suggested because the current category system may be misleading. For instance, some practitioners may believe that risk increases from category A to B to C to D to X, which is not the intent. In addition, practitioners may not be aware that some medications are categorized based on animal data, while others are based on human data. When the new labeling requirements are approved, product labeling will contain pregnancy and lactation subsections, each describing a risk summary, clinical considerations, and section for specific data.

For full descriptions of the current and proposed labeling requirements, refer to the following websites:

Labeling Requirements for Prescription Drugs and/or Insulin (Code of Federal Regulations, Title 21, Volume 4, Revised April 1, 2010). Available at http://www.accessdata.fda.gov/scripts/cdrh/cfdocs/cfCFR/CFRSearch.cfm?fr=201.57

Content and Format of Labeling for Human Prescription Drug and Biological Products; Requirements for Pregnancy and Lactation Labeling (Federal Register, May 29, 2008). Available at http://frwebgate.access.gpo.gov/cgi-bin/getdoc.cgi?dbname=2008_register&docid=fr29my08-33.pdf

REDUCING ONCOLOGY MEDICATION ERRORS

Medication errors occurring in patients receiving treatment and supportive care for cancer remain a serious problem. Risk factors are numerous, and include the multiple numbers and cycles of medication, the various routes of administration, the various locations of administration, which can progress from inpatient to ambulatory care to home administration, and to the fact that patients from the very young to the elderly are frequently administered these agents. Many of the antineoplastic agents have a narrow therapeutic index and can produce unexpected toxicities with the slightest alteration in dosage. Subtherapeutic dosing may also be detrimental, producing less toxicity, but possibly resulting in decreased efficacy and affecting patient outcomes.

The incidence of medication errors in oncology patients noted in the published literature range from 3% to 4% in adult and pediatric inpatient and ambulatory settings, and from 10% to 20% for patients receiving oral antineoplastic therapy at home. Although the numbers appear small in some settings and many of the published medication errors are caught before reaching the patient ("near misses"), the impact can be disastrous. Published literature indicates that antineoplastic agents rank second only to central nervous system medications in causing fatal medication errors.

Medication errors involving chemotherapy and supportive care have been documented in all stages of the drug therapy process, from prescribing to compounding, dispensing, and administration, including patient self-medication at home. Various risk factors for medication errors have been identified at each stage. Accordingly, institutions and healthcare organizations have developed and continue to refine various standards, consensus documents, policies/procedures, and other safeguards to minimize the safety risk. Examples are noted in the following paragraphs.

Facilities providing chemotherapy should establish and ensure that members of the oncology team have appropriate education, training, competency, credentialing, and continuing education to care for patients receiving antineoplastic therapy. Staff must also be educated on safe handling of hazardous agents. Additionally, and fundamental to most safety strategies, is the standardization of the prescribing and documentation process through established guidelines, policies, and procedures which should be followed by all healthcare professionals involved. The use of collaboratively developed preprinted order forms or predefined computer generated order sets for approved protocols or treatment plans is one method to facilitate standardization. Examples of standardizing of the ordering processes, medication nomenclature, dosing, and other elements are noted below.

MEDICATION PRESCRIBING AND VERIFICATION

- Do not permit or accept verbal orders for chemotherapy, except for withholding or discontinuation of treatment.
- While there are certain situations in which treatment is urgent, do not permit or accept "STAT" orders for chemotherapy.

- Use redundant checks and verifications (by a second individual) at different points of the chemotherapy medication use process, (eg, prescribing, preparation, dispensing, administration).
- Individuals verifying orders that contain calculations should independently perform their own calculations, rather than checking another's mathematical work.

MEDICATION NAMES

Chemotherapy agents are highly susceptible to sound-alike/look-alike confusion (eg, fluorouracil / flucytosine / fluocinonide, leucovorin / Leukine® / Alkeran® / Leukeran®) so particular precaution should be heeded to ensure correct drug identified by those interpreting the order.

- Use full generic names including descriptive terms, (eg, liposomal). Brand names should be reserved for products when they assist in further identifying the correct product (eg, combination product or liposomal vs non-liposomal formulation).
- Use full study name and/or protocol number with investigational antineoplastic treatments.
- Avoid abbreviated medication names, (eg, CTX, HN_2, MTX, VCR, or generalized generic terms [eg, "platinum" which can create confusion between CISplatin, CARBOplatin, and oxaliplatin]).
- Avoid investigational names for medications **with FDA approval** (eg, VP-16, FK-506, CBDCA).
- Utilize TALLman lettering (eg, DAUNOrubicin / DOXOrubicin, VinBLAStine / VinCRIStine).
- Omit the use of numbers within a medication name (eg, fluorouracil is correct, 5-fluorouracil is **incorrect**; mercaptopurine is correct, 6-mercaptopurine is **incorrect**).
- Avoid abbreviated names or acronyms for multidrug regimens, (eg, MOPP, ICE, ProMACE).

MEDICATION DOSE AND DURATION

- Include variables used for dosage calculations on the chemotherapy orders to allow for necessary double checks, (eg, height [centimeters], weight [kilograms], BSA, laboratory test results or creatinine clearance). It is recommended that organizations standardize equations used for BSA and creatinine clearance calculations and situations when dosing should be based on actual or ideal body weight.
- Use full weight-based dosing when appropriate (eg, for curative intent) in obese adult cancer patients to avoid underdosing.
- Provide supporting references and/or rationale when doses vary from a standard regimen or are prescribed as flat doses to allow for necessary double-checks.
- Provide complete dosing information including calculated dose with reduction noted with rationale, total volume and solution to administer dose (if applicable), route of administration, rate or number of hours or days that dose is to be administered, which specific days dose is to be administered

and total dose per treatment course, cycle or cumulative lifetime (if applicable). In some situations, clearly defining when to initiate therapy (Day 0 or Day 1) may be necessary for clarity.

Example: Patient = 1.8 m^2

Drug "X" 50 mg/m^2/day I.V. push for 3 days = 90 mg I.V. push on Days 3, 4, and 5 (Total Dose Drug "X" per cycle = 150 mg/m^2 = 270 mg)

- Always use a leading zero for numbers less than 1 (0.5 mg is correct and .5 mg is **incorrect**) and never use a trailing zero for whole numbers (2 mg is correct and 2.0 mg is **incorrect**).
- For doses that are greater than 1,000 dosing units, use properly placed commas to prevent 10-fold errors (100,000 units is correct and 100000 units is **incorrect**).
- Avoid dangerous, error-prone abbreviations (eg, regardless of letter-case: U, IU, QD, QOD, µg, cc, @, MS, MS04, MgS04). Regarding the example above, the terminology "I.V. push" is commonly used and accepted. However, consider using the complete term "intravenous push," and stating the rate of infusion for the "push" dose to minimize confusion.
- Establish regimen-specific appropriate monitoring (eg, laboratory tests) and follow-up intervals.
- Establish dosing and administration constraints including maximum single doses, maximum doses within specified time limits and acceptable routes and rates of administration.
- Consider verification of lifetime dosing limits for certain agents, including DOXOrubicin, DAUNOrubicin, EPIrubicin, IDArubicin, and bleomycin.

ORAL CHEMOTHERAPY

Medication errors involving oral chemotherapy in both adult and pediatric patients are being increasingly reported and like other routes of administration, the origin of the error ranges from prescribing to dispensing to patient self-administration. Oral chemotherapy should go through the same double-check system in which parenteral chemotherapy is processed. Patient noncompliance with the prescribed dose regimen is a concern for institutional, outpatient, and retail practices. A major risk factor for these errors is the multiple dosage strengths for many agents, which must be combined to provide the prescribed dose. The prescriber, the pharmacist, and the patient must be cautious and very clear in the process of prescribing, dispensing, and administering the desired dose. Increased emphasis on patient counseling and additional techniques such as pill counts may decrease error risk and increase adherence.

INTRATHECAL CHEMOTHERAPY

- During the admixture process, intrathecal agents should not be prepared during the preparation of any other agents.
- After preparation, keep in an isolated location or container clearly marked with a label identifying as "intrathecal" use only.
- Delivery to the patient should only be with other medications intended for administration into the central nervous system.

THE ROLE OF TECHNOLOGY

Computerized provider order entry (CPOE) and bar-code technology have been adopted by some institutions and practices in an effort to improve safety and efficiency and enhance communication between healthcare providers. Both technology tools have been shown to be useful, but certainly do not replace the need for continued surveillance and safety checks in all stages of the chemotherapy order process. For example, CPOE has been shown to decrease prescribing errors, but has little or no impact on dispensing and administration mistakes.

THE ROLE OF THE CANCER PATIENT

The patient remains the one constant in every health practitioner encounter, and could provide vigilance and support in identifying and preventing errors in his/her therapy. The majority of cancer patients are knowledgeable about their disease and their treatments, and can serve as a valuable resource in error prevention. Institutions should foster an environment which encourages patient participation. Informed consent for chemotherapy must be obtained prior to chemotherapy administration. A policy to assess adherence or oral chemotherapy should be developed.

Provide patient education, including information on:

- Medication(s), schedule, and planned duration
- Management of missed doses
- Possible short- and long-term adverse effects, including possible risks to future fertility (if applicable)
- Symptoms that should trigger notification of healthcare provider (and who to notify)
- Proper handling and storage of oral medications and proper disposal of unused medications

Medication errors are inevitable in all healthcare scenarios, including oncology. When such events occur, the issues of appropriate disclosure and follow-up are first priorities. The published literature has provided some insight to disclosure and to the support required by the patient and the healthcare team in such events. References addressing this issue are among the list at the end of the chapter.

ON-GOING INSTITUTIONAL REVIEW TO INCREASE ONCOLOGY MEDICATION SAFETY

Institutions and oncology practices should constantly review the chemotherapy order process and look for opportunities to promote a culture of safety:

- Consistent education to the healthcare team on all aspects of chemotherapy management
- Re-engineer processes if needed, as per the following examples:
  - Centralize the pharmaceutical chemotherapy compound process
  - Observe work flow: Minimize nursing interruptions during the administration of oncology medications, which has been shown to affect the incidence and severity of errors with high-risk medications

  - Restrict certain high-risk medications from specific hospital or clinic locations, such as keeping vinca alkaloids away from certain procedure areas to minimize risk of wrong route administration
  - Special packaging and warning labels for high-alert medications
  - Computer pop-up alerts
- Document, review, and discuss all oncology medication errors, including the "near misses"; not for punitive measures, but as teaching tools to improve the oncology medication process.
- Enhance communication among all healthcare team members (ie, utilize or improve the medication reconciliation process).

SELECTED READINGS

Aboumatar HJ, Winner L, Davis R, et al, "Applying Lean Sigma Solutions to Mistake-Proof the Chemotherapy Preparation Process," *Jt Comm J Qual Patient Saf*, 2010, 36(2):79-86.

ASHP Council on Professional Affairs, "ASHP Guidelines on Preventing Medication Errors With Antineoplastic Agents," *Am J Health Syst Pharm*, 2002, 59(17):1648-68.

Bartel SB, "Safe Practices and Financial Considerations in Using Oral Chemotherapeutic Agents," *Am J Health Syst Pharm*, 2007, 64(9 Suppl 5):S8-S14.

Bonnabry P, Cingria L, Ackermann M, et al, "Use of a Prospective Risk Analysis Method to Improve the Safety of the Cancer Chemotherapy Process," *Int J Qual Health Care*, 2006, 18(1):9-16.

Brunetti L, Santell JP, and Hicks RW, "The Impact of Abbreviations on Patient Safety," *Jt Comm J Qual Patient Saf*, 2007, 33(9):576-83.

Cooke DL, Dunscombe PB, and Lee RC, "Using a Survey of Incident Reporting and Learning Practices to Improve Organisational Learning at a Cancer Care Centre," *Qual Saf Health Care*, 2007, 16(5):342-8.

Crossno CL, Cartwright JA, and Hargrove FR, "Using CPOE to Improve Communication, Safety, and Policy Compliance When Ordering Pediatric Chemotherapy," *Hosp Pharm*, 2007, 42(4):368–73.

DuBeshter B, Griggs J, Angel C, et al, "Chemotherapy Dose Limits Set by Users of a Computer Order Entry System," *Hosp Pharm*, 2006, 41(2):136-42.

Griggs JJ, Mangu PB, Anderson H, et al, "Appropriate Chemotherapy Dosing for Obese Adult Patients With Cancer: American Society of Clinical Oncology Clinical Practice Guideline," *J Clin Oncol*, 2012, 30(13):1553-61.

Harris TJ and Northfelt DW, "Chemotherapy Error: Practical Approaches to Increasing Patient Safety," *J Patient Safety*, 2005,1(4):215-9.

Jacobson JO, Polovich M, Gilmore TR, et al, "Revisions to the 2009 American Society of Clinical Oncology/Oncology Nursing Society Chemotherapy Administration Safety Standards: Expanding the Scope to Include Inpatient Settings," *J Oncol Pract*, 2012, 8(1):2-6.

Jacobson JO, Polovich M, McNiff KK, et al, "American Society of Clinical Oncology/Oncology Nursing Society Chemotherapy Administration Safety Standards," *J Clin Oncol*, 2009, 27 (32):5469-75.

Kozakiewicz JM, Benis LJ, Fisher SM, et al, "Safe Chemotherapy Administration: Using Failure Mode and Effects Analysis in Computerized Prescriber Order Entry," *Am J Health Syst Pharm*, 2005, 62(17):1813-6.

Markert A, Thierry V, Kleber M, et al, "Chemotherapy Safety and Severe Adverse Events in Cancer Patients: Strategies to Efficiently Avoid Chemotherapy Errors in In- and Outpatient Treatment," *Int J Cancer*, 2009, 124(3):722-8.

Poon EG, Keohane CA, Yoon CS, et al, "Effect of Bar-Code Technology on the Safety of Medication Administration," *N Engl J Med*, 2010, 362(18):1698-707.

Rinke ML, Shore AD, Morlock L, et al, "Characteristics of Pediatric Chemotherapy Medication Errors in a National Error Reporting Database," *Cancer*, 2007, 110(1):186-95.

Schwappach DL and Wernli M, "Chemotherapy Patients' Perceptions of Drug Administration Safety," *J Clin Oncol*, 2010, 28(17):2896-901.

Schwappach DL and Wernli M, "Medication Errors in Chemotherapy: Incidence, Types and Involvement of Patients in Prevention. A Review of the Literature," *Eur J Cancer Care (Engl)*, 2010, 19(3):285-92.

Schwappach DL, Hochreutener MA, and Wernli M, "Oncology Nurses' Perceptions About Involving Patients in the Prevention of Chemotherapy Administration Errors," *Oncol Nurs Forum*, 2010, 37 (2):E84-91.

To Err is Human: Building a Safer Health System, Kohn LT, Corrigan JM, and Donaldson MS, eds, Washington, D.C.: National Academy Press, 2000.

Trbovich P, Prakash V, Stewart J, et al, "Interruptions During the Delivery of High-Risk Medications," *J Nurs Adm*, 2010, 40(5):211-8.

Walsh KE, Dodd KS, Seetharaman K, et al, "Medication Errors Among Adults and Children With Cancer in the Outpatient Setting," *J Clin Oncol*, 2009, 27(6):891-6.

Weingart SN, Price J, Duncombe D, et al, "Patient-Reported Safety and Quality of Care in Outpatient Oncology," *Jt Comm J Qual Patient Saf*, 2007, 33(2):83-94.

Weingart SN, Simchowitz B, Eng TK, et al, "The You CAN Campaign: Teamwork Training for Patients and Families in Ambulatory Oncology," *Jt Comm J Qual Patient Saf*, 2009, 35(2):63-71.

Weingart SN, Toro J, Spencer J, et al, "Medication Errors Involving Oral Chemotherapy," *Cancer*, 2010, 116(10):2455-64.

Westbrook JI, Woods A, Rob MI, et al, "Association of Interruptions With an Increased Risk and Severity of Medication Administration Errors," *Arch Intern Med*, 2010, 170(8):683-90.

ALPHABETICAL LISTING OF DRUGS

◆ **Abbott-43818** *see* Leuprolide *on page* 876
◆ **ABCD** *see* Amphotericin B Cholesteryl Sulfate Complex *on page* 78
◆ **Abelcet®** *see* Amphotericin B (Lipid Complex) *on page* 84
◆ **ABI-007** *see* PACLitaxel (Protein Bound) *on page* 1098
◆ **Abiraterone** *see* Abiraterone Acetate *on page* 26

Abiraterone Acetate (a bir A ter one AS e tate)

Related Information

Principles of Anticancer Therapy *on page* 1878

Brand Names: U.S. Zytiga™

Brand Names: Canada Zytiga™

Index Terms Abiraterone; CB7630

Generic Availability (U.S.) No

Pharmacologic Category Antiandrogen; Antineoplastic Agent, Antiandrogen

Use Treatment of metastatic, castration-resistant prostate cancer (in combination with prednisone) in patients previously treated with docetaxel

Labeled Contraindications Use in women who are or may become pregnant

Canadian labeling: Additional contraindication (not in U.S. labeling): Hypersensitivity to abiraterone acetate or any component of the formulation or container

Pregnancy Risk Factor X

Lactation Excretion in breast milk unknown/not recommended

Warnings/Precautions Hazardous agent; use appropriate precautions for handling and disposal. Significant increases in liver enzymes have been reported; may require dosage reduction or discontinuation. ALT, AST, and bilirubin should be monitored prior to treatment, every 2 weeks for 3 months and monthly thereafter; patients with hepatic impairment, elevations in liver function tests, or experiencing hepatotoxicity require more frequent monitoring (see dosage adjustment for hepatic impairment and monitoring parameters). Evaluate liver function promptly with signs or symptoms of hepatotoxicity. The safety of retreatment after significant elevations (ALT or AST >20 times the upper limit of normal [ULN] or total bilirubin >10 times ULN) has not been evaluated. Avoid use in patients with pre-existing severe hepatic impairment; dosage reduction is recommended in patients with baseline moderate impairment. Canadian labeling (not in U.S. labeling) also recommends avoiding use in patients with pre-existing moderate hepatic impairment.

Concurrent infection, stress, or interruption of daily corticosteroids is associated with reports of adrenocortical insufficiency. Monitor closely for signs and symptoms of adrenocorticoid insufficiency, which could be masked by adverse events associated with mineralocorticoid excess. Diagnostic testing for insufficiency may be clinically indicated. Increased corticosteroid doses may be required before, during, and after stress. May cause increased mineralocorticoid levels, which may result in hypertension, hypokalemia and fluid retention. Concomitant administration with corticosteroids reduces the incidence and severity of these adverse events. Due to potential for hypertension, hypokalemia, or fluid retention, use with caution in patients with cardiovascular disease (particularly heart failure, recent MI, or ventricular arrhythmia); patients with left ventricular ejection fraction (LVEF) <50% or NYHA class III or IV heart failure were excluded from clinical trials. Monitor at least monthly for hypertension, hypokalemia, and fluid retention.

Must be administered on an empty stomach (administer at least 1 hour before and 2 hours after any food). Avoid (or use caution) with concomitant CYP3A4 strong inhibitors and inducers. Avoid concurrent administration with CYP2D6 substrates with a narrow therapeutic index (eg, thioridazine); if concurrent administration cannot be avoided, consider a dose reduction of the CYP2D6 substrate.

Adverse Reactions Note: Adverse reactions reported for use in combination with prednisone.

>10%:

Cardiovascular: Edema (27%)

Endocrine & metabolic: Triglycerides increased (63%), hypokalemia (28%; grades 3/4: 5%), hypophosphatemia (24%; grades 3/4: 7%), hot flush (19%)

Gastrointestinal: Diarrhea (18%)

Genitourinary: Urinary tract infection (12%)

Hepatic: AST increased (31%; grades 3/4: 2%), ALT increased (11%; grades 3/4: 1%)

Neuromuscular & skeletal: Joint swelling/discomfort (30%), muscle discomfort (26%)

Respiratory: Cough (11%)

1% to 10%:

Cardiovascular: Hypertension (9%; grades 3/4: 1%), arrhythmia (7%), chest pain/discomfort (4%), heart failure (2%)

Gastrointestinal: Dyspepsia (6%)

Genitourinary: Polyuria (7%), nocturia (6%)

Hepatic: Bilirubin increased (7%; grades 3/4: <1%)

Neuromuscular & skeletal: Fractures (6%)

Respiratory: Upper respiratory infection (5%)

<1%, postmarketing, and/or case reports: Adrenal insufficiency

Drug Interactions

Metabolism/Transport Effects Substrate of CYP3A4 (major); **Note:** Assignment of Major/Minor substrate status based on clinically relevant drug interaction potential; **Inhibits** CYP1A2 (strong), CYP2C19 (moderate), CYP2C9 (moderate), CYP2D6 (strong), CYP3A4 (moderate), P-glycoprotein

Avoid Concomitant Use

Avoid concomitant use of Abiraterone Acetate with any of the following: Bosutinib; Clopidogrel; Conivaptan; Pimozide; Silodosin; Tamoxifen; Thioridazine; Tolvaptan; Topotecan; VinCRIStine (Liposomal)

Increased Effect/Toxicity

Abiraterone Acetate may increase the levels/effects of: ARIPiprazole; AtoMOXetine; Avanafil; Bendamustine; Bosutinib; Budesonide (Systemic, Oral Inhalation); Carvedilol; Citalopram; Colchicine; CYP1A2 Substrates; CYP2C19 Substrates; CYP2C9 Substrates; CYP2D6 Substrates; CYP3A4 Substrates; Dabigatran Etexilate; Eplerenone; Everolimus; FentaNYL; Fesoterodine; Halofantrine; Iloperidone; Ivacaftor; Lurasidone; Nebivolol; P-glycoprotein/ABCB1 Substrates; Pimecrolimus; Pimozide; Propafenone; Prucalopride; Ranolazine; Rivaroxaban; Salmeterol; Saxagliptin; Silodosin; Tetrabenazine; Thioridazine; Tolvaptan; Topotecan; Vilazodone; VinCRIStine (Liposomal); Zuclopenthixol

The levels/effects of Abiraterone Acetate may be increased by: Conivaptan; CYP3A4 Inhibitors (Moderate); CYP3A4 Inhibitors (Strong); Dasatinib; Ivacaftor; Mifepristone

Decreased Effect

Abiraterone Acetate may decrease the levels/effects of: Clopidogrel; Codeine; Ifosfamide; Iloperidone; Tamoxifen; TraMADol

The levels/effects of Abiraterone Acetate may be decreased by: CYP3A4 Inducers (Strong); Deferasirox; Herbs (CYP3A4 Inducers); Tocilizumab

Ethanol/Nutrition/Herb Interactions Food: Taking with food will increase systemic exposure. Management: Do not administer with food. Must be taken on an empty stomach, at least 1 hour before and 2 hours after food.

Storage/Stability Store at 20°C to 25°C (68°F to 77°F); excursions permitted to 15°C to 30°C (59°F to 86°F).

Mechanism of Action Selectively and irreversibly inhibits CYP17 (17 alpha-hydroxylase/C17, 20-lyase), an enzyme required for androgen biosynthesis which is expressed in testicular, adrenal, and prostatic tumor tissues. Inhibits the formation of the testosterone precursors dehydroepiandrosterone (DHEA) and androstenedione.

Pharmacodynamics/Kinetics

Distribution: V_{dss}: 19,669 ± 13,358 L

Protein binding: >99%; to albumin and alpha$_1$-acid glycoprotein

Metabolism: Abiraterone acetate is hydrolyzed to the active metabolite abiraterone; further metabolized to inactive metabolites abiraterone sulphate and N-oxide abiraterone sulphate via CYP3A4 and SULT2A1

Bioavailability: Systemic exposure is increased by food

Half-life elimination: 12 ± 5 hours

Time to peak: 2 hours

Excretion: Feces (~88%); urine (~5%)

Dosing

Adult & Geriatric Prostate cancer, metastatic, castration-resistant: Oral: 1000 mg once daily (in combination with prednisone 5 mg twice daily)

Renal Impairment No adjustment required.

Hepatic Impairment

Hepatic impairment ***prior to*** treatment initiation:

Mild (Child-Pugh class A): No adjustment required

Moderate (Child-Pugh class B): 250 mg once daily (**Note:** Canadian labeling does not recommend use). Permanently discontinue treatment if ALT and/or AST >5 times the upper limit of normal (ULN) or total bilirubin >3 times ULN.

Severe (Child-Pugh class C): Avoid use

Hepatotoxicity ***during*** treatment:

U.S. labeling:

ALT and/or AST >5 times ULN or total bilirubin >3 times ULN: Withhold treatment until liver function tests return to baseline or ALT and AST ≤2.5 times ULN and total bilirubin ≤1.5 times ULN, then reinitiate at 750 mg once daily.

Recurrent hepatotoxicity on 750 mg/day: Withhold treatment until liver function tests return to baseline or ALT and AST ≤2.5 times ULN and total bilirubin ≤1.5 times ULN, then reinitiate at 500 mg once daily.

Recurrent hepatotoxicity on 500 mg/day: Discontinue treatment

Canadian labeling:

ALT and/or AST >5 times ULN or total bilirubin >3 times ULN:

Withhold treatment until liver function tests return to baseline, then reinitiate at 500 mg once daily

Recurrent hepatotoxicity on 500 mg/day: Discontinue treatment

ALT >20 times ULN (any time during treatment): Discontinue permanently.

Adjustment for Toxicity Hepatotoxicity: Refer to Dosing: Hepatic Impairment.

Combination Regimens

Prostate cancer: Abiraterone-Prednisone (Prostate Cancer) on page 1516

Administration Administer orally on an empty stomach, at least 1 hour before and 2 hours after food. Swallow tablets whole with water.

Monitoring Parameters ALT, AST, and bilirubin prior to treatment, every 2 weeks for 3 months and monthly thereafter; if baseline moderate hepatic impairment (Child-Pugh class B), monitor ALT, AST, and bilirubin prior to treatment, weekly for the first month, every 2 weeks for 2 months then monthly thereafter. If hepatotoxicity develops during treatment (and only after therapy is interrupted and liver function tests have returned to safe levels), monitor ALT, AST, and bilirubin every 2 weeks for 3 months and monthly thereafter. Monitoring of testosterone levels is not necessary.

Monitor for signs and symptoms of adrenocorticoid insufficiency; monthly for hypertension, hypokalemia, and fluid retention.

Dietary Considerations Must be taken on an empty stomach, at least 1 hour before and 2 hours after food.

Dosage Forms Excipient information presented when available (limited, particularly for generics); consult specific product labeling.

Tablet, oral:

Zytiga™: 250 mg

References

Attard G, Reid AH, A'Hern R, et al, "Selective Inhibition of CYP17 With Abiraterone Acetate is Highly Active in the Treatment of Castration-Resistant Prostate Cancer," *J Clin Oncol*, 2009, 27(23):3742-8.

Danila DC, Morris MJ, de Bono JS, et al, "Phase II Multicenter Study of Abiraterone Acetate Plus Prednisone Therapy in Patients With Docetaxel-Treated Castration-Resistant Prostate Cancer," *J Clin Oncol*, 2010, 28(9):1496-501.

de Bono JS, Logothetis CJ, Molina A, et al, "Abiraterone and Increased Survival in Metastatic Prostate Cancer," *New Engl J Med*, 2011, 364(21):1995-2005.

Reid AH, Attard G, Danila DC, et al, "Significant and Sustained Antitumor Activity in Post-Docetaxel, Castration-Resistant Prostate Cancer With the CYP17 Inhibitor Abiraterone Acetate," *J Clin Oncol*, 2010, 28(9):1489-95

- **ABLC** *see* Amphotericin B (Lipid Complex) *on page 84*
- **Abraxane®** *see* PACLitaxel (Protein Bound) *on page 1098*
- **Abraxane® for Injectable Suspension (Can)** *see* PACLitaxel (Protein Bound) *on page 1098*
- **Absorica** *see* ISOtretinoin *on page 832*
- **Abstral®** *see* FentaNYL *on page 583*
- **Abstral™ (Can)** *see* FentaNYL *on page 583*
- **ABX-EGF** *see* Panitumumab *on page 1115*
- **Accutane** *see* ISOtretinoin *on page 832*
- **Accutane® (Can)** *see* ISOtretinoin *on page 832*
- **Acetoxymethylprogesterone** *see* MedroxyPROGESTERone *on page 916*
- **Aciclovir** *see* Acyclovir (Systemic) *on page 30*
- **Aciclovir** *see* Acyclovir (Topical) *on page 35*
- **Aclasta® (Can)** *see* Zoledronic Acid *on page 1488*

- ◆ **4-(9-Acridinylamino) Methanesulfon-m-Anisidide** *see* Amsacrine *on page 90*
- ◆ **Acridinyl Anisidide** *see* Amsacrine *on page 90*
- ◆ **ACT-D** *see* DACTINomycin *on page 371*
- ◆ **Actinomycin** *see* DACTINomycin *on page 371*
- ◆ **Actinomycin D** *see* DACTINomycin *on page 371*
- ◆ **Actinomycin CI** *see* DACTINomycin *on page 371*
- ◆ **Actiq®** *see* FentaNYL *on page 583*
- ◆ **Activase®** *see* Alteplase *on page 55*
- ◆ **Activase® rt-PA (Can)** *see* Alteplase *on page 55*
- ◆ **ACV** *see* Acyclovir (Systemic) *on page 30*
- ◆ **ACV** *see* Acyclovir (Topical) *on page 35*
- ◆ **Acycloguanosine** *see* Acyclovir (Systemic) *on page 30*
- ◆ **Acycloguanosine** *see* Acyclovir (Topical) *on page 35*

Acyclovir (Systemic) (ay SYE kloe veer)

Brand Names: U.S. Zovirax®

Brand Names: Canada Apo-Acyclovir®; Mylan-Acyclovir; Nu-Acyclovir; ratio-Acyclovir; Teva-Acyclovir; Zovirax®

Index Terms Aciclovir; ACV; Acycloguanosine

Generic Availability (U.S.) Yes

Pharmacologic Category Antiviral Agent

Use Treatment of genital herpes simplex virus (HSV) and HSV encephalitis

Unlabeled Use Prevention of HSV reactivation in HIV-positive patients; prevention of HSV reactivation in hematopoietic stem cell transplant (HSCT); prevention of HSV reactivation during periods of neutropenia in patients with cancer; prevention of varicella zoster virus (VZV) reactivation in allogenic HSCT; prevention of CMV reactivation in low-risk allogeneic HSCT; treatment of disseminated HSV or VZV in immunocompromised patients with cancer; empiric treatment of suspected encephalitis in immunocompromised patients with cancer; treatment of initial and prophylaxis of recurrent mucosal and cutaneous herpes simplex (HSV-1 and HSV-2) infections in immunocompromised patients

Labeled Contraindications Hypersensitivity to acyclovir, valacyclovir, or any component of the formulation

Pregnancy Risk Factor B

Lactation Enters breast milk/use with caution (AAP rates "compatible"; AAP 2001 update pending)

Warnings/Precautions Use with caution in immunocompromised patients; thrombocytopenic purpura/hemolytic uremic syndrome (TTP/HUS) has been reported. Use caution in the elderly, pre-existing renal disease (may require dosage modification), or in those receiving other nephrotoxic drugs. Renal failure (sometimes fatal) has been reported. Maintain adequate hydration during oral or intravenous therapy. Use I.V. preparation with caution in patients with underlying neurologic abnormalities, serious hepatic or electrolyte abnormalities, or substantial hypoxia.

Varicella-zoster: Treatment should begin within 24 hours of appearance of rash; oral route not recommended for routine use in otherwise healthy children with varicella, but may be effective in patients at increased risk of moderate-to-severe infection (>12 years of age, chronic cutaneous or pulmonary disorders, long-term salicylate therapy, corticosteroid therapy).

Ethanol/Nutrition/Herb Interactions Food: Does not affect absorption of oral acyclovir.

Storage/Stability

Capsule, tablet: Store at controlled room temperature of 15°C to 25°C (59°F to 77°F); protect from moisture.

Injection: Store powder at controlled room temperature of 15°C to 25°C (59°F to 77°F). Reconstituted solutions remain stable for 12 hours at room temperature. Do not refrigerate reconstituted solutions or solutions diluted for infusion as they may precipitate. Once diluted for infusion, use within 24 hours.

Reconstitution Powder for injection: Reconstitute acyclovir 500 mg powder with SWFI 10 mL; do not use bacteriostatic water containing benzyl alcohol or parabens. For intravenous infusion, dilute in D_5W, D_5NS, $D_5{}^1/_4NS$, $D_5{}^1/_2NS$, LR, or NS to a final concentration ≤7 mg/mL. Concentrations >10 mg/mL increase the risk of phlebitis.

Mechanism of Action Acyclovir is converted to acyclovir monophosphate by virus-specific thymidine kinase then further converted to acyclovir triphosphate by other cellular enzymes. Acyclovir triphosphate inhibits DNA synthesis and viral replication by competing with deoxyguanosine triphosphate for viral DNA polymerase and being incorporated into viral DNA.

Pharmacodynamics/Kinetics

Absorption: Oral: 15% to 30%

Distribution: V_d: 0.8 L/kg (63.6 L): Widely (eg, brain, kidney, lungs, liver, spleen, muscle, uterus, vagina, CSF)

Protein binding: 9% to 33%

Metabolism: Converted by viral enzymes to acyclovir monophosphate, and further converted to diphosphate then triphosphate (active form) by cellular enzymes

Bioavailability: Oral: 10% to 20% with normal renal function (bioavailability decreases with increased dose)

Half-life elimination: Terminal: Neonates: 4 hours; Children 1-12 years: 2-3 hours; Adults: 3 hours

Time to peak, serum: Oral: Within 1.5-2 hours

Excretion: Urine (62% to 90% as unchanged drug and metabolite)

Dosing

Adult & Geriatric Note: Obese patients should be dosed using ideal body weight

Genital herpes simplex virus (HSV) infection:

I.V.: Immunocompetent: Initial episode, severe: 5 mg/kg/dose every 8 hours for 5-7 days **or** 5-10 mg/kg/dose every 8 hours for 2-7 days, follow with oral therapy to complete at least 10 days of therapy (CDC, 2010)

Oral:

Initial episode: 200 mg every 4 hours while awake (5 times/day) for 10 days **or** 400 mg 3 times/day for 7-10 days (CDC, 2010)

Recurrence: 200 mg every 4 hours while awake (5 times/day) for 5 days (per manufacturer's labeling; begin at earliest signs of disease)

Alternatively, the following regimens are also recommended by the CDC: 400 mg 3 times/day for 5 days; 800 mg twice daily for 5 days; 800 mg 3 times/day for 2 days (CDC, 2010)

Chronic suppression: 400 mg twice daily or 200 mg 3-5 times/day, for up to 12 months followed by re-evaluation (per manufacturer's labeling)

Herpes zoster (shingles):

Oral: Immunocompetent: 800 mg every 4 hours (5 times/day) for 7-10 days

I.V.: Immunocompromised: 10 mg/kg/dose or 500 mg/m^2/dose every 8 hours for 7 days

HSV encephalitis: I.V.: 10 mg/kg/dose every 8 hours for 10 days (per manufacturer's labeling); 10-15 mg/kg/dose every 8 hours for 14-21 days also reported

Mucocutaneous HSV:

I.V.: Immunocompromised: Treatment: 5 mg/kg/dose every 8 hours for 7 days (Leflore, 2000); dosing for up to 14 days also reported

Oral (unlabeled use): Immunocompromised: 400 mg 5 times/day for 7 days (Leflore, 2000)

Orolabial HSV (unlabeled use): Oral (immunocompetent):

Treatment: 200-400 mg 5 times/day for 5 days (Cernik, 2008; Leflore, 2000; Spruance, 1990) for episodic/recurrent treatment; for initial treatment, limited data are available, 200 mg 5 times/day or 400 mg 3 times/day for 7-10 days has been recommended by some clinicians.

Chronic suppression: 400 mg 2 times/day (has been clinically evaluated for up to 1 year) (Cernik, 2008; Rooney, 1993)

Varicella-zoster (chickenpox): Begin treatment within the first 24 hours of rash onset:

Oral: >40 kg (immunocompetent): 800 mg/dose 4 times/day for 5 days

I.V.:

Manufacturer's labeling (immunocompromised): 10 mg/kg/dose every 8 hours for 7 days

CDC HIV guidelines (immunocompromised): 10-15 mg/kg/dose every 8 hours for 7-10 days

Prevention of HSV reactivation in HIV-positive patients (unlabeled use): Oral: 400-800 mg 2-3 times/day (CDC, 2010)

Prevention of HSV reactivation in HSCT (unlabeled use): *CDC recommendation:* **Note:** Start at the beginning of conditioning therapy and continue until engraftment or until mucositis resolves (~30 days)

Oral: 200 mg 3 times/day

I.V.: 250 mg/m^2/dose every 12 hours

Prevention of VZV reactivation in allogeneic HSCT (unlabeled use): *NCCN guidelines:* Oral: 800 mg twice a day

Prevention of CMV reactivation in low-risk allogeneic HSCT (unlabeled use): *NCCN guidelines:* **Note:** Requires close monitoring (due to weak activity); not for use in patients at high risk for CMV disease: Oral: 800 mg 4 times/day

Treatment of disseminated HSV or VZV or empiric treatment of suspected encephalitis in immunocompromised patients with cancer: (unlabeled use): *NCCN guidelines:* I.V.: 10-12 mg/kg/dose every 8 hours

Treatment of episodic HSV infection in HIV-positive patient (unlabeled use): Oral: 400 mg 3 times/day for 5-10 days (CDC, 2010)

Pediatric Note: Obese patients should be dosed using ideal body weight

Genital herpes simplex virus (HSV) infection:

I.V.: Children ≥12 years: Refer to adult dosing.

Oral:

Immunocompetent:

Initial episode (unlabeled use): 40-80 mg/kg/day divided into 3-4 doses for 5-10 days (maximum: 1 g/day)

Chronic suppression (unlabeled use; limited data): 80 mg/kg/day in 3 divided doses (maximum: 1 g/day), re-evaluate after 12 months of treatment

Immunocompromised (unlabeled use; CDC, 2009): Initial episode:

Children <45 kg: 60 mg/kg/day divided into 3 doses for 5-14 days (maximum: 1.2 g/day)

Adolescents: 400 mg twice daily for 5-14 days

Herpes zoster (shingles): I.V.:

Children <12 years (immunocompromised): 20 mg/kg/dose every 8 hours for 7 days

Children ≥12 years: Refer to adult dosing.

HSV encephalitis: I.V.:

Children 3 months to 12 years: 20 mg/kg/dose every 8 hours for 10 days (per manufacturer's labeling); dosing for 14-21 days also reported

Children ≥12 years: Refer to adult dosing.

Mucocutaneous HSV: I.V.:

Children <12 years (immunocompromised): Treatment: 10 mg/kg/dose every 8 hours for 7 days

Children ≥12 years (immunocompromised): Treatment: 5-10 mg/kg/dose every 8 hours for 7 days (Leflore, 2000); dosing for up to 14 days also reported

Neonatal HSV: I.V.: Infants: Birth to 3 months: 10 mg/kg/dose every 8 hours for 10 days (manufacturer's labeling); 20 mg/kg/dose every 8 hours for 14 (skin and mucous membrane disease) to 21 days (CNS disease) (CDC, 2010)

Orolabial HSV (unlabeled use): Oral: Children 1-6 years (immunocompetent, gingivostomatitis): Treatment of primary infection: 15 mg/kg/dose (maximum: 200 mg/dose) 5 times/day for 7 days, initiated within 72 hours of symptom onset (Amir, 1997)

Varicella-zoster (chickenpox): Begin treatment within the first 24 hours of rash onset:

Oral: **Note:** The CDC HIV guidelines recommended duration of therapy is 7-10 days or until no new lesions for 48 hours (for patients with mild varicella and no or moderate immune suppression).

Children ≥2 years and ≤40 kg (immunocompetent): 20 mg/kg/dose (up to 800 mg/dose) 4 times/day for 5 days

Children >40 kg: Refer to adult dosing.

I.V.:

Manufacturer's labeling (immunocompromised):

Children <12 years: 20 mg/kg/dose every 8 hours for 7 days

Children ≥12 years: 10 mg/kg/dose every 8 hours for 7 days

CDC HIV guidelines (immunocompromised):

Children <1 year: 10 mg/kg/dose every 8 hours for 7-10 days or until no new lesions for 48 hours

Children ≥1 year: 10 mg/kg/dose or 500 mg/m^2/dose every 8 hours for 7-10 days or until no new lesions for 48 hours

Adolescents: Refer to adult dosing.

Varicella-zoster acute retinal necrosis infection in HIV-exposed/-positive patients (unlabeled use; CDC, 2009): I.V.: Infants and Children: 10-15 mg/kg/dose every 8 hours for 10-14 days, followed by valacyclovir for 4-6 weeks

Prevention of HSV reactivation in HIV-exposed/-positive patients (unlabeled use; CDC, 2009): Oral: 20 mg/kg/dose twice daily (maximum: 400 mg/dose)

Prevention of HSV reactivation in HSCT (unlabeled use): *CDC recommendation:* **Note:** Start at the beginning of conditioning therapy and continue until engraftment or until mucositis resolves (~30 days): I.V.: 250 mg/m²/dose every 8 hours or 125 mg/m²/dose every 6 hours

Renal Impairment

Oral:

- Cl_{cr} 10-25 mL/minute/1.73 m²: Normal dosing regimen 800 mg every 4 hours: Administer 800 mg every 8 hours
- Cl_{cr} <10 mL/minute/1.73 m²:
  - Normal dosing regimen 200 mg every 4 hours or 400 mg every 12 hours: Administer 200 mg every 12 hours
  - Normal dosing regimen 800 mg every 4 hours: Administer 800 mg every 12 hours

I.V.:

- Cl_{cr} 25-50 mL/minute/1.73 m²: Administer recommended dose every 12 hours
- Cl_{cr} 10-25 mL/minute/1.73 m²: Administer recommended dose every 24 hours
- Cl_{cr} <10 mL/minute/1.73 m²: Administer 50% of recommended dose every 24 hours

Intermittent hemodialysis (IHD) (administer after hemodialysis on dialysis days): Dialyzable (60% reduction following a 6-hour session): I.V.: 2.5-5 mg/kg every 24 hours (Heintz, 2009). **Note:** Dosing dependent on the assumption of 3 times/week, complete IHD sessions.

Peritoneal dialysis (PD): Administer 50% of normal dose once daily; no supplemental dose needed

Continuous renal replacement therapy (CRRT) (Heintz, 2009; Trotman, 2005): Drug clearance is highly dependent on the method of renal replacement, filter type, and flow rate. Appropriate dosing requires close monitoring of pharmacologic response, signs of adverse reactions due to drug accumulation, as well as drug concentrations in relation to target trough (if appropriate). The following are general recommendations only (based on dialysate flow/ultrafiltration rates of 1-2 L/hour and minimal residual renal function) and should not supersede clinical judgment:

- CVVH: I.V.: 5-10 mg/kg every 24 hours
- CVVHD/CVVHDF: I.V.: 5-10 mg/kg every 12-24 hours
- **Note:** The higher end of dosage range (eg, 10 mg/kg every 12 hours for CVVHDF) is recommended for viral meningoencephalitis and varicella-zoster virus infections.

Administration

Oral: May be administered with or without food.

I.V.: Avoid rapid infusion; infuse over 1 hour to prevent renal damage; maintain adequate hydration of patient; check for phlebitis and rotate infusion sites. Avoid I.M. or SubQ administration.

Dosage Forms Excipient information presented when available (limited, particularly for generics); consult specific product labeling.

Capsule, oral: 200 mg
  Zovirax®: 200 mg
Injection, powder for reconstitution, as sodium [strength expressed as base]: 500 mg, 1000 mg
Injection, solution, as sodium [strength expressed as base, preservative free]: 50 mg/mL (10 mL, 20 mL)
Suspension, oral: 200 mg/5 mL (473 mL)
  Zovirax®: 200 mg/5 mL (473 mL) [banana flavor]
Tablet, oral: 400 mg, 800 mg
  Zovirax®: 400 mg
  Zovirax®: 800 mg [scored]

Acyclovir (Topical) (ay SYE kloe veer)

Brand Names: U.S. Zovirax®

Brand Names: Canada Zovirax®

Index Terms Aciclovir; ACV; Acycloguanosine

Generic Availability (U.S.) No

Pharmacologic Category Antiviral Agent, Topical

Use Treatment of herpes labialis (cold sores), mucocutaneous HSV in immunocompromised patients

Labeled Contraindications Hypersensitivity to acyclovir, valacyclovir, or any component of the formulation

Pregnancy Risk Factor B

Warnings/Precautions

Genital herpes: Physical contact should be avoided when lesions are present; transmission may also occur in the absence of symptoms. Treatment should begin with the first signs or symptoms.

Herpes labialis: For external use only to the lips and face; do not apply to eye or inside the mouth or nose. Treatment should begin with the first signs or symptoms.

Storage/Stability

Cream: Store at controlled room temperature of 15°C to 25°C (59°F to 77°F).
Ointment: Store at controlled room temperature of 15°C to 25°C (59°F to 77°F) in a dry place.

Mechanism of Action Acyclovir is converted to acyclovir monophosphate by virus-specific thymidine kinase then further converted to acyclovir triphosphate by other cellular enzymes. Acyclovir triphosphate inhibits DNA synthesis and viral replication by competing with deoxyguanosine triphosphate for viral DNA polymerase and being incorporated into viral DNA.

Pharmacodynamics/Kinetics

Absorption: Plasma concentrations following topical application of the cream were below the limit of detection in 5/6 male volunteers (<0.01μM) and 0.014 μM in one subject. Following application of the ointment to patients with varicella-zoster infection, acyclovir plasma concentrations were <0.01-0.28 mcg/mL in patients with normal renal function and <0.01-0.78 mcg/mL in a patient with renal impairment.

Excretion: Urine (0.04% of the daily dose following topical application of the cream; <0.02% to 9.4% of the daily dose following topical application of the ointment)

Dosing

Adult & Geriatric

Genital HSV: Topical: Immunocompromised: Ointment: Initial episode: 1/2" ribbon of ointment for a 4" square surface area every 3 hours (6 times/day) for 7 days

Herpes labialis (cold sores): Topical: Apply 5 times/day for 4 days

Mucocutaneous HSV: Topical: Ointment: Non-life-threatening, immunocompromised: 1/2" ribbon of ointment for a 4" square surface area every 3 hours (6 times/day) for 7 days

Pediatric Herpes labialis (cold sores): Topical: Children ≥12 years: Refer to adult dosing.

Administration Topical: Not for use in the eye. Apply using a finger cot or rubber glove to avoid transmission to other parts of the body or to other persons.

Dosage Forms Excipient information presented when available (limited, particularly for generics); consult specific product labeling.

Cream, topical:
Zovirax®: 5% (2 g, 5 g)

Ointment, topical:
Zovirax®: 5% (15 g, 30 g)

- **AD32** *see* Valrubicin *on page 1425*
- **Adcetris™** *see* Brentuximab Vedotin *on page 199*
- **ADR (error-prone abbreviation)** *see* DOXOrubicin *on page 467*
- **AdreView™** *see* Iobenguane I 123 *on page 806*
- **Adria** *see* DOXOrubicin *on page 467*
- **Adriamycin®** *see* DOXOrubicin *on page 467*
- **Adrucil®** *see* Fluorouracil (Systemic) *on page 627*
- **Advagraf® (Can)** *see* Tacrolimus (Systemic) *on page 1315*
- **Advate** *see* Antihemophilic Factor (Recombinant) *on page 103*
- **Afinitor®** *see* Everolimus *on page 552*
- **Afinitor® Disperz** *see* Everolimus *on page 552*
- **Aflibercept I.V.** *see* Ziv-Aflibercept (Systemic) *on page 1484*
- **AG-013736** *see* Axitinib *on page 135*
- **Agrylin®** *see* Anagrelide *on page 93*
- **AHF (Human)** *see* Antihemophilic Factor (Human) *on page 101*
- **AHF (Recombinant)** *see* Antihemophilic Factor (Recombinant) *on page 103*
- **Ahi-Temozolomide Capsules (Can)** *see* Temozolomide *on page 1331*
- **A-hydroCort** *see* Hydrocortisone (Systemic) *on page 713*
- **A-Hydrocort®** *see* Hydrocortisone (Systemic) *on page 713*
- **A-hydroCort** *see* Hydrocortisone (Topical) *on page 719*
- **AJ-PIP/TAZ (Can)** *see* Piperacillin and Tazobactam *on page 1175*
- **ALA** *see* Aminolevulinic Acid *on page 75*
- **5-ALA** *see* Aminolevulinic Acid *on page 75*
- **Ala-Cort** *see* Hydrocortisone (Topical) *on page 719*
- **Ala-Scalp** *see* Hydrocortisone (Topical) *on page 719*
- **Albumin-Bound Paclitaxel** *see* PACLitaxel (Protein Bound) *on page 1098*

◆ **Albumin-Stabilized Nanoparticle Paclitaxel** *see* PACLitaxel (Protein Bound) *on page 1098*

Aldesleukin (al des LOO kin)

Related Information

Management of Chemotherapy-Induced Nausea and Vomiting *on page 1786*
Principles of Anticancer Therapy *on page 1878*
Safe Handling of Hazardous Drugs *on page 1904*

Brand Names: U.S. Proleukin®

Brand Names: Canada Proleukin®

Index Terms IL-2; Interleukin 2; Interleukin-2; Lymphocyte Mitogenic Factor; Recombinant Human Interleukin-2; T-Cell Growth Factor; TCGF; Thymocyte Stimulating Factor

Generic Availability (U.S.) No

Pharmacologic Category Antineoplastic Agent, Miscellaneous; Biological Response Modulator

Use Treatment of metastatic renal cell cancer, metastatic melanoma

Unlabeled Use Treatment of acute myeloid leukemia (AML)

Labeled Contraindications Hypersensitivity to aldesleukin or any component of the formulation; patients with abnormal thallium stress or pulmonary function tests; patients who have had an organ allograft. **Retreatment is contraindicated** in patients who have experienced sustained ventricular tachycardia (≥5 beats), uncontrolled or unresponsive cardiac arrhythmias, chest pain with ECG changes consistent with angina or MI, cardiac tamponade, intubation >72 hours, renal failure requiring dialysis for >72 hours, coma or toxic psychosis lasting >48 hours, repetitive or refractory seizures, bowel ischemia/perforation, or GI bleeding requiring surgery.

Pregnancy Risk Factor C

Lactation Excretion in breast milk unknown/not recommended

Warnings/Precautions Hazardous agent - use appropriate precautions for handling and disposal.

[U.S. Boxed Warning]: High-dose aldesleukin therapy has been associated with capillary leak syndrome (CLS), characterized by vascular tone loss and extravasation of plasma proteins and fluid into extravascular space. CLS results in significant hypotension and reduced organ perfusion which may be severe and can result in death; CLS onset is immediately after treatment initiation. Cardiac arrhythmia, angina, MI, respiratory insufficiency (requiring intubation), gastrointestinal bleeding or infarction, renal insufficiency, edema and mental status changes are also associated with CLS. Monitor fluid status and organ perfusion status carefully; consider fluids and/or pressor agents to maintain organ perfusion. **[U.S. Boxed Warning]: Therapy should be restricted to patients with normal cardiac and pulmonary functions as defined by thallium stress and formal pulmonary function testing.** Extreme caution should be used in patients with a history of prior cardiac or pulmonary disease and in patients who are fluid-restricted or where edema may be poorly tolerated. Withhold treatment for signs of organ hypoperfusion, including altered mental status, reduced urine output, systolic BP <90 mm Hg or cardiac arrhythmia. Once blood pressure is normalized, may consider diuretics for excessive weight gain/edema. Recovery from CLS generally begins soon after treatment cessation. Perform a thorough clinical evaluation prior to treatment initiation; exclude patients with significant cardiac, pulmonary, renal, hepatic, or central nervous system impairment from treatment. Patients with a more favorable performance status prior to treatment initiation are more likely to respond to aldesleukin treatment, with a higher response rate and generally lower toxicity.

[U.S. Boxed Warning]: Should be administered under the supervision of an experienced cancer chemotherapy physician in a facility with cardiopulmonary or intensive specialists and intensive care facilities available. Adverse effects are frequent and sometimes fatal. May exacerbate pre-existing or initial presentation of autoimmune diseases and inflammatory disorders; exacerbation and/or new onset have been reported with aldesleukin and interferon alfa combination therapy. Patients should be evaluated and treated for CNS metastases and have a negative scan prior to treatment; new neurologic symptoms and lesions have been reported in patients without pre-existing evidence of CNS metastases (symptoms generally improve upon discontinuation, however, cases with permanent damage have been reported). Mental status changes (irritability, confusion, depression) can occur and may indicate bacteremia, sepsis, hypoperfusion, CNS malignancy, or CNS toxicity. May cause seizure; use with caution in patients with seizure disorder.

[U.S. Boxed Warning]: Impaired neutrophil function is associated with treatment; patients are at risk for disseminated infection (including sepsis and bacterial endocarditis), and central line-related gram-positive infections. Treat pre-existing bacterial infection appropriately prior to treatment initiation. Monitor for signs of infection or sepsis during treatment. Antibiotic prophylaxis which has been associated with a reduced incidence of staphylococcal infections in aldesleukin studies includes the use of oxacillin, nafcillin, ciprofloxacin, or vancomycin.

[U.S. Boxed Warning]: Withhold treatment for patients developing moderate-to-severe lethargy or somnolence; continued treatment may result in coma. Standard prophylactic supportive care during high-dose aldesleukin treatment includes acetaminophen to relieve constitutional symptoms and an H_2 antagonist to reduce the risk of GI ulceration and/or bleeding. May impair renal or hepatic function; patients must have a serum creatinine ≤1.5 mg/dL prior to treatment. Concomitant nephrotoxic or hepatotoxic agents may increase the risk of renal or hepatic toxicity. Enhancement of cellular immune function may increase the risk of allograft rejection in transplant patients. An acute array of symptoms resembling aldesleukin adverse reactions (fever, chills, nausea, rash, pruritus, diarrhea, hypotension, edema, and oliguria) were observed within 1-4 hours after iodinated contrast media administration, usually when given within 4 weeks after aldesleukin treatment, although has been reported several months after aldesleukin treatment. The incidence of dyspnea and severe urogenital toxicities is potentially increased in elderly patients.

Adverse Reactions

>10%:

Cardiovascular: Hypotension (71%; grade 4: 3%), peripheral edema (28%), tachycardia (23%), edema (15%), vasodilation (13%), supraventricular tachycardia (12%; grade 4: 1%), cardiovascular disorder (11%; includes blood pressure changes, HF and ECG changes)

Central nervous system: Chills (52%), confusion (34%; grade 4: 1%), fever (29%; grade 4: 1%), malaise (27%), somnolence (22%), anxiety (12%), pain (12%), dizziness (11%)

Dermatologic: Rash (42%), pruritus (24%), exfoliative dermatitis (18%)

Endocrine & metabolic: Acidosis (12%; grade 4: 1%), hypomagnesemia (12%), hypocalcemia (11%)

Gastrointestinal: Diarrhea (67%; grade 4: 2%), vomiting (19% to 50%; grade 4: 1%), nausea (19% to 35%), stomatitis (22%), anorexia (20%), weight gain (16%), abdominal pain (11%)

Hematologic: Thrombocytopenia (37%; grade 4: 1%), anemia (29%), leukopenia (16%)

Hepatic: Hyperbilirubinemia (40%; grade 4: 2%), AST increased (23%; grade 4: 1%)

Neuromuscular & skeletal: Weakness (23%)

Renal: Oliguria (63%; grade 4: 6%), creatinine increased (33%; grade 4: 1%)

Respiratory: Dyspnea (43%; grade 4: 1%), lung disorder (24%; includes pulmonary congestion, rales, and rhonchi), cough (11%), respiratory disorder (11%; includes acute respiratory distress syndrome, infiltrates and pulmonary changes)

Miscellaneous: Antibody formation (66% to 74%), infection (13%; grade 4: 1%)

1% to 10%:

Cardiovascular: Arrhythmia (10%), cardiac arrest (grade 4: 1%), MI (grade 4: 1%), ventricular tachycardia (grade 4: 1%)

Central nervous system: Coma (grade 4: 2%), stupor (grade 4: 1%), psychosis (grade 4: 1%)

Gastrointestinal: Abdomen enlarged (10%)

Hematologic: Coagulation disorder (grade 4: 1%; includes intravascular coagulopathy)

Hepatic: Alkaline phosphatase increased (10%)

Renal: Anuria (grade 4: 5%), acute renal failure (grade 4: 1%)

Respiratory: Rhinitis (10%), apnea (grade 4: 1%)

Miscellaneous: Sepsis (grade 4: 1%)

<1%, postmarketing, and/or case reports: Agitation, allergic interstitial nephritis, anaphylaxis, angioedema, asthma, atrial arrhythmia, AV block, blindness (transient or permanent), bowel infarction/necrosis/perforation, bradycardia, bullous pemphigoid, BUN increased, capillary leak syndrome, cardiomyopathy, cellulitis, cerebral edema, cerebral lesions, cerebral vasculitis, cholecystitis, colitis, crescentic IgA glomerulonephritis, Crohn's disease exacerbation, delirium, depression (severe; leading to suicide), diabetes mellitus, duodenal ulcer, encephalopathy, endocarditis, eosinophilia, extrapyramidal syndrome, gastritis, hematemesis, hemoptysis, hemorrhage (including cerebral, gastrointestinal, retroperitoneal, subarachnoid, subdural), hepatic failure, hepatitis, hepatosplenomegaly, hypertension, hyperuricemia, hyper-/hypoventilation, hypothermia, hyperthyroidism, hypoxia, inflammatory arthritis, injection site necrosis, insomnia, intestinal obstruction, intestinal perforation, leukocytosis, lymphocytopenia, malignant hyperthermia, meningitis, mydriasis, myocardial ischemia, myocarditis, myopathy, myositis, neuralgia, neuritis, neuropathy, neutropenia, NPN increased, oculobulbar myasthenia gravis, optic neuritis, organ perfusion decreased, pancreatitis, paranoia, pericardial effusion, pericarditis, peripheral gangrene, phlebitis, pneumonia, pneumothorax, pulmonary edema, pulmonary embolus, respiratory acidosis, respiratory arrest, respiratory failure, rhabdomyolysis, scleroderma, seizure, shock, Stevens-Johnson syndrome, stroke, syncope, thrombosis, thyroiditis, tracheoesophageal fistula, transient ischemic attack, tubular necrosis, urticaria, ventricular extrasystoles

Drug Interactions

Metabolism/Transport Effects None known.

Avoid Concomitant Use

Avoid concomitant use of Aldesleukin with any of the following: CloZAPine; Corticosteroids

Increased Effect/Toxicity

Aldesleukin may increase the levels/effects of: CloZAPine; Hypotensive Agents

The levels/effects of Aldesleukin may be increased by: Contrast Media (Non-ionic); Interferons (Alfa)

Decreased Effect

The levels/effects of Aldesleukin may be decreased by: Corticosteroids

Ethanol/Nutrition/Herb Interactions Ethanol: May increase CNS adverse effects.

Storage/Stability Store intact vials under refrigeration at 2°C to 8°C (36°F to 46°F). Protect from light. Plastic (polyvinyl chloride) bags result in more consistent drug delivery and are recommended. According to the manufacturer, reconstituted vials and solutions diluted for infusion are stable for 48 hours at room temperature or refrigerated although refrigeration is preferred because they do not contain preservatives. Do not freeze. Solution diluted with D_5W to a concentration of 220 mcg/mL and repackaged into tuberculin syringes was reported to be stable for 14 days refrigerated.

Reconstitution Reconstitute vials with 1.2 mL SWFI (preservative free) to a concentration of 18 million units (1.1 mg)/1 mL (sterile water should be injected towards the side of the vial). Gently swirl; do not shake. Further dilute with 50 mL of D_5W. Smaller volumes of D_5W should be used for doses ≤1.5 mg; avoid concentrations <30 mcg/mL and >70 mcg/mL (an increased variability in drug delivery has been seen). Plastic (polyvinyl chloride) bags result in more consistent drug delivery and are recommended. Filtration may result in loss of bioactivity. Addition of 0.1% albumin has been used to increase stability and decrease the extent of sorption if low final concentrations cannot be avoided.

Mechanism of Action Aldesleukin is a human recombinant interleukin-2 product which promotes proliferation, differentiation, and recruitment of T and B cells, natural killer (NK) cells, and thymocytes; causes cytolytic activity in a subset of lymphocytes and subsequent interactions between the immune system and malignant cells; can stimulate lymphokine-activated killer (LAK) cells and tumor-infiltrating lymphocytes (TIL) cells.

Pharmacodynamics/Kinetics

Distribution: V_d: 4-7 L; primarily in plasma and then in the lymphocytes

Metabolism: Renal (metabolized to amino acids)

Half-life elimination: I.V.: Initial: 6-13 minutes; Terminal: 80-120 minutes

Excretion: Urine (primarily as metabolites)

Dosing

Adult & Geriatric Consider premedication with an antipyretic to reduce fever, an H_2 antagonist for prophylaxis of gastrointestinal irritation/bleeding, antiemetics, and antidiarrheals; continue for 12 hours after the last aldesleukin dose. Antibiotic prophylaxis is recommended to reduce the incidence of infection.

Renal cell carcinoma: I.V.: 600,000 units/kg every 8 hours for a maximum of 14 doses; repeat after 9 days for a total of 28 doses per course; retreat if tumor shrinkage observed (and if no contraindications) at least 7 weeks after hospital discharge date

or

Unlabeled dosing: 720,000 units/kg every 8 hours for up to 12 doses; repeat with a second cycle 10-15 days later (Klapper, 2008)

Melanoma: I.V.:

Single-agent use: 600,000 units/kg every 8 hours for a maximum of 14 doses; repeat after 9 days for a total of 28 doses per course; retreat if tumor shrinkage observed (and if no contraindications) at least 7 weeks after hospital discharge date

or

Unlabeled dosing: 720,000 units/kg every 8 hours for 12-15 doses; repeat with a second cycle ~14 days after the first dose of the initial cycle (Smith, 2008)

Combination biochemotherapy (unlabeled use): 9 million units/m^2/day continuous infusion over 24 hours for 4 days every 3 weeks for up to 4 cycles (Atkins, 2008) **or** 9 million units/m^2/day continuous infusion over 24 hours days 5 to 8, 17 to 20, and 26 to 29 every 42 days for up to 5 cycles (Eton, 2002) **or** 9 million units/m^2/day continuous infusion over 24 hours for 4 days every 3 weeks for 6 cycles (Legha, 1998)

Pediatric Consider premedication with an antipyretic to reduce fever, an H_2 antagonist for prophylaxis of gastrointestinal irritation/bleeding, antiemetics, and antidiarrheals; continue for 12 hours after the last aldesleukin dose. Antibiotic prophylaxis is recommended to reduce the incidence of infection.

AML (unlabeled use): I.V.: 9 million units (9 x 10^6 units)/m^2/day continuous infusion over 24 hours daily for 4 days; repeat 4 days later with 1.6 million units (1.6 x 10^6 units)/m^2/day continuous infusion over 24 hours daily for 10 days (Lange, 2008)

Renal Impairment No specific recommendations by manufacturer. Use with caution.

Adjustment for Toxicity Withhold or interrupt a dose for toxicity; do not reduce the dose.

Cardiovascular toxicity:

Atrial fibrillation, supraventricular tachycardia, or bradycardia that is persistent, recurrent, or requires treatment: Withhold dose; may resume when asymptomatic with full recovery to normal sinus rhythm.

Systolic BP <90 mm Hg (with increasing pressor requirements): Withhold dose; may resume treatment when systolic BP ≥90 mm Hg and stable or pressor requirements improve.

Any ECG change consistent with MI, ischemia or myocarditis (with or without chest pain), or suspected cardiac ischemia: Withhold dose; may resume when asymptomatic, MI/myocarditis have been ruled out, suspicion of angina is low, or there is no evidence of ventricular hypokinesia.

CNS toxicity: Mental status change, including moderate confusion or agitation: Withhold dose; may resume when resolved completely.

Dermatologic toxicity: Bullous dermatitis or marked worsening of pre-existing skin condition: Withhold dose; may treat with antihistamines or topical products (do not use topical steroids); may resume with resolution of all signs of bullous dermatitis.

Gastrointestinal: Stool guaiac repeatedly >3-4+: Withhold dose; may resume with negative stool guaiac.

Hepatotoxicity: Signs of hepatic failure, encephalopathy, increasing ascites, liver pain, hypoglycemia: Withhold dose and discontinue treatment for balance of cycle; may initiate a new course if indicated only after at least

7 weeks past resolution of all signs of hepatic failure (including hospital discharge).

Infection: Sepsis syndrome, clinically unstable: Withhold dose; may resume when sepsis syndrome has resolved, patient is clinically stable, and infection is under treatment.

Renal toxicity:

Serum creatinine >4.5 mg/dL (or ≥4 mg/dL with severe volume overload, acidosis or hyperkalemia): Withhold dose; may resume when <4 mg/dL and fluid/electrolyte status is stable.

Persistent oliguria or urine output <10 mL/hour for 16-24 hours with rising serum creatinine: Withhold dose; may resume when urine output >10 mL/hour with serum creatinine decrease of >1.5 mg/dL or normalization.

Respiratory toxicity: Oxygen saturation <90%: Withhold dose; may resume when >90%.

Retreatment with aldesleukin is contraindicated with the following toxicities: Sustained ventricular tachycardia (≥5 beats), uncontrolled or unresponsive cardiac arrhythmias, chest pain with ECG changes consistent with angina or MI, cardiac tamponade, intubation >72 hours, renal failure requiring dialysis for >72 hours, coma or toxic psychosis lasting >48 hours, repetitive or refractory seizures, bowel ischemia/perforation, or GI bleeding requiring surgery

Combination Regimens

Melanoma: CVD-Interleukin-Interferon (Melanoma) on page 1597

Renal cell cancer: Interleukin 2-Interferon Alfa-2 (RCC) on page 1692

Administration Administer as I.V. infusion over 15 minutes (do not administer with an inline filter). Allow solution to reach room temperature prior to administration. Flush before and after with D_5W, particularly if maintenance I.V. line contains sodium chloride. May also be administered by SubQ injection (unlabeled route)

Emetic Potential

>12 million units/m^2: Moderate (30% to 90%)

≤12 million units/m^2: Low (10% to 30%)

Monitoring Parameters

Baseline and periodic: CBC with differential and platelets, blood chemistries including electrolytes, renal and hepatic function tests, and chest x-ray; pulmonary function tests and arterial blood gases (baseline), thallium stress test (prior to treatment)

Monitoring during therapy should include daily (hourly if hypotensive) vital signs (temperature, pulse, blood pressure, and respiration rate), weight and fluid intake and output; in a patient with a decreased blood pressure, especially systolic BP <90 mm Hg, cardiac monitoring for rhythm should be conducted. If an abnormal complex or rhythm is seen, an ECG should be performed; vital signs in these hypotension patients should be taken hourly and central venous pressure (CVP) checked; monitor for change in mental status, and for signs of infection.

Additional Information 18 x 10^6 units = 1.1 mg protein

Dosage Forms Excipient information presented when available (limited, particularly for generics); consult specific product labeling.

Injection, powder for reconstitution:

Proleukin®: 22 x 10^6 units [18 million units/mL = 1.1 mg/mL when reconstituted]

References

Atkins MB, Hsu J, Lee S, et al, "Phase III Trial Comparing Concurrent Biochemotherapy With Cisplatin, Vinblastine, Dacarbazine, Interleukin-2, and Interferon Alfa-2b With Cisplatin, Vinblastine, and Dacarbazine Alone in Patients With Metastatic Malignant Melanoma (E3695): A Trial Coordinated by the Eastern Cooperative Oncology Group," *J Clin Oncol*, 2008, 26(35):5748-54.

Atkins MB, Lotze MT, Dutcher JP, et al, "High-Dose Recombinant Interleukin 2 Therapy for Patients With Metastatic Melanoma: Analysis of 270 Patients Treated Between 1985 and 1993," *J Clin Oncol*, 1999, 17(7):2105-16.

Bergmann L, Heil G, Kolbe K, et al, "Interleukin-2 Bolus Infusion as Late Consolidation Therapy in 2nd Remission of Acute Myeloblastic Leukemia," *Leuk Lymphoma*, 1995, 16(3-4):271-9.

Eton O, Legha SS, Bedikian AY, et al, "Sequential Biochemotherapy Versus Chemotherapy for Metastatic Melanoma: Results From a Phase III Randomized Trial," *J Clin Oncol*, 2002, 20 (8):2045-52.

Klapper JA, Downey SG, Smith FO, et al, "High-Dose Interleukin-2 for the Treatment of Metastatic Renal Cell Carcinoma: A Retrospective Analysis of Response and Survival in Patients Treated in the Surgery Branch at the National Cancer Institute Between 1986 and 2006," *Cancer*, 2008, 113 (2):293-301.

Lange BJ, Smith FO, Feusner J, et al, "Outcomes in CCG-2961, a Children's Oncology Group Phase 3 Trial for Untreated Pediatric Acute Myeloid Leukemia: a Report From the Children's Oncology Group," *Blood*, 2008, 111(3):1044-53.

Legha SS, Ring S, Eton O, et al, "Development of a Biochemotherapy Regimen With Concurrent Administration of Cisplatin, Vinblastine, Dacarbazine, Interferon Alfa, and Interleukin-2 for Patients With Metastatic Melanoma," *J Clin Oncol*, 1998, 16(5):1752-9.

McDermott DF, Regan MM, Clark JI, et al, "Randomized Phase III Trial of High-Dose Interleukin-2 Versus Subcutaneous Interleukin-2 and Interferon in Patients With Metastatic Renal Cell Carcinoma," *J Clin Oncol*, 2005, 23(1):133-41.

Smith FO, Downey SG, Klapper JA, et al, "Treatment of Metastatic Melanoma Using Interleukin-2 Alone or in Conjunction With Vaccines," *Clin Cancer Res*, 2008, 14(17):5610-8.

Yang JC, Sherry RM, Steinberg, SM, et al, "Randomized Study of High-Dose and Low-Dose Interleukin-2 in Patients With Metastatic Renal Cancer," *J Clin Oncol*, 2003, 21(16): 3127-32.

Alemtuzumab (ay lem TU zoo mab)

Related Information

Management of Chemotherapy-Induced Nausea and Vomiting *on page 1786*

Management of Infections *on page 1809*

Principles of Anticancer Therapy *on page 1878*

Safe Handling of Hazardous Drugs *on page 1904*

Brand Names: U.S. Campath® [DSC]

Brand Names: Canada MabCampath®

Index Terms Anti-CD52 Monoclonal Antibody; Campath-1H; Humanized IgG1 Anti-CD52 Monoclonal Antibody; Lemtrada; MoAb CD52; Monoclonal Antibody Campath-1H; Monoclonal Antibody CD52

Generic Availability (U.S.) No

Pharmacologic Category Antineoplastic Agent, Monoclonal Antibody; Monoclonal Antibody

Use Campath®: Treatment (as a single agent) of B-cell chronic lymphocytic leukemia (B-CLL)

Unlabeled Use Conditioning regimen in stem cell transplant; prophylaxis of graft-versus-host disease (GVHD); treatment of steroid-refractory GVHD; treatment of T-cell prolymphocytic leukemia; treatment of autoimmune hemolytic anemia (CLL-induced); immunosuppressant in solid organ transplant (induction and steroid-refractory rejection); treatment of relapsed-remitting multiple sclerosis

Labeled Contraindications There are no contraindications listed in the manufacturer's labeling

Pregnancy Risk Factor C

Lactation Excretion in breast milk unknown/not recommended

Warnings/Precautions [U.S. Boxed Warning]: Serious infections (bacterial, viral, fungal, and protozoan) have been reported. Administer prophylactic medications against PCP pneumonia and herpes viral infections during treatment and for at least 2 months following last dose or until $CD4^+$ counts are ≥200 cells/µL (whichever is later). Severe and prolonged lymphopenia may occur; $CD4^+$ counts usually return to ≥200 cells/µL within 2-6 months; however, $CD4^+$ and $CD8^+$ lymphocyte counts may not return to baseline levels for more than 1 year. Monitor for CMV infection (during and for at least 2 months after completion of therapy). Withhold treatment during serious infections; may be reinitiated upon resolution of infection. Monitor for CMV infection (during and for at least 2 months after completion of therapy); initiate appropriate antiviral treatment and withhold alemtuzumab for CMV infection or confirmed CMV viremia (withhold alemtuzumab during CMV antiviral treatment).

[U.S. Boxed Warning]: Serious and potentially fatal infusion-related reactions may occur; monitor for infusion reaction; withhold treatment for grade 3 or 4 infusion reactions. Gradual escalation to the recommended maintenance dose is required at initiation and with treatment interruptions (for ≥7 days) to minimize infusion-related reactions. Infusion reaction symptoms may include acute respiratory distress syndrome, anaphylactic shock, angioedema, bronchospasm, cardiac arrest, cardiac arrhythmias, chills, dyspnea, fever, hypotension, myocardial infarction, pulmonary infiltrates, rash, rigors, syncope, or urticaria. The incidence of infusion reaction is highest during the first week of treatment. Premedicate with acetaminophen and an oral antihistamine. Medications for the treatment of reactions should be available for immediate use. Use caution and carefully monitor blood pressure in patients with ischemic heart disease and patients on antihypertensive therapy. Reinitiate with gradual dose escalation if treatment is withheld ≥7 days.

[U.S. Boxed Warning]: Serious and fatal cytopenias (including pancytopenia, bone marrow hypoplasia, autoimmune hemolytic anemia, and autoimmune idiopathic thrombocytopenia) have occurred. Single doses >30 mg or cumulative weekly doses >90 mg are associated with an increased incidence of pancytopenia. Severe prolonged myelosuppression, hemolytic anemia, pure red cell aplasia, bone marrow aplasia, and bone marrow hypoplasia have also been reported with use at the normal dose for the treatment of B-CLL. Discontinue for serious hematologic or other serious toxicity (except lymphopenia) until the event resolves. Permanently discontinue if autoimmune anemia or autoimmune thrombocytopenia occurs. Patients receiving blood products should only receive irradiated blood products due to the potential for transfusion-associated GVHD during lymphopenia.

Immune thrombocytopenia (ITP) or idiopathic thrombocytopenic purpura has been reported in 6 patients receiving alemtuzumab for the treatment of relapsed-remitting multiple sclerosis (RMSS); some cases were severe, with 1 fatality (Cuker, 2011). The median time to onset was 24.5 months from initial alemtuzumab exposure and 10.5 months from the last dose. In 4 cases, ITP was treated with standard ITP management and responses were observed within 1 week. After the initial case was discovered, patients in the RMSS study were instructed to report abnormal bleeding, bruising or petechial rash and blood counts were monitored monthly.

Patients should not be immunized with live, viral vaccines during or recently after treatment. The ability to respond to any vaccine following therapy is unknown.

Adverse Reactions Adverse reactions reported with Campath®:

>10%:

Cardiovascular: Hypotension (16%), hypertension (14%), dysrhythmia (14%)

Central nervous system: Fever (69%), chills (53%), headache (14%), dysthesias, fatigue

Dermatologic: Urticaria (16%), rash (13%)

Gastrointestinal: Abdominal pain, anorexia, mucositis, nausea, vomiting

Hematologic: Lymphopenia (grades 3/4: 97%), neutropenia (77%; grade 3/4: 42% to 64% [median onset: 31 days, median duration: 28-37 days]), anemia (76%; grade 3/4: 12% to 38% [median onset: 31 days, median duration 8 days]), thrombocytopenia (71%; grade 3/4: 13% to 52% [median onset: 9 days, median duration: 14-21 days])

Local: Injection site reaction (SubQ administration: 90%)

Neuromuscular & skeletal: Musculoskeletal pain

Respiratory: Dyspnea (14%)

Miscellaneous: Infection (50% to 74%; grades 3/4: 5% to 21%; includes bacterial, fungal, protozoan, viral), CMV viremia (55%), infusion reactions (grades 3/4: 10% to 35%), CMV infection (16%), sepsis (grades 3/4/5: 3% to 10%)

1% to 10%:

Cardiovascular: Tachycardia (10%)

Central nervous system: Insomnia (10%), anxiety (8%)

Dermatologic: Erythema (4%)

Gastrointestinal: Diarrhea (10%)

Hematologic: Neutropenic fever (grades 3/4: 5% to 10%)

Neuromuscular & skeletal: Tremor (3%)

Respiratory: Bronchospasm

<1%, postmarketing, and/or case reports (limited to important or life-threatening): Acute respiratory distress syndrome, anaphylactoid shock, angioedema, aplastic anemia, arrhythmia, bleeding, bone marrow aplasia, bone marrow hypoplasia, bruising, cardiac arrest, cardiac insufficiency, cardiomyopathy, chronic inflammatory demyelinating polyradiculoneuropathy (CIDP), ejection fraction decreased, Epstein-Barr virus, Epstein-Barr virus-associated lymphoproliferative disorder, Goodpasture's syndrome, Graves' disease, Guillain-Barré syndrome, hemolytic anemia, HF, idiopathic thrombocytopenic purpura (ITP), MI, optic neuropathy, pallor, petechia, *Pneumocystis jirovecii* pneumonia (PCP), progressive multifocal leukoencephalopathy (PML), pulmonary infiltrates, pure red cell aplasia, purpura, respiratory arrest, serum sickness, syncope, transfusion-associated GVHD, tumor lysis syndrome, virus reactivation (latent), weakness

Drug Interactions

Metabolism/Transport Effects None known.

Avoid Concomitant Use

Avoid concomitant use of Alemtuzumab with any of the following: BCG; Belimumab; CloZAPine; Natalizumab; Pimecrolimus; Tacrolimus (Topical); Vaccines (Live)

Increased Effect/Toxicity

Alemtuzumab may increase the levels/effects of: Belimumab; CloZAPine; Leflunomide; Natalizumab; Vaccines (Live)

The levels/effects of Alemtuzumab may be increased by: Abciximab; Denosumab; Pimecrolimus; Roflumilast; Tacrolimus (Topical); Trastuzumab

Decreased Effect

Alemtuzumab may decrease the levels/effects of: BCG; Coccidioidin Skin Test; Sipuleucel-T; Vaccines (Inactivated); Vaccines (Live)

The levels/effects of Alemtuzumab may be decreased by: Echinacea

Ethanol/Nutrition/Herb Interactions Herb/Nutraceutical: Echinacea may diminish the therapeutic effect of alemtuzumab.

Storage/Stability Campath®: Prior to dilution, store intact (30 mg/1 mL) vials at 2°C to 8°C (36°F to 46°F); do not freeze (if accidentally frozen, thaw in refrigerator prior to administration). Do not shake; protect from light. Following dilution, store at room temperature or refrigerate; protect from light; use within 8 hours. Discard unused portion in the vial.

Reconstitution Campath®: Dilute for infusion in 100 mL NS or D_5W. Compatible in polyvinylchloride (PVC) bags. Gently invert the bag to mix the solution. Do not shake prior to use.

Mechanism of Action Binds to CD52, a nonmodulating antigen present on the surface of B and T lymphocytes, a majority of monocytes, macrophages, NK cells, and a subpopulation of granulocytes. After binding to $CD52^+$ cells, an antibody-dependent lysis of malignant cells occurs.

Pharmacodynamics/Kinetics

Distribution: V_d: I.V.: 0.18 L/kg (range: 0.1-0.4 L/kg)

Metabolism: Clearance decreases with repeated dosing (due to loss of CD52 receptors in periphery), resulting in a sevenfold increase in AUC after 12 weeks of therapy.

Half-life elimination: I.V.: 11 hours (following first 30 mg dose; range: 2-32 hours); 6 days (following the last 30 mg dose; range: 1-14 days)

Dosing

Adult & Geriatric Note: Dose escalation is required; usually accomplished in 3-7 days. Single doses >30 mg or cumulative doses >90 mg/week increase the incidence of pancytopenia. Pretreatment (with acetaminophen 500-1000 mg and diphenhydramine 50 mg) is recommended prior to the first dose, with dose escalations, and as clinically indicated; I.V. hydrocortisone may be used for severe infusion-related reactions. Reinitiate with gradual dose escalation if treatment is withheld ≥7 days.

Dose escalation: Initial: 3 mg daily beginning on day 1; if tolerated (infusion reaction ≤grade 2), increase to 10 mg daily; if tolerated (infusion reaction ≤grade 2), may increase to maintenance of 30 mg per dose 3 times weekly if required for maintenance dose.

B-cell chronic lymphocytic leukemia (B-CLL): I.V.: Gradually escalate to a maintenance of 30 mg per dose 3 times weekly on alternate days for a total duration of therapy of up to 12 weeks (Hillmen, 2007; Keating, 2002)

B-CLL (unlabeled route): SubQ: Initial: 3 mg on day 1; if tolerated 10 mg on day 3; if tolerated increase to 30 mg on day 5; maintenance: 30 mg per dose 3 times weekly for a maximum of 18 weeks (Lundin, 2002) **or** 3 mg on day 1; if tolerated 10 mg on day 2; if tolerated 30 mg on day 3, followed by 30 mg per dose 3 times weekly for 4-12 weeks (Stilgenbauer, 2009)

Autoimmune cytopenias, CLL-induced, refractory (unlabeled use): I.V., SubQ: Gradually escalate to a maintenance of 10-30 mg per dose 3 times weekly for 4-12 weeks (Karlsson, 2007; Osterborg, 2009)

Graft versus host disease (GVHD), acute, steroid refractory, treatment (unlabeled use): I.V.: 10 mg daily for 5 consecutive days, then 10 mg weekly on days 8, 15, and 22 if CR not achieved (Martínez, 2009) **or** 10 mg weekly until symptom resolution (Schnitzler, 2009)

Multiple sclerosis, relapsed-remitting (RRMS; unlabeled use): I.V.: 12 mg daily for 5 consecutive days, followed 12 months later by 12 mg daily for 3 consecutive days; may receive an additional 12 mg daily for 3 consecutive days 12 months later (CAMMS223, 2008; Coles, 2012)

Renal transplant, induction (unlabeled use): I.V.: 30 mg as a single dose at the time of transplant (Hanaway, 2011)

Stem cell transplant (allogeneic) conditioning regimen (unlabeled use): I.V.: 20 mg daily for 5 days (in combination with fludarabine and melphalan) beginning 8 days prior to transplant (Mead, 2010) **or** beginning 7 days prior to transplant (Van Besien, 2009)

T-cell prolymphocytic leukemia (T-PLL; unlabeled use): I.V.: Initial test dose 3 mg or 10 mg, followed by dose escalation to 30 mg per dose 3 times weekly as tolerated until maximum response (Dearden, 2001) **or** Initial dose: 3 mg day 1, if tolerated increase to 10 mg day 2, if tolerated increase to 30 mg on day 3 (days 1, 2, and 3 are consecutive days), followed by 30 mg per dose every Monday, Wednesday, Friday for a total of 4-12 weeks (Keating, 2002)

Adjustment for Toxicity

Dosage adjustment for nonhematologic toxicity:

Note: If treatment is withheld ≥7 days, reinitiate at 3 mg with re-escalation to 10 mg and then 30 mg.

Grade 3 or 4 infusion reaction: Withhold infusion

Serious infection or other serious adverse reaction: Withhold alemtuzumab until resolution

Autoimmune anemia or autoimmune thrombocytopenia: Discontinue alemtuzumab

Dosage adjustment for hematologic toxicity (severe neutropenia or thrombocytopenia, not autoimmune):

Note: If treatment is withheld ≥7 days, reinitiate at 3 mg with re-escalation to 10 mg and then 30 mg.

ANC <250/mm³ and/or platelet count ≤25,000/mm³:

- First occurrence: Withhold treatment; resume at 30 mg per dose when ANC ≥500/mm³ and platelet count ≥50,000/mm³
- Second occurrence: Withhold treatment; resume at 10 mg per dose when ANC ≥500/mm³ and platelet count ≥50,000/mm³
- Third occurrence: Discontinue alemtuzumab.

Patients with a baseline ANC ≤250/mm³ and/or a baseline platelet count ≤25,000/mm³ at initiation of therapy: If ANC and/or platelet counts decrease to ≤50% of the baseline value:

- First occurrence: Withhold treatment; resume at 30 mg per dose upon return to baseline values
- Second occurrence: Withhold treatment; resume at 10 mg per dose upon return to baseline values
- Third occurrence: Discontinue alemtuzumab.

Combination Regimens

Leukemia, chronic lymphocytic:

Cyclophosphamide-Fludarabine-Alemtuzumab-Rituximab (CLL) on page 1601

Fludarabine-Alemtuzumab (CLL) on page 1645

Administration Administer by I.V. infusion over 2 hours. Premedicate with diphenhydramine 50 mg and acetaminophen 500-1000 mg 30 minutes before each infusion. Hydrocortisone (I.V.) has been effective in decreasing severe infusion-related events. Start anti-infective prophylaxis. Other drugs should not be added to or simultaneously infused through the same I.V. line. Do not give I.V. push or bolus. Compatible in polyvinylchloride (PVC) or polyethylene lined administration sets.

SubQ (unlabeled route): SubQ administration has been studied (Lundin, 2002; Stilgenbauer, 2009); an increased rate of injection site reactions has been observed, with only rare incidences of chills or infusion-like reactions typically observed with I.V. infusion. A longer dose escalation time (1-2 weeks) may be needed due to injection site reactions (Lundin, 2002). Premedicate with diphenhydramine 50 mg and acetaminophen 500-1000 mg 30 minutes before dose. The subQ route should **NOT** be used for the treatment of T-PLL (Deardon, 2011).

Emetic Potential Moderate (30% to 90%)

Monitoring Parameters Vital signs; carefully monitor BP especially in patients with ischemic heart disease or on antihypertensive medications; CBC with differential and platelets (weekly, more frequent if worsening); signs and symptoms of infection; CD4+ lymphocyte counts (after treatment until recovery); CMV antigen (routinely during and for 2 months after treatment). Monitor closely for infusion reactions (including hypotension, rigors, fever, shortness of breath, bronchospasm, chills, and/or rash); consider TSH at baseline and then every 2-3 months during alemtuzumab treatment (Hamnvik, 2011).

Test Interactions May interfere with diagnostic serum tests that utilize antibodies.

Prescribing and Access Restrictions As of September 4, 2012, alemtuzumab (Campath®) is no longer commercially available in the United States (or Europe); a restricted distribution program will allow access (free of charge) for appropriate patients. Information on necessary documentation and requirements is available at Campath Distribution Program (1-877-422-6728) or Genzyme Medical Information (1-800-745-4447, option 2).

Dosage Forms Excipient information presented when available (limited, particularly for generics); consult specific product labeling. [DSC] = Discontinued product

Injection, solution [preservative free]:

Campath®: 30 mg/mL (1 mL [DSC]) [contains edetate disodium, polysorbate 80]

References

CAMMS223 Trial Investigators: Coles AJ, Compston DA, Selmaj KW, et al, "Alemtuzumab vs Interferon Beta-1a in Early Multiple \Sclerosis," *N Engl J Med*, 2008, 359(17):1786-801.

Coles AJ, Fox E, Vladic A, et al, "Alemtuzumab More Effective Than Interferon B-1a at 5-Year Follow-Up of CAMMS223 Clinical Trial," Neurology, 2012, 78(14):1069-78.

Cuker A, Coles AJ, Sullivan H, et al, "A Distinctive Form of Immune Thrombocytopenia in a Phase 2 Study of Alemtuzumab for the Treatment of Relapsing-Remitting Multiple Sclerosis," *Blood*, 2011, 118(24):6299-305.

Dearden CE, Johnson R, Pettengell R, et al, "Guidelines for the Management of Mature T-Cell and NK-Cell Neoplasms (Excluding Cutaneous T-Cell Lymphoma)," *Br J Haematol*, 2011, 153 (4):451-85.

Dearden CE, Matutes E, Cazin B, et al, "High Remission Rate in T-Cell Prolymphocytic Leukemia With CAMPATH-1H," *Blood*, 2001, 98(6):1721-6.

Enblad G, Hagberg H, Erlanson M, et al, "A Pilot Study of Alemtuzumab (Anti-CD52 Monoclonal Antibody) Therapy for Patients With Relapsed or Chemotherapy-Refractory Peripheral T-cell Lymphomas," *Blood*, 2003, 103(8):2920-4.

Ferrajoli A, O'Brien SM, Cortes JE, et al, "Phase II Study of Alemtuzumab in Chronic Lymphoproliferative Disorders," *Cancer*, 2003, 98(4):773-8.

Hale G, Rebello P, Brettman LR, et al, "Blood Concentrations of Alemtuzumab and Antiglobulin Responses in Patients With Chronic Lymphocytic Leukemia Following Intravenous or Subcutaneous Routes of Administration, *Blood*, 2004, 104(4):948-55.

Hamnvik OP, Larsen PR, and Marqusee E, "Thyroid Dysfunction From Antineoplastic Agents," *J Natl Cancer Inst*, 2011, 103(21):1572-87.

Hanaway MJ, Woodle ES, Mulgaonkar S, et al, "Alemtuzumab Induction In Renal Transplantation," *N Engl J Med*, 2011, 364(20):1909-19.

Hillmen P, Skotnicki A, Robak T, et al, "Alemtuzumab Compared With Chlorambucil as First-Line Therapy for Chronic Lymphocytic Leukemia," *J Clin Oncol*, 2007, 25(35):5616-23.

Karlsson C, Hansson L, Celsing F, et al, "Treatment of Severe Refractory Autoimmune Hemolytic Anemia in B-Cell Chronic Lymphocytic Leukemia With Alemtuzumab (Humanized CD52 Monoclonal Antibody)," *Leukemia*, 2007, 21(3):511-4.

Keating MJ, Cazin B, Coutré S, et al, "Campath-1H Treatment of T-Cell Prolymphocytic Leukemia in Patients for Whom at Least One Prior Chemotherapy Regimen Has Failed," *J Clin Oncol*, 2002, 20(1):205-13.

Keating MJ, Flinn I, Jain V, et al, "Therapeutic Role of Alemtuzumab (Campath-1H) in Patients Who Have Failed Fludarabine: Results of a Large International Study," *Blood*, 2002, 99(10):3554-61.

Kennedy B and Hillmen P, "Immunological Effects and Safe Administration of Alemtuzumab (MabCampath) in Advanced B-cLL," *Med Oncol*, 2002, 19(Suppl):49-55.

Lundin J, Hagberg H, Repp R, et al, "Phase 2 Study of Alemtuzumab (Anti-CD52 Monoclonal Antibody) In Patients With Advanced Mycosis Fungoides/Sézary Syndrome," *Blood*, 2003, 101 (11):4267-72.

Lundin J, Kimby E, Bjorkholm M, et al, "Phase II Trial of Subcutaneous Anti-CD52 Monoclonal Antibody Alemtuzumab (Campath-1H) as First-Line Treatment for Patients With B-Cell Chronic Lymphocytic Leukemia (B-CLL)," *Blood*, 2002, 100(3):768-73.

Lundin J, Osterborg A, Brittinger G, et al, "CAMPATH-1H Monoclonal Antibody in Therapy for Previously Treated Low-Grade Non-Hodgkin's Lymphomas: A Phase II Multicenter Study. European Study Group of CAMPATH-1H Treatment in Low-Grade Non-Hodgkin's Lymphoma," *J Clin Oncol*, 1998, 16(10):3257-63.

Magliocca JF and Knechtle SJ, "The Evolving Role of Alemtuzumab (Campath-1H) for Immunosuppressive Therapy in Organ Transplantation," *Transpl Int*, 2006, 19(9):705-14.

Martinez C, Solano C, Ferrá C, et al, "Alemtuzumab as Treatment of Steroid-Refractory Acute Graft-Versus-Host Disease: Results From a Phase II Study," *Biol Blood Marrow Transplant*, 2009, 15(5):639-42.

Mead AJ, Thomson KJ, Morris EC, et al, "HLA-Mismatched Unrelated Donors are a Viable Alternate Graft Source for Allogeneic Transplantation Following Alemtuzumab-Based Reduced-Intensity Conditioning," *Blood*, 2010, 115(25):5147-53.

Osterborg A, Fassas AS, Anagnostopoulos A, et al, "Humanifed CD52 Monoclonal Antibody Campath-1H as First-Line Treatment in Chronic Lymphocytic Leukaemia," *Br J Haematol*, 1996, 93(1):151-3.

Osterborg A, Karlsson C, and Lundin J, "Alemtuzumab to Treat Refractory Autoimmune Hemolytic Anemia or Thrombocytopenia in Chronic Lymphocytic Leukemia," *Curr Hematol Malig Rep*, 2009, 4(1):47-53.

Rai KR, Freter CE, Mercier RJ, et al, "Alemtuzumab in Previously Treated Chronic Lymphocytic Leukemia Patients Who Also Had Received Fludarabine," *J Clin Oncol*, 2002, 20(18):3891-7.

Schnitzler M, Hasskerl J, Egger M, et al, "Successful Treatment of Severe Acute Intestinal Graft-Versus-Host Resistant to Systemic and Topical Steroids With Alemtuzumab," *Biol Blood Marrow Transplant*, 2009, 15(8):910-18.

Stilgenbauer S, Zenz T, Winkler D, et al, "Subcutaneous Alemtuzumab in Fludarabine-Refractory Chronic Lymphocytic Leukemia: Clinical Results and Prognostic Marker Analyses from the CLL2H Study of the German Chronic Lymphocytic Leukemia Study Group," *J Clin Oncol*, 2009, 27(24):3994-4001.

van Besien K, Kunavakkam R, Rondon G, et al, "Fludarabine-Melphalan Conditioning for AML and MDS: Alemtuzumab Reduces Acute and Chronic GVHD Without Affecting Long-term Outcomes," *Biol Blood Marrow Transplant*, 2009, 15(5):610-7.

Vo AA, Wechsler EA, Wang J, et al, "Analysis of Subcutaneous (SQ) Alemtuzumab Induction Therapy in Highly Sensitized Patients Desensitized With IVIG and Rituximab," *Am J Transplant*, 2008, 8(1):144-9.

◆ **Alimta®** *see* PEMEtrexed *on page 1151*

Alitretinoin (a li TRET i noyn)

Related Information

Safe Handling of Hazardous Drugs *on page 1904*

Brand Names: U.S. Panretin®

Generic Availability (U.S.) No

Pharmacologic Category Antineoplastic Agent, Miscellaneous; Retinoic Acid Derivative

Use Orphan drug: Topical treatment of cutaneous lesions in AIDS-related Kaposi's sarcoma

Unlabeled Use Cutaneous T-cell lymphomas

Labeled Contraindications Hypersensitivity to alitretinoin, other retinoids, or any component of the formulation; pregnancy

Pregnancy Risk Factor D

Lactation Excretion in breast milk unknown/not recommended

Warnings/Precautions Hazardous agent - use appropriate precautions for handling and disposal. May cause fetal harm if absorbed by a woman who is pregnant. May be photosensitizing (based on experience with other retinoids); minimize sun or other UV exposure of treated areas. Do not use concurrently with topical products containing DEET. Safety in pediatric patients or geriatric patients has not been established.

Adverse Reactions

>10%:

Central nervous system: Pain (0% to 34%)

Dermatologic: Rash (25% to 77%), pruritus (8% to 11%)

Neuromuscular & skeletal: Paresthesia (3% to 22%)

5% to 10%:

Cardiovascular: Edema (3% to 8%)

Dermatologic: Exfoliative dermatitis (3% to 9%), skin disorder (0% to 8%)

Drug Interactions

Metabolism/Transport Effects None known.

Avoid Concomitant Use

Avoid concomitant use of Alitretinoin with any of the following: Multivitamins/Minerals (with ADEK, Folate, Iron)

Increased Effect/Toxicity

Alitretinoin may increase the levels/effects of: Porfimer

The levels/effects of Alitretinoin may be increased by: Multivitamins/Minerals (with ADEK, Folate, Iron)

Decreased Effect

Alitretinoin may decrease the levels/effects of: Contraceptives (Progestins)

Storage/Stability Store at room temperature.

Mechanism of Action Binds to retinoid receptors to inhibit growth of Kaposi's sarcoma

Pharmacodynamics/Kinetics Absorption: Not extensive

Dosing

Adult & Geriatric

Kaposi's sarcoma: Topical: Apply gel twice daily to cutaneous lesions.

T-cell lymphomas (unlabeled use): Topical: Apply gel twice daily to cutaneous lesions.

Administration Do not use occlusive dressings.

Dosage Forms Excipient information presented when available (limited, particularly for generics); consult specific product labeling.

Gel, topical:
  Panretin®: 0.1% (60 g) [contains dehydrated ethanol]

- **Alkeran®** *see* Melphalan *on page 925*
- **Alloprin® (Can)** *see* Allopurinol *on page 51*

Allopurinol (al oh PURE i nole)

Related Information

Oral Mucositis/Stomatitis *on page 1814*

Brand Names: U.S. Aloprim®; Zyloprim®

Brand Names: Canada Alloprin®; Novo-Purol; Zyloprim®

Index Terms Allopurinol Sodium

Generic Availability (U.S.) Yes

Pharmacologic Category Antigout Agent; Xanthine Oxidase Inhibitor

Use

Oral: Management of primary or secondary gout (acute attack, tophi, joint destruction, uric acid lithiasis, and/or nephropathy); management of hyperuricemia associated with cancer treatment for leukemia, lymphoma, or solid tumor malignancies; management of recurrent calcium oxalate calculi (with uric acid excretion >800 mg/day in men and >750 mg/day in women)

I.V.: Management of hyperuricemia associated with cancer treatment for leukemia, lymphoma, or solid tumor malignancies

Labeled Contraindications Hypersensitivity to allopurinol or any component of the formulation

Pregnancy Risk Factor C

Lactation Enters breast milk/use caution (AAP rates "compatible"; AAP 2001 update pending)

Warnings/Precautions Do not use to treat asymptomatic hyperuricemia. Has been associated with a number of hypersensitivity reactions, including severe reactions (vasculitis and Stevens-Johnson syndrome); discontinue at first sign of rash. Reversible hepatotoxicity has been reported; use with caution in patients with pre-existing hepatic impairment. Bone marrow suppression has been reported; use caution with other drugs causing myelosuppression. Caution in renal impairment, dosage adjustments needed. Use with caution in patients taking diuretics concurrently. Risk of skin rash may be increased in patients receiving amoxicillin or ampicillin. The risk of hypersensitivity may be increased in patients receiving thiazides, and possibly ACE inhibitors. Use caution with mercaptopurine or azathioprine; dosage adjustment necessary. Full effect on serum uric acid levels in chronic gout may take several weeks to become evident; gradual titration is recommended.

Adverse Reactions

Most commonly reported:

Dermatologic: Rash

Endocrine & metabolic: Gout (acute)

Gastrointestinal: Diarrhea, nausea

Hepatic: Alkaline phosphatase increased, liver enzymes increased

<1%: Abdominal pain, agranulocytosis, alopecia, angioedema, aplastic anemia, arthralgia, bronchospasm, cataracts, cholestatic jaundice, dermatitis (eczematoid, exfoliative, vascular bullous), dyspepsia, ecchymosis, eosinophilia, epistaxis, fever, gastritis, granuloma annulare, hepatitis, gynecomastia, headache, hepatic necrosis, hepatomegaly, hyperbilirubinemia, hypersensitivity reactions, leukocytosis, leukopenia, lichen planus, loss of taste perception, macular retinitis, myopathy, necrotizing angiitis, nephritis, neuritis,

neuropathy, onycholysis, pancreatitis, paresthesia, purpura, pruritus, renal failure, somnolence, Stevens-Johnson syndrome, taste perversion, thrombocytopenia, toxic epidermal necrolysis, toxic pustuloderma, uremia, vasculitis, vomiting

Drug Interactions

Metabolism/Transport Effects None known.

Avoid Concomitant Use

Avoid concomitant use of Allopurinol with any of the following: Didanosine

Increased Effect/Toxicity

Allopurinol may increase the levels/effects of: Amoxicillin; Ampicillin; Anticonvulsants (Hydantoin); AzaTHIOprine; CarBAMazepine; ChlorproPAMIDE; Cyclophosphamide; Didanosine; Mercaptopurine; Theophylline Derivatives; Vitamin K Antagonists

The levels/effects of Allopurinol may be increased by: ACE Inhibitors; Loop Diuretics; Thiazide Diuretics

Decreased Effect

The levels/effects of Allopurinol may be decreased by: Antacids

Ethanol/Nutrition/Herb Interactions

Ethanol: May decrease effectiveness.

Iron supplements: Hepatic iron uptake may be increased.

Vitamin C: Large amounts of vitamin C may acidify urine and increase kidney stone formation.

Storage/Stability

Powder for injection: Store at controlled room temperature of 20°C to 25°C (68°F to 77°F). Following preparation, intravenous solutions should be stored at 20°C to 25°C (68°F to 77°F). Do not refrigerate reconstituted and/or diluted product. Must be administered within 10 hours of solution preparation.

Tablet: Store at controlled room temperature of 20°C to 25°C (68°F to 77°F). Protect from moisture and light.

Reconstitution Reconstitute powder for injection with SWFI. Further dilution with NS or D_5W (50-100 mL) to ≤6 mg/mL is recommended.

Mechanism of Action Allopurinol inhibits xanthine oxidase, the enzyme responsible for the conversion of hypoxanthine to xanthine to uric acid. Allopurinol is metabolized to oxypurinol which is also an inhibitor of xanthine oxidase; allopurinol acts on purine catabolism, reducing the production of uric acid without disrupting the biosynthesis of vital purines.

Pharmacodynamics/Kinetics

Onset of action: Peak effect: 1-2 weeks

Absorption: Oral: ~80%; Rectal: Poor and erratic

Distribution: V_d: ~1.6 L/kg; V_{ss}: 0.84-0.87 L/kg; enters breast milk

Protein binding: <1%

Metabolism: ~75% to active metabolites, chiefly oxypurinol

Bioavailability: 49% to 53%

Half-life elimination:

Normal renal function: Parent drug: 1-3 hours; Oxypurinol: 18-30 hours

End-stage renal disease: Prolonged

Time to peak, plasma: Oral: 30-120 minutes

Excretion: Urine (76% as oxypurinol, 12% as unchanged drug)

Allopurinol and oxypurinol are dialyzable

Dosing

Adult & Geriatric Note: Oral doses >300 mg should be given in divided doses.

Gout (chronic): Oral:

Manufacturer's labeling: Mild: 200-300 mg/day; Severe: 400-600 mg/day; to reduce the possibility of acute gouty attacks, initiate dose at 100 mg/day and increase weekly to recommended dosage, also consider using low-dose colchicine or an NSAID to reduce the risk of a gouty attack. Maximum daily dose: 800 mg/day.

Alternative recommendations (unlabeled dosing): Initial: 100 mg/day, increasing the dose gradually every 4 weeks, while monitoring plasma uric acid levels to achieve a goal of <6 mg/dL; dosages of 600 mg/day and rarely, 900 mg/day may be required (McGill, 2010) **or** Initial: 100 mg/day, increasing the dose by 100 mg/day at 2-4 weeks intervals as required to achieve desired uric acid level of ≤6 mg/dL (EULAR gout guidelines; Zhang, 2006).

Management of hyperuricemia associated with chemotherapy:

Oral:

Manufacturer's labeling: 600-800 mg/day in 2-3 divided doses

Alternative recommendations (unlabeled dosing; intermediate-risk for tumor lysis syndrome): Intermediate-risk for tumor lysis syndrome: 10 mg/kg/day (maximum dose/day: 800 mg) in 3 divided doses **or** 50-100 mg/m^2 every 8 hours (maximum dose: 300 mg/m^2/day), begin 1-2 days before initiation of induction chemotherapy; may continue for 3-7 days after chemotherapy (Coiffier, 2008)

I.V.:

Manufacturer's labeling: 200-400 mg/m^2/day (maximum: 600 mg/day) beginning 1-2 days before chemotherapy

Alternative recommendations (unlabeled dosing; intermediate-risk for tumor lysis syndrome): 200-400 mg/m^2/day (maximum dose/day: 600 mg) in 1-3 divided doses beginning 1-2 days before the start of induction chemotherapy; may continue for 3-7 days after chemotherapy (Coiffier, 2008)

Note: Intravenous daily dose can be given as a single infusion or in equally divided doses at 6-, 8-, or 12-hour intervals. A fluid intake sufficient to yield a daily urinary output of at least 2 L in adults is desirable.

Recurrent calcium oxalate stones: Oral: 200-300 mg/day in single or divided doses

Pediatric

Management of hyperuricemia associated with chemotherapy:

Oral: **Note:** Oral doses >300 mg should be given in divided doses.

Manufacturer's labeling:

Children <6 years: 150 mg/day

Children 6-10 years: 300 mg/day

Children >10 years: Refer to adult dosing.

Alternative recommendations (unlabeled dosing; intermediate-risk for tumor lysis syndrome): Intermediate-risk for tumor lysis syndrome: 10 mg/kg/day (maximum dose/day: 800 mg) in 3 divided doses **or** 50-100 mg/m^2 every 8 hours (maximum dose: 300 mg/m^2/day), begin 1-2 days before initiation of induction chemotherapy; may continue for 3-7 days after chemotherapy (Coiffier, 2008)

I.V.:

Manufacturer's labeling: Starting dose: 200 mg/m^2/day beginning 1-2 days before chemotherapy

Alternative recommendations (unlabeled dosing; intermediate-risk for tumor lysis syndrome) 200-400 mg/m²/day (maximum dose/day: 600 mg) in 1-3 divided doses beginning 1-2 days before the start of induction chemotherapy; may continue for 3-7 days after chemotherapy (Coiffier, 2008)

Note: Adequate fluid intake is desirable.

Renal Impairment

Manufacturer's labeling: Oral, I.V.: Lower doses are required in renal impairment due to potential for accumulation of allopurinol and metabolites.

Cl_{cr} 10-20 mL/minute: 200 mg/day

Cl_{cr} 3-10 mL/minute: ≤100 mg/day

Cl_{cr} <3 mL/minute: 100 mg/dose at extended intervals

Alternative recommendations (unlabeled dosing):

Management of hyperuricemia associated with chemotherapy: Dosage reduction of 50% is recommended in renal impairment (Coiffier, 2008)

Gout: Oral:

Initiate therapy with 50-100 mg daily, and gradually increase to a maintenance dose to achieve a serum uric acid level of ≤6 mg/dL (with close monitoring of serum uric acid levels and for hypersensitivity) (Dalbeth, 2007).

Hemodialysis: Initial: 100 mg alternate days given postdialysis, increase cautiously to 300 mg based on response. If dialysis is on a daily basis, an additional 50% of the dose may be required postdialysis (Dalbeth, 2007)

Administration

Oral: Do not initiate or discontinue allopurinol during an acute gout attack. Should administer oral forms after meals with plenty of fluid.

I.V.: The rate of infusion depends on the volume of the infusion; infuse maximum single daily doses (600 mg/day) over ≥30 minutes. Whenever possible, therapy should be initiated at 24-48 hours before the start of chemotherapy known to cause tumor lysis (including adrenocorticosteroids). I.V. daily dose can be administered as a single infusion or in equally divided doses at 6-, 8-, or 12-hour interval.

Extemporaneous Preparations A 20 mg/mL oral suspension may be made with tablets and either a 1:1 mixture of Ora-Sweet® and Ora-Plus® or a 1:1 mixture of Ora-Sweet® SF and Ora-Plus® or a 1:4 mixture of cherry syrup concentrate and simple syrup, NF. Crush eight 300 mg tablets in a mortar and reduce to a fine powder. Add small portions of chosen vehicle and mix to a uniform paste; mix while adding the vehicle in incremental proportions to **almost** 120 mL; transfer to a calibrated bottle, rinse mortar with vehicle, and add quantity of vehicle sufficient to make 120 mL. Label "shake well". Stable for 60 days refrigerated or at room temperature (Allen, 1996; Nahata, 2004).

Allen LV Jr and Erickson MA 3rd, "Stability of Acetazolamide, Allopurinol, Azathioprine, Clonazepam, and Flucytosine in Extemporaneously Compounded Oral Liquids," *Am J Health Syst Pharm*, 1996, 53(16):1944-9.

Nahata MC, Pai VB, and Hipple TF, *Pediatric Drug Formulations*, 5th ed, Cincinnati, OH: Harvey Whitney Books Co, 2004.

Monitoring Parameters CBC, serum uric acid levels, I & O, hepatic and renal function, especially at start of therapy; signs and symptoms of hypersensitivity

Dietary Considerations Should take oral forms after meals with plenty of fluid. Fluid intake should be administered to yield neutral or slightly alkaline urine and an output of ~2 L (in adults).

Dosage Forms Excipient information presented when available (limited, particularly for generics); consult specific product labeling.

Injection, powder for reconstitution, as sodium: 500 mg (base)
Aloprim®: 500 mg (base)
Tablet, oral: 100 mg, 300 mg
Zyloprim®: 100 mg, 300 mg [scored]

References

Coiffier B, Altman A, Pui CH, et al, "Guidelines for the Management of Pediatric and Adult Tumor Lysis Syndrome: An Evidence-Based Review," *J Clin Oncol*, 2008, 26(16):2767-78.

Dalbeth N and Stamp L, "Allopurinol Dosing in Renal Impairment: Walking the Tightrope Between Adequate Urate Lowering and Adverse Events," *Semin Dial*, 2007, 20(5):391-5.

Day RO, Graham GG, Hicks M, et al, "Clinical Pharmacokinetics and Pharmacodynamics of Allopurinol and Oxypurinol," *Clin Pharmacokinet*, 2007, 46(8):623-44.

El-Zawawy H and Mandell BF, "Managing Gout: How Is it Different in Patients With Chronic Kidney Disease?" *Cleve Clin J Med*, 2010, 77(12):919-28.

Hande KR, Noone RM, and Stone WJ, "Severe Allopurinol Toxicity," *Am J Med*, 1984, 76(1):47-56.

Stamp LK, O'Donnell JL, Zhang M, et al, "Using Allopurinol Above the Dose Based on Creatinine Clearance Is Effective and Safe in Patients With Chronic gout, Including Those With Renal Impairment," *Arthritis Rheum*, 2011, 63(2):412-21.

Zhang W, Doherty M, Bardin T, et al, "EULAR Evidence Based Recommendations for Gout. Part II: Management. Report of a Task Force of the EULAR Standing Committee for International Clinical Studies Including Therapeutics (ESCISIT)," *Ann Rheum Dis*, 2006, 65(10):1312-24.

- **Allopurinol Sodium** *see* Allopurinol *on page 51*
- **All-*trans* Retinoic Acid** *see* Tretinoin (Systemic) *on page 1405*
- **All-*trans* Vitamin A Acid** *see* Tretinoin (Systemic) *on page 1405*
- **Aloprim®** *see* Allopurinol *on page 51*
- **Aloxi®** *see* Palonosetron *on page 1106*
- **AlphaNine® SD** *see* Factor IX *on page 571*

Alteplase (AL te plase)

Brand Names: U.S. Activase®; Cathflo® Activase®

Brand Names: Canada Activase® rt-PA; Cathflo® Activase®

Index Terms Alteplase, Recombinant; Alteplase, Tissue Plasminogen Activator, Recombinant; tPA

Generic Availability (U.S.) No

Pharmacologic Category Thrombolytic Agent

Use Management of ST-elevation myocardial infarction (STEMI) for the lysis of thrombi in coronary arteries; management of acute ischemic stroke (AIS); management of acute pulmonary embolism (PE)

Recommended criteria for treatment:

STEMI: Chest pain ≥20 minutes duration, onset of chest pain within 12 hours of treatment (or within prior 12-24 hours in patients with continuing ischemic symptoms), and ST-segment elevation >0.1 mV in at least two contiguous precordial leads or two adjacent limb leads on ECG or new or presumably new left bundle branch block (LBBB)

AIS: Onset of stroke symptoms within 3 hours of treatment

Acute pulmonary embolism: Age ≤75 years: Documented massive PE (defined as acute PE with sustained hypotension [SBP <90 mm Hg for ≤15 minutes or requiring inotropic support], persistent profound bradycardia [HR <40 bpm with signs or symptoms of shock], or pulselessness); alteplase may be considered for submassive PE with clinical evidence of adverse prognosis (eg, new hemodynamic instability, worsening respiratory insufficiency, severe RV dysfunction, or major myocardial necrosis) and low risk of bleeding complications. **Note:** Not recommended for patients with low-risk PE (eg, normotensive, no RV dysfunction, normal biomarkers) or submassive acute PE with minor RV dysfunction, minor myocardial necrosis, and no clinical worsening (Jaff, 2011).

Cathflo® Activase®: Restoration of central venous catheter function

Unlabeled Use Acute ischemic stroke presenting 3-4.5 hours after symptom onset; acute peripheral arterial occlusion; infected parapneumonic effusion (with [adult] or without [pediatric] dornase alfa); prosthetic valve thrombosis

Labeled Contraindications Hypersensitivity to alteplase or any component of the formulation

Treatment of STEMI or PE: Active internal bleeding; history of CVA; ischemic stroke within 3 months (Antman, 2004; Jaff, 2011); recent intracranial or intraspinal surgery or trauma; intracranial neoplasm; prior intracranial hemorrhage (Antman, 2004; Jaff, 2011); arteriovenous malformation or aneurysm; known bleeding diathesis; severe uncontrolled hypertension (listed as a relative contraindication in STEMI [Antman, 2004] and PE [Jaff, 2011] guidelines); suspected aortic dissection (Antman, 2004; Jaff, 2011); significant closed head or facial trauma (Antman, 2004; Jaff, 2011) within 3 months with radiographic evidence of bony fracture or brain injury (Jaff, 2011)

Treatment of acute ischemic stroke: Evidence of intracranial hemorrhage or suspicion of subarachnoid hemorrhage on pretreatment evaluation; intracranial or intraspinal surgery within 3 months; stroke or serious head injury within 3 months; history of intracranial hemorrhage; uncontrolled hypertension at time of treatment (eg, >185 mm Hg systolic or >110 mm Hg diastolic); seizure at the onset of stroke; active internal bleeding; intracranial neoplasm; arteriovenous malformation or aneurysm; multilobar cerebral infarction (hypodensity >1/3 cerebral hemisphere; Adams, 2007); known bleeding diathesis including but not limited to current use of oral anticoagulants (unless INR ≤1.7 [Adams, 2007]), an INR >1.7 (or PT >15 seconds), administration of heparin within 48 hours preceding the onset of stroke with an elevated aPTT at presentation, or platelet count <100,000/mm^3. **Note:** Specific guidelines have been suggested for the patient currently receiving dabigatran (Alberts, 2012).

Additional exclusion criteria within clinical trials:

Presentation <3 hours after initial symptoms (NINDS, 1995): Time of symptom onset unknown, rapidly improving or minor symptoms, major surgery within 2 weeks, GI or urinary tract hemorrhage within 3 weeks, aggressive treatment required to lower blood pressure, glucose level <50 or >400 mg/dL, and arterial puncture at a noncompressible site or lumbar puncture within 1 week.

Presentation 3-4.5 hours after initial symptoms (del Zoppo, 2009; ECASS-III; Hacke, 2008): Age >80 years, time of symptom onset unknown, rapidly improving or minor symptoms, current use of oral anticoagulants regardless of INR, glucose level <50 or >400 mg/dL, aggressive intravenous treatment required to lower blood pressure, major surgery or severe trauma within 3 months, baseline National Institutes of Health Stroke Scale (NIHSS) score >25, and history of both stroke and diabetes.

Pregnancy Risk Factor C

Lactation Excretion in breast milk unknown/use caution

Warnings/Precautions The total dose should not exceed 90 mg for acute ischemic stroke or 100 mg for acute myocardial infarction or pulmonary embolism. Doses ≥150 mg associated with significantly increased risk of intracranial hemorrhage compared to doses ≤100 mg. Concurrent heparin anticoagulation may contribute to bleeding. In the treatment of acute ischemic stroke, concurrent use of anticoagulants was not permitted during the initial 24 hours of the <3 hour window trial (NINDS, 1995). Initiation of SubQ heparin (≤10,000 units) or equivalent doses of low molecular weight heparin for prevention of DVT during the first 24 hours of the 3-4.5 hour window trial was permitted and did not increase the incidence of intracerebral hemorrhage (Hacke, 2008). For acute PE, withhold heparin during the 2-hour infusion period. Monitor all potential bleeding sites. Intramuscular injections and non-essential handling of the patient should be avoided. Venipunctures should be performed carefully and only when necessary. If arterial puncture is necessary, use an upper extremity vessel that can be manually compressed. If serious bleeding occurs, the infusion of alteplase and heparin should be stopped. Avoid aspirin for 24 hours following administration of alteplase; administration within 24 hours increases the risk of hemorrhagic transformation.

For the following conditions, the risk of bleeding is higher with use of thrombolytics and should be weighed against the benefits of therapy: Recent major surgery (eg, CABG, obstetrical delivery, organ biopsy, pregnancy, previous puncture of noncompressible vessels), prolonged CPR with evidence of thoracic trauma, lumbar puncture within 1 week, cerebrovascular disease, recent gastrointestinal or genitourinary bleeding, recent trauma, hypertension (systolic BP >175 mm Hg and/or diastolic BP >110 mm Hg), high likelihood of left heart thrombus (eg, mitral stenosis with atrial fibrillation), acute pericarditis, subacute bacterial endocarditis, hemostatic defects including ones caused by severe renal or hepatic dysfunction, significant hepatic dysfunction, pregnancy, diabetic hemorrhagic retinopathy or other hemorrhagic ophthalmic conditions, septic thrombophlebitis or occluded AV cannula at seriously infected site, advanced age (eg, >75 years), any other condition in which bleeding constitutes a significant hazard or would be particularly difficult to manage because of location. When treating acute MI or pulmonary embolism, use with caution in patients receiving oral anticoagulants. In the treatment of acute ischemic stroke (AIS) within 3 hours of symptom onset, the current use of oral anticoagulants is a contraindication per the manufacturer. According to the AHA/ASA, the current use of oral anticoagulants producing an INR >1.7 is a contraindication (Adams, 2007). It has been suggested that alteplase should be avoided in patients who are also receiving oral anticoagulants that do not or minimally affect the INR (eg, dabigatran) unless there is clear evidence of normal renal function (Cl_{cr} >50 mL/minute), the patient has not taken dabigatran in the past 48 hours, and normal coagulation testing (aPTT, INR, platelet count) (Alberts, 2012). When treating AIS 3-4.5 hours after symptom onset, the use of alteplase should be avoided with current use of any oral anticoagulant regardless of INR (del Zoppo, 2009).

Coronary thrombolysis may result in reperfusion arrhythmias. Patients who present **within 3 hours** of stroke symptom onset should be treated with alteplase unless contraindications exist. A longer time window (**3-4.5 hours** after symptom onset) has now been formally evaluated and shown to be safe and efficacious for select individuals (del Zoppo, 2009; Hacke, 2008). Treatment of patients with minor neurological deficit or with rapidly improving symptoms is not recommended. Follow standard management for STEMI while infusing alteplase.

Cathflo® Activase®: When used to restore catheter function, use Cathflo® cautiously in those patients with known or suspected catheter infections. Evaluate catheter for other causes of dysfunction before use. Avoid excessive pressure when instilling into catheter.

Adverse Reactions As with all drugs which may affect hemostasis, bleeding is the major adverse effect associated with alteplase. Hemorrhage may occur at virtually any site. Risk is dependent on multiple variables, including the dosage administered, concurrent use of multiple agents which alter hemostasis, and patient predisposition. Rapid lysis of coronary artery thrombi by thrombolytic agents may be associated with reperfusion-related atrial and/or ventricular arrhythmia. **Note:** Lowest rate of bleeding complications expected with dose used to restore catheter function.

1% to 10%:

Cardiovascular: Hypotension
Central nervous system: Fever
Dermatologic: Bruising (1%)
Gastrointestinal: GI hemorrhage (5%), nausea, vomiting
Genitourinary: GU hemorrhage (4%)
Hematologic: Bleeding (0.5% major, 7% minor: GUSTO trial)
Local: Bleeding at catheter puncture site (15.3%, accelerated administration)

<1% (Limited to important or life-threatening): Angioedema (orolingual), intracranial hemorrhage (0.4% to 0.87% when adult dose is ≤100 mg), retroperitoneal hemorrhage, pericardial hemorrhage, gingival hemorrhage, epistaxis, allergic reaction (anaphylaxis, anaphylactoid reactions, laryngeal edema, rash, and urticaria [<0.02%])

Additional cardiovascular events associated **with use in STEMI:** AV block, cardiogenic shock, heart failure, cardiac arrest, recurrent ischemia/infarction, myocardial rupture, electromechanical dissociation, pericardial effusion, pericarditis, mitral regurgitation, cardiac tamponade, thromboembolism, pulmonary edema, asystole, ventricular tachycardia, bradycardia, ruptured intracranial AV malformation, seizure, hemorrhagic bursitis, cholesterol crystal embolization

Additional events associated **with use in pulmonary embolism:** Pulmonary re-embolization, pulmonary edema, pleural effusion, thromboembolism

Additional events associated **with use in stroke:** Cerebral edema, cerebral herniation, seizure, new ischemic stroke

Drug Interactions

Metabolism/Transport Effects None known.

Avoid Concomitant Use There are no known interactions where it is recommended to avoid concomitant use.

Increased Effect/Toxicity

Alteplase may increase the levels/effects of: Anticoagulants; Dabigatran Etexilate; Drotrecogin Alfa (Activated)

The levels/effects of Alteplase may be increased by: Antiplatelet Agents; Herbs (Anticoagulant/Antiplatelet Properties); Nonsteroidal Anti-Inflammatory Agents; Salicylates

Decreased Effect

The levels/effects of Alteplase may be decreased by: Aprotinin; Nitroglycerin

Ethanol/Nutrition/Herb Interactions Herb/Nutraceutical: Avoid cat's claw, dong quai, evening primrose, feverfew, red clover, horse chestnut, garlic, green tea, ginseng, ginkgo (all have additional antiplatelet activity).

Storage/Stability

Activase®: The lyophilized product may be stored at room temperature (not to exceed 30°C/86°F), or under refrigeration. Once reconstituted, it should be used within 8 hours.

Cathflo® Activase®: Store lyophilized product under refrigeration. Once reconstituted, it should be used within 8 hours.

Reconstitution

Activase®:

50 mg vial: Use accompanying diluent; mix by gentle swirling or slow inversion; do not shake. Vacuum is present in 50 mg vial. Final concentration: 1 mg/mL.

100 mg vial: Use transfer set with accompanying diluent (100 mL vial of sterile water for injection). No vacuum is present in 100 mg vial. Final concentration: 1 mg/mL.

Activase®: ST-elevation MI: Accelerated infusion: Bolus dose may be prepared by one of three methods:

1) Removal of 15 mL reconstituted (1 mg/mL) solution from vial
2) Removal of 15 mL from a port on the infusion line after priming
3) Programming an infusion pump to deliver a 15 mL bolus at the initiation of infusion

Activase®: Acute ischemic stroke: Bolus dose (10% of total dose) may be prepared by one of three methods:

1) Removal of the appropriate volume from reconstituted solution (1 mg/mL)
2) Removal of the appropriate volume from a port on the infusion line after priming
3) Programming an infusion pump to deliver the appropriate volume at the initiation of infusion

Cathflo® Activase®: Add 2.2 mL SWFI to vial; do not shake. Final concentration: 1 mg/mL.

Mechanism of Action Initiates local fibrinolysis by binding to fibrin in a thrombus (clot) and converts entrapped plasminogen to plasmin

Pharmacodynamics/Kinetics

Duration: >50% present in plasma cleared ~5 minutes after infusion terminated, ~80% cleared within 10 minutes

Excretion: Clearance: Rapidly from circulating plasma (550-650 mL/minute), primarily hepatic; >50% present in plasma is cleared within 5 minutes after the infusion is terminated, ~80% cleared within 10 minutes

Dosing

Adult & Geriatric

ST-elevation myocardial infarction (STEMI): I.V. (Activase®): **Note:** Manufacturer's labeling recommends 3 hour infusion regimen; however, accelerated regimen preferred by the ACC/AHA (Antman, 2004).

Accelerated regimen (weight-based):

Patients >67 kg: Total dose: 100 mg over 1.5 hours; administered as a 15 mg I.V. bolus over 1-2 minutes followed by infusions of 50 mg over 30 minutes, then 35 mg over 1 hour. Maximum total dose: 100 mg

Patients ≤67 kg: Infuse 15 mg I.V. bolus over 1-2 minutes followed by infusions of 0.75 mg/kg (not to exceed 50 mg) over 30 minutes then 0.5 mg/kg (not to exceed 35 mg) over 1 hour. Maximum total dose: 100 mg

Note: All patients should receive 162-325 mg of chewable nonenteric coated aspirin as soon as possible and then daily. Administer concurrently with heparin 60 units/kg bolus (maximum: 4000 units) followed by continuous infusion of 12 units/kg/hour (maximum: 1000 units/hour) and adjust to aPTT target of 50-70 seconds (or 1.5-2 times the upper limit of control).

Acute massive or submassive pulmonary embolism (PE): I.V. (Activase®): 100 mg over 2 hours; may be administered as a 10 mg bolus followed by 90 mg over 2 hours as was done in patients with submassive PE (Konstantinides, 2002). **Note:** Not recommended for submassive PE with minor RV dysfunction, minor myocardial necrosis, and no clinical worsening or low-risk PE (ie, normotensive, no RV dysfunction, normal biomarkers) (Jaff, 2011).

Acute ischemic stroke: I.V. (Activase®): Within 3 hours of the onset of symptom onset (labeled use) **or** within 3-4.5 hours of symptom onset (unlabeled use; del Zoppo, 2009; Hacke, 2008): **Note:** Initiation of anticoagulants (eg, heparin) or antiplatelet agents (eg, aspirin) within 24 hours after starting alteplase is not recommended; however, initiation of aspirin between 24-48 hours after stroke onset is recommended (Adams, 2007). Initiation of SubQ heparin (≤10,000 units) or equivalent doses of low molecular weight heparin for prevention of DVT during the first 24 hours of the 3-4.5 hour window trial did not increase incidence of intracerebral hemorrhage (Hacke, 2008).

Recommended total dose: 0.9 mg/kg (maximum total dose: 90 mg)

Patients ≤100 kg: Load with 0.09 mg/kg (10% of 0.9 mg/kg dose) as an I.V. bolus over 1 minute, followed by 0.81 mg/kg (90% of 0.9 mg/kg dose) as a continuous infusion over 60 minutes.

Patients >100 kg: Load with 9 mg (10% of 90 mg) as an I.V. bolus over 1 minute, followed by 81 mg (90% of 90 mg) as a continuous infusion over 60 minutes.

Central venous catheter clearance: Intracatheter (Cathflo® Activase® 1 mg/mL):

Patients <30 kg: 110% of the internal lumen volume of the catheter, not to exceed 2 mg/2 mL; retain in catheter for 0.5-2 hours; may instill a second dose if catheter remains occluded

Patients ≥30 kg: 2 mg (2 mL); retain in catheter for 0.5-2 hours; may instill a second dose if catheter remains occluded

Acute peripheral arterial occlusion (unlabeled use): Intra-arterial:

Weight-based regimen: 0.001-0.02 mg/kg/hour (maximum dose: 2 mg/hour) (Semba, 2000)

or

Fixed-dose regimen: 0.12-2 mg/hour (Semba, 2000)

Note: The ACC/AHA guidelines state that thrombolysis is an effective and beneficial therapy for those with acute limb ischemia (Rutherford categories I and IIa) of <14 days duration (Hirsch, 2006). The optimal dosage and concentration has not been established; a number of intra-arterial delivery techniques are employed with continuous infusion being the most common (Ouriel, 2004). The Advisory Panel to the Society for Cardiovascular and Interventional Radiology on Thrombolytic Therapy recommends dosing of ≤2 mg/hour and concomitant administration of subtherapeutic heparin (aPTT 1.25-1.5 times baseline) (Semba, 2000). Duration of alteplase infusion dependent upon size and location of the thrombus; typically between 6-48 hours (Disini, 2008).

Complicated parapneumonic effusion (unlabeled use): Intrapleural: 10 mg in 30 mL NS administered twice daily with a 1 hour dwell time for a total of 3 days; each dose followed in >2 hours by intrapleural dornase alfa (Rahman, 2011). Some clinicians suggest consideration of fibrinolytic use when patients have failed at least 24 hours of chest tube drainage and are poor surgical candidates (Hamblin, 2010).

Prosthetic valve thrombosis, right-sided (any size thrombus) or left-sided (thrombus area <0.8 cm^2), or left-sided (thrombus area ≥0.8 cm^2) when contraindications to surgery exist (unlabeled use) (Alpert, 2003; Guyatt, 2012; Roudaut, 2003): I.V.:

High-dose regimen: Load with 10 mg, followed by 90 mg over 90-180 minutes (without heparin during infusion)

Low dose regimen (preferred for very small adults): Load with 20 mg, followed by 10 mg/hour for 3 hours (without heparin during infusion)

Note: After successful administration of alteplase, heparin infusion should be introduced until warfarin achieves therapeutic INR (aortic: 3.0-4.0; mitral: 3.5-4.5) (Bonow, 2008). The 2012 ACCP guidelines for antithrombotic therapy make no recommendation regarding INR range after prosthetic valve thrombosis.

Pediatric

Central venous catheter clearance: Intracatheter: Patients <30 kg: 110% of the internal lumen volume of the catheter, not to exceed 2 mg/2 mL; retain in catheter for 0.5-2 hours; may instill a second dose if catheter remains occluded

Complicated parapneumonic effusion (unlabeled use): Intrapleural: Children >3 months: 4 mg in 40 mL NS, first dose at time of chest tube placement with 1 hour dwell time, repeat every 24 hours for 3 days (total of 3 doses) or 0.1 mg/kg (maximum: 3 mg) in 10-30 mL NS, first dose after pigtail catheter (chest tube) placement, 0.75-1 hour dwell time, repeat every 8 hours for 3 days (total of 9 doses) (IDSA/PIDS, 2011)

Usual Infusion Concentrations: Pediatric I.V. infusion: 0.5 mg/mL **or** 1 mg/mL

Usual Infusion Concentrations: Adult I.V. infusion: 1 mg/mL

Note: Concentrations for some indications (eg, peripheral arterial occlusion) are more dilute (eg, 0.1-0.2 mg/mL) and a usual concentration may not be established.

Administration

Activase®: ST-elevation MI or acute ischemic stroke: Administer bolus dose (prepared by one of three methods) over 1 minute followed by infusion.

Infusion: Remaining dose for STEMI, AIS, or total dose for acute pulmonary embolism may be administered as follows: Any quantity of drug not to be administered to the patient must be removed from vial(s) prior to administration of remaining dose.

50 mg vial: Either PVC bag or glass vial and infusion set

100 mg vial: Insert spike end of the infusion set through the same puncture site created by transfer device and infuse from vial

If further dilution is desired, may be diluted in equal volume of 0.9% sodium chloride or D_5W to yield a final concentration of 0.5 mg/mL.

Cathflo® Activase®: Intracatheter: Instill dose into occluded catheter. Do not force solution into catheter. After a 30-minute dwell time, assess catheter function by attempting to aspirate blood. If catheter is functional, aspirate 4-5 mL of blood in patients ≥10 kg or 3 mL in patients <10 kg to remove Cathflo® Activase® and residual clots. Gently irrigate the catheter with NS. If catheter remains nonfunctional, let Cathflo® Activase® dwell for another 90 minutes (total dwell time: 120 minutes) and reassess function. If catheter function is not restored, a second dose may be instilled.

Parapneumonic effusion (unlabeled use): Intrapleural: Instill dose into chest tube and clamp drain. Although the optimum dwell time has not been determined, clinical trials more often have used either a 45 minute (Hawkins,

2004) or 1 hour (Rahman, 2011; St. Peter, 2009) dwell time; after dwell period, release clamp and connect chest tube to continuous suction.

Monitoring Parameters

Acute ischemic stroke (AIS): Baseline: Neurologic examination, head CT (without contrast), blood pressure, CBC, aPTT, PT/INR, glucose. During and after initiation: In addition to monitoring for bleeding complications, the 2007 AHA/ASA guidelines for the early management of AIS recommends the following:

Perform neurological assessments every 15 minutes during infusion and every 30 minutes thereafter for the next 6 hours, then hourly until 24 hours after treatment.

If severe headache, acute hypertension, nausea, or vomiting occurs, discontinue the infusion and obtain emergency CT scan.

Measure BP every 15 minutes for the first 2 hours then every 30 minutes for the next 6 hours, then hourly until 24 hours after initiation of alteplase. Increase frequency if a systolic BP is ≥180 mm Hg or if a diastolic BP is ≥105 mm Hg; administer antihypertensive medications to maintain BP at or below these levels.

Obtain a follow-up CT scan at 24 hours before starting anticoagulants or antiplatelet agents.

Central venous catheter clearance: Assess catheter function by attempting to aspirate blood.

ST-elevation MI: Baseline: Blood pressure, serum cardiac biomarkers, CBC, PT/INR, aPTT. During and after initiation: Assess for evidence of cardiac reperfusion through resolution of chest pain, resolution of baseline ECG changes, preserved left ventricular function, cardiac enzyme washout phenomenon, and/or the appearance of reperfusion arrhythmias; assess for bleeding potential through clinical evidence of GI bleeding, hematuria, gingival bleeding, fibrinogen levels, fibrinogen degradation products, PT and aPTT.

Test Interactions Altered results of coagulation and fibrinolytic activity tests

Dosage Forms Excipient information presented when available (limited, particularly for generics); consult specific product labeling.

Injection, powder for reconstitution [recombinant]:

Activase®: 50 mg, 100 mg [contains polysorbate 80; derived from or manufactured using Chinese hamster ovary cells; supplied with diluent]

Cathflo® Activase®: 2 mg [contains polysorbate 80; derived from or manufactured using Chinese hamster ovary cells]

References

Adams HP Jr, del Zoppo G, Alberts MJ, et al, "Guidelines for the Early Management of Adults With Ischemic Stroke: A Guideline From the American Heart Association/American Stroke Association Stroke Council, Clinical Cardiology Council, Cardiovascular Radiology and Intervention Council, and the Atherosclerotic Peripheral Vascular Disease and Quality of Care Outcomes in Research Interdisciplinary Working Groups: The American Academy of Neurology Affirms the Value of This Guideline as an Educational Tool for Neurologists," *Stroke*, 2007, 38(5):1655-711.

Alberts MJ, Bernstein RA, Naccarelli GV, et al, "Using Dabigatran in Patients With Stroke: A Practical Guide for Clinicians," *Stroke*, 2012, 43(1):271-9.

Broderick J, Connolly S, Feldmann E, et al, "Guidelines for the Management of Spontaneous Intracerebral Hemorrhage in Adults: 2007 Update: A Guideline From the American Heart Association/American Stroke Association Stroke Council, High Blood Pressure Research Council, and the Quality of Care and Outcomes in Research Interdisciplinary Working Group," *Stroke*, 2007, 38(6):2001-23. Available at http://stroke.ahajournals.org/cgi/content/short/STROKEAHA.107.183689

del Zoppo GJ, Saver JL, Jauch EC, et al, "Expansion of the Time Window for Treatment of Acute Ischemic Stroke With Intravenous Tissue Plasminogen Activator: A Science Advisory From the American Heart Association/American Stroke Association," *Stroke*, 2009, 40(8):2945-8.

ECC Committee, Subcommittees and Task Forces of the American Heart Association, "2005 American Heart Association Guidelines for Cardiopulmonary Resuscitation and Emergency Cardiovascular Care," *Circulation*, 2005, 112(24 Suppl):IV1-203.

Field JM, Hazinski MF, Sayre MR, et al, "Part 1: Executive Summary: 2010 American Heart Association Guidelines for Cardiopulmonary Resuscitation and Emergency Cardiovascular Care," *Circulation*, 2010, 122 (18 Suppl 3):640-56.

Goodman SG, Menon V, Cannon CP, et al, "Acute ST-Segment Elevation Myocardial Infarction: American College of Chest Physicians Evidence-Based Clinical Practice," *Chest*, 2008, 133(6 Suppl):708-75.

Hacke W, Kaste M, Bluhmki E, et al, "Thrombolysis With Alteplase 3 to 4.5 Hours After Acute Ischemic Stroke," *N Engl J Med*, 2008, 359(13):1317-29.

Hirsh J, Guyatt G, Albers GW, et al, "Executive Summary: American College of Chest Physicians Evidence-Based Clinical Practice Guidelines (8th Edition)," *Chest*, 2008, 133(6 Suppl):71-109.

Jaff MR, McMurtry MS, Archer SL, et al, "Management of Massive and Submassive Pulmonary Embolism, Iliofemoral Deep Vein Thrombosis, and Chronic Thromboembolic Pulmonary Hypertension: A Scientific Statement from the American Heart Association," *Circulation*, 2011, 123 (16):1788-830.

Kearon C, Kahn SR, Agnelli G, et al, "Antithrombotic Therapy for Venous Thromboembolic Disease: American College of Chest Physicians Evidence-Based Clinical Practice Guidelines (8th Edition)," *Chest*, 2008, 33(6 Suppl):454-545.

Konstantinides S, Geibel A, Heusel G, et al, "Heparin Plus Alteplase Compared With Heparin Alone in Patients With Submassive Pulmonary Embolism," *N Engl J Med*, 2002, 347 (15):1143-50.

Ponec D, Irwin D, Haire WD, et al, "Recombinant Tissue Plasminogen Activator (Alteplase) for Restoration of Flow in Occluded Central Venous Access Devices: A Double-Blind Placebo-Controlled Trial - The Cardiovascular Thrombolytic to Open Occluded Lines (COOL) Efficacy Trial," *J Vasc Interv Radiol*, 2001, 12(8):951-5.

Semba CP, Murphy TP, Bakal CW, et al, "Thrombolytic Therapy With Use of Alteplase (rtPA) in Peripheral Arterial Occlusive Disease: Review of the Clinical Literature. The Advisory Panel," *J Vasc Interv Radiol*, 2000, 11(2 Pt 1):149-61.

Zacharias JM, Weatherston CP, Spewak CR, et al, "Alteplase Versus Urokinase for Occluded Hemodialysis Catheters," *Ann Pharmacother*, 2003, 37(1):27-33.

◆ **Alteplase, Recombinant** *see* Alteplase *on page 55*

◆ **Alteplase, Tissue Plasminogen Activator, Recombinant** *see* Alteplase *on page 55*

◆ **Alti-MPA (Can)** *see* MedroxyPROGESTERone *on page 916*

Altretamine (al TRET a meen)

Related Information

Management of Chemotherapy-Induced Nausea and Vomiting *on page 1786*

Safe Handling of Hazardous Drugs *on page 1904*

Brand Names: U.S. Hexalen®

Brand Names: Canada Hexalen®

Index Terms Hexamethylmelamine; HMM; HXM

Generic Availability (U.S.) No

Pharmacologic Category Antineoplastic Agent, Miscellaneous

Use Palliative treatment of persistent or recurrent ovarian cancer

Labeled Contraindications Hypersensitivity to altretamine or any component of the formulation; pre-existing severe bone marrow suppression or severe neurologic toxicity

Pregnancy Risk Factor D

Lactation Excretion in breast milk unknown/not recommended

Warnings/Precautions Hazardous agent - use appropriate precautions for handling and disposal. **[U.S. Boxed Warning]: Peripheral blood counts and neurologic examinations should be done routinely before each cycle and during treatment.** Dose-related bone marrow suppression is common; use with caution in patients previously treated with other myelosuppressive agents.

Peripheral neuropathy and neurotoxicity (ataxia, dizziness, vertigo, mood disorders, and disorders of consciousness) have been reported; usually occur in patients receiving continuous high-dose daily treatment and is generally reversible upon discontinuation. Has been administered safely to patients with pre-existing neuropathy (due to cisplatin); close monitoring is required. Concurrent use of altretamine and MAO inhibitors may cause severe orthostatic hypotension. **[U.S. Boxed Warning]: Should be administered under the supervision of an experienced cancer chemotherapy physician.**

Adverse Reactions

>10%:

Gastrointestinal: Nausea/vomiting (33%; severe 1%)
Hematologic: Anemia (33%), leukopenia (5% to 15%; grade 4: <1%)
Neuromuscular & skeletal: Peripheral sensory neuropathy (31%; mild: 9%; moderate-to-severe: 9%)

1% to 10%:

Central nervous system: Fatigue, seizure
Gastrointestinal: Anorexia
Hematologic: Thrombocytopenia
Hepatic: Alkaline phosphatase increased
Renal: BUN increased, serum creatinine increased

<1%, postmarketing, and/or case reports: Alopecia, ataxia, depression, dizziness, hepatotoxicity, mood disorders, neurotoxicity, pruritus, rash, vertigo

Drug Interactions

Metabolism/Transport Effects None known.

Avoid Concomitant Use

Avoid concomitant use of Altretamine with any of the following: BCG; CloZAPine; Natalizumab; Pimecrolimus; Tacrolimus (Topical); Vaccines (Live)

Increased Effect/Toxicity

Altretamine may increase the levels/effects of: CloZAPine; Leflunomide; MAO Inhibitors; Natalizumab; Tricyclic Antidepressants; Vaccines (Live)

The levels/effects of Altretamine may be increased by: Denosumab; MAO Inhibitors; Pimecrolimus; Roflumilast; Tacrolimus (Topical); Trastuzumab

Decreased Effect

Altretamine may decrease the levels/effects of: BCG; Coccidioidin Skin Test; Sipuleucel-T; Vaccines (Inactivated); Vaccines (Live)

The levels/effects of Altretamine may be decreased by: Echinacea; Multivitamins/Minerals (with ADEK, Folate, Iron); Pyridoxine

Storage/Stability Store at 25°C (77°F); excursions permitted to 15°C to 30°C (59°F to 86°F).

Mechanism of Action Altretamine structurally resembles alkylating agents, although has demonstrated activity in tumors resistant to classic alkylating agents. Cytotoxic effect not fully characterized, however it is theorized that metabolically activated oxidative N-demethylation intermediates bind to and damage DNA.

Pharmacodynamics/Kinetics

Absorption: Well absorbed
Distribution: Distributed into tissues high in lipid content and into tumor tissue
Metabolism: Hepatic; rapid and extensive oxidative N-demethylation to active metabolites (pentamethylmelamine and tetramethylmelamine)
Half-life elimination: ~7 hours (range: 2-10 hours)
Time to peak, plasma: 0.5-3 hours

Excretion: Urine (90%, <1% as unchanged drug)

Dosing

Adult & Geriatric Ovarian cancer, persistent or recurrent: Oral: 260 mg/m²/day in 4 divided doses for 14 or 21 days of a 28-day cycle

Adjustment for Toxicity Temporarily withhold for 14 days or longer, and resume dose at 200 mg/m²/day for any of the following:

Platelet count <75,000/mm³

White blood cell count <2000/mm³ or granulocyte count <1000/mm³

Progressive neurotoxicity

Gastrointestinal intolerance not responsive to antiemetic regimens

Discontinue if neurotoxicity does not stabilize at 200 mg/m²/day.

Administration Administer total daily dose orally as 4 divided doses after meals and at bedtime.

Emetic Potential Moderate (30% to 90%)

Monitoring Parameters CBC with differential (before each cycle and regularly during treatment), neurologic examination (before each cycle and regularly during treatment)

Dietary Considerations Should be taken after meals (and at bedtime).

Dosage Forms Excipient information presented when available (limited, particularly for generics); consult specific product labeling.

Capsule, oral:

Hexalen®: 50 mg

References

Alberts DS, Jiang C, Liu PY, et al, "Long-Term Follow-Up of a Phase II Trial of Oral Altretamine for Consolidation of Clinical Complete Remission in Women With Stage III Epithelial Ovarian cancer in the Southwest Oncology Group," Int J Gynecol Cancer, 2004, 14(2):224-8.

Keldsen N, Havsteen H, Vergote I, et al, "Altretamine (Hexamethylmelamine) in the Treatment of Platinum-Resistant Ovarian Cancer: A Phase II Study," *Gynecol Oncol*, 2003, 88(2):118-22.

Markman M, Blessing JA, Moore D, et al, "Altretamine (Hexamethylmelamine) in Platinum-Resistant and Platinum-Refractory Ovarian Cancer: A Gynecologic Oncology Group Phase II Trial," *Gynecol Oncol*, 1998, 69(3):226-9.

◆ **AmBisome®** *see* Amphotericin B (Liposomal) *on page 87*

◆ **AMD3100** *see* Plerixafor *on page 1180*

◆ **A-Methapred** *see* MethylPREDNISolone *on page 967*

◆ **A-Methapred®** *see* MethylPREDNISolone *on page 967*

◆ **Amethopterin** *see* Methotrexate *on page 949*

◆ **AMG 073** *see* Cinacalcet *on page 280*

◆ **AMG-162** *see* Denosumab *on page 428*

◆ **AMG 531** *see* RomiPLOStim *on page 1257*

◆ **Amicar®** *see* Aminocaproic Acid *on page 72*

Amifostine (am i FOS teen)

Related Information

Management of Chemotherapy-Induced Nausea and Vomiting *on page 1786*

Brand Names: U.S. Ethyol®

Brand Names: Canada Ethyol®

Index Terms Ethiofos; Gammaphos; WR-2721; YM-08310

Generic Availability (U.S.) Yes

Pharmacologic Category Adjuvant, Chemoprotective Agent (Cytoprotective); Antidote

Use Reduce the incidence of moderate-to-severe xerostomia in patients undergoing postoperative radiation treatment for head and neck cancer, where the radiation port includes a substantial portion of the parotid glands; reduce the cumulative renal toxicity associated with repeated administration of cisplatin

Unlabeled Use Prevention of radiation proctitis in patients with rectal cancer

Labeled Contraindications Hypersensitivity to aminothiol compounds or any component of the formulation

Pregnancy Risk Factor C

Lactation Excretion in breast milk unknown/not recommended

Warnings/Precautions Patients who are hypotensive or dehydrated should not receive amifostine. Interrupt antihypertensive therapy for 24 hours before treatment; patients who cannot safely stop their antihypertensives 24 hours before, should not receive amifostine. Adequately hydrated prior to treatment and keep in a supine position during infusion. Monitor blood pressure every 5 minutes during the infusion. If hypotension requiring interruption of therapy occurs, patients should be placed in the Trendelenburg position and given an infusion of normal saline using a separate I.V. line; subsequent infusions may require a dose reduction. Infusions >15 minutes are associated with a higher incidence of adverse effects. Use caution in patients with cardiovascular and cerebrovascular disease and any other patients in whom the adverse effects of hypotension may have serious adverse events.

Serious cutaneous reactions, including erythema multiforme, Stevens-Johnson syndrome, toxic epidermal necrolysis, toxoderma and exfoliative dermatitis have been reported with amifostine. May be delayed, developing up to weeks after treatment initiation. Cutaneous reactions have been reported more frequently when used as a radioprotectant. Discontinue treatment for severe/serious cutaneous reaction, or with fever. Withhold treatment and obtain dermatologic consultation for rash involving lips or mucosa (of unknown etiology outside of radiation port) and for bullous, edematous or erythematous lesions on hands, feet, or trunk; reinitiate only after careful evaluation.

It is recommended that antiemetic medication, including dexamethasone 20 mg I.V. and a serotonin 5-HT_3 receptor antagonist be administered prior to and in conjunction with amifostine. Rare hypersensitivity reactions, including anaphylaxis and allergic reaction, have been reported; discontinue if allergic reaction occurs; do not rechallenge. Medications for the treatment of hypersensitivity reactions should be available.

Reports of clinically-relevant hypocalcemia are rare, but serum calcium levels should be monitored in patients at risk of hypocalcemia, such as those with nephrotic syndrome; may require calcium supplementation. Should not be used (in patients receiving chemotherapy for malignancies other than ovarian cancer) where chemotherapy is expected to provide significant survival benefit or in patients receiving definitive radiotherapy, unless within the context of a clinical trial. Safety and efficacy in children have not been established.

Adverse Reactions

>10%:

Cardiovascular: Hypotension (15% to 61%; grades 3/4: 3% to 8%; dose dependent)

Gastrointestinal: Nausea/vomiting (53% to 96%; grades 3/4: 8% to 30%; dose dependent)

1% to 10%: Endocrine & metabolic: Hypocalcemia (clinically significant: 1%)

<1%, postmarketing, and/or case reports: Apnea, anaphylactoid reactions, anaphylaxis, arrhythmia, atrial fibrillation, atrial flutter, back pain, bradycardia, cardiac arrest, chest pain, chest tightness, chills, cutaneous eruptions, dizziness, erythema multiforme, exfoliative dermatitis, extrasystoles, dyspnea, fever, flushing, hiccups, hypersensitivity reactions (fever, rash, hypoxia, dyspnea, laryngeal edema), hypertension (transient), hypoxia, malaise, MI, myocardial ischemia, pruritus, rash (mild), renal failure, respiratory arrest, rigors, seizure, sneezing, somnolence, Stevens-Johnson syndrome, supraventricular tachycardia, syncope, tachycardia, toxic epidermal necrolysis, toxoderma, urticaria

Drug Interactions

Metabolism/Transport Effects None known.

Avoid Concomitant Use There are no known interactions where it is recommended to avoid concomitant use.

Increased Effect/Toxicity

The levels/effects of Amifostine may be increased by: Antihypertensives

Decreased Effect There are no known significant interactions involving a decrease in effect.

Storage/Stability Store intact vials of lyophilized powder at room temperature of 20°C to 25°C (68°F to 77°F). Reconstituted solutions (500 mg/10 mL) and solutions for infusion are chemically stable for up to 5 hours at room temperature (25°C) or up to 24 hours under refrigeration (2°C to 8°C).

Reconstitution For I.V. infusion, reconstitute intact vials with 9.7 mL 0.9% sodium chloride injection and dilute in 0.9% sodium chloride to a final concentration of 5-40 mg/mL. For SubQ administration, reconstitute with 2.5 mL NS or SWFI.

Mechanism of Action Prodrug that is dephosphorylated by alkaline phosphatase in tissues to a pharmacologically-active free thiol metabolite. The free thiol is available to bind to, and detoxify, reactive metabolites of cisplatin; and can also act as a scavenger of free radicals that may be generated (by cisplatin or radiation therapy) in tissues.

Pharmacodynamics/Kinetics

Distribution: V_d: 3.5 L

Metabolism: Hepatic dephosphorylation to two metabolites (active-free thiol and disulfide)

Half-life elimination: ~8-9 minutes

Excretion: Urine

Clearance, plasma: 2.17 L/minute

Dosing

Adult & Geriatric Note: Antiemetic medication, including dexamethasone 20 mg I.V. and a serotonin $5\text{-}HT_3$ receptor antagonist, is recommended prior to and in conjunction with amifostine.

Cisplatin-induced renal toxicity, reduction: I.V.: 910 mg/m^2 once daily over 15 minutes 30 minutes prior to cytotoxic therapy

For 910 mg/m^2 doses, the manufacturer suggests the following blood pressure-based adjustment schedule:

The infusion of amifostine should be interrupted if the systolic blood pressure decreases significantly from baseline, as defined below:

Decrease of 20 mm Hg if baseline systolic blood pressure <100
Decrease of 25 mm Hg if baseline systolic blood pressure 100-119
Decrease of 30 mm Hg if baseline systolic blood pressure 120-139
Decrease of 40 mm Hg if baseline systolic blood pressure 140-179
Decrease of 50 mm Hg if baseline systolic blood pressure ≥180

If blood pressure returns to normal within 5 minutes (assisted by fluid administration and postural management) and the patient is asymptomatic, the infusion may be restarted so that the full dose of amifostine may be administered. If the full dose of amifostine cannot be administered, the dose of amifostine for subsequent cycles should be 740 mg/m^2.

Xerostomia from head and neck cancer, reduction:

I.V.: 200 mg/m^2 over 3 minutes once daily 15-30 minutes prior to radiation therapy **or**

SubQ (unlabeled route): 500 mg once daily prior to radiation therapy

Prevention of radiation proctitis in rectal cancer (unlabeled use): I.V.: 340 mg/m^2 once daily prior to radiation therapy (Keefe, 2007; Peterson, 2008)

Administration I.V.: Administer over 3 minutes (prior to radiation therapy) or 15 minutes (prior to cisplatin); administration as a longer infusion is associated with a higher incidence of side effects. Patients should be kept in supine position during infusion. **Note:** SubQ administration (unlabeled) has been used.

Emetic Potential

>300 mg/m^2: Moderate (30% to 90%)

≤300 mg/m^2: Low (10% to 30%)

Monitoring Parameters Blood pressure should be monitored every 5 minutes during the infusion and after administration if clinically indicated; serum calcium levels (in patients at risk for hypocalcemia). Evaluate for cutaneous reactions prior to each dose.

Additional Information Oncology Comment: The American Society of Clinical Oncology (ASCO) guidelines for the use of protectants for chemotherapy and radiation (Hensley, 2008) recommend the use of amifostine for prevention of nephrotoxicity due to cisplatin-based chemotherapy and to decrease the incidence of acute and delayed radiation therapy-induced xerostomia. The ASCO guidelines do not recommend the use of amifostine to reduce the incidence of neutropenia or thrombocytopenia associated with chemotherapy or radiation therapy, neurotoxicity or ototoxicity associated with platinum-based chemotherapy, radiation therapy-induced mucositis associated with head and neck cancer, or esophagitis due to chemotherapy in patients with nonsmall cell lung cancer. Additionally, the guidelines do not support the use of amifostine in patients with head and neck cancer receiving concurrent platinum-based chemotherapy.

Dosage Forms Excipient information presented when available (limited, particularly for generics); consult specific product labeling.

Injection, powder for reconstitution: 500 mg

Ethyol®: 500 mg

References

Anne PR and Curran WJ Jr, "A Phase II Trial of Subcutaneous Amifostine and Radiation Therapy in Patients With Head and Neck Cancer," *Semin Radiat Oncol*, 2002, 12(1 Suppl 1):18-9.

Bonner HS and Shaw LM, "New Dosing Regimens for Amifostine: A Pilot Study to Compare the Relative Bioavailability of Oral and Subcutaneous Administration With Intravenous Infusion," *J Clin Pharmacol*, 2002, 42(2):166-74.

Brizel DM, Wasserman TH, Henke M, et al, "Phase III Randomized Trial of Amifostine as a Radioprotector in Head and Neck Cancer," *J Clin Oncol*, 2000, 18(19): 3339-45.

Hensley ML, Hagerty KL, Kewalramani T, et al, "American Society of Clinical Oncology 2008 Clinical Practice Guideline Update: Use of Chemotherapy and Radiotherapy Protectants," *J Clin Oncol*, 2009, 27(1): 127-45.

Keefe DM, Schubert MM, Elting LS, et al, "Updated Clinical Practice Guidelines for the Prevention and Treatment of Mucositis," *Cancer*, 2007, 109(5): 820-31.

Koukourakis MI, Kyrias G, and Kakolyris S, "Subcutaneous Administration of Amifostine During Fractionated Radiotherapy: A Randomized Phase II Study," *J Clin Oncol*, 2000, 18(11):2226-33.

Peterson DE, Bensadiun RJ, and Roila F, "Management of Oral and Gastrointestinal Mucositis: ESMO Clinical Recommendations," *Ann Oncol*, 2008, 19(Suppl 2): 122-5.

Samuels MA, Chico IM, Hirsch RL, et al, "Ongoing Prospective Multicenter Safety Study of the Cytoprotoctant Amifostine Given Subcutaneously: Overview of Trial Design," *Semin Oncol*, 2003, 30(6 Suppl 18):94-5.

Amikacin (am i KAY sin)

Brand Names: Canada Amikacin Sulfate Injection, USP; Amikin®

Index Terms Amikacin Sulfate

Generic Availability (U.S.) Yes

Pharmacologic Category Antibiotic, Aminoglycoside

Use Treatment of serious infections (bone infections, respiratory tract infections, endocarditis, and septicemia) due to organisms resistant to gentamicin and tobramycin, including *Pseudomonas*, *Proteus*, *Serratia*, and other gram-negative bacilli; documented infection of mycobacterial organisms susceptible to amikacin

Unlabeled Use Bacterial endophthalmitis; *Mycobacterium avium* complex (MAC; fibrocavitary or severe nodular/bronchiectatic disease)

Labeled Contraindications Hypersensitivity to amikacin sulfate or any component of the formulation; cross-sensitivity may exist with other aminoglycosides

Pregnancy Risk Factor D

Lactation Enters breast milk/not recommended

Warnings/Precautions [U.S. Boxed Warning]: Amikacin may cause neurotoxicity, nephrotoxicity, and/or neuromuscular blockade and respiratory paralysis; usual risk factors include pre-existing renal impairment, concomitant neuro-/nephrotoxic medications, advanced age and dehydration. Dose and/or frequency of administration must be monitored and modified in patients with renal impairment. Drug should be discontinued if signs of ototoxicity, nephrotoxicity, or hypersensitivity occur. Ototoxicity is proportional to the amount of drug given and the duration of treatment. Tinnitus or vertigo may be indications of vestibular injury and impending bilateral irreversible damage. Renal damage is usually reversible. Use with caution in patients with neuromuscular disorders, hearing loss and hypocalcemia. Prolonged use may result in fungal or bacterial superinfection, including *C. difficile*-associated diarrhea (CDAD) and pseudomembranous colitis; CDAD has been observed >2 months postantibiotic treatment. Solution contains sodium metabisulfate; use caution in patients with sulfite allergy.

Storage/Stability Store at controlled room temperature. Following admixture at concentrations of 0.25-5 mg/mL, amikacin is stable for 24 hours at room temperature and 2 days at refrigeration when mixed in D_5W, NS, and LR.

Mechanism of Action Inhibits protein synthesis in susceptible bacteria by binding to 30S ribosomal subunits

Pharmacodynamics/Kinetics

Absorption:

I.M.: Rapid

Oral: Poorly absorbed

Distribution: V_d: 0.25 L/kg; primarily into extracellular fluid (highly hydrophilic); penetrates blood-brain barrier when meninges inflamed

Relative diffusion of antimicrobial agents from blood into CSF: Good only with inflammation (exceeds usual MICs)

CSF:blood level ratio: Normal meninges: 10% to 20%; Inflamed meninges: 15% to 24%

Protein-binding: 0% to 11%

Half-life elimination (renal function and age dependent):

Infants: Low birth weight (1-3 days): 7-9 hours; Full-term >7 days: 4-5 hours

Children: 1.6-2.5 hours

Adults: Normal renal function: 1.4-2.3 hours; Anuria/end-stage renal disease: 28-86 hours

Time to peak, serum: I.M.: 45-120 minutes

Excretion: Urine (94% to 98%)

Dosing

Adult & Geriatric Individualization is critical because of the low therapeutic index

Note: Use of ideal body weight (IBW) for determining the mg/kg/dose appears to be more accurate than dosing on the basis of total body weight (TBW)

In morbid obesity, dosage requirement may best be estimated using a dosing weight of IBW + 0.4 (TBW - IBW)

Initial and periodic peak and trough plasma drug levels should be determined, particularly in critically-ill patients with serious infections or in disease states known to significantly alter aminoglycoside pharmacokinetics (eg, cystic fibrosis, burns, or major surgery). Manufacturer recommends a maximum daily dose of 15 mg/kg/day (or 1.5 g/day in heavier patients). Higher doses may be warranted based on therapeutic drug monitoring or susceptibility information.

Usual dosage range:

I.M., I.V.: 5-7.5 mg/kg/dose every 8 hours; **Note:** Some clinicians suggest a daily dose of 15-20 mg/kg for all patients with normal renal function. This dose is at least as efficacious with similar, if not less, toxicity than conventional dosing.

Intrathecal/intraventricular (unlabeled route): Meningitis (susceptible gram-negative organisms): 5-50 mg/day

Indication-specific dosing:

Endophthalmitis, bacterial (unlabeled use): Intravitreal: 0.4 mg/0.1 mL NS in combination with vancomycin

Hospital-acquired pneumonia (HAP): I.V.: 20 mg/kg/day with antipseudomonal beta-lactam or carbapenem (American Thoracic Society/ATS guidelines)

Meningitis (susceptible gram-negative organisms):

I.V.: 5 mg/kg every 8 hours (administered with another bactericidal drug)

Intrathecal/intraventricular (unlabeled route): Usual dose: 30 mg/day (IDSA, 2004); Range: 5-50 mg/day (with concurrent systemic antimicrobial therapy) (Gilbert, 1986; Guardado, 2008; IDSA, 2004; Kasiakou, 2005)

Mycobacterium avium **complex (MAC) (unlabeled use):** I.V.: Adjunct therapy (with macrolide, rifamycin, and ethambutol): 8-25 mg/kg 2-3 times weekly for first 2-3 months for severe disease (maximum single dose for age >50 years: 500 mg) (Griffith, 2007)

Mycobacterium fortuitum, M. chelonae, or M. abscessus: I.V.: 10-15 mg/kg daily for at least 2 weeks with high dose cefoxitin

Pediatric **Usual dosage range:** Infants and Children: I.M., I.V.: 5-7.5 mg/kg/dose every 8 hours

Note: Individualization is critical because of the low therapeutic index

Use of ideal body weight (IBW) for determining the mg/kg/dose appears to be more accurate than dosing on the basis of total body weight (TBW)

In morbid obesity, dosage requirement may best be estimated using a dosing weight of IBW + 0.4 (TBW - IBW)

Initial and periodic peak and trough plasma drug levels should be determined, particularly in critically-ill patients with serious infections or in disease states known to significantly alter aminoglycoside pharmacokinetics (eg, cystic fibrosis, burns, or major surgery). Manufacturer recommends a maximum daily dose of 15 mg/kg/day (or 1.5 g/day in heavier patients). Higher doses may be warranted based on therapeutic drug monitoring or susceptibility information.

Renal Impairment Some patients may require larger or more frequent doses if serum levels document the need (ie, cystic fibrosis or febrile granulocytopenic patients).

Cl_{cr} ≥60 mL/minute: Administer every 8 hours
Cl_{cr} 40-60 mL/minute: Administer every 12 hours
Cl_{cr} 20-40 mL/minute: Administer every 24 hours
Cl_{cr} <20 mL/minute: Loading dose, then monitor levels

Intermittent hemodialysis (IHD) (administer after hemodialysis on dialysis days): Dialyzable (20%; variable; dependent on filter, duration, and type of HD): 5-7.5 mg/kg every 48-72 hours. Follow levels. Redose when pre-HD concentration <10 mg/L; redose when post-HD concentration <6-8 mg/L (Heintz, 2009). **Note:** Dosing dependent on the assumption of 3 times/week, complete IHD sessions.

Peritoneal dialysis (PD): Dose as Cl_{cr} <20 mL/minute: Follow levels.

Continuous renal replacement therapy (CRRT) (Heintz, 2009; Trotman, 2005): Drug clearance is highly dependent on the method of renal replacement, filter type, and flow rate. Appropriate dosing requires close monitoring of pharmacologic response, signs of adverse reactions due to drug accumulation, as well as drug concentrations in relation to target trough (if appropriate). The following are general recommendations only (based on dialysate flow/ultrafiltration rates of 1-2 L/hour and minimal residual renal function) and should not supersede clinical judgment:

CVVH/CVVHD/CVVHDF: Loading dose of 10 mg/kg followed by maintenance dose of 7.5 mg/kg every 24-48 hours

Note: For severe gram-negative rod infections, target peak concentration of 15-30 mg/L; redose when concentration <10 mg/L (Heintz, 2009).

Administration Administer around-the-clock to promote less variation in peak and trough serum levels. Do not mix with other drugs, administer separately.

I.M.: Administer I.M. injection in large muscle mass.

I.V.: Infuse over 30-60 minutes.

Some penicillins (eg, carbenicillin, ticarcillin, and piperacillin) have been shown to inactivate *in vitro*. This has been observed to a greater extent with tobramycin and gentamicin, while amikacin has shown greater stability against inactivation. Concurrent use of these agents may pose a risk of reduced antibacterial efficacy *in vivo*, particularly in the setting of profound renal impairment. However, definitive clinical evidence is lacking. If combination penicillin/aminoglycoside therapy is desired in a patient with renal dysfunction, separation of doses (if feasible), and routine monitoring of aminoglycoside levels, CBC, and clinical response should be considered.

Intrathecal/Intraventricular (unlabeled route): Reserved solely for meningitis due to susceptible gram-negative organisms. Available formulation contains sodium metabisulfite. If possible, consider alternative therapy with gentamicin or tobramycin as both of these agents are available as preservative-free formulations.

Test Interactions Some penicillin derivatives may accelerate the degradation of aminoglycosides *in vitro*, leading to a potential underestimation of aminoglycoside serum concentration.

Dosage Forms Excipient information presented when available (limited, particularly for generics); consult specific product labeling.

Injection, solution, as sulfate: 250 mg/mL (2 mL, 4 mL)

- **Amikacin Sulfate** *see* Amikacin *on page 69*
- **Amikacin Sulfate Injection, USP (Can)** *see* Amikacin *on page 69*
- **Amikin® (Can)** *see* Amikacin *on page 69*
- **2-Amino-6-Mercaptopurine** *see* Thioguanine *on page 1354*
- **2-Amino-6-Methoxypurine Arabinoside** *see* Nelarabine *on page 1028*

Aminocaproic Acid (a mee noe ka PROE ik AS id)

Brand Names: U.S. Amicar®

Index Terms EACA; Epsilon Aminocaproic Acid

Generic Availability (U.S.) Yes

Pharmacologic Category Antifibrinolytic Agent; Antihemophilic Agent; Hemostatic Agent; Lysine Analog

Use To enhance hemostasis when fibrinolysis contributes to bleeding (causes may include cardiac surgery, hematologic disorders, neoplastic disorders, abruptio placentae, hepatic cirrhosis, and urinary fibrinolysis)

Unlabeled Use Treatment of traumatic hyphema; control bleeding in thrombocytopenia; control oral bleeding in congenital and acquired coagulation disorders; topical treatment (mouth rinse) of bleeding associated with dental procedures in patients on oral anticoagulant therapy; prevention of perioperative bleeding associated with cardiac surgery; prevention of bleeding associated with extracorporeal membrane oxygenation (ECMO); prevention of perioperative bleeding associated with spinal surgery (eg, idiopathic scoliosis)

Labeled Contraindications Disseminated intravascular coagulation (without heparin); evidence of an active intravascular clotting process

Pregnancy Risk Factor C

Lactation Excretion in breast milk unknown/use caution

Warnings/Precautions Avoid rapid I.V. administration (may induce hypotension, bradycardia, or arrhythmia); rapid injection of undiluted solution is not recommended. Use with caution in patients with renal disease; aminocaproic acid may accumulate in patients with decreased renal function. Intrarenal obstruction may occur secondary to glomerular capillary thrombosis or clots in the renal pelvis and ureters. Do not use in hematuria of upper urinary tract origin unless possible benefits outweigh risks. Do not administer without a definite diagnosis of laboratory findings indicative of hyperfibrinolysis. Inhibition of fibrinolysis may promote clotting or thrombosis; more likely due to the presence of DIC. Skeletal muscle weakness ranging from mild myalgias and fatigue to severe myopathy with rhabdomyolysis and acute renal failure has been reported with prolonged use. Monitor CPK; discontinue treatment with a rise in CPK. Benzyl alcohol is used as a preservative in the injection; therefore, these products should not be used in the neonate. Do not administer with factor IX complex concentrates or anti-inhibitor coagulant complexes; may increase risk for thrombosis.

Adverse Reactions Frequency not defined.

Cardiovascular: Arrhythmia, bradycardia, edema, hypotension, intracranial hypertension, peripheral ischemia, syncope, thrombosis

Central nervous system: Confusion, delirium, dizziness, fatigue, hallucinations, headache, malaise, seizure, stroke

Dermatologic: Rash, pruritus

Gastrointestinal: Abdominal pain, anorexia, cramps, diarrhea, GI irritation, nausea, vomiting

Genitourinary: Dry ejaculation

Hematologic: Agranulocytosis, bleeding time increased, leukopenia, thrombocytopenia

Local: Injection site necrosis, injection site pain, injection site reactions

Neuromuscular & skeletal: CPK increased, myalgia, myositis, myopathy, rhabdomyolysis (rare), weakness

Ophthalmic: Vision decreased, watery eyes

Otic: Tinnitus

Renal: BUN increased, intrarenal obstruction (glomerular capillary thrombosis), myoglobinuria (rare), renal failure (rare)

Respiratory: Dyspnea, nasal congestion, pulmonary embolism

Miscellaneous: Allergic reaction, anaphylactoid reaction, anaphylaxis

Postmarketing and/or case reports: Hepatic lesion, hyperkalemia, myocardial lesion

Drug Interactions

Metabolism/Transport Effects None known.

Avoid Concomitant Use

Avoid concomitant use of Aminocaproic Acid with any of the following: Anti-inhibitor Coagulant Complex; Factor IX; Factor IX Complex (Human)

Increased Effect/Toxicity

Aminocaproic Acid may increase the levels/effects of: Anti-inhibitor Coagulant Complex; Factor IX; Factor IX Complex (Human); Fibrinogen Concentrate (Human)

The levels/effects of Aminocaproic Acid may be increased by: Fibrinogen Concentrate (Human); Tretinoin (Systemic)

Decreased Effect There are no known significant interactions involving a decrease in effect.

Storage/Stability Store intact vials, tablets, and syrup at 15°C to 30°C (59°F to 86°F). Do not freeze injection or syrup. Solutions diluted for I.V. use in D_5W or NS to concentrations of 10-100 mg/mL are stable at 4°C (39°F) and 23°C (73°F) for 7 days (Zhang, 1997).

Reconstitution Dilute I.V. solution in D_5W, 0.9% sodium chloride, or Ringer's injection.

Mechanism of Action Binds competitively to plasminogen; blocking the binding of plasminogen to fibrin and the subsequent conversion to plasmin, resulting in inhibition of fibrin degradation (fibrinolysis).

Pharmacodynamics/Kinetics

Onset of action: ~1-72 hours

Distribution: Widely through intravascular and extravascular compartments

V_d: Oral: 23 L, I.V.: 30 L

Metabolism: Minimally hepatic

Half-life elimination: ~2 hours

Time to peak: Oral: Within 2 hours

Excretion: Urine (65% as unchanged drug, 11% as metabolite)

Dosing

Adult & Geriatric

Acute bleeding: Oral, I.V.: Loading dose: 4-5 g during the first hour, followed by 1 g/hour for 8 hours (or 1.25 g/hour using oral solution) or until bleeding controlled (maximum daily dose: 30 g)

Control of bleeding with severe thrombocytopenia (unlabeled use) (Bartholomew, 1989; Gardner, 1980):

Initial: I.V.: 100 mg/kg (maximum dose: 5 g) over 30-60 minutes

Maintenance: Oral, I.V.: 1-4 g every 4-8 hours or 1 g/hour (maximum daily dose: 24 g)

Control of oral bleeding in congenital and acquired coagulation disorder (unlabeled use): Oral: 50-60 mg/kg every 4 hours (Mannucci, 1998)

Prevention of dental procedure bleeding in patients on oral anticoagulant therapy (unlabeled use): Oral rinse: Hold 4 g/10 mL in mouth for 2 minutes then spit out. Repeat every 6 hours for 2 days after procedure (Souto, 1996). Concentration and frequency may vary by institution and product availability.

Prevention of perioperative bleeding associated with cardiac surgery (unlabeled use): I.V.: Loading dose of 75-150 mg/kg (typically 5-10 g), followed by 10-15 mg/kg/hour (typically 1 g/hour); may add 2-2.5 g/L of cardiopulmonary bypass circuit priming solution (Gravlee, 2008)

or

Loading dose of 10 g followed by 2 g/hour during surgery; no medication added to the bypass circuit (Fergusson, 2008)

or

10 g over 20-30 minutes prior to skin incision, followed by 10 g after heparin administration then 10 g at discontinuation of cardiopulmonary bypass (Vander Salm, 1996)

Traumatic hyphema (unlabeled use): Oral: 50 mg/kg/dose every 4 hours (maximum daily dose: 30 g) for 5 days (Brandt, 2001; Crouch, 1999)

Pediatric

Prevention of perioperative bleeding associated with cardiac surgery (unlabeled use): I.V.: 100 mg/kg given over 20-30 minutes after induction and prior to incision, 100 mg/kg during cardiopulmonary bypass, and 100 mg/kg after heparin reversal over 3 hours (Chauhan, 2004)

Prevention of bleeding associated with extracorporeal membrane oxygenation (ECMO) (unlabeled use): I.V.: 100 mg/kg prior to or immediately after cannulation, followed by 25-30 mg/kg/hour for up to 72 hours (Downard, 2003; Horwitz, 1998; Wilson, 1993)

Prevention of perioperative bleeding associated with spinal surgery (eg, idiopathic scoliosis) (unlabeled use): Children and Adolescents: I.V.: 100 mg/kg given over 15-20 minutes after induction, followed by 10 mg/kg/hour for the remainder of the surgery; discontinue at time of wound closure (Florentino-Pineda, 2001; Florentino-Pineda, 2004)

Traumatic hyphema (unlabeled use): Oral: Refer to adult dosing.

Renal Impairment May accumulate in patients with decreased renal function. When used during cardiopulmonary bypass in anephric patients, a normal or slightly reduced loading dose and a continuous infusion rate of 5 mg/kg/hour has been recommended (Gravlee, 2008).

Usual Infusion Concentrations: Adult I.V. infusion: 5000 mg in 250 mL (concentration: 20 mg/mL) of D_5W, NS, or Ringer's injection

Administration Rapid I.V. injection (IVP) of undiluted solution is not recommended due to possible hypotension, bradycardia, and arrhythmia.

I.V.: May administer loading dose over 15-60 minutes depending on indication; a continuous infusion may be necessary.

Monitoring Parameters Fibrinogen, fibrin split products, creatine phosphokinase (with long-term therapy), BUN, creatinine

Dosage Forms Excipient information presented when available (limited, particularly for generics); consult specific product labeling.

Injection, solution: 250 mg/mL (20 mL)

Solution, oral: 1.25 g/5 mL (237 mL, 473 mL)

Syrup, oral:

Amicar®: 1.25 g/5 mL (473 mL) [raspberry flavor]

Tablet, oral: 500 mg

Amicar®: 500 mg, 1000 mg [scored]

References

Bartholomew JR, Salgia R, and Bell WR, "Control of Bleeding in Patients With Immune and Nonimmune Thrombocytopenia With Aminocaproic Acid," *Arch Intern Med*, 1989, 149 (9):1959-61.

Brandt MT and Haug RH, "Traumatic Hyphema: A Comprehensive Review," *J Oral Maxillofac Surg*, 2001, 59(12):1462-70.

Chauhan S, Das SN, Bisoi A, et al, "Comparison of Epsilon Aminocaproic Acid and Tranexamic Acid in Pediatric Cardiac Surgery," *J Cardiothorac Vasc Anesth*, 2004, 18(2):141-43.

Crouch ER Jr and Crouch ER, "Management of Traumatic Hyphema: Therapeutic Options," *J Pediatr Ophthalmol Strabismus*, 1999, 36(5):238-50.

Douketis JD, Berger PB, Dunn AS, et al, "The Perioperative Management of Antithrombotic Therapy: American College of Chest Physicians Evidence-Based Clinical Practice Guidelines (8th Edition)," *Chest*, 2008, 133(6 Suppl):299-339.

Downard CD, Betit P, Chang RW, et al, "Impact of AMICAR on Hemorrhagic Complications of ECMO: A Ten-Year Review," *J Pediatr Surg*, 2003, 38(8):1212-6.

Fergusson DA, Hebert PC, Mazer CD, et al, "A Comparison of Aprotinin and Lysine Analogues in High-Risk Cardiac Surgery," *N Engl J Med*, 2008, 358(22):2319-31.

Florentino-Pineda I, Blakemore LC, Thompson GH, et al, "The Effect of Epsilon-Aminocaproic Acid on Perioperative Blood Loss in Patients With Idiopathic Scoliosis Undergoing Posterior Spinal Fusion: A Preliminary Prospective Study," *Spine (Phila Pa 1976)*, 2001, 26(10):1147-51.

Florentino-Pineda I, Thompson GH, Poe-Kochert C, et al, "The Effect of Amicar on Perioperative Blood Loss in Idiopathic Scoliosis: The Results of a Prospective, Randomized Double-Blind Study," *Spine (Phila Pa 1976)*, 2004, 29(3):233-8.

Gardner FH and Helmer RE 3rd, "Aminocaproic Acid. Use in Control of Hemorrhage in Patients With Amegakaryocytic Thrombocytopenia," *JAMA*, 1980, 243(1):35-7.

Gravlee GP and Spiess B, "Pharmacologic Prophylaxis for Post-Cardiopulmonary Bypass Bleeding," *Cardiopulmonary Bypass: Principles and Practice*, 3rd ed, Philadelphia, PA: Lippincott Williams & Wilkins, 2008, 522-42.

Hirsh J, Guyatt G, Albers GW, et al, "Executive Summary: American College of Chest Physicians Evidence-Based Clinical Practice Guidelines (8th Edition)," *Chest*, 2008, 133(6 Suppl):71-109.

Horwitz JR, Cofer BR, Warner BW, et al, "A Multicenter Trial of 6-Aminocaproic Acid (Amicar) in the Prevention of Bleeding in Infants on ECMO," *J Pediatr Surg*, 1998, 33(11):1610-3.

Mannucci P, "Hemostatic Drugs," *N Engl J Med*, 1998, 339(4):245-53.

Vander Salm TJ, Kaur S, Lancey RA, et al, "Reduction of Bleeding After Heart Operations Through the Prophylactic Use of Epsilon Aminocaproic Acid," *J Thorac Cardiovasc Surg*, 1996, 112 (4):1098-107.

Wilson JM, Bower LK, Fackler JC, et al, "Aminocaproic Acid Decreases the Incidence of Intracranial Hemorrhage and Other Hemorrhagic Complications of ECMO," *J Pediatr Surg*, 1993, 28 (4):536-40.

Aminolevulinic Acid (a MEE noh lev yoo lin ik AS id)

Brand Names: U.S. Levulan® Kerastick®

Brand Names: Canada Levulan® Kerastick®

Index Terms 5-ALA; 5-Aminolevulinic Acid; ALA; Amino Levulinic Acid; Aminolevulinic Acid Hydrochloride

Generic Availability (U.S.) No

Pharmacologic Category Photosensitizing Agent, Topical; Topical Skin Product

Use Treatment of minimally to moderately thick actinic keratoses (grade 1 or 2) of the face or scalp; to be used in conjunction with blue light illumination

Unlabeled Use Photodynamic treatment of low-risk superficial basal cell skin cancer and low-risk squamous cell skin cancer *in situ* (Bowen's disease)

Labeled Contraindications Hypersensitivity to aminolevulinic acid or any component of the formulation; individuals with cutaneous photosensitivity at wavelengths of 400-450 nm; porphyria; allergy to porphyrins

Pregnancy Risk Factor C

Lactation Excretion in breast milk unknown/use caution

Warnings/Precautions Treatment site will become photosensitive following application. Patients should be instructed to avoid exposure to sunlight, bright indoor lights, or tanning beds during the period prior to blue light treatment (exposure may result in lesion burning, edema, erythema and/or stinging). Sunscreen will not protect against visible light; head should be covered with light-opaque material or wide-brimmed hat. If unable to return the next day for blue light treatment, avoid sunlight/bright light exposure to treated lesions for at least 40 hours. Concomitant use of other known photosensitizing agents may increase the degree of photosensitivity reaction.

For external use only. Do not apply to eyes or mucous membranes. Excessive skin irritation may occur if applied under occlusion. Application should involve either scalp or face lesions, although not simultaneously. Should be applied by a qualified health professional to avoid application to perilesional skin. Has not been tested in individuals with coagulation defects (acquired or inherited).

Adverse Reactions Transient stinging, burning, itching, erythema, and edema result from the photosensitizing properties of this agent. Symptoms subside between 1 minute and 24 hours after turning off the blue light illuminator. Severe stinging or burning was reported in at least 50% of patients from at least 1 lesional site during treatment.

>10%: Dermatologic: Stinging or burning (most patients; severe: ≥50%), erythema (99%), scaling/crusted skin (64% to 71%), hyper-/hypopigmentation (22% to 36%), edematous lesions (35%), itching (14% to 25%), erosion (2% to 14%), skin disorder (5% to 12%)

1% to 10%:

Central nervous system: Dysesthesia (≤2%)

Dermatologic: Vesiculation (4% to 5%), skin ulceration (2% to 4%), pustular drug eruption (≤4%)

Hematologic: Bleeding/hemorrhage (2% to 4%)

Local: Wheal/flare (2% to 7%), scabbing (≤2%), tenderness (1% to 2%), edema (≤1%), excoriation (≤1%), local pain (≤1%), oozing (≤1%)

Drug Interactions

Metabolism/Transport Effects None known.

Avoid Concomitant Use There are no known interactions where it is recommended to avoid concomitant use.

Increased Effect/Toxicity There are no known significant interactions involving an increase in effect.

Decreased Effect There are no known significant interactions involving a decrease in effect.

Storage/Stability Store at 20°C to 25°C (68°F to 77°F); excursions permitted to 15°C to 30°C (59°F to 86°F). Once prepared, the topical solution should be used immediately and application must be completed within 2 hours of solution preparation.

Reconstitution Follow instructions on Kerastick® Krusher or mix manually: Prepare solution by holding applicator tube with cap pointing up, applying finger pressure to "Position A" on cardboard sleeve to crush ampul containing solution vehicle. Apply finger pressure to "Position B" to crush ampul containing aminolevulinic acid powder. Shake gently for at least 30 seconds to dissolve; point applicator cap away from face while shaking tube. Remove cap; dab dry applicator tip on gauze pad until wet with solution.

Mechanism of Action Aminolevulinic acid is a metabolic precursor of the photosensitizer protoporphyrin IX (PpIX). Photosensitization following local application of aminolevulinic acid occurs through the metabolic conversion to PpIX. When exposed to light of appropriate wavelength and energy, accumulated PpIX produces a photodynamic reaction resulting in local cytotoxicity. Precancerous and cancerous cells exhibit a higher rate of porphyrin induction compared to normal cells.

Pharmacodynamics/Kinetics

Peak fluorescence intensity of protoporphyrin IX (PpIX): Actinic keratosis: 11 hours ± 1 hour; Perilesional skin: 12 hours ± 1 hour

Half-life elimination: Mean fluorescence clearance half-life of PpIX for lesions: 30 ± 10 hours

Dosing

Adult & Geriatric Actinic keratoses: Topical: Apply to actinic keratoses (**not** perilesional skin) followed 14-18 hours later by blue light illumination. Application/treatment may be repeated at a treatment site (once) after 8 weeks.

Administration Dab lesion gently with wet applicator tip (apply enough to uniformly wet lesion without excess running or dripping). Only apply to affected skin. Do not apply to periorbital area, ocular tissue, or mucosal surfaces. Allow to dry, then reapply to same lesion. Apply to either scalp or facial lesions, but not to both simultaneously. Follow application with blue light exposure in 14-18 hours. Do not wash the application area during the time between application and photosensitization; after photosensitization, gently rinse actinic keratosis with water and pat dry. Stinging or burning may occur during blue light treatment. Following blue light treatment, the lesion will temporarily redden, swell and/or scale, which should resolve within 4 weeks after treatment.

Additional Information Use in conjunction with the BLU-U™ Blue Light Photodynamic Therapy Illuminator.

Dosage Forms Excipient information presented when available (limited, particularly for generics); consult specific product labeling.

Powder for solution, topical, as hydrochloride:

Levulan® Kerastick®: 20% (6s) [contains ethanol 48% (in diluent); supplied with diluent]

References

Braathen LR, Szeimies RM, Basset-Seguin N, et al, "Guidelines on the Use of Photodynamic Therapy for Nonmelanoma Skin Cancer: An International Consensus. International Society for Photodynamic Therapy in Dermatology, 2005," *J Am Acad Dermatol*, 2007, 56(1):125-43.

Moloney FJ and Collins P, et al, "Randomized, Double-Blind, Prospective Study to Compare Topical 5-Aminolaevulinic Acid Methylester With Topical 5-Aminolaevulinic Acid Photodynamic Therapy for Extensive Scalp Actinic Keratosis," *Br J Dermatol*, 2007, 157(1):87-91.

Tierney E, Barker A, Ahdout J, et al, "Photodynamic Therapy for the Treatment of Cutaneous Neoplasia, Inflammatory Disorders, and Photoaging," *Dermatol Surg*, 2009, 35(5):725-46.

- **Amino Levulinic Acid** *see* Aminolevulinic Acid *on page* 75
- **5-Aminolevulinic Acid** *see* Aminolevulinic Acid *on page* 75
- **Aminolevulinic Acid Hydrochloride** *see* Aminolevulinic Acid *on page* 75

◆ **AMJ 9701** *see* Palifermin *on page* 1104

◆ **AMN107** *see* Nilotinib *on page* 1031

◆ **Amnesteem®** *see* ISOtretinoin *on page* 832

◆ **Amphadase™** *see* Hyaluronidase *on page* 711

◆ **Amphotec®** *see* Amphotericin B Cholesteryl Sulfate Complex *on page* 78

Amphotericin B Cholesteryl Sulfate Complex

(am foe TER i sin bee kole LES te ril SUL fate KOM plecks)

Brand Names: U.S. Amphotec®

Brand Names: Canada Amphotec®

Index Terms ABCD; Amphotericin B Colloidal Dispersion

Generic Availability (U.S.) No

Pharmacologic Category Antifungal Agent, Parenteral

Use Treatment of invasive aspergillosis in patients who have failed amphotericin B deoxycholate treatment, or who have renal impairment or experience unacceptable toxicity which precludes treatment with amphotericin B deoxycholate in effective doses.

Unlabeled Use Effective in patients with serious *Candida* species infections

Labeled Contraindications Hypersensitivity to amphotericin B or any component of the formulation (unless the benefits outweigh the possible risk to the patient)

Pregnancy Risk Factor B

Lactation Excretion in breast milk unknown/not recommended

Warnings/Precautions Anaphylaxis has been reported with amphotericin B-containing drugs. If severe respiratory distress occurs, the infusion should be immediately discontinued; the patient should not receive further infusions. During the initial dosing, the drug should be administered under close clinical observation. Acute infusion reactions, sometimes severe, may occur 1-3 hours after starting infusion. These reactions are usually more common with the first few doses and generally diminish with subsequent doses. Pretreatment with antihistamines/corticosteroids and/or decreasing the rate of infusion can be used to manage reactions. Avoid rapid infusion.

Storage/Stability Store intact vials at 15°C to 30°C (59°F to 86°F). After reconstitution, the solution should be refrigerated at 2°C to 8°C (36°F to 46°F) and used within 24 hours. Concentrations of 0.1-2 mg/mL in D_5W are stable for 24 hours at 2°C to 8°C (36°F to 46°F).

Reconstitution Reconstitute 50 mg and 100 mg vials with 10 mL and 20 mL of SWI, respectively. The reconstituted vials contain 5 mg/mL of amphotericin B. Shake the vial gently by hand until all solid particles have dissolved. Further dilute amphotericin B colloidal dispersion with D_5W.

Mechanism of Action Binds to ergosterol altering cell membrane permeability in susceptible fungi and causing leakage of cell components with subsequent cell death. Proposed mechanism suggests that amphotericin causes an oxidation-dependent stimulation of macrophages (Lyman, 1992).

Pharmacodynamics/Kinetics

Distribution: V_d: Total volume increases with higher doses, reflects increasing uptake by tissues (with 4 mg/kg/day = 4 L/kg); predominantly distributed in the liver; concentrations in kidneys and other tissues are lower than observed with conventional amphotericin B

Half-life elimination: ~28 hours; prolonged with higher doses

Dosing

Adult & Geriatric Aspergillosis (invasive), treatment: *Usual dosage range:* 3-4 mg/kg/day. **Note:** 6 mg/kg/day has been used for treatment of life-threatening invasive aspergillosis in immunocompromised patients (Bowden, 2002).

Premedication: For patients who experience chills, fever, hypotension, nausea, or other nonanaphylactic infusion-related immediate reactions, premedicate with the following drugs 30-60 minutes prior to drug administration: A nonsteroidal with or without diphenhydramine **or** acetaminophen with diphenhydramine **or** hydrocortisone 50-100 mg with or without a nonsteroidal and diphenhydramine (Paterson, 2008).

Test dose: For patients receiving their first dose in a new treatment course, a small amount (10 mL of the final preparation, containing between 1.6-8.3 mg) infused over 15-30 minutes is recommended. The patient should then be observed for an additional 30 minutes.

Pediatric Refer to adult dosing.

Administration Initially infuse at 1 mg/kg/hour. Rate of infusion may be increased with subsequent doses as patient tolerance allows (minimum infusion time: 2 hours). For a patient who experiences chills, fever, hypotension, nausea, or other nonanaphylactic infusion-related reactions, premedicate with the following drugs 30-60 minutes prior to drug administration: A nonsteroidal with or without diphenhydramine **or** acetaminophen with diphenhydramine **or** hydrocortisone 50-100 mg with or without a nonsteroidal and diphenhydramine (Paterson, 2008). If the patient experiences rigors during the infusion, meperidine may be administered. If severe respiratory distress occurs, the infusion should be immediately discontinued.

Dosage Forms Excipient information presented when available (limited, particularly for generics); consult specific product labeling.

Injection, powder for reconstitution:

Amphotec®: 50 mg [contains edetate disodium, lactose 950 mg]

Amphotec®: 100 mg [contains edetate disodium, lactose 1900 mg]

◆ **Amphotericin B Colloidal Dispersion** *see* Amphotericin B Cholesteryl Sulfate Complex *on page* 78

Amphotericin B (Conventional)

(am foe TER i sin bee con VEN sha nal)

Brand Names: Canada Fungizone®

Index Terms Amphotericin B Deoxycholate; Amphotericin B Desoxycholate; Conventional Amphotericin B

Generic Availability (U.S.) Yes

Pharmacologic Category Antifungal Agent, Parenteral

Use Treatment of severe systemic and central nervous system infections caused by susceptible fungi such as *Candida* species, *Histoplasma capsulatum*, *Cryptococcus neoformans*, *Aspergillus* species, *Blastomyces dermatitidis*, *Torulopsis glabrata*, and *Coccidioides immitis*; fungal peritonitis; irrigant for bladder fungal infections; used in fungal infection in patients with bone marrow transplantation, amebic meningoencephalitis, ocular aspergillosis (intraocular injection), candidal cystitis (bladder irrigation), chemoprophylaxis (low-dose I.V.), immunocompromised patients at risk of aspergillosis (intranasal/nebulized), refractory meningitis (intrathecal), coccidioidal arthritis (intra-articular/I.M.).

Low-dose amphotericin B has been administered after bone marrow transplantation to reduce the risk of invasive fungal disease.

Labeled Contraindications Hypersensitivity to amphotericin or any component of the formulation

Pregnancy Risk Factor B

Lactation Excretion in breast milk unknown/not recommended

Warnings/Precautions Anaphylaxis has been reported with amphotericin B-containing drugs. During the initial dosing, the drug should be administered under close clinical observation. May cause nephrotoxicity; usual risk factors include underlying renal disease, concomitant nephrotoxic medications and daily and/or cumulative dose of amphotericin. Avoid use with other nephrotoxic drugs; drug-induced renal toxicity usually improves with interrupting therapy, decreasing dosage, or increasing dosing interval. However permanent impairment may occur, especially in patients receiving large cumulative dose (eg, >5 g) and in those also receiving other nephrotoxic drugs. Hydration and sodium repletion prior to administration may reduce the risk of developing nephrotoxicity. Frequent monitoring of renal function is recommended. Acute reactions (eg, fever, shaking chills, hypotension, anorexia, nausea, vomiting, headache, tachypnea) are most common 1-3 hours after starting the infusion and diminish with continued therapy. Avoid rapid infusion to prevent hypotension, hypokalemia, arrhythmias, and shock. If therapy is stopped for >7 days, restart at the lowest dose recommended and increase gradually. Leukoencephalopathy has been reported following administration of amphotericin. Total body irradiation has been reported to be a possible predisposition.

[U.S. Boxed Warning]: Should be used primarily for treatment of progressive, potentially life-threatening fungal infections, not noninvasive forms of infection. [U.S. Boxed warning]: Verify the product name and dosage if dose exceeds 1.5 mg/kg.

Storage/Stability Store intact vials under refrigeration. Protect from light. Reconstituted vials are stable, protected from light, for 24 hours at room temperature and 1 week when refrigerated. Parenteral admixtures are stable, protected from light, for 24 hours at room temperature and 2 days under refrigeration. Short-term exposure (<24 hours) to light during I.V. infusion does **not** appreciably affect potency.

Reconstitution Add 10 mL of SWFI (without a bacteriostatic agent) to each vial of amphotericin B. Further dilute with 250-500 mL D_5W; final concentration should not exceed 0.1 mg/mL (peripheral infusion) or 0.25 mg/mL (central infusion).

Mechanism of Action Binds to ergosterol altering cell membrane permeability in susceptible fungi and causing leakage of cell components with subsequent cell death. Proposed mechanism suggests that amphotericin causes an oxidation-dependent stimulation of macrophages (Lyman, 1992).

Pharmacodynamics/Kinetics

Distribution: Minimal amounts enter the aqueous humor, bile, CSF (inflamed or noninflamed meninges), pericardial fluid, pleural fluid, and synovial fluid

Protein binding, plasma: 90%

Half-life elimination: Biphasic: Initial: 15-48 hours; Terminal: 15 days

Time to peak: Within 1 hour following a 4- to 6-hour dose

Excretion: Urine (2% to 5% as biologically active form); ~40% eliminated over a 7-day period and may be detected in urine for at least 7 weeks after discontinued use

Dosing

Adult & Geriatric Note: Premedication: For patients who experience infusion-related immediate reactions, premedicate with the following drugs 30-60 minutes prior to drug administration: NSAID ± diphenhydramine **or** acetaminophen with diphenhydramine **or** hydrocortisone. If the patient experiences rigors during the infusion, meperidine may be administered.

Test dose: I.V.: 1 mg infused over 20-30 minutes. Many clinicians believe a test dose is unnecessary.

Susceptible fungal infections: I.V.: Adults: 0.3-1.5 mg/kg/day; 1-1.5 mg/kg over 4-6 hours every other day may be given once therapy is established; aspergillosis, rhinocerebral mucormycosis, often require 1-1.5 mg/kg/day; do not exceed 1.5 mg/kg/day

Aspergillosis, disseminated: I.V.: 0.6-0.7 mg/kg/day for 3-6 months

Bone marrow transplantation (prophylaxis): I.V.: Low-dose amphotericin B 0.1-0.25 mg/kg/day has been administered after bone marrow transplantation to reduce the risk of invasive fungal disease.

Candidemia (neutropenic or non-neutropenic): I.V.: 0.5-1 mg/kg/day until 14 days after first negative blood culture and resolution of signs and symptoms (Pappas, 2009)

Candidiasis, chronic, disseminated: I.V.: 0.5-0.7 mg/kg/day for 3-6 months and resolution of radiologic lesions (Pappas, 2009)

Dematiaceous fungi: I.V.: 0.7 mg/kg/day in combination with an azole

Endocarditis: I.V.: 0.6-1 mg/kg/day (with or without flucytosine) for 6 weeks after valve replacement; **Note:** If isolates susceptible and/or clearance demonstrated, guidelines recommend step-down to fluconazole; also for long-term suppression therapy if valve replacement is not possible (Pappas, 2009)

Endophthalmitis, fungal:

Intravitreal (unlabeled use): 10 mcg in 0.1 mL (in conjunction with systemic therapy)

I.V.: 0.7-1 mg/kg/day (with or without flucytosine) for at least 4-6 weeks (Pappas, 2009)

Esophageal candidiasis: I.V.: 0.3-0.7 mg/kg/day for 14-21 days after clinical improvement (Pappas, 2009)

Histoplasmosis: Chronic, severe pulmonary or disseminated: I.V.: 0.5-1 mg/kg/day for 7 days, then 0.8 mg/kg every other day (or 3 times/week) until total dose of 10-15 mg/kg; may continue itraconazole as suppressive therapy (lifelong for immunocompromised patients)

Meningitis:

Candidal: I.V.: 0.7-1 mg/kg/day (with or without flucytosine) for at least 4 weeks; **Note:** Liposomal amphotericin favored by IDSA guidelines based on decreased risk of nephrotoxicity and potentially better CNS penetration (Pappas, 2009)

Cryptococcal or Coccidioides: I.T.: Initial: 0.01-0.05 mg as single daily dose; may increase daily in increments of 0.025-0.1 mg as tolerated (maximum: 1.5 mg/day; most patients will tolerate a maximum dose of ~0.5 mg/treatment). Once titration to a maximum tolerated dose is achieved, that dose is administered daily. Once CSF improvement noted, may decrease frequency on a weekly basis (eg, 5 times/week, then 3 times/week, then 2 times/week, then once weekly, then once every other week, then once every 2 weeks, etc) until administration occurs once every 6 weeks. Typically, concurrent oral azole therapy is maintained (Stevens, 2001). **Note:** IDSA notes that the use of I.T. amphotericin for cryptococcal meningitis is generally discouraged and rarely necessary (Perfect, 2010).

Histoplasma: I.V.: 0.5-1 mg/kg/day for 7 days, then 0.8 mg/kg every other day (or 3 times/week) for 3 months total duration; follow with fluconazole suppressive therapy for up to 12 months

Meningoencephalitis, cryptococcal (Perfect, 2010): I.V.:

HIV positive: Induction: 0.7-1 mg/kg/day (plus flucytosine 100 mg/kg/day) for 2 weeks, then change to oral fluconazole for at least 8 weeks; alternatively, amphotericin (0.7-1 mg/kg/day) may be continued uninterrupted for 4-6 weeks; maintenance: amphotericin 1 mg/kg/week for ≥1 year may be considered, but inferior to use of azoles

HIV negative: Induction: 0.7-1 mg/kg/day (plus flucytosine 100 mg/kg/day) for 2 weeks (low-risk patients), ≥4 weeks (non-low-risk, but without neurologic complication, immunosuppression, underlying disease, and negative CSF culture at 2 weeks), >6 weeks (neurologic complication or patients intolerant of flucytosine) Follow with azole consolidation/maintenance treatment.

Oropharyngeal candidiasis: I.V.: 0.3 mg/kg/day for 7-14 days (Pappas, 2009)

Osteoarticular candidiasis: I.V.: 0.5-1 mg/kg/day for several weeks, followed by fluconazole for 6-12 months (osteomyelitis) or 6 weeks (septic arthritis) (Pappas, 2009)

Penicillium marneffei: I.V.: 0.6 mg/kg/day for 2 weeks

Pneumonia: Cryptococcal (mild-to-moderate): I.V.:

HIV positive: 0.5-1 mg/kg/day

HIV negative: 0.5-0.7 mg/kg/day (plus flucytosine) for 2 weeks

Sporotrichosis: Pulmonary, meningeal, osteoarticular or disseminated: I.V.: Total dose of 1-2 g, then change to oral itraconazole or fluconazole for suppressive therapy

Urinary tract candidiasis (Pappas, 2009):

Fungus balls: I.V.: 0.5-0.7 mg/kg/day with or without flucytosine 25 mg/kg 4 times daily

Pyelonephritis: I.V.: 0.5-0.7 mg/kg/day with or without flucytosine 25 mg/kg 4 times daily for 2 weeks

Symptomatic cystitis: I.V.: 0.3-0.6 mg/kg/day for 1-7 days

Bladder irrigation: Irrigate with 50 mcg/mL solution instilled periodically or continuously for 5-10 days or until cultures are clear for fluconazole-resistant *Candida*

Pediatric Note: Premedication: For patients who experience infusion-related immediate reactions, premedicate with the following drugs 30-60 minutes prior to drug administration: NSAID ± with or without diphenhydramine **or** acetaminophen with diphenhydramine **or** hydrocortisone. If the patient experiences rigors during the infusion, meperidine may be administered.

Test dose: I.V.: Infants and Children: 0.1 mg/kg/dose to a maximum of 1 mg; infuse over 30-60 minutes. Many clinicians believe a test dose is unnecessary.

Susceptible fungal infections: I.V.: Infants and Children: Maintenance dose: 0.25-1 mg/kg/day given once daily; infuse over 2-6 hours. Once therapy has been established, amphotericin B can be administered on an every-other-day basis at 1-1.5 mg/kg/dose; cumulative dose: 1.5-2 g over 6-10 weeks

Note: Duration of therapy varies with nature of infection: Usual duration is 4-12 weeks or cumulative dose of 1-4 g.

Indication-specific dosing: Infants and Children:

Aspergillosis (HIV-exposed/-positive): I.V.: 1-1.5 mg/kg/day once daily (CDC, 2009)

Candidiasis (HIV-exposed/-positive):

Invasive: I.V.: 0.5-1.5 mg/kg/day once daily (CDC, 2009)

Esophageal: I.V.: 0.3-0.5 mg/kg/day once daily (CDC, 2009)

Oropharyngeal, refractory: I.V.: 0.3-0.5 mg/kg/day (CDC, 2009)

Coccidioidomycosis (HIV-exposed/-positive): I.V.: 0.5-1 mg/kg/day (CDC, 2009)

***Cryptococcus*, CNS disease (HIV-exposed/-positive):** I.V.: 0.7-1 mg/kg/day plus flucytosine; **Note:** Minimum 2 week induction followed by consolidation and chronic suppressive therapy; may increase amphotericin dose to 1.5 mg/kg/day if flucytosine is not tolerated.

***Cryptococcus*, disseminated (non-CNS disease) or severe pulmonary disease (HIV-exposed/-positive):** I.V.: 0.7-1 mg/kg/day once daily with or without flucytosine

Histoplasma, CNS or severe disseminated: I.V.: 1 mg/kg/day once daily (CDC, 2009)

Renal Impairment

If renal dysfunction is due to the drug, the daily total can be decreased by 50% or the dose can be given every other day. I.V. therapy may take several months.

Renal replacement therapy: Poorly dialyzed; no supplemental dose or dosage adjustment necessary, including patients on intermittent hemodialysis or CRRT.

Peritoneal dialysis (PD): Administration in dialysate: 1-2 mg/L of peritoneal dialysis fluid either with or without low-dose I.V. amphotericin B (a total dose of 2-10 mg/kg given over 7-14 days). Precipitate may form in ionic dialysate solutions.

Administration May be infused over 4-6 hours. For a patient who experiences chills, fever, hypotension, nausea, or other nonanaphylactic infusion-related reactions, premedicate with the following drugs 30-60 minutes prior to drug administration: A nonsteroidal (eg, ibuprofen, choline magnesium trisalicylate) ± diphenhydramine **or** acetaminophen with diphenhydramine **or** hydrocortisone. If the patient experiences rigors during the infusion, meperidine may be administered. Bolus infusion of normal saline immediately preceding, or immediately preceding and following amphotericin B may reduce drug-induced nephrotoxicity. Risk of nephrotoxicity increases with amphotericin B doses >1 mg/kg/day. Infusion of admixtures more concentrated than 0.25 mg/mL should be limited to patients absolutely requiring volume contraction.

Dosage Forms Excipient information presented when available (limited, particularly for generics); consult specific product labeling.

Injection, powder for reconstitution, as desoxycholate: 50 mg

- **Amphotericin B Deoxycholate** *see* Amphotericin B (Conventional) *on page 79*
- **Amphotericin B Desoxycholate** *see* Amphotericin B (Conventional) *on page 79*

Amphotericin B (Lipid Complex)

(am foe TER i sin bee LIP id KOM pleks)

Brand Names: U.S. Abelcet®

Brand Names: Canada Abelcet®

Index Terms ABLC

Generic Availability (U.S.) No

Pharmacologic Category Antifungal Agent, Parenteral

Use Treatment of invasive fungal infection in patients who are refractory to or intolerant of conventional amphotericin B (amphotericin B deoxycholate) therapy

Labeled Contraindications Hypersensitivity to amphotericin or any component of the formulation

Pregnancy Risk Factor B

Lactation Enters breast milk/not recommended

Warnings/Precautions Anaphylaxis has been reported with amphotericin B-containing drugs. If severe respiratory distress occurs, the infusion should be immediately discontinued. During the initial dosing, the drug should be administered under close clinical observation. Acute reactions (including fever and chills) may occur 1-2 hours after starting an intravenous infusion. These reactions are usually more common with the first few doses and generally diminish with subsequent doses. Infusion has been rarely associated with hypotension, bronchospasm, arrhythmias, and shock. Acute pulmonary toxicity has been reported in patients receiving leukocyte transfusions and amphotericin B; amphotericin B lipid complex and concurrent leukocyte transfusions are not recommended. Concurrent use with antineoplastic agents may enhance the potential for renal toxicity, bronchospasm or hypotension; use with caution. Concurrent use of amphotericin B with other nephrotoxic drugs may enhance the potential for drug-induced renal toxicity.

Storage/Stability Intact vials should be stored at 2°C to 8°C (35°F to 46°F); do not freeze. Protect intact vials from exposure to light. Solutions for infusion are stable for 48 hours under refrigeration and for an additional 6 hours at room temperature.

Reconstitution Shake the vial gently until there is no evidence of any yellow sediment at the bottom. Withdraw the appropriate dose from the vial using an 18-gauge needle. Remove the 18-gauge needle and attach the provided 5-micron filter needle to filter, and dilute the dose with D_5W to a final concentration of 1 mg/mL. Each filter needle may be used to filter up to four 100 mg vials. A final concentration of 2 mg/mL may be used for pediatric patients and patients with cardiovascular disease.

Do not dilute with saline solutions or mix with other drugs or electrolytes-compatibility has not been established

Mechanism of Action Binds to ergosterol altering cell membrane permeability in susceptible fungi and causing leakage of cell components with subsequent cell death. Proposed mechanism suggests that amphotericin causes an oxidation-dependent stimulation of macrophages.

Pharmacodynamics/Kinetics Note: Exhibits nonlinear kinetics; volume of distribution and clearance from blood increases with increasing dose.

Distribution: V_d: Increases with higher doses (likely reflects increased uptake by tissues); 131 L/kg with 5 mg/kg/day

Half-life elimination: 173 hours following multiple doses

Excretion: 0.9% of dose excreted in urine over 24 hours; effects of hepatic and renal impairment on drug disposition are unknown

Dialysis: Amphotericin B (lipid complex) is not hemodialyzable

Dosing

Adult & Geriatric Note: Premedication: For patients who experience infusion-related immediate reactions, premedicate with the following drugs 30-60 minutes prior to drug administration: A nonsteroidal anti-inflammatory agent ± diphenhydramine **or** acetaminophen with diphenhydramine **or** hydrocortisone. If the patient experiences rigors during the infusion, meperidine may be administered.

Usual dose: I.V.: 5 mg/kg once daily

Manufacturer's labeling: Invasive fungal infections (when patients are intolerant or refractory to conventional amphotericin B): I.V.: 5 mg/kg/day

Indication-specific dosing:

Aspergillosis, invasive (HIV positive or HIV negative patients) (alternative to preferred therapy): I.V.: 5 mg/kg/day; duration of treatment in HIV-negative patients depends on site of infection, extent of disease and level of immunosuppression; in HIV-positive patients, treat until CD4 count >200 cells/mm^3 and evidence of clinical response (CDC [adults], 2009; Walsh, 2008)

Blastomycosis, moderately-severe-to-severe (unlabeled dose): I.V.: 3-5 mg/kg/day for 1-2 weeks or until improvement, followed by oral itraconazole (Chapman, 2008)

Candidiasis (unlabeled dose): I.V.:

Chronic disseminated candidiasis, pericarditis or myocarditis due to Candida, suppurative thrombophlebitis: 3-5 mg/kg/day. **Note:** In chronic disseminated candidiasis, transition to fluconazole after several weeks in stable patients is preferred (Pappas, 2009)

CNS candidiasis: 3-5 mg/kg/day (with or without flucytosine) for several weeks, followed by fluconazole (Pappas, 2009)

Endocarditis due to Candida, infected pacemaker, ICD, or VAD: 3-5 mg/kg/day (with or without flucytosine); continue to treat for 4-6 weeks after device removal unless device cannot be removed then chronic suppression with fluconazole is recommended (Pappas, 2009)

Coccidioidomycosis (unlabeled dose): I.V.:

Progressive, disseminated: (alternative to preferred therapy): 2-5 mg/kg/day (Galgiani, 2005)

HIV-positive patients with severe, nonmeningeal infection: 4-6 mg/kg/day until clinical improvement, then switch to fluconazole or itraconazole (CDC, 2009)

Cryptococcosis: I.V.:

Cryptococcal meningoencephalitis in HIV-positive patients (as an alternative to conventional amphotericin B in patients with renal concerns): Induction therapy: 4-6 mg/kg/day (unlabeled dose; CDC [adult], 2009) or 5 mg/kg/day (Perfect, 2010) with flucytosine for at least 2 weeks, followed by oral fluconazole. **Note:** If flucytosine is not given due to intolerance, duration of amphotericin B lipid complex therapy should be 4-6 weeks (Perfect, 2010).

Cryptococcal meningoencephalitis in HIV-negative patients and nontransplant patients (as an alternative to conventional amphotericin B): Induction therapy: 5 mg/kg/day (with flucytosine if possible) for ≥4 weeks followed by oral fluconazole. **Note:** If flucytosine is not given or treatment is interrupted, consider prolonging induction therapy for an additional 2 weeks (Perfect, 2010).

Cryptococcal meningoencephalitis in transplant recipients: Induction therapy: 5 mg/kg/day (with flucytosine) for at least 2 weeks, followed by oral fluconazole **Note:** If flucytosine is not given, duration of amphotericin B lipid complex therapy should be 4-6 weeks (Perfect, 2010).

Nonmeningeal cryptococcosis: Induction therapy: 5 mg/kg/day (with flucytosine if possible) for ≥4 weeks may be used for severe pulmonary cryptococcosis or for cryptococcemia with evidence of high fungal burden, followed by oral fluconazole. **Note:** If flucytosine is not given or treatment is interrupted, consider prolonging induction therapy for an additional 2 weeks (Perfect, 2010).

Histoplasmosis: I.V.:

Acute pulmonary (moderately-severe-to-severe): 5 mg/kg/day for 1-2 weeks, followed by oral itraconazole (Wheat, 2007)

Progressive disseminated (alternative to preferred therapy): 5 mg/kg/day for 1-2 weeks, followed by oral itraconazole (Wheat, 2007)

Sporotrichosis (unlabeled dose): I.V.:

Meningeal: 5 mg/kg/day for 4-6 weeks, followed by oral itraconazole (Kauffman, 2007)

Pulmonary, osteoarticular, and disseminated: 3-5 mg/kg/day, followed by oral itraconazole after a favorable response is seen with amphotericin initial therapy (Kauffman, 2007)

Pediatric Note: Premedication: For patients who experience infusion-related immediate reactions, premedicate with the following drugs 30-60 minutes prior to drug administration: A nonsteroidal anti-inflammatory agent ± diphenhydramine **or** acetaminophen with diphenhydramine **or** hydrocortisone. If the patient experiences rigors during the infusion, meperidine may be administered.

Usual dose: 5 mg/kg once daily

Manufacturer's labeling: Invasive fungal infections (when patients are intolerant or refractory to conventional amphotericin B): Children: I.V.: 5 mg/kg/day

Indication-specific dosing:

Aspergillosis (HIV-positive patients) (alternative to preferred therapy): Infants and Children: I.V.: 5 mg/kg/day for ≥12 weeks (CDC, [pediatric], 2009)

Candidiasis, invasive (HIV-positive patients) (alternative to preferred therapy): Infants and Children: I.V.:5 mg/kg/day; treatment duration based on clinical response, treat until 2-3 weeks after last positive blood culture (CDC [pediatric], 2009)

***Cryptococcus neoformans*, disseminated disease (non-CNS disease) (HIV-positive patients):** Infants and Children: I.V.:5 mg/kg/day (with or without flucytosine); treatment duration of non-CNS disease varies by clinical response and site/severity of infection (CDC [pediatric], 2009)

Renal Impairment

Manufacturer's recommendations: No dosage adjustment provided in manufacturer's labeling (has not been studied).

Alternate recommendations (Aronoff, 2007):

Intermittent hemodialysis: No supplemental dosage necessary.

Peritoneal dialysis: No supplemental dosage necessary.

Continuous renal replacement therapy (CRRT): No supplemental dosage necessary.

Hepatic Impairment No dosage adjustment provided in manufacturer's labeling (has not been studied).

Administration For patients who experience nonanaphylactic infusion-related reactions, premedicate 30-60 minutes prior to drug administration with a nonsteroidal anti-inflammatory agent ± diphenhydramine **or** acetaminophen with diphenhydramine **or** hydrocortisone. If the patient experiences rigors during the infusion, meperidine may be administered.

Administer at an infusion rate of 2.5 mg/kg/hour (eg, over 2 hours for 5 mg/kg). Invert infusion container several times prior to administration and every 2 hours during infusion if it exceeds 2 hours. **Do not use an in-line filter during administration.** Flush line with dextrose; normal saline may cause precipitate.

Dosage Forms Excipient information presented when available (limited, particularly for generics); consult specific product labeling.

Injection, suspension [preservative free]:

Abelcet®: 5 mg/mL (20 mL)

Amphotericin B (Liposomal) (am foe TER i sin bee lye po SO mal)

Brand Names: U.S. AmBisome®

Brand Names: Canada AmBisome®

Index Terms Amphotericin B Liposome; L-AmB

Generic Availability (U.S.) No

Pharmacologic Category Antifungal Agent, Parenteral

Use Empirical therapy for presumed fungal infection in febrile, neutropenic patients; treatment of patients with *Aspergillus* species, *Candida* species, and/or *Cryptococcus* species infections refractory to amphotericin B desoxycholate (conventional amphotericin), or in patients where renal impairment or unacceptable toxicity precludes the use of amphotericin B desoxycholate; treatment of cryptococcal meningitis in HIV-infected patients; treatment of visceral leishmaniasis

Unlabeled Use Treatment of systemic *Histoplasmosis* infection; empiric treatment of fungal meningitis or osteoarticular infections

Labeled Contraindications Hypersensitivity to amphotericin B deoxycholate or any component of the formulation

Pregnancy Risk Factor B

Lactation Excretion in breast milk unknown/not recommended

Warnings/Precautions Patients should be under close clinical observation during initial dosing. As with other amphotericin B containing products, anaphylaxis has been reported. Facilities for cardiopulmonary resuscitation should be available during administration. Acute infusion reactions (including fever and chills) may occur 1-2 hours after starting infusions; reactions are more common with the first few doses and generally diminish with subsequent doses. Immediately discontinue infusion if severe respiratory distress occurs; the patient should not receive further infusions. Concurrent use of amphotericin B with other nephrotoxic drugs may enhance the potential for drug-induced renal toxicity. Concurrent use with antineoplastic agents may enhance the potential for renal toxicity, bronchospasm or hypotension. Acute pulmonary toxicity has been reported in patients receiving simultaneous leukocyte transfusions and amphotericin B. Safety and efficacy have not been established in patients <1 month of age.

Storage/Stability Store intact vials at ≤25°C (≤77°F). Reconstituted vials are stable refrigerated at 2°C to 8°C (36°F to 46°F) for 24 hours. Do not freeze. Manufacturer's labeling states infusion should begin within 6 hours of dilution with D_5W; data on file with Astellas Pharma shows extended formulation stability when admixed in D_5W at 0.2-2 mg/mL (in polyolefin or PVC bags) for up to 11 days when stored refrigerated at 2°C to 8°C (36°F to 46°F).

Reconstitution Reconstitute with 12 mL SWFI to a concentration of 4 mg/mL. The use of any solution other than those recommended, or the presence of a bacteriostatic agent in the solution, may cause precipitation. **Shake the vial vigorously** for 30 seconds, until dispersed into a translucent yellow suspension.

Filtration and dilution: The 5-micron filter should be on the syringe used to remove the reconstituted AmBisome®. Dilute to a final concentration of 1-2 mg/mL (0.2-0.5 mg/mL for infants and small children).

Mechanism of Action Binds to ergosterol altering cell membrane permeability in susceptible fungi and causing leakage of cell components with subsequent cell death. Proposed mechanism suggests that amphotericin causes an oxidation-dependent stimulation of macrophages (Lyman, 1992).

Pharmacodynamics/Kinetics

Distribution: V_d: 131 L/kg

Half-life elimination: Terminal: 174 hours

Dosing

Adult & Geriatric

Usual dosage range: I.V.: 3-6 mg/kg/day; **Note:** Higher doses (7.5-15 mg/kg/day) have been used clinically in special cases (Walsh, 2001; CDC [parameningeal], 2012; Kauffman, 2012)

Note: Premedication: For patients who experience nonanaphylactic infusion-related immediate reactions, premedicate with the following drugs 30-60 minutes prior to drug administration: A nonsteroidal anti-inflammatory agent ± diphenhydramine; **or** acetaminophen with diphenhydramine; **or** hydrocortisone. If the patient experiences rigors during the infusion, meperidine may be administered.

Indication-specific dosing: I.V.:

Cryptococcal meningitis (HIV-positive): 6 mg/kg/day or 4-6 mg/kg/day in combination with addition of oral flucytosine 25 mg/kg 4 times daily (unlabeled combination; CDC, 2009)

Empiric candidiasis therapy: 3-5 mg/kg/day (Pappas, 2009)

Endocarditis: I.V.: 3-5 mg/kg/day (with or without flucytosine 25 mg/kg 4 times daily) for 6 weeks after valve replacement; **Note:** If isolates susceptible and/or clearance demonstrated, guidelines recommend step-down to fluconazole; also for long-term suppression therapy if valve replacement is not possible (Pappas, 2009)

Fungal sinusitis: Limited data in immunocompromised patients have shown efficacy with 3-10 mg/kg/day (Barron, 2005; Pagano, 2004; Rokicka, 2006). **Note:** An azole antifungal is recommended if causative organism is *Aspergillus* spp or *Pseudallescheria boydii* (*Scedosporium* sp).

Meningitis (secondary to contaminated [eg, *Exserohilum rostratum*] steroid products), severe or in patients not improving with voriconazole monotherapy (unlabeled use) (CDC [parameningeal], 2012; Kauffman, 2012): I.V.: 5-6 mg/kg/day in combination with voriconazole for ≥3 months; a higher dose (7.5 mg/kg/day) may be considered in patients who are not improving. **Note:** Consult an infectious disease specialist and current CDC guidelines for specific treatment recommendations.

Osteoarticular candidiasis: I.V.: 3-5 mg/kg/day for several weeks, followed by fluconazole for 6-12 months (osteomyelitis) or 6 weeks (septic arthritis) (Pappas, 2009)

Osteoarticular infection (secondary to contaminated [eg, *Exserohilum rostratum*] steroid products), severe or in patients with clinical instability (unlabeled use) (CDC [osteoarticular], 2012; Kauffman, 2012): I.V.: 5 mg/kg/day in combination with voriconazole for ≥3 months. **Note:** Consult an infectious disease specialist and current CDC guidelines for specific treatment recommendations.

Systemic fungal infections *(Aspergillus, Candida, Cryptococcus)*: 3-5 mg/kg/day

General invasive Candidal disease: 3-5 mg/kg/day with oral flucytosine 25 mg/kg 4 times daily (unlabeled combination; Pappas, 2009)

Candidal meningitis: 3-5 mg/kg/day with oral flucytosine 25 mg/kg 4 times daily (unlabeled combination; Pappas, 2009)

Histoplasmosis (unlabeled use): 3-5 mg/kg/day (CDC, 2009)

Visceral leishmaniasis:

Immunocompetent: 3 mg/kg/day on days 1-5, and 3 mg/kg/day on days 14 and 21; a repeat course may be given in patients who do not achieve parasitic clearance

Note: Alternate regimen of 2 mg/kg/day for 5 days has been reportedly effective.

Immunocompromised: 4 mg/kg/day on days 1-5, and 4 mg/kg/day on days 10, 17, 24, 31, and 38

Pediatric

Usual dosage range: Children ≥1 month: I.V.: 3-6 mg/kg/day

Note: Premedication: For patients who experience nonanaphylactic infusion-related immediate reactions, premedicate with the following drugs 30-60 minutes prior to drug administration: A nonsteroidal anti-inflammatory agent ± diphenhydramine; **or** acetaminophen with diphenhydramine; **or** hydrocortisone. If the patient experiences rigors during the infusion, meperidine may be administered.

Indication-specific dosing: Children ≥1 month: I.V.:

Empiric therapy: 3 mg/kg/day

Systemic fungal infections *(Aspergillus, Candida, Cryptococcus)*: 3-5 mg/kg/day

Systemic fungal infections (HIV-exposed/-positive [CDC, 2009; unlabeled use]):

Aspergillosis: 5 mg/kg/day once daily

Candida, invasive: 5 mg/kg/day once daily (may consider addition of oral flucytosine for severe disease)

Cryptococcal meningitis: 4-6 mg/kg/day once daily plus oral flucytosine

Cryptococcus, disseminated (non-CNS): 3-5 mg/kg/day (may consider addition of oral flucytosine)

Histoplasmosis: 3-5 mg/kg/day once daily

Visceral leishmaniasis:

Immunocompetent: 3 mg/kg/day on days 1-5, and 3 mg/kg/day on days 14 and 21; a repeat course may be given in patients who do not achieve parasitic clearance

Note: Alternate regimen of 10 mg/kg/day for 2 days has been reportedly effective.

Immunocompromised: 4 mg/kg/day on days 1-5, and 4 mg/kg/day on days 10, 17, 24, 31, and 38

Renal Impairment None necessary; effects of renal impairment are not currently known.

Poorly dialyzed; no supplemental dose or dosage adjustment necessary, including patients on intermittent hemodialysis, peritoneal dialysis, or continuous renal replacement therapy (eg, CVVHD).

Administration Administer via intravenous infusion, over a period of approximately 2 hours. Infusion time may be reduced to approximately 1 hour in patients in whom the treatment is well-tolerated. If the patient experiences discomfort during infusion, the duration of infusion may be increased. Administer at a rate of 2.5 mg/kg/hour. Existing intravenous line should be flushed with D_5W prior to infusion (if not feasible, administer through a separate line). An in-line membrane filter (not less than 1 micron) may be used.

For a patient who experiences chills, fever, hypotension, nausea, or other nonanaphylactic infusion-related reactions, premedicate with the following drugs, 30-60 minutes prior to drug administration: A nonsteroidal (eg, ibuprofen, choline magnesium trisalicylate) ± diphenhydramine **or** acetaminophen with diphenhydramine **or** hydrocortisone. If the patient experiences rigors during the infusion, meperidine may be administered.

Test Interactions

Falsely-elevated serum phosphate may occur when using the PHOSm assay.

Dosage Forms Excipient information presented when available (limited, particularly for generics); consult specific product labeling.

Injection, powder for reconstitution:

AmBisome®: 50 mg [contains soy, sucrose 900 mg]

◆ **Amphotericin B Liposome** *see* Amphotericin B (Liposomal) *on page* *87*

◆ **AMSA** *see* Amsacrine *on page* *90*

Amsacrine (AM sah kreen)

Related Information

Management of Drug Extravasations *on page* *1800*

Safe Handling of Hazardous Drugs *on page* *1904*

Brand Names: Canada AMSA PD

Index Terms 4-(9-Acridinylamino) Methanesulfon-m-Anisidide; Acridinyl Anisidide; AMSA; m-AMSA

Pharmacologic Category Antineoplastic Agent

Use Refractory acute leukemia

Unlabeled Use Acute myeloid leukemia (AML)

Labeled Contraindications Hypersensitivity to amsacrine, acridine derivatives, or any component of the formulation; pre-existing bone marrow suppression due to chemotherapy or radiation therapy

Lactation Excretion in breast milk unknown/not recommended

Warnings/Precautions Hazardous agent - use appropriate precautions for handling and disposal. Myelosuppression, including transient leukopenia, is a common toxicity; prolonged marrow aplasia may occur; may require dose reduction, therapy interruption or treatment delay. Acute cardiotoxicity, including arrhythmia, ECG changes, and rarely, cardiomyopathy and CHF, have been reported with use, although generally not considered to be a cumulative dose effect; use with caution in patients with underlying cardiovascular disease. Risk factors for cardiotoxicity may include hypokalemia and a history of anthracycline therapy; correct fluid and electrolyte imbalance prior to treatment initiation. Serum potassium should be >4 mEq/L prior to administration

(Arlin, 1998). Use with caution in patients who have received high cumulative doses of anthracyclines. Tumor lysis syndrome may occur; adequate hydration and prophylactic uric acid reduction should be considered prior to or during treatment; monitor closely. Hepatic metabolism and biliary excretion are major routes of elimination. Use with caution in patients with significant hepatic impairment (bilirubin >2 mg/dL); toxicity may be increased; dosage reductions may be required. Use with caution in patients with significant renal impairment (BUN >20 mg/dL; serum creatinine >1.2 mg/dL); toxicity may be increased; dosage reductions may be recommended. Evaluate renal and hepatic function prior to and during treatment. Avoid vaccination with live virus vaccines during treatment.

Adverse Reactions

>10%:

Gastrointestinal: Nausea (>10%), vomiting (>10%), stomatitis (>10%), diarrhea (>10%), perirectal abscess (>10%), abdominal pain (>10%)

Hematologic: Myelosuppression, leukopenia (nadir: 11-13 days; recovery: days 17-25)

Frequency not defined:

Cardiovascular: Atrial tachyarrhythmia, atrial tachycardia, atrial fibrillation, bradycardia, cardiomyopathy (rare), cardiopulmonary arrest, CHF (rare); ECG changes (QT prolongation, nonspecific ST segment or T wave changes), ejection fraction decreased, hypotension, sinus tachycardia, tachycardia, ventricular arrhythmia, ventricular extrasystoles, ventricular fibrillation, ventricular tachyarrhythmia

Central nervous system: Confusion, dizziness, emotional lability, fever, headache, hypoesthesia, lethargy, seizure

Dermatologic: Alopecia, cutaneous inflammatory reaction, dermatologic reaction, purpura, rash (purpuric or maculopapular), urticaria

Gastrointestinal: Anorexia, dysphagia, gingivitis, gum hemorrhage, hematemesis, weight changes

Genitourinary: Orange-red discoloration of the urine

Hematologic: Anemia, granulocytopenia, hemorrhage, pancytopenia, thrombocytopenia

Hepatic: Alkaline phosphatase increased, AST increased, bilirubin increased, hepatic insufficiency, hepatitis, hepatotoxicity, jaundice, progressive liver failure

Local: Injection site inflammation, phlebitis

Neuromuscular & skeletal: Musculoskeletal pain, paresthesia, weakness

Renal: BUN increased, creatinine increased, hematuria, proteinuria, renal failure

Respiratory: Dyspnea

Miscellaneous: Allergic reaction, infection

Drug Interactions

Metabolism/Transport Effects

None known.

Avoid Concomitant Use

Avoid concomitant use of Amsacrine with any of the following: BCG; CloZAPine; Natalizumab; Pimecrolimus; Tacrolimus (Topical); Vaccines (Live)

Increased Effect/Toxicity

Amsacrine may increase the levels/effects of: CloZAPine; Leflunomide; Natalizumab; Vaccines (Live); Vitamin K Antagonists

The levels/effects of Amsacrine may be increased by: Denosumab; Pimecrolimus; Roflumilast; Tacrolimus (Topical); Trastuzumab

Decreased Effect

Amsacrine may decrease the levels/effects of: BCG; Cardiac Glycosides; Coccidioidin Skin Test; Sipuleucel-T; Vaccines (Inactivated); Vaccines (Live); Vitamin K Antagonists

The levels/effects of Amsacrine may be decreased by: Echinacea

Storage/Stability Store intact ampuls and diluent vials at controlled room temperature of 15°C to 25°C (59°F to 77°F). Concentrated amsacrine should not be stored in plastic syringes for >15 minutes. Reconstituted vials may be stored at room temperature for up to 24 hours, under ambient light conditions. Solutions diluted for administration are stable for up to 7 days in glass or plastic containers, however, the manufacturer recommends use with in 24 hours when stored at room temperature and 72 hours if refrigerated.

Reconstitution Use appropriate precautions for handling and disposal. Reconstitute by adding 1.5 mL amsacrine to diluent vial (containing 13.5 mL L-lactic acid), resulting in a 5 mg/mL reconstituted solution. Glass syringes should be used, however if using plastic syringes, do not allow concentrated amsacrine to remain in plastic syringe for >15 minutes. Further dilute appropriate dose in 500 mL D_5W (the solution may be mixed in plastic bags when diluted for infusion).

Mechanism of Action Amsacrine has been shown to inhibit DNA synthesis by binding to, and intercalating with, DNA; inhibits topoisomerase II activity.

Pharmacodynamics/Kinetics

Distribution: V_d: 1.67 L/kg; minimal CNS penetration

Protein binding: 96% to 98%

Metabolism: Hepatic, to inactive metabolites (major metabolite is 5′ glutathione conjugate)

Half-life elimination: 1.4-5 hours; Terminal: 8-9 hours

Excretion: Bile; urine (35%; 20% as unchanged drug)

Dosing

Adult & Geriatric Details concerning dosing in combination regimens should also be consulted.

Acute leukemia: I.V.:

Induction: 75-125 mg/m^2/day for 5 days every 3-4 weeks (125 mg/m^2/day is preferred; two courses may be necessary to achieve induction; increase dose by 20% in second and subsequent cycles if marrow hypoplasia not achieved and in absence of significant toxicity in previous course.)

Maintenance: Once remission has been achieved, maintenance dose should be ~50% of induction dose, administered every 4-8 weeks, depending on blood counts and marrow recovery

Renal Impairment

Dosage reduction recommended; specific guidelines from the manufacturer are not available; the following guidelines have been used by some clinicians:

Hall, 1983:

Serum creatinine 1.2-1.8 mg/dL: No adjustment recommended

Serum creatinine 2-3 mg/dL, oliguric patients: Administer 60% to 70% of dose; may increase subsequent dose based on toxicity.

Hornedo, 1985: BUN >20 mg/dL or serum creatinine >1.5 mg/dL: Administer 75% of dose

Hepatic Impairment Bilirubin >2 mg/dL: Dosage reduction recommended; specific guidelines from the manufacturer are not available; the following guidelines have been used by some clinicians:

Hall, 1983: Bilirubin >2 mg/dL: Administer 60% to 70% of dose; may increase subsequent dose based on toxicity.

Hornedo, 1985: Bilirubin >2 mg/dL: Administer 75% of dose

Koren, 1992: Severe hepatic dysfunction: Administer ≤50% of dose

Adjustment for Toxicity Consider decreasing dose by 20% if life-threatening infection or hemorrhage occurred in previous cycle; delay second and subsequent cycles until recovery from myelosuppression or evidence of leukemic infiltrate is evident.

Administration I.V.: Infuse over 60-90 minutes; avoid extravasation.

Vesicant/Extravasation Risk Vesicant; see Management of Drug Extravasations on page 1800.

Monitoring Parameters CBC with differential, bone marrow studies, serum potassium, hepatic function, renal function; ECG (during and after infusion)

Product Availability Not available in U.S.

Dosage Forms: Canada Excipient information presented when available (limited, particularly for generics); consult specific product labeling.

Injection, solution [preservative free]:

AMSA PD: 50 mg/mL (1.5 mL) [supplied with L-lactic acid 0.0353 M 13.5 mL]

References

Hall SW, Friedman J, Legha SS, et al, "Human Pharmacokinetics of a New Acridine Derivative, 4'-(9-Acridinylamino)methanesulfon-m-anisidide (NSC 249992)," *Cancer Res*, 1983, 43(7):3422-6.

Hornedo J and Van Echo DA, "Amsacrine (m-AMSA): A New Antineoplastic Agent. Pharmacology, Clinical Activity and Toxicity," *Pharmacotherapy*, 1985, 5(2):78-90.

Koren G, Beatty K, Seto A, et al, "The Effects of Impaired Liver Function on the Elimination of Antineoplastic Agents," *Ann Pharmacother*, 1992, 26(3):363-71.

◆ **AMSA PD (Can)** *see* Amsacrine *on page 90*

Anagrelide (an AG gre lide)

Brand Names: U.S. Agrylin®

Brand Names: Canada Agrylin®; Dom-Anagrelide; Mylan-Anagrelide; PMS-Anagrelide; Sandoz-Anagrelide

Index Terms Anagrelide Hydrochloride; BL4162A

Generic Availability (U.S.) Yes

Pharmacologic Category Phosphodiesterase-3 Enzyme Inhibitor; Phospholipase A_2 Inhibitor

Use Treatment of thrombocythemia associated with myeloproliferative disorders (eg, chronic myelogenous leukemia, essential thrombocythemia, polycythemia vera, myeloid metaplasia with myelofibrosis, or other myeloproliferative disorder) to reduce the risk of thrombosis and reduce associated symptoms (including thrombo-hemorrhagic events)

Labeled Contraindications Severe hepatic impairment

Pregnancy Risk Factor C

Lactation Excretion in breast milk unknown/not recommended

Warnings/Precautions Use caution in patients with known or suspected heart disease; tachycardia, palpitation, vasodilation, orthostatic hypotension, and CHF; a pretreatment cardiovascular evaluation and careful monitoring during treatment is recommended. Interstitial lung disease (including allergic alveolitis, eosinophilic pneumonia, and interstitial pneumonitis) has been associated with use; onset is from 1 week to several years, usually presenting with progressive dyspnea with lung infiltrations; symptoms usually improve ▶

after discontinuation. Use caution in patients with mild-to-moderate hepatic dysfunction; dosage reduction and careful monitoring are required for moderate hepatic impairment; use is contraindicated in severe hepatic impairment; monitor liver function prior to and during treatment. Renal abnormalities (including renal failure) have been observed with anagrelide use; may be associated with pre-existing renal impairment, although dosage adjustment due to renal insufficiency was not required; monitor closely in patients with renal insufficiency.

Adverse Reactions

>10%:

Cardiovascular: Palpitation (26%), edema (21%)

Central nervous system: Headache (44%), dizziness (15%), pain (15%)

Gastrointestinal: Diarrhea (26%), nausea (17%), abdominal pain (16%)

Neuromuscular & skeletal: Weakness (23%)

Respiratory: Dyspnea (12%)

1% to 10%:

Cardiovascular: Peripheral edema (9%), chest pain (8%), tachycardia (8%), angina, arrhythmia, HF, hypertension, orthostatic hypotension, syncope, thrombosis, vasodilatation

Central nervous system: Fever (9%), malaise (6%), amnesia, chills, confusion, depression, insomnia, migraine, nervousness, somnolence

Dermatologic: Rash (8%), pruritus (6%), alopecia, bruising, photosensitivity, urticaria

Endocrine & skeletal: Dehydration

Gastrointestinal: Flatulence (10%), vomiting (10%), anorexia (8%), dyspepsia (5%), aphthous stomatitis, constipation, eructation, gastritis, GI distress, GI hemorrhage, melena

Genitourinary: Dysuria

Hematologic: Thrombocytopenia (9%; grades 3/4: 5%), anemia, hemorrhage

Neuromuscular & skeletal: Back pain (6%), paresthesia (6%), arthralgia, leg cramps, myalgia

Ocular: Amblyopia, diplopia, visual field abnormality

Otic: Tinnitus

Renal: Renal abnormality (2%), renal failure (1%), hematuria

Respiratory: Pharyngitis (7%), cough (6%), asthma, bronchitis, epistaxis, pneumonia, rhinitis, sinusitis

Miscellaneous: Flu-like syndrome, lymphadenopathy

<1%, postmarketing, and/or case reports: Atrial fibrillation, cardiomegaly, cardiomyopathy, cerebrovascular accident, complete heart block, gastric/duodenal ulceration, hepatotoxicity, interstitial lung disease (allergic alveolitis, eosinophilic pneumonia, interstitial pneumonitis); leukocyte count increased, liver enzymes (ALT, AST) increased, MI, pancreatitis, pericarditis, pericardial effusion, pleural effusion, pulmonary fibrosis, pulmonary hypertension, pulmonary infiltrates, seizure, tubulointerstitial nephritis

Drug Interactions

Metabolism/Transport Effects None known.

Avoid Concomitant Use There are no known interactions where it is recommended to avoid concomitant use.

Increased Effect/Toxicity

Anagrelide may increase the levels/effects of: Anticoagulants; Antiplatelet Agents; Collagenase (Systemic); Dabigatran Etexilate; Drotrecogin Alfa (Activated); Ibritumomab; Rivaroxaban; Salicylates; Thrombolytic Agents; Tositumomab and Iodine I 131 Tositumomab

The levels/effects of Anagrelide may be increased by: Dasatinib; Glucosamine; Herbs (Anticoagulant/Antiplatelet Properties); MAO Inhibitors; Multivitamins/Minerals (with ADEK, Folate, Iron); Nonsteroidal Anti-Inflammatory Agents; Omega-3 Fatty Acids; Pentosan Polysulfate Sodium; Pentoxifylline; Prostacyclin Analogues; Tipranavir; Vitamin E

Decreased Effect

The levels/effects of Anagrelide may be decreased by: Nonsteroidal Anti-Inflammatory Agents

Ethanol/Nutrition/Herb Interactions

Ethanol: May increase CNS adverse effects.

Food: No clinically significant effect on absorption.

Herb/Nutraceutical: Avoid herbs with anticoagulant/antiplatelet properties (alfalfa, anise, bilberry, bladderwrack, bromelain, cat's claw, celery, chamomile, coleus, cordyceps, dong quai, evening primrose oil, fenugreek, feverfew, garlic, ginger, ginkgo biloba, ginseng [American], ginseng [Panax], ginseng [Siberian], grape seed, green tea, guggul, horse chestnut seed, horseradish, licorice, prickly ash, red clover, reishi, SAMe [S-adenosylmethionine], sweet clover, turmeric, white willow); may enhance the adverse effect of antiplatelets agents.

Storage/Stability Store at 27°C (77°F); excursions permitted to 15°C to 30°C (59°F to 86°F). Protect from light.

Mechanism of Action Anagrelide appears to inhibit cyclic nucleotide phosphodiesterase and the release of arachidonic acid from phospholipase, possibly by inhibiting phospholipase A_2. It also causes a dose related reduction in platelet production, which results from decreased megakaryocyte hypermaturation (disrupts the postmitotic phase of maturation).

Pharmacodynamics/Kinetics

Onset of action: Initial: Within 7-14 days; complete response (platelets ≤600,000/mm^3): 4-12 weeks

Duration: 6-24 hours; upon discontinuation, platelet count begins to rise within 4 days

Metabolism: Hepatic, partially via CYP1A2; to two major metabolites, RL603 and 3-hydroxy anagrelide

Half-life elimination, plasma: 1.3 hours

Time to peak, serum: 1 hour

Excretion: Urine (<1% as unchanged drug)

Dosing

Adult & Geriatric Thrombocythemia: Oral: Initial: 0.5 mg 4 times/day or 1 mg twice daily (most patients will experience adequate response at dose ranges of 1.5-3 mg/day)

Note: Maintain initial dose for ≥1 week, then adjust to the lowest effective dose to reduce and maintain platelet count <600,000/mm^3 ideally to the normal range; the dose must not be increased by >0.5 mg/day in any 1 week; maximum dose: 10 mg/day or 2.5 mg/dose

Pediatric Thrombocythemia: Oral: Initial: 0.5 mg/day (range: 0.5 mg 1-4 times/day); see **"Note"** in adult dosing.

Renal Impairment No adjustment required in renal insufficiency; monitor closely.

Hepatic Impairment

Moderate impairment: Initial: 0.5 mg once daily; maintain for at least 1 week with careful monitoring of cardiovascular status; the dose must not be increased by >0.5 mg/day in any 1 week.

Severe impairment: Use is contraindicated.

Administration May be administered without regard to food.

Monitoring Parameters Platelet count (every 2 days during the first week of treatment and at least weekly until the maintenance dose is reached; continue to monitor after cessation of treatment); CBC with differential (monitor closely during first 2 weeks of treatment), liver function (ALT and AST; baseline and during treatment), BUN, and serum creatinine (monitor closely during first weeks of treatment); blood pressure; cardiovascular exam (pretreatment; monitor during therapy). Monitor for thrombosis or bleeding.

Dietary Considerations May be taken without regard to food.

Dosage Forms Excipient information presented when available (limited, particularly for generics); consult specific product labeling.

Capsule, oral: 0.5 mg, 1 mg

Agrylin®: 0.5 mg

References

Harrison CN, Campbell PJ, Buck G, et al, "Hydroxyurea Compared With Anagrelide in High-Risk Essential Thrombocythemia," *N Engl J Med*, 2005, 353(1):33-45.

Steurer M, Gastl G, Jedrzejczak WW, et al, Anagrelide for Thrombocytosis in Myeloproliferative Disorders: A Prospective Study to Assess Efficacy and Adverse Event Profile," Cancer, 2004, 101(10):2239-46.

◆ **Anagrelide Hydrochloride** *see* Anagrelide *on page 93*

◆ **Anandron® (Can)** *see* Nilutamide *on page 1037*

Anastrozole (an AS troe zole)

Related Information

Safe Handling of Hazardous Drugs *on page 1904*

Brand Names: U.S. Arimidex®

Brand Names: Canada Apo-Anastrozole®; Arimidex®; JAMP-Anastrozole; Mar-Anastrozole; PMS-Anastrozole; Riva-Anastrozole; Sandoz-Anastrozole; Taro-Anastrozole; Teva-Anastrozole

Index Terms ICI-D1033; ZD1033

Generic Availability (U.S.) Yes

Pharmacologic Category Antineoplastic Agent, Aromatase Inhibitor

Use First-line treatment of locally-advanced or metastatic breast cancer (hormone receptor-positive or unknown) in postmenopausal women; treatment of advanced breast cancer in postmenopausal women with disease progression following tamoxifen therapy; adjuvant treatment of early hormone receptor-positive breast cancer in postmenopausal women

Unlabeled Use Treatment of recurrent or metastatic endometrial or uterine cancers, treatment of recurrent ovarian cancer

Labeled Contraindications Hypersensitivity to anastrozole or any component of the formulation; use in women who are or may become pregnant

Pregnancy Risk Factor X

Lactation Excretion in breast milk unknown/not recommended

Warnings/Precautions Hazardous agent - use appropriate precautions for handling and disposal. Use is contraindicated in women who are or may become pregnant. Anastrozole offers no clinical benefit in premenopausal women with breast cancer. Patients with pre-existing ischemic cardiac disease have an increased risk for ischemic cardiovascular events.

Due to decreased circulating estrogen levels, anastrozole is associated with a reduction in bone mineral density (BMD); decreases (from baseline) in total hip and lumbar spine BMD have been reported. Patients with pre-existing osteopenia are at higher risk for developing osteoporosis (Eastell, 2008). When initiating anastrozole treatment, follow available guidelines for bone mineral density management in postmenopausal women with similar fracture risk; concurrent use of bisphosphonates may be useful in patients at risk for fractures.

Elevated total cholesterol levels (contributed to by LDL cholesterol increases) have been reported in patients receiving anastrozole; use with caution in patients with hyperlipidemias; cholesterol levels should be monitored/managed in accordance with current guidelines for patients with LDL elevations. Plasma concentrations in patients with stable hepatic cirrhosis were within the range of concentrations seen in normal subjects across all clinical trials; use has not been studied in patients with severe hepatic impairment. Safety and efficacy in children have not been established.

Adverse Reactions

>10%:

Cardiovascular: Vasodilatation (25% to 36%), ischemic cardiovascular disease (4%; 17% in patients with pre-existing ischemic heart disease), hypertension (2% to 13%), angina (2%; 12% in patients with pre-existing ischemic heart disease)

Central nervous system: Mood disturbance (19%), fatigue (19%), pain (11% to 17%), headache (9% to 13%), depression (5% to 13%)

Dermatologic: Rash (6% to 11%)

Endocrine & metabolic: Hot flashes (12% to 36%)

Gastrointestinal: Nausea (11% to 19%), vomiting (8% to 13%)

Neuromuscular & skeletal: Weakness (16% to 19%), arthritis (17%), arthralgia (2% to 15%), back pain (10% to 12%), bone pain (6% to 11%), osteoporosis (11%)

Respiratory: Pharyngitis (6% to 14%), cough increased (8% to 11%)

1% to 10%:

Cardiovascular: Peripheral edema (5% to 10%), chest pain (5% to 7%), edema (7%), venous thromboembolic events (2% to 4%), ischemic cerebrovascular events (2%), MI (1%)

Central nervous system: Insomnia (2% to 10%), dizziness (6% to 8%), anxiety (2% to 6%), fever (2% to 5%), malaise (2% to 5%), confusion (2% to 5%), nervousness (2% to 5%), somnolence (2% to 5%), lethargy (1%)

Dermatologic: Alopecia (2% to 5%), pruritus (2% to 5%)

Endocrine & metabolic: Hypercholesterolemia (9%), breast pain (2% to 8%)

Gastrointestinal: Diarrhea (8% to 9%), constipation (7% to 9%), abdominal pain (7% to 9%), weight gain (2% to 9%), anorexia (5% to 7%), xerostomia (6%), dyspepsia (7%), weight loss (2% to 5%)

Genitourinary: Urinary tract infection (2% to 8%), vulvovaginitis (6%), pelvic pain (5%), vaginal bleeding (1% to 5%), vaginitis (4%), vaginal discharge (4%), vaginal hemorrhage (2% to 4%), leukorrhea (2% to 3%), vaginal dryness (2% to 5%)

Hematologic: Anemia (2% to 5%), leukopenia (2% to 5%)

Hepatic: Liver function tests increased (1% to 10%), alkaline phosphatase increased (1% to 10%), gamma GT increased (≤5%)

Local: Thrombophlebitis (2% to 5%)

Neuromuscular & skeletal: Fracture (1% to 10%), arthrosis (7%), paresthesia (5% to 7%), joint disorder (6%), myalgia (2% to 6%), neck pain (2% to 5%), carpal tunnel syndrome (3%), hypertonia (3%)

Ocular: Cataracts (6%)

Respiratory: Dyspnea (8% to 10%), sinusitis (2% to 6%), bronchitis (2% to 5%), rhinitis (2% to 5%)

Miscellaneous: Lymphedema (10%), infection (2% to 9%), flu-like syndrome (2% to 7%), diaphoresis (2% to 5%), cyst (5%), neoplasm (5%), tumor flare (3%)

<1%, postmarketing, and/or case reports: Anaphylaxis, angioedema, bilirubin increased, CVA, cerebral ischemia, cerebral infarct, cutaneous vasculitis (including Henoch-Schönlein purpura), endometrial cancer, erythema multiforme, hepatitis, jaundice, joint pain, joint stiffness, liver inflammation, liver pain, liver swelling, myocardial ischemia, pulmonary embolus, retinal vein thrombosis; skin reactions (eg, blisters, lesions, ulcers); Stevens-Johnson syndrome, trigger finger, urticaria

Drug Interactions

Metabolism/Transport Effects Inhibits CYP1A2 (weak), CYP2C8 (weak), CYP2C9 (weak), CYP3A4 (weak)

Avoid Concomitant Use

Avoid concomitant use of Anastrozole with any of the following: Estrogen Derivatives; Pimozide

Increased Effect/Toxicity

Anastrozole may increase the levels/effects of: ARIPiprazole; Pimozide

Decreased Effect

The levels/effects of Anastrozole may be decreased by: Estrogen Derivatives; Tamoxifen

Storage/Stability Store at 20°C to 25°C (68°F to 77°F).

Mechanism of Action Potent and selective nonsteroidal aromatase inhibitor. By inhibiting aromatase, the conversion of androstenedione to estrone, and testosterone to estradiol, is prevented, thereby decreasing tumor mass or delaying progression in patients with tumors responsive to hormones. Anastrozole causes an 85% decrease in estrone sulfate levels.

Pharmacodynamics/Kinetics

Onset of estradiol reduction: 70% reduction after 24 hours; 80% after 2 weeks therapy

Duration of estradiol reduction: 6 days

Absorption: Well absorbed; extent of absorption not affected by food

Protein binding, plasma: 40%

Metabolism: Extensively hepatic (~85%) via N-dealkylation, hydroxylation, and glucuronidation; primary metabolite (triazole) inactive

Half-life elimination: ~50 hours

Time to peak, plasma: ~2 hours without food; 5 hours with food

Excretion: Feces; urine (urinary excretion accounts for ~10% of total elimination, mostly as metabolites)

Dosing

Adult & Geriatric Females: Postmenopausal:

Breast cancer, advanced: Oral: 1 mg once daily; continue until tumor progression

Breast cancer, early (adjuvant treatment): Oral: 1 mg once daily; optimal duration unknown, duration in clinical trial is 5 years

Renal Impairment Dosage adjustment is not necessary.

Hepatic Impairment

Mild-to-moderate impairment or stable hepatic cirrhosis: Dosage adjustment is not required.

Severe hepatic impairment: Has not been studied in this population.

Administration May be administered with or without food.

Monitoring Parameters Bone mineral density; total cholesterol and LDL

Dietary Considerations May be taken with or without food.

Additional Information Oncology Comment: The American Society of Clinical Oncology (ASCO) guidelines for adjuvant endocrine therapy in postmenopausal women with HR-positive breast cancer (Burstein, 2010) recommend considering aromatase inhibitor (AI) therapy at some point in the treatment course (primary, sequentially, or extended). Optimal duration at this time is not known; however, treatment with an AI should not exceed 5 years in primary and extended therapies, and 2-3 years if followed by tamoxifen in sequential therapy (total of 5 years). If initial therapy with AI has been discontinued before the 5 years, consideration should be taken to receive tamoxifen for a total of 5 years. The optimal time to switch to an AI is also not known, but data supports switching after 2-3 years of tamoxifen (sequential) or after 5 years of tamoxifen (extended). If patient becomes intolerant or has poor adherence, consideration should be made to switch to another AI or initiate tamoxifen.

Dosage Forms Excipient information presented when available (limited, particularly for generics); consult specific product labeling.

Tablet, oral: 1 mg

Arimidex®: 1 mg

References

Burstein HJ, Prestrud AA, Seidenfeld J, et al, "American Society of Clinical Oncology Clinical Practice Guideline: Update on Adjuvant Endocrine Therapy for Women with Hormone Receptor-Positive Breast Cancer," *J Clin Oncol*, 2010, 28(23):3784-96.

del Carmen MG, Fuller AF, Matulonis U, et al, "Phase II Trial of Anastrozole in Women With Asymptomatic Müllerian Cancer," *Gynecol Oncol*, 2003, 91(3):596-602.

Eastell R, Adams JE, Coleman RE, et al, "Effect of Anastrozole on Bone Mineral Density: 5-Year Results From the Anastrozole, Tamoxifen, Alone or in Combination Trial 18233230," *J Clin Oncol*, 2008, 26(7):1051-7.

National Comprehensive Cancer Network® (NCCN), "Clinical Practice Guidelines in Oncology™: Breast Cancer," Version 3.2010. Available at http://www.nccn.org/professionals/physician_gls/PDF/breast.pdf

National Comprehensive Cancer Network® (NCCN), "Clinical Practice Guidelines in Oncology™: Ovarian Cancer," Version 1.2011. Available at http://www.nccn.org/professionals/physician_gls/PDF/ovarian.pdf

National Comprehensive Cancer Network® (NCCN), "Clinical Practice Guidelines in Oncology™: Uterine Neoplasms," Version 1.2011. Available at http://www.nccn.org/professionals/physician_gls/PDF/uterine.pdf

National Osteoporosis Foundation, "Clinician's Guide to Prevention and Treatment of Osteoporosis," Washington, DC, 2010. Available at http://www.nof.org

Rose PG, Brunetto VL, VanLe L, et al, "A Phase II Trial of Anastrozole in Advanced Recurrent or Persistent Endometrial Carcinoma: A Gynecologic Oncology Group Study," *Gynecol Oncol*, 2000, 78(2):212-6.

"Third Report of the National Cholesterol Education Program (NCEP) Expert Panel on Detection, Evaluation, and Treatment of High Blood Cholesterol in Adults (Adult Treatment Panel III) Final Report," *Circulation*, 2002, 106(25):3143-21.

Winer EP, Hudis C, Burstein HJ, et al, "American Society of Clinical Oncology Technology Assessment on the Use of Aromatase Inhibitors as Adjuvant Therapy for Postmenopausal Women With Hormone Receptor-Positive Breast Cancer: Status Report 2004," *J Clin Oncol*, 2005, 23(3):619-29.

◆ **Ancobon®** *see* Flucytosine *on page 618*

◆ **Androcur® (Can)** *see* Cyproterone *on page 344*

◆ **Androcur® Depot (Can)** *see* Cyproterone *on page 344*

◆ **Androxy™** *see* Fluoxymesterone *on page 634*

Anidulafungin (ay nid yoo la FUN jin)

Brand Names: U.S. Eraxis™

Brand Names: Canada Eraxis™

Index Terms LY303366

Generic Availability (U.S.) No

Pharmacologic Category Antifungal Agent, Parenteral; Echinocandin

Use Treatment of candidemia and other forms of *Candida* infections (including those of intra-abdominal, peritoneal, and esophageal locus)

Unlabeled Use Treatment of infections due to *Aspergillus* spp.

Labeled Contraindications Hypersensitivity to anidulafungin, other echinocandins, or any component of the formulation

Pregnancy Risk Factor C

Lactation Excretion in breast milk unknown/use caution

Warnings/Precautions Histamine-mediated reactions (eg, urticaria, flushing, hypotension) have been observed; these may be related to infusion rate. Elevated liver function tests, hepatitis, and worsening hepatic failure have been reported. Monitor for progressive hepatic impairment if increased transaminase enzymes noted. Safety and efficacy in pediatric patients, neutropenic patients, or other *Candida* infections (eg, endocarditis, osteomyelitis, meningitis) have not been established.

Storage/Stability Store vials at 2°C to 8°C (36°F to 46°F); do not freeze. The reconstituted solution can be stored for up to 1 hour at 2°C to 8°C (36°F to 46°F) prior to dilution into the infusion solution; do not freeze. If the infusion solution is not used immediately, it should be stored in a refrigerator at 2°C to 8°C (36°F to 46°F) and administered within 24 hours of preparation; do not freeze.

Reconstitution Aseptically add 15 mL (50 mg vial) or 30 mL (100 mg vial) of sterile water for injection to each vial. Swirl to dissolve; do not shake. Further dilute 50 mg, 100 mg, or 200 mg in 50 mL, 100 mL, or 200 mL, respectively, of D_5W or NS.

Mechanism of Action Noncompetitive inhibitor of 1,3-beta-D-glucan synthase resulting in reduced formation of 1,3-beta-D-glucan, an essential polysaccharide comprising 30% to 60% of *Candida* cell walls (absent in mammalian cells); decreased glucan content leads to osmotic instability and cellular lysis

Pharmacodynamics/Kinetics

Distribution: 30-50 L

Protein binding: 84%

Metabolism: No hepatic metabolism observed; undergoes slow chemical hydrolysis to open-ring peptide-lacking antifungal activity

Half-life elimination: 27 hours

Excretion: Feces (30%, 10% as unchanged drug); urine (<1%)

Dosing

Adult & Geriatric

Candidemia, intra-abdominal or peritoneal candidiasis: I.V.: 200 mg loading dose on day 1, followed by 100 mg daily for at least 14 days after last positive culture

Esophageal candidiasis: I.V.: 100 mg loading dose on day 1, followed by 50 mg daily for at least 14 days and for at least 7 days after symptom resolution

Renal Impairment No adjustment necessary, including dialysis patients.

Hepatic Impairment No adjustment necessary.

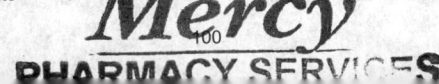

Administration For intravenous use only; infusion rate should not exceed 1.1 mg/minute

Dosage Forms Excipient information presented when available (limited, particularly for generics); consult specific product labeling. [DSC] = Discontinued product

Injection, powder for reconstitution:

Eraxis™: 50 mg [contains polysorbate 80]

Eraxis™: 100 mg [DSC] [contains dehydrated ethanol (in diluent), polysorbate 80]

Eraxis™: 100 mg [contains polysorbate 80]

◆ **Anti-D Immunoglobulin** *see* Rh$_o$(D) Immune Globulin *on page* *1237*

◆ **131 I Anti-B1 Antibody** *see* Tositumomab and Iodine I 131 Tositumomab *on page* *1379*

◆ **131 I-Anti-B1 Monoclonal Antibody** *see* Tositumomab and Iodine I 131 Tositumomab *on page* *1379*

◆ **Antibody-Drug Conjugate SGN-35** *see* Brentuximab Vedotin *on page* *199*

◆ **Anti-CD20 Monoclonal Antibody** *see* RiTUXimab *on page* *1244*

◆ **Anti-CD20-Murine Monoclonal Antibody I-131** *see* Tositumomab and Iodine I 131 Tositumomab *on page* *1379*

◆ **Anti-CD30 ADC SGN-35** *see* Brentuximab Vedotin *on page* *199*

◆ **Anti-CD30 Antibody-Drug Conjugate SGN-35** *see* Brentuximab Vedotin *on page* *199*

◆ **Anti-CD52 Monoclonal Antibody** *see* Alemtuzumab *on page* *43*

◆ **anti-c-erB-2** *see* Trastuzumab *on page* *1399*

◆ **anti-ERB-2** *see* Trastuzumab *on page* *1399*

Antihemophilic Factor (Human)

(an tee hee moe FIL ik FAK tor HYU man)

Brand Names: U.S. Hemofil M; Koāte®-DVI; Monoclate-P®

Brand Names: Canada Hemofil M

Index Terms AHF (Human); Factor VIII (Human); Kaote DVI

Generic Availability (U.S.) Yes

Pharmacologic Category Antihemophilic Agent; Blood Product Derivative

Use Prevention and treatment of hemorrhagic episodes in patients with hemophilia A (classic hemophilia); perioperative management of hemophilia A; can be of significant therapeutic value in patients with acquired factor VIII inhibitors not exceeding 10 Bethesda units/mL

Labeled Contraindications Hypersensitivity to any component of the formulation

Pregnancy Risk Factor C

Lactation Excretion in breast milk unknown/use caution

Warnings/Precautions Risk of viral transmission is not totally eradicated. Because antihemophilic factor is prepared from pooled plasma, it may contain the causative agent of viral hepatitis and other viral diseases. Hepatitis B vaccination is recommended for all patients. Hepatitis A vaccination is also recommended for seronegative patients. Antihemophilic factor contains trace amounts of blood groups A and B isohemagglutinins and when large or frequently repeated doses are given to individuals with blood groups A, B, and AB, the patient should be monitored for signs of progressive anemia and the possibility of intravascular hemolysis should be considered. The dosage requirement will vary in patients with factor VIII inhibitors; optimal treatment should be determined by clinical response. Natural rubber latex is a ▶

component of Hemofil M packaging. Hemofil M and Monoclate-P® contain trace amounts of mouse protein. Products contain naturally-occurring von Willebrand factor for stabilization, however efficacy has not been established for the treatment of von Willebrand disease. Products vary by preparation method; final formulations contain human albumin.

Adverse Reactions <1%: Acute hemolytic anemia, AHF inhibitor development, allergic reactions (rare), anaphylaxis (rare), bleeding tendency increased, blurred vision, chest tightness, chills, fever, headache, hyperfibrinogenemia, jittery feeling, lethargy, nausea, somnolence, stinging at the infusion site, stomach discomfort, tingling, urticaria, vasomotor reactions with rapid infusion, vomiting

Drug Interactions

Metabolism/Transport Effects None known.

Avoid Concomitant Use There are no known interactions where it is recommended to avoid concomitant use.

Increased Effect/Toxicity There are no known significant interactions involving an increase in effect.

Decreased Effect There are no known significant interactions involving a decrease in effect.

Storage/Stability Store under refrigeration, 2°C to 8°C (36°F to 46°F); avoid freezing. Use within 3 hours of reconstitution. Do not refrigerate after reconstitution, precipitation may occur.

Hemofil M: May also be stored at room temperature not to exceed 30°C (86°F).

Koāte®-DVI; Monoclate-P®: May also be stored at room temperature of 25°C (77°F) for ≤6 months.

Reconstitution If refrigerated, the dried concentrate and diluent should be warmed to room temperature before reconstitution. Gently swirl or rotate vial after adding diluent; do not shake vigorously.

Mechanism of Action Protein (factor VIII) in normal plasma which is necessary for clot formation and maintenance of hemostasis; activates factor X in conjunction with activated factor IX; activated factor X converts prothrombin to thrombin, which converts fibrinogen to fibrin, and with factor XIII forms a stable clot

Pharmacodynamics/Kinetics Half-life elimination: Mean: 8-27 hours

Dosing

Adult & Geriatric Hemophilia: I.V.: Individualize dosage based on coagulation studies performed prior to treatment and at regular intervals during treatment. In general, administration of factor VIII 1 unit/kg will increase circulating factor VIII levels by ~2 units/dL. (General guidelines presented; consult individual product labeling for specific dosing recommendations.)

Dosage based on desired factor VIII increase (%):

To calculate dosage needed based on desired factor VIII increase (%):

Body weight (kg) x 0.5 units/kg x desired factor VIII increase (%) = units factor VIII required

For example:

50 kg x 0.5 units/kg x 30 (% increase) = 750 units factor VIII

Dosage based on expected factor VIII increase (%):

It is also possible to calculate the **expected** % factor VIII increase:

(# units administered x 2%/units/kg) divided by body weight (kg) = expected % factor VIII increase

For example:

(1400 units x 2%/units/kg) divided by 70 kg = 40%

General guidelines:

Minor hemorrhage: 10-20 units/kg as a single dose to achieve FVIII plasma level ~20% to 40% of normal. Mild superficial or early hemorrhages may respond to a single dose; may repeat dose every 12-24 hours for 1-3 days until bleeding is resolved or healing achieved.

Moderate hemorrhage/minor surgery: 15-25 units/kg to achieve FVIII plasma level 30% to 50% of normal. If needed, may continue with a maintenance dose of 10-15 units/kg every 8-12 hours.

Major to life-threatening hemorrhage: Initial dose 40-50 units/kg, followed by a maintenance dose of 20-25 units/kg every 8-12 hours until threat is resolved, to achieve FVIII plasma level 80% to 100% of normal.

Major surgery: 50 units/kg given preoperatively to raise factor VIII level to 100% before surgery begins. May repeat as necessary after 6-12 hours initially and for a total of 10-14 days until healing is complete. Intensity of therapy may depend on type of surgery and postoperative regimen.

Bleeding prophylaxis: May be administered on a regular basis for bleeding prophylaxis. Doses of 24-40 units/kg 3 times/week have been reported in patients with severe hemophilia to prevent joint bleeding.

If bleeding is not controlled with adequate dose, test for presence of inhibitor. It may not be possible or practical to control bleeding if inhibitor titers are >10 Bethesda units/mL.

Pediatric Refer to adult dosing.

Administration Administer I.V. over 5-10 minutes (maximum: 10 mL/minute). Infuse Monoclate-P® at 2 mL/minute.

Monitoring Parameters Heart rate and blood pressure (before and during I.V. administration); AHF levels prior to and during treatment; in patients with circulating inhibitors, the inhibitor level should be monitored; hematocrit; monitor for signs and symptoms of intravascular hemolysis; bleeding

Dosage Forms Excipient information presented when available (limited, particularly for generics); consult specific product labeling. [DSC] = Discontinued product

Injection, powder for reconstitution:

Hemofil M: ~250 units, ~500 units, ~1000 units, ~1700 units [contains albumin (human), mouse protein; packaging may contain natural rubber latex]. Supplied with diluent.

Koāte®-DVI: ~250 units, ~500 units, ~1000 units [contains albumin (human), aluminum, polysorbate 80]. Supplied with diluent.

Monoclate-P®: ~250 units, ~500 units, ~1000 units, ~1500 units [contains albumin (human), mouse protein]. Supplied with diluent.

References

White GC, Rosendaal F, Aledort LM, et al, "Definitions in Hemophilia. Recommendation of the Scientific Subcommittee on Factor VIII and Factor IX of the Scientific and Standardization Committee of the International Society on Thrombosis and Haemostasis," *Thromb Haemost*, 2001, 85(3):560.

Antihemophilic Factor (Recombinant)

(an tee hee moe FIL ik FAK tor ree KOM be nant)

Brand Names: U.S. Advate; Helixate® FS; Kogenate® FS; Recombinate; Xyntha®; Xyntha® Solofuse™

Brand Names: Canada Advate; Helixate® FS; Kogenate® FS; Xyntha®

Index Terms AHF (Recombinant); Factor VIII (Recombinant); rAHF

Generic Availability (U.S.) No

Pharmacologic Category Antihemophilic Agent

Use Prevention and treatment of hemorrhagic episodes in patients with hemophilia A (classic hemophilia or congenital factor VIII deficiency); perioperative management of hemophilia A; routine prophylaxis in patients with hemophilia A to prevent bleeding episodes (Advate, Helixate® FS, Kogenate® FS)

Note: Helixate® FS and Kogenate® FS are also approved in children with hemophilia A with no pre-existing joint damage to reduce risk of joint damage. In addition, Recombinate can be of therapeutic value in patients with acquired factor VIII inhibitors ≤10 Bethesda units/mL.

Labeled Contraindications Hypersensitivity to any component of the formulation

Pregnancy Risk Factor C

Lactation Excretion in breast milk unknown/use caution

Warnings/Precautions Monitor for signs of formation of antibodies to factor VIII; may occur at anytime but more common in young children with severe hemophilia. The dosage requirement will vary in patients with factor VIII inhibitors; optimal treatment should be determined by clinical response. Allergic hypersensitivity reactions (including anaphylaxis) may occur; monitor. Products vary by preparation method. Recombinate is stabilized using human albumin. Helixate® FS and Kogenate® FS are stabilized with sucrose. Advate, Helixate® FS, Kogenate® FS, and Xyntha® may contain trace amounts of mouse or hamster protein. Recombinate may contain mouse, hamster or bovine protein. Some products may contain polysorbate 80. Products may contain von Willebrand factor for stabilization; however, efficacy has not been established for the treatment of von Willebrand's disease.

Adverse Reactions Actual frequency may vary by product.

>1%:

- Central nervous system: Chills, dizziness, fever, headache, pain
- Dermatologic: Pruritus, rash, urticaria
- Gastrointestinal: Constipation, diarrhea, nausea, taste perversion, vomiting
- Local: Injection/infusion site reactions
- Neuromuscular & skeletal: Arthralgia, joint swelling, pain in extremity, weakness
- Otic: Ear infection, ear pain
- Respiratory: Cough, nasal congestion, nasopharyngitis, pharyngolaryngeal pain, rhinorrhea, sinusitis
- Miscellaneous: Catheter thrombosis, catheter infection, factor VIII inhibitor formation, flu-like syndrome, influenza

≤1%, postmarketing, and/or case reports: Abdominal pain, adenopathy, allergic reactions, anaphylaxis, anemia, angioedema, anorexia, arthralgia, AST increased, chest discomfort, chest pain, cyanosis, depersonalization, diaphoresis, dyspnea, edema, epistaxis, erythema, facial edema, facial flushing, factor VIII decreased, fatigue, GI hemorrhage, hematoma, hives, hot flashes, hyperhidrosis, hypersensitivity reaction, hyper-/hypotension (slight), infection, laryngeal edema, lethargy, malaise, pallor, paresthesia, restlessness, rhinitis, rigors, shortness of breath, somnolence, tachycardia, tremor, urinary tract infection, vasodilation, venous catheter access complications

Drug Interactions

Metabolism/Transport Effects None known.

Avoid Concomitant Use There are no known interactions where it is recommended to avoid concomitant use.

Increased Effect/Toxicity There are no known significant interactions involving an increase in effect.

Decreased Effect There are no known significant interactions involving a decrease in effect.

Storage/Stability Prior to reconstitution, store refrigerated at 2°C to 8°C (36°F to 46°F); avoid freezing. Use within 3 hours of reconstitution. Do not refrigerate after reconstitution.

Advate: May also be stored at room temperature for up to 6 months.

Helixate® FS: May also be stored at room temperature (not to exceed 25°C [77°F]) up to 3 months; do not return to refrigerator. Avoid prolonged exposure to light during storage.

Kogenate® FS: May also be stored at room temperature (not to exceed 25°C [77°F]) up to 12 months; do not return to refrigerator. Avoid prolonged exposure to light during storage.

Recombinate: May also be stored at room temperature, not to exceed 30°C (86°F).

Xyntha®: May also be stored at room temperature (not to exceed 25°C [77°F]) up to 3 months; after room temperature storage, product may be returned to the refrigerator until the expiration date; however, do not store at room temperature and return to refrigerator temperature more than once. Avoid prolonged exposure to light during storage.

Xyntha® Solofuse™: May also be stored at room temperature not to exceed 25°C [77°F]) up to 3 months; do not return to refrigerator; after 3 months at room temperature, must use immediately or discard.

Reconstitution If refrigerated, the dried concentrate and diluent should be warmed to room temperature before reconstitution. Gently agitate or rotate vial after adding diluent, do not shake vigorously. Refer to product specific labeling for reconstitution instructions; recommendations vary by product.

Mechanism of Action Factor VIII replacement, necessary for clot formation and maintenance of hemostasis. It activates factor X in conjunction with activated factor IX; activated factor X converts prothrombin to thrombin, which converts fibrinogen to fibrin, and with factor XIII forms a stable clot.

Pharmacodynamics/Kinetics

Distribution: V_{ss}: ~0.1 dL/kg

Half-life elimination: Mean: ~11-15 hours

Dosing

Adult & Geriatric Hemophilia A: I.V.: Individualize dosage based on coagulation studies performed prior to treatment and at regular intervals during treatment. In general, administration of factor VIII 1 unit/kg will increase circulating factor VIII levels by ~2 units/dL. (General guidelines presented; consult individual product labeling for specific dosing recommendations.)

Dosage based on desired factor VIII increase (%):

To calculate dosage needed based on desired factor VIII increase (%):

[Body weight (kg) x desired factor VIII increase (%)] divided by 2(%/units/kg) = units factor VIII required

For example:

50 kg x 30 (% increase) divided by 2 = 750 units factor VIII

Dosage based on expected factor VIII increase (%):

It is also possible to calculate the **expected** % factor VIII increase:

[# units administered x 2(%/units/kg)] divided by body weight (kg) = expected % factor VIII increase

For example:
[1400 units x 2] divided by 70 kg = 40%

General guidelines (consult individual product labeling for specific dosage recommendations):

Minor hemorrhage: 10-20 units/kg as a single dose to achieve FVIII plasma level ~20% to 40% of normal. Mild superficial or early hemorrhages may respond to a single dose; may repeat dose every 12-24 hours for 1-3 days until bleeding is resolved or healing achieved.

Moderate hemorrhage/minor surgery: 15-30 units/kg to achieve FVIII plasma level 30% to 60% of normal. May repeat 1 dose at 12-24 hours if needed. Some products suggest continuing for ≥3 days until pain and disability are resolved.

Major to life-threatening hemorrhage: Initial dose 30-50 units/kg followed by a maintenance dose of 20-50 units/kg every 8-24 hours until threat is resolved, to achieve FVIII plasma level 60% to 100% of normal.

Minor surgery (including tooth extraction): 15-50 units/kg to raise factor VIII level to ~30-100% before procedure/surgery. May repeat every 12-24 hours until bleeding is resolved.

Major surgery: 40-60 units/kg given preoperatively to raise factor VIII level to ~60% to 120% before surgery begins. May repeat as necessary after 6-24 hours until wound healing. Intensity of therapy may depend on type of surgery and postoperative regimen.

If bleeding is not controlled with adequate dose, test for presence of inhibitor. It may not be possible or practical to control bleeding if inhibitor titers >10 Bethesda units/mL.

Routine prophylaxis to prevent bleeding episodes (Advate): 20-40 units/kg every other day (3-4 times weekly). Alternatively, an every-third-day dosing regimen may be used to target factor VIII trough levels of ≥1%.

Pediatric Hemophilia A: I.V.: Refer to adult dosing. **Note:** Children <6 years may require more frequent administration.

Routine prophylaxis to prevent bleeding episodes (Advate): Refer to adult dosing.

Routine prophylaxis to prevent bleeding episodes and joint damage (without pre-existing joint damage) (Helixate® FS, Kogenate® FS): 25 units/kg every other day

Administration Use administration sets/tubing provided by manufacturer (if provided).

Advate: Infuse over ≤5 minutes (maximum: 10 mL/minute)

Helixate® FS, Kogenate® FS: Infuse over 1-15 minutes; based on patient tolerability

Recombinate reconstituted with 5 mL of SWFI: Infuse at a rate of ≤5 mL/minute (maximum: 5 mL/minute)

Recombinate reconstituted with 10 mL of SWFI: Infuse at a rate of ≤10 mL/minute (maximum: 10 mL/minute)

Xyntha®, Xyntha® Solufuse™: Infuse over several minutes; adjust based on patient comfort. Do not admix or administer in same tubing as other medications.

Monitoring Parameters Heart rate and blood pressure (before and during I.V. administration); plasma factor VIII activity prior to and during treatment; development of factor VIII inhibitors; signs of bleeding; hemoglobin, hematocrit

Dietary Considerations Some products may contain sodium.

Dosage Forms Excipient information presented when available (limited, particularly for generics); consult specific product labeling.

Injection, powder for reconstitution [preservative free]:

Advate: 250 units, 500 units, 1000 units, 1500 units, 2000 units, 3000 units, 4000 units [plasma/albumin free; contains mannitol, polysorbate 80, sodium; derived from or manufactured using hamster or mouse protein; supplied with diluent]

Helixate® FS: 250 units, 500 units, 1000 units [contains polysorbate 80, sodium, sucrose 28 mg/vial; derived from or manufactured using hamster or mouse protein]

Helixate® FS: 2000 units, 3000 units [contains polysorbate 80, sodium, sucrose 52 mg/vial; derived from or manufactured using hamster or mouse protein]

Kogenate® FS: 250 units, 500 units, 1000 units [contains polysorbate 80, sodium, sucrose 28 mg/vial; derived from or manufactured using hamster or mouse protein]

Kogenate® FS: 2000 units, 3000 units [contains polysorbate 80, sodium, sucrose 52 mg/vial; derived from or manufactured using hamster or mouse protein]

Recombinate: 250 units, 500 units, 1000 units, 1500 units, 2000 units [contains albumin (human), natural rubber/natural latex in packaging, polysorbate 80, sodium; derived from or manufactured using bovine, hamster or mouse protein; supplied with diluent]

Xyntha®: 250 units, 500 units, 1000 units, 2000 units [albumin free; contains polysorbate 80, sucrose; derived from or manufactured using hamster protein; supplied with diluent]

Xyntha® Solofuse™: 1000 units, 2000 units, 3000 units [albumin free; contains polysorbate 80, sucrose; derived from or manufactured using hamster protein, dual-chamber syringe]

References

White GC, Rosendaal F, Aledort LM, et al, "Definitions in Hemophilia. Recommendation of the Scientific Subcommittee on Factor VIII and Factor IX of the Scientific and Standardization Committee of the International Society on Thrombosis and Haemostasis," *Thromb Haemost*, 2001, 85(3):560.

Antithrombin (an tee THROM bin)

Brand Names: U.S. Atryn®; Thrombate III®

Brand Names: Canada Thrombate III®

Index Terms Antithrombin Alfa; Antithrombin III; AT; AT-III; hpAT; rhAT; rhATIII

Generic Availability (U.S.) No

Pharmacologic Category Anticoagulant; Blood Product Derivative

Use Prophylaxis (ATryn®, Thrombate III®) of thromboembolic events in patients with hereditary antithrombin (AT or AT-III) deficiency undergoing surgical or obstetrical procedures (eg, childbirth); treatment (Thrombate III®) of thromboembolism in patients with hereditary AT deficiency

Labeled Contraindications

ATryn®: Hypersensitivity to goat or goat milk proteins

Thrombate III®: There are no contraindications listed in manufacturer's labeling.

Pregnancy Risk Factor B (Thrombate III®); C (ATryn®)

Lactation Enters breast milk/use caution

Warnings/Precautions

ATryn®: Recombinant-derived product may cause severe hypersensitivity reactions, including anaphylaxis; monitor closely during infusions. Antibodies against the recombinant antithrombin protein (or goat-milk protein) may theoretically develop and lead to an immunological reaction. A postmarketing patient registry has been created to monitor for antibody development; physicians are encouraged to enroll by contacting Ovation Pharmaceuticals at 1-800-455-1141. Pharmacokinetics of the recombinant derived product are influenced by pregnancy; distinct dosing recommendations are provided for pregnant women. Product is not indicated for the treatment of thromboembolic events in hereditary antithrombin deficient patients.

Thrombate III®: Product of human plasma; may potentially contain infectious agents which could transmit disease; screening of donors, as well as testing and/or inactivation or removal of certain viruses, reduces this risk. Infections thought to be transmitted by this product should be reported to Talecris Biotherapeutics at 1-800-520-2807. Safety and efficacy in children have not been established.

Half-life and clearance differ significantly (~7-9 times) between the plasma-derived (Thrombate III®) and the recombinant-derived (ATryn®) product.

Adverse Reactions

1% to 10%:
- Cardiovascular: Chest pain (≤2%)
- Central nervous system: Dizziness (2%)
- Hematologic: Hemorrhage (≥5%), hematoma (≤2%)
- Hepatic: Liver enzyme abnormalities (≤2%)
- Neuromuscular & skeletal: Hemarthrosis (≤2%)
- Renal: Hematuria (≤2%)
- Local: Infusion site reaction (≥5%)

<1%: Bowel fullness, chest tightness, chills, cramps, dyspnea, fever, film over eye, foul taste, hives, lightheadedness, nausea

Drug Interactions

Metabolism/Transport Effects None known.

Avoid Concomitant Use

Avoid concomitant use of Antithrombin with any of the following: Omacetaxine; Rivaroxaban

Increased Effect/Toxicity

Antithrombin may increase the levels/effects of: Anticoagulants; Collagenase (Systemic); Dabigatran Etexilate; Deferasirox; Drotrecogin Alfa (Activated); Ibritumomab; Omacetaxine; Rivaroxaban; Tositumomab and Iodine I 131 Tositumomab

The levels/effects of Antithrombin may be increased by: Antiplatelet Agents; Dasatinib; Herbs (Anticoagulant/Antiplatelet Properties); Nonsteroidal Anti-Inflammatory Agents; Pentosan Polysulfate Sodium; Prostacyclin Analogues; Salicylates; Thrombolytic Agents; Tipranavir; Vitamin E

Decreased Effect There are no known significant interactions involving a decrease in effect.

Ethanol/Nutrition/Herb Interactions Herb/Nutraceutical: Recent use/intake of herbs with anticoagulant or antiplatelet activity (including cat's claw, dong quai, evening primrose, garlic, ginkgo and ginseng) may increase the risk of bleeding.

Storage/Stability

ATryn®: Prior to reconstitution, store vials under refrigeration at 2°C to 8°C (38°F to 46°F). Bring vial to room temperature prior to reconstitution (≤3 hours). Do not shake; swirl to mix. Use within 8-12 hours after reconstitution when stored at room temperature. Discard any unused portion.

Thrombate III®: Prior to reconstitution, store vials refrigerated or at room temperature not exceeding 25°C (77°F); avoid freezing. Bring drug and diluent to room temperature prior to reconstitution. Administer within 3 hours after reconstitution. Do not refrigerate reconstituted product.

Reconstitution

ATryn®: Bring vial to room temperature prior to reconstitution (≤3 hours). Reconstitute with 10 mL of sterile water for injection. Do not shake; swirl to mix. May administer solution following reconstitution or may further dilute in 0.9% NS to a concentration of 100 units/mL and administer.

Thrombate III®: Bring drug and diluent to room temperature prior to reconstitution. Reconstitute with sterile water for injection. Do not shake; swirl to mix to avoid foaming. Filter through sterile filter needle provided prior to administration.

Mechanism of Action Antithrombin is the primary physiologic inhibitor of *in vivo* coagulation. It is an alpha$_2$-globulin. Its principal actions are the inactivation of thrombin, plasmin, and other active serine proteases of coagulation, including factors IXa, Xa, XIa, and XIIa. The inactivation of proteases is a major step in the normal clotting process. The strong activation of clotting enzymes at the site of every bleeding injury facilitates fibrin formation and maintains normal hemostasis. Thrombosis in the circulation would be caused by active serine proteases if they were not inhibited by antithrombin after the localized clotting process.

Pharmacodynamics/Kinetics

Plasma derived (Thrombate III®):

Half-life elimination: Biologic: 2.5 days (immunologic assay); 3.8 days (functional AT assay). Half-life may be decreased following surgery, with hemorrhage, acute thrombosis, and/or during heparin administration.

Recombinant derived (Atryn®):

Distribution: V_d: Pregnant women: 14.3 L; Nonpregnant patients: 7.7 L

Half-life elimination: 12-18 hours; surgery, childbirth hemorrhage, and/or concomitant heparin may shorten half-life

Dosing

Adult & Geriatric Antithrombin deficiency: I.V.:

Atryn®: Prophylaxis of thrombosis during surgical or obstetrical procedures:

Dosing is individualized based on pretherapy antithrombin (AT) activity levels. Therapy should begin before delivery or ~24 hours prior to surgery to obtain target AT activity levels. Dosing should be targeted to keep levels between 80% to 120% of normal. Loading dose should be given as a 15-minute infusion, followed by maintenance dose as a continuous infusion. Doses may be calculated based on the following formulas:

Surgical patients (nonpregnant):

Loading dose: [(100 - baseline AT activity level) **divided** by 2.3] x body weight (kg) = units of antithrombin required

Maintenance infusion: [(100 - baseline AT activity level) **divided** by 10.2] x body weight (kg) = units of antithrombin required/hour

Pregnant patients: **Note:** Pregnant women undergoing surgical procedures (other than a Cesarean section) should also be dosed according to the formula below.

Loading dose: [(100 - baseline AT activity level) **divided** by 1.3] x body weight (kg) = units of antithrombin required

Maintenance infusion: [(100 - baseline AT activity level) **divided** by 5.4] x body weight (kg) = units of antithrombin required/hour

Dosing adjustments: Adjustments should be made based on AT activity levels to maintain levels between 80% to 120% of normal. Surgery or delivery may rapidly decrease AT levels; check AT level just after surgery or delivery. The first AT level should be obtained 2 hours after initiation and adjusted as follows:

AT activity level <80%: Increase infusion rate by 30%; recheck AT level 2 hours after adjustment. Alternatively, an additional bolus dose (using loading dose formula) may be needed to rapidly restore AT levels. Calculate the additional bolus/loading dose using the last available AT activity result. After additional loading/bolus dose given, resume maintenance infusion at the same rate prior to bolus administration.

AT activity level 80% to 120%: No dosage adjustment needed; recheck AT level in 6 hours

AT activity level >120%: Decrease infusion rate by 30%; recheck AT level 2 hours after adjustment

Thrombate III®: Prophylaxis of thrombosis during surgical or obstetrical procedures or treatment of thromboembolism:

Initial loading dose: Dosing is individualized based on pretherapy antithrombin (AT) levels. The initial dose should raise AT levels to 120% and may be calculated based on the following formula:

[(desired AT level % - baseline AT level %) x body weight (kg)] **divided** by 1.4 = units of antithrombin required

For example, if a 70 kg adult patient had a baseline AT level of 57%, the initial dose would be

[(120% - 57%) x 70] divided by 1.4 = 3150 units

Maintenance dose: In general, subsequent dosing should be targeted to keep levels between 80% to 120% which may be achieved by administering 60% of the initial loading dose every 24 hours. Adjustments may be made by adjusting dose or interval. Maintain level within normal range for 2-8 days depending on type of procedure/situation.

Administration Administer intravenously.

ATryn®: Infuse loading dose over 15 minutes, followed immediately by a continuous maintenance infusion. Administer reconstituted solution (without further dilution) or further diluted 100 units/mL solution. Filter during administration using an infusion set with a 0.22 micron in-line filter.

Thrombate III®: Infuse over 10-20 minutes.

Monitoring Parameters

ATryn®: Monitor AT activity level at baseline, 2 hours after initiation (and each dosage adjustment), and thereafter, at least once or twice daily when predictable levels achieved (between 80% and 120%).

Thrombate III®: Initially, monitor AT at baseline, 20 minutes postinfusion (peak), 12 hours postinfusion, then preceding next infusion (trough level). Measure peak and trough AT levels with each subsequent dose until predictable levels achieved (between 80% and 120%). Some situations (eg, following surgery, hemorrhage or acute thrombosis, concurrent I.V. heparin administration), may require more frequent AT monitoring.

Dietary Considerations Some products may contain sodium.

Additional Information

Antithrombin is commercially available in two formulations. Thrombate III® is AT collected from pooled human plasma (hpAT) and ATryn® is AT manufactured using recombinant technology (rhAT). Recombinant human AT, also known as antithrombin alfa, is produced by transgenic goats expressing recombinant human AT in their milk which is then collected and purified.

Thromboembolism has been reported in children of women with hereditary antithrombin (AT) deficiency; AT levels in neonates of parents with hereditary AT deficiency should be measured immediately after birth. Plasma AT levels are typically lower in neonates and infants than in adults. Low plasma AT levels in neonates may not be indicative of deficiency; consultation with a coagulation expert is recommended.

Dosage Forms Excipient information presented when available (limited, particularly for generics); consult specific product labeling.

Injection, powder for reconstitution [human, preservative free]:
- Thrombate III®: ~500 units [contains heparin; exact potency labeled on each vial]

Injection, powder for reconstitution [recombinant, preservative free]:
- Atryn®: ~1750 units [contains goat protein; exact potency labeled on each vial]

References

Konkle BA, Bauer KA, Weinstein R, et al, "Use of Recombinant Human Antithrombin in Patients With Congenital Antithrombin Deficiency Undergoing Surgical Procedures," *Transfusion*, 2003, 43(3):390-94.

Tiede A, Tait RC, Shaffer DW, et al, "Antithrombin Alfa in Hereditary Antithrombin Deficient Patients: A Phase 3 Study of Prophylactic Intravenous Administration in High Risk Situations," *Thromb Haemost*, 2008, 99(3):616-22.

◆ **Antithrombin III** *see* Antithrombin *on page* 107

◆ **Antithrombin Alfa** *see* Antithrombin *on page* 107

Antithymocyte Globulin (Equine)

(an te THY moe site GLOB yu lin, E kwine)

Related Information

Hematopoietic Stem Cell Transplantation *on page* 1887

Brand Names: U.S. Atgam®

Brand Names: Canada Atgam®

Index Terms Antithymocyte Immunoglobulin; ATG; Horse Antihuman Thymocyte Gamma Globulin; Lymphocyte Immune Globulin

Generic Availability (U.S.) No

Pharmacologic Category Immune Globulin; Immunosuppressant Agent; Polyclonal Antibody

Use Prevention and treatment of acute renal allograft rejection; treatment of moderate-to-severe aplastic anemia in patients not considered suitable candidates for bone marrow transplantation

Unlabeled Use Prevention and treatment of other solid organ allograft rejection; prevention or treatment of graft-versus-host disease (GVHD) following allogeneic stem cell transplantation; treatment of myelodysplastic syndrome (MDS)

Labeled Contraindications History of severe systemic reaction to prior administration of antithymocyte globulin or other equine gamma globulins

Pregnancy Risk Factor C

Lactation Excretion in breast milk unknown/use caution

Warnings/Precautions For I.V. use only. Must be administered via central line due to chemical phlebitis. **[U.S. Boxed Warning]: Should only be used by physicians experienced in immunosuppressive therapy or management of solid organ or bone marrow transplant patients. Adequate**

laboratory and supportive medical resources must be readily available in the facility for patient management. Hypersensitivity and anaphylactic reactions can occur; immediate treatment (including epinephrine 1:1000) should be available. Rash, dyspnea, hypotension, tachycardia, or anaphylaxis precludes further administration of the drug. Respiratory distress, hypotension, or pain (chest, flank or back) may indicate an anaphylactoid/anaphylactic reaction. Discontinue if severe and unremitting thrombocytopenia and/or leukopenia occur in transplant patients. Clinically significant hemolysis has been reported (rarely); severe and unremitting hemolysis may require treatment discontinuation; chest, flank or back pain may indicate hemolysis. Monitor closely for signs of infection; there may be an increased incidence of cytomegalovirus (CMV) infection. Dose must be administered over at least 4 hours. Patient may need to be pretreated with an antipyretic, antihistamine, and/or corticosteroid. Intradermal skin testing is recommended prior to first-dose administration. Product of equine and human plasma; may have a risk of transmitting disease, including a theoretical risk of Creutzfeldt-Jakob disease (CJD). Product potency and activity may vary from lot to lot.

Adverse Reactions

>10%:

Central nervous system: Chills, fever, headache

Dermatologic: Pruritus, rash, urticaria, wheal/flare

Hematologic: Leukopenia, thrombocytopenia

Neuromuscular & skeletal: Arthralgia

1% to 10%:

Cardiovascular: Bradycardia, cardiac irregularity, chest pain, edema, heart failure, hyper-/hypotension, myocarditis

Central nervous system: Agitation, encephalitis, lethargy, lightheadedness, listlessness, seizure, viral encephalopathy

Gastrointestinal: Diarrhea, nausea, stomatitis, vomiting

Hepatic: Hepatosplenomegaly, liver function tests abnormal

Local: Injection site reactions (pain, redness, swelling), phlebitis, thrombophlebitis, burning soles/palms

Neuromuscular & skeletal: Aches, back pain, joint stiffness, myalgia

Ocular: Periorbital edema

Renal: Proteinuria, renal function tests abnormal

Respiratory: Dyspnea, pleural effusion, respiratory distress

Miscellaneous: Anaphylactic reaction, diaphoresis, lymphadenopathy, night sweats, serum sickness, viral infection

<1%, postmarketing, and/or case reports: Abdominal pain, acute renal failure, anaphylactoid reaction, anemia, aplasia, apnea, confusion, cough, deep vein thrombosis, disorientation, dizziness, eosinophilia, epigastric pain, epistaxis, erythema, faintness, flank pain, GI bleeding, GI perforation, granulocytopenia, hemolysis, hemolytic anemia, herpes simplex reactivation, hiccups, hyperglycemia, iliac vein obstruction, infection, involuntary movement, kidney enlarged/ruptured, laryngospasm, malaise, neutropenia, pancytopenia, paresthesia, pulmonary edema, renal artery thrombosis, rigidity, sore mouth/throat, tachycardia, toxic epidermal necrosis, tremor, vasculitis, viral hepatitis, weakness, wound dehiscence

Drug Interactions

Metabolism/Transport Effects None known.

Avoid Concomitant Use

Avoid concomitant use of Antithymocyte Globulin (Equine) with any of the following: BCG; Natalizumab; Pimecrolimus; Tacrolimus (Topical); Vaccines (Live)

Increased Effect/Toxicity

Antithymocyte Globulin (Equine) may increase the levels/effects of: Leflunomide; Natalizumab; Vaccines (Live)

The levels/effects of Antithymocyte Globulin (Equine) may be increased by: Denosumab; Pimecrolimus; Roflumilast; Tacrolimus (Topical); Trastuzumab

Decreased Effect

Antithymocyte Globulin (Equine) may decrease the levels/effects of: BCG; Coccidioidin Skin Test; Sipuleucel-T; Vaccines (Inactivated); Vaccines (Live)

The levels/effects of Antithymocyte Globulin (Equine) may be decreased by: Echinacea

Storage/Stability Refrigerate ampuls at 2°C to 8°C (36°F to 46°F); do not freeze. Diluted solution is stable for 24 hours (including infusion time) at refrigeration. Allow infusion solution to reach room temperature prior to administration.

Reconstitution Dilute into inverted bottle of sterile vehicle to ensure that undiluted lymphocyte immune globulin does not contact air. Gently rotate or swirl to mix; do not shake. Final concentration should be 4 mg/mL. May be diluted in NS, $D_5$1/4NS, $D_5$1/2NS **(do not use D_5W; low salt concentrations may result in precipitation)**.

Mechanism of Action Immunosuppressant involved in the elimination of antigen-reactive T-lymphocytes (killer cells) in peripheral blood or alteration in the function of T-lymphocytes, which are involved in humoral immunity and partly in cell-mediated immunity; induces complete or partial hematologic response in aplastic anemia

Pharmacodynamics/Kinetics

Distribution: Poorly into lymphoid tissues; binds to circulating lymphocytes, granulocytes, platelets, bone marrow cells

Half-life elimination, plasma: 1.5-12 days

Excretion: Urine (~1%)

Dosing

Adult & Geriatric Note: An intradermal skin test is recommended prior to administration of the initial dose of ATG; use 0.1 mL of a fresh 1:1000 dilution of ATG in normal saline; observe every 15-20 minutes for 1 hour. A positive skin reaction consists of a wheal ≥10 mm in diameter. If a positive skin test occurs, the first infusion should be administered in a controlled environment with intensive life support immediately available. A systemic reaction precludes further administration of the drug. The absence of a reaction does **not** preclude the possibility of an immediate sensitivity reaction.

Note: Premedication with diphenhydramine, hydrocortisone, and acetaminophen is recommended prior to first dose.

Aplastic anemia protocol: I.V.: 10-20 mg/kg/day for 8-14 days, then give every other day for 7 more doses for a total of 21 doses in 28 days **or** *Unlabeled dosing:* 40 mg/kg/day for 4 days (Rosenfeld, 1995).

Renal allograft rejection, prevention: I.V.: 15 mg/kg/day for 14 days, then give every other day for 7 more doses for a total of 21 doses in 28 days; the initial dose should be administered within 24 hours before or after transplantation.

Renal allograft rejection, treatment: I.V.: 10-15 mg/kg/day for 14 days, then administer every other day for 7 more doses for a total of 21 doses in 28 days.

Acute GVHD treatment (unlabeled use): I.V.: 30 mg/kg/dose every other day for 6 doses (MacMillan, 2007) **or** 15 mg/kg/dose twice daily for 10 doses (MacMillan, 2002)

Myelodysplastic syndrome (unlabeled use): I.V.: 40 mg/kg/dose once daily for 4 days; an intradermal test dose was administered prior to treatment (Molldrem, 2002)

Pediatric Note: See adult dosing for notes on intradermal skin testing and premedication.

Aplastic anemia protocol: I.V.: 10-20 mg/kg/day for 8-14 days; then administer every other day for 7 more doses; additional doses may be given every other day for 21 total doses in 28 days **or**

Unlabeled dosing: Children >10 kg: 40 mg/kg/day for 4 days (Rosenfeld, 1995).

Renal allograft: I.V.: 5-25 mg/kg/day

Acute GVHD treatment (unlabeled use): I.V.: 30 mg/kg/dose every other day for 6 doses (MacMillan, 2007) **or** 15 mg/kg/dose twice daily for 10 doses (MacMillan, 2002)

Adjustment for Toxicity

Anaphylaxis: Stop infusion immediately; administer epinephrine. May require corticosteroids, respiration assistance, and/or other resuscitative measures. Do not resume infusion.

Hemolysis (severe and unremitting): May require discontinuation of treatment.

Administration Infuse dose over at least 4 hours. Any severe systemic reaction to the skin test, such as generalized rash, tachycardia, dyspnea, hypotension, or anaphylaxis, should preclude further therapy. Epinephrine and resuscitative equipment should be nearby. Patient may need to be pretreated with an antipyretic, antihistamine, and/or corticosteroid. Mild itching and erythema can be treated with antihistamines. May cause vein irritation (chemical phlebitis) if administered peripherally. Infuse into a vascular shunt, arterial venous fistula, or high-flow central vein through a 0.2-1 micron in-line filter.

First dose: Premedicate with diphenhydramine orally 30 minutes prior to and hydrocortisone I.V. 15 minutes prior to infusion and acetaminophen 2 hours after start of infusion.

Monitoring Parameters Lymphocyte profile, CBC with differential and platelet count, vital signs during administration

Dosage Forms Excipient information presented when available (limited, particularly for generics); consult specific product labeling.

Injection, solution:

Atgam®: 50 mg/mL (5 mL)

References

Hardinger KL, Rhee S, Buchanan P, et al, "A Prospective, Randomized, Double-Blinded Comparison of Thymoglobulin Versus Atgam for Induction Immunosuppressive Therapy: 10 Year Results," *Transplantation*, 2008, 86(7):947-52.

MacMillan ML, Couriel D, Weisdorf DJ, et al, "A Phase 2/3 Multicenter Randomized Clinical Trial of ABX-CBL versus ATG as Secondary Therapy for Steroid-Resistant Acute Graft-Versus-Host-Disease," *Blood*, 2007, 109(6):2657-62.

MacMillan ML, Weisdorf DJ, Davies SM, et al, "Early Antithymocyte Globulin Therapy Improves Survival in Patients With Steroid-Resistant Acute Graft-Versus-Host Disease," *Biol Blood Marrow Transplant*, 2002, 8(1):40-6.

Molldrem JJ, Caples M, Mavroudis D, et al, "Antithymocyte Globulin for Patients With Myelodysplastic Syndrome," *Br J Haematol*, 1997, 99(3):699-705.

Molldrem JJ, Leifer E, Bahceci E, et al, "Antithymocyte Globulin for Treatment of Bone Marrow Failure Associated With Myelodysplastic Syndromes," *Ann Intern Med*, 2002, 137(3):156-63.
Rosenfeld SJ, Kimball J, Vining D, et al, "Intensive Immunosuppression With Antithymocyte Globulin and Cyclosporine as Treatment for Severe Acquired Aplastic Anemia," *Blood*, 1995, 85(11):3058-65.
Taylor DO, Edwards LB, Aurora P, et al, "Registry of the International Society for Heart and Lung Transplantation: Twenty-Fifth Official Adult Heart Transplant Report - 2008," *J Heart Lung Transplant*, 2008; 27(9):943-56.

Antithymocyte Globulin (Rabbit)

(an te THY moe site GLOB yu lin RAB bit)

Related Information

Hematopoietic Stem Cell Transplantation *on page* 1887

Brand Names: U.S. Thymoglobulin®

Index Terms Antithymocyte Immunoglobulin; rATG

Generic Availability (U.S.) No

Pharmacologic Category Immune Globulin; Immunosuppressant Agent; Polyclonal Antibody

Use Treatment of acute rejection of renal transplant; used in conjunction with concomitant immunosuppression

Unlabeled Use Induction therapy in renal transplant; treatment of myelodysplastic syndrome (MDS)

Labeled Contraindications Hypersensitivity to antithymocyte globulin, rabbit proteins, or any component of the formulation; acute or chronic infection

Pregnancy Risk Factor C

Lactation Excretion in breast milk unknown/use caution

Warnings/Precautions **[U.S. Boxed Warning]: Should only be used by physicians experienced in immunosuppressive therapy for the treatment of renal transplant patients.** Medical surveillance is required during the infusion. Initial dose must be administered over at least 6 hours into a high flow vein; patient may need pretreatment with an antipyretic, antihistamine, and/or corticosteroid. Hypersensitivity and fatal anaphylactic reactions can occur; immediate treatment (including epinephrine 1:1000) should be available. An increased incidence of lymphoma, post-transplant lymphoproliferative disease (PTLD), other malignancies, or severe infections may develop following concomitant use of immunosuppressants and prolonged use or overdose of antithymocyte globulin. Appropriate antiviral, antibacterial, antiprotozoal, and/or antifungal prophylaxis is recommended. Reversible neutropenia or thrombocytopenia may result from the development of cross-reactive antibodies.

Release of cytokines by activated monocytes and lymphocytes may cause fatal cytokine release syndrome (CRS) during administration of antithymocyte globulin. Rapid infusion rates of have been associated with CRS in case reports. Symptoms range from a mild, self-limiting "flu-like reaction" to severe, life-threatening reactions. Severe or life-threatening symptoms include hypotension, acute respiratory distress syndrome, pulmonary edema, myocardial infarction, and tachycardia. Patients should not be immunized with attenuated live viral vaccines during or shortly after treatment; safety of immunization following therapy has not been studied.

Adverse Reactions

>10%:

Cardiovascular: Hypertension, peripheral edema, tachycardia

Central nervous system: Chills, fever, headache, pain, malaise

Endocrine & metabolic: Hyperkalemia

Gastrointestinal: Abdominal pain, diarrhea, nausea
Genitourinary: Urinary tract infection
Hematologic: Leukopenia, thrombocytopenia
Neuromuscular & skeletal: Weakness
Respiratory: Dyspnea
Miscellaneous: Antirabbit antibody development, cytomegalovirus infection, sepsis, systemic infection

1% to 10%:
Central nervous system: Dizziness
Gastrointestinal: Gastritis, gastrointestinal moniliasis
Miscellaneous: Herpes simplex infection, oral moniliasis

Postmarketing and/or case reports: Anaphylaxis, cytokine release syndrome, PTLD, neutropenia, serum sickness (delayed)

Drug Interactions

Metabolism/Transport Effects None known.

Avoid Concomitant Use

Avoid concomitant use of Antithymocyte Globulin (Rabbit) with any of the following: BCG; Natalizumab; Pimecrolimus; Tacrolimus (Topical); Vaccines (Live)

Increased Effect/Toxicity

Antithymocyte Globulin (Rabbit) may increase the levels/effects of: Leflunomide; Natalizumab; Vaccines (Live)

The levels/effects of Antithymocyte Globulin (Rabbit) may be increased by: Denosumab; Pimecrolimus; Roflumilast; Tacrolimus (Topical); Trastuzumab

Decreased Effect

Antithymocyte Globulin (Rabbit) may decrease the levels/effects of: BCG; Coccidioidin Skin Test; Sipuleucel-T; Vaccines (Inactivated); Vaccines (Live)

The levels/effects of Antithymocyte Globulin (Rabbit) may be decreased by: Echinacea

Storage/Stability Store powder under refrigeration at 2°C to 8°C (36°F to 46°F); do not freeze. Protect from light. Reconstituted product is stable for up to 24 hours at room temperature; however, since it contains no preservatives, it should be used immediately following reconstitution.

Reconstitution Allow vials to reach room temperature, then reconstitute each vial with SWFI 5 mL. Rotate vial gently until dissolved. Prior to administration, further dilute one vial in 50 mL saline or dextrose (total volume is usually 50-500 mL depending on total number of vials needed per dose). Mix by gently inverting infusion bag once or twice.

Mechanism of Action Polyclonal antibody which appears to cause immunosuppression by acting on T-cell surface antigens and depleting CD4 lymphocytes

Pharmacodynamics/Kinetics

Duration: Lymphopenia may persist ≥1 year
Half-life elimination, plasma: 2-3 days

Dosing

Adult & Geriatric Treatment of acute rejection: I.V.: 1.5 mg/kg/day for 7-14 days

Pediatric Refer to adult dosing.

Adjustment for Toxicity

WBC count 2000-3000 cells/mm^3 or platelet count 50,000-75,000 cells/mm^3: Reduce dose by 50%

WBC count <2000 cells/mm^3 or platelet count <50,000 cells/mm^3: Consider discontinuing treatment

Administration The first dose should be infused over at least 6 hours through a high-flow vein. Subsequent doses should be administered over at least 4 hours. Administer through an in-line 0.22 micron filter. Premedication with corticosteroids, acetaminophen, and/or an antihistamine may reduce infusion-related reactions.

Monitoring Parameters Lymphocyte profile, CBC with differential and platelet count; vital signs during administration; signs and symptoms of infection

Test Interactions Potential interference with rabbit antibody-based immunoassays

Dosage Forms Excipient information presented when available (limited, particularly for generics); consult specific product labeling.

Injection, powder for reconstitution:

Thymoglobulin®: 25 mg

References

Broliden PA, Dahl IM, Hast R, et al, "Antithymocyte Globulin and Cyclosporine A as Combination Therapy for Low-Risk Non-Sideroblastic Myelodysplastic Syndromes," *Haematologica*, 2006, 91 (5):667-70.

Hardinger KL, "Rabbit Antithymocyte Globulin Induction Therapy in Adult Renal Transplantation," *Pharmacotherapy*, 2006, 26(12):1771-83.

◆ **Antithymocyte Immunoglobulin** *see* Antithymocyte Globulin (Equine) *on page* 111

◆ **Antithymocyte Immunoglobulin** *see* Antithymocyte Globulin (Rabbit) *on page* 115

◆ **Anti-VEGF Monoclonal Antibody** *see* Bevacizumab *on page* 165

◆ **Anti-VEGF rhuMAb** *see* Bevacizumab *on page* 165

◆ **Anucort-HC™** *see* Hydrocortisone (Topical) *on page* 719

◆ **Anu-med HC** *see* Hydrocortisone (Topical) *on page* 719

◆ **Anusol-HC®** *see* Hydrocortisone (Topical) *on page* 719

◆ **Anzemet®** *see* Dolasetron *on page* 462

◆ **APC8015** *see* Sipuleucel-T *on page* 1279

◆ **APO-066** *see* Deferiprone *on page* 412

◆ **Apo-Acyclovir® (Can)** *see* Acyclovir (Systemic) *on page* 30

◆ **Apo-Anastrozole® (Can)** *see* Anastrozole *on page* 96

◆ **Apo-Benzydamine® (Can)** *see* Benzydamine *on page* 164

◆ **Apo-Bicalutamide® (Can)** *see* Bicalutamide *on page* 178

◆ **Apo-Calcitonin® (Can)** *see* Calcitonin *on page* 214

◆ **Apo-Ciproflox® (Can)** *see* Ciprofloxacin (Systemic) *on page* 283

◆ **Apo-Cyclosporine® (Can)** *see* CycloSPORINE (Systemic) *on page* 333

◆ **Apo-Desmopressin® (Can)** *see* Desmopressin *on page* 434

◆ **Apo-Dexamethasone® (Can)** *see* Dexamethasone (Systemic) *on page* 440

◆ **Apo-Famciclovir® (Can)** *see* Famciclovir *on page* 580

◆ **Apo-Fluconazole® (Can)** *see* Fluconazole *on page* 612

◆ **Apo-Flutamide® (Can)** *see* Flutamide *on page* 635

◆ **Apo-Haloperidol® (Can)** *see* Haloperidol *on page* 691

◆ **Apo-Haloperidol LA® (Can)** *see* Haloperidol *on page* 691

◆ **Apo-Hydroxyurea® (Can)** *see* Hydroxyurea *on page* *731*

◆ **Apo-Hydroxyzine® (Can)** *see* HydrOXYzine *on page* *736*

◆ **Apo-Ketoconazole® (Can)** *see* Ketoconazole (Systemic) *on page* *848*

◆ **APO-Levofloxacin (Can)** *see* Levofloxacin (Systemic) *on page* *883*

◆ **Apo-Lorazepam® (Can)** *see* LORazepam *on page* *907*

◆ **Apo-Medroxy® (Can)** *see* MedroxyPROGESTERone *on page* *916*

◆ **Apo-Megestrol® (Can)** *see* Megestrol *on page* *922*

◆ **Apo-Methotrexate® (Can)** *see* Methotrexate *on page* *949*

◆ **Apo-Metoclop® (Can)** *see* Metoclopramide *on page* *974*

◆ **Apo-Metronidazole® (Can)** *see* MetroNIDAZOLE (Systemic) *on page* *978*

◆ **Apo-Mycophenolate (Can)** *see* Mycophenolate *on page* *1015*

◆ **Apo-Oflox® (Can)** *see* Ofloxacin (Systemic) *on page* *1053*

◆ **Apo-Olanzapine® (Can)** *see* OLANZapine *on page* *1056*

◆ **Apo-Olanzapine ODT® (Can)** *see* OLANZapine *on page* *1056*

◆ **Apo-Ondansetron® (Can)** *see* Ondansetron *on page* *1068*

◆ **Apo-Paclitaxel® (Can)** *see* PACLitaxel *on page* *1092*

◆ **Apo-Prednisone® (Can)** *see* PredniSONE *on page* *1199*

◆ **Apo-Prochlorperazine® (Can)** *see* Prochlorperazine *on page* *1212*

◆ **Apo-Raloxifene® (Can)** *see* Raloxifene *on page* *1222*

◆ **Apo-Sulfatrim® (Can)** *see* Sulfamethoxazole and Trimethoprim *on page* *1302*

◆ **Apo-Sulfatrim® DS (Can)** *see* Sulfamethoxazole and Trimethoprim *on page* *1302*

◆ **Apo-Sulfatrim® Pediatric (Can)** *see* Sulfamethoxazole and Trimethoprim *on page* *1302*

◆ **Apo-Tamox® (Can)** *see* Tamoxifen *on page* *1324*

◆ **Apo-Valacyclovir® (Can)** *see* Valacyclovir *on page* *1420*

Aprepitant (ap RE pi tant)

Related Information

Management of Chemotherapy-Induced Nausea and Vomiting *on page* *1786*

Palliative Care Medicine (Cancer) *on page* *1871*

Brand Names: U.S. Emend®

Brand Names: Canada Emend®

Index Terms L 754030; MK 869

Generic Availability (U.S.) No

Pharmacologic Category Antiemetic; Substance P/Neurokinin 1 Receptor Antagonist

Use Prevention of acute and delayed nausea and vomiting associated with moderately- and highly-emetogenic chemotherapy (in combination with other antiemetics); prevention of postoperative nausea and vomiting (PONV)

Labeled Contraindications Hypersensitivity to aprepitant or any component of the formulation; concurrent use with cisapride or pimozide

Pregnancy Risk Factor B

Lactation Excretion in breast milk unknown/not recommended

Warnings/Precautions Use caution with agents primarily metabolized via CYP3A4; aprepitant is a 3A4 inhibitor. Effect on orally administered 3A4 substrates is greater than those administered intravenously. Chronic continuous use is not recommended; however, a single 40 mg aprepitant oral dose is not likely to alter plasma concentrations of CYP3A4 substrates. Use caution with severe hepatic impairment; has not been studied in patients with severe hepatic impairment (Child-Pugh class C). Not studied for treatment of existing nausea and vomiting. Chronic continuous administration is not recommended.

Adverse Reactions Note: Adverse reactions reported as part of a combination chemotherapy regimen or with general anesthesia.

>10%:

Central nervous system: Fatigue (≤18%)
Gastrointestinal: Nausea (6% to 13%), constipation (9% to 10%)
Neuromuscular & skeletal: Weakness (≤18%)
Miscellaneous: Hiccups (11%)

1% to 10%:

Cardiovascular: Hypotension (≤6%), bradycardia (≤4%)
Central nervous system: Dizziness (≤7%)
Endocrine & metabolic: Dehydration (≤6%)
Gastrointestinal: Diarrhea (≤10%), dyspepsia (≤6%), abdominal pain (≤5%), epigastric discomfort (4%), gastritis (4%), stomatitis (3%)
Hepatic: ALT increased (≤6%), AST increased (3%)
Renal: Proteinuria (7%), BUN increased (5%)

>0.5%: Acid reflux, acne, albumin decreased, alkaline phosphatase increased, anemia, anxiety, appetite decreased, arthralgia, back pain, bilirubin increased, candidiasis, confusion, conjunctivitis, cough, deglutition disorder, depression, diabetes mellitus, diaphoresis, DVT, dysphagia, dyspnea, dysuria, edema, eructation, erythrocyturia, febrile neutropenia, flatulence, flushing, glucosuria, herpes simplex, hyperglycemia, hypertension, hypoesthesia, hypokalemia, hyponatremia, hypothermia, hypovolemia, hypoxia, leukocytes increased, leukocyturia, malaise, MI, muscular weakness, musculoskeletal pain, myalgia, nasal secretion, obstipation, pain, palpitation, pelvic pain, peripheral neuropathy, pharyngitis, pharyngolaryngeal pain, pneumonitis, pruritus, pulmonary embolism, rash, renal insufficiency, respiratory infection, respiratory insufficiency, rigors, salivation increased, sensory neuropathy, septic shock, syncope, tachycardia, taste disturbance, thrombocytopenia, tremor, urinary tract infection, urticaria, vocal disturbance, weight loss, xerostomia

<0.5%, postmarketing, and/or case reports: Anaphylactic reaction, angioedema, disorientation, duodenal ulcer (perforating), dysarthria, enterocolitis, hypersensitivity reaction, miosis, neutropenic sepsis, pneumonia, sensory disturbance, Stevens-Johnson syndrome, toxic epidermal necrolysis, visual acuity decreased, wheezing

Drug Interactions

Metabolism/Transport Effects Substrate of CYP1A2 (minor), CYP2C19 (minor), CYP3A4 (major); **Note:** Assignment of Major/Minor substrate status based on clinically relevant drug interaction potential; **Inhibits** CYP2C19 (weak), CYP2C9 (weak), CYP3A4 (moderate); **Induces** CYP2C9 (strong), CYP3A4 (weak/moderate)

Avoid Concomitant Use

Avoid concomitant use of Aprepitant with any of the following: Axitinib; Bosutinib; Cisapride; Conivaptan; Pimozide; Tolvaptan

Increased Effect/Toxicity

Aprepitant may increase the levels/effects of: ARIPiprazole; Avanafil; Benzodiazepines (metabolized by oxidation); Bosutinib; Budesonide (Systemic, Oral Inhalation); Cisapride; Colchicine; Corticosteroids (Systemic); CYP3A4 Substrates; Diltiazem; Eplerenone; Everolimus; FentaNYL; Halofantrine; Ivacaftor; Lurasidone; Pimecrolimus; Pimozide; Propafenone; Ranolazine; Salmeterol; Saxagliptin; Tolvaptan; Vilazodone; Zuclopenthixol

The levels/effects of Aprepitant may be increased by: Antifungal Agents (Azole Derivatives, Systemic); Conivaptan; CYP3A4 Inhibitors (Moderate); CYP3A4 Inhibitors (Strong); Dasatinib; Diltiazem; Ivacaftor; Mifepristone

Decreased Effect

Aprepitant may decrease the levels/effects of: ARIPiprazole; Axitinib; Contraceptives (Estrogens); Contraceptives (Progestins); CYP2C9 Substrates; Diclofenac (Systemic); Ifosfamide; PARoxetine; Saxagliptin; TOLBUTamide; Warfarin

The levels/effects of Aprepitant may be decreased by: CYP3A4 Inducers (Strong); Deferasirox; Herbs (CYP3A4 Inducers); PARoxetine; Rifamycin Derivatives; Tocilizumab

Ethanol/Nutrition/Herb Interactions

Food: Aprepitant serum concentration may be increased when taken with grapefruit juice; avoid concurrent use.

Herb/Nutraceutical: Avoid St John's wort (may decrease aprepitant levels).

Storage/Stability Store at room temperature of 20°C to 25°C (68°F to 77°F).

Mechanism of Action Prevents acute and delayed vomiting by inhibiting the substance P/neurokinin 1 (NK_1) receptor; augments the antiemetic activity of 5-HT_3 receptor antagonists and corticosteroids to inhibit acute and delayed phases of chemotherapy-induced emesis.

Pharmacodynamics/Kinetics

Distribution: V_d: ~70 L; crosses the blood-brain barrier

Protein binding: >95%

Metabolism: Extensively hepatic via CYP3A4 (major); CYP1A2 and CYP2C19 (minor); forms 7 metabolites (weakly active)

Bioavailability: ~60% to 65%

Half-life elimination: Terminal: ~9-13 hours

Time to peak, plasma: ~3-4 hours

Dosing

Adult & Geriatric

Prevention of chemotherapy-induced nausea/vomiting: Oral: 125 mg 1 hour prior to chemotherapy on day 1, followed by 80 mg once daily on days 2 and 3 (in combination with a corticosteroid and 5-HT_3 antagonist antiemetic)

Prevention of PONV: Oral: 40 mg within 3 hours prior to induction

Renal Impairment No dose adjustment necessary in patients with renal disease or end-stage renal disease maintained on hemodialysis.

Hepatic Impairment

Mild-to-moderate impairment (Child-Pugh class A or B): No adjustment necessary.

Severe impairment (Child-Pugh class C): Use caution; no data available.

Administration

Chemotherapy-induced nausea/vomiting: Administer with or without food. First dose should be given 1 hour prior to antineoplastic therapy; subsequent doses should be given in the morning.

PONV: Administer within 3 hours prior to induction; follow healthcare providers instructions about food/drink restrictions prior to surgery.

Extemporaneous Preparations A 20 mg/mL oral aprepitant suspension may be prepared with capsules and a 1:1 combination of Ora-Sweet® and Ora-Plus® (or Ora-Blend®). Empty the contents of four 125 mg capsules into a mortar and reduce to a fine powder (process will take 10-15 minutes). Add small portions of vehicle and mix to a uniform paste. Add sufficient vehicle to form a liquid; transfer to a graduated cylinder, rinse mortar with vehicle, and add quantity of vehicle sufficient to make 25 mL. Label "shake well" and "refrigerate". Stable for 90 days refrigerated.

Dupuis LL, Lingertat-Walsh K, and Walker SE, "Stability of an Extemporaneous Oral Liquid Aprepitant Formulation," *Support Care Cancer*, 2009, 17(6):701-6.

Dietary Considerations May be taken with or without food.

Additional Information Oncology Comment: Aprepitant is recommended in the American Society of Clinical Oncology (ASCO) oncology antiemetic guidelines for use in combination with a serotonin receptor antagonist and dexamethasone for chemotherapy with high emetic risk and for chemotherapy regimens of moderate emetic risk which contain an anthracycline and cyclophosphamide (Kris, 2006). The National Comprehensive Cancer Network® (NCCN) Clinical Practice Guidelines in Oncology for Antiemesis (version 1.2011) recommend the same use of aprepitant as is in the ASCO recommendation. In addition to the moderately emetogenic chemotherapy listed above, the NCCN guidelines suggest that aprepitant may also be used for select moderately emetogenic regimens containing carboplatin, cisplatin, doxorubicin, epirubicin, ifosfamide, irinotecan and methotrexate. Either fosaprepitant 115 mg or aprepitant (125 mg orally) are administered on day 1; for day 2 and 3, patients should receive aprepitant 80 mg orally.

Dosage Forms Excipient information presented when available (limited, particularly for generics); consult specific product labeling.

Capsule, oral:

Emend®: 40 mg, 80 mg, 125 mg

Combination package, oral [each package contains]:

Emend®: Capsule: 80 mg (2s) and Capsule: 125 mg (1s)

References

Kris MG, Hesketh PJ, Somerfield MR, et al, "American Society of Clinical Oncology Guideline for Antiemetics in Oncology: Update 2006," *J Clin Oncol*, 2006, 24(18):2932-47.

Multinational Association of Supportive Care in Cancer (MASCC), "Antiemetic Guidelines," Updated April 2010. Available at http://data.memberclicks.com/site/mascc/MASCC_Guidelines_English_2010.pdf

National Comprehensive Cancer Network® (NCCN), "Clinical Practice Guidelines in Oncology™: Antiemesis," Version 1.2011. Available at http://www.nccn.org/professionals/physician_gls/PDF/antiemesis.pdf

◆ **Aprepitant Injection** *see* Fosaprepitant *on page 640*

◆ **Aquacort® (Can)** *see* Hydrocortisone (Topical) *on page 719*

◆ **AquaMEPHYTON® (Can)** *see* Phytonadione *on page 1169*

◆ **Aquanil HC® [OTC]** *see* Hydrocortisone (Topical) *on page 719*

◆ **Aquoral™** *see* Saliva Substitute *on page 1266*

◆ **Ara-C** *see* Cytarabine (Conventional) *on page 348*

◆ **Arabinosylcytosine** *see* Cytarabine (Conventional) *on page 348*

◆ **Aranesp®** *see* Darbepoetin Alfa *on page 382*

◆ **Aranesp® SingleJect®** *see* Darbepoetin Alfa *on page 382*

◆ **Aredia®** *see* Pamidronate *on page 1109*

◆ **Arimidex®** *see* Anastrozole *on page 96*

◆ **Arixtra®** *see* Fondaparinux *on page 638*

◆ **Aromasin®** *see* Exemestane *on page 564*

◆ **Arranon®** *see* Nelarabine *on page 1028*

Arsenic Trioxide (AR se nik tri OKS id)

Related Information

Management of Chemotherapy-Induced Nausea and Vomiting *on page 1786*

Management of Drug Extravasations *on page 1800*

Safe Handling of Hazardous Drugs *on page 1904*

Brand Names: U.S. Trisenox®

Index Terms As_2O_3

Generic Availability (U.S.) No

Pharmacologic Category Antineoplastic Agent, Miscellaneous

Use Remission induction and consolidation in patients with relapsed or refractory acute promyelocytic leukemia (APL) characterized by t(15;17) translocation or PML/RAR-alpha gene expression

Unlabeled Use Initial treatment of APL, treatment of myelodysplastic syndrome (MDS)

Labeled Contraindications Hypersensitivity to arsenic or any component of the formulation

Pregnancy Risk Factor D

Lactation Enters breast milk/not recommended

Warnings/Precautions Hazardous agent - use appropriate precautions for handling and disposal. **[U.S. Boxed Warnings]: May prolong the QT interval. May lead to torsade de pointes or complete AV block.** Risk factors for torsade de pointes include extent of prolongation, HF, a history of torsade de pointes, pre-existing QT interval prolongation, patients taking medications know to prolong the QT interval or potassium-wasting diuretics, and conditions which cause hypokalemia or hypomagnesemia. If possible, discontinue all medications known to prolong the QT interval. **[U.S. Boxed Warning]: A baseline 12-lead ECG, serum electrolytes (potassium, calcium, magnesium), and creatinine should be obtained prior to treatment.** Correct electrolyte abnormalities prior to treatment and monitor potassium and magnesium levels during therapy (maintain potassium >4 mEq/dL and magnesium >1.8 mg/dL). If baseline QT_c >500 msec, correct prior to treatment. If QT_c >500 msec during treatment, reassess, correct contributing factors, and consider temporarily withholding treatment. If syncope or irregular heartbeat develop during therapy, hospitalize patient and do not reinitiate until QT_c <460 msec, electrolyte abnormalities are corrected and syncope/irregular heartbeat has resolved. Monitor ECG weekly; more frequently if clinically indicated.

[U.S. Boxed Warning]: May cause APL differentiation syndrome (formerly called retinoic-acid-APL [RA-APL] syndrome) in patients with APL, which is characterized by dyspnea, fever, weight gain, pulmonary infiltrates, and pleural or pericardial effusions. May be fatal. High-dose steroids (dexamethasone 10 mg I.V. twice daily for ≥3 days; begin at initial presentation) have been used for treatment; in general, most patients may continue arsenic trioxide during treatment of APL differentiation syndrome. May lead to the development of hyperleukocytosis (leukocytes ≥10,000/mm^3); did not correlate with baseline WBC counts and generally was not as high during consolidation as observed during induction treatment. Use with caution in patients with hepatic impairment; in patients with severe hepatic impairment, monitor closely for toxicity. Use with caution in patients with severe renal impairment; systemic exposure to metabolites may be higher; has not been studied in dialysis patients. Monitor electrolytes, CBC with differential, and coagulation parameters at least twice a week during induction and weekly during consolidation; more frequently if clinically indicated. **[U.S. Boxed Warning]: Should be administered under the supervision of a physician experienced in acute leukemia management.**

Adverse Reactions

>10%:

Cardiovascular: Tachycardia (55%), edema (40%), QT interval >500 msec (40%), chest pain (25%; grades 3/4: 5%), hypotension (25%; grades 3/4: 5%)

Central nervous system: Fatigue (63%), fever (63%), headache (60%), insomnia (43%), anxiety (30%), dizziness (23%), depression (20%), pain (15%)

Dermatologic: Dermatitis (43%), pruritus (33%), bruising (20%), dry skin (15%), erythema (13%)

Endocrine & metabolic: Hypokalemia (50%; grades 3/4: 13%), hyperglycemia (45%; grades 3/4: 13%), hypomagnesemia (45%; grades 3/4: 13%), hyperkalemia (18%; grades 3/4: 5%)

Gastrointestinal: Nausea (75%), abdominal pain (58%), vomiting (58%), diarrhea (53%), sore throat (35%), constipation (28%), anorexia (23%), appetite decreased (15%), weight gain (13%)

Genitourinary: Vaginal hemorrhage (13%)

Hematologic: Leukocytosis (50%; grades 3/4: 3%), APL differentiation syndrome (23%; grades 3/4: 8%), anemia (20%; grades 3/4: 5%), thrombocytopenia (18%; grades 3/4: 13%), febrile neutropenia (13%; grades 3/4: 8%)

Hepatic: ALT increased (20%; grades 3/4: 5%), AST increased (13%; grades 3/4: 3%)

Local: Injection site: Pain (20%), erythema (13%)

Neuromuscular & skeletal: Rigors (38%), arthralgia (33%), paresthesia (33%), myalgia (25%), bone pain (23%), back pain (18%), limb pain (13%), neck pain (13%), tremor (13%)

Respiratory: Cough (65%), dyspnea (53%; grades 3/4: 10%), epistaxis (25%), hypoxia (23%), pleural effusion (20%), sinusitis (20%), postnasal drip (13%), upper respiratory tract infection (13%), wheezing (13%)

Miscellaneous: Herpes simplex (13%), diaphoresis (13%)

1% to 10%:

Cardiovascular: Hypertension (10%), flushing (10%), pallor (10%), palpitation (10%), facial edema (8%), abnormal ECG (not QT prolongation) (8%), atrial dysrhythmia (5%), torsade de pointes (3%)

Central nervous system: Seizure (8%; grades 3/4: 5%), somnolence (8%), agitation (5%), coma (5%), confusion (5%)

Dermatologic: Hyperpigmentation (8%), petechia (8%), skin lesions (8%), urticaria (8%), local exfoliation (5%)

Endocrine & metabolic: Hypocalcemia (10%), hypoglycemia (8%), intermenstrual bleeding (8%), acidosis (5%)

Gastrointestinal: Dyspepsia (10%), loose stools (10%), abdominal distension (8%), abdominal tenderness (8%), caecitis (children: 8%), fecal incontinence (8%), gastrointestinal hemorrhage (8%), hemorrhagic diarrhea (8%), oral blistering (8%), weight loss (8%), xerostomia (8%), oral candidiasis (5%)

Genitourinary: Incontinence (5%)
Hematologic: Neutropenia (10%; grades 3/4: 10%), DIC (8%), hemorrhage (8%)
Local: Injection site edema (10%)
Neuromuscular & skeletal: Weakness (10%)
Ocular: Blurred vision (10%), eye irritation (10%), dry eye (8%), eyelid edema (5%), painful red eye (5%)
Otic: Earache (8%), tinnitus (5%)
Renal: Renal failure (8%; grades 3/4: 3%), renal impairment (8%), oliguria (5%)
Respiratory: Breath sounds decreased (10%), crepitations (10%), rales (10%), hemoptysis (8%), pulmonary edema (children: 8%), rhonchi (8%), tachypnea (8%), nasopharyngitis (5%)
Miscellaneous: Bacterial infection (8%), herpes zoster (8%), lymphadenopathy (8%), night sweats (8%), hypersensitivity (5%), sepsis (5%; grades 3/4: 5%)

<1%, postmarketing, and/or case reports: Acute respiratory distress syndrome, AV block, capillary leak syndrome, CHF, dysphagia, enuresis, heart block, hypoalbuminemia, hyponatremia, hypophosphatemia, lipase increased, mitochondrial myopathy, mucosal inflammation, neuralgia, oropharyngeal pain, pancytopenia, peripheral neuropathy, pneumonitis, pulmonary infiltrate, respiratory distress, stomatitis, ventricular extrasystoles, ventricular tachycardia

Drug Interactions

Metabolism/Transport Effects None known.

Avoid Concomitant Use

Avoid concomitant use of Arsenic Trioxide with any of the following: CloZAPine; Highest Risk QTc-Prolonging Agents; Mifepristone; Moderate Risk QTc-Prolonging Agents

Increased Effect/Toxicity

Arsenic Trioxide may increase the levels/effects of: CloZAPine; Highest Risk QTc-Prolonging Agents; Hypoglycemic Agents

The levels/effects of Arsenic Trioxide may be increased by: Herbs (Hypoglycemic Properties); MAO Inhibitors; Mifepristone; Moderate Risk QTc-Prolonging Agents; QTc-Prolonging Agents (Indeterminate Risk and Risk Modifying); Salicylates; Selective Serotonin Reuptake Inhibitors

Decreased Effect

The levels/effects of Arsenic Trioxide may be decreased by: Loop Diuretics

Ethanol/Nutrition/Herb Interactions Herb/Nutraceutical: Avoid homeopathic products (arsenic is present in some homeopathic medications). Avoid hypoglycemic herbs, including alfalfa, aloe, bilberry, bitter melon, burdock, celery, damiana, fenugreek, garcinia, garlic, ginger, ginseng, gymnema, marshmallow, and stinging nettle (may enhance the hypoglycemic effect of arsenic trioxide).

Storage/Stability Store at 25°C (77°F); excursions permitted to 15°C to 30°C (59°F to 86°F); do not freeze. Following dilution, stable for 24 hours at room temperature or 48 hours when refrigerated.

Reconstitution Dilute in 100-250 mL D_5W or 0.9% NaCl. Discard unused portion of ampul. Use appropriate precautions for handling and disposal.

Mechanism of Action Induces apoptosis in APL cells via morphological changes and DNA fragmentation; also damages or degrades the fusion protein PML-RAR alpha

Pharmacodynamics/Kinetics

Distribution: V_{dss}: As^{III}: 562 L; widely distributed throughout body tissues; orally administered arsenic trioxide distributes into the CNS

Metabolism: Arsenic trioxide is immediately hydrolyzed to the active form, arsenious acid (As^{III}) which is methylated (hepatically) to the less active pentavalent metabolites, monomethylarsonic acid (MMA^{V}) and dimethylarsinic acid (DMA^{V}) by methyltransferases; As^{III} is also oxidized to the minor metabolite, arsenic acid (As^{V})

Half-life elimination: AS^{III}: 10-14 hours; MMA^{V}: ~32 hours; DMA^{V}: ~72 hours

Time to peak: As^{III}: At the end of infusion; MMA^{V} and DMA^{V}; ~10-24 hours

Excretion: Urine (MMA^{V}, DMA^{V}, and 15% of a dose as unchanged As^{III})

Dosing

Adult

APL, relapsed or refractory: I.V.:

Induction: 0.15 mg/kg/day; administer daily until bone marrow remission; maximum induction: 60 doses

Consolidation: 0.15 mg/kg/day starting 3-6 weeks after completion of induction therapy; maximum consolidation: 25 doses over a period of up to 5 weeks

APL initial treatment (unlabeled use): I.V.:

Induction, consolidation, and maintenance (Mathews, 2006):

Induction: 10 mg/day; administer daily until bone marrow remission; maximum induction: 60 doses

Consolidation: 10 mg/day for 4 weeks, starting 4 weeks after completion of induction therapy

Maintenance: 10 mg/dose administered 10 days per month for 6 months, starting 4 weeks after completion of consolidation therapy

Consolidation therapy after remission induction with tretinoin, daunorubicin and cytarabine (Powell, 2007; Powell, 2010): Two consolidation courses (2 weeks apart): 0.15 mg/kg/day 5 days/week for 5 weeks

In combination with tretinoin (Estey, 2006; Ravandi, 2009):

Induction (beginning 10 days after initiation of tretinoin): 0.15 mg/kg/day until bone marrow remission; maximum induction: 75 doses

Consolidation: 0.15 mg/kg/day Monday through Friday for 4 weeks every 8 weeks for 4 cycles (weeks 1 to 4, 9 to 12, 17 to 20, and 25 to 28)

MDS (unlabeled uses): I.V.: 0.25 mg/kg/day 5 consecutive days/week for 2 weeks, followed by a 2-week rest period (Schiller, 2006)

Pediatric

APL, relapsed or refractory: I.V.: Children ≥4 years: Refer to adult dosing.

APL initial treatment (unlabeled use): I.V.: *Induction, consolidation, and maintenance (Mathews, 2006).*

Induction: 0.15 mg/kg/day (maximum dose: 10 mg); administer daily until bone marrow remission, maximum induction: 60 doses

Consolidation: 0.15 mg/kg/day (maximum dose: 10 mg) for 4 weeks, starting 4 weeks after completion of induction therapy

Maintenance: 0.15 mg/kg/dose (maximum dose: 10 mg) administered 10 days per month for 6 months, starting 4 weeks after completion of consolidation therapy

Renal Impairment

Severe renal impairment (Cl_{cr} <30 mL/minute): Use with caution (systemic exposure to metabolites may be higher); may require dosage reduction; monitor closely for toxicity.

Dialysis patients: Has not been studied.

Hepatic Impairment

Hepatic impairment: Use with caution.

Severe hepatic impairment (Child-Pugh class C): Monitor closely for toxicity.

Combination Regimens

Leukemia, acute promyelocytic: Tretinoin-Arsenic Trioxide (APL) on page 1761

Administration Administer as I.V. infusion over 1-2 hours. If acute vasomotor reactions occur, infuse over a maximum of 4 hours. Does not require administration via a central venous catheter.

Emetic Potential Moderate (30% to 90%)

Vesicant/Extravasation Risk May be an irritant

Monitoring Parameters Baseline then weekly 12-lead ECG; monitor electrolytes, CBC with differential, and coagulation at baseline then at least twice weekly during induction and at least weekly during consolidation; more frequent monitoring may be necessary in unstable patients

Dosage Forms Excipient information presented when available (limited, particularly for generics); consult specific product labeling.

Injection, solution [preservative free]:

Trisenox®: 1 mg/mL (10 mL)

References

Estey E, Garcia-Manero G, Ferrajoli A, et al, "Use of All-Trans Retinoic Acid Plus Arsenic Trioxide as an Alternative to Chemotherapy in Untreated Acute Promyelocytic Leukemia," *Blood*, 2006, 107(9):3469-73.

Gore SD, Gojo I, Sekeres MA, et al, "Single Cycle of Arsenic Trioxide-Based Consolidation Chemotherapy Spares Anthracycline Exposure in the Primary Management of Acute Promyelocytic Leukemia," *J Clin Oncol*, 2010, 28(6):1047-53.

Mathews V, George B, Chendamarai E, et al, "Single-Agent Arsenic Trioxide in the Treatment of Newly Diagnosed Acute Promyelocytic Leukemia: Long-Term Follow-Up Data," *J Clin Oncol*, 2010, 28(24):3866-71.

Mathews V, George B, Lakshmi KM, et al, "Single-Agent Arsenic Trioxide in the Treatment of Newly Diagnosed Acute Promyelocytic Leukemia: Durable Remissions With Minimal Toxicity," *Blood*, 2006, 107(7):2627-32.

Powell BL, Moser B, Stock W, et al, "Arsenic Trioxide Improves Event-Free and Over-All Survival for Adults With Acute Promyelocytic Leukemia: North American Leukemia Intergroup Study C9710," *Blood*, 2010, 116(19):3751-7.

Powell BL, Moser B, Stock W, et al, "Effect of Consolidation With Arsenic Trioxide (As2O3) on Event-Free Survival (EFS) and Overall Survival (OS) Among Patients With Newly Diagnosed Acute Promyelocytic Leukemia (APL): North American Intergroup Protocol C9710," *J Clin Oncol*, 2007, 25(18s):2 [abstract 2 from 2007 ASCO Annual Meeting].

Ravandi F, Estey E, Jones D, et al, "Effective Treatment of Acute Promyelocytic Leukemia With All-Trans-Retinoic Acid, Arsenic Trioxide, and Gemtuzumab Ozogamicin," *J Clin Oncol*, 2009, 27(4):504-10.

Schiller GJ, Slack J, Hainsworth JD, et al, "Phase II Multicenter Study of Arsenic Trioxide in Patients With Myelodysplastic Syndromes," *J Clin Oncol*, 2006, 24(16):2456-64.

Vey N, Bosly A, Guerci A, et al, "Arsenic Trioxide in Patients With Myelodysplastic Syndromes: A Phase II Multicenter Study," *J Clin Oncol*, 2006, 24(16):2465-71.

- **Artificial Saliva** *see* Saliva Substitute *on page 1266*
- **Arzerra™** *see* Ofatumumab *on page 1050*
- **As_2O_3** *see* Arsenic Trioxide *on page 122*
- **Asparaginase** *see* Asparaginase (*E. coli*) *on page 130*

Asparaginase (*Erwinia*) (a SPEAR a ji nase er WIN i ah)

Related Information

Management of Chemotherapy-Induced Nausea and Vomiting *on page 1786*

Brand Names: U.S. Erwinaze™

Brand Names: Canada Erwinase®

Index Terms *Erwinia chrysanthemi*; Asparaginase *Erwinia chrysanthemi*; L-asparaginase (*Erwinia*)

Generic Availability (U.S.) No

Pharmacologic Category Antineoplastic Agent, Miscellaneous; Enzyme

Use Treatment (in combination with other chemotherapy) of acute lymphoblastic leukemia (ALL) in patients with hypersensitivity to *E. coli*-derived asparaginase

Labeled Contraindications History of serious hypersensitivity reactions, including anaphylaxis to asparaginase (*Erwinia*) or any component of the formulation; history of serious pancreatitis, serious thrombosis, or serious hemorrhagic event with prior asparaginase treatment

Canadian labeling: Additional contraindications (not in the U.S. labeling): Women who are or may become pregnant

Pregnancy Risk Factor C

Lactation Excretion in breast milk unknown/not recommended

Warnings/Precautions Hazardous agent - use appropriate precautions for handling and disposal.

Serious hypersensitivity reactions, including anaphylaxis, have occurred in 5% of patients in clinical trials. Immediate treatment for hypersensitivity reactions should be available during treatment; discontinue for serious hypersensitivity (and administer appropriate treatment for reaction).

Pancreatitis has been reported in 4% of patients in clinical trials, promptly evaluate with symptoms suggestive of pancreatitis. For mild pancreatitis, withhold treatment until signs and symptoms subside and amylase returns to normal; may resume after resolution. Discontinue for severe or hemorrhagic pancreatitis characterized by abdominal pain >72 hours and amylase ≥2 x ULN. Further use is contraindicated if severe pancreatitis is diagnosed.

Serious thrombotic events, including sagittal sinus thrombosis, have been reported with asparaginase formulations. Decreases in fibrinogen, protein C activity, protein S activity, and antithrombin III have been noted following a 2-week treatment course. Discontinue for hemorrhagic or thrombotic events; may resume treatment after resolution (contraindicated with history of serious thrombosis or hemorrhagic event with prior asparaginase treatment).

In clinical trials, 2% of patients experienced glucose intolerance; may be irreversible; monitor glucose levels (baseline and periodic) during treatment; may require insulin administration.

Adverse Reactions

>10%: Miscellaneous: Allergic reaction/hypersensitivity (17%; grades 3/4: 5% to 9%; includes anaphylaxis, urticaria)

1% to 10%:

Cardiovascular: Thrombosis (2%; grades 3/4: ≤1%)

Central nervous system: Fever (3%), headache (1%), seizure (1%)

Endocrine & metabolic: Glucose intolerance (2%), hyperglycemia (2%; grades 3/4: 2%), hyperammonemia (1%)

Gastrointestinal: Pancreatitis (4%; grades 3/4: ≤1%), nausea (2%), vomiting (2%), abdominal pain (1%), diarrhea (1%)

Hematologic: Coagulation abnormalities (3%; grades 3/4: ≤1%), hemorrhage (1%; grades 3/4: <1%)

Hepatic: Transaminases increased (3%; grades 3/4: ≤2%), hyperbilirubinemia (1%)

<1%, postmarketing, and/or case reports: Acute renal failure, albumin decreased, alkaline phosphatase increased, anorexia, azotemia, bone marrow depression (rare), chills, cholesterol decreased, disseminated intravascular coagulation (DIC), hepatomegaly, injection site reactions, irritability, lipids (total) decreased/increased, malabsorption syndrome, proteinuria, transient ischemic event, weight loss

Drug Interactions

Metabolism/Transport Effects None known.

Avoid Concomitant Use There are no known interactions where it is recommended to avoid concomitant use.

Increased Effect/Toxicity

Asparaginase (Erwinia) may increase the levels/effects of: Dexamethasone (Systemic)

Decreased Effect There are no known significant interactions involving a decrease in effect.

Storage/Stability Store intact vials refrigerated at 2°C to 8°C (36°F to 48°F). Protect from light. Within 15 minutes of reconstitution, withdraw appropriate volume for dose into a polypropylene syringe. Do not freeze or refrigerate reconstituted solution; discard if not administered within 4 hours.

Reconstitution Hazardous agent; use appropriate precautions for handling and disposal. Reconstitute each vial with 1 mL of preservative free sodium chloride 0.9% (NS) to obtain a concentration of 10,000 units/mL, or with 2 mL preservative free NS to obtain a concentration of 5,000 units/mL. Gently direct the NS down the wall of the vial (do not inject forcefully into or onto the powder). Dissolve by gently swirling or mixing; do not shake or invert the vial. Resulting reconstituted solution should be clear and colorless and free of visible particles or protein aggregates. Withdraw appropriate volume for dose into a polypropylene syringe.

Mechanism of Action Asparaginase catalyzes the deamidation of asparagine to aspartic acid and ammonia, reducing circulating levels of asparagine. Leukemia cells lack asparagine synthetase and are unable to synthesize asparagine. Asparaginase reduces the exogenous asparagine source for the leukemic cells, resulting in cytotoxicity specific to leukemic cells.

Pharmacodynamics/Kinetics Half-life elimination: I.M.: ~16 hours (Asselin, 1993; Avramis, 2005)

Dosing

Adult

Acute lymphoblastic leukemia (ALL): I.M.:

As a substitute for pegaspargase: 25,000 units/m^2 3 times/week (Mon, Wed, Fri) for 6 doses for each planned pegaspargase dose

As a substitute for asparaginase (E. coli): 25,000 units/m^2 for each planned asparaginase (*E. coli*) dose

ALL induction: Canadian labeling (not in the U.S. labeling): SubQ: 10,000 units/m^2 days 1, 3, and 5 of week 4 and day 1 of week 5 (in combination with prednisolone, vincristine, mercaptopurine, and methotrexate) **or** 10,000 units/m^2 3 times/week (starting week 4) for 4 weeks (in combination with prednisolone, vincristine, and daunorubicin)

Pediatric

Acute lymphoblastic leukemia (ALL): I.M.: Refer to adult dosing.

ALL induction: *Canadian labeling (not in the U.S. labeling):*

Children <14 years: I.M.: 6000 units/m^2 3 times/week for 9 doses beginning day 4 of week 1 (in combination with vincristine, prednisone, methotrexate, and daunorubicin)

Children >14 years: SubQ: Refer to adult dosing.

Renal Impairment No dosage adjustment provided in the manufacturer's labeling.

Hepatic Impairment No dosage adjustment provided in the manufacturer's labeling.

Adjustment for Toxicity

Hemorrhagic or thrombotic event: Discontinue treatment; may resume treatment upon symptom resolution.

Pancreatitis:

Mild pancreatitis: Withhold treatment until signs and symptoms subside and amylase returns to normal; may resume after resolution.

Severe or hemorrhagic pancreatitis (abdominal pain >72 hours and amylase ≥2 x ULN): Discontinue treatment; further use is contraindicated.

Serious hypersensitivity: Discontinue treatment.

Administration

Administer I.M.; volume of each single injection site should be limited to 2 mL; use multiple injections for volumes >2 mL

Canadian labeling (additional administration routes not in the U.S. labeling): May also be administered SubQ and I.V., although I.M. and SubQ are preferred

Monitoring Parameters CBC with differential, amylase, liver enzymes, blood glucose, coagulation parameters, symptoms of hypersensitivity, symptoms of pancreatitis, thrombosis, or hemorrhage

Prescribing and Access Restrictions Erwinaze™ is distributed through Accredo Health Group, Inc. (1-877-900-9223).

Dosage Forms Excipient information presented when available (limited, particularly for generics); consult specific product labeling.

Injection, powder for reconstitution:

Erwinaze™: 10,000 units [contains glucose 5 mg/vial]

References

Asselin BL, Whitin JC, Coppola DJ, et al, "Comparative Pharmacokinetic Studies of Three Asparaginase Preparations," *J Clin Oncol*, 1993, 11(9):1780-6.

Avramis VI and Panosyan EH, "Pharmacokinetic/Pharmacodynamic Relationships of Asparaginase Formulations: The Past, the Present and Recommendations for the Future," *Clin Pharmacokinet*, 2005, 44(4):367-93.

Cheung KC, van den Bemt PM, Torringa ML, et al, "Erroneous Exchange of Asparaginase Forms in the Treatment of Acute Lymphoblastic Leukemia," *J Pediatr Hematol Oncol*, 2011, 33(3):e109-13.

Duval M, Suciu S, Ferster A, et al, "Comparison of *Escherichia Coli* -Asparaginase With *Erwinia*-Asparaginase in the Treatment of Childhood Lymphoid Malignancies: Results of a Randomized European Organisation for Research and Treatment of Cancer - Children's Leukemia Group Phase 3 Trial," *Blood*, 2002, 99(8):2734-9.

Grace RF, Dahlberg SE, Neuberg D, et al, "The Frequency and Management of Asparaginase-Related Thrombosis in Paediatric and Adult Patients With Acute Lymphoblastic Leukaemia Treated on Dana-Farber Cancer Institute Consortium Protocols," *Br J Haematol*, 2011, 152 (4):452-9.

Salzer W, Asselin B, Supko JG, et al, "Administration of Erwinia Asparaginase (Erwinase®) Following Allergy to PEG-Asparaginase In Children and Young Adults With Acute Lymphoblastic Leukemia Treated on AALL07P2 Achieves Therapeutic Nadir Serum Asparaginase Activity: A Report From the Children's Oncology Group (COG)," *Blood*, 2010, 116(21):2134 [abstract 2134 from 2010 ASH Annual Meeting].

Schrey D, Speitel K, Lanvers-Kaminsky C, et al, "Five-Year Single-Center Study of Asparaginase Therapy Within the ALL-BFM 2000 Trial," *Pediatr Blood Cancer*, 2011, 57(3):378-84.
Vrooman LM, Supko JG, Neuberg DS, et al, "*Erwinia* Asparaginase After Allergy to *E. coli* Asparaginase in Children With Acute Lymphoblastic Leukemia," Pediatr Blood Cancer, 2010, 54(2):199-205.
Zalewska-Szewczyk B, Gach A, Wyka K, et al, "The Cross-Reactivity of Anti-Asparaginase Antibodies Against Different L-Asparaginase Preparations," *Clin Exp Med*, 2009, 9(2):113-6.

Asparaginase (*E. coli*) (a SPEAR a ji nase e ko lye)

Related Information

Management of Chemotherapy-Induced Nausea and Vomiting *on page 1786*
Safe Handling of Hazardous Drugs *on page 1904*

Brand Names: U.S. Elspar®

Brand Names: Canada Kidrolase®

Index Terms *E. coli* Asparaginase; Asparaginase; L-asparaginase (*E. coli*)

Generic Availability (U.S.) No

Pharmacologic Category Antineoplastic Agent, Miscellaneous; Enzyme

Use Treatment (in combination with other chemotherapy) of acute lymphoblastic leukemia (ALL)

Unlabeled Use Treatment of lymphoblastic lymphoma

Labeled Contraindications History of serious allergic reaction to asparaginase or any *E. coli*-derived L-asparaginase; history of serious thrombosis, pancreatitis, or serious hemorrhagic events with prior L-asparaginase treatment

Pregnancy Risk Factor C

Lactation Excretion in breast milk unknown/not recommended

Warnings/Precautions Hazardous agent - use appropriate precautions for handling and disposal. Monitor for severe allergic reactions; immediate treatment for hypersensitivity reactions should be available during administration. May alter hepatic function; use caution with pre-existing liver impairment. Serious thrombosis, including sagittal sinus thrombosis may occur; discontinue with serious thrombotic events. Increased prothrombin time, partial thromboplastin time and hypofibrinogenemia may occur; cerebrovascular hemorrhage has been reported; monitor coagulation parameters; use cautiously in patients with an underlying coagulopathy. Monitor blood glucose; may cause hyperglycemia/glucose intolerance (possibly irreversible). May cause serious and possibly fatal pancreatitis; promptly evaluate patients with abdominal pain; discontinue permanently if pancreatitis develops. Appropriate measures must be taken to prevent tumor lysis syndrome and subsequent hyperuricemia and uric acid nephropathy; monitor, consider allopurinol, hydration and urinary alkalization.

Severe allergic reactions may occur; monitor; immediate treatment for hypersensitivity reactions should be available during administration. Risk factors for allergic reactions include: I.V. administration, doses >6000-12,000 units/m^2, patients who have received previous cycles of asparaginase, and intervals of even a few days between doses. Up to 33% of patients who have an allergic reaction to *E. coli* asparaginase will also react to the *Erwinia* form or pegaspargase. A test dose may be administered prior to the first dose of asparaginase, or prior to restarting therapy after a hiatus of several days. **False-negative rates of up to 80% to test doses of 2-50 units are reported.** Desensitization may be performed in patients found to be hypersensitive by the intradermal test dose or who have received previous courses of therapy with the drug.

Adverse Reactions Note: Immediate effects: Fever, chills, nausea, and vomiting occur in 50% to 60% of patients.

>10%:

Central nervous system: Fatigue, fever, chills, depression, agitation, seizure (10% to 60%), somnolence, stupor, confusion, coma (25%)

Endocrine & metabolic: Hyperglycemia/glucose intolerance (10%)

Gastrointestinal: Nausea, vomiting (50% to 60%), anorexia, abdominal cramps (70%), acute pancreatitis (15%, may be severe in some patients)

Hematologic: Hypofibrinogenemia and depression of clotting factors V and VIII, variable decrease in factors VII and IX, severe protein C deficiency and decrease in antithrombin III (may be dose limiting or fatal)

Hepatic: Transaminases, bilirubin, and alkaline phosphatase increased (transient)

Hypersensitivity: Acute allergic reactions (fever, rash, urticaria, arthralgia, hypotension, angioedema, bronchospasm, respiratory distress, anaphylaxis (15% to 35%); may be dose limiting in some patients, may be fatal)

Renal: Azotemia (66%)

1% to 10%:

Endocrine & metabolic: Hyperuricemia

Gastrointestinal: Stomatitis

Miscellaneous: Allergic reaction (including anaphylaxis), antibody formation/immunogenicity (~25%)

<1%, postmarketing case reports, and/or frequency not defined: Acute renal failure, albumin decreased, cerebrovascular hemorrhage, cerebrovascular thrombosis, cough, disorientation, drowsiness, fatty liver, fibrinogen decreased, glucosuria, hallucinations, headache, hemorrhagic pancreatitis, hyper-/hypolipidemia, hyperthermia, hypocholesterolemia, hypotension, insulin-dependent diabetes, intracranial hemorrhage, irritability, ketoacidosis, laryngospasm, malabsorption syndrome, myelosuppression (mild–to-moderate anemia, leukopenia, and thrombocytopenia; onset: 7 days; nadir: 14 days; recovery: 21 days), pancreatic pseudocyst, Parkinsonian symptoms (including tremor and increased muscle tone), partial thromboplastin time increased, peripheral edema, polyuria, proteinuria, prothrombin time increased, pruritus, rash, renal insufficiency, serum ammonia increased, serum cholesterol decreased, sagittal sinus thrombosis, stroke (hemorrhagic and thrombotic), thrombosis, urticaria, venous thrombosis, weight loss

Drug Interactions

Metabolism/Transport Effects None known.

Avoid Concomitant Use There are no known interactions where it is recommended to avoid concomitant use.

Increased Effect/Toxicity

Asparaginase (E. coli) may increase the levels/effects of: Dexamethasone (Systemic)

Decreased Effect There are no known significant interactions involving a decrease in effect.

Storage/Stability Intact vials of powder should be refrigerated at 2°C to 8°C (36°F to 48°F). Reconstituted solutions are stable 1 week refrigerated at 8°C (Stecher, 1999), although the manufacturer recommends use within 8 hours. Solutions for I.V. infusion are stable for 8 hours at room temperature or under refrigeration.

Reconstitution For I.V. administration, reconstitute lyophilized powder with 5 mL sterile water for injection or NS. For I.M. administration, the manufacturer recommends reconstitution of the lyophilized powder with 2 mL NS to a concentration of 5000 units/mL; however, some institutions reconstitute with 1 mL NS for I.M. use, resulting in a concentration of 10,000 units/mL. Shake well, but not too vigorously. A 5 micron filter may be used to remove fiber-like particles in the solution (do not use a 0.2 micron filter; has been associated with loss of potency).

Standard I.M. dilution: 5000 units/mL (10,000 units/mL has been used by some institutions)

Standard I.V. dilution: Dilute in 50-250 mL NS or D_5W

Mechanism of Action Asparaginase inhibits protein synthesis by hydrolyzing asparagine to aspartic acid and ammonia. Leukemia cells, especially lymphoblasts, require exogenous asparagine; normal cells can synthesize asparagine. Asparaginase is cycle-specific for the G_1 phase.

Pharmacodynamics/Kinetics

Absorption: I.M.: Produces peak blood levels 50% lower than those from I.V. administration

Distribution: V_d: 4-5 L/kg; 70% to 80% of plasma volume; <1% CSF penetration

Metabolism: Systemically degraded

Half-life elimination: I.M.: 39-49 hours; I.V.: 8-30 hours

Time to peak, plasma: I.M.: 14-24 hours

Dosing

Adult & Geriatric Refer to individual protocols. **Note:** Dose, frequency, number of doses, and start date may vary by protocol and treatment phase.

ALL:

I.V.:

6000 units/m²/dose 3 times/week for ~6-9 doses **or**

1000 units/kg/day for 10 days **or**

High-dose therapy (unlabeled dose): 10,000 units/m²/day for ~3-12 doses

Single-agent therapy (rare): 200 units/kg/day for 28 days

I.M.:

6000 units/m²/dose 3 times/week for ~6-9 doses **or** 6000 units/m²/dose every ~3 days for ~6-9 doses

High-dose therapy (unlabeled dose): 10,000 units/m²/day for ~3-12 doses

Test dose: A test dose is often recommended prior to the first dose of asparaginase, or prior to restarting therapy after a hiatus of several days. Most commonly, 0.1 mL of a 20 units/mL (2 units) asparaginase dilution is injected intradermally, and the patient observed for at least 1 hour. False-negative rates of up to 80% to test doses of 2-50 units are reported.

Some practitioners recommend an asparaginase desensitization regimen for patients who react to a test dose, or are being retreated following a break in therapy. Doses are doubled and given every 10 minutes until the total daily dose for that day has been administered. One schedule begins with a total of 1 unit given I.V. and doubles the dose every 10 minutes until the total amount given is the planned dose for that day. For example, if a patient was to receive a total dose of 4000 units, he/she would receive injections 1 through 12 during the desensitization. See table on next page.

Asparaginase Desensitization

Injection No.	Elspar Dose (units)	Accumulated Total Dose
1	1	1
2	2	3
3	4	7
4	8	15
5	16	31
6	32	63
7	64	127
8	128	255
9	256	511
10	512	1023
11	1024	2047
12	2048	4095
13	4096	8191
14	8192	16,383
15	16,384	32,767
16	32,768	65,535
17	65,536	131,071
18	131,072	262,143

Pediatric Refer to individual protocols. **Note:** Dose, frequency, number of doses, and start date may vary by protocol and treatment phase.

ALL:

I.V.:

6000 units/m^2/dose 3 times/week for ~6-9 doses **or**

1000 units/kg/day for 10 days **or**

High-dose therapy (unlabeled dose): 10,000 units/m^2/dose every ~3 days for ~4-8 doses

I.M.:

6000 units/m^2/dose 3 times/week **or** 6000 units/m^2/dose every ~3 days for ~6-9 doses

High-dose therapy (unlabeled dose): 10,000 units/m^2/dose every ~3 days for ~4-8 doses **or** 25,000 units/m^2/dose weekly for ~9 doses (generally used in high-risk continuation therapy)

Test dose: Refer to adult dosing.

Combination Regimens

Leukemia, acute lymphocytic:

Hyper-CVAD (Leukemia, Acute Lymphocytic) on page 1681
Larson Regimen (ALL) on page 1699
Linker Protocol (ALL) on page 1703
PVA (POG 8602) on page 1742
PVDA on page 1745

Administration May be administered I.M., I.V., or intradermal (skin test only); has been administered SubQ in specific protocols

I.M.: Doses should be given as a deep intramuscular injection into a large muscle; volumes >2 mL should be divided and administered in 2 separate sites

Note: I.V. administration greatly increases the risk of allergic reactions and should be avoided if possible.

I.V.: I.V. infusion in 50-250 mL of D_5W or NS over at least 30-60 minutes. The manufacturer recommends a test dose (0.1 mL of a dilute 20 unit/mL solution) prior to initial administration and when given after an interval of 7 days or more. Institutional policies vary. The skin test site should be observed for at least 1 hour for a wheal or erythema. Note that a negative skin test does not preclude the possibility of an allergic reaction. Desensitization may be performed in patients who have been found to be hypersensitive by the intradermal skin test or who have received previous courses of therapy with the drug. Have epinephrine, diphenhydramine, and hydrocortisone at the bedside. Have a running I.V. in place. A physician should be readily accessible.

Gelatinous fiber-like particles may develop on standing. Filtration through a 5-micron filter during administration will remove the particles with no loss of potency.

Emetic Potential Very low (<10%)

Monitoring Parameters CBC with differential, urinalysis, amylase, liver function prior to and frequently during therapy, liver enzymes, coagulation parameters (baseline and periodic), renal function tests, urine dipstick for glucose, blood glucose, uric acid. Monitor for allergic reaction, be prepared to treat anaphylaxis at each administration; monitor for onset of abdominal pain and mental status changes. Monitor vital signs during administration.

Test Interactions Decreased thyroxine and thyroxine-binding globulin

Additional Information Some institutions recommended the following pre-cautions for asparaginase administration: Parenteral epinephrine, diphenhydr-amine, and hydrocortisone available at bedside; freely running I.V. in place; physician readily accessible; monitor the patient closely for 30-60 minutes; avoid administering at night.

The *E. coli* and the *Erwinia* strains of asparaginase differ slightly in their gene sequencing, and have slight differences in their enzyme characteristics. Both are highly specific for asparagine and have <10% activity for the D-isomer.

Dosage Forms Excipient information presented when available (limited, particularly for generics); consult specific product labeling.

Injection, powder for reconstitution:

Elspar®: 10,000 units

References

Avramis VI, Sencer S, Periclou AP, et al, "A Randomized Comparison of Native Escherichia Coli Asparaginase and Polyethylene Glycol Conjugated Asparaginase for Treatment of Children With Newly Diagnosed Standard-Risk Acute Lymphoblastic Leukemia: A Children's Cancer Group Study," *Blood*, 2002, 99(6):1986-94.

Duval M, Suciu S, Ferster A, et al, "Comparison of *Escherichia Coli* -Asparaginase With *Erwinia*-Asparaginase in the Treatment of Childhood Lymphoid Malignancies: Results of a Randomized European Organisation for Research and Treatment of Cancer – Children's Leukemia Group Phase 3 Trial," *Blood*, 2002, 99(8):2734-9.

Larson RA, Dodge RK, Burns P, et al, "A Five-Drug Remission Induction Regimen With Intensive Consolidation for Adults With Acute Lymphoblastic Leukemia: Cancer and Leukemia Group B Study 8811," *Blood*, 1995, 85(8):2025-37.

Lazarus HM, Richards SM, Chopra R, et al, "Central Nervous System Involvement in Adult Acute Lymphoblastic Leukemia at Diagnosis: Results from the International ALL Trial MRC UKALL XII/ECOG E2993," *Blood*, 2006, 108(2):465-72.

Morgan C, Tillett T, Braybrooke J, et al, "Management of Uncommon Chemotherapy-Induced Emergencies," *Lancet Oncol*, 2011, 12(8):806-14.

Pession A, Valsecchi MG, Masera G, et al, "Long-Term Results of a Randomized Trial on Extended Use of High Dose L-Asparaginase for Standard Risk Childhood Acute Lymphoblastic Leukemia," *J Clin Oncol*, 2005, 23(28):7161-7.

Stecher AL, de Deus PM, Polikarpov I, et al, "Stability of L-Asparaginase: An Enzyme Used in Leukemia Treatment," *Pharm Acta Helv*, 1999, 74(1):1-9.

◆ **Asparaginase *Erwinia chrysanthemi*** *see* Asparaginase (*Erwinia*) *on page 126*
◆ **Astramorph®/PF** *see* Morphine (Systemic) *on page 1004*
◆ **AT** *see* Antithrombin *on page 107*
◆ **AT-III** *see* Antithrombin *on page 107*
◆ **Atarax® (Can)** *see* HydrOXYzine *on page 736*
◆ **ATG** *see* Antithymocyte Globulin (Equine) *on page 111*
◆ **Atgam®** *see* Antithymocyte Globulin (Equine) *on page 111*
◆ **Ativan®** *see* LORazepam *on page 907*
◆ **ATRA** *see* Tretinoin (Systemic) *on page 1405*
◆ **Atriance™ (Can)** *see* Nelarabine *on page 1028*
◆ **Atryn®** *see* Antithrombin *on page 107*
◆ **Auro-Ciprofloxacin (Can)** *see* Ciprofloxacin (Systemic) *on page 283*
◆ **Ava-Bicalutamide (Can)** *see* Bicalutamide *on page 178*
◆ **Ava-Famciclovir (Can)** *see* Famciclovir *on page 500*
◆ **Avakine** *see* InFLIXimab *on page 789*
◆ **AVA-Levofloxacin (Can)** *see* Levofloxacin (Systemic) *on page 883*
◆ **Ava-Olanzapine (Can)** *see* OLANZapine *on page 1056*
◆ **Avastin®** *see* Bevacizumab *on page 165*
◆ **AVINza®** *see* Morphine (Systemic) *on page 1004*

Axitinib (ax I ti nib)

Brand Names: U.S. Inlyta®

Brand Names: Canada Inlyta®

Index Terms AG-013736; Inlyta®

Generic Availability (U.S.) No

Pharmacologic Category Antineoplastic Agent, Tyrosine Kinase Inhibitor; Vascular Endothelial Growth Factor (VEGF) Inhibitor

Use Treatment of advanced renal cell cancer (RCC) after failure of one prior systemic treatment

Labeled Contraindications There are no contraindications listed within the manufacturer's labeling.

Pregnancy Risk Factor D

Lactation Excretion in breast milk unknown/not recommended

Warnings/Precautions May cause hypertension; the median onset is within the first month, and has been observed as early as 4 days after treatment initiation. Hypertensive crisis has been reported. Blood pressure should be well-controlled prior to treatment initiation. Monitor blood pressure and treat with standard antihypertensive therapy. Persistent hypertension (despite antihypertensive therapy) may require dose reduction; discontinue if severe and persistent despite concomitant antihypertensives (or dose reduction), or with evidence of hypertensive crisis. Monitor for hypotension if on antihypertensive therapy and axitinib is withheld or discontinued.

Gastrointestinal perforation and fistulas (including a fatality) have been reported. Monitor for signs/symptoms throughout treatment. Has not been studied in patients with recent active gastrointestinal bleeding; use is not recommended.

Arterial thrombotic events (cerebrovascular accident, MI, retinal artery occlusion, and transient ischemic attack), with fatalities, have been reported. Venous thrombotic events, including pulmonary embolism, deep vein thrombosis, retinal vein occlusion and retinal vein thrombosis, have been observed (with some fatalities). Use with caution in patients with a history of or risks for arterial or venous thrombotic events; has not been studied in patients within 12 months of an arterial thrombotic event or within 6 months of a venous thrombotic event. Hemorrhagic events (cerebral hemorrhage, gastrointestinal hemorrhage, hematuria, hemoptysis, and melena) have been reported (with some fatalities). Temporarily interrupt treatment with any hemorrhage requiring medical intervention.

Cases of reversible posterior leukoencephalopathy syndrome (RPLS) have been reported. Symptoms of RPLS include confusion, headache, hypertension (mild-to-severe), lethargy, seizure, blindness and/or other vision, or neurologic disturbances; interrupt treatment and manage hypertension. MRI is recommended to confirm RPLS diagnosis. Discontinue axitinib if RPLS is confirmed. The safety of reinitiating axitinib in patients previously experiencing RPLS is unknown.

Hypothyroidism occurs commonly with tyrosine kinase inhibitors, including axitinib. Hyperthyroidism has also been reported. Monitor thyroid function. Thyroid disorders should be treated according to standard practice to achieve/maintain euthyroid state. Proteinuria is associated with use. Monitor for proteinuria. If moderate or severe proteinuria occurs, reduce dose or temporarily withhold treatment. Although the effect on wound healing has not been studied with axitinib, vascular endothelial growth factor (VEGF) receptor inhibitors are associated with impaired wound healing. Discontinue treatment at least 24 hours prior to scheduled surgery; treatment reinitiation should be guided by clinical judgment and wound assessment. Has not been studied in patients with evidence of untreated brain metastases; use is not recommended. Systemic exposure to axitinib is increased in patients with moderate hepatic impairment; dose reductions are recommended. Has not been studied in patients with severe hepatic impairment. Increases in ALT have been observed during treatment; monitor liver function tests.

Adverse Reactions

>10%:

Cardiovascular: Hypertension (40%; grades 3/4: 16%)

Central nervous system: Fatigue (39%), dysphonia (31%), headache (14%)

Dermatologic: Palmar-plantar erythrodysesthesia syndrome (27%; grades 3/4: 5%), rash (13%; grades 3/4: <1%)

Endocrine & metabolic: Bicarbonate decreased (44%), hypocalcemia (39%), hyperglycemia (28%), hypothyroidism (19%; grades 3/4: <1%), hypernatremia (17%), hyperkalemia (15%), hypoalbuminemia (15%), hyponatremia (13%), hypophosphatemia (13%), hypoglycemia (11%)

Gastrointestinal: Diarrhea (55%; grades 3/4: 11%), appetite decreased (34%), nausea (32%; grades 3/4: 3%), lipase increased (3% to 27%), amylase increased (25%), weight loss (25%), vomiting (24%; grades 3/4: 3%), constipation (20%), mucosal inflammation (15%), stomatitis (15%), abdominal pain (8% to 14%), taste alteration (11%)

Hematologic: Anemia (4% to 35%; grades 3/4: <1%), lymphopenia (33%; grades 3/4: 3%), hemorrhage (16%; grades 3/4 1%), thrombocytopenia (15%; grades 3/4: <1%), leukopenia (11%)

Hepatic: Alkaline phosphatase increased (30%), ALT increased (22%; grades 3/4: <1%), AST increased (20%; grades 3/4: <1%)

Neuromuscular & skeletal: Weakness (21%), arthralgia (15%), limb pain (13%)

Renal: Creatinine increased (55%), proteinuria (11%; grade 3: 3%)

Respiratory: Cough (15%), dyspnea (15%)

1% to 10%:

Cardiovascular: Venous thrombotic events (grades 3/4: 3%), arterial thrombotic events (2%; grade 3/4: 1%), deep vein thrombosis (1%), transient ischemic attack (1%)

Central nervous system: Dizziness (9%)

Dermatologic: Dry skin (10%), pruritus (7%), alopecia (4%), erythema (2%)

Endocrine & metabolic: Dehydration (6%), hyperthyroidism (1%)

Gastrointestinal: Dyspepsia (10%), hemorrhoids (4%), rectal hemorrhage (2%), fistula (1%), gastrointestinal perforation (≤1%)

Hematologic: Hemoglobin increased (9%), polycythemia (1%)

Neuromuscular & skeletal: Myalgia (7%)

Ocular: Retinal vein occlusion/thrombosis (1%)

Otic: Tinnitus (3%)

Renal: Hematuria (3%)

Respiratory: Epistaxis (6%), hemoptysis (2%), pulmonary embolism (2%)

<1%, postmarketing, and/or case reports: Cerebral bleeding, cerebrovascular accident, fever, hypertensive crisis, heart failure, neutropenia, reversible posterior leukoencephalopathy syndrome (RPLS)

Drug Interactions

Metabolism/Transport Effects **Substrate** of CYP1A2 (minor), CYP2C19 (minor), CYP3A4 (major), UGT1A1; **Note:** Assignment of Major/Minor substrate status based on clinically relevant drug interaction potential

Avoid Concomitant Use

Avoid concomitant use of Axitinib with any of the following: CYP3A4 Inducers (Strong); CYP3A4 Inducers (Weakly to Moderately Effective); CYP3A4 Inhibitors (Strong); Grapefruit Juice; St Johns Wort

Increased Effect/Toxicity

Axitinib may increase the levels/effects of: Vitamin K Antagonists

The levels/effects of Axitinib may be increased by: CYP3A4 Inhibitors (Moderate); CYP3A4 Inhibitors (Strong); Dasatinib; Grapefruit Juice; Ivacaftor; Mifepristone

Decreased Effect

Axitinib may decrease the levels/effects of: Cardiac Glycosides; Vitamin K Antagonists

The levels/effects of Axitinib may be decreased by: CYP3A4 Inducers (Strong); CYP3A4 Inducers (Weakly to Moderately Effective); Deferasirox; St Johns Wort; Tocilizumab

Ethanol/Nutrition/Herb Interactions

Food: Axitinib serum concentrations may be increased when taken with grapefruit or grapefruit juice. Management: Avoid concurrent use.

Herb/Nutraceutical: St John's wort may decrease axitinib serum concentrations. Management: Avoid concurrent use.

Storage/Stability Store at 20°C to 25°C (68°F to 77°F); excursions permitted to 15°C to 30°C (59°F to 86°F).

Mechanism of Action Axitinib is a selective second generation tyrosine kinase inhibitor which blocks angiogenesis and tumor growth by inhibiting vascular endothelial growth factor receptors (VEGFR-1, VEGFR-2, and VEGFR-3).

Pharmacodynamics/Kinetics

Absorption: Rapid (Rugo, 2005)

Distribution: V_d: 160 L

Protein binding: >99%; to albumin (primarily) and to $alpha_1$ acid glycoprotein (AAG)

Metabolism: Hepatic; primarily via CYP3A4/5 and to a lesser extend via CYP1A2, CYP2C19 and UGT1A1

Bioavailability: 58%

Half-life elimination: 2.5-6 hours

Time to peak: 2.5-4 hours

Excretion: Feces (~41%; 12% as unchanged drug); urine (~23%; as metabolites)

Dosing

Adult Renal cell cancer, advanced: Oral: Initial: 5 mg twice daily (approximately every 12 hours)

Dose increases: If dose is tolerated (no adverse events above grade 2, blood pressure is normal and no antihypertensive use) for at least 2 consecutive weeks, may increase the dose to 7 mg twice daily, and then further increase (using the same tolerance criteria) to 10 mg twice daily.

Dose decreases: For adverse events, reduce dose from 5 mg twice daily to 3 mg twice daily; further reduce to 2 mg twice daily if adverse events persist.

Dosage adjustment for strong CYP3A4 inhibitors: Avoid concomitant administration with strong CYP3A4 inhibitors (eg, clarithromycin, itraconazole, ketoconazole, nefazodone, protease inhibitors, telithromycin, voriconazole, grapefruit juice); if concomitant administration with a strong CYP3A4 inhibitor cannot be avoided, ~50% dosage reduction is recommended; adjust dose based on individual tolerance and safety. When the strong CYP3A4 inhibitor is discontinued, resume previous axitinib dose after 3-5 half-lives of the inhibitor have passed.

Geriatric Refer to adult dosing. No adjustment necessary.

Renal Impairment

Mild-to-severe renal impairment (Cl_{cr} 15 to <89 mL/minute): No initial dosage adjustment necessary.

End-stage renal disease: (ESRD) No dosage adjustment provided in the manufacturer's labeling.

Hepatic Impairment

Mild impairment (Child-Pugh class A): No starting dosage adjustment necessary.

Moderate impairment (Child-Pugh class B): Reduce starting dose by ~50%; increase or decrease based on individual tolerance.

Severe impairment (Child-Pugh class C): No dosage adjustment provided in the manufacturer's labeling (has not been studied).

Adjustment for Toxicity

Adverse events: May require temporary interruption, dose decreases (reduce dose from 5 mg twice daily to 3 mg twice daily; further reduce to 2 mg twice daily) or discontinuation

Hypertension: Treat with standard antihypertensive therapy.

Persistent hypertension: May require dose reduction

Severe, persistent (despite antihypertensives and dose reduction), or evidence of hypertensive crisis: Discontinue treatment

Hemorrhage: Any bleeding requiring medical intervention: Temporarily interrupt treatment.

Proteinuria (moderate-to-severe): Reduce dose or temporarily interrupt treatment.

Administration Oral: Swallow tablet whole with a glass of water. May be taken with or without food. If a dose is missed or vomited, do not make up; resume dosing with the next scheduled dose.

Monitoring Parameters Hepatic function (ALT, AST, and bilirubin; baseline and periodic), thyroid function (baseline and periodic), urinalysis (for proteinuria; baseline and periodically); blood pressure, signs/symptoms of RPLS, gastrointestinal bleeding/perforation/fistula

Thyroid function testing recommendations (Hamnvik, 2011):

Pre-existing levothyroxine therapy: Obtain baseline TSH levels, then monitor every 4 weeks until levels and levothyroxine dose are stable, then monitor every 2 months

Without pre-existing thyroid hormone replacement: TSH at baseline, then monthly for 4 months, then every 2-3 months

Dietary Considerations May be taken without regard to food. Avoid grapefruit and grapefruit juice.

Prescribing and Access Restrictions Available from select specialty pharmacies. Further information may be obtained at 877-744-5675 or www.-inlytahcp.com.

Dosage Forms Excipient information presented when available (limited, particularly for generics); consult specific product labeling.

Tablet, oral:

Inlyta®: 1 mg, 5 mg

References

Hamnvik OP, Larsen PR, and Marqusee E, "Thyroid Dysfunction From Antineoplastic Agents," *J Natl Cancer Inst*, 2011, 103(21):1572-87.

Rini BI, Escudier B, Tomczak P, et al, "Comparative Effectiveness of Axitinib Versus Sorafenib in Advanced Renal Cell Carcinoma (AXIS): A Randomised Phase 3 Trial," *Lancet*, 2011, 378 (9807):1931-9.

Rini BI, Wilding G, Hudes G, et al, "Phase II Study of Axitinib in Sorafenib-Refractory Metastatic Renal Cell Carcinoma," *J Clin Oncol*, 2009, 27(27):4462-8.

Rixe O, Bukowski RM, Michaelson MD, et al, "Axitinib Treatment in Patients With Cytokine-Refractory Metastatic Renal-Cell Cancer: A Phase II Study," *Lancet Oncol*, 2007, 8(11):975-84.

◆ **AY-25650** *see* Triptorelin *on page 1413*

◆ **5-Aza-2'-deoxycytidine** *see* Decitabine *on page 403*

AzaCITIDine (ay za SYE ti deen)

Related Information

Management of Chemotherapy-Induced Nausea and Vomiting *on page 1786*
Safe Handling of Hazardous Drugs *on page 1904*

Brand Names: U.S. Vidaza®

Brand Names: Canada Vidaza®

Index Terms 5-Azacytidine; 5-AZC; AZA-CR; Azacytidine; Ladakamycin

Generic Availability (U.S.) No

Pharmacologic Category Antineoplastic Agent, DNA Methylation Inhibitor

Use Treatment of myelodysplastic syndrome (MDS)

Unlabeled Use Treatment of acute myelogenous leukemia (AML)

Labeled Contraindications Hypersensitivity to azacitidine, mannitol, or any component of the formulation; advanced malignant hepatic tumors

Pregnancy Risk Factor D

Lactation Excretion in breast milk unknown/not recommended

Warnings/Precautions Hazardous agent - use appropriate precautions for handling and disposal. Azacitidine may be hepatotoxic, use caution with hepatic impairment; use is contraindicated in patients with advanced malignant hepatic tumors. Progressive hepatic coma leading to death has been reported (rare) in patients with extensive tumor burden, especially those with a baseline albumin <30 g/L. Use caution with renal impairment; dose adjustment may be required. Serum creatinine elevations, renal tubular acidosis, and renal failure have been reported with combination chemotherapy; decrease or withhold dose for unexplained elevations in BUN or serum creatinine or reductions in serum bicarbonate to <20 mEq/L. Patients with renal and hepatic impairment were excluded from clinical studies. Neutropenia, thrombocytopenia, and anemia are common; may cause therapy delays and/or dosage reductions. Not FDA approved for use in children.

Adverse Reactions

>10%:

Cardiovascular: Peripheral edema (7% to 19%), chest pain (16%), pallor (16%), pitting edema (15%)

Central nervous system: Fever (30% to 52%), fatigue (13% to 36%), headache (22%), dizziness (19%), anxiety (5% to 13%), depression (12%), insomnia (9% to 11%), malaise (11%), pain (11%)

Dermatologic: Bruising (19% to 31%), petechiae (11% to 24%), erythema (7% to 17%), skin lesion (15%), rash (10% to 14%), pruritus (12%)

Endocrine & metabolic: Hypokalemia (6% to 13%)

Gastrointestinal: Nausea (48% to 71%), vomiting (27% to 54%), diarrhea (36%), constipation (34% to 50%), anorexia (13% to 21%), weight loss (16%), abdominal pain (11% to 16%), abdominal tenderness (12%)

Hematologic: Thrombocytopenia (66% to 70%; grades 3/4: 58%), anemia (51% to 70%; grades 3/4: 14%), neutropenia (32% to 66%; grades 3/4: 61%), leukopenia (18% to 48%; grades 3/4: 15%), febrile neutropenia (14% to 16%; grades 3/4: 13%), myelosuppression (nadir: days 10-17; recovery: days 28-31)

Local: Injection site reactions (14% to 29%): Erythema (35% to 43%; more common with I.V. administration), pain (19% to 23%; more common with I.V. administration), bruising (5% to 14%)

Neuromuscular & skeletal: Weakness (29%), rigors (26%), arthralgia (22%), limb pain (20%), back pain (19%), myalgia (16%)

Respiratory: Cough (11% to 30%), dyspnea (5% to 29%), pharyngitis (20%), epistaxis (16%), nasopharyngitis (15%), upper respiratory tract infection (9% to 13%), pneumonia (11%), crackles (11%)

Miscellaneous: Diaphoresis (11%)

5% to 10%:

Cardiovascular: Cardiac murmur (10%), hypertension (≤9%), tachycardia (9%), hypotension (7%), syncope (6%), chest wall pain (5%)

Central nervous system: Lethargy (7% to 8%), hypoesthesia (5%), postprocedural pain (5%)

Dermatologic: Cellulitis (8%), urticaria (6%), dry skin (5%), skin nodule (5%)

Gastrointestinal: Gingival bleeding (10%), oral mucosal petechiae (8%), stomatitis (8%), weight loss (≤8%), dyspepsia (6% to 7%), hemorrhoids (7%), abdominal distension (6%), loose stools (6%), dysphagia (5%), oral hemorrhage (5%), tongue ulceration (5%)

Genitourinary: Dysuria (8%), urinary tract infection (8% to 9%)

Hematologic: Hematoma (9%), postprocedural hemorrhage (6%)

Local: Injection site reactions: Pruritus (7%), hematoma (6%), rash (6%), granuloma (5%), induration (5%), pigmentation change (5%), swelling (5%)

Neuromuscular & skeletal: Muscle cramps (6%)

Renal: Hematuria (≤6%)

Respiratory: Rhinorrhea (10%), rales (9%), wheezing (9%), breath sounds decreased (8%), pharyngolaryngeal pain (6%), pleural effusion (6%), postnasal drip (6%), rhinitis (6%), rhonchi (6%), nasal congestion (6%), atelectasis (5%), sinusitis (5%)

Miscellaneous: Lymphadenopathy (10%), herpes simplex (9%), night sweats (9%), transfusion reaction (7%), mouth hemorrhage (5%)

<5%, postmarketing, and/or case reports: Abscess (limb, perirectal), acute febrile neutrophilic dermatosis (Sweet's syndrome), agranulocytosis, anaphylactic shock, atrial fibrillation, azotemia, blastomycosis, bone marrow depression/failure, bone pain aggravated, cardiac failure, cardiorespiratory arrest, catheter site hemorrhage, cellulitis, cerebral hemorrhage, CHF, cholecystectomy, cholecystitis, congestive cardiomyopathy, dehydration, diverticulitis, eye hemorrhage, fibrosis (interstitial and alveolar), gastrointestinal hemorrhage, glycosuria, hemoptysis, hepatic coma, hypersensitivity reaction, hypophosphatemia, infection (bacterial), injection site infection, injection site necrosis, interstitial lung disease, intracranial hemorrhage, leukemia cutis, lung infiltration, melena, neutropenic sepsis, orthostatic hypotension, pancytopenia, pneumonitis, polyuria, pyoderma gangrenosum, renal failure, renal tubular acidosis, seizure, respiratory distress, sepsis, septic shock, serum bicarbonate levels decreased, serum creatinine increased, splenomegaly, systemic inflammatory response syndrome, toxoplasmosis, tumor lysis syndrome

Drug Interactions

Metabolism/Transport Effects None known.

Avoid Concomitant Use

Avoid concomitant use of AzaCITIDine with any of the following: BCG; CloZAPine; Natalizumab; Pimecrolimus; Tacrolimus (Topical); Vaccines (Live)

Increased Effect/Toxicity

AzaCITIDine may increase the levels/effects of: CloZAPine; Leflunomide; Natalizumab; Vaccines (Live)

The levels/effects of AzaCITIDine may be increased by: Denosumab; Pimecrolimus; Roflumilast; Tacrolimus (Topical); Trastuzumab

Decreased Effect

AzaCITIDine may decrease the levels/effects of: BCG; Coccidioidin Skin Test; Sipuleucel-T; Vaccines (Inactivated); Vaccines (Live)

The levels/effects of AzaCITIDine may be decreased by: Echinacea

Storage/Stability Prior to reconstitution, store powder at room temperature of 25°C (77°F); excursions permitted to 15°C to 30°C (59°F to 86°F).

SubQ: Following reconstitution, suspension may be stored at room temperature for up to 1 hour, or immediately refrigerated at 2°C to 8°C (36°F to 46°F) and stored for up to 8 hours.

I.V.: **Solutions for I.V. administration have very limited stability and must be prepared immediately prior to each dose.** Administration must be completed within 1 hour of (vial) reconstitution.

Reconstitution Use appropriate precautions for handling and disposal.

SubQ: To prepare a 25 mg/mL suspension, slowly add 4 mL SWFI to each vial. Vigorously shake or roll vial until a suspension is formed (suspension will be cloudy).

I.V.: Reconstitute vial with 10 mL SWFI to form a 10 mg/mL solution; vigorously shake until solution is dissolved and clear. Mix in 50-100 mL of NS or lactated Ringer's injection for infusion.

Mechanism of Action Antineoplastic effects may be a result of azacitidine's ability to promote hypomethylation of DNA leading to direct toxicity of abnormal hematopoietic cells in the bone marrow.

Pharmacodynamics/Kinetics

Absorption: SubQ: Rapid and complete

Distribution: V_d: I.V.: 76 ± 26 L; does not cross blood-brain barrier

Metabolism: Hepatic; hydrolysis to several metabolites

Bioavailability: SubQ: ~89%

Half-life elimination: I.V., SubQ: ~4 hours

Time to peak, plasma: SubQ: 30 minutes

Excretion: Urine (50% to 85%); feces (minor)

Dosing

Adult

MDS: I.V., SubQ: 75 mg/m^2/day for 7 days repeated every 4 weeks. Dose may be increased to 100 mg/m^2/day if no benefit is observed after 2 cycles and no toxicity other than nausea and vomiting have occurred. Treatment is recommended for at least 4 cycles; treatment may be continued as long as patient continues to benefit.

Note: Alternate (unlabeled) schedules (which have produced hematologic response) have been used for convenience in community oncology centers (Lyons, 2009):

75 mg/m^2/day for 5 days (Mon-Fri), 2 days rest (Sat, Sun), then 75 mg/m^2/day for 2 days (Mon, Tues); repeat cycle every 28 days **or**

50 mg/m^2/day for 5 days (Mon-Fri), 2 days rest (Sat, Sun), then 50 mg/m^2/day for 5 days (Mon-Fri); repeat cycle every 28 days **or**

75 mg/m^2/day for 5 days (Mon-Fri), repeat cycle every 28 days

AML (unlabeled use): SubQ: 75 mg/m^2/day for 7 days repeated every 4 weeks (Sudan, 2006)

Dosage adjustment based on hematology: Adults: I.V., SubQ: MDS:

For baseline WBC ≥3.0 x 10^9/L, ANC ≥1.5 x 10^9/L, and platelets ≥75 x 10^9/L:

Nadir count: ANC <0.5 x 10^9/L or platelets <25 x 10^9/L: Administer 50% of dose during next treatment course

Nadir count: ANC 0.5-1.5 x 10^9/L or platelets 25-50 x 10^9/L: Administer 67% of dose during next treatment course

Nadir count: ANC >1.5 x 10^9/L or platelets >50 x 10^9/L: Administer 100% of dose during next treatment course

For baseline WBC <3 x 10^9/L, ANC <1.5 x 10^9/L, or platelets <75 x 10^9/L: Adjust dose as follows based on nadir counts and bone marrow biopsy cellularity at the time of nadir, unless clear improvement in differentiation at the time of the next cycle:

WBC or platelet nadir decreased 50% to 75% from baseline and bone marrow biopsy cellularity at time of nadir 30% to 60%: Administer 100% of dose during next treatment course

WBC or platelet nadir decreased 50% to 75% from baseline and bone marrow biopsy cellularity at time of nadir 15% to 30%: Administer 50% of dose during next treatment course

WBC or platelet nadir decreased 50% to 75% from baseline and bone marrow biopsy cellularity at time of nadir <15%: Administer 33% of dose during next treatment course

WBC or platelet nadir decreased >75% from baseline and bone marrow biopsy cellularity at time of nadir 30% to 60%: Administer 75% of dose during next treatment course

WBC or platelet nadir decreased >75% from baseline and bone marrow biopsy cellularity at time of nadir 15% to 30%: Administer 50% of dose during next treatment course

WBC or platelet nadir decreased >75% from baseline and bone marrow biopsy cellularity at time of nadir <15%: Administer 33% of dose during next treatment course

Note: If a nadir defined above occurs, administer the next treatment course 28 days after the start of the preceding course as long as WBC and platelet counts are >25% above the nadir and rising. If a >25% increase above the nadir is not seen by day 28, reassess counts every 7 days. If a 25% increase is not seen by day 42, administer 50% of the scheduled dose.

Dosage adjustment based on serum electrolytes: The manufacturer recommends that if serum bicarbonate falls to <20 mEq/L (unexplained decrease): Reduce dose by 50% for next treatment course

Geriatric Refer to adult dosing. Due to the potential for decreased renal function in the elderly, select dose carefully and closely monitor renal function.

Pediatric Refractory AML (unlabeled use): 250 mg/m^2/dose days 4 and 5 every 4 weeks (Steuber, 1996) **or** 300 mg/m^2/dose days 4 and 5 every 4 weeks (Hurwitz, 1995)

Renal Impairment Not studied in patients with renal impairment; select dose carefully (excretion is primarily renal; consider dose reduction); monitor closely for toxicity.

Hepatic Impairment Not studied in patients with hepatic impairment; use caution. Contraindicated in patients with advanced malignant hepatic tumors.

Adjustment for Toxicity Renal toxicity: If increases in BUN or serum creatinine (unexplained) occur, delay next cycle until values reach baseline or normal, then reduce dose by 50% for next treatment course.

Combination Regimens

Leukemia, acute myeloid: Azacitidine (AML Regimen) on page 1521
Myelodysplastic syndrome: Azacitidine (MDS Regimen) on page 1521

Administration

SubQ: Premedication for nausea and vomiting is recommended. The manufacturer recommends equally dividing volumes >4 mL into 2 syringes and injecting into 2 separate sites; however, policies for maximum SubQ administration volume may vary by institution; interpatient variations may also apply. Administer subsequent injections at least 1 inch from previous injection sites. Allow refrigerated suspensions to come to room temperature (up to 30 minutes) prior to administration. Resuspend by inverting the syringe 2-3 times and then rolling the syringe between the palms for 30 seconds. If azacitidine suspension comes in contact with the skin, immediately wash with soap and water.

I.V.: Premedication for nausea and vomiting is recommended. Infuse over 10-40 minutes; infusion must be completed within 1 hour of (vial) reconstitution.

Emetic Potential Moderate (30% to 90%)

Monitoring Parameters Liver function tests, electrolytes, CBC with differential and platelets, renal function tests (BUN and serum creatinine) should be obtained prior to initiation of therapy. Electrolytes, renal function (BUN and creatinine), CBC should be monitored prior to each cycle and periodically as needed to monitor response and toxicity.

Additional Information Oncology Comment: Azacitidine treatment for MDS is associated with an improvement in quality of life (including a reduction in transfusion requirements), a decrease in transformation to AML, and improved survival, when compared to best supportive care. Treatment should be continued for a minimum of 4-6 cycles (NCCN MDS guidelines v.2.2009).

Dosage Forms Excipient information presented when available (limited, particularly for generics); consult specific product labeling.

Injection, powder for suspension:

Vidaza®: 100 mg [contains mannitol]

References

Hurwitz CA, Mounce KG, and Grier HE, "Treatment of Patients With Acute Myelogenous Leukemia: Review of Clinical Trials of the Past Decade," *J Pediatr Hematol Oncol*, 1995, 17 (3):185-97.

Lyons RM, Cosgriff TM, Modi SS, et al, "Hematologic Response to Three Alternative Dosing Schedules of Azacitidine in Patients With Myelodysplastic Syndrome," *J Clin Oncol*, 2009, 27 (11):1850-6.

National Comprehensive Cancer Network® (NCCN), "Clinical Practice Guidelines in Oncology™: Myelodysplastic Syndromes," Version 2.2009. Available at http://www.nccn.org/professionals/physician_gls/PDF/mds.pdf

Silverman LR, Demakos EP, Peterson BL, et al, "Randomized Controlled Trial of Azacitidine in Patients With the Myelodysplastic Syndrome: A Study of the Cancer and Leukemia Group B," *J Clin Oncol*, 2002, 20(10):2429-40.

Silverman LR, McKenzie DR, Peterson BL, et al,"Further Analysis of Trials With Azacitidine in Patients With Myelodysplastic Syndrome: Studies 8421, 8921, and 9221 by the Cancer and Leukemia Group B," *J Clin Oncol*, 2006, 24(24):3895-903.

Steuber CP, Krischer J, Holbrook T, et al, "Therapy of Refractory or Recurrent Childhood Acute Myeloid Leukemia Using Amsacrine and Etoposide With or Without Azacitidine: A Pediatric Oncology Group Randomized Phase II Study," *J Clin Oncol*, 1996, 14(5):1521-5.

Steuber CP, Holbrook T, Camitta B, et al, "Toxicity Trials of Amsacrine (AMSA) and Etoposide ± Azacitidine (AZ) in Childhood Acute Nonlymphocytic Leukemia (ANLL): A Pilot Study," *Invest New Drugs*, 1991, 9(2):181-4.

Sudan N, Rossetti JM, Shadduck RK, et al, "Treatment of Acute Myelogenous Leukemia With Outpatient Azacitidine," *Cancer*, 2006, 107(8):1839-43.

◆ **AZA-CR** *see* AzaCITIDine *on page 140*

◆ **Azactam®** *see* Aztreonam *on page 145*

◆ **Azacytidine** *see* AzaCITIDine *on page 140*

- **5-Azacytidine** *see* AzaCITIDine *on page* 140
- **5-Aza-dCyd** *see* Decitabine *on page* 403
- **Azaepothilone B** *see* Ixabepilone *on page* 842
- **5-AZC** *see* AzaCITIDine *on page* 140
- **AZD6474** *see* Vandetanib *on page* 1435
- **Azthreonam** *see* Aztreonam *on page* 145

Aztreonam (AZ tree oh nam)

Brand Names: U.S. Azactam®; Cayston®

Brand Names: Canada Cayston®

Index Terms Azthreonam

Generic Availability (U.S.) Yes: Injection (powder for reconstitution)

Pharmacologic Category Antibiotic, Miscellaneous

Use

Injection: Treatment of patients with urinary tract infections, lower respiratory tract infections, septicemia, skin/skin structure infections, intra-abdominal infections, and gynecological infections caused by susceptible gram-negative bacilli

Inhalation: Improve respiratory symptoms in cystic fibrosis (CF) patients with *Pseudomonas aeruginosa*

Labeled Contraindications Hypersensitivity to aztreonam or any component of the formulation

Pregnancy Risk Factor B

Lactation Enters breast milk/not recommended (AAP rates "compatible"; AAP 2001 update pending)

Warnings/Precautions Rare cross-allergenicity to penicillins and cephalosporins has been reported. Use caution in renal impairment; dosing adjustment required for the injectable formulation. Prolonged use may result in fungal or bacterial superinfection, including *C. difficile*-associated diarrhea (CDAD) and pseudomembranous colitis; CDAD has been observed >2 months postantibiotic treatment. Patients colonized with *Burkholderia cepacia* have not been studied. Safety and efficacy has not been established in patients with FEV_1 <25% or >75% predicted. To reduce the development of resistant bacteria and maintain efficacy reserve use for CF patients with known *Pseudomonas aeruginosa*. Bronchospasm may occur occur following nebulization; administer a bronchodilator prior to treatment.

Adverse Reactions

Inhalation:

>10%:

Central nervous system: Fever (13%; more common in children)

Respiratory: Cough (54%), nasal congestion (16%), pharyngeal pain (12%), wheezing (16%)

1% to 10%:

Cardiovascular: Chest discomfort (8%)

Dermatologic: Rash (2%)

Gastrointestinal: Abdominal pain (7%), vomiting (6%)

Respiratory: Bronchospasm (3%)

<1%, postmarketing, and/or case reports: Arthralgia, facial edema, hypersensitivity reaction, joint swelling, throat tightness

Injection:

>10%:

Hematologic: Neutropenia (children 3% to 11%)

Hepatic: ALT/AST increased (children 4% to 6%; >3 times ULN: 15% to 20%, high dose)

Local: Pain at injection site (children 12%, adults 2%)

1% to 10%:

Central nervous system: Fever (≤1%)

Dermatologic: Rash (children 4%, adults 1%)

Gastrointestinal: Diarrhea (1%), nausea (1%), vomiting (1%)

Hematologic: Eosinophilia (children 6%, adults <1%), thrombocytosis (children 4%, adults <1%), neutropenia (adults <1%)

Local: Injection site reactions (1% to 3%) (erythema, induration; more common in children), phlebitis/thrombophlebitis (2%)

Renal: Serum creatinine increased (children 6%)

<1%: Abdominal cramps, abnormal taste, anaphylaxis, anemia, angioedema, aphthous ulcer, breast tenderness, bronchospasm, *C. difficile*-associated diarrhea, chest pain, confusion, diaphoresis, diplopia, dizziness, dyspnea, erythema multiforme, exfoliative dermatitis, flushing, halitosis, headache, hepatitis, hypotension, insomnia, jaundice, leukopenia, liver enzymes increased, muscular aches myalgia, numb tongue, pancytopenia, paresthesia, petechiae, pruritus, pseudomembranous colitis, purpura, seizure, sneezing, thrombocytopenia, tinnitus, toxic epidermal necrolysis, urticaria, vaginitis, vertigo, weakness, wheezing

Drug Interactions

Metabolism/Transport Effects None known.

Avoid Concomitant Use

Avoid concomitant use of Aztreonam with any of the following: BCG

Increased Effect/Toxicity There are no known significant interactions involving an increase in effect.

Decreased Effect

Aztreonam may decrease the levels/effects of: BCG; Sodium Picosulfate; Typhoid Vaccine

Storage/Stability

Inhalation: Prior to reconstitution, store at 2°C to 8°C (36°F to 46°F). Once removed from refrigeration, aztreonam and the diluent may be stored at room temperature (up to 25°C [77°F]) for ≤28 days. Protect from light. Use immediately after reconstitution.

Injection: Prior to reconstitution, store at room temperature; avoid excessive heat. Reconstituted solutions are colorless to light yellow straw and may turn pink upon standing without affecting potency. Use reconstituted solutions and I.V. solutions (in NS and D_5W) within 48 hours if kept at room temperature (25°C) or 7 days under refrigeration (4°C).

Infusion: Solution for infusion may be frozen at less than -2°C (less than -4°F) for up to 3 months. Thawed solution should be used within 24 hours if thawed at room temperature or within 72 hours if thawed under refrigeration. **Do not refreeze.**

Reconstitution

Inhalation: Reconstitute immediately prior to use. Squeeze diluent into opened glass vial. Replace rubber stopper and gently swirl vial until contents have completely dissolved.

I.M.: Reconstitute with at least 3 mL SWFI, sterile bacteriostatic water for injection, NS, or bacteriostatic sodium chloride.

I.V.:

Bolus injection: Reconstitute with 6-10 mL SWFI.

Infusion: Reconstitute to a final concentration ≤2%; the final concentration should not exceed 20 mg/mL.

Mechanism of Action Inhibits bacterial cell wall synthesis by binding to one or more of the penicillin-binding proteins (PBPs) which in turn inhibits the final transpeptidation step of peptidoglycan synthesis in bacterial cell walls, thus inhibiting cell wall biosynthesis. Bacteria eventually lyse due to ongoing activity of cell wall autolytic enzymes (autolysins and murein hydrolases) while cell wall assembly is arrested. Monobactam structure makes cross-allergenicity with beta-lactams unlikely.

Pharmacodynamics/Kinetics

Absorption: I.M.: Well absorbed; I.M. and I.V. doses produce comparable serum concentrations; Inhalation: Low systemic absorption

Distribution: Injection: Widely to most body fluids and tissues

V_d: Children: 0.2-0.29 L/kg; Adults: 0.2 L/kg

Relative diffusion of antimicrobial agents from blood into CSF: Good only with inflammation (exceeds usual MICs)

CSF:blood level ratio: Meninges: Inflamed: 8% to 40%; Normal: ~1%

Protein binding: 56%

Metabolism: Injection: Hepatic (minor %)

Half-life elimination: Injection:

Children 2 months to 12 years: 1.7 hours

Adults: Normal renal function: 1.7-2.9 hours

End-stage renal disease: 6-8 hours

Time to peak: I.M., I.V. push: Within 60 minutes; I.V. infusion: 1.5 hours

Excretion: Injection: Urine (60% to 70% as unchanged drug); feces (~13% to 15%)

Dosing

Adult & Geriatric

Urinary tract infection: I.M., I.V.: 500 mg to 1 g every 8-12 hours

Moderately severe systemic infections:

I.M.: 1 g every 8-12 hours

I.V.: 1-2 g every 8-12 hours

Severe systemic or life-threatening infections (especially caused by *Pseudomonas aeruginosa*): I.V.: 2 g every 6-8 hours; maximum: 8 g/day

Meningitis (gram-negative): I.V.: 2 g every 6-8 hours

***Pseudomonas aeruginosa* infection in cystic fibrosis:** Inhalation (nebulizer): 75 mg 3 times daily (at least 4 hours apart) for 28 days. Do not repeat for 28 days after completion.

Pediatric

Susceptible infections: I.M., I.V.: Children >1 month:

Mild-to-moderate infections: 30 mg/kg every 8 hours

Moderate-to-severe infections: 30 mg/kg every 6-8 hours; maximum: 120 mg/kg/day (8 g/day)

Infection in children with cystic fibrosis: I.V.: Children >1 month: 50 mg/kg/dose every 6-8 hours (ie, up to 200 mg/kg/day); maximum: 8 g/day

***Pseudomonas aeruginosa* infection in cystic fibrosis:** Inhalation (nebulizer): Children ≥7 years: 75 mg 3 times daily (at least 4 hours apart) for 28 days. Do not repeat for 28 days after completion.

Renal Impairment

Oral inhalation: Dosage adjustment not required for mild, moderate or severe renal impairment.

I.M., I.V.: Adults: Following initial dose, maintenance doses should be given as follows:

Cl_{cr} 10-30 mL/minute: 50% of usual dose at the usual interval

Cl_{cr} <10 mL/minute: 25% of usual dosage at the usual interval

Intermittent hemodialysis (IHD): Dialyzable (20% to 50%): Loading dose of 500 mg, 1 g, or 2 g, followed by 25% of initial dose at usual interval; for serious/life-threatening infections, administer one-eighth (1/8) of initial dose after each hemodialysis session (given in addition to the maintenance doses). Alternatively, may administer 500 mg every 12 hours (Heintz, 2009). **Note:** Dosing dependent on the assumption of 3 times/week, complete IHD sessions.

Peritoneal dialysis (PD): Administer as for Cl_{cr} <10 mL/minute

Continuous renal replacement therapy (CRRT) (Heintz, 2009; Trotman, 2005): Drug clearance is highly dependent on the method of renal replacement, filter type, and flow rate. Appropriate dosing requires close monitoring of pharmacologic response, signs of adverse reactions due to drug accumulation, as well as drug concentrations in relation to target trough (if appropriate). The following are general recommendations only (based on dialysate flow/ultrafiltration rates of 1-2 L/hour and minimal residual renal function) and should not supersede clinical judgment:

CVVH: Loading dose of 2 g followed by 1-2 g every 12 hours

CVVHD/CVVHDF: Loading dose of 2 g followed by either 1 g every 8 hours **or** 2 g every 12 hours (Heintz, 2009)

Administration

Inhalation: Administer using only an Altera® nebulizer system; **administer alone; do not mix with other nebulizer medications**. Administer a bronchodilator before administration of aztreonam (short-acting: 15 minutes to 4 hours before; long-acting: 30 minutes to 12 hours before). For patients on multiple inhaled therapies, administer bronchodilator first, then mucolytic, and lastly, aztreonam.

To administer Cayston®, pour reconstituted solution into the handset of the nebulizer system, turn unit on. Place the mouthpiece in the patient's mouth and encourage to breath normally through the mouth. Administration time is usually 2-3 minutes. Administer doses ≥4 hours apart.

Injection: Doses >1 g should be administered I.V.

I.M.: Administer by deep injection into large muscle mass, such as upper outer quadrant of gluteus maximus or the lateral part of the thigh

I.V.: Administer by slow I.V. push over 3-5 minutes or by intermittent infusion over 20-60 minutes.

Monitoring Parameters

Injection: Periodic liver function test; monitor for signs of anaphylaxis during first dose

Inhalation: Consider measuring FEV_1 prior to initiation of therapy

Test Interactions May interfere with urine glucose tests containing cupric sulfate (Benedict's solution, Clinitest®); positive Coombs' test

Additional Information Although marketed as an agent similar to aminoglycosides, aztreonam is a monobactam antimicrobial with almost pure gram-negative aerobic activity. It cannot be used for gram-positive infections.

Prescribing and Access Restrictions Cayston® (aztreonam inhalation solution) is only available through a select group of specialty pharmacies and cannot be obtained through a retail pharmacy. Because Cayston® may only be used with the Altera® Nebulizer System, it can only be obtained from the following specialty pharmacies: Cystic Fibrosis Services, Inc; IV Solutions; Foundation Care; and Pharmaceutical Specialties, Inc. This network of specialty pharmacies ensures proper access to both the drug and device. To obtain the medication and proper nebulizer, contact the Cayston Access Program at 1-877-7CAYSTON (1-877-722-9786) or at www.cayston.com.

Dosage Forms Excipient information presented when available (limited, particularly for generics); consult specific product labeling.

Infusion, premixed iso-osmotic solution:
 Azactam®: 1 g (50 mL); 2 g (50 mL)
Injection, powder for reconstitution: 1 g, 2 g
 Azactam®: 1 g, 2 g
Powder for reconstitution, for oral inhalation [preservative free]:
 Cayston®: 75 mg [supplied with diluent]

References

Heintz BH, Matzke GR, Dager WE, "Antimicrobial Dosing Concepts and Recommendations for Critically Ill Adult Patients Receiving Continuous Renal Replacement Therapy or Intermittent Hemodialysis," *Pharmacotherapy*, 2009, 29(5):562-77.

Retsch-Bogart GZ, Quittner AI, Gibson RL, et al, "Efficacy and Safety of Inhaled Aztreonam Lysine for Airway Pseudomonas in Cystic Fibrosis," *Chest*, 2009, 135 (5):1223-32.

Trotman RL, Williamson JC, Shoemaker DM, et al, "Antibiotic Dosing in Critically Ill Adult Patients Receiving Continuous Renal Replacement Therapy," *Clin Infect Dis*, 2005, 41(8):1159-66.

Tunkel AR, Hartman BJ, Kaplan SL, et al, "Practice Guidelines for the Management of Bacterial Meningitis," *Clin Infect Dis*, 2004, 39(9):1267-84.

◆ **B1939** *see* Eribulin *on page* 524

◆ **Bacillus Calmette-Guérin (BCG) Live** *see* BCG *on page* 153

◆ **Bactrim™** *see* Sulfamethoxazole and Trimethoprim *on page* 1302

◆ **Bactrim™ DS** *see* Sulfamethoxazole and Trimethoprim *on page* 1302

Basiliximab (ba si LIK si mab)

Related Information

Hematopoietic Stem Cell Transplantation *on page* 1887

Brand Names: U.S. Simulect®

Brand Names: Canada Simulect®

Generic Availability (U.S.) No

Pharmacologic Category Immunosuppressant Agent; Monoclonal Antibody

Use Prophylaxis of acute organ rejection in renal transplantation (in combination with cyclosporine and corticosteroids)

Unlabeled Use Treatment of refractory acute graft-versus-host disease (GVHD); prevention of liver or cardiac transplant rejection

Labeled Contraindications Hypersensitivity to basiliximab or any component of the formulation

Pregnancy Risk Factor B

Lactation Excretion in breast milk unknown/not recommended

Warnings/Precautions To be used as a component of an immunosuppressive regimen which includes cyclosporine and corticosteroids. The incidence of lymphoproliferative disorders and/or opportunistic infections may be increased by immunosuppressive therapy. Severe hypersensitivity reactions, occurring within 24 hours, have been reported. Reactions, including anaphylaxis, have occurred both with the initial exposure and/or following re-exposure after several months. Use caution during re-exposure to a subsequent course of therapy in a patient who has previously received basiliximab; patients in whom concomitant immunosuppression was prematurely discontinued due to abandoned transplantation or early graft loss are at increased risk for developing a severe hypersensitivity reaction upon re-exposure. Discontinue permanently if a severe reaction occurs. Medications for the treatment of hypersensitivity reactions should be available for immediate use. Treatment may result in the development of human antimurine antibodies (HAMA); however, limited evidence suggesting the use of muromonab-CD3 or other murine products is not precluded. **[U.S. Boxed Warning]: Should be administered under the supervision of a physician experienced in immunosuppression therapy and organ transplant management.** In renal transplant patients receiving basiliximab plus prednisone, cyclosporine, and mycophenolate, new-onset diabetes, glucose intolerance, and impaired fasting glucose were observed at rates significantly higher than observed in patients receiving prednisone, cyclosporine, and mycophenolate without basiliximab (Aasebo, 2010).

Adverse Reactions Administration of basiliximab did not appear to increase the incidence or severity of adverse effects in clinical trials. Adverse events were reported in 96% of both the placebo and basiliximab groups.

>10%:

- Cardiovascular: Hypertension, peripheral edema
- Central nervous system: Fever, headache, insomnia, pain
- Dermatologic: Acne, wound complications
- Endocrine & metabolic: Hypercholesterolemia, hyperglycemia, hyper-/hypokalemia, hyperuricemia, hypophosphatemia
- Gastrointestinal: Abdominal pain, constipation, diarrhea, dyspepsia, nausea, vomiting
- Genitourinary: Urinary tract infection
- Hematologic: Anemia
- Neuromuscular & skeletal: Tremor
- Respiratory: Dyspnea, infection (upper respiratory)
- Miscellaneous: Viral infection

3% to 10%:

- Cardiovascular: Abnormal heart sounds, angina, arrhythmia, atrial fibrillation, chest pain, generalized edema, heart failure, hypotension, tachycardia
- Central nervous system: Agitation, anxiety, depression, dizziness, fatigue, hypoesthesia, malaise
- Dermatologic: Cyst, hypertrichosis, pruritus, rash, skin disorder, skin ulceration
- Endocrine & metabolic: Acidosis, dehydration, diabetes mellitus, fluid overload, glucocorticoids increased, hyper-/hypocalcemia, hyperlipemia, hypertriglyceridemia, hypoglycemia, hypomagnesemia, hyponatremia, hypoproteinemia
- Gastrointestinal: Abdomen enlarged, esophagitis, flatulence, gastroenteritis, GI hemorrhage, gingival hyperplasia, melena, moniliasis, stomatitis (including ulcerative), weight gain
- Genitourinary: Bladder disorder, dysuria, genital edema (male), impotence, ureteral disorder, urinary frequency, urinary retention
- Hematologic: Hematoma, hemorrhage, leukopenia, polycythemia, purpura, thrombocytopenia, thrombosis
- Neuromuscular & skeletal: Arthralgia, arthropathy, back pain, cramps, fracture, hernia, leg pain, myalgia, neuropathy, paresthesia, rigors, weakness
- Ocular: Abnormal vision, cataract, conjunctivitis
- Renal: Albuminuria, hematuria, nonprotein nitrogen increased, oliguria, renal function abnormal, renal tubular necrosis

Respiratory: Bronchitis, bronchospasm, cough, pharyngitis, pneumonia, pulmonary edema, rhinitis, sinusitis

Miscellaneous: Accidental trauma, cytomegalovirus (CMV) infection, herpes infection (simplex and zoster), infection, sepsis

Postmarketing and/or case reports: Anaphylaxis, capillary leak syndrome, cytokine release syndrome, diabetes (new onset), fasting glucose impaired, glucose intolerance, hypersensitivity reaction (including heart failure, hypotension, tachycardia, bronchospasm, dyspnea, pulmonary edema, respiratory failure, sneezing, pruritus, rash, urticaria), lymphoproliferative disease

Drug Interactions

Metabolism/Transport Effects None known.

Avoid Concomitant Use

Avoid concomitant use of Basiliximab with any of the following: BCG; Belimumab; Natalizumab; Pimecrolimus; Tacrolimus (Topical); Vaccines (Live)

Increased Effect/Toxicity

Basiliximab may increase the levels/effects of: Belimumab; Hypoglycemic Agents; Leflunomide; Natalizumab; Vaccines (Live)

The levels/effects of Basiliximab may be increased by: Abciximab; Denosumab; Herbs (Hypoglycemic Properties); MAO Inhibitors; Pimecrolimus; Roflumilast; Salicylates; Selective Serotonin Reuptake Inhibitors; Tacrolimus (Topical); Trastuzumab

Decreased Effect

Basiliximab may decrease the levels/effects of: BCG; Coccidioidin Skin Test; Sipuleucel-T; Vaccines (Inactivated); Vaccines (Live)

The levels/effects of Basiliximab may be decreased by: Echinacea; Loop Diuretics

Ethanol/Nutrition/Herb Interactions Herb/Nutraceutical: Echinacea may diminish the therapeutic effect of basiliximab. Avoid hypoglycemic herbs, including alfalfa, bilberry, bitter melon, burdock, celery, damiana, fenugreek, garcinia, garlic, ginger, ginseng, gymnema, marshmallow, and stinging nettle (may enhance the hypoglycemic effect of basiliximab).

Storage/Stability Store intact vials refrigerated at 2°C to 8°C (36°F to 46°F). Should be used immediately after reconstitution; however, if not used immediately, reconstituted solution may be stored at 2°C to 8°C for up to 24 hours or at room temperature for up to 4 hours. Discard the reconstituted solution if not used within 24 hours.

Reconstitution Reconstitute with preservative free sterile water for injection (reconstitute 10 mg vial with 2.5 mL, 20 mg vial with 5 mL). Shake gently to dissolve. May further dilute reconstituted solution with 25 mL (10 mg) or 50 mL (20 mg) 0.9% sodium chloride or dextrose 5% in water. When mixing the solution, gently invert the bag to avoid foaming. Do not shake solutions diluted for infusion.

Mechanism of Action Chimeric (murine/human) immunosuppressant monoclonal antibody which blocks the alpha-chain of the interleukin-2 (IL-2) receptor complex; this receptor is expressed on activated T lymphocytes and is a critical pathway for activating cell-mediated allograft rejection

Pharmacodynamics/Kinetics

Duration: Mean: 36 days (determined by IL-2R alpha saturation)

Distribution: Mean: V_d: Children 1-11 years: 4.8 ± 2.1 L; Adolescents 12-16 years: 7.8 ± 5.1 L; Adults: 8.6 ± 4.1 L

Half-life elimination: Children 1-11 years: 9.5 days; Adolescents 12-16 years: 9.1 days; Adults: Mean: 7.2 days

Dosing

Adult & Geriatric Note: Patients previously administered basiliximab should only be re-exposed to a subsequent course of therapy with extreme caution.

Acute renal transplant rejection prophylaxis: I.V.: 20 mg within 2 hours prior to transplant surgery, followed by a second 20 mg dose 4 days after transplantation. The second dose should be withheld if complications occur (including severe hypersensitivity reactions or graft loss).

Acute cardiac transplant rejection prophylaxis (unlabeled use): I.V.: 20 mg on the day of transplant, followed by a second dose 4 days after transplantation (Mehra, 2005); usually given within the first hour postoperatively

Acute liver transplant rejection prophylaxis (unlabeled use): I.V.: 20 mg within 6 hours of organ reperfusion, followed by a second 20 mg dose 4 days after transplantation (Neuhaus, 2002)

Treatment of refractory acute GVHD (unlabeled use): I.V.: 20 mg on days 1 and 4; may repeat for recurrent acute GVHD (Schmidt-Hieber, 2005)

Pediatric Note: Patients previously administered basiliximab should only be re-exposed to a subsequent course of therapy with extreme caution.

Acute renal transplant rejection prophylaxis: I.V.:

Children <35 kg: 10 mg within 2 hours prior to transplant surgery, followed by a second 10 mg dose 4 days after transplantation; the second dose should be withheld if complications occur (including severe hypersensitivity reactions or graft loss)

Children ≥35 kg: Refer to adult dosing

Administration For intravenous administration only. Infuse as a bolus or I.V. infusion over 20-30 minutes. (Bolus dosing is associated with nausea, vomiting, and local pain at the injection site.) Administer only after assurance that patient will receive renal graft and immunosuppression. For the treatment of acute GVHD (unlabeled use), the dose was diluted in 250 mL NS and administered over 30 minutes (Schmidt-Hieber, 2005).

Monitoring Parameters Signs and symptoms of acute rejection; hypersensitivity, infection

Dosage Forms Excipient information presented when available (limited, particularly for generics); consult specific product labeling.

Injection, powder for reconstitution:

Simulect®: 10 mg [contains sucrose 10 mg/vial]

Simulect®: 20 mg [contains sucrose 20 mg/vial]

References

Aasebø W, Midtvedt K, Valderhaug TG, et al, "Impaired Glucose Homeostasis in Renal Transplant Recipients Receiving Basiliximab," *Nephrol Dial Transplant*, 2010, 25(4):1289-93.

Brennen DC, Daller JA, Lake KD, et al, "Rabbit Antithymocyte Globulin Versus Basiliximab in Renal Transplantation," *N Engl J Med*, 2006, 355(19):1967-77.

Mehra MR, Zucker MJ, Wagoner L, et al, "A Multicenter, Prospective, Randomized, Double-Blind Trial of Basiliximab in Heart Transplantation," *J Heart Lung Transplant*, 2005, 24(9):1297-304.

Neuhaus P, Clavien PA, Kittur D, et al, "Improved Treatment Response With Basiliximab Immunoprophylaxis After Transplantation: Results From a Double-Blind Randomized Placebo-Controlled Trial," *Liver Transpl*, 2002, 8(2):132-42.

Offner G, Toenshoff B, Höcker B, et al, "Efficacy and Safety of Basiliximab in Pediatric Renal Transplant Patients Receiving Cyclosporine, Mycophenolate Mofetil, and Steroids," *Transplantation*, 2008, 86(9):1241-8.

Schmidt-Hieber M, Feitz T, Knauf W, et al, "Efficacy if the Interleukin-2 Receptor Antagonist Basiliximab in Steroid-Refractory Acute Graft-Versus-Host Disease, *Br J Haematol*, 2005, 130 (4):568-74.

- **BAY 43-9006** *see* SORAfenib *on page* 1292
- **BAY 73-4506** *see* Regorafenib *on page* 1233
- **Baycadron™** *see* Dexamethasone (Systemic) *on page* 440

BCG (bee see jee)

Related Information

Safe Handling of Hazardous Drugs *on page* 1904

Brand Names: U.S. BCG Vaccine; TheraCys®; TICE® BCG

Brand Names: Canada BCG Vaccine; ImmuCyst®; Oncotice™

Index Terms Bacillus Calmette-Guérin (BCG) Live; BCG Vaccine U.S.P. *(percutaneous use product)*; BCG, Live

Generic Availability (U.S.) No

Pharmacologic Category Biological Response Modulator; Vaccine, Live (Bacterial)

Use

BCG intravesical: Treatment and prophylaxis of carcinoma *in situ* of the bladder; prophylaxis of primary or recurrent superficial or minimally invasive papillary tumors following transurethral resection

BCG vaccine: Immunization against *Mycobacterium tuberculosis* in persons not previously infected and who are at high risk for exposure

BCG vaccine is not routinely administered for the prevention of *M. tuberculosis* in the United States. The Advisory Committee on Immunization Practices (ACIP) recommends vaccination be considered for the following:

- Children with a negative tuberculin skin test who are continually exposed to (and cannot be separated from) adults who are untreated or ineffectively treated for TB disease when the child cannot be given long-term treatment for infection **or** if the adult has TB caused by strains resistant to isoniazid and rifampin.
- Healthcare workers with a high percentage of patients with *M. tuberculosis* strains resistant to both isoniazid and rifampin, if there is ongoing transmission of the resistant strains and subsequent infection is likely, or if comprehensive infection-control precautions have not been successful. In addition, healthcare workers should be counseled on the risks and benefits of vaccination and treatment of latent TB infection

Labeled Contraindications Immunosuppressed patients or persons with congenital or acquired immune deficiencies (eg, HIV infection, leukemia, lymphoma, cancer therapy, immunosuppressive therapy such as corticosteroids); active tuberculosis

BCG intravesical additional contraindications: Febrile illness, urinary tract infection, or gross hematuria; current symptoms or previous history of a systemic BCG reaction; recent (<7-14 days) biopsy, transurethral resection (TUR), or traumatic catheterization

BCG vaccine additional contraindications: Prior hypersensitivity to the vaccine or any component of the formulation

Pregnancy Risk Factor C

Lactation Excretion in breast milk unknown/not recommended

Warnings/Precautions [U.S. Boxed Warning]: Contains live, attenuated mycobacteria. Use appropriate precautions for handling and disposal. BCG is a biohazard; proper preparation technique, handling, and disposal of all equipment in contact with BCG as a biohazard material is recommended. BCG infections have been reported in healthcare workers due to accidental exposure (needlestick, skin laceration); nosocomial infections have been reported in patients receiving parenteral medications prepared in areas where BCG was prepared. To avoid cross contamination, do not prepare parenteral medications in an area where BCG has been prepared. Should be administered with caution to persons in groups at high risk for HIV. Use is contraindicated in HIV-infected persons, and HIV-infected persons thought to be infected with Mycobacterium tuberculosis should be strongly recommended for tuberculosis preventive therapy. Determine PPD status prior to use. BCG vaccination is not recommended for persons with a positive PPD reaction. Prior to intravesical instillation, patients with a positive PPD test should be further assessed for signs and/or symptoms of active or latent tuberculosis. Intravesical products should not be handled by persons with an immunodeficiency. All products are contraindicated for use in immunocompromised patients. Vaccination may not result in effective immunity in all patients. Response depends upon multiple factors (eg, type of vaccine, age of patient) and may be improved by administering the vaccine at the recommended dose, route, and interval. Vaccines may not be effective if administered during periods of altered immune competence (CDC, 2011).

[U.S. Boxed Warning]: May cause disseminated (including fatal) infections following intravesical administration. Instillation to actively bleeding mucosa may promote systemic BCG infection or sepsis; postpone treatment for ≥1 week following TUR, biopsy, traumatic catheterization, or gross hematuria. Do not use in patients with concurrent infections. Use caution in patients with aneurysms and prosthetic devices; ectopic BCG infection may occur at these sites. If signs and symptoms of a systemic BCG infection occur, permanently discontinue BCG treatment and begin therapy with ≥2 antimycobacterial agents while conducting a diagnostic evaluation. Infection from vaccine is not sensitive to pyrazinamide.

A systemic granulomatous illness occurring following exposure to BCG is referred to as a systemic BCG reaction when any of the following are present without another detectable etiology: fever ≥39.5°C for ≥12 hours or ≥ 38.5°C for ≥48 hours; pneumonitis; hepatitis; organ dysfunction outside of the GU tract with granulomatous inflammation; clinical signs of sepsis. A systemic BCG reaction is more likely to occur with intravesical administration <7 days after a biopsy, transurethral resection (TUR), or traumatic catheterization. Systemic symptoms may also occur following BCG vaccination.

Intravesical instillations should be postponed during antibiotic therapy; antibiotics may reduce the efficacy of therapy. Intravesical BCG may cause symptoms of bladder irritability which usually begin 4-6 hours after instillation and may last 24-72 hours; symptoms may increase in severity following each instillation. Intravesical instillation may be associated with increased risk of severe local reactions in the presence of small bladder capacity; use with caution. Safety and efficacy of intravesicular BCG have not been established in children. Packaging may contain natural latex rubber.

BCG vaccine should not be used for the active treatment of tuberculosis or for the prevention of cancer. Immediate treatment (including epinephrine 1:1000) for anaphylactoid and/or hypersensitivity reactions should be available during vaccine administration. Information not available for interchanging products used for intravesical administration.

Adverse Reactions Following vaccination, all serious adverse reactions must be reported to the U.S. Department of Health and Human Services (DHHS) Vaccine Adverse Event Reporting System (VAERS)

1-800-822-7967 or online at https://vaers.hhs.gov/esub/index. Adverse events following intravesicular administration should be reported to MEDWATCH (800-FDA-1088 or www.fda.gov/medwatch) or the manufacturer.

Adverse reactions associated with **intravesicular administration**:

>10%:

- Central nervous system: Malaise (7% to 40%), fever (17% to 38%), chills (9% to 34%), pain (17%)
- Gastrointestinal: Nausea/vomiting (3% to 16%), anorexia/weight loss (2% to 11%)
- Genitourinary: Dysuria (52% to 60%), bladder irritation (50% to 60%), urinary urgency/frequency (6% to 50%), hematuria (26% to 39%), cystitis (6% to 29%), urinary tract infection (2% to 18%)
- Hematological: Anemia (≤21%)
- Miscellaneous: Flu-like syndrome (24% to 33%)

1% to 10%:

- Central nervous system: Fatigue (≤7%), headache/dizziness (2% to 5%)
- Dermatologic: Rash (≤5%)
- Gastrointestinal: Diarrhea (6%), abdominal pain (2% to 5%), constipation (≤5%)
- Genitourinary: Genital pain (10%), hemorrhagic cystitis (9%), bladder cramps/pain (8%), urinary incontinence (2% to 6%), contracted bladder (≤5%), nocturia (5%), urinary debris (2% to 5%), genital inflammation/abscess (2%)
- Hematological: Leukopenia (≤5%), coagulopathy (≤5%), thrombocytopenia (≤5%)
- Neuromuscular & skeletal: Arthralgia/myalgia (3% to 7%), cramps/pain (1% to 6%), rigors (3%)
- Renal: Renal toxicity (10%)
- Respiratory: Pulmonary infection (<5%)
- Miscellaneous: Infection (3% to 5%), diaphoresis (3%), allergy (2%)

<1%: Abscesses, conjunctivitis, disseminated sepsis, epididymitis, granulomatous chorioretinitis, hepatitis, hepatic granuloma, iritis, keratitis, *M. bovis* infection (lung, liver, bone, bone marrow, kidney, lymph nodes, prostate, eye, peritoneum), orchitis, pneumonitis, prostatitis, skin ulceration, urethritis, urinary obstruction, uveitis

Adverse reactions associated with **BCG vaccination**: Axillary lymphadenopathy, cervical lymphadenopathy, disseminated BCG infection (BCG osteomyelitis, may occur from 4 months to 2 years after vaccination), local reactions (induration, itching, lesions, lymphadenitis, pustule, tenderness, ulceration). Local reactions may persist for up to 3 months; more severe manifestations may occur up to 5 months after vaccination and persist for several weeks.

Drug Interactions

Metabolism/Transport Effects None known.

Avoid Concomitant Use

Avoid concomitant use of BCG with any of the following: Antibiotics; Belimumab; Fingolimod; Hexaminolevulinate; Immunosuppressants

Increased Effect/Toxicity

The levels/effects of BCG may be increased by: AzaTHIOprine; Belimumab; Corticosteroids (Systemic); Fingolimod; Hydroxychloroquine; Immunosuppressants; Leflunomide; Mercaptopurine; Methotrexate

Decreased Effect

BCG may decrease the levels/effects of: Hexaminolevulinate; Tuberculin Tests

The levels/effects of BCG may be decreased by: Antibiotics; Fingolimod; Immune Globulins; Immunosuppressants

Storage/Stability Store vials under refrigeration at 2°C to 8°C (36°F to 46°F). Protect from light. Use within 2 hours of mixing. Do not freeze vaccine after reconstitution.

Reconstitution Prepare using aseptic technique. Do not prepare parenteral medications in an area where BCG has been prepared. Do not filter.

TheraCys®: Reconstitute with 3 mL of sterile preservative free saline and shake gently. Withdraw contents and add 50 mL of sterile preservative free saline.

TICE® BCG: Reconstitute with 1 mL sterile preservative free saline using a 3 mL syringe. Add to vial and swirl gently to form a homogenous suspension (forceful agitation may cause clumping). Dispense into a catheter tip syringe containing 49 mL of sterile preservative free saline. Mix by gently rotating the syringe. May also order reconstitution accessories from manufacturer.

BCG Vaccine U.S.P.: Reconstitute with 1 mL of SWFI; swirl gently, do not vigorously shake. For children <1 month, reconstitute with 2 mL SWFI.

Mechanism of Action BCG live is an attenuated strain of bacillus Calmette-Guérin (*Mycobacterium bovis*) used as a biological response modifier. BCG live, when used intravesicularly for treatment of bladder carcinoma *in situ*, is thought to cause a local, chronic inflammatory response involving macrophage and leukocyte infiltration of the bladder. By a mechanism not fully understood, this local inflammatory response leads to destruction of superficial tumor cells of the urothelium. BCG is active immunotherapy which stimulates the host's immune mechanism to reject the tumor. Evidence of systemic immune response is also commonly seen, manifested by a positive PPD tuberculin skin test reaction, however, its relationship to clinical efficacy is not well-established.

Dosing

Adult & Geriatric

Immunization against tuberculosis: Percutaneous: 0.2-0.3 mL (full strength dilution); conduct postvaccinal tuberculin test (5 TU of PPD) in 2-3 months; if test is negative, repeat vaccination. **Note:** Initial lesion usually appears after 10-14 days consisting of small, red papule at injection site and reaches maximum diameter of 3 mm in 4-6 weeks.

Immunotherapy for bladder cancer: Intravesicular: **Note:** Treatment should begin 7-14 days after biopsy or TUR. The contents of one vial is used for each dose.

TheraCys®: One dose instilled into bladder (retain for 2 hours) once weekly for 6 weeks followed by 1 treatment at 3, 6, 12, 18, and 24 months after initial treatment

TICE® BCG: One dose instilled into the bladder (retain for 2 hours) once weekly for 6 weeks (may repeat cycle 1 time) followed by approximately once monthly for at least 6-12 months

Pediatric

Immunization against tuberculosis: Percutaneous:

Children <1 month: 0.2-0.3 mL (half-strength dilution). Administer tuberculin test (5 TU) after 2-3 months; repeat vaccination after 1 year of age for negative tuberculin test if indications persist. **Note:** Initial lesion usually appears after 10-14 days consisting of small, red papule at injection site and reaches maximum diameter of 3 mm in 4-6 weeks.

Children >1 month: Refer to adult dosing.

Administration Should only be given intravesicularly (bladder irrigation) or percutaneously; **do not administer I.V., SubQ, I.M., or intradermally**.

Intravesicular: Empty or drain bladder. Instill BCG vaccine; retain for as long as possible, up to 2 hours. Patient should lie prone, rotating positions every 15 minutes to maximize bladder surface exposure. Following bladder instillation, patients should be instructed to void in a seated position in order to avoid the splashing of urine; burning may occur with the first void following therapy. Prior to flushing, disinfect the urine for 15 minutes with an equal amount of household bleach (this should be done for the first 6 hours after therapy). After administration, patients should drink plenty of water in order to flush the bladder.

Percutaneous: Apply vaccine with syringe and needle by dropping onto 1-2 inch area of horizontally positioned surface of cleansed, dry site (deltoid region of arm preferred); pulling skin tight, puncture skin with multiple puncture device centered over the vaccine; apply pressure for 5 seconds; spread vaccine evenly over puncture area. Apply loose covering and keep dry for 24 hours.

Simultaneous administration of vaccines helps ensure the patients will be fully vaccinated by the appropriate age. Simultaneous administration of vaccines is defined as administering >1 vaccine on the same day at different anatomic sites. Separate vaccines should not be combined in the same syringe unless indicated by product specific labeling. Separate needles and syringes should be used for each injection. The ACIP prefers each dose of a specific vaccine in a series come from the same manufacturer when possible. Adolescents and adults should be vaccinated while seated or lying down. In general, preterm infants should be vaccinated at the same chronological age as full-term infants (CDC, 2011).

Antipyretics have not been shown to prevent febrile seizures. Antipyretics may be used to treat fever or discomfort following vaccination (CDC, 2011). One study reported that routine prophylactic administration of acetaminophen to prevent fever prior to vaccination decreased the immune response of some vaccines; the clinical significance of this reduction in immune response has not been established (Prymula, 2009).

Monitoring Parameters PPD test prior to vaccination or intravesical treatment

Intravesical treatment: Signs and symptoms of toxicity/infection following every treatment. Signs that antituberculous therapy may be needed: Flu-like symptoms ≥72 hours, fever ≥101.3°F, systemic symptoms which worsen with each treatment, persistently abnormal liver function tests, prostatitis, epididymitis or orchitis of >2-3 day duration

Vaccination: Flu-like symptoms ≥72 hours, fever ≥103°F, acute local reactions lasting >2-3 days. Monitor for syncope for 15 minutes following administration. If seizure-like activity associated with syncope occurs, maintain patient in supine or Trendelenburg position to reestablish adequate cerebral perfusion.

Test Interactions PPD intradermal test: BCG results in reactive tuberculin skin test; rule out active tuberculosis prior to initiating intravesicular BCG treatment. BCG vaccine may be administered to persons with a PPD reaction of <5 mm induration; PPD should be used again 2-3 months after vaccination to ensure reactivity to vaccine (document in mm of induration). Vaccinees with a positive PPD test (>5 mm) should not be tested again unless exposed to tuberculosis. In this situation, an increase of induration may indicate a newly acquired TB infection. Vaccinees with a negative PPD test (<5 mm induration) may continue periodic skin testing as long as the results remain <5 mm (CDC, 1996).

Additional Information When used for immunization against tuberculosis, U.S. federal law requires that the name of medication, date of administration, the vaccine manufacturer, lot number of vaccine, and the administering person's name, title, and address be entered into the patient's permanent medical record. Multiple puncture device for vaccination available from Organon Teknika (1-800-662-6842).

Dosage Forms Excipient information presented when available (limited, particularly for generics); consult specific product labeling. [DSC] = Discontinued product

Injection, powder for reconstitution, intravesical:
  TICE® BCG: 50 mg
Injection, powder for reconstitution, intravesical [preservative free]:
  TheraCys®: 81 mg [contains natural rubber/natural latex in packaging; supplied with diluent]
  TheraCys®: 81 mg [contains natural rubber/natural latex in packaging, polysorbate 80 (in diluent); supplied with diluent] [DSC]
Injection, powder for reconstitution, percutaneous:
  BCG Vaccine: 50 mg

References

Bassi P, "BCG (Bacillus of Calmette Guerin) Therapy of High-Risk Superficial Bladder Cancer," *Surg Oncol*, 2002, 11(1-2):77-83.

Centers for Disease Control and Prevention (CDC), "Recommendations of the Advisory Committee on Immunization Practices (ACIP): General Recommendations on Immunization," *MMWR Recomm Rep*, 2011, 60(2):1-64.

Centers for Disease Control and Prevention,"The Role of BCG Vaccine in the Prevention and Control of Tuberculosis in the United States: A Joint Statement by the Advisory Council for the Elimination of Tuberculosis and the Advisory Committee on Immunization Practices," *MMWR Recomm Rep*, 1996, 45(RR-4):1-18. Available at http://www.cdc.gov/mmwr/PDF/rr/rr4504.pdf

National Comprehensive Cancer Network® (NCCN), "Clinical Practice Guidelines in Oncology™: Bladder Cancer," Version 2.2012. Available at http://www.nccn.org/professionals/physician_gls/PDF/bladder.pdf

Rischmann P, Desgrandchamps F, Malavaud B, et al, "BCG Intravesical Instillations: Recommendations for Side-Effects Management," *Eur Urol*, 2000, 37(Suppl 1):33-6.

◆ **BCG, Live** *see* BCG *on page* 153

◆ **BCG Vaccine** *see* BCG *on page* 153

◆ **BCG Vaccine U.S.P. *(percutaneous use product)*** *see* BCG *on page* 153

◆ **BCNU** *see* Carmustine *on page* 243

◆ **Bebulin® VH** *see* Factor IX Complex (Human) *on page* 575

Bendamustine (ben da MUS teen)

Related Information

Management of Chemotherapy-Induced Nausea and Vomiting *on page* 1786
Management of Drug Extravasations *on page* 1800
Safe Handling of Hazardous Drugs *on page* 1904

Brand Names: U.S. Treanda®

Brand Names: Canada Treanda®

Index Terms Bendamustine Hydrochloride; Cytostasan; SDX-105

Generic Availability (U.S.) No

Pharmacologic Category Antineoplastic Agent; Antineoplastic Agent, Alkylating Agent; Antineoplastic Agent, Alkylating Agent (Nitrogen Mustard)

Use Treatment of chronic lymphocytic leukemia (CLL); treatment of progressed indolent B-cell non-Hodgkin's lymphoma (NHL)

Unlabeled Use Treatment of relapsed or refractory Hodgkin lymphoma; treatment of mantle cell lymphoma; salvage therapy for relapsed multiple myeloma; first-line therapy for follicular lymphoma; treatment of Waldenström's macroglobulinemia

Labeled Contraindications Hypersensitivity to bendamustine, mannitol, or any component of the formulation

Pregnancy Risk Factor D

Lactation Excretion in breast milk unknown/not recommended

Warnings/Precautions Hazardous agent - use appropriate precautions for handling and disposal. Myelosuppression (neutropenia, thrombocytopenia, and anemia) is a common toxicity; may require therapy delay and/or dose reduction; monitor blood counts. Complications due to febrile neutropenia and severe thrombocytopenia have been reported. ANC should recover to ≥1000/mm^3 and platelets to ≥75,000/mm^3 prior to cycle initiation. Pneumonia and sepsis have been reported with use; may require hospitalization; septic shock and fatalities due to infection have occurred; patients with myelosuppression are more susceptible to infection; monitor closely.

Infusion reactions, including chills, fever, pruritus, and rash are common; rarely, anaphylactic and anaphylactoid reactions have occurred, particularly with the second or subsequent cycle(s). In general, patients who experienced grade 3 or higher allergic reactions were not rechallenged. Consider premedication with antihistamines, antipyretics, and corticosteroids for patients with a history of grade 1 or 2 infusion reaction. Discontinue for severe allergic reaction; consider discontinuation with grade 3 or 4 infusion reaction. Rash, toxic skin reactions and bullous exanthema have been reported with monotherapy and in combination with other antineoplastics; may be progressive or worsen with continued treatment; discontinue bendamustine treatment for severe or progressive skin reaction; monitor closely; discontinue bendamustine treatment for severe or progressive skin reaction. The risk for severe skin toxicity is increased with concurrent use of allopurinol and other medications known to cause skin toxicity; Stevens-Johnson syndrome and toxic epidermal necrolysis (TEN) have been reported. TEN has also been reported when used in combination with rituximab. Erythema, marked swelling, and pain have been reported with extravasation; monitor infusion site; avoid extravasation.

Tumor lysis syndrome (usually occurring in the first treatment cycle) may occur as a consequence of antineoplastic treatment, including treatment with bendamustine. May lead to life-threatening acute renal failure; adequate hydration and prophylactic measures should be instituted prior to treatment in high-risk patients; monitor closely. **Note:** Allopurinol may increase the risk for bendamustine skin toxicity. May cause hypokalemia; monitor potassium closely during therapy, particularly in patients with cardiac disease.

Per manufacturer's labeling, use with caution in patients with mild hepatic impairment. However, a pharmacokinetic study showed only slight differences in bendamustine AUC and C_{max} in patients with mild hepatic impairment (defined in the study as total bilirubin 1-1.5 times ULN or AST greater than ULN), as compared to patients with normal hepatic function (Owen, 2010). Use is not recommended in patients with moderate (AST or ALT 2.5-10 times ULN and total bilirubin 1.5-3 times ULN) or severe (total bilirubin >3 times ULN) hepatic impairment.

Use with caution in patients with mild-to-moderate renal impairment. The U.S. and Canadian product labels do not recommend use in patients with Cl_{cr} <40 mL/minute. A pharmacokinetic study illustrated only slight differences in bendamustine AUC and C_{max} in patients with mild (Cl_{cr} >50 to ≤80 mL/minute) and moderate (Cl_{cr} >30 to ≤50 mL/minute) renal dysfunction, compared to patients with normal renal function (Owen, 2010). A retrospective safety study found no significant difference in lab toxicities between CLL patients with renal impairment (Cl_{cr} <40 mL/minute) compared to those without renal impairment, although an increase in grades 3/4 thrombocytopenia and grades 3/4 BUN increases were detected in patients with renal impairment (Nordstrom, 2012); monitor blood counts and renal function. **Note:** UK labeling (Levact prescribing information, October, 2010) recommends no dosage adjustment for patients with Cl_{cr} >10 mL/minute. Malignancies (including myelodysplastic syndrome, myeloproliferative disorders, acute myeloid leukemia and bronchial cancer) and premalignant diseases have been reported in patients who have received bendamustine.

Adverse Reactions

>10%:

- Cardiovascular: Peripheral edema (≤13%)
- Central nervous system: Fatigue (9% to 57%), fever (24% to 34%), headache (≤21%), chills (6% to 14%), dizziness (≤14%), insomnia (≤13%)
- Dermatologic: Rash (8% to 16%; grades 3/4: ≤3%)
- Endocrine & metabolic: Dehydration (≤14%)
- Gastrointestinal: Nausea (20% to 75%), vomiting (16% to 40%), diarrhea (9% to 37%), constipation (≤29%), anorexia (≤23%), weight loss (7% to 18%), stomatitis (≤15%), abdominal pain (5% to 13%), appetite loss (≤13%), dyspepsia (≤11%)
- Hematologic: Myelosuppression (nadir: in week 3), lymphopenia (68% to 99%; grades 3/4: 47% to 94%), leukopenia (61% to 94%; grades 3/4: 28% to 56%), anemia (88% to 89%; grades 3/4: 11% to 13%), thrombocytopenia (77% to 86%; grades 3/4: 11% to 25%), neutropenia (75% to 86%; grades 3/4: 43% to 60%)
- Hepatic: Bilirubin increased (≤34%; grades 3/4: 3%)
- Neuromuscular & skeletal: Back pain (≤14%), weakness (8% to 11%)
- Respiratory: Cough (4% to 22%), dyspnea (≤16%)

1% to 10%:

- Cardiovascular: Tachycardia (≤7%), hypotension (≤6%), chest pain (≤6%), hypertension aggravated (≤3%)
- Central nervous system: Anxiety (≤8%), depression (≤6%), pain (≤6%)
- Dermatologic: Pruritus (5% to 6%), dry skin (≤5%)
- Endocrine & metabolic: Hypokalemia (≤9%), hyperuricemia (≤7%; grades 3/4: 2%), hyperglycemia (grades 3/4: ≤3%), hypocalcemia (grades 3/4: ≤2%), hyponatremia (grades 3/4: ≤2%)
- Gastrointestinal: Gastroesophageal reflux disease (≤10%), xerostomia (9%), taste alteration (≤7%), oral candidiasis (≤6%), abdominal distention (≤5%)
- Genitourinary: Urinary tract infection (≤10%)
- Hematologic: Febrile neutropenia (3% to 6%)
- Hepatic: ALT increased (grades 3/4: ≤3%), AST increased (grades 3/4: ≤1%)
- Local: Infusion site pain (≤6%), catheter site pain (≤5%)
- Neuromuscular & skeletal: Arthralgia (≤6%), bone pain (≤5%), limb pain (≤5%)

Renal: Creatinine increased (grades 3/4: ≤2%)

Respiratory: Upper respiratory infection (10%), sinusitis (≤9%), pharyngolaryngeal pain (≤8%), pneumonia (≤8%), nasopharyngitis (6% to 7%), wheezing (≤5%), nasal congestion (≤5%)

Miscellaneous: Herpes infection (3% to 10%), infection (≤6%; grades 3/4: 2%), hypersensitivity (≤5%; grades 3/4: 1%), diaphoresis (≤5%), night sweats (≤5%)

<1%, postmarketing, and/or case reports: Acute myeloid leukemia, acute renal failure, alopecia, anaphylaxis, bronchial carcinoma, bullous exanthema, cardiac failure, dermatitis, erythema, hemolysis, hepatitis B virus reactivation, infusion reaction, injection/infusion site reaction (erythema, irritation, pain, phlebitis, pruritus, swelling), malaise, mucosal inflammation, myelodysplastic syndrome, myeloproliferative disorders, pulmonary fibrosis, sepsis, septic shock, skin necrosis, somnolence, Stevens-Johnson syndrome, toxic epidermal necrolysis, toxic skin reactions, tumor lysis syndrome

Drug Interactions

Metabolism/Transport Effects **Substrate** of BCRP, CYP1A2 (minor), P-glycoprotein; **Note:** Assignment of Major/Minor substrate status based on clinically relevant drug interaction potential

Avoid Concomitant Use

Avoid concomitant use of Bendamustine with any of the following: CloZAPine

Increased Effect/Toxicity

Bendamustine may increase the levels/effects of: CloZAPine

The levels/effects of Bendamustine may be increased by: CYP1A2 Inhibitors (Strong)

Decreased Effect

The levels/effects of Bendamustine may be decreased by: CYP1A2 Inducers (Strong)

Storage/Stability Prior to reconstitution, store intact vials up to 25°C (77°F); excursions permitted up to 30°C (86°F). Protect from light. The solution in the vial (reconstituted with SWFI) is stable for 30 minutes (transfer to 500 mL infusion bag within that 30 minutes). The solution diluted in 500 mL for infusion is stable for 24 hours refrigerated or 3 hours at room temperature and room light. Infusion must be completed within these time frames.

Reconstitution Use appropriate precautions for handling and disposal. Reconstitute 25 mg vial with 5 mL and 100 mg vial with 20 mL of sterile water for injection to a concentration of 5 mg/mL; powder usually dissolves within 5 minutes. Prior to administration, dilute appropriate dose in 500 mL NS (or $D_{2.5}$½NS) to a final concentration of 0.2-0.6 mg/mL; mix thoroughly.

Mechanism of Action Bendamustine is an alkylating agent (nitrogen mustard derivative) with a benzimidazole ring (purine analog) which demonstrates only partial cross-resistance (*in vitro*) with other alkylating agents. It leads to cell death via single and double strand DNA cross-linking. Bendamustine is active against quiescent and dividing cells. The primary cytotoxic activity is due to bendamustine (as compared to metabolites).

Pharmacodynamics/Kinetics

Distribution: V_{ss}: ~25 L

Protein binding: 94% to 96%

Metabolism: Hepatic, via CYP1A2 to active (minor) metabolites gamma-hydroxy bendamustine (M3) and N-desmethyl-bendamustine (M4)

Half-life elimination: Bendamustine: ~40 minutes; M3: ~3 hours; M4: ~30 minutes

Time to peak, serum: At end of infusion

Excretion: Feces (~90%); urine (1% to 10%)

Dosing

Adult & Geriatric

Chronic lymphocytic leukemia (CLL): I.V.:100 mg/m² over 30 minutes on days 1 and 2 of a 28-day treatment cycle (as a single agent) for up to 6 cycles (Knauf, 2009; Knauf, 2012)

CLL, relapsed/refractory (unlabeled dosing): I.V.: 70 mg/m² on days 1 and 2 of a 28-day treatment cycle (in combination with rituximab) for up to 6 cycles (Fischer, 2011)

Non-Hodgkin lymphomas: I.V.:

Lymphoma, indolent B-cell, refractory: 120 mg/m² over 60 minutes on days 1 and 2 of a 21-day treatment cycle (as a single agent) for up to 8 cycles (Kahl, 2010)

Lymphoma, indolent B-cell, follicular, or mantle cell, first-line (unlabeled use): 90 mg/m² on days 1 and 2 of a 28-day treatment cycle (in combination with rituximab) for up to 6 cycles (Rummel, 2009)

Lymphoma, follicular, relapsed or refractory (unlabeled use): 90 mg/m² on days 1 and 2 of a 35-day treatment cycle (in combination with bortezomib and rituximab) for 5 cycles (Fowler, 2011)

Lymphoma, mantle cell, relapsed or refractory (unlabeled use): 90 mg/m² over 30 minutes on days 2 and 3 of a 28-day treatment cycle (in combination with rituximab) for up to 4 cycles (Rummel, 2005)

Hodgkin lymphoma, relapsed or refractory (unlabeled use): I.V.: 120 mg/m² on days 1 and 2 of a 28-day treatment cycle for up to 6 cycles (Moskowitz, 2009)

Multiple myeloma, salvage therapy (unlabeled use): I.V.: 90-100 mg/m² on days 1 and 2 of a 28-day treatment cycle for at least 2 cycles (Knop, 2005)

Waldenström's macroglobulinemia, refractory (unlabeled use): I.V.: 90 mg/m² on days 1 and 2 of a 28-day treatment cycle (in combination with rituximab) for 6 cycles (Treon, 2011) **or** 90 mg/m² over 30 minutes on days 2 and 3 of a 28-day treatment cycle (in combination with rituximab) for 4 cycles (Rummel, 2005)

Renal Impairment

Cl_{cr} <40 mL/minute: Use is not recommended in the U.S. and Canadian manufacturers' labeling.

Study data suggest minor changes in systemic exposure may occur with mild-to-moderate renal impairment. Based on a pharmacokinetic study (patients receiving 120 mg/m² for 2 days every 21 days), only slight differences in bendamustine AUC and C_{max} were demonstrated in patients with mild (Cl_{cr} >50 to ≤80 mL/minute) and moderate (Cl_{cr} >30 to ≤50 mL/minute) renal dysfunction, compared to patients with normal renal function (Owen, 2010). A retrospective study of bendamustine in CLL and NHL patients with renal impairment (Cl_{cr} <40 mL/minute) compared to those without (Cl_{cr} ≥60 mL/minute) found no significant difference in lab toxicities in CLL patients with renal impairment compared to those without renal impairment, although an increase in grades 3/4 thrombocytopenia was noted in NHL patients and grades 3/4 BUN increases were higher when combining data for CLL and NHL (Nordstrom, 2012).

Note: UK manufacturer's labeling (Levact [prescribing information], October, 2010) recommends no dosage adjustment for patients with Cl_{cr} >10 mL/minute.

Hepatic Impairment

Mild impairment: Per U.S. and Canadian manufacturers' labeling, use with caution. However, a pharmacokinetic study showed only slight differences in bendamustine AUC and C_{max} in patients with mild hepatic impairment (defined in the study as total bilirubin 1-1.5 times ULN or AST greater than ULN), compared to patients with normal hepatic function (Owen, 2010).

Moderate impairment (AST or ALT 2.5-10 times ULN and total bilirubin 1.5-3 times ULN): Use is not recommended.

Severe impairment (total bilirubin >3 times ULN): Use is not recommended.

Adjustment for Toxicity

Infusion reactions:

Grade 1 or 2: Consider premedication with antihistamines, antipyretics, and corticosteroids in subsequent cycles

Grade 3 or 4: Consider discontinuing treatment

Treatment delay:

Hematologic toxicity ≥grade 4: Delay treatment until resolves (ANC ≥1000/mm^3, platelets ≥75,000/mm^3)

Nonhematologic toxicity ≥grade 2 (clinically significant): Delay treatment until resolves to ≤grade 1

Dose modification CLL:

Hematologic toxicity ≥grade 3: Reduce dose to 50 mg/m^2 on days 1 and 2 of each treatment cycle. For recurrent hematologic toxicity (≥grade 3), further reduce dose to 25 mg/m^2 on days 1 and 2 of the treatment cycle. May cautiously re-escalate dose in subsequent cycles.

Nonhematologic toxicity ≥grade 3 (clinically significant): Reduce dose to 50 mg/m^2 on days 1 and 2 of the treatment cycle with discretion. May cautiously re-escalate dose in subsequent cycles.

Dose modification in NHL:

Hematologic toxicity grade 4: Reduce dose to 90 mg/m^2 on days 1 and 2 of each treatment cycle. For recurrent hematologic toxicity (grade 4), further reduce dose to 60 mg/m^2 on days 1 and 2 of each treatment cycle.

Nonhematologic toxicity ≥grade 3: Reduce dose to 90 mg/m^2 on days 1 and 2 of the treatment cycle with discretion. For recurrent toxicity ≥grade 3, further reduce dose to 60 mg/m^2 on days 1 and 2 of each treatment cycle.

Combination Regimens

Lymphoma, non-Hodgkin's: Bendamustine-Rituximab on page 1525

Lymphoma, non-Hodgkin's (Mantle Cell): Bendamustine-Rituximab on page 1525

Administration Infuse over 30 minutes for the treatment of CLL and over 60 minutes for NHL; administration times for unlabeled uses/doses vary by protocol. Consider premedication with antihistamines, antipyretics, and corticosteroids for patients with a previous grade 1 or 2 infusion reaction to bendamustine. Avoid extravasation; monitor I.V. site for redness, swelling, or pain.

Emetic Potential Moderate (30% to 90%)

Vesicant/Extravasation Risk May be an irritant; there are case reports of erythema, swelling and pain from extravasation

Monitoring Parameters CBC with differential (monitored weekly [initially] in clinical trials); serum creatinine; ALT, AST, and total bilirubin; monitor potassium and uric acid levels in patients at risk for tumor lysis syndrome; monitor for infusion reactions anaphylaxis, infection and dermatologic toxicity; monitor I.V. site during and after infusion.

Canadian labeling also recommends periodic monitoring of blood pressure, serum glucose, and ECG (in patients with cardiac disease particularly if concomitant electrolyte disturbances).

Dosage Forms Excipient information presented when available (limited, particularly for generics); consult specific product labeling.

Injection, powder for reconstitution:

Treanda®: 25 mg, 100 mg [contains mannitol]

References

Fischer K, Cramer P, Busch R, et al, "Bendamustine Combined With Rituximab in Patients With Relapsed and/or Refractory Chronic Lymphocytic Leukemia: A Multicenter Phase II Trial of the German Chronic Lymphocytic Leukemia Study Group," *J Clin Oncol*, 2011, 29(26):3559-66.

Fowler N, Kahl BS, Lee P, et al, "Bortezomib, Bendamustine, and Rituximab in Patients With Relapsed or Refractory Follicular Lymphoma: The Phase II VERTICAL Study," *J Clin Oncol*, 2011, 29(25):3389-95.

Friedberg JW, Cohen P, Chen L, et al, "Bendamustine in Patients With Rituximab-Refractory Indolent and Transformed Non-Hodgkin's Lymphoma: Results From a Phase II Multicenter, Single-Agent Study," *J Clin Oncol*, 2008, 26(2):204-10.

Kahl BS, Bartlett NL, Leonard JP, et al, "Bendamustine Is Effective Therapy in Patients With Rituximab-Refractory, Indolent B-Cell Non-Hodgkin Lymphoma: Results From a Multicenter Study," *Cancer*, 2010, 116(1):106-14.

Knauf WU, Lissitchkov T, Aldaoud A, et al, "Bendamustine Compared With Chlorambucil In Previously Untreated Patients With Chronic Lymphocytic Leukaemia: Updated Results of a Randomized Phase III Trial," *Br J Haematol*, 2012, 159(1):67-77.

Knauf WU, Lissichkov T, Aldaoud A, et al, "Phase III Randomized Study of Bendamustine Compared With Chlorambucil in Previously Untreated Patients With Chronic Lymphocytic Leukemia (B-CLL)," *J Clin Oncol*, 2009, 27(26):4378-84.

Knop S, Straka C, Haen M, et al, "The Efficacy and Toxicity of Bendamustine in Recurrent Multiple Myeloma After High-Dose Chemotherapy," *Haematologica*, 2005, 90(9):1287-8.

Moskowitz, AJ, Hamlin PA, Gerecitano J, et al, "Bendamustine is Highly Active in Heavily Pre-Treated Relapsed and Refractory Hodgkin Lymphoma and Serves as a Bridge to Allogeneic Stem Cell Transplant," *Blood*, 2009, 114(22):720 [abstract 720 from 2009 ASH Annual Meeting].

Nordstrom BL, Knopf KB, Teltsch D, et al, "Retrospective safety assessment of bendamustine in patients with renal impairment," *J Clin Oncol*, 2012, 30(15s):e13018 [abstract e13018 from 2012 ASCO Annual Meeting].

Owen JS, Melhem M, Passarell JA, et al, "Bendamustine Pharmacokinetic Profile and Exposure-Response Relationships in Patients With Indolent Non-Hodgkin's Lymphoma," *Cancer Chemother Pharmacol*, 2010, 66(6):1039-49.

Robinson KS, Williams ME, van der Jagt RH, et al, "Phase II Multicenter Study of Bendamustine Plus Rituximab in Patients With Relapsed Indolent B-Cell and Mantle Cell Non-Hodgkin's Lymphoma," *J Clin Oncol*, 2008, 26(27):4473-9.

Rummel MJ, Al-Batran SE, Kim SZ, et al, "Bendamustine Plus Rituximab is Effective and has a Favorable Toxicity Profile in the Treatment of Mantle Cell and Low-Grade Non-Hodgkin's Lymphoma," *J Clin Oncol*, 2005, 23(15):3383-9.

Rummel MJ, Niederle N, Maschmeyer G, et al, "Bendamustine Plus Rituximab is Superior in Respect of Progression Free Survival and CR Rate When Compared to CHOP Plus Rituximab as First-Line Treatment of Patients With Advanced Follicular, Indolent, and Mantle Cell Lymphomas: Final Results of a Randomized Phase III Study of the StiL (Study Group Indolent Lymphomas, Germany)," *Blood*, 2009, 114(22):405 [abstract 405 from 2009 ASH Annual Meeting]

◆ **Bendamustine Hydrochloride** *see* Bendamustine *on page* 158

◆ **BeneFix®** *see* Factor IX *on page* 571

◆ **Benzmethyzin** *see* Procarbazine *on page* 1208

Benzydamine (ben ZID a meen)

Brand Names: Canada Apo-Benzydamine®; Dom-Benzydamine; Novo-Benzydamine; PMS-Benzydamine; Tantum®

Index Terms Benzydamine Hydrochloride

Pharmacologic Category Local Anesthetic, Oral

Use Symptomatic treatment of pain associated with acute pharyngitis; treatment of pain associated with radiation-induced oropharyngeal mucositis

Labeled Contraindications Hypersensitivity to benzydamine or any component of the formulation

Lactation Excretion in breast milk unknown/use caution

Warnings/Precautions May cause local irritation and/or burning sensation in patients with altered mucosal integrity. Dilution (1:1 in warm water) may attenuate this effect. Use caution in renal impairment.

Storage/Stability Store at 15°C to 30°C; protect from freezing.

Mechanism of Action Local anesthetic and anti-inflammatory, reduces local pain and inflammation. Does not interfere with arachidonic acid metabolism.

Pharmacodynamics/Kinetics

Absorption: Oral rinse may be absorbed, at least in part, through the oral mucosa

Excretion: Urine (primarily as unchanged drug)

Dosing

Adult & Geriatric

Acute pharyngitis: Oral rinse: Gargle with 15 mL of undiluted solution every 1½-3 hours until symptoms resolve. Patient should expel solution from mouth following use; solution should not be swallowed.

Mucositis: Oral rinse: 15 mL of undiluted solution as a gargle or rinse 3-4 times/day; contact should be maintained for at least 30 seconds, followed by expulsion from the mouth.

Renal Impairment No adjustment required.

Administration Patient should not swallow the liquid. Begin treatment 1 day prior to initiation of radiation therapy and continue daily during treatment. Continue oral rinse treatments after the completion of radiation therapy until desired result/healing is achieved.

Dosage Forms: Canada Excipient information presented when available (limited, particularly for generics); consult specific product labeling.

Oral rinse: 0.15% (100 mL, 250 mL)

◆ **Benzydamine Hydrochloride** *see* Benzydamine *on page* 164

◆ **Beta-HC® [OTC]** *see* Hydrocortisone (Topical) *on page* 719

◆ **Bethkis®** *see* Tobramycin (Systemic, Oral Inhalation) *on page* 1366

Bevacizumab (be vuh SIZ uh mab)

Related Information

Management of Chemotherapy-Induced Nausea and Vomiting *on page* 1786

Principles of Anticancer Therapy *on page* 1878

Brand Names: U.S. Avastin®

Brand Names: Canada Avastin®

Index Terms Anti-VEGF Monoclonal Antibody; Anti-VEGF rhuMAb; rhuMAb-VEGF

Generic Availability (U.S.) No

Pharmacologic Category Antineoplastic Agent, Monoclonal Antibody; Vascular Endothelial Growth Factor (VEGF) Inhibitor

Use Treatment of metastatic colorectal cancer (first-or second-line treatment); treatment of unresectable, locally advanced, recurrent or metastatic nonsquamous, nonsmall cell lung cancer; treatment of progressive glioblastoma; treatment of metastatic renal cell cancer (not an approved use in Canada)

Note: Not indicated for the adjuvant treatment of colorectal cancer. For the treatment of glioblastoma, effectiveness is based on improvement in objective response rate.

Unlabeled Use Treatment of metastatic breast cancer, recurrent cervical cancer, recurrent advanced ovarian cancer, soft tissue sarcomas (angiosarcoma or hemangiopericytoma/solitary fibrous tumor), age-related macular degeneration (AMD)

Labeled Contraindications There are no contraindications listed in the FDA-approved manufacturer's labeling.

Canadian labeling: Hypersensitivity to bevacizumab, any component of the formulation, Chinese hamster ovary cell products or other recombinant human or humanized antibodies; untreated CNS metastases

Pregnancy Risk Factor C

Lactation Excretion in breast milk unknown/not recommended

Warnings/Precautions **[U.S. Boxed Warning]: Gastrointestinal (GI) perforation (sometimes fatal) has occurred in 0.3 to 2.4% of clinical study patients receiving bevacizumab; discontinue if GI perforation occurs.** Most cases occur within 50 days of treatment initiation; monitor patients for signs/symptoms (eg, fever, abdominal pain with constipation and/or nausea/vomiting). GI fistula (including enterocutaneous, esophageal, duodenal, and rectal fistulas), and intra-abdominal abscess have been reported in patients receiving bevacizumab for colorectal cancer and other cancers (not related to treatment duration). Non-GI fistula formation (including tracheoesophageal, bronchopleural, biliary, vaginal, renal, and bladder fistulas) has been observed, most commonly within the first 6 months of treatment; permanently discontinue in patients who develop internal organ fistulas. **[U.S. Boxed Warning]: The incidence of wound healing and surgical complications is increased in patients who have received bevacizumab; discontinue with wound dehiscence. Although the appropriate interval between withholding bevacizumab and elective surgery has not been defined, bevacizumab should be discontinued at least 28 days prior to surgery and should not be reinitiated for at least 28 days after surgery and until wound is fully healed.** In a retrospective review of central venous access device placements, a greater risk of wound dehiscence was observed when port placement and bevacizumab administration were separated by <14 days (Erinjeri, 2011).

Bevacizumab is associated with an increased risk for arterial thromboembolic events (ATE), including cerebral infarction, stroke, MI, TIA, angina, and other ATEs, when used in combination with chemotherapy. History of ATE or ≥65 years of age may present an even greater risk. Although patients with cancer are at risk for venous thromboembolism (VTE), a meta-analysis of 15 controlled trials has demonstrated an increased risk for VTE in patients who received bevacizumab (Nalluri, 2008). Permanently discontinue therapy in patients with severe ATE or life-threatening pulmonary embolism; the safety of treatment reinitiation after ATE has not been studied.

Use with caution in patients with cardiovascular disease. Among approved and nonapproved uses evaluated thus far, the incidence of heart failure (HF) and/or left ventricular dysfunction (including LVEF decline), is higher in patients receiving bevacizumab plus chemotherapy when compared to chemotherapy alone. Bevacizumab may potentiate the cardiotoxic effects of anthracyclines. HF is more common with prior anthracycline exposure and/or left chest wall irradiation. The safety of therapy resumption or continuation in patients with cardiac dysfunction has not been studied. In studies of patients with metastatic breast cancer (an unlabeled use), the incidence of grades 3 or 4 HF was increased in patients receiving bevacizumab plus paclitaxel, compared to the control arm. Patients with metastatic breast cancer who had received prior anthracycline therapy had a higher rate of HF compared to those receiving paclitaxel alone (3.8% vs 0.6% respectively). A meta-analysis of 5 studies which enrolled patients with metastatic breast cancer who received bevacizumab suggested an association with an increased risk of heart failure; all trials included in the analysis enrolled patients who either received prior or were receiving concurrent anthracycline therapy (Choueiri, 2011).

Bevacizumab may cause and/or worsen hypertension; use caution in patients with pre-existing hypertension and monitor BP closely in all patients. Permanent discontinuation is recommended in patients who experience a hypertensive crisis or encephalopathy. Temporarily discontinue in patients who develop uncontrolled hypertension. An increase in diastolic and systolic blood pressures were noted in a retrospective review of patients with renal insufficiency (Cl_{cr} ≤60 mL/minute) who received bevacizumab for renal cell cancer (Gupta, 2011). Cases of reversible posterior leukoencephalopathy syndrome (RPLS) have been reported. Symptoms (which include headache, seizure, confusion, lethargy, blindness and/or other vision, or neurologic disturbances) may occur from 16 hours to 1 year after treatment initiation. Resolution of symptoms usually occurs within days after discontinuation; however, neurologic sequelae may remain. RPLS may be associated with hypertension; discontinue bevacizumab and begin management of hypertension, if present.

[U.S. Boxed Warning]: Severe or fatal hemorrhage, including hemoptysis, gastrointestinal bleeding, central nervous system hemorrhage, epistaxis, and vaginal bleeding have been reported (up to 5 times more frequently if receiving bevacizumab). Avoid use in patients with serious hemorrhage or recent hemoptysis (≥2.5 mL blood). Serious pulmonary hemorrhage has been reported in patients receiving bevacizumab (primarily in patients with nonsmall cell lung cancer with squamous cell histology [not an FDA-approved indication]). Intracranial hemorrhage, including cases of grade 3 or 4 hemorrhage, has occurred in patients with previously treated glioblastoma. Treatment discontinuation is recommended in all patients with intracranial or other serious hemorrhage. Use with caution in patients with CNS metastases; once case of CNS hemorrhage was observed in an ongoing study of NSCLC patients with CNS metastases. Use in patients with untreated CNS metastases is contraindicated in the Canadian labeling. Use with caution in patients at risk for thrombocytopenia.

Infusion reactions (eg, hypertension, hypertensive crisis, wheezing, oxygen desaturation, hypersensitivity [including anaphylactic/anaphylactoid reactions], chest pain, rigors, headache, diaphoresis) may occur with the first infusion (uncommon); interrupt therapy in patients experiencing severe infusion reactions; there are no data to address routine premedication use or reinstitution of therapy in patients who experience severe infusion reactions. Proteinuria and/or nephrotic syndrome have been associated with bevacizumab; risk may be increased in patients with a history of hypertension; thrombotic microangiopathy has been associated with bevacizumab-induced proteinuria. Withhold treatment for ≥2 g proteinuria/24 hours and resume when proteinuria is <2 g/24 hours; discontinue in patients with nephrotic syndrome. Elderly patients (≥65 years of age) are at higher risk for adverse events, including thromboembolic events and proteinuria; serious adverse events occurring more frequently in the elderly also include deep thrombophlebitis, sepsis, hyper-/hypotension,

MI, CHF, leukopenia, anemia, dehydration, hypokalemia, and hyponatremia. Microangiopathic hemolytic anemia (MAHA) has been reported when bevacizumab has been used in combination with sunitinib. Concurrent therapy with sunitinib and bevacizumab is also associated with dose-limiting hypertension in patients with metastatic renal cell cancer. The incidence of hand-foot syndrome is increased in patients treated with bevacizumab plus sorafenib in comparison to those treated with sorafenib monotherapy. When used in combination with myelosuppressive chemotherapy, increased rates of severe or febrile neutropenia and neutropenic infection were reported. Bevacizumab, in combination with chemotherapy (or biologic therapy), is associated with an increased risk of treatment-related mortality; a higher risk of fatal adverse events was identified in a meta-analysis of 16 trials in which bevacizumab was used for the treatment of various cancers (breast cancer, colorectal cancer, non small cell lung cancer, pancreatic cancer, prostate cancer, and renal cell cancer) and compared to chemotherapy alone (Ranpura, 2011). When bevacizumab is used in combination with myelosuppressive chemotherapy, increased rates of severe or febrile neutropenia and neutropenic infection have been reported. In premenopausal women receiving bevacizumab in combination with mFOLFOX (fluorouracil/oxaliplatin based chemotherapy) the incidence of ovarian failure (amenorrhea ≥3 months) was higher (34%) compared to women who received mFOLFOX alone (2%); ovarian function recovered in some patients after treatment was discontinued; premenopausal women should be informed of the potential risk of ovarian failure. Serious eye infections and vision loss due to endophthalmitis have been reported from intravitreal administration (unlabeled use/route).

Adverse Reactions Percentages reported as monotherapy and as part of combination chemotherapy regimens. Some studies only reported hematologic toxicities grades ≥4 and nonhematologic toxicities grades ≥3.

>10%:

Cardiovascular: Hypertension (12% to 34%; grades 3/4: 5% to 18%), thromboembolic event (≤21%; grades 3/4: 15%; venous thrombus/embolus: 8%; grades 3/4: 5% to 7%; arterial thrombosis 6%; grades 3/4: 3%), hypotension (7% to 15%)

Central nervous system: Pain (8% to 62%), headache (24% to 37%; grades 3/4: 2% to 4%), dizziness (19% to 26%), fatigue (≤45%; grades 3/4: 4% to 19%), sensory neuropathy (grades 3/4: 1% to 17%; in combination with paclitaxel: 24%)

Dermatologic: Alopecia (6% to 32%), dry skin (7% to 20%), exfoliative dermatitis (3% to 19%), skin discoloration (2% to 16%)

Gastrointestinal: Abdominal pain (8% to 61%; grades 3/4: 8%), vomiting (47% to 52%; grades 3/4: ≤11%), anorexia (35% to 43%), constipation (4% to 40%), diarrhea (grades 3/4: 1% to 34%), stomatitis (30% to 32%), gastrointestinal hemorrhage (19% to 24%), dyspepsia (17% to 24%), taste disorder (14% to 21%), weight loss (15% to 20%), flatulence (11% to 19%), nausea (grades 3/4: ≤12%)

Hematologic: Hemorrhage (≤40%; grades 3/4: 1% to 5%), leukopenia (grades 3/4: 37%), neutropenia (grade 4: 21% to 27%)

Neuromuscular & skeletal: Myalgia (8% to 19%), back pain (≤12%)

Renal: Proteinuria (4% to 36%; grades 3/4: ≤7%; median onset: 5.6 months; median time to resolution: 6.1 months)

Respiratory: Upper respiratory infection (40% to 47%), epistaxis (19% to 35%), dyspnea (25% to 26%), rhinitis

Miscellaneous: Infection (≤55%; serious: 7% to 14%; pneumonia, catheter, or wound infections)

1% to 10%:

Cardiovascular: DVT (6% to 9%; grades 3/4: 9%), HF (grades 3/4: 1% to 4%), syncope (grades 3/4: 3%), intra-abdominal venous thrombosis (grades 3/4: 3%), cardio-/cerebrovascular arterial thrombotic event (2% to 4%), left ventricular dysfunction (grades 3/4: 1%)

Central nervous system: CNS hemorrhage (1% to 5%; grades 3/4: 1%), dysphonia (≤5%)

Dermatologic: Skin ulcer (≤6%), wound dehiscence (1% to 6%), acne (≤1%)

Endocrine & metabolic: Dehydration (grades 3/4: ≤10%), hyponatremia (grades 3/4: 4%)

Gastrointestinal: Xerostomia (4% to 7%), colitis (1% to 6%), ileus (grades 3/4: 4% to 5%), gingival bleeding (2% to 4%), fistula (1%), gastrointestinal perforation (≤4%), gastroesophageal reflux (≤2%), gingivitis (≤2%), mouth ulceration (≤2%), tooth abscess (≤2%), intra-abdominal abscess (1%), gastritis (≤1%), gingival pain (≤1%)

Genitourinary: Vaginal hemorrhage (4%)

Hematologic: Neutropenic fever/infection (5%; grades 3 and/or 4: 4% to 5%), thrombocytopenia (5%)

Neuromuscular & skeletal: Weakness (10%), neuropathy (other than sensory: grades 3/4: 1% to 5%)

Ocular: Blurred vision (≤2%)

Otic: Tinnitus (≤2%), deafness (≤1%)

Respiratory: Voice alteration (5% to 9%), pneumonitis/pulmonary infiltrates (grades 3/4: 5%), hemoptysis (nonsquamous histology 2%), pulmonary embolism (≤1%)

Miscellaneous: Infusion reactions (<3%)

<1%, postmarketing, and/or case reports (limited to important or life-threatening): Anaphylaxis, anastomotic ulceration, angina, antibody formation (anti-bevacizumab and neutralizing), bladder perforation, cerebral infarction; fistula (biliary, bladder, bronchopleural, duodenal, enterocutaneous, esophageal, gastrointestinal, rectal, renal, tracheoesophageal [TE] and vaginal); gastrointestinal ulcer, gall bladder perforation, hemorrhagic stroke, hypersensitivity, hypertensive crises, hypertensive encephalopathy, intestinal necrosis, intestinal obstruction, mesenteric venous occlusion, microangiopathic hemolytic anemia (when used in combination with sunitinib), MI, nasal septum perforation, nephrotic syndrome, osteonecrosis (jaw), ovarian failure, pancytopenia, polyserositis, pulmonary hemorrhage, pulmonary hypertension, renal failure, renal thrombotic microangiopathy, reversible posterior leukoencephalopathy syndrome (RPLS), sepsis, subarachnoid hemorrhage, toxic anterior segment syndrome (TASS), transient ischemic attack, ureteral stricture, wound healing complications

Reported from unlabeled use: Eye disorders: Endophthalmitis (infectious and sterile), hemorrhage (conjunctival, retinal or vitreous), intraocular inflammation (iritis, vitritis), intraocular pressure increased, ocular hyperemia, ocular pain/discomfort, permanent vision loss, retinal detachment, visual disturbance, vitreous floaters

Drug Interactions

Metabolism/Transport Effects None known.

Avoid Concomitant Use

Avoid concomitant use of Bevacizumab with any of the following: CloZAPine; SUNItinib

Increased Effect/Toxicity

Bevacizumab may increase the levels/effects of: Antineoplastic Agents (Anthracycline, Systemic); CloZAPine; Irinotecan; SORAfenib; SUNItinib

The levels/effects of Bevacizumab may be increased by: SUNItinib

Decreased Effect There are no known significant interactions involving a decrease in effect.

Storage/Stability Store vials at 2°C to 8°C (36°F to 46°F); do not freeze. Protect from light; do not shake. Diluted solutions are stable for up to 8 hours under refrigeration. Discard unused portion of vial.

Reconstitution Dilute in 100 mL NS prior to infusion (the manufacturer recommends a total volume of 100 mL). Do not mix with dextrose-containing solutions.

Mechanism of Action Bevacizumab is a recombinant, humanized monoclonal antibody which binds to, and neutralizes, vascular endothelial growth factor (VEGF), preventing its association with endothelial receptors, Flt-1 and KDR. VEGF binding initiates angiogenesis (endothelial proliferation and the formation of new blood vessels). The inhibition of microvascular growth is believed to retard the growth of all tissues (including metastatic tissue).

Pharmacodynamics/Kinetics

Distribution: V_d: 46 mL/kg

Half-life elimination: ~20 days (range: 11-50 days)

Excretion: Clearance: 2.75-5 mL/kg/day

Dosing

Adult & Geriatric Details concerning dosing in combination regimens should also be consulted.

Colorectal cancer, metastatic: I.V.: 5 or 10 mg/kg every 2 weeks (in combination with fluorouracil-based chemotherapy)

Canadian labeling: 5 mg/kg every 2 weeks (in combination with fluorouracil-based chemotherapy)

Glioblastoma: 10 mg/kg every 2 weeks as monotherapy **or** (unlabeled) 10 mg/kg every 2 weeks (in combination with irinotecan) (Vredenburgh, 2007)

Nonsmall cell lung cancer (nonsquamous cell histology): I.V.: 15 mg/kg every 3 weeks (in combination with carboplatin and paclitaxel) for 4-6 cycles followed by maintenance treatment (unlabeled use) of bevacizumab 15 mg/kg every 3 weeks as monotherapy until disease progression or unacceptable toxicity (Sandler, 2006)

Renal cell cancer, metastatic: 10 mg/kg every 2 weeks (in combination with interferon alfa) **or** (unlabeled) 10 mg/kg every 2 weeks as monotherapy (Yang, 2003)

Age-related macular degeneration (unlabeled use/route): Intravitreal: 1.25 mg (0.05 mL) monthly until improvement/resolution, usually ~1-3 injections (Avery, 2006) or 2.5 mg (0.1 mL) every 4 weeks for 3 doses (Bashshur, 2006)

Breast cancer, metastatic (unlabeled use): I.V.: 10 mg/kg every 2 weeks (in combination with paclitaxel) (Miller, 2007)

Ovarian cancer, advanced recurrent (unlabeled use): I.V.: 15 mg/kg every 3 weeks (Burger, 2007)

Renal Impairment There are no dosage adjustments provided in manufacturer's labeling

Hepatic Impairment There are no dosage adjustments provided in manufacturer's labeling

Adjustment for Toxicity I.V. administration (systemic): There are no recommended dosage reductions. Temporary suspension is recommended for severe infusion reactions, at least 4 weeks prior to (and after) elective surgery, in moderate-to-severe proteinuria (in most studies, treatment was withheld for ≥2 g proteinuria/24 hours), or in patients with severe hypertension which is not controlled with medical management. Permanent discontinuation is recommended (by the manufacturer) in patients who develop wound dehiscence and wound healing complications requiring intervention, fistula (gastrointestinal and nongastrointestinal), gastrointestinal perforation, intra-abdominal abscess, hypertensive crisis, hypertensive encephalopathy, serious bleeding/hemorrhage, severe arterial thromboembolic event, nephrotic syndrome, or RPLS.

Combination Regimens

Brain tumors: Bevacizumab-Irinotecan (Glioblastoma) on page 1531

Breast cancer:
- Bevacizumab-Capecitabine (Breast Cancer) on page 1528
- Docetaxel-Bevacizumab on page 1608
- Paclitaxel-Bevacizumab on page 1725

Colorectal cancer:
- Bevacizumab-Fluorouracil-Leucovorin on page 1530
- Bevacizumab + FOLFIRI (Colorectal) on page 1530
- Bevacizumab-Oxaliplatin-Fluorouracil-Leucovorin on page 1531
- Bevacizumab + XELOX (Colorectal) on page 1532

Lung cancer (nonsmall cell):
- Bevacizumab-Carboplatin-Paclitaxel (NSCLC) on page 1528
- Bevacizumab-Carboplatin-Pemetrexed (NSCLC) on page 1529
- Bevacizumab-Cisplatin-Gemcitabine (NSCLC) on page 1529

Renal cell cancer:
- Bevacizumab-Interferon Alfa (RCC) on page 1530
- Bevacizumab (RCC Regimen) on page 1532

Administration

I.V. infusion, usually after the other antineoplastic agents. Infuse the initial dose over 90 minutes. The second infusion may be shortened to 60 minutes if the initial infusion is well tolerated. The third and subsequent infusions may be shortened to 30 minutes if the 60-minute infusion is well tolerated. Monitor closely during the infusion for signs/symptoms of an infusion reaction. Some institutions use a 10-minute infusion (0.5 mg/kg/minute) for bevacizumab dosed at 5 mg/kg (after tolerance at the 90-, 60-, and 30-minute infusion rates has been established; Reidy, 2007). Do not administer I.V. push. Do not administer with dextrose solutions.

Intravitreal injection (unlabeled use/route): Adequate local anesthesia and a topical broad-spectrum antimicrobial agent should be administered prior to the procedure; administer topical ophthalmic antibiotics for 3 days after procedure (Avery, 2006; Bashshur, 2006).

Emetic Potential Very low <10%

Monitoring Parameters Monitor closely during the infusion for signs/symptoms of an infusion reaction. Monitor CBC with differential; signs/symptoms of gastrointestinal perforation, fistula, or abscess (including abdominal pain, constipation, vomiting, and fever); signs/symptoms of bleeding, including hemoptysis, gastrointestinal, and/or CNS bleeding, and/or epistaxis. Monitor blood pressure every 2-3 weeks; more frequently if hypertension develops during therapy. Continue to monitor blood pressure after discontinuing due to bevacizumab-induced hypertension. Monitor for proteinuria/nephrotic syndrome with urine dipstick; collect 24 hour urine in patients with ≥2+ reading.

AMD: Monitor intraocular pressure and retinal artery perfusion

Dosage Forms Excipient information presented when available (limited, particularly for generics); consult specific product labeling.

Injection, solution [preservative free]:

Avastin®: 25 mg/mL (4 mL, 16 mL) [derived from or manufactured using Chinese hamster ovary cells]

References

Allegra CJ, Yothers G, O'Connell MJ, et al, "Initial Safety Report of NSABP C-08: A Randomized Phase III Study of Modified FOLFOX6 With or Without Bevacizumab for the Adjuvant Treatment of Patients With Stage II or III Colon Cancer," *J Clin Oncol*, 2009, 27(20):3385-90.

Avery RL, Pieramici DJ, Rabena MD, et al, "Intravitreal Bevacizumab (Avastin) for Neovascular Age-Related Macular Degeneration," *Ophthalmology*, 2006, 113(3):363-72.

Bashshur AF, Bazarbachi A, Schakal A, et al, "Intravitreal Bevacizumab for the Management of Choroidal Neovascularization in Age-Related Macular Degeneration," *Am J Ophthalmol*, 2006, 142(1):1-9.

Bracarda S, Bellmunt J, Melichar B, et al, "Overall Survival in Patients With Metastatic Renal Cell Carcinoma Initially Treated With Bevacizumab Plus Interferon-α2a and Subsequent Therapy With Tyrosine Kinase Inhibitors: A Retrospective Analysis of the Phase III AVOREN Trial," *BJU Int*, 2011, 107(2):214-9.

Burger RA, Sill MW, Monk BJ, et al, "Phase II Trial of Bevacizumab in Persistent or Recurrent Epithelial Ovarian Cancer or Primary Peritoneal Cancer: A Gynecologic Oncology Group Study," *J Clin Oncol*, 2007, 25(33):5165-71.

Choueiri TK, Mayer EL, Je Y, et al, "Congestive Heart Failure Risk in Patients With Breast Cancer Treated With Bevacizumab," *J Clin Oncol*, 2011, 29(6):632-8.

Cloughesy TF, Prados MD, Wen PY, et al, "A Phase II, Randomized, Non-Comparative Clinical Trial of the Effect of Bevacizumab (BV) Alone or in Combination With Irinotecan (CPT) on 6-Month Progression Free Survival (PFS6) in Recurrent, Treatment-Refractory Glioblastoma (GBM)," *J Clin Oncol*, 2008, 26(Supp):2010B [abstract 2010b from 2008 ASCO Annual Meeting].

Erinjeri JP, Fong AJ, Kemeny NE, et al, "Timing of Administration of Bevacizumab Chemotherapy Affects Wound Healing After Chest Wall Port Placement," *Cancer*, 2011, 117(6):1296-301.

Escudier B, Pluzanska A, Koralewski P, et al, "Bevacizumab Plus Interferon Alfa-2a for Treatment of Metastatic Renal Cell Carcinoma: A Randomised, Double-Blind Phase III Trial," *Lancet*, 2007, 370(9605):2103-11.

Gray R, Bhattacharya S, Bowden C, et al, "Independent Review of E2100: A Phase III Trial of Bevacizumab Plus Paclitaxel Versus Paclitaxel in Women With Metastatic Breast Cancer," *J Clin Oncol*, 2009, 27(30):4966-72.

Gupta S, Parsa VB, Heilbrun LK, et al, "Safety and Efficacy of Molecularly Targeted Agents in Patients With Metastatic Kidney Cancer With Renal Dysfunction," *Anticancer Drugs*, 2011, 22 (8):794-800.

Johnson DH, Fehrenbacher L, Novotny WF, et al, "Randomized Phase II Trial Comparing Bevacizumab Plus Carboplatin and Paclitaxel With Carboplatin and Paclitaxel Alone in Previously Untreated Locally Advanced or Metastatic Non-Small-Cell Lung Cancer," *J Clin Oncol*, 2004, 22(11):2184-91.

Kreisl TN, Kim L, Moore K, et al, "Phase II Trial of Single-Agent Bevacizumab Followed by Bevacizumab Plus Irinotecan at Tumor Progression in Recurrent Glioblastoma," *J Clin Oncol*, 2009, 27(5):740-5.

Miles D, Chan A, Dirix LY, et al, "Phase III Study of Bevacizumab Plus Docetaxel Compared With Placebo Plus Docetaxel for the First-Line Treatment of Human Epidermal Growth Factor Receptor 2-Negative Metastatic Breast Cancer," *J Clin Oncol*, 2010, 28(20):3239-47.

Miller KD, "E2100: A Phase III Trial of Paclitaxel Versus Paclitaxel/Bevacizumab for Metastatic Breast Cancer," *Clin Breast Cancer*, 2003, 3(6):421-2.

Miller KD, Chap LI, Holmes FA, et al, "Randomized Phase III Trial of Capecitabine Compared With Bevacizumab Plus Capecitabine in Patients With Previously Treated Metastatic Breast Cancer," *J Clin Oncol*, 2005, 23(4):792-9.

Miller K, Wang M, Gralow J, et al, "Paclitaxel Plus Bevacizumab Versus Paclitaxel Alone for Metastatic Breast Cancer," *N Engl J Med*, 2007, 357(26):2666-76.

Monk BJ, Choi DC, Pugmire G, et al, "Activity of Bevacizumab (rhuMAB VEGF) in Advanced Refractory Epithelial Ovarian Cancer," *Gynecol Oncol*, 2005, 96(3):902-5.

Monk BJ, Sill MW, Burger RA, et al, "Phase II Trial of Bevacizumab in the Treatment of Persistent or Recurrent Squamous Cell Carcinoma of the Cervix: A Gynecologic Oncology Group Study," *J Clin Oncol*, 2009, 27(7):1069-74.

Nalluri SR, Chu D, Keresztes R, et al, "Risk of Venous Thromboembolism With the Angiogenesis Inhibitor Bevacizumab in Cancer Patients: A Meta-Analysis," *JAMA*, 2008, 300(19): 2277-85.

National Comprehensive Cancer Network® (NCCN), "Clinical Practice Guidelines in Oncology™: Soft Tissue Sarcoma," Version 2.2011. Available at http://www.nccn.org/professionals/physician_gls/PDF/sarcoma.pdf

Ranpura V, Hapani S, and Wu S, "Treatment-Related Mortality With Bevacizumab in Cancer Patients," *JAMA*, 2011, 305(5):487-94.

Reidy DL, Chung KY, Timoney JP, et al, "Bevacizumab 5 mg/kg Can be Infused Safely over 10 minutes," *J Clin Oncol*, 2007, 25(19):2691-5.

Rini BI, Halabi S, Rosenberg JE, et al, "Bevacizumab Plus Interferon Alfa Compared With Interferon Alfa Monotherapy in Patients With Metastatic Renal Cell Carcinoma: CALGB 90206," *J Clin Oncol*, 2008, 26(33):5422-8.

Robert NJ, Dieras V, Glaspy J, et al, "RIBBON-1: Randomized, Double-Blind, Placebo-Controlled, Phase III Trial of Chemotherapy With or Without Bevacizumab (B) for First-Line Treatment of HER2-Negative Locally Recurrent or Metastatic Breast Cancer (MBC)," *J Clin Oncol*, 2009, 27 (15s):1005 [abstract 1005 from 2009 ASCO Annual Meeting]

Saltz LB, Clarke S, Díaz-Rubio E, et al, "Bevacizumab in Combination With Oxaliplatin-Based Chemotherapy as First-Line Therapy in Metastatic Colorectal Cancer: A Randomized Phase III Study," *J Clin Oncol*, 2008, 26(12):2013-9.

Sandler A, Gray R, Perry MC, et al, "Paclitaxel-Carboplatin Alone or With Bevacizumab for Non-Small-Cell Lung Cancer," *N Engl J Med*, 2006, 355(24):2542-50.

Vredenburgh JJ, Desjardins A, Herndon JE 2nd, et al, "Bevacizumab Plus Irinotecan in Recurrent Glioblastoma Multiforme," *J Clin Oncol*, 2007, 25(30):4722-9.

Yang JC, Haworth L, Sherry RM, et al, "A Randomized Trial of Bevacizumab, An Antivascular Endothelial Growth Factor Antibody, for Metastatic Renal Cancer," *N Engl J Med*, 2003, 349 (5):427-34.

Bexarotene (Systemic) (beks AIR oh teen)

Related Information

Management of Chemotherapy-Induced Nausea and Vomiting *on page 1786*

Safe Handling of Hazardous Drugs *on page 1904*

Brand Names: U.S. Targretin®

Generic Availability (U.S.) No

Pharmacologic Category Antineoplastic Agent, Miscellaneous

Use Treatment of cutaneous manifestations of cutaneous T-cell lymphoma in patients who are refractory to at least one prior systemic therapy

Labeled Contraindications Hypersensitivity to bexarotene or any component of the formulation; pregnancy

Pregnancy Risk Factor X

Lactation Excretion in breast milk unknown/not recommended

Warnings/Precautions Hazardous agent - use appropriate precautions for handling and disposal. **[U.S. Boxed Warning]: Bexarotene is a retinoid, a drug class associated with birth defects in humans; do not administer during pregnancy.** Pregnancy test needed 1 week before initiation and every month thereafter. Effective contraception must be in place 1 month before initiation, during therapy, and for at least 1 month after discontinuation. Male patients with sexual partners who are pregnant, possibly pregnant, or who could become pregnant, must use condoms during sexual intercourse during treatment and for 1 month after last dose. Induces significant lipid abnormalities in a majority of patients (triglyceride, total cholesterol, and HDL); reversible on discontinuation. Use extreme caution in patients with underlying hypertriglyceridemia. Pancreatitis secondary to hypertriglyceridemia has been reported. Patients with risk factors for pancreatitis (eg, prior pancreatitis, uncontrolled hyperlipidemia, excess ethanol consumption, uncontrolled diabetes, biliary tract disease) should generally not receive bexarotene (oral).

Monitor for liver function test abnormalities and discontinue drug if tests are three times the upper limit of normal values for AST, ALT, or bilirubin. Hypothyroidism occurs in about a third of patients. Monitor for signs and symptoms of infection about 4-8 weeks after initiation (leukopenia may occur). Any new visual abnormalities experienced by the patient should be evaluated by an ophthalmologist (cataracts can form, or worsen, especially in the geriatric population). May cause photosensitization. Safety and efficacy are not established in the pediatric population. Use only with extreme caution in patients with hepatic impairment. Limit additional vitamin A intake to <15,000 units/day. Use caution with diabetic patients.

Adverse Reactions First percentage is at a dose of 300 mg/m^2/day; the second percentage is at a dose >300 mg/m^2/day.

>10%:

Cardiovascular: Peripheral edema (13% to 11%)

Central nervous system: Headache (30% to 42%), chills (10% to 13%)

Dermatologic: Rash (17% to 23%), exfoliative dermatitis (10% to 28%)

Endocrine & metabolic: Hyperlipidemia (about 79% in both dosing ranges), hypercholesteremia (32% to 62%), hypothyroidism (29% to 53%)

Hematologic: Leukopenia (17% to 47%)

Neuromuscular & skeletal: Weakness (20% to 45%)

Miscellaneous: Infection (13% to 23%)

<10%:

Cardiovascular: Hemorrhage, hypertension, angina pectoris, right heart failure, tachycardia, cerebrovascular accident, syncope

Central nervous system: Fever (5% to 17%), insomnia (5% to 11%), subdural hematoma, depression, agitation, ataxia, confusion, dizziness, hyperesthesia

Dermatologic: Dry skin (about 10% for both dosing ranges), alopecia (4% to 11%), skin ulceration, acne, skin nodule, maculopapular rash, serous drainage, vesicular bullous rash, cheilitis

Endocrine & metabolic: Hypoproteinemia, hyperglycemia, weight loss/gain, breast pain

Gastrointestinal: Abdominal pain (11% to 4%), nausea (16% to 8%), diarrhea (7% to 42%), vomiting (4% to 13%), anorexia (2% to 23%), constipation, xerostomia, flatulence, colitis, dyspepsia, gastroenteritis, gingivitis, melena, pancreatitis, serum amylase increased

Genitourinary: Albuminuria, hematuria, urinary incontinence, urinary tract infection, urinary urgency, dysuria, kidney function abnormality

Hematologic: Hypochromic anemia (4% to 13%), anemia (6% to 25%), eosinophilia, thrombocythemia, coagulation time increased, lymphocytosis, thrombocytopenia

Hepatic: LDH increased (7% to 13%), hepatic failure

Neuromuscular & skeletal: Back pain (2% to 11%), arthralgia, myalgia, bone pain, myasthenia, arthrosis, neuropathy

Ocular: Dry eyes, conjunctivitis, blepharitis, corneal lesion, visual field defects, keratitis

Otic: Ear pain, otitis externa

Renal: Creatinine increased

Respiratory: Pharyngitis, rhinitis, dyspnea, pleural effusion, bronchitis, cough increased, lung edema, hemoptysis, hypoxia

Miscellaneous: Flu-like syndrome (4% to 13%), bacterial infection (1% to 13%)

Drug Interactions

Metabolism/Transport Effects **Substrate** of CYP3A4 (minor); **Note:** Assignment of Major/Minor substrate status based on clinically relevant drug interaction potential; **Induces** CYP3A4 (weak/moderate)

Avoid Concomitant Use

Avoid concomitant use of Bexarotene (Systemic) with any of the following: Axitinib; CloZAPine; Gemfibrozil; Multivitamins/Minerals (with ADEK, Folate, Iron); Tetracycline Derivatives; Vitamin A

Increased Effect/Toxicity

Bexarotene (Systemic) may increase the levels/effects of: CloZAPine; Porfimer; Vitamin A

The levels/effects of Bexarotene (Systemic) may be increased by: CARBOplatin; Gemfibrozil; Multivitamins/Minerals (with ADEK, Folate, Iron); PACLitaxel; Tetracycline Derivatives

Decreased Effect

Bexarotene (Systemic) may decrease the levels/effects of: ARIPiprazole; AtorvaSTATin; Axitinib; Contraceptives (Estrogens); Contraceptives (Progestins); PACLitaxel; Saxagliptin

The levels/effects of Bexarotene (Systemic) may be decreased by: Tocilizumab

Ethanol/Nutrition/Herb Interactions

Food: Bioavailability is increased when administered with a fat-containing meal. Serum levels may be increased by grapefruit juice. Management: Administer with food, preferably high-fat meals (peanuts or ice cream). Avoid grapefruit juice.

Herb/Nutraceutical: Dong quai and St John's wort may cause photosensitization. St John's wort may decrease bexarotene levels. Additional vitamin A supplementation may lead to vitamin A toxicity (dry skin, irritation, arthralgias, myalgias, abdominal pain, hepatic changes). Management: Avoid St John's wort and dong quai. Avoid use of vitamin A supplements.

Storage/Stability Store at 2°C to 25°C (36°F to 77°F). Protect from light.

Mechanism of Action The exact mechanism is unknown. Binds and activates retinoid X receptor subtypes. Once activated, these receptors function as transcription factors that regulate the expression of genes which control cellular differentiation and proliferation. Bexarotene inhibits the growth *in vitro* of some tumor cell lines of hematopoietic and squamous cell origin.

Pharmacodynamics/Kinetics

Absorption: Significantly improved by a fat-containing meal

Protein binding: >99%

Metabolism: Hepatic via CYP3A4 isoenzyme; four metabolites identified; further metabolized by glucuronidation

Half-life elimination: ~7 hours

Time to peak: ~2 hours

Excretion: Primarily feces; urine (<1% as unchanged drug and metabolites)

Dosing

Adult & Geriatric Cutaneous T-cell lymphoma: Oral: 300-400 mg/m^2/day taken as a single daily dose.

Renal Impairment No studies have been conducted; however, renal insufficiency may result in significant protein binding changes and alter pharmacokinetics of bexarotene.

Hepatic Impairment No studies have been conducted; however, hepatic impairment would be expected to result in decreased clearance of bexarotene due to the extensive hepatic contribution to elimination.

Administration Administer capsule following a fat-containing meal.

Emetic Potential Low (10% to 30%)

Extemporaneous Preparations Hazardous agent: Use appropriate precautions for handling and disposal.

A 1 mg/mL oral suspension may be prepared with capsules. Cut one 75 mg capsule in half, rinse the interior contents of the capsule, and suspend with 75 mL sterile water. Administer immediately after preparation. To ensure administration of full dose, rinse empty glass with half a glass of water and administer residue.

Targretin® data on file, Eisai Inc.

Monitoring Parameters If female, pregnancy test 1 week before initiation then monthly while on bexarotene; lipid panel before initiation, then weekly until lipid response established and then at 8-week intervals thereafter; baseline LFTs, repeat at 1, 2, and 4 weeks after initiation then at 8-week intervals thereafter if stable; baseline and periodic thyroid function tests; baseline CBC with periodic monitoring

Dietary Considerations It is preferable to take the oral capsule following a fat-containing meal. Avoid grapefruit juice.

Dosage Forms Excipient information presented when available (limited, particularly for generics); consult specific product labeling.

Capsule, oral:

Targretin®: 75 mg

References

Duvic M, "Bexarotene and DAB(389)IL-2 (Denileukin Diftitox, ONTAK) in Treatment of Cutaneous T-Cell Lymphomas: Algorithms," *Clin Lymphoma*, 2000, 1(Suppl 1):51-5.

Hamnvik OP, Larsen PR, and Marqusee E, "Thyroid Dysfunction From Antineoplastic Agents," *J Natl Cancer Inst*, 2011, 103(21):1572-87.

Bexarotene (Topical) (beks AIR oh teen)

Related Information

Safe Handling of Hazardous Drugs *on page 1904*

Brand Names: U.S. Targretin®

Generic Availability (U.S.) No

Pharmacologic Category Antineoplastic Agent, Miscellaneous

Use Treatment of cutaneous lesions in patients with refractory cutaneous T-cell lymphoma (stage 1A and 1B) or who have not tolerated other therapies

Labeled Contraindications Hypersensitivity to bexarotene or any component of the formulation; pregnancy

Pregnancy Risk Factor X

Lactation Excretion in breast milk unknown/not recommended

Warnings/Precautions Hazardous agent - use appropriate precautions for handling and disposal. **Bexarotene is a retinoid, a drug class associated with birth defects in humans; do not administer during pregnancy.** Pregnancy test needed 1 week before initiation and every month thereafter. Effective contraception must be in place 1 month before initiation, during therapy, and for at least 1 month after discontinuation. Male patients with sexual partners who are pregnant, possibly pregnant, or who could become pregnant, must use condoms during sexual intercourse during treatment and for 1 month after last dose. May induce lipid abnormalities; reversible on discontinuation. Use extreme caution in patients with underlying hypertriglyceridemia. Monitor for signs and symptoms of infection about 4-8 weeks after initiation (leukopenia may occur). May cause photosensitization. Safety and efficacy are not established in the pediatric population. Use only with extreme caution in patients with hepatic impairment. Limit additional vitamin A intake to <15,000 units/day.

Adverse Reactions

Cardiovascular: Edema (10%)

Central nervous system: Headache (14%), weakness (6%), pain (30%)

Dermatologic: Rash (14% to 72%), pruritus (6% to 40%), contact dermatitis (14%), exfoliative dermatitis (6%)

Endocrine & metabolic: Hyperlipidemia (10%)

Hematologic: Leukopenia (6%), lymphadenopathy (6%)

Neuromuscular & skeletal: Paresthesia (6%)

Respiratory: Cough (6%), pharyngitis (6%)

Miscellaneous: Diaphoresis (6%), infection (18%)

Drug Interactions

Metabolism/Transport Effects Substrate of CYP3A4 (minor); **Note:** Assignment of Major/Minor substrate status based on clinically relevant drug interaction potential; **Induces** CYP3A4 (weak/moderate)

Avoid Concomitant Use

Avoid concomitant use of Bexarotene (Topical) with any of the following: Axitinib; Multivitamins/Minerals (with ADEK, Folate, Iron); Tetracycline Derivatives; Vitamin A

Increased Effect/Toxicity

Bexarotene (Topical) may increase the levels/effects of: Porfimer; Vitamin A

The levels/effects of Bexarotene (Topical) may be increased by: Multivitamins/Minerals (with ADEK, Folate, Iron); Tetracycline Derivatives

Decreased Effect

Bexarotene (Topical) may decrease the levels/effects of: ARIPiprazole; Axitinib; Contraceptives (Estrogens); Contraceptives (Progestins); Saxagliptin

The levels/effects of Bexarotene (Topical) may be decreased by: Tocilizumab

Storage/Stability Store at 2°C to 25°C (36°F to 77°F). Protect from light.

Mechanism of Action The exact mechanism is unknown. Binds and activates retinoid X receptor subtypes. Once activated, these receptors function as transcription factors that regulate the expression of genes which control cellular differentiation and proliferation.

Pharmacodynamics/Kinetics Absorption: Systemically absorbed following topical application (1% gel: <55 ng/mL)

Dosing

Adult & Geriatric Cutaneous lesions of T-cell lymphoma: Topical: Apply to lesions once every other day for first week, then increase on a weekly basis to once daily, 2 times/day, 3 times/day, and finally 4 times/day, according to tolerance.

Renal Impairment No studies have been conducted; however, renal insufficiency may result in significant protein binding changes and alter pharmacokinetics of bexarotene.

Hepatic Impairment No studies have been conducted; however, hepatic impairment would be expected to result in decreased clearance of bexarotene due to the extensive hepatic contribution to elimination.

Administration Allow gel to dry before covering with clothing. Avoid application to normal skin. Use of occlusive dressings is not recommended.

Monitoring Parameters If female, pregnancy test 1 week before initiation then monthly while on bexarotene; lipid panel before initiation, then weekly until lipid response established and then at 8-week intervals thereafter; baseline LFTs, repeat at 1, 2, and 4 weeks after initiation then at 8-week intervals thereafter if stable; baseline and periodic thyroid function tests; baseline CBC with periodic monitoring

Dosage Forms Excipient information presented when available (limited, particularly for generics); consult specific product labeling.

Gel, topical:

Targretin®: 1% (60 g) [contains dehydrated ethanol]

References

Martin AG, "Bexarotene Gel: A New Skin-Directed Treatment Option for Cutaneous T-Cell Lymphomas," *J Drugs Dermatol*, 2003, 2(2):155-67.

◆ **Bexxar®** *see* Tositumomab and Iodine I 131 Tositumomab *on page 1379*

Bicalutamide (bye ka LOO ta mide)

Related Information

Safe Handling of Hazardous Drugs *on page 1904*

Brand Names: U.S. Casodex®

Brand Names: Canada Apo-Bicalutamide®; Ava-Bicalutamide; Casodex®; CO Bicalutamide; Dom-Bicalutamide; JAMP-Bicalutamide; Mylan-Bicalutamide; Novo-Bicalutamide; PHL-Bicalutamide; PMS-Bicalutamide; PRO-Bicalutamide; ratio-Bicalutamide; Sandoz-Bicalutamide

Index Terms CDX; ICI-176334

Generic Availability (U.S.) Yes

Pharmacologic Category Antineoplastic Agent, Antiandrogen

Use Treatment of metastatic prostate cancer (in combination with an LHRH agonist)

Unlabeled Use Monotherapy for locally-advanced prostate cancer

Labeled Contraindications Hypersensitivity to bicalutamide or any component of the formulation; use in women, especially women who are or may become pregnant

Pregnancy Risk Factor X

Lactation Excretion in breast milk unknown/contraindicated

Warnings/Precautions Hazardous agent - use appropriate precautions for handling and disposal. Rare cases of death or hospitalization due to hepatitis have been reported postmarketing. Use with caution in moderate-to-severe hepatic dysfunction. Hepatotoxicity generally occurs within the first 3-4 months of use; patients should be monitored for signs and symptoms of liver dysfunction. Bicalutamide should be discontinued if patients have jaundice or ALT is >2 times the upper limit of normal. Androgen-deprivation therapy may increase the risk for cardiovascular disease (Levine, 2010). May cause gynecomastia, breast pain, or lead to spermatogenesis inhibition. When used in combination with LHRH agonists, a loss of glycemic control and decrease in glucose tolerance has been reported in patients with diabetes; monitor. May cause gynecomastia or breast pain (at higher, unlabeled doses), or lead to spermatogenesis inhibition.

Adverse Reactions Adverse reaction percentages reported as part of combination regimen with an LHRH analogue unless otherwise noted.

>10%:

Cardiovascular: Peripheral edema (13%)

Central nervous system: Pain (35%)

Endocrine & metabolic: Hot flashes (53%), breast pain (6%; monotherapy [150 mg]: 39% to 85%), gynecomastia (9%; monotherapy [150 mg]: 38% to 73%)

Gastrointestinal: Constipation (22%), nausea (15%), diarrhea (12%), abdominal pain (11%)

Genitourinary: Pelvic pain (21%), hematuria (12%), nocturia (12%)

Hematologic: Anemia (11%)

Neuromuscular & skeletal: Back pain (25%), weakness (22%)

Respiratory: Dyspnea (13%)

Miscellaneous: Infection (18%)

≥2% to 10%:

Cardiovascular: Chest pain (8%), hypertension (8%), angina pectoris (2% to <5%), cardiac arrest (2% to <5%), CHF (2% to <5%), edema (2% to <5%), MI (2% to <5%), coronary artery disorder (2% to <5%), syncope (2% to <5%)

Central nervous system: Dizziness (10%), headache (7%), insomnia (7%), anxiety (5%), depression (4%), chills (2% to <5%), confusion (2% to <5%), fever (2% to <5%), nervousness (2% to <5%), somnolence (2% to <5%)

Dermatologic: Rash (9%), alopecia (2% to <5%), dry skin (2% to <5%), pruritus (2% to <5%), skin carcinoma (2% to <5%)

Endocrine & metabolic: Hyperglycemia (6%), dehydration (2% to <5%), gout (2% to <5%), hypercholesterolemia (2% to <5%), libido decreased (2% to <5%)

Gastrointestinal: Dyspepsia (7%), weight loss (7%), anorexia (6%), flatulence (6%), vomiting (6%), weight gain (5%), dysphagia (2% to <5%), gastrointestinal carcinoma (2% to <5%), melena (2% to <5%), periodontal abscess (2% to <5%), rectal hemorrhage (2% to <5%), xerostomia (2% to <5%)

Genitourinary: Urinary tract infection (9%), impotence (7%), polyuria (6%), urinary retention (5%), urinary impairment (5%), urinary incontinence (4%), dysuria (2% to <5%), urinary urgency (2% to <5%)

Hepatic: LFTs increased (7%), alkaline phosphatase increased (5%)

Neuromuscular & skeletal: Bone pain (9%), paresthesia (8%), myasthenia (7%), arthritis (5%), pathological fracture (4%), hypertonia (2% to <5%), leg cramps (2% to <5%), myalgia (2% to <5%), neck pain (2% to <5%), neuropathy (2% to <5%)

Ocular: Cataract (2% to <5%)

Renal: BUN increased (2% to <5%), creatinine increased (2% to <5%), hydronephrosis (2% to <5%)

Respiratory: Cough (8%), pharyngitis (8%), bronchitis (6%), pneumonia (4%), rhinitis (4%), asthma (2% to <5%), epistaxis (2% to <5%), sinusitis (2% to <5%)

Miscellaneous: Flu-like syndrome (7%), diaphoresis (6%), cyst (2% to <5%), hernia (2% to <5%), herpes zoster (2% to <5%), sepsis (2% to <5%)

Postmarketing and/or case reports: Bilirubin increased, glucose tolerance decreased, hemoglobin decreased, hepatitis, hepatotoxicity, hypersensitivity reactions (including angioneurotic edema and urticaria), interstitial pneumonitis, pulmonary fibrosis, WBC decreased

Drug Interactions

Metabolism/Transport Effects Inhibits CYP3A4 (moderate)

Avoid Concomitant Use

Avoid concomitant use of Bicalutamide with any of the following: Bosutinib; Pimozide; Tolvaptan

Increased Effect/Toxicity

Bicalutamide may increase the levels/effects of: ARIPiprazole; Avanafil; Bosutinib; Budesonide (Systemic, Oral Inhalation); Colchicine; CYP3A4 Substrates; Eplerenone; Everolimus; FentaNYL; Halofantrine; Ivacaftor; Lurasidone; Pimecrolimus; Pimozide; Propafenone; Ranolazine; Salmeterol; Saxagliptin; Tolvaptan; Vilazodone; Vitamin K Antagonists; Zuclopenthixol

Decreased Effect

Bicalutamide may decrease the levels/effects of: Ifosfamide

Storage/Stability Store at room temperature of 20°C to 25°C (68°F to 77°F).

Mechanism of Action Androgen receptor inhibitor; pure nonsteroidal antiandrogen that binds to androgen receptors; specifically a competitive inhibitor for the binding of dihydrotestosterone and testosterone; prevents testosterone stimulation of cell growth in prostate cancer

Pharmacodynamics/Kinetics

Absorption: Rapid and complete; unaffected by food

Protein binding: 96%

Metabolism: Extensively hepatic; glucuronidation and oxidation of the R (active) enantiomer to inactive metabolites; the S enantiomer is inactive

Half-life elimination: Active enantiomer: ~6 days, ~10 days in severe liver disease

Time to peak, plasma: Active enantiomer: ~31 hours

Excretion: Urine (36%, as inactive metabolites); feces (42%, as unchanged drug and inactive metabolites)

Dosing

Adult & Geriatric

Prostate cancer, metastatic: Oral: 50 mg once daily (in combination with an LHRH analogue)

Prostate cancer, locally-advanced (unlabeled use): Oral: 150 mg once daily (as monotherapy) (McLeod, 2006)

Renal Impairment No adjustment required

Hepatic Impairment No adjustment required for mild, moderate, or severe hepatic impairment; use caution with moderate-to-severe impairment. Discontinue if ALT >2 times ULN or patient develops jaundice.

Combination Regimens

Prostate cancer:

Bicalutamide-Goserelin on page 1533

Bicalutamide-Leuprolide on page 1533

Administration Dose should be taken at the same time each day with or without food. Treatment for metastatic cancer should be started concomitantly with an LHRH analogue.

Monitoring Parameters Periodically monitor CBC, ECG, echocardiograms, serum testosterone, luteinizing hormone, and prostate specific antigen (PSA). Liver function tests should be obtained at baseline and repeated regularly during the first 4 months of treatment, and periodically thereafter; monitor for signs and symptoms of liver dysfunction (discontinue if jaundice is noted or ALT is >2 times the upper limit of normal). Monitor blood glucose in patients with diabetes. If initiating bicalutamide in patients who are on warfarin, closely monitor prothrombin time.

Dietary Considerations May be taken with or without food.

Dosage Forms Excipient information presented when available (limited, particularly for generics); consult specific product labeling.

Tablet, oral: 50 mg

Casodex®: 50 mg

References

Iversen, P, Johansson JE, Lodding P, et al, "Bicalutamide (150 mg) Versus Placebo as Immediate Therapy Alone or as Adjuvant to Therapy With Curative Intent for Early Nonmetastatic Prostate Cancer: 5.3 Year Median Followup from the Scandinavian Prostate Cancer Group Study Number 6," *J Urol*, 2004, 172(5 Pt 1):1871-6.

Levine GN, D'Amico AV, Berger P, et al, "Androgen-Deprivation Therapy in Prostate Cancer and Cardiovascular Risk. A Science Advisory from the American Heart Association, American Cancer Society, and American Urological Association," *Circulation*, 2010, 121:831-38.

Loblaw DA, Virgo KS, Nam R, et al, "Initial Hormonal Management of Androgen-Sensitive Metastatic, Recurrent, or Progressive Prostate Cancer: 2007 Update of an American Society of Clinical Oncology Practice Guideline," *J Clin Oncol*, 2007, 25(12):1596-605.

McLeod DG, Iversen P, See WA, et al, "Bicalutamide 150 mg Plus Standard Care vs Standard Care Alone for Early Prostate Cancer," *BJU Int*, 2005, 97(2):247-54.

McLeod DG, See WA, Klimberg I, et al, "The Bicalutamide 150 mg Early Prostate Cancer Program: Findings of the North American Trial at 7.7-Year Median Followup," *J Urol*, 2006, 176(1):75-80.

- **BiCNU®** *see* Carmustine *on page 243*
- **Bioniche Promethazine (Can)** *see* Promethazine *on page 1218*
- **Biotene® Moisturizing Mouth Spray [OTC]** *see* Saliva Substitute *on page 1266*
- **Biotene® Oral Balance® [OTC]** *see* Saliva Substitute *on page 1266*
- **bis(chloroethyl) nitrosourea** *see* Carmustine *on page 243*
- **bis-chloronitrosourea** *see* Carmustine *on page 243*
- **Bivalent Human Papillomavirus Vaccine** *see* Papillomavirus (Types 16, 18) Vaccine (Human, Recombinant) *on page 1124*
- **BL4162A** *see* Anagrelide *on page 93*
- **Blenoxane** *see* Bleomycin *on page 181*
- **Blenoxane® (Can)** *see* Bleomycin *on page 181*
- **Bleo** *see* Bleomycin *on page 181*

Bleomycin (blee oh MYE sin)

Related Information

Chemotherapy and Obesity *on page 1834*

Malignant Pleural Effusions *on page 1865*

Management of Chemotherapy-Induced Nausea and Vomiting *on page 1786*

Management of Drug Extravasations *on page 1000*

Safe Handling of Hazardous Drugs *on page 1904*

Brand Names: Canada Blenoxane®; Bleomycin Injection, USP

Index Terms Blenoxane; Bleo; Bleomycin Sulfate; BLM

Generic Availability (U.S.) Yes

Pharmacologic Category Antineoplastic Agent, Antibiotic

Use Treatment of squamous cell carcinomas of the head and neck, penis, cervix, or vulva, testicular carcinoma, Hodgkin's lymphoma, and non-Hodgkin's lymphoma; sclerosing agent for malignant pleural effusion

Unlabeled Use Treatment of ovarian germ cell tumors

Labeled Contraindications Hypersensitivity to bleomycin or any component of the formulation

Pregnancy Risk Factor D

Lactation Excretion in breast milk unknown/not recommended

Warnings/Precautions Hazardous agent - use appropriate precautions for handling and disposal. **[U.S. Boxed Warning]: Occurrence of pulmonary fibrosis (commonly presenting as pneumonitis; occasionally progressing to pulmonary fibrosis) is the most severe toxicity. Risk is higher in elderly patients or patients receiving >400 units total lifetime dose;** other possible risk factors include smoking and patients with prior radiation therapy or receiving concurrent oxygen (especially high inspired oxygen doses). A review of patients receiving bleomycin for the treatment of germ cell tumors suggests risk for pulmonary toxicity is increased in patients >40 years of age, with glomerular filtration rate <80 mL/minute, advanced disease, and cumulative doses >300 units (O'Sullivan, 2003). Pulmonary toxicity may include bronchiolitis obliterans and organizing pneumonia (BOOP), eosinophilic hypersensitivity, and interstitial pneumonitis, progressing to pulmonary fibrosis (Sleijfer, 2001); pulmonary toxicity may be due to a lack of the enzyme which inactivates bleomycin (bleomycin hydrolase) in the lungs (Morgan, 2011; Sleijfer, 2001). If pulmonary changes occur, withhold treatment and investigate if drug-related. In children, a younger age at treatment, cumulative dose ≥400 units/m^2 (combined with chest irradiation), and renal impairment are associated with a higher incidence of pulmonary toxicity (Huang, 2011).

A severe idiosyncratic reaction consisting of hypotension, mental confusion, fever, chills, and wheezing (similar to anaphylaxis) has been reported in 1% of lymphoma patients treated with bleomycin. Since these reactions usually occur after the first or second dose, careful monitoring is essential after these doses. Use caution when administering O_2 during surgery to patients who have received bleomycin; the risk of bleomycin-related pulmonary toxicity is increased. Use caution with renal impairment (Cl_{cr} <50 mL/minute), may require dose adjustment. May cause renal or hepatic toxicity. **[U.S. Boxed Warning]: Should be administered under the supervision of an experienced cancer chemotherapy physician.**

Adverse Reactions

>10%:

Dermatologic: Pain at the tumor site, phlebitis. About 50% of patients develop erythema, rash, striae, induration, hyperkeratosis, vesiculation, and peeling of the skin, particularly on the palmar and plantar surfaces of the hands and feet. Hyperpigmentation (50%), alopecia, nailbed changes may also occur. These effects appear dose related and reversible with discontinuation.

Gastrointestinal: Stomatitis and mucositis (30%), anorexia, weight loss

Respiratory: Tachypnea, rales, acute or chronic interstitial pneumonitis, and pulmonary fibrosis (5% to 10%); hypoxia and death (1%). Symptoms include cough, dyspnea, and bilateral pulmonary infiltrates. The pathogenesis is not certain, but may be due to damage of pulmonary, vascular, or connective tissue. Response to steroid therapy is variable and somewhat controversial.

Miscellaneous: Acute febrile reactions (25% to 50%)

1% to 10%:

Dermatologic: Skin thickening, diffuse scleroderma, onycholysis, pruritus

Miscellaneous: Anaphylactoid-like reactions (characterized by hypotension, confusion, fever, chills, and wheezing; onset may be immediate or delayed for several hours); idiosyncratic reactions (1% in lymphoma patients)

<1%, postmarketing, and/or case reports: Angioedema, cerebrovascular accident, cerebral arteritis, chest pain, coronary artery disease, flagellate hyperpigmentation, hepatotoxicity, malaise, MI, myelosuppression (rare),

myocardial ischemia, nausea, pericarditis, Raynaud's phenomenon, renal toxicity, scleroderma-like skin changes, Stevens-Johnson syndrome, thrombotic microangiopathy, toxic epidermal necrolysis, vomiting

Drug Interactions

Metabolism/Transport Effects None known.

Avoid Concomitant Use

Avoid concomitant use of Bleomycin with any of the following: BCG; Brentuximab Vedotin; Natalizumab; Pimecrolimus; Tacrolimus (Topical); Vaccines (Live)

Increased Effect/Toxicity

Bleomycin may increase the levels/effects of: Leflunomide; Natalizumab; Vaccines (Live)

The levels/effects of Bleomycin may be increased by: Brentuximab Vedotin; Denosumab; Filgrastim; Gemcitabine; Pimecrolimus; Roflumilast; Sargramostim; Tacrolimus (Topical); Trastuzumab

Decreased Effect

Bleomycin may decrease the levels/effects of: BCG; Cardiac Glycosides; Coccidioidin Skin Test; Sipuleucel-T; Vaccines (Inactivated); Vaccines (Live)

The levels/effects of Bleomycin may be decreased by: Echinacea

Storage/Stability Refrigerate intact vials of powder. Intact vials are stable for up to 4 weeks at room temperature. Solutions reconstituted in NS are stable for up to 28 days refrigerated and 14 days at room temperature; however, the manufacturer recommends stability of 24 hours in NS at room temperature.

Reconstitution For I.V. use, reconstitute 15-unit vial with 5 mL with NS and the 30-unit vial with 10 mL NS; for I.M. or SubQ use, reconstitute 15-unit vial with 1-5 mL of SWFI, BWFI, or NS and the 30-unit vial with 2-10 mL of SWFI, BWFI, or NS. For intrapleural use, mix in 50-100 mL of NS. Use appropriate precautions for handling and disposal.

Mechanism of Action Inhibits synthesis of DNA; binds to DNA leading to single- and double-strand breaks; also inhibits (to a lesser degree) RNA and protein synthesis

Pharmacodynamics/Kinetics

Absorption: I.M. and intrapleural administration: 30% to 50% of I.V. serum concentrations; intraperitoneal and SubQ routes produce serum concentrations equal to those of I.V.

Distribution: V_d: 22 L/m^2; highest concentrations in skin, kidney, lung, heart tissues; lowest in testes and GI tract; does not cross blood-brain barrier

Protein binding: 1%

Metabolism: Via several tissues including hepatic, GI tract, skin, pulmonary, renal, and serum

Half-life elimination: Biphasic (renal function dependent):

Normal renal function: Initial: 1.3 hours; Terminal: 9 hours

End-stage renal disease: Initial: 2 hours; Terminal: 30 hours

Time to peak, serum: I.M.: Within 30 minutes

Excretion: Urine (50% to 70% as active drug)

Dosing

Adult Note: The risk for pulmonary toxicity increases with age >70 years and cumulative lifetime dose of >400 units; 1 unit = 1 mg. Details concerning dosage in combination regimens should also be consulted.

Test dose for lymphoma patients: I.M., I.V., SubQ: Because of the possibility of an anaphylactoid reaction, the manufacturer recommends administering 1-2 units of bleomycin before the first 1-2 doses; monitor vital signs every 15 minutes; wait a minimum of 1 hour before administering remainder of dose; if no acute reaction occurs, then the regular dosage schedule may be followed. **Note:** Test doses may not be predictive of a reaction (Lam, 2005) and/or may produce false-negative results.

Hodgkin's lymphoma (unlabeled dosing; combination regimens): I.V.:
ABVD: 10 units/m² days 1 and 15 of a 28-day treatment cycle (Straus, 2004)
BEACOPP: 10 units/m² day 8 of a 21-day treatment cycle (Dann, 2007; Diehl, 2003)
Stanford V: 5 units/m²/dose in weeks 2, 4, 6, 8, 10 and 12 (Horning, 2002; Horning, 2000)

Testicular cancer (unlabeled dosing; combination therapy): I.V.: 30 units/dose days 1, 8, and 15 of a 21-day treatment cycle for 4 cycles (Culine, 2008; Nichols, 1998)

Ovarian germ cell cancer (unlabeled use; combination therapy): I.V.: 30 units/dose days 1, 8, and 15 of a 21-day treatment cycle for 3 cycles (Williams, 1994) **or** 15 units/m² day 1 of a 21-day treatment cycle for 4 cycles (Cushing, 2004)

Malignant pleural effusion: Intrapleural: 60 units as a single instillation; mix in 50-100 mL of NS

Dosing adjustment in obesity: Adults: Fixed doses (dosing which is independent of body weight or BSA), are used in some protocols (eg, testicular cancer); due to toxicity concerns, the same fixed dose should also be considered for obese patients (Griggs, 2012).

Geriatric Refer to adult dosing. The incidence of pulmonary toxicity is higher in patients >70 years of age.

Pediatric Note: The risk for pulmonary toxicity increases with age >70 years and cumulative lifetime dose of >400 units; 1 unit = 1 mg. Details concerning dosage in combination regimens should also be consulted.

Test dose for lymphoma patients: I.M., I.V., SubQ: Because of the possibility of an anaphylactoid reaction, the manufacturer recommends administering 1-2 units of bleomycin before the first 1-2 doses; monitor vital signs every 15 minutes; wait a minimum of 1 hour before administering remainder of dose; if no acute reaction occurs, then the regular dosage schedule may be followed. **Note:** Test doses may not be predictive of a reaction (Lam, 2005) and/or may produce false-negative results.

Hodgkin's lymphoma (unlabeled dosing; combination regimen): I.V.: ABVD: I.V.: 10 units/m² days 1 and 15 of a 28-day treatment cycle (Hutchinson, 1998)

Renal Impairment

The U.S. labeling recommends the following adjustments (creatinine clearance should be estimated using the Cockcroft-Gault formula):
Cl_{cr} >50 mL/minute: No dosage adjustment necessary.
Cl_{cr} 40-50 mL/minute: Administer 70% of normal dose
Cl_{cr} 30-40 mL/minute: Administer 60% of normal dose
Cl_{cr} 20-30 mL/minute: Administer 55% of normal dose
Cl_{cr} 10-20 mL/minute: Administer 45% of normal dose
Cl_{cr} 5-10 mL/minute: Administer 40% of normal dose

The Canadian labeling recommends the following adjustment: Cl_{cr} ≤40 mL/minute: Reduce dose by 40% to 75%.

The following adjustments have also been recommended:
Aronoff, 2007: Adults: Continuous renal replacement therapy (CRRT): Administer 75% of dose

Kintzel, 1995: Adults:

Cl_{cr} 46-60 mL/minute: Administer 70% of dose

Cl_{cr} 31-45 mL/minute: Administer 60% of dose

Cl_{cr} <30 mL/minute: Consider use of alternative drug

Hepatic Impairment No dosage adjustment provided in the manufacturer's labeling (has not been studied); however, adjustment for hepatic impairment is not necessary (King, 2001).

Adjustment for Toxicity

Pulmonary changes: Discontinue until determined not to be drug-related.

Pulmonary diffusion capacity for carbon monoxide (DL_{CO}) <30% to 35% of baseline: Discontinue treatment.

Combination Regimens

Lymphoma, Hodgkin:

ABVD Early Stage (Hodgkin) on page 1516

ABVD (Hodgkin) on page 1516

BEACOPP-14 (Hodgkin) on page 1522

BEACOPP Escalated (Hodgkin) on page 1522

BEACOPP Escalated Plus Standard (Hodgkin) on page 1523

BEACOPP Standard (Hodgkin) on page 1525

C-MOPP/ABV Hybrid (Hodgkin) on page 1588

MOPP/ABVD (Hodgkin) on page 1714

MOPP/ABV Hybrid (Hodgkin) on page 1715

Stanford V (Hodgkin) on page 1752

Lymphoma, non-Hodgkin:

CEPP(B) on page 1556

COP-BLAM on page 1595

MACOP-B on page 1704

m-BACOD on page 1706

Pro-MACE-CytaBOM on page 1741

Osteosarcoma: POG-8651 on page 1740

Ovarian cancer:

BEP (Ovarian Cancer) on page 1526

BEP (Ovarian Cancer, Testicular Cancer) on page 1526

Testicular cancer:

BEP (Ovarian Cancer, Testicular Cancer) on page 1526

BEP (Testicular Cancer) on page 1527

PVB on page 1744

VBP on page 1770

Administration

I.V. doses should be administered slowly over 10 minutes.

I.M. or SubQ: May cause pain at injection site

Intrapleural: 60 units in 50-100 mL NS; use of topical anesthetics or narcotic analgesia is usually not necessary

Emetic Potential Very low (<10%)

Vesicant/Extravasation Risk May be an irritant

Monitoring Parameters Pulmonary function tests, including total lung volume, forced vital capacity, diffusion capacity for carbon monoxide; vital capacity, total lung capacity and pulmonary capillary blood volume may be better indicators of changes induced by bleomycin (Sleifjer, 2001); chest x-ray, renal function, liver function, temperature initially; check body weight at regular intervals

Dosage Forms Excipient information presented when available (limited, particularly for generics); consult specific product labeling.

Injection, powder for reconstitution: 15 units, 30 units

References

Aronoff GR, Bennett WM, Berns JS, et al, *Drug Prescribing in Renal Failure: Dosing Guidelines for Adults and Children*, 5th ed. Philadelphia, PA: American College of Physicians; 2007, p 97.

Azambuja E, Fleck JF, Batista RG, et al, "Bleomycin Lung Toxicity: Who are the Patients With Increased Risk?" *Pulm Pharmacol Ther*, 2005, 18(5):363-66.

Culine S, Kramar A, Théodore C, et al, "Randomized Trial Comparing Bleomycin/Etoposide/Cisplatin With Alternating Cisplatin/Cyclophosphamide/Doxorubicin and Vinblastine/Bleomycin Regimens of Chemotherapy for Patients With Intermediate- and Poor-Risk Metastatic Nonseminomatous Germ Cell Tumors: Genito-Urinary Group of the French Federation of Cancer Centers Trial T93MP," *J Clin Oncol*, 2008, 26(3):421-7.

Cushing B, Giller R, Cullen JW, et al, "Randomized Comparison of Combination Chemotherapy With Etoposide, Bleomycin, and Either High-Dose or Standard-Dose Cisplatin in Children and Adolescents With High-Risk Malignant Germ Cell Tumors: A Pediatric Intergroup Study – Pediatric Oncology Group 9049 and Children's Cancer Group 8882," *J Clin Oncol*, 2004, 22 (13):2691-700.

Dann EJ, Bar-Shalom R, Tamir A, et al, "Risk-Adapted BEACOPP Regimen Can Reduce the Cumulative Dose of Chemotherapy for Standard and High-Risk Hodgkin Lymphoma With No Impairment of Outcome," *Blood*, 2007, 109(3):905-9.

Diehl V, Franklin J, Pfreundschuh M, et al, "Standard and Increased-Dose BEACOPP Chemotherapy Compared With COPP-ABVD for Advanced Hodgkin's Disease," *N Engl J Med*, 2003, 348(24):2386-95.

Griggs JJ, Mangu PB, Anderson H, et al, "Appropriate Chemotherapy Dosing For Obese Adult Patients With Cancer: American Society of Clinical Oncology Clinical Practice Guideline," *J Clin Oncol*, 2012, 30(13):1553-61.

Horning SJ, Hoppe RT, Breslin S, et al, "Stanford V and Radiotherapy for Locally Extensive and Advanced Hodgkin's Disease: Mature Results of a Prospective Clinical Trial," *J Clin Oncol*, 2002, 20(3):630-7.

Horning SJ, Williams J, Bartlett NL, et al, "Assessment of the Stanford V Regimen and Consolidative Radiotherapy for Bulky and Advanced Hodgkin's Disease: Eastern Cooperative Oncology Group Pilot Study E1492," *J Clin Oncol*, 2000, 18(5):972-80.

Huang TT, Hudson MM, Stokes DC, et al, "Pulmonary Outcomes in Survivors of Childhood Cancer: A Systematic Review," *Chest*, 2011, 140(4): 881-901.

Hutchinson RJ, Fryer CJ, Davis PC, et al, "MOPP or Radiation in Addition to ABVD in the Treatment of Pathologically Staged Advanced Hodgkin's Disease in Children: Results of the Children's Cancer Group Phase III Trial," *J Clin Oncol*, 1998, 16(3):897-906.

King PD and Perry MC, "Hepatotoxicity of Chemotherapy," *Oncologist*, 2001, 6(2):162-76.

Kintzel PE and Dorr RT, "Anticancer Drug Renal Toxicity and Elimination: Dosing Guidelines for Altered Renal Function," *Cancer Treat Rev*, 1995, 21(1):33-64.

Lam MS, "The Need for Routine Bleomycin Test Dosing in the 21st Century," *Ann Pharmacother*, 2005, 39(11):1897-902.

Morgan C, Tillett T, Braybrooke J, et al, "Management of Uncommon Chemotherapy-Induced Emergencies," *Lancet Oncol*, 2011, 12(8):806-14.

Nichols CR, Catalano PJ, Crawford ED, et al, "Randomized Comparison of Cisplatin and Etoposide and Either Bleomycin or Ifosfamide in Treatment of Advanced Disseminated Germ Cell Tumors: An Eastern Cooperative Oncology Group, Southwest Oncology Group, and Cancer and Leukemia Group B Study," *J Clin Oncol*, 1998, 16(4):1287-93.

O'Sullivan JM, Huddart RA, Norman AR, et al, "Predicting the Risk of Bleomycin Lung Toxicity in Patients With Germ-Cell Tumours," *Ann Oncol*, 2003, 14(1):91-6.

Sleijfer S, "Bleomycin-Induced Pneumonitis," *Chest*, 2001, 120(2):617-24.

Straus DJ, Portlock CS, Qin J, et al, "Results of aPprospective Randomized Clinical Trial of Doxorubicin, Bleomycin, Vinblastine, and Dacarbazine (ABVD) Followed by Radiation Therapy (RT) Versus ABVD Alone for stages I, II, and IIIA Nonbulky Hodgkin Disease," *Blood*, 2004, 104 (12):3483-9.

Tobias JS, Monson K, Gupta N, et al, "Chemoradiotherapy for Locally Advanced Head and Neck Cancer: 10-year Follow-Up of the UK Head and Neck (UKHAN1) Trial," *Lancet Oncol*, 2010, 11 (1):66-74.

Williams S, Blessing JA, Liao SY, et al, "Adjuvant Therapy of Ovarian Germ Cell Tumors With Cisplatin, Etoposide, and Bleomycin: A Trial of the Gynecologic Oncology Group," *J Clin Oncol*, 1994, 12(4):701-6.

- **Bleomycin Injection, USP (Can)** *see* Bleomycin *on page 181*
- **Bleomycin Sulfate** *see* Bleomycin *on page 181*
- **BLM** *see* Bleomycin *on page 181*
- **BMS-247550** *see* Ixabepilone *on page 842*
- **BMS-354825** *see* Dasatinib *on page 390*
- **Bonefos® (Can)** *see* Clodronate *on page 303*
- **Boniva®** *see* Ibandronate *on page 739*

Bortezomib (bore TEZ oh mib)

Related Information

Hypercalcemia of Malignancy *on page 1860*
Management of Chemotherapy-Induced Nausea and Vomiting *on page 1786*
Management of Drug Extravasations *on page 1800*
Management of Infections *on page 1809*
Principles of Anticancer Therapy *on page 1878*
Safe Handling of Hazardous Drugs *on page 1904*

Brand Names: U.S. Velcade®

Brand Names: Canada Velcade®

Index Terms LDP-341; MLN341; PS-341

Generic Availability (U.S.) No

Pharmacologic Category Antineoplastic Agent; Proteasome Inhibitor

Use Treatment of multiple myeloma; treatment of relapsed or refractory mantle cell lymphoma

Unlabeled Use Treatment of relapsed/refractory cutaneous T-Cell lymphomas (mycosis fungoides), relapsed/refractory follicular lymphoma, relapsed/refractory peripheral T-cell lymphoma, systemic light-chain amyloidosis, relapsed/refractory Waldenström's macroglobulinemia

Labeled Contraindications Hypersensitivity (excluding local reactions) to bortezomib, boron, mannitol, or any component of the formulation; administration via the intrathecal route

Pregnancy Risk Factor D

Lactation Excretion in breast milk unknown/not recommended

Warnings/Precautions Hazardous agent - use appropriate precautions for handling and disposal. May cause or worsen peripheral neuropathy (usually sensory but may be mixed sensorimotor); risk may be increased with previous use of neurotoxic agents or pre-existing peripheral neuropathy (patients with pre-existing neuropathy should use only after risk versus benefit assessment); monitor for signs and symptoms; adjustment of dose and/or schedule may be required. The incidence of grades 2 and 3 peripheral neuropathy may be lower with SubQ route (compared to I.V.); consider subQ administration in patients with pre-existing or at high risk for peripheral neuropathy; the majority of patients with ≥grade 2 peripheral neuropathy have improvement in or resolution of symptoms with dose adjustments or discontinuation; in a study of elderly patients receiving a weekly bortezomib schedule with combination chemotherapy, the incidence of peripheral neuropathy was significantly reduced without an effect on outcome (Boccadoro, 2010; Palumbo, 2009). May cause hypotension (including postural and orthostatic); use caution with dehydration, history of syncope, or medications associated with hypotension (may require adjustment of antihypertensive medication, hydration, and mineralocorticoids and/or sympathomimetics). Has been associated with the development or exacerbation of heart failure (HF) and decreased left ventricular ejection fraction (LVEF); monitor closely in patients with risk factors for HF or existing heart disease, although HF and decreased LVEF have been observed in patients without risk factors. Has also been associated with isolated reports of QT_c prolongation.

Pulmonary disorders (some fatal) including pneumonitis, interstitial pneumonia, lung infiltrates, and acute respiratory distress syndrome (ARDS) have been reported. Pulmonary hypertension (without left heart failure or significant pulmonary disease has been reported rarely). Promptly evaluate with new or worsening cardiopulmonary symptoms; therapy interruption may be required. Tumor lysis syndrome has been reported; risk is increased in patients with high tumor burden prior to treatment. Posterior reversible leukoencephalopathy syndrome (PRES, formerly RPLS) has been reported (rarely). Promptly evaluate with new or worsening cardiopulmonary symptoms. Symptoms of PRES include confusion, headache, hypertension, lethargy, seizure, blindness and/or other vision, or neurologic disturbances; discontinue bortezomib if PRES occurs. MRI is recommended to confirm PRES diagnosis. The safety of reinitiating bortezomib in patients previously experiencing PRES is unknown. Herpes (zoster and simplex) reactivation has been reported with bortezomib; consider antiviral prophylaxis during therapy. Hematologic toxicity, including neutropenia and severe thrombocytopenia, may occur (nadirs generally occur following the last dose of a cycle and recover prior to the next cycle); risk is increased in patients with pretreatment platelet counts <75,000/µL; frequent monitoring is required throughout treatment; may require dosage or schedule adjustments; withhold treatment for platelets <30,000/µL. Hemorrhage (gastrointestinal and intracerebral) due to low platelet count has been observed. Acute liver failure has been reported (rarely) in patients receiving multiple concomitant medications and with serious underlying conditions. Hepatitis, transaminase increases, and hyperbilirubinemia have also been reported; interrupt therapy to assess reversibility. Use caution in patients with hepatic dysfunction; reduced initial doses are recommended for moderate and severe hepatic impairment (exposure is increased); closely monitor for toxicities. Hyper- and hypoglycemia may occur in diabetic patients receiving oral hypoglycemics; may require adjustment of diabetes medications. Nausea, vomiting, diarrhea or constipation may occur; may require antiemetics or antidiarrheals; ileus may occur; administer fluid and electrolytes to prevent dehydration (monitor closely); interrupt therapy for severe symptoms.

Coadministration of strong CYP3A4 inhibitors (eg, ketoconazole, ritonavir) may increase bortezomib exposure; monitor for signs of toxicity and consider dose reduction if concurrent therapy cannot be avoided. Efficacy may be reduced when administered with strong CYP3A4 inducers (eg, rifampin); concomitant use is not recommended.

For I.V. or SubQ administration only. Intrathecal administration is contraindicated; inadvertent intrathecal administration has resulted in death. Bortezomib should **NOT** be prepared during the preparation of any intrathecal medications. After preparation, keep bortezomib in a location **away** from the separate storage location recommended for intrathecal medications. Bortezomib should **NOT** be delivered to the patient at the same time with any medications intended for central nervous system administration.

Adverse Reactions

>10%:

Cardiovascular: Edema (11% to 23%), cardiac disorder (treatment emergent; 15%), hypotension (13%; grades 3/4: 3%)

Central nervous system: Psychiatric disturbance (≤35%), fever (16% to 34%), dysesthesia (22% to 27%), headache (3% to 22%), insomnia (11% to 20%), dizziness (17%; excludes vertigo), fatigue (12% to 20%)

Dermatologic: Rash (18%)

Gastrointestinal: Nausea (18% to 55%), diarrhea (24% to 52%), constipation (14% to 41%), anorexia (36%), vomiting (12% to 33%), abdominal pain (2% to 15%), weight loss (3% to 15%), abnormal taste, dyspepsia

Hematologic: Thrombocytopenia (35% to 36%; grade 4: 5% to 8%; nadir: day 11; recovery: by day 21), anemia (29% to 36%; grade 4: ≤3%), neutropenia (17% to 29%; grade 4: 3% to 4%; nadir: day 11; recovery: by day 21), leukopenia (20% to 22%; grade 4: ≤1%)

Neuromuscular & skeletal: Weakness (16% to 64%; grades 3/4: 16%), peripheral neuropathy (38% to 53%; grade ≥2: SubQ 24%, I.V. 41%; grade ≥3: SubQ 6%, I.V. 16%; grade 4: ≤1%), neuralgia (23% to 24%; grade 3: SubQ 3%, I.V. 9%), paresthesia (22%), arthralgia (17%), limb pain (5% to 15%), bone pain (14%), back pain (11% to 13%), myalgia (12%), muscle cramps (11%), rigors (≤11%)

Respiratory: Dyspnea (7% to 21%), cough (20%), respiratory tract infection (12% to 15%), nasopharyngitis (12%), pneumonia (12%)

Miscellaneous: Herpesvirus infections (2% to 12%)

1% to 10%:

Cardiovascular: Hypertension (4% to 10%), heart failure (5%; includes acute pulmonary edema, cardiac failure, congestive cardiac failure, cardiogenic shock, pulmonary edema)

Central nervous system: Anxiety (10%)

Endocrine & metabolic: Dehydration (10%), hypercalcemia (grade 4: 2%)

Gastrointestinal: Appetite decreased (9% to 10%)

Hematologic: Bleeding events (≥grade 3: 4%)

Local: Injection site irritation (SubQ: 6%; resolved in 6 days on average; severe: 1%; I.V.: 5%)

Frequency not defined (including postmarketing and/or case reports; limited to important or life-threatening): Acute diffuse infiltrative pulmonary disease, acute respiratory distress syndrome, alkaline phosphatase increased, amyloidosis, anaphylaxis, angina, angioedema, ascites, aspergillosis, atelectasis, atrial fibrillation, atrial flutter, AV block, bacteremia, blindness, blurred vision, bronchitis, cardiac amyloidosis, cardiac arrest, cardiac tamponade, cardiopulmonary arrest, cerebral hemorrhage, cerebrovascular accident, cholestasis, coma, confusion, conjunctival infection/irritation, cranial palsy, deep venous thrombosis, diplopia, disseminated intravascular coagulation (DIC), duodenitis (hemorrhagic), DVT, dysautonomia, dysphagia, encephalopathy, embolism, epistaxis, fecal impaction, fracture, gastritis (hemorrhagic), gastroenteritis, GGT increased, glomerular nephritis, hearing impairment, hematemesis, hematuria, hemoptysis, hemorrhagic cystitis, hepatic failure, hepatic hemorrhage, hepatitis, hepatocellular damage, herpes meningoencephalitis, hyperbilirubinemia, hyper-/hypoglycemia, hyper-/hypokalemia, hyper-/hyponatremia, hypersensitivity, hyperuricemia, hypocalcemia, hypoxia, ileus, immune complex hypersensitivity, inappropriate ADH secretion, injection site reaction, interstitial pneumonia, intestinal obstruction, intestinal perforation, intracerebral hemorrhage, ischemic colitis, ischemic stroke, laryngeal edema, left ventricular ejection fraction decreased, leukocytoclastic vasculitis, leukopenia, listeriosis, lymphopenia, melena, mental status change, MI, myocardial ischemia, neuralgia, neutropenic fever, ophthalmic herpes, optic neuritis, oral candidiasis, pancreatitis, paralytic ileus, pericardial effusion, pericarditis, peritonitis, pleural effusion, pneumonitis, portal vein thrombosis, posterior reversible leukoencephalopathy syndrome (PRES), proliferative glomerular nephritis, pruritus, psychosis, pulmonary embolism, pulmonary hypertension, pulmonary infiltrate, QT_c prolongation, renal calculus, renal failure, respiratory failure, respiratory insufficiency, seizure, septic shock, sepsis, sinus arrest, spinal cord compression, Stevens-Johnson syndrome, stomatitis, stroke (hemorrhagic), subarachnoid hemorrhage, subdural hematoma, suicidal ideation, Sweet's syndrome (acute febrile neutrophilic dermatosis), syncope, tachycardia, torsade de pointes, toxic epidermal necrolysis, toxoplasmosis, transaminases increased, transient ischemic attack, tumor lysis syndrome, urinary incontinence, urinary retention, urinary tract infection, urticaria, ventricular tachycardia

Drug Interactions

Metabolism/Transport Effects **Substrate** of CYP1A2 (minor), CYP2C19 (major), CYP2C9 (minor), CYP2D6 (minor), CYP3A4 (major); **Note:** Assignment of Major/Minor substrate status based on clinically relevant drug interaction potential; **Inhibits** CYP1A2 (weak), CYP2C19 (moderate), CYP2C9 (weak), CYP2D6 (weak), CYP3A4 (weak)

Avoid Concomitant Use

Avoid concomitant use of Bortezomib with any of the following: Clopidogrel; CloZAPine; CYP3A4 Inducers (Strong); Green Tea; Pimozide; St Johns Wort

Increased Effect/Toxicity

Bortezomib may increase the levels/effects of: ARIPiprazole; Citalopram; CloZAPine; CYP2C19 Substrates; Pimozide

The levels/effects of Bortezomib may be increased by: CYP3A4 Inhibitors (Moderate); CYP3A4 Inhibitors (Strong); Dasatinib; Ivacaftor; Mifepristone

Decreased Effect

Bortezomib may decrease the levels/effects of: Clopidogrel

The levels/effects of Bortezomib may be decreased by: Ascorbic Acid; CYP3A4 Inducers (Strong); Deferasirox; Green Tea; Multivitamins/Minerals (with ADEK, Folate, Iron); Peginterferon Alfa-2b; St Johns Wort; Tocilizumab

Ethanol/Nutrition/Herb Interactions

Food: Avoid grapefruit juice (may increase bortezomib levels).

Herb/Nutraceutical: Avoid St John's wort (may decrease bortezomib levels). Avoid green tea and green tea extracts (may diminish the therapeutic effect of bortezomib) (Golden, 2009). Avoid ascorbic acid supplements, including multivitamins containing ascorbic acid (may diminish bortezomib activity) during treatment, especially 12 hours before and after bortezomib treatment (Perrone, 2009).

Storage/Stability Prior to reconstitution, store at room temperature of 25°C (77°F); excursions permitted between 15°C to 30°C (59°F to 86°F). Once reconstituted, the manufacturer recommends use within 8 hours of reconstitution. However, stability studies have demonstrated solutions of 1 mg/mL (vial or syringe) may be stored at room temperature for up to 3 days, or under refrigeration for up to 5 days(Andre, 2005); or refrigerated in the original vial for up to 15 days (Vanderloo, 2010). Protect from light. After preparation, keep bortezomib in a location away from the separate storage location recommended for intrathecal medications.

Reconstitution Note: The reconstituted concentrations for I.V. and SubQ administration are different; the manufacturer provides stickers to facilitate identification of the route for reconstituted vials. The amount contained in each vial may exceed the prescribed dose; use care with dosage and volume calculations.

Hazardous agent; use appropriate precautions for handling and disposal. Reconstitute only with normal saline (NS). Reconstituted solutions should be clear and colorless.

I.V.: Reconstitute each 3.5 mg vial with 3.5 mL NS to a concentration of 1 mg/mL.

SubQ: Reconstitute each 3.5 mg vial with 1.4 mL NS to a concentration of 2.5 mg/mL (Moreau, 2011). If injection site reaction occurs, the more dilute 1 mg/mL concentration may be used SubQ.

Mechanism of Action Bortezomib inhibits proteasomes, enzyme complexes which regulate protein homeostasis within the cell. Specifically, it reversibly inhibits chymotrypsin-like activity at the 26S proteasome, leading to activation of signaling cascades, cell-cycle arrest, and apoptosis.

Pharmacodynamics/Kinetics

Distribution: 498-1884 L/m^2; distributes widely to peripheral tissues

Protein binding: ~83%

Metabolism: Hepatic primarily via CYP2C19 and 3A4 and to a lesser extent CYP1A2; forms metabolites (inactive) via deboronization followed by hydroxylation

Half-life elimination: Single dose: I.V.: 9-15 hours; multiple dosing: 1 mg/m^2: 40-193 hours; 1.3 mg/m^2: 76-108 hours

Dosing

Adult & Geriatric Details concerning dosing in combination regimens should also be consulted. **Note:** Consecutive doses should be separated by at least 72 hours.

Multiple myeloma (first-line therapy; in combination with melphalan and prednisone): I.V., SubQ: 1.3 mg/m^2 days 1, 4, 8, 11, 22, 25, 29, and 32 of a 42-day treatment cycle for 4 cycles, followed by 1.3 mg/m^2 days 1, 8, 22, and 29 of a 42-day treatment cycle for 5 cycles.

Alternative first-line therapy (unlabeled dosing):

CyBorD regimen: I.V.: 1.5 mg/m^2 days 1, 8, 15, and 22 of a 28-day treatment cycle for 4 cycles (may continue beyond 4 cycles) in combination with cyclophosphamide and dexamethasone (Khan, 2012)

Patients ≥65 years: I.V.: 1.3 mg/m^2 days 1, 8, 15, and 22 of a 35-day treatment cycle, in combination with **either** melphalan and prednisone or melphalan, prednisone, and thalidomide (Boccadoro, 2010; Bringhen, 2010; Palumbo, 2009)

Multiple myeloma (relapsed) and mantle cell lymphoma: I.V., SubQ: 1.3 mg/m^2 twice weekly for 2 weeks on days 1, 4, 8, and 11 of a 21-day treatment cycle. Therapy extending beyond 8 cycles may be administered by the standard schedule or may be given once weekly for 4 weeks (days 1, 8, 15, and 22), followed by a 13-day rest (days 23 through 35).

Cutaneous or peripheral T-cell lymphoma, relapsed/refractory (unlabeled use): I.V.: 1.3 mg/m^2 twice weekly for 2 weeks on days 1, 4, 8, and 11 of a 21-day treatment cycle (Zinzani, 2007).

Follicular lymphoma, relapsed/refractory (unlabeled use): I.V.: 1.3 mg/m^2 days 1, 4, 8, and 11 of a 28-day treatment cycle, in combination with bendamustine and rituximab for 6 cycles (Friedberg, 2011) **or** 1.6 mg/m^2 days 1, 8, 15, and 22 of a 35-day treatment cycle, in combination with bendamustine and rituximab for 5 cycles (Fowler, 2011)

Systemic light-chain amyloidosis (unlabeled use): I.V.: 1.3 mg/m^2 days 1, 4, 8, and 11 of a 21-day treatment cycle (with or without dexamethasone) (Kastritis, 2010)

Waldenström's macroglobulinemia, relapsed/refractory (unlabeled use): I.V.: 1.3 mg/m^2 days 1, 4, 8, and 11 of a 21-day treatment cycle (Chen, 2007) **or** 1.3 mg/m^2 days 1, 4, 8, and 11 of a 21-day treatment cycle (in combination with dexamethasone and rituximab) (Treon, 2009) **or** 1.6 mg/m^2 days 1, 8, and 15 of a 28-day treatment cycle (in combination with rituximab) (Ghobrial, 2010)

Renal Impairment No dosage adjustment necessary. Dialysis may reduce bortezomib concentrations; administer postdialysis (Leal, 2011).

Hepatic Impairment

Mild impairment (bilirubin ≤1 times ULN and AST >UNL or bilirubin >1-1.5 times ULN): No initial dose adjustment necessary (LoRusso, 2012).

Moderate (bilirubin >1.5-3 times ULN) and severe impairment (bilirubin >3 times ULN): Reduce initial dose to 0.7 mg/m^2 in the first cycle; based on patient tolerance, may consider dose escalation to 1 mg/m^2 (LoRusso, 2012) or further dose reduction to 0.5 mg/m^2 in subsequent cycles

Adjustment for Toxicity

Myeloma (first-line therapy):

Platelets should be ≥70,000/mm^3, ANC should be ≥1000/mm^3, and nonhematologic toxicities should resolve to grade 1 or baseline prior to therapy initiation.

Platelets ≤30,000/mm^3 or ANC ≤750/mm^3 on bortezomib day(s) (except day 1): Withhold bortezomib; if several bortezomib doses in consecutive cycles are withheld, reduce dose 1 level (1.3 mg/m^2/dose reduced to 1 mg/m^2/dose; 1 mg/m^2/dose reduced to 0.7 mg/m^2/dose)

Grade ≥3 nonhematological toxicity (other than neuropathy): Withhold bortezomib until toxicity resolves to grade 1 or baseline. May reinitiate bortezomib at 1 dose level reduction (1.3 mg/m^2/dose reduced to 1 mg/m^2/dose; 1 mg/m^2/dose reduced to 0.7 mg/m^2/dose).

Neuropathic pain and/or peripheral sensory or motor neuropathy: See "Neuropathic pain and/or peripheral sensory or motor neuropathy" toxicity adjustment guidelines below.

Relapsed multiple myeloma and mantle cell lymphoma:

Grade 3 nonhematological (excluding neuropathy) or Grade 4 hematological toxicity: Withhold until toxicity resolved; may reinitiate with a 25% dose reduction (1.3 mg/m^2/dose reduced to 1 mg/m^2/dose; 1 mg/m^2/dose reduced to 0.7 mg/m^2/dose)

Neuropathic pain and/or peripheral sensory or motor neuropathy:

Note: Consider subQ administration in patients with pre-existing or at high risk for peripheral neuropathy.

Grade 1 (asymptomatic; deep tendon reflex loss or paresthesia) without pain or loss of function: No action needed

Grade 1 with pain or Grade 2 (moderate symptoms; limiting instrumental activities of daily living): Reduce dose to 1 mg/m^2

Grade 2 with pain or Grade 3 (severe symptoms; limiting self-care activities of daily living): Withhold until toxicity resolved, may reinitiate at 0.7 mg/m^2 once weekly

Grade 4 (life-threatening consequences with urgent intervention indicated): Discontinue therapy

Combination Regimens

Amyloidosis: Bortezomib-Dexamethasone (Amyloidosis) on page 1534

Multiple myeloma:

Bortezomib-Dexamethasone (Multiple Myeloma) on page 1534
Bortezomib-Doxorubicin-Dexamethasone on page 1535
Bortezomib-Doxorubicin (Liposomal) on page 1536
Bortezomib-Doxorubicin (Liposomal)-Dexamethasone on page 1536
Bortezomib-Melphalan-Prednisone-Thalidomide on page 1537
Cyclophosphamide-Bortezomib-Dexamethasone (Multiple Myeloma) on page 1599
Lenalidomide-Bortezomib-Dexamethasone (Multiple Myeloma) on page 1702
Melphalan-Prednisone-Bortezomib (Multiple Myeloma) on page 1708

Waldenstrom's Macroglobulinemia:

Bortezomib-Dexamethasone-Rituximab (Waldenstrom's Macroglobulinemia) on page 1535
Bortezomib-Rituximab (Waldenstrom's Macroglobulinemia) on page 1537
Bortezomib (Waldenstrom's Macroglobulinemia) on page 1537

Administration

Note: The reconstituted concentrations for I.V. and SubQ administration are different; use caution when calculating the volume for each dose. Consider SubQ administration in patients with pre-existing or at high risk for peripheral neuropathy.

I.V.: Administer via rapid I.V. push (3-5 seconds)

SubQ: Subcutaneous administration of bortezomib 1.3 mg/m^2 days 1, 4, 8, and 11 of a 21-day treatment cycle has been studied in a limited number of patients with relapsed multiple myeloma; doses were administered subcutaneously (concentration of 2.5 mg/mL) into the thigh or abdomen, rotating the injection site with each dose; injections at the same site within a single cycle were avoided (Moreau, 2010, Moreau, 2011). Response rates were similar to I.V. administration; decreased incidence of grade 3 or higher adverse events were observed with SubQ administration. Administer at least 1 inch from an old site and never administer to tender, bruised, erythematous, or indurated sites. If injection site reaction occurs, the more dilute 1 mg/mL concentration may be used SubQ (or I.V. administration of 1 mg/mL concentration may be considered).

For I.V. or SubQ administration only; fatalities have been reported with inadvertent intrathecal administration. Bortezomib should **NOT** be delivered to the patient at the same time with any medications intended for central nervous system administration.

Emetic Potential Low (10% to 30%)

Vesicant/Extravasation Risk May be an irritant; extravasation has not been associated with tissue damage

Monitoring Parameters CBC with differential and platelets (monitor frequently throughout therapy); liver function tests (in patients with existing hepatic impairment); signs/symptoms of peripheral neuropathy, dehydration, hypotension, or PRES; renal function, pulmonary function (with new or worsening pulmonary symptoms)

Dietary Considerations Green tea and green tea extracts may diminish the therapeutic effect of bortezomib and should be avoided (Golden, 2009). Avoid grapefruit juice. Avoid additional, nondietary sources of ascorbic acid supplements, including multivitamins containing ascorbic acid (may diminish bortezomib activity) during treatment, especially 12 hours before and after bortezomib treatment (Perrone, 2009).

Dosage Forms Excipient information presented when available (limited, particularly for generics); consult specific product labeling.

Injection, powder for reconstitution:

Velcade®: 3.5 mg [contains mannitol]

References

Andre P, Cisternino S, Chiadmi F, et al, "Stability of Bortezomib 1-mg/mL Solution in Plastic Syringe and Glass Vial," *Ann Pharmacother*, 2005, 39(9):1462-6.

Boccadoro M, Bringhen S, Gaidano G, et al, "Bortezomib, Melphalan, Prednisone, and Thalidomide (VMPT) Followed by Maintenance With Bortexomib and Thalidomide (VT) for Initial Treatment of Elderly Multiple Myeloma Patients," *J Clin Oncol*, 2010, 28(7s):8013 [abstract 8013 from 2010 ASCO Annual Meeting].

Bringhen S, Larocca A, Rossi D, et al, "Efficacy and Safety of Once-Weekly Bortezomib in Multiple Myeloma Patients," *Blood*, 2010, 116(23):4745-53.

Chanan-Khan AA, Kaufman JL, Mehta J, et al, "Activity and Safety of Bortezomib in Multiple Myeloma Patients With Advanced Renal Failure: A Multicenter Retrospective Study," *Blood*, 2006, 109(9):2604-6.

Chanan-Khan A, Sonneveld P, Schuster MW, et al, "Analysis of Herpes Zoster Events Among Bortezomib-Treated Patients in the Phase III APEX Study," *J Clin Oncol*, 2008, 26(29):4784-90.

Chen CI, Kouroukis CT, White D, et al, "Bortezomib is Active in Patients With Untreated or Relapsed Waldenstrom's Macroglobulinemia: A Phase II Study of the National Cancer Institute of Canada Clinical Trials Group," *J Clin Oncol*, 2007, 25(12):1570-5.

Dimopoulos MA, Mateos MV, Richardson PG, et al, "Risk Factors for, and Reversibility of, Peripheral Neuropathy Associated With Bortezomib-Melphalan-Prednisone in Newly Diagnosed Patients With Multiple Myeloma: Subanalysis of the Phase 3 VISTA Study," *Eur J Haematol*, 2011, 86(1):23-31.

Fowler N, Kahl BS, Lee P, et al, "Bortezomib, Bendamustine, and Rituximab in Patients With Relapsed or Refractory Follicular Lymphoma: The Phase II VERTICAL Study," *J Clin Oncol*, 2011, 29(25):3389-95.

Friedberg JW, Vose JM, Kelly JL, et al, "The Combination of Bendamustine, Bortezomib, and Rituximab for Patients With Relapsed/Refractory Indolent and Mantle Cell Non-Hodgkin Lymphoma," *Blood*, 2011, 117(10):2807-12.

Ghobrial IM, Hong F, Padmanabhan S, et al, "Phase II Trial of Weekly Bortezomib in Combination With Rituximab in Relapsed or Relapsed and Refractory Waldenstrom Macroglobulinemia," *J Clin Oncol*, 2010, 28(8):1422-8.

Golden EB, Lam PY, Kardosh A, et al, "Green Tea Polyphenols Block the Anticancer Effects of Bortezomib and Other Boronic Acid-Based Proteasome Inhibitors," *Blood*, 2009, 113 (23):5927-37.

Jacobson JO, Polovich M, McNiff KK, et al, "American Society of Clinical Oncology/ Oncology Nursing Society Chemotherapy Administration Safety Standards," *J Clin Oncol*, 2009, 27 (32):5469-75.

Jagannath S, Barlogie B, Berenson JR, et al, "Bortezomib in Recurrent and/or Refractory Multiple Myeloma; Initial Clinical Experience in Patients With Impaired Renal Function," *Cancer*, 2005, 103(6):1195-200.

Kastritis E, Anagnostopoulos A, Bamias A, et al, "Reversibility of Renal Failure in Newly Diagnosed Patients With Multiple Myeloma Treated With High-Dose Dexamethasone Containing Regimens and the Impact of Novel Agents," *Blood*, 2006, 108(11):3586 [abstract 3586 from 2006 ASH Annual Meeting].

Kastritis E, Wechalekar AD, Dimopoulos MA, et al, "Bortezomib With or Without Dexamethasone in Primary Systemic (Light Chain) Amyloidosis," *J Clin Oncol*, 2010, 28(6):1031-7.

Khan ML, Reeder CB, Kumar SK, et al, "A Comparison of Lenalidomide/Dexamethasone versus Cyclophosphamide/Lenalidomide/Dexamethasone versus Cyclophosphamide/Bortezomib/Dexamethasone in Newly Diagnosed Multiple Myeloma," *Br J Haematol*, 2012, 156(3):326-33.

Lamm W, Willenbacher W, Lang A, et al, "Efficacy of the Combination of Bortezomib and Dexamethasone in Systemic AL Amyloidosis," *Ann Hematol*, 2011, 90(2):201-6.

Leal TB, Remick SC, Takimoto CH, et al, "Dose-Escalating and Pharmacological Study of Bortezomib in Adult Cancer Patients With Impaired Renal Function: A National Cancer Institute Organ Dysfunction Working Group Study," *Cancer Chemother Pharamcol*, 2011, 68(6):1439-47.

LoRusso PM, Venkatakrishnan K, Ramanathan RK, et al, "Pharmacokinetics and Safety of Bortezomib in Patients With Advanced Malignancies and Varying Degrees of Liver Dysfunction: Phase I NCI Organ Dysfunction Working Group Study NCI-6432," *Clin Cancer Res*, 2012, 18 (10):2954-63.

Moreau P, Pylypenko H, Grosicki S, et al, "A Phase 3 Prospective Randomized International Study (MMY-3021) Comparing Subcutaneous and Intravenous Administration of Bortezomib In Patients With Relapsed Multiple Myeloma, *Blood*, 2010, 116(21):312 [abstract 312 from 2010 ASH Annual Meeting].

Moreau P, Pylypenko H, Grosicki S, et al, "Subcutaneous Versus Intravenous Administration of Bortezomib in Patients With Relapsed Multiple Myeloma: A Randomised, Phase 3, Non-Inferiority Study," *Lancet Oncol*, 2011, 12(5):431-40.

Mulkerin D, Remick S, Ramanathan R, et al, "A Dose-Escalating and Pharmacologic Study of Bortezomib in Adult Cancer Patients With Impaired Renal Function," *J Clin Oncol*, 24(18S):2032 [abstract 2032 from ASCO Annual Meeting Proceedings, Part I].

O'Connor OA, Wright J, Moskowitz C, et al "Phase II Clinical Experience With the Novel Proteasome Inhibitor Bortezomib in Patients With Indolent Non-Hodgkin's Lymphoma and Mantle Cell Lymphoma," *J Clin Oncol*, 2005, 23(4):676-84.

Orlowski RZ, Nagler A, Sonneveld P, et al, "Randomized Phase III Study of Pegylated Liposomal Doxorubicin Plus Bortezomib Compared With Bortezomib Alone in Relapsed or Refractory Multiple Myeloma: Combination Therapy Improves Time to Progression," *J Clin Oncol*, 2007, 25(25):3892-901.

Palumbo A, Bringhen S, Rossi D, et al, "Bortezomib, Melphalan, Prednisone and Thalidomide (VMPT) Followed by Maintenance With Bortezomib and Thalidomide for Initial Treatment of Elderly Multiple Myeloma Patients," *Blood*, 2009, 114(22):128 [abstract 128 from ASH 2009 Annual Meeting].

Pekol T, Daniels JS, Labutti J, et al, "Human Metabolism of the Proteasome Inhibitor Bortezomib: Identification of Circulating Metabolites," *Drug Metab Dispos*, 2005, 33(6):771-7.

Perrone G, Hideshima T, Ikeda H, et al, "Ascorbic Acid Inhibits Activity of Bortezomib *in vivo*," *Leukemia*, 2009, 23(9):1679-86.

Reece DE, Hegenbart U, Sanchorawala V, et al, "Efficacy and Safety of Once-Weekly and Twice-Weekly Bortezomib in Patients With Relapsed Systemic AL Amyloidosis: Results of a Phase 1/2 Study," *Blood*, 2011.

San-Miguel JF, Richardson PG, Sonneveld P, et al, "Efficacy and Safety of Bortezomib in Patients With Renal Impairment: Results from the APEX Phase 3 Study," *Leukemia*, 2008, 22(4):842-9.

San Miguel JF, Schlag R, Khuageva N, et al, "Bortezomib Plus Melphalan and Prednisone for Initial Treatment of Multiple Myeloma," *N Engl J Med*, 2008, 359(9):906-17.

Treon SP, Ioakimidis L, Soumerai JD, et al, "Primary Therapy of Waldenström Macroglobulinemia With Bortezomib, Dexamethasone, and Rituximab: WMCTG Clinical Trial 05-180," *J Clin Oncol*, 2009, 27(23):3830-5.

Vanderloo JP, Pomplun ML, Vermeulen LC, et al, "Stability of Unused Reconstituted Bortezomib in Original Manufacturer Vials," *J Oncol Pharm Pract*, 2011, 17(4):400-2.

Zinzani PL, Musuraca G, Tani M, et al, "Phase II Trial of Proteasome Inhibitor Bortezomib in Patients With Relapsed or Refractory Cutaneous T-cell Lymphoma," *J Clin Oncol*, 2007, 25 (27):4293-7.

◆ **Bosulif®** *see* Bosutinib *on page* 195

◆ **Bosulif®** *see* Bosutinib *on page* 195

Bosutinib (boe SUE ti nib)

Brand Names: U.S. Bosulif®

Index Terms Bosulif®; Bosutinib Monohydrate; SKI-606

Generic Availability (U.S.) No

Pharmacologic Category Antineoplastic Agent, Tyrosine Kinase Inhibitor

Use Treatment of chronic, accelerated or blast phase Philadelphia chromosome-positive (Ph+) chronic myelogenous leukemia (CML) patients resistant or intolerant to prior therapy

Labeled Contraindications Hypersensitivity to bosutinib or any component of the formulation

Pregnancy Risk Factor D

Lactation Excretion in breast milk unknown/not recommended

Warnings/Precautions Hazardous agent: Use appropriate precautions for handling and disposal.

Diarrhea, nausea, vomiting, and abdominal pain may occur. Monitor; may require treatment interruption, dose reduction, or discontinuation. For patients experiencing diarrhea (all grades), the median time to onset was 2 days; median duration (per event) was 1 day; manage diarrhea with antidiarrheals and/or fluid replacement. Nausea and vomiting may be managed with antiemetics and/or fluid replacement.

Anemia, neutropenia, and thrombocytopenia may occur. May require treatment interruption, dose reduction, or discontinuation. Monitor blood counts weekly during first month, then monthly thereafter (or as clinically indicated). Fluid retention, manifesting as pericardial effusion, pleural effusion, pulmonary edema and/or peripheral edema may occur; may be severe. Monitor and manage appropriately; may require treatment interruption, dose reduction, or discontinuation.

Bosutinib exposure is increased in patients with hepatic impairment; dose reduction is recommended. Hepatotoxicity has been reported during treatment; dose reductions may be necessary. Monitor liver function. ALT and AST elevations may occur, usually with an onset in the first 3 months of treatment (median onset was ~30-33 days; median duration was 21 days). Once case of drug-induced liver injury has been reported; full recovery occurred after discontinuation.

Avoid concurrent use with strong or moderate CYP3A4 inducers; may decrease bosutinib levels/effects. Avoid concurrent use with strong or moderate CYP3A4 and/or P-gp inhibitors; may increase bosutinib levels/effects. Proton pump inhibitors (PPIs) may decrease bosutinib effects; consider using short acting antacids or H_2 antagonists instead of PPIs. Separate administration of antacids or H_2 antagonists from bosutinib by at least 2 hours.

Adverse Reactions

>10%:

- Cardiovascular: Edema (14%; grades 3/4: <1%)
- Central nervous system: Fever (26%), fatigue (24%), headache (20%)
- Dermatologic: Rash (35%)
- Endocrine & metabolic: Bicarbonate decreased (31%), hypermagnesemia (25%; grades 3/4: 12%), hypomagnesemia (19%)
- Gastrointestinal: Diarrhea (82%; grades 3/4: 8%), nausea (46%; grades 3/4: 1%), vomiting (39%; grades 3/4: 32%), abdominal pain (37%; grades 3/4: 2%), appetite decreased (13%)
- Hematologic: Thrombocytopenia (41%; grades 3/4: 29% to 33%), anemia (27%; grades 3/4: 13% to 19%), neutropenia (17%; grades 3/4: 12% to 23%)
- Hepatic: ALT increased (17%; grades 3/4: 7% to 9%), AST increased (14%; grades 3/4: 3% to 4%)
- Neuromuscular & skeletal: Arthralgia (14%), back pain (11%), weakness (11%)
- Respiratory: Cough (20%), dyspnea (12%), respiratory tract infection (12%)

1% to 10%:

- Cardiovascular: Chest pain (<10%), pericardial effusion (<10%; grades 3/4: <1%)
- Central nervous system: Dizziness (10%), pain (<10%)

Dermatologic: Pruritus (10%), acne (<10%), urticaria (<10%)
Endocrine & metabolic: Dehydration (<10%), hypophosphatemia (grades 3/4: 7%), uric acid increased (grades 3/4: 6%), hypocalcemia (grades 3/4: 3% to 4%)
Gastrointestinal: Abnormal taste (<10%), gastritis (<10%), lipase increased (grades 3/4: 7%)
Hematologic: Neutropenic fever (<10%), INR increased (grades 3/4: 2%)
Hepatic: Abnormal hepatic function (<10%), hepatotoxicity (<10%), bilirubin increased (grades 3/4: 1%)
Neuromuscular & skeletal: CPK increased (<10%), myalgia (<10%), bone pain (4%), muscle spasm (2%)
Otic: Tinnitus (<10%)
Renal: Creatinine increased (<10%), renal failure (<10%)
Respiratory: Nasopharyngitis (10%), bronchitis (<10%), pleural effusion (<10%; grades 3/4: <2%), pneumonia (<10%)
Miscellaneous: Hypersensitivity reactions (<10%), influenza (<10%)

<1%, postmarketing, and/or case reports: Anaphylactic shock, erythema multiforme, exfoliative rash, fixed drug eruption, gastrointestinal hemorrhage, hemorrhage, liver injury, muscle cramping, pancreatitis, pericarditis, pulmonary edema, pulmonary hypertension, QT_c prolongation, respiratory failure

Drug Interactions

Metabolism/Transport Effects Substrate of CYP3A4 (major), P-glycoprotein; **Note:** Assignment of Major/Minor substrate status based on clinically relevant drug interaction potential; **Inhibits** P glycoprotein

Avoid Concomitant Use

Avoid concomitant use of Bosutinib with any of the following: CloZAPine; CYP3A4 Inducers (Strong); CYP3A4 Inhibitors (Moderate); CYP3A4 Inhibitors (Strong); Modafinil; P-glycoprotein/ABCB1 Inhibitors; St Johns Wort

Increased Effect/Toxicity

Bosutinib may increase the levels/effects of: CloZAPine; Highest Risk QTc-Prolonging Agents; Moderate Risk QTc-Prolonging Agents

The levels/effects of Bosutinib may be increased by: CYP3A4 Inhibitors (Moderate); CYP3A4 Inhibitors (Strong); Dasatinib; Ivacaftor; Mifepristone; P-glycoprotein/ABCB1 Inhibitors

Decreased Effect

The levels/effects of Bosutinib may be decreased by: Antacids; CYP3A4 Inducers (Strong); Deferasirox; H2-Antagonists; Modafinil; P-glycoprotein/ABCB1 Inducers; Proton Pump Inhibitors; St Johns Wort; Tocilizumab

Ethanol/Nutrition/Herb Interactions

Food: Grapefruit juice may increase imatinib plasma concentration. Management: Avoid grapefruit juice

Herb/Nutraceutical: St John's wort may increase metabolism and decrease imatinib plasma concentration. Management: Avoid St John's wort.

Storage/Stability Store at room temperature of 20°C to 25°C (68°F to 77°F); excursions permitted to 15°C to 30°C (59°F to 86°F).

Mechanism of Action BCR-ABL tyrosine kinase inhibitor (TKI); inhibits BCR-ABL kinase that promotes CML. Also inhibits SRC family (including SRC, LYN, and HCK). Bosutinib has minimal activity against c-KIT and platelet-derived growth factor receptor (PDGFR), which are nonspecific targets associated with toxicity in other TKIs (Cortes, 2012). Bosutinib has activity in 16 of 18 imatinib-resistant BCR-ABL mutations, with the exceptions of the T315I and V299L mutants (Cortes, 2011).

Pharmacodynamics/Kinetics

Onset:

Median time to complete hematologic response (in responders): 2 weeks (Cortes, 2011)

Median time to major cytogenetic response (in responders): 12.3 weeks (Cortes, 2011)

Median time to first complete cytogenic response: 12.9 weeks (Cortes, 2012)

Absorption: Slow (Abbas, 2012)

Distribution: V_d: 6080 ± 1230 L

Protein binding: 94% to plasma proteins

Metabolism: Hepatic via CYP3A4, primarily to inactive metabolites oxydechlorinated (M2) bosutinib and *N*-desmethylated (M5) bosutinib, also to bosutinib *N*-oxide (M6)

Half-life elimination: 22-27 hours (Cortes, 2011)

Time to peak: 4-6 hours

Excretion: Feces (91%); urine (3%)

Dosing

Adult & Geriatric Philadelphia chromosome-positive chronic myelogenous leukemia (Ph+CML): Oral: 500 mg once daily; continue until disease progression or unacceptable toxicity. **Note:** If complete hematologic response is not achieved by week 8 or complete cytogenetic response is not achieved by week 12, in the absence of grade 3 or higher adverse reactions, consider increasing the dose from 500 mg once daily to 600 mg once daily.

Missed doses: If a dose is missed beyond 12 hours, skip the dose and resume the usual dose the following day

Renal Impairment No dosage adjustment provided in the manufacturer's labeling; based on pharmacokinetics, the need for dosage adjustment is not likely in patients with Cl_{cr} ≥25 mL/minute (creatinine clearance had no meaningful impact on bosutinib exposure).

Hepatic Impairment

Pre-existing impairment (mild, moderate, or severe): Reduce dose to 200 mg once daily (this dose is predicted to result in an AUC similar to that of patients with normal hepatic function, however, there is no efficacy data for this dose in CML patients with hepatic impairment).

Hepatotoxicity during treatment:

ALT or AST >5 times ULN: Withhold treatment until recovery to ≤2.5 times ULN and resume at 400 mg once daily thereafter. If recovery to ≤2.5 times ULN takes >4 weeks: Discontinue bosutinib.

ALT or AST >3 times ULN in conjunction with bilirubin elevation >2 times ULN and alkaline phosphatase <2 times ULN: Discontinue bosutinib.

Adjustment for Toxicity

Hematologic toxicity: ANC <1000/mm^3 or platelets <50,000/mm^3: Withhold treatment until ANC ≥1000/mm^3 **and** platelets ≥50,000/mm^3; if recovery occurs within 2 weeks, resume treatment at the same dose. If ANC and platelets remain low for >2 weeks, upon recovery, resume treatment with the dose reduced by 100 mg. If cytopenia recurs, withhold until recovery and resume treatment with the dose reduced by an additional 100 mg. Doses <300 mg daily have not been evaluated.

Nonhematologic toxicity:

Diarrhea: Grade 3 or 4 (≥7 stools/day increase over baseline): Withhold treatment until recovery to ≤ grade 1; may resume at 400 mg once daily.

Other clinically significant nonhematologic toxicity, moderate or severe: Withhold treatment until resolved, then consider resuming at 400 mg once daily; may re-escalate dose to 500 mg once daily if clinically appropriate.

Combination Regimens

Leukemia, Chronic Myelogenous: Bosutinib (CML Regimen) on page 1538

Administration Oral: Administer with food. Swallow tablet whole; do not crush or break.

Monitoring Parameters CBC with differential and platelets (weekly during first month, then monthly thereafter, or as clinically indicated); hepatic enzymes (monthly for first 3 months or as clinically indicated; monitor more frequently with transaminase elevations); diarrhea episodes; fluid/edema status

Dietary Considerations Take with food.

Dosage Forms Excipient information presented when available (limited, particularly for generics); consult specific product labeling.

Tablet, oral:

Bosulif®: 100 mg, 500 mg

References

Cortes JE, Kantarjian HM, Brümmendorf TH, et al, "Safety and Efficacy of Bosutinib (SKI-606) in Chronic Phase Philadelphia Chromosome-Positive Chronic Myeloid Leukemia Patients With Resistance or Intolerance to Imatinib," *Blood*, 2011, 118(17):4567-76.

Cortes JE, Kim DW, Kantarjian HM, et al, "Bosutinib versus Imatinib in Newly Diagnosed Chronic-Phase Chronic Myeloid Leukemia: Results From the BELA Trial," *J Clin Oncol*, 2012, 30 (28):3486-92.

Khoury HJ, Cortes JE, Kantarjian HM, et al, "Bosutinib is Active in Chronic Phase Chronic Myeloid Leukemia After Imatinib and Dasatinib and/or Nilotinib Therapy Failure," *Blood*, 2012, 119 (15):3403-12.

Redaelli S, Piazza R, Rostagno R, et al, "Activity of Bosutinib, Dasatinib, and Nilotinib Against 18 Imatinib-Resistant BCR/ABL Mutants," *J Clin Oncol*, 2009, 27(3):469-71.

- **Bosutinib Monohydrate** *see* Bosutinib *on page 195*
- **BRAF(V600E) Kinase Inhibitor RO5185426** *see* Vemurafenib *on page 1440*
- **Brentuximab** *see* Brentuximab Vedotin *on page 199*

Brentuximab Vedotin (bren TUX i mab ve DOE tin)

Related Information

Principles of Anticancer Therapy *on page 1878*

Brand Names: U.S. Adcetris™

Index Terms Anti-CD30 ADC SGN-35; Anti-CD30 Antibody-Drug Conjugate SGN-35; Antibody-Drug Conjugate SGN-35; Brentuximab; SGN-35

Generic Availability (U.S.) No

Pharmacologic Category Antineoplastic Agent, Monoclonal Antibody

Use Treatment of Hodgkin lymphoma after failure of at least 2 prior chemotherapy regimens (in patients ineligible for transplant) or after stem cell transplant failure; treatment of systemic anaplastic large cell lymphoma (sALCL) after failure of at least 1 prior chemotherapy regimen

Labeled Contraindications Concurrent use with bleomycin

Pregnancy Risk Factor D

Lactation Excretion in breast milk unknown/not recommended

Warnings/Precautions

Hazardous agent - use appropriate precautions for handling and disposal.

[U.S. Boxed Warning]: Cases of PML and death due to JC virus infection have been reported. Immunosuppression due to prior chemotherapy treatments or underlying disease may also contribute to PML development.

New-onset signs/symptoms of central nervous system abnormalities (eg,changes in mood, memory, cognition, motor incoordination and/or weakness, speech and/or visual disturbances) should receive prompt evaluation with neurology consultation, brain MRI, and lumbar puncture or brain biopsy. Withhold treatment with new-onset symptoms suggestive of PML; discontinue if diagnosis of PML is confirmed.

Peripheral neuropathy is common and is generally cumulative; usually sensory neuropathy, although motor neuropathy has also been observed; neuropathy completely resolved in nearly half of patients; almost one-third had partial improvement. Monitor for symptoms of neuropathy; dose interruption, reduction or discontinuation may be recommended.

Neutropenia, thrombocytopenia and anemia may occur; neutropenia may be prolonged (≥1 week); monitor blood counts; may require dose interruption, reduction or discontinuation. Infusion reactions, including anaphylaxis have been reported; monitor during infusion. For anaphylaxis, immediately and permanently discontinue and administer appropriate medical intervention. For infusion-related reaction, interrupt infusion and administer appropriate medical intervention; premedicate for subsequent infusions (with acetaminophen, an antihistamine, and/or a corticosteroid).

Due to the risk for pulmonary injury, concurrent use with bleomycin is contraindicated. In a study comparing brentuximab combined with ABVD (doxorubicin, bleomycin, vinblastine, and dacarbazine) to brentuximab combined with AVD (doxorubicin, vinblastine, and dacarbazine), the occurrence of pulmonary toxicity was 40% in the brentuximab/ABVD group compared to a literature-based frequency of ≤25% for other bleomycin-containing regimens. There were no cases of pulmonary toxicity documented with brentuximab in combination with AVD. Pulmonary symptoms/toxicities reported with brentuximab in combination with ABVD consisted of cough, dyspnea, and interstitial infiltration/inflammation; most patients responded to corticosteroids.

Stevens-Johnson syndrome has been observed; discontinue and administer appropriate medical intervention. Tumor lysis syndrome (TLS) may occur; risk of TLS is higher in patients with a high tumor burden or with rapid tumor proliferation; monitor closely. A component of brentuximab vedotin, the microtubule-disrupting agent MMAE is excreted renally and hepatically; the impact of renal or hepatic impairment on MMAE pharmacokinetics is undetermined.

Adverse Reactions

>10%:

Cardiovascular: Peripheral edema (4% to 16%)

Central nervous system: Fatigue (41% to 49%), fever (29% to 38%), pain (7% to 28%), headache (16% to 19%), insomnia (14% to 16%), dizziness (11% to 16%), chills (12% to 13%), anxiety (7% to 11%)

Dermatologic: Rash (27% to 31%), pruritus (17% to 19%), alopecia (13% to 14%)

Gastrointestinal: Nausea (38% to 42%), diarrhea (29% to 36%), abdominal pain (9% to 25%), vomiting (17% to 22%), constipation (16% to 19%), appetite decreased (11% to 16%), weight loss (6% to 12%)

Hematologic: Neutropenia (54% to 55%; grade 4: 6% to 9%); anemia (33% to 52%; grade 4: ≤2%), thrombocytopenia (16% to 28%; grade 4: 2% to 5%)

Neuromuscular & skeletal: Peripheral sensory neuropathy (52% to 53%; grade 3: 8% to 10%), arthralgia (9% to 19%), myalgia (16% to 17%), peripheral motor neuropathy (7% to 16%; grade 3: 3% to 4%), back pain (10% to 14%)

Respiratory: Upper respiratory tract infection (12% to 47%), cough (17% to 25%), dyspnea (13% to 19%), oropharyngeal pain (9% to 11%)

Miscellaneous: Infusion reactions (grades 1/2: 12%), night sweats (9% to 12%), lymphadenopathy (10% to 11%)

1% to 10%:

Cardiovascular: Supraventricular arrhythmia

Dermatologic: Dry skin

Genitourinary: Urinary tract infection

Neuromuscular & skeletal: Limb pain, muscle spasms

Renal: Pyelonephritis

Respiratory: Pneumonitis, pneumothorax, pulmonary embolism

Miscellaneous: Antibrentuximab antibody formation, septic shock

<1% and/or case reports: Anaphylaxis, progressive multifocal leukoencephalopathy (PML), Stevens-Johnson syndrome, tachycardia, tumor lysis syndrome

Drug Interactions

Metabolism/Transport Effects **Substrate** of CYP3A4 (major); **Note:** Assignment of Major/Minor substrate status based on clinically relevant drug interaction potential

Avoid Concomitant Use

Avoid concomitant use of Brentuximab Vedotin with any of the following: BCG; Bleomycin; Natalizumab; Pimecrolimus; Tacrolimus (Topical); Vaccines (Live)

Increased Effect/Toxicity

Brentuximab Vedotin may increase the levels/effects of: Bleomycin; Leflunomide; Natalizumab; Vaccines (Live); Vitamin K Antagonists

The levels/effects of Brentuximab Vedotin may be increased by: CYP3A4 Inhibitors (Strong); Denosumab; Pimecrolimus; Roflumilast; Tacrolimus (Topical); Trastuzumab

Decreased Effect

Brentuximab Vedotin may decrease the levels/effects of: BCG; Cardiac Glycosides; Coccidioidin Skin Test; Sipuleucel-T; Vaccines (Inactivated); Vaccines (Live); Vitamin K Antagonists

The levels/effects of Brentuximab Vedotin may be decreased by: CYP3A4 Inducers (Strong); Deferasirox; Echinacea; Herbs (CYP3A4 Inducers); Tocilizumab

Storage/Stability Store intact vials refrigerated at 2°C to 8°C (36°F to 46°F) in the original carton. Protect from light. Reconstituted solution may be stored refrigerated for up to 24 hours; do not freeze. Solutions diluted for infusion may be stored for 24 hours refrigerated (do not freeze); use within 24 hours of initial reconstitution.

Reconstitution Use appropriate precautions for handling and disposal. Reconstitute each 50 mg vial with 10.5 mL sterile water for injection (SWFI), resulting in a concentration of 5 mg/mL. Direct SWFI toward the vial wall; do not direct toward the cake or powder. Swirl gently to dissolve, do not shake. Reconstituted solution should be clear to slightly opalescent without visible particles. Further dilute in at least 100 mL of either NS, D_5W, or lactated Ringer's to a final concentration of 0.4 to 1.8 mg/mL; gently invert bag to mix. Do not mix with other medications. Use within 24 hours of initial reconstitution.

Mechanism of Action Brentuximab vedotin is an antibody drug conjugate (ADC) directed at CD30 consisting of 3 components: 1) a CD30-specific chimeric IgG1 antibody cAC10; 2) a microtubule-disrupting agent, monomethylauristatin E (MMAE); and 3) a protease cleavable dipeptide linker (which covalently conjugates MMAE to cAC10). The conjugate binds to cells which express CD30, and forms a complex which is internalized within the cell and releases MMAE. MMAE binds to the tubules and disrupts the cellular microtubule network, inducing cell cycle arrest (G2/M phase) and apoptosis.

Pharmacodynamics/Kinetics

Distribution: V_{dss}: ADC: 6-10 L

Metabolism: MMAE: Minimal, primarily via oxidation by CYP3A4/5

Half-life elimination: Terminal: ADC: ~4-6 days

Time to peak: ADC: At end of infusion; MMAE: ~1-3 days

Excretion: MMAE: Feces (~72%, primarily unchanged); urine

Dosing

Adult & Geriatric Note: For patients weighing >100 kg, dose should be calculated using a weight of 100 kg.

Hodgkin lymphoma, refractory: I.V.: 1.8 mg/kg (maximum dose: 180 mg) every 3 weeks, continue until disease progression, unacceptable toxicities, or a maximum of 16 cycles

Systemic anaplastic large cell lymphoma (sALCL), refractory: I.V.: 1.8 mg/kg (maximum dose: 180 mg) every 3 weeks, continue until disease progression, unacceptable toxicities, or a maximum of 16 cycles

Renal Impairment No dosage adjustment provided in the manufacturer's labeling; active drug (MMAE) pharmacokinetics have not been determined in renal impairment.

Hepatic Impairment No dosage adjustment provided in the manufacturer's labeling; active drug (MMAE) pharmacokinetics have not been determined in hepatic impairment.

Adjustment for Toxicity

Hematologic toxicity:

Grade 3 or 4 neutropenia: Withhold treatment until resolves to baseline or ≤grade 2, consider growth factor support in subsequent cycles.

Recurrent grade 4 neutropenia (despite the use of growth factor support): Consider reducing the dose to 1.2 mg/kg or discontinuing treatment

Nonhematologic toxicities:

Anaphylaxis: Discontinue immediately and permanently

Infusion reaction: Interrupt infusion and administer appropriate medical intervention. Premedicate subsequent infusions with acetaminophen, an antihistamine, and/or a corticosteroid.

Peripheral neuropathy, new or worsening grade 2 or 3: Withhold treatment until improves or returns to grade 1 or baseline; then resume with dose reduced to 1.2 mg/kg

Peripheral neuropathy, grade 4: Discontinue treatment

Progressive multifocal leukoencephalopathy (PML): Withhold treatment with new-onset symptoms suggestive of PML; discontinue if PML diagnosis confirmed

Stevens-Johnson syndrome: Discontinue and administer appropriate medical intervention

Administration Infuse over 30 minutes. Do not administer as I.V. push or bolus.

Monitoring Parameters CBC with differential prior to each dose (more frequently if clinically indicated). Monitor for infusion reaction, tumor lysis syndrome, and for signs of neuropathy (hyperesthesia, paresthesia, discomfort, burning sensation, or neuropathic pain or weakness).

Dosage Forms Excipient information presented when available (limited, particularly for generics); consult specific product labeling.

Injection, powder for reconstitution:

Adcetris™: 50 mg [contains polysorbate 80; derived from or manufactured using hamster or mouse protein]

References

Chen RW, Gopal AK, Smith SE, et al, "Results From a Pivitol Phase II Study of Brentuximab Vedotin (SGN-35) in Patients With Relapsed or Refractory Hodgkin Lymphoma (HL)," *J Clin Oncol*, 2011, 29(15s):8031 [abstract 8031 from 2011 ASCO Annual Meeting].

Pro B, Avandi R, Brice P, et al, "Durable Remissions With Brentuximab Vedotin (SG-35): Updated Results of a Phase II Study in Patients With Relapsed or Refractory Systemic Anaplastic Large Cell Lymphoma (sALCL)," *J Clin Oncol*, 2011, 29(15s):8032 [abstract 8032 from 2011 ASCO Annual Meeting].

Younes A, Bartlett NL, Leonard JP, et al, "Brentuximab Vedotin (SGN-35) for Relapsed CD30-Positive Lymphomas," *N Engl J Med*, 2010, 363(19):1812-21.

Younes A, Connors JM, Park SI, et al, "Frontline Therapy With Brentuximab Vedotin Combined With ABVD or AVD in Patients With Newly Diagnosed Advanced Stage Hodgkin Lymphoma," *Blood*, 2011, 118(21):955 [abstract 955 from 2011 ASH Annual Meeting].

◆ **BRL 43694** *see* Granisetron *on page 687*

◆ **Buscopan® (Can)** *see* Scopolamine (Systemic) *on page 1274*

◆ **Bussulfam** *see* Busulfan *on page 203*

Busulfan (byoo SUL fan)

Related Information

Fertility and Cancer Therapy *on page 1782*

Hematopoietic Stem Cell Transplantation *on page 1887*

Management of Chemotherapy-Induced Nausea and Vomiting *on page 1786*

Management of Drug Extravasations *on page 1800*

Safe Handling of Hazardous Drugs *on page 1904*

Brand Names: U.S. Busulfex®; Myleran®

Brand Names: Canada Busulfex®; Myleran®

Index Terms Bussulfam; Busulfanum; Busulphan

Generic Availability (U.S.) No

Pharmacologic Category Antineoplastic Agent, Alkylating Agent

Use Palliative treatment of chronic myelogenous leukemia (CML) (oral); conditioning regimen prior to allogeneic hematopoietic progenitor cell transplantation (I.V.) for CML

Unlabeled Use Conditioning regimen prior to hematopoietic stem cell transplant (HSCT) (oral); treatment of polycythemia vera and essential thrombocytosis

Labeled Contraindications Hypersensitivity to busulfan or any component of the formulation; oral busulfan is contraindicated in patients without a definitive diagnosis of CML

Pregnancy Risk Factor D

Lactation Excretion in breast milk unknown/not recommended

Warnings/Precautions Hazardous agent - use appropriate precautions for handling and disposal. **[U.S. Boxed Warning]: Severe bone marrow suppression is common; reduce dose or discontinue oral busulfan for unusual suppression; may require bone marrow biopsy.** May result in severe neutropenia, thrombocytopenia, anemia, bone marrow failure, and/or pancytopenia; pancytopenia may be prolonged (1 month up to 2 years) and may be reversible. Use with caution in patients with compromised bone marrow reserve (due to prior treatment or radiation therapy). Monitor closely for signs of infection (due to neutropenia) or bleeding (due to thrombocytopenia) Seizures have been reported with use; use caution in patients predisposed to seizures, history of seizures or head trauma; when using as a conditioning regimen for transplant, initiate prophylactic anticonvulsant therapy (eg, phenytoin) prior to treatment. Phenytoin increases busulfan clearance by ≥15%; busulfan kinetics and dosing recommendations for high-dose HSCT conditioning were studied with concomitant phenytoin. If alternate anticonvulsants are used, busulfan clearance may be decreased and dosing should be monitored accordingly.

Bronchopulmonary dysplasia with pulmonary fibrosis ("busulfan lung") is associated with busulfan; onset is delayed with symptoms occurring at an average of 4 years (range: 4 months to 10 years) after treatment; may be fatal. Symptoms generally include a slow onset of cough, dyspnea, and fever (low-grade), although acute symptomatic onset may also occur. Diminished diffusion capacity and decreased pulmonary compliance have been noted with pulmonary function testing. Differential diagnosis should rule out opportunistic pulmonary infection or leukemic pulmonary infiltrates; may require lung biopsy. Discontinue busulfan if toxicity develops. Pulmonary toxicity may be additive if administered with other cytotoxic agents also associated with pulmonary toxicity. Cardiac tamponade as been reported in children with thalassemia treated with high-dose oral busulfan in combination with cyclophosphamide. Busulfan has been causally related to the development of secondary malignancies (tumors and acute leukemias); chromosomal alterations may also occur. Busulfan has been associated with ovarian failure (including failure to achieve puberty).

High busulfan area under the concentration versus time curve (AUC) values (>1500 micromolar•minute) are associated with increased risk of hepatic sinusoidal obstruction syndrome (SOS; formerly called veno-occlusive disease [VOD]) due to conditioning for allogenic HSCT; patients with a history of radiation therapy, prior chemotherapy (≥3 cycles), or prior stem cell transplantation are at increased risk; monitor liver function tests periodically. Oral busulfan doses above 16 mg/kg (based on IBW) and concurrent use with alkylating agents may also increase the risk for hepatic SOS. The solvent in I.V. busulfan, DMA, may impair fertility. DMA may also be associated with hepatotoxicity, hallucinations, somnolence, lethargy, and confusion. **[U.S. Boxed Warning]: Should be administered under the supervision of an experienced cancer chemotherapy physician; for the I.V. formulation, should be experienced in management of HSCT and management of patients with severe pancytopenia; according to the manufacturer, oral busulfan should not be used until CML diagnosis has been established.** Cellular dysplasia in many organs has been observed (in addition to lung dysplasia); giant hyperchromatic nuclei have been noted in adrenal glands, liver, lymph nodes, pancreas, thyroid, and bone marrow. May obscure routine diagnostic cytologic exams (eg, cervical smear).

Adverse Reactions

I.V.:

>10%:

Cardiovascular: Tachycardia (44%), hypertension (36%; grades 3/4: 7%), edema (28% to 79%), thrombosis (33%), chest pain (26%), vasodilation (25%), hypotension (11%; grades 3/4: 3%)

Central nervous system: Insomnia (84%), fever (80%), anxiety (72% to 75%), headache (69%), chills (46%), pain (44%), dizziness (30%), depression (23%), confusion (11%)
Dermatologic: Rash (57%), pruritus (28%), alopecia (17%)
Endocrine & metabolic: Hypomagnesemia (77%), hyperglycemia (66% to 67%; grades 3/4: 15%), hypokalemia (64%), hypocalcemia (49%), hypophosphatemia (17%)
Gastrointestinal: Vomiting (43% to 100%), nausea (83% to 98%), mucositis/stomatitis (79% to 97%, grades 3/4: 26%), anorexia (85%), diarrhea (84%; grades 3/4: 5%), abdominal pain (72%), dyspepsia (44%), constipation (38%), xerostomia (26%), rectal disorder (25%), abdominal fullness (23%)
Hematologic: Myelosuppression (≤100%), neutropenia (100%; onset: 4 days; median recovery: 13 days [with G-CSF support]), thrombocytopenia (98%; median onset: 5-6 days), lymphopenia (children: 79%), anemia (69%)
Hepatic: Hyperbilirubinemia (49%; grades 3/4: 30%), ALT increased (31%; grades 3/4: 7%), hepatic sinusoidal obstruction syndrome (SOS; veno-occlusive disease) (adults: 8% to 12%; children: 21%), alkaline phosphatase increased (15%), jaundice (12%)
Local: Injection site inflammation (25%), injection site pain (15%)
Neuromuscular & skeletal: Weakness (51%), back pain (23%), myalgia (16%), arthralgia (13%)
Renal: Creatinine increased (21%), oliguria (15%)
Respiratory: Rhinitis (44%), lung disorder (34%), cough (28%), epistaxis (25%), dyspnea (25%), pneumonia (children: 21%), hiccup (18%), pharyngitis (18%)
Miscellaneous: Infection (51%; includes severe bacterial, viral [CMV], and fungal infections), allergic reaction (26%)

1% to 10%:
Cardiovascular: Arrhythmia (5%), cardiomegaly (5%), atrial fibrillation (2%), ECG abnormal (2%), heart block (2%), heart failure (grade 3/4: 2%), pericardial effusion (2%), tamponade (children with thalassemia: 2%), ventricular extrasystoles (2%), hypervolemia
Central nervous system: Lethargy (7%), hallucination (5%), agitation (2%), delirium (2%), encephalopathy (2%), seizure (2%), somnolence (2%), cerebral hemorrhage (1%)
Dermatologic: Vesicular rash (10%), vesiculobullous rash (10%), skin discoloration (8%), maculopapular rash (8%), acne (7%), exfoliative dermatitis (5%), erythema nodosum (2%)
Endocrine & metabolic: Hyponatremia (2%)
Gastrointestinal: Ileus (8%), weight gain (8%), esophagitis (grade 3: 2%), hematemesis (2%), pancreatitis (2%)
Hematologic: Prothrombin time increased (2%)
Hepatic: Hepatomegaly (6%)
Renal: Hematuria (8%), dysuria (7%), hemorrhagic cystitis (grade 3/4: 7%), BUN increased (3%; grades 3/4: 2%)
Respiratory: Asthma (8%), alveolar hemorrhage (5%), hyperventilation (5%), hemoptysis (3%), pleural effusion (3%), sinusitis (3%), atelectasis (2%), hypoxia (2%)

Oral: Frequency not defined:
Dermatologic: Hyperpigmentation of skin (5% to 10%), rash
Endocrine & metabolic: Amenorrhea, ovarian suppression
Gastrointestinal: Xerostomia
Hematologic: Myelosuppression (anemia, leukopenia, thrombocytopenia)

I.V. and/or Oral: Infrequent, postmarketing, and/or case reports: Acute leukemias, adrenal insufficiency, alopecia (permanent), aplastic anemia (may be irreversible), azoospermia, bronchopulmonary dysplasia, capillary leak syndrome, cataracts (rare), cheilosis, cholestatic jaundice, corneal thinning, dry skin, endocardial fibrosis, erythema multiforme, esophageal varices, gynecomastia, hepatic dysfunction, hepatocellular atrophy, hyperuricemia, hyperuricosuria, interstitial pulmonary fibrosis, malignant tumors, myasthenia gravis, neutropenic fever, ocular (lens) changes, ovarian failure, pancytopenia, porphyria cutanea tarda, pulmonary fibrosis, radiation myelopathy, radiation recall (skin rash), sepsis, sterility, testicular atrophy, thrombotic microangiopathy (TMA), tumor lysis syndrome, urticaria

Drug Interactions

Metabolism/Transport Effects Substrate of CYP3A4 (major); **Note:** Assignment of Major/Minor substrate status based on clinically relevant drug interaction potential

Avoid Concomitant Use

Avoid concomitant use of Busulfan with any of the following: BCG; CloZAPine; Conivaptan; Natalizumab; Pimecrolimus; Tacrolimus (Topical); Vaccines (Live)

Increased Effect/Toxicity

Busulfan may increase the levels/effects of: CloZAPine; Ifosfamide; Leflunomide; Natalizumab; Vaccines (Live); Vitamin K Antagonists

The levels/effects of Busulfan may be increased by: Acetaminophen; Antifungal Agents (Azole Derivatives, Systemic); Conivaptan; CYP3A4 Inhibitors (Moderate); CYP3A4 Inhibitors (Strong); Dasatinib; Denosumab; Ivacaftor; MetroNIDAZOLE (Systemic); Mifepristone; Pimecrolimus; Roflumilast; Tacrolimus (Topical); Trastuzumab

Decreased Effect

Busulfan may decrease the levels/effects of: BCG; Coccidioidin Skin Test; Sipuleucel-T; Vaccines (Inactivated); Vaccines (Live); Vitamin K Antagonists

The levels/effects of Busulfan may be decreased by: CYP3A4 Inducers (Strong); Deferasirox; Echinacea; Fosphenytoin; Herbs (CYP3A4 Inducers); Phenytoin; Tocilizumab

Ethanol/Nutrition/Herb Interactions

Ethanol: Avoid ethanol due to GI irritation.

Food: No clear or firm data on the effect of food on busulfan bioavailability.

Herb/Nutraceutical: Avoid St John's wort (may decrease busulfan levels).

Storage/Stability

Injection: Store intact vials under refrigeration at 2°C to 8°C (36°F to 46°F). Solutions diluted in sodium chloride (NS) injection or dextrose 5% in water (D_5W) for infusion are stable for up to 8 hours at room temperature (25°C [77°F]); the infusion must also be completed within that 8-hour timeframe. Dilution of busulfan injection in NS is stable for up to 12 hours at refrigeration (2°C to 8°C); the infusion must be completed within that 12-hour timeframe.

Tablet: Store at 25°C (77°F); excursions permitted to 15°C to 30°C (59°F to 86°F).

Reconstitution Injection: Dilute NS or D_5W. The dilution volume should be 10 times the volume of busulfan injection, ensuring that the final concentration of busulfan is 0.5 mg/mL. Always add busulfan to the diluent, and not the diluent to the busulfan. Mix with several inversions. Do not use polycarbonate syringes or filters for preparation or administration.

Mechanism of Action Busulfan is an alkylating agent which reacts with the N-7 position of guanosine and interferes with DNA replication and transcription of RNA. Busulfan has a more marked effect on myeloid cells than on lymphoid cells and is also very toxic to hematopoietic stem cells. Busulfan exhibits little immunosuppressive activity. Interferes with the normal function of DNA by alkylation and cross-linking the strands of DNA.

Pharmacodynamics/Kinetics

Absorption: Rapid and complete

Distribution: V_d: ~1 L/kg; distributes into CSF with levels equal to plasma

Protein binding: 32% to plasma proteins and 47% to red blood cells

Metabolism: Extensively hepatic (may increase with multiple doses); glutathione conjugation followed by oxidation

Bioavailability: Oral: Children ≥13 years and adults: 80% ± 20%; Children 1.5-6 years: 68% ± 31%

Half-life elimination: 2-3 hours

Time to peak, serum: Oral: ~1 hour; I.V.: Within 5 minutes

Excretion: Urine (25% to 60% predominantly as metabolites; <2% as unchanged drug)

Dosing

Adult Note: Premedicate with prophylactic anticonvulsant therapy (eg, phenytoin) prior to high-dose busulfan treatment. Prophylactic antiemetics may be necessary for high-dose (HSCT) regimens.

Chronic myelogenous leukemia (CML), palliation (manufacturer's labeling): *Oral:*

Remission induction: 60 mcg/kg/day or 1.8 mg/m²/day; usual range: 4-8 mg/day; titrate dose (or withhold) to maintain leukocyte counts ≥15,000/mm³ (doses >4 mg/day should be reserved for patients with the most compelling symptoms)

Maintenance: When leukocyte count ≥50,000/mm³: Resume induction dose **or** (if remission <3 months) 1-3 mg/day (to control hematologic status and prevent relapse)

Hematopoietic stem cell (HSCT) conditioning regimen:

I.V.:

0.8 mg/kg every 6 hours for 4 days (a total of 16 doses); **Note:** Use ideal body weight or actual body weight, (whichever is lower) for dosing. For obese or severely-obese patients, use of an adjusted body weight [IBW + 0.25 x (actual – IBW)] is recommended.

Reduced intensity conditioning regimen (unlabeled dosing): 0.8 mg/kg/day for 4 days starting 6 days prior to transplant (in combinations with fludarabine) (Ho, 2009)

Oral (unlabeled use): 1 mg/kg/dose every 6 hours for 16 doses (in combination with cyclophosphamide) (Socié, 2001) **or** 1 mg/kg/dose every 6 hours for 16 doses beginning 9 days prior to transplant (in combination with cyclophosphamide) (Cassileth, 1993) **or** 0.44 mg/kg/dose every 6 hours for 16 doses (in combination with cyclophosphamide) (Anderson, 1996) **or** 1 mg/kg/dose every 6 hours for 16 doses beginning 6 days prior to transplant (in combination with melphalan) (Fermand, 2005)

Polycythemia vera and essential thrombocythemia (unlabeled uses): Oral: 2-4 mg/day (Fabris, 2009; Tefferi, 2011)

Geriatric Oral (refer to individual protocols): Start with lowest recommended doses for adults.

Pediatric Note: Premedicate with prophylactic anticonvulsant therapy (eg, phenytoin) prior to high-dose busulfan treatment. Prophylactic antiemetics may be necessary for high-dose (HSCT) regimens.

Chronic myelogenous leukemia (CML), palliation (manufacturer's labeling): *Oral:*

Remission induction: 60 mcg/kg/day or 1.8 mg/m²/day; titrate dose (or withhold) to maintain leukocyte counts ≥15,000/mm³ (doses >4 mg/day should be reserved for patients with the most compelling symptoms)

Maintenance: When leukocyte count ≥50,000/mm³: Resume induction dose **or** (if remission <3 months) 1-3 mg/day (to control hematologic status and prevent relapse)

Hematopoietic stem cell transplant (HSCT) conditioning regimen:

I.V.:

≤12 kg: 1.1 mg/kg/dose (actual body weight) every 6 hours for 16 doses

>12 kg: 0.8 mg/kg/dose (actual body weight) every 6 hours for 16 doses

Adjust dose to desired AUC (1125 micromolar•minute) using the following formula:

Adjusted dose (mg) = Actual dose (mg) x [target AUC (micromolar•minute) / actual AUC (micromolar •minute)]

Reduced intensity conditioning regimen (unlabeled dosing): 0.8 mg/kg/dose for 1 dose 7-10 days prior to transplant, followed by ~0.8 mg/kg/dose (busulfan kinetics calculated after initial dose) every 6 hours for 7 doses beginning 3-6 days prior to transplant (in combination with fludarabine and antithymocyte globulin) (Pulsipher, 2009)

Oral (unlabeled use): 1 mg/kg/dose every 6 hours for 16 doses beginning 9 days prior to transplant (in combination with cyclophosphamide) (Cassileth, 1998)

Renal Impairment

I.V.: No dosage adjustment provided in the manufacturer's labeling (has not been studied).

Oral: No dosage adjustment provided in the manufacturer's labeling (elimination appears to be independent of renal function); however, some clinicians suggest adjustment is not necessary (Aronoff, 2007).

Hepatic Impairment

I.V.: No dosage adjustment provided in the manufacturer's labeling (has not been studied).

Oral: No dosage adjustment provided in the manufacturer's labeling.

Administration Intravenous busulfan should be infused over 2 hours via central line. Flush line before and after each infusion with 5 mL D_5W or NS. Do not use polycarbonate syringes or filters for preparation or administration

HSCT only: To facilitate ingestion of high oral doses, may insert multiple tablets into gelatin capsules.

Emetic Potential

Oral ≥4 mg/day and I.V.: Moderate (30% to 90%)

Oral <4 mg/day: Very low (<10%)

Vesicant/Extravasation Risk May be an irritant

Extemporaneous Preparations Hazardous agent: Use appropriate precautions for handling and disposal.

A 2 mg/mL oral suspension can be prepared in a vertical flow hood with tablets and simple syrup. Crush one-hundred-twenty 2 mg tablets in a mortar and reduce to a fine powder. Add small portions of simple syrup and mix to a uniform paste; mix while adding the simple syrup in incremental proportions to

almost 120 mL; transfer to a graduated cylinder, rinse mortar and pestle with simple syrup, and add quantity of vehicle sufficient to make 120 mL. Transfer contents of the graduated cylinder into an amber prescription bottle. Label "shake well", "refrigerate", and "caution chemotherapy". Stable for 30 days.

Allen LV, "Busulfan Oral Suspension," *US Pharm*, 1990, 15:94-5.

Monitoring Parameters CBC with differential and platelet count (weekly for palliative treatment; daily until engraftment for HSCT); liver function tests (evaluate transaminases, alkaline phosphatase, and bilirubin daily for at least 20 days post transplant). If conducting therapeutic drug monitoring for AUC calculations in HSCT, monitor blood samples at appropriate collections times (record collection times).

Dosage Forms Excipient information presented when available (limited, particularly for generics); consult specific product labeling.

Injection, solution:

Busulfex®: 6 mg/mL (10 mL) [contains N,N-dimethylacetamide (DMA), polyethylene glycol 400]

Tablet, oral:

Myleran®: 2 mg [scored]

References

Anderson JE, Appelbaum FR, Schoch G, et al, "Allogeneic Marrow Transplantation for Myelodysplastic Syndrome With Advanced Disease Morphology: A Phase II Study of Busulfan, Cyclophosphamide, and Total Body-Irradiation and Analysis of Prognostic Factors," *J Clin Oncol*, 1996, 14(1):220-6.

Aronoff GR, Bennett WM, Berns JS, et al, *Drug Prescribing in Renal Failure: Dosing Guidelines for Adults and Children*, 5th ed. Philadelphia, PA: American College of Physicians; 2007, p 97, 169.

Booth BP, Rahman A, Dagher R, et al, "Population Pharmacokinetic-Based Dosing of Intravenous Busulfan in Pediatric Patients," *J Clin Pharmacol*, 2007, 47(1):101-11.

Cassileth PA, Andersen J, Lazarus HM, et al, "Autologous Bone Marrow Transplant in Acute Myeloid Leukemia in First Remission," *J Clin Oncol*, 1993, 11(2):314-9.

Cassileth PA, Harrington DP, Appelbaum FR, et al, "Chemotherapy Compared With Autologous or Allogeneic Bone Marrow Transplantation in the Management of Acute Myeloid Leukemia in First Remission," *N Engl J Med*, 1998, 339(23):1649-56.

Fabris F and Randi ML, "Essential Thrombocythemia: Past and Present," *Intern Emerg Med*, 2009, 4(5):381-8.

Fermand JP, Katsahian S, Divine M, et al, "High-Dose Therapy and Autologous Blood Stem-Cell Transplantation Compared With Conventional Treatment in Myeloma Patients Aged 55 to 65 years: Long-Term Results of a Randomized Control Trial From the Group Myelome-Autogreffe," *J Clin Oncol*, 2005, 23(36):9227-33.

Ho VT, Aldridge J, Kim HT, et al, Comparison of Tacrolimus and Sirolimus (Tac/Sir) Versus Tacrolimus, Sirolimus, and Mini-Methotrexate (Tac/Sir/MTX) as Acute Graft-Versus-Host Disease Prophylaxis After Reduced-Intensity Conditioning Allogeneic Peripheral Blood Stem Cell Transplantation," *Biol Blood Marrow Transplant*, 2009, 15(7):844-50.

Pulsipher MA, Boucher KM, Wall D, et al, "Reduced-Intensity Allogeneic Transplantation in Pediatric Patients Ineligible for Myeloablative Therapy: Results of the Pediatric Blood and Marrow Transplant Consortium Study ONC0313," *Blood*, 2009, 114(7):1429-36.

Radich JP, Gooley T, Bensinger W, et al, "HLA-Matched Related Hematopoietic Cell Transplantation for Chronic-Phase CML Using a Targeted Busulfan and Cyclophosphamide Preparative Regimen," *Blood*, 2003, 102(1):31-5.

Regazzi MB, Locatelli F, Buggia I, et al, "Disposition of High-Dose Busulfan in Pediatric Patients Undergoing Bone Marrow Transplantation," *Clin Pharmacol Ther*, 1993, 54(1):45-52.

Shaw PJ, Nath C, Berry A, et al, "Busulphan Given as Four Single Daily Doses of 150 mg/m^2 Is Safe and Effective in Children of All Ages," *Bone Marrow Transplant*, 2004, 34(3):197-205.

Socié G, Clift RA, Blaise D, et al, "Busulfan Plus Cyclophosphamide Compared With Total-Body Irradiation Plus Cyclophosphamide Before Marrow Transplantation for Myeloid Leukemia: Long-Term Follow-Up of 4 Randomized Studies," *Blood*, 2001, 98(13):3569-74.

Tefferi A, "Annual Clinical Updates in Hematological Malignancies: A Continuing Medical Education Series: Polycythemia Vera and Essential Thrombocythemia: 2011 Update on Diagnosis, Risk-Stratification, and Management," *Am J Hematol*, 2011, 86(3):292-301.

◆ **Busulfanum** *see* Busulfan *on page 203*

◆ **Busulfex®** *see* Busulfan *on page 203*

◆ **Busulphan** *see* Busulfan *on page* 203
◆ **C2B8 Monoclonal Antibody** *see* RiTUXimab *on page* 1244
◆ **2C4 Antibody** *see* Pertuzumab *on page* 1165
◆ **C225** *see* Cetuximab *on page* 264

Cabazitaxel (ca baz i TAKS el)

Related Information

Management of Chemotherapy-Induced Nausea and Vomiting *on page* 1786

Brand Names: U.S. Jevtana®

Brand Names: Canada Jevtana®

Index Terms RPR-116258A; XRP6258

Generic Availability (U.S.) No

Pharmacologic Category Antineoplastic Agent, Antimicrotubular; Antineoplastic Agent, Taxane Derivative

Use Treatment of hormone-refractory metastatic prostate cancer (in patients previously treated with a docetaxel-containing regimen)

Labeled Contraindications Hypersensitivity to cabazitaxel, polysorbate 80, or any component of the formulation; neutrophil count ≤1500/mm^3

Pregnancy Risk Factor D

Lactation Excretion in breast milk unknown/not recommended

Warnings/Precautions Hazardous agent - use appropriate precautions for handling and disposal. **[U.S. Boxed Warning]: Severe hypersensitivity reactions, including generalized rash, erythema, hypotension, and bronchospasm may occur; may require immediate discontinuation if hypersensitivity is severe. Premedicate with an I.V. antihistamine, corticosteroid and H2 antagonist prior to infusion. Use in patients with history of severe hypersensitivity to cabazitaxel or polysorbate 80 is contraindicated.** Observe closely during infusion, especially during the first and second infusions; reaction may occur within minutes. Do not rechallenge after severe hypersensitivity reactions.

[U.S. Boxed Warning]: Deaths due to neutropenia have been reported. Do not administer in patients with neutrophil count ≤1500/mm_3; monitor blood counts frequently. Dose reductions are recommended following neutropenic fever or prolonged neutropenia. Administration of WBC growth factors may reduce the risk of complications due to neutropenia; consider primary WBC growth factor prophylaxis in high-risk patients (eg, >65 years of age, poor performance status, history of neutropenic fever, extensive prior radiation, poor nutrition status, or other serious comorbidities); secondary prophylaxis and therapeutic WBC growth factors should be considered in all patients with increased risk for neutropenic complications. Patients ≥65 years of age are more likely to experience certain adverse reactions, including neutropenia and neutropenic fever.

Use is not recommended in patients with hepatic impairment (total bilirubin ≥ULN or AST and/or ALT ≥1.5 times ULN). Due to extensive hepatic metabolism, cabazitaxel exposure is increased in patients with hepatic impairment. Renal failure has been reported from clinical trials; generally associated with dehydration, sepsis, or obstructive uropathy; use with caution in patients with severe renal impairment (Cl_{cr} <30 mL/minute) and end-stage renal disease. Nausea, vomiting and diarrhea may occur. Diarrhea may be severe and may result in dehydration and electrolyte imbalance. Antiemetics, antidiarrhea medication, and fluid and electrolyte replacement may be necessary. Diarrhea ≥ grade 3 may require treatment delay and or dosage reduction.

Avoid concomitant use of strong CYP3A4 inducers or inhibitors; use with moderate CYP3A4 inhibitors with caution. Strong CYP3A4 inducers (eg, carbamazepine, phenobarbital, phenytoin, rifabutin rifampin, rifapentine) may decrease the levels/effects of cabazitaxel. Strong CYP3A4 inhibitors (eg, atazanavir, clarithromycin, indinavir, itraconazole, ketoconazole, nefazodone, nelfinavir, ritonavir, saquinavir, telithromycin, voriconazole) may increase the levels/effects of cabazitaxel.

Adverse Reactions **Note:** Adverse reactions reported for combination therapy with prednisone.

>10%:

Central nervous system: Fatigue (37%), fever (12%)

Gastrointestinal: Diarrhea (47%; grades 3/4: 6%), nausea (34%), vomiting (22%), constipation (20%), abdominal pain (17%), anorexia (16%), taste alteration (11%)

Hematologic: Anemia (98%; grades 3/4: 11%), leukopenia (96%; grades 3/4: 69%), neutropenia (94%; grades 3/4: 82%; nadir: 12 days [range: 4-17 days]), thrombocytopenia (48%; grades 3/4: 4%)

Neuromuscular & skeletal: Weakness (20%), back pain (16%), peripheral neuropathy (13%; grades 3/4: <1%), arthralgia (11%)

Renal: Hematuria (17%)

Respiratory: Dyspnea (12%), cough (11%)

1% to 10%:

Cardiovascular: Peripheral edema (9%), arrhythmia (5%), hypotension (5%)

Central nervous system: Dizziness (8%), headache (8%), pain (5%)

Dermatologic: Alopecia (10%)

Endocrine & metabolic: Dehydration (5%)

Gastrointestinal: Dyspepsia (10%), weight loss (9%), mucosal inflammation (6%)

Genitourinary: Urinary tract infection (8%), dysuria (7%)

Hematologic: Neutropenic fever (grades 3/4: 7%)

Hepatic: ALT increased (grades 3/4: ≤1%), AST increased (grades 3/4: ≤1%), bilirubin increased (grades 3/4: ≤1%)

Neuromuscular & skeletal: Muscle spasm (7%)

<1%, postmarketing, and/or case reports: Hypersensitivity (eg, rash, erythema, hypotension, bronchospasm), electrolyte imbalance, renal failure, sepsis, septic shock

Drug Interactions

Metabolism/Transport Effects **Substrate** of CYP2C8 (minor), CYP3A4 (major); **Note:** Assignment of Major/Minor substrate status based on clinically relevant drug interaction potential

Avoid Concomitant Use

Avoid concomitant use of Cabazitaxel with any of the following: BCG; CloZAPine; Conivaptan; Natalizumab; Pimecrolimus; Tacrolimus (Topical); Vaccines (Live)

Increased Effect/Toxicity

Cabazitaxel may increase the levels/effects of: Antineoplastic Agents (Anthracycline, Systemic); CloZAPine; DOXOrubicin; Leflunomide; Natalizumab; Vaccines (Live); Vitamin K Antagonists

The levels/effects of Cabazitaxel may be increased by: Conivaptan; CYP3A4 Inhibitors (Moderate); CYP3A4 Inhibitors (Strong); Dasatinib; Denosumab; Ivacaftor; Mifepristone; Pimecrolimus; Platinum Derivatives; Roflumilast; Tacrolimus (Topical); Trastuzumab

Decreased Effect

Cabazitaxel may decrease the levels/effects of: BCG; Cardiac Glycosides; Coccidioidin Skin Test; Sipuleucel-T; Vaccines (Inactivated); Vaccines (Live); Vitamin K Antagonists

The levels/effects of Cabazitaxel may be decreased by: CYP3A4 Inducers (Strong); Deferasirox; Echinacea; Herbs (CYP3A4 Inducers); Tocilizumab

Ethanol/Nutrition/Herb Interactions

Food: Avoid grapefruit juice (may increase the levels/effects of cabazitaxel).

Herb/Nutraceutical: Avoid St John's wort (may increase metabolism and decrease cabazitaxel concentrations).

Storage/Stability Store intact vials at 25°C (77°F); excursions permitted between 15°C and 30°C (59°F and 86°F). Do not refrigerate. Do not prepare in PVC-containing infusion containers. Initial reconstituted solution (at 10 mg/mL) is stable for 30 minutes in the vial. Solutions for infusion are stable for 8 hours at room temperature or 24 hours refrigerated. Infusion should be completed within 8 hours if stored at room temperature or 24 hours if refrigerated.

Reconstitution Use appropriate precautions for handling and disposal. Do not prepare in PVC-containing infusion containers. Cabazitaxel and diluent vials contain overfill. Preparation requires 2 steps. Slowly inject the entire contents of the provided diluent into the 60 mg/1.5 mL cabazitaxel vial, directing the diluent down the vial wall. Mix gently by inverting the vial for at least 45 seconds; do not shake. Allow vial to sit so that foam dissipates and solution appears homogeneous. This results in an intermediate reconstituted concentration of 10 mg/mL. Further dilute (within 30 minutes) into a 250 mL D_5W or NS non-PVC infusion container to final concentration of 0.1-0.26 mg/mL (total doses >65 mg will require a larger infusion volume; final concentration should not exceed 0.26 mg/mL). Gently invert to mix. Do not use infusion solutions if crystals or precipitate appear; discard.

Mechanism of Action Cabazitaxel is a taxane derivative which is a microtubule inhibitor; it binds to tubulin promoting assembly into microtubules and inhibiting disassembly which stabilizes microtubules. This inhibits microtubule depolymerization and cell division, arresting the cell cycle and inhibiting tumor proliferation. Unlike other taxanes, cabazitaxel has a poor affinity for multidrug resistance (MDR) proteins, therefore conferring activity in resistant tumors.

Pharmacodynamics/Kinetics

Distribution: V_{dss}: 4864 L; has greater CNS penetration than other taxanes

Protein binding: 89% to 92%; primarily to serum albumin and lipoproteins

Metabolism: Extensively hepatic; primarily via CYP3A4 and 3A5; also via CYP2C8 (minor)

Half-life elimination: Terminal: 95 hours

Excretion: Feces (76% as metabolites); Urine (~4%)

Dosing

Adult Note: Premedicate at least 30 minutes prior to each dose of cabazitaxel with an antihistamine (eg, diphenhydramine I.V. 25 mg or equivalent), a corticosteroid (eg, dexamethasone 8 mg I.V. or equivalent), and an H_2 antagonist (eg, ranitidine 50 mg I.V. or equivalent). Antiemetic prophylaxis is also recommended. Details concerning dosing in combination regimens should also be consulted.

Prostate cancer: I.V.: 25 mg/m^2/dose once every 3 weeks (in combination with prednisone)

Renal Impairment Severe renal impairment (Cl_{cr} <30 mL/minute) or end-stage renal disease: Use with caution.

Hepatic Impairment Hepatic impairment (total bilirubin ≥ULN or AST and/or ALT ≥1.5 times ULN): Use is not recommended.

Adjustment for Toxicity

Hematologic toxicity:

Neutropenia ≥ grade 3 for > 1 week despite WBC growth factors: Delay treatment until ANC >1500/mm^3 and then reduce dose to 20 mg/m^2 with continued WBC growth factor secondary prophylaxis.

Neutropenic fever: Delay treatment until improvement/resolution and ANC >1500/mm^3 and then reduce dose to 20 mg/m^2 with continued WBC growth factor secondary prophylaxis.

Persistent hematologic toxicity (despite dosage reduction): Discontinue treatment.

Nonhematologic toxicity:

Severe hypersensitivity: Discontinue immediately.

Diarrhea ≥grade 3 or persistent despite appropriate medication, fluids, and electrolyte replacement: Delay treatment until improves or resolves and then reduce dose to 20 mg/m^2.

Persistent diarrhea (despite dosage reduction): Discontinue treatment.

Combination Regimens

Prostate cancer: Cabazitaxel-Prednisone (Prostate Cancer) on page 1538

Administration I.V.: Infuse over 1 hour using a 0.22 micron inline filter. Do not use polyurethane-containing infusion sets for administration. Allow to reach room temperature prior to infusion. Premedicate with an antihistamine, a corticosteroid, and an H_2 antagonist at least 30 minutes prior to infusion. Observe closely during infusion (for hypersensitivity). Antiemetic prophylaxis (oral or I.V.) is also recommended.

Emetic Potential Low (10% to 30%)

Monitoring Parameters CBC with differential and platelets (weekly during first cycle, then prior to each treatment cycle); monitor for hypersensitivity

Dietary Considerations Avoid grapefruit juice.

Dosage Forms Excipient information presented when available (limited, particularly for generics); consult specific product labeling.

Injection, solution:

Jevtana®: 40 mg/mL (1.5 mL) [contains ethanol 13% (in diluent), polysorbate 80; supplied with diluent]

References

De Bono JS, Oudard S, Ozguroglu M, et al, "Cabazitaxel or Mitoxantrone With Prednisone in Patients With Metastatic Castration-Resistant Prostate Cancer (mCRPC) Previously Treated With Docetaxel: Final Results of a Multinational Phase III Trial (TROPIC)," *J Clin Oncol*, 2010, 28 (7s):4508 [abstract 4508 from 2010 ASCO Annual Meeting]

Mita AC, Denis LJ, Rowinsky Ek, et al, "Phase I and Pharmacokinetic Study of XRP6258 (RPR 116258A), a Novel Taxane, Administered as a 1-Hour Infusion Every 3 Weeks in Patients With Advanced Solid Tumors, *Clin Cancer Res*, 2009, 15(2):723-30.

Sartor AO, Oudard S, Ozguroglu M, et al, "Cabazitaxel or Mitoxantrone With Prednisone in Patients With Metastatic Castration-Resistant Prostate Cancer (mCRPC) Previously Treated With Docetaxel: Final Results of a Multinational Phase III Trial (TROPIC)," 2010:9 [abstract 9 from 2010 ASCO Genitourinary Cancers Symposium].

◆ **Caelyx® (Can)** *see* DOXOrubicin (Liposomal) *on page* 473

◆ **CAFdA** *see* Clofarabine *on page* 306

◆ **Calcijex®** *see* Calcitriol *on page* 215

◆ **Calcimar® (Can)** *see* Calcitonin *on page* 214

Calcitonin (kal si TOE nin)

Brand Names: U.S. Fortical®; Miacalcin®

Brand Names: Canada Apo-Calcitonin®; Calcimar®; Caltine®; Miacalcin® NS; PRO-Calcitonin; Sandoz-Calcitonin

Index Terms Calcitonin (Salmon)

Generic Availability (U.S.) Yes: Intranasal solution

Pharmacologic Category Antidote; Hormone

Use Treatment of Paget's disease of bone (osteitis deformans); adjunctive therapy for hypercalcemia; treatment of osteoporosis in women >5 years postmenopause

Labeled Contraindications Hypersensitivity to calcitonin salmon or any component of the formulation

Pregnancy Risk Factor C

Lactation Excretion in breast milk unknown/not recommended

Warnings/Precautions A skin test should be performed prior to initiating therapy of calcitonin salmon in patients with suspected sensitivity; have epinephrine immediately available for a possible hypersensitivity reaction. A detailed skin testing protocol is available from the manufacturers. Temporarily withdraw use of nasal spray if ulceration of nasal mucosa occurs. Discontinue for ulcerations >1.5 mm or those that penetrate below the mucosa. Patients >65 years of age may experience a higher incidence of nasal adverse events with calcitonin nasal spray.

Ethanol/Nutrition/Herb Interactions Ethanol: Avoid ethanol (may increase risk of osteoporosis).

Storage/Stability

Injection: Store under refrigeration at 2°C to 8°C (36°F to 46°F); protect from freezing. The following stability information has also been reported: May be stored at room temperature for up to 14 days (Cohen, 2007).

Nasal: Store unopened bottle under refrigeration at 2°C to 8°C (36°F to 46°F); do not freeze.

Fortical®: After opening, store for up to 30 days at 20°C to 25°C (68°F to 77°F); excursions permitted to 15°C to 30°C (59°F to 86°F). Store in upright position.

Miacalcin®: After opening, store for up to 35 days at room temperature of 15°C to 30°C (59°F to 86°F). Store in upright position.

Reconstitution Injection: NS has been recommended for the dilution to prepare a skin test in patients with suspected sensitivity.

Mechanism of Action Peptide sequence similar to human calcitonin; functionally antagonizes the effects of parathyroid hormone. Directly inhibits osteoclastic bone resorption; promotes the renal excretion of calcium, phosphate, sodium, magnesium, and potassium by decreasing tubular reabsorption; increases the jejunal secretion of water, sodium, potassium, and chloride

Pharmacodynamics/Kinetics

Onset of action:

Hypercalcemia: I.M., SubQ: ~2 hours

Paget's disease: Within a few months; may take up to 1 year for neurologic symptom improvement

Duration: Hypercalcemia: I.M., SubQ: 6-8 hours

Distribution: V_d: 0.15-0.3 L/kg

Metabolism: Metabolized in kidneys, blood and peripheral tissue

Bioavailability: I.M.: 66%; SubQ: 71%; Nasal: ~3% to 5% (relative to I.M.)

Half-life elimination (terminal): I.M. 58 minutes; SubQ 59-64 minutes; Nasal: ~18 minutes

Time to peak, plasma: SubQ ~23 minutes; Nasal: ~13 minutes

Excretion: Urine (as inactive metabolites)

Dosing

Adult & Geriatric

Paget's disease *(Miacalcin®)*: I.M., SubQ: Initial: 100 units/day; maintenance: 50 units/day or 50-100 units every 1-3 days

Hypercalcemia *(Miacalcin®)*: Initial: I.M., SubQ: 4 units/kg every 12 hours; may increase up to 8 units/kg every 12 hours; if the response remains unsatisfactory, a further increase up to a maximum of 8 units/kg every 6 hours may be considered

Postmenopausal osteoporosis:

Miacalcin®: I.M., SubQ: 100 units/every other day

Fortical®, Miacalcin®: Intranasal: 200 units (1 spray) in one nostril daily

Administration

Injection solution: May be administered I.M. or SubQ. I.M route is preferred if the injection volume is >2 mL. SubQ route is preferred for outpatient self administration unless the injection volume is >2 mL.

Nasal spray: Before first use, allow bottle to reach room temperature, then prime pump by releasing at least 5 sprays until full spray is produced. To administer, place nozzle into nostril with head in upright position. Alternate nostrils daily. Do not prime pump before each daily use. Discard after 30 doses.

Dosage Forms Excipient information presented when available (limited, particularly for generics); consult specific product labeling.

Injection, solution [calcitonin-salmon]:

Miacalcin®: 200 units/mL (2 mL)

Solution, intranasal [calcitonin-salmon/rDNA origin/spray]:

Fortical®: 200 units/actuation (3.7 mL) [contains benzyl alcohol; delivers 30 doses]

Solution, intranasal [calcitonin-salmon/spray]: 200 units/actuation (3.7 mL)

Miacalcin®: 200 units/actuation (3.7 mL) [contains benzalkonium chloride; delivers 30 doses]

◆ **Calcitonin (Salmon)** *see* Calcitonin *on page* 214

Calcitriol (kal si TRYE ole)

Brand Names: U.S. Calcijex®; Rocaltrol®; Vectical®

Brand Names: Canada Calcijex®; Rocaltrol®; Silkis™

Index Terms 1,25 Dihydroxycholecalciferol

Generic Availability (U.S.) Yes: Excludes ointment

Pharmacologic Category Vitamin D Analog

Use

Management of hypocalcemia in patients on chronic renal dialysis (oral, injection); management of secondary hyperparathyroidism in patients with chronic kidney disease (CKD) (oral); management of hypocalcemia in patients with hypoparathyroidism and pseudohypoparathyroidism (oral); management of mild-to-moderate plaque psoriasis (topical)

Canadian labeling: Additional uses (not in U.S. labeling): Vitamin D-resistant rickets (oral)

Unlabeled Use Vitamin D-dependent rickets type I/pseudovitamin D deficiency rickets (PDDR)

Labeled Contraindications

U.S. labeling:

Oral, injection: Hypersensitivity to calcitriol or any component of the formulation; hypercalcemia, vitamin D toxicity

Topical: There are no contraindications listed in the manufacturer's labeling.

Canadian labeling:

Oral, injection: Hypersensitivity to calcitriol, vitamin D or its analogues or derivatives, or any component of the formulation or container; hypercalcemia, vitamin D toxicity

Topical: Ophthalmic or internal use; hypercalcemia or a history of abnormal calcium metabolism; concurrent systemic treatment of calcium homeostasis; severe renal impairment or end-stage renal disease (ESRD)

Pregnancy Risk Factor C

Lactation Enters breast milk/not recommended

Warnings/Precautions Oral, injection: Adequate dietary (supplemental) calcium is necessary for clinical response to vitamin D. Excessive vitamin D may cause severe hypercalcemia, hypercalciuria, and hyperphosphatemia. Discontinue use immediately in patients with a calcium-phosphate product (serum calcium times phosphorus) >70 mg^2/dL^2, may resume therapy at decreased doses when levels are appropriate. Other forms of vitamin D should be withheld during therapy to avoid the potential for hypercalcemia to develop. In addition, several months may be required for ergocalciferol levels to return to baseline in patients switching from ergocalciferol therapy to calcitriol. Monitor calcium levels closely with initiation of therapy and with dose adjustments; discontinue use promptly in patients who develop hypercalcemia. Avoid abrupt dietary modifications (eg, increased intake of dairy products) which may lead to hypercalcemia; adjust calcium intake if indicated and maintain adequate hydration. Chronic hypercalcemia can result in generalized vascular and soft tissue calcification. Immobilized patients may be at a higher risk for hypercalcemia.

Use oral calcitriol with caution in patients with malabsorption syndromes (efficacy may be limited and/or response may be unpredictable). Use of calcitriol for the treatment of secondary hyperparathyroidism associated with CKD is not recommended in patients with rapidly worsening kidney function or in noncompliant patients. Increased serum phosphate levels in patients with renal failure may lead to calcification; the use of an aluminum-containing phosphate binder is recommended along with a low phosphate diet in these patients. Use with caution in patients taking cardiac glycosides; digitalis toxicity is potentiated by hypocalcemia. Concomitant use with magnesium-containing products such as antacids may lead to hypermagnesemia in patients receiving chronic renal dialysis. Products may contain coconut (capsule) or palm seed oil (oral solution). Some products may contain tartrazine.

Topical: May cause hypercalcemia; if alterations in calcium occur, discontinue treatment until levels return to normal. For external use only; not for ophthalmic, oral, or intravaginal use. Do not apply to facial skin, eyes, or lips. Absorption may be increased with occlusive dressings. Avoid or limit excessive exposure to natural or artificial sunlight, or phototherapy. The safety and effectiveness has not been evaluated in patients with erythrodermic, exfoliative, or pustular psoriasis. Canadian labeling does not recommend use in patients with hepatic or renal impairment.

Adverse Reactions

Oral, I.V.: Frequency not defined.

Cardiovascular: Cardiac arrhythmia, hypertension

Central nervous system: Apathy, headache, hyperthermia, psychosis, sensory disturbances, somnolence

Dermatologic: Erythema multiforme, erythematous skin disorders, pruritus, rash, urticaria

Endocrine & metabolic: Dehydration, growth suppression, hypercalcemia, hypercholesterolemia, libido decreased, polydipsia

Gastrointestinal: Abdominal pain, anorexia, constipation, metallic taste, nausea, pancreatitis, stomach ache, vomiting, weight loss, xerostomia

Genitourinary: Nocturia, urinary tract infection

Hepatic: ALT increased, AST increased

Local: Injection site pain (mild)

Neuromuscular & skeletal: Bone pain, myalgia, dystrophy, soft tissue calcification, weakness

Ocular: Conjunctivitis, photophobia

Renal: Albuminuria, BUN increased, creatinine increased, hypercalciuria, nephrocalcinosis, polyuria

Respiratory: Rhinorrhea

Miscellaneous: Allergic reaction, hypersensitivity reactions

Postmarketing and/or case reports: Anaphylaxis

Topical:

>10%: Endocrine: Hypercalcemia (24%)

1% to 10%:

Dermatologic: Psoriasis (4%), skin discomfort (3%), pruritus (1% to 3%)

Genitourinary: Urine abnormality (4%)

Renal: Hypercalciuria (3%)

<1%, postmarketing, and/or case reports: Dermatitis (acute; blistering), erythema, kidney stones, skin burning

Drug Interactions

Metabolism/Transport Effects Substrate of CYP3A4 (major); **Note:** Assignment of Major/Minor substrate status based on clinically relevant drug interaction potential; **Induces** CYP3A4 (weak/moderate)

Avoid Concomitant Use

Avoid concomitant use of Calcitriol with any of the following: Aluminum Hydroxide; Axitinib; Conivaptan; Multivitamins/Minerals (with ADEK, Folate, Iron); Sucralfate; Vitamin D Analogs

Increased Effect/Toxicity

Calcitriol may increase the levels/effects of: Aluminum Hydroxide; Cardiac Glycosides; Magnesium Salts; Sucralfate; Vitamin D Analogs

The levels/effects of Calcitriol may be increased by: Calcium Salts; Conivaptan; CYP3A4 Inhibitors (Moderate); CYP3A4 Inhibitors (Strong);

Danazol; Dasatinib; Ivacaftor; Mifepristone; Multivitamins/Minerals (with ADEK, Folate, Iron); Thiazide Diuretics

Decreased Effect

Calcitriol may decrease the levels/effects of: ARIPiprazole; Axitinib; Saxagliptin

The levels/effects of Calcitriol may be decreased by: Bile Acid Sequestrants; Corticosteroids (Systemic); CYP3A4 Inducers (Strong); Deferasirox; Herbs (CYP3A4 Inducers); Mineral Oil; Orlistat; Sevelamer; Tocilizumab

Storage/Stability

Injection: Store at room temperature of 15°C to 30°C (59°F to 86°F). Protect from light.

Oral capsule, solution: Store at room temperature of 15°C to 30°C (59°F to 86°F). Protect from light.

Topical: Store at room temperature of 25°C (77°F); excursions permitted to 15°C to 30°C (59°F to 86°F); do not refrigerate; do not freeze.

Mechanism of Action Calcitriol is a potent active metabolite of vitamin D. Vitamin D promotes absorption of calcium in the intestines and retention at the kidneys thereby increasing calcium levels in the serum; decreases excessive serum phosphatase levels, parathyroid hormone levels, and decreases bone resorption; increases renal tubule phosphate resorption

The mechanism by which calcitriol is beneficial in the treatment of psoriasis has not been established.

Pharmacodynamics/Kinetics

Duration: Oral, I.V.: 3-5 days

Absorption: Oral: Rapid

Protein binding: 99.9%

Metabolism: Primarily to calcitroic acid and a lactone metabolite

Half-life elimination: Children ~27 hours; Healthy adults: 5-8 hours; Hemodialysis: 16-22 hours

Time to peak, serum: Oral: 3-6 hours; Hemodialysis: 8-12 hours

Excretion: Primarily feces; urine

Dosing

Adult

Hypocalcemia in patients on chronic renal dialysis:

Oral: Initial: 0.25 mcg daily; may increase dose by 0.25 mcg daily at 4- to 8-week intervals, up to 0.5-1 mcg daily; patients with normal or mildly decreased serum calcium levels may respond to 0.25 mcg every other day

I.V.:

U.S. labeling: Initial: 1-2 mcg 3 times weekly approximately every other day. Adjust dose by 0.5-1 mcg at 2- to 4-week intervals; dosing range: 0.5-4 mcg 3 times weekly. Gradual dose reduction and discontinuation of therapy may be necessary as PTH levels decrease below target of (1.5-3 x ULN) in response to therapy.

Canadian labeling: Initial: 0.5 mcg 3 times weekly, approximately every other day. Adjust dose by 0.25-0.5 mcg at 2- to 4-week intervals; dosing range: 0.5-3 mcg 3 times weekly

Hypocalcemia in hypoparathyroidism/pseudohypoparathyroidism: Oral:

U.S. labeling: Initial: 0.25 mcg daily(may adjust dose at 2- to 4-week intervals); range: 0.5-2 mcg once daily

Canadian labeling: Initial: 0.25 mcg daily; may increase dose by 0.25 mcg daily at 2- to 4-week intervals. Discontinue use immediately for hypercalcemia; may resume therapy after calcium levels normalize.

Psoriasis: Topical: Apply twice daily to affected areas (maximum: 200 g weekly); Canadian labeling recommends maximum of 30 g daily

Secondary hyperparathyroidism associated with moderate-to-severe CKD in patients not on dialysis: Oral: 0.25 mcg daily; may increase to 0.5 mcg daily

KDOQI guidelines for vitamin D therapy in CKD (KDOQI, 2003):

CKD stage 3: Oral: 0.25 mcg daily. Treatment should only be started with serum 25(OH) D >30 ng/mL, serum iPTH >70 pg/mL, serum calcium <9.5 mg/dL and serum phosphorus <4.6 mg/dL

CKD stage 4: Oral: 0.25 mcg daily. Treatment should only be started with serum 25(OH) D >30 ng/mL, serum iPTH >110 pg/mL, serum calcium <9.5 mg/dL and serum phosphorus <4.6 mg/dL

CKD stage 5:

Peritoneal dialysis: Oral: Initial: 0.5-1 mcg 2-3 times weekly or 0.25 mcg daily

Hemodialysis: **Note:** The following initial doses are based on plasma PTH and serum calcium levels for patients with serum phosphorus <5.5 mg/dL and Ca-P product <55. Adjust dose based on serum phosphate, calcium, and PTH levels. Intermittent I.V. administration may be more effective than daily oral dosing. Administer per hemodialysis session.

Plasma PTH 300-600 pg/mL and serum Ca <9.5 mg/dL: Oral, I.V.: 0.5-1.5 mcg

Plasma PTH 600-1000 pg/mL and serum Ca <9.5 mg/dL:

Oral: 1-4 mcg

I.V.: 1-3 mcg

Plasma PTH >1000 pg/mL and serum Ca <10 mg/dL:

Oral: 3-7 mcg

I.V.: 3-5 mcg

Vitamin D-dependent rickets type 1/pseudovitamin D deficiency rickets (PDDR): *U.S. unlabeled use:* Oral: Initial: 0.5 mcg twice daily; subsequent dosing adjusted to maintain normal serum calcium and PTH levels; median dose after 2 years: 0.25 mcg daily (range: 0.1-0.5 mcg daily) (Edouard, 2011)

Vitamin D-resistant rickets: *Canadian labeling (not in U.S. labeling):* Oral: Initial: 0.25 mcg daily; may increase dose by 25 mcg daily at 2- to 4-week intervals if response is inadequate; discontinue use immediately for hypercalcemia and do not resume until calcium levels normalize.

Geriatric Refer to adult dosing. Start at the lower end of the dosage range.

Pediatric

Hypocalcemia in hypoparathyroidism/pseudohypoparathyroidism:

U.S. labeling: Oral:

Children 1-5 years: Usual dosage range: 0.25-0.75 mcg once daily (may adjust dose at 2- to 4-week intervals)

Children ≥6 years: Refer to adult dosing.

Canadian labeling: Oral: Children: Initial: 0.03-0.05 mcg/kg/day; evaluate response after 2 weeks and increase dose by 25% if response is inadequate. Dose may be increased or decreased by 25% every 2 weeks thereafter until therapeutic response is achieved. **Note:** May consider initial dose of 0.05 mcg/kg/day for severe hypocalcemia/ symptoms (hospitalization recommended with close monitoring and dose reduction as soon as clinically possible). Maintenance dose: 0.014-0.04 mcg/kg/day

Secondary hyperparathyroidism associated with moderate-to-severe CKD in patients not on dialysis: Oral:

U.S. labeling:

Children <3 years: Initial dose: 0.01-0.015 mcg/kg/day

Children ≥3 years: Refer to adult dosing.

KDOQI guidelines for vitamin D therapy in CKD: Children (KDOQI, 2005):

CKD stage 2, 3: Oral:

<10 kg: 0.05 mcg every other day

10-20 kg: 0.1-0.15 mcg daily

>20 kg: 0.25 mcg daily

Note: Treatment should only be started with serum 25(OH) D >30 ng/mL, serum iPTH >70 pg/mL, serum calcium <10 mg/dL and serum phosphorus less than or equal to the age appropriate level.

CKD stage 4: Oral:

<10 kg: 0.05 mcg every other day

10-20 kg: 0.1-0.15 mcg daily

>20 kg: 0.25 mcg daily

Note: Treatment should only be started with serum 25(OH) D >30 ng/mL, serum iPTH >110 pg/mL, serum calcium <10 mg/dL and serum phosphorus less than or equal to the age appropriate level.

CKD stage 5: Peritoneal dialysis or hemodialysis: Oral, I.V.: **Note:** The following initial doses are based on plasma PTH and serum calcium levels for patients with serum phosphorus <5.5 mg/dL in adolescents or <6.5 in infants and children, and Ca-P product <55 in adolescents or <65 in infants and children <12 years. Adjust dose based on serum phosphate, calcium and PTH levels. Administer dose with each dialysis session (3 times weekly). Intermittent I.V./oral administration is more effective than daily oral dosing.

Plasma PTH 300-500 pg/mL and serum Ca <10 mg/dL: 0.0075 mcg/kg (maximum: 0.25 mcg daily)

Plasma PTH >500-1000 pg/mL and serum Ca <10 mg/dL: 0.015 mcg/kg (maximum: 0.5 mcg daily)

Plasma PTH >1000 pg/mL and serum Ca <10.5 mg/dL: 0.025 mcg/kg (maximum: 1 mcg daily)

Vitamin D-dependent rickets type 1/pseudovitamin D deficiency rickets (PDDR): Oral:

U.S. unlabeled use: Children: Refer to adult dosing.

Canadian labeling: Children: Initial: 0.01-0.025 mcg/kg/day; evaluate response after two weeks and increase dose by 25% if response is inadequate. Dose may be increased or decreased by 25% every 2 weeks thereafter until therapeutic response is achieved. **Note:** May consider initial dose of 0.05 mcg/kg/day for severe hypocalcemia/ symptoms (hospitalization recommended with close monitoring and dose reduction as soon as clinically possible). Maintenance dose: 0.0046-0.015 mcg/kg/day.

X-linked hypophosphatemic rickets: *Canadian labeling (not in U.S. labeling):* Children: Oral: Initial: 0.01-0.02 mcg/kg/day; evaluate response after 2 weeks and increase dose by 25% if response is inadequate. Dose may be increased or decreased by 25% every two weeks thereafter until therapeutic response is achieved. **Note:** May consider initial dose of 0.05 mcg/kg/day for severe hypocalcemia/ symptoms (hospitalization recommended with close monitoring and dose reduction as soon as clinically possible). Maintenance dose: 0.01-0.05 mcg/kg/day.

Hepatic Impairment No dosage adjustment provided in manufacturer's labeling (has not been studied).

Adjustment for Toxicity

KDOQI guidelines:

Children (KDOQI, 2005): CKD stages 2-4:

Serum iPTH below target range: Hold calcitriol until levels rise above target range appropriate for CKD stage, than resume treatment at half the previous dose. If the lowest dose was being used, switch to alternate day therapy.

Corrected total calcium >10.2 mg/dL: Hold calcitriol until serum calcium returns to <9.8 mg/dL then resume treatment at half the previous dose. If the lowest dose was being used, switch to alternate day therapy.

Serum phosphorus greater than the age appropriate limits: Hold calcitriol and add/increase dose of phosphate binder until levels of phosphorous decrease to age appropriate levels, then resume at half the previous dose

Adults (KDOQI, 2003): CKD stage 3 and 4:

iPTH below target: Hold calcitriol until levels rise then resume treatment at half the previous dose. If the lowest dose was being used, switch to alternate day therapy.

Corrected total calcium >9.5 mg/dL: Hold calcitriol until serum calcium returns to <9.5 mg/dL, then resume treatment at half the previous dose. If the lowest dose was being used, switch to alternate day therapy.

Serum phosphorus >4.6 mg/dL: Hold calcitriol (or add/increase dose of phosphate binder) until levels of phosphorous decrease, then resume at half the prior dose.

Combination Regimens

Prostate cancer: Estramustine + Docetaxel + Calcitriol on page 1635

Administration

I.V.: May be administered as a bolus dose I.V. through the catheter at the end of hemodialysis.

Oral: May be administered without regard to food. Administer with meals to reduce GI problems.

Topical: Apply externally; not for ophthalmic, oral, or intravaginal use. Do not apply to eyes, lips, or facial skins. Rub in gently so that no medication remains visible. Limit application to only the areas of skin affected by psoriasis.

Monitoring Parameters

Manufacturer's labeling:

Oral therapy:

Dialysis patients: Serum calcium, phosphorus, magnesium, and alkaline phosphate monitored periodically

Hypoparathyroid patients: Serum calcium, phosphorus, 24 hour urinary calcium monitored periodically

Predialysis patients: Serum calcium, phosphorus, alkaline phosphatase, creatinine, and intact PTH, initially; then serum calcium, phosphorus, alkaline phosphatase, and creatinine monthly x 6 months, then periodically. Intact PTH should be monitored every 3-4 months.

During titration periods (all patients), monitor serum calcium levels at least twice weekly.

I.V. therapy: Serum calcium and phosphorus twice weekly (following initiation and during dosage adjustments) and periodically during therapy; periodic magnesium, alkaline phosphatase, 24 hour urinary calcium and phosphorous

KDOQI Guidelines: Oral and I.V. therapy: **Note:** More frequent monitoring may be necessary depending on the presence and magnitude of abnormalities, the rate of progression of CKD, and the use of treatments for CKD-mineral and bone disorders.

Children (KDOQI, 2005):

Serum calcium and phosphorous: CKD stages 2-4: At least monthly for first 3 months following initiation of therapy and at least every 3 months thereafter

CKD stage 5: At least every 2 weeks for one month following initiation of therapy and dose increases and monthly thereafter

Serum iPTH:

CKD stages 2-4: At least every 3 months

CKD stage 5: Monthly for at least 3 months following initiation of therapy or dose increases; once target levels are achieved monitor at least every 3 months thereafter

Adults (KDOQI, 2003):

Serum calcium and phosphorous:

CKD stages 3 and 4: At least monthly for first 3 months following initiation of therapy and every 3 months thereafter

CKD stage 5: At least every 2 weeks for one month following initiation of therapy or dose increases and monthly thereafter

Serum iPTH:

CKD stages 3 and 4: At least every 3 months for 6 months and every 3 months thereafter

CKD stage 5: Monthly for at least 3 months following initiation of therapy or dose increases and at least every 3 months once target levels are achieved

Dietary Considerations May be taken without regard to food. Give with meals to reduce GI problems. Adequate calcium intake should be maintained during therapy; dietary phosphorous may need to be restricted.

Dosage Forms Excipient information presented when available (limited, particularly for generics); consult specific product labeling.

Capsule, softgel, oral: 0.25 mcg, 0.5 mcg

Rocaltrol®: 0.25 mcg, 0.5 mcg [contains coconut oil]

Injection, solution: 1 mcg/mL (1 mL)

Calcijex®: 1 mcg/mL (1 mL) [contains aluminum]

Ointment, topical:

Vectical®: 3 mcg/g (100 g)

Solution, oral: 1 mcg/mL (15 mL)

Rocaltrol®: 1 mcg/mL (15 mL) [contains palm oil]

Dosage Forms: Canada Excipient information presented when available (limited, particularly for generics); consult specific product labeling.

Ointment, topical:

Silkis™: 3 mcg/g (5 g, 30 g, 100 g)

References

"K/DOQI Clinical Practice Guidelines for Bone Metabolism and Disease in Children With Chronic Kidney Disease." Available at http://www.kidney.org/professionals/KDOQI/guidelines_pedbone/index.htm

"K/DOQI Clinical Practice Guidelines for Bone Metabolism and Disease in Chronic Kidney Disease. Guideline 8A. Active Vitamin D Therapy in Patients With Stages 3 and 4 CKD." Available at http://www.kidney.org/professionals/KDOQI/guidelines_bone/Guide8A.htm

"K/DOQI Clinical Practice Guidelines for Bone Metabolism and Disease in Chronic Kidney Disease. Guideline 8B. Vitamin D Therapy in Patients on Dialysis (CKD Stage 5)." Available at http://www.kidney.org/professionals/KDOQI/guidelines_bone/Guide8B.htm

Kidney Disease: Improving Global Outcomes (KDIGO) CKD-MBD Work Group, "KDIGO Clinical Practice Guideline for the Diagnosis, Evaluation, Prevention, and Treatment of Chronic Kidney Disease-Mineral and Bone Disorder (CKD-MBD)," *Kidney Int Suppl*, 2009, 76(S113):1-130.

◆ **Calcium Folinate** *see* Leucovorin Calcium *on page* 870
◆ **Calcium Leucovorin** *see* Leucovorin Calcium *on page* 870
◆ **Calcium Levoleucovorin** *see* LEVOleucovorin *on page* 888
◆ **Caldecort® [OTC]** *see* Hydrocortisone (Topical) *on page* 719
◆ **Caltine® (Can)** *see* Calcitonin *on page* 214
◆ **Campath® [DSC]** *see* Alemtuzumab *on page* 43
◆ **Campath-1H** *see* Alemtuzumab *on page* 43
◆ **Camptosar®** *see* Irinotecan *on page* 813
◆ **Camptothecin-11** *see* Irinotecan *on page* 813
◆ **Cancidas®** *see* Caspofungin *on page* 249
◆ **Candistatin® (Can)** *see* Nystatin (Topical) *on page* 1042
◆ **CanesOral® (Can)** *see* Fluconazole *on page* 612
◆ **CAPE** *see* Capecitabine *on page* 223

Capecitabine (ka pe SITE a been)

Related Information

Management of Chemotherapy Induced Nausea and Vomiting *on page* 1786
Oral Mucositis/Stomatitis *on page* 1814
Safe Handling of Hazardous Drugs *on page* 1904

Brand Names: U.S. Xeloda®

Brand Names: Canada Xeloda®

Index Terms CAPE

Generic Availability (U.S.) No

Pharmacologic Category Antineoplastic Agent, Antimetabolite; Antineoplastic Agent, Antimetabolite (Pyrimidine Analog)

Use Treatment of metastatic colorectal cancer; adjuvant therapy of Dukes' C colon cancer; treatment of metastatic breast cancer

Unlabeled Use Treatment of gastric cancer, pancreatic cancer, esophageal cancer, ovarian cancer, metastatic renal cell cancer, neuroendocrine tumors, metastatic CNS lesions

Labeled Contraindications Hypersensitivity to capecitabine, fluorouracil, or any component of the formulation; known deficiency of dihydropyrimidine dehydrogenase (DPD); severe renal impairment (Cl_{cr} <30 mL/minute)

Pregnancy Risk Factor D

Lactation Excretion in breast milk unknown/not recommended

Warnings/Precautions Hazardous agent - use appropriate precautions for handling and disposal. Use with caution in patients ≥80 years of age, or with renal or hepatic dysfunction. Patients with baseline moderate renal impairment require dose reduction. Patients with mild-to-moderate renal impairment require careful monitoring and subsequent dose reduction with any grade 2 or higher adverse event. Bone marrow suppression may occur, hematologic toxicity is more common when used in combination therapy; use with caution; dosage adjustments may be required. Canadian labeling recommends that patients with baseline platelets <100,000/mm^3 and/or neutrophils <1500/mm^3 not receive capecitabine therapy and also to withhold for grade 3 or 4 hematologic toxicity during treatment. Use with caution in patients who have received extensive pelvic radiation or alkylating therapy. Use cautiously with warfarin. Rare and unexpected severe toxicity may be attributed to dihydropyrimidine dehydrogenase (DPD) deficiency. Necrotizing enterocolitis (typhlitis) has been reported.

Capecitabine can cause severe diarrhea; median time to first occurrence is 34 days. Subsequent doses should be reduced after grade 3 or 4 diarrhea or recurrence of grade 2 diarrhea. Dehydration may occur rapidly in patients with diarrhea, nausea, vomiting, anorexia, and/or weakness; adequately hydrate prior to treatment initiation. Elderly patients may be a higher risk for dehydration. Note: the Canadian labeling recommends treatment interruption for dehydration requiring I.V. hydration lasting <24 hours and dosage reduction if I.V hydration required for ≥24 hours; correct precipitating factors and ensure rehydration prior to resuming therapy.

Hand-and-foot syndrome is characterized by numbness, dysesthesia/paresthesia, tingling, painless or painful swelling, erythema, desquamation, blistering, and severe pain. If grade 2 or 3 hand-and-foot syndrome occurs, interrupt administration of capecitabine until decreases to grade 1. Following grade 3 hand-and-foot syndrome, decrease subsequent doses of capecitabine. In patients with colorectal cancer, treatment with capecitabine immediately following 6 weeks of fluorouracil/leucovorin (FU/LV) therapy has been associated with an increased incidence of grade ≥3 toxicity, when compared to patients receiving the reverse sequence, capecitabine (two 3-week courses) followed by FU/LV (Hennig, 2008).

There has been cardiotoxicity associated with fluorinated pyrimidine therapy. May be more common in patients with a history of coronary artery disease. **[U.S. Boxed Warning]: Capecitabine may increase the anticoagulant effects of warfarin; monitor closely.**

Safety and efficacy in children <18 years of age have not been established.

Adverse Reactions Frequency listed derived from monotherapy trials.

>10%:

Cardiovascular: Edema (9% to 15%)

Central nervous system: Fatigue (16% to 42%), fever (7% to 18%), pain (12%)

Dermatologic: Palmar-plantar erythrodysesthesia (hand-and-foot syndrome) (54% to 60%; grade 3: 11% to 17%; may be dose limiting), dermatitis (27% to 37%)

Gastrointestinal: Diarrhea (47% to 57%; may be dose limiting; grade 3: 12% to 13%; grade 4: 2% to 3%), nausea (34% to 53%), vomiting (15% to 37%), abdominal pain (7% to 35%), stomatitis (22% to 25%), appetite decreased (26%), anorexia (9% to 23%), constipation (9% to 15%)

Hematologic: Lymphopenia (94%; grade 4: 14%), anemia (72% to 80%; grade 4: <1% to 1%), neutropenia (2% to 26%; grade 4: 2%), thrombocytopenia (24%; grade 4: 1%)

Hepatic: Bilirubin increased (22% to 48%; grades 3/4: 11% to 23%)

Neuromuscular & skeletal: Paresthesia (21%)

Ocular: Eye irritation (13% to 15%)

Respiratory: Dyspnea (14%)

5% to 10%:

Cardiovascular: Venous thrombosis (8%), chest pain (6%)

Central nervous system: Headache (5% to 10%), lethargy (10%), dizziness (6% to 8%), insomnia (7% to 8%), mood alteration (5%), depression (5%)

Dermatologic: Nail disorder (7%), rash (7%), skin discoloration (7%), alopecia (6%), erythema (6%)

Endocrine & metabolic: Dehydration (7%)

Gastrointestinal: Motility disorder (10%), oral discomfort (10%), dyspepsia (6% to 8%), upper GI inflammatory disorders (colorectal cancer: 8%), hemorrhage (6%), ileus (6%), taste perversion (colorectal cancer: 6%)

Neuromuscular & skeletal: Back pain (10%), weakness (10%), neuropathy (10%), myalgia (9%), arthralgia (8%), limb pain (6%)

Ocular: Abnormal vision (colorectal cancer: 5%), conjunctivitis (5%)

Respiratory: Cough (7%)

Miscellaneous: Viral infection (colorectal cancer: 5%)

<5%, postmarketing, and/or case reports: Abdominal distension, angina, appetite increased, arthritis, ascites, asthma, ataxia, atrial fibrillation, bone pain, bradycardia, bronchitis, bronchopneumonia, bronchospasm, cachexia, cardiac arrest, cardiac failure, cardiomyopathy, cerebral vascular accident, cholestatic hepatitis, coagulation disorder, colitis, confusion, deep vein thrombosis, diaphoresis, duodenitis, dysarthria, dysphagia, dysrhythmia, ecchymoses, ECG changes, encephalopathy, epistaxis, esophagitis, fibrosis, fingerprint distortion (secondary to hand-and-foot syndrome), fungal infection, gastric ulcer, gastritis, gastroenteritis, gastrointestinal perforation, hematemesis, hemoptysis, hepatic failure, hepatic fibrosis, hepatitis, hoarseness, hot flushes, hypokalemia, hypomagnesemia, hyper /hypotension, hypersensitivity, hypertriglyceridemia, idiopathic thrombocytopenia purpura, ileus, impaired balance, infection, influenza-like illness, intestinal obstruction (~1%), irritability, joint stiffness, keratoconjunctivitis, lacrimal duct stenosis, laryngitis, leukopenia, loss of consciousness, lymphedema, MI, multifocal leukoencephalopathy, myocardial ischemia, myocarditis, necrotizing enterocolitis (typhlitis), nocturia, oral candidiasis, pericardial effusion, thrombocytopenic purpura, pancytopenia, photosensitivity reaction, pneumonia, proctalgia, pruritus, pulmonary embolism, radiation recall syndrome, renal impairment, respiratory distress, sedation, sepsis, skin ulceration, sore throat, Stevens-Johnson syndrome, tachycardia, thirst, thrombophlebitis, toxic epidermal necrolysis, toxic megacolon, tremor, ventricular extrasystoles, vertigo, weight gain

Drug Interactions

Metabolism/Transport Effects Inhibits CYP2C9 (strong)

Avoid Concomitant Use

Avoid concomitant use of Capecitabine with any of the following: BCG; CloZAPine; Natalizumab; Pimecrolimus; Tacrolimus (Topical); Vaccines (Live)

Increased Effect/Toxicity

Capecitabine may increase the levels/effects of: Carvedilol; CloZAPine; CYP2C9 Substrates; Diclofenac (Systemic); Fosphenytoin; Leflunomide; Natalizumab; Phenytoin; Vaccines (Live); Vitamin K Antagonists

The levels/effects of Capecitabine may be increased by: Denosumab; Leucovorin Calcium-Levoleucovorin; Pimecrolimus; Roflumilast; Tacrolimus (Topical); Trastuzumab

Decreased Effect

Capecitabine may decrease the levels/effects of: BCG; Coccidioidin Skin Test; Sipuleucel-T; Vaccines (Inactivated); Vaccines (Live)

The levels/effects of Capecitabine may be decreased by: Echinacea

Ethanol/Nutrition/Herb Interactions Food: Food reduced the rate and extent of absorption of capecitabine.

Storage/Stability Store at room temperature of 25°C (77°F); excursions permitted between 15°C and 30°C (59°F and 86°F).

Mechanism of Action Capecitabine is a prodrug of fluorouracil. It undergoes hydrolysis in the liver and tissues to form fluorouracil which is the active moiety. Fluorouracil is a fluorinated pyrimidine antimetabolite that inhibits thymidylate synthetase, blocking the methylation of deoxyuridylic acid to thymidylic acid, interfering with DNA, and to a lesser degree, RNA synthesis. Fluorouracil appears to be phase specific for the G_1 and S phases of the cell cycle.

Pharmacodynamics/Kinetics

Absorption: Rapid and extensive

Protein binding: <60%; ~35% to albumin

Metabolism:

Hepatic: Inactive metabolites: 5′-deoxy-5-fluorocytidine, 5′-deoxy-5-fluorouridine

Tissue: Active metabolite: Fluorouracil

Half-life elimination: 0.5-1 hour

Time to peak: 1.5 hours; Fluorouracil: 2 hours

Excretion: Urine (96%, 57% as α-fluoro-β-alanine); feces (<3%)

Dosing

Adult Note: Details concerning dosing in combination regimens should also be consulted. Capecitabine toxicities, particularly hand-foot syndrome, may be higher in North American populations (for the treatment of colorectal cancer); therapy initiation at doses of 1000 mg/m^2 twice daily (for 2 weeks every 21 days) may be considered (Haller, 2008; NCCN Colon Cancer Guidelines)

Metastatic breast cancer, metastatic colorectal cancer: Oral: 1250 mg/m^2 twice daily (morning and evening) for 2 weeks, every 21 days

Adjuvant therapy of Dukes' C colon cancer: Recommended for a total of 24 weeks (8 cycles of 2 weeks of drug administration and 1 week rest period).

Pancreatic cancer (unlabeled use): 1000 mg/m^2 twice daily for 2 weeks, every 21 days (NCCN Pancreatic Cancer Guidelines v.1.2009) **or** 1250 mg/m^2 twice daily for 2 weeks, every 21 days (Cartwright, 2002)

Geriatric The elderly may be more sensitive to the toxic effects of fluorouracil. Insufficient data are available to provide dosage modifications.

Renal Impairment

Cl_{cr} 51-80 mL/minute: No adjustment of initial dose.

Cl_{cr} 30-50 mL/minute: Administer 75% of normal dose.

Cl_{cr} <30 mL/minute: Use is contraindicated.

Hepatic Impairment

Mild-to-moderate impairment: No starting dose adjustment is necessary; however, carefully monitor patients.

Severe hepatic impairment: Patients have not been studied.

Adjustment for Toxicity

Dosage modification guidelines: See table on next page.

Refer to package labeling for modifications when administered in combination with docetaxel.

Recommended Dose Modifications

Toxicity NCI Grades	During a Course of Therapy (Monotherapy)	Dose Adjustment for Next Cycle (% of starting dose)
Grade 1	Maintain dose level	Maintain dose level
Grade 2		
1st appearance	Interrupt until resolved to grade 0-1	100%
2nd appearance	Interrupt until resolved to grade 0-1	75%
3rd appearance	Interrupt until resolved to grade 0-1	50%
4th appearance	Discontinue treatment permanently	
Grade 3		
1st appearance	Interrupt until resolved to grade 0-1	75%
2nd appearance	Interrupt until resolved to grade 0-1	50%
3rd appearance	Discontinue treatment permanently	
Grade 4		
1st appearance	Discontinue permanently or If physician deems it to be in the patient's best interest to continue, interrupt until resolved to grade 0-1	50%

Dosage adjustments for hematologic toxicity in combination therapy with ixabepilone:

Neutrophils <500/mm^3 for ≥7 days or neutropenic fever: Hold for concurrent diarrhea or stomatitis until neutrophils recover to >1000/mm^3, then continue at same dose

Platelets <25,000/mm^3 (or <50,000/mm^3 with bleeding): Hold for concurrent diarrhea or stomatitis until platelets recover to >50,000/mm^3, then continue at same dose

Combination Regimens

Biliary adenocarcinoma:
- CAPOX (Biliary Cancer) on page 1542
- Gemcitabine-Capecitabine (Biliary Cancer) on page 1668

Breast cancer:
- Bevacizumab-Capecitabine (Breast Cancer) on page 1528
- Capecitabine + Docetaxel (Breast Cancer) on page 1539
- Capecitabine + Lapatinib (Breast Cancer) on page 1541
- Capecitabine-Trastuzumab on page 1541
- Ixabepilone-Capecitabine on page 1698

Colorectal cancer:
- Bevacizumab + XELOX (Colorectal) on page 1532
- XELOX (Colorectal) on page 1778

Esophageal cancer:
- Cisplatin-Capecitabine (Esophageal Cancer) on page 1566
- Epirubicin-Cisplatin-Capecitabine (Esophageal Cancer) on page 1626
- Epirubicin-Oxaliplatin-Capecitabine on page 1627
- Irinotecan-Capecitabine (Esophageal Cancer) on page 1693

Gastric cancer:
Capecitabine-Docetaxel (Gastric Cancer) on page 1539
Cisplatin-Capecitabine (Gastric Cancer) on page 1566
Epirubicin-Oxaliplatin-Capecitabine on page 1627
Irinotecan-Capecitabine (Gastric Cancer) on page 1693
Trastuzumab-Cisplatin-Capecitabine (Gastric Cancer) on page 1757
Pancreatic cancer:
Capecitabine-Gemcitabine (Pancreatic) on page 1540
CAPOX (Pancreatic) on page 1543
Renal cell cancer: Gemcitabine-Capecitabine (RCC) on page 1668

Administration Usually administered in 2 divided doses taken 12 hours apart. Doses should be taken with water within 30 minutes after a meal.

Emetic Potential Low (10% to 30%)

Extemporaneous Preparations Hazardous agent: Use appropriate precautions for handling and disposal.

A 10 mg/mL oral solution may be made with tablets. Crush four 500 mg tablets in a mortar and reduce to a fine powder; add to 200 mL water. Capecitabine tablets are water soluble (data on file from Roche). Administer immediately after preparation, 30 minutes after a meal.

Judson IR, Beale PJ, Trigo JM, et al, "A Human Capecitabine Excretion Balance and Pharmacokinetic Study After Administration of a Single Oral Dose of ^{14}C-Labelled Drug," *Invest New Drugs*, 1999, 17(1):49-56.

Monitoring Parameters Renal function should be estimated at baseline to determine initial dose. During therapy, CBC with differential, hepatic function, and renal function should be monitored.

Dietary Considerations Because current safety and efficacy data are based upon administration with food, it is recommended that capecitabine be administered with food. In all clinical trials, patients were instructed to take with water within 30 minutes after a meal.

Additional Information Oncology Comment: An investigational uridine prodrug, uridine triacetate (formerly called vistonuridine), has been studied in a limited number of cases of fluorouracil overdose. Of 17 patients receiving uridine triacetate beginning within 8-96 hours after fluorouracil overdose, all patients fully recovered (von Borstel, 2009). Updated data has described a total of 28 patients treated with uridine triacetate for fluorouracil overdose (including overdoses related to continuous infusions delivering fluorouracil at rates faster than prescribed), all of whom recovered fully (Bamat, 2010). Refer to Uridine Triacetate monograph.

Dosage Forms Excipient information presented when available (limited, particularly for generics); consult specific product labeling.
Tablet, oral:
Xeloda®: 150 mg, 500 mg

References

Bamat MK, Tremmel R, O'Neil JD, et al, "Uridine Triacetate: An Orally Administered Life-Saving Antidote for 5-FU Overdose," *J Clin Oncol*, 28(15s):9084 [abstract 9084 from 2010 ASCO Annual Meeting].

Cartwright TH, Cohn A, Varkey JA, et al, "Phase II Study of Oral Capecitabine in Patients With Advanced or Metastatic Pancreatic Cancer," *J Clin Oncol*, 2002, 20(1):160-4.

Cassidy J, Tabernero J, Twelves C, et al, "XELOX (Capecitabine Plus Oxaliplatin): Active First-Line Therapy for Patients With Metastatic Colorectal Cancer," *J Clin Oncol*, 2004, 22(11):2084-91.

Haller DG, Cassidy J, Clarke S, et al, "Potential Regional Differences for the Tolerability Profiles of Fluoropyrimidines," *J Clin Oncol*, 2008, 26(13):2118-23.

Hennig IM, Naik JD, Brrown S, et al, "Severe Sequence-Specific Toxicity When Capecitabine Is Given After Fluorouracil and Leucovorin," *J Clin Oncol*, 2008, 26(20):3411-7.

Hoff PM, Ansari R, Batist G, et al, "Comparison of Oral Capecitabine Versus Intravenous Fluorouracil Plus Leucovorin as First-Line Treatment in 605 Patients With Metastatic Colorectal Cancer: Results of a Randomized Phase III Study," *J Clin Oncol*, 2001, 19(8):2282-92.

Morgan C, Tillett T, Braybrooke J, et al, "Management of Uncommon Chemotherapy-Induced Emergencies," *Lancet Oncol*, 2011, 12(8):806-14.

National Comprehensive Cancer Network® (NCCN), "Clinical Practice Guidelines in Oncology™: Prevention and Treatment of Colon Cancer," Version 2.2010. Available at http://www.nccn.org/professionals/physician_gls/PDF/colon.pdf

National Comprehensive Cancer Network® (NCCN), "Clinical Practice Guidelines in Oncology™: Prevention and Treatment of Pancreatic Adenocarcinoma," Version 1.2009. Available at http://www.nccn.org/professionals/physician_gls/PDF/pancreatic.pdf

Twelves C, Wong A, Nowacki MP, et al, "Capecitabine as Adjuvant Treatment for Stage III Colon Cancer," *N Engl J Med*, 2005, 352(26):2696-704.

Van Cutsem E, Twelves C, Cassidy J, et al, "Oral Capecitabine Compared With Intravenous Fluorouracil Plus Leucovorin in Patients With Metastatic Colorectal Cancer: Results of a Large Phase III Study," *J Clin Oncol*, 2001, 19(21):4097-106.

von Borstel R, O'Neil J, and Bamat M, "Vistonuridine: An Orally Administered, Life-Saving Antidote for 5-Fluorouracil (5FU) Overdose," *J Clin Oncol*, 2009, 27(15S):9616 [abstract from 2009 ASCO Annual Meeting].

Wong M, Choo SP, and Tan EH, "Travel Warning With Capecitabine," *Ann Oncol*, 2009, 20(7):2081.

- **Caphosol®** *see* Saliva Substitute *on page 1200*
- **Caprelsa®** *see* Vandetanib *on page 1435*
- **Carac®** *see* Fluorouracil (Topical) *on page 632*

CARBOplatin (KAR boe pla tin)

Related Information

Chemotherapy and Obesity *on page 1834*

Hematopoietic Stem Cell Transplantation *on page 1887*

Management of Chemotherapy-Induced Nausea and Vomiting *on page 1786*

Management of Drug Extravasations *on page 1800*

Safe Handling of Hazardous Drugs *on page 1904*

Brand Names: Canada Carboplatin Injection; Carboplatin Injection - LIQ IV

Index Terms CBDCA; Paraplatin

Generic Availability (U.S.) Yes

Pharmacologic Category Antineoplastic Agent, Alkylating Agent; Antineoplastic Agent, Platinum Analog

Use Initial treatment of advanced ovarian cancer in combination with other established chemotherapy agents; palliative treatment of recurrent ovarian cancer after prior chemotherapy, including cisplatin-based treatment

Unlabeled Use Treatment of bladder cancer, breast cancer (metastatic), central nervous system tumors, cervical cancer (recurrent or metastatic), endometrial cancer, esophageal cancer, head and neck cancer, Hodgkin's lymphoma (relapsed or refractory), malignant pleural mesothelioma, melanoma (advanced or metastatic), merkel cell carcinoma, neuroendocrine tumors (adrenal gland and carcinoid tumors), non-Hodgkin's lymphomas (relapsed or refractory), nonsmall cell lung cancer, retinoblastoma, sarcomas (Ewing's sarcoma and osteosarcoma), small-cell lung cancer, testicular cancer, thymic malignancies, unknown primary adenocarcinoma, and as a conditioning regimen prior to hematopoietic stem cell transplantation

Labeled Contraindications History of severe allergic reaction to carboplatin, cisplatin, other platinum-containing formulations, mannitol, or any component of the formulation; should not be used in patients with severe bone marrow depression or significant bleeding

Pregnancy Risk Factor D

Lactation Excretion in breast milk unknown/not recommended

Warnings/Precautions Hazardous agent - use appropriate precautions for handling and disposal. High doses have resulted in severe abnormalities of liver function tests. **[U.S. Boxed Warning]: Bone marrow suppression, which may be severe, is dose related; may result in infection (due to neutropenia) or bleeding (due to thrombocytopenia); anemia may require blood transfusion;** reduce dosage in patients with bone marrow suppression; cycles should be delayed until WBC and platelet counts have recovered. Patients who have received prior myelosuppressive therapy and patients with renal dysfunction are at increased risk for bone marrow suppression. Anemia is cumulative.

When calculating the carboplatin dose using the Calvert formula and an estimated glomerular filtration rate (GFR), the laboratory method used to measure serum creatinine may impact dosing. Compared to other methods, standardized isotope dilution mass spectrometry (IDMS) may underestimate serum creatinine values in patients with low creatinine values (eg, ≤0.7 mg/dL) and may overestimate GFR in patients with normal renal function. This may result in higher calculated carboplatin doses and increased toxicities. If using IDMS, the Food and Drug Administration (FDA) recommends that clinicians consider capping estimated GFR at a maximum of 125 mL/minute to avoid potential toxicity.

[U.S. Boxed Warning]: Anaphylactic-like reactions have been reported with carboplatin; may occur within minutes of administration. Epinephrine, corticosteroids and antihistamines have been used to treat symptoms. The risk of allergic reactions (including anaphylaxis) is increased in patients previously exposed to platinum therapy. Skin testing and desensitization protocols have been reported (Confina-Cohen, 2005; Lee, 2004; Markman, 2003). When administered as sequential infusions, taxane derivatives (docetaxel, paclitaxel) should be administered before the platinum derivatives (carboplatin, cisplatin) to limit myelosuppression and to enhance efficacy. Ototoxicity may occur when administered concomitantly with aminoglycosides. Clinically significant hearing loss has been reported to occur in pediatric patients when carboplatin was administered at higher than recommended doses in combination with other ototoxic agents (eg, aminoglycosides). In a study of children receiving carboplatin for the treatment of retinoblastoma, those <6 months of age at treatment initiation were more likely to experience ototoxicity; long-term audiology monitoring is recommended (Qaddoumi, 2012). Loss of vision (usually reversible within weeks of discontinuing) has been reported with higher than recommended doses.

Use caution in elderly patients; may cause or exacerbate syndrome of inappropriate antidiuretic hormone secretion or hyponatremia; monitor sodium closely with initiation or dosage adjustments in older adults (Beers Criteria). Peripheral neuropathy occurs infrequently, the incidence of peripheral neuropathy is increased patients >65 years of age and those who have previously received cisplatin treatment. Patients >65 years of age are more likely to develop severe thrombocytopenia.

Limited potential for nephrotoxicity unless administered concomitantly with aminoglycosides. **[U.S. Boxed Warning]: Vomiting may occur;** may be severe in patients who have received prior emetogenic therapy. **[U.S. Boxed**

Warning]: Should be administered under the supervision of an experienced cancer chemotherapy physician.

Adverse Reactions Percentages reported with single-agent therapy.

>10%:

Central nervous system: Pain (23%)

Endocrine & metabolic: Hyponatremia (29% to 47%), hypomagnesemia (29% to 43%), hypocalcemia (22% to 31%), hypokalemia (20% to 28%)

Gastrointestinal: Vomiting (65% to 81%), abdominal pain (17%), nausea (without vomiting: 10% to 15%)

Hematologic: Myelosuppression (dose related and dose limiting; nadir at ~21 days with single-agent therapy), anemia (71% to 90%; grades 3/4: 21%), leukopenia (85%; grades 3/4: 15% to 26%), neutropenia (67%; grades 3/4: 16% to 21%), thrombocytopenia (62%; grades 3/4: 25% to 35%)

Hepatic: Alkaline phosphatase increased (24% to 37%), AST increased (15% to 19%)

Neuromuscular & skeletal: Weakness (11%)

Renal: Creatinine clearance decreased (27%), BUN increased (14% to 22%)

Miscellaneous: Hypersensitivity/allergic reaction (2% to 16%)

1% to 10%:

Central nervous system: Neurotoxicity (5%)

Dermatologic: Alopecia (2% to 3%)

Gastrointestinal: Constipation (6%), diarrhea (6%), stomatitis/mucositis (1%), taste dysgeusia (1%)

Hematologic: Bleeding (5%), hemorrhagic complications (5%)

Hepatic: Bilirubin increased (5%)

Neuromuscular & skeletal: Peripheral neuropathy (4% to 6%)

Ocular: Visual disturbance (1%)

Otic: Ototoxicity (1%)

Renal: Creatinine increased (6% to 10%)

Miscellaneous: Infection (5%)

<1%, postmarketing, and/or case reports (limited to important or life-threatening): Anaphylactic reaction, anorexia, bronchospasm, cardiac failure, cerebrovascular accident, dehydration, embolism, erythema, hemolytic anemia (acute), hemolytic uremic syndrome (HUS), hyper-/hypotension, injection site reactions (pain, redness, swelling), limb ischemia (acute), malaise, necrosis (associated with extravasation), neutropenic fever, pruritus, rash, secondary malignancies, urticaria, vision loss

Drug Interactions

Metabolism/Transport Effects None known.

Avoid Concomitant Use

Avoid concomitant use of CARBOplatin with any of the following: BCG; CloZAPine; Natalizumab; Pimecrolimus; SORAfenib; Tacrolimus (Topical); Vaccines (Live)

Increased Effect/Toxicity

CARBOplatin may increase the levels/effects of: Bexarotene (Systemic); CloZAPine; Leflunomide; Natalizumab; Taxane Derivatives; Topotecan; Vaccines (Live)

The levels/effects of CARBOplatin may be increased by: Aminoglycosides; Denosumab; Pimecrolimus; Roflumilast; SORAfenib; Tacrolimus (Topical); Trastuzumab

Decreased Effect

CARBOplatin may decrease the levels/effects of: BCG; Coccidioidin Skin Test; Sipuleucel-T; Vaccines (Inactivated); Vaccines (Live)

The levels/effects of CARBOplatin may be decreased by: Echinacea

Ethanol/Nutrition/Herb Interactions Herb/Nutraceutical: Avoid black cohosh, dong quai in estrogen-dependent tumors.

Storage/Stability Store intact vials at room temperature at 25°C (77°F); excursions permitted to 15°C to 30°C (59°F to 86°F). Protect from light. Further dilution to a concentration as low as 0.5 mg/mL is stable at room temperature (25°C) for 8 hours in NS or D_5W. Stability has also been demonstrated for dilutions in D_5W in PVC bags at room temperature for 9 days (Benaji, 1994); however, the manufacturer recommends use within 8 hours due to lack of preservative.

Reconstitution

Solution for injection: Manufacturer's labeling states solution can be further diluted to concentrations as low as 0.5 mg/mL in NS or D_5W; however, most clinicians generally dilute dose in either 100 mL or 250 mL of NS or D_5W.

Concentrations used for desensitization vary based on protocol.

Use appropriate precautions for handling and disposal. Needles or I.V. administration sets that contain aluminum should not be used in the preparation or administration of carboplatin; aluminum can react with carboplatin resulting in precipitate formation and loss of potency.

Mechanism of Action Carboplatin is a platinum compound alkylating agent which covalently binds to DNA; interferes with the function of DNA by producing interstrand DNA cross-links

Pharmacodynamics/Kinetics

Distribution: V_d: 16 L (based on a dose of 300-500 mg/m^2); into liver, kidney, skin, and tumor tissue

Protein binding: Carboplatin: 0%; Platinum (from carboplatin): Irreversibly binds to plasma proteins

Metabolism: Minimally hepatic to aquated and hydroxylated compounds

Half-life elimination: Cl_{cr} >60 mL/minute: Carboplatin: 2.6-5.9 hours (based on a dose of 300-500 mg/m^2); Platinum (from carboplatin): ≥5 days

Excretion: Urine (~70% as carboplatin within 24 hours; 3% to 5% as platinum within 1-4 days)

Dosing

Adult Details concerning dosing in combination regimens should also be consulted. **Note:** Doses for adults are commonly calculated by the target AUC using the Calvert formula, where **Total dose (mg) = Target AUC x (GFR + 25)**. If estimating glomerular filtration rate (GFR) instead of a measured GFR, the Food and Drug Administration (FDA) recommends that clinicians consider capping estimated GFR at a maximum of 125 mL/minute to avoid potential toxicity.

Ovarian cancer, advanced: I.V.: 360 mg/m^2 every 4 weeks (as a single agent) **or** 300 mg/m^2 every 4 weeks (in combination with cyclophosphamide) **or** Target AUC 4-6 (single agent; in previously-treated patients)

Unlabeled dosing for advanced ovarian cancer: I.V.: Target AUC 5-7.5 every 3 weeks (in combination with paclitaxel) (Ozols, 2003; Parmar, 2003) **or** Target AUC 5 every 3 weeks (in combination with docetaxel) (Vasey, 2004)

Bladder cancer (unlabeled use): I.V.: Target AUC 5 every 3 weeks (in combination with gemcitabine and paclitaxel) (Hainsworth, 2005) **or** Target

AUC 5 every 3 weeks (in combination with gemcitabine) (Bamias, 2006) **or** Target AUC 6 every 3 weeks (in combination with paclitaxel) (Vaughn, 2002)

Breast cancer, metastatic (unlabeled use): I.V.: Target AUC 6 every 3 weeks (in combination with trastuzumab and paclitaxel) (Robert, 2006) **or** Target AUC 6 every 3 weeks (in combination with trastuzumab and docetaxel) (Pegram, 2004; Valero, 2011)

Cervical cancer, recurrent or metastatic (unlabeled use): I.V.: Target AUC 5 every 3 weeks (in combination with paclitaxel) (Pectasides, 2009) **or** Target AUC 5-6 every 4 weeks (in combination with paclitaxel) (Tinker, 2005) **or** 400 mg/m^2 every 28 days (as a single agent) (Weiss, 1990)

Endometrial cancer (unlabeled use): I.V.: Target AUC 5 every 3 weeks (in combination with paclitaxel) (Pectasides, 2008) **or** Target AUC 2 on days 1, 8, and 15 every 28 days (in combination with paclitaxel) (Secord, 2007)

Esophageal cancer (unlabeled use): I.V.: Target AUC 2 on days 1, 8, 15, 22, and 29 for 1 cycle (in combination with paclitaxel) (van Meerten, 2006) **or** Target AUC 5 every 3 weeks (in combination with paclitaxel) (El-Rayes, 2004)

Head and neck cancer (unlabeled use): I.V.: Target AUC 5 every 3 weeks (in combination with cetuximab) (Chan, 2005) **or** Target AUC 5 every 3 weeks (in combination with cetuximab and fluorouracil) (Vermorken, 2008) **or** 300 mg/m^2 every 4 weeks (in combination with fluorouracil) (Forastiere, 1992) **or** Target AUC 6 every 3 weeks (in combination with paclitaxel) (Clark, 2001)

Hodgkin's lymphoma, relapsed or refractory (unlabeled use): I.V.: Target AUC 5 (maximum dose 800 mg) for 2 cycles (in combination with ifosfamide and etoposide) (Moskowitz, 2001)

Malignant pleural mesothelioma (unlabeled use): I.V.: Target AUC 5 every 3 weeks (in combination with pemetrexed) (Castagneto, 2008; Ceresoli, 2006)

Melanoma, advanced or metastatic (unlabeled use): I.V.: Target AUC 2 days on 1, 8, and 15 every 4 weeks (in combination with paclitaxel) (Rao, 2006)

Non-Hodgkin's lymphomas, relapsed or refractory (unlabeled use): I.V.: Target AUC 5 (maximum dose 800 mg) per cycle for 3 cycles (in combination with rituximab, ifosfamide and etoposide) (Kewalramani, 2004)

Nonsmall cell lung cancer (unlabeled use): I.V.: Target AUC 6 every 3-4 weeks (in combination with paclitaxel) (Ramalingam, 2008; Schiller, 2002; Strauss, 2008) **or** Target AUC 6 every 3 weeks (in combination with bevacizumab and paclitaxel) (Sandler, 2006) **or** Target AUC 5 every 3 weeks (in combination with pemetrexed) (Gronberg, 2009) **or** in combination with radiation therapy and paclitaxel (Belani, 2005):

Target AUC 6 every 3 weeks for 2 cycles **or**

Target AUC 6 every 3 weeks for 2 cycles; then target AUC 2 weekly for 7 weeks **or**

Target AUC 2 every week for 7 weeks; then target AUC 6 every 3 weeks for 2 cycles

Sarcomas: Ewing's sarcoma, osteosarcoma (unlabeled uses): I.V.: 400 mg/m^2/day for 2 days every 21 days (in combination with ifosfamide and etoposide) (van Winkle, 2005)

Small cell lung cancer (unlabeled use): I.V.: Target AUC 6 every 3 weeks (in combination with etoposide) (Skarlos, 2001) **or** Target AUC 5 every 3 weeks (in combination with irinotecan) (Hermes, 2008) **or** Target AUC 5 every 28 days (in combination with irinotecan) (Schmittel, 2006)

Testicular cancer (unlabeled use): I.V.: Target AUC 7 as a one-time dose (Oliver, 2011) **or** 700 mg/m^2/day for 3 days beginning 5 days prior to peripheral stem cell infusion (in combination with etoposide) for 2 cycles (Einhorn, 2007)

Thymic malignancies (unlabeled use): I.V.: Target AUC 5 every 3 weeks (in combination with paclitaxel) (Lemma, 2008)

Unknown primary adenocarcinoma (unlabeled use): I.V.: Target AUC 6 every 3 weeks (in combination with paclitaxel) (Briasoulis, 2000) **or** Target AUC 6 every 3 weeks (in combination with docetaxel) (Greco, 2000) **or** Target AUC 6 every 3 weeks (in combination with paclitaxel and etoposide) (Hainsworth, 2006) **or** Target AUC 5 every 3 weeks (in combination with paclitaxel and gemcitabine) (Greco, 2002)

Dosing adjustment in obesity: Dosing based on GFR should be considered in obese patients (Griggs, 2012).

Geriatric The Calvert formula should be used to calculate dosing for elderly patients. Refer to adult dosing.

Pediatric Details concerning dosing in combination regimens should also be consulted.

Glioma (unlabeled use): I.V.: 175 mg/m^2 weekly for 4 weeks every 6 weeks, with a 2-week recovery period between courses (in combination with vincristine) (Packer, 1997)

Neuroblastoma, localized and unresectable (unlabeled use): I.V.: Children ≥10 kg: 200 mg/m^2/day days 1, 2, and 3 every 21 days for 2 cycles (in combination with etoposide for 2 cycles then followed by cyclophosphamide, doxorubicin and vincristine) (Rubie, 1998) **or** Children <1 year: 6.6 mg/kg/day days 1, 2, and 3 (in combination with etoposide for 2 cycles, then followed by cyclophosphamide, doxorubicin, and vincristine) (Rubie, 2001)

Sarcomas: Ewing's sarcoma, osteosarcoma (unlabeled uses): I.V.: 400 mg/m^2/day for 2 days every 21 days (in combination with ifosfamide and etoposide) (van Winkle, 2005)

Renal Impairment Note: Dose determination with Calvert formula uses GFR and, therefore, inherently adjusts for renal dysfunction.

The manufacturer's labeling recommends the following dosage adjustment guidelines for single-agent therapy: Adults:

Baseline Cl_{cr} 41-59 mL/minute: Initiate at 250 mg/m^2 and adjust subsequent doses based on bone marrow toxicity

Baseline Cl_{cr} 16-40 mL/minute: Initiate at 200 mg/m^2 and adjust subsequent doses based on bone marrow toxicity

Baseline Cl_{cr} ≤15 mL/minute: No dosage adjustment provided in manufacturer's labeling.

The following dosage adjustments have also been recommended:

Aronoff, 2007:

Children:

GFR <50 mL/minute: Use Calvert formula incorporating patient's GFR

Hemodialysis, peritoneal dialysis, continuous renal replacement therapy (CRRT): Use Calvert formula incorporating patient's GFR

Adults (**Note:** For dosing based on **mg/m^2**):

GFR >50 mL/minute: No dosage adjustment necessary

GFR 10-50 mL/minute: Administer 50% of the dose

GFR <10 mL/minute: Administer 25% of the dose

Hemodialysis: Administer 50% of dose

Continuous ambulatory peritoneal dialysis (CAPD): Administer 25% of dose

Continuous renal replacement therapy (CRRT): 200 mg/m²

Janus, 2010: Hemodialysis: Carboplatin dose (mg) = Target AUC x 25; administer on a nondialysis day, hemodialysis should occur between 12-24 hours after carboplatin dose

Hepatic Impairment No dosage adjustment provided in manufacturer's labeling; however, carboplatin undergoes minimal hepatic metabolism therefore dosage adjustment may not be needed.

Adjustment for Toxicity Platelets <50,000 cells/mm³ or ANC <500 cells/mm³: Administer 75% of dose

Combination Regimens

Bladder cancer:

Gemcitabine-Carboplatin (Bladder Cancer) on page 1668
Paclitaxel-Carboplatin (Bladder Cancer) on page 1726
Paclitaxel-Carboplatin-Gemcitabine on page 1726

Breast cancer:

Docetaxel-Trastuzumab-Carboplatin on page 1615
Trastuzumab-Paclitaxel-Carboplatin on page 1760

Cervical cancer: Carboplatin-Paclitaxel (Cervical Cancer) on page 1549

Esophageal cancer: Paclitaxel-Carboplatin (Esophageal Cancer) on page 1726

Head and neck cancer:

Carboplatin-Cetuximab (Head and Neck Cancer) on page 1543
Cetuximab-Carboplatin-Fluorouracil (Head and Neck Cancer) on page 1557
Fluorouracil-Carboplatin (Head and Neck Cancer) on page 1652

Lung cancer (nonsmall cell):

Bevacizumab-Carboplatin-Paclitaxel (NSCLC) on page 1528
Bevacizumab-Carboplatin-Pemetrexed (NSCLC) on page 1529
Carboplatin-Gemcitabine (NSCLC) on page 1547
Carboplatin-Pemetrexed (NSCLC) on page 1551
Carbo-Tax (NSCLC) on page 1552
CaT (NSCLC) on page 1553
EC (NSCLC) on page 1621
PC (NSCLC) on page 1734

Lung cancer (small cell):

Carboplatin-Etoposide (Small Cell Lung Cancer) on page 1546
Carboplatin-Irinotecan (Small Cell Lung Cancer) on page 1548

Lymphoma, Hodgkin: ICE (Hodgkin) on page 1688

Lymphoma, non-Hodgkin's:

ICE (Lymphoma, non-Hodgkin's) on page 1689
RICE on page 1747

Malignant pleural mesothelioma: Carboplatin-Pemetrexed (Mesothelioma) on page 1551

Neuroblastoma: CE-CAdO (Neuroblastoma) on page 1555

Osteosarcoma: ICE (Sarcoma) on page 1689

Ovarian cancer:

Carboplatin-Docetaxel (Ovarian) on page 1543
Carboplatin-Doxorubicin (Liposomal) (Ovarian) on page 1544
Carboplatin-Gemcitabine (Ovarian) on page 1548
Carboplatin-Paclitaxel (Ovarian) on page 1550
Etoposide-Carboplatin (Ovarian Cancer) on page 1639

Prostate cancer:
Estramustine + Docetaxel + Carboplatin on page 1636
Paclitaxel + Estramustine + Carboplatin on page 1728
Retinoblastoma:
Carboplatin-Etoposide (Retinoblastoma) on page 1545
Carboplatin-Etoposide-Vincristine (Retinoblastoma) on page 1546
Carboplatin-Vincristine (Retinoblastoma) on page 1552
Rhabdomyosarcoma: CEV on page 1562
Soft tissue sarcoma: ICE (Sarcoma) on page 1689
Testicular cancer: Carboplatin (Testicular Regimen) on page 1552
Unknown primary, adenocarcinoma:
Carboplatin-Docetaxel (Unknown Primary) on page 1544
Carboplatin-Etoposide-Paclitaxel (Unknown Primary) on page 1545
Carboplatin-Gemcitabine-Paclitaxel (Unknown Primary) on page 1548
Carboplatin-Paclitaxel (Unknown Primary) on page 1551

Administration Usually infused over 15-60 minutes, although some protocols may require infusions up to 24 hours. When administered as a part of a combination chemotherapy regimen, sequence of administration may vary by regimen; refer to specific protocol for sequence recommendation.

Needles or I.V. administration sets that contain aluminum should not be used in the preparation or administration of carboplatin; aluminum can react with carboplatin resulting in precipitate formation and loss of potency.

Emetic Potential Moderate (30% to 90%)

Vesicant/Extravasation Risk May be an irritant

Monitoring Parameters CBC (with differential and platelet count), serum electrolytes, serum creatinine and BUN, creatinine clearance, liver function tests; audiology evaluations (children <6 months of age)

Dosage Forms Excipient information presented when available (limited, particularly for generics); consult specific product labeling.

Injection, solution [preservative free]: 10 mg/mL (5 mL, 15 mL, 45 mL, 60 mL)

References

Aronoff GR, Bennett WM, Berns JS, et al, *Drug Prescribing in Renal Failure: Dosing Guidelines for Adults and Children*, 5th ed. Philadelphia, PA: American College of Physicians; 2007, p 97, 169.

Bamias A, Moulopoulos LA, Koutras A, et al, "The Combination of Gemcitabine and Carboplatin as First-Line Treatment in Patients With Advanced Urothelial Carcinoma. A Phase II Study of the Hellenic Cooperative Oncology Group," *Cancer*, 2006, 106(2):297-303.

Belani CP, Choy H, Bonomi P, et al, "Combined Chemoradiotherapy Regimens of Paclitaxel and Carboplatin for Locally Advanced Non-Small-Cell Lung Cancer: A Randomized Phase II Locally Advanced Multi-Modality Protocol," *J Clin Oncol*, 2005, 23(25):5883-91.

Benaji B, Dine T, Luyckx M, et al, "Stability and Compatibility of Cisplatin and Carboplatin With PVC Infusion Bags," *J Clin Pharm Ther*, 1994, 19(2):95-100.

Briasoulis E, Kalofonos H, Bafaloukos D, et al, "Carboplatin Plus Paclitaxel in Unknown Primary Carcinoma: A Phase II Hellenic Cooperative Oncology Group Study," *J Clin Oncol*, 2000, 18 (17):3101-7.

Calvert AH, Newell DR, Grumbell LA, et al, "Carboplatin Dosage: Prospective Evaluation of a Simple Formula Based on Renal Function," *J Clin Oncol*, 1989, 7(11):1748-56.

Castagneto B, Botta M, Aitini E, et al, "Phase II Study of Pemetrexed in Combination With Carboplatin in Patients With Malignant Pleural Mesothelioma (MPM)," *Ann Oncol*, 2008, 19 (2):370-3.

Ceresoli GL, Zucali PA, Favaretto AG, et al, "Phase II Study of Pemetrexed Plus Carboplatin in Malignant Pleural Mesothelioma," *J Clin Oncol*, 2006, 24(9):1443-8.

Chan AT, Hsu MM, Goh BC, et al, "Multicenter, Phase II Study of Cetuximab in Combination With Carboplatin in Patients With Recurrent or Metastatic Nasopharyngeal Carcinoma," *J Clin Oncol*, 2005, 23(15):3568-76.

Cheung Y-W, Cradock JC, Vishnuvajjala BR, et al, "Stability of Cisplatin, Iproplatin, Carboplatin, and Tetraplatin in Commonly Used Intravenous Solutions," *Am J Hosp Pharm*, 1987, 44:124-30.

Clark JI, Hofmeister C, Choudhury A, et al, "Phase II Evaluation of Paclitaxel in Combination With Carboplatin in Advanced Head and Neck Carcinoma," *Cancer*, 2001, 92(9):2334-40.

Confino-Cohen R, Fishman A, Altaras M, et al, "Successful Carboplatin Desensitization in Patients With Proven Carboplatin Allergy," *Cancer*, 2005, 104(3):640-3.

Donahue A, McCune JS, Faucette S, et al, "Measured Versus Estimated Glomerular Filtration Rate in the Calvert Equation: Influence on Carboplatin Dosing," *Cancer Chemother Pharmacol*, 2001, 47(5):373-9.

Einhorn LH, Williams SD, Chamness A, et al, "High-Dose Chemotherapy and Stem-Cell Rescue for Metastatic Germ-Cell Tumors," *N Engl J Med*, 2007, 357(4):340-8.

El-Rayes BF, Shields A, Zalupski M, et al, "A Phase II Study of Carboplatin and Paclitaxel in Esophageal Cancer," *Ann Oncol*, 2004, 15(6):960-5.

Forastiere AA, Metch B, Schuller DE, et al, "Randomized Comparison of Cisplatin Plus Fluorouracil and Carboplatin Plus Fluorouracil Versus Methotrexate in Advanced Squamous-Cell Carcinoma of the Head and Neck: A Southwest Oncology Group Study," *J Clin Oncol*, 1992, 10(8):1245-51.

Greco FA, Burris HA 3rd, Erland JB, et al, "Carcinoma of Unknown Primary Site," *Cancer*, 2000, 89 (12):2655-60.

Greco FA, Burris HA 3rd, Litchy S, et al, "Gemcitabine, Carboplatin, and Paclitaxel for Patients With Carcinoma of Unknown Primary Site: A Minnie Pearl Cancer Research Network Study," *J Clin Oncol*, 2002, 20(6):1651-6.

Greco FA, Erland JB, Morrissey LH, et al, "Carcinoma of Unknown Primary Site: Phase II Trials With Docetaxel Plus Cisplatin or Carboplatin," *Ann Oncol*, 2000, 11(2):211-5.

Griggs JJ, Mangu PB, Anderson H, et al, "Appropriate Chemotherapy Dosing For Obese Adult Patients With Cancer: American Society of Clinical Oncology Clinical Practice Guideline," *J Clin Oncol*, 2012, 30(13):1553-61.

Gronberg BH, Bremnes RM, Flotten O, et al, "Phase III Study by the Norwegian Lung Cancer Study Group: Pemetrexed Plus Carboplatin Compared With Gemcitabine Plus Carboplatin as First-Line Chemotherapy in Advanced Non-Small-Cell Lung Cancer, " *J Clin Oncol*, 2009, 27(19):3217-24.

Hainsworth JD, Meluch AA, Litchy S, et al, "Paclitaxel, Carboplatin, and Gemcitabine in the Treatment of Patients With Advanced Transitional Cell Carcinoma of the Urothelium," *Cancer*, 2005, 103(11):2298-303

Hainsworth JD, Spigel DR, Litchy S, et al, "Phase II Trial of Paclitaxel, Carboplatin, and Etoposide in Advanced Poorly Differentiated Neuroendocrine Carcinoma: A Minnie Pearl Cancer Research Network Study," *J Clin Oncol*, 2006, 24(22):3548-54.

Hermes A, Bergman B, Bremnes R, et al, "Irinotecan Plus Carboplatin Versus Oral Etoposide Plus Carboplatin in Extensive Small-Cell Lung Cancer: A Randomized Phase III Trial," *J Clin Oncol*, 2008, 26(26):4261-7.

Janus N, Thariat J, Boulanger H, et al, "Proposal for Dosage Adjustment and Timing of Chemotherapy in Hemodialyzed Patients," *Ann Oncol*, 2010, 21(7).1395-403.

Kewalramani T, Zelenetz AD, Nimer SD, et al, "Rituximab and ICE as Second-Line Therapy before Autologous Stem Cell Transplantation for Relapsed or Primary Refractory Diffuse Large B-Cell Lymphoma," *Blood*, 2004, 103(10):3684-8.

Lee CW, Matulonis UA, and Castells MC, "Carboplatin Hypersensitivity: A 6-h 12-Step Protocol Effective in 35 Desensitizations in Patients With Gynecological Malignancies and Mast Cell/IgE-Mediated Reactions," *Gynecol Oncol*, 2004, 95(2):370-6.

Lemma GL, Loehrer PJ, Lee JW, et al, "A Phase II Study of Carboplatin Plus Paclitaxel in Advanced Thymoma or Thymic Carcinoma: E1C99," *J Clin Oncol*, 2008, 26(15s):8018 [abstract 8018 from 2000 annual ASCO meeting].

Markman M, Zanotti K, Peterson G, et al, "Expanded Experience With an Intradermal Skin Test to Predict for the Presence or Absence of Carboplatin Hypersensitivity," *J Clin Oncol*, 2003, 21 (24):4611-4.

Morgan C, Tillett T, Braybrooke J, et al, "Management of Uncommon Chemotherapy Induced Emergencies," *Lancet Oncol*, 2011, 12(8):806-14.

Moskowitz CH, Nimer SD, Zelenetz AD, et al, "A 2-Step Comprehensive High-Dose Chemoradiotherapy Second-Line Program for Relapsed and Refractory Hodgkin Disease: Analysis by Intent to Treat and Development of a Prognostic Model," *Blood*, 2001, 97(3):616-23.

Oliver RT, Mead GM, Rustin GJ, et al, "Randomized Trial of Carboplatin versus Radiotherapy for Stage I Seminoma: Mature Results on Relapse and Contralateral Testis Cancer Rates in MRC TE19/EORTC 30982 Study (ISRCTN27163214), *J Clin Oncol*, 2011, 29(8):957-62.

Ozols RF, Bundy BN, Greer BE, et al, "Phase III Trial of Carboplatin and Paclitaxel Compared With Cisplatin and Paclitaxel in Patients With Optimally Resected Stage III Ovarian Cancer: A Gynecologic Oncology Group Study," *J Clin Oncol*, 2003, 21(17):3194-200.

Packer RJ, Ater J, Allen J, et al, "Carboplatin and Vincristine Chemotherapy for Children With Newly Diagnosed Progressive Low-Grade Gliomas," *J Neurosurg*, 1997, 86(5):747-54.

Parmar MK, Ledermann JA, Colombo N, et al, "Paclitaxel Plus Platinum-Based Chemotherapy Versus Conventional Platinum-Based Chemotherapy in Women With Relapsed Ovarian Cancer: The ICON4/AGO-OVAR-2.2 Trial," *Lancet*, 2003, 361(9375):2099-106.

Pectasides D, Fountzilas G, Papaxoinis G, et al, "Carboplatin and Paclitaxel in Metastatic or Recurrent Cervical Cancer," *Int J Gynecol Cancer*, 2009, 19(4):777-81.

Pectasides D, Xiros N, Papaxoinis G, et al, "Carboplatin and Paclitaxel in Advanced or Metastatic Endometrial Cancer," *Gynecol Oncol*, 2008, 109(2):250-4.

Pegram MD, Pienkowski T, Northfelt DW, et al, "Results of Two Open-Label, Multicenter Phase II Studies of Docetaxel, Platinum Salts, and Trastuzumab in HER2-Positive Advanced Breast Cancer," *J Natl Cancer Inst*, 2004, 96(10):759-69.

Qaddoumi I, Bass JK, Wu J, et al, "Carboplatin-Associated Ototoxicity in Children With Retinoblastoma," *J Clin Oncol*, 2012 [epub ahead of print].

Ramalingam S, Perry MC, La Rocca RV, et al, "Comparison of Outcomes for Elderly Patients Treated With Weekly Paclitaxel in Combination With Carboplatin versus the Standard 3-Weekly Paclitaxel and Carboplatin for Advanced Nonsmall Cell Lung Cancer," *Cancer*, 2008, 113 (3):542-6.

Rao D, Holtan SG, Ingle JN, et al, "Combination of Paclitaxel and Carboplatin as Second-Line Therapy for Patients With Metastatic Melanoma," *Cancer*, 2006, 106(2):375-82.

Robert N, Leyland-Jones B, Asmar L, et al, "Randomized Phase III Study of Trastuzumab, Paclitaxel, and Carboplatin Compared With Trastuzumab and Paclitaxel in Women With HER-2-Overexpressing Metastatic Breast Cancer," *J Clin Oncol*, 2006, 24(18):2786-92.

Rubie H, Michon J, Plantaz D, et al, "Unresectable Localized Neuroblastoma: Improved Survival After Primary Chemotherapy Including Carboplatin-Etoposide. Neuroblastoma Study Group of the Societe Francaise d'Oncologie Pediatrique (SFOP)," *Br J Cancer*, 1998, 77(12):2310-7.

Rubie H, Plantaz D, Coze C, et al, "Localised and Unresectable Neuroblastoma in Infants: Excellent Outcome With Primary Chemotherapy. Neuroblastoma Study Group, Société Française d'Oncologie Pédiatrique," *Med Pediatr Oncol*, 2001, 36(1):247-50.

Sandler A, Gray R, Perry MC, et al, "Paclitaxel-Carboplatin Alone or With Bevacizumab for Non-Small-Cell Lung Cancer," *N Engl J Med*, 2006, 355(24):2542-50.

Schiller JH, Harrington D, Belani CP, et al, "Comparison of Four Chemotherapy Regimens for Advanced Non-Small-Cell Lung Cancer," *N Engl J Med*, 2002, 346(2):92-8.

Schmittel A, Fischer von Weikersthal L, Sebastian M, et al, "A Randomized Phase II Trial of Irinotecan Plus Carboplatin Versus Etoposide Plus Carboplatin Treatment in Patients With Extended Disease Small-Cell Lung Cancer," *Ann Oncol*, 2006, 17(4):663-7.

Secord AA, Havrilesky LJ, Carney ME, et al, "Weekly Low-Dose Paclitaxel and Carboplatin in the Treatment of Advanced or Recurrent Cervical and Endometrial Cancer," *Int J Clin Oncol*, 2007, 12(1):31-6.

Skarlos DV, Samantas E, Briassoulis E, et al, "Randomized Comparison of Early Versus Late Hyperfractionated Thoracic Irradiation Concurrently With Chemotherapy in Limited Disease Small-Cell Lung Cancer: A Randomized Phase II Study of the Hellenic Cooperative Oncology Group (HeCOG)," *Ann Oncol*, 2001, 12(9):1231-38.

Strauss GM, Herndon JE 2nd, Maddaus AA, et al, "Adjuvant Paclitaxel Plus Carboplatin Compared With Observation in Stage IB Non-Small-Cell Lung Cancer: CALGB 9633 With the Cancer and Leukemia Group B, Radiation Therapy Oncology Group, and North Central Cancer Treatment Group Study Groups," *J Clin Oncol*, 2008, 26(31):5043-51.

Tinker AV, Bhagat K, Swenerton KD, et al, "Carboplatin and Paclitaxel for Advanced and Recurrent Cervical Carcinoma: The British Columbia Cancer Agency Experience," *Gynecol Oncol*, 2005, 98 (1):54-8.

Valero V, Forbes J, Pegram MD, et al, "Multicenter Phase III Randomized Trial Comparing Docetaxel and Trastuzumab With Docetaxel, Carboplatin, and Trastuzumab as First-Line Chemotherapy for Patients With HER2-Gene-Amplified Metastatic Breast Cancer (BCIRG 007 Study): Two Highly Active Therapeutic Regimens, *J Clin Oncol*, 2011, 29(2):149-56.

van Meerten E, Muller K, Tilanus HW, et al, "Neoadjuvant Concurrent Chemoradiation With Weekly Paclitaxel and Carboplatin for Patients With Oesophageal Cancer: A Phase II Study," *Br J Cancer*, 2006, 94(10):1389-94.

van Winkle P, Angiolillo A, Krailo M, et al, "Ifosfamide, Carboplatin, and Etoposide (ICE) Reinduction Chemotherapy in a Large Cohort of Children and Adolescents With Recurrent/Refractory Sarcoma: The Children's Cancer Group (CCG) Experience," *Pediatr Blood Cancer*, 2005, 44(4):338-47.

Vasey PA, Jayson GC, Gordon A, et al, "Phase III Randomized Trial of Docetaxel-Carboplatin Versus Paclitaxel-Carboplatin as First-Line Chemotherapy for Ovarian Carcinoma," *J Natl Cancer Inst*, 2004, 96(22):1682-91.

Vaughn DJ, Manola J, Dreicer R, et al, "Phase II Study of Paclitaxel Plus Carboplatin in Patients With Advanced Carcinoma of the Urothelium and Renal Dysfunction (E2896): A Trial of the Eastern Cooperative Oncology Group," *Cancer*, 2002, 95(5):1022-7.

Vermorken JB, Mesia R, Rivera F, et al, "Platinum-Based Chemotherapy Plus Cetuximab in Head and Neck Cancer," *N Engl J Med*, 2008, 359(11):1116-27.
Weiss GR, Green S, Hannigan EV, et al, "A Phase II Trial of Carboplatin for Recurrent or Metastatic Squamous Carcinoma of the Uterine Cervix: A Southwest Oncology Group Study," *Gynecol Oncol*, 1990, 39(3):332-6.

◆ **Carboplatin Injection (Can)** *see* CARBOplatin *on page 229*
◆ **Carboplatin Injection - LIQ IV (Can)** *see* CARBOplatin *on page 229*
◆ **Carboxypeptidase-G2** *see* Glucarpidase *on page 680*

Carfilzomib (kar FILZ oh mib)

Brand Names: U.S. Kyprolis™

Index Terms PR-171

Generic Availability (U.S.) No

Pharmacologic Category Antineoplastic Agent; Proteasome Inhibitor

Use Treatment of multiple myeloma in patients who have received at least 2 prior treatment regimens (including a proteasome inhibitor and an immunomodulator) with disease progression within 60 days after the most recent treatment

Labeled Contraindications There are no contraindications listed in the manufacturer's labeling.

Pregnancy Risk Factor D

Lactation Excretion in breast milk unknown/not recommended

Warnings/Precautions Hazardous agent – use appropriate precautions for handling and disposal. Thrombocytopenia (including grade 4) was observed in patients receiving carfilzomib, with platelet nadirs occurring around day 8 of each 28-day treatment cycle, and recovery to baseline by the start of the next cycle. Monitor platelets closely and adjust dose or withhold therapy if necessary. Anemia, lymphopenia, and neutropenia were also observed. Death caused by cardiac arrest has occurred within 24 hours of drug administration. Carfilzomib has been associated with the development or worsening of congestive heart failure (HF) and decreased left ventricular ejection fraction (LVEF). HF, pulmonary edema, and decreased LVEF were observed in clinical trials; monitor closely for cardiac complications; withhold therapy for grade 3 or 4 cardiac events until recovery. Patients with New York Heart Association Class III and IV heart failure, recent myocardial infarction (within 6 months), and conduction abnormalities not managed by medication were excluded from clinical trials. Pulmonary arterial hypertension (PAH) was observed (including grade 3) in studies; perform cardiac imaging or other testing as appropriate, and withhold carfilzomib until PAH is resolved or returns to baseline. Dyspnea (including 1 death) has been reported; monitor closely, and withhold carfilzomib until symptom resolution or return to baseline.

Infusion reactions such as chills, fever, arthralgia, myalgia, shortness of breath, hypotension, facial flushing, facial edema, vomiting, weakness, syncope, chest tightness, or angina may occur immediately following or within 24 hours of carfilzomib infusion. To lessen the incidence and intensity of infusion reactions, administer dexamethasone prior to drug administration. Tumor lysis syndrome (TLS) risk is increased in multiple myeloma patients with a high tumor burden. Adequately hydrate patients prior to carfilzomib therapy and monitor closely for signs and symptoms of tumor lysis syndrome. If TLS occurs, interrupt treatment until resolved.

Hepatic failure, including fatal cases, has been reported rarely (<1%). Increased transaminases and hyperbilirubinemia have also been observed.

Interrupt carfilzomib therapy in patients with grade 3 or higher hepatic toxicity until resolved or recovered to baseline; monitor liver enzymes closely and for signs of toxicity.

Adverse Reactions

>10%:

Cardiovascular: Peripheral edema (24%), hypertension (14%), chest wall pain (11%)

Central nervous system: Fatigue (56%), fever (30%), headache (28%), insomnia (18%), chills (16%), dizziness (13%), hypoesthesia (12%), pain (12%)

Endocrine & metabolic: Hypokalemia (14%), hypomagnesemia (14%), hyperglycemia (12%), hypercalcemia (11%), hypophosphatemia (11%)

Gastrointestinal: Nausea (45%), diarrhea (33%), vomiting (22%), constipation (21%), anorexia (12%)

Hematologic: Anemia (47%; grade 3: 21%; grade 4: 1%), thrombocytopenia (36%; grade 3: 13%; grade 4: 10%), lymphopenia (24%; grade 3: 16%; grade 4: 2%), neutropenia (21%; grade 3: 10%; grade 4: 1%), leukopenia (14%; grade 3: 5%; grade 4:<1%)

Hepatic: AST increased (13%; grade 3: 3%; grade 4: <1%)

Neuromuscular & skeletal: Back pain (20%), arthralgia (16%), muscle spasms (14%), peripheral neuropathy (14%; grade 3: 1%), weakness (14%), limb pain (13%)

Renal: Creatinine increased (24%; grade 3: 3%; grade 4: <1%)

Respiratory: Dyspnea (35%; grade 3: 5%; grade 4: <1%), upper respiratory tract infection (28%), cough (26%), pneumonia (13%; grade 3: 10%; grade 4: <1%)

1% to 10%:

Cardiovascular: Cardiac failure (7%; includes CHF, pulmonary edema, ejection fraction decrease)

Endocrine & metabolic: Hyponatremia (10%)

Renal: Renal failure (9%)

Respiratory: Pulmonary arterial hypertension (2%)

Miscellaneous: Herpes zoster reactivation (2%)

<1%, postmarketing, and/or case reports: Bilirubin increased, hepatic failure, infusion reaction, intracranial hemorrhage, multiorgan failure, myocardial ischemia, neutropenic fever, sepsis, tumor lysis syndrome

Drug Interactions

Metabolism/Transport Effects **Substrate** of P-glycoprotein; **Inhibits** CYP3A4 (weak), P-glycoprotein

Avoid Concomitant Use

Avoid concomitant use of Carfilzomib with any of the following: CloZAPine; Pimozide

Increased Effect/Toxicity

Carfilzomib may increase the levels/effects of: ARIPiprazole; CloZAPine; Pimozide

The levels/effects of Carfilzomib may be increased by: P-glycoprotein/ABCB1 Inhibitors

Decreased Effect

The levels/effects of Carfilzomib may be decreased by: P-glycoprotein/ABCB1 Inducers

Storage/Stability Store intact vials refrigerated at 2°C to 8°C (36°F to 46°F). Do not shake; store in original carton until use to protect from light.

Reconstituted drug (in the vial or in a syringe) and preparations diluted for infusion are stable for 4 hours at room temperature or for 24 hours refrigerated at 2°C to 8°C (36°F to 46°F).

Reconstitution Use appropriate precautions for handling and disposal. Reconstitute with 29 mL sterile water for injection to a concentration of 2 mg/mL (directing solution onto the inside wall of the vial to avoid foaming). Gently invert and/or swirl vial slowly for ~1 minute to mix; do not shake. If foaming results, allow solution to sit for 2-5 minutes until foaming resolves. Reconstituted solution should be clear and colorless. May further dilute dose in 50 mL D_5W. The amount contained in each vial may exceed the prescribed dose; use care with dosage and volume calculations. Discard unused portion of the vial.

Mechanism of Action Carfilzomib inhibits proteasomes, which are responsible for intracellular protein homeostasis. Specifically, it is a potent, selective, and irreversible inhibitor of chymotrypsin-like activity of the 20S proteasome, leading to cell cycle arrest and apoptosis.

Pharmacodynamics/Kinetics

Distribution: V_{dss}: 28 L

Protein binding: 97%

Metabolism: Rapid and extensive; peptidase cleavage and epoxide hydrolysis; minimal metabolism through cytochrome P450-mediated mechanisms

Half-life elimination: Doses ≥15 mg/m^2: <1 hour on day 1 of cycle 1

Dosing

Adult & Geriatric Note: Hydrate with 250-500 mL normal saline (or other appropriate I.V. fluid) predose (recommended) and postdose (if needed) during cycle 1 (continue in subsequent cycles if necessary). Premedicate with dexamethasone (4 mg orally or I.V.) prior to all doses in cycle 1, all doses during first dose escalation cycle, and as needed with future cycles to reduce the incidence and severity of infusion reaction.

Multiple myeloma, relapsed/refractory: I.V.: **Note:** Patients with a body surface area (BSA) >2.2 m^2 should be dosed based upon a maximum BSA of 2.2 m^2. Dose adjustments for weight changes of ≤20% are not necessary, per manufacturer labeling.

Cycle 1: 20 mg/m^2 on 2 consecutive days, each week for 3 weeks (days 1, 2, 8, 9, 15, and 16) of a 28-day treatment cycle

Cycle 2 and subsequent cycles (if cycle 1 is tolerated): 27 mg/m^2 on 2 consecutive days, each week for 3 weeks (days 1, 2, 8, 9, 15, and 16) of a 28-day treatment cycle. Continue until disease progression or occurrence of unacceptable toxicity.

Renal Impairment No dosage adjustment provided in manufacturer's labeling; however, results from a phase 2 trial in patients with renal impairment indicate that the pharmacokinetics and safety of carfilzomib were unchanged in this patient population; no dosage adjustment is necessary in patients with baseline dysfunction, including hemodialysis (Harvey, 2012; Niesvizky, 2011). **Note:** Dialysis clearance of carfilzomib has not been studied; per manufacturer labeling, administer postdialysis.

Hepatic Impairment No dosage adjustment provided in manufacturer's labeling (has not been studied; patients with ALT or AST ≥3 times ULN and bilirubin ≥2 times ULN were excluded from clinical trials).

Adjustment for Toxicity

Hematologic toxicity:

ANC: Grade 3 or 4 neutropenia: Withhold dose; continue at same dose level if fully recovered before next scheduled dose. If recovered to grade 2, reduce dose by one dose level (from 27 mg/m^2 to 20 mg/m^2 or from 20 mg/m^2 to 15 mg/m^2). Consider escalating to the previous dose if reduced dose is tolerated.

Platelets: Grade 4 thrombocytopenia: Withhold dose; continue at same dose level if fully recovered before next scheduled dose. If recovered to grade 3 thrombocytopenia, reduce dose by one dose level (from 27 mg/m^2 to 20 mg/m^2 or from 20 mg/m^2 to 15 mg/m^2). Consider escalating to the previous dose if reduced dose is tolerated.

Nonhematologic toxicity:

Cardiac: Grade 3 or 4, new onset or worsening of congestive heart failure, decreased left ventricular function, or myocardial ischemia: Withhold dose until resolved or at baseline. After resolution, if appropriate to reinitiate, consider restarting at a reduced dose level (from 27 mg/m^2 to 20 mg/m^2 or from 20 mg/m^2 to 15 mg/m^2). Consider escalating to the previous dose if reduced dose is tolerated.

Hepatic: Grade 3 or 4 elevation of bilirubin, transaminases, or other liver abnormalities: Withhold dose until resolved or at baseline. After resolution, if appropriate to reinitiate, consider restarting at a reduced dose level (from 27 mg/m^2 to 20 mg/m^2 or from 20 mg/m^2 to 15 mg/m^2). Consider escalating to the previous dose if reduced dose is tolerated.

Peripheral neuropathy: Grade 3 or 4: Withhold dose until resolved or at baseline. After resolution, if appropriate to reinitiate, restart at prior dose or at a reduced dose level (from 27 mg/m^2 to 20 mg/m^2 or from 20 mg/m^2 to 15 mg/m^2). Consider escalating to the previous dose if reduced dose is tolerated.

Pulmonary toxicity

Pulmonary hypertension: Withhold dose until resolved or at baseline. After resolution, if appropriate to reinitiate, restart at prior dose or at a reduced dose level (from 27 mg/m^2 to 20 mg/m^2 or from 20 mg/m^2 to 15 mg/m^2). Consider escalating to the previous dose if reduced dose is tolerated.

Grade 3 or 4 pulmonary complications: Withhold dose until resolved or at baseline. After resolution, consider restarting (at next scheduled treatment) at a reduced dose level (from 27 mg/m^2 to 20 mg/m^2 or from 20 mg/m^2 to 15 mg/m^2). Consider escalating to the previous dose if reduced dose is tolerated.

Renal: Serum creatinine ≥2 times baseline: Withhold dose until renal function has improved to grade 1 or baseline. If renal toxicity due to carfilzomib, reduce dose at the next scheduled treatment (from 27 mg/m^2 to 20 mg/m^2 or from 20 mg/m^2 to 15 mg/m^2). Consider escalating to the previous dose if reduced dose is tolerated. If toxicity not due to carfilzomib, restart at previous dose.

Tumor lysis syndrome: Interrupt treatment until resolved.

Other grade 3 or 4 nonhematologic toxicities: Withhold dose until resolved or at baseline. After resolution, consider restarting (at next scheduled treatment) at a reduced dose level (from 27 mg/m^2 to 20 mg/m^2 or from 20 mg/m^2 to 15 mg/m^2). Consider escalating to the previous dose if reduced dose is tolerated.

Combination Regimens

Multiple myeloma: Carfilzomib (Multiple Myeloma Regimen) on page 1553

Administration I.V.: Administer over 2-10 minutes. Flush line before and after carfilzomib with NS or D_5W.

Monitoring Parameters CBC with differential and platelets (monitor frequently throughout therapy); renal function, pulmonary function (with new or worsening pulmonary symptoms), liver function tests, serum creatinine. Signs/symptoms of infusion-related reactions, congestive heart failure, tumor lysis syndrome, and peripheral neuropathy.

Dosage Forms Excipient information presented when available (limited particularly for generics); consult specific product labeling.

Injection, powder for reconstitution:

Kyprolis™: 60 mg [contains cyclodextrin]

References

Harvey RD, Lonial S, Patel P, et al, "Summary of Treatment-Emergent Renal Events From Patients Treated With Single-Agent Carfilzomib From Four Phase II Studies in Relapsed and/or Refractory Multiple Myeloma," *J Clin Oncol*, 2012, 30(15S):e18569 [abstract e18569 from ASCO 2012 Annual Meeting].

Niesvizky R, Vij R, Martin T, et al, "Carfilzomib Pharmacokinetics, Safety, and Activity in Patients With Relapsed or Refractory Multiple Myeloma and Renal Dysfunction," *Haematol*, 2011, 96 (s2):370 [abstract 0890 from EHA 2011 Annual Meeting].

Siegel DS, Martin T, Wang M, et al, "A Phase 2 Study of Single-Agent Carfilzomib (PX-171-003-A1) in Patients With Relapsed and Refractory Multiple Myeloma, *Blood*, 2012 [epub ahead of print].

◆ **Carimune® NF** *see* Immune Globulin *on page* 777

Carmustine (kar MUS teen)

Related Information

Hematopoietic Stem Cell Transplantation *on page* 1887

Management of Chemotherapy-Induced Nausea and Vomiting *on page* 1786

Management of Drug Extravasations *on page* 1800

Safe Handling of Hazardous Drugs *on page* 1904

Brand Names: U.S. BiCNU®; Gliadel®

Brand Names: Canada BiCNU®; Gliadel Wafer®

Index Terms BCNU; bis(chloroethyl) nitrosourea; bis-chloronitrosourea; Carmustine Polymer Wafer; Carmustinum; WR-139021

Generic Availability (U.S.) No

Pharmacologic Category Antineoplastic Agent; Antineoplastic Agent, Alkylating Agent; Antineoplastic Agent, Alkylating Agent (Nitrosourea)

Use

Injection: Treatment of brain tumors (glioblastoma, brainstem glioma, medulloblastoma, astrocytoma, ependymoma, and metastatic brain tumors), multiple myeloma, Hodgkin's lymphoma (relapsed or refractory), non-Hodgkin's lymphomas (relapsed or refractory)

Wafer (implant): Adjunct to surgery in patients with recurrent glioblastoma multiforme; adjunct to surgery and radiation in patients with newly-diagnosed high-grade malignant glioma

Unlabeled Use Treatment of mycosis fungoides (topical)

Labeled Contraindications Hypersensitivity to carmustine or any component of the formulation

Pregnancy Risk Factor D

Lactation Excretion in breast milk unknown/not recommended

Warnings/Precautions Hazardous agent - use appropriate precautions for handling and disposal.

[U.S. Boxed Warning]: Injection: Bone marrow suppression (primarily thrombocytopenia and leukopenia) is the major carmustine toxicity; generally is delayed. Monitor blood counts weekly for at least 6 weeks after administration. Myelosuppression is cumulative. When given at the FDA-approved doses, treatment should not be administered less than 6 weeks apart. Consider nadir blood counts from prior dose for dosage adjustment. May cause bleeding (due to thrombocytopenia) or infections (due to neutropenia); monitor closely. Patients must have platelet counts >100,000/mm^3 and leukocytes >4000/mm^3 for a repeat dose. Anemia may occur (less common and less severe than leukopenia or thrombocytopenia). Long-term use is associated with the development of secondary malignancies (acute leukemias and bone marrow dysplasias).

[U.S. Boxed Warnings]: Injection: Dose-related pulmonary toxicity may occur; patients receiving cumulative doses >1400 mg/m^2 are at higher risk. Delayed onset of pulmonary fibrosis (may be fatal) has occurred in children up to 17 years after treatment; this occurred in ages 1-16 for the treatment of intracranial tumors; cumulative doses ranged from 770-1800 mg/m^2 (in combination with cranial radiotherapy). Pulmonary toxicity is characterized by pulmonary infiltrates and/or fibrosis and has been reported from 9 days to 43 months after nitrosourea treatment (including carmustine). Although pulmonary toxicity generally occurs in patients who have received prolonged treatment, pulmonary fibrosis has been reported with cumulative doses <1400 mg/m^2. In addition to high cumulative doses, other risk factors for pulmonary toxicity include history of lung disease and baseline predicted forced vital capacity (FVC) or carbon monoxide diffusing capacity (DL_{CO}) <70%. Baseline and periodic pulmonary function tests are recommended. For high-dose treatment (transplant; unlabeled dose), acute lung injury may occur ~1-3 months post transplant; advise patients to contact their transplant physician for dyspnea, cough, or fever; interstitial pneumonia may be managed with a course of corticosteroids. Children are at higher risk for delayed pulmonary toxicity.

Injection site burning and local tissue reactions, including swelling, pain, erythema, and necrosis have been reported. Monitor infusion site closely for infiltration or injection site reactions. Reversible increases in transaminases, bilirubin and alkaline phosphatase have been reported (rare); monitor liver function tests periodically during treatment. Renal failure, progressive azotemia, and decreased kidney size have been reported in patients who have received large cumulative doses or prolonged treatment (renal toxicity has also been reported in patients who have received lower cumulative doses); monitor renal function tests periodically during treatment. Unlabeled administration (intraarterial intracarotid route) has been associated with ocular toxicity. Consider initiating treatment at the lower end of the dose range in the elderly. Diluent contains ethanol. With wafer implantation, monitor closely for known craniotomy-related complications (seizure, intracranial infection, abnormal wound healing, brain edema); intracerebral mass effect (unresponsive to corticosteroids) has been reported; may lead to brain herniation; avoid communication between the resection cavity and the ventricular system to prevent wafer migration; communications larger than the wafer should be closed prior to implantation; wafer migration may cause obstructive hydrocephalus. **[U.S. Boxed Warning]: Injection: Should be administered under the supervision of an experienced cancer chemotherapy physician.**

Adverse Reactions

I.V.: Frequency not defined:

Cardiovascular: Arrhythmia (with high doses), chest pain, flushing (with rapid infusion), hypotension, tachycardia

Central nervous system: Ataxia, dizziness

Central nervous system: Ethanol intoxication (with high doses), headache

Dermatologic: Hyperpigmentation/skin burning (after skin contact)

Gastrointestinal: Nausea (common; dose related), vomiting (common; dose related), mucositis (with high doses), toxic enterocolitis (with high doses)

Hematologic: Leukopenia (common; onset: 5-6 weeks; recovery: after 1-2 weeks), thrombocytopenia (common: onset:~4 weeks; recovery: after 1-2 weeks), anemia, neutropenic fever, secondary malignancies (acute leukemia, bone marrow dysplasias)

Hepatic: Alkaline phosphatase increased, bilirubin increased, hepatic sinusoidal obstruction syndrome (SOS; veno-occlusive disease; with high doses), transaminases increased

Local: Injection site reactions (burning, erythema, necrosis, pain, swelling)

Ocular: Conjunctival suffusion (with rapid infusion), neuroretinitis

Renal: Kidney size decreased, progressive azotemia, renal failure

Respiratory: Interstitial pneumonitis (with high doses), pulmonary fibrosis, pulmonary hypoplasia, pulmonary infiltrates

Miscellaneous: Allergic reaction, infection (with high doses)

Wafer:

≥4% (percentages reported only where incidence was greater compared to placebo):

Cardiovascular: Deep thrombophlebitis (10%), facial edema (6%), chest pain (5%)

Central nervous system: Brain edema (4% to 23%), confusion (10% to 23%), depression (16%), headache (15%), somnolence (14%), fever (12%), speech disorder (11%), intracranial hypertension (9%), anxiety (7%), facial paralysis (7%), pain (7%), ataxia (6%), hypesthesia (6%), hallucination (5%), seizure (grand mal 5%), meningitis (4%)

Dermatologic: Abnormal wound healing (14% to 16%), rash (5% to 12%)

Endocrine: Diabetes (5%)

Gastrointestinal: Nausea (8% to 22%), vomiting (8% to 21%), constipation (19%), abdominal pain (8%), diarrhea (5%)

Genitourinary: Urinary tract infection (21%)

Hematologic: Hemorrhage (7%)

Local: Abscess (4% to 8%)

Neuromuscular & skeletal: Weakness (22%), back pain (7%)

<1%, postmarketing, and/or case reports: Abnormal thinking, allergic reaction, amnesia, aspiration pneumonia, cerebral hemorrhage, cerebral infarction, coma, cyst formation, diplopia, dizziness, dysphagia, eye pain, fecal incontinence, gastrointestinal hemorrhage, hydrocephalus, hyperglycemia, hyper-/hypotension, hypokalemia, hyponatremia, insomnia, leukocytosis, monoplegia, neck pain, paranoia, peripheral edema, sepsis, thrombocytopenia, urinary incontinence, visual field defect

Drug Interactions

Metabolism/Transport Effects None known.

Avoid Concomitant Use

Avoid concomitant use of Carmustine with any of the following: BCG; CloZAPine; Natalizumab; Pimecrolimus; Tacrolimus (Topical); Vaccines (Live)

Increased Effect/Toxicity

Carmustine may increase the levels/effects of: CloZAPine; Leflunomide; Natalizumab; Vaccines (Live)

The levels/effects of Carmustine may be increased by: Cimetidine; Denosumab; Melphalan; Pimecrolimus; Roflumilast; Tacrolimus (Topical); Trastuzumab

Decreased Effect

Carmustine may decrease the levels/effects of: BCG; Cardiac Glycosides; Coccidioidin Skin Test; Sipuleucel-T; Vaccines (Inactivated); Vaccines (Live)

The levels/effects of Carmustine may be decreased by: Echinacea

Storage/Stability

Injection: Store intact vials under refrigeration at 2°C to 8°C (36°F to 46°F); provided diluent may be stored in refrigerator or at room temperature; intact vials are stable for 7 days at room temperature. Reconstituted solutions are stable for 24 hours refrigerated (2°C to 8°C) and protected from light. Solutions diluted to a concentration of 0.2 mg/mL in D_5W are stable for 8 hours at room temperature (25°C) in glass or polyolefin containers and protected from light.

Wafer: Store at or below -20°C (-4°F). Unopened foil pouches may be kept at room temperature for up to 6 hours.

Reconstitution Injection: Reconstitute initially with 3 mL of supplied diluent (dehydrated alcohol injection, USP); then further dilute with SWFI (27 mL), this provides a concentration of 3.3 mg/mL in ethanol 10%; protect from light; further dilute for infusion with D_5W using a non-PVC container.

Mechanism of Action Interferes with the normal function of DNA and RNA by alkylation and cross-linking the strands of DNA and RNA, and by possible protein modification; may also inhibit enzyme processes by carbamylation of amino acids in protein

Pharmacodynamics/Kinetics

Distribution: 3.3 L/kg; readily crosses blood-brain barrier producing CSF levels >50% of blood plasma levels; highly lipid soluble

Metabolism: Rapidly hepatic; forms active metabolites

Half-life elimination: Biphasic: Initial: 1.4 minutes; Secondary: 20 minutes (active metabolites: plasma half-life of 67 hours)

Excretion: Urine (~60% to 70%) within 96 hours; lungs (6% to 10% as CO_2)

Dosing

Adult & Geriatric

Brain tumors, Hodgkin's lymphoma, multiple myeloma, non-Hodgkin's lymphoma (per manufacturer labeling): I.V.: 150-200 mg/m^2 every 6 weeks or 75-100 mg/m^2/day for 2 days every 6 weeks

Glioblastoma multiforme (recurrent), newly-diagnosed high-grade malignant glioma: Implantation (wafer): 8 wafers placed in the resection cavity (total dose 61.6 mg); should the size and shape not accommodate 8 wafers, the maximum number of wafers allowed (up to 8) should be placed

Indication-specific dosing:

Brain tumor, primary (unlabeled doses): I.V.:

80 mg/m^2/day for 3 days every 8 weeks for 6 cycles (Brandes, 2004)

200 mg/m^2 every 8 weeks [maximum cumulative dose: 1500 mg/m^2] (Selker, 2002)

Hodgkin's lymphoma, relapsed or refractory (unlabeled dose): I.V.: Mini-BEAM regimen: 60 mg/m² day 1 every 4-6 weeks (in combination with etoposide, cytarabine, and melphalan) (Colwill, 1995; Martin, 2001)

Multiple myeloma, relapsed, refractory (unlabeled dose): I.V.: VBMCP regimen: 20 mg/m² day 1 every 35 days (in combination with vincristine, melphalan, cyclophosphamide, and prednisone) (Kyle, 2006; Oken, 1997)

Mycosis fungoides, early stage (unlabeled use; Zackheim, 2003): Topical:

Ointment (10 mg/100 grams petrolatum): Apply (with gloves) once daily to affected areas

Solution (0.2% solution in alcohol; dilute 5 mL in 60 mL water): Apply (with gloves) once daily to affected areas

Stem cell or bone marrow transplant, autologous (unlabeled use): I.V.:

BEAM regimen: 300 mg/m² 6 days prior to transplant (in combination with etoposide, cytarabine, and melphalan) (Chopra, 1993; Linch, 2010)

CBV regimen: 600 mg/m² 3 days prior to transplant (in combination with cyclophosphamide and etoposide) (Reece, 1991)

Renal Impairment I.V.: The FDA-approved labeling does not contain renal dosing adjustment guidelines. The following dosage adjustments have been used by some clinicians (Kintzel, 1995):

Cl_{cr} 46-60 mL/minute: Administer 80% of dose

Cl_{cr} 31-45 mL/minute: Administer 75% of dose

Cl_{cr} ≤30 mL/minute: Consider use of alternative drug.

Hepatic Impairment Dosage adjustment may be necessary; however, no specific guidelines are available.

Adjustment for Toxicity Hematologic toxicity: Based on nadir counts with previous dose (manufacturer's labeling). I.V.:

If leukocytes >3000/mm³ and platelets >75,000/mm³: Administer 100% of dose

If leukocytes 2000-2999/mm³ or platelets 25,000-74,999/mm³: Administer 70% of dose

If leukocytes <2000/mm³ or platelets <25,000/mm³: Administer 50% of dose

Combination Regimens

Lymphoma, Hodgkin:

Dexa-BEAM (Hodgkin) on page 1607

mini-BEAM (Hodgkin) on page 1712

Multiple myeloma: VBMCP (Multiple Myeloma) on page 1769

Administration

Injection: Hazardous agent; use appropriate precautions for handling and disposal. Irritant (alcohol-based diluent). Significant absorption to PVC containers; should be prepared in either glass or polyolefin containers. Infuse over 2 hours (infusions <2 hours may lead to injection site pain or burning); infuse through a free-flowing saline or dextrose infusion, or administer through a central catheter to alleviate venous pain/irritation.

High-dose carmustine (transplant dose; unlabeled use): Infuse over a least 2 hours to avoid excessive flushing, agitation, and hypotension; was infused over 1 hour in some trials (Chopra, 1993). **High-dose carmustine may be fatal if not followed by stem cell rescue.** Monitor vital signs frequently during infusion; patients should be supine during infusion and may require the Trendelenburg position, fluid support, and vasopressor support.

Implant: Hazardous agent; use appropriate precautions for handling and disposal; double glove before handling; outer gloves should be discarded as chemotherapy waste after handling wafers. Any wafer or remnant that is removed upon repeat surgery should be discarded as chemotherapy waste. The outer surface of the external foil pouch is not sterile. Open pouch gently; avoid pressure on the wafers to prevent breakage. Wafer that are broken in half may be used, however, wafers broken into more than 2 pieces should be discarded in a biohazard container. Oxidized regenerated cellulose (Surgicel®) may be placed over the wafer to secure; irrigate cavity prior to closure.

Topical (unlabeled use): Hazardous agent; use appropriate precautions for handling and disposal. Apply solution with brush or gauze pads; ointment and solution should be applied while wearing gloves to involved areas only; avoid contact with eyes or mouth (Zackheim, 2003).

Emetic Potential

>250 mg/m^2: Very high (>90%)

≤250 mg/m^2: Moderate (30% to 90%)

Vesicant/Extravasation Risk Irritant; infiltration may result in local pain, erythema, swelling, burning and skin necrosis; the alcohol-based diluent may be an irritant, especially with high doses.

Monitoring Parameters CBC with differential and platelet count (weekly for at least 6 weeks after a dose), pulmonary function tests (FVC, DL_{CO}; at baseline and frequently during treatment), liver function (periodically), renal function tests (periodically); monitor blood pressure and vital signs during administration, monitor infusion site for possible infiltration

Wafer: Complications of craniotomy (seizures, intracranial infection, brain edema)

Dosage Forms Excipient information presented when available (limited, particularly for generics); consult specific product labeling.

Injection, powder for reconstitution:

BiCNU®: 100 mg [supplied with diluent]

Wafer, for implantation:

Gliadel®: 7.7 mg (8s)

References

Brandes AA, Tosoni A, Amistà P, et al, "How Effective is BCNU in Recurrent Glioblastoma in the Modern Era? A Phase II Trial," *Neurology*, 2004, 63(7):1281-4.

Chopra R, McMillan AK, Linch DC, et al, "The Place of High-Dose BEAM Therapy and Autologous Bone Marrow Transplantation in Poor-Risk Hodgkin's Disease. A Single-Center Eight-Year Study of 155 Patients," *Blood*, 1993, 81(5):1137-45.

Colwill R, Crump M, Couture F, et al,, "Mini-BEAM as Salvage Therapy for Relapsed or Refractory Hodgkin's Disease Before Intensive Therapy and Autologous Bone Marrow Transplantation," *J Clin Oncol*, 1995, 13(2):396-402.

Durando X, Lemaire JJ, Tortochaux J, et al, "High-Dose BCNU Followed by Autologous Hematopoietic Stem Cell Transplantation in Supratentorial High-Grade Malignant Gliomas: A Retrospective Analysis of 114 Patients," *Bone Marrow Transplant*, 2003, 31(7):559-64.

Fleming AB and Saltzman WM, "Pharmacokinetics of the Carmustine Implant," *Clin Pharmacokinet*, 2002, 41(6):403-19.

Kim JE, Lee DH, Yoo C, et al, "BEAM or BuCyE High-Dose Chemotherapy Followed by Autologous Stem Cell Transplantation in Non-Hodgkin's Lymphoma Patients: A Single Center Comparative Analysis of Efficacy and Toxicity," *Leuk Res*, 2011, 35(2):183-7.

Kintzel PE and Dorr RT, "Anticancer Drug Renal Toxicity and Elimination: Dosing Guidelines for Altered Renal Function," *Cancer Treat Rev*, 1995, 21(1):33-64.

Kyle RA, Leong T, Li S, et al, "Complete Response in Multiple Myeloma: Clinical Trial E9486, an Eastern Cooperative Oncology Group Study Not Involving Stem Cell Transplantation," *Cancer*, 2006, 106(9):1958-66.

Linch DC, Yung L, Smith P, et al, "Final Analysis of the UKLG LY02 Trial Comparing 6-8 Cycles of CHOP With 3 Cycles of CHOP Followed by a BEAM Autograft in Patients <65 Years With Poor Prognosis Histologically Aggressive NHL," *Br J Haematol*, 2010, 149(2):237-43.

Mahendra P, Johnson D, Scott MA, et al, "Peripheral Blood Progenitor Cell Transplantation: A Single Centre Experience Comparing Two Mobilisation Regimens in 67 Patients," *Bone Marrow Transplant*, 1996, 17(4):503-7.

Martín A, Fernández-Jiménez MC, Caballero MD, et al, "Long-Term Follow-Up in Patients Treated With Mini-BEAM as Salvage Therapy for Relapsed or Refractory Hodgkin's Disease," *Br J Haematol*, 2001, 113(1):161-71.

Oken MM, Harrington DP, Abramson N, et al, "Comparison of Melphalan and Prednisone With Vincristine, Carmustine, Melphalan, Cyclophosphamide, and Prednisone in the Treatment of Multiple Myeloma: Results of Eastern Cooperative Oncology Group Study E2479," *Cancer*, 1997, 79(8):1561-7.

Reece DE, Barnett MJ, Connors JM, et al, "Intensive Chemotherapy With Cyclophosphamide, Carmustine, and Etoposide Followed by Autologous Bone Marrow Transplantation for Relapsed Hodgkin's Disease," *J Clin Oncol*, 1991, 9(10):1871-9.

Selker RG, Shapiro WR, Burger P, et al, "The Brain Tumor Cooperative Group NIH Trial 87-01: A Randomized Comparison of Surgery, External Radiotherapy, and Carmustine Versus Surgery, Interstitial Radiotherapy Boost, External Radiation Therapy, and Carmustine," *Neurosurgery*, 2002, 51(2):343-55.

Zackheim HS, "Topical Carmustine (BCNU) in the Treatment of Mycosis Fungoides," *Dermatol Ther*, 2003,16(4):299-302.

◆ **Carmustine Polymer Wafer** *see* Carmustine *on page 243*

◆ **Carmustinum** *see* Carmustine *on page 243*

◆ **Casodex®** *see* Bicalutamide *on page 178*

Caspofungin (kas poe FUN jin)

Brand Names: U.S. Cancidas®

Brand Names: Canada Cancidas®

Index Terms Caspofungin Acetate

Generic Availability (U.S.) No

Pharmacologic Category Antifungal Agent, Parenteral; Echinocandin

Use Treatment of invasive *Aspergillus* infections in patients who are refractory or intolerant of other therapy; treatment of candidemia and other *Candida* infections (intra-abdominal abscesses, esophageal, peritonitis, pleural space); empirical treatment for presumed fungal infections in febrile neutropenic patient

Labeled Contraindications Hypersensitivity to caspofungin or any component of the formulation

Pregnancy Risk Factor C

Lactation Excretion in breast milk unknown/use caution

Warnings/Precautions Concurrent use of cyclosporine should be limited to patients for whom benefit outweighs risk, due to a high frequency of hepatic transaminase elevations observed during concurrent use. Use caution in hepatic impairment; increased transaminases and rare cases of liver impairment have been reported in pediatric and adult patients. Dosage reduction required in adults with moderate hepatic impairment; safety and efficacy have not been established in children with any degree of hepatic impairment and adults with severe hepatic impairment.

Storage/Stability Store vials at 2°C to 8°C (36°F to 46°F). Reconstituted solution may be stored at ≤25°C (≤77°F) for 1 hour prior to preparation of infusion solution. Infusion solutions may be stored at ≤25°C (≤77°F) and should be used within 24 hours; up to 48 hours if stored at 2°C to 8°C (36°F to 46°F).

Reconstitution Bring refrigerated vial to room temperature. Reconstitute vials using 0.9% sodium chloride for injection, SWFI, or bacteriostatic water for injection. Mix gently until clear solution is formed; do not use if cloudy or contains particles. Solution should be further diluted with 0.9%, 0.45%, or 0.225% sodium chloride or LR (do not exceed final concentration of 0.5 mg/mL).

Mechanism of Action Inhibits synthesis of β(1,3)-D-glucan, an essential component of the cell wall of susceptible fungi. Highest activity in regions of active cell growth. Mammalian cells do not require β(1,3)-D-glucan, limiting potential toxicity.

Pharmacodynamics/Kinetics

Protein binding: ~97% to albumin

Metabolism: Slowly, via hydrolysis and *N*-acetylation as well as by spontaneous degradation, with subsequent metabolism to component amino acids. Overall metabolism is extensive.

Half-life elimination: Beta (distribution): 9-11 hours; Terminal: 40-50 hours

Excretion: Urine (41%; primarily as metabolites, ~1% of total dose as unchanged drug); feces (35%; primarily as metabolites)

Dosing

Adult & Geriatric Note: Duration of caspofungin treatment should be determined by patient status and clinical response. Empiric therapy should be given until neutropenia resolves. In patients with positive cultures, treatment should continue until 14 days after last positive culture. In neutropenic patients, treatment should be given at least 7 days after both signs and symptoms of infection **and** neutropenia resolve.

Aspergillosis, invasive: I.V.: Initial dose: 70 mg on day 1; subsequent dosing: 50 mg/day. If clinical response inadequate, may increase up to 70 mg/day if tolerated, but increased efficacy not demonstrated. **Note:** Duration of therapy should be a minimum of 6-12 weeks or throughout period of immunosuppression.

Candidiasis: I.V.: Initial dose: 70 mg on day 1; subsequent dosing: 50 mg/day; higher doses (150 mg once daily infused over ~2 hours) compared to the standard adult dosing regimen (50 mg once daily) have not demonstrated additional benefit or toxicity in patients with invasive candidiasis (Betts, 2009)

Esophageal: 50 mg/day; **Note:** The majority of patients studied for this indication also had oropharyngeal involvement.

Empiric therapy: I.V.: Initial dose: 70 mg on day 1; subsequent dosing: 50 mg/day; if clinical response inadequate, may increase up to 70 mg/day if tolerated, but increased efficacy not demonstrated

Dosage adjustment with concomitant use of an enzyme inducer:

Patients receiving rifampin: 70 mg caspofungin daily

Patients receiving carbamazepine, dexamethasone, efavirenz, nevirapine, or phenytoin (and possibly other enzyme inducers) may require an increased daily dose of caspofungin (70 mg/day).

Pediatric

Aspergillosis, candidiasis, empiric therapy: Children >3 months to 17 years: I.V.: Initial dose: 70 mg/m^2 on day 1, subsequent dosing: 50 mg/m^2 once daily, may increase to 70 mg/m^2 once daily if clinical response inadequate (maximum dose: 70 mg)

Dosage adjustment with concomitant use of an enzyme inducer: Patients receiving carbamazepine, dexamethasone, efavirenz, nevirapine, phenytoin, or rifampin (and possibly other enzyme inducers): Consider 70 mg/m^2 once daily (maximum: 70 mg/day)

Renal Impairment No dosage adjustment required in renal impairment.

Poorly dialyzed; no supplemental dose or dosage adjustment necessary, including patients on intermittent hemodialysis, peritoneal dialysis, or continuous renal replacement therapy (eg, CVVHD).

Hepatic Impairment

Children: Mild-to-severe hepatic insufficiency: No clinical experience

Adults:

Mild hepatic insufficiency (Child-Pugh score 5-6): No adjustment necessary.

Moderate hepatic insufficiency (Child-Pugh score 7-9): 70 mg on day 1 (where recommended), followed by 35 mg once daily.

Severe hepatic insufficiency (Child-Pugh score >9): No clinical experience.

Administration Infuse slowly, over 1 hour; monitor during infusion. Isolated cases of possible histamine-related reactions have occurred during clinical trials (rash, flushing, pruritus, facial edema).

Dosage Forms Excipient information presented when available (limited, particularly for generics); consult specific product labeling.

Injection, powder for reconstitution, as acetate:

Cancidas®: 50 mg [contains sucrose 39 mg]

Cancidas®: 70 mg [contains sucrose 54 mg]

◆ **Caspofungin Acetate** *see* Caspofungin *on page* 249

◆ **Cathflo® Activase®** *see* Alteplase *on page* 55

◆ **Cayston®** *see* Aztreonam *on page* 145

◆ **CB-1348** *see* Chlorambucil *on page* 270

◆ **CB7630** *see* Abiraterone Acetate *on page* 26

◆ **CBDCA** *see* CARBOplatin *on page* 229

◆ **CC-5013** *see* Lenalidomide *on page* 859

◆ **CCI-779** *see* Temsirolimus *on page* 1337

◆ **CCNU** *see* Lomustine *on page* 904

◆ **2-CdA** *see* Cladribine *on page* 298

◆ **CDDP** *see* CISplatin *on page* 290

◆ **CDX** *see* Bicalutamide *on page* 178

◆ **CeeNU®** *see* Lomustine *on page* 904

Cefepime (SEF e pim)

Brand Names: U.S. Maxipime® [DSC]

Brand Names: Canada Maxipime®

Index Terms Cefepime Hydrochloride

Generic Availability (U.S.) Yes

Pharmacologic Category Antibiotic, Cephalosporin (Fourth Generation)

Use Treatment of uncomplicated and complicated urinary tract infections, including pyelonephritis caused by *Escherichia coli, Klebsiella pneumoniae,* or *Proteus mirabilis*; monotherapy for febrile neutropenia; uncomplicated skin and skin structure infections caused by *Streptococcus pyogenes* or methicillin-susceptible staphylococci; moderate-to-severe pneumonia caused by *Streptococcus pneumoniae, Pseudomonas aeruginosa, Klebsiella pneumoniae*, or *Enterobacter* species; complicated intra-abdominal infections (in combination with metronidazole) caused by *E. coli, P. aeruginosa, K. pneumoniae, Enterobacter* species, or *Bacteroides fragilis* against methicillin-susceptible staphylococci, *Enterobacter* sp, and many other gram-negative bacilli.

Children 2 months to 16 years: Empiric therapy of febrile neutropenia patients, uncomplicated skin/soft tissue infections, pneumonia, and uncomplicated/complicated urinary tract infections, including pyelonephritis.

Unlabeled Use Brain abscess (postneurosurgical prevention); malignant otitis externa; septic lateral/cavernous sinus thrombosis

Labeled Contraindications Hypersensitivity to cefepime, other cephalosporins, penicillins, other beta-lactam antibiotics, or any component of the formulation

Pregnancy Risk Factor B

Lactation Enters breast milk/use caution

Warnings/Precautions Severe neurological reactions (some fatal) have been reported, including encephalopathy, myoclonus, seizures, and nonconvulsive status epilepticus; risk may be increased in the presence of renal impairment (Cl_{cr} ≤60 mL/minute); ensure dose adjusted for renal function or discontinue therapy if patient develops neurotoxicity; effects are often reversible upon discontinuation of cefepime. Use with caution in patients with a history of penicillin or cephalosporin allergy, especially IgE-mediated reactions (eg, anaphylaxis, urticaria). Prolonged use may result in fungal or bacterial superinfection, including *C. difficile*-associated diarrhea (CDAD) and pseudomembranous colitis; CDAD has been observed >2 months postantibiotic treatment. Use with caution in patients with a history of gastrointestinal disease, especially colitis. May be associated with increased INR, especially in nutritionally-deficient patients, prolonged treatment, hepatic or renal disease. Use with caution in patients with a history of seizure disorder; high levels, particularly in the presence of renal impairment, may increase risk of seizures.

Storage/Stability

Vials: Store at 20°C to 25°C (68°F to 77°F). Protect from light. After reconstitution, stable in normal saline, D_5W, and a variety of other solutions for 24 hours at room temperature and 7 days refrigerated.

Premixed solution: Store frozen at -20°C (-4°F). Thawed solution is stable for 24 hours at room temperature or 7 days under refrigeration; do not refreeze.

Mechanism of Action Inhibits bacterial cell wall synthesis by binding to one or more of the penicillin-binding proteins (PBPs) which in turn inhibits the final transpeptidation step of peptidoglycan synthesis in bacterial cell walls, thus inhibiting cell wall biosynthesis. Bacteria eventually lyse due to ongoing activity of cell wall autolytic enzymes (autolysis and murein hydrolases) while cell wall assembly is arrested.

Pharmacodynamics/Kinetics

Absorption: I.M.: Rapid and complete

Distribution: V_d: Adults: 16-20 L; penetrates into inflammatory fluid at concentrations ~80% of serum levels and into bronchial mucosa at levels ~60% of those reached in the plasma; crosses blood-brain barrier

Protein binding, plasma: ~20%

Metabolism: Minimally hepatic

Half-life elimination: 2 hours

Time to peak: I.M.: 1-2 hours; I.V.: 0.5 hours

Excretion: Urine (85% as unchanged drug)

Dosing

Adult & Geriatric

Brain abscess, postneurosurgical prevention (unlabeled use): I.V.: 2 g every 8 hours with vancomycin

Febrile neutropenia, monotherapy: I.V: 2 g every 8 hours for 7 days or until the neutropenia resolves

Intra-abdominal infections, complicated, severe (in combination with metronidazole): I.V.: 2 g every 12 hours for 7-10 days. **Note:** 2010 IDSA guidelines recommend 2 g every 8-12 hours for 4-7 days (provided source controlled). Not recommended for hospital-acquired intra-abdominal infections (IAI) associated with multidrug-resistant gram negative organisms or in mild-to-moderate community-acquired IAIs due to risk of toxicity and the development of resistant organisms (Solomkin, [IDSA] 2010).

Otitis externa, malignant (unlabeled use): I.V.: 2 g every 12 hours

Pneumonia: I.V.:

Nosocomial (HAP/VAP): 1-2 g every 8-12 hours; **Note:** Duration of therapy may vary considerably (7-21 days); usually longer courses are required if *Pseudomonas*. In absence of *Pseudomonas*, and if appropriate empiric treatment used and patient responsive, it may be clinically appropriate to reduce duration of therapy to 7-10 days (American Thoracic Society Guidelines, 2005).

Community-acquired (including pseudomonal): 1-2 g every 12 hours for 10 days

Septic lateral/cavernous sinus thrombosis (unlabeled use): I.V.: 2 g every 8-12 hours; with metronidazole for lateral

Skin and skin structure, uncomplicated: I.V.: 2 g every 12 hours for 10 days

Urinary tract infections, complicated and uncomplicated:

Mild-to-moderate: I.M., I.V.: 0.5-1 g every 12 hours for 7-10 days

Severe: I.V.: 2 g every 12 hours for 10 days

Pediatric

Febrile neutropenia: I.V.: 50 mg/kg/dose every 8 hours for 7 days or until neutropenia resolves

Skin and skin structure infections (uncomplicated) and pneumonia: I.V.: 50 mg/kg/dose every 12 hours for 10 days

Urinary tract infections, complicated and uncomplicated: I.V., I.M.: 50 mg/kg/dose every 12 hours for 7-10 days; **Note:** I.M. may be considered for mild-to-moderate infection only.

Renal Impairment

Children: No dosage adjustment provided in the manufacturer's labeling; however, similar dosage adjustments to adults would be anticipated based on comparable pharmacokinetics between children and adults.

Adults: Recommended maintenance schedule based on creatinine clearance (may be estimated using the Cockcroft-Gault formula), compared to normal dosing schedule: See table.

Cefepime Hydrochloride

Creatinine Clearance (mL/minute)	Recommended Maintenance Schedule			
>60 (normal recommended dosing schedule)	500 mg every 12 hours	1 g every 12 hours	2 g every 12 hours	2 g every 8 hours
30-60	500 mg every 24 hours	1 g every 24 hours	2 g every 24 hours	2 g every 12 hours
11-29	500 mg every 24 hours	500 mg every 24 hours	1 g every 24 hours	2 g every 24 hours
<11	250 mg every 24 hours	250 mg every 24 hours	500 mg every 24 hours	1 g every 24 hours

Intermittent hemodialysis (IHD) (administer after hemodialysis on dialysis days): I.V.: Initial: 1 g (single dose) on day 1. Maintenance: 0.5-1 g every 24 hours **or** 1-2 g every 48-72 hours (Heintz, 2009). **Note:** Dosing dependent on the assumption of 3 times/week, complete IHD sessions.

Peritoneal dialysis (PD): Removed to a lesser extent than hemodialysis; administer normal recommended dose every 48 hours

Continuous renal replacement therapy (CRRT) (Heintz, 2009; Trotman, 2005): Drug clearance is highly dependent on the method of renal replacement, filter type, and flow rate. Appropriate dosing requires close monitoring of pharmacologic response, signs of adverse reactions due to drug accumulation, as well as drug concentrations in relation to target trough (if appropriate). The following are general recommendations only (based on dialysate flow/ultrafiltration rates of 1-2 L/hour and minimal residual renal function) and should not supersede clinical judgment:

CVVH: Loading dose of 2 g followed by 1-2 g every 12 hours

CVVHD/CVVHDF: Loading dose of 2 g followed by either 1 g every 8 hours **or** 2 g every 12 hours. **Note:** Dosage of 1 g every 8 hours results in similar steady-state concentrations as 2 g every 12 hours and is more cost effective (Heintz, 2009).

Note: Consider higher dosage of 4 g/day if treating *Pseudomonas* or life-threatening infections in order to maximize time above MIC (Trotman, 2005). Dosage of 2 g every 8 hours may be needed for gram-negative rods with MIC ≥4 mg/L (Heintz, 2009).

Administration May be administered either I.M. or I.V.

Inject deep I.M. into large muscle mass. Inject direct I.V. over 5 minutes. Infuse intermittent infusion over 30 minutes.

Test Interactions Positive direct Coombs', false-positive urinary glucose test using cupric sulfate (Benedict's solution, Clinitest®, Fehling's solution), false-positive serum or urine creatinine with Jaffé reaction, false-positive urinary proteins and steroids

Dosage Forms Excipient information presented when available (limited, particularly for generics); consult specific product labeling. [DSC] = Discontinued product

Infusion, premixed iso-osmotic dextrose solution, as hydrochloride: 1 g (50 mL); 2 g (100 mL)

Injection, powder for reconstitution, as hydrochloride: 500 mg, 1 g, 2 g

Maxipime®: 500 mg [DSC], 1 g [DSC], 2 g [DSC]

◆ **Cefepime Hydrochloride** *see* Cefepime *on page* 251

CefTAZidime (SEF tay zi deem)

Brand Names: U.S. Fortaz®; Tazicef®

Brand Names: Canada Ceftazidime For Injection; Fortaz®

Generic Availability (U.S.) Yes: Injection

Pharmacologic Category Antibiotic, Cephalosporin (Third Generation)

Use Treatment of documented susceptible *Pseudomonas aeruginosa* infection and infections due to other susceptible aerobic gram-negative organisms; empiric therapy of a febrile, granulocytopenic patient

Unlabeled Use Bacterial endophthalmitis

Labeled Contraindications Hypersensitivity to ceftazidime, any component of the formulation, or other cephalosporins

Pregnancy Risk Factor B

Lactation Enters breast milk/use caution (AAP rates "compatible"; AAP 2001 update pending)

Warnings/Precautions Modify dosage in patients with severe renal impairment. Use with caution in patients with a history of penicillin allergy, especially IgE-mediated reactions (eg, anaphylaxis, urticaria). Prolonged use may result in fungal or bacterial superinfection, including *C. difficile*-associated diarrhea (CDAD) and pseudomembranous colitis; CDAD has been observed >2 months postantibiotic treatment. May be associated with increased INR, especially in nutritionally-deficient patients, prolonged treatment, hepatic or renal disease. Use with caution in patients with a history of seizure disorder; high levels, particularly in the presence of renal impairment, may increase risk of seizures.

Storage/Stability

Fortaz®: Store dry vials at 15°C to 30°C (59°F to 86°F). Protect from light. Reconstituted solution and solution further diluted for I.V. infusion are stable for 12 hours at room temperature, for 3 days when refrigerated, or for 12 weeks when frozen at -20°C (-4°F). After freezing, thawed solution in SWFI for I.M. administration is stable for 3 hours at room temperature or for 3 days when refrigerated; thawed solution in NS in a Viaflex® small volume container for I.V. administration is stable for 12 hours at room temperature or for 3 days when refrigerated; and thawed solution in SWFI in the original container is stable for 8 hours at room temperature or for 3 days when refrigerated.

Premixed frozen solution: Store frozen at -20°C (-4°F). Thawed solution is stable for 8 hours at room temperature or for 3 days under refrigeration; do not refreeze.

Fortaz®, Tazicef®: ADD-Vantage® vials: Following dilution, may be stored for up to 12 hours at room temperature or for 3 days under refrigeration. Freezing solutions in the ADD-Vantage® system is not recommended. Joined vials that have not been activated may be used within 14 days.

Tazicef® vials: Store dry vials at 20°C to 25°C (68°F to 77°F). Protect from light. Reconstituted vials and solution further diluted for I.V. infusion are stable for 24 hours at room temperature, for 7 days when refrigerated, or for 12 weeks when frozen at -20°C (-4°F). When thawed, solution is stable for 8 hours at room temperature and 4 days when refrigerated.

Reconstitution

I.M.: Using SWFI, bacteriostatic water, lidocaine 0.5%, or lidocaine 1%, reconstitute the 500 mg vials with 1.5 mL or the 1 g vials with 3 mL; final concentration of ~*280 mg/mL*

I.V.: Using SWFI, reconstitute as follows (**Note:** After reconstitution, may dilute further with a compatible solution to administer via I.V. infusion):

Fortaz®:

~*100 mg/mL solution:*

500 mg vial: 5.3 mL SWFI (withdraw 5 mL from the reconstituted vial to obtain a 500 mg dose)

1 g vial: 10 mL SWFI (withdraw 10 mL from the reconstituted vial to obtain a 1 g dose)

6 g vial: 56 mL SWFI (withdraw 10 mL from the reconstituted vial to obtain a 1 g dose)

~*170 mg/mL solution:* 2 g vial: 10 mL SWFI (withdraw 11.5 mL from the reconstituted vial to obtain a 2 g dose)

~*200 mg/mL solution:* 6 g vial: 26 mL SWFI (withdraw 5 mL from the reconstituted vial to obtain a 1 g dose)

Tazicef®:

~95 mg/mL solution: 1 g vial: 10 mL SWFI (withdraw 10.6 mL from the reconstituted vial to obtain a 1 g dose)

~180 mg/mL solution: 2 g vial: 10 mL SWFI (withdraw 11.2 mL from the reconstituted vial to obtain a 2 g dose)

Fortaz®, Tazicef®: ADD-Vantage® vials: Dilute in 50 or 100 mL of D_5W, NS, or 0.45% sodium chloride in an ADD-Vantage® flexible diluent container only.

Mechanism of Action Inhibits bacterial cell wall synthesis by binding to one or more of the penicillin-binding proteins (PBPs) which in turn inhibits the final transpeptidation step of peptidoglycan synthesis in bacterial cell walls, thus inhibiting cell wall biosynthesis. Bacteria eventually lyse due to ongoing activity of cell wall autolytic enzymes (autolysins and murein hydrolases) while cell wall assembly is arrested.

Pharmacodynamics/Kinetics

Distribution: Widely throughout the body including bone, bile, skin, CSF (higher concentrations achieved when meninges are inflamed), endometrium, heart, pleural and lymphatic fluids

Protein binding: 17%

Half-life elimination: 1-2 hours, prolonged with renal impairment; Neonates <23 days: 2.2-4.7 hours

Time to peak, serum: I.M.: ~1 hour

Excretion: Urine (80% to 90% as unchanged drug)

Dosing

Adult

Bacterial arthritis (gram negative bacilli): I.V.: 1-2 g every 8 hours

Bone and joint infections: I.V.: 2 g every 12 hours

Cystic fibrosis, lung infection caused by *Pseudomonas* spp: I.V.: 30-50 mg/kg/dose every 8 hours (maximum: 6 g/day)

Endophthalmitis, bacterial (unlabeled use): Intravitreal: 2.25 mg/0.1 mL NS in combination with vancomycin

Intra-abdominal infection, severe (in combination with metronidazole): I.V.: 2 g every 8 hours for 4-7 days (provided source controlled). Not recommended for hospital-acquired intra-abdominal infections (IAI) associated with multidrug-resistant gram negative organisms or in mild-to-moderate community-acquired IAIs due to risk of toxicity and the development of resistant organisms (Solomkin, 2010).

Melioidosis: I.V.: 40 mg/kg/dose every 8 hours for 10 days, followed by oral therapy with doxycycline or TMP/SMX

Otitis externa: I.V.: 2 g every 8 hours

Peritonitis (CAPD):

Anuric, intermittent: 1000-1500 mg/day

Anuric, continuous (per liter exchange): Loading dose: 250 mg; maintenance dose: 125 mg

Pneumonia: I.V.:

Uncomplicated: 500 mg to 1 g every 8 hours

Complicated or severe: 2 g every 8 hours

Skin and soft tissue infections: I.V., I.M.: 500 mg to 1 g every 8 hours

Severe infections, including meningitis, complicated pneumonia, endophthalmitis, CNS infection, osteomyelitis, gynecological, skin and soft tissue: I.V.: 2 g every 8 hours

Urinary tract infections: I.V., I.M.:
Uncomplicated: 250 mg every 12 hours
Complicated: 500 mg every 8-12 hours

Geriatric I.M., I.V.: Dosage should be based on renal function with a dosing interval not more frequent then every 12 hours.

Pediatric Susceptible infections: I.V.:
Children 1 month to 12 years: 30-50 mg/kg/dose every 8 hours; maximum dose: 6 g/day (higher doses reserved for immunocompromised patients, cystic fibrosis, or meningitis)
Children ≥12 years: Refer to adult dosing

Renal Impairment
Cl_{cr} 30-50 mL/minute: Administer every 12 hours
Cl_{cr} 10-30 mL/minute: Administer every 24 hours
Cl_{cr} <10 mL/minute: Administer every 48-72 hours
Intermittent hemodialysis (IHD) (administer after hemodialysis on dialysis days): Dialyzable (50% to 100%): 0.5-1 g every 24 hours **or** 1-2 g every 48-72 hours (Heintz, 2009). **Note:** Dosing dependent on the assumption of 3 times/week, complete IHD sessions.
Peritoneal dialysis (PD): Loading dose of 1 g, followed by 500 mg every 24 hours
Continuous renal replacement therapy (CRRT) (Heintz, 2009; Trotman, 2005): Drug clearance is highly dependent on the method of renal replacement, filter type, and flow rate. Appropriate dosing requires close monitoring of pharmacologic response, signs of adverse reactions due to drug accumulation, as well as drug concentrations in relation to target trough (if appropriate). The following are general recommendations only (based on dialysate flow/ultrafiltration rates of 1-2 L/hour and minimal residual renal function) and should not supersede clinical judgment:
CVVH: Loading dose of 2 g followed by 1-2 g every 12 hours
CVVHD/CVVHDF: Loading dose of 2 g followed by either 1 g every 8 hours **or** 2 g every 12 hours. **Note:** Dosage of 1 g every 8 hours results in similar steady-state concentrations as 2 g every 12 hours and is more cost effective. Dosage of 2 g every 8 hours may be needed for gram-negative rods with MIC ≥4 mg/L (Heintz, 2009).
Note: For patients receiving CVVHDF, some recommend giving a loading dose of 2 g followed by 3 g over 24 hours as a continuous I.V. infusion to maintain concentrations ≥4 times the MIC for susceptible pathogens (Heintz, 2009).

Administration Any carbon dioxide bubbles that may be present in the withdrawn solution should be expelled prior to injection. Administer around-the-clock to promote less variation in peak and trough serum levels. Ceftazidime can be administered deep I.M. into large mass muscle, IVP over 3-5 minutes, or I.V. intermittent infusion over 15-30 minutes. Do not admix with aminoglycosides in same bottle/bag. Final concentration for I.V. administration should not exceed 100 mg/mL.

Test Interactions Positive direct Coombs', false-positive urinary glucose test using cupric sulfate (Benedict's solution, Clinitest®, Fehling's solution), false-positive serum or urine creatinine with Jaffé reaction

Dosage Forms Excipient information presented when available (limited, particularly for generics); consult specific product labeling. [DSC] = Discontinued product

Infusion, premixed iso-osmotic solution, as sodium [strength expressed as base]:
Fortaz®: 1 g (50 mL); 2 g (50 mL) [contains sodium ~54 mg (2.3 mEq)/g]
Injection, powder for reconstitution: 500 mg [DSC], 1 g, 2 g, 6 g
Fortaz®: 500 mg, 1 g, 2 g, 6 g [contains sodium ~54 mg (2.3 mEq)/g]
Tazicef®: 1 g, 2 g, 6 g [contains sodium ~54 mg (2.3 mEq)/g]

◆ **Ceftazidime For Injection (Can)** *see* CefTAZidime *on page* 254

CefTRIAXone (sef trye AKS one)

Brand Names: U.S. Rocephin®

Brand Names: Canada Ceftriaxone for Injection; Ceftriaxone Sodium for Injection BP; Rocephin®

Index Terms Ceftriaxone Sodium

Generic Availability (U.S.) Yes

Pharmacologic Category Antibiotic, Cephalosporin (Third Generation)

Use Treatment of lower respiratory tract infections, acute bacterial otitis media, skin and skin structure infections, bone and joint infections, intra-abdominal and urinary tract infections, pelvic inflammatory disease (PID), uncomplicated gonorrhea, bacterial septicemia, and meningitis; used in surgical prophylaxis

Unlabeled Use Treatment of chancroid, epididymitis, complicated gonococcal infections; sexually-transmitted diseases (STD); periorbital or buccal cellulitis; salmonellosis or shigellosis; atypical community-acquired pneumonia; acute bacterial rhinosinusitis (ABRS); epiglottitis, Lyme disease; used in chemoprophylaxis for high-risk contacts (close exposure to patients with invasive meningococcal disease); sexual assault; typhoid fever, Whipple's disease

Labeled Contraindications Hypersensitivity to ceftriaxone sodium, any component of the formulation, or other cephalosporins; **do not use in hyperbilirubinemic neonates**, particularly those who are premature since ceftriaxone is reported to displace bilirubin from albumin binding sites; concomitant use with intravenous calcium-containing solutions/products in neonates (≤28 days)

Pregnancy Risk Factor B

Lactation Enters breast milk/use caution (AAP rates "compatible"; AAP 2001 update pending)

Warnings/Precautions Use with caution in patients with a history of penicillin allergy, especially IgE-mediated reactions (eg, anaphylaxis, urticaria). Abnormal gallbladder sonograms have been reported, possibly due to cetriaxone-calcium precipitates; discontinue in patients who develop signs and symptoms of gallbladder disease. Secondary to biliary obstruction, pancreatitis has been reported rarely. Use with caution in patients with a history of GI disease, especially colitis. Severe cases (including some fatalities) of immune-related hemolytic anemia have been reported in patients receiving cephalosporins, including ceftriaxone. Prolonged use may result in fungal or bacterial superinfection, including *C. difficile*-associated diarrhea (CDAD) and pseudomembranous colitis; CDAD has been observed >2 months postantibiotic treatment.

May be associated with increased INR (rarely), especially in nutritionally-deficient patients, prolonged treatment, hepatic or renal disease. No adjustment is generally necessary in patients with renal impairment; use with caution in patients with concurrent hepatic dysfunction and significant renal disease, dosage should not exceed 2 g/day. Ceftriaxone may complex with calcium causing precipitation. Fatal lung and kidney damage associated with calcium-ceftriaxone precipitates has been observed in premature and term neonates.

Do not reconstitute, admix, or coadminister with calcium-containing solutions, even via separate infusion lines/sites or at different times in any neonatal patient. Ceftriaxone should not be diluted or administered simultaneously with any calcium-containing solution via a Y-site in any patient. However, ceftriaxone and calcium-containing solution may be administered sequentially of one another for use in patients **other than neonates** if infusion lines are thoroughly flushed, with a compatible fluid, between infusions

Storage/Stability

Powder for injection: Prior to reconstitution, store at room temperature ≤25°C (≤77°F). Protect from light.

Premixed solution (manufacturer premixed): Store at -20°C; once thawed, solutions are stable for 3 days at room temperature of 25°C (77°F) or for 21 days refrigerated at 5°C (41°F). Do not refreeze.

Stability of reconstituted solutions:

10-40 mg/mL: Reconstituted in D_5W, $D_{10}W$, NS, or SWFI: Stable for 2 days at room temperature of 25°C (77°F) or for 10 days when refrigerated at 4°C (39°F). Stable for 26 weeks when frozen at -20°C when reconstituted with D_5W or NS. Once thawed (at room temperature), solutions are stable for 2 days at room temperature of 25°C (77°F) or for 10 days when refrigerated at 4°C (39°F); does not apply to manufacturer's premixed bags. Do not refreeze.

100 mg/mL:

Reconstituted in D_5W, SWFI, or NS: Stable for 2 days at room temperature of 25°C (77°F) or for 10 days when refrigerated at 4°C (39°F).

Reconstituted in lidocaine 1% solution or bacteriostatic water: Stable for 24 hours at room temperature of 25°C (77°F) or for 10 days when refrigerated at 4°C (39°F).

250-350 mg/mL: Reconstituted in D_5W, NS, lidocaine 1% solution, bacteriostatic water, or SWFI: Stable for 24 hours at room temperature of 25°C (77°F) or for 3 days when refrigerated at 4°C (39°F).

Reconstitution

I.M. injection: Vials should be reconstituted with appropriate volume of diluent (including D_5W, NS, SWFI, bacteriostatic water, or 1% lidocaine) to make a final concentration of 250 mg/mL or 350 mg/mL.

Volume to add to create a **250 mg/mL** solution:

250 mg vial: 0.9 mL
500 mg vial: 1.8 mL
1 g vial: 3.6 mL
2 g vial: 7.2 mL

Volume to add to create a **350 mg/mL** solution:

500 mg vial: 1.0 mL
1 g vial: 2.1 mL
2 g vial: 4.2 mL

I.V. infusion: Infusion is prepared in two stages: Initial reconstitution of powder, followed by dilution to final infusion solution.

Vials: Reconstitute powder with appropriate I.V. diluent (including SWFI, D_5W, $D_{10}W$, NS) to create an initial solution of ~100 mg/mL. Recommended volume to add:

250 mg vial: 2.4 mL
500 mg vial: 4.8 mL
1 g vial: 9.6 mL
2 g vial: 19.2 mL

Note: After reconstitution of powder, further dilution into a volume of compatible solution (eg, 50-100 mL of D_5W or NS) is recommended.

Piggyback bottle: Reconstitute powder with appropriate I.V. diluent (D_5W or NS) to create a resulting solution of ~100 mg/mL. Recommended initial volume to add:

1 g bottle:10 mL

2 g bottle: 20 mL

Note: After reconstitution, to prepare the final infusion solution, further dilution to 50 mL or 100 mL volumes with the appropriate I.V. diluent (including D_5W or NS) is recommended.

Mechanism of Action Inhibits bacterial cell wall synthesis by binding to one or more of the penicillin-binding proteins (PBPs) which in turn inhibits the final transpeptidation step of peptidoglycan synthesis in bacterial cell walls, thus inhibiting cell wall biosynthesis. Bacteria eventually lyse due to ongoing activity of cell wall autolytic enzymes (autolysins and murein hydrolases) while cell wall assembly is arrested.

Pharmacodynamics/Kinetics

Absorption: I.M.: Well absorbed

Distribution: V_d: 6-14 L; widely throughout the body including gallbladder, lungs, bone, bile, CSF (higher concentrations achieved when meninges are inflamed)

Protein binding: 85% to 95%

Half-life elimination: Normal renal and hepatic function: 5-9 hours; Renal impairment (mild-to-severe): 12-16 hours

Time to peak, serum: I.M.: 2-3 hours

Excretion: Urine (33% to 67% as unchanged drug); feces (as inactive drug)

Dosing

Adult & Geriatric

Dosage range: Usual dose: 1-2 g every 12-24 hours, depending on the type and severity of infection

Acute bacterial rhinosinusitis, severe infection requiring hospitalization (unlabeled use): I.V.: 1-2 g every 12-24 hours for 5-7 days (Chow, 2012)

Arthritis, septic (unlabeled use): I.V.: 1-2 g once daily

Brain abscess (unlabeled use): I.V.: 2 g every 12 hours with metronidazole

Cavernous sinus thrombosis (unlabeled use): I.V.: 2 g once daily with vancomycin or linezolid

Chancroid (unlabeled use): I.M.: 250 mg as single dose (CDC, 2010)

Chemoprophylaxis for high-risk contacts (close exposure to patients with invasive meningococcal disease) (unlabeled use): I.M.: 250 mg in a single dose

Cholecystitis, mild-to-moderate: 1-2 g every 12-24 hours for 4-7 days (provided source controlled)

Gonococcal infections:

Uncomplicated gonorrhea of the cervix, pharynx, urethra, or rectum (unlabeled regimen): I.M.: 250 mg in a single dose with oral azithromycin (preferred) or oral doxycycline (alternative to preferred) (CDC, 2012)

Conjunctivitis, complicated (unlabeled use): I.M.: 1 g in a single dose (CDC, 2010)

Disseminated (unlabeled use): I.M., I.V.: 1 g once daily for 24-48 hours may switch to cefixime (after improvement noted) to complete a total of 7 days of therapy (CDC, 2010)

Endocarditis (unlabeled use): I.V.: 1-2 g every 12 hours for at least 28 days (CDC, 2010)

Epididymitis, acute (unlabeled use): I.M.: 250 mg in a single dose with doxycycline (CDC, 2010)
Meningitis: I.V.: 1-2 g every 12 hours for 10-14 days (CDC, 2010)

Infective endocarditis: I.M., I.V.:
Native valve: 2 g once daily for 2-4 weeks; **Note:** If using 2-week regimen, concurrent gentamicin is recommended
Prosthetic valve: I.M., I.V.: 2 g once daily for 6 weeks (with or without 2 weeks of gentamicin [dependent on penicillin MIC]); **Note:** For HACEK organisms, duration of therapy is 4 weeks
Enterococcus faecalis (resistant to penicillin, aminoglycoside, and vancomycin), native or prosthetic valve: 2 g twice daily for ≥8 weeks administered concurrently with ampicillin
Prophylaxis: I.M., I.V.: 1 g 30-60 minutes before procedure. Intramuscular injections should be avoided in patients who are receiving anticoagulant therapy. In these circumstances, orally administered regimens should be given whenever possible. Intravenously administered antibiotics should be used for patients who are unable to tolerate or absorb oral medications.
Note: American Heart Association (AHA) guidelines now recommend prophylaxis only in patients undergoing invasive procedures and in whom underlying cardiac conditions may predispose to a higher risk of adverse outcomes should infection occur. As of April 2007, routine prophylaxis for GI/GU procedures is no longer recommended by the AHA.

Intra-abdominal infection, complicated, community-acquired, mild-to-moderate (in combination with metronidazole): 1-2 g every 12-24 hours for 4-7 days (provided source controlled)

Lyme disease (unlabeled use): I.V.: 2 g once daily for 14-28 days

Mastoiditis (hospitalized; unlabeled use): I.V.: 2 g once daily; >60 years old: 1 g once daily

Meningitis (empiric treatment): I.V.: 2 g every 12 hours for 7-14 days (longer courses may be necessary for selected organisms)

Orbital cellulitis (unlabeled use) and endophthalmitis: I.V.: 2 g once daily

Pelvic inflammatory disease: I.M.: 250 mg in a single dose plus doxycycline (with or without metronidazole) (CDC, 2010)

Pneumonia, community-acquired: I.V.: 1 g once daily, usually in combination with a macrolide; consider 2 g/day for patients at risk for more severe infection and/or resistant organisms (ICU status, age >65 years, disseminated infection)

Prophylaxis against sexually-transmitted diseases following sexual assault: I.M.: 250 mg as a single dose (in combination with azithromycin and metronidazole) (CDC, 2010)

Pyelonephritis (acute, uncomplicated): Females: I.V.: 1-2 g once daily (Stamm, 1993). Many physicians administer a single parenteral dose before initiating oral therapy (Warren, 1999).

Septic/toxic shock/necrotizing fasciitis (unlabeled use): I.V.: 2 g once daily; with clindamycin for toxic shock

Surgical prophylaxis: I.V.: 1 g 30 minutes to 2 hours before surgery
Cholecystectomy: 1-2 g every 12-24 hours, discontinue within 24 hours unless infection outside gallbladder suspected

Syphilis (unlabeled use): I.M., I.V.: 1 g once daily for 10-14 days; **Note:** Alternative treatment for early syphilis, optimal dose, and duration have not been defined (CDC, 2010)

Typhoid fever (unlabeled use): I.V.: 2 g once daily for 14 days

Whipple's disease (unlabeled use): Initial: 2 g once daily for 10-14 days, then oral therapy for ~1 year.

Pediatric

Dosage range: Infants and Children: Usual dose: I.M., I.V.:

Mild-to-moderate infections: 50-75 mg/kg/day in 1-2 divided doses every 12-24 hours (maximum: 2 g/day); continue until at least 2 days after signs and symptoms of infection have resolved

Serious infections: 80-100 mg/kg/day in 1-2 divided doses (maximum: 4 g/day)

Acute bacterial rhinosinusitis, severe infection requiring hospitalization (unlabeled use): I.V.: 50 mg/kg/day divided every 12 hours for 10-14 days (Chow, 2012)

Community-acquired pneumonia (CAP) (IDSA/PIDS, 2011): Infants >3 months and Children: I.V.: 50-100 mg/kg/day once daily or divided every 12 hours. **Note:** May consider addition of vancomycin or clindamycin to empiric therapy if community-acquired MRSA suspected. Use the higher end of the range for penicillin-resistant *S. pneumoniae*; in children ≥5 years, a macrolide antibiotic should be added if atypical pneumonia cannot be ruled out; preferred in patients not fully immunized for *H. influenzae* type b and *S. pneumoniae*, or significant local resistance to penicillin in invasive pneumococcal strains

Chemoprophylaxis for high-risk contacts (close exposure to patients with invasive meningococcal disease) (unlabeled use):

Children <15 years: I.M.: 125 mg in a single dose

Children ≥15 years: Refer to adult dosing.

Epididymitis, acute: Children >8 years (≥45 kg) and Adolescents (unlabeled use): I.M.: 125 mg in a single dose

Epiglottis (unlabeled use): I.M., I.V.: 50-100 mg/kg once daily; reported duration of treatment ranged from 2-14 days

Gonococcal infections:

Arthritis (CDC, 2010): I.M., I.V.:

≤45 kg: 50 mg/kg/dose once daily (maximum: 1 g) for 7 days

>45 kg: 50 mg/kg/dose once daily (maximum: 2 g) for 7 days

Bacteremia (CDC, 2010): I.M., I.V.:

≤45 kg: 50 mg/kg/dose once daily (maximum: 1 g) for 7 days

>45 kg: 50 mg/kg/dose once daily (maximum: 2 g) for 7 days

Conjunctivitis, complicated (unlabeled use): I.M., I.V.:

<45 kg: 50 mg/kg in a single dose (maximum: 1 g)

≥45 kg: 1 g in a single dose

Disseminated (unlabeled use): I.M., I.V.:

Infants: 25-50 mg/kg/dose once daily for 7 days (10-14 days for meningitis) (CDC, 2010); **Note**: Use contraindicated in hyperbilirubinemic neonates.

Children <45 kg: 25-50 mg/k dose once daily (maximum: 1 g) for 7 days (CDC, 2010)

Children >45 kg: Refer to adult dosing.

Endocarditis (unlabeled use):

≤45 kg: I.M., I.V.: 50 mg/kg/day every 12 hours (maximum: 2 g daily) for at least 28 days

>45 kg: I.V.: 1-2 g every 12 hours, for at least 28 days

Meningitis:

≤45 kg: I.V.: 50 mg/kg/day given every 12 hours (maximum: 2 g daily); usual duration of treatment is 10-14 days

>45 kg: I.V.: 1-2 g every 12 hours; usual duration of treatment is 10-14 days

Prophylaxis (due to maternal gonococcal infection): I.M., I.V.: 25-50 mg/kg as a single dose (maximum: 125 mg) (CDC, 2010)

Uncomplicated cervicitis, pharyngitis, proctitis, urethritis, vulvovaginitis (unlabeled use) (CDC, 2010):

≤45 kg: I.M.: 125 mg as a single dose

>45 kg: Refer to adult dosing

Infective endocarditis: I.M., I.V.:

Native valve: 100 mg/kg once daily for 2-4 weeks; **Note:** If using 2-week regimen, concurrent gentamicin is recommended

Prosthetic valve: 100 mg/kg once daily for 6 weeks (with or without 2 weeks of gentamicin [dependent on penicillin MIC]); **Note:** For HACEK organisms, duration of therapy is 4 weeks

Enterococcus faecalis (resistant to penicillin, aminoglycoside, and vancomycin), native or prosthetic valve: 100 mg/kg once daily for ≥8 weeks administered concurrently with ampicillin

Prophylaxis: 50 mg/kg 30-60 minutes before procedure; maximum dose: 1 g. Intramuscular injections should be avoided in patients who are receiving anticoagulant therapy. In these circumstances, orally administered regimens should be given whenever possible. Intravenously administered antibiotics should be used for patients who are unable to tolerate or absorb oral medications.

Note: American Heart Association (AHA) guidelines now recommend prophylaxis only in patients undergoing invasive procedures and in whom underlying cardiac conditions may predispose to a higher risk of adverse outcomes should infection occur. As of April 2007, routine prophylaxis for GI/GU procedures is no longer recommended by the AHA

Lyme disease, persistent arthritis (unlabeled use): I.M., I.V.: 75-100 mg/kg (maximum: 2 g) for 2-4 weeks

Meningitis (empiric treatment): I.M., I.V.:

Uncomplicated: Loading dose of 100 mg/kg (maximum: 4 g), followed by 100 mg/kg/day divided every 12-24 hours (maximum: 4 g/day); usual duration of treatment is 7-14 days

Gonococcal, complicated:

≤45 kg: 50 mg/kg/day given every 12 hours (maximum: 2 g/day); usual duration of treatment is 10-14 days

>45 kg: I.V.: 1-2 g every 12 hours; usual duration of treatment is 10-14 days

Ophthalmia neonatorum (unlabeled use): Infants: I.M., I.V.: 25-50 mg/kg as a single dose (maximum: 125 mg) (CDC, 2010)

Otitis media: I.M.:

Acute: 50 mg/kg in a single dose (maximum: 1 g)

Persistent or relapsing (unlabeled use): 50 mg/kg once daily for 3 days

Pneumonia: I.V.: 50-75 mg/kg once daily

Prophylaxis against sexually-transmitted diseases following sexual assault (unlabeled use):

≤45 kg: I.M.: 125 mg in a single dose (in combination with azithromycin and metronidazole) (CDC, 2010)

>45 kg: Refer to adult dosing.

Skin/skin structure infections: I.M., I.V.: 50-75 mg/kg/day in 1-2 divided doses (maximum: 2 g/day)

Typhoid fever (unlabeled use): I.V.: 75-80 mg/kg once daily for 5-14 days

Renal Impairment No dosage adjustment is generally necessary in renal impairment; **Note:** Concurrent renal and hepatic dysfunction: Maximum dose: ≤2 g/day

Poorly dialyzed; no supplemental dose or dosage adjustment necessary, including patients on intermittent hemodialysis, peritoneal dialysis, or continuous renal replacement therapy (eg, CVVHD).

Hepatic Impairment No adjustment necessary unless there is concurrent renal dysfunction (see dosage adjustment in renal impairment).

Administration Do not admix with aminoglycosides in same bottle/bag. Do not reconstitute, admix, or coadminister with calcium-containing solutions. Infuse intermittent infusion over 30 minutes.

I.M.: Inject deep I.M. into large muscle mass; a concentration of 250 mg/mL or 350 mg/mL is recommended for all vial sizes except the 250 mg size (250 mg/mL is suggested); can be diluted with 1:1 water and 1% lidocaine for I.M. administration.

I.V.: Infuse intermittent infusion over 30 minutes.

Test Interactions Positive direct Coombs', false-positive urinary glucose test using cupric sulfate (Benedict's solution, Clinitest®, Fehling's solution), false-positive serum or urine creatinine with Jaffé reaction

Dosage Forms Excipient information presented when available (limited, particularly for generics); consult specific product labeling.

Infusion, premixed in D_5W: 1 g (50 mL); 2 g (50 mL)

Injection, powder for reconstitution: 250 mg, 500 mg, 1 g, 2 g, 10 g

Rocephin®: 500 mg, 1 g [contains sodium ~83 mg (3.6 mEq) per ceftriaxone 1 g]

- **Ceftriaxone for Injection (Can)** *see* CefTRIAXone *on page* 258
- **Ceftriaxone Sodium** *see* CefTRIAXone *on page* 258
- **Ceftriaxone Sodium for Injection BP (Can)** *see* CefTRIAXone *on page* 258
- **CellCept®** *see* Mycophenolate *on page* 1015
- **Cerubidine®** *see* DAUNOrubicin (Conventional) *on page* 396
- **Cervarix®** *see* Papillomavirus (Types 16, 18) Vaccine (Human, Recombinant) *on page* 1124
- **Cesamet®** *see* Nabilone *on page* 1023

Cetuximab (se TUK see mab)

Related Information

Management of Chemotherapy-Induced Nausea and Vomiting *on page* 1786

Principles of Anticancer Therapy *on page* 1878

Brand Names: U.S. Erbitux®

Brand Names: Canada Erbitux®

Index Terms C225; IMC-C225; MOAB C225

Generic Availability (U.S.) No

Pharmacologic Category Antineoplastic Agent, Monoclonal Antibody; Epidermal Growth Factor Receptor (EGFR) Inhibitor

Use Treatment of *KRAS* mutation-negative (wild-type), EGFR-expressing metastatic colorectal cancer (in combination with FOLFIRI [irinotecan, fluorouracil, and leucovorin] as first-line treatment, in combination with irinotecan [in patients refractory to irinotecan-based chemotherapy], or as a single agent in patients who have failed oxaliplatin and irinotecan based chemotherapy or who are intolerant to irinotecan); treatment of squamous cell cancer of the head and neck (as a single agent for recurrent or metastatic disease after platinum-based chemotherapy failure; in combination with radiation therapy as initial treatment of locally or regionally advanced disease; in combination with platinum and fluorouracil-based chemotherapy as first-line treatment of locoregional or metastatic disease)

Note: Cetuximab is not indicated for the treatment of *KRAS* mutation-positive colorectal cancer.

Unlabeled Use Treatment of EGFR-expressing advanced nonsmall cell lung cancer (NSCLC); treatment of unresectable squamous cell skin cancer

Labeled Contraindications There are no contraindications listed in the manufacturer's labeling

Pregnancy Risk Factor C

Lactation Excretion in breast milk is unknown/not recommended

Warnings/Precautions [U.S. Boxed Warning]: In clinical trials, serious infusion reactions have been reported in ~3% of patients; fatal outcome has been reported rarely (<1 in 1000); interrupt infusion promptly and permanently discontinue for serious infusion reactions. Reactions have included airway obstruction (bronchospasm, stridor, hoarseness), hypotension, loss of consciousness, shock, MI, and/or cardiac arrest. Premedicate with an I.V. H_1 antagonist 30-60 minutes prior to the first dose; premedication for subsequent doses is based on clinical judgement and with consideration of prior reaction to the initial infusion. The use of nebulized albuterol-based premedication to prevent infusion reaction has been reported (Tra, 2008). Approximately 90% of reactions occur with the first infusion despite the use of prophylactic antihistamines. Immediate treatment for anaphylactic/anaphylactoid reactions should be available during administration. The manufacturer recommends monitoring patients for at least 1 hour following completion of infusion, or longer if a reaction occurs. Mild-to-moderate infusion reactions are managed by slowing the infusion rate (by 50%) and administering antihistamines. Patients with pre-existing IgE antibody against cetuximab (specific for galactose-α-1,3-galactose) are reported to have a higher incidence of severe hypersensitivity reaction. Severe hypersensitivity reaction has been reported more frequently in patients living in the middle south area of the United States, including North Carolina and Tennessee (Chung, 2008; O'Neil, 2007).

[U.S. Boxed Warning]: In patients with squamous cell head and neck cancer, cardiopulmonary arrest and/or sudden death has occurred in 2% of patients receiving radiation therapy in combination with cetuximab and in 3% of patients receiving combination chemotherapy (platinum and fluorouracil-based) with cetuximab. Closely monitor serum electrolytes (magnesium, potassium, calcium) during and after cetuximab treatment (monitor for at least 8 weeks after treatment). Use with caution in patients with history of coronary artery disease, HF, and arrhythmias; fatalities have been reported. Interstitial lung disease (ILD) has been reported, use with caution in patients with pre-existing lung disease; interrupt treatment for acute onset or worsening of pulmonary symptoms; permanently discontinue with confirmed ILD.

Acneiform rash has been reported in 76% to 88% of patients (severe in 1% to 17%), usually developing within the first 2 weeks of therapy; may require dose modification; generally resolved after discontinuation in most patients, although persisted beyond 28 days in some patients; monitor for dermatologic toxicity and corresponding infections. Acneiform rash should be treated with topical and/or oral antibiotics; topical corticosteroids are not recommended. In colorectal cancer, the presence of acneiform rash correlates with treatment response and prolonged survival (Cunningham, 2004). Other dermatologic toxicities, including dry skin, fissures, hypertrichosis, paronychial inflammation, and skin infections have been reported; related ocular toxicities (blepharitis, conjunctivitis, keratitis, ulcerative keratitis with decreased visual acuity) may also occur. Sunlight may exacerbate skin reactions (limit sun exposure). Hypomagnesemia is common (may be severe); the onset of electrolyte disturbance may occur within days to months after initiation of treatment; monitor magnesium, calcium, and potassium during treatment and for at least 8 weeks after completion; may require electrolyte replacement. Non-neutralizing anti-cetuximab antibodies were detected in 5% of evaluable patients. Safety has not been established when used in combination with radiation therapy **and** cisplatin; fatalities and serious cardiotoxicity, pneumonia or other adverse events have been observed.

In patients with colorectal cancer, cetuximab is only indicated for EGFR-expressing, *KRAS* mutation-negative metastatic colorectal cancer. Determine *KRAS* mutation status prior to treatment (the therascreen KRAS RGQ PCR Kit is approved in the U.S. to determine *KRAS* gene mutation information). Patients with a codon 12 or 13 (exon 2) *KRAS* mutation are unlikely to benefit from EGFR inhibitor therapy and should not receive cetuximab treatment; cetuximab is not effective for *KRAS* mutation-positive colorectal cancer. Cetuximab is also reported to be ineffective in patients with *BRAF* V600E mutation (Di Nicolantonio, 2008). In trials for colorectal cancer, evidence of EGFR expression was required, although the response rate did not correlate with either the percentage of cells positive for EGFR or the intensity of expression. EGFR expression has been detected in nearly all patients with head and neck cancer, therefore laboratory evidence of EGFR expression is not necessary for head and neck cancers.

Adverse Reactions Except where noted, percentages reported for studies with cetuximab monotherapy.

>10%:

Central nervous system: Fatigue (91%), pain (59%), sensory neuropathy (45%; grades 3/4: 1%), headache (38%), insomnia (27%), fever (25%), confusion (18%), anxiety (14%), chills/rigors (16%), depression (14%)

Dermatologic: Rash/desquamation (95%; grades 3/4: 16%), acneiform rash (all studies: 76% to 88%; grades 3/4: 1% to 17%; onset: ≤14 days), dry skin (57%), pruritus (47%), nail changes (31%)

Endocrine & metabolic: Hypomagnesemia (all studies: 55%; grades 3/4: 6% to 17%), dehydration (13%)

Gastrointestinal: Nausea (64%), abdominal pain (59%), constipation (53%), diarrhea (42%), vomiting (37% to 40%), stomatitis (32%), xerostomia (12%)

Neuromuscular & skeletal: Bone pain (15%), arthralgia (14%)

Respiratory: Dyspnea (48% to 49%), cough (30%)

Miscellaneous: Infection (all studies: 13% to 44%; grades 3/4: 11%), infusion reaction (all studies: 15% to 21%; grades 3/4: 2% to 5%; 90% of severe reactions occurred with first infusion)

1% to 10%:

Cardiovascular: Cardiopulmonary arrest (2%; with radiation therapy; 3% with platinum/fluorouracil-based chemotherapy)

Gastrointestinal: Taste disturbance (10%)

Renal: Renal failure (all studies: 1%)

Miscellaneous: Antibody formation (5%), sepsis (all studies: 1% to 4%)

<1%, postmarketing, and/or case reports (all studies): Abscess formation, arrhythmia, aseptic meningitis, blepharitis, bronchospasm, cardiac arrest, cellulitis, cheilitis, conjunctivitis, electrolyte abnormality, hoarseness, hypertrichosis, hypotension, interstitial lung disease (occurred between the fourth and eleventh doses), keratitis, leukopenia, loss of consciousness, MI, paronychial inflammation, pulmonary embolism, radiation dermatitis, shock, skin fissure, skin infection, stridor, ulcerative keratitis

Drug Interactions

Metabolism/Transport Effects None known.

Avoid Concomitant Use There are no known interactions where it is recommended to avoid concomitant use.

Increased Effect/Toxicity There are no known significant interactions involving an increase in effect.

Decreased Effect There are no known significant interactions involving a decrease in effect.

Storage/Stability Store unopened vials refrigerated at 2°C to 8°C (36°F to 46°F); do not freeze. Preparations in infusion containers are stable for up to 12 hours refrigerated at 2°C to 8°C (36°F to 46°F) and up to 8 hours at room temperature of 20°C to 25°C (68°F to 77°F).

Reconstitution Reconstitution is not required. Appropriate dose should be added to empty sterile container (may contain a small amount of visible white, amorphous cetuximab particles); do not shake or dilute. Discard unused portion of the vial.

Mechanism of Action Recombinant human/mouse chimeric monoclonal antibody which binds specifically to the epidermal growth factor receptor (EGFR, HER1, c-ErbB-1) and competitively inhibits the binding of epidermal growth factor (EGF) and other ligands. Binding to the EGFR blocks phosphorylation and activation of receptor-associated kinases, resulting in inhibition of cell growth, induction of apoptosis, and decreased matrix metalloproteinase and vascular endothelial growth factor production. EGFR signal transduction results in *KRAS* wild-type activation; cells with *KRAS* mutations appear to be unaffected by EGFR inhibition.

Pharmacodynamics/Kinetics

Distribution: V_d: ~2-3 L/m^2

Half-life elimination: ~112 hours (range: 63-230 hours)

Dosing

Adult & Geriatric Note: Premedicate with an H_1 antagonist (eg, diphenhydramine) I.V. 30-60 minutes prior to the first dose; premedication for subsequent doses is based on clinical judgement.

Colorectal cancer, metastatic, KRAS mutation-negative (wild-type): I.V.:

Initial loading dose: 400 mg/m^2 infused over 120 minutes

Maintenance dose: 250 mg/m^2 infused over 60 minutes weekly until disease progression or unacceptable toxicity

Note: If given in combination with FOLFIRI (irinotecan, fluorouracil, and leucovorin), complete cetuximab infusion 1 hour prior to FOLFIRI.

Head and neck cancer (squamous cell): I.V.:

Initial loading dose: 400 mg/m^2 infused over 120 minutes

Maintenance dose: 250 mg/m^2 infused over 60 minutes weekly

Note: If given in combination with radiation therapy, administer loading dose 1 week prior to initiation of radiation course; weekly maintenance dose should be completed 1 hour prior to radiation for the duration of radiation therapy (6-7 weeks). If given in combination with chemotherapy, administer loading dose on the day of initiation of platinum and fluorouracil-based chemotherapy, cetuximab infusion should be completed 1 hour prior to initiation of chemotherapy; weekly maintenance dose should be completed 1 hour prior to chemotherapy; continue until disease progression or unacceptable toxicity. Monotherapy weekly doses should be continued until disease progression or unacceptable toxicity

Colorectal cancer, advanced, biweekly administration (unlabeled dosing): I.V.: 500 mg/m^2 every 2 weeks (initial dose infused over 120 minutes, subsequent doses infused over 60 minutes) in combination with irinotecan (Pfeiffer, 2008)

Nonsmall cell lung cancer (NSCLC), EGFR-expressing, advanced (unlabeled use): I.V.: Initial loading dose: 400 mg/m^2, followed by maintenance dose: 250 mg/m^2 weekly in combination with cisplatin and vinorelbine for up to 6 cycles, then as monotherapy until disease progression or unacceptable toxicity (Pirker, 2009; Pirker, 2012)

Squamous cell skin cancer, unresectable (unlabeled use): I.V.: Initial loading dose: 400 mg/m^2, followed by maintenance dose: 250 mg/m^2 weekly until disease progression (Maubec, 2011)

Adjustment for Toxicity

Infusion reactions, grade 1 or 2 and nonserious grade 3: Reduce the infusion rate by 50% and continue to use prophylactic antihistamines

Infusion reactions, severe: Immediately and permanently discontinue treatment

Pulmonary toxicity:
- Acute onset or worsening pulmonary symptoms: Hold treatment
- Interstitial lung disease: Permanently discontinue

Skin toxicity, mild-to-moderate: No dosage modification required

Acneiform rash, severe (grade 3 or 4):
- First occurrence: Delay cetuximab infusion 1-2 weeks
  - If improvement, continue at 250 mg/m^2
  - If no improvement, discontinue therapy
- Second occurrence: Delay cetuximab infusion 1-2 weeks
  - If improvement, continue at reduced dose of 200 mg/m^2
  - If no improvement, discontinue therapy
- Third occurrence: Delay cetuximab infusion 1-2 weeks
  - If improvement, continue at reduced dose of 150 mg/m^2
  - If no improvement, discontinue therapy
- Fourth occurrence: Discontinue therapy

Note: Dose adjustments are not recommended for severe **radiation** dermatitis.

Combination Regimens

Colorectal cancer:

Cetuximab Biweekly (Colorectal Regimen) on page 1556
Cetuximab (Biweekly)-Irinotecan on page 1557
Cetuximab (Colorectal Regimen) on page 1559
Cetuximab + FOLFIRI (Colorectal) on page 1559
Cetuximab-FOLFOX4 on page 1560
Cetuximab-Irinotecan (Colorectal) on page 1561

Head and neck cancer:

Carboplatin-Cetuximab (Head and Neck Cancer) on page 1543
Cetuximab-Carboplatin-Fluorouracil (Head and Neck Cancer) on page 1557
Cetuximab-Cisplatin-Fluorouracil (Head and Neck Cancer) on page 1558
Cisplatin-Cetuximab (Head and Neck Cancer) on page 1566
Paclitaxel-Cetuximab on page 1727

Lung cancer (nonsmall cell): Cetuximab-Cisplatin-Vinorelbine (NSCLC) on page 1558

Administration Administer via I.V. infusion; loading dose over 2 hours, weekly maintenance dose over 1 hour. Do not administer as I.V. push or bolus. Do not shake or dilute. Administer via infusion pump or syringe pump. Following the infusion, an observation period (1 hour) is recommended; longer observation time (following an infusion reaction) may be required. Premedication with an H_1 antagonist prior to the initial dose is recommended. The maximum infusion rate is 10 mg/minute. Administer through a low protein-binding 0.22 micrometer in-line filter. Use 0.9% NaCl to flush line at the end of infusion.

For biweekly administration (unlabeled frequency and dose), the initial dose was infused over 120 minutes and subsequent doses infused over 60 minutes (Pfeiffer, 2007; Pfeiffer, 2008).

Emetic Potential Minimal (<10%)

Monitoring Parameters Vital signs during infusion and observe for at least 1 hour postinfusion. Patients developing dermatologic toxicities should be monitored for the development of complications. Periodic monitoring of serum magnesium, calcium, and potassium are recommended to continue over an interval consistent with the half-life (8 weeks); monitor closely (during and after treatment) for cetuximab plus radiation therapy. *KRAS* genotyping of tumor tissue in patients with colorectal cancer (the therascreen *KRAS* RGQ PCR Kit is approved in the U.S. to determine *KRAS* gene mutation status [codon 12 or 13])

Additional Information Oncology Comment: The National Comprehensive Cancer Network® (NCCN) guidelines for colon cancer (v.3.2012) and the American Society of Clinical Oncology (ASCO) provisional clinical opinion (Allegra, 2009) recommend genotyping tumor tissue for *KRAS* mutation in all patients with metastatic colorectal cancer (genotyping may be done on archived specimens). Patients with known codon 12 or 13 *KRAS* gene mutations are unlikely to respond to EGFR inhibitors and should not receive cetuximab. Favorable progression-free survival and overall survival has been demonstrated with cetuximab in patients with *KRAS* wild-type (Karapetis, 2008; Van Cutsem, 2008). Cetuximab is also reported to be ineffective in patients with *BRAF* V600E mutation (Di Nicolantonio, 2008). Because EGFR testing in colorectal tumors does not correlate with response, the NCCN guidelines do not recommend routine EGFR testing in colorectal cancer. Dermatologic toxicity with cetuximab is predictive for response; the presence of acneiform rash correlates with treatment response and prolonged survival (Cunningham, 2004).

Dosage Forms Excipient information presented when available (limited, particularly for generics); consult specific product labeling.

Injection, solution [preservative free]:

Erbitux®: 2 mg/mL (50 mL, 100 mL)

References

Allegra CJ, Jessup JM, Somerfield MR, et al, "American Society of Clinical Oncology Provisional Clinical Opinion: Testing for *KRAS* Gene Mutations in Patients With Metastatic Colorectal Carcinoma to Predict Response to Anti-Epidermal Growth Factor Receptor Monoclonal Antibody Therapy, " *J Clin Oncol*, 2009, 27(12):2091-6.

Chung CH, Mirakhur B, Chan E, et al, "Cetuximab-Induced Anaphylaxis and IgE Specific for Galactose-alpha-1,3-galactose," *N Engl J Med*, 2008, 358(11):1109-17

Cunningham D, Humblet Y, Siena S, et al, "Cetuximab Monotherapy and Cetuximab Plus Irinotecan in Irinotecan-Refractory Metastatic Colorectal Cancer," *N Engl J Med*, 2004, 351 (4):337-45.

Di Nicolantonio F, Martini M, Molinari F, et al, "Wild-type BRAF is Required for Response to Panitumumab or Cetuximab in Metastatic Colorectal Cancer," *J Clin Oncol*, 2008, 26 (35):5705-12.

Karapetis CS, Khambata-Ford S, Jonker DJ, et al, "K-ras Mutations and Benefit From Cetuximab in Advanced Colorectal Cancer," *N Engl J Med*, 2008, 359(17):1757-65.

Kies MS and Harari PM, "Cetuximab (Imclone/Merck/Bristol-Myers Squibb)," *Curr Opin Investig Drugs*, 2002, 3(7):1092-100.

Maubec E, Petrow P, Scheer-Senyarich I, et al, "Phase II Study of Cetuximab as First-Line Single-Drug Therapy in Patients With Unresectable Squamous Cell Carcinoma of the Skin," *J Clin Oncol*, 2011, 29(25):3419-26.

National Comprehensive Cancer Network® (NCCN), "Clinical Practice Guidelines in Oncology™: Colon Cancer," Version 3.2012. Available at http://www.nccn.org/professionals/physician_gls/PDF/colon.pdf

O'Neil BH, Allen R, Spigel DR, et al, "High Incidence of Cetuximab-Related Infusion Reactions in Tennessee and North Carolina and the Association With Atopic History," *J Clin Oncol*, 2007, 25 (24):3644-8.

Pfeiffer P, Bjerregarrd JK, Qvortrup C, et al, "Simplification of Cetuximab (Cet) Administration: Double Dose Every Second Week as a 60 Minute Infusion," *J Clin Oncol*, 2007, 25(18S):4133 [abstract 4133 from 2007 ASCO Annual Meeting Proceedings, Part I].

Pfeiffer P, Nielsen D, Bjerregaard J, et al, "Biweekly Cetuximab and Irinotecan as Third-Line Therapy in Patients With Advanced Colorectal Cancer After Failure to Irinotecan, Oxaliplatin and 5-Fluorouracil," *Ann Oncol*, 2008, 19(6):1141-5.

Pirker R, Pereira JR, Szczesna A, et al, "Cetuximab Plus Chemotherapy in Patients With Advanced Non-Small-Cell Lung Cancer (FLEX): An Open-Label Randomised Phase III Trial," *Lancet*, 2009, 373(9674):1525-31.

Tra F, Fesen MR, Pianalto M, et al, "Albuterol-Based Premedication Therapy for the Prevention of Cetuximab Infusion-Related Reactions," *J Clin Oncol*, 2008, 26(Supp):17040 [abstract 17040 from ASCO 2008 Annual Meeting].

Van Cutsem E, Köhne CH, Láng I, et al, "Cetuximab Plus Irinotecan, Fluorouracil, and Leucovorin as First-Line Treatment for Metastatic Colorectal Cancer: Updated Analysis of Overall Survival According to Tumor *KRAS* and *BRAF* Mutation Status," *J Clin Oncol*, 2011, 29(15):2011-9.

Van Cutsem E, Lang, I, D'haens G, et al, "*KRAS* Status and Efficacy in the First-Line Treatment of Patients With Metastatic Colorectal Cancer (mCRC) Treated With FOLFIRI With or Without Cetuximab: The CRYSTAL Experience," *J Clin Oncol*, 2008, 26(Supp):2 [abstract 2 from ASCO 2008 Annual Meeting].

◆ **CGP-42446** *see* Zoledronic Acid *on page 1488*

◆ **CGP-57148B** *see* Imatinib *on page 762*

◆ **CGS-20267** *see* Letrozole *on page 867*

◆ **CGX-625** *see* Omacetaxine *on page 1064*

◆ **Chloditan** *see* Mitotane *on page 994*

◆ **Chlodithane** *see* Mitotane *on page 994*

Chlorambucil (klor AM byoo sil)

Related Information

Fertility and Cancer Therapy *on page 1782*

Management of Chemotherapy-Induced Nausea and Vomiting *on page 1786*

Safe Handling of Hazardous Drugs *on page 1904*

Brand Names: U.S. Leukeran®

Brand Names: Canada Leukeran®

Index Terms CB-1348; Chlorambucilum; Chloraminophene; Chlorbutinum; WR-139013

Generic Availability (U.S.) No

Pharmacologic Category Antineoplastic Agent, Alkylating Agent

Use Management of chronic lymphocytic leukemia (CLL), Hodgkin lymphoma, non-Hodgkin's lymphomas (NHL)

Canadian labeling: Additional uses (not in U.S. labeling): Management of Waldenström's macroglobulinemia

Unlabeled Use Treatment of nephrotic syndrome (steroid sensitive) in children; treatment of Waldenström's macroglobulinemia (unlabeled in U.S.)

Labeled Contraindications Hypersensitivity to chlorambucil or any component of the formulation; hypersensitivity to other alkylating agents (may have cross-hypersensitivity); prior (demonstrated) resistance to chlorambucil

Canadian labeling: Additional contraindications (not in U.S. labeling): Use within 4 weeks of a full course of radiation or chemotherapy

Pregnancy Risk Factor D

Lactation Excretion in breast milk unknown/not recommended

Warnings/Precautions Hazardous agent - use appropriate precautions for handling and disposal. Seizures have been observed; use with caution in patients with seizure disorder or head trauma; history of nephrotic syndrome and high pulse doses are at higher risk of seizures. **[U.S. Boxed Warning]: May cause severe bone marrow suppression;** neutropenia may be severe. Reduce initial dosage if patient has received myelosuppressive or radiation therapy within the previous 4 weeks, or has a depressed baseline leukocyte or platelet count. Irreversible bone marrow damage may occur with total doses approaching 6.5 mg/kg. Progressive lymphopenia may develop (recovery is generally rapid after discontinuation). Avoid administration of live vaccines to immunocompromised patients. Rare instances of severe skin reactions (eg, erythema multiforme, Stevens-Johnson syndrome, toxic epidermal necrolysis) have been reported; discontinue promptly if skin reaction occurs.

Chlorambucil is primarily metabolized in the liver. Dosage reductions should be considered in patients with hepatic impairment. **[U.S. Boxed Warning]: Affects human fertility; carcinogenic in humans and probably mutagenic and teratogenic as well;** chromosomal damage has been documented. Reversible and irreversible sterility (when administered to prepubertal and pubertal males), azoospermia (in adult males) and amenorrhea (in females) have been observed. **[U.S. Boxed Warning]: Carcinogenic;** acute myelocytic leukemia and secondary malignancies may be associated with chronic therapy. Duration of treatment and higher cumulative doses are associated with a higher risk for development of leukemia.

Adverse Reactions Frequency not always defined.

Central nervous system: Agitation (rare), ataxia (rare), confusion (rare), drug fever, fever, focal/generalized seizure (rare), hallucinations (rare)

Dermatologic: Angioneurotic edema, erythema multiforme (rare), rash, skin hypersensitivity, Stevens-Johnson syndrome (rare), toxic epidermal necrolysis (rare), urticaria

Endocrine & metabolic: Amenorrhea, infertility, SIADH (rare)

Gastrointestinal: Diarrhea (infrequent), nausea (infrequent), oral ulceration (infrequent), vomiting (infrequent)

Genitourinary: Azoospermia, cystitis (sterile)

Hematologic: Neutropenia (onset: 3 weeks; recovery: 10 days after last dose), bone marrow failure (irreversible), bone marrow suppression, anemia, leukemia (secondary), leukopenia, lymphopenia, pancytopenia, thrombocytopenia

Hepatic: Hepatotoxicity, jaundice

Neuromuscular & skeletal: Flaccid paresis (rare), muscular twitching (rare), myoclonia (rare), peripheral neuropathy, tremor (rare)

Respiratory: Interstitial pneumonia, pulmonary fibrosis

Miscellaneous: Allergic reactions, malignancies (secondary)

Drug Interactions

Metabolism/Transport Effects None known.

Avoid Concomitant Use

Avoid concomitant use of Chlorambucil with any of the following: BCG; CloZAPine; Natalizumab; Pimecrolimus; Tacrolimus (Topical); Vaccines (Live)

Increased Effect/Toxicity

Chlorambucil may increase the levels/effects of: CloZAPine; Leflunomide; Natalizumab; Vaccines (Live)

The levels/effects of Chlorambucil may be increased by: Denosumab; Pimecrolimus; Roflumilast; Tacrolimus (Topical); Trastuzumab

Decreased Effect

Chlorambucil may decrease the levels/effects of: BCG; Coccidioidin Skin Test; Sipuleucel-T; Vaccines (Inactivated); Vaccines (Live)

The levels/effects of Chlorambucil may be decreased by: Echinacea

Ethanol/Nutrition/Herb Interactions Food: Absorption is decreased when administered with food.

Storage/Stability Store in refrigerator at 2°C to 8°C (36°F to 46°F).

Mechanism of Action Alkylating agent; interferes with DNA replication and RNA transcription by alkylation and cross-linking the strands of DNA

Pharmacodynamics/Kinetics

Absorption: Rapid and complete (>70%); reduced with food
Distribution: V_d: ~0.3 L/kg
Protein binding: ~99%; primarily to albumin
Metabolism: Hepatic (extensively); primarily to active metabolite, phenylacetic acid mustard
Half-life elimination: ~1.5 hours; Phenylacetic acid mustard: ~1.8 hours
Time to peak, plasma: Within 1 hour; Phenylacetic acid mustard: 1.2-2.6 hours
Excretion: Urine (~20% to 60%, primarily as inactive metabolites, <1% as unchanged drug or phenylacetic acid mustard)

Dosing

Adult Note: With bone marrow lymphocytic infiltration involvement (in CLL, Hodgkin lymphoma, or NHL), the maximum dose is 0.1 mg/kg/day. While short treatment courses are preferred, if maintenance therapy is required, the maximum dose is 0.1 mg/kg/day.

Chronic lymphocytic leukemia (CLL): Oral:

U.S. labeling: 0.1 mg/kg/day for 3-6 weeks **or** 0.4 mg/kg pulsed doses administered intermittently, biweekly, or monthly (increased by 0.1 mg/kg/dose until response/toxicity observed)

Canadian labeling: Initial: 0.15 mg/kg/day until WBC is 10,000/mm^3; interrupt treatment for 4 weeks, then may resume at 0.1 mg/kg/day until response (generally ~2 years)/toxicity observed

Unlabeled dosing: 30 mg/m^2 day 1 every 2 weeks (in combination with prednisone) (Raphael, 1991) **or** 0.4 mg/kg day 1 every 2 weeks; if tolerated may increase by 0.1 mg/kg with each treatment course to a maximum dose of 0.8 mg/kg and maximum of 24 cycles (Eichhorst, 2009) **or** 40 mg/m^2 day 1 every 4 weeks until disease progression or complete remission or response plateau for up to a maximum of 12 cycles (Rai, 2000)

Hodgkin lymphoma: Oral:

U.S. labeling: 0.2 mg/kg/day for 3-6 weeks
Canadian labeling: 0.2 mg/kg/day for 4-8 weeks

Non-Hodgkin's lymphomas (NHL): Oral

U.S. labeling: 0.1 mg/kg/day for 3-6 weeks

Canadian labeling: Initial: 0.1-0.2 mg/kg/day for 4-8 weeks; for maintenance treatment, reduce dose or administer intermittently

Waldenström's macroglobulinemia (U.S. unlabeled use): Oral: 0.1 mg/kg/day (continuously) for at least 6 months **or** 0.3 mg/kg/day for 7 days every 6 weeks for at least 6 months (Kyle, 2000)

Geriatric Refer to adult dosing. Begin at the lower end of dosing range(s)

Pediatric Nephrotic syndrome, steroid sensitive (unlabeled use): Oral: 0.2 mg/kg once daily for ~8 weeks (Hodson, 2010)

Renal Impairment No dosage adjustment provided in manufacturer's labeling; however, renal elimination of unchanged chlorambucil and active metabolite (phenylacetic acid mustard) is minimal and renal impairment is not likely to affect elimination. The following adjustments have been recommended:

Adults:

Aronoff, 2007:

Cl_{cr} >50 mL/minute: No adjustment necessary.

Cl_{cr} 10-50 mL/minute: Administer 75% of dose.

Cl_{cr} <10 mL/minute: Administer 50% of dose.

Peritoneal dialysis (PD): Administer 50% of dose.

Kintzel, 1995: Based on the pharmacokinetics, dosage adjustment is not indicated

Hepatic Impairment Chlorambucil undergoes extensive hepatic metabolism. Although dosage reduction should be considered in patients with hepatic impairment, no dosage adjustment is provided in the manufacturer's labeling (data is insufficient).

Adjustment for Toxicity

Skin reactions: Discontinue treatment

Hematologic:

WBC or platelets below normal: Reduce dose.

Severely depressed WBC or platelet counts: Discontinue.

Persistently low neutrophil or platelet counts or peripheral lymphocytosis: May be suggestive of bone marrow infiltration; if infiltration confirmed, do not exceed 0.1 mg/kg/day.

Concurrent or within 4 weeks (before or after) of chemotherapy/radiotherapy: Initiate treatment cautiously; reduce dose; monitor closely.

Combination Regimens

Leukemia, chronic lymphocytic:

Chlorambucil (CLL Regimen) on page 1563

Chlorambucil-Prednisone (CLL) on page 1563

Lymphoma, Hodgkin: ChlVPP (Hodgkin) on page 1562

Administration Usually administered as a single dose; preferably on an empty stomach.

Emetic Potential Very low (<10%)

Extemporaneous Preparations Hazardous agent: Use appropriate precautions for handling and disposal.

A 2 mg/mL oral suspension may be made with tablets. Crush sixty 2 mg tablets in a mortar and reduce to a fine powder. Add small portions of methylcellulose 1% and mix to a uniform paste (total methylcellulose: 30 mL); mix while adding simple syrup in incremental proportions to **almost** 60 mL; transfer to a graduated cylinder, rinse mortar and pestle with simple syrup, and add quantity of vehicle sufficient to make 60 mL. Transfer contents of graduated cylinder to an amber prescription bottle. Label "shake well", "refrigerate", and "protect from light". Stable for 7 days refrigerated.

Dressman JB and Poust RI, "Stability of Allopurinol and of Five Antineoplastics in Suspension," *Am J Hosp Pharm*, 1983, 40(4):616-8.

Nahata MC, Pai VB, and Hipple TF, *Pediatric Drug Formulations*, 5th ed, Cincinnati, OH: Harvey Whitney Books Co, 2004.

Monitoring Parameters Liver function tests, CBC with differential (weekly, with WBC monitored twice weekly during the first 3-6 weeks of treatment)

Dosage Forms Excipient information presented when available (limited, particularly for generics); consult specific product labeling.

Tablet, oral:

Leukeran®: 2 mg

References

Aronoff GR, Bennett WM, Berns JS, et al, *Drug Prescribing in Renal Failure: Dosing Guidelines for Adults and Children*, 5th ed. Philadelphia, PA: American College of Physicians; 2007, p 98.

Eichhorst BF, Busch R, Stilgenbauer S, et al, "First-Line Therapy With Fludarabine Compared With Chlorambucil Does Not Result in a Major Benefit for Elderly Patients With Advanced Chronic Lymphocytic Leukemia," *Blood*, 2009, 114(16):3382-91.

Hodson EM, Willis NS, and Craig JC, "Non-Corticosteroid Treatment for Nephrotic Syndrome in Children (Review)," *Cochrane Database Syst Rev*, 2010, (4):CD002290.

Kintzel PE and Dorr RT, "Anticancer Drug Renal Toxicity and Elimination: Dosing Guidelines for Altered Renal Function," *Cancer Treat Rev*, 1995, 21(1):33-64.

Kyle RA, Greipp PR, Gertz MA, et al, "Waldenström's Macroglobulinemia: A Prospective Study Comparing Daily With Intermittent Oral Chlorambucil," *Br J Haematol*, 2000, 108(4):737-42.

Rai KR, Peterson BL, Appelbaum FR, et al, "Fludarabine Compared With Chlorambucil as Primary Therapy for Chronic Lymphocytic Leukemia," *N Engl J Med*, 2000, 343(24):1750-7.

Raphael B, Andersen JW, Silber R, et al, "Comparison of Chlorambucil and Prednisone Versus Cyclophosphamide, Vincristine, and Prednisone as Initial Treatment for Chronic Lymphocytic Leukemia: Long-Term Follow-Up of an Eastern Cooperative Oncology Group Randomized Clinical Trial," *J Clin Oncol*, 1991, 9(5):770-6.

Robinson RF, Nahata MC, Mahan JD, "Management of Nephrotic Syndrome in Children," *Pharmacotherapy*, 2003, 23(8):1021-36.

◆ **Chlorambucilum** *see* Chlorambucil *on page 270*

◆ **Chloraminophene** *see* Chlorambucil *on page 270*

◆ **Chlorbutinum** *see* Chlorambucil *on page 270*

◆ **Chlorethazine** *see* Mechlorethamine *on page 913*

◆ **Chlorethazine Mustard** *see* Mechlorethamine *on page 913*

◆ **Chlormeprazine** *see* Prochlorperazine *on page 1212*

◆ **2-Chlorodeoxyadenosine** *see* Cladribine *on page 298*

ChlorproMAZINE (klor PROE ma zeen)

Related Information

Hospice (End of Life) Care *on page 1857*

Management of Chemotherapy-Induced Nausea and Vomiting *on page 1786*

Palliative Care Medicine (Cancer) *on page 1871*

Brand Names: Canada Chlorpromazine Hydrochloride Inj; Teva-Chlorpromazine

Index Terms Chlorpromazine Hydrochloride; CPZ; Thorazine

Generic Availability (U.S.) Yes

Pharmacologic Category Antimanic Agent; Antipsychotic Agent, Typical, Phenothiazine

Use Management of psychotic disorders (control of mania, treatment of schizophrenia); control of nausea and vomiting; relief of restlessness and apprehension before surgery; acute intermittent porphyria; adjunct in the treatment of tetanus; intractable hiccups; combativeness and/or explosive hyperexcitable behavior in children 1-12 years of age and in short-term treatment of hyperactive children

Unlabeled Use Behavioral symptoms associated with dementia (elderly); psychosis/agitation related to Alzheimer's dementia

Labeled Contraindications Hypersensitivity to chlorpromazine or any component of the formulation (cross-reactivity between phenothiazines may occur); severe CNS depression; coma

Lactation Enters breast milk/not recommended (AAP rates "of concern"; AAP 2001 update pending)

Warnings/Precautions **[U.S. Boxed Warning]: Elderly patients with dementia-related psychosis treated with antipsychotics are at an increased risk of death compared to placebo.** Most deaths appeared to be either cardiovascular (eg, heart failure, sudden death) or infectious (eg, pneumonia) in nature. Chlorpromazine is not approved for the treatment of dementia-related psychosis. Highly sedating, use with caution in disorders where CNS depression is a feature and in patients with Parkinson's disease. Use with caution in patients with hemodynamic instability, predisposition to seizures, subcortical brain damage, severe cardiac, hepatic, or renal disease. Use caution in respiratory disease (eg, severe asthma, emphysema) due to potential for CNS effects.

Leukopenia, neutropenia, and agranulocytosis (sometimes fatal) have been reported in clinical trials and postmarketing reports with antipsychotic use; presence of risk factors (eg, pre-existing low WBC or history of drug-induced leuko/neutropenia) should prompt periodic blood count assessment. Discontinue therapy at first signs of blood dyscrasias or if absolute neutrophil count $<1000/mm^3$

Esophageal dysmotility and aspiration have been associated with antipsychotic use; use with caution in patients at risk of aspiration pneumonia (ie, Alzheimer's disease). Use associated with increased prolactin levels; clinical significance of hyperprolactinemia in patients with breast cancer or other prolactin-dependent tumors is unknown. May alter temperature regulation or mask toxicity of other drugs due to antiemetic effects. May alter cardiac conduction; life-threatening arrhythmias have occurred with therapeutic doses of neuroleptics. May cause QT prolongation and subsequent torsade de pointes; avoid use in patients with diagnosed or suspected congenital long QT syndrome. Avoid concurrent use with other drugs known to prolong QT_c interval.

Use with caution in patients at risk of hypotension (orthostasis is common) or those who would tolerate transient hypotensive episodes (cerebrovascular disease, cardiovascular disease, or other medications which may predispose). Significant hypotension may occur, particularly with parenteral administration. Injection contains sulfites.

Use with caution in patients with decreased gastrointestinal motility, urinary retention, BPH, xerostomia, or visual problems (ie, narrow-angle glaucoma), and myasthenia gravis. Relative to other neuroleptics, chlorpromazine has a moderate potency of cholinergic blockade. May cause pigmentary retinopathy, and lenticular and corneal deposits, particularly with prolonged therapy.

May cause extrapyramidal symptoms (EPS), including pseudoparkinsonism, acute dystonic reactions, akathisia, and tardive dyskinesia. Risk of dystonia (and possibly other EPS) may be greater with increased doses, use of conventional antipsychotics, males, and younger patients. May cause neuroleptic malignant syndrome (NMS).

Use in elderly patients with dementia is associated with an increased risk of mortality and cerebrovascular accidents; avoid antipsychotic use for behavioral problems associated with dementia unless alternative nonpharmacologic therapies have failed and patient may harm self or others. In addition, may cause or exacerbate syndrome of inappropriate antidiuretic hormone secretion or hyponatremia; monitor sodium closely with initiation or dosage adjustments in older adults. May be inappropriate in older adults depending on comorbidities (eg, delirium) due to its potent anticholinergic effects (Beers Criteria). Increased risk for developing tardive dyskinesia, particularly in elderly women.

Adverse Reactions Frequency not defined.

Cardiovascular: Orthostatic hypotension, tachycardia, dizziness, nonspecific QT changes

Central nervous system: Drowsiness, dystonias, akathisia, pseudoparkinsonism, tardive dyskinesia, neuroleptic malignant syndrome, seizure

Dermatologic: Photosensitivity, dermatitis, skin pigmentation (slate gray)

Endocrine & metabolic: Lactation, breast engorgement, false-positive pregnancy test, amenorrhea, gynecomastia, hyper- or hypoglycemia

Gastrointestinal: Xerostomia, constipation, nausea

Genitourinary: Urinary retention, ejaculatory disorder, impotence

Hematologic: Agranulocytosis, eosinophilia, leukopenia, hemolytic anemia, aplastic anemia, thrombocytopenic purpura

Hepatic: Jaundice

Ocular: Blurred vision, corneal and lenticular changes, epithelial keratopathy, pigmentary retinopathy

Drug Interactions

Metabolism/Transport Effects Substrate of CYP1A2 (minor), CYP2D6 (major), CYP3A4 (minor); **Note:** Assignment of Major/Minor substrate status based on clinically relevant drug interaction potential; **Inhibits** CYP2D6 (moderate), CYP2E1 (weak)

Avoid Concomitant Use

Avoid concomitant use of ChlorproMAZINE with any of the following: Aclidinium; Azelastine (Nasal); Highest Risk QTc-Prolonging Agents; Ipratropium (Oral Inhalation); Metoclopramide; Mifepristone; Paraldehyde; Tiotropium

Increased Effect/Toxicity

ChlorproMAZINE may increase the levels/effects of: Alcohol (Ethyl); Analgesics (Opioid); Anticholinergics; Antidepressants (Serotonin Reuptake Inhibitor/Antagonist); ARIPiprazole; Azelastine (Nasal); Beta-Blockers; CNS Depressants; CYP2D6 Substrates; Desmopressin; Divalproex; Fesoterodine; Haloperidol; Highest Risk QTc-Prolonging Agents; Methotrimeprazine; Methylphenidate; Moderate Risk QTc-Prolonging Agents; Paraldehyde; Porfimer; Serotonin Modulators; Tiotropium; Valproic Acid; Zolpidem

The levels/effects of ChlorproMAZINE may be increased by: Abiraterone Acetate; Acetylcholinesterase Inhibitors (Central); Aclidinium; Antidepressants (Serotonin Reuptake Inhibitor/Antagonist); Antimalarial Agents; Beta-Blockers; CYP2D6 Inhibitors (Moderate); CYP2D6 Inhibitors (Strong); Darunavir; Haloperidol; HydrOXYzine; Ipratropium (Oral Inhalation); Lithium formulations; Methotrimeprazine; Methylphenidate; Metoclopramide; Metyrosine; Mifepristone; Perampanel; Pramlintide; QTc-Prolonging Agents (Indeterminate Risk and Risk Modifying); Tetrabenazine

Decreased Effect

ChlorproMAZINE may decrease the levels/effects of: Amphetamines; Anti-Parkinson's Agents (Dopamine Agonist); Quinagolide; Tamoxifen

The levels/effects of ChlorproMAZINE may be decreased by: Antacids; Anti-Parkinson's Agents (Dopamine Agonist); Lithium formulations; Peginterferon Alfa-2b; Tocilizumab

Ethanol/Nutrition/Herb Interactions

Ethanol: May increase CNS depression; monitor for increased effects with coadministration. Caution patients about effects.

Herb/Nutraceutical: Avoid St John's wort (may decrease chlorpromazine levels, increase photosensitization, or enhance sedative effect). Avoid dong quai (may enhance photosensitization). Avoid kava kava, gotu kola, valerian (may increase CNS depression).

Storage/Stability Injection solution: Protect from light. A slightly yellowed solution does not indicate potency loss, but a markedly discolored solution should be discarded. Solution diluted with NS (1 mg/mL) and stored in 5 mL vials remains stable for 30 days.

Reconstitution Direct I.V. injection: Dilute with NS to a maximum concentration of 1 mg/mL.

I.V.: For treatment of intractable hiccups the manufacturer recommends diluting 25-50 mg of chlorpromazine in 500-1000 mL NS.

Mechanism of Action Chlorpromazine is an aliphatic phenothiazine antipsychotic which blocks postsynaptic mesolimbic dopaminergic receptors in the brain; exhibits a strong alpha-adrenergic blocking effect and depresses the release of hypothalamic and hypophyseal hormones; believed to depress the reticular activating system, thus affecting basal metabolism, body temperature, wakefulness, vasomotor tone, and emesis

Pharmacodynamics/Kinetics

Onset of action: I.M.: 15 minutes; Oral: 30-60 minutes

Absorption: Rapid

Distribution: V_d: 20 L/kg

Protein binding: 92% to 97%

Metabolism: Extensively hepatic to active and inactive metabolites

Bioavailability: 20%

Half-life, biphasic: Initial: 2 hours; Terminal: 30 hours

Excretion: Urine (<1% as unchanged drug) within 24 hours

Dosing

Adult

Schizophrenia/psychoses:

Oral: Range: 30-800 mg/day in 1-4 divided doses, initiate at lower doses and titrate as needed; usual dose: 200-600 mg/day; some patients may require 1-2 g/day

I.M., I.V.: Initial: 25 mg, may repeat (25-50 mg) in 1-4 hours, gradually increase to a maximum of 400 mg/dose every 4-6 hours until patient is controlled; usual dose: 300-800 mg/day

Intractable hiccups:

Oral, I.M.: 25-50 mg 3-4 times/day

I.V. (refractory to oral or I.M. treatment): 25-50 mg via slow I.V. infusion

Nausea and vomiting:

Oral: 10-25 mg every 4-6 hours

I.M., I.V.: 25-50 mg every 4-6 hours

Geriatric

Behavioral symptoms associated with dementia (unlabeled use): Initial: 10-25 mg 1-2 times/day; increase at 4- to 7-day intervals by 10-25 mg/day. Increase dose intervals (eg, twice daily, 3 times/day) as necessary to control behavior response or side effects; maximum daily dose: 800 mg; gradual increases (titration) may prevent some side effects or decrease their severity.

Other indications: Refer to adult dosing.

Pediatric

Schizophrenia/psychoses: Children ≥6 months:

Oral: 0.5-1 mg/kg/dose every 4-6 hours; older children may require 200 mg/day or higher.

I.M., I.V.: 0.5-1 mg/kg/dose every 6-8 hours; maximum dose for <5 years (<22.7 kg): 40 mg/day; maximum for 5-12 years (22.7-45.5 kg): 75 mg/day

Nausea and vomiting: Children ≥6 months:

Oral: 0.5-1 mg/kg/dose every 4-6 hours as needed

I.M., I.V.: 0.5-1 mg/kg/dose every 6-8 hours; maximum dose for <5 years (<22.7 kg): 40 mg/day; maximum for 5-12 years (22.7-45.5 kg): 75 mg/day

Renal Impairment Not dialyzable (0% to 5%)

Hepatic Impairment Avoid use in severe hepatic dysfunction.

Administration Do not administer SubQ (tissue damage and irritation may occur); for direct I.V. injection, administer diluted solution slow I.V. at a rate not to exceed 0.5 mg/minute in children and 1 mg/minute in adults. To reduce the risk of hypotension, patients receiving I.V. chlorpromazine must remain lying down during and for 30 minutes after the injection. **Note:** Avoid skin contact with solution; may cause contact dermatitis.

Monitoring Parameters Vital signs (especially with parenteral use); lipid profile, fasting blood glucose/Hgb A_{1c}; BMI; mental status; abnormal involuntary movement scale (AIMS); extrapyramidal symptoms (EPS); CBC in patients with risk factors for leukopenia/neutropenia

Test Interactions False-positives for phenylketonuria, amylase, uroporphyrins, urobilinogen. May cause false-positive pregnancy test. May interfere with urine detection of amphetamine/methamphetamine and methadone (false-positives).

Dosage Forms Excipient information presented when available (limited, particularly for generics); consult specific product labeling.

Injection, solution, as hydrochloride: 25 mg/mL (1 mL, 2 mL)

Tablet, oral, as hydrochloride: 10 mg, 25 mg, 50 mg, 100 mg, 200 mg

References

Gez E, Ben-Yosef R, Catane R, et al, "Chlorpromazine and Dexamethasone Versus High-Dose Metoclopramide and Dexamethasone in Patients Receiving Cancer Chemotherapy, Particularly Cis-Platinum: A Prospective Randomized Crossover Study," *Oncology*, 1989, 46(3):150-4.

Gez E, Brufman G, Kaufman B, et al, "Methylprednisolone and Chlorpromazine in Patients Receiving Cancer Chemotherapy: A Prospective Nonrandomized Study," *J Chemother*, 1989, 1(2):140-3.

Gill SS, Bronskill SE, Normand SL, et al, "Antipsychotic Drug Use and Mortality in Older Adults With Dementia," *Ann Intern Med*, 2007, 146(11):775-86.

◆ **Chlorpromazine Hydrochloride** *see* ChlorproMAZINE *on page* 274

◆ **Chlorpromazine Hydrochloride Inj (Can)** *see* ChlorproMAZINE *on page* 274

Chromic Phosphate P 32 (KROME ik FOS fate pe THUR tee too)

Brand Names: U.S. Phosphocol® P 32

Index Terms P32; Phosphorus p32

Generic Availability (U.S.) No

Pharmacologic Category Radiopharmaceutical

Use Treatment of peritoneal or pleural effusions caused by metastatic disease by intracavitary instillation; may be injected interstitially for the treatment of cancer

Labeled Contraindications Should not be used in patients with ulcerative tumors or in exposed cavities or where there is evidence of loculation, unless the extent of loculation has been determined

Lactation Excretion in breast milk unknown/not recommended

Warnings/Precautions Radiopharmaceutical: use appropriate precautions for handling, disposal, and minimizing exposure to patients and healthcare personnel. Use under supervision of experienced personnel. Use of this medication may increase risk of developing acute lymphocytic leukemia. Cases have been reported in children following intra-articular injection of this medication for hemarthroses (**not** an approved use). Intestinal fibrosis/necrosis and chronic fibrosis of the body wall may result from misplacement of the medication. Avoid placing into intrapleural or intraperitoneal loculations, bowel lumen, or body wall. May be less effective in bloody effusions. This product is not for intravascular use. Patients must be instructed in measures to minimize exposure of others. Should only be used by nuclear medicine physicians and/or radiopharmacists qualified and experienced in use and handling of radionuclides. Safety and efficacy have not been established in children.

Adverse Reactions Frequency not defined.

Gastrointestinal: Abdominal cramps, nausea

Hematologic: Bone marrow suppression

Respiratory: Pleuritis

Miscellaneous: Peritonitis, radiation sickness

Postmarketing and/or case reports: Radiation damage (interstitial or loculation injection), leukemia (children)

Drug Interactions

Metabolism/Transport Effects None known.

Avoid Concomitant Use There are no known interactions where it is recommended to avoid concomitant use.

Increased Effect/Toxicity There are no known significant interactions involving an increase in effect.

Decreased Effect There are no known significant interactions involving a decrease in effect.

Storage/Stability Store at controlled room temperature of 20°C to 25°C (68°F to 77°F).

Dosing

Adult & Geriatric Consult manufacturer potency tables when applicable. All doses should be individualized.

General dosing ranges (based on 70 kg patient):

Intraperitoneal instillation: 370-740 megabecquerels (10-20 millicuries)

Intrapleural instillation: 222-444 megabecquerels (6-12 millicuries)

Interstitial use: ~3.7-18.5 megabecquerels/g of tumor weight (0.1-0.5 millicuries/g)

Administration This product is for intraperitoneal or intrapleural instillation; **not** for intravascular use.

Dosage Forms Excipient information presented when available (limited, particularly for generics); consult specific product labeling.
Injection, suspension:
Phosphocol® P 32: 185 MBq (5mCi) per mL

◆ **Ciclosporin** *see* CycloSPORINE (Systemic) *on page* 333

Cinacalcet (sin a KAL cet)

Brand Names: U.S. Sensipar®
Brand Names: Canada Sensipar®
Index Terms AMG 073; Cinacalcet Hydrochloride
Generic Availability (U.S.) No
Pharmacologic Category Calcimimetic
Use Treatment of secondary hyperparathyroidism in patients with chronic kidney disease (CKD) on dialysis; treatment of hypercalcemia in patients with parathyroid carcinoma; treatment of severe hypercalcemia in patients with primary hyperparathyroidism who are unable to undergo parathyroidectomy
Labeled Contraindications Hypocalcemia (serum calcium lower than the lower limit of normal range)

Canadian labeling: Additional contraindications (not in U.S. labeling): Hypersensitivity to any component of the formulation
Pregnancy Risk Factor C
Lactation Excretion in breast milk unknown/not recommended
Warnings/Precautions Use is contraindicated in hypocalcemia. Monitor serum calcium and for symptoms of hypocalcemia (eg, cramps, myalgia, paresthesia, seizure, tetany); may require treatment interruption, dose reduction, or initiation (or dose increases) of calcium-based phosphate binder or vitamin D to raise serum calcium depending on calcium levels or symptoms of hypocalcemia. Use with caution in patients with a seizure disorder (seizure threshold is lowered by significant serum calcium reductions); monitor calcium levels closely. Adynamic bone disease may develop if intact parathyroid hormone (iPTH) levels are suppressed (<100 pg/mL).

Use caution in patients with moderate-to-severe hepatic impairment (Child-Pugh classes B and C); monitor serum calcium, serum phosphorus and iPTH closely. In the U.S., the long-term safety and efficacy of cinacalcet has not been evaluated in chronic kidney disease (CKD) patients with hyperparathyroidism not requiring dialysis. Not indicated for CKD patients not receiving dialysis. Although possibly related to lower baseline calcium levels, clinical studies have shown an increased incidence of hypocalcemia (<8.4 mg/dL) in patients not requiring dialysis. Monitor serum calcium and iPTH concentrations closely in patients on concurrent CYP3A4 inhibitors; dosage adjustment may be required. Cinacalcet is a strong inhibitor of CYP2D6; if on concurrent therapy with a CYP2D6 substrate, dosage adjustment of the CYP2D6 substrate may be necessary. May cause a decrease in testosterone levels (free and total); although below normal testosterone levels may occur in patients with end-stage renal disease, the clinical significance has not been determined. Use with caution in patients with cardiovascular disease; idiosyncratic hypotension, worsening of heart failure, and/or arrhythmia have been reported in patients with impaired cardiovascular function; may correlate with decreased serum calcium.

Adverse Reactions

>10%:

Central nervous system: Fatigue (12% to 21%), headache (≤21%), depression (10% to 18%)

Endocrine & metabolic: Hypocalcemia (≤66%), dehydration (≤24%), hypercalcemia (12% to 21%)

Gastrointestinal: Nausea (31% to 66%), vomiting (27% to 52%), diarrhea (≤21%), anorexia (6% to 21%), constipation (10% to 18%)

Hematologic: Anemia (6% to 17%)

Neuromuscular & skeletal: Parasthesia (14% to 29%), fracture (12% to 21%), weakness (7% to 17%), arthralgia (6% to 17%), myalgia (≤15%), limb pain (10% to 12%)

Respiratory: Upper respiratory infection (10% to 12%)

1% to 10%:

Cardiovascular: Hypertension (≤7%)

Central nervous system: Dizziness (≤10%), seizure (1%)

Endocrine & metabolic: Testosterone decreased

Neuromuscular & skeletal: Chest pain (noncardiac; ≤6%)

Postmarketing and/or case reports: Adynamic bone disease, angioedema, arrhythmia, heart failure, hypersensitivity reactions, hypotension (idiosyncratic), rash, urticaria

Drug Interactions

Metabolism/Transport Effects Substrate of CYP1A2 (minor), CYP2D6 (minor), CYP3A4 (major); **Note:** Assignment of Major/Minor substrate status based on clinically relevant drug interaction potential; **Inhibits** CYP2D6 (strong)

Avoid Concomitant Use

Avoid concomitant use of Cinacalcet with any of the following: Conivaptan; Pimozide; Tamoxifen; Thioridazine

Increased Effect/Toxicity

Cinacalcet may increase the levels/effects of: ARIPiprazole; AtoMOXetine; CYP2D6 Substrates; Fesoterodine; Iloperidone; Nebivolol; Pimozide; Propafenone; Tetrabenazine; Thioridazine; Tricyclic Antidepressants

The levels/effects of Cinacalcet may be increased by: Antifungal Agents (Azole Derivatives, Systemic); Conivaptan; CYP3A4 Inhibitors (Moderate); CYP3A4 Inhibitors (Strong); Dasatinib; Ivacaftor; Mifepristone

Decreased Effect

Cinacalcet may decrease the levels/effects of: Codeine; Iloperidone; Tacrolimus (Systemic); Tamoxifen; TraMADol

The levels/effects of Cinacalcet may be decreased by: Peginterferon Alfa-2b; Tocilizumab

Ethanol/Nutrition/Herb Interactions Food: Food increases bioavailability. Management: Administer with food or shortly after a meal.

Storage/Stability Store at 25°C (77°F); excursions permitted to 15°C to 30°C (59°F to 86°F).

Mechanism of Action Increases the sensitivity of the calcium-sensing receptor on the parathyroid gland thereby, concomitantly lowering parathyroid hormone (PTH), serum calcium, and serum phosphorus levels, preventing progressive bone disease and adverse events associated with mineral metabolism disorders.

Pharmacodynamics/Kinetics

Distribution: V_d: ~1000 L

Protein binding: ~93% to 97%

Metabolism: Hepatic (extensive) via CYP3A4, 2D6, 1A2; forms inactive metabolites

Half-life elimination: Terminal: 30-40 hours; moderate hepatic impairment: 65 hours; severe hepatic impairment: 84 hours

Time to peak, plasma: ~2-6 hours

Excretion: Urine ~80% (as metabolites); feces ~15%

Dosing

Adult Note: Do not titrate dose more frequently than every 2-4 weeks. Dosage adjustment may be required in patients on concurrent CYP3A4 inhibitors.

Secondary hyperparathyroidism: Oral: Initial: 30 mg once daily (maximum daily dose: 180 mg); increase dose incrementally (60 mg, 90 mg, 120 mg, 180 mg once daily) as necessary to maintain intact parathyroid hormone (iPTH) level between 150-300 pg/mL.

Parathyroid carcinoma, primary hyperparathyroidism: Oral: Initial: 30 mg twice daily (maximum daily dose: 360 mg daily as 90 mg 4 times/day); increase dose incrementally (60 mg twice daily, 90 mg twice daily, 90 mg 3-4 times/day) as necessary to normalize serum calcium levels.

Geriatric Refer to adult dosing. No adjustment required.

Renal Impairment No adjustment required.

Hepatic Impairment Patients with moderate-to-severe dysfunction (Child-Pugh class B or C) have an increased exposure to cinacalcet and increased half-life. Dosage adjustments may be necessary based on serum calcium, serum phosphorus and/or iPTH.

Adjustment for Toxicity Dosage adjustment for hypocalcemia:

If serum calcium >7.5 mg/dL but <8.4 mg/dL **or** if hypocalcemia symptoms occur: Use calcium-containing phosphate binders and/or vitamin D to raise calcium levels.

If serum calcium <7.5 mg/dL **or** if hypocalcemia symptoms persist and the dose of vitamin D cannot be increased: Withhold cinacalcet until serum calcium ≥8 mg/dL and/or symptoms of hypocalcemia resolve. Reinitiate cinacalcet at the next lowest dose.

If iPTH <150-300 pg/mL: Reduce dose or discontinue cinacalcet and/or vitamin D.

Administration Administer with food or shortly after a meal. Do not break or divide tablet; should be taken whole.

Monitoring Parameters

Secondary hyperparathyroidism: Serum calcium and phosphorus levels prior to initiation and within a week of initiation or dosage adjustment; iPTH should be measured 1-4 weeks after initiation or dosage adjustment. After the maintenance dose is established, monthly calcium and phosphorus levels and iPTH every 1-3 months are required. Wait at least 12 hours after dose before drawing iPTH levels.

Parathyroid carcinoma and primary hyperparathyroidism: Serum calcium levels prior to initiation and within a week of initiation or dosage adjustment; once maintenance dose is established, obtain serum calcium every 2 months.

Dietary Considerations Take with food or shortly after a meal. May be taken with vitamin D and/or phosphate binders.

Dosage Forms Excipient information presented when available (limited, particularly for generics); consult specific product labeling.

Tablet, oral:

Sensipar®: 30 mg, 60 mg, 90 mg

References

Block GA, Martin KJ, de Francisco AL, et al, "Cinacalcet for Secondary Hyperparathyroidism in Patients Receiving Hemodialysis," *N Engl J Med*, 2004, 350(15):1516-25.

Eknoyan G, Levin A, and Levin NW, "Bone Metabolism and Disease in Chronic Kidney Disease," *Am J Kidney Dis*, 2003, 42(4 Suppl 3):1-201.

Marcocci C, Chanson P, Shoback D, et al, "Cinacalcet Reduces Serum Calcium Concentrations in Patients With Intractable Primary Hyperparathyroidism," *J Clin Endocrinol Metab*, 2009, 94 (8):2766-72.

National Kidney Foundation. K/DOQI Clinical Practice Guidelines for Bone Metabolism and Disease in Chronic Kidney Disease. Guideline 13: Treatment of Bone Disease in Chronic Kidney Disease. Available at http://www.kidney.org/professionals/kdoqi/guidelines_bone/index.htm

Silverberg SJ, Rubin MR, Faiman C, et al, "Cinacalcet Hydrochloride Reduces the Serum Calcium Concentration in Inoperable Parathyroid Carcinoma," *J Clin Endocrinol Metab*, 2007, 92 (10):3803-8.

◆ **Cinacalcet Hydrochloride** *see* Cinacalcet *on page* 280

◆ **Cipro®** *see* Ciprofloxacin (Systemic) *on page* 283

◆ **Cipro® XL (Can)** *see* Ciprofloxacin (Systemic) *on page* 283

Ciprofloxacin (Systemic) (sip roe FLOKS a sin)

Brand Names: U.S. Cipro®; Cipro® I.V.

Brand Names: Canada Apo-Ciproflox®; Auro-Ciprofloxacin; Ciprofloxacin Injection; Ciprofloxacin Intravenous Infusion; Cipro®; Cipro® XL; CO Ciprofloxacin; Dom-Ciprofloxacin; JAMP-Ciprofloxacin; Mint-Ciprofloxacin; Mylan-Ciprofloxacin; Novo-Ciprofloxacin; PHL-Ciprofloxacin; PMS-Ciprofloxacin; PRO-Ciprofloxacin; RAN™-Ciprofloxacin; ratio-Ciprofloxacin; Riva-Ciprofloxacin; Sandoz-Ciprofloxacin; Taro-Ciprofloxacin

Index Terms Ciprofloxacin Hydrochloride

Generic Availability (U.S.) Yes: Excludes suspension

Pharmacologic Category Antibiotic, Quinolone

Use

Children: Complicated urinary tract infections and pyelonephritis due to *E. coli*. **Note:** Although effective, ciprofloxacin is not the drug of first choice in children.

Children and Adults: To reduce incidence or progression of disease following exposure to aerolized *Bacillus anthracis*.

Adults: Treatment of the following infections when caused by susceptible bacteria: Urinary tract infections; acute uncomplicated cystitis in females; chronic bacterial prostatitis, lower respiratory tract infections (including acute exacerbations of chronic bronchitis); acute sinusitis; skin and skin structure infections; bone and joint infections; complicated intra-abdominal infections (in combination with metronidazole); infectious diarrhea; typhoid fever due to *Salmonella typhi* (eradication of chronic typhoid carrier state has not been proven); uncomplicated cervical and urethra gonorrhea (due to *N. gonorrhoeae*); nosocomial pneumonia; empirical therapy for febrile neutropenic patients (in combination with piperacillin)

Note: As of April 2007, the CDC no longer recommends the use of fluoroquinolones for the treatment of gonococcal disease.

Unlabeled Use Acute pulmonary exacerbations in cystic fibrosis (children); cutaneous/gastrointestinal/oropharyngeal anthrax (treatment, children and adults); disseminated gonococcal infection (adults); chancroid (adults);

epididymitis (adults); prophylaxis to *Neisseria meningitidis* following close contact with an infected person; empirical therapy (oral) for febrile neutropenia in low-risk cancer patients; HACEK group endocarditis; infectious diarrhea (children); periodontitis

Labeled Contraindications Hypersensitivity to ciprofloxacin, any component of the formulation, or other quinolones; concurrent administration of tizanidine

Pregnancy Risk Factor C

Lactation Enters breast milk/not recommended (AAP rates "compatible"; AAP 2001 update pending)

Warnings/Precautions **[U.S. Boxed Warning]: There have been reports of tendon inflammation and/or rupture with quinolone antibiotics; risk may be increased with concurrent corticosteroids, organ transplant recipients, and in patients >60 years of age.** Rupture of the Achilles tendon sometimes requiring surgical repair has been reported most frequently; but other tendon sites (eg, rotator cuff, biceps) have also been reported. Strenuous physical activity, rheumatoid arthritis, and renal impairment may be an independent risk factor for tendonitis. Discontinue at first sign of tendon inflammation or pain. May occur even after discontinuation of therapy. Use with caution in patients with rheumatoid arthritis; may increase risk of tendon rupture. CNS effects may occur (tremor, restlessness, confusion, and very rarely hallucinations, increased intracranial pressure [including pseudotumor cerebri] or seizures). Use with caution in patients with known or suspected CNS disorder. Potential for seizures, although very rare, may be increased with concomitant NSAID therapy. Use with caution in individuals at risk of seizures. Fluoroquinolones may prolong QT_c interval; avoid use in patients with a history of QT_c prolongation, uncorrected hypokalemia, hypomagnesemia, or concurrent administration of other medications known to prolong the QT interval (including Class Ia and Class III antiarrhythmics, cisapride, erythromycin, antipsychotics, and tricyclic antidepressants). Prolonged use may result in fungal or bacterial superinfection, including *C. difficile*-associated diarrhea (CDAD) and pseudomembranous colitis; CDAD has been observed >2 months postantibiotic treatment. Rarely crystalluria has occurred; urine alkalinity may increase the risk. Ensure adequate hydration during therapy. Adverse effects, including those related to joints and/or surrounding tissues, are increased in pediatric patients and therefore, ciprofloxacin should not be considered as drug of choice in children (exception is anthrax treatment). Rare cases of peripheral neuropathy may occur.

Fluoroquinolones have been associated with the development of serious, and sometimes fatal, hypoglycemia, most often in elderly diabetics but also in patients without diabetes. This occurred most frequently with gatifloxacin (no longer available systemically), but may occur at a lower frequency with other quinolones.

Severe hypersensitivity reactions, including anaphylaxis, have occurred with quinolone therapy. Reactions may present as typical allergic symptoms after a single dose, or may manifest as severe idiosyncratic dermatologic, vascular, pulmonary, renal, hepatic, and/or hematologic events, usually after multiple doses. Prompt discontinuation of drug should occur if skin rash or other symptoms arise. **[U.S. Boxed Warning]: Quinolones may exacerbate myasthenia gravis; avoid use (rare, potentially life-threatening weakness of respiratory muscles may occur).** Use caution in renal impairment. Avoid excessive sunlight and take precautions to limit exposure (eg, loose fitting clothing, sunscreen); may cause moderate-to-severe phototoxicity reactions.

Discontinue use if photosensitivity occurs. Since ciprofloxacin is ineffective in the treatment of syphilis and may mask symptoms, all patients should be tested for syphilis at the time of gonorrheal diagnosis and 3 months later. Hemolytic reactions may (rarely) occur with quinolone use in patients with latent or actual G6PD deficiency.

Ciprofloxacin is a potent inhibitor of CYP1A2. Coadministration of drugs which depend on this pathway may lead to substantial increases in serum concentrations and adverse effects.

Ethanol/Nutrition/Herb Interactions

Food: Food decreases rate, but not extent, of absorption. Ciprofloxacin serum levels may be decreased if taken with divalent or trivalent cations. Ciprofloxacin may increase serum caffeine levels if taken concurrently. Rarely, crystalluria may occur. Enteral feedings may decrease plasma concentrations of ciprofloxacin probably by >30% inhibition of absorption. Management: May administer with food to minimize GI upset. Avoid or take ciprofloxacin 2 hours before or 6 hours after antacids, dairy products, or calcium-fortified juices alone or in a meal containing >800 mg calcium, oral multivitamins, or mineral supplements containing divalent and/or trivalent cations. Restrict caffeine intake if excessive cardiac or CNS stimulation occurs. Ensure adequate hydration during therapy. Ciprofloxacin should not be administered with enteral feedings. The feeding would need to be discontinued for 1-2 hours prior to and after ciprofloxacin administration. Nasogastric administration produces a greater loss of ciprofloxacin bioavailability than does nasoduodenal administration.

Herb/Nutraceutical: Dong quai and St John's wort may also cause photosensitization. Management: Avoid dong quai and St John's wort.

Storage/Stability

Injection:

Premixed infusion: Store between 5°C to 25°C (41°F to 77°F); avoid freezing. Protect from light.

Vial: Store between 5°C to 30°C (41°F to 86°F); avoid freezing. Protect from light. Diluted solutions of 0.5-2 mg/mL are stable for up to 14 days refrigerated or at room temperature.

Microcapsules for oral suspension: Prior to reconstitution, store below 25°C (77°F). Protect from freezing. Following reconstitution, store below 30°C (86°F) for up to 14 days. Protect from freezing.

Tablet:

Immediate release: Store below 30°C (86°F).

Extended release: Store at room temperature of 15°C to 30°C (59°F to 86°F).

Reconstitution Injection, vial: May be diluted with NS, D_5W, SWFI, $D_{10}W$, $D_5$1/4NS, $D_5$1/2NS, LR.

Mechanism of Action Inhibits DNA gyrase in susceptible organisms; inhibits relaxation of supercoiled DNA and promotes breakage of double-stranded DNA

Pharmacodynamics/Kinetics

Absorption: Oral: Immediate release tablet: Rapid (~50% to 85%)

Distribution: V_d: 2.1-2.7 L/kg; tissue concentrations often exceed serum concentrations especially in kidneys, gallbladder, liver, lungs, gynecological tissue, and prostatic tissue; CSF concentrations: 10% of serum concentrations (noninflamed meninges), 14% to 37% (inflamed meninges)

Protein binding: 20% to 40%

Metabolism: Partially hepatic; forms 4 metabolites (limited activity)

Half-life elimination: Children: 2.5 hours; Adults: Normal renal function: 3-5 hours
Time to peak: Oral:
Immediate release tablet: 0.5-2 hours
Extended release tablet: Cipro® XR: 1-2.5 hours
Excretion: Urine (30% to 50% as unchanged drug); feces (15% to 43%)

Dosing

Adult Note: Extended release tablets and immediate release formulations are not interchangeable. Unless otherwise specified, oral dosing reflects the use of immediate release formulations.

Anthrax:

Inhalational (postexposure prophylaxis):
Oral: 500 mg every 12 hours for 60 days
I.V.: 400 mg every 12 hours for 60 days

Cutaneous (treatment, CDC guidelines): Oral: Immediate release formulation: 500 mg every 12 hours for 60 days. **Note:** In the presence of systemic involvement, extensive edema, lesions on head/neck, refer to I.V. dosing for treatment of inhalational/gastrointestinal/oropharyngeal anthrax.

Inhalational/gastrointestinal/oropharyngeal (treatment, CDC guidelines): I.V.: 400 mg every 12 hours. **Note:** Initial treatment should include two or more agents predicted to be effective (per CDC recommendations). Continue combined therapy for 60 days.

Bone/joint infections:
Oral: 500-750 mg twice daily for 4-6 weeks
I.V.:
Mild/moderate: 400 mg every 12 hours for 4-6 weeks
Severe/complicated: 400 mg every 8 hours for 4-6 weeks

Chancroid (unlabeled use): Oral: 500 mg twice daily for 3 days (CDC, 2010)

Endocarditis due to HACEK organisms (AHA guidelines, unlabeled use): Note: Not first-line option; use only if intolerant of beta-lactam therapy:
Oral: 500 mg every 12 hours for 4 weeks
I.V.: 400 mg every 12 hours for 4 weeks

Epididymitis, chlamydial (unlabeled use): Oral: 500 mg single dose (Canadian STI Guidelines, 2008)

Febrile neutropenia: I.V.: 400 mg every 8 hours for 7-14 days (combination therapy generally recommended)

Gonococcal infections:

Urethral/cervical gonococcal infections: Oral: 250-500 mg as a single dose (CDC recommends concomitant doxycycline or azithromycin due to possible coinfection with *Chlamydia*); **Note:** As of April 2007, the CDC no longer recommends the use of fluoroquinolones for the treatment of uncomplicated gonococcal disease.

Disseminated gonococcal infection (CDC guidelines): Oral: 500 mg twice daily to complete 7 days of therapy (initial treatment with ceftriaxone 1 g I.M./I.V. daily for 24-48 hours after improvement begins); **Note:** As of April 2007, the CDC no longer recommends the use of fluoroquinolones for the treatment of more serious gonococcal disease, unless no other options exist and susceptibility can be confirmed via culture.

Granuloma inguinale (donovanosis) (unlabeled use): Oral: 750 mg twice daily for at least 3 weeks (and until lesions have healed) (CDC, 2010)

Infectious diarrhea: Oral:

Salmonella: 500 mg twice daily for 5-7 days

Shigella: 500 mg twice daily for 3 days

Traveler's diarrhea: Mild: 750 mg for one dose; Severe: 500 mg twice daily for 3 days

Vibrio cholerae: 1 g for one dose

Intra-abdominal, complicated, community-acquired (in combination with metronidazole): Note: Avoid using in settings where *E. coli* susceptibility to fluoroquinolones is <90%:

Oral: 500 mg every 12 hours for 7-14 days

I.V.: 400 mg every 12 hours for 7-14 days; **Note:** 2010 IDSA guidelines recommend treatment duration of 4-7 days (provided source controlled)

Lower respiratory tract, skin/skin structure infections:

Oral: 500-750 mg twice daily for 7-14 days

I.V.:

Mild/moderate: 400 mg every 12 hours for 7-14 days

Severe/complicated: 400 mg every 8 hours for 7-14 days

Meningococcal meningitis prophylaxis (unlabeled use): Oral: 500 mg as a single dose (CDC, 2005)

Nosocomial pneumonia: I.V.: 400 mg every 8 hours for 10-14 days

Periodontitis (unlabeled use): Oral: 500 mg every 12 hours for 8-10 days

Prostatitis (chronic, bacterial): Oral: 500 mg every 12 hours for 28 days

Sinusitis (acute): Oral: 500 mg every 12 hours for 10 days

Typhoid fever: Oral: 500 mg every 12 hours for 10 days

Urinary tract infection:

Acute uncomplicated, cystitis:

Oral:

Immediate release formulation: 250 mg every 12 hours for 3 days

Extended release formulation (Cipro® XR): 500 mg every 24 hours for 3 days

I.V.: 200 mg every 12 hours for 7-14 days

Complicated (including pyelonephritis):

Oral:

Immediate release formulation: 500 mg every 12 hours for 7-14 days

Extended release formulation (Cipro® XR): 1000 mg every 24 hours for 7-14 days

I.V.: 400 mg every 12 hours for 7-14 days

Geriatric Refer to adult dosing. Adjust dose carefully based on renal function.

Pediatric See Warnings/Precautions. **Note:** Extended release tablets and immediate release formulations are not interchangeable. Unless otherwise specified, oral dosing reflects the use of immediate release formulations.

Anthrax:

Inhalational (postexposure prophylaxis):

Oral: 15 mg/kg/dose every 12 hours for 60 days; maximum: 500 mg/dose

I.V.: 10 mg/kg/dose every 12 hours for 60 days; do **not** exceed 400 mg/dose (800 mg/day)

Cutaneous (treatment, CDC guidelines): Oral: 10-15 mg/kg every 12 hours for 60 days (maximum: 1 g/day); amoxicillin 80 mg/kg/day divided every 8 hours is an option for completion of treatment after clinical improvement. **Note:** In the presence of systemic involvement, extensive edema, lesions on head/neck, refer to I.V. dosing for treatment of inhalational/gastrointestinal/oropharyngeal anthrax.

Inhalational/gastrointestinal/oropharyngeal (treatment, CDC guidelines): I.V.: Initial: 10-15 mg/kg every 12 hours for 60 days (maximum: 500 mg/dose); switch to oral therapy when clinically appropriate; refer to adult dosing for notes on combined therapy and duration

Community-acquired pneumonia (CAP) (IDSA/PIDS, 2011): *H. influenzae,* moderate-to-severe infection (alternative to ampicillin, ceftriaxone, or cefotaxime): Infants >3 months and Children: I.V.: 30 mg/kg/day divided every 12 hours

Cystic fibrosis (unlabeled use): Children 5-17 years:

Oral: 40 mg/kg/day divided every 12 hours administered following 1 week of I.V. therapy has been reported in a clinical trial; total duration of therapy: 10-21 days

I.V.: 30 mg/kg/day divided every 8 hours for 1 week, followed by oral therapy, has been reported in a clinical trial

Urinary tract infection (complicated) or pyelonephritis: Children 1-17 years:

Oral: 20-30 mg/kg/day in 2 divided doses (every 12 hours) for 10-21 days; maximum: 1.5 g/day

I.V.: 6-10 mg/kg every 8 hours for 10-21 days (maximum: 400 mg/dose)

Renal Impairment Adults:

Manufacturer's recommendations:

Oral, immediate release:

Cl_{cr} >50 mL/minute: No dosage adjustment necessary.

Cl_{cr} 30-50 mL/minute: 250-500 mg every 12 hours

Cl_{cr} 5-29 mL/minute: 250-500 mg every 18 hours

Hemodialysis/peritoneal dialysis (PD) (administer after dialysis on dialysis days): 250-500 mg every 24 hours

Oral, extended release:

Cl_{cr} ≥30 mL/minute: No dosage adjustment necessary.

Cl_{cr} <30 mL/minute: 500 mg every 24 hours

Hemodialysis/peritoneal dialysis (PD) (administer after dialysis on dialysis days): 500 mg every 24 hours

I.V.:

Cl_{cr} ≥30 mL/minute: No dosage adjustment necessary.

Cl_{cr} 5-29 mL/minute: 200-400 mg every 18-24 hours

Alternate recommendations: Oral (immediate release), I.V.:

Cl_{cr} >50 mL/minute: No dosage adjustment necessary (Aronoff, 2007).

Cl_{cr} 10-50 mL/minute: Administer 50% to 75% of usual dose every 12 hours (Aronoff, 2007).

Cl_{cr} <10 mL/minute: Administer 50% of usual dose every 12 hours (Aronoff, 2007).

Intermittent hemodialysis (IHD) (administer after hemodialysis on dialysis days): Minimally dialyzable (<10%): Oral: 250-500 mg every 24 hours **or** I.V.: 200-400 mg every 24 hours (Heintz, 2009). **Note:** Dosing dependent on the assumption of 3 times/week, complete IHD sessions.

Continuous renal replacement therapy (CRRT) (Heintz, 2009; Trotman, 2005): Drug clearance is highly dependent on the method of renal replacement, filter type, and flow rate. Appropriate dosing requires close monitoring of pharmacologic response, signs of adverse reactions due to drug accumulation, as well as drug concentrations in relation to target trough (if appropriate). The following are general recommendations only (based on dialysate flow/ultrafiltration rates of 1-2 L/hour and minimal residual renal function) and should not supersede clinical judgment:

CVVH/CVVHD/CVVHDF: I.V.: 200-400 mg every 12-24 hours

Administration

Oral: May administer with food to minimize GI upset; avoid antacid use; maintain proper hydration and urine output. Administer immediate release ciprofloxacin and Cipro® XR at least 2 hours before or 6 hours after antacids or other products containing calcium, iron, or zinc (including dairy products or calcium-fortified juices). Separate oral administration from drugs which may impair absorption.

Oral suspension: Should not be administered through feeding tubes (suspension is oil-based and adheres to the feeding tube). Patients should avoid chewing on the microcapsules.

Nasogastric/orogastric tube: Crush immediate-release tablet and mix with water. Flush feeding tube before and after administration. Hold tube feedings at least 1 hour before and 2 hours after administration.

Tablet, extended release: Do not crush, split, or chew. May be administered with meals containing dairy products (calcium content <800 mg), but not with dairy products alone.

Parenteral: Administer by slow I.V. infusion over 60 minutes to reduce the risk of venous irritation (burning, pain, erythema, and swelling); final concentration for administration should not exceed 2 mg/mL.

Test Interactions Some quinolones may produce a false-positive urine screening result for opiates using commercially-available immunoassay kits. This has been demonstrated most consistently for levofloxacin and ofloxacin, but other quinolones have shown cross-reactivity in certain assay kits. Confirmation of positive opiate screens by more specific methods should be considered.

Medication Guide Available Yes

Dosage Forms Excipient information presented when available (limited, particularly for generics); consult specific product labeling. [DSC] = Discontinued product

Infusion, premixed in D_5W: 200 mg (100 mL); 400 mg (200 mL)

Cipro® I.V.: 200 mg (100 mL [DSC]), 400 mg (200 mL)

Infusion, premixed in D_5W [preservative free]: 200 mg (100 mL); 400 mg (200 mL)

Injection, solution: 10 mg/mL (20 mL, 40 mL)

Injection, solution [preservative free]: 10 mg/mL (20 mL)

Microcapsules for suspension, oral:

Cipro®: 250 mg/5 mL (100 mL) [contains sucrose 1.4 g/5 mL; strawberry flavor]

Cipro®: 500 mg/5 mL (100 mL) [contains sucrose 1.3 g/5 mL; strawberry flavor]

Tablet, oral, as hydrochloride [strength expressed as base]: 100 mg, 250 mg, 500 mg, 750 mg

Cipro®: 250 mg, 500 mg

Tablet, extended release, oral, as base and hydrochloride [strength expressed as base]: 500 mg, 1000 mg

- **Ciprofloxacin Hydrochloride** *see* Ciprofloxacin (Systemic) *on page* *283*
- **Ciprofloxacin Injection (Can)** *see* Ciprofloxacin (Systemic) *on page* *283*
- **Ciprofloxacin Intravenous Infusion (Can)** *see* Ciprofloxacin (Systemic) *on page* *283*
- **Cipro® I.V.** *see* Ciprofloxacin (Systemic) *on page* *283*
- **cis-DDP** *see* CISplatin *on page* *290*
- **cis-Diamminedichloroplatinum** *see* CISplatin *on page* *290*

CISplatin (SIS pla tin)

Related Information

Chemotherapy and Obesity *on page* *1834*
Fertility and Cancer Therapy *on page* *1782*
Hematopoietic Stem Cell Transplantation *on page* *1887*
Management of Chemotherapy-Induced Nausea and Vomiting *on page* *1786*
Management of Drug Extravasations *on page* *1800*
Safe Handling of Hazardous Drugs *on page* *1904*

Index Terms CDDP; cis-DDP; cis-Diamminedichloroplatinum; Platinol; Platinol-AQ

Generic Availability (U.S.) Yes

Pharmacologic Category Antineoplastic Agent, Alkylating Agent; Antineoplastic Agent, Platinum Analog

Use Treatment of advanced bladder cancer, metastatic testicular cancer, and metastatic ovarian cancer

Unlabeled Use Treatment of breast cancer (metastatic), central nervous system tumors, cervical cancer, endometrial cancer, esophageal cancer, gastric cancer, germ cell tumors, gestational trophoblastic disease (refractory), head and neck cancer, hepatobiliary cancer, hepatoblastoma, Hodgkin lymphoma, malignant pleural mesothelioma, melanoma (metastatic), multiple myeloma, neuroblastoma, neuroendocrine tumors, non-Hodgkin lymphoma (NHL), nonsmall cell lung cancer (NSCLC), osteosarcoma, pancreatic cancer (advanced), prostate cancer, small cell lung cancer (SCLC), soft tissue sarcomas, and unknown primary cancers

Labeled Contraindications Hypersensitivity to cisplatin, other platinum-containing compounds, or any component of the formulation (anaphylactic-like reactions have been reported); pre-existing renal impairment; myelosuppression; hearing impairment

Pregnancy Risk Factor D

Lactation Enters breast milk/not recommended

Warnings/Precautions Hazardous agent - use appropriate precautions for handling and disposal. **[U.S. Boxed Warning]: Doses >100 mg/m² once every 3-4 weeks are rarely used; verify with the prescriber. Exercise caution to avoid potential sound-alike/look-alike confusion between CISplatin and CARBOplatin.** Patients should receive adequate hydration, with or without diuretics, prior to and for 24 hours after cisplatin administration. **[U.S. Boxed Warning]: Cumulative renal toxicity may be severe.** Monitor serum creatinine, blood urea nitrogen, creatinine clearance, and serum electrolytes closely. According to the manufacturer's labeling, use is contraindicated in patients with preexisting renal impairment and renal function must return to normal prior to administering subsequent cycles; some literature recommends reduced doses with renal impairment. Nephrotoxicity may be potentiated by aminoglycosides.

Use caution in the elderly; may cause or exacerbate syndrome of inappropriate antidiuretic hormone secretion or hyponatremia; monitor sodium closely with initiation or dosage adjustments in older adults (Beers Criteria). Elderly patients may be more susceptible to nephrotoxicity and peripheral neuropathy; select dose cautiously and monitor closely.

[U.S. Boxed Warning]: Dose-related toxicities include myelosuppression, nausea, and vomiting. Nausea and vomiting may be immediate and/or delayed; antiemetics are recommended. Diarrhea may also occur. **[U.S. Boxed Warning]: Ototoxicity, especially pronounced in children, is manifested by tinnitus or loss of high frequency hearing and occasionally, deafness; may be significant**. Pediatric patients with certain genetic variations in the thiopurine S-methyltransferase (TPMT) gene may be at increased risk of ototoxicity, even when conventional cisplatin doses are given. Ototoxicity is cumulative; audiometric testing should be performed at baseline and prior to each dose. Pediatric patients should receive audiometric testing for several years after discontinuing therapy. Severe (and possibly irreversible) neuropathies may occur with higher than recommended doses or more frequent administration; may require therapy discontinuation. Seizures, loss of motor function, loss of taste, leukoencephalopathy, and posterior reversible leukoencephalopathy syndrome (PRES [formerly RPLS]) have also been described. Serum electrolytes, particularly magnesium and potassium, should be monitored and replaced as needed during and after cisplatin therapy.

[U.S. Boxed Warning]: Anaphylactic-like reactions have been reported, may include facial edema, bronchoconstriction, tachycardia, and hypotension and may occur within minutes of administration; may be managed with epinephrine, corticosteroids, and/or antihistamines. Hyperuricemia has been reported with cisplatin use, and is more pronounced with doses >50 mg/m^2; consider allopurinol therapy to reduce uric acid levels. Local infusion site reactions may occur; monitor infusion site during administration; avoid extravasation. Secondary malignancies have been reported with cisplatin in combination with other chemotherapy agents. **[U.S. Boxed Warning]: Should be administered under the supervision of an experienced cancer chemotherapy physician.**

Adverse Reactions

>10%:

Central nervous system: Neurotoxicity: Peripheral neuropathy is dose- and duration dependent.

Gastrointestinal: Nausea and vomiting (76% to 100%)

Hematologic: Myelosuppression (25% to 30%; nadir: day 18-23; recovery: by day 39; mild with moderate doses, mild-to-moderate with high-dose therapy)

Hepatic: Liver enzymes increased

Renal: Nephrotoxicity (acute renal failure and chronic renal insufficiency)

Otic: Ototoxicity (10% to 30%; manifested as high frequency hearing loss; ototoxicity is especially pronounced in children)

1% to 10%: Local: Tissue irritation

<1%, postmarketing, and/or case reports: Alopecia (mild), anaphylactic reaction, arrhythmias, arterial vasospasm (acute), blurred vision, bradycardia, diarrhea, heart block, heart failure, hemolytic anemia (acute), hemolytic uremic syndrome, hypercholesterolemia, hypocalcemia, hypokalemia,

hypomagnesemia, hyponatremia, hypophosphatemia, limb ischemia (acute), mesenteric ischemia (acute), MI, myocardial ischemia, mouth sores, neutropenic typhlitis, optic neuritis, orthostatic hypotension, pancreatitis, papilledema, phlebitis, reversible posterior leukoencephalopathy syndrome (RPLS), SIADH, stroke, thrombophlebitis, thrombotic thrombocytopenic purpura

Drug Interactions

Metabolism/Transport Effects None known.

Avoid Concomitant Use

Avoid concomitant use of CISplatin with any of the following: BCG; CloZAPine; Natalizumab; Pimecrolimus; Tacrolimus (Topical); Vaccines (Live)

Increased Effect/Toxicity

CISplatin may increase the levels/effects of: Aminoglycosides; CloZAPine; Leflunomide; Natalizumab; Taxane Derivatives; Topotecan; Vaccines (Live); Vinorelbine

The levels/effects of CISplatin may be increased by: Denosumab; Loop Diuretics; Pimecrolimus; Roflumilast; Tacrolimus (Topical); Trastuzumab

Decreased Effect

CISplatin may decrease the levels/effects of: BCG; Coccidioidin Skin Test; Fosphenytoin; Phenytoin; Sipuleucel-T; Vaccines (Inactivated); Vaccines (Live)

The levels/effects of CISplatin may be decreased by: Echinacea

Storage/Stability Store intact vials at room temperature 15°C to 25°C (59°F to 77°F). Protect from light. Do not refrigerate solution as a precipitate may form. Further dilution **stability is dependent on the chloride ion concentration** and should be mixed in solutions of NS (at least 0.3% NaCl). After initial entry into the vial, solution is stable for 28 days protected from light or for at least 7 days under fluorescent room light at room temperature.

Further dilutions in NS, D_5/0.45% NaCl or D_5/NS to a concentration of 0.05-2 mg/mL are stable for 72 hours at 4°C to 25°C. The infusion solution should have a final sodium chloride concentration ≥0.2%.

Reconstitution Hazardous agent; use appropriate precautions for handling and disposal. The infusion solution should have a final sodium chloride concentration ≥0.2%. Needles or I.V. administration sets that contain aluminum should not be used in the preparation or administration; aluminum can react with cisplatin resulting in precipitate formation and loss of potency.

Mechanism of Action Inhibits DNA synthesis by the formation of DNA cross-links; denatures the double helix; covalently binds to DNA bases and disrupts DNA function; may also bind to proteins; the *cis*-isomer is 14 times more cytotoxic than the *trans*-isomer; both forms cross-link DNA but cis-platinum is less easily recognized by cell enzymes and, therefore, not repaired. Cisplatin can also bind two adjacent guanines on the same strand of DNA producing intrastrand cross-linking and breakage.

Pharmacodynamics/Kinetics

Distribution: I.V.: Rapidly into tissue; high concentrations in kidneys, liver, ovaries, uterus, and lungs

Protein binding: >90% (O'Dwyer, 2000)

Metabolism: Nonenzymatic; inactivated (in both cell and bloodstream) by sulfhydryl groups; covalently binds to glutathione and thiosulfate

Half-life elimination: Initial: 14-49 minutes; Beta: 0.7-4.6 hours; Gamma: 24-127 hours (O'Dwyer, 2000)

Excretion: Urine (>90%); feces (minimal)

Dosing

Adult VERIFY ANY CISPLATIN DOSE EXCEEDING 100 mg/m² PER COURSE. Pretreatment hydration with 1-2 L of I.V. fluid is recommended. Details concerning dosing in combination regimens should also be consulted.

Bladder cancer, advanced: I.V.: 50-70 mg/m² every 3-4 weeks; heavily pretreated patients: 50 mg/m² every 4 weeks

Ovarian cancer, metastatic: I.V.:

Single agent: 100 mg/m² every 4 weeks

Combination therapy: 75-100 mg/m² every 4 weeks or (unlabeled dosing) 75 mg/m² every 3 weeks (Ozols, 2003)

Testicular cancer, metastatic: I.V.: 20 mg/m²/day for 5 days repeated every 3 weeks (Cushing, 2004; Saxman, 1998)

Cervical cancer (unlabeled use): I.V.: 75 mg/m² on day 1 every 3 weeks (in combination with fluorouracil and radiation) for 3 cycles (Morris, 1999) **or** 70 mg/m² on day 1 every 3 weeks for 4 cycles (in combination with fluorouracil; cycles 1 and 2 given concurrently with radiation) (Peters, 2000) **or** 50 mg/m² on day 1 every 4 weeks (in combination with radiation and fluorouracil) for 2 cycles (Whitney, 1999)

Endometrial carcinoma, recurrent, metastatic, or high-risk (unlabeled use): I.V.: 50 mg/m² on day 1 every 3 weeks (in combination with doxorubicin ± paclitaxel) for 7 cycles or until disease progression or unacceptable toxicity (Fleming, 2004)

Head and neck cancer (unlabeled use): I.V.:

Locally-advanced disease: 100 mg/m² every 3 weeks for 3 doses (with concurrent radiation) (Bernier, 2004; Cooper, 2004) **or** 75 mg/m² every 3 weeks (in combination with docetaxel and fluorouracil) for 4 cycles or until disease progression or unacceptable toxicity (if no disease progression after 4 cycles, chemotherapy was followed by radiation) (Vermorken, 2007) **or** 100 mg/m² every 3 weeks (in combination with docetaxel and fluorouracil) for 3 cycles or until disease progression or unacceptable toxicity (chemotherapy was followed by chemoradiation) (Posner, 2007)

Metastatic disease: 100 mg/m² every 3 weeks (in combination with fluorouracil and cetuximab) until disease progression or unacceptable toxicity or a maximum of 6 cycles (Vermorken, 2008)

Malignant pleural mesothelioma (unlabeled use): I.V.: 75 mg/m² on day 1 of each 21-day cycle (in combination with pemetrexed) (Vogelzang, 2003) **or** 100 mg/m² on day 1 of a 28-day cycle (in combination with gemcitabine) (Nowak, 2002) **or** 80 mg/m² on day 1 of a 21-day cycle (in combination with gemcitabine) (van Haarst, 2002)

NSCLC (unlabeled use): I.V.: **Note:** There are multiple cisplatin-containing regimens for the treatment of NSCLC. Listed below are several commonly used regimens.

100 mg/m² on day 1 every 4 weeks (in combination with etoposide) for 3-4 cycles; (Arriagada, 2007), or

100 mg/m² on day 1 every 4 weeks (in combination with vinorelbine) (Kelly, 2001; Wozniak, 1998), or

100 mg/m² on day 1 every 4 weeks (in combination with gemcitabine) (Comella, 2000), or

80 mg/m² on day 1 every 3 weeks (in combination with gemcitabine) (Ohe, 2007), or

75 mg/m² on day 1 every 3 weeks (in combination with pemetrexed) for up to 6 cycles or until disease progression or unacceptable toxicity (Scagliotti, 2008)

Ovarian cancer (unlabeled route): Intraperitoneal: 75-100 mg/m^2 on day 2 of a 21-day treatment cycle (in combination with I.V. and intraperitoneal paclitaxel) for 6 cycles (Armstrong, 2006; NCCN Ovarian Cancer guidelines, v.1.2013)

SCLC (unlabeled use): I.V.:

Limited-stage disease: 60 mg/m^2 on day 1 every 3 weeks for 4 cycles (in combination with etoposide and concurrent radiation) (Turrisi, 1999)

Extensive-stage disease: 80 mg/m^2 on day 1 every 3 weeks (in combination with etoposide) for 4 cycles (Lara, 2009) or a maximum of 8 cycles (Ihde, 1994) **or** 60 mg/m^2 on day 1 every 4 weeks for 4 cycles (in combination with irinotecan) (Lara, 2009)

Testicular germ cell tumor, malignant (unlabeled use): I.V.: 25 mg/m^2 on days 2-5 every 3 weeks (in combination with paclitaxel and ifosfamide) for 4 cycles (Kondagunta, 2005) **or** 20 mg/m^2 on days 1-5 every 3 weeks (in combination with bleomycin and etoposide) for 4 cycles (Nichols, 1998) **or** 20 mg/m^2 on days 1-5 every 3 weeks (in combination with etoposide and ifosfamide) for 4 cycles (Nichols, 1998)

Geriatric Refer to adult dosing. Select dose cautiously and monitor closely in the elderly; may be more susceptible to nephrotoxicity and peripheral neuropathy.

Pediatric VERIFY ANY CISPLATIN DOSE EXCEEDING 100 mg/m^2 PER COURSE. Pretreatment hydration is recommended. Details concerning dosing in combination regimens should also be consulted.

Germ cell tumors (unlabeled use; combination chemotherapy): I.V.: 20 mg/m^2/day on days 1-5 or 100 mg/m^2 on day 1 of a 21-day treatment cycle (Pinkerton, 1986)

Hepatoblastoma (unlabeled use; combination chemotherapy): I.V.: 80 mg/m^2 continuous infusion over 24 hours on day 1 of a 21-day treatment cycle (Pritchard, 2000)

Medulloblastoma (unlabeled use; combination chemotherapy): I.V.: 75 mg/m^2 on either day 0 or day 1 of each chemotherapy cycle (Packer, 2006)

Neuroblastoma, high-risk (unlabeled use; combination chemotherapy): I.V.: 50 mg/m^2/day on days 0-3 of a 21-day cycle (cycles 3 and 5) (Naranjo, 2011) **or** 50 mg/m^2/day on days 1-4 (cycles 3, 5, and 7) (Kushner, 1994)

Osteosarcoma (unlabeled use; combination chemotherapy): I.V.: 60 mg/m^2/day for 2 days weeks 2, 7, 25, and 28 (neoadjuvant) or weeks 5, 10, 25, and 28 (adjuvant) (Goorin, 2003)

Renal Impairment Note: The manufacturer(s) recommend that repeat courses of cisplatin should not be given until serum creatinine is <1.5 mg/dL and/or BUN is <25 mg/dL and use is contraindicated in pre-existing renal impairment. The following adjustments have been recommended.

Aronoff, 2007:

Cl_{cr} 10-50 mL/minute: Administer 75% of dose

Cl_{cr} <10 mL/minute: Administer 50% of dose

Hemodialysis: Partially cleared by hemodialysis

Administer 50% of dose posthemodialysis

Continuous ambulatory peritoneal dialysis (CAPD): Administer 50% of dose

Continuous renal replacement therapy (CRRT): Administer 75% of dose

Janus, 2010: Hemodialysis: Reduce initial dose by 50%; administer post hemodialysis or on nondialysis days.

Kintzel, 1995:

Cl_{cr} 46-60 mL/minute: Administer 75% of dose

Cl_{cr} 31-45 mL/minute: Administer 50% of dose

Cl_{cr} <30 mL/minute: Consider use of alternative drug

Hepatic Impairment No dosage adjustment provided in manufacturer's labeling. However, cisplatin undergoes nonenzymatic metabolism and predominantly renal elimination; therefore, dosage adjustment is likely not necessary.

Combination Regimens

Biliary adenocarcinoma: Gemcitabine-Cisplatin (Biliary Cancer) on page 1669

Bladder cancer:

- Cisplatin-Fluorouracil (Bladder Cancer) on page 1571
- CMV on page 1589
- Gemcitabine-Cisplatin (Bladder Cancer) on page 1669
- M-VAC (Bladder Cancer) on page 1718

Brain tumors:

- CDDP/VP-16 on page 1555
- COPE on page 1596

Breast Cancer: Docetaxel-Trastuzumab-Cisplatin on page 1616

Cervical cancer:

- Cisplatin-Fluorouracil (Cervical Cancer) on page 1571
- Cisplatin-Gemcitabine (Cervical Cancer) on page 1578
- Cisplatin-Paclitaxel (Cervical Cancer) on page 1581
- Cisplatin-Topotecan (Cervical Cancer) on page 1583
- Cisplatin-Vinorelbine (Cervical Cancer) on page 1585

Endometrial cancer: AP on page 1520

Esophageal cancer:

- Cisplatin-Capecitabine (Esophageal Cancer) on page 1566
- Cisplatin-Fluorouracil (Esophageal Cancer) on page 1572
- Docetaxel-Cisplatin-Fluorouracil (Gastric/Esophageal Cancer) on page 1609
- Epirubicin-Cisplatin-Capecitabine (Esophageal Cancer) on page 1626
- Epirubicin-Cisplatin-Fluorouracil (Gastric/Esophageal Cancer) on page 1626
- Irinotecan-Cisplatin (Esophageal Cancer) on page 1694
- Paclitaxel-Cisplatin (Esophageal Cancer) on page 1727
- Paclitaxel-Cisplatin-Fluorouracil (Esophageal Cancer) on page 1728

Gastric cancer:

- Cisplatin-Capecitabine (Gastric Cancer) on page 1566
- Cisplatin-Fluorouracil (Gastric Cancer) on page 1574
- Docetaxel-Cisplatin-Fluorouracil (Gastric/Esophageal Cancer) on page 1609
- Epirubicin-Cisplatin-Fluorouracil (Gastric/Esophageal Cancer) on page 1626
- Irinotecan-Cisplatin (Gastric Cancer) on page 1695
- Trastuzumab-Cisplatin-Capecitabine (Gastric Cancer) on page 1757
- Trastuzumab-Cisplatin-Fluorouracil (Gastric Cancer) on page 1758

Gestational trophoblastic tumor: EP/EMA on page 1625

Head and neck cancer:

- Cetuximab-Cisplatin-Fluorouracil (Head and Neck Cancer) on page 1558
- Cisplatin-Cetuximab (Head and Neck Cancer) on page 1566
- Cisplatin-Fluorouracil (Head and Neck Cancer) on page 1575
- Cisplatin-Paclitaxel (Head and Neck Cancer) on page 1581
- Docetaxel-Cisplatin-Fluorouracil (Head and Neck Cancer) on page 1610

Hepatoblastoma:

- IPA on page 1692
- PA-CI on page 1725

Lung cancer (nonsmall cell):
Bevacizumab-Cisplatin-Gemcitabine (NSCLC) on page 1529
Cetuximab-Cisplatin-Vinorelbine (NSCLC) on page 1558
Cisplatin-Etoposide (NSCLC) on page 1568
Cisplatin-Irinotecan (NSCLC) on page 1580
Cisplatin-Pemetrexed (NSCLC) on page 1583
Cisplatin-Vinblastine (NSCLC) on page 1585
Docetaxel-Cisplatin on page 1609
EP (NSCLC) on page 1628
EP/PE on page 1631
Gemcitabine-Cisplatin (NSCLC) on page 1670
PC (NSCLC) on page 1734
Vinorelbine-Cisplatin on page 1772
Lung cancer (small cell):
Cisplatin–Etoposide (Small Cell Lung Cancer) on page 1569
Cisplatin-Irinotecan (Small Cell Lung Cancer) on page 1580
Lymphoma, Hodgkin:
DHAP (Hodgkin) on page 1608
ESHAP (Hodgkin) on page 1634
GDP (Hodgkin) on page 1667
MINE-ESHAP (Hodgkin) on page 1711
Lymphoma, non-Hodgkin's:
Cisplatin-Cytarabine-Dexamethasone (NHL Regimen) on page 1567
ESHAP on page 1633
MINE-ESHAP (NHL) on page 1712
Malignant pleural mesothelioma:
Cisplatin-Gemcitabine (Mesothelioma) on page 1578
Cisplatin-Pemetrexed (Mesothelioma) on page 1582
Cisplatin-Raltitrexed (Mesothelioma) on page 1583
Melanoma:
Cisplatin-Vinblastine-Dacarbazine (Melanoma) on page 1584
CVD-Interleukin-Interferon (Melanoma) on page 1597
Multiple myeloma: DTPACE on page 1620
Neuroblastoma:
A3 (Neuroblastoma) on page 1515
CAV-P/VP (Neuroblastoma) on page 1554
Cisplatin-Doxorubicin-Etoposide-Cyclophosphamide (Neuroblastoma) on page 1568
New A1 (Neuroblastoma) on page 1721
Osteosarcoma:
MTX-CDDPAdr on page 1717
POG-8651 on page 1740
Ovarian cancer:
BEP (Ovarian Cancer) on page 1526
BEP (Ovarian Cancer, Testicular Cancer) on page 1526
Cisplatin-Paclitaxel Intraperitoneal (Ovarian) on page 1582
Cisplatin-Paclitaxel (Ovarian) on page 1582
PAC (CAP) on page 1725
Pancreatic cancer: Cisplatin-Gemcitabine (Pancreatic) on page 1579
Testicular cancer:
BEP (Ovarian Cancer, Testicular Cancer) on page 1526
BEP (Testicular Cancer) on page 1527
EP (Testicular Cancer) on page 1631
Paclitaxel-Ifosfamide-Cisplatin on page 1730

PVB on page 1744
VBP on page 1770
VIP (Etoposide) (Testicular Cancer) on page 1776
VIP (Vinblastine) (Testicular Cancer) on page 1777

Unknown primary, adenocarcinoma:
Cisplatin-Docetaxel (Unknown Primary) on page 1568
Cisplatin-Gemcitabine (Unknown Primary) on page 1580

Unknown primary, squamous cell:
Cisplatin-Docetaxel-Fluorouracil (Unknown Primary) on page 1568
Cisplatin-Fluorouracil-Paclitaxel (Unknown Primary) on page 1577

Administration Pretreatment hydration with 1-2 L of fluid is recommended prior to cisplatin administration; adequate post hydration and urinary output (>100 mL/hour) should be maintained for 24 hours after administration.

I.V.: Infuse over 6- 8 hours; has also been infused (unlabeled rates) over 30 minutes to 3 hours, at a rate of 1 mg/minute, or as a continuous infusion; infusion rate varies by protocol (refer to specific protocol for infusion details). Avoid extravasation.

Needles or I.V. administration sets that contain aluminum should not be used in the preparation or administration; aluminum can react with cisplatin resulting in precipitate formation and loss of potency.

Emetic Potential

≥50 mg/m^2: Very high (>90%)
<50 mg/m^2: Moderate (30% to 90%)

Vesicant/Extravasation Risk Vesicant (>0.5 mg/mL); Irritant (<0.5 mg/mL); see Management of Drug Extravasations on page 1800

Monitoring Parameters Renal function (serum creatinine, BUN, Cl_{cr}); electrolytes (particularly magnesium, calcium, potassium [periodic]); CBC with differential and platelet count (weekly); liver function tests (periodic); audiography (baseline and prior to each subsequent dose, and following treatment in children), neurologic exam (with high dose); urine output, urinalysis

Dietary Considerations Some products may contain sodium.

Dosage Forms Excipient information presented when available (limited, particularly for generics); consult specific product labeling.

Injection, solution [preservative free]: 1 mg/mL (50 mL, 100 mL, 200 mL)

References

Armstrong DK, Bundy B, Wenzel L, et al, "Intraperitoneal Cisplatin and Paclitaxel in Ovarian Cancer," *N Engl J Med*, 2006, 354(1):34-43.

Aronoff GR, Bennett WM, Berns JS, et al, *Drug Prescribing in Renal Failure: Dosing Guidelines for Adults and Children*, 5th ed. Philadelphia, PA: American College of Physicians; 2007, p 97, 170.

Bernier J, Domenge C, Ozsahin M, et al, "Postoperative Irradiation With or Without Concomitant Chemotherapy for Locally Advanced Head and Neck Cancer," *N Engl J Med*, 2004, 350 (19):1945-52.

Cooper JS, Pajak TF, Forastiere AA, et al, "Postoperative Concurrent Radiotherapy and Chemotherapy for High-Risk Squamous-Cell Carcinoma of the Head and Neck," *N Engl J Med*, 2004, 350(19):1937-44.

Goorin AM, Schwartzentruber DJ, Devidas M, et al, "Presurgical Chemotherapy Compared With Immediate Surgery and Adjuvant Chemotherapy for Nonmetastatic Osteosarcoma: Pediatric Oncology Group Study POG-8651," *J Clin Oncol*, 2003, 21(8):1574-80.

Kintzel PE and Dorr RT, "Anticancer Drug Renal Toxicity and Elimination: Dosing Guidelines for Altered Renal Function," *Cancer Treat Rev*, 1995, 21(1):33-64.

Morgan C, Tillett T, Braybrooke J, et al, "Management of Uncommon Chemotherapy-Induced Emergencies," *Lancet Oncol*, 2011, 12(8):806-14.

Nowak AK, Byrne MJ, Williamson R, et al, "A Multicentre Phase II Study of Cisplatin and Gemcitabine for Malignant Mesothelioma," *Br J Cancer*, 2002, 87(5):491-6.

Packer RJ, Gajjar A, Vezina G, et al, "Phase III Study of Craniospinal Radiation Therapy Followed by Adjuvant Chemotherapy for Newly Diagnosed Average-Risk Medulloblastoma," *J Clin Oncol*, 2006, 24(25):4202-8.

Pritchard J, Brown J, Shafford E, et al, "Cisplatin, Doxorubicin, and Delayed Surgery for Childhood Hepatoblastoma: A Successful Approach–Results of the First Prospective Study of the International Society of Pediatric Oncology," *J Clin Oncol*, 2000, 18(22):3819-28.
Saxman SB, Finch D, Gonin R, et al, "Long-Term Follow-Up of a Phase III Study of Three Versus Four Cycles of Bleomycin, Etoposide, and Cisplatin in Favorable-Prognosis Germ-Cell Tumors: The Indian University Experience," *J Clin Oncol*, 1998, 16(2):702-6.
Schuchter LM, Hensley ML, Meropol NJ, et al, "2002 Update of Recommendations for the Use of Chemotherapy and Radiotherapy Protectants: Clinical Practice Guidelines of the American Society of Clinical Oncology," *J Clin Oncol*, 2002, 20(12):2895-903.
van Haarst JM, Baas P, Manegold Ch, et al, "Multicentre Phase II Study of Gemcitabine and Cisplatin in Malignant Pleural Mesothelioma," *Br J Cancer*, 2002, 86(3):342-5.
Vogelzang NJ, Rusthoven JJ, Symanowski J, et al, "Phase III Study of Pemetrexed in Combination With Cisplatin Versus Cisplatin Alone in Patients With Malignant Pleural Mesothelioma," *J Clin Oncol*, 2003, 21(14):2636-44.

◆ ***Cis*-Retinoic Acid** *see* ISOtretinoin *on page 832*
◆ **13-*cis*-Retinoic Acid** *see* ISOtretinoin *on page 832*
◆ **13-*cis*-Vitamin A Acid** *see* ISOtretinoin *on page 832*
◆ **Citrovorum Factor** *see* Leucovorin Calcium *on page 870*
◆ **CL-118,532** *see* Triptorelin *on page 1413*
◆ **CL-184116** *see* Porfimer *on page 1183*
◆ **CL-232315** *see* MitoXANtrone *on page 996*

Cladribine (KLA dri been)

Related Information

Management of Chemotherapy-Induced Nausea and Vomiting *on page 1786*
Management of Drug Extravasations *on page 1800*
Safe Handling of Hazardous Drugs *on page 1904*

Brand Names: U.S. Leustatin® [DSC]

Index Terms 2-CdA; 2-Chlorodeoxyadenosine

Generic Availability (U.S.) Yes

Pharmacologic Category Antineoplastic Agent, Antimetabolite; Antineoplastic Agent, Antimetabolite (Purine Analog)

Use Treatment of active hairy cell leukemia

Unlabeled Use Treatment of acute myeloid leukemia (AML), chronic lymphocytic leukemia (CLL), non-Hodgkin's lymphomas (mantle cell), Waldenström's macroglobulinemia, refractory Langerhans cell histiocytosis

Labeled Contraindications Hypersensitivity to cladribine or any component of the formulation

Pregnancy Risk Factor D

Lactation Excretion in breast milk unknown/not recommended

Warnings/Precautions Hazardous agent - use appropriate precautions for handling and disposal. **[U.S. Boxed Warning]: Dose-dependent, reversible myelosuppression (neutropenia, anemia, and thrombocytopenia) is common and generally reversible;** use with caution in patients with pre-existing hematologic or immunologic abnormalities; monitor blood counts, especially during the first 4-8 weeks after treatment. **[U.S. Boxed Warning]: Serious, dose-related neurologic toxicity (including irreversible paraparesis and quadriparesis) has been reported with continuous infusions of higher doses (4-9 times the FDA-approved dose); may also occur at approved doses (rare).** Neurotoxicity may be delayed and may present as progressive, irreversible weakness; diagnostics with electromyography and nerve conduction studies were consistent with demyelinating disease. **[U.S. Boxed Warning]: Acute nephrotoxicity (eg, acidosis, anuria, increased serum**

creatinine), possibly requiring dialysis, has been reported with high doses (4-9 times the FDA-approved dose), particularly when administered with other nephrotoxic agents. Use with caution in patients with renal or hepatic impairment. Fever (>100°F) may occur, with or without neutropenia, observed more commonly in the first month of treatment. Infections (bacterial, viral, and fungal) were reported more commonly in the first month after treatment (generally mild or moderate in severity, although serious infections including sepsis have been reported); the incidence is reduced in the second month; due to neutropenia and T-cell depletion, risk versus benefit of treatment should be evaluated in patients with active infections. Administration of live vaccines is not recommended during treatment with cladribine (may increase the risk of infection due to immunosuppression). Use caution in patients with high tumor burden; tumor lysis syndrome may occur (rare). **[U.S. Boxed Warning]: Should be administered under the supervision of an experienced cancer chemotherapy physician.** Diluted product may contain benzyl alcohol which has been associated with "gasping syndrome" in neonates.

Adverse Reactions

>10%:

Central nervous system: Fever (33% to 69%; ≥100°F: 67%; ≥104°F: 11%), fatigue (11% to 45%), headache (7% to 22%)

Dermatologic: Rash (10% to 27%)

Gastrointestinal: Nausea (22% to 28%), appetite decreased (8% to 17%), vomiting (9% to 13%)

Hematologic: Neutropenia (grade 4: 70%; recovery: by week 5); anemia (1% to 37%; recovery: by week 8); myelosuppression (34%; prolonged), neutropenic fever (8% to 47%; severe: 32%), thrombocytopenia (grade 4: 12%; recovery: by day 12)

Local: Injection site reactions (9% to 19%)

Respiratory: Abnormal breath sounds (4% to 11%)

Miscellaneous: Infection (month 1: 28% [serious: 6%]; month 2: 6%)

1% to 10%:

Cardiovascular: Edema (2% to 6%), tachycardia (2% to 6%), thrombosis (2%)

Central nervous system: Chills (2% to 9%), dizziness (6% to 9%), insomnia (3% to 7%), malaise (5% to 7%), pain (6%), anxiety (1%)

Dermatologic: Purpura (10%), petechiae (2% to 8%), pruritus (2% to 6%), erythema (6%), hyperhidrosis (3%), bruising (1% to 2%)

Gastrointestinal: Diarrhea (7% to 10%), constipation (4% to 9%), abdominal pain (4% to 6%), flatulence (1%)

Local: Phlebitis (2%)

Neuromuscular & skeletal: Weakness (6% to 9%), myalgia (6% to 7%), arthralgia (3% to 5%), muscle weakness (1%)

Respiratory: Cough (7% to 10%), abnormal chest sounds (9%), dyspnea (5% to 7%), epistaxis (5%), rales (1%)

Miscellaneous: Diaphoresis (9%)

<1%, postmarketing, and/or case reports: Aplastic anemia, bacteremia, bilirubin increased, CD4 lymphocytopenia (nadir: 4-6 months), cellulitis, consciousness decreased, confusion, conjunctivitis, hemolytic anemia, hypereosinophilia, hypersensitivity, myelodysplastic syndrome, opportunistic infections (cytomegalovirus, fungal infections, herpes virus infections, listeriosis, *Pneumocystis jirovecii*), pancytopenia (prolonged), paraparesis, pneumonia, polyneuropathy (with high doses), progressive multifocal leukoencephalopathy (PML), pulmonary interstitial infiltrates, quadriparesis (reported at high doses), renal dysfunction (with high doses), renal failure,

septic shock, Stevens-Johnson syndrome, stroke, toxic epidermal necrolysis, transaminases increased, tuberculosis reactivation, tumor lysis syndrome, urticaria

Drug Interactions

Metabolism/Transport Effects None known.

Avoid Concomitant Use

Avoid concomitant use of Cladribine with any of the following: BCG; CloZAPine; Natalizumab; Pimecrolimus; Tacrolimus (Topical); Vaccines (Live)

Increased Effect/Toxicity

Cladribine may increase the levels/effects of: CloZAPine; Leflunomide; Natalizumab; Vaccines (Live)

The levels/effects of Cladribine may be increased by: Denosumab; Pimecrolimus; Roflumilast; Tacrolimus (Topical); Trastuzumab

Decreased Effect

Cladribine may decrease the levels/effects of: BCG; Coccidioidin Skin Test; Sipuleucel-T; Vaccines (Inactivated); Vaccines (Live)

The levels/effects of Cladribine may be decreased by: Echinacea

Ethanol/Nutrition/Herb Interactions Ethanol: Avoid ethanol (due to GI irritation).

Storage/Stability

Store intact vials refrigerated at 2°C to 8°C (36°F to 46°F). Protect from light. A precipitate may develop at low temperatures and may be resolubilized at room temperature or by shaking the solution vigorously. Inadvertent freezing does not affect the solution; if freezing occurs prior to dilution, allow to thaw naturally prior to reconstitution; do not heat or microwave; do not refreeze.

24-hour continuous infusion: Dilutions for infusion should be used promptly; if not used promptly, the 24-hour infusion may be stored refrigerated for up to 8 hours prior to administration.

7-day continuous infusion: Dilutions for infusion should be used promptly; if not used promptly, the 7-day infusion may be stored refrigerated for up to 8 hours prior to administration. Reconstituted solution is stable for 7 days (when diluted in bacteriostatic NS) in a CADD® medication cassette reservoir. For patients weighing >85 kg, the effectiveness of the preservative in the bacteriostatic diluent may be reduced (due to dilution).

Reconstitution Hazardous agent; use appropriate precautions for handling and disposal.

A precipitate may develop at low temperatures and may be resolubilized at room temperature or by shaking the solution vigorously. Inadvertent freezing does not affect the solution; if freezing occurs prior to dilution, allow to thaw naturally prior to reconstitution; do not heat or microwave; do not refreeze.

To prepare a 24-hour continuous infusion: Dilute in 500 mL NS. The manufacturer recommends filtering with a 0.22 micron hydrophilic syringe filter prior to adding to infusion bag.

To prepare a 7-day continuous infusion: Dilute to a total volume of 100 mL in a CADD® medication cassette reservoir using bacteriostatic NS. Filter diluent and cladribine with a 0.22 micron hydrophilic filter prior to adding to cassette/reservoir.

Mechanism of Action A purine nucleoside analogue; prodrug which is activated via phosphorylation by deoxycytidine kinase to a 5'-triphosphate derivative (2-CaAMP). This active form incorporates into DNA to result in the breakage of DNA strand and shutdown of DNA synthesis and repair. This also results in a depletion of nicotinamide adenine dinucleotide and adenosine triphosphate (ATP). Cladribine is cell-cycle nonspecific.

Pharmacodynamics/Kinetics

Distribution: V_d: ~9 L/kg; penetrates CSF (CSF concentrations are ~25% of plasma concentrations)

Protein binding: ~20%

Half-life elimination: After a 2-hour infusion (with normal renal function): 5.4 hours

Excretion: Urine (18%)

Dosing

Adult & Geriatric Details concerning dosing in combination regimens should also be consulted.

Hairy cell leukemia: I.V.: 0.09 mg/kg/day continuous infusion for 7 days for 1 cycle **or** (unlabeled dosing) 0.1 mg/kg/day continuous infusion for 7 days for 1 cycle (Goodman, 2003; Saven, 1998)

Acute myeloid leukemia, induction (unlabeled use): I.V.: CLAG or CLAG-M regimen: 5 mg/m²/day over 2 hours for 5 days; a second induction may be administered if needed (Robak, 2000; Wierzbowska, 2008; Wrzesień-Kuś, 2003)

Chronic lymphocytic leukemia (unlabeled use): I.V.: 0.1 mg/kg/day continuous infusion for 7 days every 4-5 weeks (Saven, 1995) **or** 0.14 mg/kg/day over 2 hours for 5 days every 28 days for 3-6 cycles (Byrd, 2003)

Mantle cell lymphoma (unlabeled use): I.V.: 5 mg/m²/day over 2 hours for 5 days every 4 weeks for 2-6 cycles (Inwards, 2008; Rummel, 1999) **or** 5 mg/m²/day over 2 hours for 5 days every 4 weeks for 2-6 cycles (in combination with rituximab) (Inwards, 2008)

Waldenström's macroglobulinemia (unlabeled use):

I.V.: 0.1 mg/kg/day continuous infusion for 7 days every 4 weeks for 2 cycles (Dimopoulos, 1994)

SubQ: 0.1 mg/kg/day for 5 consecutive days every month for 4 cycles (in combination with rituximab) (Laszlo, 2010)

Pediatric

Acute myeloid leukemia (unlabeled use): I.V.: 8.9 mg/m²/day continuous infusion for 5 days for 1 or 2 courses (Krance, 2001) **or** 9 mg/m²/day over 30 minutes for 5 days for 1 course (in combination with cytarabine) (Crews, 2002; Rubnitz, 2009)

Langerhans cell histiocytosis, refractory (unlabeled use): I.V.: 5 mg/m²/day over 2 hours for 5 days every 21 days for up to 6 cycles (Weitzman, 2009)

Renal Impairment No dosage adjustment provided in the manufacturer's labeling (due to inadequate data), use with caution. The following adjustments have been used (Aronoff, 2007):

Children:

- Cl_{cr} 10-50 mL/minute: Administer 50% of dose
- Cl_{cr} <10 mL/minute: Administer 30% of dose
- Hemodialysis: Administer 30% of dose
- Continuous renal replacement therapy (CRRT): Administer 50% of dose

Adults:

- Cl_{cr} 10-50 mL/minute: Administer 75% of dose
- Cl_{cr} <10 mL/minute: Administer 50% of dose
- Continuous ambulatory peritoneal dialysis (CAPD): Administer 50% of dose

Hepatic Impairment No dosage adjustment provided in the manufacturer's labeling (due to inadequate data); use with caution.

Combination Regimens

Leukemia, acute myeloid:

CLAG (AML Induction) on page 1586

CLAG-M (AML Induction) on page 1586

Administration

I.V.: Administer as a continuous infusion. May also be administered over 30 minutes or over 2 hours (unlabeled administration rates) depending on indication and/or protocol.

SubQ (unlabeled route): May also be administered SubQ (Laszlo, 2010)

Emetic Potential Very low (<10%)

Monitoring Parameters CBC with differential (particularly during the first 4-8 weeks post-treatment), renal and hepatic function; bone marrow biopsy (after CBC has normalized, to confirm treatment response); monitor for fever; monitor for signs/symptoms of neurotoxicity

Dosage Forms Excipient information presented when available (limited, particularly for generics); consult specific product labeling. [DSC] = Discontinued product

Injection, solution [preservative free]: 1 mg/mL (10 mL)

Leustatin®: 1 mg/mL (10 mL [DSC])

References

Aronoff GR, Bennett WM, Berns JS, et al, *Drug Prescribing in Renal Failure: Dosing Guidelines for Adults and Children*, 5th ed. Philadelphia, PA: American College of Physicians; 2007, p 98, 170.

Bernard F, Thomas C, Bertrand Y, et al, "Multi-Centre Pilot Study of 2-Chlorodeoxyadenosine and Cytosine Arabinoside Combined Chemotherapy in Refractory Langerhans Cell Histiocytosis With Haematological Dysfunction," *Eur J Cancer*, 2005, 41(17):2682-9.

Byrd JC, Peterson B, Piro L, et al, "A Phase II Study of Cladribine Treatment for Fludarabine Refractory B Cell Chronic Lymphocytic Leukemia: Results From CALGB Study 9211," *Leukemia*, 2003, 17(2):323-7.

Crews KR, Gandhi V, Srivastava DK, et al, "Interim Comparison of a Continuous Infusion versus a Short Daily Infusion of Cytarabine Given in Combination With Cladribine for Pediatric Acute Myeloid Leukemia," *J Clin Oncol*, 2002, 20(20):4217-24.

Dimopoulos MA, Kantarjian H, Weber D, et al, "Primary Therapy of Waldenström's Macroglobulinemia With 2-Chlorodeoxyadenosine," *J Clin Oncol*, 1994, 12(12):2694-8.

Goodman GR, Burian C, Koziol JA., et al, "Extended Follow-Up of Patients With Hairy Cell Leukemia After Treatment With Cladribine," *J Clin Oncol*, 2003, 21(5):891-6.

Inwards DJ, Fishkin PA, Hillman DW, et al, "Long-Term Results of the Treatment of Patients With Mantle Cell Lymphoma With Cladribine (2-CDA) Alone (95-80-53) or 2-CDA and Rituximab (N0189) in the North Central Cancer Treatment Group," *Cancer*, 2008, 113(1):108-16.

Krance RA, Hurwitz CA, Head DR, et al, "Experience With 2-Chlorodeoxyadenosine in Previously Untreated Children With Newly Diagnosed Acute Myeloid Leukemia and Myelodysplastic Diseases," *J Clin Oncol*, 2001, 19(11):2804-11.

Laszlo D, Andreola G, Rigacci L, et al, "Rituximab and Subcutaneous 2-Chloro-2'-Deoxyadenosine Combination Treatment for Patients With Waldenström Macroglobulinemia: Clinical and Biologic Results of a Phase II Multicenter Study," *J Clin Oncol*, 2010, 28(13):2233-8.

Robak T, Wrzesień-Kuś A, Lech-Marańda E, et al, "Combination Regimen of Cladribine (2-Chlorodeoxyadenosine), Cytarabine and G-CSF (CLAG) as Induction Therapy for Patients With Relapsed or Refractory Acute Myeloid Leukemia," *Leuk Lymphoma*, 2000, 39(1-2):121-9.

Rubnitz JE, Crews KR, Pounds S, et al, "Combination of Cladribine and Cytarabine is Effective for Childhood Acute Myeloid Leukemia: Results of the St Jude AML97 Trial," *Leukemia*, 2009, 23 (8):1410-6.

Rummel MJ, Chow KU, Jäger E, "Treatment of Mantle Cell Lymphomas With Intermittent Two-Hour Infusion of Cladribine as First-Line Therapy or in First Relapse," *Ann Oncol*, 1999, 10(1):115-7.

Saven A, Burian C, Koziol JA, et al, "Long-Term Follow-Up of Patients With Hairy Cell Leukemia After Cladribine Treatment," *Blood*, 1998, 92(6):1918-26.

Saven A, Lemon RH, Kosty M, et al, "2-Chlorodeoxyadenosine Activity in Patients With Untreated Chronic Lymphocytic Leukemia," *J Clin Oncol*, 1995, 13(3):570-4.

Stine KC, Saylors RL, Saccente S, et al, "Efficacy of Continuous Infusion 2-CDA (Cladribine) in Pediatric Patients With Langerhans Cell Histiocytosis," *Pediatr Blood Cancer*, 2004, 43(1):81-4.

Weitzman S, Braier J, Donadieu J, et al, "2'-Chlorodeoxyadenosine (2-CdA) as Salvage Therapy for Langerhans Cell Histiocytosis (LCH). Results of the LCH-S-98 Protocol of the Histiocyte Society," *Pediatr Blood Cancer*, 2009, 53(7):1271-6.

Wierzbowska A, Robak T, Pluta A, et al, "Cladribine Combined With High Doses of Arabinoside Cytosine, Mitoxantrone, and G-CSF (CLAG-M) is a Highly Effective Salvage Regimen in Patients With Refractory and Relapsed Acute Myeloid Leukemia of the Poor Risk: A Final Report of the Polish Adult Leukemia Group," *Eur J Haematol*, 2008, 80(2):115-26.

Wrzesień-Kuś A, Robak T, Lech-Marańda E, et al, "A Multicenter, Open, Non-Comparative Phase II Study of the Combination of Cladribine (2-Chlorodeoxyadenosine), Cytarabine, and G-CSF as Induction Therapy in Refractory Acute Myeloid Leukemia – a Report of the Polish Adult Leukemia Group (PALG)," *Eur J Haematol*, 2003, 71(3):155–62.

◆ **Claravis™** *see* ISOtretinoin *on page 832*

◆ **Clarus™ (Can)** *see* ISOtretinoin *on page 832*

◆ **Clasteon® (Can)** *see* Clodronate *on page 303*

Clodronate (KLOE droh nate)

Brand Names: Canada Bonefos®; Clasteon®

Index Terms Clodronate Disodium

Pharmacologic Category Bisphosphonate Derivative

Use Management of hypercalcemia of malignancy; management of osteolysis due to bone metastases of malignancy

Labeled Contraindications Hypersensitivity to clodronate, bisphosphonates, or any component of the formulation; severe GI inflammation; renal impairment (serum creatinine >5 mg/dL, SI 440 micromole/L); concomitant use with other bisphosphonates; pregnancy or breast-feeding

Lactation Excretion in breast milk unknown/contraindicated

Warnings/Precautions Use caution in patients with renal impairment; dose reductions, as well as close monitoring of serum creatinine and BUN, are necessary. Use is contraindicated when serum creatinine >5 mg/dL (SI 440 micromole/L). May cause irritation to upper gastrointestinal mucosa. Esophagitis, dysphagia, esophageal ulcers, esophageal erosions, and esophageal stricture (rare) have been reported with bisphosphonates (oral). Use with caution in patients with dysphagia, esophageal disease, gastritis, duodenitis, or ulcers (may worsen underlying condition). Discontinue use if new or worsening symptoms develop.

Bisphosphonate therapy has been associated with osteonecrosis, primarily of the jaw; this has been observed mostly in cancer patients, but also in patients with postmenopausal osteoporosis and other diagnoses. Most reported cases occurred after I.V. bisphosphonate therapy; however, cases have been reported following oral therapy. Dental exams and preventative dentistry should be performed prior to placing patients with risk factors on chronic bisphosphonate therapy. Invasive dental procedures should be avoided during treatment.

Infrequently, severe (and occasionally debilitating) bone, joint, and/or muscle pain have been reported during bisphosphonate treatment. The onset of pain ranged from a single day to several months. Consider discontinuing therapy in patients who experience severe symptoms; symptoms usually resolve upon discontinuation. Some patients experienced recurrence when rechallenged with same drug or another bisphosphonate; avoid use in patients with a history of these symptoms in association with bisphosphonate therapy. May cause hypocalcemia (increased risk with intravenous administration) or transient hypophosphatemia.

For I.V. preparation: Dilute prior to use; adequate hydration should be ensured prior to infusion; avoid infiltration/extravasation. Do not administer as bolus injection (may precipitate acute renal failure, severe local reactions, and thrombophlebitis). Monitor renal function during and after intravenous administration. Interrupt infusion in patients experiencing deteriorating renal function during therapy.

Adverse Reactions

>10%: Hepatic: Transaminases increased (≤18%; >2 x ULN: 2%)

1% to 10%:

Endocrine & metabolic: Hypocalcemia (≤3%)

Gastrointestinal: GI disturbances (≤10%; includes anorexia, diarrhea, gastric pain, nausea, vomiting)

Renal: Serum creatinine increased (1%), BUN increased

<1%, postmarketing, and/or case reports: Alkaline phosphatase increased, bronchospasm (patients with aspirin-sensitive asthma), dysphagia, erythematous rash, hypersensitivity reactions (angioedema, pruritus, rash, respiratory disorder, urticaria), hypophosphatemia (transient), leukemia/myelodysplasia (rare), macropapular rash, mouth irritation, musculoskeletal pain (severe), oliguria, osteonecrosis (primarily of jaw), parathyroid hormone increased, proteinuria, renal failure, ulcerative pharyngitis

Drug Interactions

Metabolism/Transport Effects None known.

Avoid Concomitant Use There are no known interactions where it is recommended to avoid concomitant use.

Increased Effect/Toxicity

Clodronate may increase the levels/effects of: Deferasirox; Estramustine; Phosphate Supplements; SUNItinib

The levels/effects of Clodronate may be increased by: Aminoglycosides; Nonsteroidal Anti-Inflammatory Agents

Decreased Effect

The levels/effects of Clodronate may be decreased by: Antacids; Calcium Salts; Iron Salts; Magnesium Salts; Multivitamins/Minerals (with ADEK, Folate, Iron); Proton Pump Inhibitors

Ethanol/Nutrition/Herb Interactions Food: All food and beverages may interfere with absorption. Coadministration with dairy products may decrease absorption. Beverages (especially orange juice and coffee), food, and medications (eg, antacids, calcium, iron, and multivalent cations) may reduce the absorption of bisphosphonates as much as 60%.

Storage/Stability Store capsules and undiluted ampuls at room temperature (15°C to 30°C).

Clasteon®: Diluted solution should be infused within 12 hours of preparation.

Bonefos®: Diluted solution should be infused within 24 hours of preparation. Once diluted, Bonefos® may be stored up to 24 hours at room temperature.

Reconstitution Injection must be further diluted (in 500 mL of NS or D_5W) prior to administration.

Mechanism of Action A bisphosphonate which lowers serum calcium by inhibition of bone resorption via actions on osteoclasts or on osteoclast precursors.

Pharmacodynamics/Kinetics

Onset of calcium-lowering effects: I.V.: Within 48 hours

Duration of calcium-lowering effects: 5 days to 3 weeks following discontinuation

Absorption: Oral: Rapid but low absorption (~1% to 3%)
Distribution: V_d: ~20 L; 20% of absorbed clodronate is bound to bone
Protein binding: Variable (2% to 36%)
Bioavailability: Oral: 1% to 3%
Half-life elimination: Terminal: Oral: ~6 hours; I.V.: 13 hours (serum); prolonged in bone tissue
Time to peak, plasma: Oral: 30 minutes
Excretion: Urine (60% to 80% of absorbed dose as unchanged drug); feces (as unabsorbed drug)

Dosing

Adult & Geriatric

Hypercalcemia of malignancy:

I.V.:

Clasteon®

Single infusion: 1500 mg as a single dose

Multiple infusions: 300 mg once daily; treatment duration should not exceed 10 days

Bonefos®: Multiple infusions: 300 mg once daily; treatment duration should not exceed 7 days

Oral: Recommended daily maintenance dose following I.V. therapy:

Clasteon®: Range: 1600 mg (4 capsules) to 2400 mg (6 capsules) given in a single or 2 divided doses; maximum recommended daily dose: 3200 mg (8 capsules).

Bonefos®: Range: 1600 mg (4 capsules) to 2400 mg (6 capsules) given in single or 2 divided doses; maximum recommended daily dose: 3200 mg (8 capsules).

Osteolytic bone metastases:

I.V.:

Clasteon®:

Single infusion: 1500 mg as a single dose

Multiple infusions: 300 mg once daily; treatment duration should not exceed 10 days

Bonefos®: Multiple infusions: 300 mg once daily; treatment duration should not exceed 7 days

Oral:

Clasteon®: Recommended daily maintenance dose following I.V. therapy: Range: 1600 mg (4 capsules) to 2400 mg (6 capsules) given in a single or 2 divided doses; maximum recommended daily dose: 3200 mg (8 capsules).

Bonefos®: Initial: 1600 mg/day; may be increased to a maximum of 3200 mg/day

Note: Retreatment: Limited data suggests that patients who develop hypercalcemia following discontinuation of therapy or during oral therapy may be retreated with Bonefos® or Clasteon® at a higher oral dosage (up to 3200 mg/day) or by I.V. infusion with Clasteon® (1500 mg as single dose or 300 mg once daily) or Bonefos® (300 mg once daily).

Renal Impairment

Clasteon®:

Serum creatinine (S_{cr}) >5 mg/dL: Use is contraindicated.

S_{cr} ≥2.5-5 mg/dL: Dosage reduction is recommended; however, there are no dosage adjustments provided in manufacturer's labeling.

Bonefos®: **Note:** S_{cr} >5 mg/dL: Use is contraindicated.

I.V.:
Cl_{cr}: 50-80 mL/minute: Administer 75% to 100% of normal dose.
Cl_{cr}: 12-49 mL/minute: Administer 50% to 75% of normal dose.
Cl_{cr}: <12 mL/minute: Administer 50% of normal dose.
Oral: **Note:** Daily doses >1600 mg should not be used continuously.
Cl_{cr}: >50 mL/minute: No dosage reduction recommended.
Cl_{cr}: 30-50 mL/minute: Administer 75% of normal dose.
Cl_{cr}: <30 mL/minute: Administer 50% of normal dose.

Administration

Capsules: Administer with a glass of plain water at least 2 hours (Bonefos®) or 1 hour (Clasteon®) before or after food.

Injection: Do not administer as bolus injection; for single infusion therapy administer over at least 4 hours; for multiple-infusion therapy administered once daily, infuse over 2-6 hours. Patients should be adequately hydrated with oral or I.V. fluids prior to infusion.

Monitoring Parameters Serum electrolytes including calcium, phosphorous, magnesium, and potassium; monitor for hypocalcemia for at least 2 weeks after therapy; serum creatinine, BUN, CBC with differential, hepatic function

Test Interactions Bisphosphonates may interfere with diagnostic imaging agents such as technetium-99m-diphosphonate in bone scans.

Dietary Considerations Take at least 1 hour (Clasteon®) or 2 hours (Bonefos®) before or after food.

Product Availability Not available in U.S.

Dosage Forms: Canada Excipient information presented when available (limited, particularly for generics); consult specific product labeling.

Capsule, oral:
Bonefos®, Clasteon®: 400 mg

Injection, solution:
Bonefos®: 60 mg/mL (5 mL)
Clasteon®: 30 mg/mL (10 mL)

References

Assael LA, "Oral Bisphosphonates as a Cause of Bisphosphonate-Related Osteonecrosis of the Jaws: Clinical Findings, Assessment of Risks, and Preventive Strategies," *J Oral Maxillofac Surg*, 2009, 67(5 Suppl):35-43.

Durie BG, Katz M, and Crowley J, "Osteonecrosis of the Jaw and Bisphosphonates," *N Engl J Med*, 2005, 353(1):99-102.

Maerevoet M, Martin C, and Duck L, "Osteonecrosis of the Jaw and Bisphosphonates,"*N Engl J Med*, 2005, 353(1):99-102.

◆ **Clodronate Disodium** *see* Clodronate *on page* 303

Clofarabine (klo FARE a been)

Related Information

Management of Chemotherapy-Induced Nausea and Vomiting *on page* 1786
Management of Infections *on page* 1809
Safe Handling of Hazardous Drugs *on page* 1904

Brand Names: U.S. Clolar®

Index Terms CAFdA; Clofarex

Generic Availability (U.S.) No

Pharmacologic Category Antineoplastic Agent, Antimetabolite (Purine Analog)

Use Treatment of relapsed or refractory acute lymphoblastic leukemia (ALL) in children (ages 1-21 years)

Unlabeled Use Treatment of acute myeloid leukemia (AML) in adults ≥60 years of age

Labeled Contraindications There are no contraindications listed within the manufacturer's labeling.

Pregnancy Risk Factor D

Lactation Excretion in breast milk unknown/not recommended

Warnings/Precautions Hazardous agent - use appropriate precautions for handling and disposal. Tumor lysis syndrome and cytokine release may develop into systemic inflammatory response syndrome (SIRS)/capillary leak syndrome, and organ dysfunction; discontinuation of clofarabine should be considered with the presentation of SIRS or capillary leak syndrome (see Tumor Lysis Syndrome on page 1822). Safety and efficacy have not been established with renal or hepatic dysfunction; use with caution. Safety and efficacy in pediatric patients <1 year of age or adults >21 years have not been established.

Adverse Reactions

>10%:

Cardiovascular: Tachycardia (35%), hypotension (29%; grades 3/4: 19%), flushing (19%), hypertension (13%), edema (12%)

Central nervous system: Headache (43%), fever (39%), chills (34%), fatigue (34%), anxiety (21%), pain (15%)

Dermatologic: Pruritus (43%), rash (38%), petechiae (26%), palmar-plantar erythrodysesthesia syndrome (16%), erythema (11%)

Gastrointestinal: Vomiting (78%; grades 3/4: 9%), nausea (73%; grades 3/4: 15%), diarrhea (56%), abdominal pain (8% to 35%), anorexia (30%), mucosal inflammation (16%), gingival bleeding (14%), oral candidiasis (11%)

Hematologic: Leukopenia (grades 3/4: 88%), anemia (83%; grades 3/4: 75%), lymphopenia (grades 3/4: 82%), thrombocytopenia (81%; grades 3/4: 80%), neutropenia (grades 3/4: 10% to 64%), febrile neutropenia (55%, grade 4: 3%)

Hepatic: ALT increased (81%; grades 3/4: 43% to 44%), AST increased (74%; grades 3/4: 36%), bilirubin increased (45%; grades 3/4: 13%)

Neuromuscular & skeletal: Limb pain (30%), myalgia (14%)

Renal: Creatinine increased (50%; grades 3/4: 8%), hematuria (13%)

Respiratory: Epistaxis (27%), dyspnea (13%), pleural effusion (12%)

Miscellaneous: Infection (83%; includes bacterial, fungal, and viral), catheter-related infection (12%)

1% to 10%:

Cardiovascular: Pericardial effusion (8%)

Central nervous system: Irritability (10%), lethargy (10%), somnolence (10%), agitation (5%), mental status change (1% to 4%)

Dermatologic: Cellulitis (8%), pruritic rash (8%)

Gastrointestinal: Proctalgia (8%), clostridium colitis (7%), stomatitis (7%), mouth hemorrhage (5%), oral mucosal petechiae (5%), cecitis (1% to 4%), pancreatitis (1% to 4%)

Hepatic: Jaundice (8%)

Neuromuscular & skeletal: Back pain (10%), bone pain (10%), weakness (10%), arthralgia (9%)

Respiratory: Pneumonia (10%), respiratory distress (10%), tachypnea (9%), upper respiratory tract infection (5%), pulmonary edema (1% to 4%)

Miscellaneous: Herpes simplex (10%), sepsis (10%), bacteremia (9%), candidiasis (7%), herpes zoster (7%), septic shock (7%), staphylococcus bacteremia (6%), tumor lysis syndrome (grade 3: 6%), capillary leak syndrome (4%), hypersensitivity (1% to 4%), SIRS (2%)

<1%, postmarketing, and/or case reports: Bone marrow failure, dermatitis, hallucination, hepatic sinusoidal obstruction syndrome (SOS; veno-occlusive disease), hepatomegaly, hypokalemia, hypophosphatemia, left ventricular systolic function decreased, right ventricular pressure increased, Stevens-Johnson syndrome, toxic epidermal necrolysis

Drug Interactions

Metabolism/Transport Effects None known.

Avoid Concomitant Use

Avoid concomitant use of Clofarabine with any of the following: BCG; CloZAPine; Natalizumab; Pimecrolimus; Tacrolimus (Topical); Vaccines (Live)

Increased Effect/Toxicity

Clofarabine may increase the levels/effects of: CloZAPine; Leflunomide; Natalizumab; Vaccines (Live); Vitamin K Antagonists

The levels/effects of Clofarabine may be increased by: Denosumab; Pimecrolimus; Roflumilast; Tacrolimus (Topical); Trastuzumab

Decreased Effect

Clofarabine may decrease the levels/effects of: BCG; Cardiac Glycosides; Coccidioidin Skin Test; Sipuleucel-T; Vaccines (Inactivated); Vaccines (Live); Vitamin K Antagonists

The levels/effects of Clofarabine may be decreased by: Echinacea

Storage/Stability Store intact vials at room temperature of 25°C (77°F); excursions permitted to 15°C to 30°C (59°F to 86°F). Solutions diluted for infusion in D_5W or NS are stable for 24 hours at room temperature.

Reconstitution Clofarabine should be diluted with NS or D_5W to a final concentration of 0.15-0.4 mg/mL. Manufacturer recommends the product be filtered through a 0.2 micron filter prior to dilution. Use appropriate precautions for handling and disposal.

Mechanism of Action Clofarabine, a purine (deoxyadenosine) nucleoside analog, is metabolized to clofarabine 5'-triphosphate. Clofarabine 5'-triphosphate decreases cell replication and repair as well as causing cell death. To decrease cell replication and repair, clofarabine 5'-triphosphate competes with deoxyadenosine triphosphate for the enzymes ribonucleotide reductase and DNA polymerase. Cell replication is decreased when clofarabine 5'-triphosphate inhibits ribonucleotide reductase from reacting with deoxyadenosine triphosphate to produce deoxynucleotide triphosphate which is needed for DNA synthesis. Cell replication is also decreased when clofarabine 5'-triphosphate competes with DNA polymerase for incorporation into the DNA chain; when done during the repair process, cell repair is affected. To cause cell death, clofarabine 5'-triphosphate alters the mitochondrial membrane by releasing proteins, an inducing factor and cytochrome C.

Pharmacodynamics/Kinetics

Distribution: V_d: Children: 172 L/m^2 or 5.8 L/kg (Bonate, 2011); Elderly: 268 L/kg (Bonate, 2011)

Protein binding: 47%, primarily to albumin

Metabolism: Intracellulary by deoxycytidine kinase and mono- and diphosphokinases to active metabolite clofarabine 5′-triphosphate; limited hepatic metabolism (0.2%)

Half-life elimination: Children: ~5 hours; Children and Adults: 7 hours (Bonate, 2011); half-life may be increased in elderly and in patients with renal impairment (Bonate, 2011)

Excretion: Urine (49% to 60%, as unchanged drug)

Dosing

Adult Consider prophylactic corticosteroids (hydrocortisone 100 mg/m² on days 1-3) to prevent signs/symptoms of capillary leak syndrome or systemic inflammatory response syndrome (SIRS), hydration and allopurinol (to reduce the risk of tumor lysis syndrome/hyperuricemia), and prophylactic antiemetics.

Acute lymphoblastic leukemia (ALL): Adults ≤21 years: I.V.: 52 mg/m²/day days 1 through 5; repeat every 2-6 weeks; subsequent cycles should begin no sooner than 14 days from day 1 of the previous cycle (subsequent cycles may be administered when ANC ≥750/mm³)

Acute myelocytic leukemia (AML; unlabeled use): Adults ≥60 years: I.V.:

Monotherapy (Kantarjian, 2010):

Induction: 30 mg/m²/day for 5 days; may repeat one time after day 20 (if needed) with 20 mg/m²/day for 5 days

Consolidation: 20 mg/m²/day for 5 days for up to a maximum total 6 cycles, including induction cycles

Combination therapy with cytarabine (Faderl, 2008):

Induction: 30 mg/m²/day for 5 days; may repeat one time if needed

Consolidation: 30 mg/m²/day for 3 days every 4-7 weeks for up to a total of 12 consolidation cycles

Pediatric Consider prophylactic corticosteroids (hydrocortisone 100 mg/m² on days 1-3) to prevent signs/symptoms of capillary leak syndrome or systemic inflammatory response syndrome (SIRS), hydration and allopurinol (to reduce the risk of tumor lysis syndrome/hyperuricemia), and prophylactic antiemetics.

Acute lymphoblastic leukemia (ALL): Children ≥1 year: I.V.: 52 mg/m²/day days 1 through 5; repeat every 2-6 weeks; subsequent cycles should begin no sooner than 14 days from day 1 of the previous cycle (subsequent cycles may be administered when ANC ≥750/mm³)

Renal Impairment No dosage adjustment provided in manufacturer's labeling; use with caution (has not been studied). Clofarabine undergoes renal elimination and exposure is increased as creatinine clearance decreases (Bonate, 2011).

NCCN AML guidelines (v.2.2011): Adults >60 years with creatinine clearance <60 mL/minute: Use is not recommended.

Hepatic Impairment No dosage adjustment provided in manufacturer's labeling; use with caution (has not been studied).

Adjustment for Toxicity

Hematologic toxicity: ANC <500/mm³ lasting ≥4 weeks: Reduce clofarabine dose by 25% for next cycle

Nonhematologic toxicity:

Clinically significant infection: Withhold treatment until infection is under control, then restart clofarabine at full dose

Grade 3 toxicity excluding infection, nausea and vomiting, and transient elevations in transaminases and bilirubin: Withhold treatment; may reinitiate clofarabine with a 25% dose-reduction with resolution or return to baseline

Grade ≥3 increase in creatinine or bilirubin: Discontinue clofarabine; may reinitiate with 25% dosage reduction when creatinine or bilirubin return to baseline and patient is stable; administer allopurinol for hyperuricemia

Grade 4 toxicity (noninfectious): Discontinue clofarabine treatment

Capillary leak or systemic inflammatory response syndrome (SIRS) early signs/symptoms (eg, hypotension, tachycardia, tachypnea, pulmonary edema): Discontinue clofarabine; institute supportive measures

Combination Regimens

Leukemia, acute myeloid:

Clofarabine (AML Consolidation) on page 1587
Clofarabine (AML Induction) on page 1587
Clofarabine-Cytarabine (AML Consolidation) on page 1587
Clofarabine-Cytarabine (AML Induction) on page 1587

Administration

Acute lymphoblastic leukemia (ALL): I.V. infusion: Over 2 hours. Continuous I.V. fluids are encouraged to decrease adverse events and tumor lysis effects. Hypotension may be a sign of capillary leak syndrome or systemic inflammatory response syndrome (SIRS). Discontinue if the patient becomes hypotensive during administration. Retreatment should only be considered if the hypotension is not related to capillary leak syndrome or SIRS.

Acute myelocytic leukemia (AML): Was infused over 1 hour in AML studies (Faderl, 2008; Kantarjian, 2010)

Emetic Potential Moderate (30% to 90%)

Monitoring Parameters Blood pressure, cardiac function, and respiratory status during infusion; CBC with differential (periodic; increase frequency in patients who develop cytopenias); liver and kidney function (during 5 days of clofarabine administration); signs and symptoms of tumor lysis syndrome and cytokine release syndrome (tachypnea, tachycardia, hypotension, pulmonary edema); hydration status

Dosage Forms Excipient information presented when available (limited, particularly for generics); consult specific product labeling.

Injection, solution [preservative free]:

Clolar®: 1 mg/mL (20 mL)

References

Bonate PL, Cunningham CC, Gaynon P, et al, "Population Pharmacokinetics of Clofarabine and its Metabolite 6-Ketoclofarabine in Adult and Pediatric Patients With Cancer," *Cancer Chemother Pharmacol*, 2011, 67(4):875-90.

Faderl S, Ravandi F, Huang X, et al, "A Randomized Study of Clofarabine versus Clofarabine Plus Low-Dose Cytarabine as Front-Line Therapy for Patients Aged 60 Years and Older With Acute Myeloid Leukemia and High-Risk Myelodysplastic Syndrome," *Blood*, 2008, 112(5):1638-45.

Jeha S, Gaynon PS, Razzouk BI, et al, "Phase II Study of Clofarabine in Pediatric Patients With Refractory or Relapsed Acute Lymphoblastic Leukemia," *J Clin Oncol*, 2008, 24(12):1917-23.

Kantarjian HM, Erba HP, Claxton D, et al, "Phase II Study of Clofarabine Monotherapy in Previously Untreated Older Adults With Acute Myeloid Leukemia and Unfavorable Prognostic Factors," *J Clin Oncol*, 2010, 28(4):549-55.

National Comprehensive Cancer Network® (NCCN), "Practice Guidelines in Oncology™: Acute Myeloid Leukemia," Version 2, 2011. Available at http://www.nccn.org/professionals/physician_gls/PDF/aml.pdf

◆ **Clofarex** *see* Clofarabine *on page* 306

◆ **Clolar®** *see* Clofarabine *on page* 306

Clotrimazole (Oral) (kloe TRIM a zole)

Index Terms Mycelex

Generic Availability (U.S.) Yes

Pharmacologic Category Antifungal Agent, Oral Nonabsorbed

Use Treatment of susceptible fungal infections, including oropharyngeal candidiasis; limited data suggest that clotrimazole troches may be effective for prophylaxis against oropharyngeal candidiasis in neutropenic patients

Labeled Contraindications Hypersensitivity to clotrimazole or any component of the formulation

Pregnancy Risk Factor C

Lactation Excretion in breast milk unknown

Warnings/Precautions Clotrimazole should not be used for treatment of systemic fungal infection. Safety and effectiveness of clotrimazole lozenges (troches) in children <3 years of age have not been established.

Mechanism of Action Binds to phospholipids in the fungal cell membrane altering cell wall permeability resulting in loss of essential intracellular elements

Pharmacodynamics/Kinetics

Distribution: Oral (troche): Inhibitory concentrations remain in the saliva for up to 3 hours after dissolution of the troche

Excretion: Feces (as metabolites)

Dosing

Adult & Geriatric Oropharyngeal candidiasis: Oral:

Prophylaxis: 10 mg troche dissolved 3 times/day for the duration of chemotherapy or until steroids are reduced to maintenance levels

Treatment: 10 mg troche dissolved slowly 5 times/day for 14 consecutive days

Pediatric Oropharyngeal candidiasis: Children >3 years: Refer to adult dosing.

Administration Oral: Allow troche to dissolve slowly over 15-30 minutes.

Dosage Forms Excipient information presented when available (limited, particularly for generics); consult specific product labeling.

Troche, oral: 10 mg

- **CMA-676** *see* Gemtuzumab Ozogamicin *on page 673*
- **C-Met/Hepatocyte Growth Factor Receptor Tyrosine Kinase Inhibitor PF-02341066** *see* Crizotinib *on page 317*
- **C-Met/HGFR Tyrosine Kinase Inhibitor PF-02341066** *see* Crizotinib *on page 317*
- **CMV-IGIV** *see* Cytomegalovirus Immune Globulin (Intravenous-Human) *on page 365*
- **Coagulation Factor I** *see* Fibrinogen Concentrate (Human) *on page 602*
- **Coagulation Factor VIIa** *see* Factor VIIa (Recombinant) *on page 568*
- **CO Bicalutamide (Can)** *see* Bicalutamide *on page 178*
- **CO Ciprofloxacin (Can)** *see* Ciprofloxacin (Systemic) *on page 283*

Codeine (KOE deen)

Brand Names: Canada Codeine Contin®; PMS-Codeine; ratio-Codeine

Index Terms Codeine Phosphate; Codeine Sulfate; Methylmorphine

Generic Availability (U.S.) Yes

Pharmacologic Category Analgesic, Opioid; Antitussive

Use Management of mild-to-moderately-severe pain

Unlabeled Use Short-term relief of cough in select patients

Labeled Contraindications Hypersensitivity to codeine or any component of the formulation; respiratory depression in the absence of resuscitative equipment; acute or severe bronchial asthma or hypercarbia; presence or suspicion of paralytic ileus

Canadian labeling: Additional contraindications (not in U.S. labeling): Hypersensitivity to other opioid analgesics; cor pulmonale; acute alcoholism; delirium tremens; severe CNS depression; convulsive disorders; increased cerebrospinal or intracranial pressure; head injury; suspected surgical abdomen; use with or within 14 days of MAO inhibitors.

Pregnancy Risk Factor C

Lactation Enters breast milk/use caution (AAP rates "compatible"; AAP 2001 update pending)

Warnings/Precautions May cause dose-related respiratory depression. The risk is increased in elderly patients, debilitated patients, and patients with conditions associated with hypoxia, hypercapnia, or upper airway obstruction. Use with caution in patients with pre-existing respiratory compromise (hypoxia and/or hypercapnia), COPD or other obstructive pulmonary disease, and kyphoscoliosis or other skeletal disorder which may alter respiratory function; critical respiratory depression may occur, even at therapeutic dosages.

Use may cause or aggravate constipation; chronic use may result in obstructive bowel disease, particularly in those with underlying intestinal motility disorders. Avoid use in patients with gastrointestinal obstruction, particularly paralytic ileus. May cause hypotension; use with caution in patients with hypovolemia, cardiovascular disease (including acute MI), or drugs which may exaggerate hypotensive effects (including phenothiazines or general anesthetics). May cause CNS depression, which may impair physical or mental abilities; patients must be cautioned about performing tasks which require mental alertness (eg, operating machinery or driving).

Use with extreme caution in patients with head injury, intracranial lesions, or elevated intracranial pressure; exaggerated elevation of ICP may occur. Use with caution in patients with hypersensitivity reactions to other phenanthrene-derivative opioid agonists (hydrocodone, hydromorphone, levorphanol, oxycodone, oxymorphone), adrenal insufficiency (including Addison's disease), biliary tract dysfunction, CNS depression or coma, thyroid dysfunction, morbid obesity, prostatic hyperplasia and/or urinary stricture, or severe hepatic or renal impairment. Use may obscure diagnosis or clinical course of patients with acute abdominal conditions. May induce or aggravate seizures; use with caution in patients with seizure disorders.

Use with caution in patients with a history of drug abuse or acute alcoholism; potential for drug dependency exists. Tolerance, psychological and physical dependence may occur with prolonged use. Effects may be potentiated when used with other sedative drugs or ethanol. Concurrent use of agonist/antagonist analgesics may precipitate withdrawal symptoms and/or reduced analgesic efficacy in patients following prolonged therapy with mu opioid agonists. Abrupt discontinuation following prolonged use may also lead to withdrawal symptoms.

Use caution in patients with two or more copies of the variant CYP2D6*2 allele; may have extensive conversion to morphine and thus increased opioid-mediated effects.

Some preparations contain sulfites which may cause allergic reactions. Healthcare provider should be alert to the potential for abuse, misuse, and diversion.

Ethanol/Nutrition/Herb Interactions

Ethanol: May increase CNS depression; monitor for increased effects with coadministration. Caution patients about effects.

Herb/Nutraceutical: St John's wort may decrease codeine levels. Avoid valerian, St John's wort, kava kava, gotu kola (may increase CNS depression).

Storage/Stability Oral solution, tablet: Store at controlled room temperature.

Mechanism of Action Binds to opioid receptors in the CNS, causing inhibition of ascending pain pathways, altering the perception of and response to pain; causes cough suppression by direct central action in the medulla; produces generalized CNS depression

Pharmacodynamics/Kinetics

Onset of action: Oral: Immediate release: 0.5-1 hour

Peak effect: Oral: Immediate release: 1-1.5 hours

Duration: Immediate release: 4-6 hours

Distribution: ~3-6 L/kg

Protein binding: ~7% to 25%

Metabolism: Hepatic via UGT2B7 and UGT2B4 to codeine-6-glucuronide, via CYP2D6 to morphine (active), and via CYP3A4 to norcodeine. Morphine is further metabolized via glucuronidation to morphine-3-glucuronide and morphine-6-glucuronide (active).

Bioavailability: 53%

Half-life elimination: ~3 hours

Time to peak, plasma: Immediate release: 1 hour; Controlled release (Canadian availability; not available in the U.S.): 3.3 hours

Excretion: Urine (~90%, ~10% of the total dose as unchanged drug); feces

Dosing

Adult & Geriatric Note: These are guidelines and do not represent the maximum doses that may be required in all patients. Doses should be titrated to pain relief/prevention.

Pain management (analgesic): Oral:

Immediate release (tablet, oral solution): Initial: 15-60 mg every 4 hours as needed; maximum total daily dose: 360 mg/day; patients with prior opioid exposure may require higher initial doses. **Note:** The American Pain Society recommends an initial dose of 30-60 mg for adults with moderate pain (American Pain Society, 2008).

Controlled release: Codeine Contin® (Canadian availability; not available in U.S.): **Note:** Titrate at intervals of ≥48 hours until adequate analgesia has been achieved. Daily doses >600 mg/day should not be used; patients requiring higher doses should be switched to an opioid approved for use in severe pain. In patients who receive both Codeine Contin® and an immediate release or combination codeine product for breakthrough pain, the rescue dose of immediate release codeine product should be ≤12.5% of the total daily Codeine Contin® dose.

Opioid-naive patients: Initial: 50 mg every 12 hours

Conversion from immediate release codeine preparations: Immediate release codeine preparations contain ~75% codeine base. Therefore, patients who are switching from immediate release codeine preparations may be transferred to a ~25% lower total daily dose of Codeine Contin®, equally divided into 2 daily doses.

*Conversion from a combination codeine product (eg, codeine with acetaminophen **or** aspirin):* See table:

Number of 30 mg Codeine Combination Tablets Daily	Initial Dose of Codeine Contin®	Maintenance Dose of Codeine Contin®
≤6	50 mg every 12 h	100 mg every 12 h
7-9	100 mg every 12 h	150 mg every 12 h
10-12	150 mg every 12 h	200 mg every 12 h
>12	200 mg every 12 h	200-300 every 12 h (maximum: 300 mg every 12 h)

Conversion from another opioid analgesic: Using the patient's current opioid dose, calculate an equivalent daily dose of immediate release codeine. A ~25% lower dose of Codeine Contin® should then be initiated, equally divided into 2 daily doses.

Discontinuation of therapy: **Note:** Gradual dose reduction is recommended if clinically appropriate. Initially reduce the total daily dose by 50% and administer equally divided into 2 daily doses for 2 days followed by a 25% reduction every 2 days thereafter.

Treatment of cough (unlabeled use): Oral: Reported doses vary; range: 7.5-120 mg/day as a single dose or in divided doses (Bolser, 2006; Smith, 2010); **Note:** The American College of Chest Physicians does not recommend the routine use of codeine as an antitussive in patients with upper respiratory infections (Bolser, 2006).

Pediatric Note: These are guidelines and do not represent the maximum doses that may be required in all patients. Doses should be titrated to pain relief/prevention.

Pain management (analgesic; unlabeled use): Oral: Immediate release (tablet, oral solution): Initial: 0.5-1 mg/kg/dose every 4 hours as needed; maximum: 60 mg/dose (American Pain Society, 2008)

Renal Impairment

Manufacturer's recommendations: Clearance may be reduced; active metabolites may accumulate. Initiate at lower doses or longer dosing intervals followed by careful titration.

Alternate recommendations: The following guidelines have been used by some clinicians (Aronoff, 2007):

Cl_{cr} 10-50 mL/minute: Administer 75% of dose

Cl_{cr} <10 mL/minute: Administer 50% of dose

Hepatic Impairment No dosage adjustment provided in manufacturer's labeling (has not been studied); however, initial lower doses or longer dosing intervals followed by careful titration are recommended.

Administration May administer without regard to meals. Take with food or milk to decrease adverse GI effects.

Controlled release tablets: Codeine Contin® (Canadian availability; not available in U.S.): Tablets should be swallowed whole; do not chew, dissolve, or crush. All strengths may be halved, **except** the 50 mg tablets; half tablets should also be swallowed intact.

Test Interactions Some quinolones may produce a false-positive urine screening result for opioids using commercially-available immunoassay kits. This has been demonstrated most consistently for levofloxacin and ofloxacin, but other quinolones have shown cross-reactivity in certain assay kits. Confirmation of positive opioid screens by more specific methods should be considered.

Medication Guide Available Yes

Dosage Forms Excipient information presented when available (limited, particularly for generics); consult specific product labeling. [DSC] = Discontinued product

Powder, for prescription compounding, as phosphate: USP: 100% (10 g, 25 g)
Solution, oral, as phosphate: 30 mg/5 mL (500 mL)
Solution, oral, as sulfate: 30 mg/5 mL (500 mL)
Tablet, oral, as phosphate: 30 mg [DSC], 60 mg [DSC]
Tablet, oral, as sulfate: 15 mg, 30 mg, 60 mg

Dosage Forms: Canada Excipient information presented when available (limited, particularly for generics); consult specific product labeling.

Tablet, controlled release:
Codeine Contin®: 50 mg, 100 mg, 150 mg, 200 mg

Controlled Substance C-II

- ◆ **Codeine Contin® (Can)** *see* Codeine *on page* 311
- ◆ **Codeine Phosphate** *see* Codeine *on page* 311
- ◆ **Codeine Sulfate** *see* Codeine *on page* 311
- ◆ **CO Exemestane (Can)** *see* Exemestane *on page* 564
- ◆ **CO Famciclovir (Can)** *see* Famciclovir *on page* 580
- ◆ **CO Fluconazole (Can)** *see* Fluconazole *on page* 612
- ◆ **CO Levofloxacin (Can)** *see* Levofloxacin (Systemic) *on page* 883
- ◆ **Colocort®** *see* Hydrocortisone (Topical) *on page* 719
- ◆ **Compazine** *see* Prochlorperazine *on page* 1212
- ◆ **Compound F** *see* Hydrocortisone (Systemic) *on page* 713
- ◆ **Compound F** *see* Hydrocortisone (Topical) *on page* 719
- ◆ **Compro®** *see* Prochlorperazine *on page* 1212
- ◆ **CO Mycophenolate (Can)** *see* Mycophenolate *on page* 1015
- ◆ **Conventional Amphotericin B** *see* Amphotericin B (Conventional) *on page* 79
- ◆ **Conventional Cytarabine** *see* Cytarabine (Conventional) *on page* 348
- ◆ **Conventional Daunomycin** *see* DAUNOrubicin (Conventional) *on page* 396
- ◆ **Conventional Doxorubicin** *see* DOXOrubicin *on page* 467
- ◆ **Conventional Paclitaxel** *see* PACLitaxel *on page* 1092
- ◆ **Conventional Vincristine** *see* VinCRIStine *on page* 1450
- ◆ **ConZip™** *see* TraMADol *on page* 1388

- **CO Olanzapine (Can)** *see* OLANZapine *on page* 1056
- **CO Olanzapine ODT (Can)** *see* OLANZapine *on page* 1056
- **CO Ondansetron (Can)** *see* Ondansetron *on page* 1068
- **Cortaid® Advanced [OTC]** *see* Hydrocortisone (Topical) *on page* 719
- **Cortaid® Intensive Therapy [OTC]** *see* Hydrocortisone (Topical) *on page* 719
- **Cortaid® Maximum Strength [OTC]** *see* Hydrocortisone (Topical) *on page* 719
- **Cortamed® (Can)** *see* Hydrocortisone (Topical) *on page* 719
- **Cortef®** *see* Hydrocortisone (Systemic) *on page* 713
- **Cortenema®** *see* Hydrocortisone (Topical) *on page* 719
- **CortiCool® [OTC]** *see* Hydrocortisone (Topical) *on page* 719
- **Cortifoam®** *see* Hydrocortisone (Topical) *on page* 719
- **Cortifoam™ (Can)** *see* Hydrocortisone (Topical) *on page* 719
- **Cortisol** *see* Hydrocortisone (Systemic) *on page* 713
- **Cortisol** *see* Hydrocortisone (Topical) *on page* 719
- **Cortizone-10® Hydratensive Healing [OTC]** *see* Hydrocortisone (Topical) *on page* 719
- **Cortizone-10® Hydratensive Soothing [OTC]** *see* Hydrocortisone (Topical) *on page* 719
- **Cortizone-10® Intensive Healing Eczema [OTC]** *see* Hydrocortisone (Topical) *on page* 719
- **Cortizone-10® Maximum Strength [OTC]** *see* Hydrocortisone (Topical) *on page* 719
- **Cortizone-10® Maximum Strength Cooling Relief [OTC]** *see* Hydrocortisone (Topical) *on page* 719
- **Cortizone-10® Maximum Strength Easy Relief [OTC]** *see* Hydrocortisone (Topical) *on page* 719
- **Cortizone-10® Maximum Strength Intensive Healing Formula [OTC]** *see* Hydrocortisone (Topical) *on page* 719
- **Cortizone-10® Plus Maximum Strength [OTC]** *see* Hydrocortisone (Topical) *on page* 719
- **Cosmegen®** *see* DACTINomycin *on page* 371
- **Co-Trimoxazole** *see* Sulfamethoxazole and Trimethoprim *on page* 1302
- **CO Valacyclovir (Can)** *see* Valacyclovir *on page* 1420
- **Co-Vidarabine** *see* Pentostatin *on page* 1161
- **CP358774** *see* Erlotinib *on page* 528
- **CPDG2** *see* Glucarpidase *on page* 680
- **CPG2** *see* Glucarpidase *on page* 680
- **CPM** *see* Cyclophosphamide *on page* 321
- **CPT-11** *see* Irinotecan *on page* 813
- **CPZ** *see* ChlorproMAZINE *on page* 274
- **13-CRA** *see* ISOtretinoin *on page* 832

Crizotinib (kriz OH ti nib)

Brand Names: U.S. Xalkori®

Brand Names: Canada Xalkori™

Index Terms C-Met/Hepatocyte Growth Factor Receptor Tyrosine Kinase Inhibitor PF-02341066; C-Met/HGFR Tyrosine Kinase Inhibitor PF-02341066; MET Tyrosine Kinase Inhibitor PF-02341066; PF-02341066

Generic Availability (U.S.) No

Pharmacologic Category Antineoplastic Agent, Anaplastic Lymphoma Kinase Inhibitor; Antineoplastic Agent, Tyrosine Kinase Inhibitor

Use Treatment of locally advanced or metastatic nonsmall cell lung cancer (NSCLC) that is anaplastic lymphoma kinase (ALK) positive (as detected by an approved test)

Labeled Contraindications There are no contraindications listed within the manufacturer's U.S. labeling.

Canadian labeling: Hypersensitivity to crizotinib or any component of the formulation; congenital long QT syndrome or with persistent Fridericia-corrected QT interval (QTcF) ≥500 msec

Pregnancy Risk Factor D

Lactation Excretion in breast milk unknown/not recommended

Warnings/Precautions Approved for use only in patients with locally advanced or metastatic nonsmall cell lung cancer (NSCLC) who test positive for the abnormal anaplastic lymphoma kinase (ALK) gene. The Vysis ALK break-apart FISH probe kit is approved to test for the gene abnormality.

Grade 3 or 4 ALT increases (usually asymptomatic and reversible) have been observed in clinical trials. May require dosage interruption and/or reduction; permanent discontinuation was necessary in some cases; concurrent ALT elevations >3 x ULN and total bilirubin elevations >2 x ULN (without alkaline phosphatase elevations) were observed rarely. Fatalities due to crizotinib-induced hepatotoxicity have also occurred (rare). Monitor liver function tests, including ALT and total bilirubin. Transaminase elevation onset was within 2 months of treatment initiation. Use with caution in patients with hepatic impairment (has not been studied); crizotinib is extensively metabolized in the liver and liver impairment is likely to increase crizotinib levels.

Severe, life-threatening, and potentially fatal pneumonitis has been associated with crizotinib. Onset was generally within 2 months of treatment initiation. Monitor for pulmonary symptoms which may indicate pneumonitis; exclude other potential causes (eg, disease progression, infection, other pulmonary disease, or radiation therapy). Permanently discontinue if treatment-related pneumonitis is confirmed.

QT_c prolongation has been observed; consider periodic monitoring of ECG and electrolytes in patients with heart failure, bradyarrhythmias, electrolyte abnormalities, or who are taking medications known to prolong the QT interval. May require treatment interruption, dosage reduction, or discontinuation. Avoid use in patients with congenital long QT syndrome. Canadian labeling contraindicates use in patients with congenital long QT syndrome or persistent QTcF ≥500 msec.

Ocular toxicities (eg, blurred vision, diplopia, photophobia, photopsia, visual acuity decreased, visual brightness, visual field defect, visual impairment, and/or vitreous floaters) commonly occur. Onset is generally within 2 weeks of treatment initiation; consider ophthalmology exam, especially if photopsia or vitreous floaters occur. Severe or worsening vitreous floaters or photopsia could be a sign of retinal hole or impending detachment. Use with caution in patients with severe renal impairment; only one patient with severe renal impairment was studied in clinical trials and end stage renal disease was not studied. CYP3A4 inhibitors may increase crizotinib levels; avoid concomitant use with strong CYP3A4 inhibitors and use moderate CYP3A4 inhibitors with caution. CYP3A4 inducers may decrease crizotinib levels; avoid concomitant use with strong CYP3A4 inducers. Avoid concomitant use with CYP3A4 substrates.

Adverse Reactions

>10%:

Cardiovascular: Edema (28%)

Central nervous system: Fatigue (20%), dizziness (16%)

Gastrointestinal: Nausea (53%), diarrhea (43%), vomiting (40%), constipation (27%), appetite decreased (19%), taste alteration (12%), esophageal disorder (11%; includes dyspepsia, dysphagia, epigastric burning/discomfort/pain, esophageal obstruction/pain/spasm/ulcer, esophagitis, gastroesophageal reflux, odynophagia, reflux esophagitis)

Hematologic: Lymphopenia (grades 3/4: 11%)

Hepatic: ALT increased (13%; grades 3/4: 5%)

Neuromuscular & skeletal: Neuropathy (13%; grades 3/4: <1%)

Ocular: Vision disorder (62%; onset: <2 weeks; includes blurred vision, diplopia, photophobia, photopsia, visual acuity decreased, visual brightness, visual field defect, visual impairment, vitreous floaters)

1% to 10%:

Cardiovascular: Bradycardia (5%), chest pain (1%)

Central nervous system: Headache (4%), insomnia (3%)

Dermatologic: Rash (10%)

Gastrointestinal: Abdominal pain (8%), stomatitis (6%)

Hematologic: Neutropenia (grades 3/4: 5%)

Hepatic: AST increased (9%; grades 3/4: 2%)

Neuromuscular & skeletal: Arthralgia (2%)

Renal: Renal cysts (1%)

Respiratory: Cough (4%), dyspnea (2%), pneumonitis (2%), upper respiratory infection (2%)

<1% and/or case reports: Back pain, fever, QT_c prolongation, thrombocytopenia

Drug Interactions

Metabolism/Transport Effects Substrate of CYP3A4 (major), P-glycoprotein; **Note:** Assignment of Major/Minor substrate status based on clinically relevant drug interaction potential; **Inhibits** CYP3A4 (moderate), P-glycoprotein

Avoid Concomitant Use

Avoid concomitant use of Crizotinib with any of the following: Alfentanil; Bosutinib; CycloSPORINE (Systemic); CYP3A4 Inducers (Strong); CYP3A4 Inhibitors (Strong); Dihydroergotamine; Ergotamine; FentaNYL; Grapefruit Juice; Highest Risk QTc-Prolonging Agents; Mifepristone; Pimozide; QuiNIDine; Silodosin; Sirolimus; St Johns Wort; Tacrolimus (Systemic); Tolvaptan; Topotecan; VinCRIStine (Liposomal)

Increased Effect/Toxicity

Crizotinib may increase the levels/effects of: Alfentanil; ARIPiprazole; Avanafil; Bosutinib; Budesonide (Systemic, Oral Inhalation); Colchicine; CycloSPORINE (Systemic); CYP3A4 Substrates; Dabigatran Etexilate;

Dihydroergotamine; Eplerenone; Ergotamine; Everolimus; FentaNYL; Highest Risk QTc-Prolonging Agents; Ivacaftor; Lurasidone; Moderate Risk QTc-Prolonging Agents; P-glycoprotein/ABCB1 Substrates; Pimecrolimus; Pimozide; Prucalopride; QuiNIDine; Rivaroxaban; Salmeterol; Saxagliptin; Silodosin; Sirolimus; Tacrolimus (Systemic); Tolvaptan; Topotecan; Vilazodone; VinCRIStine (Liposomal); Vitamin K Antagonists

The levels/effects of Crizotinib may be increased by: CYP3A4 Inhibitors (Moderate); CYP3A4 Inhibitors (Strong); Dasatinib; Grapefruit Juice; Ivacaftor; Mifepristone; P-glycoprotein/ABCB1 Inhibitors; QTc-Prolonging Agents (Indeterminate Risk and Risk Modifying)

Decreased Effect

Crizotinib may decrease the levels/effects of: Cardiac Glycosides; Ifosfamide; Vitamin K Antagonists

The levels/effects of Crizotinib may be decreased by: CYP3A4 Inducers (Strong); Deferasirox; P-glycoprotein/ABCB1 Inducers; St Johns Wort; Tocilizumab

Ethanol/Nutrition/Herb Interactions

Food: Grapefruit juice may increase serum crizotinib levels. Management: Avoid grapefruit and grapefruit juice.

Herb/Nutraceutical: St John's wort may decrease the serum concentration of crizotinib. Management: Avoid St John's wort.

Storage/Stability Store at room temperature of 20°C to 25°C (68°F to 77°F); excursions permitted to 15°C and 30°C (59°F and 86°F).

Mechanism of Action Tyrosine kinase receptor inhibitor, which inhibits anaplastic lymphoma kinase (ALK), Hepatocyte Growth Factor Receptor (HGFR, c-MET), and Recepteur d'Origine Nantais (RON). ALK gene abnormalities due to mutations or translocations may result in expression of oncogenic fusion proteins (eg, ALK fusion protein) which alter signaling and expression and result in increased cellular proliferation and survival in tumors which express these fusion proteins. Approximately 2% to 7% of patients with NSCLC have the abnormal echinoderm microtubule-associated protein-like 4, or EML4-ALK gene (which has a higher prevalence in never smokers or light smokers and in patients with adenocarcinoma). Crizotinib selectively inhibits ALK tyrosine kinase, which reduces proliferation of cells expressing the genetic alteration.

Pharmacodynamics/Kinetics

Distribution: V_{ss}: 1772 L

Protein binding: 91%

Metabolism: Hepatic, via CYP3A4/5

Bioavailability: 43% (range: 32% to 66%); bioavailability is reduced 14% with a high-fat meal

Half-life elimination: Terminal: 42 hours

Time to peak: 4-6 hours

Excretion: Feces (63%; 53% as unchanged drug); urine (22%; 2% as unchanged drug)

Dosing

Adult & Geriatric Nonsmall cell lung cancer, locally advanced or metastatic (ALK-positive): Oral: 250 mg twice daily, continue treatment until no longer clinically beneficial

Renal Impairment

Mild (Cl_{cr} 30-60 mL/minute) to moderate impairment (Cl_{cr} 60-90 mL/minute): No adjustment required

Severe impairment (Cl_{cr} <30 mL/minute): Data are insufficient to determine if dosage adjustment necessary; use with caution

End-stage renal disease (ESRD): Was not studied in patients with ESRD; use with caution

Hepatic Impairment Data are insufficient to determine if dosage adjustment necessary; however, crizotinib undergoes extensive hepatic metabolism and systemic exposure may be increased with impairment; use with caution

Adjustment for Toxicity Note: If dose reduction is necessary, reduce dose to 200 mg orally twice daily; if necessary, further reduce to 250 mg once daily

Hematologic toxicity (except lymphopenia, unless lymphopenia is associated with clinical events such as opportunistic infection):

Grade 3 toxicity (WBC 1000-2000/mm^3, ANC 500-1000/mm^3, platelets 25,000-50,000/mm^3), grade 3 anemia: Withhold treatment until recovery to ≤grade 2, then resume at the same dose and schedule

Grade 4 toxicity (WBC <1000/mm^3, ANC <500/mm^3, platelets <25,000/mm^3), grade 4 anemia: Withhold treatment until recovery to ≤grade 2, then resume at 200 mg twice daily

Recurrent grade 4 toxicity on 200 mg twice daily: Withhold treatment until recovery to ≤grade 2, then resume at 250 mg once daily

Recurrent grade 4 toxicity on 250 mg once daily: Permanently discontinue

Nonhematologic toxicities:

Grade 3 or 4 ALT or AST elevation (ALT or AST >5 x ULN) with ≤grade 1 total bilirubin elevation (total bilirubin ≤1.5 x ULN): Withhold treatment until recovery to ≤grade 1 (<2.5 X ULN) or baseline, then resume at 200 mg twice daily

Recurrent grade 3 or 4 ALT or AST elevation with ≤grade 1 total bilirubin elevation: Withhold treatment until recovery to ≤grade 1, then resume at 250 mg once daily

Recurrent grade 3 or 4 ALT or AST elevation on 250 mg once daily: Permanently discontinue

Grade 2, 3, or 4 ALT or AST elevation with concurrent grade 2, 3, or 4 total bilirubin elevation (>1.5 x ULN) in the absence of cholestasis or hemolysis: Permanently discontinue

Pneumonitis (any grade; not attributable to disease progression, infection, other pulmonary disease or radiation therapy): Permanently discontinue

Grade 3 QT_c prolongation (QT_c >500 msec without life-threatening signs or symptoms): Withhold treatment until recovery to ≤grade 1 (QT_c ≤470 msec), then resume at 200 mg twice daily

Recurrent grade 3 QT_c prolongation at 200 mg twice daily: Withhold treatment until recovery to ≤grade 1, then resume at 250 mg once daily

Recurrent grade 3 QT_c prolongation at 250 mg once daily: Permanently discontinue

Grade 4 QT_c prolongation: Permanently discontinue

Combination Regimens

Lung cancer (nonsmall cell): Crizotinib (NSCLC Regimen) on page 1596

Administration Swallow capsules whole (do not crush, dissolve, or open capsules). May be administered with or without food. If a dose is missed, take as soon as remembered unless it is <6 hours prior to the next scheduled dose (skip the dose if <6 hours before the next dose); do not take 2 doses at the same time to make up for a missed dose.

Monitoring Parameters ALK positivity; CBC with differential monthly and as clinically appropriate (monitor more frequently if grades 3 or 4 abnormalities observed or with fever or infection), liver function tests monthly and as clinically appropriate (monitor more frequently if grades 2, 3 or 4 abnormalities observed). Monitor pulmonary symptoms (for pneumonitis). Consider monitoring ECG and electrolytes in patients with heart failure, bradyarrhythmias, electrolyte abnormalities, or who are taking medications known to prolong the QT interval. Consider ophthalmic evaluation, especially if photopsia or vitreous floaters occur.

Dietary Considerations May be taken with or without food. Avoid grapefruit and grapefruit juice.

Prescribing and Access Restrictions Available through specialty pharmacies. Further information may be obtained from the manufacturer, Pfizer, at 1-877-744-5675, or at http://www.pfizerpro.com/resources/minisites/xalkori_-home/aval/docs/pharmacy_financial_info.pdf

Dosage Forms Excipient information presented when available (limited, particularly for generics); consult specific product labeling.

Capsule, oral:

Xalkori®: 200 mg, 250 mg

References

Butrynski JE, D'Adamo DR, Hornick JL et al, "Crizotinib in ALK-Rearranged Inflammatory Myofibroblastic Tumor," *N Engl J Med*, 2010, 363(18):1727-33.

Choi YL, Soda M, Yamashita Y, et al, "EML4-ALK Mutations in Lung Cancer that Confer Resistance to ALK Inhibitors," *N Engl J Med*, 2010, 363(18):1734-9.

Kwak EL, Bang YJ, Camidge DR, et al, "Anaplastic Lymphoma Kinase Inhibition in Non-Small-Cell Lung Cancer," *N Engl J Med*, 2010, 363(18):1693-703.

◆ **CsA** *see* CycloSPORINE (Systemic) *on page 333*

◆ **CTX** *see* Cyclophosphamide *on page 321*

◆ **CyA** *see* CycloSPORINE (Systemic) *on page 333*

Cyclophosphamide (sye kloe FOS fa mide)

Related Information

Chemotherapy and Cancer Treatment During Pregnancy *on page 1829*

Chemotherapy and Obesity *on page 1834*

Fertility and Cancer Therapy *on page 1782*

Hematopoietic Stem Cell Transplantation *on page 1887*

Management of Chemotherapy-Induced Nausea and Vomiting *on page 1786*

Management of Drug Extravasations *on page 1800*

Oral Mucositis/Stomatitis *on page 1814*

Principles of Anticancer Therapy *on page 1878*

Safe Handling of Hazardous Drugs *on page 1904*

Brand Names: Canada Procytox®

Index Terms CPM; CTX; CYT; Cytoxan; Neosar

Generic Availability (U.S.) Yes

Pharmacologic Category Antineoplastic Agent, Alkylating Agent; Antirheumatic Miscellaneous; Immunosuppressant Agent

Use

Oncology-related uses: Treatment of Hodgkin lymphoma, non-Hodgkin lymphomas (including Burkitt's lymphoma), chronic lymphocytic leukemia (CLL), chronic myelocytic leukemia (CML), acute myelocytic leukemia (AML), acute lymphoblastic leukemia (ALL), mycosis fungoides, multiple myeloma, neuroblastoma, retinoblastoma; breast cancer; ovarian adenocarcinoma

Canadian labeling: Additional use (not in U.S. labeling): Treatment of lung cancer

Nononcology uses: Treatment of refractory nephrotic syndrome in children who are unresponsive or intolerant to corticosteroid therapy

Unlabeled Use

Oncology-related uses: Ewing's sarcoma, rhabdomyosarcoma, Wilms tumor, ovarian germ cell tumors, gestational trophoblastic tumors (high-risk), small cell lung cancer, testicular cancer, pheochromocytoma, hematopoietic stem cell transplant (HSCT) conditioning regimen

Nononcology uses: Severe rheumatoid disorders, granulomatosis with polyangiitis (GPA; Wegener's granulomatosis), myasthenia gravis, multiple sclerosis, lupus nephritis, autoimmune hemolytic anemia, idiopathic thrombocytic purpura (ITP), antibody-induced pure red cell aplasia

Labeled Contraindications

U.S. labeling: Hypersensitivity to cyclophosphamide or any component of the formulation; severely depressed bone marrow function

Canadian labeling: Hypersensitivity to cyclophosphamide or its metabolites, urinary outflow obstructions, severe myelosuppression, severe renal or hepatic impairment, active infection (especially varicella zoster), severe immunosuppression

Pregnancy Risk Factor D

Lactation Enters breast milk/not recommended

Warnings/Precautions Hazardous agent - use appropriate precautions for handling and disposal.

Cyclophosphamide is associated with the development of hemorrhagic cystitis; may rarely be severe and even fatal. Discontinue cyclophosphamide with severe hemorrhagic cystitis. Bladder injury is due to excretion of cyclophosphamide metabolites in the urine and appears to be dose- and treatment duration-dependent. Bladder fibrosis may also occur, either with or without cystitis. Increased hydration and frequent voiding is recommended to help prevent cystitis; some protocols utilize mesna to protect against hemorrhagic cystitis. Monitor urinalysis for hematuria. Severe or prolonged hemorrhagic cystitis may require medical or surgical treatment. Hematuria generally resolves within a few days after treatment is withheld, although it may persist. Cyclophosphamide may potentiate the cardiotoxicity of anthracyclines.

Cardiotoxicity has been reported, usually with high doses associated with transplant conditioning regimens, although may rarely occur with lower doses. Cardiac abnormalities do not appear to persist. Cardiotoxicities reported have included arrhythmia, congestive heart failure, heart block, hemorrhagic myocarditis, hemopericardium (secondary to hemorrhagic myocarditis and myocardial necrosis), pericarditis, and tachyarrhythmias. Cardiotoxicity is related to endothelial capillary damage; symptoms may be managed with diuretics, ACE inhibitors, beta blockers, or inotropics (Floyd, 2005). Use with caution in patients with pre-existing cardiovascular disease. For patients with multiple cardiac risk factors, considering monitoring during treatment (Floyd, 2005).

Pulmonary toxicities, including pneumonitis and acute respiratory distress syndrome, have been reported. Consider pulmonary function testing to assess the severity of pneumonitis (Morgan, 2011). Cyclophosphamide-induced pneumonitis is rare and may present as early (within 1-6 months) or late onset (several months to years); early onset has been reversible with discontinuation; late onset is associated with pleural thickening and may persist chronically (Malik, 1996).

Dose-related neutropenia is common; thrombocytopenia and anemia may also occur. Monitor for infections; immunosuppression and serious infections may occur; infections may require dose reduction, or interruption or discontinuation of treatment. Nausea and vomiting commonly occur; premedication with antiemetics is recommended. Stomatitis/mucositis may also occur. Anaphylactic reactions have been reported; cross-sensitivity with other alkylating agents may occur. May interfere with wound healing. Secondary malignancies (bladder cancer, myeloproliferative, and lymphoproliferative malignancies) have been reported with both single-agent and with combination chemotherapy regimens; onset may be delayed (up to several years after treatment); bladder malignancy usually occurs in patients previously experiencing hemorrhagic cystitis. May impair fertility; interferes with oogenesis and spermatogenesis; effect on fertility is generally dependent on dose and duration of treatment and may be irreversible. The age at treatment initiation and cumulative dose were determined to be risk factors for ovarian failure in cyclophosphamide use for the treatment of systemic lupus erythematosus (SLE) (Mok, 1998). Use with caution in patients with renal and hepatic impairment; dosage adjustment may be needed (use is contraindicated in severe impairment in the Canadian labeling).

Adverse Reactions Frequency not defined.

Dermatologic: Alopecia (reversible; onset: 3-6 weeks after start of treatment)

Endocrine & metabolic: Amenorrhea, azoospermia, gonadal suppression, oligospermia, oogenesis impaired, sterility

Gastrointestinal: Abdominal pain, anorexia, diarrhea, mucositis, nausea/vomiting (dose-related), stomatitis

Genitourinary: Hemorrhagic cystitis

Hematologic: Anemia, leukopenia (dose-related; recovery: 7-10 days after cessation), myelosuppression, neutropenia, neutropenic fever, thrombocytopenia

Miscellaneous: Infection

Postmarketing and/or case reports: Acute respiratory distress syndrome, anaphylactic reactions, anaphylaxis, arrhythmias (with high-dose [HSCT] therapy), bladder/urinary fibrosis, blurred vision, cardiac tamponade (with high-dose [HSCT] therapy), cardiotoxicity, confusion, C-reactive protein increased, dizziness, dyspnea, ejection fraction decreased, erythema multiforme, gastrointestinal hemorrhage, hearing disorders, heart block, heart failure (with high-dose [HSCT] therapy), hematuria, hemopericardium, hemorrhagic colitis, hemorrhagic myocarditis (with high-dose [HSCT] therapy), hemorrhagic ureteritis, hepatic sinusoidal obstruction syndrome (SOS; formerly called veno-occlusive liver disease), hepatitis, hepatotoxicity, hypersensitivity reactions, hyperuricemia, hypokalemia, hyponatremia, interstitial pneumonitis, interstitial pulmonary fibrosis (with high doses), jaundice, latent infection reactivation, LDH increased, malaise, mesenteric ischemia (acute), methemoglobinemia (with high-dose [HSCT] therapy), multiorgan failure, myocardial necrosis (with high-dose [HSCT] therapy), neurotoxicity, neutrophilic eccrine hidradenitis, ovarian fibrosis, pancreatitis, pericarditis, pigmentation changes (skin/fingernails), pneumonia, pulmonary hypertension, pulmonary infiltrates, pulmonary veno-occlusive disease, pyelonephritis, radiation recall, rash, renal tubular necrosis, reversible posterior leukoencephalopathy syndrome (RPLS), rhabdomyolysis, secondary malignancy, septic shock, sepsis, SIADH, Stevens-Johnson syndrome, testicular atrophy, thrombocytopenia (immune mediated), thrombotic disorders (arterial and venous), toxic epidermal necrolysis, toxic megacolon, tumor lysis syndrome, weakness, wound healing impaired

Drug Interactions

Metabolism/Transport Effects **Substrate** of CYP2A6 (minor), CYP2B6 (major), CYP2C19 (minor), CYP2C9 (minor), CYP3A4 (minor); **Note:** Assignment of Major/Minor substrate status based on clinically relevant drug interaction potential; **Inhibits** CYP3A4 (weak); **Induces** CYP2B6 (weak/moderate), CYP2C9 (weak/moderate)

Avoid Concomitant Use

Avoid concomitant use of Cyclophosphamide with any of the following: BCG; Belimumab; CloZAPine; Etanercept; Natalizumab; Pimecrolimus; Pimozide; Tacrolimus (Topical); Vaccines (Live)

Increased Effect/Toxicity

Cyclophosphamide may increase the levels/effects of: ARIPiprazole; CloZAPine; Leflunomide; Natalizumab; Pimozide; Succinylcholine; Vaccines (Live); Vitamin K Antagonists

The levels/effects of Cyclophosphamide may be increased by: Allopurinol; Belimumab; CYP2B6 Inhibitors (Moderate); CYP2B6 Inhibitors (Strong); Denosumab; Etanercept; Pentostatin; Pimecrolimus; Quazepam; Roflumilast; Tacrolimus (Topical); Trastuzumab

Decreased Effect

Cyclophosphamide may decrease the levels/effects of: BCG; Cardiac Glycosides; Coccidioidin Skin Test; Sipuleucel-T; Vaccines (Inactivated); Vaccines (Live); Vitamin K Antagonists

The levels/effects of Cyclophosphamide may be decreased by: CYP2B6 Inducers (Strong); Echinacea; Tocilizumab

Ethanol/Nutrition/Herb Interactions Herb/Nutraceutical: Avoid black cohosh, dong quai in estrogen-dependent tumors.

Storage/Stability Use appropriate precautions for handling and disposal.

Injection powder for reconstitution: Store intact vials of powder at room temperature of 25°C (77°F). Reconstituted solutions in normal saline (NS) are stable for 24 hours at room temperature and for 6 days refrigerated at 2°C to 8°C (36°F to 46°F). Solutions diluted for infusion in 1/2NS are stable for 24 hours at room temperature and for 6 days refrigerated; solutions diluted in D_5W or D_5NS are stable for 24 hours at room temperature and for 36 hours refrigerated.

Tablets: Store tablets at room temperature of 25°C (77°F); excursions permitted to 15°C to 30°C (59°F to 86°F).

Reconstitution Use appropriate precautions for handling and disposal.

Injection powder for reconstitution: Store intact vials of powder at room temperature of 25°C (77°F). Use appropriate precautions for handling and disposal. For I.V. push, reconstitute with normal saline (NS) to a concentration of 20 mg/mL. For I.V. infusion, reconstitute with sterile water or NS to a concentration of 20 mg/mL; further dilute for infusion in D_5W, 1/2NS or D_5NS.

Mechanism of Action Cyclophosphamide is an alkylating agent that prevents cell division by cross-linking DNA strands and decreasing DNA synthesis. It is a cell cycle phase nonspecific agent. Cyclophosphamide also possesses potent immunosuppressive activity. Cyclophosphamide is a prodrug that must be metabolized to active metabolites in the liver.

Pharmacodynamics/Kinetics

Absorption: Oral: Well absorbed

Distribution: V_d: 0.48-0.71 L/kg; crosses into CSF (not in high enough concentrations to treat meningeal leukemia)
Protein binding: 10% to 60%
Metabolism: Hepatic to active metabolites acrolein, 4-aldophosphamide, 4-hydroperoxycyclophosphamide, and nor-nitrogen mustard
Bioavailability: >75%
Half-life elimination: 3-12 hours
Time to peak, serum: Oral: ~1 hour; I.V.: Metabolites: 2-3 hours
Excretion: Urine (<10% as unchanged drug, 85% to 90% as metabolites)

Dosing

Adult Details concerning dosing in combination regimens should also be consulted. Antiemetics may be recommended (emetogenic potential varies by dose and combination therapy).

U.S. labeling:

Single agent for solid tumors:

I.V.: 40-50 mg/kg in divided doses over 2-5 days **or** 10-15 mg/kg every 7-10 days **or** 3-5 mg/kg twice weekly

Oral: 1-5 mg/kg/day (initial and maintenance dosing)

Canadian labeling:

I.V.: Initial: 40-50 mg/kg (1500-1800 mg/m^2) administered as 10-20 mg/kg/day over 2-5 days; Maintenance: 10-15 mg/kg (350-550 mg/m^2) every 7-10 days **or** 3-5 mg/kg (110-185 mg/m^2) twice weekly

Oral: Initial 1-5 mg/kg/day (depending on tolerance); Maintenance: 1-5 mg/kg/day

Indication specific and/or unlabeled uses/dosing:

Acute lymphoblastic leukemia (unlabeled dosing): Multiple-agent regimens:

Hyper-CVAD regimen: I.V.: 300 mg/m^2 over 3 hours (with mesna) every 12 hours for 6 doses on days 1, 2, and 3 during odd-numbered cycles (cycles 1, 3, 5, 7) of an 8-cycle phase (Kantarjian, 2004)

Larson (CALGB8811) regimen: I.V.:

Adults <60 years: Induction phase: 1200 mg/m^2 on day 1 of a 4-week cycle; Early intensification phase: 1000 mg/m^2 on day 1 of a 4-week cycle (repeat once); Late intensification phase: 1000 mg/m^2 on day 29 of an 8-week cycle (Larson, 1995)

Adults ≥60 years: Induction phase: 800 mg/m^2 on day 1 of a 4-week cycle; Early intensification phase: 1000 mg/m^2 on day 1 of a 4-week cycle (repeat once); Late intensification phase: 1000 mg/m^2 on day 29 of an 8-week cycle (Larson, 1995)

Breast cancer (unlabeled dosing):

AC regimen: I.V.: 600 mg/m^2 on day 1 every 21 days (in combination with doxorubicin) for 4 cycles (Fisher, 1990)

CEF regimen: Oral: 75 mg/m^2/day days 1-14 every 28 days (in combination with epirubicin and fluorouracil) for 6 cycles (Levine, 1998)

CMF regimen: Oral: 100 mg/m^2/day days 1-14 every 28 days (in combination with methotrexate and fluorouracil) for 6 cycles (Levine, 1998) **or** I.V.: 600 mg/m^2 on day 1 every 21 days (in combination with methotrexate and fluorouracil); Goldhirsch, 1998)

Chronic lymphocytic leukemia (unlabeled dosing): I.V.: R-FC regimen: 250 mg/m^2/day for 3 days every 28 days (in combination with rituximab and fludarabine) for 6 cycles (Robak, 2010)

Ewing's sarcoma (unlabeled use): I.V.: VAC/IE regimen: VAC: 1200 mg/m^2 (plus mesna) on day 1 of a 21-day treatment cycle (in combination with vincristine and doxorubicin [then dactinomycin when maximum doxorubicin dose reached]), alternates with IE (ifosfamide and etoposide) for a total of 17 cycles (Grier, 2003)

Gestational trophoblastic tumors, high-risk (unlabeled use): I.V.: EMA/CO regimen: 600 mg/m^2 on day 8 of 2-week treatment cycle (in combination with etoposide, methotrexate, dactinomycin, and vincristine), continue for at least 2 treatment cycles after a normal hCG level (Escobar, 2003)

Granulomatosis with polyangiitis (GPA; Wegener's granulomatosis) (unlabeled use; in combination with glucocorticoids):

Low-dose: Oral: 1.5-2 mg/kg/day (Jayne, 2003; Stone, 2010) or 2 mg/kg/day until remission, followed by 1.5 mg/kg/day for 3 additional months (de Groot, 2009; Harper, 2012)

Pulse: I.V.: 15 mg/kg (maximum dose: 1200 mg) every 2 weeks for 3 doses, followed by maintenance pulses of either 15 mg/kg I.V. (maximum dose: 1200 mg) every 3 weeks or 2.5-5 mg/kg/day orally on days 1, 2, and 3 every 3 weeks for 3 months after remission achieved (de Groot, 2009; Harper, 2012)

Hodgkin lymphoma (unlabeled dosing): I.V.:

BEACOPP regimen: 650 mg/m^2 on day 1 every 3 weeks (in combination with bleomycin, etoposide, doxorubicin, vincristine, procarbazine, and prednisone) for 8 cycles (Diehl, 2003)

BEACOPP escalated regimen: 1200 mg/m^2 on day 1 every 3 weeks (in combination with bleomycin, etoposide, doxorubicin, vincristine, procarbazine, and prednisone) for 8 cycles (Diehl, 2003)

Multiple myeloma (unlabeled dosing): Oral: CyBorD regimen: 300 mg/m^2 on days 1, 8, 15, and 22 every 4 weeks (in combination with bortezomib and dexamethasone) for 4 cycles; may continue beyond 4 cycles (Khan, 2012)

Non-Hodgkin lymphoma (unlabeled dosing): I.V.:

R-CHOP regimen: 750 mg/m^2 on day 1 every 3 weeks (in combination with rituximab, doxorubicin, vincristine, and prednisone) for 8 cycles (Coiffier, 2002)

R-EPOCH (dose adjusted) regimen: 750 mg/m^2 on day 5 every 3 weeks (in combination with rituximab, etoposide, prednisone, vincristine, and doxorubicin) for 6-8 cycles (Garcia-Suarez, 2007)

CODOX-M/IVAC (Burkitt's lymphoma): Cycles 1 and 3 (CODOX-M): 800 mg/m^2 on day 1, followed by 200 mg/m^2 on days 2-5 (in combination with vincristine, doxorubicin, and methotrexate); CODOX-M alternates with IVAC (etoposide, ifosfamide, and cytarabine) for a total of 4 cycles (Magrath, 1996)

Lupus nephritis (unlabeled use): I.V.: 500 mg once every 2 weeks for 6 doses or 500-1000 mg/m^2 once every month for 6 doses (Hahn, 2012) **or** 500-1000 mg/m^2 every month every month for 6 months, then every 3 months for a total of at least 2.5 years (Austin, 1986; Gourley, 1996)

Transplant conditioning (unlabeled use): I.V.:

Nonmyeloablative transplant (allogeneic): 750 mg/m^2/day for 3 days beginning 5 days prior to transplant (in combination with fludarabine) (Khouri, 2008)

Myeloablative transplant:

100 mg/kg (based on IBW, unless actual weight <95% of IBW) as a single dose 2 days prior to transplant (in combination with total body irradiation and etoposide) (Thompson, 2008)

50 mg/kg/day for 4 days beginning 5 days before transplant (with or without antithymocyte globulin [equine]) (Champlin, 2007)

50 mg/kg/day for 4 days beginning 5 days prior to transplant (in combination with busulfan) (Cassileth, 1993)
60 mg/kg/day for 2 days (in combination with busulfan and total body irradiation) (Anderson, 1996)
1800 mg/m²/day for 4 days beginning 7 days prior to transplant (in combination with etoposide and carmustine) (Reece, 1991)

Geriatric Refer to adult dosing; adjust for renal clearance.

Pediatric Details concerning dosing in combination regimens should also be consulted. Antiemetics may be recommended (emetogenic potential varies by dose and combination therapy).

U.S. labeling:

Malignancy, solid tumor (single agent):
I.V.: 40-50 mg/kg in divided doses over 2-5 days **or** 10-15 mg/kg every 7-10 days **or** 3-5 mg/kg twice weekly
Oral: 1-5 mg/kg/day (initial and maintenance dosing)

Nephrotic syndrome, corticosteroid refractory or intolerant: Oral: 2.5-3 mg/kg/day every day for 60-90 days

Canadian labeling:

I.V.: Initial: 2-8 mg/kg (60-250 mg/m²) in divided doses for 6 or more days; Maintenance: 10-15 mg/kg every 7-10 days or 30 mg/kg every 3-4 weeks or when bone marrow function recovers
Oral: Initial: 2-8 mg/kg (60-250 mg/m²) in divided doses for 6 or more days; Maintenance: 2-5 mg/kg (50-150 mg/m²) twice weekly

Indication specific and/or unlabeled uses/dosing:

Ewing's sarcoma (unlabeled use): I.V.: VAC/IE regimen; VAC: 1200 mg/m² (plus mesna) on day 1 of a 21-day treatment cycle (in combination with vincristine and doxorubicin [then dactinomycin when maximum doxorubicin dose reached]), alternates with IE (ifosfamide and etoposide) for a total of 17 cycles (Grier, 2003)

Hodgkin lymphoma (unlabeled dosing): I.V.: BEACOPP escalated regimen: 1200 mg/m² on day 0 of a 21-day treatment cycle (in combination with bleomycin, etoposide, doxorubicin, vincristine, prednisone, and procarbazine) for 4 cycles (Kelly, 2011)

Lupus nephritis (unlabeled use): I.V.: 500-1000 mg/m² every month for 6 months, then every 3 months for a total of 2.5-3 years (Austin, 1986; Gourley, 1996; Lehman, 2000)

Neuroblastoma (unlabeled dosing): I.V.: CE-CAdO regimen, courses 3 and 4: 300 mg/m² days 1-5 every 21 days for 2 cycles (Rubie, 1998) **or** 10 mg/kg days 1-5 every 21 days for 2 cycles (Rubie, 2001). **Note:** Decreased doses may be recommended for newborns or children <10 kg.

Transplant conditioning (unlabeled use): Myeloablative transplant: I.V.: 50 mg/kg/day for 4 days beginning 5 days before transplant (with or without antithymocyte globulin [equine]) (Champlin, 2007)

Renal Impairment

U.S. labeling: No adjustment provided in the manufacturer's labeling (use with caution; elevated levels of metabolites may occur).

Canadian labeling:

Mild impairment: No dosage adjustment provided in manufacturer's labeling
Moderate impairment: Dose reduction may be necessary; manufacturer's labeling does not provide specific dosing recommendations
Severe impairment: Use is contraindicated.

The following adjustments have also been recommended:

Aronoff, 2007: Children and Adults:

Cl_{cr} ≥10 mL/minute: No dosage adjustment required.

Cl_{cr} <10 mL/minute: Administer 75% of normal dose.

Hemodialysis: Moderately dialyzable (20% to 50%); administer 50% of normal dose; administer after hemodialysis

Continuous ambulatory peritoneal dialysis (CAPD): Administer 75% of normal dose.

Continuous renal replacement therapy (CRRT): Administer 100% of normal dose.

Janus, 2010: Hemodialysis: Administer 75% of normal dose; administer after hemodialysis

Hepatic Impairment The pharmacokinetics of cyclophosphamide are not significantly altered in the presence of hepatic insufficiency.

U.S. labeling: No dosage adjustment provided in the manufacturer's labeling.

Canadian labeling:

Mild-to-moderate impairment: No dosage adjustment provided in the manufacturer's labeling.

Severe impairment: Use is contraindicated.

The following adjustments have been recommended (Floyd, 2006):

Serum bilirubin 3.1-5 mg/dL or transaminases >3 times ULN: Administer 75% of dose.

Serum bilirubin >5 mg/mL: Avoid use.

Adjustment for Toxicity

Hematologic toxicity: May require dose reduction or treatment interruption; Canadian labeling recommends reducing initial dose by 30% to 50% if bone marrow function compromised (due to prior radiation therapy, prior chemotherapy, or tumor infiltration)

Hemorrhagic cystitis, severe: Discontinue treatment.

Combination Regimens

Brain tumor: COPE on page 1596
Breast cancer:
AC on page 1517
AC/Paclitaxel (Sequential) on page 1517
AC-Paclitaxel-Trastuzumab on page 1518
CAF on page 1538
CEF on page 1556
CMF on page 1588
CMF-IV on page 1588
Docetaxel-Cyclophosphamide (TC) on page 1611
Docetaxel-FEC on page 1611
Docetaxel-Trastuzumab-FEC on page 1616
Dox-CMF (Sequential) on page 1617
FAC on page 1641
FEC on page 1642
TAC on page 1753
Vinorelbine-FEC on page 1773
Vinorelbine-Trastuzumab-FEC on page 1775
Gestational trophoblastic tumor: EMA/CO on page 1622
Leukemia, acute lymphocytic:
Hyper-CVAD + Imatinib on page 1680
Hyper-CVAD (Leukemia, Acute Lymphocytic) on page 1681

Larson Regimen (ALL) on page 1699
VAD/CVAD on page 1768
Leukemia, chronic lymphocytic:
CVP (Leukemia) on page 1598
Cyclophosphamide-Fludarabine-Alemtuzumab-Rituximab (CLL) on page 1601
Fludarabine-Cyclophosphamide (CLL) on page 1646
Fludarabine-Cyclophosphamide-Rituximab (CLL) on page 1648
PCR on page 1705
Pentostatin-Cyclophosphamide on page 1739
Lung cancer (small cell): CAV (Small Cell Lung Cancer) on page 1554
Lymphoma, Hodgkin:
BEACOPP-14 (Hodgkin) on page 1522
BEACOPP Escalated (Hodgkin) on page 1522
BEACOPP Escalated Plus Standard (Hodgkin) on page 1523
BEACOPP Standard (Hodgkin) on page 1525
C-MOPP/ABV Hybrid (Hodgkin) on page 1588
Lymphoma, non-Hodgkin's:
CEPP(B) on page 1556
CHOP (NHL) on page 1564
CNOP on page 1589
CODOX-M on page 1590
COMLA on page 1595
COP-BLAM on page 1595
COPP on page 1596
CVP (Lymphoma, non-Hodgkin's) on page 1598
EPOCH Dose-Adjusted (AIDS-Related Lymphoma) on page 1628
EPOCH Dose-Adjusted (NHL) on page 1628
EPOCH (Dose-Adjusted)-Rituximab (NHL) on page 1629
EPOCH (NHL) on page 1630
EPOCH-Rituximab (NHL) on page 1631
Fludarabine-Cyclophosphamide-Mitoxantrone-Rituximab on page 1647
Fludarabine-Cyclophosphamide-Rituximab (NHL-Follicular) on page 1649
Hyper-CVAD (Lymphoma, non-Hodgkin's) on page 1687
MACOP-B on page 1704
m-BACOD on page 1706
Pro-MACE-CytaBOM on page 1741
R-CVP on page 1745
Rituximab-CHOP (NHL) on page 1748
Lymphoma, non-Hodgkin's (Burkitt): CODOX-M/IVAC on page 1591
Lymphoma, non-Hodgkin's (Mantle cell):
Fludarabine-Cyclophosphamide (NHL-Mantle Cell) on page 1648
Hyper-CVAD + Rituximab on page 1688
Multiple myeloma:
Cyclophosphamide-Bortezomib-Dexamethasone (Multiple Myeloma) on page 1599
DTPACE on page 1620
Hyper-CVAD (Multiple Myeloma) on page 1687
VBMCP (Multiple Myeloma) on page 1769
VCAP on page 1770
Neuroblastoma:
A3 (Neuroblastoma) on page 1515
CAV-P/VP (Neuroblastoma) on page 1554
CE-CAdO (Neuroblastoma) on page 1555

Cisplatin-Doxorubicin-Etoposide-Cyclophosphamide (Neuroblastoma) on page 1568
New A1 (Neuroblastoma) on page 1721
Osteosarcoma: POG-8651 on page 1740
Ovarian cancer:
PAC (CAP) on page 1725
Vincristine-Dactinomycin-Cyclophosphamide (Ovarian Cancer) on page 1771
Rhabdomyosarcoma:
VAC Pulse on page 1767
VAC (Rhabdomyosarcoma) on page 1767
Sarcoma:
CYVADIC on page 1605
Topotecan-Cyclophosphamide (Ewing's Sarcoma) on page 1756
VAC Alternating With IE (Ewing's Sarcoma) on page 1766
Wilms' tumor: Regimen I (Wilms' Tumor) on page 1745

Administration

I.V.: Infusion rate may vary based on protocol (refer to specific protocol for infusion rate). Administer by direct I.V. injection (if reconstituted in NS), IVPB, or continuous I.V. infusion

Bladder toxicity: To minimize bladder toxicity, increase normal fluid intake during and for 1-2 days after cyclophosphamide dose. Most adult patients will require a fluid intake of at least 2 L/day. High-dose regimens should be accompanied by vigorous hydration with or without mesna therapy.

Hematopoietic stem cell transplant: Approaches to reduction of hemorrhagic cystitis include infusion of 0.9% NaCl 3 L/m^2/24 hours, infusion of 0.9% NaCl 3 L/m^2/24 hours with continuous 0.9% NaCl bladder irrigation 300-1000 mL/hour, and infusion of 0.9% NaCl 1.5-3 L/m^2/24 hours with intravenous mesna. Hydration should begin at least 4 hours before cyclophosphamide and continue at least 24 hours after completion of cyclophosphamide. The dose of daily mesna used may be 67% to 100% of the daily dose of cyclophosphamide. Mesna can be administered as a continuous 24-hour intravenous infusion or be given in divided doses every 4 hours. Mesna should begin at the start of treatment, and continue at least 24 hours following the last dose of cyclophosphamide.

Oral: Tablets are not scored and should not be cut or crushed. To minimize the risk of bladder irritation, do not administer tablets at bedtime.

Emetic Potential

>1500 mg/m^2: Very high (>90%)
≤1500 mg/m^2: Moderate (30% to 90%)
Oral: Moderate (30% to 90%)

Vesicant/Extravasation Risk May be an irritant

Extemporaneous Preparations Hazardous agent: Use appropriate precautions for handling and disposal.

Liquid solutions or oral administration may be prepared by dissolving cyclophosphamide injection in Aromatic Elixir, N.F. Store refrigerated (in glass container) for up to 14 days.

Cyclophosphamide Prescribing Information, Baxter Healthcare Corporation, Deerfield, Il, April, 2012.

A 10 mg/mL oral suspension may be prepared by reconstituting one 2 g vial for injection with 100 mL of NaCl 0.9%, providing an initial concentration of 20 mg/mL. Mix this solution in a 1:1 ratio with either Simple Syrup, NF or

Ora-Plus® to obtain a final concentration of 10 mg/mL. Label "shake well" and "refrigerate". Stable for 56 days refrigerated.

Kennedy R, Groepper D, Tagen M, et al, "Stability of Cyclophosphamide in Extemporaneous Oral Suspensions," *Ann Pharmacother*, 2010, 44(2):295-301.

Monitoring Parameters CBC with differential and platelets, BUN, UA, serum electrolytes, serum creatinine; monitor for signs/symptoms of hemorrhagic cystitis

Dietary Considerations Tablets should be administered during or after meals

Additional Information In patients with CYP2B6 G516T variant allele, cyclophosphamide metabolism is markedly increased; metabolism is not influenced by CYP2C9 and CYP2C19 isotypes.

Dosage Forms Excipient information presented when available (limited, particularly for generics); consult specific product labeling.

Injection, powder for reconstitution: 500 mg, 1 g, 2 g

Tablet, oral: 25 mg, 50 mg

Dosage Forms: Canada

Additional dosage forms available in Canada. Excipient information presented when available (limited, particularly for generics); consult specific product labeling.

Injection, powder for reconstitution: 200 mg

References

Anderson JE, Appelbaum FR, Schoch G, et al, "Allogeneic Marrow Transplantation for Myelodysplastic Syndrome With Advanced Disease Morphology: A Phase II Study of Busulfan, Cyclophosphamide, and Total Body Irradiation and Analysis of Prognostic Factors," *J Clin Oncol*, 1996, 14(1):220-6.

Aronoff GR, Bennett WM, Berns JS, et al, *Drug Prescribing in Renal Failure: Dosing Guidelines for Adults and Children*, 5th ed, Philadelphia, PA: American College of Physicians, 2007, p 97, 170.

Austin HA 3rd, Klipel JH, Balow JE, et al, "Therapy of Lupus Nephritis. Controlled Trial of Prednisone and Cytotoxic Drugs," *N Engl J Med*, 1986, 314(10):614-9.

Cassileth PA, Andersen J, Lazarus HM, et al, "Autologous Bone Marrow Transplant in Acute Myeloid Leukemia in First Remission," *J Clin Oncol*, 1993, 11(2):314-9.

Champlin RE, Perez WS, Passweg JR, et al, "Bone Marrow Transplantation for Severe Aplastic Anemia: A Randomized Controlled Study of Conditioning Regimens," *Blood*, 2007, 109 (10):4582-5.

Coiffier B, Lepage E, Briere J, et al, "CHOP Chemotherapy Plus Rituximab Compared With CHOP Alone in Elderly Patients With Diffuse Large-B-Cell Lymphoma," *N Engl J Med*, 2002, 346 (4):235-42.

de Groot K, Harper L, Jayne DR, et al, "Pulse Versus Daily Oral Cyclophosphamide for Induction of Remission in Antineutrophil Cytoplasmic Antibody-Associated Vasculitis: A Randomized Trial," *Ann Intern Med*, 2009, 150(10):670-80.

Diehl V, Franklin J, Pfreundschuh M, et al, "Standard and Increased-Dose BEACOPP Chemotherapy Compared With COPP-ABVD for Advanced Hodgkin's disease," *N Engl J Med*, 2003, 348(21):2386-95.

Escobar PF, Lurain JR, Singh DK, et al, "Treatment of High-Risk Gestational Trophoblastic Neoplasia With Etoposide, Methotrexate, Actinomycin D, Cyclophosphamide, and Vincristine Chemotherapy," *Gynecol Oncol*, 2003, 91(3):552-7.

Fisher B, Brown AM, Dimitrov NV, et al, "Two Months of Doxorubicin-Cyclophosphamide With and Without Interval Reinduction Therapy Compared With 6 Months of Cyclophosphamide, Methotrexate, and Fluorouracil in Positive-Node Breast Cancer Patients With Tamoxifen-Nonresponsive Tumors: Results From the National Surgical Adjuvant Breast and Bowel Project B-15," *J Clin Oncol*, 1990, 8(9):1483-96.

Floyd J, Mirza I, Sachs B, et al, "Hepatotoxicity of Chemotherapy," *Semin Oncol*, 2006, 33 (1):50-67.

Floyd JD, Nguyen DT, Lobins RL, et al, "Cardiotoxicity of Cancer Therapy," *J Clin Oncol*, 2005, 23 (30):7685-96.

García-Suárez J, Bañas H, Arribas I, et al, "Dose-Adjusted EPOCH Plus Rituximab is an Effective Regimen in Patients With Poor-Prognostic Untreated Diffuse Large B-Cell Lymphoma: Results From a Prospective Observational Study," *Br J Haematol*, 2007, 136(2):276-85.

Goldhirsch A, Colleoni M, Coates AS, et al, "Adding Adjuvant CMF Chemotherapy to Either Radiotherapy or Tamoxifen: Are All CMFs Alike? The International Breast Cancer Study Group (IBCSG)," *Ann Oncol*, 1998, 9(5):489-93.

Gourley MF, Austin HA 3rd, Scott D, et al, "Methylprednisolone and Cyclophosphamide, Alone or in Combination, in Patients With Lupus Nephritis. A Randomized, Controlled Trial," *Ann Intern Med*, 1996, 125(7):549-57.

Grier HE, Krailo MD, Tarbell NJ, et al, "Addition of Ifosfamide and Etoposide to Standard Chemotherapy for Ewing's Sarcoma and Primitive Neuroectodermal Tumor of Bone," *N Engl J Med*, 2003, 348(8):694-701.

Hahn BH, McMahon MA, Wilkinson A, et al, "American College of Rheumatology Guidelines for Screening, Treatment, and Management of Lupus Nephritis," *Arthritis Care Res (Hoboken)*, 2012, 64(6):797-808.

Harper L, Morgan MD, Walsh M, et al, "Pulse versus Daily Oral Cyclophosphamide for Induction of Remission in ANCA-Associated Vasculitis: Long-Term Follow-up," *Ann Rheum Dis*, 2012, 71 (6):955-60.

Hensley ML, Hagerty KL, Kewalramani T, et al, "American Society of Clinical Oncology 2008 Clinical Practice Guideline Update: Use of Chemotherapy and Radiotherapy Protectants," *J Clin Oncol*, 2008, 27(1):127-45.

Janus N, Thariat J, Boulanger H, et al, "Proposal for Dosage Adjustment and Timing of Chemotherapy in Hemodialyzed Patients," *Ann Oncol*, 2010, 21(7):1395-403.

Jayne D, Rasmussen N, Andrassy K, et al, "A randomized Trial of Maintenance Therapy for Vasculitis Associated With Antineutrophil Cytoplasmic Autoantibodies," *N Engl J Med*, 2003, 349 (1):36-44.

Kantarjian HM, O'Brien S, Smith TL, et al, "Results of Treatment With Hyper-CVAD, A Dose-Intensive Regimen, in Adult Acute Lymphocytic Leukemia," *J Clin Oncol*, 2000, 18(3): 547-61.

Kelly KM, Sposto R, Hutchinson R, et al, "BEACOPP Chemotherapy is a Highly Effective Regimen in Children and Adolescents With High-Risk Hodgkin lymphoma: A Report from the Children's Oncology Group," *Blood*, 2011, 117(9):2596-603.

Khan ML, Reeder CB, Kumar SK, et al, "A Comparison of Lenalidomide/Dexamethasone versus Cyclophosphamide/Lenalidomide/Dexamethasone versus Cyclophosphamide/Bortezomib/Dexamethasone in Newly Diagnosed Multiple Myeloma," *Br J Haematol*, 2012, 156(3):326-33.

Khouri IF, McLaughlin P, Saliba RM, et al, "Eight-Year Experience With Allogeneic Stem Cell Transplantation for Relapsed Follicular Lymphoma After Nonmyeloablative Conditioning With Fludarabine, Cyclophosphamide, and Rituximab," *Blood*, 2008, 111(12):5530-6.

Larson RA, Dodge RK, Burns CP, et al, "A Five-Drug Remission Induction Regimen With Intensive Consolidation for Adults With Acute Lymphoblastic Leukemia: Cancer and Leukemia Group B Study 8811," *Blood*, 1995, 85(8):2025-37.

Lehman TJ and Onel K, "Intermittent Intravenous Cyclophosphamide Arrests Progression of the Renal Chronicity Index in Childhood Systemic Lupus Erythematosus," *J Pediatr*, 2000, 136 (2):243-7.

Levine MN, Bramwell VH, Pritchard KI, et al, "Randomized Trial of Intensive Cyclophosphamide, Epirubicin, and Fluorouracil Chemotherapy Compared With Cyclophosphamide, Methotrexate, and Fluorouracil in Premenopausal Women With Node-Positive Breast Cancer. National Cancer Institute of Canada Clinical Trials Group," *J Clin Oncol*, 1998, 16(8):2651-8.

Magrath I, Adde M, Shad A, et al, "Adults and Children With Small Non-Cleaved-Cell Lymphoma Have a Similar Excellent Outcome When Treated With the Same Chemotherapy Regimen," *J Clin Oncol*, 1996, 14(3):925-34.

Malik SW, Myers JL, DeRemee RA, et al, "Lung Toxicity Associated With Cyclophosphamide Use. Two Distinct Patterns," *Am J Respir Crit Care Med*, 1996, 154(6 Pt 1):1851-6.

Mok CC, Lau CS, and Wong RW, "Risk Factors for Ovarian Failure in Patients With Systemic Lupus Erythematosus Receiving Cyclophosphamide Therapy," *Arthritis Rheum*, 1998, 41 (5):831-7.

Morgan C, Tillett T, Braybrooke J, et al, "Management of Uncommon Chemotherapy-Induced Emergencies," *Lancet Oncol*, 2011, 12(8):806-14.

National Comprehensive Cancer Network® (NCCN), "Clinical Practice Guidelines in Oncology™: Breast Cancer," Version 3.2012. Available at http://www.nccn.org/professionals/physician_gls/PDF/breast.pdf

Reece DE, Barnett MJ, Connors JM, et al, "Intensive Chemotherapy With Cyclophosphamide, Carmustine, and Etoposide Followed by Autologous Bone Marrow Transplantation for Relapsed Hodgkin's Disease," *J Clin Oncol*, 1991, 9(10):1871-9.

Robak T, Dmoszynska A, Solal-Céligny P, et al, "Rituximab Plus Fludarabine and Cyclophosphamide Prolongs Progression-Free Survival Compared With Fludarabine and Cyclophosphamide Alone in Previously Treated Chronic Lymphocytic Leukemia," *J Clin Oncol*, 2010, 28 (10):1756-65.

Rubie H, Michon J, Plantaz D, et al, "Unresectable Localized Neuroblastoma: Improved Survival After Primary Chemotherapy Including Carboplatin-Etoposide. Neuroblastoma Study Group of the Societe Francaise d'Oncologie Pediatrique (SFOP)," *Br J Cancer*, 1998, 77(12):2310-7.

Rubie H, Plantaz D, Coze C, et al, "Localised and Unresectable Neuroblastoma in Infants: Excellent Outcome With Primary Chemotherapy. Neuroblastoma Study Group, Société Française d'Oncologie Pédiatrique," *Med Pediatr Oncol*, 2001, 36(1):247-50.

Stone JH, Merkel PA, Spiera R, et al, "Rituximab Versus Cyclophosphamide for ANCA-Associated Vasculitis," *N Engl J Med*, 2010, 363(3):221-32.

Thompson JA, Fisher RI, Leblanc M, et al, "Total Body Irradiation, Etoposide, Cyclophosphamide, and Autologous Peripheral Blood Stem-Cell Transplantation Followed by Randomization to Therapy With Interleukin-2 Versus Observation for Patients With Non-Hodgkin Lymphoma: Results of a Phase 3 Randomized Trial by the Southwest Oncology Group (SWOG 9438)," *Blood*, 2008, 111(8):4048-54.

◆ **Cyclosporin A** *see* CycloSPORINE (Systemic) *on page* *333*

CycloSPORINE (Systemic) (SYE kloe spor een)

Related Information

Hematopoietic Stem Cell Transplantation *on page 1887*

Safe Handling of Hazardous Drugs *on page 1904*

Brand Names: U.S. Gengraf®; Neoral®; SandIMMUNE®

Brand Names: Canada Apo-Cyclosporine®; Neoral®; Rhoxal-cyclosporine; Sandimmune® I.V.; Sandoz-Cyclosporine

Index Terms Ciclosporin; CsA; CyA; Cyclosporin A

Generic Availability (U.S.) Yes: Excludes non-modified solution

Pharmacologic Category Calcineurin Inhibitor; Immunosuppressant Agent

Use Prophylaxis of organ rejection in kidney, liver, and heart transplants, has been used with azathioprine and/or corticosteroids; severe, active rheumatoid arthritis (RA) not responsive to methotrexate alone; severe, recalcitrant plaque psoriasis in nonimmunocompromised adults unresponsive to or unable to tolerate other systemic therapy

Unlabeled Use Allogenic stem cell transplants for prevention and treatment of graft-versus-host disease; also used in some cases of severe autoimmune disease (eg, SLE) that are resistant to corticosteroids and other therapy; focal segmental glomerulosclerosis; severe ulcerative colitis

Labeled Contraindications Hypersensitivity to cyclosporine or any component of the formulation. I.V. cyclosporine is contraindicated in hypersensitivity to polyoxyethylated castor oil (Cremophor® EL).

Rheumatoid arthritis and psoriasis: Abnormal renal function, uncontrolled hypertension, malignancies. Concomitant treatment with PUVA or UVB therapy, methotrexate, other immunosuppressive agents, coal tar, or radiation therapy are also contraindications for use in patients with psoriasis.

Pregnancy Risk Factor C

Lactation Enters breast milk/not recommended

Warnings/Precautions Hazardous agent - use appropriate precautions for handling and disposal. **[U.S. Boxed Warning]: Renal impairment, including structural kidney damage has occurred (when used at high doses); monitor renal function closely.** Elevations in serum creatinine and BUN generally respond to dosage reductions. Use caution with other potentially nephrotoxic drugs (eg, acyclovir, aminoglycoside antibiotics, amphotericin B, ciprofloxacin). **[U.S. Boxed Warning]: Increased risk of lymphomas and other malignancies, particularly those of the skin;** risk is related to intensity/duration of therapy and the use of >1 immunosuppressive agent; all patients should avoid excessive sun/UV light exposure. **[U.S. Boxed Warning]: Increased risk of infection; fatal infections have been reported.** ▶

Latent viral infections may be activated (including BK virus which is associated with nephropathy) and result in serious adverse effects. **[U.S. Boxed Warning]: May cause hypertension.** Use caution when changing dosage forms. **[U.S. Boxed Warning]: Cyclosporine (modified) has increased bioavailability as compared to cyclosporine (non-modified) and cannot be used interchangeably without close monitoring.** Monitor cyclosporine concentrations closely following the addition, modification, or deletion of other medications; live, attenuated vaccines may be less effective; use should be avoided. Increased hepatic enzymes and bilirubin have occurred (when used at high doses); improvement usually seen with dosage reduction.

Transplant patients: To be used initially with corticosteroids. May cause significant hyperkalemia and hyperuricemia, seizures (particularly if used with high dose corticosteroids), and encephalopathy. Other neurotoxic events (eg, optic disc edema including papilledema and visual impairment) have been reported rarely. Make dose adjustments based on cyclosporine blood concentrations. **[U.S. Boxed Warning]: Adjustment of dose should only be made under the direct supervision of an experienced physician.** Anaphylaxis has been reported with I.V. use; reserve for patients who cannot take oral form. **[U.S. Boxed Warning]: Risk of skin cancer may be increased in transplant patients.** Due to the increased risk for nephrotoxicity in renal transplantation, avoid using standard doses of cyclosporine in combination with everolimus; reduced cyclosporine doses are recommended; monitor cyclosporine concentrations closely. Cyclosporine and everolimus combination therapy may increase the risk for proteinuria. Cyclosporine combined with either everolimus or sirolimus may increase the risk for thrombotic microangiopathy/thrombotic thrombocytopenic purpura/hemolytic uremic syndrome (TMA/TTP/HUS).

Psoriasis: Patients should avoid excessive sun exposure; safety and efficacy in children <18 years of age have not been established. **[U.S. Boxed Warning]: Risk of skin cancer may be increased with a history of PUVA and possibly methotrexate or other immunosuppressants, UVB, coal tar, or radiation.**

Rheumatoid arthritis: Safety and efficacy for use in juvenile idiopathic arthritis (JIA) have not been established. If receiving other immunosuppressive agents, radiation or UV therapy, concurrent use of cyclosporine is not recommended.

Products may contain corn oil, ethanol, or propylene glycol; injection also contains Cremophor® EL (polyoxyethylated castor oil), which has been associated with rare anaphylactic reactions.

Adverse Reactions Adverse reactions reported with systemic use, including rheumatoid arthritis, psoriasis, and transplantation (kidney, liver, and heart). Percentages noted include the highest frequency regardless of indication/dosage. Frequencies may vary for specific conditions or formulation.

>10%:

- Cardiovascular: Hypertension (8% to 53%), edema (5% to 14%)
- Central nervous system: Headache (2% to 25%)
- Dermatologic: Hirsutism (21% to 45%), hypertrichosis (5% to 19%)
- Endocrine & metabolic: Triglycerides increased (15%), female reproductive disorder (9% to 11%)
- Gastrointestinal: Nausea (23%), diarrhea (3% to 13%), gum hyperplasia (2% to 16%), abdominal discomfort (<1% to 15%), dyspepsia (2% to 12%)
- Neuromuscular & skeletal: Tremor (7% to 55%), paresthesia (1% to 11%), leg cramps/muscle contractions (2% to 12%)

Renal: Renal dysfunction/nephropathy (10% to 38%), creatinine increased (16% to ≥50%)
Respiratory: Upper respiratory infection (1% to 14%)
Miscellaneous: Infection (3% to 25%)

Kidney, liver, and heart transplant only (≤2% unless otherwise noted):

Cardiovascular: Flushes (<1% to 4%), MI
Central nervous system: Convulsions (1% to 5%), anxiety, confusion, fever, lethargy
Dermatologic: Acne (1% to 6%), brittle fingernails, hair breaking, pruritus
Endocrine & metabolic: Gynecomastia (<1% to 4%), hyperglycemia
Gastrointestinal: Nausea (2% to 10%), vomiting (2% to 10%), diarrhea (3% to 8%), abdominal discomfort (<1% to 7%), cramps (0% to 4%), anorexia, constipation, gastritis, mouth sores, pancreatitis, swallowing difficulty, upper GI bleed, weight loss
Hematologic: Leukopenia (<1% to 6%), anemia, thrombocytopenia
Hepatic: Hepatotoxicity (<1% to 7%)
Neuromuscular & skeletal: Paresthesia (1% to 3%), joint pain, muscle pain, tingling, weakness
Ocular: Conjunctivitis, visual disturbance
Otic: Hearing loss, tinnitus
Renal: Hematuria
Respiratory: Sinusitis (<1% to 7%)
Miscellaneous: Lymphoma (<1% to 6%), allergic reactions, hiccups, night sweats

Rheumatoid arthritis only (1% to <3% unless otherwise noted):

Cardiovascular: Hypertension (8%), edema (5%), chest pain (4%), arrhythmia (2%), abnormal heart sounds, cardiac failure, MI, peripheral ischemia
Central nervous system: Dizziness (8%), pain (6%), insomnia (4%), depression (3%), migraine (2%), anxiety, hypoesthesia, emotional lability, impaired concentration, malaise, nervousness, paranoia, somnolence, vertigo
Dermatologic: Purpura (3%), abnormal pigmentation, angioedema, cellulitis, dermatitis, dry skin, eczema, folliculitis, nail disorder, pruritus, skin disorder, urticaria
Endocrine & metabolic: Menstrual disorder (3%), breast fibroadenosis, breast pain, diabetes mellitus, goiter, hot flashes, hyperkalemia, hyperuricemia, hypoglycemia, libido increased/decreased
Gastrointestinal: Vomiting (9%), flatulence (5%), gingivitis (4%), gum hyperplasia (2%), constipation, dry mouth, dysphagia, enanthema, eructation, esophagitis, gastric ulcer, gastritis, gastroenteritis, gingival bleeding, glossitis, peptic ulcer, salivary gland enlargement, taste perversion, tongue disorder, gum hyperplasia, weight loss/gain
Genitourinary: Leukorrhea (1%), abnormal urine, micturition urgency, nocturia, polyuria, pyelonephritis, urinary incontinence, uterine hemorrhage
Hematologic: Anemia, leukopenia
Hepatic: Bilirubinemia
Neuromuscular & skeletal: Paresthesia (8%), tremor (8%), leg cramps/muscle contractions (2%), arthralgia, bone fracture, joint dislocation, myalgia, neuropathy, stiffness, synovial cyst, tendon disorder, weakness
Ocular: Abnormal vision, cataract, conjunctivitis, eye pain
Otic: Tinnitus, deafness, vestibular disorder
Renal: BUN increased, hematuria, renal abscess
Respiratory: Cough (5%), dyspnea (5%), sinusitis (4%), abnormal chest sounds, bronchospasm, epistaxis

Miscellaneous: Infection (9%), abscess, allergy, bacterial infection, carcinoma, fungal infection, herpes simplex, herpes zoster, lymphadenopathy, moniliasis, diaphoresis increased, tonsillitis, viral infection

Psoriasis only (1% to <3% unless otherwise noted):

Cardiovascular: Chest pain, flushes

Central nervous system: Psychiatric events (4% to 5%), pain (3% to 4%), dizziness, fever, insomnia, nervousness, vertigo

Dermatologic: Hypertrichosis (5% to 7%), acne, dry skin, folliculitis, keratosis, pruritus, rash, skin malignancies

Endocrine & metabolic: Hot flashes

Gastrointestinal: Nausea (5% to 6%), diarrhea (5% to 6%), gum hyperplasia (4% to 6%), abdominal discomfort (3% to 6%), dyspepsia (2% to 3%), abdominal distention, appetite increased, constipation, gingival bleeding

Genitourinary: Micturition increased

Hematologic: Bleeding disorder, clotting disorder, platelet disorder, red blood cell disorder

Hepatic: Hyperbilirubinemia

Neuromuscular & skeletal: Paresthesia (5% to 7%), arthralgia (1% to 6%)

Ocular: Abnormal vision

Respiratory: Bronchospasm (5%), cough (5%), dyspnea (5%), rhinitis (5%), respiratory infection

Miscellaneous: Flu-like syndrome (8% to 10%)

Postmarketing and/or case reports (any indication): Anaphylaxis/anaphylactoid reaction (possibly associated with Cremophor® EL vehicle in injection formulation), benign intracranial hypertension, BK virus-associated nephropathy, cholesterol increased, death (due to renal deterioration), encephalopathy, gout, hyperbilirubinemia, hyperkalemia, hypomagnesemia (mild), impaired consciousness, neurotoxicity, papilloedema, pulmonary edema (noncardiogenic), reversible posterior leukoencephalopathy syndrome (RPLS), uric acid increased

Drug Interactions

Metabolism/Transport Effects Substrate of CYP3A4 (major), P-glycoprotein; **Note:** Assignment of Major/Minor substrate status based on clinically relevant drug interaction potential; **Inhibits** CYP2C9 (weak), CYP3A4 (moderate), P-glycoprotein

Avoid Concomitant Use

Avoid concomitant use of CycloSPORINE (Systemic) with any of the following: Aliskiren; AtorvaSTATin; BCG; Bosentan; Bosutinib; Conivaptan; Crizotinib; Dronedarone; Enzalutamide; Eplerenone; Lovastatin; Mifepristone; Natalizumab; Pimecrolimus; Pimozide; Pitavastatin; Potassium-Sparing Diuretics; Silodosin; Simvastatin; Sitaxentan; Tacrolimus (Systemic); Tacrolimus (Topical); Tolvaptan; Topotecan; Vaccines (Live); VinCRIStine (Liposomal)

Increased Effect/Toxicity

CycloSPORINE (Systemic) may increase the levels/effects of: Aliskiren; Ambrisentan; ARIPiprazole; AtorvaSTATin; Avanafil; Boceprevir; Bosentan; Bosutinib; Budesonide (Systemic, Oral Inhalation); Calcium Channel Blockers (Dihydropyridine); Calcium Channel Blockers (Nondihydropyridine); Cardiac Glycosides; Caspofungin; Colchicine; CYP3A4 Substrates; Dabigatran Etexilate; Dexamethasone (Systemic); DOXOrubicin; Dronedarone; Etoposide; Etoposide Phosphate; Everolimus; Ezetimibe; FentaNYL; Fibric Acid Derivatives; Fluvastatin; Halofantrine; Imipenem; Ivacaftor; Leflunomide; Loop Diuretics; Lovastatin; Lurasidone; Methotrexate; MethylPREDNISolone; Minoxidil (Systemic); Minoxidil (Topical); Natalizumab; Nonsteroidal

Anti-Inflammatory Agents; P-glycoprotein/ABCB1 Substrates; Pimozide; Pitavastatin; Pravastatin; PrednisoLONE (Systemic); PredniSONE; Propafenone; Protease Inhibitors; Prucalopride; Ranolazine; Repaglinide; Rivaroxaban; Rosuvastatin; Salmeterol; Saxagliptin; Silodosin; Simvastatin; Sirolimus; Sitaxentan; Tacrolimus (Systemic); Tacrolimus (Topical); Tolvaptan; Topotecan; Vaccines (Live); Vilazodone; VinCRIStine (Liposomal); Zuclopenthixol

The levels/effects of CycloSPORINE (Systemic) may be increased by: ACE Inhibitors; AcetaZOLAMIDE; Aminoglycosides; Amiodarone; Amphotericin B; Androgens; Angiotensin II Receptor Blockers; Antifungal Agents (Azole Derivatives, Systemic); Boceprevir; Bromocriptine; Calcium Channel Blockers (Nondihydropyridine); Carvedilol; Chloramphenicol; Conivaptan; Crizotinib; CYP3A4 Inhibitors (Moderate); CYP3A4 Inhibitors (Strong); Dasatinib; Denosumab; Dexamethasone (Systemic); Eplerenone; Ezetimibe; Fluconazole; GlyBURIDE; Grapefruit Juice; Imatinib; Imipenem; Ivacaftor; Macrolide Antibiotics; Melphalan; Methotrexate; MethylPREDNISolone; Metoclopramide; MetroNIDAZOLE (Systemic); Mifepristone; Nonsteroidal Anti-Inflammatory Agents; Norfloxacin; Omeprazole; P-glycoprotein/ABCB1 Inhibitors; Pimecrolimus; Potassium-Sparing Diuretics; Pravastatin; PrednisoLONE (Systemic); PredniSONE; Protease Inhibitors; Pyrazinamide; Quinupristin; Roflumilast; Sirolimus; Sulfonamide Derivatives; Tacrolimus (Systemic); Tacrolimus (Topical); Telaprevir; Temsirolimus; Trastuzumab

Decreased Effect

CycloSPORINE (Systemic) may decrease the levels/effects of: BCG; Coccidioidin Skin Test; GlyBURIDE; Ifosfamide; Mycophenolate; Sipuleucel-T; Vaccines (Inactivated); Vaccines (Live)

The levels/effects of CycloSPORINE (Systemic) may be decreased by: Adalimumab; Armodafinil; Ascorbic Acid; Barbiturates; Bosentan; CarBAMazepine; Colesevelam; CYP3A4 Inducers (Strong); Deferasirox; Dexamethasone (Systemic); Echinacea; Efavirenz; Enzalutamide; Fibric Acid Derivatives; Fosphenytoin; Griseofulvin; Imipenem; MethylPREDNISolone; Modafinil; Multivitamins/Minerals (with ADEK, Folate, Iron); Nafcillin; Orlistat; P-glycoprotein/ABCB1 Inducers; Phenytoin; PrednisoLONE (Systemic); PredniSONE; Rifamycin Derivatives; Somatostatin Analogs; St Johns Wort; Sulfinpyrazone [Off Market]; Sulfonamide Derivatives; Tocilizumab; Vitamin E

Ethanol/Nutrition/Herb Interactions

Food: Grapefruit juice increases cyclosporine serum concentrations. Management: Avoid grapefruit juice.

Herb/Nutraceutical: St John's wort may increase the metabolism of and decrease plasma levels of cyclosporine; organ rejection and graft loss have been reported. Cat's claw and echinacea have immunostimulant properties. Management: Avoid St John's wort, cat's claw, and echinacea.

Storage/Stability

Capsule: Store at controlled room temperature.

Injection: Store at controlled room temperature; do not refrigerate. Ampuls and vials should be protected from light. Stability of injection of parenteral admixture at room temperature (25°C) is 6 hours in PVC; 12-24 hours in Excel®, PAB® containers, or glass.

Oral solution: Store at controlled room temperature; do not refrigerate. Use within 2 months after opening; should be mixed in glass containers.

Reconstitution Injection: To minimize leaching of DEHP, non-PVC containers and sets should be used for preparation and administration.

Sandimmune® injection: Injection should be further diluted (1 mL [50 mg] of concentrate in 20-100 mL of D_5W or NS) for administration by intravenous infusion.

Mechanism of Action Inhibition of production and release of interleukin II and inhibits interleukin II-induced activation of resting T-lymphocytes.

Pharmacodynamics/Kinetics

Absorption: Oral:

Cyclosporine (non-modified): Erratic and incomplete; dependent on presence of food, bile acids, and GI motility; larger oral doses are needed in pediatrics due to shorter bowel length and limited intestinal absorption

Cyclosporine (modified): Erratic and incomplete; increased absorption, up to 30% when compared to cyclosporine (non-modified); less dependent on food, bile acids, or GI motility when compared to cyclosporine (non-modified)

Distribution: Widely in tissues and body fluids including the liver, pancreas, and lungs

V_{dss}: 4-6 L/kg in renal, liver, and marrow transplant recipients (slightly lower values in cardiac transplant patients; children <10 years have higher values)

Protein binding: 90% to 98% to lipoproteins

Metabolism: Extensively hepatic via CYP3A4; forms at least 25 metabolites; extensive first-pass effect following oral administration

Bioavailability: Oral:

Cyclosporine (non-modified): Dependent on patient population and transplant type (<10% in adult liver transplant patients and as high as 89% in renal transplant patients); bioavailability of Sandimmune® capsules and oral solution are equivalent; bioavailability of oral solution is ~30% of the I.V. solution

Children: 28% (range: 17% to 42%); gut dysfunction common in BMT patients and oral bioavailability is further reduced

Cyclosporine (modified): Bioavailability of Neoral® capsules and oral solution are equivalent:

Children: 43% (range: 30% to 68%)

Adults: 23% greater than with cyclosporine (non-modified) in renal transplant patients; 50% greater in liver transplant patients

Half-life elimination: Oral: May be prolonged in patients with hepatic impairment and shorter in pediatric patients due to the higher metabolism rate

Cyclosporine (non-modified): Biphasic: Alpha: 1.4 hours; Terminal: 19 hours (range: 10-27 hours)

Cyclosporine (modified): Biphasic: Terminal: 8.4 hours (range: 5-18 hours)

Time to peak, serum: Oral:

Cyclosporine (non-modified): 2-6 hours; some patients have a second peak at 5-6 hours

Cyclosporine (modified): Renal transplant: 1.5-2 hours

Excretion: Primarily feces; urine (6%, 0.1% as unchanged drug and metabolites)

Dosing

Adult Neoral®/Gengraf® and Sandimmune® are not bioequivalent and cannot be used interchangeably.

Newly-transplanted patients: Adjunct therapy with corticosteroids is recommended. Initial dose should be given 4-12 hours prior to transplant or may be given postoperatively; adjust initial dose to achieve desired plasma concentration.

Oral: Dose is dependent upon type of transplant and formulation:
Cyclosporine (modified):
Renal: 9 ± 3 mg/kg/day, divided twice daily
Liver: 8 ± 4 mg/kg/day, divided twice daily
Heart: 7 ± 3 mg/kg/day, divided twice daily
Cyclosporine (non-modified): Initial doses of 10-14 mg/kg/day have been used for renal transplants (the manufacturer's labeling includes dosing from initial clinical trials of 15 mg/kg/day [range: 14-18 mg/kg/day]; however, this higher dosing level is rarely used any longer). Continue initial dose daily for 1-2 weeks; taper by 5% per week to a maintenance dose of 5-10 mg/kg/day; some renal transplant patients may be dosed as low as 3 mg/kg/day
Note: When using the non-modified formulation, cyclosporine levels may increase in liver transplant patients when the T-tube is closed; dose may need decreased
I.V.: Cyclosporine (non-modified): Manufacturer's labeling: Initial dose: 5-6 mg/kg/day or one-third of the oral dose as a single dose, infused over 2-6 hours; use should be limited to patients unable to take capsules or oral solution; patients should be switched to an oral dosage form as soon as possible
Note: Many transplant centers administer cyclosporine as "divided dose" infusions (in 2-3 doses/day) or as a continuous (24-hour) infusion; dosages range from 3-7.5 mg/kg/day. Specific institutional protocols should be consulted.

Note: Conversion to cyclosporine (modified) from cyclosporine (non-modified): Start with daily dose previously used and adjust to obtain preconversion cyclosporine trough concentration. Plasma concentrations should be monitored every 4-7 days and dose adjusted as necessary, until desired trough level is obtained. When transferring patients with previously poor absorption of cyclosporine (non-modified), monitor trough levels at least twice weekly (especially if initial dose exceeds 10 mg/kg/day); high plasma levels are likely to occur.

Rheumatoid arthritis: Oral: Cyclosporine (modified): Initial dose: 2.5 mg/kg/day, divided twice daily; salicylates, NSAIDs, and oral glucocorticoids may be continued (refer to Drug Interactions); dose may be increased by 0.5-0.75 mg/kg/day if insufficient response is seen after 8 weeks of treatment; additional dosage increases may be made again at 12 weeks (maximum dose: 4 mg/kg/day). Discontinue if no benefit is seen by 16 weeks of therapy.
Note: Increase the frequency of blood pressure monitoring after each alteration in dosage of cyclosporine. Cyclosporine dosage should be decreased by 25% to 50% in patients with no history of hypertension who develop sustained hypertension during therapy and, if hypertension persists, treatment with cyclosporine should be discontinued.

Psoriasis: Oral: Cyclosporine (modified): Initial dose: 2.5 mg/kg/day, divided twice daily; dose may be increased by 0.5 mg/kg/day if insufficient response is seen after 4 weeks of treatment; additional dosage increases may be made every 2 weeks if needed (maximum dose: 4 mg/kg/day). Discontinue if no benefit is seen by 6 weeks of therapy. Once patients are adequately controlled, the dose should be decreased to the lowest effective dose. Doses <2.5 mg/kg/day may be effective. Treatment longer than 1 year is not recommended.
Note: Increase the frequency of blood pressure monitoring after each alteration in dosage of cyclosporine. Cyclosporine dosage should be

decreased by 25% to 50% in patients with no history of hypertension who develop sustained hypertension during therapy and, if hypertension persists, treatment with cyclosporine should be discontinued.

Focal segmental glomerulosclerosis (unlabeled use): Oral: Initial: 3.5-5 mg/kg/day divided every 12 hours (in combination with oral prednisone) (Braun, 2008; Cattran, 1999)

Lupus nephritis (unlabeled use): Oral: Initial: 4 mg/kg/day for 1 month (reduce dose if trough concentrations >200 ng/mL); reduce dose by 0.5 mg/kg every 2 weeks to a maintenance dose of 2.5-3 mg/kg/day (Moroni, 2006)

Severe ulcerative colitis (steroid-refractory) (unlabeled use):

I.V.: Cyclosporine (non-modified): 2-4 mg/kg/day, infused continuously over 24 hours. (Lichtiger, 1994; Van Assche, 2003). **Note:** Some studies suggest no therapeutic difference between low-dose (2 mg/kg) and high-dose (4 mg/kg) cyclosporine regimens (Van Assche, 2003).

Oral: Cyclosporine (modified): 2.3-3 mg/kg every 12 hours (De Saussure, 2005; Weber, 2006)

Note: Patients responsive to I.V. therapy should be switched to oral therapy when possible.

Geriatric Refer to adult dosing. **Sandimmune® and Neoral®/Gengraf® are not bioequivalent and cannot be used interchangeably.**

Pediatric Transplant: Refer to adult dosing. Children may require, and are able to tolerate, larger doses than adults.

Renal Impairment For severe psoriasis:

Serum creatinine levels ≥25% above pretreatment levels: Take another sample within 2 weeks; if the level remains ≥25% above pretreatment levels, decrease dosage of cyclosporine (modified) by 25% to 50%. If two dosage adjustments do not reverse the increase in serum creatinine levels, treatment should be discontinued.

Serum creatinine levels ≥50% above pretreatment levels: Decrease cyclosporine dosage by 25% to 50%. If two dosage adjustments do not reverse the increase in serum creatinine levels, treatment should be discontinued.

Hemodialysis: Supplemental dose is not necessary.

Peritoneal dialysis: Supplemental dose is not necessary.

Hepatic Impairment Dosage adjustment is probably necessary; monitor levels closely

Administration

Oral solution: Do not administer liquid from plastic or styrofoam cup. May dilute Neoral® oral solution with orange juice or apple juice. May dilute Sandimmune® oral solution with milk, chocolate milk, or orange juice. Avoid changing diluents frequently. Mix thoroughly and drink at once. Use syringe provided to measure dose. Mix in a glass container and rinse container with more diluent to ensure total dose is taken. Do not rinse syringe before or after use (may cause dose variation).

Combination therapy with renal transplantation:

Everolimus: Administer cyclosporine at the same time as everolimus

Sirolimus: Administer cyclosporine 4 hours prior to sirolimus

I.V.: The manufacturer recommends that following dilution, intravenous admixture be administered over 2-6 hours. However, many transplant centers administer as divided doses (2-3 doses/day) or as a 24-hour continuous infusion. Discard solution after 24 hours. Anaphylaxis has been reported with I.V. use; reserve for patients who cannot take oral form. Patients should be under continuous observation for at least the first 30 minutes of the infusion, and should be monitored frequently thereafter. Maintain patent airway; other supportive measures and agents for treating anaphylaxis should be present when I.V. drug is given. To minimize leaching of DEHP, non-PVC sets should be used for administration.

Monitoring Parameters Monitor blood pressure and serum creatinine after any cyclosporine dosage changes or addition, modification, or deletion of other medications. Monitor plasma concentrations periodically.

Transplant patients: Cyclosporine trough levels, serum electrolytes, renal function, hepatic function, blood pressure, lipid profile

Psoriasis therapy: Baseline blood pressure, serum creatinine (2 levels each), BUN, CBC, serum magnesium, potassium, uric acid, lipid profile. Biweekly monitoring of blood pressure, complete blood count, and levels of BUN, uric acid, potassium, lipids, and magnesium during the first 3 months of treatment for psoriasis. Monthly monitoring is recommended after this initial period. Also evaluate any atypical skin lesions prior to therapy. Increase the frequency of blood pressure monitoring after each alteration in dosage of cyclosporine. Cyclosporine dosage should be decreased by 25% to 50% in patients with no history of hypertension who develop sustained hypertension during therapy and, if hypertension persists, treatment with cyclosporine should be discontinued.

Rheumatoid arthritis: Baseline blood pressure, and serum creatinine (2 levels each); serum creatinine every 2 weeks for first 3 months, then monthly if patient is stable. Increase the frequency of blood pressure monitoring after each alteration in dosage of cyclosporine. Cyclosporine dosage should be decreased by 25% to 50% in patients with no history of hypertension who develop sustained hypertension during therapy and, if hypertension persists, treatment with cyclosporine should be discontinued.

Test Interactions Specific whole blood assay for cyclosporine may be falsely elevated if sample is drawn from the same central venous line through which dose was administered (even if flush has been administered and/or dose was given hours before); cyclosporine metabolites cross-react with radioimmunoassay and fluorescence polarization immunoassay

Dietary Considerations Administer this medication consistently with relation to time of day and meals. Avoid grapefruit juice with oral cyclosporine use.

Additional Information Cyclosporine (modified): Refers to the capsule dosage formulation of cyclosporine in an aqueous dispersion (previously referred to as "microemulsion"). Cyclosporine (modified) has increased bioavailability as compared to cyclosporine (non-modified) and cannot be used interchangeably without close monitoring.

Dosage Forms Excipient information presented when available (limited, particularly for generics); consult specific product labeling. [DSC] = Discontinued product

Capsule, oral [modified]:
  Gengraf®: 25 mg, 100 mg [contains ethanol 12.8%]
Capsule, oral [non-modified]: 25 mg [DSC], 100 mg
Capsule, softgel, oral [modified]: 25 mg, 50 mg, 100 mg
  Neoral®: 25 mg, 100 mg [contains corn oil, dehydrated ethanol 11.9%]
Capsule, softgel, oral [non-modified]:
  SandIMMUNE®: 25 mg, 100 mg [contains corn oil, dehydrated ethanol 12.7%]
Injection, solution [non-modified]: 50 mg/mL (5 mL)

SandIMMUNE®: 50 mg/mL (5 mL) [contains ethanol 32.9%, polyoxyethylated castor oil]

Solution, oral [modified]: 100 mg/mL (50 mL)

Gengraf®: 100 mg/mL (50 mL) [contains propylene glycol]

Neoral®: 100 mg/mL (50 mL) [contains corn oil, dehydrated ethanol 11.9%, propylene glycol]

Solution, oral [non-modified]:

SandIMMUNE®: 100 mg/mL (50 mL) [contains ethanol 12.5%]

References

Benfield MR, Tejani A, Harmon WE, et al, "A Randomized Multicenter Trial of OKT3 mAbs Induction Compared With Intravenous Cyclosporine in Pediatric Renal Transplantation," *Pediatr Transplant*, 2005, 9(3):282-92.

Braun N, Schmutzler F, Lange C, et al, "Immunosuppressive Treatment for Focal Segmental Glomerulosclerosis in Adults," *Cochrane Database Syst Rev*, 2008, (3):CD003233.

Caforio AL, Gambino A, Tona F, "Sulfinpyrazone Reduces Cyclosporine Levels: A New Drug Interaction in Heart Transplant Recipients," *J Heart Lung Transplant*, 2000, 19(12):1205-8.

Cattran DC, Appel GB, Hebert LA, et al, "A Randomized Trial of Cyclosporine in Patients With Steroid-Resistant Focal Segmental Glomerulosclerosis. North America Nephrotic Syndrome Study Group," *Kidney Int*, 1999, 56(6):2220-6.

De Saussure P, Soravia C, Morel P, et al, "Low-Dose Oral Microemulsion Ciclosporin for Severe, Refractory Ulcerative Colitis," *Aliment Pharmacol Ther*, 2005, 22(3):203-08.

Lichtenstein GR, Abreu MT, Cohen R, et al, "American Gastroenterological Association Institute Technical Review on Corticosteroids, Immunomodulators, and Infliximab in Inflammatory Bowel Disease," *Gastroenterology*, 2006, 30(3):940-87.

Lichtiger S, Present DH, Kornbluth A, et al, "Cyclosporine in Severe Ulcerative Colitis Refractory to Steroid Therapy, *N Engl J Med*, 1994, 330(26):1841-5.

Memon M, de Magalhace-Silverman M, Bloom EJ, et al, "Reversible Cyclosporine-Induced Cortical Blindness in Allogeneic Bone Marrow Transplant Recipients," *Bone Marrow Transplant*, 1995, 15 (2):283-6.

Moroni G, Doria A, Mosca M, et al, "A Randomized Pilot Trial Comparing Cyclosporine and Azathioprine for Maintenance Therapy in Diffuse Lupus Nephritis Over Four Years," *Clin J Am Soc Nephrol*, 2006, 1(5):925-32.

Ratanatharathorn V, Nash RA, Przepiorka D, et al, "Phase III Study Comparing Methotrexate and Tacrolimus (Prograf, FK506) With Methotrexate and Cyclosporine for Graft-Versus-Host Disease Prophylaxis After HLA-Identical Sibling Bone Marrow Transplantation," *Blood*, 1998, 92 (7):2303-14.

Tugwell P, Pincus T, Yocum D, et al, "Combination Therapy With Cyclosporine and Methotrexate in Severe Rheumatoid Arthritis," *N Engl J Med*, 1995, 333(3):137-41.

Van Assche G, D'Haens G, Noman M, et al, "Randomized, Double-Blind Comparison of 4 mg/kg Versus 2 mg/kg Intravenous Cyclosporine in Severe Ulcerative Colitis," *Gastroenterology*, 2003, 125(4):1025-31.

Weber A, Fein F, Koch S, et al, "Treatment of Ulcerative Colitis Refractory to Steroid Therapy by Oral Microemulsion Cyclosporin (Neoral)," *Inflamm Bowel Dis*, 2006, 12(12):1131-35.

◆ **Cyklokapron®** *see* Tranexamic Acid *on page 1392*

Cyproheptadine (si proe HEP ta deen)

Brand Names: Canada Euro-Cyproheptadine; PMS-Cyproheptadine

Index Terms Cyproheptadine Hydrochloride; Periactin

Generic Availability (U.S.) Yes

Pharmacologic Category Histamine H_1 Antagonist; Histamine H_1 Antagonist, First Generation; Piperidine Derivative

Use Perennial and seasonal allergic rhinitis and other allergic symptoms including urticaria

Unlabeled Use Migraine headache prophylaxis, pruritus, spasticity associated with spinal cord damage

Labeled Contraindications Hypersensitivity to cyproheptadine or any component of the formulation; narrow-angle glaucoma; bladder neck obstruction; pyloroduodenal obstruction; symptomatic prostatic hyperplasia; stenosing peptic ulcer; concurrent use of MAO inhibitors; use in debilitated elderly patients; use in premature and term newborns due to potential association with SIDS; breast-feeding

Pregnancy Risk Factor B

Lactation Excretion in breast milk unknown/contraindicated

Warnings/Precautions May cause CNS depression, which may impair physical or mental abilities; patients must be cautioned about performing tasks which require mental alertness (eg, operating machinery or driving). Effects may be potentiated when used with other sedative drugs or ethanol. Use with caution in patients with cardiovascular disease; increased intraocular pressure; respiratory disease; or thyroid dysfunction. In the elderly, avoid use of this potent anticholinergic agent due to increased risk of confusion, dry mouth, constipation, and other anticholinergic effects; clearance decreases in patients of advanced age (Beers Criteria). Antihistamines may cause excitation in young children.

Adverse Reactions Frequency not defined.

Cardiovascular: Extrasystoles, hypotension, palpitation, tachycardia

Central nervous system: Confusion, coordination disturbed, dizziness, excitation, euphoria, faintness, hallucinations, headache, hysteria, insomnia, irritability, nervousness, neuritis, restlessness, sedation, seizure, sleepiness, tremor, vertigo

Dermatologic: Angioedema, photosensitivity, rash, urticaria

Gastrointestinal: Abdominal pain, anorexia, appetite increased, constipation, diarrhea, nausea, vomiting, xerostomia

Genitourinary: Difficult urination, urinary frequency, urinary retention

Hematologic: Agranulocytosis, hemolytic anemia, leukopenia, thrombocytopenia

Hepatic: Cholestasis, hepatic failure, hepatitis, jaundice

Neuromuscular & skeletal: Paresthesia

Ocular: Blurred vision, diplopia

Otic: Labyrinthitis (acute), tinnitus

Respiratory: Bronchial secretions (thickening), nasal congestion, pharyngitis

Miscellaneous: Allergic reactions, anaphylactic shock, chills, diaphoresis, fatigue

Drug Interactions

Metabolism/Transport Effects None known.

Avoid Concomitant Use

Avoid concomitant use of Cyproheptadine with any of the following: Aclidinium; Azelastine (Nasal); Ipratropium (Oral Inhalation); Methadone; Mirtazapine; Paraldehyde; Tiotropium

Increased Effect/Toxicity

Cyproheptadine may increase the levels/effects of: Alcohol (Ethyl); Anticholinergics; Azelastine (Nasal); Buprenorphine; CNS Depressants; Methadone; Methotrimeprazine; Metyrosine; Mirtazapine; Paraldehyde; Pramipexole; ROPINIRole; Rotigotine; Tiotropium; Zolpidem

The levels/effects of Cyproheptadine may be increased by: Aclidinium; Droperidol; HydrOXYzine; Ipratropium (Oral Inhalation); Methotrimeprazine; Perampanel; Pramlintide

Decreased Effect

Cyproheptadine may decrease the levels/effects of: Acetylcholinesterase Inhibitors (Central); Benzylpenicilloyl Polylysine; Betahistine; Hyaluronidase; Selective Serotonin Reuptake Inhibitors

The levels/effects of Cyproheptadine may be decreased by: Acetylcholinesterase Inhibitors (Central); Amphetamines

Ethanol/Nutrition/Herb Interactions Ethanol: May increase CNS depression; monitor for increased effects with coadministration. Caution patients about effects.

Mechanism of Action A potent antihistamine and serotonin antagonist, competes with histamine for H_1-receptor sites on effector cells in the gastrointestinal tract, blood vessels, and respiratory tract

Pharmacodynamics/Kinetics

Metabolism: Primarily by hepatic glucuronidation via UGT1A (Walker, 1996)

Half-life elimination: Metabolites: ~16 hours (Paton, 1985)

Time to peak, plasma: 6-9 hours (Paton, 1985)

Excretion: Urine (~40% primarily as metabolites); feces (2% to 20%)

Dosing

Adult

Allergic conditions: Oral: 4-20 mg/day divided every 8 hours (not to exceed 0.5 mg/kg/day); some patients may require up to 32 mg/day for adequate control of symptoms

Spasticity associated with spinal cord damage (unlabeled use): Oral: Initial: 2-4 mg every 8 hours; maximum: 8 mg every 8 hours (Barbeau, 1982; Wainberg, 1990)

Geriatric Initiate therapy at the lower end of the dosage range.

Pediatric

Allergic conditions: Oral: Children: 0.25 mg/kg/day or 8 mg/m^2/day in 2-3 divided doses **or**

2-6 years: 2 mg every 8-12 hours (not to exceed 12 mg/day)

7-14 years: 4 mg every 8-12 hours (not to exceed 16 mg/day)

Migraine headache prophylaxis (unlabeled use): Oral: 4 mg every 8-12 hours

Test Interactions Diagnostic antigen skin test results may be suppressed; false positive serum TCA screen

Dosage Forms Excipient information presented when available (limited, particularly for generics); consult specific product labeling.

Syrup, oral, as hydrochloride: 2 mg/5 mL (473 mL, 480 mL)

Tablet, oral, as hydrochloride: 4 mg

References

Barbeau H, Richards CL, and Bedard PJ, "Action of Cyproheptadine in Spastic Paraparetic Patients," *J Neurol Neurosurg Psychiatry*, 1982, 45(10):926-6.

Paton DM and Webster DR, "Clinical Pharmacokinetics of H1-Receptor Antagonists (The Antihistamines)," *Clin Pharmacokinet*, 1985, 10(6):477-97.

Wainberg M, Barbeau H, and Gauthier S, "The Effects of Cyproheptadine on Locomotion and on Spasticity in Patients With Spinal Cord Injuries," *J Neurol Neurosurg Psychiatry*, 1990, 53 (9):754-63.

Walker RB and Kanfer I, "Pharmacokinetics of Cyclizine Following Intravenous Administration to Human Volunteers," *Eur J Pharm Sci*, 1996, 4(5):301-6.

◆ **Cyproheptadine Hydrochloride** *see* Cyproheptadine *on page* 342

Cyproterone (sye PROE ter one)

Brand Names: Canada Androcur®; Androcur® Depot; Novo-Cyproterone

Index Terms Cyproterone Acetate; SH 714

Pharmacologic Category Antiandrogen

Use Palliative treatment of advanced prostate cancer

Unlabeled Use Treatment of paraphilia/hypersexuality

Labeled Contraindications Hypersensitivity to cyproterone or any component of the formulation; liver disease or hepatic dysfunction; Dubin-Johnson syndrome; Rotor syndrome; previous or existing liver tumors (if not due to metastases from prostate cancer); presence or history of meningioma; wasting diseases (except inoperable prostate cancer); severe chronic depression; existing thromboembolic processes

Warnings/Precautions [Canadian Boxed Warning]: Use is associated with dose-dependent hepatotoxicity (jaundice, hepatitis, acute hepatic failure) including fatal case reports with doses ≥100 mg/day. Hepatotoxicity typically develops after a few weeks to several months of treatment initiation. Use in patients with prior or existing hepatic disease is contraindicated. Use caution with concurrent use of other hepatotoxic drugs. Monitor hepatic function and discontinue in patients with evidence of hepatic injury.

Use caution in patients with a history of depression (contraindicated in severe chronic depression). Cyproterone has been associated with an increased incidence of depression, particularly early in the course of therapy (initial 6-8 weeks). Use with caution in patients with diabetes or impaired glucose tolerance, may cause alterations in glucose metabolism and require dosage adjustments in diabetes medications. Use with caution in conditions that may be aggravated by fluid retention, or cardiovascular disease. May increase the risk of thromboembolism (particularly when used in combination with ethinyl estradiol) and/or alter lipid profiles.

Benign and malignant hepatic tumors have been observed (rarely) after use; rule out the presence of tumor in patients presenting with severe upper abdominal discomfort, hepatic enlargement or signs of intra-abdominal hemorrhage. Meningioma formation has been reported with chronic therapy (years) at doses ≥25 mg/day. Avoid initiation of therapy in patients with a history or presence of meningioma; discontinue treatment in patients diagnosed with meningioma. Hyperplasia of the breast has been reported; subsides usually within 1-3 months after therapy discontinuation and/or dose reduction. Risk of treatment failure should be considered prior to discontinuation or dose reduction.

Shortness of breath commonly observed in patients receiving doses of 300 mg/day; use caution in patients with existing pulmonary dysfunction. Adrenalcortical function suppression has been reported with use; monitor adrenal function periodically. Hypochromic anemia has been observed (rarely); monitor CBC regularly. May promote prostate cancer growth in some patients with metastatic prostate cancer; discontinue therapy immediately with increasing prostate specific antigen (PSA) levels and monitor 6-8 weeks for withdrawal response prior to initiating alternative treatment. Decreased PSA levels and/or clinical improvement have been reported following therapy discontinuation.

Lassitude, weakness, and fatigue are common during first few weeks of treatment; symptoms usually lessen ~3 months after therapy initiation. Patients must be cautioned about performing tasks which require mental alertness (eg, operating machinery or driving). Five-year survival rates may be lower when used concomitantly with a GnRH agonist or orchiectomy versus patients treated with castration alone. Antiandrogen effects in hypersexuality may be reduced with ethanol. Ethanol should be avoided during treatment.

[Canadian Boxed Warning]: Should be prescribed and managed by a clinician experienced with hormonal therapy in prostate cancer.

Adverse Reactions Frequency not defined.

Cardiovascular: Edema, heart failure, hypotension, MI, phlebitis, shock, stroke, syncope, tachycardia, thrombosis (DVT, embolus, superficial venous thrombosis)

Central nervous system: Aphasia, chills, coma, depression, dizziness, encephalopathy, fatigue, headache, hemiplegia, lassitude, malaise, meningioma (with chronic therapy), personality disorder, psychotic depression, pyrexia, restlessness, vascular headache, vasovagal reactions

Dermatologic: Dry skin (sebum reduction), eczema, erythema nodosum, exfoliative dermatitis, hirsutism, maculopapular rash, patchy loss of body hair, photosensitivity, pruritus, rash, scleroderma, skin discoloration, urticaria

Endocrine & metabolic: Adrenal suppression (dose related), benign nodular breast hyperplasia, diabetes mellitus, galactorrhea, gynecomastia, hot flashes, hypercalcemia, hyperglycemia, hypernatremia, impotence, inhibition of spermatogenesis, libido decreased, negative nitrogen balance

Gastrointestinal: Anorexia, constipation, diarrhea, dyspepsia, glossitis, nausea, pancreatitis, vomiting, weight gain/loss

Genitourinary: Bladder carcinoma, crystalluria, urinary frequency, uterine fibroids enlarged, uterine hemorrhage

Hematologic: Anemia, fibrinogen increased, hemolytic anemia, hemorrhage, hypochromic anemia, leukopenia, leukocytosis, normocytic anemia, PT decreased, thrombocytopenia

Hepatic: Ascites, cholestatic jaundice, cirrhosis, hepatic carcinoma, hepatic coma, hepatic dysfunction (dose related), hepatic failure, hepatic necrosis, hepatitis, hepatoma, hepatomegaly, transaminases increased

Local: Injection site reaction

Neuromuscular and skeletal: Gait abnormal, myasthenia, osteoporosis, weakness

Ocular: Abnormal accommodation, abnormal vision, blindness, optic neuritis, optic atrophy, retinal vascular disorder, retinal vein thrombosis

Renal: Hematuria, renal failure, serum creatinine increased

Respiratory: Asthma, cough, dyspnea, hyperventilation, pulmonary embolism, pulmonary fibrosis, pulmonary oil microembolism

Miscellaneous: Allergic reaction, diaphoresis

Drug Interactions

Metabolism/Transport Effects Substrate of CYP3A4 (major); **Note:** Assignment of Major/Minor substrate status based on clinically relevant drug interaction potential; **Inhibits** CYP2C19 (weak), CYP2C8 (weak), CYP2C9 (weak), CYP2D6 (weak), CYP3A4 (weak); **Induces** CYP1A2 (weak/moderate), CYP2E1 (weak/moderate)

Avoid Concomitant Use

Avoid concomitant use of Cyproterone with any of the following: Conivaptan; Pimozide

Increased Effect/Toxicity

Cyproterone may increase the levels/effects of: ARIPiprazole; HMG-CoA Reductase Inhibitors; Pimozide

The levels/effects of Cyproterone may be increased by: Conivaptan; CYP3A4 Inhibitors (Moderate); CYP3A4 Inhibitors (Strong); Dasatinib; Herbs (Progestogenic Properties); Ivacaftor; Mifepristone

Decreased Effect

Cyproterone may decrease the levels/effects of: CYP1A2 Substrates; CYP2E1 Substrates

The levels/effects of Cyproterone may be decreased by: Aminoglutethimide; CYP3A4 Inducers (Strong); Deferasirox; Herbs (CYP3A4 Inducers); Tocilizumab

Ethanol/Nutrition/Herb Interactions

Ethanol: May reduce the effect of cyproterone (not established in the treatment of prostatic carcinoma); avoid concurrent use.

Herb/Nutraceutical: St John's wort may decrease cyproterone levels.

Storage/Stability

Injection: Store at 15°C to 30°C (59°F to 86°F).

Tablet: Store at 15°C to 30°C (59°F to 86°F). Protect from light.

Mechanism of Action Cyproterone is a steroid with antiandrogenic, antigonadotropic, and progestin-like activity. Blocks binding of dihydrotestosterone (DHT) to prostatic cancer cells and exerts negative feedback on hypothalamic-pituitary axis by inhibiting luteinizing hormone (LH) secretion leading to decreased testosterone production.

Pharmacodynamics/Kinetics

Absorption: Oral: Complete

Metabolism: Hepatic, some metabolites have activity

Half-life elimination: Oral: 38 hours (range: 33-43 hours); Depot injection: 4 days

Time to peak, plasma: Oral: 3-4 hours; Depot injection: 3 days

Excretion: Feces (60%); urine (33%)

Dosing

Adult & Geriatric

Prostate cancer, advanced (palliative treatment): Males:

Oral: 200-300 mg daily in 2-3 divided doses (maximum: 300 mg daily); following orchiectomy, reduce dose to 100-200 mg daily

I.M.: 300 mg (3 mL) once weekly; reduce dose in orchiectomized patients to 300 mg every 2 weeks

Note: May interchange between oral and I.M. administration during chronic therapy; dosages should remain within usual ranges (oral: 100-300 mg daily; I.M.: 300 mg weekly or every 2 weeks).

Treatment of paraphilia/hypersexuality (unlabeled use; Guay, 2009; Reilly, 2000): Males (**Note:** Avoid use if active pituitary pathology, hepatic failure, or thromboembolic disease):

Oral: 50-600 mg daily

I.M.: 300-600 mg weekly or every other week

Renal Impairment Has not been studied in patients with renal impairment. Use with caution; 33% of cyproterone is excreted renally.

Hepatic Impairment Use is contraindicated with hepatic impairment or liver disease.

Administration

I.M.: Administer I.M. injections slowly and avoid intravascular injection which can lead to pulmonary microembolism.

Oral: Administer tablets at the same time each day, after meals and with liquids. Tablets may be divided into equal halves.

Monitoring Parameters Liver function tests should be performed at baseline and periodically thereafter, or with signs or symptoms suggestive of hepatotoxicity. CBC, adrenal function, electrolytes, fasting blood glucose and glucose tolerance (diabetic patients) should be monitored periodically. In patients with PSA progression, monitor for withdrawal response syndrome (eg, decrease in PSA levels) for 6-8 weeks following therapy discontinuation.

Treatment of paraphilia/hypersexuality (Guay 2009; Reilly, 2000): ECG; hepatic function test (baseline and during treatment if suspected hepatotoxicity); CBC (baseline); serum testosterone (baseline then monthly for 4 months then every 6 months); serum luteinizing hormone and prolactin (baseline and every 6 months); follicle-stimulating hormone (baseline); glucose; bone scan (baseline then annually) if serum testosterone significantly suppressed; blood pressure; weight gain

Dietary Considerations Tablets should be taken after meals.

Product Availability Not available in U.S.

Dosage Forms: Canada Excipient information presented when available (limited, particularly for generics); consult specific product labeling.

Injection, solution, as acetate: 100 mg/mL (3 mL)

Androcur® Depot: 100 mg/mL (3 mL) [contains benzyl benzoate and castor oil]

Tablet, as acetate: 50 mg

Androcur®: 50 mg

References

Guay DR, "Drug Treatment of Paraphilic and Nonparaphilic Sexual Disorders," *Clin Ther*, 2009, 31 (1):1-31.

Lukka H, Waldron T, Klotz L, et al, "Maximal Androgen Blockade for the Treatment of Metastatic Prostate Cancer– A Systematic Review," *Curr Oncol*, 2006, 13(3):81-93.

Reilly DR, Delva NJ, and Hudson RW, "Protocols for the Use of Cyproterone, Medroxyprogesterone, and Leuprolide in the Treatment of Paraphilia," *Can J Psychiatry*, 2000, 45(6):559-63.

Thibaut F, De La Barra F, Gordon H, et al, "The World Federation of Societies of Biological Psychiatry (WFSBP) Guidelines for the Biological Treatment of Paraphilias," *World J Biol Psychiatry*, 2010, 11(4):604-55.

◆ **Cyproterone Acetate** *see* Cyproterone *on page 344*

◆ **Cysview™** *see* Hexaminolevulinate *on page 705*

◆ **CYT** *see* Cyclophosphamide *on page 321*

◆ **Cytarabine** *see* Cytarabine (Conventional) *on page 348*

Cytarabine (Conventional) (sye TARE a been con VEN sha nal)

Related Information

Chemotherapy and Cancer Treatment During Pregnancy *on page 1829*

Hematopoietic Stem Cell Transplantation *on page 1887*

Management of Chemotherapy-Induced Nausea and Vomiting *on page 1786*

Safe Handling of Hazardous Drugs *on page 1904*

Brand Names: Canada Cytosar®

Index Terms Ara-C; Arabinosylcytosine; Conventional Cytarabine; Cytarabine; Cytarabine Hydrochloride; Cytosar-U; Cytosine Arabinosine Hydrochloride

Generic Availability (U.S.) Yes

Pharmacologic Category Antineoplastic Agent, Antimetabolite; Antineoplastic Agent, Antimetabolite (Pyrimidine Analog)

Use Remission induction in acute myeloid leukemia (AML), treatment of acute lymphocytic leukemia (ALL) and chronic myelocytic leukemia (CML; blast phase); prophylaxis and treatment of meningeal leukemia

Unlabeled Use AML consolidation treatment, AML salvage treatment; acute promyelocytic leukemia (APL) consolidation treatment; treatment of primary central nervous system (CNS) lymphoma; treatment of chronic lymphocytic leukemia (CLL); treatment of relapsed or refractory Hodgkin lymphoma; treatment of non-Hodgkin's lymphomas (NHL)

Labeled Contraindications Hypersensitivity to cytarabine or any component of the formulation

Pregnancy Risk Factor D

Lactation Excretion in breast milk unknown/not recommended

Warnings/Precautions Hazardous agent - use appropriate precautions for handling and disposal. **[U.S. Boxed Warning]: Myelosuppression (leukopenia, thrombocytopenia and anemia) is the major toxicity of cytarabine.** Use with caution in patients with prior drug induced bone marrow suppression. Monitor blood counts frequently; once blasts are no longer apparent in the peripheral blood, bone marrow should be monitored frequently. Monitor for signs of infection or neutropenic fever due to neutropenia or bleeding due to thrombocytopenia.

High-dose regimens are associated with CNS, gastrointestinal, ocular (reversible corneal toxicity and hemorrhagic conjunctivitis; prophylaxis with ophthalmic corticosteroid drops is recommended), pulmonary toxicities and cardiomyopathy. Neurotoxicity associated with high-dose treatment may present as acute cerebellar toxicity (with or without cerebral impairment), personality changes, or may be severe with seizure and/or coma; may be delayed, occurring up to 3-8 days after treatment has begun. Risk factors for neurotoxicity include cumulative cytarabine dose, prior CNS disease and renal impairment; high-dose therapy (>18 g/m^2 per cycle) and age >50 years also increase the risk for cerebellar toxicity (Herzig, 1987). Tumor lysis syndrome and subsequent hyperuricemia may occur with high dose cytarabine; monitor, consider allopurinol and hydrate accordingly. There have been case reports of fatal cardiomyopathy when high dose cytarabine was used in combination with cyclophosphamide as a preparation regimen for transplantation.

Use with caution in patients with impaired renal and hepatic function; may be at higher risk for CNS toxicities; dosage adjustments may be necessary. A sudden respiratory arrest syndrome is characterized by fever, myalgia, bone pain, chest pain, maculopapular rash, conjunctivitis, and malaise, and may occur 6-12 hours following administration; may be managed with corticosteroids. Anaphylaxis resulting in acute cardiopulmonary arrest has been reported (rare). There have been reports of acute pancreatitis in patients receiving continuous infusion and in patients previously treated with L-asparaginase. **[U.S. Boxed Warning]: Should be administered under the supervision of an experienced cancer chemotherapy physician. Due to the potential toxicities, induction treatment with cytarabine should be in a facility with sufficient laboratory and supportive resources.** Some products may contain benzyl alcohol; do not use products containing benzyl alcohol or products reconstituted with bacteriostatic diluent intrathecally or for high-dose cytarabine regimens. When used for intrathecal administration, should not be prepared during the preparation of any other agents; after preparation, store intrathecal medications in an isolated location or container clearly marked with a label identifying as "intrathecal" use only; delivery of intrathecal medications to the patient should only be with other medications also intended for administration into the central nervous system (Jacobson, 2009).

Adverse Reactions

Frequent:

Central nervous system: Fever

Dermatologic: Rash

Gastrointestinal: Anal inflammation, anal ulceration, anorexia, diarrhea, mucositis, nausea, vomiting

Hematologic: Myelosuppression, neutropenia (onset: 1-7 days; nadir [biphasic]: 7-9 days and at 15-24 days; recovery [biphasic]: 9-12 days and at

24-34 days), thrombocytopenia (onset: 5 days; nadir: 12-15 days; recovery 15-25 days), anemia, bleeding, leukopenia, megaloblastosis, reticulocytes decreased

Hepatic: Hepatic dysfunction, transaminases increased (acute)

Local: Thrombophlebitis

Less frequent:

Cardiovascular: Chest pain, pericarditis

Central nervous system: Dizziness, headache, neural toxicity, neuritis

Dermatologic: Alopecia, pruritus, skin freckling, skin ulceration, urticaria

Gastrointestinal: Abdominal pain, bowel necrosis, esophageal ulceration, esophagitis, pancreatitis, sore throat

Genitourinary: Urinary retention

Hepatic: Jaundice

Local: Injection site cellulitis

Ocular: Conjunctivitis

Renal: Renal dysfunction

Respiratory: Dyspnea

Miscellaneous: Allergic edema, anaphylaxis, sepsis

Infrequent and/or case reports: Acute respiratory distress syndrome, amylase increased, angina, aseptic meningitis, cardiopulmonary arrest (acute), cerebral dysfunction, cytarabine syndrome (bone pain, chest pain, conjunctivitis, fever, maculopapular rash, malaise, myalgia); exanthematous pustulosis, hepatic sinusoidal obstruction syndrome (SOS; veno-occlussive disease), hyperuricemia, injection site inflammation (SubQ injection), injection site pain (SubQ injection), interstitial pneumonitis, lipase increased, paralysis (intrathecal and I.V. combination therapy), reversible posterior leukoencephalopathy syndrome (RPLS), rhabdomyolysis, toxic megacolon

Adverse events associated with high-dose cytarabine (CNS, gastrointestinal, ocular, and pulmonary toxicities are more common with high-dose regimens):

Cardiovascular: Cardiomegaly, cardiomyopathy (in combination with cyclophosphamide)

Central nervous system: Cerebellar toxicity, coma, neurotoxicity (up to 55% in patients with renal impairment), personality change, somnolence

Dermatologic: Alopecia (complete), desquamation, rash (severe)

Gastrointestinal: Gastrointestinal ulcer, pancreatitis, peritonitis, pneumatosis cystoides intestinalis

Hepatic: Hyperbilirubinemia, liver abscess, liver damage, necrotizing colitis

Neuromuscular & skeletal: Peripheral neuropathy (motor and sensory)

Ocular: Corneal toxicity, hemorrhagic conjunctivitis

Respiratory: Pulmonary edema, syndrome of sudden respiratory distress

Miscellaneous: Sepsis

Adverse events associated with intrathecal cytarabine administration:

Central nervous system: Accessory nerve paralysis, fever, necrotizing leukoencephalopathy (with concurrent cranial irradiation, I.T. methotrexate, and I.T. hydrocortisone), neurotoxicity, paraplegia

Gastrointestinal: Dysphagia, nausea, vomiting

Ocular: Blindness (with concurrent systemic chemotherapy and cranial irradiation), diplopia

Respiratory: Cough, hoarseness

Miscellaneous: Aphonia

Drug Interactions

Metabolism/Transport Effects None known.

Avoid Concomitant Use

Avoid concomitant use of Cytarabine (Conventional) with any of the following: BCG; CloZAPine; Natalizumab; Pimecrolimus; Tacrolimus (Topical); Vaccines (Live)

Increased Effect/Toxicity

Cytarabine (Conventional) may increase the levels/effects of: CloZAPine; Leflunomide; Natalizumab; Vaccines (Live)

The levels/effects of Cytarabine (Conventional) may be increased by: Denosumab; Pimecrolimus; Roflumilast; Tacrolimus (Topical); Trastuzumab

Decreased Effect

Cytarabine (Conventional) may decrease the levels/effects of: BCG; Cardiac Glycosides; Coccidioidin Skin Test; Flucytosine; Sipuleucel-T; Vaccines (Inactivated); Vaccines (Live)

The levels/effects of Cytarabine (Conventional) may be decreased by: Echinacea

Storage/Stability Store intact vials of powder for injection at room temperature of 20°C to 25°C (68°F to 77°F); store intact vials of solution at room temperature of 15°C to 30°C (59°F to 86°F).

I.V.:

Powder for reconstitution: Reconstituted solutions should be stored at room temperature and used within 48 hours.

For I.V. infusion: Solutions for I.V. infusion diluted in D_5W or NS are stable for 7 days at room temperature, although the manufacturer recommends administration as soon as possible after preparation.

Intrathecal: Administer as soon as possible after preparation. After preparation, store intrathecal medications in an isolated location or container clearly marked with a label identifying as "intrathecal" use only.

Reconstitution Use appropriate precautions for handling and disposal. **Note:** Solutions containing bacteriostatic agents may be used for SubQ and standard-dose (100-200 mg/m^2) I.V. cytarabine preparations, but should not be used for the preparation of either intrathecal doses or high-dose I.V. therapies.

I.V.:

Powder for reconstitution: Reconstitute with bacteriostatic water for injection (for standard-dose).

For I.V. infusion: Further dilute in 250-1000 mL 0.9% NaCl or D_5W.

Intrathecal: Powder for reconstitution: Reconstitute with preservative free sodium chloride 0.9%; may further dilute to preferred final volume (volume generally based on institution or practitioner preference; may be up to 12 mL) with Elliott's B solution, sodium chloride 0.9% or lactated Ringer's. Intrathecal medications should not be prepared during the preparation of any other agents.

Triple intrathecal therapy (TIT): Cytarabine 30-50 mg with hydrocortisone sodium succinate 15-25 mg and methotrexate 12 mg; compatible together for up to 24 hours in a syringe; however, should be administered administer as soon as possible after preparation because intrathecal preparations are preservative free

Mechanism of Action Inhibits DNA synthesis. Cytosine gains entry into cells by a carrier process, and then must be converted to its active compound, aracytidine triphosphate. Cytosine is a pyrimidine analog and is incorporated into DNA; however, the primary action is inhibition of DNA polymerase resulting in decreased DNA synthesis and repair. The degree of cytotoxicity correlates linearly with incorporation into DNA; therefore, incorporation into the DNA is responsible for drug activity and toxicity. Cytarabine is specific for the S phase of the cell cycle (blocks progression from the G_1 to the S phase).

Pharmacodynamics/Kinetics

Distribution: V_d: Total body water; widely and rapidly since it enters the cells readily; crosses blood-brain barrier with CSF levels of 40% to 50% of plasma level

Metabolism: Primarily hepatic; metabolized by deoxycytidine kinase and other nucleotide kinases to aracytidine triphosphate (active); about 86% to 96% of dose is metabolized to inactive uracil arabinoside (ARA-U); intrathecal administration results in little conversion to ARA-U due to the low levels of deaminase in the cerebral spinal fluid

Half-life elimination: I.V.: Initial: 7-20 minutes; Terminal: 1-3 hours; I.T.: 2-6 hours

Time to peak, plasma: SubQ: 20-60 minutes

Excretion: Urine (~80%; 90% as metabolite ARA-U) within 24 hours

Dosing

Adult & Geriatric Details concerning dosing in combination regimens should also be consulted.

Acute myeloid leukemia (AML) remission induction: I.V.: Standard-dose (provided in the FDA-approved labeling): 100 mg/m²/day continuous infusion for 7 days **or** 200 mg/m²/day continuous infusion (as 100 mg/m² over 12 hours every 12 hours) for 7 days

Indication-specific dosing:

AML induction: I.V.:

7 + 3 regimens (a second induction course may be administered if needed; refer to specific references): 100 mg/m²/day continuous infusion for 7 days (in combination with daunorubicin **or** idarubicin **or** mitoxantrone) (Arlin, 1990; Dillman, 1991; Fernandez, 2009; Wiernick, 1992) **or** (Adults <60 years) 200 mg/m²/day continuous infusion for 7 days (in combination with daunorubicin) (Dillman, 1991)

Low intensity therapy (unlabeled dosing): Adults ≥65 years: SubQ: 20 mg/m²/day for 14 days out of every 28-day cycle for at least 4 cycles (Fenaux, 2010) **or** 10 mg/m² every 12 hours for 21 days; if complete response not achieved, may repeat a second course after 15 days (Tilly, 1990)

AML consolidation (unlabeled use): I.V.:

5 + 2 regimens: 100 mg/m²/day continuous infusion for 5 days (in combination with daunorubicin **or** idarubicin **or** mitoxantrone) (Arlin, 1990; Wiernick, 1992)

5 + 2 + 5 regimen: 100 mg/m²/day continuous infusion for 5 days (in combination with daunorubicin **and** etoposide) (Bishop, 1996)

Single-agent: Adults ≤60 years: 3000 mg/m² over 3 hours every 12 hours on days 1, 3, and 5 (total of 6 doses); repeat every 28-35 days for 4 courses (Mayer, 1994)

AML salvage treatment (unlabeled use): I.V.:

ADE regimen: Course 1: 100 mg/m² I.V push every 12 hours for 10 days (in combination with daunorubicin and etoposide) followed by Course 2: 100 mg/m² I.V push every 12 hours for 8 days (Milligan, 2006)

CLAG regimen: 2000 mg/m²/day over 4 hours for 5 days (in combination with cladribine and G-CSF); may repeat once if needed (Wrzesień-Kuś, 2003)

CLAG-M regimen: 2000 mg/m^2/day over 4 hours for 5 days (in combination with cladribine, G-CSF, and mitoxantrone); may repeat once if needed (Wierzbowska, 2008)

FLAG regimen: 2000 mg/m^2/day over 4 hours for 5 days (in combination with fludarabine and G-CSF); may repeat once if needed (Montillo, 1998)

HiDAC (high-dose cytarabine) ± an anthracycline: 3000 mg/m^2 over 1 hour every 12 hours for 12 doses (Herzig, 1985)

MEC regimen: 1000 mg/m^2/day over 6 hours for 6 days (in combination with mitoxantrone and etoposide) (Amadori, 1991) **or**

Adults <60 years: 500 mg/m^2/day continuous infusion days 1, 2, and 3 and days 8, 9, and 10 (in combination with mitoxantrone and etoposide); may administer a second course if needed (Archimbaud, 1991; Archimbaud, 1995)

Acute promyelocytic leukemia (APL) induction (unlabeled dosing): I.V.: 200 mg/m^2/day continuous infusion for 7 days beginning on day 3 of treatment (in combination with tretinoin and daunorubicin) (Ades, 2006; Powell, 2010)

APL consolidation (unlabeled use): I.V.:

In combination with idarubicin and tretinoin: High-risk patients (WBC ≥10,000/mm^3) (Sanz, 2010): Adults ≤60 years:

First consolidation course: 1000 mg/m^2/day for 4 days

Third consolidation course: 150 mg/m^2 every 8 hours for 4 days

In combination with idarubicin, tretinoin, and thioguanine: High-risk patients (WBC >10,000/mm^3) (Lo Coco, 2010): Adults ≤61 years:

First consolidation course: 1000 mg/m^2/day for 4 days

Third consolidation course: 150 mg/m^2 every 8 hours for 5 days

In combination with daunorubicin (Ades, 2006; Ades, 2008):

First consolidation course: 200 mg/m^2/day for 7 days

Second consolidation course:

Age ≤60 years and low risk (WBC <10,000/mm^3): 1000 mg/m^2 every 12 hours for 4 days (8 doses)

Age <50 years and high risk (WBC ≥10,000/mm^3): 2000 mg/m^2 every 12 hours for 5 days (10 doses)

Age 50-60 years and high risk (WBC ≥10,000/mm^3): 1500 mg/m^2 every 12 hours for 5 days (10 doses) (Ades, 2008)

Age >60 years and high risk (WBC ≥10,000/mm^3): 1000 mg/m^2 every 12 hours for 4 days (8 doses)

Acute lymphocytic leukemia (ALL; unlabeled dosing):

Induction regimen, relapsed or refractory: I.V.: 3000 mg/m^2 over 3 hours daily for 5 days (in combination with idarubicin [day 3]) (Weiss, 2002)

Dose intensive regimen: I.V.: 3000 mg/m^2 over 2 hours every 12 hours days 2 and 3 (4 doses/cycle) of even numbered cycles (in combination with methotrexate; alternates with Hyper-CVAD) (Kantarjian, 2000)

Larson regimen (Larson, 1995): SubQ:

Early intensification phase: 75 mg/m^2/dose days 1-4 and 8-11 (4-week cycle; repeat once)

Late intensification phase: 75 mg/m^2/dose days 29-32 and 36-39

Linker protocol: I.V.: 300 mg/m^2/day days 1, 4, 8, and 11 of even numbered consolidation cycles (in combination with teniposide) (Linker, 1991)

Chronic lymphocytic leukemia (CLL; unlabeled use): *OFAR regimen:* I.V.: 1000 mg/m^2/dose over 2 hours days 2 and 3 every 4 weeks for up to 6 cycles (in combination with oxaliplatin, fludarabine, and rituximab) (Tsimberidou, 2008)

Chronic myeloid leukemia (CML; unlabeled dosing): SubQ: 20 mg/m²/dose days 15-24 every month (in combination with interferon alfa-2b) (Guilhot, 1997)

CNS lymphoma, primary (unlabeled use): I.V.: 2000 mg/m² over 1 hour every 12 hours days 2 and 3 (total of 4 doses) every 3 weeks (in combination with methotrexate and followed by whole brain irradiation) for a total of 4 courses (Ferreri, 2009)

Hodgkin lymphoma, relapsed or refractory (unlabeled use): I.V.:

DHAP regimen: 2000 mg/m² over 3 hours every 12 hours day 2 (total of 2 doses/cycle) for 2 cycles (in combination with dexamethasone and cisplatin) (Josting, 2002)

ESHAP regimen: 2000 mg/m² day 5 (in combination with etoposide, methylprednisolone, and cisplatin) every 3-4 weeks for 3 or 6 cycles (Aparicio, 1999)

Mini-BEAM regimen: 100 mg/m² every 12 hours days 2-5 (total of 8 doses) every 4-6 weeks (in combination with carmustine, etoposide, and melphalan) (Colwill, 1995; Martin, 2001)

BEAM regimen (transplant preparative regimen): 200 mg/m² twice daily for 4 days beginning 5 days prior to transplant (in combination with carmustine, etoposide, and melphalan) (Chopra, 1993)

Non-Hodgkin's lymphomas (unlabeled use): I.V.:

CALGB 9251 regimen: Cycles 2, 4, and 6: 150 mg/m²/day continuous infusion days 4 and 5 (Lee, 2001; Rizzieri, 2004)

CODOX-M/IVAC regimen:

Adults ≤60 years: Cycles 2 and 4 (IVAC): 2000 mg/m² every 12 hours days 1 and 2 (total of 4 doses/cycle) (IVAC is combination with ifosfamide, mesna, and etoposide; IVAC alternates with CODOX-M) (Magrath, 1996)

Adults ≤65 years: Cycles 2 and 4 (IVAC): 2000 mg/m² over 3 hours every 12 hours days 1 and 2 (total of 4 doses/cycle) (IVAC is combination with ifosfamide, mesna, and etoposide; IVAC alternates with CODOX-M) (Mead, 2008)

Adults >65 years: Cycles 2 and 4 (IVAC): 1000 mg/m² over 3 hours every 12 hours days 1 and 2 (total of 4 doses/cycle) (IVAC is combination with ifosfamide, mesna, and etoposide; IVAC alternates with CODOX-M) (Mead, 2008)

DHAP regimen:

Adults ≤70 years: 2000 mg/m² over 3 hours every 12 hours day 2 (total of 2 doses/cycle) every 3-4 weeks for 6-10 cycles (in combination with dexamethasone and cisplatin) (Velasquez, 1988)

Adults >70 years: 1000 mg/m² over 3 hours every 12 hours day 2 (total of 2 doses/cycle) every 3-4 weeks for 6-10 cycles (in combination with dexamethasone and cisplatin) (Velasquez, 1988)

ESHAP regimen: 2000 mg/m² over 2 hours day 5 every 3-4 weeks for 6-8 cycles (in combination with etoposide, methylprednisolone, and cisplatin) (Velasquez, 1994)

BEAM regimen (transplant preparative regimen): 200 mg/m² twice daily for 3 days beginning 4 days prior to transplant (in combination with carmustine, etoposide, and melphalan) (Linch 2010) **or** 100 mg/m² over 1 hour every 12 hours for 4 days beginning 5 days prior to transplant (in combination with carmustine, etoposide, and melphalan) (van Imhoff, 2005)

Meningeal leukemia: I.T.: **Note:** Optimal intrathecal chemotherapy dosing should be based on age rather than on body surface area (BSA); CSF volume correlates with age and not to BSA (Bleyer, 1983; Kerr, 2001).

Dosing provided in the FDA-approved labeling is BSA-based (usual dose 30 mg/m^2 every 4 days; range: 5-75 mg/m^2 once daily for 4 days or once every 4 days until CNS findings normalize, followed by 1 additional treatment).

Unlabeled uses or doses for intrathecal therapy: I.T.:

CNS prophylaxis (ALL): 100 mg weekly for 8 doses, then every 2 weeks for 8 doses, then monthly for 6 doses (high-risk patients) **or** 100 mg on day 7 or 8 with each chemotherapy cycle for 4 doses (low risk patients) **or** 16 doses (high-risk patients) (Cortes, 1995)

or as part of intrathecal triple therapy (TIT): 40 mg days 0 and 14 during induction, days 1, 4, 8, and 11 during CNS therapy phase, every 18 weeks during intensification and maintenance phases (Storring, 2009)

CNS prophylaxis (APL, as part of TIT): 50 mg per dose; administer 1 dose prior to consolidation and 2 doses during each of 2 consolidation phases (total of 5 doses) (Ades, 2006; Ades, 2008)

CNS leukemia treatment (ALL, as part of TIT): 40 mg twice weekly until CSF cleared (Storring, 2009)

CNS lymphoma treatment: 50 mg twice a week for 4 weeks, then weekly for 4-8 weeks, then every other week for 4 weeks, then every 4 weeks for 4 doses (Glantz, 1999)

Leptomeningeal metastases treatment: 50 mg twice a week for 4 weeks, then weekly for 4 weeks then monthly for 4 doses (NCCN CNS cancer guidelines v.1.2010) **or** 40-60 mg per dose (DeAngelis, 2005)

Pediatric Details concerning dosing in combination regimens should also be consulted.

Acute myeloid leukemia (AML) remission induction: I.V.: Standard-dose (provided in the FDA approved labeling): 100 mg/m^2/day continuous infusion for 7 days **or** 200 mg/m^2/day continuous infusion (as 100 mg/m^2 over 12 hours every 12 hours) for 7 days

Indication-specific dosing:

AML induction: *7 + 3 regimen:* I.V.:

Children <3 years (unlabeled dosing): 3.3 mg/kg/day continuous infusion for 7 days; minimum of 2 courses (in combination with daunorubicin) (Woods, 1990)

Children ≥3 years: 100 mg/m^2/day continuous infusion for 7 days; minimum of 2 courses (in combination with daunorubicin) (Woods, 1990)

AML consolidation (unlabeled use): *5 + 2 + 5 regimen:* I.V.: Children ≥15 years: 100 mg/m^2/day continuous infusion for 5 days for 2 consolidation courses (in combination with daunorubicin and etoposide) (Bishop, 1996)

AML salvage treatment (unlabeled use):

FLAG regimen: I.V.: Children ≥11 years: 2000 mg/m^2/day over 4 hours for 5 days (in combination with fludarabine and G-CSF); may repeat once if needed (Montillo, 1998)

MEC regimen: I.V.: Children ≥5 years: 1000 mg/m^2/day over 6 hours for 6 days (in combination with etoposide and mitoxantrone) (Amadori, 1991)

Acute lymphocytic leukemia (ALL; unlabeled dosing): *POG 8602/PVA regimen, intensification phase:* I.V.: Children ≥1 year: 1000 mg/m^2 continuous infusion over 24 hours day 1 (beginning 12 hours after start of methotrexate) every 3 weeks or every 12 weeks for 6 cycles (Land, 1994)

Chronic myeloid leukemia (CML; unlabeled dosing): SubQ: Children ≥7 years: 20 mg/m^2 once daily days 15-24 every month (in combination with interferon alfa-2b) (Guilhot, 1997)

Non-Hodgkin's lymphomas (unlabeled use): *CODOX-M/IVAC regimen:* I.V.: Children ≥3 years: Cycles 2 and 4 (IVAC): 2000 mg/m² every 12 hours days 1 and 2 (total of 4 doses/cycle) (IVAC is combination with ifosfamide, mesna and etoposide; IVAC alternates with CODOX-M) (Magrath, 1996)

Meningeal leukemia: I.T.: **Note:** Optimal intrathecal chemotherapy dosing should be based on age rather than on body surface area (BSA); CSF volume correlates with age and not to BSA (Bleyer, 1983; Kerr, 2001). Dosing provided in the FDA-approved labeling is BSA-based (usual dose 30 mg/m² every 4 days; range: 5-75 mg/m² once daily for 4 days or once every 4 days until CNS findings normalize, followed by 1 additional treatment).

Age-based intrathecal dosing (unlabeled): I.T.:

CNS prophylaxis:

<1 year: 20 mg per dose
1 to 1.99 years: 30 mg per dose
2 to 2.99 years: 50 mg per dose
≥3 years: 70 mg per dose

ALL CNS prophylaxis, age-specific doses from literature:

Administer on day 0 of induction therapy (Gaynon, 1993):

1 to <2 years: 30 mg per dose
2 to <3 years: 50 mg per dose
≥3 years: 70 mg per dose

Administer as part of triple intrathecal therapy (TIT) on days 1 and 15 of induction therapy; days 1, 15, 50, and 64 (standard risk patients) or days 1, 15, 29, and 43 (high-risk patients) during consolidation therapy; day 1 of reinduction therapy, and during maintenance therapy (very high-risk patients receive on days 1, 22, 45, and 59 of induction, days 8, 22, 36, and 50 of consolidation therapy, days 8 and 38 of reinduction therapy, and during maintenance) (Lin, 2007):

<1 year: 18 mg per dose
1-2 years: 24 mg per dose
2-3 years: 30 mg per dose
≥3 years: 36 mg per dose

Administer on day 0 of induction therapy, then as part of TIT on days 7, 14, and 21 during consolidation therapy; as part of TIT on days 0, 28, and 35 for 2 cycles of delayed intensification therapy, and then maintenance treatment as part of TIT on day 0 every 12 weeks for 38 months (boys) or 26 months (girls) from initial induction treatment (Matloub, 2006):

1 to <2 years: 16 mg per dose
2 to <3 years: 20 mg per dose
≥3 years: 24-30 mg per dose

Administer on day 15 of induction therapy, days 1 and 15 of reinduction phase; and day 1 of cycle 2 of maintenance 1A phase (Pieters, 2007):

<1 year: 15 mg per dose
≥1 year: 20 mg per dose

Treatment, CNS leukemia (ALL): I.T.: Administer as part of TIT weekly until CSF remission, then every 4 weeks throughout continuation treatment (Lin, 2007):

<1 year: 18 mg per dose
1-2 years: 24 mg per dose
2-3 years: 30 mg per dose
≥3 years: 36 mg per dose

Renal Impairment The FDA-approved labeling does not contain renal dosing adjustment guidelines; the following guidelines have been used by some clinicians:

Aronoff, 2007 (cytarabine 100-200 mg/m^2): Children and Adults: No adjustment necessary

Kintzel, 1995 (high-dose cytarabine 1-3 g/m^2):

Cl_{cr} 46-60 mL/minute: Administer 60% of dose

Cl_{cr} 31-45 mL/minute: Administer 50% of dose

Cl_{cr} <30 mL/minute: Consider use of alternative drug

Smith, 1997 (high-dose cytarabine; ≥2 g/m^2/dose):

Serum creatinine 1.5-1.9 mg/dL or increase (from baseline) of 0.5-1.2 mg/dL: Reduce dose to 1 g/m^2/dose

Serum creatinine ≥2 mg/dL or increase (from baseline) of >1.2 mg/dL: Reduce dose to 0.1 g/m^2/day as a continuous infusion

Hemodialysis: In 4 hour dialysis sessions (with high flow polysulfone membrane) 6 hours after cytarabine 1 g/m^2 over 2 hours, 63% of the metabolite ARA-U was extracted from plasma (based on a single adult case report) (Radeski, 2011)

Hepatic Impairment Dose may need to be adjusted in patients with liver failure since cytarabine is partially detoxified in the liver. The FDA-approved labeling does not contain hepatic dosing adjustment guidelines; the following guideline has been used by some clinicians:

Floyd, 2006: Transaminases (any elevation): Administer 50% of dose; may increase subsequent doses in the absence of toxicities

Koren, 1992 (dose level not specified): Bilirubin >2 mg/dL: Administer 50% of dose; may increase subsequent doses in the absence of toxicities

Combination Regimens

Leukemia, acute lymphocytic:

Hyper-CVAD + Imatinib on page 1680
Hyper-CVAD (Leukemia, Acute Lymphocytic) on page 1681
Larson Regimen (ALL) on page 1699
Linker Protocol (ALL) on page 1703
PVA (POG 8602) on page 1742

Leukemia, acute myeloid:

5 + 2 (Cytarabine-Daunorubicin) (AML Induction) on page 1512
5 + 2 (Cytarabine-Daunorubicin) (AML Postremission) on page 1512
5 + 2 (Cytarabine-Idarubicin) (AML Consolidation) on page 1512
5 + 2 (Cytarabine-Mitoxantrone) (AML Consolidation) on page 1512
5 + 2 + 5 (Cytarabine-Daunorubicin-Etoposide) (AML Consolidation) on page 1513
7 + 3 (Cytarabine-Daunorubicin) (AML Induction) on page 1513
7 + 3 (Cytarabine-Idarubicin) (AML Induction) on page 1514
7 + 3 (Cytarabine-Mitoxantrone) (AML Induction) on page 1514
7 + 3 + 7 (Cytarabine-Daunorubicin-Etoposide) (AML Induction) on page 1515
CLAG (AML Induction) on page 1586
CLAG-M (AML Induction) on page 1586
Clofarabine-Cytarabine (AML Consolidation) on page 1587
Clofarabine-Cytarabine (AML Induction) on page 1587
Cytarabine (High Dose)-Daunorubicin (AML Induction) on page 1602
Cytarabine (High Dose)-Daunorubicin-Etoposide (AML Induction) on page 1602
Cytarabine (High-Dose Single-Agent AML Induction Regimen) on page 1603

Cytarabine (Single-Agent AML Consolidation Regimen) on page 1603
Cytarabine (SubQ Single-Agent AML Induction Regimen) on page 1604
FLAG (AML Induction) on page 1643
FLAG-IDA on page 1644
MEC (AML Induction) on page 1706
MEC-G (AML Induction) on page 1707
Leukemia, acute promyelocytic: Tretinoin-Daunorubicin-Cytarabine (APL) on page 1762
Leukemia, chronic lymphocytic: OFAR (CLL) on page 1722
Lymphoma, Hodgkin:
Dexa-BEAM (Hodgkin) on page 1607
DHAP (Hodgkin) on page 1608
ESHAP (Hodgkin) on page 1634
MINE-ESHAP (Hodgkin) on page 1711
mini-BEAM (Hodgkin) on page 1712
Lymphoma, non-Hodgkin's:
Cisplatin-Cytarabine-Dexamethasone (NHL Regimen) on page 1567
CODOX-M on page 1590
COMLA on page 1595
ESHAP on page 1633
Hyper-CVAD (Lymphoma, non-Hodgkin's) on page 1687
MINE-ESHAP (NHL) on page 1712
Oxaliplatin-Cytarabine-Dexamethasone (NHL Regimen) on page 1723
Pro-MACE-CytaBOM on page 1741
Lymphoma, non-Hodgkin's (Burkitt): CODOX-M/IVAC on page 1591
Lymphoma, non-Hodgkin's (Mantle cell): Hyper-CVAD + Rituximab on page 1688

Administration

I.V.: Infuse standard dose therapy for AML (100-200 mg/m^2/day) as a continuous infusion. Infuse high-dose therapy (unlabeled) over 1-3 hours (usually). Other rates have been used, refer to specific reference.

I.T.: Intrathecal doses should be administered as soon as possible after preparation.

May also be administered SubQ.

Emetic Potential

>1000 mg/m^2: Moderate (30% to 90%)

100-200 mg/m^2: Low (10% to 30%)

Monitoring Parameters Liver function tests, CBC with differential and platelet count, serum creatinine, BUN, serum uric acid

Additional Information I.V. doses ≥1.5 g/m^2 may produce conjunctivitis which can be ameliorated with prophylactic use of corticosteroid (0.1% dexamethasone) eye drops. Dexamethasone eye drops should be administered at 1-2 drops every 6 hours during and for 2-7 days after completion of cytarabine.

Dosage Forms Excipient information presented when available (limited, particularly for generics); consult specific product labeling.

Injection, powder for reconstitution: 100 mg [contains benzyl alcohol (in diluent)], 500 mg [contains benzyl alcohol (in diluent)], 1 g [contains benzyl alcohol (in diluent)], 2 g [contains benzyl alcohol (in diluent)]

Injection, solution: 20 mg/mL (25 mL) [contains benzyl alcohol]

Injection, solution [preservative free]: 20 mg/mL (5 mL, 50 mL); 100 mg/mL (20 mL)

References

Adès L, Chevret S, Raffous, et al, "Is Cytarabine Useful in the Treatment of Acute Promyelocytic Leukemia? Results of a Randomized Trial From the European Acute Promyelocytic Leukemia Group," *J Clin Oncol*, 2006, 24(36):5703-10.

Adès L, Sanz MA, Chevret S, et al, "Treatment of Newly Diagnosed Acute Promyelocytic Leukemia (APL): A Comparison of French-Belgian-Swiss and PETHEMA Results," *Blood*, 2008, 111 (3):1078-84.

Amadori S, Arcese W, Isacchi G, et al, "Mitoxantrone, Etoposide, and Intermediate-Dose Cytarabine: An Effective and Tolerable Regimen for the Treatment of Refractory Acute Myeloid Leukemia," *J Clin Oncol*, 1991, 9(7):1210-4.

Aparicio J, Segura A, Garcerá S, et al, "ESHAP is an Active Regimen for Relapsing Hodgkin's Disease," *Ann Oncol*, 1999, 10(5):593-5.

Archimbaud E, Leblond V, Michallet M, et al ""Intensive Sequential Chemotherapy With Mitoxantrone and Continuous Infusion Etoposide and Cytarabine for Previously Treated Acute Myelogenous Leukemia," *Blood*, 1991, 77(9):1894-900.

Archimbaud E, Thomas X, Leblond V, et al, "Timed Sequential Chemotherapy for Previously Treated Patients With Acute Myeloid Leukemia: Long-Term Follow-Up of the Etoposide, Mitoxantrone, and Cytarabine-86 Trial," *J Clin Oncol*, 1995, 13(1):11-8.

Arlin Z, Case DC Jr, Moore J, et al, "Randomized Multicenter Trial of Cytosine Arabinoside With Mitoxantrone or Daunorubicin in Previously Untreated Adult Patients With Acute Nonlymphocytic Leukemia (ANLL). Lederle Cooperative Group," *Leukemia*, 1990, 4(3):177-83.

Aronoff GR, Bennett WM, Berns JS, et al, *Drug Prescribing in Renal Failure: Dosing Guidelines for Adults and Children*, 5th ed. Philadelphia, PA: American College of Physicians; 2007, p 98, 170.

Bishop JF, Matthews JP, Young GA, et al, "A Randomized Study of High-Dose Cytarabine in Induction in Acute Myeloid Leukemia," *Blood*, 1996, 87(5):1710-7.

Bleyer WA, Coccia PF, Sather HN, et al, "Reduction in Central Nervous System Leukemia With a Pharmacokinetically Derived Intrathecal Methotrexate Dosage Regimen," *J Clin Oncol*, 1983, 1 (5):317-25.

Chopra R, McMillan AK, Linch DC, et al, "The Place of High-Dose BEAM Therapy and Autologous Bone Marrow Transplantation in Poor-Risk Hodgkin's Disease. A Single-Center Eight-Year Study of 155 Patients," *Blood*, 1993, 81(5):1137-45.

Colwill R, Crump M, Couture F, et al., "Mini-BEAM as Salvage Therapy for Relapsed or Refractory Hodgkin's Disease Before Intensive Therapy and Autologous Bone Marrow Transplantation," *J Clin Oncol*, 1995, 13(2):396-402.

Cortes J, O'Brien SM, Pierce S, et al, "The Value of High-Dose Systemic Chemotherapy and Intrathecal Therapy for Central Nervous System Prophylaxis in Different Risk Groups of Adult Acute Lymphoblastic Leukemia," *Blood*, 1995, 86(6):2091-7.

DeAngelis LM and Boutros D, "Leptomeningeal Metastasis," *Cancer Invest*, 2005, 23(2):145-54.

Dillman RO, Davis RB, Green MR, et al, "A Comparative Study of Two Different Doses of Cytarabine for Acute Myeloid Leukemia: A Phase III Trial of Cancer and Leukemia Group B," *Blood*, 1991, 78(10):2520-6.

Fenaux P, Mufti GJ, Hellstrom-Lindberg E, et al, "Azacitidine Prolongs Overall Survival Compared With Conventional Care Regimens in Elderly Patients With Low Bone Marrow Blast Count Acute Myeloid Leukemia, *J Clin Oncol*, 2010, 28(4):562-9.

Fernandez HF, Sun Z, Yao X, et al, "Anthracycline Dose Intensification in Acute Myeloid Leukemia," *N Engl J Med*, 2009, 361(13):1249-59.

Ferreri AJ, Reni M, Foppoli M, et al, "High-Dose Cytarabine Plus High-Dose Methotrexate Versus High-Dose Methotrexate Alone in Patients With Primary CNS Lymphoma: a Randomised Phase 2 Trial," *Lancet*, 2009, 374(9700):1512-20.

Floyd J, Mirza I, Sachs B, et al, "Hepatotoxicity of Chemotherapy," *Semin Oncol*, 2006, 33 (1):50-67.

Gaynon PS, Steinherz PG, Bleyer WA, et al, "Improved Therapy for Children With Acute Lymphoblastic Leukemia and Unfavorable Presenting Features: A Follow-Up Report of the Childrens Cancer Group Study CCG-106," *J Clin Oncol*, 1993, 11(11):2234-42.

Glantz MJ, LaFollette S, Jaeckle KA, et al, "Randomized Trial of a Slow-Release Versus a Standard Formulation of Cytarabine for the Intrathecal Treatment of Lymphomatous Meningitis," *J Clin Oncol*, 1999, 17(10):3110-6.

Guilhot F, Chastang C, Michallet M, et al, "Interferon Alfa-2b Combined With Cytarabine Versus Interferon Alone in Chronic Myelogenous Leukemia. French Chronic Myeloid Leukemia Study Group," *N Engl J Med*, 1997, 337(4):223-9.

Herzig RH, Hines JD, Herzig GP, et al, "Cerebellar Toxicity With High-Dose Cytosine Arabinoside," *J Clin Oncol*, 1987, 5(6):927-32.

Herzig RH, Lazarus HM, Wolff SN, et al, "High-Dose Cytosine Arabinoside Therapy With and Without Anthracycline Antibiotics for Remission Reinduction of Acute Nonlymphoblastic Leukemia," *J Clin Oncol*, 1985, 3(7):992-7.

Jacobson JO, Polovich M, McNiff KK, et al, "American Society of Clinical Oncology/Oncology Nursing Society Chemotherapy Administration Safety Standards," *J Clin Oncol*, 2009, 27 (32):5469-75.

Josting A, Rudolph C, Reiser M, et al, "Time-Intensified Dexamethasone/Cisplatin/Cytarabine: An Effective Salvage Therapy With Low Toxicity in Patients With Relapsed and Refractory Hodgkin's Disease," *Ann Oncol*, 2002, 13(10):1628-35.

Kantarjian HM, O'Brien S, Smith TL, et al, "Results of Treatment With Hyper-CVAD, A Dose-Intensive Regimen, in Adult Acute Lymphocytic Leukemia," *J Clin Oncol*, 2000, 18(3): 547-61.

Kerr JZ, Berg S, and Blaney SM, "Intrathecal Chemotherapy," *Crit Rev Oncol Hematol*, 2001, 37 (3):227-36.

Kintzel PE and Dorr RT, "Anticancer Drug Renal Toxicity and Elimination: Dosing Guidelines for Altered Renal Function," *Cancer Treat Rev*, 1995, 21(1):33-64.

Koren G, Beatty K, Seto A, et al, "The Effects of Impaired Liver Function on the Elimination of Antineoplastic Agents," *Ann Pharmacother*, 1992, 26(3):363-71.

Land VJ, Shuster JJ, Crist WM, et al, "Comparison of Two Schedules of Intermediate-Dose Methotrexate and Cytarabine Consolidation Therapy for Childhood B-Precursor Cell Acute Lymphoblastic Leukemia: A Pediatric Oncology Group Study," *J Clin Oncol*, 1994, 12(9):1939-45.

Larson RA, Dodge RK, Burns CP, et al, "A Five-Drug Remission Induction Regimen With Intensive Consolidation for Adults With Acute Lymphoblastic Leukemia: Cancer and Leukemia Group B Study 8811," *Blood*, 1995, 85(8):2025-37.

Lee EJ, Petroni GR, Schiffer CA, et al, "Brief-Duration High-Intensity Chemotherapy for Patients With Small Noncleaved-Cell Lymphoma or FAB L3 Acute Lymphocytic Leukemia: Results of Cancer and Leukemia Group B Study 9251," *J Clin Oncol*, 2001, 19(20):4014-22.

Lin WY, Liu HC, Yeh TC, et al, "Triple Intrathecal Therapy Without Cranial Irradiation for Central Nervous System Preventive Therapy in Childhood Acute Lymphoblastic Leukemia," *Pediatr Blood Cancer*, 2008, 50(3):523-7.

Linch DC, Yung L, Smith P, et al, "Final Analysis of the UKLG LY02 Trial Comparing 6-8 Cycles of CHOP With 3 Cycles of CHOP Followed by a BEAM Autograft in Patients <65 Years With Poor Prognosis Histologically Aggressive NHL," *Br J Haematol*, 2010, 149(2):237-43.

Linker CA, Levitt LJ, O'Donnell M, et al, "Treatment of Adult Acute Lymphoblastic Leukemia With Intensive Cyclical Chemotherapy: A Follow-up Report," *Blood*, 1991, 78(11):2814-22.

Lo Coco F, Avvisati G, Vignetti M, et al, "Front-Line Treatment of Acute Promyelocytic Leukemia With AIDA Induction Followed by Risk-Adapted Consolidation for Adults Younger Than 61 Years: Results of the AIDA-2000 Trial of the GIMEMA Group," *Blood*, 2010, 116(17):3171-9.

Magrath I, Adde M, Shad A, et al, "Adults and Children With Small Non-Cleaved-Cell Lymphoma Have a Similar Excellent Outcome When Treated With the Same Chemotherapy Regimen," *J Clin Oncol*, 1996, 14(3):925-34.

Martín A, Fernández-Jiménez MC, Caballero MD, et al. "Long-Term Follow-Up in Patients Treated With Mini-BEAM as Salvage Therapy for Relapsed or Refractory Hodgkin's Disease," *Br J Haematol*, 2001, 113(1):161-71.

Matloub Y, Lindemulder S, Gaynon PS, et al, "Intrathecal Triple Therapy Decreases Central Nervous System Relapse but Fails to Improve Event-Free Survival When Compared With Intrathecal Methotrexate: Results of the Children's Cancer Group (CCG) 1952 Study for Standard-Risk Acute Lymphoblastic Leukemia, Reported by the Children's Oncology Group," *Blood*, 2006, 108(4):1165-73.

Mayer RJ, Davis RB, Schiffer CA, et al, "Intensive Postremission Chemotherapy in Adults With Acute Myeloid Leukemia, Cancer and Leukemia Group B," *N Engl J Med*, 1994, 331 (14):896-903.

Mead GM, Barrans SL, Qian W, et al, "A Prospective Clinicopathologic Study of Dose-Modified CODOX-M/IVAC in Patients With Sporadic Burkitt Lymphoma Defined Using Cytogenetic and Immunophenotypic Criteria (MRC/NCRI LY10 Trial)," *Blood*, 2008, 112(6):2248-60.

Milligan DW, Wheatley K, Littlewood T, et al, "Fludarabine and Cytosine are Less Effective than Standard ADE Chemotherapy in High-Risk Acute Myeloid Leukemia, and Addition of G-CSF and ATRA are not Beneficial: Results of the MRC AML-HR Randomized Trial," *Blood*, 2006, 107 (12):4614-22.

Montillo M, Mirto S, Petti MC, et al, "Fludarabine, Cytarabine, and G-CSF (FLAG) for the Treatment of Poor Risk Acute Myeloid Leukemia," *Am J Hematol*, 1998, 58(2):105-9.

Morgan C, Tillett T, Braybrooke J, et al, "Management of Uncommon Chemotherapy-Induced Emergencies," *Lancet Oncol*, 2011, 12(8):806-14.

National Comprehensive Cancer Network® (NCCN), "Clinical Practice Guidelines in Oncology™: Central Nervous System Cancers," Version 1.2010. Available at http://www.nccn.org/professionals/physician_gls/PDF/cns.pdf

Pieters R, Schrappe M, De Lorenzo P, et al, "A Treatment Protocol for Infants Younger Than 1 Year With Acute Lymphoblastic Leukaemia (Interfant-99): An Observational Study and a Multicentre Randomised Trial," *Lancet*, 2007, 370(9583):240-50.

Powell BL, Moser B, Stock W, et al, "Arsenic Trioxide Improves Event-Free and Over-All Survival for Adults With Acute Promyelocytic Leukemia: North American Leukemia Intergroup Study C9710," *Blood*, 2010, 116(19):3751-7.

Radeski D, Cull GM, Cain M, et al, "Effective Clearance of Ara-U the Major Metabolite of Cytosine Arabinoside (Ara-C) by Hemodialysis in a Patient With Lymphoma and End-Stage Renal Failure," *Cancer Chemother Pharmacol*, 2011, 67(4):765-8.

Rizzieri DA, Johnson JL, Niedzwiecki D, et al, "Intensive Chemotherapy With and Without Cranial Radiation for Burkitt Leukemia and Lymphoma: Final Results of Cancer and Leukemia Group B Study 9251," *Cancer*, 2004, 100(7):1438-48.

Sanz MA, Montesinos P, Rayón C, et al, "Risk-Adapted Treatment of Acute Promyelocytic Leukemia Based on all-trans Retinoic Acid and Anthracycline With Addition of Cytarabine in Consolidation Therapy for High-Risk Patients: Further Improvements in Treatment Outcome," *Blood*, 2010, 115(25):5137-46.

Smith G, Damon LE, Rugo HS, et al. "High-Dose Cytarabine Dose Modification Reduces the Incidence of Neurotoxicity in Patients With Renal Insufficiency," *J Clin Oncol*, 1997, 15(2): 833-9.

Storring JM, Minden MD, Kao S, et al, "Treatment of Adults With BCR-ABL Negative Acute Lymphoblastic Leukaemia With a Modified Paediatric Regimen," *Br J Haematol*, 2009, 146 (1):76-85.

Tilly H, Castaigne S, Bordessoule D, et al, "Low-Dose Cytarabine Versus Intensive Chemotherapy in the Treatment of Acute Nonlymphocytic Leukemia in the Elderly," *J Clin Oncol*, 1990, 8 (2):272-9.

Tsimberidou AM, Wierda WG, Plunkett W, et al, "Phase I-II Study of Oxaliplatin, Fludarabine, Cytarabine, and Rituximab Combination Therapy in Patients With Richter's Syndrome or Fludarabine-Refractory Chronic Lymphocytic Leukemia," *J Clin Oncol*, 2008, 26(2):196-203.

van Imhoff GW, van der Holt B, MacKenzie MA, et al, "Short Intensive Sequential Therapy Followed by Autologous Stem Cell Transplantation in Adult Burkitt, Burkitt-Like and Lymphoblastic Lymphoma," *Leukemia*, 2005, 19(6):945-52.

Velasquez WS, Cabanillas F, Salvador P, et al, "Effective Salvage Therapy for Lymphoma With Cisplatin in Combination With High-Dose Ara-C and Dexamethasone (DHAP)," *Blood*, 1988, 71 (1):117-22.

Velasquez WF, McLaughlin P, Tucker S, et al, "ESHAP - An Effective Chemotherapy Regimen in Refractory and Relapsing Lymphoma: A 4-Year Follow-up Study," *J Clin Oncol*, 1994, 12 (6):1169-76.

Weiss MA, Aliff TB, Tallman MS, et al, "A Single, High Dose of Idarubicin Combined With Cytarabine as Induction Therapy for Adult Patients With Recurrent or Refractory Acute Lymphoblastic Leukemia," *Cancer*, 2002, 95(3):581-7.

Wierzbowska A, Robak T, Pluta A, et al, "Cladribine Combined With High Doses of Arabinoside Cytosine, Mitoxantrone, and G-CSF (CLAG-M) is a Highly Effective Salvage Regimen in Patients With Refractory and Relapsed Acute Myeloid Leukemia of the Poor Risk: A Final Report of the Polish Adult Leukemia Group," *Eur J Haematol* 2008; 80(2):115-26.

Wiernik PH, Banks P, Case Jr DC, et al, "Cytarabine Plus Idarubicin or Daunorubicin as Induction and Consolidation Therapy for Previously Untreated Adult Patients With Acute Myeloid Leukemia," *Blood*, 1992, 79(2):313-9.

Woods WG, Ruymann FB, Lampkin BC, et al, "The Role of Timing of High-Dose Cytosine Arabinoside Intensification and of Maintenance Therapy in the Treatment of Children With Acute Nonlymphocytic Leukemia," *Cancer*, 1990, 66(6):1106-13.

Wrzesień-Kuś A, Robak T, Lech-Marańda E, et al, "A Multicenter, Open, Non-Comparative Phase II Study of the Combination of Cladribine (2-Chlorodeoxyadenosine), Cytarabine, and G-CSF as Induction Therapy in Refractory Acute Myeloid Leukemia - A Report of the Polish Adult Leukemia Group (PALG)," *Eur J Haematol*, 2003;71(3):155-62.

Cytarabine (Liposomal) (sye TARE a been lye po SOE mal)

Related Information

Management of Chemotherapy-Induced Nausea and Vomiting *on page 1786*

Safe Handling of Hazardous Drugs *on page 1904*

Brand Names: U.S. DepoCyt®

Brand Names: Canada DepoCyt®

Index Terms Cytarabine Lipid Complex; Cytarabine Liposome; DepoFoam-Encapsulated Cytarabine; DTC 101; Liposomal Cytarabine

Generic Availability (U.S.) No

Pharmacologic Category Antineoplastic Agent, Antimetabolite (Pyrimidine Antagonist)

Use Treatment of lymphomatous meningitis

Labeled Contraindications Hypersensitivity to cytarabine or any component of the formulation; active meningeal infection

Pregnancy Risk Factor D

Lactation Excretion in breast milk unknown/not recommended

Warnings/Precautions Hazardous agent - use appropriate precautions for handling and disposal. **[U.S. Boxed Warning]: Chemical arachnoiditis (nausea, vomiting, headache, fever) occurs commonly; may be fatal if untreated. The incidence and severity of chemical arachnoiditis is reduced by coadministration with dexamethasone; dexamethasone should be administered concomitantly with cytarabine (liposomal) to diminish chemical arachnoid symptoms.** Hydrocephalus has been reported and may be precipitated by chemical arachnoiditis. May cause neurotoxicity (including myelopathy), which may lead to permanent neurologic deficit (rare); monitor for neurotoxicity; reduce subsequent doses; discontinue with persistent neurotoxicity. The risk of neurotoxicity is increased with concurrent radiation therapy or systemic chemotherapy. The risk for neurotoxicity is increased when administered with other antineoplastic agents or with cranial/spinal irradiation. Persistent (extreme) somnolence, hemiplegia, visual disturbances (including blindness; may be permanent), deafness, cranial nerve palsies, peripheral neuropathy, and even combined neurologic features (cauda equina syndrome) have been reported. CSF flow blockage may lead to increased free cytarabine concentrations in the CSF and increase the risk for neurotoxicity; assess CSF flow prior to administration. Infectious meningitis may be associated with intrathecal administration. **[U.S. Boxed Warning]: Should be administered under the supervision of an experienced cancer chemotherapy physician; facilities appropriate for diagnosis and management of complications should be readily available.** For intrathecal use only. Intrathecal medications should not be prepared during the preparation of any other agents; after preparation, store intrathecal medications in an isolated location or container clearly marked with a label identifying as "intrathecal" use only; delivery of intrathecal medications to the patient should only be with other medications intended for administration into the central nervous system (Jacobson, 2009).

Adverse Reactions

>10%:

Cardiovascular: Peripheral edema (11%)

Central nervous system: Chemical arachnoiditis (without dexamethasone premedication: 100%; with dexamethasone premedication: 33% to 42%; grade 4: 19% to 30%; onset: ≤5 days); headache (56%), confusion (33%), fever (32%), fatigue (25%), seizure (20% to 22%), dizziness (18%), lethargy (16%), insomnia (14%), memory impairment (14%), pain (14%)

Endocrine & metabolic: Dehydration (13%)

Gastrointestinal: Nausea (46%), vomiting (44%), constipation (25%), diarrhea (12%), appetite decreased (11%)

Genitourinary: Urinary tract infection (14%)

Hematologic: Anemia (12%), thrombocytopenia (3% to 11%)

Neuromuscular & skeletal: Weakness (40%), back pain (24%), abnormal gait (23%), limb pain (15%), neck pain (14%), arthralgia (11%), neck stiffness (11%)

Ocular: Blurred vision (11%)

1% to 10%:
- Cardiovascular: Tachycardia (9%), hypotension (8%), hypertension (6%), syncope (3%), edema (2%)
- Central nervous system: Agitation (10%), hypoesthesia (10%), depression (8%), anxiety (7%), sensory neuropathy (3%)
- Dermatologic: Pruritus (2%)
- Endocrine & metabolic: Hypokalemia (7%), hyponatremia (7%), hyperglycemia (6%)
- Gastrointestinal: Abdominal pain (9%), dysphagia (8%), anorexia (5%), hemorrhoids (3%), mucosal inflammation (3%)
- Genitourinary: Incontinence (7%), urinary retention (5%)
- Hematologic: Neutropenia (10%), contusion (2%)
- Neuromuscular & skeletal: Muscle weakness (10%), tremor (9%), peripheral neuropathy (3% to 4%), abnormal reflexes (3%)
- Otic: Hypoacusis (6%)
- Respiratory: Dyspnea (10%), cough (7%), pneumonia (6%)
- Miscellaneous: Diaphoresis (2%)

<1%, postmarketing, and/or case reports: Anaphylaxis, bladder control impaired, blindness, bowel control impaired, cauda equine syndrome, cranial nerve palsies, CSF protein increased, CSF WBC increased, deafness, encephalopathy, hemiplegia, hydrocephalus, infectious meningitis, intracranial pressure increased, myelopathy, neurologic deficit, numbness, papilledema, somnolence, visual disturbance

Drug Interactions

Metabolism/Transport Effects None known.

Avoid Concomitant Use There are no known interactions where it is recommended to avoid concomitant use.

Increased Effect/Toxicity There are no known significant interactions involving an increase in effect.

Decreased Effect There are no known significant interactions involving a decrease in effect.

Storage/Stability Store under refrigeration at 2°C to 8°C (36°F to 46°F); protect from freezing. Avoid aggressive agitation. Withdraw from the vial immediately prior to administration; solutions should be used within 4 hours of withdrawal from the vial.

After preparation, store intrathecal medications in an isolated location or container clearly marked with a label identifying as "intrathecal" use only.

Reconstitution Use appropriate precautions for handling and disposal. Allow vial to warm to room temperature prior to withdrawal from vial. Particles may settle in diluent over time, and may be resuspended with gentle agitation or inversion immediately prior to withdrawing from the vial. Do not further dilute or mix with any other medications. Further reconstitution or dilution is not required. Intrathecal medications should not be prepared during the preparation of any other agents.

Mechanism of Action Cytarabine liposomal is a sustained-release formulation of the active ingredient cytarabine, an antimetabolite which acts through inhibition of DNA synthesis and is cell cycle-specific for the S phase of cell division. Cytarabine is converted intracellularly to its active metabolite cytarabine-5'-triphosphate (ara-CTP). Ara-CTP also appears to be incorporated into DNA and RNA; however, the primary action is inhibition of DNA polymerase, resulting in decreased DNA synthesis and repair. The liposomal formulation allows for gradual release, resulting in prolonged exposure.

Pharmacodynamics/Kinetics

Absorption: Systemic exposure following intrathecal administration is negligible since transfer rate from CSF to plasma is slow

Half-life elimination, CSF: 6-82 hours

Time to peak, CSF: Intrathecal: <1 hour

Dosing

Adult & Geriatric Note: Initiate dexamethasone 4 mg twice daily (oral or I.V.) for 5 days, beginning on the day of cytarabine liposomal administration.

Lymphomatous meningitis: I.T.:

Induction: 50 mg every 14 days for a total of 2 doses (weeks 1 and 3)

Consolidation: 50 mg every 14 days for 3 doses (weeks 5, 7, and 9), followed by an additional dose at week 13

Maintenance: 50 mg every 28 days for 4 doses (weeks 17, 21, 25, and 29)

Adjustment for Toxicity If drug-related neurotoxicity develops, reduce dose to 25 mg. If toxicity persists, discontinue treatment.

Administration For intrathecal use only. Dose should be removed from vial immediately before administration (must be administered within 4 hours of removal). An in-line filter should **NOT** be used. Administer directly into the CSF via an intraventricular reservoir or by direct injection into the lumbar sac. Injection should be made slowly (over 1-5 minutes). Patients should lie flat for 1 hour after lumbar puncture.

Monitoring Parameters Monitor closely for signs of an immediate reaction; neurotoxicity

Test Interactions Since cytarabine liposomes are similar in appearance to WBCs, care must be taken in interpreting CSF examinations in patients receiving cytarabine liposomal.

Dosage Forms Excipient information presented when available (limited, particularly for generics); consult specific product labeling.

Injection, suspension, intrathecal [preservative free]:

DepoCyt®: 10 mg/mL (5 mL)

References

Garcia-Marco JA, Panizo C, Garcia ES, et al, "Efficacy and Safety of Liposomal Cytarabine in Lymphoma Patients With Central Nervous System Involvement From Lymphoma," *Cancer*, 2009, 115(9):1892-8.

Glantz MJ, LaFollette S, Jaeckle KA, et al, "Randomized Trial of a Slow-Release Versus a Standard Formulation of Cytarabine for the Intrathecal Treatment of Lymphomatous Meningitis," *J Clin Oncol*, 1999, 17(10):3110-6.

Jacobson JO, Polovich M, McNiff KK, et al, "American Society of Clinical Oncology/Oncology Nursing Society Chemotherapy Administration Safety Standards," *J Clin Oncol*, 2009, 27(32):5469-75.

Jaeckle KA, Batchelor T, O'Day SJ, et al, "An Open Label Trial of Sustained-Release Cytarabine (DepoCyt) for the Intrathecal Treatment of Solid Tumor Neoplastic Meningitis," *J Neurooncol*, 2002, 57(3):231-9.

Spina M, Chimienti E, Martellotta F, et al, "Phase 2 Study of Intrathecal, Long-Acting Liposomal Cytarabine in the Prophylaxis of Lymphomatous Meningitis in Human Immunodeficiency Virus-Related non-Hodgkin Lymphoma," *Cancer*, 2010, 116(6):1495-501.

◆ **Cytarabine Hydrochloride** *see* Cytarabine (Conventional) *on page 348*

◆ **Cytarabine Lipid Complex** *see* Cytarabine (Liposomal) *on page 361*

◆ **Cytarabine Liposome** *see* Cytarabine (Liposomal) *on page 361*

◆ **CytoGam®** *see* Cytomegalovirus Immune Globulin (Intravenous-Human) *on page 365*

Cytomegalovirus Immune Globulin (Intravenous-Human) (sye toe meg a low VYE rus i MYUN GLOB yoo lin in tra VEE nus HYU man)

Brand Names: U.S. CytoGam®

Brand Names: Canada CytoGam®

Index Terms CMV-IGIV

Generic Availability (U.S.) No

Pharmacologic Category Blood Product Derivative; Immune Globulin

Use Prophylaxis of cytomegalovirus (CMV) disease associated with kidney, lung, liver, pancreas, and heart transplants; concomitant use with ganciclovir should be considered in organ transplants (other than kidney) from CMV seropositive donors to CMV seronegative recipients

Unlabeled Use Adjunct therapy in the treatment of CMV disease in immunocompromised patients

Labeled Contraindications Hypersensitivity to CMV-IGIV, other immunoglobulins, or any component of the formulation; immunoglobulin A deficiency

Pregnancy Risk Factor C

Lactation Excretion in breast milk unknown

Warnings/Precautions Hypersensitivity and anaphylactic reactions can occur; immediate treatment (including epinephrine 1:1000) should be available. Aseptic meningitis syndrome (AMS) has been reported with intravenous immune globulin administration (rare); may occur with high doses (≥2 g/kg). Intravenous immune globulin has been associated with antiglobulin hemolysis; monitor for signs of hemolytic anemia. Monitor for transfusion related acute lung injury (TRALI); noncardiogenic pulmonary edema has been reported with intravenous immune globulin use. Acute renal dysfunction (increased serum creatinine, oliguria, acute renal failure) can rarely occur; usually within 7 days of use (more likely with products stabilized with sucrose). Use with caution in the elderly, patients with renal disease, diabetes mellitus, volume depletion, sepsis, paraproteinemia, and nephrotoxic medications due to risk of renal dysfunction. In patients at risk of renal dysfunction, the rate of infusion and concentration of solution should be minimized. discontinue if renal function deteriorates. Patients should not be volume depleted prior to therapy. Thrombotic events have been reported with administration of intravenous immune globulin; use with caution in patients with cardiovascular risk factors. Use with caution in patients >65 years of age. Product is stabilized with albumin. Product of human plasma; may potentially contain infectious agents which could transmit disease. Screening of donors, as well as testing and/or inactivation or removal of certain viruses, reduces the risk. Infections thought to be transmitted by this product should be reported to the manufacturer. Product is stabilized with sucrose.

Adverse Reactions

<6%:

Cardiovascular: Flushing

Central nervous system: Chills, fever

Gastrointestinal: Nausea, vomiting

Neuromuscular & skeletal: Arthralgia, back pain, muscle cramps

Respiratory: Wheezing

<1%: Blood pressure decreased

Postmarketing and/or case reports: Acute renal failure, acute tubular necrosis, anaphylactic shock, angioneurotic edema, anuria, aseptic meningitis syndrome (AMS), BUN increased, oliguria, osmotic nephrosis, proximal tubular nephropathy, serum creatinine increased

Drug Interactions

Metabolism/Transport Effects None known.

Avoid Concomitant Use There are no known interactions where it is recommended to avoid concomitant use.

Increased Effect/Toxicity There are no known significant interactions involving an increase in effect.

Decreased Effect

Cytomegalovirus Immune Globulin (Intravenous-Human) may decrease the levels/effects of: Vaccines (Live)

Storage/Stability Store between 2°C and 8°C (35.6°F and 46.4°F). Use reconstituted product within 6 hours.

Reconstitution Do not admix with other medications; do not use if turbid. Do not shake vials. Dilution is not recommended.

Mechanism of Action CMV-IGIV is a preparation of immunoglobulin G derived from pooled healthy blood donors with a high titer of CMV antibodies; administration provides a passive source of antibodies against cytomegalovirus

Dosing

Adult

Kidney transplant: I.V.:

Initial dose (within 72 hours of transplant): 150 mg/kg/dose

2, 4, 6, and 8 weeks after transplant: 100 mg/kg/dose

12 and 16 weeks after transplant: 50 mg/kg/dose

Liver, lung, pancreas, or heart transplant: I.V.:

Initial dose (within 72 hours of transplant): 150 mg/kg/dose

2, 4, 6, and 8 weeks after transplant: 150 mg/kg/dose

12 and 16 weeks after transplant: 100 mg/kg/dose

Severe CMV pneumonia: I.V.: Various regimens have been used, including 400 mg/kg CMV-IGIV in combination with ganciclovir on days 1, 2, 7, or 8, followed by 200 mg/kg CMV-IGIV on days 14 and 21

Geriatric Use with caution in patients >65 years of age; elderly may be at increased risk of renal insufficiency.

Renal Impairment Use with caution; specific dosing adjustments are not available. Infusion rate should be the minimum practical; do not exceed 180 mg/kg/hour.

Administration Administer through an I.V. line containing an in-line filter (pore size 15 micron) using an infusion pump. Do not mix with other infusions; do not use if turbid. Begin infusion within 6 hours of entering vial, complete infusion within 12 hours.

Infuse at 15 mg/kg/hour. If no adverse reactions occur within 30 minutes, may increase rate to 30 mg/kg/hour. If no adverse reactions occur within the second 30 minutes, may increase rate to 60 mg/kg/hour; maximum rate of infusion: 75 mL/hour. When infusing subsequent doses, may decrease titration interval from 30 minutes to 15 minutes. If patient develops nausea, back pain, or flushing during infusion, slow the rate or temporarily stop the infusion. Discontinue if blood pressure drops or in case of anaphylactic reaction.

Monitoring Parameters Vital signs (throughout infusion), flushing, chills, muscle cramps, back pain, fever, nausea, vomiting, wheezing, decreased blood pressure, or anaphylaxis; renal function and urine output

Dietary Considerations Some products may contain sodium.

Dosage Forms Excipient information presented when available (limited, particularly for generics); consult specific product labeling.

Injection, solution [preservative free]:
CytoGam®: 50 mg (± 10 mg)/mL (50 mL) [contains sodium 20-30 mEq/L, human albumin, and sucrose 50 mg/mL]

References

Reed EC, Bowden RA, Dandliker PS, et al, "Efficacy of Cytomegalovirus Immunoglobulin in Marrow Transplant Recipients With Cytomegalovirus Pneumonia," *J Infect Dis*, 1987, 156:641-5.
Reed EC, Bowden RA, Dandliker PS, et al, "Treatment of Cytomegalovirus Pneumonia With Ganciclovir and Intravenous Cytomegalovirus Immunoglobulin in Patients With Bone Marrow Transplants," *Ann Intern Med*, 1988, 109:783-8.

◆ **Cytosar® (Can)** *see* Cytarabine (Conventional) *on page 348*
◆ **Cytosar-U** *see* Cytarabine (Conventional) *on page 348*
◆ **Cytosine Arabinosine Hydrochloride** *see* Cytarabine (Conventional) *on page 348*
◆ **Cytostasan** *see* Bendamustine *on page 158*
◆ **Cytovene® (Can)** *see* Ganciclovir (Systemic) *on page 656*
◆ **Cytovene®-IV** *see* Ganciclovir (Systemic) *on page 656*
◆ **Cytoxan** *see* Cyclophosphamide *on page 321*
◆ **D1694** *see* Raltitrexed *on page 1226*
◆ **DAB_{389}IL-2** *see* Denileukin Diftitox *on page 425*
◆ **DAB389 Interleukin-2** *see* Denileukin Diftitox *on page 425*
◆ **DABIL2** *see* Denileukin Diftitox *on page 425*

Dacarbazine (da KAR ba zeen)

Related Information

Management of Chemotherapy-Induced Nausea and Vomiting *on page 1786*
Management of Drug Extravasations *on page 1800*
Safe Handling of Hazardous Drugs *on page 1904*

Brand Names: Canada Dacarbazine for Injection

Index Terms DIC; Dimethyl Triazeno Imidazole Carboxamide; DTIC; DTIC-Dome; Imidazole Carboxamide; Imidazole Carboxamide Dimethyltriazene; WR-139007

Generic Availability (U.S.) Yes

Pharmacologic Category Antineoplastic Agent, Alkylating Agent (Triazene)

Use Treatment of malignant melanoma, Hodgkin's disease

Unlabeled Use Treatment of soft-tissue sarcomas, islet cell tumors, pheochromocytoma, medullary carcinoma of the thyroid

Labeled Contraindications Hypersensitivity to dacarbazine or any component of the formulation

Pregnancy Risk Factor C

Lactation Excretion in breast milk unknown/not recommended

Warnings/Precautions Hazardous agent - use appropriate precautions for handling and disposal. **[U.S. Boxed Warnings]: Bone marrow suppression is a common toxicity;** leukopenia and thrombocytopenia may be severe; may result in treatment delays or discontinuation; monitor closely. **Hepatotoxicity with hepatocellular necrosis and hepatic vein thrombosis has been reported (rare),** usually with combination chemotherapy, but may occur with dacarbazine alone. The half-life is increased in patients with renal and/or hepatic impairment; use caution, monitor for toxicity and consider dosage reduction. Anaphylaxis may occur following dacarbazine administration. Extravasation may result in tissue damage and severe pain. **[U.S. Boxed**

Warnings]: May be carcinogenic and/or teratogenic. Should be administered under the supervision of an experienced cancer chemotherapy physician. Carefully evaluate the potential benefits of therapy against the risk for toxicity.

Adverse Reactions Frequency not always defined.

Dermatologic: Alopecia

Gastrointestinal: Nausea and vomiting (>90%), anorexia

Hematologic: Myelosuppression (onset: 5-7 days; nadir: 7-10 days; recovery: 21-28 days), leukopenia, thrombocytopenia

Local: Pain on infusion

Infrequent, postmarketing, and/or case reports: Anaphylactic reactions, anemia, diarrhea, eosinophilia, erythema, facial flushing, facial paresthesia, flu-like syndrome (fever, myalgia, malaise), hepatic necrosis, hepatic vein occlusion, liver enzymes increased (transient), paresthesia, photosensitivity, rash, renal functions test abnormalities, taste alteration, urticaria

Drug Interactions

Metabolism/Transport Effects Substrate of CYP1A2 (major), CYP2E1 (major); **Note:** Assignment of Major/Minor substrate status based on clinically relevant drug interaction potential

Avoid Concomitant Use

Avoid concomitant use of Dacarbazine with any of the following: BCG; CloZAPine; Natalizumab; Pimecrolimus; Tacrolimus (Topical); Vaccines (Live)

Increased Effect/Toxicity

Dacarbazine may increase the levels/effects of: CloZAPine; Leflunomide; Natalizumab; Vaccines (Live)

The levels/effects of Dacarbazine may be increased by: Abiraterone Acetate; CYP1A2 Inhibitors (Moderate); CYP1A2 Inhibitors (Strong); CYP2E1 Inhibitors (Moderate); CYP2E1 Inhibitors (Strong); Deferasirox; Denosumab; MAO Inhibitors; Pimecrolimus; Roflumilast; Tacrolimus (Topical); Trastuzumab

Decreased Effect

Dacarbazine may decrease the levels/effects of: BCG; Coccidioidin Skin Test; Sipuleucel-T; Vaccines (Inactivated); Vaccines (Live)

The levels/effects of Dacarbazine may be decreased by: CYP1A2 Inducers (Strong); Cyproterone; Echinacea; SORAfenib

Ethanol/Nutrition/Herb Interactions

Ethanol: Avoid ethanol (due to GI irritation).

Herb/Nutraceutical: Avoid dong quai, St John's wort (may also cause photosensitization).

Storage/Stability Store intact vials under refrigeration (2°C to 8°C). Protect from light. The following stability information has also been reported: Intact vials are stable for 3 months at room temperature (Cohen, 2007). Reconstituted solution is stable for 24 hours at room temperature (20°C) and 96 hours under refrigeration (4°C) when protected from light, although the manufacturer recommends use within 72 hours if refrigerated and 8 hours at room temperature. Solutions for infusion (in D_5W or NS) are stable for 24 hours at room temperature if protected from light. Decomposed drug turns pink.

Reconstitution Use appropriate precautions for handling and disposal. The manufacturer recommends reconstituting 100 mg and 200 mg vials with 9.9 mL and 19.7 mL SWFI, respectively, to a concentration of 10 mg/mL; some institutions use different standard dilutions (eg, 20 mg/mL).

Standard I.V. dilution: Dilute in 250-1000 mL D_5W or NS.

Mechanism of Action Alkylating agent which is converted to the active alkylating metabolite MTIC [(methyl-triazene-1-yl)-imidazole-4-carboxamide] via the cytochrome P450 system. The cytotoxic effects of MTIC are manifested through alkylation (methylation) of DNA at the O^6, N^7 guanine positions which lead to DNA double strand breaks and apoptosis. Non-cell cycle specific.

Pharmacodynamics/Kinetics

Distribution: V_d: 0.6 L/kg, exceeding total body water; suggesting binding to some tissue (probably liver)

Protein binding: ~5%

Metabolism: Extensively hepatic to the active metabolite MTIC [(methyl-triazene-1-yl)-imidazole-4-carboxamide]

Half-life elimination: Biphasic: Initial: 20-40 minutes, Terminal: 5 hours; Patients with renal and hepatic dysfunction: Initial: 55 minutes, Terminal: 7.2 hours

Excretion: Urine (~40% as unchanged drug)

Dosing

Adult & Geriatric Details concerning dosing in combination regimens should also be consulted.

Hodgkin's disease (combination chemotherapy): I.V.: 375 mg/m²/dose days 1 and 15 every 4 weeks (ABVD regimen)

Metastatic melanoma: I.V.: 250 mg/m²/dose days 1-5 every 3 weeks

Metastatic melanoma (unlabeled dosing; in combination with cisplatin and vinblastine): I.V:. 800 mg/m² on day 1 every 3 weeks (Atkins, 2008; Eton, 2002)

Soft tissue sarcoma (unlabeled use; MAID regimen): I.V.: 250 mg/m²/day continuous infusion for 4 days every 3 weeks (total of 1000 mg/m²/cycle) (Antman, 1993; Antman, 1990)

Pediatric Details concerning dosing in combination regimens should also be consulted.

Hodgkin's disease (combination chemotherapy): I.V.: 375 mg/m²/dose days 1 and 15 every 4 weeks (ABVD regimen; Hutchinson, 1998)

Renal Impairment The FDA-approved labeling does not contain dosage adjustment guidelines. The following guidelines have been used by some clinicians (Kintzel, 1995):

Cl_{cr} 46-60 mL/minute: Administer 80% of dose

Cl_{cr} 31-45 mL/minute: Administer 75% of dose

Cl_{cr} <30 mL/minute: Administer 70% of dose

Hepatic Impairment The FDA-approved labeling does not contain adjustment guidelines. May cause hepatotoxicity; monitor closely for signs of toxicity.

Combination Regimens

Lymphoma, Hodgkin:

ABVD Early Stage (Hodgkin) on page 1516

ABVD (Hodgkin) on page 1516

MOPP/ABVD (Hodgkin) on page 1714

Melanoma:

Cisplatin-Vinblastine-Dacarbazine (Melanoma) on page 1584

CVD-Interleukin-Interferon (Melanoma) on page 1597

Sarcoma:

CYVADIC on page 1605

MAID (Sarcoma) on page 1704

Soft tissue sarcoma: AD (Soft Tissue Sarcoma) on page 1519

Administration Infuse over 30-60 minutes; rapid infusion may cause severe venous irritation. May also be administered as a continuous infusion (unlabeled administration rate) depending on the protocol.

Extravasation management: Local pain, burning sensation, and irritation at the injection site may be relieved by local application of hot packs. If extravasation occurs, apply cold packs. Protect exposed tissue from light following extravasation.

Emetic Potential High (>90%)

Vesicant/Extravasation Risk May be an irritant

Monitoring Parameters CBC with differential, liver function

Dosage Forms Excipient information presented when available (limited, particularly for generics); consult specific product labeling.

Injection, powder for reconstitution: 100 mg, 200 mg

References

Antman K, Crowley J, Balcerzak SP, et al, "An Intergroup Phase III Randomized Study of Doxorubicin and Dacarbazine With or Without Ifosfamide and Mesna in Advanced Soft Tissue and Bone Sarcomas," *J Clin Oncol*, 1993, 11(7):1276-85.

Antman K, Crowley J, Balcerzak SP, et al, "A Southwest Oncology Group and Cancer and Leukemia Group B phase II Study of Doxorubicin, Dacarbazine, Ifosfamide, and Mesna in Adults With Advanced Osteosarcoma, Ewing's Sarcoma, and Rhabdomyosarcoma," *Cancer*, 1998, 82 (7):1288-95.

Atkins MB, Hsu J, Lee S, et al, "Phase III Trial Comparing Concurrent Biochemotherapy With Cisplatin, Vinblastine, Dacarbazine, Interleukin-2, and Interferon Alfa-2b With Cisplatin, Vinblastine, and Dacarbazine Alone in Patients With Metastatic Malignant Melanoma (E3695): A Trial Coordinated by the Eastern Cooperative Oncology Group," *J Clin Oncol*, 2008, 26(35):5748-54.

Cohen V, Jellinek SP, Teperikidis L, et al, "Room-Temperature Storage of Medications Labeled for Refrigeration," *Am J Health-Syst Pharm*, 2007, 64(16):1711-15.

Engert A, Franklin J, Eich HT, et al, "Two Cycles of Doxorubicin, Bleomycin, Vinblastine, and Dacarbazine Plus Extended-Field Radiotherapy is Superior to Radiotherapy Alone in Early Favorable Hodgkin's Lymphoma: Final Results of the GHSG HD7 Trial," *J Clin Oncol*, 2007, 25(23):3495-502.

Eton O, Legha SS, Bedikian AY, et al, "Sequential Biochemotherapy Versus Chemotherapy for Metastatic Melanoma: Results From a Phase III Randomized Trial," *J Clin Oncol*, 2002, 20 (8):2045-52.

Hutchinson RJ, Fryer CJ, Davis PC, et al, "MOPP or Radiation in Addition to ABVD in the Treatment of Pathologically Staged Advanced Hodgkin's Disease in Children: Results of the Children's Cancer Group Phase III Trial," *J Clin Oncol*, 1998, 16(3):897-906.

Kintzel PE and Dorr RT, "Anticancer Drug Renal Toxicity and Elimination: Dosing Guidelines for Altered Renal Function," *Cancer Treat Rev*, 1995, 21(1):33-64.

Marchesi F, Turriziani M, Tortorelli G, et al, "Triazene Compounds: Mechanism of Action and Related DNA Repair Systems," *Pharmacol Res*, 2007, 56(4):275-87.

Meyer RM, Gospodarowicz MK, Connors JM, et al, "Randomized Comparison of ABVD Chemotherapy With a Strategy That Includes Radiation Therapy in Patients With Limited-Stage Hodgkin's Lymphoma: National Cancer Institute of Canada Clinical Trials Group and the Eastern Cooperative Oncology Group," *J Clin Oncol*, 2005, 23(21):4634-42.

Middleton MR, Grob JJ, Aaronson N, et al, "Randomized Phase III Study of Temozolomide Versus Dacarbazine in the Treatment of Patients With Advanced Metastatic Malignant Melanoma," *J Clin Oncol*, 2000, 18(1):158-66.

Nocera M, Baudin E, Pellegriti G, et al, "Treatment of Advanced Medullary Thyroid Cancer With an Alternating Combination of Doxorubicin-Streptozocin and 5 FU-Dacarbazine, Groupe d'Etude des Tumeurs à Calcitonine (GETC)," *Br J Cancer*, 2000, 83(6):715-8.

Ramanathan RK, Cnaan A, Hahn RG, et al, "Phase II Trial of Dacarbazine (DTIC) in Advanced Pancreatic Islet Cell Carcinoma, Study of the Eastern Cooperative Oncology Group-E6282," *Ann Oncol*, 2001, 12(8):1139-43.

Straus DJ, Portlock CS, Qin J, et al, "Results of a Prospective Randomized Clinical Trial of Doxorubicin, Bleomycin, Vinblastine, and Dacarbazine (ABVD) Followed by Radiation Therapy (RT) Versus ABVD Alone for Stages I, II, and IIIA Nonbulky Hodgkin Disease," *Blood*, 2004, 104 (12):3483-9.

◆ **Dacarbazine for Injection (Can)** *see* Dacarbazine *on page* 367

◆ **Dacogen®** *see* Decitabine *on page 403*

◆ **DACT** *see* DACTINomycin *on page 371*

DACTINomycin (dak ti noe MYE sin)

Related Information

Management of Chemotherapy-Induced Nausea and Vomiting *on page 1786*
Management of Drug Extravasations *on page 1800*
Safe Handling of Hazardous Drugs *on page 1904*

Brand Names: U.S. Cosmegen®

Brand Names: Canada Cosmegen®

Index Terms ACT-D; Actinomycin; Actinomycin CI; Actinomycin D; DACT

Generic Availability (U.S.) Yes

Pharmacologic Category Antineoplastic Agent, Antibiotic

Use Treatment of Wilms' tumor, childhood rhabdomyosarcoma, Ewing's sarcoma, metastatic testicular tumors (nonseminomatous), gestational trophoblastic neoplasm; regional perfusion (palliative or adjunctive) of locally recurrent or locoregional solid tumors (sarcomas, carcinomas and adenocarcinomas)

Unlabeled Use Treatment of ovarian cancer (germ cell or stromal tumors), osteosarcoma, soft tissue sarcoma (other than rhabdomyosarcoma)

Labeled Contraindications Hypersensitivity to dactinomycin or any component of the formulation; patients with concurrent or recent chickenpox or herpes zoster

Pregnancy Risk Factor D

Lactation Excretion in breast milk unknown/not recommended

Warnings/Precautions [U.S. Boxed Warnings]. Hazardous agent - use appropriate precautions for handling and disposal. Dactinomycin is extremely irritating to tissues; if extravasation occurs during I.V. use, severe damage to soft tissues will occur; has led to contracture of the arm (rare). Avoid inhalation of vapors or contact with skin, mucous membrane, or eyes; avoid exposure during pregnancy. Recommended for I.V. administration only. The manufacturer recommends intermittent ice (15 minutes 4 times/day) for suspected extravasation. If accidental exposure occurs, immediately irrigate copiously for at least 15 minutes with water, saline, or balanced ophthalmic irrigation solution (eye exposure) and at least 15 minutes with water (skin exposure); prompt ophthalmic or medical consultation is also recommended. Contaminated clothing should be destroyed and shoes thoroughly cleaned prior to reuse.

May cause hepatic sinusoidal obstruction syndrome (SOS; formerly called veno-occlusive liver disease); use with caution in hepatobiliary dysfunction. Monitor for signs or symptoms of hepatic SOS, including bilirubin >1.4 mg/dL, unexplained weight gain, ascites, hepatomegaly, or unexplained right upper quadrant pain (Arndt, 2004). The risk of fatal SOS is increased in children <4 years of age.

Dactinomycin potentiates the effects of radiation therapy; use with caution in patients who have received radiation therapy; reduce dosages in patients who are receiving dactinomycin and radiation therapy simultaneously; combination with radiation therapy may result in increased toxicity (eg, GI toxicity, myelosuppression, severe oropharyngeal mucositis). Avoid dactinomycin use within 2 months of radiation treatment for right-sided Wilms' tumor, may increase the risk of hepatotoxicity.

Toxic effects may be delayed in onset (2-4 days following a course of treatment) and may require 1-2 weeks to reach maximum severity. Discontinue treatment with severe myelosuppression, diarrhea, or stomatitis. Long-term observation of cancer survivors is recommended due to the increased risk of second primary tumors following treatment with radiation and antineoplastic agents. Regional perfusion therapy may result in local limb edema, soft tissue damage, and possible venous thrombosis; leakage of dactinomycin into systemic circulation may result in hematologic toxicity, infection, impaired wound healing, and mucositis. Dosage is usually expressed in **MICRO**grams and should be calculated on the basis of body surface area (BSA) in obese or edematous adult patients (to relate dose to lean body mass). Avoid administration of live vaccines during dactinomycin treatment. Avoid use in infants <6 months of age (toxic effects may occur more frequently). May be associated with an increased risk of myelosuppression in the elderly; use with caution. **[U.S. Boxed Warning]: Should be administered under the supervision of an experienced cancer chemotherapy physician.**

Adverse Reactions Frequency not defined.

Central nervous system: Fatigue, fever, lethargy, malaise

Dermatologic: Acne, alopecia (reversible), cheilitis, erythema multiforme, increased pigmentation, sloughing, or erythema of previously irradiated skin; skin eruptions, Stevens-Johnson syndrome, toxic epidermal necrolysis

Endocrine & metabolic: Growth retardation, hyperuricemia, hypocalcemia

Gastrointestinal: Abdominal pain, anorexia, diarrhea, dysphagia, esophagitis, GI ulceration, mucositis, nausea, pharyngitis, proctitis, stomatitis, vomiting

Hematologic: Agranulocytosis, anemia, aplastic anemia, febrile neutropenia, leukopenia, myelosuppression (onset: 7 days, nadir: 14-21 days, recovery: 21-28 days), neutropenia, pancytopenia, reticulocytopenia, thrombocytopenia, thrombocytopenia (immune mediated)

Hepatic: Ascites, bilirubin increased, hepatic failure, hepatitis, hepatomegaly, hepatopathy thrombocytopenia syndrome, hepatotoxicity, liver function test abnormality, hepatic sinusoidal obstruction syndrome (SOS; veno-occlusive liver disease)

Local: Erythema, edema, epidermolysis, pain, tissue necrosis, and ulceration (following extravasation)

Neuromuscular & skeletal: Myalgia

Renal: Renal function abnormality

Respiratory: Pneumonitis

Miscellaneous: Anaphylactoid reaction, infection, sepsis (including neutropenic sepsis)

Drug Interactions

Metabolism/Transport Effects None known.

Avoid Concomitant Use

Avoid concomitant use of DACTINomycin with any of the following: BCG; CloZAPine; Natalizumab; Pimecrolimus; Tacrolimus (Topical); Vaccines (Live)

Increased Effect/Toxicity

DACTINomycin may increase the levels/effects of: CloZAPine; Leflunomide; Natalizumab; Vaccines (Live)

The levels/effects of DACTINomycin may be increased by: Denosumab; Pimecrolimus; Roflumilast; Tacrolimus (Topical); Trastuzumab

Decreased Effect

DACTINomycin may decrease the levels/effects of: BCG; Coccidioidin Skin Test; Sipuleucel-T; Vaccines (Inactivated); Vaccines (Live)

The levels/effects of DACTINomycin may be decreased by: Echinacea

Storage/Stability Store at controlled room temperature of 20°C to 25°C (68°F to 77°F). Protect from light and humidity. According to the manufacturer's labeling, recommended final concentrations (≥10 mcg/mL) are stable for 10 hours at room temperature but should be administered within 4 hours due to the lack of preservative.

Reconstitution Use appropriate precautions for handling and disposal. Reconstitute initially with 1.1 mL of preservative-free SWFI to yield a concentration of 500 mcg/mL (diluent containing preservatives will cause precipitation). May further dilute in D_5W or NS in glass or polyvinyl chloride (PVC) containers to a recommended concentration of ≥10 mcg/mL; final concentrations <10 mcg/mL are not recommended. Cellulose ester membrane filters may partially remove dactinomycin from solution and should not be used during preparation or administration.

Mechanism of Action Binds to the guanine portion of DNA intercalating between guanine and cytosine base pairs inhibiting DNA and RNA synthesis and protein synthesis

Pharmacodynamics/Kinetics

Distribution: Children: Extensive extravascular distribution (59-714 L) (Veal, 2005); does not penetrate blood-brain barrier

Metabolism: Minimal

Half-life elimination: ~36 hours; Children: Range: 14-43 hours (Veal, 2005)

Excretion: ~30% in urine and feces within 1week

Dosing

Adult Details concerning dosing in combination regimens should also be consulted. **Note: Medication orders for dactinomycin are commonly written in MICROgrams (eg, 150 mcg) although many regimens list the dose in MILLIgrams (eg, mg/kg or mg/m²).** The dose intensity per 2-week cycle should not exceed 15 mcg/kg/day for 5 days or 400-600 mcg/m²/day for 5 days. Some practitioners recommend calculation of the dosage for obese or edematous adult patients on the basis of body surface area in an effort to relate dosage to lean body mass.

Testicular cancer: I.V.: 1000 mcg/m² on day 1 (as part of a combination chemotherapy regimen)

Gestational trophoblastic neoplasm: I.V.: 12 mcg/kg/day for 5 days (monotherapy) **or** 500 mcg/dose days 1 and 2 (as part of a combination chemotherapy regimen)

Wilms' tumor, Ewing's sarcoma, rhabdomyosarcoma: I.V.: 15 mcg/kg/day for 5 days (in various combination regimens and schedules)

Regional perfusion (dosages and techniques may vary by institution; obese patients and patients with prior chemotherapy or radiation therapy may require lower doses): Lower extremity or pelvis: 50 mcg/kg; Upper extremity: 35 mcg/kg

Osteosarcoma (unlabeled use): I.V.: 600 mcg/m²/dose days 1, 2, and 3 of weeks 15, 31, 34, 39, and 42 (as part of a combination chemotherapy regimen) (Goorin, 2003)

Ovarian (germ cell) tumor (unlabeled use): I.V.: 500 mcg/day for 5 days every 4 weeks (in combination with vincristine and cyclophosphamide) (Gershenson, 1985) **or** 300 mcg/m²/day for 5 days every 4 weeks (in combination with vincristine and cyclophosphamide) (Slayton, 1985)

Geriatric Refer to adult dosing. Elderly patients are at increased risk of myelosuppression; dosing should begin at the low end of the dosing range.

Pediatric Details concerning dosing in combination regimens should also be consulted. **Note: Medication orders for dactinomycin are commonly written in MICROgrams (eg, 150 mcg) although many regimens list the dose in MILLIgrams (eg, mg/kg or mg/m^2).** The dose intensity per 2-week cycle should not exceed 15 mcg/kg/day for 5 days or 400-600 mcg/m^2/day for 5 days.

Wilms' tumor, rhabdomyosarcoma, Ewing's sarcoma: Children >6 months: I.V.: 15 mcg/kg/day for 5 days (in various combination regimens and schedules)

Unlabeled dosing:

Rhabdomyosarcoma: I.V.:

VAC regimen:

Children <1 year: 25 mcg/kg every 3 weeks, weeks 0 to 45 (in combination with vincristine and cyclophosphamide, and mesna); dose omission required following radiation therapy (Raney, 2011)

Children ≥1 year: 45 mcg/kg (maximum dose: 2500 mcg) every 3 weeks, weeks 0 to 45 (in combination with vincristine and cyclophosphamide, and mesna); dose omission required following radiation therapy (Raney, 2011)

Wilms' tumor: I.V.:

DD-4A regimen: 45 mcg/kg on day 1 every 6 weeks for 54 weeks (in combination with doxorubicin and vincristine) (Green, 1998)

EE-4A regimen: 45 mcg/kg on day 1 every 3 weeks for 18 weeks (in combination with vincristine) (Green, 1998)

VAD regimen:

Children <1 year: 750 mcg/m^2 every 6 weeks for 1 year (stage III disease) (in combination with vincristine and doxorubicin) (Pritchard, 1995)

Children ≥1 year: 1500 mcg/m^2 every 6 weeks for 1 year (stage III disease) (in combination with vincristine and doxorubicin) (Pritchard, 1995)

Osteosarcoma (unlabeled use): I.V.: 600 mcg/m^2/dose days 1, 2, and 3 of weeks 15, 31, 34, 39, and 42 (as part of a combination chemotherapy regimen) (Goorin, 2003)

Renal Impairment No dosage adjustment provided in the manufacturer's labeling; however, based on the amount of urinary excretion, dosage adjustments may not be necessary.

Hepatic Impairment

U.S. labeling: No dosage adjustment provided in manufacturer's labeling.

Canadian labeling:

Mild impairment: No dosage adjustment provided.

Moderate-severe impairment: Dose reduction may be considered; 33% to 50% dose reductions for patients with hyperbilirubinemia have been recommended by some clinicians.

Unlabeled dosing: Any transaminase increase: Reduce dose by 50%; may increase by monitoring toxicities (Floyd, 2006).

Combination Regimens

Gestational trophoblastic tumor:

EMA/CO on page 1622

EP/EMA on page 1625

Osteosarcoma: POG-8651 on page 1740

Ovarian cancer: Vincristine-Dactinomycin-Cyclophosphamide (Ovarian Cancer) on page 1771

Rhabdomyosarcoma:
- VAC Pulse on page 1767
- VAC (Rhabdomyosarcoma) on page 1767

Sarcoma: VAC Alternating With IE (Ewing's Sarcoma) on page 1766

Wilms' tumor:
- EE-4A (Wilms' Tumor) on page 1621
- DD-4A (Wilms' Tumor) on page 1606
- VAD (Wilms' Tumor) on page 1768

Administration I.V.: Administer by slow I.V. push or infuse over 10-15 minutes. Avoid extravasation. Do not filter with cellulose ester membrane filters. Do not administer I.M. or SubQ.

Emetic Potential Moderate (30% to 90%)

Vesicant/Extravasation Risk Vesicant; see Management of Drug Extravasations on page 1800.

Monitoring Parameters CBC with differential and platelet count, liver function tests, and renal function tests; monitor for signs/symptoms of hepatic SOS, including unexplained weight gain, ascites, hepatomegaly, or unexplained right upper quadrant pain (Arndt, 2004)

Test Interactions May interfere with bioassays of antibacterial drug levels

Dosage Forms Excipient information presented when available (limited, particularly for generics); consult specific product labeling.

Injection, powder for reconstitution: 0.5 mg

Cosmegen®: 0.5 mg [contains mannitol]

References

Arndt C, Hawkins, D, Anderson JR, et al, "Age is a Risk Factor for Chemotherapy-Induced Hepatopathy With Vincristine, Dactinomycin and Cyclophosphamide," *J Clin Oncol*, 2004, 22 (10):1894-901.

Bagshawe KD, "High-Risk Metastatic Trophoblastic Disease," *Obstet Gynecol Clin North Am*, 1988, 15(3):531-43.

Berkowitz RS and Goldstein DP, "Gestational Trophoblastic Disease," *Cancer*, 1995, 76(10 Suppl):2079-85.

Carli M, Pastore G, Perilongo G, et al, "Tumor Response and Toxicity After Single High Dose Versus Standard Five-Day Divided Dose Dactinomycin in Childhood Rhabdomyosarcoma," *J Clin Oncol*, 1988, 6(4):654-8.

Czauderna P, Katski K, Kowalczyk J, et al, "Venoocclusive Liver Disease (VOD) as a Complication of Wilms' Tumour Management in the Series of Consecutive 206 Patients," *Eur J Pediatr Surg*, 2000, 10(5):300-3.

D'Antiga L, Baker A, Pritchard J. et al, "Veno-Occlusive Disease With Multi-Organ Involvement Following Actinomycin-D," *Eur J Cancer*, 2001, 37(9):1141-8.

Floyd J, Mirza I, Sachs B, et al, "Hepatotoxicity of Chemotherapy," *Semin Oncol*, 2006, 33 (1):50-67.

Gershenson DM, Copeland LJ, Kavanagh JJ, et al, "Treatment of Malignant Nondysgerminomatous Germ Cell Tumors of the Ovary With Vincristine, Dactinomycin, and Cyclophosphamide," *Cancer*, 1985, 56(12):2756-61.

Goorin AM, Schwartzentruber DJ, Devidas M, et al, "Presurgical Chemotherapy Compared With Immediate Surgery and Adjuvant Chemotherapy for Nonmetastatic Osteosarcoma: Pediatric Oncology Group Study POG-8651," *J Clin Oncol*, 2003, 21(8):1574-80.

Green DM, Breslow NE, Beckwith JB, et al, "Effect of Duration of Treatment on Treatment Outcome and Cost of Treatment for Wilms' Tumor: A Report From the National Wilms' Tumor Study Group," *J Clin Oncol*, 1998, 16(12):3744-51.

Grier HE, Krailo MD, Tarbell NJ, et al, "Addition of Ifosfamide and Etoposide to Standard Chemotherapy for Ewing's Sarcoma and Primitive Neuroectodermal Tumor of Bone," *N Engl J Med*, 2003, 348(8):694-701.

Morgan C, Tillett T, Braybrooke J, et al, "Management of Uncommon Chemotherapy-Induced Emergencies," *Lancet Oncol*, 2011, 12(8):806-14.

Pritchard J, Imeson J, Barnes J, et al, "Results of the United Kingdom Children's Cancer Study Group First Wilms' Tumor Study," *J Clin Oncol*, 1995, 13(1):124-33.

Raney RB, Walterhouse DO, Meza JL, et al, "Results of the Intergroup Rhabdomyosarcoma Study Group D9602 Protocol, Using Vincristine and Dactinomycin With or Without Cyclophosphamide and Radiation Therapy, for Newly Diagnosed Patients With Low-Risk Embryonal Rhabdomyosarcoma: A Report From the Soft Tissue Sarcoma Committee of the Children's Oncology Group," *J Clin Oncol*, 2011, 29(10):1312-8.

Slayton RE, Park RC, Silverberg SG, et al, "Vincristine, Dactinomycin, and Cyclophosphamide in the Treatment of Malignant Germ Cell Tumors of the Ovary. A Gynecologic Oncology Group Study (A Final Report)," *Cancer*, 1985, 56(2):243-8.

Sulis ML, Bessmertny O, Granowetter L, et al, "Veno-Occlusive Disease in Pediatric Patients Receiving Actinomycin D and Vincristine Only for the Treatment of Rhabdomyosarcoma, *J Pediatr Hematol Oncol*, 2004, 26(12):843-6.

Veal GJ, Cole M, Errington J, et al, "Pharmacokinetics of Dactinomycin in a Pediatric Patient Population: A United Kingdom Children's Cancer Study Group Study," *Clin Cancer Res*, 2005, 11 (16):5893-9.

Dalteparin (dal TE pa rin)

Related Information

Venous Thromboembolism in the Cancer Patient *on page 1883*

Brand Names: U.S. Fragmin®

Brand Names: Canada Fragmin®

Index Terms Dalteparin Sodium

Generic Availability (U.S.) No

Pharmacologic Category Low Molecular Weight Heparin

Use Prevention of deep vein thrombosis (DVT) which may lead to pulmonary embolism, in patients requiring abdominal surgery who are at risk for thromboembolism complications (eg, patients >40 years of age, obesity, patients with malignancy, history of DVT or pulmonary embolism, and surgical procedures requiring general anesthesia and lasting >30 minutes); prevention of DVT in patients undergoing hip-replacement surgery; patients immobile during an acute illness; prevention of ischemic complications in patients with unstable angina or non-Q-wave myocardial infarction on concurrent aspirin therapy; in patients with cancer, extended treatment (6 months) of acute symptomatic venous thromboembolism (DVT and/or PE) to reduce the recurrence of venous thromboembolism

Canadian labeling: Additional use (unlabeled use in U.S.): Treatment of acute DVT; prevention of venous thromboembolism (VTE) in patients at risk of VTE undergoing general surgery; anticoagulant in extracorporeal circuit during hemodialysis and hemofiltration

Unlabeled Use Active treatment of deep vein thrombosis (noncancer patients)

Labeled Contraindications Hypersensitivity to dalteparin (eg, pruritus, rash, anaphylactic reactions) or any component of the formulation; history of heparin-induced thrombocytopenia (HIT) or HIT with thrombosis; hypersensitivity to heparin or pork products; active major bleeding; patients with unstable angina, non-Q-wave MI, or prolonged venous thromboembolism prophylaxis undergoing epidural/neuraxial anesthesia

Note: Use of dalteparin in patients with current HIT or HIT with thrombosis is **not** recommended and considered contraindicated due to high cross-reactivity to heparin-platelet factor-4 antibody (Guyatt [ACCP], 2012; Warkentin, 1999).

Canadian labeling: Additional contraindications (not in U.S. labeling): Septic endocarditis, major blood clotting disorders; acute gastroduodenal ulcer; cerebral hemorrhage; severe uncontrolled hypertension; diabetic or hemorrhagic retinopathy; other diseases that increase risk of hemorrhage; injuries to and operations on the CNS, eyes, and ears

Pregnancy Risk Factor B

Lactation Enters breast milk/use caution

Warnings/Precautions [U.S. Boxed Warning]: Spinal or epidural hematomas, including subsequent paralysis, may occur with recent or anticipated neuraxial anesthesia (epidural or spinal) or spinal puncture in patients anticoagulated with LMWH or heparinoids. Consider risk versus benefit prior to spinal procedures; risk is increased by the use of concomitant agents which may alter hemostasis, the use of indwelling epidural catheters for analgesia, a history of spinal deformity or spinal surgery, as well as traumatic or repeated epidural or spinal punctures. Use of dalteparin is contraindicated in patients undergoing epidural/neuraxial anesthesia. Patient should be observed closely for bleeding if enoxaparin is administered during or immediately following diagnostic lumbar puncture, epidural anesthesia, or spinal anesthesia.

Use with caution in patients with pre-existing thrombocytopenia, recent childbirth, subacute bacterial endocarditis, peptic ulcer disease, pericarditis or pericardial effusion, liver or renal function impairment, recent lumbar puncture, vasculitis, concurrent use of aspirin (increased bleeding risk), previous hypersensitivity to heparin, heparin-associated thrombocytopenia. Monitor platelet count closely. Cases of dalteparin-induced thrombocytopenia and thrombosis (similar to heparin-induced thrombocytopenia [HIT]), some complicated by organ infarction, limb ischemia, or death, have been observed. In patients with a history of HITor HIT with thrombosis, dalteparin is contraindicated. Consider discontinuation of therapy in any patient developing significant thrombocytopenia (eg, <100,000/mm^3) and/or thrombosis related to initiation of dalteparin especially when associated with a positive *in vitro* test for antiplatelet antibodies. Use caution in patients with congenital or drug-induced thrombocytopenia or platelet defects.

Monitor patient closely for signs or symptoms of bleeding. Certain patients are at increased risk of bleeding. Risk factors include bacterial endocarditis; congenital or acquired bleeding disorders; active ulcerative or angiodysplastic GI diseases; severe uncontrolled hypertension; hemorrhagic stroke; or use shortly after brain, spinal, or ophthalmology surgery; in patients treated concomitantly with platelet inhibitors; recent GI bleeding; thrombocytopenia or platelet defects; severe liver disease; hypertensive or diabetic retinopathy; or in patients undergoing invasive procedures.

Use with caution in patients with severe renal impairment; accumulation may occur with repeated dosing increasing the risk for bleeding. Multidose vials contain benzyl alcohol and should not be used in pregnant women. In neonates, large amounts of benzyl alcohol (>100 mg/kg/day) have been associated with fatal toxicity (gasping syndrome). Heparin can cause hyperkalemia by affecting aldosterone. Similar reactions could occur with dalteparin. Monitor for hyperkalemia. Do **not** administer intramuscularly. Not to be used interchangeably (unit for unit) with heparin or any other low molecular weight heparins.

There is no consensus for adjusting/correcting the weight-based dosage of LMWH for patients who are morbidly obese (BMI ≥40 kg/m^2). The American College of Chest Physicians Practice Guidelines suggest consulting with a pharmacist regarding dosing in bariatric surgery patients and other obese patients who may require higher doses of LMWH (Gould, 2012).

Adverse Reactions

Note: As with all anticoagulants, bleeding is the major adverse effect of dalteparin. Hemorrhage may occur at virtually any site. Risk is dependent on multiple variables.

>10%: Hematologic: Bleeding (3% to 14%), thrombocytopenia (including heparin-induced thrombocytopenia), <1%; cancer clinical trials: ~11%)

1% to 10%:

Hematologic: Major bleeding (up to 6%), wound hematoma (up to 3%)

Hepatic: AST >3 times upper limit of normal (5% to 9%), ALT >3 times upper limit of normal (4% to 10%)

Local: Pain at injection site (up to 12%), injection site hematoma (up to 7%)

<1% (Limited to important or life-threatening): Allergic reaction (fever, pruritus, rash, injections site reaction, bullous eruption), alopecia, anaphylactoid reaction, gastrointestinal bleeding, hemoptysis, operative site bleeding, skin necrosis, subdural hematoma, thrombosis (associated with heparin-induced thrombocytopenia). Spinal or epidural hematomas can occur following neuraxial anesthesia or spinal puncture, resulting in paralysis.

Drug Interactions

Metabolism/Transport Effects None known.

Avoid Concomitant Use

Avoid concomitant use of Dalteparin with any of the following: Omacetaxine; Rivaroxaban

Increased Effect/Toxicity

Dalteparin may increase the levels/effects of: Anticoagulants; Collagenase (Systemic); Dabigatran Etexilate; Deferasirox; Drotrecogin Alfa (Activated); Ibritumomab; Omacetaxine; Palifermin; Rivaroxaban; Tositumomab and Iodine I 131 Tositumomab

The levels/effects of Dalteparin may be increased by: 5-ASA Derivatives; Antiplatelet Agents; Dasatinib; Herbs (Anticoagulant/Antiplatelet Properties); Nonsteroidal Anti-Inflammatory Agents; Pentosan Polysulfate Sodium; Pentoxifylline; Prostacyclin Analogues; Salicylates; Thrombolytic Agents; Tipranavir; Vitamin E

Decreased Effect There are no known significant interactions involving a decrease in effect.

Ethanol/Nutrition/Herb Interactions Herb/Nutraceutical: Alfalfa, anise, bilberry, bladderwrack, bromelain, cat's claw, celery, chamomile, coleus, cordyceps, dong quai, evening primrose oil, fenugreek, feverfew, garlic, ginger, ginkgo biloba, ginseng (American), ginseng (panax), ginseng (Siberian), grapeseed, green tea, guggul, horse chestnut seed, horseradish, licorice, prickly ash, red clover, reishi, SAMe (s-adenosylmethionine), sweet clover, turmeric, white willow (all have additional antiplatelet/anticoagulant activity)

Storage/Stability Store at temperatures of 20°C to 25°C (68°F to 77°F). Multidose vials may be stored for up to 2 weeks at room temperature after entering.

Reconstitution Canadian labeling: If necessary, may dilute in isotonic sodium chloride or dextrose solutions to a concentration of 20 units/mL. Use within 24 hours of mixing.

Mechanism of Action Low molecular weight heparin analog with a molecular weight of 4000-6000 daltons; the commercial product contains 3% to 15% heparin with a molecular weight <3000 daltons, 65% to 78% with a molecular weight of 3000-8000 daltons and 14% to 26% with a molecular weight >8000 daltons; while dalteparin has been shown to inhibit both factor Xa and factor IIa (thrombin), the antithrombotic effect of dalteparin is characterized by a higher ratio of antifactor Xa to antifactor IIa activity (ratio = 4)

Pharmacodynamics/Kinetics

Onset of action: Anti-Xa activity: Within 1-2 hours

Duration: >12 hours

Distribution: V_d: 40-60 mL/kg

Protein binding: Low affinity for plasma proteins (Howard, 1997)

Bioavailability: SubQ: 81% to 93%

Half-life elimination (route dependent): Anti-Xa activity: 2-5 hours; prolonged in chronic renal insufficiency: 3.7-7.7 hours (following a single 5000 unit dose)

Time to peak, serum: Anti-Xa activity: ~4 hours

Excretion: Primarily renal (Howard, 1997)

Dosing

Adult & Geriatric Note: Each 2500 units of anti-Xa activity is equal to 16 mg of dalteparin.

Anticoagulant for hemodialysis and hemofiltration: I.V.: Canadian labeling (not in U.S. labeling):

Chronic renal failure with no other bleeding risks:

Hemodialysis/filtration ≤4 hours: I.V. bolus: 5,000 units

Hemodialysis/filtration >4 hours: I.V. bolus: 30-40 units/kg, followed by an infusion of 10-15 units/kg/hour (typically produces plasma concentrations of 0.5-1 units anti-Xa/mL)

Acute renal failure and high bleeding risk: I.V. bolus: 5-10 units/kg, followed by an infusion of 4-5 units/kg/hour (typically produces plasma concentrations of 0.2-0.4 units anti-Xa/mL)

DVT prophylaxis: Note: In morbidly obese patients (BMI ≥40 kg/m^2), increasing the prophylactic dose by 30% may be appropriate (Nutescu, 2009):

Abdominal surgery:

Low-to-moderate DVT risk: SubQ: 2500 units 1-2 hours prior to surgery, then once daily for 5-10 days postoperatively

High DVT risk: SubQ: 5000 units the evening prior to surgery and then once daily for 5-10 days postoperatively. Alternatively in patients with malignancy: 2500 units 1-2 hours prior to surgery, 2500 units 12 hours later, then 5000 units once daily for 5-10 days postoperatively.

General surgery with risk factors for VTE: Canadian labeling (not in U.S. labeling): 2500 units 1-2 hours preoperatively followed by 2500-5000 int.units every morning (may administer 2500 units no sooner than 4 hours after surgery and 8 hours after previous dose provided hemostasis has been achieved) or if other risk factors are present (eg, malignancy, heart failure), then may administer 5000 units the evening prior to surgery followed by 5000 units every evening postoperatively; continue treatment until patient is mobilized (approximately ≥5-7 days)

Total hip replacement surgery: SubQ: **Note:** Three treatment options are currently available. Dose is given for 5-10 days, although up to 14 days of treatment have been tolerated in clinical trials. The American College of Chest Physicians (ACCP) recommends a minimum duration of at least 10-14 days; extended duration of up to 35 days is suggested (Guyatt, 2012).

Postoperative regimen:

Initial: 2500 units 4-8 hours after surgery (or later if hemostasis not achieved). The ACCP recommends initiation ≥12 hours after surgery if postoperative regimen chosen (Guyatt, 2012).

Maintenance: 5000 int. units once daily; allow at least 6 hours to elapse after initial postsurgical dose (adjust administration time accordingly)

Preoperative regimen (starting day of surgery):

Initial: 2500 int. units within 2 hours **before** surgery. The ACCP recommends initiation ≥12 hours before surgery if preoperative regimen chosen (Guyatt, 2012). At 4-8 hours **after** surgery (or later if hemostasis not achieved), administer 2500 int. units.

Maintenance: 5000 units once daily; allow at least 6 hours to elpase after initial postsurgical dose (adjust administration time accordingly)

Preoperative regimen (starting evening prior to surgery):

Initial: 5000 int. units 10-14 hours **before** surgery. The ACCP recommends initiation ≥12 hours before surgery if preoperative regimen chosen (Guyatt, 2012). At 4-8 hours **after** surgery (or later if hemostasis not achieved), administer 5000 int. units.

Maintenance: 5000 int. units once daily, allowing 24 hours between doses

Immobility during acute illness: 5000 units once daily

Unstable angina or non-Q-wave myocardial infarction: SubQ: 120 units/kg body weight (maximum dose: 10,000 units) every 12 hours for up to 5-8 days with concurrent aspirin therapy. Discontinue dalteparin once patient is clinically stable.

Obesity: Use actual body weight to calculate dose; dose capping at 10,000 units recommended (Nutescu, 2009)

Venous thromboembolism, extended treatment in cancer patients: SubQ:

Initial (month 1): 200 units/kg (maximum dose: 18,000 units) once daily for 30 days

Maintenance (months 2-6): ~150 units/kg (maximum dose: 18,000 units) once daily. If platelet count between 50,000-100,000/mm^3, reduce dose by 2,500 units until platelet count recovers to ≥100,000/mm^3. If platelet count <50,000/mm^3, discontinue dalteparin until platelet count recover to >50,000/mm^3.

Obesity: Use actual body weight to calculate dose; dose capping is not recommended (Nutescu, 2009). However, the manufacturer recommends a maximum dose of 18,000 units per day for the treatment of VTE in cancer patients.

DVT (with or without PE) treatment in noncancer patients (unlabeled use in U.S.): SubQ: 200 units/kg once daily (Feissinger, 1996; Jaff, 2011; Wells, 2005) **or** 100 units/kg twice daily (Jaff, 2011). Use of once daily administration is suggested (Guyatt, 2012).

Canadian labeling: SubQ: 200 units/kg once daily (maximum dose: 18,000 units/day) **or** alternatively, may adapt dose as follows (SubQ):

46-56 kg: 10,000 units once daily

57-68 kg: 12,500 units once daily

69-82 kg: 15,000 units once daily

≥83 kg: 18,000 units once daily

Note: If increased bleeding risk, may give 100 units/kg SubQ twice daily. Concomitant treatment with a vitamin-K antagonist is usually initiated immediately.

Obesity: Use actual body weight to calculate dose; dose capping is not recommended (Nutescu, 2009). One study demonstrated similar anti-Xa levels after 3 days of therapy in obese patients (>40% above IBW; range: 82-190 kg) compared to those ≤20% above IBW or between 20% to 40% above IBW (Wilson, 2001).

Pregnant women: 200 units/kg/dose once daily or 100 units/kg/dose every 12 hours. Discontinue ≥24 hours prior to the induction of labor or cesarean section. Dalteparin therapy may be substituted with heparin near term. Continue anticoagulation therapy for ≥6 weeks postpartum (minimum duration of therapy: 3 months). LMWH or heparin therapy is preferred over warfarin during pregnancy (Bates, 2012).

Prevention of recurrent venous thromboembolism in pregnancy (unlabeled use): SubQ: 5000 units once daily. Therapy should continue for 6 weeks postpartum in high-risk women (Bates, 2012).

Renal Impairment Half-life is increased in patients with chronic renal failure, use with caution, accumulation can be expected; specific dosage adjustments have not been recommended. Accumulation was not observed in critically ill patients with severe renal insufficiency (Cl_{cr} <30 mL/minute) receiving prophylactic doses (5000 units) for a median of 7 days (Douketis, 2008). In cancer patients, receiving treatment for venous thromboembolism, if Cl_{cr} <30 mL/minute, manufacturer recommends monitoring anti-Xa levels to determine appropriate dose.

Hepatic Impairment No dosage adjustment provided in manufacturer's labeling; use with caution.

Administration

For deep SubQ injection; may be injected in a U-shape to the area surrounding the navel, the upper outer side of the thigh, or the upper outer quadrangle of the buttock. Use thumb and forefinger to lift a fold of skin when injecting dalteparin to the navel area or thigh. Insert needle at a 45- to 90-degree angle. The entire length of needle should be inserted. Do not expel air bubble from fixed-dose syringe prior to injection. Air bubble (and extra solution, if applicable) may be expelled from graduated syringes. In order to minimize bruising, do not rub injection site.

To convert from I.V. unfractionated heparin (UFH) infusion to SubQ dalteparin (Nutescu, 2007): Calculate specific dose for dalteparin based on indication, discontinue UFH and begin dalteparin within 1 hour

To convert from SubQ dalteparin to I.V. UFH infusion (Nutescu, 2007): Discontinue dalteparin; calculate specific dose for I.V. UFH infusion based on indication; omit heparin bolus/loading dose

Converting from SubQ dalteparin dosed every 12 hours: Start I.V. UFH infusion 10-11 hours after last dose of dalteparin

Converting from SubQ dalteparin dosed every 24 hours: Start I.V. UFH infusion 22-23 hours after last dose of dalteparin

I.V. (Canadian labeling; not an approved route in U.S. labeling): Administer as bolus I.V. injection or as continuous infusion. Recommended concentration for infusion: 20 units/mL.

Monitoring Parameters Periodic CBC including platelet count; stool occult blood tests; monitoring of PT and PTT is not necessary. Once patient has received 3-4 doses, anti-Xa levels, drawn 4-6 hours after dalteparin administration, may be used to monitor effect in patients with severe renal dysfunction or if abnormal coagulation parameters or bleeding should occur. For patients >190 kg, if anti-Xa monitoring is available, adjusting dose based on anti-Xa levels is recommended; if anti-Xa monitoring is unavailable, reduce dose if bleeding occurs (Nutescu, 2009).

Dosage Forms Excipient information presented when available (limited, particularly for generics); consult specific product labeling.

Injection, solution:

Fragmin®: 25,000 anti-Xa units/mL (3.8 mL) [contains benzyl alcohol]

Injection, solution [preservative free]:

Fragmin®: 10,000 anti-Xa units/mL (1 mL); 2500 anti-Xa units/0.2 mL (0.2 mL); 5000 anti-Xa units/0.2 mL (0.2 mL); 7500 anti-Xa units/0.3 mL (0.3 mL); 12,500 anti-Xa units/0.5 mL (0.5 mL); 15,000 anti-Xa units/0.6 mL (0.6 mL); 18,000 anti-Xa units/0.72 mL (0.72 mL)

References

Fiessinger JN, Lopez-Fernandez M, Gatterer E, et al, "Once-Daily Subcutaneous Dalteparin, a Low Molecular Weight Heparin, for the Initial Treatment of Acute Deep Vein Thrombosis," *Thromb Haemost*, 1996, 76(2):195-9.

Geerts WH, Bergqvist D, Pineo GF, et al, "Prevention of Venous Thromboembolism: American College of Chest Physicians Evidence-Based Clinical Practice Guidelines (8th Edition)," *Chest*, 2008, 133(6 Suppl):381S-453S.

Guyatt GH, Akl EA, Crowther M, et al, "Executive Summary: Antithrombotic Therapy and Prevention of Thrombosis, 9th ed: American College of Chest Physicians Evidence-Based Clinical Practice Guidelines," *Chest*, 2012, 141(2 Suppl):7-47.

Hirsh J, Bauer KA, Donati MB, et al, "Parenteral Anticoagulants: American College of Chest Physicians Evidence-Based Clinical Practice Guidelines (8th Edition)," *Chest*, 2008, 133(6 Suppl):141-59.

Hirsh J, Guyatt G, Albers GW, et al, "Executive Summary: American College of Chest Physicians Evidence-Based Clinical Practice Guidelines (8th Edition)," *Chest*, 2008, 133(6 Suppl):71-109.

Jaff MR, McMurtry MS, Archer SL, et al, "Management of Massive and Submassive Pulmonary Embolism, Iliofemoral Deep Vein Thrombosis, and Chronic Thromboembolic Pulmonary Hypertension: A Scientific Statement from the American Heart Association," *Circulation*, 2011, 123 (16):1788-830.

Lee AY, Levine MN, Baker RI, et al, "Low-Molecular-Weight Heparin Versus a Coumarin for the Prevention of Recurrent Venous Thromboembolism in Patients with Cancer," *N Engl J Med*, 2003, 349(2):146-53.

Lee AY, Rickels FR, Julian JA, et al, "Randomized Comparison of Low Molecular Weight Heparin and Coumarin Derivatives on the Survival of Patients With Cancer and Venous Thromboembolism," *J Clin Oncol*, 2005, 23(10):2123-9.

Mechanick JI, Kushner RF, Sugerman HJ, et al, "American Association of Clinical Endocrinologists, The Obesity Society, and American Society for Metabolic & Bariatric Surgery Medical Guidelines for Clinical Practice for the Perioperative Nutritional, Metabolic, and Nonsurgical Support of the Bariatric Surgery Patient," *Obesity*, 2009, 17(Suppl 1):1-70.

Nagge J, Crowther M, and Hirsh J, "Is Impaired Renal Function a Contraindication to the Use of Low-Molecular Weight Heparin?" *Arch Intern Med*, 2002, 162(22):2605-9.

Nutescu EA and Dager W, "Heparin, Low Molecular Weight Heparin, and Fondaparinux," *Managing Anticoagulation Patients in the Hospital*, Gulseth M ed, American Society of Health-System Pharmacists®, Bethesda, MD: 2007, 181.

Nutescu EA, Spinler SA, Wittkowsky A, et al, "Low-Molecular-Weight Heparins in Renal Impairment and Obesity: Available Evidence and Clinical Practice Recommendations Across Medical and Surgical Settings," *Ann Pharmacother*, 2009, 43(6):1064-83.

Wells PS, Anderson DR, Rodger MA, et al, "Randomized Trial Comparing 2 Low-Molecular-Weight Heparins for the Outpatient Treatment of Deep Vein Thrombosis and Pulmonary Embolism," *Arch Intern Med*, 2005, 165(7):733-8.

Wilson SJ, Wilbur K, Burton E, et al, "Effect of Patient Weight on the Anticoagulant Response to Adjusted Therapeutic Dosage of Low-Molecular-Weight Heparin for the Treatment of Venous Thromboembolism," *Haemostasis*, 2001, 31(1):42-8.

◆ **Dalteparin Sodium** *see* Dalteparin *on page* *376*

Darbepoetin Alfa (dar be POE e tin AL fa)

Brand Names: U.S. Aranesp®; Aranesp® SingleJect®

Brand Names: Canada Aranesp®

Index Terms Erythropoiesis-Stimulating Agent (ESA); Erythropoiesis-Stimulating Protein; NESP; Novel Erythropoiesis-Stimulating Protein

Generic Availability (U.S.) No

Pharmacologic Category Colony Stimulating Factor; Erythropoiesis-Stimulating Agent (ESA); Growth Factor; Recombinant Human Erythropoietin

Use Treatment of anemia due to concurrent myelosuppressive chemotherapy in patients with cancer (nonmyeloid malignancies) receiving chemotherapy (palliative intent) for a planned minimum of 2 additional months of chemotherapy; treatment of anemia due to chronic kidney disease (including patients on dialysis and not on dialysis)

Note: Darbepoetin is **not** indicated for use under the following conditions:
- Cancer patients receiving hormonal therapy, therapeutic biologic products, or radiation therapy unless also receiving concurrent myelosuppressive chemotherapy
- Cancer patients receiving myelosuppressive chemotherapy when the expected outcome is curative
- As a substitute for RBC transfusion in patients requiring immediate correction of anemia

Note: In clinical trials, darbepoetin has not demonstrated improved quality of life, fatigue, or well-being.

Unlabeled Use Treatment of symptomatic anemia in myelodysplastic syndrome (MDS)

Labeled Contraindications Hypersensitivity to darbepoetin or any component of the formulation; uncontrolled hypertension; pure red cell aplasia (due to darbepoetin or other erythropoietin protein drugs)

Pregnancy Risk Factor C

Lactation Excretion in breast milk unknown/use caution

Warnings/Precautions [U.S. Boxed Warning]: Erythropoiesis-stimulating agents (ESAs) increased the risk of serious cardiovascular events, thromboembolic events, stroke, and/or tumor progression in clinical studies when administered to target hemoglobin levels >11 g/dL (and provide no additional benefit); a rapid rise in hemoglobin (>1 g/dL over 2 weeks) may also contribute to these risks. **[U.S. Boxed Warning]: A shortened overall survival and/or increased risk of tumor progression or recurrence has been reported in studies with breast, cervical, head and neck, lymphoid, and nonsmall cell lung cancer patients.** It is of note that in these studies, patients received ESAs to a target hemoglobin of ≥12 g/dL; although risk has not been excluded when dosed to achieve a target hemoglobin of <12 g/dL. **[U.S. Boxed Warnings]: To decrease these risks, and risk of cardio- and thrombovascular events, use ESAs in cancer patients only for the treatment of anemia related to concurrent myelosuppressive chemotherapy and use the lowest dose needed to avoid red blood cell transfusions. Discontinue ESA following completion of the chemotherapy course. ESAs are <u>not</u> indicated for patients receiving myelosuppressive therapy when the anticipated outcome is curative.** A dosage modification is appropriate if hemoglobin levels rise >1 g/dL per 2-week time period during treatment (Rizzo, 2010). Use of ESAs has been associated with an increased risk of venous thromboembolism (VTE) without a reduction in transfusions in patients >65 years of age with cancer (Hershman, 2009). Improved anemia symptoms, quality of life, fatigue, or well-being have not been demonstrated in controlled clinical trials. **[U.S. Boxed Warning]: Because of the risks of decreased survival and increased risk of tumor growth or progression, all healthcare providers and hospitals are required to enroll and comply with the ESA APPRISE (Assisting Providers and Cancer Patients with Risk Information for the Safe use of ESAs) Oncology Program prior to prescribing or dispensing ESAs to**

cancer patients. Prescribers and patients will have to provide written documentation of discussed risks prior to each course.

[U.S. Boxed Warning]: An increased risk of death, serious cardiovascular events, and stroke was reported in patients with chronic kidney disease (CKD) administered ESAs to target hemoglobin levels ≥11 g/dL; use the lowest dose sufficient to reduce the need for RBC transfusions. An optimal target hemoglobin level, dose or dosing strategy to reduce these risks has not been identified in clinical trials. Hemoglobin rising >1 g/dL in a 2-week period may contribute to the risk (dosage reduction recommended). CKD patients who exhibit an inadequate hemoglobin response to ESA therapy may be at a higher risk for cardiovascular events and mortality compared to other patients. ESA therapy may reduce dialysis efficacy (due to increase in red blood cells and decrease in plasma volume); adjustments in dialysis parameters may be needed. Patients treated with epoetin may require increased heparinization during dialysis to prevent clotting of the extracorporeal circuit. CKD patients not requiring dialysis may have a better response to darbepoetin and may require lower doses. An increased risk of DVT has been observed in patients treated with epoetin undergoing surgical orthopedic procedures. Darbepoetin is **not** approved for reduction in allogeneic red blood cell transfusions in patients scheduled for surgical procedures. The risk for seizures is increased with darbepoetin use in patients with CKD; use with caution in patients with a history of seizures. Monitor closely for neurologic symptoms during the first several months of therapy. Use with caution in patients with hypertension; hypertensive encephalopathy has been reported. Use is contraindicated in patients with uncontrolled hypertension. If hypertension is difficult to control, reduce or hold darbepoetin alfa. Due to the delayed onset of erythropoiesis, darbepoetin alfa is **not** recommended for acute correction of severe anemia or as a substitute for emergency transfusion. Consider discontinuing in patients who receive a renal transplant.

Prior to treatment, correct or exclude deficiencies of iron, vitamin B_{12}, and/or folate, as well as other factors which may impair erythropoiesis (inflammatory conditions, infections, bleeding). Prior to and during therapy, iron stores must be evaluated. Supplemental iron is recommended if serum ferritin <100 mcg/L or serum transferrin saturation <20%; most patients with CKD will require iron supplementation. Poor response should prompt evaluation of these potential factors, as well as possible malignant processes and hematologic disease (thalassemia, refractory anemia, myelodysplastic disorder), occult blood loss, hemolysis, osteitis fibrosa cystic, and/or bone marrow fibrosis. Severe anemia and pure red cell aplasia (PRCA) with associated neutralizing antibodies to erythropoietin has been reported, predominantly in patients with CKD receiving SubQ darbepoetin (the I.V. route is preferred for hemodialysis patients). Cases have also been reported in patients with hepatitis C who were receiving ESAs, interferon, and ribavirin. Patients with a sudden loss of response to darbepoetin (with severe anemia and a low reticulocyte count) should be evaluated for PRCA with associated neutralizing antibodies to erythropoietin; discontinue treatment (permanently) in patients with PRCA secondary to neutralizing antibodies to erythropoietin. Antibodies may cross-react; do not switch to another ESA in patients who develop antibody-mediated anemia.

Potentially serious allergic reactions have been reported (rarely). Discontinue immediately (and permanently) in patients who experience serious allergic/anaphylactic reactions. Some products may contain albumin and the packaging of some formulations may contain latex.

Adverse Reactions

>10%:

Cardiovascular: Hypertension (31%), peripheral edema (17%), edema (6% to 13%)

Gastrointestinal: Abdominal pain (10% to 13%)

Respiratory: Dyspnea (17%), cough (12%)

1% to 10%:

Cardiovascular: Angina, fluid overload, hypotension, MI, thromboembolic events

Central nervous system: Cerebrovascular disorder

Dermatologic: Rash/erythema

Local: AV graft thrombosis, vascular access complications

Respiratory: Pulmonary embolism

<1%, postmarketing, and/or case reports: Allergic reaction, anaphylactic reactions, anemia associated with neutralizing antibodies (severe; with or without other cytopenias), angioedema, bronchospasm, hypertensive encephalopathy, pure red cell aplasia (PRCA), seizure, stroke, tumor progression/recurrence (cancer patients), urticaria

Drug Interactions

Metabolism/Transport Effects None known.

Avoid Concomitant Use There are no known interactions where it is recommended to avoid concomitant use.

Increased Effect/Toxicity There are no known significant interactions involving an increase in effect.

Decreased Effect There are no known significant interactions involving a decrease in effect.

Ethanol/Nutrition/Herb Interactions Ethanol: Should be avoided due to adverse effects on erythropoiesis.

Storage/Stability Store at 2°C to 8°C (36°F to 46°F); do not freeze. Do not shake. Protect from light. Store in original carton until use. The following stability information has also been reported. May be stored at room temperature for up to 7 days (Cohen, 2007).

Mechanism of Action Induces erythropoiesis by stimulating the division and differentiation of committed erythroid progenitor cells; induces the release of reticulocytes from the bone marrow into the bloodstream, where they mature to erythrocytes. There is a dose response relationship with this effect. This results in an increase in reticulocyte counts followed by a rise in hematocrit and hemoglobin levels. When administered SubQ or I.V., darbepoetin's half-life is ~3 times that of epoetin alfa concentrations.

Pharmacodynamics/Kinetics

Onset of action: Increased hemoglobin levels not generally observed until 2-6 weeks after initiating treatment

Absorption: SubQ: Slow

Distribution: V_d: 0.06 L/kg

Bioavailability: CKD: SubQ: Adults: ~37% (range: 30% to 50%); Children: 54% (range: 32% to 70%)

Half-life elimination:

CKD: Adults:

I.V.: 21 hours

SubQ: Nondialysis patients: 70 hours (range: 35-139 hours); Dialysis patients: 46 hours (range: 12-89 hours)

Cancer: Adults: SubQ: 74 hours (range: 24-144 hours); Children: 49 hours

Note: Darbepoetin half-life is approximately threefold longer than epoetin alfa following I.V. administration

Time to peak: SubQ:

CKD: Adults: 48 hours (range: 12-72 hours; independent of dialysis); Children: 36 hours (range: 10-58 hours)

Cancer: Adults: 71-90 hours (range: 28-123 hours); Children: 71 hours (range: 21-143 hours)

Dosing

Adult & Geriatric

Anemia associated with chronic kidney disease (CKD): Individualize dosing and use the lowest dose necessary to reduce the need for RBC transfusions.

Chronic kidney disease patients ***ON dialysis*** (I.V. route is preferred for hemodialysis patients; initiate treatment when hemoglobin is <10 g/dL; reduce dose or interrupt treatment if hemoglobin approaches or exceeds 11 g/dL): I.V., SubQ: Initial: 0.45 mcg/kg once weekly **or** 0.75 mcg/kg once every 2 weeks **or** epoetin alfa doses of <1500 to ≥90,000 units per week may be converted to doses ranging from 6.25-200 mcg darbepoetin alfa per week (see adult column in conversion table).

Chronic kidney disease patients ***NOT on dialysis*** (consider initiating treatment when hemoglobin is <10 g/dL; use only if rate of hemoglobin decline would likely result in RBC transfusion and desire is to reduce risk of alloimmunization or other RBC transfusion-related risks; reduce dose or interrupt treatment if hemoglobin exceeds 10 g/dL): I.V., SubQ: Initial: 0.45 mcg/kg once every 4 weeks

Dosage adjustments for chronic kidney disease patients (either on dialysis or not on dialysis): Do not increase dose more frequently than every 4 weeks (dose decreases may occur more frequently).

If hemoglobin increases >1 g/dL in any 2-week period: Decrease dose by ≥25%

If hemoglobin does not increase by >1 g/dL after 4 weeks: Increase dose by 25%

Inadequate or lack of response: If adequate response is not achieved over 12 weeks, further increases are unlikely to be of benefit and may increase the risk for adverse events; use the minimum effective dose that will maintain a hemoglobin level sufficient to avoid red blood cell transfusions **and** evaluate patient for other causes of anemia; discontinue treatment if responsiveness does not improve

Anemia due to chemotherapy in cancer patients: Initiate treatment only if hemoglobin <10 g/dL and anticipated duration of myelosuppressive chemotherapy is ≥2 months. Titrate dosage to use the minimum effective dose that will maintain a hemoglobin level sufficient to avoid red blood cell transfusions. Discontinue darbepoetin following completion of chemotherapy.

SubQ: Initial: 2.25 mcg/kg once weekly **or** 500 mcg once every 3 weeks until completion of chemotherapy

Dosage adjustments:

Increase dose: If hemoglobin does not increase by 1 g/dL **and** remains below 10 g/dL after initial 6 weeks (for patients receiving weekly therapy only), increase dose to 4.5 mcg/kg once weekly (no dosage adjustment if using every 3 week dosing).

Reduce dose by 40% if hemoglobin increases >1g/dL in any 2-week period **or** hemoglobin reaches a level sufficient to avoid red blood cell transfusion.

Withhold dose if hemoglobin exceeds a level needed to avoid red blood cell transfusion. Resume treatment with a 40% dose reduction when hemoglobin approaches a level where transfusions may be required.

Discontinue: On completion of chemotherapy or if after 8 weeks of therapy there is no hemoglobin response or RBC transfusions still required

Symptomatic anemia associated with MDS (unlabeled use): SubQ: 150-300 mcg once weekly (NCCN MDS guidelines v.2.2011)

Conversion from epoetin alfa to darbepoetin alfa: See table.

Conversion From Epoetin Alfa to Darbepoetin Alfa (Initial Dose)

Previous Dosage of Epoetin Alfa (units/week)	Children Darbepoetin Alfa Dosage (mcg/week)	Adults Darbepoetin Alfa Dosage (mcg/week)
<1500	Not established	6.25
1500-2499	6.25	6.25
2500-4999	10	12.5
5000-10,999	20	25
11,000-17,999	40	40
18,000-33,999	60	60
34,000-89,999	100	100
≥90,000	200	200

Note: In patients receiving epoetin alfa 2-3 times per week, darbepoetin alfa is administered once weekly. In patients receiving epoetin alfa once weekly, darbepoetin alfa is administered once every 2 weeks. The darbepoetin dose to be administered every 2 weeks is derived by adding together 2 weekly epoetin alfa doses and then converting to the appropriate darbepoetin dose. Titrate dose to hemoglobin response thereafter.

Pediatric

Anemia associated with chronic kidney disease (CKD): Individualize dosing and use the lowest dose necessary to reduce the need for RBC transfusions.

*Chronic kidney disease patients **ON dialysis*** (I.V. route is preferred for hemodialysis patients; initiate treatment when hemoglobin is <10 g/dL; reduce dose or interrupt treatment if hemoglobin approaches or exceeds 11 g/dL): Children ≥1 year: I.V., SubQ: Conversion from epoetin alfa: Initial dose: Epoetin alfa doses of 1500 to ≥90,000 units per week may be converted to doses ranging from 6.25-200 mcg darbepoetin alfa per week (see pediatric column in conversion table)

Dosage adjustments for chronic kidney disease patients: Do not increase dose more frequently than every 4 weeks (dose decreases may occur more frequently).

If hemoglobin increases >1 g/dL in any 2-week period: Decrease dose by ≥25%

If hemoglobin does not increase by >1 g/dL after 4 weeks: Increase dose by 25%

Inadequate or lack of response: If adequate response is not achieved over 12 weeks, further increases are unlikely to be of benefit and may increase the risk for adverse events; use the minimum effective dose that will maintain a hemoglobin level sufficient to avoid red blood cell transfusions **and** evaluate patient for other causes of anemia; discontinue treatment if responsiveness does not improve

Administration May be administered by SubQ or I.V. injection. The I.V. route is recommended in hemodialysis patients. Do not shake; vigorous shaking may denature darbepoetin alfa, rendering it biologically inactive. Do not dilute or administer in conjunction with other drug solutions. Discard any unused portion of the vial; do not pool unused portions.

Monitoring Parameters Hemoglobin (at least once per week until maintenance dose established and after dosage changes; monitor less frequently once hemoglobin is stabilized); CKD patients should be also be monitored at least monthly following hemoglobin stability); iron stores (transferrin saturation and ferritin) prior to and during therapy; serum chemistry (CKD patients); blood pressure; fluid balance (CKD patients); seizures (CKD patients following initiation for first few months, includes new-onset or change in seizure frequency or premonitory symptoms)

Cancer patients: Examinations recommended by the ASCO/ASH guidelines (Rizzo, 2010) prior to treatment include peripheral blood smear (in some situations a bone marrow exam may be necessary), assessment for iron, folate, or vitamin B_{12} deficiency, reticulocyte count, renal function status, and occult blood loss; during ESA treatment, assess baseline and periodic iron, total iron-binding capacity, and transferrin saturation or ferritin levels.

Dietary Considerations Supplemental iron intake may be required in patients with low iron stores.

Additional Information Oncology Comment: The American Society of Clinical Oncology (ASCO) and American Society of Hematology (ASH) 2010 updates to the clinical practice guidelines for the use of erythropoiesis-stimulating agents (ESAs) in patients with cancer indicate that ESAs are appropriate when used according to the parameters identified within the Food and Drug Administration (FDA) approved labeling for epoetin and darbepoetin (Rizzo, 2010). ESAs are an option for chemotherapy associated anemia when the hemoglobin has fallen to <10 g/dL to decrease the need for RBC transfusions. ESAs should only be used in conjunction with concurrent chemotherapy. Although the FDA label now limits ESA use to the palliative setting, the ASCO/ASH guidelines suggest using clinical judgment in weighing risks versus benefits as formal outcomes studies of ESA use defined by intent of chemotherapy treatment have not been conducted.

The ASCO/ASH guidelines continue to recommend following the FDA approved dosing (and dosing adjustment) guidelines as alternate dosing and schedules have not demonstrated consistent differences in effectiveness with regard to hemoglobin response. In patients who do not have a response within 6-8 weeks (hemoglobin rise <1-2 g/dL or no reduction in transfusions) ESA therapy should be discontinued.

Prior to the initiation of ESAs, other sources of anemia (in addition to chemotherapy or underlying hematologic malignancy) should be investigated. Examinations recommended prior to treatment include peripheral blood smear (in some situations a bone marrow exam may be necessary), assessment for iron, folate, or vitamin B_{12} deficiency, reticulocyte count, renal function status, and occult blood loss. During ESA treatment, assess baseline and periodic iron, total iron-binding capacity, and transferrin saturation or ferritin levels. Iron supplementation may be necessary.

The guidelines note that patients with an increased risk of thromboembolism (generally includes previous history of thrombosis, surgery, and/or prolonged periods of immobilization) and patients receiving concomitant medications that may increase thromboembolic risk, should begin ESA therapy only after careful consideration. With the exception of low-risk myelodysplasia-associated anemia (which has evidence supporting the use of ESAs without concurrent chemotherapy), the guidelines do not support the use of ESAs in the absence of concurrent chemotherapy.

Prescribing and Access Restrictions As a requirement of the REMS program, access to this medication is restricted. Healthcare providers and hospitals must be enrolled in the ESA APPRISE (Assisting Providers and Cancer Patients with Risk Information for the Safe use of ESAs) Oncology Program (866-284-8089; http://www.esa-apprise.com) to prescribe or dispense ESAs (ie, darbepoetin alfa, epoetin alfa) to patients with cancer.

Medication Guide Available Yes

Dosage Forms Excipient information presented when available (limited, particularly for generics); consult specific product labeling.

Injection, solution [preservative free]:

Aranesp®: 25 mcg/mL (1 mL); 40 mcg/mL (1 mL); 60 mcg/mL (1 mL), 100 mcg/mL (1 mL); 150 mcg/0.75 mL (0.75 mL); 200 mcg/mL (1 mL); 300 mcg/mL (1 mL) [contains polysorbate 80]

Aranesp® SingleJect®: 25 mcg/0.42 mL (0.42 mL); 40 mcg/0.4 mL (0.4 mL); 60 mcg/0.3 mL (0.3 mL); 100 mcg/0.5 mL (0.5 mL); 150 mcg/0.3 mL (0.3 mL); 200 mcg/0.4 mL (0.4 mL); 300 mcg/0.6 mL (0.6 mL); 500 mcg/mL (1 mL) [contains natural rubber/natural latex in packaging, polysorbate 80]

References

Andre JL, Deschenes G, Boudaillies B, et al, "Darbepoetin, Effective Treatment of Anaemia in Paediatric Patients With Chronic Renal Failure," *Pediatr Nephrol*, 2007, 22(5):708-14.

Bennett CL, Silver SM, Djulbegovic B, et al, "Venous Thromboembolism and Mortality Associated With Recombinant Erythropoietin and Darbepoetin Administration for the Treatment of Cancer-Associated Anemia," *JAMA*, 2008, 299(8):914-24.

Bristoyiannis G, Germanos N, Grekas D, et al, "Unit Dosing of Darbepoetin Alfa for the Treatment of Anemia in Patients With End-Stage Renal Disease Being Switched From Recombinant Human Erythropoetin: Results of a Phase IIIb, 27-Week, Multicenter, Open-Label Study in Greek Patients," *Curr Ther Res*, 2005, 66(3):195-211.

Canon JL, Vansteenkiste J, Bodoky G, et al, "Randomized, Double-Blind, Active-Controlled Trial of Every-3-Week Darbepoetin Alfa for the Treatment of Chemotherapy-Induced Anemia," *J Natl Cancer Inst*, 2006, 98(4):273-84.

Giraldo P, Nomdedeu B, Loscertales J, et al, "Darbepoetin Alpha for the Treatment of Anemia in Patients With Myelodysplastic Syndromes," *Cancer*, 2006, 107(12):2807-16.

Hershman DL, Buono DL, Malin J, et al, "Patterns of Use and Risks Associated With Erythropoiesis-Stimulating Agents Among Medicare Patients With Cancer," *J Natl Cancer Inst*, 2009, 101 (23):1-9.

Hesketh PJ, Arena F, Patel D, et al, "A Randomized Controlled Trial of Darbepoetin Alfa Administered as a Fixed or Weight-Based Dose Using a Front-Loading Schedule in Patients With Anemia Who Have Nonmyeloid Malignancies," *Cancer*, 2004, 100(4):859-68.

National Comprehensive Cancer Network® (NCCN), "Practice Guidelines in Oncology™: Cancer- and Chemotherapy-Induced Anemia Version 1.2011." Available at http://www.nccn.org/professionals/physician_gls/PDF/anemia.pdf

National Comprehensive Cancer Network® (NCCN), "Practice Guidelines in Oncology™: Myelodysplastic Syndromes Version 2.2011." Available at http://www.nccn.org/professionals/physician_gls/PDF/mds.pdf

National Kidney Foundation, "KDOQI Clinical Practice Guidelines and Clinical Practice Recommentaions for Anemia in Chronic Kidney Disease," *Am J Kidney Dis*, 2007, 50(3):529-30. Available at http://www.kidney.org/professionals/KDOQI/guidelines_anemiaUP/index.htm or http://www.kidney.org/professionals/KDOQI

Rizzo JD, Brouwers M, Hurley P, et al, "American Society of Clinical Oncology/American Society of Hematology Clinical Practice Guideline Update on the Use of Epoetin and Darbepoetin in Adult Patients With Cancer," *J Clin Oncol*, 2010, 28(33):4996-5010.

Rizzo JD, Somerfield MR, Hagerty LK, et al, "American Society of Hematology/American Society of Clinical Oncology 2007 Clinical Practice Guideline Update on the Use of Epoetin and Darbepoetin," *Blood*, 2008, 111(1):25-41.
Singh AJ, Szczech L, Tang KI, et al, "Correction of Anemia with Epoetin Alfa in Chronic Kidney Disease," *N Engl J Med*, 2006, 355(20):2085-98.
Warady BA, Arar MY, Lerner G, et al, "Darbepoetin Alfa for the Treatment of Anemia in Pediatric Patients With Chronic Kidney Disease," *Pediatr Nephrol*, 2006, 21(8):1144-52.

Dasatinib (da SA ti nib)

Related Information

Management of Chemotherapy-Induced Nausea and Vomiting *on page 1786*
Principles of Anticancer Therapy *on page 1878*
Safe Handling of Hazardous Drugs *on page 1904*

Brand Names: U.S. Sprycel®

Brand Names: Canada Sprycel®

Index Terms BMS-354825

Generic Availability (U.S.) No

Pharmacologic Category Antineoplastic Agent, Tyrosine Kinase Inhibitor

Use Treatment of chronic myelogenous leukemia (CML) in chronic, accelerated or blast (myeloid or lymphoid) phase resistant or intolerant to prior therapy (including imatinib); treatment of newly-diagnosed Philadelphia chromosome-positive (Ph+) CML in chronic phase; treatment of Philadelphia chromosome-positive (Ph+) acute lymphoblastic leukemia (ALL) resistant or intolerant to prior therapy

Unlabeled Use Post-stem cell transplant (allogeneic) follow-up treatment of CML; treatment of gastrointestinal stromal tumor (GIST)

Labeled Contraindications There are no contraindications listed within the FDA-approved manufacturer's labeling.

Canadian labeling: Hypersensitivity to dasatinib or any other component of the formulation

Pregnancy Risk Factor D

Lactation Excretion in breast milk unknown/not recommended

Warnings/Precautions Hazardous agent - use appropriate precautions for handling and disposal. Severe dose-related bone marrow suppression (thrombocytopenia, neutropenia, anemia) is associated with treatment; dosage adjustment or temporary interruption may be required for severe myelosuppression; the incidence of myelosuppression is higher in patients with advanced CML and Ph+ ALL. Fatal intracranial hemorrhage has been reported in association with dasatinib use; monitor blood counts. Severe hemorrhage (including CNS, GI) may occur due to thrombocytopenia; in addition to thrombocytopenia, dasatinib may also cause platelet dysfunction. Use caution with patients taking anticoagulants or medications interfering with platelet function; not studied in clinical trials. Avoid concomitant use with CYP3A4 inducers and inhibitors; if concomitant use cannot be avoided, consider dasatinib dosage adjustments.

Cardiomyopathy, diastolic dysfunction, heart failure (congestive), left ventricular dysfunction, and MI have been reported; monitor for signs and symptoms of cardiac dysfunction. Fluid retention, including pleural and pericardial effusions, severe ascites, severe pulmonary edema, and generalized edema were reported; may be dose-related. A chest x-ray is recommended for symptoms suggestive of effusion (dyspnea or dry cough). Utilizing once-daily dosing is associated with a decreased frequency of fluid retention. The risk for pleural effusion is increased in patients with hypertension, prior cardiac history and a twice a day administration schedule; interrupt treatment for grade ≥2 effusion; may consider reinitiating at a reduced dose after resolution (Quintás-Cardama, 2007). Use caution in patients where fluid accumulation may be poorly tolerated, such as in cardiovascular disease (HF or hypertension) and pulmonary disease. Elderly may be more likely to experience dyspnea and fluid retention. Pulmonary arterial hypertension (PAH) has been reported with use, sometimes after >12 months of therapy. Evaluate for underlying cardiopulmonary disease prior to therapy initiation and during therapy; evaluate and rule out alternative etiologies in patients with symptoms suggestive of PAH (eg, dyspnea, fatigue) and interrupt therapy if symptoms are severe. Discontinue permanently with confirmed PAH diagnosis.

May prolong QT interval; use caution in patients at risk for QT prolongation, including patients with long QT syndrome; patients taking antiarrhythmic medications or other medications that lead to QT prolongation or potassium-wasting diuretics; patients with cumulative high-dose anthracycline therapy, and conditions which cause hypokalemia or hypomagnesemia. Correct hypokalemia and hypomagnesemia prior to initiation of therapy. Use caution with hepatic impairment due to extensive hepatic metabolism; patients with ALT or AST >2.5 times the upper limit of normal (ULN) or total bilirubin >2 times the ULN were excluded from clinical trials.

Adverse Reactions

≥10%:

Cardiovascular: Fluid retention (21% to 35%; grades 3/4: 1% to 8%), superficial edema (3% to 19%; grades 3/4: ≤1%)

Central nervous system: Headache (12% to 33%), fatigue (8% to 24%), fever (5% to 18%)

Dermatologic: Rash (11% to 21%; includes drug eruption, erythema, erythema multiforme, erythematous rash, erythrosis, exfoliative rash, follicular rash, heat rash, macular rash, maculopapular rash, milia, papular rash, pruritic rash, pustular rash, skin exfoliation, skin irritation, urticaria vesiculosa, vesicular rash)

Endocrine & metabolic: Hypophosphatemia (grades 3/4: 5% to 10%), hypokalemia (grades 3/4: ≤15%), hypocalcemia (grades 3/4: <1% to 12%)

Gastrointestinal: Diarrhea (18% to 31%; grades 3/4: ≤5%), nausea (9% to 24%), vomiting (5% to 16%), abdominal pain (3% to 12%)

Hematologic: Thrombocytopenia (grades 3/4: 19% to 85%), neutropenia (grades 3/4: 22% to 79%), anemia (grades 3/4: 11% to 74%), hemorrhage (6% to 26%; grades 3/4: 1% to 9%), neutropenic fever (grades 3/4: 1% to 12%)

Neuromuscular & skeletal: Musculoskeletal pain (≤19%), myalgia (3% to 13%), arthralgia (≤12%)

Respiratory: Pleural effusion (12% to 24%; grades 3/4: ≤11%), dyspnea (3% to 20%; grades 3/4: 2% to 3%)

Miscellaneous: Infection (9% to 12%, includes bacterial, fungal, viral)

1% to <10%:

Cardiovascular: Generalized edema (≤1%), pericardial effusion (≤3%; grades 3/4: ≤1%), CHF/cardiac dysfunction (≤4%; includes cardiac failure, cardiomyopathy, diastolic dysfunction, ejection fraction decreased, left ventricular dysfunction, ventricular failure); arrhythmia, chest pain, flushing, hypertension, palpitation

Central nervous system: CNS bleeding (≤3%; grades 3/4: <3%), chills, depression, dizziness, insomnia, pain, somnolence

Dermatologic: Acne, alopecia, dermatitis, dry skin, eczema, hyperhydrosis, pruritus, urticaria

Gastrointestinal: Gastrointestinal bleeding (2% to 9%; grades 3/4: 1% to 7%), abdominal distention, anorexia, colitis (including neutropenic colitis), constipation, dyspepsia, enterocolitis, gastritis, mucositis/stomatitis, oral soft tissue disorder, taste alteration, weight loss/gain

Hematologic: Contusion, pancytopenia

Hepatic: Bilirubin increased (grades 3/4: ≤6%), ALT increased (grades 3/4: ≤5%), AST increased (grades 3/4: ≤4%)

Neuromuscular & skeletal: Muscle inflammation (4%), muscle weakness, neuropathy, peripheral neuropathy, weakness

Ocular: Visual disorder (blurred vision, acuity reduced, visual disturbance), xerophthalmia

Otic: Tinnitus

Renal: Serum creatinine increased (grades 3/4: ≤8%)

Respiratory: Pulmonary edema (≤4%; grades 3/4: ≤3%), cough, lung infiltration, pneumonia (bacterial, viral or fungal), pneumonitis, pulmonary hypertension, upper respiratory tract infection/inflammation

Miscellaneous: Herpes virus infection

<1%, postmarketing, and/or case reports (limited to important or life-threatening): Acute coronary syndrome, acute febrile neutrophilic dermatosis, acute respiratory distress syndrome, affect lability, amnesia, anal fissure, angina, anxiety, ascites, asthma, atrial fibrillation, atrial flutter, bronchospasm, bruising, bullous conditions, cardiomegaly, cerebrovascular accident, cholecystitis, cholestasis, confusion, conjunctivitis, cor pulmonale, creatine phosphokinase increased, deep vein thrombosis (DVT), dysphagia, ear hemorrhage, epistaxis, embolism, erythema nodosum, esophagitis, gastroenteropathy (protein wasting), gingival bleeding, gynecomastia, hand-foot syndrome (palmar-plantar erythrodysesthesia syndrome), hematoma, hematuria, hemoptysis, hepatitis, hypersensitivity, hyperuricemia, hypoalbuminemia, hypotension, interstitial lung disease, libido decreased, livedo reticularis, malaise, menstrual irregularities, MI, musculoskeletal stiffness, myocarditis, nail disorder, neutropenic colitis, ocular hemorrhage, optic neuritis, pancreatitis, panniculitis, pericarditis, petechiae, photosensitivity, pigmentation disorder, platelet aggregation abnormal, polyuria, proteinuria, pulmonary arterial hypertension, pulmonary embolism, pure red cell aplasia, QT_c prolongation, renal failure, rhabdomyolysis, seizure, sepsis, skin ulcer, syncope, temperature intolerance, tendonitis, thrombophlebitis, thrombosis, TIA, tremor, tumor lysis syndrome, upper gastrointestinal ulcer, uterine hemorrhage, vaginal hemorrhage, ventricular arrhythmia, ventricular tachycardia

Drug Interactions

Metabolism/Transport Effects **Substrate** of CYP3A4 (major); **Note:** Assignment of Major/Minor substrate status based on clinically relevant drug interaction potential; **Inhibits** CYP3A4 (weak)

Avoid Concomitant Use

Avoid concomitant use of Dasatinib with any of the following: BCG; CloZAPine; Conivaptan; H2-Antagonists; Natalizumab; Pimecrolimus; Pimozide; Proton Pump Inhibitors; St Johns Wort; Tacrolimus (Topical); Vaccines (Live)

Increased Effect/Toxicity

Dasatinib may increase the levels/effects of: Acetaminophen; Anticoagulants; Antiplatelet Agents; ARIPiprazole; CloZAPine; CYP3A4 Substrates; Highest Risk QTc-Prolonging Agents; Leflunomide; Moderate Risk QTc-Prolonging Agents; Natalizumab; Pimozide; Vaccines (Live); Vitamin K Antagonists

The levels/effects of Dasatinib may be increased by: Acetaminophen; Conivaptan; CYP3A4 Inhibitors (Moderate); CYP3A4 Inhibitors (Strong); Denosumab; Ivacaftor; Mifepristone; Pimecrolimus; Roflumilast; Tacrolimus (Topical); Trastuzumab

Decreased Effect

Dasatinib may decrease the levels/effects of: BCG; Cardiac Glycosides; Coccidioidin Skin Test; Sipuleucel-T; Vaccines (Inactivated); Vaccines (Live); Vitamin K Antagonists

The levels/effects of Dasatinib may be decreased by: Antacids; CYP3A4 Inducers (Strong); Deferasirox; Echinacea; H2-Antagonists; Proton Pump Inhibitors; St Johns Wort; Tocilizumab

Ethanol/Nutrition/Herb Interactions

Food: Dasatinib serum concentrations may be increased when taken with grapefruit or grapefruit juice. Management: Avoid concurrent use.

Herb/Nutraceutical: Avoid St John's wort (may increase metabolism and decrease dasatinib plasma concentration).

Storage/Stability Store at 25°C (77°F); excursions permitted to 15°C to 30°C (59°F to 86°F).

Mechanism of Action BCR-ABL tyrosine kinase inhibitor; targets most imatinib-resistant BCR-ABL mutations (except the T315I and F317V mutants) by distinctly binding to active and inactive ABL-kinase. Kinase inhibition halts proliferation of leukemia cells. Also inhibits SRC family (including SRC, LKC, YES, FYN); c-KIT, EPHA2 and platelet derived growth factor receptor (PDGFRβ)

Pharmacodynamics/Kinetics

Distribution: 2505 L

Protein binding: Dasatinib: 96%; metabolite (active): 93%

Metabolism: Hepatic (extensive); metabolized by CYP3A4 (primarily), flavin-containing mono-oxygenase-3 (FOM-3) and uridine diphosphate-glucuronosyltransferase (UGT) to an active metabolite and other inactive metabolites (the active metabolite plays only a minor role in the pharmacology of dasatinib)

Half-life elimination: Terminal: 3-5 hours

Time to peak, plasma: 0.5-6 hours

Excretion: Feces (~85%, 19% as unchanged drug); urine (~4%, 0.1% as unchanged drug)

Dosing

Adult & Geriatric Note: The effect of discontinuation after complete cytogenetic remission is achieved has not been studied.

Chronic myelogenous leukemia (CML), Philadelphia chromosome-positive (Ph+), newly diagnosed in chronic phase: Oral: 100 mg once daily until disease progression or unacceptable toxicity. In clinical studies, a dose escalation to 140 mg once daily was allowed in patients not achieving hematologic or cytogenetic response at recommended initial dosage.

CML, Ph+, resistant or intolerant: Oral:

Chronic phase: 100 mg once daily until disease progression or unacceptable toxicity. In clinical studies, a dose escalation to 140 mg once daily was allowed in patients not achieving hematologic or cytogenetic response at recommended initial dosage.

Accelerated or blast phase: 140 mg once daily until disease progression or unacceptable toxicity. In clinical studies, a dose escalation to 180 mg once daily was allowed in patients not achieving hematologic or cytogenetic response at recommended initial dosage.

Acute lymphoblastic leukemia (ALL), Ph+: Oral: 140 mg once daily until disease progression or unacceptable toxicity. In clinical studies, a dose escalation to 180 mg once daily was allowed in patients not achieving hematologic or cytogenetic response at recommended initial dosage.

Dosage adjustment for concomitant CYP3A4 inhibitors: Avoid concomitant administration with strong CYP3A4 inhibitors (eg, clarithromycin, itraconazole, ketoconazole, nefazodone, protease inhibitors, telithromycin, voriconazole, grapefruit juice); if concomitant administration with a strong CYP3A4 inhibitor cannot be avoided, consider reducing dasatinib from 100 mg once daily to 20 mg once daily **or** from 140 mg once daily to 40 mg once daily, with careful monitoring. If reduced dose is not tolerated, the strong CYP3A4 inhibitor must be discontinued or dasatinib therapy temporarily held until concomitant inhibitor use has ceased. When a strong CYP3A4 inhibitor is discontinued, allow a washout period (~1 week) prior to adjusting dasatinib dose upward.

Dosage adjustment for concomitant CYP3A4 inducers: Avoid concomitant administration with strong CYP3A4 inducers (eg, carbamazepine, dexamethasone, phenobarbital, phenytoin, rifampin, St John's wort); if concomitant administration with a strong CYP3A4 inducer cannot be avoided, consider increasing the dasatinib dose with careful monitoring.

Renal Impairment No dosage adjustment provided in the manufacturer's labeling; <4% of dasatinib and metabolites are renally excreted.

Hepatic Impairment No dosage adjustment necessary (use with caution).

Adjustment for Toxicity

Hematologic toxicity:

Chronic phase CML (100 mg daily starting dose): For ANC <500/mm^3 or platelets <50,000/mm^3, withhold treatment until ANC ≥1000/mm^3 and platelets ≥50,000/mm^3; then resume treatment at the original starting dose if recovery occurs in ≤7 days. If platelets <25,000/mm^3 or recurrence of ANC <500/mm^3 for >7 days, withhold treatment until ANC ≥1000/mm^3 and platelets ≥50,000/mm^3; then resume treatment at 80 mg once daily (second episode). For third episode, further reduce dose to 50 mg once daily (for newly-diagnosed patients) or discontinue (for patients resistant or intolerant to prior therapy)

Accelerated or blast phase CML and Ph+ ALL (140 mg once daily starting dose): For ANC <500/mm^3 or platelets <10,000/mm^3, if cytopenia unrelated to leukemia, withhold treatment until ANC ≥1000/mm^3 and platelets ≥20,000/mm^3; then resume treatment at the original starting dose. If cytopenia recurs, withhold treatment until ANC ≥1000/mm^3 and platelets ≥20,000/mm^3; then resume treatment at 100 mg once daily (second episode) or 80 mg once daily (third episode). For cytopenias related to leukemia (confirm with marrow aspirate or biopsy), consider dose escalation to 180 mg once daily.

Nonhematologic toxicity: Withhold treatment until toxicity improvement or resolution; if appropriate, resume treatment at a reduced dose based on the event severity. Fluid retention is managed with diuretics and supportive care. Effusions may require diuretics and/or dose interruption. Corticosteroids (eg, prednisone 20 mg/day for 3 days) may be considered for pleural or pericardial effusion with significant symptoms (hold dasatinib and reinitiate at a decreased dose when effusion resolves). Rash may be managed with steroids (topical or systemic), treatment interruption, dose reduction, or discontinuation (NCCN CML guidelines v.2.2013). Discontinue with confirmed pulmonary arterial hypertension.

Combination Regimens

Leukemia, Chronic Myelogenous: Dasatinib (CML Regimen) on page 1605

Administration Administer once daily (morning or evening). May be taken without regard to food. Swallow whole; do not break, crush, or chew tablets. Take with a meal or with a large glass of water if GI upset occurs.

Emetic Potential Very low (<10%)

Extemporaneous Preparations Hazardous agent: Use appropriate precautions for handling and disposal.

An oral suspension may be prepared by dissolving dasatinib tablet(s) for one dose in 30 mL chilled orange or apple juice (without preservatives). After 5 minutes, swirl the contents for 3 seconds and repeat the process every 5 minutes for a total of 20 minutes following addition of tablet(s). Minimize time between end of 20 minutes and administration since suspension will taste more bitter if allowed to stand longer. Swirl contents of container one last time, then administer immediately. To ensure the full dose is administered, rinse container with 15 mL juice and administer residue. May be administered orally (or by nasogastric tube). Discard any unused portion after 60 minutes.

Sprycel® data on file, Bristol-Myers Squibb

Monitoring Parameters CBC with differential (weekly for 2 months, then monthly or as clinically necessary); bone marrow biopsy; liver function tests, electrolytes including calcium, phosphorus, magnesium; monitor for fluid retention; ECG monitoring if at risk for QT_c prolongation; chest x-ray is recommended for symptoms suggestive of pleural effusion (eg, cough, dyspnea)

Thyroid function testing recommendations (Hamnvik, 2011):

- Preexisting levothyroxine therapy: Obtain baseline TSH levels, then monitor every 4 weeks until levels and levothyroxine dose are stable, then monitor every 2 months
- Without pre-existing thyroid hormone replacement: TSH at baseline, then monthly for 4 months, then every 2-3 months

Dietary Considerations May be taken without regard to food. Avoid grapefruit juice.

Additional Information Oncology Comment: In a dose finding study in chronic-phase CML, dasatinib 100 mg once daily provided comparable efficacy to the original FDA-approved dose of 70 mg twice daily. The 100 mg once daily dose was better tolerated (lower rates of pleural effusion and grades 3/4 thrombocytopenia), required fewer dose reductions, and fewer dosing interruptions or discontinuations (Shah, 2008).

Dosage Forms Excipient information presented when available (limited, particularly for generics); consult specific product labeling.

Tablet, oral:

Sprycel®: 20 mg, 50 mg, 70 mg, 100 mg

References

Apperley JF, Cortes JE, Kim DW, et al, "Dasatinib in the Treatment of Chronic Myeloid Leukemia in Accelerated Phase After Imatinib Failure: The START A Trial," *J Clin Oncol*, 2009, 27(21):3472-9.

Bradeen HA, Eide CA, O'Hare T, et al, "Comparison of Imatinib, Dasatinib (BMS-354825), and Nilotinib (AMN107) in an N-Ethyl-N-Nitrosourea (ENU)-Based Mutagenesis Screen: High Efficacy of Drug Combinations," *Blood*, 2006, 108(7):2332-8.

Cortes J, Rousselot P, Kim DW, et al, "Dasatinib Induces Complete Hematologic and Cytogenetic Responses in Patients With Imatinib-Resistant or Intolerant Chronic Myeloid Leukemia in Blast Crisis," *Blood*, 2007, 109(8):3207-13.

Guilhot F, Apperley J, Kim DW, et al, "Dasatinib Induces Significant Hematologic and Cytogenetic Responses in Patients With Imatinib-Resistant or Intolerant Chronic Myeloid Leukemia in Accelerated Phase," *Blood*, 2007, 109(10):4143-50.

Hamnvik OP, Larsen PR, and Marqusee E, "Thyroid Dysfunction From Antineoplastic Agents," *J Natl Cancer Inst*, 2011, 103(21):1572-87.

Hochhaus A, Kantarjian HM, Baccarani M, et al, "Dasatinib Induces Notable Hematologic and Cytogenetic Responses in Chronic-Phase Chronic Myeloid Leukemia After Failure of Imatinib Therapy," *Blood*, 2007, 109(6):2303-09.

Kantarjian H, Shah NP, Hochhaus A, et al, "Dasatinib Versus Imatinib in Newly Diagnosed Chronic-Phase Chronic Myeloid Leukemia," *N Engl J Med*, 2010, 362(24):2260-70.

National Comprehensive Cancer Network® (NCCN) "Practice Guidelines in Oncology™: Chronic Myelogenous Leukemia Version 2.2013." Available at http://www.nccn.org/professionals/physician_gls/PDF/cml.pdf

Ottmann O, Dombret H, Martinelli G, et al, "Dasatinib Induces Rapid Hematologic and Cytogenetic Responses in Adult Patients with Philadelphia Chromosome-Positive Acute Lymphoblastic Leukemia With Intolerance to Imatinib: Interim Results of a Phase 2 Study," *Blood*, 2007, 110 (7):2309-15.

Quintas-Cardama A, Han X, Kantarjian H, et al, "Dasatinib-Induced Platelet Dysfunction," *Blood* 2007, 110:2941 [abstract 2941 from 2007 ASH Annual Meeting].

Quintás-Cardama A, Kantarjian H, O'brien S, et al, "Pleural Effusion in Patients With Chronic Myelogenous Leukemia Treated With Dasatinib After Imatinib Failure," *J Clin Oncol*, 2007, 25 (25):3908-14.

Shah NP, Kantarjian HM, Kim DW, et al, "Intermittent Target Inhibition With Dasatinib 100 mg Once Daily Preserves Efficacy and Improves Tolerability in Imatinib-Resistant and -Intolerant Chronic-Phase Chronic Myeloid Leukemia," *J Clin Oncol*, 2008, 26(19):3204-12.

Talpaz M, Shah NP, Kantarjian H, et al, "Dasatinib in Imatinib-Resistant Philadelphia Chromosome-Positive Leukemias," *N Engl J Med*, 2006, 354(24):2531-41.

◆ **Daunomycin** *see* DAUNOrubicin (Conventional) *on page 396*

◆ **DAUNOrubicin Citrate** *see* DAUNOrubicin (Liposomal) *on page 400*

◆ **DAUNOrubicin Citrate (Liposomal)** *see* DAUNOrubicin (Liposomal) *on page 400*

◆ **DAUNOrubicin Citrate Liposome** *see* DAUNOrubicin (Liposomal) *on page 400*

DAUNOrubicin (Conventional) (daw noe ROO bi sin con VEN sha nal)

Related Information

Chemotherapy and Cancer Treatment During Pregnancy *on page 1829*

Management of Chemotherapy-Induced Nausea and Vomiting *on page 1786*

Management of Drug Extravasations *on page 1800*

Safe Handling of Hazardous Drugs *on page 1904*

Brand Names: U.S. Cerubidine®

Brand Names: Canada Cerubidine®

Index Terms Conventional Daunomycin; Daunomycin; DAUNOrubicin Hydrochloride; Rubidomycin Hydrochloride

Generic Availability (U.S.) Yes

Pharmacologic Category Antineoplastic Agent, Anthracycline

Use Treatment of acute lymphocytic leukemia (ALL) and acute myeloid leukemia (AML)

Labeled Contraindications Hypersensitivity to daunorubicin or any component of the formulation

Pregnancy Risk Factor D

Lactation Excretion in breast milk unknown/not recommended

Warnings/Precautions Hazardous agent - use appropriate precautions for handling and disposal. Use with caution in patients who have received radiation therapy; reduce dosage in patients who are receiving radiation therapy simultaneously. **[U.S. Boxed Warnings]: Use caution with renal impairment or in the presence of hepatic dysfunction; dosage reduction is recommended. Potent vesicant; if extravasation occurs, severe local**

tissue damage leading to ulceration and necrosis, and pain may occur. For I.V. administration only. Severe bone marrow suppression may occur.

[U.S. Boxed Warning]: May cause cumulative, dose-related myocardial toxicity (concurrent or delayed). Total cumulative dose should take into account previous or concomitant treatment with cardiotoxic agents or irradiation of chest. The incidence of irreversible myocardial toxicity increases as the total cumulative (lifetime) dosages approach:

550 mg/m^2 in adults
400 mg/m^2 in adults receiving chest radiation
300 mg/m^2 in children >2 years of age
10 mg/kg in children <2 years of age

Although the risk increases with cumulative dose, irreversible cardiotoxicity may occur at any dose level. Patients with pre-existing heart disease, hypertension, concurrent administration of other antineoplastic agents, prior or concurrent chest irradiation, advanced age; and infants and children are at increased risk. Monitor left ventricular (LV) function (baseline and periodic) with ECHO or MUGA scan; monitor ECG.

Secondary leukemias may occur when used with combination chemotherapy or radiation therapy. **[U.S. Boxed Warning]: Should be administered under the supervision of an experienced cancer chemotherapy physician.**

Adverse Reactions

>10%:

Cardiovascular: Transient ECG abnormalities (supraventricular tachycardia, S-T wave changes, atrial or ventricular extrasystoles); generally asymptomatic and self-limiting. CHF, dose related, may be delayed for 7-8 years after treatment

Dermatologic: Alopecia (reversible), radiation recall

Gastrointestinal: Mild nausea or vomiting, stomatitis

Genitourinary: Discoloration of urine (red)

Hematologic: Myelosuppression (onset: 7 days; nadir: 10-14 days; recovery: 21-28 days), primarily leukopenia; thrombocytopenia and anemia

1% to 10%:

Dermatologic: Skin "flare" at injection site; discoloration of saliva, sweat, or tears

Endocrine & metabolic: Hyperuricemia

Gastrointestinal: Abdominal pain, GI ulceration, diarrhea

<1%, postmarketing, and/or case reports: Anaphylactoid reaction, arrhythmia, bilirubin increased, cardiomyopathy, hepatitis, infertility; local (cellulitis, pain, thrombophlebitis at injection site); MI, myocarditis, nail banding, neutropenic typhlitis, onycholysis, pericarditis, pigmentation of nailbeds, secondary leukemia, skin rash, sterility, systemic hypersensitivity (including urticaria, pruritus, angioedema, dysphagia, dyspnea); transaminases increased

Drug Interactions

Metabolism/Transport Effects Substrate of P-glycoprotein

Avoid Concomitant Use

Avoid concomitant use of DAUNOrubicin (Conventional) with any of the following: BCG; CloZAPine; Natalizumab; Pimecrolimus; Tacrolimus (Topical); Vaccines (Live)

Increased Effect/Toxicity

DAUNOrubicin (Conventional) may increase the levels/effects of: CloZAPine; Leflunomide; Natalizumab; Vaccines (Live)

The levels/effects of DAUNOrubicin (Conventional) may be increased by: Bevacizumab; Denosumab; P-glycoprotein/ABCB1 Inhibitors; Pimecrolimus; Roflumilast; Tacrolimus (Topical); Taxane Derivatives; Trastuzumab

Decreased Effect

DAUNOrubicin (Conventional) may decrease the levels/effects of: BCG; Cardiac Glycosides; Coccidioidin Skin Test; Sipuleucel-T; Vaccines (Inactivated); Vaccines (Live)

The levels/effects of DAUNOrubicin (Conventional) may be decreased by: Cardiac Glycosides; Echinacea; P-glycoprotein/ABCB1 Inducers

Ethanol/Nutrition/Herb Interactions Ethanol: Avoid ethanol (due to GI irritation).

Storage/Stability Store intact vials of powder for injection at room temperature of 15°C to 30°C (59°F to 86°F); intact vials of solution for injection should be refrigerated at 2°C to 8°C (36°F to 46°F). Protect from light. Reconstituted solution is stable for 4 days at 15°C to 25°C. Further dilution in D_5W, LR, or NS is stable at room temperature (25°C) for up to 4 weeks if protected from light.

Reconstitution Dilute vials of powder for injection with 4 mL SWFI for a final concentration of 5 mg/mL. May further dilute in 100 mL D_5W or NS.

Mechanism of Action Inhibition of DNA and RNA synthesis by intercalation between DNA base pairs and by steric obstruction. Daunomycin intercalates at points of local uncoiling of the double helix. Although the exact mechanism is unclear, it appears that direct binding to DNA (intercalation) and inhibition of DNA repair (topoisomerase II inhibition) result in blockade of DNA and RNA synthesis and fragmentation of DNA.

Pharmacodynamics/Kinetics

Distribution: Many body tissues, particularly the liver, kidneys, lung, spleen, and heart; not into CNS; crosses placenta; V_d: 40 L/kg

Metabolism: Primarily hepatic to daunorubicinol (active), then to inactive aglycones, conjugated sulfates, and glucuronides

Half-life elimination: Distribution: 2 minutes; Elimination: 14-20 hours; Terminal: 18.5 hours; Daunorubicinol plasma half-life: 24-48 hours

Excretion: Feces (40%); urine (~25% as unchanged drug and metabolites)

Dosing

Adult Refer to individual protocols. **Note:** Cumulative dose should not exceed 550 mg/m^2 in adults without risk factors for cardiotoxicity and should not exceed 400 mg/m^2 in adults receiving chest irradiation.

Range: I.V.: 30-60 mg/m^2/day for 3 days, repeat dose in 3-4 weeks

ALL combination therapy: I.V.: 45 mg/m^2/day for 3 days

AML combination therapy (induction): I.V.: Adults <60 years: Induction: 45 mg/m^2/day for 3 days of the first course of induction therapy; subsequent courses: 45 mg/m^2/day for 2 days

Geriatric

ALL combination therapy: I.V.: 45 mg/m^2/day for 3 days

AML combination therapy (induction): Elderly ≥60 years: Induction: 30 mg/m^2/day for 3 days of the first course of induction therapy; subsequent courses: 30 mg/m^2/day for 2 days

Pediatric Refer to individual protocols. **Note:** Cumulative dose should not exceed 300 mg/m^2 in children >2 years or 10 mg/kg in children <2 years of age; maximum cumulative doses for younger children are unknown.

ALL combination therapy: I.V.:

Children <2 years or BSA <0.5 m^2: 1 mg/kg/dose per protocol, with frequency dependent on regimen employed

Children ≥2 years and BSA ≥0.5 m^2: Remission induction: 25 mg/m^2 on day 1 every week for up to 4-6 cycles

AML combination therapy (induction): Children ≥2 years and BSA ≥0.5 m^2: I.V. continuous infusion: 30-60 mg/m^2/day on days 1-3 of cycle

Renal Impairment

The FDA-approved labeling recommends the following adjustment: S_{cr} >3 mg/dL: Administer 50% of normal dose.

The following guidelines have been used by some clinicians (Aronoff, 2007):

Children:

Cl_{cr} <30 mL/minute: Administer 50% of dose.

Hemodialysis/continuous ambulatory peritoneal dialysis (CAPD): Administer 50% of dose.

Adults: No adjustment recommended.

Hepatic Impairment

The FDA-approved labeling recommends the following adjustments:

Serum bilirubin 1.2-3 mg/dL: Administer 75% of dose.

Serum bilirubin >3 mg/dL: Administer 50% of dose.

The following guidelines have been used by some clinicians (Floyd, 2006):

Serum bilirubin 1.2-3 mg/dL: Administer 75% of dose

Serum bilirubin 3.1-5 mg/dL: Administer 50% of dose

Serum bilirubin >5 mg/dL: Avoid use

Combination Regimens

Leukemia, acute lymphocytic:

DVP on page 1621

Larson Regimen (ALL) on page 1699

Linker Protocol (ALL) on page 1703

PVDA on page 1745

Leukemia, acute myeloid:

5 + 2 (Cytarabine-Daunorubicin) (AML Induction) on page 1512

5 + 2 (Cytarabine-Daunorubicin) (AML Postremission) on page 1512

5 + 2 + 5 (Cytarabine-Daunorubicin-Etoposide) (AML Consolidation) on page 1513

7 + 3 (Cytarabine-Daunorubicin) (AML Induction) on page 1513

7 + 3 + 7 (Cytarabine-Daunorubicin-Etoposide) (AML Induction) on page 1515

Cytarabine (High Dose)-Daunorubicin (AML Induction) on page 1602

Cytarabine (High Dose)-Daunorubicin-Etoposide (AML Induction) on page 1602

Leukemia, acute promyelocytic:

Tretinoin-Daunorubicin (APL) on page 1762

Tretinoin-Daunorubicin-Cytarabine (APL) on page 1762

Administration Not for I.M. or SubQ administration. Administer as slow I.V. push over 1-5 minutes into the tubing of a rapidly infusing I.V. solution of D_5W or NS or may dilute further and infuse over 15-30 minutes.

Emetic Potential Moderate (30% to 90%)

Vesicant/Extravasation Risk Vesicant; see Management of Drug Extravasations on page 1800.

Monitoring Parameters CBC with differential and platelet count, liver function test, ECG, left ventricular ejection function (echocardiography [ECHO] or multigated radionuclide angiography [MUGA] scan), renal function test

Dosage Forms Excipient information presented when available (limited, particularly for generics); consult specific product labeling.

Injection, powder for reconstitution: 20 mg

Cerubidine®: 20 mg [contains mannitol]

Injection, solution [preservative free]: 5 mg/mL (4 mL, 10 mL)

References

Aronoff GR, Bennett WM, Berns JS, et al, *Drug Prescribing in Renal Failure: Dosing Guidelines for Adults and Children*, 5th Ed. Philadelphia, PA: American College of Physicians, 2007, 98.

Floyd J, Mirza I, Sachs B, et al, "Hepatotoxicity of Chemotherapy," *Semin Oncol*, 2006, 33 (1):50-67.

Keefe DL, "Anthracycline-Induced Cardiomyopathy," *Semin Oncol*, 2001, 28(4 Suppl 12):2-7.

Masaoka T, Ogawa M, Yamada K, et al, "A Phase II Comparative Study of Idarubicin Plus Cytarabine Versus Daunorubicin Plus Cytarabine in Adult Acute Myeloid Leukemia," *Semin Hematol*, 1996, 33(4 Suppl 3):12-7.

Morgan C, Tillett T, Braybrooke J, et al, "Management of Uncommon Chemotherapy-Induced Emergencies," *Lancet Oncol*, 2011, 12(8):806-14.

Weick JK, Kopecky KJ, Appelbaum FR, et al, "A Randomized Investigation of High-Dose Versus Standard-Dose Cytosine Arabinoside With Daunorubicin in Patients With Previously Untreated Acute Myeloid Leukemia: A Southwest Oncology Group Study," *Blood*, 1996, 88(8):2841-51.

◆ **DAUNOrubicin Hydrochloride** *see* DAUNOrubicin (Conventional) *on page 396*

DAUNOrubicin (Liposomal) (daw noe ROO bi sin lye po SO mal)

Related Information

Management of Chemotherapy-Induced Nausea and Vomiting *on page 1786*

Management of Drug Extravasations *on page 1800*

Safe Handling of Hazardous Drugs *on page 1904*

Brand Names: U.S. DaunoXome®

Index Terms DAUNOrubicin Citrate; DAUNOrubicin Citrate (Liposomal); DAUNOrubicin Citrate Liposome; Liposomal DAUNOrubicin

Generic Availability (U.S.) No

Pharmacologic Category Antineoplastic Agent, Anthracycline

Use First-line treatment of advanced HIV-associated Kaposi's sarcoma (KS)

Labeled Contraindications Hypersensitivity to daunorubicin citrate (liposomal), daunorubicin, or any component of the formulation

Pregnancy Risk Factor D

Lactation Excretion in breast milk unknown/not recommended

Warnings/Precautions Hazardous agent - use appropriate precautions for handling and disposal. **[U.S. Boxed Warning]: Monitor cardiac function regularly; especially in patients with previous therapy with high cumulative doses of anthracyclines, cyclophosphamide, or thoracic radiation, or who have pre-existing cardiac disease.** Although the risk increases with cumulative dose, irreversible cardiotoxicity may occur with anthracycline treatment at any dose level. Patients with pre-existing heart disease, hypertension, concurrent administration of other antineoplastic agents, prior or concurrent chest irradiation, and advanced age are at increased risk. Evaluate left ventricular ejection fraction (LVEF) prior to treatment and periodically during treatment.

[U.S. Boxed Warning]: May cause bone marrow suppression, particularly neutropenia; monitor closely for infections. **[U.S. Boxed Warning]: Use caution with hepatic impairment;** dosage reduction is recommended. Use caution with renal impairment; may require dose adjustment. **[U.S. Boxed Warning]: The lipid component is associated with infusion-related reactions (back pain, flushing, chest tightness) usually within the first 5 minutes of infusion;** monitor, interrupt infusion, and resume at reduced infusion rate. Safety and efficacy in children and the elderly have not been established. **[U.S. Boxed Warning]: Should be administered under the supervision of an experienced cancer chemotherapy physician.**

Adverse Reactions

>10%:

- Cardiovascular: Edema (11%)
- Central nervous system: Fatigue (49%), fever (47%), headache (25%), neutropenic fever (17%)
- Gastrointestinal: Nausea (54%), diarrhea (38%), abdominal pain (23%), anorexia (23%), vomiting (23%)
- Hematologic: Myelosuppression (onset: 7 days; nadir: 14 days; recovery 21 days), neutropenia (up to 55%; grade 4: 15%), anemia (up to 55%; grade 4: 2%), thrombocytopenia (up to 12%; grade 4: 1%)
- Neuromuscular & skeletal: Rigors (19%), back pain (16%), neuropathy (13%)
- Respiratory: Cough (28%), dyspnea (26%), rhinitis (12%)
- Miscellaneous: Opportunistic infections (40%), allergic reactions (24%), diaphoresis (14%), infusion-related reactions (14%; includes back pain, flushing, chest tightness)

1% to 10%:

- Cardiovascular: Chest pain (10%), hypertension (≤5%), palpitation (≤5%), syncope (≤5%), tachycardia (≤5%), LVEF decreased (3%), CHF/cardiomyopathy
- Central nervous system: Depression (10%), malaise (10%), dizziness (8%), insomnia (6%), abnormal thinking (≤5%), amnesia (≤5%), anxiety (≤5%), ataxia (≤5%), confusion (≤5%), emotional lability (≤5%), hallucination (≤5%), meningitis (≤5%), seizure (≤5%), somnolence (≤5%)
- Dermatologic: Alopecia (8%), pruritus (7%), dry skin (≤5%), folliculitis (≤5%), seborrhea (≤5%)
- Endocrine & metabolic: Dehydration (≤5%), hot flashes (≤5%)
- Gastrointestinal: Stomatitis (10%), constipation (7%), tenesmus (5%), appetite increased (≤5%), dental caries (≤5%), dysphagia (≤5%), gastrointestinal hemorrhage (≤5%), gastritis (≤5%), gingival bleeding (≤5%), hemorrhoids (≤5%), melena (≤5%), splenomegaly (≤5%), taste perversion (≤5%), xerostomia (≤5%)
- Genitourinary: Dysuria (≤5%), nocturia (≤5%), polyuria (≤5%)
- Hepatic: Hepatomegaly (≤5%)
- Local: Injection site inflammation (≤5%)
- Neuromuscular & skeletal: Arthralgia (7%), myalgia (7%), gait abnormal (≤5%), hyperkinesia (≤5%), hypertonia (≤5%), tremor (≤5%)
- Ocular: Abnormal vision (5%) conjunctivitis (≤5%), eye pain (≤5%)
- Otic: Deafness (≤5%), earache (≤5%), tinnitus (≤5%)
- Respiratory: Sinusitis (8%), hemoptysis (≤5%), pulmonary infiltrate (≤5%), sputum increased (≤5%)
- Miscellaneous: Flu-like syndrome (5%), hiccups (≤5%), lymphadenopathy (≤5%), thirst (≤5%)

Postmarketing and/or case reports: Angina, atrial fibrillation, cardiac arrest, MI, pericardial effusion, pericardial tamponade, pulmonary hypertension, supraventricular tachycardia, ventricular extrasystoles

Drug Interactions

Metabolism/Transport Effects Substrate of P-glycoprotein

Avoid Concomitant Use

Avoid concomitant use of DAUNOrubicin (Liposomal) with any of the following: BCG; CloZAPine; Natalizumab; Pimecrolimus; Tacrolimus (Topical); Vaccines (Live)

Increased Effect/Toxicity

DAUNOrubicin (Liposomal) may increase the levels/effects of: CloZAPine; Leflunomide; Natalizumab; Vaccines (Live)

The levels/effects of DAUNOrubicin (Liposomal) may be increased by: Bevacizumab; Denosumab; P-glycoprotein/ABCB1 Inhibitors; Pimecrolimus; Roflumilast; Tacrolimus (Topical); Taxane Derivatives; Trastuzumab

Decreased Effect

DAUNOrubicin (Liposomal) may decrease the levels/effects of: BCG; Cardiac Glycosides; Coccidioidin Skin Test; Sipuleucel-T; Vaccines (Inactivated); Vaccines (Live)

The levels/effects of DAUNOrubicin (Liposomal) may be decreased by: Cardiac Glycosides; Echinacea; P-glycoprotein/ABCB1 Inducers

Storage/Stability Store intact vials of solution under refrigeration at 2°C to 8°C (36°F to 46°F); do not freeze. Protect from light. Diluted daunorubicin liposomal for infusion may be refrigerated at 2°C to 8°C (36°F to 46°F) for a maximum of 6 hours. Do not use with in-line filters.

Reconstitution Only fluid which may be mixed with DaunoXome® is D_5W. Dilute to a 1:1 solution (1 mg daunorubicin liposomal/mL D_5W). Must **not** be mixed with saline, bacteriostatic agents (such as benzyl alcohol), or any other solution.

Mechanism of Action Liposomes have been shown to penetrate solid tumors more effectively, possibly because of their small size and longer circulation time. Once in tissues, daunorubicin is released. Daunorubicin inhibits DNA and RNA synthesis by intercalation between DNA base pairs and by steric obstruction; and intercalates at points of local uncoiling of the double helix. Although the exact mechanism is unclear, it appears that direct binding to DNA (intercalation) and inhibition of DNA repair (topoisomerase II inhibition) result in blockade of DNA and RNA synthesis and fragmentation of DNA.

Pharmacodynamics/Kinetics

Distribution: V_d: 5-8 L

Metabolism: Similar to daunorubicin, but metabolite plasma levels are low

Half-life elimination: Distribution: 4.4 hours; Terminal: 3-5 hours

Excretion: Primarily feces; some urine

Clearance, plasma: 17.3 mL/minute

Dosing

Adult Refer to individual protocols.

Advanced HIV-associated Kaposi's sarcoma: I.V.: 40 mg/m^2 every 2 weeks

Geriatric Refer to adult dosing. Use with caution.

Renal Impairment

S_{cr} 1.2-3 mg/dL: Reduce dose to 75% of normal.

S_{cr} >3 mg/dL: Reduce dose to 50% of normal.

Hepatic Impairment

Serum bilirubin 1.2-3 mg/dL: Reduce to 75% of normal dose.

Serum bilirubin >3 mg/dL: Reduce to 50% of normal dose.

Adjustment for Toxicity Withhold treatment for ANC <750/mm^3

Combination Regimens

Leukemia, acute lymphocytic: Hyper-CVAD (Leukemia, Acute Lymphocytic) on page 1681

Administration Infuse over 1 hour; do not mix with other drugs. Avoid extravasation.

Vesicant/Extravasation Risk May be an irritant

Monitoring Parameters CBC with differential and platelets (prior to each dose), liver function tests, renal function tests; evaluate cardiac function (baseline left ventricular ejection fraction [LVEF] prior to treatment initiation; repeat LVEF at total cumulative doses of 320 mg/m^2, and every 160 mg/m^2 thereafter; patients with pre-existing cardiac disease, history of prior chest irradiation, or history of prior anthracycline treatment should have baseline LVEF and every 160 mg/m^2 thereafter); signs and symptoms of infection or disease progression; monitor closely for infusion reactions

Dosage Forms Excipient information presented when available (limited, particularly for generics); consult specific product labeling.

Injection, solution [preservative free]:

DaunoXome®: 2 mg/mL (25 mL) [contains sucrose 2125 mg/25 mL]

References

Eckardt JR, Campbell E, Burris HA, et al, "A Phase II Trial of DaunoXome®, Liposome-Encapsulated Daunorubicin, in Patients With Metastatic Adenocarcinoma of the Colon," *Am J Clin Oncol*, 1994, 17(6):498-501.

Gill PS, Espina BM, Muggia F, et al, "Phase I/II Clinical and Pharmacokinetic Evaluation of Liposomal Daunorubicin," *J Clin Oncol*, 1995, 13(4):996-1003.

Gill PS, Wernz J, Scadden DT, et al, "Randomized Phase III Trial of Liposomal Daunorubicin Versus Doxorubicin, Bleomycin, and Vincristine in AIDS-Related Kaposi's Sarcoma," *J Clin Oncol*, 1996, 14(8):2353-64.

◆ **DaunoXome®** *see* DAUNOrubicin (Liposomal) *on page 400*

◆ **DAVA** *see* Vindesine *on page 1464*

◆ **dCF** *see* Pentostatin *on page 1161*

◆ **DDAVP®** *see* Desmopressin *on page 434*

◆ **DDAVP® Melt (Can)** *see* Desmopressin *on page 434*

◆ **Deacetyl Vinblastine Carboxamide** *see* Vindesine *on page 1464*

◆ **1-Deamino-8-D-Arginine Vasopressin** *see* Desmopressin *on page 434*

◆ **Decadron** *see* Dexamethasone (Systemic) *on page 440*

◆ **Decapeptyl® (Can)** *see* Triptorelin *on page 1413*

Decitabine (de SYE ta been)

Related Information

Management of Chemotherapy-Induced Nausea and Vomiting *on page 1786*

Safe Handling of Hazardous Drugs *on page 1904*

Brand Names: U.S. Dacogen®

Index Terms 5-Aza-2'-deoxycytidine; 5-Aza-dCyd; Deoxyazacytidine; Dezocitidine

Generic Availability (U.S.) No

Pharmacologic Category Antineoplastic Agent, DNA Methylation Inhibitor

Use Treatment of myelodysplastic syndrome (MDS)

Unlabeled Use Treatment of acute myelogenous leukemia (AML), sickle cell anemia

Labeled Contraindications There are no contraindications listed within the manufacturer's labeling.

Pregnancy Risk Factor D

Lactation Excretion in breast milk unknown/not recommended

Warnings/Precautions Hazardous agent - use appropriate precautions for handling and disposal. The dose-limiting toxicity is bone marrow suppression; worsening neutropenia is common in first two treatment cycles and may not correlate with progression of underlying MDS; may require dosage adjustment (after the first cycle), growth factor support and/or antimicrobial agents; monitor for infection. Not studied in hepatic and renal disease; use caution.

Adverse Reactions

>10%:

Cardiovascular: Peripheral edema (25% to 27%), pallor (23%), edema (5% to 18%), cardiac murmur (16%), hypotension (6% to 11%)

Central nervous system: Fever (6% to 53%), fatigue (46%), headache (23% to 28%), insomnia (14% to 28%), dizziness (18% to 21%), chills (16%), pain (5% to 13%), confusion (8% to 12%), lethargy (12%), anxiety (9% to 11%), hypoesthesia (11%)

Dermatologic: Petechiae (12% to 39%), bruising (9% to 22%), rash (11% to 19%), erythema (5% to 14%), cellulitis (9% to 12%), lesions (5% to 11%), pruritus (9% to 11%)

Endocrine & metabolic: Hyperglycemia (6% to 33%), hypoalbuminemia (7% to 24%), hypomagnesemia (5% to 24%), hypokalemia (12% to 22%), hyperkalemia (13%), hyponatremia (19%)

Gastrointestinal: Nausea (40% to 42%), constipation (30% to 35%), diarrhea (28% to 34%), vomiting (16% to 25%), anorexia/appetite decreased (8% to 23%), abdominal pain (5% to 14%), oral mucosal petechiae (13%), stomatitis (11% to 12%), dyspepsia (10% to 12%)

Hematologic: Neutropenia (38% to 90%; grades 3/4: 37% to 87%; recovery 28-50 days), thrombocytopenia (27% to 89%; grades 3/4: 24% to 85%), anemia (31% to 82%; grades 3/4: 22%), febrile neutropenia (20% to 29%; grades 3/4: 23%), leukopenia (6% to 28%; grades 3/4: 22%), lymphadenopathy (12%)

Hepatic: Hyperbilirubinemia (6% to 14%), alkaline phosphatase increased (11%)

Local: Tenderness (11%)

Neuromuscular & skeletal: Rigors (22%), arthralgia (17% to 20%), limb pain (18% to 19%), back pain (17% to 18%), weakness (15%)

Respiratory: Cough (27% to 40%), dyspnea (29%), pneumonia (20% to 22%), pharyngitis (16%), lung crackles (14%), epistaxis (13%)

5% to 10%:

Cardiovascular: Tachycardia (8%), chest pain/discomfort (6% to 7%), facial edema (6%), hypertension (6%), heart failure (5%)

Central nervous system: Depression (9%), malaise (5%)

Dermatologic: Alopecia (8%), dry skin (8%), urticaria (6%)

Endocrine & metabolic: Hyperuricemia (10%), LDH increased (8%), bicarbonate increased (6%), dehydration (6% to 8%), hypochloremia (6%), bicarbonate decreased (5%), hypoproteinemia (5%)

Gastrointestinal: Mucosal inflammation (9%), weight loss (9%), gingival bleeding (8%), hemorrhoids (8%), loose stools (7%), tongue ulceration (7%), dysphagia (5% to 6%), oral candidiasis (6%), toothache (6%), abdominal distension (5%), gastroesophageal reflux (5%), glossodynia (5%), lip ulceration (5%), oral pain (5%), tooth abscess (5%)

Genitourinary: Urinary tract infection (7%), dysuria (6%), polyuria (5%)

Hematologic: Bacteremia (5% to 8%), hematoma (5%), pancytopenia (5%), thrombocythemia (5%)

Hepatic: Ascites (10%), AST increased (10%), hypobilirubinemia (5%)

Local: Catheter infection (8%), catheter site erythema (5%), catheter site pain (5%), injection site swelling (5%)

Neuromuscular & skeletal: Myalgia (5% to 9%), falling (8%), chest wall pain (7%), muscle spasm (7%), bone pain (6%), musculoskeletal pain/discomfort (5% to 6%), crepitation (5%)

Ocular: Blurred vision (6%)

Otic: Ear pain (6%)

Respiratory: Breath sounds abnormal (5% to 10%), hypoxia (10%), upper respiratory tract infection (10%), pharyngolaryngeal pain (8%), rales (8%), pulmonary edema (6%), sinusitis (5% to 6%), pleural effusion (5%), post-nasal drip (5%), sinus congestion (5%)

Miscellaneous: Candidal infection (10%), staphylococcal infection (7%), transfusion reaction (7%), night sweats (5%)

<5%, postmarketing, and/or case reports: Anaphylactic reaction, atrial fibrillation, bronchopulmonary aspergillosis, cardiomyopathy, cardiorespiratory arrest/failure, catheter site hemorrhage, cholecystitis, fungal infection, gastrointestinal hemorrhage, gingival pain, hemoptysis, hypersensitivity, intracranial hemorrhage, mental status change, MI, mycobacterium avium complex infection, peridiverticular abscess, pseudomonal lung infection, pulmonary embolism, pulmonary infiltrates, pulmonary mass, renal failure, respiratory arrest, sepsis, splenomegaly, supraventricular tachycardia, Sweet's syndrome (acute febrile neutrophilic dermatosis), urethral hemorrhage

Drug Interactions

Metabolism/Transport Effects None known.

Avoid Concomitant Use

Avoid concomitant use of Decitabine with any of the following: CloZAPine

Increased Effect/Toxicity

Decitabine may increase the levels/effects of: CloZAPine

Decreased Effect There are no known significant interactions involving a decrease in effect.

Storage/Stability Store vials at 25°C (77°F); excursions permitted to 15°C to 30°C (59°F to 86°F). Solutions diluted for infusion may be stored for up to 7 hours under refrigeration at 2°C to 8°C (36°F to 46°F) if prepared with cold infusion fluids.

Reconstitution Vials should be reconstituted with 10 mL SWFI to a concentration of 5 mg/mL. Immediately further dilute with 50-250 mL NS, D_5W, or lactated Ringer's to a final concentration of 0.1-1 mg/mL. Use appropriate precautions for handling and disposal. Solutions not administered within 15 minutes of preparation should be prepared with cold (2°C to 8°C [36°F to 46°F]) infusion solutions.

Mechanism of Action After phosphorylation, decitabine is incorporated into DNA and inhibits DNA methyltransferase causing hypomethylation and subsequent cell death (within the S-phase of the cell cycle).

Pharmacodynamics/Kinetics

Distribution: 63-89 L/m^2

Protein binding: <1%

Metabolism: Possibly via deamination by cytidine deaminase

Half-life elimination: ~30-35 minutes

Time to peak: At end of infusion

Dosing

Adult & Geriatric

MDS: I.V.:

15 mg/m^2 over 3 hours every 8 hours (45 mg/m^2/day) for 3 days (135 mg/m^2/cycle) every 6 weeks (treatment is recommended for at least 4 cycles and may continue until the patient no longer continues to benefit)

Adjustment for prolonged hematologic toxicity (ANC <1000/mm^3 and platelets <50,000/mm^3):

>6 weeks but <8 weeks: Delay dose for up to 2 weeks and temporarily reduce dose to 11 mg/m^2 every 8 hours (33 mg/m^2/day) for 3 days

>8 weeks but <10 weeks: Assess for disease progression; if no disease progression, delay dose for up to 2 weeks and reduce dose to 11 mg/m^2 every 8 hours (33 mg/m^2/day) for 3 days; maintain or increase dose with subsequent cycles if clinically indicated

or

20 mg/m^2 over 1 hour daily for 5 days every 28 days (delay subsequent treatment cycles until hematologic recovery (ANC ≥1000/mm^3 and platelets ≥50,000/mm^3)

AML (unlabeled use): I.V.: 20 mg/m^2 over 1 hour daily for 5 days every 28 days (Cashen, 2010)

Adjustment for Toxicity

Hematologic toxicity (ANC <1000/mm^3 and platelets <50,000/mm^3): Delay and/or reduce dose; refer to adult dosing for recommendations specific to each MDS dosing regimen

Nonhematologic toxicity: Temporarily hold treatment until resolution for any of the following toxicities:

Serum creatinine ≥2 mg/dL

ALT, bilirubin ≥2 times ULN

Active or uncontrolled infection

Combination Regimens

Leukemia, acute myeloid: Decitabine (AML Regimen) on page 1606

Myelodysplastic syndrome: Decitabine (MDS Regimen) on page 1607

Administration Infuse over 1-3 hours. Premedication with antiemetics is recommended.

Emetic Potential Very low (<10%)

Monitoring Parameters CBC with differential and platelets with each cycle, more frequently if needed; liver enzymes; serum creatinine

Dosage Forms Excipient information presented when available (limited, particularly for generics); consult specific product labeling.

Injection, powder for reconstitution:

Dacogen®: 50 mg

References

Cashen AF, Schiller GJ, O'Donnell, MR, et al, "Multicenter Phase II Study of Decitabine for the First-Line Treatment of Older Patients With Acute Myeloid Leukemia," *J Clin Oncol*, 2010, 28 (4):556-61.

Cashen AF, Shah AK, Todt L, et al, "Pharmacokinetics of Decitabine Administered as a 3-h Infusion to Patients With Acute Myeloid Leukemia (AML) or Myelodysplastic Syndrome (MDS)," *Cancer Chemother Pharmacol*, 2008, 61(5):759-66.

Kantarjian H, Issa JP, Rosenfeld CS, et al, "Decitabine Improves Patient Outcomes in Myelodysplastic Syndromes," *Cancer*, 2006, 106(8):1794-803.

Kantarjian H, Oki Y, Garcia-Manero G, et al, "Results of a Randomized Study of 3 Schedules of Low-Dose Decitabine in Higher-Risk Myelodysplastic Syndrome and Chronic Myelomonocytic Leukemia," *Blood*, 2007, 109(1):52-7.

Saunthararajah Y, Hillery CA, Lavelle D, et al, "Effects of 5-Aza-2'-Deoxycytidine on Fetal Hemoglobin Levels, Red Cell Adhesion, and Hematopoietic Differentiation in Patients With Sickle Cell Disease," *Blood*, 2003, 102(12):3865-70.
Steensma DP, Baer MR, Slack JL, et al, "Multicenter Study of Decitabine Administered Daily for 5 Days Every 4 Weeks to Adults With Myelodysplastic Syndromes: The Alternative Dosing For Outpatient Treatment (ADOPT) Trial," *J Clin Oncol*, 2009, 27(23):3842-8.

Deferasirox (de FER a sir ox)

Brand Names: U.S. Exjade®
Brand Names: Canada Exjade®
Index Terms ICL670
Generic Availability (U.S.) No
Pharmacologic Category Chelating Agent
Use Treatment of chronic iron overload due to blood transfusions (transfusional hemosiderosis)
Labeled Contraindications Hypersensitivity to deferasirox or any component of the formulation; platelet counts <50,000/mm^3; poor performance status; high-risk myelodysplastic syndromes; advanced malignancies; creatinine clearance <40 mL/minute or serum creatinine >2 x age-appropriate ULN

Canadian labeling: Additional contraindications (not in U.S. labeling): Cl_{cr} <60 mL/minute

Pregnancy Risk Factor C
Lactation Excretion in breast milk unknown/not recommended
Warnings/Precautions **[U.S. Boxed Warning]: Acute renal failure (including fatalities and cases requiring dialysis) may occur; observed more frequently in patients with comorbid conditions and advanced hematologic malignancies. Obtain serum creatinine and calculate creatinine clearance in duplicate at baseline prior to initiation, and monitor at least monthly thereafter; in patients with underlying renal dysfunction or at risk for acute renal failure, monitor creatinine weekly during the first month then at least monthly thereafter. Dose reduction, interruption, or discontinuation should be considered for serum creatinine elevations.** Use is contraindicated in patients with a creatinine clearance <40 mL/minute or serum creatinine >2 x age-appropriate ULN. May cause proteinuria; monitor monthly. Renal tubular damage, including Fanconi's syndrome, has also been reported, primarily in pediatric/adolescent patients with β-thalassemia and serum ferritin levels <1500 mcg/L.

[U.S. Boxed Warning]: Hepatotoxicity and failure (including fatalities) may occur. Monitor transaminases and bilirubin at baseline, every 2 weeks for 1 month, then at least monthly thereafter. Hepatitis and elevated transaminases have also been reported. Hepatotoxicity is more common in patients >55 years of age and in patients with significant comorbidities (eg, cirrhosis, multiorgan failure). Reduce dose or temporarily interrupt treatment for severe or persistent increases in transaminases/bilirubin. **[U.S. Boxed Warning]: Avoid use in patients with severe (Child-Pugh class C) hepatic impairment; a dose reduction is required in patients with moderate (Child-Pugh class B) hepatic impairment.** Monitor patients with mild (Child-Pugh class A) or moderate (Child-Pugh class B) impairment closely for efficacy and for adverse reactions requiring dosage reduction.

[U.S. Boxed Warning]: Gastrointestinal (GI) hemorrhage (including fatalities) may occur; observed more frequently in elderly patients with advanced hematologic malignancies and/or low platelet counts;

discontinue treatment for suspected GI hemorrhage or ulceration. Other GI effects including irritation and ulceration have been reported. Use caution with concurrent medications that may increase risk of adverse GI effects (eg, NSAIDs, corticosteroids, anticoagulants, oral bisphosphonates). Monitor patients closely for signs/symptoms of GI ulceration/bleeding.

May cause skin rash (dose-related), including erythema multiforme; mild-to-moderate rashes may resolve without treatment interruption; for severe rash, interrupt and consider restarting at a lower dose with dose escalation and oral steroids; discontinue if erythema multiforme is suspected. Hypersensitivity reactions, including severe reactions (anaphylaxis and angioedema) have been reported, onset is usually within the first month of treatment; discontinue if severe. Auditory (decreased hearing and high frequency hearing loss) or ocular disturbances (lens opacities, cataracts, intraocular pressure elevation, and retinal disorders) have been reported (rare); monitor and consider dose reduction or treatment interruption. Bone marrow suppression (including agranulocytosis, neutropenia, and thrombocytopenia) has been reported, risk may be increased in patients with preexisting hematologic disorders; monitor blood counts regularly; interrupt treatment in patients who develop cytopenias; may reinitiate once cause of cytopenia has been determined; use contraindicated if platelet count <50,000/mm^3. Potent UGT inducers (eg, rifampin) or bile acid sequestrants (eg, cholestyramine) may decrease the efficacy of deferasirox; avoid concomitant use. If coadministration necessary, dosage modifications may be needed; monitor serum ferritin and clinical response. Not approved for use in combination with other iron chelation therapies; safety of combinations has not been established. Treatment should be initiated with evidence of chronic iron overload (ie, transfusion of ≥100 mL/kg of packed RBCs [eg, ≥20 units for a 40 kg individual] and serum ferritin consistently >1000 mcg/L). Prior to use, consider risk versus anticipated benefit with respect to individual patient's life expectancy and prognosis. Use with caution in the elderly due to the higher incidence of toxicity (eg, hepatotoxicity) and fatal events during use. Overchelation of iron may increase development of toxicity; temporary interruption of treatment should be considered if serum ferritin <500 mcg/L.

Adverse Reactions

>10%:

- Central nervous system: Fever (19%), headache (16%)
- Dermatologic: Rash (dose related; 8% to 11%)
- Gastrointestinal: Abdominal pain (dose related; 21% to 28%), nausea (dose related; 11% to 23%), vomiting (dose related; 10% to 21%), diarrhea (dose related; 12% to 20%)
- Renal: Serum creatinine increased (dose related; 7% to 38%), proteinuria (19%)
- Respiratory: Cough (14%), nasopharyngitis (13%), pharyngolaryngeal pain (11%)
- Miscellaneous: Influenza (11%)

1% to 10%:

- Central nervous system: Fatigue (6%)
- Dermatologic: Urticaria (4%)
- Hepatic: ALT increased (2% to 8%), transaminitis (4%)
- Neuromuscular & skeletal: Arthralgia (7%), back pain (6%)
- Otic: Ear infection (5%)
- Respiratory: Respiratory tract infection (10%), bronchitis (9%), pharyngitis (8%), acute tonsillitis (6%), rhinitis (6%)

<1%, postmarketing, and/or case reports: Acute renal failure, agranulocytosis, anaphylaxis, angioedema, anxiety, ascites, bilirubin increased, cataract, cholecystitis, cholelithiasis, constipation, cytopenias, dizziness, drug fever, duodenal ulcer, edema, erythema multiforme, esophagitis, Fanconi's syndrome, gastric ulcer, gastritis, gastrointestinal bleeding, gastrointestinal hemorrhage, glomerulonephritis, glucosuria, hearing loss (including high frequency), hematuria, Henoch-Schönlein purpura, hepatic dysfunction, hepatic encephalopathy, hepatic failure, hepatic transaminases increased, hepatitis, hyperactivity, hypersensitivity reaction, hypocalcemia, insomnia, intraocular pressure increased, jaundice, lens opacities, leukocytoclastic vasculitis, maculopathy, neutropenia, optic neuritis, pigment disorder, purpura, renal tubular necrosis, renal tubulopathy, retinal disorder, sleep disorder, thrombocytopenia, tubulointerstitial nephritis, visual disturbance

Drug Interactions

Metabolism/Transport Effects **Substrate** of UGT1A1; **Inhibits** CYP1A2 (moderate), CYP2C8 (moderate); **Induces** CYP3A4 (weak/moderate)

Avoid Concomitant Use

Avoid concomitant use of Deferasirox with any of the following: Aluminum Hydroxide; Axitinib; Bile Acid Sequestrants; Theophylline

Increased Effect/Toxicity

Deferasirox may increase the levels/effects of: CYP1A2 Substrates; CYP2C8 Substrates; Repaglinide; Theophylline

The levels/effects of Deferasirox may be increased by: Anticoagulants; Bisphosphonate Derivatives; Corticosteroids; Corticosteroids (Systemic); Nonsteroidal Anti-Inflammatory Agents

Decreased Effect

Deferasirox may decrease the levels/effects of: ARIPiprazole; Axitinib; CYP3A4 Substrates; Saxagliptin

The levels/effects of Deferasirox may be decreased by: Aluminum Hydroxide; Bile Acid Sequestrants; Fosphenytoin; PHENobarbital; Phenytoin; Rifampin; Ritonavir

Ethanol/Nutrition/Herb Interactions Food: Bioavailability is increased variably when taken with food. Management: Take on an empty stomach at the same time each day at least 30 minutes before food. Maintain adequate hydration, unless instructed to restrict fluid intake.

Storage/Stability Store at room temperature of 25°C (77°F); excursions permitted to 15°C and 30°C (59°F and 86°F). Protect from moisture.

Mechanism of Action Selectively binds iron, forming a complex which is excreted primarily through the feces.

Pharmacodynamics/Kinetics

Distribution: Adults: 14.4 ± 2.7L

Protein binding: ~99% to serum albumin

Metabolism: Hepatic via glucuronidation by UGT1A1(primarily) and UGT1A3; minor oxidation by CYP450; undergoes enterohepatic recirculation

Bioavailability: 70%

Half-life elimination: 8-16 hours

Time to peak, plasma: ~1.5-4 hours

Excretion: Feces (84%); urine (8%)

Dosing

Adult & Geriatric Chronic iron overload due to blood transfusion: Oral: **Note:** Treatment should only be initiated with evidence of chronic iron overload (ie, transfusion of ≥100 mL/kg of packed RBCs [eg, ≥20 units for a 40 kg individual] and serum ferritin consistently >1000 mcg/L).

Initial: 20 mg/kg once daily (calculate dose to nearest whole tablet)

Maintenance: Adjust dose every 3-6 months based on serum ferritin trends; adjust by 5 or 10 mg/kg/day (calculate dose to nearest whole tablet); titrate to individual response and treatment goals. Usual range: 20-30 mg/kg/day; doses up to 40 mg/kg/day may be considered for serum ferritin levels persistently >2500 mcg/L (doses above 40 mg/kg/day are not recommended). **Note:** Consider interrupting therapy for serum ferritin <500 mcg/L (risk of toxicity may be increased).

Dosage adjustment with concomitant bile acid sequestrants (eg,cholestyramine, colesevelam, colestipol) or potent UGT inducers (eg, rifampin, phenytoin, phenobarbital, ritonavir): Avoid concomitant use; if coadministration necessary, consider increasing the initial dose of deferasirox dose by 50%; monitor serum ferritin and clinical response.

Pediatric Children ≥2 years and Adolescents: Refer to adult dosing.

Renal Impairment Creatinine clearance should be estimated using the Cockcroft-Gault formula.

Children ≥2 years, Adolescents, and Adults:

Prior to initiation:

Cl_{cr} ≥40 mL/minute **and** serum creatinine <2 times age-appropriate ULN at baseline: No initial dosage adjustment necessary. Use caution; monitor renal function closely, particularly in patients at increased risk for renal impairment (eg, concomitant nephrotoxic therapy, dehydration, severe infection); increases in serum creatinine may require alteration or discontinuation of therapy.

Cl_{cr} <40 mL/minute **or** serum creatinine >2 times age-appropriate ULN at baseline: Do not initiate therapy; use is contraindicated.

During therapy: Refer to dosage adjustment for toxicity.

Hepatic Impairment

Mild impairment (Child-Pugh class A): No dosage adjustment necessary; monitor closely for efficacy and for adverse reactions requiring dosage reduction.

Moderate impairment (Child-Pugh class B): Initial: Reduce dose by 50%; monitor closely for efficacy and for adverse reactions requiring dosage reduction.

Severe impairment (Child-Pugh class C): Avoid use.

Adjustment for Toxicity

Bone marrow suppression: Interrupt treatment; may reinitiate once cause of cytopenia has been determined; use contraindicated if platelet count <50,000/mm^3

Gastrointestinal: Discontinue treatment for suspected GI ulceration or hemorrhage.

Hearing loss or visual disturbance: Consider dose reduction or treatment interruption

Severe rash: Interrupt treatment; may reintroduce at a lower dose (with future dose escalation) and short-term oral corticosteroids. Permanently discontinue treatment if erythema multiforme is suspected.

Renal: **Note:** Discontinue treatment if serum creatinine >2 times age-appropriate ULN or Cl_{cr} <40 mL/minute (use is contraindicated).

Children ≥2 years and Adolescents <16 years: For increase in serum creatinine >33% above the average pretreatment level and above the age-appropriate ULN, reduce daily dose by 10 mg/kg.

Adolescents ≥16 years and Adults: For increase in serum creatinine ≥33% above the average pretreatment level for 2 consecutive weekly levels, reduce daily dose by 10 mg/kg.

Administration Oral: Administer tablets by making an oral suspension; **do not chew or swallow tablets whole.** Completely disperse tablets in water, orange juice, or apple juice (use 3.5 ounces for total doses <1 g; 7 ounces for doses ≥1 g); stir to form a fine suspension and drink entire contents. Rinse remaining residue with more fluid; drink. Administer at same time each day on an empty stomach, at least 30 minutes before food. Do not take simultaneously with aluminum-containing antacids.

Monitoring Parameters Serum ferritin (baseline, monthly thereafter), iron levels (baseline), CBC with differential, serum creatinine and creatinine clearance (2 baseline assessments then monthly thereafter; in patients who are at increased risk of complications [eg, pre-existing renal conditions, elderly, comorbid conditions, or receiving other potentially nephrotoxic medications]: weekly for the first month then at least monthly thereafter); urine protein (monthly); serum transaminases (ALT/AST) and bilirubin (baseline, every 2 weeks for the first month, then monthly); baseline and annual auditory and ophthalmic function (including slit lamp examinations and dilated fundoscopy); performance status (in patients with hematologic malignancies); signs and symptoms of GI ulcers or hemorrhage; cumulative number of RBC units received

Dietary Considerations Bioavailability increased variably when taken with food; take on empty stomach 30 minutes before a meal.

Additional Information Deferasirox has a low affinity for binding with zinc and copper, may cause variable decreases in the serum concentration of these trace minerals.

Oncology Comment: The National Comprehensive Cancer Network (NCCN) guidelines for myelodysplastic syndromes (MDS) recommend considering iron chelation therapy in low- or intermediate-risk MDS patients to decrease iron overload due to multiple transfusions (v.2.2011). Treatment is generally recommended in MDS patients who have received >20-30 RBC transfusions and for those with serum ferritin levels >2500 mcg/L, with a goal to decrease ferritin levels to <1000 mcg/L.

Prescribing and Access Restrictions Deferasirox (Exjade®) is only available through a restricted distribution program called EPASS™ Complete Care. Prescribers must enroll patients in this program in order to obtain the medication. For patient enrollment, contact 1-888-90-EPASS (1-888-903-7277).

Dosage Forms Excipient information presented when available (limited, particularly for generics); consult specific product labeling.

Tablet for suspension, oral:

Exjade®: 125 mg, 250 mg, 500 mg

References

Bacon BR, Adams PC, Kowdley KV, et al, "Diagnosis and Management of Hemochromatosis: 2011 Practice Guideline by the American Association for the Study of Liver Disease," *Hepatology*, 2011, 54(1):328-43.

Cappellini MD, Cohen A, Piga A, et al, "A Phase 3 Study of Deferasirox (ICL670), a Once-Daily Oral Iron Chelator, in Patients With Beta-Thalassemia," *Blood*, 2006, 107(9):3455-62.

Cappellini MD, "Long-Term Efficacy and Safety of Deferasirox," *Blood Rev*, 2008, 22(Suppl 2):35-41.

Cohen AR, Glimm E, and Porter JB, "Effect of Transfusional Iron Intake on Response to Chelation Therapy in β-Thalassemia Major," *Blood*, 2008, 111(2):583-7.

Galanello R, Piga A, Alberti D, et al, "Safety, Tolerability, and Pharmacokinetics of ICL670, a New Orally Active Iron-Chelating Agent in Patients With Transfusion-Dependent Iron Overload Due to Beta-Thalassemia," *J Clin Pharmacol*, 2003, 43(6):565-72.

National Comprehensive Cancer Network® (NCCN), "Clinical Practice Guidelines in Oncology™: Myelodysplastic Syndromes," Version 2.2011. Available at http://www.nccn.org/professionals/physician_gls/PDF/mds.pdf

Nisbet-Brown E, Oliveri NF, Giardina PJ, et al, "Effectiveness and Safety of ICL670 in Iron-Loaded Patients With Thalassaemia: A Randomised, Double-Blind, Placebo-Controlled, Dose-Escalation Trial," *Lancet*, 2003, 361(9369):1597-602.

Pennell DJ, Porter JB, Cappellini MD, et al, "Efficacy of Deferasirox in Reducing and Preventing Cardiac Iron Overload in Beta-Thalassemia," *Blood*, 2010, 115(12):2364-71.

Porter JB, "Optimizing Iron Chelation Strategies In Beta-Thalassaemia Major," *Blood Rev*, 2009, 23 (Suppl 1):3-7.

Porter J, Galanello R, Saglio G, et al, "Relative Response of Patients With Myelodysplastic Syndromes and Other Transfusion-Dependent Anaemias to Deferasirox (ICL670): A 1-Yr Prospective Study," *Eur J Haematol*, 2008, 80(2):168-76.

Raphael JL, Bernhardt MB, Mahoney DH, et al, "Oral Iron Chelation and the Treatment of Iron Overload in a Pediatric Hematology Center," *Pediatr Blood Cancer*, 2009, 52(5):616-20.

Vichinsky E, Onyekwere O, Porter J, et al, "A Randomised Comparison of Deferasirox Versus Deferoxamine for the Treatment of Transfusional Iron Overload in Sickle Cell Disease," *Br J Haematol*, 2007, 136(3):501-8.

Deferiprone (de FER i prone)

Brand Names: U.S. Ferriprox®

Index Terms APO-066; Ferriprox®

Pharmacologic Category Chelating Agent

Use Treatment of transfusional iron overload due to thalassemia syndromes with inadequate response to other chelation therapy

Labeled Contraindications Hypersensitivity to deferiprone or any component of the formulation

Pregnancy Risk Factor D

Lactation Excretion in breast milk unknown/not recommended

Warnings/Precautions [U.S. Boxed Warning]: May cause agranulocytosis, which may lead to serious infections (some fatal). Neutropenia may precede agranulocytosis; monitor absolute neutrophil count (ANC) prior to treatment initiation and weekly during therapy. If infection develops, interrupt treatment and monitor ANC more frequently. Patients should promptly report any symptoms which may indicate infection. Interrupt treatment if neutropenia (ANC <1500/mm^3) develops; withhold other medications which may also be associated with neutropenia; monitor CBC, corrected WBC, ANC, and platelets daily until ANC recovery. If ANC <500/mm^3, consider hospitalization (and other clinically appropriate management); do not resume or rechallenge unless the potential benefits outweigh potential risks. Neutropenia and agranulocytosis were generally reversible upon discontinuation. Avoid concurrent use with other agents associated with neutropenia (or agranulocytosis).

ALT elevations in have been observed; monitor ALT and consider treatment interruption for persistent elevations. Use with caution in patients at risk for QT prolongation (eg, bradycardia, cardiac hypertrophy, congestive HF, diuretic use, hypokalemia or hypomagnesemia). There has been a single case report of torsade de pointes in a patient with a history of QT prolongation. Patients should promptly report any symptoms suggestive of arrhythmias (eg, dizziness, light headedness, palpitations, seizure or syncope). Lower plasma zinc concentrations have been observed; monitor zinc levels and supplement if necessary.

Adverse Reactions

>10%:

Gastrointestinal: Nausea (13%)

Genitourinary: Chromaturia (15%)

1% to 10%:

Central nervous system: Headache (3%)

Gastrointestinal: Abdominal pain/discomfort (10%), vomiting (10%), appetite increased (4%), diarrhea (3%), dyspepsia (2%), weight gain (2%), appetite decreased (1%)

Hematologic: Neutropenia (6% to 7%), agranulocytosis (2%)

Hepatic: ALT increased (8%), AST increased (1%)

Neuromuscular and skeletal: Arthralgia (10%), back pain (2%), limb pain (2%), arthropathy (1%)

<1%, postmarketing, and/or case reports: Acute respiratory distress syndrome, anaphylactic shock, atrial fibrillation, bilirubin increased, bruxism, cardiac failure, cerebellar syndrome, cerebral hemorrhage, chills, chondropathy, CPK increased, cryptococcal cutaneous infection, dehydration, depression, diplopia, enterocolitis, enteroviral encephalitis, epistaxis, fever, furuncle, gait disturbance, gastric ulcer, glycosuria, hemoglobinuria, hemoptysis, Henoch-Schönlein purpura, hepatitis (infectious), hepatomegaly, hyperhydrosis, hyper-/hypotension, hypersensitivity, hypospadias, intracranial pressure increased, jaundice, metabolic acidosis, multiorgan failure, myositis, obsessive compulsive disorder, pancreatitis, pancytopenia, papilledema, parotid gland enlargement, periorbital edema, peripheral edema, pharyngitis, photosensitivity, pneumonia, pruritus, psychomotor skills impaired, pulmonary embolism, pustular rash, pyramidal tract syndrome, rash, rectal hemorrhage, retinal toxicity, seizure, sepsis, somnolence, subcutaneous abscess, thrombocytosis, torsade de pointes, trismus, urticaria, zinc levels decreased

Drug Interactions

Metabolism/Transport Effects **Substrate** of UGT1A6, UGT1A9, UGT2B15, UGT2B7

Avoid Concomitant Use There are no known interactions where it is recommended to avoid concomitant use.

Increased Effect/Toxicity

The levels/effects of Deferiprone may be increased by: UGT1A6 Inhibitors

Decreased Effect

The levels/effects of Deferiprone may be decreased by: Antacids; Calcium Salts; Iron Salts; Magnesium Salts; Multivitamins/Minerals (with ADEK, Folate, Iron); Zinc Salts

Ethanol/Nutrition/Herb Interactions Herb/Nutraceutical: Deferiprone may bind with polyvalent cations (eg, aluminum, zinc). Allow at least 4 hours between other medications or supplements containing polyvalent cations.

Storage/Stability Store at 20°C to 25°C (68°F to 77°F); excursions permitted to 15°C to 30°C (59°F to 86°F).

Mechanism of Action Iron-chelating agent with affinity for ferric ion (iron III); binds to ferric ion and forms a 3:1 (deferiprone:iron) complex which is excreted in the urine. Has a lower affinity for other metals such as copper, aluminum, and zinc.

Pharmacodynamics/Kinetics

Absorption: Rapid

Distribution: 1.6 L/kg (in thalassemia patients)

Protein binding: <10%

Metabolism: Primarily by UGT 1A6; major metabolite (3-O-glucuronide) lacks iron-binding capacity

Half life elimination: 1.9 hours

Time to peak: ~1-2 hours

Excretion: Urine (75% to 90%; as free deferiprone, the iron deferiprone complex, and glucuronide metabolite)

Dosing

Adult Note: Round dose to the nearest 250 mg (or 1/2 tablet). If serum ferritin falls consistently below 500 mcg/L, consider temporary treatment interruption.

Transfusional iron overload: Oral: Initial: 25 mg/kg 3 times/day (75 mg/kg/day); individualize dose based on response and therapeutic goal; maximum dose: 33 mg/kg 3 times/day (99 mg/kg/day)

Geriatric Refer to adult dosing. Begin at the low end of dosing range.

Renal Impairment No dosage adjustments are provided in the manufacturer's labeling (has not been studied).

Hepatic Impairment No dosage adjustments are provided in the manufacturer's labeling (has not been studied).

Adjustment for Toxicity

ANC <1500/mm^3: Interrupt treatment

ANC <500/mm^3: In addition to treatment interruption, consider hospitalization (and other clinically-appropriate management); do not resume or rechallenge unless the potential benefits outweigh potential risks

Infection: Interrupt treatment; monitor ANC more frequently

Administration Administer in the morning, at mid day and in the evening. Administration with food may decrease nausea.

Monitoring Parameters Serum ferritin (every 2-3 months); ANC (at baseline and weekly during treatment); if ANC <1500/mm^3, monitor CBC, WBC (corrected for nucleated RBCs), ANC, and platelets daily until ANC recovery; ALT (monthly); zinc levels; symptoms suggestive of QT prolongation; signs or symptoms of infection

Dietary Considerations May be taken with food to decrease nausea.

Medication Guide Available Yes

Dosage Forms Excipient information presented when available (limited, particularly for generics); consult specific product labeling.

Tablet, oral:

Ferriprox®: 500 mg [scored]

References

Ceci A, Baiardi P, Felisi M, et al, "The Safety and Effectiveness of Deferiprone in a Large-Scale, 3-Year Study in Italian patients," *Br J Haematol*, 2002, 118(1):330-6.

Cohen AR, Galanello R, Piga A, et al, Safety and Effectiveness of Long-Term Therapy With the Oral Iron Chelator Deferiprone," *Blood*, 2003, 102(5):1583-7.

Neufeld EJ, "Oral Chelators Deferasirox and Deferiprone for Transfusional Iron Overload in Thalassemia Major: New Data, New Questions," *Blood*, 2006, 107(9):3436-41.

Deferoxamine (de fer OKS a meen)

Brand Names: U.S. Desferal®

Brand Names: Canada Desferal®; PMS-Deferoxamine

Index Terms Deferoxamine Mesylate; Desferrioxamine; DFM

Generic Availability (U.S.) Yes

Pharmacologic Category Antidote; Chelating Agent

Use Adjunct in the treatment of acute iron intoxication; treatment of chronic iron overload secondary to multiple transfusions

Canadian labeling (unlabeled use in the U.S.): Diagnosis of aluminum overload; treatment of chronic aluminum overload in patients with end-stage renal failure undergoing maintenance dialysis

Unlabeled Use Diagnosis or treatment of aluminum induced toxicity associated with chronic kidney disease (CKD)

Labeled Contraindications Hypersensitivity to deferoxamine or any component of the formulation; patients with severe renal disease or anuria

Note: Canadian labeling does not include severe renal disease or anuria as contraindications.

Pregnancy Risk Factor C

Lactation Excretion in breast milk unknown/use caution

Warnings/Precautions Flushing of the skin, hypotension, urticaria and shock are associated with rapid I.V. infusion; administer I.M., by slow subcutaneous or slow I.V. infusion only. Auditory disturbances (tinnitus and high frequency hearing loss) have been reported following prolonged administration, at high doses, or in patients with low ferritin levels; generally reversible with early detection and immediate discontinuation. Elderly patients are at increased risk for hearing loss. Audiology exams are recommended with long-term treatment. Ocular disturbances (blurred vision, cataracts, corneal opacities, decreased visual acuity, impaired peripheral, color, and night vision, optic neuritis, retinal pigment abnormalities, scotoma, visual loss/defect) have been reported following prolonged administration, at high doses, or in patients with low ferritin levels; generally reversible with early detection and immediate discontinuation. Elderly patients are at increased risk for ocular disorders. Periodic ophthalmic exams are recommended with long-term treatment.

Deferoxamine has been associated with acute respiratory distress syndrome following excessively high-dose I.V. treatment of acute iron intoxication or thalassemia (has been reported in children and adults). High deferoxamine doses and concurrent low ferritin levels are also associated with growth retardation. Growth velocity may partially resume to pretreatment velocity rates after deferoxamine dose reduction. Patients with iron overload are at increased susceptibility to infection with *Yersinia enterocolitica* and *Yersinia pseudotuberculosis*; treatment with deferoxamine may enhance this risk; if infection develops, discontinue therapy until resolved. Rare and serious cases of mucormycosis have been reported with use; withhold treatment with signs and symptoms of mucormycosis.

Increases in serum creatinine, acute renal failure and renal tubular disorders have been reported; monitor for changes in renal function. When iron is chelated with deferoxamine, the chelate is excreted renally. Deferoxamine is readily dialyzable. Treatment with deferoxamine in patients with aluminum toxicity may cause hypocalcemia and aggravate hyperparathyroidism. Deferoxamine may cause neurological symptoms (including seizure) in patients with aluminum-related encephalopathy receiving dialysis and may precipitate dialysis dementia onset.

Deferoxamine is **not** indicated for the treatment of primary hemochromatosis (treatment of choice is phlebotomy). Patients should be informed that urine may have a reddish color. Combination treatment with ascorbic acid (>500 mg/day in adults) and deferoxamine may impair cardiac function (rare), reversible upon discontinuation of ascorbic acid. If combination treatment is warranted, initiate ascorbic acid only after one month of regular deferoxamine treatment, do not exceed ascorbic acid dose of 200 mg/day for adults (in divided doses), 100 mg/day for children ≥10 years of age, or 50 mg/day in children <10 years of age; monitor cardiac function. Do not administer deferoxamine in combination with ascorbic acid in patients with pre-existing cardiac failure.

Adverse Reactions Frequency not defined.

Cardiovascular: Flushing, hypotension, shock, tachycardia

Central nervous system: Dizziness, encephalopathy (aluminum toxicity/dialysis-related), fever, headache, seizure

Dermatologic: Angioedema, rash, urticaria

Endocrine & metabolic: Growth retardation (children), hyperparathyroidism (aggravated), hypocalcemia

Gastrointestinal: Abdominal discomfort, abdominal pain, diarrhea, nausea, vomiting

Genitourinary: Dysuria, urine discoloration (reddish color)

Hematologic: Leukopenia, thrombocytopenia

Hepatic: Hepatic dysfunction, transaminases increased

Local: Injection site: Burning, crust, edema, erythema, eschar, induration, infiltration, irritation, pain, pruritus, swelling, vesicles, wheal formation

Neuromuscular & skeletal: Arthralgia, metaphyseal dysplasia (children <3 years; dose related), muscle spasms, myalgia, neuropathy (peripheral, sensory, motor, or mixed), paresthesia

Ocular: Blurred vision, cataract, corneal opacities, dyschromatopsia, loss of vision, night blindness, optic neuritis, peripheral vision impaired, retinal pigment abnormalities, scotoma, visual acuity decreased, visual field defects

Otic: Hearing loss, tinnitus

Renal: Acute renal failure, renal tubular disorders, serum creatinine increased

Respiratory: Acute respiratory distress syndrome (dyspnea, cyanosis, and/or interstitial infiltrates), asthma

Miscellaneous: Anaphylaxis (with or without shock), hypersensitivity reaction, infections (*Yersinia*, mucormycosis)

Drug Interactions

Metabolism/Transport Effects None known.

Avoid Concomitant Use There are no known interactions where it is recommended to avoid concomitant use.

Increased Effect/Toxicity

Deferoxamine may increase the levels/effects of: Prochlorperazine

The levels/effects of Deferoxamine may be increased by: Ascorbic Acid; Multivitamins/Minerals (with ADEK, Folate, Iron)

Decreased Effect There are no known significant interactions involving a decrease in effect.

Storage/Stability Prior to reconstitution, store at ≤25°C (≤77°F). Following reconstitution, may be stored at room temperature for 24 hours, although the manufacturer recommends use begin within 3 hours of reconstitution. Do not refrigerate reconstituted solution. When stored at 30°C in polypropylene infusion pump syringes, deferoxamine 250 mg/mL in sterile water for injection retained 95% of initial concentration for 14 days (Stiles, 1996).

Reconstitution

I.M.: Reconstitute with sterile water for injection (500 mg vial with 2 mL SWFI; 2000 mg vial with 8 mL SWFI) to a final concentration of 213 mg/mL

I.V.: Reconstitute with sterile water for injection (500 mg vial with 5 mL SWFI; 2000 mg vial with 20 mL SWFI) to a final concentration of 95 mg/mL; further dilute for infusion in sodium chloride 0.9%, sodium chloride 0.45%, D_5W, or LR.

SubQ: Reconstitute with sterile water for injection (500 mg vial with 5 mL SWFI; 2000 mg vial with 20 mL SWFI) to a final concentration of 95 mg/mL

Mechanism of Action Complexes with trivalent ions (ferric ions) to form ferrioxamine, which is removed by the kidneys, slows accumulation of hepatic iron and retards or eliminates progression of hepatic fibrosis. Also known to inhibit DNA synthesis *in vitro*.

Pharmacodynamics/Kinetics

Absorption: I.M., SubQ: Well absorbed

Distribution: Distributed throughout body fluids

Protein binding: <10%

Metabolism: Plasma enzymes; binds with iron to form ferrioxamine (iron complex)

Half-life elimination: 14 hours (plasma half-life: 20-30 minutes)

Excretion: Primarily urine (as unchanged drug and ferrioxamine); feces (via bile)

Dosing

Adult

Acute iron toxicity: Note: The I.V. route is used when severe toxicity is evidenced by cardiovascular collapse or systemic symptoms (coma, shock, metabolic acidosis, or gastrointestinal bleeding) or potentially severe intoxications (peak serum iron level >500 mcg/dL) (Perrone, 2011). When severe symptoms are not present, the I.M. route may be used (per the manufacturer).

I.M., I.V.: Initial: 1000 mg, may be followed by 500 mg every 4 hours for 2 doses; subsequent doses of 500 mg have been administered every 4-12 hours based on clinical response (maximum recommended dose: 6000 mg/day [per manufacturer])

Canadian labeling:

I.M.: Initial: 90 mg/kg/dose (maximum/dose: 2000 mg) followed by 45 mg/kg every 4-12 hours as needed (maximum: 6000 mg/24 hours)

I.V.: 15 mg/kg/hour up to a maximum of 80 mg/kg/dose or maximum of 6000 mg/24 hours

Chronic iron overload:

I.M.: 500-1000 mg/day (maximum: 1000 mg/day)

I.V.: 40-50 mg/kg/day (maximum: 60 mg/kg/day) over 8-12 hours for 5-7 days per week

SubQ: 1000-2000 mg/day or 20-40 mg/kg/day over 8-24 hours

Unlabeled dosing: I.V., SubQ: 25-50 mg/kg over 8-10 hours 5-7 days per week (Brittenham, 2011)

Canadian labeling: I.V., SubQ: 1000-4000 mg/day (20-60 mg/kg/day) over ~12 hours (may further increase iron excretion with infusion at the same dose over 24 hours). SubQ infusions are administered 4-7 days per week based on the degree of iron overload.

Diagnosis of aluminum-induced toxicity with CKD (unlabeled use; K/DOQI guidelines, 2003): I.V.: Test dose: 5 mg/kg during the last hour of dialysis if serum aluminum levels are 60-200 mcg/L, or clinical signs/symptoms of toxicity, or aluminum exposure prior to parathyroid surgery. Measure aluminum just prior to deferoxamine; remeasure 2 days later (test is positive if serum aluminum is ≥50 mcg/L). Do not use if aluminum serum levels are >200 mcg/L.

Canadian labeling: **Note:** Measure serum aluminum levels prior to and after administration of deferoxamine. I.V.: Test dose: 5 mg/kg/dose (infusion rate not to exceed 15 mg/kg/hour) following hemodialysis (preferred) or during the last hour of dialysis if serum aluminum levels are >60 mcg/L in association with serum ferritin levels >100 mcg/L; continuous rise in serum aluminum over the next 24-48 hours suggests overload. Remeasure serum aluminum levels prior to next hemodialysis, test is considered positive if serum aluminum levels increase >150 mcg/L above baseline.

Treatment of aluminum toxicity with CKD (unlabeled use; K/DOQI guidelines, 2003): I.V.:

Administer after diagnostic deferoxamine test dose. **Note:** The risk for deferoxamine-associated neurotoxicity is increased if aluminum serum levels are >200 mcg/L; withhold deferoxamine and administer intensive dialysis until <200 mcg/L.

Aluminum rise ≥300 mcg/L: 5 mg/kg once a week 5 hours before dialysis for 4 months

Aluminum rise <300 mcg/L: 5 mg/kg once a week during the last hour of dialysis for 2 months

Canadian labeling: Treatment should be considered for symptomatic patients with serum aluminum levels >60 mcg/L and a positive deferoxamine test dose.

Hemodialysis: I.V.: 5 mg/kg/dose (infusion rate not to exceed 15 mg/kg/hour) once weekly for 3 months following hemodialysis (preferred) or during the last hour of dialysis administered. Withhold treatment for 1 month then perform deferoxamine test. Further treatment is not recommended if 2 consecutive tests (performed 1 month apart) yield an increase in serum aluminum levels <75 mcg/L.

Continuous ambulatory or cyclic peritoneal dialysis: Intraperitoneal (preferred), I.M., SubQ infusion (slow), or I.V. infusion (slow): 5 mg/kg/dose once weekly prior to final daily exchange

Geriatric Refer to adult dosing. May initiate at the lower end of the dosing range.

Pediatric

Acute iron toxicity: Children ≥3 years: **Note:** The I.V. route is used when severe toxicity is evidenced by cardiovascular collapse or systemic symptoms (coma, shock, metabolic acidosis, or gastrointestinal bleeding) or potentially severe intoxications (peak serum iron level >500 mcg/dL) (Perrone, 2011). When severe symptoms are not present, the I.M. route may be used (per the manufacturer).

I.M.: 90 mg/kg/dose every 8 hours (maximum: 6000 mg/24 hours)

I.V.: 15 mg/kg/hour (maximum: 6000 mg/24 hours)

Canadian labeling:

I.M.: Initial: 90 mg/kg/dose (maximum/dose: 1000 mg) followed by 45 mg/kg every 4-12 hours as needed (maximum: 6000 mg/24 hours)

I.V.: 15 mg/kg/hour up to a maximum of 80 mg/kg/dose or maximum of 6000 mg/24 hours

Chronic iron overload: Children ≥3 years:

I.V.: 20-40 mg/kg/day over 8-12 hours for 5-7 days per week; dose should not exceed 40 mg/kg/day until growth has ceased

SubQ: 20-40 mg/kg/day over 8-12 hours (maximum: 1000-2000 mg/day)

Unlabeled dosing: I.V., SubQ: 25-30 mg/kg over 8-10 hours 5-7 days per week (Brittenham, 2011)

Diagnosis of aluminum induced toxicity with CKD (unlabeled use; K/DOQI guidelines, 2003): Children: I.V.: Test dose: 5 mg/kg during the last hour of dialysis if serum aluminum levels are 60-200 mcg/L, or clinical signs/symptoms of toxicity, or aluminum exposure prior to parathyroid surgery. Measure aluminum just prior to deferoxamine; remeasure 2 days later (test is positive if serum aluminum is ≥50 mcg/L). Do not use if aluminum serum levels are >200 mcg/L.

Treatment of aluminum toxicity with CKD (unlabeled use; K/DOQI guidelines, 2003): Children: I.V.: Administer after diagnostic deferoxamine test dose. **Note:** The risk for deferoxamine-associated neurotoxicity is increased if aluminum serum levels are >200 mcg/L; withhold deferoxamine and administer intensive dialysis until <200 mcg/L.

Aluminum rise ≥300 mcg/L: 5 mg/kg once a week 5 hours before dialysis for 4 months

Aluminum rise <300 mcg/L: 5 mg/kg once a week during the last hour of dialysis for 2 months

Renal Impairment Severe renal disease or anuria: Use is contraindicated in the manufacturer's U.S. labeling.

The following adjustments have been used by some clinicians (Aronoff, 2007): Adults:

Cl_{cr} >50 mL/minute: No adjustment required

Cl_{cr} 10-50 mL/minute, CRRT: Administer 25% to 50% of normal dose

Cl_{cr} <10 mL/minute, hemodialysis, peritoneal dialysis: Avoid use

Hepatic Impairment There are no dosage adjustments provided in the manufacturer's labeling (has not been studied).

Administration

I.V.: Urticaria, flushing of the skin, hypotension, and shock have occurred following rapid I.V. administration; limiting infusion rate to 15mg/kg/hour may help avoid infusion-related adverse effects.

Acute iron toxicity: The manufacturer states that the I.M. route is preferred; however, the I.V. route is generally preferred in patients with severe toxicity (ie, patients in shock). For the first 1000 mg, infuse at 15 mg/kg/hour. Subsequent doses may be given over 4-12 hours at a rate not to exceed 125 mg/hour.

Chronic iron overload: Administer over 8-12 hours for 5-7 days per week; rate not to exceed 15 mg/kg/hour. In patients with poor compliance, deferoxamine may be administered on the same day of blood transfusion, either prior to or following transfusion; do not administer concurrently with transfusion. Longer infusion times (24 hours) and I.V. administration may be required in patients with severe cardiac iron deposition (Brittenham, 2011).

Diagnosis or treatment of aluminum-induced toxicity with CKD: Administer dose over 1 hour, during the last hour of dialysis (K/DOQI guidelines, 2003).

SubQ: When administered for chronic iron overload, administration over 8-12 hours using a portable infusion pump is generally recommended; however, longer infusion times (24 hours) may also be used. Topical anesthetic or glucocorticoid creams may be used for induration or erythema (Brittenham, 2011).

I.M.: I.M. administration may be used for patients with acute iron toxicity that do not exhibit severe symptoms (per the manufacturer); may also be used in the treatment of chronic iron toxicity.

Monitoring Parameters Serum iron, ferritin, total iron-binding capacity, CBC with differential, renal function tests (serum creatinine), liver function tests, serum chemistries; ophthalmologic exam (visual acuity tests, fundoscopy, slit-lamp exam) and audiometry with long-term treatment; growth and body weight in children (every 3 months)

Dialysis patients: Serum aluminum (yearly; every 3 months in patients on aluminum-containing medications)

Aluminum-induced bone disease: Serum aluminum 2 days following test dose; test is considered positive if serum aluminum increases ≥50 mcg/L

Test Interactions TIBC may be falsely elevated with high serum iron concentrations or deferoxamine therapy. Imaging results may be distorted due to rapid urinary excretion of deferoxamine-bound gallium-67; discontinue deferoxamine 48 hours prior to scintigraphy.

Dietary Considerations Vitamin C supplements may need to be limited. The manufacturer recommends a maximum ascorbic acid dose of 200 mg/day in adults (given in divided doses), 100 mg/day in children ≥10 years of age, or 50 mg/day in children <10 years of age. Avoid concurrent use with ascorbic acid in patients with heart failure.

Additional Information Oncology Comment: The National Comprehensive Cancer Network (NCCN) guidelines for myelodysplastic syndromes (MDS) recommend considering iron chelation therapy in low- or intermediate-risk MDS patients to decrease iron overload due to multiple transfusions (v.1.2012). Treatment (subcutaneous deferoxamine or oral deferasirox) is generally recommended in MDS patients who have received >20-30 RBC transfusions. For those with serum ferritin levels >2500 mcg/L, the goal to decrease ferritin levels to <1000 mcg/L.

Dosage Forms Excipient information presented when available (limited, particularly for generics); consult specific product labeling.

Injection, powder for reconstitution, as mesylate: 500 mg, 2 g

Desferal®: 500 mg, 2 g

References

Aronoff GR, Bennett WM, Berns JS, et al, *Drug Prescribing in Renal Failure: Dosing Guidelines for Adults and Children*, 5th ed. Philadelphia, PA: American College of Physicians; 2007, p 116.

Bacon BR, Adams PC, Kowdley KV, et al, "Diagnosis and Management of Hemochromatosis: 2011 Practice Guideline by the American Association for the Study of Liver Disease," *Hepatology*, 2011, 54(1):328-43.

Brittenham GM. "Iron-Chelating Therapy for Transfusional Iron Overload," *N Engl J Med*, 2011, 364 (2):146-56.

"K/DOQI Clinical Practice Guidelines for Bone Metabolism and Disease in Chronic Kidney Disease." Available at http://www.kidney.org/professionals/KDOQI/guidelines_bone/index.htm

National Comprehensive Cancer Network® (NCCN), "Clinical Practice Guidelines in Oncology™: Myelodysplastic Syndromes," Version 1.2012. Available at http://www.nccn.org/professionals/physician_gls/PDF/mds.pdf

Perrone J, "Iron," *Goldfrank's Toxicologic Emergencies*, 9th ed, Nelson LS, Hoffman RS, Lewin NA, et al, eds, New York, NY: McGraw-Hill Companies, Inc, 2011.

Stiles ML, Allen LV, and Prince SJ, "Stability of Deferoxamine Mesylate, Floxuridine, Fluorouracil, Hydromorphone Hydrochloride, Lorazepam, and Midazolam Hydrochloride in Polypropylene Infusion-Pump Syringes," *Am J Health Syst Pharm*, 1996, 53(13):1583-8.

◆ **Deferoxamine Mesylate** *see* Deferoxamine *on page 414*

Defibrotide (DE fib ro tide)

Index Terms DF; Prociclide

Generic Availability (U.S.) No

Pharmacologic Category Antiplatelet Agent; Thrombolytic Agent

Unlabeled Use Prevention of hepatic sinusoidal obstruction syndrome (SOS; formerly called veno-occlusive disease) in hematopoietic stem cell transplant (HSCT); treatment of hepatic SOS associated with HSCT

Warnings/Precautions Predominant exclusion criteria from studies were clinically significant bleeding, >1 pressor agent to maintain blood pressure, neurotoxicity, intubated patients, grade B to D graft versus host disease

(GVHD); grade B skin GVHD was allowed (Richardson, 2010; Richardson, 2011). Patients were excluded from studies if on prior or concurrent systemic tissue plasminogen activator use, concomitant anticoagulants (except when used for central line management or dialysis; patients on prior heparin were eligible if heparin was discontinued ≥12 hours prior to enrollment); or concomitant treatment with antithrombin III, other antithrombotics, ursodiol (unless for confirmed bile sludging), or nonsteroidal anti-inflammatory agents (Richardson, 2010). Defibrotide is derived from porcine tissue.

Adverse Reactions Frequency not defined.

Cardiovascular: Hypotension

Central nervous system: CNS hemorrhage, fever

Endocrine: Hot flashes

Gastrointestinal: Abdominal pain, cramping, diarrhea, diarrhea (hemorrhagic), gastrointestinal bleeding, hematemesis, mouth hemorrhage, nausea, vomiting

Hematologic: Hemorrhage/bleeding

Local: Thrombophlebitis

Renal: Hematuria, renal failure

Respiratory: Diffuse alveolar hemorrhage, epistaxis, pulmonary hemorrhage

Miscellaneous: Allergic reaction

Reconstitution Defibrotide was mixed in D_5W to a maximum concentration of 4 mg/mL (Richardson, 2010).

Mechanism of Action Defibrotide binds to and protects vascular hepatic endothelial cells (especially small vessels) by enhancing fibrinolysis and suppressing coagulation. Effects are local, with no significant effect on systemic coagulation. Has antithrombotic, anti-inflammatory, antiplatelet, and anti-ischemic properties.

Pharmacodynamics/Kinetics

Distribution: V_d: 0.04-0.05 L/kg (Palmer, 1993)

Excretion: Urine and feces (Palmer, 1993)

Dosing

Adult

Prevention of hepatic sinusoidal obstruction syndrome (SOS) in HSCT (unlabeled use): I.V.: 5 mg/kg twice daily for 21 days post-transplant (Dignan, 2007)

Treatment of hepatic SOS in HSCT (unlabeled use; begin treatment as soon as possible after SOS is suspected): I.V.: 6.25 mg/kg every 6 hours for at least 21 days (Richardson, 2009; Richardson, 2011)

Geriatric Refer to adult dosing.

Pediatric

Prevention of hepatic sinusoidal obstruction syndrome (SOS) in hematopoietic stem cell transplant (HSCT; unlabeled use): I.V.: 6.25 mg/kg every 6 hours beginning the same day as the conditioning regimen and continued for at least 14 and up to 30 days post-transplant (Corbacioglu, 2012)

Treatment of hepatic SOS in HSCT (unlabeled use; begin treatment as soon as possible after SOS is suspected): I.V.: Refer to adult dosing.

Administration I.V.: Infuse over 2 hours (Corbacioglu, 2012; Dignan, 2007; Richardson, 2002)

Monitoring Parameters Monitor for signs and symptoms of hepatic SOS; monitor for bleeding

Prescribing and Access Restrictions Defibrotide is an investigational agent available for the treatment of hepatic SOS through an Expanded Access

Treatment IND Protocol (protocol 2006-05). Information on access is available at http://www.gentium.com/vod/about-vod/access-to-defibrotide.

References

Corbacioglu S, Cesaro S, Faraci M, et al, "Defibrotide for Prophylaxis of Hepatic Veno-Occlusive Disease in Paediatric Haemopoietic Stem-Cell Transplantation: An Open-Label, Phase 3, Randomised Controlled Trial," *Lancet*, 2012, 379(9823):1301-9.

Corbacioglu S, Greil J, Peters C, et al, "Defibrotide in the Treatment of Children With Veno-Occlusive Disease (VOD): A Retrospective Multicentre Study Demonstrates Therapeutic Efficacy Upon Early Intervention," *Bone Marrow Transplant*, 2004, 33(2):189-95.

Dignan F, Gujral D, Ethell M, et al, "Prophylactic Defibrotide in Allogeneic Stem Cell Transplantation: Minimal Morbidity and Zero Mortality From Veno-Occlusive Disease," *Bone Marrow Transplant*, 2007, 40(1):79-82.

Palmer KJ and Goa KL, "Defibrotide: a Review of its Pharmacodynamic and Pharmacokinetic Properties and Therapeutic Use in Vascular Disorders," *Drugs*, 1993, 45(2):259-94.

Richardson PG, Murakami C, Jin Z, et al, "Multi-Institutional Use of Defibrotide in 88 Patients after Stem Cell Transplantation With Severe Veno-Occlusive Disease and Multisystem Organ Failure: Response Without Significant Toxicity in a High-Risk Population and Factors Predictive of Outcome," *Blood*, 2002, 100(13):4337-43.

Richardson PG, Smith AR, Grupp, SA, et al, "Defibrotide (DF) in the Treatment of Hepatic Veno-Occlusive Disease (VOD) in Stem Cell Transplant (SCT) and Non-SCT Patients (Pts): Early Intervention Improves Outcome - Updated Results of a Treatment IND Expanded Access Protocol," *Blood*, 2011, 118(21):487 [abstract #487 from 2011 ASH Annual Meeting]

Richardson PG, Soiffer RJ, Antin JH, et al, "Defibrotide for the Treatment of Severe Hepatic Veno-Occlusive Disease and Multiorgan Failure After Stem Cell Transplantation: A Multicenter, Randomized, Dose-Finding Trial," *Biol Blood Marrow Transplant*, 2010, 16(7):1005-17.

Richardson P, Tomblyn M, Kernan N, et al, "Defibrotide (DF) in the Treatment of Severe Hepatic Veno-Occlusive Disease (VOD) With Multi-Organ Failure (MOF) Following Stem Cell Transplantation (SCT): Results of a Phase 3 Study Utilizing a Historical Control," *Blood*, 2009, 114 (22):654 [abstract #654 from 2009 ASH Anual meeting].

Degarelix (deg a REL ix)

Related Information

Safe Handling of Hazardous Drugs *on page 1904*

Brand Names: U.S. Firmagon®

Brand Names: Canada Firmagon®

Index Terms Degarelix Acetate; FE200486

Generic Availability (U.S.) No

Pharmacologic Category Antineoplastic Agent, Gonadotropin-Releasing Hormone Antagonist; Gonadotropin Releasing Hormone Antagonist

Use Treatment of advanced prostate cancer

Labeled Contraindications Hypersensitivity to degarelix or any component of the formulation; pregnancy (or potential to become pregnant)

Pregnancy Risk Factor X

Lactation Excretion in breast milk unknown/not recommended

Warnings/Precautions Hazardous agent - use appropriate precautions for handling and disposal. Long-term androgen deprivation therapy may prolong the QT interval; use with caution in patients with a known history of QT prolongation or other risk factors for QT prolongation (eg, concomitant use of medications known to prolong QT interval, heart failure, and/or electrolyte abnormalities). Androgen-deprivation therapy may increase the risk for cardiovascular disease (Levine, 2010) and decreased bone mineral density. Androgen deprivation therapy may cause obesity and insulin resistance; the risk for diabetes is increased.

Degarelix exposure is decreased in patients with hepatic impairment, dosage adjustment is not recommended in patients with mild-to-moderate hepatic impairment, although testosterone levels should be monitored. Has not been studied in patients with severe hepatic impairment; use with caution. Data for use in patients with moderate-to-severe renal impairment (Cl_{cr} <50 mL/minute) is limited; use with caution.

Adverse Reactions

>10%:

Endocrine & metabolic: Hot flashes (26%)

Local: Injections site reactions (35%, grade 3: ≤2%; pain 28%, erythema 17%, swelling 6%, induration 4%, nodule 3%)

1% to 10%:

Cardiovascular: Hypertension (6%)

Central nervous system: Chills (5%), dizziness (1% to 5%), fever (1% to 5%), headache (1% to 5%), insomnia (1% to 5%), fatigue (3%)

Dermatologic: Hyperhydrosis

Endocrine & metabolic: Hypercholesterolemia (3%), gynecomastia, testicular atrophy

Gastrointestinal: Weight gain (9%), constipation (5%), nausea (1% to 5%), diarrhea

Genitourinary: Urinary tract infection (5%), erectile dysfunction

Hepatic: ALT increased (10%; grade 3: <1%), AST increased (5%; grade 3: <1%), GGT increased

Neuromuscular & skeletal: Back pain (6%), arthralgia (5%), weakness (1% to 5%)

Miscellaneous: Antidegarelix antibody formation (10%), night sweats (1% to 5%)

<1%, postmarketing, and/or case reports: Bone metastases worsening, cerebral stroke, depression, injection site pruritus, injection site soreness, lymphoma (malignant), mental status changes, MI, osteoarthritis, QT interval prolongation, squamous cell cancer, unstable angina

Drug Interactions

Metabolism/Transport Effects None known.

Avoid Concomitant Use

Avoid concomitant use of Degarelix with any of the following: Highest Risk QTc-Prolonging Agents; Mifepristone

Increased Effect/Toxicity

Degarelix may increase the levels/effects of: Highest Risk QTc-Prolonging Agents; Moderate Risk QTc-Prolonging Agents

The levels/effects of Degarelix may be increased by: Mifepristone; QTc-Prolonging Agents (Indeterminate Risk and Risk Modifying)

Decreased Effect There are no known significant interactions involving a decrease in effect.

Storage/Stability Store at 25°C (77°F); excursions permitted to 15°C to 30°C (59°F to 86°F).

Reconstitution Use appropriate precautions (wear gloves for preparation and administration) for handling and disposal. Reconstitute with preservative free sterile water for injection (reconstitute each 120 mg vial with 3 mL; reconstitute the 80 mg vial with 4.2 mL). Swirl gently; do not shake (to prevent foaming). Dissolution may take up to 15 minutes. Keep vial upright at all times. Tilt vial slightly, keeping needle in lowest section of vial to withdraw for administration. Administer within 1 hour of reconstitution.

Mechanism of Action Gonadotropin-releasing hormone (GnRH) antagonist which reversibly binds to GnRH receptors in the anterior pituitary gland, blocking the receptor and decreasing secretion of luteinizing hormone (LH) and follicle stimulation hormone (FSH), resulting in rapid androgen deprivation by decreasing testosterone production, thereby decreasing testosterone levels. Testosterone levels do not exhibit an initial surge, or flare, as is typical with GnRH agonists.

Pharmacodynamics/Kinetics

Onset of action: Rapid; ~96% of patients had testosterone levels ≤50 ng/dL within 3 days (Klotz, 2008)

Distribution: V_d: >1000 L

Protein binding: ~90%

Metabolism: Hepatobiliary, via peptide hydrolysis

Bioavailability: Biphasic release: Rapid release initially, then slow release from depot formed after subcutaneous injection administration (Tornoe, 2007)

Half-life elimination: Loading dose: SubQ: ~53 days

Time to peak, plasma: Loading dose: SubQ: Within 2 days

Excretion: Feces (~70% to 80%, primarily as peptide fragments); urine (~20% to 30%)

Dosing

Adult & Geriatric Prostate cancer: SubQ:

Loading dose: 240 mg administered as two 120 mg (3 mL) injections

Maintenance dose: 80 mg every 28 days (beginning 28 days after initial loading dose)

Renal Impairment Cl_{cr} <50 mL/minute: Use with caution.

Hepatic Impairment

Mild-to-moderate hepatic impairment: No adjustment required; monitor serum testosterone levels.

Severe hepatic impairment: Has not been studied; use with caution.

Administration Not for I.V. use. Administer SubQ in the abdominal area by grasping skin and elevating SubQ tissue; insert the needle deeply at an angle not ≤45 degrees. Avoid pressure exposed areas (eg, waistband, belt, or near ribs); rotate injection site. Inject loading dose as two 3 mL injections (40 mg/mL); maintenance dose should be administered as a single 4 mL injection (20 mg/mL); begin maintenance dose 28 days after initial loading dose.

Monitoring Parameters Prostate-specific antigen (PSA) periodically, serum testosterone levels (if PSA increases; in patients with hepatic impairment: monitor testosterone levels monthly until achieve castration levels, then consider monitoring every other month), liver function tests (at baseline), serum electrolytes (calcium, magnesium, potassium, sodium); bone mineral density

Screen for diabetes and cardiovascular risk prior to initiating treatment.

Test Interactions Suppression of pituitary-gonadal function may affect diagnostic tests of pituitary gonadotropic and gonadal functions.

Dietary Considerations Supplementation with 500 mg calcium and 400 units of vitamin D is recommended (due to the increased risk for osteoporosis with androgen deprivation therapy).

Dosage Forms Excipient information presented when available (limited, particularly for generics); consult specific product labeling.

Injection, powder for reconstitution, as acetate:

Firmagon®: 80 mg, 120 mg

References

Crawford ED, Tombal B, Miller K, et al, "A Phase III Extension Trial With a 1-Arm Crossover From Leuprolide to Degarelix: Comparison of Gonadotropin-Releasing Hormone Agonist and Antagonist Effect on Prostate Cancer," *J Urol*, 2011, 186(3):889-97.

Gittelman M, Pommerville PJ, Persson BE, et al, "A 1-Year, Open Label, Randomized Phase II Dose Finding Study of Degarelix for the Treatment of Prostate Cancer in North America," *J Urol*, 2008, 180(5):1986-92.

Klotz L, Boccon-Gibod L, Shore ND, et al, "The Efficacy and Safety of Degarelix: A 12-month, Comparative, Randomized, Open-Label, Parallel-Group Phase III Study in Patients With Prostate Cancer," *BJU Int*, 2008, 102(11):1531-8.

Levine GN, D'Amico AV, Berger P, et al, "Androgen-Deprivation Therapy in Prostate Cancer and Cardiovascular Risk. A Science Advisory from the American Heart Association, American Cancer Society, and American Urological Association," *Circulation*, 2010, 121:831-38.

◆ **Degarelix Acetate** *see* Degarelix *on page 422*

◆ **Dehydrobenzperidol** *see* Droperidol *on page 486*

◆ **Delta-9-tetrahydro-cannabinol** *see* Dronabinol *on page 484*

◆ **Delta-9 THC** *see* Dronabinol *on page 484*

◆ **Deltacortisone** *see* PredniSONE *on page 1199*

◆ **Deltadehydrocortisone** *see* PredniSONE *on page 1199*

◆ **Demerol®** *see* Meperidine *on page 932*

◆ **4-Demethoxydaunorubicin** *see* IDArubicin *on page 749*

Denileukin Diftitox (de ni LOO kin DIF ti toks)

Related Information

Management of Chemotherapy-Induced Nausea and Vomiting *on page 1786*
Management of Infections *on page 1809*
Principles of Anticancer Therapy *on page 1878*
Safe Handling of Hazardous Drugs *on page 1904*

Brand Names: U.S. ONTAK®

Index Terms DAB389 Interleukin-2; DAB_{389}IL-2; DABIL2

Generic Availability (U.S.) No

Pharmacologic Category Antineoplastic Agent, Miscellaneous

Use Treatment of persistent or recurrent cutaneous T-cell lymphoma (CTCL) whose malignant cells express the CD25 component of the IL-2 receptor

Unlabeled Use Treatment of relapsed or refractory peripheral T-cell lymphoma (PTCL)

Labeled Contraindications There are no contraindications listed within the manufacturer's labeling.

Lactation Excretion in breast milk unknown/not recommended

Warnings/Precautions Hazardous agent - use appropriate precautions for handling and disposal. **[U.S. Boxed Warning]: Has been associated with a potentially severe, including life-threatening, capillary leak syndrome; monitor weight, edema, blood pressure, and serum albumin prior to and during treatment.** Symptoms of capillary leak syndrome (defined as occurrence of ≥2 of the following symptoms: hypotension, edema, hypoalbuminemia) may be delayed, occurring up to 2 weeks post infusion; symptoms may persist or worsen after treatment cessation. Withhold treatment if serum albumin <3 g/dL; pre-existing low serum albumin levels may correlate with capillary leak syndrome. **[U.S. Boxed Warning]: Serious and fatal infusion reactions have occurred. Administer in a facility appropriate for cardiopulmonary resuscitation. Discontinue immediately and permanently with serious infusion reaction.** Infusion reaction symptoms usually occur within 24 hours of infusion and resolve within 48 hours of last infusion of cycle. Incidence of infusion reaction has been reported to be lower in cycles 3 and 4 (compared to cycles 1 and 2). The manufacturer recommends premedicating with an antihistamine and acetaminophen; corticosteroid (eg, dexamethasone) ▶

premedication may help to reduce the incidence of hypersensitivity and edema (Foss, 2001). **[U.S. Boxed Warning]: Loss of visual acuity, usually associated with loss of color vision (with or without retinal pigment mottling) has been reported;** most patients have persistent visual impairment.

Confirm CD25 expression on malignant cells prior to treatment. May develop immunogenicity; patients with antibodies have a two- to threefold increase in clearance; the presence of antibodies does not correlate with risk for hypersensitivity/infusion related reactions. Monitor closely for infection; may impair immune function. Use with caution in patients >65 years of age; adverse events (anemia, anorexia, confusion, hypotension, rash, nausea/vomiting) may occur more frequently.

Adverse Reactions

>10%:

Cardiovascular: Capillary leak syndrome (33%; serious: 11%), peripheral edema (20% to 26%), vasodilation (22%), hypotension (7% to 16%), chest pain (4% to 13%), tachycardia (12%), thrombosis-related events (7% to 11%)

Central nervous system: Fever (49% to 64%), fatigue (44% to 47%), headache (26% to 29%), dizziness (11% to 13%), pain (11% to 13%)

Dermatologic: Rash (20% to 24%), pruritus (16% to 18%)

Endocrine & metabolic: Hypoalbuminemia (14% to 17%)

Gastrointestinal: Nausea (47% to 60%), vomiting (13% to 35%), diarrhea (22%), anorexia (9% to 20%), taste disturbance (11% to 13%)

Hematologic: Lymphopenia (70%; 24% had lymphopenia at baseline)

Hepatic: ALT increased (84%), AST increased (84%)

Neuromuscular & skeletal: Rigors (42% to 47%), myalgia (18% to 20%), weakness (18%), back pain (16% to 18%), arthralgia (13% to 16%)

Respiratory: Cough (18% to 20%), upper respiratory infection (13%), dyspnea (11% to 13%)

Miscellaneous: Antibody formation (76% to 100%) neutralizing antibodies (45% to 97%), flu-like syndrome (≤85%), infusion reaction (71%; serious: 8%), infection (48%)

1% to 10%:

Cardiovascular: Arrhythmia (6%), hypertension (6%)

Hematologic: Leukopenia (grades 3/4: 3% to 6%), neutropenia (grades 3/4: 3%), thrombocytopenia (grades 3/4: 3%)

Local: Injection site reaction (8%)

Ocular: Visual changes (serious: 4%; includes loss of visual acuity)

Renal: Serum creatinine increased (3% to 10%), proteinuria/casts/hematuria (6%)

Postmarketing and/or case reports: Acute renal insufficiency, hyper-/hypothyroidism, oral ulcer, pancreatitis, thyroiditis, thyrotoxicosis, toxic epidermal necrolysis

Drug Interactions

Metabolism/Transport Effects
None known.

Avoid Concomitant Use

Avoid concomitant use of Denileukin Diftitox with any of the following: BCG; Belimumab; Natalizumab; Pimecrolimus; Tacrolimus (Topical); Vaccines (Live)

Increased Effect/Toxicity

Denileukin Diftitox may increase the levels/effects of: Belimumab; Leflunomide; Natalizumab; Vaccines (Live)

The levels/effects of Denileukin Diftitox may be increased by: Denosumab; Pimecrolimus; Roflumilast; Tacrolimus (Topical); Trastuzumab

Decreased Effect

Denileukin Diftitox may decrease the levels/effects of: BCG; Coccidioidin Skin Test; Sipuleucel-T; Vaccines (Inactivated); Vaccines (Live)

The levels/effects of Denileukin Diftitox may be decreased by: Echinacea

Storage/Stability Store intact vials frozen at or below -10°C (14°F); do not refreeze after thawing. Solutions (diluted for infusion) ≥15 mcg/mL in NS should be used within 6 hours.

Reconstitution Must be brought to room temperature (25°C or 77°F) before preparing the dose. Do **not** heat vials. Thaw intact vials in refrigerator for not more than 24 hours or at room temperature for 1-2 hours. Solution may be mixed by gentle swirling; avoid vigorous agitation. Dilute (for infusion) with preservative-free normal saline (PFNS) to a concentration of ≥15 mcg/mL; the concentration must be maintained at ≥15 mcg/mL during all steps of preparation. Add drug to the empty sterile I.V. bag first, then add NS. Do not add more than 9 mL of PFNS for each 1 mL of denileukin diftitox. Do not prepare with glass syringes or in glass containers. **Hazardous agent; use appropriate precautions for handling and disposal.**

Mechanism of Action Denileukin diftitox is a fusion protein (a combination of amino acid sequences from diphtheria toxin and interleukin-2) which selectively delivers the cytotoxic activity of diphtheria toxin to targeted cells. It interacts with the high-affinity IL-2 receptor on the surface of malignant cells to inhibit intracellular protein synthesis, rapidly leading to cell death.

Pharmacodynamics/Kinetics

Distribution: V_d: 0.06-0.09 L/kg

Metabolism: Hepatic via proteolytic degradation (animal studies)

Half-life elimination: Distribution: 2-5 minutes; Terminal: 70-80 minutes

Dosing

Adult & Geriatric Note: Premedicate with an antihistamine and acetaminophen prior to each infusion; corticosteroid premedication (eg, dexamethasone) may reduce the incidence of hypersensitivity and edema (Foss, 2001). Withhold treatment if serum albumin <3 g/dL.

Cutaneous T-cell lymphoma (CTCL), persistent/recurrent: I.V.: 9 or 18 mcg/kg once daily on days 1 through 5 every 21 days for 8 cycles (Olsen, 2001; Prince, 2010)

Peripheral T-cell lymphoma (PTCL), relapsed/refractory (unlabeled use): I.V.: 18 mcg/kg once daily for 5 consecutive days every 21 days for up to 8 cycles (Dang, 2007)

Renal Impairment No dosage adjustment provided in the manufacturer's labeling.

Hepatic Impairment No dosage adjustment provided in the manufacturer's labeling.

Adjustment for Toxicity

Serum albumin <3 g/dL: Withhold treatment

Severe infusion reaction: Permanently discontinue treatment

Administration For I.V. use only. Infuse over 30-60 minutes. Should **not** be given as a rapid I.V. bolus. Discontinue or reduce infusion rate for infusion related reactions; discontinue for severe infusion reaction. Do not administer through an in-line filter. Premedicate with an antihistamine and acetaminophen; consider corticosteroid premedication.

Emetic Potential Very low (<10%)

Monitoring Parameters Baseline CD25 expression (on malignant cells); serum albumin level (prior to each treatment), CBC, blood chemistry panel, renal and hepatic function tests (prior to initiation of therapy and weekly during therapy). During the infusion, the patient should be monitored for symptoms of an infusion reaction. After infusion, the patient should be monitored for the development of a delayed capillary leak syndrome (usually in the first 2 weeks), including careful monitoring of weight, edema (new or worsening), blood pressure, and serum albumin.

Thyroid function monitoring (Hamnvik, 2011): TSH and anti-TPO antibodies at baseline; then monitor TSH every month for 3 months, then every 2-3 months

Information on assay for malignant cell CD25 expression is available at 1-877-873-4724.

Additional Information Corticosteroids may be considered for prevention of hypersensitivity reaction. In a small study (Foss, 2001) reviewing denileukin diftitox and premedication with either prednisone 20 mg orally or dexamethasone 8 mg I.V. on day 1 followed by dexamethasone 8 mg I.V. on days 2-5, a reduction in adverse events was observed when compared to a previous (Olsen, 2001) phase III study. A statistically significant reduction in the incidence of edema was demonstrated. Improved response rates (compared to the phase III study) were noted, likely due to in increase in tolerability due to corticosteroid premedication. While some studies did not allow premedication with corticosteroids (Kuzel, 2007; Olsen, 2001) as part of the trial design, dexamethasone premedication has been utilized in other studies and case reports (Foss, 2005; Frankel, 2006; Gerena-Lewis, 2009; Talpur, 2002) with denileukin diftitox use for cutaneous T-cell lymphoma as well as other (unlabeled) uses.

Dosage Forms Excipient information presented when available (limited, particularly for generics); consult specific product labeling.

Injection, solution:

ONTAK®: 150 mcg/mL (2 mL) [contains edetate disodium]

References

Dang NH, Pro B, Hagemeister FB, et al, "Phase II Trial of Denileukin Diftitox for Relapsed/Refractory T-Cell Non-Hodgkin Lymphoma," *Br J Haematol*, 2007, 136(3):439-47.

Foss FM, Bacha P, Osann KE, et al, "Biological Correlates of Acute Hypersensitivity Events With DAB389IL-2 (Denileukin Diftitox, Ontak®) in Cutaneous T-Cell Lymphoma: Decreased Frequency and Severity With Steroid Premedication," *Clin Lymphoma*, 2001, 1(4):298-302.

Foss F, Demierre MF, and DiVenuti F, "A Phase-1 Trial of Bexarotene and Denileukin Diftitox in Patients With Relapsed or Refractory Cutaneous T-Cell Lymphoma," *Blood*, 2005, 106(2):454-7.

Frankel AE, Surendranathan A, Black JH, et al, "Phase II Clinical Studies of Denileukin Diftitox Diphtheria Toxin Fusion Protein in Patients With Previously Treated Chronic Lymphocytic Leukemia," *Cancer*, 2006, 106(10):2158-64.

Hamnvik OP, Larsen PR, and Marqusee E, "Thyroid Dysfunction From Antineoplastic Agents," *J Natl Cancer Inst*, 2011, 103(21):1572-87.

Kuzel TM, Li S, Eklund J, et al, "Phase II Study of Denileukin Diftitox for Previously Treated Indolent Non-Hodgkin Lymphoma: Final Results of E1497," *Leuk Lymphoma*, 2007 48(12):2397-402.

Olsen E, Duvic M, Frankel A, et al, "Pivotal Phase III Trial of Two Dose Levels of Denileukin Diftitox for the Treatment of Cutaneous T-Cell Lymphoma," *J Clin Oncol*, 2001, 19(2):376-88.

Prince HM, Duvic M, Martin A, et al, "Phase III Placebo-Controlled Trial of Denileukin Diftitox for Patients With Cutaneous T-Cell Lymphoma," *J Clin Oncol*, 2010, 28(11):1870-7.

Talpur R, Apisarnthanarax N, Ward S, et al, "Treatment of Refractory Peripheral T-Cell Lymphoma With Denileukin Diftitox (Ontak®)," *Leuk Lymphoma*, 2002, 43(1):121-6.

Denosumab (den OH sue mab)

Related Information

Hypercalcemia of Malignancy *on page 1860*

Brand Names: U.S. Prolia™; Xgeva®

Brand Names: Canada Prolia®; Xgeva®

Index Terms AMG-162

Generic Availability (U.S.) No

Pharmacologic Category Bone-Modifying Agent; Monoclonal Antibody

Use Treatment of osteoporosis in men and in postmenopausal women at high risk for fracture; treatment of bone loss in men receiving androgen deprivation therapy (ADT) for nonmetastatic prostate cancer; treatment of bone loss in women receiving aromatase inhibitor (AI) therapy for breast cancer; prevention of skeletal-related events (eg, fracture, spinal cord compression, bone pain requiring surgery/radiation therapy) in patients with bone metastases from solid tumors

Unlabeled Use Treatment of bone destruction caused by rheumatoid arthritis

Labeled Contraindications

Prolia®: Hypersensitivity to denosumab or any component of the formulation; pre-existing hypocalcemia; pregnancy

Xgeva®: There are no contraindications listed in the manufacturer's labeling.

Pregnancy Risk Factor D (Xgeva®)/X (Prolia®)

Lactation Excretion unknown/not recommended

Warnings/Precautions Denosumab may cause or exacerbate hypocalcemia; severe symptomatic cases (including fatalities) have been reported. Monitor calcium levels; correct pre-existing hypocalcemia prior to therapy. Use caution in patients with a history of hypoparathyroidism, thyroid surgery, parathyroid surgery, malabsorption syndromes, excision of small intestine, severe renal impairment/dialysis or other conditions which would predispose the patient to hypocalcemia; monitor calcium, phosphorus, and magnesium closely during therapy. Ensure adequate calcium and vitamin D intake; supplement with calcium and vitamin D, magnesium supplementation may also be necessary. Incidence of infections may be increased, including serious skin infections, abdominal, urinary, ear, or periodontal infections. Endocarditis has also been reported following use. Patients should be advised to contact healthcare provider if signs or symptoms of severe infection or cellulitis develop. Use with caution in patients with impaired immune systems or using concomitant immunosuppressive therapy; may be at increased risk for serious infections. Evaluate the need for continued treatment with serious infection.

Atypical femur fractures have been reported in patients receiving denosumab. The fractures include subtrochanteric femur (bone just below the hip joint) and diaphyseal femur (long segment of the thigh bone). Some patients experience prodromal pain weeks or months before the fracture occurs. It is unclear if denosumab therapy is the cause for these fractures. Consider interrupting therapy in patients who develop an atypical femoral fracture. Osteonecrosis of the jaw (ONJ) has been reported in patients receiving denosumab. ONJ may manifest as jaw pain, osteomyelitis, osteitis, bone erosion, tooth/periodontal infection, toothache, gingival ulceration/erosion. Risk factors include invasive dental procedures (eg, tooth extraction, dental implants, boney surgery); a diagnosis of cancer, concomitant chemotherapy or corticosteroids, poor oral hygiene, ill-fitting dentures; and comorbid disorders (anemia, coagulopathy, infection, pre-existing dental disease). Patients should maintain good oral hygiene during treatment. A dental exam and preventative dentistry should be performed prior to therapy. The benefit/risk must be assessed by the treating physician and/or dentist/surgeon prior to any invasive dental procedure; avoid invasive procedures in patients with bone metastases receiving therapy for prevention of skeletal-related events. Patients developing ONJ while on denosumab therapy should receive care by a dentist or oral surgeon; extensive dental surgery to treat ONJ may exacerbate ONJ; evaluate individually and consider discontinuing if extensive dental surgery is necessary.

Postmenopausal osteoporosis: For use in women at high risk for fracture which is defined as a history of osteoporotic fracture or multiple risk factors for fracture. May also be used in women who failed or did not tolerate other therapies.

Bone metastases: Denosumab is not indicated for the prevention of skeletal-related events in patients with multiple myeloma. In trials of with multiple myeloma patients, denosumab was noninferior to zoledronic acid in delaying time to first skeletal-related event and mortality was increased in a subset of the denosumab-treated group.

Denosumab therapy results in significant suppression of bone turnover; the long term effects of treatment are not known but may contribute to adverse outcomes such as ONJ, atypical fractures, or delayed fracture healing; monitor. Use with caution in patients with renal impairment (Cl_{cr} <30 mL/minute) or patients on dialysis; risk of hypocalcemia is increased. Dose adjustment is not needed when administered at 60 mg every 6 months (Prolia®); once-monthly dosing has not been evaluated in patients with renal impairment (Xgeva®). Dermatitis, eczema, and rash (which are not necessarily specific to the injection site) have been reported; consider discontinuing if severe symptoms occur. Packaging may contain natural latex rubber. May impair bone growth in children with open growth plates or inhibit eruption of dentition. Do not administer Prolia® and Xgeva® to the same patient for different indications.

Adverse Reactions A postmarketing safety program for Prolia® is available to collect information on adverse events; more information is available at http://www.proliasafety.com. To report adverse events for either Prolia® or Xgeva®, prescribers may also call Amgen at 800-772-6436 or FDA at 800-332-1088.

Percentages noted with Prolia® (60 mg every 6 months) unless specified as Xgeva® (120 mg every 4 weeks):

>10%:
- Central nervous system: Fatigue (Xgeva®: 45%), headache (Xgeva®: 13%)
- Dermatologic: Dermatitis (4% to 11%), eczema (4% to 11%), rash (3% to 11%)
- Endocrine & metabolic: Hypophosphatemia (Xgeva®: 32%; grade 3: 15%), hypocalcemia (2%; Xgeva®: 18%; grade 3: 3%)
- Gastrointestinal: Nausea (Xgeva®: 31%), diarrhea (Xgeva®: 20%)
- Neuromuscular & skeletal: Weakness (Xgeva®: 45%), arthralgia (7% to 14%), limb pain (10% to 12%), back pain (8% to 12%)
- Respiratory: Dyspnea (Xgeva®: 21%), cough (Xgeva®: 15%)

1% to 10%:
- Cardiovascular: Peripheral edema (5%), angina (3%)
- Endocrine & metabolic: Hypercholesterolemia (7%)
- Gastrointestinal: Flatulence (2%)
- Neuromuscular & skeletal: Musculoskeletal pain (6%), sciatica (5%), bone pain (4%), myalgia (3%), osteonecrosis of the jaw (ONJ; ≤2%)
- Ocular: Cataracts (≤5%)
- Respiratory: Nasopharyngitis (7%), upper respiratory tract infection (5%)
- Miscellaneous: New malignancies (3% to 5%), infections (nonfatal, serious; 4%)

<1%, postmarketing, and/or case reports: Antibody formation, constipation, cystitis, diaphyseal femur fracture, endocarditis, erythema, facial swelling, GERD, hypertension, hypocalcemia (severe symptomatic), influenza, pancreatitis, subtrochanteric femur fracture, urticaria

Drug Interactions

Metabolism/Transport Effects None known.

Avoid Concomitant Use There are no known interactions where it is recommended to avoid concomitant use.

Increased Effect/Toxicity

Denosumab may increase the levels/effects of: Immunosuppressants

Decreased Effect There are no known significant interactions involving a decrease in effect.

Ethanol/Nutrition/Herb Interactions Ethanol: Avoid ethanol (may increase risk of osteoporosis).

Storage/Stability Prior to use, store in original carton under refrigeration, 2°C to 8°C (36°F to 46°F). Do not freeze. Prior to use, bring to room temperature of 25°C (77°F) in original container (usually takes 15-30 minutes); do not use any other methods for warming. Use within 14 days once at room temperature. Protect from direct heat and light; do not expose to temperatures >25°C (77°F). Avoid vigorous shaking.

Mechanism of Action Denosumab is a monoclonal antibody with affinity for nuclear factor-kappa ligand (RANKL). Osteoblasts secrete RANKL; RANKL activates osteoclast precursors and subsequent osteolysis which promotes release of bone-derived growth factors, such as insulin-like growth factor-1 (IGF1) and transforming growth factor-beta (TGF-beta), and increases serum calcium levels. Denosumab binds to RANKL, blocks the interaction between RANKL and RANK (a receptor located on osteoclast surfaces), and prevents osteoclast formation, leading to decreased bone resorption and increased bone mass in osteoporosis. In solid tumors with bony metastases, RANKL inhibition decreases osteoclastic activity leading to decreased skeletal related events and tumor-induced bone destruction.

Pharmacodynamics/Kinetics

Onset of action: Decreases markers of bone resorption by ~85% within 3 days; maximal reductions observed within 1 month

Duration: Markers of bone resorption return to baseline within 12 months of discontinuing therapy

Bioavailability: SubQ: 62%

Half-life elimination: ~25-28 days

Time to peak, serum: 10 days (range: 3-21 days)

Dosing

Adult & Geriatric

Prevention of skeletal-related events in bone metastases from solid tumors (Xgeva®): SubQ: 120 mg every 4 weeks (Fizazi, 2011; Henry, 2011; Stopeck, 2010)

Treatment of androgen deprivation-induced bone loss in men with prostate cancer (Prolia®): SubQ: 60 mg as a single dose, once every 6 months (Smith, 2009)

Treatment of aromatase inhibitor-induced bone loss in women with breast cancer (Prolia®): SubQ: 60 mg as a single dose, once every 6 months (ELlis, 2008)

Treatment of osteoporosis in men or postmenopausal women (Prolia®): SubQ: 60 mg as a single dose, once every 6 months

Renal Impairment Cl_{cr} <30 mL/minute (including dialysis-dependent): No adjustment necessary when administered every 6 months (Prolia®); once-monthly dosing has not been evaluated in patients with renal impairment (Xgeva®). Monitor patients with severe impairment (Cl_{cr} <30 mL/minute or on dialysis) due to increased risk of hypocalcemia.

Hepatic Impairment No dosage adjustment provided in manufacturer's labeling (has not been studied).

Administration SubQ: Prior to administration, bring to room temperature in original container (allow to stand ~15-30 minutes); do not warm by any other method. Solution may contain trace amounts of translucent to white protein particles; do not use if cloudy, discolored (normal solution should be clear and colorless to pale yellow), or contains excessive particles or foreign matter. Avoid vigorous shaking. Administer via SubQ injection in the upper arm, upper thigh, or abdomen.

Prolia®: If a dose is missed, administer as soon as possible, then continue dosing every 6 months from the date of the last injection.

Monitoring Parameters Recommend monitoring of serum creatinine, serum calcium, phosphorus and magnesium, signs and symptoms of hypocalcemia, especially in patients predisposed to hypocalcemia (severe renal impairment, thyroid/parathyroid surgery, malabsorption syndromes, hypoparathyroidism); infection, or dermatologic reactions; routine oral exam (prior to treatment); dental exam if risk factors for ONJ

Osteoporosis: Bone mineral density as measured by central dual-energy x-ray absorptiometry (DXA) of the hip or spine (prior to initiation of therapy and at least every 2 years; annual measurements of height and weight, assessment of chronic back pain; serum calcium and 25(OH)D; may consider monitoring biochemical markers of bone turnover (National Osteoporosis Foundation Guidelines, 2010)

Dietary Considerations Ensure adequate calcium and vitamin D intake to prevent or treat hypocalcemia. Calcium 1000 mg/day and vitamin D ≥400 units/day is recommended in product labeling (Prolia®).

Women and men >50 years of age should consume elemental calcium 1200-1500 mg/day and vitamin D 800-1000 units/day (National Osteoporosis Foundation Guidelines, 2010).

Additional Information Oncology Comment: Metastatic breast cancer: The American Society of Clinical Oncology (ASCO) updated guidelines on the role of bone-modifying agents (BMAs) in the prevention and treatment of skeletal-related events for metastatic breast cancer patients (Van Poznak, 2011). The guidelines recommend initiating a BMA (denosumab, pamidronate, zoledronic acid) in patients with metastatic breast cancer to the bone. There is currently no literature indicating the superiority of one particular BMA. Optimal duration is not defined; however, the guidelines recommend continuing therapy until substantial decline in patient's performance status. In patients with normal creatinine clearance (Cl_{cr} >60 mL/minute), no dosage/interval/infusion rate changes for pamidronate or zoledronic acid are necessary. For patients with Cl_{cr} <30 mL/minute, pamidronate and zoledronic acid are not recommended. While no renal dose adjustments are recommended for denosumab, close monitoring is advised for risk of hypocalcemia in patients with Cl_{cr} <30 mL/minute or on dialysis. The ASCO guidelines are in alignment with package insert guidelines for dosing, renal dose adjustments, infusion times, prevention and management of osteonecrosis of the jaw, and monitoring of laboratory parameter recommendations. BMAs are not the first-line therapy for pain. BMAs are to be used as adjunctive therapy for cancer-related bone pain associated with bone metastasis, demonstrating a modest pain control benefit. BMAs should be used in conjunction with agents such as NSAIDs, opioid and nonopioid analgesics, corticosteroids, radiation/surgery, and interventional procedures.

Medication Guide Available Yes

Dosage Forms Excipient information presented when available (limited, particularly for generics); consult specific product labeling.

Injection, solution [preservative free]:

Prolia™: 60 mg/mL (1 mL) [contains natural rubber/natural latex in packaging]

Xgeva®: 70 mg/mL (1.7 mL)

References

Cohen SB, Dore RK, Lane NE, et al, "Denosumab Treatment Effects on Structural Damage, Bone Mineral Density, and Bone Turnover in Rheumatoid Arthritis: A Twelve-Month, Multicenter, Randomized, Double-Blind Placebo-Controlled, Phase II Clinical Trial," *Arthritis Rheum*, 2008, 58(5):1299-309.

Cummings SR, San Martin J, McClung MR, et al, "FREEDOM Trial. Denosumab for Prevention of Fractures in Postmenopausal Women With Osteoporosis," *N Engl J Med*, 2009, 361(8):756-65.

Ellis GK, Bone HG, Chlebowski R, et al, "Randomized Trial of Denosumab in Patients receiving Adjuvant Aromatase Inhibitors for Nonmetastatic Breast Cancer," *J Clin Oncol*, 2008, 26 (30):4875-82.

Fizazi K, Carducci M, Smith M, et al, "Denosumab Versus Zoledronic Acid for Treatment of Bone Metastases in Men With Castration-Resistant Prostate Cancer: A Randomised, Double-Blind Study," *Lancet*, 2011, 377(9768):813-22.

Henry DH, Costa L, Goldwasser F, et al, "Randomized, Double-Blind Study of Denosumab Verses Zoledronic Acid in the Treatment of Bone Metastases in Patients With Advanced Cancer (Excluding Breast and Prostate Cancer) or Multiple Myeloma," *J Clin Oncol*, 2011, 29(9):1125-32.

Lewiecki EM, Miller PD, McClung MR, et al, "Two-Year Treatment With Denosumab (AMG 162) in a Randomized Phase 2 Study of Postmenopausal Women With Low BMD," *J Bone Miner Res*, 2007, 22(12):1832-41.

Lipton A, Steger GG, Figueroa J, et al, "Randomized Active-Controlled Phase II Study of Denosumab Efficacy and Safety in Patients With Breast Cancer-Related Bone Metastases," *J Clin Oncol*, 2007, 25(28):4431-7.

McClung MR, Lewiecki EM, Cohen SB, et al, "Denosumab in Postmenopausal Women With Low Bone Mineral Density," *N Engl J Med*, 2006, 354(8):821-31.

National Osteoporosis Foundation, "Clinician's Guide to Prevention and Treatment of Osteoporosis," Washington, DC, 2010. Available at http://www.nof.org

Smith MR, Egerdie B, Hernández Toriz N, et al, "Denosumab in Men Receiving Androgen-Deprivation Therapy for Prostate Cancer," *N Engl J Med*, 2009, 361(8):745-55.

Stopeck AT, Lipton A, Body JJ, et al, "Denosumab Compared With Zoledronic Acid for the Treatment of Bone Metastases in Patients With Advanced Breast Cancer: A Randomized, Double-Blind Study," *J Clin Oncol*, 2010, 28(35):5132-9.

Van Poznak CH, Temin S, Yee GC, et al, "American Society of Clinical Oncology Executive Summary of the Clinical Practice Guideline Update on the Role of Bone-Modifying Agents in Metastatic Breast Cancer," *J Clin Oncol*, 2011, 29(9):1221-7.

◆ **Deoxyazacytidine** *see* Decitabine *on page 403*

◆ **2′-Deoxycoformycin** *see* Pentostatin *on page 1161*

◆ **Deoxycoformycin** *see* Pentostatin *on page 1161*

◆ **DepoCyt®** *see* Cytarabine (Liposomal) *on page 361*

◆ **DepoDur®** *see* Morphine (Liposomal) *on page 1011*

◆ **DepoFoam-Encapsulated Cytarabine** *see* Cytarabine (Liposomal) *on page 361*

◆ **Depo-Medrol®** *see* MethylPREDNISolone *on page 967*

◆ **Depo-Prevera® (Can)** *see* MedroxyPROGESTERone *on page 916*

◆ **Depo-Provera®** *see* MedroxyPROGESTERone *on page 916*

◆ **Depo-Provera® Contraceptive** *see* MedroxyPROGESTERone *on page 916*

- **depo-subQ provera 104®** *see* MedroxyPROGESTERone *on page 916*
- **Depsipeptide** *see* RomiDEPsin *on page 1254*
- **Dermarest® Eczema Medicated [OTC]** *see* Hydrocortisone (Topical) *on page 719*
- **Desacetyl Vinblastine Amide Sulfate** *see* Vindesine *on page 1464*
- **Desferal®** *see* Deferoxamine *on page 414*
- **Desferrioxamine** *see* Deferoxamine *on page 414*

Desmopressin (des moe PRES in)

Brand Names: U.S. DDAVP®; Stimate®

Brand Names: Canada Apo-Desmopressin®; DDAVP®; DDAVP® Melt; Minirin®; Novo-Desmopressin; Octostim®; PMS-Desmopressin

Index Terms 1-Deamino-8-D-Arginine Vasopressin; Desmopressin Acetate

Generic Availability (U.S.) Yes

Pharmacologic Category Antihemophilic Agent; Hemostatic Agent; Vasopressin Analog, Synthetic

Use

Injection: Treatment of diabetes insipidus; maintenance of hemostasis and control of bleeding in hemophilia A with factor VIII coagulant activity levels >5% and mild-to-moderate classic von Willebrand's disease (type 1) with factor VIII coagulant activity levels >5%

Nasal solutions (DDAVP® Nasal Spray and DDAVP® Rhinal Tube): Treatment of central diabetes insipidus

Nasal spray (Stimate®): Maintenance of hemostasis and control of bleeding in hemophilia A with factor VIII coagulant activity levels >5% and mild-to-moderate classic von Willebrand's disease (type 1) with factor VIII coagulant activity levels >5%

Tablet: Treatment of central diabetes insipidus, temporary polyuria and polydipsia following pituitary surgery or head trauma, primary nocturnal enuresis

Unlabeled Use Uremic bleeding associated with acute or chronic renal failure; prevention of surgical bleeding in patients with uremia

Labeled Contraindications Hypersensitivity to desmopressin or any component of the formulation; hyponatremia or a history of hyponatremia; moderate-to-severe renal impairment (Cl_{cr}<50 mL/minute)

Canadian labeling: Additional contraindications (not in U.S. labeling): Type 2B or platelet-type (pseudo) von Willebrand's disease (injection, intranasal, oral, sublingual); known hyponatremia, habitual or psychogenic polydipsia, cardiac insufficiency or other conditions requiring diuretic therapy (intranasal, sublingual); nephrosis, severe hepatic dysfunction (sublingual); primary nocturnal enuresis (intranasal)

Pregnancy Risk Factor B

Lactation Excretion in breast milk unknown/use caution

Warnings/Precautions Allergic reactions and anaphylaxis have been reported rarely with both the I.V. and intranasal formulations. Fluid intake should be adjusted downward in the elderly and very young patients to decrease the possibility of water intoxication and hyponatremia. Use may rarely lead to extreme decreases in plasma osmolality, resulting in seizures, coma, and death. Use caution with cystic fibrosis, heart failure, renal dysfunction, polydipsia (habitual or psychogenic [contraindicated in Canadian labeling]), or other conditions associated with fluid and electrolyte imbalance due to potential hyponatremia. Use caution with coronary artery insufficiency or hypertensive cardiovascular disease; may increase or decrease blood pressure leading to changes in heart rate. Consider switching from nasal to intravenous solution if changes in the nasal mucosa (scarring, edema) occur leading to unreliable absorption. Use caution in patients predisposed to thrombus formation; thrombotic events (acute cerebrovascular thrombosis, acute myocardial infarction) have occurred (rare).

Desmopressin (intranasal and I.V.), when used for hemostasis in hemophilia, is not for use in hemophilia B, type 2B von Willebrand disease, severe classic von Willebrand disease (type 1), or in patients with factor VIII antibodies. In general, desmopressin is also not recommended for use in patients with ≤5% factor VIII activity level, although it may be considered in selected patients with activity levels between 2% and 5%.

Consider switching from nasal to intravenous administration if changes in the nasal mucosa (scarring, edema) occur leading to unreliable absorption. Consider alternative rout of administration (I.V. or intranasal) with inadequate therapeutic response at maximum recommended oral doses. Therapy should be interrupted if patient experiences an acute illness (eg, fever, recurrent vomiting or diarrhea), vigorous exercise, or any condition associated with an increase in water consumption. Some patients may demonstrate a change in response after long term therapy (>6 months) characterized as decreased response or a shorter duration of response.

Adverse Reactions Frequency may not be defined (may be dose or route related).

Cardiovascular: Blood pressure increased/decreased (I.V.), facial flushing

Central nervous system: Headache (2% to 5%), dizziness (intranasal; ≤3%), chills (intranasal; 2%)

Dermatologic: Rash

Endocrine & metabolic: Hyponatremia, water intoxication

Gastrointestinal: Abdominal pain (intranasal; 2%), gastrointestinal disorder (intranasal; ≤2%), nausea (intranasal; ≤2%), abdominal cramps, sore throat

Hepatic: Transient increases in liver transaminases (associated primarily with tablets)

Local: Injection: Burning pain, erythema, and swelling at the injection site

Neuromuscular & Skeletal: Weakness (intranasal; ≤2%)

Ocular: Conjunctivitis (intranasal; ≤2%), eye edema (intranasal; ≤2%), lacrimation disorder (intranasal; ≤2%)

Respiratory: Rhinitis (intranasal; 3% to 8%), epistaxis (intranasal; ≤3%), nostril pain (intranasal; ≤2%), cough, nasal congestion, upper respiratory infection

<1%, postmarketing, and/or case reports: Acute cerebrovascular thrombosis (I.V.), acute MI (I.V.), agitation, allergic reactions (rare), anaphylaxis (rare), balanitis, chest pain, coma, diarrhea, dyspepsia, edema, insomnia, itching eyes, light-sensitive eyes, pain, palpitation, seizure, somnolence, tachycardia, thinking abnormal, vomiting, vulval pain, warmth

Drug Interactions

Metabolism/Transport Effects None known.

Avoid Concomitant Use There are no known interactions where it is recommended to avoid concomitant use.

Increased Effect/Toxicity

Desmopressin may increase the levels/effects of: Lithium

The levels/effects of Desmopressin may be increased by: Analgesics (Opioid); CarBAMazepine; ChlorproMAZINE; LamoTRIgine; Nonsteroidal

Anti-Inflammatory Agents; Selective Serotonin Reuptake Inhibitors; Tricyclic Antidepressants

Decreased Effect

The levels/effects of Desmopressin may be decreased by: Demeclocycline; Lithium

Ethanol/Nutrition/Herb Interactions Ethanol: Avoid ethanol (may decrease antidiuretic effect).

Storage/Stability

DDAVP®:

Nasal spray: Store at controlled room temperature of 20°C to 25°C (68°F to 77°F). Keep nasal spray in upright position.

Rhinal Tube solution: Store refrigerated at 2°C to 8°C (36°F to 46°F). May store at controlled room temperature of 20°C to 25°C (68°F to 77°F) for up to 3 weeks.

Solution for injection: Store refrigerated at 2°C to 8°C (36°F to 46°F).

Tablet: Store at controlled room temperature of 20°C to 25°C (68°F to 77°F).

DDAVP® Melt (CAN; not available in U.S.): Store at 15°C to 25°C (59°F to 77°F) in original container. Protect from moisture.

Stimate® nasal spray: Store refrigerated at 2°C to 8°C (36°F to 46°F). May store at controlled room temperature of 22°C (72°F) for up to 3 weeks.

Reconstitution DDAVP®: Dilute solution for injection in 10-50 mL NS for I.V. infusion (10 mL for children ≤10 kg: 50 mL for adults and children >10 kg).

Mechanism of Action In a dose dependent manner, desmopressin increases cyclic adenosine monophosphate (cAMP) in renal tubular cells which increases water permeability resulting in decreased urine volume and increased urine osmolality; increases plasma levels of von Willebrand factor, factor VIII, and t-PA contributing to a shortened activated partial thromboplastin time (aPTT) and bleeding time.

Pharmacodynamics/Kinetics

Onset of action:

Intranasal: Antidiuretic: 15-30 minutes; Increased factor VIII and von Willebrand factor (vWF) activity (dose related): 30 minutes

Peak effect: Antidiuretic: 1 hour; Increased factor VIII and vWF activity: 1.5 hours

I.V. infusion: Increased factor VIII and vWF activity: 30 minutes (dose related)

Peak effect: 1.5-2 hours

Oral tablet: Antidiuretic: ~1 hour

Peak effect: 4-7 hours

Duration: Intranasal, I.V. infusion, Oral tablet: ~6-14 hours

Absorption: Sublingual: Rapid

Bioavailability: Intranasal: ~3.5%; Oral tablet: 5% compared to intranasal, 0.16% compared to I.V.

Half-life elimination: Intranasal: ~3.5 hours; I.V. infusion: 3 hours; Oral tablet: 2-3 hours

Renal impairment: ≤9 hours

Excretion: Urine

Dosing

Adult & Geriatric

Diabetes insipidus:

I.V., SubQ: U.S. labeling: 2-4 mcg/day (0.5-1 mL) in 2 divided doses or one-tenth ($^1/_{10}$) of the maintenance intranasal dose. Fluid restriction should be observed.

I.M., I.V., SubQ: Canadian labeling (not in U.S. labeling): 1-4 mcg (0.25-1 mL) once daily or one-tenth (1/10) of the maintenance intranasal dose. Fluid restriction should be observed.

Intranasal (100 mcg/mL nasal solution): 10-40 mcg/day (0.1-0.4 mL) divided 1-3 times/day; adjust morning and evening doses separately for an adequate diurnal rhythm of water turnover. **Note:** The nasal spray pump can only deliver doses of 10 mcg (0.1 mL) or multiples of 10 mcg (0.1 mL); if doses other than this are needed, the rhinal tube delivery system is preferred. Fluid restriction should be observed.

Oral:

U.S. labeling: Initial: 0.05 mg twice daily; total daily dose should be increased or decreased as needed to obtain adequate antidiuresis (range: 0.1-1.2 mg divided 2-3 times/day). Fluid restriction should be observed.

Canadian labeling (not in U.S. labeling): Initial: 0.1 mg 3 times/day; total daily dose should be increased or decreased as needed to obtain adequate antidiuresis (range: 0.3-1.2 mg divided 3 times/day). Fluid restriction should be observed.

Sublingual formulation: Canadian labeling (not in U.S. labeling): Initial: 60 mcg 3 times/day; total daily dose should be increased or decreased as needed to obtain adequate antidiuresis. Usual maintenance: 60-120 mcg 3 times/day (range: 120-720 mcg divided 2-3 times/day). Fluid restriction should be observed.

Nocturnal enuresis: *Oral:* 0.2 mg at bedtime; dose may be titrated up to 0.6 mg to achieve desired response.

Hemophilia A and mild-to-moderate von Willebrand disease (type 1):

I.V.: 0.3 mcg/kg by slow infusion; if used preoperatively, administer 30 minutes before procedure

Canadian labeling (not in U.S. labeling): Maximum I.V. dose: 20 mcg

Intranasal (using high concentration spray [1.5 mg/mL]): <50 kg: 150 mcg (1 spray); >50 kg: 300 mcg (1 spray each nostril); repeat use is determined by the patient's clinical condition and laboratory work. If using preoperatively, administer 2 hours before surgery.

Uremic bleeding associated with acute or chronic renal failure (unlabeled use) (Watson, 1984): I.V.: 0.4 mcg/kg over 10 minutes

Prevention of surgical bleeding in patients with uremia (unlabeled use) (Mannucci, 1983): I.V.: 0.3 mcg/kg over 30 minutes

Pediatric

Diabetes insipidus:

I.M., I.V., SubQ: Canadian labeling (not in U.S. labeling): Infants and Children ≥3 months: 0.4 mcg (0.1 mL) once daily or one-tenth (1/10) of the maintenance intranasal dose. Fluid restriction should be observed.

I.V., SubQ:

Children <12 years: No definitive dosing available. Adult dosing should **not** be used in this age group; adverse events such as hyponatremia-induced seizures may occur. Dose should be reduced. Some have suggested an initial dosage range of 0.1-1 mcg in 1 or 2 divided doses (Cheetham, 2002). Initiate at low dose and increase as necessary. Closely monitor serum sodium levels and urine output; fluid restriction is recommended.

Children ≥12 years: Refer to adult dosing.

Intranasal (using 100 mcg/mL nasal solution):

Infants and Children 3 months to 12 years: Initial: 5 mcg/day (0.05 mL/day) divided 1-2 times/day; range: 5-30 mcg/day (0.05-0.3 mL/day) divided 1-2 times/day; adjust morning and evening doses separately for an adequate diurnal rhythm of water turnover. **Note:** The nasal spray pump can only deliver doses of 10 mcg (0.1 mL) or multiples of 10 mcg (0.1 mL); if doses other than this are needed, the rhinal tube delivery system is preferred. Fluid restriction should be observed.

Children ≥12 years: Refer to adult dosing.

Oral:

U.S. labeling: Children ≥4 years: Initial: 0.05 mg twice daily; total daily dose should be increased or decreased as needed to obtain adequate antidiuresis (range: 0.1-1.2 mg divided 2-3 times/day). Fluid restriction should be observed.

Canadian labeling (not in U.S. labeling): Children ≥5 years: Initial: 0.1 mg 3 times/day; total daily dose should be increased or decreased as needed to obtain adequate antidiuresis (range: 0.3-1.2 mg divided 3 times/day). Divide daily doses so that the evening dose is 2 times higher than the morning or afternoon dose to ensure adequate antidiuresis during the night. Fluid restriction should be observed.

Sublingual formulation: Canadian labeling (not in U.S. labeling): Infants and Children ≥3 months: Initial: 60 mcg 3 times/day; total daily dose should be increased or decreased as needed to obtain adequate antidiuresis. Usual maintenance: 60-120 mcg 3 times/day (range: 120-720 mcg divided 2-3 times/day); divide daily doses so that the evening dose is 2 times higher than the morning or afternoon dose to ensure adequate antidiuresis during the night. Fluid restriction should be observed.

Hemophilia A and von Willebrand disease (type 1):

I.V.: Infants and Children ≥3 months: 0.3 mcg/kg by slow infusion; may repeat dose if needed; if used preoperatively, administer 30 minutes before procedure

Canadian labeling (not in U.S. labeling): Maximum I.V. dose: 20 mcg

Note: Adverse events such as hyponatremia-induced seizures have been reported especially in young children using this dosing regimen (Das, 2005; Molnar, 2005; Smith, 1989; Thumfart, 2005; Weinstein, 1989). Fluid restriction and careful monitoring of serum sodium levels and urine output are necessary.

Intranasal (using high concentration spray [1.5 mg/mL]): Infants and Children ≥11 months: Refer to adult dosing.

Nocturnal enuresis:

Oral:

Children ≥6 years: 0.2 mg at bedtime. Dose may be titrated up to 0.6 mg to achieve desired response. Fluid intake should be limited 1 hour prior to dose until the next morning, or at least 8 hours after administration. **Note:** In the Canadian labeling, use is approved for patients ≥5 years.

Children >12 years: Refer to adult dosing.

Sublingual: Canadian labeling (not in U.S. labeling): Children ≥5 years: Initial: 120 mcg at bedtime; dose may be titrated up to 360 mcg to achieve desired response. Fluid intake should be limited 1 hour prior to dose until the next morning, or at least 8 hours after administration.

Renal Impairment Cl_{cr} <50 mL/minute: Use is contraindicated according to the manufacturer; however, has been used in acute and chronic renal failure patients experiencing uremic bleeding or for prevention of surgical bleeding (unlabeled uses) (Mannucci, 1983; Watson, 1984).

Administration

I.M., I.V. push, SubQ injection: Central diabetes insipidus: Withdraw dose from ampul into appropriate syringe size (eg, insulin syringe). Further dilution is not required. Administer as direct injection.

I.V. infusion:

Hemophilia A, von Willebrand disease (type 1), and prevention of surgical bleeding in patients with uremia (unlabeled) (Mannucci, 1983): Infuse over 15-30 minutes

Acute uremic bleeding (unlabeled) (Watson, 1984): May infuse over 10 minutes

Intranasal:

DDAVP®: Nasal pump spray: Delivers 0.1 mL (10 mcg); for doses <10 mcg or for other doses which are not multiples, use rhinal tube. DDAVP® Nasal spray delivers fifty 10 mcg doses. For 10 mcg dose, administer in one nostril. Any solution remaining after 50 doses should be discarded. Pump must be primed prior to first use.

DDAVP® Rhinal tube: Insert top of dropper into tube (arrow marked end) in downward position. Squeeze dropper until solution reaches desired calibration mark. Disconnect dropper. Grasp the tube 3/4 inch from the end and insert tube into nostril until the fingertips reach the nostril. Place opposite end of tube into the mouth (holding breath). Tilt head back and blow with a strong, short puff into the nostril (for very young patients, an adult should blow solution into the child's nose). Reseal dropper after use.

Monitoring Parameters Blood pressure and pulse should be monitored during I.V. infusion

Note: For all indications, fluid intake, urine volume, and signs and symptoms of hyponatremia should be closely monitored especially in high-risk patient subgroups (eg, young children, elderly, patients with heart failure).

Diabetes insipidus: Urine specific gravity, plasma and urine osmolality, serum electrolytes

Hemophilia A: Factor VIII coagulant activity, factor VIII ristocetin cofactor activity, and factor VIII antigen levels, aPTT

von Willebrand disease: Factor VIII coagulant activity, factor VIII ristocetin cofactor activity, and factor VIII von Willebrand antigen levels, bleeding time

Nocturnal enuresis: Serum electrolytes if used for >7 days

Additional Information 10 mcg of desmopressin acetate is equivalent to 40 units

Dosage Forms Excipient information presented when available (limited, particularly for generics); consult specific product labeling.

Injection, solution, as acetate: 4 mcg/mL (1 mL, 10 mL)

DDAVP®: 4 mcg/mL (1 mL)

DDAVP®: 4 mcg/mL (10 mL) [contains chlorobutanol]

Solution, intranasal, as acetate: 0.1 mg/mL (2.5 mL)

DDAVP®: 0.1 mg/mL (2.5 mL) [contains chlorobutanol; with rhinal tube]

Solution, intranasal, as acetate [spray]: 0.1 mg/mL (5 mL)

DDAVP®: 0.1 mg/mL (5 mL) [contains benzalkonium chloride; delivers 10 mcg/spray]

Stimate®: 1.5 mg/mL (2.5 mL) [contains benzalkonium chloride; delivers 150 mcg/spray]

Tablet, oral, as acetate: 0.1 mg, 0.2 mg

DDAVP®: 0.1 mg, 0.2 mg [scored]

Dosage Forms: Canada Excipient information presented when available (limited, particularly for generics); consult specific product labeling.

Tablet, as acetate, sublingual:

DDAVP® Melt: 60 mcg, 120 mcg, 240 mcg

References

Couch P and Stumpf JL, "Management of Uremic Bleeding," *Clin Pharm*, 1990, 9(9):673-81.

Das P, Carcao M, and Hitzler J, "DDAVP-Induced Hyponatremia in Young Children," *J Pediatr Hematol Oncol*, 2005, 27(6):330-2.

Das P, Carcao M, and Hitzler J, "Use of Recombinant Factor VIIa Prior to Lumbar Puncture in Pediatric Patients With Acute Leukemia," *Pediatr Blood Cancer*, 2006, 47(2):206-9.

Mannucci PM and Cattaneo M, "Desmopressin: A Nontransfusional Treatment of Hemophilia and von Willebrand Disease," *Haemostasis*, 1992, 22(5)276-80.

Mannucci PM, Remuzzi G, Pusineri F, et al, "Deamino-8-D-Arginine Vasopressin Shortens the Bleeding Time in Uremia," *N Engl J Med*, 1983, 308(1):8-12.

Molnar Z, Farkas V, Nemes L, et al, "Hyponatraemic Seizures Resulting From Inadequate Post-Operative Fluid Intake Following a Single Dose of Desmopressin," *Nephrol Dial Transplant*, 2005, 20(10):2265-7.

Smith TJ, Gill JC, Ambruso DR, et al, "Hyponatremia and Seizures in Young Children given DDAVP," *Am J Hematol*, 1989, 31(3):199-202.

Stenberg A and Läckgren G, "Desmopressin Tablets in the Treatment of Severe Nocturnal Enuresis in Adolescents," *Pediatrics*, 1994, 94(6 Pt 1):841-46.

Thumfart J, Roehr CC, Kapelari K, et al, "Desmopressin Associated Symptomatic Hyponatremic Hypervolemia in Children. Are There Predictive Factors?" *J Urol*, 2005, 174(1):294-8.

Watson AJ and Keogh JA., "1-Deamino-8-D-Arginine Vasopressin as a Therapy for the Bleeding Diathesis of Renal Failure," *Am J Nephrol*, 1984, 4(1):49-51.

Watson AJ and Keogh JA, "1-Deamino-8-d-Arginine Vasopressin (DDAVP): A Potential New Treatment for the Bleeding Diathesis of Acute Renal Failure," *Pharmatherapeutica*, 1984, 3 (9):618-22.

Weinstein RE, Bona RD, Altman AJ, et al, "Severe Hyponatremia after Repeated Intravenous Administration of Desmopressin," *Am J Hematol*, 1989, 32(4):258-61.

◆ **Desmopressin Acetate** *see* Desmopressin *on page* *434*

◆ **Detryptoreline** *see* Triptorelin *on page* *1413*

Dexamethasone (Systemic) (deks a METH a sone)

Related Information

Management of Chemotherapy-Induced Nausea and Vomiting *on page* *1786*

Management of Infections *on page* *1809*

Palliative Care Medicine (Cancer) *on page* *1871*

Brand Names: U.S. Baycadron™; Dexamethasone Intensol™; DexPak® 10 Day TaperPak®; DexPak® 13 Day TaperPak®; DexPak® 6 Day TaperPak®

Brand Names: Canada Apo-Dexamethasone®; Dexasone®; Dom-Dexamethasone; PHL-Dexamethasone; PMS-Dexamethasone; PRO-Dexamethasone; ratio-Dexamethasone

Index Terms Decadron; Dexamethasone Sodium Phosphate

Generic Availability (U.S.) Yes: Excludes concentrated oral solution

Pharmacologic Category Anti-inflammatory Agent; Antiemetic; Corticosteroid, Systemic

Use Primarily as an anti-inflammatory or immunosuppressant agent in the treatment of a variety of diseases including those of allergic, dermatologic, endocrine, hematologic, inflammatory, neoplastic, nervous system, renal, respiratory, rheumatic, and autoimmune origin; may be used in management of cerebral edema, chronic swelling, as a diagnostic agent, diagnosis of Cushing's syndrome, antiemetic

Unlabeled Use Dexamethasone suppression test as an indicator of depression and/or risk of suicide; prevention and treatment of acute mountain sickness and high altitude cerebral edema; accelerate fetal lung maturation in patients with preterm labor

Labeled Contraindications Hypersensitivity to dexamethasone or any component of the formulation; systemic fungal infections, cerebral malaria

Pregnancy Risk Factor C

Lactation Excretion in breast milk unknown/use caution

Warnings/Precautions Use with caution in patients with thyroid disease, hepatic impairment, renal impairment, cardiovascular disease, diabetes, glaucoma, cataracts, myasthenia gravis, patients at risk for osteoporosis, patients at risk for seizures, or GI diseases (diverticulitis, peptic ulcer, ulcerative colitis) due to perforation risk. Use caution following acute MI (corticosteroids have been associated with myocardial rupture). Because of the risk of adverse effects, systemic corticosteroids should be used cautiously in the elderly in the smallest possible effective dose for the shortest duration. May affect growth velocity; growth should be routinely monitored in pediatric patients. Withdraw therapy with gradual tapering of dose.

May cause hypercorticism or suppression of hypothalamic-pituitary-adrenal (HPA) axis, particularly in younger children or in patients receiving high doses for prolonged periods. HPA axis suppression may lead to adrenal crisis. Withdrawal and discontinuation of a corticosteroid should be done slowly and carefully. Particular care is required when patients are transferred from systemic corticosteroids to inhaled products due to possible adrenal insufficiency or withdrawal from steroids, including an increase in allergic symptoms. Patients receiving >20 mg per day of prednisone (or equivalent) may be most susceptible. Fatalities have occurred due to adrenal insufficiency in asthmatic patients during and after transfer from systemic corticosteroids to aerosol steroids; aerosol steroids do not provide the systemic steroid needed to treat patients having trauma, surgery, or infections. Dexamethasone does not provide adequate mineralocorticoid activity in adrenal insufficiency (may be employed as a single dose while cortisol assays are performed). The lowest possible dose should be used during treatment; discontinuation and/or dose reductions should be gradual.

Acute myopathy has been reported with high dose corticosteroids, usually in patients with neuromuscular transmission disorders; may involve ocular and/or respiratory muscles; monitor creatine kinase; recovery may be delayed. Corticosteroid use may cause psychiatric disturbances, including depression, euphoria, insomnia, mood swings, and personality changes. Pre-existing psychiatric conditions may be exacerbated by corticosteroid use. Prolonged use of corticosteroids may also increase the incidence of secondary infection, mask acute infection (including fungal infections), prolong or exacerbate viral infections, or limit response to vaccines. Exposure to chickenpox should be avoided; corticosteroids should not be used to treat ocular herpes simplex. Corticosteroids should not be used for cerebral malaria or viral hepatitis. Close observation is required in patients with latent tuberculosis and/or TB reactivity; restrict use in active TB (only in conjunction with antituberculosis treatment). Prolonged treatment with corticosteroids has been associated with the development of Kaposi's sarcoma (case reports); if noted, discontinuation of therapy should be considered. High-dose corticosteroids should not be used to manage acute head injury.

Adverse Reactions Frequency not defined.

Cardiovascular: Arrhythmia, bradycardia, cardiac arrest, cardiomyopathy, CHF, circulatory collapse, edema, hypertension, myocardial rupture (post-MI), syncope, thromboembolism, vasculitis

Central nervous system: Depression, emotional instability, euphoria, headache, intracranial pressure increased, insomnia, malaise, mood swings, neuritis, personality changes, pseudotumor cerebri (usually following discontinuation), psychic disorders, seizure, vertigo

Dermatologic: Acne, allergic dermatitis, alopecia, angioedema, bruising, dry skin, erythema, fragile skin, hirsutism, hyper-/hypopigmentation, hypertrichosis, perianal pruritus (following I.V. injection), petechiae, rash, skin atrophy, skin test reaction impaired, striae, urticaria, wound healing impaired

Endocrine & metabolic: Adrenal suppression, carbohydrate tolerance decreased, Cushing's syndrome, diabetes mellitus, glucose intolerance decreased, growth suppression (children), hyperglycemia, hypokalemic alkalosis, menstrual irregularities, negative nitrogen balance, pituitary-adrenal axis suppression, protein catabolism, sodium retention

Gastrointestinal: Abdominal distention, appetite increased, gastrointestinal hemorrhage, gastrointestinal perforation, nausea, pancreatitis, peptic ulcer, ulcerative esophagitis, weight gain

Genitourinary: Altered (increased or decreased) spermatogenesis

Hepatic: Hepatomegaly, transaminases increased

Local: Postinjection flare (intra-articular use), thrombophlebitis

Neuromuscular & skeletal: Arthropathy, aseptic necrosis (femoral and humoral heads), fractures, muscle mass loss, myopathy (particularly in conjunction with neuromuscular disease or neuromuscular-blocking agents), neuropathy, osteoporosis, parasthesia, tendon rupture, vertebral compression fractures, weakness

Ocular: Cataracts, exophthalmos, glaucoma, intraocular pressure increased

Renal: Glucosuria

Respiratory: Pulmonary edema

Miscellaneous: Abnormal fat deposition, anaphylactoid reaction, anaphylaxis, avascular necrosis, diaphoresis, hiccups, hypersensitivity, impaired wound healing, infections, Kaposi's sarcoma, moon face, secondary malignancy

Drug Interactions

Metabolism/Transport Effects **Substrate** of CYP3A4 (major), P-glycoprotein; **Note:** Assignment of Major/Minor substrate status based on clinically relevant drug interaction potential; **Inhibits** P-glycoprotein; **Induces** CYP2A6 (weak/moderate), CYP2B6 (weak/moderate), CYP2C9 (weak/moderate), CYP3A4 (strong), P-glycoprotein

Avoid Concomitant Use

Avoid concomitant use of Dexamethasone (Systemic) with any of the following: Aldesleukin; Axitinib; BCG; Bosutinib; Conivaptan; Crizotinib; Dabigatran Etexilate; Dronedarone; Enzalutamide; Everolimus; Lapatinib; Lurasidone; Mifepristone; Natalizumab; Nilotinib; Nisoldipine; Pazopanib; Perampanel; Pimecrolimus; Praziquantel; Ranolazine; Regorafenib; Rilpivirine; Rivaroxaban; RomiDEPsin; SORAfenib; Tacrolimus (Topical); Ticagrelor; Tolvaptan; Toremifene; Vandetanib; VinCRIStine (Liposomal)

Increased Effect/Toxicity

Dexamethasone (Systemic) may increase the levels/effects of: Acetylcholinesterase Inhibitors; Amphotericin B; CycloSPORINE (Systemic); Deferasirox; Ifosfamide; Leflunomide; Lenalidomide; Loop Diuretics; Natalizumab;

NSAID (COX-2 Inhibitor); NSAID (Nonselective); Thalidomide; Thiazide Diuretics; Vaccines (Live); Warfarin

The levels/effects of Dexamethasone (Systemic) may be increased by: Antifungal Agents (Azole Derivatives, Systemic); Aprepitant; Asparaginase (E. coli); Asparaginase (Erwinia); Calcium Channel Blockers (Nondihydropyridine); Conivaptan; CycloSPORINE (Systemic); CYP3A4 Inhibitors (Moderate); CYP3A4 Inhibitors (Strong); Dasatinib; Denosumab; Estrogen Derivatives; Fluconazole; Fosaprepitant; Indacaterol; Ivacaftor; Macrolide Antibiotics; Mifepristone; Neuromuscular-Blocking Agents (Nondepolarizing); P-glycoprotein/ABCB1 Inhibitors; Pimecrolimus; Quinolone Antibiotics; Roflumilast; Salicylates; Tacrolimus (Topical); Telaprevir; Trastuzumab

Decreased Effect

Dexamethasone (Systemic) may decrease the levels/effects of: Aldesleukin; Antidiabetic Agents; Apixaban; ARIPiprazole; Axitinib; BCG; Boceprevir; Bosutinib; Brentuximab Vedotin; Calcitriol; Caspofungin; Cobicistat; Coccidioidin Skin Test; Corticorelin; Crizotinib; CycloSPORINE (Systemic); CYP3A4 Substrates; Dabigatran Etexilate; Dasatinib; Dronedarone; Elvitegravir; Enzalutamide; Everolimus; Exemestane; Gefitinib; GuanFACINE; Hyaluronidase; Imatinib; Isoniazid; Ixabepilone; Lapatinib; Lurasidone; Maraviroc; NIFEdipine; Nilotinib; Nisoldipine; Pazopanib; Perampanel; P-glycoprotein/ABCB1 Substrates; Praziquantel; Ranolazine; Regorafenib; Rilpivirine; Rivaroxaban; RomiDEPsin; Salicylates; Sipuleucel-T; SORAfenib; SUNItinib; Tadalafil; Telaprevir; Ticagrelor; Tolvaptan; Toremifene; Ulipristal; Vaccines (Inactivated); Vandetanib; Vemurafenib; VinCRIStine (Liposomal); Zuclopenthixol

The levels/effects of Dexamethasone (Systemic) may be decreased by: Aminoglutethimide; Antacids; Barbiturates; Bile Acid Sequestrants; CYP3A4 Inducers (Strong); Echinacea; Herbs (CYP3A4 Inducers); Mifepristone; Mitotane; P-glycoprotein/ABCB1 Inducers; Primidone; Rifamycin Derivatives; Tocilizumab

Ethanol/Nutrition/Herb Interactions

Ethanol: Avoid ethanol (may enhance gastric mucosal irritation).

Food: Dexamethasone interferes with calcium absorption. Limit caffeine.

Herb/Nutraceutical: Avoid cat's claw, echinacea (have immunostimulant properties).

Storage/Stability Injection solution: Store at room temperature; protect from light and freezing.

Stability of injection of parenteral admixture at room temperature (25°C): 24 hours

Stability of injection of parenteral admixture at refrigeration temperature (4°C): 2 days; protect from light and freezing.

Reconstitution

Oral: Oral administration of dexamethasone for croup may be prepared using a parenteral dexamethasone formulation and mixing it with an oral flavored syrup (Bjornson, 2004).

I.V.: Injection should be diluted in 50-100 mL NS or D_5W.

Mechanism of Action Decreases inflammation by suppression of neutrophil migration, decreased production of inflammatory mediators, and reversal of increased capillary permeability; suppresses normal immune response. Dexamethasone's mechanism of antiemetic activity is unknown.

Pharmacodynamics/Kinetics

Onset of action: Acetate: Prompt

Duration of metabolic effect: 72 hours; acetate is a long-acting repository preparation
Metabolism: Hepatic
Half-life elimination: Normal renal function: 1.8-3.5 hours; Biological half-life: 36-54 hours
Time to peak, serum: Oral: 1-2 hours; I.M.: ~8 hours
Excretion: Urine and feces

Dosing

Adult

Anti-inflammatory:

Oral, I.M., I.V.: 0.75-9 mg/day in divided doses every 6-12 hours
Intra-articular, intralesional, or soft tissue: 0.4-6 mg/day

Extubation or airway edema: Oral, I.M., I.V.: 0.5-2 mg/kg/day in divided doses every 6 hours beginning 24 hours prior to extubation and continuing for 4-6 doses afterwards

Antiemetic:

Prophylaxis: Oral, I.V.: 10-20 mg 15-30 minutes before treatment on each treatment day
Continuous infusion regimen: Oral or I.V.: 10 mg every 12 hours on each treatment day
Mildly emetogenic therapy: Oral, I.M., I.V.: 4 mg every 4-6 hours

Delayed nausea/vomiting: Oral: 4-10 mg 1-2 times/day for 2-4 days **or**
8 mg every 12 hours for 2 days; then
4 mg every 12 hours for 2 days **or**
20 mg 1 hour before chemotherapy; then
10 mg 12 hours after chemotherapy; then
8 mg every 12 hours for 4 doses; then
4 mg every 12 hours for 4 doses

Multiple myeloma: Oral, I.V.: 40 mg/day, days 1 to 4, 9 to 12, and 17 to 20, repeated every 4 weeks (alone or as part of a regimen)

Cerebral edema: I.V. 10 mg stat, 4 mg I.M./I.V. (should be given as sodium phosphate) every 6 hours until response is maximized, then switch to oral regimen, then taper off if appropriate; dosage may be reduced after 2-4 days and gradually discontinued over 5-7 days

Dexamethasone suppression test (depression/suicide indicator) (unlabeled use): Oral: 1 mg at 11 PM, draw blood at 8 AM the following day for plasma cortisol determination

Cushing's syndrome, diagnostic: Oral: 1 mg at 11 PM, draw blood at 8 AM; greater accuracy for Cushing's syndrome may be achieved by the following: Dexamethasone 0.5 mg by mouth every 6 hours for 48 hours (with 24-hour urine collection for 17-hydroxycorticosteroid excretion)

Differentiation of Cushing's syndrome due to ACTH excess from Cushing's due to other causes: Oral: Dexamethasone 2 mg every 6 hours for 48 hours (with 24-hour urine collection for 17-hydroxycorticosteroid excretion)

Multiple sclerosis (acute exacerbation): Oral: 30 mg/day for 1 week, followed by 4-12 mg/day for 1 month

Treatment of shock:

Addisonian crisis/shock (eg, adrenal insufficiency/responsive to steroid therapy): I.V.: 4-10 mg as a single dose, which may be repeated if necessary

Unresponsive shock (eg, unresponsive to steroid therapy): I.V.: 1-6 mg/kg as a single I.V. dose or up to 40 mg initially followed by repeat doses every 2-6 hours while shock persists

Physiological replacement: Oral, I.M., I.V. (should be given as sodium phosphate): 0.03-0.15 mg/kg/day **or** 0.6-0.75 mg/m²/day in divided doses every 6-12 hours

Acute mountain sickness (AMS)/high altitude cerebral edema (HACE) (unlabeled use):

Prevention: Oral: 2 mg every 6 hours **or** 4 mg every 12 hours starting on the day of ascent; may be discontinued after staying at the same elevation for 2-3 days or if descent is initiated; do not exceed a 10 day duration (Luks, 2010). **Note:** In situations of rapid ascent to altitudes >3500 meters (such as rescue or military operations), 4 mg every 6 hours may be considered (Luks, 2010).

Treatment: Oral, I.M., I.V.:

AMS: 4 mg every 6 hours (Luks, 2010)

HACE: Initial: 8 mg as a single dose; Maintenance: 4 mg every 6 hours until symptoms resolve (Luks, 2010)

Geriatric Refer to adult dosing. Use cautiously in the elderly in the smallest possible dose.

Pediatric

Antiemetic (prior to chemotherapy): Refer to individual protocols and emetogenic potential: I.V.: 10 mg/m²/dose every 12-24 hours on days of chemotherapy for severely emetogenic chemotherapy courses

Anti-inflammatory and/or immunosuppressant: Oral, I.M., I.V.: 0.08-0.3 mg/kg/day **or** 2.5-10 mg/m²/day in divided doses every 6-12 hours

Extubation or airway edema: Oral, I.M., I.V.: 0.5-2 mg/kg/day in divided doses every 6 hours beginning 24 hours prior to extubation and continuing for 4-6 doses afterwards

Cerebral edema: I.V.: Loading dose: 1-2 mg/kg/dose as a single dose; maintenance: 1-1.5 mg/kg/day (maximum: 16 mg/day) in divided doses every 4-6 hours, taper off over 1-6 weeks

Croup (laryngotracheobronchitis): Oral, I.M., I.V.: 0.6 mg/kg once; usual maximum dose: 16 mg (doses as high as 20 mg have been used) (Bjornson, 2004; Hegenbarth, 2008; Rittichier, 2000); a single oral dose of 0.15 mg/kg has been shown effective in children with mild-to-moderate croup (Russell, 2004; Sparrow, 2006)

Bacterial meningitis: Infants and Children >6 weeks: I.V.: 0.15 mg/kg/dose every 6 hours for the first 2-4 days of antibiotic treatment; start dexamethasone 10-20 minutes before or with the first dose of antibiotic

Physiologic replacement: Oral, I.M., I.V.: 0.03-0.15 mg/kg/day or 0.6-0.75 mg/m²/day in divided doses every 6-12 hours

Acute mountain sickness (AMS)/high altitude cerebral edema (HACE) (unlabeled use): Oral, I.M., I.V.: 0.15 mg/kg/dose every 6 hours; consider using for high altitude pulmonary edema because of associated HACE with this condition (Luks, 2010; Pollard, 2001)

Renal Impairment Hemodialysis or peritoneal dialysis: Supplemental dose is not necessary.

Combination Regimens

Amyloidosis: Bortezomib-Dexamethasone (Amyloidosis) on page 1534

Leukemia, acute lymphocytic:

Hyper-CVAD + Imatinib on page 1680

Hyper-CVAD (Leukemia, Acute Lymphocytic) on page 1681

Larson Regimen (ALL) on page 1699

VAD/CVAD on page 1768

Lymphoma, Hodgkin:
Dexa-BEAM (Hodgkin) on page 1607
DHAP (Hodgkin) on page 1608
GDP (Hodgkin) on page 1667
VIM-D (Hodgkin) on page 1770
Lymphoma, non-Hodgkin's:
Cisplatin-Cytarabine-Dexamethasone (NHL Regimen) on page 1567
Fludarabine-Mitoxantrone-Dexamethasone (NHL) on page 1650
Fludarabine-Mitoxantrone-Dexamethasone-Rituximab on page 1650
Hyper-CVAD (Lymphoma, non-Hodgkin's) on page 1687
m-BACOD on page 1706
Oxaliplatin-Cytarabine-Dexamethasone (NHL Regimen) on page 1723
Lymphoma, non-Hodgkin's (Mantle cell): Hyper-CVAD + Rituximab on page 1688
Multiple myeloma:
Bortezomib-Dexamethasone (Multiple Myeloma) on page 1534
Bortezomib-Doxorubicin-Dexamethasone on page 1535
Bortezomib-Doxorubicin (Liposomal)-Dexamethasone on page 1536
Cyclophosphamide-Bortezomib-Dexamethasone (Multiple Myeloma) on page 1599
Doxorubicin (Liposomal) - Vincristine - Dexamethasone on page 1620
DTPACE on page 1620
Hyper-CVAD (Multiple Myeloma) on page 1687
Lenalidomide-Bortezomib-Dexamethasone (Multiple Myeloma) on page 1702
Lenalidomide-Dexamethasone on page 1702
Lenalidomide-Dexamethasone (Low Dose) on page 1703
Melphalan-Prednisone (Multiple Myeloma) on page 1709
Thalidomide-Dexamethasone (MM) on page 1754
VAD on page 1767
Waldenstrom's Macroglobulinemia: Bortezomib-Dexamethasone-Rituximab (Waldenstrom's Macroglobulinemia) on page 1535

Administration
Oral: Administer with meals to decrease GI upset.
I.V.: Administer as a 5-10 minute bolus; rapid injection is associated with a high incidence of perineal discomfort.

Monitoring Parameters Hemoglobin, occult blood loss, serum potassium, glucose, growth in children

Test Interactions May suppress the wheal and flare reactions to skin test antigens

Dietary Considerations May be taken with meals to decrease GI upset. May need diet with increased potassium, pyridoxine, vitamin C, vitamin D, folate, calcium, and phosphorus.

Additional Information Effects of inhaled/intranasal steroids on growth have been observed in the absence of laboratory evidence of HPA axis suppression, suggesting that growth velocity is a more sensitive indicator of systemic corticosteroid exposure in pediatric patients than some commonly used tests of HPA axis function. The long-term effects of this reduction in growth velocity associated with orally-inhaled and intranasal corticosteroids, including the impact on final adult height, are unknown. The potential for "catch up" growth following discontinuation of treatment with inhaled corticosteroids has not been adequately studied.

Withdrawal/tapering of therapy: Corticosteroid tapering following short-term use is limited primarily by the need to control the underlying disease state; tapering may be accomplished over a period of days. Following longer-term use, tapering over weeks to months may be necessary to avoid signs and symptoms of adrenal insufficiency and to allow recovery of the HPA axis. Testing of HPA axis responsiveness may be of value in selected patients. Subtle deficits in HPA response may persist for months after discontinuation of therapy, and may require supplemental dosing during periods of acute illness or surgical stress.

Dosage Forms Excipient information presented when available (limited, particularly for generics); consult specific product labeling.

Elixir, oral: 0.5 mg/5 mL (237 mL)

Baycadron™: 0.5 mg/5 mL (237 mL) [contains benzoic acid, ethanol 5.1%, propylene glycol; raspberry flavor]

Injection, solution, as sodium phosphate: 4 mg/mL (1 mL, 5 mL, 30 mL); 10 mg/mL (1 mL, 10 mL)

Injection, solution, as sodium phosphate [preservative free]: 10 mg/mL (1 mL)

Solution, oral: 0.5 mg/5 mL (240 mL, 500 mL)

Solution, oral [concentrate]:

Dexamethasone Intensol™: 1 mg/mL (30 mL) [dye free, sugar free; contains benzoic acid, ethanol 30%, propylene glycol]

Tablet, oral: 0.5 mg, 0.75 mg, 1 mg, 1.5 mg, 2 mg, 4 mg, 6 mg

DexPak® 6 Day TaperPak®: 1.5 mg [scored; 21 tablets on taper dose card]

DexPak® 10 Day TaperPak®: 1.5 mg [scored; 35 tablets on taper dose card]

DexPak® 13 Day TaperPak®: 1.5 mg [scored; 51 tablets on taper dose card]

References

Bjornson CL, Klassen TP, Williamson J, et al, "A Randomized Trial of a Single Dose of Oral Dexamethasone for Mild Croup," *N Engl J Med*, 2004, 351(13):1306-13.

Dellinger RP, Levy MM, Carlet JM, et al, "Surviving Sepsis Campaign: International Guidelines for Management of Severe Sepsis and Septic Shock: 2008," [published correction appears in *Crit Care Med*, 2008, 36(4):1394-6], *Crit Care Med*, 2008, 36(1):296-327.

"Dexamethasone, Granisetron, or Both for the Prevention of Nausea and Vomiting During Chemotherapy for Cancer. The Italian Group for Antiemetic Research," *N Engl J Med*, 1995, 332(1):1-5.

Goedert JJ, Vitale F, Lauria C, et al, "Risk Factors for Classical Kaposi's Sarcoma," *J Natl Cancer Inst*, 2002, 94(22):1712-8.

Hegenbarth MA and American Academy of Pediatrics Committee on Drugs, "Preparing for Pediatric Emergencies: Drugs to Consider," *Pediatrics*, 2008, 121(2):433-43.

Kris MG, Baltzer L, Pisters KM, et al, "Enhancing the Effectiveness of the Specific Serotonin Antagonists. Combination Antiemetic Therapy With Dexamethasone," *Cancer*, 1993, 72(11 Suppl):3436-42.

Kyle RA and Rajkumar SV, "Multiple Myeloma," *N Engl J Med*, 2004, 351(18): 1860-73.

Luks AM, McIntosh SE, Grissom CK, et al, "Wilderness Medical Society Consensus Guidelines for the Prevention and Treatment of Acute Altitude Illness," *Wilderness Environ Med*, 2010, 21 (2):146-55.

Peterson C, Hursti TJ, Borjeson S, et al, "Single High-Dose Dexamethasone Improves the Effect of Ondansetron on Acute Chemotherapy-Induced Nausea and Vomiting But Impairs the Control of Delayed Symptoms," *Support Care Cancer*, 1996, 4(6):440-6.

Pollard AJ, Niermeyer S, Barry P, et al, "Children at High Altitude: An International Consensus Statement by an Ad Hoc Committee of the International Society for Mountain Medicine, March 12, 2001," *High Alt Med Biol*, 2001, 2(3):389-403.

Rittichier KK and Ledwith CA, "Outpatient Treatment of Moderate Croup With Dexamethasone: Intramuscular Versus Oral Dosing," *Pediatrics*, 2000, 106(6):1344-8.

Russell K, Wiebe N, Saenz A, et al, "Glucocorticoids for Croup," *Cochrane Database Syst Rev*, 2004, (1):CD001955.

Sparrow A and Geelhoed G, "Prednisolone Versus Dexamethasone in Croup: A Randomised Equivalence Trial," *Arch Dis Child*, 2006, 91(7):580-3.

◆ **Dexamethasone Intensol™** *see* Dexamethasone (Systemic) *on page* *440*

- **Dexamethasone Sodium Phosphate** *see* Dexamethasone (Systemic) *on page 440*
- **Dexasone® (Can)** *see* Dexamethasone (Systemic) *on page 440*
- **Dexferrum®** *see* Iron Dextran Complex *on page 824*
- **Dexiron™ (Can)** *see* Iron Dextran Complex *on page 824*
- **DexPak® 6 Day TaperPak®** *see* Dexamethasone (Systemic) *on page 440*
- **DexPak® 10 Day TaperPak®** *see* Dexamethasone (Systemic) *on page 440*
- **DexPak® 13 Day TaperPak®** *see* Dexamethasone (Systemic) *on page 440*

Dexrazoxane (deks ray ZOKS ane)

Related Information

Management of Chemotherapy-Induced Nausea and Vomiting *on page 1786*

Management of Drug Extravasations *on page 1800*

Safe Handling of Hazardous Drugs *on page 1904*

Brand Names: U.S. Totect®; Zinecard®

Brand Names: Canada Zinecard®

Index Terms ICRF-187

Generic Availability (U.S.) Yes

Pharmacologic Category Antidote; Cardioprotectant

Use

Zinecard®: Reduction of the incidence and severity of cardiomyopathy associated with doxorubicin administration in women with metastatic breast cancer who have received a cumulative doxorubicin dose of 300 mg/m^2 and who would benefit from continuing therapy with doxorubicin. (Not recommended for use with initial doxorubicin therapy.)

Totect®: Treatment of anthracycline-induced extravasation.

Unlabeled Use Reduction of the incidence and severity of cardiomyopathy associated with doxorubicin administration (cumulative doses >300 mg/m^2) in patients with malignancies other than metastatic breast cancer who would benefit from continuing therapy with doxorubicin; reduction of the incidence and severity of cardiomyopathy associated with continued epirubicin administration for advanced breast cancer; prevention of doxorubicin cardiomyopathy associated with acute lymphoblastic leukemia treatment in children

Labeled Contraindications

Zinecard®: Use with chemotherapy regimens that do not contain an anthracycline

Totect®: There are no contraindications listed within the manufacturer's labeling.

Pregnancy Risk Factor D

Lactation Excretion in breast milk unknown/not recommended

Warnings/Precautions Hazardous agent - use appropriate precautions for handling and disposal. Dexrazoxane may cause mild myelosuppression activity; myelosuppression may be additive with concurrently administered chemotherapeutic agents. Does not eliminate the potential for anthracycline-induced cardiac toxicity; carefully monitor cardiac function. May interfere with the antitumor effect of chemotherapy when given concurrently with fluorouracil, doxorubicin and cyclophosphamide (FAC). Acute myeloid leukemia (AML) and myelodysplastic syndrome (MDS) have been reported in pediatric patients and some adult patients receiving dexrazoxane in combination with chemotherapy. When used for the prevention of cardiomyopathy, doxorubicin should be administered within 30 minutes after the beginning of the dexrazoxane infusion. Dosage adjustment required for moderate or severe renal insufficiency (clearance is reduced). Due to dosage adjustments for doxorubicin in hepatic impairment, a proportional dose reduction in dexrazoxane is recommended to maintain the dosage ratio of 10:1. Do not use DMSO in patients receiving dexrazoxane for anthracycline-induced extravasation; may diminish dexrazoxane efficacy. For I.V. administration; **not** for local infiltration into extravasation site.

Adverse Reactions Note: Most adverse reactions are thought to be attributed to chemotherapy, except for increased myelosuppression, pain at injection site, and phlebitis.

Prevention of doxorubicin cardiomyopathy (reactions listed are those which were greater in the dexrazoxane arm in a comparison of chemotherapy plus dexrazoxane vs chemotherapy alone):

Central nervous system: Fatigue/malaise, fever
Dermatologic: Alopecia, streaking/erythema
Gastrointestinal: Serum amylase increased
Hematologic: Granulocytopenia, leukopenia, myelosuppression, thrombocytopenia
Local: Extravasation, injection site pain, phlebitis
Neuromuscular & skeletal: Neurotoxicity
Miscellaneous: Infection, sepsis

Anthracycline extravasation:

Cardiovascular: Peripheral edema
Central nervous system: Depression, dizziness, fatigue, fever, headache, insomnia
Dermatologic: Alopecia
Endocrine & metabolic: Hypercalcemia, hyponatremia
Gastrointestinal: Abdominal pain, anorexia, constipation, diarrhea, nausea, vomiting
Hematologic: Anemia, leukopenia, neutropenia, neutropenic fever, thrombocytopenia
Hepatic: Alkaline phosphatase increased, ALT increased, AST increased, bilirubin increased, LDH increased
Local: Injection site pain/discomfort, phlebitis
Renal: Creatinine increased
Respiratory: Cough, dyspnea, pneumonia
Miscellaneous: Infection

Drug Interactions

Metabolism/Transport Effects None known.

Avoid Concomitant Use

Avoid concomitant use of Dexrazoxane with any of the following: CloZAPine; Dimethyl Sulfoxide

Increased Effect/Toxicity

Dexrazoxane may increase the levels/effects of: CloZAPine

Decreased Effect

The levels/effects of Dexrazoxane may be decreased by: Dimethyl Sulfoxide

Storage/Stability Note: Preparation and storage are product specific; refer to individual product labeling for further details. Use appropriate precautions for handling and disposal. Discard unused solutions.

Totect®: Store intact vials at room temperature of 25°C (77°F); excursions permitted to 15°C to 30°C (59°F to 86°F). Protect from light. When reconstituted with the supplied diluent to a final concentration of 10 mg/mL the reconstituted solution is stable for 2 hours. Solutions for infusion are stable for 4 hours when stored <25°C (77°F).

Zinecard®: Store intact vials at room temperature of 25°C (77°F); excursions permitted to 15°C to 30°C (59°F to 86°F). When reconstituted with sterile water for injection, the reconstituted solution is stable for 30 minutes at room temperature or 3 hours under refrigeration. Solutions for infusion are stable for 1 hour when stored at room temperature or 4 hours under refrigeration at 2°C to 8°C (36°F to 46°F).

Dexrazoxane generic formulation (Bedford Laboratories; Mylan, Inc): Store intact vials at room temperature of 20°C to 25°C (68°F to 77°F). Reconstituted solutions and solutions diluted for infusion are stable for 6 hours when stored at room temperature or under refrigeration 2°C to 8°C (36°F to 46°F).

Additional stability information: When studied as a 24-hour continuous infusion for the prevention of cardiomyopathy, solutions prepared with sodium lactate diluent and diluted to a final concentration of 0.1 or 0.5 mg/mL in D_5W were found to retain ≥90% of their initial concentration when stored at room temperature (ambient light conditions) for ≤24 hours (Tetef, 2001).

Reconstitution Note: Preparation and storage are product specific; refer to individual product labeling for further details. Use appropriate precautions for handling and disposal. Discard unused solutions.

Totect®: Reconstitute 500 mg vial with 50 mL of the supplied diluent (0.167 Molar sodium lactate injection) to a final concentration of 10 mg/mL. Prior to infusion, further dilute reconstituted dexrazoxane solution in NS 1000 mL.

Zinecard®: Reconstitute vial with sterile water for injection to a concentration of dexrazoxane 10 mg/mL. Prior to infusion, further dilute reconstituted dexrazoxane solution in lactated Ringer's injection to a final concentration of 1.3-3 mg/mL.

Dexrazoxane generic formulation (Bedford Laboratories; Mylan, Inc): Reconstitute with the supplied diluent (0.167 Molar sodium lactate injection) to a final concentration of 10 mg/mL. Prior to infusion, further dilute reconstituted dexrazoxane solution with D_5W or NS to a final concentration of 1.3-5 mg/mL.

Mechanism of Action Derivative of ethylenediaminetetraacetic acid (EDTA); potent intracellular chelating agent. The mechanism of cardioprotectant activity is not fully understood. Appears to be converted intracellularly to a ring-opened chelating agent that interferes with iron-mediated oxygen free radical generation thought to be responsible, in part, for anthracycline-induced cardiomyopathy. In the management of anthracycline-induced extravasation, dexrazoxane may act by reversibly inhibiting topoisomerase II, protecting tissue from anthracycline cytotoxicity, thereby decreasing tissue damage.

Pharmacodynamics/Kinetics

Distribution: V_d: 22 L/m^2

Protein binding: None

Half-life elimination: 2-2.5 hours

Excretion: Urine (42%)

Dosing

Adult & Geriatric

Prevention of doxorubicin cardiomyopathy: I.V.: A 10:1 ratio of dexrazoxane:doxorubicin (dexrazoxane 500 mg/m^2:doxorubicin 50 mg/m^2). **Note:** Cardiac monitoring should continue during dexrazoxane therapy; doxorubicin/dexrazoxane should be discontinued in patients who develop a decline in LVEF or clinical CHF.

Treatment of anthracycline extravasation: I.V.: 1000 mg/m² on days 1 and 2 (maximum dose: 2000 mg), followed by 500 mg/m² on day 3 (maximum dose: 1000 mg); begin treatment as soon as possible, within 6 hours of extravasation

Pediatric Prevention of doxorubicin cardiomyopathy associated with acute lymphoblastic leukemia treatment (high-risk patients; unlabeled use): I.V.: A 10:1 ratio of dexrazoxane:doxorubicin (eg, dexrazoxane 300 mg/m²:doxorubicin 30 mg/m²) was used in patients with high-risk acute lymphoblastic leukemia (Lipshultz, 2010; Moghrabi, 2007; Silverman, 2010)

Renal Impairment Note: Renal function may be estimated using the Cockcroft-Gault formula.

Moderate-to-severe (Cl_{cr}<40 mL/minute):

Prevention of cardiomyopathy: Reduce dose by 50%, using a 5:1 dexrazoxane:doxorubicin ratio (dexrazoxane 250 mg/m²:doxorubicin 50 mg/m²)

Anthracycline-induced extravasation: Reduce dose by 50%

Hepatic Impairment

Prevention of cardiomyopathy: Since doxorubicin dosage is reduced in hyperbilirubinemia, a proportional reduction in dexrazoxane dosage is recommended (maintain a 10:1 ratio of dexrazoxane:doxorubicin)

Anthracycline-induced extravasation: Use has not been evaluated in patients with hepatic dysfunction

Administration

Prevention of doxorubicin cardiomyopathy: Administer doxorubicin within 30 minutes after beginning the infusion with dexrazoxane.

Zinecard®: Administer by rapid drip infusion; do **not** administer by I.V. push

Dexrazoxane generic formulation (Bedford Laboratories, Mylan, Inc): Administer by slow I.V push or rapid drip infusion

Treatment of anthracycline extravasation: Administer I.V. over 1-2 hours; begin infusion as soon as possible, within 6 hours of extravasation. Infusion solution should be at room temperature prior to administration. Infuse in a large vein in an area remote from the extravasation. If extravasation is also being managed with cooling, withhold cooling beginning 15 minutes before dexrazoxane infusion; continue withholding cooling until 15 minutes after infusion is completed. Day 2 and 3 doses should be administered at approximately the same time (± 3 hours) as the dose on day 1. For I.V. administration; **not** for local infiltration into extravasation

Emetic Potential Very low (<10%)

Monitoring Parameters CBC with differential (frequent); liver function; serum creatinine; cardiac function (repeat monitoring at 400 mg/m², 500 mg/m² and with every 50 mg/m² of doxorubicin thereafter); monitor site of extravasation

Additional Information Oncology Comment: Guidelines from the American Society of Clinical Oncology (ASCO) for the use of chemotherapy and radio therapy protectants (Hensley, 2008 [update]; Schuchter, 2002) recommend the use of dexrazoxane as a cardioprotectant in patients with metastatic breast cancer who may benefit from further doxorubicin-based chemotherapy after a cumulative doxorubicin dose >300 mg/m² has been reached. In patients with metastatic breast cancer who had previously received >300 mg/m² doxorubicin in the adjuvant setting, the decision to use dexrazoxane should be individualized, weighing the benefits of cardioprotection against the possibility of decreased response rates (due to dexrazoxane). Dexrazoxane use is not recommended in patients with metastatic breast cancer receiving doxorubicin as initial therapy. In the adjuvant setting, dexrazoxane use is not recommended outside of a clinical trial. Dexrazoxane may be considered for reduction of the incidence and severity of cardiomyopathy associated with continued epirubicin administration in patients with advanced breast cancer. In adults with malignancies other than breast cancer, dexrazoxane may be considered in patients who have received >300 mg/m^2 of doxorubicin-based therapy. Cardiac monitoring should continue during dexrazoxane therapy; discontinue doxorubicin/dexrazoxane in patients who develop a decline in LVEF or clinical CHF.

Dosage Forms Excipient information presented when available (limited, particularly for generics); consult specific product labeling.

Injection, powder for reconstitution: 250 mg, 500 mg

Totect®: 500 mg

Zinecard®: 250 mg, 500 mg

References

Hensley ML, Hagerty KL, Kewalramani T, et al, "American Society of Clinical Oncology 2008 Clinical Practice Guideline Update: Use of Chemotherapy and Radiotherapy Protectants," *J Clin Oncol*, 2009, 27(1): 127-45.

Lipshultz SE, Scully RE, Lipsitz SR, et al, "Assessment of Dexrazoxane as a Cardioprotectant In Doxorubicin-Treated Children With High-Risk Acute Lymphoblastic Leukaemia: Long-Term Follow-Up of a Prospective, Randomised, Multicentre Trial," *Lancet Oncol*, 2010, 11(10):950-61.

Marty M, Espié M, Llombart A, et al, "Multicenter Randomized Phase III Study of the Cardioprotective Effect of Dexrazoxane (Cardioxane) in Advanced/Metastatic Breast Cancer Patients Treated With Anthracycline-Based Chemotherapy," *Ann Oncol*, 2006, 17(4):614-22.

Moghrabi A, Levy DE, Asselin B, et al, "Results of the Dana-Farber Cancer Institute ALL Consortium Protocol 95-01 for Children With Acute Lymphoblastic Leukemia," *Blood*, 2007, 109(3):896-904.

Mouridsen HT, Langer SW, Buter J, et al, "Treatment of Anthracycline Extravasation With Savene (Dexrazoxane): Results From Two Prospective Clinical Multicentre Studies," *Ann Oncol*, 2007, 18 (3):546-50.

Schuchter LM, Hensley ML, Meropol NJ, et al, "2002 Update of Recommendations for the Use of Chemotherapy and Radiotherapy Protectants: Clinical Practice Guidelines of the American Society of Clinical Oncology," *J Clin Oncol*, 2002, 20(12):2895-903.

Silverman LB, Stevenson KE, O'Brien JE, et al, "Long-Term Results of Dana-Farber Cancer Institute ALL Consortium Protocols for Children With Newly Diagnosed Acute Lymphoblastic Leukemia (1985-2000)," *Leukemia*, 2010, 24(2):320-34.

Tebbi CK, London WB, Friedman D, et al, "Dexrazoxane-Associated Risk for Acute Myeloid Leukemia/Myelodysplastic Syndrome and Other Secondary Malignancies in Pediatric Hodgkin's Disease," *J Clin Oncol*, 2007, 25(5):493-500.

Tetef ML, Synold TW, Chow W, et al, "Phase I Trial of 96-Hour Continuous Infusion of Dexrazoxane I Patients With Advanced Malignancies," *Clin Cancer Res*, 2001, 7(6):1569-76.

◆ **Dezocitidine** *see* Decitabine *on page* *403*

◆ **DF** *see* Defibrotide *on page* *420*

◆ **dFdC** *see* Gemcitabine *on page* *663*

◆ **dFdCyd** *see* Gemcitabine *on page* *663*

◆ **DFM** *see* Deferoxamine *on page* *414*

◆ **DHAD** *see* MitoXANtrone *on page* *996*

◆ **DHAQ** *see* MitoXANtrone *on page* *996*

◆ **DHPG Sodium** *see* Ganciclovir (Systemic) *on page* *656*

◆ **Diaminocyclohexane Oxalatoplatinum** *see* Oxaliplatin *on page* *1077*

◆ **DIC** *see* Dacarbazine *on page* *367*

◆ **Diflucan®** *see* Fluconazole *on page* *612*

◆ **Difluorodeoxycytidine Hydrochlorothiazide** *see* Gemcitabine *on page* *663*

◆ **Dihematoporphyrin Ether** *see* Porfimer *on page* *1183*

◆ **Dihydrohydroxycodeinone** *see* OxyCODONE *on page* *1084*

◆ **Dihydromorphinone** *see* HYDROmorphone *on page* *724*

- **Dihydroxyanthracenedione** *see* MitoXANtrone *on page 996*
- **Dihydroxyanthracenedione Dihydrochloride** *see* MitoXANtrone *on page 996*
- **1,25 Dihydroxycholecalciferol** *see* Calcitriol *on page 215*
- **Dihydroxydeoxynorvinkaleukoblastine** *see* Vinorelbine *on page 1465*
- **Dilaudid®** *see* HYDROmorphone *on page 724*
- **Dilaudid-HP®** *see* HYDROmorphone *on page 724*
- **Dimethyl Triazeno Imidazole Carboxamide** *see* Dacarbazine *on page 367*
- **Diopred® (Can)** *see* PrednisoLONE (Ophthalmic) *on page 1198*
- **Disodium Thiosulfate Pentahydrate** *see* Sodium Thiosulfate *on page 1289*
- **5071-1DL(6)** *see* Megestrol *on page 922*
- **4-DMDR** *see* IDArubicin *on page 749*
- **Docefrez™** *see* DOCEtaxel *on page 453*

DOCEtaxel (doe se TAKS el)

Related Information

Chemotherapy and Obesity *on page 1834*
Management of Chemotherapy-Induced Nausea and Vomiting *on page 1780*
Management of Drug Extravasations *on page 1800*
Oral Mucositis/Stomatitis *on page 1814*
Safe Handling of Hazardous Drugs *on page 1904*

Brand Names: U.S. Docefrez™; Taxotere®

Brand Names: Canada Docetaxel for Injection; Taxotere®

Index Terms RP 6076

Generic Availability (U.S.) Yes: Excludes injection, powder for reconstitution

Pharmacologic Category Antineoplastic Agent, Antimicrotubular; Antineoplastic Agent, Natural Source (Plant) Derivative; Antineoplastic Agent, Taxane Derivative

Use Treatment of breast cancer (locally advanced/metastatic or adjuvant treatment of operable node-positive); locally-advanced or metastatic nonsmall cell lung cancer (NSCLC); hormone refractory, metastatic prostate cancer; advanced gastric adenocarcinoma; locally-advanced squamous cell head and neck cancer

Unlabeled Use Treatment of bladder cancer (metastatic), ovarian cancer, cervical cancer (relapsed), esophageal cancer, small cell lung cancer (relapsed), soft tissue sarcoma, Ewing's sarcoma, osteosarcoma, and unknown-primary adenocarcinoma

Labeled Contraindications Severe hypersensitivity to docetaxel or any component of the formulation; severe hypersensitivity to other medications containing polysorbate 80; neutrophil count <1500/mm^3

Pregnancy Risk Factor D

Lactation Excretion in breast milk unknown/not recommended

Warnings/Precautions Hazardous agent - use appropriate precautions for handling and disposal. **[U.S. Boxed Warning]: Avoid use in patients with bilirubin exceeding upper limit of normal (ULN) or AST and/or ALT >1.5 times ULN in conjunction with alkaline phosphatase >2.5 times ULN; patients with abnormal liver function are at increased risk of treatment-related adverse events,** including grade 4 neutropenia, neutropenic fever, infections, and sever thrombocytopenia, stomatitis, skin toxicity or toxic death;

obtain liver function tests prior to each treatment cycle. **[U.S. Boxed Warnings]: Severe hypersensitivity reactions, characterized by generalized rash/erythema, hypotension, bronchospasms, or anaphylaxis may occur; minor reactions including flushing or localized skin reactions may also occur; do not administer to patients with a history of severe hypersensitivity to docetaxel or polysorbate 80. Severe fluid retention, characterized by pleural effusion (requiring immediate drainage, ascites, peripheral edema (poorly tolerated), dyspnea at rest, cardiac tamponade, and weight gain (2-15 kg) has been reported.** The incidence and severity of fluid retention increase sharply at cumulative doses ≥400 mg/m². Observe for hypersensitivity, especially with the first two infusions. Discontinue for severe reactions; do not rechallenge if severe. Patients should be premedicated with a corticosteroid (starting one day prior to administration) to prevent or reduce the severity of hypersensitivity reactions and fluid retention; severity is reduced with dexamethasone premedication starting one day prior to docetaxel administration.

[U.S. Boxed Warning]: Patients with abnormal liver function, those receiving higher doses, and patients with nonsmall cell lung cancer and a history of prior treatment with platinum derivatives who receive single-agent docetaxel at a dose of 100 mg/m² are at higher risk for treatment-related mortality.

Neutropenia is the dose-limiting toxicity. Patients with increased liver function tests experienced more episodes of neutropenia with a greater number of severe infections. **[U.S. Boxed Warning]: Patients with an absolute neutrophil count <1500/mm³ should not receive docetaxel.** Platelets should recover to >100,000/mm³ prior to treatment. When administered as sequential infusions, taxane derivatives (docetaxel, paclitaxel) should be administered before platinum derivatives (carboplatin, cisplatin) to limit myelosuppression and to enhance efficacy.

Cutaneous reactions including erythema (with edema) and desquamation have been reported; may require dose reduction. Dosage adjustment is recommended with severe neurosensory symptoms (paresthesia, dysesthesia, pain); persistent symptoms may require discontinuation; reversal of symptoms may be delayed after discontinuation. Treatment-related acute myeloid leukemia or myelodysplasia occurred in patients receiving docetaxel in combination with anthracyclines and/or cyclophosphamide. Fatigue and weakness (may be severe) have been reported; symptoms may last a few days up to several weeks; in patients with progressive disease, weakness may be associated with a decrease in performance status. Avoid concomitant use with strong CYP3A4 inhibitors; although data is limited, a 50% dose reduction is suggested if concomitant therapy with a strong CYP3A4 inhibitor is required.

Adverse Reactions Percentages reported for docetaxel monotherapy; frequency may vary depending on diagnosis, dose, liver function, prior treatment, and premedication. The incidence of adverse events was usually higher in patients with elevated liver function tests.

>10%:

Cardiovascular: Fluid retention (13% to 60%; dose dependent)

Central nervous system: Neurosensory events (20% to 58%; including neuropathy), fever (31% to 35%), neuromotor events (16%)

Dermatologic: Alopecia (56% to 76%), cutaneous events (20% to 48%), nail disorder (11% to 41%)

Gastrointestinal: Stomatitis (19% to 53%; severe 1% to 8%), diarrhea (23% to 43%; severe: 5% to 6%), nausea (34% to 42%), vomiting (22% to 23%)
Hematologic: Neutropenia (84% to 99%; grade 4: 75% to 86%; nadir (median): 7 days, duration (severe neutropenia): 7 days; dose dependent), leukopenia (84% to 99%; grade 4: 32% to 44%), anemia (65% to 94%; dose dependent; grades 3/4: 8% to 9%), thrombocytopenia (8% to 14%; grade 4: 1%; dose dependent), febrile neutropenia (6% to 12%; dose dependent)
Hepatic: Transaminases increased (4% to 19%)
Neuromuscular & skeletal: Weakness (53% to 66%; severe 13% to 18%), myalgia (3% to 23%)
Respiratory: Pulmonary events (41%)
Miscellaneous: Infection (1% to 34%; dose dependent), hypersensitivity (1% to 21%; with premedication 15%)

1% to 10%:
Cardiovascular: Left ventricular ejection fraction decreased (prostate cancer: 10%; metastatic breast cancer: 8%), hypotension (3%)
Gastrointestinal: Taste perversion (6%)
Hepatic: Bilirubin increased (9%), alkaline phosphatase increased (4% to 7%)
Local: Infusion-site reactions (4%, including hyperpigmentation, inflammation, redness, dryness, phlebitis, extravasation, swelling of the vein)
Neuromuscular and skeletal: Arthralgia (3% to 9%)
Ocular: Epiphora associated with canalicular stenosis (≤77% with weekly administration; ≤1% with every 3-week administration)

<1%, postmarketing, and/or case reports (limited to important or life-threatening): Acute myeloid leukemia (AML), acute respiratory distress syndrome (ARDS), anaphylactic shock, arrhythmia, ascites, atrial fibrillation, atrial flutter, AV block, bleeding episodes, bradycardia, bronchospasm, cardiac tamponade, chest pain, chest tightness, colitis, conjunctivitis, constipation, cutaneous lupus erythematosus, deep vein thrombosis, dehydration, disseminated intravascular coagulation (DIC), drug fever, duodenal ulcer, dyspnea, dysrhythmia, ECG abnormalities, erythema multiforme, esophagitis, gastrointestinal hemorrhage, gastrointestinal obstruction, gastrointestinal perforation, hand and foot syndrome, hearing loss, heart failure, hepatitis, hypertension, ileus, interstitial pneumonia, ischemic colitis, lacrimal duct obstruction, loss of consciousness (transient), MI, multiorgan failure, myelodysplastic syndrome, myocardial ischemia, neutropenic enterocolitis, neutropenic typhlitis, ototoxicity, pericardial effusion, pleural effusion, pruritus, pulmonary edema, pulmonary embolism, pulmonary fibrosis, radiation pneumonitis, radiation recall, renal failure, renal insufficiency, scleroderma-like changes, seizure, sepsis, sinus tachycardia, Stevens-Johnson syndrome, syncope, toxic epidermal necrolysis, tachycardia, thrombophlebitis, unstable angina, visual disturbances (transient)

Drug Interactions

Metabolism/Transport Effects Substrate of CYP3A4 (major), P-glycoprotein; **Note:** Assignment of Major/Minor substrate status based on clinically relevant drug interaction potential; **Inhibits** CYP3A4 (weak)

Avoid Concomitant Use

Avoid concomitant use of DOCEtaxel with any of the following: BCG; CloZAPine; Conivaptan; Natalizumab; Pimecrolimus; Pimozide; Tacrolimus (Topical); Vaccines (Live)

Increased Effect/Toxicity

DOCEtaxel may increase the levels/effects of: Antineoplastic Agents (Anthracycline, Systemic); ARIPiprazole; CloZAPine; Leflunomide; Natalizumab; Pimozide; Vaccines (Live)

The levels/effects of DOCEtaxel may be increased by: Antifungal Agents (Azole Derivatives, Systemic); Conivaptan; CYP3A4 Inhibitors (Moderate); CYP3A4 Inhibitors (Strong); Dasatinib; Denosumab; Dronedarone; Ivacaftor; Mifepristone; P-glycoprotein/ABCB1 Inhibitors; Pimecrolimus; Platinum Derivatives; Roflumilast; SORAfenib; Tacrolimus (Topical); Trastuzumab

Decreased Effect

DOCEtaxel may decrease the levels/effects of: BCG; Coccidioidin Skin Test; Sipuleucel-T; Vaccines (Inactivated); Vaccines (Live)

The levels/effects of DOCEtaxel may be decreased by: CYP3A4 Inducers (Strong); Deferasirox; Echinacea; Herbs (CYP3A4 Inducers); P-glycoprotein/ABCB1 Inducers; Tocilizumab

Ethanol/Nutrition/Herb Interactions

Ethanol: Avoid ethanol (due to GI irritation).

Herb/Nutraceutical: Avoid St John's wort (may decrease docetaxel levels).

Storage/Stability

Docetaxel 10 mg/mL: Store intact vials between 2°C to 25°C (36°F to 77°F) (actual recommendations may vary by generic manufacturer; consult manufacturer's labeling). Protect from bright light. Freezing does not adversely affect the product. Multi-use vials (80 mg/8 mL and 160 mg/16 mL) are stable for up to 28 days after first entry when stored between 2°C to 8°C (36°F to 46°F) and protected from light.

Docetaxel concentrate (Taxotere®) 20 mg/mL: Store intact vials between 2°C to 25°C (36°F to 77°F). Protect from bright light. Freezing does not adversely affect the product.

Docetaxel lyophilized powder (Docefrez™): Store intact vials between 2°C to 8°C (36°F to 46°F). Protect from light. Allow vials (and provided diluent) to stand at room temperature for 5 minutes prior to reconstitution. After reconstitution, may be stored refrigerated or at room temperature for up to 8 hours.

Solutions diluted for infusion should be used within 4 hours of preparation, including infusion time.

Two-vial formulation *(discontinued product):* Reconstituted solutions of the two-vial formulation are stable in the vial for 8 hours at room temperature or under refrigeration. Solutions diluted for infusion in polyolefin containers should be used within 4 hours of preparation, including infusion time.

Reconstitution Note: Multiple concentrations: Docetaxel is available as a one-vial formulation at concentrations of 10 mg/mL (generic formulation) and 20 mg/mL (concentrate; Taxotere®, and as a lyophilized powder (Docefrez™) which is reconstituted (with provided diluent) to 20 mg/0.8 mL (20 mg vial) or 24 mg/mL (80 mg vial). Admixture errors have occurred due to the availability of various concentrations. Docetaxel was previously available as a two-vial formulation which included two vials (a concentrated docetaxel vial and a diluent vial), resulting in a reconstituted concentration of 10 mg/mL; the two-vial formulation has been discontinued by the manufacturer.

Use appropriate precautions for handling and disposal.

One-vial formulations: Further dilute for infusion in 250-500 mL of NS or D_5W in a non-DEHP container (eg, glass, polypropylene, polyolefin) to a final concentration of 0.3-0.74 mg/mL. Gently rotate and invert manually to mix thoroughly; avoid shaking or vigorous agitation. **Note:** For docetaxel injection concentrate 20 mg/mL (Taxotere®), use **only** a 21 gauge needle to withdraw docetaxel from the vial (larger bore needles, such as 18 gauge or 19 gauge needles may cause stopper coring and rubber precipitates).

Lyophilized powder: Dilute with the provided diluent (contains ethanol in polysorbate 80); add 1 mL to each 20 mg vial (resulting concentration is 20 mg/0.8 mL) and 4 mL to each 80 mg vial (resulting concentration is 24 mg/mL). Shake well to dissolve completely. If air bubbles are present, allow to stand for a few minutes while air bubbles dissipate. Further dilute in 250 mL of NS or D_5W in a non-DEHP container (eg, glass, polypropylene, polyolefin) to a final concentration of 0.3-0.74 mg/mL (for doses >200 mg, use a larger volume of NS or D_5W, not to exceed a final concentration of 0.74 mg/mL). Mix thoroughly by manual agitation. Solutions diluted for infusion should be used within 4 hours of preparation, including infusion time.

Two-vial formulation *(discontinued product)*: Vials should be diluted with 13% (w/w) ethanol/water (provided with the drug) to a final concentration of 10 mg/mL. Do not shake. Further dilute for infusion in 250-500 mL of NS or D_5W in a non-DEHP container (eg, glass, polypropylene, polyolefin) to a final concentration of 0.3-0.74 mg/mL. Gently rotate to mix thoroughly. Do not use the two-vial formulation with the one-vial formulation for the same admixture product.

Mechanism of Action Docetaxel promotes the assembly of microtubules from tubulin dimers, and inhibits the depolymerization of tubulin which stabilizes microtubules in the cell. This results in inhibition of DNA, RNA, and protein synthesis. Most activity occurs during the M phase of the cell cycle.

Pharmacodynamics/Kinetics Exhibits linear pharmacokinetics at the recommended dosage range

Distribution: Extensive extravascular distribution and/or tissue binding; V_d: 80-90 L/m^2, V_{dss}: 113 L (mean steady state)

Protein binding: ~94% to 97%, primarily to alpha$_1$-acid glycoprotein, albumin, and lipoproteins

Metabolism: Hepatic; oxidation via CYP3A4 to metabolites

Half-life elimination: Terminal: ~11 hours

Excretion: Feces (~75%, <8% as unchanged drug); urine (<5%)

Dosing

Adult & Geriatric Note: Premedicate with corticosteroids, beginning the day before docetaxel administration, (administer corticosteroids for 3 days) to reduce the severity of hypersensitivity reactions and fluid retention. Details concerning dosing in combination regimens should also be consulted.

Breast cancer: I.V.:

Locally-advanced or metastatic: 60-100 mg/m^2 every 3 weeks (as a single agent)

Operable, node-positive (adjuvant treatment): 75 mg/m^2 every 3 weeks for 6 courses (in combination with doxorubicin and cyclophosphamide)

Weekly administration (unlabeled dosing): 40 mg/m^2/dose once a week (as a single agent) for 6 weeks followed by a 2-week rest, repeat until disease progression or unacceptable toxicity (Burstein, 2000) **or** 35 mg/m^2/dose once a week (in combination with trastuzumab) for 3 weeks followed by a 1-week rest; repeat until disease progression or unacceptable toxicity (Esteva, 2002)

Nonsmall cell lung cancer: I.V.: 75 mg/m^2 every 3 weeks (as monotherapy or in combination with cisplatin)

Prostate cancer: I.V.: 75 mg/m^2 every 3 weeks (in combination with prednisone)

Gastric adenocarcinoma: I.V.: 75 mg/m^2 every 3 weeks (in combination with cisplatin and fluorouracil)

Head and neck cancer: I.V.: 75 mg/m^2 every 3 weeks (in combination with cisplatin and fluorouracil) for 3 or 4 cycles, followed by radiation therapy

Bladder cancer, metastatic (unlabeled use): I.V.: 100 mg/m^2 every 3 weeks (as a single agent) (McCaffrey, 1997)

Esophageal cancer (unlabeled use): I.V.: 75 mg/m^2 every 3 weeks (in combination with cisplatin and fluorouracil) (Ajani, 2007; Van Cutsem, 2006)

Ovarian cancer (unlabeled use): I.V.: 60 mg/m^2 every 3 weeks (in combination with carboplatin) (Markman, 2001) **or** 75 mg/m^2 every 3 weeks (in combination with carboplatin) (Vasey, 2004) **or** 35 mg/m^2 (maximum dose: 70 mg) weekly for 3 weeks followed by a 1-week rest (in combination with carboplatin) (Kushner, 2007)

Soft tissue sarcoma (unlabeled use): I.V.: 100 mg/m^2 on day 8 of a 3-week treatment cycle (in combination with gemcitabine and filgrastim or pegfilgrastim) (Leu, 2004; Maki, 2007)

Unknown-primary, adenocarcinoma (unlabeled use): I.V.: 65 mg/m^2 every 3 weeks (in combination with carboplatin) (Greco, 2000) **or** 75 mg/m^2 on day 8 of a 3-week treatment cycle (in combination with gemcitabine) (Pouessel, 2004)

Dosing adjustment for concomitant CYP3A4 inhibitors: Avoid the concomitant use of strong CYP3A4 inhibitors with docetaxel. If concomitant use of a strong CYP3A4 inhibitor cannot be avoided, consider reducing the docetaxel dose by 50% (based on limited pharmacokinetic data).

Renal Impairment Renal excretion is minimal (<5%), therefore, the need for dosage adjustments for renal dysfunction is unlikely (Li, 2007). Not removed by hemodialysis, may be administered before or after hemodialysis (Janus, 2010).

Hepatic Impairment

The FDA-approved labeling recommends the following adjustments:

Total bilirubin greater than the ULN, or AST and/or ALT >1.5 times ULN concomitant with alkaline phosphatase >2.5 times ULN: Use is not recommended.

Hepatic impairment dosing adjustment specific for gastric adenocarcinoma:

AST/ALT >2.5 to ≤5 times ULN and alkaline phosphatase ≤2.5 times ULN: Administer 80% of dose

AST/ALT >1.5 to ≤5 times ULN and alkaline phosphatase >2.5 to ≤5 times ULN: Administer 80% of dose

AST/ALT >5 times ULN and /or alkaline phosphatase >5 times ULN: Discontinue docetaxel

The following guidelines have been used by some clinicians (Floyd, 2006):

Transaminases 1.6-6 times ULN: Administer 75% of dose

Transaminases >6 times ULN: Use clinical judgment

Adjustment for Toxicity Note: Toxicity includes febrile neutropenia, neutrophils ≤500/mm^3 for >1 week, severe or cumulative cutaneous reactions; in nonsmall cell lung cancer, this may also include platelets <25,000/mm^3 and other grade 3/4 nonhematologic toxicities.

Breast cancer (single agent): Patients dosed initially at 100 mg/m^2; reduce dose to 75 mg/m^2; **Note:** If the patient continues to experience these adverse reactions, the dosage should be reduced to 55 mg/m^2 or therapy should be discontinued; discontinue for peripheral neuropathy ≥ grade 3. Patients initiated at 60 mg/m^2 who do not develop toxicity may tolerate higher doses.

Breast cancer, adjuvant treatment (combination chemotherapy): TAC regimen should be administered when neutrophils are ≥1500/mm^3. Patients experiencing febrile neutropenia should receive G-CSF in all subsequent cycles. Patients with persistent febrile neutropenia (while on G-CSF), patients experiencing severe/cumulative cutaneous reactions, moderate neurosensory effects (signs/symptoms) or grade 3 or 4 stomatitis should receive a reduced dose (60 mg/m^2) of docetaxel. Discontinue therapy with persistent toxicities after dosage reduction.

Nonsmall cell lung cancer:

Monotherapy: Patients dosed initially at 75 mg/m^2 should have dose held until toxicity is resolved, then resume at 55 mg/m^2; discontinue for peripheral neuropathy ≥ grade 3.

Combination therapy (with cisplatin): Patients dosed initially at 75 mg/m^2 should have the docetaxel dosage reduced to 65 mg/m^2 in subsequent cycles; if further adjustment is required, dosage may be reduced to 50 mg/m^2

Prostate cancer: Reduce dose to 60 mg/m^2; discontinue therapy if toxicities persist at lower dose.

Gastric cancer, head and neck cancer: **Note:** Cisplatin may require dose reductions/therapy delays for peripheral neuropathy, ototoxicity, and /or nephrotoxicity. Patients experiencing febrile neutropenia, documented infection with neutropenia or neutropenia >7 days should receive G-CSF in all subsequent cycles. For neutropenic complications despite G-CSF use, further reduce dose to 60 mg/m^2. Neutropenic complications in subsequent cycles should be further dose reduced to 45 mg/m^2. Patients who experience grade 4 thrombocytopenia should receive a dose reduction from 75 mg/m^2 to 60 mg/m^2. Discontinue therapy for persistent toxicities.

Gastrointestinal toxicity for docetaxel in combination with cisplatin and fluorouracil for treatment of gastric cancer or head and neck cancer:

Diarrhea, grade 3:
- First episode: Reduce fluorouracil dose by 20%
- Second episode: Reduce docetaxel dose by 20%

Diarrhea, grade 4:
- First episode: Reduce fluorouracil and docetaxel doses by 20%
- Second episode: Discontinue treatment

Stomatitis, grade 3:
- First episode: Reduce fluorouracil dose by 20%
- Second episode: Discontinue fluorouracil for all subsequent cycles
- Third episode: Reduce docetaxel dose by 20%

Stomatitis, grade 4:
- First episode: Discontinue fluorouracil for all subsequent cycles
- Second episode: Reduce docetaxel dose by 20%

Combination Regimens

Breast cancer:

Capecitabine + Docetaxel (Breast Cancer) on page 1539
Docetaxel-Bevacizumab on page 1608
Docetaxel-Cyclophosphamide (TC) on page 1611
Docetaxel-Doxorubicin (Breast Cancer) on page 1611
Docetaxel-FEC on page 1611

Docetaxel-Pertuzumab-Trastuzumab (Breast) on page 1614
Docetaxel-Trastuzumab on page 1615
Docetaxel-Trastuzumab-Carboplatin on page 1615
Docetaxel-Trastuzumab-Cisplatin on page 1616
Docetaxel-Trastuzumab-FEC on page 1616
Docetaxel (Weekly)-Trastuzumab on page 1617
Doxorubicin (Liposomal)-Docetaxel (Breast Cancer) on page 1619
TAC on page 1753

Esophageal cancer:
Docetaxel-Cisplatin-Fluorouracil (Gastric/Esophageal Cancer) on page 1609
Docetaxel-Oxaliplatin-Fluorouracil (Esophageal Cancer) on page 1613
Docetaxel-Oxaliplatin-Leucovorin-Fluorouracil (Esophageal Cancer) on page 1613

Gastric cancer:
Capecitabine-Docetaxel (Gastric Cancer) on page 1539
Docetaxel-Cisplatin-Fluorouracil (Gastric/Esophageal Cancer) on page 1609

Head and neck cancer: Docetaxel-Cisplatin-Fluorouracil (Head and Neck Cancer) on page 1610

Lung cancer (nonsmall cell):
Docetaxel-Cisplatin on page 1609
Docetaxel (NSCLC Regimen) on page 1612

Lung cancer (small cell): Docetaxel (Small Cell Lung Cancer Regimen) on page 1614

Osteosarcoma: Gemcitabine-Docetaxel (Sarcoma) on page 1671

Ovarian cancer:
Carboplatin-Docetaxel (Ovarian) on page 1543
Docetaxel (Ovarian Regimen) on page 1612
Docetaxel-Oxaliplatin (Ovarian Cancer) on page 1613

Prostate cancer:
Docetaxel-Prednisone on page 1614
Docetaxel (Weekly Regimen) on page 1617
Estramustine + Docetaxel on page 1634
Estramustine + Docetaxel + Calcitriol on page 1635
Estramustine + Docetaxel + Carboplatin on page 1636
Estramustine + Docetaxel + Hydrocortisone on page 1636
Estramustine + Docetaxel + Prednisone on page 1636

Soft tissue sarcoma: Gemcitabine-Docetaxel (Sarcoma) on page 1671

Unknown primary, adenocarcinoma:
Carboplatin-Docetaxel (Unknown Primary) on page 1544
Cisplatin-Docetaxel (Unknown Primary) on page 1568
Docetaxel-Gemcitabine (Unknown Primary) on page 1611

Unknown primary, squamous cell: Cisplatin-Docetaxel-Fluorouracil (Unknown Primary) on page 1568

Administration Administer I.V. infusion over 1-hour through nonsorbing polyethylene lined (non-DEHP) tubing; in-line filter is not necessary (the use of a filter during administration is not recommended by the manufacturer). Infusion should be completed within 4 hours of final preparation. **Note:** Premedication with corticosteroids for 3 days, beginning the day before docetaxel administration, is recommended to prevent hypersensitivity reactions and fluid retention (see Additional Information).

Emetic Potential Low (10% to 30%)

Vesicant/Extravasation Risk May be an irritant

Monitoring Parameters CBC with differential, liver function tests, bilirubin, alkaline phosphatase, renal function; monitor for hypersensitivity reactions, neurosensory symptoms, gastrointestinal toxicity (eg, diarrhea, stomatitis), cutaneous reactions, fluid retention, epiphora, and canalicular stenosis

Additional Information Premedication with oral corticosteroids is recommended to decrease the incidence and severity of fluid retention and severity of hypersensitivity reactions. The manufacturer recommends dexamethasone 16 mg/day (8 mg twice daily) orally for 3 days, starting the day before docetaxel administration; for prostate cancer, when prednisone is part of the antineoplastic regimen, dexamethasone 8 mg orally is administered at 12 hours, 3 hours, and 1 hour prior to docetaxel.

Dosage Forms Excipient information presented when available (limited, particularly for generics); consult specific product labeling.

Injection, powder for reconstitution:

Docefrez™: 20 mg, 80 mg [contains ethanol (in diluent), polysorbate 80 (in diluent); supplied with diluent]

Injection, solution: 10 mg/mL

Injection, solution [concentrate]: 20 mg/0.5 mL

Taxotere®: 20 mg/mL [contains dehydrated ethanol 0.395 g/mL, polysorbate 80]

References

Ajani JA, Fodor MD, Tjulandin SA, et al, "Phase II Multi-Institutional Randomized Trial of Docetaxel Plus Cisplatin With or Without Fluorouracil in Patients With Untreated, Advanced Gastric, or Gastroesophageal Adenocarcinoma," *J Clin Oncol*, 2005, 23(24):5660-7.

Ajani JA, Moiseyenko VM, Tjulandin S, et al, "Clinical Benefit With Docetaxel Plus Fluorouracil and Cisplatin Compared With Cisplatin and Fluorouracil in a Phase III Trial of Advanced Gastric or Gastroesophageal Cancer Adenocarcinoma: The V 325 Study Group," *J Clin Oncol*, 2007, 25 (22):3205-9.

Blohmer JU, Schmid P, Hilfrich J, et al, "Epirubicin and Cyclophosphamide Versus Epirubicin and Docetaxel as First-Line Therapy for Women With Metastatic Breast Cancer: Final Results of a Randomised Phase III Trial," *Ann Oncol*, 2010, 21(7):1430-5.

Burstein HJ, Manola J, Younger J, et al, "Docetaxel Administered on a Weekly Basis for Metastatic Breast Cancer," *J Clin Oncol*, 2000, 18(6):1212-9.

Esteva FJ, Valero V, Booser D, et al, "Phase II Study of Weekly Docetaxel and Trastuzumab for Patients With HER-2-Overexpressing Metastatic Breast Cancer," *J Clin Oncol*, 2002, 20 (7):1800-8.

Floyd J, Mirza I, Sachs B, et al, "Hepatotoxicity of Chemotherapy," *Semin Oncol*, 2006, 33 (1):50-67.

Garcia AA, Blessing JA, Vaccarell L, et al, "Phase II Clinical Trial of Docetaxel in Refractory Squamous Cell Carcinoma of the Cervix: A Gynecologic Oncology Group Study," *Am J Clin Oncol*, 2007, 30(4):428-31.

Greco FA, Erland JB, Morrissey LH, et al, "Carcinoma of Unknown Primary Site. Phase II Trials With Docetaxel Plus Cisplatin or Carboplatin," *Ann Oncol*, 2000, 11(2):211-5.

Janus N, Thariat J, Boulanger H, et al, "Proposal for Dosage Adjustment and Timing of Chemotherapy in Hemodialyzed Patients," *Ann Oncol*, 2010, 21(7):1395-403.

Kushner DM, Connor JP, Sanchez F, et al, "Weekly Docetaxel and Carboplatin for Recurrent Ovarian and Peritoneal Cancer: A Phase II Study," *Gynecol Oncol*, 2007, 105(2):358-64.

Leu KM, Ostruszka LJ, Shewach D, et al, "Laboratory and Clinical Evidence of Synergistic Cytotoxicity of Sequential Treatment With Gemcitabine Followed by Docetaxel in the Treatment of Sarcoma," *J Clin Oncol*, 2004, 22(9):1706-12.

Li YF, Fu S, Hu W, et al, "Systemic Anticancer Therapy in Gynecological Cancer Patients With Renal Dysfunction," *Int J Gynecol Cancer*, 2007, 7(4):739-63.

Maki RG, Wathen JK, Patel SR, et al, "Randomized Phase II Study of Gemcitabine and Docetaxel Compared With Gemcitabine Alone in Patients With Metastatic Soft Tissue Sarcomas: Results of Sarcoma Alliance for Research Through Collaboration Study 002," *J Clin Oncol*, 2007, 25 (19):2755-63.

Markman M, Kennedy A, Webster K, et al, "Combination Chemotherapy With Carboplatin and Docetaxel in the Treatment of Cancers of the Ovary and Fallopian Tube and Primary Carcinoma of the Peritoneum," *J Clin Oncol*, 2001, 19(7):1901-5.

Mavroudis D, Papakotoulas P, Ardavanis A, et al, "Randomized Phase III Trial Comparing Docetaxel Plus Epirubicin Versus Docetaxel Plus Capecitabine as First-Line Treatment in Women With Advanced Breast Cancer," *Ann Oncol*, 2010, 21(1):48-54.

McCaffrey JA, Hilton S, Mazumdar M, et al, "Phase II Trial of Docetaxel in Patients With Advanced or Metastatic Transitional-Cell Carcinoma," *J Clin Oncol*, 1997, 15(5):1853-7.

Morgan C, Tillett T, Braybrooke J, et al, "Management of Uncommon Chemotherapy-Induced Emergencies," *Lancet Oncol*, 2011, 12(8):806-14.

Muro K, Hamaguchi T, Ohtsu A, et al, "A Phase II Study of Single-Agent Docetaxel in Patients With Metastatic Esophageal Cancer," *Ann Oncol*, 2004, 15(6):955-9.

Navid F, Willert JR, McCarville MB, et al, "Combination of Gemcitabine and Docetaxel in the Treatment of Children and Young Adults With Refractory Bone Sarcoma," *Cancer*, 2008, 113 (2):419-25.

Pointreau Y, Garaud P, Chapet S, et al, "Randomized Trial of Induction Chemotherapy With Cisplatin and 5-Fluorouracil With or Without Docetaxel forLlarynx Preservation," *J Natl Cancer Inst*, 2009, 101(7):498-506.

Posner MR, Glisson B, Frenette G, et al, "Multicenter Phase I-II Trial of Docetaxel, Cisplatin, and Fluorouracil Induction Chemotherapy for Patients With Locally Advanced Squamous Cell Cancer of the Head and Neck," *J Clin Oncol*, 2001, 19(4):1096-104.

Posner MR, Hershock DM, Blajman CR, et al, "Cisplatin and Fluorouracil Alone or With Docetaxel in Head and Neck Cancer," *N Engl J Med*, 2007, 357(17):1705-15.

Pouessel D, Culine S, Becht C, et al, "Gemcitabine and Docetaxel as Front-Line Chemotherapy in Patients With Carcinoma of an Unknown Primary Site," *Cancer*, 2004, 100(6):1257-61.

Schrijvers D, Van Herpen C, Kerger J, et al, "Docetaxel, Cisplatin and 5-Fluorouracil in Patients With Locally Advanced Unresectable Head and Neck Cancer: A Phase I-II Feasibility Study," *Ann Oncol*, 2004, 15(4):638-45.

Smyth JF, Smith IE, Sessa C, et al, "Activity of Docetaxel (Taxotere) in Small Cell Lung Cancer. The Early Clinical Trials Group of the EORTC," *Eur J Cancer*, 1994, 30A(8):1058-60.

Van Cutsem E, Moiseyenko VM, Tjulandin S, et al, "Phase III Study of Docetaxel and Cisplatin Plus Fluorouracil Compared With Cisplatin and Fluorouracil as First-Line Therapy for Advanced Gastric Cancer: A Report of the V325 Study Group," *J Clin Oncol*, 2006, 24(31):4991-7.

Vasey PA, Jayson GC, Gordon A, et al, "Phase III Randomized Trial of Docetaxel-Carboplatin Versus Paclitaxel-Carboplatin as First-line Chemotherapy for Ovarian Carcinoma," *J Natl Cancer Inst*, 2004, 96(22):1682-91.

Vermorken JB, Remenar E, van Herpen C, et al, "Cisplatin, Fluorouracil, and Docetaxel in Unresectable Head and Neck Cancer," *N Engl J Med*, 2007, 357(17):1695-704.

◆ **Docetaxel for Injection (Can)** *see* DOCEtaxel *on page 453*

Dolasetron (dol A se tron)

Related Information

Management of Chemotherapy-Induced Nausea and Vomiting *on page 1786*

Brand Names: U.S. Anzemet®

Brand Names: Canada Anzemet®

Index Terms Dolasetron Mesylate; MDL 73,147EF

Generic Availability (U.S.) No

Pharmacologic Category Antiemetic; Selective 5-HT_3 Receptor Antagonist

Use

U.S. labeling:

Injection: Prevention and treatment of postoperative nausea and vomiting

Oral: Prevention of nausea and vomiting associated with emetogenic cancer chemotherapy (initial and repeat courses); prevention of postoperative nausea and vomiting

Canadian labeling: Oral: Prevention of nausea and vomiting associated with emetogenic cancer chemotherapy (initial and repeat courses)

Labeled Contraindications

U.S. labeling:

Injection: Hypersensitivity to dolasetron or any component of the formulation; use for the prevention of chemotherapy induced nausea and vomiting

Tablet: Hypersensitivity to dolasetron or any component of the formulation

Canadian labeling: Hypersensitivity to dolasetron or any component of the formulation; use in children and adolescents <18 years of age; use for the prevention or treatment of postoperative nausea and vomiting

Pregnancy Risk Factor B

Lactation Excretion in breast milk unknown/use caution

Warnings/Precautions Dolasetron is associated with a number of dose-dependent increases in ECG intervals (eg, PR, QRS duration, QT/QT_c, JT), usually occurring 1-2 hours after I.V. administration and usually lasting 6-8 hours; however, may last ≥24 hours and rarely lead to heart block or arrhythmia. Clinically relevant QT-interval prolongation may occur resulting in torsade de pointes, when used in conjunction with other agents that prolong the QT interval (eg, Class I and III antiarrhythmics). Avoid use in patients at greater risk for QT prolongation (eg, patients with congenital long QT syndrome, medications known to prolong QT interval, electrolyte abnormalities, and cumulative high-dose anthracycline therapy) and/or ventricular arrhythmia. Correct potassium or magnesium abnormalities prior to initiating therapy. I.V. formulations of 5-HT_3 antagonists have more association with ECG interval changes, compared to oral formulations. Reduction in heart rate may also occur with the 5-HT_3 antagonists. Use with caution in children and adolescents who have or may develop QT_c prolongation; rare cases of supraventricular and ventricular arrhythmias, cardiac arrest, and MI have been reported in this population.

Use with caution in patients allergic to other 5-HT_3 receptor antagonists; cross-reactivity has been reported with other 5-HT_3 receptor antagonists. **For chemotherapy-associated nausea and vomiting, should be used on a scheduled basis, not on an "as needed" (PRN) basis,** since data support the use of this drug only in the prevention of nausea and vomiting (due to antineoplastic therapy) and not in the rescue of nausea and vomiting. Not intended for treatment of nausea and vomiting or for chronic continuous therapy.

Adverse Reactions Adverse events may vary according to indication

>10%:

Central nervous system: Headache (7% to 24%)

Gastrointestinal: Diarrhea (2% to 12%)

1% to 10%:

Cardiovascular: Bradycardia (4% to 5%), hypertension (≤3%), tachycardia (2% to 3%)

Central nervous system: Dizziness (1% to 6%), fatigue (3% to 6%), fever (4%), pain (≤2%), chills/shivering (1% to 2%)

Gastrointestinal: Dyspepsia (≤3%), abdominal pain (≤3%)

Hepatic: Abnormal hepatic function (4%)

Renal: Oliguria (3%)

<1%, postmarketing, and/or case reports (limited to important or life-threatening): Abnormal vision, abnormal dreams, acute renal failure, alkaline phosphatase increased, ALT increased, anaphylactic reaction, anemia, anxiety, AST increased, ataxia, bronchospasm, cardiac arrest, chest pain, confusion, constipation, diaphoresis, dyspnea, dysuria, edema, epistaxis, facial

edema, flushing, GGT increased, hematuria, hyperbilirubinemia, hypotension, ischemia (peripheral), local injection site reaction (pain/burning), MI, myocardial ischemia, orthostatic hypotension, palpitation, pancreatitis, paresthesia, peripheral edema, photophobia, polyuria, prothrombin time increased, PTT increased, purpura/hematoma, rash, syncope, taste alteration, thrombocytopenia, thrombophlebitis/phlebitis, tinnitus, tremor, twitching, urticaria, vertigo

Note: Cardiac conduction abnormalities (including arrhythmia [sinus, supraventricular and ventricular], atrial flutter/fibrillation, AV block, bundle branch block, extrasystoles, poor R wave progression, prolonged PR, QRS, JT, and QT_c intervals, ST, T and U wave changes, torsade de pointes, ventricular tachycardia, wide complex tachycardia and ventricular fibrillation) have also been reported.

Drug Interactions

Metabolism/Transport Effects Substrate of CYP2C9 (minor), CYP3A4 (minor); **Note:** Assignment of Major/Minor substrate status based on clinically relevant drug interaction potential; **Inhibits** CYP2D6 (weak)

Avoid Concomitant Use

Avoid concomitant use of Dolasetron with any of the following: Apomorphine; Highest Risk QTc-Prolonging Agents; Mifepristone

Increased Effect/Toxicity

Dolasetron may increase the levels/effects of: Apomorphine; ARIPiprazole; Highest Risk QTc-Prolonging Agents; Moderate Risk QTc-Prolonging Agents

The levels/effects of Dolasetron may be increased by: Mifepristone; QTc-Prolonging Agents (Indeterminate Risk and Risk Modifying)

Decreased Effect

Dolasetron may decrease the levels/effects of: Tapentadol; TraMADol

The levels/effects of Dolasetron may be decreased by: Tocilizumab

Ethanol/Nutrition/Herb Interactions Food: Food does not affect the bioavailability of oral doses.

Storage/Stability Store intact vials and tablets at room temperature of 20°C to 25°C (68°F to 77°F). Protect from light. Solutions diluted for infusion are stable under normal lighting conditions at room temperature for 24 hours or under refrigeration for 48 hours.

Reconstitution Dilute in 50 mL of a compatible solution (ie, 0.9% NS, D_5W, $D_5$1/2NS, D_5LR, LR, and 10% mannitol injection).

Mechanism of Action Selective serotonin receptor (5-HT_3) antagonist, blocking serotonin both peripherally (primary site of action) and centrally at the chemoreceptor trigger zone

Pharmacodynamics/Kinetics

Absorption: Oral: Rapid and complete

Distribution: Hydrodolasetron: 5.8 L/kg

Protein binding: Hydrodolasetron: 69% to 77% (50% bound to $alpha_1$-acid glycoprotein)

Metabolism: Hepatic; rapid reduction by carbonyl reductase to hydrodolasetron (active metabolite); further metabolized by CYP2D6, CYP3A, and flavin monooxygenase

Bioavailability: Oral: ~75% (not affected by food)

Half-life elimination: Dolasetron: ≤10 minutes; hydrodolasetron: Adults: 6-8 hours; Children: 4-6 hours; Severe renal impairment: 11 hours; Severe hepatic impairment: 11 hours

Time to peak, plasma: Hydrodolasetron: I.V.: 0.6 hours; Oral: ~1 hour

Excretion: Urine ~67% (53% to 61% of the total dose as active metabolite hydrodolasetron); feces ~33%

Dosing

Adult & Geriatric Note: Use of dolasetron injection is contraindicated for the prevention of chemotherapy induced nausea and vomiting. In Canada, use of dolasetron is also contraindicated in the prevention and treatment of post-operative nausea and vomiting in adults.

Prevention of chemotherapy-associated nausea and vomiting (including initial and repeat courses): Oral: 100 mg within 1 hour before chemotherapy

Postoperative nausea and vomiting: *U.S. labeling:*

Prevention:

Oral: 100 mg within 2 hours before surgery

I.V.: 12.5 mg ~15 minutes before cessation of anesthesia

Treatment: I.V.: 12.5 mg as soon as nausea or vomiting present

Pediatric Note: In Canada, use of dolasetron is contraindicated in children and adolescents <18 years of age.

Prevention of chemotherapy-associated nausea and vomiting (including initial and repeat courses): Children 2-16 years: Oral: 1.8 mg/kg within 1 hour before chemotherapy; maximum: 100 mg/dose

Postoperative nausea and vomiting: Children 2-16 years:

Prevention:

Oral: 1.2 mg/kg within 2 hours before surgery; maximum: 100 mg/dose

I.V.: 0.35 mg/kg ~15 minutes before cessation of anesthesia; maximum: 12.5 mg

Treatment: I.V.: 0.35 mg/kg as soon as nausea or vomiting present; maximum: 12.5 mg/dose

Renal Impairment No dosage adjustment necessary.

Hepatic Impairment No dosage adjustment necessary.

Administration

I.V. injection may be given either undiluted IVP over 30 seconds or diluted in 50 mL of compatible fluid and infused over 15 minutes. Flush line before and after dolasetron administration.

Oral: When unable to administer in tablet form, dolasetron injection may be diluted in apple or apple-grape juice and taken orally; this dilution is stable for 2 hours at room temperature.

Extemporaneous Preparations Dolasetron injection may be diluted in apple or apple-grape juice and taken orally; this dilution is stable for 2 hours at room temperature (Anzemet® prescribing information, 2011).

A 10 mg/mL oral suspension may be prepared with tablets and either a 1:1 mixture of Ora-Plus® and Ora-Sweet® SF or a 1:1 mixture of strawberry syrup and Ora Plus®. Crush twelve 50 mg tablets in a mortar and reduce to a fine powder. Slowly add chosen vehicle to **almost** 60 mL; transfer to a calibrated bottle, rinse mortar with vehicle, and add quantity of vehicle sufficient to make 60 mL. Label "shake well" and "refrigerate". Stable for 90 days refrigerated.

Anzemet® prescribing information, sanofi-aventis U.S. LLC, Bridgewater, NJ, 2011.

Johnson CE, Wagner DS, and Bussard WE, "Stability of Dolasetron in Two Oral Liquid Vehicles," *Am J Health Syst Pharm*, 2003, 60(21):2242-4.

Monitoring Parameters ECG (in patients with cardiovascular disease, elderly, renally impaired, those at risk of developing hypokalemia and/or hypomagnesemia); potassium, magnesium

Dietary Considerations May be taken without regard to meals.

Additional Information Efficacy of dolasetron, for chemotherapy treatment, is enhanced with concomitant administration of dexamethasone 20 mg (increases complete response by 10% to 20%). Oral administration of the intravenous solution is equivalent to tablets.

Dosage Forms Excipient information presented when available (limited, particularly for generics); consult specific product labeling.

Injection, solution, as mesylate:

Anzemet®: 20 mg/mL (0.625 mL, 5 mL, 25 mL) [contains mannitol]

Tablet, oral, as mesylate:

Anzemet®: 50 mg, 100 mg

References

Dimmitt DC, Cramer MB, Keung A, et al, "Pharmacokinetics of Dolasetron With Coadministration of Cimetidine or Rifampin in Healthy Subjects," *Cancer Chemother Pharmacol*, 1999, 43(2):126-32.

Fauser AA, Russ W, and Bischoff M, "Oral Dolasetron Mesilate (MDL 73, 147EF) for the Control of Emesis During Fractionated Total-Body Irradiation and High-Dose Cyclophosphamide in Patients Undergoing Allogeneic Bone Marrow Transplantation," *Support Care Cancer*, 1997, 5(3):219-22.

Gan TJ, Meyer TA, Apfel CC, et al, "Society for Ambulatory Anesthesia Guidelines for the Management of Postoperative Nausea and Vomiting," *Anesth Analg*, 2007, 105(6):1615-28.

Hesketh P, Navari R, Grote T, et al, "Double-Blind, Randomized Comparison of the Antiemetic Efficacy of Intravenous Dolasetron Mesylate and Intravenous Ondansetron in the Prevention of Acute Cisplatin-Induced Emesis in Patients With Cancer: Dolasetron Comparative Chemotherapy-induced Emesis Prevention Group," *J Clin Oncol*, 1996, 14(8):2242-9.

Kovac AI, Scuderi PE, et al, "Treatment of Postoperative Nausea and Vomiting With Single Intravenous Doses of Dolasetron Mesylate: A Multicenter Trial," *Anesth Analg*, 1997, 85 (3):546-52.

Kris MG, Hesketh PJ, Somerfield MR, et al, "American Society of Clinical Oncology Guideline for Antiemetics in Oncology: Update 2006," *J Clin Oncol*, 2006, 24(18):2932-47.

Kris MG, Pendergrass KB, Navari RM, et al, "Prevention of Acute Emesis in Cancer Patients Following High-Dose Cisplatin With the Combination of Oral Dolasetron and Dexamethasone," *J Clin Oncol*, 1997, 15(5):2135-8.

Multinational Association of Supportive Care in Cancer (MASCC), "Antiemetic Guidelines," Updated April 2010. Available at http://data.memberclicks.com/site/mascc/MASCC_Guidelines_English_2010.pdf

National Comprehensive Cancer Network® (NCCN), "Clinical Practice Guidelines in Oncology™: Antiemesis," Version 1.2011. Available at http://www.nccn.org/professionals/physician_gls/PDF/antiemesis.pdf

Navari RM and Koeller JM, "Electrocardiographic and Cardiovascular Effects of the 5-Hydroxytryptamine$_3$ Receptor Antagonists," *Ann Pharmacother*, 2003, 37(9):1276-86.

Sanwald P, David M, and Dow J, "Characterization of the Cytochrome P450 Enzymes Involved in the *in vitro* Metabolism of Dolasetron. Comparison With Other Indole-Containing 5-HT3 Antagonists," *Drug Metab Dispos*, 1996, 24(5):602-9.

Steiner ME, Lensmeyer G, and Vermeulen LC, "Stability and Sterility of Dolasetron Mesylate in Syringes Stored at Room Temperature," *Am J Health Syst Pharm*, 2005, 62(9):896-9.

◆ **Dolasetron Mesylate** *see* Dolasetron *on page* 462

◆ **Dolophine®** *see* Methadone *on page* 944

◆ **Doloral (Can)** *see* Morphine (Systemic) *on page* 1004

◆ **Dom-Anagrelide (Can)** *see* Anagrelide *on page* 93

◆ **Dom-Benzydamine (Can)** *see* Benzydamine *on page* 164

◆ **Dom-Bicalutamide (Can)** *see* Bicalutamide *on page* 178

◆ **Dom-Ciprofloxacin (Can)** *see* Ciprofloxacin (Systemic) *on page* 283

◆ **Dom-Dexamethasone (Can)** *see* Dexamethasone (Systemic) *on page* 440

◆ **Dom-Fluconazole (Can)** *see* Fluconazole *on page* 612

◆ **Dom-Lorazepam (Can)** *see* LORazepam *on page* 907

◆ **Dom-Medroxyprogesterone (Can)** *see* MedroxyPROGESTERone *on page* 916

◆ **Dom-Ondansetron (Can)** *see* Ondansetron *on page 1068*
◆ **DOM-Valacyclovir (Can)** *see* Valacyclovir *on page 1420*
◆ **Doxil®** *see* DOXOrubicin (Liposomal) *on page 473*

DOXOrubicin (doks oh ROO bi sin)

Related Information

Chemotherapy and Cancer Treatment During Pregnancy *on page 1829*
Chemotherapy and Obesity *on page 1834*
Management of Chemotherapy-Induced Nausea and Vomiting *on page 1786*
Management of Drug Extravasations *on page 1800*
Principles of Anticancer Therapy *on page 1878*
Safe Handling of Hazardous Drugs *on page 1904*

Brand Names: U.S. Adriamycin®

Brand Names: Canada Adriamycin®; Doxorubicin Hydrochloride Injection

Index Terms ADR (error-prone abbreviation); Adria; Conventional Doxorubicin; Doxorubicin Hydrochloride; Hydroxydaunomycin Hydrochloride; Hydroxyldaunorubicin Hydrochloride

Generic Availability (U.S.) Yes

Pharmacologic Category Antineoplastic Agent, Anthracycline

Use Treatment of acute lymphocytic leukemia (ALL), acute myeloid leukemia (AML), Hodgkin's disease, malignant lymphoma, soft tissue and bone sarcomas, thyroid cancer, small cell lung cancer, breast cancer, gastric cancer, ovarian cancer, bladder cancer, neuroblastoma, and Wilms' tumor

Unlabeled Use Treatment of multiple myeloma, endometrial carcinoma, uterine sarcoma, head and neck cancer, liver cancer, kidney cancer

Labeled Contraindications Hypersensitivity to doxorubicin, any component of the formulation, or to other anthracyclines or anthracenediones; recent MI, severe myocardial insufficiency, severe arrhythmia; previous therapy with high cumulative doses of doxorubicin, daunorubicin, idarubicin, or other anthracycline and anthracenediones; baseline neutrophil count <1500/mm^3; severe hepatic impairment

Pregnancy Risk Factor D

Lactation Enters breast milk/not recommended

Warnings/Precautions Hazardous agent - use appropriate precautions for handling and disposal. **[U.S. Boxed Warning]: May cause cumulative, dose-related, myocardial toxicity (early or delayed).** Cardiotoxicity is dose-limiting. Total cumulative dose should take into account previous or concomitant treatment with cardiotoxic agents or irradiation of chest. The incidence of irreversible myocardial toxicity increases as the total cumulative (lifetime) dosages approach 450-500 mg/m^2. Although the risk increases with cumulative dose, irreversible cardiotoxicity may occur at any dose level. Patients with pre-existing heart disease, hypertension, concurrent administration of other antineoplastic agents, prior or concurrent chest irradiation, advanced age; and infants and children are at increased risk. Alternative administration schedules (weekly or continuous infusions) have are associated with less cardiotoxicity Baseline and periodic monitoring of ECG and LVEF (with either ECHO or MUGA scan) is recommended. **[U.S. Boxed Warnings]: Reduce dose in patients with impaired hepatic function; dose-limiting severe myelosuppression (primarily leukopenia and neutropenia) may occur. Secondary acute myelogenous leukemia and myelodysplastic syndrome have been reported following treatment.** May cause tumor lysis syndrome and hyperuricemia (in patients with rapidly growing tumors).

Children are at increased risk for developing delayed cardiotoxicity; follow-up cardiac function monitoring is recommended. Doxorubicin may contribute to prepubertal growth failure in children; may also contribute to gonadal impairment (usually temporary). Radiation recall pneumonitis has been reported in children receiving concomitant dactinomycin and doxorubicin. **[U.S. Boxed Warnings]: For I.V. administration only. Potent vesicant; if extravasation occurs, severe local tissue damage leading to ulceration, necrosis, and pain may occur. Should be administered under the supervision of an experienced cancer chemotherapy physician.** Use caution when selecting product for preparation and dispensing; indications, dosages and adverse event profiles differ between conventional doxorubicin hydrochloride solution and doxorubicin liposomal. Both formulations are the same concentration. As a result, serious errors have occurred.

Adverse Reactions Frequency not defined.

Cardiovascular:

Acute cardiotoxicity: Atrioventricular block, bradycardia, bundle branch block, ECG abnormalities, extrasystoles (atrial or ventricular), sinus tachycardia, ST-T wave changes, supraventricular tachycardia, tachyarrhythmia, ventricular tachycardia

Delayed cardiotoxicity: LVEF decreased, CHF (manifestations include ascites, cardiomegaly, dyspnea, edema, gallop rhythm, hepatomegaly, oliguria, pleural effusion, pulmonary edema, tachycardia); myocarditis, pericarditis

Central nervous system: Malaise

Dermatologic: Alopecia, itching, photosensitivity, radiation recall, rash; discoloration of saliva, sweat, or tears

Endocrine & metabolic: Amenorrhea, dehydration, infertility (may be temporary), hyperuricemia

Gastrointestinal: Abdominal pain, anorexia, colon necrosis, diarrhea, GI ulceration, mucositis, nausea, vomiting

Genitourinary: Discoloration of urine

Hematologic: Leukopenia/neutropenia (75%; nadir: 10-14 days; recovery: by day 21); thrombocytopenia and anemia

Local: Skin "flare" at injection site, urticaria

Neuromuscular & skeletal: Weakness

Postmarketing and/or case reports: Anaphylaxis, azoospermia, bilirubin increased, chills, coma (when in combination with cisplatin or vincristine), conjunctivitis, fever, gonadal impairment (children), growth failure (prepubertal), hepatitis, hyperpigmentation (nail, skin & oral mucosa), infection, keratitis, lacrimation, myelodysplastic syndrome, neutropenic fever, neutropenic typhlitis, oligospermia, onycholysis, peripheral neurotoxicity (with intra-arterial doxorubicin), phlebosclerosis, radiation recall pneumonitis (children), secondary acute myelogenous leukemia, seizure (when in combination with cisplatin or vincristine), sepsis, shock, Stevens-Johnson syndrome, systemic hypersensitivity (including urticaria, pruritus, angioedema, dysphagia, and dyspnea), toxic epidermal necrolysis, transaminases increased, urticaria

Drug Interactions

Metabolism/Transport Effects Substrate of CYP2D6 (major), CYP3A4 (major), P-glycoprotein; **Note:** Assignment of Major/Minor substrate status based on clinically relevant drug interaction potential; **Inhibits** CYP2B6 (moderate), CYP2D6 (weak), CYP3A4 (weak); **Induces** P-glycoprotein

Avoid Concomitant Use

Avoid concomitant use of DOXOrubicin with any of the following: BCG; CloZAPine; Conivaptan; Dabigatran Etexilate; Natalizumab; Pimecrolimus; Pimozide; Tacrolimus (Topical); Vaccines (Live); VinCRIStine (Liposomal)

Increased Effect/Toxicity

DOXOrubicin may increase the levels/effects of: ARIPiprazole; CloZAPine; CYP2B6 Substrates; Leflunomide, Natalizumab; Pimozide; Vaccines (Live); Vitamin K Antagonists; Zidovudine

The levels/effects of DOXOrubicin may be increased by: Abiraterone Acetate; Bevacizumab; Conivaptan; CycloSPORINE (Systemic); CYP2D6 Inhibitors (Moderate); CYP2D6 Inhibitors (Strong); CYP3A4 Inhibitors (Moderate); CYP3A4 Inhibitors (Strong); Darunavir; Dasatinib; Denosumab; Ivacaftor; Mifepristone; P-glycoprotein/ABCB1 Inhibitors; Pimecrolimus; Roflumilast; SORAfenib; Tacrolimus (Topical); Taxane Derivatives; Trastuzumab

Decreased Effect

DOXOrubicin may decrease the levels/effects of: BCG; Cardiac Glycosides; Coccidioidin Skin Test; Dabigatran Etexilate; Linagliptin; P-glycoprotein/ABCB1 Substrates; Sipuleucel-T; Stavudine; Vaccines (Inactivated); Vaccines (Live); VinCRIStine (Liposomal); Vitamin K Antagonists; Zidovudine

The levels/effects of DOXOrubicin may be decreased by: Cardiac Glycosides; CYP3A4 Inducers (Strong); Deferasirox; Echinacea; Herbs (CYP3A4 Inducers); Peginterferon Alfa-2b; P-glycoprotein/ABCB1 Inducers; Tocilizumab

Ethanol/Nutrition/Herb Interactions Herb/Nutraceutical: Avoid St John's wort (may decrease doxorubicin levels). Avoid black cohosh, dong quai in estrogen-dependent tumors.

Storage/Stability Store intact vials of solution under refrigeration at 2°C to 8°C. Protected from light. Store intact vials of lyophilized powder at room temperature (15°C to 30°C). Reconstituted vials are stable for 7 days at room temperature (25°C) and 15 days under refrigeration (5°C) when protected from light. Infusions are stable for 48 hours at room temperature (25°C) when protected from light. Solutions diluted in 50-1000 mL D_5W or NS are stable for 48 hours at room temperature (25°C) when protected from light.

Reconstitution Reconstitute lyophilized powder with NS to a final concentration of 2 mg/mL (may further dilute in 50-1000 mL D_5W or NS for infusion). Unstable in solutions with a pH <3 or >7.

Mechanism of Action Inhibition of DNA and RNA synthesis by intercalation between DNA base pairs by inhibition of topoisomerase II and by steric obstruction. Doxorubicin intercalates at points of local uncoiling of the double helix. Although the exact mechanism is unclear, it appears that direct binding to DNA (intercalation) and inhibition of DNA repair (topoisomerase II inhibition) result in blockade of DNA and RNA synthesis and fragmentation of DNA. Doxorubicin is also a powerful iron chelator; the iron-doxorubicin complex can bind DNA and cell membranes and produce free radicals that immediately cleave the DNA and cell membranes.

Pharmacodynamics/Kinetics

Absorption: Oral: Poor (<50%)

Distribution: V_d: 809-1214 L/m^2; to many body tissues, particularly liver, spleen, kidney, lung, heart; does not distribute into the CNS; crosses placenta

Protein binding, plasma: 70% to 76%

Metabolism: Primarily hepatic to doxorubicinol (active), then to inactive aglycones, conjugated sulfates, and glucuronides

Half-life elimination:
- Distribution: 5-10 minutes
- Elimination: Doxorubicin: 1-3 hours; Metabolites: 3-3.5 hours
- Terminal: 17-48 hours
- Male: 54 hours; Female: 35 hours

Excretion: Feces (~40% to 50% as unchanged drug); urine (~5% to 12% as unchanged drug and metabolites)
- Clearance: Male: 113 L/hour; Female: 44 L/hour

Dosing

Adult & Geriatric Refer to individual protocols. **Note:** Lower dosage should be considered for patients with inadequate marrow reserve (due to old age, prior treatment or neoplastic marrow infiltration).

Usual or typical dosages: I.V.: 60-75 mg/m^2/dose every 21 days **or**
- 60 mg/m^2/dose every 2 weeks (dose dense) **or**
- 40-60 mg/m^2/dose every 3-4 weeks **or**
- 20-30 mg/m^2/day for 2-3 days every 4 weeks **or**
- 20 mg/m^2/dose once weekly

Pediatric Refer to individual protocols. **Note:** Lower dosage should be considered for patients with inadequate marrow reserve (due to prior treatment or neoplastic marrow infiltration).

Usual/typical dosages: Children: I.V.:
- 35-75 mg/m^2/dose every 21 days **or**
- 20-30 mg/m^2/dose once weekly **or**
- 60-90 mg/m^2 given as a continuous infusion over 96 hours every 3-4 weeks

Renal Impairment

Adjustments are not required.

Hemodialysis: Supplemental dose is not necessary.

Hepatic Impairment

The FDA-approved labeling recommends the following adjustments:
- Serum bilirubin 1.2-3 mg/dL: Administer 50% of dose
- Serum bilirubin 3.1-5 mg/dL: Administer 25% of dose
- Severe hepatic impairment: Use is contraindicated

The following guidelines have been used by some clinicians: Floyd, 2006:
- Transaminases 2-3 times ULN: Administer 75% of dose
- Transaminases >3 times ULN or serum bilirubin 1.2-3 mg/dL: Administer 50% of dose
- Serum bilirubin 3.1-5 mg/dL: Administer 25% of dose
- Serum bilirubin >5 mg/dL: Do not administer

Adjustment for Toxicity The following delays and/or dose reductions have been used:
- Neutropenic fever/infection: Consider reducing to 75% of dose in subsequent cycles
- ANC <1000/mm^3: Delay treatment until ANC recovers to ≥1000/mm^3
- Platelets <100,000/mm^3: Delay treatment until platelets recover to ≥100,000/mm^3

Combination Regimens

Bladder cancer: M-VAC (Bladder Cancer) on page 1718

Breast cancer:
- AC on page 1517
- AC/Paclitaxel (Sequential) on page 1517
- AC-Paclitaxel-Trastuzumab on page 1518
- CAF on page 1538
- Docetaxel-Doxorubicin (Breast Cancer) on page 1611

Dox-CMF (Sequential) on page 1617
FAC on page 1641
TAC on page 1753
Endometrial cancer: AP on page 1520
Hepatoblastoma:
IPA on page 1692
PA CI on page 1725
Leukemia, acute lymphocytic:
Hyper-CVAD + Imatinib on page 1680
Hyper-CVAD (Leukemia, Acute Lymphocytic) on page 1681
Larson Regimen (ALL) on page 1699
VAD/CVAD on page 1768
Lung cancer (small cell): CAV (Small Cell Lung Cancer) on page 1554
Lymphoma, Hodgkin:
ABVD Early Stage (Hodgkin) on page 1516
ABVD (Hodgkin) on page 1516
BEACOPP-14 (Hodgkin) on page 1522
BEACOPP Escalated (Hodgkin) on page 1522
BEACOPP Escalated Plus Standard (Hodgkin) on page 1523
BEACOPP Standard (Hodgkin) on page 1525
C-MOPP/ABV Hybrid (Hodgkin) on page 1588
MOPP/ABVD (Hodgkin) on page 1714
MOPP/ABV Hybrid (Hodgkin) on page 1715
Stanford V (Hodgkin) on page 1752
VAMP (Hodgkin) on page 1769
Lymphoma, non-Hodgkin's:
CHOP (NHL) on page 1564
CODOX-M on page 1590
COP-BLAM on page 1595
EPOCH Dose-Adjusted (AIDS-Related Lymphoma) on page 1628
EPOCH Dose-Adjusted (NHL) on page 1628
EPOCH (Dose-Adjusted)-Rituximab (NHL) on page 1629
EPOCH (NHL) on page 1630
EPOCH-Rituximab (NHL) on page 1631
Hyper-CVAD (Lymphoma, non-Hodgkin's) on page 1687
MACOP-B on page 1704
m-BACOD on page 1706
Pro-MACE-CytaBOM on page 1741
Rituximab-CHOP (NHL) on page 1748
Lymphoma, non-Hodgkin's (Burkitt): CODOX-M/IVAC on page 1591
Lymphoma, non-Hodgkin's (Mantle cell): Hyper-CVAD + Rituximab on page 1688
Multiple myeloma:
Bortezomib-Doxorubicin-Dexamethasone on page 1535
DTPACE on page 1620
Hyper-CVAD (Multiple Myeloma) on page 1687
VAD on page 1767
VCAP on page 1770
Neuroblastoma:
A3 (Neuroblastoma) on page 1515
CAV-P/VP (Neuroblastoma) on page 1554
CE-CAdO (Neuroblastoma) on page 1555
Cisplatin-Doxorubicin-Etoposide-Cyclophosphamide (Neuroblastoma) on page 1568

New A1 (Neuroblastoma) on page 1721
Osteosarcoma:
MTX-CDDPAdr on page 1717
POG-8651 on page 1740
Ovarian cancer: PAC (CAP) on page 1725
Prostate cancer:
Doxorubicin + Ketoconazole on page 1619
Doxorubicin + Ketoconazole/Estramustine + Vinblastine on page 1619
Sarcoma:
CYVADIC on page 1605
MAID (Sarcoma) on page 1704
VAC Alternating With IE (Ewing's Sarcoma) on page 1766
Soft tissue sarcoma:
AD (Soft Tissue Sarcoma) on page 1519
AI on page 1520
Wilms' tumor:
DD-4A (Wilms' Tumor) on page 1606
Regimen I (Wilms' Tumor) on page 1745
VAD (Wilms' Tumor) on page 1768

Administration Vesicant. Administer I.V. push over at least 3-5 minutes or by continuous infusion (infusion via central venous line recommended). Avoid extravasation associated with severe ulceration and soft tissue necrosis. Flush with 5-10 mL of I.V. solution before and after drug administration. Incompatible with heparin. Monitor for local erythematous streaking along vein and/or facial flushing (may indicate rapid infusion rate).

Emetic Potential
>60 mg/m^2: Very high (>90%)
≤60 mg/m^2: Moderate (30% to 90%)

Vesicant/Extravasation Risk Vesicant; see Management of Drug Extravasations on page 1800.

Monitoring Parameters CBC with differential and platelet count; liver function tests (bilirubin, ALT/AST, alkaline phosphatase); serum uric acid, calcium, potassium, phosphate and creatinine; cardiac function (baseline, periodic, and followup): ECG, left ventricular ejection fraction (echocardiography [ECHO] or multigated radionuclide angiography [MUGA])

Dosage Forms Excipient information presented when available (limited, particularly for generics); consult specific product labeling.
Injection, powder for reconstitution, as hydrochloride: 10 mg, 50 mg
Adriamycin®: 10 mg [contains lactose 50 mg]
Adriamycin®: 20 mg [contains lactose 100 mg]
Adriamycin®: 50 mg [contains lactose 250 mg]
Injection, solution, as hydrochloride [preservative free]: 2 mg/mL (5 mL, 10 mL, 25 mL, 75 mL, 100 mL)
Adriamycin®: 2 mg/mL (5 mL, 10 mL, 25 mL, 100 mL)

References

Floyd J, Mirza I, Sachs B, et al, "Hepatotoxicity of Chemotherapy," *Semin Oncol*, 2006, 33 (1):50-67.

Floyd JD, Nguyen DT, Lobins RL, et al, "Cardiotoxicity of Cancer Therapy," *J Clin Oncol*, 2005, 23 (30):7685-96.

King PD and Perry MC, "Hepatotoxicity of Chemotherapy," *Oncologist*, 2001, 6(2):162-76.

Lauvin R, Miglianico L, and Hellegouarc'h R, "Skin Cancer Occurring 10 Years After the Extravasation of Doxorubicin," *N Engl J Med*, 1995, 332(11):754.

Legha SS, Benjamin RS, Mackay B, et al, "Reduction of Doxorubicin Cardiotoxicity by Prolonged Continuous Intravenous Infusion," *Ann Intern Med*, 1982, 96(2):133-9.

Morgan C, Tillett T, Braybrooke J, et al, "Management of Uncommon Chemotherapy-Induced Emergencies," *Lancet Oncol*, 2011, 12(8):806-14.

National Comprehensive Cancer Network® (NCCN), "Clinical Practice Guidelines in Oncology™: Breast Cancer," Version 2.2011. Available at http://www.nccn.org/professionals/physician_gls/PDF/breast.pdf

Seifert CF, Nesser ME, and Thompson DF, "Dexrazoxane in the Prevention of Doxorubicin-Induced Cardiotoxicity," *Ann Pharmacother*, 1994, 28(9):1063-72.

◆ **Doxorubicin Hydrochloride** *see* DOXOrubicin *on page 467*

◆ **DOXOrubicin Hydrochloride Encapsulated Liposomes (Myocet™)** *see* DOXOrubicin (Liposomal) *on page 473*

◆ **Doxorubicin Hydrochloride Injection (Can)** *see* DOXOrubicin *on page 467*

◆ **DOXOrubicin Hydrochloride (Liposomal)** *see* DOXOrubicin (Liposomal) *on page 473*

◆ **DOXOrubicin Hydrochloride Liposome** *see* DOXOrubicin (Liposomal) *on page 473*

◆ **DOXOrubicin Hydrochloride Liposomes (Myocet™)** *see* DOXOrubicin (Liposomal) *on page 473*

DOXOrubicin (Liposomal) (doks oh ROO bi sin lye po SO mal)

Related Information

Management of Chemotherapy-Induced Nausea and Vomiting *on page 1786*

Management of Drug Extravasations *on page 1800*

Safe Handling of Hazardous Drugs *on page 1904*

Brand Names: U.S. Doxil®

Brand Names: Canada Caelyx®; Myocet™

Index Terms DOXOrubicin Hydrochloride (Liposomal); DOXOrubicin Hydrochloride Encapsulated Liposomes (Myocet™); DOXOrubicin Hydrochloride Liposome; DOXOrubicin Hydrochloride Liposomes (Myocet™); Lipodox; Liposomal DOXOrubicin; Pegylated DOXOrubicin Liposomal; Pegylated Liposomal DOXOrubicin; Pegylated Liposomal DOXOrubicin Hydrochloride (Doxil®, Caelyx®)

Generic Availability (U.S.) No

Pharmacologic Category Antineoplastic Agent, Anthracycline

Use

U.S. labeling: Treatment of ovarian cancer (progressive or recurrent after platinum-based treatment); multiple myeloma (in combination with bortezomib in patients who are bortezomib naïve and after failure of at least 1 prior therapy); AIDS-related Kaposi's sarcoma (after failure of or intolerance to prior systemic therapy)

Canadian labeling: Treatment of metastatic breast cancer (as monotherapy [Caelyx®] or in combination with cyclophosphamide [Myocet™]); advanced ovarian cancer (after failure of first-line treatment [Caelyx®]); AIDS-related Kaposi's sarcoma (after failure of or intolerance to prior systemic therapy [Caelyx®])

Unlabeled Use Treatment of metastatic breast cancer, Hodgkin lymphoma (salvage treatment), cutaneous T-cell lymphomas (mycosis fungoides and Sézary syndrome), advanced soft tissue sarcomas; advanced or recurrent uterine sarcoma

Labeled Contraindications Hypersensitivity to doxorubicin liposomal, conventional doxorubicin, or any component of the formulation

Canadian labeling (Caelyx®): Additional contraindications (not in U.S. labeling): Breast-feeding

Pregnancy Risk Factor D

Lactation Excretion in breast milk unknown/not recommended

Warnings/Precautions Hazardous agent - use appropriate precautions for handling and disposal.

[U.S. Boxed Warning]: Doxorubicin may cause cumulative, dose-related myocardial toxicity may lead to congestive heart failure as the cumulative (lifetime) dose of pegylated doxorubicin liposomal approaches 550 mg/m^2. When calculating cumulative doses, also include prior dose of other anthracyclines and anthracenediones. Cardiotoxicity may occur at lower cumulative doses (400 mg/m^2) in patients who have received prior mediastinal irradiation or are receiving concurrent cyclophosphamide treatment. For Myocet™ (Canadian availability), cardiotoxicity may occur as the cumulative (lifetime) dose approaches 750 mg/m^2. Anthracycline-induced cardiotoxicity may be delayed (after discontinuation of anthracycline treatment). Use only if potential benefits outweigh cardiovascular risk in patients with a history of cardiovascular disease. Monitor cardiac function with biopsy, echocardiography, or MUGA scan; evaluate left ventricular ejection fraction (LVEF) prior to treatment and periodically during treatment; if results indicate possible heart failure, carefully evaluate the potential effects of continued treatment.

[U.S. Boxed Warning]: Acute infusion reactions may occur, some may be serious/life-threatening (eg, allergic or anaphylactoid reactions). Reactions may include flushing, dyspnea, facial swelling, headache, chills, back pain, hypotension, and/or chest/throat tightness. Infusion reactions typically occur with the first dose and usually resolve with within several hours to a day after terminating the infusion; some have resolved with slowing the infusion rate. To minimize the risk of infusion reactions, infuse at an initial rate of 1 mg/minute. Medications for the treatment of reactions should be readily available in the event of severe reaction.

[U.S. Boxed Warning]: Use with caution in patients with hepatic impairment; dosage reduction is recommended. Use in patients with hepatic impairment has not been adequately studied; no dosing adjustment recommendations are available for multiple myeloma patients with hepatic impairment. **[U.S. Boxed Warning]: Severe myelosuppression may occur.** Monitor blood counts. Treatment delay, dosage modification, or discontinuation may be required. Leukopenia is usually transient, although persistent or severe neutropenia may result in superinfection or neutropenic fever; sepsis due to neutropenia has resulted in discontinuation (may rarely be fatal). Hemorrhage due to thrombocytopenia may occur. Hematologic toxicity may be more severe with combination chemotherapy. Palmar-plantar erythrodysesthesia (hand-foot syndrome) has been reported, more commonly in patients with ovarian cancer and multiple myeloma, and less commonly in patients with Kaposi's sarcoma. May occur early in treatment, but is usually seen after 2-3 treatment cycles. Dosage modification may be required; mild cases resolve within 1-2 weeks; in severe cases, treatment discontinuation may be required. Use of Caelyx® (Canadian availability) in splenectomized patients with AIDS-related Kaposi's sarcoma is not recommended (has not been studied). **[U.S. Boxed Warning]: Liposomal formulations of doxorubicin should NOT be substituted for conventional doxorubicin hydrochloride on a mg-per-mg basis.**

Doxorubicin may potentiate the toxicity of cyclophosphamide (hemorrhagic cystitis) and mercaptopurine (hepatotoxicity). Radiation recall reaction has been reported with doxorubicin liposomal treatment after radiation therapy. Radiation-induced toxicity (to the myocardium, mucosa, skin, and liver) may be increased by doxorubicin.

Adverse Reactions

>10%:

Cardiovascular: Peripheral edema (≤11%)

Central nervous system: Fever (8% to 21%), headache (≤11%), pain (≤21%)

Dermatologic: Palmar-plantar erythrodysesthesia/hand-foot syndrome (≤51% in ovarian cancer [grades 3/4: 24%]; 3% in Kaposi's sarcoma), rash (≤29% in ovarian cancer, ≤5% in Kaposi's sarcoma), alopecia (9% to 19%)

Gastrointestinal: Nausea (17% to 46%), stomatitis (5% to 41%), vomiting (8% to 33%), constipation (≤30%), diarrhea (5% to 21%), anorexia (≤20%), mucositis (≤14%), dyspepsia (≤12%), intestinal obstruction (≤11%)

Hematologic: Myelosuppression (onset: 7 days; nadir: 10-14 days; recovery: 21-28 days), thrombocytopenia (13% to 65%; grades 3/4: 1%), neutropenia (12% to 62%; grade 4: 4%), leukopenia (36%), anemia (6% to 74%; grade 4: <1%)

Neuromuscular & skeletal: Weakness (7% to 40%), back pain (≤12%)

Respiratory: Pharyngitis (≤16%), dyspnea (≤15%)

Miscellaneous: Infection (≤12%)

1% to 10%:

Cardiovascular: Cardiac arrest, chest pain, deep thrombophlebitis, edema, hypotension, pallor, tachycardia, vasodilation

Central nervous system: Agitation, anxiety, chills, confusion, depression, dizziness, emotional lability, insomnia, somnolence, vertigo

Dermatologic: Acne, bruising, dry skin (6%), exfoliative dermatitis, fungal dermatitis, furunculosis, maculopapular rash, pruritus, skin discoloration, vesiculobullous rash

Endocrine & metabolic: Dehydration, hypercalcemia, hyperglycemia, hypokalemia, hyponatremia

Gastrointestinal: Abdomen enlarged, anorexia, ascites, cachexia, dyspepsia, dysphagia, esophagitis, flatulence, gingivitis, glossitis, ileus, mouth ulceration, oral moniliasis, rectal bleeding, taste perversion, weight loss, xerostomia

Genitourinary: Cystitis, dysuria, leukorrhea, pelvic pain, polyuria, urinary incontinence, urinary tract infection, urinary urgency, vaginal bleeding, vaginal moniliasis

Hematologic: Hemolysis, prothrombin time increased

Hepatic: ALT increased, alkaline phosphatase increased, hyperbilirubinemia

Local: Thrombophlebitis

Neuromuscular & skeletal: Arthralgia, hypertonia, myalgia, neuralgia, neuritis (peripheral), neuropathy, paresthesia (≤10%), pathological fracture

Ocular: Conjunctivitis, dry eyes, retinitis

Otic: Ear pain

Renal: Albuminuria, hematuria

Respiratory: Apnea, cough (≤10%), epistaxis, pleural effusion, pneumonia, rhinitis, sinusitis

Miscellaneous: Allergic reaction; infusion-related reactions (7%; includes bronchospasm, chest tightness, chills, dyspnea, facial edema, flushing, headache, herpes simplex/zoster, hypotension, pruritus); moniliasis, diaphoresis

<1%, postmarketing, and/or case reports (limited to important or life-threatening): Abscess, acute brain syndrome, abnormal vision, acute myeloid leukemia (secondary), alkaline phosphatase increased, anaphylactic or anaphylactoid reaction, asthma, balanitis, blindness, bone pain, bronchitis, BUN increased, bundle branch block, cardiomegaly, cardiomyopathy, cellulitis, CHF, colitis, creatinine increased, cryptococcosis, diabetes mellitus, erythema multiforme, erythema nodosum, eosinophilia, fecal impaction, flu-like syndrome, gastritis, glucosuria, hemiplegia, hemorrhage, hepatic failure, hepatitis, hepatosplenomegaly, hyperkalemia, hypernatremia, hyperuricemia, hyperventilation, hypoglycemia, hypolipidemia, hypomagnesemia, hypophosphatemia, hypoproteinemia, hypothermia, injection site hemorrhage, injection site pain, jaundice, ketosis, lactic dehydrogenase increased, lymphadenopathy, lymphangitis, migraine, myositis, optic neuritis, oral cancers (squamous cell; long-term use), palpitation, pancreatitis, pericardial effusion, petechia, pneumonitis, pneumothorax, pulmonary embolism, radiation injury, reddish/orange discoloration of urine/body fluids, renal failure, sclerosing cholangitis, seizure, sepsis, skin necrosis, skin ulcer, syncope, Stevens-Johnson syndrome, tenesmus, thromboplastin decreased, thrombosis, tinnitus, toxic epidermal necrolysis, urticaria, visual field defect, ventricular arrhythmia

Drug Interactions

Metabolism/Transport Effects **Substrate** of CYP2D6 (major), CYP3A4 (major); **Note:** Assignment of Major/Minor substrate status based on clinically relevant drug interaction potential; **Inhibits** CYP2B6 (moderate)

Avoid Concomitant Use

Avoid concomitant use of DOXOrubicin (Liposomal) with any of the following: BCG; CloZAPine; Conivaptan; Natalizumab; Pimecrolimus; Tacrolimus (Topical); Vaccines (Live)

Increased Effect/Toxicity

DOXOrubicin (Liposomal) may increase the levels/effects of: CloZAPine; CYP2B6 Substrates; Leflunomide; Natalizumab; Vaccines (Live); Zidovudine

The levels/effects of DOXOrubicin (Liposomal) may be increased by: Abiraterone Acetate; Bevacizumab; Conivaptan; CYP2D6 Inhibitors (Moderate); CYP2D6 Inhibitors (Strong); CYP3A4 Inhibitors (Moderate); CYP3A4 Inhibitors (Strong); Darunavir; Dasatinib; Denosumab; Ivacaftor; Mifepristone; Pimecrolimus; Roflumilast; Tacrolimus (Topical); Taxane Derivatives; Trastuzumab

Decreased Effect

DOXOrubicin (Liposomal) may decrease the levels/effects of: BCG; Cardiac Glycosides; Coccidioidin Skin Test; Sipuleucel-T; Stavudine; Vaccines (Inactivated); Vaccines (Live); Zidovudine

The levels/effects of DOXOrubicin (Liposomal) may be decreased by: Cardiac Glycosides; CYP3A4 Inducers (Strong); Deferasirox; Echinacea; Herbs (CYP3A4 Inducers); Peginterferon Alfa-2b; Tocilizumab

Ethanol/Nutrition/Herb Interactions

Ethanol: Avoid ethanol (due to GI irritation).

Herb/Nutraceutical: St John's wort may decrease doxorubicin levels.

Storage/Stability Store intact vials refrigerated at 2°C to 8°C (36°F to 46°F); avoid freezing.

Doxil®, Caelyx®: Prolonged freezing may adversely affect liposomal drug products, however, short-term freezing (<1 month) does not appear to have a deleterious effect (Doxil®). Solutions diluted for infusion should be refrigerated at 2°C to 8°C (36°F to 46°F); administer within 24 hours. **Do not infuse with in-line filters.**

Myocet™: Refer to product labeling for detailed reconstitution and preparation information. Following reconstitution, may be stored up to 8 hours at room temperature or up to 72 hours refrigerated at 2°C to 8°C (36°F to 46°F); do not freeze.

Reconstitution Hazardous agent; use appropriate precautions for handling and disposal.

Doxil®, Caelyx®: Doses ≤90 mg must be diluted in D_5W 250 mL prior to administration. Doses >90 mg should be diluted in D_5W 500 mL. Solution is not clear, but has a red, translucent appearance due to the liposomal dispersion. Dilute only in D_5W; do not use bacteriostatic agents; do not mix with other medications.

Myocet™: Refer to product labeling for detailed reconstitution and preparation information.

Mechanism of Action Doxorubicin inhibits DNA and RNA synthesis by intercalating between DNA base pairs causing steric obstruction and inhibits topoisomerase II at the point of DNA cleavage. Doxorubicin is also a powerful iron chelator. The iron-doxorubicin complex can bind DNA and cell membranes, producing free hydroxyl (OH) radicals that cleave DNA and cell membranes. Active throughout entire cell cycle. Doxorubicin liposomal is a pegylated formulation which protects the liposomes, and thereby increases blood circulation time.

Pharmacodynamics/Kinetics

Distribution: V_{dss}: 2.7-2.8 L/m^2

Protein binding, plasma: Unknown; nonliposomal (conventional) doxorubicin: 70%

Half-life elimination: Terminal: Distribution: 4.7-5.2 hours, Elimination: 44-55 hours

Metabolism: Hepatic and in plasma to doxorubicinol and the sulfate and glucuronide conjugates of 4-demethyl,7-deoxyaglycones

Excretion: Urine (5% as doxorubicin or doxorubicinol)

Dosing

Adult & Geriatric Details concerning dosing in combination regimens should also be consulted. **Liposomal formulations of doxorubicin should NOT be substituted for conventional doxorubicin hydrochloride on a mg-per-mg basis.**

U.S. labeling:

AIDS-related Kaposi's sarcoma: I.V.: 20 mg/m^2 once every 3 weeks; continue as long as responding and tolerating

Multiple myeloma: I.V.: 30 mg/m^2 on day 4 every 3 weeks (in combination with bortezomib) for up to 8 cycles until disease progression or unacceptable toxicity

Ovarian cancer, progressive or recurrent: I.V.: 50 mg/m^2 once every 4 weeks (minimum of 4 cycles is recommended)

Canadian labeling:

AIDS-related Kaposi's sarcoma (Caelyx®): I.V.: 20 mg/m^2 once every 2-3 weeks; continue as long as responding and tolerating

Breast cancer, metastatic: I.V.:

Caelyx®: 50 mg/m^2 once every 4 weeks until disease progression or unacceptable toxicity

Myocet™: 60-75 mg/m^2 once every 3 weeks (in combination with cyclophosphamide)

Ovarian cancer, advanced (Caelyx®): I.V.: 50 mg/m^2 once every 4 weeks until disease progression or unacceptable toxicity

Unlabeled uses/doses:

Breast cancer, metastatic (unlabeled use in U.S.): I.V.: 50 mg/m^2 every 4 weeks (Keller, 2004)

Cutaneous T-cell lymphomas (unlabeled use): I.V.: 20 mg/m^2 days 1 and 15 every 4 weeks for 6 cycles (Dummer, 2012) **or** 20 mg/m^2 every 4 weeks (Wollina, 2003)

Hodgkin lymphoma, salvage treatment (unlabeled use): I.V.: GVD regimen: 10 mg/m^2 (post-transplant patients) or 15 mg/m^2 (transplant-naive patients) days 1 and 8 every 3 weeks (in combination with gemcitabine and vinorelbine) for 2-6 cycles (Bartlett, 2007)

Multiple myeloma (unlabeled dosing): I.V.: 40 mg/m^2 on day 1 every 4 weeks (in combination with vincristine and dexamethasone) for at least 4 cycles (Rifkin, 2006)

Soft tissue sarcoma, advanced (unlabeled use): I.V.: 50 mg/m^2 every 4 weeks for 6 cycles (Judson, 2001)

Uterine sarcoma, advanced or recurrent (unlabeled use): I.V.: 50 mg/m^2 every 4 weeks until disease progression or unacceptable toxicity (Sutton, 2005)

Renal Impairment No dosage adjustment provided in the manufacturer's labeling (has not been studied).

Hepatic Impairment

U.S. labeling:

Ovarian cancer and AIDS-related Kaposi's sarcoma:

Bilirubin 1.2-3 mg/dL: Administer 50% of normal dose

Bilirubin >3 mg/dL: Administer 25% of normal dose

Multiple myeloma: Dosage adjustment information is not available.

Canadian labeling:

AIDS-related Kaposi's sarcoma (Caelyx®):

Bilirubin 1.2-3 mg/dL: Administer 50% of normal dose

Bilirubin >3 mg/dL: Administer 25% of normal dose

Breast cancer:

Caelyx®:

Bilirubin 1.2-3 mg/dL: Initial dose: Administer 75% of normal dose; if tolerated and no change in bilirubin/hepatic enzymes, may increase to full dose with cycle 2

Bilirubin >3 mg/dL: Initial dose: Administer 50% of normal dose; if tolerated and no change in bilirubin/hepatic enzymes, may increase dose to 75% of normal dose for cycle 2; if cycle 2 dose tolerated, may increase to full dose for subsequent cycles.

Myocet™:
Bilirubin 1.2-3 mg/dL: Administer 50% of normal dose
Bilirubin >3 mg/dL: Administer 25% of normal dose

Ovarian cancer (Caelyx®):

Bilirubin 1.2-3 mg/dL: Initial dose: Administer 75% of normal dose; if tolerated and no change in bilirubin/hepatic enzymes, may increase to full dose with cycle 2

Bilirubin >3 mg/dL: Initial dose: Administer 50% of normal dose; if tolerated and no change in bilirubin/hepatic enzymes, may increase dose to 75% of normal dose for cycle 2; if cycle 2 dose tolerated, may increase to full dose for subsequent cycles.

Adjustment for Toxicity

Recommended Dose Modification Guidelines

Toxicity Grade	Dose Adjustment
HAND FOOT SYNDROME (HFS)	
1 (Mild erythema, swelling, or desquamation not interfering with daily activities)	Redose unless patient has experienced previous Grade 3 or 4 HFS toxicity. If so, delay up to 2 weeks and decrease dose by 25%; return to original dosing interval.
2 (Erythema, desquamation, or swelling interfering with, but not precluding, normal physical activities; small blisters or ulcerations <2 cm in diameter)	Delay dosing up to 2 weeks or until resolved to Grade 0-1. If after 2 weeks there is no resolution, discontinue liposomal doxorubicin. Otherwise, if no prior Grade 3-4 HFS, continue treatment at previous dose and dosage interval. If a prior Grade 3-4 HFS has occurred, continue prior dosage interval, but decrease dose by 25%.
3 (Blistering, ulceration, or swelling interfering with walking or normal daily activities; cannot wear regular clothing)	Delay dosing up to 2 weeks or until resolved to Grade 0-1. Decrease dose by 25% and return to original dosing interval; if after 2 weeks there is no resolution, discontinue liposomal doxorubicin.
4 (Diffuse or local process causing infectious complications, or a bedridden state or hospitalization)	Delay dosing up to 2 weeks or until resolved to Grade 0-1. Decrease dose by 25% and return to original dosing interval. If after 2 weeks there is no resolution, discontinue liposomal doxorubicin.
STOMATITIS	
1 (Painless ulcers, erythema, or mild soreness)	Redose unless patient has experienced previous Grade 3 or 4 toxicity. If so, delay up to 2 weeks and decrease by 25%. Return to original dosing interval.
2 (Painful erythema, edema, or ulcers, but can eat)	Delay dosing up to 2 weeks or until resolved to Grade 0-1. If after 2 weeks there is no resolution, discontinue liposomal doxorubicin. Otherwise, if not prior Grade 3-4 stomatitis, continue treatment at previous dose and dosage interval. If prior Grade 3-4 toxicity, continue treatment with previous dosage interval, but decrease dose by 25%.
3 (Painful erythema, edema, or ulcers, and cannot eat)	Delay dosing up to 2 weeks or until resolved to Grade 0-1. Decrease dose by 25% and return to original dosing interval. If after 2 weeks there is no resolution, discontinue liposomal doxorubicin.
4 (Requires parenteral or enteral support)	Delay dosing up to 2 weeks or until resolved to Grade 0-1. Decrease dose by 25% and return to original dosing interval. If after 2 weeks there is no resolution, discontinue liposomal doxorubicin.

Hematologic Toxicity (see below for multiple myeloma)

Grade	ANC	Platelets	Modification
1	1500-1900	75,000-150,000	Resume treatment with no dose reduction.
2	1000-<1500	50,000-<75,000	Wait until ANC ≥1500 and platelets ≥75,000; redose with no dose reduction.
3	500-999	25,000-<50,000	Wait until ANC ≥1500 and platelets ≥75,000; redose with no dose reduction.
4	<500	<25,000	Wait until ANC ≥1500 and platelets ≥75,000; redose at 25% dose reduction or continue full dose with cytokine support.

Dosing Adjustment for Toxicity in Treatment with Bortezomib (for Multiple Myeloma) (see Bortezomib monograph for bortezomib dosage reduction with toxicity guidelines):

Fever ≥38°C and ANC <1000/mm³: If prior to doxorubicin liposomal treatment (day 4), do not administer; if after doxorubicin liposomal administered, reduce dose by 25% in next cycle.

ANC <500/mm³, platelets <25,000/mm³, hemoglobin <8 g/dL: If prior to doxorubicin liposomal treatment (day 4); do not administer; if after doxorubicin liposomal administered, reduce dose by 25% in next cycle if bortezomib dose reduction occurred for hematologic toxicity.

Grade 3 or 4 nonhematologic toxicity: Delay dose until resolved to grade <2; reduce dose by 25% for all subsequent doses.

Neuropathic pain or peripheral neuropathy: No dose reductions needed for doxorubicin liposomal, refer to Bortezomib monograph for bortezomib dosing adjustment.

Canadian labeling:

Caelyx®: Nonhematologic toxicity: Breast cancer, ovarian cancer:

Caelyx®: Recommended Dose Modification Guidelines

	Week After Prior Caelyx® Dose (Breast Cancer or Ovarian Cancer)	
Toxicity Grade	**Weeks 4 and 5**	**Week 6**
HAND FOOT SYNDROME (HFS)		
1 (Mild erythema, swelling, or desquamation not interfering with daily activities)	Redose unless patient has experienced previous Grade 3 or 4 HFS toxicity. If so, wait an additional week	Decrease dose by 25%; return to 4-week interval
2 (Erythema, desquamation, or swelling interfering with, but not precluding, normal physical activities; small blisters or ulcerations <2 cm in diameter)	Wait an additional week	Decrease dose by 25%; return to 4-week interval
3 (Blistering, ulceration, or swelling interfering with walking or normal daily activities; cannot wear regular clothing)	Wait an additional week	Discontinue therapy
4 (Diffuse or local process causing infectious complications, or a bedridden state or hospitalization)	Wait an additional week	Discontinue therapy

(continued)

Caelyx®: Recommended Dose Modification Guidelines *(continued)*

	Week After Prior Caelyx® Dose (Breast Cancer or Ovarian Cancer)	
Toxicity Grade	Weeks 4 and 5	Week 6
STOMATITIS		
1 (Painless ulcers, erythema, or mild soreness)	Redose unless patient has experienced previous Grade 3 or 4 stomatitis. If so, wait an additional week.	Decrease dose by 25%; return to 4-week interval or if warranted, discontinue therapy
2 (Painful erythema, edema, or ulcers, but can eat)	Wait an additional week	Decrease dose by 25%; return to 4-week interval or if warranted, discontinue therapy
3 (Painful erythema, edema, or ulcers, and cannot eat)	Wait an additional week	Discontinue therapy
4 (Requires parenteral or enteral support)	Wait an additional week	Discontinue therapy

Caelyx®: Hematologic toxicity: Breast cancer, ovarian cancer: Refer to U.S. dosage adjustment for hematologic toxicity section.

Caelyx®: Nonhematologic toxicity: AIDS-related Kaposi's sarcoma:

Caelyx®: Recommended Dose Modification Guidelines: Hand-Foot Syndrome (HFS) (AIDS-related Kaposi's Sarcoma)

	Weeks Since Last Caelyx® Dose (AIDS-related Kaposi's Sarcoma)	
Toxicity Grade	3 Weeks	4 Weeks
HAND-FOOT SYNDROME (HFS)		
1 (Mild erythema, swelling, or desquamation not interfering with daily activities)	Redose unless patient has experienced previous Grade 3 or 4 skin toxicity. If so, wait an additional week	Decrease dose by 25%; return to 3-week interval
2 (Erythema, desquamation, or swelling interfering with, but not precluding, normal physical activities; small blisters or ulcerations <2 cm in diameter)	Wait an additional week	Decrease dose by 50%; return to 3-week interval
3 (Blistering, ulceration, or swelling interfering with walking or normal daily activities, cannot wear regular clothing)	Wait an additional week	Discontinue therapy
4 (Diffuse or local process causing infectious complications, or a bedridden state or hospitalization)	Wait an additional week	Discontinue therapy

Caelyx®: Recommended Dose Modification Guidelines: Stomatitis (AIDS-related Kaposi's Sarcoma)

STOMATITIS Toxicity grade:	Caelyx® Dosage Adjustment (AIDS-related Kaposi's Sarcoma)
1 (Painless ulcers, erythema, or mild soreness)	No dosage adjustment
2 (Painful erythema, edema, or ulcers, but can eat)	Wait 1 week and if symptoms improve, redose at 100% dose
3 (Painful erythema, edema, or ulcers, and cannot eat)	Wait 1 week and if symptoms improve, redose with a 25% dose reduction
4 (Requires parenteral or enteral support)	Wait 1 week and if symptoms improve, redose with a 50% dose reduction

Caelyx®: Hematologic toxicity: AIDS-related Kaposi's sarcoma:

Caelyx®: Hematologic Toxicity (AIDS-related Kaposi's Sarcoma)

Grade	ANC	Platelets	Modification
1	1500-1900	75,000-150,000	None
2	1000-<1500	50,000-<75,000	None
3	500-999	25,000-<50,000	Wait until ANC ≥1000 and/or platelets ≥50,000; redose with a 25% dose reduction.
4	<500	<25,000	Wait until ANC ≥1000 and/or platelets ≥50,000; redose with a 50% dose reduction.

Myocet™: Hematologic or gastrointestinal toxicity: Dosage reduction: If initial dose was 75 mg/m^2, reduce dose to 60 mg/m^2; if initial dose was 60 mg/m^2, reduce dose to 50 mg/m^2. If toxicity persists with subsequent cycles, consider reducing dose further (from 60 mg/m^2 to 50 mg/m^2 or from 50 mg/m^2 to 40 mg/m^2).

Neutropenia: If grade 4 neutropenia (ANC <500 /mm^3) without fever lasting ≥7 days or grade 4 neutropenia of any duration with concurrent fever (≥38.5°C) occurs, consider reducing dose with subsequent cycles. **Note:** Prior to dose reductions, prophylactic cytokine therapy may be considered.

Thrombocytopenia or anemia: If grade 4 thrombocytopenia or anemia occurs, hold therapy until recovery to ≤ grade 2. Reduce dose with subsequent cycles or consider discontinuing treatment.

Gastrointestinal toxicity or mucositis: Grade 3 mucositis persisting ≥3 days, or grade 4 mucositis of any duration, or grade 3 or 4 gastrointestinal toxicity not responsive to interventions and/or prophylaxis: Consider dose reduction with subsequent cycles.

Combination Regimens

Breast cancer: Doxorubicin (Liposomal)-Docetaxel (Breast Cancer) on page 1619

Lymphoma, Hodgkin: GVD (Hodgkin) on page 1679

Multiple myeloma:

Bortezomib-Doxorubicin (Liposomal) on page 1536

Bortezomib-Doxorubicin (Liposomal)-Dexamethasone on page 1536

Doxorubicin (Liposomal)-Vincristine-Dexamethasone on page 1620

Ovarian cancer:

Carboplatin-Doxorubicin (Liposomal) (Ovarian) on page 1544

Doxorubicin (Liposomal) (Ovarian Regimen) on page 1618

Trabectedin-Doxorubicin (Liposomal) (Ovarian Cancer) on page 1757

Administration Do not administer as a bolus injection or I.M. or SubQ. Avoid extravasation (irritant); monitor infusion site; extravasation may occur without stinging or burning. Monitor for infusion reaction.

Doxil®, Caelyx®: Administer IVPB over 60 minutes; manufacturer recommends administering at initial rate of 1 mg/minute to minimize risk of infusion reactions until the absence of a reaction has been established, then increase the infusion rate for completion over 1 hour. Do **NOT** administer undiluted. Do **NOT** infuse with in-line filters. Incompatible with heparin flushes; flush with 5-10 mL of D_5W solution before and after drug administration (do not rapidly flush through the I.V. line). Monitor for local erythematous streaking along vein and/or facial flushing (may indicate rapid infusion rate).

Myocet™: Infuse over 1 hour.

Emetic Potential Low (10% to 30%)

Vesicant/Extravasation Risk May be an irritant

Monitoring Parameters CBC with differential and platelet count, liver function tests (ALT/AST, bilirubin, alkaline phosphatase); monitor for infusion reactions, hand-foot syndrome, and stomatitis

Cardiac function (left ventricular ejection fraction [LVEF]; baseline and periodic); echocardiography, or MUGA scan may be used. Endomyocardial biopsy is the most definitive test for anthracycline myocardial injury.

Dosage Forms Excipient information presented when available (limited, particularly for generics); consult specific product labeling.

Injection, solution, as hydrochloride:

Doxil®: 2 mg/mL (10 mL, 25 mL) [contains soy, sucrose]

Dosage Forms: Canada

Excipient information presented when available (limited, particularly for generics); consult specific product labeling.

Injection, solution, as hydrochloride, pegylated:

Caelyx®: 2 mg/mL (10 mL, 25 mL)

Injection, encapsulated liposomes:

Myocet™: 3-vial kit (doxorubicin HCl for injection 50 mg/vial, liposomes for injection, and buffer for injection)

References

Bartlett NL, Niedzwiecki D, Johnson JL, et al, "Gemcitabine, Vinorelbine, and Pegylated Liposomal Doxorubicin (GVD), A Salvage Regimen in Relapsed Hodgkin's Lymphoma: CALGB 59804," *Ann Oncol*, 2007, 18(6):1071-9.

Biehn SE, Moore DT, Voorhees PM, et al, "Extended Follow-Up of Outcome Measures in Multiple Myeloma Patients Treated on a Phase I Study With Bortezomib and Pegylated Liposomal Doxorubicin," *Ann Hematol*, 2007, 86(3):211-6.

Dummer R, Quaglino P, Becker JC, Hasan B, et al, "Prospective International Multicenter Phase II Trial of Intravenous Pegylated Liposomal Doxorubicin Monochemotherapy in Patients With Stage IIB, IVA, or IVB Advanced Mycosis Fungoides: Final Results From EORTC 21012," *J Clin Oncol*, 2012 [epub ahead of print].

Gordon AN, Fleagle JT, Guthrie D, et al, "Recurrent Epithelial Ovarian Carcinoma: A Randomized Phase III Study of Pegylated Liposomal Doxorubicin Versus Topotecan," *J Clin Oncol*, 2001, 19(14):3312-22.

Hussein MA, Wood L, Hsi E, et al, "A Phase II Trial of Pegylated Liposomal Doxorubicin, Vincristine, and Reduced-Dose Dexamethasone Combination Therapy in Newly Diagnosed Multiple Myeloma Patients," *Cancer*, 2002, 95(10):2160-8.

Judson I, Radford JA, Harris M, et al, "Randomised Phase II Trial of Pegylated Liposomal Doxorubicin (DOXIL/CAELYX) versus Doxorubicin in the Treatment of Advanced or Metastatic

Soft Tissue Sarcoma: a Study by the EORTC Soft Tissue and Bone Sarcoma Group," *Eur J Cancer*, 2001, 37(7):870-7.

Keller AM, Mennel RG, Georgoulias VA, et al, "Randomized Phase III Trial of Pegylated Liposomal Doxorubicin Versus Vinorelbine or Mitomycin C Plus Vinblastine in Women With Taxane-Refractory Advanced Breast Cancer," *J Clin Oncol*, 2004, 22(19):3893-901.

King PD and Perry MC, "Hepatotoxicity of Chemotherapy," *Oncologist*, 2001, 6(2):162-76.

Northfelt DW, Dezebe BJ, Thommes JA, et al, "Pegylated-Liposomal Doxorubicin Versus Doxorubicin, Bleomycin, and Vincristine in the Treatment of AIDS-Related Kaposi's Sarcoma: Results of a Randomized Phase III Clinical Trial," *J Clin Oncol*, 1998, 16(7):2445-51.

O'Brien ME, Wigler N, Inbar M, et al, "Reduced Cardiotoxicity and Comparable Efficacy in a Phase III Trial of Pegylated Liposomal Doxorubicin HCl (CAELYX™/Doxil®) Versus Conventional Doxorubicin for First-Line Treatment of Metastatic Breast Cancer," *Ann Oncol*, 2004, 15(3):440-9.

O'Shaughnessy JA, "Pegylated Liposomal Doxorubicin in the Treatment of Breast Cancer," *Clin Breast Cancer*, 2003, 4(5):318-28.

Rifkin RM, Gregory SA, Mohrbacher A, et al, "Pegylated Liposomal Doxorubicin, Vincristine, and Dexamethasone Provide Significant Reduction in Toxicity Compared With Doxorubicin, Vincristine, and Dexamethasone in Patients With Newly Diagnosed Multiple Myeloma," *Cancer*, 2006, 106(4):848-58.

Sutton G, Blessing J, Hanjani P, et al, "Phase II Evaluation of Liposomal Doxorubicin (Doxil) in Recurrent or Advanced Leiomyosarcoma of the Uterus: A Gynecologic Oncology Group Study," *Gynecol Oncol*, 2005, 96(3):749-52.

Vorbiof DA, Rapoport BL, Chasen C, et al, "First Line Therapy With Paclitaxel (Taxol) and Pegylated Liposomal Doxorubicin (Caelyx) in Patients With Metastatic Breast Cancer: A Multicentre Phase II Study," *Breast*, 2004, 13(3):219-26.

Wollina U, Dummer R, Brockmeyer NH, "Multicenter Study of Pegylated Liposomal Doxorubicin in Patients With Cutaneous T-Cell Lymphoma," *Cancer*, 2003, 98(5):993-1001.

Dronabinol (droe NAB i nol)

Related Information

Management of Chemotherapy-Induced Nausea and Vomiting *on page 1786*

Brand Names: Canada Marinol®

Index Terms Delta-9 THC; Delta-9-tetrahydro-cannabinol; Tetrahydrocannabinol; THC

Generic Availability (U.S.) Yes

Pharmacologic Category Antiemetic; Appetite Stimulant

Use Chemotherapy-associated nausea and vomiting refractory to other antiemetic(s); AIDS-related anorexia

Unlabeled Use Cancer-related anorexia

Labeled Contraindications Hypersensitivity to dronabinol, cannabinoids, sesame oil, or any component of the formulation, or marijuana; should be avoided in patients with a history of schizophrenia

Pregnancy Risk Factor C

Lactation Enters breast milk/not recommended

Warnings/Precautions Use with caution in patients with hepatic disease or seizure disorders. Reduce dosage in patients with severe hepatic impairment. May cause additive CNS effects with sedatives, hypnotics or other psychoactive agents; patients must be cautioned about performing tasks which require mental alertness (eg, operating machinery or driving).

May have potential for abuse; drug is psychoactive substance in marijuana; use caution in patients with a history of substance abuse or potential. May cause withdrawal symptoms upon abrupt discontinuation. Use with caution in patients with mania, depression, or schizophrenia; careful psychiatric monitoring is recommended. Use caution in elderly; they are more sensitive to adverse effects.

Adverse Reactions Frequency not always specified.

>1%:

Cardiovascular: Palpitations, tachycardia, vasodilation/facial flushing

Central nervous system: Euphoria (8% to 24%, dose related), abnormal thinking (3% to 10%), dizziness (3% to 10%), paranoia (3% to 10%), somnolence (3% to 10%), amnesia, anxiety, ataxia, confusion, depersonalization, hallucination

Gastrointestinal: Abdominal pain (3% to 10%), nausea (3% to 10%), vomiting (3% to 10%)

Neuromuscular & skeletal: Weakness

<1%, postmarketing, and/or case reports: Conjunctivitis, depression, diarrhea, fatigue, fecal incontinence, flushing, hypotension, myalgia, nightmares, seizure, speech difficulties, tinnitus, vision difficulties

Drug Interactions

Metabolism/Transport Effects None known.

Avoid Concomitant Use

Avoid concomitant use of Dronabinol with any of the following: Azelastine (Nasal); Mirtazapine; Paraldehyde

Increased Effect/Toxicity

Dronabinol may increase the levels/effects of: Alcohol (Ethyl); Azelastine (Nasal); CNS Depressants; Methotrimeprazine; Metyrosine; Mirtazapine; Paraldehyde; Pramipexole; ROPINIRole; Rotigotine; Selective Serotonin Reuptake Inhibitors; Sympathomimetics; Zolpidem

The levels/effects of Dronabinol may be increased by: Anticholinergic Agents; Cocaine; Droperidol; HydrOXYzine; MAO Inhibitors; Methotrimeprazine; Perampanel; Ritonavir

Decreased Effect There are no known significant interactions involving a decrease in effect.

Ethanol/Nutrition/Herb Interactions

Ethanol: May increase CNS depression; monitor for increased effects with coadministration. Caution patients about effects.

Food: Administration with high-lipid meals may increase absorption.

Herb/Nutraceutical: St John's wort may decrease dronabinol levels.

Storage/Stability Store under refrigeration (or in a cool environment) between 8°C and 15°C (46°F and 59°F); protect from freezing.

Mechanism of Action Unknown, may inhibit endorphins in the brain's emetic center, suppress prostaglandin synthesis, and/or inhibit medullary activity through an unspecified cortical action. Some pharmacologic effects appear to involve sympathomimetic activity; tachyphylaxis to some effect (eg, tachycardia) may occur, but appetite-stimulating effects do not appear to wane over time. Antiemetic activity may be due to effect on cannabinoid receptors (CB1) within the central nervous system.

Pharmacodynamics/Kinetics

Onset of action: Within 1 hour

Peak effect: 2-4 hours

Duration: 24 hours (appetite stimulation)

Absorption: Oral: 90% to 95%; 10% to 20% of dose gets into systemic circulation

Distribution: V_d: 10 L/kg; dronabinol is highly lipophilic and distributes to adipose tissue

Protein binding: 97% to 99%

Metabolism: Hepatic to at least 50 metabolites, some of which are active; 11-hydroxy-delta-9-tetrahydrocannabinol (11-OH-THC) is the major metabolite; extensive first-pass effect

Half-life elimination: Dronabinol: 25-36 hours (terminal); Dronabinol metabolites: 44-59 hours

Time to peak, serum: 0.5-4 hours

Excretion: Feces (50% as unconjugated metabolites, 5% as unchanged drug); urine (10% to 15% as acid metabolites and conjugates)

Dosing

Adult & Geriatric

Antiemetic: Oral: 5 mg/m^2 1-3 hours before chemotherapy, then give 5 mg/m^2/dose every 2-4 hours after chemotherapy for a total of 4-6 doses/day; dose may be increased up to a maximum of 15 mg/m^2/dose if needed (dosage may be increased by 2.5 mg/m^2 increments).

Appetite stimulant (AIDS-related): Oral: Initial: 2.5 mg twice daily (before lunch and dinner); titrate up to a maximum of 20 mg/day.

Pediatric Antiemetic: Oral: Refer to adult dosing.

Hepatic Impairment Usual dose should be reduced in patients with severe liver failure.

Monitoring Parameters CNS effects, heart rate, blood pressure, behavioral profile

Test Interactions Decreased FSH, LH, growth hormone, and testosterone

Dietary Considerations Capsules contain sesame oil.

Dosage Forms Excipient information presented when available (limited, particularly for generics); consult specific product labeling.

Capsule, soft gelatin, oral: 2.5 mg [contains sesame oil], 5 mg [contains sesame oil], 10 mg [contains sesame oil]

Controlled Substance C-III

References

Anderson PO and Muire GG, "Delta-9-Tetrahydrocannabinol as an Antiemetic," *Am J Hosp Pharm*, 1981, 38:639-46.

Tramer MR, Carroll D, Campbell FA, et al, "Cannabinoids for Control of Chemotherapy Induced Nausea and Vomiting: Quantitative Systematic Review," *BMJ*, 2001, 323(7303):16-21.

Droperidol (droe PER i dole)

Related Information

Management of Chemotherapy-Induced Nausea and Vomiting *on page* 1786

Brand Names: Canada Droperidol Injection, USP

Index Terms Dehydrobenzperidol

Generic Availability (U.S.) Yes

Pharmacologic Category Antiemetic; Antipsychotic Agent, Typical

Use Prevention and/or treatment of nausea and vomiting from surgical and diagnostic procedures

Labeled Contraindications Hypersensitivity to droperidol or any component of the formulation; known or suspected QT prolongation, including congenital long QT syndrome (prolonged QT_c is defined as >440 msec in males or >450 msec in females)

Canadian labeling: Additional contraindications (not in U.S. labeling): Not for use in children ≤2 years of age

Pregnancy Risk Factor C

Lactation Excretion in breast milk unknown/use caution

Warnings/Precautions May alter cardiac conduction. **[U.S. Boxed Warning]: Cases of QT prolongation and torsade de pointes, including some fatal cases, have been reported.** Use extreme caution in patients with bradycardia (<50 bpm), cardiac disease, concurrent MAO inhibitor therapy, Class I and Class III antiarrhythmics or other drugs known to prolong QT interval, and electrolyte disturbances (hypokalemia or hypomagnesemia), including concomitant drugs which may alter electrolytes (diuretics).

Use with caution in patients with seizures or severe liver disease. May be sedating, use with caution in disorders where CNS depression is a feature. Caution in patients with hemodynamic instability, predisposition to seizures, subcortical brain damage, pheochromocytoma or renal disease. Esophageal dysmotility and aspiration have been associated with antipsychotic use - use with caution in patients at risk of pneumonia (ie, Alzheimer's disease). Caution in breast cancer or other prolactin-dependent tumors (may elevate prolactin levels). May alter temperature regulation or mask toxicity of other drugs due to antiemetic effects. May cause orthostatic hypotension - use with caution in patients at risk of this effect or those who would tolerate transient hypotensive episodes (cerebrovascular disease, cardiovascular disease, or other medications which may predispose). Significant hypotension may occur.

May cause anticholinergic effects (confusion, agitation, constipation, xerostomia, blurred vision, urinary retention). Therefore, they should be used with caution in patients with decreased gastrointestinal motility, urinary retention, BPH, xerostomia, or visual problems. Conditions which also may be exacerbated by cholinergic blockade include narrow-angle glaucoma (screening is recommended) and worsening of myasthenia gravis. Relative to other neuroleptics, droperidol has a low potency of cholinergic blockade.

May cause extrapyramidal symptoms (EPS), including pseudoparkinsonism, acute dystonic reactions, akathisia, and tardive dyskinesia. Risk of dystonia (and possibly other EPS) may be greater with increased doses, use of conventional antipsychotics, males, and younger patients. May be associated with neuroleptic malignant syndrome (NMS). May mask toxicity of other drugs or conditions (eg, intestinal obstruction, Reye's syndrome, brain tumor) due to antiemetic effects. Use with caution in the elderly; reduce initial dose.

Adverse Reactions Frequency not defined.

Cardiovascular: Cardiac arrest, hypertension, hypotension (especially orthostatic), QT_c prolongation (dose dependent), tachycardia, torsade de pointes, ventricular tachycardia

Central nervous system: Anxiety, chills, depression (postoperative, transient), dizziness, drowsiness (postoperative) increased, dysphoria, extrapyramidal symptoms (akathisia, dystonia, oculogyric crisis), hallucinations (postoperative), hyperactivity, neuroleptic malignant syndrome (NMS) (rare), restlessness

Respiratory: Bronchospasm, laryngospasm

Miscellaneous: Anaphylaxis, shivering

Drug Interactions

Metabolism/Transport Effects None known.

Avoid Concomitant Use

Avoid concomitant use of Droperidol with any of the following: Aclidinium; Azelastine (Nasal); Highest Risk QTc-Prolonging Agents; Ipratropium (Oral Inhalation); Metoclopramide; Mifepristone; Paraldehyde; Tiotropium

Increased Effect/Toxicity

Droperidol may increase the levels/effects of: Alcohol (Ethyl); Anticholinergics; Azelastine (Nasal); Buprenorphine; CNS Depressants; Highest Risk QTc-Prolonging Agents; Methotrimeprazine; Methylphenidate; Metoclopramide; Moderate Risk QTc-Prolonging Agents; Paraldehyde; Serotonin Modulators; Tiotropium; Zolpidem

The levels/effects of Droperidol may be increased by: Acetylcholinesterase Inhibitors (Central); Aclidinium; HydrOXYzine; Ipratropium (Oral Inhalation); Lithium formulations; MAO Inhibitors; Methotrimeprazine; Methylphenidate; Metoclopramide; Metyrosine; Mifepristone; Perampanel; Pramlintide; QTc-Prolonging Agents (Indeterminate Risk and Risk Modifying); Tetrabenazine

Decreased Effect

Droperidol may decrease the levels/effects of: Amphetamines; Anti-Parkinson's Agents (Dopamine Agonist); Quinagolide

The levels/effects of Droperidol may be decreased by: Anti-Parkinson's Agents (Dopamine Agonist); Lithium formulations

Storage/Stability Store at 20°C to 25°C (68°F to 77°F); excursions permitted to 15°C to 30°C (59°F to 86°F). Protect from light. Solutions diluted in NS or D_5W are stable at room temperature for up to 7 days in PVC bags or glass bottles. Solutions diluted in LR are stable at room temperature for 24 hours in PVC bags and up to 7 days in glass bottles.

Reconstitution I.V. infusion: Dilute in 50-100 mL NS or D_5W.

Mechanism of Action Droperidol is a butyrophenone antipsychotic; antiemetic effect is a result of blockade of dopamine stimulation of the chemoreceptor trigger zone. Other effects include alpha-adrenergic blockade, peripheral vascular dilation, and reduction of the pressor effect of epinephrine resulting in hypotension and decreased peripheral vascular resistance; may also reduce pulmonary artery pressure

Pharmacodynamics/Kinetics

Onset of action: 3-10 minutes
- Peak effect: ~30 minutes

Duration: 2-4 hours, may extend to 12 hours

Absorption: I.M.: Rapid

Distribution: Crosses blood-brain barrier and placenta
- V_d: Children: ~0.6 L/kg; Adults: ~1.5 L/kg

Protein binding: 85% to 90%

Metabolism: Hepatic, to *p*-fluorophenylacetic acid, benzimidazolone, *p*-hydroxypiperidine

Half-life elimination: ~2.3 hours

Excretion: Urine (75%, <1% as unchanged drug); feces (22%, 11% as unchanged drug)

Dosing

Adult & Geriatric Note: Titrate carefully to desired effect

Prevention of PONV: I.M., I.V.:

Manufacturer labeling: Maximum initial dose: 2.5 mg; additional doses of 1.25 mg may be administered with caution to achieve desired effect

Consensus guideline recommendations: 0.625-1.25 mg I.V. administered at the end of surgery (Gan, 2007)

Canadian labeling:

Prevention and treatment of PONV: I.V.: 0.625-1.25 mg 30 minutes prior to anticipated end of surgery, and then every 6 hours as needed for breakthrough PONV

Pediatric Note: Titrate carefully to desired effect

Prevention of postoperative nausea and vomiting (PONV): I.M., I.V.:

Children 2-12 years:

Manufacturer labeling: Maximum dose: 0.1 mg/kg; additional doses may be repeated with caution to achieve desired effect

Consensus guideline recommendations: 0.01-0.015 mg/kg (maximum: 1.25 mg) I.V. administered at the end of surgery (Gan, 2007)

Canadian labeling:

Prevention and treatment of PONV: I.V.: Children >2 years and Adolescents: 0.02-0.05 mg/kg (maximum dose: 1.25 mg) 30 minutes prior to anticipated end of surgery, and then every 6 hours as needed for breakthrough PONV

Renal Impairment

U.S. labeling: Specific dosing recommendations are not provided; use with caution.

Canadian labeling: I.V.: 0.625 mg; additional dosing should be administered with caution.

Hepatic Impairment

U.S. labeling: Specific dosing recommendations are not provided; use with caution.

Canadian labeling: I.V.: 0.625 mg; additional dosing should be administered with caution.

Administration Administer I.M. or I.V.; according to the manufacturer, I.V. push administration should be slow. For I.V. infusion, further dilute.

Monitoring Parameters To identify QT prolongation, a 12-lead ECG prior to use is recommended; continued ECG monitoring for 2-3 hours following administration is recommended. Vital signs; serum magnesium and potassium; mental status, abnormal involuntary movement scale (AIMS); observe for dystonias, extrapyramidal side effects, and temperature changes

Dosage Forms Excipient information presented when available (limited, particularly for generics); consult specific product labeling.

Injection, solution: 2.5 mg/mL (2 mL)

Injection, solution [preservative free]: 2.5 mg/mL (2 mL)

References

Gan TJ, Meyer TA, Apfel CC, et al, "Society for Ambulatory Anesthesia Guidelines for the Management of Postoperative Nausea and Vomiting," *Anesth Analg*, 2007, 105(6):1615-28.

Grunberg SM and Hesketh PJ, "Control of Chemotherapy-Induced Emesis," *N Engl J Med*, 1993, 329(24):1790-6.

Kao LW, Kirk MA, Evers SJ, et al, "Droperidol, QT Prolongation, and Sudden Death: What Is the Evidence," *Ann Emerg Med*, 2003, 41(4):546-58.

Sridhar KS and Donnelly E, "Combination Antiemetics for Cisplatin Chemotherapy," *Cancer*, 1988, 61(8):1508-17.

Tortorice PV and O'Connell MB, "Management of Chemotherapy-Induced Nausea and Vomiting," *Pharmacotherapy*, 1990, 10(2):129-45.

◆ **Droperidol Injection, USP (Can)** *see* Droperidol *on page* 486

◆ **Droxia®** *see* Hydroxyurea *on page* 731

◆ **DTC 101** *see* Cytarabine (Liposomal) *on page* 361

◆ **DTIC** *see* Dacarbazine *on page* 367

◆ **DTIC-Dome** *see* Dacarbazine *on page* 367

- **D-Trp(6)-LHRH** *see* Triptorelin *on page 1413*
- **Duragesic®** *see* FentaNYL *on page 583*
- **Duragesic® MAT (Can)** *see* FentaNYL *on page 583*
- **Duramorph** *see* Morphine (Systemic) *on page 1004*
- **Durela™ (Can)** *see* TraMADol *on page 1388*
- **DVA** *see* Vindesine *on page 1464*
- **E7389** *see* Eribulin *on page 524*
- **EACA** *see* Aminocaproic Acid *on page 72*
- ***E. coli* Asparaginase** *see* Asparaginase (*E. coli*) *on page 130*
- **Econopred** *see* PrednisoLONE (Ophthalmic) *on page 1198*
- **Ecteinascidin** *see* Trabectedin *on page 1384*
- **Ecteinascidin 743** *see* Trabectedin *on page 1384*

Eculizumab (e kue LIZ oo mab)

Brand Names: U.S. Soliris®

Brand Names: Canada Soliris®

Index Terms h5G1.1; Monoclonal Antibody 5G1.1; Monoclonal Antibody Anti-C5

Generic Availability (U.S.) No

Pharmacologic Category Monoclonal Antibody; Monoclonal Antibody, Complement Inhibitor

Use Treatment of paroxysmal nocturnal hemoglobinuria (PNH) to reduce hemolysis; treatment of atypical hemolytic uremic syndrome (aHUS) to inhibit complement-mediated thrombotic microangiopathy

Note: Not indicated for the treatment of hemolytic uremic syndrome related to Shiga toxin *E. coli* (STEC-HUS)

Labeled Contraindications Unresolved serious *Neisseria meningitidis* infection; patients not currently vaccinated against *Neisseria meningitidis* (unless risks of treatment delay outweigh risk of meningococcal infection)

Pregnancy Risk Factor C

Lactation Excretion in breast milk unknown/use caution

Warnings/Precautions **[U.S. Boxed Warning]: Meningococcal *(Neisseria meningitides)* infections have occurred in patients receiving eculizumab; may be fatal or life-threatening if not detected and treated promptly. Monitor for early signs of meningococcal infection; evaluate and treat promptly if suspected. Follow current meningococcal immunization recommendations for patients with complement deficiencies. Vaccinate with meningococcal vaccine at least 2 weeks prior to initiation of treatment;** revaccinate according to current guidelines. Polyvalent meningococcal vaccines are recommended. If urgent treatment is necessary in an unvaccinated patient, administer meningococcal vaccine as soon as possible. Although the risk/benefits of prophylactic meningococcal antibiotic therapy have not been determined, prophylactic antibiotics were administered in clinical studies until at least 2 weeks after vaccination. Meningococcal infections developed in some patients despite vaccination. Discontinue eculizumab during the treatment of serious meningococcal infections. In addition to meningitis, the risk of other infections, especially encapsulated bacteria (eg, *Streptococcus pneumoniae, H. influenzae*) is increased with eculizumab treatment (because eculizumab blocks terminal complement activation). Children should receive vaccination for prevention of *S. pneumoniae, H. influenzae* according to current ACIP guidelines. Use caution in patients with concurrent systemic infection. Patients should be up to date with all immunizations before initiating therapy. **[U.S. Boxed Warning]: Access is restricted through a REMS program. Prescribers must be enrolled in the program; enrollment information is available at 1-888-765-4747.** Counsel patients on the risk of meningococcal infection; ensure patients are vaccinated and provide educational materials.

Infusion reactions, including anaphylaxis or hypersensitivity, may occur; interrupt infusion for severe reaction. Continue monitoring for 1 hour after completion of infusion. Patients with PNH who discontinue treatment may be at increased risk for serious hemolysis; monitor closely for at least 8 weeks after treatment discontinuation. Consider RBC transfusion, exchange transfusion, anticoagulation, corticoids or reinitiation of eculizumab for serious hemolysis after discontinuation. When used for aHUS, monitor for at least 12 weeks after treatment discontinuation for signs/symptoms of thrombotic microangiopathy (TMA) complications (angina, dyspnea, mental status changes, seizure, serum creatinine elevation, serum LDH elevation, thrombocytopenia, or thrombosis). If TMA complications occur after stopping eculizumab, consider reinitiation of treatment, plasmapheresis, plasma exchange, fresh frozen plasma infusion, and/or appropriate organ-specific measures. In clinical trials, anticoagulant therapy was continued in patients who were receiving these agents (due to history of or risk for thromboembolism) prior to initiation of eculizumab. The effect of anticoagulant therapy withdrawal is unknown; treatment with eculizumab should not alter anticoagulation management

Adverse Reactions

>10%:

Cardiovascular: Hypertension (aHUS: 35%), tachycardia (aHUS: children 21%), peripheral edema (11%)

Central nervous system: Headache (30% to 44%; serious: 2%), insomnia (14%), fatigue (11% to 12%), fever (2% to 11%; children 47%), vertigo (11%)

Gastrointestinal: Diarrhea (32%), vomiting (21% to 22%), nausea (16% to 19%), abdominal pain (11%)

Genitourinary: Urinary tract infection (16%)

Hematologic: Anemia (24%; serious: 2%), leukopenia (16%)

Neuromuscular & skeletal: Back pain (19%), limb pain (7% to 11%)

Respiratory: Respiratory tract infection (7% to 35%), cough (12% to 26%), nasopharyngitis (23%), nasal congestion (aHUS: children 21%), pharyngolaryngeal pain (14%)

1% to 10%:

Gastrointestinal: Constipation (7%)

Neuromuscular & skeletal: Myalgia (7%)

Respiratory: Sinusitis (7%)

Miscellaneous: Herpes infections (7%), flu-like syndrome (5%), viral infection (serious: 2%), meningococcal infection (≤1%)

<1%, postmarketing, and/or case reports: Abdominal distention, anxiety, arthralgia, cholangitis, dizziness, endometritis, hematoma (mild), infusion reaction, pyelonephritis, renal impairment, taste alteration

Drug Interactions

Metabolism/Transport Effects None known.

Avoid Concomitant Use

Avoid concomitant use of Eculizumab with any of the following: BCG; Natalizumab; Pimecrolimus; Tacrolimus (Topical); Vaccines (Live)

Increased Effect/Toxicity

Eculizumab may increase the levels/effects of: Leflunomide; Natalizumab; Vaccines (Live)

The levels/effects of Eculizumab may be increased by: Denosumab; Pimecrolimus; Roflumilast; Tacrolimus (Topical); Trastuzumab

Decreased Effect

Eculizumab may decrease the levels/effects of: BCG; Coccidioidin Skin Test; Sipuleucel-T; Vaccines (Inactivated); Vaccines (Live)

The levels/effects of Eculizumab may be decreased by: Echinacea

Storage/Stability Prior to dilution, store vials at 2°C to 8°C (36°F to 46°F); do not freeze. Protect from light; do not shake. Allow admixture to reach room temperature prior to administration (do not use a heat source or warming). Following dilution, store at room temperature or refrigerate; protect from light; use within 24 hours.

Reconstitution Add eculizumab to an infusion bag and dilute with an equal volume of D_5W, sodium chloride 0.9%, sodium chloride 0.45%, or Ringer's injection to a final concentration of 5 mg/mL (eg, 300 mg to a total volume of 60 mL, 600 mg in a total volume of 120 mL, 900 mg in a total volume of 180 mL, or 1200 mg to a total volume of 240 mL). Gently invert bag to mix thoroughly.

Mechanism of Action Terminal complement-mediated intravascular hemolysis is a key clinical feature of paroxysmal nocturnal hemoglobinuria (PNH); blocking the formation of membrane attack complex (MAC) results in stabilization of hemoglobin and a reduction in the need for RBC transfusions. Impairment of complement activity regulation leads to uncontrolled complement activation in atypical hemolytic uremic syndrome (aHUS). Eculizumab is a humanized monoclonal IgG antibody that binds to complement protein C5, preventing cleavage into C5a and C5b. Blocking the formation of C5b inhibits the subsequent formation of terminal complex C5b-9 or MAC.

Pharmacodynamics/Kinetics

Onset of action: PNH: Reduced hemolysis: ≤1 week

Distribution: PNH: 7.7 L; aHUS: 6.14 L

Half-life elimination: PNH: ~11 days (range: ~8-15 days); aHUS: ~12 days (during plasma exchange the half-life is reduced to 1.26 hours)

Dosing

Adult & Geriatric Note: Patients must receive meningococcal vaccine at least 2 weeks prior to treatment initiation; revaccinate according to current guidelines. Treatment should be administered at the recommended time interval although administration may be varied by ±2 days.

Atypical hemolytic uremic syndrome (aHUS): I.V.: Induction: 900 mg weekly for 4 doses; Maintenance: 1200 mg at week 5, then 1200 mg every 2 weeks

Supplemental dosing for patients receiving plasmapheresis or plasma exchange: If most recent dose was ≥600 mg, administer 600 mg within 60 minutes after each plasmapheresis or plasma exchange

Supplemental dosing for patients receiving fresh frozen plasma infusion: If most recent dose was ≥300 mg, administer 300 mg within 60 minutes prior to each 1 unit of fresh frozen plasma infusion

Paroxysmal nocturnal hemoglobinuria (PNH): I.V.: 600 mg weekly for 4 doses, followed by 900 mg 1 week later; then 900 mg every 2 weeks

Pediatric Note: Patients must receive meningococcal vaccine at least 2 weeks prior to treatment initiation; revaccinate according to current guidelines. Treatment should be administered at the recommended time interval although administration may be varied by ±2 days.

Atypical hemolytic uremic syndrome (aHUS): I.V.:

Children 5 kg to <10 kg: Induction: 300 mg weekly for 1 dose; Maintenance: 300 mg at week 2, then 300 mg every 3 weeks

Children 10 kg to <20 kg: Induction: 600 mg weekly for 1 dose; Maintenance: 300 mg at week 2, then 300 mg every 2 weeks

Children 20 kg to <30 kg: Induction: 600 mg weekly for 2 doses; Maintenance: 600 mg at week 3, then 600 mg every 2 weeks

Children 30 kg to <40 kg: Induction: 600 mg weekly for 2 doses; Maintenance: 900 mg at week 3, then 900 mg every 2 weeks

Children ≥40 kg: Induction: 900 mg weekly for 4 doses; Maintenance: 1200 mg at week 5, then 1200 mg every 2 weeks

Supplemental dosing for patients receiving plasmapheresis or plasma exchange:

If most recent dose was 300 mg, administer 300 mg within 60 minutes after each plasmapheresis or plasma exchange

If most recent dose was ≥600 mg, administer 600 mg within 60 minutes after each plasmapheresis or plasma exchange

Supplemental dosing for patients receiving fresh frozen plasma infusion: If most recent dose was ≥300 mg, administer 300 mg within 60 minutes prior to each 1 unit of fresh frozen plasma infusion

Renal Impairment No dosage adjustment is recommended in the manufacturer's labeling.

Hepatic Impairment Not studied in hepatic dysfunction.

Administration I.V.: Allow to reach room temperature prior to administration. Infuse over 35 minutes. Decrease infusion rate or discontinue for infusion reactions; do not exceed a maximum 2-hour duration of infusion. Monitor for at least 1 hour following completion of infusion (for signs/symptoms of infusion reaction).

Monitoring Parameters Signs and symptoms of infusion reaction (during infusion and for 1 hour after infusion complete); CBC with differential, lactic dehydrogenase (LDH), serum creatinine, AST, urinalysis

Serum LDH levels greater than pretreatment level along with: >25% decrease in PNH clone size in ≤1 week, or hemoglobin level <5 g/dL, or a hemoglobin decrease of >4 g/dL in ≤1 week, or 50% increase in serum creatinine, or angina, mental status change, or thrombosis is indicative of serious hemolysis

After discontinuation:

aHUS: Signs/symptoms of thrombotic microangiopathy (TMA) complications (monitor for at least 12 weeks after treatment discontinuation), including angina, dyspnea, mental status changes, seizure, serum creatinine elevation, serum LDH elevation, thrombocytopenia, or thrombosis.

PNH: Signs and symptoms of intravascular hemolysis (monitor for at least 8 weeks after discontinuation), including serum LDH, hemoglobin, serum creatinine; signs of angina, mental status change, or thrombosis

Prescribing and Access Restrictions Patients and providers must enroll with Soliris® OneSource™ (1-888-765-4747) program prior to treatment initiation.

Medication Guide Available Yes

Dosage Forms Excipient information presented when available (limited, particularly for generics); consult specific product labeling.

Injection, solution [preservative free]:

Soliris®: 10 mg/mL (30 mL) [contains polysorbate 80]

References

Brodsky RA, Young NS, Antonioli E, et al, "Multicenter Phase 3 Study of the Complement Inhibitor Eculizumab for the Treatment of Patients With Paroxysmal Nocturnal Hemoglobinuria," *Blood*, 2008, 111(4):1840-7.

Centers for Disease Control and Prevention, "Prevention and Control of Meningococcal Disease Recommendations of the Advisory Committee on Immunization Practices (ACIP)," *MMWR Recomm Rep*, 2005, 54(RR-7):1-21. Available at http://www.cdc.gov/mmwr/pdf/rr/rr5407.pdf

Centers for Disease Control and Prevention (CDC), "Recommendations of the Advisory Committee on Immunization Practices (ACIP): General Recommendations on Immunization," *MMWR Recomm Rep*, 2011, 60(2):1-64.

Centers for Disease Control and Prevention (CDC), "Updated Recommendations for Use of Meningococcal Conjugate Vaccines – Advisory Committee on Immunization Practices, 2010," *MMWR Morb Mortal Wkly Rep*, 2011, 60(3):72-6. Available at http://www.cdc.gov/mmwr/preview/mmwrhtml/mm6003a3.htm

Hill A, Hillmen P, Richards SJ, et al, "Sustained Response and Long-Term Safety of Eculizumab in Paroxysmal Nocturnal Hemoglobinuria," *Blood*, 2005, 106(7):2559-65.

Hillmen P, Hall C, Marsh JC, et al, "Effect of Eculizumab on Hemolysis and Transfusion Requirements in Patients With Paroxysmal Nocturnal Hemoglobinuria," *N Engl J Med*, 2004, 350(6):552-9.

Hillmen P, Muus P, Duhrsen U, et al, "Effect of Complement Inhibitor Eculizumab on Thromboembolism in Patients With Paroxysmal Nocturnal Hemoglobinuria," *Blood*, 2007, 110(12):4123-8.

Hillmen P, Young NS, Schubert J, et al, "The Complement Inhibitor Eculizumab in Paroxysmal Nocturnal Hemoglobinuria," *N Engl J Med*, 2006, 355(12):1233-43.

Taylor CM, Machin S, Wigmore SJ, et al, "Clinical Practice Guidelines for the Management of Atypical Haemolytic Uraemic Syndrome in the United Kingdom," *Br J Haematol*, 2010, 148(1):37-47.

◆ **Efudex®** *see* Fluorouracil (Topical) *on page 632*

◆ **Eldisine Lilly 99094** *see* Vindesine *on page 1464*

◆ **Eligard®** *see* Leuprolide *on page 876*

◆ **Elitek®** *see* Rasburicase *on page 1229*

◆ **Ellence®** *see* Epirubicin *on page 510*

◆ **Eloxatin®** *see* Oxaliplatin *on page 1077*

◆ **Elspar®** *see* Asparaginase (*E. coli*) *on page 130*

Eltrombopag (el TROM boe pag)

Brand Names: U.S. Promacta®

Brand Names: Canada Revolade™

Index Terms Eltrombopag Olamine; Revolade®; SB-497115; SB-497115-GR

Generic Availability (U.S.) No

Pharmacologic Category Colony Stimulating Factor; Thrombopoietic Agent

Use Treatment of thrombocytopenia in patients with chronic immune (idiopathic) thrombocytopenic purpura (ITP) at risk for bleeding who have had insufficient response to corticosteroids, immune globulin, or splenectomy

Labeled Contraindications There are no contraindications listed within the manufacturer's labeling.

Pregnancy Risk Factor C

Lactation Excretion in breast milk unknown/not recommended

Warnings/Precautions [U.S. Boxed Warning]: May cause hepatotoxicity; obtain ALT, AST, and bilirubin prior to treatment initiation, every 2 weeks during adjustment phase, then monthly (after stable dose established); obtain fractionation for elevated bilirubin levels. Repeat abnormal liver

function tests within 3-5 days; if confirmed abnormal, monitor weekly until resolves, stabilizes, or returns to baseline. Discontinue treatment for ALT levels ≥3 times the upper limit of normal (ULN) and which are progressive, or persistent (≥4 weeks), or accompanied by Increased direct bilirubin, or accompanied by clinical signs of liver injury or evidence of hepatic decompensation. Reinitiation is not recommended; hepatotoxicity usually recurred with retreatment after therapy interruption; however, if the benefit of treatment outweighs the hepatotoxicity risk, initiate carefully, and monitor liver function tests weekly during the dose adjustment phase; permanently discontinue if hepatotoxicity recurs with rechallenge. Use with caution in patients with pre-existing hepatic impairment (clearance may be reduced); dosage reductions are recommended in patients with hepatic dysfunction; monitor closely.

May increase the risk for bone marrow reticulin formation or progression; collagen fibrosis (not associated with cytopenias) was observed in clinical trials. In an extension study, myelofibrosis (≤grade 1) was observed in a majority of bone marrow biopsies performed after 1 year of treatment. Monitor peripheral blood smear for cellular morphologic abnormalities; analyze CBC monthly; discontinue treatment with onset of new or worsening abnormalities (eg, teardrop and nucleated RBC, immature WBC) or cytopenias and consider bone marrow biopsy (with staining for fibrosis).

Thromboembolism may occur with excess increases in platelet levels. Use with caution in patients with known risk factors for thromboembolism (eg, Factor V Leiden, ATIII deficiency, antiphospholipid syndrome, chronic liver disease). Portal venous thrombosis was reported in a study of non-ITP patients with chronic liver disease (not an FDA-approved indication) receiving eltrombopag 75 mg once daily for 14 days as a preparative regimen prior to invasive procedures to reduce platelet transfusions. Stimulation of cell surface thrombopoietin (TPO) receptors may increase the risk for hematologic malignancies.

Cataract formation or worsening was observed in clinical trials. Monitor regularly for signs and symptoms of cataracts; obtain ophthalmic exam at baseline and during therapy. Use with caution in patients at risk for cataracts (eg, advanced age, long-term glucocorticoid use). Allow at least 4 hours between dosing of eltrombopag and antacids, minerals (eg, iron, calcium, aluminum, magnesium, selenium, zinc), or foods high in calcium; may reduce eltrombopag levels. Patients of East-Asian ethnicity (eg, Chinese, Japanese, Korean, Taiwanese) may have greater drug exposure (compared to non-East Asians); therapy should be initiated with lower starting doses. Use with caution in renal impairment (any degree) and monitor closely; initial dosage adjustment is not necessary.

Indicated only when the degree of thrombocytopenia and clinical conditions increase the risk for bleeding; use the lowest dose necessary to achieve and maintain platelet count ≥50,000/mm^3. Do not use to normalize platelet counts. Discontinue if platelet count does not respond to a level to avoid clinically important bleeding after 4 weeks at the maximum recommended dose.

Adverse Reactions

>10%: Hepatic: Liver function tests abnormal (11%)

1% to 10%:

Central nervous system: Headache (10%), fatigue (4%)

Dermatologic: Rash (3%), alopecia (2%)

Gastrointestinal: Diarrhea (9%), nausea (4% to 9%), vomiting (6%), xerostomia (2%)
Genitourinary: Urinary tract infection (5%)
Hematologic: Myelofibrosis (Extension study: Grade ≤1: 93%; grade 2: 7%), rebound thrombocytopenia (8%)
Hepatic: Hyperbilirubinemia (6%), ALT increased (5% to 6%), AST increased (4%), alkaline phosphatase increased (2%)
Neuromuscular & skeletal: Myalgia (5%), back pain (3%), paresthesia (3%)
Ocular: Cataract (4% to 7%)
Respiratory: Upper respiratory infection (7%), oropharyngeal pain (4%), pharyngitis (4%)
Miscellaneous: Influenza (3%)

<1%, postmarketing, and/or case reports: Anemia, arthralgia, bone marrow collagen fiber deposits, bone marrow reticulin fiber deposits, constipation, hemorrhage (due to thrombocytopenia or rebound thrombocytopenia), non-Hodgkin's lymphoma, portal vein thrombosis, thrombotic/thromboembolic complications, vertigo, visual acuity decreased

Drug Interactions

Metabolism/Transport Effects **Substrate** of CYP1A2 (minor), CYP2C8 (minor), UGT1A1, UGT1A3; **Note:** Assignment of Major/Minor substrate status based on clinically relevant drug interaction potential; **Inhibits** CYP2C8 (moderate), SLCO1B1, UGT1A1, UGT1A3, UGT1A4, UGT1A6, UGT1A9, UGT2B15, UGT2B7

Avoid Concomitant Use There are no known interactions where it is recommended to avoid concomitant use.

Increased Effect/Toxicity

Eltrombopag may increase the levels/effects of: CYP2C8 Substrates; Deferiprone; OATP1B1/SLCO1B1 Substrates; Rosuvastatin

Decreased Effect

The levels/effects of Eltrombopag may be decreased by: Aluminum Hydroxide; Calcium Salts; Iron Salts; Magnesium Salts; Multivitamins/Minerals (with ADEK, Folate, Iron); Selenium; Sucralfate; Zinc Salts

Ethanol/Nutrition/Herb Interactions Food: Food, especially dairy products, may decrease the absorption of eltrombopag. Management: Take on an empty stomach at least 1 hour before or 2 hours after a meal. Separate intake from antacids, foods high in calcium, or minerals (eg, iron, calcium, aluminum, magnesium, selenium, zinc) by at least 4 hours.

Storage/Stability Store at room temperature of 25°C (77°F); excursions permitted to 15°C to 30°C (59°F to 86°F).

Mechanism of Action Thrombopoietin (TPO) nonpeptide agonist which increases platelet counts by binding to and activating the human TPO receptor. Activates intracellular signal transduction pathways to increase proliferation and differentiation of marrow progenitor cells. Does not induce platelet aggregation or activation.

Pharmacodynamics/Kinetics

Onset of action: Platelet count increase: Within 1-2 weeks
Peak platelet count increase: 14-16 days
Duration: Platelets return to baseline: 1-2 weeks after last dose
Protein binding: >99%
Metabolism: Extensive hepatic metabolism; via CYP 1A2, 2C8 oxidation and UGT 1A1, 1A3 glucuronidation
Bioavailability: ~52%

Half-life elimination: ~21-32 hours in healthy individuals; ~26-35 hours in patients with ITP

Time to peak, plasma: 2-6 hours

Excretion: Feces (~59%, 20% as unchanged drug, 21% glutathione-related conjugates); urine (31%, 20% glucuronide of the phenypyrazole moiety)

Dosing

Adult & Geriatric Note: Use the lowest dose to achieve and maintain platelet count ≥50,000/mm^3 as needed to reduce the risk of bleeding. Adjust dose based on platelet count response; initial platelet response generally occurs within 1-2 weeks. Discontinue if platelet count does not respond to a level that avoids clinically important bleeding after 4 weeks at the maximum daily dose of 75 mg.

Immune (idiopathic) thrombocytopenic purpura (ITP): Oral: Initial: 50 mg once daily; adjust dose to achieve and maintain platelet count ≥50,000/mm^3 to reduce the risk of bleeding; maximum dose: 75 mg once daily

Initial dosage for patients of East-Asian ethnicity (eg, Chinese, Japanese, Korean, Taiwanese): Oral: 25 mg once daily

Dosage adjustment recommendations (based on platelet response):

Platelet count <50,000/mm^3 (after at least 2 weeks): Increase daily dose by 25 mg (if taking 12.5 mg once daily, increase dose to 25 mg once daily prior to increasing the dose amount by 25 mg/day); maximum dose: 75 mg/day

Platelet count ≥200,000/mm^3 and ≤400,000/mm^3 (at any time): Reduce daily dose by 25 mg; reassess in 2 weeks

Platelet count >400,000/mm^3: Withhold dose; assess platelet count twice weekly; when platelet count <150,000/mm^3, resume with the daily dose reduced by 25 mg (if taking 25 mg once daily, resume with 12.5 mg once daily)

Platelet count >400,000/mm^3 after 2 weeks at the lowest dose: Discontinue treatment

Renal Impairment No initial dosage adjustment necessary.

Hepatic Impairment

Adjustment for hepatic impairment prior to initiating treatment:

Mild, moderate, or severe impairment (Child-Pugh classes A, B, or C): Initial dose: 25 mg once daily

Patients of East-Asian ethnicity with hepatic impairment (Child-Pugh classes A, B, or C): Initial dose: 12.5 mg once daily

Adjustment for hepatic impairment during treatment:

Hepatic impairment (Child-Pugh classes A, B, or C) after treatment initiation or after dose increases: Wait 3 weeks (instead of 2 weeks) prior to increasing dose for platelet count <50,000/mm^3

ALT levels ≥3 times the upper limit of normal (ULN) **and** which are progressive, persistent (≥4 weeks), accompanied by increased direct bilirubin, or accompanied by clinical signs of liver injury or evidence of hepatic decompensation: Discontinue treatment.

Adjustment for Toxicity

Excessive platelet response (platelets >400,000/mm^3 after 2 weeks at the lowest dose): Discontinue treatment.

New or worsening cellular abnormalities or cytopenias: Discontinue treatment.

Administration Administer on an empty stomach, 1 hour before or 2 hours after a meal. Do not administer concurrently with antacids, foods high in calcium, or minerals (eg, iron, calcium, aluminum, magnesium, selenium, zinc); separate by at least 4 hours. Do not administer more than one dose within 24 hours.

Monitoring Parameters Liver tests, including ALT, AST, and bilirubin (baseline, every 2 weeks during dosage titration, then monthly; evaluate abnormal liver function tests within 3-5 days; monitor weekly if retreating [not recommended] after therapy interruption for hepatotoxicity); bilirubin fractionation (for elevated bilirubin); CBC with differential and platelet count (weekly at initiation and during dosage titration, then monthly when stable; after cessation, monitor weekly for ≥4 weeks); peripheral blood smear (baseline and monthly when stable), bone marrow biopsy with staining for fibrosis (if peripheral blood smear reveals abnormality); ophthalmic exam (baseline and during treatment)

Dietary Considerations Take on an empty stomach (1 hour before or 2 hours after a meal). Food, especially dairy products, may decrease the absorption of eltrombopag; allow at least 4 hours between dosing of eltrombopag and polyvalent cation intake (eg, dairy products, calcium-rich foods, multivitamins with minerals).

Additional Information Restricted access to Promacta® was previously a REMS requirement via the Promacta® Cares™ program. Patients, prescribers, and pharmacies were required to be enrolled in this program. However, the FDA eliminated this REMS requirement in December 2011. There is currently no restricted access to obtaining Promacta®.

Product Availability

Promacta® 12.5 mg tablets (new strength): FDA approved December 2011; expected availability currently unknown.

Product labeling for Promacta® has also been updated to include dosage adjustment recommendations utilizing the new 12.5 mg strength.

Medication Guide Available Yes

Dosage Forms Excipient information presented when available (limited, particularly for generics); consult specific product labeling.

Tablet, oral:

Promacta®: 12.5 mg, 25 mg, 50 mg, 75 mg

References

Bussel JB, Cheng G, Saleh MN, et al, "Eltrombopag for the Treatment of Chronic Idiopathic Thrombocytopenic Purpura," *N Engl J Med*, 2007, 357(22):2237-47.

Bussel JB, Provan D, Shamsi T, et al, "Effect of Eltrombopag on Platelet Counts and Bleeding During Treatment of Chronic Idiopathic Thrombocytopenic Purpura: A Randomised, Double-Blind, Placebo-Controlled Trial," *Lancet*, 2009, 373(9664):641-8.

Cheng G, Saleh MN, Marcher C, et al, "Eltrombopag for Management of Chronic Immune Thrombocytopenia (RAISE): A 6-Month, Randomised, Phase 3 Study," *Lancet*, 2011, 377 (9763):393-402.

Pecci A, Gresele P, Klersy C, et al, "Eltrombopag for the Treatment of the Inherited Thrombocytopenia Deriving From MYH9 Mutations," *Blood*, 2010, 116(26):5832-7.

◆ **Eltrombopag Olamine** *see* Eltrombopag *on page* *494*

◆ **Emcyt®** *see* Estramustine *on page* *535*

◆ **Emend®** *see* Aprepitant *on page* *118*

◆ **Emend® IV (Can)** *see* Fosaprepitant *on page* *643*

◆ **Emend® for Injection** *see* Fosaprepitant *on page* *643*

◆ **EMLA®** *see* Lidocaine and Prilocaine *on page* *894*

◆ **Emo-Cort® (Can)** *see* Hydrocortisone (Topical) *on page* *719*

Enoxaparin (ee noks a PA rin)

Related Information

Venous Thromboembolism in the Cancer Patient *on page 1883*

Brand Names: U.S. Lovenox®

Brand Names: Canada Enoxaparin Injection; Lovenox®; Lovenox® HP

Index Terms Enoxaparin Sodium

Generic Availability (U.S.) Yes

Pharmacologic Category Low Molecular Weight Heparin

Use

Acute coronary syndromes: Unstable angina (UA), non-ST-elevation (NSTEMI), and ST-elevation myocardial infarction (STEMI)

DVT prophylaxis: Following hip or knee replacement surgery, abdominal surgery, or in medical patients with severely-restricted mobility during acute illness who are at risk for thromboembolic complications

DVT treatment (acute): Inpatient treatment (patients with and without pulmonary embolism) and outpatient treatment (patients without pulmonary embolism)

Note: High-risk patients include those with one or more of the following risk factors: >40 years of age, obesity, general anesthesia lasting >30 minutes, malignancy, history of deep vein thrombosis or pulmonary embolism

Unlabeled Use Prophylaxis and treatment of thromboembolism in children; anticoagulant bridge therapy during temporary interruption of vitamin K antagonist therapy in patients at high risk for thromboembolism; DVT prophylaxis following moderate-risk general surgery, major gynecologic surgery and following higher-risk general surgery for cancer; management of venous thromboembolism (VTE) during pregnancy; anticoagulant used during percutaneous coronary intervention (PCI)

Labeled Contraindications Hypersensitivity to enoxaparin, heparin, or any component of the formulation; thrombocytopenia associated with a positive *in vitro* test for antiplatelet antibodies in the presence of enoxaparin; hypersensitivity to pork products; active major bleeding; not for I.M. use

Note: Use of enoxaparin in patients with current heparin-induced thrombocytopenia (HIT) or HIT with thrombosis is **not** recommended and considered contraindicated due to high cross-reactivity to heparin-platelet factor-4 antibody (Guyatt [ACCP], 2012; Warkentin, 1999).

Pregnancy Risk Factor B

Lactation Excretion in breast milk unknown/not recommended

Warnings/Precautions **[U.S. Boxed Warning]: Spinal or epidural hematomas, including subsequent paralysis, may occur with recent or anticipated neuraxial anesthesia (epidural or spinal anesthesia) or spinal puncture in patients anticoagulated with LMWH or heparinoids.** Consider risk versus benefit prior to spinal procedures; risk is increased by the use of concomitant agents which may alter hemostasis, the use of indwelling epidural catheters for analgesia, a history of spinal deformity or spinal surgery, as well as a history of traumatic or repeated epidural or spinal punctures. Patient should be observed closely for bleeding and signs and symptoms of neurological impairment if therapy is administered during or immediately following diagnostic lumbar puncture, epidural anesthesia, or spinal anesthesia.

Do not administer intramuscularly. Discontinue use 12-24 hours prior to CABG and dose with unfractionated heparin per institutional practice (Jneid, 2012). Not recommended for thromboprophylaxis in patients with prosthetic heart valves (especially pregnant women). Not to be used interchangeably (unit for unit) with heparin or any other low molecular weight heparins. Monitor patient closely for signs or symptoms of bleeding. Certain patients are at increased risk of bleeding. Risk factors include bacterial endocarditis; congenital or acquired bleeding disorders; active ulcerative or angiodysplastic GI diseases; severe uncontrolled hypertension; history of hemorrhagic stroke; use shortly after brain, spinal, or ophthalmic surgery; patients treated concomitantly with platelet inhibitors; recent GI bleeding; thrombocytopenia or platelet defects; severe liver disease; hypertensive or diabetic retinopathy; or in patients undergoing invasive procedures. Cases of enoxaparin-induced thrombocytopenia and thrombosis (similar to heparin-induced thrombocytopenia [HIT]), some complicated by organ infarction, limb ischemia, or death, have been observed. Use with extreme caution or avoid in patients with history of HIT, especially if administered within 100 days of HIT episode (Warkentin, 2001); monitor platelet count closely. Use is contraindicated in patients with thrombocytopenia associated with a positive *in vitro* test for antiplatelet antibodies in the presence of enoxaparin. Discontinue therapy and consider alternative treatment if platelets are <100,000/mm^3 and/or thrombosis develops. Use caution in patients with congenital or drug-induced thrombocytopenia or platelet defects. Risk of bleeding may be increased in women <45 kg and in men <57 kg. Use caution in patients with renal failure; dosage adjustment needed if Cl_{cr} <30 mL/minute. Use with caution in the elderly (delayed elimination may occur); dosage alteration/adjustment may be required (eg, omission of I.V. bolus in acute STEMI in patients ≥75 years of age). Monitor for hyperkalemia; can cause hyperkalemia possibly by suppressing aldosterone production. Multiple-dose vials contain benzyl alcohol (use caution in pregnant women). In neonates, large amounts of benzyl alcohol (>100 mg/kg/day) have been associated with fatal toxicity (gasping syndrome).

There is no consensus for adjusting/correcting the weight-based dosage of LMWH for patients who are morbidly obese (BMI ≥40 kg/m^2). The American College of Chest Physicians Practice Guidelines suggest consulting with a pharmacist regarding dosing in bariatric surgery patients and other obese patients who may require higher doses of LMWH (Gould, 2012).

Adverse Reactions As with all anticoagulants, bleeding is the major adverse effect of enoxaparin. Hemorrhage may occur at virtually any site. Risk is dependent on multiple variables. At the recommended doses, single injections of enoxaparin do not significantly influence platelet aggregation or affect global clotting time (ie, PT or aPTT).

1% to 10%:

Central nervous system: Fever (5% to 8%), confusion, pain

Dermatologic: Erythema, bruising

Gastrointestinal: Nausea (3%), diarrhea

Hematologic: Hemorrhage (major, <1% to 4%; includes cases of intracranial, retroperitoneal, or intraocular hemorrhage; incidence varies with indication/population), thrombocytopenia (moderate 1%; severe 0.1% - see "**Note**" below), anemia (<2%)

Hepatic: ALT, increased, AST increased

Local: Injection site hematoma (9%), local reactions (irritation, pain, ecchymosis, erythema)

Renal: Hematuria (<2%)

<1% and/or postmarketing case reports (limited to important or life-threatening): Allergic reaction, anaphylactoid reaction, cutaneous vasculitis

(hypersensitive), eczematous plaques, hematoma (see note on "Spinal or epidural hematomas" below), hyperkalemia, hyperlipidemia, hypertriglyceridemia, intracranial hemorrhage (up to 0.8%), erythematous pruritic patches, pruritus, purpura, retroperitoneal bleeding, skin necrosis, thrombocytopenia with thrombosis, thrombocytosis, urticaria, vesicobullous rash

Note:

Spinal or epidural hematomas: Can occur following neuraxial anesthesia or spinal puncture, resulting in paralysis. Risk is increased in patients with indwelling epidural catheters or concomitant use of other drugs affecting hemostasis. Prosthetic valve thrombosis, including fatal cases, has been reported in pregnant women receiving enoxaparin as thromboprophylaxis.

Thrombocytopenia with thrombosis: Cases of heparin-induced thrombocytopenia (some complicated by organ infarction, limb ischemia, or death) have been reported.

Drug Interactions

Metabolism/Transport Effects None known.

Avoid Concomitant Use

Avoid concomitant use of Enoxaparin with any of the following: Omacetaxine; Rivaroxaban

Increased Effect/Toxicity

Enoxaparin may increase the levels/effects of: Anticoagulants; Collagenase (Systemic); Dabigatran Etexilate; Deferasirox; Drotrecogin Alfa (Activated); Ibritumomab; Omacetaxine; Palifermin; Rivaroxaban; Tositumomab and Iodine I 131 Tositumomab

The levels/effects of Enoxaparin may be increased by: 5-ASA Derivatives; Antiplatelet Agents; Dasatinib; Herbs (Anticoagulant/Antiplatelet Properties); Nonsteroidal Anti-Inflammatory Agents; Pentosan Polysulfate Sodium; Pentoxifylline; Prostacyclin Analogues; Salicylates; Thrombolytic Agents; Tipranavir; Vitamin E

Decreased Effect There are no known significant interactions involving a decrease in effect.

Ethanol/Nutrition/Herb Interactions Herb/Nutraceutical: Avoid cat's claw, dong quai, evening primrose, feverfew, garlic, ginger, ginkgo, red clover, horse chestnut, green tea, ginseng (all have additional antiplatelet activity).

Storage/Stability Store at 25°C (77°F); excursions permitted to 15°C to 30°C (59°F to 86°F); do not freeze.

Mechanism of Action Standard heparin consists of components with molecular weights ranging from 4000-30,000 daltons with a mean of 16,000 daltons. Heparin acts as an anticoagulant by enhancing the inhibition rate of clotting proteases by antithrombin III impairing normal hemostasis and inhibition of factor Xa. Low molecular weight heparins have a small effect on the activated partial thromboplastin time and strongly inhibit factor Xa. Enoxaparin is derived from porcine heparin that undergoes benzylation followed by alkaline depolymerization. The average molecular weight of enoxaparin is 4500 daltons which is distributed as (≤20%) 2000 daltons (≥68%) 2000-8000 daltons, and (≤15%) >8000 daltons. Enoxaparin has a higher ratio of antifactor Xa to antifactor IIa activity than unfractionated heparin.

Pharmacodynamics/Kinetics

Onset of action: Peak effect: SubQ: Antifactor Xa and antithrombin (antifactor IIa): 3-5 hours

Duration: 40 mg dose: Antifactor Xa activity: ~12 hours

Distribution: 4.3 L (based on antifactor Xa activity)

Protein binding: Does not bind to heparin binding proteins
Metabolism: Hepatic, to lower molecular weight fragments (little activity)
Half-life elimination, plasma: 2-4 times longer than standard heparin, independent of dose; based on anti-Xa activity: 4.5-7 hours
Excretion: Urine (40% of dose; 10% as active fragments)

Dosing

Adult One mg of enoxaparin is equal to 100 units of anti-Xa activity (World Health Organization First International Low Molecular Weight Heparin Reference Standard).

DVT prophylaxis: Note: In morbidly obese patients (BMI ≥40 kg/m^2), increasing the prophylactic dose by 30% may be appropriate for some indications (Nutescu, 2009). For bariatric surgery, dose increases may be >30% based on clinical trial data. SubQ:

Hip replacement surgery:

Twice-daily dosing: 30 mg every 12 hours, with initial dose within 12-24 hours after surgery, and every 12 hours for at least 10 days or until risk of DVT has diminished or the patient is adequately anticoagulated on warfarin. The American College of Chest Physicians recommends initiation ≥12 hours preoperatively **or** ≥12 hours postoperatively; extended duration of up to 35 days suggested (Guyatt, 2012).

Once-daily dosing: 40 mg once daily, with initial dose within 9-15 hours before surgery, and daily for at least 10 days (or up to 35 days postoperatively) or until risk of DVT has diminished or the patient is adequately anticoagulated on warfarin. The American College of Chest Physicians recommends initiation ≥12 hours preoperatively **or** ≥12 hours postoperatively; extended duration of up to 35 days suggested (Guyatt, 2012).

Knee replacement surgery: 30 mg every 12 hours, with initial dose within 12-24 hours after surgery, and every 12 hours for at least 10 days or until risk of DVT has diminished or the patient is adequately anticoagulated on warfarin. The American College of Chest Physicians recommends initiation ≥12 hours preoperatively **or** ≥12 hours postoperatively; extended duration of up to 35 days suggested (Guyatt, 2012).

Abdominal surgery: 40 mg once daily, with initial dose given 2 hours prior to surgery; continue until risk of DVT has diminished (usually 7-10 days).

Bariatric surgery: Roux-en-Y gastric bypass: Appropriate dosing strategies have not been clearly defined (Borkgren-Okonek, 2008; Scholten, 2002):

BMI ≤50 kg/m^2: 40 mg every 12 hours

BMI >50 kg/m^2: 60 mg every 12 hours

Note: Bariatric surgery guidelines suggest initiation 30-120 minutes before surgery and postoperatively until patient is fully mobile (Mechanick, 2009). Alternatively, limiting administration to the postoperative period may reduce perioperative bleeding.

Medical patients with severely-restricted mobility during acute illness: 40 mg once daily; continue until risk of DVT has diminished (usually 6-11 days).

Prevention of recurrent venous thromboembolism in pregnancy (unlabeled use): 40 mg once daily. Therapy should continue for 6 weeks postpartum in high-risk women (Bates, 2012).

DVT treatment (acute): SubQ: **Note:** Start warfarin on the first or second treatment day and continue enoxaparin until INR is ≥2 for at least 24 hours (usually 5-7 days) (Guyatt, 2012).

Inpatient treatment (with or without pulmonary embolism): 1 mg/kg/dose every 12 hours or 1.5 mg/kg once daily.

Outpatient treatment (without pulmonary embolism): 1 mg/kg/dose every 12 hours.

Obesity: Use actual body weight to calculate dose; dose capping not recommended; use of twice daily dosing preferred (Nutescu, 2009)

Pregnant women: 1 mg/kg/dose every 12 hours. Discontinue ≥24 hours prior to the induction of labor or cesarean section. Enoxaparin therapy may be substituted with heparin near term. Continue anticoagulation therapy for ≥6 weeks postpartum (minimum duration of therapy: 3 months). LMWH or heparin therapy is preferred over warfarin during pregnancy (Bates, 2012).

Percutaneous coronary intervention (PCI), adjunctive therapy (unlabeled use): I.V.: In patients treated with multiple doses of enoxaparin undergoing PCI, if PCI occurs within 8 hours after the last SubQ enoxaparin dose, no additional dosing is needed. If PCI occurs 8-12 hours after the last SubQ enoxaparin dose or the patient received only 1 therapeutic SubQ dose (eg, 1 mg/kg), a single I.V. dose of 0.3 mg/kg should be administered. If PCI occurs >12 hours after the last SubQ dose, it is prudent to use an established anticoagulation regimen (eg, unfractionated heparin or bivalirudin) (Levine, 2011).

If patient has not received prior anticoagulant therapy: 0.5-0.75 mg/kg bolus dose (Levine, 2011)

ST-elevation MI (STEMI):

Patients <75 years of age: Initial: 30 mg I.V. single bolus plus 1 mg/kg (maximum 100 mg for the first 2 doses only) SubQ every 12 hours. The first SubQ dose should be administered with the I.V. bolus. Maintenance: After first 2 doses, administer 1 mg/kg SubQ every 12 hours.

Patients ≥75 years of age: Initial: SubQ: 0.75 mg/kg every 12 hours (**Note:** No I.V. bolus is administered in this population); a maximum dose of 75 mg is recommended for the first 2 doses. Maintenance: After first 2 doses, administer 0.75 mg/kg SubQ every 12 hours

Obesity: Use weight-based dosing; a maximum dose of 100 mg is recommended for the first 2 doses (Nutescu, 2009)

Additional notes on STEMI treatment: Therapy was continued for 8 days or until hospital discharge; optimal duration not defined. Unless contraindicated, all patients received aspirin (75-325 mg daily) in clinical trials. In patients with STEMI receiving thrombolytics, initiate enoxaparin dosing between 15 minutes before and 30 minutes after fibrinolytic therapy.

Unstable angina or non-ST-elevation MI (NSTEMI): 1 mg/kg every 12 hours in conjunction with oral aspirin therapy (100-325 mg once daily); continue until clinical stabilization (a minimum of at least 2 days)

Obesity: Use actual body weight to calculate dose; dose capping not recommended (Nutescu, 2009)

Geriatric SubQ: Refer to adult dosing. Increased incidence of bleeding with doses of 1.5 mg/kg/day or 1 mg/kg every 12 hours; injection-associated bleeding and serious adverse reactions are also increased in the elderly. Careful attention should be paid to elderly patients, particularly those <45 kg. **Note:** Dosage alteration/adjustment may be required.

Pediatric One mg of enoxaparin is equal to 100 units of anti-Xa activity (World Health Organization First International Low Molecular Weight Heparin Reference Standard).

Thromboembolism (unlabeled use; Monagle, 2012): SubQ:

Infants <2 months: Initial:

Prophylaxis: 0.75 mg/kg every 12 hours

Treatment: 1.5 mg/kg every 12 hours

Infants >2 months and Children ≤18 years: Initial:
Prophylaxis: 0.5 mg/kg every 12 hours
Treatment: 1 mg/kg every 12 hours
Maintenance: See **Dosage Titration** table:

Enoxaparin Pediatric Dosage Titration[1]

Anti-Xa Result	Dose Titration	Time to Repeat Anti-Xa Measurement
<0.35 units/mL	Increase dose by 25%	4 h after next dose
0.35-0.49 units/mL	Increase dose by 10%	4 h after next dose
0.5-1 unit/mL	Keep same dosage	Next day, then 1 wk later, then monthly (4 h after dose)
1.1-1.5 units/mL	Decrease dose by 20%	Before next dose
1.6-2 units/mL	Hold dose for 3 h and decrease dose by 30%	Before next dose, then 4 h after next dose
>2 units/mL	Hold all doses until anti-Xa is 0.5 units/mL, then decrease dose by 40%	Before next dose and every 12 h until anti-Xa <0.5 units/mL

[1]Nomogram to be used for treatment dosing.

Modified from Duplaga BA, et al, "Dosing and Monitoring of Low-Molecular-Weight Heparins in Special Populations," *Pharmacotherapy*, 2001, 21(2):218-34.

Renal Impairment

Cl_{cr} ≥30 mL/minute: No specific adjustment recommended (per manufacturer); monitor closely for bleeding.

Cl_{cr} <30 mL/minute:

DVT prophylaxis in abdominal surgery, hip replacement, knee replacement, or in medical patients during acute illness: SubQ: 30 mg once daily

DVT treatment (inpatient or outpatient treatment in conjunction with warfarin): SubQ: 1 mg/kg once daily

STEMI:

<75 years: Initial: I.V.: 30 mg as a single dose with the first dose of the SubQ maintenance regimen administered at the same time as the I.V. bolus; Maintenance: SubQ: 1 mg/kg every 24 hours

≥75 years of age: Omit I.V. bolus; Maintenance: SubQ: 1 mg/kg every 24 hours

Unstable angina, NSTEMI: SubQ: 1 mg/kg once daily

Dialysis: Enoxaparin has not been FDA approved for use in dialysis patients. It's elimination is primarily via the renal route. Serious bleeding complications have been reported with use in patients who are dialysis dependent or have severe renal failure. LMWH administration at fixed doses without monitoring has greater unpredictable anticoagulant effects in patients with chronic kidney disease. If used, dosages should be reduced and anti-Xa levels frequently monitored, as accumulation may occur with repeated doses. Many clinicians would not use enoxaparin in this population especially without timely anti-Xa levels.

Hemodialysis: Supplemental dose is not necessary.

Peritoneal dialysis: Significant drug removal is unlikely based on physiochemical characteristics.

Administration Do **not** administer I.M.; should be administered by deep SubQ injection to the left or right anterolateral and left or right posterolateral abdominal wall. A single dose may be administered I.V. as part of treatment for ST-elevation myocardial infarction (STEMI) to patients <75 years of age; no I.V. bolus is given to patients ≥75 years of age. To avoid loss of drug from the 30 mg and 40 mg syringes, do not expel the air bubble from the syringe prior to injection. In order to minimize bruising, do not rub injection site. An automatic injector (Lovenox EasyInjector™) is available with the 30 mg and 40 mg syringes to aid the patient with self-injections. **Note:** Enoxaparin is available in 100 mg/mL and 150 mg/mL concentrations.

To convert from I.V. unfractionated heparin (UFH) infusion to SubQ enoxaparin (Nutescu, 2007): Calculate specific dose for enoxaparin based on indication, discontinue UFH and begin enoxaparin within 1 hour.

To convert from SubQ enoxaparin to I.V. UFH infusion (Nutescu, 2007): Discontinue enoxaparin, calculate specific dose for I.V. UFH infusion based on indication, omit heparin bolus/loading dose:

Converting from SubQ enoxaparin dosed every 12 hours: Start I.V. UFH infusion 10-11 hours after last dose of enoxaparin

Converting from SubQ enoxaparin dosed every 24 hours: Start I.V. UFH infusion 22-23 hours after last dose of enoxaparin

Monitoring Parameters Platelets, occult blood, anti-Xa levels, serum creatinine; monitoring of PT and/or aPTT is not necessary. Routine monitoring of anti-Xa levels is not required, but has been utilized in patients with obesity and/or renal insufficiency. Monitoring anti-Xa levels is recommended in pregnant women receiving therapeutic doses of enoxaparin or when receiving enoxaparin for the prevention of thromboembolism with mechanical heart valves (Guyatt, 2012). For patients >190 kg, if anti-Xa monitoring is available, adjusting dose based on anti-Xa levels is recommended; if anti-Xa monitoring is unavailable, reduce dose if bleeding occurs (Nutescu, 2009).

Dosage Forms Excipient information presented when available (limited, particularly for generics); consult specific product labeling.

Injection, solution, as sodium: 100 mg/mL (3 mL)

Lovenox®: 100 mg/mL (3 mL) [contains benzyl alcohol; vial]

Injection, solution, as sodium [preservative free]: 30 mg/0.3 mL (0.3 mL); 40 mg/0.4 mL (0.4 mL); 60 mg/0.6 mL (0.6 mL); 80 mg/0.8 mL (0.8 mL); 100 mg/mL (1 mL); 120 mg/0.8 mL (0.8 mL); 150 mg/mL (1 mL)

Lovenox®: 30 mg/0.3 mL (0.3 mL); 40 mg/0.4 mL (0.4 mL); 60 mg/0.6 mL (0.6 mL); 80 mg/0.8 mL (0.8 mL); 100 mg/mL (1 mL); 120 mg/0.8 mL (0.8 mL); 150 mg/mL (1 mL) [prefilled syringe]

References

Antman EM, Morrow DA, McCabe CH, et al, "Enoxaparin Versus Unfractionated Heparin With Fibrinolysis for ST-Elevation Myocardial Infarction," *N Engl J Med*, 2006, 354(14):1477-88.

Bates SM, Greer IA, Middeldorp S, et al, "VTE, Thrombophilia, Antithrombotic Therapy and Pregnancy: Antithrombotic Therapy and Prevention of Thrombosis, 9th ed: American College of Chest Physicians Evidence-Based Clinical Practice Guidelines," *Chest*, 2012, 141(2 Suppl): e691-736S.

Borkgren-Okonek MJ, Hart RW, Pantano JE, et al, "Enoxaparin Thromboprophylaxis in Gastric Bypass Patients: Extended Duration, Dose Stratification, and Antifactor Xa Activity," *Surg Obes Relat Dis*, 2008, 4(5):625-31.

Duplaga BA, Rivers CW, and Nutescu E, "Dosing and Monitoring of Low-Molecular-Weight Heparins in Special Populations," *Pharmacotherapy*, 2001, 21(2):218-34.

Farooq V, Hegarty J, Chandrasekar T, et al, "Serious Adverse Incidents With the Usage of Low Molecular Weight Heparins in Patients With Chronic Kidney Disease," *Am J Kidney Dis*, 2004, 43 (3):531-7.

Geerts WH, Bergqvist D, Pineo GF, et al, "Prevention of Venous Thromboembolism: American College of Chest Physicians Evidence-Based Clinical Practice Guidelines (8th Edition)," *Chest*, 2008, 133(6 Suppl):381-453.

Gould MK, Garcia DA, Wren SM, et al, "Prevention of VTE in Nonorthopedic Surgical Patients: Antithrombotic Therapy and Prevention of Thrombosis, 9th ed: American College of Chest Physicians Evidence-Based Clinical Practice Guidelines," *Chest*, 2012, 141(2 Suppl):e227-77.

Guyatt GH, Akl EA, Crowther M, et al, "Executive Summary: Antithrombotic Therapy and Prevention of Thrombosis, 9th ed: American College of Chest Physicians Evidence-Based Clinical Practice Guidelines," *Chest*, 2012, 141(2 Suppl):7-47.

Hirsh J, Dalen J, and Guyatt G, et al, "The Sixth (2000) ACCP Guidelines for Antithrombotic Therapy for Prevention and Treatment of Thrombosis. American College of Chest Physicians," *Chest*, 2001, 119(1 Suppl):346-7.

Hirsh J, Guyatt G, Albers GW, et al, "Executive Summary: American College of Chest Physicians Evidence-Based Clinical Practice Guidelines (8th Edition)," *Chest*, 2008, 133(6 Suppl):71-109.

Jaff MR, McMurtry MS, Archer SL, et al, "Management of Massive and Submassive Pulmonary Embolism, Iliofemoral Deep Vein Thrombosis, and Chronic Thromboembolic Pulmonary Hypertension: A Scientific Statement from the American Heart Association," *Circulation*, 2011, 123 (16):1788-830.

King SB 3rd, Smith SC Jr, Hirshfeld JW JR, et al, "2007 Focused Update of the ACC/AHA/SCAI 2005 Guideline Update for Percutaneous Coronary Intervention. A Report of the American College of Cardiology/American Heart Association Task Force on Practice Guidelines: 2007 Writing Group to Review New Evidence and Update the ACC/AHA/SCAI 2005 Guideline Update for Percutaneous Coronary Intervention, Writing on Behalf of the 2005 Writing Committee," *Circulation*, 2008, 117(2):261-95.

Levine GN, Bates ER, Blankenship JC, et al, "2011 ACCF/AHA/SCAI Guideline for Percutaneous Coronary Intervention: A Report of the American College of Cardiology Foundation/American Heart Association Task Force on Practice Guidelines and the Society for Cardiovascular Angiography and Interventions," *Circulation*, 2011, 124(23):e574-651.

Mechanick JI, Kushner RF, Sugerman HJ, et al, "American Association of Clinical Endocrinologists, The Obesity Society, and American Society for Metabolic & Bariatric Surgery Medical Guidelines for Clinical Practice for the Perioperative Nutritional, Metabolic, and Nonsurgical Support of the Bariatric Surgery Patient," *Obesity*, 2009, 17(Suppl 1):1-70.

Monagle P, Chalmers E, Chan A, et al, "Antithrombotic Therapy in Neonates and Children: American College of Chest Physicians Evidence-Based Clinical Practice Guidelines (8th Edition)," *Chest*, 2008, 133(6 Suppl):887-968.

Monagle P, Chan A, Goldenberg NA, et al, "Antithrombotic Therapy in Neonates and Children: American College of Chest Physicians Evidence-Based Clinical Practice Guidelines (9th Edition)," *Chest*, 2012, 141(2 Suppl):e737-801.

Nutescu EA and Dager W, "Heparin, Low Molecular Weight Heparin, and Fondaparinux," *Managing Anticoagulation Patients in the Hospital*, Gulseth M ed, American Society of Health-System Pharmacists®, Bethesda, MD: 2007, 181.

Nutescu EA, Spinler SA, Wittkowsky A, et al, "Low-Molecular-Weight Heparins in Renal Impairment and Obesity: Available Evidence and Clinical Practice Recommendations Across Medical and Surgical Settings," *Ann Pharmacother*, 2009, 43(6):1064-83.

Sanderink GJ, Le Liboux A, Jariwala N, et al, "The Pharmacokinetic and Pharmacodynamics of Enoxaparin in Obese Volunteers," *Clin Pharmacol Ther*, 2002, 72(3):308-18.

Scholten DJ, Hoedema RM, and Scholten SE, "A Comparison of Two Different Prophylactic Dose Regimens of Low Molecular Weight Heparin in Bariatric Surgery," *Obes Surg*, 2002, 12(1):19-24.

◆ **Enoxaparin Injection (Can)** *see* Enoxaparin *on page* 499

◆ **Enoxaparin Sodium** *see* Enoxaparin *on page* 499

◆ **Entertainer's Secret® [OTC]** *see* Saliva Substitute *on page* 1266

Enzalutamide (en za LOO ta mide)

Brand Names: U.S. Xtandi®

Index Terms MDV3100

Generic Availability (U.S.) No

Pharmacologic Category Antiandrogen; Antineoplastic Agent, Antiandrogen

Use Treatment of metastatic, castration-resistant prostate cancer in patients previously treated with docetaxel

Labeled Contraindications Pregnancy

Pregnancy Risk Factor X

Lactation Excretion unknown/not recommended

Warnings/Precautions Hazardous agent: Use appropriate precautions for handling and disposal. Seizures were observed in a clinical trial (onset: ~1-20 months after treatment initiation). Therapy was permanently discontinued and patients were not rechallenged; seizures resolved upon therapy cessation. Patients with predisposing factors for seizure were excluded from the trial; factors include seizure history, underlying brain injury with loss of consciousness, transient ischemic attack within the past 12 months, cerebral vascular accident, brain metastases, brain arteriovenous malformation, or the use of concomitant medications which may lower the seizure threshold. Enzalutamide should be used with caution in patients with a history of seizure disorders or other predisposing factors. Enzalutamide may cause hypospermatogenesis and may impair male fertility. Androgen-deprivation therapy may increase the risk of cardiovascular disease (Levine, 2010).

Enzalutamide is a strong CYP3A4 and moderate CYP2C9 and CYP2C19 inducer; avoid concomitant use with narrow therapeutic index medications metabolized by CYP3A4, CYP2C9, and CYP2C19. If possible, avoid concomitant administration with moderate and strong CYP3A4 inducers (may reduce enzalutamide plasma concentrations). Avoid coadministration with strong CYP2C8 inhibitors; if concomitant use is necessary, reduce enzalutamide dose. Avoid coadministration with strong and moderate CYP2C8 inducers. If concomitant administration with warfarin cannot be avoided, additional INR monitoring is recommended.

Adverse Reactions

>10%:

Cardiovascular: Peripheral edema (15%)

Central nervous system: Fatigue (51%), headache (12%)

Endocrine & metabolic: Hot flashes (20%)

Gastrointestinal: Diarrhea (22%)

Hematologic: Neutropenia (15%; grades 3/4: 1%)

Neuromuscular & skeletal: Back pain (26%), arthralgia (21%), musculoskeletal pain (15%)

Respiratory: Upper respiratory tract infection (11%)

1% to 10%:

Cardiovascular: Hypertension (6%)

Central nervous system: Dizziness (10%), insomnia (9%), anxiety (7%), hypoesthesia (4%), mental impairment (4%), hallucinations (2%)

Dermatologic: Dry skin (4%), pruritus (4%)

Genitourinary: Hematuria (7%), pollakiuria (5%)

Hepatic: Bilirubin increased (3%)

Neuromuscular & skeletal: Muscle weakness (10%), paresthesia (7%), falling (5%), fractures (4%), stiffness (3%)

Respiratory: Lower respiratory tract infection (9%), epistaxis (3%)

Miscellaneous: Infection (≤6%; including sepsis)

<1%: Seizures

Drug Interactions

Metabolism/Transport Effects **Substrate** of CYP2C8 (major), CYP3A4 (major); **Note:** Assignment of Major/Minor substrate status based on clinically relevant drug interaction potential; **Inhibits** P-glycoprotein; **Induces** CYP2C19 (weak/moderate), CYP2C9 (weak/moderate), CYP3A4 (strong)

Avoid Concomitant Use

Avoid concomitant use of Enzalutamide with any of the following: Alfentanil; Axitinib; Bortezomib; Bosutinib; Crizotinib; CycloSPORINE (Systemic); CYP2C8 Inducers (Strong); CYP2C8 Inhibitors (Strong); CYP3A4 Inducers

(Strong); Dienogest; Dihydroergotamine; Dronedarone; Ergotamine; Everolimus; FentaNYL; Fosphenytoin-Phenytoin; Lapatinib; Lurasidone; Mifepristone; Nilotinib; Nisoldipine; Pazopanib; Perampanel; Pimozide; Praziquantel; QuiNIDine; Ranolazine; Regorafenib; Rivaroxaban; Roflumilast; RomiDEPsin; Sirolimus; SORAfenib; St Johns Wort; Tacrolimus (Systemic); Ticagrelor; Tolvaptan; Toremifene; Vandetanib; VinCRIStine (Liposomal); Warfarin

Increased Effect/Toxicity

Enzalutamide may increase the levels/effects of: Ifosfamide

The levels/effects of Enzalutamide may be increased by: CYP2C8 Inhibitors (Moderate); CYP2C8 Inhibitors (Strong); CYP3A4 Inhibitors (Strong); Deferasirox; Mifepristone

Decreased Effect

Enzalutamide may decrease the levels/effects of: Alfentanil; Apixaban; ARIPiprazole; Axitinib; Bortezomib; Bosutinib; Brentuximab Vedotin; Crizotinib; CycloSPORINE (Systemic); CYP3A4 Substrates; Dasatinib; Dienogest; Dihydroergotamine; Dronedarone; Ergotamine; Everolimus; Exemestane; FentaNYL; Fosphenytoin-Phenytoin; Gefitinib; GuanFACINE; Ixabepilone; Lapatinib; Linagliptin; Lurasidone; Maraviroc; Mifepristone; NIFEdipine; Nilotinib; Nisoldipine; Pazopanib; Perampanel; Pimozide; Praziquantel; QuiNIDine; Ranolazine; Regorafenib; Rivaroxaban; Roflumilast; RomiDEPsin; Saxagliptin; Sirolimus; SORAfenib; SUNItinib; Tacrolimus (Systemic); Tadalafil; Ticagrelor; Tolvaptan; Toremifene; Ulipristal; Vandetanib; Vemurafenib; VinCRIStine (Liposomal); Warfarin; Zuclopenthixol

The levels/effects of Enzalutamide may be decreased by: CYP2C8 Inducers (Strong); CYP3A4 Inducers (Strong); Deferasirox; St Johns Wort; Tocilizumab

Storage/Stability Store at 20°C to 25°C (68°F to 77°F); excursions permitted to 15°C to 30°C (59°F to 86°F). Protect from moisture; keep bottle tightly closed.

Mechanism of Action Enzalutamide is a pure androgen receptor signaling inhibitor; unlike other antiandrogen therapies, it has no known agonistic properties. It inhibits androgen receptor nuclear translocation, DNA binding, and coactivator mobilization, leading to cellular apoptosis and decreased prostate tumor volume.

Pharmacodynamics/Kinetics

Absorption: Rapid

Distribution: 110 L

Protein binding: Parent drug: 97% to 98% to primarily albumin; active metabolite: 95% to plasma proteins

Metabolism: Primarily hepatic via CYP2C8 (responsible for formation of active metabolite N-desmethyl enzalutamide) and CYP3A4

Half-life elimination: 5.8 days (range: 2.8-10.2 days)

Time to peak: 1 hour (range: 0.5-3 hours)

Excretion: Urine (71%); feces (14%); primarily as inactive metabolite

Dosing

Adult & Geriatric Prostate cancer, metastatic, castration-resistant: Oral: 160 mg once daily

Dosage adjustment for concomitant strong CYP2C8 inhibitors: Avoid concomitant use if possible. If coadministration is necessary, reduce enzalutamide dose to 80 mg once daily. If the strong CYP2C8 inhibitor is discontinued, adjust the enzalutamide dose back up to the dose used prior to the initiation of the inhibitor.

Renal Impairment

Pre-existing mild-to-moderate impairment (Cl_{cr} 30-89 mL/minute): No initial dosage adjustment necessary.

Pre-existing severe impairment (Cl_{cr} <30 mL/minute), including end-stage renal disease: No dosage adjustment provided in manufacturer's labeling (has not been studied).

Hepatic Impairment

Pre-existing mild-to-moderate impairment (Child-Pugh class A or B): No dosage adjustment necessary.

Pre-existing severe impairment (Child-Pugh class C): No dosage adjustment provided in manufacturer's labeling (has not been studied).

Adjustment for Toxicity If ≥grade 3 toxicity occurs, withhold treatment for 1 week or until symptom(s) improve to ≤grade 2, then resume at same dose, or reduce dose to 120 mg or 80 mg once daily, if necessary.

Seizures: Discontinue treatment.

Combination Regimens

Prostate Cancer: Enzalutamide (Prostate Regimen) on page 1625

Administration May be administered with or without food; take at the same time each day. Swallow capsules whole; do not chew, dissolve, or open the capsules.

Monitoring Parameters Monitor for signs/symptoms of seizure, loss of consciousness, dizziness, and hallucinations; CBC with differential and liver function tests (baseline and periodic); additional INR monitoring (if on warfarin)

Dietary Considerations May be taken with or without food.

Dosage Forms Excipient information presented when available (limited, particularly for generics); consult specific product labeling.

Capsule, liquid filled, oral:

Xtandi®: 40 mg

References

Baskin-Bey ES, Shore ND, Barber K, et al, "TERRAIN: A Randomized, Double-Blind, Phase II Study Comparing MDV3100 With Bicalutamide (Bic) in Men With Metastatic Castrate-Resistant Prostate Cancer (CRPC)," *J Clin Oncol*, 2012, 30(Suppl): TPS4698 [abstract TPS4698 from 2012 ASCO Annual Meeting].

Higano CS, Beer TM, Taplin M, et al, "Antitumor Activity of MDV3100 in Pre- and Post-Docetaxel Advanced Prostate Cancer: Long-Term Follow-Up of a Phase I/II Study," *J Clin Oncol*, 2011, 29 (Suppl): 134 [abstract 134 from 2011 Genitourinary Cancers Symposium].

Levine GN, D'Amico AV, Berger P, et al, "Androgen-Deprivation Therapy in Prostate Cancer and Cardiovascular Risk: A Science Advisory From the American Heart Association, American Cancer Society, and American Urological Association: Endorsed by the American Society for Radiation Oncology," *Circulation*, 2010, 121(6):833-40.

Montgomery RB, Joshua A, Hannah AL, et al, "A Randomized, Open-Label, Phase II Study of MDV3100 Alone or in Combination With Leuprolide and Dutasteride as Neoadjuvant Therapy to Prostatectomy in Intermediate and High-Risk Prostate Cancer," *J Clin Oncol*, 2012, 30(Suppl): TPS4695 [abstract TPS4695 from 2012 ASCO Annual Meeting].

Mukherji D, Eichholz A, and De Bono JS, "Management of Metastatic Castration-Resistant Prostate Cancer: Recent Advances," *Drugs*, 2012, 72(8):1011-28.

Scher HI, Beer TM, Higano CS, et al, "Antitumour Activity of MDV3100 in Castration-Resistant Prostate Cancer: A Phase 1-2 Study," *Lancet*, 2010, 375(9724):1437-46.

Scher HI, Fizazi K, Saad F, et al, "Increased Survival With Enzalutamide in Prostate Cancer After Chemotherapy," *N Engl J Med*, 2012, 367(13):1187-977.

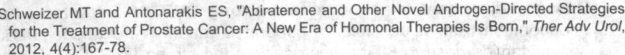

Schweizer MT and Antonarakis ES, "Abiraterone and Other Novel Androgen-Directed Strategies for the Treatment of Prostate Cancer: A New Era of Hormonal Therapies Is Born," *Ther Adv Urol*, 2012, 4(4):167-78.

◆ **EPEG** *see* Etoposide *on page 538*

◆ **Epidoxorubicin** *see* Epirubicin *on page 510*

◆ **Epipodophyllotoxin** *see* Etoposide *on page 538*

◆ **Epipodophyllotoxin** *see* Etoposide Phosphate *on page 548*

Epirubicin (ep i ROO bi sin)

Related Information

Chemotherapy and Cancer Treatment During Pregnancy *on page 1829*
Management of Chemotherapy-Induced Nausea and Vomiting *on page 1786*
Management of Drug Extravasations *on page 1800*
Safe Handling of Hazardous Drugs *on page 1904*

Brand Names: U.S. Ellence®

Brand Names: Canada Ellence®; Epirubicin for Injection; Epirubicin Hydrochloride Injection; Pharmorubicin®

Index Terms Epidoxorubicin; Epirubicin Hydrochloride; Pidorubicin; Pidorubicin Hydrochloride

Generic Availability (U.S.) Yes

Pharmacologic Category Antineoplastic Agent, Anthracycline

Use Adjuvant therapy component for primary breast cancer

Unlabeled Use Treatment of esophageal cancer, gastric cancer, soft tissue sarcoma, uterine sarcoma

Labeled Contraindications Hypersensitivity to epirubicin or any component of the formulation, other anthracyclines, or anthracenediones; previous anthracycline treatment up to maximum cumulative dose; severe myocardial insufficiency, severe arrhythmias; recent myocardial infarction

Pregnancy Risk Factor D

Lactation Excretion in breast milk unknown/not recommended

Warnings/Precautions Hazardous agent - use appropriate precautions for handling and disposal.

[U.S. Boxed Warning]: Myocardial toxicity, including heart failure (HF) may occur, particularly in patients who have received prior anthracyclines, prior or concomitant radiotherapy to the mediastinal/pericardial area, who have pre-existing cardiac disease (active or dormant), or with concomitant cardiotoxic medications. Cardiotoxicity may be concurrent or delayed (months to years after treatment). The risk of HF is ~0.9% at a cumulative dose of 550 mg/m^2, ~1.6% at a cumulative dose of 700 mg/m^2, and ~3.3% at a cumulative dose of 900 mg/m^2. Cardiotoxicity may also occur at lower cumulative doses or without risk factors. The risk of delayed cardiotoxicity increases more steeply with cumulative doses >900 mg/m^2 and this dose should be exceeded only with extreme caution. Acute toxicity, primarily sinus tachycardia and/or ECG abnormalities, including arrhythmia, and delayed toxicity, including decreased left ventricular ejection fraction (LVEF) and HF, have been described. Delayed toxicity usually develops late in the course of therapy or within 2-3 months after completion. Toxicity may be additive with other anthracyclines or anthracenediones, and may be increased in pediatric patients. Regular monitoring of LVEF and discontinuation at the first sign of impairment is recommended especially in patients with cardiac risk factors or impaired cardiac function. Discontinue treatment with signs of decreased LVEF. The half life of other cardiotoxic agents must be considered in sequential therapy; avoid epirubicin for up to 24 weeks after completing trastuzumab treatment.

[U.S. Boxed Warning]: May cause severe myelosuppression; neutropenia is the dose-limiting toxicity; severe thrombocytopenia or anemia may occur; obtain baseline and periodic blood counts. Patients should recover from myelosuppression due to prior chemotherapy treatment before beginning treatments. Thrombophlebitis and thromboembolic phenomena (including pulmonary embolism) have occurred.

[U.S. Boxed Warning]: Reduce dosage in patients with mild-to-moderate hepatic impairment (not recommended in severe hepatic impairment; predominantly hepatically eliminated) and in patients with serum creatinine >5 mg/dL (has not been studied in patients on dialysis); monitor hepatic and renal function at baseline and during treatment. May cause tumor lysis syndrome (TLS), although generally generally does not occur in patients with breast cancer; if TLS risk is suspected, consider monitoring serum uric acid, potassium, calcium, phosphate, and serum creatinine after initial administration; hydration and allopurinol prophylaxis may minimize potential TLS complications. Radiation recall (inflammatory) has been reported; epirubicin may have radiosensitizing activity. **[U.S. Boxed Warning]: Treatment with anthracyclines (including epirubicin) may increase the risk of secondary acute myelogenous leukemia (AML). AML is more common when given in combination with other antineoplastic agents, in patients who have received multiple courses of previous chemotherapy, or with escalated cumulative anthracycline doses (>720 mg/m² for epirubicin). In breast cancer patients, the risk for treatment related AML or myelodysplastic syndrome (MDS) was estimated at 0.3% at 3 years, 0.5% at 5 years, and 0.6% at 8 years after treatment.** The latency period for secondary leukemias may be short (1-3 years).

[U.S. Boxed Warning]: For I.V. administration only, severe local tissue damage and necrosis will result if extravasation occurs (vesicant); not for I.M. or SubQ use. Injection in to a small vein or repeated administration in the same vein may result in venous sclerosis. Women ≥70 years of age should be closely monitored for toxicity. **[U.S. Boxed Warning]: Should be administered under the supervision of an experienced cancer chemotherapy physician.** Epirubicin is emetogenic; consider prophylactic antiemetics prior to administration. Patients should recover from acute toxicities (stomatitis, myelosuppression, infections) prior to initiating treatment. Assess baseline labs (blood counts, bilirubin, ALT, AST, serum creatinine) and cardiac function (with LVEF). Prophylactic antibiotics should be administered with the CDF-120 regimen. Patients should not be immunized with live viral vaccines during or shortly after treatment. Inactivated vaccines may be administered (response may be diminished).

Adverse Reactions Percentages reported as part of combination chemotherapy regimens.

>10%:

Central nervous system: Lethargy (1% to 46%)

Dermatologic: Alopecia (70% to 96%)

Endocrine & metabolic: Amenorrhea (69% to 72%), hot flashes (5% to 39%)

Gastrointestinal: Nausea/vomiting (83% to 92%; grades 3/4: 22% to 25%), mucositis (9% to 59%; grades 3/4: ≤9%), diarrhea (7% to 25%)

Hematologic: Leukopenia (50% to 80%; grades 3/4: 2% to 59%), neutropenia (54% to 80%; grades 3/4: 11% to 67%; nadir: 10-14 days; recovery: by day 21), anemia (13% to 72%; grades 3/4: ≤6%), thrombocytopenia (5% to 49%; grades 3/4: ≤5%)
Local: Injection site reactions (3% to 20%; grades 3/4: <1%)
Ocular: Conjunctivitis (1% to 15%)
Miscellaneous: Infection (15% to 22%; grades 3/4: ≤2%)

1% to 10%:
Cardiovascular: LVEF decreased (asymptomatic; delayed: 1% to 2%), HF (0.4% to 1.5%)
Central nervous system: Fever (1% to 5%)
Dermatologic: Rash (1% to 9%), skin changes (1% to 5%)
Gastrointestinal: Anorexia (2% to 3%)
Hematologic: Neutropenic fever (grades 3/4: ≤6%)

<1%, postmarketing, case reports, and/or frequency not defined: Abdominal pain, acute lymphoid leukemia (ALL), acute myelogenous leukemia (AML), anaphylaxis, arrhythmia, ascites, atrioventricular block, bradycardia, bundle-branch block, cardiomyopathy, chills, dehydration, dyspnea, ECG abnormalities, esophagitis, hepatomegaly, hyperpigmentation (oral mucosa, nails, skin), hypersensitivity, myelodysplastic syndrome, myocarditis, neutropenic typhlitis, photosensitivity, premature menopause, premature ventricular contractions, pulmonary edema, pulmonary embolism, radiation recall, shock, sinus tachycardia, stomatitis, ST-T wave changes (nonspecific), tachyarrhythmias, thromboembolism, thrombophlebitis, toxic megacolon, transaminases increased, urine discoloration (red), urticaria, ventricular tachycardia

Drug Interactions

Metabolism/Transport Effects None known.

Avoid Concomitant Use

Avoid concomitant use of EPIrubicin with any of the following: BCG; Cimetidine; CloZAPine; Natalizumab; Pimecrolimus; Tacrolimus (Topical); Vaccines (Live)

Increased Effect/Toxicity

EPIrubicin may increase the levels/effects of: CloZAPine; Leflunomide; Natalizumab; Vaccines (Live)

The levels/effects of EPIrubicin may be increased by: Bevacizumab; Cimetidine; Denosumab; Pimecrolimus; Roflumilast; Tacrolimus (Topical); Taxane Derivatives; Trastuzumab

Decreased Effect

EPIrubicin may decrease the levels/effects of: BCG; Cardiac Glycosides; Coccidioidin Skin Test; Sipuleucel-T; Vaccines (Inactivated); Vaccines (Live)

The levels/effects of EPIrubicin may be decreased by: Cardiac Glycosides; Echinacea

Ethanol/Nutrition/Herb Interactions

Ethanol: Avoid ethanol (due to GI irritation).
Herb/Nutraceutical: Avoid black cohosh, dong quai in estrogen-dependent tumors.

Storage/Stability Protect from light.

Solution: Store intact vials refrigerated at 2°C to 8°C (36°F to 46°F); do not freeze. Product may "gel" at refrigerated temperatures; will return to slightly viscous solution after 2-4 hours at room temperature (15°C to 30°C). Discard unused solution from single dose vials within 24 hours of entry.

Lyophilized powder: Store at room temperature of 25°C (77°F); excursions permitted to 15°C to 30°C (59°F to 86°F). Reconstituted solutions are stable for 24 hours when stored at 2°C to 8°C (36°F to 46°F) or at room temperature.

Reconstitution Use appropriate precautions for handling and disposal. Reconstitute lyophilized powder with SWFI (25 mL for the 50 mg vial or 100 mL for the 200 mg vial) to a final concentration of 2 mg/mL.

Mechanism of Action Epirubicin is an anthracycline antineoplastic agent; known to inhibit DNA and RNA synthesis by steric obstruction after intercalating between DNA base pairs; active throughout entire cell cycle. Intercalation triggers DNA cleavage by topoisomerase II, resulting in cytocidal activity. Also inhibits DNA helicase, and generates cytotoxic free radicals.

Pharmacodynamics/Kinetics

Distribution: V_{ss}: 21-27 L/kg

Protein binding: ~77% to albumin

Metabolism: Extensively via hepatic and extrahepatic (including RBCs) routes

Half-life elimination: Triphasic; Mean terminal: 33 hours

Excretion: Feces (34% to 35%); urine (20% to 27%)

Dosing

Adult Note: Patients receiving 120 mg/m²/cycle as part of combination therapy (CEF-120 regimen) should also receive prophylactic therapy with sulfamethoxazole/trimethoprim or a fluoroquinolone. Details concerning dosing in combination regimens should also be consulted. Lower starting doses may be necessary for heavily pretreated patients, patients with pre-existing myelosuppression, or with bone marrow involvement.

Breast cancer, adjuvant treatment: I.V.: Usual dose: 100-120 mg/m² per 3- or 4-week treatment cycle as follows:

60 mg/m² on days 1 and 8 every 28 days for 6 cycles in combination with cyclophosphamide and fluorouracil (CEF-120 regimen; Levine, 2005) **or**

100 mg/m² on day 1 every 21 days for 6 cycles in combination with cyclophosphamide and fluorouracil (FEC-100 regimen; Bonneterre, 2005) **or**

Breast cancer (unlabeled regimens; as a part of combination chemotherapy): I.V.:

60 mg/m² on day 1 every 21 days for 8 cycles (EC regimen; Piccart, 2001) **or**

75 mg/m² on day 1 every 21 days for 4 cycles (FEC regimen; Buzdar, 2005) **or**

75 mg/m² on day 1 every 21 days for 8 cycles (EP and EC regimens; Langley, 2005) **or**

90 mg/m² on day 1 every 21 days for 4 or 6 cycles (FEC regimen ± paclitaxel; Martin, 2008) **or**

50 mg/m² on days 1 and 8 every 21-28 days for 6-9 cycles (CEF regimen; Ackland, 2001)

Esophageal cancer (unlabeled use; as part of combination chemotherapy): I.V.:

50 mg/m² on day 1 every 21 days for up to 8 cycles (ECF, ECX, EOF, and EOX regimens; Cunningham, 2008) **or**

50 mg/m² on day 1 every 21 days for 3 preoperative and 3 postoperative cycles (ECF regimen; Cunningham, 2006)

Gastric cancer (unlabeled use; as part of combination chemotherapy):

I.V.:

50 mg/m^2 on day 1 every 21 days for up to 8 cycles (ECF, ECX, EOF, and EOX regimens [Cunningham, 2008]; ECF regimen [Waters, 1999]) **or**

50 mg/m^2 on day 1 every 21 days for 3 preoperative and 3 postoperative cycles (ECF regimen; Cunningham, 2006)

Dosage modifications (breast cancer; labeled dosing):

Delay day 1 dose until platelets are ≥100,000/mm^3, ANC ≥1500/mm^3, and nonhematologic toxicities have recovered to ≤grade 1

Reduce day 1 dose in subsequent cycles to 75% of previous day 1 dose if patient experiences nadir platelet counts <50,000/mm^3, ANC <250/mm^3, neutropenic fever, or grade 3/4 nonhematologic toxicity during the previous cycle

For CEF-120 regimen, reduce day 8 dose to 75% of day 1 dose if platelet counts are 75,000-100,000/mm^3 and ANC is 1000-1499/mm^3; omit day 8 dose if platelets are <75,000/mm^3, ANC <1000/mm^3, or grade 3/4 nonhematologic toxicity

Dosage adjustment in bone marrow dysfunction: Heavily-treated patients, patients with pre-existing bone marrow depression or neoplastic bone marrow infiltration: Lower starting doses (75-90 mg/m^2) should be considered.

Geriatric Plasma clearance of epirubicin in elderly female patients was noted to be reduced by 35%. Although no initial dosage reduction is specifically recommended, particular care should be exercised in monitoring toxicity and adjusting subsequent dosage in elderly patients (particularly females >70 years of age).

Renal Impairment The manufacturer's labeling recommends lower doses (dose not specified) in patients with severe renal impairment (serum creatinine >5 mg/dL). Other sources (Aronoff, 2007) suggest no dosage adjustment is needed for Cl_{cr} <50 mL/minute.

Hepatic Impairment The manufacturer's labeling recommends the following adjustments (based on clinical trial information):

Bilirubin 1.2-3 mg/dL or AST 2-4 times the upper limit of normal: Administer 50% of recommended starting dose

Bilirubin >3 mg/dL or AST >4 times the upper limit of normal: Administer 25% of recommended starting dose

Severe hepatic impairment: Use is not recommended (has not been studied).

Combination Regimens

Breast cancer:

CEF on page 1556
Docetaxel-FEC on page 1611
Docetaxel-Trastuzumab-FEC on page 1616
FEC on page 1642
Vinorelbine-FEC on page 1773
Vinorelbine-Trastuzumab-FEC on page 1775

Esophageal cancer:

Epirubicin-Cisplatin-Capecitabine (Esophageal Cancer) on page 1626
Epirubicin-Cisplatin-Fluorouracil (Gastric/Esophageal Cancer) on page 1626
Epirubicin-Oxaliplatin-Capecitabine on page 1627
Epirubicin-Oxaliplatin-Fluorouracil (Esophageal Cancer) on page 1627

Gastric cancer:

Epirubicin-Cisplatin-Fluorouracil (Gastric/Esophageal Cancer) on page 1626

Epirubicin-Oxaliplatin-Capecitabine on page 1627

Rhabdomyosarcoma: CEV on page 1562

Administration I.V.: Infuse over 15-20 minutes or slow I.V. push; if lower doses due to dose reduction are administered, may reduce infusion time proportionally. Do not infuse over <3 minutes. Infuse into a free-flowing I.V. solution. Avoid the use of veins over joints or in extremities with compromised venous or lymphatic drainage. Monitor infusion site; avoid extravasation.

Emetic Potential

>90 mg/m^2: Very high (>90%)

≤90 mg/m^2: Moderate (30% to 90%)

Vesicant/Extravasation Risk Vesicant; see Management of Drug Extravasations on page 1800.

Monitoring Parameters Monitor injection site during infusion for possible extravasation or local reactions. Baseline and repeated measurements of CBC with differential, liver function tests, serum creatinine, ECG, and LVEF. The method used for assessment of LVEF (echocardiogram or MUGA) should be consistent during routine monitoring.

Dosage Forms Excipient information presented when available (limited, particularly for generics); consult specific product labeling.

Injection, powder for reconstitution, as hydrochloride: 50 mg

Injection, solution, as hydrochloride [preservative free]: 2 mg/mL (25 mL, 100 mL)

Ellence®: 2 mg/mL (25 mL, 100 mL)

References

Ackland SP, Anton A, Breitbach GP, et al, "Dose-Intensive Epirubicin-Based Chemotherapy is Superior to an Intensive Intravenous Cyclophosphamide, Methotrexate, and Fluorouracil Regimen in Metastatic Breast Cancer: A Randomized Multinational Study," *J Clin Oncol*, 2001, 19 (4):943-53.

Aronoff GR, Bennett WM, Berns JS, et al, *Drug Prescribing in Renal Failure: Dosing Guidelines for Adults and Children*, 5th ed. Philadelphia, PA: American College of Physicians; 2007, p 99.

Bonneterre J, Roche H, Kerbrat P, et al, "Epirubicin Increases Long-Term Survival in Adjuvant Chemotherapy of Patients With Poor-Prognosis, Node-Positive, Early Breast Cancer: 10-Year Follow-Up Results of the French Adjuvant Study Group 05 Randomized Trial," *J Clin Oncol*, 2005, 23(12):2686-93.

Burnell M, Levine MN, Chapman JA, et al, "Cyclophosphamide, Epirubicin, and Fluorouracil Versus Dose-Dense Epirubicin and Cyclophosphamide Followed by Paclitaxel Versus Doxorubicin and Cyclophosphamide Followed by Paclitaxel in Node-Positive or High-Risk Node-Negative Breast Cancer," *J Clin Oncol*, 2010, 28(1):77-82.

Buzdar A, Ibrahim NK, Francis D, et al, "Significantly Higher Pathologic Complete Remission Rate After Neoadjuvant Therapy With Trastuzumab, Paclitaxel, and Epirubicin Chemotherapy: Results of a Randomized Trial in Human Epidermal Growth Factor Receptor 2-Positive Operable Breast Cancer," *J Clin Oncol*, 2005, 23(16):3676-85.

Cunningham D, Allum WH, Stenning SP, et al, "Perioperative Chemotherapy Versus Surgery Alone for Resectable Gastroesophageal Cancer," *N Engl J Med*, 2006, 355(1):11-20.

Cunningham D, Starling N, Rao S, et al, "Capecitabine and Oxaliplatin for Advanced Esophagogastric Cancer," *N Engl J Med*, 2008, 358(1):36-46.

Eiermann W, Graf E, Ataseven B, et al, "Dose-Intensified Epirubicin Versus Standard-Dose Epirubicin/Cyclophosphamide Followed by CMF in Breast Cancer Patients With 10 or More Positive Lymph Nodes: Results of a Randomised Trial (GABG-IV E-93) - The German Adjuvant Breast Cancer Group," *Eur J Cancer*, 2010, 46(1):84-94.

Frustaci S, Gherlinzoni F, De Paoli A, et al, "Adjuvant Chemotherapy for Adult Soft Tissue Sarcomas of the Extremities and Girdles: Results of the Italian Randomized Cooperative Trial," *J Clin Oncol*, 2001, 19(5):1238-47.

Langley RE, Carmichael J, Jones AL, et al, "Phase III Trial of Epirubicin Plus Paclitaxel Compared With Epirubicin Plus Cyclophosphamide as First-Line Chemotherapy for Metastatic Breast Cancer: United Kingdom National Cancer Research Institute Trial AB01," *J Clin Oncol*, 2005, 23(33):8322-30.

Levine MN, Pritchard KI, Bramwell VH, et al, "Randomized Trial Comparing Cyclophosphamide, Epirubicin, and Fluorouracil With Cyclophosphamide, Methotrexate, and Fluorouracil in Premenopausal Women With Node-Positive Breast Cancer: Update of National Cancer Institute of Canada Clinical Trials Group Trial MA5," *J Clin Oncol*, 2005, 23(22):5166-70.

Martin M, Rodríguez-Lescure A, Ruiz A, et al, "Randomized Phase 3 Trial of Fluorouracil, Epirubicin, and Cyclophosphamide Alone or Followed by Paclitaxel for Early Breast Cancer," *J Natl Cancer Inst*, 2008, 100(11):805-14.

National Comprehensive Cancer Network® (NCCN), "Clinical Practice Guidelines in Oncology™: Uterine Neoplasms," Version 2.2012. Available at http://www.nccn.org/professionals/physician_gls/PDF/uterine.pdf

Peccatori FA, Azim HA Jr, Scarfone G, et al, "Weekly Epirubicin in the Treatment of Gestational Breast Cancer (GBC)," *Breast Cancer Res Treat*, 2009, 115(3):591-4.

Piccart MJ, Di Leo A, Beauduin M, et al, "Phase III Trial Comparing Two Dose Levels of Epirubicin Combined With Cyclophosphamide With Cyclophosphamide, Methotrexate, and Fluorouracil in Node-Positive Breast Cancer," *J Clin Oncol*, 2001, 19(12):3103-10

Ring AE, Smith IE, Jones A, et al, "Chemotherapy for Breast Cancer During Pregnancy: An 18-Year Experience From Five London Teaching Hospitals," *J Clin Oncol*, 2005, 23(18):4192-7.

Waters JS, Norman A, Cunningham D, et al, "Long-Term Survival After Epirubicin, Cisplatin and Fluorouracil for Gastric Cancer: Results of a Randomized Trial," *Br J Cancer*, 1999, 80 (1-2):269-72.

◆ **Epirubicin for Injection (Can)** *see* Epirubicin *on page* *510*

◆ **Epirubicin Hydrochloride** *see* Epirubicin *on page* *510*

◆ **Epirubicin Hydrochloride Injection (Can)** *see* Epirubicin *on page* *510*

◆ **EPO** *see* Epoetin Alfa *on page* *516*

Epoetin Alfa (e POE e tin AL fa)

Brand Names: U.S. Epogen®; Procrit®

Brand Names: Canada Eprex®

Index Terms *r*HuEPO; *r*HuEPO-α; EPO; Erythropoiesis-Stimulating Agent (ESA); Erythropoietin

Generic Availability (U.S.) No

Pharmacologic Category Colony Stimulating Factor; Erythropoiesis-Stimulating Agent (ESA); Growth Factor; Recombinant Human Erythropoietin

Use Treatment of anemia due to concurrent myelosuppressive chemotherapy in patients with cancer (nonmyeloid malignancies) receiving chemotherapy (palliative intent) for a planned minimum of 2 additional months of chemotherapy; treatment of anemia due to chronic kidney disease (including patients on dialysis and not on dialysis) to decrease the need for RBC transfusion; treatment of anemia associated with HIV (zidovudine) therapy when endogenous erythropoietin levels ≤500 mUnits/mL; reduction of allogeneic RBC transfusion for elective, noncardiac, nonvascular surgery when perioperative hemoglobin is >10 to ≤13 g/dL and there is a high risk for blood loss

Note: Epoetin is **not** indicated for use under the following conditions:

- Cancer patients receiving hormonal therapy, therapeutic biologic products, or radiation therapy unless also receiving concurrent myelosuppressive chemotherapy
- Cancer patients receiving myelosuppressive chemotherapy when the expected outcome is curative
- Surgery patients who are willing to donate autologous blood
- Surgery patients undergoing cardiac or vascular surgery
- As a substitute for RBC transfusion in patients requiring immediate correction of anemia

Note: In clinical trials (and one meta-analysis), epoetin has not demonstrated improved quality of life, fatigue, or well-being.

Unlabeled Use Treatment of symptomatic anemia in myelodysplastic syndrome (MDS)

Labeled Contraindications Hypersensitivity to epoetin or any component of the formulation; uncontrolled hypertension; pure red cell aplasia (due to epoetin or other epoetin protein drugs); multidose vials contain benzyl alcohol and are contraindicated in neonates, infants, pregnant women, and nursing women

Pregnancy Risk Factor C

Lactation Excretion in breast milk unknown/use caution

Warnings/Precautions **[U.S. Boxed Warning]: Erythropoiesis-stimulating agents (ESAs) increased the risk of serious cardiovascular events, thromboembolic events, stroke, mortality, and/or tumor progression in clinical studies when administered to target hemoglobin levels >11 g/dL** (and provide no additional benefit); a rapid rise in hemoglobin (>1 g/dL over 2 weeks) may also contribute to these risks. **[U.S. Boxed Warning]: A shortened overall survival and/or increased risk of tumor progression or recurrence has been reported in studies with breast, cervical, head and neck, lymphoid, and nonsmall cell lung cancer patients.** It is of note that in these studies, patients received ESAs to a target hemoglobin of ≥12 g/dL; although risk has not been excluded when dosed to achieve a target hemoglobin of <12 g/dL. **[U.S. Boxed Warnings]: To decrease these risks, and risk of cardio- and thrombovascular events, use the lowest dose needed to avoid red blood cell transfusions. Use ESAs in cancer patients only for the treatment of anemia related to concurrent myelosuppressive chemotherapy; discontinue ESA following completion of the chemotherapy course. ESAs are not indicated for patients receiving myelosuppressive therapy when the anticipated outcome is curative.** A dosage modification is appropriate if hemoglobin levels rise >1 g/dL per 2 week time period during treatment (Rizzo, 2010). Use of ESAs has been associated with an increased risk of venous thromboembolism (VTE) without a reduction in transfusions in patients with cancer (Hershman, 2009). Improved anemia symptoms, quality of life, fatigue, or well-being have not been demonstrated in controlled clinical trials. **[U.S. Boxed Warning]: Because of the risks of decreased survival and increased risk of tumor growth or progression, all healthcare providers and hospitals are required to enroll and comply with the ESA APPRISE (Assisting Providers and Cancer Patients with Risk Information for the Safe use of ESAs) Oncology Program prior to prescribing or dispensing ESAs to cancer patients.** Prescribers and patients will have to provide written documentation of discussed risks prior to each epoetin course.

[U.S. Boxed Warning]: An increased risk of death, serious cardiovascular events, and stroke was reported in chronic kidney disease (CKD) patients administered ESAs to target hemoglobin levels ≥11 g/dL; use the lowest dose sufficient to reduce the need for RBC transfusions. An optimal target hemoglobin level, dose or dosing strategy to reduce these risks has not been identified in clinical trials. Hemoglobin rising >1 g/dL in a 2-week period may contribute to the risk (dosage reduction recommended). Chronic kidney disease patients who exhibit an inadequate hemoglobin response to ESA therapy may be at a higher risk for cardiovascular events and mortality compared to other patients. ESA therapy may reduce dialysis efficacy (due to increase in red blood cells and decrease in plasma volume); adjustments in dialysis parameters may be needed. Patients treated with epoetin may require increased heparinization during dialysis to prevent clotting of the extracorporeal circuit. **[U.S. Boxed Warning]: DVT prophylaxis is recommended in perisurgery patients due to the risk of DVT.** Increased mortality was also observed in patients undergoing coronary artery bypass surgery who received epoetin alfa; these deaths were associated with thrombotic events. Epoetin is **not** approved for reduction of red blood cell transfusion in patients undergoing cardiac or vascular surgery and is **not** indicated for surgical patients willing to donate autologous blood.

Use with caution in patients with hypertension (contraindicated in uncontrolled hypertension) or with a history of seizures; hypertensive encephalopathy and seizures have been reported. If hypertension is difficult to control, reduce or hold epoetin alfa. An excessive rate of rise of hemoglobin is associated with hypertension or exacerbation of hypertension; decrease the epoetin dose if the hemoglobin increase exceeds 1 g/dL in any 2-week period. Blood pressure should be controlled prior to start of therapy and monitored closely throughout treatment. The risk for seizures is increased with epoetin use in patients with CKD; monitor closely for neurologic symptoms during the first several months of therapy. Due to the delayed onset of erythropoiesis, epoetin alfa is **not** recommended for acute correction of severe anemia or as a substitute for emergency transfusion.

Prior to treatment, correct or exclude deficiencies of iron, vitamin B_{12}, and/or folate, as well as other factors which may impair erythropoiesis (inflammatory conditions, infections). Prior to and periodically during therapy, iron stores must be evaluated. Supplemental iron is recommended if serum ferritin <100 mcg/L or serum transferrin saturation <20%; most patients with chronic kidney disease will require iron supplementation. Poor response should prompt evaluation of these potential factors, as well as possible malignant processes and hematologic disease (thalassemia, refractory anemia, myelodysplastic disorder), occult blood loss, hemolysis, ostetis fibrosa cystic, and/or bone marrow fibrosis. Severe anemia and pure red cell aplasia (PRCA) with associated neutralizing antibodies to erythropoietin has been reported, predominantly in patients with CKD receiving SubQ epoetin (the I.V. route is preferred for hemodialysis patients). Cases have also been reported in patients with hepatitis C who were receiving ESAs, interferon, and ribavirin. Patients with a sudden loss of response to epoetin alfa (with severe anemia and a low reticulocyte count) should be evaluated for PRCA with associated neutralizing antibodies to erythropoietin; discontinue treatment (permanently) in patients with PRCA secondary to neutralizing antibodies to epoetin.

Potentially serious allergic reactions have been reported (rarely). Discontinue immediately (and permanently) in patients who experience serious allergic/anaphylactic reactions. Some products may contain albumin. Multidose vials contain benzyl alcohol; do not use in premature infants.

Adverse Reactions

>10%:

Cardiovascular: Hypertension (3% to 28%)
Central nervous system: Fever (10% to 42%), headache (5% to 18%)
Dermatologic: Pruritus (12% to 21%), rash (2% to 19%)
Gastrointestinal: Nausea (35% to 56%), vomiting (12% to 28%)
Local: Injection site reaction (7% to 13%)
Neuromuscular & skeletal: Arthralgia (10% to 16%)
Respiratory: Cough (4% to 26%)

1% to 10%:

Cardiovascular: Deep vein thrombosis, edema, thrombosis
Central nervous system: Chills, depression, dizziness, insomnia
Dermatologic: Urticaria
Endocrine & metabolic: Hyperglycemia, hypokalemia
Gastrointestinal: Dysphagia, stomatitis, weight loss
Hematologic: Leukopenia
Local: Clotted vascular access
Neuromuscular & skeletal: Bone pain, muscle spasm, myalgia
Respiratory: Pulmonary embolism, respiratory congestion, upper respiratory infection

<1%, postmarketing, and/or case reports: Allergic reaction, anaphylactic reaction, angioedema, bronchospasm, erythema, hypersensitivity reactions, hypertensive encephalopathy, MI, microvascular thrombosis, neutralizing antibodies, porphyria, pure red cell aplasia (PRCA), renal vein thrombosis, retinal artery thrombosis, seizure, stroke, tachycardia, temporal vein thrombosis, thrombophlebitis, TIA, tumor progression

Drug Interactions

Metabolism/Transport Effects None known.

Avoid Concomitant Use There are no known interactions where it is recommended to avoid concomitant use.

Increased Effect/Toxicity There are no known significant interactions involving an increase in effect.

Decreased Effect There are no known significant interactions involving a decrease in effect.

Storage/Stability Vials should be stored at 2°C to 8°C (36°F to 46°F); **do not freeze or shake**. Protect from light.

Single-dose 1 mL vial contains no preservative: Use one dose per vial. Do not re-enter vial; discard unused portions.

Single-dose vials (except 40,000 units/mL vial) are stable for 2 weeks at room temperature (Cohen, 2007). Single-dose 40,000 units/mL vial is stable for 1 week at room temperature.

Multidose 1 mL or 2 mL vial contains preservative. Store at 2°C to 8°C after initial entry and between doses. Discard 21 days after initial entry.

Multidose vials (with preservative) are stable for 1 week at room temperature (Cohen, 2007).

Prefilled syringes containing the 20,000 units/mL formulation with preservative are stable for 6 weeks refrigerated (2°C to 8°C) (Naughton, 2003).

Dilutions of 1:10 and 1:20 (1 part epoetin:19 parts sodium chloride) are stable for 18 hours at room temperature (Ohls, 1996).

Prior to SubQ administration, preservative free solutions may be mixed with bacteriostatic NS containing benzyl alcohol 0.9% in a 1:1 ratio (Corbo, 1992).

Dilutions of 1:10 in $D_{10}W$ with human albumin 0.05% or 0.1% are stable for 24 hours.

Reconstitution Prior to SubQ administration, preservative free solutions may be mixed with bacteriostatic NS containing benzyl alcohol 0.9% in a 1:1 ratio.

Mechanism of Action Induces erythropoiesis by stimulating the division and differentiation of committed erythroid progenitor cells; induces the release of reticulocytes from the bone marrow into the bloodstream, where they mature to erythrocytes. There is a dose response relationship with this effect. This results in an increase in reticulocyte counts followed by a rise in hematocrit and hemoglobin levels.

Pharmacodynamics/Kinetics

Onset of action: Several days

Peak effect: Hemoglobin level: 2-6 weeks

Distribution: V_d: 9 L; rapid in the plasma compartment; concentrated in liver, kidneys, and bone marrow

Metabolism: Some degradation does occur

Bioavailability: SubQ: ~21% to 31%; intraperitoneal epoetin: 3% (Macdougall, 1989)

Half-life elimination: Cancer: SubQ: 16-67 hours; Chronic kidney disease: I.V.: 4-13 hours

Time to peak, serum: Chronic kidney disease: SubQ: 5-24 hours

Excretion: Feces (majority); urine (small amounts, 10% unchanged in normal volunteers)

Dosing

Adult & Geriatric

Anemia associated with chronic kidney disease: Individualize dosing and use the lowest dose necessary to reduce the need for RBC transfusions.

*Chronic kidney disease patients **ON dialysis*** (I.V. route is preferred for hemodialysis patients; initiate treatment when hemoglobin is <10 g/dL; reduce dose or interrupt treatment if hemoglobin approaches or exceeds 11 g/dL): I.V., SubQ: Initial dose: 50-100 units/kg 3 times/week

*Chronic kidney disease patients **NOT on dialysis*** (consider initiating treatment when hemoglobin is <10 g/dL; use only if rate of hemoglobin decline would likely result in RBC transfusion and desire is to reduce risk of alloimmunization or other RBC transfusion-related risks; reduce dose or interrupt treatment if hemoglobin exceeds 10 g/dL): I.V., SubQ: Initial dose: 50-100 units/kg 3 times/week

Dosage adjustments for chronic kidney disease patients (either on dialysis or not on dialysis):

If hemoglobin does not increase by >1 g/dL after 4 weeks: Increase dose by 25%; do not increase the dose more frequently than once every 4 weeks

If hemoglobin increases >1 g/dL in any 2-week period: Reduce dose by ≥25%; dose reductions can occur more frequently than once every 4 weeks; avoid frequent dosage adjustments

Inadequate or lack of response over a 12-week escalation period: Further increases are unlikely to improve response and may increase risks; use the minimum effective dose that will maintain a Hgb level sufficient to avoid RBC transfusions and evaluate patient for other causes of anemia. Discontinue therapy if responsiveness does not improve.

Anemia due to chemotherapy in cancer patients: Initiate treatment only if hemoglobin <10 g/dL and anticipated duration of myelosuppressive chemotherapy is ≥2 months. Titrate dosage to use the minimum effective dose that will maintain a hemoglobin level sufficient to avoid red blood cell transfusions. Discontinue erythropoietin following completion of chemotherapy. SubQ: Initial dose: 150 units/kg 3 times/week or 40,000 units once weekly until completion of chemotherapy

Dosage adjustments:

If hemoglobin does not increase by >1 g/dL **and** remains below 10 g/dL after initial 4 weeks: Increase to 300 units/kg 3 times/week or 60,000 units weekly; discontinue after 8 weeks of treatment if RBC transfusions are still required or there is no hemoglobin response

If hemoglobin exceeds a level needed to avoid red blood cell transfusion: Withhold dose; resume treatment with a 25% dose reduction when hemoglobin approaches a level where transfusions may be required.

If hemoglobin increases >1 g/dL in any 2-week period **or** hemoglobin reaches a level sufficient to avoid red blood cell transfusion: Reduce dose by 25%.

Anemia due to zidovudine in HIV-infected patients: Titrate dosage to use the minimum effective dose that will maintain a hemoglobin level sufficient to avoid red blood cell transfusions. Hemoglobin levels should not exceed 12 g/dL.

Serum erythropoietin levels ≤500 mUnits/mL and zidovudine doses ≤4200 mg/week): I.V., SubQ: Initial: 100 units/kg 3 times/week; if hemoglobin does not increase after 8 weeks, increase dose by ~50-100 units/kg at 4-8 week intervals until hemoglobin reaches a level sufficient to avoid RBC transfusion; maximum dose: 300 units/kg. Withhold dose if hemoglobin exceeds 12 g/dL, may resume treatment with a 25% dose reduction once hemoglobin <11 g/dL. Discontinue if hemoglobin increase is not achieved with 300 units/kg for 8 weeks.

Surgery patients (perioperative hemoglobin should be >10 g/dL and ≤13 g/dL; DVT prophylactic anticoagulation is recommended): SubQ: Initial dose:

300 units/kg/day beginning 10 days before surgery, on the day of surgery, and for 4 days after surgery **or**

600 units/kg once weekly for 4 doses, given 21-, 14-, and 7 days before surgery, and on the day of surgery

Symptomatic anemia associated with myelodysplastic syndrome (unlabeled use): SubQ: 40,000-60,000 units 1-3 times/week (NCCN MDS guidelines v.2.2011)

Pediatric

Anemia associated with chronic kidney disease (CKD): Individualize dosing and use the lowest dose necessary to reduce the need for RBC transfusions.

Chronic kidney disease patients ***ON dialysis*** (I.V. route is preferred for hemodialysis patients; initiate treatment when hemoglobin is <10 g/dL; reduce dose or interrupt treatment if hemoglobin approaches or exceeds 11 g/dL):

Children 1 month to 16 years: I.V., SubQ: Initial dose: 50 units/kg 3 times/week

Dosage adjustments for chronic kidney disease patients:

If hemoglobin does not increase by >1 g/dL after 4 weeks: Increase dose by 25%; do not increase the dose more frequently than once every 4 weeks

If hemoglobin increases >1 g/dL in any 2-week period: Reduce dose by ≥25%; dose reductions can occur more frequently than once every 4 weeks; avoid frequent dosage adjustments

Inadequate or lack of response over a 12-week escalation period: Further increases are unlikely to improve response and may increase risks; use the minimum effective dose that will maintain a Hgb level sufficient to avoid RBC transfusions and evaluate patient for other causes of anemia. Discontinue therapy if responsiveness does not improve.

Anemia due to chemotherapy in cancer patients: Initiate treatment only if hemoglobin <10 g/dL and anticipated duration of myelosuppressive chemotherapy is ≥2 months. Titrate dosage to use the minimum effective dose that will maintain a hemoglobin level sufficient to avoid red blood cell transfusions. Discontinue erythropoietin following completion of chemotherapy.

Children ≥5 years: I.V.: Initial dose: 600 units/kg once weekly until completion of chemotherapy.

Dosage adjustments:

If hemoglobin does not increase by >1 g/dL **and** remains <10 g/dL after initial 4 weeks: Increase to 900 units/kg (maximum dose: 60,000 units); discontinue after 8 weeks of treatment if RBC transfusions are still required or there is no hemoglobin response.

If hemoglobin exceeds a level needed to avoid red blood cell transfusion: Withhold dose; resume treatment with a 25% dose reduction when hemoglobin approaches a level where transfusions may be required.

If hemoglobin increases >1 g/dL in any 2-week period **or** hemoglobin reaches a level sufficient to avoid red blood cell transfusion: Reduce dose by 25%.

Anemia due to zidovudine in HIV-infected patients: Titrate dosage to use the minimum effective dose that will maintain a hemoglobin level sufficient to avoid red blood cell transfusions. Hemoglobin levels should not exceed 12 g/dL. Children 8 months to 17 years (based on limited data): I.V., SubQ: Reported dosing range: 50-400 units/kg 2-3 times/week

Administration

SubQ is the preferred route of administration **except** in patients with CKD on hemodialysis; 1:1 dilution with bacteriostatic NS (containing benzyl alcohol) acts as a local anesthetic to reduce pain at the injection site

Patients with CKD on hemodialysis: I.V. route preferred; it may be administered into the venous line at the end of the dialysis procedure

Monitoring Parameters Transferrin saturation and serum ferritin (prior to and during treatment); hemoglobin (weekly after initiation and following dose adjustments until stable and sufficient to minimize need for RBC transfusion, CKD patients should be also be monitored at least monthly following hemoglobin stability); blood pressure; seizures (CKD patients following initiation for first few months, includes new-onset or change in seizure frequency or premonitory symptoms)

Cancer patients: Examinations recommended by the ASCO/ASH guidelines (Rizzo, 2010) prior to treatment include: peripheral blood smear (in some situations a bone marrow exam may be necessary), assessment for iron, folate, or vitamin B_{12} deficiency, reticulocyte count, renal function status, and occult blood loss; during ESA treatment, assess baseline and periodic iron, total iron-binding capacity, and transferrin saturation or ferritin levels.

Additional Information Oncology Comment: The American Society of Clinical Oncology (ASCO) and American Society of Hematology (ASH) 2010 updates to the clinical practice guidelines for the use of erythropoiesis-stimulating agents (ESAs) in patients with cancer indicate that ESAs are most appropriate when used according to the parameters identified within the Food and Drug Administration (FDA) approved labeling for epoetin and darbepoetin (Rizzo, 2010). ESAs are an option for chemotherapy associated anemia when the hemoglobin has fallen to <10 g/dL to decrease the need for RBC transfusions. ESAs should only be used in conjunction with concurrent chemotherapy. Although the FDA label now limits ESA use to the palliative setting, the

ASCO/ASH guidelines suggest using clinical judgment in weighing risks versus benefits as formal outcomes studies of ESA use defined by intent of chemotherapy treatment have not been conducted.

The ASCO/ASH guidelines continue to recommend following the FDA approved dosing (and dosing adjustment) guidelines as alternate dosing and schedules have not demonstrated consistent differences in effectiveness with regard to hemoglobin response. In patients who do not have a response within 6-8 weeks (hemoglobin rise <1-2 g/dL or no reduction in transfusions) ESA therapy should be discontinued.

Prior to the initiation of ESAs, other sources of anemia (in addition to chemotherapy or underlying hematologic malignancy) should be investigated. Examinations recommended prior to treatment include peripheral blood smear (in some situations a bone marrow exam may be necessary), assessment for iron, folate, or vitamin B_{12} deficiency, reticulocyte count, renal function status, and occult blood loss. During ESA treatment, assess baseline and periodic iron, total iron-binding capacity, and transferrin saturation or ferritin levels. Iron supplementation may be necessary

The guidelines note that patients with an increased risk of thromboembolism (generally includes previous history of thrombosis, surgery, and/or prolonged periods of immobilization) and patients receiving concomitant medications that may increase thromboembolic risk, should begin ESA therapy only after careful consideration. With the exception of low-risk myelodysplasia-associated anemia (which has evidence supporting the use of ESAs without concurrent chemotherapy), the guidelines do not support the use of ESAs in the absence of concurrent chemotherapy.

Prescribing and Access Restrictions As a requirement of the REMS program, access to this medication is restricted. Healthcare providers and hospitals must be enrolled in the ESA APPRISE (Assisting Providers and Cancer Patients with Risk Information for the Safe use of ESAs) Oncology Program (866-284-8089; http://www.esa-apprise.com) to prescribe or dispense ESAs (ie, epoetin alfa, darbepoetin alfa) to patients with cancer.

Medication Guide Available Yes

Dosage Forms Excipient information presented when available (limited, particularly for generics); consult specific product labeling.

Injection, solution:

Epogen®: 10,000 units/mL (2 mL); 20,000 units/mL (1 mL) [contains albumin (human), benzyl alcohol]

Procrit®: 10,000 units/mL (2 mL); 20,000 units/mL (1 mL) [contains albumin (human), benzyl alcohol]

Injection, solution [preservative free]:

Epogen®: 2000 units/mL (1 mL); 3000 units/mL (1 mL); 4000 units/mL (1 mL); 10,000 units/mL (1 mL) [contains albumin (human)]

Procrit®: 2000 units/mL (1 mL); 3000 units/mL (1 mL); 4000 units/mL (1 mL); 10,000 units/mL (1 mL); 40,000 units/mL (1 mL) [contains albumin (human)]

Dosage Forms: Canada Excipient information presented when available (limited, particularly for generics); consult specific product labeling.

Injection, solution [preservative free]:

Eprex®: 1000 units/0.5 mL (0.5 mL), 2000 units/0.5 mL (0.5 mL), 3000 units/0.3 mL (0.3 mL), 4000 units/0.4 mL (0.4 mL), 5000 units/0.5 mL (0.5 mL), 6000 units/0.6 mL (0.6 mL), 8000 units/0.8 mL (0.8 mL), 10,000 units/mL (1 mL), 20,000 units/0.5 mL (0.5 mL), 30,000 units/0.75 mL (0.75 mL), 40,000 units/mL (1 mL) [contains polysorbate 80; prefilled syringe, free of human serum albumin]

References

Bennett CL, Silver SM, Djulbegovic B, et al, "Venous Thromboembolism and Mortality Associated With Recombinant Erythropoietin and Darbepoetin Administration for the Treatment of Cancer-Associated Anemia," *JAMA*, 2008, 299(8):914-24.

Cohen V, Jellinek SP, Teperikidis L, et al, "Room-temperature Storage of Medications Labeled for Refrigeration," *Am J Health-Syst Pharm*, 2007, 64(16):1711-5.

Hershman DL, Buono DL, Malin J, et al, "Patterns of Use and Risks Associated With Erythropoiesis-Stimulating Agents Among Medicare Patients With Cancer," *J Natl Cancer Inst*, 2009, 101 (23):1-9.

Macdougall IC, Roberts DE, Neubert P, et al, "Pharmacokinetics of Recombinant Human Erythropoietin in Patients on Continuous Ambulatory Peritoneal Dialysis," *Lancet*, 1989, 1 (8635):425-7.

Napolitano LM, Fabian TC, Kelly KM, et al, "Improved Survival of Critically Ill Trauma Patients Treated With Recombinant Human Erythropoietin," *J Trauma*, 2008, 65(2):285-97.

National Comprehensive Cancer Network® (NCCN), "Practice Guidelines in Oncology™: Cancer- and Chemotherapy-Induced Anemia Version 1.2012." Available at http://www.nccn.org/professionals/physician_gls/PDF/anemia.pdf

National Comprehensive Cancer Network® (NCCN), "Practice Guidelines in Oncology™: Myelodysplastic Syndromes Version 2.2011." Available at http://www.nccn.org/professionals/physician_gls/PDF/mds.pdf

National Kidney Foundation, "KDOQI Clinical Practice Guidelines and Clinical Practice Recommendations for Anemia in Chronic Kidney Disease," *Am J Kidney Dis*, 2007, 50(3):529-30. Available at http://www.kidney.org/professionals/KDOQI/guidelines_anemiaUP/index.htm or http://www.kidney.org/professionals/KDOQI

Phronmmintikul A, Haas SJ, Elsik M, et al, "Mortality and Target Haemoglobin Concentrations in Anaemic Patients with Chronic Kidney Disease Treated With Erythropoietin: A Meta-Analysis, *Lancet*, 2007, 369(9559):381-88.

Rizzo JD, Brouwers M, Hurley P, et al, "American Society of Clinical Oncology/American Society of Hematology Clinical Practice Guideline Update on the Use of Epoetin and Darbepoetin in Adult Patients With Cancer," *J Clin Oncol*, 2010, 28(33):4996-5010.

Rizzo JD, Somerfield MR, Hagerty LK, et al, "American Society of Hematology/American Society of Clinical Oncology 2007 Clinical Practice Guideline Update on the Use of Epoetin and Darbepoetin," *Blood*, 2008, 111(1):25-41.

Singh AJ, Szczech L, Tang KI, et al, "Correction of Anemia With Epoetin Alfa in Chronic Kidney Disease," *N Engl J Med*, 2006, 355(20):2085-98.

◆ **Epogen®** *see* Epoetin Alfa *on page 516*

◆ **Epothilone B Lactam** *see* Ixabepilone *on page 842*

◆ **Eprex® (Can)** *see* Epoetin Alfa *on page 516*

◆ **Epsilon Aminocaproic Acid** *see* Aminocaproic Acid *on page 72*

◆ **EPT** *see* Teniposide *on page 1342*

◆ **Eptacog Alfa (Activated)** *see* Factor VIIa (Recombinant) *on page 568*

◆ **ER-086526** *see* Eribulin *on page 524*

◆ **Eraxis™** *see* Anidulafungin *on page 99*

◆ **Erbitux®** *see* Cetuximab *on page 264*

Eribulin (er i BUE lin)

Related Information

Management of Chemotherapy-Induced Nausea and Vomiting *on page 1786*

Brand Names: U.S. Halaven™

Brand Names: Canada Halaven™

Index Terms B1939; E7389; ER-086526; Eribulin Mesylate; Halichondrin B Analog

Generic Availability (U.S.) No

Pharmacologic Category Antineoplastic Agent, Antimicrotubular

Use Treatment of metastatic breast cancer in patients who have received at least 2 prior chemotherapy regimens

Labeled Contraindications There are no contraindications listed within the manufacturer's labeling.

Canadian labeling (not in U.S. labeling): Hypersensitivity to eribulin mesylate, halichondrin B, or its chemical derivatives.

Pregnancy Risk Factor D

Lactation Excretion in breast milk unknown/not recommended

Warnings/Precautions Hazardous agent - Use appropriate precautions for handling and disposal. Hematologic toxicity, including severe neutropenia, has occurred; may require treatment delay and dosage reduction. A higher incidence of grade 4 neutropenia and neutropenic fever occurred in patients with ALT or AST >3 x ULN or bilirubin >1.5 x ULN. Monitor complete blood counts prior to each dose; more frequently if severe cytopenias develop.

Peripheral neuropathy is a common toxicity; may be prolonged (>1 year in 5% of patients); may require treatment delay. Monitor for signs of motor or sensory neuropathy. Some patients may have pre-existing neuropathy due to prior chemotherapy; monitor closely for worsening.

QT prolongation was observed on day 8 (in an uncontrolled study); monitor ECG in patients with heart failure, bradyarrhythmia, and with concomitant medication known to prolong the QT interval, correct hypokalemia and hypomagnesemia prior to treatment; monitor electrolytes periodically during treatment. Avoid use in patients with congenital long QT syndrome.

Dosage reduction required in patients with mild-to-moderate (Child-Pugh class A or B) hepatic impairment; use has not been studied in patients with severe hepatic impairment; transaminase or bilirubin elevations are associated with a higher incidence of grade 4 neutropenia and neutropenic fever. Dosage reduction required in patients with renal impairment (Cl_{cr} 30-50 mL/minute); use has not been studied in patients with Cl_{cr} <30 mL/minute.

Adverse Reactions

>10%:

- Central nervous system: Fatigue (54%), fever (21%), headache (19%)
- Dermatologic: Alopecia (45%)
- Gastrointestinal: Nausea (35%), stomatitis (5% to 18%), constipation (25%), weight loss (21%), anorexia (20%), diarrhea (18%), vomiting (18%)
- Hematologic: Neutropenia (82%; grades 3: 28%; grade 4: 29%; nadir: 13 days; recovery: 8 days), anemia (58%; grades 3/4: 2%)
- Hepatic: ALT increased (18%)
- Neuromuscular & skeletal: Weakness (54%), peripheral neuropathy (35%; grades 3/4: ≤8%), arthralgia/myalgia (22%), back pain (16%), bone pain (12%), limb pain (11%)
- Respiratory: Dyspnea (16%), cough (14%)

1% to 10%:

- Cardiovascular: Peripheral edema
- Central nervous system: Depression, dizziness, insomnia
- Dermatologic: Rash

Endocrine & metabolic: Hypokalemia
Gastrointestinal: Mucosal inflammation (9%), abdominal pain, dyspepsia, taste alteration, xerostomia
Genitourinary: Urinary tract infection (10%)
Hematologic: Neutropenic fever (5%), thrombocytopenia (grades 3/4: 1%)
Neuromuscular & skeletal: Muscle spasm
Ocular: Lacrimation increased
Respiratory: Upper respiratory infection

<1%, postmarketing, and/or case reports: Pharyngolaryngeal pain, sepsis

Drug Interactions

Metabolism/Transport Effects Substrate of CYP3A4 (minor); **Note:** Assignment of Major/Minor substrate status based on clinically relevant drug interaction potential; **Inhibits** CYP3A4 (weak)

Avoid Concomitant Use

Avoid concomitant use of EriBULin with any of the following: CloZAPine; Highest Risk QTc-Prolonging Agents; Mifepristone

Increased Effect/Toxicity

EriBULin may increase the levels/effects of: Antiarrhythmic Agents (Class Ia); Antiarrhythmic Agents (Class III); ARIPiprazole; CloZAPine; Highest Risk QTc-Prolonging Agents; Moderate Risk QTc-Prolonging Agents; Vitamin K Antagonists

The levels/effects of EriBULin may be increased by: Mifepristone; QTc-Prolonging Agents (Indeterminate Risk and Risk Modifying)

Decreased Effect

EriBULin may decrease the levels/effects of: Cardiac Glycosides; Vitamin K Antagonists

The levels/effects of EriBULin may be decreased by: Tocilizumab

Storage/Stability Store intact vials at 25°C (77°F); excursions permitted between 15°C and 30°C (59°F and 86°F); do not freeze. Store in original carton. Undiluted solutions in a syringe and solutions diluted in normal saline for infusion are stable for up to 4 hours at room temperature or up to 24 hours refrigerated.

Reconstitution No dilution required. May dilute in 100 mL normal saline.

Mechanism of Action Eribulin is a non-taxane microtubule inhibitor which is a halichondrin B analog. It inhibits the growth phase of the microtubule by inhibiting formation of mitotic spindles causing mitotic blockage and arresting the cell cycle at the G_2/M phase; suppresses microtubule polymerization yet does not affect depolymerization.

Pharmacodynamics/Kinetics

Distribution: V_d: 43-114 L/m^2
Protein binding: 49% to 65%
Metabolism: Negligible
Half-life, elimination: ~40 hours
Excretion: Feces (82%; predominantly as unchanged drug); urine (9%, primarily as unchanged drug)

Dosing

Adult & Geriatric Breast cancer, metastatic: I.V.: 1.4 mg/m^2/dose on days 1 and 8 of a 21-day treatment cycle

Renal Impairment

Cl_{cr} >50 mL/minute: No adjustment required.
Cl_{cr} 30-50 mL/minute: Reduce to 1.1 mg/m^2/dose.
Cl_{cr} <30 mL/minute: Use has not been studied.

Hepatic Impairment

Mild hepatic impairment (Child-Pugh class A): Reduce to 1.1 mg/m²/dose.

Moderate hepatic impairment (Child-Pugh class B): Reduce to 0.7 mg/m²/dose.

Severe hepatic impairment (Child-Pugh class C): Use has not been studied.

Adjustment for Toxicity

ANC <1000/mm³ or platelets <75,000/mm³ or grade 3 or 4 nonhematologic toxicity on day 1 or 8: Withhold dose; may delay day 8 dose up to 1 week. If toxicity resolves to ≤grade 2 by day 15 administer a reduced dose and wait at least 2 weeks before beginning the next cycle. Omit dose if not resolved to ≤grade 2 by day 15. Do not re-escalate dose after reduction.

Permanently reduce dose from 1.4 mg/m² to 1.1 mg/m² for the following:
- ANC <500/mm³ for >7 days
- ANC <1000/mm³ with fever or infection
- Platelets <25,000/mm³
- Platelets <50,000/mm³ requiring transfusion
- Nonhematologic toxicity of grade 3 or 4
- Dose omission or delay due to toxicity on day 8 of prior cycle

Permanently reduce dose from 1.1 mg/m² to 0.7 mg/m² for occurrence of any of the above events; discontinue treatment if the above toxicities occur at the 0.7 mg/m² dose level.

Administration I.V.: Infuse over 2-5 minutes. May be administered undiluted or diluted.

Emetic Potential Low (10% to 30%)

Monitoring Parameters CBC with differential prior to each dose; renal and liver function tests; serum electrolytes, including potassium and magnesium. Assess for peripheral neuropathy prior to each dose. Monitor ECG in patients with heart failure, bradyarrhythmia, and with concomitant medication known to prolong the QT interval, and electrolyte abnormalities (eg, hypokalemia, hypomagnesemia).

Dosage Forms Excipient information presented when available (limited, particularly for generics); consult specific product labeling.

Injection, solution, as mesylate:

Halaven™: 0.5 mg/mL (2 mL)

References

Cortes J, Vahdat L, Blum JL, et al, "Phase II Study of the Halichondrin B Analog Eribulin Mesylate in Patients With Locally Advanced or Metastatic Breast Cancer Previously Treated With an Anthracycline, a Taxane, and Capecitabine," *J Clin Oncol*, 2010, 28(25):3922-8.

Twelves C, Loesch, D, Blum JL, et al, "A Phase III Study (EMBRACE) of Eribulin Mesylate Versus Treatment of Physician's Choice in Patients With Locally Recurrent or Metastatic Breast Cancer Previously Treated With an Anthracycline and a Taxane," *J Clin Oncol*, 2010, 28 (18s):CRA1004 [abstract CRA1004 from 2010 ASCO Annual Meeting].

Twelves C, Vahdat LT, Akerele CE, et al, "Eribulin Mesylate (E7389) Versus Treatment of Physician's Choice in Patients (pts) With Metastatic Breast Cancer (MBC): A Phase III Study (EMBRACE)," *J Clin Oncol*, 2010:257 [abstract 257 from 2010 ASCO Breast Cancer Symposium].

Vahdat LT, Pruitt B, Fabian CJ, et al, "Phase II Study of Eribulin Mesylate, a Halichondrin B Analog, in Patients With Metastatic Breast Cancer Previously Treated With an Anthracycline and a Taxane," *J Clin Oncol*, 2009, 27(18):2954-61.

Witteveen P, Marchette S, Mergui-Roelvink M, et al, "Eribulin Mesylate Pharmacokinetics in Patients With Hepatic Impairment," *J Clin Oncol*, 2010, 28(15s):2582 [abstract 2582 from 2010 ASCO Annual Meeting].

◆ **Eribulin Mesylate** *see* Eribulin *on page 524*

◆ **Erivedge™** *see* Vismodegib *on page 1470*

Erlotinib (er LOE tye nib)

Related Information

Management of Chemotherapy-Induced Nausea and Vomiting *on page 1786*
Principles of Anticancer Therapy *on page 1878*
Safe Handling of Hazardous Drugs *on page 1904*

Brand Names: U.S. Tarceva®

Brand Names: Canada Tarceva®

Index Terms CP358774; Erlotinib Hydrochloride; OSI-774

Generic Availability (U.S.) No

Pharmacologic Category Antineoplastic Agent, Tyrosine Kinase Inhibitor; Epidermal Growth Factor Receptor (EGFR) Inhibitor

Use Treatment of locally advanced or metastatic nonsmall cell lung cancer (NSCLC) refractory to at least 1 prior chemotherapy regimen (as monotherapy); maintenance treatment of locally advanced or metastatic NCSLC which has not progressed after 4-6 cycles of first line platinum-based chemotherapy; locally advanced, unresectable or metastatic pancreatic cancer (first-line therapy in combination with gemcitabine)

Canadian labeling: First-line treatment of locally advanced or metastatic non-small cell lung cancer (NSCLC) with known EGFR mutation (as monotherapy); treatment of locally advanced or metastatic NSCLC refractory to at least 1 prior chemotherapy regimen and positive or unknown EGFR status (as monotherapy); maintenance treatment of locally advanced or metastatic NCSLC which has not progressed after 4 cycles of first line platinum-based chemotherapy

Unlabeled Use First-line treatment of NSCLC with known EGFR mutation (unlabeled in U.S.)

Labeled Contraindications There are no contraindications listed within the FDA-approved manufacturer's labeling.

Canadian labeling: Hypersensitivity to erlotinib or any component of the formulation

Pregnancy Risk Factor D

Lactation Excretion in breast milk unknown/not recommended

Warnings/Precautions Hazardous agent - use appropriate precautions for handling and disposal. Rare, sometimes fatal, interstitial lung disease (ILD) has occurred; symptoms include acute respiratory distress syndrome, interstitial pneumonia, obliterative bronchiolitis, pneumonitis (including radiation and hypersensitivity), pulmonary fibrosis, and pulmonary infiltrates. The onset of symptoms has been within 5 days to more than 9 months after treatment initiation (median: 39 days). Interrupt treatment for unexplained new or worsening pulmonary symptoms (dyspnea, cough, and fever); discontinue for confirmed ILD.

Liver enzyme elevations have been reported. Hepatic failure and hepatorenal syndrome have also been reported, particularly in patients with baseline hepatic impairment. Monitor liver function; patients with any hepatic impairment (total bilirubin >ULN; Child-Pugh class A, B, or C) should be closely monitored, including those with hepatic disease due to tumor burden; use with extreme caution in patients with total bilirubin >3 times ULN. Dosage reduction, interruption or discontinuation may be recommended for changes in hepatic function. Acute renal failure, renal insufficiency, and hepatorenal syndrome have been reported, either secondary to hepatic impairment at baseline or due to severe dehydration; use with caution in patients with or at risk for renal impairment. Monitor closely for dehydration; monitor renal function and electrolytes in patients at risk for dehydration. Gastrointestinal perforation has been reported with use; risk for perforation is increased with concurrent anti-angiogenic agents, corticosteroids, NSAIDs, and/or taxane based-therapy, and patients with history of peptic ulcers or diverticular disease; permanently discontinue in patients who develop perforation.

Bullous, blistering, or exfoliating skin conditions, some suggestive of Stevens-Johnson or toxic epidermal necrolysis (TEN) have been reported. An acne-like rash commonly appears on the face, back, and upper chest. Generalized or severe acneiform, erythematous or maculopapular rash may occur. Skin rash may correlate with treatment response and prolonged survival (Saif, 2008); management of skin rashes that are not serious should include alcohol-free lotions, topical antibiotics, or topical corticosteroids, or if necessary, oral antibiotics and systemic corticosteroids; avoid sunlight. Reduce dose or temporarily interrupt treatment for severe skin reactions; interrupt or discontinue treatment for bullous, blistering or exfoliative skin toxicity. Corneal perforation and ulceration have been reported with use; abnormal eyelash growth, keratoconjunctivitis sicca, or keratitis have also been reported and are known risk factors for corneal ulceration/perforation. Interrupt or discontinue treatment in patients presenting with eye pain or other acute or worsening ocular symptoms.

MI, CVA, and microangiopathic hemolytic anemia with thrombocytopenia have been reported. Elevated INR and bleeding events have been reported; monitor for INR changes. Erlotinib levels may be lower in patients who smoke; advise patients to stop smoking. Smokers treated with 300 mg/day exhibited steady-state erlotinib levels comparable to former- and never-smokers receiving 150 mg/day (Hughes, 2009). Concurrent use with CYP3A4 inhibitors and moderate or strong CYP3A4 inducers may affect erlotinib levels; consider alternative agents to CYP3A4 inducers to avoid the potential for CYP-mediated interactions; use with caution in patients taking strong CYP3A4 inhibitors. Consider erlotinib dosage modification if concurrent use with CYP3A4 inhibitors/inducers cannot be avoided. In patients with NSCLC, EGFR mutations, specifically exon 19 deletions and exon 21 mutation (L858R), are associated with better response to erlotinib (Riely, 2006); erlotinib treatment is not recommended in patients with *K-ras* mutations; they are not likely to benefit from erlotinib treatment (Eberhard, 2005; Miller, 2008). Concurrent erlotinib plus platinum based chemotherapy is not recommended for first line treatment of locally advanced or metastatic NSCLC due to a lack of clinical benefit. Product may contain lactose; avoid use in patients with Lapp lactase deficiency, glucose-galactose malabsorption, or glucose intolerance.

Adverse Reactions

Adverse reactions reported with monotherapy:

>10%:

Cardiovascular: Chest pain (≤17%)

Central nervous system: Fatigue (9% to 52%), pyrexia (≤11%)

Dermatologic: Rash (49% to 75%; grade 3: 5% to 13%; grade 4: <1%; median onset: 8 days), dry skin (4% to 17%), paronychia (4% to 16%), alopecia (14% to 15%), pruritus (7% to 13%), acne (6% to 12%)

Gastrointestinal: Diarrhea (20% to 57%; grade 3: 2% to 6%; grade 4: <1%; median onset: 12 days), anorexia (9% to 52%), nausea (23% to 33%), appetite decreased (≤28%), vomiting (13% to 23%), stomatitis (11% to 17%), mucosal inflammation (≤17%), abdominal pain (3% to 11%), constipation (≤8%)
Genitourinary: Urinary tract infection (≤4%)
Hematologic: Anemia (≤11%; grade 4: 1%)
Neuromuscular & skeletal: Weakness (≤53%), back pain (≤16%)
Ocular: Conjunctivitis (12%), keratoconjunctivitis sicca (12%)
Respiratory: Dyspnea (41%), cough (33% to 45%)
Miscellaneous: Infection (4% to 24%)

1% to 10%:
Cardiovascular: Peripheral edema (≤5%)
Central nervous system: Pain (≤9%), headache (≤7%), anxiety (≤5%), dizziness (≤4%), dysphonia (≤4%), insomnia (≤4%), neurotoxicity (≤4%)
Dermatologic: Folliculitis (≤8%), nail disorder (≤7%), exfoliative rash (5%), hypertrichosis (5%), skin fissures (5%), dermatitis acneiform (4% to 5%), erythema (≤5%), dermatitis (4%), erythematous rash (≤4%), palmar-plantar erythrodysesthesia (≤4%)
Gastrointestinal: Dyspepsia (≤5%), weight loss (4% to 5%), xerostomia (≤3%), taste disturbance (≤1%)
Hematologic: Lymphopenia (≤4%; grade 3: 1%), leukopenia (≤3%), thrombocytopenia (≤1%)
Hepatic: Hyperbilirubinemia (7%; grade 3: ≤1%), ALT increased (grade 2: 2% to 4%; grade 3: 1% to 3%), GGT increased (≤4%)
Neuromuscular & skeletal: Arthralgia (≤10%), musculoskeletal pain (≤9%), bone pain (≤4%), muscle spasms (≤4%), musculoskeletal chest pain (≤4%), paresthesia (≤4%)
Otic: Tinnitus (≤1%)
Renal: Renal failure (≤1%), serum creatinine increased (≤1%)
Respiratory: Nasopharyngitis (≤7%), epistaxis (≤4%), pulmonary embolus (≤4%), respiratory tract infection (≤4%), pneumonitis/pulmonary infiltrate (3%), pulmonary fibrosis (3%)

<1%: Interstitial lung disease-like events

Adverse reactions reported with combination (erlotinib plus gemcitabine) therapy:

>10%:
Cardiovascular: Edema (37%), thrombotic events (grades 3/4: 11%)
Central nervous system: Fatigue (73% to 79%), fever (36%), depression (19%), dizziness (15%), headache (15%), anxiety (13%)
Dermatologic: Rash (69%), alopecia (14%)
Gastrointestinal: Nausea (60%), anorexia (52%), diarrhea (48%), abdominal pain (46%), vomiting (42%), weight loss (39%), stomatitis (22%), dyspepsia (17%), flatulence (13%)
Hepatic: ALT increased (grade 2: 31%, grade 3: 13%, grade 4: <1%), AST increased (grade 2: 24%, grade 3: 10%, grade 4 <1%), hyperbilirubinemia (grade 2: 17%, grade 3: 10%, grade 4: <1%)
Neuromuscular & skeletal: Bone pain (25%), myalgia (21%), neuropathy (13%), rigors (12%)
Respiratory: Dyspnea (24%), cough (16%)
Miscellaneous: Infection (39%)

1% to 10%:

Cardiovascular: Arrhythmia (<5%), syncope (<5%), deep venous thrombosis (4%), cerebrovascular accident (2%; including cerebral hemorrhage), MI/myocardial ischemia (2%)

Gastrointestinal: Ileus (<5%), pancreatitis (<5%)

Hematologic: Hemolytic anemia (<5%), microangiopathic hemolytic anemia with thrombocytopenia (1%)

Renal: Renal insufficiency (<5%)

Respiratory: Interstitial lung disease-like events (<3%)

Mono- or combination therapy: <1%, postmarketing, and/or case reports: Acute renal failure, blistering/bullous/exfoliative skin conditions (suggesting Stevens-Johnson syndrome or TEN), bronchiolitis, corneal perforation, corneal ulcerations, episcleritis, eye lash disorders (ingrown lashes, excessive growth, thickening), gastritis, gastroduodenal ulcers, GI bleeding, GI hemorrhage, GI perforation, hearing loss, hematemesis, hematochezia, hepatic failure, hepatorenal syndrome, hepatotoxicity, hirsutism, hyperpigmentation, hypokalemia, keratitis, melena, peptic ulcer bleeding, photosensitivity, rash (acneiform; sparing prior radiation field), skin fissures, tympanic membrane perforation

Drug Interactions

Metabolism/Transport Effects Substrate of CYP1A2 (minor), CYP3A4 (major); **Note:** Assignment of Major/Minor substrate status based on clinically relevant drug interaction potential

Avoid Concomitant Use

Avoid concomitant use of Erlotinib with any of the following: Conivaptan; Proton Pump Inhibitors

Increased Effect/Toxicity

Erlotinib may increase the levels/effects of: Vitamin K Antagonists

The levels/effects of Erlotinib may be increased by: Antifungal Agents (Azole Derivatives, Systemic); Ciprofloxacin (Systemic); Conivaptan; CYP3A4 Inhibitors (Moderate); CYP3A4 Inhibitors (Strong); Dasatinib; FluvoxaMINE; Ivacaftor; Mifepristone

Decreased Effect

Erlotinib may decrease the levels/effects of: Cardiac Glycosides; Vitamin K Antagonists

The levels/effects of Erlotinib may be decreased by: Antacids; CYP3A4 Inducers (Strong); Deferasirox; H2-Antagonists; Herbs (CYP3A4 Inducers); Proton Pump Inhibitors; Rifampin; Tocilizumab

Ethanol/Nutrition/Herb Interactions

Food: Erlotinib bioavailability is increased with food. Grapefruit or grapefruit juice may decrease metabolism and increase erlotinib plasma concentrations. Management: Take on an empty stomach at least 1 hour before or 2 hours after the ingestion of food. Avoid grapefruit and grapefruit juice. Maintain adequate nutrition and hydration, unless instructed to restrict fluid intake.

Herb/Nutraceutical: St John's wort may increase metabolism and decrease erlotinib concentrations. Management: Avoid St John's wort.

Storage/Stability Store at room temperature of 25°C (77°F); excursions permitted to 15°C and 30°C (59°F and 86°F).

Mechanism of Action The mechanism of erlotinib's antitumor action is not fully characterized. It is known to inhibit overall epidermal growth factor receptor (HER1/EGFR) - tyrosine kinase. Active competitive inhibition of adenosine triphosphate inhibits downstream signal transduction of ligand dependent HER1/EGFR activation.

Pharmacodynamics/Kinetics

Absorption: Oral: 60% on an empty stomach; almost 100% on a full stomach

Distribution: 94-232 L

Protein binding: 92% to 95% to albumin and α_1-acid glycoprotein

Metabolism: Hepatic, via CYP3A4 (major), CYP1A1 (minor), CYP1A2 (minor), and CYP1C (minor)

Bioavailability: Almost 100% when given with food; 60% without food

Half-life elimination: 24-36 hours

Time to peak, plasma: 1-7 hours

Excretion: Primarily as metabolites: Feces (83%; 1% as unchanged drug); urine (8%)

Dosing

Adult & Geriatric

Nonsmall cell lung cancer (NSCLC), refractory: Oral: 150 mg once daily until disease progression or unacceptable toxicity (Shepherd, 2005)

NSCLC, maintenance therapy: Oral: 150 mg once daily until disease progression or unacceptable toxicity (Capuzzo, 2010)

Pancreatic cancer: Oral: 100 mg once daily until disease progression or unacceptable toxicity (in combination with gemcitabine) (Moore, 2007)

NSCLC, first-line therapy in patients with EGFR mutations (U.S. unlabeled use): Oral: 150 mg once daily until disease progression or unacceptable toxicity (Rosell, 2012; Zhou, 2011)

Dosage adjustment for concomitant CYP3A4 inhibitors/inducers:

CYP3A4 inhibitors: Consider dose reductions for severe adverse reactions when erlotinib is administered concomitantly with strong CYP3A4 inhibitors (eg, azole antifungals, clarithromycin, erythromycin, nefazodone, protease inhibitors, telithromycin). Dose reduction (if required) should be done in decrements of 50 mg.

Concomitant CYP3A4 and CYP1A2 inhibitor (eg, ciprofloxacin): Consider dose reductions if severe adverse reactions occur.

CYP3A4 inducers: Alternatives to the enzyme-inducing agent should be utilized first. Concomitant administration with CYP3A4 inducers (eg, carbamazepine, phenobarbital, phenytoin, rifamycins, and St John's wort) may require erlotinib increased doses (increase as tolerated at 2-week intervals); doses >150 mg/day should be considered with rifampin (the maximum erlotinib dose studied in combination with rifampin was 450 mg). Immediately reduce erlotinib dose to recommended starting dose when CYP3A4 inducer is discontinued.

Dosage adjustment for concomitant smoking: A dose increase to a maximum dose of 300 mg (with careful monitoring) may be required in patients who continue to smoke; immediately reduce erlotinib dose to recommended starting dose upon smoking cessation.

Renal Impairment No dosage adjustment provided in the manufacturer's labeling (has not been studied), although <9% of a single dose is excreted in the urine. Interrupt treatment (or discontinue) for risk of renal failure due to dehydration; may resume after euvolemia re-established.

Hepatic Impairment

U.S. labeling:

Patients with normal hepatic function at baseline: Total bilirubin >3 times ULN and/or transaminases >5 times ULN: Interrupt or discontinue treatment

Patients with baseline hepatic impairment: Total bilirubin >3 times ULN: Use extreme caution.

Canadian labeling:

Moderate impairment: No dosage adjustment provided in manufacturer's labeling; however, a reduced dose should be considered.

Severe impairment (including total bilirubin >3 times ULN and/or transaminases >5 times ULN): Use is not recommended.

The following adjustments have also been studied: A reduced starting dose (75 mg once daily) has been recommended in patients with hepatic dysfunction (AST ≥3 times ULN or direct bilirubin 1-7 mg/dL), with individualized dosage escalation if tolerated (Miller, 2007); another study determined that pharmacokinetic and safety profiles were similar between patients with normal hepatic function and moderate hepatic impairment (O'Bryant, 2012).

Adjustment for Toxicity Dose reductions should be made in 50 mg decrements.

Bullous, blistering or exfoliative skin toxicity, acute or worsening ocular toxicities, or dehydration with risk for renal failure: Interrupt or discontinue treatment

Diarrhea: Manage with loperamide; in severe diarrhea (unresponsive to loperamide) or dehydration due to diarrhea, reduce dose or temporarily interrupt treatment

Gastrointestinal perforation, hepatic failure: Discontinue treatment

Hepatotoxicity:

Worsening liver function (not yet severe): Consider treatment interruption or dose reduction.

Significant changes in liver function (eg, doubling of total bilirubin and/or tripling of transaminases from baseline): Interrupt or discontinue treatment.

Pulmonary symptoms: Acute onset (or worsening) of pulmonary symptoms (eg, dyspnea, cough, fever): Interrupt treatment and evaluate for drug-induced interstitial lung disease; discontinue permanently with development of interstitial lung disease

Severe skin reaction: Reduce dose or temporarily interrupt treatment

Combination Regimens

Lung cancer (nonsmall cell): Erlotinib (NSCLC Regimen) on page 1632

Pancreatic cancer: Erlotinib-Gemcitabine (Pancreatic) on page 1632

Administration The manufacturer recommends administration on an empty stomach (at least 1 hour before or 2 hours after the ingestion of food).

For patients unable to swallow whole, tablets may be dissolved in 100 mL water and administered orally or via feeding tube (silicone-based); to ensure full dose is received, rinse container with 40 mL water, administer residue and repeat rinse (data on file, Genentech; Siu, 2007; Soulieres, 2004).

Emetic Potential Very low (<10%)

Extemporaneous Preparations A suspension for oral or feeding tube (silicone-based) administration may be prepared by dissolving tablets needed for dose in 100 mL water. To ensure full dose is received, rinse container with 40 mL water, administer residue and repeat rinse. Administer immediately after preparation; stability of solution is unknown (Tarceva® data on file from Genentech).

Siu LL, Soulieres D, Chen EX, et al, "Phase I/II Trial of Erlotinib and Cisplatin in Patients With Recurrent or Metastatic Squamous Cell Carcinoma of the Head and Neck: A Princess Margaret Hospital Phase II Consortium and National Cancer Institute of Canada Clinical Trials Group Study," *J Clin Oncol*, 2007, 25(16):2178-83.

Soulieres D, Senzer NN, Vokes EE, et al, "Multicenter Phase II Study of Erlotinib, an Oral Epidermal Growth Factor Receptor Tyrosine Kinase Inhibitor, in Patients With Recurrent or Metastatic Squamous Cell Cancer of the Head and Neck," *J Clin Oncol*, 2004, 22(1):77-85.

Monitoring Parameters Periodic liver function tests (transaminases, bilirubin, and alkaline phosphatase); monitor more frequently with worsening liver function; periodic renal function tests and serum electrolytes (in patients at risk for dehydration); hydration status; EGFR mutation status in patients with NSCLC adenocarcinoma (Keedy, 2011)

Dietary Considerations Take this medicine an empty stomach, 1 hour before or 2 hours after a meal. Avoid grapefruit juice.

Additional Information In patients with NSCLC, some factors which correlate positively with response to EGFR-tyrosine kinase inhibitor (TKI) therapy include patients who have never smoked, EGFR mutation, and patients of Asian origin. EGFR mutations, specifically exon 19 deletions and exon 21 mutation (L858R) correlate with response to tyrosine kinase inhibitors (Riely, 2006). *K-ras* mutations correlated with poorer outcome with EGFR-TKI therapy in patients with NSCLC. (Cooley, 2008; Jackman, 2008; Masarelli, 2007; Shepherd, 2005).

Dosage Forms Excipient information presented when available (limited, particularly for generics); consult specific product labeling.

Tablet, oral:

Tarceva®: 25 mg, 100 mg, 150 mg

References

Azzoli CG, Baker S Jr, Temin S, et al, "American Society of Clinical Oncology Clinical Practice Guideline Update on Chemotherapy for Stage IV Non-Small-Cell Lung Cancer," *J Clin Oncol*, 2009, 27(36):6251-66.

Capuzzo F, Ciuleanu T, Stelmakh L, et al, "SATURN: A Double-Blind, Randomized, Phase III Study of Maintenance Erlotinib Versus Placebo Following Nonprogression With First-Line Platinum-Based Chemotherapy in Patients With Advanced NSCLC," *J Clin Oncol*, 2009, 27(15s):8001 [abstract 8001 from 2009 ASCO Annual Meeting].

Cooley ME, Emmons KM, Li, H, et al, "Smoking History, Drug Toxicity, and Survival in Non-Small Cell Lung Cancer (NSCLC) Patients Receiving Epidermal Growth Factor Receptor Tyrosine Kinase Inhibitor (EGFI-TKI) Drugs," *J Clin Oncol*, 2008, 26(15 Supp):9570 [abstract 9570 from 2008 ASCO Annual Meeting].

Eberhard DA, Johnson BE, Amler LC, et al, "Mutations in the Epidermal Growth Factor Receptor and in KRAS are Predictive and Prognostic Indicators in Patients With Non-Small-Cell Lung Cancer Treated With Chemotherapy Alone and in Combination With Erlotinib," *J Clin Oncol*, 2005, 23(25):5900-9.

Herbst RS, Prager D, Hermann R, et al, "TRIBUTE: A Phase III Trial of Erlotinib Hydrochloride (OSI-774) Combined With Carboplatin and Paclitaxel Chemotherapy in Advanced Non-Small-Cell Lung Cancer," *J Clin Oncol*, 2005, 23(25):5892-9.

Hughes AN, O'Brien ME, Petty WJ, et al, "Overcoming CYP1A1/1A2 Mediated Induction of Metabolism by Escalating Erlotinib Dose in Current Smokers," *J Clin Oncol*, 2009, 27(8):1220-6.

Jackman DM, Sequist LV, Cioffrei L, et al, "Impact of EGFR and KRAS Genotype on Outcome in a Clinical Trial Registry of NSCLC Patients Initially Treated With Erlotinib or Gefitinib," *J Clin Oncol*, 2008, 26(15 Supp) [abstract 8035 from 2008 ASCO Annual Meeting].

Keedy VL, Temin S, Somerfield MR, et al, "American Society of Clinical Oncology Provisional Clinical Opinion: Epidermal Growth Factor Receptor (EGFR) Mutation Testing for Patients With Advanced Non-Small-Cell Lung Cancer Considering First-Line EGFR Tyrosine Kinase Inhibitor Therapy," *J Clin Oncol*, 2011, 29(15):2121-7.

Massarelli E, Varella-Garcia M, Tang X, et al, "KRAS Mutation is an Important Predictor of Resistance to Therapy With Epidermal Growth Factor Receptor Tyrosine Kinase Inhibitors in Non-Small-Cell Lung Cancer," *Clin Cancer Res*, 2007, 13(10):2890-6.

Miller AA, Murry DJ, Owzar K, et al, "Phase I and Pharmacokinetic Study of Erlotinib for Solid Tumors in Patients With Hepatic or Renal Dysfunction: CALGB 60101," *J Clin Oncol*, 2007, 25 (21):3055-60.

Miller VA, Riely GJ, Zakowski MF, et al, "Molecular Characteristics of Bronchioloalveolar Carcinoma and Adenocarcinoma, Bronchioloalveolar Carcinoma Subtype, Predict Response to Erlotinib," *J Clin Oncol*, 2008, 26(9):1472-8.

Moore MJ, Goldstein D, Hamm J, et al, "Erlotinib Plus Gemcitabine Compared With Gemcitabine Alone in Patients With Advanced Pancreatic Cancer: A Phase III Trial of the National Cancer Institute of Canada Clinical Trials Group," *J Clin Oncol*, 2007, 25(15):1960-6.

O'Bryant CL, Haluska P, Rosen L, et al, "An Open-Label Study to Describe Pharmacokinetic Parameters of Erlotinib in Patients With Advanced Solid Tumors With Adequate and Moderately Impaired Hepatic Function," *Cancer Chemother Pharmacol*, 2012, 69(3):605-12.

Riely GJ, Pao W, Pham D, et al, "Clinical Course of Patients With Non-Small Cell Lung Cancer and Epidermal Growth Factor Receptor Exon 19 and Exon 21 Mutations Treated With Gefitinib or Erlotinib," *Clin Cancer Res*, 2006, 12(3 Pt 1):839-44.

Rosell R, Carcereny E, Gervais R, et al, "Erlotinib Versus Standard Chemotherapy as First-Line Treatment for European Patients With Advanced EGFR Mutation-Positive Non-Small-Cell Lung Cancer (EURTAC): A Multicentre, Open-Label, Randomised Phase 3 Trial," *Lancet Oncol*, 2012, 13(3):239-46.

Rosell R, Moran T, Queralt C, et al, "Screening for Epidermal Growth Factor Mutations in Lung Cancer," *N Engl J Med*, 2009, 361(10):958-67.

Saif MS, Merikas I, Tsimboukis S, et al, "Erlotinib-Induced Skin Rash. Pathogenesis, Clinical Significance and Management in Pancreatic Cancer Patients," *JOP*, 2008, 9(3):267-74.

Shepherd FA, Rodrigues Pereira J, Ciuleanu T, et al, "Erlotinib in Previously Treated Non-Small-Cell Lung Cancer," *N Engl J Med*, 2005, 353(2):123-32.

Siu LL, Soulieres D, Chen EX, et al, "Phase I/II Trial of Erlotinib and Cisplatin in Patients With Recurrent or Metastatic Squamous Cell Carcinoma of the Head and Neck: A Princess Margaret Hospital Phase II Consortium and National Cancer Institute of Canada Clinical Trials Group Study," *J Clin Oncol*, 2007, 25(16):2178-83.

Soulieres D, Senzer NN, Vokes EE, et al, "Multicenter Phase II Study of Erlotinib, an Oral Epidermal Growth Factor Receptor Tyrosine Kinase Inhibitor, in Patients With Recurrent or Metastatic Squamous Cell Cancer of the Head and Neck," *J Clin Oncol*, 2004, 22(1):77-85.

Zhou C, Wu YL, Chen G, et al, "Erlotinib Versus Chemotherapy as First-Line Treatment for Patients With Advanced EGFR Mutation-Positive Non-Small-Cell Lung Cancer (OPTIMAL, CTONG-0802): A Multicentre, Open-Label, Randomised, Phase 3 Study," *Lancet Oncol*, 2011,12 (8):735-42.

◆ **Erlotinib Hydrochloride** *see* Erlotinib *on page 528*

◆ **Erwinase® (Can)** *see* Asparaginase (*Erwinia*) *on page 126*

◆ **Erwinaze™** *see* Asparaginase (*Erwinia*) *on page 126*

◆ ***Erwinia chrysanthemi*** *see* Asparaginase (*Erwinia*) *on page 126*

◆ **Erythropoiesis-Stimulating Agent (ESA)** *see* Darbepoetin Alfa *on page 382*

◆ **Erythropoiesis-Stimulating Agent (ESA)** *see* Epoetin Alfa *on page 516*

◆ **Erythropoiesis-Stimulating Protein** *see* Darbepoetin Alfa *on page 382*

◆ **Erythropoietin** *see* Epoetin Alfa *on page 516*

Estramustine (es tra MUS teen)

Related Information

Management of Chemotherapy-Induced Nausea and Vomiting *on page 1786*
Safe Handling of Hazardous Drugs *on page 1904*

Brand Names: U.S. Emcyt®

Brand Names: Canada Emcyt®

Index Terms Estramustine Phosphate; Estramustine Phosphate Sodium

Generic Availability (U.S.) No

Pharmacologic Category Antineoplastic Agent, Alkylating Agent; Antineoplastic Agent, Hormone; Antineoplastic Agent, Hormone (Estrogen/Nitrogen Mustard)

Use Palliative treatment of progressive or metastatic prostate cancer

Labeled Contraindications Hypersensitivity to estramustine, estradiol, nitrogen mustard, or any component of the formulation; active thrombophlebitis or thromboembolic disorders (except where tumor mass is the cause of thromboembolic disorder and the benefit may outweigh the risk)

Canadian labeling: Additional contraindications (not in the U.S. labeling): Severe hepatic or cardiac disease

Warnings/Precautions Hazardous agent - use appropriate precautions for handling and disposal. Glucose tolerance may be decreased; use with caution in patients with diabetes. Elevated blood pressure, peripheral edema (new-onset or exacerbation), or congestive heart disease may occur; use with caution in patients where fluid accumulation may be poorly tolerated, including cardiovascular disease (HF or hypertension), migraine, seizure disorder or renal dysfunction. Estrogen treatment for prostate cancer is associated with an increased risk of thrombosis and MI; use caution with history of cardiovascular disease (eg, thrombophlebitis, thrombosis, or thromboembolic disease) and cerebrovascular or coronary artery disease. Use with caution in patients with hepatic impairment (may be metabolized poorly) or with metabolic bone diseases. Allergic reactions and angioedema, including airway involvement, have been reported with use. Patients with prostate cancer and osteoblastic metastases should have their calcium monitored regularly. Estrogen use may cause gynecomastia and/or impotence. Avoid vaccination with live vaccines during treatment (risk of infection may be increased due to immunosuppression). Although the response to vaccines may be diminished, inactivated vaccines may be administered during treatment.

Adverse Reactions

>10%:

Cardiovascular: Edema (20%)

Endocrine & metabolic: Gynecomastia (75%), breast tenderness (71%), libido decreased

Gastrointestinal: Nausea (16%), diarrhea (13%), gastrointestinal upset (12%)

Hepatic: LDH increased (2% to 33%), AST increased (2% to 33%)

Respiratory: Dyspnea (12%)

1% to 10%:

Cardiovascular: CHF (3%), MI (3%), cerebrovascular accident (2%), chest pain (1%), flushing (1%)

Central nervous system: Lethargy (4%), insomnia (3%), emotional lability (2%), anxiety (1%), headache (1%)

Dermatologic: Bruising (3%), dry skin (2%), pruritus (2%), hair thinning (1%), rash (1%), skin peeling (1%)

Gastrointestinal: Anorexia (4%), flatulence (2%), burning throat (1%), gastrointestinal bleeding (1%), thirst (1%), vomiting (1%)

Hematologic: Leukopenia (4%), thrombocytopenia (1%)

Hepatic: Bilirubin increased (1% to 2%)

Local: Thrombophlebitis (3%)

Neuromuscular & skeletal: Leg cramps (9%)

Ocular: Tearing (1%)

Respiratory: Pulmonary embolism (2%), upper respiratory discharge (1%), hoarseness (1%)

<1%, postmarketing, and/or case reports: Allergic reactions, anemia, angina, angioedema, cerebrovascular ischemia, confusion, coronary ischemia, depression, glucose tolerance decreased, hyper-/hypocalcemia, hypertension, impotence, muscle weakness, venous thrombosis

Drug Interactions

Metabolism/Transport Effects None known.

Avoid Concomitant Use

Avoid concomitant use of Estramustine with any of the following: BCG; Natalizumab; Pimecrolimus; Tacrolimus (Topical); Vaccines (Live)

Increased Effect/Toxicity

Estramustine may increase the levels/effects of: Leflunomide; Natalizumab; Vaccines (Live)

The levels/effects of Estramustine may be increased by: Clodronate; Denosumab; Pimecrolimus; Roflumilast; Tacrolimus (Topical); Trastuzumab

Decreased Effect

Estramustine may decrease the levels/effects of: BCG; Coccidioidin Skin Test; Sipuleucel-T; Vaccines (Inactivated); Vaccines (Live)

The levels/effects of Estramustine may be decreased by: Calcium Salts; Echinacea

Ethanol/Nutrition/Herb Interactions Food: Estramustine serum levels may be decreased if taken with milk or other dairy products, calcium supplements, and vitamins containing calcium. Management: Take on an empty stomach at least 1 hour before or 2 hours after eating.

Storage/Stability Refrigerate at 2°C to 8°C (36°F to 46°F).

Mechanism of Action Combines the effects of estradiol and nitrogen mustard. It appears to bind to microtubule proteins, preventing normal tubulin function. The antitumor effect may be due solely to an estrogenic effect. Estramustine causes a marked decrease in plasma testosterone and an increase in estrogen levels.

Pharmacodynamics/Kinetics

Absorption: Oral: 75%

Metabolism:

- GI tract: Initial dephosphorylation
- Hepatic: Oxidation and hydrolysis; metabolites include estramustine, estrone analog, estrone, and estradiol

Half-life elimination: Terminal: 15-24 hours

Time to peak, serum: 2-3 hours

Excretion: Feces (2.9% to 4.8% as unchanged drug)

Dosing

Adult & Geriatric Details concerning dosing in combination regimens should also be consulted.

Prostate cancer: Oral: Males: 14 mg/kg/day (range: 10-16 mg/kg/day) in 3 or 4 divided doses

Combination therapy with docetaxel (unlabeled dose): 280 mg 3 times/day for 5 days (days 1 through 5) of a 21-day treatment cycle for up to 12 cycles (Petrylak, 2004)

Combination Regimens

Prostate cancer:

Doxorubicin + Ketoconazole/Estramustine + Vinblastine on page 1619
Estramustine + Docetaxel on page 1634
Estramustine + Docetaxel + Calcitriol on page 1635
Estramustine + Docetaxel + Carboplatin on page 1636
Estramustine + Docetaxel + Hydrocortisone on page 1636
Estramustine + Docetaxel + Prednisone on page 1636
Estramustine + Etoposide on page 1636
Estramustine-Paclitaxel on page 1637

Estramustine-Vinblastine *on page* 1638
Estramustine + Vinorelbine *on page* 1638
Paclitaxel + Estramustine + Carboplatin *on page* 1728
Paclitaxel + Estramustine + Etoposide *on page* 1729

Administration Administer on an empty stomach, at least 1 hour before or 2 hours after eating.

Emetic Potential Moderate (30% to 90%)

Monitoring Parameters Serum calcium, liver function tests; blood pressure

Dietary Considerations Should be taken at least 1 hour before or 2 hours after eating. Milk products and calcium-rich foods or supplements may impair the oral absorption of estramustine phosphate sodium.

Dosage Forms Excipient information presented when available (limited, particularly for generics); consult specific product labeling.

Capsule, oral, as phosphate sodium:
Emcyt®: 140 mg

References

Bergenheim AT and Henriksson R, "Pharmacokinetics and Pharmacodynamics of Estramustine Phosphate," *Clin Pharmacokinet*, 1998, 34(2):163-72.

Lubiniecki GM, Berlin JA, Weinstein RB, et al, "Thromboembolic Events With Estramustine Phosphate-Based Chemotherapy in Patients With Hormone-Refractory Prostate Carcinoma: Results of a Meta-Analysis," *Cancer*, 2004, 101(12):2755-9.

Petrylak DP, Tangen CM, Hussain MH, et al, "Docetaxel and Estramustine Compared With Mitoxantrone and Prednisone for Advanced Refractory Prostate Cancer," *N Engl J Med*, 2004, 351(15):1513-20.

◆ **Estramustine Phosphate** *see* Estramustine *on page* 535
◆ **Estramustine Phosphate Sodium** *see* Estramustine *on page* 535
◆ **ET-743** *see* Trabectedin *on page* 1384
◆ **Ethiofos** *see* Amifostine *on page* 65
◆ **Ethoxynaphthamido Penicillin Sodium** *see* Nafcillin *on page* 1026
◆ **Ethyol®** *see* Amifostine *on page* 65
◆ **ETOP** *see* Etoposide Phosphate *on page* 548
◆ **Etopophos®** *see* Etoposide Phosphate *on page* 548

Etoposide (e toe POE side)

Related Information

Hematopoietic Stem Cell Transplantation *on page* 1887
Management of Chemotherapy-Induced Nausea and Vomiting *on page* 1786
Management of Drug Extravasations *on page* 1800
Palliative Care Medicine (Cancer) *on page* 1871
Safe Handling of Hazardous Drugs *on page* 1904

Brand Names: U.S. Toposar®

Brand Names: Canada Etoposide Injection USP; Vepesid™

Index Terms EPEG; Epipodophyllotoxin; VePesid; VP-16; VP-16-213

Generic Availability (U.S.) Yes

Pharmacologic Category Antineoplastic Agent, Podophyllotoxin Derivative; Antineoplastic Agent, Topoisomerase II Inhibitor

Use Treatment of refractory testicular tumors (injectable formulation); treatment of small cell lung cancer (SCLC)

Canadian labeling: Treatment of small cell lung cancer (SCLC; first- and second-line); treatment of nonsmall cell lung cancer (NSCLC); treatment of non-Hodgkin lymphomas (first-line); treatment of testicular cancer (first-line [injectable formulation] and refractory)

Unlabeled Use Treatment of acute lymphocytic leukemia (ALL), refractory acute myeloid leukemia (AML), recurrent or metastatic breast cancer, central nervous system tumors, Ewing's sarcoma, gestational trophoblastic disease, Hodgkin lymphoma, merkel cell cancer, refractory multiple myeloma, neuroblastoma, neuroendocrine tumors (adrenal gland and carcinoid tumors), non-Hodgkin lymphomas, nonsmall cell lung cancer (NSCLC), osteosarcoma, ovarian cancer (refractory), prostate cancer, retinoblastoma, metastatic soft tissue sarcoma, thymic malignancies (locally advanced or metastatic), unknown-primary adenocarcinoma, Wilms' tumor; conditioning regimen for hematopoietic cell transplantation

Labeled Contraindications Hypersensitivity to etoposide or any component of the formulation

Canadian labeling: Additional contraindications (not in U.S. labeling): Severe leukopenia or thrombocytopenia; severe hepatic impairment; severe renal impairment

Pregnancy Risk Factor D

Lactation Excretion in breast milk unknown/not recommended

Warnings/Precautions Hazardous agent - use appropriate precautions for handling and disposal. **[U.S. Boxed Warning]: Severe dose-limiting and dose-related myelosuppression with resulting infection or bleeding may occur.** Treatment should be withheld for platelets <50,000/mm³ or absolute neutrophil count (ANC) <500/mm³. May cause anaphylactic like reactions manifested by chills, fever, tachycardia, bronchospasm, dyspnea, and hypotension. In addition, facial/tongue swelling, coughing, chest tightness, cyanosis, laryngospasm, diaphoresis, hypertension, back pain, loss of consciousness, and flushing have also been reported less commonly. Incidence is primarily associated with intravenous administration (up to 2%) compared to oral administration (<1%). Infusion should be interrupted and medications for the treatment of anaphylaxis should be available for immediate use. High drug concentration and rate of infusion, as well as presence of polysorbate 80 and benzyl alcohol in the etoposide intravenous formulation have been suggested as contributing factors to the development of hypersensitivity reactions. Etoposide intravenous formulations may contain polysorbate 80 and/or benzyl alcohol, while etoposide phosphate (the water soluble prodrug of etoposide) intravenous formulation does not contain either vehicle. Case reports have suggested that etoposide phosphate has been used successfully in patients with previous hypersensitivity reactions to etoposide (Collier, 2008; Siderov, 2002). The use of concentrations higher than recommended were associated with higher rates of anaphylactic-like reactions in children.

Secondary acute leukemias have been reported with etoposide, either as monotherapy or in combination with other chemotherapy agents. Must be diluted; do not give I.V. push, infuse over at least 30-60 minutes; hypotension is associated with rapid infusion. If hypotension occurs, interrupt infusion and administer I.V. hydration and supportive care; decrease infusion upon reinitiation. Tissue irritation and inflammation have occurred following extravasation. Do not administer I.M. or SubQ. Dosage should be adjusted in patients with hepatic or renal impairment (Canadian labeling contraindicates use in severe hepatic and/or renal impairment). Use with caution in patients with low serum albumin; may increase risk for toxicities. Use with caution in elderly patients;

may be more likely to develop severe myelosuppression and/or GI effects (eg, nausea/vomiting). **[U.S. Boxed Warning]: Should be administered under the supervision of an experienced cancer chemotherapy physician.** Injectable formulation contains polysorbate 80; do not use in premature infants. May contain benzyl alcohol; do not use in newborn infants. Injectable formulation also contains alcohol (~33% v/v); may contribute to adverse reactions, especially with higher etoposide doses.

Adverse Reactions Note: The following may occur with higher doses used in stem cell transplantation: Alopecia, ethanol intoxication, hepatitis, hypotension (infusion-related), metabolic acidosis, mucositis, nausea and vomiting (severe), secondary malignancy, skin lesions (resembling Stevens-Johnson syndrome).

>10%:

Dermatologic: Alopecia (8% to 66%)

Gastrointestinal: Nausea/vomiting (31% to 43%), anorexia (10% to 13%), diarrhea (1% to 13%)

Hematologic: Leukopenia (60% to 91%; grade 4: 3% to 17%; nadir: 7-14 days; recovery: by day 20), thrombocytopenia (22% to 41%; grades 3/4: 1% to 20%; nadir 9-16 days; recovery: by day 20), anemia (≤33%)

1% to 10%:

Cardiovascular: Hypotension (1% to 2%; due to rapid infusion)

Gastrointestinal: Stomatitis (1% to 6%), abdominal pain (up to 2%)

Hepatic: Hepatic toxicity (up to 3%)

Neuromuscular & skeletal: Peripheral neuropathy (1% to 2%)

Miscellaneous: Anaphylactic-like reaction (I.V. infusion 1% to 2%; oral capsules <1%; including chills, fever, tachycardia, bronchospasm, dyspnea)

<1%, postmarketing, and/or case reports: Amenorrhea, back pain, blindness (transient/cortical), constipation, cough, cyanosis, diaphoresis, dysphagia, erythema, esophagitis, extravasation (induration/necrosis), facial swelling, fatigue, fever, hyperpigmentation, hypersensitivity, hypersensitivity-associated apnea, interstitial pneumonitis, laryngospasm, maculopapular rash, malaise, metabolic acidosis, MI, mucositis, myocardial ischemia, optic neuritis, ovarian failure, perivasculitis, pruritus, pulmonary fibrosis, radiation-recall dermatitis, rash, reversible posterior leukoencephalopathy syndrome (RPLS), seizure, somnolence, Stevens-Johnson syndrome, tongue swelling, toxic epidermal necrolysis, toxic megacolon, urticaria, vasospasm, weakness

Drug Interactions

Metabolism/Transport Effects Substrate of CYP1A2 (minor), CYP2E1 (minor), CYP3A4 (major), P-glycoprotein; **Note:** Assignment of Major/Minor substrate status based on clinically relevant drug interaction potential; **Inhibits** CYP2C9 (weak), CYP3A4 (weak)

Avoid Concomitant Use

Avoid concomitant use of Etoposide with any of the following: BCG; CloZAPine; Conivaptan; Natalizumab; Pimecrolimus; Pimozide; Tacrolimus (Topical); Vaccines (Live)

Increased Effect/Toxicity

Etoposide may increase the levels/effects of: ARIPiprazole; CloZAPine; Leflunomide; Natalizumab; Pimozide; Vaccines (Live); Vitamin K Antagonists

The levels/effects of Etoposide may be increased by: Atovaquone; Conivaptan; CycloSPORINE (Systemic); CYP3A4 Inhibitors (Moderate); CYP3A4 Inhibitors (Strong); Dasatinib; Denosumab; Ivacaftor; Mifepristone; P-glycoprotein/ABCB1 Inhibitors; Pimecrolimus; Roflumilast; Tacrolimus (Topical); Trastuzumab

Decreased Effect

Etoposide may decrease the levels/effects of: BCG; Coccidioidin Skin Test; Sipuleucel-T; Vaccines (Inactivated); Vaccines (Live); Vitamin K Antagonists

The levels/effects of Etoposide may be decreased by: Barbiturates; CYP3A4 Inducers (Strong); Deferasirox; Echinacea; Fosphenytoin; Herbs (CYP3A4 Inducers); P-glycoprotein/ABCB1 Inducers; Phenytoin; Tocilizumab

Ethanol/Nutrition/Herb Interactions

Ethanol: Avoid ethanol (may increase GI irritation)

Herb/Nutraceutical: Avoid concurrent St John's wort; may decrease etoposide levels.

Storage/Stability

Capsules: Store oral capsules under refrigeration at 2°C to 8°C (36°F to 46°F); do not freeze.

Injection: Store intact vials of injection at room temperature of 25°C (77°F); do not freeze. Protect from light. Diluted solutions for infusion, at room temperature, in D_5W or NS in polyvinyl chloride, are stable as follows, depending on the concentration:

0.2 mg/mL: 96 hours

0.4 mg/mL: 24 hours

Etoposide injection contains polysorbate 80 which may cause leaching of diethylhexyl phthalate (DEHP), a plasticizer contained in polyvinyl chloride (PVC) bags and tubing. Higher concentrations and longer storage time after preparation in PVC bags may increase DEHP leaching. Preparation in glass or polyolefin containers will minimize patient exposure to DEHP. When undiluted etoposide injection is stored in acrylic or ABS (acrylonitrile, butadiene and styrene) plastic containers, the containers may crack and leak.

Reconstitution Hazardous agent; use appropriate precautions for handling and disposal. Etoposide should be diluted to a concentration of 0.2-0.4 mg/mL in D_5W or NS for administration. Diluted solutions have concentration-dependent stability: More concentrated solutions have shorter stability times. Precipitation may occur with concentrations >0.4 mg/mL.

Mechanism of Action Etoposide has been shown to delay transit of cells through the S phase and arrest cells in late S or early G_2 phase. The drug may inhibit mitochondrial transport at the NADH dehydrogenase level or inhibit uptake of nucleosides into HeLa cells. It is a topoisomerase II inhibitor and appears to cause DNA strand breaks. Etoposide does not inhibit microtubular assembly.

Pharmacodynamics/Kinetics

Absorption: Oral: Significant inter- and intrapatient variation

Distribution: Average V_d: 7-17 L/m²; poor penetration across the blood-brain barrier; CSF concentrations <5% of plasma concentrations

Protein binding: 94% to 98%

Metabolism: Hepatic, via CYP3A4 and 3A5, to various metabolites; in addition, conversion of etoposide to the O-demethylated metabolites (catechol and quinine) via prostaglandin synthases or myeloperoxidase occurs, as well as glutathione and glucuronide conjugation via GSTT1/GSTP1 and UGT1A1 (Yang, 2009)

Bioavailability: Oral: ~50% (range: 25% to 75%)

Half-life elimination: Terminal: I.V.: 4-11 hours; Children: Normal renal/hepatic function: 6-8 hours

Excretion:

Children: I.V.: Urine (~55% as unchanged drug) in 24 hours

Adults: I.V.: Urine (56%; 45% as unchanged drug) within 120 hours; feces (44%) within 120 hours

Dosing

Adult & Geriatric Details concerning dosing in combination regimens should also be consulted:

U.S. labeling:

Small cell lung cancer (combination chemotherapy):

I.V.: 35 mg/m²/day for 4 days, up to 50 mg/m²/day for 5 days every 3-4 weeks

Oral: Due to poor bioavailability, oral doses should be twice the I.V. dose (and rounded to the nearest 50 mg)

Testicular cancer (combination chemotherapy): I.V.: 50-100 mg/m²/day for days 1-5 **or** 100 mg/m²/day on days 1, 3, and 5 repeated every 3-4 weeks

Canadian labeling: **Non-Hodgkin lymphoma (in combination with other agents), nonsmall cell lung cancer (alone or in combination), small cell lung cancer (first-line in combination; second-line alone or in combination), testicular cancer (in combination; oral therapy for refractory disease):**

I.V.: 50-100 mg/m²/day for 5 days

Oral: 100-200 mg/m²/day for 5 days; administer daily doses >200 mg in 2 divided doses.

Adult unlabeled uses and/or dosing:

Hematopoietic stem cell transplant conditioning regimen, lymphoid malignancies: I.V.: 60 mg/kg over 4 hours as a single dose 3 or 4 days prior to transplantation (Horning, 1994; Snyder, 1993; Weaver, 1994)

Nonsmall cell lung cancer: I.V.: 100 mg/m² days 1, 2, and 3 every 3 weeks for 4 cycles or every 4 weeks for 3-4 cycles (in combination with cisplatin) (Arriagada, 2004) **or** 50 mg/m² days 1-5 and days 29-33 (in combination with cisplatin and radiation therapy) (Albain, 2009)

Ovarian cancer, refractory: Oral: 50 mg/m² once daily for 21 days every 4 weeks until disease progression or unacceptable toxicity (Rose, 1998)

Small cell lung cancer, limited stage (combination chemotherapy): I.V.: 120 mg/m²/day on days 1, 2, and 3 every 3 weeks for 4 courses (Turrisi, 1999) **or** 100 mg/m²/day on days 1, 2, and 3 for induction therapy, followed by consolidation chemotherapy (Saito, 2006) **or** 100 mg/m²/day on days 1, 2, and 3 every 3 weeks up to a maximum of 6 cycles (Skarlos, 2001) **or** 100 mg/m²/day I.V. on day 1, followed by 200 mg/m²/day **orally** on days 2 through 4 every 3 weeks for a maximum of 5 courses (Sundstrom, 2002)

Small cell lung cancer, extensive stage (combination chemotherapy): 100 mg/m²/day I.V. on days 1, 2, and 3 every 3 weeks for 4 cycles (Lara, 2009) **or** 100 mg/m²/day I.V. on day 1, followed by 200 mg/m²/day **orally** on days 2 through 4 every 3 weeks for a maximum of 5 courses (Sundstrom, 2002) **or** I.V.: 80 mg/m²/day on days 1, 2, and 3 every 3 weeks up to 8 cycles (Ihede, 1994)

Testicular cancer (combination chemotherapy):

Nonseminoma: I.V.: 100 mg/m²/day on days 1 through 5 every 21 days for 3-4 courses (Saxman, 1998)

Nonseminoma, metastatic (high-dose regimens): I.V.: 750 mg/m²/day administered 5, 4, and 3 days before peripheral blood stem cell infusion, repeat for a second cycle after recovery of granulocyte and platelet counts (Einhorn, 2007) **or** 400 mg/m^2/day (beginning on cycle 3) on days 1, 2, and 3, with peripheral blood stem cell support, administered at 14- to 21-day intervals for 3 cycles (Kondagunta, 2007)

Thymoma, locally advanced or metastatic: I.V.: 120 mg/m^2 days 1, 2, and 3 every 3 weeks (in combination with cisplatin) for up to 8 cycles (Giaccone, 1996)

Unknown primary adenocarcinoma: Oral: 50 mg once daily on days 1, 3, 5, 7, and 9 alternating with 100 mg once daily on days 2, 4, 6, 8, and 10 every 3 weeks (in combination with paclitaxel and carboplatin) (Greco, 2000; Hainsworth, 2006)

Pediatric Details concerning dosing in combination regimens should also be consulted:

AML induction (unlabeled use; combination chemotherapy) (Woods, 1996): I.V.:

<3 years: 3.3 mg/kg/day continuous infusion for 4 days

≥3 years: 100 mg/m^2/day continuous infusion for 4 days

Central nervous system tumors (unlabeled use; combination chemotherapy): I.V.:

<3 years: 6.5 mg/kg/dose days 3 and 4 of each 28-day "B" treatment cycle (Duffner, 1993)

≥3 years: 100 mg/m^2/day on days 1, 2, and 3 of a 3-week treatment cycle (Taylor, 2003)

≥6 years: 150 mg/m^2/day on days 3 and 4 of a 3-week treatment course (Kovnar, 1990)

Hematopoietic stem cell transplantation conditioning regimen: I.V.: 60 mg/kg/dose over 4 hours as a single dose 3 or 4 days prior to transplantation (Horning, 1994; Snyder, 1993)

Hodgkin lymphoma (unlabeled use): I.V.: 200 mg/m^2/day on days 1, 2, and 3 every 3 weeks (Kelly, 2002)

Neuroblastoma (unlabeled use): I.V.:

Induction: 100 mg/m^2/day on days 1-5 of each cycle (Kaneko, 2002)

Hematopoietic stem cell transplantation conditioning regimen: 200 mg/m^2/day for 4 days beginning 8 or 9 days prior to transplantation (Kaneko, 2002)

Sarcoma, refractory (unlabeled use): I.V.: 100 mg/m^2/day on days 1-5 of cycle; repeat cycle every 21 days (Van Winkle, 2005)

Renal Impairment Oral, I.V.:

U.S. labeling recommends the following adjustments:

Cl_{cr} >50 mL/minute: No adjustment required.

Cl_{cr} 15-50 mL/minute: Administer 75% of dose

Cl_{cr} <15 mL/minute: Data not available; consider further dose reductions

The following adjustments have been recommended:

Aronoff, 2007:

Children:

Cl_{cr} 10-50 mL/minute/1.73 m^2: Administer 75% of dose.

Cl_{cr} <10 mL/minute/1.73 m^2: Administer 50% of dose.

Hemodialysis: Administer 50% of dose.

Peritoneal dialysis: Administer 50% of dose.

Continuous renal replacement therapy (CRRT): Administer 75% of dose and reduce for hyperbilirubinemia.

Adults:

Cl_{cr} 10-50 mL/minute: Administer 75% of dose.

Cl_{cr} <10 mL/minute: Administer 50% of dose.

Hemodialysis: Administer 50% of dose; supplemental posthemodialysis dose is not necessary.

Peritoneal dialysis: Administer 50% of dose; supplemental dose is not necessary.

Continuous renal replacement therapy (CRRT): Administer 75% of dose.

Janus, 2010: Hemodialysis: Reduce dose by 50%; not removed by hemodialysis so may be administered before or after dialysis

Kintzel, 1995:

Cl_{cr} 46-60 mL/minute: Administer 85% of dose

Cl_{cr} 31-45 mL/minute: Administer 80% of dose

Cl_{cr} ≤30 mL/minute: Administer 75% of dose

Hepatic Impairment

U.S. labeling: No dosage adjustment provided in manufacturer's labeling.

Canadian labeling:

Mild-to-moderate impairment: No dosage adjustment provided in manufacturer's labeling.

Severe impairment: Use is contraindicated.

The following adjustments have also been recommended:

Donelli, 1998: Liver dysfunction may reduce the metabolism and increase the toxicity of etoposide. Normal doses of I.V. etoposide should be given to patients with liver dysfunction (dose reductions may result in subtherapeutic concentrations); however, use caution with concomitant liver dysfunction (severe) and renal dysfunction as the decreased metabolic clearance cannot be compensated by increased renal clearance.

Floyd, 2006: Bilirubin 1.5-3 mg/dL or AST >3 times ULN: Administer 50% of dose

King, 2001; Koren, 1992: Bilirubin 1.5-3 mg/dL or AST >180 units/L: Administer 50% of dose

Adjustment for Toxicity Oral, I.V.:

Infusion (hypersensitivity) reactions: Interrupt infusion.

ANC <500/mm³ or platelets <50,000/mm³: Withhold treatment until recovery.

Severe adverse reactions (nonhematologic): Reduce dose or discontinue treatment.

WBC 2000-3000/mm³ or platelets 75,000-100,000/mm³: Canadian labeling (not in U.S. labeling): Reduce dose by 50%

Combination Regimens

Brain tumors:

CDDP/VP-16 on page 1555

COPE on page 1596

Gestational trophoblastic tumor:

EMA/CO on page 1622

EP/EMA on page 1625

Leukemia, acute lymphocytic: Hyper-CVAD (Leukemia, Acute Lymphocytic) on page 1681

Leukemia, acute myeloid:

5 + 2 + 5 (Cytarabine-Daunorubicin-Etoposide) (AML Consolidation) on page 1513

7 + 3 + 7 (Cytarabine-Daunorubicin-Etoposide) (AML Induction) on page 1515

Cytarabine (High Dose)-Daunorubicin-Etoposide (AML Induction) on page 1602

MEC (AML Induction) on page 1706

MEC-G (AML Induction) on page 1707

Mitoxantrone-Etoposide (AML Induction) on page 1713
Lung cancer (nonsmall cell):
Cisplatin-Etoposide (NSCLC) on page 1568
EC (NSCLC) on page 1621
EP (NSCLC) on page 1628
EP/PE on page 1631
Lung cancer (small cell):
Carboplatin-Etoposide (Small Cell Lung Cancer) on page 1546
Cisplatin–Etoposide (Small Cell Lung Cancer) on page 1569
Etoposide Oral (Small Cell Lung Cancer Regimen) on page 1640
Lymphoma, Hodgkin:
BEACOPP-14 (Hodgkin) on page 1522
BEACOPP Escalated (Hodgkin) on page 1522
BEACOPP Escalated Plus Standard (Hodgkin) on page 1523
BEACOPP Standard (Hodgkin) on page 1525
Dexa-BEAM (Hodgkin) on page 1607
ESHAP (Hodgkin) on page 1634
ICE (Hodgkin) on page 1688
MINE-ESHAP (Hodgkin) on page 1711
mini-BEAM (Hodgkin) on page 1712
Stanford V (Hodgkin) on page 1752
VIM-D (Hodgkin) on page 1770
Lymphoma, non-Hodgkin's:
CEPP(B) on page 1556
EPOCH Dose-Adjusted (AIDS-Related Lymphoma) on page 1628
EPOCH Dose-Adjusted (NHL) on page 1628
EPOCH (Dose-Adjusted)-Rituximab (NHL) on page 1629
EPOCH (NHL) on page 1630
EPOCH-Rituximab (NHL) on page 1631
ESHAP on page 1633
ICE (Lymphoma, non-Hodgkin's) on page 1689
IMVP-16 on page 1691
MINE on page 1711
MINE-ESHAP (NHL) on page 1712
Pro-MACE-CytaBOM on page 1741
RICE on page 1747
Lymphoma, non-Hodgkin's (Burkitt): CODOX-M/IVAC on page 1591
Multiple myeloma: DTPACE on page 1620
Neuroblastoma:
A3 (Neuroblastoma) on page 1515
CAV-P/VP (Neuroblastoma) on page 1554
CDDP/VP-16 on page 1555
CE-CAdO (Neuroblastoma) on page 1555
Cisplatin-Doxorubicin-Etoposide-Cyclophosphamide (Neuroblastoma) on page 1568
New A1 (Neuroblastoma) on page 1721
Osteosarcoma: ICE (Sarcoma) on page 1689
Ovarian cancer:
BEP (Ovarian Cancer) on page 1526
BEP (Ovarian Cancer, Testicular Cancer) on page 1526
Etoposide-Carboplatin (Ovarian Cancer) on page 1639
Etoposide (Ovarian Regimen) on page 1639

Prostate cancer:
- Estramustine + Etoposide on page 1636
- Paclitaxel + Estramustine + Etoposide on page 1729

Retinoblastoma:
- Carboplatin-Etoposide (Retinoblastoma) on page 1545
- Carboplatin-Etoposide-Vincristine (Retinoblastoma) on page 1546

Sarcoma: VAC Alternating With IE (Ewing's Sarcoma) on page 1766

Soft tissue sarcoma
- ICE (Sarcoma) on page 1689
- IE on page 1690

Testicular cancer:
- BEP (Ovarian Cancer, Testicular Cancer) on page 1526
- BEP (Testicular Cancer) on page 1527
- EP (Testicular Cancer) on page 1631
- VIP (Etoposide) (Testicular Cancer) on page 1776

Unknown primary, adenocarcinoma: Carboplatin-Etoposide-Paclitaxel (Unknown Primary) on page 1545

Wilms' tumor: Regimen I (Wilms' Tumor) on page 1745

Administration

Oral: Doses ≤200 mg/day as a single once daily dose; doses >200 mg should be given in 2-4 divided doses. If necessary, the injection may be used for oral administration (see Extemporaneous Preparations). Canadian labeling recommends administering capsule on an empty stomach.

I.V.: Administer standard doses over at least 30-60 minutes to minimize the risk of hypotension. Higher (unlabeled) doses used in transplantation may be infused over longer time periods depending on the protocol. Etoposide injection contains polysorbate 80 which may cause leaching of diethylhexyl phthalate (DEHP), a plasticizer contained in polyvinyl chloride (PVC) tubing. Administration through non-PVC (low sorbing) tubing will minimize patient exposure to DEHP. Tissue irritation and inflammation have occurred following extravasation.

Concentrations >0.4 mg/mL are very unstable and may precipitate within a few minutes. For large doses, where dilution to ≤0.4 mg/mL is not feasible, consideration should be given to slow infusion of the undiluted drug through a running normal saline, dextrose or saline/dextrose infusion; or use of etoposide phosphate. Etoposide solutions of 0.1-0.4 mg/mL may be filtered through a 0.22 micron filter without damage to the filter; etoposide solutions of 0.2 mg/mL may be filtered through a 0.22 micron filter without significant loss of drug.

Emetic Potential

Oral: Low (10% to 30%)

I.V.: Low (10% to 30%)

Vesicant/Extravasation Risk May be an irritant

Extemporaneous Preparations Hazardous agent: Use appropriate precautions for handling and disposal.

Etoposide 10 mg/mL oral solution: Dilute etoposide for injection 1:1 with normal saline to a concentration of 10 mg/mL. This solution is stable in plastic oral syringes for 22 days at room temperature. Prior to oral administration, further mix with fruit juice (orange, apple, or lemon; **NOT** grapefruit juice) to a concentration of <0.4 mg/mL; once mixed with fruit juice, use within 3 hours.

McLeod HL and Relling MV, "Stability of Etoposide Solution for Oral Use," *Am J Hosp Pharm*, 1992, 49(11):2784-5.

Monitoring Parameters CBC with differential; liver function (bilirubin, ALT, AST), albumin, renal function tests; vital signs (blood pressure)

Dosage Forms Excipient information presented when available (limited, particularly for generics); consult specific product labeling.

Capsule, softgel, oral: 50 mg

Injection, solution: 20 mg/mL (5 mL, 25 mL, 50 mL)

Toposar®: 20 mg/mL (5 mL, 25 mL, 50 mL) [contains dehydrated ethanol 33.2%, polyethylene glycol 300, polysorbate 80]

References

Albain KS, Swann RS, Rusch VW, et al, "Radiotherapy Plus Chemotherapy With or Without Surgical Resection for Stage III Non-Small-Cell Lung Cancer: A Phase III Randomised Controlled Trial," *Lancet*, 2009, 374(9687):379-86.

Aronoff GR, Bennett WM, Berns JS, et al, *Drug Prescribing in Renal Failure: Dosing Guidelines for Adults and Children*, 5th ed. Philadelphia, PA: American College of Physicians; 2007, p 99, 171.

Arriagada R, Bergman B, Dunant A, et al, "Cisplatin-Based Adjuvant Chemotherapy in Patients With Completely Resected Non-Small-Cell Lung Cancer," *N Engl J Med*, 2004, 350(4):351-60.

Collier K, Schink C, Young AM, et al, "Case Report: Successful Treatment With Etoposide Phosphate in Patients With Previous Etoposide Hypersensitivity," *J Oncol Pharm Pract*, 2008, 14(1):51-5.

Donelli MG, Zucchetti M, Munzone E, et al, "Pharmacokinetics of Anticancer Agents in Patients With Impaired Liver Function," *Eur J Cancer*, 1998, 34(1):33-46.

Duffner PK, Horowitz ME, Krischer JP, et al "Postoperative Chemotherapy and Delayed Radiation in Children Less Than Three Years of Age With Malignant Brain Tumors," *N Engl J Med*, 1993, 328(24):1725-31.

Einhorn LH, Williams SD, Chamness A, et al, "High-Dose Chemotherapy and Stem-Cell Rescue for Metastatic Germ-cell Tumors," *N Engl J Med*, 2007, 357(4):340-8.

Floyd J, Mirza I, Sachs B, et al, "Hepatotoxicity of Chemotherapy," *Semin Oncol*, 2006, 33 (1):50-67.

Giaccone G, Ardizzoni A, Kirkpatrick A, et al, "Cisplatin and Etoposide Combination Chemotherapy for Locally Advanced or Metastatic Thymoma. A Phase II Study of the European Organization for Research and Treatment of Cancer Lung Cancer Cooperative Group," *J Clin Oncol*, 1996, 14 (3):814-20.

Greco FA, Burris HA 3rd, Erland JB, et al, "Carcinoma of Unknown Primary Site," *Cancer*, 2000, 89 (12):2655-60.

Hainsworth JD, Spigel DR, Litchy S, et al, "Phase II Trial of Paclitaxel, Carboplatin, and Etoposide in Advanced Poorly Differentiated Neuroendocrine Carcinoma: A Minnie Pearl Cancer Research Network Study," *J Clin Oncol*, 2006, 24(22):3548-54.

Horning SJ, Negrin RS, Chao JC, et al, "Fractionated Total-Body Irradiation, Etoposide, and Cyclophosphamide and Non-Hodgkin's Lymphoma," *J Clin Oncol*, 1994, 12(12):2552-8.

Ihde DC, Mulshine JL, Kramer BS, et al, "Prospective Randomized Comparison of High-Dose and Standard-Dose Etoposide and Cisplatin Chemotherapy in Patients With Extensive-Stage Small-Cell Lung Cancer," *J Clin Oncol*, 1994, 12(10):2022-34.

Janus N, Thariat J, Boulanger H, et al, "Proposal for Dosage Adjustment and Timing of Chemotherapy in Hemodialyzed Patients," *Ann Oncol*, 2010, 21(7):1395-403.

Kaneko M, Tsuchida Y, Mugishima H, et al, "Intensified Chemotherapy Increases the Survival Rates in Patients With Stage 4 Neuroblastoma With MYCN Amplification," *J Pediatr Hematol Oncol*, 2002, 24(8):613-21.

Kelly KM, Hutchinson RJ, Sposto R, et al, "Feasibility of Upfront Dose-Intensive Chemotherapy in Children With Advanced-Stage Hodgkin's Lymphoma: Preliminary Results From the Children's Cancer Group Study CCG-59704," *Ann Oncol*, 2002, 13(Suppl 1):107-11.

King PD and Perry MC, "Hepatotoxicity of Chemotherapy," *Oncologist*, 2001, 6(2):162-76.

Kintzel PE and Dorr RT, "Anticancer Drug Renal Toxicity and Elimination: Dosing Guidelines for Altered Renal Function," *Cancer Treat Rev*, 1995, 21(1):33-64.

Kondagunta GV, Bacik J, Donadio A, et al, "Combination of Paclitaxel, Ifosfamide, and Cisplatin is an Effective Second-Line Therapy for Patients With Relapsed Testicular Germ Cell Tumors," *J Clin Oncol*, 2005, 23(27):6549-55.

Koren G, Beatty K, Seto A, et al, "The Effects of Impaired Liver Function on the Elimination of Antineoplastic Agents," *Ann Pharmacother*, 1992, 26(3):363-71.

Kovnar EH, Kellie SJ, Horowitz ME, et al, "Preirradiation Cisplatin and Etoposide in the Treatment of High-Risk Medulloblastoma and Other Malignant Embryonal Tumors of the Central Nervous System: A Phase II Study," *J Clin Oncol*, 1990, 8(2):330-6.

Lara PN Jr, Natale R, Crowley J, et al, "Phase III Trial of Irinotecan/Cisplatin Compared With Etoposide/Cisplatin in Extensive-Stage Small-Cell Lung Cancer: Clinical and Pharmacogenomic Results from SWOG S0124," *J Clin Oncol*, 2009, 27(15):2530-5.

Rose PG, Blessing JA, Mayer AR, et al, "Prolonged Oral Etoposide as Second-Line Therapy for Platinum-Resistant and Platinum-Sensitive Ovarian Carcinoma: A Gynecologic Oncology Group Study," *J Clin Oncol*, 1998, 16(2):405-10.

Saito H, Takada Y, Ichinose Y, et al, "Phase II Study of Etoposide and Cisplatin With Concurrent Twice-Daily Thoracic Radiotherapy Followed by Irinotecan and Cisplatin in Patients With Limited-Disease Small-Cell Lung Cancer: West Japan Thoracic Oncology Group 9902," *J Clin Oncol*, 2006, 24(33):5247-52.

Saxman SB, Finch D, Gonin R, et al, "Long-Term Follow-Up of a Phase III Study of Three Versus Four Cycles of Bleomycin, Etoposide, and Cisplatin in Favorable-Prognosis Germ-Cell Tumors: The Indian University Experience," *J Clin Oncol*, 1998, 16(2):702-6.

Siderov J, Prasad P, De Boer R, et al, "Safe Administration of Etoposide Phosphate After Hypersensitivity Reaction to Intravenous Etoposide," *Br J Cancer*, 2002, 86(1):12-3.

Skarlos DV, Samantas E, Briassoulis E, et al, "Randomized Comparison of Early Versus Late Hyperfractionated Thoracic Irradiation Concurrently With Chemotherapy in Limited Disease Small-Cell Lung Cancer: A Randomized Phase II Study of the Hellenic Cooperative Oncology Group (HeCOG)," *Ann Oncol*, 2001, 12(9):1231-38.

Snyder DS, Chao NJ, Amylon MD, et al, "Fractionated Total Body Irradiation and High-Dose Etoposide as a Preparatory Regimen for Bone Marrow Transplantation for 99 Patients With Acute Leukemia in First Complete Remission," *Blood*, 1993, 82(9):2920-8.

Sundstrom S, Bremnes RM, Kaasa S, et al, "Cisplatin and Etoposide Regimen is Superior to Cyclophosphamide, Epirubicin, and Vincristine Regimen in Small-Cell Lung Cancer: Results From a Randomized Phase III Trial With 5 Years' Follow-up," *J Clin Oncol*, 2002, 20(24):4665-72.

Taylor RE, Bailey CC, Robinson K, et al, "Results of a Randomized Study of Preradiation Chemotherapy Versus Radiotherapy Alone for Nonmetastatic Medulloblastoma: The International Society of Paediatric Oncology/United Kingdom Children's Cancer Study Group PNET-3 Study," *J Clin Oncol*, 2003, 21(8):1581-91.

Turrisi AT, Kim K, Blum R, et al, "Twice-daily Compared With Once-daily Thoracic Radiotherapy in Limited Small-Cell Lung Cancer Treated Concurrently With Cisplatin and Etoposide," *N Engl J Med*, 1999, 340(4):265-71.

van Winkle P, Angiolillo A, Krailo M, et al, "Ifosfamide, Carboplatin, and Etoposide (ICE) Reinduction Chemotherapy in a Large Cohort of Children and Adolescents With Recurrent/Refractory Sarcoma: The Children's Cancer Group (CCG) Experience," *Pediatr Blood Cancer*, 2005, 44(4):338-47.

Weaver CH, Petersen FB, Appelbaum FR, et al, "High-dose Fractionated Total-Body Irradiation, Etoposde, and Cyclophosphamide Followed by Autologous Stem-Cell Support in Patients With Malignant Lymphoma," *J Clin Oncol*, 1994, 12(12):2559-66.

Yang J, Bogni A, Schuetz EG, "Etoposide Pathway," *Pharmacogenet Genomics*, 2009, 19(7):552-3.

◆ **Etoposide Injection USP (Can)** *see* Etoposide *on page 538*

Etoposide Phosphate (e toe POE side FOS fate)

Related Information

Management of Drug Extravasations *on page 1800*

Safe Handling of Hazardous Drugs *on page 1904*

Brand Names: U.S. Etopophos®

Index Terms Epipodophyllotoxin; ETOP

Generic Availability (U.S.) No

Pharmacologic Category Antineoplastic Agent, Podophyllotoxin Derivative; Antineoplastic Agent, Topoisomerase II Inhibitor

Use Treatment of refractory testicular tumors; treatment of small cell lung cancer

Labeled Contraindications Hypersensitivity to etoposide, etoposide phosphate, or any component of the formulation

Pregnancy Risk Factor D

Lactation Excretion in breast milk unknown/not recommended

Warnings/Precautions Hazardous agent - use appropriate precautions for handling and disposal. **[U.S. Boxed Warning]: Severe dose-limiting and dose-related myelosuppression with resulting infection or bleeding may occur.** Treatment should be withheld for platelets <50,000/mm^3 or absolute neutrophil count (ANC) <500/mm^3. May cause anaphylactic-like reactions manifested by chills, fever, tachycardia, bronchospasm, dyspnea, and hypotension. In addition, facial/tongue swelling, coughing, throat tightness, cyanosis, laryngospasm, diaphoresis, back pain, hypertension, flushing, apnea and loss of consciousness have also been reported less commonly. Anaphylactic-type reactions have occurred with the first infusion. Infusion should be interrupted and medications for the treatment of anaphylaxis should be available for immediate use. Underlying mechanisms behind the development of hypersensitivity reactions is unknown, but have been attributed to high drug concentration and rate of infusion. Another possible mechanism may be due to the differences between available etoposide intravenous formulations. Etoposide intravenous formulation contains polysorbate 80 and benzyl alcohol, while etoposide phosphate (the water soluble prodrug of etoposide) intravenous formulation does not contain either vehicle. Case reports have suggested that etoposide phosphate has been used successfully in patients with previous hypersensitivity reactions to etoposide (Collier, 2008; Siderov, 2002).

Secondary acute leukemias have been reported with etoposide, either as monotherapy or in combination with other chemotherapy agents. Dosage should be adjusted in patients with hepatic or renal impairment. Use with caution in patients with low serum albumin; may increase risk for toxicities. Doses of etoposide phosphate >175 mg/m^2 have not been evaluated. Use caution in elderly patients (may be more likely to develop severe myelosuppression and/or GI effects. Administer by slow I.V. infusion; hypotension has been reported with etoposide phosphate administration, generally associated with rapid I.V. infusion. Injection site reactions may occur; monitor infusion site closely. **[U.S. Boxed Warning]: Should be administered under the supervision of an experienced cancer chemotherapy physician.**

Adverse Reactions Note: Also see adverse reactions for **etoposide;** etoposide phosphate is converted to etoposide, adverse reactions experienced with etoposide would also be expected with etoposide phosphate.

>10%:

- Central nervous system: Chills/fever (24%)
- Dermatologic: Alopecia (33% to 44%)
- Gastrointestinal: Nausea/vomiting (37%), anorexia (16%), mucositis (11%)
- Hematologic: Leukopenia (91%; grade 4: 17%; nadir: day 15-22; recovery: usually by day 21), neutropenia (88%; grade 4: 37%; nadir: day 12-19; recovery: usually by day 21), anemia (72%; grades 3/4: 19%), thrombocytopenia (23%; grade 4: 9%; nadir: day 10-15; recovery: usually by day 21)
- Neuromuscular & skeletal: Weakness/malaise (39%)

1% to 10%:

- Cardiovascular: Hypotension (1% to 5%), hypertension (3%), facial flushing (2%)
- Central nervous system: Dizziness (5%)
- Dermatologic: Skin rash (3%)
- Gastrointestinal: Constipation (8%), abdominal pain (7%), diarrhea (6%), taste perversion (6%)
- Local: Extravasation/phlebitis (5%; including swelling, pain, cellulitis, necrosis, and/or skin necrosis at site of infiltration)

Miscellaneous: Anaphylactic-type reactions (3%; including chills, diaphoresis, fever, rigor, tachycardia, bronchospasm, dyspnea, pruritus)

<1%, postmarketing, and/or case reports: Acute leukemia (with/without pre-leukemia phase), anaphylactic-like reactions, back pain, blindness (transient, cortical), cough, cyanosis, diaphoresis, dysphagia, erythema, facial swelling, hepatic toxicity, hyperpigmentation, hypersensitivity-associated apnea, infection, interstitial pneumonitis, laryngospasm, maculopapular rash, neutropenic fever, optic neuritis, perivasculitis, pulmonary fibrosis, radiation recall dermatitis, seizure, Stevens-Johnson syndrome, tongue swelling, toxic epidermal necrolysis, urticaria

Drug Interactions

Metabolism/Transport Effects Substrate of CYP1A2 (minor), CYP2E1 (minor), CYP3A4 (major), P-glycoprotein; **Note:** Assignment of Major/Minor substrate status based on clinically relevant drug interaction potential; **Inhibits** CYP2C9 (weak), CYP3A4 (weak)

Avoid Concomitant Use

Avoid concomitant use of Etoposide Phosphate with any of the following: BCG; CloZAPine; Conivaptan; Natalizumab; Pimecrolimus; Pimozide; Tacrolimus (Topical); Vaccines (Live)

Increased Effect/Toxicity

Etoposide Phosphate may increase the levels/effects of: ARIPiprazole; CloZAPine; Leflunomide; Natalizumab; Pimozide; Vaccines (Live)

The levels/effects of Etoposide Phosphate may be increased by: Conivaptan; CycloSPORINE (Systemic); CYP3A4 Inhibitors (Moderate); CYP3A4 Inhibitors (Strong); Dasatinib; Denosumab; Ivacaftor; Mifepristone; P-glycoprotein/ABCB1 Inhibitors; Pimecrolimus; Roflumilast; Tacrolimus (Topical); Trastuzumab

Decreased Effect

Etoposide Phosphate may decrease the levels/effects of: BCG; Coccidioidin Skin Test; Sipuleucel-T; Vaccines (Inactivated); Vaccines (Live)

The levels/effects of Etoposide Phosphate may be decreased by: Barbiturates; CYP3A4 Inducers (Strong); Deferasirox; Echinacea; Fosphenytoin; Herbs (CYP3A4 Inducers); P-glycoprotein/ABCB1 Inducers; Phenytoin; Tocilizumab

Ethanol/Nutrition/Herb Interactions

Ethanol: Avoid ethanol (may increase GI irritation).

Herb/Nutraceutical: Avoid St John's wort (may decrease etoposide levels).

Storage/Stability Store intact vials under refrigeration at 2°C to 8°C (36°F to 46°F). Protect from light. Reconstituted solution is stable refrigerated at 2°C to 8°C (36°F to 46°F) for 7 days. At room temperature of 20°C to 25°C (68°F to 77°F), reconstituted solutions are stable for 24 hours when reconstituted with SWFI, D_5W, or NS, or for 48 hours when reconstituted with bacteriostatic SWFI or bacteriostatic NS. Further diluted solutions for infusion are stable at room temperature 20°C to 25°C (68°F to 77°F) or under refrigeration 2°C to 8°C (36°F to 46°F) for up to 24 hours.

Reconstitution Reconstitute vials with 5 mL or 10 mL SWFI, D_5W, NS, bacteriostatic SWFI, or bacteriostatic NS to a concentration of 20 mg/mL or 10 mg/mL etoposide equivalent. These solutions may be administered without further dilution or may be diluted in 50-500 mL of D_5W or NS to a concentration as low as 0.1 mg/mL. Use appropriate precautions for handling and disposal.

Mechanism of Action Etoposide phosphate is converted *in vivo* to the active moiety, etoposide, by dephosphorylation. Etoposide inhibits mitotic activity;

inhibits cells from entering prophase; inhibits DNA synthesis. Initially thought to be mitotic inhibitors similar to podophyllotoxin, but actually have no effect on microtubule assembly. However, later shown to induce DNA strand breakage and inhibition of topoisomerase II (an enzyme which breaks and repairs DNA); etoposide acts in late S or early G2 phases.

Pharmacodynamics/Kinetics

Distribution: Average V_d: 7-17 L/m^2; poor penetration across blood-brain barrier; concentrations in CSF being <10% that of plasma

Protein binding: 97%

Metabolism:

Etoposide phosphate: Rapidly and completely converted to etoposide in plasma

Etoposide: Hepatic, via CYP3A4 and 3A5 to various metabolites; in addition, conversion of etoposide to the O-demethylated metabolites (catechol and quinine) via prostaglandin synthases or myeloperoxidase occurs, as well as glutathione and glucuronide conjugation via GSTT1/GSTP1 and UGT1A1 (Yang, 2009)

Half-life elimination: Terminal: 4-11 hours; Children: Normal renal/hepatic function: 6-8 hours

Excretion: Urine (56%; 45% as etoposide) within 120 hours; feces (44%) within 120 hours

Children: Urine (~55% as etoposide) in 24 hours

Dosing

Adult & Geriatric Refer to individual protocols. **Note:** Etoposide phosphate is a prodrug of etoposide, doses should be expressed as the desired **ETOPOSIDE** dose; **not** as the etoposide phosphate dose. (eg, etoposide phosphate equivalent to _____ mg etoposide). Etoposide phosphate 113.5 mg is equivalent to etoposide 100 mg.

Small cell lung cancer: I.V. (in combination with other approved chemotherapeutic drugs): Etoposide 35 mg/m^2/day for 4 days up to 50 mg/m^2/day for 5 days. Courses are repeated at 3- to 4-week intervals after adequate recovery from toxicity.

Testicular cancer: I.V. (in combination with other approved chemotherapeutic agents): Etoposide 50-100 mg/m^2/day on days 1-5 to 100 mg/m^2/day on days 1, 3, and 5. Courses are repeated at 3- to 4-week intervals after adequate recovery from toxicity.

Indication-specific unlabeled dosing: Refer to Etoposide monograph.

Renal Impairment Manufacturer recommended guidelines:

Cl_{cr} >50 mL/minute: No adjustment required.

Cl_{cr} 15-50 mL/minute: Administer 75% of dose.

Cl_{cr} <15 mL/minute: Data are not available; consider further dose reductions.

Etoposide phosphate is rapidly and completely converted to etoposide in plasma, please refer to Etoposide monograph for additional renal dosing adjustments (for etoposide).

Hepatic Impairment The FDA-approved labeling does not contain dosing adjustment guidelines. Etoposide phosphate is rapidly and completely converted to etoposide in plasma; please refer to Etoposide monograph for etoposide hepatic dosing adjustments.

Combination Regimens

Retinoblastoma: Carboplatin-Etoposide-Vincristine (Retinoblastoma) on page 1546

Administration Infuse by slow I.V. infusion over 5-210 minutes; risk of hypotension may increase with rate of infusion. Do not administer as a bolus injection.

Emetic Potential Low (10% to 30%)

Vesicant/Extravasation Risk May be an irritant

Monitoring Parameters CBC with differential and platelets (prior to initial treatment and each cycle), vital signs (blood pressure), bilirubin, AST/ALT, renal function

Additional Information Etoposide phosphate 113.5 mg is equivalent to etoposide 100 mg. Dosages should always be expressed, and calculated, as the desired **etoposide** dose.

Dosage Forms Excipient information presented when available (limited, particularly for generics); consult specific product labeling.

Injection, powder for reconstitution [strength expressed as base]:

Etopophos®: 100 mg

References

Aronoff GR, Bennett WM, Berns JS, et al, *Drug Prescribing in Renal Failure: Dosing Guidelines for Adults and Children*, 5th ed. Philadelphia, PA: American College of Physicians; 2007, p 97.

Collier K, Schink C, Young AM, et al, "Case Report: Successful Treatment with Etoposide Phosphate in Patients With Previous Etoposide Hypersensitivity," *J Oncol Pharm Pract*, 2008, 14(1):51-5.

Donelli MG, Zucchetti M, Munzone E, et al, "Pharmacokinetics of Anticancer Agents in Patients With Impaired Liver Function," *Eur J Cancer*, 1998, 34(1):33-46.

Dorr RT, Briggs A, Kintzel P, et al, "Comparative Pharmacokinetic Study of High-Dose Etoposide and Etoposide Phosphate in Patients With Lymphoid Malignancy Receiving Autologous Stem Cell Transplantation," *Bone Marrow Transplant*, 2003, 31(8):643-9.

Floyd J, Mirza I, Sachs B, et al, "Hepatotoxicity of Chemotherapy," *Semin Oncol*, 2006, 33 (1):50-67.

King PD and Perry MC, "Hepatotoxicity of Chemotherapy," *Oncologist*, 2001, 6(2):162-76.

Kintzel PE and Dorr RT, "Anticancer Drug Renal Toxicity and Elimination: Dosing Guidelines for Altered Renal Function," *Cancer Treat Rev*, 1995, 21(1):33-64.

Koren G, Beatty K, Seto A, et al, "The Effects of Impaired Liver Function on the Elimination of Antineoplastic Agents," *Ann Pharmacother*, 1992, 26(3):363-71.

Mummaneni V, Kaul S, Igwemezie LN, et al, "Bioequivalence Assessment of Etoposide Phosphate and Etoposide Using Pharmacodynamic and Traditional Pharmacokinetic Parameters," *J Pharmacokinet Biopharm*, 1996, 24(4):313-25.

Perry MC, "Hepatotoxicity of Chemotherapeutic Agents," *Semin Oncol*, 1982, 9(1):65-73.

Siderov J, Prasad P, De Boer R, et al, "Safe Administration of Etoposide Phosphate After Hypersensitivity Reaction to Intravenous Etoposide," *Br J Cancer*, 2002, 86(1):12-3.

Yang J, Bogni A, Schuetz EG, "Etoposide Pathway," *Pharmacogenet Genomics*, 2009, 19 (7):552-3.

◆ **Euflex® (Can)** *see* Flutamide *on page 635*

◆ **Eulexin** *see* Flutamide *on page 635*

◆ **Eulexin® (Can)** *see* Flutamide *on page 635*

◆ ***Euphorbia peplus* Derivative** *see* Ingenol Mebutate *on page 796*

◆ **Euro-Cyproheptadine (Can)** *see* Cyproheptadine *on page 342*

Everolimus (e ver OH li mus)

Related Information

Management of Chemotherapy-Induced Nausea and Vomiting *on page 1786*

Principles of Anticancer Therapy *on page 1878*

Brand Names: U.S. Afinitor®; Afinitor® Disperz; Zortress®

Brand Names: Canada Afinitor®

Index Terms RAD001

Generic Availability (U.S.) No

Pharmacologic Category Antineoplastic Agent, mTOR Kinase Inhibitor; Immunosuppressant Agent; mTOR Kinase Inhibitor

Use

Afinitor®: Treatment of advanced hormone receptor-positive, HER2-negative breast cancer in postmenopausal women (in combination with exemestane and after letrozole or anastrozole failure); treatment of advanced renal cell cancer (RCC), after sunitinib or sorafenib failure; treatment of renal angiomyolipoma with tuberous sclerosis complex (TSC) not requiring immediate surgery; treatment of subependymal giant cell astrocytoma (SEGA) associated with TSC which requires intervention, but cannot be curatively resected; treatment of advanced, metastatic or unresectable pancreatic neuroendocrine tumors (PNET)

Afinitor® Disperz: Treatment of subependymal giant cell astrocytoma (SEGA) associated with TSC which requires intervention, but cannot be curatively resected

Zortress®: Prophylaxis of organ rejection in renal transplantation patients at low-moderate immunologic risk

Unlabeled Use Treatment of relapsed or refractory Waldenström's macroglobulinemia (WM)

Labeled Contraindications Hypersensitivity to everolimus, sirolimus, other rapamycin derivatives, or any component of the formulation.

Pregnancy Risk Factor D (Afinitor®) / C (Zortress®)

Lactation Excretion in breast milk unknown/not recommended

Warnings/Precautions Hazardous agent - use appropriate precautions for handling and disposal. Noninfectious pneumonitis (sometimes fatal) has been observed with mTOR inhibitors including everolimus; symptoms include dyspnea, cough, hypoxia and/or pleural effusion; promptly evaluate worsening respiratory symptoms; may require treatment interruption followed by dose reduction (pneumonitis has developed even with reduced doses) and/or corticosteroid therapy; discontinue for grade 4 symptoms. Imaging may overestimate the incidence of clinical pneumonitis. **[U.S. Boxed Warning]: Everolimus has immunosuppressant properties which may result in infection;** the risk of developing bacterial (including mycobacterial), viral, fungal and protozoal infections and for local, opportunistic (including polyomavirus infection), systemic infections, and/or sepsis is increased. Polyomavirus infection in transplant patients may be serious and/or fatal. Polyoma virus-associated nephropathy (due to BK virus), which may result in serious cases of deteriorating renal function and renal graft loss, has been observed with use. JC virus-associated progressive multiple leukoencephalopathy (PML) may also be associated with everolimus use in transplantation. Reduced immunosuppression should be considered with evidence of polyoma virus infection or PML. Reactivation of hepatitis B has been observed in patients receiving everolimus. Resolve pre-existing invasive fungal infections prior to treatment initiation. Monitor for signs and symptoms of infection during treatment. Discontinue if invasive systemic fungal infection is diagnosed (and manage with appropriate antifungal therapy).

[U.S. Boxed Warning]: Immunosuppressant use may result in the development of malignancy, including lymphoma and skin cancer. The risk is associated with treatment intensity and the duration of therapy. To minimize the risk for skin cancer, limit exposure to sunlight and ultraviolet light; wear protective clothing and use effective sunscreen.

[U.S. Boxed Warning]: Due to the increased risk for nephrotoxicity in renal transplantation, avoid standard doses of cyclosporine in combination with everolimus; reduced cyclosporine doses are recommended when everolimus is used in combination with cyclosporine. Therapeutic monitoring of cyclosporine and everolimus concentrations is recommended. Monitor for proteinuria; the risk of proteinuria is increased when everolimus is used in combination with cyclosporine, and with higher serum everolimus concentrations. Everolimus and cyclosporine combination therapy may increase the risk for thrombotic microangiopathy/thrombotic thrombocytopenic purpura/hemolytic uremic syndrome (TMA/TTP/HUS); monitor blood counts. Elevations in serum creatinine (generally mild), renal failure, and proteinuria have been also observed with everolimus use; monitor renal function (BUN, creatinine, and/or urinary protein). An increased incidence of rash, infection and dose interruptions have been reported in patients with renal insufficiency (Cl_{cr} ≤60 mL/minute) who received mTOR inhibitors for the treatment of renal cell cancer (Gupta, 2011); pharmacokinetic studies have not been conducted; dosage adjustments are not required based on renal impairment. **[U.S. Boxed Warning]: An increased risk of renal arterial and venous thrombosis has been reported with use in renal transplantation, generally within the first 30 days after transplant; may result in graft loss.**

Avoid concomitant use with strong CYP3A4 inducers (eg, dexamethasone, phenytoin, carbamazepine, rifampin, rifabutin, rifapentine, phenobarbital) and strong CYP3A4 inhibitors (eg, ketoconazole, itraconazole, voriconazole, clarithromycin, telithromycin, atazanavir, saquinavir, ritonavir, indinavir, delavirdine, fosamprenavir, nelfinavir, nefazodone, grapefruit juice). Dosage modification may be needed if concomitant use with strong CYP3A4 inducers cannot be avoided. Use with caution with concomitant moderate CYP3A4 inhibitors and/or P-gp inhibitors; decreased everolimus doses are recommended. In renal transplantation, avoid the use of HMG-CoA reductase inhibitors; may increase the risk for rhabdomyolysis due to the potential interaction with cyclosporine (which is given in combination with everolimus for renal transplantation).

Use is associated with mouth ulcers, mucositis and stomatitis; manage with topical therapy; avoid the use of alcohol-, peroxide-, iodine-, or thyme-based mouthwashes (due to the high potential for drug interactions, avoid the use of systemic antifungals unless fungal infection has been diagnosed). Everolimus is associated with the development of angioedema; concomitant use with other agents known to cause angioedema (eg, ACE inhibitors) may increase the risk. Everolimus use may delay wound healing and increase the occurrence of wound-related complications (eg, wound dehiscence, infection, incisional hernia, lymphocele, seroma); may require surgical intervention. Generalized edema, including peripheral edema and lymphedema, and local fluid accumulation (eg, pericardial effusion, pleural effusion, ascites) may also occur.

Everolimus exposure is increased in patients with hepatic impairment. For patients with breast cancer, PNET, RCC, or renal angiomyolipoma with mild and moderate hepatic impairment, reduced doses are recommended; in patients with severe hepatic impairment, use is recommended (at reduced doses) if the potential benefit outweighs risks. For patients with SEGA, reduced doses may be needed for mild and moderate hepatic impairment (based on therapeutic drug monitoring), and are recommended in severe hepatic impairment; monitor trough levels. Reduced doses are also recommended in renal transplant patients with moderate hepatic impairment;

pharmacokinetic information does not exist for renal transplant patients with severe impairment, although an AUC increase greater than observed in moderate impairment is likely.

[U.S. Boxed Warning]: Increased mortality (usually associated with infections) within the first 3 months after transplant was noted in a study of patients with *de novo* heart transplant receiving immunosuppressive regimens containing everolimus (with or without induction therapy). Use in heart transplantation is not recommended. Use with caution in patients with hyperlipidemia; may increase serum lipids (cholesterol and triglycerides); higher serum concentrations are associated with an increased risk for hyperlipidemia; use has not been studied in patients with baseline cholesterol >350 mg/dL; antihyperlipidemic therapy may not normalize levels. Decreases in hemoglobin, neutrophils, platelets, and lymphocytes have been reported with use. Increases in serum glucose are common; may alter insulin and/or oral hypoglycemic therapy requirements in patients with diabetes; the risk for new onset diabetes is increased with everolimus use after transplantation; achieve optimal glucose levels prior to treatment. Patients should not be immunized with live viral vaccines during or shortly after treatment and should avoid close contact with recently vaccinated (live vaccine) individuals; consider the timing of routine immunizations prior to the start of therapy in pediatric patients treated for SEGA. Continue treatment with everolimus for renal cell cancer as long as clinical benefit is demonstrated or until occurrence of unacceptable toxicity. Safety and efficacy have not been established for the use of everolimus in the treatment of carcinoid tumors. Decreases in hemoglobin, neutrophils, platelets, and lymphocytes have been reported with use. Increases in serum glucose are common; may alter insulin and/or oral hypoglycemic therapy requirements in patients with diabetes; the risk for new onset diabetes is increased with everolimus use after transplantation. Patients should not be immunized with live viral vaccines during or shortly after treatment and should avoid close contact with recently vaccinated (live vaccine) individuals. In pediatric patients treated for SEGA, complete recommended series of live virus childhood vaccinations prior to treatment (if immediate everolimus treatment is not indicated); an accelerated vaccination schedule may be appropriate. Continue treatment with everolimus for renal cell cancer as long as clinical benefit is demonstrated or until occurrence of unacceptable toxicity. Safety and efficacy have not been established for the use of everolimus in the treatment of carcinoid tumors. Continue treatment with everolimus for renal cell cancer as long as clinical benefit is demonstrated or until occurrence of unacceptable toxicity. Safety and efficacy have not been established for the use of everolimus in the treatment of carcinoid tumors.

Tablets (Afinitor®, Zortress®) and tablets for oral suspension (Afinitor® Disperz) are not interchangeable; Afinitor® Disperz is only indicated in conjunction with therapeutic monitoring for the treatment of SEGA. Do not combine formulations to achieve desired dose. Azoospermia and oligospermia have been observed in males. Avoid use in patients with hereditary galactose intolerance, Lapp lactase deficiency, or glucose-galactose malabsorption; may result in diarrhea and malabsorption. The safety and efficacy of everolimus in renal transplantation patients with high-immunologic risk or in solid organ transplant other than renal have not been established. **[U.S. Boxed Warning]: In renal transplantation, everolimus should only be used by physicians experienced in immunosuppressive therapy and**

management of transplant patients. Adequate laboratory and supportive medical resources must be readily available.

Adverse Reactions

>10%:

Cardiovascular: Peripheral edema (4% to 45%), hypertension (4% to 30%; hypertensive crisis: 1%)

Central nervous system: Fatigue (7% to 45%), fever (15% to 32%), headache (18% to 30%), seizure (5% to 29%), anxiety/aggression/behavioral disturbance (SEGA: 21%), insomnia (6% to 17%), dizziness (7% to 14%)

Dermatologic: Rash (18% to 59%), acneiform dermatitis (3% to 25%), nail disorders (5% to 22%), acne (3% to 22%), cellulitis (SEGA: 29%), pruritus (13% to 21%), dry skin (9% to 18%), contact dermatitis (14%), excoriation (14%)

Endocrine & metabolic: Hypercholesterolemia (17% to 85%), hyperglycemia (12% to 75%; grades 3/4: <1% to 17%), hypertriglyceridemia (≤73%), bicarbonate decreased (≤56%), hypophosphatemia (9% to 49%), hypocalcemia (17% to 37%), albumin decreased (≤33%), hypoglycemia (≤32%), hypokalemia (12% to 29%), hyperlipidemia (renal transplant: 21%), hyperkalemia (renal transplant: 18%), amenorrhea (≤17%), hyponatremia (≤16%), dyslipidemia (renal transplant: 15%), hypomagnesemia (renal transplant: 14%)

Gastrointestinal: Taste alteration (1% to 88%), stomatitis (oncology uses: 44% to 86%; grade 3: 4% to 9%; grade 4: <1%; renal transplant: 8%), diarrhea (14% to 50%; grade 3: ≤5%; grade 4: <1%), constipation (10% to 38%), abdominal pain (3% to 36%), nausea (8% to 32%: grade 3: ≤2%; grade 4: <1%), appetite decreased (6% to 30%), anorexia (1% to 30%), vomiting (15% to 29%; grade 3: ≤2%; grade 4: <1%), weight loss (9% to 28%), gastroenteritis (1% to 18%), xerostomia (8% to 11%)

Genitourinary: Urinary tract infection (5% to 22%), dysuria (renal transplant: 11%)

Hematologic: Anemia (26% to 92%; grades 3/4: ≤15%; grade 4: <1%), PTT increased (SEGA: 72%), leukopenia (oncology uses: 26% to 58%; renal transplant 3%), lymphocytopenia (20% to 54%; grades 3/4: ≤18%), thrombocytopenia (19% to 54%; grade 3: ≤3%; renal transplant <10%), neutropenia (14% to 46%; grades 3/4: ≤9%)

Hepatic: AST increased (23% to 89%; grade 3: ≤4%; grade 4: <1%), alkaline phosphatase increased (32% to 74%), ALT increased (18% to 51%; grade 3: ≤4%; grade 4: <1%)

Neuromuscular & skeletal: Weakness (13% to 33%), arthralgia (≤20%), back pain (11% to 15%), limb pain (8% to 14%)

Otic: Otitis (6% to 36%)

Renal: Creatinine increased (11% to 50%), hematuria (renal transplant: 12%)

Respiratory: Upper respiratory infection (11% to 82%), sinusitis (3% to 39%), cough (7% to 30%), dyspnea (20% to 24%; grade 3: 2% to 6%; grade 4: ≤1%), epistaxis (≤22%), pneumonitis (includes alveolitis, interstitial lung disease, lung infiltrate, pulmonary alveolar hemorrhage, pulmonary toxicity; 1% to 19%; grade 3: 3% to 4%; grade 4: <1%), nasal congestion (14%), rhinitis (14%), pharyngitis (4% to 11%)

Miscellaneous: Infection (13% to 62%; grade 3: 4% to 7%; grade 4: 1% to 3%)

1% to 10%:

Cardiovascular: Chest pain (5%), tachycardia (3%), heart failure (1%), angina, atrial fibrillation, chest discomfort, deep vein thrombosis, edema (generalized), hypotension, palpitation, syncope

Central nervous system: Depression (5%), migraine (5%), chills (4%), agitation, hallucination, hemiparesis, hypesthesia, malaise, somnolence

Dermatologic: Eczema (10%), alopecia (≤10%), palmar-plantar erythrodysesthesia syndrome ([hand-foot syndrome] 5%), papule (5%), erythema 4%, onychoclasis (4%), pityriasis rosea (4%), skin lesions (4%), hirsutism, incision complications, hyperhydrosis, hypertrichosis

Endocrine & metabolic: Menorrhagia (6% to 10%), menstrual irregularities (6% to 10%), diabetes mellitus (exacerbation: 2%; new-onset: <10%), dysmenorrhea (6%), metrorrhagia (6%), cushingoid syndrome, dehydration, gout, hypercalcemia, hyperparathyroidism, hyperphosphatemia, hyperuricemia, iron deficiency, vitamin B_{12} deficiency

Gastrointestinal: Gastritis (7%), hemorrhoids (5%), dyspepsia (4%), dysphagia (4%), ageusia (1%), abdominal distention, epigastric discomfort, flatulence, gastroesophageal reflux, gingival hypertrophy, hematemesis, ileus, peritonitis

Genitourinary: Vaginal hemorrhage (8%), bladder spasm, erectile dysfunction, ovarian cysts, pollakiuria, polyuria, pyuria, scrotal edema, urinary retention, urinary urgency

Hematologic: Hemorrhage (3%), leukocytosis, lymphadenopathy, thrombocythemia

Hepatic: Bilirubin increased (3% to 10%; grades 3/4: ≤1%)

Neuromuscular & skeletal: Muscle spasm (≤10%), tremor (8%), paresthesia (5%), jaw pain (3%), joint swelling, musculoskeletal pain, myalgia, osteonecrosis, osteopenia, osteoporosis, spondylitis

Ocular: Eyelid edema (4%), ocular hyperemia (4%), conjunctivitis (2%), blurred vision, cataract

Renal: Renal failure (3%), BUN increased, hydronephrosis, interstitial nephritis, proteinuria, renal artery thrombosis, renal impairment

Respiratory: Pleural effusion (7%), nasopharyngitis (6%), pneumonia (6%), bronchitis (4%), pharyngolaryngeal pain (4%), rhinorrhea (3%), atelectasis, nasal congestion, pulmonary edema, sinus congestion, wheezing

Miscellaneous: Hypersensitivity (3%; includes anaphylaxis, dyspnea, flushing, chest pain, angioedema), BK virus infection, candidiasis, night sweats

<1%, postmarketing, and/or case reports: Aspergillosis, azoospermia, cardiac arrest, fluid accumulation, graft thrombosis, hepatic cholestasis, hepatitis B reactivation, lymphoma, oligospermia, pancreatitis, pancytopenia, polyoma virus infection (BK virus), progressive multiple leukoencephalopathy (PML), respiratory distress, sepsis, skin cancer, synovitis (severe), testosterone levels decreased, thrombotic microangiopathy/thrombotic thrombocytopenic purpura/hemolytic uremic syndrome (TMA/TTP/HUS), wound healing impaired

Drug Interactions

Metabolism/Transport Effects Substrate of CYP3A4 (major), P-glycoprotein; **Note:** Assignment of Major/Minor substrate status based on clinically relevant drug interaction potential

Avoid Concomitant Use

Avoid concomitant use of Everolimus with any of the following: BCG; CloZAPine; CYP3A4 Inducers (Strong); CYP3A4 Inhibitors (Strong); Grapefruit Juice; Natalizumab; Pimecrolimus; St Johns Wort; Tacrolimus (Topical); Vaccines (Live)

Increased Effect/Toxicity

Everolimus may increase the levels/effects of: ACE Inhibitors; CloZAPine; Leflunomide; Natalizumab; Vaccines (Live)

The levels/effects of Everolimus may be increased by: CycloSPORINE (Systemic); CYP3A4 Inhibitors (Moderate); CYP3A4 Inhibitors (Strong); Dasatinib; Denosumab; Grapefruit Juice; Ivacaftor; Mifepristone; P-glycoprotein/ABCB1 Inhibitors; Pimecrolimus; Roflumilast; Tacrolimus (Topical); Trastuzumab

Decreased Effect

Everolimus may decrease the levels/effects of: BCG; Coccidioidin Skin Test; Sipuleucel-T; Vaccines (Inactivated); Vaccines (Live)

The levels/effects of Everolimus may be decreased by: CYP3A4 Inducers (Strong); Deferasirox; Echinacea; Efavirenz; P-glycoprotein/ABCB1 Inducers; St Johns Wort; Tocilizumab

Ethanol/Nutrition/Herb Interactions

Food: Grapefruit juice may increase levels of everolimus. Absorption with food may be variable. Management: Avoid grapefruit juice. Take with or without food, but be consistent with regard to food.

Herb/Nutraceutical: St John's wort may decrease the levels of everolimus. Management: Avoid St John's wort.

Storage/Stability Tablets and tablets for suspension: Store at room temperature of 25°C (77°F); excursions permitted to 15°C to 30°C (59°F to 86°F). Protect from light; protect from moisture.

Mechanism of Action Everolimus is a macrolide immunosuppressant and an m-TOR inhibitor which has antiproliferative and antiangiogenic properties, and also reduces lipoma volume in patients with angiomyolipoma. Reduces protein synthesis and cell proliferation by binding to the FK binding protein-12 (FKBP-12), an intracellular protein, to form a complex that inhibits activation of mTOR (mammalian target of rapamycin) serine-threonine kinase activity. Also reduces angiogenesis by inhibiting vascular endothelial growth factor (VEGF) and hypoxia-inducible factor (HIF-1) expression. Angiomyolipomas may occur due to unregulated mTOR activity in TSC-associated renal angiomyolipoma (Budde, 2012); everolimus reduces lipoma volume (Bissler, 2012).

Pharmacodynamics/Kinetics

Absorption: Rapid, but moderate

Protein binding: ~74%

Metabolism: Extensively metabolized in the liver via CYP3A4; forms 6 weak metabolites

Bioavailability:

- Tablets: ~30%; systemic exposure reduced by 22% with a high-fat meal and by 32% with a light-fat meal
- Tablets for suspension: AUC equivalent to tablets although peak concentrations are 20% to 36% lower; steady state concentrations are similar

Half-life elimination: ~30 hours

Time to peak, plasma: 1-2 hours

Excretion: Feces (80%, based on solid organ transplant studies); Urine (~5%, based on solid organ transplant studies)

Dosing

Adult & Geriatric Note: Tablets (Afinitor®, Zortress®) and tablets for oral suspension (Afinitor® Disperz) are not interchangeable; Afinitor® Disperz is only indicated for the treatment of subependymal giant cell astrocytoma (SEGA), in conjunction with therapeutic monitoring. Do not combine formulations to achieve desired dose.

Breast cancer, advanced, hormone receptor-positive, HER2-negative: Oral: 10 mg once daily (in combination with exemestane), continue treatment until no longer clinically beneficial or until unacceptable toxicity

Pancreatic neuroendocrine tumors (PNET), advanced: Oral: 10 mg once daily, continue treatment until no longer clinically beneficial or until unacceptable toxicity

Renal angiomyolipoma: Oral: 10 mg once daily, continue treatment until no longer clinically beneficial or until unacceptable toxicity

Renal cell cancer, advanced (RCC): Oral: 10 mg once daily, continue treatment until no longer clinically beneficial or until unacceptable toxicity

Renal transplantation, rejection prophylaxis: Oral: Initial: 0.75 mg twice daily; adjust maintenance dose if needed at a 4- to 5-day interval (from prior dose adjustment) based on serum concentrations, tolerability, and response; administer in combination with basiliximab induction and concurrently with cyclosporine [dose adjustment required] and corticosteroids

Subependymal giant cell astrocytoma (SEGA; dosing based on body surface area [BSA]): Oral: Initial dose: 4.5 mg/m^2 once daily; round to nearest tablet (tablet or tablet for oral suspension) size. Assess trough concentrations 2 weeks after initiation or dosage modification; adjust maintenance dose if needed at 2-week intervals to achieve and maintain serum trough concentrations between 5 and 15 ng/mL; monitor trough concentrations routinely; once stable dose is attained and BSA is stable throughout treatment, monitor trough concentrations every 6-12 months; monitor every 3-6 months if BSA is changing. Continue until disease progression or unacceptable toxicity.

If trough <5 ng/mL: Increase dose by 2.5 mg/day (tablets) or 2 mg/day (tablets for oral suspension)

If trough >15 ng/mL: Reduce dose by 2.5 mg/day (tablets) or 2 mg/day (tablets for oral suspension)

If dose reduction necessary in patients receiving the lowest strength available, administer every other day.

Waldenström's macroglobulinemia, relapsed or refractory (unlabeled use): Oral: 10 mg once daily until disease progression or toxicity (Ghobrial, 2010)

Dosage adjustment for concomitant CYP3A4 inhibitors/inducers and/or P-gp inhibitors:

Breast cancer, PNET, RCC, renal angiomyolipoma:

CYP3A4 inducers: Strong inducers: Avoid concomitant administration with strong CYP3A4 inducers; if concomitant use cannot be avoided, consider adjusting everolimus dose upward in 5 mg increments up to 20 mg daily, with careful monitoring. If the strong CYP3A4 enzyme inducer is discontinued, reduce the everolimus to the dose used prior to initiation of the CYP3A4 inducer.

CYP3A4 or P-gp inhibitors:

Strong inhibitors: Avoid concomitant administration with strong CYP3A4 inhibitors.

Moderate CYP3A4 and/or P-gp inhibitors: Reduce everolimus dose to 2.5 mg once daily; may consider increasing from 2.5 mg to 5 mg once daily based on patient tolerance. When the moderate inhibitor is discontinued, allow ~2-3 days to elapse prior to adjusting the everolimus upward to the dose used prior to initiation of the moderate inhibitor.

Renal transplantation: Dosage adjustments may be necessary based on everolimus serum concentrations

SEGA:

CYP3A4 inducers: Strong inducers: Avoid concomitant administration with strong CYP3A4 inducers; if concomitant use cannot be avoided, an initial starting everolimus dose of 9 mg/m^2 once daily is recommended, or, double the everolimus dose; individualize subsequent doses based on therapeutic drug monitoring. If the strong CYP3A4 enzyme inducer is discontinued, reduce the everolimus to the dose used prior to initiation of the CYP3A4 inducer; reassess trough concentration after 2 weeks.

CYP3A4 or P-gp inhibitors:

Strong inhibitors: Avoid concomitant administration with strong CYP3A4 inhibitors.

Moderate CYP3A4 and/or P-gp inhibitors: Initial everolimus dose: 2.5 mg/m^2 once daily or reduce everolimus dose by ~50% (if dose reduction is required for patients receiving the lowest strength available, consider alternate day dosing); assess trough concentrations after 2 weeks; individualize dosing based on therapeutic drug monitoring. When the moderate inhibitor is discontinued, allow 2-3 days to elapse prior to adjusting the everolimus upward to the dose used prior to initiation of the moderate inhibitor; reassess trough concentrations after 2 weeks.

Pediatric Note: Tablets (Afinitor®, Zortress®) and tablets for oral suspension (Afinitor® Disperz) are not interchangeable. Do not combine formulations to achieve desired dose.

Subependymal giant cell astrocytoma (SEGA): Children ≥1 year: Refer to adult dosing.

Renal Impairment No dosage adjustment necessary.

Hepatic Impairment

Mild impairment (Child-Pugh class A):

Breast cancer, PNET, RCC, renal angiomyolipoma: Reduce dose to 7.5 mg once daily; if not tolerated, may further reduce to 5 mg once daily.

Renal transplantation: No adjustment necessary.

SEGA: Adjustment to initial dose may not be necessary; subsequent dosing is based on therapeutic drug monitoring (monitor 2 weeks after initiation, dosage modifications, or after any change in hepatic status; target trough concentration: 5-15 ng/mL).

Moderate impairment (Child-Pugh class B):

Breast cancer, PNET, RCC, renal angiomyolipoma: Reduce dose to 5 mg once daily; if not tolerated, may further reduce to 2.5 mg once daily.

Renal transplantation: Reduce initial dose by 50%; individualize subsequent dosing based on therapeutic drug monitoring.

SEGA: Adjustment to initial dose may not be necessary; subsequent dosing is based on therapeutic drug monitoring (monitor 2 weeks after initiation, dosage modifications, or after any change in hepatic status; target trough concentration: 5-15 ng/mL).

Severe impairment (Child-Pugh class C):

Breast cancer, PNET, RCC, renal angiomyolipoma: If potential benefit outweighs risks, a maximum dose of 2.5 mg once daily may be used.

Renal transplantation: No dosage adjustment provided in the manufacturer's labeling (pharmacokinetics have not been studied in severe hepatic impairment).

SEGA: Reduce initial dose to 2.5 mg/m^2 once daily (or current dose by ~50%); subsequent dosing is based on therapeutic drug monitoring

Adjustment for Toxicity

Breast cancer (adjustments apply to everolimus), PNET, RCC, renal angiomyolipoma, SEGA: Reduce everolimus dose by ~50% if dosage adjustment is necessary:

Noninfectious pneumonitis:

Grade 1 (asymptomatic radiological changes suggestive of pneumonitis): No dosage adjustment necessary; monitor appropriately.

Grade 2 (symptomatic but not interfering with activities of daily living [ADL]): Consider interrupting treatment, rule out infection, and consider corticosteroids until symptoms improve to ≤grade 1; reinitiate at a lower dose. (Discontinue if recovery does not occur within 4 weeks.)

Grade 3 (symptomatic, interferes with ADL; oxygen indicated): Interrupt treatment until symptoms improve to ≤grade 1; rule out infection and consider corticosteroid treatment; may reinitiate at a lower dose. If grade 3 toxicity recurs, consider discontinuing.

Grade 4 (life-threatening; ventilatory support indicated): Discontinue treatment; rule out infection; consider corticosteroid treatment.

Stomatitis (avoid the use of products containing alcohol, hydrogen peroxide, iodine, or thyme derivatives):

Grade 1 (minimal symptoms, normal diet): No dosage adjustment necessary; manage with mouth wash (nonalcoholic or salt water) several times a day

Grade 2 (symptomatic but can eat and swallow modified diet): Interrupt treatment until symptoms improve to ≤grade 1; reinitiate at same dose; if stomatitis recurs at grade 2, interrupt treatment until symptoms improve to ≤grade 1 and then reinitiate at a lower dose. Also manage with topical (oral) analgesics (eg, benzocaine, butyl aminobenzoate, tetracaine, menthol, or phenol) ± topical (oral) corticosteroids (eg, triamcinolone).

Grade 3 (symptomatic and unable to orally aliment or hydrate adequately): Interrupt treatment until symptoms improve to ≤grade 1; then reinitiate at a lower dose. Also manage with topical (oral) analgesics (eg, benzocaine, butyl aminobenzoate, tetracaine, menthol, or phenol) ± topical (oral) corticosteroids (eg, triamcinolone).

Grade 4 (life-threatening symptoms): Discontinue treatment; initiate appropriate medical intervention.

Metabolic toxicity (eg, hyperglycemia, dyslipidemia):

Grade 1: No dosage adjustment necessary; initiate appropriate medical intervention and monitor.

Grade 2: No dosage adjustment necessary; manage with appropriate medical intervention and monitor.

Grade 3: Temporarily interrupt treatment; reinitiate at a lower dose; manage with appropriate medical intervention and monitor.

Grade 4: Discontinue treatment; manage with appropriate medical intervention.

Nonhematologic toxicities (excluding pneumonitis, stomatitis, and metabolic toxicity):

Grade 1: If toxicity is tolerable, no dosage adjustment necessary; initiate appropriate medical intervention and monitor.

Grade 2: If toxicity is tolerable, no dosage adjustment necessary; initiate appropriate medical intervention and monitor. If toxicity becomes intolerable, temporarily interrupt treatment until improvement to ≤grade 1 and reinitiate at the same dose; if toxicity recurs at grade 2, temporarily interrupt treatment until improvement to ≤ grade 1 and then reinitiate at a lower dose.

Grade 3: Temporarily interrupt treatment until improvement to ≤grade 1; initiate appropriate medical intervention and monitor. May reinitiate at a lower dose; if toxicity recurs at grade 3, consider discontinuing.

Grade 4 (life-threatening symptoms): Discontinue treatment; initiate appropriate medical intervention.

Renal transplantation: Evidence of polyoma virus infection or PML: Consider reduced immunosuppression (taking into account the allograft risks associated with decreased immunosuppression)

SEGA: *Other severe/intolerable adverse reactions:* Temporarily reduce dose (by ~50% from prior dose) and/or temporarily interrupt treatment; if dose reduction is required for patients receiving the lowest available strength, consider alternate day dosing.

Combination Regimens

Breast cancer: Everolimus-Exemestane (Breast) on page 1640

Renal cell cancer: Everolimus (RCC Regimen) on page 1640

Administration May be taken with or without food; to reduce variability, take consistently with regard to food.

Tablets: Swallow whole with a glass of water. Do not break, chew, or crush (do not administer tablets that are crushed or broken). Avoid contact with or exposure to crushed or broken tablets.

Tablets for oral suspension: Administer as a suspension only. Administer immediately after preparation; discard if not administered within 60 minutes after preparation. Prepare suspension in water only. Do not break or crush tablets.

Preparation in an oral syringe: Place dose into 10 mL oral syringe (maximum 10 mg/syringe; use an additional syringe for doses >10 mg). Draw ~5 mL of water and ~4 mL of air into oral syringe; allow to sit (tip up) in a container until tablets are in suspension (3 minutes). Gently invert syringe 5 times immediately prior to administration; administer contents, then add ~5 mL water and ~4 mL of air to same syringe, swirl to suspend remaining particles and administer entire contents.

Preparation in a small glass: Place dose into a small glass (≤100 mL) containing ~25 mL water (maximum 10 mg/glass; use and additional glass for doses >10 mg); allow to sit until tablets are in suspension (3 minutes). Stir gently with spoon immediately prior to administration; administer contents, then add ~25 mL water to same glass, swirl with same spoon to suspend remaining particles and administer entire contents.

Breast cancer, pancreatic neuroendocrine tumors, renal cell cancer, renal angiolipoma, SEGA: Administer at the same time each day.

Renal transplantation: Administer consistently ~12 hours apart; administer at the same time as cyclosporine.

Emetic Potential Low (10% to 30%)

Extemporaneous Preparations

Hazardous agent: Use appropriate precautions for handling and disposal.

Tablets: An oral liquid may be prepared using tablets. Disperse tablet in ~30 mL (1 oz) of water; gently stir. Administer and rinse container with additional 30 mL (1 oz) water and administer to ensure entire dose is administered. Administer immediately after preparation.

Afinitor® prescribing information, East Hanover, NJ: Novartis Pharmaceuticals Corporation, July 2012.

Tablets for oral suspension: Administer as a suspension only. Administer immediately after preparation; discard if not administered within 60 minutes after preparation. Prepare suspension in water only. Do not break or crush tablets.

Preparation in an oral syringe: Place dose into 10 mL oral syringe (maximum 10 mg/syringe; use an additional syringe for doses >10 mg). Draw ~5 mL of water and ~4 mL of air into oral syringe; allow to sit (tip up) in a container until tablets are in suspension (3 minutes). Gently invert syringe 5 times immediately prior to administration; administer contents, then add ~5 mL water and ~4 mL of air to same syringe, swirl to suspend remaining particles and administer entire contents.

Preparation in a small glass: Place dose into a small glass (≤100 mL) containing ~25 mL water (maximum 10 mg/glass; use an additional glass for doses >10 mg); allow to sit until tablets are in suspension (3 minutes). Stir gently with spoon immediately prior to administration; administer contents, then add ~25 mL water to same glass, swirl with same spoon to suspend remaining particles and administer entire contents.

Administer immediately after preparation, discard if not administered within 60 minutes after preparation.

Afinitor® and Afinitor® Disperz prescribing information, East Hanover, NJ: Novartis Pharmaceuticals Corporation, August 2012.

Monitoring Parameters CBC with differential (baseline and periodic), liver function; serum creatinine, urinary protein, and BUN (baseline and periodic); fasting serum glucose and lipid profile (baseline and periodic); monitor for signs and symptoms of infection, noninfectious pneumonitis, or malignancy

For renal transplantation, monitor everolimus serum trough concentrations, especially in patients with hepatic impairment, with concomitant CYP3A4 inhibitors and inducers, and when cyclosporine formulations or doses are changed; dosage adjustments should be made on trough concentrations obtained 4-5 days after a previous dosage adjustment; monitor cyclosporine concentrations; monitor for proteinuria

For SEGA, monitor everolimus serum trough concentrations ~2 weeks after treatment initiation, 2 weeks after dose modifications and after initiation of dose modification of concomitant CYP3A4 and/or P-gp inducers or inhibitors.

Dietary Considerations Avoid grapefruit juice. May be taken with or without food, although should be administered consistently with regard to food.

Product Availability Afinitor Disperz (tablets for oral suspension): FDA approved August 2012; anticipated availability in November 2012. Consult prescribing information for additional information.

Medication Guide Available Yes

Dosage Forms Excipient information presented when available (limited, particularly for generics); consult specific product labeling.

Tablet, oral:

Afinitor®: 2.5 mg, 5 mg, 7.5 mg, 10 mg [contains lactose]

Zortress®: 0.25 mg, 0.5 mg, 0.75 mg [contains lactose]

References

Amato RJ, Jac J, Geissinger S, et al, "A Phase 2 Study With a Daily Regimen of the Oral mTOR Inhibitor RAD001 (Everolimus) in Patients With Metastatic Clear Cell Renal Cell Cancer," *Cancer*, 2009, 115(11):2438-46.

Baselga J, Campone M, Piccart M, et al, "Everolimus in Postmenopausal Hormone-Receptor-Positive Advanced Breast Cancer," *N Engl J Med*, 2012, 366(6):520-9.

Bissler JJ, Kingswood JC, Zonnenberg BA, et al, "Everolimus Therapy for Angiomyolipoma in Patients With Tuberous Sclerosis Complex or Sporadic Lymphangioleiomyomatosis: Results From EXIST-2," *J Clin Oncology*, 2012, 30(supp 5):356 [abstract 356 from 2012 ASCO Genitourinary Cancers Symposium].

Budde K and Gaedeke J, "Tuberous Sclerosis Complex-Associated Angiomyolipomas: Focus on mTOR Inhibition," *Am J Kidney Dis*, 2012, 59(2):276-83.

Eisen HJ, Tuzcu EM, Dorent R, et al, "Everolimus for the Prevention of Allograft Rejection and Vasculopathy in Cardiac-Transplant Recipients," *N Engl J Med*, 2003, 349(9):847-58.

Franz DN, Krueger DA, Care MM, et al, "Everolimus for Subependymal Giant-Cell Astrocytomas (SEGAs) in Tuberous Sclerosis (TS)," *J Clin Oncol*, 2010, 28(15s):2004 [abstract 2004 from 2010 ASCO Annual Meeting].

Ghobrial IM, Gertz M, Laplant B, et al, "Phase II Trial of the Oral Mammalian Target of Rapamycin Inhibitor Everolimus in Relapsed or Refractory Waldenstrom Macroglobulinemia," *J Clin Oncol*, 2010, 28(8):1408-14.

Gupta S, Parsa VB, Heilbrun LK, et al, "Safety and Efficacy of Molecularly Targeted Agents in Patients With Metastatic Kidney Cancer With Renal Dysfunction," *Anticancer Drugs*, 2011, 22 (8):794-800.

Kovarik JM, Sabia HD, Figuerierdo J, et al, "Influence of Hepatic Impairment on Everolimus Pharmacokinetics: Implications for Dose Adjustment," *Clin Pharmacol Ther*, 2001, 70(5):425-30.

Krueger DA, Care MM, Holland K, et al, "Everolimus for Subependymal Giant-Cell Astrocytomas in Tuberous Sclerosis," *N Engl J Med*, 2010, 363(19):1801-11.

Motzer RJ, Escudier B, Oudard S, et al, "Efficacy of Everolimus in Advanced Renal Cell Carcinoma: A Double-Blind, Randomised, Placebo-Controlled Phase III Trial," *Lancet*, 2008, 372(9637):449-56.

Porta C, Calvo E, Climent MA, et al, "Efficacy and Safety of Everolimus in Elderly Patients With Metastatic Renal Cell Carcinoma: An Exploratory Analysis of the Outcomes of Elderly Patients in the RECORD-1 Trial," *Eur Urol*, 2012, 61(4):826-33.

Yao JC, Lombard-Bohas C, Baudin E, et al, "Daily Oral Everolimus Activity in Patients With Metastatic Pancreatic Neuroendocrine Tumors After Failure of Cytotoxic Chemotherapy: A Phase II Trial," *J Clin Oncol*, 2010, 28(1):69-76.

Yao JC, Phan AT, Chang DZ, et al, "Efficacy of RAD001 (Everolimus) and Octreotide LAR in Advanced Low- to Intermediate-Grade Neuroendocrine Tumors: Results of a Phase II Study," *J Clin Oncol*, 2008, 26(26):4311-8.

Yao JC, Shah MH, Ito T, et al, "Everolimus for Advanced Pancreatic Neuroendocrine Tumors," *N Engl J Med*, 2011, 364(6):514-23.

Viganò M, Tuzcu M, Benza R, et al, "Prevention of Acute Rejection and Allograft Vasculopathy by Everolimus in Cardiac Transplants Recipients: A 24-Month Analysis," *J Heart Lung Transplant*, 2007, 26(6):584-92.

Zuckermann A, Manito N, Epailly E, et al, "Multidisciplinary Insights on Clinical Guidance for the Use of Proliferation Signal Inhibitors in Heart Transplantation," *J Heart Lung Transplant*, 2008, 27 (2):141-9.

◆ **Evista®** *see* Raloxifene *on page 1222*

◆ **Exalgo®** *see* HYDROmorphone *on page 724*

Exemestane (ex e MES tane)

Related Information

Safe Handling of Hazardous Drugs *on page 1904*

Brand Names: U.S. Aromasin®

Brand Names: Canada Aromasin®; CO Exemestane

Generic Availability (U.S.) Yes

Pharmacologic Category Antineoplastic Agent, Aromatase Inactivator

Use Treatment of advanced breast cancer in postmenopausal women whose disease has progressed following tamoxifen therapy; adjuvant treatment of postmenopausal estrogen receptor-positive early breast cancer following 2-3 years of tamoxifen (for a total of 5 years of adjuvant therapy)

Unlabeled Use Risk reduction for invasive breast cancer in postmenopausal women; treatment of endometrial cancer; treatment of uterine sarcoma

Labeled Contraindications Hypersensitivity to exemestane or any component of the formulation; use in women who are or may become pregnant; use in premenopausal women

Pregnancy Risk Factor X

Lactation Excretion in breast milk unknown/not recommended

Warnings/Precautions Hazardous agent - use appropriate precautions for handling and disposal. Due to decreased circulating estrogen levels, exemestane is associated with a reduction in bone mineral density; decreases (from baseline) in lumbar spine and femoral neck density have been observed. Grade 3 or 4 lymphopenia has been observed with exemestane use, although most patients had preexisting lower grade lymphopenia. Increases in bilirubin, alkaline phosphatase and serum creatinine have been observed. Not to be given with estrogen-containing agents. Dose adjustment recommended with concomitant CYP3A4 inducers.

Adverse Reactions

>10%:

Cardiovascular: Hypertension (5% to 15%)

Central nervous system: Fatigue (8% to 22%), insomnia (11% to 14%), pain (13%), headache (7% to 13%), depression (6% to 13%)

Dermatological: Hyperhidrosis (4% to 18%), alopecia (15%)

Endocrine & metabolic: Hot flashes (13% to 33%)

Gastrointestinal: Nausea (9% to 18%), abdominal pain (6% to 11%)

Hepatic: Alkaline phosphatase increased (14% to 15%)

Neuromuscular & skeletal: Arthralgia (15% to 29%)

1% to 10%:

Cardiovascular: Edema (6% to 7%); cardiac ischemic events (2%: MI, angina, myocardial ischemia), chest pain

Central nervous system: Dizziness (8% to 10%), anxiety (4% to 10%), fever (5%), confusion, hypoesthesia

Dermatologic: Dermatitis (8%), itching, rash

Endocrine & metabolic: Weight gain (8%)

Gastrointestinal: Diarrhea (4% to 10%), vomiting (7%), anorexia (6%), constipation (5%), appetite increased (3%), dyspepsia

Genitourinary: Urinary tract infection (2% to 5%)

Hepatic: Bilirubin increased (5% to 7%)

Neuromuscular & skeletal: Back pain (9%), limb pain (9%), myalgia (6%), osteoarthritis (6%), weakness (6%), osteoporosis (5%), pathological fracture (4%), paresthesia (3%), carpal tunnel syndrome (2%), cramps (2%)

Ocular: Visual disturbances (5%)

Renal: Creatinine increased (6%)

Respiratory: Dyspnea (10%), cough (6%), bronchitis, pharyngitis, rhinitis, sinusitis, upper respiratory infection

Miscellaneous: Flu-like syndrome (6%), lymphedema, infection

<1%, postmarketing, and/or case reports: Cardiac failure, cholestatic hepatitis, endometrial hyperplasia, gastric ulcer, GGT increased, hepatitis, neuropathy, osteochondrosis, thromboembolism, transaminases increased, trigger finger, uterine polyps

A dose-dependent decrease in sex hormone-binding globulin has been observed with daily doses of ≥2.5 mg. Serum luteinizing hormone and follicle-stimulating hormone levels have increased with this medicine.

Drug Interactions

Metabolism/Transport Effects Substrate of CYP3A4 (major); **Note:** Assignment of Major/Minor substrate status based on clinically relevant drug interaction potential; **Induces** CYP3A4 (weak/moderate)

Avoid Concomitant Use

Avoid concomitant use of Exemestane with any of the following: Axitinib

Increased Effect/Toxicity There are no known significant interactions involving an increase in effect.

Decreased Effect

Exemestane may decrease the levels/effects of: ARIPiprazole; Axitinib; Saxagliptin

The levels/effects of Exemestane may be decreased by: CYP3A4 Inducers (Strong); Deferasirox; Herbs (CYP3A4 Inducers); Tocilizumab

Ethanol/Nutrition/Herb Interactions

Food: Plasma levels increased by 40% when exemestane was taken with a fatty meal.

Herb/Nutraceutical: St John's wort may decrease exemestane levels. Avoid black cohosh, dong quai in estrogen-dependent tumors.

Storage/Stability Store at 25°C (77°F); excursions permitted to 15°C to 30°C (59°F to 86°F).

Mechanism of Action Exemestane is an irreversible, steroidal aromatase inactivator. It is structurally related to androstenedione, and is converted to an intermediate that irreversibly blocks the active site of the aromatase enzyme, leading to inactivation ("suicide inhibition") and thus preventing conversion of androgens to estrogens in peripheral tissues. In postmenopausal breast cancers where growth is estrogen-dependent, this medicine will lower circulating estrogens.

Pharmacodynamics/Kinetics

Absorption: Rapid and moderate (~42%) following oral administration; absorption increases ~40% following high-fat meal

Distribution: Extensive into tissues

Protein binding: 90%, primarily to albumin and α_1-acid glycoprotein

Metabolism: Extensively hepatic; oxidation (CYP3A4) of methylene group, reduction of 17-keto group with formation of many secondary metabolites; metabolites are inactive

Half-life elimination: 24 hours

Time to peak: Women with breast cancer: 1.2 hours

Excretion: Urine (<1% as unchanged drug, 39% to 45% as metabolites); feces (36% to 48%)

Dosing

Adult & Geriatric Females: Postmenopausal:

Breast cancer, advanced: Oral: 25 mg once daily; continue until tumor progression

Breast cancer, early (adjuvant treatment): Oral: 25 mg once daily (following 2-3 years of tamoxifen therapy) for a total duration of 5 years of endocrine therapy (in the absence of recurrence or contralateral breast cancer)

Breast cancer, risk reduction (unlabeled use): Oral: 25 mg once daily for up to 5 years (Goss, 2011)

Dosage adjustment with CYP3A4 inducers: U.S. labeling: 50 mg once daily when used with potent inducers (eg, rifampin, phenytoin)

Renal Impairment No adjustment necessary (although the safety of chronic doses in patients with moderate-to-severe renal impairment has not been studied, dosage adjustment does not appear necessary).

Hepatic Impairment No adjustment necessary (although the safety of chronic doses in patients with moderate-to-severe hepatic impairment has not been studied, dosage adjustment does not appear necessary).

Combination Regimens

Breast cancer: Everolimus-Exemestane (Breast) on page 1640

Administration Administer after a meal.

Dietary Considerations Take after a meal; patients on aromatase inhibitor therapy should receive vitamin D and calcium supplements.

Additional Information Oncology Comment: The American Society of Clinical Oncology (ASCO) guidelines for adjuvant endocrine therapy in postmenopausal women with HR-positive breast cancer (Burstein, 2010) recommend considering aromatase inhibitor (AI) therapy at some point in the treatment course (primary, sequentially, or extended). Optimal duration at this time is not known; however, treatment with an AI should not exceed 5 years in primary and extended therapies, and 2-3 years if followed by tamoxifen in sequential therapy (total of 5 years). If initial therapy with AI has been discontinued before the 5 years, consideration should be taken to receive tamoxifen for a total of 5 years. The optimal time to switch to an AI is also not known, but data supports switching after 2-3 years of tamoxifen (sequential) or after 5 years of tamoxifen (extended). If patient becomes intolerant or has poor adherence, consideration should be made to switch to another AI or initiate tamoxifen.

Dosage Forms Excipient information presented when available (limited, particularly for generics); consult specific product labeling.

Tablet, oral: 25 mg

Aromasin®: 25 mg

References

Bertelli G, Hall E, Ireland E, et al, "Long-Term Endometrial Effects in Postmenopausal Women With Early Breast Cancer Participating in the Intergroup Exemestane Study (IES) – A Randomised Controlled Trial of Exemestane versus Continued Tamoxifen After 2-3 Years Tamoxifen," *Ann Oncol*, 2010, 21(3):498-505.

Burstein HJ, Prestrud AA, Seidenfeld J, et al, "American Society of Clinical Oncology Clinical Practice Guideline: Update on Adjuvant Endocrine Therapy for Women with Hormone Receptor-Positive Breast Cancer," *J Clin Oncol*, 2010, 28(23):3784-96.

Chia S, Gradishar W, Mauriac L, et al, "Double-Blind, Randomized Placebo Controlled Trial of Fulvestrant Compared With Exemestane After Prior Nonsteroidal Aromatase Inhibitor Therapy in Postmenopausal Women With Hormone Receptor-Positive, Advanced Breast Cancer: Results From EFECT," *J Clin Oncol*, 2008, 26(10):1664-70.

Goss PE, Ingle JN, Ales-Martinez JE, et al, "Exemestane for Breast-Cancer Prevention in Postmenopausal Women," *N Engl J Med*, 2011, 364(25):2381-91.

Kieback DG, Harbeck N, Bauer W, et al, "Endometrial Effects of Exemestane Compared to Tamoxifen Within the Tamoxifen Exemestane Adjuvant Multicenter (TEAM) Trial: Results of a Prospective Gynecological Ultrasound Substudy," *Gynecol Oncol*, 2010, 119(3):500-5.

Morandi P, Rouzier R, Altundag K, et al, "The Role of Aromatase Inhibitors in the Adjuvant Treatment of Breast Carcinoma: The M. D. Anderson Cancer Center Evidence-Based Approach," *Cancer*, 2004, 101(7):1482-9.

National Comprehensive Cancer Network® (NCCN), "Clinical Practice Guidelines in Oncology™: Uterine Neoplasms," Version 2.2012. Available at http://www.nccn.org/professionals/physician_gls/PDF/uterine.pdf

Paridaens RJ, Dirix LY, Beex LV, et al, "Phase III Study Comparing Exemestane With Tamoxifen as First-Line Hormonal Treatment of Metastatic Breast Cancer in Postmenopausal Women: The European Organisation for Research and Treatment of Cancer Breast Cancer Cooperative Group," *J Clin Oncol*, 2008, 26(30):4883-90.

Winer EP, Hudis C, Burstein HJ, et al, "American Society of Clinical Oncology Technology Assessment on the Use of Aromatase Inhibitors as Adjuvant Therapy for Postmenopausal Women With Hormone Receptor-Positive Breast Cancer: Status Report 2004," *J Clin Oncol*, 2005, 23(3):619-29.

- **Exjade®** *see* Deferasirox *on page 407*
- **Extended Release Epidural Morphine** *see* Morphine (Liposomal) *on page 1011*

Factor VIIa (Recombinant) (FAK ter SEV en aye ree KOM be nant)

Brand Names: U.S. NovoSeven® RT

Brand Names: Canada Niastase®; Niastase® RT

Index Terms Coagulation Factor VIIa; Eptacog Alfa (Activated); rFVIIa

Generic Availability (U.S.) No

Pharmacologic Category Antihemophilic Agent

Use Treatment of bleeding episodes and prevention of bleeding in surgical interventions in patients with either hemophilia A or B with inhibitors to factor VIII or factor IX, acquired hemophilia, or congenital factor VII deficiency

Unlabeled Use Warfarin-related intracerebral hemorrhage; treatment of refractory bleeding after cardiac surgery in nonhemophiliac patients

Labeled Contraindications There are no contraindications listed within the FDA-approved labeling.

Pregnancy Risk Factor C

Lactation Excretion in breast milk unknown/not recommended

Warnings/Precautions [U.S. Boxed Warning]: Serious thrombotic events are associated with the use of factor VIIa outside labeled indications. Arterial and venous thrombotic and thromboembolic events, some fatal, following administration of factor VIIa have been reported during postmarketing surveillance. All patients receiving factor VIIa should be monitored for signs and symptoms of activation of the coagulation system or thrombosis; thrombotic events may be increased in patients with disseminated intravascular coagulation (DIC), advanced atherosclerotic disease, sepsis, crush injury, or concomitant treatment with prothrombin complex concentrates. Use with caution in patients with an increased risk of thromboembolic complications (eg, coronary heart disease, liver disease, DIC, postoperative immobilization, elderly patients, and neonates). Decreased dosage or discontinuation is warranted with confirmed intravascular coagulation or presence of clinical thrombosis. Use with caution in patients with known hypersensitivity to mouse, hamster, or bovine proteins, or factor VIIa, or any components of the product. Efficacy with prolonged infusions and data evaluating this agent's long-term adverse effects are limited.

Adverse Reactions

1% to 10%:

Cardiovascular: Hypertension (2%), bradycardia (1%), edema (1%), hypotension (1%)

Central nervous system: Fever (4%), headache (1%), pain (1%)

Dermatologic: Pruritus (1%), purpura (1%), rash (1%)

Gastrointestinal: Vomiting (1%)

Hematologic: Plasma fibrinogen decreased (2%), disseminated intravascular coagulation (1%), fibrinolysis increased (1%), prothrombin decreased (1%)

Local: Injection site reaction (1%)

Neuromuscular & skeletal: Arthrosis (1%)

Renal: Abnormal renal function (1%)

Respiratory: Pneumonia (1%)

Miscellaneous: Allergic reactions (1%)

<1%: Angina, arthralgia, cerebral artery occlusion, CVA, deep vein thrombosis, fibrin degradation products increased, hypersensitivity reaction, I.V. site thrombosis, localized phlebitis, nausea, pulmonary embolism, thrombophlebitis, thrombosis, urticaria

Postmarketing and/or case reports: Anaphylactic shock, angioedema, antibody formation, arterial thrombosis, arterial thrombosis (limb), bowel infarction, cerebral infarction and/or ischemia, consumptive coagulopathy, D-dimer elevation, flushing, hepatic artery thrombosis, hypersensitivity, injection site pain, intestinal infarction, MI, myocardial ischemia, peripheral ischemia, portal vein thrombosis, renal artery thrombosis, retinal artery embolism, retinal artery thrombosis, shock

Drug Interactions

Metabolism/Transport Effects None known.

Avoid Concomitant Use There are no known interactions where it is recommended to avoid concomitant use.

Increased Effect/Toxicity There are no known significant interactions involving an increase in effect.

Decreased Effect There are no known significant interactions involving a decrease in effect.

Storage/Stability NovoSeven® RT: Prior to reconstitution, store under refrigeration or between 2°C to 25°C (36°F to 77°F); do not freeze. Protect from light. Reconstituted solutions may be stored at room temperature or under refrigeration, but must be infused within 3 hours of reconstitution. Do not freeze reconstituted solutions. Do not store reconstituted solutions in syringes.

Reconstitution Prior to reconstitution, bring vials to room temperature. Add recommended diluent along wall of vial; do not inject directly onto powder. Gently swirl until dissolved.

NovoSeven® RT: Reconstitute each vial to a final concentration of 1 mg/mL using the provided histidine diluent as follows:

1 mg vial: 1.1 mL histidine diluent
2 mg vial: 2.1 mL histidine diluent
5 mg vial: 5.2 mL histidine diluent
8 mg vial: 8.1 mL histidine diluent

Mechanism of Action Recombinant factor VIIa, a vitamin K-dependent glycoprotein, promotes hemostasis by activating the extrinsic pathway of the coagulation cascade. It replaces deficient activated coagulation factor VII, which complexes with tissue factor and may activate coagulation factor X to Xa and factor IX to IXa. When complexed with other factors, coagulation factor Xa converts prothrombin to thrombin, a key step in the formation of a fibrin-platelet hemostatic plug.

Pharmacodynamics/Kinetics

Distribution: V_d: 103 mL/kg (range: 78-139)

Half-life elimination: 2.3 hours (range: 1.7-2.7)

Excretion: Clearance: 33 mL/kg/hour (range: 27-49)

Dosing

Adult & Geriatric For I.V. administration only:

Hemophilia A or B with inhibitors:

Bleeding episodes: 90 mcg/kg every 2 hours until hemostasis is achieved or until the treatment is judged ineffective. Doses between 35-120 mcg/kg have been used successfully in clinical trials. The dose, interval, and duration of therapy may be adjusted based upon the severity of bleeding and the degree of hemostasis achieved. For patients experiencing severe bleeds, dosing should be continued at 3- to 6-hour intervals after hemostasis has been achieved and the duration of dosing should be minimized.

Surgical interventions: 90 mcg/kg immediately before surgery; repeat at 2-hour intervals for the duration of surgery. Continue every 2 hours for 48 hours, then every 2-6 hours until healed for minor surgery; continue every 2 hours for 5 days, then every 4 hours until healed for major surgery.

Congenital factor VII deficiency: Bleeding episodes and surgical interventions: 15-30 mcg/kg every 4-6 hours until hemostasis is achieved. Doses as low as 10 mcg/kg have been effective.

Acquired hemophilia: 70-90 mcg/kg every 2-3 hours until hemostasis is achieved.

Intracerebral hemorrhage (ICH) (warfarin-related) (unlabeled use; Freeman, 2004; Ilyas, 2008): 10-100 mcg/kg (see **"Note"** below) administered concurrently with I.V. vitamin K (to correct the nonfactor VII coagulation factors).

Note: Lower doses (10-20 mcg/kg) are generally preferred given the higher risk of thromboembolic complications with higher doses; response is highly variable; monitor INR frequently after administration since rebound increases in INR occur quickly given the short half-life of rFVIIa; duration of INR correction is dose dependent. Routine use as a sole agent is not recommended for warfarin-related ICH (Morgenstern, 2010).

Treatment of refractory bleeding after cardiac surgery in nonhemophiliac patients: Dosing not established; doses in the range of 35-70 mcg/kg have been recommended based on low-quality evidence (case series, observational studies) (Chapman, 2011; Ferraris, 2011; Karkouti, 2007); in patients with a left ventricular assist device, lower doses (ie, 10-20 mcg/kg) may be preferred to reduce thromboembolic events (Bruckner, 2009).

Pediatric

Hemophilia A or B with inhibitors: Refer to adult dosing.

Congenital factor VII deficiency: Refer to adult dosing.

Acquired hemophilia: Refer to adult dosing.

Administration I.V. administration only; bolus over 2-5 minutes. Administer within 3 hours after reconstitution.

Monitoring Parameters Monitor for evidence of hemostasis; although the prothrombin time/INR, aPTT, and factor VII clotting activity have no correlation with achieving hemostasis, these parameters may be useful as adjunct tests to evaluate efficacy and guide dose or interval adjustments

Dietary Considerations Some products may contain sodium.

Additional Information The Hemophilia and Thrombosis Research Society (HTRS) Registry surveillance program is designed to collect data on the treatment of congenital and acquired bleeding disorders. All prescribers can obtain information regarding contribution of patient data to this program by calling 1-877-362-7355 or at www.novosevensurveillance.com.

Dosage Forms Excipient information presented when available (limited, particularly for generics); consult specific product labeling.

Injection, powder for reconstitution [preservative free]:

NovoSeven® RT: 1 mg [contains polysorbate 80, sodium 0.4 mEq/mg rFVIIa, sucrose 10 mg/vial; supplied with diluent]

NovoSeven® RT: 2 mg [contains polysorbate 80, sodium 0.4 mEq/mg rFVIIa, sucrose 20 mg/vial; supplied with diluent]

NovoSeven® RT: 5 mg [contains polysorbate 80, sodium 0.4 mEq/mg rFVIIa, sucrose 50 mg/vial; supplied with diluent]

NovoSeven® RT: 8 mg [contains polysorbate 80, sodium 0.4 mEq/mg rFVIIa, sucrose 80 mg/vial; supplied with diluent]

References

Bruckner BA, DiBardino DJ, Ning Q, et al, "High Incidence of Thromboembolic Events in Left Ventricular Assist Device Patients Treated With Recombinant Activated Factor VII," *J Heart Lung Transplant*, 2009, 28(8):785-90.

Chapman AJ, Blount AL, Davis AT, et al, "Recombinant Factor VIIa (NovoSeven RT) Use in High Risk Cardiac Surgery," *Eur J Cardiothorac Surg*, 2011.

Ferraris VA, Brown JR Despotis GJ, et al, "2011 Update to the Society of Thoracic Surgeons and the Society of Cardiovascular Anesthesiologists Blood Conservation Clinical Practice Guidelines," *Ann Thorac Surg*, 2011, 91(3):944-82.

Freeman WD, Brott TG, Barrett KM, et al, "Recombinant Factor VIIa for Rapid Reversal of Warfarin Anticoagulation in Acute Intracranial Hemorrhage," *Mayo Clin Proc*, 2004, 79(12):1495-500.

Ilyas C, Beyer GM, Dutton RP, et al, "Recombinant Factor VIIa for Warfarin-Associated Intracranial Bleeding," *J Clin Anesth*, 2008, 20(4):276-9.

Karkouti K, Beattie WS, Crowther MA, et al, "The Role of Recombinant Factor VIIa in On-Pump Cardiac Surgery: Proceedings of the Canadian Consensus Conference," *Can J Anaesth*, 2007, 54(7):573-82.

Morgenstern LB, Hemphill JC, Anderson C, et al, "Guidelines for the Management of Spontaneous Intracerebral Hemorrhage: A Guideline for Healthcare Professionals from the American Heart Association/American Stroke Association," *Stroke*, 2010, 41(9):2108-29.

- ◆ **Factor VIII (Human)** *see* Antihemophilic Factor (Human) *on page 101*
- ◆ **Factor VIII (Recombinant)** *see* Antihemophilic Factor (Recombinant) *on page 103*

Factor IX (FAK tor nyne)

Brand Names: U.S. AlphaNine® SD; BeneFix®; Mononine®

Brand Names: Canada BeneFix®; Immunine® VH; Mononine®

Index Terms Factor IX Concentrate

Generic Availability (U.S.) No

Pharmacologic Category Antihemophilic Agent; Blood Product Derivative

Use Prevention and control of bleeding in patients with factor IX deficiency (hemophilia B or Christmas disease)

NOTE: Contains either **nondetectable levels of factors II, VII, and X** (AlphaNine®, Mononine®) or **only factor IX** (BeneFIX®). Therefore, **NOT INDICATED** for replacement therapy of any other clotting factor besides factor IX or for reversal of anticoagulation due to either vitamin K antagonists or other anticoagulants (eg, dabigatran), hemophilia A patients with factor VIII inhibitors, or patients in a hemorrhagic state caused by reduced production of liver-dependent coagulation factors (eg, hepatitis, cirrhosis).

Labeled Contraindications Hypersensitivity to mouse protein (Mononine®) or hamster protein (BeneFix®)

Pregnancy Risk Factor C

Warnings/Precautions Hypersensitivity and anaphylactic reactions have been reported with use. Delayed reactions (up to 20 days after infusion) in previously untreated patients may also occur. Due to potential for allergic reactions, the initial ~10-20 administrations should be performed under appropriate medical supervision. The development of factor IX antibodies (or inhibitors) has been reported with factor IX therapy (usually occurs within the first 10-20 exposure days); the risk of severe hypersensitivity reactions occurring may be greater in these patients. Patients experiencing allergic reactions should be evaluated for factor IX inhibitors. When clinical response is suboptimal or patient is to undergo surgical procedure, screen for inhibitors. Patients with severe gene defects (eg, gene deletion or inversion) are more likely to develop inhibitors (WFH, 2005).

Observe closely for signs or symptoms of intravascular coagulation or thrombosis; risk is generally associated with the use of factor IX complex concentrates (containing therapeutic amounts of additional factors); however, potential risk exists with use of factor IX products (containing only factor IX). Use with caution when administering to patients with liver disease, postoperatively, neonates, or patients at risk of thromboembolic phenomena, disseminated intravascular coagulation or patients with signs of fibrinolysis due to the potential risk of thromboembolic complications.

Contains either **nondetectable levels of factors II, VII, and X** (AlphaNine®, Mononine®) or **only factor IX** (BeneFIX®). Therefore, factor IX products are **NOT INDICATED** for replacement therapy of any other clotting factor besides factor IX. Factor IX is **NOT INDICATED** for reversal of anticoagulation due to either vitamin K antagonists or other anticoagulants (eg, dabigatran), hemophilia A patients with factor VIII inhibitors, or patients in a hemorrhagic state caused by reduced production of liver-dependent coagulation factors (eg, hepatitis, cirrhosis). AlphaNine® SD and Mononine® are products of human plasma and may potentially contain infectious agents which could transmit disease. Screening of donors, as well as testing and/or inactivation or removal of certain viruses, reduces the risk. Infections thought to be transmitted by this product should be reported to the manufacturer. Safety and efficacy have not been established with factor IX products in immune tolerance induction. Nephrotic syndrome has occurred following immune tolerance induction in patients with factor IX inhibitors and a history of allergic reactions to therapy.

Adverse Reactions Frequency not defined.

Cardiovascular: Cyanosis, flushing, hypotension, chest tightness, thrombosis

Central nervous system: Chills, dizziness, drowsiness, fever (including transient fever following rapid administration), headache, lethargy, lightheadedness, somnolence

Dermatologic: Angioedema, photosensitivity reaction, rash, urticaria

Gastrointestinal: Abnormal taste, diarrhea, nausea, vomiting

Hematologic: Disseminated intravascular coagulation (DIC)

Hepatic: Alkaline phosphatase increased, ALT increased, AST increased

Local: Injection site reactions: Cellulitis, discomfort, pain, phlebitis, stinging

Neuromuscular & skeletal: Neck tightness, paresthesia, rigors

Ocular: Visual disturbance

Respiratory: Allergic rhinitis, asthma, cough, dyspnea, hypoxia, laryngeal edema, lung disorder

Miscellaneous: Allergic reaction, anaphylaxis, burning sensation in jaw/skull, factor IX inhibitor development, hypersensitivity reaction

Postmarketing and/or case reports: HAV seroconversion, inadequate response/recovery, nephrotic syndrome (associated with immune tolerance induction), parvovirus B19 seroconversion, renal infarction, superior vena cava syndrome (neonates)

Drug Interactions

Metabolism/Transport Effects None known.

Avoid Concomitant Use

Avoid concomitant use of Factor IX with any of the following: Aminocaproic Acid

Increased Effect/Toxicity

The levels/effects of Factor IX may be increased by: Aminocaproic Acid

Decreased Effect There are no known significant interactions involving a decrease in effect.

Storage/Stability When stored at refrigerator temperature, 2°C to 8°C (36°F to 46°F), factor IX is stable for the period indicated by the expiration date on its label. Avoid freezing which may damage container for the diluent.

AlphaNine® SD: May also be stored at room temperature not to exceed 30°C (86°F) for up to 1 month. Reconstituted solution should be used within 3 hours of preparation.

BeneFix®: May also be stored at room temperature not to exceed 25°C (77°F) for up to 6 months. Reconstituted solution should be at room temperature and used within 3 hours of preparation.

Mononine®: May also be stored at room temperature not to exceed 25°C (77°F) for up to 1 month. Reconstituted solution should be at room temperature and used within 3 hours of preparation.

Reconstitution Refer to instructions for individual products. Diluent and factor IX should come to room temperature before combining.

Mechanism of Action Replaces deficient clotting factor IX. Hemophilia B, or Christmas disease, is an X-linked inherited disorder of blood coagulation characterized by insufficient or abnormal synthesis of the clotting protein factor IX. Factor IX is a vitamin K-dependent coagulation factor which is synthesized in the liver. Factor IX is activated by factor XIa in the intrinsic coagulation pathway. Activated factor IX (IXa), in combination with factor VII:C activates factor X to Xa, resulting ultimately in the conversion of prothrombin to thrombin and the formation of a fibrin clot. The infusion of exogenous factor IX to replace the deficiency present in hemophilia B temporarily restores hemostasis.

Pharmacodynamics/Kinetics Half-life elimination: IX component: Adults: 21-31 hours; children: 14-28 hours

Dosing

Adult & Geriatric NOTE: Contains either **nondetectable levels of factors II, VII, and X** (AlphaNine®, Mononine®) or **only factor IX** (BeneFIX®). Therefore, **NOT INDICATED** for replacement therapy of any other clotting factor besides factor IX or for reversal of anticoagulation due to either vitamin K antagonists or other anticoagulants (eg, dabigatran), hemophilia A patients with factor VIII inhibitors, or patients in a hemorrhagic state caused by reduced production of liver-dependent coagulation factors (eg, hepatitis, cirrhosis).

Control bleeding in patients with factor IX deficiency (hemophilia B or Christmas disease): Dosage is expressed in units of factor IX activity; dosing must be individualized based on severity of factor IX deficiency, extent and location of bleeding, and clinical status of patient:

Formula for units required to raise blood level %:

AlphaNine® SD, Mononine®: I.V.:

Number of factor IX units required = body weight (in kg) x desired factor IX level increase (as %) x 1 unit/kg

For example, to attain a 100% level in a 70 kg patient who has a baseline level of 20%: Number of factor IX units needed = 70 kg x 80% x 1 unit/kg = 5600 units

BeneFix®: I.V.: Number of factor IX units required = body weight (in kg) x desired factor IX level increase (as %) x 1.3 units/kg

Guidelines: As a general rule, the level of factor IX required for different conditions is as follows; **Note:** The following recommendations may vary from those found within prescribing information or practitioner preference.

Primary prophylaxis: 25-40 units/kg twice weekly (World Federation of Hemophilia, 2005) **or** 40-100 units/kg 2 or 3 times weekly (National

Hemophilia Foundation, MASAC recommendation, 2007); however, the optimum regimen has yet to be defined.

Minor hemorrhage (eg, bruising, cuts/scrapes, uncomplicated joint hemorrhage):

Desired levels of factor IX for hemostasis: 15% to 30%

Frequency of dosing: Every 12-24 hours if necessary

Duration of treatment: 1-2 days

Moderate hemorrhage (eg, epistaxis, oropharyngeal bleeds, dental extractions, hematuria):

Desired levels of factor IX for hemostasis: 25% to 50%

Frequency of dosing: Every 12-24 hours

Duration of treatment: 2-7 days

Major hemorrhage (eg, joint and muscle [especially large muscles] hemorrhage, intracranial or intraperitoneal hemorrhage), major trauma, or surgical prophylaxis:

Desired levels of factor IX for hemostasis: 50% to 100% (depending on the clinical situation, desired factor IX level may be reduced following active treatment period for hemorrhage or >48 hours postop)

Frequency of dosing: Every 12-24 hours or every 18-30 hours, depending on half-life and measured factor IX levels (after 3-5 days, maintain at least 20% activity)

Duration of treatment: 7-10 days, depending upon nature of insult

Pediatric NOTE: Contains either **nondetectable levels of factors II, VII, and X** (AlphaNine®, Mononine®) or **only factor IX** (BeneFIX®). Therefore, **NOT INDICATED** for replacement therapy of any other clotting factor besides factor IX or for reversal of anticoagulation due to either vitamin K antagonists or other anticoagulants (eg, dabigatran), hemophilia A patients with factor VIII inhibitors, or patients in a hemorrhagic state caused by reduced production of liver-dependent coagulation factors (eg, hepatitis, cirrhosis).

Control bleeding in patients with factor IX deficiency (hemophilia B or Christmas disease): Dosage is expressed in units of factor IX activity; dosing must be individualized based on severity of factor IX deficiency, extent and location of bleeding, and clinical status of patient:

AlphaNine® SD, Mononine®: I.V.: Refer to adult dosing.

BeneFix®: I.V.:

Children <15 years:

Formula for units required to raise blood level %:

Number of factor IX units required = body weight (in kg) x desired factor IX level increase (as %) x 1.4 units/kg

Children ≥15 years: Refer to adult dosing.

Note: See **"Guidelines"** section in adult dosing.

Administration Solution should be infused at room temperature

I.V. administration only: Should be infused **slowly**: The rate of administration should be determined by the response and comfort of the patient.

AlphaNine® SD: Administer I.V. at a rate not exceeding 10 mL/minute

BeneFix®: Administer I.V. over several minutes

Mononine®: Administer I.V. at a rate of ~2 mL/minute. Administration rates of up to 225 units/minute have been regularly tolerated without incident (when reconstituted as directed to ~100 units/mL).

Monitoring Parameters Factor IX levels, aPTT; BP, HR, signs of hypersensitivity reactions; screen for factor IX inhibitors when patient is to undergo surgery or if suboptimal response to treatment occurs

Dosage Forms Excipient information presented when available (limited, particularly for generics); consult specific product labeling.

Injection, powder for reconstitution [recombinant]:

BeneFix®: ~250 units, ~500 units, ~1000 units, ~2000 units [contains polysorbate 80 and sucrose 0.8%; derived from or manufactured using Chinese hamster ovary cells; exact potency labeled on each vial]

Injection, powder for reconstitution [human derived]:

AlphaNine® SD: ~500 units, ~1000 units, ~1500 units [contains polysorbate 80 and trace amounts of factors II, VII, and X; exact potency labeled on each vial; solvent detergent treated/virus filtered]

Mononine®: ~500 units, ~1000 units [contains polysorbate 80, mouse protein, and trace amounts of factors II, VII, and X; exact potency labeled on each vial]

References

National Hemophilia Foundation, "Guidelines for Emergency Department Management of Individuals with Hemophilia," 2006. Available at http://www.hemophilia.org/NHFWeb/Resource/StaticPages/menu0/menu5/menu57/175.pdf

National Hemophilia Foundation, "MASAC Recommendations Concerning Products Licensed for the Treatment of Hemophilia and Other Bleeding Disorders," 2010. Available at http://www.hemophilia.org/NHFWeb/Resource/StaticPages/menu0/menu5/menu57/masac190.pdf

National Hemophilia Foundation, "MASAC Recommendations Concerning Prophylaxis (Regular Administration of Clotting Factor Concentrate to Prevent Bleeding)," 2007. Available at http://www.hemophilia.org/NHFWeb/Resource/StaticPages/menu0/menu5/menu57/masac179.pdf

World Federation of Hemophilia, "Guidelines for the Management of Hemophilia," 2005. Available at http://www.ehc.eu/fileadmin/dokumente/Gudelines_Mng_Hemophilia.pdf

Factor IX Complex (Human) (FAK ter nyne KOM pleks HYU man)

Brand Names: U.S. Bebulin® VH; Profilnine® SD

Index Terms PCC, Prothrombin Complex Concentrate

Generic Availability (U.S.) No

Pharmacologic Category Antihemophilic Agent; Blood Product Derivative; Prothrombin Complex Concentrate (PCC)

Use Prevention and control of bleeding in patients with factor IX deficiency (hemophilia B or Christmas disease)

Unlabeled Use Emergent correction of warfarin-induced coagulopathy (with clinically significant bleeding); **Note:** Products contain low or nontherapeutic levels of factor VII component; use of fresh frozen plasma (FFP) should be considered

Labeled Contraindications There are no contraindications listed in the manufacturer's labeling

Pregnancy Risk Factor C

Warnings/Precautions Hypersensitivity and anaphylactic reactions have been reported with use. Delayed reactions (up to 20 days after infusion) in previously untreated patients may also occur. Due to potential for allergic reactions, the initial ~10-20 administrations should be performed under appropriate medical supervision. The development of factor IX antibodies (or inhibitors) has been reported with factor IX therapy (usually occurs within the first 10-20 exposure days); the risk of severe hypersensitivity reactions occurring may be greater in these patients. Patients experiencing allergic reactions should be evaluated for factor IX inhibitors. When clinical response is suboptimal or patient is to undergo surgical procedure, screen for inhibitors. Patients with severe gene defects (eg, gene deletion or inversion) are more likely to develop inhibitors (WFH, 2005).

Observe closely for signs or symptoms of intravascular coagulation or thrombosis. Use with caution when administering to patients with liver disease, postoperatively, neonates, or patients at risk of thromboembolic phenomena, disseminated intravascular coagulation or patients with signs of fibrinolysis due to the potential risk of thromboembolic complications. Use with caution in patients with liver dysfunction; may be at increased risk of developing thrombosis or DIC. Products do not contain therapeutic levels of factor VII and should not be used for the treatment of factor VII deficiency. Product of human plasma; may potentially contain infectious agents which could transmit disease. Screening of donors, as well as testing and/or inactivation or removal of certain viruses, reduces the risk. Infections thought to be transmitted by this product should be reported to the manufacturer. Some products may contain heparin. Use with caution in patients with a history of heparin-induced thrombocytopenia. Some product packaging may contain natural rubber latex.

Adverse Reactions Frequency not defined.

Cardiovascular: Flushing, thrombosis (sometimes fatal)

Central nervous system: Chills, fever, headache, lethargy, somnolence

Dermatologic: Rash, urticaria

Gastrointestinal: Nausea, vomiting

Hematologic: DIC

Neuromuscular & skeletal: Paresthesia

Respiratory: Dyspnea

Miscellaneous: Anaphylactic shock, clotting factor antibodies (development of), heparin-induced thrombocytopenia (with products containing heparin)

Drug Interactions

Metabolism/Transport Effects None known.

Avoid Concomitant Use

Avoid concomitant use of Factor IX Complex (Human) with any of the following: Aminocaproic Acid

Increased Effect/Toxicity

The levels/effects of Factor IX Complex (Human) may be increased by: Aminocaproic Acid

Decreased Effect There are no known significant interactions involving a decrease in effect.

Storage/Stability

Bebulin® VH: Prior to use, store under refrigeration at 2°C to 8°C (36°F to 46°F); avoid freezing. Following reconstitution, do not refrigerate and use within 3 hours.

Profilnine® SD: Prior to use, store under refrigeration at 2°C to 8°C (36°F to 46°F); avoid freezing; may also stored at room temperature (not to exceed 30°C) for up to 3 months. Following reconstitution, do not refrigerate and use within 3 hours.

Reconstitution Bring diluent and concentrate to room temperature; gently rotate or agitate to dissolve.

Mechanism of Action Replaces deficient clotting factor including factor X; hemophilia B, or Christmas disease, is an X-linked recessively inherited disorder of blood coagulation characterized by insufficient or abnormal synthesis of the clotting protein factor IX. Factor IX is a vitamin K-dependent coagulation factor which is synthesized in the liver. Factor IX is activated by factor XIa in the intrinsic coagulation pathway. Activated factor IX (IXa), in combination with factor VII:C, activates factor X to Xa, resulting ultimately in the conversion of prothrombin to thrombin and the formation of a fibrin clot. The infusion of exogenous factor IX to replace the deficiency present in hemophilia B temporarily restores hemostasis.

Pharmacodynamics/Kinetics Half-life elimination: IX component: ~24 hours

Dosing

Adult & Geriatric Dosage is expressed in units of factor IX activity and must be individualized based on severity of factor IX deficiency, extent and location of bleeding, and clinical status of patient. When multiple doses are required, administer at 24-hour intervals unless otherwise specified. Administer I.V. only:

Formula for units required to raise blood level %:

Bebulin® VH: In general, factor IX 1 unit/kg will increase the plasma factor IX level by 0.8%

Number of Factor IX units required = body weight (kg) x desired factor IX increase (as %) x 1.2 units/kg

Profilnine® SD: In general, factor IX 1 unit/kg will increase the plasma factor IX level by 1%:

Number of factor IX units required = bodyweight (kg) x desired factor IX increase (as %) x 1 unit/kg

For example, to increase factor IX level to 25% of normal in a 70 kg patient: Number of factor IX units needed = 70 kg x 25 x 1 unit/kg = 1750 units

As a general rule, the level of factor IX required for treatment of different conditions is listed below:

Hemorrhage:

Minor bleeding (early hemarthrosis, minor epistaxis, gingival bleeding, mild hematuria):

Bebulin® VH: Raise factor IX level to 20% of normal [typical initial dose: 25-35 units/kg]; generally a single dose is sufficient.

Profilnine® SD: Mild-to-moderate bleeding: Raise factor IX level to 20% to 30% of normal.

Moderate bleeding (severe joint bleeding, early hematoma, major open bleeding, minor trauma, minor hemoptysis, hematemesis, melena, major hematuria):

Bebulin® VH: Raise factor IX level to 40% of normal [typical initial dose: 40-55 units/kg]; average duration of treatment is 2 days or until adequate wound healing.

Profilnine® SD: Mild-to-moderate bleeding: raise factor IX level to 20% to 30% of normal.

Major bleeding (severe hematoma, major trauma, severe hemoptysis, hematemesis, melena):

Bebulin® VH: Raise factor IX level to ≥60% of normal [typical initial dose: 60-70 units/kg]; average duration of treatment is 2-3 days or until adequate wound healing. Do not raise >60% in patients who may be predisposed to thrombosis.

Profilnine® SD: Raise factor IX level to 30% to 50% of normal.

Surgical procedures:

Dental surgery:

Bebulin® VH: Raise factor IX level to 40% to 60% of normal on day of surgery [typical dose: 50-60 units/kg]. One infusion, administered 1 hour prior to surgery, is generally sufficient for the extraction of one tooth; for the extraction of multiple teeth, replacement therapy may be required for up to 1 week (See dosing guidelines for *Minor Surgery on next page*).

Profilnine® SD: Raise factor IX level to 50% of normal immediately prior to procedure.

Minor surgery:

Bebulin® VH: Raise factor IX level to 40% to 60% of normal on day of surgery [typical initial dose: 50-60 units/kg]. Decrease factor IX level from 40% of normal to 20% of normal during initial postoperative period (1-2 weeks or until adequate wound healing) [typical dose: 55 units/kg decreasing to 25 units/kg]. The preoperative dose should be given 1 hour prior to surgery. The average dosing interval may be every 12 hours initially, then every 24 hours later in the postoperative period.

Profilnine® SD: Raise factor IX level to 30% to 50% of normal for at least 1 week following surgery.

Major surgery:

Bebulin® VH: Raise factor IX level to ≥60% of normal on day of surgery [typical initial dose: 70-95 units/kg]; do not raise >60% in patients who may be predisposed to thrombosis. Decrease factor IX level from 60% of normal to 20% of normal during initial postoperative period (1-2 weeks) [typical dose: 70 units/kg decreasing to 35 units/kg]; further decrease to maintain a factor IX level of 20% of normal during late postoperative period (≥3 weeks) and continuing until adequate wound healing is achieved [typical dose: 35 units/kg decreasing to 25 units/kg]. The preoperative dose should be given 1 hour prior to surgery. The average dosing interval may be every 12 hours initially, then every 24 hours later in the postoperative period.

Profilnine® SD: Raise Factor IX level to 30% to 50% of normal for at least 1 week following surgery.

Hemorrhage:

Long-term prophylactic treatment: Bebulin® VH: 20-30 units/kg once or twice a week may reduce frequency of spontaneous hemorrhage; dosing regimen should be individualized.

Warfarin associated hemorrhage (unlabeled use): I.V.: **Note:** Products contain low or nontherapeutic levels of factor VII component; therefore, additional fresh frozen plasma (FFP) or factor VIIa may be considered (Masotti, 2011). When immediate INR reversal is required, concomitant use of 1-2 units of FFP should be considered to ensure acute INR reversal (Baker, 2004; Chong, 2010; Holland, 2009). Administer vitamin K (phytonadione) 5-10 mg by slow I.V. infusion (Guyatt, 2012); vitamin K may be repeated every 12 hours if INR is persistently elevated.

Adjusted-dose regimen, weight based (Chong, 2010): Profilnine® SD:

INR <5: 30 units/kg

INR >5 (emergent): 50 units/kg

Note: If after administration, INR remains >1.2 consider repeating dose and administering more FFP until INR <1.2

The following 2 methods have also been suggested, but are not product specific:

Adjusted-dose regimen, weight based (Liumbruno, 2009):

INR <2.0: 20 units/kg

INR 2.0-4.0: 30 units/kg

INR >4.0: 50 units/kg

Note: If after administration, INR remains >1.5 consider repeating dose appropriate for INR.

May also determine dose based on presenting INR and estimated functional prothrombin complex (PC) expressed as percentage of normal plasma levels (see table; Masotti, 2011):

Units needed to be infused = (**target** % of functional PC to be reached – **current** estimated % of functional PC) x kg of body weight

Example:

Patient (weight: 70 kg) presents with INR of 4.5 which corresponds to an **estimated % functional PC** of 10% (see table). Target INR of 1.4 corresponds to an **estimated target % functional PC** of 40%.

Units needed to be infused = (40 - 10) x 70 kg = 2100 units

Conversion of the INR to Estimated Functional Prothrombin Complex (PC)

INR Value	Estimated Functional PC
≥5.0	5%
4-4.9	10%
2.6-3.2	15%
2.2-2.5	20%
1.9-2.1	25%
1.7-1.8	30%
1.4-1.6	40%
1.0-1.3	100%

Pediatric Refer to adult dosing.

Administration I.V. administration only; should be infused **slowly**. Rate should not exceed 2 mL/minute for Bebulin® VH or 10 mL/minute for Profilnine® SD. Slowing the rate of infusion, changing the lot of medication, or administering antihistamines may relieve some adverse reactions

Monitoring Parameters Levels of factor IX; PT, PTT; INR (when used for warfarin reversal); signs and symptoms of hypersensitivity reactions, DIC, thrombosis

Additional Information Vaccination with hepatitis A and hepatitis B vaccines are recommended at diagnosis for patients with hemophilia.

Factor IX concentrate containing only factor IX is also available and preferable for hemophilia B (or Christmas disease). Prothrombin complex concentrates also contain factor II, factor VII, and factor X and are of intermediate purity. Heparin may be present in some products to decrease thrombotic effects.

Dosage Forms Excipient information presented when available (limited, particularly for generics); consult specific product labeling. [DSC] = Discontinued product

Injection, powder for reconstitution:

Bebulin® VH: Exact potency labeled on each vial [vapor heated; contains heparin and natural rubber/natural latex in packaging]

Profilnine® SD: ~500 units, ~1000 units, ~1500 units [exact potency labeled on each vial; solvent/detergent treated]

References

Baker RI, Coughlin PB, Gallus AS, et al, "Warfarin Reversal: Consensus Guidelines, on Behalf of the Australasian Society of Thrombosis and Haemostasis," *Med J Aust*, 2004, 181(9):492-7.

Chong CT, Lew TWK, Kuperan P, et al, "Rapid Reversal of Coagulopathy in Warfarin-Related Intracranial Haemorrhages With Prothombin Complex Concentrates," *Anaesth Intensive Care*, 2010, 38(3):474-80.

Guyatt GH, Akl EA, Crowther M, et al, "Executive Summary: Antithrombotic Therapy and Prevention of Thrombosis, 9th ed: American College of Chest Physicians Evidence-Based Clinical Practice Guidelines," *Chest*, 2012, 141(2 Suppl):7-47.

Hirsh J, Guyatt G, Albers GW, et al, "Executive Summary: American College of Chest Physicians Evidence-Based Clinical Practice Guidelines (8th Edition)," *Chest*, 2008, 133(6 Suppl):71-109.

Holland L, Warkentin TE, Refaai M, et al, "Suboptimal Effect of a Three-Factor Prothrombin Complex Concentrate (Profilnine-SD) in Correcting Supratherapeutic International Normalized Ratio Due to Warfarin Overdose," *Transfusion*, 2009, 49(6):1171-7.

Makris M and Watson HG, "The Management of Coumarin-Induced Over-Anticoagulation Annotation," *Br J Haematol*, 2001, 114(2):271-80.

Makris M, Greaves M, Phillips WS, et al, "Emergency Oral Anticoagulant Reversal: The Relative Efficacy of Infusions of Fresh Frozen Plasma and Clotting Factor Concentrate on Correction of the Coagulopathy," *Thromb Haemost*, 1997, 77(3):477-80.

Masotti L, Di Napoli M, Godoy DA, et al, "The Practical Management of Intracerebral Hemorrhage Associated With Oral Anticoagulant Therapy," *Int Stroke J*, 2001, 6(3):228-40.

National Hemophilia Foundation, "Guidelines for Emergency Department Management of Individuals with Hemophilia," 2006. Available at http://www.hemophilia.org/NHFWeb/Resource/StaticPages/menu0/menu5/menu57/175.pdf

National Hemophilia Foundation, "MASAC Recommendations Concerning Products Licensed for the Treatment of Hemophilia and Other Bleeding Disorders," 2010. Available at http://www.-hemophilia.org/NHFWeb/Resource/StaticPages/menu0/menu5/menu57/masac190.pdf

National Hemophilia Foundation, "MASAC Recommendations Concerning Prophylaxis (Regular Administration of Clotting Factor Concentrate to Prevent Bleeding)," 2007. Available at http://www.hemophilia.org/NHFWeb/Resource/StaticPages/menu0/menu5/menu57/masac179.pdf

Preston FE, Laidlaw ST, Sampson B, et al, "Rapid Reversal of Oral Anticoagulation With Warfarin by a Prothrombin Complex Concentrate (Beriplex): Efficacy and Safety in 42 Patients," *Br J Haematol*, 2002, 116(3):619-24.

World Federation of Hemophilia, "Guidelines for the Management of Hemophilia," 2005. Available at http://www.ehc.eu/fileadmin/dokumente/Gudelines_Mng_Hemophilia.pdf

Yasaka M, Sakata T, Naritomi H, et al, "Optimal Dose of Prothrombin Complex Concentrate for Acute Reversal of Oral Anticoagulation," *Thromb Res*, 2005, 115(6):455-9.

◆ **Factor IX Concentrate** *see* Factor IX *on page* 571

Famciclovir (fam SYE kloe veer)

Brand Names: U.S. Famvir®

Brand Names: Canada Apo-Famciclovir®; Ava-Famciclovir; CO Famciclovir; Famvir®; PMS-Famciclovir; Sandoz-Famciclovir

Generic Availability (U.S.) Yes

Pharmacologic Category Antiviral Agent

Use Treatment of acute herpes zoster (shingles) in immunocompetent patients; treatment and suppression of recurrent episodes of genital herpes in immunocompetent patients; treatment of herpes labialis (cold sores) in immunocompetent patients; treatment of recurrent orolabial/genital (mucocutaneous) herpes simplex in HIV-infected patients

Labeled Contraindications Hypersensitivity to famciclovir, penciclovir, or any component of the formulation

Pregnancy Risk Factor B

Lactation Excretion in breast milk unknown/not recommended

Warnings/Precautions Has not been established for use in immunocompromised patients (except HIV-infected patients with orolabial or genital herpes, patients with ophthalmic or disseminated zoster or with initial episode of genital herpes, and in Black and African American patients with recurrent episodes of genital herpes. Acute renal failure has been reported with use of inappropriate high doses in patients with underlying renal disease. Dosage adjustment is required in patients with renal insufficiency. Tablets contain lactose; do not use with galactose intolerance, severe lactase deficiency, or glucose-galactose malabsorption syndromes.

Ethanol/Nutrition/Herb Interactions Food: Rate of absorption and/or conversion to penciclovir and peak concentration are reduced with food, but bioavailability is not affected.

Storage/Stability Store at 25°C (77°F); excursions permitted to 15°C to 30°C (59°F to 86°F).

Mechanism of Action Famciclovir undergoes rapid biotransformation to the active compound penciclovir (prodrug), which is phosphorylated by viral thymidine kinase in HSV-1, HSV-2, and VZV-infected cells to a monophosphate form; this is then converted to penciclovir triphosphate and competes with deoxyguanosine triphosphate to inhibit HSV-2 polymerase, therefore, herpes viral DNA synthesis/replication is selectively inhibited.

Pharmacodynamics/Kinetics

Absorption: Food decreases maximum peak penciclovir concentration and delays time to penciclovir peak; AUC remains the same

Distribution: V_d: Penciclovir: 0.91-1.25 L/kg

Protein binding: Penciclovir: <20%

Metabolism: Famciclovir is rapidly deacetylated and oxidized to penciclovir (active prodrug); *in vitro* data demonstrate that metabolism does not occur via CYP isoenzymes

Bioavailability: Penciclovir: 69% to 85%

Half-life elimination: Penciclovir: 2-4 hours; Prolonged in renal impairment: Cl_{cr} 20-39 mL/minute: 5-8 hours, Cl_{cr} <20 mL/minute: 3-24 hours

Time to peak: Penciclovir: ~1 hour

Excretion: Urine (73% primarily as penciclovir), feces (27%)

Dosing

Adult & Geriatric

Immunocompetent patients:

Acute herpes zoster: Oral: 500 mg every 8 hours for 7 days (**Note:** Initiate therapy as soon as possible after diagnosis and within 72 hours of rash onset)

Genital herpes simplex virus (HSV) infection: Oral:

Initial episode: 250 mg 3 times/day for 7-10 days (CDC, 2010)

Recurrence: 1000 mg twice daily for 1 day (**Note:** Initiate therapy as soon as possible and within 6 hours of symptoms/lesions onset)

Alternatively, the following regimens are also recommended: 125 mg twice daily for 5 days or 500 mg as a single dose, followed by 250 mg twice daily for 2 days (CDC, 2010). **Note:** Canadian labeling recommends 125 mg twice daily for 5 days.

Suppressive therapy: 250 mg twice daily for up to 1 year; **Note:** Duration not established, but efficacy/safety have been demonstrated for 1 year (CDC, 2010)

Recurrent herpes labialis (cold sores): Oral: 1500 mg as a single dose; initiate therapy at first sign or symptom such as tingling, burning, or itching (initiated within 1 hour in clinical studies)

HIV patients (**Note:** Initiate therapy as soon as possible and within 48 hours of symptoms/lesions onset):

Recurrent orolabial/genital (mucocutaneous) HSV infection: Oral: 500 mg twice daily for 7 days or 5-10 days (CDC, 2010).

Prevention of HSV reactivation: Oral: 500 mg twice daily (CDC, 2010)

Renal Impairment

Dosing adjustment in renal impairment:

Herpes zoster:

Cl_{cr} ≥60 mL/minute: No dosage adjustment necessary
Cl_{cr} 40-59 mL/minute: Administer 500 mg every 12 hours
Cl_{cr} 20-39 mL/minute: Administer 500 mg every 24 hours
Cl_{cr} <20 mL/minute: Administer 250 mg every 24 hours
Hemodialysis: Administer 250 mg after each dialysis session.

Recurrent genital herpes: Treatment:

U.S. labeling (single-day regimen):

Cl_{cr} ≥60 mL/minute: No dosage adjustment necessary
Cl_{cr} 40-59 mL/minute: Administer 500 mg every 12 hours for 1 day
Cl_{cr} 20-39 mL/minute: Administer 500 mg as a single dose
Cl_{cr} <20 mL/minute: Administer 250 mg as a single dose
Hemodialysis: Administer 250 mg as a single dose after a dialysis session.

Canadian labeling:

Cl_{cr} >20 mL/minute/1.73 m^2: No dosage adjustment necessary
Cl_{cr} <20 mL/minute/1.73 m^2: Administer 125 mg every 24 hours
Hemodialysis: Administer 125 mg after each dialysis session.

Recurrent genital herpes: Suppression:

Cl_{cr} ≥40 mL/minute: No dosage adjustment necessary
Cl_{cr} 20-39 mL/minute: Administer 125 mg every 12 hours
Cl_{cr} <20 mL/minute: Administer 125 mg every 24 hours
Hemodialysis: Administer 125 mg after each dialysis session.

Recurrent herpes labialis: Treatment (single-dose regimen):

Cl_{cr} ≥60 mL/minute: No dosage adjustment necessary
Cl_{cr} 40-59 mL/minute: Administer 750 mg as a single dose
Cl_{cr} 20-39 mL/minute: Administer 500 mg as a single dose
Cl_{cr} <20 mL/minute: Administer 250 mg as a single dose
Hemodialysis: Administer 250 mg as a single dose after a dialysis session.

Recurrent orolabial/genital (mucocutaneous) herpes in HIV-infected patients:

Cl_{cr} ≥40 mL/minute: No dosage adjustment necessary
Cl_{cr} 20-39 mL/minute: Administer 500 mg every 24 hours
Cl_{cr} <20 mL/minute: Administer 250 mg every 24 hours
Hemodialysis: Administer 250 mg after each dialysis session.

Hepatic Impairment

Mild-to-moderate impairment: No dosage adjustment is necessary

Severe impairment: No dosage adjustment provided in manufacturer's labeling; has not been studied. However, a 44% decrease in the C_{max} of penciclovir (active metabolite) was noted in patients with mild-to-moderate impairment; impaired conversion of famciclovir to penciclovir may affect efficacy.

Administration May be administered without regard to meals.

Dosage Forms Excipient information presented when available (limited, particularly for generics); consult specific product labeling.

Tablet, oral: 125 mg, 250 mg, 500 mg
Famvir®: 125 mg [contains lactose 26.9 mg/tablet]
Famvir®: 250 mg [contains lactose 53.7 mg/tablet]
Famvir®: 500 mg [contains lactose 107.4 mg/tablet]

◆ **Famvir®** *see* Famciclovir *on page* 580

◆ **2F-ara-AMP** *see* Fludarabine *on page* 619

- **Fareston®** *see* Toremifene *on page* *1376*
- **Faslodex®** *see* Fulvestrant *on page* *651*
- **Fasturtec® (Can)** *see* Rasburicase *on page* *1229*
- **5-FC** *see* Flucytosine *on page* *618*
- **FC1157a** *see* Toremifene *on page* *1376*
- **FE200486** *see* Degarelix *on page* *422*
- **Femara®** *see* Letrozole *on page* *867*

FentaNYL (FEN ta nil)

Brand Names: U.S. Abstral®; Actiq®; Duragesic®; Fentora®; Lazanda®; Onsolis®; Subsys®

Brand Names: Canada Abstral™; Actiq®; Duragesic®; Duragesic® MAT; Fentanyl Citrate Injection, USP; Novo-Fentanyl; PMS-Fentanyl MTX; RAN™-Fentanyl Matrix Patch; RAN™-Fentanyl Transdermal System; ratio-Fentanyl

Index Terms Fentanyl Citrate; Fentanyl Hydrochloride; Fentanyl Patch; OTFC (Oral Transmucosal Fentanyl Citrate)

Generic Availability (U.S.) Yes: Injection, lozenge, patch

Pharmacologic Category Analgesic, Opioid; Anilidopiperidine Opioid; General Anesthetic

Use

Injection: Relief of pain, preoperative medication, adjunct to general or regional anesthesia

Transdermal patch (eg, Duragesic®): Management of persistent moderate-to-severe chronic pain in opioid-tolerant patients when around-the clock analgesia is needed for an extended period of time

Transmucosal lozenge (eg, Actiq®), buccal tablet (Fentora®), buccal film (Onsolis®), nasal spray (Lazanda®), sublingual tablet (Abstral®), sublingual spray (Subsys®): Management of breakthrough cancer pain in opioid-tolerant patients

Note: "Opioid-tolerant" patients are defined as patients who are taking at least:
- Oral morphine 60 mg/day, **or**
- Transdermal fentanyl 25 mcg/hour, **or**
- Oral oxycodone 30 mg/day, **or**
- Oral hydromorphone 8 mg/day, **or**
- Oral oxymorphone 25 mg/day, **or**
- Equianalgesic dose of another opioid for at least 1 week

Labeled Contraindications Hypersensitivity to fentanyl or any component of the formulation

Additional contraindications for transdermal patches (eg, Duragesic®): Severe respiratory disease or depression including acute asthma (unless patient is mechanically ventilated); paralytic ileus; patients requiring short-term therapy, management of acute or intermittent pain, postoperative or mild pain, and in patients who are **not** opioid tolerant

Additional contraindications for transmucosal buccal tablets (Fentora®), buccal films (Onsolis™), lozenges (eg, Actiq®), sublingual tablets (Abstral®), sublingual spray (Subsys®), nasal spray (Lazanda®): Contraindicated in the management of acute or postoperative pain (including headache, migraine, or dental pain), and in patients who are **not** opioid tolerant. Abstral® and Onsolis™ also are contraindicated for acute pain management in the emergency room.

Canadian labeling: Additional contraindication (not in U.S. labeling): Sublingual tablets (Abstral™): Severe respiratory depression or severe obstructive lung disease

Pregnancy Risk Factor C

Lactation Enters breast milk/not recommended (AAP rates "compatible"; AAP 2001 update pending)

Warnings/Precautions An opioid-containing analgesic regimen should be tailored to each patient's needs and based upon the type of pain being treated (acute versus chronic), the route of administration, degree of tolerance for opioids (naive versus chronic user), age, weight, and medical condition. The optimal analgesic dose varies widely among patients. Doses should be titrated to pain relief/prevention. May cause CNS depression, which may impair physical or mental abilities; patients must be cautioned about performing tasks which require mental alertness (eg, operating machinery or driving). When using with other CNS depressants, reduce dose of one or both agents. Fentanyl shares the toxic potentials of opiate agonists, and precautions of opiate agonist therapy should be observed; use with caution in patients with bradycardia or bradyarrhythmias; rapid I.V. infusion may result in skeletal muscle and chest wall rigidity leading to respiratory distress and/or apnea, bronchoconstriction, laryngospasm; inject slowly over 3-5 minutes. **[U.S. Boxed Warning]: Healthcare provider should be alert to problems of abuse, misuse, and diversion.** Tolerance or drug dependence may result from extended use. The elderly may be particularly susceptible to the CNS depressant and constipating effects of narcotics. Use extreme caution in patients with COPD or other chronic respiratory conditions. Use caution with head injuries, morbid obesity, renal impairment, or hepatic dysfunction. **[U.S. Boxed Warning]: Use with strong or moderate CYP3A4 inhibitors may result in increased effects and potentially fatal respiratory depression.** Use is not recommended with MAO inhibitors or within 14 days of MAO inhibitor use; severe and unpredictable adverse effects may result. Concurrent use of agonist/antagonist analgesics may precipitate withdrawal symptoms and/or reduced analgesic efficacy in patients following prolonged therapy with mu opioid agonists. Abrupt discontinuation following prolonged use may also lead to withdrawal symptoms.

Pediatric patients: **[U.S. Boxed Warning]: Buccal film, buccal tablet, nasal spray, sublingual tablet, sublingual spray, transdermal patch, and lozenge preparations contain an amount of medication that can be fatal to children. Keep all used and unused products out of the reach of children at all times and discard products properly.** Patients and caregivers should be counseled on the dangers to children including the risk of exposure to partially-consumed products.

[U.S. Boxed Warning] Abstral®, Actiq®, Duragesic®, Fentora®, Lazanda®, Onsolis®, Subsys®: May cause potentially life-threatening hypoventilation, respiratory depression, and/or death; Abstral®, Actiq®, Duragesic®, Fentora®, Lazanda®, Onsolis®, or Subsys® should only be prescribed for opioid-tolerant patients. Risk of respiratory depression increased in elderly patients, debilitated patients, and patients with conditions associated with hypoxia or hypercapnia; usually occurs after administration of initial dose in nontolerant patients or when given with other drugs that depress respiratory function.

Transmucosal (buccal film/tablet, sublingual spray/tablet, lozenge) and nasal spray: **[U.S. Boxed Warning]: Transmucosal and nasal fentanyl**

formulations are contraindicated in the management of acute or postoperative pain and in opioid nontolerant patients. Should be used only for the care of opioid-tolerant cancer patients with breakthrough pain and is intended for use by specialists who are knowledgeable in treating cancer pain. **[U.S. Boxed Warning]: Substantial differences exist in the pharmacokinetic profile of fentanyl products. Do not convert patients on a mcg-per-mcg basis from one fentanyl product to another fentanyl product; the substitution of one fentanyl product for another fentanyl product may result in a fatal overdose. [U.S. Boxed Warning]: Available only through the TIRF REMS ACCESS program, a restricted distribution program with outpatients, prescribers who prescribe to outpatients, pharmacies (inpatient and outpatient), and distributor-required enrollment.** Avoid use of topical nasal decongestants (eg, oxymetazoline) during episodes of rhinitis when using fentanyl nasal spray; response to fentanyl may be delayed or reduced. Avoid use of sublingual spray in cancer patients with grade 2 or higher mucositis (fentanyl exposure increased); use with caution in patients with grade 1 mucositis, and closely monitor for respiratory and CNS depression.

Transdermal patch: **[U.S. Boxed Warning]: Transdermal patch is contraindicated in the management of short-term analgesia, or in the management of postoperative pain, and in patients who are opioid nontolerant. Should only be prescribed by healthcare professionals who are knowledgeable in the use of potent opioids in the management of chronic pain. Monitor closely for respiratory depression during use, particularly during first two applications after initiation of therapy or after dose increases. [U.S. Boxed Warning]: Avoid exposure of application site and surrounding area to direct external heat sources. Patients who experience fever or increase in core body temperature should be monitored closely.** Serum fentanyl concentrations may increase by approximately one-third for patients with a body temperature of 40°C (104°F) secondary to a temperature-dependent increase in fentanyl release from the patch and increased skin permeability. **[U.S. Boxed Warning]: Accidental exposure may lead to severe respiratory depression, including death, in children and adults; proper procedures for handling and disposal of patches should be followed.** Avoid unclothed/unwashed application site exposure, inadvertent person-to-person patch transfer (eg, while hugging), incidental exposure (eg, sharing same bed, sitting on patch), intentional exposure (eg, chewing), or accidental exposure by caregivers when applying/removing patch. Should be applied only to intact skin. Use of a patch that has been cut, damaged, or altered in any way may result in overdosage. Patients who experience adverse reactions should be monitored for at least 24 hours after removal of the patch. May contain conducting metal (eg, aluminum); remove patch prior to MRI.

Ethanol/Nutrition/Herb Interactions

Ethanol: Ethanol may increase CNS depression. Management: Monitor for increased effects with coadministration. Caution patients about effects.

Food: Fentanyl concentrations may be increased by grapefruit juice. Management: Avoid concurrent intake of large quantities (>1 quart/day) of grapefruit juice.

Herb/Nutraceutical: St John's wort may decrease fentanyl levels; gotu kola, valerian, and kava kava may increase CNS depression. Management: Avoid St John's wort, gotu kola, valerian, and kava kava.

Storage/Stability

Injection formulation: Store at controlled room temperature of 20°C to 25°C (68°F to 77°F). Protect from light.

Nasal spray: Do not store above 25°C (77°F); do not freeze. Protect from light. Bottle should be stored in the provided child-resistant container when not in use and kept out of the reach of children at all times.

Transdermal patch: Do not store above 25°C (77°F). Keep out of the reach of children.

Transmucosal (buccal film, buccal tablet, lozenge, sublingual spray, sublingual tablet): Store at controlled room temperature of 20°C to 25°C (68°F to 77°F). Protect from freezing and moisture. Keep out of the reach of children.

Mechanism of Action Binds with stereospecific receptors at many sites within the CNS, increases pain threshold, alters pain reception, inhibits ascending pain pathways

Pharmacodynamics/Kinetics

Onset of action: Analgesic: I.M.: 7-8 minutes; I.V.: Almost immediate; Transdermal (initial placement): 6 hours; Transmucosal: 5-15 minutes

Peak effect: Analgesic: Transdermal (initial placement): 12 hours; Transmucosal: 15-30 minutes

Duration: I.M.: 1-2 hours; I.V.: 0.5-1 hour; Transdermal (removal of patch/no replacement): 12 hours; Transmucosal: Related to blood level; respiratory depressant effect may last longer than analgesic effect

Absorption:

Transdermal: Initial application: Gradually absorbed for the first 12-24 hours, followed by a constant absorption for the remainder of the dosing interval. Absorption is decreased in cachectic patients (compared to normal size patients).

Transmucosal, buccal tablet and buccal film: Rapid, ~50% from the buccal mucosa; remaining 50% swallowed with saliva and slowly absorbed from GI tract.

Transmucosal, lozenge: Rapid, ~25% from the buccal mucosa; 75% swallowed with saliva and slowly absorbed from GI tract

Distribution: 4-6 L/kg; Highly lipophilic, redistributes into muscle and fat

Protein binding: 80% to 85%

Metabolism: Hepatic, primarily via CYP3A4

Bioavailability:

Buccal film: 71% (mucositis did not have a clinically significant effect on C_{max} and AUC; however, bioavailability is expected to decrease if film is inappropriately chewed and swallowed)

Buccal tablet: 65% (range: 45% to 85%)

Lozenge: 47% (range: 37% to 57%)

Sublingual spray: 76%

Sublingual tablet: 54%

Half-life elimination:

I.V.: 2-4 hours

Transdermal patch: 17 hours (13-22 hours, half-life is influenced by extended absorption rate)

Transmucosal products: 3-14 hours (dose dependent); Nasal spray: 15-25 hours (based on a multiple-dose pharmacokinetic study when doses are administered in the same nostril and separated by a 1-, 2-, or 4-hour time lapse)

Time to peak:
Buccal film: 0.75-4 hours (median: 1 hour)
Buccal tablet: 20-240 minutes (median: 47 minutes)
Lozenge: 20-480 minutes (median: 20-40 minutes)
Nasal spray: Median: 15-21 minutes
Sublingual spray: 10-120 minutes (median: 90 minutes)
Sublingual tablet: 15-240 minutes (median: 30-60 minutes)
Transdermal patch: 24-72 hours, after several sequential 72-hour applications, steady state serum concentrations are reached

Excretion: Urine 75% (primarily as metabolites, <7% to 10% as unchanged drug); feces ~9%

Dosing

Adult Note: Ranges listed may not represent the maximum doses that may be required in all patients. Doses and dosage intervals should be titrated to pain relief/prevention. Monitor vital signs routinely. Single I.M. doses have duration of 1-2 hours, single I.V. doses last 0.5-1 hour.

Surgery:

Premedication: I.M., slow I.V.: 50-100 mcg/dose 30-60 minutes prior to surgery

Adjunct to regional anesthesia: Slow I.V.: 25-100 mcg/dose over 1-2 minutes. **Note:** An I.V. should be in place with regional anesthesia so the I.M. route is rarely used but still maintained as an option in the package labeling.

Adjunct to general anesthesia: Slow I.V.:

Low dose: 0.5-2 mcg/kg/dose depending on the indication.

Moderate dose: Initial: 2-20 mcg/kg/dose; Maintenance (bolus or infusion): 1-2 mcg/kg/**hour**. Discontinuing fentanyl infusion 30-60 minutes prior to the end of surgery will usually allow adequate ventilation upon emergence from anesthesia. For "fast-tracking" and early extubation following major surgery, total fentanyl doses are limited to 10-15 mcg/kg.

High dose: 20-50 mcg/kg/dose; **Note:** High-dose fentanyl as an adjunct to general anesthesia is rarely used, but is still described in the manufacturer's label.

Pain management: Adults:

I.V. (unlabeled use): Bolus at start of infusion: 1-2 mcg/kg **or** 25-100 mcg/dose; continuous infusion rate: 1-2 mcg/kg/**hour or** 25-200 mcg/hour

Severe (unlabeled use): I.M, I.V.: 50-100 mcg/dose every 1-2 hours as needed; patients with prior opiate exposure may tolerate higher initial doses

Patient-controlled analgesia (PCA) (unlabeled use): I.V.:

Usual concentration: 10 mcg/mL
Demand dose: Usual: 20 mcg; range: 10-50 mcg
Lockout interval: 5-8 minutes
Usual basal rate: ≤50 mcg/hour

Critically-ill patients (unlabeled dose): Slow I.V.: 25-100 mcg (based on ~70 kg patient) **or** 0.35-1.5 mcg/kg every 30-60 minutes as needed. **Note:** More frequent dosing may be needed (eg, mechanically-ventilated patients).

Continuous infusion: 50-700 mcg/hour (based on ~70 kg patient) **or** 0.7-10 mcg/kg/**hour**

Intrathecal (I.T.) (unlabeled use; American Pain Society, 2008): **Must be preservative-free.** Doses must be adjusted for age, injection site, and patient's medical condition and degree of opioid tolerance.

Single dose: 5-25 mcg/dose; may provide adequate relief for up to 6 hours

Continuous infusion: Not recommended in acute pain management due to risk of excessive accumulation. For chronic cancer pain, infusion of very small doses may be practical (American Pain Society, 2008).

Epidural (unlabeled use; American Pain Society, 2008): **Must be preservative-free.** Doses must be adjusted for age, injection site, and patient's medical condition and degree of opioid tolerance

Single dose: 25-100 mcg/dose; may provide adequate relief for up to 8 hours

Continuous infusion: 25-100 mcg/hour

Breakthrough cancer pain: Transmucosal: For patients who are tolerant to and currently receiving opioid therapy for persistent cancer pain; dosing should be individually titrated to provide adequate analgesia with minimal side effects. Dose titration should be done if patient requires more than 1 dose/breakthrough pain episode for several consecutive episodes. Patients experiencing >4 breakthrough pain episodes/day should have the dose of their long-term opioid re-evaluated.

Lozenge: Initial dose: 200 mcg; the second dose may be started 15 minutes after completion of the first dose if pain unrelieved. A maximum of 1 additional dose can be given per pain episode; must wait at least 4 hours before treating another episode. Consumption should be limited to ≤4 units/day. Additional requirements suggest need for improved baseline therapy.

Buccal film (Onsolis®): Initial dose: 200 mcg for all patients **Note:** Patients previously using another transmucosal product should be initiated at doses of 200 mcg; do **not** switch patients using any other fentanyl product on a mcg-per-mcg basis.

Dose titration: If titration required, increase dose in 200 mcg increments once per episode using multiples of the 200 mcg film; do not redose within a single episode of breakthrough pain and separate single doses by ≥2 hours. During titration, do not exceed 4 simultaneous applications of the 200 mcg films (800 mcg). If >800 mcg required, treat next episode with one 1200 mcg film (maximum dose: 1200 mcg). Once maintenance dose is determined, all other unused films should be disposed of and that strength (using a single film) should be used. During any pain episode, if adequate relief is not achieved after 30 minutes following buccal film application, a rescue medication (as determined by healthcare provider) may be used.

Maintenance: Determined dose applied as a single film once per episode and separated by ≥2 hours (dose range: 200-1200 mcg); limit to 4 applications/day. Consider increasing the around-the-clock opioid therapy in patients experiencing >4 breakthrough pain episodes/day.

Buccal tablet (Fentora®): Initial dose: 100 mcg; a second 100 mcg dose, if needed, may be started 30 minutes after the start of the first dose. **Note:** For patients previously using the transmucosal lozenge (Actiq®), the initial dose should be selected using the conversions listed below (maximum: 2 doses per breakthrough pain episode every 4 hours).

Dose titration, if required, should be done using multiples of the 100 mcg tablets. Patient can take two 100 mcg tablets (one on each side of mouth). If that dose is not successful, can use four 100 mcg tablets (two on each side of mouth). If titration requires >400 mcg/dose, then use 200 mcg tablets.

Conversion from lozenge to buccal tablet (Fentora®):

Lozenge dose 200-400 mcg, then buccal tablet 100 mcg

Lozenge dose 600-800 mcg, then buccal tablet 200 mcg

Lozenge dose 1200-1600 mcg, then buccal tablet 400 mcg

Note: Four 100 mcg buccal tablets deliver approximately 12% and 13% higher values of C_{max} and AUC, respectively, compared to one 400 mcg buccal tablet. To prevent confusion, patient should only have one strength available at a time. Using more than four buccal tablets at a time has not been studied.

Nasal spray (Lazanda®):

Initial dose: 100 mcg (one 100 mcg spray in one nostril) for all patients. **Note:** Patients previously using another fentanyl product should be initiated at a dose of 100 mcg; do not convert patients from other fentanyl products to Lazanda® on a mcg-per-mcg basis.

Dose titration: If pain is relieved within 30 minutes, that same dose should be used to treat subsequent episodes. If pain is unrelieved, may increase to a higher dose using the recommended titration steps. **Must wait at least 2 hours before treating another episode with nasal spray.** Dose titration steps: If no relief with 100 mcg dose, increase to 200 mcg dose per episode (one 100 mcg spray in each nostril); if no relief with 200 mcg dose, increase to 400 mcg per episode (one 400 mcg spray); if no relief with 400 mcg dose, increase to 800 mcg dose per episode (one 400 mcg spray in each nostril). **Note:** Single doses >800 mcg have not been evaluated. There are no data supporting the use of a combination of dose strengths.

Maintenance dose: Once maintenance dose for breakthrough pain episode has been determined, use that dose for subsequent episodes. For pain that is not relieved after 30 minutes of Lazanda® administration or if a separate breakthrough pain episode occurs within the 2 hour window before the next Lazanda® dose is permitted, a rescue medication may be used. Limit Lazanda® use to ≤4 episodes of breakthrough pain per day. If response to maintenance dose changes (increase in adverse reactions or alterations in pain relief), dose readjustment may be necessary. If patient is experiencing >4 breakthrough pain episodes/day, consider increasing the around the clock, long-acting opioid therapy; if long-acting opioid therapy dose is altered, re-evaluate and retitrate Lazanda® dose as needed.

Sublingual spray (Subsys®):

Initial dose: 100 mcg for all patients. If pain is unrelieved, 1 additional 100 mcg dose may be given 30 minutes after administration of the first dose. A maximum of 2 doses can be given per breakthrough pain episode; must wait at least 4 hours before treating another episode. **Note:** Patients must remain on around-the-clock opioids during use. Patients previously using other fentanyl products should be initiated at a dose of 100 mcg; do not convert patients from any other fentanyl product (transmucosal, transdermal, or parenteral) to Subsys® on a mcg-per-mcg basis.

Dose titration: If pain is relieved within 30 minutes, that same dose should be used to treat subsequent episodes and no titration is necessary. If pain is unrelieved, may increase to a higher dose using the recommended titration steps. Goal is to determine the dose that provides adequate analgesia (with tolerable side effects) using a single dose per breakthrough pain episode. For each breakthrough pain episode, if pain unrelieved after 30 minutes only 1 additional dose using the same strength may be given (maximum: 2 doses per breakthrough pain episode). **Must wait at least 4 hours before treating another episode with Subsys®.**

Dose titration steps: If no relief with 100 mcg dose, increase to 200 mcg dose per episode (one 200 mcg unit); if no relief with 200 mcg dose, increase to 400 mcg per episode (one 400 mcg unit); if no relief with 400 mcg dose, increase to 600 mcg dose per episode (one 600 mcg unit); if no relief with 600 mcg dose, increase to 800 mcg dose per episode (one 800 mcg unit); if no relief with 800 mcg dose, increase to 1200 mcg dose per episode (two 600 mcg units); if no relief with 1200 mcg dose, increase to 1600 mcg per episode (two 800 mcg units).

Maintenance dose: Once maintenance dose for breakthrough pain episode has been determined, use that dose for subsequent episodes. If occasional episodes of unrelieved breakthrough pain occur following 30 minutes of Subsys® administration, 1 additional dose using the same strength may be administered (maximum: 2 doses per breakthrough pain episode); patient must wait 4 hours before treating another breakthrough pain episode with Subsys®. Once maintenance dose is determined, limit Susbsys™ use to ≤4 episodes of breakthrough pain per day. If response to maintenance dose changes (increase in adverse reactions or alterations in pain relief), dose readjustment may be necessary. If patient is experiencing >4 breakthrough pain episodes/day, consider increasing the around-the-clock, long-acting opioid therapy.

Sublingual tablet (Abstral®):

Initial dose:

U.S. labeling: 100 mcg for all patients; if pain is unrelieved, a second dose may be given 30 minutes after administration of the first dose. A maximum of 2 doses can be given per breakthrough pain episode; must wait at least 2 hours before treating another episode.

Canadian labeling: 100 mcg for all patients; if pain is unrelieved 30 minutes after administration of Abstral™, an alternative rescue medication (other than Abstral™) may be given. Administer only 1 dose of Abstral™ per breakthrough pain episode; must wait at least 2 hours before treating another episode.

Note: Patients previously using another fentanyl product should be initiated at a dose of 100 mcg; do not convert patients from other fentanyl products to Abstral® on a mcg-per-mcg basis.

Dose titration: If titration required, increase in 100 mcg increments (up to 400 mcg) over consecutive breakthrough episodes. If titration requires >400 mcg/dose, increase in increments of 200 mcg, starting with 600 mcg dose. During titration, patients may use multiples of 100 mcg and/or 200 mcg tablets for any single dose; do not exceed 4 tablets at one time; safety and efficacy of doses >800 mcg have not been evaluated.

Maintenance dose: Once maintenance dose for breakthrough pain episode has been determined, use only 1 tablet in the appropriate strength per episode; if pain is unrelieved with maintenance dose:

U.S. labeling recommendations: A second dose may be given after 30 minutes; maximum of 2 doses/episode of breakthrough pain; separate treatment of subsequent episodes by ≥2 hours; limit treatment to ≤4 breakthrough episodes/day.

Canadian labeling recommendations: Administer alternative rescue medication after 30 minutes; maximum of 1 Abstral™ dose/episode of breakthrough pain; separate treatment of subsequent episodes by ≥2 hours; limit treatment to ≤4 breakthrough episodes/day.

Consider increasing the around-the-clock long-acting opioid therapy in patients experiencing >4 breakthrough pain episodes/day; if long-acting opioid therapy dose altered, re-evaluate and retitrate Abstral® dose as needed.

Chronic pain management: Children ≥2 years and Adults (opioid-tolerant patients): Transdermal patch (Duragesic®):

Initial: To convert patients from oral or parenteral opioids to transdermal patch, a 24-hour analgesic requirement should be calculated (based on prior opiate use). Using the tables, the appropriate initial dose can be determined. The initial fentanyl dosage may be approximated from the 24-hour morphine dosage equivalent and titrated to minimize adverse effects and provide analgesia. With the initial application, the absorption of transdermal fentanyl requires several hours to reach plateau; therefore transdermal fentanyl is inappropriate for management of acute pain. Change patch every 72 hours.

Conversion from continuous infusion of fentanyl: In patients who have adequate pain relief with a fentanyl infusion, fentanyl may be converted to transdermal dosing at a rate equivalent to the intravenous rate. A two-step taper of the infusion to be completed over 12 hours has been recommended (Kornick, 2001) after the patch is applied. The infusion is decreased to 50% of the original rate six hours after the application of the first patch, and subsequently discontinued twelve hours after application.

Titration: Short-acting agents may be required until analgesic efficacy is established and/or as supplements for "breakthrough" pain. The amount of supplemental doses should be closely monitored. Appropriate dosage increases may be based on daily supplemental dosage using the ratio of 45 mg/24 hours of oral morphine to a 12.5 mcg/hour increase in fentanyl dosage.

Frequency of adjustment: The dosage should not be titrated more frequently than every 3 days after the initial dose or every 6 days thereafter. Patients should wear a consistent fentanyl dosage through two applications (6 days) before dosage increase based on supplemental opiate dosages can be estimated. **Note:** Upon discontinuation, ~17 hours are required for a 50% decrease in fentanyl levels.

Frequency of application: The majority of patients may be controlled on every 72-hour administration; however, a small number of patients require every 48-hour administration.

Dose conversion guidelines for transdermal fentanyl (see tables below and on next page).

Note: U.S. and Canadian dose conversion guidelines differ. Consult appropriate table.

U.S. Labeling: Dose Conversion Guidelines: Recommended Initial Duragesic® Dose Based Upon Daily Oral Morphine Dose[1,2]

Oral 24-Hour Morphine (mg/day)	Duragesic® Dose[3] (mcg/h)
60-134	25
135-224	50
225-314	75
315-404	100
405-494	125
495-584	150
585-674	175
675-764	200
765-854	225
855-944	250
945-1034	275
1035-1124	300

[1]The table should NOT be used to convert from transdermal fentanyl (Duragesic®) to other opioid analgesics. Rather, following removal of the patch, titrate the dose of the new opioid until adequate analgesia is achieved.

[2]Recommendations are based on U.S. product labeling for Duragesic®.

[3]Pediatric patients initiating therapy on a 25 mcg/hour Duragesic® system should be opioid-tolerant and receiving at least 60 mg oral morphine equivalents per day.

U.S. Labeling: Dose Conversion Guidelines[1,2]

Current Analgesic	Daily Dosage (mg/day)			
Morphine (I.M./I.V.)	10-22	23-37	38-52	53-67
Oxycodone (oral)	30-67	67.5-112	112.5-157	157.5-202
Codeine (oral)	150-447	-	-	-
Hydromorphone (oral)	8-17	17.1-28	28.1-39	39.1-51
Hydromorphone (I.V.)	1.5-3.4	3.5-5.6	5.7-7.9	8-10
Meperidine (I.M.)	75-165	166-278	279-390	391-503
Methadone (oral)	20-44	45-74	75-104	105-134
Fentanyl transdermal recommended dose (mcg/h)	**25 mcg/h**	**50 mcg/h**	**75 mcg/h**	**100 mcg/h**

[1]The table should NOT be used to convert from transdermal fentanyl (Duragesic®) to other opioid analgesics. Rather, following removal of the patch, titrate the dose of the new opioid until adequate analgesia is achieved.

[2]Recommendations are based on U.S. product labeling for Duragesic®.

Transdermal patch (Duragesic® MAT [Canada; not available in U.S.]): Adults:

Canadian Labeling: Dose Conversion Guidelines (Adults): Recommended Initial Duragesic® MAT Dose Based Upon Daily Oral Morphine Dose[1,2]

Oral 24-Hour Morphine (Current Dose in mg/day)	Duragesic® MAT Dose (Initial Dose in mcg/h)
45-59	12
60-134	25
135-179	37
180-224	50
225-269	62
270-314	75
315-359	87
360-404	100
405-494	125
495-584	150
585-674	175
675-764	200
765-854	225
855-944	250
945-1034	275
1035-1124	300

[1]The table should NOT be used to convert from transdermal fentanyl (Duragesic® MAT) to other opioid analgesics. Rather, following removal of the patch, titrate the dose of the new opioid until adequate analgesia is achieved.

[2]Recommendations are based on Canadian product labeling for Duragesic® MAT.

Note: The 12 mcg/hour dose included in this table is to be used for incremental dose adjustment and is generally not recommended for initial dosing, except for patients in whom lower starting doses are deemed clinically appropriate.

Canadian Labeling: Dosing Conversion Guidelines (Adults)[1,2]

Current Analgesic	Daily Dosage (mg/day)						
Morphine[3] (I.M./I.V.)	20-44	45-60	61-75	76-90	n/a[4]	n/a[4]	n/a[4]
Oxycodone (oral)	30-66	67-90	91-112	113-134	135-157	158-179	180-202
Codeine (oral)	150-447	448-597	598-747	748-897	898-1047	1048-1197	1198-1347
Hydromorphone (oral)	8-16	17-22	23-28	29-33	34-39	40-45	46-51
Hydromorphone (I.V.)	4-8.4	8.5-11.4	11.5-14.4	14.5-16.5	16.6-19.5	19.6-22.5	22.6-25.5
Fentanyl transdermal recommended dose (mcg/h)	**25 mcg/h**	**37 mcg/h**	**50 mcg/h**	**62 mcg/h**	**75 mcg/h**	**87 mcg/h**	**100 mcg/h**

[1]The table should NOT be used to convert from transdermal fentanyl (Duragesic® MAT) to other opioid analgesics. Rather, following removal of the patch, titrate the dose of the new opioid until adequate analgesia is achieved.

[2]Recommendations are based on Canadian product labeling for Duragesic® MAT.

[3]Morphine dose conversion based upon I.M to oral dose ratio of 1:3.

[4]Insufficient data available to provide specific dosing recommendations. Use caution; adjust dose conservatively.

Geriatric Elderly have been found to be twice as sensitive as younger patients to the effects of fentanyl. A wide range of doses may be used. When choosing a dose, take into consideration the following patient factors: age, weight, physical status, underlying disease states, other drugs used, type of anesthesia used, and the surgical procedure to be performed.

Transmucosal lozenge (eg, Actiq®): In clinical trials, patients who were >65 years of age were titrated to a mean dose that was 200 mcg less than that of younger patients.

Pediatric Note: Ranges listed may not represent the maximum doses that may be required in all patients. Doses and dosage intervals should be titrated to pain relief/prevention. Monitor vital signs routinely. Single I.M. doses have duration of 1-2 hours, single I.V. doses last 0.5-1 hour.

Adjunct to anesthesia (induction and maintenance): Children ≥2 years: I.V.: 2-3 mcg/kg/dose every 1-2 hours as needed

Pain management (unlabeled use): I.V.: 0.5-2 mcg/kg/dose given every 1-2 hours as needed; continuous infusion: 0.5-2 mcg/kg/**hour**; titrate to desired effects

Patient-controlled analgesia (PCA) (unlabeled use; American Pain Society, 2008): Children <50 kg: **Note:** Opiate-naive: Consider lower end of dosing range:

Usual concentration: 10 mcg/mL
Demand dose: 0.5-1 mcg/kg/dose
Lockout interval: 6-8 minutes
Usual basal rate: 0-0.5 mcg/kg/**hour**

Chronic pain management: Children ≥2 years (opioid-tolerant patients): Transdermal patch (Duragesic®): Refer to adult dosing.

Minor procedures/analgesia (unlabeled use): I.V.:

Children 1-12 years: 0.5-2 mcg/kg/dose given 3 minutes prior to procedure; may repeat every 1-2 hours

Children >12 years: 0.5-2 mcg/kg/dose (maximum: 50 mcg/dose) given 3 minutes prior to procedure; may repeat in 5 minutes if necessary; if more than 2 doses are needed, repeat with a maximum of 25 mcg/dose up to 5 times

Continuous sedation/analgesia: 0.5-2 mcg/kg/**hour**; titrate to desired effect

Breakthrough cancer pain: Children ≥16 years: Transmucosal lozenge: Refer to adult dosing.

Renal Impairment

Transdermal (patch): Degree of impairment (ie, Cl_{cr}) not defined in manufacturer's labeling.

Mild-to-moderate impairment: Initial: Reduce dose by 50%.
Severe impairment: Use not recommended.

Transmucosal (buccal film/tablet, sublingual spray/tablet, lozenge) and nasal spray: Although fentanyl pharmacokinetics may be altered in renal disease, fentanyl can be used successfully in the management of breakthrough cancer pain. Doses should be titrated to reach clinical effect with careful monitoring of patients with severe renal disease.

Hepatic Impairment

Transdermal (patch):

Mild-to-moderate impairment: Initial: Reduce dose by 50%.

Severe impairment: Use not recommended.

Transmucosal (buccal film/tablet, sublingual spray/tablet, lozenge) and nasal spray: Although fentanyl pharmacokinetics may be altered in hepatic disease, fentanyl can be used successfully in the management of breakthrough cancer pain. Doses should be titrated to reach clinical effect with careful monitoring of patients with severe hepatic disease.

Usual Infusion Concentrations: Pediatric I.V. infusion: 10 **mcg**/mL

Usual Infusion Concentrations: Adult I.V. infusion: 10 **mcg**/mL

Administration

I.V.: Administer as slow I.V. infusion over 1-2 minutes. May also be administered as continuous infusion or PCA (unlabeled use) routes. Muscular rigidity may occur with rapid I.V. administration.

Transdermal patch (eg, Duragesic®): Apply to nonirritated and nonirradiated skin, such as chest, back, flank, or upper arm. Do not shave skin; hair at application site should be clipped. Prior to application, clean site with clear water and allow to dry completely. Do not use damaged, cut or leaking patches; patch may be less effective. Skin exposure from fentanyl gel leaking from patch may lead to serious adverse effects; thoroughly wash affected skin surfaces with water (do not use soap). Firmly press in place and hold for 30 seconds. Change patch every 72 hours. Do **not** use soap, alcohol, or other solvents to remove transdermal gel if it accidentally touches skin; use copious amounts of water. Avoid exposing application site to external heat sources (eg, heating pad, electric blanket, heat lamp, hot tub). If there is difficulty with patch adhesion, the edges of the system may be taped in place with first-aid tape. If there is continued difficulty with adhesion, an adhesive film dressing (eg, Bioclusive®, Tegaderm®) may be applied over the system.

Lozenge: Foil overwrap should be removed just prior to administration. Place the unit in mouth between the cheek and gum and allow it to dissolve. Do not chew. Lozenge may be moved from one side of the mouth to the other. The unit should be consumed over a period of 15 minutes. Handle should be removed after the lozenge is consumed; early removal should be considered if the patient has achieved an adequate response and/or shows signs of respiratory depression.

Buccal film: Foil overwrap should be removed just prior to administration. Prior to placing film, wet inside of cheek using tongue or by rinsing with water. Place film inside mouth with the pink side of the unit against the inside of the moistened cheek. With finger, press the film against cheek and hold for 5 seconds. The film should stick to the inside of cheek after 5 seconds. The film should be left in place until it dissolves (usually within 15-30 minutes after application). Liquids may be consumed after 5 minutes of application. Food can be eaten after film dissolves. If using more than 1 film simultaneously (during titration period), apply films on either side of mouth (do not apply on top of each other). Do not chew or swallow film. Do not cut or tear the film. All patients must initiate therapy using the 200 mcg film.

Buccal tablet: Patient should not open blister until ready to administer. The blister backing should be peeled back to expose the tablet; tablet should not be pushed out through the blister. Immediately use tablet once removed from blister. Place entire tablet in the buccal cavity (above a rear molar, between the upper cheek and gum). Tablet should not be broken, sucked, chewed, or swallowed. Should dissolve in about 14-25 minutes when left between the cheek and the gum. If remnants remain they may be swallowed with water.

Nasal spray: Prior to initial use, prime device by spraying 4 sprays into the provided pouch (the counting window will show a green bar when the bottle is ready for use). Insert nozzle a short distance into the nose (~1/2 inch or 1 cm) and point towards the bridge of the nose (while closing off the other nostril using 1 finger). Press on finger grips until a "click" sound is heard and the number in the counting window advances by one. The "click" sound and dose counter are the only reliable methods for ensuring a dose has been administered (spray is not always felt on the nasal mucosa). Patient should remain seated for at least 1 minute following administration. Do not blow nose for ≥30 minutes after administration. Wash hands before and after use. There are 8 full therapeutic sprays in each bottle; do not continue to use bottle after "8" sprays have been used. Dispose of bottle and contents if ≥5 days have passed since last use or if it has been ≥4 days since bottle was primed. Spray the remaining contents into the provided pouch, seal in the child-resistant container, and dispose of in the trash.

Sublingual spray: Open sealed blister unit with scissors immediately prior to administration. Contents of unit should be sprayed into mouth under the tongue.

Sublingual tablet: Remove from the blister unit immediately prior to administration. Place tablet directly under the tongue on the floor of the mouth and allow to completely dissolve; do not chew, suck, or swallow. Do not eat or drink anything until tablet is completely dissolved. In patients with a dry mouth, water may be used to moisten the buccal mucosa just before administration. All patients must initiate therapy using the 100 mcg tablet.

Prescribing and Access Restrictions As a requirement of the REMS program, access is restricted.

Transmucosal immediate-release fentanyl products (eg, sublingual tablets and spray, oral lozenges, buccal tablets and soluble film, nasal spray) are only available through the Transmucosal Immediate-Release Fentanyl (TIRF) REMS ACCESS program. Enrollment in the program is required for outpatients, prescribers for outpatient use, pharmacies (inpatient and outpatient), and distributors. Enrollment is not required for inpatient administration (eg, hospitals, hospices, long-term care facilities), inpatients, and prescribers who prescribe to inpatients. Further information is available at 1-866-822-1483 or at www.TIRFREMSaccess.com

Note: Effective December, 2011, individual REMs programs for TIRF products were combined into a single access program (TIRF REMS Access). Prescribers and pharmacies that were enrolled in at least one individual REMS program for these products will automatically be transitioned to the single access program.

Medication Guide Available Yes

Dosage Forms Excipient information presented when available (limited, particularly for generics); consult specific product labeling.

Film, for buccal application, as citrate [strength expressed as base]:

Onsolis®: 200 mcg (30s); 400 mcg (30s); 600 mcg (30s); 800 mcg (30s); 1200 mcg (30s)

Injection, solution, as citrate [strength expressed as base, preservative free]: 0.05 mg/mL (2 mL, 5 mL, 10 mL, 20 mL, 50 mL)

Liquid, sublingual, as base [spray]:

Subsys®: 100 mcg (30s); 200 mcg (30s); 400 mcg (30s); 600 mcg (30s); 800 mcg (30s) [contains dehydrated ethanol 63.6%, propylene glycol]

Lozenge, oral, as citrate [strength expressed as base, transmucosal]: 200 mcg (30s); 400 mcg (30s); 600 mcg (30s); 800 mcg (30s); 1200 mcg (30s); 1600 mcg (30s)

Actiq®: 200 mcg (30s); 400 mcg (30s); 600 mcg (30s); 800 mcg (30s); 1200 mcg (30s); 1600 mcg (30s) [contains sugar 2 g/lozenge; berry flavor]

Patch, transdermal, as base: 12 [delivers 12.5 mcg/hr] (5s); 25 [delivers 25 mcg/hr] (5s); 50 [delivers 50 mcg/hr] (5s); 75 [delivers 75 mcg/hr] (5s); 100 [delivers 100 mcg/hr] (5s)

Duragesic®: 12 [delivers 12.5 mcg/hr] (5s) [contains ethanol 0.1mL/10 cm^2; 5 cm^2]

Duragesic®: 25 [delivers 25 mcg/hr] (5s) [contains ethanol 0.1 mL/10 cm^2; 10 cm^2]

Duragesic®: 50 [delivers 50 mcg/hr] (5s) [contains ethanol 0.1 mL/10 cm^2; 20 cm^2]

Duragesic®: 75 [delivers 75 mcg/hr] (5s) [contains ethanol 0.1 mL/10 cm^2; 30 cm^2]

Duragesic®: 100 [delivers 100 mcg/hr] (5s) [contains ethanol 0.1 mL/10 cm^2; 40 cm^2]

Powder, for prescription compounding, as citrate: USP: 100% (1 g)

Solution, intranasal, as citrate [strength expressed as base, spray]:

Lazanda®: 100 mcg/spray (5 mL); 400 mcg/spray (5 mL) [delivers 8 metered sprays]

Tablet, for buccal application, as citrate [strength expressed as base]:

Fentora®: 100 mcg (28s); 200 mcg (28s); 400 mcg (28s); 600 mcg (28s); 800 mcg (28s)

Tablet, sublingual, as citrate [strength expressed as base]:

Abstral®: 100 mcg (12s, 32s); 200 mcg (12s, 32s); 300 mcg (12s, 32s); 400 mcg (12s, 32s); 600 mcg (32s); 800 mcg (32s)

Dosage Forms: Canada Excipient information presented when available (limited, particularly for generics); consult specific product labeling.

Patch, transdermal, as base: 12 mcg/hr (5s); 25 mcg/hr (5s); 50 mcg/hr (5s); 75 mcg/hr (5s); 100 mcg/hr (5s)

Duragesic® MAT: 12 mcg/hr (5s) [contains ethanol 0.1 mL/10 cm^2; 5 cm^2]

Duragesic® MAT: 25 mcg/hr (5s) [contains ethanol 0.1 mL/10 cm^2; 10 cm^2]

Duragesic® MAT: 50 mcg/hr (5s) [contains ethanol 0.1 mL/10 cm^2; 20 cm^2]

Duragesic® MAT: 75 mcg/hr (5s) [contains ethanol 0.1 mL/10 cm^2; 30 cm^2]

Duragesic® MAT: 100 mcg/hr (5s) [contains ethanol 0.1 mL/10 cm^2; 40 cm^2]

Controlled Substance C-II

- **Fentanyl Citrate** *see* FentaNYL *on page 583*
- **Fentanyl Citrate Injection, USP (Can)** *see* FentaNYL *on page 583*
- **Fentanyl Hydrochloride** *see* FentaNYL *on page 583*
- **Fentanyl Patch** *see* FentaNYL *on page 583*
- **Fentora®** *see* FentaNYL *on page 583*
- **Feraheme®** *see* Ferumoxytol *on page 600*

Ferric Gluconate (FER ik GLOO koe nate)

Brand Names: U.S. Ferrlecit®; Nulecit™ [DSC]

Brand Names: Canada Ferrlecit®

Index Terms Sodium Ferric Gluconate

Generic Availability (U.S.) Yes

Pharmacologic Category Iron Salt

Use Treatment of iron-deficiency anemia in patients undergoing hemodialysis in conjunction with erythropoietin therapy

Unlabeled Use Cancer-/chemotherapy-associated anemia

Labeled Contraindications Hypersensitivity to ferric gluconate or any component of the formulation

Pregnancy Risk Factor B

Lactation Excretion in breast milk unknown/use caution

Warnings/Precautions Serious hypersensitivity reactions, including anaphylactoid reactions, have occurred. Monitor during administration and for ≥30 minutes after administration until clinically stable. Avoid rapid administration. Equipment for resuscitation and trained personnel experienced in handling medical emergencies should always be immediately available. Clinically significant hypotension may occur; usually resolves within 1-2 hours. May augment hemodialysis-induced hypotension. Use with caution in elderly patients. Use only in patients with documented iron deficiency; caution with hemoglobinopathies or other refractory anemias. Contains benzyl alcohol which has been associated with "gasping syndrome" in neonates (not indicated for use in this population).

Adverse Reactions Percentages reported in adults unless otherwise noted:

>10%:

- Cardiovascular: Hypotension (children 35%; adults 29%), hypertension (children 23%; adults 13%), tachycardia (children 17%; adults 5%)
- Central nervous system: Headache (children 24%; adults 7%), dizziness (13%)
- Gastrointestinal: Vomiting (adults ≤35%; children 11%), nausea (adults ≤35%; children 9%), diarrhea (adults ≤35%; children 8%)
- Hematologic: Erythrocytes abnormal (11% [changes in morphology, color, or number])
- Local: Injection site reaction (33%)
- Neuromuscular & skeletal: Cramps (25%)
- Respiratory: Dyspnea (11%)

1% to 10%:

- Cardiovascular: Chest pain (10%), syncope (6%), edema (5%), angina pectoris, bradycardia, hypervolemia, MI, peripheral edema, vasodilation
- Central nervous system: Pain (10%), fever (children 9%; adults 5%), fatigue (6%), agitation, chills, consciousness decreased, lightheadedness, malaise, rigors, somnolence
- Dermatologic: Pruritus (6%), rash
- Endocrine & metabolic: Hyperkalemia (6%), hypoglycemia, hypokalemia
- Gastrointestinal: Abdominal pain (children 9%; adults 6%), anorexia, dyspepsia, eructation, flatulence, GI disorder, melena, rectal disorder
- Genitourinary: Menorrhagia, UTI
- Hematologic: Thrombosis (children 6%), anemia, leukocytosis, lymphadenopathy
- Neuromuscular & skeletal: Leg cramps (10%), weakness (7%), paresthesias (6%), arm pain, arthralgia, back pain, leg edema, myalgia
- Ocular: Arcus senilis, conjunctivitis, diplopia, puffy eyelids, redness of eyes, rolling of eyes, watery eyes
- Otic: Deafness
- Respiratory: Pharyngitis (children 9%), cough (6%), rhinitis (children 6%), upper respiratory infections (6%), pneumonia, pulmonary edema
- Miscellaneous: Abscess, carcinoma, diaphoresis, flu-like symptoms, infection, sepsis

Postmarketing and/or case reports: Allergic reaction, anaphylactic reactions, convulsion, dry mouth, dysgeusia, facial flushing, hemorrhage, hypertonia, hypoesthesia, loss of consciousness, nervousness, pallor, phlebitis, shock, skin discoloration

Drug Interactions

Metabolism/Transport Effects None known.

Avoid Concomitant Use

Avoid concomitant use of Ferric Gluconate with any of the following: Dimercaprol

Increased Effect/Toxicity

The levels/effects of Ferric Gluconate may be increased by: ACE Inhibitors; Dimercaprol

Decreased Effect

Ferric Gluconate may decrease the levels/effects of: Cefdinir; Eltrombopag; Levothyroxine; Phosphate Supplements; Trientine

The levels/effects of Ferric Gluconate may be decreased by: Pancrelipase; Trientine

Storage/Stability Store at 20°C to 25°C (68°F to 77°F); do not freeze.

Reconstitution For I.V. infusion, dilute ferric gluconate in 0.9% sodium chloride (children: 25 mL NS, adults: 100 mL NS); use immediately after dilution.

Mechanism of Action Supplies a source to elemental iron necessary to the function of hemoglobin, myoglobin and specific enzyme systems; allows transport of oxygen via hemoglobin

Pharmacodynamics/Kinetics Half-life elimination: Bound iron: 1 hour

Dosing

Adult & Geriatric

Iron-deficiency anemia, hemodialysis patients: I.V.: 125 mg elemental iron per dialysis session. Most patients will require a cumulative dose of 1 g elemental iron over approximately 8 sequential dialysis treatments to achieve a favorable response.

Note: A test dose of 2 mL diluted in NS 50 mL administered over 60 minutes was previously recommended (not in current manufacturer labeling). Doses >125 mg are associated with increased adverse events.

Cancer-/chemotherapy-associated anemia (unlabeled use): I.V. infusion: 125 mg over 1 hour; maximum: 250 mg/infusion. Repeat dose every week for 8 doses. Test doses (25 mg slow I.V. push or infusion) are recommended in patients with iron dextran hypersensitivity or those with other drug allergies (NCCN guidelines, v.2.2010)

Pediatric Iron-deficiency anemia, hemodialysis patients: Children ≥6 years: I.V.: 1.5 mg/kg of elemental iron (maximum: 125 mg/dose) per dialysis session. Doses >1.5 mg/kg are associated with increased adverse events.

Renal Impairment No dosage adjustment necessary.

Hepatic Impairment No dosage adjustment necessary.

Administration I.V.: Iron-deficiency anemia

Children: Dilute dose in NS 25 mL and administer over 1 hour

Adults: Avoid rapid administration. May be diluted prior to administration and administered over 1 hour. If administered undiluted, infuse slowly at a rate of up to 12.5 mg/minute.

Monitoring Parameters Hemoglobin and hematocrit, serum ferritin, iron saturation; vital signs; signs and symptoms of hypersensitivity (monitor for ≥30 minutes following the end of administration and until clinically stable)

NKF K/DOQI guidelines recommend that iron status should be monitored monthly during initiation through the percent transferrin saturation (TSAT) and serum ferritin.

Test Interactions Serum or transferrin bound iron levels may be falsely elevated if assessed within 24 hours of ferric gluconate administration. Serum ferritin levels may be falsely elevated for 5 days after ferric gluconate administration.

Dosage Forms Excipient information presented when available (limited, particularly for generics); consult specific product labeling. [DSC] = Discontinued product

Injection, solution: Elemental iron 12.5 mg/mL (5 mL)

Ferrlecit®: Elemental iron 12.5 mg/mL (5 mL) [contains benzyl alcohol, sucrose 20%]

Nulecit™: Elemental iron 12.5 mg/mL (5 mL [DSC]) [contains benzyl alcohol, sucrose ~20%]

References

National Comprehensive Cancer Network® (NCCN), "Practice Guidelines in Oncology™: Cancer- and Chemotherapy-Induced Anemia Version 2.2010." Available at http://www.nccn.org/professionals/physician_gls/PDF/anemia.pdf

National Kidney Foundation, "KDOQI Clinical Practice Guidelines and Clinical Practice Recommendations for Anemia in Chronic Kidney Disease," *Am J Kidney Dis*, 2007, 50(3):529-30. Available at http://www.kidney.org/professionals/KDOQI/guidelines_anemiaUP/index.htm or http://www.kidney.org/professionals/KDOQI

◆ **Ferriprox®** *see* Deferiprone *on page* 412

◆ **Ferriprox®** *see* Deferiprone *on page* 412

◆ **Ferrlecit®** *see* Ferric Gluconate *on page* 597

Ferumoxytol (fer ue MOX i tol)

Brand Names: U.S. Feraheme®

Brand Names: Canada Feraheme®

Generic Availability (U.S.) No

Pharmacologic Category Iron Salt

Use Treatment of iron-deficiency anemia in chronic kidney disease

Labeled Contraindications Hypersensitivity to ferumoxytol or any component of the formulation

Canadian labeling: Additional contraindications (not in U.S. labeling): Evidence of iron overload; anemia not caused by iron deficiency

Pregnancy Risk Factor C

Lactation Excretion in breast milk unknown/not recommended

Warnings/Precautions Serious hypersensitivity reactions, including rare anaphylactic and anaphylactoid reactions, may occur, presenting with cardiac/cardiorespiratory arrest, clinically significant hypotension, syncope, or unresponsiveness; equipment for resuscitation and trained personnel experienced in handling emergencies should be immediately available during use. Monitor patients for signs/symptoms of hypersensitivity reactions for ≥30 minutes and until clinically stable following administration.

Do not administer in the presence of tissue iron overload; periodic monitoring of hemoglobin, serum ferritin, serum iron, and transferrin saturation is recommended. Serum iron and transferrin-bound iron may be overestimated in laboratory assays if level is drawn during the first 24 hours following administration. Administration may alter magnetic resonance (MR) imaging; conduct anticipated MRI studies prior to use. MR imaging alterations may persist for ≤3 months following use, with peak alterations anticipated in the first 2 days following administration. If MR imaging is required within 3 months after administration, use T1- or proton density-weighted MR pulse sequences to decrease effect on imagining. Do not use T2-weighted sequence MR imaging prior to 4 weeks following ferumoxytol administration. Ferumoxytol does not interfere with X-ray, computed tomography (CT), positron emission tomography (PET), single photon emission computed tomography (SPECT), ultrasound or nuclear medicine imaging.

Adverse Reactions

1% to 10%:

Cardiovascular: Hypotension (≤3%), edema (2%), peripheral edema (2%), chest pain (1%), hypertension (1%)

Central nervous system: Dizziness (3%), headache (2%), fever (1%)

Dermatologic: Pruritus (1%), rash (1%)

Gastrointestinal: Diarrhea (4%), nausea (3%), constipation (2%), vomiting (2%), abdominal pain (1%)

Neuromuscular & skeletal: Back pain (1%), muscle spasms (1%)

Respiratory: Cough (1%), dyspnea (1%)

Miscellaneous: Hypersensitivity reactions (≤4%; serious reactions: <1%)

<1%, postmarketing, and/or case reports: Anaphylactic/anaphylactoid reactions, angioedema, cardiac/cardiorespiratory arrest, cardiac rhythm abnormalities, congestive heart failure, cyanosis, fatigue, hypotension (clinically significant); infusion site reactions (including bruising, burning, erythema, irritation, pain, swelling, warmth); ischemic myocardial events, loss of consciousness, pulse absent, syncope, tachycardia, unresponsiveness, urticaria, wheezing

Drug Interactions

Metabolism/Transport Effects None known.

Avoid Concomitant Use

Avoid concomitant use of Ferumoxytol with any of the following: Dimercaprol

Increased Effect/Toxicity

The levels/effects of Ferumoxytol may be increased by: Dimercaprol

Decreased Effect There are no known significant interactions involving a decrease in effect.

Storage/Stability Store vials at controlled room temperature of 20°C to 25°C (68°F to 77°F); excursions permitted to 15°C to 30°C (59°F to 86°F). Do not freeze.

Mechanism of Action Superparamagnetic iron oxide coated with a low molecular weight semisynthetic carbohydrate; Iron-carbohydrate complex enters the reticuloendothelial system macrophages of the liver, spleen, and bone marrow where the iron is released from the complex. The released iron is either transported into storage pools or is transported via plasma transferrin for incorporation into hemoglobin.

Pharmacodynamics/Kinetics

Distribution: V_d: 3.16 L

Metabolism: Iron released from iron-carbohydrate complex after uptake in the reticuloendothelial system macrophages of the liver, spleen, and bone marrow

Half-life elimination: ~15 hours

Dialysis: Ferumoxytol is not removed by hemodialysis

Dosing

Adult & Geriatric Doses expressed in mg of **elemental** iron. **Note:** Test dose: Product labeling does not indicate need for a test dose.

Iron-deficiency anemia in chronic kidney disease: I.V.: 510 mg (17 mL) as a single dose, followed by a second 510 mg dose 3-8 days (U.S. labeling) or 2-8 days (Canadian labeling) after initial dose. Assess response at least 30 days following the second dose. U.S. manufacturer labeling states the recommended dose may be readministered in patients with persistent or recurrent iron-deficiency anemia.

Renal Impairment No dosage adjustment necessary.

Hepatic Impairment No dosage adjustment provided in manufacturer's labeling.

Administration Administer intravenously as an undiluted injection at a rate ≤1 mL/second (30 mg of elemental iron/second). Do not administer if solution has particulate matter or is discolored (solution is black to reddish-brown). Hemodialysis patients should receive injection after at least 1 hour of hemodialysis has been completed and once blood pressure has stabilized.

Monitoring Parameters Hemoglobin, serum ferritin, serum iron, transferrin saturation (for at least 1 month following second injection and periodically); signs/symptoms of hypotension following administration; signs/symptoms of hypersensitivity reactions (≥30 minutes following administration)

Test Interactions May interfere with MR imaging; alterations may persist for ≤3 months following use, with peak alterations anticipated in the first 2 days following administration. If MR imaging is required within 3 months after administration, use T1- or proton density-weighted MR pulse sequences to decrease effect on imaging. Do not use T2-weighted sequence MR imaging prior to 4 weeks following administration.

Serum iron and transferrin-bound iron may be overestimated in laboratory assays if level is drawn during the first 24 hours following administration (due to contribution of iron in ferumoxytol).

Dosage Forms Excipient information presented when available (limited, particularly for generics); consult specific product labeling.

Injection, solution:

Feraheme®: Elemental iron 30 mg/mL (17 mL)

References

Singh A, Patel T, Hertel J, et al, "Safety of Ferumoxytol in Patients With Anemia and CKD", *Am J of Kidney Dis*, 2008, 52(5):907-15.

Fibrinogen Concentrate (Human)

(fi BRIN o gin KON suhn trate HYU man)

Brand Names: U.S. RiaSTAP®

Index Terms Coagulation Factor I

Generic Availability (U.S.) No

Pharmacologic Category Blood Product Derivative

Use Treatment of acute bleeding episodes in patients with congenital fibrinogen deficiency (afibrinogenemia and hypofibrinogenemia)

Labeled Contraindications Severe hypersensitivity reactions to fibrinogen concentrate or any component of the formulation

Pregnancy Risk Factor C

Warnings/Precautions Hypersensitivity reactions (eg, urticaria, hives, wheezing, hypotension, anaphylaxis) may occur. In the event of hypersensitivity reactions, treatment should be discontinued immediately. Thrombosis may occur in patients with congenital fibrinogen deficiency with or without fibrinogen replacement therapy. Consider potential risk of thrombosis with use. Product of human plasma; may potentially contain infectious agents which could transmit disease. Screening of donors, as well as testing and/or inactivation or removal of certain viruses, reduces the risk. Infections thought to be transmitted by this product should be reported to the manufacturer. Not for the treatment of dysfibrinogenemia.

Adverse Reactions

>1%: Central nervous system: Fever, headache

Postmarketing and/or case reports: Allergic reactions, anaphylaxis, arterial thrombosis, chills, DVT, dyspnea, MI, nausea, pulmonary embolism, rash, thromboembolism, vomiting

Drug Interactions

Metabolism/Transport Effects None known.

Avoid Concomitant Use There are no known interactions where it is recommended to avoid concomitant use.

Increased Effect/Toxicity

Fibrinogen Concentrate (Human) may increase the levels/effects of: Antifibrinolytic Agents

The levels/effects of Fibrinogen Concentrate (Human) may be increased by: Antifibrinolytic Agents

Decreased Effect There are no known significant interactions involving a decrease in effect.

Storage/Stability Store at 2°C to 25°C (36°F to 77°F) in original carton; do not freeze. Protect from light. Stable for 24 hours after reconstitution when stored at 20°C to 25°C (68°F to 77°F). Discard partially used vials.

Reconstitution Transfer sterile water for injection 50 mL into vial. Gently swirl until dissolved; do not shake.

Mechanism of Action Fibrinogen (coagulation factor I), a protein found in normal plasma, is required to clot blood. Fibrinogen concentrate made from pooled human plasma replaces this protein which is missing or reduced in patients with a congenital fibrinogen deficiency.

Pharmacodynamics/Kinetics

Distribution: V_d: 45-60 mL/kg (range 36-68 mL/kg)

Half-life elimination: 61-97 hours (range 56-117 hours); may be decreased in children <16 years of age

Dosing

Adult & Geriatric Congenital fibrinogen deficiency: I.V.: **Note:** Adjust dose based on laboratory values and condition of patient. Maintain a target fibrinogen level of 100 mg/dL until hemostasis is achieved.

When baseline fibrinogen level is known:

Dose (mg/kg) = [Target level (mg/dL) - measured level (mg/dL)] **divided by** 1.7 (mg/dL per mg/kg body weight)

When baseline fibrinogen level is not known: 70 mg/kg

Pediatric Congenital fibrinogen deficiency: I.V.: Refer to adult dosing.

Administration For I.V. administration only; infuse at ≤5 mL/minute

Monitoring Parameters Signs and symptoms of hypersensitivity, thrombosis; fibrinogen level

Dosage Forms Excipient information presented when available (limited, particularly for generics); consult specific product labeling. [DSC] = Discontinued product

Injection, powder for reconstitution:

RiaSTAP®: 900-1300 mg [contains albumin (human); exact potency labeled on vial]

References

Acharya SS and Dimichele DM, "Rare Inherited Disorders of Fibrinogen," *Haemophilia*, 2008, 14 (6):1151-8.

Kreuz W, Meili E, Peter-Salonen K, et al. "Efficacy and Tolerability of a Pasteurised Human Fibrinogen Concentrate in Patients With Congenital Fibrinogen Deficiency," *Transfus Apher Sci*, 2005, 32(3):247-53.

Filgrastim (fil GRA stim)

Related Information

Hematopoietic Stem Cell Transplantation *on page 1887*

Brand Names: U.S. Neupogen®

Brand Names: Canada Neupogen®

Index Terms G-CSF; Granulocyte Colony Stimulating Factor

Generic Availability (U.S.) No

Pharmacologic Category Colony Stimulating Factor

Use

Cancer patients (nonmyeloid malignancies) receiving myelosuppressive chemotherapy to decrease the incidence of infection (febrile neutropenia) in regimens associated with a high incidence of neutropenia with fever

Acute myelogenous leukemia (AML) following induction or consolidation chemotherapy to shorten time to neutrophil recovery and reduce the duration of fever

Cancer patients (nonmyeloid malignancies) receiving bone marrow transplant to shorten the duration of neutropenia and neutropenia-related events (eg, neutropenic fever)

Peripheral stem cell transplantation to mobilize hematopoietic progenitor cells for apheresis collection

Severe chronic neutropenia (SCN; chronic administration) to reduce the incidence and duration of neutropenic complications (fever, infections, oropharyngeal ulcers) in symptomatic patients with congenital, cyclic, or idiopathic neutropenia

Unlabeled Use Treatment of anemia in myelodysplastic syndrome (in combination with epoetin); mobilization of hematopoietic stem cells (HSC) for collection and subsequent autologous transplantation (in combination with plerixafor) in patients with non-Hodgkin's lymphoma (NHL) and multiple myeloma (MM); treatment of neutropenia in HIV-infected patients receiving zidovudine; hepatitis C treatment-associated neutropenia

Labeled Contraindications Hypersensitivity to filgrastim, *E. coli*-derived proteins, or any component of the formulation

Pregnancy Risk Factor C

Lactation Excretion in breast milk unknown/use caution

Warnings/Precautions Do not use filgrastim in the period 24 hours before to 24 hours after administration of cytotoxic chemotherapy because of the potential sensitivity of rapidly dividing myeloid cells to cytotoxic chemotherapy. May potentially act as a growth factor for any tumor type, particularly myeloid malignancies; caution should be exercised in the usage of filgrastim in any malignancy with myeloid characteristics. Increases circulating leukocytes when used in conjunction with plerixafor for stem cell mobilization; monitor WBC; use with caution in patients with neutrophil count >50,000/mm^3; tumor cells released from marrow could be collected in leukapheresis product; potential effect of tumor cell reinfusion is unknown. Reports of alveolar hemorrhage, manifested as pulmonary infiltrates and hemoptysis, have occurred in healthy donors undergoing PBPC collection (not FDA approved for use in healthy donors); hemoptysis resolved upon discontinuation. Safety and efficacy have not been established with patients receiving radiation therapy (avoid concurrent radiation therapy with filgrastim), or chemotherapy associated with delayed myelosuppression (eg, nitrosoureas, mitomycin).

Allergic-type reactions (rash, urticaria, facial edema, wheezing, dyspnea, tachycardia, and/or hypotension) have occurred with first or subsequent doses. Reactions tended to involve ≥2 body systems and occur more frequently with intravenous administration and generally within 30 minutes of administration; may recur with rechallenge. Rare cases of acute respiratory distress syndrome (ARDS) have been reported (possibly due to influx of neutrophils to sites of lung inflammation); withhold or discontinue filgrastim if ARDS occurs; patients must be instructed to report respiratory distress; monitor for fever, infiltrates, or respiratory distress. Rare cases of splenic rupture have been reported (may be fatal); patients must be instructed to report left upper quadrant pain or shoulder tip pain. Cutaneous vasculitis has been reported, generally occurring in severe chronic neutropenia (SCN) patients on long-term therapy; symptoms generally developed with increasing absolute neutrophil count (ANC) and subsided when the ANC decreased; dose reductions may improve symptoms to allow for continued therapy. Use caution in patients with sickle cell disorders; severe sickle cell crises (sometimes resulting in fatalities) have been reported following filgrastim therapy. Filgrastim use prior to appropriate diagnosis of SCN may impair proper evaluation and treatment for neutropenia not due to SCN. Cytogenetic abnormalities, transformation to myelodysplastic syndrome (MDS) and acute myeloid leukemia (AML) have been observed in patients treated with filgrastim for congenital neutropenia; a longer duration of treatment and poorer ANC response appear to increase the risk. Carefully consider the risk of continuing filgrastim in patients who develop abnormal cytogenetics or MDS. The packaging of some forms may contain latex.

Adverse Reactions

>10%:

Central nervous system: Fever (12%)

Dermatologic: Petechiae (≤17%), rash (≤12%)

Endocrine & metabolic: LDH increased, uric acid increased

Gastrointestinal: Splenomegaly (severe chronic neutropenia: 30%; rare in other patients)

Hepatic: Alkaline phosphatase increased (21%)

Neuromuscular & skeletal: Bone/skeletal pain (22% to 33%; dose related), commonly in the lower back, posterior iliac crest, and sternum

Respiratory: Epistaxis (9% to 15%)

1% to 10%:

Cardiovascular: Hyper-/hypotension (4%), myocardial infarction/arrhythmias (3%)

Central nervous system: Headache (7%)

Gastrointestinal: Nausea (10%), vomiting (7%), peritonitis (≤2%)

Hematologic: Leukocytosis (2%)

Miscellaneous: Transfusion reaction (≤10%)

<1%, postmarketing, and/or case reports: Acute respiratory distress syndrome (ARDS), allergic reactions, alopecia, alveolar hemorrhage, arthralgia, bone density decreased, capillary leak syndrome, cerebral hemorrhage, cutaneous vasculitis, dyspnea, edema (facial), erythema nodosum, hematuria, hemoptysis, hepatomegaly, hypersensitivity reaction, injection site reaction, osteoporosis, pericarditis, proteinuria, psoriasis exacerbation, pulmonary infiltrates, renal insufficiency, sickle cell crisis, splenic rupture, Sweet's syndrome (acute febrile dermatosis), tachycardia, thrombocytopenia (in PBPC mobilization), thrombophlebitis, transient supraventricular arrhythmia, urticaria, wheezing

Drug Interactions

Metabolism/Transport Effects None known.

Avoid Concomitant Use There are no known interactions where it is recommended to avoid concomitant use.

Increased Effect/Toxicity

Filgrastim may increase the levels/effects of: Bleomycin; Topotecan

Decreased Effect There are no known significant interactions involving a decrease in effect.

Storage/Stability Intact vials and prefilled syringes should be stored under refrigeration at 2°C to 8°C (36°F to 46°F) and protected from direct sunlight. Filgrastim should be protected from freezing and temperatures >30°C to avoid aggregation.

Filgrastim vials and prefilled syringes are stable for 24 hours at 9°C to 30°C (47°F to 86°F).

Undiluted filgrastim is stable for 24 hours at 15°C to 30°C (59°F to 86°F) and for up to 14 days at 2°C to 8°C (36°F to 46°F) (data on file, Amgen Medical Information) in BD tuberculin syringes; however, sterility has only been assessed and maintained for up to 7 days when prepared under strict aseptic conditions (Jacobson, 1996; Singh, 1994). The manufacturer recommends using syringes within 24 hours due to the potential for bacterial contamination.

Filgrastim diluted with D_5W for I.V. infusion (5-15 mcg/mL) is stable for 7 days at 2°C to 8°C (36°F to 46°F), however, should be used within 24 hours due to the possibility for bacterial contamination.

Reconstitution Do not dilute with saline at any time; product may precipitate. Filgrastim may be diluted with D_5W to a concentration of 5-15 mcg/mL for I.V. infusion administration (minimum concentration: 5 mcg/mL). Concentrations 5-15 mcg/mL require addition of albumin (final albumin concentration of 2 mg/mL) to prevent adsorption to plastics. Dilution to <5 mcg/mL is not recommended. Do not shake.

Mechanism of Action Stimulates the production, maturation, and activation of neutrophils; filgrastim activates neutrophils to increase both their migration and cytotoxicity.

Pharmacodynamics/Kinetics

Onset of action: ~24 hours; plateaus in 3-5 days

Duration: Neutrophil counts generally return to baseline within 4 days

Absorption: SubQ: 100%

Distribution: V_d: 150 mL/kg; no evidence of drug accumulation over a 11- to 20-day period

Metabolism: Systemically degraded

Half-life elimination: 1.8-3.5 hours

Time to peak, serum: SubQ: 2-8 hours

Dosing

Adult & Geriatric Details concerning dosing in combination regimens and institution protocols should also be consulted. Rounding doses to the nearest vial size may enhance patient convenience and reduce costs without compromising clinical response.

Chemotherapy-induced neutropenia SubQ, I.V.: 5 mcg/kg/day; doses may be increased by 5 mcg/kg (for each chemotherapy cycle) according to the duration and severity of the neutropenia; continue for up to 14 days or until the ANC reaches 10,000/mm^3

Bone marrow transplantation (in patients with cancer; to shorten the duration of neutropenia and neutropenia-related events): SubQ, I.V.: 10 mcg/kg/day (administer ≥24 hours after chemotherapy and ≥24 hours after bone marrow infusion); adjust the dose according to the duration and severity of neutropenia; recommended steps based on neutrophil response:

When ANC >1000/mm^3 for 3 consecutive days: Reduce filgrastim dose to 5 mcg/kg/day

If ANC remains >1000/mm^3 for 3 more consecutive days: Discontinue filgrastim

If ANC decreases to <1000/mm^3: Resume at 5 mcg/kg/day.

If ANC decreases to <1000/mm^3 during the 5 mcg/kg/day dose: Increase filgrastim to 10 mcg/kg/day and follow the above steps.

Peripheral blood progenitor cell (PBPC) collection: SubQ: 10 mcg/kg daily, usually for 6-7 days. Begin at least 4 days before the first apheresis and continue until the last apheresis; consider dose adjustment for WBC >100,000/mm^3

Severe chronic neutropenia: SubQ:

Congenital: Initial: 6 mcg/kg twice daily; adjust the dose based on ANC and clinical response

Idiopathic/cyclic: Initial: 5 mcg/kg/day; adjust the dose based on ANC and clinical response

Anemia in myelodysplastic syndrome (unlabeled use; in combination with epoetin): SubQ: 30 mcg, 75 mcg, or 150 mcg once daily (Hellstrom-Lindberg, 1998) **or** 1 mcg/kg once daily (Greenberg, 2009) **or** 75 mcg, 150 mcg or 300 mcg/dose 3 times/week (Hellstrom-Lindberg, 2003) **or** 1-2 mcg/kg/dose 1-3 times/week (NCCN MDS guidelines v.2.2011)

Hematopoietic stem cell mobilization in autologous transplantation in patients with non-Hodgkin's lymphoma or multiple myeloma (in combination with plerixafor; unlabeled use): SubQ: 10 mcg/kg once daily; begin 4 days before initiation of plerixafor; continue G-CSF on each day prior to apheresis for up to 8 days (DiPersio, *JCO* 2009; DiPersio, *Blood* 2009)

Hepatitis C treatment-associated neutropenia (unlabeled use): SubQ: 150 mcg once weekly to 300 mcg 3 times/week; titrate to maintain ANC between 750-10,000/mm^3 (Younossi, 2008)

Pediatric Details concerning dosing in combination regimens and institution protocols should also be consulted.

Chemotherapy induced neutropenia, bone marrow transplantation, peripheral blood progenitor cell collection, severe chronic neutropenia: Refer to adult dosing.

Neutropenia (ANC <500/mm^3) due to zidovudine treatment for HIV-infection (unlabeled use): SubQ, I.V.: 5-10 mcg/kg once daily (AIDS*info* guidelines, 2010)

Combination Regimens

Breast cancer: AC/Paclitaxel (Sequential) on page 1517
Esophageal cancer: Paclitaxel-Cisplatin (Esophageal Cancer) on page 1727
Leukemia, acute lymphocytic: Larson Regimen (ALL) on page 1699
Leukemia, acute myeloid:
CLAG (AML Induction) on page 1586
CLAG-M (AML Induction) on page 1586
FLAG (AML Induction) on page 1643
FLAG-IDA on page 1644
MEC-G (AML Induction) on page 1707
Lymphoma, Hodgkin:
BEACOPP-14 (Hodgkin) on page 1522
BEACOPP Escalated (Hodgkin) on page 1522
BEACOPP Escalated Plus Standard (Hodgkin) on page 1523
DHAP (Hodgkin) on page 1608
ESHAP (Hodgkin) on page 1634
ICE (Hodgkin) on page 1688
IGEV (Hodgkin) on page 1690
Lymphoma, non-Hodgkin's:
CHOP (NHL) on page 1564
CODOX-M on page 1590
EPOCH Dose-Adjusted (AIDS-Related Lymphoma) on page 1628
EPOCH Dose-Adjusted (NHL) on page 1628
EPOCH (Dose-Adjusted)-Rituximab (NHL) on page 1629
ICE (Lymphoma, non-Hodgkin's) on page 1689
RICE on page 1747
Rituximab-CHOP (NHL) on page 1748
Lymphoma, non-Hodgkin's (Burkitt): CODOX-M/IVAC on page 1591
Soft tissue sarcoma: AI on page 1520
Unknown primary, adenocarcinoma Carboplatin-Paclitaxel (Unknown Primary) on page 1551
Wilms' tumor: Regimen I (Wilms' Tumor) on page 1745

Administration May be administered by SubQ injection, either as a bolus injection (chemotherapy-induced neutropenia) or as a continuous infusion (chemotherapy-induced neutropenia, bone marrow transplantation, and peripheral blood progenitor cell collection). May also be administered I.V. as a short infusion over 15-30 minutes (chemotherapy-induced neutropenia) or by continuous infusion (chemotherapy-induced neutropenia) or as a 4- or 24-hour infusion (bone marrow transplantation). Do not administer earlier than 24 hours after or in the 24 hours prior to cytotoxic chemotherapy.

Monitoring Parameters CBC with differential and platelets prior to treatment and twice weekly during filgrastim treatment for chemotherapy-induced neutropenia (3 times/week following marrow transplantation). For severe chronic neutropenia, monitor CBC with differential and platelets twice weekly during the first month of therapy and for 2 weeks following dose adjustments; once clinically stable, monthly for 1 year and quarterly thereafter; for congenital neutropenia also monitor bone marrow and karyotype prior to treatment; and monitor marrow and cytogenetics annually throughout treatment. Monitor temperature.

Test Interactions May interfere with bone imaging studies; increased hematopoietic activity of the bone marrow may appear as transient positive bone imaging changes

Dietary Considerations Some products may contain sodium.

Product Availability

Tbo-filgrastim: FDA approved August 2012; availability anticipated November 2013.

Tbo-filgrastim is a short-acting recombinant form of G-CSF (biologically similar to Neupogen®), indicated to reduce the duration of severe neutropenia in patients with nonmyeloid malignancies.

Dosage Forms Excipient information presented when available (limited, particularly for generics); consult specific product labeling.

Injection, solution [preservative free]:

Neupogen®: 300 mcg/mL (1 mL, 1.6 mL) [contains polysorbate 80, sodium 0.035 mg/mL, sorbitol; vial]

Neupogen®: 600 mcg/mL (0.5 mL, 0.8 mL) [contains natural rubber/natural latex in packaging, polysorbate 80, sodium 0.035 mg/mL, sorbitol; prefilled syringe]

References

Calandra G, McCarty J, McGuirk J, et al, "AMD3100 Plus G-CSF Can Successfully Mobilize CD34+ Cells From Non-Hodgkin's Lymphoma, Hodgkin's Disease and Multiple Myeloma Patients Previously Failing Mobilization With Chemotherapy and/or Cytokine Treatment: Compassionate Use Data," *Bone Marrow Transplant*, 2008, 41(4):331-8.

DiPersio JF, Micallef I, Stiff PJ, et al, "Phase III Prospective Randomized Double-Blinded Placebo-Controlled Trial of Plerixafor Plus Granulocyte Colony-Stimulating Factor Compared With Placebo Plus Granulocyte Stimulating Factor for Autologous Stem-Cell Mobilization and Transplantation for Patients With Non-Hodgkin's Lymphoma," *J Clin Oncol*, 2009, 27(28):4767-73.

DiPersio JF, Stadtmauer EA, Nadamanee NP, et al, "Plerixafor and G-CSF Versus Placebo and G-CSF to Moboilize Hematopoietic Stem Cells for Autologous Stem Cell Transplantation in Patients With Multiple Myeloma," *Blood*, 2009, 113(23):5720-6.

Ghany MG, Strader DB, Thomas DL, et al, "Diagnosis, Management and Treatment of Hepatitis C: An Update," *Hepatology*, 2009, 49(4):1335-74.

Greenberg PL, Sun Z, Miller KB, et al, "Treatment of Myelodysplastic Syndrome Patients With Erythropoietin With or Without Granulocyte Colony-Stimulating Factor: Results of a Prospective Randomized Phase 3 Trial by the Eastern Cooperative Oncology Group (E1996)," *Blood*, 2009, 114(12):2393-400.

"Guidelines for the Use of Antiretroviral Agents in Pediatric HIV Infection, Panel on Antiretroviral Therapy and Medical Management of HIV-Infected Children," August 16, 2010. Available at http://www.aidsinfo.nih.gov

Hellström-Lindberg E, Ahlgren T, Beguin Y, et al, "Treatment of Anemia in Myelodysplastic Syndromes With Granulocyte Colony-Stimulating Factor Plus Erythropoietin: Results from a Randomized Phase II Study and Long-Term Follow-Up of 71 Patients," *Blood*, 1998, 92(1):68-75.

Hellström-Lindberg E, Gulbrandsen N, Lindberg G, et al, "A Validated Decision Model for Treating the Anaemia of Myelodysplastic Syndromes With Erythropoietin + Granulocyte Colony-Stimulating Factor: Significant Effects on Quality of Life," *Br J Haematol*, 2003, 120(6):1037-46.

National Comprehensive Cancer Network® (NCCN), "Clinical Practice Guidelines in Oncology™: Myelodysplastic Syndromes," Version 2.2011. Available at http://www.nccn.org/professionals/physician_gls/PDF/mds.pdf

National Comprehensive Cancer Network® (NCCN), "Clinical Practice Guidelines in Oncology™: Myeloid Growth Factors," Version 1.2011. Available at http://www.nccn.org/professionals/physician_gls/PDF/myeloid_growth.pdf

Smith TJ, Khatcheressian J, Lyman GH, et al, "2006 Update of Recommendations for the Use of White Blood Cell Growth Factors: An Evidence-Based Clinical Practice Guideline," *J Clin Oncol*, 2006, 24(19):3187-205.

Younossi ZM, Nader FH, Bai C, et al, "A Phase II Dose Finding Study of Darbepoetin Alpha and Filgrastim for the Management of Anaemia and Neutropenia in Chronic Hepatitis C Ttreatment," *J Viral Hepat*, 2008, 15(5):370-8.

◆ **Firmagon®** *see* Degarelix *on page* 422

◆ **FK228** *see* RomiDEPsin *on page* 1254

◆ **FK506** *see* Tacrolimus (Systemic) *on page* 1315

◆ **Flagyl®** *see* MetroNIDAZOLE (Systemic) *on page* 978

◆ **Flagyl® 375** *see* MetroNIDAZOLE (Systemic) *on page* 978

◆ **Flagyl® ER** *see* MetroNIDAZOLE (Systemic) *on page* 978

◆ **Flebogamma® DIF** *see* Immune Globulin *on page* 777

◆ **Flo-Pred™** *see* PrednisoLONE (Systemic) *on page* 1193

◆ **Florazole® ER (Can)** *see* MetroNIDAZOLE (Systemic) *on page* 978

Floxuridine (floks YOOR i deen)

Related Information

Management of Drug Extravasations *on page* 1800

Safe Handling of Hazardous Drugs *on page* 1904

Brand Names: Canada FUDR®

Index Terms Fluorodeoxyuridine; FUDR

Generic Availability (U.S.) Yes

Pharmacologic Category Antineoplastic Agent, Antimetabolite (Pyrimidine Analog)

Use Management of hepatic metastases of colorectal and gastric cancers

Labeled Contraindications Poor nutritional states, depressed bone marrow function, potentially serious infections

Pregnancy Risk Factor D

Lactation Excretion in breast milk unknown/not recommended

Warnings/Precautions Hazardous agent - use appropriate precautions for handling and disposal. Use caution with impaired kidney or liver function. Discontinue if intractable vomiting, diarrhea, precipitous fall in leukocyte or platelet counts, myocardial ischemia, hemorrhage, gastrointestinal ulcer, or stomatitis occur. Use with caution in patients with poor nutritional status; depressed (leukocyte count <5000/mm^3 or platelet count <100,000/mm^3) bone marrow function; potentially serious infections. Use with caution in patients who have had high-dose pelvic radiation or previous use of alkylating agents. **[U.S. Boxed Warnings]: Should be administered under the supervision of an experienced cancer chemotherapy physician. Patients should be hospitalized for initiation of the first course of therapy due to the risk for severe toxic reactions.**

Adverse Reactions

>10%:

Gastrointestinal: Stomatitis, diarrhea; may be dose limiting

Hematologic: Myelosuppression, may be dose limiting; leukopenia, thrombocytopenia, anemia

Onset: 4-7 days

Nadir: 5-9 days

Recovery: 21 days

1% to 10%:

Dermatologic: Alopecia, photosensitivity, hyperpigmentation of the skin, localized erythema, dermatitis

Gastrointestinal: Anorexia

Hepatic: Biliary sclerosis, cholecystitis, jaundice

<1%: Nausea, vomiting, intrahepatic abscess

Drug Interactions

Metabolism/Transport Effects Inhibits CYP2C9 (strong)

Avoid Concomitant Use

Avoid concomitant use of Floxuridine with any of the following: BCG; CloZAPine; Natalizumab; Pimecrolimus; Tacrolimus (Topical); Vaccines (Live)

Increased Effect/Toxicity

Floxuridine may increase the levels/effects of: Carvedilol; CloZAPine; CYP2C9 Substrates; Diclofenac (Systemic); Fosphenytoin; Leflunomide; Natalizumab; Phenytoin; Vaccines (Live); Vitamin K Antagonists

The levels/effects of Floxuridine may be increased by: Denosumab; Pimecrolimus; Roflumilast; Tacrolimus (Topical); Trastuzumab

Decreased Effect

Floxuridine may decrease the levels/effects of: BCG; Cardiac Glycosides; Coccidioidin Skin Test; Sipuleucel-T; Vaccines (Inactivated); Vaccines (Live); Vitamin K Antagonists

The levels/effects of Floxuridine may be decreased by: Echinacea

Ethanol/Nutrition/Herb Interactions Ethanol: Avoid ethanol (due to GI irritation).

Storage/Stability Store intact vials at room temperature of 15°C to 30°C (59°F to 86°F). Reconstituted vials are stable for up to 2 weeks under refrigeration at 2°C to 8°C (36°F to 46°F). Further dilution in 500-1000 mL D_5W or NS is stable for 2 weeks at room temperature. Solutions in 0.9% sodium chloride are stable in some ambulatory infusion pumps for up to 21 days.

Reconstitution Reconstitute with 5 mL SWFI for a final concentration of 100 mg/mL. Further dilute in 500-1000 mL D_5W or NS for I.V. infusion.

Mechanism of Action Mechanism of action and pharmacokinetics are very similar to fluorouracil; floxuridine is the deoxyribonucleotide of fluorouracil. Floxuridine is a fluorinated pyrimidine antagonist which inhibits DNA and RNA synthesis and methylation of deoxyuridylic acid to thymidylic acid.

Pharmacodynamics/Kinetics

Metabolism: Hepatic; Active metabolites: Floxuridine monophosphate (FUDR-MP) and fluorouracil; Inactive metabolites: Urea, CO_2, α-fluoro-β-alanine, α-fluoro-β-guanidopropionic acid, α-fluoro-β-ureidopropionic acid, and dihydrofluorouracil

Excretion: Urine: Fluorouracil, urea, α-fluoro β-alanine, α-fluoro-β-guanidopropionic acid, α-fluoro-β-ureidopropionic acid, and dihydrofluorouracil; exhaled gases (CO_2)

Dosing

Adult Refer to individual protocols.

Colorectal or gastric metastases:

Intra-arterial: Primarily by an implantable pump: 0.1-0.6 mg/kg/day continuous intra-arterial administration for 14 days then heparinized saline is given for 14 days; toxicity requires dose reduction.

I.V. (unlabeled use): Many regimens in use, examples:

0.15 mg/kg/day for 7-14 days

0.5-1 mg/kg/day for 6-15 days

30 mg/kg/day for 5 days, then 15 mg/kg/day every other day, up to 11 days

Geriatric Adjust dose since elderly patients are prone to toxicity.

Renal Impairment The FDA-approved labeling does not contain dosing adjustment guidelines; use with extreme caution.

Hepatic Impairment The FDA-approved labeling does not contain dosing adjustment guidelines; use with extreme caution. The following guidelines have been used by some clinicians (Floyd, 2006):

Serum bilirubin 1.2 times ULN or alkaline phosphatase 1.2 times ULN: Administer 80% of dose

Serum bilirubin 1.5 times ULN; transaminases 3 times baseline or alkaline phosphatase 1.5 times ULN: Administer 50% of dose

Serum bilirubin 2 times ULN; transaminases >3 times baseline or alkaline phosphatase 2 times ULN: No recommendation is available

Administration Continuous intra-arterial or I.V. infusion (unlabeled use)

Vesicant/Extravasation Risk May be an irritant

Monitoring Parameters CBC, platelet count, liver function

Dosage Forms Excipient information presented when available (limited, particularly for generics); consult specific product labeling.

Injection, powder for reconstitution: 500 mg

References

Davidson BS, Izzo F, Chase JL, et al, "Alternating Floxuridine and 5-Fluorouracil Hepatic Arterial Chemotherapy for Colorectal Liver Metastases Minimizes Biliary Toxicity," *Am J Surg*, 1996, 172 (3):244-7.

de Takats PG, Kerr DJ, Poole CJ, et al, "Hepatic Arterial Chemotherapy for Metastatic Colorectal Carcinoma," *Br J Cancer*, 1994, 69(2):372-8.

Floyd J, Mirza I, Sachs B, et al, "Hepatotoxicity of Chemotherapy," *Semin Oncol*, 2006, 33 (1):50-67.

Kemeny N, Seiter K, Conti JA, et al, Hepatic Arterial Floxuridine and Leucovorin for Unresectable Liver Metastases From Colorectal Carcinoma. New Dose Schedules and Survival Update," *Cancer*, 1994, 73(4):1134-42.

Fluconazole (floo KOE na zole)

Brand Names: U.S. Diflucan®

Brand Names: Canada Apo-Fluconazole®; CanesOral®; CO Fluconazole; Diflucan®; Dom-Fluconazole; Fluconazole Injection; Fluconazole Omega; Monicure; Mylan-Fluconazole; Novo-Fluconazole; PHL-Fluconazole; PMS-Fluconazole; PRO-Fluconazole; Riva-Fluconazole; Taro-Fluconazole; ZYM-Fluconazole

Generic Availability (U.S.) Yes

Pharmacologic Category Antifungal Agent, Oral; Antifungal Agent, Parenteral

Use Treatment of candidiasis (esophageal, oropharyngeal, peritoneal, urinary tract, vaginal); systemic candida infections (eg, candidemia, disseminated candidiasis, and pneumonia); cryptococcal meningitis; antifungal prophylaxis in allogeneic bone marrow transplant recipients

Unlabeled Use Cryptococcal pneumonia; candidal intertrigo

Labeled Contraindications Hypersensitivity to fluconazole or any component of the formulation (cross-reaction with other azole antifungal agents may occur, but has not been established; use caution); coadministration of CYP3A4 substrates which may lead to QT_c prolongation (eg, cisapride, pimozide, or quinidine)

Pregnancy Risk Factor C (single dose for vaginal candidiasis)/D (all other indications)

Lactation Enters breast milk/not recommended (AAP rates "compatible"; AAP 2001 update pending)

Warnings/Precautions Should be used with caution in patients with renal and hepatic dysfunction or previous hepatotoxicity from other azole derivatives. Patients who develop abnormal liver function tests during fluconazole therapy should be monitored closely and discontinued if symptoms consistent with liver disease develop. Rare exfoliative skin disorders have been observed; monitor closely if rash develops and discontinue if lesions progress. Cases of QT_c prolongation and torsade de pointes associated with fluconazole use have been reported (usually high dose or in combination with agents known to prolong the QT interval); use caution in patients with concomitant medications or conditions which are arrhythmogenic. Use caution in patients treated with medications having a narrow therapeutic window and which are metabolized via CYP2C9 or CYP3A4 (monitor). Use with erythromycin should be avoided (may increase risk of cardiotoxicity). May occasionally cause dizziness or seizures; use caution driving or operating machines. Powder for oral suspension contains sucrose; use caution with fructose intolerance, sucrose-isomaltase deficiency, or glucose-galactose malabsorption.

Storage/Stability

Tablet: Store at <30°C (86°F).

Powder for oral suspension: Store dry powder at <30°C (86°F). Following reconstitution, store at 5°C to 30°C (41°F to 86°F). Discard unused portion after 2 weeks. Do not freeze.

Injection: Store injection in glass at 5°C to 30°C (41°F to 86°F). Store injection in Viaflex® at 5°C to 25°C (41°F to 77°F). Do not freeze. Do not unwrap unit until ready for use.

Mechanism of Action Interferes with fungal cytochrome P450 activity (lanosterol 14-α-demethylase), decreasing ergosterol synthesis (principal sterol in fungal cell membrane) and inhibiting cell membrane formation

Pharmacodynamics/Kinetics

Distribution: V_d: ~0.6 L/kg; widely throughout body with good penetration into CSF, eye, peritoneal fluid, sputum, skin, and urine

Relative diffusion blood into CSF: Adequate with or without inflammation (exceeds usual MICs)

CSF:blood level ratio: Normal meninges: 50% to 90%; Inflamed meninges: ~80%

Protein binding, plasma: 11% to 12%

Bioavailability: Oral: >90%

Half-life elimination: Normal renal function: ~30 hours (range: 20-50 hours); Elderly: ~46 hours

Time to peak, serum: Oral: 1-2 hours

Excretion: Urine (80% as unchanged drug)

Dosing

Adult & Geriatric The daily dose of fluconazole is the same for both oral and I.V. administration

Usual dosage range: Oral, I.V: 150 mg once **or** Loading dose: 200-800 mg; maintenance: 200-800 mg once daily; duration and dosage depend on location and severity of infection

Indication-specific dosing:

Blastomycosis (unlabeled use): Oral: *CNS disease:* Consolidation: 800 mg daily for ≥12 months and until resolution of CSF abnormalities (Chapman, 2008)

Candidiasis: Oral, I.V.:

Candidemia (neutropenic and non-neutropenic): Loading dose: 800 mg (12 mg/kg) on day 1, then 400 mg daily (6 mg/kg/day) for 14 days after first negative blood culture and resolution of signs/symptoms. **Note:** Not recommended for patients with recent azole exposure, critical illness, or if *C. krusei* or *C. glabrata* are suspected (Pappas, 2009).

Chronic, disseminated: 400 mg daily (6 mg/kg/day) until calcification or lesion resolution (Pappas, 2009)

CNS candidiasis (alternative therapy): 400-800 mg daily (6-12 mg/kg/day) until CSF/radiological abnormalities resolved. **Note:** Recommended as alternative therapy in patients intolerant of amphotericin B (Pappas, 2009).

Endocarditis, prosthetic valve (unlabeled use): 400-800 mg daily (6-12 mg/kg/day) for 6 weeks after valve replacement (as step-down in stable, culture-negative patients); long-term suppression in absence of valve replacement: 400-800 mg daily (Pappas, 2009)

Endophthalmitis (unlabeled use): 400-800 mg daily (6-12 mg/kg/day) for 4-6 weeks until examination indicates resolution (Pappas, 2009)

Esophageal:

Manufacturer's recommendation: Loading dose: 200 mg on day 1, then maintenance dose of 100-400 mg daily for 21 days and for at least 2 weeks following resolution of symptoms

Alternative dosing: 200-400 mg daily for 14-21 days; suppressive therapy of 100-200 mg 3 times weekly may be used for recurrent infections (Pappas, 2009)

Intertrigo (unlabeled use): 50 mg daily or 150 mg once weekly (Coldiron, 1991; Nozickova, 1998; Stengel, 1994)

Oropharyngeal:

Manufacturer's recommendation: Loading dose: 200 mg on day 1; maintenance dose 100 mg daily for ≥2 weeks. **Note:** Therapy with 100 mg daily is associated with resistance development (Rex, 1995).

Alternative dosing: 100-200 mg daily for 7-14 days for uncomplicated, moderate-to-severe disease; chronic therapy of 100 mg 3 times weekly is recommended in immunocompromised patients with history of oropharyngeal candidiasis (OPC) (Pappas, 2009)

Osteoarticular: 400 mg daily for 6-12 months (osteomyelitis) or 6 weeks (septic arthritis) (Pappas, 2009)

Pacemaker (or ICD, VAD) infection (unlabeled use): 400-800 mg daily (6-12 mg/kg/day) for 4- 6 weeks after device removal (as step-down in stable, culture-negative patients); long-term suppression when VAD cannot be removed: 400-800 mg daily (Pappas, 2009)

Pericarditis or myocarditis: 400-800 mg daily for several months (Pappas, 2009)

Peritonitis: 50-200 mg daily. **Note:** Some clinicians do not recommend using <200 mg daily (Chen, 2004).

Prophylaxis:

Bone marrow transplant: 400 mg once daily. Patients anticipated to have severe granulocytopenia should start therapy several days prior to the anticipated onset of neutropenia and continue for 7 days after the neutrophil count is >1000 mm^3.

High-risk ICU patients in units with high incidence of invasive candidiasis: 400 mg once daily (Pappas, 2009)

Neutropenic patients: 400 mg once daily for duration of neutropenia (Pappas, 2009)

Peritoneal dialysis associated infection (concurrently treated with antibiotics), prevention of secondary fungal infection: 200 mg every 48 hours (Restrepo, 2010)

Solid organ transplant: 200-400 mg once daily for at least 7-14 days (Pappas, 2009)

Thrombophlebitis, suppurative (unlabeled use): 400-800 mg daily (6-12 mg/kg/day) and as step-down in stable patients for ≥2 weeks (Pappas, 2009)

Urinary tract:

Cystitis:

Manufacturer's recommendation: UTI: 50-200 mg once daily

Asymptomatic, patient undergoing urologic procedure: 200-400 mg once daily several days before and after the procedure (Pappas, 2009)

Symptomatic: 200 mg once daily for 2 weeks (Pappas, 2009)

Fungus balls: 200-400 mg once daily (Pappas, 2009)

Pyelonephritis: 200-400 mg once daily for 2 weeks (Pappas, 2009)

Vaginal:

Uncomplicated: Manufacturer's recommendation: 150 mg as a single oral dose

Complicated: 150 mg every 72 hours for 3 doses (Pappas, 2009)

Recurrent: 150 mg once daily for 10-14 days, followed by 150 mg once weekly for 6 months (Pappas, 2009), **or** fluconazole (oral) 100 mg, 150 mg, or 200 mg every third day for a total of 3 doses (day 1, 4, and 7), then 100 mg, 150 mg, or 200 mg dose weekly for 6 months (CDC, 2010)

Coccidioidomycosis, treatment: Oral, I.V.:

HIV-infected (unlabeled use):

Meningitis: 400-800 mg once daily continued indefinitely (CDC, 2009)

Pneumonia, focal, mild or positive serology alone: 400 mg once daily continued indefinitely (CDC, 2009)

Pneumonia, diffuse or severe extrathoracic disseminated disease (after clinical improvement noted with amphotericin B): 400 mg once daily (CDC, 2009)

Non-HIV infected (unlabeled use):

Disseminated, extrapulmonary: 400 mg once daily (some experts use 2000 mg daily [Galgiani, 2005])

Meningitis: 400 mg once daily (some experts use initial doses of 800-1000 mg daily), lifelong duration (Galgiani, 2005)

Pneumonia, acute, uncomplicated: 200-400 mg daily for 3-6 months (Catanzaro, 1995; Galgiani, 2000)

Pneumonia, chronic progressive, fibrocavitary: 200-400 mg daily for 12 months (Catanzaro, 1995; Galgiani, 2000)

Pneumonia, diffuse: Consolidation after amphotericin B induction: 400 mg daily for 12 months (lifelong in chronically immunosuppressed) (Galgiani, 2005)

Coccidioidomycosis, prophylaxis: Oral:

HIV-infected, positive serology, CD4+ count <250 cells/microL (unlabeled use): 400 mg once daily (CDC, 2009)

Solid organ transplant (unlabeled use): **Note:** Prophylaxis regimens in this setting have not been established; the following regimen has been proposed for transplant recipients who maintain residence in a *Coccidioides* spp endemic area.

Previous history >12 months prior to transplant: 200 mg once daily for 6-12 months (Vikram, 2009; Vucicevic, 2011)

Previous history ≤12 months prior to transplant: 400 mg once daily, lifelong treatment (Vikram, 2009; Vucicevic, 2011)

Positive serology before or at transplant: 400 mg once daily, lifelong treatment; if serology is negative at 12 months, consider a dose reduction to 200 mg daily (Vikram, 2009; Vucicevic, 2011)

No history (at risk for *de novo* post-transplant disease): some clinicians treat with 200 mg daily for 6-12 months (Vucicevic, 2011)

Cryptococcosis: Oral, I.V.:

Meningitis: Manufacturer's recommendation: 400 mg for 1 dose, then 200-400 mg once daily for 10-12 weeks following negative CSF culture

HIV-infected:

Meningitis (in patients amphotericin B resistant or intolerant): Induction: 400-800 mg once daily for 4-6 weeks with concomitant flucytosine (CDC, 2009) **or** 800-1200 mg once daily with concomitant flucytosine for 6 weeks (Perfect, 2010)

Consolidation: 400 mg once daily for 8 weeks (CDC, 2009)

Maintenance (suppression): 200 mg once daily lifelong or until CD4+ count >200 (CDC, 2009)

Pulmonary (immunocompetent) (unlabeled use): 400 mg once daily for 6-12 months (Perfect, 2010)

Pediatric The daily dose of fluconazole is the same for oral and I.V. administration

Usual dosage range: Oral, I.V: Loading dose: 6-12 mg/kg/dose; maintenance: 3-12 mg/kg/dose once daily; duration and dosage depend on location and severity of infection

Indication-specific dosing:

Candidiasis: Oral, I.V.:

Esophageal:

Manufacturer's recommendation: Loading dose: 6 mg/kg/dose; maintenance: 3-12 mg/kg/dose once daily for 21 days and for at least 2 weeks following resolution of symptoms (maximum: 600 mg/day)

HIV-exposed/-infected: Loading dose: 6 mg/kg/dose once on day 1; maintenance: 3-6 mg/kg/dose once daily for 4-21 days (maximum: 400 mg/day) (CDC, 2009)

Relapse suppression (HIV-exposed/-infected): 3-6 mg/kg/dose once daily (maximum: 200 mg/day) (CDC, 2009)

Invasive disease (alternative therapy): 5-6 mg/kg/dose every 12 hours for ≥28 days (maximum: 600 mg/day) (CDC, 2009)

Oropharyngeal:

Manufacturer's recommendation: Loading dose: 6 mg/kg/dose; maintenance: 3 mg/kg/dose once daily for ≥2 weeks (maximum: 600 mg/day)

HIV-exposed/-infected: 3-6 mg/kg/dose once daily for 7-14 days (maximum: 400 mg/day) (CDC, 2009)

Coccidiodomycosis: Oral, I.V.: *Meningeal infection, or in a stable patient with diffuse pulmonary or disseminated disease* (HIV-exposed/-infected):

Treatment: 5-6 mg/kg/dose twice daily (maximum daily dose: 800 mg/**day**) (CDC, 2009) followed by chronic suppressive therapy (see below)

Relapse suppression: 6 mg/kg/dose once daily (maximum daily dose: 400 mg/**day**) (CDC, 2009)

Cryptococcosis: Oral, I.V.:

Meningitis: Manufacturer's recommendation:: 12 mg/kg/dose for 1 dose, then 6-12 mg/kg/day for 10-12 weeks following negative CSF culture

HIV-exposed/-infected:

CNS disease (alternative therapy in patients intolerant of amphotericin B):

Induction: 12 mg/kg/dose for 1 dose, then 6-12 mg/kg/day (maximum: 800 mg/day) for ≥2 weeks (in combination with flucytosine) (CDC, 2009)

Consolidation: 10-12 mg/kg/day for 8 weeks (Perfect, 2010) **or** 12 mg/kg/dose for 1 dose, then 6-12 mg/kg/day (maximum: 800 mg/day) for 8 weeks (CDC, 2009)

Maintenance (suppression): 6 mg/kg/day (maximum: 200 mg/day) (CDC, 2009; Perfect, 2010)

Non-CNS disease, disseminated (including severe pulmonary disease) (alternative therapy; unlabeled use): Induction: 12 mg/kg/dose for 1 dose, then 6-12 mg/kg/day (maximum: 600 mg/day) (CDC, 2009)

Non-CNS disease, localized (including isolated pulmonary disease) (unlabeled use): 12 mg/kg/dose for 1 dose, then 6-12 mg/kg/day (maximum: 600 mg/day). **Note:** Duration depends upon infection site and severity (CDC, 2009). For patients with pulmonary disease (not delineated by severity), the IDSA recommends a duration of 6-12 months (Perfect, 2010).

Renal Impairment

Manufacturer's recommendation: **Note:** Renal function estimated using the Cockcroft-Gault formula

No adjustment for vaginal candidiasis single-dose therapy

For multiple dosing in adults, administer loading dose of 50-400 mg, then adjust daily doses as follows (dosage reduction in children should parallel adult recommendations): Cl_{cr} ≤50 mL/minute (no dialysis): Administer 50% of recommended dose daily

Intermittent hemodialysis (IHD): Dialyzable (50%): May administer 100% of daily dose (according to indication) after each dialysis session. Alternatively, doses of 200-400 mg every 48-72 hours **or** 100- 200 mg every 24 hours have been recommended. **Note:** Dosing dependent on the assumption of 3 times/ week, complete IHD sessions (Heintz, 2009).

Continuous renal replacement therapy (CRRT) (Heintz, 2009; Trotman, 2005): Drug clearance is highly dependent on the method of renal replacement, filter type, and flow rate. Appropriate dosing requires close monitoring of pharmacologic response, signs of adverse reactions due to drug accumulation, as well as drug concentrations in relation to target trough (if appropriate). The following are general recommendations only (based on dialysate flow/ultrafiltration rates of 1-2 L/hour and minimal residual renal function) and should not supersede clinical judgment:

CVVH: Loading dose of 400-800 mg followed by 200-400 mg every 24 hours

CVVHD/CVVHDF: Loading dose of 400-800 mg followed by 400-800 mg every 24 hours (CVVHD or CVVHDF) **or** 800 mg every 24 hours (CVVHDF)

Note: Higher maintenance doses of 400 mg every 24 hours (CVVH), 800 mg every 24 hours (CVVHD), and 500-600 mg every 12 hours (CVVHDF) may be considered when treating resistant organisms and/or when employing combined ultrafiltration and dialysis flow rates of ≥2 L/hour for CVVHD/ CVVHDF (Heintz, 2009; Trotman, 2005).

Administration

I.V.: Do not use if cloudy or precipitated. Infuse over ~1-2 hours; do not exceed 200 mg/hour.

Oral: May be administered without regard to meals.

Dosage Forms Excipient information presented when available (limited, particularly for generics); consult specific product labeling. [DSC] = Discontinued product

Infusion, premixed iso-osmotic dextrose solution: 200 mg (100 mL); 400 mg (200 mL)

Infusion, premixed iso-osmotic sodium chloride solution: 100 mg (50 mL); 200 mg (100 mL); 400 mg (200 mL)

Diflucan®: 200 mg (100 mL [DSC]); 400 mg (200 mL [DSC])

Infusion, premixed iso-osmotic sodium chloride solution [preservative free]: 200 mg (100 mL); 400 mg (200 mL)
Powder for suspension, oral: 10 mg/mL (35 mL); 40 mg/mL (35 mL)
Diflucan®: 10 mg/mL (35 mL); 40 mg/mL (35 mL) [contains sodium benzoate, sucrose; orange flavor]
Tablet, oral: 50 mg, 100 mg, 150 mg, 200 mg
Diflucan®: 50 mg, 100 mg, 150 mg, 200 mg

◆ **Fluconazole Injection (Can)** *see* Fluconazole *on page 612*

◆ **Fluconazole Omega (Can)** *see* Fluconazole *on page 612*

Flucytosine (floo SYE toe seen)

Brand Names: U.S. Ancobon®

Brand Names: Canada Ancobon®

Index Terms 5-FC; 5-Fluorocytosine; 5-Flurocytosine

Generic Availability (U.S.) Yes

Pharmacologic Category Antifungal Agent, Oral

Use Adjunctive treatment of systemic fungal infections (eg, septicemia, endocarditis, UTI, meningitis, or pulmonary) caused by susceptible strains of *Candida* or *Cryptococcus*

Labeled Contraindications Hypersensitivity to flucytosine or any component of the formulation

Pregnancy Risk Factor C

Lactation Excretion in breast milk unknown/not recommended

Warnings/Precautions [U.S. Boxed Warning]: Use with extreme caution in patients with renal dysfunction; dosage adjustment required. Avoid use as monotherapy; resistance rapidly develops. Use with caution in patients with bone marrow depression; patients with hematologic disease or who have been treated with radiation or drugs that suppress the bone marrow may be at greatest risk. Bone marrow toxicity can be irreversible. **[U.S. Boxed Warning]: Closely monitor hematologic, renal, and hepatic status.** Hepatotoxicity and bone marrow toxicity appear to be dose related; monitor levels closely and adjust dose accordingly.

Ethanol/Nutrition/Herb Interactions Food: Food decreases the rate, but not the extent of absorption.

Storage/Stability Store at room temperature of 15°C to 30°C (59°F to 86°F). Protect from light.

Mechanism of Action Penetrates fungal cells and is converted to fluorouracil which competes with uracil interfering with fungal RNA and protein synthesis

Pharmacodynamics/Kinetics

Absorption: 76% to 89%
Distribution: Into CSF, aqueous humor, joints, peritoneal fluid, and bronchial secretions; V_d: 0.6 L/kg
Protein binding: 3% to 4%
Metabolism: Minimally hepatic; deaminated, possibly via gut bacteria, to 5-fluorouracil
Half-life elimination:
Normal renal function: 2-5 hours
Anuria: 85 hours (range: 30-250)
End stage renal disease: 75-200 hours
Time to peak, serum: ~1-2 hours
Excretion: Urine (>90% as unchanged drug)

Dosing

Adult & Geriatric

Endocarditis: Oral: 25-37.5 mg/kg every 6 hours (with amphotericin B) for at least 6 weeks after valve replacement

Meningoencephalitis, cryptococcal: Induction: Oral: 25 mg/kg/dose (with amphotericin B) every 6 hours for 2 weeks; if clinical improvement, may discontinue both amphotericin and flucytosine and follow with an extended course of fluconazole (400 mg/day); alternatively, may continue flucytosine for 6-10 weeks (with amphotericin B) without conversion to fluconazole treatment

Pediatric Unlabeled use. Refer to adult dosing.

Renal Impairment

Use lower initial dose:

Cl_{cr} 20-40 mL/minute: Administer 37.5 mg/kg every 12 hours

Cl_{cr} 10-20 mL/minute: Administer 37.5 mg/kg every 24 hours

Cl_{cr} <10 mL/minute: Administer 37.5 mg/kg every 24-48 hours, but monitor drug concentrations frequently

Hemodialysis: Dialyzable (50% to 100%); administer dose posthemodialysis

Peritoneal dialysis: Adults: Administer 0.5-1 g every 24 hours

Continuous arteriovenous or venovenous hemodiafiltration effects: Change dosing frequency to every 12-24 hours (monitor serum concentrations and adjust)

Administration Administer around-the-clock to promote less variation in peak and trough serum levels. To avoid nausea and vomiting, administer a few capsules at a time over 15 minutes until full dose is taken.

Test Interactions Flucytosine causes markedly false elevations in serum creatinine values when the Ektachem® analyzer is used. The Jaffé reaction is recommended for determining serum creatinine.

Dosage Forms Excipient information presented when available (limited, particularly for generics); consult specific product labeling.

Capsule, oral: 250 mg, 500 mg

Ancobon®: 250 mg, 500 mg

◆ **Fludara®** *see* Fludarabine *on page* 619

Fludarabine (floo DARE a been)

Related Information

Hematopoietic Stem Cell Transplantation *on page* 1887
Management of Chemotherapy-Induced Nausea and Vomiting *on page* 1786
Management of Infections *on page* 1809
Safe Handling of Hazardous Drugs *on page* 1904

Brand Names: U.S. Fludara®

Brand Names: Canada Fludara®

Index Terms 2F-ara-AMP; Fludarabine Phosphate

Generic Availability (U.S.) Yes

Pharmacologic Category Antineoplastic Agent, Antimetabolite (Purine Analog)

Use Treatment of progressive or refractory B-cell chronic lymphocytic leukemia (CLL)

Canadian labeling: Second-line treatment of chronic lymphocytic leukemia (CLL); second-line treatment of low-grade, refractory non-Hodgkin lymphoma (NHL)

Unlabeled Use Treatment of non-Hodgkin lymphomas (NHL); acute myeloid leukemia (AML), either refractory or in poor risk patients; relapsed acute lymphocytic leukemia (ALL) or AML in pediatric patients; Waldenström's macroglobulinemia (WM); reduced-intensity conditioning regimens prior to allogeneic hematopoietic stem cell transplantation (generally administered in combination with busulfan or cyclophosphamide and antithymocyte globulin or lymphocyte immune globulin, or in combination with melphalan and alemtuzumab)

Labeled Contraindications Hypersensitivity of fludarabine or any component of the formulation

Canadian labeling: Additional contraindications (not in U.S. labeling): Severe renal impairment (Cl_{cr} <30 mL/minute); decompensated hemolytic anemia; concurrent use with pentostatin

Pregnancy Risk Factor D

Lactation Excretion in breast milk unknown/not recommended

Warnings/Precautions Hazardous agent - use appropriate precautions for handling and disposal. Use with caution in patients with renal insufficiency (clearance of the primary metabolite 2-fluoro-ara-A is reduced); dosage reductions are recommended (monitor closely for excessive toxicity); use of the I.V. formulation is not recommended if Cl_{cr} <30 mL/minute. Canadian labeling contraindicates use of oral and I.V. formulations if Cl_{cr} <30 mL/minute. Use with caution in patients with pre-existing hematological disorders (particularly granulocytopenia) or pre-existing central nervous system disorder (epilepsy), spasticity, or peripheral neuropathy. **[U.S. Boxed Warning]: Higher than recommended doses are associated with severe neurologic toxicity (delayed blindness, coma, death); similar neurotoxicity (agitation, coma, confusion and seizure) has been reported with standard CLL doses.** Neurotoxicity symptoms due to high doses appear from 21-60 days following the last fludarabine dose, although neurotoxicity has been reported as early as 7 days and up to 225 days. Possible neurotoxic effects of chronic administration are unknown. Caution patients about performing tasks which require mental alertness (eg, operating machinery or driving).

[U.S. Boxed Warning]: Life-threatening (and sometimes fatal) autoimmune effects, including hemolytic anemia, autoimmune thrombocytopenia/thrombocytopenic purpura (ITP), Evans syndrome, and acquired hemophilia have occurred; monitor closely for hemolysis; discontinue fludarabine if hemolysis occurs; the hemolytic effects usually recur with fludarabine rechallenge. **[U.S. Boxed Warning]: Severe bone marrow suppression (anemia, thrombocytopenia, and neutropenia) may occur;** may be cumulative. Severe myelosuppression (trilineage bone marrow hypoplasia/aplasia) has been reported (rare) with a duration of significant cytopenias ranging from 2 months to 1 year. First-line combination therapy is associated with prolonged cytopenias, with anemia lasting up to 7 months, neutropenia up to 9 months, and thrombocytopenia up to 10 months; increased age is predictive for prolonged cytopenias (Gill, 2010).

Use with caution in patients with documented infection, fever, immunodeficiency, or with a history of opportunistic infection; prophylactic anti-infectives should be considered for patients with an increased risk for developing opportunistic infections. Progressive multifocal leukoencephalopathy (PML) due to JC virus (usually fatal) has been reported with use; usually in patients who had received prior and/or other concurrent chemotherapy; onset ranges from a few weeks to 1 year; evaluate any neurological change promptly. Avoid vaccination with live vaccines during and after fludarabine treatment. May cause tumor lysis syndrome; risk is increased in patients with large tumor burden prior to treatment. Patients receiving blood products should only receive irradiated blood products due to the potential for transfusion related GVHD. **[U.S. Boxed Warnings]: Do not use in combination with pentostatin; may lead to severe, even fatal pulmonary toxicity. Should be administered under the supervision of an experienced cancer chemotherapy physician.**

Adverse Reactions

>10%:

Cardiovascular: Edema (8% to 19%)

Central nervous system: Fever (11% to 69%), fatigue (10% to 38%), pain (5% to 22%), chills (11% to 19%)

Dermatologic: Rash (4% to 15%)

Gastrointestinal: Nausea/vomiting (1% to 36%), anorexia (≤34%), diarrhea (5% to 15%), gastrointestinal bleeding (3% to 13%)

Genitourinary: Urinary tract infection (2% to 15%)

Hematologic: Myelosuppression (nadir: 10-14 days; recovery: 5-7 weeks; dose-limiting toxicity), anemia (14% to 60%), neutropenia (grade 4: 37% to 59%; nadir: ~13 days), thrombocytopenia (17% to 55%; nadir: ~16 days)

Neuromuscular & skeletal: Weakness (9% to 65%), myalgia (4% to 16%), paresthesia (4% to 12%)

Ocular: Visual disturbance (3% to 15%)

Respiratory: Cough (≤44%), pneumonia (3% to 22%), dyspnea (1% to 22%), upper respiratory infection (2% to 16%), rhinitis (≤11%)

Miscellaneous: Infection (12% to 44%), diaphoresis (≤14%)

1% to 10%:

Cardiovascular: Peripheral edema (≤7%), angina (≤6%), chest pain (≤5%), CHF (≤3%), arrhythmia (≤3%), cerebrovascular accident (≤3%), MI (≤3%), supraventricular tachycardia (≤3%), deep vein thrombosis (1% to 3%), phlebitis (1% to 3%), aneurysm (≤1%), transient ischemic attack (≤1%)

Central nervous system: Headache (≤9%), malaise (6% to 8%), sleep disorder (1% to 3%), cerebellar syndrome (≤1%), depression (≤1%), mentation impaired (≤1%)

Dermatologic: Alopecia (≤3%), pruritus (1% to 3%), seborrhea (≤1%)

Endocrine & metabolic: Hyperglycemia (1% to 6%), LDH increased (≤6%), dehydration (≤1%)

Gastrointestinal: Abdominal pain (≤10%), stomatitis (≤9%), weight loss (≤6%), esophagitis (≤3%), constipation (1% to 3%), mucositis (≤2%), dysphagia (≤1%)

Genitourinary: Dysuria (3% to 4%), hesitancy (≤3%)

Hematologic: Hemorrhage (≤1%), myelodysplastic syndrome/acute myeloid leukemia (usually associated with prior or concurrent treatment with other anticancer agents)

Hepatic: Cholelithiasis (≤3%), liver function tests abnormal (1% to 3%), liver failure (≤1%)

Neuromuscular & skeletal: Back pain (≤9%), osteoporosis (≤2%), arthralgia (≤1%)

Otic: Hearing loss (2% to 6%)

Renal: Hematuria (2% to 3%), renal failure (≤1%), renal function test abnormal (≤1%), proteinuria (≤1%)

Respiratory: Bronchitis (≤9%), pharyngitis (≤9%), allergic pneumonitis (≤6%), hemoptysis (1% to 6%), sinusitis (≤5%), epistaxis (≤1%), hypoxia (≤1%)

Miscellaneous: Flu-like syndrome (5% to 8%), herpes simplex infection (≤8%), anaphylaxis (≤1%), tumor lysis syndrome (1%)

<1%, postmarketing, and/or case reports: Acute respiratory distress syndrome, agitation, blindness, blurred vision, bone marrow fibrosis, coma, confusion, diplopia, eosinophilia, Epstein-Barr virus (EBV) associated lymphoproliferation, EBV reactivation, erythema multiforme, Evans syndrome, flank pain, hemolytic anemia (autoimmune), hemophilia (acquired), hemorrhagic cystitis, herpes zoster reactivation, hyperkalemia, hyperphosphatemia, hyperuricemia, hypocalcemia, interstitial pneumonitis, metabolic acidosis, opportunistic infection, optic neuritis, optic neuropathy, pancreatic enzymes abnormal, pancytopenia, pemphigus, pericardial effusion, peripheral neuropathy, photophobia (primarily with high doses), progressive multifocal leukoencephalopathy (PML), pulmonary fibrosis, pulmonary hemorrhage, pulmonary infiltrate, respiratory distress, respiratory failure, Richter's syndrome, seizure, skin cancer (new onset or exacerbation), Stevens-Johnson syndrome, thrombocytopenia (autoimmune), thrombocytopenic purpura (autoimmune), toxic epidermal necrolysis, trilineage bone marrow aplasia, trilineage bone marrow hypoplasia, urate crystalluria, wrist drop

Also observed: Neurologic syndrome characterized by cortical blindness, coma, and paralysis [36% at doses >96 mg/m^2 for 5-7 days; <0.2% at doses <125 mg/m^2/cycle (onset of neurologic symptoms may be delayed for 3-4 weeks)]

Drug Interactions

Metabolism/Transport Effects None known.

Avoid Concomitant Use

Avoid concomitant use of Fludarabine with any of the following: BCG; CloZAPine; Natalizumab; Pentostatin; Pimecrolimus; Tacrolimus (Topical); Vaccines (Live)

Increased Effect/Toxicity

Fludarabine may increase the levels/effects of: CloZAPine; Leflunomide; Natalizumab; Pentostatin; Vaccines (Live)

The levels/effects of Fludarabine may be increased by: Denosumab; Pentostatin; Pimecrolimus; Roflumilast; Tacrolimus (Topical); Trastuzumab

Decreased Effect

Fludarabine may decrease the levels/effects of: BCG; Coccidioidin Skin Test; Sipuleucel-T; Vaccines (Inactivated); Vaccines (Live)

The levels/effects of Fludarabine may be decreased by: Echinacea; Imatinib

Ethanol/Nutrition/Herb Interactions Ethanol: Avoid ethanol (due to GI irritation).

Storage/Stability

I.V.: Store intact vials under refrigeration at 2°C to 8°C (36°F to 46°F). Reconstituted vials are stable for 16 days at room temperature of 15°C to 30°C (59°F to 86°F) or refrigerated, although the manufacturer recommends use within 8 hours. Solutions diluted in saline or dextrose are stable for 48 hours at room temperature or under refrigeration.

Tablet: Store at 15°C to 30°C (59°F to 86°F); should be kept within packaging until use.

Reconstitution Use appropriate precautions for handling and disposal. Reconstitute vials with SWI, NS, or D_5W to a concentration of 10-25 mg/mL. Standard I.V. dilution: 100-125 mL D_5W or NS.

Mechanism of Action Fludarabine inhibits DNA synthesis by inhibition of DNA polymerase and ribonucleotide reductase; also inhibits DNA primase and DNA ligase I

Pharmacodynamics/Kinetics

Distribution: V_d: 38-96 L/m^2; widely with extensive tissue binding

Protein binding: 2-fluoro-ara-A: ~19% to 29%

Metabolism: I.V.: Fludarabine phosphate is rapidly dephosphorylated in the plasma to 2-fluoro-ara-A (active metabolite), which subsequently enters tumor cells and is phosphorylated by deoxycytidine kinase to the active triphosphate derivative (2-fluoro-ara-ATP)

Bioavailability: Oral: 2-fluoro-ara-A: 50% to 65%

Half-life elimination: 2-fluoro-ara-A: ~20 hours

Time to peak, plasma: Oral: 1-2 hours

Excretion: Urine (60%, 23% as 2-fluoro-ara-A) within 24 hours

Dosing

Adult & Geriatric Details concerning dosing in combination regimens should also be consulted.

Chronic lymphocytic leukemia (CLL):

I.V.: 25 mg/m^2/day for 5 days every 28 days

Oral (Canadian labeling; not available in U.S.): 40 mg/m^2 once daily for 5 days every 28 days

CLL combination regimens (unlabeled dosing): I.V.:

CFAR: 20 mg/m^2/day for 3 days every 28 days for 6 cycles (in combination with cyclophosphamide, rituximab and alemtuzumab) (Wierda, 2008)

FC: 30 mg/m^2/day for 3 days every 28 days for 6 cycles (in combination with cyclophosphamide) (Eichhorst, 2006) **or** 20 mg/m^2/day for 5 days every 28 days for 6 cycles (in combination with cyclophosphamide) (Flinn, 2007)

FCR: 25 mg/m^2/day for 3 days every 28 days for 6 cycles (in combination with cyclophosphamide and rituximab) (Keating, 2005; Robak, 2010; Wierda, 2005)

FluCam: 30 mg/m^2/day for 3 days every 28 days for 4-6 cycles (in combination with alemtuzumab) (Elter, 2005)

FR: 25 mg/m^2/day for 5 days every 28 days for 6 cycles (in combination with rituximab) (Byrd, 2003)

OFAR: 30 mg/m^2/day for 2 days every 28 days for 6 cycles (in combination with oxaliplatin, cytarabine, and rituximab) (Tsimberidou, 2008)

AML, high-risk patients (unlabeled use): I.V.: 30 mg/m^2/day for 5 days induction therapy, followed by post remission therapy of 30 mg/m^2/day for 4 days every other cycle (in combination with cytarabine with or without filgrastim) (Borthakur, 2008)

AML, refractory (unlabeled use): I.V.: 30 mg/m^2/day for 5 days (in combination with cytarabine and filgrastim), may repeat once for partial remission (Montillo, 1998) **or** 30 mg/m^2/day for 5 days for 1 or 2 cycles (in combination with cytarabine, idarubicin, and filgrastim) (Virchis, 2004)

Non-Hodgkin lymphomas: I.V.:

Canadian labeling: 25 mg/m^2 for 5 days every 28 days; dosage adjustment may be necessary for hematologic or nonhematologic toxicity.

Follicular lymphoma (unlabeled use):

FCR: 25 mg/m^2/day for 3 days every 21 days for 4 cycles (in combination with cyclophosphamide and rituximab) (Sacchi, 2007)

FCMR: 25 mg/m^2/day for 3 days every 28 days for 4 cycles (in combination with cyclophosphamide, mitoxantrone, and rituximab) (Forstpointner, 2004; Forstpointner, 2006)

FND: 25 mg/m²/day for 3 days every 28 days for up to 8 cycles (in combination with mitoxantrone and dexamethasone) (McLaughlin, 1996; Tsimberidou, 2002)

FNDR: 25 mg/m²/day for 3 days every 28 days for up to 8 cycles (in combination with mitoxantrone, dexamethasone, and rituximab) (McLaughlin, 2000)

FR: 25 mg/m²/day for 5 days every 28 days for 6 cycles (in combination with rituximab) (Czuczman, 2005)

Mantle cell lymphoma (unlabeled use):

FC: 20 mg/m²/day for 4-5 days or 25 mg/m²/day for 3-5 days (in combination with cyclophosphamide) (Cohen, 2001)

FCMR: 25 mg/m²/day for 3 days every 28 days for 4 cycles (in combination with cyclophosphamide, mitoxantrone, and rituximab) (Forstpointner, 2004; Forstpointner, 2006)

Waldenstron's macroglobulinemia (unlabeled use): I.V.:25 mg/m²/day for 5 days every 28 days (Foran, 1999) **or** 25 mg/m²/day for 5 days every 28 days for 6 cycles (in combination with rituximab) (Treon, 2009)

Stem cell transplant (allogeneic) conditioning regimen, reduced-intensity, (unlabeled use): I.V.: 30 mg/m²/dose for 6 doses beginning 10 days prior to transplant **or** 30 mg/m²/dose for 5 days beginning 6 days prior to transplant (in combination with busulfan with or without antithymocyte globulin) (Schetelig, 2003)

Stem cell transplant (allogeneic) nonmyeloablative conditioning regimen (unlabeled use): I.V.: 30 mg/m²/dose for 3 doses beginning 5 days prior to transplant (in combination with cyclophosphamide and rituximab) (Khouri, 2008) **or** 30 mg/m²/dose for 3 doses beginning 4 days prior to transplant (in combination with total body irradiation) (Rezvani, 2008)

Pediatric

AML (unlabeled use): I.V.: 10.5 mg/m² bolus over 15 minutes followed by a continuous infusion of 30.5 mg/m²/day for 48 hours (Lange, 2008)

ALL or AML, relapsed (unlabeled use): I.V.: 10.5 mg/m² bolus over 15 minutes followed by a continuous infusion of 30.5 mg/m²/day for 48 hours (Avramis, 1998)

Stem cell transplant (allogeneic) conditioning regimen, reduced-intensity (unlabeled use): I.V.: 30 mg/m²/dose for 6 doses beginning 7-10 days prior to transplant (in combination with busulfan and antithymocyte globulin) (Pulsipher, 2009)

Renal Impairment

U.S. labeling: Adults: CLL: I.V.:

Cl_{cr} 50-79 mL/minute: Decrease dose to 20 mg/m².

Cl_{cr} 30-49 mL/minute: Decrease dose to 15 mg/m².

Cl_{cr} <30 mL/minute: Avoid use.

Canadian labeling: CLL (Oral, I.V.), NHL (I.V.):

Cl_{cr} 30-70 mL/minute: Reduce dose by up to 50%.

Cl_{cr} <30 mL/minute: Use is contraindicated.

The following guidelines have been used by some clinicians: Aronoff, 2007:

I.V.:

Children:

Cl_{cr} 30-50 mL/minute: Administer 80% of dose.

Cl_{cr} <30 mL/minute: Not recommended.

Hemodialysis: Administer 25% of dose

Continuous ambulatory peritoneal dialysis (CAPD): Not recommended.

Continuous renal replacement therapy (CRRT): Administer 80% of dose.

Adults:

Cl_{cr} 10-50 mL/minute: Administer 75% of dose.

Cl_{cr} <10 mL/minute: Administer 50% of dose.

Hemodialysis: Administer after dialysis

Continuous ambulatory peritoneal dialysis (CAPD): Administer 50% of dose.

Continuous renal replacement therapy (CRRT): Administer 75% of dose.

Adjustment for Toxicity

Hematologic or nonhematologic toxicity (other than neurotoxicity): Consider treatment delay or dosage reduction.

Hemolysis: Discontinue treatment.

Neurotoxicity: Consider treatment delay or discontinuation.

Combination Regimens

Leukemia, acute myeloid:

FLAG (AML Induction) on page 1643

FLAG-IDA on page 1644

Leukemia, chronic lymphocytic:

Cyclophosphamide-Fludarabine-Alemtuzumab-Rituximab (CLL) on page 1601

Fludarabine-Alemtuzumab (CLL) on page 1645

Fludarabine-Cyclophosphamide (CLL) on page 1646

Fludarabine-Cyclophosphamide-Rituximab (CLL) on page 1648

Fludarabine-Rituximab (CLL) on page 1651

OFAR (CLL) on page 1722

Lymphoma, non-Hodgkin's:

Fludarabine-Cyclophosphamide-Mitoxantrone-Rituximab on page 1647

Fludarabine-Cyclophosphamide-Rituximab (NHL-Follicular) on page 1649

Fludarabine-Mitoxantrone on page 1649

Fludarabine-Mitoxantrone-Dexamethasone (NHL) on page 1650

Fludarabine-Mitoxantrone-Dexamethasone-Rituximab on page 1650

Fludarabine-Mitoxantrone-Rituximab on page 1651

Fludarabine-Rituximab (NHL-Follicular) on page 1651

Lymphoma, non-Hodgkin's (Mantle cell): Fludarabine-Cyclophosphamide (NHL-Mantle Cell) on page 1648

Administration

Oral: Tablet may be administered with or without food; should be swallowed whole with water; do not chew, break, or crush.

I.V.: Usually administered as a 30-minute infusion; continuous infusions (unlabeled administration rate) are occasionally used

Emetic Potential

Oral: Low (10% to 30%)

I.V.: Very low (<10%)

Monitoring Parameters CBC with differential, platelet count, AST, ALT, serum creatinine, serum albumin, uric acid; monitor for signs of infection and neurotoxicity

Dosage Forms Excipient information presented when available (limited, particularly for generics); consult specific product labeling.

Injection, powder for reconstitution, as phosphate: 50 mg

Fludara®: 50 mg

Injection, solution, as phosphate [preservative free]: 25 mg/mL (2 mL)

Dosage Forms: Canada Excipient information presented when available (limited, particularly for generics); consult specific product labeling.

Tablet, as phosphate:
Fludara®: 10 mg

References

Aronoff GR, Bennett WM, Berns JS, et al, *Drug Prescribing in Renal Failure: Dosing Guidelines for Adults and Children*, 5th ed. Philadelphia, PA: American College of Physicians; 2007, p 99, 172.

Avramis VI, Wiersma S, Krailo MD, et al, "Pharmacokinetic and Pharmacodynamic Studies of Fludarabine and Cytosine Arabinoside Administered as Loading Boluses Followed by Continuous Infusions After a Phase I/II Study in Pediatric Patients With Relapsed Leukemias. The Children's Cancer Group," *Clin Cancer Res*, 1998, 4(1):45-52.

Boogaerts MA, Van Hoof A, Catovsky D, et al, "Activity of Oral Fludarabine Phosphate in Previously Treated Chronic Lymphocytic Leukemia," *J Clin Oncol*, 2001, 19(22):4252-8.

Borthakur G, Kantarjian H, Wang X, et al, "Treatment of Core-Binding-Factor in Acute Myelogenous Leukemia With Fludarabine, Cytarabine, and Granulocyte Colony-Stimulating Factor Results in Improved Event-Free Survival," *Cancer*, 2008, 113(11):3181-5.

Byrd JC, Peterson BL, Morrison VA, et al, "Randomized Phase 2 Study of Fludarabine With Concurrent vs Sequential Treatment With Rituximab in Symptomatic, Untreated Patients With B-Cell Chronic Lymphocytic Leukemia: Results From Cancer and Leukemia Group B 9712 (CALGB 9712)," *Blood*, 2003, 101(1):6-14.

Cohen BJ, Moskowitz C, Straus D, et al, "Cyclophosphamide/Fludarabine (CF) is Active in the Treatment of Mantle Cell Lymphoma," *Leuk Lymphoma*, 2001, 42(5):1015-22.

Czuczman MS, Koryzna A, Mohr A, et al, "Rituximab in Combination With Fludarabine Chemotherapy in Low-Grade or Follicular Lymphoma," *J Clin Oncol*, 2005, 23(4):694-704.

Eichhorst BF, Busch R, Hopfinger G, et al, "Fludarabine Plus Cyclophosphamide Versus Fludarabine Alone in First-Line Therapy of Younger Patients With Chronic Lymphocytic Leukemia," *Blood*, 2006, 107(3):885-91.

Elter T, Borchmann P, Schulz H, et al, "Fludarabine in Combination With Alemtuzumab Is Effective and Feasible in Patients With Relapsed or Refractory B-Cell Chronic Lymphocytic Leukemia: Results of a Phase II Trial," *J Clin Oncol*, 2005, 23(28):7024-31.

Flinn IW, Neuberg DS, Grever MR, et al, "Phase III Trial of Fludarabine Plus Cyclophosphamide Compared With Fludarabine for Patients With Previously Untreated Chronic Lymphocytic Leukemia: US Intergroup Trial E2997," *J Clin Oncol*, 2007, 25(7):793-8.

Forstpointner R, Dreyling M, Repp R, et al, "The Addition of Rituximab to a Combination of Fludarabine, Cyclophosphamide, Mitoxantrone (FCM) Significantly Increases the Response Rate and Prolongs Survival as Compared With FCM Alone in Patients With Relapsed and Refractory Follicular and Mantle Cell Lymphomas: Results of a Prospective Randomized Study of the German Low-Grade Lymphoma Study Group," *Blood*, 2004, 104(10):3064-71.

Forstpointner R, Unterhalt M, Dreyling M, et al, "Maintenance Therapy With Rituximab Leads to a Significant Prolongation of Response Duration After Salvage Therapy With a Combination of Rituximab, Fludarabine, Cyclophosphamide, and Mitoxantrone (R-FCM) in Patients With Recurring and Refractory Follicular and Mantle Cell Lymphomas: Results of a Prospective Randomized Study of the German Low Grade Lymphoma Study Group (GLSG)," *Blood*, 2006, 108 (13):4003-8.

Gill S, Carney D, Ritchie D, et al, "The Frequency, Manifestations, and Duration of Prolonged Cytopenias After First-Line Fludarabine Combination Therapy," *Ann Oncol*, 2010, 21(2):331-4.

Giralt S, Aleman A, Anagnostopoulos A, et al, "Fludarabine/Melphalan Conditioning for Allogeneic Transplantation in Patients With Multiple Myeloma," *Bone Marrow Transplant*, 2002, 30 (6):367-73.

Hagenbeek A, Eghbali H, Monfardini S, et al, "Phase III Intergroup Study of Fludarabine Phosphate Compared With Cyclophosphamide, Vincristine, and Prednisone Chemotherapy in Newly Diagnosed Patients With Stage III and IV Low-Grade Malignant Non-Hodgkin's Lymphoma," *J Clin Oncol*, 2006, 24(10):1590-6.

Keating MJ, O'Brien S, Albitar M, et al, "Early Results of a Chemoimmunotherapy Regimen of Fludarabine, Cyclophosphamide, and Rituximab as Initial Therapy for Chronic Lymphocytic Leukemia," *J Clin Oncol*, 2005, 23(18):4079-88.

Keating MJ, O'Brien S, McLaughlin P, et al, "Clinical Experience With Fludarabine in Hemato-Oncology," *Hematol Cell Ther*, 1996, 38(Suppl 2):83-91.

Khouri IF, McLaughlin P, Saliba RM, et al, "Eight-Year Experience With Allogeneic Stem Cell Transplantation for Relapsed Follicular Lymphoma After Nonmyeloablative Conditioning With Fludarabine, Cyclophosphamide, and Rituximab," *Blood*, 2008, 111(12):5530-6.

Lange BJ, Smith FO, Feusner J, et al, "Outcomes in CCG-2961, a Children's Oncology Group Phase 3 Trial for Untreated Pediatric Acute Myeloid Leukemia: A Report From the Children's Oncology Group," *Blood*, 2008, 111(3):1044-53.

McLaughlin P, Hagemeister FB, Rodriguez MA, et al, "Safety of Fludarabine, Mitoxantrone, and Dexamethasone Combined With Rituximab in the Treatment of Stage IV Indolent Lymphoma," *Semin Oncol*, 2000, 27(6 Suppl 12):37-41.

McLaughlin P, Hagemeister FB, Romaguera JE, et al, "Fludarabine, Mitoxantrone, and Dexamethasone: An Effective New Regimen for Indolent Lymphoma," *J Clin Oncol*, 1996, 14(4):1262-8.

Montillo M, Mirto S, Petti MC, et al, "Fludarabine, Cytarabine, and G-CSF (FLAG) for the Treatment of Poor Risk Acute Myeloid Leukemia," *Am J Hematol*, 1998, 58(2):105-9.

Pulsipher MA, Boucher KM, Wall D, et al, "Reduced-Intensity Allogeneic Transplantation in Pediatric Patients Ineligible for Myeloablative Therapy: Results of the Pediatric Blood and Marrow Transplant Consortium Study ONC0313," *Blood*, 2009, 114(7):1429-36.

Rezvani AR, Storer B, Maris M, et al, "Nonmyeloablative Allogeneic Hematopoietic Cell Transplantation in Relapsed, Refractory, and Transformed Indolent Non-Hodgkin's Lymphoma," *J Clin Oncol*, 2008, 26(2):211-7.

Robak T, Dmoszynska A, Solal-Céligny P, et al, "Rituximab Plus Fludarabine and Cyclophosphamide Prolongs Progression-Free Survival Compared With Fludarabine and Cyclophosphamide Alone in Previously Treated Chronic Lymphocytic Leukemia," *J Clin Oncol*, 2010, 28 (10):1756-65.

Sacchi S, Pozzi S, Marcheselli R, et al, "Rituximab in Combination With Fludarabine and Cyclophosphamide in the Treatment of Patients With Recurrent Follicular Lymphoma," *Cancer*, 2007, 110(1):121-8.

Schetelig J, Bornhauser M, Kiehl M, et al, "Reduced-Intensity Conditioning With Busulfan and Fludarabine With or Without Antithymocyte Globulin in HLA-Identical Sibling Transplantation - A Retrospective Analysis," *Bone Marrow Transplant*, 2004, 33(5):483-90.

Treon SP, Branagan AR, Ioakimidis L, et al, "Long-Term Outcomes to Fludarabine and Rituximab in Waldenström Macroglobulinemia," *Blood*, 2009, 113(16):3673-8.

Tsimberidou AM, McLaughlin P, Younes A, et al, "Fludarabine, Mitoxantrone, Dexamethasone (FND) Compared With an Alternating Triple Therapy (ATT) Regimen in Patients With Stage IV Indolent Lymphoma," *Blood*, 2002, 100(13):4351-7.

Tsimberidou AM, Wierda WG, Plunkett W, et al, "Phase I-II Study of Oxaliplatin, Fludarabine, Cytarabine, and Rituximab Combination Therapy in Patients With Richter's Syndrome or Fludarabine-Refractory Chronic Lymphocytic Leukemia," *J Clin Oncol*, 2008, 26(2):196-203.

Virchis A, Koh M, Rankin P, et al, "Fludarabine, Cytosine Arabinoside, Granulocyte-Colony Stimulating Factor With or Without Idarubicin in the Treatment of High Risk Acute Leukaemia of Myelodysplastic Syndromes," *Br J Haematol*, 2004, 124(1):26-32.

Wierda WG, O'Brien SM, Faderl SH, et al, "CFAR, An Active Frontline Regimen for High-Risk Patients With CLL, Including Those With Del 17p," *Blood*, 2008, 112(11):2095 [abstract 2095 from 2008 ASH Annual Meeting].

Wierda W, O'Brien S, Wen S, et al, "Chemoimmunotherapy With Fludarabine, Cyclophosphamide, and Rituximab for Relapsed and Refractory Chronic Lymphocytic Leukemia," *J Clin Oncol*, 2005, 23(18):4070-8.

◆ **Fludarabine Phosphate** *see* Fludarabine *on page* *619*

◆ **5-Fluorocytosine** *see* Flucytosine *on page* *618*

◆ **Fluorodeoxyuridine** *see* Floxuridine *on page* *610*

◆ **Fluoroplex®** *see* Fluorouracil (Topical) *on page* *632*

◆ **5-Fluorouracil** *see* Fluorouracil (Systemic) *on page* *627*

◆ **5-Fluorouracil** *see* Fluorouracil (Topical) *on page* *632*

Fluorouracil (Systemic) (flure oh YOOR a sil)

Related Information

Chemotherapy and Cancer Treatment During Pregnancy *on page* *1829*

Management of Chemotherapy-Induced Nausea and Vomiting *on page* *1786*

Management of Drug Extravasations *on page* *1800*

Oral Mucositis/Stomatitis *on page* *1814*

Safe Handling of Hazardous Drugs *on page* *1904*

Brand Names: U.S. Adrucil®

Index Terms 5-Fluorouracil; 5-FU; FU

Generic Availability (U.S.) Yes

Pharmacologic Category Antineoplastic Agent, Antimetabolite (Pyrimidine Analog)

Use Treatment of carcinomas of the breast, colon, rectum, pancreas, or stomach

Unlabeled Use Treatment of head and neck cancer, esophageal cancer, anal cancer, cervical cancer, bladder cancer, renal cell cancer, and unknown primary cancer

Labeled Contraindications Hypersensitivity to fluorouracil or any component of the formulation; poor nutritional states; depressed bone marrow function; potentially serious infections

Pregnancy Risk Factor D

Lactation Excretion in breast milk unknown/not recommended

Warnings/Precautions Hazardous agent - use appropriate precautions for handling and disposal. Use with caution in patients with impaired kidney or liver function. The drug should be discontinued if intractable vomiting or diarrhea, precipitous falls in leukocyte or platelet counts, gastrointestinal ulcer or bleeding, stomatitis, or esophagopharyngitis, hemorrhage, or myocardial ischemia occurs. Use with caution in patients who have had high-dose pelvic radiation or previous use of alkylating agents. Palmar-plantar erythrodysesthesia (hand-foot) syndrome has been associated with use.

Administration to patients with a genetic deficiency of dihydropyrimidine dehydrogenase (DPD) has been associated with prolonged clearance and increased toxicity following administration (diarrhea, neutropenia, and neurotoxicity); rechallenge has resulted in recurrent toxicity (despite dose reduction). **[U.S. Boxed Warning]: Should be administered under the supervision of an experienced cancer chemotherapy physician.**

Adverse Reactions Toxicity depends on duration of treatment

Cardiovascular: Angina, arrhythmia, heart failure, MI, myocardial ischemia, vasospasm, ventricular ectopy

Central nervous system: Acute cerebellar syndrome, confusion, disorientation, euphoria, headache, nystagmus, stroke

Dermatologic: Alopecia, dermatitis, dry skin, fissuring, palmar-plantar erythrodysesthesia syndrome, pruritic maculopapular rash, photosensitivity, Stevens-Johnson syndrome, toxic epidermal necrolysis, vein pigmentations

Gastrointestinal: Anorexia, bleeding, diarrhea, esophagopharyngitis, mesenteric ischemia (acute), nausea, sloughing, stomatitis, ulceration, vomiting

Hematologic: Myelosuppression (nadir: 9-14 days; recovery by day 30), agranulocytosis, anemia, leukopenia, pancytopenia, thrombocytopenia

Local: Thrombophlebitis

Ocular: Lacrimation, lacrimal duct stenosis, photophobia, visual changes

Respiratory: Epistaxis

Miscellaneous: Anaphylaxis, generalized allergic reactions, nail loss

Drug Interactions

Metabolism/Transport Effects Inhibits CYP2C9 (strong)

Avoid Concomitant Use

Avoid concomitant use of Fluorouracil (Systemic) with any of the following: BCG; CloZAPine; Natalizumab; Pimecrolimus; Tacrolimus (Topical); Vaccines (Live)

Increased Effect/Toxicity

Fluorouracil (Systemic) may increase the levels/effects of: Carvedilol; CloZAPine; CYP2C9 Substrates; Diclofenac (Systemic); Fosphenytoin; Leflunomide; Natalizumab; Phenytoin; Vaccines (Live); Vitamin K Antagonists

The levels/effects of Fluorouracil (Systemic) may be increased by: Denosumab; Gemcitabine; Leucovorin Calcium-Levoleucovorin; MetroNIDAZOLE (Systemic); Pimecrolimus; Roflumilast; SORAfenib; Tacrolimus (Topical); Trastuzumab

Decreased Effect

Fluorouracil (Systemic) may decrease the levels/effects of: BCG; Coccidioidin Skin Test; Sipuleucel-T; Vaccines (Inactivated); Vaccines (Live); Vitamin K Antagonists

The levels/effects of Fluorouracil (Systemic) may be decreased by: Echinacea; SORAfenib

Ethanol/Nutrition/Herb Interactions

Ethanol: Avoid ethanol (due to GI irritation).

Herb/Nutraceutical: Avoid black cohosh, dong quai in estrogen-dependent tumors.

Storage/Stability Store intact vials at room temperature. Protect from light. Slight discoloration does not usually denote decomposition. If exposed to cold, a precipitate may form; **gentle** heating to 60°C will dissolve the precipitate without impairing the potency. Solutions in 50-1000 mL NS or D_5W, or undiluted solutions in syringes are stable for 72 hours at room temperature.

Reconstitution Dilute in 50-1000 mL NS, D_5W, or bacteriostatic NS for infusion

Mechanism of Action A pyrimidine antimetabolite that interferes with DNA synthesis by blocking the methylation of deoxyuridylic acid; fluorouracil inhibits thymidylate synthetase (TS), or is incorporated into RNA. The reduced folate cofactor is required for tight binding to occur between the 5-FdUMP and TS.

Pharmacodynamics/Kinetics

Duration: ~3 weeks

Distribution: V_d: ~22% of total body water; penetrates extracellular fluid, CSF, and third space fluids (eg, pleural effusions and ascitic fluid)

Metabolism: Hepatic (90%); via a dehydrogenase enzyme; FU must be metabolized to be active

Half-life elimination: Biphasic: Initial: 6-20 minutes; two metabolites, FdUMP and FUTP, have prolonged half-lives depending on the type of tissue

Excretion: Lung (large amounts as CO_2); urine (5% as unchanged drug) in 6 hours

Dosing

Adult & Geriatric Details concerning dosing in combination regimens should be consulted.

I.V. bolus:

500 mg/m^2 once weekly **or**

500-600 mg/m^2 every 3 weeks **or**

500-600 mg/m^2/dose days 1 and 8 every 4 weeks **or**

500 mg/m^2/dose days 1 and 8 every 3 weeks **or**

500 mg/m^2/dose days 1 and 4 every 3 weeks **or**

500 mg/m^2/dose days 1, 8, 15, 22, 29, and 36 of an 8-week treatment cycle **or**

425 mg/m^2 on days 1-5 every 4 weeks

Continuous I.V. infusion:

500-750 mg/m^2/day for 5 days every 3 weeks **or**

1000 mg/m^2/day for 4-5 days every 3-4 weeks **or**

2600 mg/m^2 on day 1 every week **or**

1600 mg/m^2/day for 2 days every 2 weeks **or**

400 mg/m^2 bolus followed by 1200 mg/m^2/day for 2 days every 2 weeks **or**

200 mg/m^2/day for 21 days; can repeat 21-day cycle up to 8 cycles

Renal Impairment The FDA-approved labeling does not contain specific dosing adjustment guidelines; however, it is stated that extreme caution should be used in patients with renal impairment.

Hemodialysis: Administer dose following hemodialysis.

Aronoff, 2007: Recommends that dosage adjustment is not needed in adult patients with Cl_{cr} <50 mL/minute and patients receiving hemodialysis should be administered 50% of dose.

Hepatic Impairment The FDA-approved labeling does not contain specific dosing adjustment guidelines; however, it is stated that extreme caution should be used in patients with hepatic impairment. The following guidelines have been used by some clinicians:

Floyd, 2006: Bilirubin >5 mg/dL: Avoid use.

Koren, 1992: Hepatic impairment (degree not specified): Administer <50% of dose, then increase if toxicity does not occur.

Combination Regimens

Anal cancer: Fluorouracil-Mitomycin (Anal Cancer) on page 1659
Bladder cancer: Cisplatin-Fluorouracil (Bladder Cancer) on page 1571
Breast cancer:
- CAF on page 1538
- CEF on page 1556
- CMF on page 1588
- CMF-IV on page 1588
- Docetaxel-FEC on page 1611
- Docetaxel-Trastuzumab-FEC on page 1616
- Dox-CMF (Sequential) on page 1617
- FAC on page 1641
- FEC on page 1642
- Vinorelbine-FEC on page 1773
- Vinorelbine-Trastuzumab-FEC on page 1775

Cervical cancer: Cisplatin-Fluorouracil (Cervical Cancer) on page 1571
Colorectal cancer:
- Bevacizumab-Fluorouracil-Leucovorin on page 1530
- Bevacizumab + FOLFIRI (Colorectal) on page 1530
- Bevacizumab-Oxaliplatin-Fluorouracil-Leucovorin on page 1531
- Cetuximab + FOLFIRI (Colorectal) on page 1559
- Cetuximab-FOLFOX4 on page 1560
- FLOX (Colorectal) on page 1645
- Fluorouracil-Leucovorin on page 1653
- Fluorouracil-Leucovorin-Irinotecan (Saltz Regimen) on page 1656
- FOLFIRI (Colorectal Cancer) on page 1659
- FOLFOX1 (Colorectal) on page 1662
- FOLFOX2 (Colorectal) on page 1662
- FOLFOX3 (Colorectal) on page 1662
- FOLFOX4 (Colorectal) on page 1663
- FOLFOX6 and mFOLFOX6 (Colorectal) on page 1663
- FOLFOX7 (Colorectal) on page 1664
- FOLFOXIRI (Colorectal) on page 1665
- FU-LV-CPT-11 on page 1666
- Panitumumab + FOLFIRI (Colorectal) on page 1733
- Panitumumab + FOLFOX4 (Colorectal) on page 1733
- Ziv-Aflibercept + FOLFIRI (Colorectal) on page 1779

Esophageal cancer:
- Cisplatin-Fluorouracil (Esophageal Cancer) on page 1572
- Docetaxel-Cisplatin-Fluorouracil (Gastric/Esophageal Cancer) on page 1609
- Docetaxel-Oxaliplatin-Fluorouracil (Esophageal Cancer) on page 1613
- Docetaxel-Oxaliplatin-Leucovorin-Fluorouracil (Esophageal Cancer) on page 1613
- Epirubicin-Cisplatin-Fluorouracil (Gastric/Esophageal Cancer) on page 1626
- Epirubicin-Oxaliplatin-Fluorouracil (Esophageal Cancer) on page 1627
- Fluorouracil-Leucovorin-Oxaliplatin (Esophageal Cancer) on page 1656
- Irinotecan-Fluorouracil-Leucovorin (Esophageal Cancer) on page 1696
- Oxaliplatin-Fluorouracil (Esophageal Cancer) on page 1724
- Paclitaxel-Cisplatin-Fluorouracil (Esophageal Cancer) on page 1728
- Paclitaxel-Fluorouracil (Esophageal Cancer) on page 1729

Gastric cancer:
- Cisplatin-Fluorouracil (Gastric Cancer) on page 1574
- Docetaxel-Cisplatin-Fluorouracil (Gastric/Esophageal Cancer) on page 1609
- Epirubicin-Cisplatin-Fluorouracil (Gastric/Esophageal Cancer) on page 1626
- Fluorouracil-Leucovorin-Oxaliplatin (Gastric Cancer) on page 1657
- Irinotecan-Leucovorin-Fluorouracil (Gastric Cancer) on page 1697
- Trastuzumab-Cisplatin-Fluorouracil (Gastric Cancer) on page 1758

Head and neck cancer:
- Cetuximab-Carboplatin-Fluorouracil (Head and Neck Cancer) on page 1557
- Cetuximab-Cisplatin-Fluorouracil (Head and Neck Cancer) on page 1558
- Cisplatin-Fluorouracil (Head and Neck Cancer) on page 1575
- Docetaxel-Cisplatin-Fluorouracil (Head and Neck Cancer) on page 1610
- Fluorouracil-Carboplatin (Head and Neck Cancer) on page 1652
- Fluorouracil-Hydroxyurea (Head and Neck Cancer) on page 1653

Pancreatic cancer:
- Fluorouracil-Leucovorin (Pancreatic) on page 1658
- FOLFIRINOX (Pancreatic) on page 1661
- FOLFOX (Pancreatic) on page 1665

Renal cell cancer: Gemcitabine-Fluorouracil (RCC) on page 1672

Unknown primary, squamous cell:
- Cisplatin-Docetaxel-Fluorouracil (Unknown Primary) on page 1568
- Cisplatin-Fluorouracil-Paclitaxel (Unknown Primary) on page 1577

Administration I.V.: I.V. bolus as a slow push or short (5-15 minutes) bolus infusion, or as a continuous infusion. Doses >1000 mg/m^2 are usually administered as a 24 hour infusion, although some protocols may be continuous infusion with lower doses. Toxicity may be reduced by giving the drug as a constant infusion. Bolus doses may be administered by slow IVP or IVPB.

Vesicant/Extravasation Risk May be an irritant

Monitoring Parameters CBC with differential and platelet count, renal function tests, liver function tests

Dietary Considerations Increase dietary intake of thiamine.

Additional Information Oncology Comment: An investigational uridine prodrug, uridine triacetate (formerly called vistonuridine), has been studied in a limited number of cases of fluorouracil overdose. Of 17 patients receiving uridine triacetate beginning within 8-96 hours after fluorouracil overdose, all patients fully recovered (von Borstel, 2009). Updated data has described a total of 28 patients treated with uridine triacetate for fluorouracil overdose (including overdoses related to continuous infusions delivering fluorouracil at rates faster than prescribed), all of whom recovered fully (Bamat, 2010). Refer to Uridine Triacetate monograph.

Dosage Forms Excipient information presented when available (limited, particularly for generics); consult specific product labeling.

Injection, solution: 50 mg/mL (10 mL, 20 mL, 50 mL, 100 mL)

Adrucil®: 50 mg/mL (10 mL, 50 mL, 100 mL)

References

Aronoff GR, Bennett WM, Berns JS, et al, *Drug Prescribing in Renal Failure: Dosing Guidelines for Adults and Children*, 5th ed. Philadelphia, PA: American College of Physicians; 2007, p 100.

Bamat MK, Tremmel R, O'Neil JD, et al, "Uridine Triacetate: An Orally Administered Life-Saving Antidote for 5-FU Overdose," *J Clin Oncol*, 28(15s):9084 [abstract 9084 from 2010 ASCO Annual Meeting].

Diasio RB and Johnson MR, "The Role of Pharmacogenetics and Pharmacogenomics in Cancer Chemotherapy With 5-Fluorouracil," *Pharmacology*, 2000, 61(3):199-203.

Floyd J, Mirza I, Sachs B, et al, "Hepatotoxicity of Chemotherapy," *Semin Oncol*, 2006, 33 (1):50-67.

Koren G, Beatty K, Seto A, et al, "The Effects of Impaired Liver Function on the Elimination of Antineoplastic Agents," *Ann Pharmacother*, 1992, 26(3):363-71.

Morgan C, Tillett T, Braybrooke J, et al, "Management of Uncommon Chemotherapy-Induced Emergencies," *Lancet Oncol*, 2011, 12(8):806-14.

von Borstel R, O'Neil J, and Bamat M, "Vistonuridine: An Orally Administered, Life-Saving Antidote for 5-Fluorouracil (5FU) Overdose," *J Clin Oncol*, 2009, 27(15S):9616 [abstract 9616 from 2009 ASCO Annual Meeting].

Fluorouracil (Topical) (flure oh YOOR a sil)

Related Information

Safe Handling of Hazardous Drugs *on page 1904*

Brand Names: U.S. Carac®; Efudex®; Fluoroplex®

Brand Names: Canada Efudex®; Fluoroplex®

Index Terms 5-Fluorouracil; 5-FU; FU

Generic Availability (U.S.) Yes

Pharmacologic Category Antineoplastic Agent, Antimetabolite (Pyrimidine Analog); Topical Skin Product

Use Management of actinic or solar keratoses and superficial basal cell carcinomas

Labeled Contraindications Hypersensitivity to fluorouracil or any component of the formulation; dihydropyrimidine dehydrogenase (DPD) enzyme deficiency; pregnancy

Pregnancy Risk Factor X

Lactation Excretion in breast milk unknown/not recommended

Warnings/Precautions Avoid topical application to mucous membranes due to potential for local inflammation and ulceration. The use of occlusive dressings with topical preparations may increase the severity of inflammation in nearby skin areas. Avoid exposure to ultraviolet rays during and immediately following therapy. May be associated with delayed-type hypersensitivity reactions. Patch testing may not be useful in the evaluation of these reactions. Individuals lacking DPD enzyme actiivty may exhibit severe toxicity. In cases where this deficiency has not been previously recognized, symptoms of toxicity (stomatitis, diarrhea, neutropenia, and/or neurotoxicity) or other signs of DPD deficiency should prompt immediate discontinuation and evaluation.

Adverse Reactions Note: Systemic toxicity normally associated with parenteral administration (including neutropenia, neurotoxicity, and gastrointestinal toxicity) has been associated with topical use particularly in patients with a genetic deficiency of dihydropyrimidine dehydrogenase (DPD).

Central nervous system: Headache, insomnia, irritability

Dermatologic: Alopecia, photosensitivity, pruritus, rash, scarring, telangiectasia

Gastrointestinal: Medicinal taste, stomatitis

Hematologic: Leukocytosis, thrombocytopenia
Local: Application site reactions: Allergic contact dermatitis, burning, crusting, dryness, edema, erosion, erythema, hyperpigmentation, irritation, pain, soreness, ulceration
Ocular: Eye irritation (burning, watering, sensitivity, stinging, itching)
Miscellaneous: Birth defects, herpes simplex, miscarriage

Drug Interactions

Metabolism/Transport Effects Inhibits CYP2C9 (strong)

Avoid Concomitant Use

Avoid concomitant use of Fluorouracil (Topical) with any of the following: BCG; Natalizumab; Pimecrolimus; Tacrolimus (Topical); Vaccines (Live)

Increased Effect/Toxicity

Fluorouracil (Topical) may increase the levels/effects of: Carvedilol; CYP2C9 Substrates; Diclofenac (Systemic); Fosphenytoin; Leflunomide; Natalizumab; Phenytoin; Vaccines (Live); Vitamin K Antagonists

The levels/effects of Fluorouracil (Topical) may be increased by: Denosumab; Gemcitabine; Leucovorin Calcium-Levoleucovorin; Pimecrolimus; Roflumilast; SORAfenib; Tacrolimus (Topical); Trastuzumab

Decreased Effect

Fluorouracil (Topical) may decrease the levels/effects of: BCG; Coccidioidin Skin Test; Sipuleucel-T; Vaccines (Inactivated); Vaccines (Live); Vitamin K Antagonists

The levels/effects of Fluorouracil (Topical) may be decreased by: Echinacea; SORAfenib

Storage/Stability Store at controlled room temperature of 15°C to 30°C (59°F to 86°F).

Mechanism of Action A pyrimidine antimetabolite that interferes with DNA synthesis by blocking the methylation of deoxyuridylic acid; fluorouracil inhibits thymidylate synthetase (TS), or is incorporated into RNA. The reduced folate cofactor is required for tight binding to occur between the 5-FdUMP and TS.

Pharmacodynamics/Kinetics

Absorption: ~6% of a topical dose is absorbed systemically (Efudex® 5%)
Time to peak: 1 hour (Carac®)

Dosing

Adult & Geriatric

Refer to individual protocols.

Actinic keratoses: Topical:

Carac™: Apply thin film to lesions once daily for up to 4 weeks, as tolerated
Efudex®: Apply to lesions twice daily for 2-4 weeks; complete healing may not be evident for 1-2 months following treatment
Fluoroplex®: Apply to lesions twice daily for 2-6 weeks

Superficial basal cell carcinoma: Topical: Efudex® 5%: Apply to affected lesions twice daily for 3-6 weeks; treatment may be continued for up to 10-12 weeks

Administration Apply 10 minutes after washing, rinsing, and drying the affected area. Apply using fingertip (wash hands immediately after application) or nonmetal applicator. Do not cover area with an occlusive dressing. Wash hands immediately after topical application of the 5% cream. Topical preparations are for external use only; not for ophthalmic, oral, or intravaginal use.

Dosage Forms Excipient information presented when available (limited, particularly for generics); consult specific product labeling.

Cream, topical: 5% (40 g)
Carac®: 0.5% (30 g)
Efudex®: 5% (40 g)
Fluoroplex®: 1% (30 g) [contains benzyl alcohol]
Solution, topical: 2% (10 mL); 5% (10 mL)
Efudex®: 5% (10 mL)

Fluoxymesterone (floo oks i MES te rone)

Related Information

Safe Handling of Hazardous Drugs *on page 1904*

Brand Names: U.S. Androxy™

Generic Availability (U.S.) No

Pharmacologic Category Androgen

Use Replacement of endogenous testicular hormone; in females, palliative treatment of breast cancer

Unlabeled Use Stimulation of erythropoiesis, angioneurotic edema

Labeled Contraindications Males with carcinoma of the breast or the prostate (known or suspected); women who are or may become pregnant

Pregnancy Risk Factor X

Lactation Excretion in breast milk unknown/not recommended

Warnings/Precautions Prolonged use and/or high doses may cause peliosis hepatis or liver cell tumors which may not be apparent until liver failure or intra-abdominal hemorrhage develops. Discontinue in case of cholestatic hepatitis with jaundice or abnormal liver function tests. Use with caution in patients with breast cancer; may cause hypercalcemia by stimulating osteolysis. Use with caution in patients with diabetes mellitus; monitor carefully. Use with caution in patients with conditions influenced by edema (eg, cardiovascular disease, migraine, seizure disorder, renal impairment); may cause fluid retention. Discontinue with evidence of mild virilization in women. Use with caution in elderly. Use with caution in hepatic impairment. May accelerate bone maturation without producing compensatory gain in linear growth in children. In prepubertal children, perform radiographic examination of the hand and wrist every 6 months to determine the rate of bone maturation and to assess the effect of treatment on the epiphyseal centers. Product may contain tartrazine.

Adverse Reactions

>10%:
- Male: Priapism
- Female: Menstrual problems (amenorrhea), virilism, breast soreness
- Cardiovascular: Edema
- Dermatologic: Acne

1% to 10%:
- Male: Prostatic carcinoma, hirsutism (increase in pubic hair growth), impotence, testicular atrophy
- Cardiovascular: Edema
- Gastrointestinal: GI irritation, nausea, vomiting
- Genitourinary: Prostatic hyperplasia
- Hepatic: Hepatic dysfunction

<1%:
- Male: Gynecomastia
- Female: Amenorrhea
- Hypercalcemia, leukopenia, polycythemia, hepatic necrosis, cholestatic hepatitis, hypersensitivity reactions

Drug Interactions

Metabolism/Transport Effects None known.

Avoid Concomitant Use There are no known interactions where it is recommended to avoid concomitant use.

Increased Effect/Toxicity

Fluoxymesterone may increase the levels/effects of: CycloSPORINE (Systemic); Vitamin K Antagonists

Decreased Effect There are no known significant interactions involving a decrease in effect.

Storage/Stability Protect from light.

Mechanism of Action Synthetic androgenic anabolic hormone responsible for the normal growth and development of male sex hormones and development of male sex organs and maintenance of secondary sex characteristics; synthetic testosterone derivative with significant androgen activity; stimulates RNA polymerase activity resulting in an increase in protein production; increases bone development; halogenated derivative of testosterone with up to 5 times the activity of methyltestosterone

Pharmacodynamics/Kinetics

Absorption: Rapid

Protein binding: 98%

Metabolism: Hepatic; enterohepatic recirculation

Half-life elimination: 10-100 minutes

Excretion: Urine (90%)

Dosing

Adult & Geriatric

Hypogonadism (Males): Oral: 5-20 mg/day

Delayed puberty (Males): Oral: 2.5-20 mg/day for 4-6 months

Inoperable breast carcinoma (Females): Oral: 10-40 mg/day in divided doses for 1-3 months

Monitoring Parameters In prepubertal children, perform radiographic examination of the hand and wrist every 6 months

Test Interactions Decreased levels of thyroxine-binding globulin; decreased total T_4 serum levels; increased resin uptake of T_3 and T_4

Dosage Forms Excipient information presented when available (limited, particularly for generics); consult specific product labeling.

Tablet, oral:

Androxy™: 10 mg [scored]

Controlled Substance C-III

◆ **5-Flurocytosine** *see* Flucytosine *on page 618*

Flutamide (FLOO ta mide)

Related Information

Safe Handling of Hazardous Drugs *on page 1904*

Brand Names: Canada Apo-Flutamide®; Euflex®; Eulexin®; Novo-Flutamide; PMS-Flutamide; Teva-Flutamide

Index Terms 4′-Nitro-3′-Trifluoromethylisobutyrantide; Eulexin; Niftolid; SCH 13521

Generic Availability (U.S.) Yes

Pharmacologic Category Antineoplastic Agent, Antiandrogen

Use Treatment of metastatic prostatic carcinoma in combination therapy with LHRH agonist analogues

Unlabeled Use Female hirsutism

Labeled Contraindications Hypersensitivity to flutamide or any component of the formulation; severe hepatic impairment

Pregnancy Risk Factor D

Warnings/Precautions Hazardous agent - use appropriate precautions for handling and disposal. **[U.S. Boxed Warning]: Hospitalization and, rarely, death due to liver failure have been reported in patients taking flutamide.** Elevated serum transaminase levels, jaundice, hepatic encephalopathy, and acute hepatic failure have been reported. Androgen-deprivation therapy may increase the risk for cardiovascular disease (Levine, 2010). Product labeling states flutamide is not for use in women, particularly for non-life-threatening conditions. In some patients, the toxicity reverses after discontinuation of therapy. About 50% of the cases occur within the first 3 months of treatment. Serum transaminase levels should be measured prior to starting treatment, monthly for 4 months, and periodically thereafter. Liver function tests should be obtained at the first suggestion of liver dysfunction (nausea, vomiting, abdominal pain, fatigue, anorexia, "flu-like" symptoms, hyperbilirubinuria, jaundice, or right upper quadrant tenderness). Flutamide should be immediately discontinued any time a patient has jaundice, and/or an ALT level greater than twice the upper limit of normal. Flutamide should not be used in patients whose ALT values are greater than twice the upper limit of normal.

Patients with glucose-6 phosphate dehydrogenase deficiency or hemoglobin M disease or smokers are at risk of toxicities associated with aniline exposure, including methemoglobinemia, hemolytic anemia, and cholestatic jaundice. Monitor methemoglobin levels.

Adverse Reactions

>10%:

- Endocrine & metabolic: Galactorrhea (9% to 42%), breast tenderness, gynecomastia, hot flashes, impotence, libido decreased, tumor flare
- Gastrointestinal: Vomiting (11% to 12%), nausea
- Hepatic: AST increased (transient; mild), LDH increased (transient; mild)

1% to 10%:

- Cardiovascular: Hypertension (1%), edema
- Central nervous system: Anxiety, confusion, depression, dizziness, drowsiness, headache, insomnia, nervousness
- Dermatologic: Ecchymosis, photosensitivity, pruritus
- Gastrointestinal: Upset stomach (4% to 6%), anorexia, appetite increased, constipation, diarrhea, indigestion
- Hematologic: Anemia (6%), leukopenia (3%), thrombocytopenia (1%)
- Neuromuscular & skeletal: Weakness (1%)
- Miscellaneous: Herpes zoster

<1%: Discoloration of urine (yellow), hepatic failure, hepatitis, hypersensitivity pneumonitis, jaundice, malignant breast neoplasm (male), MI, pulmonary embolism, sulfhemoglobinemia, thrombophlebitis

Drug Interactions

Metabolism/Transport Effects **Substrate** of CYP1A2 (major), CYP3A4 (major); **Note:** Assignment of Major/Minor substrate status based on clinically relevant drug interaction potential; **Inhibits** CYP1A2 (weak)

Avoid Concomitant Use

Avoid concomitant use of Flutamide with any of the following: Conivaptan

Increased Effect/Toxicity

Flutamide may increase the levels/effects of: Prilocaine

The levels/effects of Flutamide may be increased by: Abiraterone Acetate; Conivaptan; CYP1A2 Inhibitors (Moderate); CYP1A2 Inhibitors (Strong); CYP3A4 Inhibitors (Moderate); CYP3A4 Inhibitors (Strong); Dasatinib; Deferasirox; Ivacaftor; Mifepristone

Decreased Effect

The levels/effects of Flutamide may be decreased by: CYP1A2 Inducers (Strong); CYP3A4 Inducers (Strong); Cyproterone; Deferasirox; Herbs (CYP3A4 Inducers); Tocilizumab

Ethanol/Nutrition/Herb Interactions

Food: No effect on bioavailability of flutamide.

Herb/Nutraceutical: St John's wort may decrease flutamide levels.

Storage/Stability Store at room temperature.

Mechanism of Action Nonsteroidal antiandrogen that inhibits androgen uptake or inhibits binding of androgen in target tissues

Pharmacodynamics/Kinetics

Absorption: Oral: Rapid and complete

Protein binding: Parent drug: 94% to 96%; 2-hydroxyflutamide: 92% to 94%

Metabolism: Extensively hepatic to more than 10 metabolites, primarily 2-hydroxyflutamide (active)

Half-life elimination: 5-6 hours (2-hydroxyflutamide)

Excretion: Primarily urine (as metabolites)

Dosing

Adult & Geriatric Refer to individual protocols.

Prostate carcinoma: Oral: 250 mg 3 times/day; alternatively, once-daily doses of 0.5-1.5 g have been used (unlabeled dosing)

Female hirsutism (unlabeled use): Oral: 250 mg daily (Moghetti, 2000)

Combination Regimens

Prostate cancer:

FL on page 1642

FZ on page 1667

Administration Usually administered orally in 3 divided doses. Contents of capsule may be opened and mixed with applesauce, pudding, or other soft foods. Mixing with a beverage is not recommended.

Monitoring Parameters Serum transaminase levels should be measured prior to starting treatment and should be repeated monthly for the first 4 months of therapy, and periodically thereafter. LFTs should be checked at the first sign or symptom of liver dysfunction (eg, nausea, vomiting, abdominal pain, fatigue, anorexia, flu-like symptoms, hyperbilirubinuria, jaundice, or right upper quadrant tenderness). Other parameters include tumor reduction, testosterone/estrogen, prostate specific antigen, and phosphatase serum levels.

Dosage Forms Excipient information presented when available (limited, particularly for generics); consult specific product labeling.

Capsule, oral: 125 mg

References

Hunter MH and Carek PJ, "Evaluation and Treatment of Women With Hirsutism," *Am Fam Physician*, 2003, 67(12):2565-72.

Levine GN, D'Amico AV, Berger P, et al, "Androgen-Deprivation Therapy in Prostate Cancer and Cardiovascular Risk. A Science Advisory from the American Heart Association, American Cancer Society, and American Urological Association," *Circulation*, 2010, 121:831-38.

Luo S, Martel C, Chen C, "Daily Dosing With Flutamide or Casodex Exerts Maximal Antiandrogenic Activity," *Urology*, 1997, 50(6):913-9.

Moghetti P, Tosi F, Tosti A, et al, "Comparison of Spironolactone, Flutamide, and Finasteride Efficacy in the Treatment of Hirsutism: A Randomized, Double Blind, Placebo-Controlled Trial," *J Clin Endocrinol Metab*, 2000, 85(1):89-94.

Thrasher JB, Deeths J, and Bennett C, "Comparative Study of the Clinical Efficacy of Two Dosing Regimens of Flutamide," *Mol Urol*, 2000, 4(3):259-63.

- **Folinate Calcium** *see* Leucovorin Calcium *on page 870*
- **Folinic Acid (error prone synonym)** *see* Leucovorin Calcium *on page 870*
- **Folotyn®** *see* PRALAtrexate *on page 1190*

Fondaparinux (fon da PARE i nuks)

Related Information

Venous Thromboembolism in the Cancer Patient *on page 1883*

Brand Names: U.S. Arixtra®

Brand Names: Canada Arixtra®

Index Terms Fondaparinux Sodium

Generic Availability (U.S.) Yes

Pharmacologic Category Factor Xa Inhibitor

Use Prophylaxis of deep vein thrombosis (DVT) in patients undergoing surgery for hip replacement, knee replacement, hip fracture (including extended prophylaxis following hip fracture surgery), or abdominal surgery (in patients at risk for thromboembolic complications); treatment of acute pulmonary embolism (PE); treatment of acute DVT without PE

Canadian labeling: Additional uses (not approved in U.S.): Unstable angina or non-ST segment elevation myocardial infarction (UA/NSTEMI) for the prevention of death and subsequent MI; ST segment elevation MI (STEMI) for the prevention of death and myocardial reinfarction

Unlabeled Use Prophylaxis of DVT in patients with a history of heparin-induced thrombocytopenia (HIT); treatment of acute thrombosis (unrelated to HIT) in patients with a past history of HIT; acute symptomatic superficial vein thrombosis (≥5 cm in length) of the legs

Labeled Contraindications Hypersensitivity to fondaparinux or any component of the formulation; severe renal impairment (Cl_{cr} <30 mL/minute); body weight <50 kg (prophylaxis); active major bleeding; bacterial endocarditis; thrombocytopenia associated with a positive *in vitro* test for antiplatelet antibody in the presence of fondaparinux

Pregnancy Risk Factor B

Lactation Excretion in breast milk unknown/use caution

Warnings/Precautions **[U.S. Boxed Warning]: Spinal or epidural hematomas, including subsequent paralysis, may occur with recent or anticipated neuraxial anesthesia (epidural or spinal anesthesia) or spinal puncture in patients anticoagulated with LMWH, heparinoids, or fondaparinux.** Consider risk versus benefit prior to spinal procedures; risk is increased by the use of concomitant agents which may alter hemostasis, the use of indwelling epidural catheters for analgesia, a history of spinal deformity or spinal surgery, as well as a history of traumatic or repeated epidural or spinal punctures. Patient should be observed closely for bleeding and signs and symptoms of neurological impairment if therapy is administered during or immediately following diagnostic lumbar puncture, epidural anesthesia, or spinal anesthesia.

Discontinue use 24 hours prior to CABG and dose with unfractionated heparin per institutional practice (Jneid, 2012). Use caution in patients with moderate renal dysfunction (Cl_{cr} 30-50 mL/minute); contraindicated in patients with Cl_{cr} <30 mL/minute. Discontinue if severe dysfunction or labile function develops.

Use caution in congenital or acquired bleeding disorders; bacterial endocarditis; renal impairment; hepatic impairment; active ulcerative or angiodysplastic gastrointestinal disease; hemorrhagic stroke; shortly after brain, spinal, or ophthalmologic surgery; or in patients taking platelet inhibitors. Risk of major bleeding may be increased if initial dose is administered earlier than recommended (initiation recommended at 6-8 hours following surgery). Discontinue agents that may enhance the risk of hemorrhage if possible. Although considered an insensitive measure of fondaparinux activity, there have been postmarketing reports of bleeding associated with elevated aPTT. Has occurred with administration, including very rare reports of thrombocytopenia with thrombosis similar to heparin-induced thrombocytopenia (HIT); however, has been used in patients with current or history of HIT due to a lack of an immune-mediated effect on platelets (Guyatt [ACCP], 2012; Savi, 2005). Use is contraindicated in patients with thrombocytopenia associated with a positive *in vitro* test for antiplatelet antibodies in the presence of fondaparinux. Monitor patients closely and discontinue therapy if platelets fall to <100,000/mm^3 and/or thrombosis develops.

For subcutaneous administration; not for I.M. administration. Do not use interchangeably (unit for unit) with low molecular weight heparins, heparin, or heparinoids. Use caution in patients <50 kg who are being treated for DVT/PE; dosage reduction recommended. Contraindicated in patients <50 kg when used for prophylactic therapy. Use with caution in the elderly. The needle guard contains natural latex rubber.

The administration of fondaparinux as the sole anticoagulant is **not recommended** during PCI due to an increased risk for guiding-catheter thrombosis. Use of an anticoagulant with antithrombin activity (eg, unfractionated heparin) is recommended as adjunctive therapy to PCI even if prior treatment with fondaparinux (must take into account whether GP IIb/IIIa antagonists have been administered) (Levine, 2011). Do not administer with other agents that increase the risk of hemorrhage unless they are essential for the management of the underlying condition (eg, warfarin for treatment of VTE).

Adverse Reactions As with all anticoagulants, bleeding is the major adverse effect. Hemorrhage may occur at any site. Risk appears increased by a number of factors including renal dysfunction, age (>75 years), and weight (<50 kg).

>10%:

- Central nervous system: Fever (4% to 14%)
- Gastrointestinal: Nausea (3% to 11%)
- Hematologic: Anemia (1% to 20%)

1% to 10%:

- Cardiovascular: Edema (9%), hypotension (4%), hypertension (2%), chest pain (1%), thrombosis PCI catheter (without heparin 1%)
- Central nervous system: Insomnia (4% to 5%), headache (2% to 5%), dizziness (4%), confusion (3%), pain (2%), anxiety (1%)
- Dermatologic: Rash (8%), purpura (4%), bullous eruption (3%), bruising (1%)
- Endocrine & metabolic: Hypokalemia (1% to 4%)
- Gastrointestinal: Constipation (5% to 9%), vomiting (1% to 6%), diarrhea (2% to 3%), dyspepsia (2%), abdominal pain (1%)
- Genitourinary: Urinary tract infection (2% to 4%), urinary retention (3%)

Hematologic: Minor bleeding (2% to 4%), moderate thrombocytopenia (50,000-100,000/mm^3: 3%), hematoma (3%), major bleeding (1% to 3%), prothrombin decreased (1%), risk of major bleeding increased as high as 5% in patients receiving initial dose <6 hours following surgery
Hepatic: ALT increased (≤3%), AST increased (≤2%)
Local: Injection site reaction (bleeding, rash, pruritus)
Neuromuscular & skeletal: Back pain (1%), leg pain (1%)
Respiratory: Cough (2%), pneumonia (2%), epistaxis (1%)
Miscellaneous: Wound drainage increased (5%)

<1%, postmarketing, and/or case reports: aPTT increased (associated with bleeding), heparin-induced thrombocytopenia (1 case report), hepatic dysfunction, severe thrombocytopenia (<50,000/mm^3)

Drug Interactions

Metabolism/Transport Effects None known.

Avoid Concomitant Use

Avoid concomitant use of Fondaparinux with any of the following: Omacetaxine; Rivaroxaban

Increased Effect/Toxicity

Fondaparinux may increase the levels/effects of: Anticoagulants; Collagenase (Systemic); Dabigatran Etexilate; Deferasirox; Ibritumomab; Omacetaxine; Rivaroxaban; Tositumomab and Iodine I 131 Tositumomab

The levels/effects of Fondaparinux may be increased by: Antiplatelet Agents; Dasatinib; Drotrecogin Alfa (Activated); Herbs (Anticoagulant/Antiplatelet Properties); Nonsteroidal Anti-Inflammatory Agents; Pentosan Polysulfate Sodium; Prostacyclin Analogues; Salicylates; Thrombolytic Agents; Tipranavir; Vitamin E

Decreased Effect There are no known significant interactions involving a decrease in effect.

Ethanol/Nutrition/Herb Interactions Herb/Nutraceutical: Avoid alfalfa, anise, bilberry, bladderwrack, bromelain, cat's claw, celery, coleus, cordyceps, dong quai, evening primrose oil, fenugreek, feverfew, garlic, ginger, ginkgo biloba, ginseng (American/Panax/Siberian), grapeseed, green tea, guggul, horse chestnut seed, horseradish, licorice, prickly ash, red clover, reishi, sweet clover, turmeric, white willow (all possess anticoagulant or antiplatelet activity and as such, may enhance the anticoagulant effects of fondaparinux).

Storage/Stability Store at 25°C (77°F); excursions permitted to 15°C to 30°C (59°F to 86°F).

Canadian labeling: For I.V. administration: Manufacturer recommends immediate use once diluted in NS, but is stable for up to 24 hours at 15°C to 30°C (59°F to 86°F).

Reconstitution Canadian labeling: For I.V. administration: May mix with 25 mL or 50 mL NS

Mechanism of Action Fondaparinux is a synthetic pentasaccharide that causes an antithrombin III-mediated selective inhibition of factor Xa. Neutralization of factor Xa interrupts the blood coagulation cascade and inhibits thrombin formation and thrombus development.

Pharmacodynamics/Kinetics

Absorption: SubQ: Rapid and complete
Distribution: V_d: 7-11 L; mainly in blood
Protein binding: ≥94% to antithrombin III
Bioavailability: SubQ: 100%
Half-life elimination: 17-21 hours; prolonged with renal impairment

Time to peak: SubQ: 2-3 hours
Excretion: Urine (~77%, unchanged drug)

Dosing

Adult & Geriatric

DVT prophylaxis: SubQ: Adults ≥50 kg: 2.5 mg once daily. **Note:** Prophylactic use contraindicated in patients <50 kg. Initiate dose after hemostasis has been established, 6-8 hours postoperatively.

DVT prophylaxis with history of HIT (unlabeled use): SubQ: 2.5 mg once daily (Blackmer, 2009; Harenberg, 2004; Parody, 2003)

Usual duration: 5-9 days (up to 10 days following abdominal surgery or up to 11 days following hip replacement or knee replacement). The American College of Chest Physicians recommends a minimum of 10-14 days for patients undergoing total hip arthroplasty, total knee arthroplasty, or hip fracture surgery; extended duration of up to 35 days suggested (Guyatt, 2012).

Acute DVT/PE treatment: SubQ: **Note:** Start warfarin on the first or second treatment day and continue fondaparinux until INR is ≥2 for at least 24 hours (usually 5-7 days) (Guyatt, 2012):

<50 kg: 5 mg once daily
50-100 kg: 7.5 mg once daily
>100 kg: 10 mg once daily

Usual duration: 5-9 days (has been administered up to 26 days)

Acute coronary syndrome (Canadian labeling; unlabeled use in U.S.):

UA/NSTEMI: SubQ: 2.5 mg once daily; initiate as soon as possible after presentation; treat for up to 8 days or until hospital discharge (Anderson, 2007; Yusuf 2006a)

STEMI: I.V.: 2.5 mg once; subsequent doses: SubQ: 2.5 mg once daily; treat for up to 8 days or until hospital discharge (Antman, 2007; Yusuf, 2006b)

Note: Discontinue fondaparinux 24 hours prior to coronary artery bypass graft (CABG) surgery; instead, administer unfractionated heparin per institutional practice (Anderson, 2007).

Acute symptomatic superficial vein thrombosis (≥5 cm in length) of the legs (unlabeled use): SubQ: 2.5 mg once daily for 45 days (Decousus, 2010; Guyatt, 2012)

Acute thrombosis (unrelated to HIT) in patients with a past history of HIT (unlabeled use; Guyatt, 2012; Warkentin, 2011): SubQ:

<50 kg: 5 mg once daily
50-100 kg: 7.5 mg once daily
>100 kg: 10 mg once daily

Renal Impairment

Cl_{cr} 30-50 mL/minute: Use caution; total clearance ~40% lower compared to patients with normal renal function. When used for thromboprophylaxis, the American College of Chest Physicians suggests a 50% reduction in dose or use of low-dose heparin instead of fondaparinux (Garcia, 2012).

Cl_{cr} <30 mL/minute: Use is contraindicated.

Hepatic Impairment

Mild-to-moderate impairment: Dosage adjustment not required; monitor for signs of bleeding.

Severe impairment: No dosage adjustment provided in manufacturer's labeling (has not been studied).

Administration Do **not** administer I.M.; intended for SubQ administration. Do not mix with other injections or infusions. Do not expel air bubble from syringe before injection. Administer according to recommended regimen; when used for DVT prophylaxis, early initiation (before 6 hours after orthopedic surgery) has been associated with increased bleeding. For STEMI patients (Canadian labeling; unlabeled use in U.S.) may administer initial dose as I.V. push or mix in 25-50 mL of NS (do not mix with other agents) and infuse over 2 minutes; flush tubing with NS after infusion to ensure complete administration for fondaparinux.

To convert from I.V. unfractionated heparin (UFH) infusion to SubQ fondaparinux (Nutescu, 2007): Calculate specific dose for fondaparinux based on indication, discontinue UFH, and begin fondaparinux within 1 hour

To convert from SubQ fondaparinux to I.V. UFH infusion (Nutescu, 2007): Discontinue fondaparinux; calculate specific dose for I.V. UFH infusion based on indication; omit heparin bolus/loading dose

For subQ fondaparinux dosed every 24 hours: Start I.V. UFH infusion 22-23 hours after last dose of fondaparinux

Monitoring Parameters Periodic monitoring of CBC, platelet count, serum creatinine, occult blood testing of stools recommended. Anti-Xa activity of fondaparinux can be measured by the assay if fondaparinux is used as the calibrator. PT and aPTT are insensitive measures of fondaparinux activity. If unexpected changes in coagulation parameters or major bleeding occur, discontinue fondaparinux (elevated aPTT associated with bleeding events have been reported in postmarketing data).

Test Interactions International standards of heparin or LMWH are not the appropriate calibrators for antifactor Xa activity of fondaparinux.

Dosage Forms Excipient information presented when available (limited, particularly for generics); consult specific product labeling.

Injection, solution, as sodium [preservative free]: 2.5 mg/0.5 mL (0.5 mL); 5 mg/0.4 mL (0.4 mL); 7.5 mg/0.6 mL (0.6 mL); 10 mg/0.8 mL (0.8 mL)

Arixtra®: 2.5 mg/0.5 mL (0.5 mL); 5 mg/0.4 mL (0.4 mL); 7.5 mg/0.6 mL (0.6 mL); 10 mg/0.8 mL (0.8 mL)

References

Anderson JL, Adams CD, Antman EM, et al, "ACC/AHA 2007 Guidelines for the Management of Patients With Unstable Angina/Non ST-Elevation Myocardial Infarction: Executive Summary. A Report of the American College of Cardiology/American Heart Association Task Force on Practice Guidelines (Writing Committee to Revise the 2002 Guidelines for the Management of Patients with Unstable Angina/Non ST-Elevation Myocardial Infarction) Developed in Collaboration With the American College of Emergency Physicians, The Society of Cardiovascular Angiography and Interventions, and the Society of Thoracic Surgeons," *Circulation*, 2007, 116(7): e148-304.

Antman EM, Hand M, Armstrong PW, et al, "2007 Focused Update of the ACC/AHA 2004 Guidelines for the Management of Patients With ST-Elevation Myocardial Infarction. A Report of the American College of Cardiology/American Heart Association Task Force on Practice Guidelines," *J Am Coll Cardiol*, 2008, 51(2):210-49.

Blackmer AB, Oertel MD, and Valgus JM, "Fondaparinux and the Management of Heparin-induced Thrombocytopenia: The Journey Continues," *Ann Pharmacother*, 2009, 43(!0):1636-46.

Decousus H, Prandoni P, Mismetti P, et al, "Fondaparinux for the Treatment of Superficial-Vein Thrombosis in the Legs," *N Engl J Med*, 2010, 363(13):1222-32.

Dempfle CE, "Minor Transplacental Passage of Fondaparinux *in vivo*," *N Engl J Med*, 2004, 350 (18):1914-5.

Garcia DA, Baglin TP, Weitz JI, et al, "Parenteral Anticoagulants: Antithrombotic Therapy and Prevention of Thrombosis, 9th ed: American College of Chest Physicians Evidence-Based Clinical Practice Guidelines," *Chest*, 2012, 141(2 Suppl):24-43.

Guyatt GH, Akl EA, Crowther M, et al, "Executive Summary: Antithrombotic Therapy and Prevention of Thrombosis, 9th ed: American College of Chest Physicians Evidence-Based Clinical Practice Guidelines," *Chest*, 2012, 141(2 Suppl):7-47.

Harenberg J, Jorg I, and Fenyvesi T, "Treatment of Heparin-induced Thrombocytopenia With Fondaparinux," *Haematologica*, 2004, 89(8):1017-8.

Jneid H, Anderson JL, Wright RS, et al, "2012 ACCF/AHA Focused Update of the Guideline for the Management of Patients With Unstable Angina/Non-ST-Elevation Myocardial Infarction (Updating the 2007 Guideline and Replacing the 2011 Focused Update): A Report of the American College of Cardiology Foundation/American Heart Association Task Force on Practice Guidelines," *Circulation*, 2012, 126(7):875-910.

Levine GN, Bates ER, Blankenship JC, et al, "2011 ACCF/AHA/SCAI Guideline for Percutaneous Coronary Intervention: A Report of the American College of Cardiology Foundation/American Heart Association Task Force on Practice Guidelines and the Society for Cardiovascular Angiography and Interventions," *Circulation*, 2011, 124(23):e574-651.

Nutescu EA and Dager W, "Heparin, Low Molecular Weight Heparin, and Fondaparinux," *Managing Anticoagulation Patients in the Hospital*, Gulseth M ed, American Society of Health System Pharmacists®, Bethesda, MD: 2007, 181.

Parody R, Oliver A, Souto JC, et al, "Fondaparinux (Arixtra®), as an Alternative Antithrombotic Prophylaxis When There is Hypersensitivity to Low Molecular Weight and Unfractionated Heparins," *Haematologica*, 2007, 88(11):ECR32.

Savi P, Chong BH, Greinacher A, et al, "Effect of Fondaparinux on Platelet Activation in the Presence of Heparin-Dependent Antibodies: A Blinded Comparative Multicenter Study With Unfractionated Heparin," *Blood*, 2005, 105(1):139-44.

Warkentin TE, Davidson BL, Buller HR, et al, "Prevalence and Risk of Preexisting Heparin-Induced Thrombocytopenia Antibodies in Patients With Acute VTE," *Chest*, 2011, 140(2):366-73.

Warkentin TE, Maurer BT, and Aster RH, "Heparin-Induced Thrombocytopenia Associated With Fondaparinux," *N Engl J Med*, 2007, 356(25):2653-55.

Yusuf S, Mehta SR, Chrolavicius S, et al, "Comparison of Fondaparinux and Enoxaparin in Acute Coronary Syndromes – The Fifth Organization to Assess Strategies in Acute Ischemic Syndromes Investigators," *N Engl J Med*, 2006a, 354(14):1464-76.

Yusuf S, Mehta SR, Chrolavicius S, et al, "Effects of Fondaparinux on Mortality and Reinfarction in Patients With Acute ST-Segment Elevation Myocardial Infarction: The OASIS-6 Randomized Trial," *JAMA*, 2006b, 295(13):1519-30.

◆ **Fondaparinux Sodium** *see* Fondaparinux *on page 638*
◆ **5-Formyl Tetrahydrofolate** *see* Leucovorin Calcium *on page 870*
◆ **Fortaz®** *see* CefTAZidime *on page 254*
◆ **Fortical®** *see* Calcitonin *on page 214*

Fosaprepitant (fos a PRE pi tant)

Related Information

Management of Chemotherapy-Induced Nausea and Vomiting *on page 1786*

Brand Names: U.S. Emend® for Injection

Brand Names: Canada Emend® IV

Index Terms Aprepitant Injection; Fosaprepitant Dimeglumine; L 758,298; MK 0517

Generic Availability (U.S.) No

Pharmacologic Category Antiemetic; Substance P/Neurokinin 1 Receptor Antagonist

Use Prevention of acute and delayed nausea and vomiting associated with moderately- and highly-emetogenic chemotherapy (in combination with other antiemetics)

Labeled Contraindications Hypersensitivity to fosaprepitant, aprepitant, polysorbate 80, or any component of the formulation; concurrent use with pimozide or cisapride

Canadian labeling: Additional contraindications (not in U.S. labeling): Concurrent use with astemizole or terfenadine

Pregnancy Risk Factor B

Lactation Excretion in breast milk unknown/not recommended

Warnings/Precautions Fosaprepitant is rapidly converted to aprepitant, which has a high potential for drug interactions. Use caution with agents primarily metabolized via CYP3A4; aprepitant is a 3A4 inhibitor. Effect on orally administered 3A4 substrates is greater than those administered intravenously. Immediate hypersensitivity has been reported (rarely) with fosaprepitant; stop infusion with hypersensitivity symptoms (dyspnea, erythema, flushing, or anaphylaxis); do not reinitiate. Use caution with hepatic impairment; has not been studied in patients with severe hepatic impairment (Child-Pugh class C). Not studied for treatment of existing nausea and vomiting. Chronic continuous administration of fosaprepitant is not recommended.

Adverse Reactions Adverse reactions reported with aprepitant and fosaprepitant (as part of a combination chemotherapy regimen) occurring at a higher frequency than standard antiemetic therapy:

1% to 10%:

Central nervous system: Fatigue (1% to 3%), headache (2%)

Gastrointestinal: Anorexia (2%), constipation 2%), dyspepsia (2%), diarrhea (1%), eructation (1%)

Hepatic: ALT increased (1% to 3%), AST increased (1%)

Local: Injection site reactions (3%; includes erythema, induration, pain, pruritus, or thrombophlebitis)

Neuromuscular & skeletal: Weakness (3%)

Miscellaneous: Hiccups (5%)

<1%, postmarketing, and/or case reports: Abdominal distention, abdominal pain, acid reflux, acne, alkaline phosphatase increased, anaphylactic reaction, anemia, angioedema, anxiety, bradycardia, candidiasis, cardiovascular disorder, chest discomfort, chills, cognitive disorder, conjunctivitis, cough, disorientation, dizziness, dream abnormality, duodenal ulcer (perforating), dysarthria, dyspnea, dysuria, edema, epigastric distress, erythema, euphoria, feces hard, flatulence, flushing, gait disturbance, gastroesophageal reflux disease, hematuria (microscopic), hot flush, hyperglycemia, hyperhydrosis, hypersensitivity reaction, hypertension, hypoesthesia, hyponatremia, insomnia, lethargy, malaise, miosis, muscle cramp, muscular weakness, myalgia, nausea, neutropenia, neutropenic colitis, neutropenic fever, obstipation, palpitation, pharyngitis, photosensitivity, pollakiuria, polydipsia, polyuria, postnasal drip, pruritus, rash, sensory disturbance, skin lesion, skin oily, sneezing, somnolence, staphylococcal infection, Stevens-Johnson syndrome, stomatitis, subileus, taste alteration, throat irritation, tinnitus, toxic epidermal necrolysis, urticaria, visual acuity decreased, vomiting, weight gain/loss, wheezing, xerostomia

Drug Interactions

Metabolism/Transport Effects Substrate of CYP1A2 (minor), CYP2C19 (minor), CYP3A4 (major); **Note:** Assignment of Major/Minor substrate status based on clinically relevant drug interaction potential; **Inhibits** CYP2C19 (weak), CYP2C9 (weak), CYP3A4 (moderate); **Induces** CYP2C9 (weak/moderate), CYP3A4 (weak/moderate)

Avoid Concomitant Use

Avoid concomitant use of Fosaprepitant with any of the following: Astemizole; Axitinib; Bosutinib; Cisapride; Conivaptan; Pimozide; Terfenadine; Tolvaptan

Increased Effect/Toxicity

Fosaprepitant may increase the levels/effects of: ARIPiprazole; Astemizole; Avanafil; Benzodiazepines (metabolized by oxidation); Bosutinib; Budesonide (Systemic, Oral Inhalation); Cisapride; Colchicine; Corticosteroids (Systemic); CYP3A4 Substrates; Diltiazem; Eplerenone; Everolimus; FentaNYL; Halofantrine; Ivacaftor; Lurasidone; Pimecrolimus; Pimozide; Propafenone; Ranolazine; Salmeterol; Saxagliptin; Terfenadine; Tolvaptan; Vilazodone; Zuclopenthixol

The levels/effects of Fosaprepitant may be increased by: Antifungal Agents (Azole Derivatives, Systemic); Conivaptan; CYP3A4 Inhibitors (Moderate); CYP3A4 Inhibitors (Strong); Dasatinib; Diltiazem; Ivacaftor; Mifepristone

Decreased Effect

Fosaprepitant may decrease the levels/effects of: ARIPiprazole; Axitinib; Contraceptives (Estrogens); Contraceptives (Progestins); Ifosfamide; PARoxetine; Saxagliptin; TOLBUTamide; Warfarin

The levels/effects of Fosaprepitant may be decreased by: CYP3A4 Inducers (Strong); Deferasirox; Herbs (CYP3A4 Inducers); PARoxetine; Rifampin; Tocilizumab

Ethanol/Nutrition/Herb Interactions

Food: Aprepitant serum concentration may be increased when taken with grapefruit juice; avoid concurrent use.

Herb/Nutraceutical: Avoid St John's wort (may decrease aprepitant levels).

Storage/Stability Store intact vials at 2°C to 8°C (36°F to 46°F). Solutions diluted for infusion are stable for 24 hours at room temperature of ≤25°C (≤77°F).

Reconstitution Reconstitute either vial size with 5 mL of sodium chloride 0.9%, directing diluent down side of vial to avoid foaming; swirl gently. Add reconstituted contents of the 150 mg vial to 145 mL sodium chloride 0.9% (add 115 mg vial to 110 mL), resulting in a final concentration of 1 mg/mL; gently invert bag to mix.

Mechanism of Action Fosaprepitant is a prodrug of aprepitant, a substance P/neurokinin 1 (NK1) receptor antagonist. It is rapidly converted to aprepitant which prevents acute and delayed vomiting by inhibiting the substance P/neurokinin 1 (NK1) receptor; augments the antiemetic activity of the 5-HT_3 receptor antagonist and corticosteroid activity and inhibits chemotherapy-induced emesis.

Pharmacodynamics/Kinetics

Distribution: Fosaprepitant: ~5 L; Aprepitant: V_d: ~70 L; crosses the blood-brain barrier

Protein binding: Aprepitant: >95%

Metabolism:

Fosaprepitant: Hepatic and extrahepatic; rapidly (within 30 minutes after the end of infusion) converted to aprepitant (nearly complete conversion)

Aprepitant: Hepatic via CYP3A4 (major); CYP1A2 and CYP2C19 (minor); forms 7 weakly-active metabolites

Half-life elimination: Fosaprepitant: ~2 minutes; Aprepitant: ~9-13 hours

Time to peak, plasma: Fosaprepitant is converted to aprepitant within 30 minutes after the end of infusion

Excretion: Urine (57%); feces (45%)

Dosing

Adult & Geriatric Prevention of chemotherapy-induced nausea/vomiting: I.V.:

Single-dose regimen (for highly-emetogenic chemotherapy): 150 mg over 20-30 minutes ~30 minutes prior to chemotherapy on day 1 only (in combination with a 5-HT_3 antagonist on day 1 and dexamethasone on days 1 to 4)

3-day regimen (for highly-emetogenic chemotherapy): 115 mg over 15 minutes 30 minutes prior to chemotherapy on day 1, followed by aprepitant 80 mg orally on days 2 and 3 (in combination with a 5-HT_3 antagonist on day 1 and dexamethasone on days 1 to 4)

3-day regimen (for moderately-emetogenic chemotherapy): 115 mg over 15 minutes 30 minutes prior to chemotherapy on day 1, followed by aprepitant 80 mg orally on days 2 and 3 (in combination with a 5-HT_3 antagonist and dexamethasone on day 1)

Renal Impairment

Mild, moderate, or severe impairment: No adjustment required.

Dialysis-dependent end-stage renal disease (ESRD): No adjustment required.

Hepatic Impairment

Child-Pugh class A or B: No adjustment required.

Child-Pugh class C: Has not been evaluated; use with caution.

Administration

115 mg: Infuse over 15 minutes 30 minutes prior to chemotherapy

150 mg: Infuse over 20-30 minutes ~30 minutes prior to chemotherapy

Additional Information Oncology Comment: Fosaprepitant is recommended in the National Comprehensive Cancer Network® (NCCN) Clinical Practice Guidelines in Oncology for Antiemesis (version 1.2011) for use on day 1 in combination with a serotonin receptor antagonist and dexamethasone for chemotherapy with high emetic risk and for select moderately emetogenic regimens (carboplatin, cisplatin, doxorubicin, epirubicin, ifosfamide, irinotecan, or methotrexate). Either fosaprepitant 115 mg or aprepitant (125 mg orally) are administered on day 1; for day 2 and 3, patients should receive aprepitant 80 mg orally. The 1-day regimen (fosaprepitant 150 mg on day 1 only) is listed in the guidelines for highly emetogenic treatments.

Dosage Forms Excipient information presented when available (limited, particularly for generics); consult specific product labeling. [DSC] = Discontinued product

Injection, powder for reconstitution:

Emend® for Injection: 115 mg [DSC] [contains edetate disodium, lactose 287.5 mg, polysorbate 80]

Emend® for Injection: 150 mg [contains edetate disodium, lactose 375 mg, polysorbate 80]

References

Multinational Association of Supportive Care in Cancer (MASCC), "Antiemetic Guidelines," Updated April 2010. Available at http://data.memberclicks.com/site/mascc/MASCC_Guidelines_English_2010.pdf

National Comprehensive Cancer Network® (NCCN), "Clinical Practice Guidelines in Oncology™: Antiemesis," Version 1.2011. Available at http://www.nccn.org/professionals/physician_gls/PDF/antiemesis.pdf

Van Belle S, Lichinitser SR, Navari RM, et al," Prevention of Cisplatin-Induced Acute and Delayed Emesis by the Selective Neurokinin-1 Antagonists, L-758,298 and MK-869," *Cancer*, 2002, 94 (11):3032-41.

◆ **Fosaprepitant Dimeglumine** *see* Fosaprepitant *on page 643*

Foscarnet (fos KAR net)

Related Information

Management of Infections *on page 1809*

Oral Mucositis/Stomatitis *on page 1814*

Brand Names: U.S. Foscavir®

Brand Names: Canada Foscavir®

Index Terms PFA; Phosphonoformate; Phosphonoformic Acid

Generic Availability (U.S.) Yes

Pharmacologic Category Antiviral Agent

Use Treatment of acyclovir-resistant mucocutaneous herpes simplex virus (HSV) infections in immunocompromised persons (eg, with advanced AIDS); treatment of CMV retinitis in persons with HIV

Unlabeled Use Other CMV infections (eg, colitis, esophagitis, neurological disease); CMV prophylaxis for cancer patients receiving alemtuzumab therapy or allogeneic stem cell transplant

Labeled Contraindications Hypersensitivity to foscarnet or any component of the formulation

Pregnancy Risk Factor C

Lactation Excretion in breast milk unknown/contraindicated

Warnings/Precautions **[U.S. Boxed Warning]: Indicated only for immunocompromised patients with CMV retinitis and mucocutaneous acyclovir-resistant HSV infection. [U.S. Boxed Warning]: Renal impairment occurs to some degree in the majority of patients treated with foscarnet;** renal impairment may occur at any time and is usually reversible within 1 week following dose adjustment or discontinuation of therapy, however, several patients have died with renal failure within 4 weeks of stopping foscarnet; therefore, renal function should be closely monitored. To reduce the risk of nephrotoxicity and the potential to administer a relative overdose, always calculate the creatine clearance even if serum creatinine is within the normal range. Adequate hydration may reduce the risk of nephrotoxicity; the manufacturer makes specific recommendations regarding this (see Administration).

Imbalance of serum electrolytes or minerals occurs in at least 15% of patients (hypocalcemia, low ionized calcium, hyper/hypophosphatemia, hypomagnesemia, or hypokalemia). Correct electrolytes before initiating therapy. Use caution when administering other medications that cause electrolyte imbalances. Patients who experience signs or symptoms of an electrolyte imbalance should be assessed immediately. **[U.S. Boxed Warning]: Seizures related to plasma electrolyte/mineral imbalance may occur;** incidence has been reported in up to 10% of HIV patients. Risk factors for seizures include impaired baseline renal function, low total serum calcium, and underlying CNS conditions. May cause anemia and granulocytopenia. May cause genital/vascular tissue irritation/ulceration; adequately hydrate and administer only into vein with adequate blood flow to minimize risk. Foscarnet is deposited in teeth and bone of young, growing animals; it has adversely affected tooth enamel development in rats.

Adverse Reactions

>10%:

Central nervous system: Fever (65%), headache (26%)

Endocrine & metabolic: Hypokalemia (16% to 48%), hypocalcemia (15% to 30%), hypomagnesemia (15% to 30%), hypophosphatemia (8% to 26%)

Gastrointestinal: Nausea (47%), diarrhea (30%), vomiting (26%)

Hematologic: Anemia (33%), granulocytopenia (17%)

Renal: Abnormal renal function/decreased creatinine clearance (12%; without adequate hydration 33%)

1% to 10%:

Cardiovascular: Chest pain (1% to 5%), edema (1% to 5%), facial edema (1% to 5%), flushing (1% to 5%), hyper-/hypotension (1% to 5%), palpitation (1% to 5%), ECG changes (1% to 5%)

Central nervous system: Seizures (8% to 10%), anxiety (≥5%), confusion (≥5%), depression (≥5%), dizziness (≥5%), fatigue (≥5%), hypoesthesia

(≥5%), malaise (≥5%), pain (≥5%), aggressiveness (1% to 5%), agitation (1% to 5%), amnesia (1% to 5%), aphasia (1% to 5%), ataxia (1% to 5%), coordination abnormal (1% to 5%), dementia (1% to 5%), EEG abnormal (1% to 5%), hallucination (1% to 5%), insomnia (1% to 5%), meningitis (1% to 5%), nervousness (1% to 5%), somnolence (1% to 5%), stupor (1% to 5%)

Dermatologic: Rash (≥5%), erythematous rash (1% to 5%), maculopapular rash (1% to 5%), pruritus (1% to 5%), seborrhea (1% to 5%), skin discoloration (1% to 5%), skin ulceration (1% to 5%)

Endocrine & metabolic: Hyperphosphatemia (6%), acidosis (1% to 5%), hyponatremia (1% to 5%)

Gastrointestinal: Abdominal pain (≥5%), anorexia (≥5%), cachexia (1% to 5%), constipation (1% to 5%), dyspepsia (1% to 5%), dysphagia (1% to 5%), flatulence (1% to 5%), melena (1% to 5%), pancreatitis (1% to 5%), rectal hemorrhage (1% to 5%), taste perversion (1% to 5%), ulcerative stomatitis (1% to 5%), weight loss (1% to 5%), xerostomia (1% to 5%)

Genitourinary: Dysuria (1% to 5%), nocturia (1% to 5%), urinary retention (1% to 5%), urinary tract infection (1% to 5%)

Hematologic: Bone marrow suppression (10%), leukopenia (≥5%), lymphadenopathy (1% to 5%), thrombocytopenia (1% to 5%), thrombosis (1% to 5%)

Hepatic: Alkaline phosphatase increased (1% to 5%), ALT increased (1% to 5%), AST increased (1% to 5%), hepatic function abnormal (1% to 5%), LDH increased (1% to 5%)

Local: Abscess (1% to 5%), injection site pain/inflammation (1% to 5%)

Neuromuscular & skeletal: Paresthesia (≥5%), involuntary muscle contractions (≥5%), rigors (≥5%), neuropathy (peripheral; ≥5%), weakness (≥5%), arthralgia (1% to 5%), back pain (1% to 5%), leg cramps (1% to 5%), myalgia (1% to 5%), tremor (1% to 5%)

Ocular: Vision abnormalities (≥5%), conjunctivitis (1% to 5%), eye pain (1% to 5%)

Renal: Acute renal failure (1% to 5%), albuminuria (1% to 5%), BUN increased (1% to 5%), polyuria (1% to 5%)

Respiratory: Cough (≥5%), dyspnea (≥5%), bronchospasm (1% to 5%), hemoptysis (1% to 5%), pharyngitis (1% to 5%), pneumonia (1% to 5%), pneumothorax (1% to 5%), pulmonary infiltrates (1% to 5%), respiratory failure (1% to 5%), rhinitis (1% to 5%), sinusitis (1% to 5%), stridor (1% to 5%)

Miscellaneous: Diaphoresis (≥5%), sepsis (≥5%), flu-like syndrome (1% to 5%), infection (includes bacterial and fungal; 1% to 5%), malignancies (lymphoma/sarcoma 1% to 5%), thirst (1% to 5%)

<1%, postmarketing, and/or case reports: Amylase increased, cardiac arrest, coma, creatine phosphokinase increased, dehydration, diabetes insipidus (usually nephrogenic), erythema multiforme, genital irritation/ulceration, GGT increased, hematuria, hypoproteinemia, muscle weakness, myopathy, myositis, neutropenia, pancytopenia, QT_c prolongation, renal calculus, rhabdomyolysis, Stevens-Johnson syndrome, syndrome of inappropriate antidiuretic hormone (SIADH), toxic epidermal necrolysis, ventricular arrhythmia, vesiculobullous eruptions

Drug Interactions

Metabolism/Transport Effects None known.

Avoid Concomitant Use There are no known interactions where it is recommended to avoid concomitant use.

Increased Effect/Toxicity

Foscarnet may increase the levels/effects of: Highest Risk QTc-Prolonging Agents; Moderate Risk QTc-Prolonging Agents

The levels/effects of Foscarnet may be increased by: Mifepristone

Decreased Effect There are no known significant interactions involving a decrease in effect.

Storage/Stability Foscarnet injection is a clear, colorless solution. Store intact bottles at room temperature of 15°C to 30°C (59°F to 86°F) and protect from temperatures >40°C and from freezing. Diluted solution is stable for 24 hours at room temperature or under refrigeration.

Reconstitution Foscarnet should be diluted in D_5W or NS. For peripheral line administration, foscarnet **must** be diluted to ≤12 mg/mL with D_5W or NS. For central line administration, foscarnet may be administered undiluted.

Mechanism of Action Pyrophosphate analogue which acts as a noncompetitive inhibitor of many viral RNA and DNA polymerases as well as HIV reverse transcriptase. Similar to ganciclovir, foscarnet is a virostatic agent. Foscarnet does not require activation by thymidine kinase.

Pharmacodynamics/Kinetics

Distribution: V_d: ~0.5 L/kg; up to 28% of cumulative I.V. dose may be deposited in bone

Protein binding: 14% to 17%

Metabolism: Biotransformation does not occur

Half-life elimination: Elimination: ~3 4 hours; terminal: ~88 hours (due to bone deposition)

Excretion: Urine (≤28% as unchanged drug)

Dosing

Adult & Geriatric

CMV retinitis: I.V.:

Induction treatment: 60 mg/kg/dose every 8 hours for 14-21 days **or** 90 mg/kg every 12 hours for 14-21 days

Maintenance therapy: 90-120 mg/kg/day as a single daily infusion

Acyclovir-resistant HSV induction treatment: I.V.: 40 mg/kg/dose every 8-12 hours for 14-21 days

Therapy of CMV infection in cancer patients (unlabeled use): I.V.:

Prophylaxis: 60 mg/kg every 8-12 hours for 7 days, followed by 90-120 mg/kg daily until day 100 after HSCT

Pre-emptive treatment: 60 mg/kg every 12 hours for 14 days; if CMV still detectable, continue with 90 mg/kg daily for 5 days/week for 2 additional weeks

Treatment: 90 mg/kg every 12 hours for 2 weeks, followed by 120 mg/kg daily for ≥2 weeks

Pediatric Adolescents: Refer to adult dosing.

Renal Impairment See tables below.

Induction Dosing of Foscarnet in Patients With Abnormal Renal Function

Cl_{cr} (mL/min/kg)	HSV Equivalent to 40 mg/kg q12h	HSV Equivalent to 40 mg/kg q8h	CMV Equivalent to 60 mg/kg q8h	CMV Equivalent to 90 mg/kg q12h
<0.4	Not recommended	Not recommended	Not recommended	Not recommended
≥0.4-0.5	20 mg/kg every 24 hours	35 mg/kg every 24 hours	50 mg/kg every 24 hours	50 mg/kg every 24 hours
>0.5-0.6	25 mg/kg every 24 hours	40 mg/kg every 24 hours	60 mg/kg every 24 hours	60 mg/kg every 24 hours
>0.6-0.8	35 mg/kg every 24 hours	25 mg/kg every 12 hours	40 mg/kg every 12 hours	80 mg/kg every 24 hours
>0.8-1.0	20 mg/kg every 12 hours	35 mg/kg every 12 hours	50 mg/kg every 12 hours	50 mg/kg every 12 hours
>1.0-1.4	30 mg/kg every 12 hours	30 mg/kg every 8 hours	45 mg/kg every 8 hours	70 mg/kg every 12 hours
>1.4	40 mg/kg every 12 hours	40 mg/kg every 8 hours	60 mg/kg every 8 hours	90 mg/kg every 12 hours

Maintenance Dosing of Foscarnet in Patients With Abnormal Renal Function

Cl_{cr} (mL/min/kg)	CMV Equivalent to 90 mg/kg q24h	CMV Equivalent to 120 mg/kg q24h
<0.4	Not recommended	Not recommended
≥0.4-0.5	50 mg/kg every 48 hours	65 mg/kg every 48 hours
>0.5-0.6	60 mg/kg every 48 hours	80 mg/kg every 48 hours
>0.6-0.8	80 mg/kg every 48 hours	105 mg/kg every 48 hours
>0.8-1.0	50 mg/kg every 24 hours	65 mg/kg every 24 hours
>1.0-1.4	70 mg/kg every 24 hours	90 mg/kg every 24 hours
>1.4	90 mg/kg every 24 hours	120 mg/kg every 24 hours

Hemodialysis:

Foscarnet is highly removed by hemodialysis (up to ~38% in 2.5 hours HD with high-flux membrane)

Doses of 50 mg/kg/dose posthemodialysis have been found to produce similar serum concentrations as doses of 90 mg/kg twice daily in patients with normal renal function

Doses of 60-90 mg/kg/dose loading dose (posthemodialysis) followed by 45-60 mg/kg/dose posthemodialysis (3 times/week) with the monitoring of weekly plasma concentrations to maintain peak plasma concentrations in the range of 400-800 µMolar have been recommended by some clinicians

Continuous arteriovenous or venovenous hemodiafiltration effects: Dose as for Cl_{cr} 10-50 mL/minute

Administration Foscarnet is administered by intravenous infusion, using an infusion pump, at a rate not exceeding 1 mg/kg/minute. Undiluted (24 mg/mL) solution can be administered without further dilution when using a central venous catheter for infusion. For peripheral vein administration, the solution **must** be diluted to a final concentration **not to exceed** 12 mg/mL. The manufacturer recommends 750-1000 mL of NS or D_5W be administered prior to first infusion to establish **diuresis**. With subsequent infusions of 90-120 mg/kg, this volume would be repeated. If the dose were 40-60 mg/kg, then the volume could be reduced to 500 mL. After the first dose, the hydration fluid should be administered concurrently with foscarnet.

Monitoring Parameters 24-hour creatinine clearance at baseline and periodically thereafter. During induction therapy: Obtain complete blood counts, and electrolytes (including serum creatinine, calcium, magnesium, potassium, and phosphorus) twice weekly and then one weekly during maintenance therapy. More frequent monitoring may be required in some patients. Check hydration status before and after infusion.

Additional Information CMV retinitis maintenance treatment may be discontinued if immune reconstitution occurs as a result of ART.

Dosage Forms Excipient information presented when available (limited, particularly for generics); consult specific product labeling. [DSC] = Discontinued product

Injection, solution, as sodium [preservative free]: 24 mg/mL (250 mL, 500 mL [DSC])

Foscavir®: 24 mg/mL (250 mL)

References

Aweeka FT, Jacobson MA, Martin-Munley S, et al, "Effect of Renal Disease and Hemodialysis on Foscarnet Pharmacokinetics and Dosing Recommendations," *J Acquir Immune Dof Syndr Hum Retrovirol*, 1999, 20(4):350-7.

Benson CA, Kaplan JE, Masur H, et al, "Treating Opportunistic Infections Among HIV-Exposed and Infected Adults and Adolescents: Recommendations from CDC, the National Institutes of Health and the HIV Medicine Association/IDSA," *MMWR Recomm Rep* 2004, 53(RR-15):1-112.

Mofenson LM, Oleske J, Serchuck L, et al, "Treating Opportunistic Infections Among HIV-Exposed and Infected Children: Recommendations from CDC, the National Institutes of Health, and the Infectious Diseases Society of America," *Clin Infect Dis*, 2005, 40 (Suppl 1):1-84.

◆ **Foscavir®** *see* Foscarnet *on page* *646*

◆ **FR901228** *see* RomiDEPsin *on page* *1254*

◆ **Fragmin®** *see* Dalteparin *on page* *376*

◆ **FU** *see* Fluorouracil (Systemic) *on page* *627*

◆ **FU** *see* Fluorouracil (Topical) *on page* *632*

◆ **5-FU** *see* Fluorouracil (Systemic) *on page* *627*

◆ **5-FU** *see* Fluorouracil (Topical) *on page* *632*

◆ **FUDR** *see* Floxuridine *on page* *610*

◆ **FUDR® (Can)** *see* Floxuridine *on page* *610*

Fulvestrant (fool VES trant)

Related Information

Safe Handling of Hazardous Drugs *on page* *1904*

Brand Names: U.S. Faslodex®

Brand Names: Canada Faslodex®

Index Terms ICI-182,780; ZD9238

Generic Availability (U.S.) No

Pharmacologic Category Antineoplastic Agent, Estrogen Receptor Antagonist

Use Treatment of hormone receptor positive metastatic breast cancer in postmenopausal women with disease progression following antiestrogen therapy

Labeled Contraindications Hypersensitivity to fulvestrant or any component of the formulation

Pregnancy Risk Factor D

Lactation Excretion in breast milk unknown/not recommended

Warnings/Precautions Hazardous agent - use appropriate precautions for handling and disposal. Use caution in hepatic impairment; dosage adjustment is recommended in patients with moderate hepatic impairment. Safety and efficacy have not been established in severe hepatic impairment. Use with caution in patients with a history of bleeding disorders (including thrombocytopenia) and/or patients on anticoagulant therapy; bleeding/hematoma may occur from I.M. administration.

Adverse Reactions Adverse reactions reported with 500 mg dose.

>10%:

- Endocrine & metabolic: Hot flushes (7% to 13%)
- Hepatic: Alkaline phosphatase increased (>15%; grades 3/4: 1% to 2%), transaminases increased (>15%; grades 3/4: 1% to 2%)
- Local: Injection site pain (12% to 14%)
- Neuromuscular & skeletal: Joint disorders (14% to 19%)

1% to 10%:

- Cardiovascular: Ischemic disorder (1%)
- Central nervous system: Fatigue (8%), headache (8%)
- Gastrointestinal: Nausea (10%), anorexia (6%), vomiting (6%), constipation (5%), weight gain (≤1%)
- Genitourinary: Urinary tract infection (2% to 4%)
- Neuromuscular & skeletal: Bone pain (9%), arthralgia (8%), back pain (8%), extremity pain (7%), musculoskeletal pain (6%), weakness (6%)
- Respiratory: Cough (5%), dyspnea (4%)

<1%, postmarketing, and/or case reports (reported with 250 mg or 500 mg dose): Angioedema, bilirubin increased, GGT increased, hepatitis, hypersensitivity reactions, leukopenia, liver failure, myalgia, osteoporosis, thrombosis, urticaria, vaginal bleeding, vertigo

Drug Interactions

Metabolism/Transport Effects Substrate of CYP3A4 (minor); **Note:** Assignment of Major/Minor substrate status based on clinically relevant drug interaction potential

Avoid Concomitant Use There are no known interactions where it is recommended to avoid concomitant use.

Increased Effect/Toxicity There are no known significant interactions involving an increase in effect.

Decreased Effect

The levels/effects of Fulvestrant may be decreased by: Tocilizumab

Storage/Stability Store in original carton under refrigeration at 2°C to 8°C (36°F to 46°F). Protect from light.

Mechanism of Action Estrogen receptor antagonist; competitively binds to estrogen receptors on tumors and other tissue targets, producing a nuclear complex that causes a dose-related down-regulation of estrogen receptors and inhibits tumor growth.

Pharmacodynamics/Kinetics

Duration: I.M.: Steady state concentrations reached within first month, when administered with additional dose given 2 weeks following the initial dose; plasma levels maintained for at least 1 month

Distribution: V_d: ~3-5 L/kg

Protein binding: 99%; to plasma proteins (VLDL, LDL and HDL lipoprotein fractions)

Metabolism: Hepatic via multiple biotransformation pathways (CYP3A4 substrate involved in oxidation pathway, although relative contribution to metabolism unknown); metabolites formed are either less active or have similar activity to parent compound

Half-life elimination: 250 mg: ~40 days

Excretion: Feces (~90%); urine (<1%)

Dosing

Adult & Geriatric Breast cancer, metastatic (postmenopausal women): I.M.: Initial: 500 mg on days 1, 15, and 29; Maintenance: 500 mg once monthly

Hepatic Impairment

Moderate impairment (Child-Pugh class B): Decrease initial and maintenance dose to 250 mg

Severe impairment (Child-Pugh class C): Use has not been evaluated.

Administration For I.M. administration only; do not administer I.V., SubQ, or intra-arterially. Administer 500 mg dose as two 5 mL injections (one in each buttocks) slowly over 1-2 minutes per injection.

Dosage Forms Excipient information presented when available (limited, particularly for generics); consult specific product labeling.

Injection, solution:

Faslodex®: 50 mg/mL (5 mL) [contains benzyl alcohol, benzyl benzoate, castor oil, ethanol 10% w/v]

References

Di Leo A, Jerusalem G, Petruzelka L, et al, "Results of the CONFIRM Phase III Trial Comparing Fulvestrant 250 mg With Fulvestrant 500 mg in Postmenopausal Women With Estrogen Receptor-Positive Advanced Breast Cancer," *J Clin Oncol*, 2010 28(30):4594-600.

Robertson JF, Llombart-Cussac A, Rolski J, et al, "Activity of Fulvestrant 500 mg Versus Anastrozole 1 mg as First-Line Treatment for Advanced Breast Cancer: Results From the FIRST Study," *J Clin Oncol*, 2009, 27(27):4530-5.

◆ **Fungizone® (Can)** *see* Amphotericin B (Conventional) *on page 79*

◆ **Fusilev®** *see* LEVOleucovorin *on page 888*

◆ **^{67}Ga-Citrate** *see* Gallium Citrate Ga-67 *on page 653*

◆ **^{67}Ga-Gallium Citrate** *see* Gallium Citrate Ga-67 *on page 653*

Gallium Citrate Ga-67 (GAL ee um SIT rate jee aye SIX tee SEV en)

Index Terms ^{67}Ga-Citrate; ^{67}Ga-Gallium Citrate

Pharmacologic Category Radiopharmaceutical

Use Diagnostic imaging of Hodgkin's disease, lymphoma, bronchogenic carcinoma, and inflammatory lesions to identify fevers of unknown origin; nonbacterial infections

Pregnancy Risk Factor C

Lactation Enters breast milk/not recommended

Warnings/Precautions Radiopharmaceutical: Use appropriate precautions for handling, disposal, and minimizing exposure to patients and healthcare personnel. Use only under supervision of individuals who have received training in the handling of radioactive materials and who are authorized by the applicable regulatory authority.

Adverse Reactions Frequency not defined.

Dermatologic: Rash

Gastrointestinal: Nausea

Miscellaneous: Hypersensitivity reactions

Storage/Stability Store at 20°C to 25°C (68°F to 77°F) in a lead-shielded container.

Dosing

Adult I.V. (based on 70 kg patient): 2-5 mCi (74-185 MBq). For tumors, dose may be 5-10 mCi (185-370 MBq).

Pediatric I.V.: 0.04-0.07 mCi/kg (1.5-2.6 MBq/kg)

References

Palestro CJ, Brown ML, Forstrom LA, et al, "Society of Nuclear Medicine Procedure Guideline for Gallium Scintigraphy in Inflammation," 2004. Available at http://interactive.snm.org/docs/Gallium_Scintigraphy_in_Inflammation_v3.pdf

Gallium Nitrate (GAL ee um NYE trate)

Related Information

Hypercalcemia of Malignancy *on page 1860*

Brand Names: U.S. Ganite™

Index Terms WR-135675

Generic Availability (U.S.) No

Pharmacologic Category Calcium-Lowering Agent

Use Treatment of symptomatic cancer-related hypercalcemia (refractory to adequate hydration)

Labeled Contraindications Severe renal dysfunction (serum creatinine >2.5 mg/dL)

Pregnancy Risk Factor C

Lactation Excretion in breast milk unknown/not recommended

Warnings/Precautions Hazardous agent - use appropriate precautions for handling and disposal. **[U.S. Boxed Warning]: Concurrent administration with other nephrotoxic drugs (eg, aminoglycosides, amphotericin B) may increase the risk for renal insufficiency in patients with cancer-related hypercalcemia; discontinue gallium nitrate during treatment with nephrotoxic drugs (monitor serum creatinine and urine output; continue hydration for several days). Discontinue with serum creatinine >2.5 mg/dL.** BUN and serum creatinine elevations have been observed with gallium nitrate use; establish and maintain adequate hydration with oral and/or I.V. (normal saline) fluids; establish urinary output ≥2 L/day prior to treatment initiation. Use with caution in patients where aggressive hydration may be poorly tolerated, such as in cardiovascular disease (HF or hypertension) and pulmonary disease. Treatment may result in mild-to-moderate hypocalcemia; may require discontinuation of gallium nitrate.

Adverse Reactions Frequency not always defined.

Cardiovascular: Edema (lower extremity), hypotension, tachycardia

Central nervous system: Coma, confusion, dreams, encephalopathy, fever, hallucinations, hypothermia, lethargy

Dermatologic: Rash

Endocrine & metabolic: Hypophosphatemia (≤79%), serum bicarbonate decreased (40% to 50%), hypocalcemia (38%), respiratory alkalosis (mild)

Gastrointestinal: Constipation, diarrhea, nausea, vomiting

Hematologic: Anemia, leukopenia

Neuromuscular & skeletal: Paresthesia, positive Cvostek's sign
Ocular: Optic neuritis (<1%), blindness (case report)
Otic: Auditory acuity decreased (<1%), tinnitus (<1%), hearing decreased
Renal: BUN increased (13%), creatinine increased (13%), acute renal failure
Respiratory: Dyspnea, pleural effusion, pulmonary infiltrates, rales, rhonchi

Drug Interactions

Metabolism/Transport Effects None known.

Avoid Concomitant Use

Avoid concomitant use of Gallium Nitrate with any of the following: Aminoglycosides; Amphotericin B; Vancomycin

Increased Effect/Toxicity

The levels/effects of Gallium Nitrate may be increased by: Aminoglycosides; Amphotericin B; Vancomycin

Decreased Effect There are no known significant interactions involving a decrease in effect.

Storage/Stability Store intact vials at room temperature of 20°C to 25°C (68°F to 77°F). Dilute in 1000 mL NS (preferred) or D_5W for infusion. Solutions in 0.9% NaCl or D_5W are stable for 48 hours at room temperature or for 7 days under refrigeration at 2°C to 8°C (36°F to 46°F).

Reconstitution Dilute in 1000 mL NS (preferred) or D_5W for infusion.

Mechanism of Action Inhibits calcium resorption from bone by inhibiting osteoclast activity. Gallium nitrate appears to be effective in parathyroid hormone-related protein (PTHrP) and non-PTHrP-associated hypercalcemia.

Pharmacodynamics/Kinetics

Onset of calcium lowering: Calcium begins to decrease within 24-48 hours; normocalcemia achieved within 5-9 days
Duration: Normocalcemia: 7-10 days
Distribution: Continuous infusion: V_{dss}: 670 L/m^2
Half-life elimination: Continuous infusion: 105 hours
Excretion: Primarily renal with no prior metabolism in the liver or kidney

Dosing

Adult & Geriatric Note: Initiate I.V. hydration prior to treatment; maintain throughout treatment.

Hypercalcemia (cancer-related): 200 mg/m^2/day continuous infusion for 5 consecutive days; treatment duration may be shortened if normocalcemia is achieved in <5 days. If hypercalcemia is mild and with limited symptoms, 100 mg/m^2/day may be used.

Renal Impairment

Moderate renal impairment (serum creatinine 2 to ≤2.5 mg/dL): There are no dosage adjustment s provided in the manufacturer's labeling; frequent monitoring of renal status is recommended.

Severe renal impairment (serum creatinine >2.5 mg/dL): Use is contraindicated

Administration The manufacturer recommends continuous I.V. infusion over 24 hours.

Monitoring Parameters Renal function (BUN, serum creatinine); serum calcium (baseline, then daily); serum phosphorus (baseline, then twice weekly); albumin; fluid intake, urine output

Additional Information In addition to the hypocalcemic effect, gallium nitrate has also been studied for its antitumor effects. Gallium nitrate was studied at higher doses infused over 30 minutes every 2 weeks in bladder cancer and lymphoma (Einhorn, 2003; Straus, 2003). Rapid infusion rates and higher doses are associated with an increased risk of toxicity, including nephrotoxicity and gastrointestinal toxicity.

Dosage Forms Excipient information presented when available (limited, particularly for generics); consult specific product labeling.

Injection, solution [preservative free]:

Ganite™: 25 mg/mL (20 mL)

References

Cvitkovic F, Armand JP, Tubiana-Hulin M, et al, "Randomized, Double-Blind, Phase II Trial of Gallium Nitrate Compared With Pamidronate for Acute Control of Cancer-Related Hypercalcemia," *Cancer J*, 2006, 12(1):47-53.

Einhorn L, "Gallium Nitrate in the Treatment of Bladder Cancer," *Sem Oncol*, 2003, 30(2 Suppl 5): 34-41.

Leyland-Jones B, "Treatment of Cancer-Related Hypercalcemia: The Role of Gallium Nitrate," *Semin Oncol*, 2003, 30(2 Suppl 5):13-9.

Straus DJ, "Gallium Nitrate in the Treatment of Lymphoma", *Sem Oncol*, 2003, 30(2 Suppl 5):25-33.

- **GamaSTAN™ S/D** *see* Immune Globulin *on page 777*
- **Gamastan S/D (Can)** *see* Immune Globulin *on page 777*
- **Gamimune® N (Can)** *see* Immune Globulin *on page 777*
- **Gammagard® Liquid** *see* Immune Globulin *on page 777*
- **Gammagard Liquid (Can)** *see* Immune Globulin *on page 777*
- **Gammagard S/D®** *see* Immune Globulin *on page 777*
- **Gammagard S/D (Can)** *see* Immune Globulin *on page 777*
- **Gamma Globulin** *see* Immune Globulin *on page 777*
- **Gammaked™** *see* Immune Globulin *on page 777*
- **Gammaphos** *see* Amifostine *on page 65*
- **Gammaplex®** *see* Immune Globulin *on page 777*
- **Gamunex®-C** *see* Immune Globulin *on page 777*

Ganciclovir (Systemic) (gan SYE kloe veer)

Brand Names: U.S. Cytovene®-IV

Brand Names: Canada Cytovene®

Index Terms DHPG Sodium; GCV Sodium; Nordeoxyguanosine

Generic Availability (U.S.) Yes

Pharmacologic Category Antiviral Agent

Use Treatment of CMV retinitis in immunocompromised individuals, including patients with acquired immunodeficiency syndrome; prophylaxis of CMV infection in transplant patients

Unlabeled Use CMV retinitis: May be given in combination with foscarnet in patients who relapse after monotherapy with either drug

Labeled Contraindications Hypersensitivity to ganciclovir, acyclovir, or any component of the formulation

Pregnancy Risk Factor C

Lactation Excretion in breast milk unknown/not recommended

Warnings/Precautions Hazardous agent - use appropriate precautions for handling and disposal. **[U.S. Boxed Warning]: Granulocytopenia (neutropenia), anemia, and thrombocytopenia may occur.** Dosage adjustment or interruption of ganciclovir therapy may be necessary in patients with neutropenia and/or thrombocytopenia and patients with impaired renal function. **[U.S. Boxed Warning]: Animal studies have demonstrated carcinogenic and teratogenic effects, and inhibition of spermatogenesis;** contraceptive precautions for female and male patients need to be followed during and for at least 90 days after therapy with the drug; take care to administer only into veins with good blood flow. **[U.S. Boxed Warning]: Indicated only for treatment of CMV retinitis in the immunocompromised patient and CMV prevention in transplant patients at risk.**

Storage/Stability Intact vials should be stored at room temperature and protected from temperatures >40°C. Reconstituted solution is stable for 12 hours at room temperature, however, conflicting data indicates that reconstituted solution is stable for 60 days under refrigeration (4°C). Stability of parenteral admixture at room temperature (25°C) and at refrigeration temperature (4°C) is 5 days.

Reconstitution Reconstitute powder with unpreserved sterile water not bacteriostatic water because parabens may cause precipitation. Dilute in 250-1000 mL D_5W or NS to a concentration ≤10 mg/mL for infusion.

Mechanism of Action Ganciclovir is phosphorylated to a substrate which competitively inhibits the binding of deoxyguanosine triphosphate to DNA polymerase resulting in inhibition of viral DNA synthesis

Pharmacodynamics/Kinetics

Distribution: V_d: 15.26 L/1.73 m^2; widely to all tissues including CSF and ocular tissue

Protein binding: 1% to 2%

Half-life elimination: 1.7-5.8 hours; prolonged with renal impairment; End-stage renal disease: 5-28 hours

Excretion: Urine (80% to 99% as unchanged drug)

Dosing

Adult

CMV CNS infection in HIV-exposed/-infected patients (unlabeled use; CDC, 2009): *I.V.:* 5 mg/kg/dose every 12 hours plus foscarnet until symptoms improve followed by chronic suppression

CMV retinitis: *I.V. (slow infusion):*

Induction therapy: 5 mg/kg/dose every 12 hours for 14-21 days followed by maintenance therapy

Maintenance therapy: 5 mg/kg/day as a single daily dose for 7 days/week or 6 mg/kg/day for 5 days/week

Prevention (secondary) of CMV disease in HIV-exposed/-infected patients (unlabeled use; CDC, 2009): *I.V.:* 5 mg/kg/dose daily

Prevention (secondary) of CMV disease in transplant patients: *I.V. (slow infusion):* 5 mg/kg/dose every 12 hours for 7-14 days, duration of maintenance therapy is dependent on clinical condition and degree of immunosuppression

Varicella zoster: Progressive outer retinal necrosis in HIV exposed/-infected patients (unlabeled use; CDC, 2009): *I.V.:* 5 mg/kg/dose every 12 hours plus systemic foscarnet and intravitreal ganciclovir or intravitreal foscarnet

Geriatric Refer to adult dosing. In general, dose selection should be cautious, reflecting greater frequency of organ impairment.

Pediatric

CMV CNS infection in HIV-exposed/-infected patients (unlabeled use; CDC, 2009): Infants and Children: *I.V.:* Refer to adult dosing.

CMV retinitis: Children: *I.V. (slow infusion):* Refer to adult dosing.

Prevention (secondary) of CMV disease in HIV-exposed/-infected patients (unlabeled use; CDC, 2009): Infants and Children: *I.V.:* Refer to adult dosing.

Prevention (secondary) of CMV disease in transplant patients: Children: *I.V. (slow infusion):* Refer to adult dosing.

Varicella zoster: Progressive outer retinal necrosis in HIV-exposed/-infected patients (unlabeled use; CDC, 2009): Infants and Children: *I.V.:* Refer to adult dosing.

Renal Impairment

I.V. (Induction):

Cl_{cr} 50-69 mL/minute: Administer 2.5 mg/kg/dose every 12 hours.

Cl_{cr} 25-49 mL/minute: Administer 2.5 mg/kg/dose every 24 hours.

Cl_{cr} 10-24 mL/minute: Administer 1.25 mg/kg/dose every 24 hours.

Cl_{cr} <10 mL/minute: Administer 1.25 mg/kg/dose 3 times/week following hemodialysis.

I.V. (Maintenance):

Cl_{cr} 50-69 mL/minute: Administer 2.5 mg/kg/dose every 24 hours.

Cl_{cr} 25-49 mL/minute: Administer 1.25 mg/kg/dose every 24 hours.

Cl_{cr} 10-24 mL/minute: Administer 0.625 mg/kg/dose every 24 hours

Cl_{cr} <10 mL/minute: Administer 0.625 mg/kg/dose 3 times/week following hemodialysis.

Intermittent hemodialysis (IHD) (administer after hemodialysis on dialysis days): Dialyzable (50%): CMV Infection: I.V.: Induction: 1.25 mg/kg every 48-72 hours; Maintenance: 0.625 mg/kg every 48-72 hours. **Note:** Dosing dependent on the assumption of 3 times/week, complete IHD sessions.

Peritoneal dialysis (PD): Dose as for Cl_{cr} <10 mL/minute.

Continuous renal replacement therapy (CRRT) (Heintz, 2009; Trotman, 2005): Drug clearance is highly dependent on the method of renal replacement, filter type, and flow rate. Appropriate dosing requires close monitoring of pharmacologic response, signs of adverse reactions due to drug accumulation, as well as drug concentrations in relation to target trough (if appropriate). The following are general recommendations only (based on dialysate flow/ultrafiltration rates of 1-2 L/hour and minimal residual renal function) and should not supersede clinical judgment: CMV Infection:

CVVH: I.V.: Induction: 2.5 mg/kg every 24 hours; Maintenance: 1.25 mg/kg every 24 hours

CVVHD/CVVHDF: I.V.: Induction: 2.5 mg/kg every 12 hours; Maintenance: 2.5 mg/kg every 24 hours

Administration Should not be administered by I.M., SubQ, or rapid IVP; administer by slow I.V. infusion over at least 1 hour. Too rapid infusion can cause increased toxicity and excessive plasma levels.

Dosage Forms Excipient information presented when available (limited, particularly for generics); consult specific product labeling.

Injection, powder for reconstitution: 500 mg

Cytovene®-IV: 500 mg

- **Ganite™** *see* Gallium Nitrate *on page* 654
- **Gardasil®** *see* Papillomavirus (Types 6, 11, 16, 18) Vaccine (Human, Recombinant) *on page* 1120
- **G-CSF** *see* Filgrastim *on page* 604
- **G-CSF (PEG Conjugate)** *see* Pegfilgrastim *on page* 1138
- **GCV Sodium** *see* Ganciclovir (Systemic) *on page* 656
- **GDC-0449** *see* Vismodegib *on page* 1470

Gefitinib (ge FI tye nib)

Related Information

Management of Chemotherapy-Induced Nausea and Vomiting *on page 1786*

Safe Handling of Hazardous Drugs *on page 1904*

Brand Names: U.S. Iressa®

Brand Names: Canada IRESSA®

Index Terms ZD1839

Generic Availability (U.S.) No

Pharmacologic Category Antineoplastic Agent, Tyrosine Kinase Inhibitor

Use Treatment of locally advanced or metastatic nonsmall cell lung cancer (NSCLC) after failure of platinum-based and docetaxel therapies. Treatment is limited to patients who are benefiting or have benefited from treatment with gefitinib.

Note: Due to the lack of improved survival data from clinical trials of gefitinib, and in response to positive survival data with another EGFR inhibitor, according to the U.S. labeling, physicians are advised to use treatment options other than gefitinib in patients with advanced nonsmall cell lung cancer following one or two prior chemotherapy regimens when they are refractory/intolerant to their most recent regimen.

Canada labeling: First-line treatment of locally advanced or metastatic NSCLC with activating mutations of EGFR-TK

Unlabeled Use First-line treatment of NSCLC with known EGFR mutation

Labeled Contraindications Hypersensitivity to gefitinib or any component of the formulation

Pregnancy Risk Factor D

Lactation Excretion in breast milk unknown/not recommended

Warnings/Precautions Hazardous agent - use appropriate precautions for handling and disposal. Rare, sometimes fatal, pulmonary toxicity, including interstitial lung disease (ILD) (eg, alveolitis, interstitial pneumonia, pneumonitis) has occurred. ILD has occurred in patients with prior radiation therapy, prior chemotherapy, and less commonly in treatment naïve patients. Therapy should be interrupted in patients with acute onset or worsening pulmonary symptoms (dyspnea, cough, fever); discontinue if interstitial pneumonitis is confirmed. An increase in mortality was observed in patients with concurrent idiopathic pulmonary fibrosis. Asymptomatic increases in transaminases have been reported; monitor liver function periodically and discontinue if elevations/changes are severe. Gefitinib exposure may be increased in patients with hepatic impairment. Interruption of therapy may be required in patients with poorly tolerated diarrhea or adverse skin reactions. Eye irritation should be promptly evaluated and therapy may be interrupted based on appropriate medical evaluation; may be reinitiated following resolution of symptoms or eye changes.

EGFR mutations, specifically exon 19 deletions and exon 21 mutation (L858R), are associated with better response to gefitinib in patients with NSCLC (Riely, 2006). There is a high potential for CYP3A4 mediated interactions with gefitinib. Concurrent use with CYP3A4 inducers may decrease gefitinib levels; consider increased gefitinib doses (to 500 mg) with close monitoring if concurrent use with inducers cannot be avoided. CYP3A4 inhibitors may increase gefitinib levels, use caution with concurrent administration.

Adverse Reactions

>10%:

Dermatologic: Rash (43% to 54%), acne (25% to 33%), dry skin (13% to 26%), paronychia (14%)

Gastrointestinal: Diarrhea (48% to 67%; grade 3: 1%), nausea (13% to 18%), vomiting (9% to 12%)

1% to 10%:

Cardiovascular: Peripheral edema (2%)

Dermatologic: Pruritus (8% to 9%)

Gastrointestinal: Anorexia (7% to 10%), weight loss (3% to 5%), mouth ulceration (1%)

Neuromuscular & skeletal: Weakness (4% to 6%)

Ocular: Amblyopia (2%), conjunctivitis (1%)

Respiratory: Dyspnea (2%), interstitial lung disease (1% to 2%; includes alveolitis, interstitial pneumonia, pneumonitis)

<1%, postmarketing, and/or case reports: Aberrant eyelash growth, angioedema, CNS hemorrhage (pediatrics), corneal erosion/ulcer, corneal membrane sloughing, epistaxis, erythema multiforme, eye pain, fever, hematuria, hemorrhage, ocular hemorrhage, ocular ischemia, pancreatitis, toxic epidermal necrolysis, urticaria, vesiculobullous rash

Drug Interactions

Metabolism/Transport Effects **Substrate** of CYP2D6 (major), CYP3A4 (major); **Note:** Assignment of Major/Minor substrate status based on clinically relevant drug interaction potential; **Inhibits** BCRP, CYP2C19 (weak), CYP2D6 (weak)

Avoid Concomitant Use

Avoid concomitant use of Gefitinib with any of the following: Conivaptan

Increased Effect/Toxicity

Gefitinib may increase the levels/effects of: ARIPiprazole; Topotecan; Vinorelbine; Vitamin K Antagonists

The levels/effects of Gefitinib may be increased by: Abiraterone Acetate; Antifungal Agents (Azole Derivatives, Systemic); Conivaptan; CYP2D6 Inhibitors (Moderate); CYP2D6 Inhibitors (Strong); CYP3A4 Inhibitors (Moderate); CYP3A4 Inhibitors (Strong); Darunavir; Dasatinib; Ivacaftor; Mifepristone

Decreased Effect

Gefitinib may decrease the levels/effects of: Cardiac Glycosides; Vitamin K Antagonists

The levels/effects of Gefitinib may be decreased by: CYP3A4 Inducers (Strong); Deferasirox; H2-Antagonists; Herbs (CYP3A4 Inducers); Peginterferon Alfa-2b; Proton Pump Inhibitors; Rifamycin Derivatives; Tocilizumab

Ethanol/Nutrition/Herb Interactions

Food: Grapefruit juice may increase serum gefitinib concentrations.

Herb/Nutraceutical: St John's wort may decrease serum gefitinib concentrations.

Storage/Stability Store tablets at controlled room temperature of 20°C to 25°C (68°F to 77°F). Protect from light and moisture.

Mechanism of Action Gefitinib is a tyrosine kinase inhibitor (TKI) which inhibits numerous tyrosine kinases associated with transmembrane cell surface receptors found on both normal and cancer cells, including the tyrosine kinase associated with the epidermal growth factor receptor, EGFR. Tyrosine kinase activity appears to be vitally important to cell proliferation and survival.

Pharmacodynamics/Kinetics

Absorption: Oral: Slow

Distribution: 1400 L

Protein binding: 90%, albumin and alpha$_1$-acid glycoprotein

Metabolism: Hepatic, primarily via CYP3A4; forms metabolites

Bioavailability: 60%

Half-life elimination: Oral: 41 hours

Time to peak, plasma: Oral: 3-7 hours

Excretion: Feces (86%); urine (<1%)

Dosing

Adult

Nonsmall cell lung cancer (NSCLC): Oral: 250 mg once daily

NSCLC, first-line therapy in patients with EGFR mutations (unlabeled use): Oral: 250 mg once daily (Maemondo, 2010; Mok, 2009; Sequist, 2008)

Dosage adjustment for concomitant CYP3A4 inducers (eg, phenytoin, rifampin): Consider increasing gefitinib dose to 500 mg once daily with close monitoring

Geriatric No adjustment necessary. Refer to adult dosing.

Renal Impairment No adjustment necessary.

Hepatic Impairment

Moderate-to-severe impairment due to metastases: No adjustment necessary.

Hepatotoxicity during treatment (elevations in transaminases): Discontinue if severe.

Adjustment for Toxicity

Worsening pulmonary symptoms (cough dyspnea, fever): Interrupt treatment and evaluate promptly; discontinue if interstitial lung disease is confirmed.

Diarrhea (poorly tolerated or associated with dehydration) or skin toxicity: Interrupt treatment for up to 14 days; may reinitiate at 250 mg once daily.

Ocular symptoms (eye pain): Evaluate and interrupt treatment based on symptoms; once symptoms or eye changes have resolved, may consider reinitiating at 250 mg once daily.

Administration May administer with or without food.

For patients unable to swallow tablets or for administration via NG tube: Tablets may be dispersed in noncarbonated drinking water. Drop whole tablet (do not crush) into 1/2 glass of water; stir until tablet is dispersed (~10 minutes). Drink immediately. Rinse glass with 1/2 glass of water and drink.

Emetic Potential Very low (<10%)

Extemporaneous Preparations Hazardous agent: Use appropriate precautions for handling and disposal.

An oral suspension may be prepared by placing one tablet (whole, do not crush) in half a glass of noncarbonated drinking water. Stir until tablet is disintegrated (~10 minutes), then administer immediately. To ensure the full dose is administered, rinse with half a glass of water and administer residue.

Iressa® prescribing information, AstraZeneca Pharmaceuticals, Wilmington, DE, 2005.

Monitoring Parameters Periodic liver function tests (ALT, AST, bilirubin and alkaline phosphatase), INR or prothrombin time (with concurrently warfarin treatment), pulmonary symptoms

Dietary Considerations Food does not affect gefitinib absorption.

Additional Information Oncology Comment: Recent studies have demonstrated a subset of patients who are more likely to respond to treatment with gefitinib. This subset includes: patients of Asian origin, never-smokers, women, patients with bronchoalveolar adenocarcinoma, and patients with EGFR-mutated tumors. Deletion in exon 19 and mutation in exon 21 are the two most commonly found EGFR mutations; both mutations correlate with clinical response, resulting in increased response rates in patients with the mutation (Riely, 2006). Studies have compared gefitinib in treatment naïve patients to combination chemotherapy in the subsets of patients described above, resulting in a longer progression free survival in the gefitinib arm (Mok, 2009). Based on these data, the 2009 ASCO guidelines recommend the first-line use of gefitinib in stage IV with the known EGFR mutation (Azzoli, 2009). The NCCN guidelines recommend erlotinib as first-line therapy for EGFR mutation positive patients with stage IV NSCLC, and also states that gefitinib could be used in place of erlotinib in areas of the world where available. In patients with a kras mutation, however, EGFR-TKI therapy is not recommended.

Prescribing and Access Restrictions As of September 15, 2005, distribution of gefitinib (IRESSA®) is limited to patients enrolled in the IRESSA® Access Program. Under this program, access to gefitinib will be limited to the following groups:

Patients who are currently receiving and benefiting from gefitinib

Patients who have previously received and benefited from gefitinib

Previously-enrolled patients or new patients in non-Investigational New Drug (IND) clinical trials involving gefitinib if these protocols were approved by an IRB prior to June 17, 2005

New patients may also receive gefitinib if the manufacturer (AstraZeneca) decides to make it available under IND, and the patients meet the criteria for enrollment under the IND

Additional information on the IRESSA® Access Program, including enrollment forms, may be obtained by calling AstraZeneca at 1-800-601-8933 or via the web at www.Iressa-access.com

Dosage Forms Excipient information presented when available (limited, particularly for generics); consult specific product labeling.

Tablet, oral:

Iressa®: 250 mg

References

Azzoli CG, Baker S Jr, Temin S, et al, "American Society of Clinical Oncology Clinical Practice Guideline Update on Chemotherapy for Stage IV Non-Small-Cell Lung Cancer," *J Clin Oncol*, 2009, 27(36):6251-66.

Inoue A, Kobayashi K, Usui K, et al, "First-Line Gefitinib for Patients With Advanced Non-Small-Cell Lung Cancer Harboring Epidermal Growth Factor Receptor Mutations Without Indication for Chemotherapy," *J Clin Oncol*, 2009, 27(9):1394-400.

Maemondo M, Inoue A, Kobayashi K, et al, "Gefitinib or Chemotherapy for Non-Small-Cell Lung Cancer With Mutated EGFR," *N Engl J Med*, 2010, 362(25):2380-8.

Mok TS, Wu YL, Thongprasert S, et al, "Gefitinib or Carboplatin-Paclitaxel in Pulmonary Adenocarcinoma," *N Engl J Med*, 2009, 361(10):947-57.

National Comprehensive Cancer Network® (NCCN), "Clinical Practice Guidelines in Oncology™: Non-Small Cell Lung Cancer," Version 3.2011. Available at http://www.nccn.org/professionals/physician_gls/PDF/nscl.pdf

Riely GJ, Pao W, Pham D, et al, "Clinical Course of Patients With Non-Small Cell Lung Cancer and Epidermal Growth Factor Receptor Exon 19 and Exon 21 Mutations Treated With Gefitinib or Erlotinib," *Clin Cancer Res*, 2006, 12(3 Pt 1):839-44.

Sequist LV, Martins RG, Spigel D, et al, "First-Line Gefitinib in Patients With Advanced Non-Small-Cell Lung Cancer Harboring Somatic EGFR Mutations," *J Clin Oncol*, 2008, 26(15):2442-9.

◆ **Gelclair®** *see* Mucosal Barrier Gel, Oral *on page 1014*

Gemcitabine (jem SITE a been)

Related Information

Management of Chemotherapy-Induced Nausea and Vomiting *on page 1786*
Management of Drug Extravasations *on page 1800*
Oral Mucositis/Stomatitis *on page 1814*
Safe Handling of Hazardous Drugs *on page 1904*

Brand Names: U.S. Gemzar®

Brand Names: Canada Gemcitabine For Injection, USP; Gemzar®

Index Terms dFdC; dFdCyd; Difluorodeoxycytidine Hydrochlorothiazide; Gemcitabine Hydrochloride; LY-188011

Generic Availability (U.S.) Yes

Pharmacologic Category Antineoplastic Agent, Antimetabolite (Pyrimidine Analog)

Use Treatment of metastatic breast cancer; inoperable locally-advanced or metastatic nonsmall cell lung cancer (NSCLC); locally advanced or metastatic pancreatic cancer; advanced, relapsed ovarian cancer

Unlabeled Use Treatment of biliary tract cancers (advanced), bladder cancer, cervical cancer (recurrent or persistent), Ewing's sarcoma (refractory), head and neck cancer (nasopharyngeal), Hodgkin lymphoma (relapsed), non-Hodgkin lymphomas (refractory), malignant pleural mesothelioma, osteosarcoma (refractory), renal cell cancer (metastatic), small cell lung cancer (refractory or relapsed), soft tissue sarcoma (advanced), testicular cancer (refractory germ cell tumors), thymic malignancies, uterine sarcoma, and unknown-primary adenocarcinoma

Labeled Contraindications Hypersensitivity to gemcitabine or any component of the formulation

Pregnancy Risk Factor D

Lactation Excretion in breast milk unknown/not recommended

Warnings/Precautions Hazardous agent - use appropriate precautions for handling and disposal. Prolongation of the infusion time >60 minutes and more frequent than weekly dosing have been shown to increase toxicity. Gemcitabine may suppress bone marrow function (leukopenia, thrombocytopenia, and anemia); myelosuppression is usually the dose-limiting toxicity; monitor blood counts; dosage adjustments are frequently required. Gemcitabine may cause fever in the absence of clinical infection. Pulmonary toxicity has occurred; discontinue if severe and institute supportive measures.

Hemolytic uremic syndrome (and/or renal failure) has been reported; monitor for evidence of microangiopathic hemolysis (elevation of bilirubin or LDH, reticulocytosis, severe thrombocytopenia, and/or renal failure); use with caution in patients with pre-existing renal impairment. Serious hepatotoxicity (including liver failure and death) has been reported (when used alone or in combination with other hepatotoxic medications). Use with caution in patients with hepatic impairment (history of cirrhosis, hepatitis, or alcoholism) or in patients with hepatic metastases; may lead to exacerbation of hepatic impairment; dose adjustments may be considered with elevated bilirubin.

Pulmonary toxicity has been observed; discontinue if severe and institute supportive measures. Use caution with concurrent radiation therapy; radiation toxicity, including tissue injury, severe mucositis, esophagitis, or pneumonitis, has been reported with concurrent and nonconcurrent administration; may have radiosensitizing activity when gemcitabine and radiation therapy are given ≤7 days apart; lower doses with concurrent radiation therapy may produce less severe toxicity; however, an optimum regimen for combination therapy has not been determined for all tumor types; radiation recall may occur when gemcitabine and radiation therapy are given >7 days apart. Prolongation of the infusion time >60 minutes and more frequent than weekly dosing have been shown to increase toxicity; has been administered at a fixed-dose rate (FDR) infusion rate of 10 mg/m^2/minute in studies (unlabeled); prolonged infusion times increase the accumulation of the active metabolite, gemcitabine triphosphate, optimizing the pharmacokinetics (Ko, 2006; Tempero, 2003); patients who receive gemcitabine FDR experience more grade 3/4 hematologic toxicity (Ko, 2006; Poplin, 2009). Use caution in the elderly; clearance is affected by age.

Adverse Reactions Frequency of adverse reactions reported for single-agent use of gemcitabine only.

>10%:

Cardiovascular: Peripheral edema (20%), edema (13%)

Central nervous system: Fever (38% to 41%), somnolence (11%)

Dermatologic: Rash (28% to 30%), alopecia (15% to 16%), pruritus (13%)

Gastrointestinal: Nausea/vomiting (69% to 71%; grade 3: 10% to 13%; grade 4: 1% to 2%), diarrhea (19% to 30%), stomatitis (10% to 11%)

Hematologic: Anemia (68% to 73%; grade 4: 1% to 2%), leukopenia (62% to 64%; grade 4: ≤1%), neutropenia (61% to 63%; grade 4: 6% to 7%), thrombocytopenia (24% to 36%; grade 4: ≤1%), hemorrhage (4% to 17%; grades 3: ≤2%; grade 4: <1%); myelosuppression is the dose-limiting toxicity

Hepatic: AST increased (67% to 78%; grade 3: 6% to 12%; grade 4: 2% to 5%), alkaline phosphatase increased (55% to 77%; grade 3: 7% to 16%; grade 4: 2% to 4%), ALT increased (68% to 72%; grade 3: 8% to 10%; grade 4: 1% to 2%), bilirubin increased (13% to 26%; grade 3: 2% to 6%; grade 4: ≤2%)

Renal: Proteinuria (32% to 45%; grades 3/4: <1%), hematuria (23% to 35%; grades 3/4: <1%), BUN increased (15% to 16%)

Respiratory: Dyspnea (10% to 23%)

Miscellaneous: Flu-like syndrome (19%), infection (10% to 16%; grade 3: 1% to 2%; grade 4: <1%)

1% to 10%:

Local: Injection site reactions (4%)

Neuromuscular & skeletal: Paresthesia (10%)

Renal: Creatinine increased (6% to 8%)

Respiratory: Bronchospasm (<2%)

<1%, postmarketing, and/or case reports (reported with single-agent use or with combination therapy): Acute/adult respiratory distress syndrome, anaphylactoid reaction, anorexia, arrhythmias, arthralgia, bullous skin eruptions, cellulitis, cerebrovascular accident, CHF, chills, constipation, cough, desquamation, diaphoresis, fulminant hepatic failure, gangrene, GGT increased, headache, hemolytic uremic syndrome (HUS), hepatic sinusoidal obstruction syndrome (SOS; veno-occlusive liver disease), hepatotoxicity (rare), hyperglycemia, hyper-/hypotension, hypermagnesemia, hypocalcemia, insomnia, interstitial pneumonitis, liver failure, malaise, MI, myalgia, neuropathy, peripheral vasculitis, petechiae, pulmonary edema, pulmonary fibrosis, radiation recall, renal failure, respiratory failure, reversible posterior leukoencephalopathy syndrome (RPLS), rhinitis, sepsis, supraventricular arrhythmia, thrombotic thrombocytopenic purpura, weakness

Drug Interactions

Metabolism/Transport Effects None known.

Avoid Concomitant Use

Avoid concomitant use of Gemcitabine with any of the following: BCG; CloZAPine; Natalizumab; Pimecrolimus; Tacrolimus (Topical); Vaccines (Live)

Increased Effect/Toxicity

Gemcitabine may increase the levels/effects of: Bleomycin; CloZAPine; Fluorouracil (Systemic); Fluorouracil (Topical); Leflunomide; Natalizumab; Vaccines (Live); Vitamin K Antagonists

The levels/effects of Gemcitabine may be increased by: Denosumab; Pimecrolimus; Roflumilast; Tacrolimus (Topical); Trastuzumab

Decreased Effect

Gemcitabine may decrease the levels/effects of: BCG; Coccidioidin Skin Test; Sipuleucel-T; Vaccines (Inactivated); Vaccines (Live); Vitamin K Antagonists

The levels/effects of Gemcitabine may be decreased by: Echinacea

Ethanol/Nutrition/Herb Interactions Ethanol: Avoid ethanol (due to GI irritation).

Storage/Stability

Lyophilized powder: Store intact vials at room temperature of 20°C to 25°C (68°F to 77°F); excursions permitted to 15°C to 30°C (59°F to 86°F). Reconstituted vials are stable for 24 hours at room temperature. Do not refrigerate (may form crystals).

Solution for injection: Store intact vials refrigerated at 2°C to 8°C (36°F to 46°F); do not freeze.

Solutions diluted for infusion in NS are stable for 24 hours at room temperature. Do not refrigerate.

Reconstitution Use appropriate precautions for handling and disposal. Reconstitute lyophilized powder with preservative free NS; add 5 mL to the 200 mg vial, add 25 mL to the 1000 mg vial, or add 50 mL to the 2000 mg vial, resulting in a reconstituted concentration of 38 mg/mL (solutions must be reconstituted to ≤40 mg/mL to completely dissolve).

Further dilute for infusion in NS 50-500 mL injection; to concentrations as low as 0.1 mg/mL.

Mechanism of Action A pyrimidine antimetabolite that inhibits DNA synthesis by inhibition of DNA polymerase and ribonucleotide reductase, cell cycle-specific for the S-phase of the cycle (also blocks cellular progression at G1/S phase). Gemcitabine is phosphorylated intracellularly by deoxycytidine kinase to gemcitabine monophosphate, which is further phosphorylated to active metabolites gemcitabine diphosphate and gemcitabine triphosphate. Gemcitabine diphosphate inhibits DNA synthesis by inhibiting ribonucleotide reductase; gemcitabine triphosphate incorporates into DNA and inhibits DNA polymerase.

Pharmacodynamics/Kinetics

Distribution: Infusions <70 minutes: 50 L/m^2; Long infusion times (70-285 minutes): 370 L/m^2

Protein binding: Negligible

Metabolism: Metabolized intracellularly by nucleoside kinases to the active diphosphate (dFdCDP) and triphosphate (dFdCTP) nucleoside metabolites

Half-life elimination:

Gemcitabine: Infusion time ≤70 minutes: 42-94 minutes; infusion time 3-4 hours: 4-10.5 hours (affected by age and gender)

Metabolite (gemcitabine triphosphate), terminal phase: 1.7-19.4 hours

Time to peak, plasma: 30 minutes after completion of infusion

Excretion: Urine (92% to 98%; primarily as inactive uracil metabolite); feces (<1%)

Dosing

Adult & Geriatric Details concerning dosing in combination regimens should also be consulted. **Note**: Prolongation of the infusion time >60 minutes and administration more frequently than once weekly have been shown to increase toxicity.

Pancreatic cancer, locally advanced or metastatic: I.V.: Initial: 1000 mg/m^2 over 30 minutes once weekly for up to 7 weeks followed by 1 week rest; then once weekly for 3 weeks out of every 4 weeks

Dose escalation: Patients who complete an entire cycle of therapy may have the dose in subsequent cycles increased by 25% as long as the absolute granulocyte count (AGC) nadir is >1500/mm^3, platelet nadir is >100,000/mm^3, and nonhematologic toxicity is less than WHO Grade 1. If the increased dose is tolerated (with the same parameters) the dose in subsequent cycles may again be increased by 20%.

Pancreatic cancer, advanced (unlabeled dosing/combinations): I.V.: 1000 mg/m^2 over 30 minutes weekly for up to 7 weeks followed by 1 week rest; then weekly for 3 weeks out of every 4 weeks (in combination with erlotinib) (Moore, 2007) **or** 1000 mg/m^2 over 30 minutes days 1, 8, and 15 every 4 weeks (in combination with capecitabine) (Cunningham, 2009) **or** 1000 mg/m^2 over 30 minutes days 1 and 15 every 4 weeks (in combination with cisplatin) (Heinemann, 2006) **or** 1000 mg/m^2 infused at 10 mg/m^2/minute every 2 weeks (in combination with oxaliplatin) (Louvet, 2005)

Nonsmall cell lung cancer, locally advanced or metastatic (in combination with cisplatin): I.V.: 1000 mg/m^2 over 30 minutes days 1, 8, and 15; repeat cycle every 28 days **or** 1250 mg/m^2 over 30 minutes days 1 and 8; repeat cycle every 21 days

Breast cancer, metastatic (AGC should be ≥1500/mm^3 and platelets ≥100,000/mm^3 prior to each cycle): I.V.: 1250 mg/m^2 over 30 minutes days 1 and 8; repeat cycle every 21 days (in combination with paclitaxel) **or** (unlabeled dosing) as a single agent: 800 mg/m^2 over 30 minutes days 1, 8, and 15 of a 28-day treatment cycle (Carmichael, 1995)

Ovarian cancer, advanced (AGC should be ≥1500/mm^3 and platelets ≥100,000/mm^3 prior to each cycle): I.V.: 1000 mg/m^2 over 30 minutes days 1 and 8; repeat cycle every 21 days (in combination with carboplatin)

Biliary tract cancer, advanced (unlabeled use): I.V.: 1000 mg/m^2 over 30 minutes days 1 and 8; repeat cycle every 21 days (in combination with cisplatin) (Valle, 2010) **or** 1000 mg/m^2 over 30 minutes days 1 and 8; repeat cycle every 21 days (in combination with capecitabine) (Knox, 2005) **or** 1000 mg/m^2 infused at 10 mg/m^2/minute over 100 minutes every 2 weeks (in combination with oxaliplatin) (Andre, 2004)

Bladder cancer (unlabeled use):

Advanced or metastatic: I.V.: 1000 mg/m^2 over 30-60 minutes days 1, 8, and 15; repeat cycle every 4 weeks (in combination with cisplatin) (von der Maase, 2000)

Transitional cell carcinoma: Intravesicular instillation: 2000 mg (in 100 mL NS; retain for 1 hour) twice weekly for 3 weeks; repeat cycle every 4 weeks for at least 2 cycles (Dalbagni, 2006)

Cervical cancer, recurrent or persistent (unlabeled use): I.V.: 1000 mg/m^2 days 1 and 8; repeat cycle every 21 days (in combination with cisplatin) (Monk, 2009) **or** 1250 mg/m^2 over 30 minutes days 1 and 8; repeat cycle every 21 days (in combination with cisplatin) (Burnett, 2000) **or** 800 mg/m^2 over 30 minutes days 1, 8, and 15; repeat cycle every 28 days (as a single-agent) (Schilder, 2005)

Head and neck cancer, nasopharyngeal (unlabeled use): I.V.: 1000 mg/m^2 over 30 minutes days 1, 8, and 15 every 4 weeks (Zhang, 2008)

Hodgkin lymphoma, relapsed (unlabeled use): I.V.: 1000 mg/m^2 (800 mg/m^2 for post-transplant patients) over 30 minutes days 1 and 8; repeat cycle every 21 days (in combination with vinorelbine and doxorubicin liposomal) (Bartlett, 2007) **or** 800 mg/m^2 days 1 and 4; repeat cycle every 21 days (in combination with ifosfamide, mesna, vinorelbine, and prednisolone) (Santoro, 2007)

Malignant pleural mesothelioma (unlabeled use; in combination with cisplatin): I.V.: 1000 mg/m^2 over 30 minutes days 1, 8 and 15 every 4 weeks for up to 6 cycles (Nowak, 2002) **or** 1250 mg/m^2 over 30 minutes days 1 and 8 every 3 weeks for up to 6 cycles (van Haarst, 2002)

Non-Hodgkin lymphoma, refractory (unlabeled use): I.V.: 1000 mg/m^2 over 30 minutes days 1 and 8; repeat cycle every 21 days (in combination with cisplatin and dexamethasone) (Crump, 2004) **or** 1000 mg/m^2 every 15-21days (in combination with oxaliplatin and rituximab) (Lopez, 2008)

Sarcoma (unlabeled uses): I.V.:

Ewing's sarcoma, refractory: 675 mg/m^2 over 90 minutes days 1 and 8; repeat cycle every 21 days (in combination with docetaxel) (Navid, 2008)

Osteosarcoma, refractory: 675 mg/m^2 over 90 minutes days 1 and 8; repeat cycle every 21 days (in combination with docetaxel) (Navid, 2008) **or** 1000 mg/m^2 weekly for 7 weeks followed by 1 week rest; then weekly for 3 weeks out of every 4 weeks (Merimsky, 2000)

Soft tissue sarcoma, advanced: I.V.: 800 mg/m^2 over 90 minutes days 1 and 8; repeat cycle every 21 days (in combination with vinorelbine) (Dileo, 2007) **or** 675 mg/m^2 over 90 minutes days 1 and 8; repeat cycle every 21 days (in combination with docetaxel) (Leu, 2004) **or** 900 mg/m^2 over 90 minutes days 1 and 8; repeat cycle every 21 days (in combination with docetaxel) (Maki, 2007)

Small cell lung cancer, refractory or relapsed (unlabeled use): I.V.: 1000-1250 mg/m^2 over 30 minutes days 1, 8, and 15 every 4 weeks (as a single agent) (Masters, 2003)

Testicular cancer, refractory germ cell (unlabeled use): I.V.: 1000 mg/m^2 over 30 minutes days 1 and 8 every 3 weeks (in combination with oxaliplatin) (Kohllmannsberger, 2004; Pectasides, 2004) **or** 1250 mg/m^2 over 30 minutes days 1 and 8 every 3 weeks (in combination with oxaliplatin) (De Giorgi, 2006) **or** 1000 mg/m^2 over 30 minutes days 1, 8 and 15 every 4 weeks for up to 6 cycles (in combination with paclitaxel) (Hinton, 2002)

Unknown-primary, adenocarcinoma (unlabeled use): I.V.: 1250 mg/m^2 days 1 and 8 every 3 weeks (in combination with cisplatin) (Culine, 2003) **or** 1000 mg/m^2 over 30 minutes days 1 and 8 every 3 weeks (in combination with docetaxel) for up to 6 cycles (Pouessel, 2004)

Uterine cancer (unlabeled use): I.V.: 900 mg/m^2 over 90 minutes days 1 and 8 every 3 weeks (in combination with docetaxel) (Hensley, 2008) **or** 1000 mg/m^2 over 30 minutes days 1, 8, and 15 every 4 weeks (Look, 2004)

Pediatric Details concerning dosing in combination regimens should also be consulted. **Note**: Prolongation of the infusion time >60 minutes and administration more frequently than once weekly have been shown to increase toxicity. Refer to specific references for ages of populations studied):

Germ cell tumor, refractory (unlabeled use): I.V.: 1000 mg/m^2 over 30 minutes days 1, 8, and 15 every 4 weeks (in combination with paclitaxel) for up to 6 cycles (Hinton, 2002)

Hodgkin lymphoma, relapsed (unlabeled use): I.V.: 1000 mg/m^2 over 100 minutes days 1 and 8; repeat cycle every 21 days (in combination with vinorelbine) (Cole; 2009) **or** 800 mg/m^2 days 1 and 4; repeat cycle every 21 days (in combination with ifosfamide, mesna, vinorelbine, and prednisolone) (Santoro, 2007)

Sarcomas (unlabeled use): I.V.:

Ewing's sarcoma, refractory: 675 mg/m^2 over 90 minutes days 1 and 8; repeat cycle every 21 days (in combination with docetaxel) (Navid, 2008)

Osteosarcoma, refractory: 675 mg/m^2 over 90 minutes days 1 and 8; repeat cycle every 21 days (in combination with docetaxel) (Navid, 2008) **or** 1000 mg/m^2 weekly for 7 weeks followed by 1 week rest; then weekly for 3 weeks out of every 4 weeks (Merimsky, 2000)

Renal Impairment The FDA-approved labeling does not contain dosing adjustment guidelines; use with caution in patients with pre-existing renal dysfunction. Discontinue if severe renal toxicity or hemolytic uremic syndrome (HUS) occur during gemcitabine treatment.

Mild-to-severe renal impairment: No adjustment required (Janus, 2010; Li, 2007).

ESRD (on hemodialysis): Hemodialysis should begin 6-12 hours after gemcitabine infusion (Janus 2010; Li, 2007).

Hepatic Impairment The FDA-approved labeling does not contain dosing adjustment guidelines; use with caution. Discontinue if severe hepatotoxicity occurs during treatment with gemcitabine. The following guidelines have been used by some clinicians:

Transaminases elevated (with normal bilirubin): No adjustment required (Venook, 2000).

Serum bilirubin >1.6 mg/dL: Use initial dose of 800 mg/m^2; may escalate if tolerated (Ecklund, 2005; Floyd, 2006; Venook, 2000).

Adjustment for Toxicity

Pancreatic cancer: Hematologic toxicity:

AGC ≥1000/mm^3 and platelet count ≥100,000/mm^3: Administer 100% of full dose

AGC 500-999/mm^3 or platelet count 50,000-99,999/mm^3: Administer 75% of full dose

AGC <500/mm^3 or platelet count <50,000/mm^3: Hold dose

Nonsmall cell lung cancer:

Hematologic toxicity: Refer to guidelines for pancreatic cancer. Cisplatin dosage may also need adjusted.

Severe (grades 3 or 4) nonhematologic toxicity (except alopecia, nausea, and vomiting): Hold or decrease dose by 50%.

Breast cancer:

Hematologic toxicity: Adjustments based on granulocyte and platelet counts on day 8:

- AGC >1200/mm³ and platelet count >75,000/mm³: Administer 100% of full dose
- AGC 1000-1199/mm³ or platelet count 50,000-75,000/mm³: Administer 75% of full dose
- AGC 700-999/mm³ and platelet count ≥50,000/mm³: Administer 50% of full dose
- AGC <700/mm³ or platelet count <50,000/mm³: Hold dose

Severe (grades 3 or 4) nonhematologic toxicity (except alopecia, nausea, and vomiting): Hold or decrease dose by 50%. Paclitaxel dose may also need adjusted.

Ovarian cancer:

Hematologic toxicity: Adjustments based on granulocyte and platelet counts on day 8:

- AGC ≥1500/mm³ and platelet count ≥100,000/mm³: Administer 100% of full dose
- AGC 1000-1499/mm³ and/or platelet count 75,000-99,999/mm³: Administer 50% of full dose
- AGC <1000/mm³ and/or platelet count <75,000/mm³: Hold dose

Severe (grades 3 or 4) nonhematologic toxicity (except nausea and vomiting): Hold or decrease dose by 50%. Carboplatin dose may also need adjusted.

Dose adjustment for subsequent cycles:

- AGC <500/mm³ for >5 days, AGC <100/mm³ for >3 days, febrile neutropenia, platelet count <25,000/mm³, cycle delay >1 week due to toxicity. Reduce gemcitabine to 800 mg/m² on days 1 and 8.
- For recurrence of any of the above toxicities after initial dose reduction: Administer gemcitabine 800 mg/m² on day 1 only for the subsequent cycle

Combination Regimens

Biliary adenocarcinoma:
- Gemcitabine-Capecitabine (Biliary Cancer) on page 1668
- Gemcitabine-Cisplatin (Biliary Cancer) on page 1669
- GEMOX (Biliary Cancer) on page 1678

Bladder cancer:
- Gemcitabine-Carboplatin (Bladder Cancer) on page 1668
- Gemcitabine-Cisplatin (Bladder Cancer) on page 1669
- Paclitaxel-Carboplatin-Gemcitabine on page 1726
- Paclitaxel-Gemcitabine on page 1729

Breast cancer: Gemcitabine-Paclitaxel (Breast Cancer) on page 1675

Cervical cancer: Cisplatin-Gemcitabine (Cervical Cancer) on page 1578

Lung cancer (nonsmall cell):
- Bevacizumab-Cisplatin-Gemcitabine (NSCLC) on page 1529
- Carboplatin-Gemcitabine (NSCLC) on page 1547
- Gemcitabine-Cisplatin (NSCLC) on page 1670
- Gemcitabine-Vinorelbine (NSCLC) on page 1677

Lung cancer (small cell): Gemcitabine (Small Cell Lung Cancer Regimen) on page 1676

Lymphoma, Hodgkin:
- GDP (Hodgkin) on page 1667
- Gemcitabine (Hodgkin Regimen) on page 1672

GVD (Hodgkin) on page 1679
IGEV (Hodgkin) on page 1690
Lymphoma, non-Hodgkins: Gemcitabine-Oxaliplatin-Rituximab (NHL) on page 1674
Malignant pleural mesothelioma:
Cisplatin-Gemcitabine (Mesothelioma) on page 1578
Gemcitabine (Mesothelioma Regimen) on page 1673
Osteosarcoma: Gemcitabine-Docetaxel (Sarcoma) on page 1671
Ovarian cancer:
Carboplatin-Gemcitabine (Ovarian) on page 1548
Gemcitabine (Ovarian Regimen) on page 1673
Gemcitabine-Paclitaxel (Ovarian Cancer) on page 1675
Pancreatic cancer:
Capecitabine-Gemcitabine (Pancreatic) on page 1540
Cisplatin-Gemcitabine (Pancreatic) on page 1579
Erlotinib-Gemcitabine (Pancreatic) on page 1632
Gemcitabine Fixed Dose Rate (Pancreatic Regimen) on page 1672
Gemcitabine-Oxaliplatin (Pancreatic) on page 1674
Gemcitabine-Paclitaxel (Protein Bound) (Pancreatic) on page 1675
Gemcitabine Standard Infusion (Pancreatic Regimen) on page 1676
Renal cell cancer:
Gemcitabine-Capecitabine (RCC) on page 1668
Gemcitabine-Fluorouracil (RCC) on page 1672
Soft tissue sarcoma:
Gemcitabine-Docetaxel (Sarcoma) on page 1671
Gemcitabine-Vinorelbine (Sarcoma) on page 1677
Testicular cancer:
Gemcitabine-Oxaliplatin-Paclitaxel (Testicular) on page 1674
Gemcitabine-Paclitaxel (Testicular) on page 1675
GEMOX (Testicular) on page 1678
Unknown primary, adenocarcinoma:
Carboplatin-Gemcitabine-Paclitaxel (Unknown Primary) on page 1548
Cisplatin-Gemcitabine (Unknown Primary) on page 1580
Docetaxel-Gemcitabine (Unknown Primary) on page 1611

Administration Infuse over 30 minutes; for unlabeled uses, infusion times may vary (refer to specific references). **Note:** Prolongation of the infusion time >60 minutes has been shown to increase toxicity. Gemcitabine has been administered at a fixed-dose rate (FDR) infusion rate of 10 mg/m^2/minute (unlabeled); prolonged infusion times increase the accumulation of the active metabolite, gemcitabine triphosphate, optimizing the pharmacokinetics (Ko, 2006; Tempero, 2003). Patients who receive gemcitabine FDR experience more grade 3/4 hematologic toxicity (Ko, 2006; Poplin, 2009).

For intravesicular (bladder) instillation, gemcitabine was diluted in 50-100 mL normal saline; patients were instructed to retain in the bladder for 1 hour (Addeo, 2010; Dalbaghi, 2006)

Emetic Potential Low (10% to 30%)

Vesicant/Extravasation Risk May be an irritant

Monitoring Parameters CBC with differential and platelet count (prior to each dose); hepatic and renal function (prior to initiation of therapy and periodically, thereafter); monitor electrolytes, including potassium, magnesium, and calcium (when in combination therapy with cisplatin)

Dosage Forms Excipient information presented when available (limited, particularly for generics); consult specific product labeling.

Injection, powder for reconstitution: 200 mg, 1 g, 2 g

Gemzar®: 200 mg, 1 g

Injection, solution: 38 mg/mL (5.26 mL, 26.3 mL, 52.6 mL)

References

Addeo R, Caraglia M, Bellini S, et al, "Randomized Phase III Trial on Gemcitabine Versus Mytomicin in Recurrent Superficial Bladder Cancer: Evaluation of Efficacy and Tolerance," *J Clin Oncol*, 2010, 28(4):543-8.

Albain KS, Nag SM, Calderillo-Ruiz G, et al, "Gemcitabine Plus Paclitaxel Versus Paclitaxel Monotherapy in Patients With Metastatic Breast Cancer and Prior Anthracycline Treatment," *J Clin Oncol*, 2008, 26(24):3950-7.

Andre T, Tournigand C, Rosmorduc O, et al, "Gemcitabine Combined With Oxaliplatin (GEMOX) in Advanced Biliary Tract Adenocarcinoma: A GERCOR Study," *Ann Oncol*, 2004, 15(9):1339-43.

Bartlett NL, Niedzwiecki D, Johnson JL, et al, "Gemcitabine, Vinorelbine, and Pegylated Liposomal Doxorubicin (GVD), a Salvage Regimen in Relapsed Hodgkin's Lymphoma: CALGB 59804," *Ann Oncol*, 2007, 18(6):1071-9.

Burnett AF, Roman LD, Garcia AA, "A Phase II Study of Gemcitabine and Cisplatin in Patients With Advanced, Persistent, or Recurrent Squamous Cell Carcinoma of the Cervix," *Gynecol Oncol*, 2000, 76(1):63-6.

Carmichael J, Possinger K, Phillip P, et al, "Advanced Breast Cancer: A Phase II Trial With Gemcitabine," *J Clin Oncol*, 1995, 13(11):2731-6.

Cole PD, Schwartz CL, Drachtman RA, et al, "Phase II Study of Weekly Gemcitabine and Vinorelbine for Children With Recurrent or Refractory Hodgkin's Disease: A Children's Oncology Group Report," *J Clin Oncol*, 2009, 27(9):1456-61.

Correale P, Cerretani D, Marsili S, et al, "Gemcitabine Increases Systemic 5-Fluorouracil Exposure in Advanced Cancer Patients," *Eur J Cancer*, 2003, 39(11):1547-51.

Crump M, Baetz T, Couban S, et al, "Gemcitabine, Dexamethasone, and Cisplatin in Patients With Recurrent or Refractory Aggressive Histology B-Cell Non-Hodgkin Lymphoma: A Phase II Study by the National Cancer Institute of Canada Clinical Trials Group (NCIC-CTG)," *Cancer*, 2004, 101 (8):1835-42.

Culine S, Lortholary A, Voigt JJ, et al, "Cisplatin in Combination With Either Gemcitabine or Irinotecan in Carcinomas of Unknown Primary Site: Results of a Randomized Phase II Study - Trial for the French Study Group on Carcinomas of Unknown Primary (GEFCAPI 01)," *J Clin Oncol*, 2003, 21(18):3479-82.

Cunningham D, Chau I, Stocken DD, et al, "Phase III Randomized Comparison of Gemcitabine Versus Gemcitabine Plus Capecitabine in Patients With Advanced Pancreatic Cancer," *J Clin Oncol*, 2009, 27(33):5513-8.

Dalbagni G, Russo P, Bochner B, et al, "Phase II Trial of Intravesical Gemcitabine in Bacille Calmette-Guerin-Refractory Transitional Cell Carcinoma of the Bladder," *J Clin Oncol*, 2006, 24 (18):2729-34.

De Giorgi U, Rosti G, Aieta M, et al, "Phase II Study of Oxaliplatin and Gemcitabine Salvage Chemotherapy in Patients With Cisplatin-Refractory Nonseminomatous Germ Cell Tumor," *Eur Urol*, 2006, 50(5):1032-8.

Dileo P, Morgan JA, Zahrieh D, et al, "Gemcitabine and Vinorelbine Combination Chemotherapy for Patients With Advanced Soft Tissue Sarcomas: Results of a Phase II Trial," *Cancer*, 2007, 109 (9):1863-9.

Ecklund JW, Trifilio S, and Mulcahy MF, "Chemotherapy Dosing in the Setting of Liver Dysfunction," *Oncology (Williston Park)*, 2005, 19(8):1057-63.

Edelman MJ, Belani CP, Socinski MA, et al, "Outcomes Associated With Brain Metastases in a Three-Arm Phase III Trial of Gemcitabine-Containing Regimens Versus Paclitaxel Plus Carboplatin for Advanced Non-Small Cell Lung Cancer," *J Thorac Oncol*, 2010, 5(1):110-6.

Floyd J, Mirza I, Sachs B, et al, "Hepatotoxicity of Chemotherapy," *Semin Oncol*, 2006, 33 (1):50-67.

Heinemann V, Quietzsch D, Gieseler F, et al, "Randomized Phase III Trial of Gemcitabine Plus Cisplatin Compared With Gemcitabine Alone in Advanced Pancreatic Cancer," *J Clin Oncol*, 2006, 24(24):3946-52.

Hensley ML, Blessing JA, Degeest K, et al, "Fixed-Dose Rate Gemcitabine Plus Docetaxel as Second-Line Therapy for Metastatic Uterine Leiomyosarcoma: A Gynecologic Oncology Group Phase II Study," *Gynecol Oncol*, 2008, 109(3):323-8.

Hinton S, Catalano P, Einhorn LH, et al, "Phase II Study of Paclitaxel Plus Gemcitabine in Refractory Germ Cell Tumors (E9897): A Trial of the Eastern Cooperative Oncology Group," *J Clin Oncol*, 2002, 20(7):1859-63.

Janus N, Thariat J, Boulanger H, et al, "Proposal for Dosage Adjustment and Timing of Chemotherapy in Hemodialyzed Patients," *Ann Oncol*, 2010, 21(7):1395-403.

Knox JJ, Hedley D, Oza A, et al, "Combining Gemcitabine and Capecitabine in Patients With Advanced Biliary Cancer: A Phase II Trial," *J Clin Oncol*, 2005, 23(10):2332-8.

Ko AH, Dito E, Schillinger B, et al, "Phase II Study of Fixed Dose Rate Gemcitabine With Cisplatin for Metastatic Adenocarcinoma of the Pancreas," *J Clin Oncol*, 2006, 24(3):379-85.

Kollmannsberger C, Beyer J, Liersch R, et al, "Combination Chemotherapy With Gemcitabine Plus Oxaliplatin in Patients With Intensively Pretreated or Refractory Germ Cell Cancer: A Study of the German Testicular Cancer Study Group," *J Clin Oncol*, 2004, 22(1):108-14.

Leu KM, Ostruszka LJ, Shewach D, et al, "Laboratory and Clinical Evidence of Synergistic Cytotoxicity of Sequential Treatment With Gemcitabine Followed by Docetaxel in the Treatment of Sarcoma," *J Clin Oncol*, 2004, 22(9):1706-12.

Li YF, Fu S, Hu W, et al, "Systemic Anticancer Therapy in Gynecological Cancer Patients With Renal Dysfunction," *Int J Gynecol Cancer*, 2007, 7(4):739-63.

Look KY, Sandler A, Blessing JA, et al, "Phase II Trial of Gemcitabine as Second-Line Chemotherapy of Uterine Leiomyosarcoma: A Gynecologic Oncology Group (GOG) Study," *Gynecol Oncol*, 2004, 92(2):644-7.

López A, Gutiérrez A, Palacios A, et al, "GEMOX-R Regimen is a Highly Effective Salvage Regimen in Patients With Refractory/Relapsing Diffuse Large-Cell Lymphoma: A Phase II Study," *Eur J Haematol*, 2008, 80(2):127-32.

Louvet C, Labianca R, Hammel P, et al, "Gemcitabine in Combination With Oxaliplatin Compared With Gemcitabine Alone in Locally Advanced or Metastatic Pancreatic Cancer: Results of a GERCOR and GISCAD Phase III Trial," *J Clin Oncol*, 2005, 23(15):3509-16.

Maki RG, Wathen JK, Patel SR, et al, "Randomized Phase II Study of Gemcitabine and Docetaxel Compared With Gemcitabine Alone in Patients With Metastatic Soft Tissue Sarcomas: Results of Sarcoma Alliance for Research Through Collaboration Study 002," *J Clin Oncol*, 2007, 25 (19):2755-63.

Masters GA, Declerck L, Blanke C, et al, "Phase II Trial of Gemcitabine in Refractory or Relapsed Small-Cell Lung Cancer: Eastern Cooperative Oncology Group Trial 1597," *J Clin Oncol*, 2003, 21(8):1550-5.

Merimsky O, Meller I, Flusser G, et al, "Gemcitabine in Soft Tissue or Bone Sarcoma Resistant to Standard Chemotherapy: A Phase II Study," *Cancer Chemother Pharmacol*, 2000, 45(2):177-81.

Monk BJ, Sill MW, McMeekin DS, et al, "Phase III Trial of Four Cisplatin-Containing Doublet Combinations in Stage IVB, Recurrent, or Persistent Cervical Carcinoma: A Gynecologic Oncology Group Study," *J Clin Oncol*, 2009, 27(28):4649-55.

Moore MJ, Goldstein D, Hamm J, et al, "Erlotinib Plus Gemcitabine Compared With Gemcitabine Alone in Patients With Advanced Pancreatic Cancer: A Phase III Trial of the National Cancer Institute of Canada Clinical Trials Group," *J Clin Oncol*, 2007, 25(15):1960-6.

Morgan C, Tillett T, Braybrooke J, et al, "Management of Uncommon Chemotherapy-Induced Emergencies," *Lancet Oncol*, 2011, 12(8):806-14.

Navid F, Willert JR, McCarville MB, et al, "Combination of Gemcitabine and Docetaxel in the Treatment of Children and Young Adults With Refractory Bone Sarcoma," *Cancer*, 2008, 113 (2):419-25.

Nowak AK, Byrne MJ, Williamson R, et al, "A Multicentre Phase II Study of Cisplatin and Gemcitabine for Malignant Mesothelioma," *Br J Cancer*, 2002, 87(5):491-6.

Palmieri G, Merola G, Federico P, et al, "Preliminary Results of Phase II Study of Capecitabine and Gemcitabine (CAP-GEM) in Patients With Metastatic Pretreated Thymic Epithelial Tumors (TETs)," *Ann Oncol*, 2010, 21(6):1168-72.

Pectasides D, Pectasides M, Farmakis D, et al, "Gemcitabine and Oxaliplatin (GEMOX) in Patients With Cisplatin-Refractory Germ Cell Tumors: A Phase II Study," *Ann Oncol*, 2004, 15(3):493-7.

Pfisterer J, Vergote I, Du Bois A, et al, "Combination Therapy with Gemcitabine and Carboplatin in Recurrent Ovarian Cancer," *Int J Gynecol Cancer*, 2005, 15 (Suppl 1):36-41.

Poplin E, Feng Y, Berlin J, et al, "Phase III, Randomized Study of Gemcitabine and Oxaliplatin Versus Gemcitabine (Fixed-Dose Rate Infusion) Compared With Gemcitabine (30-Minute Infusion) in Patients With Pancreatic Carcinoma E6201: a Trial of the Eastern Cooperative Oncology Group," *J Clin Oncol*, 2009, 27(23):3778-85.

Pouessel D, Culine S, Becht C, et al, "Gemcitabine and Docetaxel as Front-Line Chemotherapy in Patients With Carcinoma of an Unknown Primary Site," *Cancer*, 2004, 100(6):1257-61.

Santoro A, Magagnoli M, Spina M, et al, "Ifosfamide, Gemcitabine, and Vinorelbine: A New Induction Regimen for Refractory and Relapsed Hodgkin's Lymphoma," *Haematologica*, 2007, 92(1):35-41.

Schilder RJ, Blessing J, and Cohn DE, "Evaluation of Gemcitabine in Previously Treated Patients With Non-Squamous Cell Carcinoma of the Cervix: A Phase II Study of the Gynecologic Oncology Group," *Gynecol Oncol*, 2005, 96(1):103-7.

Seliger G, Mueller LP, Kegel T, et al, "Phase 2 Trial of Docetaxel, Gemcitabine, and Oxaliplatin Combination Chemotherapy in Platinum- and Paclitaxel-Pretreated Epithelial Ovarian Cancer," *Int J Gynecol Cancer*, 2009, 19(8):1446-53.

Tannir NM, Thall PF, Ng CS, et al, "A Phase II Trial of Gemcitabine Plus Capecitabine for Metastatic Renal Cell Cancer Previously Treated With Immunotherapy and Targeted Agents," *J Urol*, 2008, 180(3):867-72.

Tempero M, Plunkett W, Ruiz Van Haperen V, "Randomized Phase II Comparison of Dose-Intense Gemcitabine: Thirty-Minute Infusion and Fixed Dose Rate Infusion in Patients With Pancreatic Adenocarcinoma," *J Clin Oncol*, 2003, 21(18):3402-8.

Valle J, Wason H, Palmer DH, et al, "Cisplatin Plus Gemcitabine Versus Gemcitabine for Biliary Tract Cancer," *N Engl J Med*, 2010, 362(14):1273-81.

van Haarst JM, Baas P, Manegold Ch, et al, "Multicentre Phase II Study of Gemcitabine and Cisplatin in Malignant Pleural Mesothelioma," *Br J Cancer*, 2002, 86(3):342-5.

Venook AP, Egorin MJ, Rosner GL, et al, "Phase I and Pharmacokinetic Trial of Gemcitabine in Patients With Hepatic or Renal Dysfunction: Cancer and Leukemia Group B 9565," *J Clin Oncol*, 2000, 18(14):2780-7.

von der Maase H, Hansen SW, Roberts JT, et al, "Gemcitabine and Cisplatin Versus Methotrexate, Vinblastine, Doxorubicin, and Cisplatin in Advanced or Metastatic Bladder Cancer: Results of a Large, Randomized, Multinational, Multicenter, Phase III Study," *J Clin Oncol*, 2000, 18 (17):3068-77.

Zhang L, Zhang Y, Huang PY, et al, "Phase II Clinical Study of Gemcitabine in the Treatment of Patients With Advanced Nasopharyngeal Carcinoma After the Failure of Platinum-Based Chemotherapy," *Cancer Chemother Pharmacol*, 2008, 61(1):33-8.

◆ **Gemcitabine For Injection, USP (Can)** *see* Gemcitabine *on page* 663

◆ **Gemcitabine Hydrochloride** *see* Gemcitabine *on page* 663

Gemtuzumab Ozogamicin (gem TOO zoo mab oh zog a MY sin)

Related Information

Management of Chemotherapy-Induced Nausea and Vomiting *on page* 1786

Safe Handling of Hazardous Drugs *on page* 1904

Index Terms CMA-676; Mylotarg

Generic Availability (U.S.) No

Pharmacologic Category Antineoplastic Agent, Monoclonal Antibody

Use Due to safety concerns, as well as lack of clinical benefit demonstrated in a post-approval clinical trial, gemtuzumab was withdrawn from the U.S. commercial market in 2010.

Unlabeled Use Treatment of relapsed or refractory CD33-positive acute myeloid leukemia (AML); salvage therapy for acute promyelocytic leukemia (APL)

Labeled Contraindications Hypersensitivity to gemtuzumab ozogamicin, calicheamicin derivatives, or any component of the formulation; patients with anti-CD33 antibody

Lactation Excretion in breast milk unknown/not recommended

Warnings/Precautions Hazardous agent - use appropriate precautions for handling and disposal.

Gemtuzumab has been associated with hepatotoxicity, including severe hepatic sinusoidal obstruction syndrome (SOS; formerly called veno-occlusive disease [VOD]). Symptoms of SOS include right upper quadrant pain, rapid weight gain, ascites, hepatomegaly, and bilirubin/transaminase elevations. Risk may be increased by combination chemotherapy, underlying hepatic disease, or hematopoietic stem cell transplant.

Severe hypersensitivity reactions (including anaphylaxis) and other infusion-related reactions may occur. Infusion-related events are common, generally reported to occur with the first dose after the end of the 2-hour intravenous infusion. These symptoms usually resolved after 2-4 hours with a supportive therapy of acetaminophen, diphenhydramine, and intravenous fluids. Other severe and potentially fatal infusion related pulmonary events ▶

(including dyspnea and hypoxia) have been reported infrequently. Symptomatic intrinsic lung disease or high peripheral blast counts may increase the risk of severe reactions. Fewer infusion-related events were observed after the second dose. Postinfusion reactions (may include fever, chills, hypotension, or dyspnea) may occur during the first 24 hours after administration. Consider discontinuation in patients who develop severe infusion-related reactions. In addition to infusion-related pulmonary events, gemtuzumab therapy is also associated with acute respiratory distress syndrome, pulmonary infiltrates, pleural effusion, noncardiogenic pulmonary edema, and pulmonary insufficiency.

Severe myelosuppression occurs in all patients at recommended dosages. Tumor lysis syndrome may occur as a consequence of leukemia treatment, adequate hydration and prophylactic allopurinol must be instituted prior to use. Other methods to lower WBC <30,000 cells/mm^3 may be considered (hydroxyurea or leukapheresis) to minimize the risk of tumor lysis syndrome, and/or severe infusion reactions. An increased number of deaths have been reported in patients receiving gemtuzumab in combination with chemotherapy, compared to those receiving chemotherapy alone.

Adverse Reactions Frequency not defined.

Cardiovascular: Cerebral hemorrhage, hyper-/hypotension, peripheral edema, tachycardia

Central nervous system: Anxiety, chills, depression, dizziness, fever, headache, insomnia, intracranial hemorrhage, pain

Dermatologic: Bruising, petechiae, pruritus, rash

Endocrine & metabolic: Hyperglycemia, hypocalcemia, hypokalemia, hypomagnesemia, hypophosphatemia

Gastrointestinal: Abdominal pain, anorexia, diarrhea, dyspepsia, gingival hemorrhage, melena, mucositis, nausea, stomatitis, vomiting

Genitourinary: Vaginal bleeding, vaginal hemorrhage

Hematologic: Anemia, disseminated intravascular coagulation (DIC), hemorrhage, leukopenia, lymphopenia, neutropenia (median recovery 40-51 days), neutropenic fever, thrombocytopenia (median recovery 36-51 days)

Hepatic: Alkaline phosphatase increased, ALT increased, ascites, AST increased, hyperbilirubinemia, LDH increased, prothrombin time increased, PTT increased, sinusoidal obstruction syndrome (SOS; veno-occlusive disease; higher frequency in patients with prior history of or subsequent hematopoietic stem cell transplant)

Local: Local reaction

Neuromuscular & skeletal: Arthralgia, back pain, myalgia, weakness

Renal: Creatinine increased, hematuria

Respiratory: Cough, dyspnea, epistaxis, hypoxia, pharyngitis, pneumonia, rhinitis

Miscellaneous: Cutaneous herpes simplex, infection, infusion reaction, sepsis

Infrequent and/or case reports: Acute respiratory distress syndrome, anaphylaxis, bradycardia, Budd-Chiari syndrome, gastrointestinal hemorrhage, hepatic failure, hepatosplenomegaly, hypersensitivity reactions, jaundice, neutropenic sepsis, noncardiogenic pulmonary edema, portal vain thrombosis, pulmonary hemorrhage, renal impairment, renal failure (including renal failure secondary to tumor lysis syndrome)

Drug Interactions

Metabolism/Transport Effects None known.

Avoid Concomitant Use

Avoid concomitant use of Gemtuzumab Ozogamicin with any of the following: BCG; Belimumab; CloZAPine; Natalizumab; Pimecrolimus; Tacrolimus (Topical); Vaccines (Live)

Increased Effect/Toxicity

Gemtuzumab Ozogamicin may increase the levels/effects of: Belimumab; CloZAPine; Leflunomide; Natalizumab; Vaccines (Live)

The levels/effects of Gemtuzumab Ozogamicin may be increased by: Abciximab; Denosumab; Pimecrolimus; Roflumilast; Tacrolimus (Topical); Trastuzumab

Decreased Effect

Gemtuzumab Ozogamicin may decrease the levels/effects of: BCG; Coccidioidin Skin Test; Sipuleucel-T; Vaccines (Inactivated); Vaccines (Live)

The levels/effects of Gemtuzumab Ozogamicin may be decreased by: Echinacea

Storage/Stability Light sensitive; protect from light (including direct and indirect sunlight, and unshielded fluorescent light). The infusion container should be placed in a UV protectant bag immediately after preparation. Store intact vials under refrigeration at 2°C to 8°C (36°F to 46°F). Reconstituted solutions may be stored for up to 2 hours at room temperature or under refrigeration. Following dilution for infusion, solutions are stable for up to 16 hours at room temperature. Administration requires 2 hours; therefore, the maximum elapsed time from initial reconstitution to completion of infusion should be 20 hours.

Reconstitution Protect from light during preparation (and administration). Prepare in biologic safety hood with shielded fluorescent light; (some institutions prepare in a darkened room with the lights in the biologic safety cabinet turned off). Allow to warm to room temperature prior to reconstitution. Reconstitute each 5 mg vial with sterile water for injection to a concentration of 1 mg/mL. Dilute in 100 mL of 0.9% sodium chloride injection. Hazardous agent - use appropriate precautions for handling and disposal.

Mechanism of Action Antibody to CD33 antigen, which is expressed on leukemic blasts in 80% of AML patients. Binds to the CD33 antigen, resulting in internalization of the antibody-antigen complex. Following internalization, the calicheamicin derivative is released inside the myeloid cell. The calicheamicin derivative binds to DNA resulting in double strand breaks and cell death. Pluripotent stem cells and nonhematopoietic cells are not affected.

Pharmacodynamics/Kinetics

Distribution: V_{ss}: Adults: Initial dose: 21 L; Repeat dose: 10 L

Half-life elimination: Total calicheamicin: Initial: 41-45 hours, Repeat dose: 60-64 hours; Unconjugated: 100-143 hours (no change noted in repeat dosing)

Dosing

Adult & Geriatric Note: Patients should receive diphenhydramine 50 mg orally and acetaminophen 650-1000 mg orally 1 hour prior to administration of each dose. Acetaminophen dosage should be repeated as needed every 4 hours for 2 additional doses. Pretreatment with methylprednisolone may ameliorate infusion-related symptoms.

Acute myeloid leukemia (unlabeled/investigational use): I.V.:

<60 years: 9 mg/m² infused over 2 hours. A full treatment course is a total of 2 doses administered with 14-28 days between doses (Larson, 2005).

≥60 years: 9 mg/m² infused over 2 hours. A full treatment course is a total of 2 doses administered with 14-28 days between doses (Larson, 2002; Larson, 2005).

Acute promyelocytic leukemia (unlabeled/investigational use): I.V.:

Single-agent therapy: 6 mg/m² infused over 2 hours on days 1 and 15; for patients testing PCR negative after 2 doses, a third dose was administered (LoCoco, 2004).

Combination therapy (high-risk patients; Ravandi, 2009):

Induction: 9 mg/m² as a single dose on day 1 (in combination with arsenic trioxide and tretinoin)

Post remission therapy (if arsenic trioxide or tretinoin discontinued due to toxicity): 9 mg/m² once every 4-5 weeks until 28 weeks after complete remission.

Adjustment for Toxicity

Dyspnea or significant hypotension: Interrupt infusion; monitor

Anaphylaxis, pulmonary edema, acute respiratory distress syndrome: Strongly consider discontinuing treatment

Administration Do not administer as I.V. push or bolus. Administer via I.V. infusion, over at least 2 hours through a low protein-binding (0.2-1.2 micron) in-line filter. Protect from light during infusion. Premedicate with acetaminophen and diphenhydramine prior to each infusion.

Monitoring Parameters Monitor vital signs during the infusion and for 4 hours following the infusion. Monitor for signs/symptoms of postinfusion reaction. Monitor electrolytes, liver function, CBC with differential and platelets frequently. Monitor for signs and symptoms of hepatic sinusoidal obstruction syndrome (SOS; veno-occlusive disease; weight gain, right upper quadrant abdominal pain, hepatomegaly, ascites).

Product Availability No longer commercially available in the U.S. market for new patients. Available in Canada through a special access program.

Prescribing and Access Restrictions As of June 2010, gemtuzumab has been withdrawn from the U.S. market and is no longer commercially available to new patients; gemtuzumab is only available in the U.S. under an Investigational New Drug (IND) protocol.

In Canada, gemtuzumab is available through a special access program (access information is available from Health Canada).

References

Burnett AK, Hills RK, Milligan D, et al, "Identification of Patients With Acute Myeloblastic Leukemia who Benefit from the Addition of Gemtuzumab Ozogamicin: Results of the MRC AML15 Trial," *J Clin Oncol*, 2011, 29(4):369-77.

Larson RA, Boogaerts M, Estey E, et al, "Antibody-Targeted Chemotherapy of Older Patients With Acute Myeloid Leukemia in First Relapse Using Mylotarg (Gemtuzumab Ozogamicin)," *Leukemia*, 2002, 16(9):1627-36.

Larson RA, Sievers EL, Stadtmauer EA, et al, "Final Report of the Efficacy and Safety of Gemtuzumab Ozogamicin (Mylotarg) in Patients With CD33-Positive Acute Myeloid Leukemia in First Recurrence," *Cancer*, 2005, 104(7):1442-52.

Lo-Coco F, Cimino G, Breccia M, et al, "Gemtuzumab Ozogamicin (Mylotarg) as a Single Agent for Molecularly Relapsed Acute Promyelocytic Leukemia," *Blood*, 2004, 104(7):1995-9.

Ravandi F, Estey E, Jones D, et al, "Effective Treatment of Acute Promyelocytic Leukemia With All-Trans-Retinoic Acid, Arsenic Trioxide, and Gemtuzumab Ozogamicin," *J Clin Oncol*, 2009, 27 (4):504-10.

Sanz MA, Grimwade D, Tallman MS, et al, "Management of Acute Promyelocytic Leukemia: Recommendations From an Expert Panel on Behalf of the European LeukemiaNet," *Blood*, 2009, 113(9):1875-91.

◆ **Gemzar®** *see* Gemcitabine *on page 663*

◆ **Gengraf®** *see* CycloSPORINE (Systemic) *on page 333*

◆ **Gen-Hydroxyurea (Can)** *see* Hydroxyurea *on page 731*

◆ **Gen-Medroxy (Can)** *see* MedroxyPROGESTERone *on page 916*

Gentamicin (Systemic) (jen ta MYE sin)

Brand Names: Canada Gentamicin Injection, USP

Index Terms Gentamicin Sulfate

Generic Availability (U.S.) Yes

Pharmacologic Category Antibiotic, Aminoglycoside

Use Treatment of susceptible bacterial infections, normally gram-negative organisms, including *Pseudomonas*, *Proteus*, *Serratia*, and gram-positive *Staphylococcus*; treatment of bone infections, respiratory tract infections, skin and soft tissue infections, as well as abdominal and urinary tract infections, and septicemia; treatment of infective endocarditis

Labeled Contraindications Hypersensitivity to gentamicin or other aminoglycosides

Pregnancy Risk Factor D

Lactation Enters breast milk/use caution (AAP rates "compatible"; AAP 2001 update pending)

Warnings/Precautions **[U.S. Boxed Warning]: Aminoglycosides may cause neurotoxicity and/or nephrotoxicity;** usual risk factors include pre-existing renal impairment, concomitant neuro /nephrotoxic medications, advanced age and dehydration. Ototoxicity may be directly proportional to the amount of drug given and the duration of treatment; tinnitus or vertigo are indications of vestibular injury and impending hearing loss; renal damage is usually reversible. May cause neuromuscular blockade and respiratory paralysis; especially when given soon after anesthesia or muscle relaxants.

Not intended for long-term therapy due to toxic hazards associated with extended administration; use caution in pre-existing renal insufficiency, vestibular or cochlear impairment, myasthenia gravis, hypocalcemia, conditions which depress neuromuscular transmission. Dosage modification required in patients with impaired renal function. Prolonged use may result in fungal or bacterial superinfection, including *C. difficile*-associated diarrhea (CDAD) and pseudomembranous colitis; CDAD has been observed >2 months postantibiotic treatment.

Storage/Stability Gentamicin is a colorless to slightly yellow solution which should be stored between 2°C to 30°C, but refrigeration is not recommended. I.V. infusion solutions mixed in NS or D_5W solution are stable for 24 hours at room temperature and refrigeration. Premixed bag: Manufacturer expiration date; remove from overwrap stability: 30 days.

Mechanism of Action Interferes with bacterial protein synthesis by binding to 30S and 50S ribosomal subunits resulting in a defective bacterial cell membrane

Pharmacodynamics/Kinetics

Absorption:

Intramuscular: Rapid and complete

Oral: None

Distribution: Primarily into extracellular fluid (highly hydrophilic); high concentration in the renal cortex; minimal penetration to ocular tissues via I.V. route
V_d: Increased by edema, ascites, fluid overload; decreased with dehydration
Neonates: 0.4-0.6 L/kg
Children: 0.3-0.35 L/kg
Adults: 0.2-0.3 L/kg
Relative diffusion from blood into CSF: Minimal even with inflammation
CSF:blood level ratio: Normal meninges: Nil; Inflamed meninges: 10% to 30%
Protein binding: <30%
Half-life elimination:
Infants: <1 week: 3-11.5 hours; 1 week to 6 months: 3-3.5 hours
Adults: 1.5-3 hours; End-stage renal disease: 36-70 hours
Time to peak, serum: I.M.: 30-90 minutes; I.V.: 30 minutes after 30-minute infusion
Excretion: Urine (as unchanged drug)
Clearance: Directly related to renal function

Dosing

Adult & Geriatric Individualization is **critical** because of the low therapeutic index.

Use of ideal body weight (IBW) for determining the mg/kg/dose appears to be more accurate than dosing on the basis of total body weight (TBW). In morbid obesity, dosage requirement may best be estimated using a dosing weight of IBW + 0.4 (TBW - IBW).

Initial and periodic plasma drug levels (eg, peak and trough with conventional dosing) should be determined, particularly in critically-ill patients with serious infections or in disease states known to significantly alter aminoglycoside pharmacokinetics (eg, cystic fibrosis, burns, or major surgery).

Usual dosage ranges:
I.M., I.V.:
Conventional: 1-2.5 mg/kg/dose every 8-12 hours; to ensure adequate peak concentrations early in therapy, higher initial dosage may be considered in selected patients when extracellular water is increased (edema, septic shock, postsurgical, or trauma)
Once daily: 4-7 mg/kg/dose once daily; some clinicians recommend this approach for all patients with normal renal function; this dose is at least as efficacious with similar, if not less, toxicity than conventional dosing
Intrathecal: 4-8 mg/day

Indication-specific dosing: I.M., I.V.:
Brucellosis: 240 mg (I.M.) daily or 5 mg/kg (I.V.) daily for 7 days; either regimen recommended in combination with doxycycline
Cholangitis: 4-6 mg/kg once daily with ampicillin
Diverticulitis (complicated): 1.5-2 mg/kg every 8 hours (with ampicillin and metronidazole)
Endocarditis: Treatment: 3 mg/kg/day in 1-3 divided doses
Meningitis *Enterococcus* sp or *Pseudomonas aeruginosa*: I.V.: Loading dose 2 mg/kg, then 1.7 mg/kg/dose every 8 hours (administered with another bacteriocidal drug)
Pelvic inflammatory disease: Loading dose: 2 mg/kg, then 1.5 mg/kg every 8 hours
Alternate therapy: 4.5 mg/kg once daily
Plague (*Yersinia pestis*): Treatment: 5 mg/kg/day, followed by postexposure prophylaxis with doxycycline

Pneumonia, hospital- or ventilator-associated: 7 mg/kg/day (with anti-pseudomonal beta-lactam or carbapenem)

Synergy (for gram-positive infections): 3 mg/kg/day in 1-3 divided doses (with ampicillin)

Tularemia: 5 mg/kg/day divided every 8 hours for 1-2 weeks

Urinary tract infection: 1.5 mg/kg/dose every 8 hours

Pediatric Individualization is **critical** because of the low therapeutic index.

Use of ideal body weight (IBW) for determining the mg/kg/dose appears to be more accurate than dosing on the basis of total body weight (TBW). In morbid obesity, dosage requirement may best be estimated using a dosing weight of IBW + 0.4 (TBW - IBW).

Initial and periodic plasma drug levels (eg, peak and trough with conventional dosing) should be determined, particularly in critically-ill patients with serious infections or in disease states known to significantly alter aminoglycoside pharmacokinetics (eg, cystic fibrosis, burns, or major surgery).

Usual dosage ranges: I.M., I.V.:

Infants and Children <5 years: 2.5 mg/kg/dose every 8 hours*

Children ≥5 years: 2-2.5 mg/kg/dose every 8 hours*

***Note:** Higher individual doses and/or more frequent intervals (eg, every 6 hours) may be required in selected clinical situations (cystic fibrosis) or serum levels document the need.

Renal Impairment

Conventional dosing:

Cl_{cr} ≥60 mL/minute: Administer every 8 hours

Cl_{cr} 40-60 mL/minute: Administer every 12 hours

Cl_{cr} 20-40 mL/minute: Administer every 24 hours

Cl_{cr} <20 mL/minute: Loading dose, then monitor levels

High-dose therapy: Interval may be extended (eg, every 48 hours) in patients with moderate renal impairment (Cl_{cr} 30-59 mL/minute) and/or adjusted based on serum level determinations.

Intermittent hemodialysis (IHD) (administer after hemodialysis on dialysis days) (Heintz, 2009): Dialyzable (~50%; variable; dependent on filter, duration, and type of IHD):

Loading dose of 2-3 mg/kg loading dose followed by:

Mild UTI or synergy: 1 mg/kg every 48-72 hours; consider redosing for pre-HD or post-HD concentrations <1 mg/L

Moderate-to-severe UTI: 1-1.5 mg/kg every 48-72 hours; consider redosing for pre-HD concentrations <1.5-2 mg/L or post-HD concentrations <1 mg/L

Systemic gram-negative rod infection: 1.5-2 mg/kg every 48-72 hours; consider redosing for pre-HD concentrations <3-5 mg/L or post-HD concentrations <2 mg/L

Note: Dosing dependent on the assumption of 3 times/week, complete IHD sessions.

Peritoneal dialysis (PD):

Administration via PD fluid:

Gram-positive infection (eg, synergy): 3-4 mg/L (3-4 mcg/mL) of PD fluid

Gram-negative infection: 4-8 mg/L (4-8 mcg/mL) of PD fluid

Administration via I.V., I.M. route during PD: Dose as for Cl_{cr} <10 mL/minute and follow levels

Continuous renal replacement therapy (CRRT) (Heintz, 2009; Trotman, 2005): Drug clearance is highly dependent on the method of renal replacement, filter type, and flow rate. Appropriate dosing requires close monitoring of pharmacologic response, signs of adverse reactions due to drug accumulation, as well as drug concentrations in relation to target trough (if appropriate). The following are general recommendations only (based on dialysate flow/ultrafiltration rates of 1-2 L/hour and minimal residual renal function) and should not supersede clinical judgment:

CVVH/CVVHD/CVVHDF: Loading dose of 2-3 mg/kg followed by:

Mild UTI or synergy: 1 mg/kg every 24-36 hours (redose when concentration <1 mg/L)

Moderate-to-severe UTI: 1-1.5 mg/kg every 24-36 hours (redose when concentration <1.5-2 mg/L)

Systemic gram-negative infection: 1.5-2.5 mg/kg every 24-48 hours (redose when concentration <3-5 mg/L)

Hepatic Impairment Monitor plasma concentrations.

Administration

I.M.: Administer by deep I.M. route if possible. Slower absorption and lower peak concentrations, probably due to poor circulation in the atrophic muscle, may occur following I.M. injection; in paralyzed patients, suggest I.V. route.

Some penicillins (eg, carbenicillin, ticarcillin, and piperacillin) have been shown to inactivate aminoglycosides *in vitro*. This has been observed to a greater extent with tobramycin and gentamicin, while amikacin has shown greater stability against inactivation. Concurrent use of these agents may pose a risk of reduced antibacterial efficacy *in vivo*, particularly in the setting of profound renal impairment. However, definitive clinical evidence is lacking. If combination penicillin/aminoglycoside therapy is desired in a patient with renal dysfunction, separation of doses (if feasible), and routine monitoring of aminoglycoside levels, CBC, and clinical response should be considered.

Test Interactions Some penicillin derivatives may accelerate the degradation of aminoglycosides *in vitro*, leading to a potential underestimation of aminoglycoside serum concentration.

Dosage Forms Excipient information presented when available (limited, particularly for generics); consult specific product labeling. [DSC] = Discontinued product

Infusion, premixed in NS: 60 mg (50 mL, 100 mL [DSC]); 80 mg (50 mL, 100 mL); 100 mg (50 mL, 100 mL); 120 mg (100 mL)

Injection, solution: 40 mg/mL (2 mL, 20 mL)

Injection, solution [pediatric]: 10 mg/mL (2 mL [DSC])

Injection, solution [pediatric, preservative free]: 10 mg/mL (2 mL)

- **Gentamicin Injection, USP (Can)** *see* Gentamicin (Systemic) *on page 677*
- **Gentamicin Sulfate** *see* Gentamicin (Systemic) *on page 677*
- **Gleevec®** *see* Imatinib *on page 762*
- **Gliadel®** *see* Carmustine *on page 243*
- **Gliadel Wafer® (Can)** *see* Carmustine *on page 243*
- **Glivec** *see* Imatinib *on page 762*

Glucarpidase (gloo KAR pid ase)

Brand Names: U.S. Voraxaze®

Index Terms Carboxypeptidase-G2; CPDG2; CPG2; Voraxaze

Generic Availability (U.S.) No

Pharmacologic Category Antidote; Enzyme

Use Treatment of toxic plasma methotrexate concentrations (>1 micromole/L) in patients with delayed clearance due to renal impairment

Note: Due to the risk of subtherapeutic methotrexate exposure, glucarpidase is **NOT** indicated when methotrexate clearance is within expected range (plasma methotrexate concentration ≤2 standard deviations of mean methotrexate excretion curve specific for dose administered) **or** with normal renal function or mild renal impairment.

Unlabeled Use Rescue agent to reduce methotrexate toxicity in patients with accidental intrathecal methotrexate overdose

Labeled Contraindications There are no contraindications listed in the manufacturer's labeling.

Pregnancy Risk Factor C

Lactation Excretion in breast milk unknown/use caution

Warnings/Precautions Serious allergic reactions have been reported.

Leucovorin calcium administration should be continued after glucarpidase; the same dose as was given prior to glucarpidase should be continued for the first 48 hours after glucarpidase; after 48 hours, leucovorin doses should be based on methotrexate concentrations. A single methotrexate concentration should not determine when leucovorin should be discontinued; continue leucovorin until the methotrexate concentration remains below the threshold for leucovorin treatment for >3 days. Leucovorin calcium is a substrate for glucarpidase and may compete with methotrexate for binding sites; **do not administer leucovorin calcium within 2 hours before or after glucarpidase.** In addition to leucovorin, glucarpidase use should be accompanied with adequate hydration and urinary alkalinization. During the first 48 hours following glucarpidase administration, the only reliable method of measuring methotrexate concentrations is the chromatographic method. DAMPA, an inactive methotrexate metabolite with a half-life of 9 hours, may interfere with immunoassay and result in the overestimation of the methotrexate concentration (when collected within 48 hours of glucarpidase administration). Glucarpidase use for intrathecal methotrexate overdose (unlabeled route/use) should be used in conjunction with immediate lumbar drainage; concurrent dexamethasone (4 mg I.V. every 6 hours for 4 doses) may minimize methotrexate-induced chemical arachnoiditis; leucovorin calcium (100 mg I.V. every 6 hours for 4 doses) may prevent systemic methotrexate toxicity (Widemann, 2004).

Adverse Reactions

>10%: Miscellaneous: Antiglucarpidase antibody development (17%)

1% to 10%:

- Cardiovascular: Flushing (2%), hypotension (1%)
- Central nervous system: Headache (1%)
- Gastrointestinal: Nausea/vomiting (2%)
- Neuromuscular & skeletal: Paresthesia (2%)

<1%, postmarketing, and/or case reports: Allergic reaction, blurred vision, diarrhea, head pressure, hypersensitivity, hypertension, rash, shaking, throat irritation/tightness, tremor, warmth

Drug Interactions

Metabolism/Transport Effects None known.

Avoid Concomitant Use There are no known interactions where it is recommended to avoid concomitant use.

Increased Effect/Toxicity There are no known significant interactions involving an increase in effect.

Decreased Effect

Glucarpidase may decrease the levels/effects of: Leucovorin Calcium-Levoleucovorin

Storage/Stability Store intact vials refrigerated at 2°C to 8°C (36°F to 46°F); do not freeze. Reconstituted solutions should be used immediately or may be stored for up to 4 hours under refrigeration.

Reconstitution

I.V.: Reconstitute each vial (1000 units/vial) with 1 mL normal saline. Mix gently by rolling or tilting vial; do not shake. Upon reconstitution, solution should be clear, colorless and free of particulate matter.

Intrathecal (unlabeled route/use): Reconstitute 2000 units with 12 mL preservative-free normal saline (Widemann, 2004)

Mechanism of Action Recombinant enzyme which rapidly hydrolyzes the carboxyl-terminal glutamate residue from extracellular methotrexate into inactive metabolites (DAMPA and glutamate), resulting in a rapid reduction of methotrexate concentrations independent of renal function

Pharmacodynamics/Kinetics

Onset of action: Methotrexate toxicity: Reduces methotrexate concentrations by ≥97% within 15 minutes of I.V. administration

Duration: Methotrexate toxicity: Maintains a >95% reduction of methotrexate concentrations for up to 8 days

Distribution: V_d: I.V.: 3.6 L; distribution restricted to plasma volume

Half-life elimination: I.V.: Normal renal function: 6-9 hours; impaired renal function (Cl_{cr} <30 mL/minute): 8-10 hours (Phillips, 2008)

Dosing

Adult & Geriatric

Methotrexate toxicity: I.V.: 50 units/kg (Buchen, 2005; Widemann, 1997; Widemann, 2010)

Intrathecal methotrexate overdose (unlabeled route/use): Intrathecal: 2000 units as soon as possible after accidental overdose (Widemann, 2004)

Pediatric

Methotrexate toxicity: I.V.: Refer to adult dosing.

Intrathecal methotrexate overdose (unlabeled route/use): Intrathecal: Refer to adult dosing.

Renal Impairment No dosage adjustment necessary.

Hepatic Impairment No dosage adjustment provided in the manufacturer's labeling; has not been studied.

Administration

I.V.: Infuse over 5 minutes; flush I.V. line before and after glucarpidase administration

Intrathecal (for intrathecal methotrexate overdose; unlabeled route/use): Glucarpidase was administered within 3-9 hours of accidental intrathecal methotrexate overdose in conjunction with lumbar drainage or ventriculolumbar perfusion (Widemann, 2004). Administered over 5 minutes via lumbar route, ventriculostomy, Ommaya reservoir, or lumbar and ventriculostomy (O'Marcaigh, 1996; Widemann, 2004). In one case report, 1000 units was administered through the ventricular catheter over 5 minutes and another 1000 units was administered through the lumbar catheter (O'Marcaigh, 1996).

Monitoring Parameters

Serum methotrexate levels: Use chromatographic method if <48 hours from glucarpidase administration (DAMPA interferes with immunoassay results until >48 hours)

CBC with differential, bilirubin, ALT, AST, serum creatinine; evaluate for signs/ symptoms of methotrexate toxicity

Test Interactions Methotrexate levels: During the first 48 hours following glucarpidase administration, the only reliable method of measuring methotrexate concentrations is the chromatographic method. DAMPA, an inactive methotrexate metabolite with a half-life of 9 hours, may interfere with immunoassay and result in the overestimation of the methotrexate concentration (when collected within 48 hours of glucarpidase administration).

Additional Information The utility of more than one glucarpidase dose in reducing plasma methotrexate levels was evaluated in a study of 100 patients with high-dose methotrexate-induced nephrotoxicity (Widemann, 2010). Glucarpidase 50 units/kg I.V. was administered either as a single dose (n=65), 2 doses given 24 hours apart (n=28), or 3 doses given at 4 hour intervals (n=7). Six of the 65 patients randomized to a single dose also received a second delayed glucarpidase dose (>24 hours later) due to persistent methotrexate concentrations ≥1 micromole/L in spite of a ≥90% decrease in the plasma methotrexate concentration after the initial dose. The use of scheduled second and third glucarpidase doses did not result in additional methotrexate concentration decreases; and only 2 of the 6 patients who received a second delayed glucarpidase dose (>24 hours later) experienced a ≥50% methotrexate concentration reduction.

Prescribing and Access Restrictions

Voraxaze® is distributed through ASD Healthcare; procurement information is available (24 hours a day; 365 days a year) at 1-855-7-VORAXAZE (1-855-786-7292).

Dosage Forms Excipient information presented when available (limited, particularly for generics); consult specific product labeling.

Injection, powder for reconstitution:

Voraxaze®: 1000 units [contains lactose 10 mg/vial]

References

Buchen S, Ngampolo D, Melton RG, et al, "Carboxypeptidase G2 Rescue in Patients With Methotrexate Intoxication and Renal Failure," *Br J Cancer*, 2005, 92(3):480-7.

O'Marcaigh AS, Johnson CM, Smithson WA, et al, "Successful Treatment of Intrathecal Methotrexate Overdose by Using Ventriculolumbar Perfusion and Intrathecal Instillation of Carboxypeptidase G2," *Mayo Clin Proc*, 1996, 71(2):161-5.

Phillips M, Smith W, Balan G, et al, "Pharmacokinetics of Glucarpidase in Subjects With Normal and Impaired Renal Function," *J Clin Pharmacol*, 2008, 48(3):279-84.

Widemann BC, Balis FM, Kim A, et al, "Glucarpidase, Leucovorin, and Thymidine for High-Dose Methotrexate-Induced Renal Dysfunction: Clinical and Pharmacologic Factors Affecting Outcome," *J Clin Oncol*, 2010, 28(25):3979-86.

Widemann BC, Balis FM, Murphy RF, et al, "Carboxypeptidase-G2, Thymidine, and Leucovorin Rescue in Cancer Patients With Methotrexate-Induced Renal Dysfunction," *J Clin Oncol*, 1997, 15(5):2125-34.

Widemann BC, Balis FM, Shalabi A, et al, "Treatment of Accidental Intrathecal Methotrexate Overdose With Intrathecal Carboxypeptidase G2," *J Natl Cancer Inst*, 2004, 96(20):1557-9.

◆ **GM-CSF** *see* Sargramostim *on page* 1270

◆ **GnRH Agonist** *see* Histrelin *on page* 707

Goserelin (GOE se rel in)

Related Information

Safe Handling of Hazardous Drugs *on page* 1904

Brand Names: U.S. Zoladex®

Brand Names: Canada Zoladex®; Zoladex® LA

Index Terms Goserelin Acetate; ICI-118630; ZDX

Generic Availability (U.S.) No

Pharmacologic Category Antineoplastic Agent, Gonadotropin-Releasing Hormone Agonist; Gonadotropin Releasing Hormone Agonist

Use Treatment of locally confined prostate cancer; palliative treatment of advanced prostate cancer; palliative treatment of advanced breast cancer in pre- and perimenopausal women; treatment of endometriosis, including pain relief and reduction of endometriotic lesions; endometrial thinning agent as part of treatment for dysfunctional uterine bleeding

Labeled Contraindications Hypersensitivity to goserelin, GnRH, GnRH agonist analogues, or any component of the formulation; pregnancy (except if using for palliative treatment of advanced breast cancer)

Pregnancy Risk Factor X (endometriosis, endometrial thinning); D (advanced breast cancer)

Lactation Excretion in breast milk unknown/not recommended

Warnings/Precautions Hazardous agent - use appropriate precautions for handling and disposal. Allergic hypersensitivity reactions (including anaphylaxis) and antibody formation may occur; monitor. Androgen-deprivation therapy may increase the risk for cardiovascular disease (Levine, 2010). Transient increases in serum testosterone (in men with prostate cancer) and estrogen (in women with breast cancer) may result in a worsening of disease signs and symptoms (tumor flare) during the first few weeks of treatment. Urinary tract obstruction or spinal cord compression have been reported when used for prostate cancer; closely observe patients for weakness, paresthesias, and urinary tract obstruction in first few weeks of therapy. Decreased bone density has been reported in women and may be irreversible; use caution if other risk factors are present; evaluate and institute preventative treatment if necessary.

Women of childbearing potential should not receive therapy until pregnancy has been excluded. Nonhormonal contraception is recommended for premenopausal women during therapy and for 12 weeks after therapy is discontinued. Cervical resistance may be increased; use caution when dilating the cervix. The 3-month implant currently has no approved indications for use in women. Rare cases of pituitary apoplexy (frequently secondary to pituitary adenoma) have been observed with GnRH agonist administration (onset from 1 hour to usually <2 weeks); may present as sudden headache, vomiting, visual or mental status changes, and infrequently cardiovascular collapse; immediate medical attention required. Hyperglycemia has been reported in males and may manifest as diabetes or worsening of pre-existing diabetes. Decreased AUC may be observed when using the 3-month implant in obese patients. Monitor testosterone levels if desired clinical response is not observed. Safety and efficacy have not been established in pediatric patients.

Adverse Reactions Percentages reported with the 1-month implant:

>10%:

Cardiovascular: Peripheral edema (female 21%)

Central nervous system: Headache (female 32% to 75%; male 1% to 5%), emotional lability (female 60%), depression (female 54%; male 1% to 5%), pain (female 17%; male 8%), insomnia (female 11%; male 5%)

Dermatologic: Acne (female 42%), seborrhea (female 26%)

Endocrine & metabolic: Hot flashes (female 57% to 96%; male 62%), libido decreased (female 48% to 61%), sexual dysfunction (male 21%), breast atrophy (female 33%), breast enlargement (female 18%), erections decreased (18%), libido increased (female 12%)

Gastrointestinal: Nausea (female 8% to 11%; male 5%), abdominal pain (female 7% to 11%)

Genitourinary: Vaginitis (75%), pelvic symptoms (female 9% to 18%), dyspareunia (female 14%), lower urinary symptoms (male 13%)

Neuromuscular & skeletal: Bone mineral density decreased (female 23%; ~4% decrease from baseline in 6 months; postmarketing reports in males), weakness (female 11%)

Miscellaneous: Diaphoresis (female 16% to 45%; male 6%), tumor flare (female: 23%), infection (female 13%)

1% to 10%:

Cardiovascular: Arrhythmia, cerebrovascular accident, chest pain, edema, heart failure, hypertension, MI, palpitation, peripheral vascular disorder, tachycardia

Central nervous system: Abnormal thinking, anxiety, chills, dizziness, fever, lethargy, malaise, migraine, nervousness, somnolence

Dermatologic: Alopecia, bruising, dry skin, hair disorder, hirsutism, pruritus, rash, skin discoloration

Endocrine & metabolic: Breast pain, breast swelling/tenderness, dysmenorrhea, gout, hyperglycemia

Gastrointestinal: Anorexia, appetite increased, constipation, diarrhea, dyspepsia, flatulence, ulcer, vomiting, weight gain/loss, xerostomia

Genitourinary: Urinary frequency, urinary obstruction, urinary tract infection, vaginal hemorrhage, vulvovaginitis

Hematologic: Anemia, hemorrhage

Local: Application site reaction

Neuromuscular & skeletal: Arthralgia, back pain, hypertonia, joint disorder, leg cramps, myalgia, paresthesia

Ocular: Amblyopia, dry eyes

Renal: Renal insufficiency

Respiratory: Bronchitis, COPD, cough, epistaxis, pharyngitis, rhinitis, sinusitis, upper respiratory tract infection

Miscellaneous: Allergic reaction, flu-like syndrome, voice alteration

<1%, postmarketing, and/or case reports (with monthly or 3-month implant): ALT increased, anaphylaxis, AST increased, diabetes, glucose tolerance decreased, hypercalcemia, hypercholesterolemia, hyperlipidemia, hypersensitivity reactions, hypotension, ovarian cyst, pituitary apoplexy, psychotic disorders, urticaria

Drug Interactions

Metabolism/Transport Effects None known.

Avoid Concomitant Use There are no known interactions where it is recommended to avoid concomitant use.

Increased Effect/Toxicity There are no known significant interactions involving an increase in effect.

Decreased Effect

Goserelin may decrease the levels/effects of: Antidiabetic Agents

Storage/Stability Zoladex® should be stored at room temperature not to exceed 25°C (77°F). Protect from light.

Mechanism of Action Goserelin (a gonadotropin-releasing hormone [GnRH] analog) causes an initial increase in luteinizing hormone (LH) and follicle stimulating hormone (FSH), chronic administration of goserelin results in a sustained suppression of pituitary gonadotropins. Serum testosterone falls to levels comparable to surgical castration. The exact mechanism of this effect is unknown, but may be related to changes in the control of LH or down-regulation of LH receptors.

Pharmacodynamics/Kinetics

Onset:

Females: Estradiol suppression reaches postmenopausal levels within 3 weeks and FSH and LH are suppressed to follicular phase levels within 4 weeks of initiation

Males: Testosterone suppression reaches castrate levels within 2-4 weeks after initiation

Duration:

Females: Estradiol, LH and FSH generally return to baseline levels within 12 weeks following the last monthly implant.

Males: Testosterone levels maintained at castrate levels throughout the duration of therapy.

Absorption: SubQ: Rapid and can be detected in serum in 30-60 minutes; 3.6 mg: released slowly in first 8 days, then rapid and continuous release for 28 days

Distribution: V_d: Male: 44.1 L; Female: 20.3 L

Protein binding: 27%

Time to peak, serum: SubQ: Male: 12-15 days, Female: 8-22 days

Half-life elimination: SubQ: Male: ~4 hours, Female: ~2 hours; Renal impairment: Male: 12 hours

Excretion: Urine (>90%; 20% as unchanged drug)

Dosing

Adult & Geriatric

Prostate cancer, advanced: SubQ:

28-day implant: 3.6 mg every 28 days

12-week implant: 10.8 mg every 12 weeks

Prostate cancer, locally confined (in combination with an antiandrogen and radiotherapy; begin 8 weeks prior to radiotherapy): SubQ:

Combination 28-day/12-week implant: 3.6 mg implant, followed in 28 days by 10.8 mg implant

28-day implant (alternate dosing): 3.6 mg; repeated every 28 days for a total of 4 doses

Breast cancer, advanced: SubQ: 3.6 mg every 28 days

Endometriosis: SubQ: 3.6 mg every 28 days for 6 months

Endometrial thinning: SubQ: 3.6 mg every 28 days for 1 or 2 doses

Renal Impairment No adjustment is necessary.

Hepatic Impairment No adjustment is necessary.

Combination Regimens

Prostate cancer:

Bicalutamide-Goserelin on page 1533

FZ on page 1667

Administration SubQ: Administer implant by inserting needle at a 30-45 degree angle into the anterior abdominal wall below the navel line. Goserelin is an implant; therefore, do not attempt to eliminate air bubbles prior to injection (may displace implant). Do not attempt to aspirate prior to injection; if a large vessel is penetrated, blood will be visualized in the syringe chamber (if vessel is penetrated, withdraw needle and inject elsewhere with a new syringe). Do not penetrate into muscle or peritoneum. Implant may be detected by ultrasound if removal is required.

Monitoring Parameters Bone mineral density, serum calcium, cholesterol/lipids

Prostate cancer: Weakness, paresthesias, and urinary tract obstruction in first few weeks of therapy; screen for diabetes

Test Interactions Interferes with pituitary gonadotropic and gonadal function tests during and for up to 12 weeks after discontinued

Additional Information If removal is necessary, implant may be located by ultrasound.

Dosage Forms Excipient information presented when available (limited, particularly for generics); consult specific product labeling.

Implant, subcutaneous:

Zoladex®: 3.6 mg (1s) [1 month implant]

Zoladex®: 10.8 mg (1s) [3 month implant]

References

Baum M, Hackshaw A, Houghton J, et al, "Adjuvant Goserelin in Pre-Menopausal Patients With Early Breast Cancer: Results From the ZIPP Study," *Eur J Cancer*, 2006, 42(7):895-904.

Gnant M, Mlineritsch B, Stoeger H, et al, "Mature Results From ABCSG-12: Adjuvant Ovarian Suppression Combined With Tamoxifen or Anastrozole, Alone or in Combination With Zoledronic Acid, in Premenopausal Women With Endocrine-Responsive Early Breast Cancer," *J Clin Oncol*, 2008, 28(15s):533 [abstract 533 from 2008 ASCO Annual Meeting].

Hackshaw A, Baum M, Fornander T, et al, "Long-Term Effectiveness of Adjuvant Goserelin in Premenopausal Women With Early Breast Cancer," *J Natl Cancer Inst*, 2009, 101(5):341-9.

Horwitz EM, Bae K, Hanks GE, et al, "Ten-Year Follow-Up of Radiation Therapy Oncology Group Protocol 92-02: A Phase III Trial of the Duration of Elective Androgen Deprivation in Locally Advanced Prostate Cancer," *J Clin Oncol*, 2008, 26(15):2497-504.

Levine GN, D'Amico AV, Berger P, et al, "Androgen-Deprivation Therapy in Prostate Cancer and Cardiovascular Risk. A Science Advisory from the American Heart Association, American Cancer Society, and American Urological Association," *Circulation*, 2010, 121(6):833-40

Roach M 3rd, Bae K, Speight J, et al, "Short-Term Neoadjuvant Androgen Deprivation Therapy and External-Beam Radiotherapy for Locally Advanced Prostate Cancer: Long-Term Results of RTOG 8610," *J Clin Oncol*, 2000, 20(4):585-91.

◆ **Goserelin Acetate** *see* Goserelin *on page 683*

◆ **GR38032R** *see* Ondansetron *on page 1068*

Granisetron (gra NI se tron)

Related Information

Management of Chemotherapy-Induced Nausea and Vomiting *on page 1786*

Brand Names: U.S. Granisol™; Sancuso®

Brand Names: Canada Granisetron Hydrochloride Injection; Kytril®

Index Terms BRL 43694; Kytril

Generic Availability (U.S.) Yes: Injection, tablet

Pharmacologic Category Antiemetic; Selective 5-HT_3 Receptor Antagonist

Use Prophylaxis of nausea and vomiting associated with emetogenic chemotherapy and radiation therapy; prophylaxis and treatment of postoperative nausea and vomiting (PONV)

Unlabeled Use Breakthrough treatment of nausea and vomiting associated with chemotherapy

Labeled Contraindications Hypersensitivity to granisetron or any component of the formulation

Pregnancy Risk Factor B

Lactation Excretion in breast milk unknown/use caution

Warnings/Precautions Use with caution in patients with congenital long QT syndrome or other risk factors for QT prolongation (eg, medications known to prolong QT interval, electrolyte abnormalities, and cumulative high-dose anthracycline therapy). 5-HT_3 antagonists have been associated with a number of dose-dependent increases in ECG intervals (eg, PR, QRS duration, QT/QT_c, JT), usually occurring 1-2 hours after I.V. administration. In general, these changes are not clinically relevant, however, when used in conjunction with other agents that prolong these intervals, arrhythmia may occur. When used with agents that prolong the QT interval (eg, Class I and III antiarrhythmics), clinically relevant QT interval prolongation may occur resulting in torsade de pointes. I.V. formulations of 5-HT_3 antagonists have more association with ECG interval changes, compared to oral formulations.

For chemotherapy-related emesis, **granisetron should be used on a scheduled basis, not on an "as needed" (PRN) basis**, since data support the use of this drug in the prevention of nausea and vomiting and not in the rescue of nausea and vomiting. Granisetron should be used only in the first 24-48 hours of receiving chemotherapy or radiation. Data do not support any increased efficacy of granisetron in delayed nausea and vomiting.

Use with caution in patients allergic to other 5-HT_3 receptor antagonists; cross-reactivity has been reported. Routine prophylaxis for PONV is not recommended in patients where there is little expectation of nausea and vomiting postoperatively. In patients where nausea and vomiting must be avoided postoperatively, administer to all patients even when expected incidence of nausea and vomiting is low. Use caution following abdominal surgery or in chemotherapy-induced nausea and vomiting; may mask progressive ileus or gastric distention. Application site reactions, generally mild, have occurred with transdermal patch use; if skin reaction is severe or generalized, remove patch. Cover patch application site with clothing to protect from natural or artificial sunlight exposure while patch is applied and for 10 days following removal; granisetron may potentially be affected by natural or artificial sunlight. Do not apply patch to red, irritated, or damaged skin. Injection contains benzyl alcohol (1 mg/mL) and should not be used in neonates.

Adverse Reactions

>10%:

- Central nervous system: Headache (3% to 21%; transdermal patch: 1%)
- Gastrointestinal: Constipation (3% to 18%)
- Neuromuscular & skeletal: Weakness (5% to 18%)

1% to 10%:

- Cardiovascular: QT_c prolongation (1% to 3%), hypertension (1% to 2%)
- Central nervous system: Pain (10%), fever (3% to 9%), dizziness (4% to 5%), insomnia (<2% to 5%), somnolence (1% to 4%), anxiety (2%), agitation (<2%), CNS stimulation (<2%)
- Dermatologic: Rash (1%)
- Gastrointestinal: Diarrhea (3% to 9%), abdominal pain (4% to 6%), dyspepsia (3% to 6%), taste perversion (2%)
- Hepatic: Liver enzymes increased (5% to 6%)
- Renal: Oliguria (2%)
- Respiratory: Cough (2%)
- Miscellaneous: Infection (3%)

<1%, postmarketing, and/or case reports: Agitation, allergic reactions; anaphylaxis (including hypotension, dyspnea, urticaria); angina, application site reactions (transdermal patch), arrhythmias, atrial fibrillation, extrapyramidal syndrome, hot flashes, hypotension, hypersensitivity, syncope

Drug Interactions

Metabolism/Transport Effects Substrate of CYP3A4 (minor); **Note:** Assignment of Major/Minor substrate status based on clinically relevant drug interaction potential

Avoid Concomitant Use

Avoid concomitant use of Granisetron with any of the following: Apomorphine; Highest Risk QTc-Prolonging Agents; Mifepristone

Increased Effect/Toxicity

Granisetron may increase the levels/effects of: Apomorphine; Highest Risk QTc-Prolonging Agents; Moderate Risk QTc-Prolonging Agents

The levels/effects of Granisetron may be increased by: Mifepristone; QTc-Prolonging Agents (Indeterminate Risk and Risk Modifying)

Decreased Effect

Granisetron may decrease the levels/effects of: Tapentadol; TraMADol

The levels/effects of Granisetron may be decreased by: Tocilizumab

Storage/Stability

I.V.: Store at 15°C to 30°C (59°F to 86°F). Protect from light. Do not freeze vials. Stable when mixed in NS or D_5W for 7 days under refrigeration and for 3 days at room temperature.

Oral: Store tablet or oral solution at 15°C to 30°C (59°F to 86°F). Protect from light.

Transdermal patch: Store at 20°C to 25°C (68°F to 77°F). Keep patch in original packaging until immediately prior to use.

Mechanism of Action Selective 5-HT_3-receptor antagonist, blocking serotonin, both peripherally on vagal nerve terminals and centrally in the chemoreceptor trigger zone

Pharmacodynamics/Kinetics

Duration: Oral, I.V.: Generally up to 24 hours

Absorption: Oral: Tablets and oral solution are bioequivalent; Transdermal patch: ~66% over 7 days

Distribution: V_d: 2-4 L/kg; widely throughout body

Protein binding: 65%

Metabolism: Hepatic via N-demethylation, oxidation, and conjugation; some metabolites may have 5-HT_3 antagonist activity

Half-life elimination: Oral: 6 hours; I.V.: 9 hours

Time to peak, plasma: Transdermal patch: Maximum systemic concentrations: ~48 hours after application (range: 24-168 hours)

Excretion: Urine (12% as unchanged drug, 48% to 49% as metabolites); feces (34% to 38% as metabolites)

Dosing

Adult & Geriatric

Prophylaxis of chemotherapy-related emesis:

Oral: 2 mg once daily up to 1 hour before chemotherapy or 1 mg twice daily; the first 1 mg dose should be given up to 1 hour before chemotherapy.

I.V.:

Within U.S.: 10 mcg/kg/dose (maximum: 1 mg/dose) given 30 minutes prior to chemotherapy; for some drugs (eg, carboplatin, cyclophosphamide) with a later onset of emetic action, 10 mcg/kg every 12 hours may be necessary.

Outside U.S.: 40 mcg/kg/dose (or 3 mg/dose); maximum: 9 mg/24 hours

Breakthrough: Granisetron has not been shown to be effective in terminating nausea or vomiting once it occurs and should not be used for this purpose.

Transdermal patch: Prophylaxis of chemotherapy-related emesis: Apply 1 patch at least 24 hours prior to chemotherapy; do not apply ≥48 hours before chemotherapy. Remove patch a minimum of 24 hours after chemotherapy completion. Maximum duration: Patch may be worn up to 7 days, depending on chemotherapy regimen duration.

Prophylaxis of radiation therapy-associated emesis: Oral: 2 mg once daily given 1 hour before radiation therapy.

Postoperative nausea and vomiting (PONV): I.V.:

Prevention: 1 mg given undiluted over 30 seconds; the manufacturer recommends administration before induction of anesthesia or immediately before reversal of anesthesia. **Note:** The Society for Ambulatory Anesthesia (SAMBA) Guidelines recommend a dosage range of 0.35-1.5 mg administered at the end of surgery (Gan, 2007). However, doses ≤1 mg are generally used since doses >1 mg are not more effective. Of note, 5 mcg/kg (~0.35 mg in a 70 kg adult) has been shown to be effective; doses >5 mcg/kg were not more effective (Mikawa, 1997).

Treatment: 1 mg given undiluted over 30 seconds

Pediatric Prophylaxis associated with cancer chemotherapy: Children ≥2 years: Refer to adult dosing.

Renal Impairment No dosage adjustment required.

Hepatic Impairment Kinetic studies in patients with hepatic impairment showed that total clearance was approximately halved; however, standard doses were very well tolerated, and dose adjustments are not necessary.

Administration

Oral: Doses should be given up to 1 hour prior to initiation of chemotherapy/radiation

I.V.: Administer I.V. push over 30 seconds or as a 5- to 10-minute infusion

Prevention of PONV: Administer before induction of anesthesia or immediately before reversal of anesthesia.

Treatment of PONV: Administer undiluted over 30 seconds.

Transdermal (Sancuso®): Apply patch to clean, dry, intact skin on upper outer arm. Do not use on red, irritated, or damaged skin. Remove patch from pouch immediately before application. Do not cut patch.

Extemporaneous Preparations Note: Commercial oral solution is available (0.2 mg/mL)

A 0.2 mg/mL oral suspension may be made with tablets. Crush twelve 1 mg tablets in a mortar and reduce to a fine powder. Add 30 mL distilled water, mix well, and transfer to a bottle. Rinse the mortar with 10 mL cherry syrup and add to bottle. Add sufficient quantity of cherry syrup to make a final volume of 60 mL. Label "shake well". Stable 14 days at room temperature or refrigerated (Quercia, 1997).

A 50 mcg/mL oral suspension may be made with tablets and one of three different vehicles (Ora-Sweet®, Ora-Plus®, or a mixture of methylcellulose 1% and Simple Syrup, N.F.). Crush one 1 mg tablet in a mortar and reduce to a fine powder. Add 20 mL of the chosen vehicle and mix to a uniform paste; transfer to a calibrated bottle. Label "shake well" and "refrigerate". Stable for 91 days refrigerated (Nahata, 1998).

Nahata MC, Morosco RS, and Hipple TF, "Stability of Granisetron Hydrochloride in Two Oral Suspensions," *Am J Health Syst Pharm*, 1998, 55(23):2511-3.

Quercia RA, Zhang J, Fan C, et al, "Stability of Granisetron Hydrochloride in an Extemporaneously Prepared Oral Liquid," *Am J Health Syst Pharm*, 1997, 54(12):1404-6.

Dosage Forms Excipient information presented when available (limited, particularly for generics); consult specific product labeling.

Injection, solution: 1 mg/mL (1 mL, 4 mL)

Injection, solution [preservative free]: 0.1 mg/mL (1 mL); 1 mg/mL (1 mL)

Patch, transdermal:
Sancuso®: 3.1 mg/24 hours (1s) [52 cm^2, total granisetron 34.3 mg]
Solution, oral:
Granisol™: 2 mg/10 mL (30 mL) [contains sodium benzoate; orange flavor]
Tablet, oral: 1 mg

References

Gan TJ, Meyer TA, Apfel CC, et al, "Society for Ambulatory Anesthesia Guidelines for the Management of Postoperative Nausea and Vomiting," *Anesth Analg*, 2007, 105(6):1615-28.

Gill D and Howell J, "Pharmacokinetics and Bioavailability of Transdermal Granisetron After a Six-Day Application of Three Patch Sizes, Compared to 2 mg Once-Daily Oral Dose of Granisetron for Five Days," *Support Care Cancer*, 2008, 16(6):619-756 [abstract from 2008 International MASCC/ISOO Symposium].

Kris MG, Hesketh PJ, Somerfield MR, et al, "American Society of Clinical Oncology Guideline for Antiemetics in Oncology: Update 2006," *J Clin Oncol*, 2006, 24(18):2932-47.

Mikawa K, Takao Y, Nishina K, et al, "Optimal Dose of Granisetron for Prophylaxis Against Postoperative Emesis After Gynecological Surgery,"*Anesth Analg*, 1997, 85(3):652-6.

Multinational Association of Supportive Care in Cancer (MASCC), "Antiemetic Guidelines," Updated April 2010. Available at http://data.memberclicks.com/site/mascc/MASCC_Guidelines_English_2010.pdf

National Comprehensive Cancer Network® (NCCN), "Clinical Practice Guidelines in Oncology™: Antiemesis," Version 2.2010. Available at http://www.nccn.org/professionals/physician_gls/PDF/antiemesis.pdf

◆ **Granisetron Hydrochloride Injection (Can)** *see* Granisetron *on page* 687

◆ **Granisol™** *see* Granisetron *on page* 687

◆ **Granulocyte Colony Stimulating Factor** *see* Filgrastim *on page* 604

◆ **Granulocyte Colony Stimulating Factor (PEG Conjugate)** *see* Pegfilgrastim *on page* 1138

◆ **Granulocyte-Macrophage Colony Stimulating Factor** *see* Sargramostim *on page* 1270

◆ **GSK-580299** *see* Papillomavirus (Types 16, 18) Vaccine (Human, Recombinant) *on page* 1124

◆ **GW506U78** *see* Nelarabine *on page* 1028

◆ **GW572016** *see* Lapatinib *on page* 854

◆ **GW786034** *see* Pazopanib *on page* 1129

◆ **h5G1.1** *see* Eculizumab *on page* 490

◆ **HAL** *see* Hexaminolevulinate *on page* 705

◆ **Halaven™** *see* Eribulin *on page* 524

◆ **Haldol®** *see* Haloperidol *on page* 691

◆ **Haldol® Decanoate** *see* Haloperidol *on page* 691

◆ **Halichondrin B Analog** *see* Eribulin *on page* 524

Haloperidol (ha loe PER i dole)

Related Information

Hospice (End of Life) Care *on page* 1857
Management of Chemotherapy-Induced Nausea and Vomiting *on page* 1786

Brand Names: U.S. Haldol®; Haldol® Decanoate

Brand Names: Canada Apo-Haloperidol LA®; Apo-Haloperidol®; Haloperidol Injection, USP; Haloperidol Long Acting; Haloperidol-LA; Haloperidol-LA Omega; Novo-Peridol; PMS-Haloperidol; PMS-Haloperidol LA

Index Terms Haloperidol Decanoate; Haloperidol Lactate

Generic Availability (U.S.) Yes

Pharmacologic Category Antipsychotic Agent, Typical

Use Management of schizophrenia; control of tics and vocal utterances of Tourette's disorder in children and adults; severe behavioral problems in children

Unlabeled Use Treatment of nonschizophrenia psychosis; may be used for the emergency sedation of severely-agitated or delirious patients; adjunctive treatment of ethanol dependence; postoperative nausea and vomiting (alternative therapy); psychosis/agitation related to Alzheimer's dementia

Labeled Contraindications Hypersensitivity to haloperidol or any component of the formulation; Parkinson's disease; severe CNS depression; coma

Pregnancy Risk Factor C

Lactation Enters breast milk/not recommended (AAP rates "of concern"; AAP 2001 update pending)

Warnings/Precautions [U.S. Boxed Warning]: Elderly patients with dementia-related psychosis treated with antipsychotics are at an increased risk of death compared to placebo. Most deaths appeared to be either cardiovascular (eg, heart failure, sudden death) or infectious (eg, pneumonia) in nature. Haloperidol is not approved for the treatment of dementia-related psychosis. Hypotension may occur, particularly with parenteral administration. Although the short-acting form (lactate) is used clinically, the I.V. use of the injection is not an FDA-approved route of administration; the decanoate form should never be administered intravenously.

May alter cardiac conduction and prolong QT interval; life-threatening arrhythmias have occurred with therapeutic doses of antipsychotics but risk may be increased with doses exceeding recommendations and/or intravenous administration (unlabeled route). Use caution or avoid use in patients with electrolyte abnormalities (eg, hypokalemia, hypomagnesemia), hypothyroidism, familial long QT syndrome, concomitant medications which may augment QT prolongation, or any underlying cardiac abnormality which may also potentiate risk. Monitor ECG closely for dose-related QT effects. Adverse effects of decanoate may be prolonged. Avoid in thyrotoxicosis.

Leukopenia, neutropenia, and agranulocytosis (sometimes fatal) have been reported in clinical trials and postmarketing reports with antipsychotic use; presence of risk factors (eg, pre-existing low WBC or history of drug-induced leuko-/neutropenia) should prompt periodic blood count assessment. Discontinue therapy at first signs of blood dyscrasias or if absolute neutrophil count $<1000/mm^3$.

May be sedating, use with caution in disorders where CNS depression is a feature. Effects may be potentiated when used with other sedative drugs or ethanol. Caution in patients with severe cardiovascular disease, predisposition to seizures, subcortical brain damage, or renal disease. Esophageal dysmotility and aspiration have been associated with antipsychotic use - use with caution in patients at risk of pneumonia (eg, Alzheimer's disease). Use associated with increased prolactin levels; clinical significance of hyperprolactinemia in patients with breast cancer or other prolactin-dependent tumors is unknown. May alter temperature regulation or mask toxicity of other drugs due to antiemetic effects. May cause orthostatic hypotension; use with caution in patients at risk of this effect or those who would tolerate transient hypotensive episodes (cerebrovascular disease, cardiovascular disease, or other medications which may predispose). Some tablets contain tartrazine. Antipsychotics have been associated with pigmentary retinopathy.

May cause anticholinergic effects (confusion, agitation, constipation, xerostomia, blurred vision, urinary retention). Therefore, they should be used with caution in patients with decreased gastrointestinal motility, urinary retention, BPH, xerostomia, or visual problems. Conditions which also may be exacerbated by cholinergic blockade include narrow-angle glaucoma and worsening of myasthenia gravis. Relative to other neuroleptics, haloperidol has a low potency of cholinergic blockade.

May cause extrapyramidal symptoms (EPS), including pseudoparkinsonism, acute dystonic reactions, akathisia, and tardive dyskinesia. Risk of dystonia (and possibly other EPS) may be greater with increased doses, use of conventional antipsychotics, males, and younger patients. May be associated with neuroleptic malignant syndrome (NMS). Use in elderly patients with dementia is associated with an increased risk of mortality and cerebrovascular accidents; avoid antipsychotic use for behavioral problems associated with dementia unless alternative nonpharmacologic therapies have failed and patient may harm self or others. In addition, use may cause or exacerbate syndrome of inappropriate antidiuretic hormone secretion or hyponatremia; monitor sodium closely with initiation or dosage adjustments in older adults (Beers Criteria). Increased risk for developing tardive dyskinesia, particularly elderly women.

Adverse Reactions Frequency not defined.

Cardiovascular: Abnormal T waves with prolonged ventricular repolarization, arrhythmia, hyper-/hypotension, QT prolongation, sudden death, tachycardia, torsade de pointes

Central nervous system: Agitation, akathisia, altered central temperature regulation, anxiety, confusion, depression, drowsiness, dystonic reactions, euphoria, extrapyramidal reactions, headache, insomnia, lethargy, neuroleptic malignant syndrome (NMS), pseudoparkinsonian signs and symptoms, restlessness, seizure, tardive dyskinesia, tardive dystonia, vertigo

Dermatologic: Alopecia, contact dermatitis, hyperpigmentation, photosensitivity (rare), pruritus, rash

Endocrine & metabolic: Amenorrhea, breast engorgement, galactorrhea, gynecomastia, hyper-/hypoglycemia, hyponatremia, lactation, mastalgia, menstrual irregularities, sexual dysfunction

Gastrointestinal: Anorexia, constipation, diarrhea, dyspepsia, hypersalivation, nausea, vomiting, xerostomia

Genitourinary: Priapism, urinary retention

Hematologic: Agranulocytosis (rare), leukopenia, leukocytosis, neutropenia, anemia, lymphomonocytosis

Hepatic: Cholestatic jaundice, obstructive jaundice

Ocular: Blurred vision

Respiratory: Bronchospasm, laryngospasm

Miscellaneous: Diaphoresis, heat stroke

Drug Interactions

Metabolism/Transport Effects **Substrate** of CYP1A2 (minor), CYP2D6 (major), CYP3A4 (major); **Note:** Assignment of Major/Minor substrate status based on clinically relevant drug interaction potential; **Inhibits** CYP2D6 (moderate), CYP3A4 (moderate)

Avoid Concomitant Use

Avoid concomitant use of Haloperidol with any of the following: Aclidinium; Azelastine (Nasal); Bosutinib; Conivaptan; Highest Risk QTc-Prolonging Agents; Ipratropium (Oral Inhalation); Metoclopramide; Mifepristone; Paraldehyde; Tiotropium; Tolvaptan

Increased Effect/Toxicity

Haloperidol may increase the levels/effects of: Alcohol (Ethyl); Anticholinergics; ARIPiprazole; Avanafil; Azelastine (Nasal); Bosutinib; Budesonide (Systemic, Oral Inhalation); Buprenorphine; ChlorproMAZINE; CNS Depressants; Colchicine; CYP2D6 Substrates; CYP3A4 Substrates; Eplerenone; Everolimus; FentaNYL; Fesoterodine; Highest Risk QTc-Prolonging Agents; Ivacaftor; Lurasidone; Methotrimeprazine; Methylphenidate; Moderate Risk QTc-Prolonging Agents; Nebivolol; Paraldehyde; Pimecrolimus; QuiNIDine; Salmeterol; Saxagliptin; Serotonin Modulators; Tiotropium; Tolvaptan; Zolpidem

The levels/effects of Haloperidol may be increased by: Abiraterone Acetate; Acetylcholinesterase Inhibitors (Central); Aclidinium; ChlorproMAZINE; Conivaptan; CYP2D6 Inhibitors (Moderate); CYP2D6 Inhibitors (Strong); CYP3A4 Inhibitors (Moderate); CYP3A4 Inhibitors (Strong); Darunavir; Dasatinib; FLUoxetine; FluvoxaMINE; HydrOXYzine; Ipratropium (Oral Inhalation); Ivacaftor; Lithium formulations; Methotrimeprazine; Methylphenidate; Metoclopramide; Metyrosine; Mifepristone; Nonsteroidal Anti-Inflammatory Agents; Perampanel; Pramlintide; QTc-Prolonging Agents (Indeterminate Risk and Risk Modifying); QuiNIDine; Tetrabenazine

Decreased Effect

Haloperidol may decrease the levels/effects of: Amphetamines; Anti-Parkinson's Agents (Dopamine Agonist); Codeine; Ifosfamide; Quinagolide; Tamoxifen

The levels/effects of Haloperidol may be decreased by: Anti-Parkinson's Agents (Dopamine Agonist); CarBAMazepine; CYP3A4 Inducers (Strong); Deferasirox; Glycopyrrolate; Lithium formulations; Peginterferon Alfa-2b; Tocilizumab

Ethanol/Nutrition/Herb Interactions

Ethanol: May increase CNS depression; monitor for increased effects with coadministration. Caution patients about effects.

Herb/Nutraceutical: Avoid valerian, St John's wort, kava kava, gotu kola (may increase CNS depression).

Storage/Stability Protect oral dosage forms from light. Haloperidol lactate injection should be stored at controlled room temperature; do not freeze or expose to temperatures >40°C. Protect from light; exposure to light may cause discoloration and the development of a grayish-red precipitate over several weeks. Stability of standardized solutions is 38 days at room temperature (24°C).

Reconstitution Haloperidol lactate may be administered IVPB or I.V. infusion in D_5W solutions. NS solutions should not be used due to reports of decreased stability and incompatibility.

Standardized dose: 0.5-100 mg/50-100 mL D_5W.

Mechanism of Action Haloperidol is a butyrophenone antipsychotic which blocks postsynaptic mesolimbic dopaminergic D_1 and D_2 receptors in the brain; depresses the release of hypothalamic and hypophyseal hormones; believed to depress the reticular activating system thus affecting basal metabolism, body temperature, wakefulness, vasomotor tone, and emesis

Pharmacodynamics/Kinetics

Onset of action: Sedation: I.M., I.V.: 30-60 minutes

Duration: Decanoate: 2-4 weeks

Distribution: V_d: 8-18 L/kg

Protein binding: 90%

Metabolism: Hepatic: 50% to 60% glucuronidation (inactive); 23% CYP3A4-mediated reduction to inactive metabolites (some back-oxidation to haloperidol); and 20% to 30% CYP3A4-mediated N-dealkylation, including minor oxidation pathway to toxic pyridinium derivative (Kudo, 1999)

Bioavailability: Oral: 60% to 70%

Half-life elimination: 18 hours; Decanoate: 21 days

Time to peak, serum: Oral: 2-6 hours; I.M.: 20 minutes; Decanoate: 7 days

Excretion: Urine (30%, 1% as unchanged drug); feces (15%)

Dosing

Adult

Psychosis:

Oral: 0.5-5 mg 2-3 times/day; usual maximum: 30 mg/day

I.M. (as lactate): 2-5 mg every 4-8 hours as needed

I.M. (as decanoate): Initial: 10-20 times the daily oral dose administered at 4-week intervals. Maintenance dose: 10-15 times initial oral dose; used to stabilize psychiatric symptoms

Delirium in the intensive care unit (unlabeled use, unlabeled route; Jacobi, 2002): I.V.: Initial: 2-10 mg depending on degree of agitation; if inadequate response, may repeat bolus dose (with sequential doubling of initial bolus dose) every 15-30 minutes until calm achieved, then administer 25% of the last bolus dose every 6 hours; monitor ECG and QT_c interval. After the patient is controlled, haloperidol therapy should be tapered over several days. **Note:** QT_c prolongation may occur with cumulative doses ≥35 mg and torsade de pointes has been reported with single doses of ≥20 mg. The optimal dose and regimen of haloperidol for the treatment of severe agitation and/or delirium has not been established.

Rapid tranquilization of severely-agitated patient (unlabeled use; administer every 30-60 minutes):

Oral: 5-10 mg

I.M. (as lactate): 5 mg

Average total dose (oral or I.M.) for tranquilization: 10-20 mg

Postoperative nausea and vomiting (PONV) (unlabeled use): I.M., I.V.: 0.5-2 mg (Gan, 2007)

Geriatric Nonpsychotic patient, dementia behavior (unlabeled use): Initial: Oral: 0.25-0.5 mg 1-2 times/day; increase dose at 4- to 7-day intervals by 0.25-0.5 mg/day. Increase dosing intervals (twice daily, 3 times/day, etc) as necessary to control response or side effects.

Pediatric

Sedation/psychotic disorders: Oral:

Children 3-12 years (15-40 kg): Initial: 0.5 mg/day given in 2-3 divided doses; increase by 0.5 mg every 5-7 days; maximum: 0.15 mg/kg/day

Usual maintenance:

Nonpsychotic disorders, Tourette's disorder: 0.05-0.075 mg/kg/day in 2-3 divided doses

Psychotic disorders: 0.05-0.15 mg/kg/day in 2-3 divided doses

Children 6-12 years: Sedation/psychotic disorders: I.M. (as lactate): 1-3 mg/dose every 4-8 hours to a maximum of 0.15 mg/kg/day; convert to oral therapy as soon as able.

Renal Impairment Hemodialysis/peritoneal dialysis: Supplemental dose is not necessary.

Administration

Injection oil (decanoate): The decanoate injectable formulation should be administered I.M. only, **do not administer decanoate I.V.**

Injection solution (lactate): The lactate injectable formulation may be administered I.V. (unlabeled route) or I.M.

Oral solution (lactate): Dilute the oral concentrate with water or juice before administration. Avoid skin contact with oral solution; may cause contact dermatitis.

Monitoring Parameters Vital signs; lipid profile, fasting blood glucose/Hgb A_{1c}; BMI; mental status, abnormal involuntary movement scale (AIMS), extrapyramidal symptoms (EPS); ECG (with off-label intravenous administration)

Dosage Forms Excipient information presented when available (limited, particularly for generics); consult specific product labeling.

Injection, oil, as decanoate [strength expressed as base]: 50 mg/mL (1 mL, 5 mL); 100 mg/mL (1 mL, 5 mL)

Haldol® Decanoate: 50 mg/mL (1 mL); 100 mg/mL (1 mL) [contains benzyl alcohol, sesame oil]

Injection, solution, as lactate [strength expressed as base]: 5 mg/mL (1 mL, 10 mL)

Haldol®: 5 mg/mL (1 mL)

Solution, oral, as lactate [strength expressed as base, concentrate]: 2 mg/mL (5 mL, 15 mL, 120 mL)

Tablet, oral: 0.5 mg, 1 mg, 2 mg, 5 mg, 10 mg, 20 mg

References

Cole RM, Robinson F, Harvey L, et al, "Successful Control of Intractable Nausea and Vomiting Requiring Combined Ondansetron and Haloperidol in a Patient With Advanced Cancer," *J Pain Symptom Manage*, 1994, 9(1):48-50.

Gan TJ, Meyer TA, Apfel CC, et al, "Society for Ambulatory Anesthesia Guidelines for the Management of Postoperative Nausea and Vomiting," *Anesth Analg*, 2007, 105(6):1615-28.

Jacobi J, Fraser GL, Coursin DB, et al, "Clinical Practice Guidelines for the Sustained Use of Sedatives and Analgesics in the Critically Ill Adult," *Crit Care Med*, 2002, 30(1):119-41.

Kudo S and Ishizaki T, "Pharmacokinetics of Haloperidol: An Update," *Clin Pharmacokinet*, 1999, 73(6):435-56.

Plotkin DA, Plotkin D, and Okun R, "Haloperidol in the Treatment of Nausea and Vomiting Due to Cytotoxic Drug Administration," *Curr Ther Res Clin Exp*,1973, 15(9):599-602.

Silvey L, Carpenter JT Jr, Wheeler RH, et al, "A Randomized Comparison of Haloperidol Plus Dexamethasone Versus Prochlorperazine Plus Dexamethasone in Preventing Nausea and Vomiting in Patients Receiving Chemotherapy for Breast Cancer," *J Clin Oncol*, 1988, 6 (9):1397-400.

◆ **Haloperidol Decanoate** *see* Haloperidol *on page 691*

◆ **Haloperidol Injection, USP (Can)** *see* Haloperidol *on page 691*

◆ **Haloperidol-LA (Can)** *see* Haloperidol *on page 691*

◆ **Haloperidol Lactate** *see* Haloperidol *on page 691*

◆ **Haloperidol-LA Omega (Can)** *see* Haloperidol *on page 691*

◆ **Haloperidol Long Acting (Can)** *see* Haloperidol *on page 691*

◆ **Hecoria™** *see* Tacrolimus (Systemic) *on page 1315*

◆ **Hedgehog Antagonist GDC-0449** *see* Vismodegib *on page 1470*

◆ **Helixate® FS** *see* Antihemophilic Factor (Recombinant) *on page 103*

◆ **Hemofil M** *see* Antihemophilic Factor (Human) *on page 101*

◆ **Hemorrhoidal HC** *see* Hydrocortisone (Topical) *on page 719*

◆ **Hemril® -30** *see* Hydrocortisone (Topical) *on page 719*

◆ **Hepalean® (Can)** *see* Heparin *on page 697*

◆ **Hepalean® Leo (Can)** *see* Heparin *on page 697*

◆ **Hepalean®-LOK (Can)** *see* Heparin *on page 697*

Heparin (HEP a rin)

Related Information

Venous Thromboembolism in the Cancer Patient *on page 1883*

Brand Names: U.S. Hep-Lock; HepFlush®-10

Brand Names: Canada Hepalean®; Hepalean® Leo; Hepalean®-LOK

Index Terms Heparin Calcium; Heparin Lock Flush; Heparin Sodium

Generic Availability (U.S.) Yes

Pharmacologic Category Anticoagulant

Use Prophylaxis and treatment of thromboembolic disorders; as an anticoagulant for extracorporeal and dialysis procedures

Note: Heparin lock flush solution is intended only to maintain patency of I.V. devices and is **not** to be used for systemic anticoagulant therapy.

Unlabeled Use ST-elevation myocardial infarction (STEMI) as an adjunct to thrombolysis; unstable angina/non-STEMI (UA/NSTEMI); anticoagulant used during percutaneous coronary intervention (PCI)

Labeled Contraindications Hypersensitivity to heparin or any component of the formulation (unless a life-threatening situation necessitates use and use of an alternative anticoagulant is not possible); severe thrombocytopenia; uncontrolled active bleeding except when due to disseminated intravascular coagulation (DIC); not for use when appropriate blood coagulation tests cannot be obtained at appropriate intervals (applies to full-dose heparin only)

Note: Some products contain benzyl alcohol as a preservative; their use in neonates, infants, or pregnant or nursing mothers is contraindicated by some manufacturers.

Pregnancy Risk Factor C

Lactation Does not enter breast milk

Warnings/Precautions Hypersensitivity reactions can occur. Only in life-threatening situations when use of an alternative anticoagulant is not possible should heparin be cautiously used in patients with a documented hypersensitivity reaction. Hemorrhage is the most common complication. Monitor for signs and symptoms of bleeding. Certain patients are at increased risk of bleeding. Risk factors for bleeding include bacterial endocarditis; congenital or acquired bleeding disorders; active ulcerative or angiodysplastic GI diseases; continuous GI tube drainage; severe uncontrolled hypertension; history of hemorrhagic stroke; or use shortly after brain, spinal, or ophthalmology surgery; patient treated concomitantly with platelet inhibitors, conditions associated with increased bleeding tendencies (hemophilia, vascular purpura); recent GI bleeding; thrombocytopenia or platelet defects; severe liver disease; hypertensive or diabetic retinopathy; renal failure; or in patients undergoing invasive procedures including spinal tap or spinal anesthesia. Many concentrations of heparin are available ranging from 1 unit/mL to 20,000 units/mL. Clinicians **must** carefully examine each prefilled syringe or vial prior to use ensuring that the correct concentration is chosen; fatal hemorrhages have occurred related to heparin overdose especially in pediatric patients. A higher incidence of bleeding has been reported in patients >60 years of age, particularly women. They are also more sensitive to the dose. Discontinue heparin if hemorrhage occurs; severe hemorrhage or overdosage may require protamine.

May cause thrombocytopenia; monitor platelet count closely. Patients who develop HIT may be at risk of developing a new thrombus (heparin-induced thrombocytopenia and thrombosis [HITT]). Discontinue therapy and consider alternatives if platelets are <100,000/mm^3 and/or thrombosis develops. HIT or HITT may be delayed and can occur up to several weeks after discontinuation of heparin. Use with extreme caution (for a limited duration) or avoid in patients with history of HIT, especially if administered within 100 days of HIT episode (Dager, 2007; Warkentin, 2001); monitor platelet count closely. Osteoporosis may occur with prolonged use (>6 months) due to a reduction in bone mineral density. Monitor for hyperkalemia; can cause hyperkalemia by suppressing aldosterone production. Patients >60 years of age may require lower doses of heparin.

[U.S. Boxed Warning]: Some products contain benzyl alcohol as a preservative; use of these products is contraindicated in neonates. In neonates, large amounts of benzyl alcohol (>100 mg/kg/day) have been associated with fatal toxicity (gasping syndrome). Use in neonates, infants, or pregnant or nursing mothers is contraindicated by some manufacturers; the use of preservative-free heparin is, therefore, recommended in these populations. Some preparations contain sulfite which may cause allergic reactions.

Heparin resistance may occur in patients with antithrombin deficiency, increased heparin clearance, elevations in heparin-binding proteins, elevations in factor VIII and/or fibrinogen; frequently encountered in patients with fever, thrombosis, thrombophlebitis, infections with thrombosing tendencies, MI, cancer, and in postsurgical patients; measurement of anticoagulant effects using antifactor Xa levels may be of benefit.

Adverse Reactions Note: Thrombocytopenia has been reported to occur at an incidence between 0% and 30%. It is often of no clinical significance. However, immunologically mediated heparin-induced thrombocytopenia (HIT) has been estimated to occur in 1% to 2% of patients, and is marked by a progressive fall in platelet counts and, in some cases, thromboembolic complications (skin necrosis, pulmonary embolism, gangrene of the extremities, stroke, or MI).

Frequency not defined.

Cardiovascular: Allergic vasospastic reaction (possibly related to thrombosis), chest pain, hemorrhagic shock, shock, thrombosis

Central nervous system: Chills, fever, headache

Dermatologic: Alopecia (delayed, transient), bruising (unexplained), cutaneous necrosis, dysesthesia pedis, erythematous plaques (case reports), eczema, urticaria, purpura

Endocrine & metabolic: Adrenal hemorrhage, hyperkalemia (suppression of aldosterone synthesis), ovarian hemorrhage, rebound hyperlipidemia on discontinuation

Gastrointestinal: Constipation, hematemesis, nausea, tarry stools, vomiting

Genitourinary: Frequent or persistent erection

Hematologic: Bleeding from gums, epistaxis, hemorrhage, ovarian hemorrhage, retroperitoneal hemorrhage, thrombocytopenia (see note)

Hepatic: Liver enzymes increased

Local: Irritation, erythema, pain, hematoma, and ulceration have been rarely reported with deep SubQ injections; I.M. injection (not recommended) is associated with a high incidence of these effects

Neuromuscular & skeletal: Peripheral neuropathy, osteoporosis (chronic therapy effect)

Ocular: Conjunctivitis (allergic reaction), lacrimation
Renal: Hematuria
Respiratory: Asthma, bronchospasm (case reports), hemoptysis, pulmonary hemorrhage, rhinitis
Miscellaneous: Allergic reactions, anaphylactoid reactions, heparin resistance, hypersensitivity (including chills, fever, and urticaria)

Drug Interactions

Metabolism/Transport Effects None known.

Avoid Concomitant Use

Avoid concomitant use of Heparin with any of the following: Corticorelin; Omacetaxine; Palifermin; Rivaroxaban

Increased Effect/Toxicity

Heparin may increase the levels/effects of: Anticoagulants; Collagenase (Systemic); Corticorelin; Dabigatran Etexilate; Deferasirox; Drotrecogin Alfa (Activated); Ibritumomab; Omacetaxine; Palifermin; Rivaroxaban; Tositumomab and Iodine I 131 Tositumomab

The levels/effects of Heparin may be increased by: 5-ASA Derivatives; Antiplatelet Agents; Aspirin; Dasatinib; Herbs (Anticoagulant/Antiplatelet Properties); Nonsteroidal Anti-Inflammatory Agents; Pentosan Polysulfate Sodium; Pentoxifylline; Prostacyclin Analogues; Salicylates; Thrombolytic Agents; Tipranavir; Vitamin E

Decreased Effect

The levels/effects of Heparin may be decreased by: Nitroglycerin

Ethanol/Nutrition/Herb Interactions Herb/Nutraceutical: Avoid cat's claw, dong quai, evening primrose, feverfew, red clover, horse chestnut, garlic, green tea, ginseng, ginkgo (all have additional antiplatelet activity).

Storage/Stability Heparin solutions are colorless to slightly yellow. Minor color variations do not affect therapeutic efficacy. Heparin should be stored at controlled room temperature. Protect from freezing and temperatures >40°C.

Stability at room temperature and refrigeration:
Prepared bag: 24-72 hours (specific to solution, concentration, and/or study conditions)
Premixed bag: After seal is broken, 4 days.
Out of overwrap stability: 30 days.

Mechanism of Action Potentiates the action of antithrombin III and thereby inactivates thrombin (as well as activated coagulation factors IX, X, XI, XII, and plasmin) and prevents the conversion of fibrinogen to fibrin; heparin also stimulates release of lipoprotein lipase (lipoprotein lipase hydrolyzes triglycerides to glycerol and free fatty acids)

Pharmacodynamics/Kinetics

Onset of action: Anticoagulation: I.V.: Immediate; SubQ: ~20-30 minutes
Absorption: Oral, rectal: Erratic at best from these routes of administration; SubQ absorption is also erratic, but considered acceptable for prophylactic use
Metabolism: Hepatic; may be partially metabolized in the reticuloendothelial system
Half-life elimination:
Dose-dependent: I.V. bolus: 25 units/kg: 30 minutes; 100 units/kg: 60 minutes; 400 units/kg: 150 minutes (Hirsh, 2008)
Mean: 1.5 hours; Range: 1-2 hours; affected by obesity, renal function, malignancy, presence of pulmonary embolism, and infections

Note: At therapeutic doses, elimination occurs rapidly via nonrenal mechanisms. With very high doses, renal elimination may play more of a role; however, dosage adjustment remains unnecessary for patients with renal impairment (Hirsh, 2008).

Excretion: Urine (small amounts as unchanged drug)

Dosing

Adult Note: Many concentrations of heparin are available ranging from 1 unit/mL to 20,000 units/mL. Carefully examine each prefilled syringe or vial prior to use ensuring that the correct concentration is chosen. Heparin lock flush solution is intended only to maintain patency of I.V. devices and is not to be used for anticoagulant therapy.

Acute coronary syndromes: I.V. infusion (weight-based dosing per institutional nomogram recommended):

STEMI: Adjunct to fibrinolysis (full-dose alteplase, reteplase, or tenecteplase) (Antman, 2008): Initial bolus of 60 units/kg (maximum: 4000 units), then 12 units/kg/hour (maximum: 1000 units/hour) as continuous infusion. Check aPTT every 4-6 hours; adjust to target of 1.5-2 times the upper limit of control (50-70 seconds). Duration of heparin therapy depends on concurrent therapy and the specific patient risks for systemic or venous thromboembolism.

Unstable angina (UA)/non-ST-elevation myocardial infarction (NSTEMI) (Anderson, 2007): Initial bolus of 60 units/kg (maximum: 4000 units), followed by an initial infusion of 12 units/kg/hour (maximum: 1000 units/hour). Check aPTT every 4-6 hours; adjust to target of 1.5-2 times the upper limit of control (50-70 seconds). Continue for 48 hours in low risk patients managed with a conservative strategy (ie, no diagnostic angiography or PCI) (Jneid, 2012).

Percutaneous coronary intervention (Levine, 2011):

No prior anticoagulant therapy:

If no GPIIb/IIIa inhibitor use planned: Initial bolus of 70-100 units/kg (target ACT 250-300 seconds for HemoTec®, 300-350 seconds for Hemochron®)

or

If planning GPIIb/IIIa inhibitor use: Initial bolus of 50-70 units/kg (target ACT 200-250 seconds regardless of device)

Prior anticoagulant therapy:

If no GPIIb/IIIa inhibitor use planned: Additional heparin as needed (eg, 2000-5000 units) (target ACT 250-300 seconds for HemoTec®, 300-350 seconds for Hemochron®)

or

If planning GPIIb/IIIa inhibitor use: Additional heparin as needed (eg, 2000-5000 units) (target ACT 200-250 seconds regardless of device)

Thromboprophylaxis (low-dose heparin): SubQ: 5000 units every 8-12 hours. **Note:** The American College of Chest Physicians recommends a minimum of 10-14 days for patients undergoing total hip arthroplasty, total knee arthroplasty, or hip fracture surgery (Guyatt, 2012).

Treatment of venous thromboembolism: Note: Start warfarin on the first or second treatment day and continue heparin until INR is ≥2 for at least 24 hours (usually 5-7 days) (Guyatt, 2012).

DVT/PE (unlabeled dosing): I.V.: 80 units/kg (or alternatively 5000 units) I.V. push followed by continuous infusion of 18 units/kg/hour (or alternatively 1000 units/hour) (Guyatt, 2012)

or

DVT/PE (unlabeled dosing): SubQ: *Unmonitored dosing regimen:* Initial: 333 units/kg then 250 units/kg every 12 hours (Guyatt, 2012; Kearon, 2006)

Intermittent I.V. Anticoagulation: Intermittent I.V.: Initial: 10,000 units, then 50-70 units/kg (5000-10,000 units) every 4-6 hours

Maintenance of line patency (line flushing): When using daily flushes of heparin to maintain patency of single and double lumen central catheters, 10 units/mL is commonly used for younger infants (eg, <10 kg) while 100 units/mL is used for older infants, children, and adults. Capped PVC catheters and peripheral heparin locks require flushing more frequently (eg, every 6-8 hours). Volume of heparin flush is usually similar to volume of catheter (or slightly greater). Additional flushes should be given when stagnant blood is observed in catheter, after catheter is used for drug or blood administration, and after blood withdrawal from catheter.

Parenteral nutrition: Addition of heparin (0.5-3 unit/mL) to peripheral and central parenteral nutrition has not been shown to decrease catheter-related thrombosis. The final concentration of heparin used for TPN solutions may need to be decreased to 0.5 units/mL in small infants receiving larger amounts of volume in order to avoid approaching therapeutic amounts. Arterial lines are heparinized with a final concentration of 1 unit/mL.

Geriatric Patients >60 years of age may have higher serum levels and clinical response (longer aPTTs) as compared to younger patients receiving similar dosages. Lower dosages may be required.

Pediatric Note: Many concentrations of heparin are available ranging from 1 unit/mL to 20,000 units/mL. Carefully examine each prefilled syringe or vial prior to use ensuring that the correct concentration is chosen. Heparin lock flush solution is intended only to maintain patency of I.V. devices and is not to be used for anticoagulant therapy.

Prophylaxis for cardiac catheterization (arterial approach): I.V.: Bolus: 100 units/kg (Freed, 1974; Monagle, 2012)

Systemic heparinization:

Intermittent I.V.: Initial: 50-100 units/kg, then 50-100 units/kg every 4 hours (**Note:** Continuous I.V. infusion is preferred)

I.V. infusion: Initial loading dose: 75 units/kg given over 10 minutes, then initial maintenance dose: 20 units/kg/hour; adjust dose to maintain aPTT of 60-85 seconds (assuming this reflects an antifactor Xa level of 0.35-0.7 units/mL); see table on next page.

Pediatric Protocol For Systemic Heparin Adjustment

To be used after initial loading dose and maintenance I.V. infusion dose (see usual dosage listed above) to maintain aPTT of 60-85 seconds (assuming this reflects antifactor Xa level of 0.35-0.7 units/mL).

Obtain blood for aPTT 4 hours after heparin loading dose and 4 hours after every infusion rate change.

Obtain daily CBC and aPTT after aPTT is therapeutic.

aPTT (seconds)	Dosage Adjustment	Time to Repeat aPTT
<50	Give 50 units/kg bolus and increase infusion rate by 10%	4 h after rate change
50-59	Increase infusion rate by 10%	4 h after rate change
60-85	Keep rate the same	Next day
86-95	Decrease infusion rate by 10%	4 h after rate change
96-120	Hold infusion for 30 minutes and decrease infusion rate by 10%	4 h after rate change
>120	Hold infusion for 60 minutes and decrease infusion rate by 15%	4 h after rate change

Modified from Andrew M, et al, "Heparin Therapy in Pediatric Patients: A Prospective Cohort Study," *Pediatr Research*, 1994, 35(1):78-83.
Note: The aPTT range of 60-85 seconds corresponds to an anti-Xa level of 0.35-0.7 units/mL.

Note: Refer to adult dosing for notes on line flushing and TPN.

Renal Impairment No dosage adjustment required; adjust therapeutic heparin according to aPTT or anti-Xa activity.

Hepatic Impairment No dosage adjustment required; adjust therapeutic heparin according to aPTT or anti-Xa activity.

Usual Infusion Concentrations: Pediatric Note: Premixed solutions available

I.V. infusion: 100 units/mL

Usual Infusion Concentrations: Adult Note: Premixed solutions available

I.V. infusion: 25,000 units in 250 mL (concentration: 100 units/mL) of D_5W, 1/2NS, or NS

Administration

SubQ: Inject in subcutaneous tissue only (not muscle tissue). Injection sites should be rotated (usually left and right portions of the abdomen, above iliac crest).

I.M.: Do not administer I.M. due to pain, irritation, and hematoma formation; central venous catheters must be flushed with heparin solution when newly inserted, daily (at the time of tubing change), after blood withdrawal or transfusion, and after an intermittent infusion through an injectable cap. A volume of at least 10 mL of blood should be removed and discarded from a heparinized line before blood samples are sent for coagulation testing.

Continuous I.V. infusion: Infuse via infusion pump. If preparing solution, mix thoroughly prior to administration.

Heparin lock: Inject via injection cap using positive pressure flushing technique. Heparin lock flush solution is intended only to maintain patency of I.V. devices and is **not** to be used for anticoagulant therapy.

Monitoring Parameters Hemoglobin, hematocrit, signs of bleeding; fecal occult blood test; aPTT (or antifactor Xa activity levels) or ACT depending upon indication

Platelet counts should be routinely monitored (eg, every 2-3 days on days 4-14 of heparin therapy) when the risk of HIT is >1% (eg, receiving therapeutic dose heparin, postoperative antithrombotic prophylaxis), if the patient has received heparin or low molecular weight heparin (eg, enoxaparin) within the past 100 days, if pre-exposure history is uncertain, or if anaphylactoid reaction to heparin occurs. When the risk of HIT is <1% (eg, medical/obstetrical patients receiving heparin flushes), routine platelet count monitoring is not recommended (Guyatt, 2012).

For intermittent I.V. injections, aPTT is measured 3.5-4 hours after I.V. injection.

Note: Continuous I.V. infusion is preferred over I.V. intermittent injections. For full-dose heparin (ie, nonlow-dose), the dose should be titrated according to aPTT results. For anticoagulation, an aPTT 1.5-2.5 times normal is usually desired. Because of variation among hospitals in the control aPTT values, nomograms should be established at each institution, designed to achieve aPTT values in the target range (eg, for a control aPTT of 30 seconds, the target range [1.5-2.5 times control] would be 45-75 seconds). Measurements should be made prior to heparin therapy, 6 hours (pediatric: 4 hours) after initiation, and 6 hours (pediatric: 4 hours) after any dosage change, and should be used to adjust the heparin infusion until the aPTT exhibits a therapeutic level. When two consecutive aPTT values are therapeutic, subsequent measurements may be made every 24 hours, and if necessary, dose adjustment carried out. In addition, a significant change in the patient's clinical condition (eg, recurrent ischemia, bleeding, hypotension) should prompt an immediate aPTT determination, followed by dose adjustment if necessary. In general, may increase or decrease infusion by 2-4 units/kg/hour dependent upon aPTT.

Heparin infusion dose adjustment: A number of dose-adjustment nomograms have been developed which target an aPTT range of 1.5-2.5 times control (Cruickshank, 1991; Flaker, 1994; Hull, 1992; Raschke, 1993). However, institution-specific and indication-specific nomograms should be consulted for dose adjustment. **Note:** aPTT values vary throughout the day with maximum values occurring during the night (Decousus, 1985).

Test Interactions Increased thyroxine (competitive protein binding methods); increased PT

Aprotinin significantly increases aPTT and celite Activated Clotting Time (ACT) which may not reflect the actual degree of anticoagulation by heparin. Kaolin-based ACTs are not affected by aprotinin to the same degree as celite ACTs. While institutional protocols may vary, a minimal celite ACT of 750 seconds or kaolin-ACT of 480 seconds is recommended in the presence of aprotinin. Consult the manufacturer's information on specific ACT test interpretation in the presence of aprotinin.

Dosage Forms Excipient information presented when available (limited, particularly for generics); consult specific product labeling.

Infusion, premixed in 1/2 NS, as sodium [porcine intestinal mucosa source]: 25,000 units (250 mL, 500 mL)

Infusion, premixed in D_5W, as sodium [porcine intestinal mucosa source]: 10,000 units (250 mL); 12,500 units (250 mL); 20,000 units (500 mL); 25,000 units (250 mL, 500 mL)

Infusion, premixed in NS, as sodium [porcine intestinal mucosa source]: 1000 units (500 mL); 2000 units (1000 mL)

Infusion, premixed in NS, as sodium [porcine intestinal mucosa source, preservative free]: 1000 units (500 mL); 2000 units (1000 mL)

Injection, solution, as sodium [lock flush preparation; porcine intestinal mucosa source]: 10 units/mL (1 mL, 2 mL, 3 mL, 5 mL, 10 mL); 100 units/mL (1 mL, 2 mL, 3 mL, 5 mL, 10 mL, 30 mL)

Hep-Lock: 100 units/mL (1 mL) [contains benzyl alcohol]

Injection, solution, as sodium [lock flush preparation; porcine intestinal mucosa source, preservative free]: 1 units/mL (2 mL, 3 mL, 5 mL); 2 units/mL (3 mL); 10 units/mL (1 mL, 2 mL, 2.5 mL, 3 mL, 5 mL, 6 mL, 10 mL); 100 units/mL (1 mL, 2 mL, 2.5 mL, 3 mL, 5 mL, 10 mL)

HepFlush®-10: 10 units/mL (10 mL)

Injection, solution, as sodium [porcine intestinal mucosa source]: 1000 units/mL (1 mL, 10 mL, 30 mL); 5000 units/mL (1 mL, 10 mL); 10,000 units/mL (1 mL, 4 mL, 5 mL); 20,000 units/mL (1 mL)

Injection, solution, as sodium [porcine intestinal mucosa source, preservative free]: 1000 units/mL (2 mL); 5000 units/mL (0.5 mL); 10,000 units/mL (0.5 mL)

References

Anderson JL, Adams CD, Antman EM, et al, "2011 ACCF/AHA Focused Update Incorporated Into the ACC/AHA 2007 Guidelines for the Management of Patients With Unstable Angina/Non-ST-Elevation Myocardial Infarction: A Report of the American College of Cardiology Foundation/American Heart Association Task Force on Practice Guidelines," *Circulation*, 2011, 123(18): e426-579.

Antman EM, Anbe DT, Armstrong PW, et al,"ACC/AHA Guidelines for the Management of Patients With ST-Elevation Myocardial Infarction: A Report of the American College of Cardiology/American Heart Association Task Force on Practice Guidelines (Committee to Revise the 1999 Guidelines for the Management of Patients with Acute Myocardial Infarction)," *Circulation*, 2004, 110(9):e82-292.

Antman EM, Hand M, Armstrong PW, et al, "2007 Focused Update of the ACC/AHA 2004 Guidelines for the Management of Patients With ST-Elevation Myocardial Infarction. A Report of the American College of Cardiology/American Heart Association Task Force on Practice Guidelines," *J Am Coll Cardiol*, 2008, 51(2):210-49.

Broderick J, Connolly S, Feldmann E, et al, "Guidelines for the Management of Spontaneous Intracerebral Hemorrhage in Adults: 2007 Update: A Guideline From the American Heart Association/American Stroke Association Stroke Council, High Blood Pressure Research Council, and the Quality of Care and Outcomes in Research Interdisciplinary Working Group," *Stroke*, 2007, 38(6):2001-23. Available at http://stroke.ahajournals.org/cgi/content/short/STROKEAHA.107.183689

Cruickshank MK, Levine MN, Hirsh J, et al, "A Standard Heparin Nomogram for the Management of Heparin Therapy," *Arch Intern Med*, 1991, 151(2):333-7.

Dager WE and White RH, "Pharmacotherapy of Heparin-Induced Thrombocytopenia," *Expert Opin Pharmacother*, 2003, 4(6):919-40.

Flaker GC, Bartolozzi J, Davis V, et al, "Use of a Standardized Heparin Nomogram to Achieve Therapeutic Anticoagulation after Thrombolytic Therapy in Myocardial Infarction. TIMI 4 investigators. Thrombolysis in Myocardial Infarction," *Arch Intern Med*, 1994, 154(13):1492-6.

Francis JL, Groce JB 3rd, and the Heparin Consensus Group, "Challenges in Variation and Response of Unfractionated Heparin," *Pharmacotherapy*, 2004, 24(8 Pt 2), 108-19.

Freed MD, Keane JF, and Rosenthal A, "The Use of Heparinization to Prevent Arterial Thrombosis After Percutaneous Cardiac Catheterization in Children," *Circulation*, 1974, 50(3):565-9.

Garcia DA, Baglin TP, Weitz JI, et al, "Parenteral Anticoagulants: Antithrombotic Therapy and Prevention of Thrombosis, 9th ed: American College of Chest Physicians Evidence-Based Clinical Practice Guidelines," *Chest*, 2012, 141(2 Suppl):24-43.

Goodman SG, Menon V, Cannon CP, et al, "Acute ST-Segment Elevation Myocardial Infarction: American College of Chest Physicians Evidence-Based Clinical Practice," *Chest*, 2008, 133(6 Suppl):708-75.

Guyatt GH, Akl EA, Crowther M, et al, "Executive Summary: Antithrombotic Therapy and Prevention of Thrombosis, 9th ed: American College of Chest Physicians Evidence-Based Clinical Practice Guidelines," *Chest*, 2012, 141(2 Suppl):7-47.

Hirsh J, Bauer KA, Donati MB, et al, "Parenteral Anticoagulants: American College of Chest Physicians Evidence-Based Clinical Practice Guidelines (8th Edition)," *Chest*, 2008, 133(6 Suppl):141-59.

Hirsh J, Guyatt G, Albers GW, et al, "Executive Summary: American College of Chest Physicians Evidence-Based Clinical Practice Guidelines (8th Edition)," *Chest*, 2008, 133(6 Suppl):71-109.

Hull RD, Raskob GE, Rosenbloom D, et al, "Optimal Therapeutic Level of Heparin Therapy in Patients with Venous Thromboembolism," *Arch Intern Med*, 1992, 152(8):1589-95.

Jaff MR, McMurtry MS, Archer SL, et al, "Management of Massive and Submassive Pulmonary Embolism, Iliofemoral Deep Vein Thrombosis, and Chronic Thromboembolic Pulmonary

Hypertension: A Scientific Statement from the American Heart Association," *Circulation*, 2011, 123(16):1788-830.

Jneid H, Anderson JL, Wright RS, et al, "2012 ACCF/AHA Focused Update of the Guideline for the Management of Patients With Unstable Angina/Non-ST-Elevation Myocardial Infarction (Updating the 2007 Guideline and Replacing the 2011 Focused Update): A Report of the American College of Cardiology Foundation/American Heart Association Task Force on Practice Guidelines," *Circulation*, 2012, 126(7):875-910.

Kearon C, Kahn SR, Agnelli G, et al, "Antithrombotic Therapy for Venous Thromboembolic Disease: American College of Chest Physicians Evidence-Based Clinical Practice Guidelines (8th Edition)," *Chest*, 2008, 33(6 Suppl):454-545.

King SB 3rd, Smith SC Jr, Hirshfeld JW JR, et al, "2007 Focused Update of the ACC/AHA/SCAI 2005 Guideline Update for Percutaneous Coronary Intervention. A Report of the American College of Cardiology/American Heart Association Task Force on Practice Guidelines: 2007 Writing Group to Review New Evidence and Update the ACC/AHA/SCAI 2005 Guideline Update for Percutaneous Coronary Intervention, Writing on Behalf of the 2005 Writing Committee," *Circulation*, 2008, 117(2):261-95.

Kushner FG, Hand M, Smith SC, et al, "2009 Focused Updates: ACC/AHA Guidelines for the Management of Patients With ST-Elevation Myocardial Infarction (Updating the 2004 Guideline and 2007 Focused Update) and ACC/AHA/SCAI Guidelines on Percutaneous Coronary Intervention (Updating the 2005 Guideline and 2007 Focused Update): A Report of the American College of Cardiology Foundation/American Heart Association Task Force on Practice Guidelines," *J Am Coll Cardiol*, 2009, 54(23):2205-41.

Levine GN, Bates ER, Blankenship JC, et al, "2011 ACCF/AHA/SCAI Guideline for Percutaneous Coronary Intervention: A Report of the American College of Cardiology Foundation/American Heart Association Task Force on Practice Guidelines and the Society for Cardiovascular Angiography and Interventions," *Circulation*, 2011, 124(23):e574-651.

Monagle P, Chan A, Goldenberg NA, et al, "Antithrombotic Therapy in Neonates and Children: American College of Chest Physicians Evidence-Based Clinical Practice Guidelines (9th Edition)," *Chest*, 2012, 141(2 Suppl):e737-801.

Raschke RA, Reilly BM, Guidry JR, et al, "The Weight-Based Heparin Dosing Nomogram Compared With a "Standard Care" Nomogram: A Randomized Controlled Trial," *Ann Intern Med*, 1993, 119(9):874-81.

Warkentin TE, Greinacher A, Koster A, et al, "Treatment and Prevention of Heparin-Induced Thrombocytopenia: American College of Chest Physicians Evidence-Based Clinical Practice Guidelines (8th Edition)," *Chest*, 2008, 133(6 Suppl):340-80.

Wright RS, Anderson JL, Adams CD, et al, "2011 ACCF/AHA Focused Update of the Guidelines for the Management of Patients with Unstable Angina/Non-ST-Elevation Myocardial Infarction (Updating the 2007 Guideline): A Report of the American College of Cardiology Foundation/American Heart Association Task Force on Practice Guidelines Developed in Collaboration With the American College of Emergency Physicians, Society for Cardiovascular Angiography and Interventions, and Society of Thoracic Surgeons," *J Am Coll Cardiol*, 2011, 57(19):1920-59.

◆ **Heparin Calcium** *see* Heparin *on page 697*

◆ **Heparin Lock Flush** *see* Heparin *on page 697*

◆ **Heparin Sodium** *see* Heparin *on page 697*

◆ **HepFlush®-10** *see* Heparin *on page 697*

◆ **Hep-Lock** *see* Heparin *on page 697*

◆ **Herceptin®** *see* Trastuzumab *on page 1000*

◆ **Hexalen®** *see* Altretamine *on page 63*

◆ **Hexamethylmelamine** *see* Altretamine *on page 63*

Hexaminolevulinate (hex a mee noe LEV ue lin ate)

Brand Names: U.S. Cysview™

Index Terms HAL; Hexaminolevulinate Hydrochloride

Pharmacologic Category Contrast Agent

Use Detection of non-muscle invasive papillary cancer of the bladder; used in conjunction with the Karl Storz D-Light C Photodynamic Diagnostic (PDD) system

Labeled Contraindications Hypersensitivity to hexaminolevulinate, derivatives of aminolevulinic acid or any component of the formulation; porphyria; gross hematuria; bacillus Calmette-Guérin (BCG) immunotherapy or intravesical chemotherapy within the past 90 days

Pregnancy Risk Factor C

Lactation Excretion in breast milk is unknown/use caution

Warnings/Precautions Hypersensitivity reactions, including anaphylaxis and anaphylactoid shock, have been reported. Immediate treatment (including epinephrine 1:1000) for anaphylactoid and/or hypersensitivity reactions should be available.

Fluorescent areas detected during blue light cystoscopy may not always demonstrate a bladder mucosal lesion, especially if the mucosal area had not previously been classified as malignant during white light cystoscopy. Fluorescent areas may also result from inflammation, cystoscopic trauma, scar tissue, or bladder mucosal biopsy from previous examinations. Cystoscopic examination with hexaminolevulinate should not replace random biopsies or other procedures usually performed in the cystoscopic evaluation for cancer; hexaminolevulinate failed ot detect 10% of malignant lesions in clinical trials. Both light settings of the PDD system (white before blue) must be used for the most accurate detection of malignancies.

Adverse Reactions

1% to 10%:

Central nervous system: Headache

Genitourinary: Bladder spasm (2%), bladder pain, dysuria, hematuria

Local: Procedural pain

Postmarketing and/or case reports: Abnormal urinalysis, anaphylaxis (including anaphylactoid shock), cystitis, hypersensitivity reaction

Drug Interactions

Metabolism/Transport Effects None known.

Avoid Concomitant Use

Avoid concomitant use of Hexaminolevulinate with any of the following: BCG

Increased Effect/Toxicity There are no known significant interactions involving an increase in effect.

Decreased Effect

The levels/effects of Hexaminolevulinate may be decreased by: BCG

Storage/Stability Store kit at 20°C to 25°C (68°F to 77°F); excursions are permitted to 15°C to 30°C (59°F to 86°F). The reconstituted solution may be stored under refrigeration at 2°C to 8°C (36°F to 46°F) in the labeled syringe for up to 2 hours.

Reconstitution Reconstitute using 50 mL of the provided diluent to a final concentration of 2 mg/mL (**Note:** Although 50 mL of diluent is withdrawn into the syringe, only 10 mL is subsequently injected into the powder vial to dissolve the powder; upon dissolution, withdraw all of the dissolved solution back into the syringe).

Mechanism of Action Upon intravesical administration, hexaminolevulinate, an ester of aminolevulinic acid and a porphyrin precursor, enters urinary epithelial cells and is used in the formation of photoactive intermediate protoporphyrin IX (PpIX) and other photoactive porphyrins (PAPs). PpIX and PAPs are thought to preferentially accumulate in neoplastic cells. Following photoexcitation with the Karl Storz D-Light Photodynamic Diagnostic (PDD) system, PpIX and PAPs fluoresce and can be used to detect malignant lesions on cystoscopy; fluorescence from tumor tissue appears bright red and demarcated.

Pharmacodynamics/Kinetics

Bioavailability: Intravesical: 7%

Half-life elimination: Biphasic; Terminal: ~76 hours

Dosing

Adult Cystoscopic examination: Intravesical instillation: 50 mL (100 mg) instilled into empty bladder via urinary catheter

Administration Intravesical instillation: Slowly instill solution via intravesical catheter into empty bladder; catheter may be a straight or intermittent urethral catheter with a proximal funnel opening to accommodate a Luer Lock adapter. Catheters may be vinyl (uncoated or coated in hydrogel), latex (amber or red), or silicone; do not use catheters coated or embedded with silver or antibiotics. Indwelling catheters (eg, Foley catheters) may only be used if inserted shortly before and removed following instillation of hexaminolevulinate. Following instillation, instruct the patient to retain the solution for at least 1 hour (maximum: 3 hours); solution should be evacuated immediately prior to the initiation of the cystoscopic procedure (≤30 minutes). If the patient retained the solution for <1 hour, allow 1 hour to pass from the instillation to the initiation of cystoscopic examination. After voiding of the bladder, the perineal skin region should be washed with soap and water and dried.

Dosage Forms Excipient information presented when available (limited, particularly for generics); consult specific product labeling.

Powder for solution, Intravesical, as hydrochloride:

Cysview™: 100 mg [supplied with diluent and adapter]

References

Jocham D, Witjes F, Wagner S, et al, "Improved Detection and Treatment of Bladder Cancer Using Hexaminolevulinate Imaging: A Prospective, Phase III, Multicenter Study," *J Urology*, 2005, 174 (3):862-6.

- **Hexaminolevulinate Hydrochloride** *see* Hexaminolevulinate *on page* 705
- **HHT** *see* Omacetaxine *on page* 1064
- **High-Molecular-Weight Iron Dextran (DexFerrum®)** *see* Iron Dextran Complex *on page* 824
- **Histantil (Can)** *see* Promethazine *on page* 1218

Histrelin (his TREL in)

Related Information

Safe Handling of Hazardous Drugs *on page* 1904

Brand Names: U.S. Supprelin® LA; Vantas®

Brand Names: Canada Vantas®

Index Terms GnRH Agonist; Histrelin Acetate; LH-RH Agonist

Generic Availability (U.S.) No

Pharmacologic Category Gonadotropin Releasing Hormone Agonist

Use Palliative treatment of advanced prostate cancer; treatment of children with central precocious puberty (CPP)

Labeled Contraindications Hypersensitivity to histrelin acetate, GnRH, GnRH-agonist analogs, or any component of the formulation; females who are or may become pregnant

Pregnancy Risk Factor X

Lactation Excretion in breast milk unknown/contraindicated

Warnings/Precautions

CPP: Transient increases in estradiol serum levels (female) or testosterone levels (female and male) may occur during the first week of use. Worsening symptoms may occur, however, manifestations of puberty should decrease within 4 weeks.

Prostate cancer: Transient increases in testosterone serum levels occur during the first week of use (initial tumor flare), which may result in a worsening of disease signs and symptoms such as bone pain, hematuria, neuropathy, ureteral or bladder outlet obstruction, and spinal cord compression. Spinal cord compression may contribute to paralysis; close attention should be given during the first few weeks of therapy to both patients having metastatic vertebral lesions and/or urinary tract obstructions, and to any patients reporting weakness, paresthesias or poor urine output. Androgen-deprivation therapy may increase the risk for cardiovascular disease (Levine, 2010); an increased risk of MI, sudden cardiac death, and stroke has been reported with GNRH agonist use in men; monitor for symptoms associated with cardiovascular disease. Hyperglycemia has been reported with androgen deprivation therapy (in prostate cancer) and may manifest as diabetes or worsening of pre-existing diabetes; monitor blood glucose and/or Hb A_{1c}. Rare cases of pituitary apoplexy (frequently secondary to pituitary adenoma) have been observed with GnRH agonist administration (onset from 1 hour to usually <2 weeks); may present as sudden headache, vomiting, visual or mental status changes, and infrequently cardiovascular collapse; immediate medical attention required. Safety and efficacy have not been established in patients with hepatic dysfunction.

Adverse Reactions

CPP:

>10%: Local: Insertion site reaction (51%; includes bruising, discomfort, itching, pain, protrusion of implant area, soreness, swelling, tingling)

>2% to 10%:

Endocrine & metabolic: Metrorrhagia (4%)

Local: Keloid scar (6%), scar (6%), suture-related complication (6%), pain at the application site (4%), post procedural pain (4%)

≤2%, postmarketing, and/or case reports: Amblyopia, breast tenderness, cold feeling, disease progression, dysmenorrhea, epistaxis, erythema, flu-like syndrome, gynecomastia, headache, infection at the implant site, menorrhagia, migraine, mood swings, pituitary adenoma, pituitary apoplexy, pruritus, seizures, weight gain

Prostate cancer:

>10%:

Endocrine & metabolic: Hot flashes (66%)

Local: Implant site reaction (6% to 14%; includes bruising, erythema, pain, soreness, swelling, tenderness)

2% to 10%:

Central nervous system: Fatigue (10%), headache (3%), insomnia (3%)

Endocrine & metabolic: Gynecomastia (4%), sexual dysfunction (4%), libido decreased (2%)

Gastrointestinal: Constipation (4%), weight gain (2%)

Genitourinary: Expected pharmacological consequence of testosterone suppression: Testicular atrophy (5%)

Renal: Renal impairment (5%)

<2%: Abdominal discomfort, alopecia, anemia, appetite increased, arthralgia, AST increased, back pain, bone density decreased, bone pain, breast pain, breast tenderness, cold feeling, contusion, craving food, creatinine increased, depression, diaphoresis, dizziness, dyspnea (exertional), dysuria, fluid retention, flushing, genital pruritus, hematoma, hematuria, hepatic injury (severe), hypercalcemia, hypercholesterolemia, hyperglycemia, irritability, LDH increased, lethargy, limb pain, liver disorder, malaise, muscle twitching, myalgia, nausea, neck pain, night sweats, pain, palpitation, peripheral edema, prostatic acid phosphatase increased, pruritus, pituitary apoplexy, renal calculi, renal failure, stent occlusion, testosterone increased, tremor, urinary frequency, urinary retention, ventricular asystoles, weakness, weight loss

Drug Interactions

Metabolism/Transport Effects None known.

Avoid Concomitant Use There are no known interactions where it is recommended to avoid concomitant use.

Increased Effect/Toxicity

Histrelin may increase the levels/effects of: Vitamin K Antagonists

Decreased Effect

Histrelin may decrease the levels/effects of: Antidiabetic Agents; Cardiac Glycosides; Vitamin K Antagonists

Storage/Stability Supprelin® LA, Vantas®: Upon delivery, separate contents of implant carton. Store implant under refrigeration at 2°C to 8°C (36°F to 46°F); excursions permitted to 25°C (77°F) for 7 days (if unused within 7 days, may return to proper refrigeration until product expiration date). Keep implant wrapped in the amber pouch for protection from light; do not freeze. The implantation insertion kit does not require refrigeration.

Mechanism of Action Potent inhibitor of gonadotropin secretion; continuous administration results in, after an initiation phase, the suppression of luteinizing hormone (LH), follicle-stimulating hormone (FSH), and a subsequent decrease in testosterone and dihydrotestosterone (males) and estrone and estradiol (premenopausal females). Testosterone levels are reduced to castrate levels in males (treated for prostate cancer) within 2-4 weeks. Additionally, in patients with CPP, linear growth velocity is slowed (improves chance of attaining predicted adult height).

Pharmacodynamics/Kinetics

Onset of action: Prostate cancer: Chemical castration: Within 2-4 weeks; CPP: Progression of sexual development stops and growth is decreased within 1 month

Duration: 1 year

Distribution: Adults: V_d: ~58 L

Protein binding: Adults: 70% ± 9%

Metabolism: Hepatic via C-terminal dealkylation and hydrolysis

Bioavailability: Adults: 92%

Half-life elimination: Adults: Terminal: ~4 hours

Time to peak, serum: Adults: 12 hours

Dosing

Adult & Geriatric Prostate cancer, advanced: SubQ (Vantas®): 50 mg implant surgically inserted every 12 months

Pediatric CPP: SubQ (Supprelin® LA): Children ≥2 years: 50 mg implant surgically inserted every 12 months. Discontinue at the appropriate time for the onset of puberty.

Renal Impairment Cl_{cr}: 15-60 mL/minute: Adjustment not needed.

Administration SubQ: Surgical implantation (using a sterile field) into the inner portion of the upper arm requires the use of the implantation device provided. Use the patient's nondominant arm for placement; implant should be placed halfway between the shoulder and the elbow at the crease between the tricep and the bicep. Implant removal should occur after ~12 months; a replacement implant may be inserted if therapy is to be continued. Palpate area of incision to locate implant for removal. If not readily palpated, ultrasound, CT or MRI may be used to locate implant; plain films are not recommended because the implant is not radiopaque.

Monitoring Parameters

CPP: LH, FSH, estradiol, or testosterone (after 1 month then every 6 months); height, bone age (every 6-12 months); tanner staging

Prostate cancer: Serum testosterone levels, prostate specific antigen (PSA); bone mineral density; weakness, paresthesias, and urinary tract obstruction (especially during first few weeks of therapy); screen for diabetes; monitor for symptoms associated with cardiovascular disease

Test Interactions Results of diagnostic test of pituitary gonadotropic and gonadal functions may be affected during and after therapy

Dosage Forms Excipient information presented when available (limited, particularly for generics); consult specific product labeling. [DSC] = Discontinued product

Implant, subcutaneous:

Supprelin® LA: 50 mg (1s) [releases ~65 mcg/day over 12 months]

Vantas®: 50 mg (1s) [Releases ~50 mcg/day over 12 months; packaged with implantation kit]

Vantas®: 50 mg (1s [DSC]) [releases 50-60 mcg/day over 12 months]

References

Dineen MK, Tierney DS, Kuzma P, et al, "An Evaluation of the Pharmacokinetics and Pharmacodynamics of the Histrelin Implant for the Palliative Treatment of Prostate Cancer," *J Clin Pharmacol*, 2005, 45(11):1245-9.

Levine GN, D'Amico AV, Berger P, et al, "Androgen-Deprivation Therapy in Prostate Cancer and Cardiovascular Risk. A Science Advisory from the American Heart Association, American Cancer Society, and American Urological Association," *Circulation*, 2010, 121:831-38.

Schlegel PN, Histrelin Study Group, "Efficacy and Safety of Histrelin Subdermal Implant in Patients With Advanced Prostate Cancer," *J Urol*, 2006, 175(4):1353-8.

◆ **Histrelin Acetate** *see* Histrelin *on page 707*

◆ **Hizentra®** *see* Immune Globulin *on page 777*

◆ **HMM** *see* Altretamine *on page 63*

◆ **HN_2** *see* Mechlorethamine *on page 913*

◆ **Homoharringtonine** *see* Omacetaxine *on page 1064*

◆ **Horse Antihuman Thymocyte Gamma Globulin** *see* Antithymocyte Globulin (Equine) *on page 111*

◆ **hpAT** *see* Antithrombin *on page 107*

◆ **HPV2** *see* Papillomavirus (Types 16, 18) Vaccine (Human, Recombinant) *on page 1124*

◆ **HPV4** *see* Papillomavirus (Types 6, 11, 16, 18) Vaccine (Human, Recombinant) *on page 1120*

◆ **HPV 16/18 L1 VLP/AS04 VAC** *see* Papillomavirus (Types 16, 18) Vaccine (Human, Recombinant) *on page 1124*

◆ **HPV Vaccine** *see* Papillomavirus (Types 6, 11, 16, 18) Vaccine (Human, Recombinant) *on page 1120*

- ◆ **HPV Vaccine** *see* Papillomavirus (Types 16, 18) Vaccine (Human, Recombinant) *on page* 1124
- ◆ **Humanized IgG1 Anti-CD52 Monoclonal Antibody** *see* Alemtuzumab *on page* 43
- ◆ **Human Papillomavirus Vaccine** *see* Papillomavirus (Types 6, 11, 16, 18) Vaccine (Human, Recombinant) *on page* 1120
- ◆ **Human Papillomavirus Vaccine** *see* Papillomavirus (Types 16, 18) Vaccine (Human, Recombinant) *on page* 1124
- ◆ **Human Thyroid Stimulating Hormone** *see* Thyrotropin Alfa *on page* 1360
- ◆ **HuMax-CD20** *see* Ofatumumab *on page* 1050
- ◆ **HXM** *see* Altretamine *on page* 63

Hyaluronidase (hye al yoor ON i dase)

Related Information

Management of Drug Extravasations *on page* 1800

Brand Names: U.S. Amphadase™; Hylenex; Vitrase®

Generic Availability (U.S.) No

Pharmacologic Category Enzyme

Use Increase the dispersion and absorption of other injected drugs; increase rate of absorption of parenteral fluids given by subcutaneous administration (hypodermoclysis)

Unlabeled Use Management of drug extravasations; local anesthetic adjuvant in bupivacaine-lidocaine mixture for retrobulbar/peribulbar block

Labeled Contraindications Hypersensitivity to hyaluronidase or any component of the formulation

Pregnancy Risk Factor C

Lactation Excretion in breast milk unknown/use caution

Warnings/Precautions Do not inject in or around infected or inflamed areas; may spread localized infection. Should not be used for extravasation management of dopamine or alpha agonists, or to reduce swelling of bites or stings. Do not administer intravenously. Do not apply directly to the cornea. Discontinue if sensitization occurs.

Adverse Reactions

Frequency not defined:

Cardiovascular: Edema

Local: Injection site reactions

<1%: Allergic reactions, anaphylactic-like reactions (retrobulbar block or I.V. injections), angioedema, urticaria

Drug Interactions

Metabolism/Transport Effects None known.

Avoid Concomitant Use

Avoid concomitant use of Hyaluronidase with any of the following: Alpha-/Beta-Agonists; DOPamine; Phenylephrine (Systemic)

Increased Effect/Toxicity

Hyaluronidase may increase the levels/effects of: Alpha-/Beta-Agonists; DOPamine; Local Anesthetics; Phenylephrine (Systemic)

Decreased Effect

The levels/effects of Hyaluronidase may be decreased by: Antihistamines; Corticosteroids; Estrogen Derivatives; Salicylates

Storage/Stability

Amphadase™, Hylenex: Store unopened vials in refrigerator at 2°C to 8°C (36°F to 46°F); do not freeze.

Vitrase®: Store unopened vial in refrigerator at 2°C to 8°C (36°F to 46°F); do not freeze. Protect from light. If adding to other injectable solutions, store admixture at 15°C to 25°C (59°F to 77°F) and use within 6 hours.

Mechanism of Action Modifies the permeability of connective tissue through hydrolysis of hyaluronic acid, one of the chief components of tissue cement which offers resistance to diffusion of liquids through tissues; hyaluronidase increases both the distribution and absorption of locally injected substances.

Pharmacodynamics/Kinetics

Onset of action: SubQ: Immediate

Duration: 24-48 hours

Dosing

Adult & Geriatric

Skin test: Intradermal: 0.02 mL (3 units) of a 150 units/mL solution. Positive reaction consists of a wheal with pseudopods appearing within 5 minutes and persisting for 20-30 minutes with localized itching.

Dehydration: Hypodermoclysis: SubQ: Add 15 units to each 100 mL of replacement fluid to be administered **or** 150 units followed by subcutaneous isotonic fluid administration ≥1000 mL; rate and volume of a single clysis should not exceed those used for infusion of I.V. fluids

Extravasation (unlabeled use): SubQ: Inject 1 mL of a 150 unit/mL solution (as 5-10 injections of 0.1-0.2 mL) into affected area; doses of 15-250 units have been reported. **Note:** Do not use for extravasation of pressor agents (eg, dopamine, norepinephrine).

Pediatric

Skin test: Intradermal: 0.02 mL (3 units) of a 150 units/mL solution. Positive reaction consists of a wheal with pseudopods appearing within 5 minutes and persisting for 20-30 minutes with localized itching.

Dehydration: Hypodermoclysis: SubQ: Add 15 units to each 100 mL of replacement fluid to be administered **or** 150 units followed by subcutaneous isotonic fluid administration ≥1000 mL

Premature Infants: Volume of a single clysis/day should not exceed 25 mL/kg and the rate of administration should not exceed 2 mL/minute

Children <3 years: Volume of a single clysis should not exceed 200 mL

Children ≥3 years: Refer to adult dosing.

Subcutaneous urography: Infants and children: SubQ: 75 units over each scapula followed by injection of contrast medium at the same site; patient should be in the prone position during drug administration

Administration Do **not** administer I.V.

Additional Information

Amphadase™: pH: 6.8

Hylenex: pH: 7.4, osmolality: 290-350 mOsm

Vitrase® pH: ~6.7

Dosage Forms Excipient information presented when available (limited, particularly for generics); consult specific product labeling. [DSC] = Discontinued product

Injection, solution [preservative free]:

Hylenex: 150 units/mL (1 mL) [contains albumin (human), edetate disodium; derived from or manufactured using Chinese hamster ovary cells; recombinant]

Hylenex: 150 units/mL (1 mL [DSC]) [contains albumin (human), edetate disodium; recombinant]

Injection, solution [bovine derived]:

Amphadase™: 150 units/mL (1 mL) [contains edetate disodium, thimerosal]

Injection, solution [ovine derived, preservative free]:

Vitrase®: 200 units/mL (1.2 mL) [contains lactose 0.93 mg/mL]

References

Albanell J and Baselga J, "Systemic Therapy Emergencies," *Semin Oncol*, 2000, 27(3):347-61.

Bertelli G, "Prevention and Management of Extravasation of Cytotoxic Drugs," *Drug Saf*, 1995, 12(4):245-55.

Bertelli G, Dini D, Forno GB, et al, "Hyaluronidase as an Antidote to Extravasation of Vinca Alkaloids: Clinical Results," *J Cancer Res Clin Oncol*, 1994, 120(8):505-6.

Cochran ST, Bomyea K, and Kahn M, "Treatment of Iodinated Contrast Material Extravasation With Hyaluronidase," *Acad Radiol*, 2002, 9(Suppl 2):544-6.

Dorr RT, "Vinca Alkaloid Ulceration: Experimental Mouse Model and Effects of Local Antidotes," *Proc Am Soc Clin Oncol*, 1982, 1:428.

Elam EA, Dorr RT, Lagel KE, et al, "Cutaneous Ulceration Due to Contrast Extravasation. Experimental Assessment of Injury and Potential Antidotes," *Invest Radiol*, 1991, 26(1):13-6.

Kallio H, Paloheimo M, and Maunuksela EL, "Hyaluronidase as an Adjuvant in Bupivacaine-Lidocaine Mixture for Retrobulbar/Peribulbar Block," *Anesth Analg*, 2000, 91(4):934-7.

Kumar MM and Sprung J, "The Use of Hyaluronidase to Treat Mannitol Extravasation," *Anesth Analg*, 2003, 97(4):1199-200.

Raszka WV Jr, Kueser TK, Smith FR, et al, "The Use of Hyaluronidase in the Treatment of Intravenous Extravasation Injuries," *J Perinatol*, 19909, 10(2):146-9.

Zenk KE, "Hyaluronidase: An Antidote for Intravenous Extravasations," *CSHP Voice*, 1981, 66-8.

Zenk KE, "Management of Intravenous Extravasations," *Infusion*, 1981, 5:77-9.

Zenk KE, "Treating I.V. Extravasations With Hyaluronidase," *ASHP Signal*, 1986, 10:25,29.

◆ **Hycamptamine** *see* Topotecan *on page 1371*

◆ **Hycamtin®** *see* Topotecan *on page 1371*

◆ **Hycort™ (Can)** *see* Hydrocortisone (Topical) *on page 719*

◆ **Hydeltra T.B.A.® (Can)** *see* PrednisoLONE (Systemic) *on page 1193*

◆ **Hyderm (Can)** *see* Hydrocortisone (Topical) *on page 719*

◆ **Hydrea®** *see* Hydroxyurea *on page 731*

Hydrocortisone (Systemic) (hye droe KOR ti sone)

Related Information

Oral Mucositis/Stomatitis *on page 1814*

Brand Names: U.S. A-Hydrocort®; Cortef®; Solu-CORTEF®

Brand Names: Canada Cortef®; Solu-Cortef®

Index Terms A-hydroCort; Compound F; Cortisol; Hydrocortisone Sodium Succinate

Generic Availability (U.S.) Yes: Tablet

Pharmacologic Category Corticosteroid, Systemic

Use Management of adrenocortical insufficiency; anti-inflammatory or immunosuppressive

Unlabeled Use Management of septic shock when blood pressure is poorly responsive to fluid resuscitation and vasopressor therapy; treatment of thyroid storm

Labeled Contraindications Hypersensitivity to hydrocortisone or any component of the formulation; serious infections, except septic shock or tuberculous meningitis; viral, fungal, or tubercular skin lesions; I.M. administration contraindicated in idiopathic thrombocytopenia purpura; intrathecal administration of injection

Pregnancy Risk Factor C

Lactation Enters breast milk/use caution

Warnings/Precautions Use with caution in patients with thyroid disease, hepatic impairment, renal impairment, heart failure, hypertension, diabetes, glaucoma, cataracts, myasthenia gravis, patients at risk for osteoporosis, patients at risk for seizures, or GI diseases (diverticulitis, peptic ulcer, ulcerative colitis) due to perforation risk. Use caution following acute MI (corticosteroids have been associated with myocardial rupture). Because of the risk of adverse effects, systemic corticosteroids should be used cautiously in the elderly in the smallest possible effective dose for the shortest duration. May affect growth velocity; growth should be routinely monitored in pediatric patients. Withdraw therapy with gradual tapering of dose.

May cause hypercorticism or suppression of hypothalamic-pituitary-adrenal (HPA) axis, particularly in younger children or in patients receiving high doses for prolonged periods. HPA axis suppression may lead to adrenal crisis. Withdrawal and discontinuation of a corticosteroid should be done slowly and carefully. Particular care is required when patients are transferred from systemic corticosteroids to inhaled products due to possible adrenal insufficiency or withdrawal from steroids, including an increase in allergic symptoms. Patients receiving >20 mg per day of prednisone (or equivalent) may be most susceptible. Fatalities have occurred due to adrenal insufficiency in asthmatic patients during and after transfer from systemic corticosteroids to aerosol steroids; aerosol steroids do not provide the systemic steroid needed to treat patients having trauma, surgery, or infections.

Acute myopathy has been reported with high dose corticosteroids, usually in patients with neuromuscular transmission disorders; may involve ocular and/or respiratory muscles; monitor creatine kinase; recovery may be delayed. Corticosteroid use may cause psychiatric disturbances, including depression, euphoria, insomnia, mood swings, and personality changes. Pre-existing psychiatric conditions may be exacerbated by corticosteroid use. Prolonged use of corticosteroids may also increase the incidence of secondary infection, mask acute infection (including fungal infections), prolong or exacerbate viral infections, or limit response to vaccines. Exposure to chickenpox should be avoided; corticosteroids should not be used to treat ocular herpes simplex. Corticosteroids should not be used for cerebral malaria or viral hepatitis. Oral steroid treatment is not recommended for the treatment of acute optic neuritis. Close observation is required in patients with latent tuberculosis and/or TB reactivity; restrict use in active TB (only in conjunction with antituberculosis treatment). Prolonged treatment with corticosteroids has been associated with the development of Kaposi's sarcoma (case reports); if noted, discontinuation of therapy should be considered. High-dose corticosteroids should not be used to manage acute head injury. Some dosage forms contain benzyl alcohol which has been associated with "gasping syndrome" in neonates.

Adverse Reactions Frequency not defined.

Cardiovascular: Arrhythmias, bradycardia, cardiac arrest, cardiomegaly, circulatory collapse, congestive heart failure, edema, fat embolism, hypertension, hypertrophic cardiomyopathy (premature infants), myocardial rupture (post MI), syncope, tachycardia, thromboembolism, vasculitis

Central nervous system: Delirium, depression, emotional instability, euphoria, hallucinations, headache, insomnia, intracranial pressure increased, malaise, mood swings, nervousness, neuritis, neuropathy, personality changes, pseudotumor cerebri, psychic disorders, psychoses, seizure, vertigo

Dermatologic: Acne, allergic dermatitis, alopecia, bruising, burning/tingling, dry scaly skin, edema, erythema, hirsutism, hyper-/hypopigmentation, impaired wound healing, petechiae, rash, skin atrophy, skin test reaction impaired, sterile abscess, striae, urticaria

Endocrine & metabolic: Adrenal suppression, alkalosis, amenorrhea, carbohydrate intolerance increased, Cushing's syndrome, diabetes mellitus, glucose intolerance, growth suppression, hyperglycemia, hyperlipidemia, hypokalemia, hypokalemic alkalosis, menstrual irregularities, negative nitrogen balance, pituitary-adrenal axis suppression, potassium loss, protein catabolism, sodium and water retention, sperm motility increased/decreased, spermatogenesis increased/decreased

Gastrointestinal: Abdominal distention, appetite increased, bowel dysfunction (intrathecal administration), indigestion, nausea, pancreatitis, peptic ulcer, gastrointestinal perforation, ulcerative esophagitis, vomiting, weight gain

Genitourinary: Bladder dysfunction (intrathecal administration)

Hematologic: Leukocytosis (transient)

Hepatic: Hepatomegaly, transaminases increased

Local: Atrophy (at injection site), postinjection flare (intra-articular use), thrombophlebitis

Neuromuscular & skeletal: Arthralgia, necrosis (femoral and humoral heads), Charcot-like arthropathy, fractures, muscle mass loss, muscle weakness, myopathy, osteoporosis, tendon rupture, vertebral compression fractures

Ocular: Cataracts, exophthalmoses, glaucoma, intraocular pressure increased

Miscellaneous: Abnormal fat deposits, anaphylaxis, avascular necrosis, diaphoresis, hiccups, hypersensitivity reactions, infection, secondary malignancy

Drug Interactions

Metabolism/Transport Effects Substrate of CYP3A4 (minor), P-glycoprotein; **Note:** Assignment of Major/Minor substrate status based on clinically relevant drug interaction potential; **Induces** CYP3A4 (weak/moderate)

Avoid Concomitant Use

Avoid concomitant use of Hydrocortisone (Systemic) with any of the following: Aldesleukin; Axitinib; BCG; Mifepristone; Natalizumab; Pimecrolimus; Tacrolimus (Topical)

Increased Effect/Toxicity

Hydrocortisone (Systemic) may increase the levels/effects of: Acetylcholinesterase Inhibitors; Amphotericin B; Deferasirox; Leflunomide; Loop Diuretics; Natalizumab; NSAID (COX-2 Inhibitor); NSAID (Nonselective); Thiazide Diuretics; Vaccines (Live); Warfarin

The levels/effects of Hydrocortisone (Systemic) may be increased by: Antifungal Agents (Azole Derivatives, Systemic); Aprepitant; Calcium Channel Blockers (Nondihydropyridine), Denosumab; Estrogen Derivatives; Fluconazole; Fosaprepitant; Indacaterol; Macrolide Antibiotics; Mifepristone; Neuromuscular-Blocking Agents (Nondepolarizing); P-glycoprotein/ABCB1 Inhibitors; Pimecrolimus; Quinolone Antibiotics; Roflumilast; Salicylates; Tacrolimus (Topical); Telaprevir; Trastuzumab

Decreased Effect

Hydrocortisone (Systemic) may decrease the levels/effects of: Aldesleukin; Antidiabetic Agents; ARIPiprazole; Axitinib; BCG; Calcitriol; Coccidioidin Skin Test; Corticorelin; Hyaluronidase; Isoniazid; Salicylates; Sipuleucel-T; Telaprevir; Vaccines (Inactivated)

The levels/effects of Hydrocortisone (Systemic) may be decreased by: Aminoglutethimide; Antacids; Barbiturates; Bile Acid Sequestrants; Echinacea; Mifepristone; Mitotane; P-glycoprotein/ABCB1 Inducers; Primidone; Rifamycin Derivatives; Tocilizumab

Ethanol/Nutrition/Herb Interactions

Ethanol: Avoid ethanol (may enhance gastric mucosal irritation).

Food: Hydrocortisone interferes with calcium absorption.

Herb/Nutraceutical: St John's wort may decrease hydrocortisone levels. Avoid cat's claw, echinacea (have immunostimulant properties).

Storage/Stability Store at controlled room temperature 20°C to 25°C (68°F to 77°F). Protect from light. Hydrocortisone sodium phosphate and hydrocortisone sodium succinate are clear, light yellow solutions which are heat labile.

Sodium succinate: After initial reconstitution, hydrocortisone sodium succinate solutions are stable for 3 days at room temperature or under refrigeration when protected from light. Stability of parenteral admixture (Solu-Cortef®) at room temperature (25°C) and at refrigeration temperature (4°C) is concentration-dependent:

Stability of concentration 1 mg/mL: 24 hours.

Stability of concentration 2 mg/mL to 60 mg/mL: At least 4 hours.

Reconstitution

Sodium succinate: Reconstitute 100 mg vials with bacteriostatic water (not >2 mL). Act-O-Vial (self-contained powder for injection plus diluent) may be reconstituted by pressing the activator to force diluent into the powder compartment. Following gentle agitation, solution may be withdrawn via syringe through a needle inserted into the center of the stopper. May be administered (I.V. or I.M.) without further dilution.

Solutions for I.V. infusion: Reconstituted solutions may be added to an appropriate volume of compatible solution for infusion. Concentration should generally not exceed 1 mg/mL. However, in cases where administration of a small volume of fluid is desirable, 100-3000 mg may be added to 50 mL of D_5W or NS (stability limited to 4 hours).

Mechanism of Action Decreases inflammation by suppression of migration of polymorphonuclear leukocytes and reversal of increased capillary permeability

Pharmacodynamics/Kinetics

Onset of action: Hydrocortisone sodium succinate (water soluble): Rapid

Absorption: Rapid

Metabolism: Hepatic

Half-life elimination: Biologic: 8-12 hours

Excretion: Urine (primarily as 17-hydroxysteroids and 17-ketosteroids)

Dosing

Adult & Geriatric Dose should be based on severity of disease and patient response.

Adrenal insufficiency (acute): I.M., I.V.: 100 mg I.V. bolus, then 300 mg/day in divided doses every 8 hours or as a continuous infusion for 48 hours. Once patient is stable change to oral, 50 mg every 8 hours for 6 doses, then taper to 30-50 mg/day in divided doses.

Adrenal insufficiency (chronic), physiologic replacement (unlabeled dosing): Oral: 15-25 mg/day in 2-3 divided doses. **Note:** Studies suggest administering one-half to two-thirds of the daily dose in the morning in order to mimic the physiological cortisol secretion pattern. If the twice-daily regimen is utilized, the second dose should be administered 6-8 hours following the first dose (Arlt, 2003).

Anti-inflammatory or immunosuppressive: Oral, I.M., I.V.: 15-240 mg every 12 hours

Congenital adrenal hyperplasia (unlabeled dosing): Oral: 15-25 mg/day in 2-3 divided doses (Speiser, 2010)

Status asthmaticus: I.V.: 1-2 mg/kg/dose every 6 hours for 24 hours, then maintenance of 0.5-1 mg/kg every 6 hours

Stress dosing (surgery) in patients known to be adrenally-suppressed or on chronic systemic steroids: I.V.:

Minor stress (ie, inguinal herniorrhaphy): 25 mg/day for 1 day

Moderate stress (ie, joint replacement, cholecystectomy): 50-75 mg/day (25 mg every 8-12 hours) for 1-2 days

Major stress (pancreatoduodenectomy, esophagogastrectomy, cardiac surgery): 100-150 mg/day (50 mg every 8-12 hours) for 2-3 days

Septic shock (unlabeled use): I.V.: 50 mg every 6 hours (Annane, 2002; Marik, 2008); not to exceed 300 mg/day (Dellinger, 2008). Practice guidelines also recommend alternative dosing of 100 mg bolus, followed by continuous infusion of 10 mg/hour (240 mg/day). Taper slowly (for total of 11 days) and do not stop abruptly. **Note:** Fludrocortisone is optional with use of hydrocortisone.

Thyroid storm (unlabeled use): I.V.: 300 mg loading dose, followed by 100 mg every 8 hours (Bahn, 2011)

Pediatric Dose should be based on severity of disease and patient response.

Anti-inflammatory or immunosuppressive:

Infants and Children:

Oral: 2.5-10 mg/kg/day **or** 75-300 mg/m²/day every 6-8 hours

I.M., I.V.: 1-5 mg/kg/day **or** 30-150 mg/m²/day divided every 12-24 hours

Adolescents: Oral, I.M., I.V.: 15-240 mg every 12 hours

Congenital adrenal hyperplasia (unlabeled dosing): Oral: **Note:** Doses must be individualized by monitoring growth, bone age, and hormonal levels.

Children: 10-15 mg/m²/day in 3 divided doses; higher initial doses may be required to achieve initial target hormone serum concentrations in infancy (Speiser, 2010)

Adolescents: Refer to adult dosing.

Physiologic replacement: Children: Oral: 8-10 mg/m²/day divided every 8 hours; up to 12 mg/m²/day in some patients (Ahmet, 2011; Gupta, 2008; Maguire, 2007)

Status asthmaticus: Children: I.V.: 1-2 mg/kg/dose every 6 hours for 24 hours, then maintenance of 0.5-1 mg/kg every 6 hours.

Septic shock (unlabeled use): Children: I.V.: Initial: 1-2 mg/kg/day (intermittent or as continuous infusion); may titrate up to 50 mg/kg/day for shock reversal (Brierley, 2009); alternative dosing suggests 50 mg/m²/day (Dellinger, 2008). **Note:** Use recommended only in catecholamine-resistant shock and suspected or proven adrenal insufficiency.

Combination Regimens

Lymphoma, non-Hodgkin's: CODOX-M on page 1590

Lymphoma, non-Hodgkin's (Burkitt): CODOX-M/IVAC on page 1591

Prostate cancer:

Estramustine + Docetaxel + Hydrocortisone on page 1636

Mitoxantrone + Hydrocortisone on page 1713

Administration

Oral: Administer with food or milk to decrease GI upset

Parenteral: Hydrocortisone sodium succinate may be administered by I.M. or I.V. routes. Dermal and/or subdermal skin depression may occur at the site of injection. Avoid injection into deltoid muscle (high incidence of subcutaneous atrophy).

I.V. bolus: Dilute to 50 mg/mL and administer over 30 seconds or over 10 minutes for doses ≥500 mg

I.V. intermittent infusion: Dilute to 1 mg/mL and administer over 20-30 minutes

Extemporaneous Preparations A 2.5 mg/mL oral suspension may be made with either tablets or powder and a vehicle containing sodium carboxymethylcellulose (1 g), syrup BP (10 mL), hydroxybenzoate 0.1% preservatives (0.1 g), polysorbate 80 (0.5 mL), citric acid (0.6 g), and water. To make the vehicle, dissolve the hydroxybenzoate, citric acid, and syrup BP in hot water. Cool solution and add the carboxymethylcellulose; leave overnight. Crush twelve-and-one-half 20 mg hydrocortisone tablets (or use 250 mg of powder) in a mortar and reduce to a fine powder while adding polysorbate 80. Add small portions of vehicle and mix to a uniform paste; mix while adding the vehicle in incremental proportions to **almost** 100 mL; transfer to a calibrated bottle, rinse mortar with vehicle, and add sufficient quantity of vehicle to make 100 mL. Label "shake well" and "refrigerate". Stable for 90 days.

Fawcett JP, Boulton DW, Jiang R, et al, "Stability of Hydrocortisone Oral Suspensions Prepared From Tablets and Powder," *Ann Pharmacother*, 1995, 29(10):987-90.

Monitoring Parameters Serum glucose, electrolytes; blood pressure, weight, presence of infection; monitor IOP with therapy >6 weeks; bone mineral density, growth in children

Test Interactions Interferes with skin tests

Dietary Considerations Systemic use of corticosteroids may require a diet with increased potassium, vitamins A, B_6, C, D, folate, calcium, zinc, phosphorus, and decreased sodium. Some products may contain sodium.

Dosage Forms Excipient information presented when available (limited, particularly for generics); consult specific product labeling.

Injection, powder for reconstitution, as sodium succinate [strength expressed as base]:

A-Hydrocort®: 100 mg

Solu-CORTEF®: 100 mg

Injection, powder for reconstitution, as sodium succinate [strength expressed as base, preservative free]:

Solu-CORTEF®: 100 mg, 250 mg, 500 mg, 1000 mg [supplied with diluent]

Tablet, oral, as base: 5 mg, 10 mg, 20 mg

Cortef®: 5 mg, 10 mg, 20 mg [scored]

References

Ahmet A, Kim H, and Spier S, "Adrenal Suppression: A Practical Guide to the Screening and Management of this Under-Recognized Complication of Inhaled Corticosteroid Therapy," *Allergy Asthma Clin Immunol*, 2011, 7:13.

Arlt W and Allolio B, "Adrenal Insufficiency," *Lancet*, 2003, 361(9372):1881-93.

Bahn RS (Chair), Burch HB, Cooper DS, et al, "Hyperthyroidism and Other Causes of Thyrotoxicosis: Management Guidelines of the American Thyroid Association and American Association of Clinical Endocrinologists," *Thyroid*, 2011, 21(6):593-646.

Dellinger RP, Levy MM, Carlet JM, et al, "Surviving Sepsis Campaign: International Guidelines for Management of Severe Sepsis and Septic Shock: 2008," [published correction appears in *Crit Care Med*, 2008, 36(4):1394-6], *Crit Care Med*, 2008, 36(1):296-327.

Goedert JJ, Vitale F, Lauria C, et al, "Risk Factors for Classical Kaposi's Sarcoma," *J Natl Cancer Inst*, 2002, 94(22):1712-8.

Gupta P and Bhatia V, "Corticosteroid Physiology and Principles of Therapy," *Indian J Pediatr*, 2008, 75(10):1039-44.
Kornbluth A and Sachar DB, "Ulcerative Colitis Practice Guidelines in Adults: American College of Gastroenterology, Practice Parameters Committee," *Am J Gastroenterol*, 2010, 105(3):501-23.
Maguire AM, Ambler GR, Moore B, et al, "Prolonged Hypocortisolemia in Hydrocortisone Replacement Regimens in Adrenocorticotrophic Hormone Deficiency," *Pediatrics*, 2007, 120(1):e164-71.

Hydrocortisone (Topical) (hye droe KOR ti sone)

Brand Names: U.S. Ala-Cort; Ala-Scalp; Anu-med HC; Anucort-HC™; Anucol HC®; Aquanil HC® [OTC]; Beta-HC® [OTC]; Caldecort® [OTC]; Colocort®; Cortaid® Advanced [OTC]; Cortaid® Intensive Therapy [OTC]; Cortaid® Maximum Strength [OTC]; Cortenema®; CortiCool® [OTC]; Cortifoam®; Cortizone-10® Hydratensive Healing [OTC]; Cortizone-10® Hydratensive Soothing [OTC]; Cortizone-10® Intensive Healing Eczema [OTC]; Cortizone-10® Maximum Strength Cooling Relief [OTC]; Cortizone-10® Maximum Strength Easy Relief [OTC]; Cortizone-10® Maximum Strength Intensive Healing Formula [OTC]; Cortizone-10® Maximum Strength [OTC]; Cortizone-10® Plus Maximum Strength [OTC]; Dermarest® Eczema Medicated [OTC]; Hemril® -30; Hydrocortisone Plus [OTC]; HydroSKIN® [OTC]; Locoid Lipocream®; Locoid®; Pandel®; Pediaderm™ HC; Preparation H® Hydrocortisone [OTC]; Procto-Pak™; Proctocort®; ProctoCream®-HC; Proctosol-HC®; Proctozone-HC 2.5%™; Recort [OTC]; Scalpana [OTC]; Texacort™; U-Cort®; Westcort®

Brand Names: Canada Aquacort®; Cortamed®; Cortenema®; Cortifoam™; Emo-Cort®; Hycort™; Hyderm; HydroVal®; Locoid®; Prevex® HC; Sarna® HC; Westcort®

Index Terms A-hydroCort; Compound F; Cortisol; Hemorrhoidal HC; Hydrocortisone Acetate; Hydrocortisone Butyrate; Hydrocortisone Probutate; Hydrocortisone Valerate; Nutracort

Generic Availability (U.S.) Yes: Excludes foam (acetate), cream (probutate), gel (base), liquid (base), lotion (base), lotion (butyrate), solution (base)

Pharmacologic Category Corticosteroid, Rectal; Corticosteroid, Topical

Use Relief of inflammation of corticosteroid-responsive dermatoses (low and medium potency topical corticosteroid); adjunctive treatment of ulcerative colitis; mild-to-moderate atopic dermatitis; inflamed hemorrhoids, postirradiation (factitial) proctitis, and other inflammatory conditions of anorectum and pruritus ani

Labeled Contraindications Hypersensitivity to any component of the formulation.

Rectal enema: Systemic fungal infections; ileocolostomy during the immediate or early postoperative period

Cortifoam® is also contraindicated with obstruction, abscess, perforation, peritonitis, fresh intestinal anastomoses, extensive fistulas and sinus tracts (other enemas are labeled to be used with caution).

Pregnancy Risk Factor C

Lactation Enters breast milk/use caution

Warnings/Precautions May cause hypercorticism or suppression of hypothalamic-pituitary-adrenal (HPA) axis, particularly in younger children or in patients receiving high doses for prolonged periods. HPA axis suppression may lead to adrenal crisis. Withdrawal and discontinuation of a corticosteroid should be done slowly and carefully. Children may absorb proportionally larger amounts after topical application and may be more prone to systemic effects. HPA axis suppression, intracranial hypertension, and Cushing's syndrome have been reported in children receiving topical corticosteroids. Prolonged use may affect growth velocity; growth should be routinely monitored in pediatric patients. Rare cases of anaphylactoid reactions have been observed in patients receiving corticosteroids.

Prolonged use of corticosteroids may increase the incidence of secondary infection, mask acute infection (including fungal infections), prolong or exacerbate viral infections, or limit response to vaccines. Exposure to chickenpox should be avoided. Close observation is required in patients with latent tuberculosis and/or TB reactivity; restrict use in active TB (only in conjunction with antituberculosis treatment). Prolonged treatment with corticosteroids has been also associated with the development of Kaposi's sarcoma (case reports); if noted, discontinuation of therapy should be considered. Prolonged use of corticosteroids may produce cataracts or glaucoma and may enhance the establishment of secondary ocular infections Use caution with ocular herpes simplex.

Acute myopathy has been reported with high-dose corticosteroids, usually in patients with neuromuscular transmission disorders; may involve ocular and/or respiratory muscles; monitor creatine kinase; recovery may be delayed. Corticosteroid use may cause psychiatric disturbances, including depression, euphoria, insomnia, mood swings, and personality changes. Pre-existing psychiatric conditions may be exacerbated by corticosteroid use.

Use with caution in patients with hypertension, GI diseases (diverticulitis, peptic ulcer), hepatic impairment (including cirrhosis), osteoporosis, myasthenia gravis, osteoporosis, renal impairment, or thyroid disease. In patients with severe ulcerative colitis, it may be hazardous to delay surgery while waiting for response to treatment.

Topical corticosteroids may be absorbed percutaneously. Absorption is increased by the use of occlusive dressings, application to denuded skin, or application to large surface areas. Avoid use of topical preparations with occlusive dressings or on weeping or exudative lesions. Topical use has been associated with local sensitization (redness, irritation); discontinue if sensitization is noted. Because of the risk of adverse effects associated with systemic absorption, topical corticosteroids should be used cautiously in the elderly in the smallest possible effective dose for the shortest duration.

Rectal enema: Damage to the rectal wall may occur from improper or careless insertion of the enema tip.

Self-medication (OTC use): Contact healthcare provider if condition worsens, symptoms persist for >7 days, or rectal bleeding occurs. Consult with healthcare provider prior to use if needed for diaper rash.

Adverse Reactions Frequency not defined. Local adverse events presented. Adverse events similar to those observed with systemic absorption are also observed, especially following rectal use. Refer to the Hydrocortisone (Systemic) monograph for details.

Cream, ointment: Acneiform eruptions, burning, dryness, folliculitis, hypertrichosis, hypopigmentation, irritation, itching, maceration of skin, miliaria, perioral dermatitis, secondary infection, skin atrophy, striae

Enema: Burning, pain, rectal bleeding

Suppositories: Allergic contact dermatitis, burning, dryness, folliculitis, hypopigmentation, itching, secondary infection

Drug Interactions

Metabolism/Transport Effects **Substrate** of CYP3A4 (minor); **Note:** Assignment of Major/Minor substrate status based on clinically relevant drug interaction potential

Avoid Concomitant Use

Avoid concomitant use of Hydrocortisone (Topical) with any of the following: Aldesleukin

Increased Effect/Toxicity

Hydrocortisone (Topical) may increase the levels/effects of: Deferasirox

The levels/effects of Hydrocortisone (Topical) may be increased by: Telaprevir

Decreased Effect

Hydrocortisone (Topical) may decrease the levels/effects of: Aldesleukin; Corticorelin; Hyaluronidase; Telaprevir

The levels/effects of Hydrocortisone (Topical) may be decreased by: Tocilizumab

Storage/Stability Store at controlled room temperature.

Mechanism of Action Decreases inflammation by suppression of migration of polymorphonuclear leukocytes and reversal of increased capillary permeability

Pharmacodynamics/Kinetics Absorption: Topical corticosteroids are absorbed percutaneously. The extent is dependent on several factors, including epidermal integrity (intact vs abraded skin), formulation, and the use of occlusive dressings. Rectal absorption is more substantial than most topical preparations; therefore, systemic effects are more common.

Dosing

Adult & Geriatric

Dermatosis: Topical: Apply thin film to affected area 2-4 times/day.

Hydrocortisone probutate (Pandel®): Topical: Apply thin film to affected area 1-2 times/day

Hydrocortisone valerate (Westcort®): Topical: Apply thin film to affected area 2-3 times/day

External anal and genital itching: Topical (OTC labeling): Apply to clean dry skin up to 3-4 times/day

Hemorrhoids: Rectal: One suppository (30 mg) twice daily for 2 weeks. For severe cases of proctitis, 1 suppository 3 times/day or 2 suppositories twice daily may be needed. For factitial proctitis, duration of treatment may be up to 6-8 weeks.

Ulcerative colitis: Rectal:

Foam: One applicatorful (80 mg) 1-2 times/day for 2-3 weeks, and then every other day thereafter; use lowest dose to maintain clinical response; taper dose to discontinue long-term therapy

Suspension: One enema (100 mg) every night for 21 days or until remission (clinical improvement may precede improvement of mucosal integrity); 2-3 months of therapy may be required; taper dose to discontinue long-term therapy

Pediatric

Atopic dermatitis: Topical: Children ≥3 months: Hydrocortisone butyrate (Locoid Lipocream®): Apply thin film to affected area twice daily.

Dermatosis: Topical: Apply thin film to affected area 2-4 times/day. Products labeled for OTC use (self-medication) should not be used in children <2 years of age.

External anal and genital itching: Topical: Children ≥12 years: (OTC labeling): Refer to adult dosing.

Administration

Topical cream, lotion, ointment: Apply a thin film to clean, dry skin and rub in gently.

Rectal foam: Shake vigorously for 5-10 seconds prior to use. Do not remove cap during use. Hold container upright to fill applicator. Gently insert applicator tip into anus. Only use applicator provided by manufacturer; do not insert any part of the aerosol container in the anus. Clean applicator after each use.

Rectal suppository: Remove foil from rectal suppository and insert pointed end first. Avoid handling unwrapped suppository for too long.

Rectal suspension: Shake bottle well. Remove protective sheath from applicator tip. Lie on left side with left leg extended and right leg flexed forward. Gently insert lubricated applicator tip into rectum, pointed slightly toward navel. Grasp bottle firmly and squeeze slowly to instill the medication. After administering, withdraw and discard the used unit. Remain in position for at least 30 minutes. Retain the enema all night if possible.

Monitoring Parameters Serum glucose, electrolytes; blood pressure, weight, presence of infection; monitor IOP with therapy >6 weeks; bone mineral density, growth in children

Additional Information Hydrocortisone base topical cream, lotion, and ointments in concentrations of 0.25%, 0.5%, and 1% may be OTC or prescription depending on the product labeling.

Dosage Forms Excipient information presented when available (limited, particularly for generics); consult specific product labeling. [DSC] = Discontinued product

Aerosol, foam, rectal, as acetate:
- Cortifoam®: 10% (15 g) [90 mg/applicator]

Cream, topical, as acetate: 1% (28.4 g, 454 g); 2% (43 g)
- U-Cort®: 1% (28 g) [contains sodium metabisulfite]

Cream, topical, as acetate [strength expressed as base]: 1% (30 g)

Cream, topical, as base: 0.5% (28.4 g, 30 g); 1% (1 g, 1.5 g, 15 g, 28.4 g, 30 g, 114 g, 454 g); 2.5% (20 g, 28 g, 28.35 g, 30 g, 454 g)
- Ala-Cort: 1% (28.4 g, 85.2 g)
- Anusol-HC®: 2.5% (30 g) [contains benzyl alcohol]
- Caldecort®: 1% (28.4 g) [contains aloe]
- Cortaid® Advanced: 1% (42 g) [contains aloe]
- Cortaid® Intensive Therapy: 1% (37 g, 56 g)
- Cortaid® Maximum Strength: 1% (14 g, 28 g, 37 g, 56 g) [contains aloe]
- Cortizone-10® Maximum Strength: 1% (15 g, 28 g, 56 g) [contains aloe]
- Cortizone-10® Maximum Strength Intensive Healing Formula: 1% (28 g, 56 g) [contains aloe, benzyl alcohol]
- Cortizone-10® Plus Maximum Strength: 1% (28 g, 56 g) [contains aloe, vitamin A, vitamin E]
- Hydrocortisone Plus: 1% (28.4 g) [contains aloe, vitamin A, vitamin D, vitamin E]
- HydroSKIN®: 1% (28 g) [contains benzyl alcohol]
- Preparation H® Hydrocortisone: 1% (26 g) [contains sodium benzoate]
- Procto-Pak™: 1% (28.4 g)
- Proctocort®: 1% (28.35 g)
- ProctoCream®-HC: 2.5% (30 g) [contains benzyl alcohol]
- Proctosol-HC®: 2.5% (28.35 g)

Proctozone-HC 2.5%™: 2.5% (30 g)
Recort: 1% (30 g)
Cream, topical, as butyrate: 0.1% (15 g, 45 g)
Locoid Lipocream®: 0.1% (15 g [DSC], 45 g, 60 g)
Locoid®: 0.1% (15 g, 45 g)
Cream, topical, as probutate:
Pandel®: 0.1% (15 g, 45 g, 80 g)
Cream, topical, as valerate: 0.2% (15 g, 45 g, 60 g)
Gel, topical, as base:
CortiCool®: 1% (0.9 g, 42.5 g) [contains ethanol 20%]
Cortizone-10® Maximum Strength Cooling Relief: 1% (28 g) [contains aloe, ethanol 15%]
Liquid, topical, as base:
Cortizone-10® Maximum Strength Easy Relief: 1% (36 mL) [contains aloe, ethanol 45%]
Scalpana: 1% (85.5 mL)
Lotion, topical, as base: 1% (114 g, 118 mL); 2.5% (59 mL, 60 mL, 118 mL)
Ala-Scalp: 2% (29.6 mL)
Aquanil HC®: 1% (120 mL) [contains benzyl alcohol]
Beta-HC®: 1% (60 mL)
Cortaid® Intensive Therapy: 1% (98 g)
Cortizone-10® Hydratensive Healing: 1% (113 g) [contains aloe]
Cortizone-10® Hydratensive Soothing: 1% (113 g) [contains aloe]
Cortizone-10® Intensive Healing Eczema: 1% (99 g) [contains aloe, vitamin A, vitamin C, vitamin E]
Dermarest® Eczema Medicated: 1% (118 mL)
HydroSKIN®: 1% (118 mL) [contains benzyl alcohol]
Lotion, topical, as base [kit]:
Pediaderm™ HC: 2% (29.6 mL) [contains benzalkonium chloride, isopropyl alcohol; packaged with protective emollient]
Lotion, topical, as butyrate:
Locoid®: 0.1% (60 mL)
Ointment, topical, as acetate [strength expressed as base]: 1% (30 g)
Ointment, topical, as base: 0.5% (30 g); 1% (25 g, 30 g, 110 g, 430 g, 454 g); 2.5% (20 g, 30 g, 454 g)
Cortaid® Maximum Strength: 1% (28 g, 37 g)
Cortizone-10® Maximum Strength: 1% (28 g, 56 g)
Ointment, topical, as butyrate: 0.1% (15 g, 45 g)
Locoid®: 0.1% (15 g, 45 g)
Ointment, topical, as valerate: 0.2% (15 g, 45 g, 60 g)
Westcort®: 0.2% (15 g [DSC], 45 g, 60 g)
Powder, for prescription compounding, as acetate [micronized]: USP: 100% (10 g, 25 g, 100 g)
Solution, topical, as base:
Texacort™: 2.5% (30 mL) [contains ethanol 48.8%]
Solution, topical, as base [spray]:
Cortaid® Intensive Therapy: 1% (59 mL) [contains ethanol 45%]
Solution, topical, as butyrate: 0.1% (20 mL, 60 mL)
Locoid®: 0.1% (20 mL, 60 mL) [contains isopropyl alcohol 50%]
Suppository, rectal, as acetate: 25 mg (12s); 30 mg (12s)
Anu-med HC: 25 mg (12s)
Anucort-HC™: 25 mg (12s, 24s, 100s)
Anusol-HC®: 25 mg (12s, 24s)
Hemril® -30: 30 mg (12s, 24s)

Proctocort®: 30 mg (12s, 24s)
Suspension, rectal, as base: 100 mg/60 mL (60 mL)
Colocort®: 100 mg/60 mL (60 mL)
Cortenema®: 100 mg/60 mL (60 mL)

References

Reed, BR, "Dermatologic Drugs, Pregnancy, and Lactation. A Conservative Guide," *Arch Dermatol*, 1997, 133(7):894-8.

- **Hydrocortisone Acetate** *see* Hydrocortisone (Topical) *on page 719*
- **Hydrocortisone Butyrate** *see* Hydrocortisone (Topical) *on page 719*
- **Hydrocortisone Plus [OTC]** *see* Hydrocortisone (Topical) *on page 719*
- **Hydrocortisone Probutate** *see* Hydrocortisone (Topical) *on page 719*
- **Hydrocortisone Sodium Succinate** *see* Hydrocortisone (Systemic) *on page 713*
- **Hydrocortisone Valerate** *see* Hydrocortisone (Topical) *on page 719*
- **Hydromorph Contin® (Can)** *see* HYDROmorphone *on page 724*

HYDROmorphone (hye droe MOR fone)

Brand Names: U.S. Dilaudid-HP®; Dilaudid®; Exalgo®

Brand Names: Canada Dilaudid-HP®; Dilaudid®; Hydromorph Contin®; Hydromorphone HP; Hydromorphone HP® 10; Hydromorphone HP® 20; Hydromorphone HP® 50; Hydromorphone HP® Forte; Hydromorphone Hydrochloride Injection, USP; Jurnista™; PMS-Hydromorphone; Teva-Hydromorphone

Index Terms Dihydromorphinone; Hydromorphone Hydrochloride

Generic Availability (U.S.) Yes: Excludes extended release tablet, powder for injection

Pharmacologic Category Analgesic, Opioid

Use Management of moderate-to-severe pain

Exalgo®: Management of moderate-to-severe pain in opioid-tolerant patients (requiring around-the-clock analgesia for an extended period of time)

Labeled Contraindications Hypersensitivity to hydromorphone, any component of the formulation; acute or severe asthma, severe respiratory depression (in absence of resuscitative equipment or ventilatory support)

Additional product-specific contraindications:

Dilaudid® liquid and tablets: Obstetrical analgesia

Dilaudid® injection, Dilaudid-HP® injection: Opioid nontolerant patients; patients with risk of developing GI obstruction, especially paralytic ileus

Exalgo®: Opioid nontolerant patients, paralytic ileus (known or suspected), preexisting GI surgery or diseases resulting in narrowing of GI tract, loops in the GI tract or GI obstruction

Suppository: Intracranial lesion associated with increased intracranial pressure; whenever ventilatory function is depressed (COPD, cor pulmonale, emphysema, kyphoscoliosis, status asthmaticus)

Pregnancy Risk Factor C

Lactation Enters breast milk/not recommended

Warnings/Precautions **[U.S. Boxed Warning]: May cause potentially life-threatening respiratory depression even with therapeutic use, especially with initiation or dose increases; instruct patients on proper administration of extended release tablets. The use of ethanol, other opioids, and other CNS depressants may increase the risk of adverse outcomes,**

including death. Critical respiratory depression may occur, even at therapeutic dosages, particularly in elderly, cachectic, or debilitated patients or in patients with pre-existing respiratory compromise (hypoxia and/or hypercapnia). Use caution in COPD or other obstructive pulmonary disease.

Use with caution in patients with hypersensitivity reactions to other phenanthrene derivative opioid agonists (codeine, hydrocodone, levorphanol, oxycodone, oxymorphone). Hydromorphone shares toxic potential of opioid agonists, including CNS depression and respiratory depression. Precautions associated with opioid agonist therapy should be observed. May cause CNS depression, which may impair physical or mental abilities; patients must be cautioned about performing tasks which require mental alertness (eg, operating machinery or driving). Myoclonus and seizures have been reported with high doses; use with caution in patients with a history of seizure disorder. Use with caution in patients with kyphoscoliosis, cardiovascular disease, morbid obesity, adrenocortical insufficiency, hypothyroidism, acute alcoholism, delirium tremens, toxic psychoses, prostatic hyperplasia and/or urinary stricture, or severe liver or renal failure. Use with caution in patients with biliary tract dysfunction. Hydromorphone may increase biliary tract pressure following spasm in sphincter of Oddi. Use caution in patients with inflammatory or obstructive bowel disorder, acute pancreatitis secondary to biliary tract disease, and patients undergoing biliary surgery. Use extreme caution in patients with head injury, intracranial lesions, or elevated intracranial pressure; exaggerated elevation of ICP may occur (in addition, hydromorphone may complicate neurologic evaluation due to pupillary dilation and CNS depressant effects). Use with caution in patients with depleted blood volume or drugs which may exaggerate hypotensive effects (including phenothiazines or general anesthetics). May obscure diagnosis or clinical course of patients with acute abdominal conditions. Severe and unpredictable potentiation by MAO inhibitors has been reported with opioid analgesics; use within 14 days of MAO inhibitors is not recommended.

[U.S. Boxed Warning]: Hydromorphone has a high potential for abuse. Those at risk for opioid abuse include patients with a history of substance abuse or mental illness. Tolerance or drug dependence may result from extended use; however, concerns for abuse should not prevent effective management of pain. In general, abrupt discontinuation of therapy in dependent patients should be avoided.

An opioid-containing analgesic regimen should be tailored to each patient's needs and based upon the type of pain being treated (acute versus chronic), the route of administration, degree of tolerance for opioids (naive versus chronic user), age, weight, and medical condition. The optimal analgesic dose varies widely among patients. Doses should be titrated to pain relief/prevention. I.M. use may result in variable absorption and a lag time to peak effect.

Dosage form specific warnings:

[U.S. Boxed Warning]: Dilaudid-HP®: Extreme caution should be taken to avoid confusing the highly-concentrated (Dilaudid-HP®) injection with the less-concentrated (Dilaudid®) injectable product. Dilaudid-HP® should only be used in patients who are opioid-tolerant.

Controlled release: Capsules should only be used when continuous analgesia is required over an extended period of time. Controlled release products are not to be used on an "as needed" (PRN) basis.

Extended release tablets (Exalgo®): **[U.S. Boxed Warning]: For use in opioid tolerant patients only; fatal respiratory depression may occur in patient who are not opioid tolerant. The highest risk of fatal respiratory depression is at initiation and with dose increases. Indicated for the management of moderate-to-severe pain when around the clock pain control is needed for an extended time period. Not for use as an as-needed analgesic or for the management of acute or postoperative pain. Tablets should be swallowed whole; do not crush, break, chew, dissolve or inject; doing so may lead to rapid release and absorption of a potentially fatal dose of hydromorphone. Accidental consumption may lead to fatal overdose, especially in children.** Exalgo® tablets are nondeformable; do not administer to patients with preexisting severe gastrointestinal narrowing (eg, esophageal motility, small bowel inflammatory disease, short gut syndrome, history of peritonitis, cystic fibrosis, chronic intestinal pseudo-obstruction, Meckel's diverticulum); obstruction may occur.

Some dosage forms contain trace amounts of sodium metabisulfite which may cause allergic reactions in susceptible individuals. Vial stoppers of single-dose injectable vials may contain latex.

Ethanol/Nutrition/Herb Interactions

Ethanol: Ethanol may increase CNS depression. Management: Monitor for increased effects with coadministration. Caution patients about effects.

Herb/Nutraceutical: Gotu kola, valerian, and kava kava may increase CNS depression. Management: Avoid gotu kola, valerian, and kava kava.

Storage/Stability

Injection: Store at 15°C to 30°C (59°F to 86°F). A slightly yellowish discoloration has not been associated with a loss of potency.

Oral dosage forms: Store at 15°C to 30°C (59°F to 86°F). Protect tablets from light.

Suppository: Store in refrigerator. Protect from light.

Mechanism of Action Binds to opioid receptors in the CNS, causing inhibition of ascending pain pathways, altering the perception of and response to pain; causes cough supression by direct central action in the medulla; produces generalized CNS depression

Pharmacodynamics/Kinetics

Onset of action: Analgesic:
- Immediate release formulations:
  - Oral: 15-30 minutes; Peak effect: 30-60 minutes
  - I.V.: 5 minutes; Peak effect: 10-20 minutes
- Extended release tablet: 6 hours; Peak effect: ~9 hours (Angst, 2001)

Duration:
- Immediate release formulations: Oral, I.V.: 3-4 hours
- Extended release tablet: ~13 hours (Angst, 2001)

Absorption: Extended release tablet: Delayed; I.M.: Variable and delayed

Distribution: V_d: 4 L/kg

Protein binding: ~8% to 19%

Metabolism: Hepatic via glucuronidation; to inactive metabolites

Bioavailability: 62%

Half-life elimination:
- Immediate release formulations: 2-3 hours
- Extended release tablets: Apparent half-life: ~11 hours (range: 8-15 hours)

Time to peak, plasma:
Immediate release tablet: ≤1 hour
Extended release tablet: 12-16 hours
Excretion: Urine (primarily as glucuronide conjugates)

Dosing

Adult

Acute pain (moderate-to-severe): Note: These are guidelines and do not represent the maximum doses that may be required in all patients. Doses should be titrated to provide adequate pain relief. When changing routes of administration, oral doses and parenteral doses are **NOT** equivalent; parenteral doses are up to 5 times more potent. Therefore, when administered parenterally, one-fifth of the oral dose will provide similar analgesia.

Oral: Initial: Opioid-naive: 2-4 mg every 4-6 hours as needed; elderly/debilitated patients may require lower doses; patients with prior opioid exposure may require higher initial doses. **Note:** In adults with severe pain, the American Pain Society recommends an initial dose of 4-8 mg.

I.V.: Initial: Opioid-naive: 0.2-1 mg every 2-3 hours as needed; patients with prior opioid exposure may require higher initial doses.

Mechanically ventilated/critically ill patients (unlabeled use): 0.7-4 mg (based on 70 kg patient) every 4 hours as needed. **Note:** More frequent dosing may be needed (eg, every 1-2 hours); dose should be adjusted based on patient response; elderly patients may be more sensitive (Jacobi, 2002).

Continuous infusion: Usual dosage range: 0.5-1 mg/hour (based on 70 kg patient) or 7-15 **mcg**/kg/**hour**

Patient-controlled analgesia (PCA) (unlabeled dosing) (American Pain Society, 2008): **Note:** Opioid-naive: Consider lower end of dosing range:

Usual concentration: 0.2 mg/mL
Demand dose: Usual initial dose: 0.1-0.2 mg; range: 0.05-0.4 mg
Lockout interval: 5-10 minutes

Epidural PCA (unlabeled dosing) (de Leon-Casasola, 1996; Liu, 2010; Smith, 2009):

Usual concentration: 0.01 mg/mL
Bolus dose: 0.4-1 mg
Infusion rate: 0.03-0.3 mg/**hour**
Demand dose: 0.02-0.05 mg
Lockout interval: 10-15 minutes

I.M., SubQ: **Note:** I.M. use may result in variable absorption and lag time to peak effect; I.M. route not recommended for use (American Pain Society, 2008).

Initial: Opioid-naive: 0.8-1 mg every 3-4 hours as needed; patients with prior opioid exposure may require higher initial doses

Rectal: 3 mg every 6-8 hours as needed

Chronic pain: Note: Patients taking opioids chronically may become tolerant and require doses higher than the usual dosage range to maintain the desired effect. Tolerance can be managed by appropriate dose titration. There is no optimal or maximal dose for hydromorphone in chronic pain. The appropriate dose is one that relieves pain throughout its dosing interval without causing unmanageable side effects.

Controlled release formulation (Hydromorph Contin®, not available in U.S.): Oral: 3-30 mg every 12 hours. **Note:** A patient's hydromorphone requirement should be established using prompt release formulations; conversion to long acting products may be considered when chronic, continuous treatment is required. Higher dosages should be reserved for use only in opioid-tolerant patients.

Extended release formulation (Exalgo®): Dosing range: 8-64 mg every 24 hours. For use in opioid-tolerant patients only; discontinue all other extended release opioids when starting therapy. Suggested recommendations for converting to Exalgo® from other analgesics are presented, but when selecting the initial dose, other characteristics (eg, patient status, degree of opioid tolerance, concurrent medications, type of pain, risk factors for addiction or diversion, etc) should also be considered.

Individualization of dose: Pain relief and adverse events should be assessed frequently. Dose increases may occur not more often than every 3-4 days; consider titrating with increases of 25% to 50% of the current daily dose. If more than 2 doses of rescue medications are needed within 24 hours for 2 consecutive days, consider increasing the dose of Exalgo®. Do not administer more frequently than every 24 hours.

Conversion from other oral hydromorphone formulations to Exalgo®: Start with the equivalent total daily dose of immediate-release hydromorphone administered once daily. May titrate every 3-4 days until adequate pain relief with tolerable side effects have been achieved.

Conversion from other opioids to Exalgo®: In general, start Exalgo® at 50% of the calculated total daily dose every 24 hours (see Conversion Ratios to Exalgo®). Titrate until adequate pain relief with tolerable side effects has been achieved. The following conversion ratios may be used to convert from **oral** opioid therapy to Exalgo®.

Conversion ratios to Exalgo® (see table): Select the opioid, sum the total daily dose, then multiply by the conversion ratio to calculate the *approximate* oral hydromorphone equivalent; start Exalgo® at 50% of the calculated total daily dose every 24 hours. (**Note:** The conversion ratios and approximate equivalent doses in this conversion table are only to be used for the conversion from current opioid therapy to Exalgo®).

Conversion Ratios to Exalgo®[1]

Previous Opioid	Approximate Equivalent Oral Dose	Oral Conversion Ratio[2]
Hydromorphone	12 mg	1
Codeine	200 mg	0.06
Hydrocodone	30 mg	0.4
Methadone[3]	20 mg	0.6
Morphine	60 mg	0.2
Oxycodone	30 mg	0.4
Oxymorphone	20 mg	0.6

[1]*Approximate* equivalent doses for conversion from current opioid therapy to Exalgo®.
[2]Ratio for converting oral opioid dose to approximate hydromorphone equivalent dose.
[3]Monitor closely; ratio between methadone and other opioid agonists may vary widely as a function of previous drug exposure. Methadone has a long half-life and may accumulate in the plasma.

Conversion from transdermal fentanyl to Exalgo®: Treatment with Exalgo® can be started 18 hours after the removal of the transdermal fentanyl patch. For every fentanyl 25 mcg/hour transdermal dose, the equianalgesic dose of Exalgo® is 12 mg every 24 hours. An appropriate starting dose is 50% of the calculated total daily dose given every 24 hours.

Discontinuing Exalgo®: Taper by gradually decreasing the dose by 25% to 50% every 2-3 days to a dose of 8 mg every 24 hours before discontinuing therapy.

Geriatric Doses should be titrated to appropriate analgesic effects. When changing routes of administration, oral doses and parenteral doses are **NOT** equivalent; parenteral doses are up to 5 times more potent. Therefore, when administered parenterally, one-fifth of the oral dose will provide similar analgesia.

Acute pain, opioid-naive:

Oral: Use with caution; initiation at the low end of dosage range is recommended. For patients >70 years, The American Pain Society recommends consideration to lowering initial doses by 25% to 50% followed by upward or downward titration (APS, 2008).

I.V: Reduce initial dose to 0.2 mg

Pediatric Acute pain (moderate-to-severe): *Children >50 kg:* Refer to adult dosing.

Renal Impairment

Oral (immediate release), injectable: Initiate with 25% to 50% of the usual starting dose depending on the degree of impairment. Monitor closely for respiratory and CNS depression.

Oral (extended release; Exalgo®):

Moderate impairment (Cl_{cr} 30-60 mL/minute): Initiate with 50% of the usual starting dose for patients with normal renal function; monitor closely for respiratory and CNS depression

Severe impairment (Cl_{cr} <30 mL/minute): Initiate with 25% of the usual starting dose for patients with normal renal function; monitor closely for respiratory and CNS depression. Consider use of an alternate analgesic with better dosing flexibility.

Hepatic Impairment

Oral (immediate release), injectable:

Moderate impairment: Initiate with 25% to 50% of the usual starting dose for patients with normal hepatic function.

Severe impairment: Has not been studied; initial dose should be more conservative as compared to those with moderate impairment; use with caution.

Oral (extended release; Exalgo®):

Moderate impairment: Initiate with 25% of the usual starting dose for patients with normal hepatic function; monitor closely for respiratory and CNS depression.

Severe impairment: Use alternate analgesic.

Administration

Parenteral: **Note: Vial stopper may contain latex.** May be given SubQ or I.M.; I.M. route is not recommended (APS, 2008).

I.V.: For IVP, must be given slowly over 2-3 minutes (rapid IVP has been associated with an increase in side effects, especially respiratory depression and hypotension)

Oral: Hydromorphone is available in an 8 mg immediate release tablet and an 8 mg extended release tablet. Extreme caution should be taken to avoid confusing dosage forms.

Exalgo®: Tablets should be swallowed whole; do not crush, break, chew, dissolve or inject. May be taken with or without food.

Hydromorph Contin®: Capsule should be swallowed whole; do not crush or chew; contents may be sprinkled on soft food and swallowed

Test Interactions Some quinolones may produce a false-positive urine screening result for opioids using commercially-available immunoassay kits. This has been demonstrated most consistently for levofloxacin and ofloxacin, but other quinolones have shown cross-reactivity in certain assay kits. Confirmation of positive opioid screens by more specific methods should be considered.

Prescribing and Access Restrictions Exalgo®: As a requirement of the REMS program, healthcare providers who prescribe Exalgo® need to receive training on the proper use and potential risks of Exalgo®. For training, please refer to http://www.exalgorems.com. Prescribers will need retraining every 2 years or following any significant changes to the Exalgo® REMS program.

Medication Guide Available Yes

Dosage Forms Excipient information presented when available (limited, particularly for generics); consult specific product labeling.

Injection, powder for reconstitution, as hydrochloride:
- Dilaudid-HP®: 250 mg [contains natural rubber/natural latex in packaging, sodium metabisulfite]

Injection, solution, as hydrochloride: 1 mg/mL (1 mL); 2 mg/mL (1 mL, 20 mL); 4 mg/mL (1 mL); 10 mg/mL (1 mL, 5 mL, 50 mL)
- Dilaudid-HP®: 10 mg/mL (50 mL) [contains natural rubber/natural latex in packaging, sodium metabisulfite]
- Dilaudid-HP®: 10 mg/mL (1 mL, 5 mL) [contains sodium metabisulfite]
- Dilaudid®: 1 mg/mL (1 mL); 2 mg/mL (1 mL); 4 mg/mL (1 mL) [contains sodium metabisulfite]

Injection, solution, as hydrochloride [preservative free]: 10 mg/mL (1 mL, 5 mL, 50 mL)

Liquid, oral, as hydrochloride: 1 mg/mL (473 mL)
- Dilaudid®: 1 mg/mL (473 mL) [contains sodium metabisulfite (may have trace amounts)]

Powder, for prescription compounding, as hydrochloride: USP: 100% (972 mg)

Suppository, rectal, as hydrochloride: 3 mg (6s)

Tablet, oral, as hydrochloride: 2 mg, 4 mg, 8 mg
- Dilaudid®: 2 mg, 4 mg [contains sodium metabisulfite (may have trace amounts)]
- Dilaudid®: 8 mg [scored; contains sodium metabisulfite (may have trace amounts)]

Tablet, extended release, oral, as hydrochloride:
- Exalgo®: 8 mg, 12 mg, 16 mg, 32 mg [contains sodium metabisulfite]

Dosage Forms: Canada Excipient information presented when available (limited, particularly for generics); consult specific product labeling.

Capsule, controlled release:
- Hydromorph Contin®: 3 mg, 6 mg, 12 mg, 18 mg, 24 mg, 30 mg

Controlled Substance C-II

◆ **Hydromorphone HP (Can)** *see* HYDROmorphone *on page* 724

◆ **Hydromorphone HP® 10 (Can)** *see* HYDROmorphone *on page* 724

◆ **Hydromorphone HP® 20 (Can)** *see* HYDROmorphone *on page* 724

◆ **Hydromorphone HP® 50 (Can)** *see* HYDROmorphone *on page* 724

◆ **Hydromorphone HP® Forte (Can)** *see* HYDROmorphone *on page* 724

◆ **Hydromorphone Hydrochloride** *see* HYDROmorphone *on page* 724

◆ **Hydromorphone Hydrochloride Injection, USP (Can)** *see* HYDROmorphone *on page* 724

◆ **HydroSKIN® [OTC]** *see* Hydrocortisone (Topical) *on page* 719
◆ **HydroVal® (Can)** *see* Hydrocortisone (Topical) *on page* 719
◆ **Hydroxycarbamide** *see* Hydroxyurea *on page* 731
◆ **Hydroxydaunomycin Hydrochloride** *see* DOXOrubicin *on page* 467
◆ **Hydroxyldaunorubicin Hydrochloride** *see* DOXOrubicin *on page* 467

Hydroxyurea (hye droks ee yoor EE a)

Related Information

Management of Chemotherapy-Induced Nausea and Vomiting *on page* 1786
Safe Handling of Hazardous Drugs *on page* 1904

Brand Names: U.S. Droxia®; Hydrea®

Brand Names: Canada Apo-Hydroxyurea®; Gen-Hydroxyurea; Hydrea®; Mylan-Hydroxyurea

Index Terms Hydroxycarbamide; Hydurea

Generic Availability (U.S.) Yes

Pharmacologic Category Antineoplastic Agent, Antimetabolite

Use Treatment of melanoma, refractory chronic myelocytic leukemia (CML); recurrent, metastatic, or inoperable ovarian cancer; radiosensitizing agent in the treatment of squamous cell head and neck cancer (excluding lip cancer); adjunct in the management of sickle cell patients who have had at least three painful crises in the previous 12 months (to reduce frequency of these crises and the need for blood transfusions)

Unlabeled Use Treatment of essential thrombocythemia, polycythemia vera, hypereosinophilic syndrome; management of hyperleukocytosis due to acute myeloid leukemia; treatment of cervical cancer, treatment of meningiomas

Labeled Contraindications Hypersensitivity to hydroxyurea or any component of the formulation

Hydrea®: Marked bone marrow suppression (WBC <2500/mm^3 or platelet count <100,000/mm^3) or severe anemia

Pregnancy Risk Factor D

Lactation Enters breast milk/not recommended

Warnings/Precautions Hazardous agent - use appropriate precautions for handling and disposal; to decrease risk of exposure, wear gloves when handling and wash hands before and after contact. Leukopenia and neutropenia commonly occur (thrombocytopenia and anemia are less common); leukopenia/neutropenia occur first. Hematologic toxicity reversible (rapid) with treatment interruption. Correct severe anemia prior to initiating treatment. Hydrea® use is contraindicated in marked bone marrow suppression; should not be used in sickle cell anemia with severe bone marrow suppression (neutrophils <2000/mm^3, platelets <80,000/mm^3, hemoglobin <4.5 g/dL, or reticulocytes <80,000/mm^3 when hemoglobin <9 g/dL). Use with caution in patients with a history of prior chemotherapy or radiation therapy; myelosuppression is more common. Patients with a history of radiation therapy are also at risk for exacerbation of post irradiation erythema. Self-limiting megaloblastic erythropoiesis may be seen early in treatment (may resemble pernicious anemia, but is unrelated to vitamin B_{12} or folic acid deficiency). Plasma iron clearance may be delayed and iron utilization rate (by erythrocytes) may be reduced. When treated concurrently with hydroxyurea and antiretroviral agents (including didanosine and stavudine), HIV-infected patients are at higher risk for potentially fatal pancreatitis, hepatotoxicity, hepatic failure, and severe peripheral neuropathy; discontinue immediately if signs of these toxicities develop. Hyperuricemia may occur with antineoplastic treatment; adequate hydration and initiation or dosage adjustment of uricosuric agents (eg, allopurinol) may be necessary.

In patients with sickle cell anemia, use is not recommended if neutrophils <2000/mm^3, platelets <80,000/mm^3, hemoglobin <4.5 g/dL, or reticulocytes <80,000/mm^3 when hemoglobin <9 g/dL. May cause macrocytosis, which can mask folic acid deficiency; prophylactic fold acid supplementation is recommended. **[U.S. Boxed Warning]: Hydroxyurea is mutagenic and clastogenic; causes cellular transformation resulting in tumorigenicity; also considered genotoxic and may be carcinogenic. Treatment of myeloproliferative disorders (eg, polycythemia vera, thrombocythemia) with long-term hydroxyurea is associated with secondary leukemia;** it is unknown if this is drug-related or disease-related. Skin cancer has been reported with long-term hydroxyurea use. Cutaneous vasculitic toxicities (vasculitic ulceration and gangrene) have been reported with hydroxyurea treatment, most often in patients with a history of or receiving concurrent interferon therapy; discontinue hydroxyurea and consider alternate cytoreductive therapy if cutaneous vasculitic toxicity develops. Use caution with renal dysfunction; may require dose reductions. Elderly patients may be more sensitive to the effects of hydroxyurea; may require lower doses. **[U.S. Boxed Warning]: Should be administered under the supervision of a physician experienced in the treatment of sickle cell anemia** or in cancer chemotherapy.

Adverse Reactions Frequency not defined.

Cardiovascular: Edema

Central nervous system: Chills, disorientation, dizziness, drowsiness (dose-related), fever, hallucinations, headache, malaise, seizure

Dermatologic: Alopecia, cutaneous vasculitic toxicities, dermatomyositis-like skin changes, facial erythema, gangrene, hyperpigmentation, maculopapular rash, nail atrophy, nail discoloration, peripheral erythema, scaling, skin atrophy, skin cancer, skin ulcer, vasculitis ulcerations, violet papules

Endocrine & metabolic: Hyperuricemia

Gastrointestinal: Anorexia, constipation, diarrhea, gastrointestinal irritation and mucositis, (potentiated with radiation therapy), nausea, pancreatitis, stomatitis, vomiting

Genitourinary: Dysuria

Hematologic: Myelosuppression (anemia, leukopenia [common; reversal of WBC count occurs rapidly], thrombocytopenia); macrocytosis, megaloblastic erythropoiesis, secondary leukemias (long-term use)

Hepatic: Hepatic enzymes increased, hepatotoxicity

Neuromuscular & skeletal: Peripheral neuropathy, weakness

Renal: BUN increased, creatinine increased

Respiratory: Acute diffuse pulmonary infiltrates (rare), dyspnea, pulmonary fibrosis (rare)

Drug Interactions

Metabolism/Transport Effects None known.

Avoid Concomitant Use

Avoid concomitant use of Hydroxyurea with any of the following: BCG; CloZAPine; Didanosine; Natalizumab; Pimecrolimus; Stavudine; Tacrolimus (Topical); Vaccines (Live)

Increased Effect/Toxicity

Hydroxyurea may increase the levels/effects of: CloZAPine; Didanosine; Leflunomide; Natalizumab; Stavudine; Vaccines (Live)

The levels/effects of Hydroxyurea may be increased by: Denosumab; Didanosine; Pimecrolimus; Roflumilast; Stavudine; Tacrolimus (Topical); Trastuzumab

Decreased Effect

Hydroxyurea may decrease the levels/effects of: BCG; Coccidioidin Skin Test; Sipuleucel-T; Vaccines (Inactivated); Vaccines (Live)

The levels/effects of Hydroxyurea may be decreased by: Echinacea

Storage/Stability Store at room temperature of 25°C (77°F); excursions permitted between 15°C and 30°C (59°F and 86°F).

Mechanism of Action Antimetabolite which selectively inhibits ribonucleoside diphosphate reductase, preventing the conversion of ribonucleotides to deoxyribonucleotides, halting the cell cycle at the G1/S phase and therefore has radiation sensitizing activity by maintaining cells in the G_1 phase and interfering with DNA repair. In sickle cell anemia, hydroxyurea increases red blood cell (RBC) hemoglobin F levels, RBC water content, deformability of sickled cells, and alters adhesion of RBCs to endothelium.

Pharmacodynamics/Kinetics

Onset: Sickle cell anemia: Fetal hemoglobin increase: 4-12 weeks

Absorption: Readily (≥80%)

Distribution: Readily crosses blood-brain barrier; distributes into intestine, brain, lung, kidney tissues, effusions and ascites

Metabolism: 60% via hepatic and GI tract

Half-life elimination: 3-4 hours

Time to peak: 1-4 hours

Excretion: Urine (sickle cell anemia: 40% of administered dose)

Dosing

Adult & Geriatric

Antineoplastic uses: Titrate dose to patient response; if WBC count falls to <2500/mm^3, or the platelet count to <100,000/mm^3, therapy should be stopped for at least 3 days and resumed when values rise toward normal

Chronic myeloid leukemia (resistant): Oral: Continuous therapy: 20-30 mg/kg once daily

Solid tumors: Oral:

Intermittent therapy: 80 mg/kg as a single dose every third day

Continuous therapy: 20-30 mg/kg once daily

Concomitant therapy with irradiation (head and neck cancer): 80 mg/kg as a single dose every third day starting at least 7 days before initiation of irradiation

Sickle cell anemia: Oral: Initial: 15 mg/kg/day; if blood counts are in an acceptable range, may increase by 5 mg/kg every 12 weeks until the maximum tolerated dose of 35 mg/kg/day is achieved or the dose that does not produce toxic effects (do not increase dose if blood counts are between acceptable and toxic ranges). Monitor for toxicity every 2 weeks; if toxicity occurs, withhold treatment until the bone marrow recovers, then restart with a dose reduction of 2.5 mg/kg/day; if no toxicity occurs over the next 12 weeks, then the subsequent dose may be increased by 2.5 mg/kg/day every 12 weeks to a maximum tolerated dose (dose which does not produce hematologic toxicity for 24 consecutive weeks). If hematologic toxicity recurs a second time at a specific dose, do not retry that dose.

Acceptable hematologic ranges: Neutrophils ≥2500/mm^3; platelets ≥95,000/mm^3; hemoglobin >5.3 g/dL, and reticulocytes ≥95,000/mm^3 if the hemoglobin concentration is <9 g/dL

Toxic hematologic ranges: Neutrophils <2000/mm^3; platelets <80,000/mm^3; hemoglobin <4.5 g/dL; and reticulocytes <80,000/mm^3 if the hemoglobin concentration is <9 g/dL

Cervical cancer (unlabeled use; with concurrent radiation therapy, cisplatin and fluorouracil): Oral: 2000 mg/m^2 (2 hours prior to radiation treatment) twice a week for 6 weeks (Rose, 2007)

Essential thrombocythemia, high-risk (unlabeled use): Oral: 500-1000 mg daily; adjust dose to maintain platelets <400,000/mm^3 (Harrison, 2005)

Head and neck cancer (unlabeled dosing; with concurrent radiation therapy and fluorouracil): Oral: 1000 mg every 12 hours for 11 doses (Garden, 2004)

Hypereosinophilic syndrome (unlabeled use): Oral: 1000-3000 mg/day (Klion, 2006)

Meningioma (unlabeled use): Oral: 20 mg/kg once daily (Newton, 2000; Rosenthal, 2002)

Polycythemia vera, high-risk (unlabeled use): Oral: 15-20 mg/kg/day (Finazzi, 2007)

Pediatric Note: Doses should be based on ideal or actual body weight, whichever is less.

Sickle cell anemia (unlabeled use): Oral: 20 mg/kg once daily; increase by 5 mg/kg/day every 2-6 months to a maximum dose of 30 mg/kg/day (Ferster, 2001; Hankins, 2005; Thornburg, 2009; Wang, 2001; Zimmerman, 2004)

Renal Impairment

The FDA-approved labeling recommends the following adjustment:

Sickle cell anemia:

Cl_{cr} ≥60 mL/minute: No adjustment (of initial dose) required.

Cl_{cr} <60 mL/minute: Reduce initial dose to 7.5 mg/kg/day; titrate to response/avoidance of toxicity (refer to usual dosing).

ESRD: Reduce initial dose to 7.5 mg/kg/dose (administer after dialysis on dialysis days); titrate to response/avoidance of toxicity.

Other approved indications: It is recommended to reduce the initial dose; however, no specific guidelines are available.

The following guidelines have been used by some clinicians:

Aronoff, 2007: Adults:

Cl_{cr} 10-50 mL/minute: Administer 50% of dose.

Cl_{cr} <10 mL/minute: Administer 20% of dose.

Hemodialysis: Administer dose after dialysis on dialysis days; supplemental dose is not necessary. Hydroxyurea is a low molecular weight compound with high aqueous solubility that may be freely dialyzable, however, clinical studies confirming this hypothesis have not been performed.

Continuous renal replacement therapy (CRRT): Administer 50% of dose.

Kintzel, 1995:

Cl_{cr} 46-60 mL/minute: Administer 85% of dose.

Cl_{cr} 31-45 mL/minute: Administer 80% of dose.

Cl_{cr} <30 mL/minute: Administer 75% of dose.

Hepatic Impairment Specific guidelines are not available for dosage adjustment in hepatic impairment. The FDA-approved labeling recommends closely monitoring for bone marrow toxicity in patients with hepatic impairment.

Combination Regimens

Head and neck cancer: Fluorouracil-Hydroxyurea (Head and Neck Cancer) on page 1653

Leukemia, acute myeloid: Hydroxyurea (AML Regimen) on page 1680

Administration The manufacturer does not recommend opening the capsules; observe proper handling procedures (eg, wear gloves)

Emetic Potential Very low (<10%)

Extemporaneous Preparations Hazardous agent: Use appropriate precautions for handling and disposal.

A 40 mg/mL oral suspension may be prepared with capsules and either a 1:1 mixture of Ora-Sweet® and Ora-Plus® or a 1:1 mixture of methylcellulose 1% and simple syrup NF. Empty the contents of eight 500 mg capsules into a mortar. Add small portions of chosen vehicle and mix to a uniform paste; mix while incrementally adding the vehicle to **almost** 100 mL; transfer to a calibrated bottle, rinse mortar with vehicle, and add sufficient quantity of vehicle to make 100 mL. Label "shake well" and "refrigerate". Store in plastic prescription bottles. Stable for 14 days at room temperature or refrigerated (preferred) (Nahata, 2003).

A 100 mg/mL oral solution may be prepared with capsules. Mix the contents of twenty 500 mg capsules with enough room temperature sterile water (~50 mL) to initially result in a 200 mg/mL concentration. Stir vigorously using a magnetic stirrer for several hours, then filter to remove insoluble contents. Add 50 mL Syrpalta® (flavored syrup, HUMCO) to filtered solution, resulting in 100 mL of a 100 mg/mL hydroxyurea solution. Stable for 1 month at room temperature in amber plastic bottle (Heeney, 2004).

Heeney MM, Whorton MR, Howard TA, et al, "Chemical and Functional Analysis of Hydroxyurea Oral Solutions," *J Pediatr Hematol Oncol*, 2004, 26(3):179-84.

Nahata MC, Morosco RS, Boster EA, et al, "Stability of Hydroxyurea in Two Extemporaneously Prepared Oral Suspensions Stored at Two Temperatures," 2003, 38:P-161(E) [abstract from 2003 ASHP Midyear Clinical Meeting].

Monitoring Parameters CBC with differential and platelets, renal function and liver function tests, serum uric acid

Sickle cell disease: Monitor for toxicity every 2 weeks. If toxicity occurs, stop treatment until the bone marrow recovers; restart at 2.5 mg/kg/day less than the dose at which toxicity occurs. If no toxicity occurs over the next 12 weeks, then the subsequent dose should be increased by 2.5 mg/kg/day. Reduced dosage of hydroxyurea alternating with erythropoietin may decrease myelotoxicity and increase levels of fetal hemoglobin in patients who have not been helped by hydroxyurea alone.

Acceptable range: Neutrophils ≥2500 cells/mm³, platelets ≥95,000/mm³, hemoglobin >5.3 g/dL, and reticulocytes ≥95,000/mm³ if the hemoglobin concentration is <9 g/dL

Toxic range: Neutrophils <2000 cells/mm³, platelets <80,000/mm³, hemoglobin <4.5 g/dL, and reticulocytes <80,000/mm³ if the hemoglobin concentration is <9 g/dL

Test Interactions False-negative triglyceride measurement by a glycerol oxidase method

Dietary Considerations In sickle cell patients, supplemental administration of folic acid is recommended; hydroxyurea may mask development of folic acid deficiency.

Dosage Forms Excipient information presented when available (limited, particularly for generics); consult specific product labeling.

Capsule, oral: 500 mg

Droxia®: 200 mg, 300 mg, 400 mg

Hydrea®: 500 mg

References

Aronoff GR, Bennett WM, Berns JS, et al, *Drug Prescribing in Renal Failure: Dosing Guidelines for Adults and Children*, 5th ed. Philadelphia, PA: American College of Physicians; 2007, p 100.

Ferster A, Tahriri P, Vermylen C, et al, "Five Years of Experience With Hydroxyurea in Children and Young Adults With Sickle Cell Disease," *Blood*, 2001, 97(11):3628-32.

Finazzi G and Barbui T, "How I Treat Patients With Polycythemia Vera," *Blood*, 2007, 109 (12):5104-11.

Garden AS, Harris J, Vokes EE, et al, "Preliminary Results of Radiation Therapy Oncology Group 97-03: A Randomized Phase II Trial of Concurrent Radiation and Chemotherapy for Advanced Squamous Cell Carcinomas of the Head and Neck," *J Clin Oncol*, 2004, 22(14):2856-64.

Hankins JS, Ware RE, Rogers ZR, et al, "Long-Term Hydroxyurea Therapy for Infants With Sickle Cell Anemia: The HUSOFT Extension Study," *Blood*, 2005, 106(7):2269-75.

Harrison CN, Campbell PJ, Buck G, et al, "Hydroxyurea Compared With Anagrelide in High-Risk Essential Thrombocythemia," *N Engl J Med*, 2005, 353(1):33-45.

Heeney MM, Whorton MR, Howard TA, et al, "Chemical and Functional Analysis of Hydroxyurea Oral Solutions," *J Pediatr Hematol Oncol*, 2004, 26(3):179-84.

Kintzel PE and Dorr RT, "Anticancer Drug Renal Toxicity and Elimination: Dosing Guidelines for Altered Renal Function," *Cancer Treat Rev*, 1995, 21(1):33-64.

Klion AD, Bochner BS, Gleich GJ, et al, "Approaches to the Treatment of Hypereosinophilic Syndromes: A Workshop Summary Report," *J Allergy Clin Immunol*, 2006, 117(6):1292-302.

Newton HB, Slivka MA, and Stevens C, "Hydroxyurea Chemotherapy for Unresectable or Residual Meningioma," *J Neurooncol*, 2000, 49(2):165-70.

Rose PG, Ali S, Watkins E, et al, "Long-Term Follow-Up of a Randomized Trial Comparing Concurrent Single Agent Cisplatin, Cisplatin-Based Combination Chemotherapy, or Hydroxyurea During Pelvic Irradiation for Locally Advanced Cervical Cancer: A Gynecologic Oncology Group Study," *J Clin Oncol*, 2007, 25(19):2804-10.

Rosenthal MA, Ashley DL, and Cher L. "Treatment of High Risk or Recurrent Meningiomas With Hydroxyurea," *J Clin Neurosci*, 2002, 9(2):156-8.

Thornburg CD, Dixon N, Burgett S, et al, "A Pilot Study of Hydroxyurea to Prevent Chronic Organ Damage in Young Children With Sickle Cell Anemia," *Pediatr Blood Cancer*, 2009, 52(5):609-15.

Wang WC, Wynn LW, Rogers ZR, et al, "A Two-Year Pilot Trial of Hydroxyurea in Very Young Children With Sickle Cell Anemia," *J Pediatr*, 2001, 139(6):790-6.

Zimmerman SA, Schultz WH, Davis JS, et al, "Sustained Long-Term Hematologic Efficacy of Hydroxyurea at Maximum Tolerated Dose in Children With Sickle Cell Disease," *Blood*, 2004, 103 (6):2039-45.

HydrOXYzine (hye DROKS i zeen)

Related Information

Management of Chemotherapy-Induced Nausea and Vomiting *on page 1786*

Management of Drug Extravasations *on page 1800*

Brand Names: U.S. Vistaril®

Brand Names: Canada Apo-Hydroxyzine®; Atarax®; Hydroxyzine Hydrochloride Injection, USP; Novo-Hydroxyzin; Nu-Hydroxyzine; PMS-Hydroxyzine; Riva-Hydroxyzine

Index Terms Hydroxyzine Hydrochloride; Hydroxyzine Pamoate

Generic Availability (U.S.) Yes

Pharmacologic Category Antiemetic; Histamine H_1 Antagonist; Histamine H_1 Antagonist, First Generation; Piperazine Derivative

Use Treatment of anxiety/agitation (including adjunctive therapy in alcoholism); adjunct to pre- and postoperative analgesia and anesthesia; antipruritic; antiemetic

Labeled Contraindications Hypersensitivity to hydroxyzine or any component of the formulation; early pregnancy; SubQ, intra-arterial, or I.V. injection

Lactation Excretion in breast milk unknown/not recommended

Warnings/Precautions Causes sedation, caution must be used in performing tasks which require alertness (eg, operating machinery or driving). Sedative effects of CNS depressants or ethanol are potentiated. SubQ, I.V., and intra-arterial administration are contraindicated since tissue damage, intravascular hemolysis, thrombosis, and digital gangrene can occur. Use with caution with narrow-angle glaucoma, prostatic hyperplasia, bladder neck obstruction, asthma, or COPD. In the elderly, avoid use of this potent anticholinergic agent due to increased risk of confusion, dry mouth, constipation, and other anticholinergic effects; clearance decreases in patients of advanced age (Beers Criteria).

Adverse Reactions Frequency not defined.

Central nervous system: Dizziness, drowsiness, fatigue, hallucination, headache, nervousness, seizure

Dermatologic: Pruritus, rash, urticaria

Gastrointestinal: Xerostomia

Neuromuscular & skeletal: Involuntary movements, paresthesia, tremor

Ocular: Blurred vision

Respiratory: Respiratory depression (at higher than recommended doses)

Miscellaneous: Allergic reaction

Drug Interactions

Metabolism/Transport Effects Inhibits CYP2D6 (weak)

Avoid Concomitant Use

Avoid concomitant use of HydrOXYzine with any of the following: Aclidinium; Azelastine (Nasal); Ipratropium (Oral Inhalation); Methadone; Mirtazapine; Paraldehyde; Tiotropium

Increased Effect/Toxicity

HydrOXYzine may increase the levels/effects of: Alcohol (Ethyl); Anticholinergics; ARIPiprazole; Azelastine (Nasal); Barbiturates; Buprenorphine; CNS Depressants; Meperidine; Methadone; Methotrimeprazine; Metyrosine; Mirtazapine; Paraldehyde; Pramipexole; ROPINIRole; Rotigotine; Selective Serotonin Reuptake Inhibitors; Tiotropium; Zolpidem

The levels/effects of HydrOXYzine may be increased by: Aclidinium; Droperidol; Ipratropium (Oral Inhalation); Methotrimeprazine; Perampanel; Pramlintide

Decreased Effect

HydrOXYzine may decrease the levels/effects of: Acetylcholinesterase Inhibitors (Central); Benzylpenicilloyl Polylysine; Betahistine; Hyaluronidase

The levels/effects of HydrOXYzine may be decreased by: Acetylcholinesterase Inhibitors (Central); Amphetamines

Ethanol/Nutrition/Herb Interactions

Ethanol: May increase CNS depression; monitor for increased effects with coadministration. Caution patients about effects.

Herb/Nutraceutical: Avoid valerian, St John's wort, kava kava, gotu kola (may increase CNS depression).

Storage/Stability

Injection: Store at 20°C to 25°C (68°F to 77°F); excursions permitted to 15°C to 30°C (59°F to 86°F). Protect from light.

Tablets: Store at 20°C to 25°C (68°F to 77°F).

Mechanism of Action Competes with histamine for H_1-receptor sites on effector cells in the gastrointestinal tract, blood vessels, and respiratory tract. Possesses skeletal muscle relaxing, bronchodilator, antihistamine, antiemetic, and analgesic properties.

Pharmacodynamics/Kinetics

Onset of action: Oral: 15-30 minutes; Injection: Rapid

Duration: Decreased histamine-induced wheal and flare areas: 2 to ≥36 hours; Suppression of pruritus: 1-12 hours (Simons, 1984)

Absorption: Oral: Rapid

Distribution: Adults: V_d ~16 L/kg (Simons, 1984); Elderly: ~23 L/kg (Simons K, 1989); Hepatic dysfunction: ~23 L/kg (Simons F, 1989)

Metabolism: Hepatic to multiple metabolites, including cetirizine (active) (Simons F, 1989)

Half-life elimination: Adults: ~20 hours (Simons, 1984); Elderly: ~29 hours (Simons K, 1989); Hepatic dysfunction: ~37 hours (Simons F, 1989)

Time to peak: Oral administration: Serum: ~2 hours; Peak suppression of antihistamine-induced wheal and flare: 4-12 hours (Simons, 1984)

Excretion: Urine

Dosing

Adult

Note: Adjust dose based on patient response.

Antiemetic: I.M.: 25-100 mg/dose

Anxiety:

Oral: 50-100 mg 4 times/day

I.M.: Initial: 50-100 mg, then every 4-6 hours as needed

Preoperative sedation:

Oral: 50-100 mg

I.M.: 25-100 mg

Pruritus: Oral: 25 mg 3-4 times/day

Geriatric Initiate dosing using the lower end of the recommended dosage range due to an increased potential for anticholinergic side effects. Refer to adult dosing.

Pediatric

Note: Adjust dose based on patient response.

Antiemetic: I.M.: 1.1 mg/kg/dose

Preoperative sedation:

Oral: 0.6 mg/kg/dose

I.M.: 1.1 mg/kg/dose

Pruritus, anxiety: Oral:

<6 years: 50 mg daily in divided doses

≥6 years: 50-100 mg daily in divided dose

Renal Impairment No dosage adjustment provided in the manufacturer's labeling; however, the following guidelines have been used by some clinicians (Aronoff, 2007): Adults:

GFR >50 mL/minute: No adjustment recommended.

GFR ≤50 mL/minute: Administer 50% of normal dose.

Continuous renal replacement therapy (CRRT), hemodialysis, peritoneal dialysis: Administer 50% of the normal dose.

Hepatic Impairment Change dosing interval to every 24 hours in patients with primary biliary cirrhosis (Simons F, 1989)

Administration

Injection: For I. M. use only. Do not administer I.V., SubQ, or intra-arterially. Administer I.M. deep in large muscle. In adults, the preferred site is the upper outer quadrant of the buttock or midlateral thigh. In children, the preferred site is the midlateral thigh. The upper outer quadrant of the gluteal region should be used only when necessary to minimize potential damage to the sciatic nerve. With I.V. administration, extravasation can result in sterile abscess and marked tissue induration.

Oral: Shake suspension vigorously prior to use.

Vesicant/Extravasation Risk Vesicant

Monitoring Parameters Relief of symptoms, mental status, blood pressure

Test Interactions May cause false-positive serum TCA screen.

Dosage Forms Excipient information presented when available (limited, particularly for generics); consult specific product labeling.

Capsule, oral, as pamoate: 25 mg, 50 mg, 100 mg

Vistaril®: 25 mg, 50 mg

Injection, solution, as hydrochloride: 25 mg/mL (1 mL); 50 mg/mL (1 mL, 2 mL, 10 mL)

Solution, oral, as hydrochloride: 10 mg/5 mL (473 mL)

Syrup, oral, as hydrochloride: 10 mg/5 mL (118 mL, 473 mL)

Tablet, oral, as hydrochloride: 10 mg, 25 mg, 50 mg

References

Aronoff GR, Bennett WM, Berns JS, et al, *Drug Prescribing in Renal Failure: Dosing Guidelines for Adults and Children*, 5th ed. Philadelphia, PA: American College of Physicians; 2007, p 97.

Simons FE, Simons KJ, and Frith EM, "The Pharmacokinetics and Antihistaminic of the H_1 Receptor Antagonist Hydroxyzine," *J Allergy Clin Immunol*, 1984, 73(1 Pt 1):69-75.

Simons FE, Watson WT, Chen XY, et al, "The Pharmacokinetics and Pharmacodynamics of Hydroxyzine in Patients With Primary Biliary Cirrhosis," *J Clin Pharmacol*, 1989, 29(9):809-15.

Simons KJ, Watson WT, Chen XY, et al, "Pharmacokinetic and Pharmacodynamic Studies of the H_1-Receptor Antagonist Hydroxyzine in the Elderly," *Clin Pharmacol Ther*, 1989, 45(1):9-14.

◆ **Hydroxyzine Hydrochloride** *see* HydrOXYzine *on page 736*

◆ **Hydroxyzine Hydrochloride Injection, USP (Can)** *see* HydrOXYzine *on page 736*

◆ **Hydroxyzine Pamoate** *see* HydrOXYzine *on page 736*

◆ **Hydurea** *see* Hydroxyurea *on page 731*

◆ **Hylenex** *see* Hyaluronidase *on page 711*

◆ **Hyoscine Butylbromide** *see* Scopolamine (Systemic) *on page 1274*

◆ **HyperRHO™ S/D Full Dose** *see* Rh_o(D) Immune Globulin *on page 1237*

◆ **HyperRHO™ S/D Mini-Dose** *see* Rh_o(D) Immune Globulin *on page 1237*

◆ **I^{123} Iobenguane** *see* Iobenguane I 123 *on page 806*

◆ **I-123 MIBG** *see* Iobenguane I 123 *on page 806*

Ibandronate (eye BAN droh nate)

Related Information

Hypercalcemia of Malignancy *on page 1000*

Brand Names: U.S. Boniva®

Index Terms Ibandronate Sodium; Ibandronic Acid

Generic Availability (U.S.) Yes: Tablet

Pharmacologic Category Bisphosphonate Derivative

Use Treatment and prevention of osteoporosis in postmenopausal females

Unlabeled Use Hypercalcemia of malignancy; reduce bone pain and skeletal complications from metastatic bone disease due to breast cancer

Labeled Contraindications Hypersensitivity to ibandronate or any component of the formulation; hypocalcemia; oral tablets are also contraindicated in patients unable to stand or sit upright for at least 60 minutes and in patients with abnormalities of the esophagus which delay esophageal emptying, such as stricture or achalasia

Pregnancy Risk Factor C

Lactation Excretion in breast milk unknown/use caution

Warnings/Precautions Hypocalcemia must be corrected before therapy initiation. Ensure adequate calcium and vitamin D intake. Osteonecrosis of the jaw (ONJ) has been reported in patients receiving bisphosphonates. Risk factors include invasive dental procedures (eg, tooth extraction, dental implants, boney surgery); a diagnosis of cancer, with concomitant chemotherapy or corticosteroids; poor oral hygiene, ill-fitting dentures; and comorbid disorders (anemia, coagulopathy, infection, pre-existing dental disease). Most reported cases occurred after I.V. bisphosphonate therapy; however, cases have been reported following oral therapy. A dental exam and preventative dentistry should be performed prior to placing patients with risk factors on chronic bisphosphonate therapy. The manufacturer's labeling states that discontinuing bisphosphonates in patients requiring invasive dental procedures may reduce the risk of ONJ. However, other experts suggest that there is no evidence that discontinuing therapy reduces the risk of developing ONJ (Assael, 2009). The benefit/risk must be assessed by the treating physician and/or dentist/surgeon prior to any invasive dental procedure. Patients developing ONJ while on bisphosphonates should receive care by an oral surgeon.

Atypical femur fractures have been reported in patients receiving bisphosphonates for treatment/prevention of osteoporosis. The fractures include subtrochanteric femur (bone just below the hip joint) and diaphyseal femur (long segment of the thigh bone). Some patients experience prodromal pain weeks or months before the fracture occurs. It is unclear if bisphosphonate therapy is the cause for these fractures, although the majority have been reported in patients taking bisphosphonates. Patients receiving long-term (>3-5 years) therapy may be at an increased risk. Discontinue bisphosphonate therapy in patients who develop a femoral shaft fracture.

Infrequently, severe (and occasionally debilitating) bone, joint, and/or muscle pain have been reported during bisphosphonate treatment. The onset of pain ranged from a single day to several months. Consider discontinuing therapy in patients who experience severe symptoms; symptoms usually resolve upon discontinuation. Some patients experienced recurrence when rechallenged with same drug or another bisphosphonate; avoid use in patients with a history of these symptoms in association with bisphosphonate therapy.

Oral bisphosphonates may cause dysphagia, esophagitis, esophageal or gastric ulcer; risk may increase in patients unable to comply with dosing instructions; discontinue use if new or worsening symptoms develop. Intravenous bisphosphonates may cause transient decreases in serum calcium and have also been associated with renal toxicity.

Use not recommended with severe renal impairment (Cl_{cr} <30 mL/minute).

Adverse Reactions Percentages vary based on frequency of administration (daily vs monthly). Unless specified, percentages are reported with oral use.

>10%:

- Gastrointestinal: Dyspepsia (6% to 12%)
- Neuromuscular & skeletal: Back pain (4% to 14%)

1% to 10%:

- Cardiovascular: Hypertension (6% to 7%)
- Central nervous system: Headache (3% to 7%), dizziness (1% to 4%), insomnia (1% to 2%)
- Dermatologic: Rash (1% to 2%)

Endocrine & metabolic: Hypercholesterolemia (5%)

Gastrointestinal: Abdominal pain (5% to 8%), diarrhea (4% to 7%), nausea (5%), constipation (3% to 4%), vomiting (3%)

Genitourinary: Urinary tract infection (2% to 6%)

Hepatic: Alkaline phosphatase decreased (frequency not defined)

Local: Injection site reaction (<2%)

Neuromuscular & skeletal: Pain in extremity (1% to 8%), arthralgia (4% to 6%), myalgia (1% to 6%), joint disorder (4%), osteonecrosis of the jaw (4%), weakness (4%), osteoarthritis (localized, 1% to 3%), muscle cramp (2%)

Respiratory: Bronchitis (3% to 10%), pneumonia (6%), pharyngitis/nasopharyngitis (3% to 4%), upper respiratory infection (2%)

Miscellaneous: Acute phase reaction (I.V. 10%; oral 3% to 9%), infection (4%), flu-like syndrome (1% to 4%), allergic reaction (3%)

Postmarketing and/or case reports: Anaphylaxis; angioedema; bronchospasm; diaphyseal femur fracture; esophageal cancer; hypocalcemia; incapacitating bone, joint, or muscle pain; iritis; ocular inflammation; scleritis; subtrochanteric femur fracture; uveitis

Drug Interactions

Metabolism/Transport Effects None known.

Avoid Concomitant Use There are no known interactions where it is recommended to avoid concomitant use.

Increased Effect/Toxicity

Ibandronate may increase the levels/effects of: Deferasirox; Phosphate Supplements; SUNItinib

The levels/effects of Ibandronate may be increased by: Aminoglycosides; Nonsteroidal Anti-Inflammatory Agents

Decreased Effect

The levels/effects of Ibandronate may be decreased by: Antacids; Calcium Salts; Iron Salts; Magnesium Salts; Multivitamins/Minerals (with ADEK, Folate, Iron); Proton Pump Inhibitors

Ethanol/Nutrition/Herb Interactions

Ethanol: Ethanol may increase risk of osteoporosis. Management: Avoid ethanol.

Food: May reduce absorption; mean oral bioavailability is decreased up to 90% when given with food. Management: Take with a full glass (6-8 oz) of plain water, at least 60 minutes prior to any food, beverages, or medications. Mineral water with a high calcium content should be avoided. Wait at least 60 minutes after taking ibandronate before taking anything else.

Storage/Stability Store at controlled room temperature of 25°C (77°F); excursions permitted to 15°C to 30°C (59°F to 86°F).

Mechanism of Action A bisphosphonate which inhibits bone resorption via actions on osteoclasts or on osteoclast precursors; decreases the rate of bone resorption, leading to an indirect increase in bone mineral density.

Pharmacodynamics/Kinetics

Distribution: Terminal V_d: 90 L; 40% to 50% of circulating ibandronate binds to bone

Protein binding: 85.7% to 99.5%

Metabolism: Not metabolized

Bioavailability: Oral: Minimal; reduced ~90% following standard breakfast

Half-life elimination:

Oral: 150 mg dose: Terminal: 37-157 hours

I.V.: Terminal: ~5-25 hours

Time to peak, plasma: Oral: 0.5-2 hours
Excretion: Urine (50% to 60% of absorbed dose, excreted as unchanged drug); feces (unabsorbed drug)

Dosing

Adult & Geriatric

Postmenopausal osteoporosis (treatment): Patients should receive supplemental calcium and vitamin D if dietary intake is inadequate
Oral: 150 mg once a month
I.V.: 3 mg every 3 months

Postmenopausal osteoporosis (prevention): Patients should receive supplemental calcium and vitamin D if dietary intake is inadequate: Oral: 150 mg once a month

Hypercalcemia of malignancy (unlabeled use): I.V.: 2-6 mg over 1-2 hours (Pecherstorfer, 2003; Ralston, 1997)

Metastatic bone disease due to breast cancer (unlabeled use): I.V.: 6 mg every 3-4 weeks (Diel, 2004)

Renal Impairment

Osteoporosis: Oral, I.V.:
Cl_{cr} ≥30 mL/minute: No dosage adjustment necessary.
Cl_{cr} <30 mL/minute: Use not recommended.
Oncologic uses (unlabeled): I.V.: Cl_{cr} <30 mL/minute: 2 mg every 3-4 weeks (von Moos, 2005)

Hepatic Impairment No dosage adjustment necessary.

Administration

Oral: Administer 60 minutes before the first food or drink of the day (other than water) and prior to taking any oral medications or supplements (eg, calcium, antacids, vitamins). Ibandronate should be taken in an upright position with a full glass (6-8 oz) of plain water and the patient should avoid lying down for 60 minutes to minimize the possibility of GI side effects. Mineral water with a high calcium content should be avoided. The tablet should be swallowed whole; do not chew or suck. Do not eat or drink anything (except water) for 60 minutes following administration of ibandronate.

Take on the same date each month. In case of a missed dose, do not take two 150 mg tablets within the same week. If the next scheduled dose is 1-7 days away, wait until the next scheduled dose to take the tablet. If the next scheduled dose is >7 days away, take the dose the morning it is remembered, and then resume taking the once-monthly dose on the originally scheduled day.

I.V.: Administer as a 15-30 second bolus. Do not mix with calcium-containing solutions or other drugs. For osteoporosis, do not administer more frequently than every 3 months. Infuse over 1 hour for metastatic bone disease due to breast cancer (Diel, 2004) and over 1-2 hours for hypercalcemia of malignancy (Pecherstorfer, 2003; Ralston, 1997).

Monitoring Parameters

Osteoporosis: Bone mineral density as measured by central dual-energy x-ray absorptiometry (DXA) of the hip or spine (prior to initiation of therapy and at least every 2 years); annual measurements of height and weight, assessment of chronic back pain; serum calcium and 25(OH)D; may consider measuring biochemical markers of bone turnover

Serum creatinine prior to each I.V. dose

Test Interactions Bisphosphonates may interfere with diagnostic imaging agents such as technetium-99m-diphosphonate in bone scans.

Dietary Considerations Ensure adequate calcium and vitamin D intake; women and men >50 years of age should consume 1200-1500 mg/day of elemental calcium and 800-1000 units/day of vitamin D. Ibandronate tablet should be taken with a full glass (6-8 oz) of plain water, at least 60 minutes prior to any food, beverages, or medications. Mineral water with a high calcium content should be avoided.

Medication Guide Available Yes

Dosage Forms Excipient information presented when available (limited, particularly for generics); consult specific product labeling.

Injection, solution:
  Boniva®: 1 mg/mL (3 mL)
Tablet, oral: 150 mg
  Boniva®: 150 mg [once-monthly formulation]

References

American Dental Association Council on Scientific Affairs, "Dental Management of Patients Receiving Oral Bisphosphonate Therapy: Expert Panel Recommendations," *J Am Dent Assoc*, 2006, 137(8):1144-50. Available at http://jada.ada.org/cgi/content/full/137/8/1144

Assael LA, "Oral Bisphosphonates as a Cause of Bisphosphonate-Related Osteonecrosis of the Jaws: Clinical Findings, Assessment of Risks, and Preventive Strategies," *J Oral Maxillofac Surg*, 2009, 67(5 Suppl):35-43.

Diel IJ, Body JJ, Lichinitser MR, et al, "Improved Quality of Life After Long-Term Treatment With the Bisphosphonate Ibandronate in Patients With Metastatic Bone Disease Due to Breast Cancer," *Eur J Cancer*, 2004, 40(11):1704-12.

Hillner BE, Ingle JN, Chlebowski RT, et al, "American Society of Clinical Oncology 2003 Update on the Role of Bisphosphonates and Bone Health Issues in Women With Breast Cancer," *J Clin Oncol*, 2003, 21(21):4042-57.

"Management of Osteoporosis in Postmenopausal Women: 2010 Position Statement of The North American Menopause Society," *Menopause*, 2010, 17(1):25-54.

Marx RE, Sawatari Y, Fortin M, et al, "Bisphosphonate-Induced Exposed Bone (Osteonecrosis/Osteopetrosis) of the Jaws: Risk Factors, Recognition, Prevention, and Treatment," *J Oral Maxillofac Surg*, 2005, 63(11):1567-75.

Mavrokokki T, Cheng A, Stein B, et al, "Nature and Frequency of Bisphosphonate-Associated Osteonecrosis of the Jaws in Australia," *J Oral Maxillofac Surg*, 2007, 65(3):415-23.

McCormack PL and Plosker GL, "Ibandronic Acid: A Review of its Use in the Treatment of Bone Metastases of Breast Cancer," *Drugs*, 2006, 66(5):711-28.

National Osteoporosis Foundation, "Clinician's Guide to Prevention and Treatment of Osteoporosis," Washington, DC, 2010. Available at http://www.nof.org

Pecherstorfer M, Steinhauer EU, Rizzoli R, et al, " Efficacy and Safety of Ibandronate in the Treatment of Hypercalcemia of Malignancy: A Randomized Multicentric Comparison to Pamidronate," *Support Care Cancer*, 2003, 11(8):539-47.

Ralston SH, Thiébaud D, Herrmann Z, et al, "Dose-Response Study of Ibandronate in the Treatment of Cancer-Associated Hypercalcaemia," *Br J Cancer*, 1997, 75(2):295-300.

Tripathy D, Body JJ, and Bergstrom B, "Review of Ibandronate in the Treatment of Metastatic Bone Disease: Experience From Phase III Trials," *Clin Ther*, 2004, 26(12):1947-59.

Van Poznak CH, Temin S, Yee GC, et al, "American Society of Clinical Oncology Executive Summary of the Clinical Practice Guideline Update on the Role of Bone-Modifying Agents in Metastatic Breast Cancer," *J Clin Oncol*, 2011, 29(9):1221-7.

Von Moos R, "Bisphosphonate Treatment Recommendations for Oncologists," *Oncologist*, 2005, 10 (Suppl 1):19-24.

Woitge HW, Oberwittler H, Heichel S, et al, "Short- and Long-Term Effects of Ibandronate Treatment on Bone Turnover in Paget Disease of Bone," *Clin Chem*, 2000, 46(5):684-90.

Wysowski DK, "Reports of Esophageal Cancer With Oral Bisphosphonate Use," *N Engl J Med*, 2009, 360(1):89-90.

◆ **Ibandronate Sodium** *see* Ibandronate *on page 739*

◆ **Ibandronic Acid** *see* Ibandronate *on page 739*

Ibritumomab (ib ri TYOO mo mab)

Related Information

Management of Drug Extravasations *on page 1800*

Safe Handling of Hazardous Drugs *on page 1904*

Brand Names: U.S. Zevalin®

Brand Names: Canada Zevalin®

Index Terms Ibritumomab Tiuxetan; IDEC-Y2B8; Y-90 Ibritumomab; Y-90 Zevalin

Generic Availability (U.S.) No

Pharmacologic Category Antineoplastic Agent, Monoclonal Antibody; Radiopharmaceutical

Use Treatment of relapsed or refractory low-grade or follicular B-cell non-Hodgkin's lymphoma (NHL); treatment of follicular NHL in patients (previously untreated) who achieve a response (partial or complete) to first-line chemotherapy

Labeled Contraindications There are no contraindications listed within the manufacturer's labeling.

Pregnancy Risk Factor D

Lactation Excretion in breast milk unknown/not recommended

Warnings/Precautions Radiopharmaceutical - use appropriate precautions for handling and disposal. **[U.S. Boxed Warning]: Severe cutaneous and mucocutaneous skin reactions have been reported (with fatalities) in postmarketing experience. Discontinue all components of the therapeutic regimen in patients experiencing severe cutaneous or mucocutaneous skin reactions,** including erythema multiforme, Stevens-Johnson syndrome, toxic epidermal necrolysis, bullous dermatitis, and exfoliative dermatitis. Onset may occur within days to 4 months following infusion.

To be used as part of the Zevalin® therapeutic regimen (in combination with rituximab). **[U.S. Boxed Warning]: Do not exceed the Y-90 ibritumomab maximum allowable dose of 32 mCi (1184 MBq).** Use should be reserved to physicians and other professionals qualified and experienced in the safe handling of radiopharmaceuticals, and in monitoring and emergency treatment of infusion reactions. The contents of the kit are not radioactive until radiolabeling occurs. During and after radiolabeling, adequate shielding should be used with this product, minimize radiation exposure (to patient and healthcare professionals) in accordance with institutional radiation safety practices.

[U.S. Boxed Warning]: Serious fatal infusion reactions may occur with the rituximab component of the therapeutic regimen; immediately stop infusion and discontinue in patients who develop severe infusion reactions. Fatalities due to rituximab infusion were associated with acute respiratory distress syndrome, hypoxia, pulmonary infiltrates, cardiogenic shock, MI, or ventricular fibrillation. Infusion reactions typically occur with the first rituximab infusion (onset within 30-120 minutes). Reactions may also include angioedema, bronchospasm, and urticaria. Less severe reactions may be managed by slowing or interrupting infusion.

[U.S. Boxed Warning]: Delayed, prolonged, and severe cytopenias (thrombocytopenia and neutropenia) are common. Do not administer to patients with ≥25% lymphoma marrow involvement, patients with impaired bone marrow reserve (eg, prior myeloablative treatment, platelet count <100,000/mm^3, neutrophil count <1500/mm^3, hypocellular marrow), or to patients with prior stem cell collection failure. Cytopenias may persist beyond

12 weeks. Patients with mild baseline thrombocytopenia may experience higher incidences of severe neutropenia and thrombocytopenia. Hemorrhage may occur due to thrombocytopenia; avoid concomitant use of medications interfering with coagulation or platelet function. Closely monitor patients for complications of cytopenias (eg, febrile neutropenia, hemorrhage) for up to 3 months after administration.

Secondary malignancies (acute myelogenous leukemia and/or myelodysplastic syndrome) have been reported following use; the median time to diagnosis (secondary malignancy) following ibritumomab treatment was 1.9 years (range: 0.4-6.3 years). Product contains albumin, which confers a theoretical risk of transmission of viral disease or Creutzfeldt-Jakob disease. The safety of immunization with live vaccines following ibritumomab therapy has not been studied; do not administer live viral vaccines to patients who have recently received ibritumomab treatment; the ability to generate a response to any vaccine after receiving treatment has not been studied. Infusion site erythema and ulceration have been reported following extravasation; monitor infusion site; promptly terminate infusion with symptoms/signs of extravasation (restart in another limb). There is a case report of (delayed) erythema and ulceration, which is described as radiation necrosis following yttrium-90-ibritumomab extravasation (Williams, 2006). Delayed (up to 1 month) radiation injury has occurred in or near areas of lymphomatous involvement.

Adverse Reactions

>10%:

- Central nervous system: Fatigue (33%), fever (10%)
- Gastrointestinal: Nausea (18%), abdominal pain (17%), diarrhea (11%)
- Hematologic: Thrombocytopenia (62% to 95%; grades 3/4: 51% to 63%; nadir: 49-53 days; median duration: 24 days; median time to recovery: 13 days), neutropenia (45% to 77%; grades 3/4: 41% to 60%; nadir: 61-62 days; median duration: 22 days; median time to recovery: 12 days), anemia (22% to 61%; grades 3/4: 5% to 17%; nadir: 68-69 days), leukopenia (43%; grades 3/4: 36%), lymphopenia (26%; grades 3/4: 18%)
- Neuromuscular & skeletal: Weakness (15%)
- Respiratory: Nasopharyngitis (19%), cough (11%)
- Miscellaneous: Infection (29%; serious 1% to 3%)

1% to 10%:

- Cardiovascular: Hypertension (7%)
- Central nervous system: Dizziness (7%)
- Dermatologic: Petechiae (8%), bruising (7%), pruritus (7%), rash (7%)
- Gastrointestinal: Anorexia (8%)
- Genitourinary: Urinary tract infection (7%)
- Hematologic: Secondary malignancies (1% to 8%; includes acute myelogenous leukemia and myelodysplastic syndrome), prolonged cytopenia (severe: 5%)
- Neuromuscular & skeletal: Myalgia (9%)
- Respiratory: Bronchitis (8%), rhinitis (8%), pharyngolaryngeal pain (7%), sinusitis (7%), epistaxis (5%)
- Miscellaneous: Flu-like syndrome (8%), night sweats (8%), HAMA antibody formation (1% to 3%), biodistribution altered (1%)

<1%, postmarketing, and/or case reports: Acute respiratory distress syndrome, angioedema, cardiogenic shock, chills, cutaneous and mucocutaneous reactions (eg, erythema multiforme, Stevens-Johnson syndrome, toxic epidermal necrolysis, bullous dermatitis and exfoliative dermatitis); dyspnea, headache, hypoxia, infusion reaction, infusion site erythema/ulceration (following

extravasation), MI, neutropenic fever, pain, pulmonary infiltrates, radiation injury/complications (delayed [~1 month]; in tissues in or near areas of lymphomatous involvement); radiation necrosis (following Yttrium-90-ibritumomab extravasation), sepsis, ventricular fibrillation, vomiting

Drug Interactions

Metabolism/Transport Effects None known.

Avoid Concomitant Use

Avoid concomitant use of Ibritumomab with any of the following: BCG; CloZAPine; Natalizumab; Pimecrolimus; Tacrolimus (Topical); Vaccines (Live)

Increased Effect/Toxicity

Ibritumomab may increase the levels/effects of: CloZAPine; Leflunomide; Natalizumab; Vaccines (Live); Vitamin K Antagonists

The levels/effects of Ibritumomab may be increased by: Anticoagulants; Antiplatelet Agents; Denosumab; Pimecrolimus; Roflumilast; Tacrolimus (Topical); Trastuzumab

Decreased Effect

Ibritumomab may decrease the levels/effects of: BCG; Cardiac Glycosides; Coccidioidin Skin Test; Sipuleucel-T; Vaccines (Inactivated); Vaccines (Live); Vitamin K Antagonists

The levels/effects of Ibritumomab may be decreased by: Echinacea

Ethanol/Nutrition/Herb Interactions Herb/Nutraceutical: Avoid echinacea (may diminish therapeutic effect). Avoid cat's claw, dong quai, evening primrose, feverfew, garlic, ginger, ginkgo, red clover, horse chestnut, green tea, ginseng (all have antiplatelet activity).

Storage/Stability Store at 2°C to 8°C (36°F to 46°F); do not freeze. Administer Y-90 ibritumomab within 8 hours of radiolabeling.

Reconstitution To prepare radiolabeled injection, follow preparation guidelines provided by manufacturer.

Mechanism of Action Ibritumomab is a monoclonal antibody directed against the CD20 antigen found on pre-B and mature B lymphocytes (normal and malignant). Ibritumomab binding induces apoptosis in B lymphocytes *in vitro*. It is combined with the chelator tiuxetan, which acts as a specific chelation site for Yttrium-90 (Y-90). The monoclonal antibody acts as a delivery system to direct the radioactive isotope to the targeted cells, however, binding has been observed in lymphoid cells throughout the body and in lymphoid nodules in organs such as the large and small intestines. Beta-emission induces cellular damage through the formation of free radicals (in both target cells and surrounding cells).

Pharmacodynamics/Kinetics

Duration: B cell recovery begins in ~12 weeks; generally in normal range within 9 months

Distribution: To lymphoid cells throughout the body and in lymphoid nodules in organs such as the large and small intestines, spleen, testes, and liver

Metabolism: Has not been characterized; the product of yttrium-90 radioactive decay is zirconium-90 (nonradioactive)

Half-life elimination: Y-90 ibritumomab: 30 hours; Yttrium-90 decays with a physical half-life of 64 hours

Excretion: A median of 7.2% of the radiolabeled activity was excreted in urine over 7 days

Dosing

Adult & Geriatric Note: Premedication with oral acetaminophen 650 mg and oral diphenhydramine 50 mg is recommended prior to **each** rituximab infusion. Ibritumomab is administered **only** as part of the Zevalin® therapeutic regimen (a combined treatment regimen with rituximab). Allow at least 6 weeks, but no more than 12 weeks following first-line chemotherapy before treatment initiation; platelets should recover to ≥150,000/mm^3 prior to initiation of treatment regimen. The regimen consists of two steps:

Non-Hodgkin's lymphoma, B-cell (relapsed or refractory low-grade, follicular): I.V.: Ibritumomab is administered **only** as part of the Zevalin® therapeutic regimen (a combined treatment regimen with rituximab). The regimen consists of two steps:

Day 1:

Rituximab: 250 mg/m^2 at an initial rate of 50 mg/hour. If hypersensitivity or infusion-related events do not occur, increase infusion in increments of 50 mg/hour every 30 minutes, to a maximum of 400 mg/hour. Stop rituximab and discontinue regimen for severe infusion reaction. For less severe infusion reactions, temporarily slow or interrupt; the infusion may be resumed at one-half the previous rate upon improvement of symptoms.

Day 7, 8, or 9 of treatment:

Rituximab: 250 mg/m^2 at an initial rate of 100 mg/hour (50 mg/hour if infusion-related events occurred with the day 1 infusion). If hypersensitivity or infusion-related events do not occur, increase infusion in increments of 100 mg/hour every 30 minutes, to a maximum of 400 mg/hour, as tolerated (increase in 50 mg/hour increments if initial infusion rate was 50 mg/hour).

Y-90 ibritumomab: Within 4 hours of the completion of rituximab infusion:

Platelet count ≥150,000 cells/mm^3: Inject 0.4 mCi/kg (14.8 MBq/kg) actual body weight over 10 minutes; maximum dose: 32 mCi (1184 MBq)

Platelet count between 100,000-149,000 cells/mm^3 (in relapsed or refractory patients): Inject 0.3 mCi/kg (11.1 MBq/kg) actual body weight over 10 minutes; maximum dose: 32 mCi (1184 MBq)

Platelet count <100,000 cells/mm^3: Do **not** administer

Maximum dose: The prescribed, measured, and administered dose of Y-90 ibritumomab must not exceed 32 mCi (1184 MBq), regardless of the patient's body weight

Administration

Rituximab: Administer the first infusion of rituximab at an initial rate of 50 mg/hour. If hypersensitivity or infusion-related events do not occur, escalate the infusion rate in 50 mg/hour increments every 30 minutes, to a maximum of 400 mg/hour. Immediately stop infusion for severe infusion reaction (discontinue ibritumomab regimen); less severe reactions may be managed by slowing or interrupting infusion. For less severe reactions, infusion may continue at one-half the previous rate upon improvement of patient symptoms. If infusion reaction did not occur in initial rituximab infusion, subsequent rituximab infusion can be administered at an initial rate of 100 mg/hour and increased in 100 mg/hour increments at 30-minute intervals, to a maximum of 400 mg/hour as tolerated. If infusion reaction occurred with initial rituximab infusion, initiate at 50 mg/hour with increases of 50 mg/hour increments.

Y-90 ibritumomab: Inject slowly, over 10 minutes through a 0.22 micron low protein binding in-line filter (filter placed between syringe and infusion port). After injection, flush line with at least 10 mL normal saline. Establish free-flowing I.V. line prior to administration. Avoid extravasation; closely monitor infusion site; if signs or symptoms of extravasation occur, stop infusion and restart in another limb.

Vesicant/Extravasation Risk May be an irritant; there is an isolated case report of (delayed) erythema and ulceration, which is described as radiation necrosis following yttrium-90-ibritumomab extravasation (Williams, 2006).

Monitoring Parameters Patients must be monitored for infusion-related allergic reactions (typically within 30-120 minutes of administration). Monitor for extravasation during ibritumomab infusion. Obtain CBC with differential and platelet counts weekly until recovery, or as clinically indicated. Platelet count must be obtained prior to Day 7, 8, or 9. Monitor for cytopenias (and related complications) for up to 3 months after use.

Additional Information Ibritumomab tiuxetan is produced in Chinese hamster ovary cell cultures. Kit is not radioactive. Radiolabeling of ibritumomab with Yttrium-90 must be performed by appropriate personnel in a specialized facility.

Dosage Forms Excipient information presented when available (limited, particularly for generics); consult specific product labeling.

Injection, solution [preservative free]:

Zevalin®: 1.6 mg/mL (2 mL)

References

Czuczman MS, Emmanouilides C, Darif M, et al, "Treatment-Related Myelodysplastic Syndrome and Acute Myelogenous Leukemia in Patients Treated With Ibritumomab Tiuxetan Radioimmunotherapy," *J Clin Oncol*, 2007, 25(27):4285-92.

Gordon LI, Molina A, Witzig T, et al, "Durable Responses after Ibritumomab Tiuxetan Radioimmunotherapy for CD20+ B-Cell Lymphoma: Long-Term Follow-Up of a Phase 1/2 Study," *Blood*, 2004, 103(12):4429-31.

Williams G, Palmer MR, Parker JA, et al, "Extravasation of Therapeutic Yttrium-90-Ibritumomab Tiuxetan (Zevalin®): A Case Report," *Cancer Biother Radiopharm*, 2006, 21(2):101-5.

Witzig TE, Gordon LI, Cabanillas F, et al, "Randomized Controlled Trial of Yttrium-90-Labeled Ibritumomab Tiuxetan Radioimmunotherapy Versus Rituximab Immunotherapy for Patients With Relapsed or Refractory Low-Grade, Follicular, or Transformed B-Cell Non-Hodgkin's Lymphoma," *J Clin Oncol*, 2002, 20(10):2453-63.

Witzig TE, White CA, Gordon LI, et al, "Safety of Yttrium-90 Ibritumomab Tiuxetan Radioimmunotherapy for Relapsed Low-Grade, Follicular, or Transformed Non-Hodgkin's Lymphoma," *J Clin Oncol*, 2003, 21(7):1263-70.

Witzig TE, White CA, Wiseman GA, et al, "Phase I/II Trial of IDEC-Y2B8 Radioimmunotherapy for Treatment of Relapsed or Refractory CD20(+) B-Cell Non-Hodgkin's Lymphoma," *J Clin Oncol*, 1999, 17(12):3793-803.

◆ **Ibritumomab Tiuxetan** *see* Ibritumomab *on page* 744

◆ **ICI-182,780** *see* Fulvestrant *on page* 651

◆ **ICI-46474** *see* Tamoxifen *on page* 1324

◆ **ICI-118630** *see* Goserelin *on page* 683

◆ **ICI-176334** *see* Bicalutamide *on page* 178

◆ **ICI-D1033** *see* Anastrozole *on page* 96

◆ **ICI-D1694** *see* Raltitrexed *on page* 1226

◆ **ICL670** *see* Deferasirox *on page* 407

◆ **ICRF-187** *see* Dexrazoxane *on page* 448

◆ **Idamycin® (Can)** *see* IDArubicin *on page* 749

◆ **Idamycin PFS®** *see* IDArubicin *on page* 749

IDArubicin (eye da ROO bi sin)

Related Information

Management of Chemotherapy-Induced Nausea and Vomiting *on page 1786*
Management of Drug Extravasations *on page 1800*
Safe Handling of Hazardous Drugs *on page 1904*

Brand Names: U.S. Idamycin PFS®

Brand Names: Canada Idamycin®

Index Terms 4-Demethoxydaunorubicin; 4-DMDR; Idarubicin Hydrochloride; IDR; IMI 30; SC 33428

Generic Availability (U.S.) Yes

Pharmacologic Category Antineoplastic Agent, Anthracycline; Antineoplastic Agent, Antibiotic

Use Treatment of acute myeloid leukemia (AML)

Unlabeled Use Acute lymphocytic leukemia (ALL)

Labeled Contraindications Hypersensitivity to idarubicin, other anthracyclines, or any component of the formulation; bilirubin >5 mg/dL

Pregnancy Risk Factor D

Lactation Excretion in breast milk unknown/not recommended

Warnings/Precautions Hazardous agent - use appropriate precautions for handling and disposal. **[U.S. Boxed Warning]: May cause myocardial toxicity (HF, arrhythmias or cardiomyopathies) and is more common in patients who have previously received anthracyclines or have pre-existing cardiac disease.** The risk of myocardial toxicity is also increased in patients with concomitant or prior mediastinal/pericardial irradiation, patients with anemia, bone marrow depression, infections, leukemic pericarditis or myocarditis. Monitor cardiac function during treatment.

[U.S. Boxed Warnings]: May cause severe myelosuppression; use caution in patients with pre-existing myelosuppression from prior treatment or radiation. Use caution with renal or hepatic impairment; may required dosage reductions. For I.V. administration only; may cause severe local tissue damage and necrosis if extravasation occurs. Rapid lysis of leukemic cells may lead to hyperuricemia. Systemic infections should be managed prior to initiation of treatment. **[U.S. Boxed Warning]: Should be administered under the supervision of an experienced cancer chemotherapy physician. Safety and efficacy in children have not been established.**

Adverse Reactions

>10%:

Cardiovascular: CHF (dose related), transient ECG abnormalities (supraventricular tachycardia, S-T wave changes, atrial or ventricular extrasystoles), generally asymptomatic and self-limiting. The relative cardiotoxicity of idarubicin compared to doxorubicin is unclear. Some investigators report no increase in cardiac toxicity for adults at cumulative oral idarubicin doses up to 540 mg/m^2; other reports suggest a maximum cumulative intravenous dose of 150 mg/m^2.

Central nervous system: Headache

Dermatologic: Alopecia (25% to 30%), radiation recall, skin rash (11%), urticaria

Gastrointestinal: Nausea, vomiting (30% to 60%); diarrhea (9% to 22%); stomatitis (11%); GI hemorrhage (30%)

Genitourinary: Discoloration of urine (darker yellow)

Hematologic: Myelosuppression (nadir: 10-15 days; recovery: 21-28 days), primarily leukopenia; thrombocytopenia and anemia. Effects are generally less severe with oral dosing.

Hepatic: Bilirubin and transaminases increased (44%)

1% to 10%:

Central nervous system: Seizure

Neuromuscular & skeletal: Peripheral neuropathy

<1%, postmarketing, and/or case reports: Cardiomyopathy, hyperuricemia, myocarditis, neutropenic typhlitis

Drug Interactions

Metabolism/Transport Effects Substrate of P-glycoprotein

Avoid Concomitant Use

Avoid concomitant use of IDArubicin with any of the following: BCG; CloZAPine; Natalizumab; Pimecrolimus; Tacrolimus (Topical); Vaccines (Live)

Increased Effect/Toxicity

IDArubicin may increase the levels/effects of: CloZAPine; Leflunomide; Natalizumab; Vaccines (Live)

The levels/effects of IDArubicin may be increased by: Bevacizumab; Denosumab; P-glycoprotein/ABCB1 Inhibitors; Pimecrolimus; Roflumilast; Tacrolimus (Topical); Taxane Derivatives; Trastuzumab

Decreased Effect

IDArubicin may decrease the levels/effects of: BCG; Cardiac Glycosides; Coccidioidin Skin Test; Sipuleucel-T; Vaccines (Inactivated); Vaccines (Live)

The levels/effects of IDArubicin may be decreased by: Cardiac Glycosides; Echinacea; P-glycoprotein/ABCB1 Inducers

Storage/Stability Store intact vials of solution under refrigeration at 2°C to 8°C (36°F to 46°F). Protect from light. Solutions diluted in D_5W or NS for infusion are stable for 4 weeks at room temperature, protected from light. Syringe and IVPB solutions are stable for 72 hours at room temperature and 7 days under refrigeration.

Mechanism of Action Similar to doxorubicin and daunorubicin; inhibition of DNA and RNA synthesis by intercalation between DNA base pairs

Pharmacodynamics/Kinetics

Absorption: Oral: Variable (4% to 77%; mean: ~30%)

Distribution: V_d: 64 L/kg (some reports indicate 2250 L); extensive tissue binding; CSF

Protein binding: 94% to 97%

Metabolism: Hepatic to idarubicinol (pharmacologically active)

Half-life elimination: Oral: 14-35 hours; I.V.: 12-27 hours

Time to peak, serum: 1-5 hours

Excretion:

Oral: Urine (~5% of dose; 0.5% to 0.7% as unchanged drug, 4% as idarubicinol); hepatic (8%)

I.V.: Urine (13% as idarubicinol, 3% as unchanged drug); hepatic (17%)

Dosing

Adult & Geriatric Refer to individual protocols.

AML: I.V.:

Induction: 12 mg/m^2/day for 3 days

Consolidation: 10-12 mg/m^2/day for 2 days

Pediatric AML (unlabeled use): I.V.: 10-12 mg/m^2 once daily for 3 days every 3 weeks.

Renal Impairment The FDA-approved labeling does not contain specific dosing adjustment guidelines; however, it does reccomend that dosage reductions be made. Patients with S_{cr}: ≥2 mg/dL did not receive treatment in many clinical trials. The following guidelines have been used by some clinicians (Aronoff, 2007):

Children:

- Cl_{cr} <50 mL/minute: Administer 75% of dose.
- Hemodialysis: Administer 75% of dose.
- Continuous ambulatory peritoneal dialysis (CAPD): Administer 75% of dose.
- Continuous renal replacement therapy (CRRT): Administer 75% of dose.

Adults:

- Cl_{cr} 10-50 mL/minute: Administer 75% of dose.
- Cl_{cr} <10 mL/minute: Administer 50% of dose.
- Hemodialysis: Supplemental dose not needed.
- Continuous ambulatory peritoneal dialysis (CAPD): Supplemental dose not needed.

Hepatic Impairment

Bilirubin 2.6-5 mg/dL: Administer 50% of dose

Bilirubin >5 mg/dL: Avoid use

Combination Regimens

Leukemia, acute myeloid:

- 5 + 2 (Cytarabine-Idarubicin) (AML Consolidation) on page 1512
- 7 + 3 (Cytarabine-Idarubicin) (AML Induction) on page 1514
- FLAG-IDA on page 1641

Leukemia, acute promyelocytic: Tretinoin-Idarubicin (APL) on page 1764

Administration Do not administer I.M. or SubQ; administer as slow push over 3-5 minutes, preferably into the side of a freely-running saline or dextrose infusion **or** as intermittent infusion over 10-15 minutes into a free-flowing I.V. solution of NS or D_5W; also occasionally administered as a bladder lavage.

Extravasation management: Topical cooling may be achieved using ice packs or cooling pad with circulating ice water. Cooling of site for 24 hours as tolerated by the patient. Elevate and rest extremity 24-48 hours, then resume normal activity as tolerated. Application of cold inhibits vesicant's cytotoxicity. **Application of heat can be harmful and is contraindicated.** If pain, erythema, and/or swelling persist beyond 48 hours, refer patient immediately to plastic surgeon for consultation and possible debridement.

Emetic Potential Moderate (30% to 90%)

Vesicant/Extravasation Risk Vesicant; see Management of Drug Extravasations on page 1800.

Monitoring Parameters CBC with differential, platelet count, cardiac function, serum electrolytes, creatinine, uric acid, ALT, AST, bilirubin, signs of extravasation

Dosage Forms Excipient information presented when available (limited, particularly for generics); consult specific product labeling.

Injection, solution, as hydrochloride [preservative free]: 1 mg/mL (5 mL, 10 mL, 20 mL)

Idamycin PFS®: 1 mg/mL (5 mL, 10 mL, 20 mL)

References

Aronoff GR, Bennett WM, Berns JS, et al, *Drug Prescribing in Renal Failure: Dosing Guidelines for Adults and Children*, 5th ed. Philadelphia, PA: American College of Physicians; 2007, p 100, 172.

Berman E, "A Review of Idarubicin in Acute Leukemia," *Oncology*, 1993, 7(10):91-8, 104.

Blijlevens NM, Donnelly JP, and de Pauw BE, "Prospective Evaluation of Gut Mucosal Barrier Injury Following Various Myeloablative Regimens for Haematopoietic Stem Cell Transplant," *Bone Marrow Transplant*, 2005, 35:707-11.

Ferrara F, Palmieri S, Annunziata M, et al, "Continuous Infusion Idarubicin and Oral Busulfan as Conditioning for Patients With Acute Myeloid Leukemia Aged Over 60 Years Undergoing Autologous Stem Cell Transplantation," *Bone Marrow Transplant*, 2004, 34(7):73-576.

Mengarelli A, Iori AP, Guglielmi C, et al, "Idarubicin Intensified BUCY2 Regimen in Allogeneic Unmanipulated Transplant for High-Risk Hematological Malignancies," *Leukemia*, 2000, 14 (12):2052-8.

Morgan C, Tillett T, Braybrooke J, et al, "Management of Uncommon Chemotherapy-Induced Emergencies," *Lancet Oncol*, 2011, 12(8):806-14.

◆ **Idarubicin Hydrochloride** *see* IDArubicin *on page 749*

◆ **IDEC-C2B8** *see* RiTUXimab *on page 1244*

◆ **IDEC-Y2B8** *see* Ibritumomab *on page 744*

◆ **IDR** *see* IDArubicin *on page 749*

◆ **Ifex** *see* Ifosfamide *on page 752*

Ifosfamide (eye FOSS fa mide)

Related Information

Management of Chemotherapy-Induced Nausea and Vomiting *on page 1786*

Management of Drug Extravasations *on page 1800*

Safe Handling of Hazardous Drugs *on page 1904*

Brand Names: U.S. Ifex

Brand Names: Canada Ifex

Index Terms Isophosphamide; Z4942

Generic Availability (U.S.) Yes

Pharmacologic Category Antineoplastic Agent, Alkylating Agent; Antineoplastic Agent, Alkylating Agent (Nitrogen Mustard)

Use

U.S. labeling: Treatment (third-line) of germ cell testicular cancer (in combination with other chemotherapy drugs and with concurrent mesna)

Canadian labeling (not approved indications in the U.S.): Treatment of soft tissue sarcoma, pancreatic cancer (relapsed or refractory), cervical cancer (advanced or recurrent; as monotherapy or in combination with cisplatin and bleomycin)

Unlabeled Use Treatment of bladder cancer (metastatic), cervical cancer (recurrent or metastatic), head and neck cancers (recurrent or metastatic), ovarian cancer, small cell lung cancer (relapsed), Hodgkin lymphoma (relapsed or refractory), non-Hodgkin lymphomas, thymomas and thymic cancers (advanced), sarcomas (Ewing's sarcoma, osteosarcoma, and soft tissue sarcoma)

Labeled Contraindications Hypersensitivity to ifosfamide or any component of the formulation; urinary outflow obstruction

Canadian labeling: Additional contraindications (not in U.S. labeling): Severe myelosuppression; severe renal or hepatic impairment; active infection (bacterial, fungal, viral); severe immunosuppression; urinary tract disease (eg, cystitis); advanced cerebral arteriosclerosis

Pregnancy Risk Factor D

Lactation Enters breast milk/not recommended

Warnings/Precautions Hazardous agent: Use appropriate precautions for handling and disposal. **[U.S. Boxed Warning]: Hemorrhagic cystitis may occur; concomitant mesna reduces the risk of hemorrhagic cystitis.**

Hydration (at least 2 L/day), dose fractionation, and/or mesna administration will reduce the incidence of hematuria and protect against hemorrhagic cystitis. Obtain urinalysis prior to each dose; if microscopic hematuria is detected, withhold until complete resolution. Exclude or correct urinary tract obstructions prior to treatment. Use with caution (if at all) in patients with active urinary tract infection. Hemorrhagic cystitis is dose-dependent and is increased with high single doses (compared with fractionated doses); past or concomitant bladder radiation or busulfan treatment may increase the risk for hemorrhagic cystitis. **[U.S. Boxed Warning]: May cause severe nephrotoxicity, resulting in renal failure.** Acute and chronic renal failure as well as renal parenchymal and tubular necrosis (including acute) have been reported; tubular damage may be delayed and may persist. Renal manifestations include decreased glomerular rate, increased creatinine, proteinuria, enzymuria, cylindruria, aminoaciduria, phosphaturia, and glycosuria. Syndrome of inappropriate antidiuretic hormone (SIADH), renal rickets, and Fanconi syndrome have been reported. Evaluate renal function prior to and during treatment; monitor urine for erythrocytes and signs of urotoxicity.

[U.S. Boxed Warning]: May cause CNS toxicity which may be severe, resulting in encephalopathy and death; monitor for CNS toxicity; discontinue for encephalopathy. Symptoms of CNS toxicity (somnolence, confusion, dizziness, disorientation, hallucinations, cranial nerve dysfunction, psychotic behavior, extrapyramidal symptoms, seizures, coma blurred vision, and/or incontinence) have been observed within a few hours to a few days after initial dose and generally resolve within 2-3 days of treatment discontinuation (although may persist longer); maintain supportive care until complete resolution. Risk factors may include hypoalbuminemia, renal dysfunction, and prior history of ifosfamide-induced encephalopathy. Concomitant centrally-acting medications may result in additive CNS effects. Peripheral neuropathy has been reported.

[U.S. Boxed Warning]: Severe bone marrow suppression may occur (dose-limiting toxicity); monitor blood counts before and after each cycle. Leukopenia, neutropenia, thrombocytopenia and anemia are associated with ifosfamide. Myelosuppression is dose dependent, increased with single high doses (compared to fractionated doses) and increased with decreased renal function. Severe myelosuppression may occur when administered in combination with other chemotherapy agents or radiation therapy. Use with caution in patients with compromised bone marrow reserve. Unless clinically necessary, avoid administering to patients with WBC $<2000/mm^3$ and platelets $<50,000/mm^3$. Antimicrobial prophylaxis may be necessary in some neutropenic patients; Administer antibiotics and/or antifungal agents for neutropenic fever. May cause significant suppression of the immune responses; may lead to serious infection, sepsis or septic shock; reported infections have included bacterial, viral, fungal, and parasitic; latent infections may be reactivated; use with caution with other immunosuppressants or in patients with infection.

Arrhythmias, ST-segment or T-wave changes, cardiomyopathy, pericardial effusion, pericarditis, and epicardial fibrosis have been observed; the risk for cardiotoxicity is dose-dependent; concomitant cardiotoxic agents (eg, anthracyclines), irradiation of the cardiac region, and renal impairment may also increase the risk; use with caution in patients with cardiac risk factors or preexisting cardiac disease. Interstitial pneumonitis, pulmonary fibrosis, and pulmonary toxicity leading to respiratory failure have been reported; monitor for signs and symptoms of pulmonary toxicity.

Anaphylactic/anaphylactoid reactions have been associated with ifosfamide; cross sensitivity with similar agents may occur. Hepatic sinusoidal obstruction syndrome (SOS), formerly called veno-occlusive disease (VOD), has been reported with ifosfamide-containing regimens. Secondary malignancies may occur; the risk for myelodysplastic syndrome (which may progress to acute leukemia) is increased with treatment. May interfere with wound healing. Use with caution in patients with prior radiation therapy.

Adverse Reactions

>10%:

Central nervous system: CNS toxicity or encephalopathy (12% to 15%)
Dermatologic: Alopecia (83% to 90%; 100% with combination therapy)
Endocrine & metabolic: Metabolic acidosis (31%)
Gastrointestinal: Nausea/vomiting (47% to 58%)
Hematologic: Leukopenia (50% to ≤100%; grade 4: ≤50%; nadir: 8-14 days), anemia (38%), thrombocytopenia (20%; grades 3/4: ≤8%)
Renal: Hematuria (6% to 92%; reduced with mesna; grade 2 [gross hematuria]: 8% to 12%)

1% to 10%:

Central nervous system: Fever (1%)
Gastrointestinal: Anorexia (1%)
Hematologic: Neutropenic fever (1%)
Hepatic: Bilirubin increased (2% to 3%), liver dysfunction (2% to 3%), transaminases increased (2% to 3%)
Local: Phlebitis (2% to 3%)
Renal: Renal impairment (6%)
Miscellaneous: Infection (8% to 10%)

<1%, postmarketing, and/or case reports: Abdominal pain, acute renal failure, acute respiratory distress syndrome, acute tubular necrosis, agranulocytosis, alkaline phosphatase increased, allergic reaction, alveolitis (allergic), amenorrhea, aminoaciduria, amnesia, anaphylactic reaction, angina, angioedema, anuria, arrhythmia, arthralgia, asterixis, atrial ectopy, atrial fibrillation, atrial flutter, azoospermia, bladder irritation, bleeding, blurred vision, bone marrow failure, bradycardia, bradyphrenia, bronchospasm, bundle branch block, BUN increased, capillary leak syndrome, cardiac arrest, cardiogenic shock, cardiomyopathy, cardiotoxicity, catatonia, cecitis, chest pain, chills, cholestasis, chronic renal failure, coagulopathy, colitis, conjunctivitis, constipation, cough, creatinine clearance decreased/increased, creatinine increased, cylindruria, cytolytic hepatitis, delirium, delusion, dermatitis, diarrhea, disseminated intravascular coagulation, DVT, dysarthria, dysesthesia, dyspnea, dysuria, echolalia, edema, ejection fraction decreased, enterocolitis, enuresis, enzymuria, erythema, estrogen decreased, extrapyramidal disorder, facial swelling, Fanconi syndrome, fatigue, fecal incontinence, flushing, gait disturbance, gastrointestinal hemorrhage, GGT increased, glycosuria, gonadotropin increased, granulocytopenia, growth retardation (children), hearing loss, heart failure, hemolytic anemia, hemolytic uremic syndrome, hemorrhagic cystitis, hepatic failure, hepatic sinusoidal obstruction syndrome (SOS; formerly veno-occlusive disease [VOD]), hepatitis fulminant, hepatitis (viral), hepatorenal syndrome, herpes zoster, hyperglycemia, hyperhidrosis, hyper-/hypotension, hyperpigmentation, hypersensitivity reactions, hypesthesia, hypocalcemia, hypokalemia, hyponatremia, hypophosphatemia, hypoxia, ileus, immunosuppression, infertility, infusion site reactions (erythema, inflammation, pain, pruritus, swelling, tenderness), interstitial lung disease, interstitial pneumonitis, jaundice, LDH increased,

leukoencephalopathy, limb pain, logorrhea, lymphopenia, malaise, mania, mental status change, methemoglobinemia, MI, mucosal inflammation/ulceration, multiorgan failure, muscle twitching, mutism, myalgia, myocardial hemorrhage, myocarditis, nail disorder, nephrogenic diabetes insipidus, neuralgia, neutropenia, oligospermia, oliguria, osteomalacia (adults), ovarian failure, ovulation disorder, pain, palmar-plantar erythrodysesthesia syndrome, pancreatitis, pancytopenia, panic attack, paranoia, paresthesia, pericardial effusion, pericarditis, peripheral neuropathy, petechiae, phosphaturia, physical deterioration (general), pleural effusion, *Pneumocystis jiroveci* pneumonia, pneumonia, pneumonitis, pollakiuria, polydipsia, polyneuropathy, polyuria, portal vein thrombosis, premature atrial contractions, premature menopause, progressive multifocal leukoencephalopathy, proteinuria, pruritus, pulmonary edema, pulmonary embolism, pulmonary fibrosis, pulmonary hypertension, QRS complex abnormal, radiation recall dermatitis, rash (including macular and papular), renal parenchymal damage, renal tubular acidosis, respiratory failure, reversible posterior leukoencephalopathy syndrome (RPLS), rhabdomyolysis, rickets, salivation, secondary malignancy (including ALL, AML, APL, lymphoma, MDS, RCC, sarcomas, thyroid cancer), seizures, sepsis, septic shock, SIADH, skin necrosis, spermatogenesis impaired, status epilepticus, sterility, Stevens-Johnson syndrome, stomatitis, ST-segment abnormal, supraventricular extrasystoles, tachycardia, tinnitus, toxic epidermal necrolysis, tubulointerstitial nephritis, tumor lysis syndrome, T-wave inversion, uremia, urticaria, vasculitis, ventricular extrasystoles, ventricular failure, ventricular fibrillation, ventricular tachycardia, vertigo, visual impairment, wound healing impairment

Drug Interactions

Metabolism/Transport Effects **Substrate** of CYP2A6 (major), CYP2B6 (minor), CYP2C19 (major), CYP2C8 (minor), CYP2C9 (minor), CYP3A4 (major); **Note:** Assignment of Major/Minor substrate status based on clinically relevant drug interaction potential; **Inhibits** CYP3A4 (weak); **Induces** CYP2C9 (weak/moderate)

Avoid Concomitant Use

Avoid concomitant use of Ifosfamide with any of the following: BCG; CloZAPine; Natalizumab; Pimecrolimus; Pimozide; Tacrolimus (Topical); Vaccines (Live)

Increased Effect/Toxicity

Ifosfamide may increase the levels/effects of: ARIPiprazole; CloZAPine; Leflunomide; Natalizumab; Pimozide; Vaccines (Live); Vitamin K Antagonists

The levels/effects of Ifosfamide may be increased by: Busulfan; CYP2A6 Inhibitors (Moderate); CYP2A6 Inhibitors (Strong); CYP2C19 Inhibitors (Moderate); CYP2C19 Inhibitors (Strong); CYP3A4 Inducers (Strong); Dasatinib; Denosumab; Ivacaftor; Mifepristone; Pimecrolimus; Roflumilast; Tacrolimus (Topical); Trastuzumab

Decreased Effect

Ifosfamide may decrease the levels/effects of: BCG; Coccidioidin Skin Test; Sipuleucel-T; Vaccines (Inactivated); Vaccines (Live); Vitamin K Antagonists

The levels/effects of Ifosfamide may be decreased by: CYP2A6 Inducers (Strong); CYP3A4 Inhibitors (Moderate); CYP3A4 Inhibitors (Strong); Deferasirox; Echinacea; Herbs (CYP3A4 Inducers); Tocilizumab

Ethanol/Nutrition/Herb Interactions Herb/Nutraceutical: St John's wort may decrease ifosfamide levels.

Storage/Stability Store intact vials of powder for injection at room temperature of 20°C to 25°C (68°F to 77°F); avoid temperatures >30°C (86°F). Store intact vials of solution under refrigeration at 2°C to 8°C (36°F to 46°F). Reconstituted solutions and solutions diluted for administration are stable for 24 hours refrigerated.

Reconstitution Reconstitute powder with SWFI or bacteriostatic SWFI (1 g in 20 mL or 3 g in 60 mL) to a concentration of 50 mg/mL. Further dilution in 50-1000 mL D_5W, NS, or lactated Ringer's (to a final concentration of 0.6-20 mg/mL) is recommended for I.V. infusion (may also dilute in $D_{2.5}W$, 1/2 NS, or D_5NS).

Mechanism of Action Causes cross-linking of strands of DNA by binding with nucleic acids and other intracellular structures; inhibits protein synthesis and DNA synthesis

Pharmacodynamics/Kinetics Pharmacokinetics are dose dependent

Distribution: V_d: Approximates total body water; penetrates CNS, but not in therapeutic levels

Protein binding: Negligible

Metabolism: Hepatic to active metabolites isofosforamide mustard, 4-hydroxy-ifosfamide, acrolein, and inactive dichloroethylated and carboxy metabolites; acrolein is the agent implicated in development of hemorrhagic cystitis

Half-life elimination (increased in the elderly):

High dose (3800-5000 mg/m^2): ~15 hours

Lower dose (1600-2400 mg/m^2): ~7 hours

Excretion:

High dose (5000 mg/m^2): Urine (70% to 86%; 61% as unchanged drug)

Lower dose (1600-2400 mg/m^2): Urine (12% to 18% as unchanged drug)

Dosing

Adult & Geriatric Also consult details concerning dosing in combination regimens. **Note:** To prevent bladder toxicity, ifosfamide should be given with the urinary protector mesna and hydration of at least 2 L of oral or I.V. fluid per day.

Testicular cancer: I.V.:

U.S. manufacturer's labeling; as part of combination chemotherapy and with mesna: 1200 mg/m^2/day for 5 days every 3 weeks or after hematologic recovery

VIP regimen: 1200 mg/m^2/day for 5 days every 3 weeks for 4 cycles (in combination with etoposide, mesna, and cisplatin) (Nichols, 1998)

VeIP regimen: 1200 mg/m^2/day for 5 days every 3 weeks for 4 cycles (in combination with vinblastine, mesna, and cisplatin) (Loehrer, 1998)

Canadian labeling: **Soft tissue sarcoma, cervical cancer (advanced or recurrent), pancreatic cancer (relapsed or refractory):** I.V.: 2000-2400 mg/m^2/day for 5 consecutive days (with mesna), may repeat after 3-4 weeks (or longer depending on patient status) or if lower daily dosage or total dosage over a longer time period is indicated, administer every other day (eg, days 1, 3, 5, 7, 9) or over 10 consecutive days at reduced doses.

High **single-dose** infusions of up to 5000-8000 mg/m^2/24 hour with continuous mesna may also be feasible; may repeat after 3-4 weeks (or longer depending on patient's condition).

Adult unlabeled uses and/or dosing:

Testicular cancer: I.V.:

TIP regimen (unlabeled dosing): 1500 mg/m^2/day for 4 days (days 2-5) every 3 weeks for 4 cycles (in combination with paclitaxel, mesna, and cisplatin) (Kondagunta, 2005)

TICE regimen (unlabeled dosing): 2000 mg/m^2/day for 3 days (days 2-4) over 4 hours every 2 weeks for 2 cycles (in combination with paclitaxel and mesna; followed by carboplatin and etoposide) (Kondagunta, 2007)

Cervical cancer, recurrent or metastatic: I.V.: 1500 mg/m^2/day for 5 days every 3 weeks (with mesna) (Coleman, 1986; Sutton, 1993)

Hodgkin lymphoma, relapsed or refractory: I.V.:

ICE regimen: 5000 mg/m^2 (over 24 hours) beginning on day 2 every 2 weeks for 2 cycles (in combination with mesna, carboplatin, and etoposide) (Moskowitz, 2001)

IGEV regimen: 2000 mg/m^2/day for 4 days every 3 weeks for 4 cycles (in combination with mesna, gemcitabine, vinorelbine, and prednisolone) (Santoro, 2007)

MINE-ESHAP regimen: 1500 mg/m^2/day for 3 days every 4 weeks for up to 2 cycles (MINE is combination with mesna, mitoxantrone, and etoposide; MINE alternates with ESHAP for up to 2 cycles of each) (Fernandez, 2010)

Non-Hodgkin lymphomas: I.V.:

CODOX-M/IVAC regimen:

Adults ≤65 years: Cycles 2 and 4 (IVAC): 1500 mg/m^2/day for 5 days (IVAC is combination with cytarabine, mesna, and etoposide, IVAC alternates with CODOX-M) (Mead, 2008)

Adults >65 years: Cycles 2 and 4 (IVAC): 1000 mg/m^2/day for 5 days (IVAC is combination with cytarabine, mesna, and etoposide; IVAC alternates with CODOX-M) (Mead, 2008)

MINE-ESHAP regimen: 1330 mg/m^2/day for 3 days every 3 weeks for 6 cycles (MINE is combination with mesna, mitoxantrone, and etoposide; followed by ESHAP) (Rodriguez, 1995)

RICE regimen: 5000 mg/m^2 (over 24 hours) beginning on day 4 every 2 weeks for 3 cycles (in combination with mesna, carboplatin, etoposide, and rituximab) (Kewalramani, 2004)

Ewing sarcoma: I.V.:

VAC/IE regimen: Adults ≤30 years: IE: 1800 mg/m^2/day for 5 days (in combination with mesna and etoposide) alternate with VAC (vincristine, doxorubicin, and cyclophosphamide) every 3 weeks for a total of 17 courses (Grier, 2003)

VAIA regimen: 3000 mg/m^{2}day on days 1, 2, 22, 23, 43, and 44 for 4 courses (in combination with vincristine, doxorubicin, dactinomycin and mesna) (Paulussen, 2001) **or** Adults ≤35 years: 2000 mg/m^2/day for 3 days every 3 weeks for 14 courses (in combination with vincristine, doxorubicin, dactinomycin, and mesna) (Paulussen, 2008)

VIDE regimen: Adults ≤50 years: 3000 mg/m^2/day over 1-3 hours for 3 days every 3 weeks for 6 courses (in combination with vincristine, doxorubicin, etoposide, and mesna) (Juergens, 2006)

IE regimen: 1800 mg/m^2/day over 1 hour for 5 days every 3 weeks for 12 cycles (in combination with etoposide and mesna) (Miser, 1987)

ICE regimen: Adults ≤22 years: 1800 mg/m^2/day for 5 days every 3 weeks for up to 12 cycles (in combination with carboplatin and etoposide [and mesna]) (van Winkle, 2005)

Osteosarcoma: I.V.:

Ifosfamide/cisplatin/doxorubicin/HDMT regimen: Adults <40 years: 3000 mg/m²/day continuous infusion for 5 days during weeks 4 and 10 (preop) and during weeks 16, 25, and 34 (postop) (in combination with cisplatin, doxorubicin, methotrexate [high-dose], and mesna) (Bacci, 2003)

Ifosfamide/cisplatin/epirubicin regimen: 2000 mg/m²/day over 4 hours for 3 days (days 2, 3, and 4) every 3 weeks for 3 cycles (preop) and every 4 weeks for 3 cycles (postop) (in combination with cisplatin, epirubicin, and mesna) (Basaran, 2007)

ICE regimen (adults ≤22 years): 1800 mg/m²/day for 5 days every 3 weeks for up to 12 cycles (in combination with carboplatin and etoposide [and mesna]) (van Winkle, 2005)

Soft tissue sarcoma: I.V.:

Single-agent ifosfamide: 3000 mg/m²/day over 4 hours for 3 days every 3 weeks for at least 2 cycles or until disease progression (van Oosterom, 2002)

ICE regimen: 1500 mg/m²/day for 4 days every 4 weeks for 4-6 cycles (in combination with carboplatin, etoposide, and regional hyperthermia) (Nickenig, 2009)

MAID regimen: 2000 mg/m²/day continuous infusion for 3 days every 3 weeks (in combination with mesna, doxorubicin, and dacarbazine) (Antman, 1993) **or** 2500 mg/m²/day continuous infusion for 3 days every 3 weeks (in combination with mesna, doxorubicin, and dacarbazine); reduce ifosfamide to 1500mg/m²/day if prior pelvic irradiation (Elias, 1989)

Ifosfamide/epirubicin: 1800 mg/m²/day over 1 hour for 5 days every 3 weeks for 5 cycles (in combination with mesna and epirubicin) (Frustaci, 2001)

AIM regimens: 1500 mg/m²/day over 2 hours for 4 days every 3 weeks for 4-6 cycles (in combination with mesna and doxorubicin) (Worden, 2005) **or** 2000-3000 mg/m²/day over 3 hours for 3 days (in combination with mesna and doxorubicin) (Grobmyer, 2004)

Pediatric Also consult details concerning dosing in combination regimens. **Note:** To prevent bladder toxicity, ifosfamide should be given with the urinary protector mesna and hydration of at least 2 L of oral or I.V. fluid per day.

Ewing sarcoma (unlabeled use): I.V.:

VAC/IE regimen: IE: 1800 mg/m²/day for 5 days (in combination with mesna and etoposide) alternate with VAC (vincristine, doxorubicin, and cyclophosphamide) every 3 weeks for a total of 17 courses (Grier, 2003)

ICE-CAV regimen: ICE: 1800 mg/m²/day for 5 days every 3-4 weeks for 2 courses (in combination with carboplatin and etoposide [and mesna]), followed by CAV (cyclophosphamide, doxorubicin, and vincristine) (Milano, 2006)

VAIA regimen: 3000 mg/m²/day on days 1, 2, 22, 23, 43, and 44 for 4 courses (in combination with vincristine, doxorubicin, dactinomycin, and mesna) (Paulussen, 2001) **or** 2000 mg/m²/day for 3 days every 3 weeks for 14 courses (in combination with vincristine, doxorubicin, dactinomycin, and mesna) (Paulussen, 2008)

VIDE regimen: 3000 mg/m²/day over 1-3 hours for 3 days every 3 weeks for 6 courses (in combination with vincristine, doxorubicin, etoposide, and mesna) (Juergens, 2006)

IE regimen: 1800 mg/m²/day over 1 hour for 5 days every 3 weeks for 12 cycles (in combination with etoposide and mesna) (Miser, 1987)

ICE regimen: 1800 mg/m²/day for 5 days every 3 weeks for up to 12 cycles (in combination with carboplatin and etoposide [and mesna]) (van Winkle, 2005)

Osteosarcoma (unlabeled use): I.V.:

Ifosfamide/cisplatin/doxorubicin/HDMT regimen: 3000 mg/m²/day continuous infusion for 5 days during weeks 4 and 10 (preop) and during weeks 16, 25, and 34 (postop) (in combination with cisplatin, doxorubicin, methotrexate [high-dose], and mesna) (Bacci, 2003)

Ifosfamide/cisplatin/epirubicin regimen: Children ≥15 years: 2000 mg/m²/day over 4 hours for 3 days (days 2, 3, and 4) every 3 weeks for 3 cycles (preop) and every 4 weeks for 3 cycles (postop) (in combination with cisplatin, epirubicin, and mesna) (Basaran, 2007)

IE regimen: 3000 mg/m²/day over 3 hours for 4 days every 3-4 weeks (in combination with etoposide and mesna) (Gentet, 1997)

ICE regimen: Children ≥1 year: 1800 mg/m²/day for 5 days every 3 weeks for up to 12 cycles (in combination with carboplatin and etoposide [and mesna]) (van Winkle, 2005)

Ifosfamide/HDMT/etoposide regimen: 3000 mg/m²/day over 3 hours for 4 days during weeks 4 and 9 (3 additional postop courses were administered in good responders) (in combination with methotrexate [high-dose], etoposide, and mesna) (Le Deley, 2007)

Renal Impairment

U.S. labeling: Consider dosage reduction in patients with renal impairment; however, no dosage adjustment is provided in the manufacturer's labeling; ifosfamide (and metabolites) are excreted renally and may accumulate in patients with renal dysfunction. Ifosfamide and metabolites are dialyzable.

Canadian labeling:

Mild-to-moderate impairment: No dosage adjustment provided in the manufacturer's labeling.

Severe impairment: Use is contraindicated.

The following adjustments have also been recommended:

Aronoff, 2007:

Cl_{cr} ≥10 mL/minute: Children and Adults: No dosage adjustment necessary.

Cl_{cr} <10 mL/minute: Children and Adults: Administer 75% of dose.

Hemodialysis (supplement for dialysis):

Children: 1 g/m² followed by hemodialysis 6-8 hours later

Adults: No supplemental dose needed

Kintzel, 1995:

Cl_{cr} 46-60 mL/minute: Administer 80% of dose

Cl_{cr} 31-45 mL/minute: Administer 75% of dose

Cl_{cr} <30 mL/minute: Administer 70% of dose

Hepatic Impairment No dosage adjustment provided in the manufacturer's labeling; however, ifosfamide is extensively hepatically metabolized to both active and inactive metabolites; use with caution. The following adjustments have been recommended:

Floyd, 2006: Bilirubin >3 mg/dL: Administer 25% of dose.

Canadian labeling:

Mild-to-moderate impairment: No dosage adjustment provided in manufacturer labeling; use with caution.

Severe impairment: Use is contraindicated.

Combination Regimens

Hepatoblastoma: IPA on page 1692

Lymphoma, Hodgkin:
ICE (Hodgkin) on page 1688
IGEV (Hodgkin) on page 1690
MINE-ESHAP (Hodgkin) on page 1711
VIM-D (Hodgkin) on page 1770
Lymphoma, non-Hodgkin's:
ICE (Lymphoma, non-Hodgkin's) on page 1689
IMVP-16 on page 1691
MINE on page 1711
MINE-ESHAP (NHL) on page 1712
RICE on page 1747
Lymphoma, non-Hodgkin's (Burkitt): CODOX-M/IVAC on page 1591
Osteosarcoma: ICE (Sarcoma) on page 1689
Sarcoma:
MAID (Sarcoma) on page 1704
VAC Alternating With IE (Ewing's Sarcoma) on page 1766
Soft tissue sarcoma:
AI on page 1520
ICE (Sarcoma) on page 1689
IE on page 1690
Testicular cancer:
Paclitaxel-Ifosfamide-Cisplatin on page 1730
VIP (Etoposide) (Testicular Cancer) on page 1776
VIP (Vinblastine) (Testicular Cancer) on page 1777

Administration Administer I.V. over at least 30 minutes (infusion times may vary by protocol; refer to specific protocol for infusion duration)

Emetic Potential
$\geq$10 g/m^2: Very high (>90%)
<10 g/m^2: Moderate (30% to 90%)

Vesicant/Extravasation Risk May be an irritant

Monitoring Parameters CBC with differential (prior to each dose), urine output, urinalysis (prior to each dose), liver function, and renal function tests; signs and symptoms of neurotoxicity, pulmonary toxicity, and/or hemorrhagic cystitis

Dosage Forms Excipient information presented when available (limited, particularly for generics); consult specific product labeling.
Injection, powder for reconstitution: 1 g, 3 g
Ifex: 1 g, 3 g
Injection, solution: 50 mg/mL (20 mL, 60 mL)

References

Antman K, Crowley J, Balcerzak SP, et al, "An Intergroup Phase III Randomized Study of Doxorubicin and Dacarbazine With or Without Ifosfamide and Mesna in Advanced Soft Tissue and Bone Sarcomas," *J Clin Oncol*, 1993, 11(7):1276-85.

Aronoff GR, Bennett WM, Berns JS, et al, *Drug Prescribing in Renal Failure: Dosing Guidelines for Adults and Children*, 5th ed. Philadelphia, PA: American College of Physicians; 2007, p 100, 172.

Bacci G, Briccoli A, Rocca M, et al, "Neoadjuvant Chemotherapy for Osteosarcoma of the Extremities With Metastases at Presentation: Recent Experience at the Rizzoli Institute in 57 Patients Treated With Cisplatin, Doxorubicin, and a High Dose of Methotrexate and Ifosfamide," *Ann Oncol*, 2003, 14(7):1126-34.

Basaran M, Bavbek ES, Saglam S, et al, "A Phase II Study of Cisplatin, Ifosfamide and Epirubicin Combination Chemotherapy in Adults With Nonmetastatic and Extremity Osteosarcomas," *Oncology*, 2007, 72(3-4):255-60.

Coleman RE, Harper PG, Gallagher C, et al, "A Phase II Study of Ifosfamide in Advanced and Relapsed Carcinoma of the Cervix," *Cancer Chemother Pharmacol*, 1986, 18(3):280-3.

David KA and Picus J, "Evaluating Risk Factors for the Development of Ifosfamide Encephalopathy," *Am J Clin Oncol*, 2005, 28(3):277-80.

Elias A, Ryan L, Sulkes A, et al, "Response to Mesna, Doxorubicin, Ifosfamide, and Dacarbazine in 108 Patients With Metastatic or Unresectable Sarcoma and No Prior Chemotherapy," *J Clin Oncol*, 1989, 7(9):1208-16.

Fernandez de Larrea C, Martinez C, Gaya A, et al, "Salvage Chemotherapy With Alternating MINE-ESHAP Regimen in Relapsed or Refractory Hodgkin's Lymphoma Followed By Autologous Stem-Cell Transplantation," *Ann Oncol*, 2010, 21(6):1211-6.

Floyd J, Mirza I, Sachs B, et al, "Hepatotoxicity of Chemotherapy," *Semin Oncol*, 2006, 33 (1):50-67.

Frustaci S, Gherlinzoni F, De Paoli A, et al, "Adjuvant Chemotherapy for Adult Soft Tissue Sarcomas of the Extremities and Girdles: Results of the Italian Randomized Cooperative Trial," *J Clin Oncol*, 2001, 19(5):1238-47.

Gentet JC, Brunat-Mentigny M, Demaille MC, et al, "Ifosfamide and Etoposide in Childhood Osteosarcoma. A Phase II Study of the French Society of Paediatric Oncology," *Eur J Cancer*, 1997, 33(2):232-7.

Grier HE, Krailo MD, Tarbell NJ, et al, "Addition of Ifosfamide and Etoposide to Standard Chemotherapy for Ewing's Sarcoma and Primitive Neuroectodermal Tumor of Bone," *N Engl J Med*, 2003, 348(8):694-701.

Grobmyer ST, Maki RG, Demetri GD, et al, "Neo-Adjuvant Chemotherapy for Primary High-Grade Extremity Soft Tissue Sarcoma," *Ann Oncol*, 2004, 15(11):1667-72.

Juergens C, Weston C, Lewis I, et al, "Safety Assessment of Intensive Induction With Vincristine, Ifosfamide, Doxorubicin, and Etoposide (VIDE) in the Treatment of Ewing Tumors in the EURO-E.W.I.N.G. 99 Clinical Trial," *Pediatr Blood Cancer*, 2006, 47(1):22-9.

Kewalramani T, Zelenetz AD, Nimer SD, et al, "Rituximab and ICE as Second-Line Therapy before Autologous Stem Cell Transplantation for Relapsed or Primary Refractory Diffuse Large B-Cell Lymphoma," *Blood*, 2004, 103(10):3684-8.

Kintzel PE and Dorr RT, "Anticancer Drug Renal Toxicity and Elimination: Dosing Guidelines for Altered Renal Function," *Cancer Treat Rev*, 1995, 21(1):33-64.

Kondagunta GV, Bacik J, Donadio A, et al, "Combination of Paclitaxel, Ifosfamide, and Cisplatin is an Effective Second-Line Therapy for Patients With Relapsed Testicular Germ Cell Tumors," *J Clin Oncol*, 2005, 23(27):6549-55.

Kondagunta GV, Bacik J, Sheinfeld J, et al, "Paclitaxel Plus Ifosfamide Followed by High-Dose Carboplatin Plus Etoposide in Previously Treated Germ Cell Tumors," *J Clin Oncol*, 2007, 25 (1):85-90.

Le Deley MC, Guinebretière JM, Gentet JC, et al, "SFOP OS94: a Randomised Trial Comparing Preoperative High-Dose Methotrexate Plus Doxorubicin to High-Dose Methotrexate Plus Etoposide and Ifosfamide in Osteosarcoma Patients," *Eur J Cancer*, 2007, 43(4):752-61.

Loehrer PJ Sr, Gonin R, Nichols CR, et al, "Vinblastine Plus Ifosfamide Plus Cisplatin as Initial Salvage Therapy in Recurrent Germ Cell Tumor," *J Clin Oncol*, 1998, 16(7):2500-4.

Mead GM, Barrans SL, Qian W, et al, "A Prospective Clinicopathologic Study of Dose-Modified CODOX-M/IVAC in Patients With Sporadic Burkitt Lymphoma Defined Using Cytogenetic and Immunophenotypic Criteria (MRC/NCRI LY10 Trial)," *Blood*, 2008, 112(6):2248-60.

Milano GM, Cozza R, Ilari I, et al, "High Histologic and Overall Response to Dose Intensification of Ifosfamide, Carboplatin, and Etoposide With Cyclophosphamide, Doxorubicin, and Vincristine in Patients With High-Risk Ewing Sarcoma Family Tumors: The Bambino Gesù Children's Hospital Experience," *Cancer*, 2006, 106(8):1838-45.

Miser JS, Kinsella TJ, Triche TJ, et al, "Ifosfamide With Mesna Uroprotection and Etoposide: An Effective Regimen in the Treatment of Recurrent Sarcomas and Other Tumors of Children and Young Adults," *J Clin Oncol*, 1987, 5(8):1191-8.

Morgan C, Tillett T, Braybrooke J, et al, "Management of Uncommon Chemotherapy-Induced Emergencies," *Lancet Oncol*, 2011, 12(8):806-14.

Moskowitz CH, Nimer SD, Zelenetz AD, et al, "A 2-Step Comprehensive High-Dose Chemoradiotherapy Second-Line Program for Relapsed and Refractory Hodgkin Disease: Analysis by Intent to Treat and Development of a Prognostic Model," *Blood*, 2001, 97(3):616-23.

Nichols CR, Catalano PJ, Crawford ED, et al, "Randomized Comparison of Cisplatin and Etoposide and Either Bleomycin or Ifosfamide in Treatment of Advanced Disseminated Germ Cell Tumors: An Eastern Cooperative Oncology Group, Southwest Oncology Group, and Cancer and Leukemia Group B Study," *J Clin Oncol*, 1998, 16(4):1287-93.

Nickenig C, Buecklein L, Lindner LH, et al, "Ifosfamide, Carboplatin, and Etoposide (ICE) in Combination With Regional Hyperthermia (RHT) in Chemotherapy-Pretreated Nonresponders With Locally Advanced High-Risk Soft Tissue Sarcoma (HR-STS)," *J Clin Oncol*, 2009, 27(15s): 10581 [abstract 10581 from 2009 ASCO Annual Meeting].

Paulussen M, Ahrens S, Dunst J, et al, "Localized Ewing Tumor of Bone: Final Results of the Cooperative Ewing's Sarcoma Study CESS 86," *J Clin Oncol*, 2001, 19(6):1818-29.

Paulussen M, Craft AW, Lewis I, et al, "Results of the EICESS-92 Study: Two Randomized Trials of Ewing's Sarcoma Treatment–Cyclophosphamide Compared With Ifosfamide in Standard-Risk

Patients and Assessment of Benefit of Etoposide Added to Standard Treatment in High-Risk Patients," *J Clin Oncol*, 2008, 26(27):4385-93.

Pelgrims J, DeVos F, Van den Brande J, et al, "Methylene Blue in the Treatment and Prevention of Ifosfamide-Induced Encephalopathy: Report of 12 Cases and a Review of the Literature," *Br J Cancer*, 2000, 82(2) 291-4.

Rodriguez MA, Cabanillas FC, Velasquez W, et al, "Results of a Salvage Treatment Program for Relapsing Lymphoma: MINE Consolidated With ESHAP," *J Clin Oncol*, 1995, 13(7):1734-41.

Santoro A, Magagnoli M, Spina M, et al, "Ifosfamide, Gemcitabine, and Vinorelbine: A New Induction Regimen for Refractory and Relapsed Hodgkin's Lymphoma," *Haematologica*, 2007, 92(1):35-41.

Sutton GP, Blessing JA, DiSaia PJ, et al, "Phase II Study of Ifosfamide and Mesna in Non-squamous Carcinoma of the Cervix: A Gynecologic Oncology Group Study," *Gynecol Oncol*, 1993, 49(1):48-50.

van Oosterom AT, Mouridsen HT, Nielsen OS, et al, "Results of Randomised Studies of the EORTC Soft Tissue and Bone Sarcoma Group (STBSG) With Two Different Ifosfamide Regimens in First- and Second-Line Chemotherapy in Advanced Soft Tissue Sarcoma Patients," *Eur J Cancer*, 2002, 38(18):2397-406.

van Winkle P, Angiolillo A, Krailo M, et al, "Ifosfamide, Carboplatin, and Etoposide (ICE) Reinduction Chemotherapy in a Large Cohort of Children and Adolescents With Recurrent/Refractory Sarcoma: The Children's Cancer Group (CCG) Experience," *Pediatr Blood Cancer*, 2005, 44(4):338-47.

Worden FP, Taylor JM, Biermann JS, et al, "Randomized Phase II Evaluation of 6 g/m^2 of Ifosfamide Plus Doxorubicin and Granulocyte Colony-Stimulating Factor (G-CSF) Compared With 12 g/m^2 of Ifosfamide Plus Doxorubicin and G-CSF in the Treatment of Poor-Prognosis Soft Tissue Sarcoma," *J Clin Oncol*, 2005, 23(1):105-12.

◆ **IG** *see* Immune Globulin *on page 777*

◆ **IGIM** *see* Immune Globulin *on page 777*

◆ **IGIV** *see* Immune Globulin *on page 777*

◆ **IGIVnex® (Can)** *see* Immune Globulin *on page 777*

◆ **IL-2** *see* Aldesleukin *on page 37*

◆ **IL-11** *see* Oprelvekin *on page 1074*

Imatinib (eye MAT eh nib)

Related Information

Chemotherapy and Cancer Treatment During Pregnancy *on page 1829*
Management of Chemotherapy-Induced Nausea and Vomiting *on page 1786*
Principles of Anticancer Therapy *on page 1878*
Safe Handling of Hazardous Drugs *on page 1904*

Brand Names: U.S. Gleevec®

Brand Names: Canada Gleevec®

Index Terms CGP-57148B; Glivec; Imatinib Mesylate; STI-571

Generic Availability (U.S.) No

Pharmacologic Category Antineoplastic Agent, Tyrosine Kinase Inhibitor

Use Treatment of:

Gastrointestinal stromal tumors (GIST) kit-positive (CD117), including unresectable and/or metastatic malignant and adjuvant treatment following complete resection

Philadelphia chromosome-positive (Ph+) chronic myeloid leukemia (CML) in chronic phase (newly-diagnosed)

Ph+ CML in blast crisis, accelerated phase, or chronic phase after failure of interferon therapy

Ph+ acute lymphoblastic leukemia (ALL) (relapsed or refractory)

Aggressive systemic mastocytosis (ASM) without D816V c-Kit mutation (or c-Kit mutation status unknown)

Dermatofibrosarcoma protuberans (DFSP) (unresectable, recurrent and/or metastatic)

Hypereosinophilic syndrome (HES) and/or chronic eosinophilic leukemia (CEL)

Myelodysplastic/myeloproliferative disease (MDS/MPD) associated with platelet-derived growth factor receptor (PDGFR) gene rearrangements

Canadian labeling (not an approved indication in the U.S.): Ph+ ALL induction therapy (newly diagnosed)

Unlabeled Use Treatment of desmoid tumors or chordoma (soft tissue sarcomas); post-stem cell transplant (allogeneic) follow-up treatment for recurrence in CML; treatment of Ph+ acute lymphoblastic lymphoma

Labeled Contraindications There are no contraindications listed within the FDA-approved manufacturer's labeling.

Canadian labeling: Hypersensitivity to imatinib or any component of the formulation

Pregnancy Risk Factor D

Lactation Enters breast milk/not recommended

Warnings/Precautions Hazardous agent - use appropriate precautions for handling and disposal. Often associated with fluid retention, weight gain, and edema (probability increases with higher doses and age >65 years); occasionally serious and may lead to significant complications, including pleural effusion, pericardial effusion, pulmonary edema, and ascites. Monitor for rapid weight gain or other signs/symptoms of fluid retention. Use with caution in patients where fluid accumulation may be poorly tolerated, such as in cardiovascular disease (heart failure [HF] or hypertension) and pulmonary disease. Severe HF and left ventricular dysfunction (LVD) have been reported occasionally, usually in patients with comorbidities and/or risk factors; carefully monitor patients with pre-existing cardiac disease or risk factors for HF or history of renal failure. With initiation of imatinib treatment, cardiogenic shock and/or LVD have been reported in patients with hypereosinophilic syndrome and cardiac involvement (reversible with systemic steroids, circulatory support and temporary cessation of imatinib). Patients with high eosinophil levels and an abnormal echocardiogram or abnormal serum troponin level may benefit from prophylactic systemic steroids (for 1-2 weeks) with the initiation of imatinib.

Severe bullous dermatologic reactions (including erythema multiforme and Stevens-Johnson syndrome) have been reported; recurrence has been described with rechallenge. Case reports of successful resumption at a lower dose (with corticosteroids and/or antihistamine) have been described; however, some patients may experience recurrent reactions.

Hepatotoxicity may occur (may be severe); fatal hepatic failure and severe hepatic injury have been reported with both short- and long-term use; monitor; therapy interruption or dose reduction may be necessary. Transaminase and bilirubin elevations, and acute liver failure have been observed with imatinib in combination with chemotherapy. Use with caution in patients with pre-existing hepatic impairment; dosage adjustment recommended in patients with severe impairment. Use with caution in renal impairment; dosage adjustment recommended for moderate and severe impairment. Tumor lysis syndrome (TLS), including fatalities, has been reported in patients with ALL, CML eosinophilic leukemias, and GIST; risk for TLS is higher in patients with a high tumor burden or high proliferation rate; monitor closely; correct clinically significant dehydration and treat high uric acid levels prior to initiation of imatinib.

May cause GI irritation, severe hemorrhage (grades 3 and 4; including gastrointestinal hemorrhage and/or tumor hemorrhage; hemorrhage incidence is higher in patients with GIST [gastrointestinal tumors may have been hemorrhage source]), or hematologic toxicity (anemia, neutropenia, and thrombocytopenia); monitor blood counts; median duration of neutropenia is 2-3 weeks; median duration of thrombocytopenia is 3-4 weeks; in CML, cytopenias are more common in accelerated or blast phase than in chronic phase. Hypothyroidism has been reported in patients who were receiving thyroid hormone replacement therapy prior to the initiation of imatinib; monitor thyroid function; the average onset for imatinib-induced hypothyroidism is 2 weeks; consider doubling levothyroxine doses upon initiation of imatinib (Hamnvik, 2011). Use with caution in patients receiving concurrent therapy with drugs which alter cytochrome P450 activity or require metabolism by these isoenzymes; avoid concomitant use of strong CYP3A4 inducers. Imatinib exposure may be reduced in patients who have had gastric surgery (eg, bypass, major gastrectomy, or resection); monitor imatinib trough concentrations (Liu, 2011; Pavlovsky, 2009; Yoo, 2010). Growth retardation has been reported in children receiving imatinib for the treatment of CML; generally where treatment was initiated in prepubertal children; growth velocity was usually restored as pubertal age was reached (Shima, 2010); monitor growth closely. Reports of accidents have been received but it is unclear if imatinib has been the direct cause in any case; use caution when driving/operating motor vehicles and heavy machinery.

Adverse Reactions Note: Adverse reactions listed as a composite of data across many trials, except where noted for a specific indication.

>10%:

Cardiovascular: Edema/fluid retention (11% to 86%; grades 3/4: 3% to 13%; includes aggravated edema, anasarca, ascites, pericardial effusion, peripheral edema, pleural effusion, pulmonary edema and superficial edema); facial edema (≤17%), chest pain (7% to 11%)

Central nervous system: Fatigue (29% to 75%), pain (≤47%), fever (6% to 41%), headache (8% to 37%), dizziness (5% to 19%), insomnia (10% to 15%), depression (≤15%), anxiety (8% to 12%), chills (≤11%)

Dermatologic: Rash (9% to 50%; grades 3/4: 1% to 9%), dermatitis (GIST ≤39%), pruritus (8% to 26%), alopecia (GIST 10% to 15%)

Endocrine & metabolic: LDH increased (GIST ≤60%), hypoproteinemia (≤32%), albumin decreased (≤21%; grade 3: ≤4%), hypokalemia (6% to 13%)

Gastrointestinal: Nausea (42% to 73%), diarrhea (25% to 59%), vomiting (11% to 58%), abdominal pain (3% to 57%), anorexia (≤36%), weight gain (5% to 32%), dyspepsia (11% to 27%), flatulence (≤25%), abdominal distension (≤19%), constipation (9% to 16%), taste disturbance (≤13%)

Hematologic: Anemia (25% to 80%; grade 3: 1% to 42%; grade 4: ≤11%), leukopenia (GIST 5% to 47%), hemorrhage (3% to 53%; grades 3/4: ≤19%), neutropenia (grade 3: 7% to 27%; grade 4: 3% to 48%), thrombocytopenia (grade 3: 1% to 31%; grade 4: <1% to 33%)

Hepatic: AST increased (≤38%; grade 3: 2% to 5%; grade 4: ≤3%), ALT increased (≤34%; grade 3: 2% to 7%; grade 4: <3%), alkaline phosphatase increased (≤17%; grade 3: ≤6%; grade 4: <1%), bilirubin increased (≤13%; grade 3: 1% to 4%; grade 4: ≤3%)

Neuromuscular & skeletal: Muscle cramps (16% to 62%), arthralgia (≤40%), joint pain (11% to 31%), myalgia (9% to 32%), weakness (≤21%), musculoskeletal pain (children 21%; adults 38% to 47%), rigors (10% to 12%), paresthesia (≤12%), bone pain (≤11%)

Ocular: Periorbital edema (DFSP 33%; MPD 29%; GIST ≤74%), lacrimation increased (DFSP 25%; GIST ≤18%), blurred vision (≤11%)

Renal: Serum creatinine increased (≤44%; grade 3: ≤3%; DFSP: grade 4: 8%)

Respiratory: Nasopharyngitis (1% to 31%), cough (11% to 27%), dyspnea (≤21%), upper respiratory tract infection (3% to 21%), pharyngolaryngeal pain (≤18%), rhinitis (DFSP 17%), pharyngitis (CML 10% to 15%), pneumonia (CML 4% to 13%), sinusitis (4% to 11%)

Miscellaneous: Infection (GIST ≤28%), night sweats (CML 13% to 17%), influenza (1% to 14%), diaphoresis (GIST ≤13%)

1% to 10%:

Cardiovascular: Flushing, palpitation (≤5%)

Central nervous system: CNS/cerebral hemorrhage (≤9%), depression (≤8%), hypoesthesia

Dermatologic: Dry skin, erythema, photosensitivity reaction

Endocrine & metabolic: Hyperglycemia (≤10%), hypocalcemia (GIST ≤6%)

Gastrointestinal: Stomatitis/mucositis (≤10%), weight loss (≤10%), gastrointestinal hemorrhage (2% to 8%), gastritis, gastroesophageal reflux, xerostomia

Hematologic: Lymphopenia (GIST ≤10%), neutropenic fever, pancytopenia

Neuromuscular & skeletal: Back pain (GIST ≤7%), limb pain (GIST ≤7%), peripheral neuropathy, joint swelling

Ocular: Conjunctival hemorrhage, conjunctivitis, dry eyes, eyelid edema

Respiratory: Epistaxis

<1%, postmarketing, and/or case reports (limited to important or life-threatening): Acute febrile neutropenic dermatosis (Sweet's syndrome), amylase increased, anaphylactic shock, angina, angioedema, aplastic anemia, arrhythmia, ascites, atrial fibrillation, avascular necrosis, blepharitis, breast enlargement, bullous eruption, cardiac arrest, cardiac failure, cardiac tamponade, cardiogenic shock, cataract, cellulitis, cerebral edema, cheilitis, CHF (severe), colitis, confusion, CPK increased, dehydration, diverticulitis, dysphagia, embolism, eosinophilia, erythema multiforme, esophagitis, exanthematous pustulosis (acute generalized), exfoliative dermatitis, fungal infection, gastric ulcer, gastroenteritis, gastrointestinal obstruction, gastrointestinal perforation, glaucoma, gout, growth retardation (children), hearing loss, hematoma, hematemesis, hematuria, hemolytic anemia, hemorrhagic corpus luteum, hemorrhagic ovarian cyst, hepatic failure, hepatic necrosis, hepatitis, hepatotoxicity, herpes simplex, herpes zoster, hip osteonecrosis, hypercalcemia, hyperkalemia, hyperuricemia, hyper-/hypotension, hypomagnesemia, hyponatremia, hypophosphatemia, hypothyroidism, ileus, inflammatory bowel disease, interstitial lung disease, interstitial pneumonitis, intracranial pressure increased, jaundice, left ventricular dysfunction, leukocytoclastic vasculitis, libido decreased, lichen planus, lichenoid keratosis, lymphadenopathy, macular edema, melena, memory impairment, menorrhagia, MI, migraine, myopathy, optic neuritis, ovarian cyst (hemorrhagic), palmar-plantar erythrodysesthesia syndrome, pancreatitis, papilledema, pericarditis, petechiae, pleural effusion, pleuritic pain, pulmonary fibrosis, pulmonary hemorrhage, pulmonary hypertension, purpura, pustular rash, Raynaud's phenomenon, renal failure, respiratory failure, respiratory tract (lower) infection, retinal hemorrhage, rhabdomyolysis, sciatica, scleral

hemorrhage, seizure, sepsis, sexual dysfunction, skin pigment changes, somnolence, Stevens-Johnson syndrome, syncope, tachycardia, thrombocythemia, thrombosis, tinnitus, toxic epidermal necrolysis, tremor, tumor hemorrhage (GIST), tumor lysis syndrome, tumor necrosis, urinary tract infection, urticaria, vertigo, vesicular rash, vitreous hemorrhage

Drug Interactions

Metabolism/Transport Effects Substrate of CYP1A2 (minor), CYP2C19 (minor), CYP2C9 (minor), CYP2D6 (minor), CYP3A4 (major), P-glycoprotein; **Note:** Assignment of Major/Minor substrate status based on clinically relevant drug interaction potential; **Inhibits** BCRP, CYP2C9 (weak), CYP2D6 (moderate), CYP3A4 (strong), P-glycoprotein

Avoid Concomitant Use

Avoid concomitant use of Imatinib with any of the following: Alfuzosin; Avanafil; Axitinib; BCG; Bosutinib; CloZAPine; Conivaptan; Crizotinib; Dronedarone; Eplerenone; Everolimus; Fluticasone (Oral Inhalation); Halofantrine; Lapatinib; Lovastatin; Lurasidone; Natalizumab; Nilotinib; Nisoldipine; Pimecrolimus; Pimozide; Ranolazine; Red Yeast Rice; Regorafenib; Rivaroxaban; RomiDEPsin; Salmeterol; Silodosin; Simvastatin; Tacrolimus (Topical); Tamsulosin; Thioridazine; Ticagrelor; Tolvaptan; Toremifene; Vaccines (Live); VinCRIStine (Liposomal)

Increased Effect/Toxicity

Imatinib may increase the levels/effects of: Acetaminophen; Alfuzosin; Almotriptan; Alosetron; ARIPiprazole; Avanafil; Axitinib; Bortezomib; Bosutinib; Brentuximab Vedotin; Brinzolamide; Budesonide (Nasal); Budesonide (Systemic, Oral Inhalation); CloZAPine; Colchicine; Conivaptan; Corticosteroids (Orally Inhaled); Crizotinib; CycloSPORINE (Systemic); CYP2D6 Substrates; CYP3A4 Substrates; Dienogest; Dronedarone; Dutasteride; Enzalutamide; Eplerenone; Everolimus; FentaNYL; Fesoterodine; Fluticasone (Nasal); Fluticasone (Oral Inhalation); GuanFACINE; Halofantrine; Iloperidone; Ivacaftor; Ixabepilone; Lapatinib; Leflunomide; Lovastatin; Lumefantrine; Lurasidone; Maraviroc; MethylPREDNISolone; Mifepristone; Natalizumab; Nebivolol; Nilotinib; Nisoldipine; Paricalcitol; Pazopanib; Pimecrolimus; Pimozide; Propafenone; Ranolazine; Red Yeast Rice; Regorafenib; Rivaroxaban; RomiDEPsin; Ruxolitinib; Salmeterol; Saxagliptin; Sildenafil; Silodosin; Simvastatin; SORAfenib; Tadalafil; Tamsulosin; Thioridazine; Ticagrelor; Tolterodine; Tolvaptan; Topotecan; Toremifene; Vaccines (Live); Vardenafil; Vemurafenib; Vilazodone; VinCRIStine (Liposomal); Vitamin K Antagonists; Warfarin; Zuclopenthixol

The levels/effects of Imatinib may be increased by: Acetaminophen; Antifungal Agents (Azole Derivatives, Systemic); CYP3A4 Inhibitors (Moderate); CYP3A4 Inhibitors (Strong); Dasatinib; Denosumab; Lansoprazole; P-glycoprotein/ABCB1 Inhibitors; Pimecrolimus; Roflumilast; Tacrolimus (Topical); Trastuzumab

Decreased Effect

Imatinib may decrease the levels/effects of: BCG; Cardiac Glycosides; Coccidioidin Skin Test; Codeine; Fludarabine; Ifosfamide; Prasugrel; Sipuleucel-T; Tamoxifen; Ticagrelor; TraMADol; Vaccines (Inactivated); Vaccines (Live); Vitamin K Antagonists

The levels/effects of Imatinib may be decreased by: CYP3A4 Inducers (Strong); Deferasirox; Echinacea; Ibuprofen; Peginterferon Alfa-2b; P-glycoprotein/ABCB1 Inducers; Rifamycin Derivatives; St Johns Wort; Tocilizumab

Ethanol/Nutrition/Herb Interactions

Ethanol: Management: Avoid ethanol.

Food: Food may reduce GI irritation. Grapefruit juice may increase imatinib plasma concentration. Management: Take with a meal and a large glass of water. Avoid grapefruit juice. Maintain adequate hydration, unless instructed to restrict fluid intake.

Herb/Nutraceutical: St John's wort may increase metabolism and decrease imatinib plasma concentration. Management: Avoid St John's wort.

Storage/Stability Store at 25°C (77°F); excursions permitted between 15°C to 30°C (59°F to 86°F). Protect from moisture.

Mechanism of Action Inhibits Bcr-Abl tyrosine kinase, the constitutive abnormal gene product of the Philadelphia chromosome in chronic myeloid leukemia (CML). Inhibition of this enzyme blocks proliferation and induces apoptosis in Bcr-Abl positive cell lines as well as in fresh leukemic cells in Philadelphia chromosome positive CML. Also inhibits tyrosine kinase for platelet-derived growth factor (PDGF), stem cell factor (SCF), c-Kit, and cellular events mediated by PDGF and SCF.

Pharmacodynamics/Kinetics

Absorption: Rapid

Protein binding: Parent drug and metabolite: ~95% to albumin and alpha$_1$-acid glycoprotein

Metabolism: Hepatic via CYP3A4 (minor metabolism via CYP1A2, CYP2D6, CYP2C9, CYP2C19); primary metabolite (active): N-demethylated piperazine derivative (CGP74588); severe hepatic impairment (bilirubin >3-10 times ULN) increases AUC by 45% to 55% for imatinib and its active metabolite, respectively

Bioavailability: 98%; may be decreased in patients who have had gastric surgery (eg, bypass, total or partial resection)

Half-life elimination: Adults: Parent drug: ~18 hours; N-desmethyl metabolite: ~40 hours; Children: Parent drug: ~15 hours

Time to peak: 2-4 hours

Excretion: Feces (68% primarily as metabolites, 20% as unchanged drug); urine (13% primarily as metabolites, 5% as unchanged drug)

Dosing

Adult & Geriatric Note: Doses ≤600 mg/day should be administered once daily, 800 mg/day doses should be administered as 400 mg twice daily. Treatment may be continued until disease progression or unacceptable toxicity. The optimal duration of therapy for CML in complete remission is not yet determined. Discontinuing treatment is not recommended unless part of a clinical trial (Baccarani, 2009; NCCN CML guidelines v.2.2012).

Ph+ CML: Oral:

Chronic phase: 400 mg once daily; may be increased to 600 mg/day, if tolerated, for disease progression, lack of hematologic response after 3 months, lack of cytogenetic response after 6-12 months, or loss of previous hematologic or cytogenetic response; a range of up to 800 mg/day is included in the NCCN CML guidelines (v.2.2012)

Canadian labeling: 400 mg once daily; may be increased to 600-800 mg/day

Accelerated phase or blast crisis: 600 mg once daily; may be increased to 800 mg/day (400 mg twice daily), if tolerated, for disease progression, lack of hematologic response after 3 months, lack of cytogenetic response after 6-12 months, or loss of previous hematologic or cytogenetic response

Ph+ ALL (relapsed or refractory): Oral: 600 mg once daily

GIST (adjuvant treatment following complete resection): Oral: 400 mg once daily; recommended treatment duration: 3 years

GIST (unresectable and/or metastatic malignant): Oral: 400 mg once daily; may be increased up to 800 mg/day (400 mg twice daily), if tolerated, for disease progression. **Note:** Significant improvement (progression-free survival, objective response rate) was demonstrated in patients with KIT exon 9 mutation with 800 mg (versus 400 mg), although overall survival (OS) was not impacted. The higher dose did not demonstrate a difference in time to progression or OS patients with Kit exon 11 mutation or wild-type status (Debiec-Rychter, 2006; Heinrich, 2009).

Canadian labeling: 400-600 mg/day (depending on disease stage/progression); may be increased to 600-800 mg/day

ASM with eosinophilia: Oral: Initiate at 100 mg once daily; titrate up to a maximum of 400 mg once daily (if tolerated) for insufficient response to lower dose

ASM without D816V c-Kit mutation or c-Kit mutation status unknown: Oral: 400 mg once daily

DFSP: Oral: 400 mg twice daily

HES/CEL: Oral: 400 mg once daily

HES/CEL with FIP1L1-PDGFRα fusion kinase: Oral: Initiate at 100 mg once daily; titrate up to a maximum of 400 mg once daily (if tolerated) if insufficient response to lower dose

MDS/MPD: Oral: 400 mg once daily

Ph+ ALL (induction, newly diagnosed): *Canadian labeling (not an approved use in the U.S.):* Oral: 600 mg once daily

Dosage adjustment with concomitant strong CYP3A4 inducers: Avoid concomitant use of strong CYP3A4 inducers (eg, dexamethasone, carbamazepine, phenobarbital, phenytoin, rifampin); if concomitant use cannot be avoided, increase imatinib dose by at least 50% with careful monitoring.

Pediatric Notes: May be administered once daily or in 2 divided doses. Treatment may be continued until disease progression or unacceptable toxicity. The optimal duration of therapy for CML is not yet determined.

Ph+ CML, chronic phase, newly diagnosed: Children ≥2 years: Oral: 340 mg/m^2/day; maximum: 600 mg /day

Dosage adjustment with concomitant strong CYP3A4 inducers: Avoid concomitant use of strong CYP3A4 inducers (eg, dexamethasone, carbamazepine, phenobarbital, phenytoin, rifampin); if concomitant use cannot be avoided, increase imatinib dose by at least 50% with careful monitoring.

Dosage adjustment for hepatotoxicity or other nonhematologic adverse reactions: Refer to "Hepatic Impairment" dosing.

Dosage adjustment for hematologic adverse reactions: Refer to dosing adjustment for toxicity.

Renal Impairment

U.S. labeling:

Mild impairment (Cl_{cr} 40-59 mL/minute): Maximum recommended dose: 600 mg

Moderate impairment (Cl_{cr} 20-39 mL/minute): Decrease recommended starting dose by 50%; dose may be increased as tolerated; maximum recommended dose: 400 mg.

Severe impairment (Cl_{cr} <20 mL/minute): Use caution; a dose of 100 mg/day has been tolerated in a limited number of patients with severe impairment (Gibbons, 2008).

Canadian labeling:

Mild impairment (Cl_{cr} 40-59 mL/minute): Initial dose: 400 mg once daily (minimum effective dose); titrate to efficacy and tolerability.

Moderate impairment (Cl_{cr} 20-39 mL/minute): Initial dose: 400 mg once daily (minimum effective dose); titrate to efficacy and tolerability; the use of 800 mg dose is not recommended.

Severe impairment (Cl_{cr} <20 mL/minute): Use is not recommended.

Hepatic Impairment

U.S. labeling:

Mild to moderate impairment: No dosage adjustment necessary.

Severe impairment: Reduce dose by 25%.

Canadian labeling:

Mild-to-moderate impairment: Initial dose: 400 mg once daily (minimum effective dose).

Severe impairment: Initial dose: 200 mg once daily; may increase up to 300 mg once daily in the absence of severe toxicity; decrease dose with unacceptable toxicity.

Hepatotoxicity (during therapy) or other nonhematologic adverse reactions (eg, severe edema): Withhold treatment until toxicity resolves; may resume if appropriate (depending on initial severity of adverse event)

If elevations of bilirubin >3 times upper limit of normal (ULN) or transaminases >5 times ULN occur, withhold treatment until bilirubin <1.5 times ULN and transaminases <2.5 times ULN. Resume treatment at a reduced dose as follows:

Children ≥2 years: If current dose 340 mg/m²/day, reduce dose to 260 mg/m²/day.

Adults:

If current dose 400 mg/day, reduce dose to 300 mg/day.

If current dose 600 mg/day, reduce dose to 400 mg/day.

If current dose 800 mg/day, reduce dose to 600 mg/day.

Adjustment for Toxicity

Chronic phase CML (initial dose 400 mg/day in adults or 340 mg/m²/day in children), ASM, MDS/MPD, and HES/CEL (initial dose 400 mg/day), or GIST (initial dose 400 mg/day [U.S. labeling] or 400-600 mg/day [Canadian labeling]): If ANC <1 x 10^9/L and/or platelets <50 x 10^9/L: Withhold until ANC ≥1.5 x 10^9/L and platelets ≥75 x 10^9/L; resume treatment at original starting dose. For recurrent neutropenia or thrombocytopenia, withhold until recovery, and reinstitute treatment at a reduced dose as follows:

Children ≥2 years: If initial dose 340 mg/m²/day, reduce dose to 260 mg/m²/day.

Adults:

If initial dose 400 mg/day, reduce dose to 300 mg/day.

If initial dose 600 mg/day (Canadian labeling; not in U.S. labeling), reduce dose to 400 mg/day.

CML (accelerated phase or blast crisis) and PH+ ALL: Adults (initial dose 600 mg/day): If ANC <0.5 x 10^9/L and/or platelets <10 x 10^9/L, establish whether cytopenia is related to leukemia (bone marrow aspirate or biopsy). If unrelated to leukemia, reduce dose to 400 mg/day. If cytopenia persists for an additional 2 weeks, further reduce dose to 300 mg/day. If cytopenia persists for 4 weeks and is still unrelated to leukemia, withhold treatment until ANC ≥1 x 10^9/L and platelets ≥20 x 10^9/L, then resume treatment at 300 mg/day.

ASM associated with eosinophilia and HES/CEL with FIP1L1-PDGFRα fusion kinase (starting dose 100 mg/day): If ANC <1 x 10^9/L and/or platelets <50 x 10^9/L: Withhold until ANC ≥1.5 x 10^9/L and platelets ≥75 x 10^9/L; resume treatment at previous dose.

DFSP (initial dose 800 mg/day): If ANC <1 x 10^9/L and/or platelets <50 x 10^9/L, withhold until ANC ≥1.5 x 10^9/L and platelets ≥75 x 10^9/L; resume treatment at reduced dose of 600 mg/day. If depression in neutrophils or platelets recurs, withhold until recovery, and reinstitute treatment with a further dose reduction to 400 mg/day.

Combination Regimens

Leukemia, acute lymphocytic: Hyper-CVAD + Imatinib on page 1680

Leukemia, chronic myelogenous: Imatinib (CML Regimen) on page 1690

Administration Should be administered with a meal and a large glass of water. Tablets may be dispersed in water or apple juice (using ~50 mL for 100 mg tablet, ~200 mL for 400 mg tablet); stir until dissolved and use immediately. For daily dosing ≥800 mg, the 400 mg tablets should be used in order to reduce iron exposure.

Emetic Potential Moderate (30% to 60%)

Extemporaneous Preparations Hazardous agent: Use appropriate precautions for handling and disposal.

An oral suspension may be prepared by placing tablets (whole, do not crush) in a glass of water or apple juice. Use ~50 mL for 100 mg tablet, or ~200 mL for 400 mg tablet. Stir until tablets are disintegrated, then administer immediately. To ensure the full dose is administered, rinse the glass and administer residue.

Gleevec® prescribing information, Novartis Pharmaceuticals Corporation, East Hanover, NJ, 2009.

Monitoring Parameters CBC (weekly for first month, biweekly for second month, then periodically thereafter), liver function tests (at baseline and monthly or as clinically indicated; more frequently [at least weekly] in patients with moderate-to-severe hepatic impairment [Ramanathan, 2008]), renal function, serum electrolytes (including calcium, phosphorus, potassium and sodium levels); bone marrow cytogenetics (in CML; at 6-, 12-, and 18 months); fatigue, weight, and edema/fluid status; consider echocardiogram and serum troponin levels in patients with HES/CEL, and in patients with MDS/MPD or ASM with high eosinophil levels; in pediatric patients, also monitor serum glucose, albumin, and growth

Gastric surgery (eg, bypass, major gastrectomy, or resection) patients: Monitor imatinib trough concentrations (Liu, 2011; Pavlovsky, 2009, Yoo, 2010)

Thyroid function testing (Hamnvik, 2011):

Preexisting levothyroxine therapy: Obtain baseline TSH levels, then monitor every 4 weeks until levels and levothyroxine dose are stable, then monitor every 2 months

Without pre-existing thyroid hormone replacement: TSH at baseline, then every 4 weeks for 4 months, then every 2-3 months

Monitor for signs/symptoms of CHF in patients with at risk for cardiac failure or patients with pre-existing cardiac disease. In Canada, a baseline evaluation of left ventricular ejection fraction is recommended prior to initiation of imatinib therapy in all patients with known underlying heart disease or in elderly patients.

Dietary Considerations Should be taken with food and a large glass of water to decrease gastrointestinal irritation. Avoid grapefruit juice.

Dosage Forms Excipient information presented when available (limited, particularly for generics); consult specific product labeling.

Tablet, oral:

Gleevec®: 100 mg, 400 mg [scored]

References

Atallah E, Durand JB, Kantarjian H, et al, "Congestive Heart Failure is a Rare Event in Patients Receiving Imatinib Therapy," *Blood*, 2007, 110(4):1233-7.

Ault P, Kantarjian H, O'Brien S, et al, "Pregnancy Among Patients with Chronic Myeloid Leukemia Treated With Imatinib," *J Clin Oncol*, 2006, 24(7):1204-8.

Baccarani M, Cortes J, Pane F, et al, "Chronic Myeloid Leukemia: An Update of Concepts and Management Recommendations of European LeukemiaNet," *J Clin Oncol*, 2009, 27 (35):6041-51.

Berman E, Nicolaides M, Maki RG, et al, "Altered Bone and Mineral Metabolism in Patients Receiving Imatinib Mesylate," *N Engl J Med*, 2006, 354(19):2006-13.

Carpenter PA, Snyder DS, Flowers ME, et al, "Prophylactic Administration of Imatinib After Hematopoietic Cell Transplantation for High-Risk Philadelphia Chromosome-Positive Leukemia," *Blood*, 2007, 109(7):2791-3.

Debiec-Rychter M, Sciot R, Le Cesne A, et al, "KIT mutations and Dose Selection for Imatinib in Patients With Advanced Gastrointestinal Stromal Tumors," *Eur J Cancer*, 2006, 42(8):1093-103.

de Groot JW, Zonnenberg BA, Plukker JT, et al, "Imatinib Induces Hypothyroidism in Patients Receiving Levothyroxine," *Clin Pharmacol Ther*, 2005, 78(4):433-8.

DeMatteo R, Owzar K, Maki R, et al, "Adjuvant Imatinib Mesylate Increases Recurrence Free Survival (RFS) in Patients With Completely Resected Localized Primary Gastrointestinal Stromal Tumor (GIST): North American Intergroup Phase III Trial ACOSOG Z9001," *J Clin Oncol*, 2007, 28(18 Supp):10079 [abstract 10079 from 2007 ASCO Annual Meeting].

Droogendijk HJ, Kluin-Nelemans HJ, van Doormaal JJ, et al, "Imatinib Mesylate in the Treatment of Systemic Mastocytosis: A Phase II Trial," *Cancer*, 2006, 107(2):345-51

Druker BJ, Sawyers CL, Kantarjian H, et al, "Activity of a Specific Inhibitor of the BCR-ABL Tyrosine Kinase in the Blast Crisis of Chronic Myeloid Leukemia and Acute Lymphoblastic Leukemia With the Philadelphia Chromosome," *N Engl J Med*, 2001, 344(14):1038-42.

Druker BJ, Talpaz M, Resta DJ, et al, "Efficacy and Safety of a Specific Inhibitor of the BCR-ABL Tyrosine Kinase in Chronic Myeloid Leukemia," *N Engl J Med*, 2001, 344(14):1031-7.

Gibbons J, Egorin MJ, Ramanathan RK, et al, "Phase I and Pharmacokinetic Study of Imatinib Mesylate in Patients With Advanced Malignancies and Varying Degrees of Renal Dysfunction: A Study by the National Cancer Institute Organ Dysfunction Working Group," *J Clin Oncol*, 2008, 26 (4):570-6.

Gotlib J, Cools J, Malone JM 3rd, et al, "The FIP1L1-PDGFRalpha Fusion Tyrosine Kinase in Hypereosinophilic Syndrome and Chronic Eosinophilic Leukemia: Implications for Diagnosis, Classification, and Management," *Blood*, 2004, 103(8):2879-91.

Hamnvik OP, Larsen PR, and Marqusee E, "Thyroid Dysfunction From Antineoplastic Agents," *J Natl Cancer Inst*, 2011, 103(21):1572-87.

Heinrich MC, Owzar K, Corless CL, et al, "Correlation of Kinase Genotype and Clinical Outcome in the North American Intergroup Phase III Trial of Imatinib Mesylate for Treatment of Advanced Gastrointestinal Stromal Tumor: CALGB 150105 Study by Cancer and Leukemia Group B and Southwest Oncology Group," *J Clin Oncol*, 2008, 26(33):5360-7.

Hess G, Bunjes D, Siegert W, et al, "Sustained Complete Molecular Remissions After Treatment With Imatinib-Mesylate in Patients With Failure After Allogeneic Stem Cell Transplantation for Chronic Myelogenous Leukemia: Results of a Prospective Phase II Open-Label Multicenter Study," *J Clin Oncol*, 2005, 23(30):7583-93.

Kantarjian H, Sawyers C, Hochhaus A, et al, "Hematologic and Cytogenetic Responses to Imatinib Mesylate in Chronic Myelogenous Leukemia," *N Engl J Med*, 2002, 346:645-52.

Kerkela R, Grazette L, Yacobi R, et al, "Cardiotoxicity of the Cancer Therapeutic Agent Imatinib Mesylate," *Nat Med*, 2006, 12(8):908-16.

Liu H and Artz AS, "Reduction of Imatinib Absorption After Gastric Bypass Surgery," *Leuk Lymphoma*, 2011, 52(2):310-3.

McArthur GA, Demetri GD, van Oosterom A, et al, "Molecular and Clinical Analysis of Locally Advanced Dermatofibrosarcoma Protuberans Treated with Imatinib: Imatinib Target Exploration Consortium Study B2225," *J Clin Oncol*, 2005, 23(4):866-73.

National Comprehensive Cancer Network® (NCCN) "Practice Guidelines in Oncology™: Chronic Myelogenous Leukemia Version 2.2012." Available at http://www.nccn.org/professionals/physician_gls/PDF/cml.pdf

Ottmann OG, Wassmann B, Pfeifer H, et al, "Imatinib Compared With Chemotherapy as Front-Line Treatment of Elderly Patients With Philadelphia Chromosome-Positive Acute Lymphoblastic Leukemia (Ph+ALL)," *Cancer*, 2007, 109(10):2068-76.

Pavlovsky C, Egorin MJ, Shah DD, et al, "Imatinib Mesylate Pharmacokinetics Before and After Sleeve Gastrectomy in a Morbidly Obese Patient With Chronic Myeloid Leukemia," *Pharmacotherapy*, 2009, 29(9):1152-6.

Pye SM, Cortes J, Ault P, et al, "The Effects of Imatinib on Pregnancy Outcome," *Blood*, 2008, 111 (12):5505-8.

Ramanathan RK, Egorin MJ, Takimoto CH, et al, "Phase I and Pharmacokinetic Study of Imatinib Mesylate in Patients With Advanced Malignancies and Varying Degrees of Liver Dysfunction: A Study by the National Cancer Institute Organ Dysfunction Working Group," *J Clin Oncol*, 2008, 26 (4):563-9.

Shima H, Tokuyama M, Tanizawa A, et al, "Distinct Impact of Imatinib on Growth at Prepubertal and Pubertal Ages of Children With Chronic Myeloid Leukemia," *J Pediatr*, 2011, 159(4):676-81.

Thomas DA, Faderl S, Cortes J, et al, "Treatment of Philadelphia Chromosome-Positive Acute Lymphocytic Leukemia With Hyper-CVAD and Imatinib Mesylate," *Blood*, 2004, 103 (12):4396-407.

Yanada M, Takeuchi J, Sugiura I, et al, "High Complete Remission Rate and Promising Outcome by Combination of Imatinib and Chemotherapy for Newly Diagnosed BCR-ABL-Positive Acute Lymphoblastic Leukemia: A Phase II Study by the Japan Adult Leukemia Study Group," *J Clin Oncol*, 2006, 24(3):460-6.

Yoo C, Ryu MH, Kang BW, et al, "Cross-Sectional Study of Imatinib Plasma Trough Levels in Patients With Advanced Gastrointestinal Stromal Tumors: Impact of Gastrointestinal Resection on Exposure to Imatinib," *J Clin Oncol*, 2010, 28(9):1554-9.

◆ **Imatinib Mesylate** *see* Imatinib *on page* *762*

◆ **IMC-C225** *see* Cetuximab *on page* *264*

◆ **123I-Metaiodobenzylguanidine (MIBG)** *see* Iobenguane I 123 *on page* *806*

◆ **Imferon** *see* Iron Dextran Complex *on page* *824*

◆ **IMI 30** *see* IDArubicin *on page* *749*

◆ **IMid-1** *see* Lenalidomide *on page* *859*

- **Imidazole Carboxamide** *see* Dacarbazine *on page 367*
- **Imidazole Carboxamide Dimethyltriazene** *see* Dacarbazine *on page 367*
- **Imipemide** *see* Imipenem and Cilastatin *on page 773*

Imipenem and Cilastatin (i mi PEN em & sye la STAT in)

Brand Names: U.S. Primaxin® I.V.

Brand Names: Canada Imipenem and Cilastatin for Injection; Primaxin® I.V. Infusion; RAN™-Imipenem Cilastatin

Index Terms Imipemide; Primaxin® I.M. [DSC]

Generic Availability (U.S.) Yes

Pharmacologic Category Antibiotic, Carbapenem

Use Treatment of lower respiratory tract, urinary tract, intra-abdominal, gynecologic, bone and joint, skin and skin structure, endocarditis (caused by *Staphylococcus aureus*) and polymicrobic infections as well as bacterial septicemia. Antibacterial activity includes gram-positive bacteria (methicillin-sensitive *S. aureus* and *Streptococcus* spp), resistant gram-negative bacilli (including extended spectrum beta-lactamase-producing *Escherichia coli* and *Klebsiella* spp, *Enterobacter* spp, and *Pseudomonas aeruginosa*), and anaerobes.

Unlabeled Use Hepatic abscess; neutropenic fever; melioidosis

Labeled Contraindications Hypersensitivity to imipenem/cilastatin or any component of the formulation

Pregnancy Risk Factor C

Lactation Enters breast milk/use caution

Warnings/Precautions Dosage adjustment required in patients with impaired renal function; elderly patients often require lower doses (adjust to renal function). Prolonged use may result in fungal or bacterial superinfection, including *C. difficile*-associated diarrhea (CDAD) and pseudomembranous colitis; CDAD has been observed >2 months postantibiotic treatment. Carbapenems have been associated with CNS adverse effects, including confusional states and seizures (myoclonic); use caution with CNS disorders (eg, brain lesions and history of seizures) and adjust dose in renal impairment to avoid drug accumulation, which may increase seizure risk. Use with caution in patients with hypersensitivity to beta-lactams (including penicillins or cephalosporins); patients with impaired renal function are at increased risk of seizures if not properly dose adjusted. May decrease divalproex sodium/valproic acid concentrations leading to breakthrough seizures; concomitant use is not recommended. Not recommended in pediatric CNS infections due to seizure risk. Serious hypersensitivity reactions, including anaphylaxis, have been reported (some without a history of previous allergic reactions to beta-lactams).

Storage/Stability Imipenem/cilastatin powder for injection should be stored at <25°C (77°F).

I.V.: Reconstituted I.V. solutions are stable for 4 hours at room temperature and 24 hours when refrigerated. Do not freeze.

Reconstitution I.V.: Prior to use, dilute dose into 100-250 mL of an appropriate solution. Imipenem is inactivated at acidic or alkaline pH. Final concentration should not exceed 5 mg/mL.

Mechanism of Action Inhibits bacterial cell wall synthesis by binding to one or more of the penicillin-binding proteins (PBPs); which in turn inhibits the final transpeptidation step of peptidoglycan synthesis in bacterial cell walls, thus inhibiting cell wall biosynthesis. Bacteria eventually lyse due to ongoing activity of cell wall autolytic enzymes (autolysins and murein hydrolases) while cell wall assembly is arrested. Cilastatin prevents renal metabolism of imipenem by competitive inhibition of dehydropeptidase along the brush border of the renal tubules.

Pharmacodynamics/Kinetics

Distribution: Rapidly and widely to most tissues and fluids including sputum, pleural fluid, peritoneal fluid, interstitial fluid, bile, aqueous humor, and bone; highest concentrations in pleural fluid, interstitial fluid, and peritoneal fluid; low concentrations in CSF

Protein binding: Imipenem: 20%; cilastatin: 40%

Metabolism: Imipenem is metabolized in the kidney by dehydropeptidase I; cilastatin prevents imipenem metabolism by this enzyme; cilastatin is partially metabolized renally

Half-life elimination: I.V.: Both drugs: 60 minutes; prolonged with renal impairment

Excretion: Both drugs: Urine (~70% as unchanged drug)

Dosing

Adult & Geriatric Doses based on **imipenem** content.

Usual dosage range: Weight ≥70 kg: 250-1000 mg every 6-8 hours; maximum: 4 g/day. **Note:** For adults weighing <70 kg, refer to Dosing Adjustment in Renal Impairment.

Indication-specific dosing:

***Burkholderia pseudomallei* (melioidosis) (unlabeled use):** I.V.: Initial: 20 mg/kg every 8 hours for at least 10 days (White, 2003) **or** 25 mg/kg (up to 1 g) every 6 hours for at least 10 days (Currie, 2003); continue parenteral therapy until clinical improvement then switch to oral therapy if tolerated and/or appropriate.

Intra-abdominal infections: I.V.:

Mild infection: 250-500 mg every 6 hours

Severe infection: 500 mg every 6 hours **or** 1 g every 8 hours for 4-7 days (provided source controlled). **Note:** Not recommended for mild-to-moderate, community-acquired intra-abdominal infections due to risk of toxicity and the development of resistant organisms (Solomkin, 2010)

Liver abscess (unlabeled use): I.V.: 500 mg every 6 hours for 4-6 weeks (Ulug, 2010)

Moderate infections: I.V.:

Fully-susceptible organisms: 500 mg every 6-8 hours

Moderately-susceptible organisms: 500 mg every 6 hours or 1 g every 8 hours

Neutropenic fever (unlabeled use): I.V.: 500 mg every 6 hours (Paul, 2006)

***Pseudomonas* infections:** I.V.: 500 mg every 6 hours; **Note:** Higher doses may be required based on organism sensitivity.

Severe infections: I.V.:

Fully-susceptible organisms: 500 mg every 6 hours

Moderately-susceptible organisms: 1 g every 6-8 hours

Maximum daily dose should not exceed 50 mg/kg or 4 g/day, whichever is lower

Urinary tract infection, uncomplicated: I.V.: 250 mg every 6 hours

Urinary tract infection, complicated: I.V.: 500 mg every 6 hours

Mild infections: Note: Rarely a suitable option in mild infections; normally reserved for moderate-severe cases: I.V.:

Fully-susceptible organisms: 250 mg every 6 hours

Moderately-susceptible organisms: 500 mg every 6 hours

Pediatric Dosage based on **imipenem** content:

Non-CNS infections: I.V.: Children: >3 months: 15-25 mg/kg every 6 hours

Maximum dosage: Susceptible infections: 2 g/day; moderately-susceptible organisms: 4 g/day

Burkholderia pseudomallei (melioidosis) (unlabeled use): I.V.: Initial: 20 mg/kg every 8 hours for at least 10 days (White, 2003) **or** 25 mg/kg (up to 1 g) every 6 hours for at least 10 days (Currie, 2003); continue parenteral therapy until clinical improvement, then switch to oral therapy if tolerated and/or appropriate

Cystic fibrosis: I.V.: Infants, Children, and Adolescents: Up to 100 mg/kg/day divided every 6 hours; maximum dose: 4 g daily has been used. **Note:** Efficacy in exacerbations may be limited due to rapid development of resistance (Zobell, 2012).

Renal Impairment I.V.:

Patients with a Cl_{cr} ≤5 mL/minute/1.73 m^2 should not receive imipenem/cilastatin unless hemodialysis is instituted within 48 hours.

Patients weighing <30 kg with impaired renal function should not receive imipenem/cilastatin.

Reduced I.V. dosage regimen based on creatinine clearance and/or body weight: See table.

Intermittent hemodialysis (IHD) (administer after hemodialysis on dialysis days): Use the dosing recommendation for patients with a Cl_{cr} 6-20 mL/minute; administer dose after dialysis session and every 12 hours thereafter **or** 250-500 mg every 12 hours (Heintz, 2009). **Note:** Dosing dependent on the assumption of 3 times/week, complete IHD sessions.

Peritoneal dialysis (unlabeled dosing): Dose as for Cl_{cr} 6-20 mL/minute (Somani, 1988)

Continuous renal replacement therapy (CRRT) (Heintz, 2009; Trotman, 2005): Drug clearance is highly dependent on the method of renal replacement, filter type, and flow rate. Appropriate dosing requires close monitoring of pharmacologic response, signs of adverse reactions due to drug accumulation, as well as drug concentrations in relation to target trough (if appropriate). The following are general recommendations only (based on dialysate flow/ultrafiltration rates of 1-2 L/hour and minimal residual renal function) and should not supersede clinical judgment:

CVVH: Loading dose of 1 g followed by either 250 mg every 6 hours **or** 500 mg every 8 hours

CVVHD: Loading dose of 1 g followed by either 250 mg every 6 hours **or** 500 mg every 6-8 hours

CVVHDF: Loading dose of 1 g followed by either 250 mg every 6 hours **or** 500 mg every 6 hours

Note: Data suggest that 500 mg every 8-12 hours may provide sufficient time above MIC to cover organisms with MIC values ≤2 mg/L; however, a higher dose of 500 mg every 6 hours is recommended for resistant organisms (particularly *Pseudomonas* spp) with MIC ≥4 mg/L or deep-seated infections (Fish, 2005).

Reduced I.V. dosage regimen based on creatinine clearance and/or body weight:

U.S. labeling: See table.

Imipenem and Cilastatin Dosage in Renal Impairment

Reduced I.V. Dosage Regimen Based on Creatinine Clearance (mL/minute/1.73 m²) and/or Body Weight <70 kg					
	Body Weight (kg)				
	≥70	60	50	40	30
Total daily dose for normal renal function: 1 g/day					
Cl_{cr} ≥71	250 mg q6h	250 mg q8h	125 mg q6h	125 mg q6h	125 mg q8h
Cl_{cr} 41-70	250 mg q8h	125 mg q6h	125 mg q6h	125 mg q8h	125 mg q8h
Cl_{cr} 21-40	250 mg q12h	250 mg q12h	125 mg q8h	125 mg q12h	125 mg q12h
Cl_{cr} 6-20	250 mg q12h	125 mg q12h	125 mg q12h	125 mg q12h	125 mg q12h
Total daily dose for normal renal function: 1.5 g/day					
Cl_{cr} ≥71	500 mg q8h	250 mg q6h	250 mg q6h	250 mg q8h	125 mg q6h
Cl_{cr} 41-70	250 mg q6h	250 mg q8h	250 mg q8h	125 mg q6h	125 mg q8h
Cl_{cr} 21-40	250 mg q8h	250 mg q8h	250 mg q12h	125 mg q8h	125 mg q8h
Cl_{cr} 6-20	250 mg q12h	250 mg q12h	250 mg q12h	125 mg q12h	125 mg q12h
Total daily dose for normal renal function: 2 g/day					
Cl_{cr} ≥71	500 mg q6h	500 mg q8h	250 mg q6h	250 mg q6h	250 mg q8h
Cl_{cr} 41-70	500 mg q8h	250 mg q6h	250 mg q6h	250 mg q8h	125 mg q6h
Cl_{cr} 21-40	250 mg q6h	250 mg q8h	250 mg q8h	250 mg q12h	125 mg q8h
Cl_{cr} 6-20	250 mg q12h	250 mg q12h	250 mg q12h	250 mg q12h	125 mg q12h
Total daily dose for normal renal function: 3 g/day					
Cl_{cr} ≥71	1000 mg q8h	750 mg q8h	500 mg q6h	500 mg q8h	250 mg q6h
Cl_{cr} 41-70	500 mg q6h	500 mg q8h	500 mg q8h	250 mg q6h	250 mg q8h
Cl_{cr} 21-40	500 mg q8h	500 mg q8h	250 mg q6h	250 mg q8h	250 mg q8h
Cl_{cr} 6-20	500 mg q12h	500 mg q12h	250 mg q12h	250 mg q12h	250 mg q12h
Total daily dose for normal renal function: 4 g/day					
Cl_{cr} ≥71	1000 mg q6h	1000 mg q8h	750 mg q8h	500 mg q6h	500 mg q8h
Cl_{cr} 41-70	750 mg q8h	750 mg q8h	500 mg q6h	500 mg q8h	250 mg q6h
Cl_{cr} 21-40	500 mg q6h	500 mg q8h	500 mg q8h	250 mg q6h	250 mg q8h
Cl_{cr} 6-20	500 mg q12h	500 mg q12h	500 mg q12h	250 mg q12h	250 mg q12h

Canadian labeling: Reduced I.V. dosage regimen based on creatinine clearance (mL/minute/1.73 m²) and body weight ≥70 kg (**Note:** The manufacturer labeling recommends further proportionate dose reductions for patients <70 kg, but does not provide specific dosing recommendations):

Mild renal impairment (Cl_{cr} 31-70 mL/minute/1.73 m²):

- Fully-susceptible organisms: Maximum dosage: 500 mg every 8 hours
- Less susceptible organisms (primarily some *Pseudomonas* strains): Maximum dosage: 500 mg every 6 hours

Moderate renal impairment (Cl_{cr} 21-30 mL/minute/1.73 m²):

- Fully-susceptible organisms: Maximum dosage: 500 mg every 12 hours
- Less susceptible organisms (primarily some *Pseudomonas* strains): Maximum dosage: 500 mg every 8 hours

Severe renal impairment (Cl_{cr} 0-20 mL/minute/1.73 m^2):
Fully-susceptible organisms: Maximum dosage: 250 mg every 12 hours
Less susceptible organisms (primarily some *Pseudomonas* strains): Maximum dosage: 500 mg every 12 hours
Note: Patients with Cl_{cr} 6-20 mL/minute/1.73 m^2 should receive 250 mg every 12 hours or 3.5 mg/kg (whichever is lower) every 12 hours for most pathogens; seizure risk may increase with higher dosing.

Hepatic Impairment Hepatic dysfunction may further impair cilastatin clearance in patients receiving chronic renal replacement therapy; consider decreasing the dosing frequency.

Administration I.V.: Do not administer I.V. push. Infuse doses ≤500 mg over 20-30 minutes; infuse doses ≥750 mg over 40-60 minutes.

Test Interactions Interferes with urinary glucose determination using Clinitest®; positive Coombs' [direct]

Dosage Forms Excipient information presented when available (limited, particularly for generics); consult specific product labeling.
Injection, powder for reconstitution: Imipenem 250 mg and cilastatin 250 mg; imipenem 500 mg and cilastatin 500 mg
Primaxin® I.V.: Imipenem 250 mg and cilastatin 250 mg [contains sodium 18.8 mg (0.8 mEq)]; imipenem 500 mg and cilastatin 500 mg [contains sodium 37.5 mg (1.6 mEq)]

◆ **Imipenem and Cilastatin for Injection (Can)** *see* Imipenem and Cilastatin *on page 773*

◆ **ImmuCyst® (Can)** *see* BCG *on page 153*

Immune Globulin (i MYUN GLOB yoo lin)

Related Information
Hematopoietic Stem Cell Transplantation *on page 1887*
Immune Globulin Product Comparison *on page 1934*
Management of Infections *on page 1809*

Brand Names: U.S. Carimune® NF; Flebogamma® DIF; GamaSTAN™ S/D; Gammagard S/D®; Gammagard® Liquid; Gammaked™; Gammaplex®; Gamunex®-C; Hizentra®; Octagam®; Privigen®

Brand Names: Canada Gamastan S/D; Gamimune® N; Gammagard Liquid; Gammagard S/D; Hizentra®; IGIVnex®; Privigen®

Index Terms Gamma Globulin; IG; IGIM; IGIV; Immune Globulin Subcutaneous (Human); Immune Serum Globulin; ISG; IV Immune Globulin; IVIG; Panglobulin; SCIG

Generic Availability (U.S.) No

Pharmacologic Category Blood Product Derivative; Immune Globulin

Use
Treatment of primary humoral immunodeficiency syndromes (congenital agammaglobulinemia, severe combined immunodeficiency syndromes [SCIDS], common variable immunodeficiency, X-linked immunodeficiency, Wiskott-Aldrich syndrome) (Carimune® NF, Flebogamma® DIF, Gammagard® Liquid, Gammagard S/D®, Gammaked™, Gammaplex®, Gamunex®-C, Hizentra®, Octagam®, Privigen®)
Treatment of acute and chronic immune (idiopathic) thrombocytopenic purpura (ITP) (Carimune® NF, Gammagard S/D®, Gammaked™, Gamunex®-C, Privigen® [chronic only])
Treatment of chronic inflammatory demyelinating polyneuropathy (CIDP) (Gammaked™, Gamunex®-C)

Treatment of multifocal motor neuropathy (MMN) (Gammagard® Liquid)
Prevention of coronary artery aneurysms associated with Kawasaki syndrome (in combination with aspirin) (Gammagard S/D®)
Prevention of bacterial infection in patients with hypogammaglobulinemia and/or recurrent bacterial infections with B-cell chronic lymphocytic leukemia (CLL) (Gammagard S/D®)
Prevention of serious infection in immunoglobulin deficiency (select agammaglobulinemias) (GamaSTAN™ S/D)
Provision of passive immunity in the following susceptible individuals (GamaSTAN™ S/D):
Hepatitis A: Pre-exposure prophylaxis; postexposure: within 14 days and/or prior to manifestation of disease
Measles: For use within 6 days of exposure in an unvaccinated person, who has not previously had measles
Rubella: Postexposure prophylaxis (within 72 hours) to reduce the risk of infection and fetal damage in exposed pregnant women who will not consider therapeutic abortion
Varicella: For immunosuppressed patients when varicella zoster immune globulin is not available

Unlabeled Use Acquired hypogammaglobulinemia secondary to malignancy; Guillain-Barré syndrome; hematopoietic stem cell transplantation (HSCT), to prevent bacterial infections among allogeneic recipients with severe hypogammaglobulinemia (IgG <400 mg/dL) at <100 days post transplant (CDC guidelines); HIV-associated thrombocytopenia; multiple sclerosis (relapsing, remitting when other therapies cannot be used); Lambert-Eaton myasthenic syndrome (LEMS); myasthenia gravis; refractory dermatomyositis/polymyositis

Labeled Contraindications Hypersensitivity to immune globulin or any component of the formulation; selective IgA deficiency; hyperprolinemia (Hizentra®, Privigen®); severe thrombocytopenia or coagulation disorders; severe thrombocytopenia or coagulation disorders where IM injections are contraindicated

Pregnancy Risk Factor C

Lactation Excretion in breast milk unknown/use caution

Warnings/Precautions [U.S. Boxed Warning]: I.V. formulation only: Acute renal dysfunction (increased serum creatinine, oliguria, acute renal failure, osmotic nephrosis) can rarely occur; usually within 7 days of use (more likely with products stabilized with sucrose). Use with caution in the elderly, patients with renal disease, diabetes mellitus, volume depletion, sepsis, paraproteinemia, and nephrotoxic medications due to risk of renal dysfunction. In patients at risk of renal dysfunction, the rate of infusion and concentration of solution should be minimized. Discontinue if renal function deteriorates. High-dose regimens (1 g/kg for 1-2 days) are not recommended for individuals with fluid overload or where fluid volume may be of concern. Hypersensitivity and anaphylactic reactions can occur; a severe fall in blood pressure may rarely occur with anaphylactic reaction; immediate treatment (including epinephrine 1:1000) should be available. Product of human plasma; may potentially contain infectious agents which could transmit disease. Screening of donors, as well as testing and/or inactivation or removal of certain viruses, reduces the risk. Infections thought to be transmitted by this product should be reported to the manufacturer. Aseptic meningitis may occur with high doses (≥1-2 g/kg [product-dependent]) and/or rapid infusion; syndrome usually appears within several hours to 2 days following treatment; usually resolves within several days after product is discontinued; patients with a migraine history may be at higher risk for AMS. Increased risk of hypersensitivity, especially in patients with anti-IgA antibodies. Increased risk of hematoma formation when administered subcutaneously for the treatment of ITP.

Intravenous immune globulin has been associated with antiglobulin hemolysis; monitor for signs of hemolytic anemia. Risk factors include high doses (≥2 g/kg) and non-O blood type. In chronic ITP, assess risk versus benefit of high-dose regimen in patients with increased risk of thrombosis, hemolysis, acute kidney injury, or volume overload.

Patients should be adequately hydrated prior to initiation of therapy. Hyperproteinemia, increased serum viscosity and hyponatremia may occur; distinguish hyponatremia from pseudohyponatremia to prevent volume depletion, a further increase in serum viscosity, and a higher risk of thrombotic events. Use caution in patients with a history of thrombotic events or a history of atherosclerosis or cardiovascular disease or patients with known/suspected hyperviscosity; there is clinical evidence of a possible association between thrombotic events and administration of intravenous immune globulin and subcutaneous immune globulin. Consider a baseline assessment of blood viscosity in patients at risk for hyperviscosity. Patients should be monitored for adverse events during and after the infusion. Stop administration with signs of infusion reaction (fever, chills, nausea, vomiting, and rarely shock). Risk may be increased with initial treatment, when switching brands of immune globulin, and with treatment interruptions of >8 weeks. Monitor for transfusion related acute lung injury (TRALI); noncardiogenic pulmonary edema has been reported with intravenous immune globulin use. TRALI is characterized by severe respiratory distress, pulmonary edema, hypoxemia, and fever (in the presence of normal left ventricular function) and usually occurs within 1-6 hours after infusion. Response to live vaccinations may be impaired. Some clinicians may administer intravenous immune globulin products as a subcutaneous infusion based on patient tolerability and clinical judgment. SubQ infusion should begin 1 week after the last I.V. dose; dose should be individualized based on clinical response and serum IgG trough concentrations; consider premedicating with acetaminophen and diphenhydramine.

Some products may contain maltose, which may result in falsely-elevated blood glucose readings; maltose-containing products are contraindicated in patients with an allergy to corn. Some products may contain polysorbate 80, sodium, and/or sucrose. Some products may contain sorbitol; do not use in patients with fructose intolerance. Hizentra® and Privigen® contain the stabilizer L-proline and are contraindicated in patients with hyperprolinemia. Packaging of some products may contain natural latex/natural rubber; skin testing should not be performed with GamaSTAN™ S/D as local irritation can occur and be misinterpreted as a positive reaction.

Adverse Reactions Frequency not always defined.

Cardiovascular: Chest tightness (7%), hypertension (5%), angioedema, edema, flushing of the face, hypotension, palpitation, tachycardia

Central nervous system: Headache (16% to 48%), fever (6%), chills (3%), dizziness (1%), malaise (1%), anxiety, aseptic meningitis syndrome, drowsiness, fatigue, irritability, lethargy, lightheadedness, migraine, pain

Dermatologic: Bruising, contact dermatitis, eczema, erythema, hyperhidrosis, petechiae, pruritus, purpura, rash, urticaria

Endocrine & metabolic: Hyperglycemia (neuromuscular disease: 1%)

Gastrointestinal: Nausea (3% to 18%), anorexia (neuromuscular disease: 1%), abdominal cramps, abdominal pain, diarrhea, discomfort, dyspepsia, gastroenteritis, sore throat, toothache, vomiting

Hematologic: Anemia, autoimmune hemolytic anemia, hematocrit decreased, hematoma, hemolysis (mild), hemorrhage, thrombocytopenia

Hepatic: Bilirubin increased, LDH increased, liver function test increased

Local: Muscle stiffness at I.M. site; pain, swelling, redness or irritation at the infusion site

Neuromuscular & skeletal: Muscle spasm (MMN 7%), weakness (1%; MMN: 7%), arthralgia (1%), back or hip pain, leg cramps, muscle cramps, myalgia, neck pain, rigors

Ocular: Conjunctivitis

Otic: Ear pain

Renal: Acute renal failure, acute tubular necrosis, anuria, BUN increased, creatinine increased, oliguria, proximal tubular nephropathy, osmotic nephrosis

Respiratory: Oropharyngeal pain (7%), asthma aggravated, bronchitis, cough, dyspnea, epistaxis, nasal congestion, pharyngeal pain, pharyngitis, rhinitis, rhinorrhea, sinus headache, sinusitis, upper respiratory infection, wheezing

Miscellaneous: Anaphylaxis, diaphoresis, flu-like syndrome, hypersensitivity reactions, infusion reaction, thermal burn

<1%, postmarketing, and/or case reports: Apnea, ARDS, autoimmune pure red cell aplasia (PRCA) exacerbation, blurred vision, bronchopneumonia, bronchospasm, bullous dermatitis, cardiac arrest, chest pain, coma, Coombs' test positive, cyanosis, epidermolysis, erythema multiforme, heart failure, hepatic dysfunction, hypoxemia, leukopenia, loss of consciousness, MI, pancytopenia, papular rash, phlebitis, pulmonary edema, pulmonary embolism, seizures, Stevens-Johnson syndrome, stroke, syncope, thromboembolism, transfusion-related acute lung injury (TRALI), tremor, vascular collapse

Drug Interactions

Metabolism/Transport Effects None known.

Avoid Concomitant Use There are no known interactions where it is recommended to avoid concomitant use.

Increased Effect/Toxicity There are no known significant interactions involving an increase in effect.

Decreased Effect

Immune Globulin may decrease the levels/effects of: Vaccines (Live)

Storage/Stability Stability is dependent upon the manufacturer and brand. Do not freeze.

Carimune® NF: Prior to reconstitution, store at or below 30°C (86°F). Reconstitute with NS, D_5W, or SWFI. Following reconstitution in a sterile laminar air flow environment, store under refrigeration. Begin infusion within 24 hours.

Flebogamma® DIF: Store at 2°C to 25°C (36°F to 77°F); do not freeze.

GamaSTAN™ S/D: Store under refrigeration at 2°C to 8°C (36°F to 46°F). The following stability information has also been reported for GamaSTAN™ S/D: May be exposed to room temperature for a cumulative 7 days (Cohen, 2007).

Gammagard® Liquid: Prior to use, store at 2°C to 8°C (36°F to 46°F); do not freeze. May store at room temperature of 25°C (77°F) within the first 24 months of manufacturing. Storage time at room temperature varies with length of time previously refrigerated; refer to product labeling for details.

Gammagard S/D®: Store at ≤25°C (≤77°F). May store diluted solution under refrigeration at 2°C to 8°C (36°F to 46°F) for up to 24 hours if originally prepared in a sterile laminar air flow environment.

Gammaked™: Store at 2°C to 8°C (36°F to 46°F); may be stored at ≤25°C (≤77°F) for up to 6 months.
Gammaplex®: Store at 2°C to 25°C (36°F to 77°F); do not freeze. Protect from light.
Gamunex®-C: Store at 2°C to 8°C (36°F to 46°F); may be stored at ≤25°C (≤77°F) for up to 6 months.
Hizentra®: Store at ≤25°C (≤77°F); do not freeze or use product if previously frozen. Do not shake.
Octagam®: Store at 2°C to 25°C (36°F to 77°F).
Privigen®: Store at ≤25°C (≤77°F); do not freeze (do not use if previously frozen). Protect from light.

Reconstitution Dilution is dependent upon the manufacturer and brand. Gently swirl; do not shake; avoid foaming. Do not mix products from different manufacturers together. Discard unused portion of vials.

Carimune® NF: In a sterile laminar air flow environment, reconstitute with NS, D_5W, or SWFI. Complete dissolution may take up to 20 minutes. Begin infusion within 24 hours.
Flebogamma® DIF: Dilution is not recommended.
Gammagard® Liquid: May dilute in D_5W only.
Gammagard S/D®: Reconstitute with SWFI.
Gammaked™: May dilute in D_5W only.
Gamunex®-C: May dilute in D_5W only.
Privigen®: If necessary to further dilute, D_5W may be used

Mechanism of Action Replacement therapy for primary and secondary immunodeficiencies, and IgG antibodies against bacteria, viral, parasitic and mycoplasma antigens; interference with F_c receptors on the cells of the reticuloendothelial system for autoimmune cytopenias and ITP; provides passive immunity by increasing the antibody titer and antigen-antibody reaction potential

Pharmacodynamics/Kinetics

Onset of action: I.V.: Provides immediate antibody levels
Duration: I.M., I.V.: Immune effect: 3-4 weeks (variable)
Distribution: V_d: 0.09-0.13 L/kg
Intravascular portion (primarily): Healthy subjects: 41% to 57%; Patients with congenital humoral immunodeficiencies: ~70%
Half-life elimination: I.M.: ~23 days; I.V.: IgG (variable among patients): Healthy subjects: 14-24 days; Patients with congenital humoral immunodeficiencies: 26-40 days; hypermetabolism associated with fever and infection have coincided with a shortened half-life
Time to peak:
Plasma: SubQ: Gammagard® Liquid: 2.9 days; Hizentra®: 2.9 days
Serum: I.M.: ~48 hours

Dosing

Adult & Geriatric Note: Some clinicians may administer IVIG formulations FDA approved only for intravenous administration as a subcutaneous infusion based on clinical judgment and patient tolerability. Also, some clinicians dose IVIG on ideal body weight or an adjusted ideal body weight in morbidly obese patients (Siegel, 2010).

B-cell chronic lymphocytic leukemia (CLL) (Gammagard S/D®): I.V.: 400 mg/kg every 3-4 weeks

Chronic inflammatory demyelinating polyneuropathy (CIDP) (Gammaked™, Gamunex-C®): I.V.: Loading dose: 2000 mg/kg (given in divided doses over 2-4 consecutive days); Maintenance: 1000 mg/kg every 3 weeks. Alternatively, administer 500 mg/kg/day for 2 consecutive days every 3 weeks.

Hepatitis A (GamaSTAN™ S/D): I.M.:

Pre-exposure prophylaxis upon travel into endemic areas (hepatitis A vaccine preferred):

0.02 **mL**/kg for anticipated risk of exposure <3 months

0.06 **mL**/kg for anticipated risk of exposure ≥3 months; repeat every 4-6 months.

Postexposure prophylaxis: 0.02 **mL**/kg given within 14 days of exposure and/or prior to manifestation of disease; not needed if at least 1 dose of hepatitis A vaccine was given at ≥1 month before exposure

Immunoglobulin deficiency (GamaSTAN™ S/D): I.M.: 0.66 **mL**/kg (minimum dose should be 100 mg/kg) every 3-4 weeks. Administer a double dose at onset of therapy; some patients may require more frequent injections.

Immune (idiopathic) thrombocytopenic purpura (ITP):

Carimune® NF: I.V.: Initial: 400 mg/kg/day for 2-5 days; Maintenance: 400 mg/kg as needed to maintain platelet count ≥30,000/mm^3 and/or to control significant bleeding; may increase dose if needed (range: 800-1000 mg/kg)

Gammagard S/D®: I.V.: 1000 mg/kg; up to 3 additional doses may be given based on patient response and/or platelet count. **Note:** Additional doses should be given on alternate days.

Gammaked™, Gamunex-C®: I.V.: 1000 mg/kg/day for 2 consecutive days (second dose may be withheld if adequate platelet response in 24 hours) **or** 400 mg/kg once daily for 5 consecutive days

Privigen®: I.V.: 1000 mg/kg/day for 2 consecutive days

Kawasaki syndrome (Gammagard S/D®): I.V.:

Gammagard S/D®: 1000 mg/kg as a single dose **or** 400 mg/kg/day for 4 consecutive days. Begin within 7 days of onset of fever.

AHA guidelines (2004): 2000 mg/kg as a single dose within 10 days of disease onset

Note: Must be used in combination with aspirin: 80-100 mg/kg/day orally, divided every 6 hours for up to 14 days (until fever resolves for at least 48 hours); then decrease dose to 3-5 mg/kg/day once daily. In patients without coronary artery abnormalities, give lower dose for 6-8 weeks. In patients with coronary artery abnormalities, low-dose aspirin should be continued indefinitely.

Measles:

GamaSTAN™ S/D: I.M.:

Immunocompetent: 0.25 **mL**/kg given within 6 days of exposure followed by live attenuated measles vaccine in 5-6 months when indicated (CDC, 1998)

Immunocompromised children: 0.5 **mL**/kg (maximum dose: 15 **mL**) immediately following exposure

Gammaked™, Gamunex-C®, Octagam®: I.V.:

Prophylaxis in patients with primary humoral immunodeficiency (**ONLY** if routine dose is <400 mg/kg): ≥400 mg/kg immediately before expected exposure

Treatment in patients with primary immunodeficiency: 400 mg/kg administered as soon as possible after exposure

Hizentra®: SubQ infusion: Measles exposure in patients with primary humoral immunodeficiency: Weekly dose: ≥200 mg/kg for 2 consecutive weeks for patients at risk of measles exposure (eg, during an outbreak; travel to endemic area). In patients who have been exposed to measles, administer the minimum dose as soon as possible following exposure.

Multifocal motor neuropathy (MMN) (Gammagard® liquid): I.V.: 500-2400 mg/kg/month based upon response

Primary humoral immunodeficiency disorders:

I.V. infusion dosing:

Carimune® NF: I.V.: 400-800 mg/kg every 3-4 weeks

Flebogamma® DIF, Gammagard® Liquid, Gammagard S/D®, Gammaked™, Gamunex-C®, Octagam®: I.V.: 300-600 mg/kg every 3-4 weeks; adjusted based on dosage and interval in conjunction with monitored serum IgG concentrations and clinical response

Gammaplex®: I.V.: 300-800 mg/kg every 3-4 weeks

Privigen®: I.V.: 200-800 mg/kg every 3-4 weeks; adjusted based on dosage and interval in conjunction with monitored serum IgG concentrations and clinical response

Switching to weekly subcutaneous infusion dosing:

Gammagard® Liquid, Gammaked™, Gamunex-C®: SubQ infusion: Begin 1 week after last I.V. dose. Use the following equation to calculate initial dose:

Initial weekly dose (g) = [1.37 x IGIV dose (g)] divided by [I.V. dose interval (weeks)]

Note: For subsequent dose adjustments, refer to product labeling.

Hizentra®: SubQ infusion: Begin 1 week after last I.V. dose. **Note:** Patient should have received an I.V. immune globulin routinely for at least 3 months before switching to SubQ. Use the following equation to calculate initial dose:

Initial weekly dose (g) = [1.53 x IGIV dose (g)] divided by [I.V. dose interval (weeks)]

Note: For subsequent dose adjustments, refer to product labeling.

Rubella (GamaSTAN™ S/D): I.M.: Prophylaxis during pregnancy: 0.55 **mL**/kg within 72 hours of exposure (CDC, 1998)

Varicella (GamaSTAN™ S/D): I.M.: Prophylaxis: 0.6-1.2 **mL**/kg (varicella zoster immune globulin preferred) within 72 hours of exposure

Unlabeled uses: I.V.:

Acquired hypogammaglobulinemia secondary to malignancy (unlabeled use): Adults: 400 mg/kg/dose every 3 weeks; reevaluate every 4-6 months (Anderson, 2007)

Guillain-Barré syndrome (unlabeled use): Children and Adults: Various regimens have been used, including:

400 mg/kg/day for 5 days (Hughes, 2003)

or

400 mg/kg/day for 6 days (Patwa, 2012)

or

2000 mg/kg in divided doses administered over 2-5 days (Feasby, 2007)

Hematopoietic stem cell transplantation with hypogammaglobulinemia (CDC guidelines, 2000; unlabeled use):

Children: 400 mg/kg per month; increase dose or frequency to maintain IgG levels >400 mg/dL

Adolescents and Adults: 500 mg/kg/week

HIV-associated thrombocytopenia (unlabeled use): Adults: 1000 mg/kg/day for 2 days (Anderson, 2007)

Lambert-Eaton myasthenic syndrome (LEMS) (unlabeled use): Adults: 1000 mg/kg/day for 2 days (Bain, 1996; Patwa, 2012)

Multiple sclerosis (relapsing-remitting, when other therapies cannot be used) (unlabeled use): Children and Adults: 1000 mg/kg per month, with or without an induction of 400 mg/kg/day for 5 days (Feasby, 2007)

Myasthenia gravis (severe exacerbation) (unlabeled use): Children and Adults: 2000 mg/kg per treatment course over 2-5 days (Feasby, 2007; Patwa, 2012)

Refractory dermatomyositis/polymyositis (unlabeled uses): Children and Adults: 2000 mg/kg per treatment course administered over 2-5 days (Feasby, 2007)

Pediatric Refer to adult dosing.

Renal Impairment I.V.: Cl_{cr} <10 mL/minute: Avoid use; in patients at risk of renal dysfunction, consider infusion at a rate less than maximum.

Administration Note: If plasmapheresis employed for treatment of condition, administer immune globulin **after** completion of plasmapheresis session.

I.M.: Administer I.M. in the anterolateral aspects of the upper thigh or deltoid muscle of the upper arm. Avoid gluteal region due to risk of injury to sciatic nerve. Divide doses >10 mL and inject in multiple sites.

GamaSTAN™ S/D is for I.M. administration only.

I.V. infusion: Infuse over 2-24 hours; administer in separate infusion line from other medications; if using primary line, flush with NS or D_5W (product specific; consult product prescribing information) prior to administration. Decrease dose, rate and/or concentration of infusion in patients who may be at risk of renal failure. Decreasing the rate or stopping the infusion may help relieve some adverse effects (flushing, changes in pulse rate, changes in blood pressure). Epinephrine should be available during administration. For initial treatment or in the elderly, a lower concentration and/or a slower rate of infusion should be used. Initial rate of administration and titration is specific to each IVIG product. Consult specific product prescribing information for detailed recommendations. Refrigerated product should be warmed to room temperature prior to infusion. Some products require filtration; refer to individual product labeling. Antecubital veins should be used, especially with concentrations ≥10% to prevent injection site discomfort.

SubQ infusion: Initial dose should be administered in a healthcare setting capable of providing monitoring and treatment in the event of hypersensitivity. Using aseptic technique, follow the infusion device manufacturer's instructions for filling the reservoir and preparing the pump. Remove air from administration set and needle by priming. Appropriate injection sites include the abdomen, thigh, upper arm, lower back, and/or lateral hip; dose may be infused into multiple sites (spaced ≥2 inches apart) simultaneously. After the sites are clean and dry, insert subcutaneous needle and prime administration set. Attach sterile needle to administration set, gently pull back on the syringe to assure a blood vessel has not been inadvertently accessed (do not use needle and tubing if blood present). Repeat for each injection site; deliver the dose following instructions for the infusion device. Rotate the site(s) weekly. Treatment may be transitioned to the home/home care setting in the absence of adverse reactions.

Gammagard® Liquid:
Injection sites: ≤8 simultaneous injection sites
Initial infusion rate:
<40 kg: 15 mL/hour per injection site (maximum volume: 20 mL per injection site)
≥40 kg: 20 mL/hour per injection site (maximum volume: 30 mL per injection site)
Maintenance infusion rate:
<40 kg: 15-20 mL/hour per injection site (maximum volume: 20 mL per injection site)
≥40 kg: 20-30 mL/hour per injection site (maximum volume: 30 mL per injection site)
Gammaked™, Gamunex-C®:
Injection sites: ≤8 simultaneous injection sites
Recommended infusion rate: 20 mL/hour per injection site
Hizentra®:
Injection sites: ≤4 simultaneous injection sites
Maximum infusion rate: First infusion: 15 mL/hour per injection site; subsequent infusions: 25 mL/hour per injection site (maximum: 50 mL/hour for all simultaneous sites combined)
Maximum infusion volume: First 4 infusions: 15 mL per injection site; subsequent infusions: 20 mL per injection site (maximum: 25 mL per site as tolerated)

Monitoring Parameters Renal function, urine output, IgG concentrations, hemoglobin and hematocrit, platelets (in patients with ITP); infusion- or injection-related adverse reactions, anaphylaxis, signs and symptoms of hemolysis; blood viscosity (in patients at risk for hyperviscosity); presence of antineutrophil antibodies (if TRALI is suspected); volume status; neurologic symptoms (if AMS suspected); clinical response

For patients at high risk of hemolysis (dose ≥2 g/kg, given as a single dose or divided over several days, and non-O blood type): Hemoglobin or hematocrit prior to and 36 to 96 hours postinfusion.

SubQ infusion: Monitor IgG trough levels every 2-3 months before/after conversion from I.V.; subcutaneous infusions provide more constant IgG levels than usual I.V. immune globulin treatments.

Test Interactions Octagam® contains maltose. Falsely-elevated blood glucose levels may occur when glucose monitoring devices and test strips utilizing the glucose dehydrogenase pyrroloquinolinequinone (GDH-PQQ) based methods are used. Glucose monitoring devices and test strips which utilize the glucose specific method are recommended. Passively-transferred antibodies may yield false-positive serologic testing results; may yield false-positive direct and indirect Coombs' test. Skin testing should not be performed with GamaSTAN™ S/D as local irritation can occur and be misinterpreted as a positive reaction.

Dietary Considerations Some products may contain sodium.

Additional Information I.M.: When administering immune globulin for hepatitis A prophylaxis, use should be considered for the following close contacts of persons with confirmed hepatitis A: unvaccinated household and sexual contacts, persons who have shared illicit drugs, regular babysitters, staff and attendees of child care centers, food handlers within the same establishment (CDC, 2006).

All household contacts of measles patients should be evaluated to receive immune globulin unless the measles vaccine has been given on or after the first birthday, unless immunocompromised (CDC, 1998).

For travelers, immune globulin is not an alternative to careful selection of foods and water; immune globulin can interfere with the antibody response to parenterally administered live virus vaccines. Frequent travelers should be tested for hepatitis A antibody, immune hemolytic anemia, and neutropenia (with ITP, I.V. route is usually used).

IgA content:
- Carimune® NF: 720 mcg/mL
- Flebogamma® 5% DIF: 2.9 ± 0.1 mcg/mL
- Flebogamma® 10% DIF: <100 mcg/mL
- Gammagard® Liquid: 37 mcg/mL
- Gammagard S/D® 5% solution: <1 mcg/mL or <2.2 mcg/mL (product dependent)
- Gammaked™: 46 mcg/mL
- Gammaplex®: <10 mcg/mL
- Gamunex-C®: 46 mcg/mL
- Hizentra®: ≤50 mcg/mL
- Octagam®: ≤200 mcg/mL
- Privigen®: ≤25 mcg/mL

Dosage Forms Excipient information presented when available (limited, particularly for generics); consult specific product labeling.

Injection, powder for reconstitution [preservative free]:
- Carimune® NF: 3 g, 6 g, 12 g [contains sucrose]
- Gammagard S/D®: 2.5 g [contains albumin (human), glucose, glycine, natural rubber/natural latex in packaging, polyethylene glycol, polysorbate 80; IgA <2.2 mcg/mL]
- Gammagard S/D®: 5 g [contains albumin (human), glucose, glycine, natural rubber/natural latex in packaging, polyethylene glycol, polysorbate 80; IgA <1 mcg/mL]
- Gammagard S/D®: 5 g [contains albumin (human), glucose, glycine, natural rubber/natural latex in packaging, polyethylene glycol, polysorbate 80; IgA <2.2 mcg/mL]
- Gammagard S/D®: 10 g [contains albumin (human), glucose, glycine, natural rubber/natural latex in packaging, polyethylene glycol, polysorbate 80; IgA <1 mcg/mL]
- Gammagard S/D®: 10 g [contains albumin (human), glucose, glycine, natural rubber/natural latex in packaging, polyethylene glycol, polysorbate 80; IgA <2.2 mcg/mL]

Injection, solution [preservative free]:
- Flebogamma® DIF: 5% [50 mg/mL] (10 mL, 50 mL, 100 mL, 200 mL, 400 mL); 10% [100 mg/mL] (100 mL, 200 mL) [contains polyethylene glycol, sorbitol]
- GamaSTAN™ S/D: 15% to 18% [150 to 180 mg/mL] (2 mL, 10 mL)
- Gammagard® Liquid: 10% [100 mg/mL] (10 mL, 25 mL, 50 mL, 100 mL, 200 mL, 300 mL) [sucrose free; contains glycine]
- Gammaked™: 10% [100 mg/mL] (10 mL, 25 mL, 50 mL, 100 mL, 200 mL) [sucrose free; contains glycine]
- Gammaplex®: 5% [50 mg/mL] (50 mL, 100 mL, 200 mL) [sucrose free; contains glycine, natural rubber/natural latex in packaging, polysorbate 80, sorbitol]

Gamunex®-C: 10% [100 mg/mL] (10 mL, 25 mL, 50 mL, 100 mL, 200 mL) [contains glycine]
Hizentra®: 200 mg/mL (5 mL, 10 mL, 20 mL) [contains L-proline, polysorbate 80]
Octagam®: 5% [50 mg/mL] (20 mL, 50 mL, 100 mL, 200 mL) [sucrose free; contains maltose, sodium 30 mmol/L]
Privigen®: 10% [100 mg/mL] (50 mL, 100 mL, 200 mL) [sucrose free; contains L-proline]

References

Anderson D, Ali K, Blanchette V, et al, "Guidelines on the Use of Intravenous Immune Globulin for Hematologic Conditions," *Transfus Med Rev*, 2007, 21(2 Suppl 1):9-56.

Bain PG, Motomura M, Newsom-Davis J, et al, "Effects of Intravenous Immunoglobulin on Muscle Weakness and Calcium-Channel Autoantibodies in the Lambert-Eaton Myasthenic Syndrome," *Neurology*, 1996, 47(3):678-83.

Centers for Disease Control and Prevention, "Guidelines for Preventing Opportunistic Infections Among HIV-Infected Persons - 2002 Recommendations of the U.S. Public Health Service and the Infectious Diseases Society of America," *MMWR Recomm Rep*, 2002, 51(RR-8):1-52.

Centers for Disease Control and Prevention, "Guidelines for Preventing Opportunistic Infections Among Hematopoietic Stem Cell Transplant Recipients: Recommendations of CDC, the Infectious Disease Society of America, and the American Society of Blood and Marrow Transplantation," *MMWR Recomm Rep*, 2000, 49(RR-10):1-125.

Centers for Disease Control and Prevention (CDC), "Measles, Mumps, and Rubella - Vaccine Use and Strategies for Elimination of Measles, Rubella, and Congenital Rubella Syndrome and Control of Mumps: Recommendations of the Advisory Committee on Immunization Practices (ACIP)," *MMWR Recomm Rep*, 1998, 47(RR-8):1-57. Available at http://www.cdc.gov/mmwr/PDF/rr/rr4708.pdf

Centers for Disease Control and Prevention (CDC), "Prevention of Hepatitis A Through Active or Passive Immunization: Recommendations of the Advisory Committee on Immunization Practices (ACIP)," *MMWR Recomm Rep*, 2006, 55(RR-7):1-23. Available at http://www.cdc.gov/mmwr/PDF/rr/rr5507.pdf

Feasby T, Banwell B, Benstead T, et al, "Guidelines on the Use of Intravenous Immune Globulin for Neurologic Conditions," *Transfus Med Rev*, 2007, 21(2 Suppl 1):57-107.

Gurcan HM and Ahmed AR, "Efficacy of Various Intravenous Immunoglobulin Therapy Protocols in Autoimmune and Chronic Inflammatory Disorders," *Ann Pharmacother*, 2007, 41(5):812-23.

Hughes RA, Bouche P, Cornblath DR, et al, "European Federation of Neurological Societies/Peripheral Nerve Society Guideline on Management of Chronic Inflammatory Demyelinating Polyradiculoneuropathy: Report of a Joint Task Force of the European Federation of Neurological Societies and the Peripheral Nerve Society," *Eur J Neurol*, 2006, 13(4):326-32.

Hughes RA, Wijdicks EF, Barohn R, et al, "Practice Parameter: Immunotherapy for Guillain-Barré Syndrome: Report of the Quality Standards Subcommittee of the American Academy of Neurology," *Neurology*, 2003, 61(6):736-40.

Newburger JW, Takahashi M, Gerber MA, et al, "Diagnosis, Treatment, and Long-Term Management of Kawasaki Disease: A Statement for Health Professionals From the Committee on Rheumatic Fever, Endocarditis, and Kawasaki Disease, Council on Cardiovascular Disease in the Young, American Heart Association," *Pediatrics*, 2004, 114(6):1708-33.

Orange JS, Hossny EM, Weller CR, et al, "Use of Intravenous Immunoglobulin in Human Disease: A Review of Evidence by Members of the Primary Immunodeficiency Committee of the American Academy of Allergy, Asthma and Immunology," *J Allergy Clin Immunol*, 2006, 117(4 Suppl):525-53.

Patwa HS, Chaudhry V, Katzberg H, et al, "Evidence-Based Guideline: Intravenous Immunoglobulin in the Treatment of Neuromuscular Disorders: Report of the Therapeutics and Technology Assessment Subcommittee of the American Academy of Neurology," *Neurology*, 2012, 78 (13):1009-15.

Siegel J, "Immunoglobulins and Obesity," *Pharmacy Practice News*, 2010, 37:1.

Skvaril F and Gardi A, "Differences Among Available Immunoglobulin Preparations for Intravenous Use," *Pediatr Infect Dis J*, 1988, 7:543-48.

◆ **Immune Globulin Subcutaneous (Human)** *see* Immune Globulin *on page 777*

◆ **Immune Serum Globulin** *see* Immune Globulin *on page 777*

◆ **Immunine® VH (Can)** *see* Factor IX *on page 571*

- **INCB424** *see* Ruxolitinib *on page 1261*
- **INCB 18424** *see* Ruxolitinib *on page 1261*
- **Indium In-111 Pentetreotide Kit** *see* Indium In-111 Pentetreotide *on page 788*

Indium In-111 Pentetreotide

(IN dee um eye en won e LEV en pen te TREE oh tide)

Brand Names: U.S. OctreoScan®

Index Terms ^{111}In-Pentetreotide; Indium In-111 Pentetreotide Kit; OctreoScan® (Prep Kit)

Pharmacologic Category Radiopharmaceutical

Use Scintigraphic localization of primary and metastatic neuroendocrine tumors with somatostatin receptors

Pregnancy Risk Factor C

Lactation Excretion in breast milk unknown/not recommended

Warnings/Precautions Radiopharmaceutical: Use appropriate precautions for handling, disposal, and minimizing exposure to patients and healthcare personnel. Use under supervision of individuals who have received training in the handling of radioactive materials and who are authorized by the applicable regulatory authority.

May cause severe hypoglycemia in patients with insulinomas; use with caution. Administer glucose before and during indium In-111 pentetreotide administration. Sensitivity of scintigraphy may be reduced with concurrent octreotide; consider temporarily withdrawing octreotide prior to scintigraphy. Use with caution in patients with renal impairment.

Storage/Stability Store kit under refrigeration at 2°C to 8°C (36°F to 46°F). After reconstitution, store at or below 25°C (77°F). Use the reconstituted product within 6 hours of preparation.

Reconstitution Preparation: Remove the contents of the indium In-111 chloride vial using the needle provided and a shielded, sterile syringe. Inject indium In-111 solution into the reaction vial. Gently swirl. Incubate at ≤25°C (77°F) for at least 30 minutes. Assay the solution and record the date, time, total activity, and patient's ID. Solution can be diluted to a maximum volume of 3 mL with normal saline immediately prior to injection.

Dosing

Adult

Planar imaging: I.V.: 3 mCi (111 MBq)

Single photon emission computed tomograph (SPECT) imaging: I.V.: 6 mCi (222 MBq)

Pediatric I.V.: 0.14 mCi/kg (5 MBq/kg)

Administration Patient should be well-hydrated before and after administration. Laxatives should be used before and for 48 hours after receiving indium In-111 pentetreotide.

Additional Information OctreoScan® is the kit for the preparation of the product, indium In-111 pentetreotide, not the final product itself.

Dosage Forms Excipient information presented when available (limited, particularly for generics); consult specific product labeling.

Kit, [preservative free]:

OctreoScan®:

Injection, powder for reconstitution: Pentetreotide 10 mcg

Injection, solution: Indium In-111 chloride 111 MBq (3.0 mCi) per 1 mL (1.1 mL)

References

Balon HR, Goldsmith SJ, Siegel BA, et al, "Society of Nucelar Medicine Procedure Guideline for Somatostatin Receptor Scintigraphy with IN-111 Pentetreotide," J Nucl Med, 2001, 42(7):1134-8. Available at http://interactive.snm.org/docs/pg_ch27_0403.pdf. Last accessed April 27, 2010.

Rubow SM and Ellman A, "Indium-111 Scintigraphy and Breastfeeding," *Eur J Nucl Med*, 2000, 27 (8):1057.

◆ **INF-alpha 2** *see* Interferon Alfa-2b *on page* 798

◆ **INFeD®** *see* Iron Dextran Complex *on page* 824

InFLIXimab (in FLIKS e mab)

Related Information

Hematopoietic Stem Cell Transplantation *on page* 1887

Brand Names: U.S. Remicade®

Brand Names: Canada Remicade®

Index Terms Avakine; Infliximab, Recombinant

Generic Availability (U.S.) No

Pharmacologic Category Antirheumatic, Disease Modifying; Gastrointestinal Agent, Miscellaneous; Immunosuppressant Agent; Monoclonal Antibody; Tumor Necrosis Factor (TNF) Blocking Agent

Use

Treatment of moderately- to severely-active rheumatoid arthritis (with methotrexate) (to reduce signs/symptoms of active arthritis and inhibit progression of structural damage and improve physical function)

Treatment of moderately- to severely-active Crohn's disease with inadequate response to conventional therapy (to reduce signs/symptoms and induce and maintain clinical remission) or to reduce the number of draining enterocutaneous and rectovaginal fistulas and maintain fistula closure

Treatment of psoriatic arthritis (to reduce signs/symptoms of active arthritis and inhibit progression of structural damage and improve physical function)

Treatment of chronic severe (extensive and/or disabling) plaque psoriasis as an alternative to other systemic therapy

Treatment of active ankylosing spondylitis (to reduce signs/symptoms)

Treatment of moderately- to severely-active ulcerative colitis with inadequate response to conventional therapy (to reduce signs/symptoms and induce and maintain clinical remission, mucosal healing and eliminate corticosteroid use)

Labeled Contraindications Hypersensitivity to infliximab, murine proteins or any component of the formulation; doses >5 mg/kg in patients with moderate or severe heart failure (NYHA Class III/IV)

Canadian labeling: Additional contraindications (not in U.S. labeling): Severe infections (eg, sepsis, abscesses, tuberculosis, and opportunistic infections)

Pregnancy Risk Factor B

Lactation Excretion in breast milk unknown/not recommended

Warnings/Precautions **[U.S. Boxed Warning]: Patients receiving infliximab are at increased risk for serious infections which may result in hospitalization and/or fatality; infections usually developed in patients receiving concomitant immunosuppressive agents (eg, methotrexate or corticosteroids) and may present as disseminated (rather than local) disease. Active tuberculosis (or reactivation of latent tuberculosis), invasive fungal (including aspergillosis, blastomycosis, candidiasis, coccidioidomycosis, histoplasmosis, and pneumocystosis) and bacterial, viral or other opportunistic infections (including legionellosis and listeriosis) have been reported in patients receiving TNF-blocking agents,**

including infliximab. Monitor closely for signs/symptoms of infection. Discontinue for serious infection or sepsis. Consider risks versus benefits prior to use in patients with a history of chronic or recurrent infection. Consider empiric antifungal therapy in patients who are at risk for invasive fungal infection and develop severe systemic illness. Caution should be exercised when considering use the elderly or in patients with conditions that predispose them to infections (eg, diabetes) or residence/travel from areas of endemic mycoses (blastomycosis, coccidioidomycosis, histoplasmosis), or with latent or localized infections. Do not initiate infliximab therapy with an active infection, including clinically important localized infection. Patients who develop a new infection while undergoing treatment should be monitored closely. Serious infections have been reported when anakinra or abatacept have been used concurrently with other TNF-blocking agents; concurrent use of infliximab with anakinra or abatacept is not recommended. Use caution when switching from one biologic disease-modifying antirheumatic drug (DMARD) to another; overlapping biological activities may further increase the risk of infection.

[U.S. Boxed Warning]: Infliximab treatment has been associated with active tuberculosis (may be disseminated or extrapulmonary) or reactivation of latent infections; evaluate patients for tuberculosis risk factors and latent tuberculosis infection (with a tuberculin skin test) prior to and during therapy; treatment of latent tuberculosis should be initiated before use. Patients with initial negative tuberculin skin tests should receive continued monitoring for tuberculosis throughout treatment. Most cases of reactivation have been reported within the first 3-6 months of treatment. Caution should be exercised when considering the use of infliximab in patients who have been exposed to tuberculosis.

Patients should be brought up to date with all immunizations before initiating therapy. Live vaccines should not be given concurrently; there is no data available concerning secondary transmission of live vaccines in patients receiving therapy. Rare reactivation of hepatitis B virus (HBV) has occurred in chronic virus carriers; use with caution; evaluate prior to initiation and during treatment.

[U.S. Boxed Warning]: Lymphoma and other malignancies have been reported in children and adolescent patients receiving TNF-blocking agents including infliximab. Half the cases are lymphomas (Hodgkin's and non-Hodgkin's). **[U.S. Boxed Warning]: Hepatosplenic T-cell lymphoma has been reported in patients with Crohn's disease or ulcerative colitis treated with infliximab and concurrent or prior azathioprine or mercaptopurine use, usually reported in adolescent and young adult males.** The impact of infliximab on the development and course of malignancies is not fully defined, but may be dose dependent. As compared to the general population, an increased risk of lymphoma has been noted in clinical trials; however, rheumatoid arthritis alone has been previously associated with an increased rate of lymphoma. Use caution in patients with a history of COPD, higher rates of malignancy were reported in COPD patients treated with infliximab. Psoriasis patients with a history of phototherapy had a higher incidence of nonmelanoma skin cancers.

Severe hepatic reactions (including hepatitis, jaundice, acute hepatic failure, and cholestasis) have been reported during treatment; discontinue with jaundice or marked increase in liver enzymes (≥5 times ULN). Use caution with heart failure; if a decision is made to use with heart failure, monitor closely and discontinue if exacerbated or new symptoms occur. Doses >5 mg/kg should not be administered in patients with moderate-to-severe heart failure (NYHA Class III/IV). Use caution with history of hematologic abnormalities; hematologic toxicities (eg, leukopenia, neutropenia, thrombocytopenia, pancytopenia) have been reported; discontinue if significant abnormalities occur. Autoimmune antibodies and a lupus-like syndrome have been reported. If antibodies to double-stranded DNA are confirmed in a patient with lupus-like symptoms, infliximab should be discontinued. Rare cases of optic neuritis and demyelinating disease (including multiple sclerosis, systemic vasculitis, and Guillain-Barré syndrome) have been reported; use with caution in patients with pre-existing or recent onset CNS demyelinating disorders, or seizures; discontinue if significant CNS adverse reactions develop.

Acute infusion reactions may occur. Hypersensitivity reaction may occur within 2 hours of infusion. Medication and equipment for management of hypersensitivity reaction should be available for immediate use. Interruptions and/or reinstitution at a slower rate may be required (consult protocols). Pretreatment may be considered, and may be warranted in all patients with prior infusion reactions. Serum sickness-like reactions have occurred; may be associated with a decreased response to treatment. The development of antibodies to infliximab may increase the risk of hypersensitivity and/or infusion reactions; concomitant use of immunosuppressants may lessen the development of anti-infliximab antibodies. The risk of infusion reactions may be increased with retreatment after an interruption or discontinuation of prior maintenance therapy. Retreatment in psoriasis patients should be resumed as a scheduled maintenance regimen without any induction doses; use of an induction regimen should be used cautiously for retreatment of all other patients.

Efficacy was not established in a study to evaluate infliximab use in juvenile idiopathic arthritis (JIA). Safety and efficacy for use in pediatric plaque psoriasis or pediatric ulcerative colitis have not been established. **Note:** For use in Crohn's disease: Safety and efficacy have not been established in children <6 years of age (U.S. labeling) and in children <9 years of age (Canadian labeling).

Adverse Reactions Although profile is similar, frequency of adverse effects may vary with disease state. Except where noted, percentages reported in adults with rheumatoid arthritis:

>10%:

Central nervous system: Headache (18%)

Gastrointestinal: Nausea (21%), diarrhea (12%), abdominal pain (12%; Crohn's 26%)

Hepatic: ALT increased (risk increased with concomitant methotrexate)

Respiratory: Upper respiratory tract infection (32%), sinusitis (14%), cough (12%), pharyngitis (12%)

Miscellaneous: Development of antinuclear antibodies (~50%), infection (36%), infusion reactions (20%; severe <1%), development of antibodies to double-stranded DNA (20%), development of new abscess (Crohn's patients with fistulizing disease: 15%), anti-infliximab antibodies (variable; ~10% to 15% [range: 6% to 61%]; Mayer, 2006)

5% to 10%:
  Cardiovascular: Hypertension (7%)
  Central nervous system: Fatigue (9%), pain (8%), fever (7%)
  Dermatologic: Rash (1% to 10%), pruritus (7%)
  Gastrointestinal: Dyspepsia (10%)
  Genitourinary: Urinary tract infection (8%)
  Neuromuscular & skeletal: Arthralgia (1% to 8%), back pain (8%)
  Respiratory: Bronchitis (10%), rhinitis (8%), dyspnea (6%)
  Miscellaneous: Moniliasis (5%)

<5%: Abscess, adult respiratory distress syndrome, allergic reaction, anemia, arrhythmia, basal cell carcinoma, biliary pain, bradycardia, brain infarction, breast cancer, cardiac arrest, cellulitis, cholecystitis, cholelithiasis, circulatory failure, confusion, constipation, dehydration, delayed hypersensitivity (plaque psoriasis), diaphoresis increased, dizziness, edema, gastrointestinal hemorrhage, heart failure, hemolytic anemia, hepatitis, hypersensitivity reactions, hypotension, ileus, intervertebral disk herniation, intestinal obstruction, intestinal perforation, intestinal stenosis, leukopenia, lupus-like syndrome, lymphadenopathy, lymphoma, malignancies, meningitis, menstrual irregularity, MI, myalgia, neuritis, pancreatitis, pancytopenia, peripheral neuropathy, peritonitis, pleural effusion, pleurisy, proctalgia, pulmonary edema, pulmonary embolism, renal calculus, renal failure, respiratory insufficiency, sarcoidosis, seizure, sepsis, serum sickness, suicide attempt, syncope, tachycardia, tendon disorder, thrombocytopenia, thrombophlebitis (deep), ulceration

The following adverse events were reported in children with Crohn's disease and were found more frequently in children than adults:

>10%:
  Hepatic: Liver enzymes increased (18%; ≥5 times ULN: 1%)
  Hematologic: Anemia (11%)
  Miscellaneous: Infections (56%; more common with every 8-week versus every 12-week infusions)

1% to 10%:
  Central nervous system: Flushing (9%)
  Gastrointestinal: Blood in stool (10%)
  Hematologic: Leukopenia (9%), neutropenia (7%)
  Neuromuscular & skeletal: Bone fracture (7%)
  Respiratory: Respiratory tract allergic reaction (6%)
  Miscellaneous: Viral infection (8%), bacterial infection (6%), antibodies to infliximab (3%)

Postmarketing and/or case reports (adults or children): Agranulocytosis, anaphylactic reactions, anaphylactic shock, angina, angioedema, autoimmune hepatitis, bronchospasm, central demyelinating disorders (eg, multiple sclerosis, optic neuritis); cholestasis, drug-induced lupus-like syndrome, erythema multiforme, heart failure (worsening), hepatic carcinoma, hepatitis B reactivation, hepatocellular damage, hepatosplenic T-cell lymphoma (HSTCL), Hodgkin's disease, idiopathic thrombocytopenia purpura, interstitial fibrosis, interstitial pneumonitis, jaundice, laryngeal/pharyngeal edema, latent tuberculosis reactivation, leiomyosarcoma, leukemias, liver failure, liver function tests increased, melanoma, neuropathy, numbness, opportunistic infection, pericardial effusion, peripheral demyelinating disorders (eg, Guillain-Barré syndrome, chronic inflammatory demyelinating polyneuropathy, multifocal motor neuropathy); pneumonia, psoriasis (including new onset, palmoplantar, pustular, or exacerbation), renal cell carcinoma, seizure, Stevens-Johnson syndrome, thrombotic thrombocytopenia purpura, taste abnormal, tingling, toxic epidermal necrolysis, transverse myelitis, tuberculosis, urticaria, vasculitis (systemic and cutaneous)

Drug Interactions

Metabolism/Transport Effects None known.

Avoid Concomitant Use

Avoid concomitant use of InFLIXimab with any of the following: Abatacept; Anakinra; BCG; Belimumab; Canakinumab; Certolizumab Pegol; Natalizumab; Pimecrolimus; Rilonacept; Tacrolimus (Topical); Vaccines (Live)

Increased Effect/Toxicity

InFLIXimab may increase the levels/effects of: Abatacept; Anakinra; Belimumab; Canakinumab; Certolizumab Pegol; Leflunomide; Natalizumab; Rilonacept; Vaccines (Live)

The levels/effects of InFLIXimab may be increased by: Abciximab; Denosumab; Pimecrolimus; Roflumilast; Tacrolimus (Topical); Trastuzumab

Decreased Effect

InFLIXimab may decrease the levels/effects of: BCG; Coccidioidin Skin Test; Sipuleucel-T; Vaccines (Inactivated); Vaccines (Live)

The levels/effects of InFLIXimab may be decreased by: Echinacea

Ethanol/Nutrition/Herb Interactions Herb/Nutraceutical: Avoid echinacea (may diminish the therapeutic effect of infliximab).

Storage/Stability Store vials at 2°C to 8°C (36°F to 46°F).

Reconstitution Reconstitute vials with 10 mL sterile water for injection. Swirl vial gently to dissolve powder; do not shake. Allow solution to stand for 5 minutes. Total dose of reconstituted product should be further diluted to 250 mL of 0.9% sodium chloride injection to a final concentration of 0.4-4 mg/mL. Infusion of dose should begin within 3 hours of preparation.

Mechanism of Action Infliximab is a chimeric monoclonal antibody that binds to human tumor necrosis factor alpha (TNFα), thereby interfering with endogenous TNFα activity. Elevated TNFα levels have been found in involved tissues/fluids of patients with rheumatoid arthritis, ankylosing spondylitis, psoriatic arthritis, plaque psoriasis, Crohn's disease and ulcerative colitis. Biological activities of TNFα include the induction of proinflammatory cytokines (interleukins), enhancement of leukocyte migration, activation of neutrophils and eosinophils, and the induction of acute phase reactants and tissue degrading enzymes. Animal models have shown TNFα expression causes polyarthritis, and infliximab can prevent disease as well as allow diseased joints to heal.

Pharmacodynamics/Kinetics

Onset of action: Crohn's disease: ~2 weeks

Distribution: V_d: 3-6 L

Half-life elimination: 7-12 days

Dosing

Adult & Geriatric **Note:** Premedication with antihistamines (H_1-antagonist +/- H_2-antagonist), acetaminophen, and/or corticosteroids may be considered to prevent and/or manage infusion-related reactions:

Crohn's disease: I.V.: 5 mg/kg at 0, 2, and 6 weeks, followed by 5 mg/kg every 8 weeks thereafter; dose may be increased to 10 mg/kg in patients who respond but then lose their response. If no response by week 14, consider discontinuing therapy.

Psoriatic arthritis (with or without methotrexate): I.V.: 5 mg/kg at 0,2, and 6 weeks, followed by 5 mg/kg every 8 weeks thereafter

Rheumatoid arthritis (in combination with methotrexate therapy): I.V. 3 mg/kg at 0, 2, and 6 weeks, followed by 3 mg/kg every 8 weeks thereafter; doses have ranged from 3-10 mg/kg repeated at 4- to 8-week intervals

Ankylosing spondylitis: I.V.: 5 mg/kg at 0, 2, and 6 weeks, followed by 5 mg/kg every 6 weeks thereafter (Canadian labeling recommends every 6-8 weeks thereafter)

Plaque psoriasis: I.V.: 5 mg/kg at 0, 2, and 6 weeks, followed by 5 mg/kg every 8 weeks thereafter

Ulcerative colitis: I.V.: 5 mg/kg at 0, 2, and 6 weeks, followed by 5 mg/kg every 8 weeks thereafter

Dosage adjustment with heart failure (HF): Weigh risk versus benefits for individual patient:

Moderate-to-severe (NYHA Class III or IV): ≤5 mg/kg

Pediatric Note: Premedication with antihistamines (H_1-antagonist +/- H_2-antagonist), acetaminophen, and/or corticosteroids may be considered to prevent and/or manage infusion-related reactions:

Crohn's disease: I.V.: Children and Adolescents: U.S. labeling ≥6 years, Canadian labeling ≥9 years: 5 mg/kg at 0, 2, and 6 weeks, followed by 5 mg/kg every 8 weeks thereafter; if no response by week 14, consider discontinuing therapy

Ulcerative colitis: I.V.: Children ≥6 years and Adolescents: 5 mg/kg at 0, 2, and 6 weeks, followed by 5 mg/kg every 8 weeks thereafter

Renal Impairment No dosage adjustment provided in manufacturer's labeling.

Hepatic Impairment No dosage adjustment provided in manufacturer's labeling.

Administration The infusion should begin within 3 hours of reconstitution and dilution. Infuse over at least 2 hours; do not infuse with other agents; use in-line low protein binding filter (≤1.2 micron). Temporarily discontinue or decrease infusion rate with infusion-related reactions. Antihistamines (H_1-antagonist +/- H_2-antagonist), acetaminophen and/or corticosteroids may be used to manage reactions. Infusion may be reinitiated at a lower rate upon resolution of mild-to-moderate symptoms.

Canadian labeling (not approved in U.S. labeling): Infusion of doses ≤6 mg/kg over not less than 1 hour may be considered in patients treated for rheumatoid arthritis who have initially tolerated 3 infusions each over 2 hours. Safety of shortened infusion has not been studied with doses >6 mg/kg.

Guidelines for the treatment and prophylaxis of infusion reactions: (**Note:** Limited to adult patients and dosages used in Crohn's; prospective data for other populations [pediatrics, other indications/dosing] are not available).

A protocol for the treatment of infusion reactions, as well as prophylactic therapy for repeat infusions, has been published (Mayer, 2006).

Treatment of infusion reactions: Medications for the treatment of hypersensitivity reactions should be available for immediate use. For mild reactions, the rate of infusion should be decreased to 10 mL/hour. Initiate a normal saline infusion (500-1000 mL/hour) and appropriate symptomatic treatment (eg, acetaminophen and diphenhydramine); monitor vital signs every 10 minutes until normal. After 20 minutes, the infusion may be increased at 15-minute intervals, as tolerated, to completion (initial increase to 20 mL/hour, then 40 mL/hour, then 80 mL/hour, etc [maximum of 125 mL/hour]). For moderate reactions, the infusion should be stopped or slowed.

Initiate a normal saline infusion (500-1000 mL/hour) and appropriate symptomatic treatment. Monitor vital signs every 5 minutes until normal. After 20 minutes, the infusion may be reinstituted at 10 mL/hour; then increased at 15-minute intervals, as tolerated, to completion (initial increase 20 mL/hour, then 40 mL/hour, then 80 mL/hour, etc [maximum of 125 mL/hour]). For severe reactions, the infusion should be stopped with administration of appropriate symptomatic treatment (eg, hydrocortisone/methylprednisolone, diphenhydramine and epinephrine) and frequent monitoring of vitals (consult institutional policies, if available). Retreatment after a severe reaction should only be done if the benefits outweigh the risks and with appropriate prophylaxis. Delayed infusion reactions typically occur 1-7 days after an infusion. Treatment should consist of appropriate symptomatic treatment (eg, acetaminophen, antihistamine, methylprednisolone).

Prophylaxis of infusion reactions: Premedication with acetaminophen and diphenhydramine 90 minutes prior to infusion may be considered in all patients with prior infusion reactions, and in patients with severe reactions corticosteroid administration is recommended. Steroid dosing may be oral (prednisone 50 mg orally every 12 hours for 3 doses prior to infusion) or intravenous (a single dose of hydrocortisone 100 mg or methylprednisolone 20-40 mg administered 20 minutes prior to the infusion). On initiation of the infusion, begin with a test dose at 10 mL/hour for 15 minutes. Thereafter, the infusion may be increased at 15-minute intervals, as tolerated, to completion (initial increase 20 mL/hour, then 40 mL/hour, then 80 mL/hour, etc). A maximum rate of 125 mL/hour is recommended in patients who experienced prior mild-moderate reactions and 100 mL/hour is recommended in patients who experienced prior severe reactions. In patients with cutaneous flushing, aspirin may be considered (Becker, 2004). For delayed infusion reactions, premedicate with acetaminophen and diphenhydramine 90 minutes prior to infusion. On initiation of the infusion, begin with a test dose at 10 mL/hour for 15 minutes. Thereafter, the infusion may be increased to infuse over 3 hours. Postinfusion therapy with acetaminophen for 3 days and an antihistamine for 7 days is recommended.

Monitoring Parameters Monitor improvement of symptoms and physical function assessments. During infusion, if reaction is noted, monitor vital signs every 2-10 minutes, depending on reaction severity, until normal. Latent TB screening prior to initiating and during therapy; signs/symptoms of infection (prior to, during, and following therapy); CBC with differential; signs/symptoms/worsening of heart failure; HBV screening prior to initiating (all patients), HBV carriers (during and for several months following therapy); signs and symptoms of hypersensitivity reaction; symptoms of lupus-like syndrome; LFTs (discontinue if >5 times ULN); signs and symptoms of malignancy (eg, splenomegaly, hepatomegaly, abdominal pain, persistent fever, night sweats, weight loss).

Psoriasis patients with history of phototherapy should be monitored for nonmelanoma skin cancer.

Medication Guide Available Yes

Dosage Forms Excipient information presented when available (limited, particularly for generics); consult specific product labeling.

Injection, powder for reconstitution:

Remicade®: 100 mg [contains polysorbate 80, sucrose 500 mg]

References

Becker M, Rose CD, and McIlvain-Simpson G, "Niacin-Like Reaction to Infliximab Infusion in Systemic Juvenile Rheumatoid Arthritis," *J Rheumatol*, 2004, 31(12):2529-30.

Buch MH, Bryer D, Lindsay S, et al, "Shortening Infusion Times for Infliximab Administration," *Rheumatology (Oxford)*, 2006, 45(4):485-6.

Carpenter PA and Sanders JE, "Steroid-Refractory Graft-vs-Host Disease: Past, Present and Future," *Pediatr Transplant.* 2003, 7(Suppl 3):19-31.

Centers for Disease Control, "Testing and Treatment of Latent Tuberculosis Infection," *MMWR Recomm Rep*, 2000, 49(RR-6).

Couriel D, Saliba R, Hicks K, et al, "Tumor Necrosis Factor-Alpha Blockade for the Treatment of Acute GVHD," *Blood*, 2004, 104(3):649-54.

Dommasch E and Gelfand JM, "Is There Truly a Risk of Lymphoma From Biologic Therapies?" *Dermatol Ther*, 2009, 22 (5):418-30.

Kornbluth A and Sachar DB, "Ulcerative Colitis Practice Guidelines in Adults: American College of Gastroenterology, Practice Parameters Committee," *Am J Gastroenterol*, 2010, 105(3):501-23.

Lichtenstein GR, Hanauer SB, and Sandborn WJ, "Management of Crohn's Disease in Adults," *Am J Gastroenterol*, 2009, 104(2):465-83.

Mayer L and Young Y, "Infusion Reactions and Their Management," *Gastroenterol Clin North Am*, 2006, 35(4):857-66.

Thayu M, Markowitz JE, Mamula P, et al, "Hepatosplenic T-Cell Lymphoma in an Adolescent Patient After Immunomodulator and Biologic Therapy for Crohn Disease," *J Pediatr Gastroenterol Nutr*, 2005, 40(2):220-2.

◆ **Infliximab, Recombinant** *see* InFLIXimab *on page* *789*

◆ **Infufer® (Can)** *see* Iron Dextran Complex *on page* *824*

◆ **Infumorph 200** *see* Morphine (Systemic) *on page* *1004*

◆ **Infumorph 500** *see* Morphine (Systemic) *on page* *1004*

Ingenol Mebutate (IN je nol MEB u tate)

Brand Names: U.S. Picato®

Index Terms *Euphorbia peplus* Derivative; PEP005

Generic Availability (U.S.) No

Pharmacologic Category Topical Skin Product

Use Topical treatment of actinic keratosis

Labeled Contraindications There are no contraindications listed in the manufacturer's labeling.

Pregnancy Risk Factor C

Warnings/Precautions Severe dermatologic reactions including erythema, crusting, swelling, vesiculation/pustulation, and erosion/ulceration can occur. Severe eye pain, eyelid edema, eyelid ptosis, and periorbital edema can occur after exposure; avoid contact with the periocular area (patients should wash hands immediately after applying and avoid transferring to the eye area).

Apply to intact and nonirritated skin only. Instruct patients to wash hands well after applying and to avoid contact with the periocular area during and after application. Avoid touching the treated area for 6 hours after application. If inadvertent exposure to other area(s) occurs, flush the area with water and seek medical care as soon as possible. Avoid inadvertent transfer to other individuals. Administration of ingenol mebutate gel is not recommended until the skin is healed from any previous drug or surgical treatment. For topical use only; not for oral, ophthalmic, or intravaginal use.

Adverse Reactions

>10%: Dermatologic: Erythema (92% to 94%), flaking/scaling (85% to 90%), crusting (74% to 80%), swelling (64% to 79%), vesiculation/pustulation (44% to 56%), erosion/ulceration (26% to 32%), application site pain (2% to 15%)

1% to 10%:

Central nervous system: Headache (2%)

Dermatologic: Application site pruritus (8%), application site irritation (4%), application site infection (3%)

Ocular: Periorbital edema (3%)
Respiratory: Nasopharyngitis (2%)
<1%, postmarketing, and/or case reports: Eyelid edema, eye pain, conjunctivitis

Drug Interactions

Metabolism/Transport Effects None known.

Avoid Concomitant Use There are no known interactions where it is recommended to avoid concomitant use.

Increased Effect/Toxicity There are no known significant interactions involving an increase in effect.

Decreased Effect There are no known significant interactions involving a decrease in effect.

Storage/Stability Store in a refrigerator at 2°C to 8°C (36°F to 46°F); excursions are permitted to 0°C to 15°C (32°F to 59°F); do not freeze. Discard tubes after single use.

Mechanism of Action Ingenol mebutate appears to induce primary necrosis of actinic keratosis with a subsequent neutrophil-mediated inflammatory response with antibody-dependent cytotoxicity of residual disease cells; killing residual disease cells may prevent future relapse.

Pharmacodynamics/Kinetics Absorption: Absorption through the skin is minimal (with proper use); expected systemic exposure is <0.1 ng/mL.

Dosing

Adult & Geriatric Actinic keratoses: Topical:

Face and scalp: Apply 0.015% gel once daily to affected area for 3 consecutive days

Trunk/extremities: Apply 0.05% gel once daily to affected area for 2 consecutive days

Administration Apply to one contiguous affected area of skin using one unit-dose tube; one unit-dose tube will cover ~5 cm x 5 cm (~25 cm^2 or ~2 inch x 2 inch). Spread evenly then allow gel to dry for 15 minutes. Do not cover with bandages or occlusive dressings. Wash hands immediately after applying and avoid transferring gel to any other areas. Avoid washing or touching the treatment area for at least 6 hours, and following this period of time, patients may wash the area with a mild soap. Not for oral, ophthalmic, or intravaginal use.

Dosage Forms Excipient information presented when available (limited, particularly for generics); consult specific product labeling.

Gel, topical:

Picato®: 0.015% (3s); 0.05% (2s) [contains benzyl alcohol, isopropyl alcohol]

References

Lebwohl M, Swanson N, Anderson LL, et al, "Ingenol Mebutate Gel for Actinic Keratosis," *N Engl J Med*, 2012, 366(11):1010-9.

Ramsay JR, Suhrbier A, Aylward JH, et al, "The Sap From *Euphorbia peplus* is Effective Against Human Nonmelanoma Skin Cancers," *Br J Dermatol*, 2011, 164(3):633-6.

Siler G, Rosen R, Freeman M, et al, "PEP005 (Ingenol Mebutate) Gel for the Topical Treatment of Superficial Basal Cell Carcinoma: Results of a Randomized Phase IIa Trial," *Australas J Dermatol*, 2010, 51(2):99–105.

◆ **Inlyta®** *see* Axitinib *on page* 135

◆ **Inlyta®** *see* Axitinib *on page* 135

◆ **[111]In-Pentetreotide** *see* Indium In-111 Pentetreotide *on page* 788

◆ **α-2-interferon** *see* Interferon Alfa-2b *on page* 798

◆ **Interferon Alfa-2b (PEG Conjugate)** *see* Peginterferon Alfa-2b *on page 1140*

Interferon Alfa-2b (in ter FEER on AL fa too bee)

Related Information

Malignant Pleural Effusions *on page 1865*

Management of Chemotherapy-Induced Nausea and Vomiting *on page 1786*

Safe Handling of Hazardous Drugs *on page 1904*

Brand Names: U.S. Intron® A

Brand Names: Canada Intron® A

Index Terms INF-alpha 2; Interferon Alpha-2b; rLFN-α2; α-2-interferon

Generic Availability (U.S.) No

Pharmacologic Category Interferon

Use

Patients ≥1 year of age: Chronic hepatitis B

Patients ≥3 years of age: Chronic hepatitis C (in combination with ribavirin)

Patients ≥18 years of age: Condyloma acuminata, chronic hepatitis B, chronic hepatitis C, hairy cell leukemia, malignant melanoma (high-risk of recurrence), AIDS-related Kaposi's sarcoma, follicular non-Hodgkin lymphoma

Unlabeled Use Treatment of cutaneous ulcerations of Behçet's disease, neuroendocrine tumors (including carcinoid syndrome and islet cell tumor), cutaneous T-cell lymphoma, desmoid tumor, hepatitis D, chronic myelogenous leukemia (CML), non-Hodgkin lymphomas (other than follicular lymphoma, see approved use), multiple myeloma, renal cell carcinoma, West Nile virus

Labeled Contraindications Hypersensitivity to interferon alfa or any component of the formulation; decompensated liver disease; autoimmune hepatitis

Combination therapy with interferon alfa-2b and ribavirin is also contraindicated in pregnancy, males with pregnant partners; hemoglobinopathies (eg, thalassemia major, sickle-cell anemia); renal dysfunction (Cl_{cr} <50 mL/minute)

Pregnancy Risk Factor C / X in combination with ribavirin

Lactation Enters breast milk/not recommended (AAP rates "compatible"; AAP 2001 update pending)

Warnings/Precautions **[U.S. Boxed Warning]: May cause or aggravate fatal or life-threatening autoimmune disorders, neuropsychiatric symptoms (including depression and/or suicidal thoughts/behaviors), ischemic, and/or infectious disorders; monitor closely with clinical and lab evaluations (periodic); discontinue treatment for severe persistent or worsening symptoms; some cases may resolve with discontinuation.**

Neuropsychiatric disorders: May cause neuropsychiatric events, including depression, psychosis, mania, suicidal behavior/ideation, homicidal ideation; may occur in patients with or without previous psychiatric symptoms. Careful neuropsychiatric monitoring is recommended during and for 6 months after treatment in patients who develop psychiatric disorders (including clinical depression). New or exacerbated neuropsychiatric or substance abuse disorders are best managed with early intervention. Use with caution in patients with a history of psychiatric disorders. Drug screening and periodic health evaluation (including monitoring of psychiatric symptoms) is recommended if initiating treatment in patients with coexisting psychiatric condition or substance abuse disorders. Suicidal ideation or attempts may occur more frequently in pediatric patients when compared to adults. Higher doses in elderly patients, or diseases other than hairy cell leukemia, may result in increased CNS toxicity.

Hepatic disease: May cause hepatotoxicity; monitor closely if abnormal liver function tests develop. A transient increase in ALT (≥2 times baseline) may occur in patients treated with interferon alfa-2b for chronic hepatitis B. Therapy generally may continue; monitor. Worsening and potentially fatal liver disease, including jaundice, hepatic encephalopathy, and hepatic failure have been reported in patients receiving interferon alfa for chronic hepatitis B and C with decompensated liver disease, autoimmune hepatitis, history of autoimmune disease, and immunosuppressed transplant recipients; avoid use in these patients. Chronic hepatitis B or C patients with a history of autoimmune disease or who are immunosuppressed transplant recipients should not receive interferon alfa-2b. Discontinue treatment (if appropriate) in any patient developing signs or symptoms of liver failure.

Bone marrow suppression: Causes bone marrow suppression, including potentially severe cytopenias, and very rarely, aplastic anemia. Discontinue treatment for severe neutropenia (ANC <500/mm^3) or thrombocytopenia (platelets <25,000/mm^3). Hemolytic anemia (hemoglobin <10 g/dL) was observed when combined with ribavirin; anemia occurred within 1-2 weeks of initiation of therapy. Use caution in patients with pre-existing myelosuppression and in patients with concomitant medications which cause myelosuppression.

Autoimmune disorders: Avoid use in patients with history of autoimmune disorders; development of autoimmune disorders (thrombocytopenia, vasculitis, Raynaud's disease, rheumatoid arthritis, lupus erythematosus and rhabdomyolysis) has been associated with use. Monitor closely; consider discontinuing. Worsening of psoriasis and sarcoidosis (and the development of new sarcoidosis) have been reported; use caution.

Cardiovascular disease/coagulation disorders: Use caution and monitor closely in patients with cardiovascular disease (ischemic or thromboembolic), arrhythmias, hypertension, and in patients with a history of MI or prior therapy with cardiotoxic drugs. Patients with pre-existing cardiac disease and/or advanced cancer should have baseline and periodic ECGs. May cause hypotension (during administration or delayed), arrhythmia, tachycardia, cardiomyopathy (~2% in AIDS-related Kaposi's Sarcoma patients) and/or MI. Hemorrhagic cerebrovascular events have been observed with therapy. Use caution in patients with coagulation disorders.

Endocrine disorders: Thyroid disorders (possibly reversible) have been reported; use caution in patients with pre-existing thyroid disease. TSH levels should be within normal limits prior to initiating interferon. Discontinue interferon use in patients who cannot maintain normal ranges with thyroid medication. Diabetes mellitus has been reported; discontinue if cannot effectively manage with medication. Use with caution in patients with a history of diabetes mellitus, particularly if prone to DKA. Hypertriglyceridemia has been reported; discontinue if persistent and severe, and/or combined with symptoms of pancreatitis.

Pulmonary disease: Dyspnea, pulmonary infiltrates, pulmonary hypertension, interstitial pneumonitis, pneumonia, bronchiolitis obliterans, and sarcoidosis may be induced or aggravated by treatment, sometimes resulting in respiratory failure or fatality. Has been reported more in patients being treated for chronic hepatitis C, although has also occurred with use for oncology indications. Patients with fever, cough, dyspnea or other respiratory symptoms should be evaluated with a chest x-ray; monitor closely and consider discontinuing treatment with evidence of impaired pulmonary function. Use with caution in patients with a history of pulmonary disease.

Ophthalmic disorders: Decreased or loss of vision, macular edema, optic neuritis, retinal hemorrhages, cotton wool spots, papilledema, retinal detachment (serous), and retinal artery or vein thrombosis have occurred (or been aggravated) in patients receiving alpha interferons. Use caution in patients with pre-existing eye disorders; monitor closely; a complete eye exam should be done promptly in patients who develop ocular symptoms; discontinue with new or worsening ophthalmic disorders.

Commonly associated with fever and flu-like symptoms; rule out other causes/ infection with persistent fever; use with caution in patients with debilitating conditions. Acute hypersensitivity reactions have been reported. Do not treat patients with visceral AIDS-related Kaposi's sarcoma associated with rapidly-progressing or life-threatening disease. Some formulations contain albumin, which may carry a remote risk of viral transmission. Due to differences in dosage, patients should not change brands of interferons without the concurrence of their healthcare provider. Combination therapy with ribavirin is associated with birth defects and/or fetal mortality and hemolytic anemia. Do not use combination therapy with ribavirin in patients with renal dysfunction (Cl_{cr} <50 mL/minute).

Adverse Reactions Note: In a majority of patients, a flu-like syndrome (fever, chills, tachycardia, malaise, myalgia, headache), occurs within 1-2 hours of administration; may last up to 24 hours and may be dose limiting.

>10%:

Cardiovascular: Chest pain (≤28%)

Central nervous system: Fatigue (8% to 96%), fever (34% to 94%; more common in children), headache (21% to 62%), chills (≤54%), depression (3% to 40%; grades 3/4: 2%), somnolence (≤33%), dizziness (≤24%), irritability (≤22%), pain (≤18%), amnesia (≤14%), concentration impaired (≤14%), malaise (≤14%), confusion (≤12%), insomnia (≤12%)

Dermatologic: Alopecia (≤38%), rash (≤25%), pruritus (≤11%)

Endocrine & metabolic: Amenorrhea (≤12%)

Gastrointestinal: Anorexia (1% to 69%), nausea, (17% to 66%), diarrhea (2% to 45%), xerostomia (≤28%), vomiting (children 27%; adults 7% to 10%), taste alteration (≤24%), abdominal pain (1% to 23%), constipation (≤14%), gingivitis (≤14%), weight loss (<1% to 13%)

Hematologic: Neutropenia (≤92%; grade 4: 1% to 4%), leukopenia (≤68%), anemia (≤32%), thrombocytopenia (≤15%)

Hepatic: AST increased (≤63%; grades 3/4: 14%), ALT increased (≤15%), pain (upper right quadrant: up to 15%); alkaline phosphatase increased (≤13%)

Local: Injection site reaction (≤20%)

Neuromuscular & skeletal: Myalgia (28% to 75%), weakness (≤63%), rigors (≤42%), paresthesia (1% to 21%), skeletal pain (≤21%), arthralgia (≤19%), back pain (≤19%)

Renal: BUN increased (≤12%)

Respiratory: Dyspnea (≤34%), cough (≤31%), pharyngitis (≤31%), sinusitis (≤21%)

Miscellaneous: Flu-like syndrome (≤79%), diaphoresis (1% to 21%), moniliasis (≤17%)

5% to 10%:

Cardiovascular: Edema (≤10%), hypertension (≤9%)

Central nervous system: Hypoesthesia (≤10%), anxiety (≤9%), vertigo (≤8%), agitation (≤7%)

Dermatologic: Dry skin (≤10%), dermatitis (≤8%), purpura (≤5%)

Endocrine & metabolic: Libido decreased (≤5%)

Gastrointestinal: Loose stools (≤10%), dyspepsia (≤8%)

Genitourinary: Urinary tract infection (≤5%)

Renal: Polyuria (≤10%), serum creatinine increased (≤6%)

Respiratory: Bronchitis (≤10%), nasal congestion (≤10%), epistaxis (≤7%)

Miscellaneous: Infection (≤7%), herpes virus infections (≤5%)

<5%, postmarketing, and/or case reports (limited to important or life-threatening):

Cardiovascular: Angina, arrhythmia, arteritis, atrial fibrillation, bradycardia, cardiac failure, cardiomegaly, cardiomyopathy, coronary artery disorder, ejection fraction decreased, extrasystoles, flushing, heart valve disorder, hypotension, MI, palpitation, peripheral ischemia, polyarteritis, Raynaud's disease, syncope, tachycardia, thrombosis, vasculitis

Central nervous system: Nervousness (≤3%), aggression, alcohol intolerance, aphasia, ataxia, Bell's palsy, coma, extrapyramidal disorder, hallucination, homicidal ideation, hypothermia, mania, migraine, neurosis, paranoia, psychosis, stroke, suicidal attempt/ideation, seizure

Dermatologic: Angioedema, cellulitis, dermatitis lichenoides, eczema, epidermal necrolysis, erythema, erythema multiforme, erythematous rash, folliculitis, hirsutism, lipoma, maculopapular rash, photosensitivity, psoriasis, psoriasis exacerbation, sebaceous cyst, Stevens-Johnson syndrome, toxic epidermal necrolysis, urticaria

Endocrine & metabolic: Dehydration, diabetes mellitus, goiter, hot flashes, hypercalcemia, hyperglycemia, hyper-/hypothyroidism, hypertriglyceridemia, hypopituitarism, mastitis, menorrhagia, sexual dysfunction

Gastrointestinal: Colitis, dysphasia, esophagitis, gastritis, gastrointestinal hemorrhage, mucositis, pancreatitis, rectal bleeding/hemorrhage, stomatitis, ulcerative stomatitis

Genitourinary: Cystitis, dysuria, incontinence, impotence, leukorrhea, nocturia, pelvic pain, uterine bleeding

Hematologic: Aplastic anemia (rarely), granulocytopenia, hemolytic anemia, hypochromic anemia, lymphopenia, lymphadenitis, lymphadenopathy, lymphocytosis, pancytopenia, pure red cell aplasia, thrombocytopenia purpura (idiopathic and thrombotic)

Hepatic: Ascites, biliary pain, bilirubinemia, hepatic encephalopathy, hepatic failure, hepatitis, hepatotoxicity, jaundice, lactate dehydrogenase increased (up to 1%), liver function test abnormal

Local: Injection site necrosis

Neuromuscular & skeletal: Arthritis, carpal tunnel syndrome, hyporeflexia, leg cramps, muscle atrophy, myositis, neuralgia, neuropathy, peripheral neuropathy, rhabdomyolysis, rheumatoid arthritis, spondylitis, tendonitis, tremor

Ocular: Blurred vision, conjunctivitis, cotton wool spots, macular edema, nystagmus, optic neuritis, papilledema, photophobia, retinal artery thrombosis, retinal detachment (serous), retinal vein thrombosis

Otic: Hearing impairment, hearing loss

Renal: Albuminuria, hematuria, nephrotic syndrome, proteinuria, renal failure, renal insufficiency

Respiratory: Asthma, bronchiolitis obliterans, bronchoconstriction, bronchospasm, cyanosis, hemoptysis, hypoventilation, pleural effusion, pneumonia, pneumonitis (interstitial), pneumothorax, pulmonary embolism, pulmonary fibrosis, pulmonary hypertension, pulmonary infiltrates, respiratory insufficiency, upper respiratory tract infection, wheezing

Miscellaneous: Abscess, acute hypersensitivity reaction, allergic reactions, anaphylaxis, fungal infection, sarcoidosis, sarcoidosis exacerbation, sepsis, systemic lupus erythematosus, Vogt-Koyanagi-Harada syndrome

Drug Interactions

Metabolism/Transport Effects **Inhibits** CYP1A2 (weak)

Avoid Concomitant Use

Avoid concomitant use of Interferon Alfa-2b with any of the following: CloZAPine; Telbivudine

Increased Effect/Toxicity

Interferon Alfa-2b may increase the levels/effects of: Aldesleukin; CloZAPine; Methadone; Ribavirin; Telbivudine; Theophylline Derivatives; Zidovudine

Decreased Effect There are no known significant interactions involving a decrease in effect.

Storage/Stability Store powder and solution for injection (vials and pens) under refrigeration at 2°C to 8°C (36°F to 46°F); do not freeze.

Powder for injection: Following reconstitution, should be used immediately, but may be stored under refrigeration for up to 24 hours.

Prefilled pens: After first use, discard unused portion after 4 weeks.

Reconstitution Powder for injection: The manufacturer recommends reconstituting vial with the diluent provided (SWFI). When reconstituted with SWFI 1 mL, the 10 million unit vial concentration is 10 million units/mL, the 18 million unit vial concentration is 18 million units/mL, and the 50 million unit vial concentration is 50 million units/mL. Swirl gently. To prepare solution for infusion, further dilute appropriate dose in NS 100 mL. Final concentration should be ≥10 million units/100 mL.

Mechanism of Action Binds to a specific receptor on the cell wall to initiate intracellular activity; multiple effects can be detected including induction of gene transcription. Inhibits cellular growth, alters the state of cellular differentiation, interferes with oncogene expression, alters cell surface antigen expression, increases phagocytic activity of macrophages, and augments cytotoxicity of lymphocytes for target cells

Pharmacodynamics/Kinetics

Distribution: V_d: 31 L; but has been noted to be much greater (370-720 L) in leukemia patients receiving continuous infusion IFN; IFN does not penetrate the CSF

Metabolism: Primarily renal

Bioavailability: I.M.: 83%; SubQ: 90%

Half-life elimination: I.V.: ~2 hours; I.M., SubQ: ~2-3 hours

Time to peak, serum: I.M., SubQ: ~3-12 hours; I.V.: By the end of a 30-minute infusion

Dosing

Adult & Geriatric Details concerning dosing in combination regimens should also be consulted. Consider premedication with acetaminophen prior to administration to reduce the incidence of some adverse reactions. Not all dosage forms and strengths are appropriate for all indications; refer to product labeling for details.

Hairy cell leukemia: I.M., SubQ: 2 million units/m^2 3 times weekly for up to 6 months (may continue treatment with sustained treatment response); discontinue for disease progression or failure to respond after 6 months

Lymphoma (follicular): SubQ: 5 million units 3 times weekly for up to 18 months

Malignant melanoma: Induction: 20 million units/m^2 I.V. for 5 consecutive days per week for 4 weeks, followed by maintenance dosing of 10 million units/m^2 SubQ 3 times weekly for 48 weeks

AIDS-related Kaposi's sarcoma: I.M., SubQ: 30 million units/m^2 3 times weekly; continue until disease progression or until maximal response has been achieved after 16 weeks

Chronic hepatitis B: I.M., SubQ: 5 million units/ daily or 10 million units 3 times weekly for 16 weeks

Chronic hepatitis C: I.M., SubQ: 3 million units 3 times weekly. In patients with normalization of ALT at 16 weeks, continue treatment (if tolerated) for 18-24 months; consider discontinuation if normalization does not occur at 16 weeks. **Note:** May be used in combination therapy with ribavirin in previously untreated patients or in patients who relapse following alpha interferon therapy.

Condyloma acuminata: Intralesionally: 1 million units/lesion (maximum: 5 lesions per treatment) 3 times weekly (on alternate days) for 3 weeks. May administer a second course at 12-16 weeks.

Pediatric Details concerning dosing in combination regimens should also be consulted.

Note: The following dosing may also be used in **infants** in the setting of HIV-exposure/-infection (CDC, 2009).

Chronic hepatitis B (including HIV coinfection): SubQ: Children 1-17 years: 3 million units/m^2 3 times weekly for 1 week, followed by 6 million units/m^2 3 times weekly (maximum: 10 million units per dose); total duration of therapy 16-24 weeks (treat for 24 weeks in HIV-exposure/-infection)

Chronic hepatitis C with HIV coinfection: I.M., SubQ: Children 1-17 years: 3-5 million units/m^2 3 times weekly (maximum: 3 million units per dose) with ribavirin for 48 weeks, regardless of HCV genotype (CDC, 2009)

Renal Impairment Combination therapy with ribavirin (hepatitis C) should not be used in patients with reduced renal function (Cl_{cr} <50 mL/minute).

Adjustment for Toxicity

Hematologic toxicity (also refer to indication specified adjustments below): ANC <500/mm^3 or platelets < 25,000/mm^3: Discontinue treatment.

Hypersensitivity reaction (acute, serious), ophthalmic disorders (new or worsening), thyroid abnormality development (which cannot be normalized with medication), signs or symptoms of liver failure: Discontinue treatment

Liver function abnormality, pulmonary infiltrate development, evidence of pulmonary function impairment, or autoimmune disorder development, triglycerides >1000 mg/dL: Monitor closely and discontinue if appropriate.

Neuropsychiatric disorders (during treatment):

Clinical depression or other psychiatric problem: Monitor closely during and for 6 months after treatment.

Severe depression or other psychiatric disorder: Discontinue treatment.

Persistent or worsening psychiatric symptoms, suicidal ideation, aggression towards others: Discontinue treatment and follow with appropriate psychiatric intervention.

Manufacturer-recommended adjustments, listed according to indication:

Lymphoma (follicular):

Neutrophils >1000/mm^3 to <1500/mm^3: Reduce dose by 50%; may re-escalate to starting dose when neutrophils return to >1500/mm^3

Severe toxicity (neutrophils <1000/mm^3 or platelets <50,000/mm^3): Temporarily withhold.

AST >5 times ULN or serum creatinine >2 mg/dL: Permanently discontinue.

Hairy cell leukemia:

Platelet count <50,000/mm^3: Do not administer intramuscularly (administer SubQ instead).

Severe toxicity: Reduce dose by 50% or temporarily withhold and resume with 50% dose reduction; permanently discontinue if persistent or recurrent severe toxicity is noted.

Chronic hepatitis B:

WBC <1500/mm^3, granulocytes <750/mm^3, or platelet count <50,000/mm^3, or other laboratory abnormality or severe adverse reaction: Reduce dose by 50%; may re-escalate to starting dose upon resolution of hematologic toxicity. Discontinue for persistent intolerance.

WBC <1000/mm^3, granulocytes <500/mm^3, or platelet count <25,000/mm^3: Permanently discontinue

Chronic hepatitis C: Severe toxicity: Reduce dose by 50% or temporarily withhold until subsides; permanently discontinue for persistent toxicities after dosage reduction.

AIDS-related Kaposi sarcoma: Severe toxicity: Reduce dose by 50% or temporarily withhold; may resume at reduced dose with toxicity resolution; permanently discontinue for persistent/recurrent toxicities.

Malignant melanoma (induction and maintenance):

Severe toxicity including neutrophils >250/mm^3 to <500/mm^3 or ALT/AST >5-10 times ULN: Temporarily withhold; resume with a 50% dose reduction when adverse reaction abates.

Neutrophils <250/mm^3, ALT/AST >10 times ULN, or severe/persistent adverse reactions: Permanently discontinue.

Combination Regimens

Lymphoma, non-Hodgkin's: Fludarabine-Mitoxantrone-Dexamethasone-Rituximab on page 1650

Melanoma: CVD-Interleukin-Interferon (Melanoma) on page 1597

Renal cell cancer: Bevacizumab-Interferon Alfa (RCC) on page 1530

Administration Administer dose in the evening (if possible) to enhance tolerability. Not all dosage forms are recommended for all administration routes; refer to manufacturer's labeling.

I.M.: Rotate injection sites. Some patients may be appropriate for self-administration with appropriate training. Allow to reach room temperature prior to injection. In hairy cell leukemia treatment, if platelets are <50,000/mm^3, do not administer intramuscularly (administer SubQ instead).

I.V.: Infuse over ~20 minutes

SubQ: Suggested for those who are at risk for bleeding or are thrombocytopenic. Rotate SubQ injection site. Patient should be well hydrated. Some patients may be appropriate for self-administration with appropriate training. Allow to reach room temperature prior to injection.

Intralesional: Inject at an angle nearly parallel to the plane of the skin, directing the needle to center of the base of the wart to infiltrate the lesion core and cause a small wheal. Only infiltrate the keratinized layer; avoid administration which is too deep or shallow. Allow to reach room temperature prior to injection.

Emetic Potential

>10,000 units/m^2: Moderate (30% to 90%)

5,000-10,000 units/m^2: Low (10% to 30%)

Monitoring Parameters CBC with differential (baseline and periodic during treatment), liver function tests (baseline and periodic), electrolytes (baseline and periodic), serum creatinine (baseline), albumin, prothrombin time, triglycerides, thyroid-stimulating hormone (TSH) baseline and periodically during treatment (in patients with pre-existing thyroid disorders, repeat TSH at 3 months and 6 months); chest x-ray (baseline), weight; ophthalmic exam (baseline and periodic, or with new ocular symptoms); ECG (baseline and during treatment; in patients with pre-existing cardiac abnormalities or in advanced stages of cancer); neuropsychiatric changes during and for 6 months after therapy

Chronic hepatitis B: CBC with differential and platelets and liver function tests: Baseline, weeks 1, 2, 4, 8, 12, and 16, at the end of treatment, and then 3 and 6 months post treatment

Chronic hepatitis C:

CBC with differential and platelets: Baseline, weeks 1 and 2, then monthly

Liver function: Every 3 months

TSH: Baseline and periodically during treatment: In patients with pre-existing thyroid disorders also repeat at 3 months and 6 months

Malignant melanoma: CBC with differential and platelets and liver function tests: Weekly during induction phase, then monthly during maintenance

Oncology patients: Thyroid function monitoring (Hamnvik, 2011): TSH and anti-TPO antibodies at baseline; if TPO antibody positive, monitor TSH every 2 months; if TPO antibody negative, monitor TSH every 6 months

Medication Guide Available Yes

Dosage Forms Excipient information presented when available (limited, particularly for generics); consult specific product labeling.

Injection, powder for reconstitution [preservative free]:

Intron® A: 10 million units, 18 million units, 50 million units [contains albumin (human)]

Injection, solution:

Intron® A: 6 million units/mL (3 mL); 10 million units/mL (2.5 mL) [contains edetate disodium, polysorbate 80; vial]

Intron® A: 3 million units/0.2 mL (1.2 mL) [contains edetate disodium, polysorbate 80; delivers 6 doses of 0.2 mL each; 18 million units total per prefilled pen]

Intron® A: 5 million units/0.2 mL (1.2 mL) [contains edetate disodium, polysorbate 80; delivers 6 doses of 0.2 mL each; 30 million units total per prefilled pen]

Intron® A: 10 million units/0.2 mL (1.2 mL) [contains edetate disodium, polysorbate 80; delivers 6 doses of 0.2 mL each; 60 million units total per prefilled pen]

References

Atkins MB, Hsu J, Lee S, et al, "Phase III Trial Comparing Concurrent Biochemotherapy With Cisplatin, Vinblastine, Dacarbazine, Interleukin-2, and Interferon Alfa-2b With Cisplatin, Vinblastine, and Dacarbazine Alone in Patients With Metastatic Malignant Melanoma (E3695): A Trial Coordinated by the Eastern Cooperative Oncology Group," *J Clin Oncol*, 2008, 26(35):5748-54.

Centers for Disease Control and Prevention, "Guidelines for the Prevention and Treatment of Opportunistic Infections Among HIV-Exposed and HIV-Infected Children: Recommendations from CDC, the National Institutes of Health, the HIV Medicine Association of the Infectious Diseases Society of America, the Pediatric Infectious Diseases Society, and the American Academy of Pediatrics," *MMWR Recomm Rep*, 2009, 58(RR-11):1-166. Available at http://aidsinfo.nih.gov/contentfiles/Pediatric_OI.pdf

Centers for Disease Control and Prevention, "Sexually Transmitted Diseases Treatment Guidelines, 2006," *MMWR*, 2006, 55(RR-11):1-94.

Hamnvik OP, Larsen PR, and Marqusee E, "Thyroid Dysfunction From Antineoplastic Agents," *J Natl Cancer Inst*, 2011, 103(21):1572-87.

Legha SS, "The Role of Interferon Alfa in the Treatment of Metastatic Melanoma," *Semin Oncol*, 1997, 24(1 Suppl 4):24-31.

Musselman DL, Lawson DH, Gumnick JF, et al, "Paroxetine for the Prevention of Depression Induced by High-Dose Interferon Alfa," *N Engl J Med*, 2001, 344(13):961-6.

Pectasides D, Dafni U, Bafaloukos D, et al, "Randomized Phase III Study of 1 Month Versus 1 Year of Adjuvant High-Dose Interferon Alfa-2b in Patients With Resected High-Risk Melanoma," *J Clin Oncol*, 2009, 27(6):939-44.

◆ **Interferon Alpha-2b** *see* Interferon Alfa-2b *on page 798*

◆ **Interleukin 2** *see* Aldesleukin *on page 37*

◆ **Interleukin-11** *see* Oprelvekin *on page 1074*

◆ **Intrapleural Talc** *see* Talc (Sterile) *on page 1323*

◆ **Intron® A** *see* Interferon Alfa-2b *on page 798*

Iobenguane I 123 (eye oh BEN gwane eye one TWEN tee three)

Brand Names: U.S. AdreView™

Index Terms 123 Meta-Iodobenzlyguanidine Sulfate; 123I-Metaiodobenzylguanidine (MIBG); I-123 MIBG; I^{123} Iobenguane; Iobenguane Sulfate I 123

Generic Availability (U.S.) No

Pharmacologic Category Radiopharmaceutical

Use As an adjunct to other diagnostic tests, in the detection of primary or metastatic pheochromocytoma or neuroblastoma

Labeled Contraindications Hypersensitivity to iobenguane or any component of the formulation

Pregnancy Risk Factor C

Lactation Excretion in breast milk unknown/not recommended

Warnings/Precautions Radiopharmaceutical; use appropriate precautions for handling, disposal and minimizing exposure to patients and healthcare personnel. Use under supervision of experienced personnel. Hypersensitivity reactions have been reported. Use extreme caution in patients with iodine or iodine-contrast agent hypersensitivity. Appropriate equipment and emergency medications should be available during use. Use with caution in patients with hypertension; may increase blood pressure and heart rate. Use with caution in patients with severe renal impairment; safety and efficacy have not been established. Patients with severe renal impairment may have delayed elimination, therefore, decreasing quality of images. Not dialyzable. If possible, discontinue medications that inhibit norepinephrine uptake prior to iobenguane I 123 administration; allow at least 5 half-lives to elapse. These medications may interfere with the uptake of iobenguane I 123 in neuroendocrine tumors leading to false-negative results. Administer thyroid blocking medications (eg, potassium iodide oral solution, potassium perchlorate) at least 1 hour prior to administration; long-term risk for thyroid neoplasia can occur from failure to block thyroid uptake of iodine 123. Patients should be adequately hydrated prior to dosing instruct patients to void frequently for 48 hours following administration to decrease radiation exposure. Contains benzyl alcohol which has been associated with "gasping syndrome" in neonates. Safety and efficacy have not been established in infants <1 month of age.

Adverse Reactions <1%, postmarketing, and/or case reports: Dizziness, flushing, hypersensitivity (rare), injection site hemorrhage, pruritus, rash

Drug Interactions

Metabolism/Transport Effects None known.

Avoid Concomitant Use

Avoid concomitant use of Iobenguane I 123 with any of the following: Alpha2-Agonists; Antidepressants (Selective Norepinephrine Reuptake Inhibitor); Cocaine; Methyldopa; Reserpine; Selective Serotonin Reuptake Inhibitors; Serotonin/Norepinephrine Reuptake Inhibitors; Sympathomimetics; Tricyclic Antidepressants

Increased Effect/Toxicity There are no known significant interactions involving an increase in effect.

Decreased Effect

The levels/effects of Iobenguane I 123 may be decreased by: Alpha2-Agonists; Antidepressants (Selective Norepinephrine Reuptake Inhibitor); Cocaine; Methyldopa; Reserpine; Selective Serotonin Reuptake Inhibitors; Serotonin/Norepinephrine Reuptake Inhibitors; Sympathomimetics; Tricyclic Antidepressants

Storage/Stability Store at controlled room temperature of 20°C to 25°C (68°F to 77°F). Should be stored in original lead container or adequate radiation shield.

Mechanism of Action Iobenguane is structurally similar to norepinephrine and therefore is taken up and stored in adrenergic tissue such as adrenal medulla, heart, liver, lungs, salivary glands, and spleen. Iobenguane is bound to radioactive iodine in order to obtain organ and tissue images.

Pharmacodynamics/Kinetics

Distribution: Increased in adrenergically innervated tissues (eg, heart, salivary glands, adrenal medulla)

Metabolism: Has not been characterized

Half-life elimination: Iodine 123: 13.2 hours

Excretion: Urine (70 % to 90%) within 4 days (normal renal function); feces <1%

Dosing

Adult & Geriatric Note: Thyroid protective agents (SSKI, Lugol's solution or potassium iodide), should be given at least 1 hour prior to administration. Perform whole body planar scintigraphy imaging 18-30 hours after Iobenguane I 123 administration.

Radioimaging: I.V.: 10 mCi (370 MBq)

Pediatric Note: Thyroid protective agents (SSKI, Lugol's solution or potassium iodide), should be given at least 1 hour prior to administration. Perform whole body planar scintigraphy imaging 18-30 hours after Iobenguane I 123 administration.

Radioimaging: I.V.:

Children 1 month to 16 years and <70 kg: Dose according to body weight; see table.

Children <16 years and ≥70 kg: 10 mCi (370 MBq)

Children ≥16 years: Refer to adult dosing

Iobenguane I 123 Pediatric Dosing by Body Weight

(Children 1 Month to 16 Years and <70 kg)

Weight (kg)	mCi Dose	MBq Dose
3	1	37
4	1.4	52
6	1.9	70
8	2.3	85.1
10	2.7	99.9
12	3.2	118.4
14	3.6	133.2
16	4	148
18	4.4	162.8
20	4.6	170.2
22	5	185
24	5.3	196.1
26	5.6	207.2
28	5.8	214.6
30	6.2	229.4
32	6.5	240.5
34	6.8	251.6
36	7.1	262.7
38	7.3	270.1
40	7.6	281.2
42	7.8	288.6
44	8	296
46	8.2	303.4
48	8.5	314.5
50	8.8	325.6
52-54	9	333
56-58	9.2	340.4
60-62	9.6	355.2
64-66	9.8	362.6
68	9.9	366.3

Administration Administer intravenously over 1-2 minutes. May flush with NS to ensure full delivery of dose. Prior to administration, a thyroid-protective agent should be started. Ensure adequate hydration before and after treatment.

Monitoring Parameters Pulse and blood pressure prior to administration and intermittently for 30 minutes following; monitor for hypersensitivity reaction

Dietary Considerations Some dietary sources of iodine include cow's milk and dairy products, fish, seaweed, eggs, chocolate, and iodized salt.

Dosage Forms Excipient information presented when available (limited, particularly for generics); consult specific product labeling.

Injection, solution:

AdreView™: Iobenguane sulfate 0.08 mg and I 123 74 MBq (2 mCi) per mL (5 mL) [contains benzyl alcohol]

◆ **Iobenguane Sulfate I 123** *see* Iobenguane I 123 *on page 806*

◆ **Iodine I 131 Tositumomab and Tositumomab** *see* Tositumomab and Iodine I 131 Tositumomab *on page 1379*

Ipilimumab (ip i LIM u mab)

Related Information

Management of Chemotherapy-Induced Nausea and Vomiting *on page 1786*

Principles of Anticancer Therapy *on page 1878*

Brand Names: U.S. Yervoy™

Brand Names: Canada Yervoy™

Index Terms MDX-010; MDX-CTLA-4; MOAB-CTLA-4

Generic Availability (U.S.) No

Pharmacologic Category Antineoplastic Agent, Monoclonal Antibody; Monoclonal Antibody

Use Treatment of unresectable or metastatic melanoma

Labeled Contraindications There are no contraindications listed within the manufacturer's labeling

Canadian labeling: Hypersensitivity to ipilimumab or any component of the formulation; active life-threatening autoimmune disease, or with organ transplantation graft where further immune activation is potentially imminently life-threatening

Pregnancy Risk Factor C

Lactation Excretion in breast milk unknown/not recommended

Warnings/Precautions [U.S. Boxed Warning]: Severe and fatal immune-mediated adverse effects due to T-cell activation and proliferation may occur. While any organ system may be involved, common severe effects include dermatitis (including toxic epidermal necrolysis), endocrine disorder, enterocolitis, hepatitis, and neuropathy. Reactions generally occur during treatment, although some reactions have occurred weeks to months after treatment discontinuation. Discontinue treatment (permanently) and initiate high-dose corticosteroid treatment for severe immune mediated reactions. Evaluate liver function and thyroid function tests at baseline and prior to each dose. Assess for signs and symptoms of enterocolitis, dermatitis, neuropathy, and endocrine disorder at baseline and prior to each dose. Initiate prednisone 1-2 mg/kg/day (or equivalent) for severe reactions. Uncommon immune-mediated adverse effects reported include hemolytic anemia, iritis, meningitis, nephritis, pericarditis, pneumonitis, and uveitis. Administer corticosteroid ophthalmic drops in patients who develop episcleritis, iritis, or uveitis; permanently discontinue ipilimumab if unresponsive to topical ophthalmic immunosuppressive treatments.

Immune-mediated enterocolitis was reported to occur at a median onset of 6-7 weeks. Monitor for signs and symptoms of enterocolitis (abdominal pain, blood in stool, diarrhea, or mucous in stool; with or without fever) and intestinal perforation (peritoneal signs, ileus). If enterocolitis develops, infectious causes should be ruled out; consider endoscopy for persistent or severe symptoms. Withhold ipilimumab treatment and administer antidiarrheals for moderate enterocolitis (diarrhea with ≤6 stools over baseline abdominal pain, mucous or blood in stool); if persists for >1 week, initiate prednisone at 0.5 mg/kg/day (or equivalent). If severe enterocolitis (diarrhea ≥7 stools above baseline, fever, ileus, peritoneal signs) develops, permanently discontinue ipilimumab and initiate prednisone 1-2 mg/kg/day (or equivalent); when resolved to ≤grade 1, taper corticosteroids slowly over ≥1 month (rapid tapering may worsen symptoms).

Severe, life-threatening or fatal hepatotoxicity and immune-mediated hepatitis have been observed. Monitor liver function tests (LFTs) and evaluate for signs of hepatotoxicity prior to each dose; if hepatotoxicity develops, infectious or malignant causes should be ruled out and liver function should be monitored more frequently until resolves. Withhold treatment for grade 2 hepatotoxicity (ALT or AST 2.5-5 times ULN or total bilirubin 1.5-3 times ULN). If severe hepatotoxicity develops (ALT or AST >5 times ULN or total bilirubin >3 times ULN), permanently discontinue ipilimumab and initiate prednisone 1-2 mg/kg/day (or equivalent); may begin tapering corticosteroid (over 1 month) when LFTs show sustained improvement or return to baseline.

Severe, life-threatening, or fatal dermatitis has been reported. The median time to onset for dermatologic toxicity is 3 weeks (range: ≤17 weeks). Monitor for rash and pruritus; dermatitis should be considered immune-mediated unless identified otherwise. Mild-to-moderate dermatitis (localized rash and pruritus) should be treated symptomatically; topical or systemic corticosteroids should be administered if not resolved within 1 week. Withhold treatment for moderate to severe dermatologic symptoms. Permanently discontinue and initiate prednisone 1-2 mg/kg/day (or equivalent) for Stevens-Johnson syndrome, toxic epidermal necrolysis, or rash complicated by dermal ulceration (full thickness) or necrotic, bullous, or hemorrhagic manifestations; when dermatitis is controlled, taper corticosteroid over at least 1 month.

Severe or life-threatening endocrine disorders (hypopituitarism, adrenal insufficiency, hypogonadism and hypothyroidism) have been reported; may require hospitalization. Endocrine disorders of moderate severity (including hypothyroidism, adrenal insufficiency, hypopituitarism, and less commonly hyperthyroidism and Cushing's syndrome) which have required hormone replacement therapy or medical intervention have also been reported. The median onset for moderate-to-severe endocrine disorders was 11 weeks (range: ≤19 weeks); long-term hormone replacement therapy has been required in many cases. Monitor thyroid function tests and serum chemistries prior to each dose; also monitor for signs of hypophysitis, adrenal insufficiency and thyroid disorders (eg, abdominal pain, fatigue, headache, hypotension, mental status changes, unusual bowel habits); rule out other potential causes such as brain metastases. Endocrine disorders should be considered immune-mediated unless identified otherwise. If symptomatic, withhold ipilimumab treatment and initiate prednisone 1-2 mg/kg/day (or equivalent) and appropriate hormone replacement therapy.

One case each of severe peripheral motor neuropathy and fatal Guillain-Barré syndrome have been reported. Monitor for signs of motor or sensory neuropathy (unilateral or bilateral weakness, sensory changes or paresthesia). Withhold treatment in patients with neuropathy that does not interfere with daily activities (moderate neuropathy). Permanently discontinue for severe neuropathy (interferes with daily activities, including symptoms similar to Guillain-Barré syndrome). Consider initiating prednisone 1-2 mg/kg/day (or equivalent) for severe neuropathies.

Adverse Reactions

>10%:

Central nervous system: Fatigue (41% to 42%; grades 3-5: 7%), headache (15%), fever (12%)

Dermatologic: Pruritus (24% to 31%), rash (19% to 29%; grades 3-5: 2%), dermatitis (grade 2: 12%; grades 3-5: 2% to 3% [includes Stevens-Johnson syndrome, toxic epidermal necrolysis, dermal ulceration, necrotic, bullous or hemorrhagic dermatitis])

Gastrointestinal: Nausea (35%), diarrhea (32% to 33%; grades 3-5: 5%), appetite decreased (27%), vomiting (24%), constipation (21%), abdominal pain (15%)

Hematologic: Anemia (12%)

Respiratory: Cough (16%), dyspnea (15%)

1% to 10%:

Dermatologic: Urticaria (2%), vitiligo (2%)

Endocrine & metabolic: Hypopituitarism (grade 2: 2%; grades 3-5: 4%), hypothyroidism (≤2%), hypophysitis (2%), adrenal insufficiency (≤2%)

Gastrointestinal: Colitis (8%; grades 3-5: 5%), enterocolitis (grade 2: 5%; grades 3-5: 7%), intestinal perforation (1%)

Hematologic: Eosinophilia (grades 3-5: 1%)

Hepatic: Hepatotoxicity (grade 2: 3%; grades 3-5: 1% to 2%), ALT increased (2%)

Renal: Nephritis (grades 3-5: 1%)

<1%, postmarketing, and/or case reports: Acute respiratory distress syndrome, angiopathy, arthritis, AST increased, bilirubin increased, blepharitis, conjunctivitis, corticotrophin decreased, Cushing's syndrome, episcleritis, erythema multiforme, esophagitis, gastrointestinal ulcer, Guillain-Barré syndrome, hemolytic anemia, hepatic failure, hepatitis (immune-mediated), hypogonadism, hyperthyroidism, infusion reaction, iritis, leukocytoclastic vasculitis, meningitis, myasthenia gravis, myelofibrosis, myocarditis, neuropathy (sensory and motor), pancreatitis, pericarditis, peritonitis, pneumonitis, polymyalgia rheumatica, psoriasis, renal failure, sarcoidosis (pulmonary), scleritis, sepsis, temporal arteritis, thyroiditis (autoimmune), thyrotropin increased, uveitis, vascular leak syndrome, vasculitis

Drug Interactions

Metabolism/Transport Effects None known.

Avoid Concomitant Use There are no known interactions where it is recommended to avoid concomitant use.

Increased Effect/Toxicity

Ipilimumab may increase the levels/effects of: Vitamin K Antagonists

Decreased Effect

Ipilimumab may decrease the levels/effects of: Cardiac Glycosides; Vitamin K Antagonists

Storage/Stability Store intact vials refrigerated at 2°C to 8°C (36°F to 46°C); do not freeze. Protect from light. Prior to preparation, allow vials to sit at room temperature for ~5 minutes. Solutions diluted for infusion are stable for up to 24 hours refrigerated or at room temperature.

Reconstitution Prior to preparation, allow vials to sit at room temperature for ~5 minutes. Withdraw appropriate ipilimumab volume and transfer to I.V. bag, dilute with NS or D_5W to a final concentration between 1-2 mg/mL. Mix by gently inverting, do not shake.

Mechanism of Action Ipilimumab is a recombinant human IgG1 immunoglobulin monoclonal antibody which binds to the cytotoxic T-lymphocyte associated antigen 4 (CTLA-4). CTLA-4 is a down-regulator of T-cell activation pathways. Blocking CTLA-4, allows for enhanced T-cell activation and proliferation. In melanoma, ipilimumab may indirectly mediate T-cell immune responses against tumors.

Pharmacodynamics/Kinetics

Distribution: V_{ss}: 7.21 L

Half-life elimination: Terminal: 14.7 days

Dosing

Adult Melanoma, unresectable or metastatic: I.V.: 3 mg/kg every 3 weeks for 4 doses

Adjustment for Toxicity

Temporarily withhold scheduled dose for the following:

Moderate immune-mediated reactions

Symptomatic endocrine disorder

Grade 2 hepatotoxicity (AST or ALT >2.5 to ≤5 x ULN or bilirubin >1.5 to ≤3 x ULN)

Note: If receiving less than prednisone 7.5 mg/day (or equivalent), may resume with complete or partial resolution (to ≤grade 1) of symptoms. Resume ipilimumab treatment at 3 mg/kg every 3 weeks until all 4 planned doses have been administered or until 16 weeks from initial dose, whichever occurs first.

Permanently discontinue for the following:

Failure to complete treatment course within 16 weeks of initial dose

Persistent moderate adverse reactions or unable to reduce corticosteroid dose to prednisone 7.5 mg/day (or equivalent)

Severe or life-threatening adverse reactions including:

Central nervous system or neuromuscular toxicity: Severe motor or sensory neuropathy, Guillain-Barré syndrome, or myasthenia gravis

Dermatologic toxicities: Stevens-Johnson syndrome, toxic epidermal necrolysis, or rash complicated by full thickness dermal ulceration, or necrotic, bullous, or hemorrhagic manifestations

Gastrointestinal toxicities: Colitis with abdominal pain, fever, ileus, or peritoneal symptoms, increase in stool frequency (≥7 over baseline), stool incontinence, require I.V. hydration for >24 hours, or GI hemorrhage or perforation

Hepatotoxicities: ALT or AST >5 times ULN, or total bilirubin >3 times ULN

Ophthalmic toxicities: Immune-mediated ocular disease unresponsive to topical immunosuppressive treatment

Severe immune-mediated reactions involving any organ system (eg, myocarditis [noninfectious], nephritis, pancreatitis, pneumonitis)

Combination Regimens

Melanoma: Ipilimumab (Melanoma Regimen) on page 1692

Administration I.V.: Infuse over 90 minutes through a low protein-binding in-line filter. Flush with NS or D_5W at the end of infusion

Emetic Potential Very low (<10%)

Monitoring Parameters Monitor liver function and evaluate for signs of hepatotoxicity prior to each dose, if hepatotoxicity develops, liver function should be monitored more frequently until resolves. Monitor serum chemistrics prior to each dose. Monitor for signs of hypophysitis, adrenal insufficiency and thyroid disorders (eg, abdominal pain, fatigue, headache, hypotension, mental status changes, unusual bowel habits). Monitor TSH, free T_4 and cortisol levels (morning) at baseline and every 2-3 months; monitor sooner if symptoms (headache, nausea, vomiting, lethargy, or constipation) occur (Hamnvik, 2011). Monitor for signs and symptoms of enterocolitis (abdominal pain, blood or mucus in stool or diarrhea, and intestinal perforation (peritoneal signs, ileus). Monitor for rash and pruritus. Monitor for signs of motor or sensory neuropathy (unilateral or bilateral weakness, sensory changes or paresthesia).

Medication Guide Available Yes

Dosage Forms Excipient information presented when available (limited, particularly for generics); consult specific product labeling.

Injection, solution [preservative free]:

Yervoy™: 5 mg/mL (10 mL, 40 mL) [contains polysorbate 80, derived from or manufactured using Chinese hamster ovary cells]

References

Hodi FS, O'Day SJ, McDermott DF, et al, "Improved Survival with Ipilimumab in Patients with Metastatic Melanoma," *N Engl J Med*, 2010, 363(8):711-23.

Lynch TJ, Bondarenko IN, Luft A, et al, "Phase II Trial of Ipilimumab (IPI) and Paclitaxel/Carboplatin (P/C) in First-Line Stage IIIb/IV Non-Small Cell Lung Cancer," *J Clin Oncol*, 2010, 28(15s):7531 [abstract 7531 from 2010 ASCO Annual Meeting].

O'Day S, Hodi FS, McDermott DF, et al, "A Phase III, Randomized, Double-Blind, Multicenter Study Comparing Monotherapy With Ipilimumab or GP100 Peptide Vaccine and the Combination in Patients With Previously Treated, Unresectable Stage III or IV Melanoma," *J Clin Oncol*, 2010, 28 (15s):4 [abstract 4 from 2010 ASCO Annual Meeting].

Wolchok JD, Neyns B, Linette G, et al, "Ipilimumab Monotherapy in Patients With Pretreated Advanced Melanoma: A Randomised, Double-Blind, Multicentre, Phase 2, Dose-Ranging Study," *Lancet Oncol*, 2010, 11(2):155-64.

Wolchok JD, Weber JS, Hamid O, et al, "Ipilimumab Efficacy and Safety in Patients With Advanced Melanoma: A Retrospective Analysis of HLA Subtype From Four Trials," *Cancer Immun*, 2010, 10:9.

◆ **Iressa®** *see* Gefitinib *on page 659*

◆ **IRESSA® (Can)** *see* Gefitinib *on page 659*

Irinotecan (eye rye no TEE kan)

Related Information

Chemotherapy and Obesity *on page 1834*

Management of Chemotherapy-Induced Nausea and Vomiting *on page 1786*

Management of Drug Extravasations *on page 1800*

Oral Mucositis/Stomatitis *on page 1814*

Safe Handling of Hazardous Drugs *on page 1904*

Brand Names: U.S. Camptosar®

Brand Names: Canada Camptosar®; Irinotecan Hydrochloride Trihydrate

Index Terms Camptothecin-11; CPT-11; Irinotecan HCl; Irinotecan Hydrochloride

Generic Availability (U.S.) Yes

Pharmacologic Category Antineoplastic Agent, Camptothecin; Antineoplastic Agent, Natural Source (Plant) Derivative; Antineoplastic Agent, Topoisomerase I Inhibitor

Use Treatment of metastatic carcinoma of the colon or rectum

Unlabeled Use Treatment of cervical cancer (recurrent or metastatic), central nervous system tumors (recurrent glioblastoma), esophageal cancer, Ewing's sarcoma (recurrent or progressive), gastric cancer (metastatic or locally advanced), nonsmall cell lung cancer (advanced), ovarian cancer (recurrent), pancreatic cancer (advanced), small cell lung cancer (extensive stage)

Labeled Contraindications Hypersensitivity to irinotecan or any component of the formulation

Pregnancy Risk Factor D

Lactation Excretion in breast milk unknown/not recommended

Warnings/Precautions Hazardous agent - use appropriate precautions for handling and disposal. Severe hypersensitivity reactions (including anaphylaxis) have occurred. For I.V. use only; monitor infusion site; may cause local tissue necrosis or thrombophlebitis if extravasation occurs (the manufacturer recommends flushing the site with sterile water and ice application).

[U.S. Boxed Warning]: Severe diarrhea may be dose-limiting and potentially fatal; early-onset and late-onset diarrhea may occur. Early diarrhea occurs during or within 24 hours of receiving irinotecan and is characterized by cholinergic symptoms (eg, increased salivation, rhinitis, miosis, diaphoresis, flushing, abdominal cramping, lacrimation); may be prevented or treated with atropine. Late diarrhea occurs more than 24 hours after treatment which may lead to dehydration, electrolyte imbalance, or sepsis; may be life-threatening and should be promptly treated with loperamide; dose reductions may be recommended for future doses within the current cycle. Antibiotics may be necessary if patient develops ileus, fever, or severe neutropenia. Patients with diarrhea should be carefully monitored and treated promptly; may require fluid and electrolyte therapy. Colitis, complicated by ulceration, bleeding, ileus, and infection has been reported; initiate antibiotics promptly in patients with ileus.

[U.S. Boxed Warning]: May cause severe myelosuppression. Deaths due to sepsis following severe neutropenia have been reported. Complications due to neutropenia should be promptly managed with antibiotics. Therapy should be temporarily discontinued if neutropenic fever occurs or if the absolute neutrophil count is <1000/mm^3. The dose of irinotecan should be reduced if there is a clinically significant decrease in the total WBC (<200/mm^3), neutrophil count (<1500/mm^3), hemoglobin (<8 g/dL), or platelet count (<100,000/mm^3). Routine administration of a colony-stimulating factor is generally not necessary, but may be considered for patients experiencing significant neutropenia. Fatal cases of interstitial pulmonary disease (IPD)-like events have been reported with single-agent and combination therapy. Promptly evaluate changes in baseline pulmonary symptoms or any new-onset pulmonary symptoms. Discontinue all chemotherapy if IPD is diagnosed.

Patients with even modest elevations in total serum bilirubin levels (1-2 mg/dL) have a significantly greater likelihood of experiencing first-course grade 3 or 4 neutropenia than those with bilirubin levels that were <1 mg/dL. Patients with abnormal glucuronidation of bilirubin, such as those with Gilbert's syndrome, may also be at greater risk of myelosuppression when receiving therapy with irinotecan. Use caution when treating patients with known hepatic dysfunction or hyperbilirubinemia exposure to the active metabolite (SN-38) is increased; toxicities may be increased. Dosage adjustments should be considered.

Patients homozygous for the UGT1A1*28 allele are at increased risk of neutropenia; initial one-level dose reduction should be considered for both single-agent and combination regimens. Heterozygous carriers of the UGT1A1*28 allele may also be at increased risk; however, most patients have tolerated normal starting doses. Avoid vaccination with live vaccines during treatment (risk of infection may be increased due to immunosuppression). Although the response to vaccines may be diminished, inactivated vaccines may be administered during treatment.

Renal impairment and acute renal failure have been reported, possibly due to dehydration secondary to diarrhea. Use with caution in patients with renal impairment; not recommended in patients on dialysis. Patients with bowel obstruction should not be treated with irinotecan until resolution of obstruction. Use caution in patients who previously received pelvic/abdominal radiation, elderly patients with comorbid conditions, or baseline performance status of 2; close monitoring and dosage adjustments are recommended. Contains sorbitol; do not use in patients with hereditary fructose intolerance. Thromboembolic events have been reported. **[U.S. Boxed Warning]: Should be administered under the supervision of an experienced cancer chemotherapy physician.** Except as part of a clinical trial, use in combination with fluorouracil and leucovorin "Mayo Clinic" regimen is not recommended. Increased toxicity has also been noted in patients with a baseline performance status of 2 in other combination regimens containing irinotecan, leucovorin, and fluorouracil. High potential for CYP-mediated drug interactions; enzyme inducers may decrease exposure to irinotecan and SN-38 (active metabolite); enzyme inhibitors may increase exposure; for use in patients with CNS tumors (unlabeled use), selection of antiseizure medications which are not enzyme inducers is preferred.

Adverse Reactions Frequency of adverse reactions reported for single-agent use of irinotecan only.

>10%:

Cardiovascular: Vasodilation (9% to 11%)

Central nervous system: Cholinergic toxicity (47% - includes rhinitis, increased salivation, miosis, lacrimation, diaphoresis, flushing and intestinal hyperperistalsis); fever (44% to 45%), pain (23% to 24%), dizziness (15% to 21%), insomnia (19%), headache (17%), chills (14%)

Dermatologic: Alopecia (46% to 72%), rash (13% to 14%)

Endocrine & metabolic: Dehydration (15%)

Gastrointestinal: Diarrhea, late (83% to 88%; grade 3/4: 14% to 31%), diarrhea, early (43% to 51%; grade 3/4: 7% to 22%), nausea (70% to 86%), abdominal pain (57% to 68%), vomiting (62% to 67%), cramps (57%), anorexia (44% to 55%), constipation (30% to 32%), mucositis (30%), weight loss (30%), flatulence (12%), stomatitis (12%)

Hematologic: Anemia (60% to 97%; grades 3/4: 5% to 7%), leukopenia (63% to 96%, grades 3/4: 14% to 28%), thrombocytopenia (96%, grades 3/4: 1% to 4%), neutropenia (30% to 96%; grades 3/4: 14% to 31%)

Hepatic: Bilirubin increased (84%), alkaline phosphatase increased (13%)

Neuromuscular & skeletal: Weakness (69% to 76%), back pain (14%)

Respiratory: Dyspnea (22%), cough (17% to 20%), rhinitis (16%)

Miscellaneous: Diaphoresis (16%), infection (14%)

1% to 10%:

Cardiovascular: Edema (10%), hypotension (6%), thromboembolic events (5%)

Central nervous system: Somnolence (9%), confusion (3%)

Gastrointestinal: Abdominal fullness (10%), dyspepsia (10%)

Hematologic: Neutropenic fever (grades 3/4: 2% to 6%), hemorrhage (grades 3/4: 1% to 5%), neutropenic infection (grades 3/4: 1% to 2%)

Hepatic: AST increased (10%), ascites and/or jaundice (grades 3/4: 9%)

Respiratory: Pneumonia (4%)

<1%, postmarketing, and/or case reports: ALT increased, amylase increased, anaphylactoid reaction, anaphylaxis, angina, arterial thrombosis, bleeding, bradycardia, cardiac arrest, cerebral infarct, cerebrovascular accident, circulatory failure, colitis, deep thrombophlebitis, dysarthria, dysrhythmia, embolus, gastrointestinal bleeding, gastrointestinal obstruction, hepatomegaly, hiccups, hyperglycemia, hypersensitivity, hyponatremia, ileus, interstitial pulmonary disease (IPD), intestinal perforation, ischemic colitis, lipase increased, lymphocytopenia, megacolon, MI, muscle cramps, myocardial ischemia, neutropenic typhlitis, pancreatitis, paresthesia, peripheral vascular disorder, pulmonary embolus; pulmonary toxicity (dyspnea, fever, reticulonodular infiltrates on chest x-ray); renal failure (acute), renal impairment, syncope, thrombocytopenia (immune mediated), thrombophlebitis, thrombosis, typhlitis, ulceration, ulcerative colitis, vertigo

Note: In limited pediatric experience, dehydration (often associated with severe hypokalemia and hyponatremia) was among the most significant grade 3/4 adverse events, with a frequency up to 29%. In addition, grade 3/4 infection was reported in 24%.

Drug Interactions

Metabolism/Transport Effects **Substrate** of CYP2B6 (major), CYP3A4 (major), P-glycoprotein, SLCO1B1, UGT1A1; **Note:** Assignment of Major/Minor substrate status based on clinically relevant drug interaction potential

Avoid Concomitant Use

Avoid concomitant use of Irinotecan with any of the following: Atazanavir; BCG; CloZAPine; Conivaptan; Natalizumab; Pimecrolimus; St Johns Wort; Tacrolimus (Topical); Vaccines (Live)

Increased Effect/Toxicity

Irinotecan may increase the levels/effects of: CloZAPine; Leflunomide; Natalizumab; Vaccines (Live)

The levels/effects of Irinotecan may be increased by: Antifungal Agents (Azole Derivatives, Systemic); Atazanavir; Bevacizumab; Conivaptan; CYP2B6 Inhibitors (Moderate); CYP2B6 Inhibitors (Strong); CYP3A4 Inhibitors (Moderate); CYP3A4 Inhibitors (Strong); Dasatinib; Denosumab; Eltrombopag; Ivacaftor; Mifepristone; P-glycoprotein/ABCB1 Inhibitors; Pimecrolimus; Quazepam; Regorafenib; Roflumilast; SORAfenib; Tacrolimus (Topical); Trastuzumab

Decreased Effect

Irinotecan may decrease the levels/effects of: BCG; Coccidioidin Skin Test; Sipuleucel-T; Vaccines (Inactivated); Vaccines (Live)

The levels/effects of Irinotecan may be decreased by: CarBAMazepine; CYP2B6 Inducers (Strong); CYP3A4 Inducers (Strong); Deferasirox; Echinacea; Fosphenytoin; P-glycoprotein/ABCB1 Inducers; PHENobarbital; Phenytoin; St Johns Wort; Tocilizumab

Ethanol/Nutrition/Herb Interactions Herb/Nutraceutical: Avoid St John's wort (decreases the efficacy of irinotecan).

Storage/Stability Store intact vials at room temperature. Protect from light. Solutions diluted in NS may precipitate if refrigerated. Solutions diluted in D_5W are stable for 24 hours at room temperature or 48 hours under refrigeration at 2°C to 8°C, although the manufacturer recommends use within 24 hours if refrigerated, within 6 hours at room temperature, and/or within 12 hours at room temperature (including infusion time) only if prepared under strict aseptic conditions (eg, laminar flow hood). Do not freeze.

Reconstitution Use appropriate precautions for handling and disposal. Dilute in 250-500 mL D_5W (preferred) or NS to a final concentration of 0.12-2.8 mg/mL. Due to the relatively acidic pH, irinotecan appears to be more stable in D_5W than NS.

Mechanism of Action Irinotecan and its active metabolite (SN-38) bind reversibly to topoisomerase I-DNA complex preventing religation of the cleaved DNA strand. This results in the accumulation of cleavable complexes and double-strand DNA breaks. As mammalian cells cannot efficiently repair these breaks, cell death consistent with S-phase cell cycle specificity occurs, leading to termination of cellular replication.

Pharmacodynamics/Kinetics

Distribution: V_d: 33-150 L/m^2

Protein binding, plasma: Predominantly albumin; Irinotecan: 30% to 68%, SN-38 (active metabolite): ~95%

Metabolism: Primarily hepatic to SN-38 (active metabolite) by carboxylesterase enzymes; SN-38 undergoes conjugation by UDP- glucuronosyl transferase 1A1 (UGT1A1) to form a glucuronide metabolite. Conversion of irinotecan to SN-38 is decreased and glucuronidation of SN-38 is increased patients who smoke cigarettes, resulting in lower levels of the metabolite and overall decreased systemic exposure. SN-38 is increased by UGT1A1*28 polymorphism (10% of North Americans are homozygous for UGT1A1*28 allele). The lactones of both irinotecan and SN-38 undergo hydrolysis to inactive hydroxy acid forms.

Half-life elimination: Irinotecan: 6-12 hours; SN-38: ~10-20 hours

Time to peak: SN-38: Following 90-minute infusion: ~1 hour

Excretion: Urine: Irinotecan (11% to 20%), metabolites (SN-38 <1%, SN-38 glucuronide, 3%)

Dosing

Adult Note: A reduction in the starting dose by one dose level should be considered for prior pelvic/abdominal radiotherapy, performance status of 2, or known homozygosity for UGT1A1*28 allele. Consider premedication of atropine 0.25-1 mg I.V. or SubQ in patients with cholinergic symptoms (eg, increased salivation, rhinitis, miosis, diaphoresis, abdominal cramping) or early onset diarrhea. Details concerning dosage in combination regimens should also be consulted.

Colorectal cancer, metastatic (single-agent therapy): I.V.:

Weekly regimen: 125 mg/m^2 over 90 minutes on days 1, 8, 15, and 22 of a 6-week treatment cycle (may adjust upward to 150 mg/m^2 if tolerated)

Adjusted dose level -1: 100 mg/m^2

Adjusted dose level -2: 75 mg/m^2

Further adjust to 50 mg/m^2 (in decrements of 25-50 mg/m^2) if needed

Once-every-3-week regimen: 350 mg/m^2 over 90 minutes, once every 3 weeks

Adjusted dose level -1: 300 mg/m^2

Adjusted dose level -2: 250 mg/m^2

Further adjust to 200 mg/m^2 (in decrements of 25-50 mg/m^2) if needed

Colorectal cancer, metastatic (in combination with fluorouracil and leucovorin): I.V.: Six-week (42-day) cycle:

Regimen 1: 125 mg/m^2 over 90 minutes on days 1, 8, 15, and 22; to be given in combination with bolus leucovorin and fluorouracil (leucovorin administered immediately following irinotecan; fluorouracil immediately following leucovorin)

Adjusted dose level -1: 100 mg/m^2

Adjusted dose level -2: 75 mg/m^2

Further adjust if needed in decrements of ~20%

Regimen 2: 180 mg/m^2 over 90 minutes on days 1, 15, and 29; to be given in combination with infusional leucovorin and bolus/infusion fluorouracil (leucovorin administered immediately following irinotecan; fluorouracil immediately following leucovorin)

Adjusted dose level -1: 150 mg/m^2

Adjusted dose level -2: 120 mg/m^2

Further adjust if needed in decrements of ~20%

Colorectal cancer, metastatic (unlabeled dosing): I.V.: FOLFOXIRI regimen: 165 mg/m^2 over 1 hour once every 2 weeks (Falcone, 2007)

Cervical cancer, recurrent or metastatic (unlabeled use): I.V.: 125 mg/m^2 over 90 minutes once weekly for 4 consecutive weeks followed by a 2-week rest during each 6 week treatment cycle (Verschraegen, 1997)

CNS tumor, recurrent glioblastoma (unlabeled use): I.V.: 125 mg/m^2 over 90 minutes once every 2 weeks (in combination with bevacizumab). **NOTE:** in patients taking concurrent antiepileptic enzyme-inducing medications irinotecan dose was increased to 340 mg/m^2 (Friedman, 2009; Vredenburgh, 2007).

Esophageal cancer, metastatic or locally advanced (unlabeled use): I.V.: 65 mg/m^2/dose over 90 minutes days 1, 8, 15, and 22 of a 6-week treatment cycle (in combination with cisplatin) (Ajani, 2002; Ilson, 1999) **or** 80 mg/m^2/dose weekly for 6 weeks of a 7-week treatment cycle (in combination with leucovorin and fluorouracil) (Dank, 2008) **or** 250 mg/m^2/dose every 3 weeks (in combination with capecitabine) (Leary, 2009; Moehler, 2010)

Ewing's sarcoma, recurrent or progressive (unlabeled use): I.V.: 20 mg/m^2/dose days 1-5 and days 8-12 every 3 weeks (in combination with temozolomide) (Casey, 2009)

Gastric cancer, metastatic or locally advanced (unlabeled use): I.V.: 65 mg/m^2/dose over 90 minutes days 1, 8, 15, and 22 of a 6-week treatment cycle (in combination with cisplatin) (Ajani, 2002) **or** 180 mg/m^2/dose over 90 minutes every 2 weeks (in combination with leucovorin and fluorouracil) (Bouche, 2004) **or** 80 mg/m^2/dose weekly for 6 weeks of a 7-week treatment cycle (in combination with leucovorin and fluorouracil) (Dank, 2008) **or** 250 mg/m²/dose every 3 weeks (in combination with capecitabine) (Moehler, 2010)

Nonsmall cell lung cancer, advanced (unlabeled use): I.V.: 60 mg/m² days 1, 8, and 15 every 4 weeks (in combination with cisplatin) (Ohe, 2007)

Pancreatic cancer, advanced (unlabeled use): I.V.: FOLFIRINOX regimen: 180 mg/m²/dose over 90 minutes every 2 weeks (Conroy, 2005; Conroy, 2010)

Small cell lung cancer, extensive stage (unlabeled use): I.V.: 60 mg/m² days 1, 8, and 15 every 4 weeks (in combination with cisplatin) (Noda, 2002) **or** 65 mg/m² days 1 and 8 every 3 weeks (in combination with cisplatin) (Hanna, 2006) **or** 175 mg/m² day 1 every 3 weeks (in combination with carboplatin) (Hermes, 2008) **or** 50 mg/m² days 1, 8 and 15 every 4 weeks (in combination with carboplatin) (Schmittel, 2006)

Geriatric

Weekly dosing schedule: No dosing adjustment is recommended

Every 3 week dosing colorectal cancer schedule: Recommended initial dose is 300 mg/m²/dose for patients ≥70 years

Pediatric See **"Note"** in adult dosing.

Ewing's sarcoma, recurrent or progressive (unlabeled use): I.V.: Refer to adult dosing.

Renal Impairment

Renal impairment: No dosage adjustment provided in manufacturer's labeling (has not been studied); use with caution.

Dialysis: Use in patients with dialysis is not recommended by the manufacturer; however, literature suggests reducing weekly dose from 125 mg/m² to 50 mg/m² and administer after hemodialysis or on nondialysis days (Janus, 2010).

Hepatic Impairment

Manufacturer's recommendations:

Liver metastases with normal hepatic function: No dosage adjustment necessary.

Bilirubin >ULN to ≤2 mg/dL: Consider reducing initial dose by one dose level

Bilirubin >2 mg/dL: Use is not recommended

Alternate recommendations: The following adjustments have been used by some clinicians:

Bilirubin 1.5-3 mg/dL: Administer 75% of dose (Floyd, 2006)

Bilirubin 1.51 to 3 times ULN: Reduce dose from 350 mg/m² every 3 weeks to 200 mg/m² every 3 weeks (Raymond, 2002)

Adjustment for Toxicity It is recommended that new courses begin only after the granulocyte count recovers to ≥1500/mm³, the platelet counts recover to ≥100,000/mm³, and treatment-related diarrhea has fully resolved. Depending on the patient's ability to tolerate therapy, doses should be adjusted in increments of 25-50 mg/m². Treatment should be delayed 1-2 weeks to allow for recovery from treatment-related toxicities. If the patient has not recovered after a 2-week delay, consider discontinuing irinotecan. See tables on following pages.

Colorectal Cancer: Single-Agent Schedule: Recommended Dosage Modifications[1]

Toxicity NCI Grade[2] (Value)	During a Cycle of Therapy	At Start of Subsequent Cycles of Therapy (After Adequate Recovery), Compared to Starting Dose in Previous Cycle[1]	
	Weekly	Weekly	Once Every 3 Weeks
No toxicity	Maintain dose level	↑ 25 mg/m² up to a maximum dose of 150 mg/m²	Maintain dose level
Neutropenia			
1 (1500-1999/mm³)	Maintain dose level	Maintain dose level	Maintain dose level
2 (1000-1499/mm³)	↓ 25 mg/m²	Maintain dose level	Maintain dose level
3 (500-999/mm³)	Omit dose until resolved to ≤ grade 2, then ↓ 25 mg/m²	↓ 25 mg/m²	↓ 50 mg/m²
4 (<500/mm³)	Omit dose until resolved to ≤ grade 2, then ↓ 50 mg/m²	↓ 50 mg/m²	↓ 50 mg/m²
Neutropenic Fever (grade 4 neutropenia and ≥ grade 2 fever)	Omit dose until resolved, then ↓ 50 mg/m²	↓ 50 mg/m²	↓ 50 mg/m²
Other Hematologic Toxicities	Dose modifications for leukopenia, thrombocytopenia, and anemia during a course of therapy and at the start of subsequent courses of therapy are also based on NCI toxicity criteria and are the same as recommended for neutropenia above.		
Diarrhea			
1 (2-3 stools/day > pretreatment)	Maintain dose level	Maintain dose level	Maintain dose level
2 (4-6 stools/day > pretreatment)	↓ 25 mg/m²	Maintain dose level	Maintain dose level
3 (7-9 stools/day > pretreatment)	Omit dose until resolved to ≤ grade 2, then ↓ 25 mg/m²	↓ 25 mg/m²	↓ 50 mg/m²
4 (≥10 stools/day > pretreatment)	Omit dose until resolved to ≤ grade 2, then ↓ 50 mg/m²	↓ 50 mg/m²	↓ 50 mg/m²
Other Nonhematologic Toxicities[3]			
1	Maintain dose level	Maintain dose level	Maintain dose level
2	↓ 25 mg/m²	↓ 25 mg/m²	↓ 50 mg/m²
3	Omit dose until resolved to ≤ grade 2, then ↓ 25 mg/m²	↓ 25 mg/m²	↓ 50 mg/m²
4	Omit dose until resolved to ≤ grade 2, then ↓ 50 mg/m²	↓ 50 mg/m²	↓ 50 mg/m²

[1]All dose modifications should be based on the worst preceding toxicity.

[2]National Cancer Institute Common Toxicity Criteria (version 1.0).

[3]Excludes alopecia, anorexia, asthenia.

Colorectal Cancer: Combination Schedules: Recommended Dosage Modifications[1]

Toxicity NCI[2] Grade (Value)	During a Cycle of Therapy	At the Start of Subsequent Cycles of Therapy (After Adequate Recovery), Compared to the Starting Dose in the Previous Cycle[1]
No toxicity	Maintain dose level	Maintain dose level
Neutropenia		
1 (1500-1999/mm^3)	Maintain dose level	Maintain dose level
2 (1000-1499/mm^3)	↓ 1 dose level	Maintain dose level
3 (500-999/mm^3)	Omit dose until resolved to ≤ grade 2, then ↓ 1 dose level	↓ 1 dose level
4 (<500/mm^3)	Omit dose until resolved to ≤ grade 2, then ↓ 2 dose levels	↓ 2 dose levels
Neutropenic Fever (grade 4 neutropenia and ≥ grade 2 fever)	Omit dose until resolved, then ↓ 2 dose levels	
Other Hematologic Toxicities	Dose modifications for leukopenia or thrombocytopenia during a course of therapy and at the start of subsequent courses of therapy are also based on NCI toxicity criteria and are the same as recommended for neutropenia above.	
Diarrhea		
1 (2-3 stools/day > pretreatment)	Delay dose until resolved to baseline, then give same dose	Maintain dose level
2 (4-6 stools/day > pretreatment)	Omit dose until resolved to baseline, then ↓ 1 dose level	Maintain dose level
3 (7-9 stools/day > pretreatment)	Omit dose until resolved to baseline, then ↓ by 1 dose level	↓ 1 dose level
4 (≥10 stools/day > pretreatment)	Omit dose until resolved to baseline, then ↓ 2 dose levels	↓ 2 dose levels
Other Nonhematologic Toxicities[3]		
1	Maintain dose level	Maintain dose level
2	Omit dose until resolved to ≤ grade 1, then ↓ 1 dose level	Maintain dose level
3	Omit dose until resolved to ≤ grade 2, then ↓ 1 dose level	↓ 1 dose level
4	Omit dose until resolved to ≤ grade 2, then ↓ 2 dose levels	↓ 2 dose levels
Mucositis and/or stomatitis	Decrease only 5-FU, not irinotecan	Decrease only 5-FU, not irinotecan

[1]All dose modifications should be based on the worst preceding toxicity.

[2]National Cancer Institute Common Toxicity Criteria (version 1.0).

[3]Excludes alopecia, anorexia, asthenia.

Combination Regimens

Brain tumors: Bevacizumab-Irinotecan (Glioblastoma) on page 1531
Colorectal cancer:
Bevacizumab + FOLFIRI (Colorectal) on page 1530
Cetuximab (Biweekly)-Irinotecan on page 1557

Cetuximab + FOLFIRI (Colorectal) on page 1559
Cetuximab-Irinotecan (Colorectal) on page 1561
Fluorouracil-Leucovorin-Irinotecan (Saltz Regimen) on page 1656
FOLFIRI (Colorectal Cancer) on page 1659
FOLFOXIRI (Colorectal) on page 1665
FU-LV-CPT-11 on page 1666
Irinotecan (Colorectal Regimen) on page 1695
Panitumumab + FOLFIRI (Colorectal) on page 1733
Ziv-Aflibercept + FOLFIRI (Colorectal) on page 1779

Esophageal cancer:
Irinotecan-Capecitabine (Esophageal Cancer) on page 1693
Irinotecan-Cisplatin (Esophageal Cancer) on page 1694
Irinotecan-Fluorouracil-Leucovorin (Esophageal Cancer) on page 1696

Gastric cancer:
Irinotecan-Capecitabine (Gastric Cancer) on page 1693
Irinotecan-Cisplatin (Gastric Cancer) on page 1695
Irinotecan-Leucovorin-Fluorouracil (Gastric Cancer) on page 1697

Pancreatic cancer: FOLFIRINOX (Pancreatic) on page 1661

Lung cancer (nonsmall cell): Cisplatin-Irinotecan (NSCLC) on page 1580

Lung cancer, small cell:
Carboplatin-Irinotecan (Small Cell Lung Cancer) on page 1548
Cisplatin-Irinotecan (Small Cell Lung Cancer) on page 1580
Irinotecan (Small Cell Lung Cancer Regimen) on page 1697

Sarcoma: Irinotecan-Temozolomide (Ewing's Sarcoma) on page 1697

Administration Administer by I.V. infusion, usually over 90 minutes. Premedication with dexamethasone and a 5-HT_3 blocker is recommended 30 minutes prior to administration; prochlorperazine may be considered for subsequent use (if needed). Consider atropine 0.25-1 mg I.V. or SubQ as premedication for or treatment of cholinergic symptoms (eg, increased salivation, rhinitis, miosis, diaphoresis, abdominal cramping) or early onset diarrhea.

The recommended regimen to manage late diarrhea is loperamide 4 mg orally at onset of late diarrhea, followed by 2 mg every 2 hours (or 4 mg every 4 hours at night) until 12 hours have passed without a bowel movement. If diarrhea recurs, then repeat administration. Loperamide should not be used for more than 48 consecutive hours.

Emetic Potential Moderate (30% to 90%)

Vesicant/Extravasation Risk May be an irritant

Monitoring Parameters CBC with differential, platelet count, and hemoglobin with each dose; bilirubin, electrolytes (with severe diarrhea); bowel movements and hydration status; monitor infusion site for signs of inflammation and avoid extravasation

A test is available for genotyping of UGT1A1; however, guidelines for use are not established and not recommended in patients who have experienced toxicity as a dose reduction is already recommended (NCCN Colon Cancer Guidelines v.1.2011)

Dietary Considerations Contains sorbitol; do not use in patients with hereditary fructose intolerance.

Additional Information Patients who are homozygous for the UGT1A1*28 allele are at increased risk for neutropenia; a decreased dose is recommended. Clinical research of patients who are heterozygous for UGT1A1*28 have been variable for increased neutropenic risk and such patients have tolerated normal starting doses. An FDA-approved test (Invader® Molecular Assay) is available for clinical determination of UGT phenotype.

Dosage Forms Excipient information presented when available (limited, particularly for generics); consult specific product labeling.

Injection, solution, as hydrochloride: 20 mg/mL (2 mL, 5 mL, 25 mL)

Injection, solution, as hydrochloride [preservative free]: 20 mg/mL (2 mL, 5 mL)

Camptosar®: 20 mg/mL (2 mL, 5 mL, 15 mL) [contains sorbitol]

References

Ajani JA, Baker J, Pisters PW, et al, "CPT-11 Plus Cisplatin in Patients With Advanced, Untreated Gastric or Gastroesophageal Junction Carcinoma: Results of a Phase II Study," *Cancer*, 2002, 94 (3):641-6.

Bouché O, Raoul JL, Bonnetain F, et al, "Randomized Multicenter Phase II Trial of a Biweekly Regimen of Fluorouracil and Leucovorin (LV5FU2), LV5FU2 Plus Cisplatin, or LV5FU2 Plus Irinotecan in Patients With Previously Untreated Metastatic Gastric Cancer: A Federation Francophone de Cancerologie Digestive Group Study–FFCD 9803," *J Clin Oncol*, 2004, 22 (21):4319-28.

Casey DA, Wexler LH, Merchant MS, et al, "Irinotecan and Temozolomide for Ewing Sarcoma: The Memorial Sloan-Kettering Experience," *Pediatr Blood Cancer*, 2009, 53(6):1029-34.

Conroy Y, Desseigne F, Ychou M, et al, "Randomized Phase III Trial Comparing FOLFIRINOX (F: 5FU/Leucovorin [LV], Irinotecan [I], and Oxaliplatin [O]) Versus Gemcitabine (G) as First-Line Treatment for Metastatic Pancreatic Adenocarcinoma (MPA): Preplanned Interim Analysis Results of the PRODIGE 4/ACCORD 11 Trial," *J Clin Oncol*, 2010, 28(15s):4010 [abstract #4010 from the 2010 American Society of Clinical Oncology Meeting].

Conroy T, Paillot B, François E, et al, "Irinotecan Plus Oxaliplatin and Leucovorin-Modulated Fluorouracil in Advanced Pancreatic Cancer–A Groupe Tumeurs Digestives of the Federation Nationale des Centres de Lutte Contre le Cancer Study," *J Clin Oncol*, 2005, 23(6):1228-36.

Dank M, Zaluski J, Barone C, et al, "Randomized Phase III Study Comparing Irinotecan Combined With 5-Fluorouracil and Folinic Acid to Cisplatin Combined With 5-Fluorouracil in Chemotherapy Naive Patients With Advanced Adenocarcinoma of the Stomach or Esophagogastric Junction," *Ann Oncol*, 2008, 19(8):1450-7.

Falcone A, Ricci S, Brunetti I, et al, "Phase III Trial of Infusional Fluorouracil, Leucovorin, Oxaliplatin, and Irinotecan (FOLFOXIRI) Compared With Infusional Fluorouracil, Leucovorin, and Irinotecan (FOLFIRI) as First-Line Treatment for Metastatic Colorectal Cancer: The Gruppo Oncologico Nord Ovest," *J Clin Oncol*, 2007, 25(13):1670-6.

Floyd J, Mirza I, Sachs B, et al, "Hepatotoxicity of Chemotherapy," *Semin Oncol*, 2006, 33 (1):50-67.

Friedman HS, Prados MD, Wen PY, et al, "Bevacizumab Alone and in Combination With Irinotecan in Recurrent Glioblastoma," *J Clin Oncol*, 2009, 27(28):4733-40.

Hanna N, Bunn PA Jr, Langer C, et al, "Randomized Phase III Trial Comparing Irinotecan/Cisplatin With Etoposide/Cisplatin in Patients With Previously Untreated Extensive-Stage Disease Small-Cell Lung Cancer," *J Clin Oncol*, 2006, 24(13):2038-43.

Hermes A, Bergman B, Bremnes R, et al, "Irinotecan Plus Carboplatin Versus Oral Etoposide Plus Carboplatin in Extensive Small-Cell Lung Cancer: A Randomized Phase III Trial," *J Clin Oncol*, 2008, 26(26):4261-7.

Ilson DH, Saltz L, Enzinger P, et al, "Phase II Trial of Weekly Irinotecan Plus Cisplatin in Advanced Esophageal Cancer," *J Clin Oncol*, 1999, 17(10):3270-5.

Janus N, Thariat J, Boulanger H, et al, "Proposal for Dosage Adjustment and Timing of Chemotherapy in Hemodialyzed Patients," *Ann Oncol*, 2010, 21(7):1395-403.

Leary A, Assersohn L, Cunningham D, et al, "A Phase II Trial Evaluating Capecitabine and Irinotecan as Second Line Treatment in Patients With Oesophago-Gastric Cancer Who Have Progressed On, or Within 3 Months of Platinum-Based Chemotherapy," *Cancer Chemother Pharmacol*, 2009, 64(3):455-62.

Marsh S and McLeod HL, "Pharmacogenetics of Irinotecan Toxicity," *Pharmacogenomics*, 2004, 5 (7):835-43.

Moehler M, Kanzler S, Geissler M, et al, "A Randomized Multicenter Phase II Study Comparing Capecitabine With Irinotecan or Cisplatin in Metastatic Adenocarcinoma of the Stomach or Esophagogastric Junction," *Ann Oncol*, 2010 21(1):71-7.

Morgan C, Tillett T, Braybrooke J, et al, "Management of Uncommon Chemotherapy-Induced Emergencies," *Lancet Oncol*, 2011, 12(8):806-14.

National Comprehensive Cancer Network® (NCCN), "Clinical Practice Guidelines in Oncology™: Colon Cancer," Version 3.2010. Available at http://www.nccn.org/professionals/physician_gls/PDF/colon.pdf

Noda K, Nishiwaki Y, Kawahara M, et al, "Irinotecan Plus Cisplatin Compared With Etoposide Plus Cisplatin for Extensive Small-Cell Lung Cancer," *N Engl J Med*, 2002, 346(2):85-91.
Ohe Y, Ohashi Y, Kubota K, et al, "Randomized Phase III Study of Cisplatin Plus Irinotecan Versus Carboplatin Plus Paclitaxel, Cisplatin Plus Gemcitabine, and Cisplatin Plus Vinorelbine for Advanced Non-Small-Cell Lung Cancer: Four-Arm Cooperative Study in Japan," *Ann Oncol*, 2007, 18(2):317-23.
Raymond E, Boige V, Faivre S, et al, "Dosage Adjustment and Pharmacokinetic Profile of Irinotecan in Cancer Patients With Hepatic Dysfunction," *J Clin Oncol*, 2002, 20(21):4303-12.
Schmittel A, Fischer von Weikersthal L, Sebastian M, et al, "A Randomized Phase II Trial of Irinotecan Plus Carboplatin Versus Etoposide Plus Carboplatin Treatment in Patients With Extended Disease Small-Cell Lung Cancer," *Ann Oncol*, 2006, 17(4):663-7.
Verschraegen CF, Levy T, Kudelka AP, et al, "Phase II Study of Irinotecan in Prior Chemotherapy-Treated Squamous Cell Carcinoma of the Cervix," *J Clin Oncol*, 1997, 5(2):625-31.
Vredenburgh JJ, Desjardins A, Herndon JE 2nd, et al, "Bevacizumab Plus Irinotecan in Recurrent Glioblastoma Multiforme," *J Clin Oncol*, 2007, 25(30):4722-9.

- **Irinotecan HCl** *see* Irinotecan *on page 813*
- **Irinotecan Hydrochloride** *see* Irinotecan *on page 813*
- **Irinotecan Hydrochloride Trihydrate (Can)** *see* Irinotecan *on page 813*
- **Iron Dextran** *see* Iron Dextran Complex *on page 824*

Iron Dextran Complex (EYE ern DEKS tran KOM pleks)

Brand Names: U.S. Dexferrum®; INFeD®

Brand Names: Canada Dexiron™; Infufer®

Index Terms High-Molecular-Weight Iron Dextran (DexFerrum®); Imferon; Iron Dextran; Low-Molecular-Weight Iron Dextran (INFeD®)

Generic Availability (U.S.) No

Pharmacologic Category Iron Salt

Use Treatment of iron deficiency in patients in whom oral administration is infeasible or ineffective

Unlabeled Use Cancer-/chemotherapy-associated anemia

Labeled Contraindications Hypersensitivity to iron dextran or any component of the formulation; any anemia not associated with iron deficiency

Pregnancy Risk Factor C

Lactation Enters breast milk/use caution

Warnings/Precautions [U.S. Boxed Warning]: Deaths associated with parenteral administration following anaphylactic-type reactions have been reported (use only where resuscitation equipment and personnel are available). A test dose should be administered to all patients prior to the first therapeutic dose. Fatal reactions have occurred even in patients who tolerated the test dose. Monitor patients for signs/symptoms of anaphylactic reactions during any iron dextran administration. A history of drug allergy (including multiple drug allergies) and/or the concomitant use of an ACE inhibitor may increase the risk of anaphylactic-type reactions. Adverse events (including life-threatening) associated with iron dextran usually occur with the high-molecular-weight formulation (Dexferrum®), compared to low-molecular-weight (INFeD®) (Chertow, 2006). Delayed (1-2 days) infusion reaction (including arthralgia, back pain, chills, dizziness, and fever) may occur with large doses (eg, total dose infusion) of I.V. iron dextran; usually subsides within 3-4 days. Delayed reaction may also occur (less commonly) with I.M. administration; subsiding within 3-7 days. Use with caution in patients with a history of significant allergies, asthma, serious hepatic impairment, pre-existing cardiac disease (may exacerbate cardiovascular complications), and rheumatoid arthritis (may exacerbate joint pain and swelling). Avoid use during acute kidney infection.

In patients with chronic kidney disease (CKD) requiring iron supplementation, the I.V. route is preferred for hemodialysis patients; either oral iron or I.V. iron may be used for nondialysis and peritoneal dialysis CKD patients. In patients with cancer-related anemia (either due to cancer or chemotherapy-induced) requiring iron supplementation, the I.V. route is superior to oral therapy; I.M. administration is not recommended for parenteral iron supplementation.

[U.S. Boxed Warning]: Use only in patients where the iron deficient state is not amenable to oral iron therapy. Discontinue oral iron prior to initiating parenteral iron therapy. Exogenous hemosiderosis may result from excess iron stores; patients with refractory anemias and/or hemoglobinopathies may be prone to iron overload with unwarranted iron supplementation. Anemia in the elderly is often caused by "anemia of chronic disease" or associated with inflammation rather than blood loss. Iron stores are usually normal or increased, with a serum ferritin >50 ng/mL and a decreased total iron binding capacity. I.V. administration of iron dextran is often preferred over I.M. in the elderly secondary to a decreased muscle mass and the need for daily injections. Intramuscular injections of iron-carbohydrate complexes may have a risk of delayed injection site tumor development. Iron dextran products differ in chemical characteristics. The high-molecular-weight formulation (Dexferrum®) and the low-molecular-weight formulation (INFeD®) are not clinically interchangeable. Not recommended in children <4 months of age. Intramuscular iron dextran use in neonates may be associated with an increased incidence of gram-negative sepsis.

Adverse Reactions Frequency not defined. **Note:** Adverse event risk is reported to be higher with the high-molecular-weight iron dextran formulation.

Cardiovascular: Arrhythmia, bradycardia, cardiac arrest, chest pain, chest tightness, cyanosis, flushing, hyper-/hypotension, shock, syncope, tachycardia

Central nervous system: Chills, disorientation, dizziness, fever, headache, malaise, seizure, unconsciousness, unresponsiveness

Dermatologic: Pruritus, purpura, rash, urticaria

Gastrointestinal: Abdominal pain, diarrhea, nausea, taste alteration, vomiting

Genitourinary: Discoloration of urine

Hematologic: Leukocytosis, lymphadenopathy

Local: Injection site reactions (cellulitis, inflammation, pain, phlebitis, soreness, swelling), muscle atrophy/fibrosis (with I.M. injection), skin/tissue staining (at the site of I.M. injection), sterile abscess

Neuromuscular & skeletal: Arthralgia, arthritis/arthritis exacerbation, back pain, myalgia, paresthesia, weakness

Respiratory: Bronchospasm, dyspnea, respiratory arrest, wheezing

Renal: Hematuria

Miscellaneous: Anaphylactic reactions (sudden respiratory difficulty, cardiovascular collapse), diaphoresis

Postmarketing and/or case reports: Angioedema, tumor formation (at former injection site)

Drug Interactions

Metabolism/Transport Effects None known.

Avoid Concomitant Use

Avoid concomitant use of Iron Dextran Complex with any of the following: Dimercaprol

Increased Effect/Toxicity

The levels/effects of Iron Dextran Complex may be increased by: ACE Inhibitors; Dimercaprol

Decreased Effect There are no known significant interactions involving a decrease in effect.

Storage/Stability Store at controlled room temperature.

Reconstitution Solutions for infusion should be diluted in 250-1000 mL NS.

Mechanism of Action The released iron, from the plasma, eventually replenishes the depleted iron stores in the bone marrow where it is incorporated into hemoglobin

Pharmacodynamics/Kinetics

Onset of action: I.V.: Serum ferritin peak: 7-9 days after dose

Absorption:

I.M.: 50% to 90% is promptly absorbed, balance is slowly absorbed over month

I.V.: Uptake of iron by the reticuloendothelial system appears to be constant at about 10-20 mg/hour

Excretion: Urine and feces via reticuloendothelial system

Dosing

Adult & Geriatric

Note: A 0.5 mL test dose should be given prior to starting iron dextran therapy.

Iron-deficiency anemia: I.M. (INFeD®), I.V. (Dexferrum®, INFeD®):

Dose (mL) = 0.0442 (desired Hgb - observed Hgb) x LBW + (0.26 x LBW)

Desired hemoglobin: Usually 14.8 g/dL

LBW = Lean body weight in kg

Iron replacement therapy for blood loss: (INFeD®), I.V. (Dexferrum®, INFeD®): Replacement iron (mg) = blood loss (mL) x Hct

Maximum daily dosage: Manufacturer's labeling: **Note:** Replacement of larger estimated iron deficits may be achieved by serial administration of smaller incremental dosages. Daily dosages should be limited to 100 mg iron (2 mL)

Total dose infusion (unlabeled): The entire dose (estimated iron deficit) may be diluted and administered as a one-time I.V. infusion.

Cancer-/chemotherapy-associated anemia (NCCN guidelines v.2.2010) (unlabeled use): I.V.: Test dose: 25 mg slow I.V. slow push, followed 1 hour later by 100 mg over 5 minutes; larger doses (unlabeled), up to total dose infusion (over several hours) may be administered. Low-molecular-weight iron dextran preferred.

Pediatric Note: A 0.5 mL test dose (0.25 mL in infants) should be given prior to starting iron dextran therapy.

Iron-deficiency anemia: I.M. (INFeD®), I.V. (Dexferrum®, INFeD®):

Children 5-15 kg: Should not normally be given in the first 4 months of life:

Dose (mL) = 0.0442 (desired Hgb - observed Hgb) x W + (0.26 x W)

Desired hemoglobin: Usually 12 g/dL

W = Total body weight in kg

Children >15 kg: Refer to adult dosing.

Iron replacement therapy for blood loss: Refer to adult dosing.

Maximum daily dose:

Children <5 kg: 25 mg iron (0.5 mL)

Children 5-10 kg: 50 mg iron (1 mL)

Children ≥10 kg: Refer to adult dosing.

Administration Note: Test dose: A test dose should be given on the first day of therapy; patient should be observed for 1 hour for hypersensitivity reaction, then the remaining dose (dose minus test dose) should be given. Resuscitation equipment and trained personnel should be available. An uneventful test dose does not ensure an anaphylactic-type reaction will not occur during administration of the therapeutic dose.

I.M. (INFeD®): Use Z-track technique (displacement of the skin laterally prior to injection); injection should be deep into the upper outer quadrant of buttock; alternate buttocks with subsequent injections. Administer test dose at same recommended site using the same technique.

I.V.: Test dose should be given gradually over at least 30 seconds (INFeD®) or 5 minutes (Dexferrum®). Subsequent dose(s) may be administered by I.V. bolus undiluted at a rate not to exceed 50 mg/minute or diluted in 250-1000 mL NS and infused over 1-6 hours (initial 25 mL should be given slowly and patient should be observed for allergic reactions); avoid dilutions with dextrose (increased incidence of local pain and phlebitis)

Monitoring Parameters Hemoglobin, hematocrit, reticulocyte count, serum ferritin, serum iron, TIBC; monitor for anaphylaxis/hypersensitivity reaction (during test dose and therapeutic dose)

Test Interactions May cause falsely elevated values of serum bilirubin and falsely decreased values of serum calcium. Residual iron dextran may remain in reticuloendothelial cells; may affect accuracy of examination of bone marrow iron stores. Bone scans with 99m Tc-labeled bone seeking agents may show reduced bony uptake, marked renal activity, and excess blood pooling and soft tissue accumulation following I.V. iron dextran infusion or with high serum ferritin levels. Following I.M. iron dextran, bone scans with 99m Tc-diphosphonate may show dense activity in the buttocks.

Dosage Forms Excipient information presented when available (limited, particularly for generics); consult specific product labeling.

Injection, solution:

Dexferrum®: Elemental iron 50 mg/mL (1 mL, 2 mL) [high-molecular-weight iron dextran]

INFeD®: Elemental iron 50 mg/mL (2 mL) [low-molecular-weight iron dextran]

References

Auerbach M, Ballard H, Trout JR, et al, "Intravenous Iron Optimizes the Response to Recombinant Human Erythropoietin in Cancer Patients With Chemotherapy-Associated Anemia: A Multicenter, Open-Label, Randomized Trial," *J Clin Oncol*, 2004, 22(7):1301-7.

Chertow GM, Mason PD, Vaage-Nilsen O, et al, "Update on Adverse Drug Events Associated With Parenteral Iron," *Nephrol Dial Transplant*, 2006, 21(2):378-82.

National Comprehensive Cancer Network® (NCCN), "Practice Guidelines in Oncology™: Cancer- and Chemotherapy-Induced Anemia Version 1.2013." Available at http://www.nccn.org/professionals/physician_gls/PDF/anemia.pdf

National Kidney Foundation, "KDOQI Clinical Practice Guidelines and Clinical Practice Recommendations for Anemia in Chronic Kidney Disease," *Am J Kidney Dis*, 2007, 50(3):529-30. Available at http://www.kidney.org/professionals/KDOQI/guidelines_anemiaUP/index.htm or http://www.kidney.org/professionals/KDOQI

Rizzo JD, Somerfield MR, Hagerty LK, et al, "American Society of Hematology/American Society of Clinical Oncology 2007 Clinical Practice Guideline Update on the Use of Epoetin and Darbepoetin," *Blood*, 2008, 111(1):25-41.

Iron Sucrose (EYE ern SOO krose)

Brand Names: U.S. Venofer®

Brand Names: Canada Venofer®

Generic Availability (U.S.) No

Pharmacologic Category Iron Salt

Use Treatment of iron-deficiency anemia in chronic kidney disease (CKD), including nondialysis-dependent and dialysis-dependent patients

Unlabeled Use Cancer-/chemotherapy-associated anemia

Labeled Contraindications Hypersensitivity to iron sucrose or any component of the formulation

Pregnancy Risk Factor B

Lactation Excretion in breast milk unknown/use caution

Warnings/Precautions Hypersensitivity reactions, including rare postmarketing anaphylactic and anaphylactoid reactions (some fatal), have been reported; monitor patients during and for ≥30 minutes postadministration; discontinue immediately for signs/symptoms of a hypersensitivity reaction (shock, hypotension, loss of consciousness). Equipment for resuscitation and trained personnel experienced in handling medical emergencies should always be immediately available. Significant hypotension has been reported frequently in hemodialysis-dependent patients. Hypotension has also been reported in peritoneal dialysis and nondialysis patients. Hypotension may be related to total dose or rate of administration (avoid rapid I.V. injection), follow recommended guidelines. Withhold iron in the presence of tissue iron overload; periodic monitoring of hemoglobin, hematocrit, serum ferritin, and transferrin saturation is recommended.

Adverse Reactions Events and incidences are associated with use in adults unless otherwise specified.

>10%:

Cardiovascular: Hypotension (2% to 3%; children 2%; 39% in hemodialysis patients; may be related to total dose or rate of administration)

Central nervous system: Headache (3% to 13%; children 6%)

Gastrointestinal: Nausea (5% to 15%; children 3%)

Neuromuscular & skeletal: Muscle cramps (1% to 3%; 29% in hemodialysis patients)

Respiratory: Nasopharyngitis (2% to 16%), pharyngitis (2% to 16%), sinusitis (2% to 16%), upper respiratory infection (2% to 16%; children 4%)

1% to 10%:

Cardiovascular: Hypertension (7% to 8%; children 2%), peripheral edema (3% to 7%), chest pain (1% to 6%), arteriovenous fistula thrombosis (children 2%), heart failure (>1%)

Central nervous system: Dizziness (1% to 7%; children 4%), fever (1% to 3%; children 4%)

Dermatologic: Pruritus (2% to 4%)

Endocrine & metabolic: Hypoglycemia (≤4%), fluid overload (1% to 3%), gout (≤3%), hyperglycemia (≤3%)

Gastrointestinal: Vomiting (5% to 9%; children 4%), diarrhea (5% to 8%), taste perversion (≤8%), peritonitis (children 4%), abdominal pain (1% to 4%)

Local: Injection site reaction (≤6%)

Neuromuscular & skeletal: Extremity pain (3% to 6%), arthralgia (1% to 4%), myalgia (≤4%), weakness (1% to 3%), back pain (1% to 2%)

Ocular: Conjunctivitis (≤3%)

Otic: Ear pain (≤2%)

Respiratory: Dyspnea (1% to 6%), cough (1% to 3%; children 4%), nasal congestion (≤1%)

Miscellaneous: Graft complication (≤10%), sepsis (>1%)

<1%, postmarketing, and/or case reports: Anaphylactic shock, anaphylactoid reactions, angioedema, bradycardia, bronchospasm, cardiovascular collapse, confusion, facial rash, hyperhidrosis, hypersensitivity (including wheezing), hypoesthesia, injection site discoloration (following extravasation), joint swelling, lightheadedness, loss of consciousness, necrotizing

enterocolitis (reported in premature infants, no causal relationship established), paresthesia, seizure, shock, urine discoloration, urticaria

Drug Interactions

Metabolism/Transport Effects None known.

Avoid Concomitant Use

Avoid concomitant use of Iron Sucrose with any of the following: Dimercaprol

Increased Effect/Toxicity

The levels/effects of Iron Sucrose may be increased by: Dimercaprol

Decreased Effect There are no known significant interactions involving a decrease in effect.

Storage/Stability Store intact vials at controlled room temperature of 20°C to 25°C (68°F to 77°F); excursions permitted to 15°C to 30°C (59°F to 86°F); do not freeze. Iron sucrose is stable for 7 days at room temperature or under refrigeration when undiluted in a plastic syringe or following dilution in normal saline in a plastic syringe (2-10 mg/mL) or I.V. bag (1-2 mg/mL).

Reconstitution

Children: May administer undiluted or diluted in 25 mL of NS. Do not dilute to concentrations <1 mg/mL.

Adults: Doses ≤200 mg may be administered undiluted or diluted in a maximum of 100 mL NS. Doses >200 mg should be diluted in a maximum of 250 mL NS. Do not dilute to concentrations <1 mg/mL.

Mechanism of Action Iron sucrose is dissociated by the reticuloendothelial system into iron and sucrose. The released iron increases serum iron concentrations and is incorporated into hemoglobin.

Pharmacodynamics/Kinetics

Distribution: V_{dss}: Healthy adults: 7.9 L

Metabolism: Dissociated into iron and sucrose by the reticuloendothelial system

Half-life elimination: Healthy adults: 6 hours; Nondialysis-dependent adolescents: 8 hours

Excretion: Healthy adults: Urine (5%) within 24 hours

Dosing

Adult & Geriatric Doses expressed in mg of **elemental** iron. **Note:** Test dose: Product labeling does not indicate need for a test dose in product-naive patients.

Iron-deficiency anemia in chronic kidney disease (CKD): I.V.:

Hemodialysis-dependent patient: 100 mg administered during consecutive dialysis sessions to a cumulative total dose of 1000 mg (10 doses); may repeat treatment if clinically indicated.

Peritoneal dialysis-dependent patient: Two infusions of 300 mg administered 14 days apart, followed by a single 400 mg infusion 14 days later (total cumulative dose of 1000 mg in 3 divided doses); may repeat treatment if clinically indicated.

Nondialysis-dependent patient: 200 mg administered on 5 different occasions within a 14-day period (total cumulative dose: 1000 mg in 14-day period); may repeat treatment if clinically indicated. **Note:** Dosage has also been administered as 2 infusions of 500 mg on day 1 and day 14 (limited experience).

Cancer-/chemotherapy-associated anemia (unlabeled use): I.V.: 200 mg I.V. infusion (maximum: 300 mg/infusion) over 1 hour every 2-3 weeks **or** 200 mg slow I.V. injection over 2-5 minutes every 1-4 weeks. Total cumulative dose: 1000 mg. Test doses (25 mg slow I.V. push) are recommended in patients with a history of hypersensitivity to any I.V. iron preparation (eg, dextran) or those with other drug allergies (NCCN guidelines, v.1.2013).

Pediatric Doses expressed in mg of **elemental** iron. **Note:** Test dose: Product labeling does not indicate need for a test dose in product-naive patients.

Iron-deficiency anemia in chronic kidney disease (CKD): Children ≥2 years and Adolescents: I.V.: **Note:** Not indicated for iron replacement treatment in children and adolescents.

Hemodialysis-dependent patient: Maintenance therapy: 0.5 mg/kg/dose (maximum: 100 mg) every 2 weeks for 6 doses; may repeat if clinically indicated.

Nondialysis-dependent patient: Maintenance therapy: 0.5 mg/kg/dose (maximum: 100 mg) every 4 weeks for 3 doses; may repeat if clinically indicated

Peritoneal dialysis-dependent patient: Maintenance therapy: 0.5 mg/kg/dose (maximum: 100 mg) every 4 weeks for 3 doses; may repeat if clinically indicated

Administration Administer intravenously as a slow I.V. injection (**not** for rapid I.V. injection) or as an I.V. infusion. Can be administered through dialysis line.

Children and Adolescents:

Slow I.V. injection: Administer undiluted over 5 minutes

Infusion: Dilute dose in 25 mL of NS; infuse over 5-60 minutes

Adults:

Slow I.V. injection: May administer doses ≤200 mg undiluted by slow I.V. injection over 2-5 minutes. When administering to hemodialysis dependent patients, give iron sucrose early during the dialysis session.

Infusion: Dilute doses ≤200 mg in maximum of 100 mL NS and infuse over at least 15 minutes; Dilute 300 mg in a maximum of 250 mL NS and infuse over 1.5 hours; Dilute 400 mg in a maximum of 250 mL NS and infuse over 2.5 hours; Dilute 500 mg in a maximum of 250 mL NS and infuse over 3.5-4 hours (limited experience). When administering to hemodialysis-dependent patients, give iron sucrose early during the dialysis session.

Monitoring Parameters Hematocrit, hemoglobin, serum ferritin, serum iron, transferrin, percent transferrin saturation, TIBC (takes ~4 weeks of treatment to see increased serum iron and ferritin, and decreased TIBC); iron status should be assessed ≥48 hours after last dose (due to rapid increase in values following administration); signs/symptoms of hypersensitivity reactions (during and ≥30 minutes following infusion); hypotension (following infusion)

Dosage Forms Excipient information presented when available (limited, particularly for generics); consult specific product labeling.

Injection, solution [preservative free]:

Venofer®: Elemental iron 20 mg/mL (2.5 mL, 5 mL, 10 mL)

References

American College of Obstetricians and Gynecologists, "ACOG Practice Bulletin No. 95: Anemia in Pregnancy," *Obstet Gynecol*, 2008, 112(1):201-7.

Aronoff GR, Bennett WM, Blumenthal S, et al, "Iron Sucrose in Hemodialysis Patients: Safety of Replacement and Maintenance Regimens," *Kidney Int*, 2004, 66(3):1193-8.

Baker WF Jr, "Iron Deficiency in Pregnancy, Obstetrics, and Gynecology," *Hematol Oncol Clin North Am*, 2000, 14(5):1061-77.

Leijn E, Monnens LA, and Cornelissen EA, "Intravenous Iron Supplementation in Children on Hemodialysis," *J Nephrol*, 2004, 17(3):423-6.

National Comprehensive Cancer Network® (NCCN), "Practice Guidelines in Oncology™: Cancer- and Chemotherapy-Induced Anemia Version 1.2013." Available at http://www.nccn.org/professionals/physician_gls/f_guidelines.asp

National Kidney Foundation, "KDOQI Clinical Practice Guidelines and Clinical Practice Recommendations for Anemia in Chronic Kidney Disease," *Am J Kidney Dis*, 2007, 50(3):529-30.

Available at http://www.kidney.org/professionals/KDOQI/guidelines_anemiaUP/index.htm or http://www.kidney.org/professionals/KDOQI

Van Damme-Lombaerts R and Herman J, "Erythropoietin Treatment In Children With Renal Failure," *Predfiatr Nephrol*, 1999, 13(2):148-52.

- **ISG** *see* Immune Globulin *on page* 777
- **Isonipecaine Hydrochloride** *see* Meperidine *on page* 932
- **Isophosphamide** *see* Ifosfamide *on page* 752

Isosulfan Blue (eye soe SUL fan bloo)

Brand Names: U.S. Lymphazurin™

Generic Availability (U.S.) Yes

Pharmacologic Category Contrast Agent

Use Adjunct to lymphography for visualization of the lymphatic system; sentinel node identification

Labeled Contraindications Hypersensitivity to isosulfan, triphenylmethane, or any component of the formulation

Pregnancy Risk Factor C

Lactation Excretion in breast milk is unknown/use caution

Warnings/Precautions Hypersensitivity reactions, including anaphylactic reactions (rare), may occur; appropriate equipment and emergency medications should be available during use. Competent personnel and emergency facilities should be available during and for at least 60 minutes after administration, since severe delayed reactions may occur. Risk likely higher risk in patients with history of asthma, allergies, drug reactions, including previous sensitivity to triphenylmethane dyes. Peripheral oxygenation measurements may be falsely depressed due to discoloration of serum caused by isosulfan blue; (peak interference 30 minutes after administration; minimal effect by 4 hours postdose); direct determination of arterial blood gases (ABG) may be required. Methemoglobin levels via ABG may be falsely elevated; co-oximetry may be required to accurately assess. Safety and efficacy have not been established in children.

Adverse Reactions

1% to 10%:

Dermatologic: Pruritus (2%; affecting hands, abdomen and neck)

Local: Administration site swelling (2%)

Miscellaneous: Hypersensitivity reactions (2%)

Postmarketing and/or case reports: Anaphylaxis; body fluid discoloration (urine, serum; may lead to falsely low oximetry readings); skin discoloration (including blue urticaria)

Drug Interactions

Metabolism/Transport Effects None known.

Avoid Concomitant Use There are no known interactions where it is recommended to avoid concomitant use.

Increased Effect/Toxicity There are no known significant interactions involving an increase in effect.

Decreased Effect There are no known significant interactions involving a decrease in effect.

Storage/Stability Store at room temperature. Avoid prolonged exposure to elevated temperatures.

Mechanism of Action Following subcutaneous administration, isosulfan blue binds to interstitial proteins; these proteins/extracellular fluids are drained by the regional lymphatic system, resulting in concentration of the dye within the lymph. Bright blue coloration imparted by the dye permits delineation of the vessels against the surrounding tissue.

Pharmacodynamics/Kinetics

Absorption: 34% absorbed in 30 minutes; 69% and 100% in 1 and 24 hours, respectively

Protein binding: ~50%

Excretion: Urine (10%; as unchanged drug); feces (~90%; via biliary excretion)

Dosing

Adult Lymphography: SubQ: Inject 0.5 mL into 3 interdigital spaces of each extremity per study; maximum: 3 mL (30 mg)

Administration SubQ: Single patient use only; do not mix with local anesthetics (in same syringe)

Test Interactions Peripheral oxygenation measurements may be falsely depressed (peak interference 30 minutes after administration; minimal effect by 4 hours postdose). Methemoglobin levels via arterial blood gas analyzer may be falsely elevated.

Additional Information May cause blue discoloration of urine for 24 hours.

Dosage Forms Excipient information presented when available (limited, particularly for generics); consult specific product labeling.

Injection, solution [preservative free]: 1% (5 mL)

Lymphazurin™: 1% (5 mL)

References

Hoskin RW and Granger R, "Intraoperative Decrease in Pulse Oximeter Readings Following Injection of Isosulfan Blue," *Can J Anesth*, 2001, 48(1):38-40.

Kern KA, "Sentinel Lymph Node Mapping in Breast Cancer Using Subareolar Injection of Blue Dye," *J Am Coll Surg*, 1999, 189(6):539-45.

Sadiq TS, Burns WW, Taber DJ et al, "Blue Urticaria: A Previously Unreported Adverse Event Associated With Isosulfan Blue," *Arch Surg*, 2001, 136(12): 1433-5.

Sprung J, Tully MJ, and Ziser A, "Anaphylactic Reactions to Isosulfan Blue Dye During Sentinel Node Lymphadenectomy for Breast Cancer," *Anesth Analg*, 2003, 96(4):1051-3.

ISOtretinoin (eye soe TRET i noyn)

Brand Names: U.S. Amnesteem®; Claravis™; Myorisan™; Sotret®

Brand Names: Canada Accutane®; Clarus™

Index Terms 13-*cis*-Retinoic Acid; 13-*cis*-Vitamin A Acid; 13-CRA; *Cis*-Retinoic Acid; Absorica; Accutane; Isotretinoinum

Generic Availability (U.S.) No

Pharmacologic Category Acne Products; Antineoplastic Agent, Miscellaneous; Retinoic Acid Derivative

Use Treatment of severe recalcitrant nodular acne unresponsive to conventional therapy

Unlabeled Use Management of moderate degrees of treatment-resistant acne, management of acne that produces physical or psychological scarring; treatment of cutaneous T-cell lymphomas (mycosis fungoides and Sézary syndrome); prevention of squamous cell skin cancers (in high-risk patients); treatment of high-risk neuroblastoma in children

Labeled Contraindications Hypersensitivity to isotretinoin or any component of the formulation; sensitivity to parabens, vitamin A, or other retinoids; pregnant women or those who may become pregnant

Pregnancy Risk Factor X

Lactation Excretion in breast milk unknown/not recommended

Warnings/Precautions This medication should only be prescribed by prescribers competent in treating severe recalcitrant nodular acne and experienced with the use of systemic retinoids. Anaphylaxis and other types of allergic reactions, including cutaneous reactions and allergic vasculitis, have been reported. **[U.S. Boxed Warnings]: Birth defects (facial, eye, ear, skull, central nervous system, cardiovascular, thymus and parathyroid gland abnormalities) have been noted following isotretinoin exposure during pregnancy and the risk for severe birth defects is high, with any dose or even with short treatment duration. Low IQ scores have also been reported. The risk for spontaneous abortion and premature births is increased. Because of the high likelihood of teratogenic effects, all patients (male and female), prescribers, wholesalers, and dispensing pharmacists must register and be active in the iPLEDGE™ risk evaluation and mitigation strategy (REMS) program; do not prescribe isotretinoin for women who are or who are likely to become pregnant while using the drug. If pregnancy occurs during therapy, isotretinoin should be discontinued immediately and the patient referred to an obstetrician-gynecologist specializing in reproductive toxicity (see Additional Information).** Women of childbearing potential must be capable of complying with effective contraceptive measures. Patients must select and commit to two forms of contraception. Therapy is begun after two negative pregnancy tests; effective contraception must be used for at least 1 month before beginning therapy, during therapy, and for 1 month after discontinuation of therapy. Prescriptions should be written for no more than a 30-day supply, and pregnancy testing and counseling should be repeated monthly.

May cause depression, psychosis, aggressive or violent behavior, and changes in mood; use with extreme caution in patients with psychiatric disorders. Rarely, suicidal thoughts and actions have been reported during isotretinoin usage. All patients should be observed closely for symptoms of depression or suicidal thoughts. Discontinuation of treatment alone may not be sufficient, further evaluation may be necessary. Cases of pseudotumor cerebri (benign intracranial hypertension) have been reported, some with concomitant use of tetracycline (avoid using together). Patients with papilledema, headache, nausea, vomiting, and visual disturbances should be referred to a neurologist and treatment with isotretinoin discontinued. Hearing impairment, which can continue after therapy is discontinued, may occur. Clinical hepatitis, elevated liver enzymes, inflammatory bowel disease, skeletal hyperostosis, premature epiphyseal closure, vision impairment, corneal opacities, decreased tolerance to contact lenses (due to dry eyes), and decreased night vision have also been reported with the use of isotretinoin. Rare postmarketing cases of severe skin reactions (eg, Stevens-Johnson syndrome, erythema multiforme) have been reported with use.

Use with caution in patients with diabetes mellitus; impaired glucose control has been reported. Use caution in patients with hypertriglyceridemia; acute pancreatitis and fatal hemorrhagic pancreatitis (rare) have been reported. Bone mineral density may decrease; use caution in patients with a genetic predisposition to bone disorders (ie osteoporosis, osteomalacia) and with disease states or concomitant medications that can induce bone disorders. Patients may be at risk when participating in activities with repetitive impact (such as sports). Patients should be instructed not to donate blood during therapy and for 1 month following discontinuation of therapy due to risk of donated blood being given to a pregnant female. Safety of long-term use is not established and is not recommended.

Absorica™: Absorption is ~83% greater than Accutane® when administered under fasting conditions; they are bioequivalent when taken with a high-fat meal. Absorica™ is not interchangeable with other generic isotretinoin products

Adverse Reactions Frequency not always defined.

Cardiovascular: Chest pain, edema, flushing, palpitation, stroke, syncope, tachycardia, vascular thrombotic disease

Central nervous system: Aggressive behavior, depression, dizziness, drowsiness, emotional instability, fatigue, headache, insomnia, lethargy, malaise, nervousness, paresthesia, pseudotumor cerebri, psychosis, seizure, stroke, suicidal ideation, suicide attempts, suicide, violent behavior

Dermatologic: Abnormal wound healing acne fulminans, alopecia, bruising, cheilitis, cutaneous allergic reactions, dry nose, dry skin, eczema, eruptive xanthomas, facial erythema, fragility of skin, hair abnormalities, hirsutism, hyperpigmentation, hypopigmentation, increased sunburn susceptibility, nail dystrophy, paronychia, peeling of palms, peeling of soles, photoallergic reactions, photosensitizing reactions, pruritus, purpura, rash

Endocrine & metabolic: Triglycerides increased (25%), abnormal menses, blood glucose increased, cholesterol increased, HDL decreased, hyperuricemia

Gastrointestinal: Bleeding and inflammation of the gums, colitis, esophagitis, esophageal ulceration, inflammatory bowel disease, nausea, nonspecific gastrointestinal symptoms, pancreatitis, weight loss, xerostomia

Genitourinary: Nonspecific urogenital findings

Hematologic: Agranulocytosis (rare), anemia, neutropenia, pyogenic granuloma, thrombocytopenia

Hepatic: Alkaline phosphatase increased, ALT increased, AST increased, GGTP increased, hepatitis, LDH increased

Neuromuscular & skeletal: Back pain (29% in pediatric patients), arthralgia, arthritis, bone abnormalities, bone mineral density decreased, calcification of tendons and ligaments, CPK increased, myalgia, premature epiphyseal closure, skeletal hyperostosis, tendonitis, weakness

Ocular: Conjunctivitis (4%), blepharitis (1%), chalazion (1%), hordeolum (1%), cataracts, color vision disorder, corneal opacities, eyelid inflammation, keratitis, night vision decreased, optic neuritis, photophobia, visual disturbances

Otic: Hearing impairment, tinnitus

Renal: Glomerulonephritis, hematuria, proteinuria, pyuria, vasculitis

Respiratory: Bronchospasms, epistaxis, respiratory infection, voice alteration, Wegener's granulomatosis

Miscellaneous: Allergic reactions, anaphylactic reactions, disseminated herpes simplex, diaphoresis, infection, lymphadenopathy

<1%, postmarketing, and/or case reports: Abnormal meibomian gland secretion, contact lens intolerance, dry eyes, erythema multiforme, eye pain, meibomian gland atrophy, myopia, ocular sicca, pseudotumor cerebri, Stevens-Johnson syndrome, tear osmolarity increased, toxic epidermal necrolysis, visual acuity decreased

Drug Interactions

Metabolism/Transport Effects None known.

Avoid Concomitant Use

Avoid concomitant use of ISOtretinoin with any of the following: Multivitamins/Minerals (with ADEK, Folate, Iron); Tetracycline Derivatives; Vitamin A

Increased Effect/Toxicity

ISOtretinoin may increase the levels/effects of: Porfimer; Vitamin A

The levels/effects of ISOtretinoin may be increased by: Alcohol (Ethyl); Multivitamins/Minerals (with ADEK, Folate, Iron); Tetracycline Derivatives

Decreased Effect

ISOtretinoin may decrease the levels/effects of: Contraceptives (Estrogens); Contraceptives (Progestins)

Ethanol/Nutrition/Herb Interactions

Ethanol: Avoid or limit ethanol (may increase triglyceride levels if taken in excess).

Food: Isotretinoin bioavailability increased if taken with food or milk.

Herb/Nutraceutical: Avoid dong quai, St John's wort (may also cause photosensitization and may decrease the effectiveness of oral contraceptives). Additional vitamin A supplements may lead to vitamin A toxicity (dry skin, irritation, arthralgias, myalgias, abdominal pain, hepatic changes); avoid use.

Storage/Stability Store at room temperature of 59°F to 86°F (15°C to 30°C). Protect from light.

Mechanism of Action Reduces sebaceous gland size and reduces sebum production in acne treatment; in neuroblastoma, decreases cell proliferation and induces differentiation

Pharmacodynamics/Kinetics

Absorption: Enhanced with a high-fat meal; Absorica™ absorption is ~83% greater than Accutane® when administered under fasting conditions; they are bioequivalent when taken with a high-fat meal.

Protein binding: 99% to 100%; primarily albumin

Metabolism: Hepatic via CYP2B6, 2C8, 2C9, 2D6, 3A4; forms metabolites; major metabolite: 4-oxo-isotretinoin (active)

Half-life elimination: Terminal: Parent drug: 21 hours; Metabolite: 21-24 hours

Time to peak, serum: 3-5 hours

Excretion: Urine and feces (equal amounts)

Dosing

Adult & Geriatric

Acne, severe recalcitrant nodular: Oral: 0.5-1 mg/kg/day in 2 divided doses for 15-20 weeks; may discontinue earlier if the total cyst count decreases by 70%. Adults with very severe disease/scarring or primarily involves the trunk may require dosage adjustment up to 2 mg/kg/day. A second course of therapy may be initiated after a period of ≥2 months off therapy. A dose of ≤0.5 mg/kg/day may be used to minimize initial flaring (Strauss, 2007).

Acne, moderate (unlabeled use): Oral: 20 mg/day (~0.3-0.4 mg/kg/day) for 6 months (Amichai, 2006)

Pediatric

Acne, severe recalcitrant nodular: Children 12-17 years: Oral: 0.5-1 mg/kg/day in 2 divided doses for 15-20 weeks; may discontinue earlier if the total cyst count decreases by 70%. A second course of therapy may be initiated after a period of ≥2 months off therapy. A dose of ≤0.5 mg/kg/day may be used to minimize initial flaring (Strauss, 2007).

Acne, moderate (unlabeled use): Children 12-17 years: Oral: 20 mg/day (~0.3-0.4 mg/kg/day) for 6 months (Amichai, 2006)

Neuroblastoma, high-risk (unlabeled use): Children 1-17 years: Oral: 160 mg/m^2/day (in 2 divided doses) days 1 through 14 every 28 days for 6 cycles, beginning after continuation chemotherapy or transplantation (Matthay, 1999)

Renal Impairment No dosage adjustment provided in the manufacturer's labeling.

Hepatic Impairment

Hepatic impairment prior to treatment: No dosage adjustment provided in the manufacturer's labeling.

Hepatotoxicity during treatment: Liver enzymes may normalize with dosage reduction or with continued treatment; discontinue if normalization does not readily occur or if hepatitis is suspected.

Administration Administer orally with a meal (except Absorica™ which may be taken without regard to meals). According to the manufacturers' labeling, capsules should be swallowed whole with a full glass of liquid. For patients unable to swallow capsule whole, an oral liquid may be prepared; may irritate esophagus if contents are removed from the capsule.

Extemporaneous Preparations Hazardous agent: Use appropriate precautions for handling and disposal of teratogenic capsule contents.

For patients unable to swallow the capsules whole, an oral liquid may be prepared with softgel capsules (not recommended by the manufacturers) by one of the following methods:

Place capsules (softgel formulations only) in small container and add warm (~37°C [97°F]) water or milk to cover capsule(s); wait 2-3 minutes until capsule is softened and then drink the milk or water with the softened capsule, or swallow softened capsule.

Puncture capsule (softgel formulations only) with needle or cut with scissors; squeeze capsule contents into 5-10 mL of milk or tube feed formula; draw mixture up into oral syringe and administer via feeding tube; flush feeding tube with ≥30 mL additional milk or tube feeding formula.

Puncture capsule (softgel formulations only) with needle or cut with scissors and draw contents into oral syringe; add 1-5 mL of medium chain triglyceride, soybean, or safflower oil to the oral syringe; mix gently and administer via feeding tube; flush feeding tube with ≥30 mL milk or tube feeding formula.

Lam MS, "Extemporaneous Compounding of Oral Liquid Dosage Formulations and Alternative Drug Delivery Methods for Anticancer Drugs," *Pharmacotherapy*, 2011, 31(2):164-92.

Monitoring Parameters CBC with differential and platelet count, baseline sedimentation rate, glucose, CPK; signs of depression, mood alteration, psychosis, aggression, severe skin reactions

Pregnancy test (for all female patients of childbearing potential): Two negative tests with a sensitivity of at least 25 mIU/mL prior to beginning therapy (the second performed at least 19 days after the first test and performed during the first 5 days of the menstrual period immediately preceding the start of therapy); monthly tests to rule out pregnancy prior to refilling prescription.

Lipids: Prior to treatment and at weekly or biweekly intervals until response to treatment is established. Test should not be performed <36 hours after consumption of ethanol.

Liver function tests: Prior to treatment and at weekly or biweekly intervals until response to treatment is established.

Dietary Considerations Should be taken with food, except Absorbica™ which may be taken without regard to meals. Limit intake of vitamin A; avoid use of other vitamin A products. Some formulations may contain soybean oil.

Additional Information All patients (male and female), must be registered in the iPLEDGE™ risk management program. Females of childbearing potential must receive oral and written information reviewing the hazards of therapy and the effects that isotretinoin can have on a fetus. Therapy should not begin without two negative pregnancy tests at least 19 days apart. Two forms of contraception (a primary and secondary form as described in the iPLEDGE™ program materials) must be used simultaneously beginning 1 month prior to treatment, during treatment, and for 1 month after therapy is discontinued; limitations to their use must be explained. Micro-dosed progesterone products that do not contain an estrogen ("mini-pills") are not an acceptable form of contraception during isotretinoin treatment. Prescriptions should be written for no more than a 30-day supply, and pregnancy testing and counseling should be repeated monthly. During therapy, pregnancy tests must be conducted by a CLIA-certified laboratory. Prescriptions must be filled and picked up from the pharmacy within 7 days of specimen collection for pregnancy test for women of childbearing potential. Prescriptions for males and females of nonchildbearing potential must be filled and picked up within 30 days of prescribing.

Any cases of accidental pregnancy should be reported to the iPLEDGE™ program or FDA MedWatch. All patients (male and female) must read and sign the informed consent material provided in the pregnancy prevention program.

Product Availability

Absorica™: FDA approved May 2012; availability expected in the fourth quarter of 2012. Consult prescribing information for additional information.

Prescribing and Access Restrictions As a requirement of the REMS program, access to this medication is restricted. All patients (male and female), prescribers, wholesalers, and dispensing pharmacists must register and be active in the iPLEDGE™ risk management program, designed to eliminate fetal exposures to isotretinoin. This program covers all isotretinoin products (brand and generic). The iPLEDGE™ program requires that all patients meet qualification criteria and monthly program requirements (eg, pregnancy testing). Healthcare providers can only prescribe a maximum 30-day supply at each monthly visit and must counsel patients on the iPLEDGE™ program requirements and confirm counseling via the iPLEDGE™ automated system. Registration, activation, and additional information are provided at www.-ipledgeprogram.com or by calling 866-495-0654.

Medication Guide Available Yes

Dosage Forms Excipient information presented when available (limited, particularly for generics); consult specific product labeling.

Capsule, oral:

- Claravis™: 10 mg, 20 mg, 30 mg, 40 mg [contains soybean oil]
- Myorisan™: 10 mg, 20 mg, 40 mg [contains soybean oil]

Capsule, softgel, oral:

- Amnesteem®: 10 mg, 20 mg, 40 mg [contains soybean oil]
- Sotret®: 10 mg, 20 mg, 30 mg, 40 mg [contains parabens, soybean oil]

References

American Academy of Pediatrics Committee on Drugs, "Retinoid Therapy for Severe Dermatological Disorders," *Pediatrics*, 1992, 90(1 Pt 1):119-20.

Amichai B, Shemer A, and Grunwald MH, "Low-Dose Isotretinoin in the Treatment of Acne Vulgaris," *J Am Acad Dermatol*, 2006, 54(4):644-6.

Castleberry RP, Emanuel PD, Zuckerman KS, et al, "A Pilot Study of Isotretinoin in the Treatment of Juvenile Chronic Myelogenous Leukemia," *N Engl J Med*, 1994, 331(25):1680-4.

Hendrix CW, Jackson KA, Whitmore E, et al, "The Effect of Isotretinoin on the Pharmacokinetics and Pharmacodynamics of Ethinyl Estradiol and Norethindrone," *Clin Pharmacol Ther*, 2004, 75 (5):464-75.

Lotan R, Xu XC, Lippman SM, et al, "Suppression of Retinoic Acid Receptor-Beta in Premalignant Oral Lesions and Its Up-Regulation by Isotretinoin," *N Engl J Med*, 1995, 332(21):1405-10.

Matthay KK, Villablanca JG, Seeger RC, et al, "Treatment of High-Risk Neuroblastoma With Intensive Chemotherapy, Radiotherapy, Autologous Bone Marrow Transplantation, and 13-*cis*-Retinoic Acid. Children's Cancer Group," *N Engl J Med*, 1999, 341(16):1165-73.

Mitchell AA, Van Bennekom CM, Louik C, et al, "A Pregnancy-Prevention Program in Women of Childbearing Age Receiving Isotretinoin," *N Engl J Med*, 1995, 333(2):101-6.

Neudorfer M, Goldshtein I, Shamai-Lubovitz O, et al, "Ocular Adverse Effects of Systemic Treatment With Isotretinoin," *Arch Dermatol*, 2012.

Strauss JS, Krowchuk DP, Leyden JJ, et al, "Guidelines of Care for Acne Vulgaris Management," *J Am Acad Dermatol*, 2007, 56(4):651-63.

Yu AL, Gilman AL, Ozkaynak MF, et al, "Anti-GD2 Antibody With GM-CSF, Interleukin-2, and Isotretinoin for Neuroblastoma," *N Engl J Med*, 2010, 363(14):1324-34.

Zhang C and Duvic M, "Treatment of Cutaneous T-Cell Lymphoma With Retinoids," *Dermatol Ther*, 2006, 19(5):264-71.

◆ **Isotretinoinum** *see* ISOtretinoin *on page 832*

◆ **Istodax®** *see* RomiDEPsin *on page 1254*

Itraconazole (i tra KOE na zole)

Brand Names: U.S. Sporanox®

Brand Names: Canada Sporanox®

Generic Availability (U.S.) Yes: Capsule

Pharmacologic Category Antifungal Agent, Oral

Use

Oral capsules: Treatment of susceptible fungal infections in immunocompromised and immunocompetent patients including blastomycosis and histoplasmosis; indicated for aspergillosis (in patients intolerant/refractory to amphotericin B), and onychomycosis of the toenail and fingernail (in non-immunocompromised patients)

Oral solution: Treatment of oral and esophageal candidiasis

Labeled Contraindications Hypersensitivity to itraconazole (use caution in patients with a history of hypersensitivity to other azoles), any component of the formulation; concurrent administration with cisapride, dofetilide, ergot derivatives, felodipine, levomethadyl, lovastatin, methadone, midazolam (oral), nisoldipine, pimozide, quinidine, simvastatin, or triazolam; treatment of onychomycosis (or other non-life-threatening indications) in patients with evidence of ventricular dysfunction, heart failure (HF) or a history of HF; treatment of onychomycosis in patients who are pregnant or intend on becoming pregnant

Pregnancy Risk Factor C

Lactation Enters breast milk/not recommended

Warnings/Precautions [U.S. Boxed Warning]: Negative inotropic effects have been observed following intravenous administration. Discontinue or reassess use if signs or symptoms of HF (heart failure) occur during treatment. [U.S. Boxed Warning]: Use is contraindicated for treatment of onychomycosis in patients with ventricular dysfunction or a history of HF. HF has been reported, particularly in patients receiving a total daily oral dose of 400 mg. Use with caution in patients with risk factors for HF (COPD, renal failure, edematous disorders, ischemic or valvular disease). Discontinue if signs or symptoms of HF or neuropathy occur during treatment. Due to potential toxicity, the manufacturer recommends confirmation of diagnosis testing of nail specimens prior to treatment of onychomycosis.

[U.S. Boxed Warning]: Serious cardiovascular adverse events including, QT prolongation, ventricular tachycardia, torsade de pointes, cardiac arrest and/or sudden death have been observed due to itraconazole-induced increased serum concentrations of the following: cisapride, dofetilide, ergot alkaloids (dihydroergotamine, ergonovine, ergotamine, methylergonovine), felodipine, levomethadyl, lovastatin, methadone, midazolam (oral), nisoldipine, pimozide, simvastatin, quinidine, or triazolam; concurrent use contraindicated.

Calcium channel blockers (CCBs) may cause additive negative inotropic effects when used concurrently with itraconazole. Itraconazole may also inhibit the metabolism of CCBs. Use caution with concurrent use of itraconazole and CCBs due to an increased risk of HF. Concurrent use of itraconazole and nisoldipine is contraindicated.

Use with caution in patients with renal impairment. Rare cases of serious hepatotoxicity (including liver failure and death) have been reported (including some cases occurring within the first week of therapy); hepatotoxicity was reported in some patients without pre-existing liver disease or risk factors. Use with caution in patients with pre-existing hepatic impairment; monitor liver function closely and dosage adjustment may be warranted. Not recommended for use in patients with active liver disease, elevated liver enzymes, or prior hepatotoxic reactions to other drugs unless the expected benefit exceeds the risk of hepatotoxicity. Transient or permanent hearing loss has been reported. Quinidine (a contraindicated drug) was used concurrently in several of these cases. Hearing loss usually resolves after discontinuation, but may persist in some patients.

Large differences in itraconazole pharmacokinetic parameters have been observed in cystic fibrosis patients receiving the solution; if a patient with cystic fibrosis does not respond to therapy, alternate therapies should be considered. Due to differences in bioavailability, oral capsules and oral solution cannot be used interchangeably. Only the oral solution has proven efficacy for oral and esophageal candidiasis. Initiation of treatment with oral solution is not recommended in patients at immediate risk for systemic candidiasis (eg, patients with severe neutropenia).

Ethanol/Nutrition/Herb Interactions

Food:

Capsules: Absorption enhanced by food and possibly by gastric acidity. Cola drinks have been shown to increase the absorption of the capsules in patients with achlorhydria or those taking H_2-receptor antagonists or other gastric acid suppressors. Grapefruit/grapefruit juice may increase serum levels. Management: Take capsules immediately after meals. Avoid grapefruit juice.

Solution: Food decreases the bioavailability and increases the time to peak concentration. Management: Take solution on an empty stomach 1 hour before or 2 hours after meals.

Herb/Nutraceutical: St John's wort may decrease itraconazole levels.

Storage/Stability

Capsule: Store at room temperature, 15°C to 25°C (59°F to 77°F). Protect from light and moisture.

Oral solution: Store at ≤25°C (77°F); do not freeze.

Mechanism of Action Interferes with cytochrome P450 activity, decreasing ergosterol synthesis (principal sterol in fungal cell membrane) and inhibiting cell membrane formation

Pharmacodynamics/Kinetics

Absorption: Requires gastric acidity; capsule better absorbed with food, solution better absorbed on empty stomach

Distribution: V_d (average): 796 ± 185 L or 10 L/kg; highly lipophilic and tissue concentrations are higher than plasma concentrations. The highest concentrations: adipose, omentum, endometrium, cervical and vaginal mucus, and skin/nails. Aqueous fluids (eg, CSF and urine) contain negligible amounts.

Protein binding, plasma: 99.8%; metabolite hydroxy-itraconazole: 99.5%

Metabolism: Extensively hepatic via CYP3A4 into >30 metabolites including hydroxy-itraconazole (major metabolite); appears to have *in vitro* antifungal activity. Main metabolic pathway is oxidation; may undergo saturation metabolism with multiple dosing.

Bioavailability: Variable, ~55% (oral solution) in 1 small study; **Note:** Oral solution has a higher degree of bioavailability (149% ± 68%) relative to oral capsules; should not be interchanged

Half-life elimination: Oral: Single dose: ~21 hours, steady state: 64 hours; Cirrhosis (single dose): 37 hours (range: 20-54 hours)

Time to peak, plasma: Capsules: 3-5 hours; Oral solution: 2-3 hours

Excretion: Urine (<0.03% active drug, 40% as inactive metabolites); feces (~3% to 18%)

Dosing

Adult & Geriatric

Usual dosage ranges: Adults: 100-400 mg/day; doses >200 mg/day are given in 2 divided doses; length of therapy varies from 1 day to >6 months depending on the condition and mycological response

Aspergillosis, invasive (salvage therapy): Duration of therapy should be a minimum of 6-12 weeks or throughout period of immunosuppression: Oral: 200-400 mg/day; **Note:** 2008 IDSA guidelines recommend 600 mg/day for 3 days, followed by 400 mg/day (Walsh, 2008).

Appropriate use: Itraconazole should **NOT** be used for voriconazole-refractory aspergillosis since the same antifungal and/or resistance mechanism(s) may be shared by both agents. Itraconazole oral solution and capsule formulations are not bioequivalent or interchangeable. Due to variable bioavailability of oral preparations, therapeutic drug monitoring is advisable (Walsh, 2008).

Aspergillosis, allergic (ABPA, sinusitis): Oral: 200 mg/day; may be used in conjunction with corticosteroids (Walsh, 2008)

Blastomycosis: Oral: 200 mg 3 times/day for 3 days, then 200 mg twice daily for 6-12 months; in moderately-severe to severe infection, therapy should be initiated with ~2 weeks of amphotericin B (Chapman, 2008)

Candidiasis: Oral:

Oropharyngeal: Oral solution: 200 mg once daily for 1-2 weeks; in patients unresponsive or refractory to fluconazole: 100 mg twice daily (clinical response expected in 2-4 weeks)

Esophageal: Oral solution: 100-200 mg once daily for a minimum of 3 weeks; continue dosing for 2 weeks after resolution of symptoms

Coccidioidomycosis (nonprogressive, nondisseminated disease): 200 mg twice daily or 3 times/day (Galgiani, 2005)

Histoplasmosis: Oral: 200 mg 3 times/day for 3 days, then 200 mg twice daily (or once daily in mild-moderate disease) for 6-12 weeks in mild-moderate disease or ≥12 months in progressive disseminated or chronic cavitary pulmonary histoplasmosis; in moderately-severe to severe infection, therapy should be initiated with ~2 weeks of a lipid formation of amphotericin B (Wheat, 2007)

Long-term suppression therapy: 200 mg/day (CDC, 2009b)

Meningitis: Oral:

Coccidioides: 400-600 mg/day (Galgiani, 2005)

Coccidioides, HIV-positive (unlabeled use): 200 mg 3 times/day for 3 days, then 200 mg twice daily; maintenance: 200 mg twice daily life-long (CDC, 2009b)

Appropriate use: Fluconazole is preferred for meningeal infections (CDC, 2009b; Galgiani, 2005).

Onychomycosis: Oral: 200 mg once daily for 12 consecutive weeks; alternative "pulse-dosing" may be considering for fingernail involvement only: 200 mg twice daily for 1 week; repeat 1-week course after 3-week off-time

Penicilliosis, HIV-positive (unlabeled use): Oral: 400 mg daily for 8 weeks (mild disease) or 10 weeks (severe infections). In severely ill patients, initiate therapy with 2 weeks of amphotericin B. Maintenance: 200 mg/day (CDC, 2009b)

Pneumonia: Oral:

Coccidioides: Mild to moderate: 200 mg twice daily

Coccidioides, HIV-positive (focal pneumonia): 200 mg 3 times/day for 3 days, then 200 mg twice daily (CDC, 2009b)

Sporotrichosis: Oral:

Lymphocutaneous: 100-200 mg/day for 3-6 months (Kauffman, 2007)

Osteoarticular and pulmonary: 200 mg twice daily for ≥1 years (may use amphotericin B initially for stabilization) (Kauffman, 2007)

Pediatric

Usual dosage ranges: A small number of patients 3-16 years of age have been treated with 100 mg/day for systemic fungal infections with no serious adverse effects reported. A dose of 5 mg/kg once daily was used in a pharmacokinetic study using the oral solution in patients 6 months to 12 years; duration of study was 2 weeks.

Infants and Children (HIV-exposed/-positive, unlabeled use; CDC, 2009a):

Candidiasis:

Oropharyngeal: Oral solution: 2.5 mg/kg/dose twice daily (maximum: 200 mg/day [400 mg/day if fluconazole-refractory]) for 7-14 days

Esophageal: Oral solution: 5 mg/kg/day once daily or divided twice daily for 4-21 days

Coccidioidomycosis:

Treatment: Oral: 5-10 mg/kg/dose twice daily for 3 days, followed by 2-5 mg/kg/dose orally twice daily (maximum: 400 mg/day)

Relapse prevention: Oral: 2-5 mg/kg/dose twice daily (maximum: 400 mg/day)

Cryptococcus: *Relapse prevention:* Oral solution: 5 mg/kg/dose once daily (maximum: 200 mg/day)

Histoplasmosis:

Treatment of mild disseminated disease: Oral solution: 2-5 mg/kg/dose 3 times daily for 3 days (9 doses), followed by twice daily for 12 months (maximum: 200 mg/dose)

Consolidation treatment for moderate-severe to severe disseminated disease, including CNS infection (following appropriate induction therapy): 2-5 mg/kg/dose 3 times daily for 3 days, followed by 2-5 mg/kg/dose (maximum: 200 mg/dose) twice daily for 12 months for non-CNS-disseminated disease or for ≥12 months for CNS infection

Relapse prevention: Oral solution: 5 mg/kg/dose twice daily (maximum: 400 mg/day)

Renal Impairment The FDA-approved labeling states to use with caution in patients with renal impairment; wide variations observed in plasma concentrations versus time profiles in patients with uremia, or receiving hemodialysis or continuous ambulatory peritoneal dialysis. The following guidelines have been used by some clinicians:

Aronoff, 2007:

Cl_{cr} >10 mL/minute: No adjustment recommended.

Cl_{cr} <10 mL/minute: Administer 50% of normal dose.

Poorly dialyzed; no supplemental dose or dosage adjustment necessary, including patients on intermittent hemodialysis, peritoneal dialysis, or continuous renal replacement therapy (eg, CVVHD).

Hepatic Impairment No dosage adjustment provided in manufacturer's labeling; however, use caution and monitor closely for signs/symptoms of toxicity.

Administration Doses >200 mg/day are given in 2 divided doses; do not administer with antacids. Capsule and oral solution formulations are not bioequivalent and thus are not interchangeable. Capsule absorption is best if taken with food, therefore, it is best to administer itraconazole after meals; solution should be taken on an empty stomach. When treating oropharyngeal and esophageal candidiasis, solution should be swished vigorously in mouth (10 mL at a time), then swallowed.

Dosage Forms Excipient information presented when available (limited, particularly for generics); consult specific product labeling.

Capsule, oral: 100 mg

Sporanox®: 100 mg

Solution, oral:

Sporanox®: 10 mg/mL (150 mL) [contains propylene glycol; cherry-caramel flavor]

◆ **IVIG** *see* Immune Globulin *on page* *777*

◆ **IV Immune Globulin** *see* Immune Globulin *on page* *777*

Ixabepilone (ix ab EP i lone)

Related Information

Management of Chemotherapy-Induced Nausea and Vomiting *on page* *1786*

Safe Handling of Hazardous Drugs *on page* *1904*

Brand Names: U.S. Ixempra®

Index Terms Azaepothilone B; BMS-247550; Epothilone B Lactam

Generic Availability (U.S.) No

Pharmacologic Category Antineoplastic Agent, Antimicrotubular; Antineoplastic Agent, Epothilone B Analog

Use Treatment of metastatic or locally-advanced breast cancer (refractory or resistant)

Unlabeled Use Treatment (second-line) of endometrial cancer

Labeled Contraindications History of severe hypersensitivity to polyoxyethylated castor oil or its derivatives (eg, Cremophor® EL); neutrophil count <1500/mm^3 or platelet count <100,000/mm^3; combination therapy with ixabepilone and capecitabine in patients with AST or ALT >2.5 times ULN or bilirubin >1 times ULN

Pregnancy Risk Factor D

Lactation Excretion in breast milk unknown/not recommended

Warnings/Precautions Hazardous agent - use appropriate precautions for handling and disposal. **[U.S. Boxed Warning]: Due to increased risk of toxicity and neutropenia-related mortality, combination therapy with capecitabine is contraindicated in patients with AST or ALT >2.5 times ULN or bilirubin >1 times ULN.** Use (as monotherapy) is not recommended if AST or ALT >10 times ULN or bilirubin >3 times ULN; use caution in patients with AST or ALT >5 times ULN. Toxicities and serious adverse reactions are increased (in mono- and combination therapy) with hepatic dysfunction; dosage reductions are necessary. Diluent contains Cremophor® EL, which is associated with hypersensitivity reactions; use is contraindicated in patients with a history of severe hypersensitivity to Cremophor® EL or its derivatives. Medications for the treatment of reaction should be available for immediate use; reactions may also be managed with a reduction of infusion rate. Premedicate with an H_1- and H_2-antagonist 1 hour prior to infusion; patients who experience hypersensitivity (eg, bronchospasm, dyspnea, flushing, rash) should also be premedicated with a corticosteroid for all subsequent cycles if treatment is continued.

Dose-dependent myelosuppression, particularly neutropenia, may occur with mono- or combination therapy. Neutropenic fever and infection have been reported with use. The risk for neutropenia is increased with hepatic dysfunction, especially when used in combination with capecitabine. Severe neutropenia and/or thrombocytopenia may require dosage adjustment and/or treatment delay. Peripheral (sensory and motor) neuropathy occurs commonly; may require dose reductions, treatment delays or discontinuation. Usually occurs during the first 3 cycles. Use with caution in patients with pre-existing neuropathy. Patients with diabetes may have an increased risk for severe peripheral neuropathy. Use with caution in patients with a history of cardiovascular disease; the incidence of MI, ventricular dysfunction, and supraventricular arrhythmias is higher when ixabepilone is used in combination with capecitabine (as compared to capecitabine alone). Consider discontinuing ixabepilone in patients who develop cardiac ischemia or impaired cardiac function.

Avoid concurrent use with strong CYP3A4 inhibitors (eg, itraconazole, ketoconazole, voriconazole, clarithromycin, telithromycin, nefazodone, amprenavir, atazanavir, delavirdine, indinavir, nelfinavir, ritonavir, saquinavir); dosage reductions are recommended if concurrent use cannot be avoided; allow ~1 week to elapse prior to adjusting ixabepilone dose upward after a strong CYP3A4 inhibitor is discontinued. Avoid strong CYP3A4 inducers (eg, dexamethasone, phenytoin, carbamazepine, rifampin, phenobarbital); may decrease the ixabepilone level, alternative agents should be considered, dosage increases of ixabepilone (with careful monitoring) may be recommended if concomitant administration with CYP3A4 inducers cannot be avoided. Due to the ethanol content in the diluent, may cause cognitive impairment; patients must be cautioned about performing tasks which require mental alertness (eg, operating machinery or driving). Toxicities or serious adverse events with combination therapy may be increased in the elderly.

Adverse Reactions

Percentages reported with monotherapy:

>10%:

Central nervous system: Headache (11%)

Dermatologic: Alopecia (48%)

Gastrointestinal: Nausea (42%), vomiting (29%), mucositis/stomatitis (29%), diarrhea (22%), anorexia (19%), constipation (16%), abdominal pain (13%)
Hematologic: Leukopenia (grade 3: 36%; grade 4: 13%), neutropenia (grade 3: 31%; grade 4: 23%)
Neuromuscular & skeletal: Peripheral neuropathy (63%; grades 3/4: 14%; grade 3/4 median onset: cycle 4), sensory neuropathy (62%; grades 3/4: 14%), weakness (56%), myalgia/arthralgia (49%), musculoskeletal pain (20%)

1% to 10%:
Cardiovascular: Edema (9%), chest pain (5%)
Central nervous system: Fever (8%), pain (8%), dizziness (7%), insomnia (5%)
Dermatologic: Nail disorder (9%), rash (9%), palmar-plantar erythrodysesthesia/hand-and-foot syndrome (8%), pruritus (6%), skin exfoliation (2%), hyperpigmentation (2%)
Endocrine & metabolic: Hot flush (6%), dehydration (2%)
Gastrointestinal: Gastroesophageal reflux disease (6%), taste perversion (6%), weight loss (6%)
Hematologic: Anemia (grade 3: 6%; grade 4: 2%), neutropenic fever (3%; grade 3: 3%), thrombocytopenia (grade 3: 5%; grade 4: 2%)
Neuromuscular & skeletal: Motor neuropathy (10%; grade 3: 1%)
Ocular: Lacrimation increased (4%)
Respiratory: Dyspnea (9%), upper respiratory tract infection (6%), cough (2%)
Miscellaneous: Hypersensitivity (5%; grade 3: 1%), infection (5%)

Mono- and combination therapy: <1%, postmarketing, and/or case reports (limited to important or life-threatening): Alkaline phosphatase increased, angina, atrial flutter, autonomic neuropathy, cardiomyopathy, cerebral hemorrhage, coagulopathy, colitis, dysphagia, dysphonia, embolism, enterocolitis, erythema multiforme, gastrointestinal hemorrhage, gastroparesis, GGT increased, hemorrhage, hepatic failure (acute), hypokalemia, hyponatremia, hypotension, hypovolemia, hypovolemic shock, hypoxia, ileus, interstitial pneumonia, jaundice, left ventricular dysfunction, metabolic acidosis, MI, nephrolithiasis, neutropenic infection, orthostatic hypotension, pneumonia, pneumonitis, pulmonary edema (acute), radiation recall, renal failure, respiratory failure, sepsis, septic shock, supraventricular arrhythmia, syncope, thrombosis, transaminases increased, trismus, urinary tract infection, vasculitis

Drug Interactions

Metabolism/Transport Effects Substrate of CYP3A4 (major); **Note:** Assignment of Major/Minor substrate status based on clinically relevant drug interaction potential

Avoid Concomitant Use

Avoid concomitant use of Ixabepilone with any of the following: CloZAPine; St Johns Wort

Increased Effect/Toxicity

Ixabepilone may increase the levels/effects of: CloZAPine

The levels/effects of Ixabepilone may be increased by: CYP3A4 Inhibitors (Moderate); CYP3A4 Inhibitors (Strong); Dasatinib; Ivacaftor; Mifepristone

Decreased Effect

The levels/effects of Ixabepilone may be decreased by: CYP3A4 Inducers (Strong); Deferasirox; St Johns Wort; Tocilizumab

Ethanol/Nutrition/Herb Interactions

Food: Grapefruit juice may increase plasma concentrations of ixabepilone. Management: Avoid grapefruit juice.

Herb/Nutraceutical: St John's wort may decrease ixabepilone levels. Management: Avoid St John's wort.

Storage/Stability Store intact vials under refrigeration at 2°C to 8°C (36°F to 46°F); protect from light. Reconstituted solution (in the vial) is stable for 1 hour at room temperature; infusion solution diluted in appropriate solution for infusion is stable for 6 hours at room temperature if a pH range of 6-9 is maintained.

Reconstitution Allow to reach room temperature for ~30 minutes prior to reconstitution. Diluent vial may contain a white precipitate which should dissolve upon reaching room temperature. **Reconstitute only with the provided diluent.** Dilute the 15 mg vial with 8 mL and the 45 mg vial with 23.5 mL (using provided diluent) to a concentration of 2 mg/mL (contains overfill). Gently swirl and invert vial until dissolved completely. Prior to administration, further dilute using a non-DEHP container (eg, glass, polypropylene or polyolefin), to a final concentration of 0.2-0.6 mg/mL in ~250 mL lactated Ringer's, adjusted sodium chloride 0.9% (pH adjusted prior to ixabepilone addition with 2 mEq sodium bicarbonate per 250-500 mL sodium chloride) or PLASMA-LYTE A Injection pH 7.4®. Mix thoroughly. Use appropriate precautions for handling and disposal.

Mechanism of Action Epothilone B analog; binds to the beta-tubulin subunit of the microtubule, stabilizing microtubular promoting tubulin polymerization and stabilizing microtubular function, thus arresting the cell cycle (at the G2/M phase) and inducing apoptosis. Activity in taxane-resistant cells has been demonstrated.

Pharmacodynamics/Kinetics

Distribution: >1000 L

Protein binding: 67% to 77%

Metabolism: Extensively hepatic, via CYP3A4; >30 metabolites (inactive) formed

Half-life elimination: ~52 hours

Time to peak, plasma: At the end of infusion (3 hours)

Excretion: Feces (65%; 2% of the total dose as unchanged drug); urine (21%; 6% of the total dose as unchanged drug)

Dosing

Adult & Geriatric Details concerning dosing in combination regimens should also be consulted. **Note:** Premedicate with an H_1-antagonist (eg, oral diphenhydramine 50 mg) and H_2-antagonist (eg, oral ranitidine 150-300 mg) ~1 hour prior to infusion. Patients with a history of hypersensitivity should also be premedicated with corticosteroids (orally 1 hour before or I.V. 30 minutes before infusion). For dose calculation, body surface area (BSA) is capped at a maximum of 2.2 m^2.

Breast cancer (metastatic or locally advanced): I.V.: 40 mg/m^2/dose over 3 hours every 3 weeks (maximum dose: 88 mg) either as monotherapy or in combination with capecitabine

Endometrial cancer (unlabeled use): 40 mg/m^2/dose over 3 hours every 3 weeks (Dizon, 2009)

Dosage adjustment with concomitant strong CYP3A4 inhibitors/inducers:

CYP3A4 inhibitors: Avoid concomitant administration with strong CYP3A4 inhibitors; if concomitant administration with a strong CYP3A4 inhibitor cannot be avoided, consider a dose reduction to 20 mg/m^2. When a strong CYP3A4 inhibitor is discontinued, allow ~1 week to elapse prior to adjusting ixabepilone dose upward to the indicated dose.

CYP3A4 inducers: Avoid concomitant administration with strong CYP3A4 inducers; if concomitant administration with a strong CYP3A4 inducer cannot be avoided and after maintenance on the strong CYP3A4 inducer is established, consider adjusting the ixabepilone dose gradually up to 60 mg/m^2 (as a 4-hour infusion), with careful monitoring. If the strong CYP3A4 enzyme inducer is discontinued, reduce ixabepilone dose to the dose used prior to initiation of the CYP3A4 inducer.

Renal Impairment Pharmacokinetics (monotherapy) are not affected in patients with mild-to-moderate renal insufficiency (Cl_{cr} >30 mL/minute); monotherapy has not been studied in patients with serum creatinine >1.5 times ULN. Combination therapy with capecitabine has not been studied in patients with Cl_{cr} <50 mL/minute.

Hepatic Impairment

Ixabepilone monotherapy (initial cycle; adjust doses for subsequent cycles based on toxicity):

AST and ALT ≤2.5 times ULN and bilirubin ≤1 times ULN: No adjustment necessary

AST and ALT >2.5 to ≤10 times ULN and bilirubin >1 to ≤1.5 times ULN: Reduce dose to 32 mg/m^2

AST and ALT ≤10 times ULN and bilirubin >1.5 to ≤3 times ULN: Reduce dose to 20-30 mg/m^2 (initiate treatment at 20 mg/m^2, may escalate up to a maximum of 30 mg/m^2 in subsequent cycles if tolerated)

AST or ALT >10 times ULN or bilirubin >3 times ULN: Use is not recommended

Combination therapy of ixabepilone with capecitabine:

AST and ALT ≤2.5 times ULN and bilirubin ≤1 times ULN: No adjustment necessary

AST or ALT >2.5 times ULN or bilirubin >1 times ULN: Use is contraindicated

Adjustment for Toxicity

Hematologic:

Neutrophils <500/mm^3 for ≥7 days: Reduce dose by 20%

Neutropenic fever: Reduce dose by 20%

Platelets <25,000/mm^3 (or <50,000/mm^3 with bleeding): Reduce dose by 20%

Nonhematologic:

Neuropathy:

- Grade 2 (moderate) for ≥7 days: Reduce dose by 20%
- Grade 3 (severe) for <7 days: Reduce dose by 20%
- Grade 3 (severe or disabling) for ≥7 days: Discontinue treatment

Grade 3 toxicity (severe; other than neuropathy): Reduce dose by 20%

Grade 3 arthralgia/myalgia or fatigue (transient): Continue at current dose

Grade 3 hand-foot syndrome: Continue at current dose

Grade 4 toxicity (disabling): Discontinue treatment

Note: Adjust dosage at the start of a cycle are based on toxicities (hematologic and nonhematologic) from the previous cycle; delay new cycles until neutrophils have recovered to ≥1500/mm^3, platelets have recovered to ≥100,000/mm^3 and nonhematologic toxicities have resolved or improved to at least grade 1. If toxicities persist despite initial dose reduction, reduce dose an additional 20%.

Capecitabine dosage adjustments for combination therapy with ixabepilone:

Hematologic:

Neutrophils <500/mm^3 for ≥7 days or neutropenic fever: Hold for concurrent diarrhea or stomatitis until neutrophils recover to >1000/mm^3, then continue at same dose

Platelets <25,000/mm^3 (or <50,000/mm^3 with bleeding): Hold for concurrent diarrhea or stomatitis until platelets recover to >50,000/mm^3, then continue at same dose

Nonhematologic: Refer to Capecitabine monograph.

Combination Regimens

Breast cancer: Ixabepilone-Capecitabine on page 1698

Administration I.V.: Infuse over 3 hours. Use non-DEHP administration set (eg, polyethylene); filter with a 0.2-1.2 micron inline filter. Administration should be completed within 6 hours of preparation. If the dose is increased (above 40 mg/m^2) due to concomitant CYP3A4 inducer use, infuse over 4 hours.

Emetic Potential Low (10% to 30%)

Monitoring Parameters CBC with differential; hepatic function (ALT, AST, bilirubin); monitor for hypersensitivity, neuropathy

Dietary Considerations Avoid grapefruit juice (may increase plasma concentrations of ixabepilone).

Dosage Forms Excipient information presented when available (limited, particularly for generics); consult specific product labeling.

Injection, powder for reconstitution:

Ixempra®: 15 mg, 45 mg [contains dehydrated ethanol (in diluent), polyoxyethylated castor oil (in diluent)]

References

Denduluri N, Low JA, Lee JJ, et al, "Phase II Trial of Ixabepilone, an Epothilone B Analog, in Patients With Metastatic Breast Cancer Previously Untreated With Taxanes," *J Clin Oncol*, 2007, 25(23):3421-7.

Dizon DS, Blessing JA, McMeekin DS, et al, "Phase II Trial of Ixabepilone As Second-Line Treatment in Advanced Endometrial Cancer: Gynecologic Oncology Group Trial 129-P," *J Clin Oncol*, 2009, 27(19):3104-8.

Low JA, Wedam SB, Lee JJ, et al, "Phase II Clinical Trial of Ixabepilone (BMS-247550), an Epothilone B Analog, in Metastatic and Locally Advanced Breast Cancer," *J Clin Oncol*, 2005, 23 (12):2726-34.

Perez EA, Lerzo G, Pivot X, et al, "Efficacy and Safety of Ixabepilone (BMS-247550), in a Phase II Study of Patients With Advanced Breast Cancer Resistant to an Anthracycline, a Taxane and Capecitabine," *J Clin Oncol*, 2007, 25(23):3407-14.

Pivot XB, Li RK, Thomas ES, et al, "Activity of Ixabepilone in Oestrogen Receptor-Negative and Oestrogen-Receptor-Progesterone Receptor-Human Epidermal Growth Factor 2-Negative Metastatic Breast Cancer," *Eur J Cancer*, 2009, 45(17):2940-6.

Roché H, Yelle L, Cognetti F, et al, "Phase II Clinical Trial of Ixabepilone (BMS-247550), an Epothilone B Analog, as First-Line Therapy in Patients With Metastatic Breast Cancer Previously Treated With Anthracycline Chemotherapy," *J Clin Oncol*, 2007, 25(23):3415-20.

Sparano JA, Vrdoljak E, Rixe O, et al, "Randomized Phase III Trial of Ixabepilone Plus Capecitabine Versus Capecitabine in Patients With Metastatic Breast Cancer Previously Treated With an Anthracycline and a Taxane," *J Clin Oncol*, 2010, 28(20):3256-63.

Takimoto CH, Liu PY, Lenz H, et al, "A Phase I Pharmacokinetic (PK) Study of the Epothilone B Analogue, Ixabepilone (BMS-247550) in Patients (pts) With Advanced Malignancies and Varying Degrees of Hepatic Impairment: A SWOG Early Therapeutics Committee and NCI Organ Dysfunction Working Group Trial," *J Clin Oncol*, 2006, 24(18S):2004 [abstract 2004 from 2006 ASCO Annual Meeting].

Thomas ES, Gomez HL, Li RK, et al, "Ixabepilone Plus Capecitabine for Metastatic Breast Cancer Progressing After Anthracycline and Taxane Treatment," *J Clin Oncol*, 2007, 25(33):5210-7.

Thomas E, Tabernero J, Fornier M, et al, "Phase II Clinical Trial of Ixabepilone (BMS-247550), an Epothilone B Analog, in Patients With Taxane-Resistant Metastatic Breast Cancer," *J Clin Oncol*, 2007, 25(23):3399-406.

- **Ixempra®** *see* Ixabepilone *on page 842*
- **Jakafi™** *see* Ruxolitinib *on page 1261*
- **Jakavi™ (Can)** *see* Ruxolitinib *on page 1261*
- **JAMP-Anastrozole (Can)** *see* Anastrozole *on page 96*
- **JAMP-Bicalutamide (Can)** *see* Bicalutamide *on page 178*
- **JAMP-Ciprofloxacin (Can)** *see* Ciprofloxacin (Systemic) *on page 283*
- **JAMP-Letrozole (Can)** *see* Letrozole *on page 867*
- **JAMP-Mycophenolate (Can)** *see* Mycophenolate *on page 1015*
- **JAMP-Ondansetron (Can)** *see* Ondansetron *on page 1068*
- **Jevtana®** *see* Cabazitaxel *on page 210*
- **Jurnista™ (Can)** *see* HYDROmorphone *on page 724*
- **Kadian®** *see* Morphine (Systemic) *on page 1004*
- **Kaote DVI** *see* Antihemophilic Factor (Human) *on page 101*
- **Keoxifene Hydrochloride** *see* Raloxifene *on page 1222*
- **Kepivance®** *see* Palifermin *on page 1104*
- **Keratinocyte Growth Factor, Recombinant Human** *see* Palifermin *on page 1104*

Ketoconazole (Systemic) (kee toe KOE na zole)

Brand Names: Canada Apo-Ketoconazole®; Novo-Ketoconazole

Generic Availability (U.S.) Yes

Pharmacologic Category Antifungal Agent, Oral

Use Treatment of susceptible fungal infections, including candidiasis, oral thrush, blastomycosis, histoplasmosis, paracoccidioidomycosis, coccidioidomycosis, chromomycosis, candiduria, chronic mucocutaneous candidiasis, as well as certain recalcitrant cutaneous dermatophytoses

Unlabeled Use Treatment of prostate cancer (androgen synthesis inhibitor)

Labeled Contraindications Hypersensitivity to ketoconazole or any component of the formulation; CNS fungal infections (due to poor CNS penetration); coadministration with ergot derivatives, cisapride, or triazolam is contraindicated due to risk of potentially fatal cardiac arrhythmias

Pregnancy Risk Factor C

Lactation Enters breast milk/not recommended

Warnings/Precautions **[U.S. Boxed Warning]: Ketoconazole has been associated with hepatotoxicity, including some fatalities;** use with caution in patients with impaired hepatic function and perform periodic liver function tests. **[U.S. Boxed Warning]: Concomitant use with cisapride is contraindicated due to the occurrence of ventricular arrhythmias.** High doses of ketoconazole may depress adrenocortical function.

Adverse Reactions

1% to 10%:

Dermatologic: Pruritus (2%)

Gastrointestinal: Nausea/vomiting (3% to 10%), abdominal pain (1%)

<1%: Bulging fontanelles, chills, depression, diarrhea, dizziness, fever, gynecomastia, headache, hemolytic anemia, hepatotoxicity, impotence, leukopenia, photophobia, somnolence, thrombocytopenia

Drug Interactions

Metabolism/Transport Effects **Substrate** of CYP3A4 (major); **Note:** Assignment of Major/Minor substrate status based on clinically relevant drug interaction potential; **Inhibits** CYP1A2 (strong), CYP2A6 (moderate), CYP2B6 (weak), CYP2C19 (moderate), CYP2C8 (weak), CYP2C9 (strong), CYP2D6 (moderate), CYP3A4 (strong), P-glycoprotein

Avoid Concomitant Use

Avoid concomitant use of Ketoconazole (Systemic) with any of the following: Alfuzosin; Apixaban; Avanafil; Axitinib; Bosutinib; Cisapride; Clopidogrel; Conivaptan; Crizotinib; Dihydroergotamine; Dofetilide; Domperidone; Dronedarone; Eplerenone; Ergoloid Mesylates; Ergonovine; Ergotamine; Everolimus; Fluticasone (Oral Inhalation); Halofantrine; Lapatinib; Lovastatin; Lurasidone; Methylergonovine; Nevirapine; Nilotinib; Nisoldipine; Pimozide; QuiNIDine; Ranolazine; Red Yeast Rice; Regorafenib; Rivaroxaban; RomiDEPsin; Salmeterol; Silodosin; Simvastatin; Tamsulosin; Thioridazine; Ticagrelor; Tipranavir; Tolvaptan; Topotecan; Toremifene; VinCRIStine (Liposomal)

Increased Effect/Toxicity

Ketoconazole (Systemic) may increase the levels/effects of: Alfentanil; Alfuzosin; Aliskiren; Almotriptan; Alosetron; Apixaban; Aprepitant; ARIPiprazole; AtorvaSTATin; Avanafil; Axitinib; Bendamustine; Benzodiazepines (metabolized by oxidation); Boceprevir; Bortezomib; Bosentan; Bosutinib; Brentuximab Vedotin; Brinzolamide; Budesonide (Nasal); Budesonide (Systemic, Oral Inhalation); BusPIRone; Busulfan; Calcium Channel Blockers; CarBAMazepine; Carvedilol; Cilostazol; Cinacalcet; Cisapride; Citalopram; Cobicistat; Colchicine; Conivaptan; Corticosteroids (Orally Inhaled); Corticosteroids (Systemic); Crizotinib; CycloSPORINE (Systemic); CYP1A2 Substrates; CYP2A6 Substrates; CYP2C19 Substrates; CYP2C9 Substrates; CYP2D6 Substrates; CYP3A4 Substrates; Dabigatran Etexilate; Darunavir; Diclofenac (Systemic); Dienogest; Dihydroergotamine; DOCEtaxel; Dofetilide; Domperidone; Dronedarone; Dutasteride; Eletriptan; Elvitegravir; Enzalutamide; Eplerenone; Ergoloid Mesylates; Ergonovine; Ergotamine; Erlotinib; Eszopiclone; Etravirine; Everolimus; FentaNYL; Fesoterodine; Fexofenadine; Fingolimod; Fluticasone (Nasal); Fluticasone (Oral Inhalation); Fosamprenavir; Fosaprepitant; Fosphenytoin; Gefitinib; GuanFACINE; Halofantrine; Highest Risk QTc-Prolonging Agents; Iloperidone; Imatinib; Indinavir; Irinotecan; Ivacaftor; Ixabepilone; Lapatinib; Lopinavir; Losartan; Lovastatin; Lumefantrine; Lurasidone; Macrolide Antibiotics; Maraviroc; Methadone; Methylergonovine; MethylPREDNISolone; Mifepristone; Mirabegron; Moderate Risk QTc-Prolonging Agents; Nebivolol; Nilotinib; Nisoldipine; Paricalcitol; Pazopanib; P-glycoprotein/ABCB1 Substrates; Phenytoin; Pimecrolimus; Pimozide; Praziquantel; Propafenone; Proton Pump Inhibitors; Prucalopride; QuiNIDine; Ramelteon; Ranolazine; Red Yeast Rice; Regorafenib; Repaglinide; Rifamycin Derivatives; Rilpivirine; Rivaroxaban; RomiDEPsin; Ruxolitinib; Salmeterol; Saquinavir; Saxagliptin; Sildenafil; Silodosin; Simvastatin; Sirolimus; Solifenacin; SORAfenib; SUNItinib; Tacrolimus (Systemic); Tacrolimus (Topical); Tadalafil; Tamsulosin; Telaprevir; Temsirolimus; Thioridazine; Ticagrelor; Tolterodine; Tolvaptan; Topotecan; Toremifene; Vardenafil; Vemurafenib; Vilazodone; VinCRIStine (Liposomal); Vitamin K Antagonists; Ziprasidone; Zolpidem; Zuclopenthixol

The levels/effects of Ketoconazole (Systemic) may be increased by: AtorvaSTATin; Boceprevir; Cobicistat; Darunavir; Domperidone; Etravirine; Fosamprenavir; Grapefruit Juice; Indinavir; Lopinavir; Macrolide Antibiotics; Ritonavir; Saquinavir; Telaprevir; Tipranavir

Decreased Effect

Ketoconazole (Systemic) may decrease the levels/effects of: Amphotericin B; Clopidogrel; Codeine; Ifosfamide; Prasugrel; Saccharomyces boulardii; Tamoxifen; Ticagrelor; TraMADol

The levels/effects of Ketoconazole (Systemic) may be decreased by: Antacids; CYP3A4 Inducers (Strong); Deferasirox; Didanosine; Etravirine; Fosphenytoin; H2-Antagonists; Herbs (CYP3A4 Inducers); Isoniazid; Nevirapine; Phenytoin; Proton Pump Inhibitors; Rifamycin Derivatives; Rilpivirine; Sucralfate; Tocilizumab

Ethanol/Nutrition/Herb Interactions

Food: Ketoconazole peak serum levels may be prolonged if taken with food.

Herb/Nutraceutical: St John's wort may decrease ketoconazole levels.

Storage/Stability Store at 15°C to 25°C (59°F to 77°F).

Mechanism of Action Alters the permeability of the cell wall by blocking fungal cytochrome P450; inhibits biosynthesis of triglycerides and phospholipids by fungi; inhibits several fungal enzymes that results in a build-up of toxic concentrations of hydrogen peroxide; also inhibits androgen synthesis

Pharmacodynamics/Kinetics

Absorption: Rapid (~75%)

Distribution: Well into inflamed joint fluid, saliva, bile, urine, sebum, cerumen, feces, tendons, skin and soft tissue, and testes; crosses blood-brain barrier poorly; only negligible amounts reach CSF

Protein binding: 93% to 96%

Metabolism: Partially hepatic via CYP3A4 to inactive compounds

Bioavailability: Decreases as gastric pH increases

Half-life elimination: Biphasic: Initial: 2 hours; Terminal: 8 hours

Time to peak, serum: 1-2 hours

Excretion: Feces (57%); urine (13%)

Dosing

Adult & Geriatric

Fungal infections: Oral: 200-400 mg/day as a single daily dose

Prostate cancer (unlabeled use): Oral: 400 mg 3 times/day

Pediatric Fungal infections: Oral: Children ≥2 years: 3.3-6.6 mg/kg/day as a single dose for 1-2 weeks for candidiasis, for at least 4 weeks in recalcitrant dermatophyte infections, and for up to 6 months for other systemic mycoses

Renal Impairment Hemodialysis: Not dialyzable (0% to 5%)

Hepatic Impairment Dose reductions should be considered in patients with severe liver disease.

Combination Regimens

Prostate cancer:

Doxorubicin + Ketoconazole on page 1619

Doxorubicin + Ketoconazole/Estramustine + Vinblastine on page 1619

Administration Administer oral tablets 2 hours prior to antacids to prevent decreased absorption due to the high pH of gastric contents.

Extemporaneous Preparations A 20 mg/mL oral suspension may be made with tablets and one of three different vehicles (a 1:1 mixture of Ora-Sweet® and Ora-Plus®, a 1:1 mixture of Ora-Sweet® SF and Ora-Plus®, or a 1:4 mixture of cherry syrup and Simple Syrup, NF). Crush twelve 200 mg tablets in a mortar and reduce to a fine powder. Add 20 mL of chosen vehicle and mix to a uniform paste; mix while adding the vehicle in incremental proportions to **almost** 120 mL; transfer to a calibrated bottle, rinse mortar with vehicle, and add quantity of vehicle sufficient to make 120 mL. Label "shake well" and "refrigerate". Stable for 60 days.

Nahata MC, Pai VB, and Hipple TF, *Pediatric Drug Formulations*, 5th ed, Cincinnati, OH: Harvey Whitney Books Co, 2004.

Monitoring Parameters Liver function tests

Dietary Considerations May be taken with food or milk to decrease GI adverse effects.

Dosage Forms Excipient information presented when available (limited, particularly for generics); consult specific product labeling.

Tablet, oral: 200 mg

References

Ginsburg AM, McCracken GH Jr, and Olsen K, "Pharmacology of Ketoconazole Suspension in Infants and Children," *Antimicrob Agents Chemother*, 1983, 23(5):787-9.

Herrod HG, "Chronic Mucocutaneous Candidiasis in Childhood and Complications of non-*Candida* Infection: A Report of the Pediatric Immunodeficiency Collaborative Study Group," *J Pediatr*, 1990, 116(3):377-82.

Small EJ, Halabi S, Dawson NA, et al, "Antiandrogen Withdrawal Alone or in Combination With Ketoconazole in Androgen-Independent Prostate Cancer Patients: A Phase III Trial (CALGB 9583)," *J Clin Oncol*, 2004, 22(6):1025-33.

◆ **Khloditan** *see* Mitotane *on page 994*

◆ **Kidrolase® (Can)** *see* Asparaginase (*E. coli*) *on page 130*

◆ **Kogenate® FS** *see* Antihemophilic Factor (Recombinant) *on page 103*

◆ **Konakion (Can)** *see* Phytonadione *on page 1169*

◆ **Korlym™** *see* Mifepristone *on page 983*

◆ **Koāte®-DVI** *see* Antihemophilic Factor (Human) *on page 101*

◆ **Kyprolis™** *see* Carfilzomib *on page 239*

◆ **Kytril** *see* Granisetron *on page 687*

◆ **Kytril® (Can)** *see* Granisetron *on page 687*

◆ **L-758,298** *see* Fosaprepitant *on page 643*

◆ **L 754030** *see* Aprepitant *on page 118*

◆ **Ladakamycin** *see* AzaCITIDine *on page 140*

◆ **L-AmB** *see* Amphotericin B (Liposomal) *on page 87*

Lanreotide (lan REE oh tide)

Brand Names: U.S. Somatuline® Depot

Brand Names: Canada Somatuline® Autogel®

Index Terms Lanreotide Acetate

Pharmacologic Category Somatostatin Analog

Use Long-term treatment of acromegaly in patients who are not candidates for or are unresponsive to surgery and/or radiotherapy

Labeled Contraindications U.S. labeling: There are no contraindications listed in the manufacturer's labeling.

Canadian labeling: Hypersensitivity to lanreotide, somatostatin (or related peptides), or any component of the formulation; complicated, untreated lithiasis of the bile ducts

Pregnancy Risk Factor C

Lactation Excretion into breast milk unknown/not recommended

Warnings/Precautions Inhibition of insulin and glucagon secretion may affect glucose regulation, leading to hyper-/hypoglycemia, especially in patients with diabetes. Monitor serum glucose levels with the initiation of therapy and with dosage changes; dose adjustments in antidiabetic medications may be necessary. May reduce gall bladder motility, leading to cholelithiasis (may be dose- or duration-related); Canadian labeling recommends ultrasonography when initiating therapy and periodically thereafter. Slight decreases in thyroid function have been observed during therapy; may require monitoring of thyroid function tests.

Bradycardia, sinus bradycardia and hypertension have been observed with therapy; use with caution in patients with preexisting cardiac disease. Patients without preexisting cardiac disease may experience a decrease in heart rate though not to the level of bradycardia. Concurrent use with cyclosporine may lead to decreased levels of cyclosporine; monitor cyclosporine levels during therapy. Use with caution in patients with renal and hepatic impairment; lower doses are recommended at therapy initiation in patients with moderate-to-severe impairment. The packaging (needle cover) may contain latex.

Adverse Reactions

>10%:

Cardiovascular: Bradycardia (5% to 18%)

Gastrointestinal: Diarrhea (26% to 65%; dose related), abdominal pain (7% to 19%; dose related), flatulence (≤14%; dose related), nausea (11%), weight loss (5% to 11%)

Hematologic: Anemia (3% to 14%)

Hepatic: Cholelithiasis/gall bladder sludge (2% to 20%)

Local: Injection site reaction (6% to 22%; induration 5%; pain 4%; mass 2%)

1% to 10%:

Cardiovascular: Hypertension (5%), sinus bradycardia (3%)

Central nervous system: Headache (7%)

Endocrine & metabolic: Hyper-/hypoglycemia/diabetes (7%)

Gastrointestinal: Constipation (8%), vomiting (7%), loose stools (6%)

Neuromuscular & skeletal: Arthralgia (7%)

<1%, postmarketing, and/or case reports: Allergic skin reaction, aortic valve regurgitation, dysautonomia, injection site pruritus, mitral valve regurgitation, pancreatitis, steatorrhea

Drug Interactions

Metabolism/Transport Effects None known.

Avoid Concomitant Use There are no known interactions where it is recommended to avoid concomitant use.

Increased Effect/Toxicity

Lanreotide may increase the levels/effects of: Codeine; Hypoglycemic Agents; Pegvisomant

The levels/effects of Lanreotide may be increased by: Herbs (Hypoglycemic Properties); MAO Inhibitors; Salicylates; Selective Serotonin Reuptake Inhibitors

Decreased Effect

Lanreotide may decrease the levels/effects of: CycloSPORINE (Systemic)

The levels/effects of Lanreotide may be decreased by: Loop Diuretics

Ethanol/Nutrition/Herb Interactions Herb/Nutraceutical: Some herbal medications may enhance the hypoglycemic effect of lanreotide. Management: Avoid alfalfa, aloe, bilberry, bitter melon, burdock, celery, damiana, fenugreek, garcinia, garlic, ginger, ginseng, gymnema, marshmallow, and stinging nettle.

Storage/Stability Store under refrigeration 2°C to 8°C (36°F to 46°F). Protect from light. Allow to reach room temperature by removing sealed pouch from refrigerator 30 minutes prior to administration; keep in sealed pouch until just prior to administration.

Mechanism of Action Synthetic octapeptide analogue of somatostatin which is a peptide inhibitor of multiple endocrine, neuroendocrine, and exocrine mechanisms. Displays a greater affinity for somatostatin type 2 (SSTR2) and type 5 (SSTR5) receptors found in pituitary gland, pancreas, and growth hormone (GH) secreting neoplasms of pituitary gland and a lesser affinity for somatostatin receptors 1, 3, and 4. Reduces GH secretion and also reduces the levels of insulin-like growth factor 1.

Pharmacodynamics/Kinetics

Distribution: V_{ss}: ~0.2 L/kg

Protein binding: 79% to 83%

Metabolism: Extensively within GI tract after biliary excretion

Bioavailability: 69% to 83%

Half-life, elimination: 23-36 days

Time to peak, plasma: Mean: 7-12 hours

Excretion: Urine (<1% to 5% as unchanged drug); feces (<0.5% as unchanged drug)

Dosing

Adult & Geriatric Acromegaly: Adults (per U.S. labeling) **or** Children ≥16 years and Adults (per Canadian labeling): SubQ: 90 mg once every 4 weeks for 3 months; after initial 90 days of therapy, adjust dose based on clinical response of patient, growth hormone (GH) levels, and/or insulin-like growth factor 1 (IGF-1) levels as follows:

GH ≤1 ng/mL, IGF-1 normal, symptoms stable: 60 mg once every 4 weeks; once stabilized on 60 mg every 4 weeks, may consider regimen of 120 mg every 6-8 weeks (extended interval dosing)

GH >1-2.5 ng/mL, IGF-1 normal, symptoms stable: 90 mg once every 4 weeks; once stabilized on 90 mg every 4 weeks, may consider regimen of 120 mg every 6-8 weeks (extended-interval dosing)

GH >2.5 ng/mL, IGF-1 elevated and/or uncontrolled symptoms: 120 mg once every 4 weeks

Pediatric

Acromegaly: Children ≥16 years (*Canadian labeling*): Refer to adult dosing.

Renal Impairment

U.S. labeling: Moderate-to-severe impairment: Recommended starting dose: 60 mg; use of an extended-interval dose of 120 mg every 6-8 weeks should be done with caution.

Canadian labeling: Moderate-to-severe impairment: Recommended starting dose: 60 mg every 4 weeks for 3 months then adjust dose based on clinical response of patient, growth hormone (GH) levels, and/or insulin-like growth factor 1 (IGF-1) levels as described in adult dosing; however, extendedinterval dosing is **not** recommended.

Hepatic Impairment

U.S. labeling: Moderate-to-severe impairment: Recommended starting dose: 60 mg; use of an extended-interval dose of 120 mg every 6-8 weeks should be done with caution.

Canadian labeling: Moderate-to-severe impairment: Recommended starting dose: 60 mg every 4 weeks for 3 months then adjust dose based on clinical response of patient, growth hormone (GH) levels, and/or insulin-like growth factor 1 (IGF-1) levels as described in adult dosing; however, extended-interval dosing is **not** recommended.

Administration Administer by deep subcutaneous injection into superior outer quadrant of buttocks. Do not fold skin. Alternate injection sites.

Monitoring Parameters Serum GH and IGF-1 (in patients switched to extended-interval dosing; obtain initial levels 6 weeks after dose) glucose levels, thyroid function (where clinically indicated); heart rate, gall bladder ultrasonography (prior to initiation and periodically during therapy)

Dosage Forms Excipient information presented when available (limited, particularly for generics); consult specific product labeling.

Injection, solution:

Somatuline® Depot: 60 mg/0.4 mL (0.4 mL); 90 mg/0.4 mL (0.4 mL); 120 mg/0.5 mL (0.5 mL) [contains natural rubber/natural latex in packaging; volume is expressed as an approximate value]

Dosage Forms: Canada Excipient information presented when available (limited, particularly for generics); consult specific product labeling.

Injection, solution:

Somatuline® Autogel®: 60 mg/~0.3 mL (~0.3 mL); 90 mg/~0.4 mL (~0.4 mL); 120 mg/~0.5 mL (~0.5 mL) [packaging contains natural rubber/natural latex]

References

Caron P, Beckers A, Cullen DR, et al, "Efficacy of the New Long-Acting Formulation of Lanreotide (Lanreotide Autogel) in the Management of Acromegaly," *J Clin Endocrinol Metab*, 2002, 87 (1):99-104.

◆ **Lanreotide Acetate** *see* Lanreotide *on page* *851*

◆ **Lanvis® (Can)** *see* Thioguanine *on page* *1354*

Lapatinib (la PA ti nib)

Related Information

Management of Chemotherapy-Induced Nausea and Vomiting *on page* *1786*

Principles of Anticancer Therapy *on page* *1878*

Safe Handling of Hazardous Drugs *on page* *1904*

Brand Names: U.S. Tykerb®

Brand Names: Canada Tykerb®

Index Terms GW572016; Lapatinib Ditosylate

Generic Availability (U.S.) No

Pharmacologic Category Antineoplastic Agent, Anti-HER2; Antineoplastic Agent, Tyrosine Kinase Inhibitor; Epidermal Growth Factor Receptor (EGFR) Inhibitor

Use Treatment of HER2 overexpressing advanced or metastatic breast cancer (in combination with capecitabine) in patients who have received prior therapy (with an anthracycline, a taxane, and trastuzumab) and HER2 overexpressing hormone receptor positive metastatic breast cancer in postmenopausal women where hormone therapy is indicated (in combination with letrozole)

Unlabeled Use Treatment (in combination with trastuzumab) of HER2 over-expressing metastatic breast cancer which had progressed on prior trastuzumab containing therapy; treatment of HER2 overexpressing metastatic breast cancer with brain metastases

Labeled Contraindications Hypersensitivity to lapatinib or any component of the formulation

Pregnancy Risk Factor D

Lactation Excretion in breast milk unknown/not recommended

Warnings/Precautions Decreases in left ventricular ejection fraction (LVEF) have been reported (usually within the first 3 months of treatment); baseline and periodic LVEF evaluations are recommended; interrupt treatment or decrease dose with decreased LVEF ≥grade 2 or LVEF <LLN. QT_c prolongation has been observed; use caution in patients with a history of QT_c prolongation or with medications known to prolong the QT interval; a baseline and periodic 12-lead ECG should be considered; correct electrolyte (potassium, calcium and magnesium) abnormalities prior to and during treatment. Use with caution in conditions which may impair left ventricular function and in patients with a history of or predisposed to (prior treatment with anthracyclines, chest wall irradiation) left ventricular dysfunction. Interstitial lung disease (ILD) and pneumonitis have been reported (with lapatinib monotherapy and with combination chemotherapy); monitor for pulmonary symptoms which may indicate ILD or pneumonitis; discontinue treatment for grade 3 (or higher) pulmonary symptoms indicative of ILD or pneumonitis (eg, dyspnea, dry cough).

[U.S. Boxed Warning]: Hepatotoxicity (ALT or AST >3 times ULN and total bilirubin >2 times ULN) has been reported with lapatinib; may be severe and/or fatal. Onset of hepatotoxicity may occur within days to several months after treatment initiation; monitor (at baseline and during treatment); discontinue with severe changes in liver function; do not retreat. Use caution in patients with hepatic dysfunction; Dose reductions should be considered in patients with severe (Child-Pugh class C) preexisting hepatic impairment. Avoid concurrent use with strong CYP3A4 inhibitors or inducers; if concomitant therapy cannot be avoided, lapatinib dosage adjustments should be considered. May cause diarrhea (may be severe); instruct patients to immediately report any bowel pattern changes. After first unformed stool, administer antidiarrheal agents; severe diarrhea may require hydration, electrolytes, and/or treatment interruption (or discontinuation).

Adverse Reactions Percentages reported for combination therapy.

>10%:

Central nervous system: Fatigue (10% to 20%), headache (≤14%)

Dermatologic: Palmar-plantar erythrodysesthesia (hand-and foot syndrome) (with capecitabine: 53%; grade 3: 12%), rash (28% to 44%), dry skin (10% to 13%), alopecia (≤13%), pruritus (≤12%), nail disorder (≤11%)

Gastrointestinal: Diarrhea (64% to 65%; grade 3: 9% to 13%; grade 4: ≤1%), nausea (31% to 44%), vomiting (17% to 26%), abdominal pain (≤15%), mucosal inflammation (≤15%), stomatitis (≤14%), anorexia (≤11%), dyspepsia (≤11%)

Hematologic: Anemia (with capecitabine: 56%; grade 3: <1%), neutropenia (with capecitabine: 22%; grade 3: 3%; grade 4: <1%), thrombocytopenia (with capecitabine: 18%; grade 3: <1%)

Hepatic: AST increased (49% to 53%; grade 3: 2% to 6%; grade 4: <1%), ALT increased (37% to 46%; grade 3: 2% to 5%; grade 4<1%) total bilirubin increased (22% to 45%; grade 3: ≤4%; grade 4: <1%)

Neuromuscular & skeletal: Limb pain (≤12%), weakness (≤12%), back pain (≤11%)

Respiratory:Dyspnea (≤12%), epistaxis (≤11%)

1% to 10%:

Cardiovascular: LVEF decreased (grades 1/2: 2% to 4%; grades 3/4: <1%)

Central nervous system: Insomnia (≤10%)

<1%, postmarketing, and/or case reports: Anaphylaxis, hepatotoxicity, hypersensitivity, interstitial lung disease, paronychia, pneumonitis, Prinzmetal's angina, QTc prolongation

Drug Interactions

Metabolism/Transport Effects Substrate of CYP3A4 (major), P-glycoprotein; **Note:** Assignment of Major/Minor substrate status based on clinically relevant drug interaction potential; **Inhibits** BCRP, CYP2C8 (moderate), CYP3A4 (weak), P-glycoprotein

Avoid Concomitant Use

Avoid concomitant use of Lapatinib with any of the following: Bosutinib; CYP3A4 Inducers (Strong); CYP3A4 Inhibitors (Strong); Grapefruit Juice; Highest Risk QTc-Prolonging Agents; Mifepristone; Silodosin; St Johns Wort; VinCRIStine (Liposomal)

Increased Effect/Toxicity

Lapatinib may increase the levels/effects of: ARIPiprazole; Bosutinib; Colchicine; CYP2C8 Substrates; Dabigatran Etexilate; Everolimus; Highest Risk QTc-Prolonging Agents; Moderate Risk QTc-Prolonging Agents; Pazopanib; P-glycoprotein/ABCB1 Substrates; Prucalopride; Rivaroxaban; Silodosin; Topotecan; VinCRIStine (Liposomal); Vitamin K Antagonists

The levels/effects of Lapatinib may be increased by: CYP3A4 Inhibitors (Moderate); CYP3A4 Inhibitors (Strong); Dasatinib; Grapefruit Juice; Ivacaftor; Mifepristone; P-glycoprotein/ABCB1 Inhibitors; QTc-Prolonging Agents (Indeterminate Risk and Risk Modifying)

Decreased Effect

Lapatinib may decrease the levels/effects of: Cardiac Glycosides; Vitamin K Antagonists

The levels/effects of Lapatinib may be decreased by: CYP3A4 Inducers (Strong); Deferasirox; P-glycoprotein/ABCB1 Inducers; St Johns Wort; Tocilizumab

Ethanol/Nutrition/Herb Interactions

Food: Systemic exposure of lapatinib is increased when administered with food (AUC three- to fourfold higher). Grapefruit juice may increase the levels/effects of lapatinib. Management: Administer once daily on an empty stomach, 1 hour before or 1 hour after a meal at the same time each day. Avoid grapefruit juice. Maintain adequate hydration, unless instructed to restrict fluid intake.

Herb/Nutraceutical: St John's wort may increase metabolism and decrease lapatinib concentrations. Management: Avoid St John's wort.

Storage/Stability Store at room temperature of 25°C (77°F); excursions permitted between 15°C and 30°C (59°F and 86°F).

Mechanism of Action Tyrosine kinase (dual kinase) inhibitor; inhibits EGFR (ErbB1) and HER2 (ErbB2) by reversibly binding to tyrosine kinase, blocking phosphorylation and activation of downstream second messengers (Erk1/2 and Akt), regulating cellular proliferation and survival in ErbB- and ErbB2-expressing tumors. Combination therapy with lapatinib and endocrine therapy may overcome endocrine resistance occurring in HER2+ and hormone receptor positive disease.

Pharmacodynamics/Kinetics

Absorption: Incomplete and variable

Protein binding: >99% to albumin and $alpha_1$-acid glycoprotein

Metabolism: Hepatic; extensive via CYP3A4 and 3A5, and to a lesser extent via CYP2C19 and 2C8 to oxidized metabolites

Half-life elimination: ~24 hours

Time to peak, plasma: ~4 hours (Burris, 2009)

Excretion: Feces (27% as unchanged drug; range 3% to 67%); urine (<2%)

Dosing

Adult & Geriatric Details concerning dosing in combination regimens should also be consulted.

Breast cancer, metastatic, HER2+ (with prior anthracycline, taxane and trastuzumab therapy): Oral: 1250 mg once daily (in combination with capecitabine) until disease progression or unacceptable toxicity (Geyer, 2006)

Breast cancer, metastatic, HER2+, hormonal therapy indicated: Oral: 1500 mg once daily (in combination with letrozole) until disease progression (Johnston, 2009)

Breast cancer, metastatic, HER2+ with brain metastases, first-line therapy (unlabeled use): Oral: 1250 mg once daily (in combination with capecitabine) until disease progression or unacceptable toxicity (Bachelot; 2011)

Breast cancer, metastatic, HER2+, with progression on prior trastuzumab therapy (unlabeled use): Oral: 1000 mg once daily (in combination with trastuzumab) (Blackwell, 2010; Blackwell, 2012)

Missed doses: If a dose is missed, do not double the dose the next day.

Dosage adjustment for concomitant CYP3A4 inhibitors/inducers:

CYP3A4 inhibitors: Avoid the use of concomitant strong CYP3A4 inhibitors. If concomitant use cannot be avoided, consider reducing lapatinib to 500 mg once daily with careful monitoring. When a strong CYP3A4 inhibitor is discontinued, allow ~1 week to elapse prior to adjusting the lapatinib dose upward.

CYP3A4 inducers: Avoid the use of concomitant strong CYP3A4 inhibitors. If concomitant use cannot be avoided, consider gradually titrating lapatinib from 1250 mg/day up to 4500 mg/day (in combination with capecitabine) **or** from 1500 mg/day up to 5500 mg/day (in combination with letrozole), based on tolerability and with careful monitoring. If the strong CYP3A4 enzyme inducer is discontinued, reduce the lapatinib dose to the indicated dose.

Renal Impairment No dosage adjustment provided in the manufacturer's labeling (has not been studied); however, due to the minimal renal elimination (<2%), dosage adjustments may not be necessary.

Hepatic Impairment

Severe preexisting impairment (Child-Pugh class C):

In combination with capecitabine: Reduce dose from 1250 mg once daily to 750 mg once daily.

In combination with letrozole: Reduce dose from 1500 mg once daily to 1000 mg once daily.

Severe hepatotoxicity during treatment: Discontinue treatment; do not retreat.

Adjustment for Toxicity

Cardiac toxicity: Discontinue treatment for at least 2 weeks for decreased LVEF ≥grade 2 or LVEF < LLN; may be restarted at 1000 mg once daily (in combination with capecitabine) **or** 1250 mg once daily (in combination with letrozole) if LVEF recovers to normal and patient is asymptomatic.

Pulmonary toxicity: Discontinue treatment with pulmonary symptoms indicative of interstitial lung disease or pneumonitis which are ≥grade 3

Other toxicities: Withhold for any toxicity (other than cardiac) ≥grade 2 until toxicity resolves to ≤grade 1 and reinitiate at 1250 mg once daily; for persistent toxicity, reduce dosage to 1000 mg once daily (in combination with capecitabine) **or** 1250 mg once daily (in combination with letrozole)

Combination Regimens

Breast cancer:

Capecitabine + Lapatinib (Breast Cancer) on page 1541
Lapatinib-Letrozole (Breast Cancer) on page 1698
Lapatinib-Trastuzumab (Breast Cancer) on page 1698

Administration Administer once daily, on an empty stomach, 1 hour before or 1 hour after a meal. Take at the same time each day; dividing doses is not recommended.

Emetic Potential Low (10% to 30%)

Monitoring Parameters LVEF (baseline and periodic), CBC with differential, liver function tests, including transaminases, bilirubin, and alkaline phosphatase (baseline and every 4-6 weeks during treatment); electrolytes including calcium, potassium, magnesium; monitor for fluid retention; ECG monitoring if at risk for QT_c prolongation; symptoms of ILD or pneumonitis

Dietary Considerations Take on an empty stomach, 1 hour before or 1 hour after a meal. (**Note:** For combination with capecitabine treatment, capecitabine should be taken with food, or within 30 minutes after a meal.) Avoid grapefruit juice.

Additional Information Oncology Comment: In a randomized phase III study (Geyer, 2006) of lapatinib plus capecitabine versus capecitabine alone in HER2-positive advanced breast cancer, the addition of lapatinib was associated with a 51% reduction in the risk of disease progression in heavily pretreated patients. Lapatinib shows activity in HER2-positive metastatic breast cancer that has progressed after trastuzumab treatment.

Prescribing and Access Restrictions Lapatinib is available **only** at specialty pharmacies through a restricted-access program, Tykerb® CARES. Information is available at www.tykerbcares.com or 1-866-489-5372.

Dosage Forms Excipient information presented when available (limited, particularly for generics); consult specific product labeling.

Tablet, oral:

Tykerb®: 250 mg

References

Bachelot TD, Romieu G, Campone M, et al, "LANDSCAPE: An FNCLCC Phase II Study With Lapatinib (L) and Capecitabine (C) in Patients With Brain Metastases (BM) From HER2-Positive (+) Metastatic Breast Cancer (MBC) Before Whole-Brain Radiotherapy (WBR)," *J Clin Oncol*, 2011, 29(15s):509 [abstract 509 from 2011 ASCO Annual Meeting].

Blackwell KL, Burstein HJ, Storniolo AM, et al, "Overall Survival Benefit With Lapatinib in Combination With Trastuzumab for Patients With Human Epidermal Growth Factor Receptor 2-Positive Metastatic Breast Cancer: Final Results From the EGF104900 Study," *J Clin Oncol*, 2012, 30(21):2585-92.

Blackwell KL, Burstein HJ, Storniolo AM, et al, "Randomized Study of Lapatinib Alone or in Combination With Trastuzumab in Women With ErbB2-Positive, Trastuzumab-Refractory Metastatic Breast Cancer," *J Clin Oncol*, 2010, 28(7):1124-30.

Burris HA 3rd, Taylor CW, Jones SF, et al, "A Phase I and Pharmacokinetic Study of Oral Lapatinib Administered Once or Twice Daily in Patients With Solid Malignancies," *Clin Cancer Res*, 2009, 15(21):6702-8.

Geyer CE, Forster J, Lindquist D, et al "Lapatinib Plus Capecitabine for HER2-Positive Advanced Breast Cancer," *N Engl J Med*, 2006, 355(26):2733-43.

Johnston S, Pippen J Jr, Pivot X, et al, "Lapatinib Combined With Letrozole Versus Letrozole and Placebo as First-Line Therapy for Postmenopausal Hormone Receptor-Positive Metastatic Breast Cancer," *J Clin Oncol*, 2009, 27(33):5538-46.

National Comprehensive Cancer Network® (NCCN), "Clinical Practice Guidelines in Oncology™: Breast Cancer," Version 1.2010. Available at http://www.nccn.org/professionals/physician_gls/PDF/breast.pdf

O'Shaughnessy J, Blackwell KL, Burstein H, et al, "A Randomized Study of Lapatinib Alone or in Combination With Trastuzumab in Heavily Pretreated HER2+ Metastatic Breast Cancer Progressing on Trastuzumab Therapy," *J Clin Oncol*, 2008, 26(15s):1015 [abstract 1015 from 2008 ASCO Annual Meeting].

◆ **Lapatinib Ditosylate** *see* Lapatinib *on page 854*
◆ **L-asparaginase (*E. coli*)** *see* Asparaginase (*E. coli*) *on page 130*
◆ **L-asparaginase (*Erwinia*)** *see* Asparaginase (*Erwinia*) *on page 126*
◆ **L-asparaginase with Polyethylene Glycol** *see* Pegaspargase *on page 1105*
◆ **Lazanda®** *see* FentaNYL *on page 583*
◆ **LDP-341** *see* Bortezomib *on page 187*
◆ **Lederle Leucovorin (Can)** *see* Leucovorin Calcium *on page 870*
◆ **Lemtrada** *see* Alemtuzumab *on page 43*

Lenalidomide (le na LID oh mide)

Related Information

Chemotherapy and Cancer Treatment During Pregnancy *on page 1829*
Management of Chemotherapy-Induced Nausea and Vomiting *on page 1786*
Principles of Anticancer Therapy *on page 1878*
Safe Handling of Hazardous Drugs *on page 1904*

Brand Names: U.S. Revlimid®

Brand Names: Canada Revlimid®

Index Terms CC-5013; IMid-1

Generic Availability (U.S.) No

Pharmacologic Category Angiogenesis Inhibitor; Antineoplastic Agent; Immunomodulator, Systemic

Use Treatment of low- or intermediate-1-risk myelodysplastic syndrome (MDS) in patients with deletion 5q (del 5q) cytogenetic abnormality with transfusion-dependent anemia (with or without other cytogenetic abnormalities); treatment of multiple myeloma (in combination with dexamethasone) in patients who have received at least one prior therapy

Unlabeled Use Treatment of non-Hodgkin's lymphomas; systemic light chain amyloidosis; lower-risk myelodysplastic syndrome (MDS) in transfusion-dependent patients without deletion 5q (del 5q); maintenance treatment for multiple myeloma (after response to primary treatment or following autologous stem cell transplant)

Labeled Contraindications Hypersensitivity (eg, angioedema, Stevens-Johnson syndrome, toxic epidermal necrolysis) to lenalidomide or any component of the formulation; pregnancy or women capable of becoming pregnant

Canadian labeling: Additional contraindications (not in U.S. labeling): Platelet count <50,000/mm^3 (in MDS patients); hypersensitivity to thalidomide; breast-feeding women

Pregnancy Risk Factor X

Lactation Excretion in breast milk unknown/not recommended

Warnings/Precautions Hazardous agent - use appropriate precautions for handling and disposal. **[U.S. Boxed Warning]: Hematologic toxicity (neutropenia and thrombocytopenia) occurs in a majority of patients (grade 3/4: 80% in patients with del 5q myelodysplastic syndrome) and may require dose reductions and/or delays; the use of blood product support and/or growth factors may be needed. CBC should be monitored weekly for the first 8 weeks and at least monthly thereafter in patients being**

treated for del 5q myelodysplastic syndromes. In patients being treated for multiple myeloma, monitor CBC every 2 weeks for 12 weeks and monthly thereafter. **[U.S. Boxed Warning]: Lenalidomide has been associated with a significant increase in risk for thrombosis and embolism in multiple myeloma patients treated with dexamethasone combination therapy. Deep vein thrombosis (DVT) and pulmonary embolism (PE) have occurred; monitor for signs and symptoms of thromboembolism (shortness of breath, chest pain, or arm or leg swelling) and seek prompt medical attention with development of these symptoms.** The NCCN multiple myeloma guidelines (v1.2012) recommend anticoagulant prophylaxis when used in combination with dexamethasone. Anticoagulant prophylaxis should be individualized and selected based on the venous thromboembolism risk of the combination treatment regimen, using the safest and easiest to administer (Palumbo, 2008).

Second primary malignancies (SPMs), including hematologic (AML and lymphoma) and solid tumor malignancies, and skin cancers, have been reported with lenalidomide when used for the treatment of MDS and multiple myeloma; the incidence may be higher when lenalidomide is used in combination with an alkylating agent.

Angioedema, Stevens-Johnson syndrome (SJS), and toxic epidermal necrolysis (TEN) have been reported; may be fatal. Consider interrupting or discontinuing treatment with grade 2 or 3 skin rash; discontinue and do not reinitiate treatment with grade 4 rash, exfoliative or bullous rash, or for suspected SJS or TEN. Patients with a history of grade 4 rash with thalidomide should not receive lenalidomide. Discontinue treatment with angioedema. Use caution in renal impairment; may experience an increased rate of toxicities (due to reduced clearance and increased half-life); initial dosage adjustments are recommended for moderate-to-severe and dialysis-dependent renal impairment. Tumor lysis syndrome (with fatalities) has been reported with lenalidomide; patients with a high tumor burden may be at risk for tumor lysis syndrome; monitor closely. Tumor flare reaction has been observed in studies of lenalidomide for the treatment of chronic lymphocytic leukemia (CLL) and lymphoma; clinical presentation includes low grade fever, pain, rash, and tender lymph node swelling. Transient abnormal hepatic laboratory findings (eg, increased transaminases) have been reported; interrupt therapy in patients with abnormal hepatic function tests; may resume treatment upon return to baseline; successful rechallenge has been reported.

[U.S. Boxed Warning]: Lenalidomide is an analogue of thalidomide (a human teratogen) and could potentially cause birth defects in humans; do not use during pregnancy (contraindication); avoid pregnancy while taking lenalidomide. Obtain 2 negative pregnancy testes prior to initiation of treatment; 2 forms of contraception (or abstain from heterosexual intercourse) must be used at least 4 weeks prior to, during and for 4 weeks after lenalidomide treatment (and during treatment interruptions). Distribution is restricted; physicians, pharmacists, and patients must be registered with the RevAssist® program. Patients should be advised not to donate blood during therapy and for 4 weeks following completion of therapy. May cause dizziness or fatigue; caution patients about performing tasks which require mental alertness (eg, operating machinery or driving). Formulation contains lactose; avoid use in patients with Lapp lactase deficiency, glucose-galactose malabsorption, or glucose intolerance. Lenalidomide should only be prescribed to patients (male and female) who can understand and comply with the conditions of the RevAssist® program. If used in patients between 12-18 years of age, the parent or legal guardian must agree to ensure compliance with the RevAssist® program.

Adverse Reactions

>10%:

Cardiovascular: Peripheral edema (8% to 26%)

Central nervous system: Fatigue (31% to 44%), fever (21% to 28%), dizziness (20% to 23%), headache (20%)

Dermatologic: Pruritus (8% to 42%), rash (21% to 36%; grades 3/4: 7%), dry skin (9% to 14%)

Endocrine & metabolic: Hypokalemia (11% to 14%)

Gastrointestinal: Diarrhea (39% to 49%), constipation (24% to 41%), nausea (24% to 26%), weight loss (20%), anorexia (10% to 16%), taste perversion (6% to 15%), vomiting (10% to 12%), abdominal pain (8% to 12%)

Genitourinary: Urinary tract infection (9% to 11%)

Hematologic: Thrombocytopenia (22% to 62%; grades 3/4: 12% to 50%; MDS: onset: 28 days [range 8-290 days]; recovery: 22 days [range: 5-224 days]), neutropenia (42% to 59%; grades 3/4: 33% to 53%; MDS: onset: 42 days [range 14-411 days]; recovery: 17 days [range: 2-170 days]), anemia (12% to 31%; grades 3/4: 6% to 10%)

Neuromuscular & skeletal: Muscle cramp (18% to 33%), weakness (15%), arthralgia (22%), back pain (21% to 26%), tremor (21%), bone pain (14%), limb pain (11% to 12%)

Ocular: Blurred vision (17%)

Respiratory: Upper respiratory infection (15% to 25%), nasopharyngitis (18% to 23%), cough (≤20%), dyspnea (7% to 24%), pharyngitis (14% to 16%), epistaxis (15%), pneumonia (9% to 14%), bronchitis (6% to 11%)

1% to 10%:

Cardiovascular: Edema (10%), deep vein thrombosis (≤9%; grades 3/4: ≤8%), hypertension (6% to 8%), hypotension (7%), chest pain (5% to 8%), palpitation (5%), atrial fibrillation (grades 3/4: ≤4%), syncope (grade 3/4: 1% to 3%), cerebrovascular accident (2%), tachycardia (grades 3/4: 2%), angina pectoris (≥1%), bradycardia (≥1%), cerebral ischemia (≥1%), MI (≥1%), heart failure (1%)

Central nervous system: Insomnia (10%), hypoesthesia (7% to 10%), lethargy (7%), pain (7%), depression (5%), hallucinations (≥1%), malaise (≥1%), mood swings (>1%)

Dermatologic: Bruising (5% to 8%), cellulitis (5%), erythema (5%), exanthem (≥1%), hirsutism (≥1%), hyperpigmentation (≥1%)

Endocrine & metabolic: Hypothyroidism (7%), hypomagnesemia (6% to 7%), hypocalcemia (9%), dehydration (7%), hypophosphatemia (grades 3/4: 3%), loss of libido (≥1%)

Gastrointestinal: Appetite decreased (7%), xerostomia (7%), loose stools (6%), glossodynia (≥1%), GI hemorrhage (≥1%)

Genitourinary: Dysuria (7%), erectile dysfunction (≥1%)

Hematologic: Leukopenia (8%; grade 3/4: 4% to 5%), febrile neutropenia (5%; grades 3/4: 2% to 4%), granulocytopenia (grades 3/4: 2%), lymphopenia (5%; grade 3: 3%), pancytopenia (grades 3/4: 2%), autoimmune hemolytic anemia (≥1%)

Hepatic: ALT increased (8%), liver function tests abnormal (≥1%)

Neuromuscular & skeletal: Myalgia (9%), neuropathy (5% to 7%), rigors (6%)

Ocular: Cataract (grades 3/4: 1% to 2%), blindness (≥1%), ocular hypertension (≥1%),

Respiratory: Sinusitis (7% to 8%), rhinitis (7%), pulmonary embolism (≤4%; grades 3/4: 2% to 4%), respiratory distress (grades 3/4: 1% to 2%), hoarseness (≥1%), hypoxia (grades 3/4: 1%), pleural effusion (grades 3/4: 1%), pneumonitis (grades 3/4: 1%), pulmonary hypertension (grades 3/4: 1%)

Miscellaneous: Diaphoresis (7% to 10%), night sweats (8%), sepsis (grades 3/4: 3%)

<1%, postmarketing, and/or case reports (limited to important or life-threatening): Acute febrile neutrophilic dermatosis, acute leukemia, acute myeloid leukemia (AML), adrenal insufficiency, angioedema, atrial flutter, azotemia, Basedow's disease, biliary obstruction, blindness, bone marrow depression, brain edema, cardiac failure, cardiogenic shock, cardiomyopathy, cardiopulmonary arrest, cholecystitis, chondrocalcinosis, chronic obstructive airway disease, circulatory collapse, coagulopathy, colonic polyp, delirium, diabetes mellitus, diabetic ketoacidosis, diverticulitis, dysphagia, encephalitis, erythema multiforme, Fanconi syndrome, gout, hematuria, hemolysis, hemolytic anemia, hemorrhage, hepatic failure, hepatitis, herpesvirus infection, hyperbilirubinemia, hypernatremia, hypersensitivity, hypoglycemia, infection, interstitial lung disease, intestinal perforation, intracranial hemorrhage, ischemia, ischemic colitis, leukoencephalopathy, liver failure, lung cancer, lung infiltration, lymphoma, myopathy, neutropenic sepsis, orthostatic hypotension, pancreatitis, peripheral ischemia, pseudomembraneous colitis, pulmonary edema, refractory anemia, renal calculus, renal failure, renal mass, renal tubular necrosis, respiratory failure, secondary malignancy (AML, lymphomas, solid tumors, skin cancers), septic shock, serum creatinine increased, skin desquamation, small bowel obstruction, spinal cord compression, splenic infarction, Stevens-Johnson syndrome, stomatitis, supraventricular arrhythmia, tachyarrhythmia, thrombophlebitis, toxic epidermal necrolysis, troponin I increased, tumor flare, tumor lysis syndrome, urinary retention, urosepsis, urticaria, ventricular dysfunction

Drug Interactions

Metabolism/Transport Effects **Substrate** of P-glycoprotein

Avoid Concomitant Use

Avoid concomitant use of Lenalidomide with any of the following: Abatacept; Anakinra; BCG; Canakinumab; Certolizumab Pegol; CloZAPine; Natalizumab; Pimecrolimus; Rilonacept; Tacrolimus (Topical); Vaccines (Live)

Increased Effect/Toxicity

Lenalidomide may increase the levels/effects of: Abatacept; Anakinra; Canakinumab; Certolizumab Pegol; CloZAPine; Digoxin; Leflunomide; Natalizumab; Rilonacept; Vaccines (Live)

The levels/effects of Lenalidomide may be increased by: Denosumab; Dexamethasone (Systemic); Pimecrolimus; Roflumilast; Tacrolimus (Topical); Trastuzumab

Decreased Effect

Lenalidomide may decrease the levels/effects of: BCG; Coccidioidin Skin Test; Sipuleucel-T; Vaccines (Inactivated); Vaccines (Live)

The levels/effects of Lenalidomide may be decreased by: Echinacea

Ethanol/Nutrition/Herb Interactions Herb/Nutraceutical: Avoid echinacea (has immunostimulant properties; consider therapy modifications).

Storage/Stability Store at 25°C (77°F); excursions permitted to 15°C and 30°C (59°F and 86°F).

Mechanism of Action Immunomodulatory, antiangiogenic, and antineoplastic characteristics via multiple mechanisms. Selectively inhibits secretion of proinflammatory cytokines (potent inhibitor of tumor necrosis factor-alpha secretion); enhances cell-mediated immunity by stimulating proliferation of anti-CD3 stimulated T cells (resulting in increased IL-2 and interferon gamma secretion); inhibits trophic signals to angiogenic factors in cells. Inhibits the growth of myeloma cells by inducing cell cycle arrest and cell death.

Pharmacodynamics/Kinetics

Absorption: Rapid

Protein binding: ~30%

Half-life elimination: 3-5 hours; Moderate-to-severe renal impairment: Increased threefold; Hemodialysis patients: Increased ~4.5-fold

Time, to peak, plasma: MDS or myeloma patients: 0.5-6 hours

Excretion: Urine (~82%; as unchanged drug)

Hemodialysis effect: ~40% of a dose is removed in a single dialysis session

Dosing

Adult

Multiple myeloma: Oral: 25 mg once daily for 21 days of a 28-day treatment cycle (in combination with dexamethasone)

Myelodysplastic syndrome (MDS) with deletion 5q: Oral: 10 mg once daily

Diffuse large B-cell lymphoma (unlabeled use): Oral: 25 mg once daily for 21 days of a 28-day treatment cycle for up to 1 year (Wiernik, 2008)

Mantle cell lymphoma, relapsed or refractory (unlabeled use): Oral: 25 mg once daily for 21 days of a 28-day treatment cycle for up to 1 year (Habermann, 2009)

Multiple myeloma, maintenance (following autologous stem cell transplant; unlabeled use): Oral: 10-15 mg once daily until relapse (Attal, 2009; McCarthy, 2009) **or** 10 mg once daily for 21 days of a 28-day treatment cycle until relapse (Palumbo, 2010)

Myelodysplastic syndrome (MDS), lower risk, without deletion 5q (unlabeled use): Oral: 10 mg once daily (Raza, 2008)

Geriatric Refer to adult dosing. Due to the potential for decreased renal function in the elderly, select dose carefully and closely monitor renal function.

Renal Impairment

Recommended initial dose adjustment in the FDA approved labeling:

MDS:

Cl_{cr} >60 mL/minute: No adjustment required

Cl_{cr} 30-60 mL/minute: 5 mg once daily

Cl_{cr} <30 mL/minute (nondialysis dependent): 2.5 mg once daily

Cl_{cr} <30 mL/minute (dialysis dependent): 2.5 mg once daily (administer after dialysis on dialysis days)

Multiple myeloma:

Cl_{cr} >60 mL/minute: No adjustment required

Cl_{cr} 30-60 mL/minute: 10 mg once daily

Cl_{cr} <30 mL/minute (nondialysis dependent): 15 mg every 48 hours

Cl_{cr} <30 mL/minute (dialysis dependent): 5 mg once daily (administer after dialysis on dialysis days)

Recommended adjustment in Canadian labeling:

MDS:

Cl_{cr} ≥60 mL/minute: No adjustment required

Cl_{cr} 30-59 mL/minute: 5 mg once daily

Cl_{cr} <30 mL/minute (nondialysis dependent): 5 mg every 48 hours

Cl_{cr} <30 mL/minute (dialysis dependent): 5 mg 3 times/week (administer after each dialysis)

Multiple myeloma:

Cl_{cr} ≥60 mL/minute: No adjustment required

Cl_{cr} 30-59 mL/minute: 10 mg once daily; (may increase to 15 mg once daily after 2 cycles if nonresponsive but tolerating treatment; Chen, 2007)

Cl_{cr} <30 mL/minute (nondialysis dependent): 15 mg every 48 hours

Cl_{cr} <30 mL/minute (dialysis dependent): 5 mg once daily (administer after dialysis on dialysis days)

Adjustment for Toxicity

NONHEMATOLOGIC toxicities:

Dermatologic toxicities:

Skin rash, grade 2 or 3: Consider interrupting or discontinuing treatment

Angioedema, grade 4 rash, exfoliative or bullous rash, or suspected Stevens-Johnson syndrome or toxic epidermal necrolysis: Discontinue treatment

Other toxicities: For additional treatment-related grade 3/4 toxicities, hold treatment and restart at next lower dose level when toxicity has resolved to ≤grade 2.

HEMATOLOGIC toxicities:

Adjustment for thrombocytopenia in MDS:

Thrombocytopenia developing within 4 weeks of beginning treatment at 10 mg/day:

Baseline platelets ≥100,000/mm^3:

If platelets <50,000/mm^3: Hold treatment

When platelets return to ≥50,000/mm^3: Resume treatment at 5 mg/day

Baseline platelets <100,000/mm^3:

If platelets fall to 50% of baseline: Hold treatment

If baseline ≥60,000/mm^3 and platelet level returns to ≥50,000/mm^3: Resume at 5 mg/day

If baseline <60,000/mm^3 and platelet level returns to ≥30,000/mm^3: Resume at 5 mg/day

Thrombocytopenia developing after 4 weeks of beginning treatment at 10 mg/day:

Platelets <30,000/mm^3 **or** <50,000/mm^3 with platelet transfusions: Hold treatment

Platelets ≥30,000/mm^3 (without hemostatic failure): Resume at 5 mg/day

Thrombocytopenia developing with treatment at 5 mg/day:

Platelets <30,000/mm^3 **or** <50,000/mm^3 with platelet transfusions: Hold treatment

Platelets ≥30,000/mm^3 (without hemostatic failure):

U.S. labeling: Resume at 2.5 mg once daily

Canadian labeling: Resume at 5 mg every other day

Adjustment for neutropenia in MDS:

Neutropenia developing within 4 weeks of beginning treatment at 10 mg/day:

For baseline absolute neutrophil count (ANC) ≥1000/mm^3:

ANC <750/mm^3: Hold treatment

When ANC returns to ≥1000/mm^3: Resume at 5 mg/day

For baseline absolute neutrophil count (ANC) <1000/mm^3:

ANC <500/mm^3: Hold treatment

When ANC returns to ≥500/mm^3: Resume at 5 mg/day

Neutropenia developing after 4 weeks of beginning treatment at 10 mg/day:

ANC <500/mm^3 for ≥7 days or associated with fever: Hold treatment

When ≥500/mm^3: Resume at 5 mg/day

Neutropenia developing with treatment at 5 mg/day:

ANC <500/mm^3 for ≥7 days or associated with fever: Hold treatment

When ≥500/mm^3:

U.S. labeling: Resume at 2.5 mg once daily

Canadian labeling: Resume at 5 mg every other day

Adjustment for thrombocytopenia in multiple myeloma:

Platelets <30,000/mm^3: Hold treatment, check CBC weekly

When platelets ≥30,000/mm^3: Resume at 15 mg daily

Additional occurrence of platelets <30,000/mm^3: Hold treatment

When platelets ≥30,000/mm^3: Resume treatment at 5 mg below previous dose; do not dose below 5 mg daily

Adjustment for neutropenia in multiple myeloma:

ANC <1000/mm^3: Hold treatment, add G-CSF, check CBC weekly

When ≥1000/mm^3 (with neutropenia as only toxicity): Resume at 25 mg/day

When ≥1000/mm^3 (with additional toxicities): Resume at 15 mg/day

Additional occurrence of ANC <1000/mm^3: Hold treatment

When ≥1000/mm^3: Resume treatment at 5 mg below previous dose; do not dose below 5 mg daily.

Combination Regimens

Multiple myeloma:

Lenalidomide-Bortezomib-Dexamethasone (Multiple Myeloma) on page 1702

Lenalidomide-Dexamethasone on page 1702

Lenalidomide-Dexamethasone (Low Dose) on page 1703

Administration Administer at about the same time each day. Administer with water. Swallow capsule whole; do not break, open, or chew. May administer a missed dose if within 12 hours of usual dosing time. If greater than 12 hours, patient should skip dose for that day and resume usual dosing the following day. Patient should **not** take 2 doses to make up for a missed dose. Use appropriate precautions for handling and disposal.

Emetic Potential Low (10% to 30%)

Monitoring Parameters CBC with differential (MDS: weekly for first 8 weeks; multiple myeloma: every 2 weeks for the first 3 months), then monthly thereafter; serum creatinine, liver function tests, thyroid function tests (TSH at baseline then every 2-3 months during lenalidomide treatment [Hamnvik, 2011]); ECG when clinically indicated; monitor for signs and symptoms of thromboembolism or tumor lysis syndrome

Women of childbearing potential: Pregnancy test 10-14 days **and** 24 hours prior to initiating therapy, weekly during the first 4 weeks of treatment, then every 2-4 weeks through 4 weeks after therapy discontinued

Additional Information Pregnancy tests are required prior to beginning therapy, throughout treatment and during therapy interruptions for all women of childbearing age. The pregnancy test must be verified by the prescriber and the pharmacist prior to dispensing. Effective contraception with at least two reliable forms of contraception (IUD, hormonal contraception, tubal ligation or partner's vasectomy plus latex condom, diaphragm, or cervical cap) should be used for 4 weeks prior to beginning therapy, during therapy, and for 4 weeks following discontinuance of therapy. Women who have undergone a hysterectomy or have been postmenopausal for at least 24 consecutive months are the only exception. Do not prescribe, administer, or dispense to women of childbearing age or males who may have intercourse with women of childbearing age unless both female and male are capable of complying with contraceptive measures. Even males who have undergone vasectomy must acknowledge these risks in writing, and must use a latex condom during any sexual contact with women of childbearing age. Oral and written warnings concerning contraception and the hazards of thalidomide must be conveyed to females and males and they must acknowledge their understanding in writing. Parents or guardians must consent and sign acknowledgment for patients 12-18 years of age following therapy. A maximum 28-day supply should be dispensed.

Prescribing and Access Restrictions As a requirement of the REMS program, access to this medication is restricted. Lenalidomide is approved for marketing in the U.S. only under a Food and Drug Administration (FDA) approved, restricted distribution program called RevAssist® (www.REVLIMID.com or 1-888-423-5436). In Canada, distribution is restricted through RevAid® (www.RevAid.ca or 1-888-738-2431). Physicians, pharmacies, and patients must be registered; a maximum 28-day supply may be dispensed; a new prescription is required each time it is filled; pregnancy testing is required for females of childbearing potential.

Medication Guide Available Yes

Dosage Forms Excipient information presented when available (limited, particularly for generics); consult specific product labeling.

Capsule, oral:

Revlimid®: 2.5 mg, 5 mg, 10 mg, 15 mg, 25 mg

References

Attal M, Harousseau JL, Gerald Marit, et al, "Lenalidomide After Autologous Transplantation for Myeloma: First Analysis of a Prospective, Randomized Study of the Intergroupe Francophone Du Myelome (IFM 2005 02)," *Blood*, 2009, 114(22):529 [abstract 529 from 2009 ASH Annual Meeting].

Chanan-Khan A, Miller KC, Musial L, et al, "Clinical Efficacy of Lenalidomide in Patients With Relapsed or Refractory Chronic Lymphocytic Leukemia: Results of a Phase II Study," *J Clin Oncol*, 2006, 24(34):5343-9.

Chen N, Lau H, Kong L, et al, "Pharmacokinetics of Lenalidomide in Subjects With Various Degrees of Renal Function," *J Clin Oncol*, 2007, 25(18S):2520 [abstract 2520 from ASCO Annual Meeting Proceedings, Part I].

Chen N, Lau H, Kong L, et al, "Pharmacokinetics of Lenalidomide in Subjects With Various Degrees of Renal Impairment and in Subjects on Hemodialysis," *J Clin Pharmacol*, 2007, 47(12):1466-75.

Dimopoulos M, Spencer A, Attal M, et al, "Lenalidomide Plus Dexamethasone for Relapsed or Refractory Multiple Myeloma," *N Engl J Med*, 2007, 357(21):2123-32.

Ferrajoli A, Lee BN, Schlette EJ, et al, "Lenalidomide Induces Complete and Partial Remissions in Patients With Relapsed and Refractory Chronic Lymphocytic Leukemia," *Blood*, 2008, 111(11):5291-7.

Giagounidis AA, Germing U, Strupp C, et al, "Prognosis of Patients with del(5q) MDS and Complex Karotype and the Possible Role of Lenalidomide in this Patient Subgroup," *Ann Hematol*, 2005, 84(9):569-71.

Habermann TM, Lossos IS, Justice G, et al, "Lenalidomide Oral Monotherapy Produces a High Response Rate in Patients With Relapsed or Refractory Mantle Cell Lymphoma," *Br J Haematol*, 2009, 145(3):344-9.

List A, Dewald G, Bennett J, et al, "Lenalidomide in Myelodysplastic Syndrome With Chromosome 5q Deletion," *N Engl J Med*, 2006, 355(14):1456-65.

McCarthy PL, Owzar K, Stadtmauer EA, et al, "Phase III Intergroup Study of Lenalidomide (CC-5013) Versus Placebo Maintenance Therapy Following Single Autologous Stem Cell Transplant for Multiple Myeloma (CALGB 100104): Initial Report of Patient Accrual and Adverse Events," *Blood*, 2009, 114(22):3416 [abstract 3416 from 2009 ASH Annual Meeting].

National Comprehensive Cancer Network® (NCCN), "Clinical Practice Guidelines in Oncology™: Multiple Myeloma," Version 1.2013. Available at http://www.nccn.org/professionals/physician_gls/PDF/myeloma.pdf

Palumbo A, Gay F, Falco P, et al, "Bortezomib as Induction Before Autologous Transplantation, Followed by Lenalidomide as Consolidation-Maintenance in Untreated Multiple Myeloma Patients," *J Clin Oncol*, 2010, 28(5):800-7.

Palumbo A, Rajkumar SV, Dimopoulos MA, et al, "Prevention of Thalidomide- and Lenalidomide-Associated Thrombosis in Myeloma," *Leukemia*, 2008, 22(2): 414-23.

Rajkumar SV, Hayman SR, Lacy MQ, et al, "Combination Therapy With Lenalidomide Plus Dexamethasone (Rev/Dex) for Newly Diagnosed Myeloma," *Blood*, 2005, 106(13):4050-3.

Raza A, Reeves JA, Feldman JA, et al, "Phase 2 Study of Lenalidomide in Transfusion-Dependent, Low-Risk, and Intermediate-1 Risk Myelodysplastic Syndromes With Karyotypes Other than Deletion 5q," *Blood*, 2008, 111(1):86-93.

Weber DM, Chen C, Niesvizky R, et al, "Lenalidomide Plus Dexamethasone for Relapsed Multiple Myeloma in North America," *N Engl J Med*, 2007, 357(21):2133-42.

Wiernik PH, Lossos IS, Tuscano JM, et al, "Lenalidomide Monotherapy in Relapsed or Refractory Aggressive Non-Hodgkin's Lymphoma," *J Clin Oncol*, 2008, 26(30):4952-7

Letrozole (LET roe zole)

Related Information

Safe Handling of Hazardous Drugs *on page 1904*

Brand Names: U.S. Femara®

Brand Names: Canada Femara®; JAMP-Letrozole; Letrozole Tablets, USP; MED-Letrozole; Myl-Letrozole; PMS-Letrozole; Sandoz-Letrozole

Index Terms CGS-20267

Generic Availability (U.S.) Yes

Pharmacologic Category Antineoplastic Agent, Aromatase Inhibitor

Use For use in postmenopausal women in the adjuvant treatment of hormone receptor positive early breast cancer, extended adjuvant treatment of early breast cancer after 5 years of tamoxifen, advanced breast cancer with disease progression following antiestrogen therapy, hormone receptor positive or hormone receptor unknown, locally-advanced, or first-line (or second-line) treatment of advanced or metastatic breast cancer

Unlabeled Use Treatment of ovarian (epithelial) cancer, endometrial cancer

Labeled Contraindications Use in women who are or may become pregnant

Canadian labeling: Additional contraindications (not in U.S. labeling): Hypersensitivity to letrozole, other aromatase inhibitors, or any component of the formulation; use in patients <18 years of age; breast-feeding

Pregnancy Risk Factor X

Lactation Excretion in breast milk unknown/not recommended

Warnings/Precautions Hazardous agent - use appropriate precautions for handling and disposal. Use caution with hepatic impairment; dose adjustment recommended in patients with cirrhosis or severe hepatic dysfunction. May cause dizziness, fatigue, and somnolence; patients should be cautioned before performing tasks which require mental alertness (eg, operating machinery or driving). May increase total serum cholesterol; in patients treated with adjuvant therapy and cholesterol levels within normal limits, an increase of >1.5 x ULN in total cholesterol has been demonstrated in 8.2% of letrozole-treated patients (25% requiring lipid-lowering medications) vs 3.2% of tamoxifen-treated patients (16% requiring medications); monitor cholesterol panel; may require antihyperlipidemics. May cause decreases in bone mineral density (BMD); a decrease in hip BMD by 3.8% from baseline in letrozole-treated patients vs 2% in placebo at 2 years has been demonstrated; however, there was no statistical difference in changes to the lumbar spine BMD scores; monitor BMD.

Adverse Reactions

>10%:

Cardiovascular: Edema (7% to 18%)

Central nervous system: Headache (4% to 20%), dizziness (3% to 14%), fatigue (8% to 13%)

Endocrine & metabolic: Hypercholesterolemia (3% to 52%), hot flashes (6% to 50%)

Gastrointestinal: Nausea (9% to 17%), weight gain (2% to 13%), constipation (2% to 11%)

Neuromuscular & skeletal: Weakness (4% to 34%), arthralgia (8% to 25%), arthritis (7% to 25%), bone pain (5% to 22%), back pain (5% to 18%), bone mineral density decreased/osteoporosis (5% to 15%), bone fracture (10% to 14%)

Respiratory: Dyspnea (6% to 18%), cough (6% to 13%)

Miscellaneous: Diaphoresis (≤24%), night sweats (15%)

1% to 10%:

Cardiovascular: Chest pain (6% to 8%), hypertension (5% to 8%), chest wall pain (6%), peripheral edema (5%); cerebrovascular accident including hemorrhagic stroke, thrombotic stroke (2% to 3%); thromboembolic event including venous thrombosis, thrombophlebitis, portal vein thrombosis, pulmonary embolism (2% to 3%); MI (1% to 2%), angina (1% to 2%), transient ischemic attack

Central nervous system: Insomnia (6% to 7%), pain (5%), anxiety (<5%), depression (<5%), vertigo (<5%), somnolence (3%)

Dermatologic: Rash (5%), alopecia (3% to 5%), pruritus (1%)

Endocrine & metabolic: Breast pain (2% to 7%), hypercalcemia (<5%)

Gastrointestinal: Diarrhea (5% to 8%), vomiting (3% to 7%), weight loss (6% to 7%), abdominal pain (6%), anorexia (1% to 5%), dyspepsia (3%)

Genitourinary: Urinary tract infection (6%), vaginal bleeding (5%), vaginal dryness (5%), vaginal hemorrhage (5%), vaginal irritation (5%)

Neuromuscular & skeletal: Limb pain (4% to 10%), myalgia (7% to 9%)

Ocular: Cataract (2%)

Renal: Renal disorder (5%)

Respiratory: Pleural effusion (<5%)

Miscellaneous: Infection (7%), influenza (6%), viral infection (6%), secondary malignancy (2% to 4%)

<1%, postmarketing, and/or case reports: Anaphylactic reaction, angioedema, appetite increased, arterial thrombosis, blurred vision, cardiac failure, carpal tunnel syndrome, dry skin, dysesthesia, endometrial cancer, endometrial hyperplasia, endometrial proliferation, erythema multiforme, eye irritation, fever, hepatitis, hypoesthesia, irritability, leukopenia, liver enzymes increased, memory impairment, nervousness, palpitations, paresthesia, stomatitis, tachycardia, taste disturbance, thirst, thrombocytopenia, toxic

epidermal necrolysis, trigger finger, urinary frequency increased, urticaria, vaginal discharge, xerostomia

Drug Interactions

Metabolism/Transport Effects **Substrate** of CYP2A6 (minor), CYP3A4 (minor); **Note:** Assignment of Major/Minor substrate status based on clinically relevant drug interaction potential; **Inhibits** CYP2A6 (strong), CYP2C19 (weak)

Avoid Concomitant Use There are no known interactions where it is recommended to avoid concomitant use.

Increased Effect/Toxicity

Letrozole may increase the levels/effects of: CYP2A6 Substrates

Decreased Effect

The levels/effects of Letrozole may be decreased by: Tamoxifen; Tocilizumab

Storage/Stability Store at room temperature of 25°C (77°F); excursions permitted to 15°C to 30°C (59°F to 86°F).

Mechanism of Action Nonsteroidal competitive inhibitor of the aromatase enzyme system which binds to the heme group of aromatase, a cytochrome P450 enzyme which catalyzes conversion of androgens to estrogens (specifically, androstenedione to estrone and testosterone to estradiol). This leads to inhibition of the enzyme and a significant reduction in plasma estrogen (estrone, estradiol and estrone sulfate) levels. Does not affect synthesis of adrenal or thyroid hormones, aldosterone, or androgens.

Pharmacodynamics/Kinetics

Absorption: Rapid and well absorbed; not affected by food

Distribution: V_d: ~1.9 L/kg

Protein binding, plasma: Weak

Metabolism: Hepatic via CYP3A4 and 2A6 to an inactive carbinol metabolite

Half-life elimination: Terminal: ~2 days

Time to steady state, plasma: 2-6 weeks

Excretion: Urine (90%; 6% as unchanged drug, 75% as glucuronide carbinol metabolite, 9% as unidentified metabolites)

Dosing

Adult & Geriatric Females: Postmenopausal:

Breast cancer, advanced (first- or second-line treatment): Oral: 2.5 mg once daily; continue until tumor progression

Breast cancer, early (adjuvant treatment): Oral: 2.5 mg once daily; optimal duration unknown, duration in clinical trial is 5 years; discontinue at relapse

Breast cancer, early (extended adjuvant treatment): Oral: 2.5 mg once daily; optimal duration unknown, duration in clinical trials is 5 years (after 5 years of tamoxifen); discontinue at relapse

Ovarian (epithelial) cancer (unlabeled use): Oral: 2.5 mg once daily; continue until disease progression (Ramirez, 2008)

Renal Impairment No dosage adjustment is required in patients with renal impairment if Cl_{cr} is ≥10 mL/minute.

Hepatic Impairment

Mild-to-moderate impairment (Child-Pugh class A or B): No adjustment recommended.

Severe impairment (Child-Pugh class C) and cirrhosis: 2.5 mg every other day.

Combination Regimens

Breast cancer: Lapatinib-Letrozole (Breast Cancer) on page 1698

Administration Administer with or without food.

Monitoring Parameters Monitor periodically during therapy: Complete blood counts, thyroid function tests; serum electrolytes, cholesterol, transaminases, and creatinine; blood pressure; bone density

Dietary Considerations May be taken without regard to meals. Calcium and vitamin D supplementation are recommended.

Additional Information **Oncology Comment:** The American Society of Clinical Oncology (ASCO) guidelines for adjuvant endocrine therapy in postmenopausal women with HR-positive breast cancer (Burstein, 2010) recommend considering aromatase inhibitor (AI) therapy at some point in the treatment course (primary, sequentially, or extended). Optimal duration at this time is not known; however, treatment with an AI should not exceed 5 years in primary and extended therapies, and 2-3 years if followed by tamoxifen in sequential therapy (total of 5 years). If initial therapy with AI has been discontinued before the 5 years, consideration should be taken to receive tamoxifen for a total of 5 years. The optimal time to switch to an AI is also not known, but data supports switching after 2-3 years of tamoxifen (sequential) or after 5 years of tamoxifen (extended). If patient becomes intolerant or has poor adherence, consideration should be made to switch to another AI or initiate tamoxifen.

Dosage Forms Excipient information presented when available (limited, particularly for generics); consult specific product labeling.

Tablet, oral: 2.5 mg

Femara®: 2.5 mg

References

Burstein HJ, Prestrud AA, Seidenfeld J, et al, "American Society of Clinical Oncology Clinical Practice Guideline: Update on Adjuvant Endocrine Therapy for Women with Hormone Receptor-Positive Breast Cancer," *J Clin Oncol*, 2010, 28(23):3784-96.

Coates AS, Keshaviah A, Thurlimann B, et al, "Five Years of Letrozole Compared With Tamoxifen as Initial Adjuvant Therapy for Postmenopausal Women With Endocrine-Responsive Early Breast Cancer: Update of Study BIG 1-98," *J Clin Oncol*, 2007, 25(5):486-92.

Ramirez PT, Schmeler EM, Milam MR, et al, "Efficacy of Letrozole in the Treatment of Recurrent Platinum- and Taxane-Resistant High-Grade Cancer of the Ovary or Peritoneum," *Gynecol Oncol*, 2008, 110(1):56-9.

Winer EP, Hudis C, Burstein HJ, et al, "American Society of Clinical Oncology Technology Assessment on the Use of Aromatase Inhibitors as Adjuvant Therapy for Postmenopausal Women With Hormone Receptor-Positive Breast Cancer: Status Report 2004," *J Clin Oncol*, 2005, 23(3):619-29.

◆ **Letrozole Tablets, USP (Can)** *see* Letrozole *on page 867*

◆ **Leucovorin** *see* Leucovorin Calcium *on page 870*

Leucovorin Calcium (loo koe VOR in KAL see um)

Related Information

Oral Mucositis/Stomatitis *on page 1814*

Brand Names: Canada Lederle Leucovorin

Index Terms 5-Formyl Tetrahydrofolate; Calcium Folinate; Calcium Leucovorin; Citrovorum Factor; Folinate Calcium; Folinic Acid (error prone synonym); Leucovorin

Generic Availability (U.S.) Yes

Pharmacologic Category Antidote; Chemotherapy Modulating Agent; Rescue Agent (Chemotherapy); Vitamin, Water Soluble

Use Antidote for folic acid antagonists (methotrexate, trimethoprim, pyrimethamine) and rescue therapy following high-dose methotrexate; in combination with fluorouracil in the treatment of colon cancer; treatment of megaloblastic anemias when folate is deficient as in infancy, sprue, pregnancy, and nutritional deficiency when oral folate therapy is not possible

Unlabeled Use Adjunctive cofactor therapy in methanol toxicity; prevention of pyrimethamine hematologic toxicity in HIV-positive patients

Labeled Contraindications Pernicious anemia or vitamin B_{12}-deficient megaloblastic anemias

Pregnancy Risk Factor C

Lactation Excretion in breast milk unknown/use caution

Warnings/Precautions When used for the treatment of accidental weak folic acid antagonist overdose, administer as soon as possible. When used for the treatment of a methotrexate overdose, administer as soon as possible. Do not wait for the results of a methotrexate level before initiating therapy. It is important to adjust the leucovorin dose once a methotrexate level is known. When used for methotrexate rescue therapy, methotrexate serum concentrations should be monitored to determine dose and duration of leucovorin therapy. The dose may need to be increased or administration prolonged in situations where methotrexate excretion may be delayed (eg, ascites, pleural effusion, renal insufficiency, inadequate hydration); **never administer leucovorin intrathecally.** Combination of leucovorin and sulfamethoxazole-trimethoprim for the acute treatment of PCP in patients with HIV infection has been reported to cause increased rates of treatment failure. Leucovorin may increase the toxicity of 5-fluorouracil; dose of 5-fluorouracil may need decreased.

Powder for injection: When doses >10 mg/m^2 are required, reconstitute using sterile water for injection, not a solution containing benzyl alcohol.

Injection: Due to calcium content, do not administer I.V. solutions at a rate >160 mg/minute. Not intended for intrathecal use.

Adverse Reactions Frequency not defined. Toxicities (especially gastrointestinal toxicity) of fluorouracil is higher when used in combination with leucovorin.

Dermatologic: Rash, pruritus, erythema, urticaria
Hematologic: Thrombocytosis
Respiratory: Wheezing
Miscellaneous: Allergic reactions, anaphylactoid reactions

Drug Interactions

Metabolism/Transport Effects None known.

Avoid Concomitant Use

Avoid concomitant use of Leucovorin Calcium with any of the following: Raltitrexed; Trimethoprim

Increased Effect/Toxicity

Leucovorin Calcium may increase the levels/effects of: Capecitabine; Fluorouracil (Systemic); Fluorouracil (Topical)

Decreased Effect

Leucovorin Calcium may decrease the levels/effects of: Fosphenytoin; PHENobarbital; Phenytoin; Primidone; Raltitrexed; Trimethoprim

The levels/effects of Leucovorin Calcium may be decreased by: Glucarpidase

Storage/Stability

Powder for injection: Store at room temperature of 25°C (77°F). Protect from light. Solutions reconstituted with bacteriostatic water for injection U.S.P., must be used within 7 days. Solutions reconstituted with SWFI must be used immediately. Parenteral admixture is stable for 24 hours stored at room temperature (25°C) and for 4 days when stored under refrigeration (4°C).

Solution for injection: Prior to dilution, store vials under refrigeration at 2°C to 8°C (36°F to 46°F). Protect from light.

Tablet: Store at room temperature of 15°C to 30°C (59°F to 86°F).

Reconstitution Powder for injection: Reconstitute with SWFI or BWFI; dilute in 100-1000 mL NS, D_5W for infusion. When doses >10 mg/m^2 are required, reconstitute using sterile water for injection, not a solution containing benzyl alcohol.

Mechanism of Action A reduced form of folic acid, leucovorin supplies the necessary cofactor blocked by methotrexate. Leucovorin actively competes with methotrexate for transport sites, displaces methotrexate from intracellular binding sites, and restores active folate stores required for DNA/RNA synthesis. Stabilizes the binding of 5-dUMP and thymidylate synthetase, enhancing the activity of fluorouracil. When administered with pyrimethamine for the treatment of opportunistic infections, leucovorin reduces the risk for hematologic toxicity.

Methanol toxicity treatment: Formic acid (methanol's toxic metabolite) is normally metabolized to carbon dioxide and water by 10-formyltetrahydrofolate dehydrogenase after being bound to tetrahydrofolate. Administering a source of tetrahydrofolate may aid the body in eliminating formic acid.

Pharmacodynamics/Kinetics

Absorption: Oral, I.M.: Well absorbed

Metabolism: Intestinal mucosa and hepatically to 5-methyl-tetrahydrofolate (5MTHF; active)

Bioavailability: Saturable at oral doses >25 mg; 25 mg (97%), 50 mg (75%), 100 mg (37%)

Half-life elimination: ~4-8 hours

Time to peak: Oral: ~2 hours; I.V.: Total folates: 10 minutes; 5MTHF: ~1 hour

Excretion: Urine (primarily); feces

Dosing

Adult & Geriatric

Treatment of weak folic acid antagonist overdosage (eg, trimethoprim, pyrimethamine): Oral: 5-15 mg/day

Folate-deficient megaloblastic anemia: I.M.: ≤1 mg/day

High-dose methotrexate-rescue dose: Initial: Oral, I.M., I.V.: 15 mg (~10 mg/m^2); start 24 hours after beginning methotrexate infusion; continue every 6 hours for 10 doses, until methotrexate level is <0.05 micromole/L. Adjust dose as follows:

Normal methotrexate elimination: Oral, I.M., I.V.: 15 mg every 6 hours

Delayed early methotrexate elimination: I.V.: 150 mg every 3 hours until methotrexate level is <1 micromole/L, then 15 mg every 3 hours until methotrexate level is <0.05 micromole/L

Colorectal cancer (also refer to Combination Regimens):

I.V.: 200 mg/m^2 over at least 3 minutes (used in combination with fluorouracil 370 mg/m^2)

or

I.V.: 20 mg/m^2 (used in combination with fluorouracil 425 mg/m^2)

Methotrexate overdose: Note: The amount of leucovorin administered should equal the amount of methotrexate inadvertently administered.

I.V.: 1 mg per mg of methotrexate inadvertently administered; 100-1000 mg/m^2 every 3-6 hours has been used; administer until methotrexate levels decrease to goal level or longer if methotrexate levels are unavailable or if patient has renal dysfunction or third-space storage (ascites, pleural effusion)

A nomogram for leucovorin rescue in cancer patients receiving high-dose methotrexate based upon a 48-hour methotrexate level may be helpful (Widemann, 2006). Methotrexate level:

≥80 micromole/L: 1000 mg/m^2 every 6 hours

≥8 to <80 micromole/L: 100 mg/m^2 every 3 hours

≥2 to <8 micromole/L: 10 mg/m^2 every 3 hours

≥0.1 to <2 micromole/L: 10 mg/m^2 every 6 hours

Use of I.T. leucovorin is not advised (Jardine, 1996; Smith, 2008).

Pemetrexed toxicity (unlabeled dose): I.V.: 100 mg/m^2 once, followed by 50 mg/m^2 every 6 hours for 8 days (used in clinical trial for CTC grade 4 leukopenia ≥3 days; CTC grade 4 neutropenia ≥3 days; immediately for CTC grade 4 thrombocytopenia, bleeding associated with grade 3 thrombocytopenia, or grade 3 or 4 mucositis)

Cofactor therapy in methanol toxicity (unlabeled use): I.V.: 1 mg/kg (maximum dose: 50 mg) over 30-60 minutes every 4-6 hours. Therapy should continue until methanol and formic acid have been completely eliminated (Barceloux, 2002)

Prevention of pyrimethamine hematologic toxicity in HIV-positive patients (unlabeled uses; CDC, 2009): Oral:

Isosporiasis (*Isospora belli*):

Treatment: 10-25 mg once daily (in combination with pyrimethamine)

Chronic maintenance (secondary prophylaxis): 5-10 mg once daily (in combination with pyrimethamine)

Pneumocystis jirovecii pneumonia (PCP): Prophylaxis (primary and secondary): 25 mg once weekly (in combination with pyrimethamine [with dapsone]) **or** 10 mg once daily (in combination with pyrimethamine [with atovaquone])

Toxoplasmosis (*Toxoplasma gondii*):

Primary prophylaxis: 25 mg once weekly (in combination with pyrimethamine [with dapsone]) **or** 10 mg once daily (in combination with pyrimethamine [with atovaquone])

Treatment: 10-25 mg once daily (in combination with pyrimethamine [with either sulfadiazine, clindamycin, atovaquone, or azithromycin]). **Note:** May increase leucovorin to 50-100 mg/day in divided doses in cases of pyrimethamine toxicity (rash, nausea, bone marrow suppression).

Chronic maintenance (secondary prophylaxis): 10-25 mg once daily (in combination with pyrimethamine [with either sulfadiazine or clindamycin]) **or** 10 mg once daily (in combination with pyrimethamine [with atovaquone])

Pediatric

Treatment of weak folic acid antagonist overdosage (eg, trimethoprim, pyrimethamine): Refer to adult dosing.

Folate-deficient megaloblastic anemia: Refer to adult dosing.

High-dose methotrexate-rescue dose: Refer to adult dosing.

Cofactor therapy in methanol toxicity (unlabeled use): Refer to adult dosing.

Prevention of pyrimethamine hematologic toxicity in HIV-positive patients (unlabeled uses; CDC, 2009): Infants and Children >1 month of age: **Note:** Leucovorin should continue for 1 week after pyrimethamine is discontinued.

Toxoplasmosis (*Toxoplasma gondii*):

Primary prophylaxis: Oral: 5 mg once every 3 days (in combination with pyrimethamine [with either dapsone or atovaquone])

Secondary prophylaxis: Oral: 5 mg once every 3 days (in combination with pyrimethamine [with either sulfadiazine, atovaquone, or clindamycin])

Treatment (congenital): Oral or I.M.: 10 mg with every pyrimethamine dose (in combination with either sulfadiazine or clindamycin); treatment duration: 12 months

Treatment (acquired): Oral: Acute induction: 10-25 mg once daily (in combination with pyrimethamine [with either sulfadiazine, clindamycin, or atovaquone]) for ≥6 weeks

Combination Regimens

Bladder cancer: M-VAC (Bladder Cancer) on page 1718
Colorectal cancer:
Bevacizumab-Fluorouracil-Leucovorin on page 1530
Bevacizumab + FOLFIRI (Colorectal) on page 1530
Bevacizumab-Oxaliplatin-Fluorouracil-Leucovorin on page 1531
Cetuximab + FOLFIRI (Colorectal) on page 1559
Cetuximab-FOLFOX4 on page 1560
FLOX (Colorectal) on page 1645
Fluorouracil-Leucovorin on page 1653
Fluorouracil-Leucovorin-Irinotecan (Saltz Regimen) on page 1656
FOLFIRI (Colorectal Cancer) on page 1659
FOLFOX1 (Colorectal) on page 1662
FOLFOX2 (Colorectal) on page 1662
FOLFOX3 (Colorectal) on page 1662
FOLFOX4 (Colorectal) on page 1663
FOLFOX6 and mFOLFOX6 (Colorectal) on page 1663
FOLFOX7 (Colorectal) on page 1664
FOLFOXIRI (Colorectal) on page 1665
FU-LV-CPT-11 on page 1666
Panitumumab + FOLFIRI (Colorectal) on page 1733
Panitumumab + FOLFOX4 (Colorectal) on page 1733
Ziv-Aflibercept + FOLFIRI (Colorectal) on page 1779
Esophageal Cancer:
Docetaxel-Oxaliplatin-Leucovorin-Fluorouracil (Esophageal Cancer) on page 1613
Fluorouracil-Leucovorin-Oxaliplatin (Esophageal Cancer) on page 1656
Irinotecan-Fluorouracil-Leucovorin (Esophageal Cancer) on page 1696
Gastric cancer:
Fluorouracil-Leucovorin-Oxaliplatin (Gastric Cancer) on page 1657
Irinotecan-Leucovorin-Fluorouracil (Gastric Cancer) on page 1697
Gestational trophoblastic tumor:
EMA/CO on page 1622
EP/EMA on page 1625
Leukemia, acute lymphocytic:
Hyper-CVAD + Imatinib on page 1680
Hyper-CVAD (Leukemia, Acute Lymphocytic) on page 1681
Linker Protocol (ALL) on page 1703
PVA (POG 8602) on page 1742
Lymphoma, non-Hodgkin's:
CODOX-M on page 1590
COMLA on page 1595

Hyper-CVAD (Lymphoma, non-Hodgkin's) on page 1687
MACOP-B on page 1704
m-BACOD on page 1706
Pro-MACE-CytaBOM on page 1741

Lymphoma, non-Hodgkin's (Burkitt): CODOX-M/IVAC on page 1591

Lymphoma, non-Hodgkin's (Mantle cell): Hyper-CVAD + Rituximab on page 1688

Osteosarcoma:
HDMTX on page 1679
MTX-CDDPAdr on page 1717
POG-8651 on page 1740

Pancreatic cancer:
Fluorouracil-Leucovorin (Pancreatic) on page 1658
FOLFIRINOX (Pancreatic) on page 1661
FOLFOX (Pancreatic) on page 1665

Administration Due to calcium content, do not administer I.V. solutions at a rate >160 mg/minute; not intended for intrathecal use.

Refer to individual protocols. Should be administered I.M., I.V. push, or I.V. infusion (15 minutes to 2 hours). Leucovorin should not be administered concurrently with methotrexate. It is commonly initiated 24 hours after the start of methotrexate. Toxicity to normal tissues may be irreversible if leucovorin is not initiated by ~40 hours after the start of methotrexate.

As a rescue after folate antagonists: Administer by I.V. bolus, I.M., or orally. Do not administer orally in the presence of nausea or vomiting. Doses >25 mg should be administered parenterally.

In combination with fluorouracil: Fluorouracil activity, the fluorouracil is usually given after, or at the midpoint, of the leucovorin infusion. Leucovorin is usually administered by I.V. bolus injection or short (10-120 minutes) I.V. infusion. Other administration schedules have been used; refer to individual protocols.

Extemporaneous Preparations A 5 mg/mL oral suspension may be prepared with tablets, Cologel®, and a 2:1 mixture of simple syrup and wild cherry syrup. Crush twenty-four 25 mg tablets in a glass mortar and reduce to a fine powder; transfer powder to amber bottle. Add 30 mL Cologel® and shake mixture thoroughly. Add a quantity of syrup mixture sufficient to make 120 mL. Label "shake well" and "refrigerate". Stable for 28 days refrigerated.

Lam MS, "Extemporaneous Compounding of Oral Liquid Dosage Formulations and Alternative Drug Delivery Methods for Anticancer Drugs," *Pharmacotherapy*, 2011, 31(2):164-92.

Monitoring Parameters

High-dose methotrexate therapy: Plasma methotrexate concentration; leucovorin is continued until the plasma methotrexate level <0.05 micromole/L. With 4- to 6-hour high dose methotrexate infusions, plasma drug values in excess of 50 and 1 micromole/L at 24 and 48 hours after starting the infusion, respectively, are often predictive of delayed methotrexate clearance.

Fluorouracil therapy: CBC with differential and platelets, liver function tests, electrolytes

Dietary Considerations Solutions for injection contain calcium 0.004 mEq per leucovorin 1 mg

Dosage Forms Excipient information presented when available (limited, particularly for generics); consult specific product labeling.

Injection, powder for reconstitution [strength expressed as base]: 50 mg, 100 mg, 200 mg, 350 mg, 500 mg

Injection, solution [strength expressed as base, preservative free]: 10 mg/mL (50 mL)

Tablet, oral [strength expressed as base]: 5 mg, 10 mg, 15 mg, 25 mg

References

Barceloux DG, Bond GR, Krenzelok EP, et al, "American Academy of Clinical Toxicology Practice Guidelines on the Treatment of Methanol Poisoning," *J Toxicol Clin Toxicol*, 2002, 40(4):415-46.

Bleyer WA, "New Vistas for Leucovorin in Cancer Chemotherapy," *Cancer*, 1989, 63(6 Suppl):995-1007.

Centers for Disease Control and Prevention, "Guidelines for Prevention and Treatment of Opportunistic Infections in HIV-Infected Adults and Adolescents: Recommendations From CDC, the National Institutes of Health, and the HIV Medicine Association of the Infectious Diseases Society of America," *MMWR Recomm Rep*, 2009, 58(RR-4):1-207.

Centers for Disease Control and Prevention, "Guidelines for the Prevention and Treatment of Opportunistic Infections Among HIV-Exposed and HIV-Infected Children: Recommendations from CDC, the National Institutes of Health, the HIV Medicine Association of the Infectious Diseases Society of America, the Pediatric Infectious Diseases Society, and the American Academy of Pediatrics," *MMWR Recomm Rep*, 2009, 58(RR-11):1-166. Available at http://aidsinfo.nih.gov/contentfiles/Pediatric_OI.pdf

Jardine LF, Ingram LC, and Bleyer WA, "Intrathecal Leucovorin After Intrathecal Methotrexate Overdose," *J Pediatr Hematol Oncol*, 1996, 18(3):302-4.

Smith SW and Nelson LS, "Case Files of the New York City Poison Control Center: Antidotal Strategies for the Management of Methotrexate Toxicity," *J Med Toxicol*, 2008, 4(2):132-40.

Van Delden C and Hirschel B, "Folinic Acid Supplements to Pyrimethamine-Sulfadiazine for *Toxoplasma encephalitis* Are Associated With Better Outcome," *J Infect Dis*, 1996, 173 (5):1294-5.

Widemann BC and Adamson PC, "Understanding and Managing Methotrexate Nephrotoxicity," *Oncologist*, 2006, 11(6):694-703.

◆ **Leukeran®** *see* Chlorambucil *on page 270*

◆ **Leukine®** *see* Sargramostim *on page 1270*

Leuprolide (loo PROE lide)

Related Information

Safe Handling of Hazardous Drugs *on page 1904*

Brand Names: U.S. Eligard®; Lupron Depot-Ped®; Lupron Depot®

Brand Names: Canada Eligard®; Lupron®; Lupron® Depot®

Index Terms Abbott-43818; Leuprolide Acetate; Leuprorelin Acetate; TAP-144

Generic Availability (U.S.) Yes: Injection (solution)

Pharmacologic Category Antineoplastic Agent, Gonadotropin-Releasing Hormone Agonist; Gonadotropin Releasing Hormone Agonist

Use Palliative treatment of advanced prostate cancer; management of endometriosis; treatment of anemia caused by uterine leiomyomata (fibroids); central precocious puberty

Unlabeled Use Treatment of breast cancer; infertility; treatment of paraphilia/hypersexuality

Labeled Contraindications Hypersensitivity to leuprolide, GnRH, GnRH-agonist analogs, or any component of the formulation; undiagnosed abnormal vaginal bleeding; pregnancy; breast-feeding

Lupron Depot® 22.5 mg, 30 mg, and 45 mg are also not indicated for use in women

Pregnancy Risk Factor X

Lactation Excretion in breast milk unknown/contraindicated

Warnings/Precautions Hazardous agent - use appropriate precautions for handling and disposal. Transient increases in testosterone serum levels (~50% above baseline) occur at the start of treatment. Androgen-deprivation therapy (ADT) may increase the risk for cardiovascular disease (Levine, 2010); sudden cardiac death and stroke have been reported in men receiving GnRH agonists; long-term ADT may prolong the QT interval; consider the benefits of ADT versus the risk for QT prolongation in patients with a history of QT_c prolongation, with medications known to prolong the QT interval, or with pre-existing cardiac disease. Tumor flare, bone pain, neuropathy, urinary tract obstruction, and spinal cord compression have been reported when used for prostate cancer; closely observe patients for weakness, paresthesias, hematuria, and urinary tract obstruction in first few weeks of therapy. Observe patients with metastatic vertebral lesions or urinary obstruction closely. Exacerbation of endometriosis or uterine leiomyomata may occur initially. Decreased bone density has been reported when used for ≥6 months; use caution in patients with additional risk factors for bone loss (eg, chronic alcohol use, corticosteroid therapy). In patients with prostate cancer, androgen deprivation therapy may increase the risk for cardiovascular disease, diabetes, insulin resistance, obesity, alterations in lipids, and fractures. Use caution in patients with a history of psychiatric illness; alteration in mood, memory impairment, and depression have been associated with use. Rare cases of pituitary apoplexy (frequently secondary to pituitary adenoma) have been observed with GnRH agonist administration (onset from 1 hour to usually <2 weeks); may present as sudden headache, vomiting, visual or mental status changes, and infrequently cardiovascular collapse; immediate medical attention required. Females treated for precocious puberty may experience menses or spotting during the first 2 months of treatment; notify healthcare provider if bleeding continues after the second month.

Some dosage forms may contain benzyl alcohol which has been associated with "gasping syndrome" in neonates; patients with benzyl alcohol allergy may demonstrate a hypersensitivity reaction (usually local) in the form of erythema and induration at the injection site. Vehicle used in depot injectable formulations (polylactide-co-glycolide microspheres) has rarely been associated with retinal artery occlusion in patients with abnormal arteriovenous anastomosis. Due to different release properties, combinations of dosage forms or fractions of dosage forms should not be interchanged.

Adverse Reactions

Children (percentages based on 1-month and 3-month pediatric formulations combined):

>10%: Local: Injection site pain (≤20%)

2% to 10%:

- Cardiovascular: Vasodilation (2%)
- Central nervous system: Emotional lability (5%), mood altered (5%), headache (3% to 5%), pain (3%)
- Dermatologic: Acne (3%), rash (3% including erythema multiforme), seborrhea (3%)
- Gastrointestinal: Weight gain (≤7%)
- Genitourinary: Vaginal bleeding (3%), vaginal discharge (3%), vaginitis (3%)
- Local: Injection site reaction (≤9%)

<2%: Allergic reaction, alopecia, appetite decreased/increased, arthralgia, asthma, body odor, bradycardia, cervix disorder, constipation, cough, crying, depression, dizziness, dysmenorrhea, dyspepsia, dysphagia, epistaxis, extremity pain, feminization, fever, flu-like syndrome, gait disturbance, gingivitis, goiter, growth retarded, gynecomastia, hirsutism, hyperhidrosis, hyperkinesias, hypertension, infection, leukoderma, musculoskeletal pain, myalgia, myopathy, nausea, nervousness, obesity, pallor, peripheral edema, personality disorder, pharyngitis, purpura, rhinitis, sexual maturity accelerated, sinusitis, skin striae, somnolence, syncope, tearfulness, urinary incontinence, vision decreased, vomiting, weakness

Adults: Note: For prostate cancer treatment, an initial rise in serum testosterone concentrations may cause "tumor flare" or worsening of symptoms, including bone pain, neuropathy, hematuria, or ureteral or bladder outlet obstruction during the first 2 weeks. Similarly, an initial increase in estradiol levels, with a temporary worsening of symptoms, may occur in women treated with leuprolide.

Delayed release formulations:

>10%:

Cardiovascular: Edema (≤14%)

Central nervous system: Headache (≤65%), pain (<2% to 33%), depression (≤31%), insomnia (≤31%), fatigue (≤17%), dizziness/vertigo (≤16%)

Dermatologic: Skin reaction (≤12%)

Endocrine & metabolic: Hot flashes (25% to 98%), testicular atrophy (≤20%), hyperlipidemia (≤12%), libido decreased (≤11%)

Gastrointestinal: Nausea/vomiting (≤25%), bowel function altered (≤14%), weight gain/loss (≤13%)

Genitourinary: Vaginitis (11% to 28%), urinary disorder (13% to 15%)

Local: Injection site burning/stinging (transient: ≤35%)

Neuromuscular & skeletal: Weakness (≤18%), joint disorder (≤12%)

Miscellaneous: Flu-like syndrome (≤12%)

1% to 10% (limited to important or life-threatening):

Cardiovascular: Angina (<5%), arrhythmia (<5%), atrial fibrillation (<5%), bradycardia (<5%), CHF (<5%), deep thrombophlebitis (<5%), hyper-/hypotension (<5%), palpitation (<5%), syncope (<5%), tachycardia (<5%)

Central nervous system: Nervousness (≤8%), anxiety (≤6%), confusion (<5%), delusions (<5%), dementia (<5%), fever (<5%), seizure (<5%)

Dermatologic: Acne (≤10%), alopecia (≤5%), bruising (≤5%), cellulitis (<5%), pruritus (≤3%), rash (≤2%), hirsutism (<2%)

Endocrine & metabolic: Dehydration (≤8%), gynecomastia (≤7%), breast tenderness/pain (≤6%), bicarbonate decreased (≥5%), hyper-/hypocholesterolemia (≥5%), hyperglycemia (≥5%), hyperphosphatemia (≥5%), hyperuricemia (≥5%), hypoalbuminemia (≥5%), hypoproteinemia (≥5%), lactation (<5%), testicular pain (≤4%), menstrual disorder (≤2%)

Gastrointestinal: Dysphagia (<5%), gastrointestinal hemorrhage (<5%), intestinal obstruction (<5%), ulcer (<5%), constipation (≤3%), gastroenteritis/colitis (≤3%), diarrhea (≤2%)

Genitourinary: Prostatic acid phosphatase increased/decreased (≥5%), urine specific gravity increased/decreased (≥5%), impotence (≤5%), balanitis (<5%), incontinence (<5%), penile/testis disorder (<5%), urinary tract infection (<5%), nocturia (≤4%), polyuria (2% to 4%), dysuria (≤2%), bladder spasm (<2%), erectile dysfunction (<2%), hematuria (<2%), urinary retention (<2%), urinary urgency (<2%)

Hematologic: Eosinophilia (≥5%), leukopenia (≥5%), platelets increased (≥5%), anemia

Hepatic: Liver function tests abnormal (≥5%), partial thromboplastin time increased (≥5%), prothrombin time increased (≥5%), hepatomegaly (<5%)

Local: Injection site pain (2% to 5%), injection site erythema (1% to 3%)

Neuromuscular & skeletal: Myalgia (≤8%), paresthesia (≤8%), neuropathy (<5%), paralysis (<5%), pathologic fracture (<5%), bone pain (<2%), arthralgia (≤1%)

Renal: BUN increased (≥5%), creatinine increased (≥5%)

Respiratory: Emphysema (<5%), epistaxis (<5%), hemoptysis (<5%), pleural effusion (<5%), pulmonary edema (<5%), dyspnea (≤2%), cough (≤1%)

Miscellaneous: Diaphoresis (≤5%), allergic reaction (<5%), infection (5%), lymphadenopathy (<5%)

Immediate release formulation:

>10%:

Cardiovascular: ECG changes/ischemia (19%), peripheral edema (12%)

Central nervous system: Pain (13%)

Endocrine & metabolic: Hot flashes (55%)

1% to 10% (limited to important or life-threatening):

Cardiovascular: Hypertension (8%), murmur (3%), thrombosis/phlebitis (2%), CHF (1%), angina, arrhythmia, MI, syncope

Central nervous system: Headache (7%), insomnia (7%), dizziness/lightheadedness (5%), anxiety, depression, fatigue, fever, nervousness

Dermatologic: Dermatitis (5%), alopecia, bruising, itching, lesions, pigmentation

Endocrine & metabolic: Gynecomastia/breast tenderness/pain (7%), testicular size decreased (7%), diabetes, hypercalcemia, hypoglycemia, libido decreased, thyroid enlarged

Gastrointestinal: Constipation (7%), anorexia (6%), nausea/vomiting (5%), diarrhea, dysphagia, gastrointestinal bleeding, peptic ulcer, rectal polyps

Genitourinary: Urinary frequency/urgency (6%), impotence (4%), urinary tract infection (3%), bladder spasm, dysuria, incontinence, testicular pain, urinary obstruction

Hematologic: Anemia (5%)

Local: Injection site reaction

Neuromuscular & skeletal: Weakness (10%), bone pain (5%), peripheral neuropathy

Ocular: Blurred vision

Renal: Hematuria (6%), BUN increased, creatinine increased

Respiratory: Dyspnea (2%), cough, pneumonia, pulmonary embolus, pulmonary fibrosis

Miscellaneous: Infection, inflammation

Children and Adults: *Any formulations:* Postmarketing and/or case reports: Abdominal pain, anaphylactic/anaphylactoid reactions, asthmatic reactions, bone density decreased, coronary artery disease, diabetes; fibromyalgia-like symptoms (arthralgia/myalgia, headaches, GI distress); flushing, hemoptysis, hepatic dysfunction, hypokalemia, hypoproteinemia, injection site induration/abscess, interstitial lung disease, liver injury, MI, pelvic fibrosis, penile swelling, peripheral neuropathy, photosensitivity; pituitary apoplexy (cardiovascular collapse, mental status altered, ophthalmoplegia, sudden headache, visual changes, vomiting); prostate pain, pulmonary embolism, pulmonary infiltrate, seizure, spinal fracture/paralysis, stroke, suicidal ideation/attempt (rare), tenosynovitis-like symptoms, thrombocytopenia, transient ischemic attack, uric acid increased, urticaria, WBC decreased/increased

Drug Interactions

Metabolism/Transport Effects None known.

Avoid Concomitant Use There are no known interactions where it is recommended to avoid concomitant use.

Increased Effect/Toxicity There are no known significant interactions involving an increase in effect.

Decreased Effect

Leuprolide may decrease the levels/effects of: Antidiabetic Agents

Storage/Stability

Eligard®: Store at 2°C to 8°C (36°F to 46°C). Allow to reach room temperature prior to using; once mixed, must be administered within 30 minutes.

Lupron Depot®, Lupron Depot-Ped®: Store at room temperature of 25°C (77°F); excursions permitted to 15°C to 30°C (59°F to 86°F). Upon reconstitution, the suspension does not contain a preservative and should be used immediately; discard if not used within 2 hours.

Leuprolide acetate 5 mg/mL solution: Store at 20°C to 25°C (68°F to 77°F); excursions permitted to 15°C to 30°C (59°F to 86°F). Protect from light and store vial in carton until use. Do not freeze.

Reconstitution

Eligard®: Packaged in two syringes; one contains the Atrigel® polymer system and the second contains leuprolide acetate powder; follow package instructions for mixing

Lupron Depot®, Lupron Depot-Ped®: Reconstitute only with diluent provided

Mechanism of Action Leuprolide, is an agonist of luteinizing hormone-releasing hormone (LHRH). Acting as a potent inhibitor of gonadotropin secretion; continuous administration results in suppression of ovarian and testicular steroidogenesis due to decreased levels of LH and FSH with subsequent decrease in testosterone (male) and estrogen (female) levels. In males, testosterone levels are reduced to below castrate levels. Leuprolide may also have a direct inhibitory effect on the testes, and act by a different mechanism not directly related to reduction in serum testosterone.

Pharmacodynamics/Kinetics

Onset of action: Following transient increase, testosterone suppression occurs in ~2-4 weeks of continued therapy

Distribution: Males: V_d: 27 L

Protein binding: 43% to 49%

Metabolism: Major metabolite, pentapeptide (M-1)

Bioavailability: SubQ: 94%

Excretion: Urine (<5% as parent and major metabolite)

Dosing

Adult & Geriatric

Advanced prostate cancer:

I.M.:

Lupron Depot® 7.5 mg (monthly): 7.5 mg every month **or**

Lupron Depot® 22.5 mg (3 month): 22.5 mg every 12 weeks **or**

Lupron Depot® 30 mg (4 month): 30 mg every 16 weeks **or**

Lupron Depot® 45 mg (6 month): 45 mg every 24 weeks

SubQ:

Eligard®: 7.5 mg monthly **or** 22.5 mg every 3 months **or** 30 mg every 4 months **or** 45 mg every 6 months

Leuprolide acetate 5 mg/mL solution: 1 mg/day

Endometriosis: I.M.: Initial therapy may be with leuprolide alone or in combination with norethindrone; if retreatment for an additional 6 months is necessary, concomitant norethindrone should be used. Retreatment is not recommended for longer than one additional 6-month course.

Lupron Depot®: 3.75 mg every month for up to 6 months **or**

Lupron Depot®-3 month: 11.25 mg every 3 months for up to 2 doses (6 months total duration of treatment)

Uterine leiomyomata (fibroids): I.M. (in combination with iron):

Lupron Depot®: 3.75 mg every month for up to 3 months **or**

Lupron Depot®-3 month: 11.25 mg as a single injection

Breast cancer, premenopausal ovarian ablation (unlabeled use):
Lupron Depot®: 3.75 mg every 28 days for up to 24 months (Boccardo, 1999) **or**
Lupron Depot®-3 month: 11.25 mg every 3 months for up to 24 months (Boccardo, 1999; Schmid, 2007)

Treatment of paraphilia/hypersexuality (unlabeled use; Guay, 2009; Reilly, 2000): Males: I.M.:
Note: May cause an initial increase in androgen concentrations which may be treated with an antiandrogen (eg, flutamide, cyproterone) for 1-2 months (Guay, 2009). Avoid use in patients with osteoporosis or active pituitary pathology.
SubQ: Test dose: 1 mg (observe for hypersensitivity)
Depot I.M.: 3.75-7.5 mg monthly

Pediatric

Precocious puberty (consider discontinuing by age 11 for females and by age 12 for males):
I.M.:
Lupron Depot-Ped® (monthly):
≤25 kg: 7.5 mg every month
>25-37.5 kg: 11.25 mg every month
>37.5 kg: 15 mg every month
Titrate dose upward in increments of 3.75 mg every 4 weeks if down-regulation is not achieved.
Lupron Depot-Ped® (3 month): 11.25 mg or 30 mg every 12 weeks
SubQ (leuprolide acetate 5 mg/mL solution): Initial: 50 mcg/kg/day; titrate dose upward by 10 mcg/kg/day if down-regulation is not achieved. **Note:** Higher mg/kg doses may be required in younger children.

Combination Regimens

Prostate cancer:
Bicalutamide-Leuprolide on page 1533
FL on page 1642

Administration

I.M.: Lupron Depot®, Lupron Depot-Ped®: Administer as a single injection. Vary injection site periodically
SubQ:
Eligard®: Vary injection site; choose site with adequate subcutaneous tissue (eg, upper or mid-abdomen, upper buttocks); avoid areas that may be compressed or rubbed (eg, belt or waistband)
Leuprolide acetate 5 mg/mL solution: Vary injection site; if an alternate syringe from the syringe provided is required, insulin syringes should be used

Monitoring Parameters Bone mineral density

Precocious puberty: GnRH testing (blood LH and FSH levels), measurement of height and bone age every 6-12 months, testosterone in males and estradiol in females (I.M. [monthly] and SubQ formulations: 1-2 months after initiation of therapy or with dosage change; I.M. [3 month] formulation: 2-3 months after initiation of therapy, month 6, and as clinically indicated thereafter); Tanner staging

Prostatic cancer: LH and FSH levels, serum testosterone (~4 weeks after initiation of therapy), PSA; weakness, paresthesias, and urinary tract obstruction in first few weeks of therapy. Screen for diabetes (blood glucose and Hb A_{1c}) and cardiovascular risk prior to initiating and periodically during treatment.

Treatment of paraphilia/hypersexuality (unlabeled use; Reilly, 2000): CBC (baseline, monthly for 4 months then every 6 months); serum testosterone (baseline, monthly for 4 months then every 6 months); serum LH (baseline and every 6 months), FSH (baseline), serum BUN and creatinine (baseline and every 6 months); bone density (baseline and yearly); ECG (baseline)

Test Interactions Interferes with pituitary gonadotropic and gonadal function tests during and up to 3 months after monthly administration of leuprolide therapy.

Additional Information

Eligard® Atrigel®: A nongelatin-based, biodegradable, polymer matrix

Oncology Comment: Guidelines from the American Society of Clinical Oncology (ASCO) for hormonal management of advanced prostate cancer which is androgen-sensitive (Loblaw, 2007) recommend either orchiectomy or luteinizing hormone-releasing hormone (LHRH) agonists as initial treatment for androgen deprivation.

Dosage Forms Excipient information presented when available (limited, particularly for generics); consult specific product labeling.

Injection, powder for reconstitution, as acetate [depot formulation, preservative free]:

Eligard®: 7.5 mg (monthly), 22.5 mg (3 month), 30 mg (4 month), 45 mg (6 month) [contains polylactide-co-glycolide; supplied with diluent]

Lupron Depot-Ped®: 7.5 mg (monthly), 11.25 mg (3 month), 11.25 mg (monthly), 15 mg (monthly), 30 mg (3 month) [contains polylactide-co-glycolide, polysorbate 80]

Lupron Depot®: 3.75 mg (monthly), 7.5 mg (monthly), 11.25 mg (3 month), 22.5 mg (3 month), 30 mg (4 month), 45 mg (6 month) [contains polylactide-co-glycolide, polysorbate 80]

Injection, solution, as acetate: 5 mg/mL (2.8 mL)

References

Adjuvant Breast Cancer Trials Collaborative Group, "Ovarian Ablation or Suppression in Premenopausal Early Breast Cancer: Results From the International Adjuvant Breast Cancer Ovarian Ablation or Suppression Randomized Trial," *J Natl Cancer Inst*, 2007, 99(7):516-25.

Boccardo F, Rubagotti A, Amoroso D, et al, "Endocrinological and Clinical Evaluation of Two Depot Formulations of Leuprolide Acetate in Pre- and Perimenopausal Breast Cancer Patients," *Cancer Chemother Pharmacol*, 1999, 43(6):461-6.

Guay DR, "Drug Treatment of Paraphilic and Nonparaphilic Sexual Disorders," *Clin Ther*, 2009, 31 (1):1-31.

Keating NL, O'Malley AJ, and Smith MR, "Diabetes and Cardiovascular Disease During Androgen Deprivation Therapy for Prostate Cancer," *J Clin Oncol*, 2006, 24(27):4448-56.

Levine GN, D'Amico AV, Berger P, et al, "Androgen-Deprivation Therapy in Prostate Cancer and Cardiovascular Risk. A Science Advisory from the American Heart Association, American Cancer Society, and American Urological Association," *Circulation*, 2010, 121:831-38.

Loblaw DA, Virgo KS, Nam R, et al, "Initial Hormonal Management of Androgen-Sensitive Metastatic, Recurrent, or Progressive Prostate Cancer: 2006 Update of an American Society of Clinical Oncology Practice Guideline," *J Clin Oncol*, 2007, 25(12):1596-605.

Reilly DR, Delva NJ, and Hudson RW, "Protocols for the Use of Cyproterone, Medroxyprogesterone, and Leuprolide in the Treatment of Paraphilia," *Can J Psychiatry*, 2000, 45(6):559-63.

Schmid P, Untch M, Kossé V, et al, "Leuprorelin Acetate Every-3-Months Depot versus Cyclophosphamide, Methotrexate, and Fluorouracil as Adjuvant Treatment in Premenopausal Patients With Node-Positive Breast Cancer: the TABLE Study," *J Clin Oncol*, 2007, 25(18):2509-15.

Schmid P, Untch M, Wallwiener D, et al, "Cyclophosphamide, Methotrexate and Fluorouracil (CMF) Versus Hormonal Ablation With Leuprorelin Acetate as Adjuvant Treatment of Node-Positive, Premenopausal Breast Cancer Patients: Preliminary Results of the TABLE-Study (Takeda Adjuvant Breast Cancer Study With Leuprorelin Acetate)," *Anticancer Res*, 2002, 22(4):2325-32.

Spry NA, Galvão DA, Davies R, et al, "Long-Term Effects of Intermittent Androgen Suppression on Testosterone Recovery and Bone Mineral Density: Results of a 33-Month Observational Study," *BJU Int*, 2009, 104(6):806-12.

- **Leuprolide Acetate** *see* Leuprolide *on page* *876*
- **Leuprorelin Acetate** *see* Leuprolide *on page* *876*
- **Leurocristine Sulfate** *see* VinCRIStine *on page* *1450*
- **Leustatin® [DSC]** *see* Cladribine *on page* *298*
- **Levaquin®** *see* Levofloxacin (Systemic) *on page* *883*
- **Levo-Dromoran** *see* Levorphanol *on page* *892*

Levofloxacin (Systemic) (lee voe FLOKS a sin)

Brand Names: U.S. Levaquin®

Brand Names: Canada APO-Levofloxacin; AVA-Levofloxacin; CO Levofloxacin; Levaquin®; Mylan-Levofloxacin; Novo-Levofloxacin; PMS-Levofloxacin; Sandoz-Levofloxacin

Generic Availability (U.S.) Yes

Pharmacologic Category Antibiotic, Quinolone; Respiratory Fluoroquinolone

Use Treatment of community-acquired pneumonia, including multidrug resistant strains of *S. pneumoniae* (MDRSP); nosocomial pneumonia; chronic bronchitis (acute bacterial exacerbation); acute bacterial rhinosinusitis (ABRS); prostatitis (chronic bacterial), urinary tract infection (uncomplicated or complicated); acute pyelonephritis; skin or skin structure infections (uncomplicated or complicated); reduce incidence or disease progression of inhalational anthrax (postexposure); prophylaxis and treatment of plague (pneumonic and septicemic) due to *Y. pestis*

Unlabeled Use Diverticulitis, enterocolitis (*Shigella* spp), epididymitis (nongonococcal), urethritis (nongonococcal), complicated intra-abdominal infections (in combination with metronidazole), Legionnaires' disease, peritonitis, PID (alternative therapy); traveler's diarrhea

Note: As of April 2007, the CDC no longer recommends the use of fluoroquinolones for the treatment of gonococcal disease due to increased prevalence of fluoroquinolone-resistant *Neisseria gonorrhoeae*.

Labeled Contraindications Hypersensitivity to levofloxacin, any component of the formulation, or other quinolones

Canadian labeling: Additional contraindications (not in U.S. labeling): History of tendonitis or tendon rupture associated with use of any quinolone antimicrobial agent

Pregnancy Risk Factor C

Lactation Enters breast milk/not recommended

Warnings/Precautions **[U.S. Boxed Warning]: There have been reports of tendon inflammation and/or rupture with quinolone antibiotics; risk may be increased with concurrent corticosteroids, organ transplant recipients, and in patients >60 years of age.** Rupture of the Achilles tendon sometimes requiring surgical repair has been reported most frequently; but other tendon sites (eg, rotator cuff, biceps) have also been reported. Strenuous physical activity, rheumatoid arthritis, and renal impairment may be an independent risk factor for tendonitis. Discontinue at first sign of tendon inflammation or pain. May occur even after discontinuation of therapy. Use with caution in patients with rheumatoid arthritis; may increase risk of tendon rupture. Safety of use in pediatric patients for >14 days of therapy has not been studied; increased incidence of musculoskeletal disorders (eg, arthralgia, tendon rupture) has been observed in children. CNS effects may occur (toxic psychoses, tremor, restlessness, anxiety, lightheadedness, paranoia, depression, nightmares, confusion, and very rarely hallucinations increased intracranial pressure (including pseudotumor cerebri, seizures, or toxic psychosis). Potential for seizures, although very rare, may be increased with concomitant NSAID therapy. Use with caution in individuals at risk of seizures, with known or suspected CNS disorders or renal dysfunction. Avoid excessive sunlight and take precautions to limit exposure (eg, loose fitting clothing, sunscreen); may cause moderate-to-severe phototoxicity reactions. Discontinue use if photosensitivity occurs.

Rare cases of torsade de pointes have been reported in patients receiving levofloxacin. Use caution in patients with known prolongation of QT interval, bradycardia, hypokalemia, hypomagnesemia, or in those receiving concurrent therapy with Class Ia or Class III antiarrhythmics.

Severe hypersensitivity reactions, including anaphylaxis, have occurred with quinolone therapy. Reactions may present as typical allergic symptoms after a single dose, or may manifest as severe idiosyncratic dermatologic, vascular, pulmonary, renal, hepatic, and/or hematologic events, usually after multiple doses. Prompt discontinuation of drug should occur if skin rash or other symptoms arise. Prolonged use may result in fungal or bacterial superinfection, including *C. difficile*-associated diarrhea (CDAD) and pseudomembranous colitis; CDAD has been observed >2 months postantibiotic treatment. Peripheral neuropathies have been linked to levofloxacin use; discontinue if numbness, tingling, or weakness develops. **[U.S. Boxed Warning]: Quinolones may exacerbate myasthenia gravis; avoid use (rare, potentially life-threatening weakness of respiratory muscles may occur).** Unrelated to hypersensitivity, severe hepatotoxicity (including acute hepatitis and fatalities) has been reported. Elderly patients may be at greater risk. Discontinue therapy immediately if signs and symptoms of hepatitis occur. Hemolytic reactions may (rarely) occur with quinolone use in patients with latent or actual G6PD deficiency.

Fluoroquinolones have been associated with the development of serious, and sometimes fatal, hypoglycemia, most often in elderly diabetics, but also in patients without diabetes. This occurred most frequently with gatifloxacin (no longer available systemically) but may occur at a lower frequency with other quinolones.

Storage/Stability

Solution for injection:

Vial: Store at room temperature. Protect from light. Diluted solution (5 mg/mL) is stable for 72 hours when stored at room temperature; stable for 14 days when stored under refrigeration. When frozen, stable for 6 months; do not refreeze. Do not thaw in microwave or by bath immersion.

Premixed: Store at ≤25°C (77°F); do not freeze. Brief exposure to 40°C (104°F) does not affect product. Protect from light.

Tablet, oral solution: Store at 25°C (77°F); excursions permitted to 15°C to 30°C (59°F to 86°F).

Reconstitution Solution for injection: Single-use vials must be further diluted in compatible solution to a final concentration of 5 mg/mL prior to infusion.

Mechanism of Action As the S(-) enantiomer of the fluoroquinolone, ofloxacin, levofloxacin, inhibits DNA-gyrase in susceptible organisms thereby inhibits relaxation of supercoiled DNA and promotes breakage of DNA strands. DNA gyrase (topoisomerase II), is an essential bacterial enzyme that maintains the superhelical structure of DNA and is required for DNA replication and transcription, DNA repair, recombination, and transposition.

Pharmacodynamics/Kinetics

Absorption: Rapid and complete

Distribution: V_d: 74-112 L; CSF concentrations ~15% of serum levels; high concentrations are achieved in prostate, lung, and gynecological tissues, sinus, saliva

Protein binding: ~24% to 38%; primarily to albumin

Metabolism: Minimally hepatic

Bioavailability: ~99%

Half-life elimination: ~6-8 hours

Time to peak, serum: Oral: 1-2 hours

Excretion: Urine (~87% as unchanged drug, <5% as metabolites); feces (<4%)

Dosing

Adult & Geriatric Note: Sequential therapy (intravenous to oral) may be instituted based on prescriber's discretion.

Acute bacterial rhinosinusitis: Oral, I.V.:

Manufacturer's recommendations: 750 mg every 24 hours for 5 days or 500 mg every 24 hours for 10-14 days

Alternate recommendations: 500 mg every 24 hours for 5-7 days (Chow, 2012)

Anthrax (inhalational): 500 mg every 24 hours for 60 days, beginning as soon as possible after exposure

***Chlamydia trachomatis* sexually-transmitted infections (unlabeled use) (CDC, 2010):** Oral: 500 mg every 24 hours for 7 days

Chronic bronchitis (acute bacterial exacerbation): Oral: 500 mg every 24 hours for 7 days; Canadian labeling (not in U.S. labeling) also includes a dosage regimen of 750 mg every 24 hours for 5 days

Diverticulitis, peritonitis (unlabeled use) (Solomkin, [IDSA] 2010): Oral, I.V.: 750 mg every 24 hours for 7-10 days; use adjunctive metronidazole therapy

Epididymitis, nongonococcal (unlabeled use) (CDC, 2010): Oral: 500 mg once daily for 10 days

Gonococcal infection (unlabeled use) (CDC, 2010): As of April 2007, the CDC no longer recommends the use of fluoroquinolones for the treatment of uncomplicated or more serious gonococcal disease, unless no other options exist and susceptibility can be confirmed via culture.

Intra-abdominal infection, complicated, community-acquired (in combination with metronidazole) (unlabeled use) (Solomkin, [IDSA] 2010): I.V.: 750 mg once daily for 4-7 days (provided source controlled). **Note:** Avoid using in settings where *E. coli* susceptibility to fluoroquinolones is <90%.

Pelvic inflammatory disease (unlabeled use) (CDC, 2010): Oral: 500 mg once daily for 14 days with or without concomitant metronidazole; **Note:** The CDC recommends use as an alternative therapy only if standard parenteral cephalosporin therapy is not feasible and community prevalence of quinolone-resistant gonococcal organisms is low. Culture sensitivity must be confirmed.

Plague (prophylaxis and treatment): Oral, I.V.: 500 mg every 24 hours for 10-14 days, beginning as soon as possible after exposure. **Note:** Dose of 750 mg once daily may be considered if clinically warranted.

Pneumonia: Oral, I.V.:

Community-acquired (CAP): 500 mg every 24 hours for 7-14 days or 750 mg every 24 hours for 5 days (efficacy of 5-day regimen for MDRSP not established)

Healthcare-associated (HAP): 750 mg every 24 hours for 7-14 days

Prostatitis (chronic bacterial): Oral, I.V.: 500 mg every 24 hours for 28 days

Skin and skin structure infections: Oral, I.V.:

Uncomplicated: 500 mg every 24 hours for 7-10 days

Complicated: 750 mg every 24 hours for 7-14 days

Traveler's diarrhea (unlabeled use): Oral: 500 mg for one dose (Sanders, 2007)

Tuberculosis, drug-resistant tuberculosis, or intolerance to first-line agents (unlabeled use): Oral: 500-1000 mg every 24 hours (CDC, 2003)

Urethritis, nongonococcal (unlabeled use) (CDC, 2010): Oral: 500 mg every 24 hours for 7 days

Urinary tract infections:

Uncomplicated: 250 mg once daily for 3 days

Complicated, including pyelonephritis: 250 mg once daily for 10 days **or** 750 mg once daily for 5 days

Pediatric

Acute bacterial rhinosinusitis (unlabeled use): Oral, I.V.: 10-20 mg/kg/day divided every 12-24 hours for 10-14 days (maximum: 500 mg daily). **Note:** Recommended in patients with a type I penicillin allergy, after failure of initial therapy or in patients at risk for antibiotic resistance (eg, daycare attendance, age <2 years, recent hospitalization, antibiotic use within the past month) (Chow, 2012).

Anthrax (inhalational, postexposure): Oral, I.V.

Infants ≥6 months and Children ≤50 kg: 8 mg/kg every 12 hours for 60 days (do not exceed 250 mg/dose), beginning as soon as possible after exposure

Children >50 kg: 500 mg every 24 hours for 60 days, beginning as soon as possible after exposure

Community-acquired pneumonia (CAP) (IDSA/PIDS, 2011): Note: May consider addition of vancomycin or clindamycin to empiric therapy if community-acquired MRSA suspected; alternative to ceftriaxone or cefotaxime in patients not fully immunized for *H. influenzae* type b and *S. pneumoniae*, or significant local resistance to penicillin in invasive pneumococcal strains.

Infants ≥6 months and Children ≤4 years:

S. pneumoniae (MICs to penicillin ≤2.0 mcg/mL), mild infection or step-down therapy (alternative to amoxicillin): Oral: 8-10 mg/kg/dose every 12 hours (maximum: 750 mg daily)

S. pneumoniae (MICs to penicillin ≥4.0 mcg/mL):

Moderate-to-severe infection (alternative to ceftriaxone): I.V.: 8-10 mg/kg/dose every 12 hours (maximum: 750 mg daily)

Mild infection, step-down therapy (preferred): Oral: 8-10 mg/kg/dose every 12 hours (maximum: 750 mg daily)

H. influenzae, moderate-to-severe infection (alternative to ampicillin, ceftriaxone, or cefotaxime): I.V.: 8-10 mg/kg/dose every 12 hours (maximum: 750 mg daily)

Atypical pathogens, moderate-to-severe infection (alternative to azithromycin) or empiric treatment (alternative to azithromycin +/- beta-lactam; should be limited to macrolide allergic/intolerant patients): Oral, I.V.: 8-10 mg/kg/dose every 12 hours (maximum: 750 mg daily)

Children 5-16 years:

S. pneumoniae (MICs to penicillin ≤2.0 mcg/mL), mild infection or step-down therapy (alternative to amoxicillin): Oral: 8-10 mg/kg/dose once daily (maximum: 750 mg daily)

S. pneumoniae (MICs to penicillin ≥4.0 mcg/mL):

Moderate-to-severe infection (alternative to ceftriaxone): I.V.: 8-10 mg/kg/dose once daily (maximum: 750 mg daily)

Mild infection, step-down therapy (preferred): Oral: 8-10 mg/kg/dose once daily (maximum: 750 mg daily)

H. influenzae, moderate-to-severe infection (alternative to ampicillin, ceftriaxone, or cefotaxime): I.V.: 8-10 mg/kg/dose once daily (maximum: 750 mg daily)

Atypical pathogens:

Moderate-to-severe infection (alternative to azithromycin): Oral, I.V.: 8-10 mg/kg/dose once daily (maximum: 750 mg daily)

Mild infection, step-down therapy (alternative to azithromycin in adolescents with skeletal maturity): Oral: 500 mg once daily

Plague (prophylaxis and treatment): Oral, I.V.: Infants ≥6 months and Children:

<50 kg: 8 mg/kg every 12 hours for 10-14 days (do not exceed 250 mg/dose), beginning as soon as possible after exposure

>50 kg: 500 mg every 24 hours for 10-14 days, beginning as soon as possible after exposure. **Note:** Dose of 750 mg once daily may be considered if clinically warranted.

Renal Impairment Adults:

Normal renal function dosing of 750 mg daily:

Cl_{cr} 20-49 mL/minute: Administer 750 mg every 48 hours.

Cl_{cr} 10-19 mL/minute: Administer 750 mg initial dose, followed by 500 mg every 48 hours.

Hemodialysis/chronic ambulatory peritoneal dialysis (CAPD): Administer 750 mg initial dose, followed by 500 mg every 48 hours; supplemental doses are not required following either hemodialysis or CAPD.

Normal renal function dosing of 500 mg daily:

Cl_{cr} 20-49 mL/minute: Administer 500 mg initial dose, followed by 250 mg every 24 hours.

Cl_{cr} 10-19 mL/minute: Administer 500 mg initial dose, followed by 250 mg every 48 hours.

Hemodialysis/chronic ambulatory peritoneal dialysis (CAPD): Administer 500 mg initial dose, followed by 250 mg every 48 hours; supplemental doses are not required following either hemodialysis or CAPD

Normal renal function dosing of 250 mg daily:

Cl_{cr} 20-49 mL/minute: No dosage adjustment required.

Cl_{cr} 10-19 mL/minute: Administer 250 mg every 48 hours (except in uncomplicated UTI, where no dosage adjustment is required).

Hemodialysis/chronic ambulatory peritoneal dialysis (CAPD): No information available.

Continuous renal replacement therapy (CRRT) (Heintz, 2009; Trotman, 2005): Drug clearance is highly dependent on the method of renal replacement, filter type, and flow rate. Appropriate dosing requires close monitoring of pharmacologic response, signs of adverse reactions due to drug accumulation, as well as drug concentrations in relation to target trough (if appropriate). The following are general recommendations only (based on dialysate flow/ultrafiltration rates of 1-2 L/hour and minimal residual renal function) and should not supersede clinical judgment:

CVVH: Loading dose of 500-750 mg followed by 250 mg every 24 hours.

CVVHD: Loading dose of 500-750 mg followed by 250-500 mg every 24 hours.

CVVHDF: Loading dose of 500-750 mg followed by 250-750 mg every 24 hours.

Hepatic Impairment No dosage adjustment provided in manufacturer's labeling; however, levofloxacin has limited metabolism and is not expected to be affected by hepatic impairment.

Administration

Oral: Tablets may be administered without regard to meals. Oral solution should be administered 1 hour before or 2 hours after meals. Maintain adequate hydration of patient to prevent crystalluria.

I.V.: Infuse 250-500 mg I.V. solution over 60 minutes; infuse 750 mg I.V. solution over 90 minutes. Too rapid of infusion can lead to hypotension. Avoid administration through an intravenous line with a solution containing multivalent cations (eg, magnesium, calcium). Maintain adequate hydration of patient to prevent crystalluria or cylindruria.

Test Interactions Some quinolones may produce a false-positive urine screening result for opiates using commercially-available immunoassay kits. This has been demonstrated most consistently for levofloxacin and ofloxacin, but other quinolones have shown cross-reactivity in certain assay kits. Confirmation of positive opiate screens by more specific methods should be considered.

Medication Guide Available Yes

Dosage Forms Excipient information presented when available (limited, particularly for generics); consult specific product labeling. [DSC] = Discontinued product

Infusion, premixed in D_5W [preservative free]: 250 mg (50 mL); 500 mg (100 mL); 750 mg (150 mL)

Levaquin®: 250 mg (50 mL); 500 mg (100 mL); 750 mg (150 mL)

Injection, solution [preservative free]: 25 mg/mL (20 mL, 30 mL)

Levaquin®: 25 mg/mL (20 mL [DSC], 30 mL [DSC])

Solution, oral: 25 mg/mL (100 mL, 200 mL, 480 mL)

Levaquin®: 25 mg/mL (480 mL) [contains benzyl alcohol, propylene glycol]

Tablet, oral: 250 mg, 500 mg, 750 mg

Levaquin®: 250 mg, 500 mg, 750 mg

◆ **Levo-folinic Acid** *see* LEVOleucovorin *on page 888*

LEVOleucovorin (lee voe loo koe VOR in)

Brand Names: U.S. Fusilev®

Index Terms 6S-leucovorin; Calcium Levoleucovorin; L-leucovorin; Levo-folinic Acid; Levo-leucovorin; Levoleucovorin Calcium Pentahydrate; S-leucovorin

Generic Availability (U.S.) No

Pharmacologic Category Antidote; Chemotherapy Modulating Agent; Rescue Agent (Chemotherapy)

Use Treatment of advanced, metastatic colorectal cancer (palliative) in combination with fluorouracil; rescue agent after high-dose methotrexate therapy in osteosarcoma; antidote for impaired methotrexate elimination and for inadvertent overdosage of folic acid antagonists

Labeled Contraindications History of prior allergic reaction to folic acid or leucovorin calcium (folinic acid)

Pregnancy Risk Factor C

Lactation Excretion in breast milk unknown/not recommended

Warnings/Precautions For I.V. administration only; do not administer intrathecally. Due to calcium content, do not administer I.V. solutions at a rate >160 mg levoleucovorin/minute. Levoleucovorin is not approved for and should not be used to treat pernicious anemia or megaloblastic anemias secondary to vitamin B_{12} deficiency; improper use may induce hematologic remission with progressive neurologic manifestations. Methotrexate serum concentrations should be monitored to determine dose and duration of levoleucovorin therapy; dose may need to be increased or administration prolonged in situations where methotrexate excretion may be delayed (eg, ascites, pleural effusion, renal insufficiency, inadequate hydration). When used for the treatment of accidental folic acid antagonist overdose, administer as soon as possible.

The toxicity of fluorouracil is enhanced by leucovorin calcium and levoleucovorin. Deaths due to severe enterocolitis, diarrhea, and dehydration have been reported in elderly patients receiving weekly leucovorin calcium in combination with fluorouracil. Levoleucovorin is indicated in combination with fluorouracil for the palliative treatment of colorectal cancer; when administered together, the fluorouracil dose is reduced (compared to fluorouracil dosing without levoleucovorin). The typical fluorouracil gastrointestinal toxicities (eg, diarrhea, stomatitis) may be of greater severity or longer duration with fluorouracil and levoleucovorin combination therapy. Symptoms of gastrointestinal toxicity should be completely resolved prior to treatment. Elderly and/or debilitated patients are at higher risk for severe gastrointestinal toxicity. Concomitant use of leucovorin calcium and sulfamethoxazole-trimethoprim for the acute treatment of PCP in patients with HIV infection has been associated with increased rates of treatment failure and morbidity; may also occur with levoleucovorin. Seizures and/or syncope have been reported with leucovorin calcium; generally in patients with CNS metastases or other underlying risk factors.

Adverse Reactions Note: Adverse reactions reported with levoleucovorin either as a part of combination chemotherapy or following chemotherapy.

>10%:

- Central nervous system: Fatigue (≤29%)
- Dermatologic: Dermatitis (6% to 29%), alopecia (≤26%)
- Gastrointestinal: Stomatitis (38% to 72%; grades 3/4: 6% to 12%), diarrhea (6% to 70%; grades 3/4: ≤19%), nausea (19% to 62%), vomiting (38% to 40%), anorexia/appetite decreased (≤24%), abdominal pain (≤14%)
- Neuromuscular & skeletal: Weakness/malaise (≤29%)

1% to 10%:

- Central nervous system: Confusion (6%)
- Gastrointestinal: Dyspepsia (6%), taste perversion (6%), typhlitis (6%)
- Neuromuscular & skeletal: Neuropathy (6%)
- Renal: Renal function abnormal (6%)
- Respiratory: Dyspnea (6%)

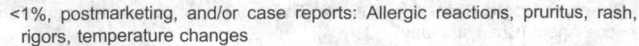

<1%, postmarketing, and/or case reports: Allergic reactions, pruritus, rash, rigors, temperature changes

Drug Interactions

Metabolism/Transport Effects None known.

Avoid Concomitant Use

Avoid concomitant use of LEVOleucovorin with any of the following: Raltitrexed; Trimethoprim

Increased Effect/Toxicity

LEVOleucovorin may increase the levels/effects of: Capecitabine; Fluorouracil (Systemic); Fluorouracil (Topical)

Decreased Effect

LEVOleucovorin may decrease the levels/effects of: Fosphenytoin; PHENobarbital; Phenytoin; Primidone; Raltitrexed; Trimethoprim

The levels/effects of LEVOleucovorin may be decreased by: Glucarpidase

Storage/Stability

Lyophilized powder: Prior to reconstitution, store intact vials at 25°C (77°F); excursions permitted from 15°C to 30°C (59°F to 86°F). Protect from light. Initial reconstituted solution in the vial may be stored for 12 hours at room temperature. Solutions further diluted for infusion in NS are stable for 12 hours at room temperature. Solutions further diluted for infusion in D_5W are stable for 4 hours at room temperature.

Solution for injection: Store intact vials refrigerated at 2°C to 8°C (36°F to 46°F). Protect from light. Store in original carton. Solutions further diluted for infusion in D_5W or NS are stable for 4 hours at room temperature. Do not use if solution appears cloudy or contains a precipitate.

Reconstitution

Lyophilized powder: Reconstitute the 50 mg vial with 5.3 mL NS (preservative free) to a concentration of 10 mg/mL. Do not use if solution appears cloudy or contains a precipitate. May further dilute for infusion in NS or D_5W to a final concentration of 0.5-5 mg/mL. Do not prepare with other products in the same admixture; may cause precipitation.

Solution for injection: May further dilute for infusion in NS or D_5W to a final concentration of 0.5 mg/mL. Do not use if solution appears cloudy or contains a precipitate.

Mechanism of Action Levoleucovorin counteracts the toxic (and therapeutic) effects of folic acid antagonists (eg, methotrexate) which act by inhibiting dihydrofolate reductase. Levoleucovorin is the levo isomeric and pharmacologic active form of leucovorin (levoleucovorin does not require reduction by dihydrofolate reductase). A reduced derivative of folic acid, leucovorin supplies the necessary cofactor blocked by methotrexate.

Leucovorin enhances the activity (and toxicity) of fluorouracil by stabilizing the binding of 5-fluoro-2'-deoxyuridine-5'-monophosphate (FdUMP; a fluorouracil metabolite) to thymidylate synthetase resulting in inhibition of this enzyme.

Pharmacodynamics/Kinetics

Metabolism: Converted to the active reduced form of folate, 5-methyl-tetrahydrofolate (5-methyl-THF; active)

Half-life elimination: 15 mg: 5-7 hours; 300 mg: elimination half life: 16-30 hours

Time to peak, serum: I.V.: 0.9 hours

Dosing

Adult & Geriatric Note: Levoleucovorin, when substituted in place of leucovorin calcium (the racemic form), is dosed at **one-half** the usual dose of leucovorin calcium:

Colorectal cancer: I.V.: The following regimens have been used (in combination with fluorouracil; fluorouracil doses may need to be adjusted for toxicity; no adjustment required for the levoleucovorin dose):

100 mg /m²/day over at least 3 minutes (followed by fluorouracil 370 mg/m²/day) for 5 days every 4 weeks for 2 cycles, then every 4-5 weeks depending on recovery from toxicities, **or**

10 mg /m²/day (followed by fluorouracil 425 mg/m²/day) for 5 days every 4 weeks for 2 cycles, then every 4-5 weeks depending on recovery from toxicities, **or**

Alternative dosing: Levoleucovorin, when substituted in place of leucovorin calcium within a chemotherapy regimen, is dosed at **one-half** the usual dose of leucovorin calcium (Goldberg, 1997; NCCN colon cancer guidelines v.3.2011)

High-dose methotrexate rescue: I.V.: Usual dose: 7.5 mg (~5 mg/m²) every 6 hours for 10 doses, beginning 24 hours after the start of the methotrexate infusion (based on a methotrexate dose of 12 g/m² I.V. over 4 hours). Levoleucovorin (and hydration and urinary alkalinization) should be continued and/or adjusted until the methotrexate level is <0.05 micromolar (5×10^{-8} M) as follows:

Normal methotrexate elimination (serum methotrexate levels ~10 micromolar at 24 hours post administration, 1 micromolar at 48 hours and <0.2 micromolar at 72 hours post infusion): 7.5 mg I.V. every 6 hours for 10 doses

Delayed late methotrexate elimination (serum methotrexate levels >0.2 micromolar at 72 hours and >0.05 micromolar at 96 hours post methotrexate infusion): Continue 7.5 mg I.V. every 6 hours until methotrexate level is <0.05 micromolar

Delayed early methotrexate elimination and/or evidence of acute renal injury (serum methotrexate level ≥50 micromolar at 24 hours, ≥5 micromolar at 48 hours or a doubling or more of the serum creatinine level at 24 hours post methotrexate infusion): 75 mg I.V. every 3 hours until methotrexate level is <1 micromolar, followed by 7.5 mg I.V. every 3 hours until methotrexate level is <0.05 micromolar

Significant clinical toxicity in the presence of less severe abnormalities in methotrexate elimination or renal function (as described above): Extend levoleucovorin treatment for an additional 24 hours (total of 14 doses) in subsequent treatment cycles.

Delayed methotrexate elimination due to third space fluid accumulation, renal insufficiency, or inadequate hydration: May require higher levoleucovorin doses or prolonged administration.

Methotrexate overdose (inadvertent): I.V.: 7.5 mg (~5 mg/m²) every 6 hours; continue until the methotrexate level is <0.01 micromolar (10^{-8} M). Initiate treatment as soon as possible after methotrexate overdose. Increase the levoleucovorin dose to 50 mg/m² I.V. every 3 hours if the 24-hour serum creatinine has increased 50% over baseline, or if the 24 hour methotrexate level is >5 micromolar (5×10^{-6} M), or if the 48-hour methotrexate level is >0.9 micromolar (9×10^{-7} M); continue levoleucovorin until the methotrexate level is <0.01 micromolar (10^{-8} M). Hydration (aggressive) and urinary alkalinization (with sodium bicarbonate) should also be maintained.

Pediatric Note: Levoleucovorin, when substituted in place of leucovorin calcium (the racemic form), is dosed at **one-half** the usual dose of leucovorin calcium:

High-dose methotrexate rescue: Refer to adult dosing.

Methotrexate overdose (inadvertent): Refer to adult dosing.

Administration For I.V. administration only; do not administer intrathecally. Administer by slow I.V. push or infusion over at least 3 minutes, not to exceed 160 mg/minute (due to calcium content).

For colorectal cancer: Levoleucovorin has also been administered (unlabeled administration rate) as I.V. infusion over 2 hours (Comella, 2000; Tournigand, 2006).

Monitoring Parameters High-dose methotrexate therapy or methotrexate overdose (inadvertent): Serum methotrexate and creatinine levels at least once daily. Monitor fluid and electrolyte status in patients with delayed methotrexate elimination (likely to experience renal toxicity).

Product Availability

Fusilev® solution for injection: FDA approved April 2011; availability expected in the third quarter of 2011

Fusilev® solution for injection is a ready-to-use formulation and will be available in 175 mg/17.5 mL and 250 mg/25 mL presentations.

Dosage Forms Excipient information presented when available (limited, particularly for generics); consult specific product labeling.

Injection, powder for reconstitution:

Fusilev®: 50 mg

References

Comella P, De Vita F, Mancarella S, et al, "Biweekly Irinotecan or Raltitrexed Plus 6S-Leucovorin and Bolus 5-Fluorouracil in Advanced Colorectal Carcinoma: A Southern Italy Cooperative Oncology Group Phase II-III Randomized Trial," *Ann Oncol*, 2000, 11(10):1323-33.

Goldberg RM, Hatfield AK, Kahn M, et al, "Prospectively Randomized North Central Cancer Treatment Group Trial of Intensive-Course Fluorouracil Combined With the l-Isomer of Intravenous Leucovorin, Oral Leucovorin, or Intravenous Leucovorin for the Treatment of Advanced Colorectal Cancer," *J Clin Oncol*, 1997, 15(11):3320-9.

Goorin A, Strother D, Poplack D, et al, "Safety and Efficacy of l-leucovorin Rescue Following High-Dose Methotrexate for Osteosarcoma," *Med Pediatr Oncol*, 1995, 24(6):362-7.

Hempel G, Lingg R, and Boos J, "Interactions of Carboxypeptidase G2 With 6S-Leucovorin and 6R-Leucovorin *in vitro*: Implications for the Application in Case of Methotrexate Intoxications," *Cancer Chemother Pharmacol*, 2005, 55(4):347-53.

Jaffe N, Jorgensen K, Robertson R, et al, "Substitution of l-leucovorin for d,l-leucovorin in the Rescue from High-Dose Methotrexate Treatment in Patients With Osteosarcoma," *Anticancer Drugs*, 1993, 4(5):559-64.

Labianca R, Cascinu S, Frontini L, et al, "High-Versus Low-Dose Levo-Leucovorin as a Modulator of 5-Fluorouracil in Advanced Colorectal Cancer: A 'GISCAD' Phase III Study," *Ann Oncol*, 1997, 8(2):169-74.

Scheithauer W, Kornek G, Marczell A, et al, "Fluorouracil Plus Racemic Leucovorin Versus Fluorouracil Combined With the Pure L-Isomer of Leucovorin for the Treatment of Advanced Colorectal Cancer: A Randomized Phase III Study," *J Clin Oncol*, 1997, 15(3):908-14.

Tournigand C, Cervantes A, Figer A, et al, "OPTIMOX1: A Randomized Study of FOLFOX4 or FOLFOX7 With Oxaliplatin in a Stop-and-Go Fashion in Advanced Colorectal Cancer–A GERCOR Study," *J Clin Oncol*, 2006, 24(3):394-400.

◆ **Levo-leucovorin** *see* LEVOleucovorin *on page* *888*

◆ **Levoleucovorin Calcium Pentahydrate** *see* LEVOleucovorin *on page* *888*

Levorphanol (lee VOR fa nole)

Index Terms Levo-Dromoran; Levorphan Tartrate; Levorphanol Tartrate

Generic Availability (U.S.) Yes: Tablet

Pharmacologic Category Analgesic, Opioid

Use Relief of moderate-to-severe pain; preoperative sedation/analgesia; management of chronic pain (eg, cancer) requiring opioid therapy

Labeled Contraindications Hypersensitivity to levorphanol or any component of the formulation; pregnancy (prolonged use or high doses at term)

Pregnancy Risk Factor C

Lactation Excretion in breast milk unknown/not recommended

Warnings/Precautions An opioid-containing analgesic regimen should be tailored to each patient's needs and based upon the type of pain being treated (acute versus chronic), the route of administration, degree of tolerance for opioids (naive versus chronic user), age, weight, and medical condition. The optimal analgesic dose varies widely among patients. Doses should be titrated to pain relief/prevention.

May cause CNS depression, which may impair physical or mental abilities; patients must be cautioned about performing tasks which require mental alertness (eg, operating machinery or driving). Effects may be potentiated when used with other sedative drugs or ethanol. Use with caution in patients with hypersensitivity reactions to other phenanthrene derivative opioid agonists (morphine, hydrocodone, hydromorphone, oxycodone, oxymorphone); respiratory diseases including asthma, emphysema, COPD, hypothyroidism, head trauma, morbid obesity, adrenal insufficiency, prostatic hyperplasia/urinary stricture, or severe liver or renal insufficiency. Use with caution in patients with biliary tract dysfunction; acute pancreatitis may cause constriction of sphincter of Oddi. May be habit-forming. May cause hypotension; use with caution in patients with depleted blood volume or drugs which may exaggerate hypotensive effects (including phenothiazines or general anesthetics). May obscure diagnosis or clinical course of patients with acute abdominal conditions. Concurrent use of agonist/antagonist analgesics may precipitate withdrawal symptoms and/or reduced analgesic efficacy in patients following prolonged therapy with mu opioid agonists. Abrupt discontinuation following prolonged use may also lead to withdrawal symptoms. Elderly and debilitated patients may be particularly susceptible to the adverse effects of narcotics

Ethanol/Nutrition/Herb Interactions

Ethanol: May increase CNS depression; monitor for increased effects with coadministration. Caution patients about effects.

Herb/Nutraceutical: Avoid valerian, St John's wort, kava kava, gotu kola (may increase CNS depression).

Storage/Stability Store at 25°C (77°F); excursions permitted to 15°C to 30°C (59°F to 86°F).

Mechanism of Action Levorphanol tartrate is a synthetic opioid agonist that is classified as a morphinan derivative. Opioids interact with stereospecific opioid receptors in various parts of the central nervous system and other tissues. Analgesic potency parallels the affinity for these binding sites. These drugs do not alter the threshold or responsiveness to pain, but the perception of pain.

Pharmacodynamics/Kinetics

Onset of action: Oral: 10-60 minutes

Duration: 4-8 hours

Metabolism: Hepatic

Half-life elimination: 11-16 hours

Excretion: Urine (as inactive metabolite)

Dosing

Adult & Geriatric Note: These are guidelines and do not represent the maximum doses that may be required in all patients. Doses should be titrated to pain relief/prevention.

Acute pain (moderate-to-severe): *Oral:* Initial: Opiate-naive: 2 mg every 6-8 hours as needed; patients with prior opiate exposure may require higher initial doses; usual dosage range: 2-4 mg every 6-8 hours as needed

Note: The American Pain Society recommends an initial dose of 4 mg for severe pain in adults (APS, 6th ed)

Chronic pain: Patients taking opioids chronically may become tolerant and require doses higher than the usual dosage range to maintain the desired effect. Tolerance can be managed by appropriate dose titration. **There is no optimal or maximal dose for levorphanol in chronic pain. The appropriate dose is one that relieves pain throughout its dosing interval without causing unmanageable side effects.**

Renal Impairment Use with caution; initial dose should be reduced in severe renal impairment.

Hepatic Impairment Use with caution; initial dose should be reduced in severe hepatic impairment.

Dosage Forms Excipient information presented when available (limited, particularly for generics); consult specific product labeling.

Tablet, oral, as tartrate: 2 mg,

Controlled Substance C-II

- **Levorphanol Tartrate** *see* Levorphanol *on page* 892
- **Levorphan Tartrate** *see* Levorphanol *on page* 892
- **Levulan® Kerastick®** *see* Aminolevulinic Acid *on page* 75
- **LH-RH Agonist** *see* Histrelin *on page* 707

Lidocaine and Prilocaine (LYE doe kane & PRIL oh kane)

Brand Names: U.S. EMLA®; Oraqix®

Brand Names: Canada EMLA®

Index Terms Prilocaine and Lidocaine

Generic Availability (U.S.) Yes: Cream

Pharmacologic Category Local Anesthetic

Use

Topical anesthetic for use on normal intact skin to provide local analgesia for minor procedures such as I.V. cannulation or venipuncture; has also been used for painful procedures such as lumbar puncture and skin graft harvesting; for superficial minor surgery of genital mucous membranes and as an adjunct for local infiltration anesthesia in genital mucous membranes.

Periodontal gel: Topical anesthetic for use in periodontal pockets during scaling or root planning procedures

Labeled Contraindications Hypersensitivity to amide-type anesthetic agents; hypersensitivity to any component of the formulation selected; application on mucous membranes or broken or inflamed skin; infants <1 month of age if gestational age is <37 weeks; infants <12 months of age receiving therapy with methemoglobin-inducing agents; children with congenital or idiopathic methemoglobinemia, or in children who are receiving medications associated with drug-induced methemoglobinemia (eg, acetaminophen [overdosage], benzocaine, chloroquine, dapsone, nitrofurantoin, nitroglycerin, nitroprusside, phenazopyridine, phenelzine, phenobarbital, phenytoin, quinine, sulfonamides)

Pregnancy Risk Factor B

Lactation Lidocaine enters breast milk/use caution

Warnings/Precautions Use with caution in patients with severe hepatic impairment. Use with caution in the debilitated or acutely ill patients and the elderly. Use with caution in patients receiving class I and III antiarrhythmic drugs, since systemic absorption occurs and synergistic toxicity is possible. Although the incidence of systemic adverse reactions with EMLA® is very low, caution should be exercised, particularly when applying over large areas and leaving on for longer than 2 hours. Avoid use on open wounds or near the eyes.

When topical anesthetics are used prior to cosmetic or medical procedures, the lowest amount of anesthetic necessary for pain relief should be applied. High systemic levels and toxic effects (eg, methemoglobinemia, irregular heart beats, respiratory depression, seizures, death) have been reported in patients who (without supervision of a trained professional) have applied topical anesthetics in large amounts (or to large areas of the skin), left these products on for prolonged periods of time, or have used wraps/dressings to cover the skin following application.

Adverse Reactions

Cream/patch: Frequency not defined.

Cardiovascular: Angioedema, hypotension
Central nervous system: Shock
Dermatologic: Burning, erythema, hyperpigmentation, itching, rash, urticaria
Genitourinary: Blistering of foreskin (rare)
Local: Burning, edema, stinging
Respiratory: Bronchospasm
Miscellaneous: Alteration in temperature sensation, hypersensitivity reactions

Periodontal gel:

>10%: Local: Application site reaction (1%, includes abscess, edema, irritation, numbness, pain, ulceration, vesicles)

1% to 10%:

Central nervous system: Fatigue (1%)
Gastrointestinal: Bitter taste (2%), nausea (1%)
Respiratory: Infection (1%)
Miscellaneous: Flu-like syndrome (1%), allergic reactions

Drug Interactions

Metabolism/Transport Effects Refer to individual components.

Avoid Concomitant Use

Avoid concomitant use of Lidocaine and Prilocaine with any of the following: Conivaptan

Increased Effect/Toxicity

Lidocaine and Prilocaine may increase the levels/effects of: Antiarrhythmic Agents (Class III); Prilocaine

The levels/effects of Lidocaine and Prilocaine may be increased by: Abiraterone Acetate; Antiarrhythmic Agents (Class III); Beta-Blockers; Conivaptan; CYP1A2 Inhibitors (Moderate); CYP1A2 Inhibitors (Strong); CYP3A4 Inhibitors (Moderate); CYP3A4 Inhibitors (Strong); Darunavir; Dasatinib; Deferasirox; Disopyramide; Hyaluronidase; Ivacaftor; Methemoglobinemia Associated Agents; Mifepristone

Decreased Effect

The levels/effects of Lidocaine and Prilocaine may be decreased by: CYP1A2 Inducers (Strong); CYP3A4 Inducers (Strong); Cyproterone; Deferasirox; Herbs (CYP3A4 Inducers); Tocilizumab

Storage/Stability

Cream/patch: Store at room temperature.

Periodontal gel: Store at 25°C (77°F); excursion permitted to 15°C to 30°C (59°F to 86°F); do not freeze. May turn opaque at temperature ≤5°C. Do not use dental cartridge warmers; heat will cause product to gel.

Mechanism of Action Local anesthetic action occurs by stabilization of neuronal membranes and inhibiting the ionic fluxes required for the initiation and conduction of impulses

Pharmacodynamics/Kinetics

EMLA®:

Onset of action: 1 hour

Peak effect: 2-3 hours

Duration: 1-2 hours after removal

Absorption: Related to duration of application and area where applied

3-hour application: 3.6% lidocaine and 6.1% prilocaine

24-hour application: 16.2% lidocaine and 33.5% prilocaine

Oraqix®: Duration: ~20 minutes

Dosing

Adult & Geriatric

Anesthetic: Topical:

Cream: Apply a thick layer to intact skin and cover with an occlusive dressing.

Transdermal patch (CAN; not available in U.S.): Apply patch or patches to intact skin.

Note: Dermal analgesia can be expected to increase for up to 3 hours under occlusive dressing and persist for 1-2 hours after removal of the cream

Minor dermal procedures (eg, I.V. cannulation or venipuncture): Topical:

Cream: Apply 2.5 g of cream (1/2 of the 5 g tube) over 20-25 cm^2 of skin surface area, or 1 anesthetic disc (1 g over 10 cm^2) for at least 1 hour.

Transdermal patch: (Canadian labeling; not available in U.S.): Apply 1 or more patches to skin surface area <10 cm^2 for at least 1 hour (maximum application time: 5 hours)

Major dermal procedures (eg, more painful dermatological procedures involving a larger skin area such as split thickness skin graft harvesting): Topical: Apply 2 g of cream per 10 cm^2 of skin and allow to remain in contact with the skin for at least 2 hours.

Adult male genital skin (eg, pretreatment prior to local anesthetic infiltration): Apply a thick layer of cream (1 g/10 cm^2) to the skin surface for 15 minutes. Local anesthetic infiltration should be performed immediately after removal of cream.

Adult female genital mucous membranes: Minor procedures (eg, removal of condylomata acuminata, pretreatment for local anesthetic infiltration): Apply 5-10 g (thick layer) of cream for 5-10 minutes

Periodontal gel (Oraqix®): Apply on gingival margin around selected teeth using the blunt-tipped applicator included in package. Wait 30 seconds, then fill the periodontal pockets using the blunt-tipped applicator until gel becomes visible at the gingival margin. Wait another 30 seconds before starting treatment. May reapply; maximum recommended dose: One treatment session: 5 cartridges (8.5 g)

Pediatric Although the incidence of systemic adverse effects is very low, caution should be exercised, particularly when applying over large areas and leaving on for >2 hours

Local anesthetic (procedures): Topical (to intact skin):

Cream: Should **not** be used in neonates with a gestation age <37 weeks nor in infants <12 months of age who are receiving treatment with methemoglobin-inducing agents

Dosing is based on child's age and weight:

Age 0-3 months or <5 kg: Apply a maximum of 1 g over no more than 10 cm^2 of skin; leave on for no longer than 1 hour.

Age 3 months to 12 months and >5 kg: Apply no more than a maximum 2 g total over no more than 20 cm^2 of skin; leave on for no longer than 4 hours.

Age 1-6 years and >10 kg: Apply no more than a maximum of 10 g total over no more than 100 cm^2 of skin; leave on for no longer than 4 hours.

Age 7-12 years and >20 kg: Apply no more than a maximum 20 g total over no more than 200 cm^2 of skin; leave on for no longer than 4 hours.

Note: If a patient >3 months of age does not meet the minimum weight requirement, the maximum total dose should be restricted to the corresponding maximum based on patient weight.

Transdermal patch: Canadian labeling (not available in U.S.): **Note:** Should not be used in neonates with a gestation age <37 weeks nor in infants <12 months of age who are receiving treatment with methemoglobin-inducing agents.

Dosing is based on child's age and weight: Apply patch(es) to skin area(s) ≤10 cm^2:

Age 0-3 months or <5 kg: Apply 1 patch and leave on for ~1 hour (do not exceed 1-hour application time); do not apply more than 1 patch at same time; safety of repeated dosing not established

Age 3 months to 12 months and >5 kg: Apply 1-2 patches for ~1 hour (maximum application time: 4 hours); do not apply more than 2 patches at the same time

Age 1-6 years and >10 kg: Apply 1 or more patches for minimum of 1 hour (maximum application time: 5 hours); maximum dose: 10 patches

Age 7-12 years and >20 kg: Apply 1 or more patches for a minimum of 1 hour (maximum application time: 5 hours); maximum dose: 20 patches

Note: If a patient >3 months of age does not meet the minimum weight requirement, the maximum total dose of EMLA® Patch should be restricted to that which corresponds to the patient's weight

Renal Impairment Smaller areas of treatment are recommended for patients with renal dysfunction.

Hepatic Impairment Smaller areas of treatment are recommended for patients with hepatic dysfunction.

Administration

Cream: For external use only. Avoid application to open wounds or near the eyes. In small infants and children, observe patient to prevent accidental ingestion of cream or dressing. Apply a thick layer (2.5 g/site ~1/2 of a 5 g tube) of cream to designated site of intact skin. Cover site with occlusive dressing. Mark the time on the dressing. **Allow at least 1 hour for optimum therapeutic effect.** Remove the dressing and wipe off excess cream (gloves should be worn). **Smaller areas of treatment are recommended for debilitated patients.**

Transdermal patch (CAN; not available in U.S.): Apply patch or patches to intact skin. **Allow at least 1 hour for optimum therapeutic effect.** After removing patch or patches, clean treated areas thoroughly prior to procedure.

Oraqix® is a viscous liquid. Make sure it is in the liquid form before administration; if gel forms refrigerate until becomes liquid again. Do not use dental cartridge warmers; heat will cause product to gel. Apply slowly and evenly on gingival margin around selected teeth. Not to be used with standard dental syringes; use Oraqix® Dispenser to apply.

Dosage Forms Excipient information presented when available (limited, particularly for generics); consult specific product labeling.

Cream, topical: Lidocaine 2.5% and prilocaine 2.5% (5 g, 30 g)

EMLA®: Lidocaine 2.5% and prilocaine 2.5% (5 g, 30 g)

Gel, periodontal:

Oraqix®: Lidocaine 2.5% and prilocaine 2.5% (1.7 g)

Dosage Forms: Canada Excipient information presented when available (limited, particularly for generics); consult specific product labeling.

Patch, transdermal:

EMLA® Patch: Lidocaine 2.5% and prilocaine 2.5% per patch (2s, 20s) [active contact surface area of each 1 g patch:10 cm^2; surface area of entire patch: 40 cm^2]

References

Broadman LM, Soliman IE, Hannallah RS, et al, "Analgesic Efficacy of Eutectic Mixture of Local Anesthetics (EMLA®) Vs Intradermal Infiltration Prior to Venous Cannulation in Children," *Am J Anaesthesiol*, 1987, 34:S56.

Halperin DL, Koren G, Attias D, et al, "Topical Skin Anesthesia for Venous Subcutaneous Drug Reservoir and Lumbar Puncture in Children," *Pediatrics*, 1989, 84(2):281-4.

Robieux I, Kumar R, Radhakrishnan S, et al, "Assessing Pain and Analgesia With a Lidocaine-Prilocaine Emulsion in Infants and Toddlers During Venipuncture," *J Pediatr*, 1991, 118(6):971-3.

◆ **Lilly CT-3231** *see* Vindesine *on page* 1464

Linezolid (li NE zoh lid)

Brand Names: U.S. Zyvox®

Brand Names: Canada Zyvoxam®

Generic Availability (U.S.) No

Pharmacologic Category Antibiotic, Oxazolidinone

Use Treatment of vancomycin-resistant *Enterococcus faecium* (VRE) infections, nosocomial pneumonia caused by *Staphylococcus aureus* (including MRSA) or *Streptococcus pneumoniae* (including multidrug-resistant strains [MDRSP]), complicated and uncomplicated skin and skin structure infections (including diabetic foot infections without concomitant osteomyelitis), and community-acquired pneumonia caused by susceptible gram-positive organisms

Labeled Contraindications Hypersensitivity to linezolid or any other component of the formulation; concurrent use or within 2 weeks of MAO inhibitors; patients with uncontrolled hypertension, pheochromocytoma, thyrotoxicosis, and/or taking sympathomimetics (eg, pseudoephedrine), vasopressive agents (eg, epinephrine, norepinephrine), or dopaminergic agents (eg, dopamine, dobutamine) unless closely monitored for increased blood pressure; patients with carcinoid syndrome and/or taking SSRIs, tricyclic antidepressants, serotonin 5-$HT_{1B,1D}$ receptor agonists, meperidine, or buspirone unless closely monitored for sign/symptoms of serotonin syndrome

Pregnancy Risk Factor C

Lactation Excreted in breast milk/use caution

Warnings/Precautions Myelosuppression has been reported and may be dependent on duration of therapy (generally >2 weeks of treatment); use with caution in patients with pre-existing myelosuppression, in patients receiving other drugs which may cause bone marrow suppression, or in chronic infection (previous or concurrent antibiotic therapy). Weekly CBC monitoring is recommended. Consider discontinuation in patients developing myelosuppression (or in whom myelosuppression worsens during treatment).

Lactic acidosis has been reported with use. Linezolid exhibits mild MAO inhibitor properties and has the potential to have the same interactions as other MAO inhibitors; use with caution and monitor closely in patients with uncontrolled hypertension, pheochromocytoma, carcinoid syndrome, or untreated hyperthyroidism; use is contraindicated in the absence of close monitoring. Hypoglycemic episodes have been reported; use with caution and closely monitor glucose in diabetic patients. Dose reductions/discontinuation of concurrent hypoglycemic agents or discontinuation of linezolid may be required. Symptoms of agitation, confusion, hallucinations, hyper-reflexia, myoclonus, shivering, and tachycardia may occur with concomitant proserotonergic drugs (eg, SSRIs/SNRIs or triptans) or agents which reduce linezolid's metabolism; concurrent use with these medications is contraindicated unless patient is closely monitored for signs/symptoms of serotonin syndrome. Unnecessary use may lead to the development of resistance to linezolid; consider alternatives before initiating outpatient treatment.

Peripheral and optic neuropathy (with vision loss) has been reported and may occur primarily with extended courses of therapy >28 days; any symptoms of visual change or impairment warrant immediate ophthalmic evaluation and possible discontinuation of therapy. Seizures have been reported; use with caution in patients with a history of seizures. Prolonged use may result in fungal or bacterial superinfection, including *C. difficile*-associated diarrhea (CDAD) and pseudomembranous colitis; CDAD has been observed >2 months postantibiotic treatment.

Due to inconsistent concentrations in the CSF, empiric use in pediatric patients with CNS infections is not recommended by the manufacturer; however, there are multiple case reports describing successful treatment of documented VRE and *Staphylococcus aureus* CNS and shunt infections in the literature. Linezolid should not be used in the empiric treatment of catheter-related blood stream infection (CRBSI), but may be appropriate for targeted therapy (Mermel, 2009). Oral suspension contains phenylalanine.

Ethanol/Nutrition/Herb Interactions

Ethanol: May cause additional CNS depressant effects and provide potential source of additional tyramine content. Management: Avoid ethanol.

Food: Concurrent ingestion of foods rich in tyramine may cause sudden and severe high blood pressure (hypertensive crisis). Food's freshness is also an important concern; improperly stored or spoiled food can create an environment where tyramine concentrations may increase. Management: Avoid tyramine-containing foods with MAOIs.

Herb/Nutraceutical: Ingestion of large quantities of supplements containing caffeine, tyrosine, tryptophan, or phenylalanine. May increase the risk of severe side effects (eg, hypertensive reactions, serotonin syndrome). Management: Avoid supplements containing caffeine, tyrosine, tryptophan, or phenylalanine.

Storage/Stability

Infusion: Store at 25°C (77°F); excursions permitted to 15°C to 30°C (59°F to 86°F). Protect from light. Keep infusion bags in overwrap until ready for use. Protect infusion bags from freezing.

Oral suspension: Following reconstitution, store at 25°C (77°F); excursions permitted to 15°C to 30°C (59°F to 86°F). Use reconstituted suspension within 21 days. Protect from light.

Tablet: Store at 25°C (77°F); excursions permitted to 15°C to 30°C (59°F to 86°F). Protect from light; protect from moisture.

Reconstitution Oral suspension: Reconstitute with 123 mL of distilled water (in 2 portions); shake vigorously. Concentration is 100 mg/5 mL. Prior to administration mix gently by inverting bottle; do not shake.

Mechanism of Action Inhibits bacterial protein synthesis by binding to bacterial 23S ribosomal RNA of the 50S subunit. This prevents the formation of a functional 70S initiation complex that is essential for the bacterial translation process. Linezolid is bacteriostatic against enterococci and staphylococci and bactericidal against most strains of streptococci.

Pharmacodynamics/Kinetics

Absorption: Rapid and extensive

Distribution: V_{dss}: Adults: 40-50 L

Protein binding: Adults: 31%

Metabolism: Hepatic via oxidation of the morpholine ring, resulting in two inactive metabolites (aminoethoxyacetic acid, hydroxyethyl glycine); minimally metabolized, may be mediated by cytochrome P450

Bioavailability: Oral: ~100%

Half-life elimination: Children ≥1 week (full-term) to 11 years: 1.5-3 hours; Adults: 4-5 hours

Time to peak: Adults: Oral: 1-2 hours

Excretion: Urine (~30% of total dose as parent drug, ~50% of total dose as metabolites); feces (~9% of total dose as metabolites)

Nonrenal clearance: Adults: ~65%

Dosing

Adult & Geriatric

Usual dosage: Oral, I.V.: 600 mg every 12 hours

Indication-specific dosing:

Pneumonia:

Community-acquired pneumonia (CAP):

Manufacturer's recommendation (includes concurrent bacteremia): Oral, I.V.: 600 mg every 12 hours for 10-14 days. **Note**: May consider 7-day treatment course (versus manufacturer recommended 10-14 days) in patients with healthcare-, hospital-, and ventilator-associated pneumonia who have demonstrated good clinical response (ATS/IDSA, 2005).

Alternate recommendation (Liu, 2011): Oral, I.V.: *S. aureus* (methicillin-resistant): 600 mg every 12 hours for 7-21 days

Healthcare-associated (HA) pneumonia:

Manufacturer's recommendation: Oral, I.V.: 600 mg every 12 hours for 10-14 days.

Note: May consider 7-day treatment course (versus manufacturer recommended 10-14 days) in patients with healthcare-, hospital-, and ventilator-associated pneumonia who have demonstrated good clinical response (ATS/IDSA, 2005).

Alternate recommendations (Liu, 2011): Oral, I.V.: *S. aureus* (methicillin-resistant): 600 mg every 12 hours for 7-21 days

Skin and skin structure infections, complicated: Oral, I.V.: 600 mg every 12 hours for 10-14 days. **Note:** For diabetic foot infections, initial treatment duration is up to 4 weeks depending on severity of infection and response to therapy (Lipsky, 2012).

Skin and skin structure infections, uncomplicated: Oral: 400 mg every 12 hours for 10-14 days. **Note:** 400 mg dose is recommended in the product labeling; however, 600 mg dose is commonly employed clinically; consider 5- to 10-day treatment course as opposed to the manufacturer recommended 10-14 days (Liu, 2011; Stevens, 2005). For diabetic foot infections, may extend treatment duration up to 4 weeks if slow to resolve (Lipsky, 2012).

VRE infections including concurrent bacteremia: Oral, I.V.: 600 mg every 12 hours for 14-28 days

Brain abscess, subdural empyema, spinal epidural abscess (*S. aureus* [methicillin-resistant]) (unlabeled use; Liu, 2011): Oral, I.V.: 600 mg every 12 hours for 4-6 weeks

Meningitis (*S. aureus* [methicillin-resistant]) (unlabeled use; Liu, 2011): Oral, I.V.: 600 mg every 12 hours for 2 weeks

Osteomyelitis (*S. aureus* [methicillin-resistant]) (unlabeled use; Liu, 2011): Oral, I.V.: 600 mg every 12 hours for a minimum of 8 weeks (some experts combine with rifampin)

Septic arthritis (*S. aureus* [methicillin-resistant]) (unlabeled use; Liu, 2011): Oral, I.V.: 600 mg every 12 hours for 3-4 weeks

Septic thrombosis of cavernous or dural venous sinus (*S. aureus* [methicillin-resistant]) (unlabeled use; Liu, 2011): Oral, I.V.: 600 mg every 12 hours for 4-6 weeks

Pediatric

Usual dosage: Oral, I.V.:

Children ≤11 years: 10 mg/kg (maximum: 600 mg/dose) every 8 hours

Children ≥12 years: Refer to adult dosing.

Indication-specific dosing:

Pneumonia:

Community-acquired pneumonia (CAP):

Manufacturer's recommendation (includes concurrent bacteremia): Oral, I.V.:

Infants (excluding preterm neonates <1 week) and Children ≤11 years: 10 mg/kg/dose every 8 hours for 10-14 days

Children ≥12 years: Refer to adult dosing.

Alternate recommendations:

Infants >3 months and Children ≤11 years (IDSA/PIDS, 2011):

S. pneumoniae (MICs to penicillin ≤2.0 mcg/mL), mild infection or step-down therapy (alternative to amoxicillin): Oral: 10 mg/kg/dose every 8 hours

S. pneumoniae (MICs to penicillin ≥4.0 mcg/mL):

Severe infection (alternative to ceftriaxone): I.V.: 10 mg/kg/dose every 8 hours

Mild infection, step-down therapy (preferred): Oral: 10 mg/kg/dose every 8 hours

S. aureus (methicillin-resistant/clindamycin-susceptible):

Severe infection (alternative to vancomycin or clindamycin): I.V.: 10 mg/kg/dose every 8 hours

Mild infection, step-down therapy (alternative to clindamycin): Oral: 10 mg/kg/dose every 8 hours

S. aureus (methicillin- and clindamycin-resistant):
Severe infection (alternative to vancomycin): I.V.: 10 mg/kg/dose every 8 hours
Mild infection, step-down therapy (preferred): Oral: 10 mg/kg/dose every 8 hours
Children ≤11 years (Liu, 2011): Oral, I.V.: *S. aureus* (methicillin-resistant): 10 mg/kg/dose every 8 hours for 7-21 days (maximum: 600 mg/dose)
Children ≥12 years (IDSA/PIDS, 2011):
S. pneumoniae (MICs to penicillin ≤2.0 mcg/mL), mild infection or step-down therapy (alternative to amoxicillin): Oral: 10 mg/kg/dose every 12 hours
S. pneumoniae (MICs to penicillin ≥4.0 mcg/mL)
Severe infection (alternative to ceftriaxone): I.V.: 10 mg/kg/dose every 12 hours
Mild infection, step-down therapy (preferred): Oral: 10 mg/kg/dose every 12 hours
S. aureus (methicillin-resistant/clindamycin-susceptible):
Severe infection (alternative to vancomycin/clindamycin): I.V.: 10 mg/kg/dose every 12 hours
Mild infection, step-down therapy (alternative to clindamycin): Oral: 10 mg/kg/dose every 12 hours
S. aureus (methicillin- and clindamycin-resistant):
Severe infection (alternative to vancomycin): I.V.: 10 mg/kg/dose every 12 hours
Mild infection, step-down therapy (preferred): Oral: 10 mg/kg/dose every 12 hours
Children ≥12 years (Liu, 2011): *S. aureus* (methicillin-resistant): Refer to adult dosing.
Healthcare-associated (HA) pneumonia: Oral, I.V.:
Manufacturer's recommendation:
Infants (excluding preterm neonates <1 week) and Children ≤11 years: 10 mg/kg every 8 hours for 10-14 days
Children ≥12 years: Refer to adult dosing.
Note: May consider 7-day treatment course (versus manufacturer recommended 10-14 days) in patients with healthcare-, hospital-, and ventilator- associated pneumonia who have demonstrated good clinical response (ATS/IDSA, 2005).
Alternate recommendations (Liu, 2011): *S. aureus* (methicillin-resistant):
Children ≤11 years: 10 mg/kg/dose every 8 hours for 7-21 days (maximum: 600 mg/dose)
Children ≥12 years: Refer to adult dosing.
Skin and skin structure infections, complicated: Oral, I.V.:
Infants (excluding preterm neonates <1 week) and Children ≤11 years: 10 mg/kg every 8 hours for 10-14 days
Children ≥12 years: Refer to adult dosing.
Skin and skin structure infections, uncomplicated: Oral:
Infants (excluding preterm neonates <1 week) and Children <5 years: 10 mg/kg every 8 hours for 10-14 days
Children 5-11 years: 10 mg/kg every 12 hours for 10-14 days
Children ≥12-18 years: 600 mg every 12 hours for 10-14 days
VRE infections including concurrent bacteremia: Oral, I.V.:
Infants (excluding preterm neonates <1 week) and Children ≤11 years: 10 mg/kg every 8 hours for 14-28 days
Children ≥12 years: Refer to adult dosing.

Brain abscess, subdural empyema, spinal epidural abscess (*S. aureus* [methicillin-resistant]) (unlabeled use; Liu, 2011): Oral, I.V.:

Children ≤ 11 years: 10 mg/kg every 8 hours for 4-6 weeks (maximum: 600 mg/dose)

Children ≥12 years: Refer to adult dosing.

Meningitis (*S. aureus* [methicillin-resistant]) (unlabeled use; Liu, 2011): Oral, I.V.: Children ≥12 years: Refer to adult dosing.

Osteomyelitis (*S. aureus* [methicillin-resistant]) (unlabeled use; Liu, 2011): Oral, I.V.:

Infants (excluding preterm neonates <1 week) and Children ≤11 years: 10 mg/kg every 8 hours for a minimum of 4-6 weeks (maximum: 600 mg/dose)

Children ≥12 years: Refer to adult dosing.

Septic arthritis (*S. aureus* [methicillin-resistant]) (unlabeled use; Liu, 2011): Oral, I.V.:

Infants (excluding preterm neonates <1 week) and Children ≤11 years: 10 mg/kg every 8 hours for 3-4 weeks (maximum: 600 mg/dose)

Children ≥12 years: Refer to adult dosing.

Septic thrombosis of cavernous or dural venous sinus (*S. aureus* [methicillin-resistant]) (unlabeled use; Liu, 2011): Oral, I.V.:

Children ≤11 years: 10 mg/kg every 8 hours for 4-6 weeks (maximum: 600 mg/dose)

Children ≥12 years: Refer to adult dosing.

Renal Impairment No adjustment is recommended. The two primary metabolites may accumulate in patients with renal impairment but the clinical significance is unknown. Weigh the risk of accumulation of metabolites versus the benefit of therapy. Monitor for hematopoietic (eg, anemia, leukopenia, thrombocytopenia) and neuropathic (eg, peripheral neuropathy) adverse events when administering for extended periods.

Intermittent hemodialysis (administer after hemodialysis on dialysis days): Dialyzable (~30% removed during 3-hour dialysis session): If administration time is not immediately after dialysis session, may consider administration of a supplemental dose especially early in the treatment course to maintain levels above the MIC (Brier, 2003). Others have recommended no supplemental dose or dosage adjustment for patients on intermittent hemodialysis, peritoneal dialysis, or continuous renal replacement therapy (eg, CVVHD) (Heintz, 2009; Trotman, 2005).

Hepatic Impairment

Mild-to-moderate hepatic impairment (Child-Pugh class A or B): No dosage adjustment required.

Severe hepatic impairment (Child-Pugh class C): Use has not been adequately evaluated.

Administration

I.V.: Administer intravenous infusion over 30-120 minutes. Do not mix or infuse with other medications. When the same intravenous line is used for sequential infusion of other medications, flush line with D_5W, NS, or LR before and after infusing linezolid. The yellow color of the injection may intensify over time without affecting potency.

Oral suspension: Invert gently to mix prior to administration, do not shake. Administer without regard to meals.

Dosage Forms Excipient information presented when available (limited, particularly for generics); consult specific product labeling.

Infusion, premixed:
Zyvox®: 200 mg (100 mL); 600 mg (300 mL) [contains sodium 0.38 mg/mL]
Powder for suspension, oral:
Zyvox®: 100 mg/5 mL (150 mL) [contains phenylalanine 20 mg/5 mL, sodium 8.52 mg (0.4 mEq)/5 mL, sodium benzoate; orange flavor]
Tablet, oral:
Zyvox®: 600 mg [contains sodium 2.92 mg (0.1 mEq)/tablet]

- **Lipodox** *see* DOXOrubicin (Liposomal) *on page 473*
- **Liposomal Cytarabine** *see* Cytarabine (Liposomal) *on page 361*
- **Liposomal DAUNOrubicin** *see* DAUNOrubicin (Liposomal) *on page 400*
- **Liposomal DOXOrubicin** *see* DOXOrubicin (Liposomal) *on page 473*
- **Liposomal Vincristine** *see* VinCRIStine (Liposomal) *on page 1459*
- **Liposome Vincristine** *see* VinCRIStine (Liposomal) *on page 1459*
- **L-leucovorin** *see* LEVOleucovorin *on page 888*
- **LM3100** *see* Plerixafor *on page 1180*
- **Locoid®** *see* Hydrocortisone (Topical) *on page 719*
- **Locoid Lipocream®** *see* Hydrocortisone (Topical) *on page 719*
- **L-OHP** *see* Oxaliplatin *on page 1077*

Lomustine (loe MUS teen)

Related Information

Management of Chemotherapy-Induced Nausea and Vomiting *on page 1786*
Safe Handling of Hazardous Drugs *on page 1904*

Brand Names: U.S. CeeNU®

Brand Names: Canada CeeNU®

Index Terms CCNU; Lomustinum

Generic Availability (U.S.) No

Pharmacologic Category Antineoplastic Agent; Antineoplastic Agent, Alkylating Agent; Antineoplastic Agent, Alkylating Agent (Nitrosourea)

Use Treatment of primary and metastatic brain tumors (after surgery and/or radiation therapy); treatment of relapsed or refractory Hodgkin's disease (as part of a combination chemotherapy regimen)

Unlabeled Use Treatment of gastric cancer, metastatic melanoma

Labeled Contraindications Hypersensitivity to lomustine or any component of the formulation

Pregnancy Risk Factor D

Lactation Enters breast milk/not recommended

Warnings/Precautions Hazardous agent - use appropriate precautions for handling and disposal. **[U.S. Boxed Warnings]: Cumulative and delayed bone marrow suppression, particularly thrombocytopenia and leukopenia, commonly occur; may lead to bleeding and overwhelming infections in an already compromised patient.** Do not administer courses more frequently than every 6 weeks due to delayed myelotoxicity. Use with caution in patients with depressed platelet, leukocyte, or erythrocyte counts. Because bone marrow toxicity is cumulative, dose adjustments should be based on nadir counts from prior dose.

May cause delayed pulmonary toxicity (infiltrates and/or fibrosis); usually related to cumulative doses >1100 mg/m^2; may be delayed (has been reported up to 17 years after childhood administration in combination with radiation therapy); patients with baseline below 70% of predicted forced vital capacity or carbon monoxide diffusing capacity are in increased risk. Long-term use may be associated with the development of secondary malignancies. Reversible hepatotoxicity (transaminase, alkaline phosphatase and bilirubin elevations) has been reported; use with caution in patients with hepatic impairment. Kidney damage has been observed and azotemia, decreased kidney size and renal failure have been reported with long-term use; use with caution in patients with renal impairment; may require dosage adjustment. **[U.S. Boxed Warning]: Should be administered under the supervision of an experienced cancer chemotherapy physician.** Lomustine should only be administered as a single dose once every 6 weeks; serious errors have occurred when lomustine was inadvertently administered daily.

Adverse Reactions

>10%:

Gastrointestinal: Nausea and vomiting, (onset: 3-6 hours after oral administration; duration: <24 hours)

Hematologic: Myelosuppression (dose-limiting, delayed, cumulative); leukopenia (65%; nadir: 5-6 weeks; recovery 6-8 weeks); thrombocytopenia (nadir: 4 weeks; recovery 5-6 weeks)

Frequency not defined: Acute leukemia, alkaline phosphatase increased, alopecia, anemia, ataxia, azotemia (progressive), bilirubin increased, blindness, bone marrow dysplasia, disorientation, dysarthria, hepatotoxicity, kidney size decreased, lethargy, optic atrophy, pulmonary fibrosis, pulmonary infiltrates, renal damage, renal failure, stomatitis, transaminases increased, visual disturbances

Drug Interactions

Metabolism/Transport Effects **Substrate** of CYP2D6 (minor); **Note:** Assignment of Major/Minor substrate status based on clinically relevant drug interaction potential; **Inhibits** CYP2D6 (weak), CYP3A4 (weak)

Avoid Concomitant Use

Avoid concomitant use of Lomustine with any of the following: BCG; CloZAPine; Natalizumab; Pimecrolimus; Pimozide; Tacrolimus (Topical); Vaccines (Live)

Increased Effect/Toxicity

Lomustine may increase the levels/effects of: ARIPiprazole; CloZAPine; Leflunomide; Natalizumab; Pimozide; Vaccines (Live)

The levels/effects of Lomustine may be increased by: Denosumab; Pimecrolimus; Roflumilast; Tacrolimus (Topical); Trastuzumab

Decreased Effect

Lomustine may decrease the levels/effects of: BCG; Coccidioidin Skin Test; Sipuleucel-T; Vaccines (Inactivated); Vaccines (Live)

The levels/effects of Lomustine may be decreased by: Echinacea; Peginterferon Alfa-2b

Ethanol/Nutrition/Herb Interactions Ethanol: Avoid ethanol (due to GI irritation).

Storage/Stability Store at room temperature of 25°C (77°F); excursions permitted to 15°C to 30°C (59°F to 86°F).

Mechanism of Action Inhibits DNA and RNA synthesis via carbamylation of DNA polymerase, alkylation of DNA, and alteration of RNA, proteins, and enzymes

Pharmacodynamics/Kinetics

Duration: Marrow recovery: ~5-8 weeks

Absorption: Complete

Distribution: Crosses blood-brain barrier to a greater degree than BCNU; CNS concentrations are ≥50% of plasma concentrations

Metabolism: Rapidly hepatic via hydroxylation producing at least two active metabolites; enterohepatically recycled

Half-life elimination: Parent drug: 16-24 hours; Active metabolite: 16-48 hours

Time to peak, serum: Active metabolite: ~3 hours

Excretion: Urine (~50%, as metabolites); feces (<5%); expired air (<10%)

Dosing

Adult & Geriatric Note: Repeat courses should only be administered after adequate recovery of leukocytes to >4000/mm^3 and platelets to >100,000/mm^3. Details concerning dosage in combination regimens should also be consulted.

Brain tumors, Hodgkin's lymphoma: Oral: 130 mg/m^2 as a single dose once every 6 weeks (dosage reductions may be recommended for combination chemotherapy regimens)

Compromised marrow function: Reduce dose to 100 mg/m^2 as a single dose once every 6 weeks

Dosing adjustment (based on nadir) for subsequent cycles:

Leukocytes >3000/mm^3, platelets >75,000/mm^3: No adjustment required

Leukocytes 2000-2999/mm^3, platelets 25,000-74,999/mm^3: Administer 70% of prior dose

Leukocytes <2000/mm^3, platelets <25,000/mm^3: Administer 50% of prior dose

Pediatric Note: Repeat courses should only be administered after adequate recovery of leukocytes to >4000/mm^3 and platelets to >100,000/mm^3. Details concerning dosage in combination regimens should also be consulted.

Brain tumors, Hodgkin's lymphoma: Oral: 130 mg/m^2 as a single dose once every 6 weeks (dosage reductions may be recommended for combination chemotherapy regimens)

Compromised marrow function: Reduce dose to 100 mg/m^2 as a single dose once every 6 weeks

Dosing adjustment (based on nadir) for subsequent cycles: Refer to adult dosing.

Renal Impairment

The FDA-approved labeling does not contain renal dosing adjustment guidelines. The following guidelines have been used by some clinicians:

Aronoff, 2007: Adults:

Cl_{cr} 10-50 mL/minute: Administer 75% of dose

Cl_{cr} <10 mL/minute: Administer 25% to 50% of dose

Hemodialysis: Supplemental dose is not necessary

Continuous ambulatory peritoneal dialysis (CAPD): Administer 25% to 50% of dose

Kintzel, 1995:

Cl_{cr} 46-60 mL/minute: Administer 75% of normal dose

Cl_{cr} 31-45 mL/minute: Administer 70% of normal dose

Cl_{cr} ≤30 mL/minute: Avoid use

Hepatic Impairment The FDA-approved labeling does not contain hepatic adjustment guidelines; lomustine is hepatically metabolized and caution should be used in patients with hepatic dysfunction.

Combination Regimens

Brain tumors:

PCV (Brain Tumor Regimen) on page 1736

POC on page 1740

Administration Oral: Administer with fluids on an empty stomach; no food or drink for 2 hours after administration. Administering on an empty stomach will reduce the incidence of nausea and vomiting. Standard antiemetics may be administered if needed. Varying strengths of capsules may be required to obtain necessary dose.

Do not break capsules; use appropriate precautions (eg, gloves) when handling; avoid exposure to broken capsules.

Emetic Potential Moderate (30% to 90%)

Monitoring Parameters CBC with differential and platelet count (for at least 6 weeks after dose), hepatic and renal function tests (periodic), pulmonary function tests (baseline and periodic)

Dietary Considerations Should be taken with fluids on an empty stomach; no food or drink for 2 hours after administration to decrease nausea.

Dosage Forms Excipient information presented when available (limited, particularly for generics); consult specific product labeling.

Capsule, oral:

CeeNU®: 10 mg, 40 mg, 100 mg

References

Aronoff GR, Bennett WM, Berns JS, et al, *Drug Prescribing in Renal Failure: Dosing Guidelines for Adults and Children*, 5th ed. Philadelphia, PA: American College of Physicians; 2007, p 101.

Cullinan SA, Moertel CG, Wieand HS, et al, "Controlled Evaluation of Three Drug Combination Regimens Versus Fluorouracil Alone for the Therapy of Advanced Gastric Cancer. North Central Cancer Treatment Group," *J Clin Oncol*, 1994, 12(2):412-6.

Federico M, Luminari S, Iannitto E, et al, "ABVD Compared With BEACOPP Compared With CEC for the Initial Treatment of Patients With Advanced Hodgkin's Lymphoma: Results From the HD2000 Gruppo Italiano per lo Studio dei Linfomi Trial," *J Clin Oncol*, 2009, 27(5):805-11.

Kintzel PE and Dorr RT, "Anticancer Drug Renal Toxicity and Elimination: Dosing Guidelines for Altered Renal Function," *Cancer Treat Rev*, 1995, 21(1):33-64.

Medical Research Council Brain Tumor Working Party, "Randomized Trial of Procarbazine, Lomustine, and Vincristine in the Adjuvant Treatment of High-Grade Astrocytoma: A Medical Research Council Trial," *J Clin Oncol*, 2001, 19(2):509-18.

National Comprehensive Cancer Network® (NCCN), "Clinical Practice Guidelines in Oncology™: Central Nervous System Cancers," Version 2.2011. Available at http://www.nccn.org/professionals/physician_gls/PDF/cns.pdf

Pendergrass TW, Milstein JM, Geyer JR, et al, "Eight Drugs in One Day Chemotherapy for Brain Tumors: Experience in 107 Children and Rationale for Preradiation Chemotherapy," *J Clin Oncol*, 1987, 5(8):1221-31.

◆ **Lomustinum** see Lomustine *on page 904*

◆ **Longastatin** see Octreotide *on page 1043*

LORazepam (lor A ze pam)

Related Information

Management of Chemotherapy-Induced Nausea and Vomiting *on page 1786*

Palliative Care Medicine (Cancer) *on page 1871*

Brand Names: U.S. Ativan®; Lorazepam Intensol™

Brand Names: Canada Apo-Lorazepam®; Ativan®; Dom-Lorazepam; Lorazepam Injection, USP; Novo-Lorazem; Nu-Loraz; PHL-Lorazepam; PMS-Lorazepam; PRO-Lorazepam

Generic Availability (U.S.) Yes

Pharmacologic Category Benzodiazepine

Use

Oral: Management of anxiety disorders or short-term (≤4 months) relief of the symptoms of anxiety, anxiety associated with depressive symptoms, or insomnia due to anxiety or transient stress

I.V.: Status epilepticus, amnesia, sedation

Unlabeled Use Ethanol detoxification; psychogenic catatonia; partial complex seizures; agitation (I.V.); antiemetic for chemotherapy; rapid tranquilization of the agitated patient

Labeled Contraindications Hypersensitivity to lorazepam or any component of the formulation (cross-sensitivity with other benzodiazepines may exist); acute narrow-angle glaucoma; sleep apnea (parenteral); intra-arterial injection of parenteral formulation; severe respiratory insufficiency (except during mechanical ventilation)

Pregnancy Risk Factor D

Lactation Enters breast milk/not recommended (AAP rates "of concern"; AAP 2001 update pending)

Warnings/Precautions Use with caution in elderly or debilitated patients, patients with hepatic disease (including alcoholics) or renal impairment. In older adults, benzodiazepines increase the risk of impaired cognition, delirium, falls, fractures, and motor vehicle accidents. Due to increased sensitivity in this age group, avoid use for treatment of insomnia, agitation, or delirium. (Beers Criteria). Use with caution in patients with respiratory disease (COPD or sleep apnea) or limited pulmonary reserve, or impaired gag reflex. Initial doses in elderly or debilitated patients should be at the lower end of the dosing range. May worsen hepatic encephalopathy.

Causes CNS depression (dose-related) resulting in sedation, dizziness, confusion, or ataxia which may impair physical and mental capabilities. Patients must be cautioned about performing tasks which require mental alertness (eg, operating machinery or driving). Use with caution in patients receiving other CNS depressants or psychoactive agents. Effects with other sedative drugs or ethanol may be potentiated. Benzodiazepines have been associated with falls and traumatic injury and should be used with extreme caution in patients who are at risk of these events.

Lorazepam may cause anterograde amnesia. Paradoxical reactions, including hyperactive or aggressive behavior have been reported with benzodiazepines, particularly in adolescent/pediatric or psychiatric patients. Does not have analgesic, antidepressant, or antipsychotic properties.

Use caution in patients with depression, particularly if suicidal risk may be present. Pre-existing depression may worsen or emerge during therapy. Not recommended for use in primary depressive or psychotic disorders. Use with caution in patients with a history of drug dependence, alcoholism, or significant personality disorders. Benzodiazepines have been associated with dependence and acute withdrawal symptoms on discontinuation or reduction in dose. Acute withdrawal, including seizures, may be precipitated after administration of flumazenil to patients receiving long-term benzodiazepine therapy.

As a hypnotic agent, should be used only after evaluation of potential causes of sleep disturbance. Failure of sleep disturbance to resolve after 7-10 days may indicate psychiatric or medical illness. A worsening of insomnia or the emergence of new abnormalities of thought or behavior may represent unrecognized psychiatric or medical illness and requires immediate and careful evaluation.

Parenteral formulation of lorazepam contains polyethylene glycol which has resulted in toxicity during high-dose and/or longer-term infusions. Parenteral formulation also contains propylene glycol (PG); may be associated with dose-related toxicity and can occur >48 hours after initiation of lorazepam. Limited data suggest increased risk of PG accumulation at doses of ≥6 mg/hour for 48 hours or more (Nelson, 2008). Consider monitoring for signs of toxicity which may include acute renal failure, lactic acidosis, and/or osmol gap. In high-risk patients requiring higher doses/extended treatment durations, use of enteral delivery of lorazepam tablets may be beneficial (Jacobi, 2002). Also contains benzyl alcohol; avoid in neonates.

Adverse Reactions

>10%:

Central nervous system: Sedation

Respiratory: Respiratory depression

1% to 10%:

Cardiovascular: Hypotension

Central nervous system: Akathisia, amnesia, ataxia, confusion, depression, disorientation, dizziness, headache

Dermatologic: Dermatitis, rash

Gastrointestinal: Changes in appetite, nausea, weight gain/loss

Neuromuscular & skeletal: Weakness

Ocular: Visual disturbances

Respiratory: Apnea, hyperventilation, nasal congestion

<1% or frequency not defined: Asthenia, blood dyscrasias, disinhibition, euphoria, fatigue, increased salivation, menstrual irregularities, physical and psychological dependence (with prolonged use), reflex slowing, polyethylene glycol or propylene glycol poisoning (prolonged I.V. infusion), suicidal ideation, seizure, vertigo

Drug Interactions

Metabolism/Transport Effects None known.

Avoid Concomitant Use

Avoid concomitant use of LORazepam with any of the following: Azelastine (Nasal); Methadone; Mirtazapine; OLANZapine; Paraldehyde

Increased Effect/Toxicity

LORazepam may increase the levels/effects of: Alcohol (Ethyl); Azelastine (Nasal); Buprenorphine; CloZAPine; CNS Depressants; Fosphenytoin; Methadone; Methotrimeprazine; Metyrosine; Mirtazapine; Paraldehyde; Phenytoin; Pramipexole; ROPINIRole; Rotigotine; Selective Serotonin Reuptake Inhibitors; Zolpidem

The levels/effects of LORazepam may be increased by: Divalproex; Droperidol; HydrOXYzine; Loxapine; Methotrimeprazine; OLANZapine; Perampanel; Probenecid; Valproic Acid

Decreased Effect

The levels/effects of LORazepam may be decreased by: Theophylline Derivatives; Yohimbine

Ethanol/Nutrition/Herb Interactions

Ethanol: May increase CNS depression; monitor for increased effects with coadministration. Caution patients about effects.

Herb/Nutraceutical: Avoid valerian, St John's wort, kava kava, gotu kola (may increase CNS depression).

Storage/Stability

I.V.: Intact vials should be refrigerated. Protect from light. Do not use discolored or precipitate-containing solutions. May be stored at room temperature for up to 3 months [data on file (Hospira Inc, 2010)]. Parenteral admixture is stable at room temperature (25°C) for 24 hours.

Tablet: Store at room temperature.

Reconstitution

Injection: Dilute with equal volume of compatible diluent (D_5W, NS, SWFI).

Infusion: Use 2 mg/mL injectable vial to prepare; there may be decreased stability when using 4 mg/mL vial. Dilute ≤1 mg/mL and mix in glass bottle. Precipitation may develop. Can also be administered undiluted via infusion.

Mechanism of Action Binds to stereospecific benzodiazepine receptors on the postsynaptic GABA neuron at several sites within the central nervous system, including the limbic system, reticular formation. Enhancement of the inhibitory effect of GABA on neuronal excitability results by increased neuronal membrane permeability to chloride ions. This shift in chloride ions results in hyperpolarization (a less excitable state) and stabilization.

Pharmacodynamics/Kinetics

Onset of action:

Hypnosis: I.M.: 20-30 minutes

Sedation: I.V.: 5-20 minutes

Anticonvulsant: I.V.: 5 minutes, oral: 30-60 minutes

Duration: 6-8 hours

Absorption: Oral, I.M.: Prompt

Distribution: V_d: Neonates: 0.76 L/kg, Adults: 1.3 L/kg

Protein binding: 85%; free fraction may be significantly higher in elderly

Metabolism: Hepatic to inactive compounds

Bioavailability: Oral: 90%

Half-life elimination: Neonates: 40.2 hours; Older children: 10.5 hours; Adults: 12.9 hours; Elderly: 15.9 hours; End-stage renal disease: 32-70 hours

Time to peak: Oral: 2 hours

Excretion: Urine; feces (minimal)

Dosing

Adult

Antiemetic: Oral, I.V. (**Note:** May be administered sublingually; not a labeled route): 0.5-2 mg every 4-6 hours as needed

Anxiety, sedation, and procedural amnesia:

Oral: 1-10 mg/day in 2-3 divided doses; usual dose: 2-6 mg/day in divided doses or 1-2 mg 1 hour before procedure

I.M.: 0.05 mg/kg administered 2 hours before surgery (maximum: 4 mg/dose)

I.V.: 0.044 mg/kg 15-20 minutes before surgery (usual dose: 2 mg; maximum: 4 mg/dose)

Insomnia: Oral: 2-4 mg at bedtime

Status epilepticus: I.V.: 4 mg/dose slow I.V. (maximum rate: 2 mg/minute); may repeat in 10-15 minutes; usual maximum dose: 8 mg. May be given I.M, but I.V. preferred.

Rapid tranquilization of agitated patient (unlabeled use): Oral, I.M.: 1-2 mg administered every 30-60 minutes; may be administered with an antipsychotic (eg, haloperidol) (Battaglia, 2005; De Fruyt, 2004)

Average total dose for tranquilization: 4-8 mg

Agitation in the ICU patient (unlabeled):

I.V.: 0.02-0.06 mg/kg every 2-6 hours or 0.01-0.1 mg/kg/hour (Jacobi, 2002)

Dosage adjustment for lorazepam with concomitant medications: *Probenecid or valproic acid:* Reduce lorazepam dose by 50%

Alcohol withdrawal syndrome (unlabeled use): Oral: 2 mg every 6 hours for 4 doses, then 1 mg every 6 hours for 8 additional doses (Mayo-Smith, 1997)

Alcohol withdrawal delirium (unlabeled use) (Mayo-Smith, 2004):

I.V.: 1-4 mg every 5-15 minutes until calm, then every hour as needed to maintain light somnolence

I.M.: 1-4 mg every 30-60 minutes until calm, then every hour as needed to maintain light somnolence

Geriatric

Anxiety, sedation, and procedural amnesia: Oral: Initial: 1-2 mg/day in divided doses; Beers Criteria: Avoid maintenance doses >3 mg/day

Other indications: Refer to adult dosing. Dose selection should generally be on the low end of the dosage range (ie, initial dose not to exceed 2 mg).

Pediatric

Antiemetic: Children 2-15 years (unlabeled): I.V.: 0.05 mg/kg (up to 2 mg/dose) prior to chemotherapy

Anxiety, sedation, and procedural amnesia: Infants and Children (unlabeled except for oral use in children >12 years):

Oral, I.M.: Usual: 0.05 mg/kg/dose (range: 0.02-0.09 mg/kg) every 4-8 hours

I.V.: Usual: 0.05 mg/kg/dose (range: 0.02-0.09 mg/kg) every 4-8 hours; may use smaller doses (eg, 0.01-0.03 mg/kg) and repeat every 20 minutes, as needed to titrate to effect

Status epilepticus:

Infants and Children (unlabeled): I.V.: 0.05-0.1 mg/kg (maximum: 4 mg/dose) slow I.V. (maximum rate: 2 mg/minute); may repeat every 10-15 minutes as needed (Hegenbarth, 2008; Sabo-Graham, 1998)

Adolescents: Refer to adult dosing.

Renal Impairment I.V.: Risk of propylene glycol toxicity. Monitor closely if using for prolonged periods or at high doses.

Hepatic Impairment No dose reduction necessary.

Administration

I.M.: Should be administered deep into the muscle mass

I.V.: Do not exceed 2 mg/minute or 0.05 mg/kg over 2-5 minutes; dilute I.V. dose with equal volume of compatible diluent (D_5W, NS, SWFI). Continuous infusion solutions should have an in-line filter and the solution should be checked frequently for possible precipitation. Avoid intra-arterial administration. Monitor I.V. site for extravasation

Extemporaneous Preparations Note: Commercial oral solution is available (2 mg/mL)

Two different 1 mg/mL oral suspensions may be made from different generic lorazepam tablets (Mylan Pharmaceuticals or Watson Laboratories), sterile water, Ora-Sweet®, and Ora-Plus®.

Mylan tablets: Place one-hundred-eighty 2 mg tablets in a 12-ounce amber glass bottle; add 144 mL of sterile water to disperse the tablets; shake until slurry is formed. Add 108 mL Ora-Plus® in incremental proportions; then add a quantity of Ora-Sweet® sufficient to make 360 mL. Label "shake well" and "refrigerate". Stable for 91 days when stored in amber glass prescription bottles at room temperature or refrigerated (preferred).

Watson tablets: Place one-hundred-eighty 2 mg tablets in a 12-ounce amber glass bottle; add 48 mL sterile water to disperse the tablets; shake until slurry is formed. Add 156 mL of Ora-Plus® in incremental proportions; then add a quantity of Ora-Sweet® sufficient to make 360 mL. Label "shake well" and "refrigerate". Store in amber glass prescription bottles. Stable for 63 days at room temperature or 91 days refrigerated.

Lee ME, Lugo RA, Rusho WJ, et al, "Chemical Stability of Extemporaneously Prepared Lorazepam Suspension at Two Temperatures," *J Pediatr Pharmacol Ther*, 2004, 9(4):254-58.

Monitoring Parameters Respiratory and cardiovascular status, blood pressure, heart rate, symptoms of anxiety

Clinical signs of propylene glycol toxicity (for continuous high-dose and/or long duration intravenous use): Serum creatinine, BUN, serum lactate, osmol gap

Additional Information Oral doses >0.09 mg/kg produced increased ataxia without increased sedative benefit vs lower doses; preferred anxiolytic when I.M. route needed. Abrupt discontinuation after sustained use (generally >10 days) may cause withdrawal symptoms.

Dosage Forms Excipient information presented when available (limited, particularly for generics); consult specific product labeling. [DSC] = Discontinued product

Injection, solution: 2 mg/mL (1 mL, 10 mL); 4 mg/mL (1 mL, 10 mL)

Ativan®: 2 mg/mL (1 mL [DSC], 10 mL [DSC]); 4 mg/mL (1 mL [DSC], 10 mL [DSC]) [contains benzyl alcohol, polyethylene glycol 400, propylene glycol]

Solution, oral [concentrate]: 2 mg/mL (30 mL)

Lorazepam Intensol™: 2 mg/mL (30 mL) [dye free, ethanol free, sugar free; contains propylene glycol]

Tablet, oral: 0.5 mg, 1 mg, 2 mg

Ativan®: 0.5 mg

Ativan®: 1 mg, 2 mg [scored]

Controlled Substance C-IV

References

Battaglia J, "Pharmacological Management of Acute Agitation," *Drugs*, 2005, 65(9):1207-22.

De Fruyt J and Demyttenaere K, "Rapid Tranquilization: New Approaches in the Emergency Treatment of Behavioral Disturbances," *Eur Psychiatry*, 2004, 19(5):243-9.

Hegenbarth MA and the American Academy of Pediatrics Committee on Drugs, "Preparing for Pediatric Emergencies: Drugs to Consider," *Pediatrics*, 2008, 121(2):433-43.

Jacobi J, Fraser GL, Coursin DB, et al, "Clinical Practice Guidelines for the Sustained Use of Sedatives and Analgesics in the Critically Ill Adult," *Crit Care Med*, 2002, 30(1):119-41.

Laszlo J, Clark RA, Hanson DC, et al, "Lorazepam in Cancer Patients Treated With Cisplatin: A Drug Having Antiemetic, Amnesic, and Anxiolytic Effects," *J Clin Oncol*, 1985, 3(6):864-9.

Malik IA, Khan WA, Qazilbash M, et al, "Clinical Efficacy of Lorazepam in Prophylaxis of Anticipatory, Acute, and Delayed Nausea and Vomiting Induced by High Doses of Cisplatin. A Prospective Randomized Trial," *Am J Clin Oncol*, 1995, 18(2):170-5.

Mayo-Smith MF, Beecher LH, Fischer TL, et al, "Management of Alcohol Withdrawal Delirium. An Evidence-Based Practice Guideline," *Arch Intern Med*, 2004, 164(13):1405-12; published erratum appears in *Arch Intern Med*, 2004, 164(18):2068.

Sabo-Graham T and Seay AR, "Management of Status Epilepticus in Children," *Pediatr Rev*, 1998, 19(9):306-9.

- **Lorazepam Injection, USP (Can)** *see* LORazepam *on page 907*
- **Lorazepam Intensol™** *see* LORazepam *on page 907*
- **Lovenox®** *see* Enoxaparin *on page 499*
- **Lovenox® HP (Can)** *see* Enoxaparin *on page 499*
- **Low-Molecular-Weight Iron Dextran (INFeD®)** *see* Iron Dextran Complex *on page 824*
- **L-PAM** *see* Melphalan *on page 925*

- **L-Phenylalanine Mustard** *see* Melphalan *on page 925*
- **L-Sarcolysin** *see* Melphalan *on page 925*
- **Lupron® (Can)** *see* Leuprolide *on page 876*
- **Lupron Depot®** *see* Leuprolide *on page 876*
- **Lupron® Depot® (Can)** *see* Leuprolide *on page 876*
- **Lupron Depot-Ped®** *see* Leuprolide *on page 876*
- **LY170053** *see* OLANZapine *on page 1056*
- **LY-188011** *see* Gemcitabine *on page 663*
- **LY231514** *see* PEMEtrexed *on page 1151*
- **LY303366** *see* Anidulafungin *on page 99*
- **Lymphazurin™** *see* Isosulfan Blue *on page 831*
- **Lymphocyte Immune Globulin** *see* Antithymocyte Globulin (Equine) *on page 111*
- **Lymphocyte Mitogenic Factor** *see* Aldesleukin *on page 37*
- **Lysodren®** *see* Mitotane *on page 994*
- **Lysteda™** *see* Tranexamic Acid *on page 1392*
- **MabCampath® (Can)** *see* Alemtuzumab *on page 43*
- **m-AMSA** *see* Amsacrine *on page 90*
- **Mar-Anastrozole (Can)** *see* Anastrozole *on page 96*
- **Marinol® (Can)** *see* Dronabinol *on page 484*
- **Marqibo®** *see* VinCRIStine (Liposomal) *on page 1459*
- **Matulane®** *see* Procarbazine *on page 1208*
- **Maxipime® [DSC]** *see* Cefepime *on page 251*
- **Maxipime® (Can)** *see* Cefepime *on page 251*
- **MDL 73,147EF** *see* Dolasetron *on page 462*
- **MDV3100** *see* Enzalutamide *on page 506*
- **MDX-010** *see* Ipilimumab *on page 809*
- **MDX-CTLA-4** *see* Ipilimumab *on page 809*

Mechlorethamine (me klor ETH a meen)

Related Information

Fertility and Cancer Therapy *on page 1782*
Management of Chemotherapy-Induced Nausea and Vomiting *on page 1786*
Management of Drug Extravasations *on page 1800*
Safe Handling of Hazardous Drugs *on page 1904*

Brand Names: U.S. Mustargen®

Index Terms Chlorethazine; Chlorethazine Mustard; HN_2; Mechlorethamine Hydrochloride; Mustine; Nitrogen Mustard

Generic Availability (U.S.) No

Pharmacologic Category Antineoplastic Agent, Alkylating Agent (Nitrogen Mustard)

Use Hodgkin's disease; non-Hodgkin's lymphoma; intracavitary injection for treatment of metastatic tumors; pleural and other malignant effusions

Unlabeled Use Topical treatment of mycosis fungoides

Labeled Contraindications Hypersensitivity to mechlorethamine or any component of the formulation; presence of known infection

Pregnancy Risk Factor D

Lactation Excretion in breast milk unknown/not recommended

Warnings/Precautions **[U.S. Boxed Warnings]: Hazardous agent - use appropriate precautions for handling and disposal. Avoid contact with skin or eyes; avoid exposure during pregnancy. Mechlorethamine is a potent vesicant; if extravasation occurs, severe tissue damage (leading to ulceration and necrosis) and pain may occur.** Sodium thiosulfate should be available for treatment of extravasation. May cause lymphopenia, granulocytopenia, thrombocytopenia and anemia. Hyperuricemia may occur, especially with lymphomas; ensure adequate hydration. **[U.S. Boxed Warning]: Should be administered under the supervision of an experienced cancer chemotherapy physician.**

Adverse Reactions Frequency not defined.

Central nervous system: Drowsiness, encephalopathy (high dose), fever, headache, lethargy, sedation, vertigo

Dermatologic: Alopecia, erythema multiforme, maculopapular rash, petechiae, rash

Endocrine & metabolic: Amenorrhea, hyperuricemia, oligomenorrhea, spermatogenesis decreased

Gastrointestinal: Anorexia, diarrhea, metallic taste, mucositis, nausea, vomiting

Hepatic: Jaundice

Hematologic: Agranulocytosis, granulocytopenia (onset 6-8 days, recovery 10-21 days), hemolytic anemia, leukopenia, lymphocytopenia, pancytopenia, secondary leukemias, thrombocytopenia

Local: Thrombophlebitis, tissue necrosis (extravasation)

Neuromuscular & skeletal: Weakness

Ocular: Lacrimation

Otic: Deafness, tinnitus

Miscellaneous: Anaphylaxis, diaphoresis, herpes zoster infection, hypersensitivity reactions

Drug Interactions

Metabolism/Transport Effects None known.

Avoid Concomitant Use

Avoid concomitant use of Mechlorethamine with any of the following: BCG; CloZAPine; Natalizumab; Pimecrolimus; Tacrolimus (Topical); Vaccines (Live)

Increased Effect/Toxicity

Mechlorethamine may increase the levels/effects of: CloZAPine; Leflunomide; Natalizumab; Vaccines (Live)

The levels/effects of Mechlorethamine may be increased by: Denosumab; Pimecrolimus; Roflumilast; Tacrolimus (Topical); Trastuzumab

Decreased Effect

Mechlorethamine may decrease the levels/effects of: BCG; Coccidioidin Skin Test; Sipuleucel-T; Vaccines (Inactivated); Vaccines (Live)

The levels/effects of Mechlorethamine may be decreased by: Echinacea

Ethanol/Nutrition/Herb Interactions Ethanol: Avoid ethanol (due to GI irritation).

Storage/Stability Store intact vials at room temperature of 15°C to 30°C (59°F to 86°F). Protect from light. Solution is stable for only 15-60 minutes after dilution

Reconstitution Must be prepared immediately before use. Use appropriate precautions for handling. Dilute powder with 10 mL SWFI or 0.9% sodium chloride to a final concentration of 1 mg/mL. May be diluted in up to 100 mL NS for intracavitary or topical administration.

Mechanism of Action Bifunctional alkylating agent that inhibits DNA and RNA synthesis via formation of carbonium ions; cross-links strands of DNA, causing miscoding, breakage, and failure of replication; produces interstrand and intrastrand cross-links in DNA resulting in miscoding, breakage, and failure of replication. Although not cell phase-specific *per se,* mechlorethamine effect is most pronounced in the S phase, and cell proliferation is arrested in the G_2 phase.

Pharmacodynamics/Kinetics

Duration: Unchanged drug is undetectable in blood within a few minutes

Absorption: Intracavitary administration: Incomplete secondary to rapid deactivation by body fluids

Metabolism: Rapid hydrolysis and demethylation, possibly in plasma

Half-life elimination: <1 minute

Excretion: Urine (50% as metabolites, <0.01% as unchanged drug)

Dosing

Adult & Geriatric Details concerning dosing in combination regimens should also be consulted. Dosage should be based on ideal dry weight (evaluate the presence of edema or ascites so that dosage is based on actual weight unaugmented by edema/ascites).

Lymphoma: *I.V.:* 0.4 mg/kg as a single dose or in divided doses of 0.1 mg/kg/day (for 4 days) or 0.2 mg/kg/day (for 2 days) per treatment course; repeat treatment course after hematologic recovery

MOPP: Unlabeled dosing: I.V.: 6 mg/m^2 on days 1 and 8 of a 28-day cycle

Intracavitary: 0.4 mg/kg as a single dose; although 0.2 mg/kg (10-20 mg) as a single dose has been used by the *intrapericardial* route

Mycosis fungoides (unlabeled use): Topical mechlorethamine has been used in the treatment of cutaneous lesions of mycosis fungoides. A skin test should be performed prior to treatment with the topical preparation to detect sensitivity and possible irritation (use fresh mechlorethamine 0.1 mg/mL and apply over a 3 x 5 cm area of normal skin).

Pediatric Details concerning dosing in combination regimens should also be consulted. Dosage should be based on ideal dry weight (evaluate the presence of edema or ascites so that dosage is based on actual weight unaugmented by edema/ascites).

MOPP (unlabeled use): Children: I.V.: 6 mg/m^2 on days 1 and 8 of a 28-day cycle

Renal Impairment

Hemodialysis: Not removed; supplemental dosing is not necessary.

Peritoneal dialysis: Not removed; supplemental dosing is not necessary.

Combination Regimens

Brain tumors: MOPP (Medulloblastoma) on page 1717

Lymphoma, Hodgkin:

MOPP/ABVD (Hodgkin) on page 1714

MOPP/ABV Hybrid (Hodgkin) on page 1715

MOPP (Hodgkin) on page 1716

Stanford V (Hodgkin) on page 1752

Administration

I.V.: Administer as a slow I.V. push over a few minutes into a free-flowing I.V. solution. Must be prepared immediately prior to administration. Due to the limited stability of the drug, and the increased risk of phlebitis and venous irritation and blistering with increased contact time, infusions of the drug are not recommended.

Intracavitary: May further dilute in 50-100 mL of normal saline prior to instillation; rotate patient position every 5-10 minutes for 1 hour after instillation to obtain uniform distribution.

Mechlorethamine may cause extravasation. Use within 1 hour of preparation. Avoid extravasation since mechlorethamine is a potent vesicant.

Emetic Potential Very high (>90%)

Vesicant/Extravasation Risk Vesicant; see Management of Drug Extravasations on page 1800.

Monitoring Parameters CBC with differential, hemoglobin, and platelet count

Dosage Forms Excipient information presented when available (limited, particularly for generics); consult specific product labeling.

Injection, powder for reconstitution, as hydrochloride:

Mustargen®: 10 mg

References

Bonadonna G, Valagussa P, and Santoro A, "Alternating Non-Cross-Resistant Combination Chemotherapy or MOPP in Stage IV Hodgkin's Disease. A Report of 8-Year Results," *Ann Intern Med*, 1986, 104(6):739-46.

DeVita VT, Serpick A, and Carbone PP, "Combination Chemotherapy in the Treatment of Advanced Hodgkin's Disease," *Ann Intern Med*, 1970, 73:881-95.

Dorr RT, Soble M, and Alberts DS, "Efficacy of Sodium Thiosulfate as a Local Antidote to Mechlorethamine Skin Toxicity in the Mouse," *Cancer Chemother Pharmacol*, 1988, 22 (4):299-302.

Price NM, Hoppe RT, and Deneau DG, "Ointment Based Mechlorethamine Treatment for Mycosis Fungoides," *Cancer*, 1983, 52:2214-9.

Taylor JR, Halprin KM, Levine V, et al, "Mechlorethamine Hydrochloride Solutions and Ointments," *Arch Dermatol*, 1980, 116:783-5.

Vonderheid EC, "Topical Mechlorethamine Chemotherapy: Considerations on its Use in Mycosis Fungoides," *Int J Dermatol*, 1984, 23(3):180-6.

- **Mechlorethamine Hydrochloride** *see* Mechlorethamine *on page 913*
- **MED-Letrozole (Can)** *see* Letrozole *on page 867*
- **Medrol®** *see* MethylPREDNISolone *on page 967*
- **Medrol Dose Pack** *see* MethylPREDNISolone *on page 967*
- **Medrol® Dosepak™** *see* MethylPREDNISolone *on page 967*
- **Medroxy (Can)** *see* MedroxyPROGESTERone *on page 916*

MedroxyPROGESTERone (me DROKS ee proe JES te rone)

Related Information

Safe Handling of Hazardous Drugs *on page 1904*

Brand Names: U.S. Depo-Provera®; Depo-Provera® Contraceptive; depo-subQ provera 104®; Provera®

Brand Names: Canada Alti-MPA; Apo-Medroxy®; Depo-Prevera®; Depo-Provera®; Dom-Medroxyprogesterone; Gen-Medroxy; Medroxy; Medroxyprogesterone Acetate Injectable Suspension USP; Novo-Medrone; PMS-Medroxyprogesterone; Provera-Pak; Provera®; Teva-Medroxyprogesterone

Index Terms Acetoxymethylprogesterone; Medroxyprogesterone Acetate; Methylacetoxyprogesterone; MPA

Generic Availability (U.S.) Yes

Pharmacologic Category Contraceptive; Progestin

Use Secondary amenorrhea or abnormal uterine bleeding due to hormonal imbalance; reduction of endometrial hyperplasia in nonhysterectomized postmenopausal women receiving conjugated estrogens; prevention of pregnancy; management of endometriosis-associated pain; adjunctive therapy and palliative treatment of recurrent and metastatic endometrial carcinoma

Unlabeled Use Treatment of low-grade endometrial stromal sarcoma; treatment of paraphilia/hypersexuality

Labeled Contraindications Hypersensitivity to medroxyprogesterone or any component of the formulation; history of or current thrombophlebitis or venous thromboembolic disorders (including DVT, PE); cerebral vascular disease; severe hepatic dysfunction or disease; carcinoma of the breast or other estrogen- or progesterone-dependent neoplasia; undiagnosed vaginal bleeding; missed abortion, diagnostic test for pregnancy, pregnancy

Pregnancy Risk Factor X

Lactation Enters breast milk

Warnings/Precautions **[U.S. Boxed Warning]: Prolonged use of medroxyprogesterone contraceptive injection may result in a loss of bone mineral density (BMD). It is not known if use during adolescence or early adulthood will decrease peak bone mass accretion or increase the risk for osteoporotic fractures later in life. Loss is related to the duration of use, may not be completely reversible on discontinuation of the drug,** and incidence is not significantly different between the SubQ and I.M. dosage forms. The impact on peak bone mass in adolescents should be weighed against the potential for unintended pregnancies in treatment decision. Consider alternative contraceptive methods in patients at risk for osteoporosis (eg, metabolic bone disease, family history of osteoporosis, chronic use of medications associated with osteoporosis such as corticosteroids). **[U.S. Boxed Warning]: Long-term use (ie, >2 years) should be limited to situations where other birth control methods are inadequate.** Consider other methods of birth control in women with (or at risk for) osteoporosis. **[U.S. Boxed Warning]: Inform patients that injectable contraceptives do not protect against HIV infection or other sexually-transmitted diseases.** When used for contraception, the possibility of ectopic pregnancy should be considered in patients with abdominal pain. Anaphylaxis or anaphylactoid reactions have been reported with use of the injection; medication for the treatment of hypersensitivity reactions should be available for immediate use.

[U.S. Boxed Warning]: Estrogens with or without progestin should not be used to prevent cardiovascular disease. Using data from the Women's Health Initiative (WHI) studies, an increased risk of deep vein thrombosis (DVT) and stroke has been reported with CE and an increased risk of DVT, stroke, pulmonary emboli (PE) and myocardial infarction (MI) has been reported with CE with MPA in postmenopausal women. Additional risk factors include diabetes mellitus, hypercholesterolemia, hypertension, SLE, obesity, tobacco use, and/or history of venous thromboembolism (VTE). Risk factors should be managed appropriately; discontinue use if adverse cardiovascular events occur or are suspected. If thrombosis develops with contraceptive treatment, discontinue treatment (unless no other acceptable contraceptive alternative). Whenever possible, progestins in combination with estrogens should be discontinued at least 4-6 weeks prior to and for 2 weeks following elective surgery associated with an increased risk of thromboembolism or during periods of prolonged immobilization.

[U.S. Boxed Warning]: Estrogens with or without progestin should not be used to prevent dementia. In the Women's Health Initiative Memory Study (WHIMS), an increased incidence of dementia was observed in women ≥65 years of age taking CE alone or in combination with MPA.

[U.S. Boxed Warning]: Based on data from the Women's Health Initiative (WHI) studies, an increased risk of invasive breast cancer was observed in postmenopausal women using conjugated estrogens (CE) in combination with medroxyprogesterone acetate (MPA). This risk may be associated with duration of use and declines once combined therapy is discontinued (Chlebowski, 2009). The risk of invasive breast cancer was decreased in postmenopausal women with a hysterectomy using CE only, regardless of weight. However, the risk was not significantly decreased in women at high risk for breast cancer (family history of breast cancer, personal history of benign breast disease) (Anderson, 2012). An increase in abnormal mammogram findings has also been reported with estrogen alone or in combination with progestin therapy. Use is contraindicated in patients with known or suspected breast cancer.

MPA is used to reduce the risk of endometrial hyperplasia in nonhysterectomized postmenopausal women receiving conjugated estrogens. The use of unopposed estrogen in women with an intact uterus is associated with an increased risk of endometrial cancer. The addition of a progestin to estrogen therapy may decrease the risk of endometrial hyperplasia, a precursor to endometrial cancer. Adequate diagnostic measures, including endometrial sampling if indicated, should be performed to rule out malignancy in postmenopausal women with undiagnosed abnormal vaginal bleeding. Estrogens may exacerbate endometriosis. Malignant transformation of residual endometrial implants has been reported posthysterectomy with unopposed estrogen therapy. Consider adding a progestin in women with residual endometriosis posthysterectomy. Postmenopausal estrogen therapy and combined estrogen/progesterone therapy may increase the risk of ovarian cancer; however, the absolute risk to an individual woman is small. Although results from various studies are not consistent, risk does not appear to be significantly associated with the duration, route, or dose of therapy. In one study, the risk decreased after 2 years following discontinuation of therapy (Mørch, 2009). Although the risk of ovarian cancer is rare, women who are at an increased risk (eg, family history) should be counseled about the association (NAMS, 2012).

[U.S. Boxed Warning]: Estrogens with or without progestin should be used for the shortest duration possible at the lowest effective dose consistent with treatment goals. Before prescribing estrogen therapy to postmenopausal women, the risks and benefits must be weighed for each patient. Women should be informed of these risks and benefits, as well as possible effects of progestin when added to estrogen therapy. Patients should be reevaluated as clinically appropriate to determine if treatment is still necessary. Available data related to treatment risks are from Women's Health Initiative (WHI) studies, which evaluated oral CE 0.625 mg with or without MPA 2.5 mg relative to placebo in postmenopausal women. Other combinations and dosage forms of estrogens and progestins were not studied. **Outcomes reported from clinical trials using CE with or without MPA should be assumed to be similar for other doses and other dosage forms of estrogens and progestins until comparable data becomes available.**

Discontinue pending examination in cases of sudden partial or complete vision loss, sudden onset of proptosis, diplopia, or migraine; discontinue permanently if papilledema or retinal vascular lesions are observed on examination. Use with caution in patients with diseases that may be exacerbated by fluid retention (including asthma, epilepsy, migraine, cardiac, or renal dysfunction). Contraceptive therapy with medroxyprogesterone commonly results in an average weight gain of ~2.5 kg after 1 year and ~3.7 kg after 2 years of treatment. Use caution with history of depression.

May have adverse effects on glucose tolerance; use caution in women with diabetes. MPA is extensively metabolized in the liver. Discontinue if jaundice develops or if acute or chronic hepatic disturbances occur. Use is contraindicated with severe hepatic disease. Unscheduled bleeding/spotting may occur. Presentation of irregular, unresolving vaginal bleeding following previously regular cycles warrants further evaluation including endometrial sampling, if indicated, to rule out malignancy. Not for use prior to menarche. The use of estrogens and/or progestins may change the results of some laboratory tests (eg, coagulation factors, lipids, glucose tolerance, binding proteins). The dose, route, and the specific estrogen/progestin influences these changes. In addition, personal risk factors (eg, cardiovascular disease, smoking, diabetes, age) also contribute to adverse events; use of specific products may be contraindicated in women with certain risk factors.

Adverse Reactions Adverse effects as reported with any dosage form; percent ranges presented are noted with the MPA I.M. contraceptive injection:

>5%:

- Central nervous system: Dizziness, headache, nervousness
- Endocrine & metabolic: Libido decreased, menstrual irregularities (includes bleeding, amenorrhea, or both)
- Gastrointestinal: Abdominal pain/discomfort, weight gain (>10 lbs at 24 months: 38%)

1% to 5%:

- Cardiovascular: Edema
- Central nervous system: Depression, fatigue, insomnia
- Dermatologic: Acne, alopecia, rash
- Endocrine & metabolic: Breast pain, hot flashes
- Gastrointestinal: Bloating, nausea
- Genitourinary: Dysmenorrhea, leukorrhea, vaginitis
- Local: Injection site reaction (SubQ administration): Atrophy, induration, pain
- Neuromuscular & skeletal: Arthralgia, backache, leg cramp, weakness

<1%, postmarketing, and/or case reports: Allergic reaction, anaphylaxis, anaphylactoid reactions, anemia, angioedema, anxiety, appetite changes, asthma, axillary swelling, blood dyscrasia, body odor, BMD loss, breast cancer, breast changes, cervical cancer, chest pain, chills, chloasma, cholestatic jaundice, deep vein thrombosis, diaphoresis, diarrhea, drowsiness, dry skin, dyspareunia, dyspnea, facial palsy, fainting, fever, galactorrhea, genitourinary infections, glucose tolerance decreased, hirsutism, hoarseness, jaundice, lack of return to fertility, lactation decreased, libido increased, melasma, nipple bleeding, oligomenorrhea, optic neuritis, osteoporosis, osteoporotic fractures, paralysis, paresthesia, pruritus, pulmonary embolus, rectal bleeding, retinal thrombosis, scleroderma, seizure, somnolence, syncope, tachycardia, thirst, thrombophlebitis, urticaria, uterine hyperplasia, vaginal cysts, varicose veins

In addition: Depo-Provera® aqueous suspension: Residual lump, sterile abscess, or skin discoloration at the injection

Drug Interactions

Metabolism/Transport Effects **Substrate** of CYP3A4 (major); **Note:** Assignment of Major/Minor substrate status based on clinically relevant drug interaction potential; **Induces** CYP3A4 (weak/moderate)

Avoid Concomitant Use

Avoid concomitant use of MedroxyPROGESTERone with any of the following: Axitinib; Griseofulvin

Increased Effect/Toxicity

MedroxyPROGESTERone may increase the levels/effects of: Benzodiazepines (metabolized by oxidation); Selegiline; Tranexamic Acid; Voriconazole

The levels/effects of MedroxyPROGESTERone may be increased by: Boceprevir; Cobicistat; Herbs (Progestogenic Properties); Mifepristone; Voriconazole

Decreased Effect

MedroxyPROGESTERone may decrease the levels/effects of: ARIPiprazole; Axitinib; Saxagliptin; Vitamin K Antagonists

The levels/effects of MedroxyPROGESTERone may be decreased by: Acitretin; Aminoglutethimide; Aprepitant; Artemether; Barbiturates; Bexarotene (Systemic); Bile Acid Sequestrants; Bosentan; CarBAMazepine; Clobazam; CYP3A4 Inducers (Strong); Deferasirox; Felbamate; Fosaprepitant; Fosphenytoin; Griseofulvin; LamoTRIgine; Mifepristone; Mycophenolate; Nevirapine; OXcarbazepine; Perampanel; Phenytoin; Prucalopride; Retinoic Acid Derivatives; Rifamycin Derivatives; St Johns Wort; Telaprevir; Tocilizumab; Topiramate

Ethanol/Nutrition/Herb Interactions

Ethanol: Avoid ethanol (may increase risk of osteoporosis).

Food: Bioavailability of the oral tablet is increased when taken with food; half-life is unchanged.

Herb/Nutraceutical: St John's wort may diminish the therapeutic effect of progestin contraceptives (contraceptive failure is possible).

Storage/Stability Store at controlled room temperature.

Mechanism of Action Inhibits secretion of pituitary gonadotropins, which prevents follicular maturation and ovulation; causes endometrial thinning

Pharmacodynamics/Kinetics

Absorption: Oral: Well absorbed; I.M.: Slow

Protein binding: 86% to 90% primarily to albumin; does not bind to sex hormone-binding globulin

Metabolism: Extensively hepatic via hydroxylation and conjugation; forms metabolites

Half-life elimination: Oral: 12-17 hours; I.M. (Depo-Provera® Contraceptive): ~50 days; SubQ: ~40 days

Time to peak: Oral: 2-4 hours; I.M. (Depo-Provera® Contraceptive): ~3 weeks; SubQ: ~1 week

Excretion: Urine

Dosing

Adult & Geriatric

Amenorrhea: Oral: 5-10 mg/day for 5-10 days

Abnormal uterine bleeding: Oral: 5-10 mg for 5-10 days starting on day 16 or 21 of cycle

Contraception:

Depo-Provera® Contraceptive: I.M.: 150 mg every 3 months

depo-subQ provera 104™: SubQ: 104 mg every 3 months (every 12-14 weeks)

Endometriosis (depo-subQ provera 104™): SubQ: 104 mg every 3 months (every 12-14 weeks)

Endometrial carcinoma, recurrent or metastatic (adjunctive/palliative treatment) (Depo-Provera®): I.M.: 400-1000 mg/week

Accompanying cyclic estrogen therapy, postmenopausal: Oral: 5-10 mg for 12-14 consecutive days each month, starting on day 1 or day 16 of the cycle; lower doses may be used if given with estrogen continuously throughout the cycle

Treatment of paraphilia/hypersexuality (unlabeled use; Reilly, 2000): Males (**Note:** Avoid use if active pituitary pathology, hepatic failure or thromboembolic disease):

I.M. (Depo-Provera®): 100-600 mg weekly

Oral: 100-500 mg daily

Pediatric Adolescents:

Amenorrhea: Refer to adult dosing.

Abnormal uterine bleeding: Refer to adult dosing.

Contraception: Refer to adult dosing.

Endometriosis: Refer to adult dosing.

Hepatic Impairment Use is contraindicated with severe impairment. Discontinue with jaundice or if liver function disturbances occur. Consider lower dose or less frequent administration with mild-to-moderate impairment. Use of the contraceptive injection has not been studied in patients with hepatic impairment; consideration should be given to not readminister if jaundice develops

Administration

I.M.: Depo-Provera® Contraceptive: Administer first dose during the first 5 days of menstrual period, or within the first 5 days postpartum if not breast-feeding, or at the sixth week postpartum if breast-feeding exclusively. Shake vigorously prior to administration. Administer by deep I.M. injection in the gluteal or deltoid muscle.

When switching from combined hormonal contraceptives (estrogen plus progestin), the first injection should be on the day after the last active tablet or (at the latest) the day after the final inactive tablet. When switching from other contraceptive methods, ensure continuous contraceptive coverage.

SubQ: depo-subQ provera 104™: Administer first dose during the first 5 days of menstrual period, or at the sixth week postpartum if breast-feeding. Shake vigorously prior to administration. Administer by SubQ injection in the anterior thigh or abdomen; avoid boney areas and the umbilicus. Administer over 5-7 seconds. Do not rub the injection area. When switching from combined hormonal contraceptives (estrogen plus progestin), the first injection should be within 7 days after the last active pill, or removal of patch or ring. If switching from the I.M. to SubQ formulation, the next dose should be given within the prescribed dosing period for the I.M. injection to assure continuous coverage.

Monitoring Parameters Before starting therapy, a physical exam with reference to the breasts and pelvis are recommended, including a Papanicolaou smear. Exam may be deferred if appropriate prior to administration of MPA contraceptive injection; pregnancy should be ruled out prior to use. Monitor patient closely for loss of vision; sudden onset of proptosis, diplopia, or migraine; signs and symptoms of thromboembolic disorders; signs or symptoms of depression; glucose in patients with diabetes; or blood pressure. BMD with long-term use (per manufacturer).

Adequate diagnostic measures, including endometrial sampling, if indicated, should be performed to rule out malignancy in all cases of undiagnosed abnormal vaginal bleeding.

Treatment of paraphilia/hypersexuality (Guay 2009; Reilly, 2000): Hepatic function test (baseline and during treatment if suspected hepatotoxicity); CBC (baseline); serum testosterone (baseline then monthly for 4 months then every 6 months); serum LH and prolactin (baseline and every 6 months); FSH (baseline); glucose; bone scan (baseline then annually) if serum testosterone significantly suppressed; gallbladder function; blood pressure; weight gain

Dietary Considerations Ensure adequate calcium and vitamin D intake

Dosage Forms Excipient information presented when available (limited, particularly for generics); consult specific product labeling.

Injection, suspension, as acetate: 150 mg/mL (1 mL)

Depo-Provera®: 400 mg/mL (2.5 mL)

Depo-Provera® Contraceptive: 150 mg/mL (1 mL) [contains polysorbate 80]

depo-subQ provera 104®: 104 mg/0.65 mL (0.65 mL) [contains polysorbate 80]

Tablet, oral, as acetate: 2.5 mg, 5 mg, 10 mg

Provera®: 2.5 mg, 5 mg, 10 mg [scored]

References

Anderson GL, Chlebowski RT, Aragaki AK, et al, "Conjugated Equine Oestrogen and Breast Cancer Incidence and Mortality in Postmenopausal Women With Hysterectomy: Extended Follow-Up of the Women's Health Initiative Randomised Placebo-Controlled Trial," *Lancet Oncol*, 2012 [epub ahead of print].

Chlebowski RT, Kuller LH, Prentice RL, et al, "Breast Cancer After Use of Estrogen Plus Progestin in Postmenopausal Women," *N Engl J Med*, 2009, 360(6):573-87.

National Comprehensive Cancer Network® (NCCN), "Clinical Practice Guidelines in Oncology™: Uterine Neoplasms," Version 3.2012. Available at http://www.nccn.org/professionals/physician_gls/PDF/uterine.pdf

North American Menopause Society [NAMS], "The 2012 Hormone Therapy Position Statement of The North American Menopause Society," *Menopause*, 2012, 19(3):257-71.

Reilly DR, Delva NJ, and Hudson RW, "Protocols for the Use of Cyproterone, Medroxyprogesterone, and Leuprolide in the Treatment of Paraphilia," *Can J Psychiatry*, 2000, 45(6):559-63.

Thigpen JT, Brady MF, Alvarez RD, et al, "Oral Medroxyprogesterone Acetate in the Treatment of Advanced or Recurrent Endometrial Carcinoma: A Dose-Response Study by the Gynecologic Oncology Group," *J Clin Oncol*, 1999, 17(6):1736-44.

◆ **Medroxyprogesterone Acetate** *see* MedroxyPROGESTERone *on page* 916

◆ **Medroxyprogesterone Acetate Injectable Suspension USP (Can)** *see* MedroxyPROGESTERone *on page* 916

◆ **Megace®** *see* Megestrol *on page* 922

◆ **Megace® ES** *see* Megestrol *on page* 922

◆ **Megace® OS (Can)** *see* Megestrol *on page* 922

Megestrol (me JES trole)

Related Information

Palliative Care Medicine (Cancer) *on page* 1871

Safe Handling of Hazardous Drugs *on page* 1904

Brand Names: U.S. Megace®; Megace® ES

Brand Names: Canada Apo-Megestrol®; Megace®; Megace® OS; Nu-Megestrol

Index Terms 5071-1DL(6); Megestrol Acetate

Generic Availability (U.S.) Yes: Excludes Megace® ES

Pharmacologic Category Antineoplastic Agent, Hormone; Appetite Stimulant; Progestin

Use Palliative treatment of breast and endometrial carcinoma; treatment of anorexia, cachexia, or unexplained significant weight loss in patients with AIDS

Labeled Contraindications Hypersensitivity to megestrol or any component of the formulation; pregnancy (suspension)

Pregnancy Risk Factor D (tablet) / X (suspension)

Lactation Enters breast milk/not recommended

Warnings/Precautions Hazardous agent - use appropriate precautions for handling and disposal. May suppress hypothalamic-pituitary-adrenal (HPA) axis during chronic administration; consider the possibility of adrenal suppression in any patient receiving or being withdrawn from chronic therapy when signs/symptoms suggestive of hypoadrenalism are noted (during stress or in unstressed state). Laboratory evaluation and replacement/stress doses of rapid-acting glucocorticoid should be considered. New-onset diabetes and exacerbation of pre-existing diabetes have been reported with long-term use. Use with caution in patients with a history of thromboembolic disease. Avoid use in older adults due to minimal effect on weight, and an increased risk of thrombosis and possibly death (Beers Criteria). Vaginal bleeding or discharge may occur in females. Megace® ES suspension is not equivalent to other formulations on a mg per mg basis; Megace® ES suspension 625 mg/5 mL is equivalent to megestrol acetate suspension 800 mg/20 mL.

Adverse Reactions

Frequency not always defined.

Cardiovascular: Hypertension (≤8%), cardiomyopathy (1% to 3%), chest pain (1% to 3%), edema (1% to 3%), palpitation (1% to 3%), peripheral edema (1% to 3%), heart failure

Central nervous system: Headache (≤10%), insomnia (≤6%), fever (1% to 6%), pain (≤6%, similar to placebo), abnormal thinking (1% to 3%), confusion (1% to 3%), depression (1% to 3%), hypoesthesia (1% to 3%), seizure (1% to 3%), mood changes, malaise, lethargy

Dermatologic: Rash (2% to 12%), alopecia (1% to 3%), pruritus (1% to 3%), vesiculobullous rash (1% to 3%)

Endocrine & metabolic: Hyperglycemia (≤6%), gynecomastia (1% to 3%), adrenal insufficiency, amenorrhea, breakthrough bleeding, cervical erosion and secretions (changes), breast tenderness increased, Cushing's syndrome, diabetes, glucose intolerance, HPA axis suppression, hot flashes, hypercalcemia, menstrual flow changes, spotting, vaginal bleeding pattern changes

Gastrointestinal: Diarrhea (6% to 15%, similar to placebo), flatulence (≤10%), vomiting (≤6%), nausea (≤5%), dyspepsia (≤4%), abdominal pain (1% to 3%), constipation (1% to 3%), salivation increased (1% to 3%), xerostomia (1% to 3%), weight gain (not attributed to edema or fluid retention)

Genitourinary: Impotence (4% to 14%), decreased libido (≤5%), urinary incontinence (1% to 3%), urinary tract infection (1% to 3%), urinary frequency (≤2%)

Hematologic: Anemia (≤5%), leukopenia (1% to 3%)

Hepatic: Hepatomegaly (1% to 3%), LDH increased (1% to 3%), cholestatic jaundice, hepatotoxicity

Neuromuscular & skeletal: Weakness (2% to 6%), neuropathy (1% to 3%), paresthesia (1% to 3%), carpal tunnel syndrome

Ocular: Amblyopia (1% to 3%)
Renal: Albuminuria (1% to 3%)
Respiratory: Dyspnea (1% to 3%), cough (1% to 3%), pharyngitis (1% to 3%), pneumonia (≤2%), hyperpnea
Miscellaneous: Diaphoresis (1% to 3%), herpes infection (1% to 3%), infection (1% to 3%), moniliasis (1% to 3%), tumor flare
Postmarketing and/or case reports: Thromboembolic phenomena (including deep vein thrombosis, pulmonary embolism, thrombophlebitis)

Drug Interactions

Metabolism/Transport Effects None known.

Avoid Concomitant Use

Avoid concomitant use of Megestrol with any of the following: Dofetilide

Increased Effect/Toxicity

Megestrol may increase the levels/effects of: Dofetilide

The levels/effects of Megestrol may be increased by: Herbs (Progestogenic Properties)

Decreased Effect

The levels/effects of Megestrol may be decreased by: Aminoglutethimide

Ethanol/Nutrition/Herb Interactions Herb/Nutraceutical: Avoid herbs with progestogenic properties (eg, bloodroot, chasteberry, damiana, oregano, and yucca); may enhance the adverse/toxic effect of megestrol.

Storage/Stability

Suspension: Store at 15°C to 25°C (59°F to 77°F); protect from heat.
Tablet: Store at 25°C (77°F); excursions permitted to 15°C to 30°C (59°F to 86°F); protect from heat (temperatures >40°C [>104°F])

Mechanism of Action A synthetic progestin with antiestrogenic properties which disrupt the estrogen receptor cycle. Megestrol interferes with the normal estrogen cycle and results in a lower LH titer. May also have a direct effect on the endometrium. Megestrol is an antineoplastic progestin thought to act through an antileutenizing effect mediated via the pituitary. May stimulate appetite by antagonizing the metabolic effects of catabolic cytokines.

Pharmacodynamics/Kinetics

Absorption: Well absorbed orally
Metabolism: Hepatic (to free steroids and glucuronide conjugates)
Half-life elimination: 13-105 hours
Time to peak, serum: 1-3 hours
Excretion: Urine (57% to 78%; 5% to 8% as metabolites); feces (8% to 30%)

Dosing

Adult & Geriatric Note: Megace® ES suspension is not equivalent to other formulations on a mg-per-mg basis.

Breast carcinoma (females): Refer to individual protocols: Oral: Tablet: 40 mg 4 times/day

Endometrial carcinoma: Refer to individual protocols: Oral: Tablet: 40-320 mg/day in divided doses; use for 2 months to determine efficacy; maximum doses used have been up to 800 mg/day.

HIV-related cachexia (males/females): Oral: Suspension:

Megace®: Initial dose: 800 mg/day; daily doses of 400 and 800 mg/day were found to be clinically effective
Megace® ES: 625 mg/day

Renal Impairment No data available; however, the urinary excretion of megestrol acetate administered in doses of 4-90 mg ranged from 57% to 78% within 10 days.

Administration Megestrol acetate (Megace®) oral suspension is compatible with water, orange juice, apple juice, or Sustacal H.C. for immediate consumption. Shake suspension well before use.

Monitoring Parameters Observe for signs of thromboembolic events; blood pressure, weight; serum glucose

Test Interactions Altered thyroid and liver function tests

Dosage Forms Excipient information presented when available (limited, particularly for generics); consult specific product labeling.

Suspension, oral, as acetate: 40 mg/mL (10 mL, 20 mL, 237 mL, 240 mL, 473 mL, 480 mL)

Megace®: 40 mg/mL (240 mL) [contains ethanol 0.06%, sodium benzoate; lemon-lime flavor]

Megace® ES: 125 mg/mL (150 mL) [contains ethanol 0.06%, sodium benzoate; lemon-lime flavor]

Tablet, oral, as acetate: 20 mg, 40 mg

References

Fietkau R, Riepl M, Kettner H, et al, "Supportive Use of Megestrol Acetate in Patients With Head and Neck Cancer During Radio(Chemo)Therapy," *Eur J Cancer*, 1997, 33(1):75-9.

Lentz SS, Brady MF, Major FJ, et al, "High-Dose Megestrol Acetate in Advanced or Recurrent Endometrial Carcinoma: A Gynecologic Oncology Group Study," *J Clin Oncol*, 1996, 14(2):357-61.

Strang P, "The Effect of Megestrol Acetate on Anorexia, Weight Loss and Cachexia in Cancer and AIDS Patients," *Anticancer Res*, 1997, 17(1B):657-62.

◆ **Megestrol Acetate** *see* Megestrol *on page 922*

Melphalan (MEL fa lan)

Related Information

Hematopoietic Stem Cell Transplantation *on page 1887*

Management of Chemotherapy-Induced Nausea and Vomiting *on page 1786*

Management of Drug Extravasations *on page 1800*

Oral Mucositis/Stomatitis *on page 1814*

Safe Handling of Hazardous Drugs *on page 1904*

Brand Names: U.S. Alkeran®

Brand Names: Canada Alkeran®

Index Terms L-PAM; L-Phenylalanine Mustard; L-Sarcolysin; Phenylalanine Mustard

Generic Availability (U.S.) Yes: Excludes tablet

Pharmacologic Category Antineoplastic Agent, Alkylating Agent

Use Palliative treatment of multiple myeloma and nonresectable epithelial ovarian carcinoma

Unlabeled Use Treatment of Hodgkin lymphoma, light chain amyloidosis; conditioning regimen for autologous hematopoietic stem cell transplantation in adults with hematologic disorders (eg, multiple myeloma) and autologous marrow or stem cell transplantation in pediatric neuroblastoma and Ewing's sarcoma

Labeled Contraindications Hypersensitivity to melphalan or any component of the formulation; patients whose disease was resistant to prior melphalan therapy

Pregnancy Risk Factor D

Lactation Excretion in breast milk unknown/not recommended

Warnings/Precautions **[U.S. Boxed Warning]: Bone marrow suppression is common; may be severe and result in infection or bleeding; has been demonstrated more with the I.V. formulation (compared to oral);** ▶

myelosuppression is dose-related. Monitor blood counts; may require treatment delay or dose modification for thrombocytopenia or neutropenia. Use with caution in patients with prior bone marrow suppression, impaired renal function (consider dose reduction), or who have received prior (or concurrent) chemotherapy or irradiation. Myelotoxicity is generally reversible, although irreversible bone marrow failure has been reported. In patients who are candidates for autologous transplantation, avoid melphalan-containing regimens prior to transplant (due to the effects on stem cell reserve). Signs of infection, such as fever and WBC rise, may not occur; lethargy and confusion may be more prominent signs of infection.

[U.S. Boxed Warning]: Hypersensitivity reactions (including anaphylaxis) have occurred in ~2% of patients receiving I.V. melphalan, usually after multiple treatment cycles. Discontinue infusion and treat symptomatically. Hypersensitivity may also occur (rarely) with oral melphalan. Do not readminister (oral or I.V.) in patients who experience hypersensitivity to melphalan.

Gastrointestinal toxicities, including nausea, vomiting, diarrhea and mucositis, are common. When administering high-dose melphalan in autologous transplantation, cryotherapy is recommended to prevent mucositis (Keefe, 2007). Abnormal liver function tests may occur; hepatitis and jaundice have also been reported; hepatic sinusoidal obstruction syndrome (SOS; formerly called veno-occlusive disease) has been reported with I.V. melphalan. Pulmonary fibrosis (some fatal) and interstitial pneumonitis have been observed with treatment. Dosage reduction is recommended with I.V. melphalan in patients with renal impairment; reduced initial doses may also be recommended with oral melphalan. Closely monitor patients with azotemia.

[U.S. Boxed Warning]: Produces chromosomal changes and is leukemogenic and potentially mutagenic; secondary malignancies (including acute myeloid leukemia, myeloproliferative disease, and carcinoma) have been reported reported (some patients were receiving combination chemotherapy or radiation therapy); the risk is increased with increased treatment duration and cumulative doses. Suppresses ovarian function and produces amenorrhea; may also cause testicular suppression.

Extravasation may cause local tissue damage; administration by slow injection into a fast running I.V. solution into an injection port or via a central line is recommended; do not administer directly into a peripheral vein. **[U.S. Boxed Warning]: Should be administered under the supervision of an experienced cancer chemotherapy physician.** Avoid vaccination with live vaccines during treatment if immunocompromised. Toxicity may be increased in elderly; start with lowest recommended adult doses.

Adverse Reactions

>10%:

- Gastrointestinal: Nausea/vomiting, diarrhea, oral ulceration
- Hematologic: Myelosuppression, leukopenia (nadir: 14-21 days; recovery: 28-35 days), thrombocytopenia (nadir: 14-21 days; recovery: 28-35 days), anemia
- Miscellaneous: Secondary malignancy (<2% to 20%; cumulative dose and duration dependent, includes acute myeloid leukemia, myeloproliferative syndrome, carcinoma)

1% to 10%: Miscellaneous: Hypersensitivity (I.V.: 2%; includes bronchospasm, dyspnea, edema, hypotension, pruritus, rash, tachycardia, urticaria)

Infrequent, frequency undefined, postmarketing, and/or case reports: Agranulocytosis, allergic reactions, alopecia, amenorrhea, anaphylaxis (rare), bleeding (with high-dose therapy), bone marrow failure (irreversible), BUN increased, cardiac arrest, cardiotoxicity (angina, arrhythmia, hypertension, MI; with high-dose therapy), encephalopathy, hemolytic anemia, hemorrhagic cystitis, hepatic sinusoidal obstruction syndrome (SOS; veno-occlusive disease; high-dose I.V. melphalan), hepatitis, infection, injection site reactions (ulceration, necrosis), interstitial pneumonitis, jaundice, mucositis (with high-dose therapy), ovarian suppression, paralytic ileus (with high-dose therapy), pruritus, pulmonary fibrosis, radiation myelopathy, rash (maculopapular), renal toxicity (with high-dose therapy), seizure (with high-dose therapy), sepsis, SIADH, skin hypersensitivity, sterility, stomatitis, testicular suppression, tingling sensation, transaminases increased, vasculitis, warmth sensation

Drug Interactions

Metabolism/Transport Effects None known.

Avoid Concomitant Use

Avoid concomitant use of Melphalan with any of the following: BCG; CloZAPine; Nalidixic Acid; Natalizumab; Pimecrolimus; Tacrolimus (Topical); Vaccines (Live)

Increased Effect/Toxicity

Melphalan may increase the levels/effects of: Carmustine; CloZAPine; CycloSPORINE (Systemic); Leflunomide; Natalizumab; Vaccines (Live); Vitamin K Antagonists

The levels/effects of Melphalan may be increased by: Denosumab; Nalidixic Acid; Pimecrolimus; Roflumilast; Tacrolimus (Topical); Trastuzumab

Decreased Effect

Melphalan may decrease the levels/effects of: BCG; Cardiac Glycosides; Coccidioidin Skin Test; Sipuleucel-T; Vaccines (Inactivated); Vaccines (Live); Vitamin K Antagonists

The levels/effects of Melphalan may be decreased by: Echinacea

Ethanol/Nutrition/Herb Interactions

Ethanol: Avoid ethanol (due to GI irritation).

Food: Food interferes with oral absorption.

Storage/Stability

Tablet: Store in refrigerator at 2°C to 8°C (36°F to 46°F). Protect from light.

Injection: Store at room temperature of 15°C to 30°C (59°F to 86°F). Protect from light. Stability is limited; must be prepared fresh. A 5 mg/mL concentration is chemically and physically stable for ≤90 minutes when stored at room temperature, although the manufacturer recommends administration be completed within 60 minutes of reconstitution; **immediately** dilute dose in NS. Do not refrigerate solution; precipitation occurs.

Reconstitution Use appropriate precautions for handling and disposal.

Injection: Stability is limited; must be prepared fresh. **The time between reconstitution/dilution and administration of parenteral melphalan must be kept to a minimum (manufacturer recommends <60 minutes) because reconstituted and diluted solutions are unstable.** Dissolve powder initially with 10 mL of supplied diluent to a concentration of 5 mg/mL; shake immediately and vigorously to dissolve. **Immediately** dilute dose in NS to a concentration of ≤0.45 mg/mL (manufacturer recommended concentration). Do not refrigerate solution; precipitation occurs. The manufacturer recommends administration within 60 minutes of reconstitution.

Mechanism of Action Alkylating agent which is a derivative of mechlorethamine that inhibits DNA and RNA synthesis via formation of carbonium ions; cross-links strands of DNA; acts on both resting and rapidly dividing tumor cells.

Pharmacodynamics/Kinetics Note: Pharmacokinetics listed are for FDA-approved doses.

Absorption: Oral: Variable and incomplete

Distribution: V_d: 0.5 L/kg; low penetration into CSF

Protein binding: 53% to 92%; primarily to albumin (40% to 60%), ~20% to α_1-acid glycoprotein

Metabolism: Hepatic; chemical hydrolysis to monohydroxymelphalan and dihydroxymelphalan

Bioavailability: Oral: Variable; 56% to 93%; exposure is reduced with a high-fat meal

Half-life elimination: Terminal: I.V.: 75 minutes; Oral: 1-2 hours

Time to peak, serum: Oral: ~1-2 hours

Excretion: Oral: Feces (20% to 50%); urine (~10% as unchanged drug)

Dosing

Adult

Details regarding dosing in combination regimens should also be consulted. Adjust dose based on patient response and weekly blood counts.

Multiple myeloma (palliative treatment): Note: Response is gradual; may require repeated courses to realize benefit:

Oral: Usual dose (as described in the manufacturer's labeling):

6 mg once daily for 2-3 weeks initially, followed by up to 4 weeks rest, then a maintenance dose of 2 mg daily as hematologic recovery begins **or**

10 mg daily for 7-10 days; institute 2 mg daily maintenance dose after WBC >4000 cells/mm^3 and platelets >100,000 cells/mm^3 (~4-8 weeks); titrate maintenance dose to hematologic response **or**

0.15 mg/kg/day for 7 days, with a 2-6 week rest, followed by a maintenance dose of ≤0.05 mg/kg/day as hematologic recovery begins **or**

0.25 mg/kg/day for 4 days (or 0.2 mg/kg/day for 5 days); repeat at 4- to 6-week intervals as ANC and platelet counts return to normal

Other dosing regimens in ***combination therapy*** *(unlabeled doses):*

4 mg/m^2/day for 7 days every 4 weeks (in combination with prednisone **or** with prednisone and thalidomide) (Palumbo, 2006; Palumbo, 2008) **or**

6 mg/m^2/day for 7 days every 4 weeks (in combination with prednisone) (Palumbo, 2004) **or**

0.25 mg/kg/day for 4 days every 6 weeks (in combination with prednisone [Facon, 2006; Facon, 2007] **or** with prednisone and thalidomide [Facon, 2007]) **or**

9 mg/m^2/day for 4 days every 6 weeks (in combination with prednisone **or** with prednisone and bortezomib) (Dimopoulos, 2009; San Miguel, 2008)

I.V.: 16 mg/m^2 administered at 2-week intervals for 4 doses, then administer at 4-week intervals after adequate hematologic recovery.

Ovarian carcinoma: Oral: 0.2 mg/kg/day for 5 days, repeat every 4-5 weeks **or**

Unlabeled dosing: 7 mg/m^2/day in 2 divided doses for 5 days, repeat every 28 days (Wadler, 1996)

Amyloidosis, light chain (unlabeled use): Oral: 0.22 mg/kg/day for 4 days every 28 days (in combination with oral dexamethasone) (Palladini, 2004)

or 10 mg/m^2/day for 4 days every month (in combination with oral dexamethasone) for 12-18 treatment cycles (Jaccard, 2007)

Hodgkin lymphoma (unlabeled use): I.V.: 30 mg/m^2 on day 6 of combination chemotherapy (mini-BEAM) regimen (Colwill, 1995; Martin, 2001)

Conditioning regimen for autologous hematopoietic stem cell transplantation (unlabeled use): I.V.:

200 mg/m^2 alone 2 days prior to transplantation (Fermand, 2005; Moreau, 2002) **or**

140 mg/m^2 2 days prior to transplantation (combined with busulfan) (Fermand, 2005) **or**

140 mg/m^2 2 days prior to transplantation (combined with total body irradiation [TBI]) (Moreau, 2002) **or**

140 mg/m^2 5 days prior to transplantation (combined with TBI) (Barlogie, 2006)

Geriatric Refer to adult dosing. Use caution and begin at the lower end of dosing range.

Pediatric Details regarding dosing in combination regimens should also be consulted.

Conditioning regimen for autologous hematopoietic stem cell transplantation (unlabeled use): I.V.:

140 mg/m^2 2 days prior to transplantation (combined with busulfan) (Canete, 2009; Oberlin, 2006) **or**

180 mg/m^2 (with pre- and posthydration) 12-30 hours prior to transplantation (Pritchard, 2005) **or**

45 mg/m^2/day for 4 days starting 8 days prior to transplantation (combined with busulfan or etoposide and carboplatin) (Berthold, 2005)

Renal Impairment

The FDA-approved labeling contains the following adjustment recommendations (for approved dosing levels) based on route of administration:

Oral: Moderate-to-severe renal impairment: Consider a reduced dose initially.

I.V.: BUN ≥30 mg/dL: Reduce dose by up to 50%.

The following guidelines have been used by some clinicians:

Aronoff, 2007 (route of administration not specified): Adults (based on a 6 mg once-daily dose):

Cl_{cr} 10-50 mL/minute: Administer 75% of dose.

Cl_{cr} <10 mL/minute: Administer 50% of dose.

Hemodialysis: Administer dose after hemodialysis.

Continuous ambulatory peritoneal dialysis (CAPD): Administer 50% of dose.

Continuous renal replacement therapy (CRRT): Administer 75% of dose.

Carlson, 2005: Oral (for melphalan-prednisone combination therapy; based on a study evaluating toxicity with melphalan dosed at 0.25 mg/kg/day for 4 days/cycle):

Cl_{cr} >10 to <30 mL/minute: Administer 75% of dose

Cl_{cr} ≤10 mL/minute: Data is insufficient for a recommendation

Kintzel, 1995:

Oral: Adjust dose in the presence of hematologic toxicity

I.V.:

Cl_{cr} 46-60 mL/minute: Administer 85% of normal dose.

Cl_{cr} 31-45 mL/minute: Administer 75% of normal dose.

Cl_{cr} <30 mL/minute: Administer 70% of normal dose.

Badros, 2001: I.V.: Autologous stem cell transplant (single-agent conditioning regimen; no busulfan or irradiation): Serum creatinine >2 mg/dL: Reduce dose from 200 mg/m^2 over 2 days (as 100 mg/m^2/day for 2 days) to 140 mg/m^2 given as a single-dose infusion

Hepatic Impairment Melphalan is hepatically metabolized; however, dosage adjustment does not appear to be necessary (King, 2001).

Adjustment for Toxicity

Oral:

WBC <3000/mm^3: Withhold treatment until recovery

Platelets <100,000/mm^3: Withhold treatment until recovery

I.V.: Adjust dose based on nadir blood cell counts

Combination Regimens

Lymphoma, Hodgkin:

Dexa-BEAM (Hodgkin) on page 1607
mini-BEAM (Hodgkin) on page 1712

Multiple myeloma:

Bortezomib-Melphalan-Prednisone-Thalidomide on page 1537
Melphalan-Prednisone-Bortezomib (Multiple Myeloma) on page 1708
Melphalan-Prednisone (Multiple Myeloma) on page 1709
Melphalan-Prednisone-Thalidomide (Multiple Myeloma) on page 1710
VBMCP (Multiple Myeloma) on page 1769

Administration

Oral: Administer on an empty stomach (1 hour prior to or 2 hours after meals)

Parenteral: Due to limited stability, complete administration of I.V. dose should occur within 60 minutes of reconstitution

I.V.: Infuse over 15-30 minutes. Extravasation may cause local tissue damage; administration by slow injection into a fast running I.V. solution into an injection port or via a central line is recommended; do not administer by direct injection into a peripheral vein.

Emetic Potential

I.V.: >50 mg/m^2: Moderate (30% to 90%)

Oral, low dose: Very low (<10%)

Vesicant/Extravasation Risk May be an irritant

Monitoring Parameters CBC with differential and platelet count, serum electrolytes, serum uric acid

Test Interactions False-positive Coombs' test [direct]

Dietary Considerations Should be taken on an empty stomach (1 hour prior to or 2 hours after meals).

Dosage Forms Excipient information presented when available (limited, particularly for generics); consult specific product labeling.

Injection, powder for reconstitution: 50 mg

Alkeran®: 50 mg [contains ethanol (in diluent), propylene glycol (in diluent)]

Tablet, oral:

Alkeran®: 2 mg

References

Aronoff GR, Bennett WM, Berns JS, et al, *Drug Prescribing in Renal Failure: Dosing Guidelines for Adults and Children*, 5th ed. Philadelphia, PA: American College of Physicians; 2007, p 100.

Badros A, Barlogie B, Siegel E, et al, "Results of Autologous Stem Cell Transplant in Multiple Myeloma Patients With Renal Failure," *Br J Haematol*, 2001, 114(4):822-9.

Barlogie B, Kyle RA, Anderson KC, et al, "Standard Chemotherapy Compared With High-Dose Chemoradiotherapy for Multiple Myeloma: Final Results of Phase III US Intergroup Trial S9321," *J Clin Oncol*, 2006, 24(6):929-36.

Berthold F, Boos J, Burdach S, et al, "Myeloablative Megatherapy With Autologous Stem-Cell Rescue Versus Oral Maintenance Chemotherapy as Consolidation Treatment in Patients With High-Risk Neuroblastoma: A Randomised Controlled Trial," *Lancet Oncol*, 2005, 6(9):649-58.

Canete A, Gerrard M. Rubie H, et al, "Poor Survival for Infants with MYCN-Amplified Metastatic Neuroblastoma Despite Intensified Treatment: The International Society for Paediatric Oncology European Neuroblastoma Experience," *J Clin Oncol*, 2009, 27(7):1014-9.

Carlson K, Hjorth M, Knudsen LM, et al, "Toxicity in Standard Melphalan-Prednisone Therapy Among Myeloma Patients With Renal Failure - A Retrospective Analysis and Recommendations for Dose Adjustment," *Br J Haematol*, 2005, 128(5):631-5.

Colwill R, Crump M, Couture F, et al, "Mini-BEAM as Salvage Therapy for Relapsed or Refractory Hodgkin's Disease Before Intensive Therapy or Autologous Bone Marrow Transplantation," *J Clin Oncol*, 1995, 13(2):396-402.

Dimopoulos MA, Richardson PG, Schlag R, et al, "VMP (Bortezomib, Melphalan, and Prednisone) is Active and Well Tolerated in Newly Diagnosed Patients With Multiple Myeloma With Moderately Impaired Renal Function, and Results in Reversal of Renal Impairment: Cohort Analysis of the Phase III VISTA Study," *J Clin Oncol*, 2009, 27(36):6086-93.

Facon T, Mary JY, Hulin C, et al, "Melphalan and Prednisone Plus Thalidomide Versus Melphalan and Prednisone Alone or Reduced-Intensity Autologous Stem Cell Transplantation in Elderly Patients With Multiple Myeloma (IFM 99-06): A Randomised Trial," *Lancet*, 2007, 370 (9594):1209-18.

Facon T, Mary JY, Pegourie B, et al, "Dexamethasone-Based Regimens versus Melphalan-Prednisone for Elderly Multiple Myeloma Patients Ineligible for High-Dose Therapy," *Blood*, 2006, 107(4):1292-8.

Fermand JP, Katsahian S, Divine M, et al, "High-Dose Therapy and Autologous Blood Stem-Cell Transplantation Compared With Conventional Treatment in Myeloma Patients Aged 55 to 65 years: Long-Term Results of a Randomized Control Trial From the Group Myelome-Autogreffe," *J Clin Oncol*, 2005, 23(36):9227-33.

Jaccard A, Moreau P, Leblond V, et al, "High-Dose Melphalan versus Melphalan Plus Dexamethasone for AL Amyloidosis," *N Engl J Med*, 2007, 357(11):1083-93.

Keefe DM, Schubert MM, Elting LS, et al, "Updated Clinical Practice Guidelines for the Prevention and Treatment of Mucositis," *Cancer*, 2007, 109(5):820-31.

King PD and Perry MC, "Hepatotoxicity of Chemotherapy," *Oncologist*, 2001, 6(2):162-76.

Kintzel PE and Dorr RT, "Anticancer Drug Renal Toxicity and Elimination: Dosing Guidelines for Altered Renal Function," *Cancer Treat Rev*, 1995, 21(1):33-64.

Martin A, Fernandez-Jimenez MC, Caballero MD, et al, "Long-Term Follow-Up in Patients Treated with Mini-BEAM as Salvage Therapy for Relapsed or Refractory Hodgkin's Disease," *Br J Haematol*, 2001, 113(1):161-71.

Moreau P, Facon T, Attal M, et al, "Comparison of 200 mg/m^2 Melphalan and 8 Gy Total Body Irradiation Plus 140 mg/m^2 Melphalan as Conditioning Regimens for Peripheral Blood Stem Cell Transplantation in Patients With Newly Diagnosed Multiple Myeloma: Final Analysis of the Intergroupe Francophone du Myélome 9502 Randomized Trial," *Blood*, 2002, 99(3):731-5.

Nath CE, Shaw PJ, Trotman J, et al, "Population Pharmacokinetics of Melphalan in Patients With Multiple Myeloma Undergoing High Dose Therapy," *Br J Clin Pharmacol*, 2010, 69(5):484-97.

Oberlin O, Rey A, Desfachelles AS, et al, "Impact of High-Dose Busulfan Plus Melphalan as Consolidation in Metastatic Ewing Tumors: A Study by the Societe Francaise des Cancers de l'Enfant," *J Clin Oncol*, 2006, 24(24):3997-4002.

Palladini G, Perfetti V, Obici L, et al, "Association of Melphalan and High-Dose Dexamethasone is Effective and Well Tolerated in Patients With AL (Primary) Amyloidosis Who are Ineligible for Stem Cell Transplantation," *Blood*, 2004, 103(8):2936-8.

Palumbo A, Bringhen S, Caravita T, et al, "Oral Melphalan and Prednisone Chemotherapy Plus Thalidomide Compared With Melphalan and Prednisone Alone in Elderly Patients With Multiple Myeloma: Randomised Controlled Trial," *Lancet*, 2006, 367(9513):825-31.

Palumbo A, Bringhen S, Liberati AM, et al, "Oral Melphalan, Prednisone, and Thalidomide in Elderly Patients With Multiple Myeloma: Updated Results of a Randomized Controlled Trial," *Blood*, 2008, 112(8):3107-14.

Palumbo A, Bringhen S, Petrucci MT, et al, "Intermediate-Dose Melphalan Improves Survival of Myeloma Patients Aged 50 to 70: Results of a Randomized Controlled Trial," *Blood*, 2004, 104 (10):3052-7.

Pritchard J, Cotterill SJ, Germond SM, et al, "High Dose Melphalan in the Treatment of Advanced Neuroblastoma: Results of a Randomised Trial (ENSG-1) by the European Neuroblastoma Study Group," *Pediatr Blood Cancer*, 2005, 44(4):348-57.

San Miguel JF, Schlag R, Khuageva NK, et al, "Bortezomib Plus Melphalan and Prednisone for Initial Treatment of Multiple Myeloma," *New Engl J Med*, 2008, 359(9):906-17.

Schuh A, Dandridge J, Haydon P, et al, "Encephalopathy Complicating High-Dose Melphalan," *Bone Marrow Transplant*, 1999, 24(10):1141-3.

Wadler S, Yeap B, Vogl S, et al, "Randomized Trial of Initial Therapy With Melphalan Versus Cisplatin-Based Combination Chemotherapy in Patients With Advanced Ovarian Carcinoma: Initial and Long Term Results – Eastern Cooperative Oncology Group Study E2878," *Cancer*, 1996, 77(40):733-42.

Meperidine (me PER i deen)

Brand Names: U.S. Demerol®

Brand Names: Canada Demerol®

Index Terms Isonipecaine Hydrochloride; Meperidine Hydrochloride; Pethidine Hydrochloride

Generic Availability (U.S.) Yes

Pharmacologic Category Analgesic, Opioid

Use Management of moderate-to-severe pain; adjunct to anesthesia and preoperative sedation

Unlabeled Use Reduce postoperative shivering; reduce rigors from amphotericin B (conventional)

Labeled Contraindications Hypersensitivity to meperidine or any component of the formulation; use with or within 14 days of MAO inhibitors; severe respiratory insufficiency

Pregnancy Risk Factor C

Lactation Enters breast milk/not recommended (AAP rates "compatible"; AAP 2001 update pending)

Warnings/Precautions Oral meperidine is not recommended for acute/chronic pain management. Meperidine should not be used for acute/cancer pain because of the risk of neurotoxicity. Normeperidine (an active metabolite and CNS stimulant) may accumulate and precipitate anxiety, tremors, or seizures; risk increases with CNS or renal dysfunction, prolonged use (>48 hours), and cumulative dose (>600 mg/24 hours). The Institute for Safe Medication Practice recommends avoiding the use of meperidine for pain control, especially in the elderly and renally-impaired (ISMP, 2007). In the elderly; meperidine is not an effective oral analgesic at commonly used doses; may cause neurotoxicity; other agents are preferred in the elderly (Beers Criteria).

May cause CNS depression, which may impair physical or mental abilities; patients must be cautioned about performing tasks which require mental alertness (eg, operating machinery or driving). Effects (eg, sedation, respiratory depression, hypotension) may be potentiated when used with other sedative/hypnotic drugs, general anesthetics, phenothiazines, or ethanol; consider reduced dose of meperidine if using concomitantly. Use only with extreme caution (if at all) in patients with head injury or increased intracranial pressure (ICP). Use caution with pulmonary, hepatic, or renal disorders, supraventricular tachycardias (including atrial flutter), acute abdominal conditions, delirium tremens, hypothyroidism, myxedema, toxic psychosis, kyphoscoliosis, morbid obesity, Addison's disease, seizure disorders, pheochromocytoma, BPH, or urethral stricture. Use with caution in patients with biliary tract dysfunction; acute pancreatitis may cause constriction of sphincter of Oddi. May cause hypotension (including orthostatic hypotension); use with caution in patients with depleted blood volume or drugs which may exaggerate hypotensive effects (including phenothiazines or general anesthetics).

An opioid-containing analgesic regimen should be tailored to each patient's needs and based upon the type of pain being treated (acute versus chronic), the route of administration, degree of tolerance for opioids (naive versus chronic user), age, weight, and medical condition. The optimal analgesic dose varies widely among patients. Some preparations contain sulfites which may cause allergic reaction. Tolerance or drug dependence may result from extended use. Healthcare provider should be alert to problems of abuse, misuse, and diversion. Concurrent use of agonist/antagonist analgesics may precipitate withdrawal symptoms and/or reduced analgesic efficacy in patients following prolonged therapy with mu opioid agonists. Abrupt discontinuation following prolonged use may also lead to withdrawal symptoms. Avoid use in the elderly.

Ethanol/Nutrition/Herb Interactions

Ethanol: May increase CNS depression; monitor for increased effects with coadministration. Caution patients about effects.

Herb/Nutraceutical: Avoid valerian, St John's wort, kava kava, gotu kola (may increase CNS depression).

Storage/Stability

Injection solution: Store at 20°C to 25°C (68°F to 77°F); excursions permitted to 15°C to 30°C (59°F to 86°F).

Tablets: Store at 25°C (77°F); excursions permitted to 15°C to 30°C (59°F to 86°F).

Mechanism of Action Binds to opioid receptors in the CNS, causing inhibition of ascending pain pathways, altering the perception of and response to pain; produces generalized CNS depression

Pharmacodynamics/Kinetics

Onset of action: Analgesic: Oral, SubQ: 10-15 minutes; I.V.: ~5 minutes

Peak effect: SubQ.: ~1 hour; Oral: 2 hours

Duration: Oral, SubQ.: 2-4 hours

Absorption: I.M.: Erratic and highly variable

Protein binding: 65% to 75%

Metabolism: Hepatic; hydrolyzed to meperidinic acid (inactive) or undergoes N-demethylation to normeperidine (active; has 1/2 the analgesic effect and 2-3 times the CNS effects of meperidine)

Bioavailability: ~50% to 60%; increased with liver disease

Half-life elimination:

Parent drug: Terminal phase: Adults: 2.5-4 hours, Liver disease: 7-11 hours

Normeperidine (active metabolite): 15-30 hours; can accumulate with high doses (>600 mg/day) or with decreased renal function

Excretion: Urine (as metabolites)

Dosing

Adult Note: The American Pain Society (2008) and ISMP (2007) do not recommend meperidine's use as an analgesic. If use in acute pain (in patients without renal or CNS disease) cannot be avoided, treatment should be limited to ≤48 hours and doses should not exceed 600 mg/24 hours. Oral route is not recommended for treatment of acute or chronic pain. If I.V. route is required, consider a reduced dose. Patients with prior opioid exposure may require higher initial doses.

Pain (analgesic): Oral, I.M., SubQ: 50-150 mg every 3-4 hours as needed

Preoperatively: I.M., SubQ: 50-150 mg given 30-90 minutes before the beginning of anesthesia

Obstetrical analgesia: I.M., SubQ: 50-100 mg when pain becomes regular; may repeat at every 1-3 hours

Postoperative shivering (unlabeled use): I.V.: 25-50 mg once (Crowley, 2008; Kranke, 2002; Mercandante, 1994; Wang, 1999)

Geriatric Avoid use (American Pain Society, 2008; ISMP, 2007).

Pediatric Note: The American Pain Society (2008) and ISMP (2007) do not recommend meperidine's use as an analgesic. If use in acute pain (in patients without renal or CNS disease) cannot be avoided, treatment should be limited to ≤48 hours and doses should not exceed 600 mg/24 hours. Oral route is not recommended for treatment of acute or chronic pain. If I.V. route is required, consider a reduced dose. Patients with prior opioid exposure may require higher initial doses.

Pain (analgesic): Oral, I.M., SubQ: 1.1-1.8 mg/kg/dose every 3-4 hours as needed (maximum: 50-150 mg/dose)

Preoperatively: I.M., SubQ: 1.1-2.2 mg/kg given 30-90 minutes before the beginning of anesthesia (maximum: 50-150 mg/dose)

Renal Impairment Avoid use in renal impairment (American Pain Society, 2008; ISMP, 2007).

Hepatic Impairment Use with caution in severe hepatic impairment; consider a lower initial dose when initiating therapy. An increased opioid effect may be seen in patients with cirrhosis; dose reduction is more important for the oral than I.V. route.

Administration

Solution for injection: Meperidine may be administered I.M., SubQ, or I.V.; I.V. push should be administered slowly using a diluted solution, use of a 10 mg/mL concentration has been recommended.

Oral solution: Administer solution in 1/2 glass of water; undiluted solution may exert topical anesthetic effect on mucous membranes

Test Interactions Increased amylase (S), increased BSP retention, increased CPK (I.M. injections)

Dosage Forms Excipient information presented when available (limited, particularly for generics); consult specific product labeling. [DSC] = Discontinued product

Injection, solution, as hydrochloride: 25 mg/mL (1 mL); 50 mg/mL (1 mL [DSC]); 100 mg/mL (1 mL [DSC])

Demerol®: 25 mg/mL (1 mL); 25 mg/0.5 mL (0.5 mL); 50 mg/mL (1 mL, 1.5 mL, 2 mL, 30 mL); 75 mg/mL (1 mL); 100 mg/mL (1 mL, 20 mL)

Injection, solution, as hydrochloride [for PCA pump]: 10 mg/mL (30 mL)

Solution, oral, as hydrochloride: 50 mg/5 mL (500 mL)

Tablet, oral, as hydrochloride: 50 mg, 100 mg

Demerol®: 50 mg [scored]

Demerol®: 100 mg

Controlled Substance C-II

◆ **Meperidine Hydrochloride** *see* Meperidine *on page* 932

◆ **Mephyton®** *see* Phytonadione *on page* 1169

◆ **Mercaptoethane Sulfonate** *see* Mesna *on page* 940

Mercaptopurine (mer kap toe PURE een)

Related Information

Management of Chemotherapy-Induced Nausea and Vomiting *on page* 1786

Safe Handling of Hazardous Drugs *on page* 1904

Brand Names: U.S. Purinethol®

Brand Names: Canada Purinethol®

Index Terms 6-Mercaptopurine (error-prone abbreviation); 6-MP (error-prone abbreviation)

Generic Availability (U.S.) Yes

Pharmacologic Category Antineoplastic Agent, Antimetabolite; Antineoplastic Agent, Antimetabolite (Purine Analog); Immunosuppressant Agent

Use Maintenance treatment component of acute lymphoblastic leukemia (ALL)

Unlabeled Use Steroid-sparing agent for corticosteroid-dependent Crohn's disease (CD) and ulcerative colitis (UC); maintenance of remission in CD; fistulizing Crohn's disease; maintenance treatment in acute promyelocytic leukemia (APL); treatment component for non Hodgkin lymphoma (NHL), treatment of autoimmune hepatitis

Labeled Contraindications Hypersensitivity to mercaptopurine or any component of the formulation; patients whose disease showed prior resistance to mercaptopurine

Pregnancy Risk Factor D

Lactation Enters breast milk/not recommended

Warnings/Precautions Hazardous agent - use appropriate precautions for handling and disposal.

Hepatotoxicity has been reported, including jaundice, ascites, hepatic necrosis (may be fatal), intrahepatic cholestasis, parenchymal cell necrosis, and/or hepatic encephalopathy; may be due to direct hepatic cell damage or hypersensitivity. While hepatotoxicity or hepatic injury may occur at any dose, dosages >2.5 mg/kg/day are associated with a higher incidence. Signs of jaundice generally appear early in treatment, after ~1-2 months (range: 1 week to 8 years) and may resolve following discontinuation; recurrence with rechallenge has been noted. Monitor liver function tests (monitor more frequently if used in combination with other hepatotoxic drugs or in patients with pre-existing hepatic impairment. Consider a reduced dose in patients with hepatic impairment. Withhold treatment for clinical signs of jaundice (hepatomegaly, anorexia, tenderness), deterioration in liver function tests, toxic hepatitis, or biliary stasis until hepatotoxicity is ruled out.

Dose-related leukopenia, thrombocytopenia, and anemia are common; however, may be indicative of disease progression. Hematologic toxicity may be delayed. Bone marrow may appear hypoplastic (could also appear normal). Monitor for bleeding (due to thrombocytopenia) or infection (due to neutropenia). Patients with homozygous genetic defect of thiopurine methyltransferase (TPMT) are more sensitive to myelosuppressive effects; generally associated with rapid myelosuppression. Significant mercaptopurine dose reductions will be necessary (possibly with continued concomitant chemotherapy at normal doses). Patients who are heterozygous for TPMT defects will have intermediate activity; may have increased toxicity (primarily myelosuppression) although will generally tolerate normal mercaptopurine doses. Consider TPMT testing for severe toxicities/excessive myelosuppression. Patients on concurrent therapy with drugs which may inhibit TPMT (eg, olsalazine) or xanthine oxidase (eg, allopurinol) may be sensitive to myelosuppressive effects.

May increase the risk for secondary malignancies; hepatic T-cell lymphoma (HTCL) has been reported with mercaptopurine when used for the treatment of irritable bowel disease (an unlabeled use). Because azathioprine is metabolized to mercaptopurine, concomitant use with azathioprine may result in profound myelosuppression and should be avoided. Mercaptopurine is immunosuppressive; the risk for infection is increased; common signs of infection, such as fever and leukocytosis may not occur; lethargy and confusion may be more prominent signs of infection. Immune response to vaccines may be diminished. Consider adjusting dosage in patients with renal impairment. To avoid potentially serious dosage errors, the terms "6-mercaptopurine" or "6-MP" should be avoided; use of these terms has been associated with sixfold overdosages.

Adverse Reactions Frequency not defined.

Central nervous system: Drug fever

Dermatologic: Alopecia, hyperpigmentation, rash

Endocrine & metabolic: Hyperuricemia

Gastrointestinal: Anorexia, diarrhea, intestinal ulcers, mucositis/oral lesions (rare), nausea (minimal), pancreatitis, sprue-like symptoms, stomach pain, vomiting (minimal)

Genitourinary: Oligospermia

Hematologic: Myelosuppression (onset 7-10 days; nadir 14 days; recovery: 21 days); anemia, bleeding, granulocytopenia, leukopenia, marrow hypoplasia, thrombocytopenia

Hepatic: Hepatotoxicity, ascites, biliary stasis, hepatic damage/injury, hepatic encephalopathy, hepatic necrosis, hepatomegaly, intrahepatic cholestasis, jaundice, parenchymal cell necrosis, toxic hepatitis

Renal: Hyperuricosuria, renal toxicity

Miscellaneous: Hepatosplenic T cell lymphoma, immunosuppression, infection, secondary malignancy

Drug Interactions

Metabolism/Transport Effects None known.

Avoid Concomitant Use

Avoid concomitant use of Mercaptopurine with any of the following: AzaTHIOprine; BCG; CloZAPine; Febuxostat; Natalizumab; Pimecrolimus; Tacrolimus (Topical)

Increased Effect/Toxicity

Mercaptopurine may increase the levels/effects of: CloZAPine; Leflunomide; Natalizumab; Vaccines (Live); Vitamin K Antagonists

The levels/effects of Mercaptopurine may be increased by: 5-ASA Derivatives; Allopurinol; AzaTHIOprine; Denosumab; Febuxostat; Pimecrolimus; Roflumilast; Sulfamethoxazole; Tacrolimus (Topical); Trastuzumab; Trimethoprim

Decreased Effect

Mercaptopurine may decrease the levels/effects of: BCG; Coccidioidin Skin Test; Sipuleucel-T; Vaccines (Inactivated); Vitamin K Antagonists

The levels/effects of Mercaptopurine may be decreased by: Echinacea

Ethanol/Nutrition/Herb Interactions Food: Absorption is variable with food. Management: Take on an empty stomach at the same time each day 1 hour before or 2 hours after a meal. Maintain adequate hydration, unless instructed to restrict fluid intake.

Storage/Stability Store at room temperature of 15°C to 25°C (59°F to 77°F). Protect from moisture.

Mechanism of Action Purine antagonist which inhibits DNA and RNA synthesis; acts as false metabolite and is incorporated into DNA and RNA, eventually inhibiting their synthesis; specific for the S phase of the cell cycle

Pharmacodynamics/Kinetics

Absorption: Variable and incomplete (~50%)

Distribution: V_d: > total body water; CNS penetration is poor

Protein binding: ~19%

Metabolism: Hepatic and in GI mucosa; hepatically via xanthine oxidase and methylation via TPMT to sulfate conjugates, 6-thiouric acid, and other inactive compounds; first-pass effect

Half-life elimination (age dependent): Children: 21 minutes; Adults: 47 minutes

Time to peak, serum: ~2 hours

Excretion: Urine (46% as mercaptopurine and metabolites)

Dosing

Adult Also consult details concerning dosing in combination regimens.

Acute lymphoblastic leukemia (ALL): Maintenance: Oral: 1.5-2.5 mg/kg/day **or**

Unlabeled ALL dosing (combination chemotherapy; refer to specific reference for combinations):

Early intensification (two 4-week courses): 60 mg/m²/day days 1-14 (Larson, 1995; Larson, 1998)

Interim maintenance (12-week course): 60 mg/m²/day days 1-70 (Larson, 1995; Larson, 1998)

Maintenance (prolonged): 50 mg 3 times/day for 2 years (Kantarjian, 2000; Thomas, 2004) **or** 60 mg/m²/day for 2 years from diagnosis (Larson, 1995; Larson, 1998)

Acute promyelocytic leukemia (APL) maintenance (unlabeled use): 60 mg/m²/day for 1 year (in combination with tretinoin and methotrexate) (Powell, 2010)

Crohn's disease, remission maintenance or reduction of steroid use (unlabeled use): Oral: 1-1.5 mg/kg/day (Lichtenstein, 2009)

Ulcerative colitis (unlabeled use): Oral:

Initial: 50 mg once daily; titrate dose up if clinical remission not achieved or down if leukopenia occurs (Lobel, 2004) **or**

Initial: 50 mg (25 mg if heterozygous for TPMT activity) once daily; titrate up to goal of 1.5 mg/kg (0.75 mg/kg if heterozygous for TPMT activity) if WBC >4000/mm³ (and at least 50% of baseline) and LFTs and amylase are stable (Siegel, 2005) **or**

Maintenance: 1-1.5 mg/kg/day (Carter, 2004) **or**

Remission maintenance: 1.5 mg/kg/day (Danese, 2011)

Dosage adjustment with concurrent allopurinol: Reduce mercaptopurine dosage to 25% to 33% of the usual dose.

Dosage adjustment in TPMT-deficiency: Not always established; substantial reductions are generally required only in homozygous deficiency.

Geriatric Due to renal decline with age, initiate treatment at the low end of recommended dose range.

Pediatric Also consult details concerning dosing in combination regimens.

Acute lymphoblastic leukemia (ALL): Maintenance: Oral: 1.5-2.5 mg/kg/day **or**

Unlabeled ALL dosing *(combination chemotherapy; refer to specific reference for combinations):* Adolescents ≥15 years:

Consolidation phase: 60 mg/m²/day days 0-27 days (5-week course) (Stock, 2008) **or** 60 mg/m²/day days 0-13 and days 28-41 (9-week course) (Stock, 2008)

Early intensification (two 4-week courses): 60 mg/m²/day days 1-14 (Larson, 1995; Larson, 1998; Stock, 2008)

Interim maintenance: 60 mg/m²/day days 0-41 (8-week course) (Stock, 2008) **or** 60 mg/m²/day days 1-70 (12-week course) (Larson, 1995; Larson, 1998; Stock, 2008)

Maintenance (prolonged): 50 mg 3 times/day for 2 years (Kantarjian, 2000; Thomas, 2004) **or** 60 mg/m^2/day for 2 years from diagnosis (Larson, 1995; Larson, 1998; Stock, 2008) **or** 75 mg/m^2/day for 2 years (girls) or 3 years (boys) from first interim maintenance (Stock, 2008)

APL maintenance (unlabeled use): Oral: Adolescents ≥15 years: 60 mg/m^2/day for 1 year (in combination with tretinoin and methotrexate) (Powell, 2010)

Autoimmune hepatitis (unlabeled use): Oral: 1.5 mg/kg/day (in combination with prednisone) (Manns, 2010)

Dosage adjustment with concurrent allopurinol: Reduce mercaptopurine dosage to 25% to 33% of the usual dose.

Dosage adjustment in TPMT-deficiency: Not always established; substantial reductions are generally required only in homozygous deficiency.

Renal Impairment The manufacturer's labeling recommends starting with reduced doses in patients with renal impairment to avoid accumulation; however, no specific dosage adjustment is provided. The following adjustments have been used by some clinicians (Aronoff, 2007): Children:

Cl_{cr} <50 mL/minute/1.73m^2: Administer every 48 hours

Hemodialysis: Administer every 48 hours

Continuous ambulatory peritoneal dialysis (CAPD): Administer every 48 hours

Continuous renal replacement therapy (CRRT): Administer every 48 hours

Hepatic Impairment The manufacturer's labeling recommends considering a reduced dose in patients with hepatic impairment; however, no specific dosage adjustment is provided.

Combination Regimens

Leukemia, acute lymphocytic:

Hyper-CVAD (Leukemia, Acute Lymphocytic) on page 1681
Larson Regimen (ALL) on page 1699
MTX/6-MP/VP (Maintenance) on page 1717
POMP on page 1741
PVA (POG 8602) on page 1742

Leukemia, acute promyelocytic:

Tretinoin-Daunorubicin (APL) on page 1762
Tretinoin-Daunorubicin-Cytarabine (APL) on page 1762
Tretinoin-Idarubicin (APL) on page 1764

Administration Preferably on an empty stomach (1 hour before or 2 hours after meals)

For the treatment of ALL in children (Schmiegelow, 1997): Administration in the evening has demonstration superior outcome; administration with food did not significantly affect outcome.

Emetic Potential Very low (<10%)

Extemporaneous Preparations Hazardous agent: Use appropriate precautions for handling and disposal.

A 50 mg/mL oral suspension may be prepared in a vertical flow hood with tablets and a 1:1 mixture of methylcellulose 1% and simple syrup. Crush thirty 50 mg tablets in a mortar and reduce to a fine powder. Add small portions of the vehicle and mix to a uniform paste; mix while adding the vehicle in incremental proportions to a final volume of 30 mL; transfer to a calibrated bottle. **Note:** May use ultrasonication dispersal. Label "shake well" and "caution chemotherapy". Stable for 35 days at room temperature.

Dressman JB and Poust RI, "Stability of Allopurinol and of Five Antineoplastics in Suspension," *Am J Hosp Pharm*, 1983, 40(4):616-8.

Monitoring Parameters CBC with differential (weekly initially, although clinical status may require increased frequency), bone marrow exam (to evaluate marrow status), liver function tests (weekly initially, then monthly; monitor more frequently if on concomitant hepatotoxic agents), renal function, urinalysis; consider TPMT genotyping to identify TPMT defect (if severe toxicity occurs)

For use as immunomodulatory therapy in CD or UC, monitor CBC with differential weekly for 1 month, then biweekly for 1 month, followed by monitoring every 1-2 months throughout the course of therapy. LFTs should be assessed every 3 months. Monitor for signs/symptoms of malignancy (eg, splenomegaly, hepatomegaly, abdominal pain, persistent fever, night sweats, weight loss).

Test Interactions TPMT testing: Recent transfusions may result in a misinterpretation of the actual TPMT activity. Concomitant drugs may influence TPMT activity in the blood.

Dietary Considerations Should not be administered with meals.

Dosage Forms Excipient information presented when available (limited, particularly for generics); consult specific product labeling.

Tablet, oral: 50 mg

Purinethol®: 50 mg [scored]

References

Aronoff GR, Bennett WM, Berns JS, et al, *Drug Prescribing in Renal Failure: Dosing Guidelines for Adults and Children*, 5th ed. Philadelphia, PA: American College of Physicians; 2007, p 173.

Carter MJ, Lobo AJ and Travis SP, "Guidelines for the Management of Inflammatory Bowel Disease in Adults," *Gut*, 2004, 53(Suppl 5):1-16.

Danese M and Fiocchi C, "Ulcerative Colitis," *New Engl J Med*, 2011, 365(18):1713-25.

Gremse DA and Crissinger KD, "Ulcerative Colitis in Children: Medical Management," *Paediatr Drugs*, 2002, 4(12):807-15.

Kantarjian HM, O'Brien S, Smith TL, et al, "Results of Treatment With Hyper-CVAD, A Dose-Intensive Regimen, in Adult Acute Lymphocytic Leukemia," *J Clin Oncol*, 2000, 18(3):547-61.

Kornbluth A and Sachar DB, "Ulcerative Colitis Practice Guidelines in Adults: American College of Gastroenterology, Practice Parameters Committee," *Am J Gastroenterol*, 2010, 105(3):501-23.

Larson RA, Dodge RK, Burns CP, et al, "A Five-Drug Remission Induction Regimen With Intensive Consolidation for Adults With Acute Lymphoblastic Leukemia: Cancer and Leukemia Group B Study 8811," *Blood*, 1995, 85(8):2025-37.

Larson RA, Dodge RK, Linker CA, et al, "A Randomized Controlled Trial of Filgrastim During Remission Induction and Consolidation Chemotherapy for Adults With Acute Lymphoblastic Leukemia: CALGB Study 9111," *Blood*, 1998, 92(5):1556-64.

Lichtenstein GR, Abreu MT, Cohen R, et al, "American Gastroenterological Association Institute Medical Position Statement on Corticosteroids, Immunomodulators, and Infliximab in Inflammatory Bowel Disease," *Gastroenterology*, 2006, 130(3):935-9.

Lichtenstein GR, Hanauer SB, and Sandborn WJ, "Management of Crohn's Disease in Adults," *Am J Gastroenterol*, 2009, 104(2):465-83.

Lobel EZ, Korelitz BI, Xuereb MA, et al, "A Search for the Optimal Duration of Treatment With 6-Mercaptopurine for Ulcerative Colitis," *Am J Gastroenterol*, 2004, 99(3):462-5.

Manns MP, Czaja AJ, Gorham JD, et al, "Diagnosis and Management of Autoimmune Hepatitis," *Hepatology*, 2010, 51(6):2193-213.

Markowitz J, Grancher K, Kohn N, et al, "A Multicenter Trial of 6-Mercaptopurine and Prednisone in Children With Newly Diagnosed Crohn's Disease," *Gastroenterology*, 2000, 119(4):895-902.

Mosesso P and Palitti F, "The Genetic Toxicology of 6-Mercaptopurine," *Mutat Res*, 1993, 296(3):279-94.

Parakkal D, Sifuentes H, Semer R, et al, "Hepatosplenic T-Cell Lymphoma in Patients Receiving TNF-α Inhibitor Therapy: Expanding the Groups at Risk," *Eur J Gastroenterol Hepatol*, 2011, 23(12):1150-6.

Powell BL, Moser B, Stock W, et al, "Arsenic Trioxide Improves Event-Free and Over-All Survival for Adults With Acute Promyelocytic Leukemia: North American Leukemia Intergroup Study C9710," *Blood*, 2010, 116(19):3751-7.

Sandborn WJ, "A Review of Immune Modifier Therapy for Inflammatory Bowel Disease: Azathioprine, 6-mercaptopurine, Cyclosporine, and Methotrexate," *Am J Gastroenterol*, 1996, 91 (3):423-33.

Schmiegelow K, Glomstein A, Kristinsson J, et al, "Impact of Morning versus Evening Schedule for Oral Methotrexate and 6-Mercaptopurine on Relapse Risk for Children With Acute Lymphoblastic Leukemia. Nordic Society for Pediatric Hematology and Oncology (NOPHO)," *J Pediatr Hematol Oncol*, 1997, 19(2):102-9.

Siegel CA and Sands BE, "Review Article: Practical Management of Inflammatory Bowel Disease Patients Taking Immunomodulators," *Aliment Pharmacol Ther*, 2005, 22(1):1-16.

Stock W, La M, Sanford B, et al, "What Determines the Outcomes for Adolescents and Young Adults With Acute Lymphoblastic Leukemia Treated on Cooperative Group Protocols? A Comparison of Children's Cancer Group and Cancer and Leukemia Group B Studies," *Blood*, 2008, 112(5):1646-54.

Thomas DA, O'Brien S, Cortes J, et al, "Outcome With the Hyper-CVAD Regimens in Lymphoblastic Lymphoma," *Blood*, 2004, 104(6):1624-30.

Zimm S, Ettinger LJ, Holcenberg JS, et al, "Phase I and Clinical Pharmacological Study of Mercaptopurine Administered as a Prolonged Intravenous Infusion," *Cancer Res*, 1988, 45 (4):1869-73.

◆ **6-Mercaptopurine (error-prone abbreviation)** *see* Mercaptopurine *on page 934*

◆ **M-Eslon® (Can)** *see* Morphine (Systemic) *on page 1004*

Mesna (MES na)

Brand Names: U.S. Mesnex®

Brand Names: Canada Mesna for injection; Uromitexan

Index Terms Mercaptoethane Sulfonate; Sodium 2-Mercaptoethane Sulfonate

Generic Availability (U.S.) Yes: Solution for injection

Pharmacologic Category Antidote; Uroprotectant

Use Preventative agent to reduce the incidence of ifosfamide-induced hemorrhagic cystitis

Unlabeled Use Preventative agent to reduce the incidence of cyclophosphamide-induced hemorrhagic cystitis with high-dose cyclophosphamide

Labeled Contraindications Hypersensitivity to mesna or other thiol compounds, or any component of the formulation

Pregnancy Risk Factor B

Lactation Excretion in breast milk unknown/not recommended

Warnings/Precautions Examine morning urine specimen for hematuria prior to ifosfamide or cyclophosphamide treatment; if hematuria (>50 RBC/HPF) develops, reduce the ifosfamide/cyclophosphamide dose or discontinue the drug; will not prevent or alleviate other toxicities associated with ifosfamide or cyclophosphamide and will not prevent hemorrhagic cystitis in all patients. Mesna will not reduce the risk of thrombocytopenia-related hematuria. Allergic reactions have been reported; symptoms ranged from mild hypersensitivity to systemic anaphylactic reactions and may include fever, hypotension, and/or tachycardia; patients with autoimmune disorders receiving cyclophosphamide and mesna may be at increased risk. Patients should receive adequate hydration during treatment. I.V. formulation contains benzyl alcohol; do not use in neonates or infants (associated with "gasping syndrome").

Adverse Reactions

Mesna alone (frequency not defined):

Cardiovascular: Flushing

Central nervous system: Dizziness, fever, headache, hyperesthesia, somnolence

Dermatologic: Rash
Gastrointestinal: Anorexia, constipation, diarrhea, flatulence, nausea, taste alteration/bad taste (with oral administration), vomiting
Local: Injection site reactions
Neuromuscular: Arthralgia, back pain, rigors
Ocular: Conjunctivitis
Respiratory: Cough, pharyngitis, rhinitis
Miscellaneous: Flu-like syndrome

Mesna alone or in combination: Postmarketing and/or case reports: Allergic reaction, anaphylactic reaction, hypersensitivity, hyper-/hypotension, injection site erythema, injection site pain, limb pain, malaise, myalgia, platelets decreased, ST-segment increased, tachycardia, tachypnea, transaminases increased

Drug Interactions

Metabolism/Transport Effects None known.

Avoid Concomitant Use There are no known interactions where it is recommended to avoid concomitant use.

Increased Effect/Toxicity There are no known significant interactions involving an increase in effect.

Decreased Effect There are no known significant interactions involving a decrease in effect.

Storage/Stability Store intact vials and tablets at room temperature of 20°C to 25°C (68°F to 77°F). Opened multidose vials may be stored and used for use to 8 days after opening. Solutions diluted for infusion are stable for at least 24 hours at room temperature. Solutions in plastic syringes are stable for 9 days under refrigeration, or at room or body temperature. Solutions of mesna and ifosfamide in lactated Ringer's are stable for 7 days in a PVC ambulatory infusion pump reservoir. Solutions of mesna (0.5-3.2 mg/mL) and cyclophosphamide (1.8-10.8 mg/mL) in D_5W are stable for 48 hours refrigerated or 6 hours at room temperature (Menard, 2003). Mesna injection is stable for at least 7 days when diluted 1:2 or 1:5 with grape- and orange-flavored syrups or 11:1 to 1:100 in carbonated beverages for oral administration.

Reconstitution Dilute in 50-1000 mL D_5W, NS, D_5¼NS, D_5⅓NS, D_5½NS, or lactated Ringer's (the manufacturer recommends a final concentration of 20 mg/mL).

Mechanism of Action In blood, mesna is oxidized to dimesna which in turn is reduced in the kidney back to mesna, supplying a free thiol group which binds to and inactivates acrolein, the urotoxic metabolite of ifosfamide and cyclophosphamide

Pharmacodynamics/Kinetics

Distribution: No tissue penetration
Protein binding: 69% to 75%
Metabolism: Rapidly oxidized intravascularly to mesna disulfide (dimesna); dimesna is reduced in renal tubules back to mesna following glomerular filtration
Bioavailability: Oral: 45% to 79%
Half-life elimination:
I.V.: Mesna: ~22 minutes; Dimesna: ~70 minutes
I.V. followed by oral: 1-8 hours
Time to peak, plasma: 2-3 hours
Excretion: Urine (18% to 32% as mesna; 33% as dimesna)

Dosing

Adult & Geriatric Note: Details concerning dosing in combination regimens should also be consulted. Mesna dosing schedule should be repeated each day ifosfamide is received. If ifosfamide dose is adjusted, the mesna dose should also be modified to maintain the mesna-to-ifosfamide ratio.

Prevention of ifosfamide-induced hemorrhagic cystitis:

I.V.:

Short infusion standard-dose ifosfamide (<2.5 g/m^2/day): Mesna dose is equal to 60% of the ifosfamide dose given in 3 divided doses (0, 4, and 8 hours after the start of ifosfamide)

Continuous infusion standard-dose ifosfamide (<2.5 g/m^2/day): ASCO guidelines: Mesna dose (as an I.V. bolus) is equal to 20% of the ifosfamide dose, followed by a continuous infusion of mesna at 40% of the ifosfamide dose, continue mesna infusion for 12-24 hours after completion of ifosfamide infusion (Hensley, 2008)

High-dose ifosfamide (>2.5 g/m^2/day): ASCO guidelines: Evidence for use is inadequate; more frequent and prolonged mesna administration regimens may be required.

I.V. followed by oral (for ifosfamide doses ≤2 g/m^2/day): Mesna dose is equal to 100% of the ifosfamide dose, given as 20% of the ifosfamide dose I.V. at hour 0, followed by 40% of the ifosfamide dose given orally 2- and 6 hours after start of ifosfamide

Pediatric Refer to adult dosing.

Combination Regimens

Leukemia, acute lymphocytic:

Hyper-CVAD + Imatinib on page 1680
Hyper-CVAD (Leukemia, Acute Lymphocytic) on page 1681

Lymphoma, Hodgkin:

ICE (Hodgkin) on page 1688
IGEV (Hodgkin) on page 1690
MINE-ESHAP (Hodgkin) on page 1711
VIM-D (Hodgkin) on page 1770

Lymphoma, non-Hodgkin's:

ICE (Lymphoma, non-Hodgkin's) on page 1689
IMVP-16 on page 1691
MINE on page 1711
MINE-ESHAP (NHL) on page 1712
RICE on page 1747

Lymphoma, non-Hodgkin's (Burkitt): CODOX-M/IVAC on page 1591
Lymphoma, non-Hodgkin's (Mantle cell): Hyper-CVAD + Rituximab on page 1688
Multiple myeloma: Hyper-CVAD (Multiple Myeloma) on page 1687
Osteosarcoma: ICE (Sarcoma) on page 1689
Sarcoma: MAID (Sarcoma) on page 1704

Soft tissue sarcoma:

AI on page 1520
ICE (Sarcoma) on page 1689
IE on page 1690

Testicular cancer:

Paclitaxel-Ifosfamide-Cisplatin on page 1730
VIP (Etoposide) (Testicular Cancer) on page 1776
VIP (Vinblastine) (Testicular Cancer) on page 1777
Wilms' tumor: Regimen I (Wilms' Tumor) on page 1745

Administration

Oral: Administer orally in tablet formulation or parenteral solution diluted in water, milk, juice, or carbonated beverages; patients who vomit within 2 hours after taking oral mesna should repeat the dose or receive I.V. mesna

I.V.: Administer by short (15-30 minutes) infusion or continuous infusion (maintain continuous infusion for 12-24 after completion of ifosfamide infusion) (Hensley, 2008)

Emetic Potential When administered orally, the unpleasant taste may result in vomiting.

Monitoring Parameters Urinalysis

Test Interactions False-positive urinary ketones with Chemstrip®, Multistix®, or Labstix®

Additional Information Oncology Comment: Guidelines from the American Society of Clinical Oncology (ASCO) for the use of chemotherapy and radiotherapy protectants (Hensley, 2008 [update]; Schuchter, 2002) recommend mesna to decrease the incidence of ifosfamide-induced urotoxicity associated with short infusion and continuous infusion standard-dose ifosfamide (<2.5 g/m^2/day). Although evidence is inadequate regarding mesna's uroprotective effects in high-dose ifosfamide (>2.5 g/m^2/day), the guidelines suggest more frequent and prolonged mesna administration times may be required. For prevention high-dose cyclophosphamide-induced urotoxicity (associated with stem cell transplantation), the guidelines recommend mesna in conjunction with saline diuresis (or forced saline diuresis alone).

Dosage Forms Excipient information presented when available (limited, particularly for generics); consult specific product labeling.

Injection, solution: 100 mg/mL (10 mL)

Mesnex®: 100 mg/mL (10 mL)

Tablet, oral:

Mesnex®: 400 mg [scored]

Dosage Forms: Canada Excipient information presented when available (limited, particularly for generics); consult specific product labeling.

Injection, solution:

Mesna for injection: 100 mg/mL (10 mL)

References

Hensley ML, Hagerty KL, Kewalramani T, et al, "American Society of Clinical Oncology 2008 Clinical Practice Guideline Update: Use of Chemotherapy and Radiotherapy Protectants," *J Clin Oncol*, 2008, 27(1):127-45.

Khaw SL, Downie PA, Waters KD, et al, "Adverse Hypersensitivity Reactions to Mesna as Adjunctive Therapy for Cyclophosphamide," *Pediatr Blood Cancer*, 2007, 49(3):341-3.

Mace JR, Keohan ML, Bernardy H, et al, "Crossover Randomized Comparison of Intravenous Versus Intravenous/Oral Mesna in Soft Tissue Sarcoma Treated With High Dose Ifosfamide," *Clin Cancer Res*, 2003, 9(16 Pt 1):5829-34.

Menard C, Bourguignon C, Schlatter J, et al, "Stability of Cyclophosphamide and Mesna Admixtures in Polyethylene Infusion Bags," *Ann Pharmacother*, 2003, 37(12):1789-92.

Schuchter LM, Hensley ML, Meropol NJ, et al, "2002 Update of Recommendations for the Use of Chemotherapy and Radiotherapy Protectants: Clinical Practice Guidelines of the American Society of Clinical Oncology," *J Clin Oncol*, 2002, 20(12):2895-903.

◆ **Mesna for injection (Can)** *see* Mesna *on page* *940*

◆ **Mesnex®** *see* Mesna *on page* *940*

◆ **Metadol™ (Can)** *see* Methadone *on page* *944*

◆ **Metadol-D™ (Can)** *see* Methadone *on page* *944*

◆ **123 Meta-Iodobenzlyguanidine Sulfate** *see* Iobenguane I 123 *on page* *806*

◆ **Metastron®** *see* Strontium-89 *on page* *1300*

Methadone (METH a done)

Brand Names: U.S. Dolophine®; Methadone Diskets®; Methadone Intensol™; Methadose®

Brand Names: Canada Metadol-D™; Metadol™

Index Terms Methadone Hydrochloride

Generic Availability (U.S.) Yes

Pharmacologic Category Analgesic, Opioid

Use Management of moderate-to-severe pain when a continuous, around-the-clock opioid analgesic is needed for an extended period of time; detoxification and maintenance treatment of opioid addiction through a certified program

Labeled Contraindications Hypersensitivity to methadone or any component of the formulation; significant respiratory depression (in the absence of resuscitative equipment or in an unmonitored setting); acute or severe bronchial asthma (in the absence of resuscitative equipment or in an unmonitored setting) or hypercarbia; known or suspected paralytic ileus; concurrent use of selegiline (Ensam® product labeling)

Methadone is not to be used on an as-needed basis; it is not for pain that is mild or not expected to persist; it is not for acute pain or postoperative pain.

Pregnancy Risk Factor C

Lactation Enters breast milk/not recommended (AAP rates "compatible"; AAP 2001 update pending)

Warnings/Precautions The optimal analgesic dose varies widely among patients. Doses should be titrated to pain relief/prevention. Patients maintained on stable doses of methadone may need rescue doses of a immediate release analgesic in case of acute pain (eg, postoperative pain, physical trauma). Methadone is ineffective for the relief of anxiety.

[U.S. Boxed Warning]: QT_c interval prolongation and serious arrhythmias (eg, torsade de pointes) have occurred during treatment. Patients should be informed of the potential arrhythmia risk, evaluated for any history of structural heart disease, arrhythmia, syncope, and for existence of potential drug interactions including drugs that possess QT_c interval-prolonging properties, promote hypokalemia, hypomagnesemia, or hypocalcemia, or reduce elimination of methadone (eg, CYP3A4 inhibitors). Obtain baseline ECG for all patients and risk stratify according to QT_c interval; QT_c interval prolongation and torsade de pointes may be associated with doses >200 mg/day, but have also been observed with lower doses. May cause severe hypotension; use caution with severe volume depletion or other conditions which may compromise maintenance of normal blood pressure. Use caution with cardiovascular disease or patients predisposed to dysrhythmias.

[U.S. Boxed Warning]: Fatal respiratory depression may occur with the highest risk at initiation and with dose increases. Use caution in patients with respiratory disease or pre-existing respiratory conditions (eg, severe obesity, asthma, COPD, sleep apnea, CNS depression) and kyphoscoliosis or other skeletal disorder which may alter respiratory function. Because the respiratory effects last longer than the analgesic effects, slow titration is required. Use extreme caution during treatment initiation, dose titration and conversion from other opioid agonists. Incomplete cross tolerance may occur; patients tolerant to other mu opioid agonists may not be tolerant to methadone. Abrupt cessation may precipitate withdrawal symptoms. Gradually taper dose.

May cause CNS depression, which may impair physical or mental abilities. Patients must be cautioned about performing tasks which require mental alertness (eg, operating machinery or driving). Effects with other sedative drugs or ethanol may be potentiated. Use with caution in patients with depression or suicidal tendencies, or in patients with a history of drug or ethanol abuse. Tolerance or psychological and physical dependence may occur with prolonged use. **[U.S. Boxed Warning]: Monitor for signs of misuse, abuse and addiction during therapy.**

Use with caution in patients with head injury or increased intracranial pressure; reduced respiratory drive and resultant CO_2 retention may increase intracranial pressure. May obscure diagnosis or clinical course of patients with acute abdominal conditions. Avoid use in gastrointestinal obstruction.

Elderly may be more susceptible to adverse effects (eg, CNS, respiratory, gastrointestinal). Decrease initial dose and use caution in the elderly or debilitated; with hyper/hypothyroidism, morbid obesity, adrenal insufficiency, prostatic hyperplasia, or urethral stricture; or with severe renal or hepatic failure. Use with caution in patients with biliary tract dysfunction including acute pancreatitis; may cause constriction of sphincter of Oddi. **[U.S. Boxed Warning]: For oral administration only;** excipients to deter use by injection are contained in tablets.

[U.S. Boxed Warning]: When used for treatment of opioid addiction: May only be dispensed by certified opioid treatment programs. Exceptions include inpatient treatment of other conditions and emergency period (not >3 days) while definitive substance abuse treatment is being sought. **[U.S. Boxed Warning]: Accidental ingestion can result in fatal overdose, especially in children. [U.S. Boxed Warning]: Should only be prescribed by healthcare professionals who are knowledgeable in the use of potent opioids for chronic pain management.**

Ethanol/Nutrition/Herb Interactions

Ethanol: Ethanol may increase CNS depression. Management: Avoid ethanol.

Food: Grapefruit/grapefruit juice may increase levels of methadone. Management: Avoid concurrent use of grapefruit juice.

Herb/Nutraceutical: St John's wort may decrease methadone levels and increase CNS depression; valerian, kava kava, and gotu kola may increase CNS depression. Management: Avoid St John's wort, valerian, kava kava, and gotu kola.

Storage/Stability

Injection: Store at controlled room temperature of 15°C to 30°C (59°F to 86°F). Protect from light.

Oral concentrate, oral solution, tablet: Store at controlled room temperature of 15°C to 30°C (59°F to 86°F).

Mechanism of Action Binds to opiate receptors in the CNS, causing inhibition of ascending pain pathways, altering the perception of and response to pain; produces generalized CNS depression

Pharmacodynamics/Kinetics

Onset of action: Oral: Analgesic: 0.5-1 hour; Parenteral: 10-20 minutes

Peak effect: Parenteral: 1-2 hours; Oral: Continuous dosing: 3-5 days

Duration of analgesia: Oral: 4-8 hours (single-dose studies), increases to 22-48 hours with repeated doses; slow release from the liver and other tissues may prolong duration of action

Distribution: Lipophilic; V_{dss}: 1-8 L/kg

Protein binding: 85% to 90% primarily to alpha-1 acid glycoprotein

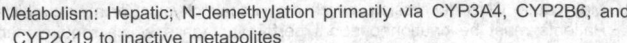

Metabolism: Hepatic; N-demethylation primarily via CYP3A4, CYP2B6, and CYP2C19 to inactive metabolites

Bioavailability: Oral: 36% to 100%

Half-life elimination: Terminal: 8-59 hours; may be prolonged with alkaline pH, decreased during pregnancy

Time to peak, plasma: 1-7.5 hours

Excretion: Urine (<10% as unchanged drug); increased with urine pH <6

Dosing

Adult Regulations regarding methadone use may vary by state and/or country. Obtain advice from appropriate regulatory agencies and/or consult with pain management/palliative care specialists. **Note:** These are guidelines and do not represent the maximum doses that may be required. Consider total daily dose, potency, prior opioid use, degree of opioid experience and tolerance, conversion from previous opioid, patient's general condition, concurrent medications, and type and severity of pain during prescribing process. Other factors to consider:

- Interpatient variability in absorption, metabolism, and relative analgesic potency.
- Population-based equianalgesic conversion ratios between methadone and other opioids may not be completely accurate.
- Duration of analgesic action is much shorter than plasma elimination half-life.
- Steady-state plasma concentrations and full analgesic effects are not attained until 3-5 days after initiation.
- Methadone has a narrow therapeutic index.

Note: When pain management is no longer required, do not abruptly discontinue. Reduce dose every 2-4 days to prevent signs or symptoms of withdrawal. With detoxification treatment, abrupt discontinuation may lead to relapse of illicit drug use in susceptible patients.

Chronic pain (moderate-to-severe): Opioid-naive:

Oral: Initial: 2.5-10 mg every 8-12 hours; more frequent administration may be required during initiation to maintain adequate analgesia (manufacturer's labeling)

I.V.: Initial: 2.5 mg every 8-12 hours; titrate slowly to effect; may also be administered by SubQ or I.M. injection (manufacturer's labeling)

Chronic pain (CPSO, 2000; VA/DoD, 2003): Oral:

Opioid-naive:

Gradual titration (for chronic noncancer pain and situations where frequent monitoring is unnecessary): Initial: 2.5 mg every 8 hours; may increase dosing interval to every 12 hours (in about 4-5 days); may increase dose by 2.5 mg per dose every 5-7 days

Faster titration (for cancer pain and situations where frequent monitoring is possible): Initial: 2.5 mg every 6-8 hours; may increase dosing interval to every 8-12 hours (in about 4-5 days); may increase dose by 2.5 mg per dose as often as every day over about 4 days.

Opioid-tolerant: ***Conversion from oral morphine to oral methadone:***

Note: 1) There is not a linear relationship when converting to methadone from oral morphine. The higher the daily morphine equivalent dose the more potent methadone is, and 2) conversion to methadone is more of a process than a calculation. In general, the starting methadone dose should not exceed 30-40 mg/day, even in patients on high doses of other opioids. Patient response to methadone needs to be monitored closely throughout the process of the conversion. There are several proposed ratios for converting from oral morphine to oral methadone (Ayonrinde, 2000; Mercadente, 2001; Ripamonti, 1998). The manufacturer of Dolophine® recommends the following conversion for chronic administration:

Daily oral morphine dose <100 mg: Estimated daily oral methadone dose: 20% to 30% of total daily morphine dose

Daily oral morphine dose 100-300 mg: Estimated daily oral methadone dose: 10% to 20% of total daily morphine dose

Daily oral morphine dose 300-600 mg: Estimated daily oral methadone dose: 8% to 12% of total daily morphine dose

Daily oral morphine dose 600-1000 mg: Estimated daily oral methadone dose: 5% to 10% of total daily morphine dose.

Daily oral morphine dose >1000 mg: Estimated daily oral methadone dose: <5% of total daily morphine dose.

Note: The estimated total daily methadone dose should then be divided to reflect the intended dosing schedule (eg, divide by 3 and administer every 8 hours).

Conversion from oral to parenteral dose: Initial dose: Parenteral:Oral ratio: 1:2 (eg, 5 mg parenteral methadone equals 10 mg oral methadone)

Detoxification: *Oral:*

Initial: A single dose of 20-30 mg is usually sufficient to suppress symptoms. Should not exceed 30 mg; lower doses should be considered in patients with low tolerance at initiation (eg, absence of opioids ≥5 days); an additional 5-10 mg of methadone may be provided if withdrawal symptoms have not been suppressed or if symptoms reappear after 2-4 hours; total daily dose on the first day should not exceed 40 mg. Do not increase dose without waiting for steady-state to be achieved. Levels will accumulate over the first few days. Reassure the patient that duration of effect will increase as methadone accumulates.

Maintenance: Titrate to a dosage which prevents craving, attenuates euphoric effect of self-administered opiates, and tolerance to sedative effects of methadone. Usual range: 80-120 mg/day (titration should occur cautiously)

Withdrawal: Dose reductions should be <10% of the maintenance dose, every 10-14 days

Detoxification (short-term): *Oral:*

Initial: Titrate to ~40 mg/day in divided doses to achieve stabilization. May continue 40 mg dose for 2-3 days

Maintenance: Titrate to a dosage which prevents/attenuates euphoric effects of self-administered opioids, reduces drug craving, and withdrawal symptoms are prevented for 24 hours.

Withdrawal: Requires individualization. Decrease daily or every other day, keeping withdrawal symptoms tolerable; hospitalized patients may tolerate a 20% reduction/day; ambulatory patients may require a slower reduction

Dosage adjustment during pregnancy: Methadone dose may need to be increased, or the dosing interval decreased; use should be reserved for cases where the benefits clearly outweigh the risks

Geriatric Oral, I.M.: 2.5 mg every 8-12 hours; refer to adult dosing.

Renal Impairment Unlabeled dosing (Aronoff, 2007): Adults:

Cl_{cr} ≥10 mL/minute: No dosage adjustment necessary

Cl_{cr} <10 mL/minute: Administer 50% to 75% of normal dose

Hepatic Impairment No dosage adjustment provided in manufacturer's labeling; however, undergoes hepatic metabolism and systemic exposure may be increased after repeated dosing. Avoid in severe liver disease.

Adjustment for Toxicity

Excessive opioid-related adverse events: Reduce next dose. Assess and reduce both the maintenance dose and dosing interval if necessary.

QT_c prolongation (Krantz, 2009):

QT_c >450-499 msecs: Monitor QT_c more frequently

QT_c ≥500 msecs: Consider discontinuation or reducing methadone dose **or** eliminate factors promoting QT_c prolongation (eg, potassium-wasting drugs) **or** use alternative therapy (eg, buprenorphine)

Administration Oral dose for detoxification and maintenance may be administered in fruit juice or water. Dispersible tablet should not be chewed or swallowed; add to liquid and allow to dissolve before administering. May rinse if residual remains. Injectable solution can be administered I.M., SubQ, or I.V.; rate of I.V. administration not defined.

Test Interactions Some quinolones may produce a false-positive urine screening result for opiates using commercially-available immunoassay kits. This has been demonstrated most consistently for levofloxacin and ofloxacin, but other quinolones have shown cross-reactivity in certain assay kits. Confirmation of positive opiate screens by more specific methods should be considered.

Prescribing and Access Restrictions When used for treatment of opioid addiction: May only be dispensed in accordance to guidelines established by the Substance Abuse and Mental Health Services Administration's (SAMHSA) Center for Substance Abuse Treatment (CSAT). Regulations regarding methadone use may vary by state and/or country. Obtain advice from appropriate regulatory agencies and/or consult with pain management/palliative care specialists.

Note: Regulatory Exceptions to the General Requirement to Provide Opioid Agonist Treatment (per manufacturer's labeling):

1. During inpatient care, when the patient was admitted for any condition other than concurrent opioid addiction, to facilitate the treatment of the primary admitting diagnosis.
2. During an emergency period of no longer than 3 days while definitive care for the addiction is being sought in an appropriately licensed facility.

Medication Guide Available Yes

Dosage Forms Excipient information presented when available (limited, particularly for generics); consult specific product labeling.

Injection, solution, as hydrochloride: 10 mg/mL (20 mL)

Solution, oral, as hydrochloride: 5 mg/5 mL (500 mL); 10 mg/5 mL (500 mL)

Solution, oral, as hydrochloride [concentrate]: 10 mg/mL (946 mL, 1000 mL, 1000s)

Methadone Intensol™: 10 mg/mL (30 mL) [dye free, sugar free; contains sodium benzoate; unflavored]

Methadose®: 10 mg/mL (1000 mL) [contains propylene glycol; cherry flavor]
Methadose®: 10 mg/mL (1000 mL) [dye free, sugar free; contains sodium benzoate; unflavored]
Tablet, oral, as hydrochloride: 5 mg, 10 mg
Dolophine®: 5 mg, 10 mg [scored]
Tablet, dispersible, oral, as hydrochloride: 40 mg
Methadone Diskets®: 40 mg [scored; orange-pineapple flavor]
Methadose®: 40 mg [scored]

Controlled Substance C II

- **Methadone Diskets®** *see* Methadone *on page 944*
- **Methadone Hydrochloride** *see* Methadone *on page 944*
- **Methadone Intensol™** *see* Methadone *on page 944*
- **Methadose®** *see* Methadone *on page 944*

Methotrexate (meth oh TREKS ate)

Related Information

Chemotherapy and Cancer Treatment During Pregnancy *on page 1829*
Hematopoietic Stem Cell Transplantation *on page 1887*
Management of Chemotherapy-Induced Nausea and Vomiting *on page 1786*
Oral Mucositis/Stomatitis *on page 1814*
Safe Handling of Hazardous Drugs *on page 1904*

Brand Names: U.S. Rheumatrex®; Trexall™

Brand Names: Canada Apo-Methotrexate®; ratio-Methotrexate

Index Terms Amethopterin; Methotrexate Sodium; Methotrexatum; MTX (error-prone abbreviation)

Generic Availability (U.S.) Yes

Pharmacologic Category Antineoplastic Agent, Antimetabolite (Antifolate); Antirheumatic, Disease Modifying; Immunosuppressant Agent

Use

Oncology-related uses: Acute lymphoblastic leukemia (ALL) maintenance treatment, ALL meningeal leukemia (prophylaxis and treatment); treatment of trophoblastic neoplasms (gestational choriocarcinoma, chorioadenoma destruens and hydatidiform mole), breast cancer, head and neck cancer (epidermoid), cutaneous T-Cell lymphoma (advanced mycosis fungoides), lung cancer (squamous cell and small cell), advanced non-Hodgkin's lymphomas (NHL), osteosarcoma

Nononcology uses: Treatment of psoriasis (severe, recalcitrant, disabling) and severe rheumatoid arthritis (RA), including polyarticular course juvenile idiopathic arthritis (JIA)

Unlabeled Use Treatment and maintenance of remission in Crohn's disease, management of ectopic pregnancy; dermatomyositis/polymyositis; treatment of bladder cancer, central nervous system tumors (including nonleukemic meningeal cancers), acute promyelocytic leukemia (maintenance treatment), soft tissue sarcoma (desmoid tumors); acute graft-versus-host disease (GVHD) prophylaxis; medical management of abortion; systemic lupus erythematosus; Takayasu arteritis

Labeled Contraindications Hypersensitivity to methotrexate or any component of the formulation; breast-feeding

Additional contraindications for patients with psoriasis or rheumatoid arthritis: Pregnancy, alcoholism, alcoholic liver disease or other chronic liver disease, immunodeficiency syndrome (overt or laboratory evidence); pre-existing blood dyscrasias (eg, bone marrow hypoplasia, leukopenia, thrombocytopenia, significant anemia)

Pregnancy Risk Factor X (psoriasis, rheumatoid arthritis)

Lactation Enters breast milk/contraindicated

Warnings/Precautions Hazardous agent - use appropriate precautions for handling and disposal.

[U.S. Boxed Warning]: Methotrexate has been associated with acute (elevated transaminases) and potentially fatal chronic (fibrosis, cirrhosis) hepatotoxicity. Risk is related to cumulative dose (≥1.5 g) and prolonged exposure. Monitor closely (with liver function tests, including serum albumin) for liver toxicities. Liver enzyme elevations may be noted, but may not be predictive of hepatic disease in long term treatment for psoriasis (but generally is predictive in rheumatoid arthritis [RA] treatment). With long-term use, liver biopsy may show histologic changes, fibrosis, or cirrhosis; periodic liver biopsy is recommended with long-term use for psoriasis patients with risk factors for hepatotoxicity and for persistent abnormal liver function tests in psoriasis patients without risk factors for hepatotoxicity and in RA patients; discontinue methotrexate with moderate-to-severe change in liver biopsy. Risk factors for hepatotoxicity include history of above moderate ethanol consumption, persistent abnormal liver chemistries, history of chronic liver disease (including hepatitis B or C), family history of inheritable liver disease, diabetes, obesity, hyperlipidemia, lack of folate supplementation during methotrexate therapy, cumulative methotrexate dose exceeding 1.5 g, continuous daily dosing of methotrexate and history of significant exposure to hepatotoxic drugs. Use caution with preexisting liver impairment; may require dosage reduction. Use caution when used with other hepatotoxic agents (azathioprine, retinoids, sulfasalazine). **[U.S. Boxed Warning]: Methotrexate elimination is reduced in patients with ascites and pleural effusions;** resulting in prolonged half-life and toxicity; may require dose reduction or discontinuation. Monitor closely for toxicity.

[U.S. Boxed Warning]: May cause renal damage leading to acute renal failure, especially with high-dose methotrexate; monitor renal function and methotrexate levels closely, maintain adequate hydration and urinary alkalinization. Use caution in osteosarcoma patients treated with high-dose methotrexate in combination with nephrotoxic chemotherapy (eg, cisplatin). **[U.S. Boxed Warning]: Methotrexate elimination is reduced in patients with renal impairment;** may require dose reduction or discontinuation; monitor closely for toxicity. **[U.S. Boxed Warning]: Tumor lysis syndrome may occur in patients with high tumor burden;** use appropriate prevention and treatment.

[U.S. Boxed Warning]: May cause potentially life-threatening pneumonitis (may occur at any time during therapy and at any dosage); monitor closely for pulmonary symptoms, particularly dry, nonproductive cough. Other potential symptoms include fever, dyspnea, hypoxemia, or pulmonary infiltrate. **[U.S. Boxed Warning]: Methotrexate elimination is reduced in patients with pleural effusions;** may require dose reduction or discontinuation. Monitor closely for toxicity.

[U.S. Boxed Warning]: Bone marrow suppression may occur, resulting in anemia, aplastic anemia, pancytopenia, leukopenia, neutropenia, and/or thrombocytopenia. Use caution in patients with pre-existing bone marrow suppression. Discontinue treatment (immediately) in RA or psoriasis if a significant decrease in hematologic components is noted. **[U.S. Boxed Warning]: Use of low dose methotrexate has been associated with the development of malignant lymphomas;** may regress upon treatment discontinuation; treat lymphoma appropriately if regression is not induced by cessation of methotrexate.

[U.S. Boxed Warning]: Diarrhea and ulcerative stomatitis may require treatment interruption; death from hemorrhagic enteritis or intestinal perforation has been reported. Use with caution in patients with peptic ulcer disease, ulcerative colitis.

May cause neurotoxicity including seizures (usually in pediatric ALL patients receiving intermediate-dose (1 g/m^2 methotrexate), leukoencephalopathy (usually with concurrent cranial irradiation) and stroke-like encephalopathy (usually with high-dose regimens). Chemical arachnoiditis (headache, back pain, nuchal rigidity, fever), myelopathy and chronic leukoencephalopathy may result from intrathecal administration.

[U.S. Boxed Warning]: Any dose level or route of administration may cause severe and potentially fatal dermatologic reactions, including toxic epidermal necrolysis, Stevens-Johnson syndrome, exfoliative dermatitis, skin necrosis, and erythema multiforme. Radiation dermatitis and sunburn may be precipitated by methotrexate administration. Psoriatic lesions may be worsened by concomitant exposure to ultraviolet radiation.

[U.S. Boxed Warning]: Concomitant administration with NSAIDs may cause severe bone marrow suppression, aplastic anemia, and GI toxicity. Do not administer NSAIDs prior to or during high dose methotrexate therapy; may increase and prolong serum methotrexate levels. Doses used for psoriasis may still lead to unexpected toxicities; use caution when administering NSAIDs or salicylates with lower doses of methotrexate for RA. Methotrexate may increase the levels and effects of mercaptopurine; may require dosage adjustments. Vitamins containing folate may decrease response to systemic methotrexate; folate deficiency may increase methotrexate toxicity. Concomitant use of proton pump inhibitors with methotrexate (primarily high-dose methotrexate) may elevate and prolong serum methotrexate and metabolite (hydroxymethotrexate) levels; may lead to toxicities; use with caution. Immunization may be ineffective during methotrexate treatment. Immunization with live vaccines is not recommended; cases of disseminated vaccinia infections due to live vaccines have been reported. **[U.S. Boxed Warning]: Concomitant methotrexate administration with radiotherapy may increase the risk of soft tissue necrosis and osteonecrosis.**

[U.S. Boxed Warnings]: Should be administered under the supervision of a physician experienced in the use of antimetabolite therapy; serious and fatal toxicities have occurred at all dose levels. Immune suppression may lead to potentially fatal opportunistic infections. Use methotrexate with extreme caution in patients with an active infection (contraindicated in patients with immunodeficiency syndrome). **[U.S. Boxed Warnings]: For rheumatoid arthritis and psoriasis, immunosuppressive therapy should only be used when disease is active and less toxic, traditional therapy is ineffective. Methotrexate formulations and/or diluents containing preservatives should not be used for intrathecal or high-dose methotrexate therapy. May cause fetal death or congenital abnormalities; do not use for psoriasis or RA treatment in pregnant women.** May cause impairment of fertility, oligospermia, and menstrual dysfunction. Toxicity from methotrexate or any immunosuppressive is increased in the elderly. Methotrexate injection may contain benzyl alcohol and should not be used in neonates. Errors have occurred (some resulting in death) when methotrexate was administered as "daily" dose instead of an intended "weekly" dose.

When used for intrathecal administration, should not be prepared during the preparation of any other agents; after preparation, store intrathecal medications in an isolated location or container clearly marked with a label identifying as "intrathecal" use only; delivery of intrathecal medications to the patient should only be with other medications intended for administration into the central nervous system (Jacobson, 2009).

Adverse Reactions Note: Adverse reactions vary by route and dosage. Hematologic and/or gastrointestinal toxicities may be common at dosages used in chemotherapy; these reactions are much less frequent when used at typical dosages for rheumatic diseases.

>10%:

Central nervous system (with intrathecal administration or very high-dose therapy):

Arachnoiditis: Acute reaction manifested as severe headache, nuchal rigidity, vomiting, and fever; may be alleviated by reducing the dose

Subacute toxicity: 10% of patients treated with 12-15 mg of intrathecal methotrexate may develop this in the second or third week of therapy; consists of motor paralysis of extremities, cranial nerve palsy, seizure, or coma. This has also been seen in pediatric cases receiving very high-dose I.V. methotrexate.

Demyelinating encephalopathy: Seen months or years after receiving methotrexate; usually in association with cranial irradiation or other systemic chemotherapy

Dermatologic: Reddening of skin

Endocrine & metabolic: Hyperuricemia, oligospermia

Gastrointestinal: Ulcerative stomatitis, glossitis, gingivitis, nausea, vomiting, diarrhea, intestinal perforation, mucositis (dose dependent; appears in 3-7 days after therapy, resolving within 2 weeks)

Hematologic: Leukopenia, myelosuppression (nadir: 7-10 days), thrombocytopenia

Renal: Renal failure, azotemia, nephropathy

Respiratory: Pharyngitis

Miscellaneous: Immunosuppression

1% to 10%:

Cardiovascular: Vasculitis

Central nervous system: Dizziness, malaise, fever, chills

Dermatologic: Alopecia, rash, photosensitivity, depigmentation or hyperpigmentation of skin, pruritus, dermatitis

Endocrine & metabolic: Diabetes

Genitourinary: Cystitis

Hematologic: Hemorrhage

Hepatic: Cirrhosis (chronic therapy), liver function tests increased (chronic therapy), portal fibrosis (chronic therapy)

Neuromuscular & skeletal: Arthralgia

Ocular: Blurred vision

Renal: Renal dysfunction: Manifested by an abrupt rise in serum creatinine and BUN and a fall in urine output; more common with high-dose methotrexate, and may be due to precipitation of the drug.

Respiratory: Pneumonitis: Associated with fever, cough, and interstitial pulmonary infiltrates; treatment is to withhold methotrexate during the acute reaction; interstitial pneumonitis has been reported to occur with an incidence of 1% in patients with RA (dose 7.5-15 mg/week)

Miscellaneous: Infection

<1%, postmarketing, and/or case reports: Abdominal distress, acne, acute neurologic syndrome (at high dosages; symptoms include confusion, hemiparesis, transient blindness, and coma); acute respiratory distress syndrome, agranulocytosis, albumin decreased, alveolitis, anaphylaxis, anemia, aphasia, aplastic anemia, arterial occlusion (acute), arrhythmia, arterial thrombosis, bruising, cerebral thrombosis, cerebrovascular accident, chest pain, chronic leukoencephalopathy, cognitive dysfunction (has been reported at low dosage), conjunctivitis, cryptococcosis, cytomegalovirus infection (including cytomegaloviral pneumonia, sepsis, nocardiosis), deep vein thrombosis, disseminated vaccinia (following smallpox immunization), drowsiness, dysarthria, dysuria, eye pain, enteritis, eosinophilia, epistaxis, erythema multiforme, exfoliative dermatitis, fatigue, fractures, furunculosis, GI bleeding, gynecomastia, headache, hematemesis, hematuria, hepatic failure, hepatitis, herpes simplex, herpes zoster, histoplasmosis, hypogammaglobulinemia, hypotension, impotence, infertility, intestinal perforation, leukoencephalopathy (especially following craniospinal irradiation or repeated high-dose therapy), libido decreased, lymphoma (may regress with discontinuation), lymphoproliferative disorders, melena, menstrual irregularities, mesenteric ischemia (acute), MI, mood changes, myocardial ischemia, nasal septum perforation, neutropenia, nodulosis, osteonecrosis and soft tissue necrosis (with radiotherapy), osteoporosis, pancreatitis, paresis, pericardial effusion, pericarditis, plaque erosions (psoriasis), *Pneumocystis carinii* pneumonia, pneumonia, proteinuria, pulmonary embolism, pulmonary fibrosis, radiation recall dermatitis, respiratory failure, retinal vein thrombosis, reversible posterior leukoencephalopathy syndrome (RPLS), seizure (more frequent in pediatric patients with ALL), skin ulceration, Stevens-Johnson syndrome, stroke, supraventricular arrythmia, sweating, syncope, telangiectasia, thromboembolism, thrombophlebitis, tinnitus, toxic epidermal necrolysis, tumor lysis syndrome, upper respiratory tract infection, urticaria, vaginal discharge, ventricular arrythmia, vision changes

Drug Interactions

Metabolism/Transport Effects Substrate of P-glycoprotein, SLCO1B1

Avoid Concomitant Use

Avoid concomitant use of Methotrexate with any of the following: Acitretin; BCG; CloZAPine; Natalizumab; Pimecrolimus; Tacrolimus (Topical)

Increased Effect/Toxicity

Methotrexate may increase the levels/effects of: CloZAPine; CycloSPORINE (Systemic); Leflunomide; Loop Diuretics; Natalizumab; Theophylline Derivatives; Vaccines (Live); Vitamin K Antagonists

The levels/effects of Methotrexate may be increased by: Acitretin; Ciprofloxacin (Systemic); CycloSPORINE (Systemic); Denosumab; Eltrombopag; Loop Diuretics; Nonsteroidal Anti-Inflammatory Agents; Penicillins; P-glycoprotein/ABCB1 Inhibitors; Pimecrolimus; Probenecid; Proton Pump Inhibitors; Roflumilast; Salicylates; SulfaSALAzine; Sulfonamide Derivatives; Tacrolimus (Topical); Trastuzumab; Trimethoprim

Decreased Effect

Methotrexate may decrease the levels/effects of: BCG; Cardiac Glycosides; Coccidioidin Skin Test; Loop Diuretics; Sapropterin; Sipuleucel-T; Vaccines (Inactivated); Vitamin K Antagonists

The levels/effects of Methotrexate may be decreased by: Bile Acid Sequestrants; Echinacea; P-glycoprotein/ABCB1 Inducers

Ethanol/Nutrition/Herb Interactions

Ethanol: Ethanol may be associated with increased liver injury. Management: Avoid ethanol.

Food: Methotrexate peak serum levels may be decreased if taken with food. Milk-rich foods may decrease methotrexate absorption. Folate may decrease drug response.

Herb/Nutraceutical: Echinacea has immunostimulant properties. Management: Avoid echinacea.

Storage/Stability Store tablets and intact vials at room temperature (15°C to 25°C). Protect from light.

I.M., I.V., SubQ: Solution diluted in D_5W or NS is stable for 24 hours at room temperature (21°C to 25°C). Reconstituted solutions with a preservative may be stored under refrigeration for up to 3 months, and up to 4 weeks at room temperature.

Intrathecal: Intrathecal dilutions are preservative free and should be used as soon as possible after preparation. After preparation, store intrathecal medications (until use) in an isolated location or container clearly marked with a label identifying as "intrathecal" use only.

Reconstitution Use appropriate precautions for handling and disposal. **Use preservative-free preparations for intrathecal or high-dose methotrexate administration.**

I.M., I.V., SubQ: Dilute powder with D_5W or NS to a concentration of ≤25 mg/mL (20 mg and 50 mg vials) and 50 mg/mL (1 g vial). May further dilute in D_5W or NS.

Intrathecal: Prepare intrathecal solutions with preservative-free NS, lactated Ringer's, or Elliot's B solution to a final volume of up to 12 mL (volume generally based on institution or practitioner preference). Intrathecal methotrexate concentrations may be institution specific or based on practitioner preference, generally ranging from a final concentration of 1 mg/mL (per prescribing information; Grossman, 1993; Lin, 2008) up to ~2-4 mg/mL (de Lemos, 2009; Glantz, 1999). For triple intrathecal therapy (methotrexate 12 mg/hydrocortisone 24 mg/cytarabine 36 mg), preparation to final volume of 12 mL is reported (Lin, 2008). Intrathecal medications should **NOT** be prepared during the preparation of any other agents.

Mechanism of Action Methotrexate is a folate antimetabolite that inhibits DNA synthesis, repair, and cellular replication. Methotrexate irreversibly binds to dihydrofolate reductase, inhibiting the formation of reduced folates, and thymidylate synthetase, resulting in inhibition of purine and thymidylic acid synthesis. Methotrexate is cell cycle specific for the S phase of the cycle.

The MOA in the treatment of rheumatoid arthritis is unknown, but may affect immune function. In psoriasis, methotrexate is thought to target rapidly proliferating epithelial cells in the skin.

In Crohn's disease, it may have immune modulator and anti-inflammatory activity.

Pharmacodynamics/Kinetics

Onset of action: Antirheumatic: 3-6 weeks; additional improvement may continue longer than 12 weeks

Absorption:

Oral: Highly variable; dose dependent

I.M. injection: Complete

Distribution: Penetrates slowly into 3rd space fluids (eg, pleural effusions, ascites), exits slowly from these compartments (slower than from plasma); sustained concentrations retained in kidney and liver

V_d: I.V.: 0.18 L/kg (initial); 0.4-0.8 L/kg (steady state)

Protein binding: ~50%

Metabolism: Partially metabolized by intestinal flora (after oral administration) to DAMPA by carboxypeptidase; hepatic aldehyde oxidase converts methotrexate to 7-hydroxy methotrexate; polyglutamates are produced intracellularly and are just as potent as methotrexate; their production is dose- and duration-dependent and they are slowly eliminated by the cell once formed. Polyglutamated forms can be converted back to methotrexate.

Bioavailability: Oral: ~20% to 95%; in general, bioavailability is dose dependent and decreases as the dose increases (especially at doses ≥80 mg/m^2)

Half-life elimination: Low dose: 3-10 hours; High dose: 8-15 hours

Time to peak, serum: Oral: 1-2 hours; I.M.: 30-60 minutes

Excretion: Dose and route dependent; I.V.: Urine (80% to 90% as unchanged drug; 5% to 7% as 7-hydroxy methotrexate); feces (<10%)

Dosing

Adult Details concerning dosing in combination regimens should also be consulted.

Note: Doses between 100-500 mg/m^2 **may require** leucovorin calcium rescue. Doses >500 mg/m^2 **require** leucovorin calcium rescue: I.V., I.M., Oral: Leucovorin calcium 10-15 mg/m^2 every 6 hours for 8 or 10 doses, starting 24 hours after the start of methotrexate infusion. Continue until the methotrexate level is ≤0.1 micromolar (10^{-7} M). Some clinicians continue leucovorin calcium until the methotrexate level is <0.05 micromolar (5×10^{-8} M) or 0.01 micromolar (10^{-8} M).

If the 48-hour methotrexate level is >1 micromolar (10^{-6} M) or the 72-hour methotrexate level is >0.2 micromolar (2×10^{-7} M): I.V., I.M, Oral: Leucovorin calcium 100 mg/m^2 every 6 hours until the methotrexate level is ≤0.1 micromolar (10^{-7} M). Some clinicians continue leucovorin calcium until the methotrexate level is <0.05 micromolar (5×10^{-8} M) or 0.01 micromolar (10^{-8} M).

Antineoplastic dosage range: I.V.: Range is wide from 30-40 mg/m^2/week to 100-12,000 mg/m^2 with leucovorin calcium rescue

Breast cancer: I.V.: 30-60 mg/m^2 Day 1 and 8 every 3-4 weeks

Head and neck cancer: Oral, I.M., I.V.: 25-50 mg/m^2 once weekly

Lymphoma, non-Hodgkin's: I.V.:

30 mg/m^2 days 3 and 10 every 3 weeks **or**

120 mg/m^2 day 8 and 15 every 3-4 weeks **or**

200 mg/m^2 day 8 and 15 every 3 weeks **or**

400 mg/m^2 every 4 weeks for 3 cycles **or**

1 g/m^2 every 3 weeks **or**

1.5 g/m^2 every 4 weeks

Meningeal leukemia: I.T.: Usual dose: 12 mg/dose. **Note:** Optimal intrathecal chemotherapy dosing should be based on age rather than on body surface area (BSA); CSF volume correlates with age and not to BSA (Bleyer, 1983; Kerr, 2001).

Mycosis fungoides (cutaneous T-cell lymphoma): Oral, I.M.: Initial (early stages):

5-50 mg once weekly **or**

15-37.5 mg twice weekly

Osteosarcoma: I.V.: 8-12 g/m^2 weekly for 2-4 weeks

Psoriasis: Some experts recommend concomitant folic acid 1-5 mg/day (except the day of methotrexate) to reduce hematologic, gastrointestinal, and hepatic adverse events related to methotrexate.

Oral: 2.5-5 mg/dose every 12 hours for 3 doses given weekly **or**

Oral, I.M., SubQ: 10-25 mg/dose given once weekly; titrate to lowest effective dose

Note: An initial test dose of 2.5-5 mg is recommended in patients with risk factors for hematologic toxicity or renal impairment. (Kalb, 2009).

Rheumatoid arthritis: Some experts recommend concomitant folic acid at a dose of least 5 mg/week (except the day of methotrexate) to reduce hematologic, gastrointestinal, and hepatic adverse events related to methotrexate.

Oral (manufacturer labeling): 7.5 mg once weekly or 2.5 mg every 12 hours for 3 doses/week (dosage exceeding 20 mg/week may cause a higher incidence and severity of adverse events); *alternatively,* 10-15 mg once weekly, increased by 5 mg every 2-4 weeks to a maximum of 20-30 mg once weekly has been recommended by some experts (Visser, 2009)

I.M., SubQ (unlabeled route): 15 mg once weekly (dosage varies, similar to oral) (Braun, 2008)

Trophoblastic neoplasms:

Oral, I.M.: 15-30 mg/day for 5 days; repeat in 7 days for 3-5 courses

I.V.: 11 mg/m^2 days 1 through 5 every 3 weeks

Unlabeled uses:

Bladder cancer (unlabeled use): I.V.:

30 mg/m^2 day 1 and 8 every 3 weeks **or**

30 mg/m^2 day 1, 15, and 22 every 4 weeks

Crohn's disease, mild/moderate, corticosteroid-dependent or refractory (unlabeled use):

Remission induction or reduction of steroid use: I.M., SubQ: 25 mg once weekly (Lichtenstein, 2009)

Remission maintenance: I.M.: 15 mg once weekly (Feagan, 2000; Lichtenstein, 2009)

Dermatomyositis/polymyositis (unlabeled uses):

Oral: Initial: 7.5-15 mg/week, often adjunctively with high-dose corticosteroid therapy; may increase in weekly 2.5 mg increments to target dose of 10-25 mg/week (**Note:** Administration of folate 5-7 mg/week has been used to reduce side effects) (Briemberg, 2003; Newman, 1995; Wiendl, 2008).

I.V., I.M.: Doses of 20-60 mg/week have been employed if failure with oral therapy (doses >50 mg/week may require leucovorin calcium rescue) (Briemberg, 2003)

Ectopic pregnancy (unlabeled use): I.M.:

Single-dose regimen: Methotrexate 50 mg/m^2 on day 1; Measure serum hCG levels on days 4 and 7; if needed, repeat dose on day 7 (Barnhart, 2009)

Two-dose regimen: Methotrexate 50 mg/m^2 on day 1; Measure serum hCG levels on day 4 and administer a second dose of methotrexate 50 mg/m^2; Measure serum hCG levels on day 7 and if needed, administer a third dose of 50 mg/m^2 (Barnhart, 2009)

Multidose regimen: Methotrexate 1 mg/kg on day 1, leucovorin calcium 0.1 mg/kg I.M. on day 2; measure serum hCG on day 2; methotrexate 1 mg/kg on day 3; leucovorin calcium 0.1 mg/kg on day 4; measure serum hCG on day 4; continue up to a total of 4 courses based on hCG concentrations (Barnhart, 2009)

GVHD (acute) prophylaxis: I.V.: 15 mg/m^2/dose on day 1 and 10 mg/m^2/dose on days 3 and 6 after allogeneic transplant (in combination with cyclosporine and prednisone) (Chao, 1993; Chao, 2000; Ross, 1999) **or** 15 mg/m^2/dose on day 1 and 10 mg/m^2/dose on days 3, 6, and 11 after allogeneic transplant (in combination with cyclosporine) (Chao, 2000)

Nonleukemic meningeal cancer (unlabeled uses): I.T.: 10-12 mg/dose twice weekly for 4 weeks, then weekly for 4 weeks, then monthly (NCCN CNS cancer guidelines v.2.2009) **or** 12 mg/dose twice weekly for 4 weeks, then weekly for 4 doses, then monthly for 4 doses (Glantz, 1998) **or** 10 mg twice weekly for 4 weeks, then weekly for 1 month, then every 2 weeks for 2 months (Glantz, 1999)

Takayasu arteritis, refractory or relapsing disease (unlabeled use): Oral: Initial dose: 0.3 mg/kg/week (maximum: 15 mg/week), titrated by 2.5 mg increments every 1-2 weeks until reaching a maximum tolerated weekly dose of 25 mg (use in combination with a corticosteroid; Hoffman, 1994)

Geriatric Refer to individual protocols; adjust for renal impairment.

Meningeal leukemia: I.T.: Consider a dose reduction (CSF volume and turnover may decrease with age)

Rheumatoid arthritis/psoriasis: Oral: Initial: 5-7.5 mg/week, not to exceed 20 mg/week

Pediatric Details concerning dosing in combination regimens should also be consulted.

Note: Doses between 100-500 mg/m^2 **may require** leucovorin calcium rescue. Doses >500 mg/m^2 **require** leucovorin calcium rescue: I.V., I.M., Oral: Leucovorin calcium 10-15 mg/m^2 every 6 hours for 8 or 10 doses, starting 24 hours after the start of methotrexate infusion. Continue until the methotrexate level is ≤0.1 micromolar (10^{-7} M). Some clinicians continue leucovorin calcium until the methotrexate level is <0.05 micromolar (5×10^{-8} M) or 0.01 micromolar (10^{-8} M).

If the 48-hour methotrexate level is >1 micromolar (10^{-6} M) or the 72-hour methotrexate level is >0.2 micromolar (2×10^{-7} M): I.V., I.M, Oral: Leucovorin calcium 100 mg/m^2 every 6 hours until the methotrexate level is ≤0.1 micromolar (10^{-7} M). Some clinicians continue leucovorin calcium until the methotrexate level is <0.05 micromolar (5×10^{-8} M) or 0.01 micromolar (10^{-8} M).

Dermatomyositis (unlabeled use): Oral: 15-20 mg/m^2/week as a single dose once weekly **or** 0.3-1 mg/kg/dose once weekly

GVHD (acute) prophylaxis (unlabeled use): I.V.: Refer to adult dosing.

Juvenile idiopathic arthritis (JIA): Oral, I.M.:10 mg/m^2 once weekly, then 5-15 mg/m^2/week as a single dose **or** as 3 divided doses given 12 hours apart

Antineoplastic dosage range:

Oral, I.M.: 7.5-30 mg/m^2/week **or** every 2 weeks

I.V.: 10-18,000 mg/m^2 bolus dosing **or** continuous infusion over 6-42 hours

Pediatric solid tumors (high-dose): I.V.:

<12 years: 12-25 g/m^2

≥12 years: 8 g/m^2

Acute lymphocytic leukemia (intermediate-dose): I.V.: Loading: 100 mg/m^2 bolus dose, followed by 900 mg/m^2/day infusion over 23-41 hours.

Meningeal leukemia: I.T.: 6-12 mg/dose based on age. **Note**: Optimal intrathecal chemotherapy dosing should be based on age rather than on body surface area (BSA); CSF volume correlates with age and not to BSA (Bleyer, 1983; Kerr, 2001):

<1 year: 6 mg/dose

1 year: 8 mg/dose

2 years: 10 mg/dose

≥3 years: 12 mg/dose

Renal Impairment No dosage adjustment provided in the manufacturer's labeling. The following adjustments have been recommended:

Aronoff, 2007:

Children:

Cl_{cr} 10-50 mL/minute/1.73m^2: Administer 50% of dose

Cl_{cr} <10 mL/minute/1.73m^2: Administer 30% of dose

Hemodialysis: Administer 30% of dose

Continuous ambulatory peritoneal dialysis (CAPD): Administer 30% of dose

Continuous renal replacement therapy (CRRT): Administer 50% of dose

Adults:

Cl_{cr} 10-50 mL/minute: Administer 50% of dose

Cl_{cr} <10 mL/minute: Avoid use

Hemodialysis: Administer 50% of dose

Continuous renal replacement therapy (CRRT): Administer 50% of dose

Kintzel, 1995:

Cl_{cr} 46-60 mL/minute: Administer 65% of normal dose

Cl_{cr} 31-45 mL/minute: Administer 50% of normal dose

Cl_{cr} <30 mL/minute: Avoid use

Hepatic Impairment No dosage adjustment provided in the manufacturer's labeling; use with caution. The following adjustments have been recommended (Floyd, 2006):

Bilirubin 3.1-5 mg/dL **or** transaminases >3 times ULN: Administer 75% of dose

Bilirubin >5 mg/dL: Avoid use

Adjustment for Toxicity

Nonhematologic toxicity: Diarrhea, stomatitis, or vomiting which may lead to dehydration: Discontinue until recovery

Hematologic toxicity:

Psoriasis, rheumatoid arthritis: Significant blood count decrease: Discontinue immediately.

Oncologic uses: Profound granulocytopenia and fever: Evaluate immediately; consider broad-spectrum parenteral antimicrobial coverage

Combination Regimens

Bladder cancer:
- CMV on page 1589
- M-VAC (Bladder Cancer) on page 1718

Breast cancer:
- CMF on page 1588
- CMF-IV on page 1588
- Dox-CMF (Sequential) on page 1617

Gestational trophoblastic tumor:
- EMA/CO on page 1622
- EP/EMA on page 1625

Leukemia, acute lymphocytic:
- Hyper-CVAD + Imatinib on page 1680
- Hyper-CVAD (Leukemia, Acute Lymphocytic) on page 1681
- Larson Regimen (ALL) on page 1699
- Linker Protocol (ALL) on page 1703
- MTX/6-MP/VP (Maintenance) on page 1717
- POMP on page 1741
- PVA (POG 8602) on page 1742

Leukemia, acute promyelocytic:
- Tretinoin-Daunorubicin (APL) on page 1762
- Tretinoin-Daunorubicin-Cytarabine (APL) on page 1762
- Tretinoin-Idarubicin (APL) on page 1764

Lymphoma, Hodgkin: VAMP (Hodgkin) on page 1769

Lymphoma, non-Hodgkin's:
- CODOX-M on page 1590
- COMLA on page 1595
- Hyper-CVAD (Lymphoma, non-Hodgkin's) on page 1687
- IMVP-16 on page 1691
- MACOP-B on page 1704
- m-BACOD on page 1706
- Pro-MACE-CytaBOM on page 1741

Lymphoma, non-Hodgkin's (Burkitt): CODOX-M/IVAC on page 1591

Lymphoma, non-Hodgkin's (Mantle cell): Hyper-CVAD + Rituximab on page 1688

Osteosarcoma:
- HDMTX on page 1679
- MTX-CDDPAdr on page 1717
- POG-0051 on page 1740

Soft tissue sarcoma: Methotrexate-Vinblastine (Desmoid tumor) on page 1710

Administration Methotrexate may be administered I.M., I.V., or I.T.; I.V. administration may be as slow push, short bolus infusion, or 24- to 42-hour continuous infusion

Specific dosing schemes vary, but high dose should be followed by leucovorin calcium to prevent toxicity; refer to Leucovorin monograph on page 870

Emetic Potential

≥250 mg/m^2: Moderate (30% to 90%)

50-250 mg/m^2: Low (10% to 30%)

≤50 mg/m^2: Very low (<10%)

Oral: Very low (<10%)

Monitoring Parameters

Laboratory tests should be performed on day 5 or day 6 of the weekly methotrexate cycle (eg, psoriasis, RA) to detect the leukopenia nadir and to avoid elevated LFTs 1-2 days after taking dose.

Patients with psoriasis:

CBC with differential and platelets (baseline, 7-14 days after initiating therapy or dosage increase, every 2-4 weeks for first few months, then every 1-3 months); BUN and serum creatinine (baseline and every 2-3 months); consider PPD for latent TB screening (baseline); LFTs (baseline, monthly for first 6 months, then every 1-2 months); chest x-ray (baseline if underlying lung disease)

Liver biopsy for patients **with** risk factors for hepatotoxicity: Baseline or after 2-6 months of therapy and with each 1-1.5 g cumulative dose interval

Liver biopsy for patients **without** risk factors for hepatotoxicity: If persistent elevations in 5 of 9 AST levels during a 12-month period, or decline of serum albumin below the normal range with normal nutritional status. Consider biopsy after cumulative dose of 3.5-4 g and after each additional 1.5 g.

Patients with rheumatoid arthritis and Crohn's disease:

CBC with differential and platelets, serum creatinine and LFTs (baseline then every 2-4 weeks for initial 3 months of therapy, then every 8-12 weeks for 3-6 months of therapy and then every 12 weeks after 6 months of therapy); chest x-ray (baseline); pulmonary function test (if methotrexate-induced lung disease suspected); hepatitis B or C testing (baseline)

Liver biopsy: Baseline (if persistent abnormal baseline LFTs, history of alcoholism, or chronic hepatitis B or C) or during treatment if persistent LFT elevations (6 of 12 tests abnormal over 1 year or 5 of 9 results when LFTs performed at 6-week intervals)

Patients with cancer: Baseline and frequently during treatment: CBC with differential and platelets, serum creatinine, BUN, LFTs; chest x-ray (baseline); methotrexate levels and urine pH (with high-dose therapy); pulmonary function test (if methotrexate-induced lung disease suspected)

Ectopic pregnancy (unlabeled use): Prior to therapy, measure serum hCG, CBC with differential, liver function tests, serum creatinine. Serum hCG concentrations should decrease between treatment days 4 and 7. If hCG decreases by >15%, additional courses are not needed however, continue to measure hCG weekly until no longer detectable. If <15% decrease is observed, repeat dose per regimen (Barnhart, 2009).

Dietary Considerations Some products may contain sodium.

Additional Information Oncology Comment: Methotrexate overexposure: The rescue agent, glucarpidase, is an enzyme which rapidly hydrolyzes extracellular methotrexate into inactive metabolites, resulting in a rapid reduction of methotrexate concentrations. Glucarpidase is approved for the treatment of toxic plasma methotrexate concentrations (>1 micromole/L) in patients with delayed clearance due to renal impairment. Glucarpidase has also been administered intrathecally (unlabeled use/route) for inadvertent intrathecal methotrexate overexposure. Refer to Glucarpidase monograph.

Dosage Forms Excipient information presented when available (limited, particularly for generics); consult specific product labeling.

Injection, powder for reconstitution: 1 g

Injection, solution: 25 mg/mL (2 mL, 10 mL)

Injection, solution [preservative free]: 25 mg/mL (2 mL, 4 mL, 8 mL, 10 mL, 40 mL)

Tablet, oral: 2.5 mg

Trexall™: 5 mg, 7.5 mg, 10 mg, 15 mg [scored]

Tablet, oral [dose-pack]:

Rheumatrex®: 2.5 mg [scored]

References

Adès L, Sanz MA, Chevret S, et al, "Treatment of Newly Diagnosed Acute Promyelocytic Leukemia (APL): A Comparison of French Belgian-Swiss and PETHEMA Results," *Blood*, 2008, 111 (3):1078-84.

American College of Rheumatology Subcommittee on Rheumatoid Arthritis Guidelines, "Guidelines for the Management of Rheumatoid Arthritis: 2002 Update," *Arthritis Rheum*, 2002, 46 (2):328–46.

Aronoff GR, Bennett WM, Berns JS, et al, *Drug Prescribing in Renal Failure: Dosing Guidelines for Adults and Children*, 5th ed. Philadelphia, PA: American College of Physicians; 2007, p 101.

Azzarelli A, Gronchi A, Bertulli R, et al, "Low-Dose Chemotherapy With Methotrexate and Vinblastine for Patients With Advanced Aggressive Fibromatosis," *Cancer*, 2001, 92(5):1259-64.

Barnhart KT, "Clinical Practice. Ectopic Pregnancy," *N Engl J Med*, 2009, 361(4):379-87.

Bartz D and Goldberg A, "Medication Abortion," *Clin Obstet Gynecol*, 2009, 52(2):140-50.

Bleyer WA, Coccia PF, Sather HN, et al, "Reduction in Central Nervous System Leukemia With a Pharmacokinetically Derived Intrathecal Methotrexate Dosage Regimen," *J Clin Oncol*, 1983, 1 (5):317-25.

Braun J, Kästner P, Flaxenberg P, et al, "Comparison of the Clinical Efficacy and Safety of Subcutaneous Versus Oral Administration of Methotrexate in Patients With Active Rheumatoid Arthritis: Results of a Six-Month, Multicenter, Randomized, Double-Blind, Controlled, Phase IV Trial," *Arthritis Rheum*, 2008, 58(1):73-81.

Briemberg HR and Amato AA, "Dermatomyositis and Polymyositis," *Curr Treat Options Neurol*, 2003, 5(5):349-56.

Chao NJ, Schmidt GM, Niland JC, et al, "Cyclosporine, Methotrexate, and Prednisone Compared with Cyclosporine and Prednisone for Prophylaxis of Acute Graft-versus-Host Disease," *N Engl J Med*, 1993, 329(17):1225-30.

Chao NJ, Snyder DS, Jain M, et al, "Equivalence of 2 Effective Graft Versus-Host Disease Prophylaxis Regimens: Results of a Prospective Double-Blind Randomized Trial," *Biol Blood Marrow Transplant*, 2000, 6(3):254-61.

deLemos ML, Monfared S, Denyssevych T, et al. "Evaluation of Osmolality and pH of Various Concentrations of Methotrexate, Cytarabine, and Thiotepa Prepared in Normal Saline, Sterile Water for Injection, and Lactated Ringer's Solution for Intrathecal Administration," *J Oncol Pharm Pract*, 2009, 15(1):45-52.

Feagan BG, Fedorak RN, Irvine EJ, et al, "A Comparison of Methotrexate With Placebo for the Maintenance of Remission in Crohn's Disease. North American Crohn's Study Group Investigators," *N Engl J Med*, 2000, 342(22):1627-32.

Floyd J, Mirza I, Sachs B, et al, "Hepatotoxicity of Chemotherapy," *Semin Oncol*, 2006, 33 (1):50-67.

Glantz MJ, Cole BF, Recht L, Akerley W, et al, "High-Dose Intravenous Methotrexate for Patients With Nonleukemic Leptomeningeal Cancer: Is Intrathecal Chemotherapy Necessary?" *J Clin Oncol*, 1998, 16(4):1561-7.

Glantz MJ, Jaeckle KA, Chamberlain MC, et al, "A Randomized Controlled Trial Comparing Intrathecal Sustained-Release Cytarabine (DepoCyt) to Intrathecal Methotrexate in Patients With Neoplastic Meningitis from Solid Tumors," *Clin Cancer Res*, 1999, 5(11):3394-402.

Grossman SA, Finkelstein DM, Ruckdeschel JC, et al, "Randomized Prospective Comparison of Intraventricular Methotrexate and Thiotepa in Patients With Previously Untreated Neoplastic Meningitis. Eastern Cooperative Oncology Group," *J Clin Oncol*, 1993, 11(3):561-9.

Hoffman GS, Leavitt RY, Kerr GS, et al, "Treatment of Glucocorticoid-Resistant or Relapsing Takayasu Arteritis With Methotrexate," *Arthritis Rheum*, 1994, 37(4):578-82.

Jacobson JO, Polovich M, McNiff KK, et al, "American Society of Clinical Oncology/Oncology Nursing Society Chemotherapy Administration Safety Standards," *J Clin Oncol*, 2009, 27 (32):5469-75.

Kalb RE, Strober B, Weinstein G, et al, "Methotrexate and Psoriasis: 2009 National Psoriasis Foundation Consensus Conference," *J Am Acad Dermatol*, 2009, 60(5):824-37.

Kerr JZ, Berg S, and Blaney SM, "Intrathecal Chemotherapy," *Crit Rev Oncol Hematol*, 2001, 37 (3):227-36.

Kintzel PE and Dorr RT, "Anticancer Drug Renal Toxicity and Elimination: Dosing Guidelines for Altered Renal Function," *Cancer Treat Rev*, 1995, 21(1):33-64.

Lichtenstein GR, Hanauer SB, and Sandborn WJ, "Management of Crohn's Disease in Adults," *Am J Gastroenterol*, 2009, 104(2):465-83.

Lin WY, Liu HC, Yeh TC, et al, "Triple Intrathecal Therapy Without Cranial Irradiation for Central Nervous System Preventive Therapy in Childhood Acute Lymphoblastic Leukemia," *Pediatr Blood Cancer*, 2008, 50(3):523-7.

Menter A, Korman NJ, Elmets CA, et al, "Guidelines of Care for the Management of Psoriasis and Psoriatic Arthritis: Section 4. Guidelines of Care for the Management and Treatment of Psoriasis With Traditional Systemic Agents," *J Am Acad Dermatol*, 2009, 61(3):451-85.

Morgan C, Tillett T, Braybrooke J, et al, "Management of Uncommon Chemotherapy-Induced Emergencies," *Lancet Oncol*, 2011, 12(8):806-14.

National Comprehensive Cancer Network® (NCCN), "Clinical Practice Guidelines in Oncology™: Central Nervous System Cancers," Version 1.2010. Available at http://www.nccn.org/professionals/physician_gls/PDF/cns.pdf

Newman ED and Scott DW, "The Use of Low-dose Oral Methotrexate in the Treatment of Polymyositis and Dermatomyositis," *J Clin Rheumatol*, 1995, 1(2):99-102.

Ross M, Schmidt GM, Niland JC, et al, "Cyclosporine, Methotrexate, and Prednisone Compared With Cyclosporine and Prednisone for Prevention of Acute Graft-vs.-Host Disease: Effect on Chronic Graft-vs.-Host Disease and Long-Term Survival," *Biol Blood Marrow Transplant*, 1999, 5 (5):285-91.

Saag KG, Teng GG, Patkar NM, et al, "American College of Rheumatology 2008 Recommendations for the Use of Nonbiologic and Biologic Disease-Modifying Antirheumatic Drugs in Rheumatoid Arthritis," *Arthritis Rheu*, 2008, 59(6):762-84.

Schwartz S, Borner K, Muller K, et al, "Glucarpidase (Carboxypeptidase G2) Intervention in Adult and Elderly Cancer Patients With Renal Dysfunction and Delayed Methotrexate Elimination After High-Dose Methotrexate Therapy," *Oncologist*, 2007 12(11):1299-308.

Visser K, Katchamart W, Loza A, et al, "Multinational Evidence-Based Recommendations for the Use of Methotrexate in Rheumatic Disorders With a Focus on Rheumatoid Arthritis: Integrating Systematic Literature Research and Expert Opinion of a Broad International Panel of Rheumatologists in the 3E Initiative," *Ann Rheum Dis*, 2009, 68(7):1086–93.

Widemann BC, Balis FM, Murphy RF, et al, "Carboxypeptidase-G2, Thymidine, and Leucovorin Rescue in Cancer Patients With Methotrexate-Induced Renal Dysfunction," *J Clin Oncol*, 1997, 15(5):2125-34.

Widemann BC, Balis FM, Shalabi A, et al, "Treatment of Accidental Intrathecal Methotrexate Overdose With Intrathecal Carboxypeptidase G2," *J Natl Cancer Inst*, 2004, 96(20):1557-9.

Wiendl H, "Idiopathic Inflammatory Myopathies: Current and Future Therapeutic Options," *Neurotherapeutics*, 2008, 5(4):548-57.

◆ **Methotrexate Sodium** *see* Methotrexate *on page 949*

◆ **Methotrexatum** *see* Methotrexate *on page 949*

◆ **Methylacetoxyprogesterone** *see* MedroxyPROGESTERone *on page 916*

Methylene Blue (METH i leen bloo)

Index Terms Methylthionine Chloride

Generic Availability (U.S.) Yes

Pharmacologic Category Antidote

Use Antidote for cyanide poisoning and drug-induced methemoglobinemia, indicator dye

Unlabeled Use Treatment/prevention of ifosfamide-induced encephalopathy; topically, in conjunction with polychromatic light to photoinactivate viruses such as herpes simplex; alone or in combination with vitamin C for the management of chronic urolithiasis; vasoplegia syndrome associated with cardiac surgery

Labeled Contraindications Hypersensitivity to methylene blue or any component of the formulation; intraspinal injection; renal insufficiency; pregnancy

Pregnancy Risk Factor X

Warnings/Precautions Do not inject SubQ or intrathecally; use with caution in young patients and in patients with G6PD deficiency; continued use can cause profound anemia. At high doses or in patients with G6PD-deficiency and infants, methylene blue may catalyze the oxidation of ferrous iron in hemoglobin to ferric iron causing paradoxical methemoglobinemia; monitor methemoglobin concentrations regularly during administration. Use with caution in patients with severe renal impairment. Avoid concomitant use with serotonin modulators (eg, serotonin reuptake inhibitors, tricyclic antidepressants) and allow a washout period of at least 4-5 half-lives of the serotonin reuptake inhibitor prior to intravenous methylene blue use. Methylene blue should not be added to enteral feeding products (Durfee, 2006; Wessel, 2005); safety and efficacy have not been established.

Adverse Reactions Frequency not defined.

Cardiovascular: Angina, arrhythmia, hypertension, precordial pain
Central nervous system: Dizziness, headache, fever, mental confusion
Dermatologic: Staining of skin
Gastrointestinal: Abdominal pain, fecal discoloration (blue-green), nausea, vomiting
Genitourinary: Bladder irritation, discoloration of urine (blue-green)
Hematologic: Anemia, transient reduction in oxygen saturation as read by pulse oximetry
Miscellaneous: Diaphoresis
Postmarketing and/or case reports: Serotonin syndrome

Drug Interactions

Metabolism/Transport Effects None known.

Avoid Concomitant Use

Avoid concomitant use of Methylene Blue with any of the following: BuPROPion; BusPIRone; MAO Inhibitors; Maprotiline; Mirtazapine; Nefazodone; Selective Serotonin Reuptake Inhibitors; Serotonin/Norepinephrine Reuptake Inhibitors; TraZODone; Tricyclic Antidepressants

Increased Effect/Toxicity

Methylene Blue may increase the levels/effects of: Metoclopramide; Serotonin Modulators

The levels/effects of Methylene Blue may be increased by: Antipsychotics; BuPROPion; BusPIRone; MAO Inhibitors; Maprotiline; Mirtazapine; Nefazodone; Selective Serotonin Reuptake Inhibitors; Serotonin/Norepinephrine Reuptake Inhibitors; TraZODone; Tricyclic Antidepressants

Decreased Effect There are no known significant interactions involving a decrease in effect.

Mechanism of Action Weak germicide in low concentrations, hastens the conversion of methemoglobin to hemoglobin; has opposite effect at high concentrations by converting ferrous ion of reduced hemoglobin to ferric ion to form methemoglobin; in cyanide toxicity, it combines with cyanide to form cyanmethemoglobin preventing the interference of cyanide with the cytochrome system

Pharmacodynamics/Kinetics

Onset of action: Reduction of methemoglobin: I.V.: 30-60 minutes
Absorption: Oral: 53% to 97%
Metabolism: Peripheral reduction to leukomethylene blue
Excretion: In bile, feces, and urine as leukomethylene blue

Dosing

Adult & Geriatric

Methemoglobinemia: I.V.: 1-2 mg/kg or 25-50 mg/m^2 over 5-10 minutes; may be repeated in 1 hour if necessary

Ifosfamide-induced encephalopathy (unlabeled use): I.V.: **Note:** Treatment may not be necessary; encephalopathy may improve spontaneously:
Prevention: 50 mg every 6-8 hours
Treatment: 50 mg as a single dose or every 4-8 hours until symptoms resolve

Vasoplegia syndrome associated with cardiac surgery (unlabeled use): I.V.: 1.5-2 mg/kg over 20-60 minutes administered once (Levin, 2004; Leyh, 2003). **Note:** Improvement of vasoplegia (eg, increased systemic vascular resistance, reduced vasopressor dosage) has been in observed 1-2 hours following methylene blue administration.

Pediatric

Methemoglobinemia: Children: Refer to adult dosing.

Renal Impairment No dosage adjustment recommendations available; however, caution should be used in severe renal impairment.

Administration I.V.: Administer undiluted by direct I.V. injection over 5-10 minutes. For the treatment of ifosfamide-induced encephalopathy, methylene blue may be administered either undiluted as a slow I.V. push over at least 5 minutes or diluted in 50 mL NS or D_5W and infused over at least 5 minutes. Consider concomitant dextrose administration, especially in patients who are hypoglycemic, to ensure efficacy of methylene blue.

Monitoring Parameters Arterial blood gases; cardiac monitoring (patients with pre-existing pulmonary and/or cardiac disease); CBC; methemoglobin levels (co-oximetry yields a direct and accurate measure of methemoglobin levels); pulse oximeter (will not provide accurate measurement of oxygenation when methemoglobin levels are >35% or following methylene blue administration); renal function; signs and symptoms of methemoglobinemia such as pallor, cyanosis, nausea, muscle weakness, dizziness, confusion, agitation, dyspnea, and tachycardia; transcutaneous O_2 saturation

Additional Information Skin stains may be removed using a hypochlorite solution.

Dosage Forms Excipient information presented when available (limited, particularly for generics); consult specific product labeling.

Injection, solution: 10 mg/mL (1 mL, 10 mL)

References

David KA and Picus J, "Evaluating Risk Factors for the Development of Ifosfamide Encephalopathy," *Am J Clin Oncol*, 2005, 28(3):277-80.

Durfee SM, Gallagher-Allred C, Pasquale JA, "Standards for Specialized Nutrition Support for Adult Residents of Long-Term Care Facilities," *Nutr Clin Pract*, 2006, 21(1):96-104.

Levin RL, Degrange MA, Bruno GF, et al, "Methylene Blue Reduces Mortality and Morbidity in Vasoplegic Patients After Cardiac Surgery," *Ann Thorac Surg*, 2004, 77(2):496-9.

Leyh RG, Kofidis T, Strüber M, et al, "Methylene Blue: The Drug of Choice for Catecholamine-Refractory Vasoplegia After Cardiopulmonary Bypass?" *J Thorac Cardiovasc Surg*, 2003, 125 (6):1426-31.

Patel PN, "Methylene Blue for Management of Ifosfamide-Induced Encephalopathy," *Ann Pharmacother*, 2006, 40(2):299-303.

Pelgrims J, DeVos F, Van den Brande J, et al, "Methylene Blue in the Treatment and Prevention of Ifosfamide-Induced Encephalopathy: Report of 12 Cases and a Review of the Literature," *Br J Cancer*, 2000, 82(2) 291-4.

Turner AR, Duong CD, and Good DJ, "Methylene Blue for the Treatment and Prophylaxis of Ifosfamide-Induced Encephalopathy," *Clin Oncol (R Coll Radiol)*, 2003, 15(7):435-9.

Wessel J, Balint J, Crill C, et al, "Standards for Specialized Nutrition Support: Hospitalized Pediatric Patients," *Nutr Clin Pract*, 2005, 20(1):103-116.

Zulian GB, Tullen E, and Maton B, "Methylene Blue for Ifosfamide-Associated Encephalopathy," *N Engl J Med*, 1995, 332(18):1239-40.

◆ **Methylmorphine** *see* Codeine *on page* 311

Methylnaltrexone (meth il nal TREKS one)

Brand Names: U.S. Relistor®

Brand Names: Canada Relistor®

Index Terms Methylnaltrexone Bromide; N-methylnaltrexone Bromide

Generic Availability (U.S.) No

Pharmacologic Category Gastrointestinal Agent, Miscellaneous; Opioid Antagonist, Peripherally-Acting

Use Treatment of opioid-induced constipation in patients with advanced illness receiving palliative care with inadequate response to conventional laxative regimens

Labeled Contraindications Known or suspected mechanical bowel obstruction

Canadian labeling: Additional contraindications (not in U.S. labeling): Hypersensitivity to methylnaltrexone or any component of the formulation

Pregnancy Risk Factor B

Lactation Excretion in breast milk unknown/use caution

Warnings/Precautions Discontinue treatment for severe or persistent diarrhea. Gastrointestinal perforation of the colon, duodenum, and stomach has been reported (rarely) in patients with advanced illnesses associated with impaired structural integrity of the GI wall (eg, cancer, Ogilvie's syndrome, peptic ulcer). Use caution in patients with known or history of GI tract lesions; discontinue therapy if persistent, severe, or worsening abdominal symptoms occur. Use with caution in patients with renal impairment; dosage adjustment recommended for severe renal impairment (Cl_{cr} <30 mL/minute). Has not been studied in patients with end-stage renal impairment requiring dialysis. Discontinue methylnaltrexone if opioids are discontinued. Use has not been studied in patients with peritoneal catheters. Use beyond 4 months has not been studied.

Adverse Reactions

>10%: Gastrointestinal: Abdominal pain (29%), flatulence (13%), nausea (12%)

1% to 10%:

Central nervous system: Dizziness (7%)

Dermatologic: Hyperhidrosis (7%)

Gastrointestinal: Diarrhea (6%)

<1%, postmarketing, and/or case reports: Abdominal cramps, body temperature increased, diaphoresis, flushing, GI perforation, malaise, muscle spasm, pain, syncope, vomiting

Drug Interactions

Metabolism/Transport Effects **Substrate** of CYP2D6 (minor); **Note:** Assignment of Major/Minor substrate status based on clinically relevant drug interaction potential

Avoid Concomitant Use There are no known interactions where it is recommended to avoid concomitant use.

Increased Effect/Toxicity There are no known significant interactions involving an increase in effect.

Decreased Effect

The levels/effects of Methylnaltrexone may be decreased by: Peginterferon Alfa-2b

Storage/Stability Store intact vials and prefilled syringes at room temperature of 20°C to 25°C (68°F to 77°F); excursions permitted to 15°C to 30°C (59°F to 86°F); do not freeze. Protect from light. Solution withdrawn from the single-use vial is stable in a syringe for 24 hours at room temperature (protection from light during this 24 hours is not necessary).

Mechanism of Action An opioid receptor antagonist which blocks opioid binding at the mu receptor, methylnaltrexone is a quaternary derivative of naltrexone with restricted ability to cross the blood-brain barrier. It therefore functions as a peripheral acting opioid antagonist, including actions on the gastrointestinal tract to inhibit opioid-induced decreased gastrointestinal motility and delay in gastrointestinal transit time, thereby decreasing opioid-induced constipation. Does not affect opioid analgesic effects or induce opioid withdrawal symptoms.

Pharmacodynamics/Kinetics

Onset of action: Usually within 30-60 minutes (in responding patients)

Absorption: SubQ: Rapid

Distribution: V_{dss}: ~1.1 L/kg

Protein binding: 11% to 15%

Metabolism: Metabolized to methyl-6-naltrexol isomers, methylnaltrexone sulfate, and other minor metabolites

Half-life elimination: Terminal: ~8 hours

Time to peak, plasma: SubQ: 30 minutes

Excretion: Urine (~50%, primarily as unchanged drug); feces (<50%, primarily as unchanged drug)

Dosing

Adult & Geriatric Opioid-induced constipation: SubQ: Dosing is according to body weight: Administer 1 dose every other day as needed; maximum: 1 dose/24 hours

<38 kg: 0.15 mg/kg (round dose up to nearest 0.1 mL of volume)

38 to <62 kg: 8 mg

62-114 kg: 12 mg

>114 kg: 0.15 mg/kg (round dose up to nearest 0.1 mL of volume)

Renal Impairment

Mild-to-moderate renal impairment: No adjustment required.

Severe renal impairment (Cl_{cr} <30 mL/minute): Administer 50% of normal dose.

End-stage renal impairment (dialysis-dependent): Has not been studied.

Hepatic Impairment

Mild-to-moderate hepatic impairment (Child-Pugh class A or B): No adjustment required.

Severe hepatic impairment: Has not been studied.

Administration SubQ: Administer subcutaneously into upper arm, abdomen, or thigh. Rotate injection site. Do not use tender, bruised, red, or hard areas.

Additional Information In some clinical trials, patients who received methylnaltrexone were on a palliative opioid therapy equivalent to a mean daily oral morphine dose of 172 mg, at a stable dose for ≥3 days. Constipation was defined as <3 bowel movements/week or no bowel movement for >2 days. Patients maintained their regular laxative regimen for at least 3 days prior to treatment and throughout the study.

Dosage Forms Excipient information presented when available (limited, particularly for generics); consult specific product labeling.

Injection, solution:

Relistor®: 8 mg/0.4 mL (0.4 mL); 12 mg/0.6 mL (0.6 mL) [contains edetate calcium disodium; prefilled syringe]

Relistor®: 12 mg/0.6 mL (0.6 mL) [contains edetate calcium disodium; vial]

References

Portenoy RK, Thomas J, Moehl Boatwright ML, et al, "Subcutaneous Methylnaltrexone for the Treatment of Opioid-Induced Constipation in Patients With Advanced Illness: A Double-Blind Randomized, Parallel Group, Dose-Ranging Study," *J Pain Symptom Manage*, 2008, 35 (5):458-68.

Thomas J, "Opioid-Induced Bowel Dysfunction," *J Pain Symptom Manage*, 2008, 35(1):103-13.

Thomas J, Karver S, Cooney GA, et al, "Methylnaltrexone for Opioid-Induced Constipation in Advanced Illness," *N Engl J Med*, 2008, 358(22):2332-43.
Yuan CS, "Methylnaltrexone Mechanisms of Action and Effects on Opioid Bowel Dysfunction and Other Opioid Adverse Effects," *Ann Pharmacother*, 2007, 41(6):984-93.

◆ **Methylnaltrexone Bromide** *see* Methylnaltrexone *on page* 964

◆ **Methylphytyl Napthoquinone** *see* Phytonadione *on page* 1169

MethylPREDNISolone (meth il pred NIS oh lone)

Related Information

Hematopoietic Stem Cell Transplantation *on page* 1887
Management of Chemotherapy-Induced Nausea and Vomiting *on page* 1786
Management of Infections *on page* 1809

Brand Names: U.S. A-Methapred®; Depo-Medrol®; Medrol®; Medrol® Dosepak™; Solu-MEDROL®

Brand Names: Canada Depo-Medrol®; Medrol®; Methylprednisolone Acetate; Solu-Medrol®

Index Terms 6-α-Methylprednisolone; A-Methapred; Medrol Dose Pack; Methylprednisolone Acetate; Methylprednisolone Sodium Succinate; Solumedrol

Generic Availability (U.S.) Yes: Excludes preservative free injection

Pharmacologic Category Corticosteroid, Systemic

Use Primarily as an anti-inflammatory or immunosuppressant agent in the treatment of a variety of diseases including those of hematologic, allergic, inflammatory, neoplastic, and autoimmune origin. Prevention and treatment of graft-versus-host disease following allogeneic bone marrow transplantation.

Unlabeled Use Acute spinal cord injury

Labeled Contraindications Hypersensitivity to methylprednisolone or any component of the formulation; systemic fungal infection (except intra-articular injection in localized joint conditions); administration of live virus vaccines. methylprednisolone formulations containing benzyl alcohol preservative are contraindicated in premature infants; I.M. administration in idiopathic thrombocytopenia purpura; intrathecal administration

Lactation Enters breast milk/use caution

Warnings/Precautions Use with caution in patients with thyroid disease, hepatic impairment, renal impairment, cardiovascular disease, diabetes, glaucoma, cataracts, myasthenia gravis, patients at risk for osteoporosis, patients at risk for seizures, or GI diseases (diverticulitis, peptic ulcer, ulcerative colitis) due to perforation risk. Not recommended for the treatment of optic neuritis; may increase frequency of new episodes. Use caution following acute MI (corticosteroids have been associated with myocardial rupture). Cardiomegaly and congestive heart failure have been reported following concurrent use of amphotericin B and hydrocortisone for the management of fungal infections.

Because of the risk of adverse effects, systemic corticosteroids should be used cautiously in the elderly in the smallest possible effective dose for the shortest duration. May affect growth velocity; growth should be routinely monitored in pediatric patients. Withdraw therapy with gradual tapering of dose.

May cause hypercorticism or suppression of hypothalamic-pituitary-adrenal (HPA) axis, particularly in younger children or in patients receiving high doses for prolonged periods. HPA axis suppression may lead to adrenal crisis. Withdrawal and discontinuation of a corticosteroid should be done slowly and carefully. Particular care is required when patients are transferred from systemic corticosteroids to inhaled products due to possible adrenal ▶

insufficiency or withdrawal from steroids, including an increase in allergic symptoms. Patients receiving >20 mg per day of prednisone (or equivalent) may be most susceptible. Fatalities have occurred due to adrenal insufficiency in asthmatic patients during and after transfer from systemic corticosteroids to aerosol steroids; aerosol steroids do not provide the systemic steroid needed to treat patients having trauma, surgery, or infections.

Acute myopathy has been reported with high dose corticosteroids, usually in patients with neuromuscular transmission disorders; may involve ocular and/or respiratory muscles; monitor creatine kinase; recovery may be delayed. Corticosteroid use may cause psychiatric disturbances, including depression, euphoria, insomnia, mood swings, and personality changes. Pre-existing psychiatric conditions may be exacerbated by corticosteroid use. Prolonged use of corticosteroids may also increase the incidence of secondary infection, cause activation of latent infections, mask acute infection (including fungal infections), prolong or exacerbate viral or parasitic infections, or limit response to vaccines. Exposure to chickenpox or measles should be avoided; corticosteroids should not be used to treat ocular herpes simplex. Corticosteroids should not be used for cerebral malaria or viral hepatitis. Close observation is required in patients with latent tuberculosis and/or TB reactivity; restrict use in active TB (only in conjunction with antituberculosis treatment). Amebiasis should be ruled out in any patient with recent travel to tropic climates or unexplained diarrhea prior to initiation of corticosteroids. Prolonged treatment with corticosteroids has been associated with the development of Kaposi's sarcoma (case reports); discontinuation may result in clinical improvement.

High-dose corticosteroids should not be used to manage acute head injury. Rare cases of anaphylactoid reactions have been observed in patients receiving corticosteroids. Avoid injection or leakage into the dermis; dermal and/or subdermal skin depression may occur at the site of injection. Avoid deltoid muscle injection; subcutaneous atrophy may occur. Some dosage forms contain benzyl alcohol which has been associated with "gasping syndrome" in neonates.

Adverse Reactions Frequency not defined.

Cardiovascular: Arrhythmias, bradycardia, cardiac arrest, cardiomegaly, circulatory collapse, congestive heart failure, edema, fat embolism, hypertension, hypertrophic cardiomyopathy in premature infants, myocardial rupture (post MI), syncope, tachycardia, thromboembolism, vasculitis

Central nervous system: Delirium, depression, emotional instability, euphoria, hallucinations, headache, intracranial pressure increased, insomnia, malaise, mood swings, nervousness, neuritis, personality changes, psychic disorders, pseudotumor cerebri (usually following discontinuation), seizure, vertigo

Dermatologic: Acne, allergic dermatitis, alopecia, dry scaly skin, ecchymoses, edema, erythema, hirsutism, hyper-/hypopigmentation, hypertrichosis, impaired wound healing, petechiae, rash, skin atrophy, sterile abscess, skin test reaction impaired, striae, urticaria

Endocrine & metabolic: Adrenal suppression, amenorrhea, carbohydrate intolerance increased, Cushing's syndrome, diabetes mellitus, fluid retention, glucose intolerance, growth suppression (children), hyperglycemia, hyperlipidemia, hypokalemia, hypokalemic alkalosis, menstrual irregularities, negative nitrogen balance, pituitary-adrenal axis suppression, protein catabolism, sodium and water retention

Gastrointestinal: Abdominal distention, appetite increased, bowel/bladder dysfunction (after intrathecal administration), gastrointestinal hemorrhage, gastrointestinal perforation, nausea, pancreatitis, peptic ulcer, perforation of the small and large intestine, ulcerative esophagitis, vomiting, weight gain

Hematologic: Leukocytosis (transient)

Hepatic: Hepatomegaly, transaminases increased

Local: Postinjection flare (intra-articular use), thrombophlebitis

Neuromuscular & skeletal: Arthralgia, arthropathy, aseptic necrosis (femoral and humoral heads), fractures, muscle mass loss, muscle weakness, myopathy (particularly in conjunction with neuromuscular disease or neuromuscular-blocking agents), neuropathy, osteoporosis, paresthesia, tendon rupture, vertebral compression fractures, weakness

Ocular: Cataracts, exophthalmoses, glaucoma, intraocular pressure increased

Renal: Glycosuria

Respiratory: Pulmonary edema

Miscellaneous: Abnormal fat disposition, anaphylactoid reaction, anaphylaxis, angioedema, avascular necrosis, diaphoresis, hiccups, hypersensitivity reactions, infections, secondary malignancy

Drug Interactions

Metabolism/Transport Effects **Substrate** of CYP3A4 (minor); **Note:** Assignment of Major/Minor substrate status based on clinically relevant drug interaction potential; **Inhibits** CYP2C8 (weak), CYP3A4 (weak)

Avoid Concomitant Use

Avoid concomitant use of MethylPREDNISolone with any of the following: Aldesleukin; BCG; Mifepristone; Natalizumab; Pimecrolimus, Pimozide; Tacrolimus (Topical)

Increased Effect/Toxicity

MethylPREDNISolone may increase the levels/effects of: Acetylcholinesterase Inhibitors; Amphotericin B; ARIPiprazole; CycloSPORINE (Systemic); Deferasirox; Leflunomide; Loop Diuretics; Natalizumab; NSAID (COX-2 Inhibitor); NSAID (Nonselective); Pimozide; Thiazide Diuretics; Vaccines (Live); Warfarin

The levels/effects of MethylPREDNISolone may be increased by: Antifungal Agents (Azole Derivatives, Systemic); Aprepitant; Calcium Channel Blockers (Nondihydropyridine); CycloSPORINE (Systemic); CYP3A4 Inhibitors (Strong); Denosumab; Estrogen Derivatives; Fluconazole; Fosaprepitant, Indacaterol; Macrolide Antibiotics; Mifepristone; Neuromuscular-Blocking Agents (Nondepolarizing); Pimecrolimus; Quinolone Antibiotics; Roflumilast; Salicylates; Tacrolimus (Topical); Telaprevir; Trastuzumab

Decreased Effect

MethylPREDNISolone may decrease the levels/effects of: Aldesleukin; Antidiabetic Agents; BCG; Calcitriol; Coccidioidin Skin Test; Corticorelin; CycloSPORINE (Systemic); Hyaluronidase; Isoniazid; Salicylates; Sipuleucel-T, Telaprevir; Vaccines (Inactivated)

The levels/effects of MethylPREDNISolone may be decreased by: Aminoglutethimide; Antacids; Barbiturates; Bile Acid Sequestrants; CarBAMazepine; Echinacea; Fosphenytoin; Mifepristone; Mitotane; Phenytoin; Primidone; Rifamycin Derivatives; Tocilizumab

Ethanol/Nutrition/Herb Interactions

Ethanol: Ethanol may increase gastric mucosal irritation. Management: Avoid ethanol.

Food: Methylprednisolone interferes with calcium absorption. May cause GI upset. Management: Administer with food. Limit caffeine.

Herb/Nutraceutical: St John's wort may decrease methylprednisolone levels. Cat's claw and echinacea have immunostimulant properties. Management: Avoid St John's wort, cat's claw, and echinacea.

Storage/Stability Intact vials of methylprednisolone sodium succinate should be stored at controlled room temperature of 20°C to 25°C (68°F to 77°F). Protect from light. Reconstituted solutions of methylprednisolone sodium succinate should be stored at room temperature of 20°C to 25°C (68°F to 77°F) and used within 48 hours. Stability of parenteral admixture at room temperature (25°C) and at refrigeration temperature (4°C) is 48 hours.

Reconstitution

Standard diluent (Solu-Medrol®): 40 mg/50 mL D_5W; 125 mg/50 mL D_5W.

Minimum volume (Solu-Medrol®): 50 mL D_5W.

Mechanism of Action In a tissue-specific manner, corticosteroids regulate gene expression subsequent to binding specific intracellular receptors and translocation into the nucleus. Corticosteroids exert a wide array of physiologic effects including modulation of carbohydrate, protein, and lipid metabolism and maintenance of fluid and electrolyte homeostasis. Moreover cardiovascular, immunologic, musculoskeletal, endocrine, and neurologic physiology are influenced by corticosteroids. Decreases inflammation by suppression of migration of polymorphonuclear leukocytes and reversal of increased capillary permeability.

Pharmacodynamics/Kinetics

Onset of action: Peak effect (route dependent): Oral: 1-2 hours; I.M.: 4-8 days; Intra-articular: 1 week; methylprednisolone sodium succinate is highly soluble and has a rapid effect by I.M. and I.V. routes

Duration (route dependent): Oral: 30-36 hours; I.M.: 1-4 weeks; Intra-articular: 1-5 weeks; methylprednisolone acetate has a low solubility and has a sustained I.M. effect

Distribution: V_d: 0.7-1.5 L/kg

Half-life elimination: 3-3.5 hours; reduced in obese

Excretion: Clearance: Reduced in obese

Dosing

Adult & Geriatric Only sodium succinate may be given I.V.; methylprednisolone sodium succinate is highly soluble and has a rapid effect by I.M. and I.V. routes. Methylprednisolone acetate has a low solubility and has a sustained I.M. effect.

Acute spinal cord injury (unlabeled use): I.V. (sodium succinate): 30 mg/kg over 15 minutes, followed in 45 minutes by a continuous infusion of 5.4 mg/kg/hour for 23 hours. **Note:** Due to insufficient evidence of clinical efficacy (ie, preserving or improving spinal cord function), the routine use of methylprednisolone in the treatment of acute spinal cord injury is no longer recommended. If used in this setting, methylprednisolone should not be initiated >8 hours after the injury; not effective in penetrating trauma (eg, gunshot) (Consortium for Spinal Cord Medicine, 2008).

Allergic conditions: Oral: Tapered-dosage schedule (eg, dose-pack containing 21 x 4 mg tablets):

Day 1: 24 mg on day 1 administered as 8 mg (2 tablets) before breakfast, 4 mg (1 tablet) after lunch, 4 mg (1 tablet) after supper, and 8 mg (2 tablets) at bedtime **OR** 24 mg (6 tablets) as a single dose or divided into 2 or 3 doses upon initiation (regardless of time of day)

Day 2: 20 mg on day 2 administered as 4 mg (1 tablet) before breakfast, 4 mg (1 tablet) after lunch, 4 mg (1 tablet) after supper, and 8 mg (2 tablets) at bedtime

Day 3: 16 mg on day 3 administered as 4 mg (1 tablet) before breakfast, 4 mg (1 tablet) after lunch, 4 mg (1 tablet) after supper, and 4 mg (1 tablet) at bedtime

Day 4: 12 mg on day 4 administered as 4 mg (1 tablet) before breakfast, 4 mg (1 tablet) after lunch, and 4 mg (1 tablet) at bedtime

Day 5: 8 mg on day 5 administered as 4 mg (1 tablet) before breakfast and 4 mg (1 tablet) at bedtime

Day 6: 4 mg on day 6 administered as 4 mg (1 tablet) before breakfast

Anti-inflammatory or immunosuppressive:

Oral: 2-60 mg/day in 1-4 divided doses to start, followed by gradual reduction in dosage to the lowest possible level consistent with maintaining an adequate clinical response.

I.M. (sodium succinate): 10-80 mg/day once daily

I.M. (acetate): 10-80 mg every 1-2 weeks

I.V. (sodium succinate): 10-40 mg over a period of several minutes and repeated I.V. or I.M. at intervals depending on clinical response; when high dosages are needed, give 30 mg/kg over a period ≥30 minutes and may be repeated every 4-6 hours for 48 hours.

Arthritis: Intra-articular (acetate): Administer every 1-5 weeks.

Large joints (eg, knee, ankle): 20-80 mg

Medium joints (eg, elbow, wrist): 10-40 mg

Small joints: 4-10 mg

Asthma exacerbations, including status asthmaticus (emergency medical care or hospital doses): Oral, I.V.: 40-80 mg/day in 1- 2 divided doses until peak expiratory flow is 70% of predicted or personal best (NIH Asthma Guidelines, NAEPP, 2007)

Asthma, severe persistent, long-term control: Oral: 7.5-60 mg/day (or on alternate days) (NIH Asthma Guidelines, NAEPP, 2007)

Dermatitis, acute severe: I.M. (acetate): 80-120 mg as a single dose

Dermatitis, chronic: I.M. (acetate): 40-120 mg every 5-10 days

Dermatologic conditions (eg, keloids, lichen planus): Intralesional (acetate): 20-60 mg

Dermatomyositis/polymyositis: I.V. (sodium succinate): 1 g/day for 3-5 days for severe muscle weakness, followed by conversion to oral prednisone (Drake, 1996)

Lupus nephritis: High-dose "pulse" therapy: I.V. (sodium succinate): 0.5-1 g/day for 3 days (Ponticelli, 2010)

***Pneumocystis* pneumonia in AIDS patients:** I.V.: 30 mg twice daily for 5 days, then 30 mg once daily for 5 days, then 15 mg once daily for 11 days

Pediatric Dosing should be based on the lesser of ideal body weight or actual body weight. **Only sodium succinate may be given I.V.**, methylprednisolone sodium succinate is highly soluble and has a rapid effect by I.M. and I.V. routes. Methylprednisolone acetate has a low solubility and has a sustained I.M. effect.

Acute spinal cord injury (unlabeled use): I.V. (sodium succinate): 30 mg/kg over 15 minutes, followed in 45 minutes by a continuous infusion of 5.4 mg/kg/hour for 23 hours. **Note:** Due to insufficient evidence of clinical efficacy (ie, preserving or improving spinal cord function), the routine use of methylprednisolone in the treatment of acute spinal cord injury is no longer recommended. If used in this setting, methylprednisolone should not be initiated >8 hours after the injury; not effective in penetrating trauma (eg, gunshot) (Consortium for Spinal Cord Medicine, 2008).

Anti-inflammatory or immunosuppressive: Oral, I.M., I.V. (sodium succinate): 0.5-1.7 mg/kg/day **or** 5-25 mg/m²/day in divided doses every 6-12 hours; "Pulse" therapy: 15-30 mg/kg/dose over ≥30 minutes given once daily for 3 days

Asthma exacerbations, including status asthmaticus (emergency medical care or hospital doses) (NIH Asthma Guidelines, NAEPP, 2007): Children <12 years: Oral, I.V.: 1-2 mg/kg/day in 2 divided doses (maximum: 60 mg/day) until peak expiratory flow is 70% of predicted or personal best

Lupus nephritis: I.V. (sodium succinate): 30 mg/kg over ≥30 minutes every other day for 6 doses

Renal Impairment

Hemodialysis effects: Slightly dialyzable (5% to 20%)

Administer dose posthemodialysis.

Combination Regimens

Leukemia, acute lymphocytic: Hyper-CVAD (Leukemia, Acute Lymphocytic) on page 1681

Lymphoma, Hodgkin:

ESHAP (Hodgkin) on page 1634

MINE-ESHAP (Hodgkin) on page 1711

Lymphoma, non-Hodgkin's:

ESHAP on page 1633

MINE-ESHAP (NHL) on page 1712

Administration

Administer with meals to decrease GI upset.

Parenteral: Methylprednisolone sodium succinate may be administered I.M. or I.V.; I.V. administration may be IVP over one to several minutes or IVPB or continuous I.V. infusion. **Acetate salt should not be given I.V.** Avoid injection into the deltoid muscle due to a high incidence of subcutaneous atrophy. Avoid injection or leakage into the dermis; dermal and/or subdermal skin depression may occur at the site of injection.

I.V.: Succinate:

Low dose: ≤1.8 mg/kg or ≤125 mg/dose: I.V. push over 3-15 minutes

Moderate dose: ≥2 mg/kg or 250 mg/dose: I.V. over 15-30 minutes

High dose: 15 mg/kg or ≥500 mg/dose: I.V. over ≥30 minutes

Doses >15 mg/kg or ≥1 g: Administer over 1 hour

Do **not** administer high-dose I.V. push; hypotension, cardiac arrhythmia, and sudden death have been reported in patients given high-dose methylprednisolone I.V. push (>0.5 g over <10 minutes); intermittent infusion over 15-60 minutes; maximum concentration: I.V. push 125 mg/mL

I.M.: Avoid injection into the deltoid muscle due to a high incidence of subcutaneous atrophy. Avoid injection or leakage into the dermis; dermal and/or subdermal skin depression may occur at the site of injection. Do not inject into areas that have evidence of acute local infection.

Monitoring Parameters Blood pressure, blood glucose, electrolytes, growth in children

Test Interactions Interferes with skin tests

Dietary Considerations Take with meals to decrease GI upset.; need diet rich in pyridoxine, vitamin C, vitamin D, folate, calcium, phosphorus, and protein.

Additional Information Sodium content of 1 g sodium succinate injection: 2.01 mEq; 53 mg of sodium succinate salt is equivalent to 40 mg of methylprednisolone base

Methylprednisolone acetate: Depo-Medrol®
Methylprednisolone sodium succinate: Solu-Medrol®

Dosage Forms Excipient information presented when available (limited, particularly for generics); consult specific product labeling.

Injection, powder for reconstitution, as sodium succinate [strength expressed as base]: 40 mg, 125 mg, 500 mg, 1 g
- A-Methapred®: 40 mg [contains benzyl alcohol (in diluent), lactose 25 mg/vial]
- A-Methapred®: 40 mg [contains lactose 25 mg/vial]
- A-Methapred®: 125 mg
- A-Methapred®: 125 mg [contains benzyl alcohol (in diluent)]
- Solu-MEDROL®: 500 mg, 1 g
- Solu-MEDROL®: 2 g [contains benzyl alcohol (in diluent)]

Injection, powder for reconstitution, as sodium succinate [strength expressed as base, preservative free]:
- Solu-MEDROL®: 40 mg [contains lactose 25 mg/vial; supplied with diluent]
- Solu-MEDROL®: 125 mg, 500 mg, 1 g [supplied with diluent]

Injection, suspension, as acetate: 40 mg/mL (1 mL, 5 mL, 10 mL); 80 mg/mL (1 mL, 5 mL)
- Depo-Medrol®: 20 mg/mL (5 mL) [contains benzyl alcohol, polysorbate 80]
- Depo-Medrol®: 40 mg/mL (1 mL)
- Depo-Medrol®: 40 mg/mL (5 mL, 10 mL); 80 mg/mL (5 mL) [contains benzyl alcohol, polysorbate 80]

Injection, suspension, as acetate [preservative free]:
- Depo-Medrol®: 80 mg/mL (1 mL)

Tablet, oral: 4 mg, 8 mg, 16 mg, 32 mg
- Medrol®: 2 mg, 4 mg, 8 mg, 16 mg, 32 mg [scored]

Tablet, oral [dose-pack]: 4 mg [21s]
- Medrol® Dosepak™: 4 mg [scored; 21s]

References

Benson CA, Kaplan JE, Masur H, et al, "Treating Opportunistic Infections Among HIV-Exposed and Infected Adults and Adolescents: Recommendations from CDC, the National Institutes of Health and the HIV Medicine Association/IDSA," *MMWR Recomm Rep*, 2004, 53(RR-15):1-112

Consortium for Spinal Cord Medicine, "Early Acute Management in Adults With Spinal Cord Injury: A Clinical Practice Guideline for Health-Care Professionals," *J Spinal Cord Med*, 2008, 31(4):403-79.

Dellinger RP, Levy MM, Carlet JM, et al, "Surviving Sepsis Campaign: International Guidelines for Management of Severe Sepsis and Septic Shock: 2008," *Intensive Care Med*, 2008, 34(1):17-60. Available at http://www.ncbi.nlm.nih.gov/pmc/articles/PMC2249616/pdf/134_2007_Article_934.pdf

Drake LA, Dinehart SM, Farmer ER, et al, "Guidelines of Care for Dermatomyositis. American Academy of Dermatology," *J Am Acad Dermatol*, 1996, 34(5 Pt 1):824-9.

Marik PE, Pastores SM, Annane D, et al, "Recommendations for the Diagnosis and Management of Corticosteroid Insufficiency in Critically Ill Adult Patients: Consensus Statements From an International Task Force by the American College of Critical Care Medicine," *Crit Care Med*, 2008, 36(6):1937-49.

McGee S and Hirschmann J, "Use of Corticosteroids in Treating Infectious Diseases," *Arch Intern Med*, 2008, 168(10):1034-46.

National Asthma Education and Prevention Program (NAEPP), "Expert Panel Report 3 (EPR-3): Guidelines for the Diagnosis and Management of Asthma," Clinical Practice Guidelines, National Institutes of Health, National Heart, Lung, and Blood Institute, NIH Publication No. 08-4051, prepublication 2007. Available at http://www.nhlbi.nih.gov/guidelines/asthma/asthgdln.htm

Ponticelli C, Glassock RJ, and Moroni G, "Induction and Maintenance Therapy in Proliferative Lupus Nephritis," *J Nephrol*, 2010, 23(1):9-16.

◆ **6-α-Methylprednisolone** *see* MethylPREDNISolone *on page 967*

◆ **Methylprednisolone Acetate** *see* MethylPREDNISolone *on page 967*

◆ **Methylprednisolone Sodium Succinate** *see* MethylPREDNISolone *on page 967*

◆ **Methylthionine Chloride** *see* Methylene Blue *on page 962*

Metoclopramide (met oh KLOE pra mide)

Related Information

Management of Chemotherapy-Induced Nausea and Vomiting *on page 1786*
Palliative Care Medicine (Cancer) *on page 1871*

Brand Names: U.S. Metozolv™ ODT; Reglan®

Brand Names: Canada Apo-Metoclop®; Metoclopramide Hydrochloride Injection; Metoclopramide Omega; Nu-Metoclopramide; PMS-Metoclopramide

Generic Availability (U.S.) Yes: Excludes oral-disintegrating tablet

Pharmacologic Category Antiemetic; Gastrointestinal Agent, Prokinetic

Use

Oral: Symptomatic treatment of diabetic gastroparesis; gastroesophageal reflux

I.V., I.M.: Symptomatic treatment of diabetic gastroparesis; postpyloric placement of enteral feeding tubes; prevention and/or treatment of nausea and vomiting associated with chemotherapy, or postsurgery; to stimulate gastric emptying and intestinal transit of barium during radiological examination of the stomach/small intestine

Labeled Contraindications Hypersensitivity to metoclopramide or any component of the formulation; GI obstruction, perforation or hemorrhage; pheochromocytoma; history of seizures or concomitant use of other agents likely to increase extrapyramidal reactions

Pregnancy Risk Factor B

Lactation Enters breast milk/use caution

Warnings/Precautions [U.S. Boxed Warning]: May cause tardive dyskinesia, which is often irreversible; duration of treatment and total cumulative dose are associated with an increased risk. Therapy durations >12 weeks should be avoided (except in rare cases following risk:benefit assessment). Risk appears to be increased in the elderly, women, and diabetics; however, it is not possible to predict which patients will develop tardive dyskinesia. Therapy should be discontinued in any patient if signs/symptoms of tardive dyskinesia appear.

May cause extrapyramidal symptoms, generally manifested as acute dystonic reactions within the initial 24-48 hours of use. Risk of these reactions is increased at higher doses, and in pediatric patients, and adults <30 years of age. Pseudoparkinsonism (eg, bradykinesia, tremor, rigidity) may also occur (usually within first 6 months of therapy) and is generally reversible following discontinuation. Use with caution or avoid in patients with Parkinson's disease. Avoid use in older adults (except for gastroparesis) due to risk of extrapyramidal effects, including tardive dyskinesia; risk potentially even greater in frail older adults (Beers Criteria). In addition, risk of tardive dyskinesia may be increased in older women. Neuroleptic malignant syndrome (NMS) has been reported (rarely) with metoclopramide.

May cause transient increase in serum aldosterone; use caution in patients who are at risk of fluid overload (HF, cirrhosis). Use caution in patients with hypertension or following surgical anastomosis/closure. Use caution with a history of mental illness; has been associated with depression. Abrupt discontinuation may (rarely) result in withdrawal symptoms (dizziness, headache, nervousness). Use caution and adjust dose in renal impairment. Patients with NADH-cytochrome b5 reductase deficiency are at increased risk of methemoglobinemia and/or sulfhemoglobinemia. Neonates may have an increased risk of methemoglobinemia due to decreased levels of NADH-cytochrome b5 reductase deficiency and prolonged clearance of metoclopramide.

Adverse Reactions Frequency not always defined.

Cardiovascular: AV block, bradycardia, HF, fluid retention, flushing (following high I.V. doses), hyper-/hypotension, supraventricular tachycardia

Central nervous system: Drowsiness (~10% to 70%; dose related), acute dystonic reactions (<1% to 25%; dose and age related), fatigue (2% to 10%), lassitude (~10%), restlessness (~10%), headache (4% to 5%), dizziness (1% to 4%), somnolence (2% to 3%), akathisia, confusion, depression, hallucinations (rare), insomnia, neuroleptic malignant syndrome (rare), Parkinsonian-like symptoms, suicidal ideation, seizure, tardive dyskinesia

Dermatologic: Angioneurotic edema (rare), rash, urticaria

Endocrine & metabolic: Amenorrhea, galactorrhea, gynecomastia, hyperprolactinemia, impotence

Gastrointestinal: Nausea (4% to 6%), vomiting (1% to 2%), diarrhea

Genitourinary: Incontinence, urinary frequency

Hematologic: Agranulocytosis, leukopenia, neutropenia, porphyria

Hepatic: Hepatotoxicity (rare)

Ocular: Visual disturbance

Respiratory: Bronchospasm, laryngeal edema (rare), laryngospasm (rare)

Miscellaneous: Allergic reactions, methemoglobinemia, sulfhemoglobinemia

Drug Interactions

Metabolism/Transport Effects **Substrate** of CYP1A2 (minor), CYP2D6 (minor); **Note:** Assignment of Major/Minor substrate status based on clinically relevant drug interaction potential; **Inhibits** CYP2D6 (weak)

Avoid Concomitant Use

Avoid concomitant use of Metoclopramide with any of the following: Antipsychotics; Droperidol; Promethazine; Tetrabenazine

Increased Effect/Toxicity

Metoclopramide may increase the levels/effects of: Antipsychotics; CycloSPORINE (Systemic); Prilocaine; Promethazine; Selective Serotonin Reuptake Inhibitors; Tetrabenazine; Tricyclic Antidepressants; Venlafaxine

The levels/effects of Metoclopramide may be increased by: Droperidol; Metyrosine; Serotonin Modulators

Decreased Effect

Metoclopramide may decrease the levels/effects of: Anti-Parkinson's Agents (Dopamine Agonist); Posaconazole; Quinagolide

The levels/effects of Metoclopramide may be decreased by: Peginterferon Alfa-2b

Ethanol/Nutrition/Herb Interactions Ethanol: Avoid ethanol (may increase CNS depression).

Storage/Stability

Injection: Store intact vial at controlled room temperature; injection is photosensitive and should be protected from light during storage; parenteral admixtures in D_5W or NS are stable for at least 24 hours and do not require light protection if used within 24 hours.

Tablet: Store at controlled room temperature of 20°C to 25°C (68°F to 77°F).

Mechanism of Action Blocks dopamine receptors and (when given in higher doses) also blocks serotonin receptors in chemoreceptor trigger zone of the

CNS; enhances the response to acetylcholine of tissue in upper GI tract causing enhanced motility and accelerated gastric emptying without stimulating gastric, biliary, or pancreatic secretions; increases lower esophageal sphincter tone

Pharmacodynamics/Kinetics

Onset of action: Oral: 30-60 minutes; I.V.: 1-3 minutes; I.M.: 10-15 minutes

Duration: Therapeutic: 1-2 hours, regardless of route

Absorption: Oral: Rapid

Distribution: V_d: ~3.5 L/kg

Protein binding: ~30%

Bioavailability: Oral: Range: 65% to 95%

Half-life elimination: Normal renal function: Children: ~4 hours; Adults: 5-6 hours (may be dose dependent)

Time to peak, serum: Oral: 1-2 hours

Excretion: Urine (~85%)

Dosing

Adult

Gastroesophageal reflux: Oral: 10-15 mg/dose up to 4 times/day 30 minutes before meals or food and at bedtime; single doses of 20 mg are occasionally needed prior to provoking situations. Treatment >12 weeks is not recommended.

Diabetic gastroparesis:

Oral: 10 mg/dose up to 4 times/day 30 minutes before meals or food and at bedtime for 2-8 weeks

I.M., I.V. (for severe symptoms): 10 mg over 1-2 minutes; 10 days of I.V. therapy may be necessary before symptoms are controlled to allow transition to oral administration

Chemotherapy-induced emesis prophylaxis: I.V.: 1-2 mg/kg 30 minutes before chemotherapy and repeated every 2 hours for 2 doses, then every 3 hours for 3 doses (manufacturer labeling); pretreatment with diphenhydramine will decrease risk of extrapyramidal reactions

Alternate dosing: **Note:** Metoclopramide is considered an antiemetic with a low therapeutic index; use is generally reserved for agents with low emetogenic potential or in patients intolerant/refractory to first line antiemetics.

Low-risk chemotherapy (unlabeled): I.V., Oral: 10-40 mg prior to dose, then every 4-6 hours as needed (NCCN Antiemesis guidelines, v.4.2009)

Breakthrough treatment (unlabeled): I.V., Oral: 10-40 mg every 4-6 hours (NCCN Antiemesis guidelines, v.4.2009)

Delayed-emesis prophylaxis (unlabeled): Oral: 20-40 mg/dose (or 0.5 mg/kg/dose) 2-4 times/day for 3-4 days (in combination with dexamethasone [ASCO guidelines, 2006])

Refractory or intolerant to antiemetics with a higher therapeutic index (unlabeled; Hesketh, 2008):

I.V.: 1-2 mg/kg/dose before chemotherapy and repeat 2 hours after chemotherapy

Oral: 0.5 mg/kg every 6 hours on days 2-4

Postoperative nausea and vomiting prophylaxis: I.M., I.V. (unlabeled route): 10-20 mg near end of surgery. **Note:** Guidelines discourage use of 10 mg metoclopramide as being ineffective (Gan, 2007); comparative study indicates higher dose (20 mg) may be efficacious (Quaynor, 2002).

Postpyloric feeding tube placement, radiological exam: I.V.: 10 mg as a single dose

Geriatric Initial: Dose at the lower end of the recommended range. Refer to adult dosing.

Pediatric

Gastroesophageal reflux (unlabeled use): Oral: 0.1-0.2 mg/kg/dose 4 times/day (maximum: 5 doses/day); pretreatment with diphenhydramine will decrease risk of extrapyramidal reactions to this dosage

Chemotherapy-induced emesis (unlabeled use): I.V.: 1-2 mg/kg 30 minutes before chemotherapy and every 2-4 hours

Postpyloric feeding tube placement: I.V.:

<6 years: 0.1 mg/kg as a single dose

6-14 years: 2.5-5 mg as a single dose

>14 years: Refer to adult dosing.

Renal Impairment

Cl_{cr} <40 mL/minute: Administer 50% of normal dose.

Not dialyzable (0% to 5%); supplemental dose is not necessary.

Administration

Injection solution: May be given I.M., direct I.V. push, short infusion (15-30 minutes), or continuous infusion; lower doses (≤10 mg) of metoclopramide can be given I.V. push undiluted over 1-2 minutes; higher doses (>10 mg) to be diluted in 50 mL of compatible solution (preferably NS) and given IVPB over at least 15 minutes; continuous SubQ infusion and rectal administration have been reported. **Note:** Rapid I.V. administration may be associated with a transient (but intense) feeling of anxiety and restlessness, followed by drowsiness.

Orally-disintegrating tablets: Administer on an empty stomach at least 30 minutes prior to food. Do not remove from packaging until time of administration. If tablet breaks or crumbles while handling, discard and remove new tablet. Using dry hands, place tablet on tongue and allow to dissolve. Swallow with saliva.

Monitoring Parameters Dystonic reactions; signs of hypoglycemia in patients using insulin and those being treated for gastroparesis; agitation, and confusion

Test Interactions Increased aminotransferase [ALT/AST] (S), increased amylase (S)

Medication Guide Available Yes

Dosage Forms Excipient information presented when available (limited, particularly for generics); consult specific product labeling. [DSC] = Discontinued product

Injection, solution [preservative free]: 5 mg/mL (2 mL)

Reglan®: 5 mg/mL (2 mL [DSC], 10 mL [DSC], 30 mL [DSC])

Solution, oral: 5 mg/5 mL (0.9 mL, 10 mL, 473 mL)

Tablet, oral: 5 mg, 10 mg

Reglan®: 5 mg

Reglan®: 10 mg [scored]

Tablet, orally disintegrating, oral:

Metozolv™ ODT: 5 mg, 10 mg [mint flavor]

References

Gan TJ, Meyer TA, Apfel CC, et al, "Society for Ambulatory Anesthesia Guidelines for the Management of Postoperative Nausea and Vomiting," *Anesth Analg*, 2007, 105(6):1615-28.

Hesketh PJ, "Chemotherapy-Induced Nausea and Vomiting," *N Engl J Med*, 2008, 358 (23):2482-94.

Kris MG, Hesketh PJ, Somerfield MR, et al, "American Society of Clinical Oncology Guideline for Antiemetics in Oncology: Update 2006," *J Clin Oncol*, 2006, 24(18):2932-46.

Martindale RG, McClave SA, Vanek VW, et al, "Guidelines for the Provision and Assessment of Nutrition Support Therapy in the Adult Critically Ill Patient: Society of Critical Care Medicine and American Society for Parenteral and Enteral Nutrition (A.S.P.E.N.)," *JPEN J Parenter Enteral Nutr*, 2007, 33(3):277-316.

Matok I, Gorodischer R, Koren G, et al, "The Safety of Metoclopramide Use in the First Trimester of Pregnancy," *N Engl J Med*, 2009, 360(24):2528-35.

Multinational Association of Supportive Care in Cancer (MASCC), "Antiemetic Guidelines," Updated April 2010. Available at http://data.memberclicks.com/site/mascc/MASCC_Guidelines_English_2010.pdf

National Comprehensive Cancer Network® (NCCN), "Clinical Practice Guidelines in Oncology™: Antiemesis," Version 1.2012. Available at http://www.nccn.org/professionals/physician_gls/PDF/antiemesis.pdf

Quaynor H and Raeder JC, "Incidence and Severity of Postoperative Nausea and Vomiting are Similar After Metoclopramide 20 mg and Ondansetron 8 mg Given by the End of Laparoscopic Cholecystectomies," *Acta Anaesthesiol Scand*, 2002, 46(1):109-13.

- **Metoclopramide Hydrochloride Injection (Can)** *see* Metoclopramide *on page* 974
- **Metoclopramide Omega (Can)** *see* Metoclopramide *on page* 974
- **Metozolv™ ODT** *see* Metoclopramide *on page* 974

MetroNIDAZOLE (Systemic) (met roe NYE da zole)

Brand Names: U.S. Flagyl®; Flagyl® 375; Flagyl® ER

Brand Names: Canada Apo-Metronidazole®; Flagyl®; Florazole® ER

Index Terms Metronidazole Hydrochloride

Generic Availability (U.S.) Yes: Excludes extended release tablet

Pharmacologic Category Amebicide; Antibiotic, Miscellaneous; Antiprotozoal, Nitroimidazole

Use Treatment of susceptible anaerobic bacterial and protozoal infections in the following conditions: Amebiasis, symptomatic and asymptomatic trichomoniasis; skin and skin structure infections, bone and joint infections, CNS infections, endocarditis, gynecologic infections, intra-abdominal infections (as part of combination regimen), respiratory tract infections (lower), systemic anaerobic infections; treatment of antibiotic-associated pseudomembranous colitis (AAPC); as part of a multidrug regimen for *H. pylori* eradication to reduce the risk of duodenal ulcer recurrence; surgical prophylaxis (colorectal); useful as single agent or in combination with amoxicillin, amoxicillin/clavulanic acid, or ciprofloxacin in the treatment of periodontitis associated with the presence of *Actinobacillus actinomycetemcomitans* (AA).

Unlabeled Use Crohn's disease

Labeled Contraindications Hypersensitivity to metronidazole, nitroimidazole derivatives, or any component of the formulation; pregnancy (first trimester)

Pregnancy Risk Factor B

Lactation Enters breast milk/not recommended (AAP rates "of concern"; AAP 2001 update pending)

Warnings/Precautions Use with caution in patients with severe liver impairment due to potential accumulation, blood dyscrasias; history of seizures, CHF or other sodium-retaining states; reduce dosage in patients with severe liver impairment, CNS disease, and consider dosage reduction in longer-term therapy with severe renal failure (Cl_{cr} <10 mL/minute); if *H. pylori* is not eradicated in patients being treated with metronidazole in a regimen, it should be assumed that metronidazole-resistance has occurred and it should not again be used; aseptic meningitis, encephalopathy, seizures, and neuropathies have been reported especially with increased doses and chronic treatment; monitor and consider discontinuation of therapy if symptoms occur.

[U.S. Boxed Warning]: Possibly carcinogenic based on animal data. Prolonged use may result in fungal or bacterial superinfection, including *C. difficile*-associated diarrhea (CDAD) and pseudomembranous colitis; CDAD has been observed >2 months postantibiotic treatment. The Infectious Disease Society of America (IDSA) recommends the use of oral metronidazole for initial treatment of mild-to-moderate *C. difficile* infection and the use of oral vancomycin for initial treatment of severe *C. difficile* infection with or without I.V. metronidazole depending on the presence of complications. May treat recurrent mild-to-moderate infection once with oral metronidazole; avoid use beyond first reoccurrence due to potential cumulative neurotoxicity (Cohen, 2010). Candidiasis infection (known or unknown) maybe more prominent during metronidazole treatment, antifungal treatment required. Disulfiram-like reactions to ethanol have been reported with oral metronidazole; avoid alcoholic beverages during therapy

Ethanol/Nutrition/Herb Interactions

Ethanol: The manufacturer recommends to avoid all ethanol or any ethanol-containing drugs (may cause disulfiram-like reaction characterized by flushing, headache, nausea, vomiting, sweating, or tachycardia).

Food: Peak antibiotic serum concentration lowered and delayed, but total drug absorbed not affected.

Storage/Stability

Injection: Store at controlled room temperature of 15°C to 30°C (59°F to 8F°C). Protect from light. Keep in overwrap until ready to use. Product may be refrigerated but crystals may form. Crystals redissolve on warming to room temperature. Prolonged exposure to light will cause a darkening of the product. However, short-term exposure to normal room light does not adversely affect metronidazole stability. Direct sunlight should be avoided. Stability of parenteral admixture at room temperature (25°C); Out of overwrap stability: 30 days.

Tablets: Store at room temperature. Protect from light and moisture.

Reconstitution Standard diluent: 500 mg/100 mL NS.

Mechanism of Action After diffusing into the organism, interacts with DNA to cause a loss of helical DNA structure and strand breakage resulting in inhibition of protein synthesis and cell death in susceptible organisms

Pharmacodynamics/Kinetics

Absorption: Oral: Well absorbed

Distribution: To saliva, bile, seminal fluid, bone, liver, and liver abscesses, lung and vaginal secretions; crosses blood-brain barrier

CSF:blood level ratio: Normal meninges: 16% to 43%; Inflamed meninges: 100%

Protein binding: <20%

Metabolism: Hepatic (30% to 60%)

Half-life elimination: Neonates: 25-75 hours; Others: 6-8 hours, prolonged with hepatic impairment; End-stage renal disease: 21 hours

Time to peak, serum: Oral: Immediate release: 1-2 hours

Excretion: Urine (60% to 80% as unchanged drug); feces (6% to 15%)

Dosing

Adult

Anaerobic infections (diverticulitis, intra-abdominal, peritonitis, cholangitis, or abscess): Oral, I.V.: 500 mg every 6-8 hours, not to exceed 4 g/day; **Note:** Initial: 1 g I.V. loading dose may be administered

Amebiasis: Oral: 500-750 mg every 8 hours for 5-10 days

Antibiotic-associated pseudomembranous colitis: IDSA Guidelines (Cohen, 2010):

Mild-to-moderate infection: Oral: 500 mg 3 times/day for 10-14 days

Severe complicated infection: I.V.: 500 mg 3 times/day with oral vancomycin (recommended agent) for 10-14 days

Note: Due to the emergence of a new strain of *C. difficile*, some clinicians recommend converting to oral vancomycin therapy if the patient does not show a clear clinical response after 2 days of metronidazole therapy.

Giardiasis: 500 mg twice daily for 5-7 days

Intra-abdominal infection, complicated, community-acquired, mild-to-moderate (in combination with cephalosporin or fluoroquinolone): I.V.: 500 mg every 8-12 hours **or** 1.5 g every 24 hours for for 4-7 days (provided source controlled)

Peptic ulcer disease: *Helicobacter pylori* eradication: Oral: 250-500 mg with meals and at bedtime for 14 days; requires combination therapy with at least one other antibiotic and an acid-suppressing agent (proton pump inhibitor or H_2 blocker)

Bacterial vaginosis or vaginitis due to *Gardnerella*, *Mobiluncus*: Oral: 500 mg twice daily (regular release) or 750 mg once daily (extended release tablet) for 7 days

Pelvic inflammatory disease (unlabeled use): Oral: 500 mg twice daily for 14 days (in combination with a cephalosporin and doxycycline) (CDC, 2010)

Periodontitis treatment (monotherapy or combination) associated with presence of *Actinobacillus actinomycetemcomitans* (AA): Oral: 250-500 mg every 8 hours for 8-10 days used in addition to scaling and root planing (Varela, 2011)

Trichomoniasis: Oral: 250 mg every 8 hours for 7 days **or** 375 mg twice daily for 7 days **or** 2 g as a single dose **or** 1 g twice daily for 2 doses (on same day)

Urethritis (unlabeled use): Oral: 2 g as a single dose with azithromycin (CDC, 2010)

Surgical prophylaxis (colorectal): I.V. 15 mg/kg 1 hour prior to surgery; followed by 7.5 mg/kg 6 and 12 hours after initial dose

Geriatric Refer to adult dosing. Use the lower end of the dosing recommendations for adults; do not administer as single dose as efficacy has not been established.

Pediatric Infants and Children:

Anaerobic infections:

Oral: 15-35 mg/kg/day in divided doses every 8 hours

I.V.: 30 mg/kg/day in divided doses every 6 hours

Colitis due to *Clostridium difficile*: Oral: 30 mg/kg/day divided every 6 hours for 7-10 days; maximum dose: 2 g/day

Amebiasis: Oral: 35-50 mg/kg/day in divided doses every 8 hours for 10 days

Trichomoniasis: Oral: 15-30 mg/kg/day in divided doses every 8 hours for 7 days

Renal Impairment Cl_{cr} <10 mL/minute (not on dialysis): Recommendations vary: To reduce possible accumulation in patients receiving multiple doses, consider reduction to 50% of dose or administer normal dose every 12 hours; **Note:** Dosage reduction is unnecessary in short courses of therapy. Some references do not recommend reduction at any level of renal impairment (Lamp, 1999).

Intermittent hemodialysis (IHD) (administer after hemodialysis on dialysis days): Dialyzable (50% to 100%): 500 mg every 8-12 hours. **Note:** Dosing regimen highly dependent on clinical indication (trichomoniasis vs *C. difficile* colitis) (Heintz, 2009). **Note:** Dosing dependent on the assumption of thrice weekly, complete IHD sessions.

Peritoneal dialysis (PD): Dose as for Cl_{cr} <10 mL/minute

Continuous renal replacement therapy (CRRT) (Heintz, 2009; Trotman, 2005): Drug clearance is highly dependent on the method of renal replacement, filter type, and flow rate. Appropriate dosing requires close monitoring of pharmacologic response, signs of adverse reactions due to drug accumulation, as well as drug concentrations in relation to target trough (if appropriate). The following are general recommendations only (based on dialysate flow/ultrafiltration rates of 1-2 L/hour and minimal residual renal function) and should not supersede clinical judgment:

CVVH/CVVHD/CVVHDF: 500 mg every 6-12 hours (or per clinical indication; dosage reduction generally not necessary)

Hepatic Impairment Unchanged in mild liver disease; reduce dosage in severe liver disease.

Administration

I.V.: Infuse intravenously over 30-60 minutes. Avoid contact of drug solution with equipment containing aluminum.

Oral: May be taken with food to minimize stomach upset. Extended release tablets should be taken on an empty stomach (1 hour before or 2 hours after meals).

Test Interactions May interfere with AST, ALT, triglycerides, glucose, and LDH testing

Dosage Forms Excipient information presented when available (limited, particularly for generics); consult specific product labeling.

Capsule, oral: 375 mg

Flagyl® 375: 375 mg

Infusion, premixed iso-osmotic sodium chloride solution: 500 mg (100 mL)

Tablet, oral: 250 mg, 500 mg

Flagyl®: 250 mg, 500 mg

Tablet, extended release, oral:

Flagyl® ER: 750 mg

◆ **Metronidazole Hydrochloride** *see* MetroNIDAZOLE (Systemic) *on page 978*

◆ **MET Tyrosine Kinase Inhibitor PF-02341066** *see* Crizotinib *on page 317*

◆ **Miacalcin®** *see* Calcitonin *on page 214*

◆ **Miacalcin® NS (Can)** *see* Calcitonin *on page 214*

Micafungin (mi ka FUN gin)

Brand Names: U.S. Mycamine®

Brand Names: Canada Mycamine®

Index Terms Micafungin Sodium

Generic Availability (U.S.) No

Pharmacologic Category Antifungal Agent, Parenteral; Echinocandin

Use Treatment of esophageal candidiasis; *Candida* prophylaxis in patients undergoing hematopoietic stem cell transplant (HSCT); treatment of candidemia, acute disseminated candidiasis, and other *Candida* infections (peritonitis and abscesses)

Unlabeled Use Treatment of infections due to *Aspergillus* spp; prophylaxis of HIV-related esophageal candidiasis

Labeled Contraindications Hypersensitivity to micafungin, other echinocandins, or any component of the formulation

Pregnancy Risk Factor C

Lactation Excretion in breast milk unknown/use caution

Warnings/Precautions Anaphylactic reactions, including shock, have been reported. New onset or worsening hepatic failure has been reported; use caution in pre-existing mild-moderate hepatic impairment; safety in severe liver failure has not been evaluated. Hemolytic anemia and hemoglobinuria have been reported. Increased BUN, serum creatinine, renal dysfunction, and/or acute renal failure has been reported; use with caution in patients with pre-existing renal impairment and monitor closely.

Storage/Stability Store at controlled room temperature of 25°C (77°F). Reconstituted and diluted solutions are stable for 24 hours at room temperature. Protect from light.

Reconstitution Aseptically add 5 mL of NS (preservative-free) to each 50 or 100 mg vial. Swirl to dissolve; do not shake. Further dilute 50-150 mg in 100 mL NS. Protect from light. Alternatively, D_5W may be used for reconstitution and dilution.

Mechanism of Action Concentration-dependent inhibition of 1,3-beta-D-glucan synthase resulting in reduced formation of 1,3-beta-D-glucan, an essential polysaccharide comprising 30% to 60% of *Candida* cell walls (absent in mammalian cells); decreased glucan content leads to osmotic instability and cellular lysis

Pharmacodynamics/Kinetics

Distribution: 0.28-0.5 L/kg

Protein binding: >99%; primarily to albumin

Metabolism: Hepatic; forms M-1 (catechol) and M-2 (methoxy) metabolites (activity unknown)

Half-life elimination: 11-21 hours

Excretion: Primarily feces (71%); urine (<15%)

Dosing

Adult & Geriatric

Candidemia, acute disseminated candidiasis, and *Candida* peritonitis and abscesses: I.V.: 100 mg daily; mean duration of therapy (from clinical trials) was 15 days (range: 10-47 days)

Esophageal candidiasis: I.V.: 150 mg daily; mean duration of therapy (from clinical trials) was 15 days (range: 10-30 days)

Prophylaxis of *Candida* infection in hematopoietic stem cell transplantation: 50 mg daily

Renal Impairment No dosage adjustment required in renal impairment.

Poorly dialyzed; no supplemental dose or dosage adjustment necessary, including patients on intermittent hemodialysis, peritoneal dialysis, or continuous renal replacement therapy (eg, CVVHD).

Hepatic Impairment No dosage adjustment required for hepatic impairment.

Administration For intravenous use only; infuse over 1 hour. Flush line with NS prior to administration.

Dosage Forms Excipient information presented when available (limited, particularly for generics); consult specific product labeling.

Injection, powder for reconstitution, as sodium:

Mycamine®: 50 mg, 100 mg [contains lactose 200 mg]

- **Micafungin Sodium** *see* Micafungin *on page* 981
- **MICRhoGAM® UF Plus** *see* Rh_o(D) Immune Globulin *on page* 1237
- **Mifeprex®** *see* Mifepristone *on page* 983

Mifepristone (mi FE pris tone)

Related Information

Safe Handling of Hazardous Drugs *on page* 1904

Brand Names: U.S. Korlym™; Mifeprex®

Index Terms RU-38486; RU-486

Generic Availability (U.S.) No

Pharmacologic Category Abortifacient; Antineoplastic Agent, Hormone Antagonist; Antiprogestin; Cortisol Receptor Blocker

Use

Korlym™: To control hyperglycemia occurring secondary to hypercortisolism in patients with endogenous Cushing's syndrome who have type 2 diabetes mellitus or glucose intolerance and who failed surgery or who are not surgical candidates

Mifeprex®: Medical termination of intrauterine pregnancy, through day 49 of pregnancy. Patients may need treatment with misoprostol and possibly surgery to complete therapy.

Unlabeled Use Treatment of unresectable meningioma; has been studied in the treatment of breast cancer and ovarian cancer; termination of pregnancy ≤63 days of pregnancy

Labeled Contraindications Hypersensitivity to mifepristone or any component of the formulation

Korlym™ (additional contraindications): Concomitant use of lovastatin, simvastatin, or CYP3A substrates with a narrow therapeutic range (eg, cyclosporine, dihydroergotamine, ergotamine, fentanyl, pimozide, quinine, sirolimus, tacrolimus); concomitant use of systemic corticosteroids for serious medical conditions (eg, immunosuppression following organ transplant); women with a history of unexplained vaginal bleeding, or endometrial hyperplasia with atypia or endometrial carcinoma; pregnancy

Mifeprex® (additional contraindications): Hypersensitivity to misoprostol; chronic adrenal failure; porphyrias; hemorrhagic disorder or concurrent anticoagulant therapy; pregnancy termination >49 days; intrauterine device (IUD) in place; ectopic pregnancy or undiagnosed adnexal mass; concurrent long-term corticosteroid therapy; inadequate or lack of access to emergency medical services; inability to understand effects and/or comply with treatment

Pregnancy Risk Factor X

Lactation Enters breast milk/not recommended

Warnings/Precautions Regardless of indication, endometrial proliferation is promoted by mifepristone resulting in endometrial thickening, cystic dilation of endometrial glands, and vaginal bleeding. **[U.S. Boxed Warning]:** When used for the termination of pregnancy, **patients should be counseled to seek medical attention in cases of excessive bleeding. Bleeding occurs and should be expected (average 9-16 days, may be ≥30 days). In some cases, bleeding may be prolonged and heavy and may be a sign of incomplete abortion or other complications,** potentially leading to hypovolemic shock; the manufacturer cites soaking through 2 thick sanitary pads per hour for 2 consecutive hours as an example of excessive bleeding. Bleeding may require blood transfusion (rare), curettage, saline infusions, and/or vasoconstrictors.

Patients should be instructed to seek medical attention if prolonged heavy vaginal bleeding occurs. When used for termination of pregnancy, use is contraindicated in women with hemorrhagic disorders or those using anti-coagulants; use caution in women with severe anemia, hypocoagulability or hemostatic disorders. When used for the treatment of hyperglycemia in patients with Cushing's syndrome, use caution in women with hemorrhagic disorders or women using anticoagulants and evaluate unexplained vaginal bleeding; use is contraindicated with a history of unexplained vaginal bleeding.

[U.S. Boxed Warning]: When used for the termination of pregnancy, **bacterial infections have been reported following use of this product and may have an atypical presentation. In rare cases, these infections may be serious and/or fatal,** with septic shock as a potential complication. A causal relationship has not been established. Sustained fever, abdominal pain, or pelvic tenderness should prompt evaluation; however, healthcare professionals are warned that atypical presentations of serious infection without these symptoms have also been noted. Patients presenting with nausea, vomiting, diarrhea, or weakness, with or without abdominal pain or fever, should be evaluated for serious bacterial infection when symptoms occur >24 hours after taking misoprostol. Treatment with antibiotics, including coverage for anaerobic bacteria (eg, *Clostridium sordellii*) should be initiated. Patients with Cushing's syndrome may be at risk for opportunistic infections such as *Pneumocystis jiroveci* pneumonia.

High potential for drug interactions exists when used for the treatment of hyperglycemia in patients with Cushing's syndrome. Refer to drug interactions for detailed information. The potential for drug interactions was not specifically studied following a single dose for the termination of pregnancy. May prolong the QT_c interval (dose related); use caution with other QT-prolonging agents. A large variability in exposure to mifepristone and its metabolites was observed at doses of 600 mg/day in patients with hepatic or renal impairment. Safety and efficacy have not been established for use in women with hepatic or impairment when used as a single dose for the termination of pregnancy; dose adjustment required when treating hyperglycemia in patients with Cushing's syndrome. Safety and efficacy have not been established for use in insulin-dependent diabetes mellitus.

Treatment of hyperglycemia in patients with Cushing's syndrome: [U.S. Boxed Warning]: Use of mifepristone will result in termination of pregnancy. Pregnancy must be excluded prior initiation of therapy. Non-hormonal contraception must be used during therapy and for 1 month after discontinuation of therapy unless the patient has had surgical sterilization. Pregnancy must be excluded if treatment is interrupted for ≥14 days. Adrenal insufficiency may occur. Serum cortisol concentrations remain elevated and may increase, and cannot be used for monitoring. If signs and symptoms of adrenal insufficiency occur (eg, fatigue, hypoglycemia, hypotension, nausea, weakness), discontinue mifepristone and administer glucocorticoids (high doses may be needed). Following resolution, treatment may be resumed at a lower dose; evaluate patient for precipitating causes (eg, infection, trauma). Hypokalemia ay occur at any time during therapy; correct hypokalemia prior to initiation of treatment. Use of mifepristone for the treatment of hyperglycemia in patients with Cushing's syndrome may antagonize the effects of steroids used for other conditions. Use is contraindicated when steroids are required for lifesaving indications. Because mifepristone does not reduce serum cortisol concentrations, mineralocorticoid receptors in cardiac tissue may be activated; use caution in patients with Cushing's syndrome who also have heart failure or coronary vascular disease.

Termination of pregnancy: [U.S. Boxed Warning]: Patients undergoing treatment with mifepristone should be instructed to bring their medication guide with them when an obtaining treatment from an emergency room or healthcare provider that did not prescribe the medication initially in order to identify that they are undergoing a medical abortion. Patient must be instructed of the treatment procedure and expected effects. A signed agreement form must be kept in the patient's file. Physicians may obtain patient agreement forms, physician enrollment forms, and medical consultation directly from Danco Laboratories at 1-877-432-7596. Prescriber should also give the patient clear instructions on whom to call and what to do in the event of an emergency following administration of therapy. Pregnancy is dated from day 1 of last menstrual period (presuming a 28-day cycle, ovulation occurring midcycle). Pregnancy duration can be determined using menstrual history and clinical examination. Ultrasound should be used if duration of pregnancy is uncertain. Confirmation of pregnancy termination by clinical exam or ultrasound must be made 14 days following treatment. Manufacturer recommends surgical termination of pregnancy when medical termination fails or is not complete. Prescriber should determine in advance whether they will provide such care themselves or through other providers. Preventative measures to prevent rhesus immunization must be taken prior to surgical abortion. Ultrasound should be used if an ectopic pregnancy is suspected or if duration of pregnancy is uncertain. Ultrasonography may not identify all ectopic pregnancies, and healthcare providers should be alert for signs and symptoms which may be related to undiagnosed ectopic pregnancy in any patient who receives mifepristone. Mifepristone is not effective in terminating ectopic pregnancies. To be administered only by physicians who can date pregnancy, diagnose ectopic pregnancies, provide access to surgical abortion (if needed), and can provide access to emergency care. Medication will be distributed directly to these physicians following signed agreement with the distributor. Must be administered under supervision by the qualified physician. Adverse effects (including blood transfusions, hospitalization, ongoing pregnancy, and other major complications) must be reported in writing to the medication distributor. Safety and efficacy have not been established for use in women with chronic cardiovascular disease, hypertension, or respiratory disease. Use with caution in patients who are heavy smokers (>10 cigarettes/day) or in women >35 years of age; these patients were excluded from clinical trials.

Adverse Reactions

Adverse events associated with treatment of hyperglycemia in patients with Cushing's syndrome:

>10%:

- Cardiovascular: Peripheral edema (26%), hypertension (24%)
- Central nervous system: Fatigue (48%), headache (44%), dizziness (22%), pain (14%)
- Endocrine & metabolic: Hypokalemia (34% to 44%), endometrial hypertrophy (38%), thyroid function tests abnormal (18%)
- Gastrointestinal: Nausea (48%), vomiting (26%), appetite decreased (20%), xerostomia (18%), diarrhea (12%)
- Genitourinary: Vaginal bleeding (14%)
- Neuromuscular & skeletal: Arthralgia (30%), back pain (16%), myalgia (14%), extremity pain (12%)
- Respiratory: Dyspnea (16%), sinusitis (14%), nasopharyngitis (12%)

5% to 10%:
- Cardiovascular: Edema, pitting edema
- Central nervous system: Anxiety (10%), somnolence (10%), insomnia, malaise
- Endocrine & metabolic: Hypoglycemia, triglycerides increased
- Gastrointestinal: Anorexia (10%), constipation (10%), abdominal pain, GI reflux
- Genitourinary: Vaginal hemorrhage, metrorrhagia
- Neuromuscular & skeletal: Flank pain, malaise, musculoskeletal chest pain, weakness
- Miscellaneous: Thirst

<5% or frequency not defined: Adrenal insufficiency (4%), pruritus (4%), rash (4%), HDL cholesterol decreased

Adverse events associated with treatment for termination of pregnancy:
Note: Vaginal bleeding and uterine cramping are expected to occur when this medication is used to terminate a pregnancy; ~90% of women using this medication for this purpose also report adverse reactions on day 3 after the procedure. Bleeding or spotting occurs in most women for a period of 9-16 days. Up to 8% of women will experience some degree of bleeding or spotting for 30 days or more. In some cases, bleeding may be prolonged and heavy, potentially leading to hypovolemic shock.

>10%:
- Central nervous system: Headache (2% to 31%), dizziness (1% to 12%)
- Gastrointestinal: Abdominal pain (cramping) (96%), nausea (43% to 61%), vomiting (18% to 26%), diarrhea (12% to 20%)
- Genitourinary: Uterine cramping (83%)

1% to 10%:
- Cardiovascular: Syncope (1%)
- Central nervous system: Fatigue (10%), fever (4%), insomnia (3%), anxiety (2%), fainting (2%)
- Gastrointestinal: Dyspepsia (3%)
- Genitourinary: Uterine hemorrhage (5%), vaginitis (3%), pelvic pain (2%), endometriosis/salpingitis/pelvic inflammatory disease (1%)
- Hematologic: Decreased hemoglobin >2 g/dL (6%), anemia (2%), leukorrhea (2%)
- Neuromuscular & skeletal: Back pain (9%), rigors (3%), leg pain (2%), weakness (2%)
- Respiratory: Sinusitis (2%)
- Miscellaneous: Viral infection (4%)

<1%: Significant ALT/AST, alkaline phosphatase, and GT changes have been reported rarely

Postmarketing and/or case reports: Adult respiratory distress syndrome (ADRS), allergic reaction including urticaria and hives, bacterial infection (including an ectopic bacteria such as *Clostridium sordellii*), Crohn's disease (exacerbation), disseminated intravascular coagulopathy (DIC), dyspnea, hematometra, hypotension, lightheadedness, loss of consciousness, MI, pancreatitis (acute), pelvic infection, postabortal infection, QT prolongation, ruptured ectopic pregnancy, sepsis, septic shock, sickle cell crisis (exacerbation), tachycardia, toxic shock syndrome

Unresectable meningioma trials: Most common adverse effects included breast tenderness or gynecomastia, fatigue, hair thinning, hot flashes, and rash. In premenopausal women, vaginal bleeding may be seen shortly after beginning therapy and cessation of menses is common. Thyroiditis and effects related to antiglucocorticoid activity have also been noted.

Drug Interactions

Metabolism/Transport Effects **Substrate** of CYP3A4 (major); **Note:** Assignment of Major/Minor substrate status based on clinically relevant drug interaction potential; **Inhibits** BCRP, CYP1A2 (weak), CYP2A6 (weak), CYP2B6 (weak), CYP2C19 (weak), CYP2C8 (weak), CYP2C9 (weak), CYP2D6 (weak), CYP2E1 (weak), CYP3A4 (weak), P-glycoprotein

Avoid Concomitant Use

Avoid concomitant use of Mifepristone with any of the following: Corticosteroids (Systemic); CycloSPORINE (Systemic); CYP3A4 Inducers (Strong); Dihydroergotamine; Ergotamine; FentaNYL; Highest Risk QTc-Prolonging Agents; Lovastatin; Moderate Risk QTc-Prolonging Agents; Pimozide; QuiNIDine; Simvastatin; Sirolimus; St Johns Wort; Tacrolimus (Systemic)

Increased Effect/Toxicity

Mifepristone may increase the levels/effects of: ARIPiprazole; BuPROPion; Contraceptives (Estrogens); Contraceptives (Progestins); Corticosteroids (Systemic); CycloSPORINE (Systemic); CYP2C8 Substrates; CYP2C9 Substrates; CYP3A4 Substrates; Digoxin; Dihydroergotamine; Efavirenz; Ergotamine; FentaNYL; Fluvastatin; Highest Risk QTc-Prolonging Agents; Lovastatin; Moderate Risk QTc-Prolonging Agents; Pimozide; QTc-Prolonging Agents (Indeterminate Risk and Risk Modifying); QuiNIDine; Simvastatin; Sirolimus; Tacrolimus (Systemic)

The levels/effects of Mifepristone may be increased by: CYP3A4 Inhibitors (Moderate); CYP3A4 Inhibitors (Strong); Dasatinib; Ivacaftor; Moderate Risk QTc-Prolonging Agents; QTc-Prolonging Agents (Indeterminate Risk and Risk Modifying)

Decreased Effect

Mifepristone may decrease the levels/effects of: Contraceptives (Estrogens); Contraceptives (Progestins); Corticosteroids (Systemic)

The levels/effects of Mifepristone may be decreased by: CYP3A4 Inducers (Strong); Deferasirox; St Johns Wort; Tocilizumab

Ethanol/Nutrition/Herb Interactions

Food: Grapefruit juice may inhibit mifepristone metabolism, leading to increased levels. Management: Do not take with grapefruit juice.

Herb/Nutraceutical: St John's wort may induce mifepristone metabolism, leading to decreased levels. Management: Avoid St John's wort.

Storage/Stability Store at room temperature of 25°C (77°F); excursions permitted to 15°C to 30°C (59°F to 86°F) .

Mechanism of Action Mifepristone is a synthetic steroid. At low doses, it competitively binds to the intracellular progesterone receptor, blocking the effects of progesterone. When used for the termination of pregnancy, this leads to contraction-inducing activity in the myometrium. In the absence of progesterone, mifepristone acts as a partial progesterone agonist. At high doses used for the treatment of hyperglycemia in patients with Cushing's syndrome, mifepristone blocks the effect of cortisol at the glucocorticoid receptor (antagonizes the effects of cortisol on glucose metabolism) while at the same time increasing circulating cortisol concentrations.

Pharmacodynamics/Kinetics

Absorption: Oral: rapid

Protein binding: 98% to albumin and α_1-acid glycoprotein

Metabolism: Hepatic via CYP3A4 to three metabolites (active)

Bioavailability: Oral: 69%

Half-life elimination: Single dose: Terminal: 18 hours following a slower phase where 50% eliminated between 12-72 hours; Multiple doses (600 mg/day): 85 hours

Time to peak: Oral: 90 minutes; Range: Single dose: 1-2 hours, Multiple doses: 1-4 hours

Excretion: Feces (83%); urine (9%)

Dosing

Adult

Hyperglycemia in patients with Cushing's syndrome (Korlym™): Oral: Initial dose: 300 mg once daily. Dose may be increased in 300 mg increments at intervals of ≥2-4 weeks based on tolerability and symptom control. Maximum dose: 1200 mg once daily, not to exceed 20 mg/kg/day. If treatment is interrupted, reinitiate at 300 mg/day or a dose lower than the dose that caused the treatment to be stopped if interruption due to adverse reactions

Dosage adjustment with concurrent use of strong CYP450 inhibitor therapy (eg, ketoconazole): Maximum dose 300 mg/day

Termination of pregnancy (Mifeprex®): Oral: Treatment consists of 3 office visits by the patient; the patient must read medication guide and sign patient agreement prior to treatment:

Day 1 (mifepristone administration): 600 mg (three 200 mg tablets) taken as a single dose under physician supervision

Day 3 (misoprostol administration): Patient must return to the healthcare provider 2 days following administration of mifepristone; unless abortion has occurred (confirmed using ultrasound or clinical examination): Misoprostol 400 mcg (two 200 mcg tablets); **Note:** Patient may need treatment for cramps or gastrointestinal symptoms at this time

Day 14 (post-treatment exam): Patient must return to the healthcare provider ~14 days after administration of mifepristone; confirm complete termination of pregnancy by ultrasound or clinical exam. Surgical termination is recommended to manage treatment failures.

Termination of pregnancy (unlabeled dosing): Mifepristone 200 mg orally followed by misoprostol 800 mcg vaginally 24-48 hours later (ACOG, 2005; FIGO, 2011).

Meningioma, unresectable (unlabeled use; refer to individual protocols): Oral: Mifepristone 200 mg/day, continue based on toxicity and response (Grunberg, 1991)

Geriatric Hyperglycemia in patients with Cushing's syndrome: Refer to adult dosing.

Renal Impairment

Hyperglycemia in patients with Cushing's syndrome: Maximum dose 600 mg/day; **Note:** Following doses of 1200 mg/day for 7 days in patients with severe renal impairment (Cl_{cr} <30 mL/minute), exposure to mifepristone and its metabolites was increased and a large variability in exposure was observed.

Termination of pregnancy: No dosage adjustment provided in manufacturer's labeling (has not been studied)

Hepatic Impairment

Hyperglycemia in patients with Cushing's syndrome:

Mild-to-moderate impairment: Maximum dose 600 mg/day

Severe impairment: Use is not recommended

Note: Following single and multiple doses of 600 mg/day in patients with moderate hepatic impairment (Child-Pugh class B), a large variability in exposure to mifepristone and its metabolites was observed.

Termination of pregnancy: No dosage adjustment provided in manufacturer's labeling (has not been studied); use with caution due to CYP3A4 metabolism.

Administration

Hyperglycemia in patients with Cushing's syndrome: Administer as a single daily dose with a meal. Tablets should be swallowed whole, not crushed, split, or chewed.

Termination of pregnancy: To be taken as a single dose under physician supervision

Monitoring Parameters

Treatment of hyperglycemia in patients with Cushing's syndrome: Signs and symptoms of adrenal insufficiency (serum cortisol concentrations will not be accurate); thyroid function; serum potassium (1-2 weeks after initiating dose or dose increase, then periodically thereafter); serum glucose and psychiatric symptoms (may show response to therapy within 6 weeks); cushingoid appearance (acne, hirsutism, striae, weight may take >2 months of therapy to show improvement); vaginal ultrasound in women (annually)

Termination of pregnancy: Clinical exam and/or ultrasound to confirm complete termination of pregnancy; hemoglobin, hematocrit, and red blood cell count in cases of heavy bleeding. Consider CBC in any patient who reports nausea, vomiting, or diarrhea and weakness with or without abdominal pain, and without fever or other signs of infection more than 24 hours after administration of misoprostol.

Test Interactions

hCG levels will not be useful to confirm pregnancy termination until at least 10 days following mifepristone treatment

When used for the treatment of hyperglycemia in patients with Cushing's syndrome, serum cortisol concentrations remain elevated and may increase, and cannot be used for monitoring.

Additional Information Mifeprex®: Medication will be distributed directly to qualified physicians following signed agreement with the distributor, Danco Laboratories. It will not be available through pharmacies. Major adverse reactions (hospitalization, blood transfusion, ongoing pregnancy, etc) should be reported to Danco Laboratories.

Prescribing and Access Restrictions

Korlym™ is only available through a restricted access program. For prescriber registration and patient enrollment forms, please refer to https://www.-korlymspark.com/login.aspx?ReturnUrl=%2fdefault.aspx or call 1-855-4Korlym (1 855 456-7596).

Mifeprex®: As a requirement of the REMS program, a medication guide must be given to the patient prior to receiving the medication. In addition, the manufacturer recommends distributing a patient agreement form which must be signed by the patient and prescriber confirming the patient's agreement to terminate her pregnancy. A signed copy of the patient agreement should be kept in the patient's medical record.

Mifeprex® is only available direct from Danco Laboratories' distributor. To obtain the product, please refer to, http://www.earlyoptionpill.com, or call 1-877-432-7596.

Investigators wishing to obtain the agent for use in oncology patients must apply for a patient-specific IND from the FDA.

Medication Guide Available Yes

Dosage Forms Excipient information presented when available (limited, particularly for generics); consult specific product labeling.

Tablet, oral:

Korlym™: 300 mg

Mifeprex®: 200 mg

References

ACOG, ACOG Practice Bulletin, Clinical Management Guidelines of Obstetrician-Gynecologists, Number 67, October 2005, "Medical Management of Abortion," *Obstet Gynecol*, 2005, 106 (4):871-82.

FIGO Working Group on Prevention of Unsafe Abortion and its Consequences, "The Combination of Mifepristone and Misoprostol for the Termination of Pregnancy," *Int J Gynaecol Obstet*, 2011, 115(1):1-4.

Grunberg SM, Weiss MH, Spitz IM, et al, "Treatment of Unresectable Meningiomas With the Antiprogesterone Agent Mifepristone," *J Neurosurg*, 1991, 74(6):861-6.

Perrault D, Eisenhauer EA, Pritchard KI, et al, "Phase II Study of the Progesterone Antagonist Mifepristone in Patients With Untreated Metastatic Breast Carcinoma: A National Cancer Institute of Canada Clinical Trials Group Study," *J Clin Oncol*, 1996, 14(10):2709-12.

Rocereto TF, Saul HM, Aikins JA, et al, "Phase II Study of Mifepristone (RU486) in Refractory Ovarian Cancer," *Gynecol Oncol*, 2000, 77(3):429-32.

Spitz IM and Bardin CW, "Mifepristone (RU486) - A Modulator of Progestin and Glucocorticoid Action," *N Engl J Med*, 1993, 329(6):404-12.

◆ **Millipred™** *see* PrednisoLONE (Systemic) *on page* *1193*

◆ **Millipred™ DP** *see* PrednisoLONE (Systemic) *on page* *1193*

◆ **Minirin® (Can)** *see* Desmopressin *on page* *434*

◆ **Mint-Ciprofloxacin (Can)** *see* Ciprofloxacin (Systemic) *on page* *283*

◆ **Mint-Ondansetron (Can)** *see* Ondansetron *on page* *1068*

◆ **MITC** *see* MitoMYcin (Systemic) *on page* *990*

◆ **MITO** *see* MitoMYcin (Systemic) *on page* *990*

◆ **MITO-C** *see* MitoMYcin (Systemic) *on page* *990*

◆ **Mitomycin-X** *see* MitoMYcin (Systemic) *on page* *990*

◆ **Mitomycin-C** *see* MitoMYcin (Systemic) *on page* *990*

MitoMYcin (Systemic) (mye toe MYE sin)

Related Information

Management of Chemotherapy-Induced Nausea and Vomiting *on page* *1786*

Management of Drug Extravasations *on page* *1800*

Oral Mucositis/Stomatitis *on page* *1814*

Safe Handling of Hazardous Drugs *on page* *1904*

Brand Names: Canada Mitomycin For Injection; Mitomycin For Injection USP; Mutamycin®

Index Terms MITC; MITO; MITO-C; Mitomycin-C; Mitomycin-X; MMC; MTC; Mutamycin

Generic Availability (U.S.) Yes

Pharmacologic Category Antineoplastic Agent, Antibiotic

Use Treatment of adenocarcinoma of stomach or pancreas

Unlabeled Use Treatment of anal carcinoma (nonmetastatic), bladder cancer, cervical cancer (recurrent or metastatic), esophageal cancer, gastric cancer, non small cell lung cancer (NSCLC)

Labeled Contraindications Hypersensitivity to mitomycin or any component of the formulation; thrombocytopenia; coagulation disorders, or other increased bleeding tendency

Lactation Excretion in breast milk unknown/not recommended

Warnings/Precautions Hazardous agent - use appropriate precautions for handling and disposal. **[U.S. Boxed Warning]: Bone marrow suppression (thrombocytopenia and leukopenia) is common and may be severe and/or contribute to infections.** Fatalities due to sepsis have been reported; monitor for infections. Myelosuppression is dose-limiting, delayed in onset, and cumulative; therefore, monitor blood counts closely during and for ≥8 weeks following treatment; treatment delay or dosage adjustment may be required for significant thrombocytopenia (platelets <100,000/mm^3) or leukopenia (WBC<4000/mm^3) or a progressive decline in either value. Use with caution in patients who have received radiation therapy or in the presence of hepatobiliary dysfunction; reduce dosage in patients who are receiving radiation therapy simultaneously. Monitor for renal toxicity; do not administer if serum creatinine is >1.7 mg/dL. **[U.S. Boxed Warning]: Hemolytic-uremic syndrome (HUS) has been reported (incidence not defined); condition usually involves microangiopathic hemolytic anemia (hematocrit ≤5%), thrombocytopenia (≤100,000/mm^3), and irreversible renal failure (serum creatinine ≥1.6 mg/dL). HUS may occur at any time, is generally associated with single doses ≥60 mg, and HUS symptoms may be exacerbated by blood transfusion.** Other less common effects may include pulmonary edema, neurologic abnormalities, and hypertension. High mortality from HUS development has been reported, and is largely the result of renal failure. HUS may also be associated with cumulative doses ≥50 mg/m^2. Bladder fibrosis/contraction has been reported with intravesical administration (unapproved administration route). **Mitomycin is a potent vesicant, may cause ulceration, necrosis, cellulitis, and tissue sloughing if infiltrated.**

Cases of acute respiratory distress syndrome (ARDS) have been reported in patients receiving mitomycin in combination with other chemotherapy who were maintained at FIO_2 concentrations >50% perioperatively; use caution to provide only enough oxygen to maintain adequate arterial saturation and avoid overhydration. Pulmonary toxicity has also been reported as dyspnea with nonproductive cough and appearance of pulmonary infiltrates on radiograph; discontinue therapy if pulmonary toxicity occurs and other potential etiologies have been ruled out. Shortness of breath and bronchospasm have been reported in patients receiving vinca alkaloids in combination with mitomycin or who received mitomycin previously; this acute respiratory distress has occurred within minutes to hours following the vinca alkaloid; may be managed with bronchodilators, steroids and/or oxygen. **[U.S. Boxed Warning]: Should be administered under the supervision of an experienced cancer chemotherapy physician.**

Adverse Reactions

>10%:

- Central nervous system: Fever (14%)
- Gastrointestinal: Nausea, vomiting and anorexia (14%)
- Hematologic: Myelosuppression (64%; onset: 4 weeks; recovery: 8-10 weeks)
- Miscellaneous: Thrombotic thrombocytopenic purpura (TTP)/hemolytic uremic syndrome (HUS) (≤15%)

1% to 10%:
- Dermatologic: Alopecia, mucous membrane toxicity (4%)
- Gastrointestinal: Stomatitis (4%)
- Renal: Serum creatinine increased (2%)

<1%, postmarketing, and/or case reports: Adult respiratory distress syndrome (ARDS), bladder fibrosis/contraction (intravesical administration), dyspnea, extravasation reactions, heart failure, hepatic sinusoidal obstruction syndrome (SOS, veno-occlusive liver disease), interstitial fibrosis, malaise, nonproductive cough, pulmonary infiltrates, rash, renal failure (irreversible), weakness

Drug Interactions

Metabolism/Transport Effects **Substrate** of P-glycoprotein

Avoid Concomitant Use

Avoid concomitant use of MitoMYcin (Systemic) with any of the following: BCG; CloZAPine; Natalizumab; Pimecrolimus; Tacrolimus (Topical); Vaccines (Live)

Increased Effect/Toxicity

MitoMYcin (Systemic) may increase the levels/effects of: CloZAPine; Leflunomide; Natalizumab; Vaccines (Live)

The levels/effects of MitoMYcin (Systemic) may be increased by: Antineoplastic Agents (Vinca Alkaloids); Denosumab; P-glycoprotein/ABCB1 Inhibitors; Pimecrolimus; Roflumilast; Tacrolimus (Topical); Trastuzumab

Decreased Effect

MitoMYcin (Systemic) may decrease the levels/effects of: BCG; Coccidioidin Skin Test; Sipuleucel-T; Vaccines (Inactivated); Vaccines (Live)

The levels/effects of MitoMYcin (Systemic) may be decreased by: Echinacea; P-glycoprotein/ABCB1 Inducers

Ethanol/Nutrition/Herb Interactions Herb/Nutraceutical: Avoid black cohosh, dong quai in estrogen-dependent tumors.

Storage/Stability Store intact vials at controlled room temperature; avoid exposure to temperatures >40°C (104°F). Reconstituted solution is stable for 7 days at room temperature and 14 days when refrigerated. Protect reconstituted solution from light. Solution of 0.5 mg/mL in a syringe is stable for 7 days at room temperature and 28 days when refrigerated and protected from light.

Further dilution to 20-40 mcg/mL:
- In normal saline: Stable for 12 hours at room temperature.
- In sodium lactate: Stable for 24 hours at room temperature.

Reconstitution Dilute powder with SWFI to a concentration of 0.5 mg/mL. May further dilute in NS or sodium lactate to 20-40 mcg/mL.

Mechanism of Action Acts like an alkylating agent and produces DNA cross-linking (primarily with guanine and cytosine pairs); cell-cycle nonspecific; inhibits DNA and RNA synthesis; degrades preformed DNA, causes nuclear lysis and formation of giant cells. While not phase-specific *per se*, mitomycin has its maximum effect against cells in late G and early S phases.

Pharmacodynamics/Kinetics

Metabolism: Hepatic

Half-life elimination: 17-78 minutes; Terminal: 50 minutes

Excretion: Urine (~10% as unchanged drug)

Dosing

Adult & Geriatric Details concerning dosing in combination regimens should also be consulted.

Stomach or pancreas adenocarcinoma (manufacturer's labeling): I.V.: 20 mg/m² every 6-8 weeks

Anal carcinoma (unlabeled use): I.V.: 10 mg/m² as an I.V. bolus on days 1 and 29 (maximum: 20 mg/dose) in combination with fluorouracil and radiation therapy (Ajani, 2008)

Bladder cancer, nonmuscle invasive (unlabeled use/route): Intravesicular instillation:

Low risk of recurrence (uncomplicated): 40 mg as a single dose post-operatively, retain in bladder for 2 hours (Hall, 2007)

Increased risk of recurrence: 20 mg weekly for 6 weeks, followed by 20 mg monthly for 3 years; retain in bladder for 1-2 hours (Friedrich, 2007)

Renal Impairment The manufacturer's labeling states to avoid use in patients with serum creatine >1.7 mg/dL, but no dosage adjustments are provided. The following adjustments have been used by some clinicians (Aronoff, 2007): Adults:

Cl_{cr} <10 mL/minute: Administer 75% of dose.

Continuous ambulatory peritoneal dialysis (CAPD): Administer 75% of dose.

Hepatic Impairment No dosage adjustment provided in manufacturer's labeling (has not been studied).

Adjustment for Toxicity

Leukocytes 2000 to <3000/mm³: Hold therapy until leukocyte count ≥4000/mm³; reduce to 70% of dose in subsequent cycles

Leukocytes <2000/mm³: Hold therapy until leukocyte count ≥4000/mm³; reduce to 50% of dose in subsequent cycles

Platelets 25,000 to <75,000/mm³: Hold therapy until platelets ≥100,000/mm³; reduce to 70% of dose in subsequent cycles

Platelets <25,000/mm³: Hold therapy until platelets ≥100,000 mm³; reduce to 50% of dose in subsequent cycles

Combination Regimens

Anal cancer: Fluorouracil-Mitomycin (Anal Cancer) on page 1659

Administration

I.V.: Administer slow I.V. push or by slow (15-30 minute) infusion via a freely-running saline infusion. Consider using a central venous catheter.

Intravesicular (unlabeled route): Instill into bladder and retain for up to 2 hours (Friedrich, 2007; Hall, 2007); rotate patient every 15-30 minutes

Emetic Potential Low (10% to 30%)

Vesicant/Extravasation Risk Vesicant; see Management of Drug Extravasations on page 1800.

Monitoring Parameters Monitor CBC with differential (repeatedly during therapy and for ≥8 weeks following therapy); serum creatinine; pulmonary function tests; monitor for signs/symptoms of HUS

Dosage Forms Excipient information presented when available (limited, particularly for generics); consult specific product labeling.

Injection, powder for reconstitution: 5 mg, 20 mg, 40 mg

References

Ajani JA, Winter KA, Gunderson LL, et al, "Fluorouracil, Mitomycin, and Radiotherapy vs Fluorouracil, Cisplatin, and Radiotherapy for Carcinoma of the Anal Canal: A Randomized Controlled Trial," *JAMA*, 2008, 299(16):1914-21.

Aronoff GR, Bennett WM, Berns JS, et al, *Drug Prescribing in Renal Failure: Dosing Guidelines for Adults and Children*, 5th ed. Philadelphia, PA: American College of Physicians; 2007, p 101.

Friedrich MG, Pichlmeier U, Schwaibold H, et al, "Long-Term Intravesical Adjuvant Chemotherapy Further Reduces Recurrence Rate Compared With Short-Term Intravesical Chemotherapy and Short-Term Therapy With Bacillus Calmette-Guérin (BCG) in Patients With Non-Muscle-Invasive Bladder Carcinoma," Eur Urol, 2007, 52(4):1123-29. PMID: 17383080

Hall MC, Chang SS, Dalbagni G, et al, "Guideline for the Management of Nonmuscle Invasive Bladder Cancer (stages Ta, T1, and Tis): 2007 Update," *J Urol*, 2007, 178(6):2314-30.
Rodriguez JA, Ferrari C, and Hernandez GA, "Intraoperative Application of Topical Mitomycin C 0.05% for Pterygium Surgery," *Bol Asoc Med P R*, 2004, 96(2):100-2.
Wilkins M, Indar A, and Wormald R, "Intra-Operative Mitomycin C for Glaucoma Surgery," *Cochrane Database Syst Rev*, 2001, (1):CD002897.

◆ **Mitomycin For Injection (Can)** *see* MitoMYcin (Systemic) *on page 990*
◆ **Mitomycin For Injection USP (Can)** *see* MitoMYcin (Systemic) *on page 990*

Mitotane (MYE toe tane)

Related Information
Safe Handling of Hazardous Drugs *on page 1904*

Brand Names: U.S. Lysodren®

Brand Names: Canada Lysodren®

Index Terms Chloditan; Chlodithane; Khloditan; Mytotan; o,p'-DDD; Ortho, para-DDD

Generic Availability (U.S.) No

Pharmacologic Category Antineoplastic Agent, Miscellaneous

Use Treatment of inoperable adrenocortical carcinoma

Unlabeled Use Treatment of Cushing's syndrome

Labeled Contraindications Hypersensitivity to mitotane or any component of the formulation

Pregnancy Risk Factor C

Lactation Excretion in breast milk unknown/not recommended

Warnings/Precautions Hazardous agent - use appropriate precautions for handling and disposal. Patients treated with mitotane may develop adrenal insufficiency; steroid replacement with glucocorticoid, and sometimes mineralocorticoid, is necessary. It has been recommended that steroid replacement therapy be initiated at the start of therapy, rather than waiting for evidence of adrenal insufficiency. **[U.S. Boxed Warning]: Because the primary action of mitotane is through adrenal suppression, discontinue mitotane temporarily with onset of shock or severe trauma; administer appropriate steroid coverage.** Because mitotane can increase the metabolism of exogenous steroids, higher than usual replacement steroid doses may be required. Surgically remove tumor tissues from metastatic masses prior to initiation of treatment; rapid cytotoxic effect may cause tumor hemorrhage. Observe patients for neurotoxicity with long-term (>2 years) use. Use caution with hepatic impairment; metabolism may be decreased. Other CNS adverse effects, including lethargy, sedation, and vertigo may occur; patients must be cautioned about performing tasks which require mental alertness (eg, operating machinery or driving). The manufacturer recommends initiating treatment within a hospital environment until a stabilized dose is achieved. Continue treatment as long as clinical benefit (maintenance of clinical status or metastatic lesion grown slowing) is observed. Clinical benefit is usually observed within 3 months at maximum tolerated dose, although 10% of patients may require more than 3 months for benefit. Continuous treatment at the maximum tolerated dose is generally the best approach. Some patients have been treated intermittently, restarting when severe symptoms reappear, although often response is no longer observed after 3 or 4 courses of intermittent treatment. **[U.S. Boxed Warnings]: Should be administered under the supervision of an experienced cancer chemotherapy physician.** Safety and efficacy in children have not been established.

Adverse Reactions The majority of adverse events are dose-dependent.

>10%:

Central nervous system: CNS depression (32%), lethargy/somnolence (25%), dizziness/vertigo (15%)

Dermatologic: Skin rash (15%)

Gastrointestinal: Anorexia (24%), nausea (39%), vomiting (37%), diarrhea (13%)

Neuromuscular & skeletal: Weakness (12%)

1% to 10%:

Central nervous system: Headache (5%), confusion (3%)

Neuromuscular & skeletal: Muscle tremor (3%)

<1%, postmarketing, and/or case reports: Aches (generalized), adrenal insufficiency, albuminuria, anemia, ataxia, autoimmune hepatitis, bleeding time prolonged, blurred vision, cataract, diplopia, flushing, GGT increased, gynecomastia, hematuria, hemorrhagic cystitis, hormone binding globulins increased, hypercholesterolemia, hyperpyrexia, hypertension, hypertriglyceridemia, lens opacity, leukopenia, macular edema, memory decreased, mucositis, myalgia, neuropathy, orthostatic hypotension, primary hypogonadism, protein bound iodine decreased, thrombocytopenia, thyroid function tests altered, toxic retinopathy, transaminases increased

Drug Interactions

Metabolism/Transport Effects None known.

Avoid Concomitant Use There are no known interactions where it is recommended to avoid concomitant use.

Increased Effect/Toxicity

Mitotane may increase the levels/effects of: Vitamin K Antagonists

The levels/effects of Mitotane may be increased by: MAO Inhibitors

Decreased Effect

Mitotane may decrease the levels/effects of: Corticosteroids (Systemic); Vitamin K Antagonists

The levels/effects of Mitotane may be decreased by: Spironolactone

Ethanol/Nutrition/Herb Interactions Ethanol: Avoid ethanol (may increase CNS depression).

Storage/Stability Store at room temperature of 25°C (77°F); excursions permitted to 15°C to 30°C (59°F to 86°F).

Mechanism of Action Adrenolytic agent which causes adrenal cortical atrophy; affects mitochondria in adrenal cortical cells and decreases production of cortisol; also alters the peripheral metabolism of steroids

Pharmacodynamics/Kinetics

Absorption: Oral: ~5% to 40%

Distribution: Stored mainly in fat tissue but is found in all body tissues

Metabolism: Hepatic and other tissues

Half-life elimination: 18-159 days

Time to peak, serum: 3-5 hours

Excretion: Urine (~10%, as metabolites); feces (1% to 17%, as metabolites)

Dosing

Adult & Geriatric

Adrenocortical carcinoma: Oral: Start at 2-6 g/day in 3-4 divided doses, then increase incrementally to 9-10 g/day in 3-4 divided doses (maximum tolerated range: 2-16 g/day, usually 9-10 g/day; maximum dose studied: 18-19 g/day)

Cushing's syndrome (unlabeled use): Oral: Initial dose: 500 mg 3 times/day; maximum dose: 3000 mg 3 times/day (Biller, 2008)

Pediatric Adrenocortical carcinoma (unlabeled use): Oral: 1-2 g/day in divided doses, increasing gradually to a maximum of 5-7 g/day

Hepatic Impairment Dose may need to be decreased in patients with liver disease.

Adjustment for Toxicity

Severe side effects: Reduce dose until achieve a maximum tolerated dose.

Significant neuropsychiatric adverse effects: Withhold treatment for at least 1 week and restart at a lower dose (Allolio, 2006).

Administration Oral: Administer in 3-4 divided doses/day. Do not crush tablets; wear gloves when handling; avoid exposure to crushed or broken tablets.

Monitoring Parameters Adrenal function; neurologic assessments (including behavioral) at regular intervals with chronic (>2 years) use

Dosage Forms Excipient information presented when available (limited, particularly for generics); consult specific product labeling.

Tablet, oral:

Lysodren®: 500 mg [scored]

References

Allolio B and Fassnacht M, "Clinical Review: Adrenocortical Carcinoma: Clinical Update," *J Clin Endocrinol Metab*, 2006, 91(6):2027-37.

Biller BM, Grossman AB, Stewart PM, et al, "Treatment of Adrenocorticotropin-Dependent Cushing's Syndrome: A Consensus Statement," *J Clin Endocrinol Metab*, 2008, 93(7):2454-62.

Boscaro M, Barzon L, Fallo F, et al, "Cushing's Syndrome," *Lancet*, 2001, 357(9258):783-91.

De Leon DD, Lange BJ, Walterhouse D, et al, "Long-Term (15 years) Outcome in an Infant with Metastatic Adrenocortical Carcinoma," *J Clin Endocrinol Metab*, 2002, 87(10):4452-6.

National Comprehensive Cancer Network® (NCCN) "Practice Guidelines in Oncology™: Neuroendocrine Tumors," Version 1.2008. Available at http://www.nccn.org/professionals/physician_gls/PDF/neuroendocrine.pdf

Newell-Price J, Bertagna X, Grossman AB, et al, "Cushing's Syndrome," *Lancet*, 2006, 367(9522):1605-17.

Rodriguez-Galindo C, Figueiredo BC, Zambetti GP, et al, "Biology, Clinical Characteristics, and Management of Adrenocortical Tumors in Children," *Pediatr Blood Cancer*, 2005, 45(3):265-73.

Terzolo M, Angeli A, Fassnacht M, et al, "Adjuvant Mitotane Treatment for Adrenal Carcinoma," *N Engl J Med*, 2007, 356(23): 2372-80.

MitoXANtrone (mye toe ZAN trone)

Related Information

Hematopoietic Stem Cell Transplantation *on page 1887*

Management of Chemotherapy-Induced Nausea and Vomiting *on page 1786*

Management of Drug Extravasations *on page 1800*

Safe Handling of Hazardous Drugs *on page 1904*

Brand Names: Canada Mitoxantrone Injection®

Index Terms CL-232315; DHAD; DHAQ; Dihydroxyanthracenedione; Dihydroxyanthracenedione Dihydrochloride; Mitoxantrone Dihydrochloride; Mitoxantrone HCl; Mitoxantrone Hydrochloride; Mitozantrone; Novantrone

Generic Availability (U.S.) Yes

Pharmacologic Category Antineoplastic Agent, Anthracenedione

Use Initial treatment of acute nonlymphocytic leukemias (ANLL [includes myelogenous, promyelocytic, monocytic and erythroid leukemias]); treatment of advanced hormone-refractory prostate cancer; secondary progressive or relapsing-remitting multiple sclerosis (MS)

Canadian labeling: Additional uses (not in U.S. labeling): Treatment of metastatic breast cancer, relapsed leukemia (adults), lymphoma, and hepatocellular carcinoma

Unlabeled Use Treatment of Hodgkin lymphoma (refractory), non-Hodgkin lymphomas (NHL), acute lymphocytic leukemia (ALL), relapsed acute myeloid leukemia (AML), breast cancer (metastatic), pediatric acute myelogenous leukemia (AML), pediatric acute promyelocytic leukemia (APL); part of a conditioning regimen for autologous hematopoietic stem cell transplantation (HSCT)

Labeled Contraindications Hypersensitivity to mitoxantrone or any component of the formulation

Canadian labeling: Additional contraindications (not in U.S. labeling): Prior hypersensitivity to anthracyclines; prior substantial anthracycline exposure and abnormal cardiac function prior to initiation of mitoxantrone therapy; presence of severe myelosuppression due to prior chemo- and/or radiotherapy; severe hepatic impairment; intrathecal administration

Pregnancy Risk Factor D

Lactation Enters breast milk/not recommended

Warnings/Precautions Hazardous agent - use appropriate precautions for handling and disposal.

[U.S. Boxed Warning]: Usually should not be administered if baseline neutrophil count <1500 cells/mm^3 (except for treatment of ANLL). Monitor blood counts and monitor for infection due to neutropenia. Treatment may lead to severe myelosuppression; unless the expected benefit outweighs the risk, use is generally not recommended in patients with pre-existing myelosuppression from prior chemotherapy.

[U.S. Boxed Warning]: May cause myocardial toxicity and potentially-fatal heart failure (HF); risk increases with cumulative dosing. Effects may occur during therapy or may be delayed (months or years after completion of therapy). Predisposing factors for mitoxantrone-induced cardiotoxicity include prior anthracycline or anthracenedione therapy, prior cardiovascular disease, concomitant use of cardiotoxic drugs, and mediastinal/pericardial irradiation, although may also occur in patients without risk factors. Prior to therapy initiation, evaluate all patients for cardiac-related signs/symptoms, including history, physical exam, and ECG; and evaluate baseline left ventricular ejection fraction (LVEF) with echocardiogram or multigated radionuclide angiography (MUGA) or MRI. Not recommended for use in MS patients when LVEF <50%, or baseline LVEF below the lower limit of normal (LLN). Evaluate for cardiac signs/symptoms (by history, physical exam, and ECG) and evaluate LVEF (using same method as baseline LVEF) in MS patients prior to each dose and if signs/symptoms of HF develop. Use in MS should be limited to a cumulative dose of ≤140 mg/m^2, and discontinued if LVEF falls below LLN or a significant decrease in LVEF is observed; decreases in LVEF and HF have been observed in patients with MS who have received cumulative doses <100 mg/m^2. Patients with MS should undergo annual LVEF evaluation following discontinuation of therapy to monitor for delayed cardiotoxicity.

[U.S. Boxed Warnings]: For I.V. administration only, into a free-flowing I.V.; may cause severe local tissue damage if extravasation occurs; do not administer subcutaneously, intramuscularly, or intra-arterially. Do not administer intrathecally; may cause serious and permanent neurologic damage. Extravasation resulting in burning, erythema, pain, swelling and skin discoloration (blue) has been reported; extravasation may result in tissue necrosis and require debridement for skin graft. May cause urine, saliva, tears, and sweat to turn blue-green for 24 hours postinfusion. Whites of eyes may have blue-green tinge. **[U.S. Boxed Warning]: Treatment with mitoxantrone increases the risk of developing secondary acute myelogenous leukemia (AML) in patients with cancer and in patients with MS;** acute promyelocytic leukemia (APL) has also been observed. Symptoms of acute leukemia include excessive bruising, bleeding and recurrent infections. The risk for secondary leukemia is increased in patients who are heavily pretreated, with higher doses, and with combination chemotherapy.

[U.S. Boxed Warning]: Should be administered under the supervision of a physician experienced in cancer chemotherapy agents. Dosage should be reduced in patients with impaired hepatobiliary function (clearance is reduced). Canadian labeling contraindicates use in severe hepatic impairment. Not for treatment of multiple sclerosis in patients with concurrent hepatic impairment. Not for treatment of primary progressive multiple sclerosis. Rapid lysis of tumor cells may lead to hyperuricemia.

Adverse Reactions Includes events reported with any indication; incidence varies based on treatment, dose, and/or concomitant medications

>10%:

Cardiovascular: Edema (10% to 30%), arrhythmia (3% to 18%), cardiac function changes (≤18%), ECG changes (≤11%)

Central nervous system: Fever (6% to 78%), pain (8% to 41%), fatigue (≤39%), headache (6% to 13%)

Dermatologic: Alopecia (20% to 61%), nail bed changes (≤11%), petechiae/bruising (6% to 11%)

Endocrine & metabolic: Menstrual disorder (26% to 61%), amenorrhea (28% to 53%), hyperglycemia (10% to 31%)

Gastrointestinal: Nausea (26% to 76%), vomiting (6% to 72%), diarrhea (14% to 47%), mucositis (10% to 29%; onset: ≤1 week), stomatitis (8% to 29%; onset: ≤1 week), anorexia (22% to 25%), weight gain/loss (13% to 17%), constipation (10% to 16%), GI bleeding (2% to 16%), abdominal pain (9% to 15%), dyspepsia (5% to 14%)

Genitourinary: Urinary tract infection (7% to 32%), abnormal urine (5% to 11%)

Hematologic: Neutropenia (79% to 100%; onset: ≤3 weeks; grade 4: 23% to 54%), leukopenia (9% to 100%), lymphopenia (72% to 95%), anemia/hemoglobin decreased (5% to 75%) thrombocytopenia (33% to 39%; grades 3/4: 3% to 4%), neutropenic fever (≤11%)

Hepatic: Alkaline phosphatase increased (≤37%), transaminases increased (5% to 20%), GGT increased (3% to 15%)

Neuromuscular & skeletal: Weakness (≤24%)

Renal: BUN increased (≤22%), creatinine increased (≤13%), hematuria (≤11%)

Respiratory: Upper respiratory tract infection (7% to 53%), pharyngitis (≤19%), dyspnea (6% to 18%), cough (5% to 13%)

Miscellaneous: Infection (4% to 60%), sepsis (ANLL 31% to 34%), fungal infection (9% to 15%)

1% to 10%:

Cardiovascular: CHF (≤5%), ischemia (≤5%), LVEF decreased (≤5%), hypertension (≤4%)

Central nervous system: Chills (≤5%), anxiety (5%), depression (5%), seizure (2% to 4%)

Dermatologic: Cutaneous mycosis (≤10%), skin infection (≤5%)

Endocrine & metabolic: Hypocalcemia (10%), hypokalemia (7% to 10%), hyponatremia (9%), menorrhagia (7%)

Gastrointestinal: Aphthosis (≤10%)

Genitourinary: Impotence (≤7%), sterility (≤5%)

Hematologic: Granulocytopenia (6%), hemorrhage (5% to 6%), secondary acute leukemias (≤3%; includes AML, APL)

Hepatic: Jaundice (3% to 7%)

Neuromuscular & skeletal: Back pain (6% to 8%), myalgia (≤5%), arthralgia (≤5%)

Ocular: Conjunctivitis (≤5%), blurred vision (≤3%)

Renal: Renal failure (≤8%), proteinuria (≤6%)

Respiratory: Rhinitis (10%), pneumonia (≤9%), sinusitis (≤6%)

Miscellaneous: Systemic infection (≤10%), diaphoresis (≤9%)

<1%, postmarketing, and/or case reports: Allergic reaction, anaphylactoid reactions, anaphylaxis, chest pain, dehydration; extravasation at injection site (may result in burning, erythema, pain, skin discoloration, swelling, or tissue necrosis); interstitial pneumonitis (with combination chemotherapy), hyperuricemia, hypotension, phlebitis at the infusion site, rash, sclera discoloration (blue), tachycardia, urine discoloration (blue-green), urticaria

Drug Interactions

Metabolism/Transport Effects Inhibits CYP3A4 (weak)

Avoid Concomitant Use

Avoid concomitant use of MitoXANtrone with any of the following: BCG; CloZAPine; Natalizumab; Pimecrolimus; Pimozide; Tacrolimus (Topical); Vaccines (Live)

Increased Effect/Toxicity

MitoXANtrone may increase the levels/effects of: ARIPiprazole; CloZAPine; Leflunomide; Natalizumab; Pimozide; Vaccines (Live)

The levels/effects of MitoXANtrone may be increased by: Denosumab; Pimecrolimus; Roflumilast; Tacrolimus (Topical); Trastuzumab

Decreased Effect

MitoXANtrone may decrease the levels/effects of: BCG; Coccidioidin Skin Test; Sipuleucel-T; Vaccines (Inactivated); Vaccines (Live)

The levels/effects of MitoXANtrone may be decreased by: Echinacea

Ethanol/Nutrition/Herb Interactions Herb/Nutraceutical: Avoid echinacea (may diminish the immunosuppressant effect).

Storage/Stability Store intact vials at 15°C to 25°C (59°F to 77°F); do not freeze. Opened vials may be stored at room temperature for 7 days or under refrigeration for up to 14 days. Solutions diluted for administration are stable for 7 days at room temperature or under refrigeration, although the manufacturer recommends immediate use.

Reconstitution Hazardous agent; use appropriate precautions for handling and disposal. Dilute in at least 50 mL of NS or D_5W.

Mechanism of Action Related to the anthracyclines, mitoxantrone intercalates into DNA resulting in cross-links and strand breaks; binds to nucleic acids and inhibits DNA and RNA synthesis by template disordering and steric obstruction; replication is decreased by binding to DNA topoisomerase II and seems to inhibit the incorporation of uridine into RNA and thymidine into DNA; active throughout entire cell cycle (cell-cycle nonspecific)

Pharmacodynamics/Kinetics

Absorption: Oral: Poor

Distribution: V_d: 14 L/kg; V_{dss}: >1000 L/m^2; distributes extensively into tissue (pleural fluid, kidney, thyroid, liver, heart) and red blood cells

Protein binding: 78%

Metabolism: Hepatic; pathway not determined

Half-life elimination: Terminal: 23-215 hours (median: ~75 hours); may be prolonged with hepatic impairment

Excretion: Feces (25%); urine (6% to 11%; 65% as unchanged drug)

Dosing

Adult & Geriatric Details concerning dosing in combination regimens should also be consulted.

U.S. labeling:

Acute nonlymphocytic leukemias (ANLL):

Acute myeloid leukemia (AML) induction: 12 mg/m^2 once daily for 3 days (in combination with cytarabine); for incomplete response, may repeat (7-10 days later) at 12 mg/m^2 once daily for 2 days (in combination with cytarabine) (Arlin, 1990)

AML consolidation (beginning ~6 weeks after initiation of the final induction course): 12 mg/m^2 once daily for 2 days (in combination with cytarabine), repeat in 4 weeks (Arlin, 1990)

Multiple sclerosis: 12 mg/m^2 every 3 months (maximum lifetime cumulative dose: 140 mg/m^2; discontinue use with LVEF <50% or clinically significant reduction in LVEF)

Prostate cancer (advanced, hormone-refractory): 12-14 mg/m^2 every 3 weeks (in combination with corticosteroids)

Canadian labeling:

Acute nonlymphocytic leukemias (ANLL):

AML induction: 10-12 mg/m^2 once daily for 3 days (in combination with cytarabine); for incomplete response, may repeat at 10-12 mg/m^2 once daily for 2 days (in combination with cytarabine)

AML consolidation (beginning ~6 weeks after initiation of the final induction course): 12 mg/m^2 once daily for 2 days (in combination with cytarabine), repeat in 4 weeks

Acute leukemias (relapsed): Induction: 12 mg/m^2 once daily for 5 consecutive days; may repeat once if needed (at the same dose and duration)

Breast cancer (metastatic), lymphoma: Initial: Single agent: 14 mg/m^2 every 21 days; reduce initial dose to ≤12 mg/m^2 for myelosuppression due to previous treatment or for poor general health. When used in combination with other agents, reduce initial dose to 10-12 mg/m^2.

Hepatocellular cancer: Initial: Single agent: 14 mg/m^2 every 21 days; reduce initial dose to ≤12 mg/m^2 for myelosuppression due to previous treatment or for poor general health

Adult unlabeled uses and/or dosing:

AML, refractory:

CLAG-M regimen: 10 mg/m^2 once daily for 3 days (in combination with cladribine, cytarabine, and filgrastim), may repeat once if needed (Wierzbowska, 2008)

MEC or EMA regimen: 6 mg/m^2 once daily for 6 days (in combination with cytarabine and etoposide) (Amadori, 1991)

Mitoxantrone/Etoposide: 10 mg/m^2 once daily for 5 days (in combination with etoposide) (Ho, 1988)

APL consolidation phase (second course): 10 mg/m^2 once daily for 5 days (Sanz, 2004)

Hodgkin lymphoma, refractory:

MINE-ESHAP regimen: 10 mg/m^2 on day 1 every 28 days for up to 2 cycles (MINE is combination with mesna, ifosfamide, mitoxantrone, and etoposide; MINE alternates with ESHAP for up to 2 cycles of each) (Fernandez, 2010)

VIM-D regimen: 10 mg/m^2 on day 1 every 28 days (in combination with etoposide, ifosfamide, mesna, and dexamethasone) (Phillips, 1990)

Non-Hodgkin lymphoma (as part of combination chemotherapy regimens):

CNOP regimen: 10 mg/m^2 every 21 days (Bessell, 2003)

FCMR regimen: 8 mg/m^2 every 28 days (Forstpointner, 2004)

FMR regimen: 10 mg/m^2 every 21 days (Zinzani, 2004)

FND regimen: 10 mg/m^2 every 28 days (Tsimberidou, 2002)

MINE-ESHAP regimen: 8 mg/m^2 every 21 days for 6 cycles (MINE is combination with mesna, ifosfamide, mitoxantrone, and etoposide; followed by ESHAP) (Rodriguez, 1995)

Stem cell transplantation, autologous: 60 mg/m^2 administered 4-5 days prior to autografting (as 3 divided doses over 1 hour each at 1-2 hour intervals on the same day; in combination with other chemotherapeutic agent[s]) (Oyan, 2006; Tarella, 2001)

Pediatric Details concerning dosing in combination regimens should also be consulted.

Acute nonlymphocytic leukemias: I.V.:

Acute myeloid leukemia (AML) consolidation phase (second course; unlabeled use): 10 mg/m^2 once daily for 5 days (in combination with cytarabine) (Stevens, 1998)

Acute promyelocytic leukemia (APL) consolidation phase (second course; unlabeled use): 10 mg/m^2 once daily for 5 days (Ortega, 2005; Sanz, 2004)

Renal Impairment Safety and efficacy have not been established.

Hemodialysis: Supplemental dose is not necessary

Peritoneal dialysis: Supplemental dose is not necessary

Elderly: Clearance is decreased in elderly patients; use with caution

Hepatic Impairment

U.S. labeling: No dosage adjustment provided in the manufacturer's labeling; however, clearance is reduced in hepatic dysfunction. Patients with severe hepatic dysfunction (bilirubin >3.4 mg/dL) have an AUC of 3 times greater than patients with normal hepatic function; consider dose adjustments. **Note:** MS patients with hepatic impairment should not receive mitoxantrone.

Canadian labeling:

Mild-to-moderate impairment: No specific dosage adjustment provided; consider dose adjustments and monitor closely.

Severe impairment: Use is contraindicated.

Adjustment for Toxicity

ANLL patients: Severe or life-threatening nonhematologic toxicity: Withhold treatment until toxicity resolves

MS patients:

Neutrophils <1500/mm^3: Use is not recommended.

Signs/symptoms of HF: Evaluate for cardiac signs/symptoms and LVEF.

LVEF <50% or baseline LVEF below the lower limit of normal (LLN): Use is not recommended.

Canadian labeling (not in U.S. labeling): **Hepatocellular cancer, lymphoma, or breast cancer (metastatic):**

WBC nadir >1500/mm^3 **and** platelet nadir >50,000/mm^3 and recovery ≤21 days: Repeat previous dose or increase dose by 2 mg/m^2 if myelosuppression is inadequate.

WBC nadir >1500/mm^3 **and** platelet nadir >50,000/mm^3 and recovery >21 days: Withhold treatment until recovery then resume at previous dose.

WBC nadir <1500/mm^3 **or** platelet nadir <50,000/mm^3 (regardless of recovery time): Withhold treatment until recovery then decrease previous dose by 2 mg/m^2.

WBC nadir <1000/mm^3 **or** platelet nadir <25,000/mm^3 (regardless of recovery time): Withhold treatment until recovery then decrease previous dose by 4 mg/m^2.

Combination Regimens

Leukemia, acute myeloid:
CLAG-M (AML Induction) on page 1586
5 + 2 (Cytarabine-Mitoxantrone) (AML Consolidation) on page 1512
7 + 3 (Cytarabine-Mitoxantrone) (AML Induction) on page 1514
MEC (AML Induction) on page 1706
MEC-G (AML Induction) on page 1707
Mitoxantrone-Etoposide (AML Induction) on page 1713
Leukemia, acute promyelocytic: Tretinoin-Idarubicin (APL) on page 1764
Lymphoma, Hodgkin:
MINE-ESHAP (Hodgkin) on page 1711
VIM-D (Hodgkin) on page 1770
Lymphoma, non-Hodgkin's:
CNOP on page 1589
Fludarabine-Cyclophosphamide-Mitoxantrone-Rituximab on page 1647
Fludarabine-Mitoxantrone on page 1649
Fludarabine-Mitoxantrone-Dexamethasone (NHL) on page 1650
Fludarabine-Mitoxantrone-Dexamethasone-Rituximab on page 1650
Fludarabine-Mitoxantrone-Rituximab on page 1651
MINE on page 1711
MINE-ESHAP (NHL) on page 1712
Prostate cancer:
Mitoxantrone + Hydrocortisone on page 1713
Mitoxantrone-Prednisone (Prostate Cancer) on page 1713

Administration Irritant (is considered a vesicant by some institutions). For I.V. administration only; do not administer intrathecally, subcutaneously, intramuscularly or intra-arterially. Must be diluted prior to use. Avoid extravasation; may cause severe local tissue damage if extravasation occurs. Usually administered as a short I.V. infusion over 5-15 minutes; do not infuse over <3-5 minutes.

High doses for bone marrow transplant (unlabeled use) are usually given as 3 divided doses over 1 hour each at 1-2 hour intervals on the same day (Oyan, 2006; Tarella, 2001).

Emetic Potential Low (10% to 30%)

Vesicant/Extravasation Risk Vesicant; see Management of Drug Extravasations on page 1800.

Monitoring Parameters CBC with differential, serum uric acid (for leukemia treatment), liver function tests; for the treatment of multiple sclerosis, obtain pregnancy test; monitor injection site for extravasation

Cardiac monitoring: Prior to initiation, evaluate all patients for cardiac-related signs/symptoms, including history, physical exam, and ECG; evaluate baseline and periodic left ventricular ejection fraction (LVEF) with echocardiogram or multigated radionuclide angiography (MUGA) or MRI. In patients with MS, evaluate for cardiac signs/symptoms (by history, physical exam, and ECG) and evaluate LVEF (using same method as baseline LVEF) prior to each dose and if signs/symptoms of HF develop. Patients with MS should undergo annual LVEF evaluation following discontinuation of therapy to monitor for delayed cardiotoxicity.

Medication Guide Available Yes

Dosage Forms Excipient information presented when available (limited, particularly for generics); consult specific product labeling.

Injection, solution [concentrate, preservative free]: 2 mg/mL (10 mL, 12.5 mL, 15 mL)

References

Amadori S, Arcese W, Isacchi G, et al, "Mitoxantrone, Etoposide, and Intermediate-Dose Cytarabine: An Effective and Tolerable Regimen for the Treatment of Refractory Acute Myeloid Leukemia," *J Clin Oncol*, 1991, 9(7):1210-4.

Arlin Z, Case DC Jr, Moore J, et al, "Randomized Multicenter Trial of Cytosine Arabinoside With Mitoxantrone or Daunorubicin in Previously Untreated Adult Patients With Acute Nonlymphocytic Leukemia (ANLL). Lederle Cooperative Group," *Leukemia*, 1990, 4(3):177-83.

Bessell EM, Burton A, Haynes AP, et al, "A Randomised Multicentre Trial of Modified CHOP Versus MCOP in Patients Aged 65 Years and Over With Aggressive Non-Hodgkin's Lymphoma, *Ann Oncol*, 2003, 14(2):258-67.

Fernandez de Larrea C, Martinez C, Gaya A, et al, "Salvage Chemotherapy With Alternating MINE-ESHAP Regimen in Relapsed or Refractory Hodgkin's Lymphoma Followed By Autologous Stem-Cell Transplantation," *Ann Oncol*, 2010, 21(6):1211-6.

Forstpointner R, Dreyling M, Repp R, et al, "The Addition of Rituximab to a Combination of Fludarabine, Cyclophosphamide, Mitoxantrone (FCM) Significantly Increases the Response Rate and Prolongs Survival as Compared With FCM Alone in Patients With Relapsed and Refractory Follicular and Mantle Cell Lymphomas: Results of a Prospective Randomized Study of the German Low-Grade Lymphoma Study Group," *Blood*, 2004, 104(10):3064-71.

Ho AD, Lipp T, Ehninger G, et al, "Combination of Mitoxantrone and Etoposide in Refractory Acute Myelogenous Leukemia an Active and Well-Tolerated Regimen," *J Clin Oncol*, 1988, 6(2):213-17.

Ortega JJ, Madero L, Martin G, et al, "Treatment With All-*Trans* Retinoic Acid and Anthracycline Monochemotherapy for Children With Acute Promyelocytic Leukemia: A Multicenter Study by the PETHEMA Group," *J Clin Oncol*, 2005, 23(30):7632-40.

Oyan B, Koc Y, Ozdemir E, et al, "High Dose Sequential Chemotherapy and Autologous Stem Cell Transplantation in Patients With Relapsed/Refractory Lymphoma," *Leuk Lymphoma*, 2006, 47(8):1545-52.

Petrylak DP, Tangen CM, Hussain MH, et al, "Docetaxel and Estramustine Compared With Mitoxantrone and Prednisone for Advanced Refractory Prostate Cancer," *N Engl J Med*, 2004, 351(15):1513-20.

Phillips JK, Spearing RL, Davies JM, et al, "VIM-D Salvage Chemotherapy in Hodgkin's Disease," *Cancer Chemother Pharmacol*, 1990, 27(2):161-3.

Rodriguez MA, Cabanillas FC, Velasquez W, et al, "Results of a Salvage Treatment Program for Relapsing Lymphoma: MINE Consolidated With ESHAP," *J Clin Oncol*, 1995, 13(7):1734-41.

Sanz MA, Martin G, Gonzalez M, et al, "Risk-Adapted Treatment of Acute Promyelocytic Leukemia With All-*Trans*-Retinoic Acid and Anthracycline Monochemotherapy: A Multicenter Study by the PETHEMA Group," *Blood*, 2004, 103(4):1237-43.

Scott LJ and Figgitt DP, "Mitoxantrone: A Review of its Use in Multiple Sclerosis," *CNS Drugs*, 2004, 18(6):379-96.

Stevens RF, Hann IM, Wheatley K, et al, "Marked Improvements in Outcome With Chemotherapy Alone in Paediatric Acute Myeloid Leukemia: Results of the United Kingdom Medical Research Council's 10th AML Trial: MRC Childhood Leukaemia Working Party," *Br J Haematol*, 1998, 101 (1):130-40.

Tannock IF, de Wit R, Berry WR, et al, "Docetaxel Plus Prednisone or Mitoxantrone Plus Prednisone for Advanced Prostate Cancer," *N Engl J Med*, 2004, 351(15):1502-12.

Tarella C, Zallio F, Caracciolo D, et al, "High-Dose Mitoxantrone + Melphalan (MITO/L-PAM) as Conditioning Regimen Supported by Peripheral Blood Progenitor Cell (PBPC) Autograft in 113 Lymphoma Patients: High Tolerability With Reversible Cardiotoxicity," *Leukemia*, 2001, 15 (2):256-63.

Tsimberidou AM, McLaughlin P, Younes A, et al, "Fludarabine, Mitoxantrone, Dexamethasone (FND) Compared With an Alternating Triple Therapy (ATT) Regimen in Patients With Stage IV Indolent Lymphoma," *Blood*, 2002, 100(13):4351-7.

Wierzbowska A, Robak T, Pluta A, et al, "Cladribine Combined With High Doses of Arabinoside Cytosine, Mitoxantrone, and G-CSF (CLAG-M) is a Highly Effective Salvage Regimen in Patients With Refractory and Relapsed Acute Myeloid Leukemia of the Poor Risk: A Final Report of the Polish Adult Leukemia Group," *Eur J Haematol*, 2008; 80(2):115-26.

Zinzani PL, Pulsoni A, Perrotti A, et al, "Fludarabine Plus Mitoxantrone With and Without Rituximab Versus CHOP With and Without Rituximab as Front-Line Treatment for Patients With Follicular Lymphoma," *J Clin Oncol*, 2004, 22(13):2654-61.

◆ **Mitoxantrone Dihydrochloride** *see* MitoXANtrone *on page 996*

◆ **Mitoxantrone HCl** *see* MitoXANtrone *on page 996*

◆ **Mitoxantrone Hydrochloride** *see* MitoXANtrone *on page 996*

◆ **Mitoxantrone Injection® (Can)** *see* MitoXANtrone *on page 996*

◆ **Mitozantrone** *see* MitoXANtrone *on page 996*

◆ **MK 0517** *see* Fosaprepitant *on page 643*

◆ **MK 869** *see* Aprepitant *on page 118*

◆ **MLN341** *see* Bortezomib *on page 187*

◆ **MMC** *see* MitoMYcin (Systemic) *on page 990*

◆ **MMF** *see* Mycophenolate *on page 1015*

◆ **MOAB 2C4** *see* Pertuzumab *on page 1165*

◆ **MOAB ABX-EGF** *see* Panitumumab *on page 1115*

◆ **MOAB C225** *see* Cetuximab *on page 264*

◆ **MoAb CD52** *see* Alemtuzumab *on page 43*

◆ **MOAB-CTLA-4** *see* Ipilimumab *on page 809*

◆ **MOAB HER2** *see* Trastuzumab *on page 1399*

◆ **Moi-Stir® [OTC]** *see* Saliva Substitute *on page 1266*

◆ **Monicure (Can)** *see* Fluconazole *on page 612*

◆ **Monoclate-P®** *see* Antihemophilic Factor (Human) *on page 101*

◆ **Monoclonal Antibody 2C4** *see* Pertuzumab *on page 1165*

◆ **Monoclonal Antibody 5G1.1** *see* Eculizumab *on page 490*

◆ **Monoclonal Antibody ABX-EGF** *see* Panitumumab *on page 1115*

◆ **Monoclonal Antibody Anti-C5** *see* Eculizumab *on page 490*

◆ **Monoclonal Antibody Campath-1H** *see* Alemtuzumab *on page 43*

◆ **Monoclonal Antibody CD52** *see* Alemtuzumab *on page 43*

◆ **Mononine®** *see* Factor IX *on page 571*

Morphine (Systemic) (MOR feen)

Brand Names: U.S. Astramorph®/PF; AVINza®; Duramorph; Infumorph 200; Infumorph 500; Kadian®; MS Contin®; Oramorph® SR

Brand Names: Canada Doloral; Kadian®; M-Eslon®; M.O.S.-SR®; M.O.S.-Sulfate®; M.O.S.® 10; M.O.S.® 20; M.O.S.® 30; Morphine Extra Forte Injection; Morphine Forte Injection; Morphine HP®; Morphine LP® Epidural; Morphine SR; Morphine-EPD; MS Contin SRT; MS Contin®; MS-IR®; Novo-Morphine SR; PMS-Morphine Sulfate SR; ratio-Morphine; ratio-Morphine SR; Sandoz-Morphine SR; Statex®; Teva-Morphine SR

Index Terms MS (error-prone abbreviation and should not be used); MSO_4 (error-prone abbreviation and should not be used); Roxanol

Generic Availability (U.S.) Yes. Excludes controlled release tablet, sustained release tablet

Pharmacologic Category Analgesic, Opioid

Use Relief of moderate-to-severe acute and chronic pain; relief of pain of myocardial infarction; relief of dyspnea of acute left ventricular failure and pulmonary edema; preanesthetic medication

Infumorph®: Used in continuous microinfusion devices for intrathecal or epidural administration in treatment of intractable chronic pain

Controlled, extended, or sustained release products: Only intended/indicated for use when repeated doses for an extended period of time are required. The 100 mg and 200 mg tablets or capsules of Kadian®, MS Contin®, and morphine sulfate controlled-release tablets and the 60 mg, 90 mg, and 120 mg capsules of Avinza® should only be used in opioid-tolerant patients.

Labeled Contraindications Note: Some contraindications are product specific. For details, please see detailed product prescribing information.

Hypersensitivity to morphine sulfate or any component of the formulation; severe respiratory depression (without resuscitative equipment); acute or severe asthma; known or suspected paralytic ileus; sustained release products are not recommended with gastrointestinal obstruction or in acute/postoperative pain. Oral solutions contraindicated in patients with heart failure due to chronic lung disease, cardiac arrhythmias, head injuries, brain tumors, acute alcoholism, deliriums tremens, seizure disorders. Injectable solution contraindicated during labor when a premature birth is anticipated. Some products contraindicated in patients with head injuries or increased intracranial pressure. MS Contin® and Kadian® contraindicated in patients with hypercarbia. Some immediate release formulations (tablets and solution) contraindicated in post biliary tract surgery, suspected surgical abdomen, surgical anastomosis, MAO inhibitor use (concurrent or within 14 days), general CNS depression.

Pregnancy Risk Factor C

Lactation Enters breast milk/use caution (AAP rates "compatible"; AAP 2001 update pending)

Warnings/Precautions An opioid-containing analgesic regimen should be tailored to each patient's needs and based upon the type of pain being treated (acute versus chronic), the route of administration, degree of tolerance for opioids (naive versus chronic user), age, weight, and medical condition. The optimal analgesic dose varies widely among patients. Doses should be titrated to pain relief/prevention. When used as an epidural injection, monitor for delayed sedation. **[U.S. Boxed Warning]: Healthcare provider should be alert to problems of abuse, misuse, and diversion.**

May cause respiratory depression; use with caution in patients (particularly elderly or debilitated) with impaired respiratory function, morbid obesity, adrenal insufficiency, prostatic hyperplasia, urinary stricture, renal impairment, or severe hepatic dysfunction and in patients with hypersensitivity reactions to other phenanthrene derivative opioid agonists (codeine, hydrocodone, hydromorphone, levorphanol, oxycodone, oxymorphone). Use with caution in patients with biliary tract dysfunction including acute pancreatitis. Use may cause constriction of sphincter of Oddi. Some preparations contain sulfites which may cause allergic reactions; infants <3 months of age are more susceptible to respiratory depression, use with caution and generally in reduced doses in this age group.

May cause CNS depression, which may impair physical or mental abilities; patients must be cautioned about performing tasks which require mental alertness (eg, operating machinery or driving). Effects may be potentiated when used with other sedative drugs or ethanol. May cause hypotension in patients with acute myocardial infarction, volume depletion, or concurrent drug therapy which may exaggerate vasodilation. Use with extreme caution in patients with head injury, intracranial lesions, or elevated intracranial pressure; exaggerated elevation of ICP may occur. May cause seizures if high doses are used; use with caution in patients with seizure disorders. Tolerance or drug dependence may result from extended use. Concurrent use of agonist/antagonist analgesics may precipitate withdrawal symptoms and/or reduced analgesic efficacy in patients following prolonged therapy with mu opioid agonists. Abrupt discontinuation following prolonged use may also lead to withdrawal symptoms. Elderly may be particularly susceptible to adverse effects of narcotics. May obscure diagnosis or clinical course of patients with acute abdominal conditions.

Extended or sustained-release formulations:

[U.S. Boxed Warning]: Extended or sustained release dosage forms should not be crushed or chewed. Controlled-, extended-, or sustained-release products are not intended for "as needed (PRN)" use. **MS Contin® 100 or 200 mg tablets and Kadian® 100 mg or 200 mg capsules are for use only in opioid-tolerant patients.** Avinza®, Kadian®, MS Contin®: **[U.S. Boxed Warning]: Indicated for the management of moderate-to-severe pain when around the clock pain control is needed for an extended time period.**

[U.S. Boxed Warning]: Avinza®: Do not administer with alcoholic beverages or ethanol-containing products, which may disrupt extended-release characteristic of product.

Highly concentrated oral solutions: [U.S. Boxed Warning]: Check doses carefully when using highly concentrated oral solutions.

Injections: Note: Products are designed for administration by specific routes (I.V., intrathecal, epidural). Use caution when prescribing, dispensing, or administering to use formulations only by intended route(s).

[U.S. Boxed Warning]: Duramorph®: Due to the risk of severe and/or sustained cardiopulmonary depressant effects of Duramorph® must be administered in a fully equipped and staffed environment. Naloxone injection should be immediately available. Patient should remain in this environment for at least 24 hours following the initial dose.

[U.S. Boxed Warning]: Intrathecal dosage is usually 1/10 that of epidural dosage.

Infumorph® solutions are **for use in microinfusion devices only**; not for I.V., I.M., or SubQ administration, or for single-dose administration.

When used as an epidural injection, monitor for delayed sedation.

Ethanol/Nutrition/Herb Interactions

Ethanol: Alcoholic beverages or ethanol-containing products may disrupt extended-release formulation resulting in rapid release of entire morphine dose. Ethanol may also increase CNS depression. Management: Avoid alcohol.

Food: Administration of oral morphine solution with food may increase bioavailability (ie, a report of 34% increase in morphine AUC when morphine oral solution followed a high-fat meal). The bioavailability of Avinza®, Oramorph SR®, or Kadian® does not appear to be affected by food. Management: Take consistently with or without meals.

Herb/Nutraceutical: Gotu kola, valerian, and kava kava may increase CNS depression. Management: Avoid gotu kola, valerian, and kava kava.

Storage/Stability

Capsule, sustained release (Avinza®, Kadian®): Store at 25°C (77°F); excursions permitted to 15°C to 30°C (59°F to 86°F). Protect from light and moisture.

Injection: Store at controlled room temperature of 20°C to 25°C (68°F to 77°F); do not freeze. Protect from light. Degradation depends on pH and presence of oxygen; relatively stable in pH ≤4; darkening of solutions indicate degradation.

Oral solution: Store at controlled room temperature of 25°C (68°F to 77°F); do not freeze.

Suppositories: Store at controlled room temperature 25°C (77°F). Protect from light.

Tablet, extended release: Store at controlled room temperature of 25°C (77°F).

Tablet, immediate release: Store at controlled room temperature of 25°C (77°F). Protect from moisture.

Reconstitution Injection: Usual concentration for continuous I.V. infusion: 0.1-1 mg/mL in D_5W.

Mechanism of Action Binds to opiate receptors in the CNS, causing inhibition of ascending pain pathways, altering the perception of and response to pain; produces generalized CNS depression

Pharmacodynamics/Kinetics

Onset of action (patient dependent; dosing must be individualized): Oral (Immediate release): ~30 minutes; I.V.: 5-10 minutes

Duration (patient dependent; dosing must be individualized): Pain relief:

Immediate release formulations: 4 hours

Extended release capsule and tablet: 8-24 hours (formulation dependent)

Absorption: Variable

Distribution: V_d: 3-4 L/kg; binds to opioid receptors in the CNS and periphery (eg, GI tract)

Protein binding: 30% to 35%

Metabolism: Hepatic via conjugation with glucuronic acid primarily to morphine-6-glucoronide (active analgesic) morphine-3-glucuronide (inactive as analgesic); minor metabolites include morphine-3-6-diglucuronide; other minor metabolites include normorphine (active) and morphine 3-ethereal sulfate

Bioavailability: Oral: 17% to 33% (first-pass effect limits oral bioavailability; oral:parenteral effectiveness reportedly varies from 1:6 in opioid naive patients to 1:3 with chronic use)

Half-life elimination: Adults: 2-4 hours (immediate release forms)

Time to peak, plasma: Avinza®: 30 minutes (maintained for 24 hours); Kadian®: ~10 hours; Oramorph® SR: ~4 hours

Excretion: Urine (primarily as morphine-3-glucuronide, ~2% to 12% excreted unchanged); feces (~7% to 10%). It has been suggested that accumulation of morphine-6-glucuronide might cause toxicity with renal insufficiency. All of the metabolites (ie, morphine-3-glucuronide, morphine-6-glucuronide, and normorphine) have been suggested as possible causes of neurotoxicity (eg, myoclonus).

Dosing

Adult These are guidelines and do not represent the doses that may be required in all patients. Doses and dosage intervals should be titrated to pain relief/prevention.

Acute pain (moderate-to-severe):

Oral (immediate release formulations): Opiate-naive: Initial: 10 mg every 4 hours as needed; patients with prior opiate exposure may require higher initial doses: usual dosage range: 10-30 mg every 4 hours as needed

I.M., SubQ: **Note:** Repeated SubQ administration causes local tissue irritation, pain, and induration.

Initial: Opiate-naive: 5-10 mg every 4 hours as needed; patients with prior opiate exposure may require higher initial doses; usual dosage range: 5-20 mg every 4 hours as needed

Rectal: 10-20 mg every 3-4 hours

I.V.: Initial: Opiate-naive: 2.5-5 mg every 3-4 hours; patients with prior opiate exposure may require higher initial doses. **Note:** Repeated doses (up to every 5 minutes if needed) in small increments (eg, 1-4 mg) may be preferred to larger and less frequent doses.

Acute myocardial infarction, analgesia (ACC/AHA 2004 Guidelines): Initial management: 2-4 mg, give 2-8 mg every 5-15 minutes as needed

Critically-ill patients (unlabeled dose): 0.7-10 mg (based on 70 kg patient) **or** 0.01-0.15 mg/kg every 1-2 hours as needed. **Note:** More frequent dosing may be needed (eg, mechanically-ventilated patients).

I.V., SubQ continuous infusion: 0.8-10 mg/hour; usual range: Up to 80 mg/hour

Continuous infusion: Usual dosage range: 5-35 mg/hour (based on 70 kg patient) **or** 0.07-0.5 mg/kg/hour

Patient-controlled analgesia (PCA): (Opiate-naive: Consider lower end of dosing range):

Usual concentration: 1 mg/mL

Demand dose: Usual: 1 mg; range: 0.5-2.5 mg

Lockout interval: 5-10 minutes

Intrathecal (I.T.): **Note: Must be preservative-free.** Administer with extreme caution and in reduced dosage to geriatric or debilitated patients. I.T. dose is usually 1/10 that of epidural dosage.

Opioid-naive: 0.2-1 mg/dose (may provide adequate relief for up to 24 hours); repeat doses are **not** recommended. **Note:** The American Pain Society recommends 0.1-0.3 mg/dose; adjust dose for age, injection site, and patient's medical condition and degree of opioid tolerance.

Continuous microinfusion (Infumorph®): Initial: 0.2-1 mg/day

Opioid-tolerant: 1-10 mg/day

Continuous microinfusion (Infumorph®): Initial: 1-10 mg/day, titrate to effect; usual maximum is ~20 mg/day

Epidural: Pain management: **Note: Must be preservative-free.** Administer with extreme caution and in reduced dosage to geriatric or debilitated patients. Vigilant monitoring is particularly important in these patients.

Single-dose (Astromorph/PF™, Duramorph®): Initial: 5 mg, if pain relief not achieved in 1 hour, careful administration of 1-2 mg at intervals sufficient to assess effectiveness may be given; maximum: 10 mg/24 hours (single doses may provide adequate relief for up to 24 hours)

Infusion: Bolus dose: 1-6 mg; infusion rate: 0.1-0.2 mg/hour; maximum dose: 10 mg/24 hours.

Note: The American Pain Society recommends 1-6 mg/dose as a single dose or an infusion of 0.1-1 mg/hour; adjust dose for age, injection site, and patient's medical condition and degree of opioid tolerance.

Continuous microinfusion (Infumorph®):

Opioid-naive: Initial: 0.2-1 mg/day

Opioid-tolerant: Initial: 1-10 mg/day, titrate to effect; usual maximum is ~20 mg/day

Chronic pain: Note: Patients taking opioids chronically may become tolerant and require doses higher than the usual dosage range to maintain the desired effect. Tolerance can be managed by appropriate dose titration. There is no optimal or maximal dose for morphine in chronic pain. The appropriate dose is one that relieves pain throughout its dosing interval without causing unmanageable side effects.

Oral: Controlled-, extended-, or sustained-release formulations: A patient's morphine requirement should be established using prompt-release formulations. Conversion to long-acting products may be considered when chronic, continuous treatment is required. Higher dosages should be reserved for use only in opioid-tolerant patients.

Capsules, extended release (Avinza®): Daily dose administered once daily (for best results, administer at same time each day)

Capsules, sustained release (Kadian®): Daily dose administered once daily or in 2 divided doses daily (every 12 hours)

Tablets, controlled release (MS Contin®), sustained release (Oramorph SR®), or extended release: Daily dose divided and administered every 8 or every 12 hours

Geriatric Refer to adult dosing. Use with caution; may require reduced dosage in the elderly and debilitated patients.

Pediatric These are guidelines and do not represent the doses that may be required in all patients. Doses and dosage intervals should be titrated to pain relief/prevention.

Acute pain (moderate-to-severe): Children >6 months and <50 kg:

Oral (prompt release): 0.15-0.2 mg/kg every 3-4 hours as needed

I.M., I.V.: 0.1-0.2 mg/kg every 3-4 hours as needed

I.V. infusion: Range: 10-60 mcg/kg/**hour**

Renal Impairment

Cl_{cr} 10-50 mL/minute: Children and Adults: Administer at 75% of normal dose

Cl_{cr} <10 mL/minute: Children and Adults: Administer at 50% of normal dose

Intermittent HD:

Children: Administer 50% of normal dose

Adults: No dosage adjustment necessary

Peritoneal dialysis: Children: Administer 50% of normal dose
CRRT: Children and Adults: Administer 75% of normal dose, titrate

Hepatic Impairment Unchanged in mild liver disease; substantial extrahepatic metabolism may occur. Excessive sedation may occur in cirrhosis.

Usual Infusion Concentrations: Pediatric I.V. infusion: 0.1 mg/mL, 0.5 mg/mL, **or** 1 mg/mL

Usual Infusion Concentrations: Adult I.V. infusion: 1 mg/mL

Administration

Oral: Do not crush controlled release drug product, swallow whole. Kadian® and Avinza® can be opened and sprinkled on applesauce; do not crush or chew the beads. Contents of Kadian® capsules may be opened and sprinkled over 10 mL water and flushed through prewetted 16F gastrostomy tube; do not administer Kadian® through nasogastric tube.

I.V.: When giving morphine I.V. push, it is best to first dilute with sterile water or NS for a final concentration of 1-2 mg/mL and then administer slowly.

Epidural: Use preservative-free solutions for intrathecal or epidural use.

Test Interactions Some quinolones may produce a false-positive urine screening result for opiates using commercially-available immunoassay kits. This has been demonstrated most consistently for levofloxacin and ofloxacin, but other quinolones have shown cross-reactivity in certain assay kits. Confirmation of positive opiate screens by more specific methods should be considered.

Medication Guide Available Yes

Dosage Forms Excipient information presented when available (limited, particularly for generics); consult specific product labeling.

Capsule, extended release, oral, as sulfate: 10 mg, 20 mg, 30 mg, 50 mg, 60 mg, 80 mg, 100 mg, 200 mg
AVINza®: 30 mg, 45 mg, 60 mg, 75 mg, 90 mg, 120 mg
Kadian®: 10 mg, 20 mg, 30 mg, 40 mg, 50 mg, 60 mg, 70 mg, 80 mg, 100 mg, 130 mg, 150 mg, 200 mg

Injection, solution, as sulfate: 1 mg/mL (10 mL); 2 mg/mL (1 mL); 4 mg/mL (1 mL); 5 mg/mL (1 mL); 8 mg/mL (1 mL); 10 mg/mL (1 mL, 10 mL); 10 mg/0.7 mL (0.7 mL); 15 mg/mL (1 mL, 20 mL); 25 mg/mL (4 mL, 10 mL); 50 mg/mL (20 mL, 50 mL)

Injection, solution, as sulfate [preservative free]: 0.5 mg/mL (10 mL); 1 mg/mL (10 mL); 25 mg/mL (10 mL)

Injection, solution, as sulfate [epidural or intrathecal infusion via microinfusion device, preservative free]:
Infumorph 200: 10 mg/mL (20 mL)
Infumorph 500: 25 mg/mL (20 mL)

Injection, solution, as sulfate [epidural, intrathecal, or I.V. infusion, preservative free]:
Astramorph®/PF: 0.5 mg/mL (2 mL, 10 mL); 1 mg/mL (2 mL, 10 mL)
Duramorph: 0.5 mg/mL (10 mL); 1 mg/mL (10 mL)

Injection, solution, as sulfate [for PCA pump]: 1 mg/mL (30 mL)

Injection, solution, as sulfate [for PCA pump, preservative free]: 1 mg/mL (30 mL); 5 mg/mL (30 mL)

Solution, oral, as sulfate: 10 mg/5 mL (5 mL, 100 mL, 500 mL); 20 mg/5 mL (100 mL, 500 mL)

Solution, oral, as sulfate [concentrate]: 100 mg/5 mL (15 mL, 30 mL, 120 mL, 240 mL)

Suppository, rectal, as sulfate: 5 mg (12s); 10 mg (12s); 20 mg (12s); 30 mg (12s)

Tablet, oral, as sulfate: 15 mg, 30 mg
Tablet, controlled release, oral, as sulfate:
MS Contin®: 15 mg, 30 mg, 60 mg, 100 mg, 200 mg
Tablet, extended release, oral, as sulfate: 15 mg, 30 mg, 60 mg, 100 mg, 200 mg
Tablet, sustained release, oral, as sulfate:
Oramorph® SR: 15 mg, 30 mg, 60 mg, 100 mg

Dosage Forms: Canada Excipient information presented when available (limited, particularly for generics); consult specific product labeling.
Solution, oral, as sulfate:
Doloral: 1 mg/mL (10 mL, 250 mL, 500 mL); 5 mg/mL (10 mL, 250 mL, 500 mL)

Controlled Substance C-II

Morphine (Liposomal) (MOR feen)

Brand Names: U.S. DepoDur®

Index Terms Extended Release Epidural Morphine; MS (error-prone abbreviation and should not be used); MSO_4 (error-prone abbreviation and should not be used)

Generic Availability (U.S.) No

Pharmacologic Category Analgesic, Opioid

Use Epidural (lumbar) single-dose management of surgical pain

Labeled Contraindications Hypersensitivity to morphine sulfate or any component of the formulation; severe respiratory depression (without resuscitative equipment); acute or severe asthma; known or suspected paralytic ileus; patients with head injuries or increased intracranial pressure; circulatory shock; upper airway obstruction. Not for use in vaginal labor and delivery.

Pregnancy Risk Factor C

Lactation Enters breast milk/use caution (AAP rates "compatible"; AAP 2001 update pending)

Warnings/Precautions

May cause respiratory depression. Risk increased in elderly patients, debilitated patients, and patients with conditions associated with hypoxia or hypercapnia. Prolonged, serious respiratory depression has been associated with nonapproved routes of administration (subarachnoid puncture and intrathecal). Although respiratory depression is reversible with naloxone, patients must be monitored for at least 48 hours due to the duration of action of the liposomal formulation and the potential for rebound sedation. Use with caution in patients with pre-existing respiratory compromise (hypoxia and/or hypercapnia), COPD or other obstructive pulmonary disease, and kyphoscoliosis or other skeletal disorder which may alter respiratory function.

May cause CNS depression and/or hypotension; use with caution in patients with hypovolemia, cardiovascular disease (including acute MI), circulatory shock, or drugs which may exaggerate hypotensive effects (including phenothiazines or general anesthetics). Use with caution in patients with CNS depression or coma. May cause orthostatic hypotension and syncope in ambulatory patients.

Use with caution in patients with hypersensitivity reactions to other phenanthrene derivative opioid agonists (codeine, hydrocodone, hydromorphone, levorphanol, oxycodone, oxymorphone). Use with caution in patients with biliary tract dysfunction including acute pancreatitis. Use may cause constriction of sphincter of Oddi diminishing biliary and pancreatic secretions. May obscure diagnosis or clinical course of patients with acute abdominal conditions. May worsen gastrointestinal ileus due to the effects on GI motility. Use with caution in patients with adrenal insufficiency, including Addison's disease. Use with caution in patients with severe hepatic impairment, renal impairment, prostatic hyperplasia, and/or urinary stricture. Use with caution in patients with seizure disorders or thyroid disease.

Use with caution in the elderly; may be more sensitive to adverse effects. Safety and efficacy have not been established in children <18 years of age.

For lumbar administration only. Monitor for delayed sedation. Physician should evaluate patient for contraindications for epidural injection (eg, anticoagulant therapy, bleeding, diathesis). Intrathecal administration has resulted in prolonged respiratory depression. Freezing may adversely affect modified-release mechanism of drug; check freeze indicator within carton prior to administration. To minimize the pharmacokinetic interaction resulting in higher peak serum concentrations of morphine, administer the test dose of the local anesthetic at least 15 minutes prior to administration. Use of DepoDur® with epidural local anesthetics has not been studied. Other medications should not be administered into the epidural space for at least 48 hours after administration.

Storage/Stability DepoDur®: Store under refrigeration at 2°C to 8°C (36°F to 46°F); keep vials in carton during refrigeration; do not freeze. Check freeze indicator before administration; do not administer if bulb is pink or purple. May store at room temperature for up to 30 days in sealed, unopened vials. Gently invert to suspend particles prior to removal from vial. Once vial is opened, use within 4 hours.

Reconstitution DepoDur® may be diluted in preservative-free NS to a volume of 5 mL.

Mechanism of Action Binds to opiate receptors in the CNS, causing inhibition of ascending pain pathways, altering the perception of and response to pain; produces generalized CNS depression

Pharmacodynamics/Kinetics

Duration (patient dependent; dosing must be individualized): >48 hours

Distribution: V_d: 3-4 L/kg; binds to opioid receptors in the CNS and periphery (eg, GI tract)

Protein binding: 30% to 35%

Metabolism: Hepatic via conjugation with glucuronic acid primarily to morphine-6-glucoronide (active analgesic) morphine-3-glucuronide (inactive as analgesic); minor metabolites include morphine-3-6-diglucuronide; other minor metabolites include normorphine (active) and morphine 3-ethereal sulfate

Excretion: Urine (primarily as morphine-3-glucuronide, ~2% to 12% excreted unchanged); feces (~7% to 10%). It has been suggested that accumulation of morphine-6-glucuronide might cause toxicity with renal insufficiency. All of the metabolites (ie, morphine-3-glucuronide, morphine-6-glucuronide, and normorphine) have been suggested as possible causes of neurotoxicity (eg, myoclonus).

Dosing

Adult Surgical anesthesia: Epidural: Single-dose (extended release, DepoDur®): Lumbar epidural only; not recommended in patients <18 years of age:

Cesarean section: 10 mg (after clamping umbilical cord)

Lower abdominal/pelvic surgery: 10-15 mg

Major orthopedic surgery of lower extremity: 15 mg; **Note:** Some patients may benefit from a 20 mg dose; however, the incidence of adverse effects may be increased.

To minimize the pharmacokinetic interaction resulting in higher peak serum concentrations of morphine, administer the test dose of the local anesthetic at least 15 minutes prior to administration. Use with epidural local anesthetics has not been studied. Other medications should not be administered into the epidural space for at least 48 hours after administration.

Geriatric Refer to adult dosing. Use with caution; may require reduced dosage in the elderly and debilitated patients.

Renal Impairment Dosing adjustment is not required.

Hepatic Impairment Dosing adjustment is not required.

Administration Epidural: Intended for lumbar administration only. Thoracic administration has not been studied. May be administered undiluted or diluted up to 5 mL total volume in preservative-free NS. Do not use an in-line filter during administration. Not for I.V., I.M., or intrathecal administration.

Resedation may occur following epidural administration; this may be delayed ≥48 hours in patients receiving extended-release injections.

Administration of an epidural test dose (lidocaine 1.5% and epinephrine 1:200,000) may affect the release of morphine from the liposomal preparation. Delaying the dose for an interval of at least 15 minutes following the test dose minimizes this pharmacokinetic interaction. Except for a test dose, other epidural local anesthetics or medications should not be administered epidurally before or after this product for a minimum of 48 hours.

Dosage Forms Excipient information presented when available (limited, particularly for generics); consult specific product labeling.

Injection, extended release liposomal suspension, as sulfate [lumbar epidural injection, preservative free]:

DepoDur®: 10 mg/mL (1 mL, 1.5 mL)

Controlled Substance C-II

◆ **Morphine-EPD (Can)** *see* Morphine (Systemic) *on page* *1004*

◆ **Morphine Extra Forte Injection (Can)** *see* Morphine (Systemic) *on page* *1004*

◆ **Morphine Forte Injection (Can)** *see* Morphine (Systemic) *on page* *1004*

◆ **Morphine HP® (Can)** *see* Morphine (Systemic) *on page* *1004*

◆ **Morphine LP® Epidural (Can)** *see* Morphine (Systemic) *on page* *1004*

◆ **Morphine SR (Can)** *see* Morphine (Systemic) *on page* *1004*

◆ **M.O.S.® 10 (Can)** *see* Morphine (Systemic) *on page* *1004*

◆ **M.O.S.® 20 (Can)** *see* Morphine (Systemic) *on page* *1004*

◆ **M.O.S.® 30 (Can)** *see* Morphine (Systemic) *on page* *1004*

◆ **M.O.S.-SR® (Can)** *see* Morphine (Systemic) *on page* *1004*

◆ **M.O.S.-Sulfate® (Can)** *see* Morphine (Systemic) *on page* *1004*

◆ **Mouth Kote® [OTC]** *see* Saliva Substitute *on page* *1266*

◆ **Mozobil™** *see* Plerixafor *on page* *1180*

◆ **MPA** *see* MedroxyPROGESTERone *on page* *916*

◆ **MPA** *see* Mycophenolate *on page* *1015*

◆ **6-MP (error-prone abbreviation)** *see* Mercaptopurine *on page* *934*

◆ **MS Contin®** *see* Morphine (Systemic) *on page* *1004*

- **MS Contin SRT (Can)** *see* Morphine (Systemic) *on page 1004*
- **MS (error-prone abbreviation and should not be used)** *see* Morphine (Liposomal) *on page 1011*
- **MS (error-prone abbreviation and should not be used)** *see* Morphine (Systemic) *on page 1004*
- **MS-IR® (Can)** *see* Morphine (Systemic) *on page 1004*
- **MSO_4 (error-prone abbreviation and should not be used)** *see* Morphine (Liposomal) *on page 1011*
- **MSO_4 (error-prone abbreviation and should not be used)** *see* Morphine (Systemic) *on page 1004*
- **MTC** *see* MitoMYcin (Systemic) *on page 990*
- **MTX (error-prone abbreviation)** *see* Methotrexate *on page 949*

Mucosal Barrier Gel, Oral (myoo KOH sul BAR ee er GEL, OR al)

Brand Names: U.S. Gelclair®

Index Terms Mucosal Bioadherent Gel

Pharmacologic Category Gastrointestinal Agent, Miscellaneous

Use Management of oral mucosal pain caused by oral mucositis/stomatitis (resulting from chemotherapy or radiation therapy), irritation due to oral surgery, traumatic ulcers caused by braces/ill-fitting dentures or disease, diffuse aphthous ulcers (canker sores)

Labeled Contraindications Hypersensitivity to any component of the formulation

Warnings/Precautions Patients should avoid eating or drinking for a minimum of 1 hour following treatment. Consult a physician if no improvement is seen after 7 days of use.

Adverse Reactions Postmarketing and/or case reports: Burning sensation in the mouth, mild inflammation and stinging of the oral cavity

Storage/Stability Store at room temperature away from direct sunlight. The gel may become thicker and darker over time; however, this has not been shown to affect its safety or efficacy.

Mechanism of Action Mechanical action for the management and relief of pain by adhering to the mucosal surface of mouth forming a protective film over the irritated areas and lesions

Dosing

Adult & Geriatric Mucosal protection: Oral: Gargle and spit the mixture of 1 single-use packet (15 mL) and water 3 times daily, or as needed. See Administration for specific dilution and administration instructions. May be used undiluted if water is unavailable.

Administration Pour the contents of a single-use packet (15 mL) into a glass and mix with 15 mL of water. May dilute with an additional 15-30 mL of water to achieve desired thickness. Stir well and use immediately. Mixture should be rinsed around the mouth for a minimum of 1 minute (as long as possible) to coat the tongue, palate, throat, inside of cheeks, and all oral tissue thoroughly. Mixture should be gargled and spit out. Accidental ingestion is not expected to cause adverse effects. The gel may become thicker and darker over time; however, this has not been shown to affect its safety or efficacy. Any packet that is not intact should not be used. **Note:** Studies have instructed patients to use 30-60 minutes prior to meals to gain maximum benefit (Barber, 2007; Hita-Iglesias, 2006)

Monitoring Parameters Consult a physician if improvement is not seen after 7 days of use.

Dosage Forms Excipient information presented when available (limited, particularly for generics); consult specific product labeling.

Gel, oral [concentrate]:

Gelclair®: 15 mL/packet (15s) [contains benzalkonium chloride, castor oil, propylene glycol, sodium benzoate]

References

Barber C, Powell R, Ellis A, et al, "Comparing Pain Control and Ability to Eat and Drink With Standard Therapy vs Gelclair: A Preliminary, Double Centre, Randomized Controlled Trial on Patients With Radiotherapy-Induced Oral Mucositis," *Support Care Cancer*, 2007, 15(4):427-40.

Hita-Iglesias P, Torres-Lagares D, and Gutiérrez-Pérez JL, "Evaluation of the Clinical Behavior of a Polyvinylpyrrolidone and Sodium Hyalonurate gel (Gelclair) in Patients Subjected to Surgical Treatment With CO2 Laser," *Int J Oral Maxillofac Surg*, 2006, 35(6):514-7.

◆ **Mucosal Bioadherent Gel** *see* Mucosal Barrier Gel, Oral *on page* 1014

◆ **Mustargen®** *see* Mechlorethamine *on page* 913

◆ **Mustine** *see* Mechlorethamine *on page* 913

◆ **Mutamycin** *see* MitoMYcin (Systemic) *on page* 990

◆ **Mutamycin® (Can)** *see* MitoMYcin (Systemic) *on page* 990

◆ **Mycamine®** *see* Micafungin *on page* 981

◆ **Mycelex** *see* Clotrimazole (Oral) *on page* 311

Mycophenolate (mye koe FEN oh late)

Related Information

Hematopoietic Stem Cell Transplantation *on page* 1887

Safe Handling of Hazardous Drugs *on page* 1904

Brand Names: U.S. CellCept®; Myfortic®

Brand Names: Canada Apo-Mycophenolate; CellCept®; CO Mycophenolate; JAMP-Mycophenolate; Myfortic®, Mylan-Mycophenolate; Novo-Mycophenolate; Sandoz-Mycophenolate; Sandoz-Mycophenolate Mofetil

Index Terms MMF; MPA; Mycophenolate Mofetil; Mycophenolate Sodium; Mycophenolic Acid

Generic Availability (U.S.) Yes: Capsule, tablet

Pharmacologic Category Immunosuppressant Agent

Use Prophylaxis of organ rejection concomitantly with cyclosporine and corticosteroids in patients receiving allogeneic renal (CellCept®, Myfortic®), cardiac (CellCept®), or hepatic (CellCept®) transplants

Unlabeled Use Treatment of rejection in liver transplant patients unable to tolerate tacrolimus or cyclosporine due to toxicity; treatment of recurrent or persistent rejection in heart transplant patients; treatment of moderate-severe psoriasis; treatment of lupus nephritis; treatment of myasthenia gravis; prevention of graft-versus-host disease (GVHD); treatment of refractory acute GVHD and chronic GVHD; treatment of refractory autoimmune hepatitis

Labeled Contraindications Hypersensitivity to mycophenolate mofetil, mycophenolic acid, mycophenolate sodium, or any component of the formulation

Cellcept®: Intravenous formulation is also contraindicated in patients who are allergic to polysorbate 80

Pregnancy Risk Factor D

Lactation Excretion in breast milk unknown/not recommended

Warnings/Precautions Hazardous agent - use appropriate precautions for handling and disposal. **[U.S. Boxed Warning]: Risk for infection and development of lymphoma and skin malignancy is increased.** Opportunistic infections, sepsis, and/or fatal infections may occur with immunosuppressive therapy. Patients should be monitored appropriately. Instruct patients to limit exposure to sunlight/UV light to decrease the risk of skin cancer and give supportive treatment should these conditions occur. Pure red cell aplasia (PRCA), progressive multifocal leukoencephalopathy (PML), or BK virus-associated nephropathy (BKVAN) may occur rarely, particularly in immunosuppressed patients or those receiving immunosuppressant therapy; monitor for signs of PRCA (anemia, fatigue, lethargy, pallor, dyspnea), PML (neurologic impairment, apathy, ataxia, cognitive deficiencies, confusion, and hemiparesis), or BKVAN (deterioration of renal function, renal graft loss); may require dosage reduction or discontinuation of therapy. Neutropenia (including severe neutropenia) may occur, requiring dose reduction or interruption of treatment (risk greater from day 31-180 post-transplant). Use may rarely be associated with gastric or duodenal ulcers, GI bleeding and/or perforation. Use caution in patients with active serious digestive system disease; patients with active peptic ulcers were not included in clinical studies. Use caution in renal impairment as toxicity may be increased; may require dosage adjustment in severe impairment.

[U.S. Boxed Warning]: Mycophenolate is associated with an increased risk of congenital malformations and first trimester pregnancy loss when used by pregnant women. Females of reproductive potential must be counseled about pregnancy prevention and planning. Alternative agents should be considered for women planning a pregnancy. Females of reproductive potential should have a negative pregnancy test with a sensitivity of ≥25 mIU/mL immediately before therapy and the test should be repeated 8-10 days later. Pregnancy tests should be repeated during routine follow-up visits. Acceptable forms of contraception should be used during treatment and for 6 weeks after therapy is discontinued. Females of childbearing potential should have a negative pregnancy test within 1 week prior to beginning therapy. Two reliable forms of contraception should be used beginning 4 weeks prior to, during, and for 6 weeks after therapy. Because mycophenolate mofetil has demonstrated teratogenic effects in rats and rabbits, tablets should not be crushed, and capsules should not be opened or crushed. Avoid inhalation or direct contact with skin or mucous membranes of the powder contained in the capsules and the powder for oral suspension. Caution should be exercised in the handling and preparation of solutions of intravenous mycophenolate. Avoid skin contact with the intravenous solution and reconstituted suspension. If such contact occurs, wash thoroughly with soap and water, rinse eyes with plain water.

Theoretically, use should be avoided in patients with the rare hereditary deficiency of hypoxanthine-guanine phosphoribosyltransferase (such as Lesch-Nyhan or Kelley-Seegmiller syndrome). Intravenous solutions should be given over at least 2 hours; never administer intravenous solution by rapid or bolus injection. **[U.S. Boxed Warning]: Should be administered under the supervision of a physician experienced in immunosuppressive therapy.**

Note: CellCept® and Myfortic® dosage forms should not be used interchangeably due to differences in absorption. Some dosage forms may contain phenylalanine. The intravenous formulation contains polysorbate 80.

Adverse Reactions Data for incidence >20% as reported in adults following oral dosing of CellCept® alone in renal, cardiac, and hepatic allograft rejection studies. Profile in 3% to <20% range reflects use in combination with cyclosporine and corticosteroids. In general, lower doses used in renal rejection patients had less adverse effects than higher doses. Rates of adverse effects were similar for each indication, except for those unique to the specific organ involved. The type of adverse effects observed in pediatric patients was similar to those seen in adults, with the exception of abdominal pain, anemia, diarrhea, fever, hypertension, infection, pharyngitis, respiratory tract infection, sepsis, and vomiting; lymphoproliferative disorder was the only type of malignancy observed. Percentages of adverse reactions were similar in studies comparing CellCept® to Myfortic® in patients following renal transplant.

>20%:

Cardiovascular: Hypertension (28% to 78%), hypotension (33%), peripheral edema (27% to 64%), edema (27% to 28%), chest pain (26%), tachycardia (20% to 22%)

Central nervous system: Pain (31% to 76%), headache (16% to 54%), insomnia (41% to 52%), fever (21% to 52%), dizziness (29%), anxiety (28%)

Dermatologic: Rash (22%)

Endocrine & metabolic: Hyperglycemia (44% to 47%), hypercholesterolemia (41%), hypomagnesemia (39%), hypokalemia (32% to 37%), hypocalcemia (30%), hyperkalemia (22%)

Gastrointestinal: Abdominal pain (25% to 63%), nausea (20% to 55%), diarrhea (31% to 51%), constipation (19% to 41%), vomiting (33% to 34%), anorexia (25%), dyspepsia (22%)

Genitourinary: Urinary tract infection (37%)

Hematologic: Leukopenia (23% to 46%), anemia (26% to 43%; hypochromic 25%), leukocytosis (22% to 41%), thrombocytopenia (24% to 38%)

Hepatic: Liver function tests abnormal (25%), ascites (24%)

Neuromuscular & skeletal: Back pain (35% to 47%), weakness (35% to 43%), tremor (24% to 34%), paresthesia (21%)

Renal: Creatinine increased (39%), BUN increased (35%), kidney function abnormal (22% to 26%)

Respiratory: Dyspnea (31% to 37%), respiratory tract infection (22% to 37%), pleural effusion (34%), cough (31%), lung disorder (22% to 30%), sinusitis (26%)

Miscellaneous: Infection (18% to 27%), sepsis (27%), lactate dehydrogenase increased (23%), *Candida* (17% to 22%), herpes simplex (10% to 21%)

3% to <20%:

Cardiovascular: Angina, arrhythmia, arterial thrombosis, atrial fibrillation, atrial flutter, bradycardia, cardiac arrest, cardiac failure, CHF, extrasystole, facial edema, hyper-/hypovolemia, orthostatic hypotension, pallor, palpitation, pericardial effusion, peripheral vascular disorder, supraventricular extrasystoles, supraventricular tachycardia, syncope, thrombosis, vasodilation, vasospasm, venous pressure increased, ventricular extrasystole, ventricular tachycardia

Central nervous system: Agitation, chills with fever, confusion, delirium, depression, emotional lability, hallucinations, hypoesthesia, malaise, nervousness, psychosis, seizure, somnolence, thinking abnormal, vertigo

Dermatologic: Acne, alopecia, bruising, cellulitis, fungal dermatitis, hirsutism, petechia, pruritus, skin carcinoma, skin hypertrophy, skin ulcer, vesiculobullous rash

Endocrine & metabolic: Acidosis, alkalosis, Cushing's syndrome, dehydration, diabetes mellitus, gout, hypercalcemia, hyper-hypophosphatemia, hyperlipemia, hyperuricemia, hypochloremia, hypoglycemia, hyponatremia, hypoproteinemia, hypothyroidism, parathyroid disorder

Gastrointestinal: Abdomen enlarged, dysphagia, esophagitis, flatulence, gastritis, gastroenteritis, gastrointestinal hemorrhage, gastrointestinal moniliasis, gingivitis, gum hyperplasia, ileus, melena, mouth ulceration, oral moniliasis, stomach disorder, stomach ulcer, stomatitis, xerostomia, weight gain/loss

Genitourinary: Impotence, nocturia, pelvic pain, prostatic disorder, scrotal edema, urinary frequency, urinary incontinence, urinary retention, urinary tract disorder

Hematologic: Coagulation disorder, hemorrhage, neutropenia, pancytopenia, polycythemia, prothrombin time increased, thromboplastin time increased

Hepatic: Alkaline phosphatase increased, bilirubinemia, cholangitis, cholestatic jaundice, GGT increased, hepatitis, jaundice, liver damage, transaminases increased

Local: Abscess

Neuromuscular & skeletal: Arthralgia, hypertonia, joint disorder, leg cramps, myalgia, myasthenia, neck pain, neuropathy, osteoporosis

Ocular: Amblyopia, cataract, conjunctivitis, eye hemorrhage, lacrimation disorder, vision abnormal

Otic: Deafness, ear disorder, ear pain, tinnitus

Renal: Albuminuria, creatinine increased, dysuria, hematuria, hydronephrosis, oliguria, pyelonephritis, renal failure, renal tubular necrosis

Respiratory: Apnea, asthma, atelectasis, bronchitis, epistaxis, hemoptysis, hiccup, hyperventilation, hypoxia, respiratory acidosis, pharyngitis, pneumonia, pneumothorax, pulmonary edema, pulmonary hypertension, respiratory moniliasis, rhinitis, sputum increased, voice alteration

Miscellaneous: *Candida* (mucocutaneous 16% to 18%), CMV viremia/syndrome (12% to 14%), CMV tissue invasive disease (6% to 12%), herpes zoster cutaneous disease (4% to 10%), cyst, diaphoresis, flu-like syndrome, healing abnormal, hernia, ileus infection, neoplasm, peritonitis, thirst

Postmarketing and/or case reports: Atypical mycobacterial infection, BK virus-associated nephropathy, colitis, gastrointestinal perforation, infectious endocarditis, interstitial lung disorder, intestinal villous atrophy, lymphoma, lymphoproliferative disease, malignancy, meningitis, pancreatitis, progressive multifocal leukoencephalopathy (sometimes fatal), pulmonary fibrosis (fatal), pure red cell aplasia, tuberculosis

Drug Interactions

Metabolism/Transport Effects None known.

Avoid Concomitant Use

Avoid concomitant use of Mycophenolate with any of the following: BCG; Cholestyramine Resin; Natalizumab; Pimecrolimus; Rifamycin Derivatives; Tacrolimus (Topical); Vaccines (Live)

Increased Effect/Toxicity

Mycophenolate may increase the levels/effects of: Acyclovir-Valacyclovir; Ganciclovir-Valganciclovir; Leflunomide; Natalizumab; Vaccines (Live)

The levels/effects of Mycophenolate may be increased by: Acyclovir-Valacyclovir; Belatacept; Denosumab; Ganciclovir-Valganciclovir; Pimecrolimus; Probenecid; Roflumilast; Tacrolimus (Topical); Trastuzumab

Decreased Effect

Mycophenolate may decrease the levels/effects of: BCG; Coccidioidin Skin Test; Contraceptives (Estrogens); Contraceptives (Progestins); Sipuleucel-T; Vaccines (Inactivated); Vaccines (Live)

The levels/effects of Mycophenolate may be decreased by: Antacids; Cholestyramine Resin; CycloSPORINE (Systemic); Echinacea; Magnesium Salts; MetroNIDAZOLE (Systemic); Penicillins; Proton Pump Inhibitors; Quinolone Antibiotics; Rifamycin Derivatives; Sevelamer

Ethanol/Nutrition/Herb Interactions

Food: Food decreases C_{max} of MPA by 40% following CellCept® administration and 33% following Myfortic® use; the extent of absorption is not changed. Management: Take CellCept® or Myfortic® on an empty stomach to decrease variability; however, Cellcept® may be taken with food if necessary in stable renal transplant patients.

Herb/Nutraceutical: Cat's claw and echinacea have immunostimulant properties. Management: Avoid cat's claw and echinacea.

Storage/Stability

Capsules: Store at 25°C (77°F); excursions permitted to 15°C to 30°C (59°F to 86°F).

Tablets: Store at 25°C (77°F); excursions permitted to 15°C to 30°C (59°F to 86°F). Protect from moisture and light.

Oral suspension: Store powder for oral suspension at 25°C (77°F); excursions permitted to 15°C to 30°C (59°F to 86°F). Once reconstituted, the oral solution may be stored at room temperature or under refrigeration. Do not freeze. The mixed suspension is stable for 60 days.

Injection: Store intact vials and diluted solutions at 25°C (77°F); excursions permitted to 15°C to 30°C (59°F to 86°F). Begin infusion within 4 hours of reconstitution.

Reconstitution Use appropriate precautions for handling and disposal (hazardous agent).

Oral suspension: Should be constituted prior to dispensing to the patient and **not** mixed with any other medication. Add 47 mL of water to the bottle and shake well for ~1 minute. Add another 47 mL of water to the bottle and shake well for an additional minute. Final concentration is 200 mg/mL of mycophenolate mofetil.

I.V.: Reconstitute the contents of each vial with 14 mL of 5% dextrose injection; dilute the contents of a vial with 5% dextrose in water to a final concentration of 6 mg mycophenolate mofetil per mL. **Note:** Vial is vacuum-sealed; if a lack of vacuum is noted during preparation, the vial should not be used.

Mechanism of Action MPA exhibits a cytostatic effect on T and B lymphocytes. It is an inhibitor of inosine monophosphate dehydrogenase (IMPDH) which inhibits *de novo* guanosine nucleotide synthesis. T and B lymphocytes are dependent on this pathway for proliferation.

Pharmacodynamics/Kinetics

Onset of action: Peak effect: Correlation of toxicity or efficacy is still being developed, however, one study indicated that 12-hour AUCs >40 mcg/mL/hour were correlated with efficacy and decreased episodes of rejection

Absorption: AUC values for MPA are lower in the early post-transplant period versus later (>3 months) post-transplant period. The extent of absorption in pediatrics is similar to that seen in adults, although there was wide variability reported.

Oral: Myfortic®: 93%

Distribution:
CellCept®: MPA: Oral: 4 L/kg; I.V.: 3.6 L/kg
Myfortic®: MPA: Oral: 54 L (at steady state); 112 L (elimination phase)
Protein binding: MPA: >97%, MPAG 82%
Metabolism: Hepatic and via GI tract; CellCept® is completely hydrolyzed in the liver to mycophenolic acid (MPA; active metabolite); enterohepatic recirculation of MPA may occur; MPA is glucuronidated to MPAG (inactive metabolite)
Bioavailability: Oral: CellCept®: 94%; Myfortic®: 72%
Half-life elimination:
CellCept®: MPA: Oral: 18 hours; I.V.: 17 hours
Myfortic®: MPA: Oral: 8-16 hours; MPAG: 13-17 hours
Time to peak, plasma: Oral: MPA:
CellCept®: 1-1.5 hours
Myfortic®: 1.5-2.75 hours
Excretion:
CellCept®: MPA: Urine (<1%), feces (6%); MPAG: Urine (87%)
Myfortic®: MPA: Urine (3%), feces; MPAG: Urine (>60%)

Dosing

Adult Note: May be used I.V. for up to 14 days; transition to oral therapy as soon as tolerated.

Renal transplant:

CellCept®:
Oral: 1 g twice daily. Doses >2 g daily are not recommended.
I.V.: 1 g twice daily
Myfortic®: Oral: 720 mg twice daily (1440 mg daily)

Cardiac transplantation: *CellCept®:*
Oral: 1.5 g twice daily
I.V.: 1.5 g twice daily

Hepatic transplantation: *CellCept®:*
Oral: 1.5 g twice daily
I.V.: 1 g twice daily

Autoimmune hepatitis, refractory (unlabeled use): *CellCept®:* Oral: 2 g daily (Manns, 2010)

Lupus nephritis (unlabeled use): CellCept®: Oral:
Induction: 1 g twice daily for 6 months in combination with a glucocorticoid (Ong, 2005) **or** 2-3 g daily for 6 months in combination with glucocorticoids (Hahn, 2012)
Maintenance: 0.5-3 g daily (Contreras, 2004) **or** 1 g twice daily (Dooley, 2011) **or** 1-2 g daily (Hahn, 2012)

Myasthenia gravis (unlabeled use): *CellCept®:* Oral: 1 g twice daily (range: 1-3 g daily) (Cahoon, 2006; Ciafaloni, 2001; Merriggioli, 2003)

Psoriasis, moderate-to-severe (unlabeled use): *CellCept®:* Oral: 2-3 g daily (Menter, 2009)

Geriatric Dosage is the same as younger patients, however, dosing should be cautious due to possibility of increased hepatic, renal, or cardiac dysfunction. Elderly patients may be at an increased risk of certain infections, gastrointestinal hemorrhage, and pulmonary edema, as compared to younger patients.

Pediatric

Renal transplant: Oral:
CellCept® suspension: 600 mg/m^2/dose twice daily; maximum dose: 1 g twice daily

Alternatively, may use solid dosage forms according to BSA as follows:
BSA 1.25-1.5 m^2: 750 mg capsule twice daily
BSA >1.5 m^2: 1 g capsule or tablet twice daily

Myfortic®: 400 mg/m^2/dose twice daily; maximum dose: 720 mg twice daily
BSA <1.19 m^2: Use of this formulation is not recommended
BSA 1.19-1.58 m^2: 540 mg twice daily (maximum: 1080 mg daily)
BSA >1.58 m^2: 720 mg twice daily (maximum: 1440 mg daily)

Renal Impairment

Renal transplant: GFR <25 mL/minute/1.73 m^2 in patients outside the immediate post-transplant period:

CellCept®: Doses of >1 g administered twice daily should be avoided; patients should also be carefully observed; no dose adjustments are needed in renal transplant patients experiencing delayed graft function postoperatively

Myfortic®: No dose adjustments are needed in renal transplant patients experiencing delayed graft function postoperatively; however, monitor carefully for potential concentration dependent adverse events

Cardiac or liver transplant: No data available; mycophenolate may be used in cardiac or hepatic transplant patients with severe chronic renal impairment if the potential benefit outweighs the potential risk.

Hemodialysis: Not removed; supplemental dose is not necessary.

Peritoneal dialysis: Supplemental dose is not necessary.

Hepatic Impairment No dosage adjustment is recommended for renal patients with severe hepatic parenchymal disease; however, it is not currently known whether dosage adjustments are necessary for hepatic disease with other etiologies.

Adjustment for Toxicity Neutropenia (ANC <1.3 x 10^3/μL): Dosing should be interrupted or the dose reduced, appropriate diagnostic tests performed and patients managed appropriately

Administration

Oral dosage formulations (tablet, capsule, suspension) should be administered on an empty stomach to avoid variability in MPA absorption. The oral solution may be administered via a nasogastric tube (minimum 8 French, 1.7 mm interior diameter); oral suspension should not be mixed with other medications. Delayed release tablets should not be crushed, cut, or chewed. Cellcept® may be administered with food in stable renal transplant patients when necessary.

Intravenous solutions should be administered over at least 2 hours (either peripheral or central vein); do **not** administer intravenous solution by rapid or bolus injection.

Extemporaneous Preparations Hazardous agent. Use appropriate precautions for handling and disposal.

A 50 mg/mL oral suspension may be made with mycophenolate mofetil capsules, Ora-Plus®, and cherry syrup. In a vertical flow hood, empty six 250 mg capsules into a mortar; add 7.5 mL Ora-Plus® and mix to a uniform paste. Mix while adding 15 mL of cherry syrup in incremental proportions; transfer to a calibrated bottle, rinse mortar with cherry syrup, and add sufficient quantity of cherry syrup to make 30 mL. Label "shake well". Stable for 210 days at 5°C, for 28 days at 25°C to 37°C, and for 11 days at 45°C.

Venkataramanan R, McCombs JR, Zuckerman S, et al, "Stability of Mycophenolate Mofetil as an Extemporaneous Suspension," *Ann Pharmacother*, 1998, 32(7-8):755-7.

Monitoring Parameters Complete blood count (weekly for first month, twice monthly during months 2 and 3, then monthly thereafter through the first year);

renal and liver function; signs and symptoms of infection; pregnancy test (immediately prior to initiation and 8-10 days later in females of childbearing potential, followed by repeat tests during therapy); monitor skin (for lesions suspicious of skin cancer); monitor for signs of lymphoma

Dietary Considerations Oral dosage formulations should be taken on an empty stomach to avoid variability in MPA absorption. However, in stable renal transplant patients, Cellcept® may be administered with food if necessary. Some products may contain phenylalanine.

Additional Information Females of reproductive potential are required to have contraceptive counseling and use acceptable birth control unless heterosexual intercourse is completely avoided. Use of an intrauterine device (IUD), tubal sterilization, or vasectomy of her partner are acceptable contraceptive methods that can be used alone. If a hormonal contraceptive is used (eg, combination oral contraceptive pills, transdermal patches, vaginal rings, or progestin only products), then one barrier method must also be used (eg, diaphragm or cervical cap with spermicide, contraceptive sponge, male or female condom). Alternatively, the use of two barrier methods is also acceptable (eg, diaphragm or cervical cap with spermicide, or contraceptive sponge **PLUS** male or female condom). Refer to manufacturer's labeling for full details.

Medication Guide Available Yes

Dosage Forms Excipient information presented when available (limited, particularly for generics); consult specific product labeling.

Capsule, oral, as mofetil: 250 mg
  CellCept®: 250 mg
Injection, powder for reconstitution, as mofetil hydrochloride:
  CellCept®: 500 mg [contains polysorbate 80]
Powder for suspension, oral, as mofetil:
  CellCept®: 200 mg/mL (175 mL) [contains phenylalanine 0.56 mg/mL, soybean lecithin; mixed fruit flavor]
Tablet, oral, as mofetil: 500 mg
  CellCept®: 500 mg [contains ethanol (may have trace amounts)]
Tablet, oral, as mycophenolic acid: 500 mg
Tablet, delayed release, oral, as mycophenolic acid:
  Myfortic®: 180 mg, 360 mg [formulated as a sodium salt]

References

Bertsias G, Ioannidis JP, Boletis J, et al, "EULAR Recommendations for the Management of Systemic Lupus Erythematosus. Report of a Task Force of the EULAR Standing Committee for International Clinical Studies Including Therapeutics," *Ann Rheum Dis*, 2008, 67(2):195-205.

Cahoon WD Jr and Kockler DR, "Mycophenolate Mofetil Treatment of Myasthenia Gravis," *Ann Pharmacother*, 2006, 40(2):295-8.

Ciafaloni E, Massey JM, Tucker-Lipscomb B, et al, "Mycophenolate Mofetil for Myasthenia Gravis: An Open-Label Pilot Study," *Neurology*, 2001, 56(1):97-9.

Contreras G, Pardo V, Leclercq B, et al, "Sequential Therapies for Proliferative Lupus Nephritis," *N Engl J Med*, 2004, 350(10):971-80.

Hahn BH, McMahon MA, Wilkinson A, et al, "American College of Rheumatology Guidelines for Screening, Treatment, and Management of Lupus Nephritis," *Arthritis Care Res (Hoboken)*, 2012, 64(6):797-808.

Manns MP, Czaja AJ, Gorham JD, et al, "Diagnosis and Management of Autoimmune Hepatitis," *Hepatology*, 2010, 51(6):2193-213.

Menter A, Korman NJ, Elmets CA, et al, "Guidelines of Care for the Management of Psoriasis and Psoriatic Arthritis: Section 4. Guidelines of Care for the Management and Treatment of Psoriasis With Traditional Systemic Agents," *J Am Acad Dermatol*, 2009, 61(3):451-85.

Meriggioli MN, Ciafaloni E, Al-Hayk KA, et al, "Mycophenolate Mofetil for Myasthenia Gravis: An Analysis of Efficacy, Safety, and Tolerability," *Neurology*, 2003, 61(10):1438-40.

Ong LM, Hooi LS, Lim TO, et al, "Randomized Controlled Trial of Pulse Intravenous Cyclophosphamide versus Mycophenolate Mofetil in the Induction Therapy of Proliferative Lupus Nephritis," *Nephrology (Carlton)*, 2005, 10(5):504-10.

Vogelsang GB, and Arai S, "Mycophenolate Mofetil for the Prevention and Treatment of Graft-Versus-Host Disease Following Stem Cell Transplantation: Preliminary Findings," *Bone Marrow Transplant*, 2001, 27(12):1255-62.

Zhu B, Chen N, Lin Y, et al, "Mycophenolate Mofetil in Induction and Maintenance Therapy of Severe Lupus Nephritis: A Meta-Analysis of Randomized Controlled Trials," *Nephrol Dial Transplant*, 2007, 22(7):1933-42.

- **Mycophenolate Mofetil** *see* Mycophenolate *on page 1015*
- **Mycophenolate Sodium** *see* Mycophenolate *on page 1015*
- **Mycophenolic Acid** *see* Mycophenolate *on page 1015*
- **Myfortic®** *see* Mycophenolate *on page 1015*
- **Mylan-Acyclovir (Can)** *see* Acyclovir (Systemic) *on page 30*
- **Mylan-Anagrelide (Can)** *see* Anagrelide *on page 93*
- **Mylan-Bicalutamide (Can)** *see* Bicalutamide *on page 178*
- **Mylan-Ciprofloxacin (Can)** *see* Ciprofloxacin (Systemic) *on page 283*
- **Mylan-Fluconazole (Can)** *see* Fluconazole *on page 612*
- **Mylan-Hydroxyurea (Can)** *see* Hydroxyurea *on page 731*
- **Mylan-Levofloxacin (Can)** *see* Levofloxacin (Systemic) *on page 883*
- **Mylan-Mycophenolate (Can)** *see* Mycophenolate *on page 1015*
- **Mylan-Olanzapine (Can)** *see* OLANZapine *on page 1056*
- **Mylan-Ondansetron (Can)** *see* Ondansetron *on page 1068*
- **Mylan-Tamoxifen (Can)** *see* Tamoxifen *on page 1324*
- **Mylan-Valacyclovir (Can)** *see* Valacyclovir *on page 1420*
- **Myleran®** *see* Busulfan *on page 203*
- **Myl-Letrozole (Can)** *see* Letrozole *on page 867*
- **Mylotarg** *see* Gemtuzumab Ozogamicin *on page 673*
- **Myocet™ (Can)** *see* DOXOrubicin (Liposomal) *on page 473*
- **Myorisan™** *see* ISOtretinoin *on page 832*
- **Mytotan** *see* Mitotane *on page 994*

Nabilone (NA bi lone)

Related Information

Management of Chemotherapy-Induced Nausea and Vomiting *on page 1786*

Brand Names: U.S. Cesamet®

Brand Names: Canada Cesamet®; PMS-Nabilone; RAN™-Nabilone; Teva-Nabilone

Generic Availability (U.S.) No

Pharmacologic Category Antiemetic

Use Treatment of refractory nausea and vomiting associated with cancer chemotherapy

Labeled Contraindications Hypersensitivity to nabilone, other cannabinoids, or any component of the formulation

Pregnancy Risk Factor C

Lactation Excretion in breast milk unknown/not recommended

Warnings/Precautions May cause tachycardia and orthostatic hypotension; use caution with cardiovascular disease. May affect CNS function (dizziness, drowsiness, ataxia, depression, hallucinations, and psychosis have been reported); use with caution in the elderly and those with pre-existing CNS depression. May cause additive CNS effects with sedatives, hypnotics, or other psychoactive agents; patients must be cautioned about performing tasks which require mental alertness (eg, operating machinery or driving). Use caution in patients with mania, depression, or schizophrenia; cannabinoid use may reveal symptoms of psychiatric disorders. Careful psychiatric monitoring is recommended; psychiatric adverse reactions may persist for up to 3 days after discontinuing treatment. Has potential for abuse and or dependence, use caution in patients with substance abuse history or potential.

Adverse Reactions

>10%:

Central nervous system: Drowsiness (52% to 66%), dizziness (59%), vertigo (52% to 59%), euphoria (11% to 38%), ataxia (13% to 14%), depression (14%), concentration decreased (12%), sleep disturbance (11%)

Gastrointestinal: Xerostomia (22% to 36%)

Ocular: Visual disturbance (13%)

1% to 10%:

Cardiovascular: Hypotension (8%)

Central nervous system: Dysphoria (9%), headache (6% to 7%), sedation (3%), depersonalization (2%), disorientation (2%)

Gastrointestinal: Anorexia (8%), nausea (4%), appetite increased (2%)

Neuromuscular & skeletal: Weakness (8%)

<1%, postmarketing, or frequency not reported: Abdominal pain, abnormal dreams, akathisia, allergic reaction, amblyopia, anemia, anhydrosis, anxiety, apathy, aphthous ulcer, arrhythmia, back pain, cerebral vascular accident, chest pain, chills, confusion, constipation, cough, diaphoresis, diarrhea, dyspepsia, dyspnea, dystonia, emotional disorder, emotional lability, epistaxis, equilibrium dysfunction, eye irritation, fatigue, fever, flushing, gastritis, hallucinations, hot flashes, hyperactivity, hypertension, infection, insomnia, joint pain, leukopenia, lightheadedness, malaise, memory disturbance, mood swings, mouth irritation, muscle pain, nasal congestion, neck pain, nervousness, neurosis (phobic), numbness, orthostatic hypotension, pain, palpitation, panic disorder, paranoia, paresthesia, perception disturbance, pharyngitis, photophobia, photosensitivity, polyuria, pruritus, psychosis (including toxic), pupil dilation, rash, seizure, sinus headache, speech disorder, stupor, syncope, tachycardia, taste perversion, thirst, thought disorder, tinnitus, tremor, urination decreased/increased, urinary retention, visual field defect, voice change, vomiting, wheezing, withdrawal, xerophthalmia

Drug Interactions

Metabolism/Transport Effects None known.

Avoid Concomitant Use

Avoid concomitant use of Nabilone with any of the following: Azelastine (Nasal); Mirtazapine; Paraldehyde

Increased Effect/Toxicity

Nabilone may increase the levels/effects of: Alcohol (Ethyl); Azelastine (Nasal); CNS Depressants; Methotrimeprazine; Metyrosine; Mirtazapine; Paraldehyde; Pramipexole; ROPINIRole; Rotigotine; Selective Serotonin Reuptake Inhibitors; Sympathomimetics; Zolpidem

The levels/effects of Nabilone may be increased by: Anticholinergic Agents; Cocaine; Droperidol; HydrOXYzine; Methotrimeprazine; Perampanel

Decreased Effect There are no known significant interactions involving a decrease in effect.

Ethanol/Nutrition/Herb Interactions Ethanol: May increase CNS depression; monitor for increased effects with coadministration. Caution patients about effects.

Storage/Stability Store at 25°C (77°F); excursion permitted to 15°C and 30°C (59°F and 86°F).

Mechanism of Action Antiemetic activity may be due to effect on cannabinoid receptors (CB1) within the central nervous system.

Pharmacodynamics/Kinetics

Absorption: Rapid and complete

Distribution: ~12.5 L/kg

Metabolism: Extensively metabolized to several active metabolites by oxidation and stereospecific enzyme reduction; CYP450 enzymes may also be involved

Half-life elimination: Parent compound: ~2 hours; Metabolites: ~35 hours

Time to peak, serum: Within 2 hours

Excretion: Feces (~60%); renal (~24%)

Dosing

Adult Nausea and vomiting associated with cancer chemotherapy: Oral: 1-2 mg twice daily (maximum: 6 mg divided in 3 doses daily); begin with the lower dose in the range and increase if needed. May administer 2 or 3 times per day during the entire chemotherapy course; continue for up to 48 hours after the last chemotherapy dose. A dose of 1-2 mg the night before chemotherapy may also be of benefit.

Geriatric Refer to adult dosing. Use the lower end of the dosing range (to minimize adverse events).

Pediatric Nausea and vomiting associated with cancer chemotherapy (unlabeled use; Dupuis, 2003): Oral: Children >4 years:

<18 kg: 0.5 mg every 12 hours

18-30 kg: 1 mg every 12 hours

>30 kg: 1 mg every 8-12 hours

Renal Impairment No dosage adjustment provided in manufacturer's labeling.

Hepatic Impairment No dosage adjustment provided in manufacturer's labeling.

Administration Initial dose should be given 1-3 hours before chemotherapy.

Emetic Potential Very low (<10%)

Monitoring Parameters Blood pressure, heart rate; signs and symptoms of excessive use, abuse, or misuse

Dosage Forms Excipient information presented when available (limited, particularly for generics); consult specific product labeling.

Capsule, oral:

Cesamet®: 1 mg

Controlled Substance C-II

References

Dupuis LL and Nathan PC, "Options for the Prevention and Management of Acute Chemotherapy-Induced Nausea and Vomiting in Children," *Pediatr Drug*, 2003, 5(9):597-613.

Tramer MR, Carroll D, Campbell FA, et al, "Cannabinoids for Control of Chemotherapy Induced Nausea and Vomiting: Quantitative Systematic Review," *BMJ*, 2001, 323(7303):16-21.

Ward A and Holmes B, "Nabilone: A Preliminary Review of Its Pharmacological Properties and Therapeutic Use," *Drugs*, 1985, 30(2):127-44.

◆ **nab-Paclitaxel** *see* PACLitaxel (Protein Bound) *on page 1098*

Nafcillin (naf SIL in)

Brand Names: Canada Nallpen®; Unipen®

Index Terms Ethoxynaphthamido Penicillin Sodium; Nafcillin Sodium; Nallpen; Sodium Nafcillin

Generic Availability (U.S.) Yes

Pharmacologic Category Antibiotic, Penicillin

Use Treatment of infections such as osteomyelitis, septicemia, endocarditis, and CNS infections caused by susceptible strains of staphylococci species

Labeled Contraindications Hypersensitivity to nafcillin, or any component of the formulation, or penicillins; premixed injection may contain corn-derived dextrose and its use is contraindicated in patients with allergy to corn-related products

Pregnancy Risk Factor B

Lactation Enters breast milk/use caution

Warnings/Precautions Serious and occasionally severe or fatal hypersensitivity (anaphylactoid) reactions have been reported in patients on penicillin therapy, especially with a history of beta-lactam hypersensitivity, history of sensitivity to multiple allergens, or previous IgE-mediated reactions (eg, anaphylaxis, angioedema, urticaria). Use with caution in asthmatic patients. Extravasation of I.V. infusions should be avoided. Modification of dosage is necessary in patients with both severe renal and hepatic impairment. Elimination rate will be slow in neonates. Prolonged use may result in fungal or bacterial superinfection, including *C. difficile*-associated diarrhea (CDAD) and pseudomembranous colitis; CDAD has been observed >2 months postantibiotic treatment.

Storage/Stability

Premixed infusions: Store in a freezer at -20°C (4°F). Thaw at room temperature or under refrigeration only. Thawed bags are stable for 21 days under refrigeration or 72 hours at room temperature. Do not refreeze.

Vials: Reconstituted parenteral solution is stable for 3 days at room temperature and 7 days when refrigerated or 12 weeks when frozen. For I.V. infusion in NS or D_5W, solution is stable for 24 hours at room temperature and 96 hours when refrigerated.

Mechanism of Action Interferes with bacterial cell wall synthesis during active multiplication, causing cell wall death and resultant bactericidal activity against susceptible bacteria

Pharmacodynamics/Kinetics

Distribution: Widely distributed; CSF penetration is poor but enhanced by meningeal inflammation

Protein binding: ~90%; primarily to albumin

Metabolism: Primarily hepatic; undergoes enterohepatic recirculation

Half-life elimination:

- Neonates: <3 weeks: 2.2-5.5 hours; 4-9 weeks: 1.2-2.3 hours
- Children 3 months to 14 years: 0.75-1.9 hours
- Adults: Normal renal/hepatic function: 30-60 minutes

Time to peak, serum: I.M.: 30-60 minutes

Excretion: Primarily feces; urine (10% to 30% as unchanged drug)

Dosing

Adult & Geriatric

Susceptible infections:

I.M.: 500 mg every 4-6 hours

I.V.: 500-2000 mg every 4-6 hours

Endocarditis: MSSA:

Native valve: I.V.: 12 g/24 hours in 4-6 divided doses for 6 weeks

Prosthetic valve: I.V.: 12 g/24 hours in 6 divided doses for ≥6 weeks (use with rifampin and gentamicin)

Joint:

Bursitis, septic: I.V.: 2 g every 4 hours

Prosthetic: I.V.: 2 g every 4-6 hours with rifampin for 6 weeks

***Staphylococcus aureus*, methicillin-susceptible infections, including brain abscess, empyema, erysipelas, mastitis, myositis, orbital cellulitis, osteomyelitis, pneumonia, splenic abscess, toxic shock, urinary tract (perinephric abscess):** I.V.: 2 g every 4 hours

Pediatric Children:

I.M.: 25 mg/kg twice daily

I.V.:

Mild-to-moderate infections: 50-100 mg/kg/day in divided doses every 6 hours

Severe infections: 100-200 mg/kg/day in divided doses every 4-6 hours (maximum: 12 g/day)

Staphylococcal endocarditis:

Native valve: 200 mg/kg/day in divided doses every 4-6 hours for 6 weeks

Prosthetic valve: 200 mg/kg/day in divided doses every 4-6 hours for ≥6 weeks (use with rifampin and gentamicin)

Renal Impairment Not necessary unless renal impairment is in the setting of concomitant hepatic impairment.

Poorly dialyzed; no supplemental dose or dosage adjustment necessary, including patients on intermittent hemodialysis, peritoneal dialysis, or continuous renal replacement therapy (eg, CVVHD).

Hepatic Impairment In patients with both hepatic and renal impairment, modification of dosage may be necessary; no data available.

Administration

I.M.: Rotate injection sites

I.V.: Vesicant. Administer around-the-clock to promote less variation in peak and trough serum levels; infuse over 30-60 minutes

Extravasation management: Use cold packs. Hyaluronidase: Add 1 mL NS to 150 unit vial to make 150 units/mL of concentration; mix 0.1 mL of above with 0.9 mL NS in 1 mL syringe to make final concentration = 15 units/mL

Test Interactions Positive Coombs' test (direct), false-positive urinary and serum proteins; may inactivate aminoglycosides *in vitro*

Dosage Forms Excipient information presented when available (limited, particularly for generics); consult specific product labeling

Infusion, premixed iso-osmotic dextrose solution: 1 g (50 mL); 2 g (100 mL)

Injection, powder for reconstitution: 1 g, 2 g, 10 g

- **Nafcillin Sodium** *see* Nafcillin *on page* 1026
- **Nallpen** *see* Nafcillin *on page* 1026
- **Nallpen® (Can)** *see* Nafcillin *on page* 1026
- **Nanoparticle Albumin-Bound Paclitaxel** *see* PACLitaxel (Protein Bound) *on page* 1098
- **Natulan® (Can)** *see* Procarbazine *on page* 1208
- **Navelbine®** *see* Vinorelbine *on page* 1465
- **Nebupent®** *see* Pentamidine *on page* 1156

Nelarabine (nel AY re been)

Related Information

Management of Chemotherapy-Induced Nausea and Vomiting *on page 1786*
Management of Infections *on page 1809*
Safe Handling of Hazardous Drugs *on page 1904*

Brand Names: U.S. Arranon®

Brand Names: Canada Atriance™

Index Terms 2-Amino-6-Methoxypurine Arabinoside; 506U78; GW506U78

Generic Availability (U.S.) No

Pharmacologic Category Antineoplastic Agent, Antimetabolite; Antineoplastic Agent, Antimetabolite (Purine Analog)

Use Treatment of relapsed or refractory T-cell acute lymphoblastic leukemia (ALL) and T-cell lymphoblastic lymphoma

Labeled Contraindications There are no contraindications listed within the manufacturer's labeling.

Pregnancy Risk Factor D

Lactation Excretion in breast milk unknown/not recommended

Warnings/Precautions Hazardous agent - use appropriate precautions for handling and disposal. **[U.S. Boxed Warning]: Severe neurotoxicity, including mental status changes, severe somnolence, seizure, and peripheral neuropathy (ranging from numbness to motor weakness or paralysis), has been reported. Observe closely for signs and symptoms of neurotoxicity; discontinue if ≥ grade 2. Adverse effects associated with demyelination or similar to Guillain-Barré syndrome (ascending peripheral neuropathies) have also been reported. Neurologic toxicities may not fully return to baseline after treatment cessation.** Neurologic toxicity is dose-limiting. Risk of neurotoxicity may increase in patients with concurrent or previous intrathecal chemotherapy or history of craniospinal irradiation. Tumor lysis syndrome (TLS) may occur as a consequence of leukemia treatment. May lead to life threatening acute renal failure; adequate hydration and prophylactic allopurinol should be instituted prior to treatment to prevent hyperuricemia and TLS; monitor closely. Bone marrow suppression, including leukopenia, thrombocytopenia, anemia, neutropenia and febrile neutropenia are associated with treatment; monitor blood counts regularly. Avoid administration of live vaccines. Use caution in patients with renal impairment; ara-G clearance may be reduced with renal dysfunction. Use caution with severe hepatic impairment; risk of adverse reactions may be higher with hepatic dysfunction.

Adverse Reactions Note: Pediatric adverse reactions fell within a range similar to adults except where noted.

>10%:

Cardiovascular: Peripheral edema (15%), edema (11%)

Central nervous system: Fatigue (50%), fever (23%), somnolence (7% to 23%; grades 2-4: 1% to 6%), dizziness (21%; grade 2: 8% adults), headache (15% to 17%; grades 2-4: 4% to 8%), hypoesthesia (6% to 17%; grades 2/3: children 5%, adults 12%), pain (11%)

Dermatologic: Petechiae (12%)

Endocrine & metabolic: Hypokalemia (11%)

Gastrointestinal: Nausea (41%), diarrhea (22%), vomiting (10% to 22%), constipation (21%)

Hematologic: Anemia (95% to 99%; grade 4: 10% to 14%), neutropenia (81% to 94%; grade 4: children 62%, adults 49%), thrombocytopenia (86% to

88%; grade 4: 22% to 32%), leukopenia (38%; grade 4: 7%), neutropenic fever (12%; grade 4: 1%)
Hepatic: Transaminases increased (12%; grade 3: 4%)
Neuromuscular & skeletal: Peripheral neuropathy (12% to 21%; grades 2/3: 11% to 14%), weakness (6% to 17%; grade 4: 1%), paresthesia (4% to 15%; grades 2/3: 3% to 4%), myalgia (13%)
Respiratory: Cough (25%), dyspnea (7% to 20%)

1% to 10%:

Cardiovascular: Hypotension (8%), sinus tachycardia (8%), chest pain (5%)
Central nervous system: Ataxia (2% to 9%; grades 2/3: children 1%, adults 8%), confusion (8%), insomnia (7%), depressed level of consciousness (6%; grades 2-4: 2%), depression (6%), seizure (grade 3: 1% adults; grade 4: 6% children), motor dysfunction (4%; grades 2/3: 2%), amnesia (3%; grade 2: 1%), balance disorder (2%; grade 2: 1%), sensory loss (1% to 2%), aphasia (grade 3: 1%), attention disturbance (1%), cerebral hemorrhage (grade 4: 1%), coma (grade 4: 1%), encephalopathy (grade 4: 1%), hemiparesis (grade 3: 1%), hydrocephalus (1%), intracranial hemorrhage (grade 4: 1%), lethargy (1%), leukoencephalopathy (grade 4: 1%), loss of consciousness (grade 3: 1%), mental impairment (1%), nerve paralysis (1%), neuropathic pain (1%), nerve palsy (1%), paralysis (1%), sciatica (1%), sensory disturbance (1%), speech disorder (1%)
Endocrine & Metabolic: Hypocalcemia (8%), dehydration (7%), hyper-/hypoglycemia (6%), hypomagnesemia (6%)
Gastrointestinal: Abdominal pain (9%), anorexia (9%), stomatitis (8%), abdominal distension (6%), taste perversion (3%)
Hepatic: Albumin decreased (10%), bilirubin increased (10%; grade 3: 7%, grade 4: 2%), AST increased (6%)
Neuromuscular & skeletal: Arthralgia (9%), back pain (8%), muscle weakness (8%), rigors (8%), limb pain (7%), abnormal gait (6%), noncardiac chest pain (5%), tremor (4% to 5%; grade 2: 2% to 3%), dysarthria (1%), hyporeflexia (1%), hypertonia (1%), incoordination (1%)
Ocular: Blurred vision (4%), nystagmus (1%)
Renal: Creatinine increased (6%)
Respiratory: Pleural effusion (10%), epistaxis (8%), pneumonia (8%), sinusitis (7%), wheezing (5%), sinus headache (1%)
Miscellaneous: Infection (5% to 9%)

<1%, postmarketing, and/or case reports: CPK increased, craniospinal demyelination, neuropathy (peripheral) (similar to Guillain-Barré syndrome), opportunistic infection, pneumothorax, progressive multifocal leukoencephalopathy (PML), respiratory arrest, rhabdomyolysis, tumor lysis syndrome

Drug Interactions

Metabolism/Transport Effects None known.

Avoid Concomitant Use

Avoid concomitant use of Nelarabine with any of the following: BCG; CloZAPine; Natalizumab; Pentostatin; Pimecrolimus; Tacrolimus (Topical); Vaccines (Live)

Increased Effect/Toxicity

Nelarabine may increase the levels/effects of: CloZAPine; Leflunomide; Natalizumab; Vaccines (Live)

The levels/effects of Nelarabine may be increased by: Denosumab; Pimecrolimus; Roflumilast; Tacrolimus (Topical); Trastuzumab

Decreased Effect

Nelarabine may decrease the levels/effects of: BCG; Coccidioidin Skin Test; Sipuleucel-T; Vaccines (Inactivated); Vaccines (Live)

The levels/effects of Nelarabine may be decreased by: Echinacea; Pentostatin

Storage/Stability Store unopened vials at 25°C (77°F); excursions permitted to 15°C to 30°C (59°F to 86°F). Stable in plastic (PVC) or glass containers for up to 8 hours at room temperature.

Reconstitution Reconstitution is not required; do not dilute; the appropriate dose should be added to empty plastic (PVC) bag or glass container. Use appropriate precautions for handling and disposal.

Mechanism of Action Nelarabine, a prodrug of ara-G, is demethylated by adenosine deaminase to ara-G and then converted to ara-GTP. Ara-GTP is incorporated into the DNA of the leukemic blasts, leading to inhibition of DNA synthesis and inducing apoptosis. Ara-GTP appears to accumulate at higher levels in T-cells, which correlates to clinical response.

Pharmacodynamics/Kinetics

Distribution: V_{ss}:

Nelarabine: Children: ~213 L/m^2; Adults: ~197 L/m^2

Ara-G: Children: ~33 L/m^2; Adults: ~50 L/m^2

Protein binding: Nelarabine and ara-G: <25%

Metabolism: Hepatic; demethylated by adenosine deaminase to form ara-G (active); also hydrolyzed to form methylguanine. Both ara-G and methylguanine metabolized to guanine. Guanine is deaminated into xanthine, which is further oxidized to form uric acid, which is then oxidized to form allantoin.

Half-life elimination: Children: Nelarabine: 13 minutes, Ara-G: 2 hours; Adults: Nelarabine: 18 minutes, Ara-G: 3 hours

Time to peak: Ara-G: Adults: 3-25 hours (of day 1)

Excretion: Urine (nelarabine 5% to 10%, ara-G 20% to 30%)

Dosing

Adult & Geriatric T-cell acute lymphoblastic leukemia (ALL), T-cell lymphoblastic lymphoma: I.V.: 1500 mg/m^2/dose on days 1, 3, and 5; repeat every 21 days until transplant, disease progression, or unacceptable toxicity.

Pediatric T-cell acute lymphoblastic leukemia (ALL), T-cell lymphoblastic lymphoma: I.V.: 650 mg/m^2/dose on days 1 through 5; repeat every 21 days until transplant, disease progression, or unacceptable toxicity.

Renal Impairment

Cl_{cr} ≥50 mL/minute: No dosage adjustment necessary.

Cl_{cr} <50 mL/minute: No dosage adjustment provided in manufacturer's labeling, (although ARA-G clearance is decreased as renal function declines, data is insufficient for a dosing recommendation); monitor closely.

Hepatic Impairment No dosage adjustment provided in manufacturer's labeling (has not been studied); closely monitor with severe impairment (total bilirubin >3 times ULN).

Adjustment for Toxicity

Neurologic toxicity ≥ grade 2: Discontinue treatment.

Hematologic or other (non-neurologic) toxicity: Consider treatment delay.

Administration Adequate I.V. hydration recommended to prevent tumor lysis syndrome; allopurinol may be used if hyperuricemia is anticipated.

Children: Infuse over 1 hour daily for 5 consecutive days

Adults: Infuse over 2 hours on days 1, 3, and 5

Emetic Potential Very low (<10%)

Monitoring Parameters Closely monitor for neurologic toxicity (severe somnolence, seizure, peripheral neuropathy, confusion, ataxia, paresthesia, hypoesthesia, coma, or craniospinal demyelination); signs and symptoms of tumor lysis syndrome; hydration status; CBC with differential, liver and kidney function

Dosage Forms Excipient information presented when available (limited, particularly for generics); consult specific product labeling.

Injection, solution:

Arranon®: 5 mg/mL (50 mL)

Dosage Forms: Canada Excipient information presented when available (limited, particularly for generics); consult specific product labeling.

Injection, solution:

Atriance™: 5 mg/mL (50 mL)

References

Berg SL, Blaney SM, Devidas M, et al, "Phase II Study of Nelarabine (Compound 506U78) in Children and Young Adults With Refractory T-Cell Malignancies: A Report from the Children's Oncology Group," *J Clin Oncol*, 2005, 23(15):3376-82.

DeAngelo DJ, Yu D, Johnson JL, et al, "Nelarabine Induces Complete Remissions in Adults With Relapsed or Refractory T-Lineage Acute Lymphoblastic Leukemia or Lymphoblastic Lymphoma: Cancer and Leukemia Group B Study 19801," *Blood*, 2007, 109(12):5136-42.

Gandhi V, Plunkett W, Weller S, et al, "Evaluation of the Combination of Nelarabine and Fludarabine in Leukemias: Clinical Response, Pharmacokinetics, and Pharmacodynamics in Leukemia Cells," *J Clin Oncol*, 2001, 19(8):2142-52.

◆ **Neoral®** *see* CycloSPORINE (Systemic) *on page* 333

◆ **Neosar** *see* Cyclophosphamide *on page* 321

◆ **NESP** *see* Darbepoetin Alfa *on page* 382

◆ **Neulasta®** *see* Pegfilgrastim *on page* 1138

◆ **Neumega®** *see* Oprelvekin *on page* 1074

◆ **Neupogen®** *see* Filgrastim *on page* 604

◆ **NeutraSal®** *see* Saliva Substitute *on page* 1266

◆ **NexAVAR®** *see* SORAfenib *on page* 1292

◆ **Nexavar® (Can)** *see* SORAfenib *on page* 1292

◆ **Niastase® (Can)** *see* Factor VIIa (Recombinant) *on page* 568

◆ **Niastase® RT (Can)** *see* Factor VIIa (Recombinant) *on page* 568

◆ **Niftolid** *see* Flutamide *on page* 635

◆ **Nilandron®** *see* Nilutamide *on page* 1037

Nilotinib (nye LOE ti nib)

Related Information

Management of Chemotherapy-Induced Nausea and Vomiting *on page* 1786

Principles of Anticancer Therapy *on page* 1878

Safe Handling of Hazardous Drugs *on page* 1904

Brand Names: U.S. Tasigna®

Brand Names: Canada Tasigna®

Index Terms AMN107; Nilotinib Hydrochloride Monohydrate

Generic Availability (U.S.) No

Pharmacologic Category Antineoplastic Agent, Tyrosine Kinase Inhibitor

Use Treatment of newly-diagnosed Philadelphia chromosome-positive chronic myelogenous leukemia (Ph+ CML) in chronic phase; treatment of chronic and accelerated phase Ph+ CML refractory or intolerant to prior therapy (including imatinib)

Unlabeled Use Treatment of refractory gastrointestinal stromal tumor (GIST)

Labeled Contraindications Use in patients with hypokalemia, hypomagnesemia, or long QT syndrome

Canadian labeling: Additional contraindication (not in U.S. labeling): Hypersensitivity to nilotinib or any component of the formulation

Pregnancy Risk Factor D

Lactation Excretion in breast milk unknown/not recommended

Warnings/Precautions Hazardous agent - use appropriate precautions for handling and disposal. **[U.S. Boxed Warnings]: May prolong the QT interval; sudden deaths have been reported. Use in patients with hypokalemia, hypomagnesemia, or long QT syndrome is contraindicated. Correct hypomagnesemia and hypokalemia prior to initiating therapy; monitor electrolytes periodically. Monitor ECG and QT_c (baseline, at 7 days, with dose change, and periodically). Avoid the use of QT-prolonging agents.** Avoid concurrent use with antiarrhythmics and other drugs which may prolong QT interval; may increase the risk of potentially-fatal arrhythmias. Sudden deaths appear to be related to dose-dependent ventricular repolarization abnormalities. Prolonged QT interval may result in torsade de pointes, which may cause syncope, seizure, and/or death. Patients with uncontrolled or significant cardiovascular disease were excluded from studies. **[U.S. Boxed Warning]: Avoid concurrent use with strong CYP3A4 inhibitors** (including grapefruit juice); interrupt nilotinib treatment if a strong CYP3A4 inhibitor is required; if coadministration cannot be avoided, consider nilotinib dose reductions. CYP3A4 inducers (including St John's wort) should also be avoided.

Dosage reduction is recommended in patients with hepatic impairment, along with close monitoring of the QT interval. Nilotinib metabolism is primarily hepatic (exposure is increased in patients with hepatic impairment). May cause hepatotoxicity, including dose-limiting elevations in bilirubin, transaminases, and alkaline phosphatase; monitor liver function.

Reversible myelosuppression, including grades 3 and 4 thrombocytopenia, neutropenia, and anemia may occur; may require dose reductions and/or treatment delay; monitor blood counts. **[U.S. Boxed Warning]: Administer on an empty stomach, at least 1 hour before and 2 hours after food;** administration with food may prolong the QT_c. Use with caution in patients with a history of pancreatitis, may cause dose-limiting elevations of serum lipase and amylase; monitor. In patients with abdominal symptoms in conjunction with lipase increases, withhold treatment and consider diagnostics to exclude pancreatitis. Tumor lysis syndrome (TLS) has been reported in patients with resistant or intolerant CML; the majority of cases had malignant disease progression, high WBC counts, and/or dehydration; maintain adequate hydration and treat high uric acid levels prior to nilotinib. Consider alternative therapy or a dosage increase (with more frequent monitoring) in patients with total gastrectomy (nilotinib exposure is reduced). Capsules contain lactose; do not use with galactose intolerance, severe lactase deficiency, or glucose-galactose malabsorption syndromes.

Adverse Reactions

>10%:

Cardiovascular: Peripheral edema (8% to 15%), hypertension (10% to 11%)

Central nervous system: Headache (20% to 35%), fatigue (21% to 32%), fever (11% to 28%), insomnia (7% to 12%)
Dermatologic: Rash (29% to 37%), pruritus (20% to 32%), alopecia (11% to 12%)
Endocrine & metabolic: Hypophosphatemia (grades 3/4: 5% to 17%), hyperglycemia (grades 3/4: 6% to 12%)
Gastrointestinal: Nausea (20% to 37%), vomiting (11% to 29%), diarrhea (14% to 28%), constipation (17% to 26%), lipase increased (grades 3/4: 7% to 18%), abdominal pain (12% to 16%), anorexia (12% to 15%)
Hematologic: Neutropenia (grades 3/4: 12% to 42%; median duration: 15 days), thrombocytopenia (grade 3/4: 10% to 42%; median duration: 22 days), anemia (grades 3/4: 4% to 27%)
Neuromuscular & skeletal: Arthralgia (16% to 26%), limb pain (11% to 20%), myalgia (14% to 19%), back pain (14% to 17%), weakness (11% to 16%), bone pain (14% to 15%), muscle spasm (11% to 15%), musculoskeletal pain (11% to 12%)
Respiratory: Cough (14% to 27%), nasopharyngitis (15% to 24%), dyspnea (9% to 15%), upper respiratory tract infection (≤14%), oropharyngeal pain (7% to 11%)
Miscellaneous: Night sweats (12% to 27%)

1% to 10%:
Cardiovascular: Angina, arrhythmia (including AV block, atrial fibrillation, bradycardia, cardiac flutter, extrasystoles, and tachycardia), chest pain, flushing, palpitation, pericardial effusion, QT interval prolonged
Central nervous system: Anxiety, depression, dizziness, dysphonia, hypoesthesia, malaise, pain, vertigo
Dermatologic: Acne, bruising, dry skin, dermatitis (allergic and acneiform), eczema, erythema, folliculitis, hyperhidrosis, skin papilloma, urticaria
Endocrine & metabolic: Hypokalemia (grades 3/4: ≤9%), hyponatremia (grades 3/4: ≤7%), hyperkalemia (grades 3/4: 2% to 6%), hypocalcemia (grades 3/4: ≤5%), albumin decreased (grades 3/4: ≤4%), diabetes mellitus, hypercalcemia, hypercholesterolemia, hyperlipidemia, hyperphosphatemia, hypomagnesemia
Gastrointestinal: Dyspepsia (4% to 10%), abdominal discomfort, abnormal taste, amylase increased, flatulence, pancreatitis, weight gain/loss
Genitourinary: Pollakuria
Hematologic: Lymphopenia, neutropenic fever, pancytopenia
Hepatic: Hyperbilirubinemia (grades 3/4: 4% to 9%), ALT increased (grades 3/4: 4%), AST increased (grades 3/4: 1% to 3%), alkaline phosphatase increased (grades 3/4: ≤1%), GGT increased
Neuromuscular & skeletal: Paresthesia, peripheral neuropathy
Ocular: Conjunctivitis, dry eye, eye hemorrhage, eyelid edema (1%), periorbital edema, pruritus
Respiratory: Dyspnea (exertional), epistaxis, pleural effusion (≤1%), pneumonia

<1%, postmarketing, and/or case reports (limited to important or life-threatening): Abscess, candidiasis, cardiac failure, cardiac murmur, cardiomegaly, cholestasis, chorioretinopathy, confusion, coronary artery disease, creatinine elevated, cyanosis, dehydration, diplopia, dysuria, ejection fraction decreased, eosinophilia, erectile dysfunction, erythema multiforme, erythema nodosum, exfoliative rash, facial edema, gastroenteritis, gastrointestinal hemorrhage, gastrointestinal ulcer perforation, gout, gynecomastia, hematemesis, hematoma, hematuria, hemorrhagic shock, hepatitis, hepatomegaly, hepatotoxicity, herpes simplex infection, hyperparathyroidism (secondary),

hyper-/hypothyroidism, hypersensitivity, hypertensive crisis, hyperuricemia, hypoglycemia, hypotension, influenza-like illness, interstitial lung disease, intracranial hemorrhage, jaundice, joint swelling, lactic dehydrogenase increased, leukocytosis, loss of consciousness, melena, MI, migraine, mouth ulceration, optic neuritis, palmar-plantar erythrodysesthesia syndrome, papilledema, pericarditis, peripheral arterial occlusive disease, petechiae, pulmonary edema, pulmonary hypertension, rectal hemorrhage, renal failure, restless leg syndrome (RLS), retroperitoneal hemorrhage, sepsis, sinusitis, skin hyperpigmentation, stomatitis, subileus, sudden death, syncope, thrombocytosis, thrombosis, thyroiditis, tinnitus, troponin increased, tumor lysis syndrome, ulcerative esophagitis, urinary tract infection, ventricular dysfunction, visual acuity decreased, wheezing

Drug Interactions

Metabolism/Transport Effects **Substrate** of CYP3A4 (major), P-glycoprotein; **Note:** Assignment of Major/Minor substrate status based on clinically relevant drug interaction potential; **Inhibits** CYP2C8 (moderate), CYP2C9 (moderate), CYP2D6 (moderate), CYP3A4 (weak), P-glycoprotein, UGT1A1; **Induces** CYP2B6 (weak/moderate), CYP2C8 (weak/moderate), CYP2C9 (weak/moderate)

Avoid Concomitant Use

Avoid concomitant use of Nilotinib with any of the following: BCG; Bosutinib; CloZAPine; CYP3A4 Inducers (Strong); CYP3A4 Inhibitors (Strong); Highest Risk QTc-Prolonging Agents; Mifepristone; Moderate Risk QTc-Prolonging Agents; Natalizumab; Pimecrolimus; Silodosin; Tacrolimus (Topical); Topotecan; Vaccines (Live); VinCRIStine (Liposomal)

Increased Effect/Toxicity

Nilotinib may increase the levels/effects of: ARIPiprazole; Bosutinib; Carvedilol; CloZAPine; Colchicine; CYP2C8 Substrates; CYP2C9 Substrates; CYP2D6 Substrates; Dabigatran Etexilate; Everolimus; Fesoterodine; Highest Risk QTc-Prolonging Agents; Leflunomide; Natalizumab; Nebivolol; P-glycoprotein/ABCB1 Substrates; Prucalopride; Rivaroxaban; Silodosin; Topotecan; Vaccines (Live); VinCRIStine (Liposomal); Vitamin K Antagonists

The levels/effects of Nilotinib may be increased by: CYP3A4 Inhibitors (Moderate); CYP3A4 Inhibitors (Strong); Dasatinib; Denosumab; Ivacaftor; Mifepristone; Moderate Risk QTc-Prolonging Agents; Pimecrolimus; QTc-Prolonging Agents (Indeterminate Risk and Risk Modifying); Roflumilast; Tacrolimus (Topical); Trastuzumab

Decreased Effect

Nilotinib may decrease the levels/effects of: BCG; Cardiac Glycosides; Coccidioidin Skin Test; Codeine; Sipuleucel-T; Tamoxifen; TraMADol; Vaccines (Inactivated); Vaccines (Live); Vitamin K Antagonists

The levels/effects of Nilotinib may be decreased by: Antacids; CYP3A4 Inducers (Strong); Deferasirox; Echinacea; H2-Antagonists; Herbs (CYP3A4 Inducers); Proton Pump Inhibitors; Tocilizumab

Ethanol/Nutrition/Herb Interactions

Food: Grapefruit juice may result in increased concentrations of nilotinib and potentiate QT prolongation. Management: Avoid grapefruit juice.

Herb/Nutraceutical: St John's wort may decrease nilotinib levels. Administration with grapefruit juice may result in increased concentrations of nilotinib and potentiate QT prolongation. Management: Avoid St John's wort and grapefruit juice.

Storage/Stability Store at 25°C (77°F); excursions permitted to 15°C to 30°C (59°F to 86°F).

Mechanism of Action Selective tyrosine kinase inhibitor that targets BCR-ABL kinase, c-KIT and platelet derived growth factor receptor (PDGFR); does not have activity against the SRC family. Inhibits BCR-ABL mediated proliferation of leukemic cell lines by binding to the ATP-binding site of BCR-ABL and inhibiting tyrosine kinase activity. Nilotinib has activity in imatinib-resistant BCR-ABL kinase mutations.

Pharmacodynamics/Kinetics

Protein binding: ~98%

Metabolism: Hepatic; oxidation and hydroxylation, via CYP3A4 to primarily inactive metabolites

Bioavailability: Capsule: ~50% (when compared to oral solution with pH of 1.2-1.3); two 200 mg capsules sprinkled on applesauce was determined to be bioequivalent to two 200 mg intact capsules; bioavailability is increased 82% when administered 30 minutes after a high-fat meal

Half-life elimination: ~15-17 hours

Time to peak: 3 hours

Excretion: Feces (93%; 69% as parent drug)

Dosing

Adult & Geriatric

Chronic myeloid leukemia (CML), Ph+, newly-diagnosed in chronic phase: Oral: 300 mg twice daily

CML, Ph+, resistant or intolerant in chronic or accelerated phase: Oral: 400 mg twice daily

Gastrointestinal stromal tumor (GIST), refractory (unlabeled use): Oral: 400 mg twice daily (Montemurro, 2009)

Dosage adjustment for concomitant CYP3A4 inhibitors/inducers:

CYP3A4 inhibitors: Avoid the concomitant use of a strong CYP3A4 inhibitor with nilotinib. If a strong CYP3A4 inhibitor is required, interruption of nilotinib treatment is recommended; if therapy cannot be interrupted and concurrent use cannot be avoided, consider reducing the nilotinib dose to 300 mg once daily in patients with resistant or intolerant Ph+ CML (chronic or accelerated phase) or to 200 mg once daily in newly-diagnosed chronic phase Ph+ CML, with careful monitoring, especially of the QT interval. When a strong CYP3A4 inhibitor is discontinued, allow a washout period prior to adjusting nilotinib dose upward.

CYP3A4 inducers: Avoid the concomitant use of a strong CYP3A4 inducer with nilotinib (based on pharmacokinetic parameters, an increased nilotinib dose is not likely to compensate for decreased exposure).

Renal Impairment Not studied in patients with serum creatinine >1.5 times ULN, however, nilotinib and its metabolites have minimal renal excretion; dosage adjustments for renal dysfunction may not be necessary.

Hepatic Impairment Note: Dosage adjustment for impairment at treatment initiation (if possible, consider alternative therapies first); recommendations vary by indication.

Newly-diagnosed Ph+ CML in chronic phase: Mild-to-severe impairment (Child-Pugh class A, B, or C): Initial: 200 mg twice daily; may increase to 300 mg twice daily based on patient tolerability

Resistant or intolerant Ph+ CML in chronic or accelerated phase:

Mild-to-moderate impairment (Child-Pugh class A or B): Initial: 300 mg twice daily; may increase to 400 mg twice daily based on patient tolerability

Severe impairment (Child-Pugh class C): Initial: 200 mg twice daily; may increase to 300 mg twice daily and then further increased to 400 mg twice daily based on patient tolerability

For hepatotoxicity during treatment:

If bilirubin >3 times ULN (≥grade 3): Withhold treatment, monitor bilirubin, resume treatment at 400 mg once daily when bilirubin returns to ≤1.5 times ULN (≤grade 1)

If ALT or AST >5 times ULN (≥grade 3): Withhold treatment, monitor transaminases, resume treatment at 400 mg once daily when ALT or AST returns to ≤2.5 times ULN (≤grade 1)

Adjustment for Toxicity

Dosage adjustment for hematologic toxicity:

ANC <1000/mm^3 and/or platelets <50,000/mm^3: Withhold treatment, monitor blood counts

If ANC >1000/mm^3 and platelets >50,000/mm^3 within 2 weeks: Resume at prior dose

If ANC <1000/mm^3 and/or platelets <50,000/mm^3 for >2 weeks: Reduce dose to 400 mg once daily

Dosage adjustment for nonhematologic toxicity:

Amylase or lipase >2 times ULN (≥grade 3): Withhold treatment, monitor serum amylase or lipase, resume treatment at 400 mg once daily when lipase or amylase returns to ≤1.5 times ULN (≤grade 1)

Lipase increases in conjunction with abdominal symptoms: Withhold treatment and consider diagnostics to exclude pancreatitis.

Clinically-significant moderate or severe nonhematologic toxicity: Withhold treatment, upon resolution of toxicity, resume at 400 mg once daily; may escalate back to initial dose (300 mg twice daily or 400 mg twice daily depending on indication) if clinically appropriate.

Dosage adjustment for QT prolongation: Note: Repeat ECG ~7 days after any dosage adjustment.

QT_c >480 msec: Withhold treatment, monitor and correct potassium and magnesium levels; review concurrent medications.

If QT_cF returns to <450 msec and to within 20 msec of baseline within 2 weeks: Resume at prior dose.

If QT_cF returns to 450-480 msec after 2 weeks: Reduce dose to 400 mg once daily.

If QT_cF >480 msec after dosage reduction to 400 mg once daily: Discontinue treatment.

Combination Regimens

Leukemia, Chronic Myelogenous: Nilotinib (CML Regimen) on page 1722

Administration Administer twice daily doses ~12 hours apart. Administer on an empty stomach, at least 1 hour before or 2 hours after food. Capsules should be swallowed whole with water. If unable to swallow whole, may empty contents into 5 mL applesauce and administer within 15 minutes (do not save for later use). If a dose is missed, do not make up, resume with next scheduled dose.

Emetic Potential Low (10% to 30%)

Monitoring Parameters CBC with differential (every 2 weeks for first 2 months, then monthly); electrolytes (including potassium and magnesium; baseline and periodic); lipid profile (periodic), hepatic function (ALT/AST, bilirubin, alkaline phosphatase; baseline and monthly or as clinically indicated); serum lipase/amylase (baseline and monthly or as clinically indicated); bone marrow assessments; ECG and QT_c (baseline, 7 days after treatment initiation or dosage adjustments, and periodically thereafter)

Thyroid function testing (Hamnvik, 2011):

Pre-existing levothyroxine therapy: Obtain baseline TSH levels, then monitor every 4 weeks until levels and levothyroxine dose are stable, then monitor every 2 months

Without pre-existing thyroid hormone replacement: TSH at baseline, then monthly for 4 months, then every 2-3 months

Dietary Considerations The bioavailability of nilotinib is increased with food. Take on an empty stomach, at least 1 hour before or 2 hours after food. Avoid grapefruit juice.

Additional Information If clinically indicated, may be administered in combination with hematopoietic growth factors (eg, erythropoietin, filgrastim) and with hydroxyurea or anagrelide.

Medication Guide Available Yes

Dosage Forms Excipient information presented when available (limited, particularly for generics); consult specific product labeling.

Capsule, oral:

Tasigna®: 150 mg, 200 mg

References

Hamnvik OP, Larsen PR, and Marqusee E, "Thyroid Dysfunction From Antineoplastic Agents," *J Natl Cancer Inst*, 2011, 103(21):1572-87.

Kantarjian HM, Giles F, Gattermann N, et al, "Nilotinib (Formerly AMN107), a Highly Selective Bcr-Abl Tyrosine Kinase Inhibitor, is Effective in Patients With Philadelphia Chromosome-Positive Chronic Myelogenous Leukemia in Chronic Phase Following Imatinib Resistance and Intolerance," *Blood*, 2007, 110(10):3540-6.

Kantarjian H, Giles F, Wunderle L, et al, "Nilotinib in Imatinib-Resistant CML and Philadelphia Chromosome-Positive ALL," *N Engl J Med*, 2006, 354(24):2542-51.

Montemurro M, Schöffski P, Reichardt P, et al, "Nilotinib in the Treatment of Advanced Gastrointestinal Stromal Tumours Resistant to Both Imatinib and Sunitinib," *Eur J Cancer*, 2009, 45 (13):2293-7.

Saglio G, Kim DW, Issaragrisil S, et al, "Nilotinib Versus Imatinib for Newly Diagnosed Chronic Myeloid Leukemia," *N Engl J Med*, 2010, 362(24):2251-9.

◆ **Nilotinib Hydrochloride Monohydrate** *see* Nilotinib *on page 1031*

Nilutamide (ni LOO to mide)

Related Information

Safe Handling of Hazardous Drugs *on page 1904*

Brand Names: U.S. Nilandron®

Brand Names: Canada Anandron®

Index Terms RU-23908

Generic Availability (U.S.) No

Pharmacologic Category Antiandrogen; Antineoplastic Agent, Antiandrogen

Use Treatment of metastatic prostate cancer (in combination with surgical castration)

Labeled Contraindications Hypersensitivity to nilutamide or any component of the formulation; severe hepatic impairment; severe respiratory insufficiency

Pregnancy Risk Factor C

Warnings/Precautions Hazardous agent - use appropriate precautions for handling and disposal. **[U.S. Boxed Warning]: Interstitial pneumonitis has been reported in 2% of patients exposed to nilutamide.** Symptoms typically include exertional dyspnea, cough, chest pain and fever; interstitial changes (including pulmonary fibrosis) leading to hospitalization and fatalities have been reported (rarely). The suggestive signs of pneumonitis most often occurred within the first 3 months of treatment. X-rays showed interstitial or alveolo-interstitial changes; pulmonary function tests revealed a restrictive pattern with decreased DLco. Consider baseline pulmonary function testing. Discontinue if signs and/or symptoms of interstitial pneumonitis are noted.

Hepatitis or marked increases in liver enzymes leading to drug discontinuation occurred in 1% of nilutamide patients; rare cases of hospitalization or deaths due to severe liver injury have been reported. Discontinue treatment for jaundice or ALT >2 times the upper limit of normal (ULN).

A delay in adaptation to dark has been reported; in clinical studies, this was reported by 13% to 57% of patients; the delay ranged from seconds to a few minutes after passing from a light to a dark area (this may not abate with continued treatment although may be alleviated by wearing tinted sunglasses); caution patients who experience adaptation delay about driving at night or through tunnels. Not indicated for use in women. Patients with disease progression while receiving antiandrogen therapy may experience clinical improvement with discontinuation of the antiandrogen.

Adverse Reactions

>10%:

Central nervous system: Insomnia (16%), headache (14%)
Endocrine & metabolic: Hot flashes (28% to 67%)
Gastrointestinal: Nausea (10% to 24%), constipation (7% to 20%), anorexia (11%), abdominal pain (10%)
Genitourinary: Testicular atrophy (16%), libido decreased (11%)
Hepatic: AST increased (8% to 13%), ALT increased (8% to 9%)
Ocular: Impaired dark adaptation (13% to 57%)
Respiratory: Dyspnea (6% to 11%)

1% to 10%:

Cardiovascular: Hypertension (5% to 9%), chest pain (7%), heart failure (3%), angina (2%), edema (2%), syncope (2%)
Central nervous system: Dizziness (7% to 10%), depression (9%), hypoesthesia (5%), malaise (2%), nervousness (2%)
Dermatologic: Alopecia (6%), dry skin (5%), rash (5%), pruritus (2%)
Endocrine & metabolic: Alcohol intolerance (5%), hyperglycemia (4%)
Gastrointestinal: Vomiting (6%), diarrhea (2%), GI hemorrhage (2%), melena (2%), weight loss (2%), xerostomia (2%), dyspepsia
Genitourinary: Nocturia (7%)
Hematologic: Anemia (7%), haptoglobin increased (2%), leukopenia (2%)
Hepatic: Alkaline phosphatase increased (3%)
Neuromuscular & skeletal: Bone pain (6%), arthritis (2%), paresthesia (2%)
Ocular: Chromatopsia (9%), impaired light adaptation (8%), abnormal vision (6% to 7%), cataract (2%), photophobia (2%)
Renal: Hematuria (8%), BUN increased (2%), creatinine increased (2%)
Respiratory: Pneumonia (5%), cough (2%), interstitial pneumonitis (2%), rhinitis (2%)
Miscellaneous: Flu-like syndrome (7%), diaphoresis (6%)

<1%, postmarketing, and/or case reports: Aplastic anemia, hepatitis

Drug Interactions

Metabolism/Transport Effects **Substrate** of CYP2C19 (major); **Note:** Assignment of Major/Minor substrate status based on clinically relevant drug interaction potential; **Inhibits** CYP2C19 (weak)

Avoid Concomitant Use There are no known interactions where it is recommended to avoid concomitant use.

Increased Effect/Toxicity

The levels/effects of Nilutamide may be increased by: CYP2C19 Inhibitors (Moderate); CYP2C19 Inhibitors (Strong)

Decreased Effect

The levels/effects of Nilutamide may be decreased by: CYP2C19 Inducers (Strong)

Ethanol/Nutrition/Herb Interactions Ethanol: Approximately 5% of patients experience an intolerance (facial flushing, hypotension, malaise) when ethanol is combined with nilutamide. Management: Avoid ethanol.

Storage/Stability Store at room temperature of 25°C (77°F); excursions permitted between 15°C to 30°C (59°F to 86°F). Protect from light.

Mechanism of Action Nonsteroidal antiandrogen which blocks testosterone effects at the androgen receptor level, preventing androgen response.

Pharmacodynamics/Kinetics

Absorption: Rapid and complete

Metabolism: Hepatic (extensive), forms active metabolites

Half-life elimination: Terminal: 38-59 hours; Metabolites: 59-126 hours

Excretion: Urine (62%; <2% as unchanged drug); feces (1% to 7%)

Dosing

Adult & Geriatric Prostate cancer, metastatic: Oral: 300 mg once daily (starting the same day or day after surgical castration) for 30 days, followed by 150 mg once daily

Hepatic Impairment

Prior to treatment initiation: Severe hepatic impairment: Use is contraindicated.

During treatment: ALT >2 times ULN or jaundice: Discontinue treatment.

Administration Administer without regard to meals.

Monitoring Parameters Hepatic enzymes (at baseline, regularly during the first 4 months of treatment, periodically thereafter); chest x-ray (at baseline); consider pulmonary function testing (at baseline)

Dietary Considerations May be taken without regard to meals.

Dosage Forms Excipient information presented when available (limited, particularly for generics); consult specific product labeling.

Tablet, oral:

Nilandron®: 150 mg

References

Bertagna C, DeGery A, Hucher M, et al, "Efficacy of the Combination of Nilutamide Plus Orchidectomy in Patients With Metastatic Prostatic Cancer, A Meta-Analysis of Seven Randomized Double Blind Trials (1056 Patients)," *Br J Urol*, 1994, 73(4):396-402.

Dijkman GA, Janknegt RA, De Reijke TM, et al, "Long-Term Efficacy and Safety of Nilutamide Plus Castration in Advanced Prostate Cancer, and the Significance of Early Prostate Specific Antigen Normalization. International Anandron Study Group," *J Urol*, 1997, 158(1):160-3

Du Plessis DJ, "Castration Plus Nilutamide Vs Castration Plus Placebo in Advanced Prostate Cancer. A Review, *Urology*, 1991, 37(2 Suppl):20-4.

◆ **Nipent®** *see* Pentostatin *on page 1161*

◆ **Nitrogen Mustard** *see* Mechlorethamine *on page 913*

◆ **4'-Nitro-3'-Trifluoromethylisobutyrantide** *see* Flutamide *on page 635*

◆ **N-Methylhydrazine** *see* Procarbazine *on page 1208*

◆ **N-methylnaltrexone Bromide** *see* Methylnaltrexone *on page 964*

◆ **Nolvadex** *see* Tamoxifen *on page 1324*

- **Nolvadex®-D (Can)** *see* Tamoxifen *on page 1324*
- **Nordeoxyguanosine** *see* Ganciclovir (Systemic) *on page 656*
- **Novantrone** *see* MitoXANtrone *on page 996*
- **Novel Erythropoiesis-Stimulating Protein** *see* Darbepoetin Alfa *on page 382*
- **Novo-Benzydamine (Can)** *see* Benzydamine *on page 164*
- **Novo-Bicalutamide (Can)** *see* Bicalutamide *on page 178*
- **Novo-Ciprofloxacin (Can)** *see* Ciprofloxacin (Systemic) *on page 283*
- **Novo-Cyproterone (Can)** *see* Cyproterone *on page 344*
- **Novo-Desmopressin (Can)** *see* Desmopressin *on page 434*
- **Novo-Fentanyl (Can)** *see* FentaNYL *on page 583*
- **Novo-Fluconazole (Can)** *see* Fluconazole *on page 612*
- **Novo-Flutamide (Can)** *see* Flutamide *on page 635*
- **Novo-Hydroxyzin (Can)** *see* HydrOXYzine *on page 736*
- **Novo-Ketoconazole (Can)** *see* Ketoconazole (Systemic) *on page 848*
- **Novo-Levofloxacin (Can)** *see* Levofloxacin (Systemic) *on page 883*
- **Novo-Lorazem (Can)** *see* LORazepam *on page 907*
- **Novo-Medrone (Can)** *see* MedroxyPROGESTERone *on page 916*
- **Novo-Morphine SR (Can)** *see* Morphine (Systemic) *on page 1004*
- **Novo-Mycophenolate (Can)** *see* Mycophenolate *on page 1015*
- **Novo-Ofloxacin (Can)** *see* Ofloxacin (Systemic) *on page 1053*
- **Novo-Peridol (Can)** *see* Haloperidol *on page 691*
- **Novo-Prednisolone (Can)** *see* PrednisoLONE (Systemic) *on page 1193*
- **Novo-Prednisone (Can)** *see* PredniSONE *on page 1199*
- **Novo-Purol (Can)** *see* Allopurinol *on page 51*
- **Novo-Raloxifene (Can)** *see* Raloxifene *on page 1222*
- **NovoSeven® RT** *see* Factor VIIa (Recombinant) *on page 568*
- **Novo-Trimel (Can)** *see* Sulfamethoxazole and Trimethoprim *on page 1302*
- **Novo-Trimel D.S. (Can)** *see* Sulfamethoxazole and Trimethoprim *on page 1302*
- **Noxafil®** *see* Posaconazole *on page 1187*
- **Nplate®** *see* RomiPLOStim *on page 1257*
- ***N*-trifluoroacetyladriamycin-14-valerate** *see* Valrubicin *on page 1425*
- **Nu-Acyclovir (Can)** *see* Acyclovir (Systemic) *on page 30*
- **Nu-Cotrimox (Can)** *see* Sulfamethoxazole and Trimethoprim *on page 1302*
- **Nu-Hydroxyzine (Can)** *see* HydrOXYzine *on page 736*
- **Nulecit™ [DSC]** *see* Ferric Gluconate *on page 597*
- **Nu-Loraz (Can)** *see* LORazepam *on page 907*
- **Nu-Megestrol (Can)** *see* Megestrol *on page 922*
- **Nu-Metoclopramide (Can)** *see* Metoclopramide *on page 974*
- **Numoisyn™** *see* Saliva Substitute *on page 1266*
- **Nu-Prochlor (Can)** *see* Prochlorperazine *on page 1212*
- **Nutracort** *see* Hydrocortisone (Topical) *on page 719*

◆ **Nyaderm (Can)** *see* Nystatin (Topical) *on page* 1042

◆ **Nyamyc®** *see* Nystatin (Topical) *on page* 1042

Nystatin (Oral) (nye STAT in)

Brand Names: Canada PMS-Nystatin

Generic Availability (U.S.) Yes

Pharmacologic Category Antifungal Agent, Oral Nonabsorbed

Use Treatment of susceptible cutaneous, mucocutaneous, and oral cavity fungal infections normally caused by the *Candida* species

Labeled Contraindications Hypersensitivity to nystatin or any component of the formulation

Pregnancy Risk Factor C

Lactation Excretion in breast milk unknown/use caution

Storage/Stability

Tablet and suspension: Store at controlled room temperature of 15°C to 25°C (59°F to 77°F).

Powder for suspension: Store under refrigeration at 2°C to 8°C (36°F to 46°F).

Mechanism of Action Binds to sterols in fungal cell membrane, changing the cell wall permeability allowing for leakage of cellular contents

Pharmacodynamics/Kinetics

Onset of action: Symptomatic relief from candidiasis: 24-72 hours

Absorption: Poorly absorbed

Excretion: Feces (as unchanged drug)

Dosing

Adult & Geriatric

Oral candidiasis: Suspension (swish and swallow): 400,000-600,000 units 4 times/day; swish in the mouth and retain for as long as possible (several minutes) before swallowing

Intestinal infections: Oral tablets: 500,000-1,000,000 units every 8 hours

Note: Powder for compounding: 1/8 teaspoon (500,000 units) to equal approximately 1/2 cup of water; give 4 times/day

Pediatric Oral candidiasis:

Suspension:

Premature infants: 100,000 units 4 times/day; paint suspension into recesses of the mouth

Infants: 200,000 units 4 times/day or 100,000 units to each side of mouth 4 times/day; paint suspension into recesses of the mouth

Children: 400,000-600,000 units 4 times/day; swish in the mouth and retain for as long as possible (several minutes) before swallowing

Powder for compounding: Children: Refer to adult dosing.

Administration Suspension: Shake well before using. Should be swished about the mouth and retained in the mouth for as long as possible (several minutes) before swallowing. For neonates and infants, paint nystatin suspension into recesses of the mouth.

Dosage Forms Excipient information presented when available (limited, particularly for generics); consult specific product labeling.

Powder, for prescription compounding: 50 million units (10 g); 150 million units (30 g); 500 million units (100 g)

Suspension, oral: 100,000 units/mL (5 mL, 60 mL, 473 mL, 480 mL)

Tablet, oral: 500,000 units

Nystatin (Topical) (nye STAT in)

Brand Names: U.S. Nyamyc®; Nystop®; Pedi-Dri®; Pediaderm™ AF

Brand Names: Canada Candistatin®; Nyaderm

Generic Availability (U.S.) Yes

Pharmacologic Category Antifungal Agent, Topical; Antifungal Agent, Vaginal

Use Treatment of susceptible cutaneous and mucocutaneous fungal infections normally caused by the *Candida* species

Labeled Contraindications Hypersensitivity to nystatin or any component of the formulation

Pregnancy Risk Factor A (vaginal)/C (topical)

Lactation Excretion in breast milk unknown/not recommended

Storage/Stability

Cream: Store at room temperature; avoid excessive heat (40°C/104°F).

Ointment: Store at controlled room temperature of 15°C to 30°C (59°F to 86°F). Do not freeze.

Topical powder: Store at 20°C to 25°C (68°F to 77°F); avoid excessive heat (40°C/104°F).

Vaginal tablet: Store at 20°C to 25°C (68°F to 77°F).

Mechanism of Action Binds to sterols in fungal cell membrane, changing the cell wall permeability allowing for leakage of cellular contents

Pharmacodynamics/Kinetics

Onset of action: Symptomatic relief from candidiasis: 24-72 hours

Absorption: None through mucous membranes or intact skin

Excretion: Feces (as unchanged drug)

Dosing

Adult & Geriatric

Mucocutaneous infections: Topical: Apply 2-3 times/day to affected areas; very moist topical lesions are treated best with powder.

Vaginal infections: Vaginal tablets: Insert 1 tablet/day at bedtime for 2 weeks. (May also be given orally.)

Pediatric Mucocutaneous infections: Children: Refer to adult dosing.

Dosage Forms Excipient information presented when available (limited, particularly for generics); consult specific product labeling. [DSC] = Discontinued product

Cream, topical: 100,000 units/g (15 g, 30 g)

Cream, topical [kit]:

Pediaderm™ AF: 100,000 units/g (30 g) [packaged with protective emollient]

Ointment, topical: 100,000 units/g (15 g, 30 g)

Powder, topical: 100,000 units/g (15 g, 30 g, 60 g)

Nyamyc®: 100,000 units/g (15 g, 30 g, 60 g) [contains talc]

Nystop®: 100,000 units/g (15 g, 30 g, 60 g) [contains talc]

Pedi-Dri®: 100,000 units/g (56.7 g) [contains talc]

Tablet, vaginal: 100,000 units [DSC]

◆ **Nystop®** *see* Nystatin (Topical) *on page 1042*

◆ **Oasis®** *see* Saliva Substitute *on page 1266*

◆ **Octagam®** *see* Immune Globulin *on page 777*

◆ **Octostim® (Can)** *see* Desmopressin *on page 434*

◆ **OctreoScan®** *see* Indium In-111 Pentetreotide *on page 788*

◆ **OctreoScan® (Prep Kit)** *see* Indium In-111 Pentetreotide *on page 788*

Octreotide (ok TREE oh tide)

Brand Names: U.S. SandoSTATIN LAR®; SandoSTATIN®

Brand Names: Canada Octreotide Acetate Injection; Octreotide Acetate Omega; Sandostatin LAR®; Sandostatin®

Index Terms Longastatin; Octreotide Acetate

Generic Availability (U.S.) Yes: Excludes depot formulation

Pharmacologic Category Antidiarrheal; Antidote; Somatostatin Analog

Use Control of symptoms (diarrhea and flushing) in patients with metastatic carcinoid tumors; treatment of watery diarrhea associated with vasoactive intestinal peptide-secreting tumors (VIPomas); treatment of acromegaly

Unlabeled Use Treatment of AIDS-associated diarrhea (including *Cryptosporidiosis*), chemotherapy-induced diarrhea, graft-versus-host disease (GVHD) associated diarrhea, postgastrectomy dumping syndrome; control of bleeding of esophageal varices; second-line treatment for thymic malignancies; Cushing's syndrome (ectopic); insulinomas; small bowel fistulas; islet cell tumors; Zollinger-Ellison syndrome; congenital hyperinsulinism; hypothalamic obesity; treatment of hypoglycemia secondary to sulfonylurea poisoning; treatment of malignant bowel obstruction

Labeled Contraindications Hypersensitivity to octreotide or any component of the formulation

Pregnancy Risk Factor B

Lactation Excretion in breast milk unknown/use caution

Warnings/Precautions May impair gallbladder function; monitor patients for cholelithiasis. The incidence of gallbladder stone or biliary sludge increases with a duration of therapy of ≥12 months. In patients with neuroendocrine tumors, the NCCN guidelines (v.1.2011) recommend considering prophylactic cholecystectomy in patients undergoing abdominal surgery if octreotide treatment is planned. Use with caution in patients with renal and/or hepatic impairment; dosage adjustment is required in patients receiving dialysis and in patients with established cirrhosis. Somatostatin analogs may affect glucose regulation. In type I diabetes, severe hypoglycemia may occur; in type II diabetes or patients without diabetes, hyperglycemia may occur. Insulin and other hypoglycemic medication requirements may change. Octreotide may worsen hypoglycemia in patients with insulinomas; use with caution. Do not use depot formulation for the treatment of sulfonylurea-induced hypoglycemia. Bradycardia, conduction abnormalities, and arrhythmia have been observed in acromegalic and carcinoid syndrome patients; use caution with CHF or concomitant medications that alter heart rate or rhythm. Cardiovascular medication requirements may change. Octreotide may enhance the adverse/toxic effects of other QT_c-prolonging agents. May alter absorption of dietary fats; monitor for pancreatitis. May reduce excessive fluid loss in patients with conditions that cause such loss; monitor for elevations in zinc levels in such patients that are maintained on total parenteral nutrition (TPN). Chronic treatment has been associated with abnormal Schillings test; monitor vitamin B_{12} levels. Suppresses secretion of TSH; monitor for hypothyroidism.

Postmarketing cases of serious and fatal events, including hypoxia and necrotizing enterocolitis, have been reported with octreotide use in children (usually with serious underlying conditions), particularly in children <2 years of age. In studies with octreotide depot, the incidence of cholelithiasis in children is higher than the reported incidences for adults and efficacy was not demonstrated. Therapy may restore fertility; females of childbearing potential should use adequate contraception. Dosage adjustment may be necessary in the elderly; significant increases in elimination half-life have been observed in older adults. Vehicle used in depot injection (polylactide-co-glycolide microspheres) has rarely been associated with retinal artery occlusion in patients with abnormal arteriovenous anastomosis.

Adverse Reactions Adverse reactions vary by route of administration and dosage form. Frequency of cardiac, endocrine, and gastrointestinal adverse reactions was generally higher in acromegalics.

>16%:

Cardiovascular: Sinus bradycardia (19% to 25%), chest pain (≤20%; non-depot formulations)

Central nervous system: Fatigue (1% to 32%), headache (6% to 30%), malaise (16% to 20%), fever (16% to 20%), dizziness (5% to 20%)

Dermatologic: Pruritus (≤18%)

Endocrine & metabolic: Hyperglycemia (2% to 27%)

Gastrointestinal: Abdominal pain (5% to 61%), loose stools (5% to 61%), nausea (5% to 61%), diarrhea (34% to 61%), flatulence (≤38%), cholelithiasis (13% to 38%; length of therapy dependent), biliary sludge (24%; length of therapy dependent), constipation (9% to 21%), vomiting (4% to 21%), biliary duct dilatation (12%)

Local: Injection site pain (2% to 50%; dose and formulation related)

Neuromuscular & skeletal: Back pain (1% to 27%), arthropathy (8% to 19%), myalgia (≤18%)

Respiratory: Upper respiratory infection (10% to 23%), dyspnea (≤20%; non-depot formulations)

Miscellaneous: Antibodies to octreotide (up to 25%; no efficacy change), flu symptoms (1% to 20%)

5% to 15%:

Cardiovascular: Hypertension (≤13%), conduction abnormalities (9% to 10%), arrhythmia (3% to 9%), palpitation, peripheral edema

Central nervous system: Pain (4% to 15%), anxiety, confusion, hypoesthesia, insomnia

Dermatologic: Rash (15%; depot formulation), alopecia (≤13%)

Endocrine & metabolic: Hypothyroidism (≤12%; non-depot formulations), goiter (≤8%; non-depot formulations)

Gastrointestinal: Dyspepsia (4% to 6%), feces discoloration (4% to 6%), steatorrhea (4% to 6%), tenesmus (4% to 6%), anorexia, cramping

Hematologic: Anemia (≤15%; non-depot formulations: <1%)

Neuromuscular & skeletal: Arthralgia, myalgia, paresthesia, rigors, weakness

Otic: Earache

Renal: Renal calculus

Respiratory: Cough, pharyngitis, rhinitis, sinusitis

Miscellaneous: Allergy, diaphoresis

1% to 4%:

Cardiovascular: Angina, cardiac failure, edema, flushing, hematoma, phlebitis

Central nervous system: Abnormal gait, amnesia, depression, dysphonia, hallucinations, nervousness, neuralgia, somnolence, vertigo

Dermatologic: Acne, bruising, cellulitis

Endocrine & metabolic: Hypoglycemia (2% to 4%), hypokalemia, hypoproteinemia, gout, cachexia, breast pain, impotence

Gastrointestinal: Colitis, diverticulitis, dysphagia, fat malabsorption, gastritis, gastroenteritis, gingivitis, glossitis, melena, stomatitis, taste perversion, xerostomia

Genitourinary: Incontinence, pollakiuria (non-depot formulations), urinary tract infection

Local: Injection site hematoma

Neuromuscular & skeletal: Hyperkinesia, hypertonia, joint pain, neuropathy, tremor

Ocular: Blurred vision, visual disturbance

Otic: Tinnitus

Renal: Albuminuria, renal abscess

Respiratory: Bronchitis, epistaxis

Miscellaneous: Bacterial infection, cold symptoms, moniliasis

<1%, postmarketing, and/or case reports: Amenorrhea, anaphylactic shock, anaphylactoid reactions, aneurysm, aphasia, appendicitis, arthritis, ascending cholangitis, ascites, atrial fibrillation, basal cell carcinoma, Bell's palsy, biliary obstruction, breast carcinoma, cardiac arrest, cerebral vascular disorder, CHF, cholecystitis, cholestatic hepatitis, CK increased, creatinine increased, deafness, diabetes insipidus, diabetes mellitus, facial edema, fatty liver, galactorrhea, gallbladder polyp, GI bleeding, GI hemorrhage, GI ulcer, glaucoma, gynecomastia, hearing impairment, hematuria, hemiparesis, hemorrhoids, hepatitis, hyperesthesia, hypertensive reaction, hypoadrenalism, hypoxia (children), intestinal obstruction, intracranial hemorrhage, intraocular pressure increased, iron deficiency, ischemia, jaundice, joint effusion, LFTs increased, libido decreased, malignant hyperpyrexia, MI, migraine, necrotizing enterocolitis (neonates), nephrolithiasis, neuritis, oligomenorrhea, orthostatic hypotension, pancreatitis, pancytopenia, paranoia, paresis, petechiae, pituitary apoplexy, pleural effusion, pneumonia, pneumothorax, polymenorrhea, pulmonary embolism, pulmonary hypertension, pulmonary nodule, QT prolongation, Raynaud's syndrome, rectal bleeding, renal failure, renal insufficiency, retinal vein thrombosis, scotoma, seizures, status asthmaticus, suicide attempt, syncope, tachycardia, thrombocytopenia, thrombophlebitis, thrombosis, urticaria, vaginitis, visual field defect, vitamin B_{12} deficiency, weight loss, wheal/erythema

Drug Interactions

Metabolism/Transport Effects None known.

Avoid Concomitant Use There are no known interactions where it is recommended to avoid concomitant use.

Increased Effect/Toxicity

Octreotide may increase the levels/effects of: Codeine; Highest Risk QTc-Prolonging Agents; Hypoglycemic Agents; Moderate Risk QTc-Prolonging Agents; Pegvisomant

The levels/effects of Octreotide may be increased by: Herbs (Hypoglycemic Properties); MAO Inhibitors; Mifepristone; Salicylates; Selective Serotonin Reuptake Inhibitors

Decreased Effect

Octreotide may decrease the levels/effects of: CycloSPORINE (Systemic)

The levels/effects of Octreotide may be decreased by: Loop Diuretics

Ethanol/Nutrition/Herb Interactions

Food: Octreotide may alter absorption of dietary fats. Management: Administer injections between meals to decrease GI effects.

Herb/Nutraceutical: Some herbal medications may enhance the hypoglycemic effect of octreotide. Management: Avoid hypoglycemic herbs, including alfalfa, aloe, bilberry, bitter melon, burdock, celery, damiana, fenugreek, garcinia, garlic, ginger, ginseng (American), gymnema, marshmallow, and stinging nettle.

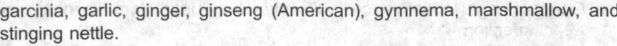

Storage/Stability

Solution: Octreotide is a clear solution and should be stored at refrigerated temperatures between 2°C and 8°C (36°F and 46°F). Protect from light. May be stored at room temperature of 20°C to 30°C (68°F and 86°F) for up to 14 days when protected from light. Stable as a parenteral admixture in NS for 96 hours at room temperature (25°C) and in D_5W for 24 hours. Stable for up to 7 days in a polypropylene syringe. Discard multidose vials within 14 days after initial entry.

Suspension: Prior to dilution, store at refrigerated temperatures between 2°C and 8°C (36°F and 46°F). Protect from light. Additionally, the manufacturer reports that octreotide suspension may be stored at room temperature of 20°C to 25°C (68°F and 77°F) for up to 10 days when protected from light (data on file [Novartis, 2011]). Depot drug product kit may be at room temperature for 30-60 minutes prior to use. Use suspension immediately after preparation.

Mechanism of Action Mimics natural somatostatin by inhibiting serotonin release, and the secretion of gastrin, VIP, insulin, glucagon, secretin, motilin, and pancreatic polypeptide. Decreases growth hormone and IGF-1 in acromegaly. Octreotide provides more potent inhibition of growth hormone, glucagon, and insulin as compared to endogenous somatostatin. Also suppresses LH response to GnRH, secretion of thyroid-stimulating hormone and decreases splanchnic blood flow.

Pharmacodynamics/Kinetics

Duration: SubQ: 6-12 hours

Absorption: SubQ: Rapid and complete; I.M. (depot formulation): Released slowly (via microsphere degradation in the muscle)

Distribution: V_d: 14 L (13-30 L in acromegaly)

Protein binding: 65%, primarily to lipoprotein (41% in acromegaly)

Metabolism: Extensively hepatic

Bioavailability: SubQ: 100%; I.M: 60% to 63% of SubQ dose

Half-life elimination: 1.7-1.9 hours; Increased in elderly patients; Cirrhosis: Up to 3.7 hours; Fatty liver disease: Up to 3.4 hours; Renal impairment: Up to 3.1 hours

Time to peak, plasma: SubQ: 0.4 hours (0.7 hours acromegaly); I.M.: 1 hour

Excretion: Urine (32% as unchanged drug)

Dosing

Adult

Acromegaly:

SubQ, I.V.: Initial: 50 mcg 3 times/day; titrate to achieve growth hormone levels <5 ng/mL or IGF-I (somatomedin C) levels <1.9 units/mL in males and <2.2 units/mL in females. Usual effective dose 100-200 mcg 3 times/day; range 300-1500 mcg/day. **Note:** Should be withdrawn yearly for a 4-week interval (8 weeks for depot injection) in patients who have received irradiation. Resume if levels increase and signs/symptoms recur.

I.M. depot injection: Patients must be stabilized on subcutaneous octreotide for at least 2 weeks before switching to the long-acting depot. Upon switch: 20 mg I.M. intragluteally every 4 weeks for 3 months, then the dose may be modified based upon response.

Dosage adjustment for acromegaly: After 3 months of depot injections, the dosage may be continued or modified as follows:

GH ≤1 ng/mL, IGF-1 normal, and symptoms controlled: Reduce octreotide depot to 10 mg I.M. every 4 weeks

GH ≤2.5 ng/mL, IGF-1 normal, and symptoms controlled: Maintain octreotide depot at 20 mg I.M. every 4 weeks

GH >2.5 ng/mL, IGF-1 elevated, and/or symptoms uncontrolled: Increase octreotide depot to 30 mg I.M. every 4 weeks

Note: Patients not adequately controlled at a dose of 30 mg may increase dose to 40 mg every 4 weeks. Dosages >40 mg are not recommended.

Carcinoid tumors:

Manufacturer labeling:

SubQ, I.V.: Initial 2 weeks: 100-600 mcg/day in 2-4 divided doses; usual range: 50-750 mcg/day (some patients may require up to 1500 mcg/day)

I.M. depot injection: Patients must be stabilized on subcutaneous octreotide for at least 2 weeks before switching to the long-acting depot. Upon switch: 20 mg I.M. intragluteally every 4 weeks for 2 months, then the dose may be modified based upon response.

NCCN guidelines (Neuroendocrine Tumor v.1.2011):

SubQ: 150-250 mcg 3 times/day; dose and frequency may be increased if needed for symptom control

I.M. depot Injection: 20-30 mg every 4 weeks; dose and frequency may be increased if needed for symptom control; SubQ octreotide may be used for breakthrough symptoms

Note: Patients should continue to receive their SubQ injections for the first 2 weeks at the same dose in order to maintain therapeutic levels (some patients may require 3-4 weeks of continued SubQ injections). Patients who experience periodic exacerbations of symptoms may require temporary SubQ injections in addition to depot injections (at their previous SubQ dosing regimen) until symptoms have resolved.

Dosage adjustment for carcinoid tumors: After 2 months of depot injections, the dosage may be continued or modified as follows:

Increase to 30 mg I.M. every 4 weeks if symptoms are inadequately controlled

Decrease to 10 mg I.M. every 4 weeks, for a trial period, if initially responsive to 20 mg dose

Dosage >30 mg is not recommended

VIPomas:

Manufacturer labeling:

SubQ, I.V.: Initial 2 weeks: 200-300 mcg/day in 2-4 divided doses; titrate dose based on response/tolerance. Range: 150-750 mcg/day (doses >450 mcg/day are rarely required)

I.M. depot injection: Patients must be stabilized on subcutaneous octreotide for at least 2 weeks before switching to the long acting depot. Upon switch: 20 mg I.M. intragluteally every 4 weeks for 2 months, then the dose may be modified based upon response.

NCCN guidelines (Neuroendocrine Tumor, v.1.2011):

SubQ: 150-250 mcg 3 times/day; dose and frequency may be increased if needed for symptom control

I.M. depot injection: 20-30 mg every 4 weeks dose and frequency may be increased if needed for symptom control; SubQ octreotide may be used for breakthrough symptoms

Note: Patients receiving depot injection should continue to receive their SubQ injections for the first 2 weeks at the same dose in order to maintain therapeutic levels (some patients may require 3-4 weeks of continued SubQ injections). Patients who experience periodic exacerbations of symptoms may require temporary SubQ injections in addition to depot injections (at their previous SubQ dosing regimen) until symptoms have resolved.

Dosage adjustment for VIPomas: After 2 months of depot injections, the dosage may be continued or modified as follows:

Increase to 30 mg I.M. every 4 weeks if symptoms are inadequately controlled

Decrease to 10 mg I.M. every 4 weeks, for a trial period, if initially responsive to 20 mg dose

Dosage >30 mg is not recommended

Diarrhea (unlabeled use): I.V.: Initial: 50-100 mcg every 8 hours; increase by 100 mcg/dose at 48-hour intervals; maximum dose: 500 mcg every 8 hours

Diarrhea associated with chemotherapy (unlabeled use):

Low grade or uncomplicated: SubQ: 100-150 mcg every 8 hours (Benson, 2004; Kornblau, 2000)

Severe: Initial: SubQ: 100-150 mcg every 8 hours; may increase to 500-1500 mcg I.V. or SubQ every 8 hours (Kornblau, 2000)

Complicated: I.V., SubQ: Initial: 100-150 mcg 3 times/day or I.V. Infusion: 25-50 mcg/hour; may escalate to 500 mcg 3 times/day until controlled (Benson, 2004)

Diarrhea associated with GVHD (unlabeled use): I.V.: 500 mcg every 8 hours; discontinue within 24 hours of resolution; Maximum duration of therapy if diarrhea is not resolved: 7 days (Kornblau, 2000)

Esophageal varices bleeding (unlabeled use): I.V. bolus: 25-100 mcg (usual bolus dose: 50 mcg) followed by continuous I.V. infusion of 25-50 mcg/hour for 2-5 days; may repeat bolus in first hour if hemorrhage not controlled (Corley, 2001; Erstad, 2001; Garcia-Tsao, 2010)

Hypoglycemia in sulfonylurea poisoning (unlabeled use): SubQ is the preferred route of administration; repeat dosing, dose escalation, or initiation of a continuous infusion may be required in patients who experience recurrent hypoglycemia. Duration of treatment may exceed 24 hours. Optimal care decisions should be made based upon patient-specific details:

SubQ: 50-100 mcg; repeat in 6-12 hours as needed based upon blood glucose concentrations (Braatvedt, 1997; Carr, 2002; Graudins, 1997; Hung, 1997)

I.V.: Doses up to 100-125 mcg/hour have been used successfully (McLaughlin, 2000)

Islet cell tumors (unlabeled use): SubQ: 150-250 mcg 3 times/day or I.M. (depot): 20-30 mg every 4 weeks dose and frequency may be increased if needed for symptom control; SubQ octreotide may be used for breakthrough symptoms (NCCN Neuroendocrine Tumor guidelines v.1.2011)

Malignant bowel obstruction (unlabeled use):

SubQ: 100-300 mcg 2-3 times/day (Mercadante, 2007; NCCN Palliative Care guidelines v.2.2011)

Continuous SubQ/I.V. infusion: 10-40 mcg/hour (NCCN Palliative Care guidelines v.2.2011)

Geriatric Refer to adult dosing. Elimination half-life is increased by 46% and clearance is decreased by 26%; dose adjustment may be required. Dosing should generally begin at the lower end of dosing range.

Pediatric Infants and Children:

Secretory diarrhea (unlabeled use): I.V., SubQ: Doses of 1-10 mcg/kg every 12 hours have been used in children beginning at the low end of the range and increasing by 0.3 mcg/kg/dose at 3-day intervals. Suppression of growth hormone (animal data) is of concern when used as long-term therapy.

Congenital hyperinsulinism (unlabeled use): SubQ: Initial: 2-10 mcg/kg/day; up to 40 mcg/kg/day have been used (Stanley, 1997).

Hypoglycemia in sulfonylurea poisoning (unlabeled use): SubQ is the preferred route of administration; repeat dosing, dose escalation, or initiation of a continuous infusion may be required in patients who experience recurrent hypoglycemia. Duration of treatment may exceed 24 hours. Optimal care decisions should be made based upon patient-specific details: SubQ: 1-1.5 mcg/kg; repeat in 6-12 hours as needed based upon blood glucose concentrations (Calello, 2005; Glatstein, 2009).

Renal Impairment

Nondialysis-dependent renal impairment: No dosage adjustment required

Dialysis-dependent renal impairment: Depot injection: Initial dose: 10 mg I.M. every 4 weeks; titrate based upon response (clearance is reduced by ~50%)

Hepatic Impairment Patients with established cirrhosis of the liver: Depot injection: Initial dose: 10 mg I.M. every 4 weeks; titrate based upon response.

Usual Infusion Concentrations: Adult I.V. infusion: 500 mcg in 250 mL (concentration: 2 **mcg**/mL) of D_5W or NS

Administration

Regular injection formulation (do not use if solution contains particles or is discolored): Administer SubQ or I.V.; I.V. administration may be I.V. push (undiluted over 3 minutes), intermittent I.V. infusion (over 15-30 minutes), or continuous I.V. infusion (unlabeled route).

SubQ: Use the concentration with smallest volume to deliver dose to reduce injection site pain. Rotate injection site; may bring to room temperature prior to injection.

Depot formulation: Administer I.M. intragluteal (avoid deltoid administration); alternate gluteal injection sites to avoid irritation. **Do not** administer Sandostatin LAR® intravenously or subcutaneously; must be administered immediately after mixing.

Monitoring Parameters

Acromegaly: Growth hormone, somatomedin C (IGF-1)

Carcinoid: 5 HIAA, plasma serotonin and plasma substance P

VIPomas: Vasoactive intestinal peptide

Chronic therapy: Thyroid function (baseline and periodic), vitamin B_{12} level, blood glucose, glycemic control and antidiabetic regimen (patients with diabetes mellitus), cardiac function (heart rate, ECG), zinc level (patients with excessive fluid loss maintained on TPN)

Dietary Considerations Schedule injections between meals to decrease GI effects. May alter absorption of dietary fats.

Dosage Forms Excipient information presented when available (limited, particularly for generics); consult specific product labeling.

Injection, microspheres for suspension [depot formulation]:

SandoSTATIN LAR®: 10 mg, 20 mg, 30 mg [contains polylactide-co-glycolide; supplied with diluent]

Injection, solution: 100 mcg/mL (1 mL); 200 mcg/mL (5 mL); 1000 mcg/mL (5 mL)

SandoSTATIN®: 200 mcg/mL (5 mL); 1000 mcg/mL (5 mL)

Injection, solution [preservative free]: 50 mcg/mL (1 mL); 100 mcg/mL (1 mL); 200 mcg/mL (5 mL); 500 mcg/mL (1 mL)

SandoSTATIN®: 50 mcg/mL (1 mL); 100 mcg/mL (1 mL); 500 mcg/mL (1 mL)

References

Benson AB 3rd, Ajani JA, Catalano RB, et al, "Recommended Guidelines for the Treatment of Cancer Treatment-Induced Diarrhea," *J Clin Oncol*, 2004, 22(14):2918-26.

Braatvedt GD, "Octreotide for the Treatment of Sulphonylurea Induced Hypoglycaemia in Type 2 Diabetes," *N Z Med J*, 1997, 110(1044):189-90.

Calello DP, Osterhoudt KC, Henretig FM, et al, "Octreotide for Pediatric Sulfonylurea Overdose: Review of 5 Cases," *Clin Toxicol*, 2005, 43:671.

Carr R and Zed PJ, "Octreotide for Sulfonylurea-Induced Hypoglycemia Following Overdose," *Ann Pharmacother*, 2002, 36(11):1727-32.

Corley DA, Cello JP, Adkisson W, et al, "Octreotide for Acute Esophageal Variceal Bleeding: A Meta-analysis," *Gastroenterology*, 2001, 120(4):946-54.

Erstad BL, "Octreotide for Acute Variceal Bleeding," *Ann Pharmacother*, 2001, 35(5):618-26.

Garcia-Tsao G and Bosch J, "Management of Varices and Variceal Hemorrhage in Cirrhosis," *N Engl J Med*, 2010, 362(9):823-32.

Glatstein M, Garcia-Bournissen F, Scolnik D, et al, "Hypoglycemia in a Healthy Toddler," *Ther Drug Monit*, 2009, 31(2):173-7.

Graudins A, Linden CH, and Ferm RP, "Diagnosis and Treatment of Sulfonylurea-Induced Hyperinsulinemic Hypoglycemia," *Am J Emerg Med*, 1997, 15(1):95-6.

Hung O, Eng J, Ho J, "Octreotide as an Antidote for Refractory Sulfonylurea Hypoglycemia," *Clin Toxicol*, 1997, 35(5), 540-1.

Kornblau S, Benson AB, Catalano R, et al, "Management of Cancer Treatment-Related Diarrhea. Issues and Therapeutic Strategies," *J Pain Symptom Manage*, 2000, 19(2):118-29.

Maroun JA, Anthony LB, Blais N, et al, 'Prevention and Management of Chemotherapy-Induced Diarrhea in Patients With Colorectal Cancer: A Consensus Statement by the Canadian Working Group on Chemotherapy-Induced Diarrhea," *Curr Oncol*, 2007, 14(1):13-20.

McLaughlin SA, Crandall CS, and McKinney PE, "Octreotide: An Antidote for Sulfonylurea-Induced Hypoglycemia," *Ann Emerg Med*, 2000, 36(2):133-6.

Mercadante S, Casuccio A, and Mangione S, "Medical Treatment for Inoperable Malignant Bowel Obstruction: A Qualitative Systematic Review," *J Pain Symptom Manage*, 2007, 33(2):217-23.

National Comprehensive Cancer Network® (NCCN), "Clinical Practice Guidelines in Oncology™: Neuroendocrine Tumors," Version 1.2011. Available at http://www.nccn.org/professionals/physician_gls/PDF/neuroendocrine.pdf

National Comprehensive Cancer Network® (NCCN), "Clinical Practice Guidelines in Oncology™: Palliative Care," Version 2.2011. Available at http://www.nccn.org/professionals/physician_gls/PDF/palliative.pdf

Rinke A, Müller HH, Schade-Brittinger C, et al, "Placebo-Controlled, Double-Blind, Prospective, Randomized Study on the Effect of Octreotide LAR in the Control of Tumor Growth in Patients With Metastatic Neuroendocrine Midgut Tumors: A Report From the PROMID Study Group," *J Clin Oncol*, 2009, 27(28):4656-63.

Stanley CA, "Hyperinsulinism in Infants and Children," *Pediatr Clin North Am*, 1997, 44(2):363-74.

◆ **Octreotide Acetate** *see* Octreotide *on page 1043*

◆ **Octreotide Acetate Injection (Can)** *see* Octreotide *on page 1043*

◆ **Octreotide Acetate Omega (Can)** *see* Octreotide *on page 1043*

Ofatumumab (oh fa TOOM yoo mab)

Related Information

Management of Chemotherapy-Induced Nausea and Vomiting *on page 1786*

Principles of Anticancer Therapy *on page 1878*

Brand Names: U.S. Arzerra™

Index Terms HuMax-CD20

Generic Availability (U.S.) No

Pharmacologic Category Antineoplastic Agent, Monoclonal Antibody; Monoclonal Antibody

Use Treatment of refractory chronic lymphocytic leukemia (CLL)

Labeled Contraindications There are no contraindications listed within the manufacturer's labeling.

Pregnancy Risk Factor C

Lactation Excretion in breast milk unknown/use caution

Warnings/Precautions May cause serious infusion reaction; reactions may include bronchospasm, dyspnea, laryngeal edema, pulmonary edema, flushing, hypertension, hypotension, syncope, cardiac ischemia/infarction, back pain, abdominal pain, fever, rash, urticaria, and/or angioedema. Premedicate prior to infusion; interrupt infusion for reaction (and institute appropriate treatment) for reaction; may require subsequent rate modification.

Severe and prolonged (≥1 week) cytopenias (neutropenia and thrombocytopenia) may occur. Monitor blood counts during treatment; more frequently if grade 3 or 4 cytopenias develop. Progressive multifocal leukoencephalopathy (PML) may occur with treatment and should be considered in any patient with new onset or worsening neurological symptoms; if PML is suspected, discontinue and evaluate promptly. Small intestine obstruction may occur with treatment; evaluate if suspected.

Reactivation of hepatitis B (including fulminant hepatitis and death) has occurred with ofatumumab; patients at high risk for hepatitis B should be screened prior to treatment initiation. Hepatitis B carriers should be closely monitored for signs of active hepatitis B infection during and for 6-12 months after completion of treatment. Use in patients with active viral hepatitis has not been sufficiently studied; discontinue (and institute appropriate treatment) in patients who develop viral hepatitis or reactivation of viral hepatitis.

Live vaccines should not be given concurrently with ofatumumab; there is no data concerning secondary transmission; the ability to generate an immune response to any vaccine following treatment is unknown.

Adverse Reactions

>10%:

Central nervous system: Fever (20%), fatigue (15%)

Dermatologic: Rash (14%)

Gastrointestinal: Diarrhea (18%), nausea (11%)

Hematologic: Neutropenia (≥grade 3: 42%; grade 4: 18%; may be prolonged >2 weeks), anemia (16%; grades 3/4: 5%)

Respiratory: Pneumonia (23%), cough (19%), dyspnea (14%), bronchitis (11%), upper respiratory tract infection (11%)

Miscellaneous: Infection (70%; includes bacterial, fungal or viral; ≥grade 3: 29%), infusion reaction (first infusion [300 mg]: 44%; second infusion [2000 mg]: 29%)

1% to 10%:

Cardiovascular: Peripheral edema (9%), hypertension (5%), hypotension (5%), tachycardia (5%)

Central nervous system: Chills (8%), insomnia (7%), headache (6%)

Dermatologic: Urticaria (8%), hyperhidrosis (5%)

Neuromuscular & skeletal: Back pain (8%), muscle spasm (5%)

Respiratory: Nasopharyngitis (8%), sinusitis (5%)

Miscellaneous: Sepsis (8%), herpes zoster (6%)

<1%, postmarketing, and/or case reports: Abdominal pain, angina, bacteremia, cytolytic hepatitis, hemolytic anemia, hypoxia, interstitial lung disease (infectious), laryngeal edema, neutropenic sepsis, peritonitis, pharyngolaryngeal pain, pruritus, rigors, septic shock, throat tightness, thrombocytopenia

Drug Interactions

Metabolism/Transport Effects None known.

Avoid Concomitant Use

Avoid concomitant use of Ofatumumab with any of the following: BCG; Belimumab; Natalizumab; Pimecrolimus; Tacrolimus (Topical); Vaccines (Live)

Increased Effect/Toxicity

Ofatumumab may increase the levels/effects of: Belimumab; Leflunomide; Natalizumab; Vaccines (Live); Vitamin K Antagonists

The levels/effects of Ofatumumab may be increased by: Abciximab; Denosumab; Pimecrolimus; Roflumilast; Tacrolimus (Topical); Trastuzumab

Decreased Effect

Ofatumumab may decrease the levels/effects of: BCG; Cardiac Glycosides; Coccidioidin Skin Test; Sipuleucel-T; Vaccines (Inactivated); Vaccines (Live); Vitamin K Antagonists

The levels/effects of Ofatumumab may be decreased by: Echinacea

Storage/Stability Store intact vials at 2°C to 8°C (36°F to 46°F); do not freeze. Protect from light. Diluted solutions for infusion must be administered within 12 hours of preparation (may store at 2°C to 8°C [36°F to 46°F] if not used immediately); discard any remaining solution 24 hours after preparation.

Reconstitution

300 mg dose: Withdraw 15 mL from a 1000 mL NS bag. Add contents of three ofatumumab 100 mg vials (total volume = 15 mL) to NS bag (final concentration of 0.3 mg/mL). Gently invert to mix; do not shake. Begin infusion within 12 hours of preparation.

2000 mg dose: Withdraw 100 mL from a 1000 mL NS bag. Add contents of two ofatumumab 1000 mg vials (total volume = 100 mL) to NS bag (final concentration of 2 mg/mL). Gently invert to mix; do not shake. Begin infusion within 12 hours of preparation.

Mechanism of Action Ofatumumab is a monoclonal antibody which binds specifically the extracellular (large and small) loops of the CD20 molecule (which is expressed on normal B lymphocytes and in B-cell CLL) resulting in potent complement-dependent cell lysis and antibody-dependent cell-mediated toxicity in cells that overexpress CD20.

Pharmacodynamics/Kinetics

Distribution: V_{dss}: 1.7-5.1 L

Half-life elimination: Between dose 4 and dose 12: ~14 days (range: 2-62 days)

Dosing

Adult & Geriatric Note: Premedicate with acetaminophen, an antihistamine, and a corticosteroid 30-120 minutes prior to treatment (see Administration).

CLL: I.V. Initial dose: 300 mg week 1, followed 1 week later by 2000 mg once weekly for 7 doses (doses 2-8), followed 4 weeks later by 2000 mg once every 4 weeks for 4 doses (doses 9-12; for a total of 12 doses)

Renal Impairment When studied in patients with creatinine clearances ranging from 33-287 mL/minute, baseline creatinine clearance did not have a clinically relevant effect.

Adjustment for Toxicity Infusion reaction: Interrupt infusion for infusion reaction (any severity).

Grade 1 or 2 infusion reaction: Resume at one-half of the previous rate; may increase (see Administration) based on patient tolerance.

Grade 3: Resume infusion at 12 mL/hour; may increase (see Administration) based on patient tolerance.

Grade 4: Do not resume.

Administration **Do not administer I.V. push or as a bolus.** Premedicate with acetaminophen, an antihistamine, and a corticosteroid 30-120 minutes prior to administration. Administer with an in-line filter (supplied) and polyvinyl chloride (PVC) administration sets. Do not mix with or infuse with other medications. Flush line before and after infusion with NS. Begin infusion within 12 hours of preparation. The final concentration of dose 1 is 0.3 mg/mL and final concentration of doses 2-12 is 2 mg/mL.

Premedication: Premedicate with oral acetaminophen (1000 mg), an oral or I.V. antihistamine (eg, cetirizine 10 mg orally or equivalent), and an I.V. corticosteroid. Full dose corticosteroid is recommended for doses 1, 2, and 9; in the absence of infusion reaction ≥grade 3, may gradually reduce corticosteroid dose for doses 3-8; administer full or half corticosteroid dose with doses 10-12 if ≥grade 3 did not occur with dose 9.

Doses 1 and 2: Initiate infusion at 12 mL/hour for 30 minutes, if tolerated (no infusion reaction) increase to 25 mL/hour for 30 minutes, if tolerated, increase to 50 mL/hour for 30 minutes, if tolerated, increase to 100 mL/hour for 30 minutes, if tolerated, increase to 200 mL/hour for duration of infusion.

Doses 3-12: Initiate infusion at 25 mL/hour for 30 minutes, if tolerated (no infusion reaction) increase to 50 mL/hour for 30 minutes, if tolerated, increase to 100 mL/hour for 30 minutes, if tolerated, increase to 200 mL/hour for 30 minutes, if tolerated, increase to 400 mL/hour for remainder of infusion.

Emetic Potential Very low (<10%)

Monitoring Parameters CBC with differential, hepatitis B screening (in patients at high-risk; prior to therapy initiation); signs of active hepatitis B infection (in hepatitis B carriers; during and for 6-12 months after therapy completion); signs or symptoms of infusion reaction, signs of infection

Dosage Forms Excipient information presented when available (limited, particularly for generics); consult specific product labeling.

Injection, solution [concentrate, preservative free]:

Arzerra™: 20 mg/mL (5 mL, 50 mL) [contains edetate disodium, polysorbate 80]

References

Coiffier B, Lepretre S, Pedersen LM, et al, "Safety and Efficacy of Ofatumumab, a Fully Human Monoclonal Anti-CD20 Antibody, in Patients With Relapsed or Refractory B-Cell Chronic Lymphocytic Leukemia: A Phase 1-2 Study," *Blood*, 2008, 111(3):1094-100.

Hagenbeek A, Gadeberg O, Johnson P, et al, "First Clinical Use of Ofatumumab, a Novel Fully Human Anti-CD20 Monoclonal Antibody in Relapsed or Refractory Follicular Lymphoma: Results of a Phase 1/2 Trial," *Blood*, 2008, 111(12):5486-95.

Kipps TJ, Osterborg A, Mayer J, et al, "Clinical Improvement With a Novel CD20 mAb, Ofatumumab, in Fludarabine-Refractory Chronic Lymphocytic Leukemia (CLL) Also Refractory to Alemtuzumab or With Bulky Lymphadenopathy," *J Clin Oncol*, 2009, 27(15s):7043 [abstract 7043 from 2009 ASCO Annual Meeting].

Osterborg A, Kipps TJ, Mayer J, et al, "Ofatumumab (HuMax-CD20), a Novel CD20 Monoclonal Antibody, is an Active Treatment for Patients With CLL Refractory to Both Fludarabine and Alemtuzumab or Bulky Fludarabine Refractory Disease: Results from the Planned Interim Analysis of an International Pivotal Trial," *Blood*, 2008, 112(11):328 [abstract 328 from 2008 ASH Annual Meeting].

Wierda WG, Kipps T, Mayer J, et al, "Activity of Ofatumumab, a Novel CD20 mAb, and Prior Rituximab Exposure in Patients With Fludarabine-and Alemtuzumab-Refractory or Bulky Fludarabine-Refractory Chronic Lymphocytic Leukemia (CLL)," *J Clin Oncol*, 2009, 27(15s):7044 [abstract 7044 from ASCO Annual Meeting].

Ofloxacin (Systemic) (oh FLOKS a sin)

Brand Names: Canada Apo-Oflox®; Novo-Ofloxacin

Generic Availability (U.S.) Yes

Pharmacologic Category Antibiotic, Quinolone

Use Quinolone antibiotic for the treatment of acute exacerbations of chronic bronchitis, community-acquired pneumonia, skin and skin structure infections (uncomplicated), urethral and cervical gonorrhea (acute, uncomplicated), urethritis and cervicitis (nongonococcal), mixed infections of the urethra and cervix, pelvic inflammatory disease (acute), cystitis (uncomplicated), urinary tract infections (complicated), prostatitis

Note: As of April 2007, the CDC no longer recommends the use of fluoroquinolones for the treatment of gonococcal disease.

Unlabeled Use Epididymitis (nongonococcal), leprosy, Traveler's diarrhea

Labeled Contraindications Hypersensitivity to ofloxacin or other members of the quinolone group, such as oxolinic acid, cinoxacin, norfloxacin, and ciprofloxacin; hypersensitivity to any component of the formulation

Pregnancy Risk Factor C

Lactation Enters breast milk/not recommended (AAP rates "compatible"; AAP 2001 update pending)

Warnings/Precautions [U.S. Boxed Warning]: There have been reports of tendon inflammation and/or rupture with quinolone antibiotics; risk may be increased with concurrent corticosteroids, organ transplant recipients, and in patients >60 years of age. Rupture of the Achilles tendon sometimes requiring surgical repair has been reported most frequently; but other tendon sites (eg, rotator cuff, biceps) have also been reported. Strenuous physical activity, rheumatoid arthritis, and renal impairment may be an independent risk factor for tendonitis. Discontinue at first sign of tendon inflammation or pain. May occur even after discontinuation of therapy. Use with caution in patients with rheumatoid arthritis; may increase risk of tendon rupture. CNS effects may occur (tremor, restlessness, confusion, and very rarely hallucinations, increased intracranial pressure [including pseudotumor cerebri] or seizures). Use with caution in patients with known or suspected CNS disorder. Potential for seizures, although very rare, may be increased with concomitant NSAID therapy. Use with caution in individuals at risk of seizures. Use with caution in patients with renal or hepatic impairment. Peripheral neuropathies have been linked to ofloxacin use; discontinue if numbness, tingling, or weakness develops.

Fluoroquinolones have been associated with the development of serious, and sometimes fatal, hypoglycemia, most often in elderly diabetics, but also in patients without diabetes. This occurred most frequently with gatifloxacin (no longer available systemically) but may occur at a lower frequency with other quinolones.

Rare cases of torsade de pointes have been reported in patients receiving ofloxacin and other quinolones. Risk may be minimized by avoiding use in patients with known prolongation of the QT interval, bradycardia, hypokalemia, hypomagnesemia, cardiomyopathy, or in those receiving concurrent therapy with Class Ia or Class III antiarrhythmics.

Severe hypersensitivity reactions, including anaphylaxis, have occurred with quinolone therapy. Reactions may present as typical allergic symptoms after a single dose, or may manifest as severe idiosyncratic dermatologic, vascular, pulmonary, renal, hepatic, and/or hematologic events, usually after multiple doses. Prompt discontinuation of drug should occur if skin rash or other symptoms arise. Prolonged use may result in fungal or bacterial superinfection, including *C. difficile*-associated diarrhea (CDAD) and pseudomembranous colitis; CDAD has been observed >2 months postantibiotic treatment. **[U.S. Boxed Warning]: Quinolones may exacerbate myasthenia gravis; avoid**

use (rare, potentially life-threatening weakness of respiratory muscles may occur). Avoid excessive sunlight and take precautions to limit exposure (eg, loose fitting clothing, sunscreen); may cause moderate-to-severe phototoxicity reactions. Discontinue use if photosensitivity occurs. Since ofloxacin is ineffective in the treatment of syphilis and may mask symptoms, all patients should be tested for syphilis at the time of gonorrheal diagnosis and 3 months later. Hemolytic reactions may (rarely) occur with quinolone use in patients with latent or actual G6PD deficiency. Safety and efficacy have not been established in children.

Ethanol/Nutrition/Herb Interactions

Food: Ofloxacin average peak serum concentrations may be decreased by 20% if taken with food.

Herb/Nutraceutical: Avoid dong quai, St John's wort (may also cause photosensitization).

Storage/Stability Store at 25°C (77°F); excursions permitted to 15°C to 30°C (59°F to 86°F).

Mechanism of Action Ofloxacin is a DNA gyrase inhibitor. DNA gyrase is an essential bacterial enzyme that maintains the superhelical structure of DNA. DNA gyrase is required for DNA replication and transcription, DNA repair, recombination, and transposition; bactericidal

Pharmacodynamics/Kinetics

Absorption: Well absorbed; food causes only minor alterations

Distribution: V_d: 2.4-3.5 L/kg

Protein binding: 32%

Bioavailability: 98%

Half-life elimination: Biphasic: 4-5 hours and 20-25 hours (accounts for <5%); prolonged with renal impairment

Excretion: Primarily urine (as unchanged drug)

Dosing

Adult

Cervicitis/urethritis (nongonococcal): Oral:

Nongonococcal: 300 mg every 12 hours for 7 days

Gonococcal (acute, uncomplicated): 400 mg as a single dose; **Note:** As of April 2007, the CDC no longer recommends the use of fluoroquinolones for the treatment of uncomplicated gonococcal disease.

Chronic bronchitis (acute exacerbation), community-acquired pneumonia, skin and skin structure infections (uncomplicated): Oral: 400 mg every 12 hours for 10 days

Epididymitis, nongonococcal (unlabeled use): Oral: 300 mg twice daily for 10 days (CDC, 2010); 200 mg twice daily for 14 days (Canadian STI Guidelines, 2008)

Leprosy (unlabeled use): Oral: 400 mg once daily

Pelvic inflammatory disease (acute): Oral: 400 mg every 12 hours for 10-14 days; **Note:** The CDC recommends use only if standard cephalosporin therapy is not feasible and community prevalence of quinolone-resistant gonococcal organisms is low. Culture sensitivity must be confirmed.

Prostatitis: Oral:

Acute: 400 mg for 1 dose, then 300 mg twice daily for 10 days

Chronic: 200 mg every 12 hours for 6 weeks

Traveler's diarrhea (unlabeled use): Oral: 300 mg twice daily for 3 days

UTI: Oral:

Uncomplicated: 200 mg every 12 hours for 3-7 days

Complicated: 200 mg every 12 hours for 10 days

Geriatric Oral: 200-400 mg every 12-24 hours (based on estimated renal function) for 7 days to 6 weeks depending on indication.

Renal Impairment Adults: Oral: After a normal initial dose, adjust as follows:

Cl_{cr} 20-50 mL/minute: Administer usual dose every 24 hours

Cl_{cr} <20 mL/minute: Administer half the usual dose every 24 hours

Continuous arteriovenous or venovenous hemodiafiltration effects: Administer 300 mg every 24 hours

Hepatic Impairment Severe impairment: Maximum dose: 400 mg/day

Administration Do not take within 2 hours of food or any antacids which contain zinc, magnesium, or aluminum.

Test Interactions Some quinolones may produce a false-positive urine screening result for opiates using commercially-available immunoassay kits. This has been demonstrated most consistently for levofloxacin and ofloxacin, but other quinolones have shown cross-reactivity in certain assay kits. Confirmation of positive opiate screens by more specific methods should be considered.

Medication Guide Available Yes

Dosage Forms Excipient information presented when available (limited, particularly for generics); consult specific product labeling.

Tablet, oral: 200 mg, 300 mg, 400 mg

OLANZapine (oh LAN za peen)

Related Information

Management of Chemotherapy-Induced Nausea and Vomiting *on page 1786*

Brand Names: U.S. ZyPREXA®; ZyPREXA® IntraMuscular; ZyPREXA® Relprevv™; ZyPREXA® Zydis®

Brand Names: Canada Apo-Olanzapine ODT®; Apo-Olanzapine®; Ava-Olanzapine; CO Olanzapine; CO Olanzapine ODT; Mylan-Olanzapine; Olanzapine ODT; PHL-Olanzapine; PHL-Olanzapine ODT; PMS-Olanzapine; PMS-Olanzapine ODT; Riva-Olanzapine; Riva-Olanzapine ODT; Sandoz-Olanzapine; Sandoz-Olanzapine ODT; Teva-Olanzapine; Teva-Olanzapine OD; Zyprexa®; Zyprexa® Intramuscular; Zyprexa® Zydis®

Index Terms LY170053; Olanzapine Pamoate; Zyprexa Zydis

Generic Availability (U.S.) Yes: Excludes Injection (powder for suspension, extended release)

Pharmacologic Category Antimanic Agent; Antipsychotic Agent, Atypical

Use

Oral: Treatment of the manifestations of schizophrenia; treatment of acute or mixed mania episodes associated with bipolar I disorder (as monotherapy or in combination with lithium or valproate); maintenance treatment of bipolar disorder; in combination with fluoxetine for treatment-resistant or bipolar I depression

I.M., extended-release (Zyprexa® Relprevv™): Treatment of schizophrenia

I.M., short-acting (Zyprexa® IntraMuscular): Treatment of acute agitation associated with schizophrenia and bipolar I mania

Unlabeled Use Treatment of psychosis/schizophrenia in children; chronic pain; prevention of chemotherapy-associated delayed nausea or vomiting; psychosis/agitation related to Alzheimer's dementia; acute treatment of delirium

Labeled Contraindications There are no contraindications listed in the manufacturer's labeling.

Canadian labeling: Hypersensitivity to olanzapine or any component of the formulation

Pregnancy Risk Factor C

Lactation Enters breast milk/not recommended

Warnings/Precautions [U.S. Boxed Warning]: Elderly patients with dementia-related psychosis treated with antipsychotics are at an increased risk of death compared to placebo. Most deaths appeared to be either cardiovascular (eg, heart failure, sudden death) or infectious (eg, pneumonia) in nature. In addition, an increased incidence of cerebrovascular effects (eg, transient ischemic attack, stroke) has been reported in studies of placebo-controlled trials of olanzapine in elderly patients with dementia-related psychosis. Olanzapine is not approved for the treatment of dementia-related psychosis.

Moderate to highly sedating, use with caution in disorders where CNS depression is a feature; patients must be cautioned about performing tasks which require mental alertness (eg, operating machinery or driving). Use caution in patients with cardiac disease. Use with caution in Parkinson's disease, predisposition to seizures, or severe hepatic or renal disease. Life-threatening arrhythmias have occurred with therapeutic doses of some neuroleptics. May induce orthostatic hypotension; use caution with history of cardiovascular disease, hemodynamic instability, prior myocardial infarction, or ischemic heart disease. Increases in cholesterol and triglycerides have been noted. Use with caution in patients with pre-existing abnormal lipid profile. Esophageal dysmotility and aspiration have been associated with antipsychotic use; use with caution in patients at risk of aspiration pneumonia. May increase prolactin levels; clinical significance of hyperprolactinemia in patients with breast cancer or other prolactin-dependent tumors is unknown. Significant weight gain (>7% of baseline weight) may occur; monitor waist circumference and BMI. Impaired core body temperature regulation may occur; caution with strenuous exercise, heat exposure, dehydration, and concomitant medication possessing anticholinergic effects.

Leukopenia, neutropenia, and agranulocytosis (sometimes fatal) have been reported in clinical trials and postmarketing reports with antipsychotic use; presence of risk factors (eg, pre-existing low WBC or history of drug-induced leuko-/neutropenia) should prompt periodic blood count assessment. Discontinue therapy at first signs of blood dyscrasias or if absolute neutrophil count <1000/mm^3.

May cause anticholinergic effects; use with caution in patients with decreased gastrointestinal motility, urinary retention, BPH, xerostomia, or narrow-angle glaucoma. Relative to other neuroleptics, olanzapine has a moderate potency of cholinergic blockade. May cause extrapyramidal symptoms (EPS), although risk of these reactions is lower relative to other neuroleptics. Risk of dystonia (and probably other EPS) may be greater with increased doses, use of conventional antipsychotics, males, and younger patients. May be associated with neuroleptic malignant syndrome (NMS). May cause extreme and life-threatening hyperglycemia; use with caution in patients with diabetes or other disorders of glucose regulation; monitor. Olanzapine levels may be lower in patients who smoke; the manufacturer does not require dosage adjustments, although dosage adjustments may be considered. Use in adolescent patients

≥13 years of age may result in increased weight gain and sedation, as well as greater increases in LDL cholesterol, total cholesterol, triglycerides, prolactin, and liver transaminase levels when compared to adults. Adolescent patients should be maintained on the lowest dose necessary.

Use in elderly patients with dementia is associated with an increased risk of mortality and cerebrovascular accidents; avoid antipsychotic use for behavioral problems associated with dementia unless alternative nonpharmacologic therapies have failed and patient may harm self or others. In addition, use may cause or exacerbate syndrome of inappropriate antidiuretic hormone secretion or hyponatremia; monitor sodium closely with initiation or dosage adjustments in older adults. May also be inappropriate in older adults depending on comorbidities (eg, dementia, delirium) due to its potent anticholinergic effects (Beers Criteria).

The possibility of a suicide attempt is inherent in psychotic illness or bipolar disorder; use caution in high-risk patients during initiation of therapy. Prescriptions should be written for the smallest quantity consistent with good patient care.

There are two Zyprexa® formulations for intramuscular injection: Zyprexa® Relprevv™ is an extended-release formulation and Zyprexa® Intramuscular is short-acting:

Extended-release I.M. injection (Zyprexa® Relprevv™): Monitor for post injection delirium/sedation syndrome; patients should be continuously watched (≥3 hours) for symptoms of olanzapine overdose. Only available through a restricted drug distribution program.

Short-acting I.M. injection (Zyprexa® IntraMuscular): Patients should remain recumbent if drowsy/dizzy until hypotension, bradycardia, and/or hypoventilation have been ruled out. Concurrent use of I.M./I.V. benzodiazepines is not recommended (fatalities have been reported, though causality not determined).

Adverse Reactions

Oral: Unless otherwise noted, adverse events are reported for placebo-controlled trials in adult patients on monotherapy:

>10%:

Central nervous system: Somnolence (dose dependent; 20% to 39%; adolescents 39% to 48%), extrapyramidal symptoms (dose dependent; ≤32%), dizziness (11% to 18%), headache (adolescents 17%), fatigue (adolescents 3% to 14%), insomnia (12%)

Endocrine & metabolic: Prolactin increased (30%; adolescents 47%)

Gastrointestinal: Weight gain (5% to 6%, has been reported as high as 40%; adolescents 29% to 31%), appetite increased (3% to 6%; adolescents 17% to 29%), xerostomia (dose dependent; 3% to 22%), constipation (9% to 11%), dyspepsia (7% to 11%)

Hepatic: ALT increased ≥3 x ULN (adolescents 12%; adults 5%)

Neuromuscular & skeletal: Weakness (dose dependent; 8% to 20%)

Miscellaneous: Accidental injury (12%)

1% to 10%:

Cardiovascular: Chest pain, hypertension, orthostatic hypotension, peripheral edema, tachycardia

Central nervous system: Fever, personality changes, restlessness (adolescents)

Dermatologic: Bruising

Endocrine & metabolic: Breast-related events ([adolescents] discharge, enlargement, galactorrhea, gynecomastia, lactation disorder); menstrual-related events (amenorrhea, hypomenorrhea, menstruation delayed, oligomenorrhea); sexual function-related events (anorgasmia, ejaculation delayed, erectile dysfunction, changes in libido, abnormal orgasm, sexual dysfunction)

Gastrointestinal: Abdominal pain (adolescents), diarrhea (adolescents), flatulence, nausea (dose dependent), vomiting

Genitourinary: Incontinence, UTI

Hepatic: Hepatic enzymes increased

Neuromuscular & skeletal: Abnormal gait, akathisia, articulation impairment, back pain, falling, hypertonia, joint/extremity pain, muscle stiffness (adolescents), tremor (dose dependent)

Ocular: Amblyopia

Respiratory: Cough, epistaxis (adolescents), pharyngitis, respiratory tract infection (adolescents), rhinitis, sinusitis (adolescents)

<1%, postmarketing, and/or case reports (limited to important or life-threatening): Acidosis, accommodation abnormal, agranulocytosis, akinesia, albuminuria, alopecia, anaphylactoid reaction, angioedema, apnea, arteritis, asthma, ataxia, atelectasis, atrial fibrillation, cerebrovascular accident, coma, confusion, congestive heart failure, deafness, diabetes mellitus, diabetic ketoacidosis, diabetic coma, dysarthria, dyskinesia, dysphagia, dystonia, dysuria, encephalopathy, facial paralysis, glaucoma, heart arrest, heart failure, hematuria, hemoptysis, hemorrhage (eye, rectal, subarachnoid, vaginal), hepatitis, hypercholesterolemia, hyper-/hypoglycemia, hyper-/hypokalemia, hyperlipemia, hyper-/hyponatremia, hypertriglyceridemia, hyperuricemia, hyper-/hypoventilation, hypoesthesia, hypokinesia, hypoproteinemia, hypoxia, jaundice, ileus, ketosis, leukocytosis (eosinophilia), leukopenia, liver damage (cholestatic or mixed), liver fatty deposit, lung edema, lymphadenopathy, migraine, myasthenia, myopathy, neuralgia, neuroleptic malignant syndrome, neuropathy, neutropenia, osteoporosis, pancreatitis, paralysis, priapism, pruritus, pulmonary embolus, rash, rhabdomyolysis, seizure, stridor, stroke, sudden death, suicide attempt, syncope, tardive dyskinesia, thrombocythemia, thrombocytopenia, tongue edema, transient ischemic attack, urticaria, venous thrombotic events, withdrawal syndrome

Injection: Unless otherwise noted, adverse events are reported for placebo-controlled trials in adult patients on extended-release I.M. injection (Zyprexa® Relprevv™). Also refer to adverse reactions noted with oral therapy.

>10%: Central nervous system: Headache (13% to 18%), sedation (8% to 13%)

1% to 10%:

Cardiovascular: Hypertension, hypotension (short-acting), orthostatic hypotension (short-acting), QT prolongation

Central nervous system: Abnormal dreams, abnormal thinking, auditory hallucination, dizziness, dysarthria, extrapyramidal symptoms, fatigue, fever, pain, restlessness, somnolence

Dermatologic: Acne

Gastrointestinal: Abdominal pain, appetite increased, diarrhea, flatulence, nausea, vomiting, weight gain, xerostomia

Genitourinary: Vaginal discharge

Hepatic: Liver enzymes increased

Local: Injection site pain

- Neuromuscular & skeletal: Arthralgia, back pain, muscle spasms, stiffness, tremor, weakness (short-acting)
- Otic: Ear pain
- Respiratory: Cough, nasal congestion, nasopharyngitis, pharyngolaryngeal pain, sneezing, upper respiratory tract infection
- Miscellaneous: Toothache, tooth infection, viral infection

<1%, postmarketing, and/or case reports (limited to important or life-threatening): CPK increased, post-injection delirium/sedation syndrome, syncope (short-acting)

Drug Interactions

Metabolism/Transport Effects Substrate of CYP1A2 (major), CYP2D6 (minor); **Note:** Assignment of Major/Minor substrate status based on clinically relevant drug interaction potential; **Inhibits** CYP1A2 (weak), CYP2C19 (weak), CYP2C9 (weak), CYP2D6 (weak), CYP3A4 (weak)

Avoid Concomitant Use

Avoid concomitant use of OLANZapine with any of the following: Aclidinium; Azelastine (Nasal); Benzodiazepines; Ipratropium (Oral Inhalation); Methadone; Metoclopramide; Paraldehyde; Pimozide; Tiotropium

Increased Effect/Toxicity

OLANZapine may increase the levels/effects of: Alcohol (Ethyl); Anticholinergics; ARIPiprazole; Azelastine (Nasal); Benzodiazepines; Buprenorphine; CNS Depressants; Methadone; Methotrimeprazine; Methylphenidate; Paraldehyde; Pimozide; Serotonin Modulators; Tiotropium; Zolpidem

The levels/effects of OLANZapine may be increased by: Abiraterone Acetate; Acetylcholinesterase Inhibitors (Central); Aclidinium; CYP1A2 Inhibitors (Moderate); CYP1A2 Inhibitors (Strong); Deferasirox; Droperidol; FluvoxaMINE; HydrOXYzine; Ipratropium (Oral Inhalation); LamoTRIgine; Lithium formulations; Methotrimeprazine; Methylphenidate; Metoclopramide; Metyrosine; Perampanel; Pramlintide; Tetrabenazine

Decreased Effect

OLANZapine may decrease the levels/effects of: Amphetamines; Anti-Parkinson's Agents (Dopamine Agonist); Quinagolide

The levels/effects of OLANZapine may be decreased by: CYP1A2 Inducers (Strong); Cyproterone; Lithium formulations; Peginterferon Alfa-2b

Ethanol/Nutrition/Herb Interactions

Ethanol: May increase CNS depression; monitor for increased effects with coadministration. Caution patients about effects.

Herb/Nutraceutical: Avoid dong quai, St John's wort (may also cause photosensitization). Avoid kava kava, gotu kola, valerian, St John's wort (may increase CNS depression).

Storage/Stability

Injection, extended-release: Store at 20°C to 25°C (68°F to 77°F); excursions permitted to 15°C to 30°C (59°F to 86°F).

Injection, short-acting: Store at 20°C to 25°C (68°F to 77°F); excursions permitted to 15°C to 30°C (59°F to 86°F); do not freeze. Protect from light.

Tablet and orally-disintegrating tablet: Store at 20°C to 25°C (68°F to 77°F); excursions permitted to 15°C to 30°C (59°F to 86°F). Protect from light and moisture.

Reconstitution

Injection, extended-release: Dilute as directed to final concentration of 150 mg/mL. Shake vigorously to mix; will form yellow, opaque suspension. Following reconstitution, suspension may be stored at room temperature and used within 24 hours. Shake vigorously to resuspend prior to administration. Use immediately once suspension is in syringe. Suspension may be irritating to skin; wear gloves during reconstitution.

Injection, short-acting: Reconstitute 10 mg vial with 2.1 mL SWFI. Resulting solution is ~5 mg/mL. Use immediately (within 1 hour) following reconstitution. Discard any unused portion.

Mechanism of Action Olanzapine is a second generation thienobenzodiazepine antipsychotic which displays potent antagonism of serotonin 5-HT_{2A} and 5-HT_{2C}, dopamine D_{1-4}, histamine H_1 and alpha$_1$-adrenergic receptors. Olanzapine shows moderate antagonism of 5-HT_3 and muscarinic M_{1-5} receptors, and weak binding to GABA-A, BZD, and beta-adrenergic receptors. Although the precise mechanism of action in schizophrenia and bipolar disorder is not known, the efficacy of olanzapine is thought to be mediated through combined antagonism of dopamine and serotonin type 2 receptor sites.

Pharmacodynamics/Kinetics

Absorption:

Oral: Well absorbed; not affected by food; tablets and orally-disintegrating tablets are bioequivalent

Short-acting injection: Rapidly absorbed

Distribution: V_d: Extensive, 1000 L

Protein binding, plasma: 93% bound to albumin and alpha$_1$-glycoprotein

Metabolism: Highly metabolized via direct glucuronidation and cytochrome P450 mediated oxidation (CYP1A2, CYP2D6); 40% removed via first pass metabolism

Half-life elimination: 21-54 hours; ~1.5 times greater in elderly; Extended-release injection: ~30 days

Time to peak, plasma: Maximum plasma concentrations after I.M. administration are 5 times higher than maximum plasma concentrations produced by an oral dose.

Extended-release injection: ~7 days

Short-acting injection: 15-45 minutes

Oral: ~6 hours

Excretion: Urine (57%, 7% as unchanged drug), feces (30%)

Clearance: 40% increase in olanzapine clearance in smokers; 30% decrease in females

Dosing

Adult & Geriatric

Schizophrenia:

Oral: Initial: 5-10 mg once daily (increase to 10 mg once daily within 5-7 days); thereafter, adjust by 5 mg/day at 1-week intervals, up to a recommended maximum of 20 mg/day. Maintenance: 10-20 mg once daily. Doses of 30-50 mg/day have been used; however, doses >10 mg/day have not demonstrated better efficacy, and safety and efficacy of doses >20 mg/day have not been evaluated.

Extended-release I.M. injection: **Note:** Establish tolerance to oral olanzapine prior to changing to extended-release I.M. injection. Maximum dose: 300 mg/2 weeks or 405 mg/4 weeks

Patients established on oral olanzapine 10 mg/day: Initial dose: 210 mg every 2 weeks for 4 doses or 405 mg every 4 weeks for 2 doses; Maintenance dose: 150 mg every 2 weeks or 300 mg every 4 weeks

Patients established on oral olanzapine 15 mg/day: Initial dose: 300 mg every 2 weeks for 4 doses; Maintenance dose: 210 mg every 2 weeks or 405 mg every 4 weeks

Patients established on oral olanzapine 20 mg/day: Initial and maintenance dose: 300 mg every 2 weeks

Acute mania associated with bipolar disorder: Oral:

Monotherapy: Initial: 10-15 mg once daily; increase by 5 mg/day at intervals of not less than 24 hours. Maintenance: 5-20 mg/day; recommended maximum dose: 20 mg/day.

Combination therapy (with lithium or valproate): Initial: 10 mg once daily; dosing range: 5-20 mg/day

Agitation (acute, associated with bipolar disorder or schizophrenia): Short-acting I.M. injection: Initial dose: 10 mg (a lower dose of 5-7.5 mg may be considered when clinical factors warrant); additional doses (up to 10 mg) may be considered; however, 2-4 hours should be allowed between doses to evaluate response (maximum total daily dose: 30 mg, per manufacturer's recommendation)

Depression:

Depression associated with bipolar disorder (in combination with fluoxetine): Oral: Initial: 5 mg in the evening; adjust as tolerated to usual range of 5-12.5 mg/day. See **"Note."**

Treatment-resistant depression (in combination with fluoxetine): Oral: Initial: 5 mg in the evening; adjust as tolerated to range of 5-20 mg/day. See **"Note."**

Note: When using individual components of fluoxetine with olanzapine rather than fixed dose combination product (Symbyax®), approximate dosage correspondence is as follows:

Olanzapine 2.5 mg + fluoxetine 20 mg = Symbyax® 3/25
Olanzapine 5 mg + fluoxetine 20 mg = Symbyax® 6/25
Olanzapine 12.5 mg + fluoxetine 20 mg = Symbyax® 12/25
Olanzapine 5 mg + fluoxetine 50 mg = Symbyax® 6/50
Olanzapine 12.5 mg + fluoxetine 50 mg = Symbyax® 12/50

Delirium (unlabeled use): Oral: 5 mg once daily for up to 5 days (NICE, 2010)

Prevention of chemotherapy-associated delayed nausea or vomiting (unlabeled use; in combination with a corticosteroid and serotonin [5-HT$_3$] antagonist): Oral: 10 mg once daily for 3-5 days, beginning on day 1 of chemotherapy **or** 5 mg once daily for 2 days before chemotherapy, followed by 10 mg once daily (beginning on the day of chemotherapy) for 3-8 days

Pediatric Schizophrenia/bipolar disorder: Adolescents ≥13 years: Oral: Initial: 2.5-5 mg once daily; adjust by 2.5-5 mg/day to target dose of 10 mg/day; dosing range: 2.5-20 mg/ day

Renal Impairment No dosage adjustment required. Not removed by dialysis.

Hepatic Impairment Dosage adjustment may be necessary; however, there are no specific recommendations. Monitor closely.

Administration

Short-acting I.M. injection: **For I.M. administration only**; do not administer injection intravenously or subcutaneously; inject slowly, deep into muscle. If dizziness and/or drowsiness are noted, patient should remain recumbent until examination indicates postural hypotension and/or bradycardia are not a problem.

Extended-release I.M. injection: **For I.M. gluteal injection only**; do not administer I.V. or subcutaneously. After needle insertion into muscle, aspirate to verify that no blood appears. Do not massage injection site. Use diluent, syringes, and needles provided in convenience kit; obtain a new kit if aspiration of blood occurs.

Tablet: May be administered without regard to meals.

Orally-disintegrating: Remove from foil blister by peeling back (do not push tablet through the foil); place tablet in mouth immediately upon removal; tablet dissolves rapidly in saliva and may be swallowed with or without liquid. May be administered with or without food/meals.

Monitoring Parameters Vital signs; fasting lipid profile and fasting blood glucose/Hgb A_{1c} (prior to treatment, at 3 months, then annually); periodic assessment of hepatic transaminases (in patients with hepatic disease); BMI, waist circumference; orthostatic blood pressure; mental status, abnormal involuntary movement scale (AIMS), extrapyramidal symptoms (EPS). Weight should be assessed prior to treatment, at 4 weeks, 8 weeks, 12 weeks, and then at quarterly intervals. Consider titrating to a different antipsychotic agent for a weight gain ≥5% of the initial weight.

Extended-release I.M. injection: Sedation/delirium for 3 hours after each dose

Dietary Considerations Tablets may be taken without regard to meals. Some products may contain phenylalanine.

Prescribing and Access Restrictions As a requirement of the REMS program, only prescribers, healthcare facilities, and pharmacies registered with the Zyprexa® Relprevv™ Patient Care Program are able to prescribe, distribute, or dispense Zyprexa® Relprevv™ for patients who are enrolled in and meet all conditions of the program. Zyprexa® Relprevv™ must be administered at a registered healthcare facility. Prescribers will need to be recertified every 3 years. Contact the Zyprexa® Relprevv™ Patient Care Program at 1-877-772-9390.

Medication Guide Available Yes

Dosage Forms Excipient information presented when available (limited, particularly for generics); consult specific product labeling.

Injection, powder for reconstitution: 10 mg
- ZyPREXA® IntraMuscular: 10 mg [contains lactose 50 mg]

Injection, powder for suspension, extended release:
- ZyPREXA® Relprevv™: 210 mg, 300 mg, 405 mg [contains polysorbate 80 (in diluent); supplied with diluent]

Tablet, oral: 2.5 mg, 5 mg, 7.5 mg, 10 mg, 15 mg, 20 mg
- ZyPREXA®: 2.5 mg, 5 mg, 7.5 mg, 10 mg, 15 mg, 20 mg

Tablet, orally disintegrating, oral: 5 mg, 10 mg, 15 mg, 20 mg
- ZyPREXA® Zydis®: 5 mg [contains phenylalanine 0.34 mg/tablet]
- ZyPREXA® Zydis®: 10 mg [contains phenylalanine 0.45 mg/tablet]
- ZyPREXA® Zydis®: 15 mg [contains phenylalanine 0.67 mg/tablet]
- ZyPREXA® Zydis®: 20 mg [contains phenylalanine 0.9 mg/tablet]

References

American Diabetes Association; American Psychiatric Association; American Association of Clinical Endocrinologists; North American Association for the Study of Obesity, "Consensus Development Conference on Antipsychotic Drugs and Obesity and Diabetes," *Diabetes Care*, 2004, 27(2):596-601.

Dixon L, Perkins D, and Calmes C, *Guideline Watch (September 2009): Practice Guideline for the Treatment of Schizophrenia*, Arlington, Va: American Psychiatric Association, 2009. Available at http://www.psychiatryonline.com/content.aspx?aid=501001

Khojainova N, Santiago-Palma J, Kornick C, et al, "Olanzapine in the Management of Cancer Pain," *J Pain Symptom Manage*, 2002, 23(4):346-50.

Lauriello J, Lambert T, Andersen S, et al, "An 8-Week, Double-Blind, Randomized, Placebo-Controlled Study of Olanzapine Long-Acting Injection in Acutely Ill Patients With Schizphrenia," *J Clin Psychiatry*, 2008, 69(5):790-9.

Moore TA, "Schizophrenia Treatment Guidelines in the United States," *Clin Schizophr Relat Psychoses*, 2011, 5(1):40-9.

National Institute for Health and Clinical Excellence (NICE), National Clinical Guideline Centre, "Delirium: Diagnosis, Prevention and Management," National Clinical Practice Guideline Number 103, 2010. Available at http://www.nice.org.uk/CG103

National Institute for Health and Clinical Excellence (NICE), National Collaborating Centre for Mental Health, "Schizophrenia. Core Interventions in the Treatment and Management of Schizophrenia in Primary and Secondary Care (Updated)," National Clinical Practice Guideline Number 82, 2009:1-399. Available at www.nice.org.uk/cg082

Navari RM, Einhorn LH, Loehrer PJ, et al, "A Phase II Trial of Olanzapine, Dexamethasone, and Palonosetron for the Prevention of Chemotherapy-Induced Nausea and Vomiting: A Hoosier Oncology Group Study," *Support Care Cancer*, 2007, 15(11):1285-91.

Navari RM, Einhorn LH, Passik SD, et al, "A Phase II Trial of Olanzapine for the Prevention of Chemotherapy-Induced Nausea and Vomiting: A Hoosier Oncology Group Study," *Support Care Cancer*, 2005, 13(7):529-34.

Passick SD, Navari RM, Jung SH, et al, "A Phase I Trial of Olanzapine (Zyprexa) for the Prevention of Delayed Emesis in Cancer Patients: A Hoosier Oncology Group Study," *Cancer Invest*, 2004, 22(3):383-8.

Sultzer DL, Davis SM, Tariot PN, et al, "Clinical Symptom Responses to Atypical Antipsychotic Medications in Alzheimer's Disease: Phase 1 Outcomes from the CATIE-AD Effectiveness Trial," *Am J Psychiatry*, 2008, 165(7):844-54.

Thangadurai P, Jyothi KS, Gopalakrishman R, et al, "Reversible Neutropenia With Olanzapine Following Clozapine-Induced Neutropenia," *Am J Psychiatry*, 2006, 163(7):1298.

Thinn SS, Liew E, May AL, et al, "Reversible Delayed Onset Olanzapine-Associated Leukopenia and Neutropenia in a Clozapine-Naive Patient on Concomitant Depot Antipsychotic," *J Clin Psychopharmacol*, 2007, 27(4):394-5.

◆ **Olanzapine ODT (Can)** *see* OLANZapine *on page 1056*

◆ **Olanzapine Pamoate** *see* OLANZapine *on page 1056*

Omacetaxine (oh ma se TAX een)

Brand Names: U.S. Synribo™

Index Terms CGX-625; HHT; Homoharringtonine; Omacetaxine Mepesuccinate

Generic Availability (U.S.) No

Pharmacologic Category Antineoplastic Agent, Cephalotaxine; Antineoplastic Agent, Protein Synthesis Inhibitor

Use Treatment of chronic or accelerated phase chronic myelogenous leukemia (CML) in patients resistant and/or intolerant to ≥2 tyrosine kinase inhibitors

Labeled Contraindications There are no contraindications listed in the manufacturer's labeling.

Pregnancy Risk Factor D

Lactation Excretion in breast milk unknown/not recommended

Warnings/Precautions Hazardous agent; use appropriate precautions for handling and disposal. Grade 3/4 neutropenia, thrombocytopenia, and anemia commonly occur; generally reversible, although may require treatment delay and/or a reduction in the number of treatment days with future cycles. Myelosuppression may rarely be fatal. Monitor blood counts (in induction and maintenance cycles). Neutropenia may increase the risk for infection. Thrombocytopenia may increase the risk of bleeding; cerebrovascular hemorrhages have been reported (some fatal); gastrointestinal hemorrhages have occurred. Due to the increased risk of bleeding, avoid the use of anticoagulants, aspirin, and NSAIDs when the platelet count is <50,000/mm^3. Patients ≥65 years of age are more likely to experience hematologic toxicity. Omacetaxine may induce glucose intolerance; hyperglycemia has been observed;

hyperosmolar nonketotic hyperglycemia has been reported (case report). Monitor blood glucose frequently, especially in patients with diabetes or with risk factors for diabetes. Avoid use in patients with poorly controlled diabetes; may initiate after glycemic control has been established.

Adverse Reactions

>10%:

Cardiovascular: Peripheral edema (13%)

Central nervous system: Fatigue (26% to 31%), fever (24% to 29%), headache (13% to 19%), chills (13%)

Dermatologic: Alopecia (15%)

Endocrine & metabolic: Uric acid increased (grades 3/4: 56% to 57%), hyperglycemia (grades 3/4: 10% to 15%; hyperosmolar nonketotic hyperglycemia: <1%)

Gastrointestinal: Diarrhea (35% to 42%), nausea (27% to 32%), constipation (15%), vomiting (12% to 15%), abdominal pain (13% to 14%), anorexia (13%)

Hematologic: Thrombocytopenia (grades 3/4: 49% to 88%), neutropenia (grades 3/4: 18% to 81%), anemia (grades 3/4: 36% to 80%), leukocytes decreased (grades 3/4: 61% to 72%), neutropenic fever (10% to 20%; grades 3/4: 10% to 16%), lymphopenia (17%; grades 3/4: 16%)

Local: Injection site reactions (22% to 34%)

Neuromuscular & skeletal: Weakness (23% to 24%), arthralgia (19%), limb pain (11% to 13%), back pain (11%)

Renal: Creatinine increased (grades 3/4: 9% to 16%)

Respiratory: Cough (≤16%), epistaxis (11% to 15%), dyspnea (11%)

Miscellaneous: Infection (46% to 56%; grades 3/4: 11% to 20%)

1% to 10%:

Cardiovascular: Acute coronary syndrome, angina pectoris, arrhythmia, bradycardia, cerebral hemorrhage, chest pain, edema, hyper-/hypotension, palpitations, tachycardia, ventricular extrasystoles

Central nervous system: Insomnia (10%), anxiety, agitation, confusion, depression, dizziness, dysphonia, hyperthermia, hypoesthesia, lethargy, malaise, mental status change, pain, seizures

Dermatologic: Bruising, burning sensation, dry skin, erythema, hyperhidrosis, hyperpigmentation, petechiae, pruritus, purpura, rash, skin exfoliation, skin lesions, skin ulceration

Endocrine & metabolic: Glucose decreased (grades 3/4: 6% to 8%), dehydration, diabetes mellitus, gout, hot flashes

Gastrointestinal: Abdominal distension, abnormal taste, anal fissure, aphthous stomatitis, appetite decreased, dyspepsia, dysphagia, gastritis, gastroesophageal reflux disease, GI bleeding, gingival bleeding, gingival pain, gingivitis, hemorrhoids, melena, mouth ulceration, mouth hemorrhage, mucosal inflammation, oral pain, stomatitis, xerostomia

Genitourinary: Dysuria

Hematologic: Bone marrow failure (10%; grades 3/4: 10%), hematoma

Hepatic: Bilirubin increased (grades 3/4: 6% to 9%), ALT increased (grades 3/4: 2% to 6%)

Neuromuscular & skeletal: Bone pain, muscle spasms, muscle weakness, musculoskeletal chest pain, musculoskeletal discomfort, musculoskeletal pain, myalgia, paresthesia, sciatica, stiffness, tremor

Ocular: Blurred vision, cataract, conjunctival hemorrhage, conjunctivitis, diplopia, dry eyes, eye pain, eyelid edema, lacrimation increased

Otic: Ear hemorrhage, ear pain, tinnitus

Respiratory: Hemoptysis, nasal congestion, pharyngolaryngeal pain, rales, rhinorrhea, sinus congestion

Miscellaneous: Flu-like syndrome, hypersensitivity reactions, night sweats, transfusion reaction

Drug Interactions

Metabolism/Transport Effects Substrate of P-glycoprotein

Avoid Concomitant Use

Avoid concomitant use of Omacetaxine with any of the following: Anticoagulants; Aspirin; BCG; Natalizumab; Nonsteroidal Anti-Inflammatory Agents; Pimecrolimus; Tacrolimus (Topical); Vaccines (Live)

Increased Effect/Toxicity

Omacetaxine may increase the levels/effects of: Leflunomide; Natalizumab; Vaccines (Live); Vitamin K Antagonists

The levels/effects of Omacetaxine may be increased by: Anticoagulants; Aspirin; Denosumab; Nonsteroidal Anti-Inflammatory Agents; Pimecrolimus; Roflumilast; Tacrolimus (Topical); Trastuzumab

Decreased Effect

Omacetaxine may decrease the levels/effects of: BCG; Cardiac Glycosides; Coccidioidin Skin Test; Sipuleucel-T; Vaccines (Inactivated); Vaccines (Live); Vitamin K Antagonists

The levels/effects of Omacetaxine may be decreased by: Echinacea

Storage/Stability Store intact vials at 20°C to 25°C (68°F to 77°F); excursions permitted between 15°C to 30°C (59°F to 86°F). Protect from light (intact vial and reconstituted solutions). Reconstituted solution should be used within 12 hours if stored at room temperature or within 24 hours if refrigerated at 2°C to 8°C (36°F to 46°F).

Reconstitution Hazardous agent; use appropriate precautions for handling and disposal. Reconstitute each 3.5 mg vial with sodium chloride 0.9% (NS) 1 mL, resulting in a concentration of 3.5 mg/mL. Gently swirl until solution is clear (lyophilized powder dissolves completely in <1 minute).

Mechanism of Action Omacetaxine is a reversible protein synthesis inhibitor which binds to the A-site cleft of the ribosomal subunit to interfere with chain elongation and inhibit protein synthesis. It acts independently of BCR-ABL1 kinase-binding activity, and has demonstrated activity against tyrosine kinase inhibitor-resistant BCR-ABL mutations.

Pharmacodynamics/Kinetics

Onset:

- Chronic phase CML: Mean time to major cytogenetic response: 3.5 months
- Accelerated phase CML: Mean time to complete hematologic response: 2.3 months

Duration:

- Chronic phase CML: Median duration of major cytogenetic response: 12.5 months
- Accelerated phase CML: Median duration of complete hematologic response: 4.7 months

Absorption: SubQ: Rapid (Nemunaitis, 2012)

Distribution: V_{dss}: 141 ± 93 L

Protein binding: ≤50%

Metabolism: Hydrolyzed by plasma esterases to 4'-DMHHT; minimal hepatic metabolism

Half-life elimination: ~6 hours
Time to peak: SubQ: ~30 minutes
Excretion: Urine (<15%)

Dosing

Adult & Geriatric Chronic myelogenous leukemia (CML), chronic or accelerated phase: SubQ:

Induction: 1.25 mg/m^2 twice daily for 14 consecutive days of a 28-day treatment cycle; continue until hematologic response is achieved

Maintenance: 1.25 mg/m^2 twice daily for 7 consecutive days of a 28-day treatment cycle; continue until no longer achieving clinical treatment benefit

Renal Impairment No dosage adjustment provided in the manufacturer's labeling (has not been studied). Based on the minimal amount of unchanged drug excreted in the urine, dosage adjustment is not likely necessary (Nemunaitis, 2012).

Hepatic Impairment No dosage adjustment provided in the manufacturer's labeling (has not been studied).

Adjustment for Toxicity

Hematologic toxicity: May delay treatment cycles and/or reduce the number of treatment days during a cycle for hematologic toxicities.

Neutropenia grade 4 (ANC <500/mm^3) or thrombocytopenia ≥ grade 3 (platelets <50,000/mm^3) during a cycle: Delay the start of the next cycle until ANC ≥1000/mm^3 and platelets ≥50,000/mm^3 **AND** reduce the number of treatment days by 2 days (eg, reduce from 14 days to 12 days or reduce from 7 days to 5 days)

Nonhematologic toxicity: Manage symptomatically; interrupt and/or delay treatment until toxicity resolves.

Administration Administer subcutaneously.

Monitoring Parameters CBC with differential (weekly during induction and maintenance cycles, then every 2 weeks or as clinically indicated after initial maintenance cycles); blood glucose (frequently); signs/symptoms of infection; signs of bleeding

References

Cortes J, Lipton JH, Rea D, et al, "Phase 2 Study of Subcutaneous Omacetaxine Mepesuccinate After TKI Failure in Patients With Chronic-Phase CML With T315I Mutation," *Blood*, 2012, 120 (13):2573-80.

Cortes, JE, Nicolini FE, Wetzler M, et al, "Subcutaneous Omacetaxine in Chronic or Accelerated Chronic Myeloid Leukemia Resistant to Two or More Tyrosine-Kinase Inhibitors Including Imatinib," *Blood*, 2011, 118(21):3761 [abstract 3761 from 2011 ASH Annual Meeting].

Nemunaitis J, Mita A, Stephenson J, et al, "Pharmacokinetic Study of Omacetaxine Mepesuccinate Administered Subcutaneously to Patients With Advanced Solid and Hematologic Tumors," *Cancer Chemother Pharmacol*, 2012 [epub ahead of print].

Wetzler M, Kantarjian H, Nicolini FE, et al, "Pooled Safety Analysis of Omacetaxine Mepesuccinate in Patients With Chronic Myeloid Leukemia (CML) Resistant to Tyrosine-Kinase Inhibitors (TKIs)," *J Clin Oncol*, 2012, 30(152):6604 [abstract 6604 from 2012 ASCO Annual Meeting].

◆ **Omacetaxine Mepesuccinate** *see* Omacetaxine *on page 1064*
◆ **Omnipred™** *see* PrednisoLONE (Ophthalmic) *on page 1198*
◆ **Omnitarg** *see* Pertuzumab *on page 1165*
◆ **Oncaspar®** *see* Pegaspargase *on page 1135*
◆ **Oncotice™ (Can)** *see* BCG *on page 153*
◆ **Oncovin** *see* VinCRIStine *on page 1450*

Ondansetron (on DAN se tron)

Related Information

Management of Chemotherapy-Induced Nausea and Vomiting *on page 1786*

Brand Names: U.S. Zofran®; Zofran® ODT; Zuplenz®

Brand Names: Canada Apo-Ondansetron®; CO Ondansetron; Dom-Ondansetron; JAMP-Ondansetron; Mint-Ondansetron; Mylan-Ondansetron; Ondansetron Injection; Ondansetron Injection USP; Ondansetron-Odan; Ondansetron-Omega; PHL-Ondansetron; PMS-Ondansetron; RAN™-Ondansetron; ratio-Ondansetron; Sandoz-Ondansetron; Teva-Ondansetron; Zofran®; Zofran® ODT; ZYM-Ondansetron

Index Terms GR38032R; Ondansetron Hydrochloride; Zuplenz®

Generic Availability (U.S.) Yes: Excludes oral soluble film

Pharmacologic Category Antiemetic; Selective 5-HT_3 Receptor Antagonist

Use

I.V.: Prevention of nausea and vomiting associated with initial and repeat courses of emetogenic cancer chemotherapy (including high-dose cisplatin); prevention of postoperative nausea and/or vomiting (PONV); treatment of PONV if no prophylactic dose of ondansetron received

Oral: Prevention of nausea and vomiting associated with highly emetogenic cancer chemotherapy (including high-dose cisplatin); prevention of nausea and vomiting associated with initial and repeat courses of moderately emetogenic cancer chemotherapy; prevention of nausea and vomiting associated with radiotherapy (either total body irradiation, single high-dose fraction to the abdomen, or daily fractions to the abdomen); prevention of PONV

Unlabeled Use Hyperemesis gravidarum (severe or refractory); breakthrough treatment of nausea and vomiting associated with chemotherapy

Labeled Contraindications Hypersensitivity to ondansetron or any component of the formulation; concomitant use of apomorphine

Pregnancy Risk Factor B

Lactation Excretion in breast milk unknown/use caution

Warnings/Precautions **Ondansetron should be used on a scheduled basis, not on an "as needed" (PRN) basis,** since data support the use of this drug only in the prevention of nausea and vomiting (due to antineoplastic therapy) and not in the rescue of nausea and vomiting. Ondansetron should only be used in the first 24-48 hours of chemotherapy. Data do not support any increased efficacy of ondansetron in delayed nausea and vomiting. Does not stimulate gastric or intestinal peristalsis; may mask progressive ileus and/or gastric distension. Use with caution in patients allergic to other 5-HT_3 receptor antagonists; cross-reactivity has been reported.

Dose-dependent QT interval prolongation occurs with ondansetron use. Cases of torsade de pointes have also been reported to the manufacturer. Selective 5-HT_3 antagonists, including ondansetron, have been associated with a number of dose-dependent increases in ECG intervals (eg, PR, QRS duration, QT/QT_c, JT), usually occurring 1-2 hours after I.V. administration. Single doses >16 mg ondansetron I.V. are no longer recommended due to the potential for an increased risk of QT prolongation. In most patients, these changes are not clinically relevant; however, when used in conjunction with other agents that prolong these intervals or in those at risk for QT prolongation, arrhythmia may occur. When used with agents that prolong the QT interval (eg, Class I and III antiarrhythmics) or in patients with cardiovascular disease, clinically relevant QT interval prolongation may occur resulting in torsade de pointes. Avoid ondansetron use in patients with congenital long QT syndrome. Use caution and monitor ECG in patients with other risk factors for QT prolongation (eg, medications known to prolong QT interval, electrolyte abnormalities [hypokalemia or hypomagnesemia], heart failure, bradyarrhythmias, and cumulative high-dose anthracycline therapy). I.V. formulations of 5-HT_3 antagonists have more association with ECG interval changes, compared to oral formulations. Dose limitations are recommended for patients with severe hepatic impairment (Child-Pugh class C); use with caution in mild-moderate hepatic impairment; clearance is decreased and half-life increased in hepatic impairment.

Orally-disintegrating tablets contain phenylalanine.

Adverse Reactions Note: Percentages reported in adult patients.

>10%:

Central nervous system: Headache (9% to 27%), malaise/fatigue (9% to 13%)

Gastrointestinal: Constipation (6% to 11%)

1% to 10%:

Central nervous system: Drowsiness (8%), fever (2% to 8%), dizziness (7%), anxiety (6%), cold sensation (2%)

Dermatologic: Pruritus (2% to 5%), rash (1%)

Gastrointestinal: Diarrhea (2% to 7%)

Genitourinary: Gynecological disorder (7%), urinary retention (5%)

Hepatic: ALT increased (>2 times ULN: 1% to 5%), AST increased (>2 times ULN: 1% to 5%)

Local: Injection site reaction (4%; pain, redness, burning)

Neuromuscular & skeletal: Paresthesia (2%)

Respiratory: Hypoxia (9%)

<1%, postmarketing, and/or case reports: Abnormal hepatic function, anaphylactoid reactions, anaphylaxis, angina, angioedema, arrhythmia, arthralgia, atrial fibrillation, AV block, blindness (transient/following infusion; lasting ≤48 hours), blurred vision (transient/following infusion), bradycardia, bronchospasm, cardiopulmonary arrest, chest discomfort, chills, dyspnea, dystonic reaction, electrocardiographic alterations (second-degree heart block and ST-segment depression), extrapyramidal symptoms, flushing, hepatic failure, hepatic necrosis, hepatitis, hiccups, hyperhidrosis, hypersensitivity reaction, hypokalemia, hypotension, jaundice, laryngeal edema, laryngospasm, lethargy, oculogyric crisis, palpitation, premature ventricular contractions (PVC), QT interval increased, seizure, shock, stridor, supraventricular tachycardia, syncope, tachycardia, torsade de pointes, urticaria, vascular occlusive events, ventricular arrhythmia, ventricular fibrillation, ventricular tachycardia

Drug Interactions

Metabolism/Transport Effects Substrate of CYP1A2 (minor), CYP2C9 (minor), CYP2D6 (minor), CYP2E1 (minor), CYP3A4 (major), P-glycoprotein; **Note:** Assignment of Major/Minor substrate status based on clinically relevant drug interaction potential; **Inhibits** CYP1A2 (weak), CYP2C9 (weak), CYP2D6 (weak)

Avoid Concomitant Use

Avoid concomitant use of Ondansetron with any of the following: Apomorphine; Highest Risk QTc-Prolonging Agents; Mifepristone

Increased Effect/Toxicity

Ondansetron may increase the levels/effects of: Apomorphine; ARIPiprazole; Highest Risk QTc-Prolonging Agents; Moderate Risk QTc-Prolonging Agents

The levels/effects of Ondansetron may be increased by: Mifepristone; P-glycoprotein/ABCB1 Inhibitors; QTc-Prolonging Agents (Indeterminate Risk and Risk Modifying)

Decreased Effect

Ondansetron may decrease the levels/effects of: Tapentadol; TraMADol

The levels/effects of Ondansetron may be decreased by: CYP3A4 Inducers (Strong); Deferasirox; Herbs (CYP3A4 Inducers); Peginterferon Alfa-2b; P-glycoprotein/ABCB1 Inducers; Rifamycin Derivatives; Tocilizumab

Ethanol/Nutrition/Herb Interactions

Food: Tablet: Food slightly increases the extent of absorption.

Herb/Nutraceutical: St John's wort may decrease ondansetron levels.

Storage/Stability

Oral soluble film: Store between 20°C and 25°C (68°F and 77°F). Store pouches in cartons; keep film in individual pouch until ready to use.

Oral solution: Store between 15°C and 30°C (59°F and 86°F). Protect from light.

Tablet: Store between 2°C and 30°C (36°F and 86°F).

Vial: Store between 2°C and 30°C (36°F and 86°F). Protect from light. Stable when mixed in D_5W or NS for 48 hours at room temperature.

Reconstitution Prior to I.V. infusion, dilute in 50 mL D_5W or NS.

Mechanism of Action Selective 5-HT_3-receptor antagonist, blocking serotonin, both peripherally on vagal nerve terminals and centrally in the chemoreceptor trigger zone

Pharmacodynamics/Kinetics

Onset of action: ~30 minutes

Absorption: Oral: Well absorbed from GI tract

Distribution: V_d: Children: 1.7-3.7 L/kg; Adults: 2.2-2.5 L/kg

Protein binding, plasma: 70% to 76%

Metabolism: Extensively hepatic via hydroxylation, followed by glucuronide or sulfate conjugation; CYP1A2, CYP2D6, and CYP3A4 substrate; some demethylation occurs

Bioavailability: Oral: 56% to 71% (some first pass metabolism); Rectal: 58% to 74%

Half-life elimination: Children <15 years: 2-7 hours; Adults: 3-6 hours

Mild-to-moderate hepatic impairment (Child-Pugh classes A and B): Adults: 12 hours

Severe hepatic impairment (Child-Pugh class C): Adults: 20 hours

Time to peak: Oral: ~2 hours; Oral soluble film: ~1 hour

Excretion: Urine (44% to 60% as metabolites, ~5% as unchanged drug); feces (~25%)

Dosing

Adult & Geriatric

Prevention of nausea and vomiting associated with emetogenic chemotherapy:

Manufacturer's labeling:

I.V.: 0.15 mg/kg/dose (maximum: 16 mg/dose) over 15 minutes for 3 doses, beginning 30 minutes prior to chemotherapy, followed by subsequent doses 4 and 8 hours after the first dose

Highly-emetogenic agents/single-day therapy: Oral: 24 mg given as three 8 mg tablets 30 minutes prior to the start of therapy

Moderately-emetogenic agents: Oral: 8 mg beginning 30 minutes before chemotherapy; repeat dose 8 hours after initial dose, then 8 mg every 12 hours for 1-2 days after chemotherapy completed

Alternate recommendations (unlabeled dose): American Society of Clinical Oncology Antiemetic Guidelines (Basch, 2011): High emetic risk: Day(s) of chemotherapy:

I.V.: 8 mg or 0.15 mg/kg. **Note:** Single I.V. doses >16 mg are no longer recommended by the manufacturer due to the potential for QT prolongation.

Oral: 8 mg twice daily

Prevention of nausea and vomiting associated with radiation therapy:

Manufacturer's labeling:

Total body irradiation: Oral: 8 mg 1-2 hours before each daily fraction of radiotherapy

Single high-dose fraction radiotherapy to abdomen: Oral: 8 mg 1-2 hours before irradiation, then 8 mg every 8 hours after first dose for 1-2 days after completion of radiotherapy

Daily fractionated radiotherapy to abdomen: Oral: 8 mg 1-2 hours before irradiation, then 8 mg every 8 hours after first dose for each day of radiotherapy

Alternate recommendations: American Society of Clinical Oncology Antiemetic Guidelines (Basch, 2011): Give before each fraction throughout radiation therapy (for high emetic risk, continue for at least 24 hours after completion; for low emetic risk, may give either as prevention or rescue; for minimal emetic risk, give as rescue; if rescue used for either low or minimal emetic risk, then prophylaxis should be given until the end of radiation therapy):

I.V. (unlabeled route): 8 mg or 0.15 mg/kg. **Note:** Single I.V. doses >16 mg are no longer recommended by the manufacturer due to the potential for QT prolongation.

Oral (unlabeled regimen): 8 mg twice daily

Postoperative nausea and vomiting (PONV):

Oral: 16 mg given 1 hour prior to induction of anesthesia

I.M., I.V.: 4 mg as a single dose (over 2-5 minutes if giving I.V.) administered ~30 minutes before the end of anesthesia (see Note below) or as treatment if vomiting occurs after surgery (Gan, 2007).

Note: The manufacturer recommends administration immediately before induction of anesthesia; however, this has been shown not to be as effective as administration at the end of surgery (Gan, 2007). Repeat doses given in response to inadequate control of nausea/vomiting from preoperative doses are generally ineffective.

Treatment of severe or refractory hyperemesis gravidum (unlabeled use):

Oral: 8 mg every 12 hours (Levichek, 2002)

I.V.: 8 mg administered over 15 minutes every 12 hours (ACOG, 2004)

Pediatric

Prevention of nausea and vomiting associated with emetogenic chemotherapy: I.V.: Children 6 months to 18 years: 0.15 mg/kg/dose (maximum: 16 mg/dose) over 15 minutes for 3 doses, beginning with the first dose administered 30 minutes prior to chemotherapy, followed by subsequent doses administered 4 and 8 hours after the first dose

Prevention of nausea and vomiting associated with moderately-emetogenic chemotherapy: Oral:

4-11 years: 4 mg 30 minutes before chemotherapy; repeat 4 and 8 hours after initial dose, then 4 mg every 8 hours for 1-2 days after chemotherapy completed

≥12 years: Refer to adult dosing.

Prevention of postoperative nausea and vomiting (PONV): I.V.: Children 1 month to 12 years:

≤40 kg: 0.1 mg/kg as a single dose over 2-5 minutes

>40 kg: 4 mg as a single dose over 2-5 minutes

Renal Impairment No dosage adjustment necessary (there is no experience for oral ondansetron beyond day 1)

Hepatic Impairment Severe impairment (Child-Pugh C):

I.V.: Day 1: Maximum dose: 8 mg (there is no experience beyond day 1)

Oral: Maximum daily dose: 8 mg

Administration

Oral: Oral dosage forms should be administered 30 minutes prior to chemotherapy; 1-2 hours before radiotherapy; 1 hour prior to the induction of anesthesia.

Orally-disintegrating tablets: Do not remove from blister until needed. Peel backing off the blister, do not push tablet through. Using dry hands, place tablet on tongue and allow to dissolve. Swallow with saliva.

Oral soluble film: Do not remove from pouch until immediately before use. Using dry hands, place film on top of tongue and allow to dissolve (4-20 seconds). Swallow with or without liquid. If using more than one film, each film should be allowed to dissolve completely before administering the next film.

I.M.: Should be administered undiluted.

I.V.:

IVPB: Dilute in 50 mL D_5W or NS. Infuse over 15-30 minutes; 24-hour continuous infusions have been reported, but are rarely used.

Chemotherapy-induced nausea and vomiting: Give first dose 30 minutes prior to beginning chemotherapy.

I.V. push: Prevention of postoperative nausea and vomiting: Single doses may be administered I.V. injection over 2-5 minutes as undiluted solution.

Extemporaneous Preparations Note: Commercial oral solution is available (0.8 mg/mL)

If commercial oral solution is unavailable, a 0.8 mg/mL syrup may be made with ondansetron tablets, Ora-Plus® (Paddock), and any of the the following syrups: Cherry syrup USP, Syrpalta® (HUMCO), Ora-Sweet® (Paddock), or Ora-Sweet® Sugar-Free (Paddock). Crush ten 8 mg tablets in a mortar and reduce to a fine powder (flaking of the tablet coating occurs). Add 50 mL Ora-Plus® in 5 mL increments, mixing thoroughly; mix while adding the chosen syrup in incremental proportions to **almost** 100 mL; transfer to a calibrated bottle, rinse mortar with syrup, and add sufficient quantity of syrup to make 100 mL. Label "shake well" and "refrigerate". Stable for 42 days refrigerated (Trissel, 1996).

Rectal suppositories: Calibrate a suppository mold for the base being used. Determine the displacement factor (DF) for ondansetron for the base being used (Fattibase® = 1.1; Polybase® = 0.6). Weigh the ondansetron tablet(s). Divide the tablet weight by the DF; this result is the weight of base displaced by the drug. Subtract the weight of base displaced from the calculated weight of base required for each suppository. Grind the ondansetron tablets in a mortar and reduce to a fine powder. Weigh out the appropriate weight of suppository base. Melt the base over a water bath (<55°C). Add the ondansetron powder to the suppository base and mix well. Pour the mixture into the suppository mold and cool. Stable for at least 30 days refrigerated (Tenjarla, 1998).

Tenjarla SN, Ward ES, and Fox JL, "Ondansetron Suppositories: Extemporaneous Preparation, Drug Release, Stability and Flux Through Rabbit Rectal Membrane," *Int J Pharm Compound*, 1998, 2(1):83-8.

Trissel LA, *Trissel's Stability of Compounded Formulations*, Washington, DC: American Pharmaceutical Association, 1996

Monitoring Parameters ECG (if applicable in high risk patients); potassium, magnesium

Dietary Considerations Take without regard to meals. Some products may contain phenylalanine.

Dosage Forms Excipient information presented when available (limited, particularly for generics); consult specific product labeling. [DSC] = Discontinued product

Film, soluble, oral:
- Zuplenz®: 4 mg (10s); 8 mg (10s) [peppermint flavor]

Infusion, premixed in D_5W [preservative free]: 32 mg (50 mL)
- Zofran®: 32 mg (50 mL [DSC])

Infusion, premixed in NS [preservative free]: 32 mg (50 mL)

Injection, solution: 2 mg/mL (2 mL, 20 mL)
- Zofran®: 2 mg/mL (20 mL)

Injection, solution [preservative free]: 2 mg/mL (2 mL)

Solution, oral: 4 mg/5 mL (5 mL, 50 mL)
- Zofran®: 4 mg/5 mL (50 mL) [contains sodium benzoate; strawberry flavor]

Tablet, oral: 4 mg, 8 mg
- Zofran®: 4 mg, 8 mg

Tablet, orally disintegrating, oral: 4 mg, 8 mg
- Zofran® ODT: 4 mg, 8 mg [contains phenylalanine <0.03 mg/tablet; strawberry flavor]

References

American College of Obstetrics and Gynecology, ACOG (American College of Obstetricians and Gynecologists) Practice Bulletin: "Nausea and Vomiting of Pregnancy," *Obstet Gynecol*, 2004, 103(4):803-14.

Basch E, Prestrud AA, Hesketh PJ, et al, "Antiemetics: American Society of Clinical Oncology Clinical Practice Guideline Update," *J Clin Oncol*, 2011, 29(31):4189-98.

Gan TJ, Meyer TA, Apfel CC, et al, "Society for Ambulatory Anesthesia Guidelines for the Management of Postoperative Nausea and Vomiting," *Anesth Analg*, 2007, 105(6):1615-28.

Kris MG, Hesketh PJ, Somerfield MR, et al, "American Society of Clinical Oncology Guideline for Antiemetics in Oncology: Update 2006," *J Clin Oncol*, 2006, 24(18):2932-47.

Levichek Z, Atanackovic G, Oepkes D, et al, "Nausea and Vomiting of Pregnancy. Evidence-Based Treatment Algorithm," *Can Fam Physician*, 2002, 48:267-8, 277.

Multinational Association of Supportive Care in Cancer (MASCC), "Antiemetic Guidelines," Updated April 2011. Available at http://data.memberclicks.com/site/mascc/MASCC Guidelines_English_2011.pdf

National Comprehensive Cancer Network® (NCCN), "Clinical Practice Guidelines in Oncology™: Antiemesis," Version 1.2012. Available at http://www.nccn.org/professionals/physician_gls/PDF/antiemesis.pdf

Sun R, Klein KW, and White PF, "The Effect of Timing of Ondansetron Administration in Outpatients Undergoing Otolaryngologic Surgery," *Anesth Analg*, 1997, 84(2):331-6.

- ◆ **Ondansetron Hydrochloride** *see* Ondansetron *on page* 1068
- ◆ **Ondansetron Injection (Can)** *see* Ondansetron *on page* 1068
- ◆ **Ondansetron Injection USP (Can)** *see* Ondansetron *on page* 1068
- ◆ **Ondansetron-Odan (Can)** *see* Ondansetron *on page* 1068

◆ **Ondansetron-Omega (Can)** *see* Ondansetron *on page* 1068
◆ **Onsolis®** *see* FentaNYL *on page* 583
◆ **ONTAK®** *see* Denileukin Diftitox *on page* 425
◆ **Opana®** *see* Oxymorphone *on page* 1088
◆ **Opana® ER** *see* Oxymorphone *on page* 1088
◆ **o,p'-DDD** *see* Mitotane *on page* 994
◆ **Ophtho-Tate® (Can)** *see* PrednisoLONE (Ophthalmic) *on page* 1198

Oprelvekin (oh PREL ve kin)

Brand Names: U.S. Neumega®

Index Terms IL-11; Interleukin-11; Recombinant Human Interleukin-11; Recombinant Interleukin-11; rhIL-11

Generic Availability (U.S.) No

Pharmacologic Category Biological Response Modulator; Human Growth Factor

Use Prevention of severe thrombocytopenia; reduce the need for platelet transfusions following myelosuppressive chemotherapy for nonmyeloid malignancy

Labeled Contraindications Hypersensitivity to oprelvekin or any component of the formulation

Pregnancy Risk Factor C

Lactation Excretion in breast milk unknown/not recommended

Warnings/Precautions [U.S. Boxed Warning]: Allergic or hypersensitivity reactions, including anaphylaxis have been reported. Permanently discontinue in any patient developing an allergic or hypersensitivity reaction. May occur with the first or with subsequent doses. May cause serious fluid retention (reversible) which may result in peripheral edema, capillary leak syndrome, arrhythmias, or exacerbation of pleural effusion. Use cautiously in patients with conditions where expansion of plasma volume should be avoided (eg, left ventricular dysfunction, HF, hypertension). Monitor fluid balance. Closely monitor fluid and electrolytes in patient on chronic diuretic therapy; severe hypokalemia contributing to sudden death have been reported in these patients. Reversible dilutional anemia may occur due to increased plasma volume; generally appears within 3-5 days of initiation of therapy and resolves over ~1 week following discontinuation. Atrial arrhythmias, pulmonary edema, and cardiac arrest have been reported; use in patients with a history of atrial arrhythmia only if the potential benefit exceeds possible risks. Patients experiencing arrhythmia may be at risk for stroke; use caution in patients with a history of transient ischemic attack or stroke. Ventricular arrhythmia has also been reported, occurring within 2-7 days of treatment initiation. Use caution in patients with conduction defects; history of thromboembolic problems; pre-existing pericardial effusions or ascites. May cause exacerbation of effusion; consider drainage if indicated. Use with caution in renal dysfunction; dosage adjustment required in severe renal impairment; monitor fluid balance.

Not indicated following myeloablative chemotherapy; increased toxicities were reported when used following myeloablative therapy. A higher incidence of adverse events has been reported when used following bone marrow transplantation. Begin 6-24 hours following completion of chemotherapy; use has not been adequately studied immediately before or during chemotherapy. Efficacy has not been established with chemotherapy regimens >5 days duration or with regimens associated with delayed myelosuppression (eg, nitrosoureas, mitomycin). Safety and efficacy have not been established with chronic administration. Papilledema, more frequently associated with use in children, has occurred (usually following repeated cycles); use caution in patients with pre-existing papilledema or with tumors involving the central nervous system; may worsen pre-existing papilledema. Papilledema is dose limiting. Patients experiencing oprelvekin-related papilledema may be at risk for visual acuity changes, including blurred vision or blindness. Although used in children in clinical trials, safety and efficacy have not been established in pediatric patients. The incidence of certain adverse events may be higher in children. Use in children, especially <12 years of age, should be as part of a clinical trial.

Adverse Reactions

>10%:

Cardiovascular: Tachycardia (children 84%; adults 20%), edema (59%), cardiomegaly (children 21%), vasodilation (19%), atrial arrhythmia (12% to 15%), palpitation (14%), syncope (13%)

Central nervous system: Neutropenic fever (48%), headache (41%), dizziness (38%), fever (36%), insomnia (33%)

Dermatologic: Rash (25%)

Endocrine & metabolic: Fluid retention

Gastrointestinal: Nausea/vomiting (77%), diarrhea (43%), mucositis (43%), oral moniliasis (14%), weight gain (due to fluid retention)

Hematologic: Anemia (dilutional; onset: 3-5 days; duration: ≤1 week)

Neuromuscular & skeletal: Weakness (severe 14%), periostitis (children 11%), arthralgia

Ocular: Conjunctival injection/redness/swelling (children 57%; adults 19%), papilledema (children 16%; adults 1%)

Respiratory: Dyspnea (48%), rhinitis (42%), cough (29%), pharyngitis (25%)

1% to 10%: Respiratory: Pleural effusion (10%)

<1%, postmarketing, and/or case reports: Allergic reaction, amblyopia, anaphylaxis/anaphylactoid reactions, blindness, blurred vision, capillary leak syndrome, cardiac arrest, chest pain, dehydration, dysarthria, exfoliative dermatitis, eye hemorrhage, facial edema, fibrinogen increased, fluid overload, HF, hypoalbuminemia, hypocalcemia, hypokalemia, hypotension, injection site reactions (dermatitis, pain, discoloration), loss of consciousness, mental status changes, optic neuropathy, paresthesia, pericardial effusion, peripheral edema, pneumonia, pulmonary edema, renal failure, shock, skin discoloration, stroke, urticaria, ventricular arrhythmia, visual acuity changes, visual field defect, von Willebrand factor concentration increased, wheezing

Drug Interactions

Metabolism/Transport Effects None known.

Avoid Concomitant Use There are no known interactions where it is recommended to avoid concomitant use.

Increased Effect/Toxicity There are no known significant interactions involving an increase in effect.

Decreased Effect There are no known significant interactions involving a decrease in effect.

Storage/Stability Store vials under refrigeration between 2°C to 8°C (36°F to 46°F); do not freeze. Protect from light. Use reconstituted oprelvekin within 3 hours of reconstitution; store reconstituted solution in the vial at either 2°C to 8°C (36°F to 46°F) or room temperature of ≤25°C (77°F). Do not freeze or shake reconstituted solution.

Reconstitution Reconstitute to a final concentration of 5 mg/mL with SWFI; direct diluent down side of vial, swirl gently, do not shake.

Mechanism of Action Oprelvekin is a thrombopoietic growth factor which stimulates multiple stages of megakaryocytopoiesis and thrombopoiesis, resulting in proliferation of megakaryocyte progenitors and megakaryocyte maturation, thereby increasing platelet production.

Pharmacodynamics/Kinetics

Bioavailability: >80%

Half-life elimination: Terminal: 5-9 hours

Time to peak, serum: 1-6 hours

Excretion: Urine (primarily as metabolites)

Dosing

Adult & Geriatric

Prevention of thrombocytopenia: SubQ: 50 mcg/kg once daily for ~10-21 days (until postnadir platelet count ≥50,000/mm^3)

Administer first dose ~6-24 hours after the end of chemotherapy. Discontinue at least 48 hours before beginning the next cycle of chemotherapy.

Renal Impairment Cl_{cr} <30 mL/minute: 25 mcg/kg once daily for ~10-21 days (until postnadir platelet count ≥50,000/mm^3).

Administration Subcutaneously in the abdomen, thigh, hip, or upper arm.

Monitoring Parameters Monitor electrolytes and fluid balance during therapy; obtain a CBC at regular intervals during therapy; monitor platelet counts until adequate recovery has occurred; renal function (at baseline)

Dosage Forms Excipient information presented when available (limited, particularly for generics); consult specific product labeling.

Injection, powder for reconstitution [preservative free]:

Neumega®: 5 mg [supplied with diluent]

References

Tepler I, Elias L, Smith JW 2d, et al, "A Randomized Placebo-Controlled Trial of Recombinant Human Interleukin-11 in Cancer Patients With Severe Thrombocytopenia Due to Chemotherapy," *Blood*, 1996, 87(9):3607-14.

Teramura M, Kobayashi S, Yoshinaga K, et al, "Effect of Interleukin 11 on Normal and Pathological Thrombopoiesis," *Cancer Chemother Pharmacol*, 1996, 38 (Suppl):99-102.

◆ **Oramorph® SR** *see* Morphine (Systemic) *on page 1004*

◆ **Orapred®** *see* PrednisoLONE (Systemic) *on page 1193*

◆ **Orapred ODT®** *see* PrednisoLONE (Systemic) *on page 1193*

◆ **Oraqix®** *see* Lidocaine and Prilocaine *on page 894*

◆ **Ortho,para-DDD** *see* Mitotane *on page 994*

◆ **Orzel® [DSC]** *see* UFT *on page 1418*

◆ **OSI-774** *see* Erlotinib *on page 528*

◆ **OTFC (Oral Transmucosal Fentanyl Citrate)** *see* FentaNYL *on page 583*

◆ **Oxalatoplatin** *see* Oxaliplatin *on page 1077*

◆ **Oxalatoplatinum** *see* Oxaliplatin *on page 1077*

Oxaliplatin (ox AL i pla tin)

Related Information

Management of Chemotherapy-Induced Nausea and Vomiting *on page 1786*
Management of Drug Extravasations *on page 1800*
Oral Mucositis/Stomatitis *on page 1814*
Safe Handling of Hazardous Drugs *on page 1904*

Brand Names: U.S. Eloxatin®

Brand Names: Canada Eloxatin®

Index Terms Diaminocyclohexane Oxalatoplatinum; L-OHP; Oxalatoplatin; Oxalatoplatinum

Generic Availability (U.S.) Yes

Pharmacologic Category Antineoplastic Agent, Alkylating Agent; Antineoplastic Agent, Platinum Analog

Use Treatment of stage III colon cancer (adjuvant) after complete resection of primary tumor; treatment of advanced colorectal cancer

Unlabeled Use Treatment of esophageal cancer, gastric cancer, hepatobiliary cancer (advanced), non-Hodgkin's lymphoma (refractory), ovarian cancer (advanced, platinum-pretreated), pancreatic cancer (advanced), testicular cancer (refractory)

Labeled Contraindications Hypersensitivity to oxaliplatin, other platinum-containing compounds, or any component of the formulation

Canadian labeling: Additional contraindications (not in U.S. labeling): Pregnancy, breast-feeding; severe renal impairment (Cl_{cr} <30 mL/minute)

Pregnancy Risk Factor D

Lactation Excretion in breast milk unknown/not recommended

Warnings/Precautions Hazardous agent - use appropriate precautions for handling and disposal. **[U.S. Boxed Warning]: Anaphylactic/anaphylactoid reactions have been reported with oxaliplatin (may occur within minutes of administration); symptoms may be managed with epinephrine, corticosteroids, antihistamines,** and discontinuation; oxygen and bronchodilators have also been used (Kim, 2009). Grade 3 or 4 hypersensitivity has been observed. Allergic reactions are similar to reactions reported with other platinum analogs, and may occur with any cycle. Reactions typically occur after multiple cycles; in retrospective reviews, reaction occurred at a median of 7-9 cycles, with an onset of 5-70 minutes (Kim, 2009; Polyzos, 2009). Symptoms may include bronchospasm (rare), erythema, hypotension (rare), pruritus, rash, and/or urticaria; previously-untreated patients have also experienced flushing, diaphoresis, diarrhea, shortness of breath, chest pain, hypotension, syncope, and disorientation. According to the manufacturer, rechallenge is contraindicated (deaths due to anaphylaxis have been associated with platinum derivatives). In patients rechallenged after mild hypersensitivity, reaction recurred at a higher level of severity; for patients with severe hypersensitivity, rechallenge (with 2-3 days of antihistamine and corticosteroid premedication, and prolongation of infusion time) allowed for 2-4 additional oxaliplatin cycles; however, rechallenge was not feasible in nearly two-thirds of patients due to the severity of the initial reaction (Polyzos, 2009).

Two different types of peripheral sensory neuropathy may occur: First, an acute (within hours to 1-2 days), reversible (resolves within 14 days), with primarily peripheral symptoms that are often exacerbated by cold (may include pharyngolaryngeal dysesthesia); commonly recur with subsequent doses;

avoid mucositis prophylaxis with ice chips during oxaliplatin infusion. Secondly, a more persistent (>14 days) presentation that often interferes with daily activities (eg, writing, buttoning, swallowing), these symptoms may improve in some patients upon discontinuing treatment. In a retrospective evaluation of patients treated with oxaliplatin for colorectal cancer, the incidence of peripheral sensory neuropathy was similar between diabetic and nondiabetic patients (Ramanathan, 2010).

Cases of reversible posterior leukoencephalopathy syndrome (RPLS) have been reported. Signs/symptoms include headache, mental status changes, seizure, blurred vision, blindness and/or other vision changes; may be associated with hypertension; diagnosis is confirmed with brain imaging. May cause pulmonary fibrosis; withhold treatment for unexplained pulmonary symptoms (eg, crackles, dyspnea, nonproductive cough, pulmonary infiltrates) until interstitial lung disease or pulmonary fibrosis are excluded. Hepatotoxicity (including rare cases of hepatitis and hepatic failure) has been reported. Liver biopsy has revealed peliosis, nodular regenerative hyperplasia, sinusoidal alterations, perisinusoidal fibrosis, and veno-occlusive lesions; the presence of hepatic vascular disorders (including veno-occlusive disease) should be considered, especially in individuals developing portal hypertension or who present with increased liver function tests. Use caution with renal dysfunction; increased toxicity may occur; reduce initial dose in severe impairment. When administered as sequential infusions, taxane derivatives (docetaxel, paclitaxel) should be administered before platinum derivatives (carboplatin, cisplatin, oxaliplatin) to limit myelosuppression and enhance efficacy. Concomitant use with 5-FU may increase risk for adverse hematologic or GI effects. Elderly patients are more sensitive to some adverse events including diarrhea, dehydration, hypokalemia, leukopenia, fatigue and syncope.

Adverse Reactions Percentages reported with monotherapy.

>10%:
- Central nervous system: Fatigue (61%), fever (25%), pain (14%), headache (13%), insomnia (11%)
- Gastrointestinal: Nausea (64%), diarrhea (46%), vomiting (37%), abdominal pain (31%), constipation (31%), anorexia (20%), stomatitis (14%)
- Hematologic: Anemia (64%; grades 3/4: 1%), thrombocytopenia (30%; grades 3/4: 3%), leukopenia (13%)
- Hepatic: AST increased (54%; grades 3/4: 4%), ALT increased (36%; grades 3/4: 1%), total bilirubin increased (13%; grades 3/4: 5%)
- Neuromuscular & skeletal: Peripheral neuropathy (may be dose limiting; 76% to 92%; acute 65%; grades 3/4: 5%; persistent 43%; grades 3/4: 3%), back pain (11%)
- Respiratory: Dyspnea (13%), cough (11%)

1% to 10%:
- Cardiovascular: Edema (10%), chest pain (5%), peripheral edema (5%), flushing (3%), thromboembolism (2%)
- Central nervous system: Dizziness (7%)
- Dermatologic: Rash (5%), alopecia (3%), hand-foot syndrome (1%)
- Endocrine & metabolic: Dehydration (5%), hypokalemia (3%)
- Gastrointestinal: Dyspepsia (7%), taste perversion (5%), flatulence (3%), mucositis (2%), gastroesophageal reflux (1%), dysphagia (acute 1% to 2%)
- Genitourinary: Dysuria (1%)
- Hematologic: Neutropenia (7%)
- Local: Injection site reaction (9%; redness/swelling/pain)
- Neuromuscular & skeletal: Rigors (9%), arthralgia (7%)

Ocular: Abnormal lacrimation (1%)
Renal: Serum creatinine increased (5% to 10%)
Respiratory: URI (7%), rhinitis (6%), epistaxis (2%), pharyngitis (2%), pharyngolaryngeal dysesthesia (grades 3/4: 1% to 2%)
Miscellaneous: Allergic reactions (3%); hypersensitivity (includes urticaria, pruritus, facial flushing, shortness of breath, bronchospasm, diaphoresis, hypotension, syncope: grades 3/4: 2% to 3%); hiccup (2%)

<1%, postmarketing, and/or case reports (reported with mono- and combination therapy): Acute renal failure, alkaline phosphatase increased, anaphylactic/anaphylactoid reactions, anaphylactic shock, angioedema, aphonia, ataxia, colitis, cranial nerve palsies, deep tendon reflex loss, deafness, diplopia, dysarthria, dysphonia, eosinophilic pneumonia, extravasation (including necrosis), fasciculations, gait abnormal, hematuria, hemolysis, hemolytic anemia (immuno-allergic), hemolytic uremia syndrome, hemorrhage, hepatic failure, hepatic sinusoidal obstruction syndrome (SOS; veno-occlusive disease), hepatitis, hepatotoxicity, hypertension, hypomagnesemia, hypoxia, ileus, INR increased, interstitial lung disease, interstitial nephritis (acute), intestinal obstruction, intracerebral bleeding, Lhermittes' sign, metabolic acidosis, muscle spasm, myoclonus, neutropenic fever, neutropenic sepsis, neutropenic typhlitis, nodular regenerative hyperplasia, optic neuritis, pancreatitis, peliosis, prothrombin time increased, ptosis, rectal hemorrhage, reversible posterior leukoencephalopathy syndrome (RPLS), rhabdomyolysis, seizure, sepsis, thrombocytopenia (immuno-allergic), trigeminal neuralgia, tubular necrosis (acute), visual disturbance (acuity decreased, field disturbance, transient loss)

Drug Interactions

Metabolism/Transport Effects None known.

Avoid Concomitant Use

Avoid concomitant use of Oxaliplatin with any of the following: BCG; CloZAPine; Natalizumab; Pimecrolimus; Tacrolimus (Topical); Vaccines (Live)

Increased Effect/Toxicity

Oxaliplatin may increase the levels/effects of: CloZAPine; Leflunomide; Natalizumab; Taxane Derivatives; Topotecan; Vaccines (Live); Vitamin K Antagonists

The levels/effects of Oxaliplatin may be increased by: Denosumab; Pimecrolimus; Roflumilast; Tacrolimus (Topical); Trastuzumab

Decreased Effect

Oxaliplatin may decrease the levels/effects of: BCG; Cardiac Glycosides; Coccidioidin Skin Test; Sipuleucel-T; Vaccines (Inactivated); Vaccines (Live); Vitamin K Antagonists

The levels/effects of Oxaliplatin may be decreased by: Echinacea

Storage/Stability Store intact vials at room temperature of 25°C (77°F); excursions permitted to 15°C to 30°C (59°F to 86°F); do not freeze. Protect concentrated solution from light (store in original outer carton). According to the manufacturer, solutions diluted for infusion are stable up to 6 hours at room temperature of 20°C to 25°C (68°F to 77°F) or up to 24 hours under refrigeration at 2°C to 8°C (36°F to 46°F). Oxaliplatin solution diluted with D_5W to a final concentration of 0.7 mg/mL (polyolefin container) has been shown to retain >90% of the original concentration for up to 30 days when stored at room temperature or refrigerated; artificial light did not affect the concentration (Andre, 2007). As this study did not examine sterility, refrigeration would be preferred to limit microbial growth. Solutions diluted for infusion do not require protection from light.

Reconstitution **Do not prepare using a chloride-containing solution such as NaCl** due to rapid conversion to monochloroplatinum, dichloroplatinum, and diaquoplatinum; all highly reactive in sodium chloride (Takimoto, 2007). Use appropriate precautions for handling and disposal. Do not use needles or administration sets containing aluminum during preparation.

Aqueous solution: Dilution with D_5W (250 or 500 mL) is required prior to administration.

Lyophilized powder: Use only SWFI or D_5W to reconstitute powder. To obtain final concentration of 5 mg/mL add 10 mL of diluent to 50 mg vial or 20 mL diluent to 100 mg vial. Gently swirl vial to dissolve powder. Dilution with D_5W (250 or 500 mL) is required prior to administration. Discard unused portion of vial.

Mechanism of Action Oxaliplatin, a platinum derivative, is an alkylating agent. Following intracellular hydrolysis, the platinum compound binds to DNA forming cross-links which inhibit DNA replication and transcription, resulting in cell death. Cytotoxicity is cell-cycle nonspecific.

Pharmacodynamics/Kinetics

Distribution: V_d: 440 L

Protein binding: >90% primarily albumin and gamma globulin (irreversible binding to platinum)

Metabolism: Nonenzymatic (rapid and extensive), forms active and inactive derivatives

Half-life elimination: Terminal: 391 hours

Excretion: Urine (~54%); feces (~2%)

Dosing

Adult Details concerning dosing in combination regimens should also be consulted.

Advanced colorectal cancer: I.V.: 85 mg/m² every 2 weeks until disease progression or unacceptable toxicity (in combination with fluorouracil/leucovorin)

Stage III colon cancer (adjuvant): I.V.: 85 mg/m² every 2 weeks for 6 months (12 cycles; in combination with fluorouracil/leucovorin)

Colon/colorectal cancer (unlabeled doses or combinations): I.V.: 85 mg/m²/dose on days 1, 15, and 29 of an 8-week treatment cycle in combination with fluorouracil/leucovorin (Kuebler, 2007) **or** 85 mg/m² every 2 weeks in combination with fluorouracil/leucovorin/irinotecan (Falcone, 2007) **or** 130 mg/m² every 3 weeks in combination with capecitabine (Cassidy, 2008; Haller, 2011)

Esophageal/gastric cancers (unlabeled use; as part of a combination chemotherapy regimen): I.V.: 85 mg/m² every 2 weeks (Al-Batran, 2008; Conroy, 2010) **or** 130 mg/m² every 3 weeks (Cunningham, 2008)

or

Gastric cancer: 100 mg/m² every 2 weeks (Louvet, 2002)

Hepatobiliary cancer, advanced (unlabeled use; as part of a combination chemotherapy regimen): I.V.: 100 mg/m² every 2 weeks (Andre, 2004) **or** 130 mg/m² every 3 weeks (Nehls, 2008)

Non-Hodgkin's lymphoma, refractory (unlabeled use; as part of a combination chemotherapy regimen): I.V.: 25 mg/m²/day for 4 days every 4 weeks (Tsimberidou, 2008) **or** 100 mg/m² every 3 weeks (Lopez, 2008; Rodriguez, 2007) **or** 130 mg/m² every 3 weeks (Chau, 2001)

Ovarian cancer, advanced (unlabeled use): I.V.: 130 mg/m^2 every 3 weeks (Dieras, 2002; Piccart, 2000)

Pancreatic cancer, advanced (unlabeled use; as part of a combination chemotherapy regimen): I.V.: 85 mg/m^2 every 2 weeks (Conroy, 2005; Conroy, 2011; Pelzer, 2011) **or** 100 mg/m^2 every 2 weeks (Louvet, 2005) **or** 110-130 mg/m^2 every 3 weeks (Xiong, 2008)

Testicular cancer, refractory (unlabeled use; in combination with gemcitabine): I.V.: 130 mg/m^2 every 3 weeks (Bokemeyer, 2008; Kollmannsberger, 2004; Pectasides, 2004)

Geriatric No dosage adjustment necessary. Refer to adult dosing.

Renal Impairment

Manufacturer's recommendations:

U.S. labeling:

Cl_{cr} ≥30 mL/minute: No dosage adjustment necessary.

Cl_{cr} <30 mL/minute: Reduce dose from 85 mg/m^2 to 65 mg/m^2.

Canadian labeling: Cl_{cr} <30 mL/minute: Use is contraindicated.

Alternate recommendations: Cl_{cr} ≥20 mL/minute: In a study with a limited number of patients with mild-to-moderate impairment, defined by the authors as Cl_{cr} 20-59 mL/minute (determined using 24-hour urine collection), oxaliplatin was well-tolerated, suggesting a dose reduction may not be necessary in patients with Cl_{cr} ≥20 mL/minute receiving every-3-week dosing (dose range: 80-130 mg/m^2 every 3 weeks) (Takimoto, 2003).

Hepatic Impairment Mild, moderate, or severe impairment: No dosage adjustment necessary (Doroshow, 2003; Synold, 2007).

Adjustment for Toxicity Acute toxicities: Longer infusion time (6 hours) may mitigate acute toxicities.

Neurosensory events:

Persistent (>7 days) grade 2 neurosensory events:

Adjuvant treatment of stage III colon cancer: Reduce dose to 75 mg/m^2

Advanced colorectal cancer: Reduce dose to 65 mg/m^2

Consider withholding oxaliplatin for grade 2 neuropathy lasting >7 days despite dose reduction.

Persistent grade 3 neurosensory events: Consider discontinuing oxaliplatin

Other toxicities (grade 3/4 gastrointestinal toxicity, grade 4 neutropenia, or grade 3/4 thrombocytopenia): After recovery from toxicity, oxaliplatin dose reductions are recommended:

Adjuvant treatment of stage III colon cancer: Reduce dose to 75 mg/m^2; delay next dose until neutrophils recover to ≥1500/mm^3 and platelets recover to ≥75,000/mm^3

Advanced colorectal cancer: Reduce dose to 65 mg/m^2; delay next dose until neutrophils recover to ≥1500/mm^3 and platelets recover to ≥75,000/mm^3

Pulmonary toxicity (unexplained respiratory symptoms including nonproductive cough, dyspnea, crackles, pulmonary infiltrates): Discontinue until interstitial lung disease or pulmonary fibrosis have been excluded.

Combination Regimens

Biliary adenocarcinoma:

CAPOX (Biliary Cancer) on page 1542

GEMOX (Biliary Cancer) on page 1678

Colorectal cancer:

Bevacizumab-Oxaliplatin-Fluorouracil-Leucovorin on page 1531

Bevacizumab + XELOX (Colorectal) on page 1532

Cetuximab-FOLFOX4 on page 1560

FLOX (Colorectal) on page 1645
FOLFOX1 (Colorectal) on page 1662
FOLFOX2 (Colorectal) on page 1662
FOLFOX3 (Colorectal) on page 1662
FOLFOX4 (Colorectal) on page 1663
FOLFOX6 and mFOLFOX6 (Colorectal) on page 1663
FOLFOX7 (Colorectal) on page 1664
FOLFOXIRI (Colorectal) on page 1665
Panitumumab + FOLFOX4 (Colorectal) on page 1733
XELOX (Colorectal) on page 1778

Esophageal cancer:
Docetaxel-Oxaliplatin-Fluorouracil (Esophageal Cancer) on page 1613
Docetaxel-Oxaliplatin-Leucovorin-Fluorouracil (Esophageal Cancer) on page 1613
Epirubicin-Oxaliplatin-Capecitabine on page 1627
Epirubicin-Oxaliplatin-Fluorouracil (Esophageal Cancer) on page 1627
Fluorouracil-Leucovorin-Oxaliplatin (Esophageal Cancer) on page 1656
Oxaliplatin-Fluorouracil (Esophageal Cancer) on page 1724

Gastric cancer:
Epirubicin-Oxaliplatin-Capecitabine on page 1627
Fluorouracil-Leucovorin-Oxaliplatin (Gastric Cancer) on page 1657

Leukemia, chronic lymphocytic: OFAR (CLL) on page 1722

Lymphoma, non-Hodgkin's:
Gemcitabine-Oxaliplatin-Rituximab (NHL) on page 1674
Oxaliplatin-Cytarabine-Dexamethasone (NHL Regimen) on page 1723

Ovarian cancer: Docetaxel-Oxaliplatin (Ovarian Cancer) on page 1613

Pancreatic cancer:
CAPOX (Pancreatic) on page 1543
FOLFIRINOX (Pancreatic) on page 1661
FOLFOX (Pancreatic) on page 1665
Gemcitabine-Oxaliplatin (Pancreatic) on page 1674

Testicular cancer:
Gemcitabine-Oxaliplatin-Paclitaxel (Testicular) on page 1674
GEMOX (Testicular) on page 1678

Administration Administer as I.V. infusion over 2 hours; extend infusion time to 6 hours for acute toxicities. Flush infusion line with D_5W prior to administration of any concomitant medication. Patients should receive an antiemetic premedication regimen. Avoid mucositis prophylaxis with ice chips during oxaliplatin infusion (may exacerbate acute neurological symptoms). Do not use needles or administration sets containing aluminum.

Emetic Potential Moderate (30% to 90%)

Vesicant/Extravasation Risk Vesicant; see Management of Drug Extravasations on page 1800.

Cool compress may be used for immediate management of extravasation, with consideration of potential for peripheral neuropathy exacerbated by cold. Warm compresses will avoid peripheral neuropathy, however, while possibly increasing drug removal through local vasodilation, may increase cellular uptake and injury.

Monitoring Parameters CBC with differential, blood chemistries (including serum creatinine, ALT, AST, and bilirubin); INR and prothrombin time (in patients on oral anticoagulant therapy); signs of neuropathy, hypersensitivity, respiratory effects, and/or RPLS

Additional Information Cold temperature may exacerbate acute neuropathy. Do not use ice for mucositis prophylaxis.

Dosage Forms Excipient information presented when available (limited, particularly for generics); consult specific product labeling.

Injection, powder for reconstitution: 50 mg, 100 mg

Injection, solution [concentrate, preservative free]: 5 mg/mL (10 mL, 20 mL)

Eloxatin®: 5 mg/mL (10 mL, 20 mL, 40 mL)

References

Al-Batran SE, Hartmann JT, Probst S, et al, "Phase III Trial in Metastatic Gastroesophageal Adenocarcinoma With Fluorouracil, Leucovorin Plus Either Oxaliplatin or Cisplatin: A Study of the Arbeitsgemeinschaft Internistische Onkologie," *J Clin Oncol*, 2008, 26(9):1435-42.

Andre P, Cisternino S, Roy AL, et al, "Stability of Oxaliplatin in Infusion Bags Containing 5% Dextrose Injection," *Am J Health Syst Pharm*, 2007, 64(18):1950-4.

Andre T, Boni C, Mounedji-Boudiaf L, et al, "Oxaliplatin, Fluorouracil, and Leucovorin as Adjuvant Treatment for Colon Cancer," *N Engl J Med*, 2004, 350(23):2343-51.

Andre T, Boni C, Navarro M, et al, "Improved Overall Survival With Oxaliplatin, Fluorouracil, and Leucovorin as Adjuvant Treatment in Stage II or III Colon Cancer in the MOSAIC Trial," *J Clin Oncol*, 2009, 27(19):3109-16.

Andre T, Tournigand C, Rosmorduc O, et al, "Gemcitabine Combined With Oxaliplatin (GEMOX) in Advanced Biliary Tract Adenocarcinoma: A GERCOR Study," *Ann Oncol*, 2004, 15(9):1339-43.

Cassidy J, Clarke S, Díaz-Rubio E, et al, "Randomized Phase III Study of Capecitabine Plus Oxaliplatin Compared With Fluorouracil/Folinic Acid Plus Oxaliplatin as First-Line Therapy for Metastatic Colorectal Cancer," *J Clin Oncol*, 2008, 26(12):2006-12.

Chau I, Webb A, Cunningham D, et al, "An Oxaliplatin-Based Chemotherapy in Patients With Relapsed or Refractory Intermediate and High-Grade Non-Hodgkin's Lymphoma," *Br J Haematol*, 2001, 115(4):786-92.

Conroy T, Desseigne F, Ychou M, et al, "FOLFIRINOX Versus Gemcitabine for Metastatic Pancreatic Cancer," *N Engl J Med*, 2011, 364(19):1817-25.

Conroy T, Paillot B, François E, et al, "Irinotecan Plus Oxaliplatin and Leucovorin-Modulated Fluorouracil in Advanced Pancreatic Cancer – A Groupe Tumeurs Digestives of the Federation Nationale des Centres de Lutte Contre le Cancer Study," *J Clin Oncol*, 2005, 23(6):1228-36.

Cunningham D, Starling N, Rao S, et al, "Capecitabine and Oxaliplatin for Advanced Esophagogastric Cancer," *N Engl J Med*, 2008, 358(1):36-46.

de Lemos ML and Walisser S, "Management of Extravasation of Oxaliplatin,"*J Oncol Pharm Pract*, 2005, 11(4):159-62.

Dieras V, Bougnoux P, Petit T, et al, "Multicentre Phase II Study of Oxaliplatin as a Single-Agent in Cisplatin/Carboplatin +/- Taxane-Pretreated Ovarian Cancer Patients," *Ann Oncol*, 2002, 13 (2):258-66.

Doroshow JH, Synold TW, Gandara D, et al, "Pharmacology of Oxaliplatin in Solid Tumor Patients With Hepatic Dysfunction: A Preliminary Report of the National Cancer Institute Organ Dysfunction Working Group," *Semin Oncol*, 2003, 30(4 Suppl 15):14-9.

Falcone A, Ricci S, Brunetti I, et al, "Phase III Trial of Infusional Fluorouracil, Leucovorin, Oxaliplatin, and Irinotecan (FOLFOXIRI) Compared With Infusional Fluorouracil, Leucovorin, and Irinotecan (FOLFIRI) as First-Line Treatment for Metastatic Colorectal Cancer: The Gruppo Oncologico Nord Ovest," *J Clin Oncol*, 2007, 25(13):1670-6.

Haller DG, Tabernero J, Maroun J, et al, "Capecitabine Plus Oxaliplatin Compared With Fluorouracil and Folinic Acid as Adjuvant Therapy for Stage III Colon Cancer," *J Clin Oncol*, 2011, 29 (11):1465-71.

Kim BH, Bradley T, Tai J, et al, "Hypersensitivity to Oxaliplatin: An Investigation of Incidence and Risk Factors, and Literature Review," *Oncology*, 2009, 76(4):231-8.

Kollmannsberger C, Beyer J, Liersch R, et al, "Combination Chemotherapy With Gemcitabine Plus Oxaliplatin in Patients With Intensively Pretreated or Refractory Germ Cell Cancer: A Study of the German Testicular Cancer Study Group," *J Clin Oncol*, 2004, 22(1):108-14.

KueblerJP, Wieand HS, O'Connell MJ, et al, "Oxaliplatin Combined With Weekly Bolus Fluorouracil and Leucovorin as Surgical Adjuvant Chemotherapy for Stage II and III Colon Cancer: Results From NSABP C-07," *J Clin Oncol*, 2007, 25(16):2198-204.

López A, Gutiérrez A, Palacios A, et al, "GEMOX-R Regimen is a Highly Effective Salvage Regimen in Patients With Refractory/Relapsing Diffuse Large-Cell Lymphoma: A Phase II Study," *Eur J Haematol*, 2008, 80(2):127-32.

Louvet C, André T, Tigaud JM, et al, "Phase II Study of Oxaliplatin, Fluorouracil, and Folinic Acid in Locally Advanced or Metastatic Gastric Cancer Patients," *J Clin Oncol*, 2002, 20(23):4543-8.

Louvet C, Labianca R, Hammel P, et al, "Gemcitabine in Combination With Oxaliplatin Compared With Gemcitabine Alone in Locally Advanced or Metastatic Pancreatic Cancer: Results of a GERCOR and GISCAD Phase III Trial," *J Clin Oncol*, 2005, 23(15):3509-16.

Morgan C, Tillett T, Braybrooke J, et al, "Management of Uncommon Chemotherapy-Induced Emergencies," *Lancet Oncol*, 2011, 12(8):806-14.

Nehls O, Oettle H, Hartmann JT, et al, "Capecitabine Plus Oxaliplatin as First-Line Treatment in Patients With Advanced Biliary System Adenocarcinoma: A Prospective Multicentre Phase II Trial," *Br J Cancer*, 2008, 98(2):309-15.

Pectasides D, Pectasides M, Farmakis D, et al, "Gemcitabine and Oxaliplatin (GEMOX) in Patients With Cisplatin-Refractory Germ Cell Tumors: A Phase II Study," *Ann Oncol*, 2004, 15(3):493-7.

Pelzer U, Schwaner I, Stieler J, et al, "Best Supportive Care (BSC) Versus Oxaliplatin, Folinic Acid and 5-Fluorouracil (OFF) Plus BSC in Patients for Second-Line Advanced Pancreatic Cancer: A Phase III-Study from the German CONKO-Study Group," *Eur J Cancer*, 2011, 47(11):1676-81.

Piccart MJ, Green JA, Lacave AJ, et al, "Oxaliplatin or Paclitaxel in Patients With Platinum-Pretreated Advanced Ovarian Cancer: A Randomized Phase II Study of the European Organization for Research and Treatment of Cancer Gynecology Group," *J Clin Oncol*, 2000, 18 (6):1193-202.

Polyzos A, Tsavaris N, Gogas H, et al, "Clinical Features of Hypersensitivity Reactions to Oxaliplatin: A 10-Year Experience," *Oncology*, 2009, 76(1):36-41.

Ramanathan PK, Rothenberg ML, de Gramont A, et al, "Incidence and Evolution of Oxaliplatin-Induced Peripheral Sensory Neuropathy in Diabetic Patients With Colorectal Cancer: A Pooled Analysis of Three Phase III Studies," *Ann Oncol*, 2010, 21(4):754-8.

Rodríguez J, Gutierrez A, Palacios A, et al, "Rituximab, Gemcitabine and Oxaliplatin: An Effective Regimen in Patients With Refractory and Relapsing Mantle Cell Lymphoma," *Leuk Lymphoma*, 2007, 48(11):2172-8.

Synold TW, Takimoto CH, Doroshow JH, et al, "Dose-Escalating and Pharmacologic Study of Oxaliplatin in Adult Cancer Patients With Impaired Hepatic Function: A National Cancer Institute Organ Dysfunction Working Group Study," *Clin Cancer Res*, 2007, 13(12):3660-6.

Takimoto CH, Graham MA, Lockwood G, et al, "Oxaliplatin Pharmacokinetics and Pharmacodynamics in Adult Cancer patients With Impaired Renal Function," *Clin Cancer Res*, 2007, 13 (16):4832-9.

Takimoto CH, Remick SC, Sharma S, et al, "Dose-Escalating and Pharmacological Study of Oxaliplatin in Adult Cancer Patients With Impaired Renal Function: A National Cancer Institute Organ Dysfunction Working Group Study," *J Clin Oncol*, 2003, 21(14):2664-72.

Tsimberidou AM, Wierda WG, Plunkett W, et al, "Phase I-II Study of Oxaliplatin, Fludarabine, Cytarabine, and Rituximab Combination Therapy in Patients With Richter's Syndrome or Fludarabine-Refractory Chronic Lymphocytic Leukemia," *J Clin Oncol*, 2008, 26(2):196-203.

Xiong HQ, Varadhachary GR, Blais JC, et al, "Phase 2 Trial of Oxaliplatin Plus Capecitabine (XELOX) as Second-Line Therapy for Patients With Advanced Pancreatic Cancer," *Cancer*, 2008, 113(8):2046-52.

◆ **Oxecta™** *see* OxyCODONE *on page 1084*

◆ **Oxecta™** *see* OxyCODONE *on page 1084*

OxyCODONE (oks i KOE done)

Brand Names: U.S. Oxecta™; OxyCONTIN®; Roxicodone®

Brand Names: Canada Oxy.IR®; OxyContin®; OxyNEO™; PMS-Oxycodone; Supeudol®

Index Terms Dihydrohydroxycodeinone; Oxecta™; Oxycodone Hydrochloride

Generic Availability (U.S.) Yes: Excludes controlled release tablet

Pharmacologic Category Analgesic, Opioid

Use Management of moderate-to-severe pain, normally used in combination with nonopioid analgesics

OxyContin® is indicated for around-the-clock management of moderate-to-severe pain when a continuous analgesic is needed for an extended period of time.

Labeled Contraindications Hypersensitivity to oxycodone or any component of the formulation; significant respiratory depression; hypercarbia; acute or severe bronchial asthma; paralytic ileus (known or suspected); GI obstruction

Pregnancy Risk Factor B

Lactation Enters breast milk/not recommended

Warnings/Precautions May cause CNS depression, which may impair physical or mental abilities; patients must be cautioned about performing tasks which require mental alertness (eg, operating machinery or driving). Effects may be potentiated when used with other sedative drugs or ethanol. Use with caution in patients with hypersensitivity reactions to other phenanthrene derivative opioid agonists (morphine, hydrocodone, hydromorphone, levorphanol, oxymorphone), respiratory diseases including asthma, emphysema, or COPD. Use with caution in pancreatitis or biliary tract disease, acute alcoholism (including delirium tremens), morbid obesity, adrenocortical insufficiency, history of seizure disorders, CNS depression/coma, kyphoscoliosis (or other skeletal disorder which may alter respiratory function), hypothyroidism (including myxedema), prostatic hyperplasia, urethral stricture, and toxic psychosis. May obscure diagnosis or clinical course of patients with acute abdominal conditions.

Use with caution in the elderly, debilitated, or cachectic patients, and hepatic or renal dysfunction. Hemodynamic effects (hypotension, orthostasis) may be exaggerated in patients with hypovolemia, concurrent vasodilating drugs, or in patients with head injury. Monitor for symptoms of hypotension following initiation or dose titration. Respiratory depressant effects and capacity to elevate CSF pressure may be exaggerated in presence of head injury, other intracranial lesion, or pre-existing intracranial pressure.

Concomitant use with CYP3A4 inhibitors may result in increased effects and potentially fatal respiratory depression. Concurrent use of agonist/antagonist analgesics may precipitate withdrawal symptoms and/or reduced analgesic efficacy in patients following prolonged therapy with mu opioid agonists. Abrupt discontinuation following prolonged use may also lead to withdrawal symptoms. Healthcare provider should be alert to problems of abuse, misuse, and diversion; abuse of products by crushing, chewing, snorting, or injecting may result in severe overdose, adverse effects, or death.

Controlled-release tablets: OxyContin® is not intended for use as an "as needed" analgesic or for the treatment of mild pain, acute pain, or postoperative pain requiring short-term analgesia (should be used postoperatively only if the patient has received it prior to surgery or if severe, persistent pain is anticipated). **[U.S. Boxed Warning]: May cause potentially life-threatening respiratory depression even with therapeutic use. Ensure proper dosing and titration; monitor for respiratory depression especially within the first 24-72 hours of initiation or dose escalation. Oxycodone controlled-release tablets should only be prescribed by healthcare professionals familiar with the use of potent opioids for chronic pain. Do NOT crush, break, chew or dissolve controlled-release tablets (may result in a potentially fatal overdose);** 60 mg and 80 mg strengths, a single dose >40 mg, or a total dose of >80 mg/day are for use only in opioid-tolerant patients. Tablets may be difficult to swallow and could become lodged in throat; patients with swallowing difficulties may be at increased risk. Cases of intestinal obstruction or diverticulitis exacerbation have also been reported, including cases requiring medical intervention to remove the tablet; patients with an underlying GI disease (eg, esophageal cancer, colon cancer) may be at increased risk. **[U.S. Boxed Warning]: Accidental exposure may result in fatal overdose of oxycodone, especially in children. [U.S. Boxed Warning]: Healthcare provider should be alert to problems of abuse, misuse, and diversion. Tolerance or drug dependence may result from extended**

use. Patients should be assessed for risk of abuse or addiction prior to therapy and all patients should be monitored for signs of misuse, abuse, and addiction. Risk of opioid abuse is increased in patients with a history or family history of alcohol or drug abuse or mental illness.

Oral solutions: **[U.S. Boxed Warning]: Highly concentrated oral solution (20 mg/mL) should only be used in opioid tolerant patients (taking ≥30 mg/day of oxycodone or equivalent for ≥1 week). [U.S. Boxed Warning]: Orders for oxycodone oral solutions (20 mg/mL or 5 mg/5 mL) should be clearly written to include the intended dose (in mg vs mL) and the intended product concentration to be dispensed to avoid potential dosing errors. Products should be stored out of reach of children; seek immediate medical care in the event of accidental ingestion.**

Ethanol/Nutrition/Herb Interactions

Ethanol: May increase CNS depression; monitor for increased effects with coadministration. Caution patients about effects.

Herb/Nutraceutical: Avoid valerian, St John's wort, kava kava, gotu kola (may increase CNS depression).

Storage/Stability Store at 25°C (77°F); excursions permitted between 15°C to 30°C (59°F to 86°F). Protect from light.

Mechanism of Action Binds to opiate receptors in the CNS, causing inhibition of ascending pain pathways, altering the perception of and response to pain; produces generalized CNS depression

Pharmacodynamics/Kinetics

Onset of action: Pain relief: Immediate release: 10-15 minutes

Peak effect: Immediate release: 0.5-1 hour

Duration: Immediate release: 3-6 hours; Controlled release: ≤12 hours

Distribution: V_d: 2.6 L/kg; distributed to skeletal muscle, liver, intestinal tract, lungs, spleen, and brain

Protein binding: ~45%

Metabolism: Hepatically via CYP3A4 to noroxycodone (has weak analgesic), noroxymorphone, and alpha- and beta-noroxycodol. CYP2D6 mediated metabolism produces oxymorphone (has analgesic activity; low plasma concentrations), alpha- and beta-oxymorphol.

Bioavailability: Controlled release, immediate release: 60% to 87%

Half-life elimination: Immediate release: 2-4 hours; controlled release: ~5 hours

Time to peak, plasma: Immediate release: 1.2-1.9 hours; Controlled release: 4-5 hours

Excretion: Urine (~19% as parent; >64% as metabolites)

Dosing

Adult & Geriatric Management of pain: Oral:

Regular or immediate release formulations: Initial: 5-15 mg every 4-6 hours as needed; dosing range: 5-20 mg per dose (APS 6th edition). For severe chronic pain, administer on a regularly scheduled basis, every 4-6 hours, at the lowest dose that will achieve adequate analgesia.

Controlled release: **Note:** 60 mg and 80 mg strengths, a single dose >40 mg, or a total dose of >80 mg daily are for use only in opioid-tolerant patients.

Opioid naive: Initial: 10 mg every 12 hours

Concurrent CNS depressants: Reduce usual initial oxycodone dose by one-third (1/3) to one-half (1/2)

Conversion from transdermal fentanyl: For each 25 mcg/hour transdermal dose, substitute 10 mg controlled release oxycodone every 12 hours; should be initiated 18 hours after the removal of the transdermal fentanyl patch

Currently on opioids: Use standard conversion chart to convert daily opioid dose to oxycodone equivalent. Initiate controlled release oxycodone with one-half (1/2) the estimated oxycodone daily dose (mg/day) and provide rescue medication in the form of immediate release oxycodone. Divide the initial controlled release oxycodone daily dose in 2 (for twice-daily dosing, usually every 12 hours) and round down to nearest dosage form.

Dose adjustment: Doses may be adjusted by changing the total daily dose (not by changing the dosing interval). Doses may be adjusted every 1-2 days and may be increased by 25% to 50%. Dose should be gradually tapered when no longer required in order to prevent withdrawal.

Multiplication factors for converting the daily dose of current oral opioid to the daily dose of oral oxycodone:

Current opioid mg/day dose x factor = Oxycodone mg/day dose

Codeine mg/day oral dose **x** 0.15 = Oxycodone mg/day dose
Hydrocodone mg/day oral dose **x** 0.9 = Oxycodone mg/day dose
Hydromorphone mg/day oral dose **x** 4 = Oxycodone mg/day dose
Levorphanol mg/day oral dose **x** 7.5 = Oxycodone mg/day dose
Meperidine mg/day oral dose **x** 0.1 = Oxycodone mg/day dose
Methadone mg/day oral dose **x** 1.5 = Oxycodone mg/day dose
Morphine mg/day oral dose **x** 0.5 = Oxycodone mg/day dose

Note: Divide the oxycodone mg/day dose into the appropriate dosing interval for the specific form being used.

Pediatric Management of pain (unlabeled use): Immediate release, initial dose: 0.1-0.2 mg/kg/dose (moderate pain) or 0.2 mg/kg/dose (severe pain) (APS 6th edition). For severe chronic pain, administer on a regularly scheduled basis, every 4-6 hours, at the lowest dose that will achieve adequate analgesia.

Renal Impairment Serum concentrations are increased ~50% in patients with Cl_{cr} <60 mL/minute; adjust dose based on clinical situation.

Hepatic Impairment

Immediate release: Reduced initial doses may be necessary (use a conservative approach to initial dosing); adjust dose based on clinical situation.

Controlled release: Decrease initial dose to one-third (1/3) to one-half (1/2) the usual starting dose; titrate carefully.

Administration

Controlled release: Swallow tablet whole. Do not moisten, dissolve, cut, crush, break, or chew controlled release tablets. Controlled release tablets are not indicated for rectal administration; increased risk of adverse events due to better rectal absorption. Controlled release tablets should be administered one at a time and each followed with water immediately after placing in the mouth.

Immediate release (Oxecta™): Must be swallowed whole with enough water to ensure complete swallowing immediately after placing in the mouth. The tablet should not be wet prior to placing in the mouth. Do not crush, chew, or dissolve the tablets. Do not administer via feeding tubes (eg, gastric, NG) due to potential for obstruction. The formulation uses technology designed to discourage common methods of tampering to prevent misuse/abuse.

Appropriate laxatives should be administered to avoid the constipating side effects associated with use. Antiemetics may be needed for persistent nausea.

Test Interactions Some quinolones may produce a false-positive urine screening result for opiates using commercially-available immunoassay kits. This has been demonstrated most consistently for levofloxacin and ofloxacin, but other quinolones have shown cross-reactivity in certain assay kits. Confirmation of positive opiate screens by more specific methods should be considered.

Prescribing and Access Restrictions As a requirement of the REMS program, healthcare providers who prescribe OxyContin® need to receive training on the proper use and potential risks of OxyContin®. For training, please refer to http://www.oxycontinrems.com. Prescribers will need retraining every 2 years or following any significant changes to the OxyContin® REMS program.

Medication Guide Available Yes

Dosage Forms Excipient information presented when available (limited, particularly for generics); consult specific product labeling. [DSC] = Discontinued product

Capsule, oral, as hydrochloride: 5 mg
Solution, oral, as hydrochloride: 5 mg/5 mL (5 mL, 500 mL)
Solution, oral, as hydrochloride [concentrate]: 20 mg/mL (30 mL)
Tablet, oral, as hydrochloride: 5 mg, 10 mg, 15 mg, 20 mg, 30 mg
  Oxecta™: 5 mg, 7.5 mg
  Roxicodone®: 5 mg [DSC], 15 mg, 30 mg [scored]
Tablet, controlled release, oral, as hydrochloride:
  OxyCONTIN®: 10 mg, 15 mg, 20 mg, 30 mg, 40 mg, 60 mg, 80 mg

Controlled Substance C-II

◆ **Oxycodone Hydrochloride** *see* OxyCODONE *on page 1084*
◆ **OxyCONTIN®** *see* OxyCODONE *on page 1084*
◆ **OxyContin® (Can)** *see* OxyCODONE *on page 1084*
◆ **Oxy.IR® (Can)** *see* OxyCODONE *on page 1084*

Oxymorphone (oks i MOR fone)

Brand Names: U.S. Opana®; Opana® ER

Index Terms Oxymorphone Hydrochloride

Generic Availability (U.S.) Yes: Excludes injection solution

Pharmacologic Category Analgesic, Opioid

Use

Parenteral: Management of moderate-to-severe acute pain; analgesia during labor; preoperative medication; anesthesia support; relief of anxiety in patients with dyspnea associated with pulmonary edema secondary to acute left ventricular failure

Oral, regular release: Management of moderate-to-severe acute pain

Oral, extended release: Management of moderate-to-severe pain in patients requiring around-the-clock opioid treatment for an extended period of time

Labeled Contraindications Hypersensitivity to oxymorphone, other morphine analogs (phenanthrene derivatives), or any component of the formulation; paralytic ileus (known or suspected); moderate-to-severe hepatic impairment; severe respiratory depression (unless using immediate release or parenteral formulation in monitored setting with resuscitative equipment); acute/severe bronchial asthma; hypercarbia

Note: Parenteral formulation is also contraindicated in the treatment of upper airway obstruction and pulmonary edema due to a chemical respiratory irritant.

Pregnancy Risk Factor C

Lactation Excretion in breast milk unknown/use caution

Warnings/Precautions An opioid-containing analgesic regimen should be tailored to each patient's needs and based upon the type of pain being treated (acute versus chronic), the route of administration, degree of tolerance for opioids (naive versus chronic user), age, weight, and patient comorbidities. The optimal analgesic dose varies widely among patients. Doses should be titrated to pain relief/prevention.

May cause CNS depression, which may impair physical or mental abilities; patients must be cautioned about performing tasks which require mental alertness (eg, operating machinery or driving). Effects may be potentiated when used with other sedative drugs or ethanol. Use not recommended within 14 days of MAO inhibitors. Due to structural similarities, hypersensitivity to other phenanthrene-derivative opioid agonists (codeine, hydrocodone, hydromorphone, levorphanol, morphine) may result in similar hypersensitivity reaction if oxymorphone is used; therefore, the use of oxymorphone is contraindicated in patients with previous hypersensitivity to other phenanthrene derivatives. May cause respiratory depression. Use extreme caution in patients with COPD or other chronic respiratory conditions characterized by hypoxia, hypercapnia, or diminished respiratory reserve (myxedema, cor pulmonale, kyphoscoliosis, obstructive sleep apnea, severe obesity). Use with caution in patients (particularly elderly or debilitated) with impaired respiratory function, adrenal disease, morbid obesity, seizure disorders, toxic psychosis, thyroid dysfunction, prostatic hyperplasia, or renal impairment. Use caution in mild hepatic dysfunction; use is contraindicated in moderate-to-severe hepatic impairment. Use only with extreme caution (if at all) in patients with head injury or increased intracranial pressure (ICP); potential to elevate ICP and/or blunt papillary response may be greatly exaggerated in these patients. Use with caution in patients with biliary tract dysfunction including acute pancreatitis; may cause constriction of sphincter of Oddi. May obscure diagnosis or clinical course of patients with acute abdominal conditions.

Oxymorphone shares the toxic potential of opiate agonists and usual precautions of opiate agonist therapy should be observed; may cause hypotension in patients with acute myocardial infarction, volume depletion, or concurrent drug therapy which may exaggerate vasodilation. The elderly may be particularly susceptible to adverse effects of narcotics.

[U.S. Boxed Warning]: Healthcare provider should be alert to problems of abuse, misuse, and diversion. Tolerance or drug dependence may result from extended use. Use caution in patients with a history of drug dependence or abuse. Abrupt discontinuation may precipitate withdrawal syndrome.

Extended release formulation:

[U.S. Boxed Warnings]: Opana® ER is an extended release oral formulation of oxymorphone and is not suitable for use as an "as needed" analgesic. Tablets should not be broken, chewed, dissolved, or crushed; tablets should be swallowed whole. Opana® ER is intended for use in long-term, continuous management of moderate-to-severe chronic pain. It is not indicated for use in the immediate postoperative period (12-24 hours). Cases of thrombotic thrombocytopenic purpura (TTP) resulting in kidney failure (requiring dialysis) and death have been reported as a result of misuse by drug abusers injecting the extended-release tablets intravenously; tablets are intended for oral administration only. **[U.S. Boxed Warning]: The coingestion of ethanol or ethanol-containing medications with Opana® ER may result**

in accelerated release of drug from the dosage form, abruptly increasing plasma levels, which may have fatal consequences.

Ethanol/Nutrition/Herb Interactions

Ethanol: Ethanol ingestion with extended-release tablets is specifically contraindicated due to possible accelerated release and potentially fatal overdose. Ethanol may also increase CNS depression; monitor for increased effects with coadministration. Caution patients about effects.

Food: When taken orally with a high-fat meal, peak concentration is 38% to 50% greater. Both immediate-release and extended-release tablets should be taken 1 hour before or 2 hours after eating.

Herb/Nutraceutical: Avoid valerian, St John's wort, kava kava, gotu kola (may increase CNS depression).

Storage/Stability Injection solution, tablet: Store at 25°C (77°F); excursions permitted to 15°C to 30°C (59°F to 86°F). Protect injection from light.

Mechanism of Action Oxymorphone hydrochloride is a potent narcotic analgesic with uses similar to those of morphine. The drug is a semisynthetic derivative of morphine (phenanthrene derivative) and is closely related to hydromorphone chemically (Dilaudid®).

Pharmacodynamics/Kinetics

Onset of action: Parenteral: 5-10 minutes

Duration: Analgesic: Parenteral: 3-6 hours

Distribution: V_d: I.V.: 1.94-4.22 L/kg

Protein binding: 10% to 12%

Metabolism: Hepatic via glucuronidation to active and inactive metabolites

Bioavailability: Oral: ~10%

Half-life elimination: Oral: Immediate release: 7-9 hours; Extended release: 9-11 hours

Excretion: Urine (<1% as unchanged drug); feces

Dosing

Adult Analgesia: Note: Dosage must be individualized.

I.M., SubQ: Initial: 1-1.5 mg; may repeat every 4-6 hours as needed

Labor analgesia: I.M.: 0.5-1 mg

I.V.: Initial: 0.5 mg

Oral:

Immediate release: Acute pain:

Opioid-naive: Initial: 5-10 mg every 4-6 hours as needed (American Pain Society, 2008). Dosage adjustment should be based on level of analgesia, side effects, pain intensity, and patient comorbidities.

Currently on stable dose of parenteral oxymorphone: Approximately 10 times the total daily parenteral requirement. The calculated total oral daily amount should be given in 4-6 equally divided doses.

Currently on other opioids: Use standard conversion chart to convert total daily dose of current opioid to oxymorphone equivalent. Generally start with one-half (1/2) the calculated total daily oxymorphone dosage and administer in divided doses every 4-6 hours.

Extended release (Opana® ER): Chronic pain:

Opioid-naive: Initial: 5 mg every 12 hours. Supplemental doses of immediate-release oxymorphone may be used as "rescue" medication as dosage is titrated.

Note: Continued requirement for supplemental dosing may be used to titrate the dose of extended-release continuous therapy. Adjust therapy incrementally, by 5-10 mg every 12 hours at intervals of every 3-7 days. Ideally, scheduled (basal) dosage may be titrated to generally mild pain or no pain with the regular use of fewer than 2 supplemental doses per 24 hours.

Currently on stable dose of parenteral oxymorphone: Approximately 10 times the total daily parenteral requirement. The calculated total oral daily amount should be given in 2 divided doses (for every 12-hour oxymorphone extended release dosing).

Currently on opioids: Use conversion chart (see **"Note"**) to convert daily dose of current opioid to oxymorphone equivalent. Generally start with one-half (1/2) the calculated daily oxymorphone dosage. Divide daily dose in 2 (for every 12-hour oxymorphone extended release dosing) and round down to nearest dosage strength. **Note:** Per manufacturer, the following approximate oral dosages are equivalent to a daily dose of oxymorphone 10 mg:

Hydrocodone 20 mg

Oxycodone 20 mg

Methadone 20 mg (methadone has a long half-life and accumulates; ratio can vary widely)

Morphine 30 mg

Conversion of stable dose of immediate-release oxymorphone to extended-release oxymorphone: Use same total daily dose. Administer one-half (1/2) of the daily dose of immediate-release oxymorphone (Opana®) as the extended-release formulation (Opana® ER) every 12 hours

Geriatric Refer to adult dosing. **Note:** Initiate dosing at the lower end of the dosage range.

Renal Impairment Cl_{cr} <50 mL/minute: Reduce initial dosage of oral and parenteral formulations (bioavailability increased 57% to 65%). Begin therapy at lowest dose and titrate slowly with careful monitoring.

Hepatic Impairment

Mild impairment: Initiate with lowest possible dose and titrate slowly with careful monitoring.

Moderate-to-severe impairment: Use is contraindicated.

Administration Oral: Administer immediate release and extended release tablets 1 hour before or 2 hours after eating. Opana® ER tablet should be swallowed whole; do not break, crush, dissolve, or chew.

Test Interactions Some quinolones may produce a false-positive urine screening result for opiates using commercially-available immunoassay kits. This has been demonstrated most consistently for levofloxacin and ofloxacin, but other quinolones have shown cross-reactivity in certain assay kits. Confirmation of positive opiate screens by more specific methods should be considered. May cause elevation in amylase (due to constriction of the sphincter of Oddi).

Medication Guide Available Yes

Dosage Forms Excipient information presented when available (limited, particularly for generics); consult specific product labeling.

Injection, solution, as hydrochloride:

Opana®: 1 mg/mL (1 mL)

Tablet, oral, as hydrochloride: 5 mg, 10 mg

Opana®: 5 mg, 10 mg

Tablet, extended release, oral, as hydrochloride: 7.5 mg, 15 mg

Opana® ER: 5 mg, 10 mg, 20 mg, 30 mg, 40 mg

Controlled Substance C-II

- **Oxymorphone Hydrochloride** *see* Oxymorphone *on page 1088*
- **OxyNEO™ (Can)** *see* OxyCODONE *on page 1084*
- **P32** *see* Chromic Phosphate P 32 *on page 279*

PACLitaxel (pac li TAKS el)

Related Information

Chemotherapy and Obesity *on page 1834*
Chronic Pain Management (Cancer) *on page 1840*
Management of Chemotherapy-Induced Nausea and Vomiting *on page 1786*
Management of Drug Extravasations *on page 1800*
Oral Mucositis/Stomatitis *on page 1814*
Principles of Anticancer Therapy *on page 1878*
Safe Handling of Hazardous Drugs *on page 1904*

Brand Names: Canada Apo-Paclitaxel®; Paclitaxel for Injection; Paclitaxel Injection USP

Index Terms Conventional Paclitaxel; Paclitaxel (Conventional); Taxol

Generic Availability (U.S.) Yes

Pharmacologic Category Antineoplastic Agent, Antimicrotubular; Antineoplastic Agent, Natural Source (Plant) Derivative; Antineoplastic Agent, Taxane Derivative

Use Treatment of breast, nonsmall cell lung, and ovarian cancers; treatment of AIDS-related Kaposi's sarcoma (KS)

Unlabeled Use Treatment of bladder, cervical, small cell lung, and head and neck cancers; treatment of (unknown primary) adenocarcinoma

Labeled Contraindications Hypersensitivity to paclitaxel, Cremophor® EL (polyoxyethylated castor oil), or any component of the formulation

Pregnancy Risk Factor D

Lactation Excretion in breast milk unknown/contraindicated

Warnings/Precautions Hazardous agent - use appropriate precautions for handling and disposal. **[U.S. Boxed Warning]: Severe hypersensitivity reactions have been reported;** premedication may minimize this effect. Stop infusion and do not rechallenge for severe hypersensitivity reactions (hypotension requiring treatment, dyspnea requiring bronchodilators, angioedema, urticaria). Minor hypersensitivity reactions (flushing, skin reactions, dyspnea, hypotension, or tachycardia) do not require interruption of treatment. **[U.S. Boxed Warning]: Bone marrow suppression is the dose-limiting toxicity; do not administer if baseline absolute neutrophil count (ANC) is <1500 cells/mm^3 (<1000 cells/mm^3 for patients with AIDS-related KS);** reduce future doses by 20% for severe neutropenia (<500 cells/mm^3 for 7 days or more) and consider the use of supportive therapy, including growth factor treatment.

Use extreme caution with hepatic dysfunction (myelotoxicity may be worsened); dose reductions are recommended. Peripheral neuropathy may occur; patients with pre-existing neuropathies from chemotherapy or coexisting conditions (eg, diabetes mellitus) may be at a higher risk; reduce dose by 20% for severe neuropathy. Paclitaxel formulations contain dehydrated alcohol; may cause adverse CNS effects. Infusion-related hypotension, bradycardia, and/or hypertension may occur; frequent monitoring of vital signs is recommended, especially during the first hour of the infusion. Rare but severe conduction abnormalities have been reported; conduct cardiac monitoring during subsequent infusions for these patients. When administered as sequential infusions, taxane derivatives (docetaxel, paclitaxel) should be administered before platinum derivatives (carboplatin, cisplatin) to limit myelosuppression. Elderly patients have an increased risk of toxicity (neutropenia, neuropathy). **[U.S. Boxed Warning]: Should be administered under the supervision of an experienced cancer chemotherapy physician.** Safety and efficacy in children have not been established.

Adverse Reactions Percentages reported with single-agent therapy. **Note:** Myelosuppression is dose related, schedule related, and infusion-rate dependent (increased incidences with higher doses, more frequent doses, and longer infusion times) and, in general, rapidly reversible upon discontinuation.

>10%:

Cardiovascular: Flushing (28%), ECG abnormal (14% to 23%), edema (21%), hypotension (4% to 12%)

Dermatologic: Alopecia (87%), rash (12%)

Gastrointestinal: Nausea/vomiting (52%), diarrhea (38%), mucositis (17% to 35%; grades 3/4: up to 3%), stomatitis (15%; most common at doses >390 mg/m^2), abdominal pain (with intraperitoneal paclitaxel)

Hematologic: Neutropenia (78% to 98%; grade 4: 14% to 75%; onset 8-10 days, median nadir 11 days, recovery 15-21 days), leukopenia (90%; grade 4: 17%), anemia (47% to 90%; grades 3/4: 2% to 16%), thrombocytopenia (4% to 20%; grades 3/4: 1% to 7%), bleeding (14%)

Hepatic: Alkaline phosphatase increased (22%), AST increased (19%)

Local: Injection site reaction (erythema, tenderness, skin discoloration, swelling: 13%)

Neuromuscular & skeletal: Peripheral neuropathy (42% to 70%; grades 3/4: up to 7%), arthralgia/myalgia (60%), weakness (17%)

Renal: Creatinine increased (observed in KS patients only: 18% to 34%; severe: 5% to 7%)

Miscellaneous: Hypersensitivity reaction (31% to 45%; grades 3/4: up to 2%), infection (15% to 30%)

1% to 10%:

Cardiovascular: Bradycardia (3%), tachycardia (2%), hypertension (1%), rhythm abnormalities (1%), syncope (1%), venous thrombosis (1%)

Dermatologic: Nail changes (2%)

Hematologic: Febrile neutropenia (2%)

Hepatic: Bilirubin increased (7%)

Respiratory: Dyspnea (2%)

<1%, postmarketing, and/or case reports: Anaphylaxis, arrhythmia, ataxia, atrial fibrillation, AV block, back pain, cardiac conduction abnormalities, cellulitis, CHF, chills, conjunctivitis, dehydration, enterocolitis, extravasation recall, hepatic encephalopathy, hepatic necrosis, induration, intestinal obstruction, intestinal perforation, interstitial pneumonia, ischemic colitis, lacrimation increased, maculopapular rash, malaise, MI, myocardial ischemia, necrotic changes and ulceration following extravasation, neuroencephalopathy, neutropenic enterocolitis, neutropenic typhlitis, ototoxicity (tinnitus and hearing loss), pancreatitis, paralytic ileus, phlebitis, pneumonitis, pruritus, pulmonary embolism, pulmonary fibrosis, radiation recall, radiation pneumonitis, renal insufficiency, scleroderma exacerbation, seizure, skin edema (diffuse), skin exfoliation, skin fibrosis, skin necrosis, skin sclerosis, skin thickening, Stevens-Johnson syndrome, supraventricular tachycardia, toxic epidermal necrolysis, ventricular tachycardia (asymptomatic), visual disturbances (scintillating scotomata)

Drug Interactions

Metabolism/Transport Effects **Substrate** of CYP2C8 (major), CYP3A4 (major), P-glycoprotein; **Note:** Assignment of Major/Minor substrate status based on clinically relevant drug interaction potential; **Induces** CYP3A4 (weak/moderate)

Avoid Concomitant Use

Avoid concomitant use of PACLitaxel with any of the following: Axitinib; BCG; CloZAPine; Conivaptan; Natalizumab; Pimecrolimus; SORAfenib; Tacrolimus (Topical); Vaccines (Live)

Increased Effect/Toxicity

PACLitaxel may increase the levels/effects of: Antineoplastic Agents (Anthracycline, Systemic); Bexarotene (Systemic); CloZAPine; DOXOrubicin; Leflunomide; Natalizumab; Trastuzumab; Vaccines (Live); Vinorelbine

The levels/effects of PACLitaxel may be increased by: Conivaptan; CYP2C8 Inhibitors (Moderate); CYP2C8 Inhibitors (Strong); CYP3A4 Inhibitors (Moderate); CYP3A4 Inhibitors (Strong); Dasatinib; Deferasirox; Denosumab; Ivacaftor; Mifepristone; P-glycoprotein/ABCB1 Inhibitors; Pimecrolimus; Platinum Derivatives; Reverse Transcriptase Inhibitors (Non-Nucleoside); Roflumilast; SORAfenib; Tacrolimus (Topical); Trastuzumab

Decreased Effect

PACLitaxel may decrease the levels/effects of: ARIPiprazole; Axitinib; BCG; Coccidioidin Skin Test; Saxagliptin; Sipuleucel-T; Vaccines (Inactivated); Vaccines (Live)

The levels/effects of PACLitaxel may be decreased by: Bexarotene (Systemic); CYP2C8 Inducers (Strong); CYP3A4 Inducers (Strong); Deferasirox; Echinacea; Herbs (CYP3A4 Inducers); P-glycoprotein/ABCB1 Inducers; Tocilizumab; Trastuzumab

Ethanol/Nutrition/Herb Interactions Herb/Nutraceutical: Avoid black cohosh, dong quai in estrogen-dependent tumors. Avoid valerian, St John's wort (may decrease paclitaxel levels), kava kava, gotu kola (may increase CNS depression).

Storage/Stability Store intact vials at room temperature of 20°C to 25°C (68°F to 77°F). Protect from light. Solutions diluted for infusion in D_5W and NS are stable for up to 3 days at room temperature (25°C).

Paclitaxel should be dispensed in either glass or non-PVC containers (eg, Excel™/PAB™). Use **nonpolyvinyl** (non-PVC) tubing (eg, polyethylene) to minimize leaching. Formulated in a vehicle known as Cremophor® EL (polyoxyethylated castor oil). Cremophor® EL has been found to leach the plasticizer DEHP from polyvinyl chloride infusion bags or administration sets. Contact of the undiluted concentrate with plasticized polyvinyl chloride (PVC) equipment or devices is not recommended.

Reconstitution Hazardous agent; use appropriate precautions for handling and disposal. Dilute for infusion in 250-1000 mL D_5W, D_5LR, D_5NS, or NS to a concentration of 0.3-1.2 mg/mL, use a non-PVC container (glass or polyethylene). Chemotherapy dispensing devices (eg, Chemo Dispensing Pin™) should not be used to withdraw paclitaxel from the vial.

Mechanism of Action Paclitaxel promotes microtubule assembly by enhancing the action of tubulin dimers, stabilizing existing microtubules, and inhibiting their disassembly, interfering with the late G_2 mitotic phase, and inhibiting cell replication. In addition, the drug can distort mitotic spindles, resulting in the breakage of chromosomes. Paclitaxel may also suppress cell proliferation and modulate immune response.

Pharmacodynamics/Kinetics

Distribution:

V_d: Widely distributed into body fluids and tissues; affected by dose and duration of infusion

V_{dss}:

1- to 6-hour infusion: 67.1 L/m²

24-hour infusion: 227-688 L/m²

Protein binding: 89% to 98%

Metabolism: Hepatic via CYP2C8 and 3A4; forms metabolites (primarily 6α-hydroxypaclitaxel)

Half-life elimination:

1- to 6-hour infusion: Mean (beta): 6.4 hours

3-hour infusion: Mean (terminal): 13.1-20.2 hours

24-hour infusion: Mean (terminal): 15.7-52.7 hours

Excretion: Feces (~70%, 5% as unchanged drug); urine (14%)

Clearance: Mean: Total body: After 1- and 6-hour infusions: 5.8-16.3 L/hour/m²; After 24-hour infusions: 14.2-17.2 L/hour/m²

Dosing

Adult & Geriatric Note: Premedication with dexamethasone (20 mg orally or I.V. at 12 and 6 hours **or** 14 and 7 hours before the dose; reduce dexamethasone dose to 10 mg orally with advanced HIV disease), diphenhydramine (50 mg I.V. 30-60 minutes prior to the dose), and cimetidine, famotidine, or ranitidine (I.V. 30-60 minutes prior to the dose) is recommended.

Ovarian carcinoma:

I.V.: 135-175 mg/m² over 3 hours every 3 weeks **or**

135 mg/m² over 24 hours every 3 weeks **or**

50-80 mg/m² over 1-3 hours weekly **or**

1.4-4 mg/m²/day continuous infusion for 14 days every 4 weeks

Intraperitoneal (unlabeled route): 60 mg/m² on day 8 of a 21-day treatment cycle for 6 cycles, in combination with I.V. paclitaxel and intraperitoneal cisplatin. **Note:** Administration of intraperitoneal paclitaxel should include the standard paclitaxel premedication regimen.

Metastatic breast cancer: I.V.: 175-250 mg/m² over 3 hours every 3 weeks **or**

50-80 mg/m² weekly **or**

1.4-4 mg/m²/day continuous infusion for 14 days every 4 weeks

Nonsmall cell lung carcinoma: I.V.: 135 mg/m² over 24 hours every 3 weeks

AIDS-related Kaposi's sarcoma: I.V.: 135 mg/m² over 3 hours every 3 weeks

or 100 mg/m² over 3 hours every 2 weeks

Renal Impairment There are no FDA-approved labeling guidelines for dosage adjustment in patients with renal impairment. Aronoff (2007) recommends no dosage adjustment necessary for adults with Cl_{cr} <50 mL/minute.

Hepatic Impairment Note: The FDA-approved labeling recommendations are based upon the patient's first course of therapy where the usual dose would be 135 mg/m² dose over 24 hours or the 175 mg/m² dose over 3 hours in patients with normal hepatic function. Dosage in subsequent courses should be based upon individual tolerance. Adjustments for other regimens are not available.

24-hour infusion:

Transaminases <2 times upper limit of normal (ULN) and bilirubin level ≤1.5 mg/dL: 135 mg/m²

Transaminases 2-<10 times ULN and bilirubin level ≤1.5 mg/dL: 100 mg/m²

Transaminases <10 times ULN and bilirubin level 1.6-7.5 mg/dL: 50 mg/m²

Transaminases ≥10 times ULN or bilirubin level >7.5 mg/dL: Avoid use

3-hour infusion:

Transaminases <10 times ULN and bilirubin level ≤1.25 times ULN: 175 mg/m²

Transaminases <10 times ULN and bilirubin level 1.26-2 times ULN: 135 mg/m²

Transaminases <10 times ULN and bilirubin level 2.01-5 times ULN: 90 mg/m²

Transaminases ≥10 times ULN or bilirubin level >5 times ULN: Avoid use

Adjustment for Toxicity

Dosage modification for toxicity (solid tumors, including ovary, breast, and lung carcinoma): Courses of paclitaxel should not be repeated until the neutrophil count is ≥1500 cells/mm³ and the platelet count is ≥100,000 cells/mm³; reduce dosage by 20% for patients experiencing severe peripheral neuropathy or severe neutropenia (neutrophil <500 cells/mm³ for a week or longer)

Dosage modification for immunosuppression in advanced HIV disease: Paclitaxel should not be given to patients with HIV if the baseline or subsequent neutrophil count is <1000 cells/mm³. Additional modifications include: Reduce dosage of dexamethasone in premedication to 10 mg orally; reduce dosage by 20% in patients experiencing severe peripheral neuropathy or severe neutropenia (neutrophil <500 cells/mm³ for a week or longer); initiate concurrent hematopoietic growth factor (G-CSF) as clinically indicated

Combination Regimens

Bladder cancer:

Paclitaxel-Carboplatin (Bladder Cancer) on page 1726
Paclitaxel-Carboplatin-Gemcitabine on page 1726
Paclitaxel-Gemcitabine on page 1729

Breast cancer:

AC/Paclitaxel (Sequential) on page 1517
AC-Paclitaxel-Trastuzumab on page 1518
Gemcitabine-Paclitaxel (Breast Cancer) on page 1675
Paclitaxel-Bevacizumab on page 1725
Paclitaxel-Vinorelbine on page 1732
Trastuzumab-Paclitaxel on page 1759
Trastuzumab-Paclitaxel-Carboplatin on page 1760
Trastuzumab-Paclitaxel (Weekly) on page 1760

Cervical cancer:

Carboplatin-Paclitaxel (Cervical Cancer) on page 1549
Cisplatin-Paclitaxel (Cervical Cancer) on page 1581

Esophageal cancer:

Paclitaxel-Carboplatin (Esophageal Cancer) on page 1726
Paclitaxel-Cisplatin (Esophageal Cancer) on page 1727
Paclitaxel-Cisplatin-Fluorouracil (Esophageal Cancer) on page 1728
Paclitaxel-Fluorouracil (Esophageal Cancer) on page 1729

Head and neck cancer:
Cisplatin-Paclitaxel (Head and Neck Cancer) on page 1581
Paclitaxel-Cetuximab on page 1727
Lung cancer (nonsmall cell):
Bevacizumab-Carboplatin-Paclitaxel (NSCLC) on page 1528
Carbo-Tax (NSCLC) on page 1552
CaT (NSCLC) on page 1553
PC (NSCLC) on page 1734
Lung cancer (small cell): Paclitaxel (Small Cell Lung Cancer Regimen) on page 1732
Ovarian cancer:
Carboplatin-Paclitaxel (Ovarian) on page 1550
Cisplatin-Paclitaxel Intraperitoneal (Ovarian) on page 1582
Cisplatin-Paclitaxel (Ovarian) on page 1582
Gemcitabine-Paclitaxel (Ovarian Cancer) on page 1675
Paclitaxel Maintenance (Ovarian Cancer) on page 1730
Paclitaxel (Ovarian Regimen) on page 1730
Prostate cancer:
Estramustine-Paclitaxel on page 1637
Paclitaxel + Estramustine + Carboplatin on page 1720
Paclitaxel + Estramustine + Etoposide on page 1729
Testicular cancer:
Gemcitabine-Oxaliplatin-Paclitaxel (Testicular) on page 1674
Gemcitabine-Paclitaxel (Testicular) on page 1675
Paclitaxel-Ifosfamide-Cisplatin on page 1730
Unknown primary, adenocarcinoma:
Carboplatin-Etoposide-Paclitaxel (Unknown Primary) on page 1545
Carboplatin-Gemcitabine-Paclitaxel (Unknown Primary) on page 1548
Carboplatin-Paclitaxel (Unknown Primary) on page 1551
Unknown primary, squamous cell: Cisplatin-Fluorouracil-Paclitaxel (Unknown Primary) on page 1577

Administration

I.V.: Infuse over 1-96 hours. When administered as sequential infusions, taxane derivatives should be administered before platinum derivatives (cisplatin, carboplatin) to limit myelosuppression and to enhance efficacy.

Premedication with dexamethasone (20 mg orally or I.V. at 12 and 6 hours **or** 14 and 7 hours before the dose; reduce to 10 mg with advanced HIV disease), diphenhydramine (50 mg I.V. 30-60 minutes prior to the dose), and cimetidine 300 mg, famotidine 20 mg, or ranitidine 50 mg (I.V. 30-60 minutes prior to the dose) is recommended.

Administer I.V. infusion over 1-24 hours; infuse through a 0.22 micron in-line filter and nonsorbing administration set.

Intraperitoneal: 1- to 2-hour infusion

Emetic Potential Low (10% to 30%)

Vesicant/Extravasation Risk May be an irritant

Monitoring Parameters CBC with differential and platelet count, liver and kidney function; monitor for hypersensitivity reactions, vital signs (frequently during the first hour of infusion), continuous cardiac monitoring (patients with conduction abnormalities)

Additional Information Sensory neuropathy is almost universal at doses >250 mg/m^2; motor neuropathy is uncommon at doses <250 mg/m^2. Myopathic effects are common with doses >200 mg/m^2, generally occur within 2-3 days of treatment, and resolve over 5-6 days. Intraperitoneal administration of paclitaxel is associated with a higher incidence of chemotherapy related toxicity.

Dosage Forms Excipient information presented when available (limited, particularly for generics); consult specific product labeling.

Injection, solution: 6 mg/mL (5 mL, 16.7 mL, 25 mL, 50 mL)

References

Armstrong DK, Bundy B, Wenzel L, et al, "Intraperitoneal Cisplatin and Paclitaxel in Ovarian Cancer," *N Engl J Med*, 2006, 354(1):34-43.

Aronoff GR, Bennett WM, Berns JS, et al, *Drug Prescribing in Renal Failure: Dosing Guidelines for Adults and Children*, 5th ed. Philadelphia, PA: American College of Physicians; 2007, p 101.

Miller K, Wang M, Gralow J, et al, "Paclitaxel Plus Bevacizumab Versus Paclitaxel Alone for Metastatic Breast Cancer," *N Engl J Med*, 2007, 357(26):2666-76.

Morgan C, Tillett T, Braybrooke J, et al, "Management of Uncommon Chemotherapy-Induced Emergencies," *Lancet Oncol*, 2011, 12(8):806-14.

◆ **Paclitaxel, Albumin-Bound** *see* PACLitaxel (Protein Bound) *on page 1098*

◆ **Paclitaxel (Conventional)** *see* PACLitaxel *on page 1092*

◆ **Paclitaxel for Injection (Can)** *see* PACLitaxel *on page 1092*

◆ **Paclitaxel Injection USP (Can)** *see* PACLitaxel *on page 1092*

◆ **Paclitaxel (Nanoparticle Albumin Bound)** *see* PACLitaxel (Protein Bound) *on page 1098*

PACLitaxel (Protein Bound) (pac li TAKS el PROE teen bownd)

Related Information

Management of Drug Extravasations *on page 1800*

Safe Handling of Hazardous Drugs *on page 1904*

Brand Names: U.S. Abraxane®

Brand Names: Canada Abraxane® for Injectable Suspension

Index Terms ABI-007; Albumin-Bound Paclitaxel; Albumin-Stabilized Nanoparticle Paclitaxel; nab-Paclitaxel; Nanoparticle Albumin-Bound Paclitaxel; Paclitaxel (Nanoparticle Albumin Bound); Paclitaxel, Albumin-Bound; Protein-Bound Paclitaxel

Generic Availability (U.S.) No

Pharmacologic Category Antineoplastic Agent, Antimicrotubular; Antineoplastic Agent, Natural Source (Plant) Derivative; Antineoplastic Agent, Taxane Derivative

Use Treatment of refractory (metastatic) or relapsed (within 6 months of adjuvant therapy) breast cancer; first-line treatment of locally advanced or metastatic nonsmall cell lung cancer (NSCLC) (in combination with carboplatin) in patients ineligible for curative surgery or radiation therapy

Unlabeled Use Treatment of recurrent or persistent ovarian, fallopian tube, or primary peritoneal cancers; metastatic pancreatic cancer

Labeled Contraindications Patients with a baseline neutrophil count of <1500/mm^3; severe hypersensitivity reaction to paclitaxel (protein bound)

Pregnancy Risk Factor D

Lactation Excretion in breast milk unknown/not recommended

Warnings/Precautions Hazardous agent - use appropriate precautions for handling and disposal.

[U.S. Boxed Warning]: Paclitaxel (protein-bound) is not interchangeable with other forms of paclitaxel, including Cremophor®-based or unbound paclitaxel.

[U.S. Boxed Warning]: Bone marrow suppression, primarily neutropenia, may occur; monitor peripheral blood counts frequently. Baseline neutrophils should be ≥1500/mm^3 for administration on day 1 of each cycle; platelets should recover to >100,000/mm^3 prior to day 1 of the next treatment cycle. Hematologic toxicity is dose-dependent, dose-limiting, and reversible. For severe neutropenia, dose reductions may be recommended for subsequent cycles. Dose-related, cumulative sensory neuropathy is common; severe sensory neuropathy may occur. If ≥ grade 3 sensory neuropathy occurs, withhold therapy until resolution to grade 1 or 2 (breast cancer) or ≤ grade 1 (NSCLC). Upon recovery, subsequent cycles should be dose reduced. Prior therapy with neurotoxic agents may influence the frequency and severity of neurologic toxicity. Severe hypersensitivity reactions (including anaphylaxis) have been reported; do not rechallenge after severe hypersensitivity reaction. Premedication is not generally necessary prior to paclitaxel (protein bound), but may be needed in patient's with prior mild-to-moderate hypersensitivity reactions. Use has not been studied in patients with a prior hypersensitivity reaction to conventional paclitaxel or albumin.

Use with caution in patients with hepatic impairment; monitor closely; the risk of toxicities is increased. Reduced initial dosages are recommended for moderate and severe hepatic impairment; withhold treatment in patients with AST >10 times ULN or bilirubin >5 times ULN. Has not been studied in renal impairment. Product contains albumin, which confers a remote risk of viral disease transmission and a theoretical risk of transmission of Creutzfeldt-Jakob disease. Certain adverse events (myelosuppression, peripheral neuropathy, arthralgia) occurred more frequently in older adults ≥65 years of age compared to younger adults in NSCLC trials.

Adverse Reactions Adverse reactions and incidences reported are associated with monotherapy unless otherwise stated.

>10%:

Cardiovascular: ECG abnormal (60%; 35% in patients with a normal baseline)

Central nervous system: Fatigue (25% combination therapy for NSCLC)

Dermatologic: Alopecia (56% [combination therapy for NSCLC] to 90%)

Gastrointestinal: Nausea (27% to 30%; grades 3/4: 3%), diarrhea (15% to 27%, grades 3/4: <1%), vomiting (12% to 18%; grades 3/4: 4%), appetite decreased (17% combination therapy for NSCLC), constipation (16% combination therapy for NSCLC)

Hematologic: Neutropenia (80%; grades 3/4: 34%; combination therapy for NSCLC: 85%; grades 3/4: 47%), anemia (33%; grades 3/4: 1%; combination therapy for NSCLC: 98%; grades 3/4: 28%), thrombocytopenia (2%; grades 3/4: <1%; combination therapy for NSCLC: 68%; grades 3/4: 18%), myelosuppression (dose related)

Hepatic: AST increased (39%), alkaline phosphatase increased (36%), GGT increased (grades 3/4: 14%)

Neuromuscular & skeletal: Sensory neuropathy (71%; grades 3/4: 10%; dose dependent; cumulative), weakness (47%; severe 8%; combination therapy for NSCLC: 16%), myalgia/arthralgia (44%; combination therapy for NSCLC: 10% to 13%)

Ocular: Vision disturbance (13%; severe [keratitis, blurred vision]: 1%)

Renal: Creatinine increased (11%; severe 1%)

Respiratory: Dyspnea (12%)

Miscellaneous: Infection (24%; primarily included oral candidiasis, respiratory tract infection, and pneumonia)

1% to 10%:
- Cardiovascular: Edema /fluid retention (10%), peripheral edema (10% combination therapy for NSCLC), hypotension (5%), cardiovascular events (grades 3/4: 3%; included chest pain, cardiac arrest, supraventricular tachycardia, thrombosis, pulmonary thromboembolism, pulmonary emboli, and hypertension)
- Dermatologic: Rash (10% combination therapy NSCLC)
- Gastrointestinal: Mucositis (7%; grades 3/4: <1%)
- Hematologic: Bleeding (2%), neutropenic fever (2%)
- Hepatic: Bilirubin increased (7%)
- Neuromuscular & skeletal: Peripheral neuropathy (grade 3: 10%; combination therapy for NSCLC: 3%)
- Respiratory: Cough (7%), epistaxis (7% combination therapy for NSCLC)
- Miscellaneous: Hypersensitivity reaction (4%, includes anaphylactic reactions, chest pain, dyspnea, flushing, hypotension; severe: <1%)

<1%, postmarketing, and/or case reports: Arrhythmia, autonomic neuropathy, bradycardia, cardiac ischemia, cerebrovascular attack, congestive heart failure, cranial nerve palsies, cystoid macular edema (transient), dehydration, embolism, erythema, fever, hand-foot syndrome (in patients previously exposed to capecitabine), injection site reaction (mild), interstitial pneumonia, intestinal obstruction, intestinal perforation, ischemic colitis, left ventricular dysfunction, maculopapular rash, MI, motor neuropathy, nail discoloration, nail pigmentation changes, optic nerve damage (rare), pancreatitis, pancytopenia, paralytic ileus, photosensitivity reaction, pneumonitis, pneumothorax, pruritus, pulmonary embolism, radiation pneumonitis with concurrent radiation therapy, radiation recall, rash (generalized), Stevens-Johnson syndrome, stroke, thrombosis, toxic epidermal necrolysis, transient ischemic attack, ventricular dysfunction, visual acuity decreased, vocal cord paresis

Adverse reactions reported with paclitaxel, which may occur with paclitaxel (protein bound): Cellulitis, conjunctivitis, extravasation recall, hepatic encephalopathy, hepatic necrosis, induration, lacrimation increased, lung fibrosis, neutropenic enterocolitis (typhlitis), optic nerve damage (persistent), phlebitis, pulmonary embolism, skin exfoliation, skin fibrosis, skin necrosis

Drug Interactions

Metabolism/Transport Effects **Substrate** of CYP2C8 (major), CYP3A4 (major), P-glycoprotein; **Note:** Assignment of Major/Minor substrate status based on clinically relevant drug interaction potential; **Induces** CYP3A4 (weak/moderate)

Avoid Concomitant Use

Avoid concomitant use of PACLitaxel (Protein Bound) with any of the following: Axitinib; BCG; CloZAPine; Conivaptan; Natalizumab; Pimecrolimus; Tacrolimus (Topical); Vaccines (Live)

Increased Effect/Toxicity

PACLitaxel (Protein Bound) may increase the levels/effects of: Antineoplastic Agents (Anthracycline, Systemic); CloZAPine; DOXOrubicin; Leflunomide; Natalizumab; Vaccines (Live); Vinorelbine; Vitamin K Antagonists

The levels/effects of PACLitaxel (Protein Bound) may be increased by: Conivaptan; CYP2C8 Inhibitors (Moderate); CYP2C8 Inhibitors (Strong); CYP3A4 Inhibitors (Moderate); CYP3A4 Inhibitors (Strong); Dasatinib; Deferasirox; Denosumab; Ivacaftor; Mifepristone; P-glycoprotein/ABCB1 Inhibitors; Pimecrolimus; Platinum Derivatives; Roflumilast; Tacrolimus (Topical); Trastuzumab

Decreased Effect

PACLitaxel (Protein Bound) may decrease the levels/effects of: ARIPiprazole; Axitinib; BCG; Cardiac Glycosides; Coccidioidin Skin Test; Saxagliptin; Sipuleucel-T; Vaccines (Inactivated); Vaccines (Live); Vitamin K Antagonists

The levels/effects of PACLitaxel (Protein Bound) may be decreased by: CYP2C8 Inducers (Strong); CYP3A4 Inducers (Strong); Deferasirox; Echinacea; Herbs (CYP3A4 Inducers); P-glycoprotein/ABCB1 Inducers; Tocilizumab

Ethanol/Nutrition/Herb Interactions

Food: Paclitaxel (protein bound) serum concentrations may be increased when taken with grapefruit or grapefruit juice. Management: Avoid concurrent use.

Herb/Nutraceutical: St John's wort may decrease paclitaxel (protein bound) serum concentrations; avoid concurrent use. Avoid echinacea.

Storage/Stability Store intact vial at room temperature of 20°C to 25°C (68°F to 77°F) and protect from bright light. Reconstituted solution may be stored under refrigeration 2°C to 8°C (36°F to 46°F) for up to 8 hours, although the manufacturer recommends immediate use. The solution for administration is stable for up to 4 hours at room temperature and ambient light.

Reconstitution Hazardous agent; use appropriate precautions for handling and disposal. Reconstitute vial with 20 mL NS to a concentration of 5 mg/mL. Add NS slowly (over a minimum of 1 minute), directing it along inside vial wall; allow vial to sit for 5 minutes, then gently swirl for 2 minutes; avoid foaming. If foaming or clumping occurs, allow solution to stand for at least 15 minutes until foaming subsides. Place dose without further dilution into an empty sterile container. **Note:** Use of DEHP-free containers or administration sets is not necessary. **Do not use an in-line filter.**

Mechanism of Action Albumin-bound paclitaxel nanoparticle formulation; paclitaxel promotes microtubule assembly by enhancing the action of tubulin dimers, stabilizing existing microtubules, and inhibiting their disassembly, interfering with the late G_2 mitotic phase, and inhibiting cell replication. May also distort mitotic spindles, resulting in the breakage of chromosomes. Paclitaxel may also suppress cell proliferation and modulate immune response.

Pharmacodynamics/Kinetics

Distribution: V_d: 632 L/m^2 (extensive extravascular distribution and/or tissue binding)

Protein binding: 89% to 98%

Metabolism: Hepatic primarily via CYP2C8 to 6-alpha-hydroxypaclitaxel; also to minor metabolites via CYP3A4

Half-life elimination: Terminal: 27 hours

Excretion: Feces (~20%); urine (4% as unchanged drug, <1% as metabolites)

Dosing

Adult & Geriatric Note: When administered as part of a combination chemotherapy regimen, sequence of administration may vary by regimen; refer to specific protocol for sequence of administration. Premedication is not generally necessary prior to paclitaxel (protein bound), but may be needed in patients with prior mild-to-moderate hypersensitivity reactions.

Breast cancer, metastatic: I.V.: 260 mg/m^2 every 3 weeks

Nonsmall cell lung cancer (NSCLC), locally advanced or metastatic: I.V.: 100 mg/m^2 on days 1, 8, and 15 of each 21-day cycle (in combination with carboplatin)

Breast cancer (unlabeled dosing): I.V.: 100-150 mg/m^2 on days 1, 8, and 15 of a 28-day cycle (Gradishar, 2009)

Ovarian, fallopian tube, or primary peritoneal cancer (recurrent; unlabeled use): I.V.: 260 mg/m^2 on day 1 of a 21-day cycle for 6-8 cycles (Teneriello, 2009) **or** 100 mg/m^2 on days 1, 8, and 15 of a 28-day cycle until disease progression or unacceptable toxicity (Coleman, 2011)

Pancreatic cancer, metastatic (unlabeled use): I.V.: 125 mg/m^2 on days 1, 8, and 15 of a 28-day cycle (in combination with gemcitabine) until disease progression or unacceptable toxicity (Von Hoff, 2011)

Renal Impairment No dosage adjustment provided in manufacturer's labeling (has not been studied).

Hepatic Impairment

Breast cancer (every 3 week regimen):

Mild impairment (AST <10 times ULN and bilirubin ≤1.25 times ULN): No adjustment required.

Moderate impairment (AST <10 times ULN and bilirubin 1.26-2 times ULN): Reduce dose to 200 mg/m^2

Severe impairment:

AST <10 times ULN and bilirubin 2.01-5 times ULN: Reduce dose to 130 mg/m^2; may increase up to 200 mg/m^2 in subsequent cycles (based on individual tolerance)

AST >10 times ULN or bilirubin >5 times ULN: Use is not recommended

Nonsmall cell lung cancer (NSCLC) regimen:

Mild impairment (AST <10 times ULN and bilirubin ≤1.25 times ULN): No dosage adjustment necessary.

Moderate impairment (AST <10 times ULN and bilirubin 1.26-2 times ULN): Reduce dose to 75 mg/m^2

Severe impairment:

AST <10 times ULN and bilirubin 2.01-5 times ULN: Reduce dose to 50 mg/m^2; may increase up to 75 mg/m^2 in subsequent cycles (based on individual tolerance)

AST >10 times ULN or bilirubin >5 times ULN: Use is not recommended.

Adjustment for Toxicity

Breast cancer (every 3 week regimen):

Severe neutropenia (<500 cells/mm^3) ≥1 week: Reduce dose to 220 mg/m^2 for subsequent courses

Recurrent severe neutropenia: Reduce dose to 180 mg/m^2 for subsequent courses

Sensory neuropathy

Grade 1 or 2: Dosage adjustment generally not required

Grade 3: Hold treatment until resolved to grade 1 or 2, then resume with reduced dose for all subsequent cycles

Severe sensory neuropathy: Reduce dose to 220 mg/m^2 for subsequent courses

Recurrent severe sensory neuropathy: Reduce dose to 180 mg/m^2 for subsequent courses

Nonsmall cell lung cancer (NSCLC):

Neutropenia: ANC <1500 cells/mm³: Withhold therapy until ANC is ≥1500 cells/mm³ on day 1 or ≥500 cells/mm³ on days 8 or 15. Reduce dose upon therapy reinitiation if:

Neutropenic fever (ANC < 500 cells/mm³ with fever >38°C) **or** delay of next cycle by >7 days due to ANC <1500 cells/mm³ **or** ANC <500 cells/mm³ for >7 days:

First occurrence: Permanently reduce dose to 75 mg/m²

Second occurrence: Permanently reduce dose to 50 mg/m²

Third occurrence: Discontinue therapy.

Thrombocytopenia: Platelet count <100,000 cells/mm³: Withhold therapy until platelet count is ≥100,000 cells/mm³ on day 1 or ≥50,000 cells/mm³ on days 8 or 15. Reduce dose upon therapy reinitiation if:

Platelet count <50,000 cells/mm³:

First occurrence: Permanently reduce dose to 75 mg/m²

Second occurrence: Discontinue therapy.

Sensory neuropathy: Withhold therapy for grade 3-4 peripheral neuropathy. Resume therapy at reduced doses when neuropathy resolves completely or improves to grade 1:

First occurrence: Permanently reduce dose to 75 mg/m²

Second occurrence: Permanently reduce dose to 50 mg/m²

Third occurrence: Discontinue therapy.

Combination Regimens

Lung cancer (nonsmall cell): Paclitaxel (Protein Bound) (NSCLC Regimen) on page 1731

Pancreatic cancer: Gemcitabine-Paclitaxel (Protein Bound) (Pancreatic) on page 1675

Administration I.V.: Administer over 30 minutes (limiting the infusion rate to 30 minutes reduces the risk for infusion-related reaction); do not use an in-line filter. Monitor infusion site; avoid extravasation. When given on a weekly (unlabeled) schedule, infusions were administered over ~30 minutes (Gradishar, 2009; Rizvi, 2008). When administered as part of a combination chemotherapy regimen, sequence of administration may vary by regimen; refer to specific protocol for sequence of administration.

Emetic Potential Low (10% to 30%)

Vesicant/Extravasation Risk May be an irritant

Monitoring Parameters CBC with differential (prior to day 1 of cycle for metastatic breast cancer and prior to days 1, 8, and 15 for NSCLC), hepatic function; monitor infusion site; monitor for neuropathy

Dosage Forms Excipient information presented when available (limited, particularly for generics); consult specific product labeling.

Injection, powder for reconstitution:

Abraxane®: 100 mg [contains albumin (human)]

References

Coleman RL, Brady WE, McMeekin DS, et al, "A Phase II Evaluation of Nanoparticle, Albumin-Bound (Nab) Paclitaxel in the Treatment of Recurrent or Persistent Platinum-Resistant Ovarian, Fallopian Tube, or Primary Peritoneal Cancer: A Gynecologic Oncology Group Study," *Gynecol Oncol*, 2011, 122(1):111-5.

Gardner ER, Dahut WL, Scripture CD, et al, "Randomized Crossover Pharmacokinetic Study of Solvent-Based Paclitaxel and nab-Paclitaxel," *Clin Cancer Res*, 2008, 14(13):4200-5.

Gradishar WJ, Krasnojon D, Cheporov S, et al, "Significantly Longer Progression-Free Survival With nab-paclitaxel Compared With Docetaxel as First-Line Therapy for Metastatic Breast Cancer," *J Clin Oncol*, 2009, 27(22):3611-9.

Gradishar WJ, Tjulandin S, Davidson N, et al, "Phase III Trial of Nanoparticle Albumin-Bound Paclitaxel Compared With Polyethylated Castor Oil-Based Paclitaxel in Women With Breast Cancer," *J Clin Oncol*, 2005, 23(31):7794-803.

Green MR, Manikhas GM, Orlov S, et al, "Abraxane®, a Novel Cremophor®-Free, Albumin-Bound Particle Form of Paclitaxel for the Treatment of Advanced Non-Small-Cell Lung Cancer," *Ann Oncol*, 2006, 17(8):1263-8.

Ibrahim NK, Samuels B, Page R, et al, "Multicenter Phase II Trial of ABI-007, an Albumin-Bound Paclitaxel, in Women With Metastatic Breast Cancer," *J Clin Oncol*, 2005, 23(25):6019-26.

Rizvi NA, Riely GJ, Azzoli CG, et al, "Phase I/II Trial of Weekly Intravenous 130-nm Albumin-Bound Paclitaxel as Initial Chemotherapy in Patients With Stage IV Non-Small-Cell Lung Cancer," *J Clin Oncol*, 2008, 26(4):639-43.

Teneriello MG, Tseng PC, Crozier M, et al, "Phase II Evaluation of Nanoparticle Albumin-Bound Paclitaxel in Platinum-Sensitive Patients With Recurrent Ovarian, Peritoneal, or Fallopian Tube Cancer," *J Clin Oncol*, 2009, 27(9):1426-31.

Von Hoff DD, Ramanathan RK, Borad MJ, et al, "Gemcitabine Plus Nab-Paclitaxel Is an Active Regimen in Patients With Advanced Pancreatic Cancer: A Phase I/II Trial," *J Clin Oncol*, 2011, 29 (34):4548-54.

Palifermin (pal ee FER min)

Related Information

Oral Mucositis/Stomatitis *on page 1814*

Brand Names: U.S. Kepivance®

Brand Names: Canada Kepivance®

Index Terms AMJ 9701; Keratinocyte Growth Factor, Recombinant Human; rhKGF; rhu Keratinocyte Growth Factor; rHu-KGF

Generic Availability (U.S.) No

Pharmacologic Category Keratinocyte Growth Factor

Use Decrease the incidence and duration of severe oral mucositis associated with hematologic malignancies in patients receiving myelotoxic therapy requiring hematopoietic stem cell support (when the preparative regimen is expected to result in mucositis ≥grade 3 in most patients)

Note: Use (safety and efficacy) is not established for nonhematologic malignancies; use is not recommended with conditioning regimens containing melphalan 200 mg/m^2

Labeled Contraindications There are no contraindications listed within the manufacturer's U.S. product labeling.

Canadian labeling: Hypersensitivity to palifermin, *E. coli*-derived proteins, or any component of the formulation

Pregnancy Risk Factor C

Lactation Excretion in breast milk unknown/not recommended

Warnings/Precautions Hazardous agent - use appropriate precautions for handling and disposal. Edema, erythema, pruritus, rash, oral/perioral dysesthesia, taste alteration, tongue discoloration, and tongue thickening may occur (median onset of cutaneous toxicities following initial dose is 6 days; median duration is 5 days); instruct patients to report mucocutaneous effects. Safety and efficacy have not been established with nonhematologic malignancies; effect on the growth of keratinocyte growth factor (KGF) receptor expressing, nonhematopoietic human tumors is not known. Palifermin has been shown to enhance epithelial tumor cell lines *in vitro*. Do not administer within 24 hours before, during, or after myelotoxic chemotherapy. If administered during or within 24 hours of (before or after) chemotherapy, palifermin may increase the severity and duration of mucositis due to the increased sensitivity of rapidly-dividing epithelial cells.

Adverse Reactions

>10%:

Cardiovascular: Edema (28%)

Central nervous system: Fever (39%); pain (16%); dysesthesia (oral hyperesthesia, hypoesthesia, and paresthesia 12%)

Dermatologic: Rash (62%; grade 3: 3%), pruritus (35%), erythema (32%)

Gastrointestinal: Serum amylase increased (62%, grades 3/4: 38%), serum lipase increased (28%, grades 3/4: 11%), mouth/tongue discoloration or thickness (17%), taste alteration (16%)

1% to 10%:

Neuromuscular & skeletal: Arthralgia (10%)

Miscellaneous: Antibody formation (2%)

<1%, postmarketing, and/or case reports: Cataracts, cough, flexural hyperpigmentation, palmar-plantar erythrodysesthesia syndrome (hand-foot syndrome), perianal pain, rhinitis, vaginal edema, vaginal erythema

Drug Interactions

Metabolism/Transport Effects None known.

Avoid Concomitant Use

Avoid concomitant use of Palifermin with any of the following: Heparin

Increased Effect/Toxicity

The levels/effects of Palifermin may be increased by: Heparin; Heparin (Low Molecular Weight)

Decreased Effect There are no known significant interactions involving a decrease in effect.

Storage/Stability Store intact vials under refrigeration at 2°C to 8°C (36°F to 46°F). Protect from light. Although the manufacturer recommends immediate use, reconstituted vials are stable for up to 24 hours refrigerated. Bring to room temperature for up to 1 hour prior to administration; however, do not use if left at room temperature >1 hour. Protect reconstituted solution from light. Do not freeze reconstituted product.

Reconstitution To reconstitute, slowly add 1.2 mL SWFI, to a final concentration of 5 mg/mL. Swirl gently; do not shake or vigorously agitate. May take up to 3 minutes to dissolve; reconstituted solution should be clear and colorless. Do not filter during preparation or administration.

Mechanism of Action Palifermin is a recombinant keratinocyte growth factor (KGF) produced in *E. coli*. Endogenous KGF is produced by mesenchymal cells in response to epithelial tissue injury. KGF binds to the KGF receptor resulting in proliferation, differentiation and migration of epithelial cells in multiple tissues, including (but not limited to) the tongue, buccal mucosa, esophagus, and salivary gland.

Pharmacodynamics/Kinetics

Onset of action: Epithelial cell proliferation (dose-dependent): 48 hours

Half-life elimination: 4.5 hours (range: 3.3-5.7 hours)

Dosing

Adult & Geriatric Oral mucositis associated with hematopoietic stem cell transplant (HSCT) conditioning regimens: I.V.: 60 mcg/kg/day for 3 consecutive days before and 3 consecutive days after myelotoxic therapy; total of 6 doses (Spielberger, 2004)

Note: Administer first 3 doses prior to myelotoxic therapy, with the 3rd dose given 24-48 hours before beginning the myelotoxic conditioning regimen. Administer the last 3 doses after completion of the conditioning regimen, with the first of these doses after but on the same day as HSCT infusion and at least 4 days after the most recent dose of palifermin.

Renal Impairment No adjustment necessary.

Hepatic Impairment No dosage adjustment provided in the manufacturer's labeling (has not been studied).

Administration Administer by I.V. bolus. If heparin is used to maintain the patency of the I.V. line, flush line with saline prior to and after palifermin administration. Do not administer palifermin during or within 24 hours before or after chemotherapy. Allow solution to reach room temperature prior to administration; do not use if at room temperature >1 hour. Do not filter.

Monitoring Parameters Monitor for oral mucositis

Additional Information Oncology Comment: The Multinational Association of Supportive Care in Cancer and the International Society for Oral Oncology (MASCC/ISOO) guidelines for the prevention and treatment of mucositis recommend palifermin (at the FDA-approved dose) for the prevention of oral mucositis in patients with hematologic malignancies who are receiving high-dose chemotherapy and total body irradiation with autologous stem cell transplantation (Keefe, 2007).

Guidelines from the American Society of Clinical Oncology (ASCO) for the use of chemotherapy and radiotherapy protectants (Hensley, 2008) recommend the use of palifermin to decrease the incidence of severe mucositis in patients undergoing autologous stem-cell transplantation with a total body irradiation (TBI) conditioning regimen. According to the ASCO guidelines, data are insufficient to recommend palifermin when the conditioning regimen is chemotherapy only. Palifermin may be considered in patients undergoing myeloablative allogeneic stem-cell transplantation with a TBI conditioning regimen, however data are again insufficient to recommend palifermin when the conditioning regimen is chemotherapy only. Due to a lack of appropriate data, the guidelines also do not recommend palifermin use in non-stem-cell transplantation treatment regimens or for use when treating solid tumors.

Dosage Forms Excipient information presented when available (limited, particularly for generics); consult specific product labeling.

Injection, powder for reconstitution [preservative free]:

Kepivance®: 6.25 mg [contains mannitol, sucrose 25 mg]

References

Hensley ML, Hagerty KL, Kewalramani T, et al, "American Society of Clinical Oncology 2008 Clinical Practice Guideline Update: Use of Chemotherapy and Radiotherapy Protectants," *J Clin Oncol*, 2009, 27(1): 127-45.

Keefe DM, Schubert MM, Elting LS, et al, "Updated Clinical Practice Guidelines for the Prevention and Treatment of Mucositis," *Cancer*, 2007, 109(5):820-31.

Spielberger R, Stiff P, Bensinger W, et al, "Palifermin for Oral Mucositis After Intensive Therapy for Hematologic Cancers," *N Engl J Med*, 2004, 351(25):2590-8.

Palonosetron (pal oh NOE se tron)

Related Information

Management of Chemotherapy-Induced Nausea and Vomiting *on page 1786*

Brand Names: U.S. Aloxi®

Index Terms Palonosetron Hydrochloride; RS-25259; RS-25259-197

Generic Availability (U.S.) No

Pharmacologic Category Antiemetic; Selective 5-HT_3 Receptor Antagonist

Use Prevention of chemotherapy-associated nausea and vomiting; indicated for prevention of acute (highly-emetogenic therapy) as well as acute and delayed (moderately-emetogenic therapy) nausea and vomiting; prevention of postoperative nausea and vomiting (PONV)

Labeled Contraindications Hypersensitivity to palonosetron or any component of the formulation

Pregnancy Risk Factor B

Lactation Excretion in breast milk unknown/not recommended

Warnings/Precautions Hypersensitivity has been observed rarely with I.V. palonosetron. Use caution in patients allergic to other 5-HT_3 receptor antagonists; cross-reactivity is possible. Some selective 5-HT_3 receptor antagonists have been associated with dose-dependent increases in ECG intervals (eg, PR, QRS duration, QT/QT_c, JT), usually occurring 1-2 hours after I.V. administration. In general, these changes are not clinically relevant, however, when these agents are used in conjunction with other agents that prolong these intervals, arrhythmia may occur. When used with agents that prolong the QT interval (eg, Class I and III antiarrhythmics), clinically relevant QT interval prolongation could result in torsade de pointes. A number of trials have shown that 5-HT_3 antagonists produce QT interval prolongation to variable degrees. Use with caution in patients at risk of QT prolongation and/or ventricular arrhythmia. Reduction in heart rate may also occur with the 5-HT_3 antagonists. Use with caution in patients with congenital long QT syndrome or other risk factors for QT prolongation (eg, medications known to prolong QT interval, electrolyte abnormalities, and cumulative high dose anthracycline therapy).

Not intended for treatment of nausea and vomiting or for chronic continuous therapy. **For chemotherapy, should be used on a scheduled basis, not on an "as needed" (PRN) basis,** since data support the use of this drug only in the prevention of nausea and vomiting (due to antineoplastic therapy) and not in the rescue of nausea and vomiting. For PONV, may use for low expectation of PONV if it is essential to avoid nausea and vomiting in the postoperative period; use is not recommended if there is little expectation of nausea and vomiting.

Adverse Reactions Adverse events may vary according to indication.

1% to 10%:

- Cardiovascular: QT prolongation (chemotherapy-associated <1%; PONV 1% to 5%), bradycardia (chemotherapy-associated 1%; PONV 4%), hypotension (≤1%), sinus bradycardia (≤1%), tachycardia (nonsustained) (≤1%)
- Central nervous system: Headache (chemotherapy-associated 5% to 9%; PONV 3%), anxiety (1%), dizziness (≤1%)
- Dermatologic: Pruritus (≤1%)
- Endocrine & metabolic: Hyperkalemia (1%)
- Gastrointestinal: Constipation (2% to 5%), diarrhea (≤1%), flatulence (≤1%)
- Genitourinary: Urinary retention (≤1%)
- Hepatic: ALT increased (≤1%; transient), AST increased (≤1%; transient)
- Neuromuscular & skeletal: Weakness (1%)

<1%, postmarketing, and/or case reports: Abdominal pain, allergic dermatitis, amblyopia, anemia, anorexia, appetite decreased, arrhythmia, arthralgia, bilirubin increased (transient), chills, dyspepsia, edema (generalized), electrolyte fluctuations, epistaxis, erythema, euphoric mood, extrasystoles, eye irritation, fatigue, fever, flu-like syndrome, glycosuria, hiccups, hot flash, hyperglycemia, hypersensitivity (rare), hypersomnia, hypertension, hypokalemia, hypoventilation, injection site reactions (burning/discomfort/induration/pain; rare), insomnia, intestinal hypomotility, laryngospasm, metabolic acidosis, motion sickness, myocardial ischemia, pain in extremities, paresthesia, platelets decreased, rash, salivation increased, seizure, sinus arrhythmia,

sinus tachycardia, somnolence, supraventricular extrasystoles, tinnitus, T-wave amplitude decreased, vein discoloration, vein distention, ventricular extrasystoles, xerostomia

Drug Interactions

Metabolism/Transport Effects Substrate of CYP1A2 (minor), CYP2D6 (minor), CYP3A4 (minor); **Note:** Assignment of Major/Minor substrate status based on clinically relevant drug interaction potential

Avoid Concomitant Use

Avoid concomitant use of Palonosetron with any of the following: Apomorphine

Increased Effect/Toxicity

Palonosetron may increase the levels/effects of: Apomorphine

Decreased Effect

Palonosetron may decrease the levels/effects of: Tapentadol; TraMADol

The levels/effects of Palonosetron may be decreased by: Peginterferon Alfa-2b; Tocilizumab

Storage/Stability Store intact vials at room temperature of 20°C to 25°C (68°F to 77°F); excursions permitted to 15°C to 30°C (59°F to 86°F); do not freeze. Protect from light. Solutions of 5 mcg/mL and 30 mcg/mL in NS, D_5W, $D_5{}^{1/2}NS$, and D_5LR injection are stable for 48 hours at room temperature and 14 days under refrigeration (Trissel, 2004).

Mechanism of Action Selective 5-HT_3 receptor antagonist, blocking serotonin, both on vagal nerve terminals in the periphery and centrally in the chemoreceptor trigger zone

Pharmacodynamics/Kinetics

Distribution: V_d: 8.3 ± 2.5 L/kg

Protein binding: ~62%

Metabolism: ~50% metabolized via CYP enzymes (and likely other pathways) to relatively inactive metabolites (N-oxide-palonosetron and 6-S-hydroxy-palonosetron); CYP1A2, 2D6, and 3A4 contribute to its metabolism

Half-life elimination: I.V.: Terminal: ~40 hours

Excretion: Urine (80% to 93%, 40% as unchanged drug); feces (5% to 8%)

Dosing

Adult

Chemotherapy-associated nausea and vomiting: I.V.: 0.25 mg 30 minutes prior to the start of chemotherapy administration

Breakthrough: Palonosetron has not been shown to be effective in terminating nausea or vomiting once it occurs and should not be used for this purpose.

PONV: I.V.: 0.075 mg immediately prior to anesthesia induction

Geriatric No dosage adjustment necessary.

Renal Impairment No dosage adjustment necessary.

Hepatic Impairment No dosage adjustment necessary.

Administration Flush I.V. line with NS prior to and following administration.

Chemotherapy-associated nausea and vomiting: Infuse over 30 seconds, 30 minutes prior to the start of chemotherapy

PONV: Infuse over 10 seconds immediately prior to anesthesia induction

Dosage Forms Excipient information presented when available (limited, particularly for generics); consult specific product labeling.

Injection, solution:

Aloxi®: 0.05 mg/mL (5 mL) [contains edetate disodium]

References

Aapro MS, Grunberg SM, Manikhas GM, et al, "A Phase III, Double-Blind, Randomized Trial of Palonosetron Compared With Ondansetron in Preventing Chemotherapy-Induced Nausea and Vomiting Following Highly Emetogenic Chemotherapy," *Ann Oncol*, 2006, 17(9):1441-9.

Boccia RV, Gonzalez EF, Pluzanska AG, et al, "Palonosetron (PALO), Administered Orally or Intravenously (IV), Plus Dexamethasone for Prevention of Chemotherapy-Induced Nausea and Vomiting (CINV)," *J Clin Oncol*, 2008, 26(15 Supp):20608 [abstract 20608 from 2008 ASCO Annual Meeting].

Kris MG, Hesketh PJ, Somerfield MR, et al, "American Society of Clinical Oncology Guideline for Antiemetics in Oncology: Update 2006," *J Clin Oncol*, 2006, 24(18):2932-47.

Multinational Association of Supportive Care in Cancer (MASCC), "Antiemetic Guidelines," Updated April 2010. Available at http://data.memberclicks.com/site/mascc/MASCC_Guidelines_English_2010.pdf

National Comprehensive Cancer Network® (NCCN), "Clinical Practice Guidelines in Oncology™: Antiemesis," Version 2.2010. Available at http://www.nccn.org/professionals/physician_gls/PDF/antiemesis.pdf

◆ **Palonosetron Hydrochloride** *see* Palonosetron *on page 1106*

Pamidronate (pa mi DROE nate)

Related Information

Chronic Pain Management (Cancer) *on page 1840*

Hypercalcemia of Malignancy *on page 1860*

Safe Handling of Hazardous Drugs *on page 1904*

Brand Names: U.S. Aredia®

Brand Names: Canada Aredia®; Pamidronate Disodium Omega; Pamidronate Disodium®; PMS-Pamidronate

Index Terms Pamidronate Disodium

Generic Availability (U.S.) Yes

Pharmacologic Category Antidote; Bisphosphonate Derivative

Use Treatment of moderate or severe hypercalcemia associated with malignancy (in conjunction with adequate hydration) with or without bone metastases; treatment of osteolytic bone lesions associated with multiple myeloma or metastatic breast cancer; moderate-to-severe Paget's disease of bone

Unlabeled Use Treatment of osteogenesis imperfecta; treatment of symptomatic bone metastases of thyroid cancer; prevention of bone loss associated with androgen deprivation treatment in prostate cancer

Labeled Contraindications Hypersensitivity to pamidronate, other bisphosphonates, or any component of the formulation

Pregnancy Risk Factor D

Lactation Excretion in breast milk unknown/not recommended

Warnings/Precautions Osteonecrosis of the jaw (ONJ) has been reported in patients receiving bisphosphonates. Risk factors include invasive dental procedures (eg, tooth extraction, dental implants, boney surgery); a diagnosis of cancer, with concomitant chemotherapy, radiotherapy, or corticosteroids; poor oral hygiene, ill-fitting dentures, and comorbid disorders (anemia, coagulopathy, infection, pre-existing dental disease). Most reported cases occurred after I.V. bisphosphonate therapy; however, cases have been reported following oral therapy. A dental exam and preventative dentistry should be performed prior to placing patients with risk factors on chronic bisphosphonate therapy. There is no evidence that discontinuing therapy reduces the risk of developing ONJ (Assael, 2009). The benefit/risk must be assessed by the treating physician and/or dentist/surgeon prior to any invasive dental procedure. Patients developing ONJ while on bisphosphonates should receive care by an oral surgeon.

Atypical femur fractures (after minimal or no trauma) have been reported. The fractures include subtrochanteric femur (bone just below the hip joint) and diaphyseal femur (long segment of the thigh bone). Some patients experience prodromal pain weeks or months before the fracture occurs. It is unclear if bisphosphonate therapy is the cause for these fractures. Patients receiving long-term (>3-5 years) bisphosphonate therapy may be at an increased risk. Consider discontinuing pamidronate in patients with a suspected femoral shaft fracture. Patients who present with thigh or groin pain in the absence of trauma should be evaluated. Infrequently, severe (and occasionally debilitating) musculoskeletal (bone, joint, and/or muscle) pain have been reported during bisphosphonate treatment. The onset of pain ranged from a single day to several months. Consider discontinuing therapy in patients who experience severe symptoms; symptoms usually resolve upon discontinuation. Some patients experienced recurrence when rechallenged with same drug or another bisphosphonate; avoid use in patients with a history of these symptoms in association with bisphosphonate therapy.

Initial or single doses have been associated with renal deterioration, progressing to renal failure and dialysis. Withhold pamidronate treatment (until renal function returns to baseline) in patients with evidence of renal deterioration. Glomerulosclerosis (focal segmental) with or without nephrotic syndrome has also been reported. Longer infusion times (>2 hours) may reduce the risk for renal toxicity, especially in patients with pre-existing renal insufficiency. Single pamidronate doses should not exceed 90 mg. Patients with serum creatinine >3 mg/dL were not studied in clinical trials; limited data are available in patients with Cl_{cr} <30 mL/minute. Evaluate serum creatinine prior to each treatment. For the treatment of bone metastases, use is not recommended in patients with severe renal impairment; for renal impairment in indications other than bone metastases, use clinical judgment to determine if benefits outweigh potential risks.

Use has been associated with asymptomatic electrolyte abnormalities (including hypophosphatemia, hypokalemia, hypomagnesemia, and hypocalcemia). Rare cases of symptomatic hypocalcemia, including tetany have been reported. Patients with a history of thyroid surgery may have relative hypoparathyroidism; predisposing them to pamidronate-related hypocalcemia. Patients with pre-existing anemia, leukopenia, or thrombocytopenia should be closely monitored during the first 2 weeks of treatment.

Multiple myeloma: According to the American Society of Clinical Oncology (ASCO) guidelines for bisphosphonates in multiple myeloma, treatment with pamidronate is not recommended for asymptomatic (smoldering) or indolent myeloma or with solitary plasmacytoma (Kyle, 2007). The National Comprehensive Cancer Network® (NCCN) multiple myeloma guidelines (v.1.2012) also do not recommend pamidronate use in stage 1 or smoldering disease, unless part of a clinical trial. Patients with Bence-Jones proteinuria and dehydration should be adequately hydrated prior to therapy.

Hypercalcemia of malignancy (HCM): Adequate hydration is required during treatment (urine output ~2 L/day); avoid overhydration, especially in patients with heart failure.

Adverse Reactions Note: Actual percentages may vary by indication; treatment for multiple myeloma is associated with higher percentage.

>10%:

Central nervous system: Fever (18% to 39%; transient), fatigue (≤37%), headache (≤26%), insomnia (≤22%)

Endocrine & metabolic: Hypophosphatemia (≤18%), hypokalemia (4% to 18%), hypomagnesemia (4% to 12%), hypocalcemia (≤12%)

Gastrointestinal: Nausea (≤54%), vomiting (≤36%), anorexia (≤26%), abdominal pain (≤23%), dyspepsia (≤23%)

Genitourinary: Urinary tract infection (≤19%)

Hematologic: Anemia (≤43%), granulocytopenia (≤20%)

Local: Infusion site reaction (≤18%; includes induration, pain, redness and swelling)

Neuromuscular & skeletal: Myalgia (≤26%), weakness (≤22%), arthralgia (≤14%), osteonecrosis of the jaw (cancer patients: 1% to 11%)

Renal: Serum creatinine increased (≤19%)

Respiratory: Dyspnea (≤30%), cough (≤26%), upper respiratory tract infection (≤24%), sinusitis (≤16%), pleural effusion (≤11%)

1% to 10%:

Cardiovascular: Atrial fibrillation (≤6%), hypertension (≤6%), syncope (≤6%), tachycardia (≤6%), atrial flutter (≤1%), cardiac failure (≤1%), edema (≤1%)

Central nervous system: Somnolence (≤6%), psychosis (≤4%), seizure (≤2%)

Endocrine & metabolic: Hypothyroidism (≤6%)

Gastrointestinal: Constipation (≤6%), gastrointestinal hemorrhage (≤6%), diarrhea (≤1%), stomatitis (≤1%)

Hematologic: Leukopenia (≤4%), neutropenia (≤1%), thrombocytopenia (≤1%)

Neuromuscular & skeletal: Back pain, bone pain

Renal: Uremia (≤4%)

Respiratory: Rales (≤6%), rhinitis (≤6%)

Miscellaneous: Moniliasis (≤6%)

<1%, postmarketing, and/or case reports: Acute renal failure, adult respiratory distress syndrome, allergic reaction, anaphylactic shock, angioedema, bone/joint/muscle pain (severe and occasionally incapacitating), bronchospasm, CHF, confusion, conjunctivitis, electrolyte/mineral abnormality, episcleritis, femoral fractures (atypical subtrochanteric, diaphyseal femoral), fluid overload, flu-like syndrome, focal segmental glomerulosclerosis (including collapsing variant), glomerulonephropathies, hallucinations (visual), hematuria, herpes virus reactivation, hyperkalemia, hypernatremia, hypotension, injection site phlebitis/thrombophlebitis, interstitial pneumonitis, iridocyclitis, iritis, joint and/or muscle pain (sometimes severe and/or incapacitating), left ventricular failure, lymphocytopenia, malaise, nephrotic syndrome, orbital inflammation, osteonecrosis (other than jaw), paresthesia, pruritus, rash, renal deterioration, renal failure, renal tubular disorders, scleritis, tetany, tubulointerstitial nephritis, uveitis, xanthopsia

Drug Interactions

Metabolism/Transport Effects None known.

Avoid Concomitant Use There are no known interactions where it is recommended to avoid concomitant use.

Increased Effect/Toxicity

Pamidronate may increase the levels/effects of: Deferasirox; Phosphate Supplements; SUNItinib

The levels/effects of Pamidronate may be increased by: Aminoglycosides; Nonsteroidal Anti-Inflammatory Agents; Thalidomide

Decreased Effect

The levels/effects of Pamidronate may be decreased by: Proton Pump Inhibitors

Storage/Stability

Powder for reconstitution: Store below 30°C (86°F). The reconstituted solution is stable for 24 hours stored under refrigeration at 2°C to 8°C (36°F to 46°F).

Solution for injection: Store at 20°C to 25°C (68°F to 77°F).

Pamidronate solution for infusion is stable at room temperature for up to 24 hours.

Reconstitution Powder for injection: Reconstitute by adding 10 mL of SWFI to each vial of lyophilized pamidronate disodium powder, the resulting solution will be 30 mg/10 mL or 90 mg/10 mL.

Pamidronate may be further diluted in 250-1000 mL of 0.45% or 0.9% sodium chloride or 5% dextrose. (The manufacturer recommends dilution in 1000 mL for hypercalcemia of malignancy, 500 mL for Paget's disease and bone metastases of myeloma, and 250 mL for bone metastases of breast cancer.)

Mechanism of Action Nitrogen-containing bisphosphonate; inhibits bone resorption and decreases mineralization by disrupting osteoclast activity (Gralow, 2009; Rogers, 2011)

Pharmacodynamics/Kinetics

Onset of action:

Hypercalcemia of malignancy (HCM): ≤24 hours for decrease in albumin-corrected serum calcium; maximum effect: ≤7 days

Paget's disease: ~1 month for ≥50% decrease in serum alkaline phosphatase

Duration: HCM: 7-14 days; Paget's disease: 1-372 days

Absorption: Oral: Poor

Metabolism: Not metabolized

Half-life elimination: 21-35 hours

Excretion: Biphasic; urine (30% to 62% as unchanged drug; lower in patients with renal dysfunction) within 120 hours

Dosing

Adult Note: Single doses should not exceed 90 mg.

Hypercalcemia of malignancy: I.V.:

Moderate cancer-related hypercalcemia (corrected serum calcium: 12-13.5 mg/dL): 60-90 mg, as a single dose over 2-24 hours

Severe cancer-related hypercalcemia (corrected serum calcium: >13.5 mg/dL): 90 mg, as a single dose over 2-24 hours

Retreatment in patients who show an initial complete or partial response (allow at least 7 days to elapse prior to retreatment): May retreat at the same dose if serum calcium does not return to normal or does not remain normal after initial treatment.

Multiple myeloma, osteolytic bone lesions: I.V.: 90 mg over 4 hours monthly

Lytic disease: American Society of Clinical Oncology (ASCO) guidelines: 90 mg over at least 2 hours every 3-4 weeks for 2 years; discontinue after 2 years in patients with responsive and/or stable disease; resume therapy with new-onset skeletal-related events (Kyle, 2007)

Newly-diagnosed, symptomatic (unlabeled dose): 30 mg over 2.5 hours monthly for at least 3 years (Gimsing, 2010)

Breast cancer, osteolytic bone metastases: I.V.: 90 mg over 2 hours every 3-4 weeks

Paget's disease (moderate-to-severe): I.V.: 30 mg over 4 hours daily for 3 consecutive days (total dose = 90 mg); may retreat at initial dose if clinically indicated

Prevention of androgen deprivation-induced osteoporosis (unlabeled use): I.V.: 60 mg over 2 hours every 3 months (Smith, 2001)

Geriatric Refer to adult dosing. Begin at lower end of adult dosing range.

Renal Impairment Patients with serum creatinine >3 mg/dL were excluded from clinical trials; there are only limited pharmacokinetic data in patients with Cl_{cr} <30 mL/minute.

Manufacturer recommends the following guidelines:

Treatment of bone metastases: Use is not recommended in patients with severe renal impairment.

Renal impairment in indications other than bone metastases: Use clinical judgment to determine if benefits outweigh potential risks.

Multiple myeloma: American Society of Clinical Oncology (ASCO) guidelines (Kyle, 2007):

Severe renal impairment (serum creatinine >3 mg/dL **or** Cl_{cr} <30 mL/minute) and extensive bone disease: 90 mg over 4-6 hours. However, a reduced initial dose should be considered if renal impairment was pre-existing.

Albuminuria >500 mg/24 hours (unexplained): Withhold dose until returns to baseline, then recheck every 3-4 weeks; consider reinitiating at a dose not to exceed 90 mg every 4 weeks and with a longer infusion time of at least 4 hours

Dosing adjustment in renal toxicity: In patients with bone metastases, treatment should be withheld for deterioration in renal function (increase of serum creatinine ≥0.5 mg/dL in patients with normal baseline or ≥1.0 mg/dL in patients with abnormal baseline). Resumption of therapy may be considered when serum creatinine returns to within 10% of baseline.

Hepatic Impairment No dosage adjustment necessary in patients with mild-to-moderate hepatic impairment; not studied in patients with severe hepatic impairment.

Administration I.V.: Infusion rate varies by indication. Longer infusion times (>2 hours) may reduce the risk for renal toxicity, especially in patients with pre-existing renal insufficiency. The manufacturer recommends infusing over 2-24 hours for hypercalcemia of malignancy; over 2 hours for osteolytic bone lesions with metastatic breast cancer; and over 4 hours for Paget's disease and for osteolytic bone lesions with multiple myeloma. The ASCO guidelines for bisphosphonate use in multiple myeloma recommend infusing pamidronate over at least 2 hours; if therapy is withheld due to renal toxicity, infuse over at least 4 hours upon reintroduction of treatment after renal recovery (Kyle, 2007).

Monitoring Parameters Serum creatinine (prior to each treatment); serum electrolytes, including calcium, phosphate, magnesium, and potassium; CBC with differential; monitor for hypocalcemia for at least 2 weeks after therapy; dental exam and preventative dentistry prior to therapy for patients at risk of osteonecrosis, including all cancer patients; patients with pre-existing anemia, leukopenia, or thrombocytopenia should be closely monitored during the first 2 weeks of treatment; in addition, monitor urine albumin every 3-6 months in multiple myeloma patients

Test Interactions Bisphosphonates may interfere with diagnostic imaging agents such as technetium-99m-diphosphonate in bone scans.

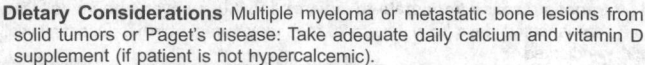

Dietary Considerations Multiple myeloma or metastatic bone lesions from solid tumors or Paget's disease: Take adequate daily calcium and vitamin D supplement (if patient is not hypercalcemic).

Additional Information

Oncology Comment:

Metastatic breast cancer: The American Society of Clinical Oncology (ASCO) updated guidelines on the role of bone-modifying agents (BMAs) in the prevention and treatment of skeletal-related events for metastatic breast cancer patients (Van Poznak, 2011). The guidelines recommend initiating a BMA (denosumab, pamidronate, zoledronic acid) in patients with metastatic breast cancer to the bone. There is currently no literature indicating the superiority of one particular BMA. Optimal duration is not defined; however, the guidelines recommend continuing therapy until substantial decline in patient's performance status. In patients with normal Cl_{cr} (>60 mL/minute), no dosage/interval/infusion rate changes for pamidronate or zoledronic acid are necessary. For patients with Cl_{cr} <30 mL/minute, pamidronate and zoledronic acid are not recommended. While no renal dose adjustments are recommended for denosumab, close monitoring is advised for risk of hypocalcemia in patients with Cl_{cr} <30 mL/minute or on dialysis. The ASCO guidelines are in alignment with package insert guidelines for dosing, renal dose adjustments, infusion times, prevention and management of osteonecrosis of the jaw, and monitoring of laboratory parameter recommendations. BMAs are not the first-line therapy for pain. BMAs are to be used as adjunctive therapy for cancer-related bone pain associated with bone metastasis, demonstrating a modest pain control benefit. BMAs should be used in conjunction with agents such as NSAIDs, opioid and nonopioid analgesics, corticosteroids, radiation/surgery, and interventional procedures.

Multiple myeloma: The American Society of Clinical Oncology (ASCO) has also published guidelines on the use of bisphosphonates for prevention and treatment of bone disease in multiple myeloma (Kyle, 2007). Pamidronate or zoledronic acid use is recommended in multiple myeloma patients with lytic bone destruction or compression spine fracture from osteopenia. Clodronate (not available in the U.S.; available in Canada), administered orally or I.V., is an alternative treatment. The use of the bisphosphonates pamidronate and zoledronic acid may be considered in patients with pain secondary to osteolytic disease, adjunct therapy to stabilize fractures or impending fractures, and I.V. bisphosphonates for multiple myeloma patients with osteopenia but no radiographic evidence of lytic bone disease. Bisphosphonates are not recommended in patients with solitary plasmacytoma, smoldering (asymptomatic) or indolent myeloma, or monoclonal gammopathy of undetermined significance. The guidelines recommend monthly treatment for a period of 2 years. At that time, physicians need to consider discontinuing in responsive and stable patients, and reinitiate if a new-onset skeletal-related event occurs. The ASCO guidelines are in alignment with package insert guidelines for dosing, renal dose adjustments, infusion times, prevention and management of osteonecrosis of the jaw, and monitoring of laboratory parameter recommendations. The guidelines also recommend in patients with extensive bone disease with existing severe renal disease (a serum creatinine >3 mg/dL or Cl_{cr} <30 mL/minute) pamidronate at a dose of 90 mg over 4-6 hours (unless pre-existing renal disease in which a reduced initial dose should be considered). ASCO also recommends monitoring for albuminuria every 3-6 months. In patients with unexplained albuminuria >500 mg/24 hours, withhold the dose until level returns to baseline, then recheck every 3-4 weeks. Pamidronate may be reinitiated at a dose not to exceed 90 mg every 4 weeks with a longer infusion time of at least 4 hours.

Dosage Forms Excipient information presented when available (limited, particularly for generics); consult specific product labeling. [DSC] = Discontinued product

Injection, powder for reconstitution, as disodium: 30 mg, 90 mg

Aredia®: 30 mg, 90 mg [DSC]

Injection, solution, as disodium: 3 mg/mL (10 mL); 6 mg/mL (10 mL); 9 mg/mL (10 mL)

Injection, solution, as disodium [preservative free]: 3 mg/mL (10 mL); 9 mg/mL (10 mL)

References

Assael LA, "Oral Bisphosphonates as a Cause of Bisphosphonate-Related Osteonecrosis of the Jaws: Clinical Findings, Assessment of Risks, and Preventive Strategies," *J Oral Maxillofac Surg*, 2009, 67(5 Suppl):35-43.

Bamias A, Kastritis E, Bamia C, et al, "Osteonecrosis of the Jaw in Cancer After Treatment With Bisphosphonates: Incidence and Risk Factors," *J Clin Oncol*, 2005, 23(34):8580-7.

Diamond TH, Winters J, Smith A, et al, "The Antiosteoporotic Efficacy of Intravenous Pamidronate in Men With Prostate Carcinoma Receiving Combined Androgen Blockade: A Double Blind, Randomized, Placebo-Controlled Crossover Study," *Cancer*, 2001, 92(6):1444-50.

Gimsing P, Carlson K, Turesson I, et al, "Effect of Pamidronate 30 mg Versus 90 mg on Physical Function in Patients With Newly Diagnosed Multiple Myeloma (Nordic Myeloma Study Group): A Double-Blind, Randomised Controlled Trial," *Lancet Oncol*, 2010, 11(10):973-82.

Gralow JR, Biermann JS, Farooki A, et al, "NCCN Task Force Report: Bone Health in Cancer Care," *J Natl Compr Canc Netw*, 2009, 7(Suppl 3):1-32.

Hillner BE, Ingel JN, Chlebowski RT, et al, "American Society of Clinical Oncology 2003 Update on the Role of Bisphosphonates and Bone Health Issues in Women With Breast Cancer," *J Clin Oncol*, 2003, 21(21):4042-57.

Kyle RA, Yee GC, Somerfield MR, et al, "American Society of Clinical Oncology 2007 Clinical Practice Guideline Update on the Role of Bisphosphonates in Multiple Myeloma," *J Clin Oncol*, 2007, 25(17):2464-72.

National Comprehensive Cancer Network® (NCCN), "Clinical Practice Guidelines in Oncology™: Multiple Myeloma," Version 1.2011. Available at http://www.nccn.org/professionals/physician_gls/PDF/myeloma.pdf

Rogers MJ, Crockett JC, Coxon FP, et al, "Biochemical and Molecular Mechanisms of Action of Bisphosphonates," *Bone*, 2011, 49(1):34-41.

Smith MR, McGovern FJ, Zietman AL, et al, "Pamidronate to Prevent Bone Loss During Androgen-Deprivation Therapy For Prostate Cancer," *N Engl J Med*, 2001, 345(13):948-55.

Stathopoulos IP, Liakou CG, Katsalira A, et al, "The Use of Bisphosphonates in Women Prior to or During Pregnancy and Lactation," *Hormones (Athens)*, 2011, 10(4):280-91.

Van Poznak CH, Temin S, Yee GC, et al, "American Society of Clinical Oncology Executive Summary of the Clinical Practice Guideline Update on the Role of Bone-Modifying Agents in Metastatic Breast Cancer," *J Clin Oncol*, 2011, 29(9):1221-7.

◆ **Pamidronate Disodium** *see* Pamidronate *on page* 1109

◆ **Pamidronate Disodium® (Can)** *see* Pamidronate *on page* 1109

◆ **Pamidronate Disodium Omega (Can)** *see* Pamidronate *on page* 1109

◆ **Pandel®** *see* Hydrocortisone (Topical) *on page* 719

◆ **Panglobulin** *see* Immune Globulin *on page* 777

Panitumumab (pan i TOOM yoo mab)

Related Information

Management of Chemotherapy-Induced Nausea and Vomiting *on page* 1786

Principles of Anticancer Therapy *on page* 1878

Brand Names: U.S. Vectibix®

Brand Names: Canada Vectibix®

Index Terms ABX-EGF; MOAB ABX-EGF; Monoclonal Antibody ABX-EGF; rHuMAb-EGFr

Generic Availability (U.S.) No

Pharmacologic Category Antineoplastic Agent, Monoclonal Antibody; Epidermal Growth Factor Receptor (EGFR) Inhibitor

Use Monotherapy in treatment of EGFR-expressing refractory metastatic colorectal cancer with disease progression on or following fluoropyrimidine-, oxaliplatin-, and irinotecan-based regimens

Panitumumab is not indicated for the treatment of patients with *KRAS* mutation-positive metastatic colorectal cancer or patients in which *KRAS* mutation status is unknown. Subset analyses (retrospective) in metastatic colorectal cancer trials have not shown a benefit with EGFR inhibitor treatment in patients whose tumors have codon 12 or 13 *KRAS* mutations.

Unlabeled Use Treatment of metastatic colorectal cancer (KRAS wild-type) in combination with other chemotherapy agents

Labeled Contraindications There are no contraindications listed in the manufacturer's labeling.

Pregnancy Risk Factor C

Lactation Excretion in breast milk unknown/not recommended

Warnings/Precautions [U.S. Boxed Warning]: Dermatologic toxicities have been reported in ~90% of patients receiving single agent panitumumab and were severe (grade 3 or higher) in ~12% of patients); may include dermatitis acneiform, pruritus, erythema, rash, skin exfoliation, paronychia, dry skin and skin fissures. Severe skin toxicities may be complicated by infection, sepsis, or abscesses. The median time to development of skin (or ocular) toxicity was 2 weeks, with resolution ~12 weeks after discontinuation. Monitor all dermatologic toxicities for development of inflammation or infection. Withhold treatment for severe or life-threatening dermatologic toxicities; may require dose reduction or permanent discontinuation. The severity of dermatologic toxicity is predictive for response; grades 2-4 skin toxicity correlates with improved progression free survival and overall survival, compared to grade 1 skin toxicity (Peeters, 2009; Van Cutsem, 2007). Patients should minimize sunlight exposure; may exacerbate skin reactions. Keratitis and ulcerative keratitis (known risk factors for corneal perforation) have occurred. Monitor for evidence of ocular toxicity; interrupt or discontinue treatment for acute or worsening keratitis. Gastric mucosal and nail toxicities have also been reported.

[U.S. Boxed Warning]: Severe infusion reactions (anaphylactic reaction, bronchospasm, fever, chills, and hypotension) have been reported in ~1% of patients; fatal infusion reactions have been reported with post-marketing surveillance. Discontinue infusion for severe reactions; permanently discontinue in patients with persistent severe infusion reactions. Appropriate medical support for the management of infusion reactions should be readily available. Mild-to-moderate infusion reactions are managed by slowing the infusion rate.

Pulmonary fibrosis has been observed (rarely) in clinical trials; fatalities have been reported. Interrupt treatment for acute onset or worsening of pulmonary symptoms; permanently discontinue treatment if interstitial lung disease is confirmed. Patients with a history of or evidence of interstitial pneumonitis or pulmonary fibrosis were excluded from most clinical trials. May cause diarrhea; the incidence and severity of chemotherapy-induced diarrhea and other toxicities (rash, electrolyte abnormalities, stomatitis) is increased with combination chemotherapy; severe diarrhea and dehydration (which may lead to acute renal failure) has been observed with panitumumab in combination with chemotherapy. In a study of bevacizumab with combination chemotherapy ± panitumumab, the use of panitumumab resulted in decreased progression-free survival and significantly increased toxicity compared to regimens without panitumumab (Hecht, 2009). Toxicities included rash, diarrhea/dehydration, electrolyte disturbances, stomatitis, infection, and an increased incidence of pulmonary embolism. Magnesium and/or calcium depletion may occur during treatment (may be delayed; hypomagnesemia occurred ≥6 weeks after panitumumab initiation) and after treatment is discontinued; electrolyte repletion may be necessary; monitor for hypomagnesemia and hypocalcemia during treatment and for at least 8 weeks after completion.

Patients with colorectal cancer with tumors with a codon 12 or 13 *KRAS* mutation are unlikely to benefit from EGFR inhibitor therapy. Panitumumab is not indicated patients with *KRAS* mutation-positive metastatic colorectal cancer or patients in which *KRAS* mutation status is unknown. In a study of FOLFOX4 (fluorouracil, leucovorin and oxaliplatin) ± panitumumab, patients with a *KRAS* mutation who received panitumumab with FOLFOX4 experienced a significantly shortened progression-free survival (Douillard, 2010); panitumumab should not be used in combination with oxaliplatin-based regimens in patients with *KRAS* mutation or if mutation status is unknown. Panitumumab is also reported to be ineffective in patients with BRAF V600E mutation (Di Nicolantonio, 2008). According to the manufacturer, evidence of EGFR expression is necessary to determine patient selection (the Dako EGFR pharmDX® kit has been used).

Adverse Reactions

>10%:

Cardiovascular: Peripheral edema (12%)

Central nervous system: Fatigue (26%)

Dermatologic: Skin toxicity (90%; grades 3/4: 14% to 16%), erythema (65%; grades 3/4: 5%), acneiform rash (57%; grades 3/4: 7%), pruritus (57%; grades 3/4: 2%), nail toxicity (29%; grades 3/4: 2%), exfoliation (25%; grades 3/4: 2%), paronychia (25%), rash (22%; grades 3/4: 1%), fissures (20%; grades 3/4: 1%), acne (13%; grades 3/4: 1%)

Endocrine & metabolic: Hypomagnesemia (38%; grades 3/4: 4%)

Gastrointestinal: Abdominal pain (25%), nausea (23%), diarrhea (21%; grades 3/4: 2%), constipation (21%), vomiting (19%)

Ocular: Ocular toxicity (15%)

Respiratory: Cough (14%)

1% to 10%:

Dermatologic: Dry skin (10%)

Gastrointestinal: Stomatitis (7%), mucositis (6%)

Ocular: Eyelash growth (6%), conjunctivitis (4%), ocular hyperemia (3%), lacrimation increased (2%), eye/eye lid irritation (1%)

Miscellaneous: Antibody formation (≤5%), infusion reactions (3%; grades 3/4: 1%)

<1%, postmarketing, and/or case reports: Abscess, allergic reaction, anaphylactoid reaction, angioedema, chills, dyspnea, fever, hypocalcemia, hypoxia, keratitis, keratitis ulcerative, pulmonary embolism, pulmonary fibrosis, pulmonary infiltrate, sepsis, septic death, skin necrosis

Drug Interactions

Metabolism/Transport Effects None known.

Avoid Concomitant Use There are no known interactions where it is recommended to avoid concomitant use.

Increased Effect/Toxicity There are no known significant interactions involving an increase in effect.

Decreased Effect There are no known significant interactions involving a decrease in effect.

Storage/Stability Store intact vials refrigerated at 2°C to 8°C (36°F to 46°F). Do not freeze; do not shake; protect from direct sunlight. Preparations diluted for infusion are stable for 6 hours at room temperature or for 24 hours refrigerated at 2°C to 8°C (36°F to 46°F); do not freeze.

Reconstitution Dilute in 100 mL (for doses ≤1000 mg) or 150 mL (doses >1000 mg) of normal saline to a final concentration of ≤10 mg/mL. Gently invert to mix; do not shake.

Mechanism of Action Recombinant human IgG2 monoclonal antibody which binds specifically to the epidermal growth factor receptor (EGFR, HER1, c-ErbB-1) and competitively inhibits the binding of epidermal growth factor (EGF) and other ligands. Binding to the EGFR blocks phosphorylation and activation of intracellular tyrosine kinases, resulting in inhibition of cell survival, growth, proliferation and transformation. EGFR signal transduction results in *KRAS* wild-type activation; cells with *KRAS* mutations appear to be unaffected by EGFR inhibition.

Pharmacodynamics/Kinetics Half-life elimination: ~7.5 days (range: 4-11 days)

Dosing

Adult & Geriatric

Colorectal cancer, metastatic, *KRAS* mutation-negative: I.V.: 6 mg/kg every 14 days as a single agent

Colorectal cancer, metastatic (*KRAS* wild-type), in combination with FOLFIRI (unlabeled use): I.V.: 6 mg/kg every 14 days in combination with fluorouracil, leucovorin, and irinotecan (Peeters, 2010)

Renal Impairment No dosage adjustment provided in the manufacturer's labeling (has not been studied).

Hepatic Impairment No dosage adjustment provided in the manufacturer's labeling (has not been studied).

Adjustment for Toxicity

Infusion reactions, mild-to-moderate (grade 1 or 2): Reduce the infusion rate by 50% for the duration of infusion.

Infusion reactions, severe (grade 3 or 4): Stop infusion; consider permanent discontinuation (depending on severity or persistence of reaction).

Dermatologic toxicity (≥grade 3, or intolerable): Withhold treatment; if skin toxicity does not improve to ≤grade 2 within 1 month, permanently discontinue. If skin toxicity improves to ≤grade 2 within 1 month (with patient missing ≤2 doses), resume treatment at 50% of the original dose. Dose may be increased in increments of 25% of the original dose (up to 6 mg/kg) if skin toxicities do not recur. For recurrent skin toxicity, permanently discontinue.

Ocular toxicity (acute or worsening keratitis): Interrupt or discontinue treatment.

Pulmonary toxicity:

Acute onset or worsening pulmonary symptoms: Interrupt treatment.

Interstitial lung disease: Permanently discontinue treatment.

Combination Regimens

Colorectal cancer:

Panitumumab (Colorectal Regimen) on page 1733
Panitumumab + FOLFIRI (Colorectal) on page 1733

Panitumumab + FOLFOX4 (Colorectal) on page 1733

Administration I.V.: Doses ≤1000 mg, infuse over 1 hour; doses >1000 mg, infuse over 90 minutes (via infusion pump); do not administer I.V. push or as a bolus. Administer through a low protein-binding 0.2 or 0.22 micrometer in-line filter. Flush with NS before and after infusion. Reduce infusion rate by 50% for mild-to-moderate infusion reactions (grades 1 and 2); stop infusion for severe infusion reactions (grades 3 and 4) and consider permanent discontinuation.

Emetic Potential Low (10% to 30%)

Monitoring Parameters *KRAS* genotyping of tumor tissue. Monitor serum electrolytes, including magnesium and calcium (periodically during and for at least 8 weeks after therapy). Monitor vital signs and temperature before, during, and after infusion. Monitor for skin toxicity, for evidence of ocular toxicity, and for acute onset or worsening pulmonary symptoms.

Additional Information Oncology Comment: The National Comprehensive Cancer Network® (NCCN) guidelines for colon cancer (v.3.2012) and the American Society of Clinical Oncology (ASCO) provisional clinical opinion (Allegra, 2009) recommend genotyping tumor tissue for *KRAS* mutation in all patients with metastatic colorectal cancer (genotyping may be done on archived specimens). Patients with known codon 12 or 13 *KRAS* gene mutations are unlikely to respond to EGFR inhibitors and should not receive panitumumab. Favorable progression-free survival and higher response rates have been demonstrated with panitumumab in patients with *KRAS* wild type; patients with the *KRAS* mutation did not respond to panitumumab (Amado, 2008). Panitumumab is also reported to be ineffective in patients with BRAF V600E mutation (Di Nicolantonio, 2008). Because EGFR testing in colorectal tumors does not correlate with response, the NCCN guidelines do not recommend routine EGFR testing in colorectal cancer. Severity of dermatologic toxicity associated with panitumumab is predictive for response, grades 2-4 skin toxicity correlates with improved progression free survival and overall survival, compared to patients with grade 1 skin toxicity (Peeters, 2009; Van Cutsem, 2007). The association between dermatologic toxicity and progression free survival was not noted in patients with *KRAS* mutation (Peeters, 2009). The NCCN guidelines do not recommend the use of panitumumab after failure of cetuximab therapy.

Dosage Forms Excipient information presented when available (limited, particularly for generics); consult specific product labeling. [DSC] = Discontinued product

Injection, solution [preservative free]:

Vectibix®: 20 mg/mL (5 mL, 10 mL [DSC], 20 mL)

References

Allegra CJ, Jessup JM, Somerfield MR, et al, "American Society of Clinical Oncology Provisional Clinical Opinion: Testing for *KRAS* Gene Mutations in Patients With Metastatic Colorectal Carcinoma to Predict Response to Anti-Epidermal Growth Factor Receptor Monoclonal Antibody Therapy," *J Clin Oncol*, 2009, 27(12):2091-6.

Amado RG, Wolf M, Peeters M, et al, "Wild-Type KRAS is Required for Panitumumab Efficacy in Patients With Metastatic Colorectal Cancer," *J Clin Oncol*, 2008, 26(10):1626-34.

Di Nicolantonio F, Martini M, Molinari F, et al, "Wild-type BRAF is Required for Response to Panitumumab or Cetuximab in Metastatic Colorectal Cancer," *J Clin Oncol*, 2008, 26 (35):5705-12.

National Comprehensive Cancer Network® (NCCN), "Clinical Practice Guidelines in Oncology™: Colon Cancer," Version 2, 2009. Available at http://www.nccn.org/professionals/physician_gls/PDF/colon.pdf

Peeters M, Price TJ, Cervantes A, et al, "Randomized Phase III Study of Panitumumab With Fluorouracil, Leucovorin, and Irinotecan (FOLFIRI) Compared With FOLFIRI Alone as Second-Line Treatment in Patients With Metastatic Colorectal Cancer," *J Clin Oncol*, 2010, 28 (31):4706-13.

Peeters M, Siena S, Van Cutsem E, et al, "Association of Progression-Free Survival, Overall Survival, and Patient-Reported Outcomes by Skin Toxicity and KRAS Status in Patients Receiving Panitumumab Monotherapy," *Cancer*, 2009, 115(7):1544-54.
Segaert S and Van Cutsem E, "Clinical Signs, Pathophysiology and Management of Skin Toxicity During Therapy with Epidermal Growth Factor Receptor Inhibitors," *Ann Oncol*, 2005, 16(9): 1425-33.
Van Cutsem E, Peeters M, Siena S, et al, "Open-Label Phase III Trial of Panitumumab Plus Best Supportive Care Compared With Best Supportive Care Alone in Patients With Chemotherapy-Refractory Metastatic Colorectal Cancer," *J Clin Oncol*, 2007, 25(13): 1658-64.

◆ **Panretin®** *see* Alitretinoin *on page 50*

Papillomavirus (Types 6, 11, 16, 18) Vaccine (Human, Recombinant)

(pap ih LO ma VYE rus typs six e LEV en SIX teen AYE teen vak SEEN YU man ree KOM be nant)

Brand Names: U.S. Gardasil®

Brand Names: Canada Gardasil®

Index Terms HPV Vaccine; HPV4; Human Papillomavirus Vaccine; Papillomavirus Vaccine, Recombinant; Quadrivalent Human Papillomavirus Vaccine

Generic Availability (U.S.) No

Pharmacologic Category Vaccine, Inactivated (Viral)

Use

U.S. labeling:

Females ≥9 years and ≤26 years of age: Prevention of cervical, vulvar, vaginal, and anal cancer caused by HPV types 16 and 18; genital warts caused by HPV types 6 and 11; cervical adenocarcinoma *in situ*, and vulvar, vaginal, cervical, or anal intraepithelial neoplasia caused by HPV types 6, 11, 16, and 18

Males ≥9 years and ≤26 years of age: Prevention of genital warts caused by human papillomavirus (HPV) types 6 and 11; anal cancer caused by HPV types 16 and 18, and anal intraepithelial neoplasia caused by HPV types 6, 11, 16, and 18

Canadian labeling:

Females ≥9 years and ≤26 years of age: Prevention of anal cancer caused by HPV types 16 and 18; anal intraepithelial neoplasia caused by HPV types 6, 11, 16, and 18

Females ≥9 years and ≤45 years of age: Prevention of cervical, vulvar, and vaginal cancer caused by HPV types 16 and 18; genital warts caused by HPV types 6 and 11; cervical adenocarcinoma *in situ*, vulvar, vaginal, or cervical intraepithelial neoplasia caused by HPV types 6, 11, 16, and 18

Males ≥9 years and ≤26 years of age: Prevention of anal cancer caused by HPV types 16 and 18; anal intraepithelial neoplasia caused by HPV types 6, 11, 16, and 18; genital warts caused by HPV types 6 and 11

The Advisory Committee on Immunization Practices (ACIP) recommends routine vaccination for females and males 11-12 years of age; catch-up vaccination is recommended for females 13-26 years of age and males 13-21 years of age. Males 22-26 years may also be vaccinated. The ACIP also recommends routine vaccination for men who have sex with men (MSM) through 26 years of age (CDC, 59[20], 2010; CDC, 60[50], 2011). Vaccination is also recommended for immunocompromised persons or MSM through 26 years of age who were not previously vaccinated when they were younger. Although not specifically recommended for their profession, health care providers within the recommended age groups should also receive the HPV vaccine (CDC, 61[4], 2012).

Labeled Contraindications Hypersensitivity to papillomavirus recombinant vaccine or any component of the formulation

Pregnancy Risk Factor B

Lactation Excretion in breast milk unknown/use caution

Warnings/Precautions Immediate treatment for anaphylactoid reaction should be available during vaccine use. Patients who develop hypersensitivity after administration should not receive further dosing. There is no evidence that individuals already infected with HPV will be protected; those already infected with 1 or more HPV types were protected from disease in the remaining HPV types. Not for the treatment of active disease; will not protect against diseases not caused by human papillomavirus (HPV) vaccine types 6, 11, 16, and 18. May administer with mild concurrent febrile illness; consider deferring vaccination with serious illness.Vaccination may not result in effective immunity in all patients. Response depends upon multiple factors (eg, type of vaccine, age of patient) and may be improved by administering the vaccine at the recommended dose, route, and interval. Vaccines may not be effective if administered during periods of altered immune competence (CDC 60[2], 2011). Immunocompromised patients may have a reduced response to vaccination. In general, household and close contacts of persons with altered immunocompetence may receive all age appropriate vaccines. Administered I.M., therefore use caution in patients at risk for bleeding. The entire 3-dose regimen should be completed for maximum efficacy. Not recommended for use during pregnancy. Syncope has been reported with use of injectable vaccines and may be accompanied by transient visual disturbances, weakness, or tonic-clonic movements. Procedures should be in place to avoid injuries from falling and to restore cerebral perfusion if syncope occurs. Safety and efficacy in children <9 years of age have not been established. Product may contain yeast. In order to maximize vaccination rates, the ACIP recommends simultaneous administration of all age-appropriate vaccines (live or inactivated) for which a person is eligible at a single clinic visit, unless contraindications exist.

Adverse Reactions All serious adverse reactions must be reported to the U.S. Department of Health and Human Services (DHHS) Vaccine Adverse Event Reporting System (VAERS) 1-800-822-7967 or online at https://vaers.hhs.gov/esub/index. In Canada, adverse reactions may be reported to local provincial/territorial health agencies or to the Vaccine Safety Section at Public Health Agency of Canada (1-866-844-0018).

>10%:

Central nervous system: Headache (12% to 28%), fever (8% to 13%)

Local: Injection site: Pain (61% to 84%), erythema (17% to 25%), swelling (14% to 25%)

1% to 10%:

Central nervous system: Dizziness (1% to 4%), malaise (1%), insomnia (1%)

Gastrointestinal: Nausea (2% to 7%), diarrhea (3% to 4%), vomiting (1% to 2%), toothache (2%)

Local: Injection site: Bruising (3%), pruritus (3%), hematoma (1%)

Neuromuscular & skeletal: Arthralgia (1%), myalgia (≤1%)

Respiratory: Pharyngolaryngeal pain (3%), cough (2%), nasal congestion (1%)

<1%, postmarketing, and/or case reports: Acute disseminated encephalomyelitis, alopecia areata, anaphylactic/anaphylactoid reaction, appendicitis, arrhythmia, arthritis, asthma, autoimmune hemolytic anemia and other autoimmune diseases, bronchospasm, cellulitis, cerebrovascular accident, chills, DVT, fatigue, gastroenteritis, Guillain-Barré syndrome, hypersensitivity

reaction, hyper-/hypothyroidism, injection site joint movement impairment, ITP, JIA, lymphadenopathy, motor neuron disease, pancreatitis, paralysis, pelvic inflammatory disease, pulmonary embolus, RA, renal failure (acute), seizure, sepsis, syncope (may result in falls with injury or be associated with tonic-clonic movements), transverse myelitis, urticaria, weakness

Drug Interactions

Metabolism/Transport Effects None known.

Avoid Concomitant Use There are no known interactions where it is recommended to avoid concomitant use.

Increased Effect/Toxicity There are no known significant interactions involving an increase in effect.

Decreased Effect

The levels/effects of Papillomavirus (Types 6, 11, 16, 18) Vaccine (Human, Recombinant) may be decreased by: Belimumab; Fingolimod; Immunosuppressants

Storage/Stability Store at 2°C to 8°C (36°F to 46°F); do not freeze. Protect from light. May be stored at temperatures ≤25°C (≤77°F) for a total time of ≤72 hours.

Mechanism of Action Contains inactive human papillomavirus (HPV) proteins HPV 6 L1, HPV 11 L1, HPV 16 L1, and HPV 18 L1 which produce neutralizing antibodies to prevent cervical cancer, cervical adenocarcinoma, cervical, vaginal and vulvar neoplasia, and genital warts caused by HPV.

Pharmacodynamics/Kinetics

Onset: Peak seroconversion was observed 1 month following the last dose of vaccine

Duration: Not well defined; at least 5 years

Dosing

Adult Immunization regimen:

U.S. labeling: I.M.: Children ≥9 years and Adults ≤26 years: 0.5 mL followed by 0.5 mL at 2 and 6 months after initial dose

Canadian labeling: I.M. Children ≥9 years and Adults ≤45 years: 0.5 mL followed by 0.5 mL at 2 and 6 months after initial dose

CDC recommended immunization schedule: Administer first dose at age 11-12 years; begin series in females aged 13-26 years or males 13-21 years if not previously vaccinated. Males may also be vaccinated through 26 years of age. Minimum interval between first and second doses is 4 weeks; the minimum interval between first and third doses is 24 weeks. Inadequate doses or doses received following a shorter than recommended dosing interval should be repeated. The HPV vaccine series should be completed with the same product whenever possible (CDC, 2007; CDC, 60 [50] 2011).

Pediatric Immunization regimen: Children ≥9 years: Refer to adult dosing.

Administration Shake suspension well before use. Inject the entire dose I.M. into the deltoid region of the upper arm or higher anterolateral thigh area. Observe for syncope for 15 minutes following administration. If the vaccine series is interrupted and only one dose was given, administer the second dose as soon as possible and give the third dose ≥12 weeks later. If the vaccine series is interrupted and the first two doses were given, administer the third dose as soon as possible. The HPV vaccine series should be completed with the same product whenever possible.

For patients at risk of hemorrhage following intramuscular injection, the ACIP recommends "it should be administered intramuscularly if, in the opinion of the physician familiar with the patient's bleeding risk, the vaccine can be administered by this route with reasonable safety. If the patient receives antihemophilia or other similar therapy, intramuscular vaccination can be scheduled shortly after such therapy is administered. A fine needle (23 gauge or smaller) can be used for the vaccination and firm pressure applied to the site (without rubbing) for at least 2 minutes. The patient should be instructed concerning the risk of hematoma from the injection." Patients on anticoagulant therapy should be considered to have the same bleeding risks and treated as those with clotting factor disorders (CDC, 2011).

Simultaneous administration of vaccines helps ensure the patients will be fully vaccinated by the appropriate age. Simultaneous administration of vaccines is defined as administering >1 vaccine on the same day at different anatomic sites. Separate vaccines should not be combined in the same syringe unless indicated by product specific labeling. Separate needles and syringes should be used for each injection. The ACIP prefers each dose of a specific vaccine in a series come from the same manufacturer when possible. Adolescents and adults should be vaccinated while seated or lying down. In general, preterm infants should be vaccinated at the same chronological age as full-term infants (CDC, 2011).

Antipyretics have not been shown to prevent febrile seizures. Antipyretics may be used to treat fever or discomfort following vaccination (CDC, 2011). One study reported that routine prophylactic administration of acetaminophen to prevent fever prior to vaccination decreased the immune response of some vaccines; the clinical significance of this reduction in immune response has not been established (Prymula, 2009).

Monitoring Parameters Gynecologic screening exam, papillomavirus test as per current guidelines; screening for HPV is not required prior to vaccination and screening for cervical cancer should continue as recommended following vaccination. Monitor for syncope for 15 minutes following administration. If seizure-like activity associated with syncope occurs, maintain patient in supine or Trendelenburg position to reestablish adequate cerebral perfusion.

Females: Gynecologic screening exam, papillomavirus test; screening for cervical cancer should continue per current guidelines following vaccination

Additional Information U.S. federal law requires that the name of medication, date of administration, the vaccine manufacturer, lot number of vaccine, and the administering person's name, title and address be entered into the patient's permanent medical record. Ideally, administration of vaccine should occur prior to potential HPV exposure. Benefits of vaccine decrease once infected with >1 of the HPV vaccine types, although patients are protected from precancerous cervical lesions and external genital lesions caused by other HPV vaccine types.

Comparison of HPV vaccines: Cervarix® and Gardasil® are both vaccines formulated to protect against infection with the human papillomavirus. Both are inactive vaccines which contain proteins HPV16 L1 and HPV 18 L1, the cause of >70% of invasive cervical cancer. The vaccines differ in that Gardasil® also contains HPV 6 L1 and HPV 11 L1 proteins which protect against 75% to 90% of genital warts. The vaccines also differ in their preparation and adjuvants used. The viral proteins in Cervarix® are prepared using *Trichoplusia ni* (insect cells) which are adsorbed on to an aluminum salt which is also combined with a monophosphoryl lipid. The viral proteins in Gardasil® are prepared using *S. cerevisiae* (baker's yeast) which are then adsorbed onto an aluminum salt.

Results from a short term study (measurements obtained 1 month following the third vaccination in the series) have shown that the immune response to HPV 16 and HPV 18 may be greater with Cervarix®; although the clinical significance of this differences is not known, local adverse events may also occur more frequently with this preparation. Both vaccines were effective and results from long term studies are pending.

Dosage Forms Excipient information presented when available (limited, particularly for generics); consult specific product labeling.

Injection, suspension [preservative free]:

Gardasil®: HPV 6 L1 protein 20 mcg, HPV 11 L1 protein 40 mcg, HPV 16 L1 protein 40 mcg, and HPV 18 L1 protein 20 mcg per 0.5 mL (0.5 mL) [contains aluminum, polysorbate 80; manufactured using *S. cerevisiae* (baker's yeast)]

References

Centers for Disease Control and Prevention, "FDA Licensure of Bivalent Human Papillomavirus Vaccine (HPV2, Cervarix) for Use in Females and Updated HPV Vaccination Recommendations from the Advisory Committee on Immunization Practices (ACIP)," *MMWR Morb Mortal Wkly Rep*, 2010, 59(20):626-9. Available at http://www.cdc.gov/mmwr/preview/mmwrhtml/mm5920a4.htm?s_cid=mm5920a4_e

Centers for Disease Control and Prevention, "Quadrivalent Human Papillomavirus Vaccine. Recommendations of the Advisory Committee on Immunization Practices (ACIP)," *MMWR Recomm Rep*, 2007, 56(RR-2):1-24.

Centers for Disease Control and Prevention (CDC), "Recommendations of the Advisory Committee on Immunization Practices (ACIP): General Recommendations on Immunization," *MMWR Recomm Rep*, 2011, 60(2):1-64.

Centers for Disease Control and Prevention (CDC), "Recommendations on the Use of Quadrivalent Human Papillomavirus Vaccine in Males - Advisory Committee on Immunization Practices (ACIP), 2011," *MMWR Morb Mortal Wkly Rep*, 2011, 60(50):1705-8.

Centers for Disease Control and Prevention (CDC), "Recommended Adult Immunization Schedule – United States, 2012," *MMWR Morb Mortal Wkly Rep*, 2012, 61(4). Available at http://www.cdc.gov/vaccines/recs/schedules/downloads/adult/mmwr-adult-schedule.pdf

Einstein MH, Baron M, Levin MJ, et al, "Comparison of the Immunogenicity and Safety of Cervarix® and Gardasil® Human Papillomavirus (HPV) Cervical Cancer Vaccines in Healthy Women Aged 18-45 Years," *Hum Vaccin*, 2009, 5(10):507-19.

FUTURE II Study Group, "Quadrivalent Vaccine Against Human Papillomavirus to Prevent High-Grade Cervical Lesions," *N Engl J Med*, 2007, 356(19):1915-27.

Garland SM, Hernandez-Avila M, Wheeler CM, et al, "Quadrivalent Vaccine Against Human Papillomavirus to Prevent Anogenital Diseases," *N Engl J Med*, 2007, 356(19):1928-43.

Giuliano AR, Palefsky JM, Goldstone S, et al, "Efficacy of Quadrivalent HPV Vaccine Against HPV Infection and Disease in Males," *N Eng J Med*, 2011, 364(5):401-11.

Mao C, Koutsky LA, Ault KA, et al, "Efficacy of Human Papillomavirus-16 Vaccine to Prevent Cervical Intraepithelial Neoplasia: A Randomized Controlled Trial," *Obstet Gynecol*, 2006, 107(1):18-27.

Saslow D, Castle PE, Cox JT, et al, "American Cancer Society Guideline for Human Papillomavirus (HPV) Vaccine Use to Prevent Cervical Cancer and Its Precursors," *CA Cancer J Clin*, 2007, 57(1):7-28.

Steinbrook R, "The Potential of Human Papillomavirus Vaccines," *N Engl J Med*, 2006, 354(11):1109-11.

Papillomavirus (Types 16, 18) Vaccine (Human, Recombinant)

(pap ih LO ma VYE rus typs SIX teen AYE teen vak SEEN YU man ree KOM be nant)

Brand Names: U.S. Cervarix®

Brand Names: Canada Cervarix®

Index Terms Bivalent Human Papillomavirus Vaccine; GSK-580299; HPV 16/18 L1 VLP/AS04 VAC; HPV Vaccine; HPV2; Human Papillomavirus Vaccine; Papillomavirus Vaccine, Recombinant

Generic Availability (U.S.) No

Pharmacologic Category Vaccine, Inactivated (Viral)

Use Females 9 through 25 years of age: Prevention of cervical cancer, cervical adenocarcinoma *in situ*, and cervical intraepithelial neoplasia caused by human papillomavirus (HPV) types 16, 18

The Advisory Committee on Immunization Practices (ACIP) recommends routine vaccination for females 11-12 years of age; catch-up vaccination is recommended for females 13-25 years of age (CDC, 59[20], 2010). Vaccination is also recommended for immunocompromised females through 26 years of age who were not previously vaccinated when they were younger. Although not specifically recommended for their profession, female health care providers within the recommended age groups should also receive the HPV vaccine (CDC, 61[4], 2012).

Labeled Contraindications Hypersensitivity to papillomavirus recombinant vaccine or any component of the formulation

Pregnancy Risk Factor B

Lactation Excretion in breast milk unknown/use caution

Warnings/Precautions Immediate treatment (including epinephrine 1:1000) for anaphylactoid and/or hypersensitivity reactions should be available during vaccine use. May consider deferring administration in patients with moderate or severe acute illness (with or without fever); may administer to patients with mild acute illness (with or without fever). Vaccination may not result in effective immunity in all patients. Response depends upon multiple factors (eg, type of vaccine, age of patient) and may be improved by administering the vaccine at the recommended dose, route, and interval. Vaccines may not be effective if administered during periods of altered immune competence (CDC, 2011). Use with caution in patients with a history of bleeding disorders (including thrombocytopenia) and/or patients on anticoagulant therapy; bleeding/hematoma may occur from I.M. administration. There is no evidence that individuals already exposed to or infected with HPV will be protected; those already infected with 1 or more HPV types were protected from disease in the remaining HPV types. Not for the treatment of active disease; will not protect against diseases not caused by HPV vaccine types 16 and 18. Use with caution in severely immunocompromised patients (eg, patients receiving chemo/radiation therapy or other immunosuppressive therapy [including high-dose corticosteroids]); may have a reduced response to vaccination. In general, household and close contacts of persons with altered immunocompetence may receive all age appropriate vaccines. Syncope has been reported with use of injectable vaccines and may be accompanied by transient visual disturbances, weakness, or tonic-clonic movements. Procedures should be in place to avoid injuries from falling and to restore cerebral perfusion if syncope occurs.

Packaging may contain natural rubber/natural latex. Safety and efficacy have not been established in males or in females <9 years of age. Not recommended for use during pregnancy. The entire 3-dose regimen should be completed for maximum efficacy. In order to maximize vaccination rates, the ACIP recommends simultaneous administration of all age-appropriate vaccines (live or inactivated) for which a person is eligible at a single clinic visit, unless contraindications exist.

Adverse Reactions **All serious adverse reactions must be reported to the U.S. Department of Health and Human Services (DHHS) Vaccine Adverse Event Reporting System (VAERS) 1-800-822-7967 or online at https://vaers.hhs.gov/esub/index.** In Canada, adverse reactions may be reported to local provincial/territorial health agencies or to the Vaccine Safety Section at Public Health Agency of Canada (1-866-844-0018).

>10%:
- Central nervous system: Fatigue (55%)
- Local: Injection site reactions: Pain (92%), redness (48%), swelling (44%)
- Neuromuscular & skeletal: Myalgia (49%), arthralgia (21%)

1% to 10%:
- Dermatologic: Urticaria (7%)
- Local: Injection site: Pruritus (1%)
- Respiratory: Nasopharyngitis (4%), pharyngolaryngeal pain (3%), upper respiratory tract infection (2%), pharyngitis (1%)
- Miscellaneous: Influenza (3%), chlamydia infection (2%), vaginal infection (1%)

<1%, postmarketing, and/or case reports: Allergic reactions, anaphylactic/anaphylactoid reactions, angioedema, erythema multiforme, lymphadenopathy, syncope (may be associated with tonic-clonic movements), vasovagal response

Note: The following occurred more often with the placebo (percentages reported with Cervarix®): Headache (5% to 53%); gastrointestinal symptoms (abdominal pain, diarrhea, nausea, vomiting) (28%); fever (13%); rash (10%); dizziness (2%); dysmenorrhea (2%); back pain (1%); injection site bruising (1%)

Drug Interactions

Metabolism/Transport Effects None known.

Avoid Concomitant Use There are no known interactions where it is recommended to avoid concomitant use.

Increased Effect/Toxicity There are no known significant interactions involving an increase in effect.

Decreased Effect

The levels/effects of Papillomavirus (Types 16, 18) Vaccine (Human, Recombinant) may be decreased by: Belimumab; Fingolimod; Immunosuppressants

Storage/Stability Store under refrigeration at 2°C to 8°C (36°F to 46°F); do not freeze; discard if frozen. May develop a fine, white deposit with a clear, colorless supernatant during storage (not a sign of deterioration).

Mechanism of Action Contains inactive human papillomavirus (HPV) proteins HPV 16 L1, and HPV 18 L1 which produce neutralizing antibodies to prevent cervical cancer, cervical adenocarcinoma, and cervical neoplasia cause by HPV.

Pharmacodynamics/Kinetics

Onset: Peak seroconversion was observed 1 month following the last dose of vaccine

Duration: Not well defined; >5 years

Dosing

Adult Immunization: I.M.: Females ≤25 years: 0.5 mL followed by 0.5 mL at 1 and 6 months after initial dose

CDC recommended immunization schedule: Administer first dose to females at age 11-12 years; begin series in females aged 13-25 years if not previously vaccinated. Minimum interval between first and second doses is 4 weeks; the minimum interval between first and third doses is 24 weeks. Inadequate doses or doses received following a shorter than recommended dosing interval should be repeated. The HPV vaccine series should be completed with the same product whenever possible.

Pediatric Immunization: I.M.: Females ≥9 years: 0.5 mL followed by 0.5 mL at 1 and 6 months after initial dose

CDC recommended immunization schedule: Administer first dose to females at age 11-12 years; begin series in females aged 13-25 years if not previously vaccinated. Minimum interval between first and second doses is 4 weeks; the minimum interval between first and third doses is 24 weeks. Inadequate doses or doses received following a shorter than recommended dosing interval should be repeated. The HPV vaccine series should be completed with the same product whenever possible.

Administration Shake well prior to use. Do not use if discolored or if containing particulate matter, or if vial or syringe is cracked. Inject I.M. into the deltoid region of the upper arm. Do not administer I.V., SubQ, or intradermally.

For patients at risk of hemorrhage following intramuscular injection, the ACIP recommends "it should be administered intramuscularly if, in the opinion of the physician familiar with the patient's bleeding risk, the vaccine can be administered by this route with reasonable safety. If the patient receives antihemophilia or other similar therapy, intramuscular vaccination can be scheduled shortly after such therapy is administered. A fine needle (23 gauge or smaller) can be used for the vaccination and firm pressure applied to the site (without rubbing) for at least 2 minutes. The patient should be instructed concerning the risk of hematoma from the injection." Patients on anticoagulant therapy should be considered to have the same bleeding risks and treated as those with clotting factor disorders (CDC, 2011).

Simultaneous administration of vaccines helps ensure the patients will be fully vaccinated by the appropriate age. Simultaneous administration of vaccines is defined as administering >1 vaccine on the same day at different anatomic sites. Separate vaccines should not be combined in the same syringe unless indicated by product specific labeling. Separate needles and syringes should be used for each injection. The ACIP prefers each dose of a specific vaccine in a series come from the same manufacturer when possible. Adolescents and adults should be vaccinated while seated or lying down. In general, preterm infants should be vaccinated at the same chronological age as full-term infants (CDC, 2011).

Antipyretics have not been shown to prevent febrile seizures. Antipyretics may be used to treat fever or discomfort following vaccination (CDC, 2011). One study reported that routine prophylactic administration of acetaminophen to prevent fever prior to vaccination decreased the immune response of some vaccines; the clinical significance of this reduction in immune response has not been established (Prymula, 2009).

Monitoring Parameters Gynecologic screening exam, papillomavirus test as per current guidelines; screening for HPV is not required prior to vaccination and screening for cervical cancer should continue as recommended following vaccination. Monitor for syncope for 15 minutes following administration. If seizure-like activity associated with syncope occurs, maintain patient in supine or Trendelenburg position to reestablish adequate cerebral perfusion.

Additional Information U.S. federal law requires that the name of medication, date of administration, the vaccine manufacturer, lot number of vaccine, and the administering person's name, title and address be entered into the patient's permanent medical record. Ideally, administration of vaccine should occur prior to potential HPV exposure.

Comparison of HPV vaccines: Cervarix® and Gardasil® are both vaccines formulated to protect against infection with the human papillomavirus. Both are inactive vaccines which contain proteins HPV16 L1 and HPV 18 L1, the cause of >70% of invasive cervical cancer. The vaccines differ in that Gardasil® also contains HPV 6 L1 and HPV 11 L1 proteins which protect against 75% to 90% of genital warts. The vaccines also differ in their preparation and adjuvants used. The viral proteins in Cervarix® are prepared using *Trichoplusia ni* (insect cells) which are adsorbed on to an aluminum salt which is also combined with a monophosphoryl lipid. The viral proteins in Gardasil® are prepared using *S. cerevisiae* (baker's yeast) which are then adsorbed onto an aluminum salt. Results from a short-term study (measurements obtained 1 month following the third vaccination in the series) have shown that the immune response to HPV 16 and HPV 18 may be greater with Cervarix®; although the clinical significance of this differences is not known, local adverse events may also occur more frequently with this preparation. Both vaccines were effective and results from long-term studies are pending.

Dosage Forms Excipient information presented when available (limited, particularly for generics); consult specific product labeling. [DSC] = Discontinued product

Injection, suspension [preservative free]:

Cervarix®: HPV 16 L1 protein 20 mcg and HPV 18 L1 protein 20 mcg per 0.5 mL (0.5 mL [DSC]) [contains aluminum; manufactured using *Trichoplusia ni* (insect cells)]

Cervarix®: HPV 16 L1 protein 20 mcg and HPV 18 L1 protein 20 mcg per 0.5 mL (0.5 mL) [contains aluminum, natural rubber/natural latex in prefilled syringe; manufactured using *Trichoplusia ni* (insect cells)]

References

Centers for Disease Control and Prevention, "FDA Licensure of Bivalent Human Papillomavirus Vaccine (HPV2, Cervarix) for Use in Females and Updated HPV Vaccination Recommendations from the Advisory Committee on Immunization Practices (ACIP)," *MMWR Morb Mortal Wkly Rep*, 2010, 59(20):626-9.

Centers for Disease Control and Prevention (CDC), "Recommendations of the Advisory Committee on Immunization Practices (ACIP): General Recommendations on Immunization," *MMWR Recomm Rep*, 2011, 60(2):1-64.

Centers for Disease Control and Prevention (CDC), "Recommended Adult Immunization Schedule – United States, 2012," *MMWR Morb Mortal Wkly Rep*, 2012, 61(4). Available at http://www.cdc.gov/vaccines/recs/schedules/downloads/adult/mmwr-adult-schedule.pdf

Einstein MH, Baron M, Levin MJ, et al, "Comparison of the Immunogenicity and Safety of Cervarix® and Gardasil® Human Papillomavirus (HPV) Cervical Cancer Vaccines in Healthy Women Aged 18-45 Years," *Hum Vaccin*, 2009, 5(10):507-19.

Saslow D, Castle PE, Cox JT, et al, "American Cancer Society Guideline for Human Papillomavirus (HPV) Vaccine Use to Prevent Cervical Cancer and Its Precursors," *CA Cancer J Clin*, 2007, 57 (1):7-28.

◆ **Papillomavirus Vaccine, Recombinant** *see* Papillomavirus (Types 6, 11, 16, 18) Vaccine (Human, Recombinant) *on page 1120*

◆ **Papillomavirus Vaccine, Recombinant** *see* Papillomavirus (Types 16, 18) Vaccine (Human, Recombinant) *on page 1124*

◆ **Paraplatin** *see* CARBOplatin *on page 229*

Pazopanib (paz OH pa nib)

Related Information

Management of Chemotherapy-Induced Nausea and Vomiting *on page* 1786
Principles of Anticancer Therapy *on page* 1878

Brand Names: U.S. Votrient™

Brand Names: Canada Votrient™

Index Terms GW786034; Pazopanib Hydrochloride

Generic Availability (U.S.) No

Pharmacologic Category Antineoplastic Agent, Tyrosine Kinase Inhibitor; Vascular Endothelial Growth Factor (VEGF) Inhibitor

Use Treatment of advanced renal cell cancer (RCC); treatment of advanced soft tissue sarcoma (STS) (in patients previously treated with chemotherapy)

Unlabeled Use Treatment of advanced, differentiated thyroid cancer

Labeled Contraindications There are no contraindications listed within the manufacturer's labeling.

Pregnancy Risk Factor D

Lactation Excretion in breast milk unknown/not recommended

Warnings/Precautions Hazardous agent - use appropriate precautions for handling and disposal. **[U.S. Boxed Warning]: Severe and fatal hepatotoxicity (transaminase and bilirubin elevations) has been reported with use; monitor hepatic function; may require dosage interruption, reduction, or discontinuation.** Transaminase elevations usually occur early in the treatment course. Use is not recommended in patients with pre-existing severe hepatic impairment (bilirubin >3 times ULN with any ALT level); dosage reductions is recommended for pre-existing moderate hepatic impairment (bilirubin >1.5-3 times ULN). Patients >60 years of age may be at higher risk for ALT >3 times ULN. Mild indirect (unconjugated) hyperbilirubinemia may occur in patients with Gilbert's syndrome; for patients with known Gilbert's syndrome (only a mild indirect bilirubin elevation) and ALT >3 times ULN, follow isolated ALT elevation dosage modification recommendations.

Venous and arterial thromboembolism have been reported. DVT, pulmonary embolism, angina, transient ischemic attack, MI, and ischemic stroke were observed more frequently in the pazopanib group (versus placebo) in clinical trials. Fatalities were observed. Use with caution in patients with a history of or an increased risk for these events. Use in patients with recent arteriothrombotic event (within 6 months) has not been studied and is not recommended. Hemorrhagic events (including fatal) have been reported; use is not recommended in patients with a history of hemoptysis, cerebral hemorrhage or clinically significant gastrointestinal hemorrhage within 6 months (these populations were excluded from clinical trials).

May cause and/or worsen hypertension (hypertensive crisis has been observed); monitor; blood pressure should be controlled prior to treatment initiation; antihypertensive therapy should be used if needed. Hypertension usually occurs early in the treatment course. Dosage reduction may be necessary for persistent hypertension (despite antihypertensive therapy); discontinue for hypertensive crisis, or for severe and persistent hypertension which is refractory to dose reduction and antihypertensive therapy. May cause new-onset or worsening of existing heart failure; baseline and periodic LVEF monitoring is recommended in patients at increased risk of heart failure (eg, prior anthracycline treatment). Concurrent hypertension may increase the risk for cardiac dysfunction. QT_c prolongation, including torsade de pointes, has been observed; use caution in patients with a history of QT_c prolongation, with medications known to prolong the QT interval, or with pre-existing cardiac disease. Obtain baseline and periodic ECGs; correct electrolyte (potassium, calcium, and magnesium) abnormalities prior to and during treatment.

Gastrointestinal perforation and fistula (including fatal) have been reported; monitor for symptoms of gastrointestinal perforation and fistula. Proteinuria has been reported with use. Obtain baseline and periodic urinalysis and 24-hour urine protein when clinically indicated. Dosage reduction may be necessary for significant proteinuria (≥3 g/24 hours); discontinue for recurrent proteinuria. Hypothyroidism has been reported with use; monitor thyroid function tests. Vascular endothelial growth factor (VEGF) receptor inhibitors are associated with impaired wound healing. Discontinue treatment at least 7 days prior to scheduled surgery; treatment reinitiation should be guided by clinical judgment. Discontinue if wound dehiscence occurs.

Patients with mild-to-moderate renal impairment (Cl_{cr} ≥30 mL/minute) were included in trials. There are no pharmacokinetic data in patients with severe renal impairment undergoing dialysis (peritoneal and hemodialysis); however, renal impairment is not expected to significantly influence pazopanib pharmacokinetics or exposure. Avoid use with strong CYP3A4 inhibitors or inducers. If pazopanib must be administered concomitantly with a potent enzyme inhibitor, dose reductions are recommended. Use is not recommended in situations where the use of a strong CYP3A4 inducer is required. Pazopanib inhibits UGT1A1 and OATP1B1; pazopanib may increase concentration of drugs eliminated by UGT1A1 and OATP1B1. Concurrent use with other drugs which may prolong QT_c interval may increase the risk of potentially-fatal arrhythmias. Increased toxicity and mortality has been observed in trials evaluating concurrent use of pazopanib with other chemotherapeutic agents (pemetrexed, lapatinib). Pazopanib is not approved for use in combination with other chemotherapy.

Reversible posterior leukoencephalopathy syndrome (RPLS) has been reported (rarely); may be fatal. Monitor for neurological changes or symptoms (blindness, confusion, headache, lethargy, seizure, visual or neurologic disturbances); discontinue pazopanib in patients who develop RPLS. Serious, including fatal, infections have been reported; monitor for signs and symptoms of infection. Temporarily or permanently discontinue therapy for serious infections as clinically indicated. Patients ≥65 years of age may be at higher risk of fatigue (grade 3 or 4), hypertension, and decreased appetite.

Adverse Reactions

>10%:

Cardiovascular: Hypertension (40% to 42%; grade 3: 4% to 7%), peripheral edema (14%)

Central nervous system: Fatigue (19% to 65%), headache (10% to 23%), dizziness (11%)

Dermatologic: Hair color change (38% to 39%), rash (8% to 18%), alopecia (8% to 12%), palmar-plantar erythrodysesthesia (6% to 11%), skin depigmentation (3% to 11%)

Endocrine & metabolic: Hyperglycemia (41% to 45%), hypophosphatemia (34%), hyponatremia (31%), thyroid-stimulating hormone (TSH) increased (27%), hypomagnesemia (26%), hypoglycemia (17%), hyperkalemia (16%)

Gastrointestinal: Diarrhea (52% to 59%; grade 3: 3% to 5%; grade 4: <1%), nausea (26% to 56%), weight loss (9% to 48%), anorexia (22% to 40%),

vomiting (21% to 33%), taste alteration (8% to 28%), lipase increased (4% to 27%), abdominal pain (11% to 23%), mucositis (12%), stomatitis (11%)
Hematologic: Leukopenia (37% to 44%; grade 3: ≤1%), lymphocytopenia (31% to 43%; grade 3: 4% to 10%; grade 4: <1%), thrombocytopenia (32% to 36%; grade 3: ≤3%; grade 4: ≤1%), neutropenia (33% to 34%; grade 3: 1% to 4%; grade 4: <1%)
Hepatic: AST increased (51% to 53%; grade 3: 5% to 7%; grade 4: <3%), ALT increased (46% to 53%; grade 3: 8% to 10%; grade 4: 2%), bilirubin increased (29% to 36%; grade 3: ≤3%; grade 4: <1%), albumin decreased (34%), alkaline phosphatase increased (32%)
Neuromuscular & skeletal: Musculoskeletal pain (23%), myalgia (23%), weakness (14%)
Respiratory: Dyspnea (20%), cough (17%)
Miscellaneous: Tumor pain (29%)

1% to 10%:
Cardiovascular: Chest pain (5% to 10%), left ventricular dysfunction (≤8%), venous thrombosis (≤5%), MI/ischemia (2%), QT prolongation (1% to 2%), facial edema (1%), transient ischemic event (≤1%)
Central nervous system: Insomnia (9%), dysphonia (4% to 8%), chills (5%)
Dermatologic: Dry skin (6%), nail disorder (5%)
Endocrine & metabolic: Hypothyroidism (4% to 8%)
Gastrointestinal: Dyspepsia (5% to 7%), mouth hemorrhage (3%), rectal hemorrhage (1% to 2%)
Ocular: Blurred vision (5%)
Renal: Proteinuria (1% to 9%), hematuria (4%)
Respiratory: Epistaxis (2% to 8%), pneumothorax (≤3%), hemoptysis (2%), PE (fatal; 1%)

<1%, postmarketing, and/or case reports: Cardiac dysfunction, cerebral hemorrhage, cerebrovascular event, extrapyramidal symptoms, gastrointestinal fistula, gastrointestinal perforation, HF, hepatotoxicity, hypertensive crisis, intracranial hemorrhage, ischemic stroke, nephrotic syndrome, pancreatitis, reversible posterior leukoencephalopathy syndrome (RPLS), torsade de pointes, tumor hemorrhage

Drug Interactions

Metabolism/Transport Effects Substrate of CYP1A2 (minor), CYP2C8 (minor), CYP3A4 (major), P-glycoprotein; **Note:** Assignment of Major/Minor substrate status based on clinically relevant drug interaction potential; **Inhibits** CYP2C8 (weak), CYP2D6 (weak), CYP3A4 (weak), SLCO1B1, UGT1A1

Avoid Concomitant Use

Avoid concomitant use of Pazopanib with any of the following: BCG; CYP3A4 Inducers (Strong); Grapefruit Juice; Highest Risk QTc-Prolonging Agents; Mifepristone; Natalizumab; Pimecrolimus; Tacrolimus (Topical); Vaccines (Live)

Increased Effect/Toxicity

Pazopanib may increase the levels/effects of: ARIPiprazole; Highest Risk QTc-Prolonging Agents; Leflunomide; Moderate Risk QTc-Prolonging Agents; Natalizumab; Vaccines (Live); Vitamin K Antagonists

The levels/effects of Pazopanib may be increased by: CYP3A4 Inhibitors (Moderate); CYP3A4 Inhibitors (Strong); Dasatinib; Denosumab; Grapefruit Juice; HMG-CoA Reductase Inhibitors; Ivacaftor; Lapatinib; Mifepristone; P-glycoprotein/ABCB1 Inhibitors; Pimecrolimus; QTc-Prolonging Agents

(Indeterminate Risk and Risk Modifying); Roflumilast; Tacrolimus (Topical); Trastuzumab

Decreased Effect

Pazopanib may decrease the levels/effects of: BCG; Cardiac Glycosides; Coccidioidin Skin Test; Sipuleucel-T; Vaccines (Inactivated); Vaccines (Live); Vitamin K Antagonists

The levels/effects of Pazopanib may be decreased by: CYP3A4 Inducers (Strong); Deferasirox; Echinacea; Herbs (CYP3A4 Inducers); P-glycoprotein/ABCB1 Inducers; Tocilizumab

Ethanol/Nutrition/Herb Interactions

Food: Systemic exposure of pazopanib is increased when administered with food (AUC twofold higher with a meal). Grapefruit juice may increase the levels/effects of pazopanib. Management: Maintain adequate nutrition and hydration, unless instructed to restrict fluid intake. Take on an empty stomach 1 hour before or 2 hours after a meal. Avoid grapefruit/grapefruit juice.

Herb/Nutraceutical: St John's wort may increase metabolism and decrease pazopanib concentrations. Echinacea may diminish the therapeutic effect. Management: Avoid St John's wort. Consider avoiding echinacea.

Storage/Stability Store at room temperature, 20°C to 25°C (68°F to 77°F); excursions permitted between 15°C and 30°C (59°F and 86°F).

Mechanism of Action Tyrosine kinase (multikinase) inhibitor; limits tumor growth via inhibition of angiogenesis angiogenesis by inhibiting cell surface vascular endothelial growth factor receptors (VEGFR-1, VEGFR-2, VEGFR-3), platelet-derived growth factor receptors (PDGFR-alpha and -beta), fibroblast growth factor receptor (FGFR-1 and -3), cytokine receptor (cKIT), interleukin-2 receptor inducible T-cell kinase, leukocyte-specific protein tyrosine kinase (Lck), and transmembrane glycoprotein receptor tyrosine kinase (c-Fms)

Pharmacodynamics/Kinetics

Protein binding: >99%

Metabolism: Hepatic; primarily via CYP3A4, minor metabolism via CYP1A2 and CYP2C8

Bioavailability: Rate and extent of bioavailability are increased with food and increased if tablets are crushed (do not crush tablets)

Half-life elimination: ~31 hours

Time to peak, plasma: 2-4 hours

Excretion: Feces (primarily); urine (<4%)

Dosing

Adult & Geriatric

Renal cell cancer (RCC): Oral: 800 mg once daily (Sternberg, 2010)

Soft tissue sarcoma (STS), advanced refractory: Oral: 800 mg once daily (Van Der Graaf, 2011)

Thyroid cancer, advanced differentiated (unlabeled use): Oral: 800 mg once daily until disease progression or unacceptable toxicity (Bible, 2010)

Concomitant CYP3A4 inhibitors/inducers:

CYP3A4 inhibitors: Avoid concomitant strong CYP3A4 inhibitors (may increase pazopanib concentrations). If pazopanib must be administered concomitantly with a potent enzyme inhibitor, reduce pazopanib to 400 mg once daily with careful monitoring; further dosage reductions may be needed if adverse events occur.

CYP3A4 inducers: Avoid concomitant strong CYP3A4 inducers (may decrease pazopanib concentrations); use of pazopanib is not recommended in situations where the use of a strong CYP3A4 inducer is required.

Renal Impairment No adjustment necessary (renal impairment is not likely to significantly influence pazopanib pharmacokinetics).

Hepatic Impairment

Pre-existing impairment:

Mild (bilirubin ≤1.5 times ULN or ALT >ULN): No adjustment required (Shibata, 2010)

Moderate (bilirubin >1.5-3 times ULN). Consider alternative therapy or reduce to 200 mg once daily (maximum tolerated dose in moderate hepatic impairment) (Shibata, 2010)

Severe (bilirubin >3 times ULN with any ALT level): Use is not recommended

During treatment:

Isolated ALT elevations 3-8 times ULN: Continue treatment, monitor liver function weekly until ALT returns to grade 1 or baseline.

Isolated ALT elevations >8 times ULN: Interrupt treatment until ALT returns to grade 1 or baseline. If therapy benefit is greater than the risk of hepatotoxicity, may reinitiate treatment at ≤400 mg once daily (with liver function monitored weekly for 8 weeks); permanently discontinue if ALT >3 times ULN occurs with reinitiation.

ALT >3 times ULN concurrently with bilirubin >2 times ULN: Permanently discontinue; monitor until resolution.

Gilbert's syndrome with mild indirect bilirubin elevation and ALT >3 times ULN. Refer to Isolated ALT elevations dosage recommendations.

Adjustment for Toxicity

Initial dosage reduction: Note: Prior to dose reduction, temporarily discontinue therapy if 24-hour urine protein ≥3 g or for other toxicities when clinically indicated.

RCC: Reduce to 400 mg once daily

STS: Reduce to 600 mg once daily

Further modification: *RCC, STS:* Adjust dose in 200 mg increments or decrements based on individual tolerance; maximum dose: 800 mg

Proteinuria (recurrent 24-hour urine protein ≥3 g refractory to dose reduction), hypertension (severe, persistent, and refractory to antihypertensives and dose reduction), wound dehiscence, reversible posterior leukoencephalopathy syndrome (RPLS): Discontinue treatment.

Infection, serious: Consider treatment interruption or discontinuation.

Combination Regimens

Renal cell cancer: Pazopanib (RCC Regimen) on page 1734

Soft tissue sarcoma: Pazopanib (Soft Tissue Sarcoma Regimen) on page 1734

Thyroid cancer: Pazopanib (Thyroid Cancer Regimen) on page 1734

Administration Administer on an empty stomach, 1 hour before or 2 hours after a meal. Do not crush tablet. If a dose is missed, do not take if <12 hours until the next dose.

Emetic Potential Very low (<10%)

Monitoring Parameters Monitor liver function tests at baseline and at least every 4 weeks for the first 4 months (more frequently if clinically indicated) and periodically thereafter; serum electrolytes (eg, calcium, magnesium, potassium); urinalysis (for proteinuria; baseline and periodic), 24-hour urine protein (if clinically indicated); thyroid function (TSH and T_4 at baseline and TSH every 6-8 weeks during treatment [Appleby, 2011]); blood pressure; ECG (baseline and periodic); LVEF (if at risk for cardiac dysfunction; baseline and periodic); signs/symptoms of gastrointestinal perforation or fistula, infection, heart failure, or neurological changes.

Dietary Considerations Take on an empty stomach, 1 hour before or 2 hours after a meal. Avoid grapefruit juice.

Additional Information **Hand-foot skin reaction (Appleby, 2011):** Hand-foot skin reaction (HFSR) observed with tyrosine kinase inhibitors (TKIs) is distinct from hand-foot syndrome (palmar-plantar erythrodysesthesia) associated with traditional chemotherapy agents. HFSR due to TKIs is localized with defined hyperkeratotic lesions; symptoms include burning, dysesthesia, paresthesia, or tingling of the palms/soles, and generally occur within the first 2-4 weeks of treatment. Pressure and flexor areas may develop blisters (callus-like), dry/cracked skin, edema, erythema, desquamation, or hyperkeratosis. The incidence of hand-foot skin reaction (HFSR) is lower with pazopanib (compared to other tyrosine kinase inhibitors). Examine skin at baseline (remove calluses with pedicure prior to treatment) and with each visit; apply an emollient based moisturizer twice daily during treatment. If HSFR develops, consider changing moisturizer to a urea-based product; topical steroids may be utilized for the anti-inflammatory effect; avoid excessive friction or pressure to affected areas and avoid restrictive footwear. Temporary dose reduction or treatment interruption may be necessary.

Medication Guide Available Yes

Dosage Forms Excipient information presented when available (limited, particularly for generics); consult specific product labeling.

Tablet, oral:

Votrient™: 200 mg

References

Bible KC, Suman VJ, Molina JR, et al, "Efficacy of Pazopanib in Progressive, Radioiodine-Refractory, Metastatic Differentiated Thyroid Cancers: Results of a Phase 2 Consortium Study," *Lancet Oncol*, 2010, 11(10):962-72.

Hutson TE, Davis ID, Machiels JP, et al, "Efficacy and Safety of Pazopanib in Patients With Metastatic Renal Cell Carcinoma," *J Clin Oncol*, 2010, 28(3):475-80.

Shibata S, Longmate J, Chung VM, et al, "A Phase I and Pharmacokinetic Single Agent Study of Pazopanib (P) in Patients (Pts) With Advanced Malignancies and Varying Degrees of Liver Dysfunction (LD)," *J Clin Oncol*, 2010, 28(Suppl 15):2571 [abstract 2571 from 2010 ASCO Annual Meeting].

Sleijfer S, Ray-Coquard I, Papai Z, et al, "Pazopanib, a Multikinase Angiogenesis Inhibitor, in Patients With Relapsed or Refractory Advanced Soft Tissue Sarcoma: A Phase II Study from the European Organisation for Research and Treatment of Cancer-Soft Tissue and Bone Sarcoma Group (EORTC Study 62043)," *J Clin Oncol*, 2009, 27(19):3126-32.

Sternberg CN, Davis ID, Mardiak J, et al, "Pazopanib in Locally Advanced or Metastatic Renal Cell Carcinoma: Results of a Randomized Phase III Trial," *J Clin Oncol*, 2010, 28(6):1061-8.

Sternberg CN, Szczylik C, Lee E, et al, "A Randomized, Double-Blind Phase III Study of Pazopanib in Treatment-Naive and Cytokine-Pretreated Patients With Advanced Renal Cell Carcinoma (RCC)," *J Clin Oncol*, 2009, 27(15s):5021 [abstract 5021 from 2009 ASCO Annual Meeting].

Van Der Graaf WT, Blay J, Chawla SP, et al, "PALETTE: A Randomized, Double-Blind, Phase III Trial of Pazopanib Versus Placebo in Patients (pts) With Soft-Tissue Sarcoma (STS) Whose Disease has Progressed During or Following Prior Chemotherapy – An EORTC STBSG Global Network Study (EORTC 62072)," *J Clin Oncol*, 2011, 29(Suppl 18):LBA10002 [abstract LBA10002 from 2011 ASCO Annual Meeting].

◆ **Pazopanib Hydrochloride** *see* Pazopanib *on page* 1129

◆ **PCC** *see* Factor IX Complex (Human) *on page* 575

◆ **PDX** *see* PRALAtrexate *on page* 1190

◆ **Pediaderm™ AF** *see* Nystatin (Topical) *on page* 1042

◆ **Pediaderm™ HC** *see* Hydrocortisone (Topical) *on page* 719

◆ **Pediapred®** *see* PrednisoLONE (Systemic) *on page* 1193
◆ **Pedi-Dri®** *see* Nystatin (Topical) *on page* 1042
◆ **PEG-L-asparaginase** *see* Pegaspargase *on page* 1135
◆ **PEG-ASP** *see* Pegaspargase *on page* 1135
◆ **PEG-asparaginase** *see* Pegaspargase *on page* 1135

Pegaspargase (peg AS par jase)

Related Information

Management of Chemotherapy-Induced Nausea and Vomiting *on page* 1786
Safe Handling of Hazardous Drugs *on page* 1904

Brand Names: U.S. Oncaspar®

Index Terms L-asparaginase with Polyethylene Glycol; PEG-ASP; PEG-asparaginase; PEG-L-asparaginase; PEGLA; Polyethylene Glycol-L-asparaginase

Generic Availability (U.S.) No

Pharmacologic Category Antineoplastic Agent, Miscellaneous; Enzyme

Use Treatment of acute lymphocytic leukemia (ALL); treatment of ALL with previous hypersensitivity to native L-asparaginase

Labeled Contraindications History of serious allergic reactions to pegaspargase; history of any of the following with prior L-asparaginase treatment: pancreatitis, serious hemorrhagic events, serious thrombosis

Pregnancy Risk Factor C

Lactation Excretion in breast milk unknown/not recommended

Warnings/Precautions Hazardous agent - use appropriate precautions for handling and disposal. Serious allergic reactions may occur; discontinue in patients with serious allergic reaction. Observe patients for at least 1 hour after administration; immediate treatment for hypersensitivity reactions should be available during administration. Pegaspargase is indicated for use in patients who have had hypersensitivity reactions to native L-asparaginase; however, in one study, 32% of patients with a history of allergic reaction to *E. coli* asparaginase products also experienced allergic reaction to pegaspargase.

Serious thrombotic events, including sagittal sinus thrombosis may occur; discontinue with serious thrombotic event. Pancreatitis may occur; promptly evaluate patients with abdominal pain; discontinue if pancreatitis occurs during treatment. May cause glucose intolerance; irreversible in some cases; use with caution in patients with hyperglycemia, or diabetes. Coagulopathy has been reported; monitor coagulation parameters; severe or symptomatic coagulopathy may require treatment with fresh-frozen plasma; use with caution in patients with underlying coagulopathy. Reversible hepatotoxicity (hyperbilirubinemia and liver enzyme elevation) may occur; use with caution in patients with hepatic dysfunction or concomitant hepatotoxic medications. Use cautiously in patients with previous hematologic complications from asparaginase.

Adverse Reactions

>5%:

Cardiovascular: Edema
Central nervous system: Fever, malaise
Dermatologic: Rash
Gastrointestinal: Nausea, vomiting
Hematologic: Coagulopathy (7%; grades 3/4: 2%)
Hepatic: Transaminases increased (11%; grades 3/4: 3%)

Miscellaneous: Allergic reactions (including bronchospasm, chills, dyspnea, edema, erythema, hypotension, rash, swelling, urticaria; no prior asparaginase hypersensitivity: 1% to 10%; grades 3/4: 2%; prior asparaginase hypersensitivity: 32%; grades 3/4: 8%)

1% to 5%:

Cardiovascular: Hypotension, peripheral edema, tachycardia, thrombosis (4%)

Central nervous system: Chills, CNS thrombosis (2% to 4%; grades 3/4: 3%), CNS hemorrhage (2%), headache, seizure

Dermatologic: Lip edema, urticaria

Endocrine & metabolic: Hyperglycemia (3% to 5%; grades 3/4: ≤5%), hyperuricemia, hypoglycemia, hypoproteinemia

Gastrointestinal: Abdominal pain, anorexia, diarrhea, pancreatitis (1% to 2%; grades 3/4: 2%)

Hematologic: Anticoagulant effect decreased, disseminated intravascular coagulation (DIC), fibrinogen decreased, hemolytic anemia, leukopenia, pancytopenia, thrombocytopenia, thromboplastin increased, myelosuppression

Hepatic: Liver function tests abnormal (grades 3/4: 5%), hyperbilirubinemia (grades 3/4: 2%), jaundice

Local: Injection site hypersensitivity, pain or reaction

Neuromuscular & skeletal: Arthralgia, limb pain, myalgia, paresthesia

Respiratory: Dyspnea

Miscellaneous: Anaphylactic reactions, night sweats

<1%, postmarketing, and/or case reports (limited to important or life-threatening): Abnormal renal function, alopecia, amylase increased, anemia, antithrombin III decreased, ascites, bacteremia, bone pain, bronchospasm, bruising, BUN increased, chest pain, coagulation time increased, colitis, coma, confusion, constipation, cough, creatinine increased, dizziness, DVT, emotional lability, endocarditis, epistaxis, excessive thirst, face edema, fatigue, fatty liver deposits, gastrointestinal pain, hematuria, hemorrhagic cystitis, hepatomegaly, hyperammonemia, hypertension, hypoalbuminemia, hyponatremia, lipase increased, liver failure, metabolic acidosis, mucositis, petechial rash, proteinuria, prothrombin time increased, purpura, renal failure, sagittal sinus thrombosis, sepsis, septic shock, subacute bacterial endocarditis, superficial venous thrombosis, uric acid nephropathy

Drug Interactions

Metabolism/Transport Effects None known.

Avoid Concomitant Use

Avoid concomitant use of Pegaspargase with any of the following: BCG; Natalizumab; Pimecrolimus; Tacrolimus (Topical); Vaccines (Live)

Increased Effect/Toxicity

Pegaspargase may increase the levels/effects of: Leflunomide; Natalizumab; Vaccines (Live)

The levels/effects of Pegaspargase may be increased by: Denosumab; Pimecrolimus; Roflumilast; Tacrolimus (Topical); Trastuzumab

Decreased Effect

Pegaspargase may decrease the levels/effects of: BCG; Coccidioidin Skin Test; Sipuleucel-T; Vaccines (Inactivated); Vaccines (Live)

The levels/effects of Pegaspargase may be decreased by: Echinacea; Pegloticase

Storage/Stability Refrigerate unused vials at 2°C to 8°C (36°F to 46°F); do not freeze. Do not shake; protect from light. Discard vial if previously frozen, stored at room temperature for >48 hours, excessively shaken/agitated, or if cloudy, discolored, or if precipitate is present. If not used immediately, solutions for infusion should be refrigerated at 2°C to 8°C (36°F to 46°F) and used within 48 hours (including administration time).

Reconstitution I.V.: Dilute in 100 mL NS or D_5W.

Mechanism of Action Pegaspargase is a modified version of asparaginase. Leukemic cells, especially lymphoblasts, require exogenous asparagine; normal cells can synthesize asparagine. Asparaginase contains L-asparaginase amidohydrolase type EC-2 which inhibits protein synthesis by deaminating asparagine to aspartic acid and ammonia in the plasma and extracellular fluid and therefore deprives tumor cells of the amino acid for protein synthesis. Asparaginase is cycle-specific for the G_1 phase of the cell cycle.

Pharmacodynamics/Kinetics

Onset: Asparagine depletion: I.M.: Within 4 days

Duration: Asparagine depletion: I.M.: ~21 days; I.V. (in asparaginase naive adults): 2-4 weeks

Absorption: I.M.: Slow

Distribution: I.M.: Children: 1.5 L/m^2; I.V.: Adults (asparaginase naive): 2.4 L/m^2

Metabolism: Systemically degraded

Half-life elimination: I.M.: ~5.5-6 days; unaffected by age, renal or hepatic function; half life decreased to 1.8-3.2 days in patients with previous hypersensitivity to native L-asparaginase; I.V.: Adults (asparaginase naive): 7 days

Time to peak: I.M.: 3-4 days

Excretion: Urine (trace amounts)

Dosing

Adult & Geriatric Details concerning dosing in combinations regimens should also be consulted.

Acute lymphoblastic leukemia (ALL): I.M., I.V.: 2500 units/m^2 (as part of a combination chemotherapy regimen), do not administer more frequently than every 14 days

Pediatric Details concerning dosing in combinations regimens should also be consulted.

Acute lymphoblastic leukemia: I.M., I.V.: Refer to adult dosing.

Renal Impairment Hemodialysis, peritoneal dialysis: Significant drug removal is unlikely based on physiochemical characteristics

Combination Regimens

Leukemia, acute lymphocytic: Hyper-CVAD (Leukemia, Acute Lymphocytic) on page 1881

Administration Have available appropriate agents for maintenance of an adequate airway and treatment of a hypersensitivity reaction (antihistamine, epinephrine, oxygen, I.V. corticosteroids). Be prepared to treat anaphylaxis at each administration.

I.M.: Must only be administered as a deep intramuscular injection into a large muscle. Do not exceed 2 mL per injection site; use multiple injection sites for I.M. injection volume >2 mL.

I.V.: Administer over 1-2 hours through a running I.V. infusion line; **do not administer I.V. push.**

Emetic Potential Very low (<10%)

Monitoring Parameters Vital signs during administration, CBC with differential, platelets, amylase, liver enzymes, fibrinogen, PT, PTT (coagulation parameters [baseline and periodic]), renal function tests, urine glucose, blood glucose; monitor for onset of abdominal pain; observe for allergic reaction (for 1 hour after administration)

Dosage Forms Excipient information presented when available (limited, particularly for generics); consult specific product labeling.

Injection, solution [preservative free]:

Oncaspar®: 750 units/mL (5 mL)

References

Abshire TC, Pollock BH, Billett AL, et al, "Weekly Polyethylene Glycol Conjugated L-Asparaginase Compared With Biweekly Dosing Produces Superior Induction Remission Rates in Childhood Relapsed Acute Lymphoblastic Leukemia: A Pediatric Oncology Group Study," *Blood*, 2000, 96 (5):1709-15.

Avramis VI, Sencer S, Periclou AP, et al, "A Randomized Comparison of Native *Escherichia Coli* Asparaginase and Polyethylene Glycol Conjugated Asparaginase for Treatment of Children With Newly Diagnosed Standard-Risk Acute Lymphoblastic Leukemia: A Children's Cancer Group Study," *Blood*, 2002, 99(6):1986-94.

Douer D, Yampolsky H, Cohen LJ, et al, "Pharmacodynamics and Safety of Intravenous Pegaspargase During Remission Induction in Adults Aged 55 Years or Younger With Newly Diagnosed Acute Lymphoblastic Leukemia," *Blood*, 2007, 109(7):2744-50.

Pegfilgrastim (peg fil GRA stim)

Brand Names: U.S. Neulasta®

Brand Names: Canada Neulasta®

Index Terms G-CSF (PEG Conjugate); Granulocyte Colony Stimulating Factor (PEG Conjugate); Pegylated G-CSF; SD/01

Generic Availability (U.S.) No

Pharmacologic Category Colony Stimulating Factor

Use To decrease the incidence of infection, by stimulation of granulocyte production, in patients with nonmyeloid malignancies receiving myelosuppressive therapy associated with a significant risk of febrile neutropenia

Labeled Contraindications Hypersensitivity to pegfilgrastim, filgrastim, or any component of the formulation

Pregnancy Risk Factor C

Lactation Excretion in breast milk unknown/use caution

Warnings/Precautions Do not use pegfilgrastim in the period 14 days before to 24 hours after administration of cytotoxic chemotherapy because of the potential sensitivity of rapidly dividing myeloid cells to cytotoxic chemotherapy. Benefit has not been demonstrated with regimens under a two-week duration. Administration on the same day as chemotherapy is not recommended (NCCN Myeloid Growth Factor Guidelines, v.1.2011). Pegfilgrastim can potentially act as a growth factor for any tumor type, particularly myeloid malignancies. Caution should be exercised in the usage of pegfilgrastim in any malignancy with myeloid characteristics. Tumors of nonhematopoietic origin may have surface receptors for pegfilgrastim. Pegfilgrastim has not been evaluated with patients receiving radiation therapy, or with chemotherapy associated with delayed myelosuppression (nitrosoureas, mitomycin). Safety and efficacy have not been evaluated for peripheral blood progenitor cell (PBPC) mobilization.

Allergic-type reactions (anaphylaxis, angioedema, erythema, skin rash, urticaria) have occurred primarily with the initial dose and may recur (possibly delayed) after discontinuation; close follow up for several days and permanent discontinuation are recommended for severe reactions. Rare cases of splenic rupture have been reported; patients must be instructed to report left upper quadrant pain or shoulder tip pain. Acute respiratory distress syndrome (ARDS) has been associated with use; evaluate patients with pulmonary symptoms such as fever, lung infiltrates, or respiratory distress; discontinue or withhold pegfilgrastim if ARDS occurs. May precipitate sickle cell crises in patients with sickle cell disease; carefully evaluate potential risks and benefits. The packaging (needle cover) contains latex. The 6 mg fixed dose should not be used in infants, children, and adolescents weighing <45 kg.

Adverse Reactions

>10%:

Cardiovascular: Peripheral edema (12%)

Central nervous system: Headache (16%)

Gastrointestinal: Vomiting (13%)

Neuromuscular & skeletal: Bone pain (31% to 57%), myalgia (21%), arthralgia (16%), weakness (13%)

1% to 10%:

Gastrointestinal: Constipation (10%)

Miscellaneous: Antibody formation (1% to 6%)

<1%, postmarketing, and/or case reports: Acute respiratory distress syndrome (ARDS), allergic reaction, anaphylaxis, cutaneous vasculitis, erythema, fever, flushing, hyperleukocytosis, hypoxia, injection site reactions (erythema, induration, pain), leukocytosis, rash, sickle cell crisis, splenic rupture, Sweet's syndrome (acute febrile dermatosis), urticaria. Cytopenias resulting from an antibody response to exogenous growth factors have been reported on rare occasions in patients treated with other recombinant growth factors.

Drug Interactions

Metabolism/Transport Effects None known.

Avoid Concomitant Use There are no known interactions where it is recommended to avoid concomitant use.

Increased Effect/Toxicity There are no known significant interactions involving an increase in effect.

Decreased Effect

The levels/effects of Pegfilgrastim may be decreased by: Pegloticase

Storage/Stability Store under refrigeration 2°C to 8°C (36°F to 46°F); do not freeze. If inadvertently frozen, allow to thaw in refrigerator; discard if frozen more than one time. Protect from light. Do not shake. Allow to reach room temperature prior to injection. May be kept at room temperature for up to 48 hours.

Mechanism of Action Stimulates the production, maturation, and activation of neutrophils, pegfilgrastim activates neutrophils to increase both their migration and cytotoxicity. Pegfilgrastim has a prolonged duration of effect relative to filgrastim and a reduced renal clearance.

Pharmacodynamics/Kinetics Half-life elimination: SubQ: **Adults:** 15-80 hours; Children (100 mcg/kg dose): ~20-30 hours (range: up to 68 hours)

Dosing

Adult & Geriatric Do not administer in the period between 14 days before and 24 hours after administration of cytotoxic chemotherapy. According to the NCCN guidelines, efficacy has been demonstrated with every-2-week chemotherapy regimens, however, benefit has not been demonstrated with regimens under a two-week duration (NCCN Myeloid Growth Factor Guidelines, v.1.2011)

Prevention of chemotherapy-induced neutropenia: SubQ: 6 mg once per chemotherapy cycle, beginning 24-72 hours after completion of chemotherapy

Pediatric Note: Do not administer in the period between 14 days before and 24 hours after administration of cytotoxic chemotherapy.

Prevention of chemotherapy-induced neutropenia:

Children (unlabeled dose): SubQ: 100 mcg/kg (maximum dose: 6 mg) once per chemotherapy cycle, beginning 24-72 hours after completion of chemotherapy

Adolescents >45 kg: Refer to adult dosing.

Renal Impairment No adjustment necessary.

Combination Regimens

Leukemia, chronic lymphocytic: Cyclophosphamide-Fludarabine-Alemtuzumab-Rituximab (CLL) on page 1601

Administration Administer subcutaneously. Do not use 6 mg fixed dose in infants, children, or adolescents <45 kg. Engage/activate needle guard following use to prevent accidental needlesticks.

Monitoring Parameters Complete blood count (with differential) and platelet count should be obtained prior to chemotherapy. Leukocytosis (white blood cell counts 100,000/mm^3) has been observed in <1% of patients receiving pegfilgrastim. Monitor platelets and hematocrit regularly. Evaluate fever, pulmonary infiltrates, and respiratory distress; evaluate for left upper abdominal pain, shoulder tip pain, or splenomegaly. Monitor for sickle cell crisis (in patients with sickle cell anemia).

Test Interactions May interfere with bone imaging studies; increased hematopoietic activity of the bone marrow may appear as transient positive bone imaging changes

Dosage Forms Excipient information presented when available (limited, particularly for generics); consult specific product labeling.

Injection, solution [preservative free]:

Neulasta®: 6 mg/0.6 mL (0.6 mL) [contains natural rubber/natural latex in packaging]

References

Andre N, Milano E, Rome A, et al, "Safety of Pegfilgrastim in Children", *Ann Pharmacother*, 2008, 42(2):290.

Fox E, Jayaprakash N, Widemann BC, et al, "Randomized Trial and Pharmacokinetic Study of Pegfilgrastim vs. Filgrastim in Children and Young Adults With Newly Diagnosed Sarcoma Treated With Dose Intensive Chemotherapy," *J Clin Oncol*, 2006, 24(18S):9020 [abstract 9020 from 2006 ASCO Annual Meeting Proceedings, Part I].

Holmes FA, O'Shaughnessy JA, Vukelja S, et al, "Blinded, Randomized, Multicenter Study to Evaluate Single Administration Pegfilgrastim Once Per Cycle Versus Daily Filgrastim as an Adjunct to Chemotherapy in Patients With High-Risk Stage II or Stage III/IV Breast Cancer," *J Clin Oncol*, 2002, 20(3): 727-31.

National Comprehensive Cancer Network® (NCCN), "Clinical Practice Guidelines in Oncology™: Myeloid Growth Factors," Version 1.2012. Available at http://www.nccn.org/professionals/physician_gls/PDF/myeloid_growth.pdf

Smith TJ, Khatcheressian J, Lyman GH, et al, "2006 Update of Recommendations for the Use of White Blood Cell Growth Factors: An Evidence-Based Clinical Practice Guideline," *J Clin Oncol*, 2006, 24(19):3187-205.

◆ **PEG-IFN Alfa-2b** *see* Peginterferon Alfa-2b *on page 1140*

Peginterferon Alfa-2b (peg in ter FEER on AL fa too bee)

Related Information

Management of Chemotherapy-Induced Nausea and Vomiting *on page 1786*

Brand Names: U.S. PegIntron®; PegIntron™ Redipen®; Sylatron™

Brand Names: Canada PegIntron®

Index Terms Interferon Alfa-2b (PEG Conjugate); PEG-IFN Alfa-2b; Pegylated Interferon Alfa-2b; Polyethylene Glycol Interferon Alfa-2b

Generic Availability (U.S.) No

Pharmacologic Category Interferon

Use

PegIntron®: Treatment of chronic hepatitis C (CHC; in combination with ribavirin) in patients who have compensated liver disease; treatment of chronic hepatitis C (as monotherapy) in adult patients with compensated liver disease who have never received alfa interferons and are intolerant to ribavirin or have contraindications to ribavirin. **Note:** Combination therapy with ribavirin provides better response rates than peginterferon monotherapy

Sylatron™: Adjuvant treatment of melanoma (with microscopic or gross nodal involvement within 84 days of definitive surgical resection, including complete lymphadenectomy)

Labeled Contraindications Hypersensitivity (including urticaria, angioedema, bronchoconstriction, anaphylaxis, Stevens Johnson syndrome and toxic epidermal necrolysis) to peginterferon alfa-2b, interferon alfa-2b, other alfa interferons, or any component of the formulation; autoimmune hepatitis; decompensated liver disease (Child-Pugh score >6, classes B and C)

Combination therapy with peginterferon alfa-2b and ribavirin is also contraindicated in pregnancy, women who may become pregnant, males with pregnant partners; hemoglobinopathies (eg, thalassemia major, sickle-cell anemia); renal dysfunction (Cl_{cr} <50 mL/minute)

Pregnancy Risk Factor C / X in combination with ribavirin

Lactation Excretion in breast milk unknown/not recommended

Warnings/Precautions **[U.S. Boxed Warnings]: May cause or aggravate severe depression or other neuropsychiatric adverse events (including suicide and suicidal ideation) in patients with and without a history of psychiatric disorder; monitor closely with clinical evaluations (periodic); discontinue treatment with worsening or persistently severe signs/symptoms of neuropsychiatric disorders (eg, depression, encephalopathy, psychosis). Many cases resolve upon discontinuation, although some cases may persist. May cause or aggravate fatal or life-threatening autoimmune disorders, infectious disorders, ischemic disorders; monitor closely with clinical evaluations (periodic); discontinue treatment in patients with worsening or persistently severe signs/symptoms of infectious disorders; may resolve with discontinuation.** May also cause hemorrhagic cerebrovascular events.

Neuropsychiatric disorders: Neuropsychiatric effects may occur in patients with and without a history of psychiatric disorder; addiction relapse, aggression, depression, homicidal ideation and suicidal behavior/ideation have been observed with peginterferon alfa-2b; bipolar disorder, encephalopathy, hallucinations, mania, and psychosis have been observed with other alfa interferons. Onset may be delayed (up to 6 months after discontinuation). Higher doses may be associated with the development of encephalopathy (higher risk in elderly patients). Use with caution in patients with a history of psychiatric disorders, including depression or substance abuse history. New or exacerbated neuropsychiatric or substance abuse disorders are best managed with early intervention. Drug screening and periodic health evaluation (including monitoring of psychiatric symptoms) is recommended if initiating treatment in patients with coexisting psychiatric condition or substance abuse disorders. Monitor all patients for evidence of depression and other psychiatric symptoms; patients being treated for melanoma should be monitored for depression and psychiatric symptoms every 3 weeks during the first 8 weeks of treatment and every 6 months thereafter; permanently discontinue treatment if psychiatric symptoms persist, worsen or if suicidal behavior develops. Patients should continue to be monitored for 6 months after completion of therapy.

Bone marrow suppression: Causes bone marrow suppression, including potentially severe cytopenias; alfa interferons may (rarely) cause aplastic anemia. Use with caution in patients who are chronically immunosuppressed, with low peripheral blood counts or myelosuppression, including concurrent use of myelosuppressive therapy. Dosage modification may be necessary for hematologic toxicity. Combination therapy with ribavirin may potentiate the neutropenic effects of alfa interferons. When used in combination with ribavirin, an increased incidence of anemia was observed when using ribavirin weight-based dosing, as compared to flat-dose ribavirin.

Hepatic disease: Use is contraindicated in patients with hepatic decompensation or autoimmune hepatitis. Discontinue treatment immediately with hepatic decompensation (Child Pugh score >6) or evidence of severe hepatic injury. Patients with chronic hepatitis C (CHC) with cirrhosis receiving peginterferon alfa-2b are at risk for hepatic decompensation. CHC patients coinfected with human immunodeficiency virus (HIV) are at increased risk for hepatic decompensation when receiving highly active antiretroviral therapy (HAART); monitor closely. A transient increase in ALT (2-5 times above baseline) which is not associated with deterioration of liver function may occur with peginterferon alfa-2b use (for the treatment of chronic hepatitis C); therapy generally may continue with monitoring.

Gastrointestinal disorders: Pancreatitis (including fatal cases) has been observed with alfa interferon therapy; discontinue therapy if known or suspected pancreatitis develops. Ulcerative or hemorrhagic/ischemic colitis has been observed with alfa interferons (within 12 weeks of initiation); withhold treatment for suspected pancreatitis; discontinue therapy for known pancreatitis. Ulcerative or hemorrhagic/ischemic colitis has been observed with alfa interferons; discontinue therapy if signs of colitis (abdominal pain, bloody diarrhea, fever) develop; symptoms typically resolve within 1-3 weeks.

Autoimmune disorders: Thyroiditis, thrombotic thrombocytopenic purpura, idiopathic thrombocytopenic purpura, rheumatoid arthritis, interstitial nephritis, systemic lupus erythematosus, and psoriasis have been reported with therapy; use with caution in patients with autoimmune disorders.

Cardiovascular disease: Use with caution in patients with cardiovascular disease or a history of cardiovascular disease; hypotension, arrhythmia, bundle branch block, tachycardia, cardiomyopathy, angina pectoris and MI have been observed with treatment. Patients with pre-existing cardiac abnormalities should have baseline ECGs prior to combination treatment with ribavirin; closely monitor patients with a history of MI or arrhythmia. Patients with a history of significant or unstable cardiac disease should not receive combination treatment with ribavirin. Discontinue treatment (permanently) for new-onset ventricular arrhythmia or cardiovascular decompensation.

Endocrine disorders: Diabetes mellitus (including new-onset type I diabetes), hyperglycemia, and thyroid disorders have been reported; discontinue peginterferon alfa-2b if cannot be effectively managed with medication. Use caution in patients with a history of diabetes mellitus, particularly if prone to DKA. Use with caution in patients with thyroid disorders; may cause or aggravate hyper- or hypothyroidism.

Pulmonary disease: May cause or aggravate dyspnea, pulmonary infiltrates, pneumonia, bronchiolitis obliterans, interstitial pneumonitis, pulmonary hypertension, and sarcoidosis which may result in respiratory failure; may recur upon rechallenge with treatment; monitor closely. Use with caution in patients with existing pulmonary disease (eg, chronic obstructive pulmonary disease). Withhold combination therapy with ribavirin for development of pulmonary infiltrate or pulmonary function impairment.

Ophthalmic disorders: Ophthalmologic disorders (including decreased visual acuity, blindness, macular edema, retinal hemorrhages, optic neuritis, papilledema, cotton wool spots, retinal detachment [serous], and retinal artery or vein thrombosis) have occurred with peginterferon alfa-2b and/or with other alfa interferons. Prior to start of therapy, ophthalmic exams are recommended for all patients; patients with diabetic or hypertensive retinopathy should have periodic ophthalmic exams during treatment; a complete eye exam should be done promptly in patients who develop ocular symptoms. Permanently discontinue treatment with new or worsening ophthalmic disorder.

[U.S. Boxed Warning]: Combination treatment with ribavirin may cause birth defects and/or fetal mortality (avoid pregnancy in females and female partners of male patients); hemolytic anemia (which may worsen cardiac disease), genotoxicity, mutagenicity, and may possibly be carcinogenic. Interferon therapy is commonly associated with flu-like symptoms, including fever; rule out other causes/infection with persistent or high fever. Acute hypersensitivity reactions (eg, urticaria, angioedema, bronchoconstriction, anaphylaxis) and cutaneous reactions (eg, Stevens-Johnson syndrome, toxic epidermal necrolysis) have been reported (rarely) with alfa interferons; prompt discontinuation is recommended; transient rashes do not require interruption of therapy. Hypertriglyceridemia has been reported (may result in pancreatitis); periodically monitor and manage with appropriate treatment; consider discontinuing peginterferon if persistent and severe (triglycerides >1000 mg/dL), particularly if combined with symptoms of pancreatitis. Interferons are commonly associated with flu-like symptoms. Use with caution in patients with debilitating conditions. Use with caution in patients with renal impairment (Cl_{cr} <50 mL/minute); monitor closely for signs of interferon toxicity. For the treatment of chronic hepatitis C, dosage adjustments are recommended with monotherapy in patients with moderate-to-severe impairment; do not use combination therapy with ribavirin in adult patients renal dysfunction (Cl_{cr} <50 mL/minute); discontinue if serum creatinine >2 mg/dL in children. Has not been studied in melanoma patients with renal impairment. Serum creatinine increases have been reported in patients with renal insufficiency. Use with caution in the elderly; the potential adverse effects (eg, neuropsychiatric events, cardiac events, systemic effects) may be more pronounced. Encephalopathy has also been observed in primarily elderly patients treated with higher doses of peginterferon alfa-2b. For the treatment of hepatitis, elderly patients generally do not respond to interferon treatment as well as younger patients. When used in combination with ribavirin, closely monitor adults >50 years of age for the development of anemia. Dental/periodontal disorders have been reported with combination therapy; dry mouth may affect teeth and mucous membranes; instruct patients to brush teeth twice daily; encourage regular dental exams; rinse mouth thoroughly after vomiting.

Combination therapy with ribavirin is preferred over monotherapy for the treatment of chronic hepatitis C. Safety and efficacy have not been established in patients who have received organ transplants or are coinfected with HIV or hepatitis B. Patients with significant bridging fibrosis or cirrhosis, genotype 1 infection or who have not responded to prior therapy, including previous pegylated interferon treatment are less likely to benefit from combination therapy with peginterferon alfa-2b and ribavirin. Growth velocity (height and weight) was decreased in children on combination treatment with ribavirin, particularly during the first 6 months of treatment. **[U.S. Boxed Warning]: Combination therapy with ribavirin is contraindicated in pregnancy.** Due to differences in dosage, patients should not change brands of interferon.

Adverse Reactions Note: Percentages reported for adults receiving monotherapy unless noted:

>10%:

Central nervous system: Fatigue (52% to 94%), fever (22% to 75%), headache (56% to 70%), chills (≤63%), depression (29% to 59%; may be severe), dizziness (12% to 35%), anxiety/emotional liability/irritability (28%), insomnia (23%), olfactory nerve disorder (≤23%)

Dermatologic: Rash (6% to 36%), alopecia (22% to 34%), pruritus (12%), dry skin (11%)

Gastrointestinal: Anorexia (20% to 69%), nausea (26% to 64%), taste perversion (≤38%), diarrhea (18% to 37%), vomiting (7% to 26%), abdominal pain (8% to 15%), weight loss (11%)

Hematologic: Neutropenia (6% to 70%; grade 4: 1%), thrombocytopenia (7% to 20%; grades 3/4: <4%), anemia (6%; in combination with ribavirin: 12% to 47%)

Hepatic: ALT/AST increased (10% to 77%), alkaline phosphatase increased (≤23%)

Local: Injection site inflammation/reaction (23% to 62%)

Neuromuscular & skeletal: Myalgia (54% to 68%), weakness (52%), arthralgia (23% to 51%), musculoskeletal pain (28%), rigors (23%), paresthesia (21%)

Miscellaneous: Viral infection (11%)

1% to 10%:

Cardiovascular: Chest pain (6%), flushing (6%), bundle branch block (4%), myocardial infarction (4%), supraventricular arrhythmia (4%), ventricular tachycardia (4%)

Central nervous system: Concentration impaired (10%), malaise (7%), nervousness (4%), agitation (2%), suicidal behavior (ideation/attempt/suicide ≤2%)

Endocrine & metabolic: Hypothyroidism (5%), menstrual disorder (4%), hyperthyroidism (3%)

Gastrointestinal: Dyspepsia (6%), xerostomia (6%), constipation (1%)

Hepatic: GGT increased (8%), hepatomegaly (6%)

Local: Injection site pain (2% to 3%)

Ocular: Conjunctivitis (4%), blurred vision (2%)

Renal: Proteinuria (≤7%)

Respiratory: Pharyngitis (10%), cough (5% to 8%), sinusitis (7%), dyspnea (4% to 6%), rhinitis (2%)

Miscellaneous: Diaphoresis (6%), neutralizing antibodies (2%)

<1%, postmarketing, and/or case reports: Addiction (drug) relapse, aggressive behavior, anaphylaxis, angina, angioedema, aphthous stomatitis, aplastic anemia, arrhythmia, autoimmune thrombocytopenia (with or without purpura), bacterial infection, bipolar disorders, blindness, bronchiolitis obliterans, bronchoconstriction, cardiac arrest, cardiomyopathy, cellulitis, colitis, cotton wool spots, cytopenia, dehydration, diabetes mellitus, diabetic ketoacidosis, drug

overdose, emphysema, encephalopathy, erythema multiforme, fungal infection, gastroenteritis, gout, hallucinations, hearing impairment/loss, hemorrhagic colitis, homicidal ideation, hyperglycemia, hyper-/hypotension, hypersensitivity reactions, hypertriglyceridemia, idiopathic thrombocytopenic purpura, injection site necrosis, interstitial nephritis, interstitial pneumonitis, ischemic colitis, leukopenia, loss of consciousness, lupus-like syndrome, macular edema, mania, memory loss, migraine, myositis, nerve palsy (facial/oculomotor), optic neuritis, palpitation, pancreatitis, papilledema, pericardial effusion, peripheral neuropathy, phototoxicity, pleural effusion, pneumonia, psoriasis, psychosis, pulmonary hypertension, pulmonary infiltrates, pure red cell aplasia, renal failure, renal insufficiency, retinal artery or vein thrombosis, retinal detachment (serous), retinal hemorrhage, retinal ischemia, retinopathy, rhabdomyolysis, rheumatoid arthritis, sarcoidosis, seizure, sepsis, serum creatinine increased, Stevens-Johnson syndrome, stroke, systemic lupus erythematosus, tachycardia, thrombotic thrombocytopenic purpura, thyroiditis, toxic epidermal necrolysis, transient ischemic attack, ulcerative colitis, urticaria, vasculitis, vertigo, vision decrease/loss, visual acuity decreased, Vogt-Koyanagi-Harada syndrome

Drug Interactions

Metabolism/Transport Effects Inhibits CYP1A2 (weak)

Avoid Concomitant Use

Avoid concomitant use of Peginterferon Alfa-2b with any of the following: CloZAPine; Telbivudine

Increased Effect/Toxicity

Peginterferon Alfa-2b may increase the levels/effects of: Aldesleukin; CloZAPine; Methadone; Ribavirin; Telbivudine; Theophylline Derivatives; Zidovudine

Decreased Effect

Peginterferon Alfa-2b may decrease the levels/effects of: CYP2C9 Substrates; CYP2D6 Substrates; FLUoxetine

The levels/effects of Peginterferon Alfa-2b may be decreased by: Pegloticase

Ethanol/Nutrition/Herb Interactions Ethanol: Avoid use in patients with hepatitis C virus.

Storage/Stability Prior to reconstitution, store Redipen® at 2°C to 8°C (36°F to 46°F). Store intact vials at 25°C (77°F); excursions permitted to 15°C to 30°C (59°F to 86°F). Do not freeze. Once reconstituted each product should be used immediately or may be stored for ≤24 hours at 2°C to 8°C (36°F to 46°F); do not freeze. Do not shake. Keep away from heat. Products do not contain preservative (single use; do not reuse).

Reconstitution

Redipen®: Hold cartridge upright and press the two halves together until there is a "click". Gently invert to mix; do not shake; do not reuse (single use).

PegIntron® (vial): Add 0.7 mL sterile water for injection, USP (supplied single-use diluent) to the vial. Gently swirl. Do not re-enter vial after dose removed.

Sylatron™ (vial): Add 0.7 mL sterile water for injection and swirl gently (do not withdraw more than 0.5 mL), resulting in the following concentrations:

296 mcg vial: 40 mcg/0.1 mL

444 mcg vial: 60 mcg/0.1 mL

888 mcg vial: 120 mcg/0.1 mL

Mechanism of Action Alpha interferons are a family of proteins, produced by nucleated cells, that have antiviral, antiproliferative, and immune-regulating activity. There are 16 known subtypes of alpha interferons. Interferons interact with cells through high affinity cell surface receptors. Following activation, multiple effects can be detected including induction of gene transcription. Inhibits cellular growth, alters the state of cellular differentiation, interferes with oncogene expression, alters cell surface antigen expression, increases phagocytic activity of macrophages, and augments cytotoxicity of lymphocytes for target cells.

Pharmacodynamics/Kinetics

Bioavailability: Increases with chronic dosing

Half-life elimination: CHC: ~40 hours (range: 22-60 hours); Melanoma: ~43-51 hours

Time to peak: CHC: 15-44 hours

Excretion: Urine (~30%)

Dosing

Adult & Geriatric

Melanoma: SubQ: 6 mcg/kg/week for 8 doses, followed by 3 mcg/kg/week for up to 5 years. **Note:** Premedicate with acetaminophen (500-1000 mg orally) 30 minutes prior to the first dose and as needed for subsequent doses thereafter.

Chronic hepatitis C (CHC): SubQ: Administer dose once weekly; **Note:** Discontinue after 12 weeks in patients with HCV (genotype 1) if HCV RNA does not decrease by at least 2 log (compared to pretreatment) or if detectable HCV RNA present at 24. Discontinuation is also recommended in patients who previously failed therapy (regardless of genotype) if detectable HCV RNA present at 12 or 24 weeks.

Monotherapy (duration of treatment is 1 year): Initial dose (based on average weekly dose of 1 mcg/kg):

≤45 kg: 40 mcg once weekly
46-56 kg: 50 mcg once weekly
57-72 kg: 64 mcg once weekly
73-88 kg: 80 mcg once weekly
89-106 kg: 96 mcg once weekly
107-136 kg: 120 mcg once weekly
137-160 kg: 150 mcg once weekly

Combination therapy with ribavirin(treatment duration is 48 weeks for genotype 1, 24 weeks for genotypes 2 and 3, or 48 weeks for patients who previously failed therapy [regardless of genotype]): Initial dose (based on an average weekly dose of 1.5 mcg/kg):

<40 kg: 50 mcg once weekly (with ribavirin 800 mg/day)
40-50 kg: 64 mcg once weekly (with ribavirin 800 mg/day)
51-60 kg: 80 mcg once weekly (with ribavirin 800 mg/day)
61-65 kg: 96 mcg once weekly (with ribavirin 800 mg/day)
66-75 kg: 96 mcg once weekly (with ribavirin 1000 mg/day)
76-80 kg: 120 mcg once weekly (with ribavirin 1000 mg/day)
81-85 kg: 120 mcg once weekly (with ribavirin 1200 mg/day)
86-105 kg: 150 mcg once weekly (with ribavirin 1200 mg/day)
>105 kg: 1.5 mcg/kg once weekly (with ribavirin 1400 mg/day)

Note: *American Association for the Study of Liver Diseases (AASLD) guidelines recommendation:* Adults with chronic HCV infection: Treatment of choice: Ribavirin plus **peginterferon**; clinical condition and ability of patient to tolerate therapy should be evaluated to determine length and/or likely benefit of therapy. Recommended treatment duration (AASLD guidelines; Ghany, 2009): Genotypes 1,4: 48 weeks; Genotypes 2,3: 24 weeks; Coinfection with HIV: 48 weeks.

Pediatric Chronic hepatitis C (CHC):

Manufacturer labeling: Children ≥3 years: SubQ: Combination therapy with ribavirin: 60 mcg/m^2 once weekly; **Note:** Children who reach their 18th birthday during treatment should remain on the pediatric regimen. Treatment duration is 48 weeks for genotype 1, 24 weeks for genotypes 2 and 3. Discontinue combination therapy in patients with HCV (genotype 1) at 12 weeks if HCV-RNA does not decrease by at least 2 log (compared to pretreatment) or if detectable HCV-RNA present at 24 weeks.

American Association for the Study of Liver Diseases (AASLD) guideline recommendations (Ghany, 2009): Children 2-17 years: SubQ: Treatment of choice: Peginterferon alfa-2b 60 mcg/m^2 once weekly in combination with oral ribavirin 15 mg/kg/day for 48 weeks

Renal Impairment Chronic hepatitis C:

Peginterferon alfa-2b monotherapy:

Cl_{cr} 30-50 mL/minute: Reduce dose by 25%

Cl_{cr} 10-29 mL/minute: Reduce dose by 50%

Hemodialysis: Reduce dose by 50%

Discontinue use if renal function declines during treatment.

Peginterferon alfa-2b combination with ribavirin:

Children: Serum creatinine >2 mg/dL: Discontinue treatment.

Adults: Cl_{cr} <50 mL/minute: Combination therapy with ribavirin is not recommended.

Hepatic Impairment

Decompensated liver disease or autoimmune hepatitis: Use is contraindicated.

Hepatic decompensation or severe hepatic injury during treatment (Child-Pugh score >6 [class B or C]): Discontinue immediately.

Adjustment for Toxicity

Melanoma:

Discontinue for any of the following: Persistent or worsening severe neuropsychiatric disorders (depression, psychosis, encephalopathy), grade 4 nonhematologic toxicity, new or worsening retinopathy, new-onset ventricular arrhythmia or cardiovascular decompensation, evidence of hepatic injury (severe) or hepatic decompensation (Child-Pugh score >6 [Class B or C]), development of hyper- or hypothyroidism or diabetes that cannot be effectively managed with medication, or inability to tolerate a dose of 1 mcg/kg/week

Temporarily withhold for any of the following: ANC <500/mm^3, platelets <50,000/mm^3, ECOG performance status (PS) ≥2, nonhematologic toxicity ≥ grade 3

May reinitiate at a reduced dose once ANC ≥500/mm^3, platelets ≥50,000/mm^3, ECOG PS at 0-1, and nonhematologic toxicity completely resolved or improved to grade 1.

Reduced dose schedule, Weeks 1-8:

First dose reduction (if prior dose 6 mcg/kg/week): 3 mcg/kg/week

Second dose reduction (if prior dose 3 mcg/kg/week): 2 mcg/kg/week

Third dose reduction (if prior dose 2 mcg/kg/week): 1 mcg/kg/week

Discontinue permanently if unable to tolerate 1 mcg/kg/week

Reduced dose schedule, Weeks 9-260:

First dose reduction (if prior dose 3 mcg/kg/week): 2 mcg/kg/week

Second dose reduction (if prior dose 2 mcg/kg/week): 1 mcg/kg/week

Discontinue permanently if unable to tolerate 1 mcg/kg/week

Chronic hepatitis C: **Dosage adjustment for depression (severity based upon DSM-IV criteria):**

Mild depression: No dosage adjustment required; evaluate once weekly by visit/phone call. If depression remains stable, continue weekly visits. If depression improves, resume normal visit schedule. For worsening depression, see "Moderate depression" or "Severe depression" below.

Moderate depression: **Note:** Evaluate once weekly (visit or phone) with an office visit at least every other week. If depression remains stable, consider psychiatric evaluation and continue with reduced dosing. If symptoms improve and remain stable for 4 weeks, resume normal visit schedule; continue reduced dosing or return to normal dose. For worsening depression, see "Severe depression" below.

Children: Decrease peginterferon alfa-2b dose to 40 mcg/m^2/week, may further decrease to 20 mcg/m^2/week if needed

Adults:

Peginterferon alfa-2b monotherapy: Refer to adult weight-based dosage reduction with monotherapy for depression below

Peginterferon alfa-2b combination therapy: Refer to adult weight-based dosage reduction with combination therapy for depression below

Severe depression: Discontinue peginterferon alfa-2b and ribavirin permanently. Obtain immediate psychiatric consultation. Utilize followup psychiatric therapy as needed.

Chronic hepatitis C: **Dosage adjustment in hematologic toxicity:**

Children:

Hemoglobin decrease ≥2 g/dL in any 4-week period in patients with preexisting cardiac disease: Monitor and evaluate weekly

Hemoglobin <10 g/dL: Decrease ribavirin dose to 12 mg/kg/day; may further reduce to 8 mg/kg/day

WBC <1500/mm^3, neutrophils <750/mm^3, or platelets <70,000/mm^3: Reduce peginterferon alfa-2b dose to 40 mcg/m^2/week; may further reduce to 20 mcg/m^2/week

Hemoglobin <8.5 g/dL, WBC <1000/mm^3, neutrophils <500/mm^3, or platelets <50,000/mm^3: Permanently discontinue peginterferon alfa-2b and ribavirin

Adults:

Hemoglobin decrease >2 g/dL in any 4-week period and stable cardiac disease: Decrease peginterferon alfa-2b dose by 50%; decrease ribavirin dose by 200 mg/day. Hemoglobin <12 g/dL after dose reductions: Permanently discontinue both peginterferon alfa-2b and ribavirin

Hemoglobin <10 g/dL in patients with cardiac disease: Reduce peginterferon alfa-2b dose by 50%; decrease ribavirin dose by 200 mg/day (patients receiving 1400 mg/day should decrease dose by 400 mg/day [ie, first dose reduction to 1000 mg/day]); may further reduce ribavirin dose by additional 200 mg/day if needed

WBC <1500/mm^3, neutrophils <750/mm^3, or platelets <50,000/mm^3:

Peginterferon alfa-2b monotherapy: Refer to adult weight-based dosage reduction monotherapy for hematologic toxicity below

Peginterferon alfa-2b combination therapy: Refer to adult weight-based dosage reduction with combination therapy for hematologic toxicity below

Hemoglobin <8.5 g/dL, WBC <1000/mm^3, neutrophils <500/mm^3, or platelets <25,000/mm^3: Permanently discontinue peginterferon alfa-2b and ribavirin

Chronic hepatitis C: **Adult weight-based dosage reduction for depression or hematologic toxicity:**

Peginterferon alfa-2b monotherapy: Reduce to average weekly dose of 0.5 mcg/kg as follows:

≤45 kg: 20 mcg once weekly
46-56 kg: 25 mcg once weekly
57-72 kg: 30 mcg once weekly
73-88 kg: 40 mcg once weekly
89-106 kg: 50 mcg once weekly
107-136 kg: 64 mcg once weekly
≥137 kg: 80 mcg once weekly

Peginterferon alfa-2b combination therapy: Initially reduce to average weekly dose of 1 mcg/kg; may further reduce to average weekly dose of 0.5 mcg/kg if needed as follows:

<40 kg: 35 mcg once weekly; may further reduce to 20 mcg once weekly if needed
40-50 kg: 45 mcg once weekly; may further reduce to 25 mcg once weekly if needed
51-60 kg: 50 mcg once weekly; may further reduce to 30 mcg once weekly if needed
61-75 kg: 64 mcg once weekly; may further reduce to 35 mcg once weekly if needed
76-85 kg: 80 mcg once weekly; may further reduce to 45 mcg once weekly if needed
86-104 kg: 96 mcg once weekly; may further reduce to 50 mcg once weekly if needed
105-125 kg: 108 mcg once weekly; may further reduce to 64 mcg once weekly if needed
>125 kg: 135 mcg once weekly; may further reduce to 72 mcg once weekly if needed

Administration For SubQ administration; rotate injection site; thigh, outer surface of upper arm, and abdomen are preferred injection sites; do not inject near navel or waistline; patients who are thin should only use thigh or upper arm. Do not inject into bruised, infected, irritated, red, or scarred skin. The weekly dose may be administered at bedtime to reduce flu-like symptoms. For the treatment of CHC, the administration volume depends on the patient's weight and the peginterferon concentration used.

Emetic Potential Very low (<10%)

Monitoring Parameters Baseline and periodic TSH (for patients being treated for melanoma, obtain baseline within 4 weeks prior to treatment initiation, and then at 3 and 6 months, and every 6 months thereafter during treatment); CBC with differential and platelets; serum chemistries, liver function tests (for patients with melanoma, monitor serum bilirubin, ALT, AST, alkaline phosphatase, and LDH at 2 and 8 weeks, and 2 and 3 months following initiation, then every 6 months during therapy), renal function, triglycerides; serum glucose or Hb A_{1c} (for patients with diabetes mellitus). Clinical studies (for combination therapy) tested as follows: CBC (including hemoglobin, WBC, and platelets) and chemistries (including liver function tests and uric acid) measured at weeks 2, 4, 8, and 12, and then every 6 weeks; TSH measured every 12 weeks during treatment. ECG at baseline for patients with pre-existing cardiac abnormalities (for combination therapy with ribavirin).

Hepatitic C: Serum HCV RNA levels (pretreatment, 12 and 24 weeks after therapy initiation, 24 weeks after completion of therapy). **Note:** Discontinuation of therapy may be considered after 12 weeks in patients with HCV (genotype 1) who fail to achieve an early virologic response (EVR) (defined as ≥2-log decrease in HCV RNA compared to pretreatment) or after 24 weeks with detectable HCV RNA. Treat patients with HCV (genotypes 2,3) for 24 weeks (if tolerated) and then evaluate HCV RNA levels (Ghany, 2009).

Evaluate for depression and other psychiatric symptoms before and after initiation of therapy; patients being treated for melanoma should be monitored for depression and psychiatric symptoms every 3 weeks during the first eight weeks of treatment and every 6 months thereafter, and continued monitoring for 6 months after the last dose; baseline ophthalmic eye examination; periodic ophthalmic exam in patients with diabetic or hypertensive retinopathy; baseline ECG in patients with cardiac disease; serum glucose or Hb A_{1c} (for patients with diabetes mellitus). In combination therapy with ribavirin, pregnancy tests (for women of childbearing age who are receiving treatment or who have male partners who are receiving treatment), continue monthly up to 6 months after discontinuation of therapy.

Medication Guide Available Yes

Dosage Forms Excipient information presented when available (limited, particularly for generics); consult specific product labeling.

Injection, powder for reconstitution:

Sylatron™: 296 mcg [contains polysorbate 80, sucrose 59.2 mg; supplied with diluent]

Sylatron™: 444 mcg [contains polysorbate 80, sucrose 59.2 mg; supplied with diluent]

Sylatron™: 888 mcg [contains polysorbate 80, sucrose 59.2 mg; supplied with diluent]

Injection, powder for reconstitution [preservative free]:

PegIntron®: 50 mcg, 80 mcg, 120 mcg, 150 mcg [contains polysorbate 80, sucrose 59.2 mg; supplied with diluent]

PegIntron™ Redipen®: 50 mcg, 80 mcg, 120 mcg, 150 mcg [contains polysorbate 80, sucrose 54 mg; supplied with diluent]

References

Bottomley A, Coens C, Suciu S, et al, "Adjuvant Therapy With Pegylated Interferon Alfa-2b Versus Observation in Resected Stage III Melanoma: A Phase III Randomized Controlled Trial of Health-Related Quality of Life and Symptoms by the European Organisation for Research and Treatment of Cancer Melanoma Group," *J Clin Oncol*, 2009, 27(18):2916-23.

Centers for Disease Control and Prevention, "Sexually Transmitted Diseases Treatment Guidelines, 2006," *MMWR*, 2006, 55(RR-11):1-94.

Dienstag JL and McHutchinson JG, "American Gastroenterological Association Medical Position Statement on the Management of Hepatitis C," *Gastroenterology*, 2006, 130(1):225-30.

Eggermont AM, Suciu S, Santinami M, et al, "EORTC18991: Long-Term Adjuvant Pegylated Interferon-Alpha2b (PEG-IFN) Compared to Observation in Resected Stage III Melanoma, Final Results of a Randomized Phase III Trial," *J Clin Onc*, 2007, 25(18S):8504 [abstract 8504 from 2007 ASCO Annual Meeting].

Eggermont AM, Suciu S, Santinami M, et al, "Adjuvant Therapy With Pegylated Interferon Alfa-2b Versus Observation Alone in Resected Stage III Melanoma: Final Results of EORTC 18991, A Randomised Phase III Trial," *Lancet*, 2008, 372(9633):117-26

Ghany MG, Strader DB, Thomas DL, et al, "Diagnosis, Management And Treatment Of Hepatitis C: An Update," *Hepatology*, 2009, 49(4):1335-74.

McHutchison JG, Lawitz EJ, Shiffman ML, et al, "Peginterferon Alfa-2b or Alfa-2a With Ribavirin for Treatment of Hepatitis C Infection," *N Engl J Med*, 2009, 361(6):580-93.

◆ **PegIntron®** *see* Peginterferon Alfa-2b *on page* *1140*

◆ **PegIntron™ Redipen®** *see* Peginterferon Alfa-2b *on page* *1140*

◆ **PEGLA** *see* Pegaspargase *on page* *1135*

- **Pegylated DOXOrubicin Liposomal** *see* DOXOrubicin (Liposomal) *on page 473*
- **Pegylated G-CSF** *see* Pegfilgrastim *on page 1138*
- **Pegylated Interferon Alfa-2b** *see* Peginterferon Alfa-2b *on page 1140*
- **Pegylated Liposomal DOXOrubicin** *see* DOXOrubicin (Liposomal) *on page 473*
- **Pegylated Liposomal DOXOrubicin Hydrochloride (Doxil®, Caelyx®)** *see* DOXOrubicin (Liposomal) *on page 473*

PEMEtrexed (pem e TREKS ed)

Related Information

Management of Chemotherapy-Induced Nausea and Vomiting *on page 1786*

Brand Names: U.S. Alimta®

Brand Names: Canada Alimta®

Index Terms LY231514; Pemetrexed Disodium

Generic Availability (U.S.) No

Pharmacologic Category Antineoplastic Agent, Antimetabolite; Antineoplastic Agent, Antimetabolite (Antifolate)

Use Treatment of unresectable malignant pleural mesothelioma (in combination with cisplatin); treatment of locally advanced or metastatic **non**squamous nonsmall cell lung cancer (NSCLC; as initial treatment in combination with cisplatin, as single-agent maintenance treatment after 4 cycles of initial platinum-based double therapy, and single-agent treatment after prior chemotherapy)

Note: Not indicated for the treatment of **squamous** cell NSCLC

Unlabeled Use Treatment of bladder cancer (metastatic), cervical cancer (recurrent or metastatic), ovarian cancer (recurrent or persistent), thymic malignancies; treatment of malignant pleural mesothelioma (either as a single agent or in combination with carboplatin)

Labeled Contraindications Severe hypersensitivity to pemetrexed or any component of the formulation

Canadian labeling (additional contraindications; not in U.S. labeling): Concomitant yellow fever vaccine

Pregnancy Risk Factor D

Lactation Excretion in breast milk unknown/not recommended

Warnings/Precautions Hazardous agent - use appropriate precautions for handling and disposal. Hypersensitivity (including anaphylaxis) has been reported with use. May cause bone marrow suppression (anemia, neutropenia, thrombocytopenia and/or pancytopenia); frequent laboratory monitoring is necessary (myelosuppression is often dose-limiting). Dose reductions in subsequent cycles may be required. Prophylactic folic acid and vitamin B_{12} supplements are necessary to reduce hematologic and gastrointestinal toxicity and infection; initiate supplementation 1 week before the first dose of pemetrexed. Pretreatment with dexamethasone is necessary to reduce the incidence and severity of cutaneous reactions. Rarely, Stevens-Johnson syndrome and toxic epidermal necrolysis have been reported. Although the effect of third space fluid is not fully defined, studies have determined pemetrexed concentrations in patients with mild-to-moderate ascites/pleural effusions were similar to concentrations in trials of patients without third space fluid accumulation. Drainage of fluid from ascites/effusions may be considered, but is not likely necessary. Use caution with hepatic dysfunction not due to metastases; may require dose adjustment. Interstitial pneumonitis with respiratory insufficiency has been observed with use; interrupt therapy and evaluate promptly with progressive dyspnea and cough.

The manufacturer does not recommend use in patients with Cl_{cr} <45 mL/minute. Decreased renal function results in increased toxicity. Use caution in patients receiving concurrent nephrotoxins; may result in delayed pemetrexed clearance. NSAIDs may reduce the clearance of pemetrexed. In patients with Cl_{cr} 45-79 mL/minute, interruption of NSAID therapy may be necessary prior to, during, and immediately after pemetrexed therapy. Not indicated for use in patients with squamous cell NSCLC.

Adverse Reactions

>10%:

Central nervous system: Fatigue (18% to 34%; dose-limiting)

Dermatologic: Rash/desquamation (10% to 14%)

Gastrointestinal: Nausea (12% to 31%), anorexia (19% to 22%), vomiting (6% to 16%), stomatitis (5% to 15%), diarrhea (5% to 13%)

Hematologic: Anemia (15% to 19%; grades 3/4: 3% to 5%), leukopenia (6% to 12%; grades 3/4: 2% to 4%), neutropenia (6% to 11%; grades 3/4: 3% to 5%; dose-limiting; nadir: 8-10 days; recovery: 4-8 days after nadir)

Respiratory: Pharyngitis (15%)

1% to 10%:

Cardiovascular: Edema (1% to 5%)

Central nervous system: Fever (1% to 8%)

Dermatologic: Pruritus (1% to 7%), alopecia (1% to 6%), erythema multiforme (≤5%)

Gastrointestinal: Constipation (1% to 6%), weight loss (1%), abdominal pain (≤5%)

Hematologic: Thrombocytopenia (1% to 8%; grades 3/4: 2%; dose-limiting), febrile neutropenia (grades 3/4: 2%)

Hepatic: ALT increased (8% to 10%; grades 3/4: ≤2%), AST increased (7% to 8%; grades 3/4: ≤1%)

Neuromuscular & skeletal: Sensory neuropathy (≤9%), motor neuropathy (≤5%)

Ocular: Conjunctivitis (≤5%), lacrimation increased (≤5%)

Renal: Creatinine increased/creatinine clearance decreased (1% to 5%)

Miscellaneous: Allergic reaction/hypersensitivity (≤5%), infection (≤5%), sepsis (1%)

<1%, postmarketing, and/or case reports: Arrhythmia, chest pain, colitis, dehydration, depression, esophagitis, gastrointestinal obstruction, GGT increased, hemolytic anemia, hepatobiliary failure, hypertension, interstitial pneumonitis, pain, pancreatitis, pancytopenia, peripheral ischemia, pulmonary embolism, radiation recall (median onset: 6 days; range: 1-35 days), renal failure, Stevens-Johnson syndrome, supraventricular arrhythmia, syncope, thrombosis/embolism, toxic epidermal necrolysis, ventricular tachycardia

Drug Interactions

Metabolism/Transport Effects None known.

Avoid Concomitant Use

Avoid concomitant use of PEMEtrexed with any of the following: BCG; CloZAPine; Natalizumab; Pimecrolimus; Tacrolimus (Topical); Vaccines (Live)

Increased Effect/Toxicity

PEMEtrexed may increase the levels/effects of: CloZAPine; Leflunomide; Natalizumab; Vaccines (Live)

The levels/effects of PEMEtrexed may be increased by: Denosumab; NSAID (Nonselective); Pimecrolimus; Roflumilast; Tacrolimus (Topical); Trastuzumab

Decreased Effect

PEMEtrexed may decrease the levels/effects of: BCG; Coccidioidin Skin Test; Sipuleucel-T; Vaccines (Inactivated); Vaccines (Live)

The levels/effects of PEMEtrexed may be decreased by: Echinacea

Ethanol/Nutrition/Herb Interactions Lower ANC nadirs occur in patients with elevated baseline cystathionine or homocysteine concentrations. Levels of these substances can be reduced by folic acid and vitamin B_{12} supplementation.

Storage/Stability Store intact vials at room temperature of 25°C (77°F); excursions permitted to 15°C to 30°C (59°F to 86°F). Reconstituted solution in NS and infusion solutions (in D_5W or NS) are stable for 24 hours when refrigerated at 2°C to 8°C (36°F to 46°F) or stored at room temperature of 15°C to 30°C (59°F to 86°F). Concentrations at 25 mg/mL are stable in polypropylene syringes for 2 days at room temperature (23°C) (Zhang, 2005).

Reconstitution Reconstitute with NS (preservative free); add 4.2 mL to the 100 mg vial and 20 mL to the 500 mg vial, resulting in a 25 mg/mL concentration. Gently swirl. Solution may be colorless to green-yellow. Further dilute in 100 mL NS for infusion; may also dilute in D_5W (Zhang, 2006), although the manufacturer recommends NS. Use appropriate precautions for handling and disposal

Mechanism of Action Antifolate; disrupts folate-dependent metabolic processes essential for cell replication. Inhibits thymidylate synthase (TS), dihydrofolate reductase (DHFR), glycinamide ribonucleotide formyltransferase (GARFT), and aminoimidazole carboxamide ribonucleotide formyltransferase (AICARFT), the enzymes involved in folate metabolism and DNA synthesis, resulting in inhibition of purine and thymidine nucleotide and protein synthesis.

Pharmacodynamics/Kinetics

Distribution: V_{dss}: 16.1 L

Protein binding: ~73% to 81%

Metabolism: Minimal

Half-life elimination: Normal renal function: 3.5 hours; Cl_{cr} 40-59 mL/minute: 5.3-5.8 hours

Excretion: Urine (70% to 90% as unchanged drug)

Dosing

Adult & Geriatric Details concerning dosing in combination regimens should also be consulted. **Note:** Start vitamin supplements 1 week before initial pemetrexed dose: Folic acid 400-1000 mcg daily orally (begin 7 days prior to treatment initiation; continue daily during treatment and for 21 days after last pemetrexed dose) and vitamin B_{12} 1000 mcg I.M. 7 days prior to treatment initiation and then every 3 cycles. Give dexamethasone 4 mg orally twice daily for 3 days, beginning the day before treatment to minimize cutaneous reactions. New treatment cycles should not begin unless ANC ≥1500/mm^3, platelets ≥100,000/mm^3, and Cl_{cr} ≥45 mL/minute.

Malignant pleural mesothelioma: I.V.: 500 mg/m^2 on day 1 of each 21-day cycle (in combination with cisplatin) **or** (unlabeled) in combination with carboplatin (Castagneto, 2008; Ceresoli, 2006) **or** (unlabeled) as single-agent therapy (Jassem, 2008; Taylor, 2008)

Nonsmall cell lung cancer: I.V:

Initial treatment: 500 mg/m^2 on day 1 of each 21-day cycle (in combination with cisplatin)

Maintenance or second-line treatment: 500 mg/m^2 on day 1 of each 21-day cycle (as a single-agent)

Bladder cancer (unlabeled use): I.V.: 500 mg/m^2 on day 1 of each 21-day cycle (Sweeney, 2006)

Cervical cancer, persistent or recurrent (unlabeled use): I.V.: 500 mg/m^2 on day 1 of each 21-day cycle until disease progression or unacceptable toxicity occurs (Lorusso, 2010) **or** 900 mg/m^2 on day 1 of each 21-day cycle (Miller, 2008)

Ovarian cancer, platinum-resistant (unlabeled use): I.V.: 500 mg/m^2 on day 1 of each 21-day cycle (Vergote, 2009)

Thymic malignancies, metastatic (unlabeled use): I.V.: 500 mg/m^2 on day 1 of each 21-day cycle for 6 cycles or until disease progression or unacceptable toxicity occurs (Loehrer, 2006)

Renal Impairment

Renal function may be estimated using the Cockcroft-Gault formula (using actual body weight) or glomerular filtration rate (GFR) measured by Tc99m-DPTA serum clearance.

Cl_{cr} ≥45 mL/minute: No dosage adjustment necessary.

Cl_{cr} <45 mL/minute: Use not recommended (an insufficient number of patients have been studied for dosage recommendations).

Concomitant NSAID use with renal dysfunction:

Cl_{cr} ≥80 mL/minute: No dosage adjustment necessary.

Cl_{cr} 45 to 79 mL/minute and NSAIDs with short half-lives (eg, ibuprofen, indomethacin, ketoprofen, ketorolac): Avoid NSAID for 2 days before, the day of, and for 2 days following a dose of pemetrexed.

Any creatinine clearance and NSAIDs with long half-lives (eg, nabumetone, naproxen, oxaprozin, piroxicam): Avoid NSAID for 5 days before, the day of, and 2 days following a dose of pemetrexed.

Hepatic Impairment Grade 3 (5.1-20 times ULN) **or** 4 (>20 times ULN) transaminase elevation during treatment: Reduce pemetrexed dose to 75% of previous dose (and cisplatin).

Adjustment for Toxicity

Toxicity: Discontinue if patient develops grade 3 or 4 toxicity after two dose reductions or immediately if grade 3 or 4 neurotoxicity develops

Hematologic toxicity: Upon recovery, reinitiate therapy

Nadir ANC <500/mm^3 and nadir platelets ≥50,000/mm^3: Reduce dose to 75% of previous dose of pemetrexed (and cisplatin)

Nadir platelets <50,000/mm^3 **without bleeding** (regardless of nadir ANC): Reduce dose to 75% of previous dose of pemetrexed (and cisplatin)

Nadir platelets <50,000/mm^3 **with bleeding** (regardless of nadir ANC): Reduce dose to 50% of previous dose of pemetrexed (and cisplatin)

Nonhematologic toxicity ≥grade 3 (excluding neurotoxicity): Withhold treatment until recovery to baseline; upon recovery, reinitiate therapy as follows:

Grade 3 or 4 toxicity (excluding mucositis): Reduce dose to 75% of previous dose of pemetrexed (and cisplatin)

Grade 3 or 4 diarrhea or any diarrhea requiring hospitalization: Reduce dose to 75% of previous dose of pemetrexed (and cisplatin)

Grade 3 or 4 mucositis: Reduce pemetrexed dose to 50% of previous dose (continue cisplatin at 100% of previous dose)

Neurotoxicity:

Grade 0-1: Continue pemetrexed at 100% of previous dose (and cisplatin)

Grade 2: Continue pemetrexed at 100% of previous dose; reduce cisplatin dose to 50% of previous dose

Combination Regimens

Bladder cancer: Pemetrexed (Bladder Cancer Regimen) on page 1737

Lung cancer (nonsmall cell):

- Bevacizumab-Carboplatin-Pemetrexed (NSCLC) on page 1529
- Carboplatin-Pemetrexed (NSCLC) on page 1551
- Cisplatin-Pemetrexed (NSCLC) on page 1583
- Pemetrexed (NSCLC Regimen) on page 1738

Malignant pleural mesothelioma:

- Carboplatin-Pemetrexed (Mesothelioma) on page 1551
- Cisplatin-Pemetrexed (Mesothelioma) on page 1582
- Pemetrexed (Mesothelioma Regimen) on page 1738

Ovarian cancer: Pemetrexed (Ovarian Regimen) on page 1739

Administration I.V.: Infuse over 10 minutes.

Emetic Potential Low (10% to 30%)

Monitoring Parameters CBC with differential and platelets (before each dose; monitor for nadir and recovery); serum creatinine, creatinine clearance, BUN, total bilirubin, ALT, AST (periodic); signs/symptoms of mucositis and diarrhea

Dietary Considerations Initiate folic acid supplementation 1 week before first dose of pemetrexed, continue for full course of therapy, and for 21 days after last dose. Institute vitamin B_{12} 1 week before the first dose; administer every 9 weeks thereafter.

Dosage Forms Excipient information presented when available (limited, particularly for generics); consult specific product labeling.

Injection, powder for reconstitution:

Alimta®: 100 mg, 500 mg

References

Castagneto B, Botta M, Aitini E, et al, "Phase II Study of Pemetrexed in Combination With Carboplatin in Patients With Malignant Pleural Mesothelioma (MPM)," *Ann Oncol*, 2008, 19 (2):370-3.

Ceresoli GL, Zucali PA, Favaretto AG, et al, "Phase II Study of Pemetrexed Plus Carboplatin in Malignant Pleural Mesothelioma," *J Clin Oncol*, 2006, 24(9):1443-8.

Ciuleanu T, Brodowicz T, Zielinski C, et al, "Maintenance Pemetrexed Plus Best Supportive Care Versus Placebo Plus Best Supportive Care for Non-Small Cell Lung Cancer: A Randomised, Double-Blind, Phase 3 Study," *Lancet*, 2009, 374(9699):1432-40.

Grønberg BH, Bremnes RM, Fløtten O, et al, "Phase III Study by the Norwegian Lung Cancer Study Group: Pemetrexed Plus Carboplatin Compared With Gemcitabine Plus Carboplatin as First-Line Chemotherapy in Advanced Non-Small-Cell Lung Cancer," *J Clin Oncol*, 2009, 27 (19):3217-24.

Hanna N, Shepherd FA, Fossella FV, et al, "Randomized Phase III Trial of Pemetrexed versus Docetaxel in Patients With Non-Small-Cell Lung Cancer Previously Treated With Chemotherapy," *J Clin Oncol*, 2004, 22(9):1589-97.

Jassem J, Ramlau R, Santoro A, et al, "Phase III Trial of Pemetrexed Plus Best Supportive Care Compared With Best Supportive Care in Previously Treated Patients With Advanced Malignant Pleural Mesothelioma," *J Clin Oncol*, 2008, 26(10):1698-704.

Loehrer PJ, Yiannoutsos CT, Dropcho S, et al, "A Phase II Trial of Pemetrexed in Patients With Recurrent Thymoma or Thymic Carcinoma," *J Clin Oncol*, 2006, 24(suppl):7079 [abstract 7079 from 2006 ASCO Annual Meeting].

Lorusso D, Ferrandina G, Pignata S, et al, "Evaluation of Pemetrexed (Alimta, LY231514) as Second-Line Chemotherapy in Persistent or Recurrent Carcinoma of the Cervix: The CERVIX 1 Study of the MITO (Multicentre Italian Trials in Ovarian Cancer and Gynecologic Malignancies) Group," *Ann Oncol*, 2010, 21(1):61-6.

Miller DS, Blessing JA, Bodurka DC, et al, "Evaluation of Pemetrexed (Alimta, LY231514) as Second Line Chemotherapy in Persistent or Recurrent Carcinoma of the Cervix: A Phase II Study of the Gynecologic Oncology Group," *Gynecol Oncol*, 2008, 110(1):65-70.

Miller DS, Blessing JA, Krasner CN, et al, "Phase II Evaluation of Pemetrexed in the Treatment of Recurrent or Persistent Platinum-Resistant Ovarian or Primary Peritoneal Carcinoma: A Study of the Gynecologic Oncology Group," *J Clin Oncol*, 2009, 27(16):2686-91.

Mita AC, Sweeney CJ, Baker SD, et al, "Phase I and Pharmacokinetic Study of Pemetrexed Administered Every 3 Weeks to Advanced Cancer Patients With Normal and Impaired Renal Function," *J Clin Oncol*, 2006, 24(4):552-62.

Ouellet D, Periclou AP, Johnson RD, et al, "Population Pharmacokinetics of Pemetrexed Disodium (ALIMTA) in Patients With Cancer," *Cancer Chemother Pharmacol*, 2000, 46(3):227-34.

Paz-Ares L, Bezares S, Tabernero JM, et al, "Review of a Promising New Agent - Pemetrexed Disodium," *Cancer*, 2003, 97(8 Suppl):2056-63.

Rusch VW, "Pemetrexed and Cisplatin for Malignant Pleural Mesothelioma: A New Standard of Care?" *J Clin Oncol*, 2003, 21(14):2629-30.

Scagliotti GV, Parikh P, von Pawel J, et al, "Phase III Study Comparing Cisplatin Plus Gemcitabine With Cisplatin Plus Pemetrexed in Chemotherapy-Naive Patients With Advanced-Stage Non-Small-Cell Lun Cancer,"*J Clin Oncol*, 2008, 26(21):3543-51.

Schmitt J and Loehrer PJ Sr, "The Role of Chemotherapy in Advanced Thymoma," *J Thorac Oncol*, 2010, 5(10 Suppl 4):357-60.

Socinski MA, Smit EF, Lorigan P, et al, "Phase III study of Pemetrexed Plus Carboplatin Compared With Etoposide Plus Carboplatin in Chemotherapy-Naive Patients With Extensive-Stage Small-Cell Lung Cancer," *J Clin Oncol*, 2009, 27(28):4787-92.

Sweeney CJ, Roth BJ, Kabbinavar FF, et al, "Phase II Study of Pemetrexed for Second-Line Treatment of Transitional Cell Cancer of the Urothelium," *J Clin Oncol*, 2006, 24(21):3451-7.

Sweeney CJ, Takimoto CH, Latz JE, et al, "Two Drug Interaction Studies Evaluating the Pharmacokinetics and Toxicity of Pemetrexed When Coadministered With Aspirin or Ibuprofen in Patients With Advanced Cancer," *Clin Cancer Res*, 2006, 12(2):536-42.

Taylor P, Castagneto B, Dark G, et al, "Single-Agent Pemetrexed for Chemonaïve and Pretreated Patients With Malignant Pleural Mesothelioma: Results of an International Expanded Access Program," *J Thorac Oncol*, 2008, 3(7):764-71

Trissel LA, Saenz CA, Ogundele AB, et al, "Physical Compatibility of Pemetrexed Disodium With Other Drugs During Simulated Y-Site Administration," *Am J Health Syst Pharm*, 2004, 61 (21):2289-93.

Urba S, van Herpen CM, Sahoo TP, et al, "Pemetrexed in Combination With Cisplatin versus Cisplatin Monotherapy in Patients With Recurrent or Metastatic Head and Neck Cancer: Final Results of a Randomized, Double-Blind, Placebo-Controlled, Phase 3 Study," *Cancer*, 2012, 118 (19):4694-705.

Vergote I, Calvert H, Kania M, et al, "A Randomised, Double-Blind, Phase II Study of Two Doses of Pemetrexed in the Treatment of Platinum-Resistant, Epithelial Ovarian or Primary Peritoneal Cancer," *Eur J Cancer*, 2009, 45(8):1415-23.

Zhang Y and Trissel LA, "Physical and Chemical Stability of Pemetrexed in Infusion Solutions," *Ann Pharmacother*, 2006, 40(6):1082-5.

Zhang Y and Trissel LA, "Physical and Chemical Stability of Pemetrexed Solutions in Plastic Syringes," *Ann Pharmacother*, 2005, 39(12):2026-8.

◆ **Pemetrexed Disodium** *see* PEMEtrexed *on page 1151*

◆ **Pentahydrate** *see* Sodium Thiosulfate *on page 1289*

◆ **Pentam® 300** *see* Pentamidine *on page 1156*

Pentamidine (pen TAM i deen)

Related Information

Hematopoietic Stem Cell Transplantation *on page 1887*

Safe Handling of Hazardous Drugs *on page 1904*

Brand Names: U.S. Nebupent®; Pentam® 300

Index Terms Pentamidine Isethionate

Generic Availability (U.S.) No

Pharmacologic Category Antifungal Agent; Antiprotozoal

Use

I.M., I.V.: Treatment of pneumonia caused by *Pneumocystis jirovecii* pneumonia (PCP)

Inhalation: Prevention of PCP in high-risk, HIV-infected patients either with a history of PCP or with a CD4+ count ≤200/mm^3

Unlabeled Use Prevention of PCP in nonHIV-infected patients; treatment of African trypanosomiasis, cutaneous leishmaniasis, and amebic meningoencephalitis

Labeled Contraindications Hypersensitivity to pentamidine isethionate or any component of the formulation

Pregnancy Risk Factor C

Lactation Excretion in breast milk unknown/not recommended

Warnings/Precautions Hazardous agent - use appropriate precautions for handling and disposal. Severe hypotension (some fatalities) has been observed (even after a single dose); may occur with either I.V. or I.M administration, although more common with rapid I.V. administration; monitor blood pressure during (and after) infusion. May cause QT prolongation and subsequent torsade de pointes; avoid use in patients with diagnosed or suspected congenital long QT syndrome. Use with caution in patients with pre-existing cardiovascular disease; hyper-/hypotension and arrhythmia, including ventricular tachycardia (eg, torsade de pointes) have been reported.

Use with caution in patients with diabetes mellitus or hypocalcemia; hyper-/hypoglycemia and pancreatic islet cell necrosis with hyperinsulinemia has been reported. Symptoms may occur months after therapy; monitor blood glucose daily on therapy and periodically thereafter. Use with caution in patients with a history of pancreatic disease or elevated amylase/lipase levels; acute pancreatitis (with fatality) has been reported. Discontinue if signs/symptoms of acute pancreatitis occur. Concurrent use with other bone marrow suppressants may increase the risk for myelotoxicity; use with caution in patients with current evidence and/or prior history of hematologic disorders; anemia, leukopenia and/or thrombocytopenia have been reported. Use with caution in patients with hepatic or renal disease. Concurrent use with other nephrotoxic drugs may increase the risk for nephrotoxicity. Avoid concurrent use with other drugs known to prolong QT_c interval. Stevens-Johnson syndrome has been reported with use. Avoid extravasation; may cause tissue ulceration, necrosis, and/or sloughing; if extravasation occurs, treat symptomatically. Assess catheter position before and during infusion.

Aerosolized pentamidine may induce bronchospasm or cough, especially in patients with a smoking or asthma history (an inhaled bronchodilator prior to pentamidine may ameliorate symptoms). Use appropriate precautions to minimize exposure to healthcare personnel; refer to individual institutional policy. Acute PCP may develop despite aerosolized pentamidine prophylaxis. Although rare, extrapulmonary PCP disease may occur and has been associated with aerosolized pentamidine.

Adverse Reactions

Aerosol:

>10%:

Central nervous system: Fatigue (66%), fever (51%), dizziness/lightheadedness (45%)

Gastrointestinal: Appetite decreased (50%)

Respiratory: Cough (1% to 63%), dyspnea (48%), wheezing (32%)

Miscellaneous: Infection (15%)

1% to 10%:

Central nervous system: Headache

Gastrointestinal: Diarrhea, nausea, oral candida, taste alteration

Hematologic: Anemia

Respiratory: Bronchitis, chest pain, pharyngitis, sinusitis, upper respiratory tract infection

Miscellaneous: Herpes infection, influenza, night sweats

Injection:

>10%:

Local: Local reactions at I.M. injection site (11%; includes sterile abscess, necrosis, pain, induration)

Renal: Renal function impaired (29%), creatinine increased (24%)

1% to 10%:

Cardiovascular: Hypotension (5%)

Central nervous system: Confusion/hallucinations (2%)

Dermatologic: Rash (3%)

Endocrine & metabolic: Hypoglycemia (6%)

Gastrointestinal: Nausea/anorexia (6%), taste alteration (2%)

Hematologic: Leukopenia (10%), thrombocytopenia (3%), anemia (1%)

Hepatic: Liver function tests increased (9%)

Renal: Azotemia (9%), BUN increased (7%)

Aerosol or injection: <1%, postmarketing, and/or case reports (limited to important or life-threatening): Abdominal pain, allergic reaction, anaphylaxis, anxiety, arthralgia, asthma, blepharitis, blurred vision, bronchitis, bronchospasm, cardiac arrhythmia, central venous line related sepsis, cerebrovascular accident, chest tightness, chills, clotting time prolonged, CMV infection, colitis, confusion, congestion (chest, nasal), conjunctivitis, cough, cryptococcal meningitis, cyanosis, defibrination, depression, dermatitis, desquamation, diabetes mellitus, diabetic ketoacidosis, diarrhea, dizziness, drowsiness, dyspepsia, dyspnea, emotional lability, eosinophilia, erythema, esophagitis, extrapulmonary pneumocystosis, extravasation (tissue ulceration, necrosis, and/or sloughing), facial edema, flank pain, gait unsteady, gagging, gingivitis, headache, hearing loss, hematochezia, hematuria, hemoptysis, hepatic dysfunction, hepatitis, hepatomegaly, histoplasmosis, hyperglycemia, hyperkalemia, hypersalivation, hypertension, hyperventilation, hypesthesia, hypocalcemia, hypomagnesemia, incontinence, insomnia, laryngitis, laryngospasm, leg edema, melena, memory loss, nephritis, nervousness, neuralgia, neuropathy, neutropenia, night sweats, palpitation, pancreatitis, pancytopenia, paranoia, paresthesia, peripheral neuropathy, phlebitis, pleuritis, pneumonitis (eosinophilic or interstitial), pneumothorax, pruritus, rales, renal dysfunction, renal failure, rhinitis, seizure, splenomegaly, Stevens-Johnson syndrome, ST segment abnormal, syncope, syndrome of inappropriate antidiuretic hormone (SIADH), tachycardia, tachypnea, temperature abnormal, torsade de pointes, tremor, vasodilation, vasculitis, ventricular tachycardia, vertigo, vomiting, urticaria, xerostomia

Drug Interactions

Metabolism/Transport Effects Substrate of CYP2C19 (major); **Note:** Assignment of Major/Minor substrate status based on clinically relevant drug interaction potential; **Inhibits** CYP2C19 (weak), CYP2C9 (weak), CYP2D6 (weak), CYP3A4 (weak)

Avoid Concomitant Use

Avoid concomitant use of Pentamidine with any of the following: BCG; Highest Risk QTc-Prolonging Agents; Mifepristone

Increased Effect/Toxicity

Pentamidine may increase the levels/effects of: ARIPiprazole; Highest Risk QTc-Prolonging Agents; Moderate Risk QTc-Prolonging Agents

The levels/effects of Pentamidine may be increased by: CYP2C19 Inhibitors (Moderate); CYP2C19 Inhibitors (Strong); Mifepristone; QTc-Prolonging Agents (Indeterminate Risk and Risk Modifying)

Decreased Effect

Pentamidine may decrease the levels/effects of: BCG; Sodium Picosulfate; Typhoid Vaccine

The levels/effects of Pentamidine may be decreased by: CYP2C19 Inducers (Strong)

Ethanol/Nutrition/Herb Interactions Ethanol: Avoid ethanol (may increase CNS depression or aggravate hypoglycemia).

Storage/Stability Store intact vials at 20°C to 25°C (68°F to 77°F); protect from light. Do not use sodium chloride for initial reconstitution (sodium chloride will cause precipitation).

Aerosol: The manufacturer recommends the use of freshly prepared solutions for inhalation; however, may be stored for up to 48 hours in the vial at room temperature if protected from light.

Injection: Reconstituted solution is stable for 48 hours in the vial at room temperature and protected from light. Solutions for injection (1-2.5 mg/mL) in D_5W are stable for at least 24 hours at room temperature. Store at room temperature to avoid crystallization.

Reconstitution Do not use sodium chloride for initial reconstitution (sodium chloride will cause precipitation).

Aerosol: Reconstitute with 6 mL SWFI. Do not mix with other nebulizer solutions.

Injection: I.M.: Reconstitute with 3 mL SWFI; I.V.: Reconstitute with 3-5 mL SWFI or D_5W; the manufacturer recommends further dilution in 50-250 mL D_5W; however, stability with further dilution in NS has also been documented.

Mechanism of Action Interferes with microbial RNA/DNA, phospholipids and protein synthesis, through inhibition of oxidative phosphorylation and/or interference with incorporation of nucleotides and nucleic acids into RNA and DNA

Pharmacodynamics/Kinetics

Absorption: I.M.: Well absorbed; Inhalation: Limited systemic absorption

Distribution: V_{dss}: I.V.: 286-1356 L; I.M.: 1658-3790 L

Half-life elimination: I.V.: 5-8 hours; I.M.: 7-11 hours; may be prolonged with severe renal impairment

Excretion: Urine (I.V.: ≤12% as unchanged drug)

Dosing

Adult & Geriatric

PCP:

FDA-approved labeling:

Prevention: Inhalation: 300 mg every 4 weeks via Respirgard® II nebulizer

Treatment: I.M., I.V.: 4 mg/kg once daily for 14-21 days

CDC recommendation:

Prevention: Inhalation: 300 mg monthly via Respirgard® II nebulizer

Treatment: I.V.: 3-4 mg/kg once daily for 21 days

AIDSinfo guidelines (2009):
Prevention: Inhalation: 300 mg/dose monthly via Respirgard® II nebulizer
Treatment: I.V.: 4 mg/kg once daily, 3 mg/kg may be used by some clinicians

Cutaneous leishmaniasis (unlabeled use; CDC recommendation): I.M., I.V.: 2-3 mg/kg once daily or every second day for 4-7 doses

Trypanosomiasis (unlabeled use; CDC recommendation): I.M.: 4 mg/kg once daily for 7 days

Pediatric

PCP:

FDA-approved labeling: Children >4 months: Treatment: I.M., I.V.: 4 mg/kg once daily for 14-21 days

CDC recommendation:
Prevention (children ≥5 years): Inhalation: 300 mg/dose monthly via Respirgard® II nebulizer
Treatment: I.V.: 3-4 mg/kg once daily for 21 days

AIDSinfo guidelines (2009):
Prevention: Children ≥5 years: Inhalation: 300 mg/dose monthly via Respirgard® II nebulizer
Treatment: I.V.: 4 mg/kg once daily, if clinical improvement may change to atovaquone after 7-10 days

PCP prevention in pediatric oncology patients (age <5 years, intolerant to trimethoprim-sulfamethoxazole; unlabeled use): 4 mg/kg I.V. once monthly (Kim, 2008; Prasad, 2007)

Cutaneous leishmaniasis (unlabeled use; CDC recommendation): I.M., I.V.: 2-3 mg/kg once daily or every second day for 4-7 doses

Trypanosomiasis (unlabeled use; CDC recommendation): I.M.: 4 mg/kg once daily for 7 days

Renal Impairment I.V.: The FDA-approved labeling recommends that caution should be used in patients with renal impairment; however, no specific dosage adjustment guidelines are available. The following guidelines have been used by some clinicians (Aronoff, 2007):

Children:
Cl_{cr} >30 mL/minute: No adjustment required.
Cl_{cr} 10-30 mL/minute: Administer 4 mg/kg every 36 hours.
Cl_{cr} <10 mL/minute and peritoneal dialysis: Administer 4 mg/kg every 48 hours.
Hemodialysis: Administer 4 mg/kg every 48 hours, after dialysis on dialysis days.

Adults:
Cl_{cr} ≥10 mL/minute: No adjustment required.
Cl_{cr} <10 mL/minute: Administer 4 mg/kg every 24-36 hours.

Administration Do not use NS to reconstitute.

Inhalation: Deliver via Respirgard® II nebulizer until nebulizer is emptied (30-45 minutes). Administer at a flow rate of 5-7 L/minute from a 40-50 pound-per-square inch (PSI) oxygen or air source. A 40-50 PSI air compressor can be used alternatively, with a set flow rate at 5-7 L/minute or a set pressure of 22-25 PSI. Air compressors <20 PSI should not be used. Use appropriate precautions to minimize exposure to healthcare personnel; refer to individual institutional policy.

I.V.: Infuse slowly over 60-120 minutes. Avoid extravasation; assess catheter position before and during infusion.

I.M.: Administer deep I.M.

Vesicant/Extravasation Risk Ulceration, tissue necrosis and/or sloughing have been reported with extravasation

Monitoring Parameters Liver function tests, renal function tests, blood glucose, serum potassium and calcium, CBC and platelets; ECG, blood pressure

Dosage Forms Excipient information presented when available (limited, particularly for generics); consult specific product labeling.

Injection, powder for reconstitution, as isethionate:
  Pentam® 300: 300 mg

Powder for solution, for nebulization, as isethionate:
  Nebupent®: 300 mg

References

Aronoff GR, Bennett WM, Berns JS, et al, *Drug Prescribing in Renal Failure: Dosing Guidelines for Adults and Children*, 5th ed. Philadelphia, PA: American College of Physicians; 2007, p 73, 160.

Centers for Disease Control and Prevention, "Amebic Meningoencephalitis, Primary and Granulomatous." Available at http://www.dpd.cdc.gov/dpdx/HTML/PDF_Files/MedLetter/AmebicMeningoencephalitis.pdf. Last accessed September 15, 2009.

Centers for Disease Control, "Guidelines for Prevention and Treatment of Opportunistic Infections Among HIV-Exposed and HIV-Infected Children," *MMWR Recomm Rep*, 2009, 58(RR-11):1-176. Available at http://aidsinfo.nih.gov/contentfiles/OI_Guidelines_Pediatrics.pdf

Centers for Disease Control, "Guidelines for Prevention and Treatment of Opportunistic Infections in HIV-Infected Adults and Adolescents," *MMWR Recomm Rep*, 2009, 58(RR-4):1-194. Available at http://aidsinfo.nih.gov/contentfiles/Adult_OI_041009.pdf

Centers for Disease Control and Prevention, "Leishmania." Available at http://www.dpd.cdc.gov/dpdx/HTML/PDF_Files/MedLetter/Leishmania.pdf. Last accessed September 15, 2009.

Centers for Disease Control and Prevention, "*Pneumocystis jiroveci* (formerly *carinii*) Pneumonia (PCP)." Available at http://www.dpd.cdc.gov/dpdx/HTML/PDF_Files/MedLetter/Pneumocystis_jiroveci.pdf. Last accessed September 15, 2009.

Centers for Disease Control and Prevention, "Trypanosomiasis." Available at http://www.dpd.cdc.gov/dpdx/HTML/PDF_Files/MedLetter/Trypanosomiasis.pdf. Last accessed September 15, 2009.

Ito S and Koren G, "Estimation of Fetal Risk From Aerosolized Pentamidine in Pregnant Healthcare Workers," *Chest*, 1994, 106(5):1460-2.

Kim SY, Dabb AA, Glenn DJ, et al, "Intravenous Pentamidine is Effective as Second Line Pneumocystis Pneumonia Prophylaxis in Pediatric Oncology Patients," *Pediatr Blood Cancer*, 2008, 50(4):779-83.

Prasad P, Nania JJ, and Shankar SM, "Pneumocystis Pneumonia in Children Receiving Chemotherapy," *Pediatr Blood Cancer*, 2008, 50(4):896-8.

Tomblyn M, Chiller T, Einsele H, et al, "Guidelines for Preventing Infectious Complications Among Hematopoietic Cell Transplantation Recipients: A Global Perspective," *Biol Blood Marrow Transplant*, 2009, 15(10):1143-238.

◆ **Pentamidine Isethionate** *see* Pentamidine *on page* *1156*

Pentostatin (pen toe STAT in)

Related Information

Hematopoietic Stem Cell Transplantation *on page* *1887*
Management of Chemotherapy-Induced Nausea and Vomiting *on page* *1786*
Safe Handling of Hazardous Drugs *on page* *1904*

Brand Names: U.S. Nipent®

Brand Names: Canada Nipent®

Index Terms 2′-Deoxycoformycin; Co-Vidarabine; dCF; Deoxycoformycin

Generic Availability (U.S.) Yes

Pharmacologic Category Antineoplastic Agent, Antibiotic; Antineoplastic Agent, Antimetabolite (Purine Analog)

Use Treatment of hairy cell leukemia

Unlabeled Use Treatment of cutaneous T-cell lymphoma, chronic lymphocytic leukemia (CLL), and acute and chronic graft-versus-host-disease (GVHD)

Labeled Contraindications Hypersensitivity to pentostatin or any component of the formulation

Pregnancy Risk Factor D

Lactation Excretion in breast milk unknown/not recommended

Warnings/Precautions Hazardous agent - use appropriate precautions for handling and disposal. **[U.S. Boxed Warnings]: Severe renal, liver, pulmonary and CNS toxicities have occurred with doses higher than recommended; do not exceed the recommended dose. Do not administer concurrently with fludarabine; concomitant use has resulted in serious or fatal pulmonary toxicity.** Bone marrow suppression may occur, primarily early in treatment; if neutropenia persists beyond early cycles, evaluate for disease status. In patients who present with infections prior to treatment, infections should be resolved, if possible, prior to initiation of treatment; treatment should be temporarily withheld for active infections during therapy. Use cautiously in patients with renal dysfunction (the half-life is prolonged); appropriate dosing guidelines in renal insufficiency have not been determined. May cause elevations (reversible) in liver function tests. Withhold treatment for CNS toxicity or severe rash. Fatal pulmonary edema and hypotension have been reported in patients treated with pentostatin in combination with carmustine, etoposide, or high-dose cyclophosphamide as part of a myeloablative regimen for bone marrow transplant. **[U.S. Boxed Warning]: Should be administered under the supervision of an experienced cancer chemotherapy physician.** Safety and efficacy in children have not been established.

Adverse Reactions

>10%:

Central nervous system: Fever (42% to 46%), fatigue (29% to 42%), pain (8% to 20%), chills (11% to 19%), headache (13% to 17%), CNS toxicity (1% to 11%)

Dermatologic: Rash (26% to 43%), pruritus (10% to 21%), skin disorder (4% to 17%)

Gastrointestinal: Nausea/vomiting (22% to 63%), diarrhea (15% to 17%), anorexia (13% to 16%), abdominal pain (4% to 16%), stomatitis (5% to 12%)

Hematologic: Myelosuppression (nadir: 7 days; recovery: 10-14 days), leukopenia (22% to 60%), anemia (8% to 35%), thrombocytopenia (6% to 32%)

Hepatic: Transaminases increased (2% to 19%)

Neuromuscular & skeletal: Myalgia (11% to 19%), weakness (10% to 12%)

Respiratory: Cough (17% to 20%), upper respiratory infection (13% to 16%), rhinitis (10% to 11%), dyspnea (8% to 11%)

Miscellaneous: Infection (7% to 36%), allergic reaction (2% to 11%)

1% to 10%:

Cardiovascular: Chest pain (3% to 10%), facial edema (3% to 10%), hypotension (3% to 10%), peripheral edema (3% to 10%), angina (<3%), arrhythmia (<3%), AV block (<3%), bradycardia (<3%), cardiac arrest (<3%), deep thrombophlebitis (<3%), heart failure (<3%), hypertension (<3%), pericardial effusion (<3%), sinus arrest (<3%), syncope (<3%), tachycardia (<3%), vasculitis (<3%), ventricular extrasystoles (<3%)

Central nervous system: Anxiety (3% to 10%), confusion (3% to 10%), depression (3% to 10%), dizziness (3% to 10%), insomnia (3% to 10%), nervousness (3% to 10%), somnolence (3% to 10%), abnormal dreams/thinking (<3%), amnesia (<3%), ataxia (<3%), emotional lability (<3%), encephalitis (<3%), hallucination (<3%), hostility (<3%), meningism (<3%), neuritis (<3%), neurosis (<3%), seizure (<3%), vertigo (<3%)

Dermatologic: Cellulitis (6%), furunculosis (4%), dry skin (3% to 10%), urticaria (3% to 10%), acne (<3%), alopecia (<3%), eczema (<3%), petechial rash (<3%), photosensitivity (<3%), abscess (2%)

Endocrine & metabolic: Amenorrhea (<3%), hypercalcemia (<3%), hyponatremia (<3%), gout (<3%), libido decreased/loss (<3%)

Gastrointestinal: Dyspepsia (3% to 10%) flatulence (3% to 10%), gingivitis (3% to 10%), constipation (<3%), dysphagia (<3%), glossitis (<3%), ileus (<3%), taste perversion (<3%), oral moniliasis (2%)

Genitourinary: Urinary tract infection (3%), impotence (<3%)

Hematologic: Agranulocytosis (3% to 10%), hemorrhage (3% to 10%), acute leukemia (<3%), aplastic anemia (<3%), hemolytic anemia (<3%)

Local: Phlebitis (<3%)

Neuromuscular & skeletal: Arthralgia (3% to 10%), paresthesia (3% to 10%), arthritis (<3%), dysarthria (<3%), hyperkinesia (<3%), neuralgia (<3%), neuropathy (<3%), paralysis (<3%), twitching (<3%), osteomyelitis (1%)

Ocular: Conjunctivitis (4%), amblyopia (<3%), eyes nonreactive (<3%), lacrimation disorder (<3%), photophobia (<3%), retinopathy (<3%), vision abnormal (<3%), watery eyes (<3%), xerophthalmia (<3%)

Otic: Deafness (<3%), earache (<3%), labyrinthitis (<3%), tinnitus (<3%)

Renal: Creatinine increased (3% to 10%), nephropathy (<3%), renal failure (<3%), renal insufficiency (<3%), renal function abnormal (<3%), renal stone (<3%)

Respiratory: Pharyngitis (8% to 10%), sinusitis (6%), pneumonia (5%), asthma (3% to 10%), bronchitis (3%), bronchospasm (<3%), laryngeal edema (<3%), pulmonary embolus (<3%)

Miscellaneous: Diaphoresis (8% to 10%), herpes zoster (8%), viral infection (≤8%), bacterial infection (5%), herpes simplex (4%), sepsis (3%), flu-like syndrome (<3%)

<1%, postmarketing, and/or case reports: Dysuria, fungal infection (skin), hematuria, lethargy, pulmonary edema, pulmonary toxicity (fatal; in combination with fludarabine), uveitis/vision loss

Drug Interactions

Metabolism/Transport Effects None known.

Avoid Concomitant Use

Avoid concomitant use of Pentostatin with any of the following: BCG; CloZAPine; Fludarabine; Natalizumab; Nelarabine; Pegademase Bovine; Pimecrolimus; Tacrolimus (Topical); Vaccines (Live)

Increased Effect/Toxicity

Pentostatin may increase the levels/effects of: CloZAPine; Cyclophosphamide; Fludarabine; Leflunomide; Natalizumab; Vaccines (Live)

The levels/effects of Pentostatin may be increased by: Denosumab; Fludarabine; Pimecrolimus; Roflumilast; Tacrolimus (Topical); Trastuzumab

Decreased Effect

Pentostatin may decrease the levels/effects of: BCG; Coccidioidin Skin Test; Nelarabine; Pegademase Bovine; Sipuleucel-T; Vaccines (Inactivated); Vaccines (Live)

The levels/effects of Pentostatin may be decreased by: Echinacea; Pegademase Bovine

Storage/Stability Store intact vials under refrigeration at 2°C to 8°C (36°F to 46°F); reconstituted vials, or further dilutions, are stable at room temperature for 8 hours in D_5W or 48 hours in NS.

Reconstitution Reconstitute with 5 mL SWFI to a concentration of 2 mg/mL. The solution may be further diluted in 25-50 mL NS or D_5W for infusion.

Mechanism of Action Pentostatin is a purine antimetabolite that inhibits adenosine deaminase, preventing the deamination of adenosine to inosine. Accumulation of deoxyadenosine (dAdo) and deoxyadenosine 5′-triphosphate (dATP) results in a reduction of purine metabolism and DNA synthesis and cell death.

Pharmacodynamics/Kinetics

Distribution: I.V.: V_d: 36.1 L (20.1 L/m^2); rapidly to body tissues

Protein binding: ~4%

Half-life elimination:

- Distribution half-life: 11-85 minutes
- Terminal: 3-7 hours
- Renal impairment (Cl_{cr} <50 mL/minute): 4-18 hours

Excretion: Urine (~50% to 96%) within 24 hours (30% to 90% as unchanged drug)

Dosing

Adult & Geriatric Refer to individual protocols.

- **Hairy cell leukemia:** I.V.: 4 mg/m^2 every 2 weeks
- **CLL (unlabeled use):** I.V.: 4 mg/m^2 weekly for 3 weeks, then every 2 weeks
- **Cutaneous T-cell lymphoma (unlabeled use):** I.V.: 3.75-5 mg/m^2 daily for 3 days every 3 weeks
- **Acute GVHD (unlabeled use):** I.V.: 1.5 mg/m^2 daily for 3 days; may repeat after 2 weeks if needed
- **Chronic GVHD (unlabeled use):** I.V.: 4 mg/m^2 every 2 weeks for 12 doses; then 4 mg/m^2 every 3-4 weeks (if still improving)

Renal Impairment The FDA-approved labeling does not contain renal dosage adjustment guidelines; use with caution in patients with Cl_{cr} <60 mL/minute. Two patients with Cl_{cr} 50-60 mL/minute achieved responses when treated with 2 mg/m^2/dose. The following guidelines have been used by some clinicians:

Kintzel, 1995:

- Cl_{cr} 46-60 mL/minute: Administer 70% of dose
- Cl_{cr} 31-45 mL/minute: Administer 60% of dose
- Cl_{cr} <30 mL/minute: Consider use of alternative drug

Lathia, 2002:

- Cl_{cr} 40-59 mL/minute: Administer 3 mg/m^2/dose
- Cl_{cr} 20-39 mL/minute: Administer 2 mg/m^2/dose

Combination Regimens

Leukemia, chronic lymphocytic:

PCR on page 1735

Pentostatin-Cyclophosphamide on page 1739

Administration Administer I.V. 20- to 30-minute infusion or I.V. bolus over 5 minutes. Hydrate with 500-1000 mL fluid prior to infusion and 500 mL after infusion.

Emetic Potential Low (10% to 30%)

Monitoring Parameters CBC with differential, platelet count, liver function, serum uric acid, renal function (creatinine clearance), bone marrow evaluation

Dosage Forms Excipient information presented when available (limited, particularly for generics); consult specific product labeling.

Injection, powder for reconstitution:
Nipent®: 10 mg [contains mannitol]
Injection, powder for reconstitution [preservative free]: 10 mg

References

Bolanos-Meade J, Jacobsohn DA, Margolis J, et al, "Pentostatin in Steroid-Refractory Acute Graft-Versus-Host Disease," *J Clin Oncol*, 2005, 23(12):2661-8.

Dillman RO, Mick R and McIntyre OR, "Pentostatin in Chronic Lymphocytic Leukemia: A Phase II Trial of Cancer and Leukemia Group B," *J Clin Oncol*, 1989, 7(4):433-8.

Jacobsohn DA, Chen AR, Zahurak M, et al, "Phase II Study of Pentostatin in Patients With Corticosteroid-Refractory Chronic Graft-Versus-Host Disease," *J Clin Oncol*, 2007, 25 (27):4255-61.

Kane BJ, Kuhn JG, and Roush MK, "Pentostatin: An Adenosine Deaminase Inhibitor For the Treatment of Hairy Cell Leukemia," *Ann Pharmacother*, 1992, 26(7-8):939-47.

Kintzel PE and Dorr RT, "Anticancer Drug Renal Toxicity and Elimination: Dosing Guidelines for Altered Renal Function," *Cancer Treat Rev*, 1995, 21(1):33-64.

Kurzrock R, Pilat S, and Duvic M, "Pentostatin Therapy of T-Cell Lymphomas With Cutaneous Manifestations," *J Clin Oncol*, 1999, 17(10):3117-21.

Lathia C, Fleming GF, Meyer M, et al, "Pentostatin Pharmacokinetics and Dosing Recommendations in Patients With Mild Renal Impairment," *Cancer Chemother Pharmacol*, 2002, 50(2):121-6.

Margolis J and Grever MR, "Pentostatin (Nipent): A Review of Potential Toxicity and its Management," *Semin Oncol*, 2000, 27(2 Suppl 5):9-14.

Tsimberidou AM, Giles F, Duvic M, et al, "Phase II Study of Pentostatin in Advanced T-Cell Lymphoid Malignancies: Update of an M.D. Anderson Cancer Center Series," *Cancer*, 2004, 100 (2):342-9.

◆ **PEP005** *see* Ingenol Mebutate *on page 796*

◆ **Periactin** *see* Cyproheptadine *on page 342*

◆ **Perjeta™** *see* Pertuzumab *on page 1165*

Pertuzumab (per TU zoo mab)

Brand Names: U.S. Perjeta™

Index Terms 2C4 Antibody; MOAB 2C4; Monoclonal Antibody 2C4; Omnitarg; rhuMAb-2C4

Generic Availability (U.S.) No

Pharmacologic Category Antineoplastic Agent, Anti-HER2; Antineoplastic Agent, Monoclonal Antibody

Use Treatment of HER2-positive metastatic breast cancer (in combination with trastuzumab and docetaxel) in patients who have not received prior anti-HER2 therapy or chemotherapy to treat metastatic disease

Labeled Contraindications There are no contraindications listed in the manufacturer's labeling.

Pregnancy Risk Factor D

Lactation Excretion in breast milk unknown/not recommended

Warnings/Precautions Hazardous agent. Use appropriate precautions for handling and disposal. Decreases in left ventricular ejection fraction (LVEF) are associated with HER-2 inhibitors, including pertuzumab. Patients who received prior anthracycline therapy or chest irradiation may be at an increased risk for cardiotoxicity. In studies of pertuzumab (versus placebo) in combination with trastuzumab and docetaxel, the rate of cardiotoxicity (LVEF decline or symptomatic LV systolic dysfunction) was not increased in the pertuzumab group when compared to placebo. However, patients with pretreatment LVEF ≤50%, CHF, LVEF decreases to <50% during prior trastuzumab treatment, or conditions which could impair LV function (eg, uncontrolled hypertension, recent MI, serious arrhythmia requiring treatment, or cumulative lifetime anthracycline exposure >360 mg/m^2 doxorubicin or its equivalent) were excluded from studies. Assess LVEF at baseline and every 3 months during treatment.

Withhold pertuzumab and trastuzumab if LVEF <40% **or** 40% to 45% with a 10% absolute decline from baseline; repeat LVEF assessment in ~3 weeks; discontinue if LVEF has not improved or has declined further (unless potential benefits outweigh risks).

Infusion reactions (either during or on the day of infusion) have been associated with pertuzumab; commonly described as fever, chills, fatigue, headache, weakness, myalgia, hypersensitivity, abnormal taste or vomiting. The incidence of hypersensitivity/anaphylaxis was slightly higher in the group receiving pertuzumab (compared to placebo) in combination with trastuzumab and docetaxel. Monitor for 1 hour after the first infusion and for 30 minutes after subsequent infusions. For significant infusion reactions, interrupt or slow infusion rate; for severe infusion reactions, consider permanently discontinuing. May cause fetal harm is administered during pregnancy. **[U.S. Boxed Warning]: Pertuzumab exposure during pregnancy may result in embryo-fetal mortality and birth defects. Oligohydramnios has been observed in animal reproduction studies. Advise patients of the risks and the need for effective contraception.** Verify pregnancy status prior to treatment initiation. Effective contraception should be used during therapy and for 6 months after treatment. Effects during pregnancy are likely to occur in any trimester. Establish HER2 status prior to treatment; has only been studied in patients with evidence of HER2 overexpression, either as 3+ IHC (Dako Herceptest™) or FISH amplification ratio ≥2 (Dako *HER*2 FISH pharmDx™ test).

Adverse Reactions Note: Reactions reported in combination therapy with trastuzumab and docetaxel unless otherwise noted.

>10%:

Central nervous system: Fatigue (38%), headache (21%), fever (19%; grades 3/4: 1%), dizziness (13%)

Dermatologic: Rash (34%; grades 3/4: <1%), pruritus (14%), dry skin (11%)

Gastrointestinal: Diarrhea (67%; grades 3/4: 8%), appetite decreased (29%), mucosal inflammation (28%), nausea (monotherapy 24%), stomatitis (19%), abnormal taste (18%), vomiting (monotherapy 15%), abdominal pain (monotherapy 12%)

Hematologic: Neutropenia (53%; grades 3/4: 49%), anemia (23%; grades 3/4: 3%), neutropenic fever (14%; grades 3/4: 13%)

Respiratory: Upper respiratory tract infection (17%; grades 3/4: <1%)

Miscellaneous: Infusion reactions (13%; grades 3/4: <1%), hypersensitivity reactions (10% to 11%; grades 3/4: 2%)

1% to 10%:

Dermatologic: Paronychia (7%)

Gastrointestinal: Anorexia (monotherapy 5%)

<1% and/or case reports with combination therapy: Alopecia, arthralgia, dyspnea, heart failure, insomnia, left ventricular ejection fraction decreased, myalgia, peripheral edema, leukopenia, peripheral neuropathy, pleural effusion, sepsis

Drug Interactions

Metabolism/Transport Effects None known.

Avoid Concomitant Use

Avoid concomitant use of Pertuzumab with any of the following: Belimumab

Increased Effect/Toxicity

Pertuzumab may increase the levels/effects of: Belimumab

The levels/effects of Pertuzumab may be increased by: Abciximab

Decreased Effect There are no known significant interactions involving a decrease in effect.

Storage/Stability Store intact vials refrigerated at 2°C to 8°C (36°F to 46°F); do not freeze. Protect from light. Do not shake. Use immediately after preparation for infusion; if not used immediately, may be stored for up to 24 hours refrigerated at 2°C to 8°C (36°F to 46°F).

Reconstitution Dilute in 250 mL NS only (do not use dextrose 5% solutions) in PVC or non-PVC (polyolefin) bags. Gently invert to mix; do not shake. Do not mix with other medications.

Mechanism of Action Pertuzumab is a recombinant humanized monoclonal antibody which targets the extracellular human epidermal growth factor receptor 2 protein (HER2) dimerization domain. Inhibits HER2 dimerization and blocks HER downstream signaling halting cell growth and initiating apoptosis. Pertuzumab binds to a different HER2 epitope than trastuzumab so that when pertuzumab is combined with trastuzumab, a more complete inhibition of HER2 signaling occurs (Baselga, 2012).

Pharmacodynamics/Kinetics

Distribution: V_d: 5.12 L (Gianni, 2010)

Half-life elimination: Terminal: 18 days

Dosing

Adult & Geriatric Breast cancer, metastatic HER2+: I.V.: Initial: 840 mg over 60 minutes followed by a maintenance dose of 420 mg over 30-60 minutes every 3 weeks until disease progression or unacceptable toxicity (in combination with trastuzumab and docetaxel) (Baselga, 2012)

Missed doses or delays: If <6 weeks has elapsed, administer the 420 mg maintenance dose; do not wait until the next planned dose. If ≥6 weeks has elapsed, readminister the 840 mg initial dose (over 60 minutes), and then follow with a maintenance dose of 420 mg (over 30-60 minutes) every 3 weeks.

Renal Impairment

Cl_{cr} ≥30 mL/minute: No dosage adjustment necessary.

Cl_{cr} <30 mL/minute: No dosage adjustment provided in the manufacturer's labeling (has not been studied).

Hepatic Impairment No dosage adjustment provided in the manufacturer's labeling (has not been studied).

Adjustment for Toxicity Note: Dose reductions are not recommended for pertuzumab; if trastuzumab is withheld, pertuzumab should also be withheld, pertuzumab and trastuzumab may be continued if docetaxel is discontinued.

Infusion-related reaction: Slow or interrupt the infusion

Serious hypersensitivity: Discontinue immediately

Cardiotoxicity: Left ventricular ejection fraction (LVEF) declines to <40% **or** LVEF between 40% to 45% with ≥10% absolute decrease from pretreatment values: Withhold treatment (pertuzumab and trastuzumab) for at least 3 weeks; may resume if LVEF returns to >45% **or** to 40% to 45% with <10% absolute decrease below pretreatment values. If after a repeat assessment within ~3 weeks, LVEF has not improved (or has declined further), consider discontinuing pertuzumab and trastuzumab (unless the benefit of treatment outweighs risks).

Combination Regimens

Breast cancer: Docetaxel-Pertuzumab-Trastuzumab (Breast) on page 1614

Administration For I.V. infusion only, as a short infusion; infuse initial dose (840 mg) over 60 minutes; infuse maintenance dose (420 mg) over 30-60 minutes. Do not administer I.V. push or as a rapid bolus. Do not mix with other medications.

Monitoring Parameters HER2 expression (either as 3+ IHC [Dako HercepTest™] or FISH amplification ratio ≥2 [Dako *HER*2 FISH pharmDx™ test]); pregnancy test; assess LVEF at baseline and every 3 months during treatment (more frequently for declines); monitor for infusion reaction and hypersensitivity

Dosage Forms Excipient information presented when available (limited, particularly for generics); consult specific product labeling.

Injection, solution [preservative free]:

Perjeta™: 30 mg/mL (14 mL) [contains sucrose 120 mM/vial; derived from or manufactured using Chinese hamster ovary cells]

References

Baselga J, Cortés J, Kim SB, et al, "Pertuzumab Plus Trastuzumab Plus Docetaxel for Metastatic Breast Cancer," *N Engl J Med*, 2012, 366(2):109-19.

Baselga J and Swain SM, "CLEOPATRA: A Phase III Evaluation of Pertuzumab and Trastuzumab for HER2-Positive Metastatic Breast Cancer," *Clin Breast Cancer*, 2010, 10(6):489-91.

Gianni L, Lladó A, Bianchi G, et al, "Open-Label, Phase II, Multicenter, Randomized Study of the Efficacy and Safety of Two Dose Levels of Pertuzumab, a Human Epidermal Growth Factor Receptor 2 Dimerization Inhibitor, in Patients With Human Epidermal Growth Factor Receptor 2-Negative Metastatic Breast Cancer," *J Clin Oncol*, 2010, 28(7):1131-7.

Gianni L, Pienkowski T, Im YH, et al, "Efficacy and Safety of Neoadjuvant Pertuzumab and Trastuzumab in Women With Locally Advanced, Inflammatory, or Early HER2-Positive Breast Cancer (Neosphere): A Randomised Multicentre, Open-Label, Phase 2 Trial," *Lancet Oncol*, 2012, 13(1):25-32.

Portera CC, Walshe JM, Rosing DR, et al, "Cardiac Toxicity and Efficacy of Trastuzumab Combined With Pertuzumab in Patients With [Corrected] Human Epidermal Growth Factor Receptor 2-Positive Metastatic Breast Cancer," *Clin Cancer Res*, 2008, 14(9):2710-6.

◆ **Pethidine Hydrochloride** *see* Meperidine *on page* *932*

◆ **PF-02341066** *see* Crizotinib *on page* *317*

◆ **PFA** *see* Foscarnet *on page* *646*

◆ **Pharmorubicin® (Can)** *see* Epirubicin *on page* *510*

◆ **Phenadoz®** *see* Promethazine *on page* *1218*

◆ **Phenergan** *see* Promethazine *on page* *1218*

◆ **Phenylalanine Mustard** *see* Melphalan *on page* *925*

◆ **PHL-Bicalutamide (Can)** *see* Bicalutamide *on page* *178*

◆ **PHL-Ciprofloxacin (Can)** *see* Ciprofloxacin (Systemic) *on page* *283*

◆ **PHL-Dexamethasone (Can)** *see* Dexamethasone (Systemic) *on page* *440*

◆ **PHL-Fluconazole (Can)** *see* Fluconazole *on page* *612*

◆ **PHL-Lorazepam (Can)** *see* LORazepam *on page* *907*

◆ **PHL-Olanzapine (Can)** *see* OLANZapine *on page* *1056*

◆ **PHL-Olanzapine ODT (Can)** *see* OLANZapine *on page* *1056*

◆ **PHL-Ondansetron (Can)** *see* Ondansetron *on page* *1068*

◆ **PHL-Valacyclovir (Can)** *see* Valacyclovir *on page* *1420*

◆ **Phosphocol® P 32** *see* Chromic Phosphate P 32 *on page* *279*

◆ **Phosphonoformate** *see* Foscarnet *on page* *646*

◆ **Phosphonoformic Acid** *see* Foscarnet *on page* *646*

◆ **Phosphorus p32** *see* Chromic Phosphate P 32 *on page 279*
◆ **Photofrin®** *see* Porfimer *on page 1183*
◆ **Phylloquinone** *see* Phytonadione *on page 1169*
◆ **Phytomenadione** *see* Phytonadione *on page 1169*

Phytonadione (fye toe na DYE one)

Brand Names: U.S. Mephyton®

Brand Names: Canada AquaMEPHYTON®; Konakion; Mephyton®

Index Terms Methylphytyl Napthoquinone; Phylloquinone; Phytomenadione; Vitamin K; Vitamin K_1

Generic Availability (U.S.) Yes

Pharmacologic Category Vitamin, Fat Soluble

Use Prevention and treatment of hypoprothrombinemia caused by vitamin K antagonist (VKA)-induced (eg, warfarin-induced) or other drug-induced vitamin K deficiency, altered activity, or altered metabolism; hypoprothrombinemia caused by malabsorption or inability to synthesize vitamin K; prophylaxis and treatment of hemorrhagic disease of the newborn

Unlabeled Use Treatment of hypoprothrombinemia caused by long-acting anticoagulant rodenticides (LAARs)

Labeled Contraindications Hypersensitivity to phytonadione or any component of the formulation

Pregnancy Risk Factor C

Lactation Enters breast milk/use caution (AAP rates "compatible"; AAP 2001 update pending)

Warnings/Precautions [U.S. Boxed Warning]: Severe reactions resembling hypersensitivity reactions (eg, anaphylaxis) have occurred rarely during or immediately after I.V. administration (even with proper dilution and rate of administration); some patients had no previous exposure to phytonadione. Anaphylactoid reactions typically occurred when patients received large I.V. doses administered rapidly with formulations containing polyethoxylated castor oil; proper dosing, dilution, and administration will minimize risk (Ageno, 2012; Riegert-Johnson, 2002). Limit I.V. administration to situations where an alternative route of administration is not feasible and the benefit of therapy outweighs the risk of hypersensitivity reactions. Allergic reactions have also occurred with I.M. and SubQ injections, albeit less frequently. In obstructive jaundice or with biliary fistulas concurrent administration of bile salts is necessary. Manufacturers recommend the SubQ route over other parenteral routes. SubQ is less predictable when compared to the oral route. The American College of Chest Physicians recommends the I.V. route in patients with major bleeding secondary to warfarin. The I.V. route should be restricted to emergency situations where oral phytonadione cannot be used. Efficacy is delayed regardless of route of administration; patient management may require other treatments in the interim. In patients receiving a therapeutic vitamin K antagonist (VKA) (eg, warfarin), administer a dose of phytonadione that will quickly lower the INR into a safe range without causing resistance to warfarin. High phytonadione doses may lead to warfarin resistance for at least one week. Patients with LAAR-induced coagulopathy require much larger doses and longer treatment durations (up to months) after exposure compared to that needed to reverse VKA-induced coagulopathy. Use caution in newborns especially premature infants; hemolysis, jaundice and hyperbilirubinemia have been reported with larger than recommended doses. Some dosage forms contain benzyl alcohol which has been associated with "gasping syndrome" in premature infants. In liver disease, if initial doses do not reverse coagulopathy then higher doses are unlikely to have any effect. Ineffective in hereditary hypoprothrombinemia. Injectable products may contain aluminum; may result in toxic levels following prolonged administration. Product may contain polysorbate 80. Some dosage forms contain Cremophor® EL which has been associated with anaphylactoid reactions; use these formulations with caution.

Adverse Reactions Frequency not defined.

Cardiovascular: Cyanosis, flushing, hyper-/hypotension

Central nervous system: Dizziness

Dermatologic: Erythematous skin eruptions, pruritus, scleroderma-like lesions

Endocrine & metabolic: Hyperbilirubinemia (newborn; greater than recommended doses)

Gastrointestinal: Abnormal taste

Local: Injection site reactions

Respiratory: Dyspnea

Miscellaneous: Diaphoresis, hypersensitivity reactions, nonimmunologic anaphylaxis (formerly known as anaphylactoid reaction), sweating

Drug Interactions

Metabolism/Transport Effects None known.

Avoid Concomitant Use There are no known interactions where it is recommended to avoid concomitant use.

Increased Effect/Toxicity There are no known significant interactions involving an increase in effect.

Decreased Effect

Phytonadione may decrease the levels/effects of: Vitamin K Antagonists

The levels/effects of Phytonadione may be decreased by: Mineral Oil; Orlistat

Storage/Stability

Injection: Store at 15°C to 30°C (59°F to 86°F). Protect from light. **Note:** Store Hospira product at 20°C to 25°C (68°F to 77°F).

Oral: Store tablets at 15°C to 30°C (59°F to 86°F). Protect from light.

Reconstitution Dilute injection solution in preservative-free NS, D_5W, or D_5NS. To reduce the incidence of anaphylactoid reaction upon I.V. administration, dilute dose in a minimum of 50 mL of compatible solution and administer using an infusion pump over at least 20 minutes (Ageno, 2012).

Mechanism of Action Promotes liver synthesis of clotting factors (II, VII, IX, X); however, the exact mechanism as to this stimulation is unknown. Menadiol is a water soluble form of vitamin K; phytonadione has a more rapid and prolonged effect than menadione; menadiol sodium diphosphate (K_4) is half as potent as menadione (K_3).

Pharmacodynamics/Kinetics

Onset of action: Increased coagulation factors: Oral: 6-10 hours; I.V.: 1-2 hours

Peak effect: INR values return to normal: Oral: 24-48 hours; I.V.: 12-14 hours

Absorption: Oral: From intestines in presence of bile; SubQ: Variable

Metabolism: Rapidly hepatic

Excretion: Urine and feces

Dosing

Adult & Geriatric Note: According to the manufacturer, SubQ is the preferred parenteral route; I.M. route should be avoided due to the risk of hematoma formation; I.V. route should be restricted for emergency use only. The American College of Chest Physicians (ACCP) recommends the I.V.

route in patients with major bleeding secondary to use of vitamin K antagonists (VKAs).

Adequate intake (AI): Oral: Males: 120 **mcg**/day; Females: 90 **mcg**/day

Hypoprothrombinemia due to drugs (other than coumarin derivatives) or factors limiting absorption or synthesis: Oral, SubQ, I.M., I.V.: Initial: 2.5-25 mg (rarely up to 50 mg)

Vitamin K deficiency (supratherapeutic INR) secondary to VKAs (eg, warfarin) (unlabeled dose):

If INR above therapeutic range to <4.5 (no evidence of bleeding): Lower or hold next VKA dose and monitor frequently; when INR approaches desired range, resume VKA dosing with a lower dose (Patriquin, 2011).

If INR 4.5-10 (no evidence of bleeding): The 2012 ACCP guidelines recommend against routine phytonadione (aka, vitamin K) administration in this setting (Guyatt, 2012). Previously, the 2008 ACCP guidelines recommended if no risk factors for bleeding exist, to omit next 1 or 2 VKA doses, monitor INR more frequently, and resume with an appropriately adjusted VKA dose when INR in desired range; may consider administering vitamin K orally 1-2.5 mg if other risk factors for bleeding exist (Hirsh, 2008). Others have recommended consideration of vitamin K 1 mg orally or 0.5 mg I.V. (Patriquin, 2011).

If INR >10 (no evidence of bleeding): The 2012 ACCP guidelines recommend administration of oral vitamin K (dose not specified) in this setting (Guyatt, 2012). Previously, the 2008 ACCP guidelines recommended to hold warfarin, administer vitamin K orally 2.5-5 mg, expect INR to be reduced within 24-48 hours, monitor INR more frequently and give additional vitamin K at an appropriate dose if necessary; resume warfarin at an appropriately adjusted dose when INR is in desired range (Hirsh, 2008). Others have recommended consideration of vitamin K 2-2.5 mg orally or 0.5-1 mg I.V. (Patriquin, 2011).

If minor bleeding at any INR elevation: Hold warfarin, may administer vitamin K orally 2.5-5 mg, monitor INR more frequently, may repeat dose after 24 hours if INR correction incomplete; resume warfarin at an appropriately adjusted dose when INR is in desired range (Patriquin, 2011).

If major bleeding at any INR elevation: The 2012 ACCP guidelines recommend administration of four-factor prothrombin complex concentrate (PCC) and I.V. vitamin K 5-10 mg in this setting (Guyatt, 2012); however, in the U.S., the available PCCs (Bebulin®VH and Profilnine® SD) are **three**-factor PCCs and do not contain adequate levels of factor VII. Four-factor PCCs include Beriplex® P/N, Cofact®, Konyne®, or Octaplex® all of which **are not** available in the U.S. Previously, the 2008 ACCP guidelines recommended to hold warfarin, administer vitamin K 10 mg by slow I.V. infusion and supplement with PCC depending on the urgency of the situation; I.V. vitamin K may be repeated every 12 hours (Hirsh, 2008).

Note: Use of high doses of vitamin K (eg, 10-15 mg) may cause warfarin resistance for ≥1 week. During this period of resistance, heparin or low-molecular-weight heparin (LMWH) may be given until INR responds (Ansell, 2008).

Preprocedural/surgical INR normalization in patients receiving warfarin (routine use): Oral: 1-2.5 mg once administered on the day before surgery; recheck INR on day of procedure/surgery (Douketis, 2012). Others have recommended the use of vitamin K 1 mg orally for mild INR elevations (ie, INR 3.0-4.5) (Patriquin, 2011).

Pediatric Note: According to the manufacturer, SubQ is the preferred parenteral route; I.M. route should be avoided due to the risk of hematoma formation; I.V. route should be restricted for emergency use only. The American College of Chest Physicians (ACCP) recommends the I.V. route in patients with major bleeding secondary to use of vitamin K antagonists (VKAs).

Adequate intake (AI): Oral:

Infants:

0-6 months: 2 **mcg**/day

7-12 months: 2.5 **mcg**/day

Children:

1-3 years: 30 **mcg**/day

4-8 years: 55 **mcg**/day

9-13 years: 60 **mcg**/day

14-18 years: 75 **mcg**/day

Hemorrhagic disease of the newborn:

Prophylaxis: I.M.: 0.5-1 mg within 1 hour of birth

Treatment: I.M., SubQ: 1 mg/dose/day; higher doses may be necessary if mother has been receiving oral anticoagulants

Vitamin K deficiency (supratherapeutic INR) secondary to vitamin K antagonists (VKAs) (eg, warfarin) (unlabeled use): Infants and Children: *Excessively prolonged INR (usually INR >8; no significant bleeding):* **Note:** Limited data available: I.V.: 0.03 mg/kg/dose; maximum dose: 1 mg (Bolton-Maggs, 2002); if significant bleeding, consider use of fresh frozen plasma, prothrombin complex concentrates, or recombinant factor VIIa (Monagle, 2012).

Administration

I.V. administration: Infuse slowly; rate of infusion should not exceed 1 mg/minute (3 mg/m^2/minute in children and infants). Alternatively, dilute dose in a minimum of 50 mL of compatible solution and administer using an infusion pump over at least 20 minutes (Ageno, 2012). The injectable route should be used only if the oral route is not feasible or there is a greater urgency to reverse anticoagulation.

Oral: The parenteral formulation may also be used for small oral doses (eg, 1 mg) or situations in which tablets cannot be swallowed (Crowther, 2000; O'Connor, 1986).

Extemporaneous Preparations A 1 mg/mL oral suspension may be made with tablets. Crush six 5 mg tablets in a mortar and reduce to a fine powder. Add 5 mL each of water and methylcellulose 1% and mix to a uniform paste. Mix while adding sorbitol in incremental proportions to **almost** 30 mL; transfer to a calibrated bottle, rinse mortar with sorbitol, and add quantity of sorbitol sufficient to make 30 mL. Label "shake well" and "refrigerate". Stable for 3 days.

Nahata MC and Hipple TF, *Pediatric Drug Formulations*, 3rd ed, Cincinnati, OH: Harvey Whitney Books Co, 1997.

Note: The parenteral formulation may also be used for small oral doses (eg, 1 mg) or situations in which tablets cannot be swallowed (Crowther, 2000; O'Connor, 1986).

Monitoring Parameters PT, INR

Dosage Forms Excipient information presented when available (limited, particularly for generics); consult specific product labeling.

Injection, aqueous colloidal: 1 mg/0.5 mL (0.5 mL) [contains benzyl alcohol, polyoxyethylated castor oil]; 10 mg/mL (1 mL) [contains benzyl alcohol, polyoxyethylated castor oil]

Injection, aqueous colloidal [preservative free]: 1 mg/0.5 mL (0.5 mL) [contains polysorbate 80, propylene glycol 10.4 mg/0.5 mL]

Tablet, oral: 100 mcg

Mephyton®: 5 mg [scored]

References

Ansell J, Hirsh J, Hylek E, et al, "Pharmacology and Management of the Vitamin K Antagonists: American College of Chest Physicians Evidence-Based Clinical Practice Guidelines (8th Edition)," *Chest*, 2008, 133(6 Suppl):160-98.

Broderick J, Connolly S, Feldmann E, et al, "Guidelines for the Management of Spontaneous Intracerebral Hemorrhage in Adults: 2007 Update: A Guideline From the American Heart Association/American Stroke Association Stroke Council, High Blood Pressure Research Council, and the Quality of Care and Outcomes in Research Interdisciplinary Working Group," *Stroke*, 2007, 38(6):2001-23.

Crowther MA, Douketis JD, Schnurr T, et al, "Oral Vitamin K Lowers the International Normalized Ratio More Rapidly Than Subcutaneous Vitamin K in the Treatment of Warfarin-Associated Coagulopathy. A Randomized, Controlled Trial," *Ann Intern Med*, 2002, 137(4):251-4.

Crowther MA, Julian J, McCarty D, et al, "Treatment of Warfarin-associated Coagulopathy With Oral Vitamin K: A Randomised Controlled Trial", *Lancet*, 2000, 356(9241):1551-3.

Douketis JD, Spyropoulos AC, Spencer FA, et al, "Perioperative Management of Antithrombotic Therapy: Antithrombotic Therapy and Prevention of Thrombosis, 9th ed: American College of Chest Physicians Evidence-Based Clinical Practice Guidelines," *Chest*, 2012, 141(2 Suppl):326-50.

Hirsh J, Guyatt G, Albers GW, et al, "Executive Summary: American College of Chest Physicians Evidence-Based Clinical Practice Guidelines (8th Edition)," *Chest*, 2008, 133(6 Suppl):71-109.

Monagle P, Chan A, Goldenberg NA, et al, "Antithrombotic Therapy in Neonates and Children: American College of Chest Physicians Evidence-Based Clinical Practice Guidelines (9th Edition)," *Chest*, 2012, 141(2 Suppl):e737-801.

O'Connor ME and Addiego JE, "Use of Oral Vitamin K1 to Prevent Hemorrhagic Disease of the Newborn Infant," *J Pediatr*, 1986, 108(4):616-9.

Patriquin C and Crowther M, "Treatment of Warfarin-associated Coagulopathy With Vitamin K," *Expert Rev Hematol*, 2011, 4(6):657-67.

◆ **Picato®** *see* Ingenol Mebutate *on page 796*

◆ **Pidorubicin** *see* Epirubicin *on page 510*

◆ **Pidorubicin Hydrochloride** *see* Epirubicin *on page 510*

Pilocarpine (Systemic) (pye loe KAR peen)

Related Information

Oral Mucositis/Stomatitis *on page 1814*

Brand Names: U.S. Salagen®

Brand Names: Canada Salagen®

Index Terms Pilocarpine Hydrochloride

Generic Availability (U.S.) Yes

Pharmacologic Category Cholinergic Agonist

Use Symptomatic treatment of xerostomia caused by salivary gland hypofunction resulting from radiotherapy for cancer of the head and neck or Sjögren's syndrome

Labeled Contraindications Hypersensitivity to pilocarpine or any component of the formulation; uncontrolled asthma; angle-closure glaucoma, severe hepatic impairment

Pregnancy Risk Factor C

Lactation Excretion in breast milk unknown/not recommended

Warnings/Precautions Use caution with cardiovascular disease; patients may have difficulty compensating for transient changes in hemodynamics or rhythm induced by pilocarpine. Use caution with controlled asthma, chronic bronchitis, or COPD; may increase airway resistance, bronchial smooth muscle tone, and bronchial secretions. Use caution with cholelithiasis, biliary tract disease, and nephrolithiasis; adjust dose with moderate hepatic impairment.

Adverse Reactions

>10%:

Cardiovascular: Flushing (8% to 13%)

Central nervous system: Chills (3% to 15%), dizziness (5% to 12%), headache (11%)

Gastrointestinal: Nausea (6% to 15%)

Genitourinary: Urinary frequency (9% to 12%)

Neuromuscular & skeletal: Weakness (2% to 12%)

Respiratory: Rhinitis (5% to 14%)

Miscellaneous: Diaphoresis (29% to 68%)

1% to 10%:

Cardiovascular: Edema (<1% to 5%), facial edema, hypertension (3%), palpitation, tachycardia

Central nervous system: Pain (4%), fever, somnolence

Dermatologic: Pruritus, rash

Gastrointestinal: Diarrhea (4% to 7%), dyspepsia (7%), vomiting (3% to 4%), constipation, flatulence, glossitis, salivation increased, stomatitis, taste perversion

Genitourinary: Vaginitis, urinary incontinence

Neuromuscular & skeletal: Myalgias, tremor

Ocular: Lacrimation (6%), amblyopia (4%), abnormal vision, blurred vision, conjunctivitis

Otic: Tinnitus

Respiratory: Cough increased, dysphagia, epistaxis, sinusitis

Miscellaneous: Allergic reaction, voice alteration

<1%: Abnormal dreams, abnormal thinking, alopecia, angina pectoris, anorexia, anxiety, aphasia, appetite increased, arrhythmia, arthralgia, arthritis, bilirubinemia, body odor, bone disorder, bradycardia, breast pain, bronchitis, cataract, cholelithiasis, colitis, confusion, contact dermatitis, cyst, deafness, depression, dry eyes, dry mouth, dry skin, dyspnea, dysuria, ear pain, ECG abnormality, eczema, emotional lability, eructation, erythema nodosum, esophagitis, exfoliative dermatitis, eye hemorrhage, eye pain, gastritis, gastroenteritis, gastrointestinal disorder, gingivitis, glaucoma, hematuria, hepatitis, herpes simplex, hiccup, hyperkinesias, hypoesthesia, hypoglycemia, hypotension, hypothermia, insomnia, intracranial hemorrhage, laryngismus, laryngitis, leg cramps, leukopenia, liver function test abnormal, lymphadenopathy, mastitis, melena, menorrhagia, metrorrhagia, migraine, moniliasis, myasthenia, MI, neck pain, photosensitivity reaction, nervousness, ovarian disorder, pancreatitis, paresthesia, parotid gland enlargement, peripheral edema, platelet abnormality, pneumonia, pyuria, salivary gland enlargement, salpingitis, seborrhea, skin ulcer, speech disorder, sputum increased, stridor, syncope, taste loss, tendon disorder, tenosynovitis, thrombocythemia, thrombocytopenia, thrombosis, tongue disorder, twitching, urethral pain, urinary impairment, urinary urgency, vaginal hemorrhage, vaginal moniliasis, vesiculobullous rash, WBC abnormality, yawning

Drug Interactions

Metabolism/Transport Effects Inhibits CYP2A6 (weak), CYP2E1 (weak), CYP3A4 (weak)

Avoid Concomitant Use

Avoid concomitant use of Pilocarpine (Systemic) with any of the following: Pimozide

Increased Effect/Toxicity

Pilocarpine (Systemic) may increase the levels/effects of: ARIPiprazole; Pimozide

The levels/effects of Pilocarpine (Systemic) may be increased by: Acetylcholinesterase Inhibitors; Beta-Blockers

Decreased Effect There are no known significant interactions involving a decrease in effect.

Ethanol/Nutrition/Herb Interactions Food: Avoid administering with high-fat meal; fat decreases the rate of absorption, maximum concentration and increases the time it takes to reach maximum concentration.

Storage/Stability Store at controlled room temperature of 15°C to 30°C (59°F to 86°F).

Pharmacodynamics/Kinetics

Onset of action: 20 minutes

Duration: 3-5 hours

Half-life elimination: 0.76-1.35 hours; increased with hepatic impairment

Excretion: Urine

Dosing

Adult & Geriatric Xerostomia: Oral:

Following head and neck cancer: 5 mg 3 times/day, titration up to 10 mg 3 times/day may be considered for patients who have not responded adequately; do not exceed 2 tablets/dose

Sjogren's syndrome: 5 mg 4 times/day

Hepatic Impairment

Moderate impairment: 5 mg 2 times/day regardless of indication; adjust dose based on response and tolerability

Severe impairment (Child-Pugh score >10): Contraindicated

Administration Avoid administering with high-fat meal.

Monitoring Parameters Intraocular pressure, funduscopic exam, visual field testing

Dietary Considerations Avoid taking with a high-fat meal.

Dosage Forms Excipient information presented when available (limited, particularly for generics); consult specific product labeling.

Tablet, oral, as hydrochloride: 5 mg, 7.5 mg

Salagen®: 5 mg, 7.5 mg

References

Hawthorne M and Sullivan K, "Pilocarpine for Radiation-Induced Xerostomia in Head and Neck Cancer," *Int J Palliat Nurs*, 2000, 6(5):228-32.

Jacobs CD and van der Pas M, "A Multicenter Maintenance Study of Oral Pilocarpine Tablets for Radiation-Induced Xerostomia," *Oncology*, 1996, 10(3 Suppl):16-20.

◆ **Pilocarpine Hydrochloride** *see* Pilocarpine (Systemic) *on page* 1173

Piperacillin and Tazobactam (pi PER a sil in & ta zoe BAK tam)

Brand Names: U.S. Zosyn®

Brand Names: Canada AJ-PIP/TAZ; Piperacillin and Tazobactam for Injection; Tazocin®

Index Terms Piperacillin and Tazobactam Sodium; Piperacillin Sodium and Tazobactam Sodium; Tazobactam and Piperacillin

Generic Availability (U.S.) Yes: Excludes infusion

Pharmacologic Category Antibiotic, Penicillin

Use Treatment of moderate-to-severe infections caused by susceptible organisms, including infections of the lower respiratory tract (community-acquired pneumonia, nosocomial pneumonia); uncomplicated and complicated skin and skin structures (including diabetic foot infections); gynecologic (endometritis, pelvic inflammatory disease); and intra-abdominal infections (appendicitis with rupture/abscess, peritonitis). Tazobactam expands activity of piperacillin to include beta-lactamase producing strains of *S. aureus*, *H. influenzae*, *E. coli*, *Bacteroides* spp, and other gram-positive and gram-negative aerobic and anaerobic bacteria.

Unlabeled Use Treatment of moderate-to-severe infections caused by susceptible organisms, including urinary tract infections, bone and joint infections, septicemia, endocarditis, and cystic fibrosis exacerbations

Labeled Contraindications Hypersensitivity to penicillins, cephalosporins, beta-lactamase inhibitors, or any component of the formulation

Pregnancy Risk Factor B

Lactation Enters breast milk/use caution

Warnings/Precautions Serious and occasionally severe or fatal hypersensitivity (anaphylactic/anaphylactoid) reactions have been reported in patients on penicillin therapy, especially with a history of beta-lactam hypersensitivity, history of sensitivity to multiple allergens, or previous IgE-mediated reactions (eg, anaphylaxis, angioedema, urticaria). Bleeding disorders have been observed, particularly in patients with renal impairment; discontinue if thrombocytopenia or bleeding occurs. Due to sodium load and to the adverse effects of high serum concentrations of penicillins, dosage modification is required in patients with impaired or underdeveloped renal function; use with caution in patients with seizures or in patients with history of beta-lactam allergy; associated with an increased incidence of rash and fever in cystic fibrosis patients. Use may result in fungal or bacterial superinfection, including *C. difficile*-associated diarrhea (CDAD) and pseudomembranous colitis; CDAD has been observed >2 months postantibiotic treatment.

Storage/Stability

Vials: Store at controlled room temperature of 20°C to 25°C (68°F to 77°F). Use single-dose vials immediately after reconstitution (discard unused portions after 24 hours at room temperature and 48 hours if refrigerated). After reconstitution, vials or solution are stable in NS or D_5W for 24 hours at room temperature and 48 hours (vials) or 7 days (solution) when refrigerated.

Premixed solution: Store frozen at -20°C (-4°F). Thawed solution is stable for 24 hours at room temperature or 14 days under refrigeration; do not refreeze.

Reconstitution Reconstitute with 5 mL of diluent per 1 g of piperacillin and then further dilute.

Mechanism of Action Piperacillin inhibits bacterial cell wall synthesis by binding to one or more of the penicillin-binding proteins (PBPs); which in turn inhibits the final transpeptidation step of peptidoglycan synthesis in bacterial cell walls, thus inhibiting cell wall biosynthesis. Bacteria eventually lyse due to ongoing activity of cell wall autolytic enzymes (autolysins and murein hydrolases) while cell wall assembly is arrested. Piperacillin exhibits time-dependent killing. Tazobactam inhibits many beta-lactamases, including staphylococcal penicillinase and Richmond-Sykes types 2, 3, 4, and 5, including extended spectrum enzymes; it has only limited activity against class 1 beta-lactamases other than class 1C types.

Pharmacodynamics/Kinetics Both AUC and peak concentrations are dose proportional; hepatic impairment does not affect kinetics

Distribution: Well into lungs, intestinal mucosa, uterus, ovary, fallopian tube, interstitial fluid, gallbladder, and bile; penetration into CSF is low in subjects with noninflamed meninges

Protein binding: Piperacillin and tazobactam: ~30%

Metabolism:

Piperacillin: 6% to 9% to desethyl metabolite (weak activity)

Tazobactam: ~26% to inactive metabolite

Bioavailability:

Piperacillin: I.M.: 71%

Tazobactam: I.M.: 84%

Half-life elimination: Piperacillin and tazobactam: 0.7-1.2 hours (unaffected by dose or duration of infusion)

Time to peak, plasma: Immediately following completion of 30-minute infusion

Excretion: Clearance of both piperacillin and tazobactam are directly proportional to renal function

Piperacillin: Urine (68% as unchanged drug); feces (10% to 20%)

Tazobactam: Urine (80% as unchanged drug; remainder as inactive metabolite)

Dialysis: Hemodialysis removes 30% to 40% of a piperacillin/tazobactam dose; peritoneal dialysis removes 6% of piperacillin and 21% of tazobactam

Dosing

Adult & Geriatric Note: Dosing presented is based on traditional infusion method (I.V. infusion over 30 minutes) unless otherwise specified as the extended infusion method (I.V. infusion over 4 hours [unlabeled method]).

Usual dosage range: I.V.: 3.375 g every 6 hours **or** 4.5 g every 6-8 hours; maximum: 18 g/day

Extended infusion method (unlabeled dosing): 3.375-4.5 g I.V. over 4 hours every 8 hours (Kim, 2007; Shea, 2009); an alternative regimen of 4.5 g I.V. over 3 hours every 6 hours has also been described (Kim, 2007)

Indication-specific dosing: I.V.: **Note:** Dosing based on piperacillin component:

Diverticulitis, intra-abdominal abscess, peritonitis: I.V.: 3.375 g every 6 hours; **Note:** Some clinicians use 4.5 g every 8 hours for empiric coverage since the % time >MIC is similar between the regimens for most pathogens; however, this regimen is NOT recommended for nosocomial pneumonia or *Pseudomonas* coverage.

Intra-abdominal infection, complicated: I.V.: 3.375 g every 6 hours for 4-7 days (provided source controlled). **Note:** Increase to 3.375 g every 4 hours or 4.5 g every 6 hours if *P. aeruginosa* is suspected. Not recommended for mild to moderate, community-acquired intra-abdominal infections due to risk of toxicity and the development of resistant organisms (Solomkin, 2010).

Pneumonia (nosocomial): I.V.: 4.5 g every 6 hours for 7-14 days (when used empirically, combination with an aminoglycoside or antipseudomonal fluoroquinolone is recommended; consider discontinuation of additional agent if *P. aeruginosa* is not isolated)

Severe infections: I.V.: 3.375 g every 6 hours for 7-10 days; **Note:** Some clinicians use 4.5 g every 8 hours for empiric coverage since the % time >MIC is similar between the regimens for most pathogens; however, this regimen is NOT recommended for nosocomial pneumonia or *Pseudomonas* coverage.

Skin and soft tissue infection: I.V.: 3.375 g every 6-8 hours for 7-14 days. **Notes:** When used for necrotizing infection of skin, fascia, or muscle, combination with clindamycin and ciprofloxacin is recommended (Stevens, 2005); for severe diabetic foot infections, recommended treatment duration is up to 4 weeks depending on severity of infection and response to therapy (Lipsky, 2012).

Pediatric Note: Dosing presented is based on traditional infusion method (I.V. infusion over 30 minutes) unless otherwise specified as the extended infusion method (I.V. infusion over 4 hours [unlabeled method]).

Usual dosage range: Children: I.V.:

2-8 months: 80 mg of piperacillin component/kg every 8 hours

≥9 months and ≤40 kg: 100 mg of piperacillin component/kg every 8 hours

Indication-specific dosing: I.V.: **Note:** Dosing based on piperacillin component:

Appendicitis, peritonitis: Children:

2-8 months: 80 mg/kg every 8 hours

≥9 months and ≤40 kg: 100 mg/kg every 8 hours

>40 kg: refer to adult dosing

Cystic fibrosis, pseudomonal infections (unlabeled use): 350-450 mg/kg/day in divided doses

Intra-abdominal infection, complicated: 200-300 mg/kg/day divided every 6-8 hours

Renal Impairment

Traditional infusion method (ie, I.V. infusion over 30 minutes): Manufacturer's labeling:

Cl_{cr} >40 mL/minute: No dosage adjustment required.

Cl_{cr} 20-40 mL/minute: Administer 2.25 g every 6 hours (3.375 g every 6 hours for nosocomial pneumonia)

Cl_{cr} <20 mL/minute: Administer 2.25 g every 8 hours (2.25 g every 6 hours for nosocomial pneumonia)

Note: Some clinicians suggest adjusting the dose at Cl_{cr} ≤20 mL/minute (rather than Cl_{cr} <40 mL/minute) in patients receiving either traditional or extended-infusion methods, particularly if treating serious gram-negative infections (empirically or definitively) (Patel, 2010).

Extended infusion method (unlabeled dosing): Cl_{cr} ≤20 mL/minute: 3.375 g I.V. over 4 hours every 12 hours (Patel, 2010)

Intermittent hemodialysis (IHD)/peritoneal dialysis (PD): 2.25 g every 12 hours (2.25 g every 8 hours for nosocomial pneumonia). **Note:** Dosing dependent on the assumption of 3 times/week, complete IHD sessions. Administer scheduled doses after hemodialysis on dialysis days; if next regularly scheduled dose is not due right after dialysis session, administer an additional dose of 0.75 g after the dialysis session.

Continuous renal replacement therapy (CRRT) (Heintz, 2009; Trotman, 2005): Drug clearance is highly dependent on the method of renal replacement, filter type, and flow rate. Appropriate dosing requires close monitoring of pharmacologic response, signs of adverse reactions due to drug accumulation, as well as drug concentrations in relation to target trough (if appropriate). The following are general recommendations only (based on dialysate flow/ultrafiltration rates of 1-2 L/hour and minimal residual renal function) and should not supersede clinical judgment (Trotman, 2005):

CVVH: 2.25-3.375 g every 6-8 hours

CVVHD: 2.25-3.375 g every 6 hours

CVVHDF: 3.375 g every 6 hours

Note: Higher dose of 3.375 g should be considered when treating resistant pathogens (especially *Pseudomonas* spp); alternative recommendations suggest dosing of 4.5 g every 8 hours (Valtonen, 2001); regardless of regimen, there is some concern of tazobactam (TAZ) accumulation, given its lower clearance relative to piperacillin (PIP). Some clinicians advocate dosing with PIP to alternate with PIP/TAZ, particularly in CVVH-dependent patients, to lessen this concern.

Hepatic Impairment No dosage adjustment necessary.

Administration Administer by I.V. infusion over 30 minutes. For extended infusion administration (unlabeled dosing), administer over 3-4 hours (Kim 2007; Shea, 2009).

Some penicillins (eg, carbenicillin, ticarcillin, and piperacillin) have been shown to inactivate aminoglycosides *in vitro*. This has been observed to a greater extent with tobramycin and gentamicin, while amikacin has shown greater stability against inactivation. Concurrent use of these agents may pose a risk of reduced antibacterial efficacy *in vivo*, particularly in the setting of profound renal impairment. However, definitive clinical evidence is lacking. If combination penicillin/aminoglycoside therapy is desired in a patient with renal dysfunction, separation of doses (if feasible), and routine monitoring of aminoglycoside levels, CBC, and clinical response should be considered. **Note:** Reformulated Zosyn® containing EDTA (applies only to specific concentrations and diluents and varies by product; consult manufacturer's labeling) has been shown to be compatible *in vitro* for Y-site infusion with amikacin and gentamicin, but not compatible with tobramycin.

Test Interactions Positive Coombs' [direct] test; false positive reaction for urine glucose using copper-reduction method (Clinitest®); may result in false positive results with the Platelia® *Aspergillus* enzyme immunoassay (EIA)

Some penicillin derivatives may accelerate the degradation of aminoglycosides *in vitro*, leading to a potential underestimation of aminoglycoside serum concentration. **Note:** Reformulated Zosyn® containing EDTA (applies only to specific concentrations and diluents and varies by product; consult manufacturer's labeling) has been shown to be compatible *in vitro* for Y-site infusion with amikacin and gentamicin, but not compatible with tobramycin.

Dosage Forms Excipient information presented when available (limited, particularly for generics); consult specific product labeling.

Note: 8:1 ratio of piperacillin sodium/tazobactam sodium

Infusion [premixed iso-osmotic solution]:

Zosyn®: 2.25 g: Piperacillin 2 g and tazobactam 0.25 g (50 mL) [contains edetate disodium, sodium 128 mg (5.58 mEq)]

Zosyn®: 3.375 g: Piperacillin 3 g and tazobactam 0.375 g (50 mL) [contains edetate disodium, sodium 192 mg (8.38 mEq)]

Zosyn®: 4.5 g: Piperacillin 4 g and tazobactam 0.5 g (100 mL) [contains edetate disodium, sodium 256 mg (11.17 mEq)]

Injection, powder for reconstitution: 2.25 g: Piperacillin 2 g and tazobactam 0.25 g; 3.375 g: Piperacillin 3 g and tazobactam 0.375 g; 4.5 g: Piperacillin 4 g and tazobactam 0.5 g; 40.5 g: Piperacillin 36 g and tazobactam 4.5 g

Zosyn®: 2.25 g: Piperacillin 2 g and tazobactam 0.25 g [contains edetate disodium, sodium 128 mg (5.58 mEq)]

Zosyn®: 3.375 g: Piperacillin 3 g and tazobactam 0.375 g [contains edetate disodium, sodium 192 mg (8.38 mEq)]

Zosyn®: 4.5 g: Piperacillin 4 g and tazobactam 0.5 g [contains edetate disodium, sodium 256 mg (11.17 mEq)]

Zosyn®: 40.5 g: Piperacillin 36 g and tazobactam 4.5 g [contains edetate disodium, sodium 2304 mg (100.4 mEq); bulk pharmacy vial]

◆ **Piperacillin and Tazobactam for Injection (Can)** *see* Piperacillin and Tazobactam *on page 1175*

◆ **Piperacillin and Tazobactam Sodium** *see* Piperacillin and Tazobactam *on page 1175*

◆ **Piperacillin Sodium and Tazobactam Sodium** *see* Piperacillin and Tazobactam *on page 1175*

◆ **Platinol** *see* CISplatin *on page 290*

◆ **Platinol-AQ** *see* CISplatin *on page 290*

Plerixafor (pler IX a fore)

Related Information

Hematopoietic Stem Cell Transplantation *on page 1887*

Brand Names: U.S. Mozobil™

Index Terms AMD3100; LM3100

Generic Availability (U.S.) No

Pharmacologic Category Hematopoietic Stem Cell Mobilizer

Use Mobilization of hematopoietic stem cells (HSC) for collection and subsequent autologous transplantation (in combination with filgrastim) in patients with non-Hodgkin's lymphoma (NHL) and multiple myeloma (MM)

Labeled Contraindications There are no contraindications listed within the manufacturer's labeling.

Pregnancy Risk Factor D

Lactation Excretion in breast milk unknown/not recommended

Warnings/Precautions Hazardous agent - use appropriate precautions for handling and disposal. Increases circulating leukocytes when used in conjunction with filgrastim; monitor WBC; use with caution in patients with neutrophil count >50,000/mm^3. Thrombocytopenia has been observed with use; monitor platelet count. Not intended for mobilization in patients with leukemia; may contaminate apheresis product by mobilizing leukemic cells. When used in combination with filgrastim, tumor cells released from marrow could be collected in leukapheresis product; potential effect of tumor cell reinfusion is unknown. Splenomegaly and splenic rupture have been reported (rarely) with filgrastim use; instruct patients to report left upper quadrant pain or scapular/shoulder tip pain; promptly evaluate in any patient who report these symptoms.

Primary route of elimination is urinary; dosage reduction is recommended in patients with moderate-severe renal impairment (Cl_{cr} ≤50 mL/minute). Medications that may reduce renal function or compete for active tubular secretion may increase serum concentrations of plerixafor. Use has not been studied in patients weighing >175% of ideal body weight. Safety and efficacy have not been established in children.

Adverse Reactions Adverse reactions reported with filgrastim combination therapy.

>10%:

Central nervous system: Fatigue (27%), headache (22%), dizziness (11%)

Gastrointestinal: Diarrhea (37%), nausea (34%)

Local: Injection site reactions (34%, including erythema, hematoma, hemorrhage, induration, inflammation, irritation, pain, paresthesia, pruritus, rash, swelling, urticaria)

Neuromuscular & skeletal: Arthralgia (13%)

5% to 10%:

Central nervous system: Insomnia (7%)

Gastrointestinal: Vomiting (10%), flatulence (7%)

<5%, postmarketing, and/or case reports: Abdominal discomfort, abdominal distension, abdominal pain, constipation, diaphoresis, dyspepsia, dyspnea, erythema, hypesthesia (oral), hypoxia, leukocytes increased, malaise, musculoskeletal pain, orthostatic hypotension, periorbital swelling, syncope, thrombocytopenia, urticaria, vasovagal reaction, xerostomia

Drug Interactions

Metabolism/Transport Effects None known.

Avoid Concomitant Use There are no known interactions where it is recommended to avoid concomitant use.

Increased Effect/Toxicity There are no known significant interactions involving an increase in effect.

Decreased Effect There are no known significant interactions involving a decrease in effect.

Storage/Stability Use appropriate precautions for handling and disposal. Store at 25°C (77°F); excursions permitted to 15°C to 30°C (59°F to 86°F). The manufacturer recommends discarding unused drug remaining in the vial after use.

Mechanism of Action Reversibly inhibits binding of stromal cell-derived factor-1-alpha (SDF-1α), expressed on bone marrow stromal cells, to the CXC chemokine receptor 4 (CXCR4), resulting in mobilization of hematopoietic stem and progenitor cells from bone marrow into peripheral blood. Plerixafor used in combination with filgrastim results in synergistic increase in CD34+ cell mobilization. Mobilized CD34+ cells are capable of engrafting with extended repopulating capacity.

Pharmacodynamics/Kinetics

Onset of action: Peak CD34+ mobilization: Plerixafor monotherapy: 6-9 hours after administration; Plerixafor + filgrastim: 10-14 hours

Duration: WBC counts return toward baseline at ~24 after administration

Absorption: SubQ: Rapid

Distribution: 0.3 L/kg; primarily to extravascular fluid space

Protein binding: ≤58%

Metabolism: Not metabolized

Half-life elimination: Terminal: 3-6 hours

Time to peak, plasma: SubQ: 30-60 minutes

Excretion: Urine (~70%; as parent drug)

Dosing

Adult & Geriatric Note: Dosing is based on actual body weight. Begin plerixafor after patient has received filgrastim 10 mcg/kg once daily for 4 days; plerixafor, filgrastim, and apheresis should be continued daily until sufficient cell collection up to a maximum of 4 days.

HSC mobilization: SubQ: 0.24 mg/kg once daily ~11 hours prior to apheresis for up to 4 consecutive days; maximum dose: 40 mg/day

Renal Impairment

Cl_{cr} >50 mL/minute: No adjustment required.

Cl_{cr} ≤50 mL/minute: 0.16 mg/kg; maximum dose: 27 mg/day.

Hemodialysis: Insufficient information for dosing recommendation

Administration Administer subcutaneously, ~11 hours prior to initiation of apheresis. In some clinical trials, plerixafor administration began in the evening prior to apheresis. (filgrastim was begun on day 1, plerixafor initiated in the evening on day 4 and apheresis in the morning on day 5; with filgrastim, plerixafor and apheresis then continued daily until sufficient cell collection for autologous transplant.)

Monitoring Parameters CBC with differential and platelets

Dosage Forms Excipient information presented when available (limited, particularly for generics); consult specific product labeling.

Injection, solution [preservative free]:

Mozobil™: 20 mg/mL (1.2 mL)

References

Calandra G, McCarty J, McGuirk J, et al, "AMD3100 Plus G-CSF Can Successfully Mobilize CD34+ Cells From Non-Hodgkin's Lymphoma, Hodgkin's Disease and Multiple Myeloma Patients Previously Failing Mobilization With Chemotherapy and/or Cytokine Treatment: Compassionate Use Data," *Bone Marrow Transplant*, 2008, 41(4):331-8.

Cashen A, Lopez S, Gao F, et al, "A Phase II Study of Plerixafor (AMD3100) Plus G-CSF for Autologous Hematopoietic Progenitor Cell Mobilization in Patients With Hodgkin Lymphoma," *Biol Blood Marrow Transplant*, 2008, 14(11):1253-61.

Devine SM, Flomenberg N, Vesole DH, et al, "Rapid Mobilization of CD34+ Cells Following Administration of the CXCR4 Antagonist AMD3100 to Patients With Multiple Myeloma and Non-Hodgkin's Lymphoma," *J Clin Oncol*, 2004, 22(6):1095-102.

Flomenberg N, Devine SM, DiPersio JF, et al, "The Use of AMD3100 Plus G-CSF for Autologous Hematopoietic Progenitor Cell Mobilization is Superior to G-CSF Alone," *Blood*, 2005, 106 (5):1867-74.

◆ **PLX4032** *see* Vemurafenib *on page* 1440
◆ **PMS-Anagrelide (Can)** *see* Anagrelide *on page* 93
◆ **PMS-Anastrozole (Can)** *see* Anastrozole *on page* 96
◆ **PMS-Benzydamine (Can)** *see* Benzydamine *on page* 164
◆ **PMS-Bicalutamide (Can)** *see* Bicalutamide *on page* 178
◆ **PMS-Ciprofloxacin (Can)** *see* Ciprofloxacin (Systemic) *on page* 283
◆ **PMS-Codeine (Can)** *see* Codeine *on page* 311
◆ **PMS-Cyproheptadine (Can)** *see* Cyproheptadine *on page* 342
◆ **PMS-Deferoxamine (Can)** *see* Deferoxamine *on page* 414
◆ **PMS-Desmopressin (Can)** *see* Desmopressin *on page* 434
◆ **PMS-Dexamethasone (Can)** *see* Dexamethasone (Systemic) *on page* 440
◆ **PMS-Famciclovir (Can)** *see* Famciclovir *on page* 580
◆ **PMS-Fentanyl MTX (Can)** *see* FentaNYL *on page* 583
◆ **PMS-Fluconazole (Can)** *see* Fluconazole *on page* 612
◆ **PMS-Flutamide (Can)** *see* Flutamide *on page* 635
◆ **PMS-Haloperidol (Can)** *see* Haloperidol *on page* 691
◆ **PMS-Haloperidol LA (Can)** *see* Haloperidol *on page* 691
◆ **PMS-Hydromorphone (Can)** *see* HYDROmorphone *on page* 724
◆ **PMS-Hydroxyzine (Can)** *see* HydrOXYzine *on page* 736
◆ **PMS-Letrozole (Can)** *see* Letrozole *on page* 867
◆ **PMS-Levofloxacin (Can)** *see* Levofloxacin (Systemic) *on page* 883
◆ **PMS-Lorazepam (Can)** *see* LORazepam *on page* 907
◆ **PMS-Medroxyprogesterone (Can)** *see* MedroxyPROGESTERone *on page* 916
◆ **PMS-Metoclopramide (Can)** *see* Metoclopramide *on page* 974
◆ **PMS-Morphine Sulfate SR (Can)** *see* Morphine (Systemic) *on page* 1004
◆ **PMS-Nabilone (Can)** *see* Nabilone *on page* 1023

◆ **PMS-Nystatin (Can)** *see* Nystatin (Oral) *on page* 1041
◆ **PMS-Olanzapine (Can)** *see* OLANZapine *on page* 1056
◆ **PMS-Olanzapine ODT (Can)** *see* OLANZapine *on page* 1056
◆ **PMS-Ondansetron (Can)** *see* Ondansetron *on page* 1068
◆ **PMS-Oxycodone (Can)** *see* OxyCODONE *on page* 1084
◆ **PMS-Pamidronate (Can)** *see* Pamidronate *on page* 1109
◆ **PMS-Prochlorperazine (Can)** *see* Prochlorperazine *on page* 1212
◆ **PMS-Promethazine (Can)** *see* Promethazine *on page* 1218
◆ **PMS-Tamoxifen (Can)** *see* Tamoxifen *on page* 1324
◆ **PMS-Valacyclovir (Can)** *see* Valacyclovir *on page* 1420
◆ **PMS-Vancomycin (Can)** *see* Vancomycin *on page* 1428
◆ **PN401** *see* Uridine Triacetate *on page* 1419
◆ **Polyethylene Glycol-L-asparaginase** *see* Pegaspargase *on page* 1135
◆ **Polyethylene Glycol Interferon Alfa-2b** *see* Peginterferon Alfa-2b *on page* 1140

Porfimer (POR fi mer)

Related Information

Safe Handling of Hazardous Drugs *on page* 1904

Brand Names: U.S. Photofrin®

Brand Names: Canada Photofrin®

Index Terms CL-184116; Dihematoporphyrin Ether; Porfimer Sodium

Generic Availability (U.S.) No

Pharmacologic Category Antineoplastic Agent, Miscellaneous

Use Palliation in patients with obstructing (partial or complete) esophageal cancer; treatment of microinvasive endobronchial nonsmall cell lung cancer (NSCLC); reduction of obstruction and palliation in patients with obstructing (partial or complete) NSCLC; ablation of high-grade dysplasia in Barrett's esophagus

Canadian labeling (additional use; not in U.S. labeling): Second-line treatment of recurrent, superficial papillary bladder cancer

Unlabeled Use Treatment of actinic keratoses and low-risk basal and squamous cell skin cancers

Labeled Contraindications Porphyria

Photodynamic therapy (PDT) is contraindicated in patients with current tracheoesophageal or bronchoesophageal fistula; tumors eroding into a major blood vessel; emergency treatment of severe acute respiratory distress when caused by endobronchial lesion; esophageal or gastric varices; esophageal ulcers >1 cm in diameter

Canadian labeling: Additional contraindications (not in U.S. labeling): Hypersensitivity to porphyrins; photodynamic therapy is contraindicated in patients with papillary bladder cancer who have received prior total bladder radiation or whose functional bladder capacity is <200 mL and in patients with coexisting bladder tumors of stage greater than stage 1 (T1) who have invasive cancer

Pregnancy Risk Factor C

Lactation Excretion in breast milk unknown/not recommended

Warnings/Precautions Hazardous agent - use appropriate precautions for handling and disposal. Treatment-induced inflammation may obstruct airway; use with caution in patients with endobronchial tumors, especially if in areas where main airway may be obstructed (long or surrounding tumors); necrotic debris or mucositis may also cause airway obstruction; monitor closely between laser therapy and debridement for respiratory distress; may require urgent bronchoscopy to remove secretions or debris. Not suited for treatment of patients with esophageal or gastric varices due to the high risk for hemorrhage; patients with esophageal varices or tumors eroding into pulmonary blood vessels are at increased risk for hemorrhage, including fatal massive pulmonary hemoptysis (FMH); other risk factors for FMH include large, centrally-located tumors, cavitating tumors, or extensive tumor extrinsic to the bronchus. In patients with Barrett's esophagus, conduct rigorous surveillance (endoscopic biopsy every 3 months until 4 consecutive negative results for high-grade dysplasia followed by further follow-up per physician judgment); the long-term effects of photodynamic therapy in patients with Barrett's esophagus is not known. Esophageal strictures may occur, usually within 6 months of treatment; esophageal dilation may be required; the risk for strictures is increased with nodule pretreatment or with retreatment of the same area. Serious and potentially fatal gastrointestinal and esophageal necrosis and perforation may occur following treatment; due to the high risk for fistula, do not use in patients with esophageal tumors eroding into the trachea or bronchial tree; use is contraindicated in patients with existing tracheoesophageal or bronchoesophageal fistula.

Photosensitivity reactions are common in patients are exposed to direct sunlight or bright indoor light (eg fluorescent lights, unshaded light bulbs, examination/operating lights). Photosensitivity may last 30-90 days. Encourage ambient indoor light exposure (aids in gradually inactivating residual porfimer); re-exposure to general sunlight should be gradual (expose small area of skin [not the face] for 10 minutes, if no photosensitivity after 24 hours, may gradually resume normal outdoor activities; if photosensitivity occurs then wait 2 weeks and retest). Ocular discomfort has been reported with sun or bright light exposure; for at least 30 days (and until ocular sensitivity resolves), when outdoors, patients should wear dark sunglasses which have an average white light transmittance of <4%. Patients should be educated to test for residual photosensitivity before resuming exposure to direct sunlight. Conventional sunscreens are **not** protective against photosensitivity reactions caused by visible light. Allow 2-4 weeks to elapse after phototherapy prior to initiating radiation therapy; 4 weeks should elapse after radiation therapy prior to initiating phototherapy. Concurrent use with other photosensitizing agents may increase the risk for photosensitivity reactions. Avoid extravasation; if occurs, protect affected area from light.

Thromboembolic events may occur, generally in patients with additional risk factors for thromboembolism. Inflammatory responses within the treatment area may result in substernal chest pain. Avoid extravasation; if occurs, protect affected area from light; use of antidotes is of unknown benefit. Elimination may be prolonged in hepatic and renal impairment; toxicities may be increased; photosensitivity may be increased beyond 90 days in patients mild-to-severe hepatic impairment and in patients with severe renal impairment.

Adverse Reactions

>10%:

Cardiovascular: Chest pain (5% to 31%), edema (3% to 18%)

Central nervous system: Fever (8% to 31%), pain (1% to 22%), insomnia (5% to 14%)

Dermatologic: Photosensitivity reaction (19% to 69%)

Gastrointestinal: Esophageal stricture/stenosis (6% to 38%), nausea (24% to 37%), vomiting (17% to 31%), constipation (5% to 24%), dysphagia (10% to 24%), mucositis (≤20%), abdominal pain (5% to 20%)

Hematologic: Anemia (32% in esophageal cancer patients)

Neuromuscular & skeletal: Back pain (3% to 11%)

Respiratory: Pleural effusion (5% to 32%), dyspnea (7% to 30%), bronchial obstruction/mucus plug (21%), pneumonia (6% to 18%), hemoptysis (7% to 16%), cough (5% to 15%), bronchostenosis (11%), pharyngitis (11%)

5% to 10%:

Cardiovascular: Atrial fibrillation, cardiac failure (esophageal cancer), hyper-/hypotension, tachycardia

Central nervous system: Anxiety, confusion, dysphonia

Endocrine & metabolic: Dehydration

Gastrointestinal: Anorexia, diarrhea, dyspepsia, eructation, esophageal edema, esophageal pain, esophagitis, hematemesis, melena, odynophagia, weight loss

Genitourinary: Urinary tract infection

Neuromuscular & skeletal: Weakness

Respiratory: Bronchial ulceration, bronchitis, fatal massive hemoptysis, respiratory insufficiency, tracheoesophageal fistula

Miscellaneous: Hiccups, moniliasis, tumor hemorrhage, surgical complication

Common adverse reactions observed in papillary bladder cancer (Canadian labeling; not an approved use in the U.S.):

Cardiovascular: Peripheral edema

Central nervous system: Anxiety, insomnia, pain

Gastrointestinal: Constipation, nausea

Genitourinary: Bladder contracture (irreversible), dysuria, genital edema, micturition frequency, nocturia, suprapubic pain, urinary incontinence, urinary tract infection, urinary urgency

Renal: Hematuria

<5%, postmarketing, and/or case reports (limited to important or life-threatening): Abnormal vision, airway obstruction, angina, bradycardia, bronchospasm, cardiac failure, cataracts, cerebrovascular accident, diplopia, dizziness, erythema, esophageal perforation, eye pain, fluid imbalance, gastric ulcer, gastroesophageal fistula/perforation, hair growth increased, hemorrhage, ileus, infusion reactions, jaundice, laryngotracheal edema, lung abscess, MI, ocular sensitivity, peritonitis, photophobia, pneumonitis, pruritus, pseudoporphyria state, pulmonary edema, pulmonary embolism, pulmonary hemorrhage, pulmonary thrombosis, respiratory distress/failure, sepsis, sick sinus syndrome, skin blistering, skin discoloration, skin fragility, skin nodules, skin wrinkles, stridor, supraventricular tachycardia, thromboembolic events, urticaria

Drug Interactions

Metabolism/Transport Effects None known.

Avoid Concomitant Use There are no known interactions where it is recommended to avoid concomitant use.

Increased Effect/Toxicity

The levels/effects of Porfimer may be increased by: Photosensitizing Agents

Decreased Effect There are no known significant interactions involving a decrease in effect.

Storage/Stability Store intact vials at 20°C to 25°C (68°F to 77°F). Reconstituted solutions should be protected from light and used immediately after preparation.

Reconstitution

U.S. labeling: Reconstitute each 75 mg vial with 31.8 mL of either D_5W or NS injection resulting in a final concentration of 2.5 mg/mL.

Canadian labeling: Reconstitute each 75 mg vial with 31.8 mL of D_5W (only) resulting in a final concentration of 2.5 mg/mL. Reconstitute each 15 mg vial with 6.6 mL of D_5W only resulting in a final concentration of 2.5 mg/mL.

Shake well until dissolved. Protect the reconstituted product from bright light and use immediately. Use appropriate precautions for handling and disposal.

Mechanism of Action Porfimer's cytotoxic activity is dependent on light and oxygen. Following administration, the drug is selectively retained in neoplastic tissues. Exposure of the drug to laser light at wavelengths >630 nm results in the production of oxygen free-radicals. Release of thromboxane A_2, leading to vascular occlusion and ischemic necrosis, may also occur.

Pharmacodynamics/Kinetics

Distribution: V_{dss}: 0.49 L/kg

Protein binding, plasma: ~90%

Half-life elimination: First dose: 17 days; Second dose: 30 days

Dosing

Adult & Geriatric

Photodynamic therapy in esophageal cancer or endobronchial non-small cell lung cancer: I.V.: 2 mg/kg, followed by endoscopic exposure to the appropriate laser light and debridement; repeat courses must be separated by at least 30 days (delay subsequent treatment for insufficient healing) for a maximum of 3 courses

Photodynamic therapy in Barrett's esophagus dysplasia: I.V.: 2 mg/kg, followed by endoscopic exposure to the appropriate laser light; repeat courses must be separated by at least 90 days (delay subsequent treatment for insufficient healing) for a maximum of 3 courses

Photodynamic therapy in papillary bladder cancer (Canadian labeling; not in U.S. labeling): I.V.: 2 mg/kg, followed by cystoscopic exposure to the appropriate laser light. **Note:** Repeat dosing is not recommended due to increased risk of bladder contracture.

Administration Administer slow I.V. injection over 3-5 minutes. Avoid contact with skin during administration. Avoid extravasation.

Dosage Forms Excipient information presented when available (limited, particularly for generics); consult specific product labeling.

Injection, powder for reconstitution, as sodium:

Photofrin®: 75 mg

Dosage Forms: Canada Excipient information presented when available (limited, particularly for generics); consult specific product labeling.

Injection, powder for reconstitution, as sodium:

Photofrin®: 15 mg

References

National Comprehensive Cancer Network® (NCCN), "Clinical Practice Guidelines in Oncology™: Basal Cell and Squamous Cell Skin Cancers," Version 2.2011. Available at http://www.nccn.org/professionals/physician_gls/PDF/nmsc.pdf

Oseroff AR, Blumenson LR, Wilson BD, et al, "A Dose Ranging Study of Photodynamic Therapy With Porfimer Sodium (Photofrin) for Treatment of Basal Cell Carcinoma," *Lasers Surg Med*, 2006, 38(5):417-26.

Overholt BF, Wang KK, Burdick JS, et al, "Five-Year Efficacy and Safety of Photodynamic Therapy With Photofrin in Barrett's High-Grade Dysplasia," *Gastrointest Endosc*, 2007, 66(3):460-8.

◆ **Porfimer Sodium** *see* Porfimer *on page* 1183

Posaconazole (poe sa KON a zole)

Brand Names: U.S. Noxafil®

Brand Names: Canada Posanol™

Index Terms SCH 56592

Generic Availability (U.S.) No

Pharmacologic Category Antifungal Agent, Oral

Use

U.S. labeling: Prophylaxis of invasive *Aspergillus* and *Candida* infections in severely-immunocompromised patients (eg, hematopoietic stem cell transplant [HSCT] recipients with graft-versus-host disease [GVHD] or those with prolonged neutropenia secondary to chemotherapy for hematologic malignancies); treatment of oropharyngeal candidiasis (including patients refractory to itraconazole and/or fluconazole)

Canadian labeling: Prophylaxis of invasive *Aspergillus* and *Candida* infections in severely-immunocompromised patients (eg, hematopoietic stem cell transplant [HSCT] recipients with graft-versus-host disease [GVHD] or those with prolonged neutropenia); treatment of invasive aspergillosis in patients refractory to or intolerant of itraconazole or amphotericin B; treatment of oropharyngeal candidiasis

Unlabeled Use Salvage therapy of refractory or relapsed invasive fungal infections; mucormycosis; pulmonary infection (nonimmunosuppressed)

Labeled Contraindications Hypersensitivity to posaconazole, other azole antifungals, or any component of the formulation; coadministration of sirolimus, cisapride, ergot alkaloids, pimozide, quinidine, or a HMG-CoA reductase inhibitor metabolized by CYP3A4 (eg, atorvastatin, lovastatin, simvastatin)

Pregnancy Risk Factor C

Lactation Excretion in breast milk unknown/not recommended

Warnings/Precautions Hepatic dysfunction has occurred, ranging from reversible mild/moderate increases of ALT, AST, alkaline phosphatase, total bilirubin, and/or clinical hepatitis to severe reactions (cholestasis, hepatic failure including death). Consider discontinuation of therapy in patients who develop clinical evidence of liver disease that may be secondary to posaconazole. Use caution in patients with an increased risk of arrhythmia (long QT syndrome, concurrent QT_c-prolonging drugs, hypokalemia). Correct electrolyte abnormalities (eg, potassium, magnesium, and calcium) before initiating therapy. Concurrent use with cyclosporine or tacrolimus may significantly increase cyclosporine/tacrolimus concentrations and may result in rare serious adverse events (eg, nephrotoxicity, leukoencephalopathy, and death); dose reduction and close monitoring are recommended with initiation of posaconazole therapy. Concurrent use with midazolam may increase midazolam concentrations and potentiate midazolam-related adverse effects.

U.S. labeling contraindicates use in patients with hypersensitivity to other azole antifungal agents; Canadian labeling does not contraindicate use, but recommends using caution in hypersensitivity with other azole antifungal agents; cross-reaction may occur, but has not been established. Consider alternative therapy or closely monitor for breakthrough fungal infections in patients receiving drugs that decrease absorption or increase the metabolism of posaconazole or in any patient unable to eat or tolerate an oral liquid nutritional supplement. Use caution in severe renal impairment or GI disturbances; monitor for breakthrough fungal infections.

Ethanol/Nutrition/Herb Interactions Food: Bioavailability increased ~3 times when posaconazole is administered with a nonfat meal or an oral liquid nutritional supplement; increased ~4 times when administered with a high-fat meal. Grapefruit juice may decrease the levels/effects of posaconazole. Management: Must be administered with or within 20 minutes of a full meal or an oral liquid nutritional supplement, or may be administered with an acidic carbonated beverage (eg, ginger ale). Consider alternative antifungal therapy in patients with inadequate oral intake or severe diarrhea/vomiting. Avoid concurrent use of grapefruit juice.

Storage/Stability Store at 25°C (77°F); excursions permitted to 15°C to 30°C (59°F to 86°F). Do not freeze.

Mechanism of Action Interferes with fungal cytochrome P450 (latosterol-14α-demethylase) activity, decreasing ergosterol synthesis (principal sterol in fungal cell membrane) and inhibiting fungal cell membrane formation.

Pharmacodynamics/Kinetics

Absorption: Coadministration with food, liquid nutritional supplements, and/or acidic carbonated beverages (eg, ginger ale) increases absorption; fasting states do not provide sufficient absorption to ensure adequate plasma concentrations.

Distribution: V_d: 465-1774 L

Protein binding: >98%; predominantly bound to albumin

Metabolism: Not significantly metabolized; ~15% to 17% undergoes non-CYP-mediated metabolism, primarily via hepatic glucuronidation into metabolites

Half-life elimination: 35 hours (range: 20-66 hours)

Time to peak, plasma: ~3-5 hours

Excretion: Feces 71% to 77% (~66% of the total dose as unchanged drug); urine 13% to 14% (<0.2% of the total dose as unchanged drug)

Dosing

Adult & Geriatric

Aspergillosis, invasive: Oral:

Prophylaxis: 200 mg 3 times daily; duration of therapy is based on recovery from neutropenia or immunosuppression; initiate posaconazole in patients with acute myelogenous leukemia (AML) or myelodysplastic syndromes (MDS) several days before the anticipated onset of neutropenia (eg, at the time of chemotherapy initiation) and discontinue once neutropenia is resolved (Cornely, 2007; NCCN, 2009).

Treatment (refractory to or intolerant of conventional therapy):

U.S. unlabeled use: 200 mg 4 times daily initially; after disease stabilization, may decrease frequency to 400 mg twice daily (Walsh, 2007). **Note:** Duration of therapy should be a minimum of 6-12 weeks or throughout period of immunosuppression and until lesions have resolved (Walsh, 2008).

Canadian labeling: 400 mg twice daily; in patients unable to tolerate food or nutritional supplement, administer 200 mg 4 times daily; duration of therapy is based on severity of underlying disease, recovery from immunosuppresion, and clinical response.

Candidal infections: Oral:

U.S. labeling:

Prophylaxis: 200 mg 3 times daily; duration of therapy is based on recovery from neutropenia or immunosuppression

Treatment:

Oropharyngeal infection: Initial: 100 mg twice daily for 1 day; maintenance: 100 mg once daily for 13 days

Refractory oropharyngeal infection: 400 mg twice daily; duration of therapy is based on underlying disease and clinical response

Canadian labeling:

Prophylaxis: 200 mg 3 times daily; duration of therapy is based on recovery from neutropenia or immunosuppression

Treatment: Oropharyngeal infection: Initial: 100 mg twice daily for 1 day; maintenance: 100 mg once daily for 13 days

Mucormycosis (unlabeled use): Oral: 800 mg daily in 2 or 4 divided doses; duration of therapy is based on response and risk of relapse due to immunosuppression (Greenburg, 2006)

Cryptococcal infections: Oral:

Pulmonary, nonimmunosuppressed (unlabeled use): 400 mg twice daily. **Note:** Fluconazole is considered first-line treatment (Perfect, 2010).

Salvage treatment of relapsed infection (unlabeled use): 400 mg twice daily (or 200 mg 4 times daily) for 10-12 weeks. **Note:** Salvage treatment should only be started after an appropriate course of an induction regimen (Perfect, 2010).

Pediatric

Aspergillosis, invasive: Oral: Children ≥13 years and Adolescents: Refer to adult dosing.

Candidal infections: Oral: Children ≥13 years and Adolescents: Refer to adult dosing.

Renal Impairment

Mild-to-moderate renal insufficiency (Cl_{cr} 20-80 mL/minute/1.73 m^2): No adjustment necessary

Severe renal insufficiency (Cl_{cr} <20 mL/minute/1.73 m^2): No adjustment necessary; however, monitor for breakthrough fungal infections due to variability in posaconazole exposure.

Hepatic Impairment

Mild-to-severe hepatic insufficiency (Child-Pugh class A, B, or C): No adjustment necessary.

Clinical signs and symptoms of liver disease due to posaconazole: Consider discontinuing therapy.

Administration Oral: Shake well before use. Must be administered during or within 20 minutes following a full meal or an oral liquid nutritional supplement; alternatively, posaconazole may be administered with an acidic carbonated beverage (eg, ginger ale). In patients able to swallow, administer oral suspension using dosing spoon provided by the manufacturer; spoon should be rinsed clean with water after each use and before storage.

Dosage Forms Excipient information presented when available (limited, particularly for generics); consult specific product labeling.

Suspension, oral:

Noxafil®: 40 mg/mL (123 mL) [contains sodium benzoate; cherry flavor; delivers 105 mL of suspension]

◆ **Posanol™ (Can)** *see* Posaconazole *on page 1187*

◆ **PR-171** *see* Carfilzomib *on page 239*

PRALAtrexate (pral a TREX ate)

Related Information

Management of Chemotherapy-Induced Nausea and Vomiting *on page 1786*
Safe Handling of Hazardous Drugs *on page 1904*

Brand Names: U.S. Folotyn®

Index Terms PDX

Generic Availability (U.S.) No

Pharmacologic Category Antineoplastic Agent, Antimetabolite (Antifolate)

Use Treatment of relapsed or refractory peripheral T-cell lymphoma (PTCL)

Unlabeled Use Treatment of relapsed or refractory cutaneous T-cell lymphomas (mycosis fungoides [MF] and Sézary syndrome [SS])

Labeled Contraindications There are no contraindications listed within the manufacturer's labeling.

Pregnancy Risk Factor D

Lactation Excretion in breast milk unknown/not recommended

Warnings/Precautions Hazardous agent - use appropriate precautions for handling and disposal. May cause bone marrow suppression (thrombocytopenia, neutropenia and anemia); may require dosage modification; monitor blood counts. Mucositis, including stomatitis or mucosal inflammation of gastrointestinal and genitourinary tracts, may occur; monitor weekly; may require dosage modification. Prophylactic folic acid and vitamin B_{12} supplements are necessary to reduce hematologic toxicity and treatment-related mucositis. Severe and potentially fatal dermatologic reactions, including skin exfoliation, ulceration, and toxic epidermal necrolysis (TEN) have been reported. Skin reaction may be progressive; severity may increase with continued treatment; may also involve skin and subcutaneous tissues which are affected by lymphoma; monitor all dermatologic reactions closely; withhold or discontinue treatment for severe dermatologic reaction.

Pralatrexate may cause tumor lysis syndrome (TLS); monitor closely, if TLS develops, treat for associated complications. Use with caution in patients with moderate-to-severe renal impairment (has not been studied in patients with renal impairment); monitor renal function and for systemic toxicity due to increased exposure. Concurrent use with drugs with substantial renal clearance (eg, NSAIDs, sulfamethoxazole/trimethoprim) may result in delayed pralatrexate clearance. Liver function test abnormalities have been observed with use; monitor liver function; persistent abnormalities may indicate hepatotoxicity and may require dosage modification.

Patients with moderate-to-severe renal impairment are at risk for increased exposure and toxicity. Avoid use in patients with end-stage renal disease (ESRD), including patients undergoing dialysis (unless the potential benefit outweighs potential risks); serious adverse reactions, including toxic epidermal necrolysis and mucositis were reported in patients with ESRD undergoing dialysis. Monitor renal function and for systemic toxicity due to increased exposure.

Adverse Reactions

>10%:

Cardiovascular: Edema (30%)

Central nervous system: Fatigue (36%), fever (32%)

Dermatologic: Rash (15%; grades 3/4: 0%), pruritus (14%; grade 3: 2%; grade 4: 0%)

Endocrine & metabolic: Hypokalemia (15%)

Gastrointestinal: Mucositis (70%; grade 3: 17%; grade 4: 4%), nausea (40%), constipation (33%), vomiting (25%), diarrhea (21%), anorexia (15%), abdominal pain (12%)

Hematologic: Thrombocytopenia (41%; grade 3: 14%; grade 4: 19%), anemia (34%; grade 3: 15%; grade 4: 2%), neutropenia (24%; grade 3: 13%; grade 4: 7%), leukopenia (11%; grade 3: 3%; grade 4: 4%)

Hepatic: Transaminases increased (13%; grade 3: 5%; grade 4: 0%)

Neuromuscular & skeletal: Limb pain (12%), back pain (11%)

Respiratory: Cough (28%), epistaxis (26%), dyspnea (19%), pharyngolaryngeal pain (14%)

Miscellaneous: Night sweats (11%), infection

1% to 10%:

Cardiovascular: Tachycardia (10%)

Endocrine & metabolic: Dehydration (serious >3%)

Hematologic: Neutropenic fever (serious >3%)

Neuromuscular & skeletal: Weakness (10%)

Respiratory: Upper respiratory infection (10%)

Miscellaneous: Sepsis (serious >3%)

<1%, postmarketing, and/or case reports: Bowel obstruction, cardiopulmonary arrest, lymphopenia, odynophagia, pancytopenia, skin exfoliation, skin ulceration, toxic epidermal necrolysis (TEN), tumor lysis syndrome (TLS)

Drug Interactions

Metabolism/Transport Effects Substrate of BCRP

Avoid Concomitant Use

Avoid concomitant use of PRALAtrexate with any of the following: BCG; Natalizumab; Pimecrolimus; Tacrolimus (Topical); Vaccines (Live)

Increased Effect/Toxicity

PRALAtrexate may increase the levels/effects of: Leflunomide; Natalizumab; Vaccines (Live); Vitamin K Antagonists

The levels/effects of PRALAtrexate may be increased by: Denosumab; Nonsteroidal Anti-Inflammatory Agents; Pimecrolimus; Probenecid; Roflumilast; Salicylates; Sulfamethoxazole; Tacrolimus (Topical); Trastuzumab; Trimethoprim

Decreased Effect

PRALAtrexate may decrease the levels/effects of: BCG; Cardiac Glycosides; Coccidioidin Skin Test; Sapropterin; Sipuleucel-T; Vaccines (Inactivated); Vaccines (Live); Vitamin K Antagonists

The levels/effects of PRALAtrexate may be decreased by: Echinacea

Storage/Stability Store intact vials refrigerated at 2°C to 8°C (36°F to 46°F). Store in original carton to protect from light until use. Unopened vials (stored in the original carton) are stable for up to 72 hours at room temperature (discard after 72 hours).

Reconstitution Use appropriate precautions for handling (hazardous agent). Withdraw into syringe for administration; do not dilute (manufacturer recommends immediate use after placing in syringe). Discard unused portion in the vial.

Mechanism of Action Antifolate analog; inhibits DNA, RNA, and protein synthesis by selectively entering cells expressing reduced folate carrier (RFC-1), is polyglutamylated by folylpolyglutamate synthetase (FPGS) and then competes for the DHFR-folate binding site to inhibit dihydrofolate reductase (DHFR)

Pharmacodynamics/Kinetics

Distribution: *S*-diastereomer: 105 L; *R*-diastereomer: 37 L

Protein binding: ~67%

Half-life elimination: 12-18 hours

Excretion: Urine (~34% as unchanged drug)

Dosing

Adult & Geriatric Note: Initiate vitamin supplements before initial pralatrexate dose: Folic acid 1-1.25 mg/day orally beginning 10 days prior to initial pralatrexate dose; continue during treatment and for 30 days after last pralatrexate dose; vitamin B_{12} 1000 mcg I.M. within 10 weeks prior to initial pralatrexate dose and every 8-10 weeks thereafter (after initial dose, B_{12} may be administered on the same day as pralatrexate).

Prior to administering any dose, mucositis should be ≤grade 1 and absolute neutrophil count (ANC) should be ≥1000/mm^3; platelets should be ≥100,000/mm^3 for the first dose and ≥50,000/mm^3 for subsequent doses

Peripheral T-cell lymphoma (PTCL), relapsed or refractory: I.V.: 30 mg/m^2 once weekly for 6 weeks of a 7-week treatment cycle; continue until disease progression or unacceptable toxicity (O'Connor, 2011)

Cutaneous T-cell lymphoma, relapsed or refractory (unlabeled use): I.V.: 15 mg/m^2 once weekly for 3 weeks of a 4-week treatment cycle (Horwitz, 2012)

Renal Impairment

Moderate-to-severe renal impairment: Exposure and toxicities may be increased; monitor for toxicities and adjust dose accordingly.

End-stage renal disease (ESRD), including dialysis-dependent: Avoid use (unless the potential benefit outweighs risks).

Hepatic Impairment Patients with total bilirubin >1.5 mg/dL, AST or ALT >2.5 times the upper limit of normal (ULN), or ALT or AST >5 times ULN if documented hepatic lymphoma involvement were excluded from clinical trials. Persistent abnormalities may indicate hepatotoxicity requiring dosage modification:

Grade 3 (AST or ALT >5-20 times ULN or bilirubin >3-10 times ULN): Omit dose; decrease to 20 mg/m^2 when recovers to ≤grade 2

Grade 4 (AST or ALT >20 times ULN or bilirubin >10 times ULN): Discontinue treatment.

Adjustment for Toxicity Severe or intolerable adverse events may require dose omission, reduction or interruption. Do not make up omitted doses at the end of a cycle; do not re-escalate dose after a reduction due to toxicity.

Hematologic toxicity:

Platelets:

<50,000/mm^3 (for 1-week duration): Omit dose; continue at previous dose if platelets recover within 1 week

<50,000/mm^3 (for 2-week duration): Omit dose; decrease to 20 mg/m^2 if platelets recover within 2 weeks

<50,000/mm^3 (for 3-week duration): Discontinue treatment.

ANC:

500-1000/mm^3 without fever (for 1-week duration): Omit dose; continue at previous dose if ANC recovers within 1 week

500-1000/mm^3 with fever **or** ANC <500/mm^3 (for 1-week duration): Omit dose, give filgrastim or sargramostim support; continue at previous dose (with growth factor support) if ANC recovers within 1 week

500-1000/mm^3 with fever **or** ANC <500/mm^3 (recurrent or for 2-week duration): Omit dose and give filgrastim or sargramostim support; decrease to 20 mg/m^2 (with growth factor support) if ANC recovers within 2 weeks

500-1000/mm^3 with fever **or** ANC <500/mm^3 (second recurrence or for 3 week duration): Discontinue treatment.

Nonhematologic toxicity: Mucositis (on day of treatment):

Grade 2: Omit dose; continue at previous dose when recovers to ≤grade 1

Grade 3 or recurrent grade 2: Omit dose and decrease to 20 mg/m^2 when recovers to ≤grade 1

Grade 4: Discontinue treatment.

Nonhematologic toxicity (other than mucositis):

Grade 3: Omit dose; decrease to 20 mg/m^2 when recovers to ≤grade 2

Grade 4: Discontinue treatment.

Administration Administer I.V. push (undiluted) over 3-5 minutes into the line of a free-flowing normal saline I.V.

Emetic Potential Low (10% to 30%)

Monitoring Parameters CBC with differential (baseline and weekly), serum chemistries, including renal and liver function tests (prior to the first and fourth doses in each cycle); mucositis severity (baseline and weekly); monitor for signs of tumor lysis syndrome

Dosage Forms Excipient information presented when available (limited, particularly for generics); consult specific product labeling.

Injection, solution [preservative free]:

Folotyn®: 20 mg/mL (1 mL, 2 mL)

References

Foss FM, Horwitz SM, Pinter-Brown L, et al, "Pralatrexate is an Effective Treatment for Heavily Pretreated Patients With Relapsed/Refractory Transformed Mycosis Fungoides (tMF)," *Blood*, 2010, 116(21):1762 [abstract 1762 from ASH 2010 Annual Meeting].

Goy A, Pro B, Savage KJ, et al, "Pralatrexate is Effective in Patients With Relapsed or Refractory Peripheral T-Cell Lymphoma (PTCL) With Prior Ifosfamide, Carboplatin, and Etoposide (ICE)-Based Regimens," *Blood*, 2010, 116(21):1753 [abstract 1753 from ASH 2010 Annual Meeting].

Horwitz SM, Kim YH, Foss F, et al, "Identification of an Active, Well-Tolerated Dose of Pralatrexate in Patients With Relapsed or Refractory Cutaneous T-cell Lymphoma," *Blood*, 2012, 119 (18):4115-22.

O'Connor OA, Horwitz S, Hamlin P, et al, "Phase II-I-II Study of Two Different Doses and Schedules of Pralatrexate, a High-Affinity Substrate for the Reduced Folate Carrier, in Patients With Relapsed or Refractory Lymphoma Reveals Marked Activity in T-Cell Malignancies," *J Clin Oncol*, 2009, 27(26):4357-64.

O'Connor OA, Pro B, Pinter-Brown L, et al, "Pralatrexate in Patients With Relapsed or Refractory Peripheral T-Cell Lymphoma: Results from the Pivotal PROPEL Study," *J Clin Oncol*, 2011, 29 (9):1182-9.

◆ **Pred Forte®** *see* PrednisoLONE (Ophthalmic) *on page* *1198*

◆ **Pred Mild®** *see* PrednisoLONE (Ophthalmic) *on page* *1198*

PrednisoLONE (Systemic) (pred NISS oh lone)

Brand Names: U.S. Flo-Pred™; Millipred™; Millipred™ DP; Orapred ODT®; Orapred®; Pediapred®; Veripred™ 20

Brand Names: Canada Hydeltra T.B.A.®; Novo-Prednisolone; Pediapred®

Index Terms Prednisolone Sodium Phosphate

Generic Availability (U.S.) Yes: Excludes orally disintegrating tablet, oral suspension, tablet

Pharmacologic Category Corticosteroid, Systemic

Use Treatment of endocrine disorders, rheumatic disorders, collagen diseases, allergic states, respiratory diseases, hematologic disorders, neoplastic diseases, edematous states, and gastrointestinal diseases; resolution of acute exacerbations of multiple sclerosis; management of fulminating or disseminated tuberculosis and trichinosis; acute or chronic solid organ rejection

Unlabeled Use Severe alcoholic hepatitis; Bell's palsy

Labeled Contraindications Hypersensitivity to prednisolone or any component of the formulation; acute superficial herpes simplex keratitis; live or attenuated virus vaccines (with immunosuppressive doses of corticosteroids); systemic fungal infections; varicella

Pregnancy Risk Factor C/D (Flo-Pred™)

Lactation Enters breast milk/use caution (AAP rates "compatible"; AAP 2001 update pending)

Warnings/Precautions May cause hypercorticism or suppression of hypothalamic-pituitary-adrenal (HPA) axis, particularly in younger children or in patients receiving high doses for prolonged periods. HPA axis suppression may lead to adrenal crisis. Withdrawal and discontinuation of a corticosteroid should be done slowly and carefully. Particular care is required when patients are transferred from systemic corticosteroids to inhaled products due to possible adrenal insufficiency or withdrawal from steroids, including an increase in allergic symptoms. Patients receiving >20 mg per day of prednisone (or equivalent) may be most susceptible. Fatalities have occurred due to adrenal insufficiency in asthmatic patients during and after transfer from systemic corticosteroids to aerosol steroids; aerosol steroids do **not** provide the systemic steroid needed to treat patients having trauma, surgery, or infections.

Acute myopathy has been reported with high dose corticosteroids, usually in patients with neuromuscular transmission disorders; may involve ocular and/or respiratory muscles; monitor creatine kinase; recovery may be delayed. Corticosteroid use may cause psychiatric disturbances, including depression, euphoria, insomnia, mood swings, and personality changes. Pre-existing psychiatric conditions may be exacerbated by corticosteroid use. Prolonged use of corticosteroids may also increase the incidence of secondary infection, mask acute infection (including fungal infections), prolong or exacerbate viral infections, or limit response to vaccines. Exposure to chickenpox should be avoided; corticosteroids should not be used to treat ocular herpes simplex. Corticosteroids should not be used for cerebral malaria or viral hepatitis. Close observation is required in patients with latent tuberculosis and/or TB reactivity; restrict use in active TB (only in conjunction with antituberculosis treatment). Prolonged use of corticosteroids may result in glaucoma; cataract formation may occur. Prolonged treatment with corticosteroids has been associated with the development of Kaposi's sarcoma (case reports); if noted, discontinuation of therapy should be considered.

Use with caution in patients with thyroid disease, hepatic impairment, renal impairment, cardiovascular disease, diabetes, glaucoma, cataracts, myasthenia gravis, patients at risk for osteoporosis, patients at risk for seizures, or GI diseases (diverticulitis, peptic ulcer, ulcerative colitis) due to perforation risk. Use caution following acute MI (corticosteroids have been associated with myocardial rupture). Because of the risk of adverse effects, systemic corticosteroids should be used cautiously in the elderly in the smallest possible effective dose for the shortest duration. Withdraw therapy with gradual tapering of dose. May affect growth velocity; growth should be routinely monitored in pediatric patients.

Adverse Reactions Frequency not defined.

Cardiovascular: Cardiomyopathy, CHF, edema, facial edema, hypertension

Central nervous system: Headache, insomnia, malaise, nervousness, pseudotumor cerebri, psychic disorders, seizure, vertigo

Dermatologic: Bruising, facial erythema, hirsutism, petechiae, skin test reaction suppression, thin fragile skin, urticaria

Endocrine & metabolic: Carbohydrate tolerance decreased, Cushing's syndrome, diabetes mellitus, growth suppression, hyperglycemia, hypernatremia, hypokalemia, hypokalemic alkalosis, menstrual irregularities, negative nitrogen balance, pituitary adrenal axis suppression

Gastrointestinal: Abdominal distention, increased appetite, indigestion, nausea, pancreatitis, peptic ulcer, ulcerative esophagitis, weight gain

Hepatic: LFTs increased (usually reversible)

Neuromuscular & skeletal: Arthralgia, aseptic necrosis (humeral/femoral heads), fractures, muscle mass decreased, muscle weakness, osteoporosis, steroid myopathy, tendon rupture, weakness

Ocular: Cataracts, exophthalmus, eyelid edema, glaucoma, intraocular pressure increased, irritation

Respiratory: Epistaxis

Miscellaneous: Diaphoresis increased, impaired wound healing

Drug Interactions

Metabolism/Transport Effects Substrate of CYP3A4 (minor); **Note:** Assignment of Major/Minor substrate status based on clinically relevant drug interaction potential; **Inhibits** CYP3A4 (weak)

Avoid Concomitant Use

Avoid concomitant use of PrednisoLONE (Systemic) with any of the following: Aldesleukin; BCG; Mifepristone; Natalizumab; Pimecrolimus; Pimozide; Tacrolimus (Topical)

Increased Effect/Toxicity

PrednisoLONE (Systemic) may increase the levels/effects of: Acetylcholinesterase Inhibitors; Amphotericin B; ARIPiprazole; CycloSPORINE (Systemic); Deferasirox; Leflunomide; Loop Diuretics; Natalizumab; NSAID (COX-2 Inhibitor); NSAID (Nonselective); Pimozide; Thiazide Diuretics; Vaccines (Live); Warfarin

The levels/effects of PrednisoLONE (Systemic) may be increased by: Antifungal Agents (Azole Derivatives, Systemic); Aprepitant; Calcium Channel Blockers (Nondihydropyridine); CycloSPORINE (Systemic); Denosumab; Estrogen Derivatives; Fluconazole; Fosaprepitant; Indacaterol; Macrolide Antibiotics; Mifepristone; Neuromuscular-Blocking Agents (Nondepolarizing); Pimecrolimus; Quinolone Antibiotics; Ritonavir; Roflumilast; Salicylates; Tacrolimus (Topical); Telaprevir; Trastuzumab

Decreased Effect

PrednisoLONE (Systemic) may decrease the levels/effects of: Aldesleukin; Antidiabetic Agents; BCG; Calcitriol; Coccidioidin Skin Test; Corticorelin; CycloSPORINE (Systemic); Hyaluronidase; Isoniazid; Salicylates; Sipuleucel-T; Telaprevir; Vaccines (Inactivated)

The levels/effects of PrednisoLONE (Systemic) may be decreased by: Aminoglutethimide; Antacids; Barbiturates; Bile Acid Sequestrants; Echinacea; Fosphenytoin; Mifepristone; Mitotane; Phenytoin; Primidone; Rifamycin Derivatives; Tocilizumab

Ethanol/Nutrition/Herb Interactions

Ethanol: Avoid ethanol (may increase gastric mucosal irritation).

Food: Prednisolone interferes with calcium absorption. Limit caffeine.

Herb/Nutraceutical: St John's wort may decrease prednisolone levels. Avoid cat's claw, echinacea (have immunostimulant properties).

Storage/Stability

Flo-Pred™: Store at 20°C to 25°C (68°F to 77°F). Flo-Pred™ should be dispensed in the original container (to avoid loss of formulation during transfer).

Millipred™: Store at 20°C to 25°C (68°F to 77°F).

Orapred ODT®: Store at 20°C to 25°C (68°F to 77°F) in blister pack. Protect from moisture.

Orapred®, Veripred™ 20: 2°C to 8°C (36°F to 46°F).

Pediapred®: 4°C to 25°C (39°F to 77°F); may be refrigerated.

Mechanism of Action Decreases inflammation by suppression of migration of polymorphonuclear leukocytes and reversal of increased capillary permeability; suppresses the immune system by reducing activity and volume of the lymphatic system

Pharmacodynamics/Kinetics

Duration: 18-36 hours

Protein binding (concentration dependent): 65% to 91%; decreased in elderly

Metabolism: Primarily hepatic, but also metabolized in most tissues, to inactive compounds

Half-life elimination: 3.6 hours; End-stage renal disease: 3-5 hours

Excretion: Primarily urine (as glucuronides, sulfates, and unconjugated metabolites)

Dosing

Adult Dose depends upon condition being treated and response of patient. Oral dosage expressed in terms of prednisolone base. Consider alternate day therapy for long-term therapy. Discontinuation of long-term therapy requires gradual withdrawal by tapering the dose. Patients undergoing unusual stress while receiving corticosteroids, should receive increased doses prior to, during, and after the stressful situation.

Usual dose (range): Oral: 5-60 mg daily

Rheumatoid arthritis: Oral: Initial: 5-7.5 mg daily, adjust dose as necessary

Multiple sclerosis: Oral: 200 mg daily for 1 week followed by 80 mg every other day for 1 month

Bell's palsy (unlabeled use): Oral: 60 mg daily for 5 days, followed by 10 mg daily for 5 days (Berg, 2012)

Severe alcoholic hepatitis (Maddrey Discriminant Function [MDF] score ≥32) (unlabeled use): Oral: 40 mg daily for 28 days, followed by a 2-week taper (O'Shea, 2010)

Dosing adjustment in hyperthyroidism: Prednisolone dose may need to be increased to achieve adequate therapeutic effects.

Geriatric Use lowest effective adult dose. Dose depends upon condition being treated and response of patient; alternate day dosing may be attempted in some disease states.

Pediatric Dose depends upon condition being treated and response of patient; dosage for infants and children should be based on severity of the disease and response of the patient rather than on strict adherence to dosage indicated by age, weight, or body surface area. Oral dosage expressed in terms of prednisolone base. Consider alternate day therapy for long-term therapy. Discontinuation of long-term therapy requires gradual withdrawal by tapering the dose. Patients undergoing unusual stress while receiving corticosteroids, should receive increased doses prior to, during, and after the stressful situation.

Acute asthma: Oral: 1-2 mg/kg/day in divided doses 1-2 times daily for 3-5 days

Anti-inflammatory or immunosuppressive dose: Oral: 0.1-2 mg/kg/day in divided doses 1-4 times daily

Nephrotic syndrome: Oral:

Initial (first 3 episodes): 2 mg/kg/day **or** 60 mg/m^2/day (maximum: 80 mg/day) in divided doses 3-4 times daily until urine is protein free for 3 consecutive days (maximum: 28 days); followed by 1-1.5 mg/kg/dose **or** 40 mg/m^2/dose given every other day for 4 weeks

Maintenance (for frequent relapses): 0.5-1 mg/kg/dose given every other day for 3-6 months

Dosing adjustment in hyperthyroidism: Refer to adult dosing.

Renal Impairment

Hemodialysis: Slightly dialyzable (5% to 20%); administer dose posthemodialysis

Peritoneal dialysis: Supplemental dose is not necessary

Combination Regimens

Lymphoma, Hodgkin:

ChlVPP (Hodgkin) on page 1562
IGEV (Hodgkin) on page 1690

Administration Administer oral formulation with food or milk to decrease GI effects.

Flo-Pred™: Administer using the provided calibrated syringe (supplied by manufacturer) to accurately measure the dose. Syringe should be washed prior to next use.

Orapred ODT®: Do not break or use partial tablet. Remove tablet from blister pack just prior to use. May swallow whole or allow to dissolve on tongue.

Monitoring Parameters Blood pressure; blood glucose, electrolytes; intraocular pressure (use >6 weeks); bone mineral density; growth in children

Test Interactions Response to skin tests

Dietary Considerations Should be taken after meals or with food or milk to decrease GI effects; increase dietary intake of pyridoxine, vitamin C, vitamin D, folate, calcium, and phosphorus.

Dosage Forms Excipient information presented when available (limited, particularly for generics); consult specific product labeling.

Solution, oral, as base: 15 mg/5 mL (240 mL, 480 mL)

Solution, oral, as sodium phosphate [strength expressed as base]: 5 mg/5 mL (120 mL); 15 mg/5 mL (237 mL, 473 mL); 25 mg/5 mL (237 mL)

Millipred™: 10 mg/5 mL (237 mL) [dye free, ethanol free; grape flavor]

Orapred®: 15 mg/5 mL (20 mL, 237 mL) [dye free; contains ethanol 2%, sodium benzoate; grape flavor]

Pediapred®: 5 mg/5 mL (120 mL) [dye free; raspberry flavor]

Veripred™ 20: 20 mg/5 mL (237 mL) [dye free, ethanol free; grape flavor]

Suspension, oral, as acetate [strength expressed as base]:
Flo-Pred™: 15 mg/5 mL (52 mL) [contains propylene glycol; cherry flavor]
Tablet, oral, as base:
Millipred™: 5 mg [scored]
Tablet, oral, as base [dose-pack]:
Millipred™ DP: 5 mg [scored; 12-day pack/48s]
Millipred™ DP: 5 mg [scored; 6-day pack/21s]
Tablet, orally disintegrating, oral, as sodium phosphate [strength expressed as base]:
Orapred ODT®: 10 mg, 15 mg, 30 mg [grape flavor]

References

Berg T, Bylund N, Marsk E, et al, "The Effect of Prednisolone on Sequelae in Bell's Palsy," *Arch Otolaryngol Head Neck Surg*, 2012, 138(5):445-9.

Cooper MS and Stewart PM, "Corticosteroid Insufficiency in Acutely Ill Patients," *N Engl J Med*, 2003, 348(8):727-34.

Hotchkiss RS and Karl IE, "The Pathophysiology and Treatment of Sepsis," *N Engl J Med*, 2003, 348(2):138-50.

McGee S and Hirschmann J, "Use of Corticosteroids in Treating Infectious Diseases," *Arch Intern Med*, 2008, 168(10):1034-46.

O'Shea R, Dasarathy S, McCullough A, et al, "Alcoholic Liver Disease," *Hepatology*, 2010, 51 (1):307-28.

Report of a Workshop by the British Association for Paediatric Nephrology and Research Unit, Royal College of Physicians, "Consensus Statement on Management and Audit Potential for Steroid Responsive Nephrotic Syndrome," *Arch Dis Child*, 1994, 70(2):151-7.

PrednisoLONE (Ophthalmic) (pred NISS oh lone)

Brand Names: U.S. Omnipred™; Pred Forte®; Pred Mild®

Brand Names: Canada Diopred®; Ophtho-Tate®; Pred Forte®; Pred Mild®

Index Terms Econopred; Prednisolone Acetate, Ophthalmic; Prednisolone Sodium Phosphate, Ophthalmic

Generic Availability (U.S.) Yes

Pharmacologic Category Corticosteroid, Ophthalmic

Use Treatment of palpebral and bulbar conjunctivitis; corneal injury from chemical, radiation, thermal burns, or foreign body penetration; steroid-responsive inflammatory ophthalmic diseases

Labeled Contraindications Hypersensitivity to prednisolone or any component of the formulation; viral diseases of the cornea and conjunctiva (eg, acute superficial herpes simplex keratitis); mycobacterial or fungal infections of the eye

Pregnancy Risk Factor C

Warnings/Precautions Prolonged use of corticosteroids may result in posterior subcapsular cataract formation. Use following cataract surgery may delay healing or increase the incidence of bleb formation. Prolonged use of corticosteroids may result in elevated intraocular pressure (IOP) and glaucoma; damage to the optic nerve (not indicated for treatment of optic neuritis); and defects in visual acuity and fields of vision. Monitor IOP in any patient receiving treatment for ≥10 days.

Prolonged use of corticosteroids may increase the incidence of secondary infection, mask acute infection (including fungal infections), or prolong or exacerbate viral infections. Corticosteroids should not be used to treat ocular herpes simplex. Fungal infection should be suspected in any patient with persistent corneal ulceration who has received corticosteroids. Various ophthalmic disorders, as well as prolonged use of corticosteroids, may result in corneal and scleral thinning. Continued use in a patient with thinning may result in rupture.

Not effective in Sjogren's keratoconjunctivitis or mustard gas keratitis. Withdraw therapy with gradual tapering of dose.

Adverse Reactions Frequency not defined: Ocular: Conjunctival hyperemia, conjunctivitis, corneal ulcers, delayed wound healing, glaucoma, intraocular pressure increased, keratitis, loss of accommodation, optic nerve damage, mydriasis, posterior subcapsular cataract formation, ptosis, secondary ocular infection

Drug Interactions

Metabolism/Transport Effects **Substrate** of CYP3A4 (minor); **Note:** Assignment of Major/Minor substrate status based on clinically relevant drug interaction potential

Avoid Concomitant Use There are no known interactions where it is recommended to avoid concomitant use.

Increased Effect/Toxicity There are no known significant interactions involving an increase in effect.

Decreased Effect

The levels/effects of PrednisoLONE (Ophthalmic) may be decreased by: Tocilizumab

Dosing

Adult & Geriatric Conjunctivitis: Ophthalmic (suspension/solution): Instill 1-2 drops in the eye 2-4 times daily

Pediatric Conjunctivitis: Ophthalmic (suspension/solution): Children: Refer to adult dosing.

Dosage Forms Excipient information presented when available (limited, particularly for generics); consult specific product labeling. [DSC] = Discontinued product

Solution, ophthalmic, as sodium phosphate [drops]: 1% (5 mL [DSC], 10 mL, 15 mL [DSC])

Suspension, ophthalmic, as acetate [drops]: 1% (5 mL, 10 mL, 15 mL)

Omnipred™: 1% (5 mL, 10 mL) [contains benzalkonium chloride]

Pred Forte®: 1% (1 mL, 5 mL, 10 mL, 15 mL) [contains benzalkonium chloride, sodium bisulfite]

Pred Mild®: 0.12% (5 mL, 10 mL) [contains benzalkonium chloride, sodium bisulfite]

- ◆ **Prednisolone Acetate, Ophthalmic** *see* PrednisoLONE (Ophthalmic) *on page 1198*
- ◆ **Prednisolone Sodium Phosphate** *see* PrednisoLONE (Systemic) *on page 1193*
- ◆ **Prednisolone Sodium Phosphate, Ophthalmic** *see* PrednisoLONE (Ophthalmic) *on page 1198*

PredniSONE (PRED ni sone)

Brand Names: U.S. PredniSONE Intensol™; Rayos®

Brand Names: Canada Apo-Prednisone®; Novo-Prednisone; Winpred™

Index Terms Deltacortisone; Deltadehydrocortisone; Rayos®

Generic Availability (U.S.) Yes

Pharmacologic Category Corticosteroid, Systemic

Use Treatment of a variety of diseases, including:

Allergic conditions: Atopic dermatitis, drug hypersensitivity reactions, allergic rhinitis, serum sickness, adjunctive treatment of anaphylaxis

Dermatologic diseases: Bullous dermatitis herpetiformis, contact dermatitis, exfoliative erythroderma, mycosis fungoides, pemphigus, severe erythema multiforme (Stevens-Johnson syndrome)

Endocrine conditions: Congenital adrenal hyperplasia, hypercalcemia of malignancy, nonsuppurative thyroiditis, adrenocortical insufficiency

Gastrointestinal diseases: Crohn's disease, ulcerative colitis

Hematologic diseases: Acquired (autoimmune) hemolytic anemia, Diamond-Blackfan anemia, idiopathic thrombocytopenic purpura, pure red cell aplasia, secondary thrombocytopenia

Infectious diseases: Trichinosis with neurologic or myocardial involvement, tuberculosis meningitis with subarachnoid block or impending block

Neoplastic conditions: Acute leukemia, aggressive lymphomas

Nervous system conditions: Acute exacerbations of multiple sclerosis, cerebral edema associated with primary or metastatic brain tumor, craniotomy or head injury

Ophthalmic conditions: Sympathetic ophthalmia, uveitis, and ocular inflammatory conditions

Organ transplantation-related conditions: Solid organ rejection

Pulmonary diseases: Acute exacerbations of chronic obstructive pulmonary disease (COPD), allergic bronchopulmonary aspergillosis, aspiration pneumonitis, asthma, pulmonary tuberculosis, hypersensitivity pneumonitis, idiopathic bronchiolitis obliterans with organizing pneumonia, idiopathic eosinophilic pneumonias, idiopathic pulmonary fibrosis, *Pneumocystis jiroveci* (formerly *carinii*) pneumonia (PCP), symptomatic sarcoidosis

Renal conditions: Nephrotic syndrome (idiopathic or related to lupus erythematosus), without uremia

Rheumatologic conditions: Acute gouty arthritis, ankylosing spondylitis, dermatomyositis/polymyositis, polymyalgia rheumatica, psoriatic arthritis, relapsing polychondritis, rheumatoid and juvenile arthritis, Sjogren's syndrome, systemic lupus erythematosus, vasculitis

Unlabeled Use Autoimmune hepatitis; adjunctive therapy for pain management in immunocompetent patients with herpes zoster; Takayasu arteritis; giant cell arteritis; Grave's ophthalmopathy prophylaxis; subacute thyroiditis; thyrotoxicosis (type II amiodarone-induced)

Labeled Contraindications Hypersensitivity to any component of the formulation; systemic fungal infections; administration of live or live attenuated vaccines with immunosuppressive doses of prednisone

Lactation Enters breast milk/AAP rates "compatible" (AAP 2001 update pending)

Warnings/Precautions May cause hypercorticism or suppression of hypothalamic-pituitary-adrenal (HPA) axis, particularly in younger children or in patients receiving high doses for prolonged periods. HPA axis suppression may lead to adrenal crisis. Withdrawal and discontinuation of a corticosteroid should be done slowly and carefully. Particular care is required when patients are transferred from systemic corticosteroids to inhaled products due to possible adrenal insufficiency or withdrawal from steroids, including an increase in allergic symptoms. Patients receiving >20 mg per day of prednisone (or equivalent) may be most susceptible. Fatalities have occurred due to adrenal insufficiency in asthmatic patients during and after transfer from systemic corticosteroids to aerosol steroids; aerosol steroids do **not** provide the systemic steroid needed to treat patients having trauma, surgery, or infections.

Acute myopathy has been reported with high dose corticosteroids, usually in patients with neuromuscular transmission disorders; may involve ocular and/or respiratory muscles; monitor creatine kinase; recovery may be delayed. Prolonged use of corticosteroids may increase the incidence of secondary infection, mask acute infection (including fungal infections), prolong or exacerbate viral infections, or limit response to vaccines. Exposure to chickenpox should be avoided. Corticosteroids should not be used to treat ocular herpes simplex or cerebral malaria. Close observation is required in patients with latent tuberculosis and/or TB reactivity; restrict use in active TB (only in conjunction with antituberculosis treatment). Prolonged treatment with corticosteroids has been associated with the development of Kaposi's sarcoma (case reports); if noted, discontinuation of therapy should be considered. Prolonged use may cause posterior subcapsular cataracts, glaucoma (with possible nerve damage) and may increase the risk for ocular infections. Corticosteroid use may cause psychiatric disturbances, including depression, euphoria, insomnia, mood swings, and personality changes. Pre-existing psychiatric conditions may be exacerbated by corticosteroid use.

Use with caution in patients with HF, diabetes, GI diseases (diverticulitis, peptic ulcer, ulcerative colitis; due to risk of perforation), hepatic impairment, myasthenia gravis, MI, patients with or who are at risk for osteoporosis, seizure disorders or thyroid disease. May affect growth velocity; growth should be routinely monitored in pediatric patients.

Prior to use, the dose and duration of treatment should be based on the risk versus benefit for each individual patient. In general, use the smallest effective dose for the shortest duration of time to minimize adverse events. A gradual tapering of dose may be required prior to discontinuing therapy.

Adverse Reactions Frequency not defined.

Cardiovascular: Congestive heart failure (in susceptible patients), hypertension

Central nervous system: Emotional instability, headache, intracranial pressure increased (with papilledema), psychic derangements (including euphoria, insomnia, mood swings, personality changes, severe depression), seizure, vertigo

Dermatologic: Bruising, facial erythema, petechiae, thin fragile skin, urticaria, wound healing impaired

Endocrine & metabolic: Adrenocortical and pituitary unresponsiveness (in times of stress), carbohydrate intolerance, Cushing's syndrome, diabetes mellitus, fluid retention, growth suppression (in children), hypokalemic alkalosis, hypothyroidism enhanced, menstrual irregularities, negative nitrogen balance due to protein catabolism, potassium loss, sodium retention

Gastrointestinal: Abdominal distension, pancreatitis, peptic ulcer (with possible perforation and hemorrhage), ulcerative esophagitis

Hepatic: ALT increased, AST increased, alkaline phosphatase increased

Neuromuscular & skeletal: Aseptic necrosis of femoral and humeral heads, muscle mass loss, muscle weakness, osteoporosis, pathologic fracture of long bones, steroid myopathy, tendon rupture (particularly Achilles tendon), vertebral compression fractures

Ocular: Exophthalmos, glaucoma, intraocular pressure increased, posterior subcapsular cataracts

Miscellaneous: Allergic reactions, anaphylactic reactions, diaphoresis, hypersensitivity reactions, infections, Kaposi's sarcoma

Drug Interactions

Metabolism/Transport Effects **Substrate** of CYP3A4 (minor); **Note:** Assignment of Major/Minor substrate status based on clinically relevant drug interaction potential; **Induces** CYP2C19 (weak/moderate), CYP3A4 (weak/moderate)

Avoid Concomitant Use

Avoid concomitant use of PredniSONE with any of the following: Aldesleukin; Axitinib; BCG; Mifepristone; Natalizumab; Pimecrolimus; Tacrolimus (Topical)

Increased Effect/Toxicity

PredniSONE may increase the levels/effects of: Acetylcholinesterase Inhibitors; Amphotericin B; CycloSPORINE (Systemic); Deferasirox; Leflunomide; Loop Diuretics; Natalizumab; NSAID (COX-2 Inhibitor); NSAID (Nonselective); Thiazide Diuretics; Vaccines (Live); Warfarin

The levels/effects of PredniSONE may be increased by: Antifungal Agents (Azole Derivatives, Systemic); Aprepitant; Calcium Channel Blockers (Nondihydropyridine); CycloSPORINE (Systemic); Denosumab; Estrogen Derivatives; Fluconazole; Fosaprepitant; Indacaterol; Macrolide Antibiotics; Mifepristone; Neuromuscular-Blocking Agents (Nondepolarizing); Pimecrolimus; Quinolone Antibiotics; Ritonavir; Roflumilast; Salicylates; Tacrolimus (Topical); Telaprevir; Trastuzumab

Decreased Effect

PredniSONE may decrease the levels/effects of: Aldesleukin; Antidiabetic Agents; ARIPiprazole; Axitinib; BCG; Calcitriol; Coccidioidin Skin Test; Corticorelin; CycloSPORINE (Systemic); Hyaluronidase; Isoniazid; Salicylates; Sipuleucel-T; Telaprevir; Vaccines (Inactivated)

The levels/effects of PredniSONE may be decreased by: Aminoglutethimide; Antacids; Barbiturates; Bile Acid Sequestrants; Echinacea; Fosphenytoin; Mifepristone; Mitotane; Phenytoin; Primidone; Rifamycin Derivatives; Somatropin; Tesamorelin; Tocilizumab

Ethanol/Nutrition/Herb Interactions

Ethanol: Avoid ethanol (may increase gastric mucosal irritation)

Food: Prednisone interferes with calcium absorption. Limit caffeine.

Herb/Nutraceutical: St John's wort may decrease prednisone levels. Avoid cat's claw, echinacea (have immunostimulant properties).

Mechanism of Action Decreases inflammation by suppression of migration of polymorphonuclear leukocytes and reversal of increased capillary permeability; suppresses the immune system by reducing activity and volume of the lymphatic system; suppresses adrenal function at high doses. Antitumor effects may be related to inhibition of glucose transport, phosphorylation, or induction of cell death in immature lymphocytes. Antiemetic effects are thought to occur due to blockade of cerebral innervation of the emetic center via inhibition of prostaglandin synthesis.

Pharmacodynamics/Kinetics

Absorption: 50% to 90% (may be altered in IBS or hyperthyroidism)

Protein binding (concentration dependent): 65% to 91%

Metabolism: Hepatically converted from prednisone (inactive) to prednisolone (active); may be impaired with hepatic dysfunction

Half-life elimination: Normal renal function: ~3.5 hours

Time to peak: Oral:

Immediate release tablet: 2 hours; Delayed release tablet (Rayos®): 6-6.5 hours

Excretion: Urine (small portion)

Dosing

Adult General dosing range: Oral: Initial: 5-60 mg/day: **Note:** Dose depends upon condition being treated and response of patient; dosage for infants and children should be based on severity of the disease and response of the patient rather than on strict adherence to dosage indicated by age, weight, or body surface area. Consider alternate day therapy for long-term therapy. Discontinuation of long-term therapy requires gradual withdrawal by tapering the dose

Prednisone taper (other regimens also available):

Day 1: 30 mg divided as 10 mg before breakfast, 5 mg at lunch, 5 mg at dinner, 10 mg at bedtime

Day 2: 5 mg at breakfast, 5 mg at lunch, 5 mg at dinner, 10 mg at bedtime

Day 3: 5 mg 4 times/day (with meals and at bedtime)

Day 4: 5 mg 3 times/day (breakfast, lunch, bedtime)

Day 5: 5 mg 2 times/day (breakfast, bedtime)

Day 6: 5 mg before breakfast

Indication-specific dosing:

Acute asthma (NIH guidelines, 2007): Oral: 40-60 mg per day for 3-10 days; administer as single or 2 divided doses

Anaphylaxis, adjunctive treatment (Lieberman, 2005): Oral: 0.5 mg/kg

Antineoplastic: Oral: Usual range: 10 mg/day to 100 mg/m²/day (depending on indication). **Note:** Details concerning dosing in combination regimens should also be consulted.

Autoimmune hepatitis (unlabeled use; Czaja, 2002): Oral: Initial treatment: 60 mg/day for 1 week, *followed by* 40 mg/day for 1 week, *then* 30 mg/day for 2 weeks, *then* 20 mg/day. Half this dose should be given when used in combination with azathioprine

Crohn's disease, moderate/severe (unlabeled use): Oral: 40-60 mg daily until resolution of symptoms and resumption of weight gain (usual duration: 7-28 days) (Lichtenstein, 2009)

Dermatomyositis/polymyositis: Oral: 1 mg/kg daily (range: 0.5-1.5 mg/kg/day), often in conjunction with steroid-sparing therapies; depending on response/tolerance, consider slow tapering after 2-8 weeks depending on response; taper regimens vary widely, but often involve 5-10 mg decrements per week and may require 6-12 months to reach a low once-daily or every-other-day dose to prevent disease flare (Briemberg, 2003; Hengstman, 2009; Iorizzo, 2008; Wiendl, 2008)

Giant cell arteritis (unlabeled use): Oral: Initial: 40-60 mg/day; typically requires 1-2 years of treatment, but may begin to taper after 2-3 months; alternative dosing of 30-40 mg/day has demonstrated similar efficacy (Hiratzka, 2010)

Graves' ophthalmopathy prophylaxis (unlabeled use): Oral: 0.4-0.5 mg/kg/day, starting 1-3 days after radioactive iodine treatment, and continued for 1 month, then gradually taper over 2 months (Bahn, 2011)

Herpes zoster (unlabeled use; Dworkin, 2007): Oral: 60 mg/day for 7 days, *followed by* 30 mg/day for 7 days, *then* 15 mg/day for 7 days

Idiopathic thrombocytopenia purpura (American Society of Hematology, 1997): Oral: 1-2 mg/kg/day

Lupus nephritis, induction (Hahn, 2012): Oral:

Class III-IV lupus nephritis: 0.5-1 mg/kg/day (after glucocorticoid pulse) tapered after a few weeks to lowest effective dose, in combination with an immunosuppressive agent

Class V lupus nephritis: 0.5 mg/kg/day for 6 months in combination mycophenolate mofetil; if not improved after 6 months, use 0.5-1 mg/kg/day (after a glucocorticoid pulse) for an additional 6 months in combination with cyclophosphamide

PCP pneumonia (AIDS*info* guidelines, 2008): Note: Begin within 72 hours of PCP therapy: 40 mg twice daily for 5 days, *followed by* 40 mg once daily for 5 days, *followed by* 20 mg once daily for 11 days or until antimicrobial regimen is completed

Rheumatoid arthritis (American College of Rheumatology, 2002): Oral: ≤10 mg/day

Subacute thyroiditis (unlabeled use): Oral: 40 mg/day for 1-2 weeks; gradually taper over 2-4 weeks or longer depending on clinical response. **Note:** NSAIDs should be considered first-line therapy in such patients (Bahn, 2011).

Takayasu arteritis (unlabeled use): Oral: Initial: 40-60 mg/day; taper to lowest effective dose when ESR and CRP levels are normal; usual duration: 1-2 years (Hiratzka, 2010)

Thyrotoxicosis (type II amiodarone-induced; unlabeled use): Oral: 40 mg/day for 14-28 days; gradually taper over 2-3 months depending on clinical response (Bahn, 2011)

Tuberculosis, severe, paradoxical reactions (unlabeled dose, AIDS*info* guidelines, 2008): Oral: 1 mg/kg/day, gradually reduce after 1-2 weeks

Geriatric Refer to adult dosing; use the lowest effective dose. Oral dose depends upon condition being treated and response of patient. Alternate day dosing may be attempted.

Pediatric

General dosing range: Oral: Refer to adult dosing. **Note:** Dose depends upon condition being treated and response of patient; dosage for infants and children should be based on severity of the disease and response of the patient rather than on strict adherence to dosage indicated by age, weight, or body surface area. Consider alternate day therapy for long-term therapy. Discontinuation of long-term therapy requires gradual withdrawal by tapering the dose.

Indication-specific dosing:

Acute asthma (NIH guidelines, 2007): Oral:

0-11 years 1-2 mg/kg/day for 3-10 days (maximum: 60 mg/day)

≥12 years: Refer to Adults dosing

Autoimmune hepatitis (unlabeled use; Czaja, 2002): Oral: Initial treatment: 2 mg/kg/day for 2 weeks (maximum: 60 mg/day), followed by a taper over 6-8 weeks to a dose of 0.1-0.2 mg/kg/day or 5 mg/day

Nephrotic syndrome (Pediatric Nephrology Panel recommendations [Hogg, 2000]): Oral: Initial: 2 mg/kg/day or 60 mg/m^2/day given every day in 1-3 divided doses (maximum: 80 mg/day) until urine is protein free or for 4-6 weeks; followed by maintenance dose: 2 mg/kg/dose or 40 mg/m^2/dose given every other day in the morning; gradually taper and discontinue after 4-6 weeks. **Note:** No definitive treatment guidelines exist. Dosing is dependent on institution protocols and individual response.

PCP pneumonia (AIDS*info* guidelines, 2008): Oral:

Children: 1 mg/kg twice daily for 5 days, *followed by* 0.5-1 mg/kg twice daily for 5 days, *followed by* 0.5 mg/kg once daily for 11-21 days

Adolescents: Refer to adult dosing.

Renal Impairment Hemodialysis effects: Supplemental dose is not necessary.

Combination Regimens Note: In the U.S. prednisone is the preferred corticosteroid. However, in the British literature prednisolone is often used. The oral doses of these two agents are equivalent (ie, 1 mg prednisone = 1 mg prednisolone). Also, early clinical trials gave prednisone only with the first and fourth cycles. Some clinicians give prednisone with every cycle.

Brain tumors:
MOPP (Medulloblastoma) on page 1717
POC on page 1740

Leukemia, acute lymphocytic:
DVP on page 1621
Hyper-CVAD + Imatinib on page 1680
Hyper-CVAD (Leukemia, Acute Lymphocytic) on page 1681
Larson Regimen (ALL) on page 1699
Linker Protocol (ALL) on page 1703
MTX/6-MP/VP (Maintenance) on page 1717
POMP on page 1741
PVA (POG 8602) on page 1742
PVDA on page 1745

Leukemia, chronic lymphocytic:
Chlorambucil-Prednisone (CLL) on page 1563
CVP (Leukemia) on page 1598

Lymphoma, Hodgkin:
BEACOPP-14 (Hodgkin) on page 1522
BEACOPP Escalated (Hodgkin) on page 1522
BEACOPP Escalated Plus Standard (Hodgkin) on page 1523
BEACOPP Standard (Hodgkin) on page 1525
ChlVPP (Hodgkin) on page 1562
C-MOPP/ABV Hybrid (Hodgkin) on page 1588
MOPP/ABVD (Hodgkin) on page 1714
MOPP/ABV Hybrid (Hodgkin) on page 1715
MOPP (Hodgkin) on page 1716
Stanford V (Hodgkin) on page 1752
VAMP (Hodgkin) on page 1769

Lymphoma, non-Hodgkin's:
CEPP(B) on page 1556
CHOP (NHL) on page 1564
CNOP on page 1589
COP-BLAM on page 1595
COPP on page 1596
CVP (Lymphoma, non-Hodgkin's) on page 1598
EPOCH Dose-Adjusted (AIDS-Related Lymphoma) on page 1628
EPOCH Dose-Adjusted (NHL) on page 1628
EPOCH (Dose-Adjusted) Rituximab (NHL) on page 1629
EPOCH (NHL) on page 1630
EPOCH-Rituximab (NHL) on page 1631
MACOP-B on page 1704
Pro-MACE-CytaBOM on page 1741
R-CVP on page 1745
Rituximab-CHOP (NHL) on page 1748

Multiple myeloma:
Bortezomib-Melphalan-Prednisone-Thalidomide on page 1537
Melphalan-Prednisone-Bortezomib (Multiple Myeloma) on page 1708
Melphalan-Prednisone (Multiple Myeloma) on page 1709

Melphalan-Prednisone-Thalidomide (Multiple Myeloma) on page 1710
VBMCP (Multiple Myeloma) on page 1769
VCAP on page 1770
Prostate cancer:
Abiraterone-Prednisone (Prostate Cancer) on page 1516
Cabazitaxel-Prednisone (Prostate Cancer) on page 1538
Docetaxel-Prednisone on page 1614
Estramustine + Docetaxel + Prednisone on page 1636
Mitoxantrone-Prednisone (Prostate Cancer) on page 1713

Administration Administer with food to decrease GI upset. Delayed release tablet (Rayos®) should be swallowed whole; do not crush or chew.

Monitoring Parameters Blood pressure, blood glucose, electrolytes

Following prolonged use: Bone mass density, growth in children, signs and symptoms of infection, cataract formation, intraocular pressure (use >6 weeks)

Test Interactions Decreased response to skin tests

Dietary Considerations Should be taken after meals or with food or milk; may require increased dietary intake of pyridoxine, vitamin C, vitamin D, folate, calcium, and phosphorus; may require decreased dietary intake of sodium

Additional Information Tapering of corticosteroids after a short course of therapy (<7-10 days) is generally not required unless the disease/inflammatory process is slow to respond. Tapering after prolonged exposure is dependent upon the individual patient, duration of corticosteroid treatments, and size of steroid dose. Recovery of the HPA axis may require several months. Subtle but important HPA axis suppression may be present for as long as several months after a course of as few as 10-14 days duration. Testing of HPA axis (cosyntropin) may be required, and signs/symptoms of adrenal insufficiency should be monitored in patients with a history of use.

Dosage Forms Excipient information presented when available (limited, particularly for generics); consult specific product labeling.
Solution, oral: 1 mg/mL (5 mL, 120 mL, 500 mL)
Solution, oral [concentrate]:
PredniSONE Intensol™: 5 mg/mL (30 mL) [dye free, sugar free; contains ethanol 30%, propylene glycol]
Tablet, oral: 1 mg, 2.5 mg, 5 mg, 10 mg, 20 mg, 50 mg
Tablet, delayed release, oral:
Rayos®: 1 mg, 2 mg, 5 mg

References

American College of Rheumatology Subcommittee on Rheumatoid Arthritis Guidelines, "Guidelines for the Management of Rheumatoid Arthritis: 2002 Update," *Arthritis Rheum*, 2002, 46 (2):328-46.

Bahn RS (Chair), Burch HB, Cooper DS, et al, "Hyperthyroidism and Other Causes of Thyrotoxicosis: Management Guidelines of the American Thyroid Association and American Association of Clinical Endocrinologists," *Thyroid*, 2011, 21(6):593-646.

Bogazzi F, Bartalena L, Cosci C, et al, "Treatment of Type II Amiodarone-Induced Thyrotoxicosis by Either Iopanoic Acid or Glucocorticoids: A Prospective, Randomized Study," *J Clin Endocrinol Metab*, 2003, 88(5):1999-2002.

Bogazzi F, Bartalena L, Tomisti L, et al, "Glucocorticoid Response in Amiodarone-Induced Thyrotoxicosis Resulting From Destructive Thyroiditis is Predicted by Thyroid Volume and Serum Free Thyroid Hormone Concentrations," *J Clin Endocrinol Metab*, 2007, 92(2):556-62.

Boot AM, Nauta J, Hokken-Koelega AC, et al, "Renal Transplantation and Osteoporosis," *Arch Dis Child*, 1995, 72(6):502-6.

Bowman H and Lennard TW, "Immunosuppressive Drugs," *Br J Hosp Med*, 1992, 48(9):570-3.

Briemberg HR and Amato AA, "Dermatomyositis and Polymyositis," *Curr Treat Options Neurol*, 2003, 5(5):349-56.

Coursin DB and Wood KE, "Corticosteroid Supplementation for Adrenal Insufficiency," *JAMA*, 2002, 287(2):236-40.

Czaja AJ and Freese DK, "Diagnosis and Treatment of Autoimmune Hepatitis," *Hepatology*, 2002, 36(2):479-97.

Dollinger RP, Levy MM, Carlet JM, et al, "Surviving Sepsis Campaign: International Guidelines for Management of Severe Sepsis and Septic Shock: 2008," *Intensive Care Med*, 2008, 34(1):17-60. Available at http://www.ncbi.nlm.nih.gov/pmc/articles/PMC2249616/pdf/134_2007_Article_934.pdf

"Diagnosis and Treatment of Idiopathic Thrombocytopenic Purpura: Recommendations of the American Society of Hematology. The American Society of Hematology ITP Practice Guideline Panel," *Ann Intern Med*, 1997, 126(4):319-26.

Dworkin RH, Johnson RW, Breuer J, et al, "Recommendations for the management of herpes zoster," *Clin Infect Dis*, 2007, 44(Suppl 1):1-26.

Frey BM and Frey FJ, "Clinical Pharmacokinetics of Prednisone and Prednisolone," *Clin Pharmacokinet*, 1990, 19(2):126-46.

Expert Panel Report 3, "Guidelines for the Diagnosis and Management of Asthma," *Clinical Practice Guidelines*, National Institutes of Health, National Heart, Lung, and Blood Institute, NIH Publication No. 08-4051, prepublication 2007. Available at http://www.nhlbi.nih.gov/guidelines/asthma/asthgdln.htm

"Guidelines for Prevention and Treatment of Opportunistic Infections in HIV-Infected Adults and Adolescents – June 18, 2008." Available at http://aidsinfo.nih.gov/contentfiles/Adult_OI.pdf

"Guidelines for Prevention and Treatment of Opportunistic Infections Among HIV-Exposed and HIV-Infected Children – June 20, 2008." Available at http://aidsinfo.nih.gov/contentfiles/Pediatric_OI.pdf.

"Guidelines for Referral and Management of Systemic Lupus Erythematosus in Adults. American College of Rheumatology Ad Hoc Committee on Systemic Lupus Erythematosus Guidelines," *Arthritis Rheum*, 1999, 42(9):1785-96.

Hengstman GJ, van den Hoogen FH, and van Engelen BG, "Treatment of the Inflammatory Myopathies: Update and Practical Recommendations," *Expert Opin Pharmacother*, 2009, 10(7):1183-90.

Hiratzka LF, Bakris GL, Beckman JA, et al, "2010 ACCF/AHA/AATS/ACR/ASA/SCA/SCAI/SIR/STS/SVM Guidelines for the Diagnosis and Management of Patients With Thoracic Aortic Disease. A Report of the American College of Cardiology Foundation/American Heart Association Task Force on Practice Guidelines, American Association for Thoracic Surgery, American College of Radiology, American Stroke Association, Society of Cardiovascular Anesthesiologists, Society for Cardiovascular Angiography and Interventions, Society of Interventional Radiology, Society of Thoracic Surgeons, and Society for Vascular Medicine," *J Am Coll Cardiol*, 2010, 55(14):e27-129.

Hogg RJ, Portman RJ, Milliner D, et al, "Evaluation and Management of Proteinuria and Nephrotic Syndrome in Children: Recommendations From a Pediatric Nephrology Panel Established at the National Kidney Foundation Conference on Proteinuria, Albuminuria, Risk, Assessment, Detection, and Elimination (PARADE)," *Pediatrics*, 2000, 105(6):1242-9.

Iorizzo LJ 3rd and Jorizzo JL, "The Treatment and Prognosis of Dermatomyositis: An Updated Review," *J Am Acad Dermatol*, 2008, 59(1):99-112.

Ito S, Blajchman A, Stephenson M, et al, "Prospective Follow-up of Adverse Reactions in Breast-Fed Infants Exposed to Maternal Medication," *Am J Obstet Gynecol*, 1993, 168(5):1393-9.

Kornbluth A and Sachar DB, "Ulcerative Colitis Practice Guidelines in Adults: American College of Gastroenterology, Practice Parameters Committee," *Am J Gastroenterol*, 2010, 105(3):501-23.

Lichtenstein GR, Hanauer SB, and Sandborn WJ, "Management of Crohn's Disease in Adults," *Am J Gastroenterol*, 2009, 104(2):465-83.

Lieberman P, Kemp SF, Oppenheimer J, et al, "The Diagnosis and Management of Anaphylaxis: An Updated Practice Parameter," *J Allergy Clin Immunol*, 2005, 115(3 Suppl 2):483-523.

McGee S and Hirschmann J, "Use of Corticosteroids in Treating Infectious Diseases," *Arch Intern Med*, 2008, 168(10):1034-46.

Moxley RT 3rd, Ashwal S, Pandya S, et al, "Practice Parameter: Corticosteroid Treatment of Duchenne Dystrophy: Report of the Quality Standards Subcommittee of the American Academy of Neurology and the Practice Committee of the Child Neurology Society," *Neurology*, 2005, 64(1):13-20.

Wallace DV, Dykewicz MS, Bernstein DI, et al, "The Diagnosis and Management of Anaphylaxis: An Updated Practice Parameter," *J Allergy Clin Immunol*, 2005, 115(3 Suppl 2):483-523.

Wiendl H, "Idiopathic Inflammatory Myopathies: Current and Future Therapeutic Options," *Neurotherapeutics*, 2008, 5(4):548-57.

◆ **PredniSONE Intensol™** *see* PredniSONE *on page 1199*

◆ **Preparation H® Hydrocortisone [OTC]** *see* Hydrocortisone (Topical) *on page 719*

◆ **Prevex® HC (Can)** *see* Hydrocortisone (Topical) *on page 719*

◆ **Prialt®** *see* Ziconotide *on page 1481*

◆ **Prilocaine and Lidocaine** *see* Lidocaine and Prilocaine *on page 894*

◆ **Primaxin® I.M. [DSC]** *see* Imipenem and Cilastatin *on page 773*

◆ **Primaxin® I.V.** *see* Imipenem and Cilastatin *on page 773*

◆ **Primaxin® I.V. Infusion (Can)** *see* Imipenem and Cilastatin *on page 773*

◆ **Privigen®** *see* Immune Globulin *on page 777*

◆ **PRO-Bicalutamide (Can)** *see* Bicalutamide *on page 178*

◆ **PRO-Calcitonin (Can)** *see* Calcitonin *on page 214*

Procarbazine (proe KAR ba zeen)

Related Information

Chemotherapy and Cancer Treatment During Pregnancy *on page 1829*
Fertility and Cancer Therapy *on page 1782*
Management of Chemotherapy-Induced Nausea and Vomiting *on page 1786*
Safe Handling of Hazardous Drugs *on page 1904*

Brand Names: U.S. Matulane®

Brand Names: Canada Matulane®; Natulan®

Index Terms Benzmethyzin; N-Methylhydrazine; Procarbazine Hydrochloride

Generic Availability (U.S.) No

Pharmacologic Category Antineoplastic Agent, Alkylating Agent

Use Treatment of Hodgkin's disease

Unlabeled Use Treatment of non-Hodgkin's lymphoma, brain tumors

Labeled Contraindications Hypersensitivity to procarbazine or any component of the formulation; pre-existing bone marrow aplasia; ethanol ingestion; pregnancy

Pregnancy Risk Factor D

Lactation Excretion in breast milk unknown/not recommended

Warnings/Precautions Hazardous agent - use appropriate precautions for handling and disposal. Use with caution in patients with pre-existing renal or hepatic impairment. Procarbazine possesses MAO inhibitor activity and has potential for severe drug and food interactions; follow MAO-I diet. Avoid ethanol consumption, may cause disulfiram-like reaction. May cause hemolysis and/or presence of Heinz inclusion bodies in erythrocytes. Bone marrow depression may occur 2-8 weeks after treatment initiation. Allow ≥1 month interval between radiation therapy or myelosuppressive chemotherapy and initiation of treatment. Withhold treatment for CNS toxicity, leukopenia (WBC $<4000/mm^3$), thrombocytopenia (platelets $<100{,}000/mm^3$), hypersensitivity, stomatitis, diarrhea, or hemorrhage. Procarbazine is a carcinogen which may cause acute leukemia. May cause infertility. **[U.S. Boxed Warning]: Should be administered under the supervision of an experienced cancer chemotherapy physician.**

Adverse Reactions Most frequencies not defined.

Cardiovascular: Edema, flushing, hypotension, syncope, tachycardia

Central nervous system: Apprehension, ataxia, chills, coma, confusion, depression, dizziness, drowsiness, fatigue, fever, hallucination, headache, insomnia, lethargy, nervousness, nightmares, pain, seizure, slurred speech

Dermatologic: Alopecia, dermatitis, hyperpigmentation, petechiae, pruritus, purpura, rash, urticaria

Endocrine & metabolic: Gynecomastia (in prepubertal and early pubertal males)
Hematologic: Eosinophilia; hemolysis (in patients with G6PD deficiency); hemolytic anemia; myelosuppression (leukopenia, anemia, thrombocytopenia); pancytopenia
Gastrointestinal: Abdominal pain, anorexia, constipation, diarrhea, dysphagia, hematemesis, melena; nausea and vomiting ([60% to 90%], increasing the dose in a stepwise fashion over several days may minimize); stomatitis, xerostomia
Genitourinary: Azoospermia (reported with combination chemotherapy), hematuria, nocturia, polyuria, reproductive dysfunction (>10%)
Hepatic: Hepatic dysfunction, jaundice
Neuromuscular & skeletal: Arthralgia, falling, foot drop, myalgia, neuropathy, paresthesia, reflex diminished, tremor, unsteadiness, weakness
Ocular: Diplopia, inability to focus, nystagmus, papilledema, photophobia, retinal hemorrhage
Otic: Hearing loss
Respiratory: Cough, epistaxis, hemoptysis, hoarseness, pleural effusion, pneumonitis, pulmonary toxicity (<1%)
Miscellaneous: Allergic reaction, diaphoresis, herpes, infection, secondary malignancies (2% to 15%; reported with combination therapy)

Drug Interactions

Metabolism/Transport Effects Inhibits Monoamine Oxidase

Avoid Concomitant Use

Avoid concomitant use of Procarbazine with any of the following: Alpha-/Beta-Agonists (Indirect-Acting); Alpha1-Agonists; Alpha2-Agonists (Ophthalmic); Amphetamines; Anilidopiperidine Opioids; Antidepressants (Serotonin Reuptake Inhibitor/Antagonist); AtoMOXetine; BCG; Bezafibrate; Buprenorphine; BuPROPion; BusPIRone; CarBAMazepine; CloZAPine; Cyclobenzaprine; Dexmethylphenidate; Dextromethorphan; Diethylpropion; HYDROmorphone; Linezolid; Maprotiline; Meperidine; Methyldopa; Methylene Blue; Methylphenidate; Mirtazapine; Natalizumab; Oxymorphone; Pimecrolimus; Pizotifen; Selective Serotonin Reuptake Inhibitors; Serotonin 5-HT1D Receptor Agonists; Serotonin/Norepinephrine Reuptake Inhibitors; Tacrolimus (Topical); Tapentadol; Tetrabenazine; Tetrahydrozoline (Nasal); Tricyclic Antidepressants; Tryptophan; Vaccines (Live)

Increased Effect/Toxicity

Procarbazine may increase the levels/effects of: Alpha-/Beta-Agonists (Direct-Acting); Alpha-/Beta-Agonists (Indirect-Acting); Alpha1-Agonists; Alpha2-Agonists (Ophthalmic); Amphetamines; Antidepressants (Serotonin Reuptake Inhibitor/Antagonist); Antihypertensives; AtoMOXetine; Beta2-Agonists; Bezafibrate; BuPROPion; CloZAPine; Dexmethylphenidate; Dextromethorphan; Diethylpropion; Doxapram; HYDROmorphone; Hypoglycemic Agents; Leflunomide; Linezolid; Lithium; Meperidine; Methadone; Methyldopa; Methylene Blue; Methylphenidate; Metoclopramide; Mirtazapine; Natalizumab; Orthostatic Hypotension Producing Agents; Pizotifen; Reserpine; Selective Serotonin Reuptake Inhibitors; Serotonin 5-HT1D Receptor Agonists; Serotonin Modulators; Serotonin/Norepinephrine Reuptake Inhibitors; Tetrahydrozoline (Nasal); Tricyclic Antidepressants; Vaccines (Live); Vitamin K Antagonists

The levels/effects of Procarbazine may be increased by: Altretamine; Anilidopiperidine Opioids; Antipsychotics; Buprenorphine; BusPIRone; CarBAMazepine; COMT Inhibitors; Cyclobenzaprine; Denosumab; Levodopa; MAO

Inhibitors; Maprotiline; Oxymorphone; Pimecrolimus; Roflumilast; Tacrolimus (Topical); Tapentadol; Tetrabenazine; TraMADol; Trastuzumab; Tryptophan

Decreased Effect

Procarbazine may decrease the levels/effects of: BCG; Cardiac Glycosides; Coccidioidin Skin Test; Sipuleucel-T; Vaccines (Inactivated); Vaccines (Live); Vitamin K Antagonists

The levels/effects of Procarbazine may be decreased by: Echinacea

Ethanol/Nutrition/Herb Interactions

Ethanol: Ethanol may enhance the adverse/toxic effects of procarbazine or cause a disulfiram reaction. Management: Avoid ethanol.

Food: Concurrent ingestion of foods rich in tyramine may cause sudden and severe high blood pressure (hypertensive crisis or serotonin syndrome). Management: Avoid tyramine-containing foods (aged or matured cheese, air-dried or cured meats including sausages and salamis; fava or broad bean pods, tap/draft beers, Marmite concentrate, sauerkraut, soy sauce, and other soybean condiments). Food's freshness is also an important concern; improperly stored or spoiled food can create an environment in which tyramine concentrations may increase.

Herb/Nutraceutical: Supplements containing caffeine, tyrosine, tryptophan, or phenylalanine may increase the risk of severe side effects (eg, hypertensive reactions, serotonin syndrome). Echinacea may diminish the therapeutic effect of immunosuppressants. Management: Avoid supplements containing caffeine, tyrosine, tryptophan, or phenylalanine. Consider avoiding echinacea.

Storage/Stability Protect from light.

Mechanism of Action Mechanism of action is not clear, methylating of nucleic acids; inhibits DNA, RNA, and protein synthesis; may damage DNA directly and suppresses mitosis; metabolic activation required by host

Pharmacodynamics/Kinetics

Absorption: Rapid and complete

Distribution: Crosses blood-brain barrier; equilibrates between plasma and CSF

Metabolism: Hepatic and renal

Half-life elimination: 1 hour

Time to peak, plasma: 1 hour

Excretion: Urine and respiratory tract (<5% as unchanged drug, 70% as metabolites)

Dosing

Adult Refer to individual protocols.

Chemotherapy: Oral: Initial: 2-4 mg/kg/day in single or divided doses for 7 days then increase dose to 4-6 mg/kg/day until response is obtained or leukocyte count decreased <4000/mm^3 or the platelet count decreased <100,000/mm^3; maintenance: 1-2 mg/kg/day

Geriatric Refer to adult dosing; use with caution. Adjust for renal impairment.

Pediatric Refer to individual protocols. Manufacturer states that the dose is based on patient's ideal weight if the patient is obese or has abnormal fluid retention. Other studies suggest that ideal body weight may not be necessary. Oral (may be given as a single daily dose or in 2-3 divided doses): Children:

BMT aplastic anemia conditioning regimen (unlabeled use): 12.5 mg/kg/day every other day for 4 doses

Hodgkin's disease: MOPP/IC-MOPP regimens: 100 mg/m²/day for 14 days and repeated every 4 weeks

Neuroblastoma and medulloblastoma (unlabeled use): Doses as high as 100-200 mg/m²/day once daily have been used.

Renal Impairment The FDA-approved labeling does not contain dosing adjustment guidelines; use with caution; may result in increased toxicity.

Hepatic Impairment The FDA-approved labeling does not contain dosing adjustment guidelines; use with caution; may result in increased toxicity. The following guidelines have been used by some clinicians:

Floyd, 2006:

Transaminases 1.6-6 times ULN: Administer 75% of dose

Transaminases >6 times ULN: Use clinical judgment

Serum bilirubin >5 mg/dL or transaminases >3 times ULN: Avoid use

King, 2001: Serum bilirubin >5 mg/dL or transaminases >180 units/L: Avoid use

Combination Regimens

Brain tumors:

MOPP (Medulloblastoma) on page 1717
PCV (Brain Tumor Regimen) on page 1736

Lymphoma, Hodgkin:

BEACOPP-14 (Hodgkin) on page 1522
BEACOPP Escalated (Hodgkin) on page 1522
BEACOPP Escalated Plus Standard (Hodgkin) on page 1523
BEACOPP Standard (Hodgkin) on page 1525
ChIVPP (Hodgkin) on page 1562
C-MOPP/ABV Hybrid (Hodgkin) on page 1588
MOPP/ABVD (Hodgkin) on page 1714
MOPP/ABV Hybrid (Hodgkin) on page 1715
MOPP (Hodgkin) on page 1716

Lymphoma, non-Hodgkin's:

CEPP(B) on page 1566
COP-BLAM on page 1595
COPP on page 1596

Administration May be given as a single daily dose or in 2-3 divided doses.

Emetic Potential High (>90%)

Extemporaneous Preparations Hazardous agent: Use appropriate precautions for handling and disposal.

A 10 mg/mL oral suspension may be prepared using capsules, glycerin, and strawberry syrup. Empty the contents of ten 50 mg capsules into a mortar. Add 2 mL glycerin and mix to a thick uniform paste. Add 10 mL strawberry syrup in incremental proportions; mix until uniform. Transfer the mixture to an amber glass bottle and rinse mortar with small amounts of strawberry syrup; add rinses to the bottle in sufficient quantity to make 50 mL. Label "shake well" and "protect from light". Stable for 7 days at room temperature.

Matulane® data on file, Sigma Tau Pharmaceuticals, Inc.

Monitoring Parameters CBC with differential, platelet and reticulocyte count, urinalysis, liver function test, renal function test.

Dietary Considerations Avoid tyramine-containing foods/beverages. Some examples include aged or matured cheese, air-dried or cured meats (including sausages and salamis), fava or broad bean pods, tap/draft beers, Marmite concentrate, sauerkraut, soy sauce and other soybean condiments.

Dosage Forms Excipient information presented when available (limited, particularly for generics); consult specific product labeling.

Capsule, oral, as hydrochloride:
Matulane®: 50 mg

References

Floyd J, Mirza I, Sachs B, et al, "Hepatotoxicity of Chemotherapy," *Semin Oncol*, 2006, 33 (1):50-67.
King PD and Perry MC, "Hepatotoxicity of Chemotherapy," *Oncologist*, 2001, 6(2):162-76.

◆ **Procarbazine Hydrochloride** *see* Procarbazine *on page 1208*

Prochlorperazine (proe klor PER a zeen)

Related Information

Management of Chemotherapy-Induced Nausea and Vomiting *on page 1786*

Brand Names: U.S. Compro®

Brand Names: Canada Apo-Prochlorperazine®; Nu-Prochlor; PMS-Prochlorperazine; Sandoz-Prochlorperazine

Index Terms Chlormeprazine; Compazine; Prochlorperazine Edisylate; Prochlorperazine Maleate; Prochlorperazine Mesylate

Generic Availability (U.S.) Yes

Pharmacologic Category Antiemetic; Antipsychotic Agent, Typical, Phenothiazine

Use Management of nausea and vomiting; psychotic disorders, including schizophrenia and anxiety; nonpsychotic anxiety

Unlabeled Use Behavioral syndromes in dementia; psychosis/agitation related to Alzheimer's dementia

Labeled Contraindications Hypersensitivity to prochlorperazine or any component of the formulation (cross-reactivity between phenothiazines may occur); coma or presence of large amounts of CNS depressants (eg, alcohol, narcotics, barbiturates); pediatric surgery; children <2 years of age or <9 kg

Canadian labeling: Additional contraindications (not in U.S. labeling): Presence of circulatory collapse; severe cardiovascular disorders; altered state of consciousness; concomitant use of high dose hypnotics; severe depression; presence of blood dyscrasias, hepatic or renal impairment, or pheochromocytoma; suspected or established subcortical brain damage with or without hypothalamic damage

Lactation Excretion in breast milk unknown/use caution

Warnings/Precautions [U.S. Boxed Warning]: Elderly patients with dementia-related psychosis treated with antipsychotics are at an increased risk of death compared to placebo. Most deaths appeared to be either cardiovascular (eg, heart failure, sudden death) or infectious (eg, pneumonia) in nature. Prochlorperazine is not approved for the treatment of dementia-related psychosis. May cause extrapyramidal symptoms (EPS), including pseudoparkinsonism, acute dystonic reactions, akathisia, and tardive dyskinesia. Risk of dystonia (and possibly other EPS) may be greater with increased doses, use of conventional antipsychotics, males, and younger patients. Risk of tardive dyskinesia and potential for irreversibility often associated with total cumulative dose and therapy duration and may also be increased in elderly patients (particularly elderly women); antipsychotics may also mask signs/symptoms of tardive dyskinesia. Consider therapy discontinuation with signs/symptoms of tardive dyskinesia. Antipsychotic use has been associated with esophageal dysmotility and aspiration; use with caution in patients at risk of pneumonia (ie, Alzheimer's disease).

May be sedating and impair physical or mental abilities; use with caution in disorders where CNS depression is a feature. Effects with other sedative drugs or ethanol may be potentiated. Use with caution in Parkinson's disease; hemodynamic instability; predisposition to seizures; subcortical brain damage; and in severe cardiac, hepatic, or renal disease. Canadian labeling contraindicates use in patients with severe cardiac disease, hepatic or renal impairment, subcortical brain damage, and circulatory collapse. May alter temperature regulation, obscure intestinal obstruction or brain tumor or mask toxicity of other drugs. May alter cardiac conduction. Hypotension may occur following administration, particularly when parenteral form is used or in high dosages. May cause orthostatic hypotension; use with caution in patients at risk of this effect or in those who would not tolerate transient hypotensive episodes (cerebrovascular disease, cardiovascular disease, hypovolemia, or concurrent medication use which may predispose to hypotension/bradycardia).

Leukopenia, neutropenia, and agranulocytosis (sometimes fatal) have been reported in clinical trials and postmarketing reports with antipsychotic use; presence of risk factors (eg, pre-existing low WBC or history of drug-induced leuko-/neutropenia) should prompt periodic blood count assessment. Discontinue therapy at first signs of blood dyscrasias or if absolute neutrophil count <1000/mm^3.

Due to its potent anticholinergic effects, may be inappropriate in older adults depending on comorbidities (eg, dementia, delirium) (Beers Criteria). Use with caution in patients with decreased gastrointestinal motility, urinary retention, BPH, xerostomia, or visual problems. Conditions which also may be exacerbated by cholinergic blockade include narrow-angle glaucoma and worsening of myasthenia gravis. Use caution with exposure to heat. May cause pigmentary retinopathy, and lenticular and corneal deposits, particularly with prolonged therapy. Use associated with increased prolactin levels; clinical significance of hyperprolactinemia in patients with breast cancer or other prolactin-dependent tumors is unknown. Avoid use in patients with signs/symptoms suggestive of Reye's syndrome. Children with acute illness or dehydration are more susceptible to neuromuscular reactions; use cautiously. May be associated with neuroleptic malignant syndrome (NMS). Some dosage forms may contain benzyl alcohol which has been associated with "gasping syndrome" in neonates. Some dosage forms may contain sodium sulfite.

Adverse Reactions Reported with prochlorperazine or other phenothiazines. Frequency not defined.

Cardiovascular: Cardiac arrest, cerebral edema, hypotension, peripheral edema, Q-wave distortions, sudden death, T-wave distortions

Central nervous system: Agitation, altered cerebrospinal fluid proteins, catatonia, coma, cough reflex suppressed, dizziness, drowsiness, fever (mild [I.M.]), headache, hyperpyrexia, impairment of temperature regulation, insomnia, neuroleptic malignant syndrome (NMS), oculogyric crisis, opisthotonos, restlessness, seizure, somnolence, tremulousness

Dermatologic: Angioedema, contact dermatitis, epithelial keratopathy, erythema, eczema, exfoliative dermatitis, itching, photosensitivity, skin pigmentation, urticaria

Endocrine & metabolic: Amenorrhea, galactorrhea, gynecomastia, glucosuria, hyper-/hypoglycemia, lactation, libido (changes in), menstrual irregularity

Gastrointestinal: Appetite increased, atonic colon, constipation, ileus, nausea, obstipation, vomiting, weight gain, xerostomia

Genitourinary: Ejaculating dysfunction, ejaculatory disturbances, impotence, priapism, urinary retention
Hematologic: Agranulocytosis, aplastic anemia, eosinophilia, hemolytic anemia, leukopenia, pancytopenia, thrombocytopenic purpura
Hepatic: Biliary stasis, cholestatic jaundice, hepatotoxicity
Neuromuscular & skeletal: Dystonias (torticollis, carpopedal spasm, trismus, protrusion of tongue); extrapyramidal symptoms (pseudoparkinsonism, akathisia, dystonias, tardive dyskinesia, hyperreflexia); SLE-like syndrome, tremor
Ocular: Blurred vision, lenticular/corneal deposits, miosis, mydriasis, pigmentary retinopathy
Respiratory: Asthma, laryngeal edema, nasal congestion
Miscellaneous: Allergic reactions, asphyxia, diaphoresis

Drug Interactions

Metabolism/Transport Effects None known.

Avoid Concomitant Use

Avoid concomitant use of Prochlorperazine with any of the following: Aclidinium; Azelastine (Nasal); Dofetilide; Ipratropium (Oral Inhalation); Metoclopramide; Paraldehyde; Tiotropium

Increased Effect/Toxicity

Prochlorperazine may increase the levels/effects of: Alcohol (Ethyl); Analgesics (Opioid); Anticholinergics; Antidepressants (Serotonin Reuptake Inhibitor/Antagonist); Azelastine (Nasal); Beta-Blockers; CNS Depressants; Dofetilide; Methotrimeprazine; Methylphenidate; Paraldehyde; Porfimer; Serotonin Modulators; Tiotropium; Zolpidem

The levels/effects of Prochlorperazine may be increased by: Acetylcholinesterase Inhibitors (Central); Aclidinium; Antidepressants (Serotonin Reuptake Inhibitor/Antagonist); Antimalarial Agents; Beta-Blockers; Deferoxamine; Droperidol; HydrOXYzine; Ipratropium (Oral Inhalation); Lithium formulations; Methotrimeprazine; Methylphenidate; Metoclopramide; Metyrosine; Perampanel; Pramlintide; Tetrabenazine

Decreased Effect

Prochlorperazine may decrease the levels/effects of: Amphetamines; Anti-Parkinson's Agents (Dopamine Agonist); Quinagolide

The levels/effects of Prochlorperazine may be decreased by: Antacids; Anti-Parkinson's Agents (Dopamine Agonist); Lithium formulations

Ethanol/Nutrition/Herb Interactions

Ethanol: May increase CNS depression; monitor for increased effects with coadministration. Caution patients about effects.
Herb/Nutraceutical: Avoid dong quai, St John's wort (may also cause photosensitization). Avoid kava kava, gotu kola, valerian, St John's wort (may increase CNS depression).

Storage/Stability

Injection:
Edisylate: Store at 20°C to 25°C (68°F to 77°F); do not freeze. Protect from light. Clear or slightly yellow solutions may be used.
Mesylate (Canadian availability; not available in U.S.): Store at 15°C to 30°C (59°F to 86°F). Protect from light. Do not use if solution is discolored or hazy.
I.V. infusion: Injection may be diluted in 50-100 mL NS or D_5W.
Suppository: Store at 20°C to 25°C (68°F to 77°F). Protect from light.
Tablet: Store at 20°C to 25°C (68°F to 77°F). Protect from light.

Mechanism of Action Prochlorperazine is a piperazine phenothiazine antipsychotic which blocks postsynaptic mesolimbic dopaminergic D_1 and D_2 receptors in the brain, including the chemoreceptor trigger zone; exhibits a strong alpha-adrenergic and anticholinergic blocking effect and depresses the release of hypothalamic and hypophyseal hormones; believed to depress the reticular activating system, thus affecting basal metabolism, body temperature, wakefulness, vasomotor tone and emesis

Pharmacodynamics/Kinetics

Onset of action: Oral: 30-40 minutes; I.M.: 10-20 minutes; Rectal: ~60 minutes
Peak antiemetic effect: I.V.: 30-60 minutes

Duration: Rectal: 3-12 hours; I.M., Oral: 3-4 hours

Distribution: V_d: 1400-1548 L (Taylor, 1987); crosses placenta; enters breast milk

Metabolism: Primarily hepatic; N-desmethyl prochlorperazine (major active metabolite)

Bioavailability: Oral: 12.5% (Isah, 1991)

Half-life elimination: Oral: 6-10 hours (single dose), 14-22 hours (repeated dosing) (Isah, 1991); I.V.: 6-10 hours (Isah, 1991; Taylor, 1987)

Excretion: Mainly in feces

Dosing

Adult Note: Injection solution mesylate formulation has Canadian availability (not available in U.S.).

Antiemetic:

Oral (tablet): 5-10 mg 3-4 times/day; usual maximum: 40 mg/day; larger doses may rarely be required

I.M. (as edisylate): 5-10 mg every 3-4 hours; usual maximum: 40 mg/day

I.M. (as mesylate): 5-10 mg 2-3 times/day; usual maximum: 40 mg/day

I.V. (as edisylate): 2.5-10 mg; maximum: 10 mg/dose or 40 mg/day; may repeat dose every 3-4 hours as needed

Rectal:

U.S. labeling: 25 mg twice daily

Canadian labeling: 5-10 mg 3-4 times/day

Surgical nausea/vomiting: Note: Should not exceed 40 mg/day

I.M. (as edisylate): 5-10 mg 1-2 hours before anesthesia induction or to control symptoms during or after surgery; may repeat once if necessary

I.M. (as mesylate): 5-10 mg 1-2 hours before anesthesia induction; may repeat once if needed during surgery; postoperatively: 5-10 mg every 3-4 hours as needed up to maximum of 40 mg daily

I.V. (as edisylate): 5-10 mg 15-30 minutes before anesthesia induction or to control symptoms during or after surgery; may repeat once if necessary

I.V. (as mesylate): 20 mg/L of I.V. solution during surgery or postoperatively, usual maximum: 30 mg daily

Rectal (unlabeled use; Golembiewski, 2005): 25 mg

Antipsychotic:

Oral: 5-10 mg 3-4 times/day; titrate dose slowly every 2-3 days; doses up to 150 mg/day may be required in some patients for treatment of severe disturbances

I.M. (as edisylate): Initial: 10-20 mg; if necessary repeat initial dose every 2-4 hours to gain control; more than 3-4 doses are rarely needed. If parenteral administration is still required; give 10-20 mg every 4-6 hours; convert to oral therapy as soon as possible.

I.M. (as mesylate): Initial: 10-20 mg; if necessary repeat initial dose every 2-4 hours to gain control; more than 3-4 doses are rarely needed; convert to oral therapy as soon as possible.

Nonpsychotic anxiety: *Oral (tablet):* Usual dose: 5 mg 3-4 times/day; do not exceed 20 mg/day or administer >12 weeks

Geriatric Initiate at lower end of dosage range; titrate slowly and cautiously. Refer to adult dosing.

Pediatric Note: Injection solution mesylate formulation has Canadian availability (not available in U.S.).

Use is contraindicated in children <9 kg or <2 years.

Antiemetic:

Oral, rectal (therapy >1 day usually not required):

9-13 kg: 2.5 mg 1-2 times/day as needed (maximum: 7.5 mg/day)

>13-18 kg: 2.5 mg 2-3 times/day as needed (maximum: 10 mg/day)

>18-39 kg: 2.5 mg 3 times/day or 5 mg 2 times/day as needed (maximum: 15 mg/day)

I.M. (as edisylate): 0.13 mg/kg/dose; convert to oral therapy as soon as possible

I.M. (as mesylate): 0.14 mg/kg/dose; convert to oral therapy at equivalent or greater dose (if necessary) as soon as possible

Antipsychotic: Children 2-12 years:

Oral, rectal: 2.5 mg 2-3 times/day; do not give more than 10 mg the first day; increase dosage as needed to maximum daily dose of 20 mg for 2-5 years and 25 mg for 6-12 years

I.M. (as edisylate): 0.13 mg/kg/dose; convert to oral therapy as soon as possible

I.M. (as mesylate): 0.14 mg/kg/dose; convert to oral therapy at equivalent or greater dose (if necessary) as soon as possible

Renal Impairment

U.S. labeling: No dosage adjustment provided in manufacturer's labeling.

Canadian labeling: Use is contraindicated.

Hepatic Impairment

U.S. labeling: No dosage adjustment provided in manufacturer's labeling; systemic exposure may be increased as drug undergoes hepatic metabolism.

Canadian labeling: Use is contraindicated.

Administration

I.M.: Inject by deep I.M. into outer quadrant of buttocks.

I.V.: May be administered by slow I.V. push at a rate not exceeding 5 mg/minute or by I.V. infusion. Do not administer as a bolus injection. To reduce the risk of hypotension, patients receiving I.V. prochlorperazine must remain lying down and be observed for at least 30 minutes following administration. Avoid skin contact with injection solution, contact dermatitis has occurred. Do not dilute with any diluent containing parabens as a preservative.

Oral: Administer tablet without regard to meals.

Monitoring Parameters Vital signs; CBC (baseline, frequently during first few months of therapy, periodically thereafter); lipid profile; fasting blood glucose/ Hgb A_{1c}; BMI; mental status; abnormal involuntary movement scale (AIMS); periodic ophthalmic exams (if chronically used); extrapyramidal symptoms (EPS)

Test Interactions False-positives for phenylketonuria, pregnancy

Dietary Considerations Increase dietary intake of riboflavin; should be administered with food or water. Rectal suppositories may contain coconut and palm oil.

Additional Information Not recommended as an antipsychotic due to inferior efficacy compared to other phenothiazines.

Dosage Forms Excipient information presented when available (limited, particularly for generics); consult specific product labeling.

Injection, solution, as edisylate [strength expressed as base]: 5 mg/mL (2 mL, 10 mL)

Suppository, rectal: 25 mg (12s)

Compro®: 25 mg (12s) [contains coconut oil, palm oil]

Tablet, oral, as maleate [strength expressed as base]: 5 mg, 10 mg

Dosage Forms: Canada Excipient information presented when available (limited, particularly for generics); consult specific product labeling.

Injection, solution, as mesylate [strength expressed as base]: 5 mg/mL (2 mL)

Suppository, rectal: 10 mg (10s)

References

Gan TJ, Meyer TA, Apfel CC, et al, "Society for Ambulatory Anesthesia Guidelines for the Management of Postoperative Nausea and Vomiting," *Anesth Analg*, 2007, 105(6):1615-28.

Golembiewski J, Chernin E, and Chopra T, "Prevention and Treatment of Postoperative Nausea and Vomiting," *Am J Health-Syst Pharm*, 2005, 62(12):1247-60.

Hesketh PJ, Gandara DR, Hesketh AM, et al, "Improved Control of High-Dose-Cisplatin-Induced Acute Emesis With the Addition of Prochlorperazine to Granisetron/Dexamethasone," *Cancer J Sci Am*, 1997, 3(3):180-3.

Isah AO, Rawlins MD, and Bateman DN, "Clinical Pharmacology of Prochlorperazine in Healthy Young Males," *Br J Clin Pharmacol*, 1991, 32(6):677-84.

National Institute for Health and Clinical Excellence (NICE), National Collaborating Centre for Mental Health, "Schizophrenia. Core Interventions in the Treatment and Management of Schizophrenia in Primary and Secondary Care (Updated)," National Clinical Practice Guideline Number 82, 2009:1-399. Available at www.nice.org.uk/cg082

Rabins PV, Blacker D, Rovner BW, et al, "Practice Guideline for the Treatment of Patients With Alzheimer's Disease and Other Dementias," October, 2007. Available at http://www.psych.org/psych_pract/treatg/pg/prac_guide.cfm

Taylor WB and Bateman DN, "Preliminary Studies of the Pharmacokinetics and Pharmacodynamics of Prochlorperazine in Healthy Volunteers," *Br J Clin Pharmacol*, 1987, 23(2): 137-42.

◆ **Prochlorperazine Edisylate** *see* Prochlorperazine *on page* 1212
◆ **Prochlorperazine Maleate** *see* Prochlorperazine *on page* 1212
◆ **Prochlorperazine Mesylate** *see* Prochlorperazine *on page* 1212
◆ **Prociclide** *see* Defibrotide *on page* 420
◆ **PRO-Ciprofloxacin (Can)** *see* Ciprofloxacin (Systemic) *on page* 283
◆ **Procrit®** *see* Epoetin Alfa *on page* 516
◆ **Proctocort®** *see* Hydrocortisone (Topical) *on page* 719
◆ **ProctoCream®-HC** *see* Hydrocortisone (Topical) *on page* 719
◆ **Procto-Pak™** *see* Hydrocortisone (Topical) *on page* 719
◆ **Proctosol-HC®** *see* Hydrocortisone (Topical) *on page* 719
◆ **Proctozone-HC 2.5%™** *see* Hydrocortisone (Topical) *on page* 719
◆ **Procytox® (Can)** *see* Cyclophosphamide *on page* 321
◆ **PRO-Dexamethasone (Can)** *see* Dexamethasone (Systemic) *on page* 440
◆ **Profilnine® SD** *see* Factor IX Complex (Human) *on page* 575
◆ **PRO-Fluconazole (Can)** *see* Fluconazole *on page* 612
◆ **Prograf®** *see* Tacrolimus (Systemic) *on page* 1315

- **Proleukin®** *see* Aldesleukin *on page* *37*
- **Prolia™** *see* Denosumab *on page* *428*
- **Prolia® (Can)** *see* Denosumab *on page* *428*
- **PRO-Lorazepam (Can)** *see* LORazepam *on page* *907*
- **Promacta®** *see* Eltrombopag *on page* *494*

Promethazine (proe METH a zeen)

Related Information

Management of Chemotherapy-Induced Nausea and Vomiting *on page* *1786*
Management of Drug Extravasations *on page* *1800*

Brand Names: U.S. Phenadoz®; Phenergan; Promethegan™

Brand Names: Canada Bioniche Promethazine; Histantil; Phenergan; PMS-Promethazine

Index Terms Promethazine Hydrochloride

Generic Availability (U.S.) Yes

Pharmacologic Category Antiemetic; Histamine H_1 Antagonist; Histamine H_1 Antagonist, First Generation; Phenothiazine Derivative

Use Symptomatic treatment of various allergic conditions; antiemetic; motion sickness; sedative; adjunct to postoperative analgesia and anesthesia

Unlabeled Use Treatment of nausea and vomiting of pregnancy (NVP)

Labeled Contraindications Hypersensitivity to promethazine or any component of the formulation (cross-reactivity between phenothiazines may occur); coma; treatment of lower respiratory tract symptoms, including asthma; children <2 years of age; intra-arterial or subcutaneous administration

Pregnancy Risk Factor C

Lactation Excretion in breast milk unknown/not recommended

Warnings/Precautions [U.S. Boxed Warning]: Respiratory fatalities have been reported in children <2 years of age. Contraindicated in children <2 years of age. In children ≥2 years, use the lowest possible dose; other drugs with respiratory depressant effects should be avoided.

[U.S. Boxed Warning]: Promethazine injection can cause severe tissue injury (including gangrene) regardless of the route of administration. Tissue irritation and damage may result from perivascular extravasation, unintentional intra-arterial administration, and intraneuronal or perineuronal infiltration. In addition to gangrene, adverse events reported include tissue necrosis, abscesses, burning, pain, erythema, edema, paralysis, severe spasm of distal vessels, phlebitis, thrombophlebitis, venous thrombosis, sensory loss, paralysis, and palsies. Surgical intervention including fasciotomy, skin graft, and/or amputation have been necessary in some cases. The preferred route of administration is by deep intramuscular (I.M.) injection. Subcutaneous administration is contraindicated. Discontinue intravenous injection immediately with onset of pain and evaluate for arterial injection or perivascular extravasation. Although there is no proven successful management of unintentional intra-arterial injection or perivascular extravasation, sympathetic block and heparinization have been used in the acute management of unintentional intra-arterial injection based on results from animal studies.

May be sedating; use with caution in disorders where CNS depression is a feature. May impair physical or mental abilities; patients must be cautioned about performing tasks which require mental alertness. Use with caution in hemodynamic instability; bone marrow suppression; subcortical brain damage; and in severe cardiac, hepatic or respiratory disease. Avoid use in Reye's syndrome. May lower seizure threshold; use caution in persons with seizure disorders or in persons using narcotics or local anesthetics which may also affect seizure threshold. May alter temperature regulation or mask toxicity of other drugs due to antiemetic effects. May alter cardiac conduction (life-threatening arrhythmias have occurred with therapeutic doses of phenothiazines). May cause orthostatic hypotension; use with caution in patients at risk of hypotension or where transient hypotensive episodes would be poorly tolerated (cardiovascular disease or cerebrovascular disease).

Phenothiazines may cause anticholinergic effects; therefore, they should be used with caution in patients with decreased gastrointestinal motility, GI or GU obstruction, urinary retention, BPH, xerostomia, or visual problems. Conditions which also may be exacerbated by cholinergic blockade include narrow-angle glaucoma (screening is recommended) and worsening of myasthenia gravis. Use with caution in Parkinson's disease. May cause extrapyramidal symptoms, including pseudoparkinsonism, acute dystonic reactions, akathisia, and tardive dyskinesia. May be associated with neuroleptic malignant syndrome (NMS). May cause photosensitivity. In the elderly, avoid use of this potent anticholinergic agent due to increased risk of confusion, dry mouth, constipation, and other anticholinergic effects; clearance decreases in patients of advanced age (Beers Criteria). Injection may contain sodium metabisulfite.

Adverse Reactions Frequency not defined.

Cardiovascular: Bradycardia, hyper-/hypotension, nonspecific QT changes, orthostatic hypotension, tachycardia,

Central nervous system: Agitation akathisia, catatonic states, confusion, delirium, disorientation, dizziness, drowsiness, dystonias, euphoria, excitation, extrapyramidal symptoms, faintness, fatigue, hallucinations, hysteria, insomnia, lassitude, pseudoparkinsonism, tardive dyskinesia, nervousness, neuroleptic malignant syndrome, nightmares, sedation, seizure, somnolence

Dermatologic: Angioneurotic edema, dermatitis, photosensitivity, skin pigmentation (slate gray), urticaria

Endocrine & metabolic: Amenorrhea, breast engorgement, gynecomastia, hyperglycemia, lactation

Gastrointestinal: Constipation, nausea, vomiting, xerostomia

Genitourinary: Ejaculatory disorder, impotence, urinary retention

Hematologic: Agranulocytosis, leukopenia, thrombocytopenia, thrombocytopenic purpura

Hepatic: Jaundice

Local: Abscess, distal vessel spasm, gangrene, injection site reactions (burning, edema, erythema, pain), palsies, paralysis, phlebitis, sensory loss, thrombophlebitis, tissue necrosis, venous thrombosis

Neuromuscular & skeletal: Incoordination, tremor

Ocular: Blurred vision, corneal and lenticular changes, diplopia, epithelial keratopathy, pigmentary retinopathy

Otic: Tinnitus

Respiratory: Apnea, asthma, nasal congestion, respiratory depression

Drug Interactions

Metabolism/Transport Effects Substrate of CYP2B6 (major), CYP2D6 (major); **Note:** Assignment of Major/Minor substrate status based on clinically relevant drug interaction potential; **Inhibits** CYP2D6 (weak)

Avoid Concomitant Use

Avoid concomitant use of Promethazine with any of the following: Aclidinium; Azelastine (Nasal); Ipratropium (Oral Inhalation); Methadone; Metoclopramide; Paraldehyde; Tiotropium

Increased Effect/Toxicity

Promethazine may increase the levels/effects of: Alcohol (Ethyl); Anticholinergics; Azelastine (Nasal); Buprenorphine; CNS Depressants; Methadone; Metoclopramide; Paraldehyde; Pramipexole; ROPINIRole; Rotigotine; Serotonin Modulators; Tiotropium; Zolpidem

The levels/effects of Promethazine may be increased by: Abiraterone Acetate; Aclidinium; Antipsychotics; CYP2B6 Inhibitors (Moderate); CYP2B6 Inhibitors (Strong); CYP2D6 Inhibitors (Moderate); CYP2D6 Inhibitors (Strong); Darunavir; HydrOXYzine; Ipratropium (Oral Inhalation); MAO Inhibitors; Metoclopramide; Metyrosine; Perampanel; Pramlintide; Quazepam

Decreased Effect

Promethazine may decrease the levels/effects of: Acetylcholinesterase Inhibitors (Central); EPINEPHrine (Nasal); Epinephrine (Racemic); EPINEPHrine (Systemic, Oral Inhalation)

The levels/effects of Promethazine may be decreased by: Acetylcholinesterase Inhibitors (Central); CYP2B6 Inducers (Strong); Peginterferon Alfa-2b

Ethanol/Nutrition/Herb Interactions

Ethanol: Avoid ethanol (may increase CNS depression).

Herb/Nutraceutical: Avoid valerian, St John's wort, kava kava, gotu kola (may increase CNS depression).

Storage/Stability

Injection: Prior to dilution, store at 20°C to 25°C (68°F to 77°F). Protect from light. Solutions in NS or D_5W are stable for 24 hours at room temperature.

Oral solution: Store at 15°C to 25°C (59°F to 77°F). Protect from light.

Suppositories: Store refrigerated at 2°C to 8°C (36°F to 46°F).

Tablets: Store at 20°C to 25°C (68°F to 77°F). Protect from light.

Mechanism of Action Phenothiazine derivative; blocks postsynaptic mesolimbic dopaminergic receptors in the brain; exhibits a strong alpha-adrenergic blocking effect and depresses the release of hypothalamic and hypophyseal hormones; competes with histamine for the H_1-receptor; muscarinic-blocking effect may be responsible for antiemetic activity; reduces stimuli to the brainstem reticular system

Pharmacodynamics/Kinetics

Onset of action: Oral, I.M.: ~20 minutes; I.V.: ~5 minutes

Duration: Usually 4-6 hours (up to 12 hours)

Absorption: Oral: Rapid and complete; large first pass effect limits systemic bioavailability (Sharma, 2003)

Distribution: V_d: Syrup: 98 L/kg (range: 17-277 L/kg) (Strenkoski-Nox, 2000)

Metabolism: Hepatic; hydroxylation via CYP2D6 and N-demethylation via CYP2B6; significant first-pass effect (Sharma, 2003)

Bioavailability: Oral: ~25% (Sharma, 2003)

Half-life elimination: I.M.: ~10 hours; I.V.: 9-16 hours; Suppositories, syrup: 16-19 hours (range: 4-34 hours) (Strenkoski-Nox, 2000)

Time to maximum serum concentration: Suppositories: 6.7-8.6 hours; Syrup: 4.4 hours (Strenkoski-Nox, 2000)

Excretion: Urine

Dosing

Adult & Geriatric

Allergic conditions (including allergic reactions to blood or plasma):

Oral, rectal: 25 mg at bedtime **or** 12.5 mg before meals and at bedtime (range: 6.25-12.5 mg 3 times/day)

I.M., I.V.: 25 mg, may repeat in 2 hours when necessary; switch to oral route as soon as feasible

Antiemetic: Oral, I.M., I.V., rectal: 12.5-25 mg every 4-6 hours as needed

Motion sickness: Oral, rectal: 25 mg 30-60 minutes before departure, then every 12 hours as needed

Obstetrics (labor) analgesia adjunct: I.M., I.V.: Early labor: 50 mg; Established labor: 25-75 mg in combination with analgesic at reduced dosage; may repeat every 4 hours for up to 2 additional doses (maximum: 100 mg/day while in labor)

Pre-/postoperative analgesia/hypnotic adjunct: I.M., I.V.: 25-50 mg in combination with analgesic or hypnotic (at reduced dosage)

Sedation: Oral, I.M., I.V., rectal: 12.5-50 mg/dose

Pediatric

Allergic conditions: Children ≥2 years: Oral, rectal: 0.1 mg/kg/dose (maximum: 12.5 mg) every 6 hours during the day and 0.5 mg/kg/dose (maximum: 25 mg) at bedtime as needed

Antiemetic: Children ≥2 years: Oral, I.M., I.V., rectal: 0.25-1 mg/kg 4-6 times/day as needed (maximum: 25 mg/dose)

Motion sickness: Children ≥2 years: Oral, rectal: 0.5 mg/kg/dose 30 minutes to 1 hour before departure, then every 12 hours as needed (maximum dose: 25 mg twice daily)

Preoperative analgesia/hypnotic adjunct: Children ≥2 years: I.M., I.V.: 1.1 mg/kg in combination with an analgesic or hypnotic (at reduced dosage) and with an atropine-like agent (at appropriate dosage). **Note:** Promethazine dosage should not exceed half of suggested adult dosage.

Sedation: Children ≥2 years: Oral, I.M., I.V., rectal: 0.5-1 mg/kg/dose every 6 hours as needed (maximum: 50 mg/dose)

Administration Formulations available for oral, rectal, I.M./I.V.; not for SubQ or intra-arterial administration. Administer I.M. into deep muscle (preferred route of administration). I.V. administration is **not** the preferred route; severe tissue damage may occur. Solution for injection should be administered in a maximum concentration of 25 mg/mL (more dilute solutions are recommended). Administer via running I.V. line at port farthest from patient's vein, or through a large bore vein (not hand or wrist). Consider administering over 10-15 minutes (maximum: 25 mg/minute). Discontinue immediately if burning or pain occurs with administration.

Vesicant/Extravasation Risk Vesicant; see Management of Drug Extravasations on page 1800.

Monitoring Parameters Relief of symptoms, mental status; signs and symptoms of tissue injury (burning or pain at injection site, phlebitis, edema) with I.V. administration

Test Interactions May interfere with urine detection of amphetamine/methamphetamine (false-positive); alters the flare response in intradermal allergen tests; hCG-based pregnancy tests may result in false-negatives or false-positives

Dietary Considerations Increase dietary intake of riboflavin.

Dosage Forms Excipient information presented when available (limited, particularly for generics); consult specific product labeling.

Injection, solution, as hydrochloride: 25 mg/mL (1 mL); 50 mg/mL (1 mL)
Phenergan: 25 mg/mL (1 mL); 50 mg/mL (1 mL) [contains edetate disodium, sodium metabisulfite]
Suppository, rectal, as hydrochloride: 12.5 mg (12s); 25 mg (12s)
Phenadoz®: 12.5 mg (12s); 25 mg (12s)
Promethegan™: 12.5 mg (12s); 25 mg (12s); 50 mg (12s)
Syrup, oral, as hydrochloride: 6.25 mg/5 mL (118 mL, 473 mL)
Tablet, oral, as hydrochloride: 12.5 mg, 25 mg, 50 mg

References

Institute for Safe Medication Practice, "Action Needed to Prevent Serious Tissue Injury With I.V. Promethazine." Available at http://www.ismp.org/Newsletters/acutecare/articles/20060810.asp
Parkman HP, Hasler WL, Fisher RS, "American Gastroenterological Association Medical Position Statement: Diagnosis and Treatment of Gastroparesis," Gastroenterology, 2004, 127(5):1589-91.
Sharma A and Hamelin BA, "Classic Histamine H1 Receptor Antagonists: A Critical Review of Their Metabolic and Pharmacokinetic Fate from a Bird's Eye View," *Curr Drug Metab*, 2003, 4 (2):105-29.
Starke PR, Weaver J, and Chowdhury BA, "Boxed Warning Added to Promethazine Labeling for Pediatric Use," *N Engl J Med*, 2005, 352(25):2653.
Strenkoski-Nix LC, Ermer J, DeCleene S, et al, "Pharmacokinetics of Promethazine Hydrochloride After Administration of Rectal Suppositories and Oral Syrup to Healthy Subjects," *Am J Health Syst Pharm*, 2000, 57(16):1499-505.

◆ **Promethazine Hydrochloride** *see* Promethazine *on page 1218*
◆ **Promethegan™** *see* Promethazine *on page 1218*
◆ **Prostate Cancer Vaccine, Cell-Based** *see* Sipuleucel-T *on page 1279*
◆ **Protein-Bound Paclitaxel** *see* PACLitaxel (Protein Bound) *on page 1098*
◆ **Prothrombin Complex Concentrate** *see* Factor IX Complex (Human) *on page 575*
◆ **PRO-Valacyclovir (Can)** *see* Valacyclovir *on page 1420*
◆ **Provenge®** *see* Sipuleucel-T *on page 1279*
◆ **Provera®** *see* MedroxyPROGESTERone *on page 916*
◆ **Provera-Pak (Can)** *see* MedroxyPROGESTERone *on page 916*
◆ **PS-341** *see* Bortezomib *on page 187*
◆ **PTG** *see* Teniposide *on page 1342*
◆ **Purinethol®** *see* Mercaptopurine *on page 934*
◆ **Quadramet®** *see* Samarium Sm 153 Lexidronam *on page 1268*
◆ **Quadrivalent Human Papillomavirus Vaccine** *see* Papillomavirus (Types 6, 11, 16, 18) Vaccine (Human, Recombinant) *on page 1120*
◆ **RAD001** *see* Everolimus *on page 552*
◆ **rAHF** *see* Antihemophilic Factor (Recombinant) *on page 103*
◆ **Ralivia™ (Can)** *see* TraMADol *on page 1388*

Raloxifene (ral OKS i feen)

Related Information

Safe Handling of Hazardous Drugs *on page 1904*

Brand Names: U.S. Evista®

Brand Names: Canada Apo-Raloxifene®; Evista®; Novo-Raloxifene; Teva-Raloxifene

Index Terms Keoxifene Hydrochloride; Raloxifene Hydrochloride

Generic Availability (U.S.) No

Pharmacologic Category Selective Estrogen Receptor Modulator (SERM)

Use Prevention and treatment of osteoporosis in postmenopausal women; risk reduction for invasive breast cancer in postmenopausal women with osteoporosis and in postmenopausal women with high risk for invasive breast cancer

Labeled Contraindications History of or current venous thromboembolic disorders (including DVT, PE, and retinal vein thrombosis); pregnancy or women who could become pregnant; breast-feeding

Pregnancy Risk Factor X

Lactation Excretion in breast milk unknown/contraindicated

Warnings/Precautions Hazardous agent - use appropriate precautions for handling and disposal. **[U.S. Boxed Warning]: May increase the risk for DVT or PE; use contraindicated in patients with history of or current venous thromboembolic disorders.** Use with caution in patients at high risk for venous thromboembolism; the risk for DVT and PE are higher in the first 4 months of treatment. Discontinue at least 72 hours prior to and during prolonged immobilization (postoperative recovery or prolonged bedrest). **[U.S. Boxed Warning]: The risk of death due to stroke may be increased in women with coronary heart disease or in women at risk for coronary events;** use with caution in patients with cardiovascular disease. Not be used for the prevention of cardiovascular disease. Use caution with moderate-to-severe renal dysfunction, hepatic impairment, unexplained uterine bleeding, and in women with a history of elevated triglycerides in response to treatment with oral estrogens (or estrogen/progestin). Safety with concomitant estrogen therapy has not been established. Safety and efficacy in premenopausal women or men have not been established. Not indicated for treatment of invasive breast cancer, to reduce the risk of recurrence of invasive breast cancer or to reduce the risk of noninvasive breast cancer. The efficacy (for breast cancer risk reduction) in women with inherited BRCA1 and BRCA1 mutations has not been established.

Adverse Reactions Note: Raloxifene has been associated with increased risk of thromboembolism (DVT, PE) and superficial thrombophlebitis; risk is similar to reported risk of HRT

>10%:

- Cardiovascular: Peripheral edema (3% to 14%)
- Endocrine & metabolic: Hot flashes (8% to 29%)
- Neuromuscular & skeletal: Arthralgia (11% to 16%), leg cramps/muscle spasm (6% to 12%)
- Miscellaneous: Flu syndrome (14% to 15%), infection (11%)

1% to 10%:

- Cardiovascular: Chest pain (3%), venous thromboembolism (1% to 2%)
- Central nervous system: Insomnia (6%)
- Dermatologic: Rash (6%)
- Endocrine & metabolic: Breast pain (4%)
- Gastrointestinal: Weight gain (9%), abdominal pain (7%), vomiting (5%), flatulence (2% to 3%), cholelithiasis (≤3%), gastroenteritis (≤3%)
- Genitourinary: Vaginal bleeding (6%), leukorrhea (3%), urinary tract disorder (3%), uterine disorder (3%), vaginal hemorrhage (3%), endometrial disorder (≤3%)
- Neuromuscular & skeletal: Myalgia (8%), tendon disorder (4%)
- Respiratory: Bronchitis (10%), sinusitis (10%), pharyngitis (8%), pneumonia (3%), laryngitis (≤2%)
- Miscellaneous: Diaphoresis (3%)

<1%, postmarketing, and/or case reports: Apolipoprotein A-1 increased, apolipoprotein B decreased, death related to VTE, fibrinogen decreased,

hypertriglyceridemia (in women with a history of increased triglycerides in response to oral estrogens), intermittent claudication, LDL cholesterol decreased, lipoprotein decreased, retinal vein occlusion, stroke related to VTE, superficial thrombophlebitis, total serum cholesterol decreased

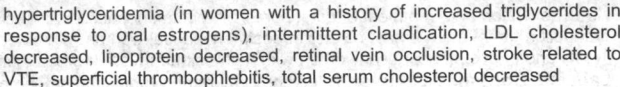

Drug Interactions

Metabolism/Transport Effects None known.

Avoid Concomitant Use There are no known interactions where it is recommended to avoid concomitant use.

Increased Effect/Toxicity There are no known significant interactions involving an increase in effect.

Decreased Effect

Raloxifene may decrease the levels/effects of: Levothyroxine

The levels/effects of Raloxifene may be decreased by: Bile Acid Sequestrants

Ethanol/Nutrition/Herb Interactions Ethanol: Avoid ethanol (may increase risk of osteoporosis).

Storage/Stability Store at controlled room temperature of 20°C to 25°C (68°F to 77°F); excursions permitted to 15°C to 30°C (59°F to 86°F).

Mechanism of Action A selective estrogen receptor modulator (SERM), meaning that it affects some of the same receptors that estrogen does, but not all, and in some instances, it antagonizes or blocks estrogen; it acts like estrogen to prevent bone loss and has the potential to block some estrogen effects in the breast and uterine tissues. Raloxifene decreases bone resorption, increasing bone mineral density and decreasing fracture incidence.

Pharmacodynamics/Kinetics

Onset of action: 8 weeks

Absorption: Rapid; ~60%

Distribution: 2348 L/kg

Protein binding: >95% to albumin and α-glycoprotein; does not bind to sex-hormone-binding globulin

Metabolism: Hepatic, extensive first-pass effect; metabolized to glucuronide conjugates

Bioavailability: ~2%

Half-life elimination: 28-33 hours

Excretion: Primarily feces; urine (<0.2% as unchanged drug; <6% as glucuronide conjugates)

Dosing

Adult & Geriatric

Osteoporosis: Females: Oral: 60 mg once daily

Invasive breast cancer risk reduction: Female: Oral: 60 mg once daily for 5 years per ASCO guidelines (Visvanathan, 2009)

Renal Impairment Moderate-to-severe impairment: Use caution; safety and efficacy have not been established.

Hepatic Impairment Mild impairment (Child-Pugh class A): Plasma concentrations were higher and correlated with total bilirubin. Safety and efficacy in hepatic insufficiency have not been established.

Administration May be administered without regard to meals.

Monitoring Parameters Bone mineral density (BMD), lipid profile; adequate diagnostic measures, including endometrial sampling, if indicated, should be performed to rule out malignancy in all cases of undiagnosed abnormal vaginal bleeding

Dietary Considerations May be taken without regard to meals. Osteoporosis prevention or treatment: Ensure adequate calcium and vitamin D intake; postmenopausal women should consume ~1500 mg/day of elemental calcium and 400-800 units/day of vitamin D.

Additional Information The decrease in estrogen-related adverse effects with the selective estrogen-receptor modulators in general and raloxifene in particular should improve compliance and decrease the incidence of cardiovascular events and fractures while not increasing breast cancer

Oncology Comment: The American Society of Clinical Oncology (ASCO) guidelines for breast cancer risk reduction (Visvanathan, 2009) recommend raloxifene (for 5 years) as an option to reduce the risk of ER-positive invasive breast cancer in postmenopausal women with a 5-year projected risk (based on NCI trial model) of ≥1.66%, or with lobular carcinoma *in situ*. Raloxifene should not be used in premenopausal women. Women with osteoporosis may use raloxifene beyond 5 years of treatment. According to the NCCN breast cancer risk reduction guidelines (v.2.2009), raloxifene is only recommended for postmenopausal women (≥35 years of age), and is equivalent to tamoxifen although, raloxifene has a better adverse event profile; however, tamoxifen is superior in reducing the risk on noninvasive breast cancer.

Medication Guide Available Yes

Dosage Forms Excipient information presented when available (limited, particularly for generics); consult specific product labeling.

Tablet, oral, as hydrochloride:

Evista®: 60 mg

References

Barrett-Connor E, Mosca L, Collins P, et al, "Raloxifene Use for The Heart (RUTH) Trial Investigators. Effects of Raloxifene on Cardiovascular Events and Breast Cancer in Postmenopausal Women," *N Engl J Med*, 2006, 355(2):125-37.

Chlebowski RT, Col N, Winer EP, et al, "American Society of Clinical Oncology Technology Assessment of Pharmacologic Interventions for Breast Cancer Risk Reduction Including Tamoxifen, Raloxifene, and Aromatase Inhibition," *J Clin Oncol*, 2002, 20(15):3328-43

Cummings SR, Eckert S, Krueger KA, et al, "The Effect of Raloxifene on Risk of Breast Cancer in Postmenopausal Women: Results from the MORE Randomized Trial," *JAMA*, 1999, 281(23) 2189-97.

Land SR, Wickerham DL, Costantino JP, et al, "Patient-Reported Symptoms and Quality of Life During Treatment With Tamoxifen or Raloxifene for Breast Cancer Prevention: The NSABP Study of Tamoxifen and Raloxifene (STAR) P-2 Trial," *JAMA*, 2006, 295(23):2742-51.

Martino S, Cauley JA, Barrett-Connor E, et al, "Continuing Outcomes Relevant to Evista: Breast Cancer Incident in Postmenopausal Women in a Randomized Trial of Raloxifene," *J Natl Cancer Inst*, 2004, 96(23):1751-61.

National Comprehensive Cancer Network® (NCCN), "Clinical Practice Guidelines in Oncology™: Breast Cancer," Version 3.2012. Available at http://www.nccn.org/professionals/physician_gls/PDF/breast.pdf

National Comprehensive Cancer Network® (NCCN), "Clinical Practice Guidelines in Oncology™: Breast Cancer Risk Reduction," Version 1.2012. Available at http://www.nccn.org/professionals/physician_gls/PDF/breast_risk.pdf

Siris ES, Harris ST, Eastell R, et al, "Skeletal Effects of Raloxifene After 8 Years: Results From the Continuing Outcomes Relevant to Evista (CORE) Study," *J Bone Miner Res*, 2005, 20 (9):1514-24.

Visvanathan K, Chlebowski RT, Hurley P, et al, "American Society of Clinical Oncology Clinical Practice Guideline Update on the Use of Pharmacologic Interventions Including Tamoxifen, Raloxifene, and Aromatase Inhibition for Breast Cancer Risk Reduction," *J Clin Oncol*, 2009, 27(19):3235-58.

Vogel VG, Costantino JP, Wickerham DL, "Effects of Tamoxifen vs Raloxifene on the Risk of Developing Invasive Breast Cancer and Other Disease Outcomes: The NSABP Study of Tamoxifen and Raloxifene (STAR) P-2 Trial," *JAMA*, 2006, 295(23):2727-41.

◆ **Raloxifene Hydrochloride** *see* Raloxifene *on page* 1222

Raltitrexed (ral ti TREX ed)

Related Information

Safe Handling of Hazardous Drugs *on page 1904*

Brand Names: Canada Tomudex®

Index Terms D1694; ICI-D1694; Raltitrexed Disodium; TDX; ZD1694

Pharmacologic Category Antineoplastic Agent, Antimetabolite

Use Treatment of advanced colorectal cancer

Unlabeled Use Treatment of malignant pleural mesothelioma (in combination with cisplatin)

Labeled Contraindications Hypersensitivity to raltitrexed or any component of the formulation; severe renal or hepatic impairment; pregnancy or breast-feeding

Lactation Excretion in breast milk unknown/contraindicated

Warnings/Precautions Hazardous agent - use appropriate precautions for handling and disposal. Neutropenia, leukopenia, anemia, and thrombocytopenia may occur. Use with caution in patients with pre-existing marrow suppression. Nausea, vomiting and diarrhea are common; mucositis and stomatitis may also occur. Severe diarrhea with concomitant hematologic toxicity (neutropenia) may be life-threatening and may require discontinuation or subsequent dose reduction.

Use caution in elderly, mild-to-moderate hepatic or renal dysfunction (use in severe hepatic or renal impairment is contraindicated). Use is not recommended in clinical jaundice or decompensated hepatic disease. Therapy interruption is required in patients with hepatotoxicity; may reintroduce therapy only with decrease in hepatic enzymes to grade 2. Asymptomatic and self-limiting increases (reversible) in ALT and AST may occur. Use caution in patients who have received prior radiation therapy.

Folinic acid (leucovorin calcium), folic acid, or folate-containing medications (eg, multivitamins) may interfere with raltitrexed; do not administer immediately prior to or concurrently with raltitrexed. May cause malaise/weakness (caution patients concerning operation of machinery/driving). Use in pediatric patients is not recommended by the manufacturer.

Adverse Reactions

>10%:

Central nervous system: Fever (2% to 23%)

Dermatologic: Rash (14%)

Gastrointestinal: Nausea (58%; grades 3/4: 12%), diarrhea (38%; grades 3/4: 11%), vomiting (38%; grades 3/4: 12%), anorexia (26% to 28%), abdominal pain (18%), constipation (13% to 15%), mucositis/stomatitis (12%; grades 3/4: 2%)

Hematologic: Leukopenia (20% to 22%; grade 3/4: 12% to 13%; nadir within 7-14 days, recovery by 21 days); anemia (15% to 18%; grades 3/4: 7% to 8%)

Hepatic: Transaminases increased (14% to 18%; grades 3/4: 10%)

Neuromuscular & skeletal: Weakness (46% to 49%)

1% to 10%:

Cardiovascular: Peripheral edema (10%), arrhythmias (3%), CHF (2%)

Central nervous system: Headache (6%), dizziness (4% to 5%), chills (4%), malaise (4%), pain (4%), insomnia (3% to 4%), depression (3%)

Dermatologic: Alopecia (6%), cellulitis (3%), pruritus (3%)

Endocrine & metabolic: Dehydration (6% to 7%), hypokalemia (2%)

Gastrointestinal: Dyspepsia (6%), taste perversion (6%), weight loss (6%), flatulence (2% to 3%), xerostomia (2% to 3%)
Genitourinary: Urinary tract infection (3%)
Hematologic: Thrombocytopenia (5% to 6%; grades 3/4: 4%)
Hepatic: Alkaline phosphatase increased (2% to 3%), bilirubin increased (2% to 3%; grades 3/4: 2%)
Neuromuscular & skeletal: Paresthesia (2% to 3%), myalgia (3%), arthralgia (<2%), hypertonia (<2%)
Ocular: Conjunctivitis (2% to 3%)
Renal: Serum creatinine increased (2% to 3%)
Respiratory: Cough (5%), dyspnea (4% to 5%), pharyngitis (4% to 5%)
Miscellaneous: Flu-like syndrome (6% to 8%), diaphoresis (3% to 4%), infection (3%), sepsis (2% to 3%)

<1%: Desquamation

Drug Interactions

Metabolism/Transport Effects None known.

Avoid Concomitant Use

Avoid concomitant use of Raltitrexed with any of the following: CloZAPine; Folic Acid; Leucovorin Calcium-Levoleucovorin; Levomefolate; Methylfolate; Multivitamins/Minerals (with ADEK, Folate, Iron)

Increased Effect/Toxicity

Raltitrexed may increase the levels/effects of: CloZAPine

Decreased Effect

The levels/effects of Raltitrexed may be decreased by: Folic Acid; Leucovorin Calcium-Levoleucovorin; Levomefolate; Methylfolate; Multivitamins/Minerals (with ADEK, Folate, Iron)

Ethanol/Nutrition/Herb Interactions Herb/Nutraceutical: Avoid folic acid and multivitamins with folic acid close to and during administration.

Storage/Stability Intact vials should be refrigerated at 2°C to 25°C (36°F to 77°F). Protect from light. Reconstituted and subsequent I.V. admixture solutions (saline or dextrose) are stable for up to 24 hours under refrigeration at 2°C to 8°C (36°F to 46°F), although the manufacturer recommends use as soon as possible after preparation.

Reconstitution Use appropriate precautions for handling and disposal. Reconstitute 2 mg vial with 4 mL SWFI to produce 0.5 mg/mL solution; volume required for dose should be further diluted by adding to 50-250 mL NS or D_5W.

Mechanism of Action Raltitrexed is a folate analogue that inhibits thymidylate synthase, blocking purine synthesis. This results in an overall inhibition of DNA synthesis.

Pharmacodynamics/Kinetics

Distribution: V_{ss}: 548 L
Protein binding: 93%
Metabolism: Undergoes extensive intracellular metabolism to active polyglutamate forms; appears to be little or no systemic metabolism of the drug
Half-life elimination: Triphasic; Beta: 2 hours; Terminal: 198 hours
Excretion: Urine (~50% as unchanged drug); feces (~15%)

Dosing

Adult & Geriatric Note: Treatment should be administered only if WBC >4000/mm^3, ANC >2000/mm^3, and platelets >100,000/mm^3

Colorectal cancer, advanced: I.V.: 3 mg/m^2 every 3 weeks

Malignant pleural mesothelioma (unlabeled use): I.V.: 3 mg/m^2 every 3 weeks (in combination with cisplatin) (van Meerbeeck, 2005)

Renal Impairment

Cl_{cr} >65 mL/minute: No adjustment required.

Cl_{cr} 55-65 mL/minute: Administer 75% of dose every 4 weeks.

Cl_{cr} 25-54 mL/minute: Administer percentage of dose equivalent to Cl_{cr} every 4 weeks (eg, 25% of dose for Cl_{cr} of 25 mL/minute).

Cl_{cr} <25 mL/minute: Do not administer (use is contraindicated in severe renal impairment).

Hepatic Impairment No adjustment required for mild-to-moderate hepatic insufficiency. Use is contraindicated in severe hepatic impairment and not recommended in clinical jaundice or decompensated liver disease. Patients who develop hepatic toxicity should have treatment held until returns to grade 2.

Adjustment for Toxicity Delay dose in subsequent cycles until recovery from toxicity.

Grade 4 gastrointestinal toxicity (diarrhea or mucositis) or grade 3 gastrointestinal toxicity in combination with grade 4 hematologic toxicity: Discontinue therapy and manage with supportive measures.

Grade 3 hematologic toxicity (neutropenia or thrombocytopenia) or grade 2 gastrointestinal toxicity (diarrhea or mucositis): Reduce dose by 25%.

Grade 4 hematologic toxicity (neutropenia or thrombocytopenia) or grade 3 gastrointestinal toxicity (diarrhea or mucositis): Reduce dose by 50%.

Combination Regimens

Malignant pleural mesothelioma: Cisplatin-Raltitrexed (Mesothelioma) on page 1583

Administration Administer via I.V. infusion over 15 minutes.

Monitoring Parameters CBC with differential (at baseline, prior to each treatment, or weekly if GI toxicity observed); hepatic function tests and serum creatinine (at baseline and prior to each treatment); signs of GI toxicity

Dietary Considerations Avoid folic acid, folinic acid (leucovorin calcium), and multivitamins with folic acid close to and during administration.

Product Availability Not available in U.S.

Dosage Forms: Canada Excipient information presented when available (limited, particularly for generics); consult specific product labeling.

Injection, powder for reconstitution, as disodium:

Tomudex®: 2 mg

References

Bottomley A, Coens C, Efficace F, et al, "Symptoms and Patient-Reported Well-Being: Do They Predict Survival in Malignant Pleural Mesothelioma? A Prognostic Factor Analysis of EORTC-NCIC 08983: Randomized Phase III Study of Cisplatin With or Without Raltitrexed in Patients With Malignant Pleural Mesothelioma," *J Clin Oncol*, 2007, 25(36):5770-6.

Bottomley A, Gaafar R, Manegold C, et al, "Short-Term Treatment-Related Symptoms and Quality of Life: Results From an International Randomized Phase III Study of Cisplatin With or Without Raltitrexed in Patients With Malignant Pleural Mesothelioma: An EORTC Lung-Cancer Group and National Cancer Institute, Canada, Intergroup Study," *J Clin Oncol*, 2006, 24(9):1435-42.

van Meerbeeck JP, Gaafar R, Manegold C, et al, "Randomized Phase III Study of Cisplatin With or Without Raltitrexed in Patients With Malignant Pleural Mesothelioma: An Intergroup Study of the European Organisation for Research and Treatment of Cancer Lung Cancer Group and the National Cancer Institute of Canada," *J Clin Oncol*, 2005, 23(28):6881-9.

◆ **Raltitrexed Disodium** *see* Raltitrexed *on page* 1226

◆ **RAN™-Ciprofloxacin (Can)** *see* Ciprofloxacin (Systemic) *on page* 283

◆ **RAN™-Fentanyl Matrix Patch (Can)** *see* FentaNYL *on page* 583

◆ **RAN™-Fentanyl Transdermal System (Can)** *see* FentaNYL *on page* 583

◆ **RAN™-Imipenem-Cilastatin (Can)** *see* Imipenem and Cilastatin *on page 773*

◆ **RAN™-Nabilone (Can)** *see* Nabilone *on page 1023*

◆ **RAN™-Ondansetron (Can)** *see* Ondansetron *on page 1068*

◆ **Rapamune®** *see* Sirolimus *on page 1282*

◆ **Rapamycin** *see* Sirolimus *on page 1282*

Rasburicase (ras BYOOR i kayse)

Brand Names: U.S. Elitek®

Brand Names: Canada Fasturtec®

Index Terms Recombinant Urate Oxidase; Urate Oxidase

Generic Availability (U.S.) No

Pharmacologic Category Enzyme; Enzyme, Urate-Oxidase (Recombinant)

Use Initial management of uric acid levels in patients with leukemia, lymphoma, and solid tumor malignancies receiving chemotherapy expected to result in tumor lysis and elevation of plasma uric acid

Labeled Contraindications History of anaphylaxis or severe hypersensitivity to rasburicase or any component of the formulation; history of hemolytic reaction or methemoglobinemia associated with rasburicase; glucose-6-phosphatase dehydrogenase (G6PD) deficiency

Pregnancy Risk Factor C

Lactation Excretion in breast milk unknown/not recommended

Warnings/Precautions **[U.S. Boxed Warning]: Severe hypersensitivity reactions (including anaphylaxis) have been reported; immediately and permanently discontinue in patients developing serious hypersensitivity reaction;** reactions may occur at any time during treatment, including the initial dose. Signs and symptoms of hypersensitivity may include bronchospasm, chest pain/tightness, dyspnea, hypotension, hypoxia, shock, or urticaria. The safety and efficacy of more than one course of administration has not been established. **[U.S. Boxed Warning]: Due to the risk for hemolysis (<1%), rasburicase is contraindicated in patients with G6PD deficiency; discontinue immediately and permanently in any patient developing hemolysis. Patients at higher risk for G6PD deficiency (eg, African, Mediterranean, or Southeast Asian descent) should be screened prior to therapy;** severe hemolytic reactions occurred within 2-4 days of rasburicase initiation. **[U.S. Boxed Warning]: Methemoglobinemia has been reported (<1%). Discontinue immediately and permanently in any patient developing methemoglobinemia;** initiate appropriate treatment (eg, transfusion, methylene blue) if methemoglobinemia occurs.

[U.S. Boxed Warning]: Enzymatic degradation of uric acid in blood samples will occur if left at room temperature, which may interfere with serum uric acid measurements; specific guidelines for the collection of plasma uric acid samples must be followed, including collection in prechilled tubes with heparin anticoagulant, immediate ice water bath immersion and assay within 4 hours. Patients at risk for tumor lysis syndrome should receive appropriate I.V. hydration as part of uric acid management; however, alkalinization (with sodium bicarbonate) concurrently with rasburicase is not recommended (Coiffier, 2008). Rasburicase is immunogenic and can elicit an antibody response; efficacy may be reduced with subsequent courses of therapy.

Adverse Reactions

>10%:

Cardiovascular: Peripheral edema (≤50%), fluid overload (≤12%)

Central nervous system: Fever (46%; serious: 5%), headache (26%), anxiety (≤24%)

Dermatologic: Rash (13%; serious: 1%)

Endocrine & metabolic: Hypophosphatemia (≤17%)

Gastrointestinal: Vomiting (50%), nausea (27%), abdominal pain (20%), constipation (20%), diarrhea (20%), mucositis (15%; serious: 2%)

Hepatic: Hyperbilirubinemia (≤16%), ALT increased (≤11%)

Respiratory: Pharyngolaryngeal pain (≤14%)

Miscellaneous: Antibody formation (healthy volunteers: 61% to 64%; patients with malignancies: 11%), sepsis (≤12%; serious: 3% to 5%)

1% to 10%:

Cardiovascular: Ischemic coronary disorder, supraventricular arrhythmia

Endocrine & metabolic: Hyperphosphatemia (≤10%)

Gastrointestinal: Abdominal/gastrointestinal infection

Hematologic: Neutropenic fever (serious: 4%), neutropenia (serious: 2%)

Respiratory: Respiratory distress (serious: 3%), pulmonary hemorrhage, respiratory failure

Miscellaneous: Hypersensitivity (≤4%)

<1%, postmarketing, and/or case reports: Acute renal failure, anaphylaxis, arrhythmia, cardiac arrest, cardiac failure, cellulitis, cerebrovascular disorder, chest pain, cyanosis, dehydration, hemolysis, hemorrhage, hot flashes, ileus, infection, intestinal obstruction, liver enzymes increased, methemoglobinemia, MI, pancytopenia, paresthesia, pneumonia, pulmonary edema, pulmonary hypertension, retinal hemorrhage, rigors, seizure, thrombosis, thrombophlebitis

Drug Interactions

Metabolism/Transport Effects None known.

Avoid Concomitant Use There are no known interactions where it is recommended to avoid concomitant use.

Increased Effect/Toxicity There are no known significant interactions involving an increase in effect.

Decreased Effect There are no known significant interactions involving a decrease in effect.

Storage/Stability Prior to reconstitution, store with diluent at 2°C to 8°C (36°F to 46°F); do not freeze. Protect from light. Reconstituted and final solution may be stored up to 24 hours at 2°C to 8°C (36°F to 46°F). Discard unused product.

Reconstitution Reconstitute with provided diluent (use 1 mL diluent for the 1.5 mg vial and 5 mL diluent for the 7.5 mg vial). Mix by gently swirling; do **not** shake or vortex. Discard if discolored or containing particulate matter. Total dose should be further diluted in NS to a final volume of 50 mL.

Mechanism of Action Rasburicase is a recombinant urate-oxidase enzyme, which converts uric acid to allantoin (an inactive and soluble metabolite of uric acid); it does not inhibit the formation of uric acid.

Pharmacodynamics/Kinetics

Onset: Uric acid levels decrease within 4 hours of initial administration

Distribution: Children: 110-127 mL/kg; Adults: 76-138 mL/kg

Half-life elimination: ~16-23 hours

Dosing

Adult & Geriatric Hyperuricemia associated with malignancy: I.V.: 0.2 mg/kg once daily for up to 5 days (manufacturer-recommended dose) **or**

Alternate dosing (unlabeled; Coiffier, 2008): 0.05-0.2 mg/kg once daily for 1-7 days (average of 2-3 days) with the duration of treatment dependent on plasma uric acid levels and clinical judgment (patients with significant tumor burden may require an increase to twice daily); the following dose levels are recommended based on risk of tumor lysis syndrome (TLS):

High risk: 0.2 mg/kg once daily (duration is based on plasma uric acid levels)

Intermediate risk: 0.15 mg/kg once daily (duration is based on plasma uric acid levels)

Low risk: 0.1 mg/kg once daily (duration is based on clinical judgment); a dose of 0.05 mg/kg was used effectively in one trial

Single-dose rasburicase (unlabeled use; based on limited data): 0.15 mg/kg (Campara, 2009; Liu, 2005) **or** 3-7.5 mg as a single dose (Hutcherson, 2006; McDonnell, 2006; Reeves, 2008; Trifilio, 2006); repeat doses (1.5-6 mg) may be needed based on serum uric acid levels

Pediatric Hyperuricemia associated with malignancy: I.V.: 0.2 mg/kg once daily for up to 5 days (manufacturer-recommended dose) **or**

Alternate dosing (unlabeled; Coiffier, 2008): 0.05-0.2 mg/kg once daily for 1-7 days (average of 2-3 days) with the duration of treatment dependent on plasma uric acid levels and clinical judgment (patients with significant tumor burden may require an increase to twice daily), the following dose levels are recommended based on risk of tumor lysis syndrome (TLS):

High risk: 0.2 mg/kg once daily (duration is based on plasma uric acid levels)

Intermediate risk: 0.15 mg/kg once daily (duration is based on plasma uric acid levels); may consider managing initially with a single dose

Low risk: 0.1 mg/kg once daily (duration is based on clinical judgment); a dose of 0.05 mg/kg was used effectively in one trial

Single-dose rasburicase (unlabeled use; based on limited data): 0.15 mg/kg; additional doses may be needed based on serum uric acid levels (Liu, 2005)

Administration I.V. infusion over 30 minutes; do **not** administer as a bolus infusion. Do **not** filter during infusion. If not possible to administer through a separate line, I.V. line should be flushed with at least 15 mL saline prior to and following rasburicase infusion. The optimal timing of rasburicase administration (with respect to chemotherapy administration) is not specified in the manufacturer's labeling. In some studies, chemotherapy was administered 4-24 hours after the first rasburicase dose (Cortes, 2010; Kikuchi, 2009, Vadhan-Raj, 2012); however, rasburicase generally may be administered irrespective of chemotherapy timing.

Monitoring Parameters Plasma uric acid levels (4 hours after rasburicase administration, then every 6-8 hours until TLS resolution), CBC, G6PD deficiency screening (in patients at high risk for deficiency); monitor for hypersensitivity

Test Interactions Specific handling procedures must be followed to prevent the degradation of uric acid in plasma samples. Blood must be collected in prechilled tubes containing heparin anticoagulant. Samples must then be **immediately** immersed in an ice water bath. Prepare samples by centrifugation in a precooled centrifuge (4°C). Samples must be kept in ice water bath and analyzed within 4 hours of collection.

Additional Information Specific handling procedures must be followed to prevent the degradation of uric acid in plasma samples. Blood must be collected in prechilled tubes containing heparin anticoagulant. Samples must then be **immediately** immersed in an ice water bath. Prepare samples by centrifugation in a precooled centrifuge (4°C). Samples must be kept in ice water bath and analyzed within 4 hours of collection.

Dosage Forms Excipient information presented when available (limited, particularly for generics); consult specific product labeling.

Injection, powder for reconstitution:

Elitek®: 1.5 mg, 7.5 mg [supplied with diluent]

References

Arnold TM, Reuter JP, Delman BS, et al, "Use of Single-Dose Rasburicase in an Obese Female," *Ann Pharmacother*, 2004, 38(9):1428-31.

Campara M, Shord SS, and Haaf CM, "Single-Dose Rasburicase for Tumour Lysis Syndrome in Adults: Weight-Based Approach," *J Clin Pharm Ther*, 2009, 34(2):207-13.

Coiffier B, Altman A, Pui CH, et al, "Guidelines for the Management of Pediatric and Adult Tumor Lysis Syndrome: An Evidence-Based Review," *J Clin Oncol*, 2008, 26(16):2767-78.

Coiffier B, Mounier N, Bologna S, et al, "Efficacy and Safety of Rasburicase (Recombinant Urate Oxidase) for the Prevention and Treatment of Hyperuricemia During Induction Chemotherapy of Aggressive Non-Hodgkin's Lymphoma: Results of GRAALI (Groupe d'Etude des Lymphomes de l'Adulte Trial on Rasburicase Activity in Adult Lymphoma) Study," *J Clin Oncol*, 2003, 21 (23):4402-6.

Hutcherson DA, Gammon DC, Bhatt MS, et al, "Reduced-Dose Rasburicase in the Treatment of Adults With Hyperuricemia Associated With Malignancy," *Pharmacother*, 2006, 26(2):242-7.

Liu CY, Sims-McCallum RP, and Schiffer CA, "A Single Dose of Rasburicase is Sufficient for the Treatment of Hyperuricemia in Patients Receiving Chemotherapy," *Leuk Res*, 2005, 29(4):463-5.

McDonnell AM, Lenz KL, Frei-Lahr DA, et al, "Single-Dose Rasburicase 6 mg in the Management of Tumor Lysis Syndrome in Adults," *Pharmacother*, 2006, 26(6):806-12.

Reeves DJ and Bestul DJ, "Evaluation of a Single Fixed Dose of Rasburicase 7.5 mg for the Treatment of Hyperuricemia in Adults With Cancer," *Pharmacother*, 2008; 28(6):685–90.

Trifilio S, Gordon L, Singhall S, et al, "Reduced Dose Rasburicase (Recombinant Xanthine Oxidase) in Adult Cancer Patients With Hyperuricemia," *Bone Marrow Transplant*, 2006, 37 (11):997-1001.

◆ **rATG** *see* Antithymocyte Globulin (Rabbit) *on page* *115*

◆ **ratio-Acyclovir (Can)** *see* Acyclovir (Systemic) *on page* *30*

◆ **ratio-Bicalutamide (Can)** *see* Bicalutamide *on page* *178*

◆ **ratio-Ciprofloxacin (Can)** *see* Ciprofloxacin (Systemic) *on page* *283*

◆ **ratio-Codeine (Can)** *see* Codeine *on page* *311*

◆ **ratio-Dexamethasone (Can)** *see* Dexamethasone (Systemic) *on page* *440*

◆ **ratio-Fentanyl (Can)** *see* FentaNYL *on page* *583*

◆ **ratio-Methotrexate (Can)** *see* Methotrexate *on page* *949*

◆ **ratio-Morphine (Can)** *see* Morphine (Systemic) *on page* *1004*

◆ **ratio-Morphine SR (Can)** *see* Morphine (Systemic) *on page* *1004*

◆ **ratio-Ondansetron (Can)** *see* Ondansetron *on page* *1068*

◆ **Rayos®** *see* PredniSONE *on page* *1199*

◆ **Rayos®** *see* PredniSONE *on page* *1199*

◆ **Reclast®** *see* Zoledronic Acid *on page* *1488*

◆ **Recombinant Human Interleukin-2** *see* Aldesleukin *on page* *37*

◆ **Recombinant Human Interleukin-11** *see* Oprelvekin *on page* *1074*

◆ **Recombinant Human Thyrotropin** *see* Thyrotropin Alfa *on page* *1360*

◆ **Recombinant Interleukin-11** *see* Oprelvekin *on page* *1074*

◆ **Recombinant Urate Oxidase** *see* Rasburicase *on page* *1229*

◆ **Recombinate** *see* Antihemophilic Factor (Recombinant) *on page* 103

◆ **Recort [OTC]** *see* Hydrocortisone (Topical) *on page* 719

◆ **Reglan®** *see* Metoclopramide *on page* 974

Regorafenib (re goe RAF e nib)

Brand Names: U.S. Stivarga®

Index Terms BAY 73-4506

Generic Availability (U.S.) No

Pharmacologic Category Antineoplastic Agent, Tyrosine Kinase Inhibitor; Vascular Endothelial Growth Factor (VEGF) Inhibitor

Use Treatment of metastatic colorectal cancer in patients previously treated with fluoropyrimidine-, oxaliplatin-, and irinotecan-based chemotherapy, anti-VEGF therapy, or anti-EGFR therapy (if *KRAS* wild type)

Labeled Contraindications There are no contraindications listed in the manufacturer's labeling

Pregnancy Risk Factor D

Lactation Excretion in breast milk unknown/not recommended

Warnings/Precautions Hazardous agent: Use appropriate precautions for handling and disposal. Myocardial ischemia and infarction were observed at a higher incidence than placebo in a clinical trial. Interrupt therapy in patients who develop new or acute onset ischemia or infarction; resume if the benefit of therapy outweighs the cardiovascular risk. Hand-foot skin reaction (HFSR), also known as palmar-plantar erythrodysesthesia (PPE), and rash were commonly seen in clinical trials; therapy interruptions, dosage reductions, and/or discontinuation may be necessary depending on the severity and persistence. Onset typically occurs in the first cycle of treatment. Gastrointestinal perforation or fistula has occurred in a small number of patients treated with regorafenib. Monitor for signs/symptoms of perforation (fever, abdominal pain with constipation, and/or nausea/vomiting); permanently discontinue therapy if perforation or fistula develop. Hemorrhage of the respiratory, gastrointestinal, or genitourinary tracts was observed in trials; some cases were fatal. Permanently discontinue in patients who experience severe or life-threatening bleeding. In patients receiving concomitant warfarin, monitor INR frequently.

[U.S. Boxed Warning]: Severe liver toxicity and hepatic failure (sometimes resulting in death) have been observed in clinical trials. Monitor hepatic function at baseline and during treatment. Interrupt therapy for hepatotoxicity; dose reductions or discontinuation are necessary depending on the severity and persistence.

Elevated blood pressure was observed in clinical trials (onset typically in the first cycle of therapy); ensure blood pressure is adequately controlled prior to initiation. Monitor blood pressure closely; if hypertension develops, interrupt therapy or permanently discontinue for severe or uncontrolled hypertension. Hypertensive crisis has occurred in some patients. Reversible posterior leukoencephalopathy syndrome (RPLS) occurred very rarely in regorafenib-treated patients; discontinue if diagnosis is confirmed. Regorafenib inhibits vascular endothelial growth factor, which may lead to impaired wound healing. Stop therapy at least 2 weeks prior to scheduled surgery; resume regorafenib postsurgery based on clinical judgment of wound healing; discontinue therapy if wound dehiscence occurs.

Adverse Reactions

>10%:

Cardiovascular: Hypertension (30%; grade ≥3: 8%)

Central nervous system: Fatigue (64%), dysphonia (30%), pain (29%), fever (28%)

Dermatologic: Palmar-plantar erythrodysesthesia (45%; grade ≥3: 17%), rash (26%; grade ≥3: 6%)

Endocrine & metabolic: Hypocalcemia (59%), hypophosphatemia (57%), hyponatremia (30%), hypokalemia (26%)

Gastrointestinal: Appetite decreased (47%), lipase increased (46%), diarrhea (43%), mucositis (33%), weight loss (32%), amylase increased (26%)

Hematologic: Anemia (79%; grade 3: 5%; grade 4: 1%), lymphopenia (54%; grade 3: 9%), thrombocytopenia (41%; grade 3: 2%; grade 4: <1%), INR increased (24%), hemorrhage (21%; grade ≥3: 2%)

Hepatic: AST increased (65%; grade 3: 5%; grade 4: 1%), ALT increased (45%; grade 3: 5%; grade 4: 1%), hyperbilirubinemia (45%)

Renal: Proteinuria (60%)

Miscellaneous: Infection (31%; grade ≥3: 9%)

1% to 10%:

Cardiovascular: Myocardial ischemia and infarction (1%)

Central nervous system: Headache (10%)

Dermatologic: Alopecia (8%)

Endocrine & metabolic: Hypothyroidism (4%)

Gastrointestinal: Taste disturbance (8%), xerostomia (5%), gastroesophageal reflux (1%)

Hematologic: Neutropenia (3%; grade 3: 1%)

Neuromuscular & skeletal: Stiffness (6%), tremor (2%)

<1%: Gastrointestinal fistula, hypertensive crisis, liver injury (severe), reversible posterior encephalopathy syndrome (RPLS), skin cancer (keratoacanthoma, squamous cell carcinoma)

Drug Interactions

Metabolism/Transport Effects **Substrate** of CYP3A4 (major), UGT1A9; **Note:** Assignment of Major/Minor substrate status based on clinically relevant drug interaction potential; **Inhibits** BCRP, P-glycoprotein, UGT1A1, UGT1A9

Avoid Concomitant Use

Avoid concomitant use of Regorafenib with any of the following: CYP3A4 Inducers (Strong); CYP3A4 Inhibitors (Strong); Grapefruit Juice; St Johns Wort

Increased Effect/Toxicity

Regorafenib may increase the levels/effects of: Irinotecan; Vitamin K Antagonists

The levels/effects of Regorafenib may be increased by: CYP3A4 Inhibitors (Moderate); CYP3A4 Inhibitors (Strong); Dasatinib; Grapefruit Juice; Ivacaftor; Mifepristone; Warfarin

Decreased Effect

Regorafenib may decrease the levels/effects of: Cardiac Glycosides; Vitamin K Antagonists

The levels/effects of Regorafenib may be decreased by: CYP3A4 Inducers (Strong); Deferasirox; St Johns Wort; Tocilizumab

Ethanol/Nutrition/Herb Interactions

Food: Regorafenib serum concentrations may be altered when taken with grapefruit or grapefruit juice. Management: Avoid concurrent use.

Herb/Nutraceutical: St John's wort may alter the levels/effects of regorafenib. Management: Avoid St John's wort.

Storage/Stability Store at 25°C (77°F); excursions permitted to 15°C to 30°C (59°F to 86°F). Store tablets in the original bottle and protect from moisture (do not remove the desiccant); keep container tightly closed. Any unused tablets remaining 28 days after opening the bottle should be discarded.

Mechanism of Action Regorafenib is a multikinase inhibitor; it targets kinases involved with tumor angiogenesis, oncogenesis, and maintenance of the tumor microenvironment which results in inhibition of tumor growth. Specifically, it inhibits VEGF receptors 1-3, KIT, PDGFR-alpha, PDGFR-beta, RET, FGFR, TIE2, DDR2, Trk2A, Eph2A, RAF-1. BRAF, SAPK2, PTK5, and Abl.

Pharmacodynamics/Kinetics

Absorption: A high-fat meal increased the mean AUC of the parent drug by 48% compared to the fasted state and decreased the mean AUC of the M-2 (N-oxide) and M-5 (N-oxide and N-desmethyl) active metabolites by 20% and 51%, respectively. A low-fat meal increased the mean AUC of regorafenib, M-2, and M-5 by 36%, 40% and 23%, respectively (as compared to the fasted state).

Protein binding: 99.5% (active metabolites M-2 and M-5 are also highly protein bound)

Metabolism: Hepatic via CYP3A4 and UGT1A9, primarily to active metabolites M-2 (N-oxide) and M-5 (N-oxide and N-desmethyl)

Bioavailability: Tablets: 69%; Oral solution: 83%

Half-life elimination: Regorafenib: 28 hours (range: 14-58 hours); M-2 metabolite: 25 hours (range: 14-32 hours); M-5 metabolite: 51 hours (range: 32-70 hours)

Time to peak: 4 hours

Excretion: Feces (71%; 47% as parent compound; 24% as metabolites); Urine (19%)

Dosing

Adult & Geriatric Colorectal cancer, metastatic: Oral: 160 mg once daily for the first 21 days of each 28-day cycle; continue until disease progression or unacceptable toxicity

Missed doses: Do not take 2 doses on the same day to make up for a missed dose from the previous day.

Renal Impairment

Pre-existing mild impairment (Cl_{cr} 60-89 mL/minute): No dosage adjustment necessary.

Pre-existing moderate impairment (Cl_{cr} 30-59 mL/minute): No dosage adjustment provided in manufacturer's labeling (limited pharmacokinetic data available).

Pre-existing severe impairment (Cl_{cr} <30 mL/minute): No dosage adjustment provided in manufacturer's labeling (has not been studied).

Hepatic Impairment

Pre-existing mild or moderate impairment (Child-Pugh Class A or B): No dosage adjustment necessary; closely monitor for adverse effects.

Pre-existing severe impairment (Child-Pugh Class C): Not recommended for use (has not been studied).

Hepatotoxicity during treatment:

Grade 3 AST and/or ALT elevation: Withhold dose until recovery. If benefit of treatment outweighs toxicity risk, resume therapy at a reduced dose of 120 mg once daily.

AST or ALT >20 times ULN: Discontinue permanently.

AST or ALT >3 times ULN **and** bilirubin >2 times ULN: Discontinue permanently.

Recurrence of AST or ALT >5 times ULN despite dose reduction to 120 mg: Discontinue permanently.

Adjustment for Toxicity

Dermatologic:

Grade 2 hand-foot skin reaction (HFSR; palmar-plantar erythrodysesthesia [PPE]) of any duration: Reduce dose to 120 mg once daily for first occurrence. If grade 2 HFSR recurs at this dose, further reduce the dose to 80 mg once daily. Interrupt therapy for grade 2 HFSR that is recurrent or fails to improve within 7 days in spite of dosage reduction.

Grade 3 HFSR: Interrupt therapy for a minimum of 7 days. Upon recovery, reduce dose to 120 mg once daily. If grade 2-3 toxicity recurs at this dose, further reduce dose to 80 mg once daily upon recovery. Interrupt therapy for grade 2-3 HFSR that is recurrent or fails to improve within 7 days in spite of dosage reduction.

Hypertension: Grade 2 (symptomatic): Interrupt therapy.

Other toxicity: Any grade 3 or 4 adverse reaction (other than hepatotoxicity): Interrupt therapy; upon recovery, reduce dose to 120 mg once daily. If any grade 3 or 4 adverse reaction occurs while on this reduced dose, may further reduce regorafenib to 80 mg once daily upon recovery. For any grade 4 adverse reaction, only resume therapy if the benefit outweighs the risk. Permanently discontinue therapy if unable to tolerate 80 mg once daily.

Gastrointestinal perforation: Discontinue permanently.

Hemorrhage (severe or life-threatening): Discontinue permanently.

Reversible posterior leukoencephalopathy syndrome (RPLS): Discontinue.

Wound dehiscence: Discontinue.

Combination Regimens

Colorectal cancer: Regorafenib (Colorectal Regimen) on page 1747

Administration Take at the same time each day with a low-fat (<30% fat) breakfast; swallow tablets whole.

Monitoring Parameters Monitor for hand-foot skin reaction (HFSR)/palmar-plantar erythrodysesthesia (PPE); signs/symptoms of cardiac ischemia or infarction; bleeding; signs/symptoms of GI perforation or fistula; signs/symptoms of reversible posterior leukoencephalopathy syndrome (severe headaches, seizure, confusion, or change in vision). Monitor for impaired wound healing. Obtain liver function tests at baseline, every 2 weeks during the first 2 months of treatment, then monthly or more frequently if clinically necessary (weekly until improvement if liver function tests are elevated). Monitor blood pressure weekly for the first 6 weeks of therapy and with every subsequent cycle, or more frequently if indicated. CBC with differential and platelets and serum electrolytes (baseline and periodic). Monitor INR more frequently if receiving warfarin.

Dietary Considerations Take with a low-fat breakfast (<30% fat)

Dosage Forms Excipient information presented when available (limited, particularly for generics); consult specific product labeling.

Tablet, oral:

Stivarga®: 40 mg [contains soy lecithin]

References

Grothey A, Sobrero AF, Siena S, at el, "Results of a Phase III Randomized, Double-Blind, Placebo-Controlled, Multicenter Trial (CORRECT) of Regorafenib Plus Best Supportive Care (BSC) Versus Placebo Plus BSC in Patients (Pts) With Metastatic Colorectal Cancer (mCRC) Who Have Progressed After Standard Therapies," *J Clin Oncol*, 2012, 30(suppl 4):LBA385 [abstract LBA385 from 2012 ASCO Gastrointestinal Cancers Symposium].

Mross K, Frost A, Steinbild S, et al, "A Phase I Dose-Escalation Study of Regorafenib (BAY 73-4506), an Inhibitor of Oncogenic, Angiogenic, and Stromal Kinases, in Patients With Advanced Solid Tumors," *Clin Cancer Res*, 2012, 18(9):2658-67.

Strumberg D, Scheulen ME, Schultheis B, et al, "Regorafenib (BAY 73-4506) in Advanced Colorectal Cancer: A Phase I Study," *Br J Cancer*, 2012, 106(11):1722-7.

◆ **Relistor®** *see* Methylnaltrexone *on page 964*

◆ **Remicade®** *see* InFLIXimab *on page 789*

◆ **Revlimid®** *see* Lenalidomide *on page 859*

◆ **Revolade®** *see* Eltrombopag *on page 494*

◆ **Revolade™ (Can)** *see* Eltrombopag *on page 494*

◆ **rFVIIa** *see* Factor VIIa (Recombinant) *on page 568*

◆ **RG7204** *see* Vemurafenib *on page 1440*

◆ **rhAT** *see* Antithrombin *on page 107*

◆ **rhATIII** *see* Antithrombin *on page 107*

◆ **Rheumatrex®** *see* Methotrexate *on page 949*

◆ **RhIG** *see* Rh_o(D) Immune Globulin *on page 1237*

◆ **rhIL-11** *see* Oprelvekin *on page 1074*

◆ **rhKGF** *see* Palifermin *on page 1104*

◆ **Rho(D) Immune Globulin (Human)** *see* Rh_o(D) Immune Globulin *on page 1237*

Rh_o(D) Immune Globulin (ar aych oh (dee) i MYUN GLOB yoo lin)

Brand Names: U.S. HyperRHO™ S/D Full Dose; HyperRHO™ S/D Mini-Dose; MICRhoGAM® UF Plus; RhoGAM® UF Plus; Rhophylac®; WinRho® SDF

Brand Names: Canada WinRho® SDF

Index Terms Anti-D Immunoglobulin; RhIG; Rho(D) Immune Globulin (Human); RhoIGIV; RhoIVIM

Generic Availability (U.S.) No

Pharmacologic Category Blood Product Derivative; Immune Globulin

Use

Suppression of Rh Isoimmunization: Use in the following situations when an Rh_o(D)-negative individual is exposed to Rh_o(D)-positive blood: During delivery of an Rh_o(D)-positive infant, abortion, amniocentesis; chorionic villus sampling; ruptured tubal pregnancy, abdominal trauma, hydatidiform mole; transplacental hemorrhage. Used when the mother is Rh_o(D)-negative, the father of the child is either Rh_o(D)-positive or Rh_o(D)-unknown, or the baby is either Rh_o(D)-positive or Rh_o(D)-unknown.

Transfusion: Suppression of Rh isoimmunization in Rh_o(D)-negative individuals transfused with Rh_o(D) antigen-positive RBCs or blood components containing Rh_o(D) antigen-positive RBCs

Treatment of idiopathic thrombocytopenic purpura (ITP): Used intravenously in the following nonsplenectomized Rh_o(D)-positive individuals: Children with acute or chronic ITP, adults with chronic ITP, and children and adults with ITP secondary to HIV infection

Labeled Contraindications Hypersensitivity to immune globulins or any component of the formulation; prior sensitization to Rh_o(D)

WinRho® SDF product labeling: Patients with autoimmune hemolytic anemia; patients with pre-existing hemolysis or at high risk for hemolysis; IgA-deficient patients with antibodies against IgA; suppression of isoimmunization in infants

WinRho® SDF Canadian labeling: Additional contraindications (not in U.S. labeling):

Rh immunization prophylaxis: Rh_o(D)-negative women who are not pregnant or have had a recent delivery or abortion and who are Rh sensitized

Treatment of ITP: Patients who are Rh_o(D)-negative or have had splenectomy, ITP secondary to conditions including leukemia, lymphoma, or active infections with Epstein-Barr virus (EBV) or hepatits C virus (HCV), elderly with comorbidities predisposing to acute hemolytic reaction (AHR), evidence of autoimmune hemolytic anemia (Evan's syndrome), systemic lupus erythematosus (SLE) or antiphospholipid antibody syndrome

Pregnancy Risk Factor C

Lactation Does not enter breast milk

Warnings/Precautions [U.S. Boxed Warning]: May cause IVH in patients treated for immune thrombocytopenic purpura (WinRho® SDF product labeling). Rare but serious signs and symptoms (eg, back pain, shaking, chills, fever, discolored urine; onset within 4 hours of infusion) of intravascular hemolysis (IVH) have been reported in postmarketing experience in patients treated for ITP and may result in clinically-compromising anemia and multi-organ system failure including acute respiratory distress syndrome. Acute renal insufficiency and disseminated intravascular coagulation (DIC) have also been reported. ITP patients should be advised of the signs and symptoms of IVH and instructed to report them immediately.

Product of human plasma; may potentially contain infectious agents which could transmit disease. Screening of donors, as well as testing and/or inactivation or removal of certain viruses, reduces the risk. Infections thought to be transmitted by this product should be reported to the manufacturer. Not for replacement therapy in immune globulin deficiency syndromes. Pulmonary edema may occur following IVIG treatment in patients being treated for ITP. Symptoms are usually present within 1-6 hours after administration; monitor patients for pulmonary reactions. Use caution with IgA deficiency, may contain trace amounts of IgA; patients who are IgA deficient may have the potential for developing IgA antibodies, anaphylactic reactions may occur. Administer I.M. injections with caution in patients with thrombocytopenia or coagulation disorders. Some products may contain maltose, which may result in falsely-elevated blood glucose readings. Use caution with renal dysfunction. Thrombotic events have been reported with administration of intravenous immune globulins (IVIG); use with caution in patients with a history of atherosclerosis or cardiovascular and/or thrombotic risk factors or patients with known/suspected hyperviscosity. Consider a baseline assessment of blood viscosity in patients at risk for hyperviscosity.

Administer at the minimum practical infusion rate in patients with renal impairment or in patients at risk for thrombotic events. Monitor for signs and symptoms of transfusion-related acute lung injury.

ITP: Do not administer I.M. or SubQ for the treatment of ITP; administer dose I.V. only. Safety and efficacy not established in Rh_o(D) negative, non-ITP thrombocytopenia, or splenectomized patients. When using WinRho® SDF, decrease dose with hemoglobin <10 g/dL; use with extreme caution if hemoglobin <8 g/dL. Safety and efficacy have not been established for Rhophylac® in patients with anemia.

Rh_o(D) suppression: For use in the mother; do not administer to the neonate.

Adverse Reactions Frequency not defined.

Cardiovascular: Hyper-/hypotension, pallor, vasodilation

Central nervous system: Chills, dizziness, fever, headache, malaise, somnolence

Dermatologic: Pruritus, rash

Gastrointestinal: Abdominal pain, diarrhea, nausea, vomiting

Hematologic: Haptoglobin decreased, hemoglobin decreased (patients with ITP), intravascular hemolysis (patients with ITP)

Hepatic: Bilirubin increased, LDH increased

Local: Injection site reaction: Discomfort, induration, mild pain, redness, swelling

Neuromuscular & skeletal: Arthralgia, back pain, hyperkinesia, myalgia, weakness

Renal: Acute renal insufficiency

Miscellaneous: Anaphylaxis, diaphoresis, infusion-related reactions, positive anti-C antibody test (transient), shivering

Postmarketing and/or case reports: Anemia (clinically-compromising), anuria, ARDS, cardiac arrest, cardiac failure, chest pain, chromaturia, DIC, edema, erythema, fatigue, hematuria, hemoglobinemia, hemoglobinuria (transient in patients with ITP), hyperhidrosis, hypersensitivity, injection site irritation, jaundice, myocardial infarction, muscle spasm, nausea, pain in extremities, renal failure, renal impairment, tachycardia, transfusion-related acute lung injury

Drug Interactions

Metabolism/Transport Effects None known.

Avoid Concomitant Use There are no known interactions where it is recommended to avoid concomitant use.

Increased Effect/Toxicity There are no known significant interactions involving an increase in effect.

Decreased Effect

Rho(D) Immune Globulin may decrease the levels/effects of: Vaccines (Live)

Storage/Stability Store at 2°C to 8°C (35°F to 46°F); do not freeze.

RhoGAM® UF Plus, MICRhoGAM® UF Plus: May be stored at 25°C (77°F) for up to 10 days (data on file [Ortho Clinical Diagnostics, 2011]). However, the manufacturer recommends storage under refrigeration. Room temperature stability information should only be utilized in situations where the drug has been inadvertently exposed to prolonged room temperature.

HyperRHO™ SD may be stored at 25°C (77°F) for ~2 weeks (data on file [Talecris Biotherapeutics, 2011]). However, the manufacturer recommends storage under refrigeration. Room temperature stability information should only be utilized in situations where the drug has been inadvertently exposed to prolonged room temperature.

Rhophylac®: Protect from light.

WinRho® SDF: After reconstitution, store at room temperature for no longer than 12 hours. Do not shake or freeze.

Mechanism of Action

Rh suppression: Prevents isoimmunization by suppressing the immune response and antibody formation by Rh$_o$(D) negative individuals to Rh$_o$(D) positive red blood cells.

ITP: Not completely characterized; Rh$_o$(D) immune globulin is thought to form anti-D-coated red blood cell complexes which bind to macrophage Fc receptors within the spleen; blocking or saturating the spleens ability to clear antibody-coated cells, including platelets. In this manner, platelets are spared from destruction.

Pharmacodynamics/Kinetics

Onset of platelet increase: ITP: Platelets should rise within 1-2 days
  Peak effect: In 7-14 days

Duration: Suppression of Rh isoimmunization: ~12 weeks; Treatment of ITP: 30 days (variable)

Distribution: V_d: I.M.: 8.59 L

Bioavailability: I.M.: Rhophylac®: 69%

Half-life elimination: ~24-30 days

Time to peak, plasma: I.M.: 5-10 days; I.V. (WinRho® SDF): ≤2 hours

Dosing

Adult

ITP:

Rhophylac®: I.V.: 50 mcg/kg

WinRho® SDF: I.V.:

Initial: 50 mcg/kg as a single injection, or can be given as a divided dose on separate days. If hemoglobin is <10 g/dL: Dose should be reduced to 25-40 mcg/kg

Subsequent dosing: 25-60 mcg/kg can be used if required to increase platelet count

Maintenance dosing if patient **did respond** to initial dosing: 25-60 mcg/kg based on platelet count and hemoglobin concentration

Maintenance dosing if patient **did not respond** to initial dosing:

Hemoglobin <8 g/dL: Alternative treatment should be used

Hemoglobin 8-10 g/dL: Redose between 25-40 mcg/kg

Hemoglobin >10 g/dL: Redose between 50-60 mcg/kg

Rh$_o$(D) suppression: Note: One "full dose" (300 mcg) provides enough antibody to prevent Rh sensitization if the volume of RBC entering the circulation is ≤15 mL. When >15 mL is suspected, a fetal red cell count should be performed to determine the appropriate dose.

Pregnancy:

Antepartum prophylaxis: In general, dose is given at 28 weeks. If given early in pregnancy, administer every 12 weeks to ensure adequate levels of passively acquired anti-Rh

HyperRHO™ S/D Full Dose, RhoGAM®: I.M.: 300 mcg

Rhophylac®, WinRho® SDF: I.M., I.V.: 300 mcg

Postpartum prophylaxis: In general, dose is administered as soon as possible after delivery, preferably within 72 hours. Can be given up to 28 days following delivery

HyperRHO™ S/D Full Dose, RhoGAM®: I.M.: 300 mcg

Rhophylac®: I.M., I.V.: 300 mcg

WinRho® SDF: I.M., I.V.: 120 mcg

Threatened abortion, any time during pregnancy (with continuation of pregnancy):

HyperRHO™ S/D Full Dose, RhoGAM®: I.M.: 300 mcg; administer as soon as possible

Rhophylac®, WinRho® SDF: I.M./I.V.: 300 mcg; administer as soon as possible

Abortion, miscarriage, termination of ectopic pregnancy:

RhoGAM®: I.M.: ≥13 weeks gestation: 300 mcg.

HyperRHO™ S/D Mini Dose, MICRhoGAM®: <13 weeks gestation: I.M.: 50 mcg

Rhophylac®: I.M., I.V.: 300 mcg

WinRho® SDF: I.M., I.V.: After 34 weeks gestation: 120 mcg; administer immediately or within 72 hours

Amniocentesis, chorionic villus sampling:

HyperRHO™ S/D Full Dose, RhoGAM®: I.M.: At 15-18 weeks gestation or during the 3rd trimester: 300 mcg. If dose is given between 13-18 weeks, repeat at 26-28 weeks and within 72 hours of delivery.

Rhophylac®: I.M., I.V.: 300 mcg

WinRho® SDF: I.M., I.V.:

Before 34 weeks gestation: 300 mcg; administer immediately, repeat dose every 12 weeks during pregnancy

After 34 weeks gestation: 120 mcg, administered immediately or within 72 hours

Excessive fetomaternal hemorrhage (>15 mL): Rhophylac®: I.M., I.V.: 300 mcg within 72 hours plus 20 mcg/mL fetal RBCs in excess of 15 mL if excess transplacental bleeding is quantified **or** 300 mcg/dose if bleeding cannot be quantified

Abdominal trauma, manipulation:

HyperRHO™ S/D Full Dose, RhoGAM®: I.M.: 2nd or 3rd trimester: 300 mcg. If dose is given between 13-18 weeks, repeat at 26-28 weeks and within 72 hours of delivery.

Rhophylac®: I.M., I.V.: 300 mcg within 72 hours

WinRho® SDF: I.M., I.V.: After 34 weeks gestation: 120 mcg; administer immediately or within 72 hours

Transfusion:

HyperRHO™ S/D Full Dose, RhoGAM®: I.M.: Multiply the volume of Rh positive whole blood administered by the hematocrit of the donor unit to equal the volume of RBCs transfused. The volume of RBCs is then divided by 15 mL, providing the number of 300 mcg doses (vials/syringes) to administer. If the dose calculated results in a fraction, round up to the next higher whole 300 mcg dose (vial/syringe).

WinRho® SDF: Administer within 72 hours after exposure of incompatible blood transfusions or massive fetal hemorrhage.

I.V.: Calculate dose as follows; administer 600 mcg every 8 hours until the total dose is administered:

Exposure to Rh_o(D) positive whole blood: 9 mcg/mL blood

Exposure to Rh_o(D) positive red blood cells: 18 mcg/mL cells

I.M.: Calculate dose as follows; administer 1200 mcg every 12 hours until the total dose is administered:

Exposure to Rh_o(D) positive whole blood: 12 mcg/mL blood

Exposure to Rh_o(D) positive red blood cells: 24 mcg/mL cells

Rhophylac®: I.M., I.V.:20 mcg per 2 mL transfused blood or 1 mL erythrocyte concentrate

Geriatric Refer to adult dosing. Patients >65 years of age with a concurrent comorbid condition (eg, infection, malignancy, autoimmune disorders) may be at increased risk of developing acute hemolytic reactions. Fatal outcomes associated with IVH have occurred most frequently in those >65 years. Careful consideration should be used when selecting dosage for elderly patients due to a higher probability of decreased hepatic, renal, or cardiac function; consider starting at lower doses.

Pediatric ITP, transfusion: Rhophylac®, WinRho® SDF: Refer to adult dosing.

Renal Impairment I.V. infusion: Use caution; may require infusion rate reduction or discontinuation.

Administration The total volume can be administered in divided doses at different sites at one time or may be divided and given at intervals, provided the total dosage is given within 72 hours of the fetomaternal hemorrhage or transfusion.

I.M.: Administer into the deltoid muscle of the upper arm or anterolateral aspect of the upper thigh; avoid gluteal region due to risk of sciatic nerve injury. If large doses (>5 mL) are needed, administration in divided doses at different sites is recommended. **Note:** Do not administer I.M. Rh_o(D) immune globulin for ITP.

I.V.:

Rhophylac®: ITP: Infuse at 2 mL per 15-60 seconds

WinRho® SDF: Infuse over at least 3-5 minutes; do not administer with other medications

Note: If preparing dose using liquid formulation, withdraw the entire contents of the vial to ensure accurate calculation of the dosage requirement.

Monitoring Parameters Signs and symptoms of intravascular hemolysis (IVH), anemia, renal insufficiency, back pain, shaking, chills, discolored urine, or hematuria; observe patient for side effects for 8 hours following administration

Patients with suspected IVH: CBC, haptoglobin, plasma hemoglobin, urine dipstick, BUN, serum creatinine, liver function tests, DIC-specific tests (D-dimer, fibrin degradation products [FDP] or fibrin split products [FSP]) for differential diagnosis. In patients at increased risk of developing acute renal failure, periodically monitor renal function and urine output. Clinical response may be determined by monitoring platelets, red blood cell (RBC) counts, hemoglobin, and reticulocyte levels.

ITP: Check blood type, CBC, reticulocyte count, DAT, urine dipstick before initiating treatment with WinRho® SDF, repeat urine dipstick at 2 and 4 hours after administration and prior to end of the 8-hour monitoring period.

Test Interactions Some infants born to women given Rh_o(D) antepartum have a weakly positive Coombs' test at birth. Fetal-maternal hemorrhage may cause false blood-typing result in the mother; when there is any doubt to the patients' Rh type, Rh_o(D) immune globulin should be administered. WinRho® SDF liquid contains maltose; may result in falsely elevated blood glucose levels with dehydrogenase pyrroloquinolinequinone or glucose-dye-oxidoreductase testing methods. WinRho® SDF contains trace amounts of anti-A, B, C and E; may alter Coombs' tests following administration.

Additional Information A "full dose" of Rh_o(D) immune globulin has previously been referred to as a 300 mcg dose. It is not the actual anti-D content. Although dosing has traditionally been expressed in mcg, potency is listed in units (1 mcg = 5 units). ITP patients requiring transfusions should be transfused with Rho-negative blood cells to avoid exacerbating hemolysis; platelet products may contain red blood cells; caution should be exercised if platelets are from Rh_o-positive donors.

Dosage Forms Excipient information presented when available (limited, particularly for generics); consult specific product labeling.

Injection, solution [preservative free]:

HyperRHO™ S/D Full Dose: ≥300 mcg/mL (1 mL) [solvent/detergent treated; ≥1500 units; for I.M. use only]

HyperRHO™ S/D Mini-Dose: ≥50 mcg/0.17 mL (0.17 mL) [solvent/detergent treated; ≥250 units; for I.M. use only]

MICRhoGAM® UF Plus: ~50 mcg/0.75 mL (0.75 mL) [contains polysorbate 80; 250 units; for I.M. use only; volume is expressed as an approximate value]

RhoGAM® UF Plus: ~300 mcg/0.75 mL (0.75 mL) [contains polysorbate 80; 1500 units; for I.M. use only; volume is expressed as an approximate value]

Rhophylac®: ≥ 300 mcg/2 mL (2 mL) [contains albumin (human); 1500 units; for I.M. or I.V. use]

WinRho® SDF: 3000 mcg/~13 mL (13 mL) [contains maltose, polysorbate 80; 15,000 units; for I.M. or I.V. use; volume is expressed as an approximate value]

WinRho® SDF: 300 mcg/~1.3 mL (1.3 mL) [contains maltose, polysorbate 80; 1500 units; for I.M. or I.V. use; volume is expressed as an approximate value]

WinRho® SDF: 500 mcg/~2.2 mL (2.2 mL) [contains maltose, polysorbate 80; 2500 units; for I.M. or I.V. use; volume is expressed as an approximate value]

WinRho® SDF: 1000 mcg/~4.4 mL (4.4 mL) [contains maltose, polysorbate 80; 5000 units; for I.M. or I.V. use; volume is expressed as an approximate value]

References

Gaines AR, "Disseminated Intravascular Coagulation Associated with Acute Hemoglobinemia or Hemoglobinuria Following Rho(D) Immune Globulin Intravenous Administration for Immune Thrombocytopenic Purpura," *Blood*, 2005, 106(5):1532-37.

George JN, Woolf SH, Raskob GE, et al, "Clinical Guideline: Diagnosis and Treatment of Idiopathic Thrombocytopenic Purpura: Recommendations of the American Society of Hematology," *Ann Intern Med*, 1997, 126(4):319-26.

Hartwell EA, "Use of Rh Immune Globulin: ASCP Practice Parameter. American Society of Clinical Pathologists," *Am J Clin Pathol*, 1998, 110(3):281-92.

"Rh_o(D) Immune Globulin I.V. for Prevention of Rh Isoimmunization and for Treatment of ITP," *Med Lett Drugs Ther*, 1996, 38(966):6-8.

Simpson KN, Coughlin CM, Eron J, et al, "Idiopathic Thrombocytopenia Purpura: Treatment Patterns and an Analysis of Cost Associated With Intravenous Immunoglobulin and Anti-D Therapy," *Semin Hematol*, 1998, 35(1 Suppl 1):58-64.

◆ **RhoGAM® UF Plus** *see* Rh_o(D) Immune Globulin *on page 1237*

◆ **RhoIGIV** *see* Rh_o(D) Immune Globulin *on page 1237*

◆ **RhoIVIM** *see* Rh_o(D) Immune Globulin *on page 1237*

◆ **Rhophylac®** *see* Rh_o(D) Immune Globulin *on page 1237*

◆ **Rhoxal-cyclosporine (Can)** *see* CycloSPORINE (Systemic) *on page 333*

◆ **Rh-TSH** *see* Thyrotropin Alfa *on page 1360*

◆ ***r*HuEPO** *see* Epoetin Alfa *on page 516*

◆ **rhuGM-CSF** *see* Sargramostim *on page 1270*

◆ **rhu Keratinocyte Growth Factor** *see* Palifermin *on page 1104*

◆ **rHu-KGF** *see* Palifermin *on page 1104*

- **rhuMAb-2C4** *see* Pertuzumab *on page 1165*
- **rHuMAb-EGFr** *see* Panitumumab *on page 1115*
- **rhuMAb HER2** *see* Trastuzumab *on page 1399*
- **rhuMAb-VEGF** *see* Bevacizumab *on page 165*
- **RiaSTAP®** *see* Fibrinogen Concentrate (Human) *on page 602*
- **Rituxan®** *see* RiTUXimab *on page 1244*

RiTUXimab (ri TUK si mab)

Related Information

Hematopoietic Stem Cell Transplantation *on page 1887*
Management of Chemotherapy-Induced Nausea and Vomiting *on page 1786*
Management of Infections *on page 1809*
Principles of Anticancer Therapy *on page 1878*

Brand Names: U.S. Rituxan®

Brand Names: Canada Rituxan®

Index Terms Anti-CD20 Monoclonal Antibody; C2B8 Monoclonal Antibody; IDEC-C2B8

Generic Availability (U.S.) No

Pharmacologic Category Antineoplastic Agent, Monoclonal Antibody; Antirheumatic Miscellaneous; Immunosuppressant Agent; Monoclonal Antibody

Use

Treatment of CD20-positive non-Hodgkin lymphomas (NHL):

Relapsed or refractory, low-grade or follicular B-cell NHL (as a single agent)

Follicular B-cell NHL, previously untreated (in combination with first-line chemotherapy, and as single-agent maintenance therapy if response to first-line rituximab with chemotherapy)

Nonprogressing, low-grade B-cell NHL (as a single agent after first-line CVP treatment)

Diffuse large B-cell NHL, previously untreated (in combination with CHOP chemotherapy [or other anthracycline-based regimen])

Treatment of CD20-positive chronic lymphocytic leukemia (CLL) (in combination with fludarabine and cyclophosphamide)

Treatment of moderately- to severely-active rheumatoid arthritis (in combination with methotrexate) in adult patients with inadequate response to one or more TNF antagonists

Treatment of granulomatosis with polyangiitis (GPA; Wegener's granulomatosis) (in combination with glucocorticoids)

Treatment of microscopic polyangiitis (MPA) (in combination with glucocorticoids)

Unlabeled Use Treatment of Burkitt's lymphoma, central nervous system lymphoma, Hodgkin's lymphoma (lymphocyte predominant); mucosal associated lymphoid tissue (MALT) lymphoma (gastric and nongastric), splenic marginal zone lymphoma; Waldenström's macroglobulinemia (WM); post-transplant lymphoproliferative disorder (PTLD); autoimmune hemolytic anemia (AIHA) in children; chronic immune thrombocytopenic purpura (ITP); refractory pemphigus vulgaris; treatment of steroid-refractory chronic graft-versus-host disease (GVHD); refractory lupus nephritis; relapsed/refractory thrombotic thrombocytopenic purpura-hemolytic uremic syndrome (TTP-HUS), resistant idiopathic membranous nephropathy (IMN), refractory nephrotic syndrome (children)

Labeled Contraindications There are no contraindications listed in the FDA-approved manufacturer's labeling.

Canadian labeling (not in U.S. labeling): Type 1 hypersensitivity or anaphylactic reaction to murine proteins, Chinese Hamster Ovary (CHO) cell proteins, or any component of the formulation; patients who have or have had progressive multifocal leukoencephalopathy (PML)

Pregnancy Risk Factor C

Lactation Excretion in breast milk unknown/not recommended

Warnings/Precautions **[U.S. Boxed Warning]: Severe (occasionally fatal) infusion-related reactions have been reported, usually with the first infusion; fatalities have been reported within 24 hours of infusion; monitor closely during infusion; discontinue with grades 3 or 4 infusion reactions.** Reactions usually occur within 30-120 minutes and may include hypotension, angioedema, bronchospasm, hypoxia, urticaria, and in more severe cases pulmonary infiltrates, acute respiratory distress syndrome, myocardial infarction, ventricular fibrillation, cardiogenic shock and/or anaphylaxis. Risk factors associated with fatal outcomes include chronic lymphocytic leukemia, female gender, mantle cell lymphoma, or pulmonary infiltrates. Closely monitor patients with a history of prior cardiopulmonary reactions or with pre-existing cardiac or pulmonary conditions and patients with high numbers of circulating malignant cells (>25,000/mm^3). Prior to infusion, premedicate patients with acetaminophen and an antihistamine (and methylprednisolone for patients with RA). Discontinue infusion for severe reactions; treatment is symptomatic. Medications for the treatment of hypersensitivity reactions (eg, bronchodilators, epinephrine, antihistamines, corticosteroids) should be available for immediate use. Discontinue infusion for serious or life-threatening cardiac arrhythmias; subsequent doses should include cardiac monitoring during and after the infusion. Mild-to-moderate infusion-related reactions (eg, chills, fever, rigors) occur frequently and are typically managed through slowing or interrupting the infusion. Infusion may be resumed at a 50% infusion rate reduction upon resolution of symptoms. Due to the potential for hypotension, consider withholding antihypertensives 12 hours prior to treatment.

[U.S. Boxed Warning]: Progressive multifocal leukoencephalopathy (PML) due to JC virus infection has been reported with rituximab use; may be fatal. Cases were reported in patients with hematologic malignancies receiving rituximab either with combination chemotherapy, or with hematopoietic stem cell transplant. Cases were also reported in patients receiving rituximab for autoimmune diseases who had received prior or concurrent immunosuppressant therapy. Onset may be delayed, although most cases were diagnosed within 12 months of the last rituximab dose. A retrospective analysis of patients (n=57) diagnosed with PML following rituximab therapy, found a median of 16 months (following rituximab initiation), 5.5 months (following last rituximab dose), and 6 rituximab doses preceded PML diagnosis. Clinical findings included confusion/disorientation, motor weakness/hemiparesis, altered vision/speech, and poor motor coordination with symptoms progressing over weeks to months (Carson, 2009). Promptly evaluate any patient presenting with neurological changes; consider neurology consultation, brain MRI and lumbar puncture for suspected PML. Discontinue rituximab in patients who develop PML; consider reduction/discontinuation of concurrent chemotherapy or immunosuppressants. Avoid use if severe active infection is present. Serious and potentially fatal bacterial, fungal, and either new or reactivated viral infections may occur during treatment, and up to 1 year after completing rituximab. Infections have been observed in patients with prolonged hypogammaglobulinemia, defined as hypogammaglobulinemia >11 months after rituximab exposure; monitor immunoglobulin levels as necessary. Associated new or reactivated viral infections have included cytomegalovirus, herpes simplex virus, parvovirus B19, varicella zoster virus, West Nile virus, and hepatitis B and C. Rarely, reactivation of hepatitis B (with fulminant hepatitis, hepatic failure, and death) has been reported in association with rituximab; median time to hepatitis diagnosis was ~4 months after initiation of therapy and 1 month following last dose; screen high-risk patients prior to therapy initiation; monitor for several months following completion of therapy. Discontinue rituximab (and concomitant chemotherapy) in patients who develop viral hepatitis and initiate antiviral therapy. Discontinue rituximab in patients who develop other serious infections and initiate appropriate anti-infective treatment.

[U.S. Boxed Warning]: Tumor lysis syndrome leading to acute renal failure requiring dialysis may occur 12-24 hours following the first dose when used as a single agent in the treatment of NHL. Hyperkalemia, hypocalcemia, hyperuricemia, and/or hyperphosphatemia may occur. Administer prophylaxis (allopurinol, hydration) in patients at high risk (high numbers of circulating malignant cells ≥25,000/mm^3 or high tumor burden). May cause fatal renal toxicity in patients with hematologic malignancies. Patients who received combination therapy with cisplatin and rituximab for NHL experienced renal toxicity during clinical trials; this combination is not an approved treatment regimen. Monitor for signs of renal failure; discontinue rituximab with increasing serum creatinine or oliguria. Correct electrolyte abnormalities; monitor hydration status.

[U.S. Boxed Warning]: Severe and sometimes fatal mucocutaneous reactions (lichenoid dermatitis, paraneoplastic pemphigus, Stevens-Johnson syndrome, toxic epidermal necrolysis and vesiculobullous dermatitis) have been reported, occurring from 1-13 weeks following exposure. Discontinue in patients experiencing severe mucocutaneous skin reactions; the safety of re-exposure following mucocutaneous reactions has not been evaluated. Use caution with pre-existing cardiac or pulmonary disease, or prior cardiopulmonary events. Rheumatoid arthritis patients are at increased risk for cardiovascular events; monitor closely during and after each infusion. Elderly patients are at higher risk for cardiac (supraventricular arrhythmia) and pulmonary adverse events (pneumonia, pneumonitis). Abdominal pain, bowel obstruction, and perforation (rarely fatal) have been reported with an average onset of symptoms of ~6 days (range: 1-77 days); complaints of abdominal pain should be evaluated, especially if early in the treatment course. Live vaccines should not be given concurrently with rituximab; there is no data available concerning secondary transmission of live vaccines with or following rituximab treatment. RA patients should be brought up to date with nonlive immunizations (following current guidelines) at least 4 weeks before initiating therapy; evaluate risks of therapy delay versus benefit (of nonlive vaccines) for NHL patients. Safety and efficacy of rituximab in combination with biologic agents or disease-modifying antirheumatic drugs (DMARD) other than methotrexate have not been established. Rituximab is not recommended for use in RA patients who have not had prior inadequate response to TNF antagonists. Safety and efficacy of retreatment for RA have not been established. The safety of concomitant immunosuppressants other than corticosteroids has not been evaluated in patients with granulomatosis with polyangiitis (GPA; Wegener's granulomatosis) or microscopic polyangiitis (MPA) after rituximab-induced B-cell depletion. There are only limited data on subsequent courses of rituximab for GPA or MPA; safety and efficacy of retreatment have not been established.

Adverse Reactions Note: Patients treated with rituximab for rheumatoid arthritis (RA) may experience fewer adverse reactions.

>10%:

Cardiovascular: Peripheral edema (8% to 16%), hypertension (6% to 12%)

Central nervous system: Fever (5% to 53%), fatigue (13% to 39%), chills (3% to 33%), headache (17% to 19%), insomnia (≤14%), pain (12%)

Dermatologic: Rash (10% to 17%; grades 3/4: 1%), pruritus (5% to 17%), angioedema (11%; grades 3/4: 1%)

Gastrointestinal: Nausea (8% to 23%), diarrhea (10% to 17%), abdominal pain (2% to 14%), weight gain (11%)

Hematologic: Cytopenias (grades 3/4: ≤48%; may be prolonged), lymphopenia (48%; grades 3/4: 40%; median duration 14 days), anemia (8% to 35%; grades 3/4: 3%), leukopenia (NHL: 14%; grades 3/4: 4%; CLL: grades 3/4: 23%; GPA/MPA: 10%), neutropenia (NHL: 14%; grades 3/4: 4% to 6%; median duration 13 days; CLL: grades 3/4: 30% to 49%), neutropenic fever (CLL: grades 3/4: 9% to 15%), thrombocytopenia (12%; grades 3/4: 2% to 11%)

Hepatic: ALT increased (≤13%)

Neuromuscular & skeletal: Neuropathy (≤30%), weakness (2% to 26%), muscle spasm (≤17%), arthralgia (6% to 13%)

Respiratory: Cough (13%), rhinitis (3% to 12%), epistaxis (≤11%)

Miscellaneous: Infusion-related reactions (lymphoma: first dose 77%; decreases with subsequent infusions; may include angioedema, bronchospasm, chills, dizziness, fever, headache, hyper-/hypotension, myalgia, nausea, pruritus, rash, rigors, urticaria, and vomiting; reactions reported are lower [first infusion: 32%] in RA; CLL: 59%; grades 3/4: 7% to 9%; GPA/MPA: 12%); infection (19% to 62%; grades 3/4: 4%; bacterial: 19%; viral 10%; fungal: 1%), human antichimeric antibody (HACA) positive (1% to 23%), night sweats (15%)

1% to 10%:

Cardiovascular: Hypotension (10%; grades 3/4: 2%), flushing (5%)

Central nervous system: Dizziness (10%), anxiety (2% to 5%), migraine (RA: 2%)

Dermatologic: Urticaria (2% to 8%)

Endocrine & metabolic: Hyperglycemia (9%)

Gastrointestinal: Vomiting (10%), dyspepsia (RA: 3%)

Neuromuscular & skeletal: Back pain (10%), myalgia (10%), paresthesia (2%)

Respiratory: Dyspnea (≤10%), throat irritation (2% to 9%), bronchospasm (8%), dyspnea (7%), upper respiratory tract infection (RA: 7%), sinusitis (6%)

Miscellaneous: LDH increased (7%)

Postmarketing and/or case reports: Acute renal failure, anaphylactoid reaction/anaphylaxis, angina, aplastic anemia, ARDS, arrhythmia, bowel obstruction/perforation, bronchiolitis obliterans, cardiac failure, cardiogenic shock, disease progression (Kaposi's sarcoma), encephalomyelitis, fatal infusion-related reactions, fulminant hepatitis, gastrointestinal perforation, hemolytic anemia, hepatic failure, hepatitis, hepatitis B reactivation, hyperviscosity syndrome (in Waldenström's macroglobulinemia), hypogammaglobulinemia (prolonged), hypoxia, interstitial pneumonitis, laryngeal edema, lichenoid dermatitis, lupus-like syndrome, marrow hypoplasia, MI, mucositis, mucocutaneous reaction, neutropenia (late-onset occurring >40 days after last dose), optic neuritis, pancytopenia (prolonged), paraneoplastic pemphigus (uncommon), pleuritis, pneumonia, pneumonitis, polyarticular arthritis, polymyositis, posterior reversible encephalopathy syndrome (PRES), progressive multifocal leukoencephalopathy (PML), pure red cell aplasia, renal toxicity, reversible posterior leukoencephalopathy syndrome (RPLS), serum sickness, Stevens-Johnson syndrome, supraventricular arrhythmia, systemic vasculitis, toxic epidermal necrolysis, tuberculosis reactivation, tumor lysis syndrome, uveitis, vasculitis with rash, ventricular fibrillation, ventricular tachycardia, vesiculobullous dermatitis, viral reactivation (includes JC virus, cytomegalovirus, herpes simplex virus, parvovirus B19, varicella zoster virus, West Nile virus, and hepatitis C), wheezing

Drug Interactions

Metabolism/Transport Effects None known.

Avoid Concomitant Use

Avoid concomitant use of RiTUXimab with any of the following: BCG; Belimumab; Certolizumab Pegol; CloZAPine; Natalizumab; Pimecrolimus; Tacrolimus (Topical); Vaccines (Live)

Increased Effect/Toxicity

RiTUXimab may increase the levels/effects of: Belimumab; Certolizumab Pegol; CloZAPine; Leflunomide; Natalizumab; Vaccines (Live)

The levels/effects of RiTUXimab may be increased by: Abciximab; Antihypertensives; Denosumab; Pimecrolimus; Roflumilast; Tacrolimus (Topical); Trastuzumab

Decreased Effect

RiTUXimab may decrease the levels/effects of: BCG; Coccidioidin Skin Test; Sipuleucel-T; Vaccines (Inactivated); Vaccines (Live)

The levels/effects of RiTUXimab may be decreased by: Echinacea

Ethanol/Nutrition/Herb Interactions Herb/Nutraceutical: Avoid echinacea (may diminish the therapeutic effect of immunosuppressants). Avoid hypoglycemic herbs, including alfalfa, aloe, bilberry, bitter melon, burdock, celery, damiana, fenugreek, garcinia, garlic, ginger, ginseng (American), gymnema, marshmallow, and stinging nettle (may enhance the hypoglycemic effect of rituximab).

Storage/Stability Store intact vials refrigerated at 2°C to 8°C (36°F to 46°F); do not freeze. Do not shake. Protect vials from direct sunlight. Solutions for infusion are stable at 2°C to 8°C (36°F to 46°F) for 24 hours and at room temperature for an additional 24 hours.

Reconstitution Withdraw necessary amount of rituximab and dilute to a final concentration of 1-4 mg/mL with 0.9% sodium chloride or 5% dextrose in water. Gently invert the bag to mix the solution. Do not shake.

Mechanism of Action Rituximab is a monoclonal antibody directed against the CD20 antigen on B-lymphocytes. CD20 regulates cell cycle initiation; and, possibly, functions as a calcium channel. Rituximab binds to the antigen on the cell surface, activating complement-dependent B-cell cytotoxicity; and to human Fc receptors, mediating cell killing through an antibody-dependent cellular toxicity. B-cells are believed to play a role in the development and progression of rheumatoid arthritis. Signs and symptoms of RA are reduced by targeting B-cells and the progression of structural damage is delayed.

Pharmacodynamics/Kinetics

Duration: Detectable in serum 3-6 months after completion of treatment; B-cell recovery begins ~6 months following completion of treatment; median B-cell levels return to normal by 12 months following completion of treatment

Absorption: I.V.: Immediate and results in a rapid and sustained depletion of circulating and tissue-based B cells

Distribution: RA: 3.1 L; GPA/MPA: 4.5 L

Half life elimination:

CLL: Median terminal half-life: 32 days (range: 14-62 days)

NHL: Median terminal half-life: 22 days (range: 6-52 days)

RA: Mean terminal half-life: 18 days (range: 5-78 days)

GPA/MPA: 23 days (range: 9-49 days)

Excretion: Uncertain; may undergo phagocytosis and catabolism in the reticuloendothelial system (RES)

Dosing

Adult & Geriatric Note: Details concerning dosing in combination regimens should also be consulted. Pretreatment with acetaminophen and an antihistamine is recommended for all indications. For oncology uses, a uricostatic agent (eg, allopurinol) and aggressive hydration is recommended for patients at risk for tumor lysis syndrome (high tumor burden or lymphocytes >25,000/mm^3). In patients with CLL, *Pneumocystis jirovecii* pneumonia (PCP) and antiherpetic viral prophylaxis is recommended during treatment (and for up to 12 months following treatment). In patients with granulomatosis with polyangiitis (GPA) and microscopic polyangiitis (MPA), PCP prophylaxis is recommended during and for 6 months after rituximab treatment. For patients with RA, premedication with methylprednisolone 100 mg I.V. (or equivalent) is recommended 30 minutes prior to each dose.

Chronic lymphocytic leukemia (CLL): I.V. infusion: 375 mg/m^2 on the day prior to fludarabine/cyclophosphamide in cycle 1, then 500 mg/m^2 on day 1 (every 28 days) of cycles 2-6

Granulomatosis with polyangiitis (GPA; Wegener's granulomatosis): I.V. infusion: 375 mg/m^2 once weekly for 4 doses (in combination with methylprednisolone I.V. for 1-3 days followed by daily prednisone)

Non-Hodgkin lymphoma (NHL; relapsed/refractory, low-grade or follicular CD20-positive, B-cell): I.V. infusion: 375 mg/m^2 once weekly for 4 or 8 doses

Retreatment following disease progression: 375 mg/m^2 once weekly for 4 doses

NHL (diffuse large B-cell): I.V. infusion: 375 mg/m^2 given on day 1 of each chemotherapy cycle for up to 8 doses

NHL (follicular, CD20-positive, B-cell, previously untreated): I.V. infusion: 375 mg/m^2 given on day 1 of each chemotherapy cycle for up to 8 doses

Maintenance therapy (as a single agent, in patients with partial or complete response to rituximab plus chemotherapy; begin 8 weeks after completion of combination chemotherapy): I.V. infusion: 375 mg/m^2 every 8 weeks for 12 doses

NHL (nonprogressing, low-grade, CD20-positive, B-cell, after 6-8 cycles of first line CVP are completed): I.V. infusion: 375 mg/m^2 once weekly for 4 doses every 6 months for a maximum of 16 doses

NHL: Combination therapy with ibritumomab: I.V. infusion: 250 mg/m^2 I.V. day 1; repeat in 7-9 days with ibritumomab (also see Ibritumomab monograph)

Canadian labeling: **NHL, low grade or follicular:** I.V. infusion:
Initial: 375 mg/m^2 once weekly for 4 doses (as a single agent) **or** 375 mg/m^2 on day 1 of each 21-day cycle for 8 cycles (in combination with CVP chemotherapy)
Maintenance (responding to induction therapy): 375 mg/m^2 every 3 months until disease progression or up to a maximum of 2 years

Rheumatoid arthritis: I.V. infusion: 1000 mg on days 1 and 15 in combination with methotrexate; subsequent courses may be administered every 24 weeks (based on clinical evaluation), if necessary may be repeated no sooner than every 16 weeks

Microscopic polyangiitis (MPA): I.V. infusion: 375 mg/m^2 once weekly for 4 doses (in combination with methylprednisolone I.V. for 1-3 days followed by daily prednisone)

Chronic graft-versus-host disease (GVHD), refractory (unlabeled use): I.V. infusion: 375 mg/m^2 once weekly for 4 doses (Cutler, 2006)

Chronic immune thrombocytopenic purpura (ITP; unlabeled use): I.V. infusion: 375 mg/m^2 once weekly for 4 doses (Arnold, 2007; Godeau, 2008)

Hodgkin's lymphoma (unlabeled use): I.V. infusion: 375 mg/m^2 once weekly for 4 weeks (Ekstrand, 2003; Schulz, 2008)

Idiopathic membranous nephropathy (IMN), resistant (unlabeled use): I.V. infusion: 375 mg/m^2 once weekly for 4 doses with retreatment at 6 months (Fervenza, 2010) **or** 1000 mg on days 1 and 15 (Fervenza, 2008) **or** 375 mg/m^2 single doses titrated to B cell response (Cravedi, 2007)

Lupus nephritis, refractory (unlabeled use): I.V. infusion: 375 mg/m^2 once weekly for 4 doses (Melander, 2009) **or** 500-1000 mg on days 1 and 15 (Vigna-Perez, 2006)

Pemphigus vulgaris, refractory (unlabeled use): I.V. infusion: 375 mg/m^2 once weekly of weeks 1, 2, and 3 of a 4-week cycle, repeat for 1 additional cycle, then 1 dose per month for 4 months (total of 10 doses in 6 months) (Ahmed, 2006)

Post-transplant lymphoproliferative disorder (unlabeled use): I.V. infusion: 375 mg/m^2 once weekly for 4 doses (Choquet, 2006)

Thrombotic thrombocytopenic purpura (TTP), relapsed/refractory (unlabeled use): I.V. infusion: 375 mg/m^2 once weekly for 4 doses (Scully, 2007; Scully, 2011)

Waldenström's macroglobulinemia (unlabeled use): I.V. infusion: 375 mg/m^2 once weekly for 4 weeks (Dimopoulos, 2002)

Pediatric Note: Pretreatment with acetaminophen and an antihistamine is recommended.

Autoimmune hemolytic anemia (AIHA; unlabeled use): I.V. infusion: 375 mg/m^2 once weekly for 2-4 doses (Zecca, 2003)

Chronic immune thrombocytopenic purpura (ITP; unlabeled use): I.V. infusion: 375 mg/m^2 once weekly for 4 doses (Parodi, 2009; Wang, 2005)

Nephrotic syndrome, severe, refractory (unlabeled use): I.V. infusion: 375 mg/m^2 once weekly for 1-4 doses has been used in small case series, case reports, and retrospective analyses, including reports of successful remission induction of severe or refractory nephrotic syndromes that are poorly responsive to standard therapies (Dello Strologo, 2009; Fujinaga, 2010; Guigonis, 2008; Prytula, 2010)

Combination Regimens

Leukemia, chronic lymphocytic:

Cyclophosphamide-Fludarabine-Alemtuzumab-Rituximab (CLL) on page 1601
Fludarabine-Cyclophosphamide-Rituximab (CLL) on page 1648
Fludarabine-Rituximab (CLL) on page 1651
OFAR (CLL) on page 1722
PCR on page 1735

Lymphoma, non-Hodgkin's:

Bendamustine-Rituximab on page 1525
EPOCH (Dose-Adjusted)-Rituximab (NHL) on page 1629
EPOCH-Rituximab (NHL) on page 1631
Fludarabine-Cyclophosphamide-Mitoxantrone-Rituximab on page 1647
Fludarabine-Cyclophosphamide-Rituximab (NHL-Follicular) on page 1649
Fludarabine-Mitoxantrone-Dexamethasone-Rituximab on page 1650
Fludarabine-Mitoxantrone-Rituximab on page 1651
Fludarabine-Rituximab (NHL-Follicular) on page 1651
Gemcitabine-Oxaliplatin-Rituximab (NHL) on page 1674
R-CVP on page 1745
RICE on page 1747
Rituximab-CHOP (NHL) on page 1748

Lymphoma, non-Hodgkin's (Mantle cell):

Bendamustine-Rituximab on page 1525
Hyper-CVAD + Rituximab on page 1688

Primary CNS Lymphoma: Temozolomide-Rituximab (CNS Lymphoma) on page 1754

Waldenstrom's Macroglobulinemia:

Bortezomib-Dexamethasone-Rituximab (Waldenstrom's Macroglobulinemia) on page 1535
Bortezomib-Rituximab (Waldenstrom's Macroglobulinemia) on page 1537

Administration Do **not** administer I.V. push or bolus. If a reaction occurs, slow or stop the infusion. If the reaction abates, restart infusion at 50% of the previous rate. Discontinue infusion in the event of serious or life-threatening cardiac arrhythmias.

I.V.: Initial infusion: Start rate of 50 mg/hour; if there is no reaction, increase the rate by 50 mg/hour increments every 30 minutes, to a maximum rate of 400 mg/hour.

Subsequent infusions:

Standard infusion rate: If patient tolerated initial infusion, start at 100 mg/hour; If there is no reaction, increase the rate by 100 mg/hour increments every 30 minutes, to a maximum rate of 400 mg/hour.

Accelerated infusion rate (90 minutes): For patients with previously untreated follicular NHL and diffuse large B-cell NHL who are receiving a corticosteroid as part of their combination chemotherapy regimen, have a circulating lymphocyte count <5000/mm^3, or have no significant cardiovascular disease. After tolerance has been established (no grade 3 or 4 infusion-related event) at the recommended infusion rate in cycle 1, a rapid infusion rate may be used beginning with cycle 2. The daily corticosteroid, acetaminophen, and diphenhydramine are administered prior to treatment, then the rituximab dose is administered over 90 minutes, with 20% of the dose administered over the first 30 minutes and the remaining 80% is given over 60 minutes (Sehn, 2007). If the 90-minute infusion in cycle 2 is tolerated, the same rate may be used for the remainder of the treatment regimen (through cycles 6 or 8).

Emetic Potential Very low (<10%)

Monitoring Parameters CBC with differential and platelets (obtain at weekly to monthly intervals and more frequently in patients with cytopenias, or at 2-4 month intervals in rheumatoid arthritis patients, GPA and MPA), peripheral CD20^{+} cells; HAMA/HACA titers (high levels may increase the risk of allergic reactions); renal function, fluid balance; vital signs; monitor for infusion reactions, cardiac monitoring during and after infusion in rheumatoid arthritis patients and in patients with pre-existing cardiac disease or if arrhythmias develop during or after subsequent infusions

Consider screening for hepatitis B in high-risk patients prior to initiation of rituximab therapy. The NCCN NHL guidelines v.3.2012 recommend screening **all** NHL patients prior to therapy. The ASCO provisional opinion states that screening may be considered in patients receiving rituximab, but such screening and/or treatment of hepatitis B should not delay initiation of therapy (Artz, 2010). In addition, carriers and patients with evidence of recovery from prior hepatitis B infection should be monitored closely for clinical and laboratory signs of HBV infection during therapy and for up to a year following completion of treatment. High-risk patients should be screened for hepatitis C (per NCCN NHL guidelines v.3.2012).

Complaints of abdominal pain, especially early in the course of treatment, should prompt a thorough diagnostic evaluation and appropriate treatment. Signs or symptoms of progressive multifocal leukoencephalopathy (focal neurologic deficits, which may present as hemiparesis, visual field deficits, cognitive impairment, aphasia, ataxia, and/or cranial nerve deficits). If PML is suspected, obtain brain MRI scan and lumbar puncture.

Medication Guide Available Yes

Dosage Forms Excipient information presented when available (limited, particularly for generics); consult specific product labeling.

Injection, solution [preservative free]:

Rituxan®: 10 mg/mL (10 mL, 50 mL) [contains polysorbate 80]

References

Ahmed AR, Spigelman Z, Cavacini LA, et al, "Treatment of Pemphigus Vulgaris With Rituximab and Intravenous Immune Globulin," *N Engl J Med*, 2006, 355(17):1772-9.

Arnold DM, Dentali F, Crowther MA, et al, "Systematic Review: Efficacy and Safety of Rituximab for Adults With Idiopathic Thrombocytopenic Purpura," *Ann Intern Med*, 2007, 146(1):25-33.

Carson KR, Evens AM, Richey EA, et al, "Progressive Multifocal Leukoencephalopathy After Rituximab Therapy in HIV-Negative Patients: A Report of 57 Cases From the Research on Adverse Drug Events and Reports Project," *Blood*, 2009, 113(20):4834-40.

Chakravarty EF, Murray ER, Kelman A, et al, "Pregnancy Outcomes Following Maternal Exposure to Rituximab," *Blood*, 2011, 117(5):1499-506.

Choquet S, Leblond V, Herbrecht R, et al, "Efficacy and Safety of Rituximab in B-Cell Post-Transplantation Lymphoproliferative Disorders: Results of a Prospective Multicenter Phase 2 Study," *Blood*, 2006, 107(8):3053-7.

Coiffier B, Haioun C, Ketterer N, et al, "Rituximab (Anti-CD20 Monoclonal Antibody) for the Treatment of Patients With Relapsing or Refractory Aggressive Lymphoma: A Multicenter Phase II Study," *Blood*, 1998, 92(6):1927-32.

Coiffier B, Lepage E, Briere J, "CHOP Chemotherapy Plus Rituximab Compared With CHOP Alone in Elderly Patients With Diffuse Large-B-Cell Lymphoma," *N Engl J Med*, 2002, 346(4):235-42.

Cutler C, Miklos D, Kim HT, et al, "Rituximab for Steroid-Refractory Chronic Graft-Versus-Host Disease," *Blood*, 2006, 108(2):756-62.

Dimopoulos MA, Kyle RA, Anagnostopoulos A, et al, "Diagnosis and Management of Waldenstrom's Macroglobulinemia," *J Clin Oncol*, 2005, 23(7):1564-77.

Dimopoulos MA, Zervas C, Zomas A, et al, "Treatment of Waldenstrom's Macroglobulinemia With Rituximab," *J Clin Oncol*, 2002, 20(9):2327-33.

Edwards JC, Szczepanski L, Szechinski J, et al, "Efficacy of B-Cell-Targeted Therapy With Rituximab in Patients With Rheumatoid Arthritis," *N Engl J Med*, 2004, 350(25):2572-81.

Ekstrand BC, Lucas JB, Horwitz SM, et al, "Rituximab in Lymphocyte-Predominant Hodgkin Disease: Results of a Phase 2 Trial," *Blood*, 101(11):4285-9.

Garcia-Suarez J, de Miguel D, Krsnik I, et al, "Changes in the Natural History of Progressive Multifocal Leukoencephalopathy in HIV-Negative Lymphoproliferative Disorders: Impact of Novel Therapies," *Am J Hematol*, 2005, 80(4):271-81.

Gisselbrecht C, Glass B, Mounier N, et al, "Salvage Regimens With Autologous Transplantation for Relapsed Large B-Cell Lymphoma in the Rituximab Era," *J Clin Oncol*, 2010, 28(27):4184-90.

Godeau B, Porcher R, Fain O, et al, "Rituximab Efficacy and Safety in Adult Splenectomy Candidates With Chronic Immune Thrombocytopenic Purpura: Results of a Prospective Multicenter Phase 2 Study," *Blood*, 2008, 112(4):999-1004.

Higashida J, Wun T, Schmidt S, et al, "Safety and Efficacy of Rituximab in Patients With Rheumatoid Arthritis Refractory to Disease Modifying Antirheumatic Drugs and Anti-Tumor Necrosis Factor-Alpha Treatment," *J Rheumatol*, 2005, 32(11):2109-15.

Jones RB, Tervaert JW, Hauser T, et al, "Rituximab Versus Cyclophosphamide in ANCA-Associated Renal Vasculitis," *N Engl J Med*, 2010, 363(3):211-20.

Keating MJ, O'Brien S, Albitar M, et al, "Early Results of a Chemoimmunotherapy Regimen of Fludarabine, Cyclophosphamide, and Rituximab as Initial Therapy for Chronic Lymphocytic Leukemia," *J Clin Oncol*, 2005, 23(18):4079-88.

Kim SJ, Lee JW, Jung CW, et al, "Weekly Rituximab Followed by Monthly Rituximab Treatment for Steroid-Refractory Chronic Graft-Versus-Host Disease: Results From a Prospective, Multicenter, Phase II Study," *Haematologica*, 2010, 95(11):1935-42.

Marcus R, Imrie K, Belch A, et al, "CVP Chemotherapy Plus Rituximab Compared With CVP as First-Line Treatment for Advanced Follicular Lymphoma," *Blood*, 2005, 105(4):1417-23.

Moore J, Ma D, Will R, et al, "A phase II Study of Rituximab in Rheumatoid Arthritis Patients With Recurrent Disease Following Haematopoietic Stem Cell Transplantation," *Bone Marrow Transplant*, 2004, 34(3):241-7

National Comprehensive Cancer Network® (NCCN), "Clinical Practice Guidelines in Oncology™: Central Nervous System Cancers," Version 2.2011. Available at http://www.nccn.org/professionals/physician_gls/PDF/cns.pdf

National Comprehensive Cancer Network® (NCCN), "Clinical Practice Guidelines in Oncology™: Non-Hodgkin's Lymphomas," Version 1.2011. Available at http://www.nccn.org/professionals/physician_gls/PDF/nhl.pdf

Parodi E, Rivetti E, Amendola G, et al, "Long-Term Follow-Up Analysis After Rituximab Therapy in Children With Refractory Symptomatic ITP: Identification of Factors Predictive of a Sustained Response," *Br J Haematol*, 2009, 144(4):552-8.

Provan D, Stasi R, Newland AC, et al, "International Consensus Report on the Investigation and Management of Primary Immune Thrombocytopenia," *Blood*, 2010, 115(2):168-86.

Rubbert-Roth A, Tak PP, Zerbini C, et al, "Efficacy and Safety of Various Repeat Treatment Dosing Regimens of Rituximab in Patients With Active Rheumatoid Arthritis: Results of a Phase III Randomized Study (MIRROR)," *Rheumatology (Oxford)*, 2010, 49(9):1683-93.

Saag KG, Teng GG, Patkar NM, et al, "American College of Rheumatology 2008 Recommendations for the Use of Nonbiologic and Biologic Disease-Modifying Antirheumatic Drugs in Rheumatoid Arthritis," Arthritis Rheum, 2008, 59(6):762-84.

Schulz H, Rehwald U, Morschhauser F, et al, "Rituximab in Relapsed Lymphocyte-Predominant Hodgkin Lymphoma: Long-Term Results of a Phase 2 Trial by the German Hodgkin Lymphoma Study Group (GHSG)," *Blood*, 2008, 111(1):109-11.

Sehn LH, Donaldson J, Filewich A, et al, "Rapid Infusion Rituximab in Combination With Corticosteroid-Containing Chemotherapy or as Maintenance Therapy Is Well Tolerated and Can Safely be Delivered in the Community Setting," *Blood*, 2007, 109(10):4171-3.

Stone JH, Merkel PA, Spiera R, et al, "Rituximab Versus Cyclophosphamide for ANCA-Associated Vasculitis," *N Engl J Med*, 2010, 363(3):221-32.

Tak PP, Rigby WF, Rubbert-Roth A, et al, "Inhibition of Joint Damage and Improved Clinical Outcomes With Rituximab Plus Methotrexate in Early Active Rheumatoid Arthritis: The IMAGE Trial," *Ann Rheum Dis*, 2011, 70(1):39-46.

Tam CS, O'Brien S, Wierda W, et al, "Long-Term Results of the Fludarabine, Cyclophosphamide, and Rituximab Regimen as Initial Therapy of Chronic Lymphocytic Leukemia," *Blood*, 2008, 112 (4):975-80.

Wang J, Wiley JM, Luddy R, et al, "Chronic Immune Thrombocytopenic Purpura in Children: Assessment of Rituximab Treatment," *J Pediatr*, 2005, 146(2):217-21.

Zaja F, Vianelli N, Volpetti S, et al, "Low-Dose Rituximab in Adult Patients With Primary Immune Thrombocytopenia," *Eur J Haematol*, 2010, 85(4):329-34.

Zecca M, Nobili B, Ramenghi U, et al, "Rituximab In the Treatment of Refractory Autoimmune Hemolytic Anemia in Children," *Blood*, 2003, 101(10): 3857-61.

- ◆ **Riva-Anastrozole (Can)** *see* Anastrozole *on page 96*
- ◆ **Riva-Ciprofloxacin (Can)** *see* Ciprofloxacin (Systemic) *on page 283*
- ◆ **Riva-Fluconazole (Can)** *see* Fluconazole *on page 612*
- ◆ **Riva-Hydroxyzine (Can)** *see* HydrOXYzine *on page 736*
- ◆ **Riva-Olanzapine (Can)** *see* OLANZapine *on page 1056*
- ◆ **Riva-Olanzapine ODT (Can)** *see* OLANZapine *on page 1056*
- ◆ **Riva-Valacyclovir (Can)** *see* Valacyclovir *on page 1420*
- ◆ **rLFN-α2** *see* Interferon Alfa-2b *on page 798*
- ◆ **Ro 5488** *see* Tretinoin (Systemic) *on page 1405*
- ◆ **RO5185426** *see* Vemurafenib *on page 1440*
- ◆ **Rocaltrol®** *see* Calcitriol *on page 215*
- ◆ **Rocephin®** *see* CefTRIAXone *on page 258*

RomiDEPsin (roe mi DEP sin)

Related Information

Management of Chemotherapy-Induced Nausea and Vomiting *on page 1786*

Principles of Anticancer Therapy *on page 1878*

Brand Names: U.S. Istodax®

Index Terms Depsipeptide; FK228; FR901228

Generic Availability (U.S.) No

Pharmacologic Category Antineoplastic Agent, Histone Deacetylase Inhibitor

Use Treatment of refractory cutaneous T-cell lymphoma (CTCL) and refractory peripheral T-cell lymphoma (PTCL)

Labeled Contraindications There are no contraindications listed within the manufacturer's labeling.

Pregnancy Risk Factor D

Lactation Excretion in breast milk unknown/not recommended

Warnings/Precautions Hazardous agent - use appropriate precautions for handling and disposal. Anemia, leukopenia, neutropenia, lymphopenia and thrombocytopenia may occur; may require dosage modification; monitor blood counts during treatment. Serious infections (occasionally fatal), including pneumonia and sepsis have occurred during or within 30 days of treatment; the risk of life-threatening infection is increased in patients who have received prior intensive or extensive chemotherapy. QT_C prolongation has been observed; use caution in patients with a history of QT_C prolongation, congenital long QT syndrome, with medications known to prolong the QT interval, or with pre-existing cardiac disease. Obtain baseline and periodic ECG (12-lead); monitor and correct electrolyte (potassium, magnesium, and calcium) abnormalities prior to and during treatment. T-wave and ST-segment changes have also been reported. Use with caution in patients with moderate-to-severe hepatic impairment or end-stage renal disease. Avoid use with strong CYP3A4 inhibitors or inducers. Use with caution with moderate CYP3A4 inhibitors and P-glycoprotein inhibitors. Tumor lysis syndrome (TLS) has been observed; closely monitor patients with advanced disease and/or with a high tumor burden; if TLS occurs, initiate appropriate treatment.

Adverse Reactions

>10%:

Cardiovascular: ST-T wave changes (2% to 63%), hypotension (7% to 23%)

Central nervous system: Fatigue (53% to 77%), fever (20% to 47%), headache (15% to 34%), chills (11% to 17%)

Dermatologic: Pruritus (7% to 31%), dermatitis/exfoliative dermatitis (4% to 27%)

Endocrine & metabolic: Hypocalcemia (4% to 52%), hyperglycemia (2% to 51%), hypoalbuminemia (3% to 48%), hyperuricemia (≤33%), hypomagnesemia (22% to 28%), hypermagnesemia (≤27%), hypophosphatemia (≤27%), hypokalemia (6% to 20%), hyponatremia (≤20%)

Gastrointestinal: Nausea (56% to 86%; grades 3/4: 2% to 6%), anorexia (23% to 54%), vomiting (34% to 52%; grades 3/4: ≤10%), taste alteration (15% to 40%), constipation (12% to 40%), diarrhea (20% to 36%), weight loss (10% to 15%), abdominal pain (13% to 14%)

Hematologic: Anemia (19% to 72%; grades 3/4: 3% to 28%), thrombocytopenia (17% to 72%; grades 3/4: ≤36%), neutropenia (11% to 66%; grades 3/4: 4% to 47%), lymphopenia (4% to 57%; grades 3/4: ≤37%), leukopenia (4% to 55%; grades 3/4: ≤45%)

Hepatic: AST increased (3% to 28%), ALT increased (3% to 22%)

Neuromuscular & skeletal: Weakness (53% to 77%)

Respiratory: Cough (18% to 21%), dyspnea (13% to 21%)

Miscellaneous: Infection (46% to 54%; grades 3/4: 11% to 33%)

1% to 10%:

Cardiovascular: Peripheral edema (6% to 10%), tachycardia (≤10%), chest pain, DVT, edema, QT prolongation, supraventricular arrhythmia, syncope, ventricular arrhythmia

Dermatologic: Cellulitis

Endocrine & metabolic: Dehydration

Gastrointestinal: Stomatitis (6% to 10%)

Hematologic: Neutropenic fever

Hepatic: Hyperbilirubinemia

Respiratory: Hypoxia, pneumonia, pneumonitis, pulmonary embolism

Miscellaneous: Central line infection, hypersensitivity, sepsis, tumor lysis syndrome (1% to 2%)

<1%, postmarketing, and/or case reports: Acute renal failure, acute respiratory distress syndrome, atrial fibrillation, bacteremia, candida infection, cardiopulmonary failure, cardiogenic shock, Epstein Barr virus reactivation, multiorgan failure, myocardial ischemia, septic shock

Drug Interactions

Metabolism/Transport Effects Substrate of CYP3A4 (major), P-glycoprotein; **Note:** Assignment of Major/Minor substrate status based on clinically relevant drug interaction potential

Avoid Concomitant Use

Avoid concomitant use of RomiDEPsin with any of the following: CYP3A4 Inducers (Strong); CYP3A4 Inhibitors (Strong); Highest Risk QTc-Prolonging Agents; Mifepristone

Increased Effect/Toxicity

RomiDEPsin may increase the levels/effects of: Highest Risk QTc-Prolonging Agents; Moderate Risk QTc-Prolonging Agents; Warfarin

The levels/effects of RomiDEPsin may be increased by: CYP3A4 Inhibitors (Moderate); CYP3A4 Inhibitors (Strong); Dasatinib; Ivacaftor; Mifepristone; P-glycoprotein/ABCB1 Inhibitors; QTc-Prolonging Agents (Indeterminate Risk and Risk Modifying)

Decreased Effect

The levels/effects of RomiDEPsin may be decreased by: CYP3A4 Inducers (Strong); Deferasirox; Herbs (CYP3A4 Inducers); P-glycoprotein/ABCB1 Inducers; Tocilizumab

Ethanol/Nutrition/Herb Interactions

Food: Avoid grapefruit juice (may increase the levels/effects of romidepsin).

Herb/Nutraceutical: Avoid St John's wort (may increase metabolism and decrease romidepsin concentrations).

Storage/Stability Store intact vials at room temperature of 20°C to 25°C (68°F to 77°F); excursions permitted between 15°C and 30°C (59°F and 86°F). The reconstituted solution is stable for 8 hours at room temperature. Solutions diluted for infusion are stable for 24 hours at room temperature; however, the manufacturer recommends use as soon as possible after dilution.

Reconstitution Use appropriate precautions for handling and disposal. Reconstitute each 10 mg vial with 2 mL of supplied diluent to a reconstituted concentration of 5 mg/mL; swirl until dissolved. (**Note:** Although the reconstituted vial contains a final volume of 2 mL, due to the viscosity of the reconstituted solution, a total volume <2 mL [usually ~1.6-1.8 mL] can be withdrawn from each vial.) Further dilute in 500 mL normal saline; compatible with polyvinyl chloride (PVC), ethylene vinyl acetate (EVA), polyethylene (PE) and glass infusion containers.

Mechanism of Action Histone deacetylase inhibitor; catalyzes acetyl group removal from protein lysine residues (including histone and transcription factors). Inhibition of histone deacetylase results in accumulation of acetyl groups, leading to alterations in chromatin structure and transcription factor activation causing termination of cell growth (induces arrest in cell cycle at G_1 and G_2/M phases) leading to cell death.

Pharmacodynamics/Kinetics

Protein binding: 92% to 94%; primarily to α_1-acid glycoprotein

Metabolism: Hepatic, primarily via CYP3A4, minor metabolism from CYP3A5, 1A1, 2B6, and 2C19

Half-life elimination: ~3 hours

Dosing

Adult & Geriatric

Cutaneous T-cell lymphoma: I.V.: 14 mg/m^2 days 1, 8, and 15 of a 28-day treatment cycle; repeat cycle as long as benefit continues and treatment is tolerated.

Peripheral T-cell lymphoma: I.V.: 14 mg/m^2 days 1, 8, and 15 of a 28-day treatment cycle; repeat cycle as long as benefit continues and treatment is tolerated.

Renal Impairment The pharmacokinetics of romidepsin are unaffected by mild, moderate, or severe renal impairment (based on pharmacokinetic analysis). Use with caution in patients with end-stage renal disease (has not been studied).

Hepatic Impairment Mild hepatic impairment does not significantly influence the pharmacokinetics of romidepsin. The effect of moderate or severe impairment is unknown; use with caution.

Adjustment for Toxicity

Nonhematologic toxicity (excluding alopecia):

Grade 2 or 3: Delay treatment until toxicity returns to ≤grade 1 or baseline, may restart at 14 mg/m^2

Grade 4 or recurrent grade 3 toxicity: Delay treatment until toxicity returns to ≤grade 1 or baseline, permanently reduce dose to 10 mg/m^2

Recurrent grade 3 or 4 toxicity despite dosage reduction: Discontinue treatment

Hematologic toxicity:

Grade 3 or 4 neutropenia or thrombocytopenia: Delay treatment until ANC ≥1500/mm^3 and/or platelets ≥75,000/mm^3 or baseline, may restart at 14 mg/m^2

Grade 4 febrile neutropenia or thrombocytopenia requiring platelet transfusion: Delay treatment until toxicity returns to ≤grade 1 or baseline, permanently reduce dose to 10 mg/m^2

Administration Infuse over 4 hours. Antiemetics to prevent nausea and vomiting were used in clinical trials (Piekarz, 2009; Piekarz, 2011).

Emetic Potential Low (10% to 30%)

Monitoring Parameters Serum electrolytes (baseline and periodic; especially potassium and magnesium); CBC with differential and platelets, ECG (baseline and periodic; in patients with significant cardiovascular disease, congenital long QT syndrome, and in patients taking QT-prolonging medications); signs/symptoms of infection or tumor lysis syndrome

Dietary Considerations Avoid grapefruit juice.

Dosage Forms Excipient information presented when available (limited, particularly for generics); consult specific product labeling.

Injection, powder for reconstitution:

Istodax®: 10 mg [contains dehydrated ethanol (in diluent), propylene glycol (in diluent); supplied with diluent]

References

Coiffier B, Pro B, Prince HM, et al, "Final Results From a Pivotal, Multicenter, International, Open-Label, Phase 2 Study of Romidepsin in Progressive or Relapsed Peripheral T-Cell Lymphoma (PTCL) Following Prior Systemic Therapy," *Blood*, 2010, 116(21):114 [abstract 114 from 2010 ASH Annual Meeting].

Piekarz RL, Frye AR, Wright JJ, et al, "Cardiac Studies in Patients Treated With Depsipeptide, FK228, in a Phase II Trial for T-Cell Lymphoma," *Clin Cancer Res*, 2006, 12(12):3762-73.

Piekarz RL, Frye R, Prince HM, et al, "Phase 2 Trial of Romidepsin in Patients With Peripheral T-Cell Lymphoma," *Blood*, 2011, 117(22):5827-34.

Piekarz RL, Frye R, Turner M, et al, "Phase II Multi-Institutional Trial of the Histone Deacetylase Inhibitor Romidepsin as Monotherapy for Patients With Cutaneous T-Cell Lymphoma," *J Clin Oncol*, 2009, 27(32):5410-7.

Piekarz R, Wright J, Frye R, et al, "Results of a Phase 2 NCI Multicenter Study of Romidepsin in Patients With Relapsed Peripheral T-Cell Lymphoma (PTCL)," *Blood*, 2008, 112(11):1567 [abstract 1567 from 2008 ASH Annual Meeting].

RomiPLOStim (roe mi PLOE stim)

Brand Names: U.S. Nplate®

Brand Names: Canada Nplate®

Index Terms AMG 531

Generic Availability (U.S.) No

Pharmacologic Category Colony Stimulating Factor; Thrombopoietic Agent

Use Treatment of thrombocytopenia in patients with chronic immune (idiopathic) thrombocytopenia purpura (ITP) who have had insufficient response to corticosteroids, immune globulin, or splenectomy

Note: Should be used only when the degree of thrombocytopenia and clinical condition increase the risk for bleeding; should not be used in attempt to normalize platelet counts; **not** indicated for the treatment of thrombocytopenia due to myelodysplastic syndrome.

Labeled Contraindications There are no contraindications listed within the manufacturer's labeling.

Pregnancy Risk Factor C

Lactation Excretion in breast milk unknown/ not recommended.

Warnings/Precautions May increase the risk for bone marrow reticulin formation or progression. In patients where reticulin formation occurred, doses were ≥5 mcg/kg. A baseline peripheral blood smear is recommended prior to treatment to establish baseline level of cellular morphologic abnormalities, then monthly (after stable dose achieved) for new or worsening abnormalities (teardrop or nucleated RBC, immature WBCs) or cytopenias. Progression to marrow fibrosis with cytopenias was not observed in clinical trials, although the risk has not been excluded. Onset of new or worsening cellular abnormalities or cytopenias may warrant therapy discontinuation and subsequent bone marrow biopsy. Thromboembolism or thrombotic complications may occur with increased platelets; maintain appropriate platelet levels with dosage adjustments; portal vein thrombosis has been reported in patients with chronic liver disease; use with caution in patients with a history of cerebrovascular disease. Progression of underlying myelodysplastic syndrome (MDS) to acute myeloid leukemia (AML) has been observed in MDS clinical trials (not indicated for the treatment of thrombocytopenia due to MDS). An increase in the percentage of circulating myeloblasts in peripheral blood smears was also noted (both in patients who progressed to AML and in those who did not); blast cells decreased to baseline after discontinuation in some patients.

Inadequate platelet response may be due to neutralizing antibodies (to romiplostim or TPO) or bone marrow fibrosis. Indicated only when the degree of thrombocytopenia and clinical conditions increase the risk for bleeding; use the lowest dose necessary to achieve and maintain platelet count ≥50,000/mm^3. Do not use to normalize platelet counts. Discontinue if platelet count does not respond to a level to avoid clinically important bleeding after 4 weeks at the maximum recommended dose. May be used in combination with other therapies for ITP, including corticosteroids, danazol, azathioprine, immune globulin, or Rho(D) immune globulin. Reduce dose or discontinue ITP medications when platelet count ≥50,000/mm^3.

Upon discontinuation of therapy, thrombocytopenia may worsen. Severity may be greater than pretreatment level. Risk of bleeding is increased, particularly in patients receiving anticoagulants or antiplatelet agents; monitor closely. Rebound thrombocytopenia generally resolves within 14 days.

Use with caution in patients with hepatic and renal impairment (has not been studied).

Adverse Reactions

>10%:

Central nervous system: Headache (35%), dizziness (17%), insomnia (16%)
Gastrointestinal: Abdominal pain (11%)
Hematologic: Circulating myeloblasts increased (MDS patients: 17%)
Neuromuscular & skeletal: Arthralgia (26%), myalgia (14%), limb pain (13%)

1% to 10%:

Gastrointestinal: Dyspepsia (7%)

Hematologic: Rebound thrombocytopenia (7%), AML (MDS patients: 4% to 6%), bone marrow reticulin formation/deposition (4%)
Neuromuscular & skeletal: Shoulder pain (8%), paresthesia (6%)
Miscellaneous: Antibody formation (romiplostim 6%; TPO 4%)

<1%, postmarketing, and/or case reports: Angioedema, erythromelalgia, hypersensitivity, marrow fibrosis with collagen, thromboembolism, thrombotic complications

Drug Interactions

Metabolism/Transport Effects None known.

Avoid Concomitant Use There are no known interactions where it is recommended to avoid concomitant use.

Increased Effect/Toxicity There are no known significant interactions involving an increase in effect.

Decreased Effect There are no known significant interactions involving a decrease in effect.

Storage/Stability Store intact vials refrigerated at 2°C to 8°C (36°F to 46°F); do not freeze. Protect from light. Store in original carton until use. Reconstituted solution may be stored at room temperature of 25°C (77°F) or refrigerated at 2°C to 8°C (36°F to 46°F) for up to 24 hours prior to administration. Protect reconstituted solution from light; discard any unused portion.

Reconstitution Reconstitute with preservative free SWFI (add 0.72 mL to 250 mcg vial or 1.2 mL to 500 mcg vial) to a final concentration of 500 mcg/mL. Gently invert vial and swirl; do not shake. Usually dissolves within 2 minutes.

Mechanism of Action Thrombopoietin (TPO) peptide mimetic which increases platelet counts in ITP by binding to and activating the human TPO receptor.

Pharmacodynamics/Kinetics

Onset of action: Platelet count increase: SubQ: 4-9 days; Peak platelet count increase: Days 12-16
Duration: Platelet counts return to baseline by day 28
Absorption: SubQ: Slow
Half-life elimination: Median: 3.5 days (range: 1-34 days)
Time to peak, plasma: SubQ: Median: 14 hours (range: 7-50 hours)

Dosing

Adult & Geriatric Note: Initial dose is based on actual body weight. Use the lowest dose sufficient to maintain platelet count ≥50,000/mm^3 as necessary to reduce the risk of bleeding. Discontinue if platelet count does not respond to a level that avoids clinically important bleeding after 4 weeks at the maximum recommended dose.

Chronic immune thrombocytopenic purpura (ITP): SubQ: Initial: 1 mcg/kg once weekly; adjust dose by 1 mcg/kg/week to achieve platelet count ≥50,000/mm^3 and to reduce the risk of bleeding; Maximum: 10 mcg/kg/week (median dose needed to achieve response in clinical trials: 2 mcg/kg)

Dosage adjustment recommendations:

Platelet count <50,000/mm^3: Increase dose by 1 mcg/kg
Platelet count >200,000/mm^3 for 2 consecutive weeks: Reduce dose by 1 mcg/kg
Platelet count >400,000/mm^3: Withhold dose; assess platelet count weekly; when platelet count <200,000/mm^3, resume with the dose reduced by 1 mcg/kg

Renal Impairment No dosage adjustment provided in manufacturer's labeling (has not been studied).

Hepatic Impairment No dosage adjustment provided in manufacturer's labeling (has not been studied).

Administration Administer SubQ. Administration volume may be small; use appropriate syringe (with graduations to 0.01 mL) for administration.

Monitoring Parameters CBC with differential and platelets (baseline, during treatment [weekly until platelet response stable for at least 4 weeks then monthly] and weekly for at least 2 weeks following completion of treatment)

Evaluate for neutralizing antibodies in patients with inadequate response (blood samples may be submitted to Amgen for assay [1-800-772-6436]).

Dietary Considerations Some products may contain sucrose.

Additional Information Restricted access to Nplate® was previously a REMS requirement via the Nplate® NEXUS (Network of Experts Understanding and Supporting Nplate® and Patients) program. Patients, prescribers, and pharmacies were required to be enrolled in this program. However, the FDA eliminated this REMS requirement in December 2011. There is currently no restricted access to obtaining Nplate®.

Medication Guide Available Yes

Dosage Forms Excipient information presented when available (limited, particularly for generics); consult specific product labeling.

Injection, powder for reconstitution:

Nplate®: 250 mcg [contains sucrose 15 mg/vial]

Nplate®: 500 mcg [contains sucrose 25 mg/vial]

References

Bussel JB, Kuter DJ, George JN, et al, "AMG 531, a Thrombopoiesis-Stimulating Protein, for Chronic ITP," *N Engl J Med*, 2006, 355(16):1672-81.

Bussel JB, Kuter DJ, Pullarkat V, et al, "Safety and Efficacy of Long-Term Treatment With Romiplostim in Thrombocytopenic Patients With Chronic ITP," *Blood*, 2009, 113(10):2161-71.

Kuter DJ, "New Thrombopoietic Growth Factors," *Blood*, 2007, 109(11):4607-16.

Kuter DJ, Bussel JB, Lyons RM, et al, "Efficacy of Romiplostim in Patients With Chronic Immune Thrombocytopenic Purpura: A Double-Blind Randomised Controlled Trial," *Lancet*, 2008, 371 (9610):395-403.

Kuter DJ, Mufti GJ, Bain BJ, et al, "Evaluation of Bone Marrow Reticulin Formation in Chronic Immune Thrombocytopenia Patients Treated With Romiplostim," *Blood*, 2009, 114(18):3748-56.

Kuter DJ, Rummel M, Boccia R, et al, "Romiplostim or Standard of Care in Patients With Immune Thrombocytopenia," *N Engl J Med*, 2010, 363(20):1889-99.

Wang B, Nichol JL, and Sullivan JT, "Pharmacodynamics and Pharmacokinetics of AMG 531, a Novel Thrombopoietin Receptor Ligand," *Clin Pharmacol Ther*, 2004, 76(6):628-38.

◆ **Roxanol** *see* Morphine (Systemic) *on page 1004*

◆ **Roxicodone®** *see* OxyCODONE *on page 1084*

◆ **RP-6976** *see* DOCEtaxel *on page 453*

◆ **RPR-116258A** *see* Cabazitaxel *on page 210*

◆ **RS-25259** *see* Palonosetron *on page 1106*

◆ **RS-25259-197** *see* Palonosetron *on page 1106*

◆ **RU-486** *see* Mifepristone *on page 983*

◆ **RU-23908** *see* Nilutamide *on page 1037*

◆ **RU-38486** *see* Mifepristone *on page 983*

◆ **Rubidomycin Hydrochloride** *see* DAUNOrubicin (Conventional) *on page 396*

Ruxolitinib (rux oh LI ti nib)

Brand Names: U.S. Jakafi™

Brand Names: Canada Jakavi™

Index Terms INCB 18424; INCB018424; INCB424; Ruxolitinib Phosphate

Generic Availability (U.S.) No

Pharmacologic Category Antineoplastic Agent, Janus Associated Kinase Inhibitor; Antineoplastic Agent, Tyrosine Kinase Inhibitor; Janus Associated Kinase Inhibitor

Use Treatment of intermediate or high-risk myelofibrosis, including primary myelofibrosis, post-polycythemia vera (post-PV) myelofibrosis and post-essential thrombocythemia (post-ET) myelofibrosis

Labeled Contraindications There are no contraindications listed within the manufacturer's U.S. labeling.

Canadian labeling: Hypersensitivity to ruxolitinib or any component of the formulation or container

Pregnancy Risk Factor C

Lactation Excretion in breast milk unknown/ not recommended

Warnings/Precautions Hematologic toxicity, including thrombocytopenia, anemia and neutropenia may occur; may require dosage modification; monitor complete blood counts. Patients with baseline platelets <200,000/mm^3 are more likely to develop thrombocytopenia during treatment. Thrombocytopenia is generally reversible with treatment interruption or dose reduction; platelet transfusions may be administered during treatment if clinically indicated. Anemia may require blood transfusion; may consider dose modification. Neutropenia (ANC <500/mm^3) is generally reversible and managed by treatment interruption.

Assess for risk of developing serious bacterial, mycobacterial, fungal or viral infection; monitor for infections during treatment. Active serious infections should be resolved prior to treatment initiation. Prompt treatment is recommended if symptoms of herpes zoster infection develop. May require initial dosage reduction for hepatic impairment; avoid use if platelets <100,000/mm^3 and with hepatic impairment (any degree). May require initial dosage reduction for renal impairment; avoid use if platelets <100,000/mm^3 and with moderate-to-severe renal impairment or in patients with ESRD not requiring dialysis. Ruxolitinib is not removed by dialysis, however, some active metabolites may be removed. On dialysis days, patients are advised to take their dose following dialysis sessions. Reduced initial doses are recommended with concomitant use of strong CYP3A4 inhibitors (eg, clarithromycin, conivaptin, itraconazole, ketoconazole, nefazodone, posaconazole, protease inhibitors, telithromycin, voriconazole, grapefruit juice); if platelets <100,000/mm^3, avoid concomitant use with strong CYP3A4 inhibitors. No adjustment is recommended with concomitant use of mild or moderate CYP3A4 inhibitors or with CYP3A4 inducers (monitor closely for efficacy and titrate dose appropriately). Discontinue treatment after 6 months if no reduction in spleen size or no improvement in symptoms. Consider gradually tapering off if discontinuing for reasons other than thrombocytopenia. Within ~1 week after discontinuation, symptoms of myelofibrosis generally return to pretreatment levels. Acute relapse of myelofibrosis symptoms, splenomegaly, worsening cytopenias, hemodynamic compensation, and septic shock-like syndrome have been reported with treatment discontinuation (Tefferi, 2011); consider gradually tapering off if discontinuing for reasons other than thrombocytopenia.

Use with caution in patients with a history of bradycardia, conduction disturbances, ischemic heart disease, heart failure and/or receiving other drugs that also affect heart rate/conduction; decreased heart rate (mean change 6-8 bpm) and prolongation of the PR interval (mean change 6-9 msec) and of the QT interval (mean 4-5 msec) were observed during some clinical trials. Canadian labeling recommends obtaining an ECG at baseline and periodically; monitor heart rate and blood pressure during treatment.

Adverse Reactions

>10%:

- Cardiovascular: Peripheral edema (22%)
- Central nervous system: Dizziness (15% to 18%), headache (10% to 15%), insomnia (12%)
- Dermatologic: Bruising (19% to 23%)
- Endocrine & metabolic: Cholesterol increased (17%; grade 2: <1%)
- Gastrointestinal: Diarrhea (23%), constipation (13%), nausea (13%), vomiting (12%)
- Hematologic: Anemia (96%; grade 3: 34%; grade 4: 11%), thrombocytopenia (70%; grade 3: 9%; grade 4: 4%), neutropenia (19%; grade 3: 5%; grade 4: 2%)
- Hepatic: ALT increased (25%; grades 2/3: 2%), AST increased (17%; grade 2: <1%)
- Respiratory: Dyspnea (16%), nasopharyngitis (16%)

1% to 10%:

- Gastrointestinal: Flatulence (5%)
- Genitourinary: Urinary tract infection (9%)
- Miscellaneous: Herpes zoster infection (2%)

<1%, postmarketing, and/or case reports: Anxiety, cardiac murmur, edema, epistaxis, limb pain, musculoskeletal pain, peripheral neuropathy, withdrawal syndrome (acute relapse of myelofibrosis symptoms, splenomegaly, worsening cytopenias, hemodynamic compensation, and septic shock-like syndrome)

Drug Interactions

Metabolism/Transport Effects Substrate of CYP3A4 (major); **Note:** Assignment of Major/Minor substrate status based on clinically relevant drug interaction potential

Avoid Concomitant Use

Avoid concomitant use of Ruxolitinib with any of the following: BCG; CloZAPine; Natalizumab; Pimecrolimus; Tacrolimus (Topical); Vaccines (Live)

Increased Effect/Toxicity

Ruxolitinib may increase the levels/effects of: CloZAPine; Leflunomide; Natalizumab; Vaccines (Live)

The levels/effects of Ruxolitinib may be increased by: CYP3A4 Inhibitors (Moderate); CYP3A4 Inhibitors (Strong); Dasatinib; Denosumab; Grapefruit Juice; Ivacaftor; Mifepristone; Pimecrolimus; Roflumilast; Tacrolimus (Topical); Trastuzumab

Decreased Effect

Ruxolitinib may decrease the levels/effects of: BCG; Coccidioidin Skin Test; Sipuleucel-T; Vaccines (Inactivated); Vaccines (Live)

The levels/effects of Ruxolitinib may be decreased by: CYP3A4 Inducers (Strong); Deferasirox; Echinacea; Herbs (CYP3A4 Inducers); Tocilizumab

Ethanol/Nutrition/Herb Interactions Food: Avoid grapefruit juice (may increase the effects of ruxolitinib).

Storage/Stability Store at room temperature of 20°C to 25°C (68°F to 77°F); excursions permitted to 15°C to 30°C (59°F to 86°F).

Mechanism of Action Kinase inhibitor which selectively inhibits Janus Associated Kinases (JAKs), JAK1 and JAK2. JAK1 and JAK2 mediate signaling of cytokine and growth factors responsible for hematopoiesis and immune function. JAK mediated signaling involves recruitment of STATs (signal transducers and activators of transcription) to cytokine receptors which leads to modulation of gene expression. In myelofibrosis, JAK1/2 activity is dysregulated; ruxolitinib modulates the affected JAK1/2 activity.

Pharmacodynamics/Kinetics

Absorption: Rapid

Distribution: V_d: 53-65 L

Protein binding: ~97%; primarily to albumin

Metabolism: Hepatic, primarily via CYP3A4; forms active metabolites responsible for 20% to 50% of activity

Half-life elimination: Ruxolitinib: 2.8-3 hours (hepatic impairment: 5 hours); Ruxolitinib + metabolites: ~6 hours

Time to peak: Within 1-2 hours

Excretion: Urine (74%, <1% as unchanged drug); feces (22%, <1% as unchanged drug)

Dosing

Adult

Myelofibrosis: Oral: Initial dose (based on platelet count, titrate dose thereafter based on efficacy and safety):

U.S. labeling:

Platelets >200,000/mm³: 20 mg twice daily

Platelets 100,000-200,000/mm³: 15 mg twice daily

Canadian labeling:

Platelets >200,000/mm³: 20 mg twice daily

Platelets 100,000-200,000/mm³: 15 mg twice daily

Platelets 50,000-100,000/ mm³: Initial dose should not exceed 5 mg twice daily; titrate dose cautiously

Dosage modification based on response: For insufficient response (with adequate platelet and neutrophil counts), may increase the dose in 5 mg twice daily increments to a maximum dose of 25 mg twice daily. Do not increase during initial 4 weeks and no more frequently than every 2 weeks. Discontinue treatment after 6 months if no reduction in spleen size or no improvement in symptoms. When discontinuing for reasons other than thrombocytopenia, consider gradual tapering by ~5 mg twice daily per week.

Dose increases may be considered if meet all of the following situations:

- Failure to achieve either a 50% reduction (from baseline) in palpable spleen length or a 35% reduction (from baseline) in spleen volume (measured by CT or MRI)
- Platelet count >125,000/mm³ at 4 weeks (and never <100,000/mm³)
- Absolute neutrophil count (ANC) >750/mm³

Dosage adjustment with concomitant strong CYP3A4 inhibitors: Initial dose: 10 mg twice daily (if platelet count ≥100,000/mm³); additional dose adjustments should be made with careful monitoring. Avoid concomitant use if platelet count <100,000/mm³.

Renal Impairment

U.S. labeling:

Cl_{cr} 15-59 mL/minute and platelets >150,000/mm^3: No dosage adjustment provided in manufacturer's labeling.

Cl_{cr} 15-59 mL/minute and platelets 100,000-150,000/mm^3: Initial dose: 10 mg twice daily; additional dose adjustments should be made with careful monitoring.

Cl_{cr} 15-59 mL/minute and platelets <100,000/mm^3: Avoid use.

End-stage renal disease (ESRD) on dialysis and platelets 100,000-200,000/mm^3: Initial dose: 15 mg; administer subsequent doses after dialysis on dialysis days. Additional dose adjustments should be made with careful monitoring.

ESRD on dialysis and platelets >200,000/mm^3: Initial dose: 20 mg; administer subsequent doses after dialysis on dialysis days. Additional dose adjustments should be made with careful monitoring.

ESRD not requiring dialysis: Avoid use.

Canadian labeling:

Cl_{cr} <50 mL/minute and platelets ≥100,000/mm^3: Initial dose: 10 mg twice daily; additional dose adjustments should be made with careful monitoring

Cl_{cr} <50 mL/minute and platelets <100,000/mm^3: Avoid use

ESRD on dialysis and platelets 100,000-200,000/mm^3: Initial dose: 15 mg; administer subsequent doses after dialysis on dialysis days. Additional dose adjustments should be made with careful monitoring.

ESRD on dialysis and platelets >200,000/mm^3: Initial dose: 20 mg; administer subsequent doses after dialysis on dialysis days. Additional dose adjustments should be made with careful monitoring.

Hepatic Impairment

U.S. labeling:

Hepatic impairment and platelets >150,000/mm^3: No dosage adjustment provided in manufacturer's labeling.

Hepatic impairment and platelets 100,000-150,000/mm^3: Initial dose: 10 mg twice daily; additional dose adjustments should be made with careful monitoring.

Hepatic impairment and platelets <100,000/mm^3: Avoid use.

Canadian labeling:

Hepatic impairment and platelets >100,000/mm^3: Initial dose: 10 mg twice daily; additional dose adjustments should be made with careful monitoring.

Hepatic impairment and platelets <100,000/mm^3: Avoid use.

Adjustment for Toxicity

Dosage modification for treatment interruption:

U.S. labeling:

Platelets <50,000/mm^3: Interrupt treatment; upon platelet recovery (to ≥50,000/mm^3), dosing may be restarted or increased based on the following platelet levels and **maximum allowable doses** (when restarting, begin with a dose that is at least 5 mg twice daily below the dose at treatment interruption):

Platelets ≥125,000/mm^3: 20 mg twice daily

Platelets 100,000 to <125,000/mm^3: 15 mg twice daily

Platelets 75,000 to <100,000/mm^3: 10 mg twice daily for at least 2 weeks; may increase to 15 mg twice daily if stable

Platelets 50,000 to <75,000/mm^3: 5 mg twice daily for at least 2 weeks; may increase to 10 mg twice daily if stable

Platelets <50,000/mm^3: Continue to withhold treatment

Note: Long-term maintenance at 5 mg twice daily has not demonstrated responses; limit use of the dose level to patients where the benefits outweigh risks

Canadian labeling: Platelets <50,000/mm^3 or ANC <500 mm^3: Interrupt treatment; upon recovery of platelets to ≥50,000/mm^3 or ANC to ≥500/mm^3, dosing may be restarted at 5 mg twice daily and then gradually titrated based on blood cell counts.

Dosage reduction for thrombocytopenia:

Platelet Count	Dose at Time of Thrombocytopenia				
	25 mg twice/day	20 mg twice/day	15 mg twice/day	10 mg twice/day	5 mg twice/day
	New Dose	New Dose	New Dose	New Dose	New Dose
100,000 to <125,000/mm^3	20 mg twice/day	15 mg twice/day	No change	No change	No change
75,000 to <100,000/mm^3	10 mg twice/day	10 mg twice/day	10 mg twice/day	No change	No change
50,000 to <75,000/mm^3	5 mg twice/day	5 mg twice/day	5 mg twice/day	5 mg twice/day	No change
<50,000/mm^3	Hold dose	Hold dose	Hold dose	Hold dose	Hold dose

Note: Long-term maintenance at 5 mg twice daily has not demonstrated responses, limit use of the dose level to patients where the benefits outweigh risks

Administration May be administered orally with or without food. If a dose is missed, return to the usual dosing schedule and do **not** administer an additional dose.

If unable to ingest tablets, may administer through a nasogastric (NG) tube (≥8 Fr): Suspend 1 tablet in ~40 mL water and stir for ~10 minutes and administer (within 6 hours after dispersion) with appropriate syringe; rinse NG tube with ~75 mL water (effect of enteral tube feeding on ruxolitinib exposure has not been evaluated)

Extemporaneous Preparations A suspension for nasogastric administration may be prepared with tablets. Place one tablet into ~40 mL water; stir for approximately 10 minutes. Administer within 6 hour after preparation.

Jakafi™ prescribing information November, 2011. Incyte Corporation, Wilmington, DE.

Monitoring Parameters CBC (baseline, every 2-4 weeks until dose stabilized, then as clinically indicated), renal function, hepatic function. Canadian labeling recommends obtaining an ECG at baseline and then periodically during therapy; monitor heart rate and blood pressure during therapy.

Dietary Considerations May be taken with or without food. Avoid grapefruit juice (may increase the effects of ruxolitinib).

Prescribing and Access Restrictions Available through specialty/network pharmacies. Further information may be obtained from the manufacturer, Incyte, at 1-855-452-5234 or at www.Jakafi.com.

Dosage Forms Excipient information presented when available (limited, particularly for generics); consult specific product labeling.

Tablet, oral:

Jakafi™: 5 mg, 10 mg, 15 mg, 20 mg, 25 mg

References

Harrison C, Kiladjian JJ, Al-Ali HK, et al, "JAK Inhibition With Ruxolitinib versus Best Available Therapy for Myelofibrosis," *N Engl J Med*, 2012, 366(9):787-98.

Shilling AD, Nedza FM, Emm T, et al, "Metabolism, Excretion, and Pharmacokinetics of [14C] INCB018424, a Selective Janus Tyrosine Kinase 1/2 Inhibitor, in Humans," *Drug Metab Dispos*, 2010, 38(11):2023-31.

Tefferi A and Pardanani A, "Serious Adverse Events During Ruxolitinib Treatment Discontinuation in Patients With Myelofibrosis," *Mayo Clin Proc*, 2011, 86(12):1188-91.

Tefferi A, Litzow MR, and Pardanani A, Long-Term Outcome of Treatment With Ruxolitinib in Myelofibrosis," *N Engl J Med*, 2011, 365(15):1455-7.

Verstovsek S, Mesa RA, Gotlib J, et al, "A Double Blind, Placebo-Controlled Trial of Ruxolitinib for Myelofibrosis," *N Engl J Med*, 2012, 366(9):799-807.

◆ **Ruxolitinib Phosphate** *see* Ruxolitinib *on page* *1261*

◆ **Rybix™ ODT** *see* TraMADol *on page* *1388*

◆ **Ryzolt™** *see* TraMADol *on page* *1388*

◆ **SAHA** *see* Vorinostat *on page* *1478*

◆ **Salagen®** *see* Pilocarpine (Systemic) *on page* *1173*

Saliva Substitute (sa LYE va SUB stee tute)

Brand Names: U.S. Aquoral™; Biotene® Moisturizing Mouth Spray [OTC]; Biotene® Oral Balance® [OTC]; Caphosol®; Entertainer's Secret® [OTC]; Moi-Stir® [OTC]; Mouth Kote® [OTC]; NeutraSal®; Numoisyn™; Oasis®; Saliva-Sure™ [OTC]

Index Terms Artificial Saliva

Generic Availability (U.S.) No

Pharmacologic Category Gastrointestinal Agent, Miscellaneous

Use Relief of dry mouth and throat in xerostomia or hyposalivation; adjunct to standard oral care in relief of symptoms associated with chemotherapy or radiation therapy-induced mucositis

Labeled Contraindications

Numoisyn™ liquid: Hypersensitivity to saliva substitute or any component of the formulation.

Numoisyn™ lozenges: Fructose intolerance

Adverse Reactions Frequency not defined.

Central nervous system: Altered speech

Gastrointestinal: Abnormal taste, digestive problems (minor), dysphagia

Drug Interactions

Metabolism/Transport Effects None known.

Avoid Concomitant Use There are no known interactions where it is recommended to avoid concomitant use.

Increased Effect/Toxicity There are no known significant interactions involving an increase in effect.

Decreased Effect There are no known significant interactions involving a decrease in effect.

Storage/Stability Store at room temperature.

Caphosol®: Do not refrigerate. Use immediately after mixing.

NeutraSal®: Avoid excess heat or moisture. Use immediately after mixing.

Numoisyn™ liquid: Do not refrigerate. Use within 3 months after opening.

Reconstitution

Caphosol®: Mix contents of 1 blue (A) and 1 clear (B) ampul in clean container; use immediately after mixing.

NeutraSal®: Mix contents of packet with 1 ounce of water in clean container; use immediately after mixing.

Mechanism of Action Protein or electrolyte mixtures which restore/replace saliva, lubricate, moisten, clean, and/or provide a coating on oral mucosa

Dosing

Adult & Geriatric

Mucositis (due to high-dose chemotherapy or radiation therapy): Oral: Caphosol®, NeutraSal®: Swish and spit 4-10 doses daily (use for the duration of chemo- or radiation therapy)

Xerostomia: Oral: Use as needed, or product specific dosing:

Aquoral™: 2 sprays 3-4 times daily

Biotene® Oral Balance® gel: Apply one-half inch length onto tongue and spread evenly; repeat as often as needed

Caphosol®, NeutraSal®: Swish and spit 2-10 doses daily

Entertainer's Secret®: Spray as often as needed

Mouth Kote® spray: Spray 3-5 times, swish for 8-10 seconds, then spit or swallow; use as often as needed

Numoisyn™ liquid: Use 2 mL as needed

Numoisyn™ lozenges: Dissolve 1 lozenge slowly; maximum 16 lozenges daily

Oasis® mouthwash: Rinse mouth with ~30 mL twice daily or as needed; do not swallow

Oasis® spray: 1-2 sprays as needed; maximum 60 sprays daily

SalivaSure™: Dissolve 1 lozenge slowly as needed; for severe symptoms, 1 lozenge per hour is recommended

Administration Oral:

Biotene® Oral Balance® gel: Apply on tongue and spread evenly.

Biotene® spray: Spray directly into mouth; spray is safe to swallow.

Caphosol®: Mix contents of 1 blue (A) and 1 clear (B) ampul in clean container, swish thoroughly with 1/2 of mixture (15 mL) for 1 minute and spit; repeat. Avoid eating or drinking for at least 15 minutes after use.

Entertainer's Secret®: Tilt head back and spray into throat or nostril while inhaling sharply.

Mouth Kote® spray: Spray into mouth and swirl for 8-10 seconds; spray may be swallowed or spit out.

NeutraSal®: For each dose, swish 1/2 the prepared solution around the mouth for 1 minute and spit out; repeat with the remaining solution. Avoid eating or drinking for at least 15 minutes after use.

Numoisyn™ liquid: Rinse in mouth before swallowing.

Numoisyn™ lozenges: Dissolve slowly in mouth; move lozenge around mouth for optimal effect.

Oasis® mouthwash: Rinse for 30 seconds.

Oasis® spray: Spray into mouth holding bottle upright; do not rinse.

SalivaSure® lozenges: Allow lozenge to move around and slowly dissolve in mouth.

Dietary Considerations

Caphosol®: Contains sodium 75 mg/30 mL dose

Moi-Stir®: Contains sodium: 6.47 mEq/120 mL, potassium: 1.93 mEq/120 mL, magnesium: 0.128 mEq/120 mL

Dosage Forms Excipient information presented when available (limited, particularly for generics); consult specific product labeling.

Liquid, oral:

Biotene® Oral Balance®: Water, starch, sunflower oil, propylene glycol, xylitol, glycerine, purified milk extract (45 mL) [sugar-free]

Numoisyn™: Water, sorbitol, linseed extract, *Chondrus crispus*, methylparaben, sodium benzoate, potassium sorbate, dipotassium phosphate, propylparaben (300 mL)

Lozenge, oral:

Numoisyn™: Sorbitol 0.3 g/lozenge, polyethylene glycol, malic acid, sodium citrate, calcium phosphate dibasic, hydrogenated cottonseed oil, citric acid, magnesium stearate, silicon dioxide (100s)

SalivaSure™: Xylitol, citric acid, apple acid, sodium citrate dihydrate, sodium carboxymethylcellulose, dibasic calcium phosphate, silica colloidal, magnesium stearate, stearic acid (90s)

Powder, for reconstitution, oral:

NeutraSal®: Sodium, phosphates, calcium, chloride, bicarbonate, silicon dioxide (30s, 120s)

Solution, oral:

Caphosol®: Dibasic sodium phosphate 0.032%, monobasic sodium phosphate 0.009%, calcium chloride 0.052%, sodium chloride 0.569%, purified water (30 mL) [packaged in two 15 mL ampuls when mixed together provide one 30 mL dose]

Entertainer's Secret®: Sodium carboxymethylcellulose, aloe vera gel, glycerin (60 mL) [ethanol free; honey-apple flavor]

Solution, oral [mouthwash/gargle]:

Oasis®: Water, glycerin, sorbitol, poloxamer 338, PEG-60, hydrogenated castor oil, copovidone, sodium benzoate, carboxymethylcellulose (473 mL) [ethanol free, sugar free; mild mint flavor]

Solution, oral [spray]:

Aquoral™: Oxidized glycerol triesters and silicon dioxide (40 mL) [contains aspartame; delivers 400 sprays, citrus flavor]

Biotene® Moisturizing Mouth Spray: Water, polyglycitol, propylene glycol, sunflower oil, xylitol, milk protein extract, potassium sorbate, acesulfame K, potassium thiocyanate, lysozyme, lactoferrin, lactoperoxidase (45 mL)

Moi-Stir®: Water, sorbitol, sodium carboxymethylcellulose, methylparaben, propylparaben, potassium chloride, dibasic sodium phosphate, calcium chloride, magnesium chloride, sodium chloride (120 mL)

Mouth Kote®: Water, xylitol, sorbitol, yerba santa, citric acid, ascorbic acid, sodium saccharin, sodium benzoate (5 mL, 60 mL, 240 mL) [ethanol free, sugar free; lemon-lime flavor]

Oasis®: Glycerin, cetylpyridinium, copovidone (30 mL) [ethanol free, sugar free; contains sodium benzoate; delivers ~150 sprays, mild mint flavor]

References

Papas AS, Clark RE, Martuscelli G, et al, "A Prospective, Randomized Trial for the Prevention of Mucositis in Patients Undergoing Hematopoietic Stem Cell Transplantation," *Bone Marrow Transplant*, 2003, 31(8): 705-12.

Sweeney MP and Bagg J, "The Mouth and Palliative Care," *Am J Palliat Care*, 2000, 17(2):118-24.

◆ **SalivaSure™ [OTC]** *see* Saliva Substitute *on page* 1266

Samarium Sm 153 Lexidronam

(sa MAR ee um es em won fif tee three lex ID roe nam)

Brand Names: U.S. Quadramet®

Index Terms ^{153}Sm-Lexidronam

Pharmacologic Category Radiopharmaceutical

Use Relief of pain associated with osteoblastic metastatic bone lesions that demonstrate increased localization on radionuclide bone scans

Labeled Contraindications Known hypersensitivity to ethylenediaminetetramethylenephosphonic acid (EDTMP) or similar phosphonate compounds

Pregnancy Risk Factor D

Lactation Excretion in breast milk unknown/not recommended

Warnings/Precautions Radiopharmaceutical: Use appropriate precautions for handling, disposal, and minimizing exposure to patients and healthcare personnel. Use under supervision of individuals who have received training in the handling of radioactive materials and who are authorized by the applicable regulatory authority.

Can cause myelosuppression (leukopenia, thrombocytopenia, and anemia); consider current hematologic status and history of myelosuppressive response to other myelotoxic agents prior to therapy. Evaluate the risk:benefit when combining with other myelotoxic therapies. Avoid myelosuppressive therapies for 4-8 weeks before and for 12 weeks after samarium Sm 153 lexidronam. Active DIC may be a risk factor for severe thrombocytopenia following therapy; deaths have occurred in patients with DIC receiving β-emitting radiopharmaceuticals. Not indicated for the treatment of SCC; SCC has been reported in patients receiving samarium Sm 153 lexidronam. Incontinent patients may require urinary catheterization to reduce the risk of radioactive contamination of clothes or bed linens. May cause fetal harm if administered during pregnancy.

Adverse Reactions

>10%: Hematologic: Thrombocytopenia (69%), leukopenia (59%), anemia (41%)

1% to 10%:

Cardiovascular: Arrhythmias, hypertension, stroke

Central nervous system: Dizziness

Dermatologic: Ecchymosis

Gastrointestinal: Diarrhea

Neuromuscular & skeletal: Bone pain, spinal cord compression

Renal: Hematuria

Respiratory: Bronchitis, epistaxis

Storage/Stability Store frozen at -20°C to -10°C (-4°F to 14°F) in a lead-shielded container.

Dosing

Adult Palliation of osteoblastic metastatic bone lesions: I.V.: 1 mCi/kg (37 MBq/kg)

Administration Note: Give 500 mL of fluids (I.V. or orally) prior to administration

References

Henkin RE, Harford AC, Del Rowe JD, et al, "ACR–ASTRO Practice Guideline for the Performance of Therapy with Unsealed Radiopharmaceutical Sources," 2010. Available at http://www.acr.org/secondarymainmenucategories/quality_safety/guidelines/nuc_med/unsealed_radiopharmaceuticals.aspx . Last accessed August 26, 2011.

Silberstein EB, Buscombe JR, McEwan A, et al, "Society of Nuclear Medicine Procedure Guideline for Palliative Treatment of Painful Bone Metastases," 2003. Available at http://interactive.snm.org/docs/pg_ch25_0403.pdf. Last accessed August 26, 2011.

U.S. Nuclear Regulatory Commission, "Regulatory Guide 8.39. Release of Patients Administered Radioactive Materials," 1977.

◆ **Sancuso®** *see* Granisetron *on page* 687

◆ **SandIMMUNE®** *see* CycloSPORINE (Systemic) *on page* 333

◆ **Sandimmune® I.V. (Can)** *see* CycloSPORINE (Systemic) *on page* 333

- **SandoSTATIN®** *see* Octreotide *on page 1043*
- **Sandostatin® (Can)** *see* Octreotide *on page 1043*
- **SandoSTATIN LAR®** *see* Octreotide *on page 1043*
- **Sandostatin LAR® (Can)** *see* Octreotide *on page 1043*
- **Sandoz-Anagrelide (Can)** *see* Anagrelide *on page 93*
- **Sandoz-Anastrozole (Can)** *see* Anastrozole *on page 96*
- **Sandoz-Bicalutamide (Can)** *see* Bicalutamide *on page 178*
- **Sandoz-Calcitonin (Can)** *see* Calcitonin *on page 214*
- **Sandoz-Ciprofloxacin (Can)** *see* Ciprofloxacin (Systemic) *on page 283*
- **Sandoz-Cyclosporine (Can)** *see* CycloSPORINE (Systemic) *on page 333*
- **Sandoz-Famciclovir (Can)** *see* Famciclovir *on page 580*
- **Sandoz-Letrozole (Can)** *see* Letrozole *on page 867*
- **Sandoz-Levofloxacin (Can)** *see* Levofloxacin (Systemic) *on page 883*
- **Sandoz-Morphine SR (Can)** *see* Morphine (Systemic) *on page 1004*
- **Sandoz-Mycophenolate (Can)** *see* Mycophenolate *on page 1015*
- **Sandoz-Mycophenolate Mofetil (Can)** *see* Mycophenolate *on page 1015*
- **Sandoz-Olanzapine (Can)** *see* OLANZapine *on page 1056*
- **Sandoz-Olanzapine ODT (Can)** *see* OLANZapine *on page 1056*
- **Sandoz-Ondansetron (Can)** *see* Ondansetron *on page 1068*
- **Sandoz-Prochlorperazine (Can)** *see* Prochlorperazine *on page 1212*

Sargramostim (sar GRAM oh stim)

Related Information

Hematopoietic Stem Cell Transplantation *on page 1887*

Oral Mucositis/Stomatitis *on page 1814*

Brand Names: U.S. Leukine®

Brand Names: Canada Leukine®

Index Terms GM-CSF; Granulocyte-Macrophage Colony Stimulating Factor; rhuGM-CSF

Generic Availability (U.S.) No

Pharmacologic Category Colony Stimulating Factor

Use

Acute myelogenous leukemia (AML) following induction chemotherapy in older adults (≥55 years of age) to shorten time to neutrophil recovery and to reduce the incidence of severe and life-threatening infections and infections resulting in death

Bone marrow transplant (allogeneic or autologous) failure or engraftment delay

Myeloid reconstitution after allogeneic bone marrow transplantation

Myeloid reconstitution after autologous bone marrow transplantation: Non-Hodgkin's lymphoma (NHL), acute lymphoblastic leukemia (ALL), Hodgkin's lymphoma

Peripheral stem cell transplantation: Mobilization and myeloid reconstitution following autologous peripheral stem cell transplantation

Labeled Contraindications Hypersensitivity to sargramostim, yeast-derived products, or any component of the formulation; concurrent (24 hours preceding/following) myelosuppressive chemotherapy or radiation therapy; patients with excessive (≥10%) leukemic myeloid blasts in bone marrow or peripheral blood

Pregnancy Risk Factor C

Lactation Excretion in breast milk unknown/use caution

Warnings/Precautions Simultaneous administration, or administration 24 hours preceding/following cytotoxic chemotherapy or radiotherapy is not recommended. Use with caution in patients with pre-existing cardiac problems or HF; supraventricular arrhythmias have been reported in patients with history of arrhythmias. Edema, capillary leak syndrome, pleural and/or pericardial effusion have been reported; use with caution in patients with pre-existing fluid retention; may worsen. Use with caution in patients with hepatic or renal impairment; monitor hepatic and/or renal function in patients with history of hepatic or renal dysfunction. Elevations in bilirubin, transaminases, and serum creatinine have been observed with use. Dyspnea may occur; monitor respiratory symptoms during and following infusion; use with caution in patients with hypoxia or pulmonary infiltrates.

With rapid increase in blood counts (ANC >20,000/mm^3, WBC >50,000/mm^3, or platelets >500,000/mm^3); decrease dose by 50% or discontinue drug (counts will fall to normal within 3-7 days after discontinuing drug). May potentially act as a growth factor for any tumor type, particularly myeloid malignancies; caution should be exercised when using in any malignancy with myeloid characteristics; tumors of nonhematopoietic origin may have surface receptors for sargramostim. Discontinue use if disease progression occurs during treatment.

There is a "first-dose effect" (refer to Adverse Reactions for details) which is seen (rarely) with the first dose of a cycle and does not usually occur with subsequent doses within that cycle. Anaphylaxis or other serious allergic reactions have been reported; discontinue immediately if occur. Solution contains benzyl alcohol; do not use in premature infants or neonates.

Adverse Reactions

>10%:

Cardiovascular: Hypertension (34%), pericardial effusion (4% to 25%), edema (13% to 25%), chest pain (15%), peripheral edema (11%), tachycardia (11%)

Central nervous system: Fever (81%), malaise (57%), headache (26%), chills (25%), anxiety (11%), insomnia (11%)

Dermatologic: Rash (44%), pruritus (23%)

Endocrine & metabolic: Hyperglycemia (25%), hypercholesterolemia (17%), hypomagnesemia (15%)

Gastrointestinal: Diarrhea (≤89%), nausea (58% to 70%), vomiting (46% to 70%), abdominal pain (38%), weight loss (37%), anorexia (13%), hematemesis (13%), dysphagia (11%), gastrointestinal hemorrhage (11%)

Genitourinary: Urinary tract disorder (14%)

Hepatic: Hyperbilirubinemia (30%)

Neuromuscular & skeletal: Weakness (66%), bone pain (21%), arthralgia (11% to 21%) myalgia (18%)

Ocular: Eye hemorrhage (11%)

Renal: BUN increased (23%), serum creatinine increased (15%)

Respiratory: Pharyngitis (23%), epistaxis (17%), dyspnea (15%)

Miscellaneous: Antibody formation (2%)

1% to 10%: Respiratory: Pleural effusion (1%)

<1%, postmarketing, and/or case reports: Allergic reaction, anaphylaxis, arrhythmia, capillary leak syndrome, constipation, dizziness, eosinophilia; first-dose effect (syndrome with respiratory distress, hypoxia, flushing, hypotension, syncope, and/or tachycardia occurring with the first dose of a treatment cycle); injection site reaction, lethargy, leukocytosis, liver function abnormalities (transient), pain, pericarditis, prothrombin time prolonged, rigors, sore throat, supraventricular arrhythmia (transient), thrombocytosis, thrombophlebitis, thrombosis

Drug Interactions

Metabolism/Transport Effects None known.

Avoid Concomitant Use There are no known interactions where it is recommended to avoid concomitant use.

Increased Effect/Toxicity

Sargramostim may increase the levels/effects of: Bleomycin

Decreased Effect There are no known significant interactions involving a decrease in effect.

Storage/Stability Store at 2°C to 8°C (36°F to 46°F); do not freeze. Do not shake.

Solution for injection: May be stored for up to 20 days at 2°C to 8°C (36°F to 46°F) once the vial has been entered. Discard remaining solution after 20 days.

Powder for injection: Preparations made with SWFI should be administered as soon as possible, and discarded within 6 hours of reconstitution. Preparations made with bacteriostatic water may be stored for up to 20 days at 2°C to 8°C (36°F to 46°F).

I.V. infusion administration: Preparations diluted with NS are stable for 48 hours at room temperature and refrigeration.

Reconstitution

Powder for injection: May be reconstituted with preservative free SWFI or bacteriostatic water for injection (with benzyl alcohol 0.9%). Gently swirl to reconstitute; do not shake.

Sargramostim may also be further diluted in 25-50 mL NS to a concentration ≥10 mcg/mL for I.V. infusion administration.

If the final concentration of sargramostim is <10 mcg/mL, 1 mg of human albumin/1 mL of NS (eg, 1 mL of 5% human albumin/50 mL of NS) should be added.

Mechanism of Action Stimulates proliferation, differentiation and functional activity of neutrophils, eosinophils, monocytes, and macrophages, as indicated.

Pharmacodynamics/Kinetics

Onset of action: Increase in WBC: 7-14 days

Duration: WBCs return to baseline within 1 week of discontinuing drug

Half-life elimination: I.V.: 60 minutes; SubQ: 2.7 hours

Time to peak, serum: SubQ: 1-3 hours

Dosing

Adult & Geriatric

I.V. infusion over ≥2 hours or SubQ: **Rounding the dose to the nearest vial size enhances patient convenience and reduces costs without clinical detrement.**

Myeloid reconstitution after allogeneic or autologous bone marrow transplant: I.V.: 250 mcg/m²/day (over 2 hours), begin 2-4 hours after the marrow infusion and ≥24 hours after chemotherapy or radiotherapy, when the post marrow infusion ANC is <500 cells/mm^3, and continue until ANC >1500 cells/mm^3 for 3 consecutive days

If a severe adverse reaction occurs, reduce the dose by 50% or temporarily discontinue until the reaction abates

If blast cells appear or progression of the underlying disease occurs, discontinue treatment

If ANC >20,000 cells/mm^3, interrupt treatment or reduce the dose by 50%

Neutrophil recovery following chemotherapy in AML: I.V.: 250 mcg/m^2/day (over 4 hours) starting approximately on day 11 or 4 days following the completion of induction chemotherapy, if day 10 bone marrow is hypoplastic with <5% blasts

If a second cycle of chemotherapy is necessary, administer ~4 days after the completion of chemotherapy if the bone marrow is hypoplastic with <5% blasts

Continue sargramostim until ANC is >1500 cells/mm^3 for 3 consecutive days or a maximum of 42 days

Discontinue sargramostim immediately if leukemic regrowth occurs

If a severe adverse reaction occurs, reduce the dose by 50% or temporarily discontinue the dose until the reaction abates

If ANC >20,000 cells/mm^3, interrupt treatment or reduce the dose by 50%

Mobilization of peripheral blood progenitor cells: I.V., SubQ: 250 mcg/m^2/day I.V. over 24 hours or SubQ once daily

Continue the same dose through the period of PBPC collection

The optimal schedule for PBPC collection has not been established (usually begun by day 5 and performed daily until protocol specified targets are achieved)

If WBC >50,000 cells/mm^3, reduce the dose by 50%

If adequate numbers of progenitor cells are not collected, consider other mobilization therapy

Postperipheral blood progenitor cell transplantation: I.V., SubQ: 250 mcg/m^2/day I.V. over 24 hours or SubQ once daily beginning immediately following infusion of progenitor cells and continuing until ANC is >1500 cells/mm^3 for 3 consecutive days is attained

BMT failure or engraftment delay: I.V.: 250 mcg/m^2/day over 2 hours for 14 days

May be repeated after 7 days off therapy if engraftment has not occurred

If engraftment still has not occurred, a third course of 500 mcg/m^2/day for 14 days may be tried after another 7 days off therapy; if there is still no improvement, it is unlikely that further dose escalation will be beneficial

If a severe adverse reaction occurs, reduce the dose by 50% or temporarily discontinue the dose until the reaction abates

If blast cells appear or disease progression occurs, discontinue treatment

If ANC >20,000 cells/mm^3, interrupt treatment or reduce the dose by 50%

Pediatric Dosage not established in children (unlabeled use). Refer to adult dosing.

Combination Regimens

Leukemia, acute myeloid: MEC-G (AML Induction) on page 1707

Lymphoma, non-Hodgkin's (Burkitt): CODOX-M/IVAC on page 1591

Administration Can premedicate with analgesics and antipyretics (eg, acetaminophen) to control adverse events (eg, fever, chills, myalgia, etc); control bone pain with non-narcotic analgesics. Sargramostim is administered as a subcutaneous injection or intravenous infusion; intravenous infusion should be over 2-24 hours; continuous infusions may be more effective than short infusion or bolus injection. An in-line membrane filter should **NOT** be used for intravenous administration. When administering GM-CSF subcutaneously, rotate injection sites.

Monitoring Parameters Vital signs, hydration status, weight, CBC with differential twice weekly during therapy, renal/liver function tests at least biweekly during therapy (in patients displaying renal or hepatic dysfunction prior to initiation of treatment), pulmonary function

Test Interactions May interfere with bone imaging studies; increased hematopoietic activity of the bone marrow may appear as transient positive bone imaging changes

Additional Information Reimbursement Hotline (Leukine®): 1-800-321-4669

Dosage Forms Excipient information presented when available (limited, particularly for generics); consult specific product labeling.

Injection, powder for reconstitution:

Leukine®: 250 mcg [contains sucrose 10 mg/mL]

Injection, solution:

Leukine®: 500 mcg/mL (1 mL) [contains benzyl alcohol, sucrose 10 mg/mL]

References

Mayer D and Bednarczyk EM, "Interaction of Colony-Stimulating Factors and Fluorodeoxyglucose F^{18} Positron Emission Tomography," *Ann Pharmacother*, 2002, 36(11):1796-9.

Smith TJ, Khatcheressian J, Lyman GH, et al, "2006 Update of Recommendations for the Use of White Blood Cell Growth Factors: An Evidence-Based Clinical Practice Guideline," *J Clin Oncol*, 2006, 24(19):3187-205.

Working Group on Antiretroviral Therapy and Medical Management of HIV-Infected Children, "Guidelines for the Use of Antiretroviral Agents in Pediatric HIV Infection," August 16, 2010. Available at http://www.aidsinfo.nih.gov

◆ **Sarna® HC (Can)** *see* Hydrocortisone (Topical) *on page 719*

◆ **SB-497115** *see* Eltrombopag *on page 494*

◆ **SB-497115-GR** *see* Eltrombopag *on page 494*

◆ **SC 33428** *see* IDArubicin *on page 749*

◆ **Scalpana [OTC]** *see* Hydrocortisone (Topical) *on page 719*

◆ **SCH 13521** *see* Flutamide *on page 635*

◆ **SCH 52365** *see* Temozolomide *on page 1331*

◆ **SCH 56592** *see* Posaconazole *on page 1187*

◆ **SCIG** *see* Immune Globulin *on page 777*

◆ **Sclerosol®** *see* Talc (Sterile) *on page 1323*

Scopolamine (Systemic) (skoe POL a meen)

Related Information

Hospice (End of Life) Care *on page 1857*

Management of Chemotherapy-Induced Nausea and Vomiting *on page 1786*

Brand Names: U.S. Transderm Scōp®

Brand Names: Canada Buscopan®; Scopolamine Hydrobromide Injection; Transderm-V®

Index Terms Hyoscine Butylbromide; Scopolamine Base; Scopolamine Butylbromide; Scopolamine Hydrobromide

Generic Availability (U.S.) Yes: Injection

Pharmacologic Category Anticholinergic Agent

Use

Scopolamine base: Transdermal: Prevention of nausea/vomiting associated with motion sickness and recovery from anesthesia and surgery

Scopolamine hydrobromide: Injection: Preoperative medication to produce amnesia, sedation, tranquilization, antiemetic effects, and decrease salivary and respiratory secretions

Scopolamine butylbromide [not available in the U.S.]: Oral/injection: Treatment of smooth muscle spasm of the genitourinary or gastrointestinal tract; injection may also be used prior to radiological/diagnostic procedures to prevent spasm

Unlabeled Use Scopolamine base: Transdermal: Breakthrough treatment of nausea and vomiting associated with chemotherapy

Labeled Contraindications

Transdermal, oral: Hypersensitivity to scopolamine, other belladonna alkaloids, or any component of the formulation; narrow-angle glaucoma

Injection: Hypersensitivity to scopolamine, other belladonna alkaloids, or any component of the formulation; narrow-angle glaucoma; chronic lung disease (repeated administration)

Canadian labeling: Additional contraindications (not in U.S. labeling):

Oral: Glaucoma, megacolon, myasthenia gravis, obstructive prostatic hypertrophy

Injection:

Hyoscine butylbromide: Untreated narrow-angle glaucoma; megacolon, prostatic hypertrophy with urinary retention; stenotic lesions of the GI tract; myasthenia gravis; tachycardia, angina, or heart failure; I.M. administration in patients receiving anticoagulant therapy

Scopolamine hydrobromide: Glaucoma or predisposition to narrow-angle glaucoma; paralytic ileus, prostatic hypertrophy; pyloric obstruction; tachycardia secondary to cardiac insufficiency or thyrotoxicosis

Pregnancy Risk Factor C

Lactation Enters breast milk/use caution (AAP rates "compatible"; AAP 2001 update pending)

Warnings/Precautions Use with caution in patients with coronary artery disease, tachyarrhythmias, heart failure, hypertension, or hyperthyroidism; evaluate tachycardia prior to administration. Use caution in hepatic or renal impairment; adverse CNS effects occur more often in these patients. Use injectable and transdermal products with caution in patients with prostatic hyperplasia or urinary retention. Discontinue if patient reports unusual visual disturbances or pain within the eye. Use caution in GI obstruction, hiatal hernia, reflux esophagitis, and ulcerative colitis. Use with caution in patients with a history of seizure or psychosis; may exacerbate these conditions.

Anaphylaxis including episodes of shock has been reported following parenteral administration; observe for signs/symptoms of hypersensitivity following parenteral administration. Patients with a history of allergies or asthma may be at increased risk of hypersensitivity reactions. Adverse events (including dizziness, headache, nausea, vomiting) may occur following abrupt discontinuation of large doses or in patients with Parkinson's disease; adverse events may also occur following removal of the transdermal patch although symptoms may not appear until ≥24 hours after removal.

Idiosyncratic reactions may rarely occur; patients may experience acute toxic psychosis, agitation, confusion, delusions, hallucinations, paranoid behavior, and rambling speech. May cause CNS depression, which may impair physical or mental abilities; patients must be cautioned about performing tasks which require mental alertness (eg, operating machinery or driving).

Transdermal patch may contain conducting metal (eg, aluminum); remove patch prior to MRI. Use of the transdermal product in patients with open-angle glaucoma may necessitate adjustments in glaucoma therapy.

Scopolamine (hyoscine) hydrobromide should not be interchanged with scopolamine butylbromide formulations; dosages are not equivalent.

Avoid use in the elderly due to potent anticholinergic adverse effects and uncertain effectiveness (Beers Criteria). Use with caution in infants and children since they may be more susceptible to adverse effects of scopolamine. Safety and efficacy have not been established for the use of transdermal and oral scopolamine in children. Tablets may contain sucrose; avoid use of tablets in patients who are fructose intolerant.

Adverse Reactions Frequency not defined.

Cardiovascular: Bradycardia, flushing, orthostatic hypotension, tachycardia

Central nervous system: Acute toxic psychosis (rare), agitation (rare), ataxia, confusion, delusion (rare), disorientation, dizziness, drowsiness, fatigue, hallucination (rare), headache, irritability, loss of memory, paranoid behavior (rare), restlessness, sedation

Dermatologic: Drug eruptions, dry skin, dyshidrosis, erythema, pruritus, rash, urticaria

Endocrine & metabolic: Thirst

Gastrointestinal: Constipation, diarrhea, dry throat, dysphagia, nausea, vomiting, xerostomia

Genitourinary: Dysuria, urinary retention

Neuromuscular & skeletal: Tremor, weakness

Ocular: Accommodation impaired, blurred vision, conjunctival infection, cycloplegia, dryness, glaucoma (narrow-angle), increased intraocular pain, itching, photophobia, pupil dilation, retinal pigmentation

Respiratory: Dry nose, dyspnea

Miscellaneous: Anaphylaxis (rare), anaphylactic shock (rare), angioedema, diaphoresis decreased, heat intolerance, hypersensitivity reactions

Drug Interactions

Metabolism/Transport Effects None known.

Avoid Concomitant Use

Avoid concomitant use of Scopolamine (Systemic) with any of the following: Aclidinium; Azelastine (Nasal); Ipratropium (Oral Inhalation); Methadone; Mirtazapine; Paraldehyde; Tiotropium

Increased Effect/Toxicity

Scopolamine (Systemic) may increase the levels/effects of: AbobotulinumtoxinA; Alcohol (Ethyl); Anticholinergics; Azelastine (Nasal); Buprenorphine; Cannabinoids; CNS Depressants; Methadone; Methotrimeprazine; Metyrosine; Mirabegron; Mirtazapine; OnabotulinumtoxinA; Paraldehyde; Potassium Chloride; Pramipexole; RimabotulinumtoxinB; ROPINIRole; Rotigotine; Selective Serotonin Reuptake Inhibitors; Tiotropium; Topiramate; Zolpidem

The levels/effects of Scopolamine (Systemic) may be increased by: Aclidinium; Droperidol; HydrOXYzine; Ipratropium (Oral Inhalation); Methotrimeprazine; Perampanel; Pramlintide

Decreased Effect

Scopolamine (Systemic) may decrease the levels/effects of: Acetylcholinesterase Inhibitors (Central); Secretin

The levels/effects of Scopolamine (Systemic) may be decreased by: Acetylcholinesterase Inhibitors (Central)

Ethanol/Nutrition/Herb Interactions Ethanol: May increase CNS depression; monitor for increased effects with coadministration. Caution patients about effects.

Storage/Stability

Injection:

Butylbromide (Canadian availability): Store at room temperature. Do not freeze. Protect from light and heat. Stable in D_5W, $D_{10}W$, NS, Ringer's solution, and LR for up to 8 hours.

Hydrobromide: Store at room temperature of 20°C to 25°C (68°F to 77°F). Protect from light. Avoid acid solutions; hydrolysis occurs at pH <3.

Tablet (Canadian availability): Store at room temperature. Protect from light and heat.

Transdermal system: Store at 20°C to 25°C (68°F to 77°F).

Mechanism of Action Blocks the action of acetylcholine at parasympathetic sites in smooth muscle, secretory glands and the CNS; increases cardiac output, dries secretions, antagonizes histamine and serotonin

Pharmacodynamics/Kinetics

Onset of action: Oral, I.M.: 0.5-1 hour; I.V.: 10 minutes; Transdermal: 6-8 hours

Duration: I.M., I.V., SubQ: 4 hours

Absorption: I.M., SubQ: Rapid; Oral: Quaternary salts (butylbromide) are poorly absorbed (local concentrations in the GI tract following oral dosing may be high)

Distribution: V_d: Butylbromide: 128 L

Protein binding: Butylbromide: ~4% (albumin)

Metabolism: Hepatic

Bioavailability: Oral: 8%

Half-life elimination: Butylbromide: ~5-11 hours; Hydrobromide: ~1-4 hours; Scopolamine base: 9.5 hours

Time to peak: Hydrobromide: I.M.: ~20 minutes, SubQ: ~15 minutes; Butylbromide: Oral: ~2 hours; Scopolamine base: Transdermal: 24 hours

Excretion: Urine (<10%, as parent drug and metabolites); I.V.: Butylbromide: Urine (42% to 61% [half as parent drug]), feces (28% to 37%)

Dosing

Adult Note: Scopolamine (hyoscine) hydrobromide should not be interchanged with scopolamine butylbromide formulations. Dosages are not equivalent.

Scopolamine base:

Preoperative: Transdermal patch: Apply 1 patch to hairless area behind ear the night before surgery or 1 hour prior to cesarean section (apply no sooner than 1 hour before surgery to minimize newborn exposure); remove 24 hours after surgery

Motion sickness: Transdermal patch: Apply 1 patch to hairless area behind the ear at least 4 hours prior to exposure and every 3 days as needed; effective if applied as soon as 2-3 hours before anticipated need, best if 12 hours before

Chemotherapy-induced nausea and vomiting, breakthrough (unlabeled use): Apply 1 patch every 72 hours (NCCN Antiemesis guidelines v.1.2012)

Scopolamine hydrobromide:

Antiemetic: SubQ: 0.6-1 mg

Preoperative: I.M., I.V., SubQ: 0.3-0.65 mg

Sedation, tranquilization: I.M., I.V., SubQ:
U.S. labeling: 0.6 mg 3-4 times/day
Canadian labeling: 0.3-0.6 mg 3-4 times/day
Scopolamine butylbromide: *Gastrointestinal/genitourinary spasm* (Buscopan® [CAN]; not available in the U.S.):
Oral: Acute therapy: 10-20 mg daily (1-2 tablets); prolonged therapy: 10 mg (1 tablet) 3-5 times/day; maximum: 60 mg/day
I.M., I.V., SubQ: 10-20 mg; maximum: 100 mg/day

Geriatric Lower dosages may be required. Refer to adult dosing.

Pediatric Scopolamine hydrobromide:
Antiemetic: SubQ: 0.006 mg/kg
Preoperative: I.M., I.V., SubQ:
Children 6 months to 3 years: 0.1-0.15 mg
Children 3-6 years: 0.2-0.3 mg

Renal Impairment There are no dosage adjustments in the manufacturer labeling; however, caution is recommended due to increased risks of adverse effects.

Hepatic Impairment There are no dosage adjustments in the manufacturer labeling; however, caution is recommended due to increased risks of adverse effects.

Administration Note: Butylbromide or hydrobromide may be administered by I.M., I.V., or SubQ injection.
I.M.: **Butylbromide:** Intramuscular injections should be administered 10-15 minutes prior to radiological/diagnostic procedures.
I.V.:
Butylbromide: No dilution is necessary prior to injection; inject at a rate of 1 mL/minute
Hydrobromide: Dilute with an equal volume of sterile water and administer by direct I.V.; inject over 2-3 minutes
Oral: Tablet should be swallowed whole and taken with a full glass of water.
Transdermal: Apply to hairless area of skin behind the ear. Wash hands before and after applying the disc to avoid drug contact with eyes. Do not use any patch that has been damaged, cut, or manipulated in any way. Topical patch is programmed to deliver 1 mg over 3 days. Once applied, do not remove the patch for 3 full days (motion sickness). When used postoperatively for nausea/vomiting, the patch should be removed 24 hours after surgery. If patch becomes displaced, discard and apply a new patch.

Monitoring Parameters Body temperature, heart rate, urinary output, intraocular pressure

Test Interactions Interferes with gastric secretion test

Dosage Forms Excipient information presented when available (limited, particularly for generics); consult specific product labeling.
Injection, solution, as hydrobromide: 0.4 mg/mL (1 mL)
Patch, transdermal:
Transderm Scōp®: 1.5 mg (4s, 10s, 24s) [contains metal; releases ~1 mg over 72 hours]

Dosage Forms: Canada Excipient information presented when available (limited, particularly for generics); consult specific product labeling.
Tablet, oral, as butylbromide:
Buscopan®: 10 mg

References

Gan TJ, Sinha AC, Kovac AL, et al, "A Randomized, Double-Blind, Multicenter Trial Comparing Transdermal Scopolamine Plus Ondansetron to Ondansetron Alone for the Prevention of Post-operative Nausea and Vomiting in the Outpatient Setting," *Anesth Analg*, 2009, 108(5):1498-504.

National Comprehensive Cancer Network® (NCCN), "Clinical Practice Guidelines in Oncology™: Antiemesis," Version 1.2012. Available at http://www.nccn.org/professionals/physician_gls/PDF/antiemesis.pdf

Sah N, Ramesh V, Kaul B, et al, "Transdermal Scopolamine Patch in Addition to Ondansetron for Postoperative Nausea and Vomiting Prophylaxis in Patients Undergoing Ambulatory Cosmetic Surgery," *J Clin Anesth*, 2009, 21(4):249-52.

- **Scopolamine Base** *see* Scopolamine (Systemic) *on page 1274*
- **Scopolamine Butylbromide** *see* Scopolamine (Systemic) *on page 1274*
- **Scopolamine Hydrobromide** *see* Scopolamine (Systemic) *on page 1274*
- **Scopolamine Hydrobromide Injection (Can)** *see* Scopolamine (Systemic) *on page 1274*
- **SD/01** *see* Pegfilgrastim *on page 1138*
- **SDX-105** *see* Bendamustine *on page 158*
- **Sensipar®** *see* Cinacalcet *on page 280*
- **Septra** *see* Sulfamethoxazole and Trimethoprim *on page 1302*
- **Septra® DS** *see* Sulfamethoxazole and Trimethoprim *on page 1302*
- **Septra® Injection (Can)** *see* Sulfamethoxazole and Trimethoprim *on page 1302*
- **SGN-35** *see* Brentuximab Vedotin *on page 199*
- **SH 714** *see* Cyproterone *on page 344*
- **Silkis™ (Can)** *see* Calcitriol *on page 215*
- **Simulect®** *see* Basiliximab *on page 149*

Sipuleucel-T (ci pu LOO sel tee)

Brand Names: U.S. Provenge®

Index Terms APC8015; Prostate Cancer Vaccine, Cell-Based

Generic Availability (U.S.) No

Pharmacologic Category Cellular Immunotherapy, Autologous

Use Treatment of metastatic hormone-refractory prostate cancer in patients who are asymptomatic or minimally symptomatic

Labeled Contraindications There are no contraindications listed within the FDA-approved manufacturer's labeling.

Warnings/Precautions For autologous use only; patient identity must be matched to the patient identifiers on the infusion bag and on the Cell Product Disposition Form (provided by manufacturer) prior to infusion; confirmation of product release must be received from the manufacturer prior to infusion.

Acute infusion reactions may occur within 1 day of infusion and are usually mild or moderate for most patients; the incidence of severe reaction may be higher with the second infusion, while the third infusion is associated with a decrease in the incidence of severe reactions. Premedication with oral acetaminophen and diphenhydramine is recommended. Depending on the severity of infusion reaction, interrupt or slow infusion rate; in clinical trials, acetaminophen, I.V. H_1 and/or H_2 antagonists, and low-dose meperidine were used to manage acute symptoms. Symptoms of acute infusion reaction may include chills, fever, bronchospasm, dyspnea, hypoxia, hypertension, tachycardia, joint or muscle aches, nausea, vomiting, fatigue, headache, and weakness; fever and chills usually resolved within 2 days.

Closely monitor during infusion in patients with cardiac pr pulmonary conditions. Concurrent use with immunosuppressives (eg, corticosteroids) has not been studied; may alter the efficacy and/or safety of sipuleucel-T. Concurrent use with chemotherapy has not been studied. In clinical trials, patients who had androgen deprivation therapy without prior bilateral orchiectomy were continued on gonadal suppression with a luteinizing hormone-releasing hormone (LHRH) agonist (Higano, 2009).

Apply universal precautions for product handling; sipuleucel-T is not routinely tested for transmissible infectious diseases; patient specific leukapheresis collection and activated product may have a risk for infectious disease transmission. Preliminary sterility testing is done based on a 2-day incubation period; final (7-day incubation) testing is not available until after administration; physicians will be notified if 7-day sterility tests are positive for microbial contamination. If unable to receive a scheduled reinfusion, an additional leukapheresis procedure may be required; advise patients of this possibility before treatment initiation.

Adverse Reactions Note: Initial infusion-related events usually present within the first 24 hours after administration.

>10%:

Central nervous system: Chills (53%), fatigue (41%), fever (31%), headache (18%), dizziness (12%), pain (12%)

Gastrointestinal: Nausea (22%), vomiting (13%)

Hematologic: Anemia (13%)

Neuromuscular & skeletal: Back pain (30%), myalgia (12%), weakness (11%)

Miscellaneous: Acute infusion reaction (71%; grade 3: 4%), citrate toxicity (15%)

1% to 10%:

Cardiovascular: Hypertension (8%)

Central nervous system: Stroke (hemorrhagic or ischemic: 4%)

Dermatologic: Rash (5%)

Neuromuscular & skeletal: Muscle spasm (8%), neck pain (6%), tremor (5%)

Renal: Hematuria (8%)

Respiratory: Dyspnea (9%), cough (6%), upper respiratory tract infection (6%)

Miscellaneous: Flu-like syndrome (10%), diaphoresis (5%)

<1%, postmarketing, and/or case reports: Eosinophilia, groin pain, incontinence, myasthenia gravis, myositis, nocturia obstructive voiding symptoms, rhabdomyolysis, tumor flare, urinary urgency

Drug Interactions

Metabolism/Transport Effects None known.

Avoid Concomitant Use There are no known interactions where it is recommended to avoid concomitant use.

Increased Effect/Toxicity There are no known significant interactions involving an increase in effect.

Decreased Effect

The levels/effects of Sipuleucel-T may be decreased by: Immunosuppressants

Storage/Stability Do not remove the infusion bag from the insulated polyurethane container within the shipping box until administration. Product may only remain at room temperature for ≤3 hours once removed from shipping container; after removal from shipping container, do not return product to container. Infusion must begin prior to product expiration.

Reconstitution Sipuleucel-T will arrive as a prepared patient-specific 250 mL suspension in lactated Ringer's injection. Contents may appear slightly cloudy and will be a cream-to-pink color. If clumps or clots are present, gently mix to resuspend.

Mechanism of Action Autologous cellular immunotherapy which stimulates an immune response against an antigen (PAP) expressed in most prostate cancer tissues. Peripheral blood is collected (~3 days prior to infusion) from the patient via leukapheresis, from which peripheral blood mononuclear cells (PBMCs) are isolated. Antigen presenting cell (APC) precursors, consisting of CD54-positive cells that include dendritic cells, are isolated from the PBMCs. The APCs are then activated (*in vitro*) with a recombinant human fusion protein, PAP-GM-CSF (also termed PA2024), composed of an antigen specific for prostate cancer, prostatic acid phosphatase (PAP) linked to granulocyte-macrophage colony-stimulating factor (GM-CSF) and cultured for ~40 hours. The final product, sipuleucel-T, is reinfused into the patient, inducing T-cell immunity to tumors that express PAP.

Dosing

Adult & Geriatric Note: Premedicate with oral acetaminophen 650 mg and an antihistamine (eg, diphenhydramine 50 mg) ~30 minutes prior to infusion. For autologous use only. Do not infuse until confirmation of product release has been received from the company.

Prostate cancer, metastatic: I.V.: Each dose contains ≥50 million autologous CD54+ cells (obtained through leukapheresis) activated with PAP-GM-CSF, administer doses at ~2 week intervals for a total of 3 doses (Kantoff, 2010)

Adjustment for Toxicity Acute infusion reaction: Interrupt or slow infusion rate (depending on the severity of infusion reaction); may require acetaminophen, I.V. H_1 and/or H_2 antagonists, or low-dose meperidine to manage acute symptoms.

Administration For autologous use only; the identity of the patient must be matched to the patient identifiers on the infusion bag and on the "Cell Product Disposition Form" prior to infusion. Do not infuse until confirmation of product release has been received from the company. Prior to infusion, inspect bag for signs of leaks (do not administer if leaking). Gently mix to resuspend contents; inspect for clumps or clotting; small clumps should disperse with the gentle mixing; do not administer if clumps remain. A cell filter should **NOT** be used for administration. If product is expired, do NOT infuse. For I.V. infusion only.

Infuse over ~60 minutes; infuse the entire contents of the bag. If infusion is interrupted, do not resume if bag is retained at room temperature for >3 hours. Observe patient for at least 30 minutes after infusion.

Monitoring Parameters Monitor for infusion reaction for at least 30 minutes after infusion

Prescribing and Access Restrictions Patients may receive Sipuleucel-T at a participating site. Physicians must go through an inservice and register to prescribe the treatment; patients must also complete an enrollment form. Information on registration and enrollment is available at 1-877-336-3736.

Dosage Forms Excipient information presented when available (limited, particularly for generics); consult specific product labeling.

Infusion, premixed in LR [preservative free]:
Provenge®: ≥50 million autologous CD54+ cells activated with PAP-GM-CSF (250 mL)

References

Burch PA, Croghan GA, Gastineau DA, et al, "Immunotherapy (APC8015, Provenge®) Targeting Prostatic Acid Phosphatase Can Induce Durable Remission of Metastatic Androgen-Independent Prostate Cancer: A Phase 2 Trial," *Prostate*, 2004, 60(3):197-204.

Higano CS, Schellhammer PF, Small EJ, et al, "Integrated Data From 2 Randomized, Double-Blind, Placebo-Controlled, Phase 3 Trials of Active Cellular Immunotherapy With Sipuleucel-T in Advanced Prostate Cancer," *Cancer*, 2009, 115(16):3670-9.

Kantoff PW, Higano CS, Shore ND, et al, "Sipuleucel-T Immunotherapy for Castration-Resistant Prostate Cancer," *N Engl J Med*, 2010, 363(5):411-22.

Small EJ, Schellhammer PF, Higano CS, et al, "Placebo-Controlled Phase III Trial of Immunologic Therapy With Sipuleucel-T (APC8015) in Patients With Metastatic, Asymptomatic Hormone Refractory Prostate Cancer," *J Clin Oncol*, 2006, 24(19):3089-94.

Sirolimus (sir OH li mus)

Related Information

Hematopoietic Stem Cell Transplantation *on page* 1887

Brand Names: U.S. Rapamune®

Brand Names: Canada Rapamune®

Index Terms Rapamycin

Generic Availability (U.S.) No

Pharmacologic Category Immunosuppressant Agent; mTOR Kinase Inhibitor

Use Prophylaxis of organ rejection in patients receiving renal transplants

Unlabeled Use Prophylaxis of organ rejection in heart transplant recipients; prevention acute graft-versus-host disease (GVHD) in allogeneic stem cell transplantation; treatment of refractory acute or chronic GVHD; treatment of soft tissue sarcoma (chordoma, angiomyolipoma, or lymphangioleiomyomatosis)

Labeled Contraindications Hypersensitivity to sirolimus or any component of the formulation

Pregnancy Risk Factor C

Lactation Excretion in breast milk unknown/not recommended

Warnings/Precautions Hazardous agent - use appropriate precautions for handling and disposal. **[U.S. Boxed Warning]: Immunosuppressive agents, including sirolimus, increase the risk of infection and may be associated with the development of lymphoma.** Immune suppression may also increase the risk of opportunistic infections (including activation of latent viral infections including BK virus-associated nephropathy), fatal infections, and sepsis. Prophylactic treatment for *Pneumocystis jirovecii* pneumonia (PCP) should be administered for 1 year post-transplant; prophylaxis for cytomegalovirus (CMV) should be taken for 3 months post-transplant in patients at risk for CMV. Progressive multifocal leukoencephalopathy (PML), an opportunistic CNS infection caused by reactivation of the JC virus, has been reported in patients receiving immunosuppressive therapy, including sirolimus. Clinical findings of PML include apathy, ataxia, cognitive deficiency, confusion, and hemiparesis; promptly evaluate any patient presenting with neurological changes; consider decreasing the degree of immunosuppression with consideration to the risk of organ rejection in transplant patients.

[U.S. Boxed Warning]: Sirolimus is not recommended for use in liver or lung transplantation. Bronchial anastomotic dehiscence cases have been reported in lung transplant patients when sirolimus was used as

part of an immunosuppressive regimen; most of these reactions were fatal. Studies indicate an association with an increase risk of hepatic artery thrombosis (HAT), graft failure, and increased mortality (with evidence of infection) in liver transplant patients when sirolimus is used in combination with cyclosporine and/or tacrolimus. Most cases of HAT occurred within 30 days of transplant.

In renal transplant patients, *de novo* use without cyclosporine has been associated with higher rates of acute rejection. Sirolimus should be used in combination with cyclosporine (and corticosteroids) initially. Cyclosporine may be withdrawn in low-to-moderate immunologic risk patients after 2-4 months, in conjunction with an increase in sirolimus dosage. In high immunologic risk patients, use in combination with cyclosporine and corticosteroids is recommended for the first year. Safety and efficacy of combination therapy with cyclosporine in high immunologic risk patients has not been studied beyond 12 months of treatment; adjustment of immunosuppressive therapy beyond 12 months should be considered based on clinical judgement. Monitor renal function closely when combined with cyclosporine; consider dosage adjustment or discontinue in patients with increasing serum creatinine.

May increase serum creatinine and decrease GFR. Use caution when used concurrently with medications which may alter renal function. May delay recovery of renal function in patients with delayed allograft function. Increased urinary protein excretion has been observed when converting renal transplant patients from calcineurin inhibitors to sirolimus during maintenance therapy. A higher level of proteinuria prior to sirolimus conversion correlates with a higher degree of proteinuria after conversion. In some patients, proteinuria may reach nephrotic levels; nephrotic syndrome (new onset) has been reported. Increased risk of BK viral-associated nephropathy which may impair renal function and cause graft loss; consider decreasing immunosuppressive burden if evidence of deteriorating renal function.

Use caution with hepatic impairment; a reduction in the maintenance dose is recommended. Has been associated with an increased risk of fluid accumulation and lymphocele; peripheral edema, lymphedema, ascites, and pleural and pericardial effusions (including significant effusions and tamponade) were reported; use with caution in patients in whom fluid accumulation may be poorly tolerated, such as in cardiovascular disease (heart failure or hypertension) and pulmonary disease. Cases of interstitial lung disease (eg, pneumonitis, bronchiolitis obliterans organizing pneumonia [BOOP], pulmonary fibrosis) have been observed; risk may be increased with higher trough levels. Avoid concurrent use of strong CYP3A4 and/or P-glycoprotein (P-gp) inhibitors (eg, clarithromycin, erythromycin, telithromycin, itraconazole, ketoconazole, voriconazole) and strong inducers of CYP3A4 and/or P-gp (eg, rifampin, rifabutin). Concurrent use with a calcineurin inhibitor (cyclosporine, tacrolimus) may increase the risk of calcineurin inhibitor-induced hemolytic uremic syndrome/thrombotic thrombocytopenic purpura/thrombotic microangiopathy (HUS/TTP/TMA).

Hypersensitivity reactions, including anaphylactic/anaphylactoid reactions, angioedema, exfoliative dermatitis, and hypersensitivity vasculitis have been reported. Concurrent use with other drugs known to cause angioedema (eg, ACE inhibitors) may increase risk. Immunosuppressant therapy is associated with an increased risk of skin cancer; limit sun and ultraviolet light exposure; use appropriate sun protection. May increase serum lipids (cholesterol and triglycerides); use with caution in patients with hyperlipidemia. May be associated with wound dehiscence and impaired healing; use caution in the perioperative period. Patients with a body mass index (BMI) >30 kg/m^2 are at increased risk for abnormal wound healing.

Sirolimus tablets and oral solution are not bioequivalent, due to differences in absorption. Clinical equivalence was seen using 2 mg tablet and 2 mg solution. It is not known if higher doses are also clinically equivalent. Monitor sirolimus levels if changes in dosage forms are made. **[U.S. Boxed Warning]: Should only be used by physicians experienced in immunosuppressive therapy and management of transplant patients. Adequate laboratory and supportive medical resources must be readily available.** Sirolimus concentrations are dependent on the assay method (eg, chromatographic and immunoassay) used; assay methods are not interchangeable. Variations in methods to determine sirolimus whole blood concentrations, as well as interlaboratory variations, may result in improper dosage adjustments, which may lead to subtherapeutic or toxic levels. Determine the assay method used to assure consistency (or accommodations if changes occur), and for monitoring purposes, be aware of alterations to assay method or reference range. The manufacturer recommends high performance liquid chromatography (HPLC) as the reference standard to determine sirolimus trough concentrations.

Adverse Reactions Incidence of many adverse effects is dose related.

>20%:

Cardiovascular: Peripheral edema (54% to 58%), hypertension (45% to 49%), edema (18% to 20%)

Central nervous system: Headache (34%), pain (29% to 33%), insomnia (13% to 22%)

Dermatologic: Acne (22%)

Endocrine & metabolic: Hypertriglyceridemia (45% to 57%), hypercholesterolemia (43% to 46%)

Gastrointestinal: Constipation (36% to 38%), abdominal pain (29% to 36%), diarrhea (25% to 36%), nausea (25% to 31%)

Genitourinary: Urinary tract infection (26% to 33%)

Hematologic: Anemia (23% to 33%), thrombocytopenia (14% to 30%)

Neuromuscular & skeletal: Arthralgia (25% to 31%)

Renal: Serum creatinine increased (39% to 40%)

3% to 20%:

Cardiovascular: Atrial fibrillation, CHF, DVT, facial edema, hypervolemia, hypotension, orthostatic hypotension, palpitation, peripheral vascular disorder, syncope, tachycardia, thrombosis, vasodilation

Central nervous system: Anxiety, chills, confusion, depression, dizziness, emotional lability, hypoesthesia, malaise, neuropathy, somnolence

Dermatologic: Rash (10% to 20%), skin carcinoma (up to 3%; includes basal cell carcinoma, squamous cell carcinoma, melanoma), cellulitis, dermal ulcer, dermatitis (fungal), ecchymosis, hirsutism, pruritus, skin hypertrophy, wound healing abnormal

Endocrine & metabolic: Acidosis, Cushing's syndrome, dehydration, diabetes mellitus, glycosuria, hypercalcemia, hyperglycemia, hyperphosphatemia, hypocalcemia, hypoglycemia, hypokalemia, hypomagnesemia, hyponatremia

Gastrointestinal: Abdomen enlarged, anorexia, dysphagia, eructation, esophagitis, flatulence, gastritis, gastroenteritis, gingival hyperplasia, gingivitis, ileus, mouth ulceration, oral moniliasis, stomatitis, weight loss

Genitourinary: Impotence, pelvic pain, scrotal edema, testis disorder

Hematologic: Hemolytic-uremic syndrome, hemorrhage, leukopenia, leukocytosis, polycythemia, TTP
Hepatic: Abnormal liver function tests, alkaline phosphatase increased, LDH increased
Local: Thrombophlebitis
Neuromuscular & skeletal: Arthrosis, bone necrosis, CPK increased, hyper-/hypotonia, leg cramps, myalgia, osteoporosis, paresthesia, tetany
Ocular: Abnormal vision, cataract, conjunctivitis
Otic: Ear pain, otitis media, tinnitus
Renal: Albuminuria, bladder pain, BUN increased, dysuria, hematuria, hydronephrosis, kidney pain, nephropathy (toxic), nocturia, oliguria, pyelonephritis, pyuria, tubular necrosis, urinary frequency, urinary incontinence, urinary retention
Respiratory: Asthma, atelectasis, bronchitis, cough, epistaxis, hypoxia, lung edema, pleural effusion, pneumonia, pulmonary embolism, rhinitis, sinusitis
Miscellaneous: Lymphoproliferative disease/lymphoma (1% to 3%), abscess, diaphoresis, flu-like syndrome, hernia, herpesvirus infection, infection (including opportunistic), lymphadenopathy, lymphocele, peritonitis, sepsis

<3%, postmarketing, and/or case reports: ALT increased, alveolar proteinosis, anaphylactoid reaction, anaphylaxis, anastomotic disruption, angioedema, ascites, AST increased, azoospermia, *Clostridium difficile* colitis, cytomegalovirus, Epstein-Barr virus, exfoliative dermatitis, fascial dehiscence, focal segmental glomerulosclerosis, hepatic necrosis, hepatotoxicity, hypersensitivity reaction, hypersensitivity vasculitis, hypophosphatemia, incisional hernia; interstitial lung disease (dose-related; includes pneumonitis, pulmonary fibrosis, and bronchiolitis obliterans organizing pneumonia [BOOP] with no identified infectious etiology); joint disorders, lymphedema, myocardial infarction, mycobacterial infection, nephropathy (BK virus-associated), nephrotic syndrome, neutropenia, pancreatitis, pancytopenia, pericardial effusion, *Pneumocystis* pneumonia, progressive multifocal leukoencephalopathy (PML), proteinuria, pulmonary hemorrhage, reversible posterior leukoencephalopathy syndrome (RPLS), tamponade, tuberculosis, wound dehiscence

Note: Hepatic artery thrombosis (HAT) and graft failure have been reported in liver transplant patients (not an approved use); bronchial anastomotic dehiscence has been reported in lung transplant patients (not an approved use)

Drug Interactions

Metabolism/Transport Effects Substrate of CYP3A4 (major), P-glycoprotein; **Note:** Assignment of Major/Minor substrate status based on clinically relevant drug interaction potential; **Inhibits** CYP3A4 (weak)

Avoid Concomitant Use

Avoid concomitant use of Sirolimus with any of the following: BCG; CloZAPine; Conivaptan; Crizotinib; Enzalutamide; Mifepristone; Natalizumab; Pimecrolimus; Pimozide; Posaconazole; Tacrolimus (Topical); Vaccines (Live); Voriconazole

Increased Effect/Toxicity

Sirolimus may increase the levels/effects of: ACE Inhibitors; ARIPiprazole; CloZAPine; CycloSPORINE (Systemic); Leflunomide; Natalizumab; Pimozide; Tacrolimus (Systemic); Tacrolimus (Topical); Vaccines (Live)

The levels/effects of Sirolimus may be increased by: Boceprevir; Conivaptan; Crizotinib; CycloSPORINE (Systemic); CYP3A4 Inhibitors (Moderate); CYP3A4 Inhibitors (Strong); Dasatinib; Denosumab; Fluconazole; Itraconazole; Ivacaftor; Ketoconazole (Systemic); Macrolide Antibiotics; Mifepristone; P-glycoprotein/ABCB1 Inhibitors; Pimecrolimus; Posaconazole; Protease

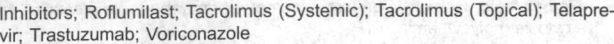

Inhibitors; Roflumilast; Tacrolimus (Systemic); Tacrolimus (Topical); Telaprevir; Trastuzumab; Voriconazole

Decreased Effect

Sirolimus may decrease the levels/effects of: BCG; Coccidioidin Skin Test; Sipuleucel-T; Tacrolimus (Systemic); Vaccines (Inactivated); Vaccines (Live)

The levels/effects of Sirolimus may be decreased by: CYP3A4 Inducers (Strong); Deferasirox; Echinacea; Efavirenz; Enzalutamide; Fosphenytoin; Herbs (CYP3A4 Inducers); P-glycoprotein/ABCB1 Inducers; Phenytoin; Rifampin; Tocilizumab

Ethanol/Nutrition/Herb Interactions

Food: Grapefruit juice may decrease clearance of sirolimus. Ingestion with high-fat meals decreases peak concentrations but increases AUC by 23% to 35%. Management: Avoid grapefruit juice. Take consistently (either with or without food) to minimize variability.

Herb/Nutraceutical: St John's wort may decrease sirolimus levels. Some herbal medications have immunostimulant properties (eg, echinacea). Herbs with hypoglycemic properties may increase the risk of sirolimus-induced hypoglycemia (eg, alfalfa). Management: Avoid St John's wort, cat's claw, and echinacea. Avoid alfalfa, aloe, bilberry, bitter melon, burdock, celery, damiana, fenugreek, garcinia, garlic, ginger, ginseng (American), gymnema, marshmallow, and stinging nettle.

Storage/Stability

Oral solution: Store under refrigeration, 2°C to 8°C (36°F to 46°F). Protect from light. A slight haze may develop in refrigerated solutions, but the quality of the product is not affected. After opening, solution should be used in 1 month. If necessary, may be stored at temperatures up to 25°C (77°F) for ≤15 days after opening. Product may be stored in amber syringe for a maximum of 24 hours (at room temperature or refrigerated). Discard syringe after single use. Solution should be used immediately following dilution.

Tablet: Store at room temperature of 20°C to 25°C (68°F to 77°F). Protect from light.

Mechanism of Action Sirolimus inhibits T-lymphocyte activation and proliferation in response to antigenic and cytokine stimulation and inhibits antibody production. Its mechanism differs from other immunosuppressants. Sirolimus binds to FKBP-12, an intracellular protein, to form an immunosuppressive complex which inhibits the regulatory kinase, mTOR (mammalian target of rapamycin). This inhibition suppresses cytokine mediated T-cell proliferation, halting progression from the G1 to the S phase of the cell cycle. It inhibits acute rejection of allografts and prolongs graft survival.

Pharmacodynamics/Kinetics

Absorption: Rapid

Distribution: 12 L/kg (range: 4-20 L/kg)

Protein binding: ~92%, primarily to albumin

Metabolism: Extensive; in intestinal wall via P-glycoprotein and hepatic via CYP3A4; to 7 major metabolites

Bioavailability: Oral solution: 14%; Oral tablet: 18%

Half-life elimination: Mean: 62 hours (range: 46-78 hours); extended in hepatic impairment (Child-Pugh class A or B) to 113 hours

Time to peak: Oral solution: 1-3 hours; Tablet: 1-6 hours

Excretion: Feces (91% due to P-glycoprotein-mediated efflux into gut lumen); urine (2%)

Dosing

Adult & Geriatric

Low-to-moderate immunologic risk renal transplant patients: Oral:

<40 kg: Loading dose: 3 mg/m^2 on day 1, followed by maintenance dosing of 1 mg/m^2 once daily

≥40 kg: Loading dose: 6 mg on day 1; maintenance: 2 mg once daily

High immunologic risk renal transplant patients: Oral: Loading dose: Up to 15 mg on day 1; maintenance: 5 mg/day; obtain trough concentration between days 5-7 and adjust accordingly. Continue concurrent cyclosporine/sirolimus therapy for 1 year following transplantation. Further adjustment of the regimen must be based on clinical status.

Dosage adjustment: Sirolimus dosages should be adjusted to maintain trough concentrations within desired range based on risk and concomitant therapy. Maximum daily dose: 40 mg. Dosage should be adjusted at intervals of 7-14 days to account for the long half-life of sirolimus. In general, dose proportionality may be assumed. New sirolimus dose **equals** current dose **multiplied by** (target concentration **divided by** current concentration). **Note:** If large dose increase is required, consider loading dose calculated as:

Loading dose **equals** (new maintenance dose **minus** current maintenance dose) **multiplied by** 3

Maximum dose in 1 day: 40 mg; if required dose is >40 mg (due to loading dose), divide loading dose over 2 days. Whole blood concentrations should not be used as the sole basis for dosage adjustment (monitor clinical signs/symptoms, tissue biopsy, and laboratory parameters).

Maintenance therapy after withdrawal of cyclosporine: Cyclosporine withdrawal is not recommended in high immunological risk patients. Following 2-4 months of combined therapy, withdrawal of cyclosporine may be considered in low-to-moderate immunologic risk patients. Cyclosporine should be discontinued over 4-8 weeks, and a necessary increase in the dosage of sirolimus (up to fourfold) should be anticipated due to removal of metabolic inhibition by cyclosporine and to maintain adequate immunosuppressive effects. Dose-adjusted trough target concentrations are typically 16-24 ng/mL for the first year post-transplant and 12-20 ng/mL thereafter (measured by chromatographic methodology).

GVHD prophylaxis (unlabeled use): Oral: 12 mg loading dose on day -3, followed by 4 mg daily (target trough level: 3-12 ng/mL); taper off after 6-9 months (Armand, 2008; Cutler, 2007)

Treatment of refractory acute GVHD (unlabeled use): Oral: 4-5 mg/m^2 for 14 days (no loading dose) (Benito, 2001)

Treatment of chronic GVHD (unlabeled use): Oral: 6 mg loading dose, followed by 2 mg daily (target trough level: 7-12 ng/mL) for 6-9 months (Couriel, 2005)

Pediatric

Immunosuppression: Children ≥13 years: Oral: Refer to adult dosing.

Renal Impairment No dosage adjustment (in loading or maintenance dose) is necessary in renal impairment. However, adjustment of regimen (including discontinuation of therapy) should be considered when used concurrently with cyclosporine and elevated or increasing serum creatinine is noted.

Hepatic Impairment

Loading dose: No adjustment required

Maintenance dose:

Mild-to-moderate hepatic impairment: reduce maintenance dose by ~33%.

Severe hepatic impairment: reduce maintenance dose by ~50%.

Administration Initial dose should be administered as soon as possible after transplant. Sirolimus should be taken 4 hours after oral cyclosporine (Neoral® or Gengraf®). Should be administered consistently (with or without food).

Solution: Mix (by stirring vigorously) with at least 2 ounces of water or orange juice. No other liquids should be used for dilution. Patient should drink diluted solution immediately. The cup should then be refilled with an additional 4 ounces of water or orange juice, stirred vigorously, and the patient should drink the contents at once.

Tablet: Do not crush, split, or chew.

Monitoring Parameters Monitor LFTs and CBC during treatment. Monitor sirolimus levels in all patients (especially in pediatric patients, patients ≥13 years of age weighing <40 kg, patients with hepatic impairment, or on concurrent potent inhibitors or inducers of CYP3A4 or P-gp, and/or if cyclosporine dosing is markedly reduced or discontinued), and when changing dosage forms of sirolimus. Also monitor serum cholesterol and triglycerides, blood pressure, serum creatinine, and urinary protein. Serum drug concentrations should be determined 3-4 days after loading doses and 7-14 days after dosage adjustments; however, these concentrations should not be used as the sole basis for dosage adjustment, especially during withdrawal of cyclosporine (monitor clinical signs/symptoms, tissue biopsy, and laboratory parameters). **Note:** Concentrations and ranges are dependent on and will vary with assay methodology (chromatographic or immunoassay); assay methods are not interchangeable.

Dietary Considerations Take consistently (with or without food) to minimize variability of absorption.

Additional Information Sirolimus tablets and oral solution are not bioequivalent, due to differences in absorption. Clinical equivalence was seen using 2 mg tablet and 2 mg solution. It is not known if higher doses are also clinically equivalent. Monitor sirolimus levels if changes in dosage forms are made.

Sirolimus solution may cause irritation if administered undiluted.

High-risk renal transplant patients are defined (per the manufacturer's labeling) as African-American transplant recipients and/or repeat renal transplant recipients who lost a previous allograft based on an immunologic process and/or patients with high PRA (panel-reactive antibodies; peak PRA level >80%). Individual transplant centers may have differences in their definitions. For example, some centers would consider a PRA >50% to be at higher risk of rejection.

Medication Guide Available Yes

Dosage Forms Excipient information presented when available (limited, particularly for generics); consult specific product labeling.

Solution, oral:

Rapamune®: 1 mg/mL (60 mL) [contains ethanol 1.5%-2.5%, propylene glycol, soy]

Tablet, oral:

Rapamune®: 0.5 mg, 1 mg, 2 mg

References

Antin J, Kim H, Cutler C, et al, "Sirolimus, Tacrolimus, and Low-Dose Methotrexate for Graft-Versus-Host Disease Prophylaxis in Mismatched Related Donor or Unrelated Donor Transplantation," *Blood*, 2003, 102(5):1601-5.

Armand P, Gannamaneni S, Kim HT, et al, "Improved Survival in Lymphoma Patients Receiving Sirolimus for Graft-Versus-Host Disease Prophylaxis After Allogeneic Hematopoietic Stem-Cell Transplantation With Reduced-Intensity Conditioning," *J Clin Oncol*, 2008, 26(35):5767-74.

Benito AI, Furlong T, Martin PJ, et al, "Sirolimus (Rapamycin) for the Treatment of Steroid-Refractory Acute Graft-Versus-Host Disease," *Transplantation*, 2001, 72(12):1924-9.

Bissler JJ, McCormack FX, Young LR, et al, "Sirolimus for Angiomyolipoma in Tuberous Sclerosis Complex or Lymphangioleiomyomatosis," *N Engl J Med*, 2008, 358(2):140-51.

Couriel DR, Saliba R, Escalon MP, et al, "Sirolimus in Combination With Tacrolimus and Corticosteroids for the Treatment of Resistant Chronic Graft-Versus-Host Disease," *Br J Haematol*, 2005, 130(3):409-17.

Cutler C, Kim H, Hochberg E, et al, "Sirolimus and Tacrolimus Without Methotrexate as Graft-Versus-Host Disease Prophylaxis After Matched Related Donor Peripheral Blood Stem Cell Transplantation," *Biol Blood Marrow Transplant*, 2004, 10(5):328-36.

Cutler C, Li S, Ho VT, et al, "Extended Follow-Up of Methotrexate-Free Immunosuppression Using Sirolimus and Tacrolimus in Related and Unrelated Donor Peripheral Blood Stem Cell Transplantation," *Blood*, 2007, 109(7):3108-14.

Kahan BD, "Efficacy of Sirolimus Compared With Azathioprine for Reduction of Acute Renal Allograft Rejection: A Randomised Multicentre Study. The Rapamune US Study Group," *Lancet*, 2000, 356(9225):194-202.

McDonald AS, "A Worldwide, Phase III, Randomized, Controlled, Safety and Efficacy Study of a Sirolimus/Cyclosporine Regimen for Prevention of Acute Rejection in Recipients of Primary Mismatched Renal Allografts. RAPAMUNE Global Study Group," *Transplantation*, 2001, 71 (2):271-80.

National Comprehensive Cancer Network® (NCCN), "Clinical Practice Guidelines in Oncology™: Soft Tissue Sarcoma," Version 2.2010. Available at http://www.nccn.org/professionals/physician_gls/PDF/sarcoma.pdf

Raichlin E, Bae JH, Khalpey Z, et al, "Conversion to Sirolimus as Primary Immunosuppression Attenuates the Progression of Allograft Vasculopathy After Cardiac Transplantation," *Circulation*, 2007, 116(23):2726-33.

- **SKF 104864** *see* Topotecan *on page 1371*
- **SKF 104864-A** *see* Topotecan *on page 1371*
- **SKI-606** *see* Bosutinib *on page 195*
- **S-leucovorin** *see* LEVOleucovorin *on page 888*
- **6S-leucovorin** *see* LEVOleucovorin *on page 888*
- **153Sm-Lexidronam** *see* Samarium Sm 153 Lexidronam *on page 1268*
- **SMX-TMP** *see* Sulfamethoxazole and Trimethoprim *on page 1302*
- **SMZ-TMP** *see* Sulfamethoxazole and Trimethoprim *on page 1302*
- **Sodium 2-Mercaptoethane Sulfonate** *see* Mesna *on page 940*
- **Sodium Ferric Gluconate** *see* Ferric Gluconate *on page 597*
- **Sodium Hyposulfate** *see* Sodium Thiosulfate *on page 1289*
- **Sodium Nafcillin** *see* Nafcillin *on page 1026*

Sodium Thiosulfate (SOW dee um thye oh SUL fate)

Related Information

Management of Drug Extravasations *on page 1800*

Index Terms Disodium Thiosulfate Pentahydrate; Pentahydrate; Sodium Hyposulfate; Sodium Thiosulphate; Thiosulfuric Acid Disodium Salt

Generic Availability (U.S.) Yes

Pharmacologic Category Antidote

Use Treatment of cyanide poisoning

Unlabeled Use Management of mechlorethamine extravasation

Labeled Contraindications There are no contraindications listed within the manufacturer's labeling.

Pregnancy Risk Factor C

Warnings/Precautions Due to the risk for serious adverse effects, use with caution in patients where the diagnosis of cyanide poisoning is uncertain. However, if clinical suspicion of cyanide poisoning is high, treatment should not be delayed. Treatment of cyanide poisoning should include decontamination and supportive therapy. Collection of pretreatment blood cyanide concentrations does not preclude administration and should not delay administration in the emergency management of highly suspected or confirmed cyanide toxicity. Pretreatment levels may be useful as postinfusion levels may be inaccurate. Monitor patients for return of symptoms for 24-48 hours; repeat treatment should be administered if symptoms return. Fire victims may present with both cyanide and carbon monoxide poisoning. In this scenario, sodium thiosulfate may be used alone to promote the clearance of cyanide. Hydroxocobalamin, however, may be considered because sodium thiosulfate has a slow onset of action. Consider consultation with a poison control center at 1-800-222-1222.

The presence of sulfite hypersensitivity should not preclude the use of this medication.

Adverse Reactions Frequency not defined

Cardiovascular: Hypotension

Central nervous system: Disorientation, headache

Gastrointestinal: Nausea, salty taste, vomiting

Hematologic: Bleeding time prolonged

Miscellaneous: Warmth

Drug Interactions

Metabolism/Transport Effects None known.

Avoid Concomitant Use There are no known interactions where it is recommended to avoid concomitant use.

Increased Effect/Toxicity There are no known significant interactions involving an increase in effect.

Decreased Effect There are no known significant interactions involving a decrease in effect.

Storage/Stability Store at 20°C to 25°C (68°F to 77°F); excursions permitted to 15°C to 30°C (59°F to 86°F).

Store the 1/6 M solution for SubQ administration (unlabeled route) at 15°C to 30°C (59°F to 86°F) (Polovich, 2009).

Reconstitution To prepare a 1/6 M solution for SubQ administration (unlabeled route), add 4 mL of a 10% sodium thiosulfate solution to 6 mL SWFI or 1.6 mL of a 25% sodium thiosulfate solution to 8.4 mL SWFI.

Mechanism of Action

Cyanide toxicity: Serves as a sulfur donor in rhodanese-catalyzed formation of thiocyanate (much less toxic than cyanide)

Mechlorethamine extravasation: Neutralizes the reactive species of mechlorethamine; reduces the formation of hydroxyl radicals

Pharmacodynamics/Kinetics

Half-life elimination: Thiosulfate: ~3 hours; Thiocyanate: ~3 days; Renal impairment: ≤9 days

Excretion: Urine (~20% to 50% as unchanged drug)

Dosing

Adult & Geriatric

Cyanide poisoning: I.V.: **Note:** Usually given in conjunction with sodium nitrite. Administer sodium nitrite first, followed immediately by the administration of sodium thiosulfate: 12.5 g (50 mL of a 25% solution); may repeat at one-half the original dose if symptoms of cyanide toxicity return

Note: Monitor the patient for 24-48 hours; if symptoms return, repeat both sodium nitrite and sodium thiosulfate at one-half the original doses.

Mechlorethamine extravasation (unlabeled route/use): SubQ: 1/6 M (~4%) solution: Inject 2 mL for each mg of mechlorethamine suspected to have extravasated (Polovich, 2009)

Pediatric

Cyanide poisoning: I.V.: **Note:** Usually given in conjunction with sodium nitrite. Administer sodium nitrite first, followed immediately by the administration of sodium thiosulfate. 7 g/m^2 or 250 mg/kg (1 mL/kg or 28-40 mL/m^2 of a 25% solution); maximum dose: 12.5 g (50 mL of a 25% solution); may repeat at one-half the original dose if symptoms of cyanide toxicity return

Note: Monitor the patient for 24-48 hours; if symptoms return, repeat both sodium nitrite and sodium thiosulfate at one-half the original doses.

Mechlorethamine extravasation (unlabeled route/use): SubQ: Refer to adult dosing.

Renal Impairment No dosage adjustment provided in the manufacturer's labeling; however, renal elimination of sodium thiosulfate is significant and risk of adverse effects may be increased in patients with renal impairment.

Hepatic Impairment No dosage adjustment provided in the manufacturer's labeling (has not been studied).

Administration

I.V.: Administer over 10-20 minutes using a 0.22 micron in-line filter

SubQ (unlabeled route): Inject into the extravasation site using ≤25-gauge needle; change needle with each injection (Polovich, 2009)

Monitoring Parameters

Cyanide poisoning: Monitor for at least 24-48 hours after administration; blood pressure and heart rate during and after infusion; hemoglobin/hematocrit; co-oximetry; serum lactate levels; venous-arterial PO_2 gradient; serum methemoglobin and oxyhemoglobin. Pretreatment cyanide levels may be useful diagnostically.

Mechlorethamine extravasation: Monitor extravasation site for pain, blister formation, skin sloughing, arm/hand swelling/stiffness; monitor for fever, chills, or worsening pain

Dosage Forms Excipient information presented when available (limited, particularly for generics); consult specific product labeling.

Injection, solution [preservative free]: 100 mg/mL (10 mL); 250 mg/mL (50 mL)

Injection, solution: 250 mg/mL (50 mL)

References

Bailey B, "Are There Teratogenic Risks Associated With Antidotes Used in the Acute Management of Poisoned Pregnant Women?" *Birth Defects Res A Clin Mol Teratol*, 2003, 67(2):133-40.

Bertelli G, "Prevention and Management of Extravasation of Cytotoxic Drugs," *Drug Saf*, 1995, 12 (4):245-55.

Dorr RT, "Antidotes to Vesicant Chemotherapy Extravasations," *Blood Rev*, 1990, 4(1):41-60.

Eckstein M, "Enhancing Public Health Preparedness for a Terrorist Attack Involving Cyanide," *J Emerg Med*, 2008, 35(1):59-62.

Ener RA, Meglathery SB, and Styler M, "Extravasation of Systemic Hemato-Oncological Therapies," *Ann Oncol*, 2004, 15(6):858-62.

Geller RJ, Barthold C, Saiers JA, et al, "Pediatric Cyanide Poisoning: Causes, Manifestations, Management, and Unmet Needs," *Pediatrics*, 2006, 118(5):2146-58.

Mullin S, Beckwith MC, Tyler LS, "Prevention and Management of Antineoplastic Extravasation Injury," *Hospital Pharmacy*, 2000, 35(1):57-76.

Polovich M, Whitford JN and Olsen M, *Chemotherapy and Biotherapy Guidelines and Reccomendations for Practice*, 3rd ed, Pittsburgh, PA: Oncology Nursing Society, 2009.

- **Sodium Thiosulphate** *see* Sodium Thiosulfate *on page* 1289
- **Soliris®** *see* Eculizumab *on page* 490
- **Soltamox™** *see* Tamoxifen *on page* 1324
- **Solu-CORTEF®** *see* Hydrocortisone (Systemic) *on page* 713
- **Solu-Cortef® (Can)** *see* Hydrocortisone (Systemic) *on page* 713
- **Solumedrol** *see* MethylPREDNISolone *on page* 967
- **Solu-MEDROL®** *see* MethylPREDNISolone *on page* 967
- **Solu-Medrol® (Can)** *see* MethylPREDNISolone *on page* 967
- **Somatuline® Autogel® (Can)** *see* Lanreotide *on page* 851
- **Somatuline® Depot** *see* Lanreotide *on page* 851

SORAfenib (sor AF e nib)

Related Information

Management of Chemotherapy-Induced Nausea and Vomiting *on page* 1786
Principles of Anticancer Therapy *on page* 1878
Safe Handling of Hazardous Drugs *on page* 1904

Brand Names: U.S. NexAVAR®

Brand Names: Canada Nexavar®

Index Terms BAY 43-9006; Sorafenib Tosylate

Generic Availability (U.S.) No

Pharmacologic Category Antineoplastic Agent, Tyrosine Kinase Inhibitor; Vascular Endothelial Growth Factor (VEGF) Inhibitor

Use Treatment of advanced renal cell cancer (RCC); treatment of unresectable hepatocellular cancer (HCC)

Unlabeled Use Treatment of advanced thyroid cancer, recurrent or metastatic angiosarcoma, resistant gastrointestinal stromal tumor (GIST)

Labeled Contraindications Hypersensitivity to sorafenib or any component of the formulation; use in combination with carboplatin and paclitaxel in patients with squamous cell lung cancer

Pregnancy Risk Factor D

Lactation Excretion in breast milk unknown/not recommended

Warnings/Precautions Hazardous agent - use appropriate precautions for handling and disposal. May cause hypertension (generally mild-to-moderate), especially in the first 6 weeks of treatment; monitor; use caution in patients with underlying or poorly-controlled hypertension; consider discontinuing (temporary or permanent) in patients who develop severe or persistent hypertension while on appropriate antihypertensive therapy. May cause cardiac ischemia or infarction; consider discontinuing (temporarily or permanently) in patients who develop these; use in patients with unstable coronary artery disease or recent myocardial infarction has not been studied. QT prolongation has been observed; may increase the risk for ventricular arrhythmia. Avoid use in patients with congenital long QT syndrome; use with caution and monitor closely in patients with heart failure, bradyarrhythmias, concurrent medications know to prolong the QT interval, and electrolyte (calcium, magnesium, potassium) imbalances.

Serious bleeding events may occur (consider permanently discontinuing if serious); monitor PT/INR in patients on warfarin therapy. May complicate wound healing; temporarily withhold treatment for patients undergoing major surgical procedures (the appropriate timing for reinitiation after surgical procedures has not been determined). Gastrointestinal perforation has been reported (rare); monitor patients for signs/symptoms (abdominal pain, constipation, or vomiting); discontinue treatment if gastrointestinal perforation occurs. Avoid concurrent use with strong CYP3A4 inducers (eg, carbamazepine, dexamethasone, phenobarbital, phenytoin, rifampin, St John's wort); may decrease sorafenib levels/effects. Use caution when administering sorafenib with compounds that are metabolized predominantly via UGT1A1 (eg, irinotecan). Use in combination with carboplatin and paclitaxel in patients with squamous cell lung cancer is contraindicated.

Hand-foot skin reaction and rash are the most common adverse events and typically appear within the first 6 weeks of treatment; usually managed with topical treatment, treatment delays, and/or dose reductions. Consider permanently discontinuing with severe or persistent dermatological toxicities. The risk for hand-foot syndrome increased with cumulative doses of sorafenib. The incidence of hand-foot syndrome is also increased in patients treated with sorafenib plus bevacizumab in comparison to those treated with sorafenib monotherapy. Severe dermatologic toxicities, including Stevens-Johnson syndrome (SJS) and toxic epidermal necrolysis (TEN) have been reported; may be life-threatening; discontinue sorafenib for suspected SJS or TEN.

Sorafenib levels in patients with mild-to-moderate hepatic impairment (Child-Pugh classes A and B) were similar to levels observed in patients without hepatic impairment; has not been studied in patients with severe hepatic impairment. In a small study of Asian patients with advanced HCC, sorafenib demonstrated efficacy with adequate tolerability in a hepatitis B-endemic area (Yau, 2009). There have been reports of sorafenib-induced hepatitis (including hepatic failure and death) which is characterized by hepatocellular liver damage and transaminase increases (significant), increased bilirubin and INR may also occur. Monitor hepatic function regularly; discontinue sorafenib for unexplained significant transaminase increases.

Adverse Reactions

>10%:

Cardiovascular: Hypertension (9% to 17%; grade 3: 3% to 4%; grade 4: <1%; onset: ~3 weeks)

Central nervous system: Fatigue (37% to 46%), sensory neuropathy (≤13%), pain (11%)

Dermatologic: Rash/desquamation (19% to 40%; grade 3: ≤1%), hand-foot syndrome (21% to 30%; grade 3: 6% to 8%), alopecia (14% to 27%), pruritus (14% to 19%), dry skin (10% to 11%), erythema

Endocrine & metabolic: Hypoalbuminemia (≤59%), hypophosphatemia (35% to 45%; grade 3: 11% to 13%; grade 4: <1%), hypocalcemia (12% to 27%)

Gastrointestinal: Diarrhea (43% to 55%; grade 3: 2% to 10%; grade 4: <1%), lipase increased (40% to 41% [usually transient]), amylase increased (30% to 34% [usually transient]), abdominal pain (11% to 31%), weight loss (10% to 30%), anorexia (16% to 29%), nausea (23% to 24%), vomiting (15% to 16%), constipation (14% to 15%)

Hematologic: Lymphopenia (23% to 47%; grades 3/4: ≤13%), thrombocytopenia (12% to 46%; grades 3/4: 1% to 4%), INR increased (≤42%), neutropenia (≤18%; grades 3/4: ≤5%), hemorrhage (15% to 18%; grade 3: 2% to 3%; grade 4: ≤2%), leukopenia

Hepatic: Liver dysfunction (≤11%; grade 3: 2%; grade 4: 1%)

Neuromuscular & skeletal: Muscle pain, weakness

Respiratory: Dyspnea (≤14%), cough (≤13%)

1% to 10%:

Cardiovascular: Cardiac ischemia/infarction (≤3%), heart failure (2%, congestive), flushing

Central nervous system: Headache (≤10%), depression, fever

Dermatologic: Acne, exfoliative dermatitis

Gastrointestinal: Appetite decreased, dyspepsia, dysphagia, esophageal varices bleeding (2%), glossodynia, mucositis, stomatitis, xerostomia

Genitourinary: Erectile dysfunction

Hematologic: Anemia

Hepatic: Transaminases increased (transient)

Neuromuscular & skeletal: Joint pain (≤10%), arthralgia, myalgia

Renal: Renal failure

Respiratory: Hoarseness

Miscellaneous: Flu-like syndrome

<1%, postmarketing, and/or case reports: Acute renal failure, alkaline phosphatase increased, anaphylactic reaction, angioedema, aortic dissection, arrhythmia, bilirubin increased, bone pain, cardiac failure, cerebral hemorrhage, cholangitis, cholecystitis, dehydration, eczema, epistaxis, erythema multiforme, folliculitis, gastritis, gastrointestinal hemorrhage, gastrointestinal perforation, gastrointestinal reflux, gynecomastia, hepatic failure, hepatitis, hypersensitivity (skin reaction, urticaria), hypertensive crisis, hyper-/hypothyroidism, hyponatremia, infection, interstitial lung disease (acute respiratory distress, interstitial pneumonia, lung inflammation, pneumonitis, pulmonitis, radiation pneumonitis), jaundice, MI, mouth pain, muscle wasting, myocardial ischemia, nephrotic syndrome, osteonecrosis of the jaw, pancreatitis, pleural effusion, preeclampsia-like syndrome (reversible hypertension and proteinuria), QT prolongation, respiratory hemorrhage, reversible posterior leukoencephalopathy syndrome (RPLS), rhabdomyolysis, rhinorrhea, skin cancer (squamous cell/keratoacanthomas), Stevens-Johnson syndrome, thromboembolism, tinnitus, toxic epidermal necrolysis (TEN), transient ischemic attack, tumor lysis syndrome, tumor pain, voice alteration

Drug Interactions

Metabolism/Transport Effects **Substrate** of CYP3A4 (minor), UGT1A9; **Note:** Assignment of Major/Minor substrate status based on clinically relevant drug interaction potential; **Inhibits** CYP2B6 (moderate), CYP2C8 (strong), CYP2C9 (moderate), UGT1A1, UGT1A9

Avoid Concomitant Use

Avoid concomitant use of SORAfenib with any of the following: BCG; CARBOplatin; CloZAPine; CYP3A4 Inducers (Strong); Enzalutamide; Natalizumab; PACLitaxel; Pimecrolimus; St Johns Wort; Tacrolimus (Topical); Vaccines (Live)

Increased Effect/Toxicity

SORAfenib may increase the levels/effects of: Acetaminophen; CARBOplatin; Carvedilol; CloZAPine; CYP2B6 Substrates; CYP2C8 Substrates; CYP2C9 Substrates; DOCEtaxel; DOXOrubicin; Enzalutamide; Fluorouracil (Systemic); Fluorouracil (Topical); Irinotecan; Leflunomide; Natalizumab; PACLitaxel; Pioglitazone; Treprostinil; Vaccines (Live); Vitamin K Antagonists; Warfarin

The levels/effects of SORAfenib may be increased by: Acetaminophen; Bevacizumab; CYP3A4 Inhibitors (Strong); Denosumab; Pimecrolimus; Roflumilast; Tacrolimus (Topical); Trastuzumab

Decreased Effect

SORAfenib may decrease the levels/effects of: BCG; Cardiac Glycosides; Coccidioidin Skin Test; Dacarbazine; Fluorouracil (Systemic); Fluorouracil (Topical); Sipuleucel-T; Vaccines (Inactivated); Vaccines (Live); Vitamin K Antagonists

The levels/effects of SORAfenib may be decreased by: CYP3A4 Inducers (Strong); Echinacea; Herbs (CYP3A4 Inducers); Neomycin; St Johns Wort; Tocilizumab

Ethanol/Nutrition/Herb Interactions

Food: Bioavailability is decreased 29% with a high-fat meal (bioavailability is similar to fasting state when administered with a moderate-fat meal). Management: Administer on an empty stomach 1 hour before or 2 hours after eating.

Herb/Nutraceutical: St John's wort may decrease the levels/effects of sorafenib. Management: Avoid St John's wort.

Storage/Stability Store at room temperature of 25°C (77°F); excursions permitted to 15°C and 30°C (59°F and 86°F). Protect from moisture.

Mechanism of Action Multikinase inhibitor; inhibits tumor growth and angiogenesis by inhibiting intracellular Raf kinases (CRAF, BRAF, and mutant BRAF), and cell surface kinase receptors (VEGFR-1, VEGFR-2, VEGFR-3, PDGFR-beta, cKIT, FLT-3, and RET)

Pharmacodynamics/Kinetics

Protein binding: 99.5%

Metabolism: Hepatic, via CYP3A4 (primarily oxidated to the pyridine N-oxide; active, minor) and UGT1A9 (glucuronidation)

Bioavailability: 38% to 49%; reduced when administered with a high-fat meal

Half-life elimination: 25-48 hours

Time to peak, plasma: ~3 hours

Excretion: Feces (77%, 51% of dose as unchanged drug); urine (19%, as metabolites)

Dosing

Adult & Geriatric

Advanced renal cell carcinoma: Oral: 400 mg twice daily; continue until no longer clinically benefiting or until unacceptable toxicity

Hepatocellular cancer: Oral: 400 mg twice daily; continue until no longer clinically benefiting or until unacceptable toxicity

Angiosarcoma (unlabeled use): Oral: 400 mg twice daily (Maki, 2009)

Gastrointestinal stromal tumor (GIST) (unlabeled use): Oral: 400 mg twice daily (Wiebe, 2008)

Thyroid cancer (unlabeled use): Oral: 400 mg twice daily (Gupta-Abramson, 2008)

Dosage adjustment for concomitant CYP3A4 inducers: Avoid the concomitant use of a strong CYP3A4 inducer (eg, carbamazepine, dexamethasone, phenobarbital, phenytoin, rifampin, St. John's wort) with sorafenib.

Renal Impairment

Manufacturer's recommendations: No dosage adjustment necessary for mild, moderate, or severe renal impairment (not dependent on dialysis); has not been studied in dialysis patients.

Alternate recommendations: Safety and pharmacokinetics were studied in varying degrees of renal dysfunction with the following empiric dose levels recommended based on patient tolerance (Miller, 2009):

Mild renal dysfunction (Cl_{cr} 40-59 mL/minute): 400 mg twice daily

Moderate renal dysfunction (Cl_{cr} 20-39 mL/minute): 200 mg twice daily
Severe renal dysfunction (Cl_{cr} <20 mL/minute): Data inadequate to define dose
Hemodialysis (any Cl_{cr}): 200 mg once daily

Hepatic Impairment

Manufacturer's recommendations: No adjustment is required for mild (Child-Pugh class A) to moderate (Child-Pugh class B) hepatic impairment at baseline; not studied in severe hepatic impairment (Child-Pugh class C). Discontinue treatment for unexplained significant increases in transaminases.

Alternate recommendations: Safety and pharmacokinetics were studied in varying degrees of hepatic dysfunction with the following empiric dose levels recommended based on patient tolerance (Miller, 2009):

Mild hepatic dysfunction (bilirubin >1 to ≤1.5 times ULN and/or AST >ULN): 400 mg twice daily
Moderate hepatic dysfunction (bilirubin >1.5 to ≤3 times ULN; any AST): 200 mg twice daily
Severe hepatic dysfunction:
Bilirubin >3-10 x ULN (any AST): 200 mg every 3 days was **not** tolerated
Albumin <2.5 g/dL (any bilirubin and any AST): 200 mg once daily

Adjustment for Toxicity Temporary interruption and/or dosage reduction may be necessary for management of adverse drug reactions. The dose may be reduced to 400 mg once daily and then further reduced to 400 mg every other day.

Dose modification for severe/persistent hypertension (despite antihypertensive therapy) or cardiac ischemia/infarction: Consider temporarily or permanently discontinuing treatment.

Dose modification for gastrointestinal perforation: Permanently discontinue treatment.

Dose modification for hemorrhage requiring medical intervention: Consider permanently discontinuing treatment.

Dose modification for skin toxicity:

Grade 1 (numbness, dysesthesia, paresthesia, tingling, painless swelling, erythema, or discomfort of the hands or feet which do not disrupt normal activities): Continue sorafenib and consider symptomatic treatment with topical therapy.

Grade 2 (painful erythema and swelling of the hands or feet and/or discomfort affecting normal activities):

1st occurrence: Continue sorafenib and consider symptomatic treatment with topical therapy. **Note:** If no improvement within 7 days, see dosing for 2nd or 3rd occurrence.
2nd or 3rd occurrence (or no improvement after 7 days of 1st occurrence): Hold treatment until resolves to grade 0-1; resume treatment with dose reduced by one dose level (400 mg daily or 400 mg every other day)
4th occurrence: Discontinue treatment

Grade 3 (moist desquamation, ulceration, blistering, or severe pain of the hands or feet or severe discomfort that prevents working or performing daily activities):

1st or 2nd occurrence: Hold treatment until resolves to grade 0-1; resume treatment with dose reduced by one dose level (400 mg daily or 400 mg every other day)
3rd occurrence: Discontinue treatment

Suspected Stevens-Johnson syndrome or toxic epidermal necrolysis: Discontinue treatment.

Combination Regimens

Renal cell cancer: Sorafenib (RCC Regimen) on page 1751

Administration Administer on an empty stomach (1 hour before or 2 hours after eating).

Emetic Potential Very low (<10%)

Extemporaneous Preparations Hazardous agent: Use appropriate precautions for handling and disposal.

An oral suspension may be prepared with tablets. Place two 200 mg tablets into a glass containing 60 mL (2 oz) water; let stand 5 minutes before stirring. Stir until tablets are completely disintegrated, forming a uniform suspension. Administer within 1 hour after preparation. Stir suspension again immediately before administration. To ensure the full dose is administered, rinse glass several times with a total of 180 mL (6 oz) water and administer residue. **Note:** Brown tablet coating may initially form a thin film but has no effect on the dosing accuracy.

Nexavar® data on file, Bayer Healthcare Pharmaceuticals.

Monitoring Parameters

CBC with differential, electrolytes, phosphorus, lipase and amylase levels; liver function tests; blood pressure (baseline, weekly for the first 6 weeks, then periodic); monitor for hand-foot syndrome

Thyroid function testing (Hamnvik, 2011):

- Pre-existing levothyroxine therapy: Obtain baseline TSH levels, then monitor every 4 weeks until levels and levothyroxine dose are stable, then monitor every 2 months
- Without pre-existing thyroid hormone replacement: TSH at baseline, then every 4 weeks for 4 months, then every 2-3 months

Dietary Considerations Take without food (1 hour before or 2 hours after eating).

Additional Information Hand-foot skin reaction (HFSR) management (Lacouture, 2008): The following treatments may be used in addition to the recommended dosage modifications. Prior to treatment initiation, a pedicure is recommended to remove hyperkeratotic areas/calluses, which may predispose to HFSR; avoid vigorous exercise/activities which may stress hands or feet. During therapy, patients should reduce exposure to hot water (may exacerbate hand-foot symptoms); avoid constrictive footwear and excessive skin friction. Patients may also wear thick cotton gloves or socks and should wear shoes with padded insoles. Grade 1 HFSR may be relieved with moisturizing creams, cotton gloves and socks (at night) and/or keratolytic creams such as urea (20% to 40%) or salicylic acid (6%). Apply topical steroid (eg, clobetasol ointment) twice daily to erythematous areas of Grade 2 HFSR; topical anesthetics (eg, lidocaine 2%) and then systemic analgesics (if appropriate) may be used for pain control. Resolution of acute erythema may result in keratotic areas which may be softened with keratolytic agents.

Dosage Forms Excipient information presented when available (limited, particularly for generics); consult specific product labeling.

Tablet, oral:

NexAVAR®: 200 mg

References

Escudier B, Eisen T, Stadler WM, et al, "Sorafenib in Advanced Clear-Cell Renal Cell Carcinoma," *N Engl J Med*, 2007, 356(2):125-34.

Gupta-Abramson V, Troxel AB, Nellore A, et al, "Phase II Trial of Sorafenib in Advanced Thyroid Cancer," *J Clin Oncol*, 2008, 26(29):4714-9.

Hamnvik OP, Larsen PR, and Marqusee E, "Thyroid Dysfunction From Antineoplastic Agents," *J Natl Cancer Inst*, 2011, 103(21):1572-87.

Lacouture ME, Wu S, Robert C, et al, "Evolving Strategies for the Management of Hand-Foot Skin Reaction Associated With the Multitargeted Kinase Inhibitors Sorafenib and Sunitinib," *Oncologist*, 2008, 13(9):1001-11.

Lam ET, Ringel MD, Kloos RT, et al, "Phase II Clinical Trial of Sorafenib in Metastatic Medullary Thyroid Cancer," *J Clin Oncol*, 2010, 28(14):2323-30.

Llovet J Ricci S, Mazzaferro V, et al, "Sorafenib in Advanced Hepatocellular Carcinoma," *N Engl J Med*, 2008 Jul 24;359(4):378-90.

Maki RG, D'Adamo DR, Keohan ML, et al, "Phase II Study of Sorafenib in Patients With Metastatic or Recurrent Sarcomas," *J Clin Oncol*, 2009, 27(19):3133-40.

Miller AA, Murry DJ, Owzar K, et al, "Phase I and Pharmacokinetic Study of Sorafenib in Patients With Hepatic or Renal Dysfunction: CALGB 60301," *J Clin Oncol*, 2009, 27(11):1800-5.

Veronese ML, Mosenkis A, Flaherty KT, et al, "Mechanisms of Hypertension Associated With BAY 43-9006," *J Clin Oncol*, 2006, 24(9):1363-9.

Wiebe L, Kasza KE, Maki RG, et al, "Activity of Sorafenib (SOR) in Patients (pts) With Imatinib (IM) and Sunitinib (SU)-Resistant (RES) Gastrointestinal Stromal Tumors (GIST): A Phase II Trial of the University of Chicago Phase II Consortium," *J Clin Oncol*, 2008, 26(15s):10502 [abstract 10502 from the 2008 ASCO Annual Meeting].

Yau T, Chan P, Ng KK, et al, "Phase 2 Open-Label Study of Single Agent Sorafenib in Treating Advanced Hepatocellular Carcinoma in a Hepatitis B–Endemic Asian Population," *Cancer*, 2009, 115(2):428-36.

◆ **Sorafenib Tosylate** *see* SORAfenib *on page 1292*

◆ **Sotret®** *see* ISOtretinoin *on page 832*

◆ **Sporanox®** *see* Itraconazole *on page 838*

◆ **Sprycel®** *see* Dasatinib *on page 390*

◆ **SR-89** *see* Strontium-89 *on page 1300*

◆ **Statex® (Can)** *see* Morphine (Systemic) *on page 1004*

◆ **Sterile Talc** *see* Talc (Sterile) *on page 1323*

◆ **Sterile Talc Powder™** *see* Talc (Sterile) *on page 1323*

◆ **Sterile Vancomycin Hydrochloride, USP (Can)** *see* Vancomycin *on page 1428*

◆ **STI-571** *see* Imatinib *on page 762*

◆ **Stimate®** *see* Desmopressin *on page 434*

◆ **Stivarga®** *see* Regorafenib *on page 1233*

Streptozocin (strep toe ZOE sin)

Related Information

Management of Chemotherapy-Induced Nausea and Vomiting *on page 1786*

Management of Drug Extravasations *on page 1800*

Safe Handling of Hazardous Drugs *on page 1904*

Brand Names: U.S. Zanosar®

Brand Names: Canada Zanosar®

Generic Availability (U.S.) No

Pharmacologic Category Antineoplastic Agent, Alkylating Agent

Use Treatment of metastatic islet cell carcinoma of the pancreas

Unlabeled Use Treatment of adrenal tumors

Labeled Contraindications There are no contraindications listed within the manufacturer's labeling.

Pregnancy Risk Factor D

Lactation Enters breast milk/not recommended

Warnings/Precautions Hazardous agent - use appropriate precautions for handling and disposal. **[U.S. Boxed Warnings]: Renal toxicity is dose-related and cumulative and may be severe or fatal; other major toxicities include liver dysfunction, diarrhea, nausea, vomiting, and hematologic changes. Should be administered under the supervision of an experienced cancer chemotherapy physician.** There may be an acute release of insulin during treatment. Keep syringe of $D_{50}W$ at bedside during administration. Local tissue irritation may occur; extravasation may cause local tissue lesions and necrosis.

Adverse Reactions

>10%:

Gastrointestinal: Nausea and vomiting (100%)

Hepatic: LFTs increased

Miscellaneous: Hypoalbuminemia

Renal: BUN increased, Cl_{cr} decreased, hypophosphatemia, nephrotoxicity (25% to 75%), proteinuria, renal dysfunction (65%), renal tubular acidosis

1% to 10%:

Endocrine & metabolic: Hypoglycemia (6%)

Gastrointestinal: Diarrhea (10%)

Local: Pain at injection site

<1%: Confusion, lethargy, depression, leukopenia, thrombocytopenia, liver dysfunction, secondary malignancy

Myelosuppressive:

WBC: Mild

Platelets: Mild

Onset: 7 days

Nadir: 14 days

Recovery: 21 days

Drug Interactions

Metabolism/Transport Effects None known.

Avoid Concomitant Use

Avoid concomitant use of Streptozocin with any of the following: BCG; CloZAPine; Natalizumab; Pimecrolimus; Tacrolimus (Topical); Vaccines (Live)

Increased Effect/Toxicity

Streptozocin may increase the levels/effects of: CloZAPine; Hypoglycemic Agents; Leflunomide; Natalizumab; Vaccines (Live)

The levels/effects of Streptozocin may be increased by: Denosumab; Herbs (Hypoglycemic Properties); MAO Inhibitors; Pimecrolimus; Roflumilast; Salicylates; Selective Serotonin Reuptake Inhibitors; Tacrolimus (Topical); Trastuzumab

Decreased Effect

Streptozocin may decrease the levels/effects of: BCG; Coccidioidin Skin Test; Sipuleucel-T; Vaccines (Inactivated); Vaccines (Live)

The levels/effects of Streptozocin may be decreased by: Echinacea; Loop Diuretics

Storage/Stability Store intact vials under refrigeration. Vials are stable for 1 year at room temperature. Solution reconstituted with SWFI or NS is stable for 48 hours at room temperature and 96 hours under refrigeration. Further dilution in D_5W or NS is stable for 48 hours at room temperature and 96 hours under refrigeration when protected from light. Manufacturer recommends that reconstituted solution be used within 12 hours; vial does not contain a preservative

Reconstitution Dilute powder with 9.5 mL SWFI or NS to a concentration of 100 mg/mL.

Mechanism of Action Interferes with the normal function of DNA by alkylation and cross-linking the strands of DNA, and by possible protein modification

Pharmacodynamics/Kinetics

Duration: Disappears from serum in 4 hours

Distribution: Concentrates in liver, intestine, pancreas, and kidney

Metabolism: Rapidly hepatic

Half-life elimination: 35-40 minutes

Excretion: Urine (60% to 70% as metabolites); exhaled gases (5%); feces (1%)

Dosing

Adult & Geriatric Antineoplastic: Refer to individual protocols.

Single agent therapy: I.V.: 1-1.5 g/m^2 weekly for 6 weeks followed by a 4-week rest period

Combination therapy: I.V.: 0.5-1 g/m^2 for 5 consecutive days followed by a 4- to 6-week rest period

Pediatric Refer to adult dosing.

Renal Impairment The FDA-approved labeling does not contain dosing adjustments; however, it is recommended to use clinical judgment weighing benefit vs risk of renal toxicity in patients with pre-existing renal impairment. The following dosing adjustments have been used by some clinicians (Aronoff, 2007): Adults:

Cl_{cr} 10-50 mL/minute: Administer 75% of dose

Cl_{cr} <10 mL/minute: Administer 50% of dose

Hepatic Impairment There are no specific guidelines on dosage adjustment in patients with hepatic impairment. Streptozocin is rapidly hepatically metabolized; dose should be decreased in patients with severe liver disease.

Administration Administer as short (30-60 minutes) or 6-hour infusion; may be given by rapid I.V. push

Emetic Potential Very high (>90%)

Vesicant/Extravasation Risk Vesicant; see Management of Drug Extravasations on page 1800.

Monitoring Parameters Liver function tests, CBC, renal function, tests (BUN, serum creatinine) at baseline and weekly during therapy

Dosage Forms Excipient information presented when available (limited, particularly for generics); consult specific product labeling.

Injection, powder for reconstitution:

Zanosar®: 1 g

References

Aronoff GR, Bennett WM, Berns JS, et al, *Drug Prescribing in Renal Failure: Dosing Guidelines for Adults and Children*, 5th ed. Philadelphia, PA: American College of Physicians; 2007, p 101.

◆ **Strontium-89 Chloride** *see* Strontium-89 *on page* 1300

Strontium-89 (STRON shee um atey nine)

Related Information

Chronic Pain Management (Cancer) *on page* 1840

Brand Names: U.S. Metastron®

Brand Names: Canada Metastron®

Index Terms SR-89; Sr89; Strontium Chloride SR 89; Strontium-89 Chloride

Generic Availability (U.S.) No

Pharmacologic Category Radiopharmaceutical

Use Relief of bone pain in patients with skeletal metastases

Labeled Contraindications There are no contraindications listed within the manufacturer's labeling.

Pregnancy Risk Factor D

Lactation Excretion is breast milk unknown/not recommended

Warnings/Precautions Bone marrow suppression (thrombocytopenia and leukopenia) is likely to occur. Use is not recommended in patients with seriously compromised bone marrow function from prior therapies or from disease infiltration (unless potential benefit outweighs risks). Monitor CBC weekly. Use with caution in patients whose platelet counts fall <60,000/mm^3 or whose white blood cell counts fall <2400/mm^3. Carefully evaluate bone marrow status and toxicity of initial treatment if considering repeat administration. Incontinent patients may require urinary catheterization (to minimize radioactive contamination). Body fluids may remain radioactive up to one week after injection. Not indicated for use in patients with cancer not involving bone or in patients with a short life expectancy (due to delayed onset of pain relief). A small number of patients have experienced a transient increase in bone pain at 36-72 hours postdose; this reaction is generally mild and self-limiting. Patients may experience a flushing sensation following rapid (<30 seconds) injection.

Primarily eliminated renally; possible risk versus benefit should be evaluated. Handle cautiously, in a similar manner to other radioactive drugs; appropriate safety measures to minimize radiation to personnel should be instituted. Should only be used under the supervision of nuclear medicine physicians and/or radiopharmacists qualified and experienced in use and handling of radionuclides.

Adverse Reactions Frequency not defined.

Cardiovascular: Flushing (after rapid injection)

Central nervous system: Chills (case report), fever (case report)

Hematologic: Leukopenia, thrombocytopenia (nadir: 12-16 weeks; recovery: 6 months)

Neuromuscular & skeletal: Bone pain (transient increase; duration: 36-72 hours)

Miscellaneous: Septicemia (case report)

Drug Interactions

Metabolism/Transport Effects None known.

Avoid Concomitant Use There are no known interactions where it is recommended to avoid concomitant use.

Increased Effect/Toxicity There are no known significant interactions involving an increase in effect.

Decreased Effect There are no known significant interactions involving a decrease in effect.

Storage/Stability Store vial and its contents inside its transportation container at room temperature of 15°C to 25°C (59°F to 77°F)

Mechanism of Action Selectively (locally) irradiates primary and metastatic bone lesions to reduce pain.

Pharmacodynamics/Kinetics

Onset: Pain relief: 7-20 days

Distribution: Retained in bone mineral (preferentially to metastatic bone lesions)

Excretion: In patients with bone metastases: Urine (67%); feces (33%)

Dosing

Adult & Geriatric Note: Measure dose by a suitable radioactivity calibration system immediately prior to administration.

Bone pain due to skeletal metastases: I.V.: 148 megabecquerel (4 millicurie) **or** 1.5-2.2 megabecquerel (40-60 microcurie)/kg; repeat doses are generally not recommended at intervals <90 days

Administration Administer intravenously slowly over 1-2 minutes.

Monitoring Parameters CBC with differential (every other week)

Additional Information Patients should the following precautions (Silberstein, 2003):

1. Avoid soiling underclothing or areas around toilet bowls for 2 weeks after injection.
2. Wash any underclothing separately if significantly stained with urine.
3. Where a normal toilet is available, use in preference to a urinal.
4. Flush toilet twice after use.
5. Wash hands thoroughly after urination.

Dosage Forms Excipient information presented when available (limited, particularly for generics); consult specific product labeling.

Injection, solution, as chloride [preservative free]:

Metastron®: 1 mCi/mL (4 mL) [37 megabecquerel per mL]

References

Robinson RG, Preston DF, Schiefelbein M, et al, "Strontium 89 Therapy for the Palliation of Pain Due to Osseous Metastases," *JAMA*, 1995, 274(5):420-4.

Silberstein EB, Buscombe JR, McEwan A, et al, "Clinical Guidelines: Society of Nuclear Medicine Procedure Guideline for Palliative Treatment of Painful Bone Metastases 3.0," 2003. Available at http://interactive.snm.org/docs/pg_ch25_0403.pdf. Last accessed May 13, 2010.

◆ **Strontium Chloride SR 89** *see* Strontium-89 *on page 1300*

◆ **SU011248** *see* SUNItinib *on page 1308*

◆ **Suberoylanilide Hydroxamic Acid** *see* Vorinostat *on page 1478*

◆ **Subsys®** *see* FentaNYL *on page 583*

Sulfamethoxazole and Trimethoprim

(sul fa meth OKS a zole & trye METH oh prim)

Brand Names: U.S. Bactrim™; Bactrim™ DS; Septra® DS

Brand Names: Canada Apo-Sulfatrim®; Apo-Sulfatrim® DS; Apo-Sulfatrim® Pediatric; Novo-Trimel; Novo-Trimel D.S.; Nu-Cotrimox; Septra® Injection

Index Terms Co-Trimoxazole; Septra; SMX-TMP; SMZ-TMP; Sulfatrim; TMP-SMX; TMP-SMZ; Trimethoprim and Sulfamethoxazole

Generic Availability (U.S.) Yes

Pharmacologic Category Antibiotic, Miscellaneous; Antibiotic, Sulfonamide Derivative

Use

Oral treatment of urinary tract infections due to *E. coli*, *Klebsiella* and *Enterobacter* sp, *M. morganii*, *P. mirabilis* and *P. vulgaris*; acute otitis media in children; acute exacerbations of chronic bronchitis in adults due to susceptible strains of *H. influenzae* or *S. pneumoniae*; treatment and prophylaxis of *Pneumocystis jirovecii* pneumonia (PCP); traveler's diarrhea due to enterotoxigenic *E. coli*; treatment of enteritis caused by *Shigella flexneri* or *Shigella sonnei*

I.V. treatment of severe or complicated infections when oral therapy is not feasible, for documented PCP, empiric treatment of PCP in immune compromised patients; treatment of documented or suspected shigellosis, typhoid fever, or other infections caused by susceptible bacteria

Unlabeled Use Cholera and *Salmonella*-type infections and nocardiosis; chronic prostatitis; as prophylaxis in neutropenic patients with *P. jirovecii*

infections, in leukemia patients, and in patients following renal transplantation, to decrease incidence of PCP; treatment of *Cyclospora* infection, typhoid fever, *Nocardia asteroides* infection; prophylaxis against urinary tract infection; alternative treatment for MRSA infections

Labeled Contraindications Hypersensitivity to any sulfa drug, trimethoprim, or any component of the formulation; megaloblastic anemia due to folate deficiency; infants <2 months of age; marked hepatic damage or severe renal disease (if patient not monitored); pregnancy (at term); breast-feeding

Pregnancy Risk Factor C

Lactation Enters breast milk/contraindicated (AAP rates "compatible"; AAP 2001 update pending)

Warnings/Precautions Use with caution in patients with G6PD deficiency, impaired renal or hepatic function or potential folate deficiency (malnourished, chronic anticonvulsant therapy, or elderly); maintain adequate hydration to prevent crystalluria; adjust dosage in patients with renal impairment. Injection vehicle contains benzyl alcohol and sodium metabisulfite.

Chemical similarities are present among sulfonamides, sulfonylureas, carbonic anhydrase inhibitors, thiazides, and loop diuretics (except ethacrynic acid). Use in patients with sulfonamide allergy is specifically contraindicated in product labeling, however, a risk of cross-reaction exists in patients with allergy to any of these compounds; avoid use when previous reaction has been severe.

Fatalities associated with severe reactions including Stevens-Johnson syndrome, toxic epidermal necrolysis, hepatic necrosis, agranulocytosis, aplastic anemia, and other blood dyscrasias; discontinue use at first sign of rash or serious adverse reactions. Elderly patients appear at greater risk for more severe adverse reactions. May cause hypoglycemia, particularly in malnourished, or patients with renal or hepatic impairment. Use with caution in patients with porphyria or thyroid dysfunction. Slow acetylators may be more prone to adverse reactions. Caution in patients with allergies or asthma. May cause hyperkalemia (associated with high doses of trimethoprim). Incidence of adverse effects appears to be increased in patients with AIDS. Prolonged use may result in fungal or bacterial superinfection, including *C. difficile*-associated diarrhea (CDAD) and pseudomembranous colitis; CDAD has been observed >2 months postantibiotic treatment. Avoid concomitant use with leucovorin when treating *Pneumocystis jirovecii* pneumonia (PCP) in HIV patients; may increase risk of treatment failure and death.

Ethanol/Nutrition/Herb Interactions Herb/Nutraceutical: Avoid dong quai; St John's wort (may diminish effects and also cause photosensitization).

Storage/Stability

Injection: Store at room temperature; do not refrigerate. Less soluble in more alkaline pH. Protect from light. Solution must be diluted prior to administration. Following dilution, store at room temperature; do not refrigerate. Manufacturer recommended dilutions and stability of parenteral admixture at room temperature (25°C):

5 mL/125 mL D_5W; stable for 6 hours.

5 mL/100 mL D_5W; stable for 4 hours.

5 mL/75 mL D_5W; stable for 2 hours.

Studies have also confirmed limited stability in NS; detailed references should be consulted.

Suspension, tablet: Store at controlled room temperature of 15°C to 25°C (59°F to 77°F). Protect from light.

Mechanism of Action Sulfamethoxazole interferes with bacterial folic acid synthesis and growth via inhibition of dihydrofolic acid formation from para-aminobenzoic acid; trimethoprim inhibits dihydrofolic acid reduction to tetrahydrofolate resulting in sequential inhibition of enzymes of the folic acid pathway

Pharmacodynamics/Kinetics

Absorption: Oral: Almost completely, 90% to 100%

Protein binding: SMX: 68%, TMP: 45%

Metabolism: SMX: N-acetylated and glucuronidated; TMP: Metabolized to oxide and hydroxylated metabolites

Half-life elimination: SMX: 9 hours, TMP: 6-17 hours; both are prolonged in renal failure

Time to peak, serum: Within 1-4 hours

Excretion: Both are excreted in urine as metabolites and unchanged drug

Effects of aging on the pharmacokinetics of both agents has been variable; increase in half-life and decreases in clearance have been associated with reduced creatinine clearance

Dosing

Adult & Geriatric Dosage recommendations are based on the trimethoprim component. double-strength tablets are equivalent to sulfamethoxazole 800 mg and trimethoprim 160 mg.

General dosing guidelines:

Oral: 1-2 double-strength tablets (sulfamethoxazole 800 mg; trimethoprim 160 mg) every 12-24 hours

I.V.: 8-20 mg TMP/kg/day divided every 6-12 hours

Chronic bronchitis (acute): Oral: One double-strength tablet every 12 hours for 10-14 days

Cyclosporiasis (unlabeled use): Oral, I.V.: 160 mg TMP twice daily for 7-10 days. **Note:** AIDS patients: Oral: One double-strength tablet 2-4 times/day for 10 days, then 1 double-strength tablet 3 times/week for 10 weeks (Pape, 1994; Verdier, 2000).

Granuloma inguinale (donovanosis) (unlabeled use): Oral: One double-strength tablet every 12 hours for at least 3 weeks and until lesions have healed (CDC, 2010)

Isosporiasis (*Isospora belli* infection) in HIV-positive patients (unlabeled use; CDC, 2009):

Treatment: Oral, I.V.: 160 mg TMP 4 times/day for 10 days **or** 160 mg TMP 2 times/day for 7-10 days. May increase dose and/or duration up to 3-4 weeks if symptoms worsen or persist

Secondary prophylaxis (in patients with CD4+ count <200 /microL): Oral: 160 mg TMP 3 times/week (preferred) **or** alternatively, 160 mg TMP daily **or** 320 mg TMP 3 times/week

Meningitis (bacterial): I.V.: 10-20 mg TMP/kg/day in divided doses every 6-12 hours

Nocardia (unlabeled use): Oral, I.V.:

Cutaneous infections: 5-10 mg TMP/kg/day in 2-4 divided doses

Severe infections (pulmonary/cerebral): 15 mg TMP/kg/day in 2-4 divided doses for 3-4 weeks, then 10 mg TMP/kg/day in 2-4 divided doses. Treatment duration is controversial; an average of 7 months has been reported.

Note: Therapy for severe infection may be initiated I.V. and converted to oral therapy (frequently converted to approximate dosages of oral solid dosage forms: 2 DS tablets every 8-12 hours). Although not widely available, sulfonamide levels should be considered in patients with questionable absorption, at risk for dose-related toxicity, or those with poor therapeutic response.

Osteomyelitis due to MRSA (unlabeled use): Oral, I.V.: 3.5-4 mg TMP/kg/dose every 8-12 hours for a minimum of 8 weeks with rifampin 600 mg once daily (Liu, 2011)

***Pneumocystis jirovecii* pneumonia (PCP):** Oral: Manufacturer's labeling:
- Prophylaxis: 160 mg TMP daily
- Treatment: 15-20 mg TMP/kg/day divided every 6 hours for 14-21 days

***Pneumocystis jirovecii* pneumonia (PCP) prophylaxis and treatment in HIV-positive patients (CDC, 2009): Note:** Sulfamethoxazole and trimethoprim is the preferred regimen for this indication.
- Prophylaxis: Oral: 80-160 mg TMP daily **or** alternatively, 160 mg TMP 3 times/week
- Treatment:
  - Mild-to-moderate: Oral: 15-20 mg TMP/kg/day in 3 divided doses for 21 days **or** alternatively, 320 mg TMP 3 times/day for 21 days
  - Moderate-to-severe: Oral, I.V.: 15-20 mg TMP/kg/day in 3-4 divided doses for 21 days

Sepsis: I.V.: 20 TMP/kg/day divided every 6 hours

Septic arthritis due to MRSA (unlabeled use): Oral, I.V.: 3.5-4 mg TMP/kg/dose every 8-12 hours for 3-4 weeks (some experts combine with rifampin) (Liu, 2011)

Shigellosis:
- Oral: One double-strength tablet every 12 hours for 5 days
- I.V.: 8-10 mg TMP/kg/day in divided doses every 6, 8, or 12 hours for up to 5 days

Skin/soft tissue infection due to community-acquired MRSA (unlabeled use): Oral: 1-2 double-strength tablets every 12 hours for 5-10 days (Liu, 2011); **Note:** If beta-hemolytic *Streptococcus* spp are also suspected, a beta-lactam antibiotic should be added to the regimen (Liu, 2011)

***Stenotrophomonas maltophilia* (ventilator-associated pneumonia):** I.V.: Most clinicians have utilized 12-15 mg TMP/kg/day for the treatment of VAP caused by *Stenotrophomonas maltophilia*. Higher doses (up to 20 mg TMP/kg/day) have been mentioned for treatment of severe infection in patients with normal renal function (Looney, 2009; Vartivarian, 1989; Wood, 2010)

***Toxoplasma gondii* encephalitis (unlabeled use; CDC, 2009):** Oral:
- Primary prophylaxis: Oral: 160 mg TMP daily (preferred) **or** 160 mg TMP 3 times/week **or** 80 mg TMP daily
- Treatment (alternative to sulfadiazine, pyrimethamine and leucovorin calcium): Oral, I.V.: 5 mg/kg TMP twice daily

Travelers' diarrhea: Oral: One double-strength tablet every 12 hours for 5 days

Urinary tract infection:
- Oral: One double-strength tablet every 12 hours
  - Duration of therapy: Uncomplicated: 3-5 days; Complicated: 7-10 days
    - Pyelonephritis: 14 days
    - Prostatitis: Acute: 2 weeks; Chronic: 2-3 months
- I.V.: 8-10 mg TMP/kg/day in divided doses every 6, 8, or 12 hours for up to 14 days with severe infections

Pediatric Recommendations are based on the trimethoprim component.

General dosing guidelines: Children >2 months: Manufacturer's labeling:

Mild-to-moderate infections: Oral: 8 mg TMP/kg/day in divided doses every 12 hours

Serious infection:
Oral: 15-20 mg TMP/kg/day in divided doses every 6 hours
I.V.: 8-12 mg TMP/kg/day in divided doses every 6-12 hours

Acute otitis media: Oral: 8 mg TMP/kg/day in divided doses every 12 hours for 10 days. **Note:** Recommended by the American Academy of Pediatrics as an alternative agent in penicillin allergic patients at a dose of 6-10mg TMP/kg/day (AOM guidelines, 2004).

Cyclosporiasis (unlabeled use): Oral, I.V.: 5 mg TMP/kg twice daily for 7-10 days (*Red Book*, 2009)

Pneumocystis:
Treatment: Oral, I.V.: 15-20 mg TMP/kg/day in divided doses every 6-8 hours for 21 days
Prophylaxis: Oral: 150 mg TMP/m^2/day in divided doses every 12 hours and administered for 3 days/week on consecutive or alternate days; an alternative dosing regimen allows for same dose to be administered in 2 divided doses daily (maximum: trimethoprim 320 mg and sulfamethoxazole 1600 mg daily) (CDC, 2009)

Shigellosis:
Oral: 8 mg TMP/kg/day in divided doses every 12 hours for 5 days
I.V.: 8-10 mg TMP/kg/day in divided doses every 6, 8, or 12 hours for up to 5 days

Skin/soft tissue infection due to community-acquired MRSA (unlabeled use): Oral: 4-6 mg TMP/kg/dose every 12 hours for 5-10 days (Liu, 2011); **Note:** If beta-hemolytic *Streptococcus* spp are also suspected, a beta-lactam antibiotic should be added to the regimen (Liu, 2011)

Toxoplasmosis primary prophylaxis in HIV-exposed/infected patients (unlabeled use; CDC, 2009): Oral: 150 mg TMP/m^2/day in 2 divided doses (preferred) or 150 mg TMP/m^2/day in a single dose 3 times/week on consecutive days or 150 mg TMP/m^2/day in 2 divided doses 3 times/week on alternate days

Urinary tract infection:
Treatment:
Oral: 8 mg TMP/kg/day in divided doses every 12 hours
I.V.: 8-10 mg TMP/kg/day in divided doses every 6, 8, or 12 hours for up to 14 days with serious infections
Prophylaxis: Oral: 2 mg TMP/kg/dose daily or 5 mg TMP/kg/dose twice weekly

Renal Impairment Oral, I.V.:
Manufacturer's recommendation: Children and Adults:
Cl_{cr} >30 mL/minute: No dosage adjustment required
Cl_{cr} 15-30 mL/minute: Administer 50% of recommended dose
Cl_{cr} <15 mL/minute: Use is not recommended
Alternate recommendations:
Cl_{cr} 15-30 mL/minute:
Treatment: Administer full daily dose (divided every 12 hours) for 24-48 hours, then decrease daily dose by 50% and administer every 24 hours (**Note:** For serious infections including *Pneumocystis jirovecii* pneumonia (PCP), full daily dose is given in divided doses every 6-8 hours for 2 days, followed by reduction to 50% daily dose divided every 12 hours) (Nahata, 1995).
PCP prophylaxis: One-half single-strength tablet (40 mg trimethoprim) daily **or** 1 single-strength tablet (80 mg trimethoprim) daily or 3 times weekly (Masur, 2002).

Cl_{cr} <15 mL/minute:

Treatment: Administer full daily dose every 48 hours (Nahata, 1995)

PCP prophylaxis: One-half single-strength tablet (40 mg trimethoprim) daily **or** 1 single-strength tablet (80 mg trimethoprim) 3 times weekly (Masur, 2002). While the guidelines do acknowledge the alternative of giving 1 single-strength tablet daily, this may be inadvisable in the uremic/ESRD patient.

Intermittent Hemodialysis (IHD) (administer after hemodialysis on dialysis days).

Treatment: Full daily dose before dialysis and 50% dose after dialysis (Nahata, 1995)

Children: GFR <10 mL/minute/1.73 m^2: Not recommended, but if required 5-10 mg TMP/kg every 24 hours (Aronoff, 2007)

PCP prophylaxis: One single-strength tablet (80 mg trimethoprim) after each dialysis session (Masur, 2002)

Note: Dosing dependent on the assumption of 3 times/week, complete IHD sessions.

Peritoneal dialysis (PD):

Use Cl_{cr} <15 mL/minute dosing recommendations. Not significantly removed by PD; supplemental dosing is not required (Aronoff, 2007):

Exit-site and tunnel infections: Oral: One single-strength tablet daily (Li, 2010)

Peritonitis: Oral: One double-strength tablet twice daily (Li, 2010)

Children: GFR <10 mL/minute/1.73 m^2: Not recommended, but if required 5-10 mg TMP/kg every 24 hours. Intraperitoneal: Loading dose: TMP-SMX 320/1600 mg/L; Maintenance: TMP-SMX 80/400 mg/L (Aronoff, 2007; Warady, 2000)

Continuous renal replacement therapy (CRRT) (Heintz, 2009; Trotman, 2005): Drug clearance is highly dependent on the method of renal replacement, filter type, and flow rate. Appropriate dosing requires close monitoring of pharmacologic response, signs of adverse reactions due to drug accumulation, as well as drug concentrations in relation to target trough (if appropriate). The following are general recommendations only (based on dialysate flow/ultrafiltration rates of 1-2 L/hour and minimal residual renal function) and should not supersede clinical judgment:

CVVH/CVVHD/CVVHDF: 2.5-7.5 mg/kg of TMP every 12 hours. **Note:** Dosing regimen dependent on clinical indication. Critically-ill patients with *P. jirovecii* pneumonia receiving CVVHDF may require up to 10 mg/kg every 12 hours (Heintz, 2009).

Administration

I.V.: Infuse over 60-90 minutes, must dilute well before giving (ie, 1:15 to 1:25, which equates to 5 mL of drug solution diluted in 75-125 mL base solution); not for I.M. injection

Oral: Administer without regard to meals. Administer with at least 8 ounces of water.

Test Interactions Increased creatinine (Jaffé alkaline picrate reaction); increased serum methotrexate by dihydrofolate reductase method

Dosage Forms Excipient information presented when available (limited, particularly for generics); consult specific product labeling. **Note:** The 5:1 ratio (SMX:TMP) remains constant in all dosage forms.

Injection, solution: Sulfamethoxazole 80 mg and trimethoprim 16 mg per mL (5 mL, 10 mL, 30 mL) [contains benzyl alcohol, ethanol 12.2%, propylene glycol 400 mg/mL, sodium metabisulfite]

Suspension, oral: Sulfamethoxazole 200 mg and trimethoprim 40 mg per 5 mL (480 mL)
Tablet: Sulfamethoxazole 400 mg and trimethoprim 80 mg
Bactrim™: Sulfamethoxazole 400 mg and trimethoprim 80 mg
Tablet, double-strength: Sulfamethoxazole 800 mg and trimethoprim 160 mg
Bactrim™ DS: Sulfamethoxazole 800 mg and trimethoprim 160 mg
Septra® DS: Sulfamethoxazole 800 mg and trimethoprim 160 mg

◆ **Sulfatrim** *see* Sulfamethoxazole and Trimethoprim *on page 1302*

SUNItinib (su NIT e nib)

Related Information

Management of Chemotherapy-Induced Nausea and Vomiting *on page 1786*
Principles of Anticancer Therapy *on page 1878*
Safe Handling of Hazardous Drugs *on page 1904*

Brand Names: U.S. Sutent®

Brand Names: Canada Sutent®

Index Terms SU011248; SU11248; Sunitinib Malate

Generic Availability (U.S.) No

Pharmacologic Category Antineoplastic Agent, Tyrosine Kinase Inhibitor; Vascular Endothelial Growth Factor (VEGF) Inhibitor

Use Treatment of gastrointestinal stromal tumor (GIST) intolerant to or with disease progression on imatinib; treatment of advanced renal cell cancer (RCC); treatment of advanced, metastatic or unresectable pancreatic neuroendocrine tumors (PNET)

Unlabeled Use Treatment of advanced thyroid cancer; treatment of non-GIST soft tissue sarcomas

Labeled Contraindications There are no contraindications listed within the FDA-approved manufacturer's labeling.

Canadian labeling: Hypersensitivity to sunitinib or any component of the formulation; pregnancy

Pregnancy Risk Factor D

Lactation Excretion in breast milk unknown/not recommended

Warnings/Precautions Hazardous agent - use appropriate precautions for handling and disposal. **[U.S. Boxed Warning]: Hepatotoxicity, which may be severe and/or result in fatal liver failure, has been observed in clinical trials and in postmarketing surveillance.** Signs of liver failure include jaundice, elevated transaminases, and/or hyperbilirubinemia, in conjunction with encephalopathy, coagulopathy and/or renal failure. Monitor liver function tests at baseline, with each treatment cycle and if clinically indicated. Withhold treatment for grade 3 or 4 hepatotoxicity; discontinue if hepatotoxicity does not resolve. Do not reinitiate in patients with severe changes in liver function tests or other signs/symptoms of liver failure. Sunitinib has not been studied in patients with ALT or AST >2.5 times ULN (or >5 times ULN if due to liver metastases).

May cause a decrease in left ventricular ejection fraction (LVEF), including grade 3 reductions; consider obtaining LVEF evaluation prior to treatment. Mean onset of symptomatic heart failure (HF) is 22 days from treatment initiation. Interrupt therapy or decrease dose with LVEF <50% or >20% reduction from baseline. Discontinue with clinical signs and symptoms of HF. Cardiovascular events (some fatal), including symptomatic HF, myocardial disorders and cardiomyopathy have been reported with use. QT_c prolongation and torsade de pointes have been observed (dose dependent); a baseline and periodic ECG should be obtained; correct electrolyte abnormalities prior to treatment and monitor and correct potassium, calcium and magnesium levels during therapy; use caution in patients with a history of QT_c prolongation, with medications known to prolong the QT_c interval, or patients with pre-existing (relevant) cardiac disease, bradycardia, or electrolyte imbalance. Use with caution in patients with cardiac dysfunction; monitor for clinical signs/symptoms of HF, obtain baseline and periodic LVEF evaluation patients with MI, bypass grafts, symptomatic HF, vascular diseases (including CVA and TIA), and PE were excluded from clinical trials. May cause hypertension; monitor and control with antihypertensives if needed; interrupt therapy until hypertension is controlled for severe hypertension. Use caution and closely monitor in patients with underlying or poorly-controlled hypertension. Use with caution in patients concurrently taking strong CYP3A4 inhibitors (may increase sunitinib levels; eg, ketoconazole) or inducers (may decrease sunitinib levels; eg, rifampin); dosage adjustments of sunitinib may be required.

Hemorrhagic events have been reported including epistaxis, rectal, gingival, upper GI, urinary tract, genital, brain, wound bleeding, tumor-related, and hemoptysis/pulmonary hemorrhage; may be serious and/or fatal. Proteinuria and (rare) cases of nephrotic syndrome have been reported; discontinue treatment in patients with nephrotic syndrome. Microangiopathic hemolytic anemia (MAHA) and dose-limiting hypertension have been reported when sunitinib has been used in combination with bevacizumab. Impaired wound healing has been reported with sunitinib; temporarily withhold treatment for patients undergoing major surgical procedures; the optimal time to resume treatment after a procedure has not been determined. Serious and fatal gastrointestinal complications, including gastrointestinal perforation, have occurred (rarely). Pancreatitis has been observed in RCC patients; discontinue sunitinib if symptoms are present. Hypothyroidism may occur; the risk for hypothyroidism appears to increase with therapy duration; hyperthyroidism, sometimes followed by hypothyroidism has also been reported; monitor thyroid function at baseline and if symptomatic. Adrenal function abnormalities have been reported; monitor for adrenal insufficiency for patients with stress such as trauma, severe infection, or undergoing surgery. May cause skin and/or hair depigmentation or discoloration. Reversible posterior leukoencephalopathy syndrome (RPLS) has been reported (rarely); symptoms include confusion, headache, hypertension, lethargy, seizure, blindness and/or other vision, or neurologic disturbances; interrupt treatment and begin hypertension management. Tumor lysis syndrome (TLS), including fatalities, has been reported, predominantly in patients with RCC or GIST; risk for TLS is higher in patients with a high tumor burden prior to treatment; monitor closely; correct clinically significant dehydration and treat high uric acid levels prior to initiation of treatment. An increased incidence of fatigue, thyroid dysfunction and treatment-induced hypertension was reported in patients with renal insufficiency (Cl_{cr} ≤60 mL/minute) who received sunitinib for the treatment of renal cell cancer (Gupta, 2011). Osteonecrosis of the jaw (ONJ) has been observed with sunitinib; concurrent bisphosphonate use or dental disease may increase the risk for ONJ. If possible, avoid invasive dental procedures in patients with current or prior bisphosphonate use. Consider a dental exam and appropriate prophylactic dentistry prior to treatment initiation Dosing schedules vary by indication; some treatment regimens are continuous daily dosing; other treatment schedules are daily dosing for 4 weeks of a 6-week cycle (4 weeks on, 2 weeks off).

Adverse Reactions

>10%:

Cardiovascular: Hypertension (15% to 34%; grade 3: 4% to 13%), peripheral edema (24%), LVEF decreased (11% to 16%; grades 3/4: 1% to 3%), heart failure (≤15%), chest pain (13%)

Central nervous system: Fatigue (33% to 62%), headache (≤23%), fever (≤22%), insomnia (15% to 18%), chills (14%), depression (11%), dizziness (11%)

Dermatologic: Skin discoloration (25% to 30%), rash (14% to 29%), hand-foot syndrome (14% to 29%; grades 3/4: 4% to 8%), hair color changes (7% to 29%), dry skin (≤23%), alopecia (5% to 14%), erythema (12%), pruritus (12%)

Endocrine & metabolic: Hyperglycemia (23% to 71%), hyperuricemia (≤46%), hypocalcemia (34% to 42%), hypoalbuminemia (28% to 41%), hypophosphatemia (≤36%), hyponatremia (≤29%), hypoglycemia (17% to 22%), hypokalemia (12% to 21%), hypomagnesemia (≤19%), hyperkalemia (≤18%), hypothyroidism (4% to 16%; grades 3/4: ≤2%), hypercalcemia (13%), hypernatremia (10% to 13%)

Gastrointestinal: Diarrhea (40% to 66%), nausea (45% to 58%), lipase increased (17% to 56%), anorexia (33% to 48%), mucositis/stomatitis (29% to 48%), taste perversion (21% to 47%), abdominal pain (39%), vomiting (34% to 39%), amylase increased (17% to 35%), dyspepsia (15% to 34%), constipation (20% to 23%), weight loss (16%), flatulence (14%), oral pain (6% to 14%), xerostomia (13%), GERD/reflux (12%), glossodynia (11%)

Hematologic: Anemia (26% to 79%; grades 3/4: ≤8%), leukopenia (78%; grades 3/4: 8%), neutropenia (53% to 77%; grades 3/4: 10% to 17%), lymphopenia (38% to 68%; grades 3/4: ≤18%), thrombocytopenia (38% to 68%; grades 3/4: 5% to 9%), hemorrhage/bleeding (18% to 37%)

Hepatic: AST increased (39% to 72%; grades 3/4: 2% to 5%), alkaline phosphatase increased (24% to 63%; grades 3/4: 2% to 10%), ALT increased (39% to 61%; grades 3/4: 2% to 4%), hyperbilirubinemia (10% to 37%; grades 3/4 ≤1%)

Neuromuscular & skeletal: Creatine kinase increased (49%), limb pain (14% to 40%), weakness (22% to 34%), arthralgia (15% to 30%), back pain (≤28%), myalgia (14%)

Renal: Creatinine increased (12% to 70%)

Respiratory: Cough (27%), dyspnea (26%), epistaxis (21%), nasopharyngitis (14%), upper respiratory tract infection (11%)

1% to 10%:

Cardiovascular: Venous thrombotic events (1% to 3%), DVT (2% to 3%)

Gastrointestinal: Hemorrhoids (10%), pancreatitis (1%)

Respiratory: Pulmonary embolism (2%)

Miscellaneous: Flu-like syndrome (5%)

<1%, postmarketing, and/or case reports: Acute renal failure, adrenal dysfunction, angioedema, aortic dissection, arterio thrombotic events, atrial flutter, cardiomyopathy, cerebral infarction, cerebral hemorrhage, cerebrovascular accident, coma, epistaxis, febrile neutropenia, fistula formation, gastrointestinal perforation, glomerular sclerosis (segmental), hepatic failure, hepatotoxicity, hypersensitivity, hyperthyroidism, hypotension, infection, macrocytosis, microangiopathic hemolytic anemia (when used in combination with bevacizumab), MI, myocardial disorders, myopathy, myxedema coma, nephrotic syndrome, neutropenic infection, osteonecrosis of the jaw (ONJ),

pneumonitis (recall), preeclampsia-like syndrome (proteinuria and reversible hypertension), proteinuria, pulmonary hemorrhage, QT_c prolongation, renal impairment, reversible posterior leukoencephalopathy syndrome (RPLS), rhabdomyolysis, seizure, septic shock, thrombotic microangiopathy, torsade de pointes, transient ischemic attack, tumor hemorrhage, tumor lysis syndrome, tumor necrosis, ventricular arrhythmia, wound healing complications

Drug Interactions

Metabolism/Transport Effects **Substrate** of CYP3A4 (major); **Note:** Assignment of Major/Minor substrate status based on clinically relevant drug interaction potential; **Inhibits** BCRP, P-glycoprotein

Avoid Concomitant Use

Avoid concomitant use of SUNItinib with any of the following: BCG; Bevacizumab; Bosutinib; Conivaptan; Highest Risk QTc-Prolonging Agents; Mifepristone; Natalizumab; Pimecrolimus; Silodosin; St Johns Wort; Tacrolimus (Topical); Temsirolimus; Vaccines (Live); VinCRIStine (Liposomal)

Increased Effect/Toxicity

SUNItinib may increase the levels/effects of: Bevacizumab; Bosutinib; Colchicine; Dabigatran Etexilate; Everolimus; Highest Risk QTc-Prolonging Agents; Leflunomide; Moderate Risk QTc-Prolonging Agents; Natalizumab; P-glycoprotein/ABCB1 Substrates; Prucalopride; Rivaroxaban; Silodosin; Topotecan; Vaccines (Live); VinCRIStine (Liposomal); Vitamin K Antagonists

The levels/effects of SUNItinib may be increased by: Antifungal Agents (Azole Derivatives, Systemic); Bevacizumab; Bisphosphonate Derivatives; Conivaptan; CYP3A4 Inhibitors (Moderate); CYP3A4 Inhibitors (Strong); Dasatinib; Denosumab; Ivacaftor; Mifepristone; Pimecrolimus; QTc-Prolonging Agents (Indeterminate Risk and Risk Modifying); Roflumilast; Tacrolimus (Topical); Temsirolimus; Trastuzumab

Decreased Effect

SUNItinib may decrease the levels/effects of: BCG; Cardiac Glycosides; Coccidioidin Skin Test; Sipuleucel-T; Vaccines (Inactivated); Vaccines (Live); Vitamin K Antagonists

The levels/effects of SUNItinib may be decreased by: CYP3A4 Inducers (Strong); Deferasirox; Echinacea; St Johns Wort; Tocilizumab

Ethanol/Nutrition/Herb Interactions

Food: Grapefruit juice may increase the levels/effects of sunitinib. Food has no effect on the bioavailability of sunitinib. Management: Avoid grapefruit juice.

Herb/Nutraceutical: St John's wort may increase metabolism and decrease sunitinib concentrations. Management: Avoid St John's wort.

Storage/Stability Store at room temperature of 25°C (77°F); excursions permitted to 15°C to 30°C (59°F to 86°F).

Mechanism of Action Exhibits antitumor and antiangiogenic properties by inhibiting multiple receptor tyrosine kinases, including platelet-derived growth factors (PDGFRα and PDGFRβ), vascular endothelial growth factors (VEGFR1, VEGFR2, and VEGFR3), FMS-like tyrosine kinase-3 (FLT3), colony-stimulating factor type 1 (CSF-1R), and glial cell-line-derived neurotrophic factor receptor (RET).

Pharmacodynamics/Kinetics

Distribution: V_d/F: 2230 L

Protein binding: Sunitinib: 95%; SU12662: 90%

Metabolism: Hepatic; primarily metabolized by CYP3A4 to the N-desethyl metabolite SU12662 (active)

Half-life elimination: Terminal: Sunitinib: 40-60 hours; SU12662: 80-110 hours

Time to peak, plasma: 6-12 hours
Excretion: Feces (61%); urine (16%)

Dosing

Adult & Geriatric Note: Dosage modifications should be done in increments or decrements of 12.5 mg; individualize based on safety and tolerability.

Gastrointestinal stromal tumor (GIST): Oral: 50 mg once daily for 4 weeks of a 6-week treatment cycle (4 weeks on, 2 weeks off)

GIST unlabeled dosing: Oral: 37.5 mg once daily, continuous daily dosing (George, 2009, *EJC*)

Pancreatic neuroendocrine tumors, advanced (PNET): Oral: 37.5 mg once daily, continuous daily dosing (maximum daily dose used in clinical trials: 50 mg)

Renal cell cancer, advanced (RCC): Oral: 50 mg once daily for 4 weeks of a 6-week treatment cycle (4 weeks on, 2 weeks off)

Soft tissue sarcoma, non-GIST (unlabeled use): Oral: 37.5 mg once daily, continuous daily dosing (George, 2009, *JCO*)

Thyroid cancer, refractory (unlabeled use): Oral: 50 mg once daily for 4 weeks of a 6-week treatment cycle (4 weeks on, 2 weeks off) (Cohen, 2008; Ravaud, 2008)

Dosage adjustment with concurrent CYP3A4 inhibitor: Avoid concomitant administration with strong CYP3A4 inhibitors (eg, clarithromycin, erythromycin, itraconazole, ketoconazole, nefazodone, protease inhibitors, telithromycin, voriconazole); if concomitant administration with a strong CYP3A4 inhibitor cannot be avoided, consider a dose reduction to a minimum of 37.5 mg/day (GIST, RCC) or 25 mg/day (PNET).

Dosage adjustment with concurrent CYP3A4 inducer: Avoid concomitant administration with strong CYP3A4 inducers (eg, carbamazepine, dexamethasone, phenobarbital, phenytoin, rifampin, St John's wort); if concomitant administration with a strong CYP3A4 inducer cannot be avoided, consider a dosage increase (with careful monitoring) to a maximum of 87.5 mg/day (GIST, RCC) or 62.5 mg/day (PNET).

Renal Impairment

Mild, moderate, or severe impairment: No initial adjustment required; subsequent adjustments may be needed based on safety and tolerance.

ESRD on hemodialysis: No initial adjustment required; subsequent dosage **increases** (up to 2 fold) may be required due to reduced (47%) exposure

Hepatic Impairment No adjustment is necessary with mild-to-moderate (Child-Pugh class A or B) hepatic impairment; not studied in patients with severe (Child-Pugh class C) hepatic impairment. Studies excluded patients with ALT or AST >2.5 x ULN, or if due to liver metastases, ALT or AST >5 x ULN.

Adjustment for Toxicity Dosage modifications should be done in increments or decrements of 12.5 mg; individualize based on safety and tolerability.

Cardiac toxicity:

Ejection fraction <50% and >20% below baseline without evidence of CHF: Interrupt treatment and/or reduce dose

LV dysfunction with CHF clinical manifestations: Discontinue treatment

Hepatotoxicity: Hepatic adverse events ≥ grade 3 or 4: Withhold treatment; discontinue if hepatotoxicity does not resolve. Do not reinitiate in patients with severe changes in liver function tests or other signs/symptoms of liver failure.

Severe hypertension: Temporarily interrupt treatment until hypertension is controlled

Nephrotic syndrome or pancreatitis: Discontinue treatment

Reversible posterior leukoencephalopathy (RPLS) or thrombotic microangiopathy: Temporarily withhold treatment; after resolution, may resume with discretion.

Combination Regimens

Renal cell cancer: Sunitinib (RCC Regimen) on page 1753

Administration May be administered with or without food.

Emetic Potential Low (10% to 30%)

Extemporaneous Preparations Hazardous agent: Use appropriate precautions for handling and disposal.

A 10 mg/mL sunitinib oral suspension may be made with capsules and a 1:1 mixture of Ora-Sweet® and Ora-Plus®. Empty the contents of three 50 mg sunitinib capsules into a mortar; add small portions of vehicle and mix to a uniform paste. Mix while adding vehicle in incremental proportions to 15 mL. Transfer to amber plastic bottle and label "shake well". This suspension maintains an average concentration of 96% to 106% (of the original concentration) at room temperature or refrigerated for up to 60 days in plastic amber prescription bottles.

Navid F, Christensen R, Minkin P, et al, "Stability of Sunitinib in Oral Suspension," *Ann Pharmacother*, 2008, 42(7):962-6.

Monitoring Parameters LVEF, baseline (and periodic with cardiac risk factors), ECG (12-lead; baseline and periodic), blood pressure; adrenal function CBC with differential and platelets (prior to each treatment cycle), liver function tests (baseline, with each cycle and if clinically indicated), serum chemistries including magnesium, phosphate, and potassium (prior to each treatment cycle), urinalysis (for proteinuria development or worsening); consider dental exam prior to treatment initiation; symptoms of hypothyroidism

Thyroid function testing (Hamnvik, 2011):

Pre-existing levothyroxine therapy: Obtain baseline TSH levels, then monitor every 4 weeks until levels and levothyroxine dose are stable, then monitor every 2 months

Without pre-existing thyroid hormone replacement: TSH at baseline, then every 4 weeks for 4 months, then every 2-3 months

Dietary Considerations May be taken with or without food. Avoid grapefruit juice.

Additional Information Hand-foot skin reaction (HFSR) observed with tyrosine kinase inhibitors (TKIs) is distinct from hand-foot syndrome (palmar-plantar erythrodysesthesia) associated with traditional chemotherapy agents; HFSR due to TKIs is localized with defined hyperkeratotic lesions; symptoms include burning, dysesthesia, paresthesia, or tingling on the palms/soles, and generally occur within the first 2-4 weeks of treatment; pressure and flexor areas may develop blisters (callus-like), dry/cracked skin, edema, erythema, desquamation, or hyperkeratosis (Appleby, 2011).

HFSR management (Lacouture, 2008): The following treatments may be used in addition to the recommended dosage modifications. Prior to treatment initiation, a pedicure is recommended to remove hyperkeratotic areas/calluses, which may predispose to HFSR; avoid vigorous exercise/activities which may stress hands or feet. During therapy, patients should reduce exposure to hot water (may exacerbate hand-foot symptoms); avoid constrictive footwear and excessive skin friction. Patients may also wear thick cotton gloves or socks and should wear shoes with padded insoles. Grade 1 HFSR may be relieved with moisturizing creams, cotton gloves and socks (at night) and/or keratolytic creams such as urea (20% to 40%) or salicylic acid (6%). Apply topical steroid (eg, clobetasol ointment) twice daily to erythematous areas of Grade 2 HFSR; topical anesthetics (eg, lidocaine 2%) and then systemic analgesics (if appropriate) may be used for pain control. Resolution of acute erythema may result in keratotic areas which may be softened with keratolytic agents.

Medication Guide Available Yes

Dosage Forms Excipient information presented when available (limited, particularly for generics); consult specific product labeling.

Capsule, oral:

Sutent®: 12.5 mg, 25 mg, 50 mg

References

Appleby L, Morrissey S, Bellmunt J, et al, "Management of Treatment-Related Toxicity With Targeted Therapies for Renal Cell Carcinoma: Evidence-Based Practice and Best Practices," *Hematol Oncol Clin North Am*, 2011, 25(4):893-915.

Castellano D, del Muro XG, Pérez-Gracia JL, et al, "Patient-Reported Outcomes in a Phase III, Randomized Study of Sunitinib Versus Interferon-{alpha} as First-Line Systemic Therapy for Patients With Metastatic Renal Cell Carcinoma in a European Population," *Ann Oncol*, 2009, 20 (11):1803-12.

Cohen EE, Needles BM, Cullen KJ, et al, "Phase 2 Study of Sunitinib in Refractory Thyroid Cancer," *J Clin Oncol*, 2008, 26(Supp):6025 [abstract 6025 from 2008 ASCO Annual Meeting].

Demetri GD, van Oosterom AT, Garret CR, et al, "Efficacy and Safety of Sunitinib in Patients With Advanced Gastrointestinal Stromal Tumour After Failure of Imatinib: A Randomised Controlled Trial," *Lancet*, 2006, 368(9544):1329-38.

George S, Blay JY, Casali PG, et al, "Clinical Evaluation of Continuous Daily Dosing of Sunitinib Malate in Patients With Advanced Gastrointestinal Stromal Tumour After Imatinib Failure," *Eur J Cancer*, 2009, 45(11):1959-68.

George S, Merriam P, Maki RG, et al, "Multicenter Phase II Trial of Sunitinib in the Treatment of Nongastrointestinal Stromal Tumor Sarcomas," *J Clin Oncol*, 2009, 27(19):3154-60.

Gupta S, Parsa VB, Heilbrun LK, et al, "Safety and Efficacy of Molecularly Targeted Agents in Patients With Metastatic Kidney Cancer With Renal Dysfunction," *Anticancer Drugs*, 2011, 22 (8):794-800.

Hamnvik OP, Larsen PR and Marqusee E, "Thyroid Dysfunction From Antineoplastic Agents," *J Natl Cancer Inst*, 2011 [epub ahead of print].

Lacouture ME, Wu S, Robert C, et al, "Evolving Strategies for the Management of Hand-Foot Skin Reaction Associated With the Multitargeted Kinase Inhibitors Sorafenib and Sunitinib," *Oncologist*, 2008, 13(9):1001-11.

Motzer RJ, Hutson TE, Tomczak P, et al, "Sunitinib Versus Interferon Alfa in Metastatic Renal-Cell Cancer," *N Engl J Med*, 2007, 356(2):115-24.

Moltzer RJ, Michaelson MD, and Redman BG, "Activity of SU11248, a Multitargeted Inhibitor of Vascular Endothelial Growth Factor Receptor, in Patients With Metastatic Renal Cell Cancer," *J Clin Oncol*, 2006, 24(1):16-24.

Niccoli P, Raoul J, Bang Y, et al, "Updated Safety and Efficacy Results of the Phase III Trial of Sunitinib (SU) Versus Placebo (PBO) for Treatment of Pancreatic Neuroendocrine Tumors (NET)," *J Clin Oncol*, 2010, 28(15s):4000 [abstract 4000 from 2010 ASCO Annual Meeting].

Ravaud A, de la Fouchardiere C, Courbon F, et al, "Sunitinib in Patients With Refractory Advanced Thyroid Cancer: The THYSU Phase II Trial," *J Clin Oncol*, 2008, 26(Supp):6058 [abstract 6058 from 2008 ASCO Annual Meeting].

Raymond E, Dahan L, Raoul JL, et al, "Sunitinib Malate for the Treatment of Pancreatic Neuroendocrine Tumors," *N Engl J Med*, 2011, 364(6):501-13.

Zastrow S, Froehner M, Platzek I, et al, "Treatment of Metastatic Renal Cell Cancer With Sunitinib During Chronic Hemodialysis," *Urology*, 2009, 73(4):868-70.

◆ **Sunitinib Malate** *see* SUNItinib *on page* 1308

◆ **Supeudol® (Can)** *see* OxyCODONE *on page* 1084

◆ **Supprelin® LA** *see* Histrelin *on page* 707

◆ **Sutent®** *see* SUNItinib *on page* 1308

◆ **Sylatron™** *see* Peginterferon Alfa-2b *on page* 1140

- **Synribo™** *see* Omacetaxine *on page* 1064
- **Tabloid®** *see* Thioguanine *on page* 1354

Tacrolimus (Systemic) (ta KROE li mus)

Related Information

Hematopoietic Stem Cell Transplantation *on page* 1887

Safe Handling of Hazardous Drugs *on page* 1904

Brand Names: U.S. Hecoria™; Prograf®

Brand Names: Canada Advagraf®; Prograf®

Index Terms FK506

Generic Availability (U.S.) Yes: Capsule

Pharmacologic Category Calcineurin Inhibitor; Immunosuppressant Agent

Use

U.S. labeling: Prevention of organ rejection in heart (Prograf® only), and kidney or liver (Hecoria™, Prograf®) transplant recipients

Canadian labeling:

Prograf®: Prevention of organ rejection in heart, kidney, or liver transplant recipients; treatment of refractory rejection in kidney or liver transplant recipients; treatment of active rheumatoid arthritis in adult patients non-responsive to disease-modifying antirheumatic drug (DMARD) therapy or when DMARD therapy is inappropriate

Advagraf®: Prevention of organ rejection in kidney transplant recipients

Unlabeled Use Prevention of organ rejection in lung, small bowel transplant recipients; prevention and treatment of graft-versus-host disease (GVHD) in allogenic hematopoietic stem cell transplantation

Labeled Contraindications Hypersensitivity to tacrolimus or any component of the formulation

Pregnancy Risk Factor C

Lactation Enters breast milk/not recommended

Warnings/Precautions Hazardous agent - use appropriate precautions for handling and disposal. **[U.S. Boxed Warning]: Risk of developing infections (including bacterial, viral [including CMV], fungal, and protozoal infections [including opportunistic infections]) is increased.** Latent viral infections may be activated, including BK virus (associated with polyoma virus-associated nephropathy [PVAN]) and JC virus (associated with progressive multifocal leukoencephalopathy [PML]); may result in serious adverse effects. The risk of CMV disease is increased for patients who are CMV-seronegative prior to transplant and receive a graft from a CMV-seropositive donor. Consider reduction in immunosuppression if PVAN, PML, CMV viremia and/or CMV disease occurs. **[U.S. Boxed Warning]: Immunosuppressive therapy may result in the development of lymphoma and other malignancies (predominantly skin malignancies).** The risk for new-onset diabetes and insulin-dependent post-transplant diabetes mellitus (PTDM) is increased with tacrolimus use after transplantation, including in patients without pretransplant history of diabetes mellitus; insulin dependence may be reversible; increased risk in African-American and Hispanic kidney transplant patients. Nephrotoxicity has has been reported, especially with higher doses; to avoid excess nephrotoxicity do not administer simultaneously with other nephrotoxic drugs (eg sirolimus, cyclosporine). Neurotoxicity may occur especially when used in high doses; tremor headache, coma and delirium have been reported and are associated with serum concentrations. Seizures may also occur. Posterior reversible encephalopathy syndrome (PRES) may also occur; symptoms (altered mental status, headache, hypertension, seizures, and visual disturbances) are reversible with dose reduction or discontinuation of therapy; stabilize blood pressure and reduce dose with suspected or confirmed PRES diagnosis.

Pure red cell aplasia (PRCA) has been reported in patients receiving tacrolimus. Use with caution in patients with risk factors for PRCA including parvovirus B19 infection, underlying disease, or use of concomitant medications associated with PRCA (eg, mycophenolate). Discontinuation of therapy should be considered with diagnosis of PRCA. Monitoring of serum concentrations (trough for oral therapy) is essential to prevent organ rejection and reduce drug-related toxicity. A period of ≥24 hours should elapse between discontinuation of cyclosporine and the initiation of tacrolimus. Delay initiation further with persistently elevated tacrolimus/cyclosporine levels. Use caution in renal or hepatic dysfunction, dosing adjustments may be required. Delay initiation of therapy in kidney transplant patients if postoperative oliguria occurs; begin therapy no sooner than 6 hours and within 24 hours post-transplant, but may be delayed until renal function has recovered. Use may be associated with the development of hypertension (common); hyperkalemia has been reported; avoid use of potassium-sparing diuretics. Myocardial hypertrophy has been reported (rare). Concurrent use with strong CYP3A4 inhibitors (eg, ritonavir, ketoconazole, itraconazole, voriconazole, clarithromycin) or inducers (eg, rifampin, rifabutin) is not recommended without close monitoring of tacrolimus trough concentrations.

Each mL of injection contains polyoxyl 60 hydrogenated castor oil (HCO-60) (200 mg) and dehydrated alcohol USP 80% v/v. Anaphylaxis has been reported with the injection, use should be reserved for those patients not able to take oral medications. Patients should not be immunized with live vaccines during or shortly after treatment and should avoid close contact with recently vaccinated (live vaccine) individuals. Oral formulations contain lactose; the Canadian labeling does not recommend use of these products in patients who may be lactose intolerant (eg, Lapp lactase deficiency, glucose-galactose malabsorption, galactose intolerance). **[U.S. Boxed Warning]: Should be administered under the supervision of a physician experienced in immunosuppressive therapy and organ transplantation in a facility appropriate for monitoring and managing therapy.**

Adverse Reactions As reported for kidney, liver, and heart transplantation:

≥15%:

Cardiovascular: Hypertension (13% to 62%), edema (peripheral 11% to 36%), chest pain (19%), edema (18%), pericardial effusion (heart transplant 15%)

Central nervous system: Headache (24% to 64%), insomnia (30% to 64%), pain (24% to 63%), fever (19% to 48%), postprocedural pain (kidney transplant 29%), dizziness (19%)

Dermatologic: Pruritus (15% to 36%), rash (10% to 24%)

Endocrine & metabolic: New-onset diabetes after transplant (kidney transplant 75%), hypophosphatemia (28% to 49%), hypomagnesemia (16% to 48%), hyperglycemia (21% to 47%), hyperkalemia (13% to 45%), hyperlipemia (10% to 31%), hypokalemia (13% to 29%), diabetes mellitus (24% to 26%), post-transplant diabetes mellitus (heart transplant 13% to 22%; kidney transplant 20%; liver transplant 11% to 18%)

Gastrointestinal: Diarrhea (25% to 72%), abdominal pain (29% to 59%), nausea (32% to 46%), constipation (23% to 36%), anorexia (7% to 34%), vomiting (14% to 29%), dyspepsia (18% to 28%)
Genitourinary: Urinary tract infection (16% to 34%)
Hematologic: Anemia (5% to 50%), leukopenia (13% to 48%), leukocytosis (8% to 32%), thrombocytopenia (14% to 24%)
Hepatic: Liver function tests abnormal (6% to 36%), ascites (7% to 27%)
Local: Incision site complication (kidney transplant 28%)
Neuromuscular & skeletal: Tremor (15% to 56%; heart transplant 15%), weakness (11% to 52%), paresthesia (17% to 40%), back pain (17% to 30%), arthralgia (25%)
Renal: Abnormal kidney function (36% to 56%), creatinine increased (23% to 45%), BUN increased (12% to 30%), oliguria (18% to 19%)
Respiratory: Atelectasis (5% to 28%), pleural effusion (30% to 36%), dyspnea (5% to 29%), cough increased (18%), bronchitis (17%)
Miscellaneous: Infection (24% to 45%), CMV infection (heart transplant 32%), graft dysfunction (kidney transplant 24%)

<15%:

Cardiovascular: Abnormal ECG (QRS or ST segment abnormal), arrhythmia, atrial fibrillation, atrial flutter, bradycardia, cardiopulmonary failure, deep thrombophlebitis, heart failure, heart rate decreased, hemorrhage, hemorrhagic stroke, hypervolemia, hypotension, orthostatic hypotension, peripheral vascular disorder, phlebitis, syncope, tachycardia, thrombosis, vasodilation
Central nervous system: Abnormal dreams, abnormal thinking, agitation, amnesia, anxiety, chills, confusion, depression, emotional lability, encephalopathy, flaccid paralysis, hallucinations, mood elevated, nervousness, psychosis, quadriparesis, seizure, somnolence, vertigo
Dermatologic: Acne, alopecia, bruising, cellulitis, exfoliative dermatitis, fungal dermatitis, hirsutism, photosensitivity reaction, skin discoloration, skin disorder, skin neoplasm, skin ulcer, wound healing impaired
Endocrine & metabolic: Acidosis, alkalosis, bicarbonate decreased, Cushing's syndrome, dehydration, gout, hypercholesterolemia, hyper-/hypocalcemia, hyponatremia, hyperphosphatemia, hyperuricemia, hypoproteinemia, serum iron decreased
Gastrointestinal: Appetite increased, cramps, duodenitis, dysphagia, enlarged abdomen, esophagitis (including ulcerative), flatulence, gastritis, gastroesophagitis, GI perforation/hemorrhage, ileus, oral moniliasis, pancreatic pseudocyst, rectal disorder, stomatitis, weight gain
Genitourinary: Bladder spasm, cystitis, dysuria, nocturia, urge incontinence, urinary frequency, urinary incontinence, urinary retention, vaginitis
Hematologic: Coagulation disorder, decreased prothrombin, hypochromic anemia, polycythemia
Hepatic: Alkaline phosphatase increased, bilirubinemia, cholangitis, cholestatic jaundice, GGT increased, hepatitis (including granulomatous), jaundice, LDH increased, liver damage
Local: Phlebitis
Neuromuscular & skeletal: Hypertonia, incoordination, joint disorder, leg cramps, monoparesis, myalgia, myasthenia, myoclonus, nerve compression, neuropathy, osteoporosis, quadriparesis
Ocular: Abnormal vision, amblyopia
Otic: Ear pain, otitis media, tinnitus
Renal: Acute renal failure, albuminuria, BK nephropathy, hematuria, hydronephrosis, renal tubular necrosis, toxic nephropathy

Respiratory: Asthma, emphysema, lung disorder, lung function decreased, pharyngitis, pneumonia, pneumothorax, pulmonary edema, respiratory disorder, rhinitis, sinusitis, voice alteration

Miscellaneous: Abscess, abnormal healing, allergic reaction, crying, diaphoresis, flu-like syndrome, generalized spasm, hernia, herpes simplex, hiccups, peritonitis, sepsis, writing impaired

Postmarketing and/or case reports: Agranulocytosis, anaphylaxis, anaphylactoid reaction, angioedema, ARDS, atrial flutter, basal cell carcinoma, bile duct stenosis, blindness, cardiac arrest, cerebral infarction, cerebrovascular accident, deafness, delirium, DIC, hemiparesis, hemolytic anemia, hemolytic-uremic syndrome, hemorrhagic cystitis, hepatic necrosis, hepatotoxicity, interstitial lung disease, leukoencephalopathy, lymphoproliferative disorder (related to EBV), malignant melanoma, myocardial hypertrophy (associated with ventricular dysfunction; reversible upon discontinuation), MI, neutropenia, osteomyelitis, pancreatitis (hemorrhagic and necrotizing), pancytopenia, posterior reversible encephalopathy syndrome (PRES), progressive multifocal leukoencephalopathy (PML), quadriplegia, QT_c prolongation, respiratory failure, septicemia, squamous cell carcinoma, Stevens-Johnson syndrome, toxic epidermal necrolysis, thrombocytopenic purpura, torsade de pointes, TTP, veno-occlusive hepatic disease, venous thrombosis, ventricular fibrillation

Note: Calcineurin inhibitor-induced hemolytic uremic syndrome/thrombotic thrombocytopenic purpura/thrombotic microangiopathy (HUS/TTP/TMA) have been reported (with concurrent sirolimus).

Drug Interactions

Metabolism/Transport Effects **Substrate** of CYP3A4 (major), P-glycoprotein; **Note:** Assignment of Major/Minor substrate status based on clinically relevant drug interaction potential; **Inhibits** CYP3A4 (weak), P-glycoprotein

Avoid Concomitant Use

Avoid concomitant use of Tacrolimus (Systemic) with any of the following: BCG; Bosutinib; CloZAPine; Conivaptan; Crizotinib; CycloSPORINE (Systemic); Enzalutamide; Eplerenone; Grapefruit Juice; Mifepristone; Natalizumab; Pimecrolimus; Pimozide; Potassium-Sparing Diuretics; Silodosin; Tacrolimus (Topical); Temsirolimus; Topotecan; Vaccines (Live); VinCRIStine (Liposomal)

Increased Effect/Toxicity

Tacrolimus (Systemic) may increase the levels/effects of: ARIPiprazole; Bosutinib; CloZAPine; Colchicine; CycloSPORINE (Systemic); Dabigatran Etexilate; Everolimus; Fenofibrate; Fenofibric Acid; Fosphenytoin; Highest Risk QTc-Prolonging Agents; Leflunomide; Moderate Risk QTc-Prolonging Agents; Natalizumab; P-glycoprotein/ABCB1 Substrates; Phenytoin; Pimozide; Prucalopride; Rivaroxaban; Silodosin; Sirolimus; Temsirolimus; Topotecan; Vaccines (Live); VinCRIStine (Liposomal)

The levels/effects of Tacrolimus (Systemic) may be increased by: Antidepressants (Serotonin Reuptake Inhibitor/Antagonist); Boceprevir; Calcium Channel Blockers (Dihydropyridine); Calcium Channel Blockers (Nondihydropyridine); Chloramphenicol; Clotrimazole (Oral); Conivaptan; Crizotinib; CycloSPORINE (Systemic); CYP3A4 Inhibitors (Moderate); CYP3A4 Inhibitors (Strong); Danazol; Dasatinib; Denosumab; Eplerenone; Fluconazole; Grapefruit Juice; Itraconazole; Ivacaftor; Ketoconazole (Systemic); Macrolide Antibiotics; MetroNIDAZOLE (Systemic); Mifepristone; P-glycoprotein/ABCB1 Inhibitors; Pimecrolimus; Posaconazole; Potassium-Sparing

Diuretics; Protease Inhibitors; Proton Pump Inhibitors; Ranolazine; Roflumilast; Sirolimus; Tacrolimus (Topical); Telaprevir; Temsirolimus; Trastuzumab; Voriconazole

Decreased Effect

Tacrolimus (Systemic) may decrease the levels/effects of: BCG; Coccidioidin Skin Test; Sipuleucel-T; Vaccines (Inactivated); Vaccines (Live)

The levels/effects of Tacrolimus (Systemic) may be decreased by: Caspofungin; Cinacalcet; CYP3A4 Inducers (Strong); Deferasirox; Echinacea; Efavirenz; Enzalutamide; Fosphenytoin; P-glycoprotein/ABCB1 Inducers; Phenytoin; Rifamycin Derivatives; Sirolimus; St Johns Wort; Temsirolimus; Tocilizumab

Ethanol/Nutrition/Herb Interactions

Food: Food decreases rate and extent of absorption. High-fat meals have most pronounced effect (37% decrease in AUC, 77% decrease in C_{max}). Grapefruit juice, a CYP3A4 inhibitor, may increase serum level and/or toxicity of tacrolimus. Management: Administer with or without food, but be consistent. Avoid concurrent use of grapefruit juice.

Herb/Nutraceutical: St John's wort may reduce tacrolimus serum concentrations. Management: Avoid St John's wort.

Storage/Stability

Injection: Prior to dilution, store at 5°C to 25°C (41°F to 77°F). Following dilution, stable for 24 hours in D_5W or NS in glass or polyethylene containers.

Capsules: Store at controlled room temperature.

Reconstitution Dilute with 5% dextrose injection or 0.9% sodium chloride injection to a final concentration between 0.004 mg/mL and 0.02 mg/mL.

Mechanism of Action Suppresses cellular immunity (inhibits T-lymphocyte activation), by binding to an intracellular protein, FKBP-12 and complexes with calcineurin dependent proteins to inhibit calcineurin phosphatase activity

Pharmacodynamics/Kinetics

Absorption: Better in resected patients with a closed stoma; unlike cyclosporine, clamping of the T-tube in liver transplant patients does not alter trough concentrations or AUC; Oral: Incomplete and variable; the rate and extent of absorption is affected by food and may be most pronounced with a high fat meal. Oral absorption may be variable in stem cell transplant patients with mucositis due to the conditioning regimen.

Distribution: V_d: Children: 0.5-4.7 L/kg; Adults: 0.55-2.47 L/kg

Protein binding: ~99% primarily to albumin and alpha$_1$-acid glycoprotein glycoprotein

Metabolism: Extensively hepatic via CYP3A4 to eight possible metabolites (major metabolite, 31-demethyl tacrolimus, shows same activity as tacrolimus *in vitro*)

Bioavailability: Oral: Children: 7% to 55%, Adults: 7% to 32%; Absolute: Unknown

Half-life elimination: Variable, 23-46 hours in healthy volunteers; 2.1-36 hours in transplant patients

Time to peak: 0.5-6 hours

Excretion: Feces (~93%); urine (<1% as unchanged drug)

Dosing

Adult & Geriatric

Prevention of organ rejection in transplant recipients: Note: The initial dose of tacrolimus should begin no sooner than 6 hours after liver and heart transplant and within 24 hours of kidney transplant (but may be delayed until renal function has recovered). Adjunctive therapy with corticosteroids is recommended early post-transplant. I.V. route should only be used in patients not able to take oral medications and continued only until oral medication can be tolerated; anaphylaxis has been reported with I.V. administration. If switching from I.V. to oral, the oral dose should be started 8-12 hours after stopping the infusion.

Liver transplant:

Oral: Initial dose: 0.1-0.15 mg/kg/day in 2 divided doses, given every 12 hours

I.V.: Initial dose: 0.03-0.05 mg/kg/day as a continuous infusion

Heart transplant: Use in combination with azathioprine or mycophenolate mofetil is recommended.

Oral: Initial dose: 0.075 mg/kg/day in 2 divided doses, given every 12 hours

I.V.: Initial dose: 0.01 mg/kg/day as a continuous infusion

Kidney transplant: Use in combination with azathioprine or mycophenolate mofetil is recommended.

Oral:

U.S. labeling: Initial dose: 0.2 mg/kg/day in combination with azathioprine **or** 0.1 mg/kg/day in combination with mycophenolate mofetil. Administer in 2 divided doses, given every 12 hours; African-American patients may require larger doses to maintain trough concentration.

Canadian labeling:

Prograf®: Initial: 0.2-0.3 mg/kg/day in 2 divided doses, given every 12 hours in combination with corticosteroids and other immunosuppressive agents.

Advagraf®: Initial: 0.15-0.2 mg/kg/day. Administer once daily in combination with corticosteroids and mycophenolate mofetil (MMF) in *de novo* kidney transplant recipients. Antibody induction therapy should also be used.

Conversion from Prograf® to Advagraf®: Initiate Advagraf® therapy using previously established total daily dose of Prograf®. Administer once daily.

I.V.: Initial dose: 0.03-0.05 mg/kg/day as a continuous infusion

Prevention of graft-versus-host disease (unlabeled use):

Oral: Convert from I.V. to oral dose (1:4 ratio): Multiply total daily I.V. dose times 4 and administer in 2 divided oral doses per day, every 12 hours (Uberti, 1999; Yanik, 2000).

I.V.: Initial: 0.03 mg/kg/day (based on lean body weight) as continuous infusion. Treatment should begin at least 24 hours prior to stem cell infusion and continued only until oral medication can be tolerated (Przepiorka, 1999; Yanik, 2000)

Rheumatoid arthritis: Canadian labeling (not in U.S. labeling): *Oral:* 3 mg once daily; carefully monitor serum creatinine during therapy

Treatment of graft-versus-host disease (unlabeled use):

Oral: 0.06 mg/kg twice daily (Furlong, 2000; Przepiorka, 1999)

I.V.: Initial: 0.03 mg/kg/day (based on lean body weight) as continuous infusion (Furlong, 2000; Przepiorka, 1999)

Pediatric

Liver transplant:

Oral: Initial dose: 0.15-0.20 mg/kg/day in 2 divided doses, given every 12 hours

I.V.: Initial dose: 0.03-0.05 mg/kg/day as a continuous infusion.

Note: The initial dose of tacrolimus should begin no sooner than 6 hours after liver and heart transplant and within 24 hours of kidney transplant (but may be delayed until renal function has recovered). Adjunctive therapy with corticosteroids is recommended early post-transplant. I.V. route should only be used in patients not able to take oral medications and continued only until oral medication can be tolerated; anaphylaxis has been reported with I.V. administration. If switching from I.V. to oral, the oral dose should be started 8-12 hours after stopping the infusion. Patients without pre-existing renal or hepatic dysfunction have required (and tolerated) higher doses than adults to achieve similar blood concentrations. It is recommended that therapy be initiated at the ***high end*** of the recommended adult I.V. and oral dosing ranges; dosage adjustments may be required.

Prevention of graft-vs-host disease (unlabeled use): Oral, I.V.: Refer to adult dosing.

Renal Impairment Evidence suggests that lower doses should be used; patients should receive doses at the lowest value of the recommended I.V. and oral dosing ranges; further reductions in dose below these ranges may be required.

Kidney transplant: Tacrolimus therapy in patients with postoperative oliguria should begin no sooner than 6 hours and within 24 hours post-transplant, but may be delayed until renal function has recovered.

Hemodialysis: Not removed by hemodialysis; supplemental dose is not necessary.

Peritoneal dialysis: Significant drug removal is unlikely based on physiochemical characteristics.

Hepatic Impairment Use of tacrolimus in liver transplant recipients experiencing post-transplant hepatic impairment may be associated with increased risk of developing renal insufficiency related to high whole blood levels of tacrolimus. The presence of moderate-to-severe hepatic dysfunction (serum bilirubin >2 mg/dL; Child-Pugh score ≥10) appears to affect the metabolism of tacrolimus. The half-life of the drug was prolonged and the clearance reduced after I.V. administration. The bioavailability of tacrolimus was also increased after oral administration. The higher plasma concentrations as determined by ELISA, in patients with severe hepatic dysfunction are probably due to the accumulation of metabolites of lower activity. These patients should be monitored closely and dosage adjustments should be considered. Some evidence indicates that lower doses could be used in these patients.

Administration

I.V.: If I.V. administration is necessary, administer by continuous infusion only. Do not use PVC tubing when administering diluted solutions. Tacrolimus is usually intended to be administered as a continuous infusion over 24 hours. Do not mix with solutions with a pH ≥9 (eg, acyclovir or ganciclovir) due to chemical degradation of tacrolimus (use different ports in multilumen lines). Do not alter dose with concurrent T-tube clamping. Adsorption of the drug to PVC tubing may become clinically significant with low concentrations.

Oral: Administer with or without food; be consistent with timing and composition of meals if GI intolerance occurs and administration with food becomes necessary (per manufacturer). If dosed once daily, administer in the morning. If dosed twice daily, doses should be 12 hours apart. If the morning and evening doses differ, the larger dose (differences are never >0.5-1 mg) should be given in the morning. If dosed 3 times/day, separate doses by 8 hours.

Advagraf®: Canadian labeling recommends that missed doses may be taken up to 14 hours after scheduled time; if >14 hours, resume at next regularly scheduled time.

Extemporaneous Preparations Hazardous agent: Use appropriate precautions for handling and disposal.

A 0.5 mg/mL tacrolimus oral suspension may be made with capsules and a 1:1 mixture of Ora-Plus® and Simple Syrup, N.F. Mix the contents of six 5 mg tacrolimus capsules with quantity of vehicle sufficient to make 60 mL. Store in glass or plastic amber prescription bottles; label "shake well". Stable for 56 days at room temperature (Esquivel, 1996; Foster, 1996).

A 1 mg/mL tacrolimus oral suspension may be made with capsules, sterile water, Ora-Plus®, and Ora-Sweet®. Pour the contents of six 5 mg capsules into a plastic amber prescription bottle. Add ~5 mL of sterile water and agitate bottle until drug disperses into a slurry. Add equal parts Ora-Plus® and Ora-Sweet® in sufficient quantity to make 30 mL. Store in plastic amber prescription bottles; label "shake well". Stable for 4 months at room temperature (Elefante, 2006).

Elefante A, Muindi J, West K, et al, "Long-Term Stability of a Patient-Convenient 1 mg/mL Suspension of Tacrolimus for Accurate Maintenance of Stable Therapeutic Levels," *Bone Marrow Transplant*, 2006, 37(8):781-4.

Esquivel C, So S, McDiarmid S, Andrews W, and Colombani PM, "Suggested Guidelines for the Use of Tacrolimus in Pediatric Liver Transplant Patients," *Transplantation*, 1996, 61(5):847-8.

Foster JA, Jacobson PA, Johnson CE, et al, "Stability of Tacrolimus in an Extemporaneously Compounded Oral Liquid (Abstract of Meeting Presentation)," *American Society of Health-System Pharmacists Annual Meeting*, 1996, 53:P-52(E).

Monitoring Parameters Renal function, hepatic function, serum electrolytes (especially potassium), glucose and blood pressure, measure 3 times/week for first few weeks, then gradually decrease frequency as patient stabilizes. Whole blood concentrations should be used for monitoring (trough for oral therapy). Signs/symptoms of anaphylactic reactions during infusion should also be monitored. Patients should be monitored during the first 30 minutes of the infusion, and frequently thereafter.

Tacrolimus serum levels may be falsely elevated in infected liver transplant patients due to interference from β-galactosidase antibodies.

Dietary Considerations Capsule: Administer with or without food; be consistent with timing and composition of meals, food decreases bioavailability. Avoid grapefruit juice.

Medication Guide Available Yes

Dosage Forms Excipient information presented when available (limited, particularly for generics); consult specific product labeling.

Capsule, oral: 0.5 mg, 1 mg, 5 mg

- Hecoria™: 0.5 mg, 1 mg, 5 mg
- Prograf®: 0.5 mg, 1 mg, 5 mg

Injection, solution:

- Prograf®: 5 mg/mL (1 mL) [contains dehydrated ethanol 80%, polyoxyl 60 hydrogenated castor oil]

Dosage Forms: Canada Excipient information presented when available (limited, particularly for generics); consult specific product labeling.

Capsule, oral:

- Advagraf®: 0.5 mg, 1 mg, 3 mg, 5 mg

References

Furlong T, Storb R, Anasetti C, et al, "Clinical Outcome After Conversion to FK 506 (Tacrolimus) Therapy for Acute Graft-Versus-Host Disease Resistant to Cyclosporine or for Cyclosporine-Associated Toxicities," *Bone Marrow Transplant*, 2000, 26(9):985-91.

Grimer M and Caring for Australians with Renal Impairment (CARI), "The CARI Guidelines. Calcineurin Inhibitors in Renal Transplantation: Pregnancy, Lactation and Calcineurin Inhibitors," Nephrology (Carlton), 2007, 12(Suppl 1):98-105.

Kaufman DB, Kaplan B, Kanwar YS, et al, "The Successful Use of Tacrolimus (FK506) in a Pancreas/Kidney Transplant Recipient With Recurrent Cyclosporine-Associated Hemolytic Uremic Syndrome," *Transplantation*, 1995, 59(12):1737-9.

McDiarmid SV, Colonna JO, Shaked A, et al, "Differences in Oral FK506 Dose Requirements Between Adults and Pediatric Liver Transplant Patients," *Transplantation*, 1993, 55(6):1328-32.

Messina C, Faraci M, de Fazio V, et al, "Paediatric Working Party. Prevention and Treatment of Acute GvHD," *Bone Marrow Transplant*, 2008, 41(Suppl 2):65-70.

Podesser BK, Rinaldi M, Yona NA, et al, "Comparison of Low and High Initial Tacrolimus Dosing in Primary Heart Transplant Recipients: A Prospective European Multicenter Study," *Transplantation*, 2005, 79(1):65-71.

Przepiorka D, Devine S, Fay J, et al, "Practical Considerations in the Use of Tacrolimus for Allogeneic Marrow Transplantation," *Bone Marrow Transplant*, 1999, 24(10):1053-6.

Przepiorka D, Suzuki J, Ippoliti C, et al, "Blood Tacrolimus Concentration Unchanged by Plasmapheresis," *Am J Hosp Pharm*, 1994, 51(13):1708.

Starzl TE, Fung J, Jordan M, et al, "Kidney Transplantation Under FK506," *JAMA*, 1990, 264(1):63-7.

Uberti JP, Cronin S, and Ratanatharathorn V, "Optimum Use of Tacrolimus in the Prophylaxis of Graft Versus Host Disease," *BioDrugs*, 1999, 11(5):343-58.

Yanik G, Levine JE, Ratanatharathorn V, et al, "Tacrolimus (FK506) and Methotrexate as Prophylaxis for Acute Graft-Versus-Host Disease in Pediatric Allogeneic Stem Cell Transplantation," *Bone Marrow Transplant*, 2000, 26(2):161-7.

◆ **Talc** *see* Talc (Sterile) *on page* 1323

◆ **Talc for Pleurodesis** *see* Talc (Sterile) *on page* 1323

Talc (Sterile) (talk STARE il)

Related Information

Malignant Pleural Effusions *on page* 1865

Brand Names: U.S. Sclerosol®; Sterile Talc Powder™

Index Terms Intrapleural Talc; Sterile Talc; Talc; Talc for Pleurodesis

Pharmacologic Category Sclerosing Agent

Use Prevention of recurrence of malignant pleural effusion in symptomatic patients

Labeled Contraindications There are no contraindications listed within the manufacturer's labeling.

Pregnancy Risk Factor B

Warnings/Precautions Acute pneumonitis and acute respiratory distress syndrome (including one death) have rarely been reported with higher doses (10 g). Should not be used to treat malignancies; does not have antineoplastic activity. Clinicians should evaluate need for future diagnostic procedures before use; sclerosis of pleural space may preclude subsequent procedures (eg, pneumonectomy for transplantation). Sclerosol® contents under pressure and should be kept away from any heat source.

Adverse Reactions Frequency not defined.

Cardiovascular: Asystolic arrest, chest pain, hypotension (transient), hypovolemia, MI, tachycardia

Central nervous system: Fever (generally lasting <24 hours)

Local: Bleeding (localized), infection at administration site, pain

Respiratory: ARDS, bronchopleural fistula, dyspnea, empyema, hemoptysis, hypoxemia, pneumonia, pulmonary edema, pulmonary embolism, subcutaneous emphysema

Storage/Stability

Sclerosol® Intrapleural Aerosol: Store at room temperature 15°C to 30°C (59°F to 86°F); do not freeze. Protect from heat and light.

Sterile Talc Powder™: Store at controlled room temperature of 18°C to 25°C (64°F to 77°F). Protect from light. Use within 12 hours of slurry preparation.

Reconstitution Sterile Talc Powder™: Vent bottle with needle; slowly add 50 mL of NS to bottle using aseptic technique. For doses >5 g, use a second bottle. Swirl the bottle to disperse talc and avoid settling. Divide the contents of each bottle into two 60 mL irrigation syringes (25 mL of talc slurry in each). Add an additional 25 mL of NS to each syringe for a total of 50 mL (2.5 g/50 mL). If not used immediately, label "For IntraPleural Use Only."

Mechanism of Action Induces an inflammatory reaction that promotes adherence of the visceral to the parietal pleura, therefore, preventing reaccumulation of pleural fluid.

Dosing

Adult Pleural effusion:

Intrapleural aerosol: 4-8 g (1-2 cans) as a single dose

Intrapleural instillation: 5 g

Administration Administer after adequate drainage of the effusion.

Sclerosol® Intrapleural Aerosol: Shake well and attach delivery tube. Insert delivery tube through pleural trocar, manually press on actuator button of canister to release; point in several different directions to distribute to all pleural surfaces. Keep canister in an upright position. Rate of delivery is 0.4 g per second.

Sterile Talc Powder™: Administer as a slurry. Shake well before instillation. Empty contents of each syringe into chest cavity through the chest tube by gently applying pressure to syringe plunger. After administration, flush with 10-25 mL of NS. Clamp chest tube and have patient rotate from supine to alternating decubitus positions at 20-30 minute intervals for 2 hours. For intrapleural use only; **not for I.V. administration.**

Dosage Forms Excipient information presented when available (limited, particularly for generics); consult specific product labeling.

Aerosol, powder, intrapleural:

Sclerosol®: 4 g (4 g) [contains chlorofluorocarbon]

Powder, intrapleural:

Sterile Talc Powder™: USP: 100% (5 g)

References

Dresler CM, Olak J, Herndon JE, et al, "Phase III Intergroup Study of Talc Poudrage Vs Talc Slurry Sclerosis for Malignant Pleural Effusion," *Chest*, 2005, 127(3):909-15.

Kvale PA, Seleecky PA, and Prakash UB, "Palliative Care in Lung Cancer: ACCP Evidence-Based Clinical Practice Guidelines (2nd Edition)," *Chest*, 2007, 132(3 Suppl):368-403.

Tamoxifen (ta MOKS i fen)

Related Information

Chemotherapy and Cancer Treatment During Pregnancy *on page 1829*

Hypercalcemia of Malignancy *on page 1860*

Safe Handling of Hazardous Drugs *on page 1904*

Brand Names: U.S. Soltamox™

Brand Names: Canada Apo-Tamox®; Mylan-Tamoxifen; Nolvadex®-D; PMS-Tamoxifen; Teva-Tamoxifen

Index Terms ICI-46474; Nolvadex; Tamoxifen Citras; Tamoxifen Citrate

Generic Availability (U.S.) Yes

Pharmacologic Category Antineoplastic Agent, Estrogen Receptor Antagonist; Selective Estrogen Receptor Modulator (SERM)

Use Treatment of metastatic (female and male) breast cancer; adjuvant treatment of breast cancer after primary treatment with surgery and radiation; reduce risk of invasive breast cancer in women with ductal carcinoma *in situ* (DCIS) after surgery and radiation; reduce the incidence of breast cancer in women at high risk

Unlabeled Use Treatment of mastalgia, gynecomastia, ovarian cancer, endometrial cancer, uterine sarcoma, and desmoid tumors; risk reduction in women with Paget's disease of the breast (with DCIS or without associated cancer); induction of ovulation; treatment of precocious puberty in females, secondary to McCune-Albright syndrome

Labeled Contraindications Hypersensitivity to tamoxifen or any component of the formulation; concurrent warfarin therapy or history of deep vein thrombosis or pulmonary embolism (when tamoxifen is used for cancer risk reduction in women at high risk for breast cancer and in women with DCIS)

Pregnancy Risk Factor D

Lactation Excretion in breast milk unknown/not recommended

Warnings/Precautions Hazardous agent - use appropriate precautions for handling and disposal. **[U.S. Boxed Warning]: Serious and life-threatening events (including stroke, pulmonary emboli, and uterine malignancy) have occurred at an incidence greater than placebo during use for breast cancer risk reduction in women at high-risk for breast cancer and in women with DCIS;** these events are rare, but require consideration in risk: benefit evaluation. An increased incidence of thromboembolic events, including DVT and pulmonary embolism, has been associated with use for breast cancer; risk is increased with concomitant chemotherapy; use with caution in individuals with a history of thromboembolic events. Thrombocytopenia and/or leukopenia may occur; neutropenia and pancytopenia have been reported rarely. Although the relationship to tamoxifen therapy is uncertain, rare hemorrhagic episodes have occurred in patients with significant thrombocytopenia. Use with caution in patients with hyperlipidemias; infrequent postmarketing cases of hyperlipidemias have been reported. Decreased visual acuity, retinal vein thrombosis, retinopathy, corneal changes, color perception changes, and increased incidence of cataracts (and the need for cataract surgery), have been reported. Hypercalcemia has occurred in patients with bone metastasis, usually within a few weeks of therapy initiation; institute appropriate hypercalcemia management; discontinue if severe. Local disease flare and increased bone and tumor pain may occur in patients with metastatic breast cancer; may be associated with (good) tumor response.

Tamoxifen is associated with a high potential for drug interactions, including CYP- and Pgp-mediated interactions. Decreased efficacy and an increased risk of breast cancer recurrence has been reported with concurrent moderate or strong CYP2D6 inhibitors (Aubert, 2009; Dezentje, 2009). Concomitant use with select SSRIs may result in decreased tamoxifen efficacy. Strong CYP2D6 inhibitors (eg, fluoxetine, paroxetine) and moderate CYP2D6 inhibitors (eg, sertraline) are reported to interfere with transformation to the active metabolite endoxifen. Weak CYP2D6 inhibitors (eg, venlafaxine, citalopram) have minimal effect on the conversion to endoxifen (Jin, 2005; NCCN Breast Cancer Risk Reduction Guidelines v.2.2010); escitalopram is also a weak CYP2D6 inhibitor. Lower plasma concentrations of endoxifen (active metabolite) have been observed in patients associated with reduced CYP2D6 activity (Jin, 2005) and may be associated with reduced efficacy. In a retrospective analysis of breast cancer patients taking tamoxifen and SSRIs, concomitant use of paroxetine and tamoxifen was associated with an increased risk of death due to breast cancer (Kelly, 2010).

Tamoxifen use may be associated with changes in bone mineral density (BMD) and the effects may be dependent upon menstrual status. In postmenopausal women, tamoxifen use is associated with a protective effect on bone mineral density (BMD), preventing loss of BMD which lasts over the 5-year treatment period. In premenopausal women, a decline (from baseline) in BMD mineral density has been observed in women who continued to menstruate; may be associated with an increased risk of fractures. Liver abnormalities such as cholestasis, fatty liver, hepatitis, and hepatic necrosis have occurred. Hepatocellular carcinomas have been reported in some studies; relationship to treatment is unclear. Tamoxifen is associated with an increased incidence of uterine or endometrial cancers. Endometrial hyperplasia, polyps, endometriosis, uterine fibroids, and ovarian cysts have occurred. Monitor and promptly evaluate any report of abnormal vaginal bleeding. Amenorrhea and menstrual irregularities have been reported with tamoxifen use.

Adverse Reactions

>10%:

Cardiovascular: Vasodilation (41%), flushing (33%), hypertension (11%), peripheral edema (11%)

Central nervous system: Mood changes (12% to 18%), pain (3% to 16%), depression (2% to 12%)

Dermatologic: Skin changes (6% to 19%), rash (13%)

Endocrine & metabolic: Hot flashes (3% to 80%), fluid retention (32%), altered menses (13% to 25%), amenorrhea (16%)

Gastrointestinal: Nausea (5% to 26%), weight loss (23%), vomiting (12%)

Genitourinary: Vaginal discharge (13% to 55%), vaginal bleeding (2% to 23%)

Neuromuscular & skeletal: Weakness (18%), arthritis (14%), arthralgia (11%)

Respiratory: Pharyngitis (14%)

Miscellaneous: Lymphedema (11%)

1% to 10%:

Cardiovascular: Chest pain (5%), venous thrombotic events (5%), edema (4%), cardiovascular ischemia (3%), angina (2%), deep venous thrombus (≤2%), MI (1%)

Central nervous system: Insomnia (9%), dizziness (8%), headache (8%), anxiety (6%), fatigue (4%)

Dermatologic: Alopecia (≤5%)

Endocrine & metabolic: Oligomenorrhea (9%), breast pain (6%), menstrual disorder (6%), breast neoplasm (5%), hypercholesterolemia (4%)

Gastrointestinal: Abdominal pain (9%), weight gain (9%), constipation (4% to 8%), diarrhea (7%), dyspepsia (6%), throat irritation (oral solution 5%), abdominal cramps (1%), anorexia (1%)

Genitourinary: Urinary tract infection (10%), leukorrhea (9%), vaginal hemorrhage (6%), vaginitis (5%), vulvovaginitis (5%), ovarian cyst (3%)

Hematologic: Thrombocytopenia (≤10%), anemia (5%)

Hepatic: AST increased (5%), serum bilirubin increased (2%)

Neuromuscular & skeletal: Back pain (10%), bone pain (6% to 10%), osteoporosis (7%), fracture (7%), arthrosis (5%), joint disorder (5%), myalgia (5%), paresthesia (5%), musculoskeletal pain (3%)

Ocular: Cataract (7%)

Renal: Serum creatinine increased (≤2%)

Respiratory: Cough (4% to 9%), dyspnea (8%), bronchitis (5%), sinusitis (5%)

Miscellaneous: Infection/sepsis (≤9%), diaphoresis (6%), flu-like syndrome (6%), cyst (5%), neoplasm (5%), allergic reaction (3%)

<1%, infrequent, or frequency not defined: Cholestasis, corneal changes, endometriosis, endometrial cancer, endometrial hyperplasia, endometrial polyps, fatty liver, hepatic necrosis, hepatitis, hypercalcemia, hyperlipidemia, lightheadedness, phlebitis, pruritus vulvae, pulmonary embolism, retinal vein thrombosis, retinopathy, second primary tumors, stroke, superficial phlebitis, taste disturbances, tumor pain and local disease flare (including increase in lesion size and erythema) during treatment of metastatic breast cancer (generally resolves with continuation), uterine fibroids, vaginal dryness

Postmarketing and/or case reports: Angioedema, bullous pemphigoid, erythema multiforme, hypersensitivity reactions, hypertriglyceridemia, impotence (males), interstitial pneumonitis, loss of libido (males), pancreatitis, Stevens-Johnson syndrome, visual color perception changes

Drug Interactions

Metabolism/Transport Effects **Substrate** of CYP2A6 (minor), CYP2B6 (minor), CYP2C9 (major), CYP2D6 (major), CYP2E1 (minor), CYP3A4 (major); **Note:** Assignment of Major/Minor substrate status based on clinically relevant drug interaction potential; **Inhibits** CYP2B6 (weak), CYP2C8 (moderate), CYP2C9 (weak), CYP3A4 (weak), P-glycoprotein

Avoid Concomitant Use

Avoid concomitant use of Tamoxifen with any of the following: Bosutinib; Conivaptan; CYP2D6 Inhibitors (Strong); Pimozide; Silodosin; Topotecan; VinCRIStine (Liposomal); Vitamin K Antagonists

Increased Effect/Toxicity

Tamoxifen may increase the levels/effects of: ARIPiprazole; Bosutinib; Colchicine; CYP2C8 Substrates; Dabigatran Etexilate; Everolimus; Highest Risk QTc-Prolonging Agents; Moderate Risk QTc-Prolonging Agents; P-glycoprotein/ABCB1 Substrates; Pimozide; Prucalopride; Rivaroxaban; Silodosin; Topotecan; VinCRIStine (Liposomal); Vitamin K Antagonists

The levels/effects of Tamoxifen may be increased by: Abiraterone Acetate; Conivaptan; CYP2C9 Inhibitors (Moderate); CYP2C9 Inhibitors (Strong); CYP3A4 Inhibitors (Moderate); CYP3A4 Inhibitors (Strong); Darunavir; Dasatinib; Ivacaftor; Mifepristone

Decreased Effect

Tamoxifen may decrease the levels/effects of: Anastrozole; Letrozole

The levels/effects of Tamoxifen may be decreased by: Aminoglutethimide; CYP2C9 Inducers (Strong); CYP2D6 Inhibitors (Moderate); CYP2D6 Inhibitors (Strong); CYP3A4 Inducers (Strong); Deferasirox; Herbs (CYP3A4 Inducers); Peginterferon Alfa-2b; Rifamycin Derivatives; Tocilizumab

Ethanol/Nutrition/Herb Interactions

Food: Grapefruit juice may decrease the metabolism of tamoxifen. Management: Avoid grapefruit juice.

Herb/Nutraceutical: Black cohosh and dong quai have estrogenic properties. St John's wort may decrease levels/effects of tamoxifen. Management: Avoid black cohosh and dong quai in estrogen-dependent tumors. Avoid St John's wort.

Storage/Stability

Oral solution: Store at ≤25°C (77°F); do not freeze or refrigerate. Protect from light. Discard opened bottle after 3 months.

Tablets: Store at 20°C to 25°C (68°F to 77°F). Protect from light.

Mechanism of Action Competitively binds to estrogen receptors on tumors and other tissue targets, producing a nuclear complex that decreases DNA synthesis and inhibits estrogen effects; nonsteroidal agent with potent anti-estrogenic properties which compete with estrogen for binding sites in breast and other tissues; cells accumulate in the G_0 and G_1 phases; therefore, tamoxifen is cytostatic rather than cytocidal.

Pharmacodynamics/Kinetics

Absorption: Well absorbed

Distribution: High concentrations found in uterus, endometrial and breast tissue

Protein binding: 99%

Metabolism: Hepatic; via CYP2D6 to 4-hydroxytamoxifen and via CYP3A4/5 to N-desmethyl-tamoxifen. Each is then further metabolized into endoxifen (4-hydroxy-tamoxifen via CYP3A4/5 and N-desmethyl-tamoxifen via CYP2D6); both 4-hydroxy-tamoxifen and endoxifen are 30- to 100-fold more potent than tamoxifen

Half-life elimination: Tamoxifen: ~5-7 days; N-desmethyl tamoxifen: ~14 days

Time to peak, serum: ~5 hours

Excretion: Feces (26% to 51%); urine (9% to 13%)

Dosing

Adult & Geriatric Note: For the treatment of breast cancer, patients receiving both tamoxifen and chemotherapy, should receive treatment sequentially, with tamoxifen following completion of chemotherapy.

Breast cancer treatment:

Adjuvant therapy (females): 20 mg once daily for 5 years

Metastatic (males and females): 20-40 mg/day (doses >20 mg should be given in 2 divided doses). **Note:** Although the FDA-approved labeling recommends dosing up to 40 mg/day, clinical benefit has not been demonstrated with doses above 20 mg/day (Bratherton, 1984).

Premenopausal women: Duration of treatment is 5 years (NCCN Breast Cancer guidelines v.1.2011)

Postmenopausal women: Duration of tamoxifen treatment is 2-3 years followed by an aromatase inhibitor (AI) to complete 5 years; if contra-indications or intolerant to AI, may take tamoxifen for the full 5 years **or** extended therapy: 4.5-6 years of tamoxifen followed by 5 years of an AI (NCCN Breast Cancer guidelines v.1.2011)

DCIS (females), to reduce the risk for invasive breast cancer: 20 mg once daily for 5 years

Breast cancer risk reduction (pre- and postmenopausal high-risk females): 20 mg once daily for 5 years

Induction of ovulation (unlabeled use): 20 mg once daily (range: 20-80 mg once daily) for 5 days (Steiner, 2005)

Paget's disease of the breast (risk reduction; with DCIS or without associated cancer): 20 mg once daily for 5 years (NCCN Breast Cancer Guidelines, v.1.2011)

Dosage adjustment for DVT, pulmonary embolism, cerebrovascular accident, or prolonged immobilization: Discontinue tamoxifen (NCCN Breast Cancer Risk Reduction Guidelines, v.2.2010)

Pediatric Females: Precocious puberty and McCune-Albright syndrome (unlabeled use): Oral: A dose of 20 mg/day has been reported in patients 2-10 years of age; safety and efficacy have not been established for treatment of longer than 1 year duration (Eugster, 2003)

Administration Administer tablets or oral solution orally with or without food. Use supplied dosing cup for oral solution.

Extemporaneous Preparations Hazardous agent: Use appropriate precautions for handling and disposal.

A 0.5 mg/mL oral suspension may be prepared with tablets. Place two 10 mg tablets into 40 mL purified water and let stand ~2-5 minutes. Stir until tablets are completely disintegrated (dispersion time for each 10 mg tablet is ~2-5 minutes). Administer immediately after preparation. To ensure the full dose is administered, rinse glass several times with water and administer residue.

Lam MS, "Extemporaneous Compounding of Oral Liquid Dosage Formulations and Alternative Drug Delivery Methods for Anticancer Drugs," *Pharmacotherapy*, 2011, 31(2):164-92.

Monitoring Parameters CBC with platelets, serum calcium, LFTs; triglycerides and cholesterol (in patients with pre-existing hyperlipidemias); INR and PT (in patients on vitamin K antagonists); abnormal vaginal bleeding; breast and gynecologic exams (baseline and routine), mammogram (baseline and routine); signs/symptoms of DVT (leg swelling, tenderness) or PE (shortness of breath); ophthalmic exam (if vision problem or cataracts); bone mineral density (premenopausal women)

Test Interactions T_4 elevations (which may be explained by increases in thyroid-binding globulin) have been reported; not accompanied by clinical hyperthyroidism

Dietary Considerations Tablets and oral solution may be taken with or without food. Avoid grapefruit and grapefruit juice.

Additional Information Estrogen receptor status may predict if adjuvant treatment with tamoxifen is of benefit. In metastatic breast cancer, patients with estrogen receptor positive tumors are more likely to benefit from tamoxifen treatment. With tamoxifen use to reduce the incidence of breast cancer in high risk-women, high risk is defined as women ≥35 years of age with a 5 year NCI Gail model predicted risk of breast cancer ≥1.67%.

Oncology Comment: The American Society of Clinical Oncology (ASCO) guidelines for adjuvant endocrine therapy in postmenopausal women with HR-positive breast cancer (Burstein, 2010) recommend considering aromatase inhibitor (AI) therapy at some point in the treatment course (primary, sequentially, or extended). Optimal duration at this time is not known; however, treatment with an AI should not exceed 5 years in primary and extended therapies, and 2-3 years if followed by tamoxifen in sequential therapy (total of 5 years). If initial therapy with AI has been discontinued before the 5 years, consideration should be taken to receive tamoxifen for a total of 5 years. The optimal time to switch to an AI is also not known; but data supports switching after 2-3 years of tamoxifen (sequential) or after 5 years of tamoxifen (extended). If patient becomes intolerant or has poor adherence, consideration should be made to switch to another AI or initiate tamoxifen.

The adjuvant endocrine therapy of choice is tamoxifen for men with breast cancer and for pre- or perimenopausal women at diagnosis. CYP2D6 genotyping is not recommended, however, due to the potential for drug-drug interactions use caution and consider avoiding concomitant therapy with tamoxifen and known CYP2D6 inhibitors.

Medication Guide Available Yes

Dosage Forms Excipient information presented when available (limited, particularly for generics); consult specific product labeling.

Solution, oral:

Soltamox™: 10 mg/5 mL (150 mL) [sugar free; contains ethanol, propylene glycol; licorice flavor]

Tablet, oral: 10 mg, 20 mg

References

Aubert RE, Stanek EJ, Yao J, et al, "Risk of Breast Cancer Recurrence in Women Initiating Tamoxifen With CYP2D6 Inhibitors," *J Clin Oncol*, 2009, 27(18S):CRA508 [abstract CRA508 from 2009 ASCO Annual Meeting].

Bratherton DG, Brown CH, Bucha a R, et al, "A Comparison of Two Doses of Tamoxifen (Nolvadex) in Postmenopausal Women With Advanced Breast Cancer: 10 mg bd Versus 20 mg bd," *Br J Cancer*, 1984, 50(2):199-205.

Burstein HJ, Prestrud AA, Seidenfeld J, et al, "American Society of Clinical Oncology Clinical Practice Guideline: Update on Adjuvant Endocrine Therapy for Women with Hormone Receptor-Positive Breast Cancer," *J Clin Oncol*, 2010, 28(23):3784-96.

Dezentje V, Van Blijderveen NJ, Gelderblom H, et al, "Concomitant CYP2D6 Inhibitor Use and Tamoxifen Adherence in Early-Stage Breast Cancer: A Pharmacoepidemiologic Study," *J Clin Oncol*, 2009, 27(18S):CRA509 [abstract CRA509 from 2009 ASCO Annual Meeting].

Eastell R, Adams JE, Coleman RE, et al, "Effect of Anastrozole on Bone Mineral Density: 5-Year Results From the Anastrozole, Tamoxifen, Alone or in Combination Trial 18233230," *J Clin Oncol*, 2008, 26(7):1051-7.

Eugster EA, Rubin SD, Reiter EO, et al, "Tamoxifen Treatment for Precocious Puberty in McCune-Albright Syndrome: A Multicenter Trial," *J Pediatr*, 2003, 143(1):60-6.

Jin Y, Desta Z, Stearns V, et al, "CYP2D6 Genotype, Antidepressant Use, and Tamoxifen Metabolism During Adjuvant Breast Cancer Treatment," *J Natl Cancer Inst*, 2005, 97(1):30-9.

Kelly CM, Juurlink DN, Gomes T, et al, "Selective Serotonin Reuptake Inhibitors and Breast Cancer Mortality in Women Receiving Tamoxifen: A Population Based Cohort Study," *BMJ*, 2010, 340: c693.

Khatcheressian JL, Wolff AC, Smith TJ, et al, "American Society of Clinical Oncology 2006 Update of the Breast Cancer Follow-Up and Management Guidelines in the Adjuvant Setting," *J Clin Oncol*, 2006, 24(31):5091-7.

National Comprehensive Cancer Network® (NCCN), "Clinical Practice Guidelines in Oncology™: Breast Cancer," Version 1.2011. Available at http://www.nccn.org/professionals/physician_gls/PDF/breast.pdf

National Comprehensive Cancer Network® (NCCN), "Clinical Practice Guidelines in Oncology™: Breast Cancer Risk Reduction, Version 2.2010." Available at http://www.nccn.org/professionals/physician_gls/PDF/breast_risk.pdf

National Comprehensive Cancer Network® (NCCN), "Clinical Practice Guidelines in Oncology™: Ovarian Cancer," Version 2.2011. Available at http://www.nccn.org/professionals/physician_gls/PDF/ovarian.pdf

National Comprehensive Cancer Network® (NCCN), "Clinical Practice Guidelines in Oncology™: Uterine Neoplasms," Version 1.2011. Available at http://www.nccn.org/professionals/physician_gls/PDF/uterine.pdf

Sideras K, Ingle JN, Ames MM, et al, "Coprescription of Tamoxifen and Medications That Inhibit CYP2D6," *J Clin Oncol*, 2010, 28(16):2768-76.

Steiner AZ, Terplan M, and Paulson RJ, "Comparison of Tamoxifen and Clomifene Citrate for Ovulation Induction: A Meta-Analysis," *Hum Reprod*, 2005, 20(6):1511-5.

Vehmanen L, Elomaa I, Blomqvist C, et al, "Tamoxifen Treatment After Adjuvant Chemotherapy Has Opposite Effects on Bone Mineral Density in Premenopausal Patients Depending on Menstrual Status," *J Clin Oncol*, 2006, 24(4):675-80.

Visvanathan K, Chlebowski RT, Hurley P, et al, "American Society of Clinical Oncology Clinical Practice Guideline Update on the Use of Pharmacologic Interventions Including Tamoxifen, Raloxifene, and Aromatase Inhibition for Breast Cancer Risk Reduction," *J Clin Oncol*, 2009, 27(19):3235-58.

Winer EP, Hudis C, Burstein HJ, et al, "American Society of Clinical Oncology Technology Assessment on the Use of Aromatase Inhibitors as Adjuvant Therapy for Postmenopausal Women With Hormone Receptor-Positive Breast Cancer: Status Report 2004," *J Clin Oncol*, 2005, 23(3):619-29.

◆ **Tamoxifen Citras** *see* Tamoxifen *on page 1324*

◆ **Tamoxifen Citrate** *see* Tamoxifen *on page 1324*

◆ **Tantum® (Can)** *see* Benzydamine *on page 164*

◆ **TAP-144** *see* Leuprolide *on page 876*

- **Tarceva®** *see* Erlotinib *on page 528*
- **Targretin®** *see* Bexarotene (Systemic) *on page 173*
- **Targretin®** *see* Bexarotene (Topical) *on page 176*
- **Taro-Anastrozole (Can)** *see* Anastrozole *on page 96*
- **Taro-Ciprofloxacin (Can)** *see* Ciprofloxacin (Systemic) *on page 283*
- **Taro-Fluconazole (Can)** *see* Fluconazole *on page 612*
- **Tasigna®** *see* Nilotinib *on page 1031*
- **Taxol** *see* PACLitaxel *on page 1092*
- **Taxotere®** *see* DOCEtaxel *on page 453*
- **Tazicef®** *see* CefTAZidime *on page 254*
- **Tazobactam and Piperacillin** *see* Piperacillin and Tazobactam *on page 1175*
- **Tazocin® (Can)** *see* Piperacillin and Tazobactam *on page 1175*
- **T-Cell Growth Factor** *see* Aldesleukin *on page 37*
- **TCGF** *see* Aldesleukin *on page 37*
- **TDX** *see* Raltitrexed *on page 1226*
- **Temodal® (Can)** *see* Temozolomide *on page 1331*
- **Temodar®** *see* Temozolomide *on page 1331*

Temozolomide (te moe ZOE loe mide)

Related Information

Management of Chemotherapy-Induced Nausea and Vomiting *on page 1786*

Safe Handling of Hazardous Drugs *on page 1904*

Brand Names: U.S. Temodar®

Brand Names: Canada Ahi-Temozolomide Capsules; Temodal®

Index Terms SCH 52365; TMZ

Generic Availability (U.S.) No

Pharmacologic Category Antineoplastic Agent, Alkylating Agent (Triazene)

Use Treatment of newly-diagnosed glioblastoma multiforme (initially in combination with radiotherapy, then as maintenance treatment); treatment of refractory anaplastic astrocytoma

Canadian labeling (not an approved indication in the U.S.): Treatment of recurrent or progressive glioblastoma multiforme

Unlabeled Use Treatment of recurrent glioblastoma multiforme, low-grade astrocytoma, low-grade oligodendroglioma, anaplastic oligodendroglioma, metastatic CNS lesions, refractory primary CNS lymphoma, advanced or metastatic melanoma, cutaneous T-cell lymphomas (mycosis fungoides [MF] and Sézary syndrome [SS]), advanced neuroendocrine tumors (carcinoid or islet cell), Ewing's sarcoma (recurrent or progressive), soft tissue sarcomas (extremity/retroperitoneal/intra-abdominal or hemangiopericytoma/solitary fibrous tumor), treatment of pediatric neuroblastoma

Labeled Contraindications Hypersensitivity (eg, allergic reaction, anaphylaxis, urticaria, Stevens-Johnson syndrome, toxic epidermal necrolysis) to temozolomide or any component of the formulation; hypersensitivity to dacarbazine (both drugs are metabolized to MTIC)

Canadian labeling: Additional contraindications (not in U.S. labeling): Not recommended in patients with severe myelosuppression

Pregnancy Risk Factor D

Lactation Excretion in breast milk unknown/not recommended

Warnings/Precautions Hazardous agent - use appropriate precautions for handling and disposal. *Pneumocystis jirovecii* pneumonia (PCP) may occur; risk is increased in those receiving steroids or longer dosing regimens; PCP prophylaxis is required in patients receiving radiotherapy in combination with the 42-day temozolomide regimen. Myelosuppression may occur; an increased incidence has been reported in geriatric and female patients. Prolonged pancytopenia resulting in aplastic anemia has been reported; concurrent use of temozolomide with medications associated with aplastic anemia (eg, carbamazepine, co-trimoxazole, phenytoin) may obscure assessment for development of aplastic anemia. Rare cases of myelodysplastic syndrome and secondary malignancies, including acute myeloid leukemia have been reported. Use caution in patients with severe hepatic or renal impairment; has not been studied in dialysis patients.

Increased MGMT (O-6-methylguanine-DNA methyltransferase) activity/levels within tumor tissue is associated with temozolomide resistance. Glioblastoma patients with decreased levels (due to methylated MGMT promoter) may be more likely to benefit from the combination of radiation therapy and temozolomide (Hegi, 2008; Stupp, 2009). Determination of MGMT status may be predictive for response to alkylating agents.

Adverse Reactions Note: With CNS malignancies, it may be difficult to distinguish between CNS adverse events caused by temozolomide versus the effects of progressive disease.

>10%:

- Cardiovascular: Peripheral edema (11%)
- Central nervous system: Fatigue (34% to 61%), headache (23% to 41%), seizure (6% to 23%), hemiparesis (18%), fever (13%), dizziness (5% to 12%), coordination abnormality (11%)
- Dermatologic: Alopecia (55%), rash (8% to 13%)
- Gastrointestinal: Nausea (49% to 53%; grades 3/4: 1% to 10%), vomiting (29% to 42%; grades 3/4: 2% to 6%), constipation (22% to 33%), anorexia (9% to 27%), diarrhea (10% to 16%)
- Hematologic: Lymphopenia (grades 3/4: 55%), thrombocytopenia (grades 3/4: adults: 4% to 19%; children: 25%), neutropenia (grades 3/4: adults: 8% to 14%; children: 20%), leukopenia (grades 3/4: 11%)
- Neuromuscular & skeletal: Weakness (7% to 13%)
- Miscellaneous: Viral infection (11%)

1% to 10%:

- Central nervous system: Amnesia (10%), insomnia (4% to 10%), somnolence (9%), ataxia (8%), paresis (8%), anxiety (7%), memory impairment (7%), depression (6%), confusion (5%)
- Dermatologic: Pruritus (5% to 8%), dry skin (5%), radiation injury (2% maintenance phase after radiotherapy), erythema (1%)
- Endocrine & metabolic: Hypercorticism (8%), breast pain (females 6%)
- Gastrointestinal: Stomatitis (9%), abdominal pain (5% to 9%), dysphagia (7%), taste perversion (5%), weight gain (5%)
- Genitourinary: Incontinence (8%), urinary tract infection (8%), urinary frequency (6%)
- Hematologic: Anemia (grades 3/4: 4%)
- Neuromuscular & skeletal: Paresthesia (9%), back pain (8%), abnormal gait (6%), arthralgia (6%), myalgia (5%)
- Ocular: Blurred vision (5% to 8%), diplopia (5%), vision abnormality (visual deficit/vision changes 5%)

Respiratory: Pharyngitis (8%), upper respiratory tract infection (8%), cough (5% to 8%), sinusitis (6%), dyspnea (5%)

Miscellaneous: Allergic reaction (≤3%)

<1%, postmarketing, and/or case reports (limited to important or life-threatening): Agitation, alkaline phosphatase increased, alveolitis, anaphylaxis, apathy, aplastic anemia, cholestasis, emotional lability, erythema multiforme, febrile neutropenia, flu-like syndrome, hallucination, hematoma, hemorrhage, hepatitis, hepatotoxicity, herpes simplex, herpes zoster, hyperbilirubinemia, hyperglycemia, hypokalemia, injection site reactions (erythema, irritation, pain, pruritus, swelling, warmth), interstitial pneumonia/pneumonitis, myelodysplastic syndrome, neuropathy, opportunistic infection (eg, PCP), oral candidiasis, pancytopenia (may be prolonged), peripheral neuropathy, petechiae, pneumonitis, pulmonary fibrosis, secondary malignancies (including myeloid leukemia), Stevens-Johnson syndrome, toxic epidermal necrolysis, transaminases increased, weight loss

Drug Interactions

Metabolism/Transport Effects None known.

Avoid Concomitant Use

Avoid concomitant use of Temozolomide with any of the following: BCG; CloZAPine; Natalizumab; Pimecrolimus; Tacrolimus (Topical); Vaccines (Live)

Increased Effect/Toxicity

Temozolomide may increase the levels/effects of: CloZAPine; Leflunomide; Natalizumab; Vaccines (Live)

The levels/effects of Temozolomide may be increased by: Denosumab; Divalproex; Pimecrolimus; Roflumilast; Tacrolimus (Topical); Trastuzumab; Valproic Acid

Decreased Effect

Temozolomide may decrease the levels/effects of: BCG; Coccidioidin Skin Test; Sipuleucel-T; Vaccines (Inactivated); Vaccines (Live)

The levels/effects of Temozolomide may be decreased by: Echinacea

Ethanol/Nutrition/Herb Interactions Food: Food reduces rate and extent of absorption.

Storage/Stability

Injection: Store intact vials refrigerated at 2°C to 8°C (36°F to 46°F). Reconstituted vials may be stored for up to 14 hours at room temperature of 25°C (77°F); infusion must be completed within 14 hours of reconstitution.

Capsule: Store at room temperature of 25°C (77°F); excursions permitted to 15°C to 30°C (59°F to 86°F).

Reconstitution Bring to room temperature prior to reconstitution. Reconstitute each 100 mg vial with 41 mL sterile water for injection to a final concentration of 2.5 mg/mL. Swirl gently; do not shake. Place dose without further dilution into a 250 mL empty sterile infusion bag. Infusion must be completed within 14 hours of reconstitution. Use appropriate precautions for handling and disposal.

Mechanism of Action Temozolomide is a prodrug which is rapidly and nonenzymatically converted to the active alkylating metabolite MTIC [(methyl-triazene-1-yl)-imidazole-4-carboxamide]; this conversion is spontaneous, nonenzymatic, and occurs under physiologic conditions in all tissues to which it distributes. The cytotoxic effects of MTIC are manifested through alkylation (methylation) of DNA at the O^6, N^7 guanine positions which lead to DNA double strand breaks and apoptosis. Non-cell cycle specific.

Pharmacodynamics/Kinetics

Absorption: Oral: Rapid and complete

Distribution: V_d: Parent drug: 0.4 L/kg; penetrates blood-brain barrier; CSF levels are ~35% to 39% of plasma levels

Protein binding: 15%

Metabolism: Prodrug, hydrolyzed to the active form, MTIC; MTIC is eventually eliminated as CO_2 and 5-aminoimidazole-4-carboxamide (AIC), a natural constituent in urine; CYP isoenzymes play only a minor role in metabolism (of temozolomide and MTIC)

Bioavailability: Oral: 100% (on a mg-per-mg basis, I.V. temozolomide, infused over 90 minutes, is bioequivalent to an oral dose)

Half-life elimination: Mean: Parent drug: 1.8 hours

Time to peak: Oral: Empty stomach: 1 hour; with food (high-fat meal): 2.25 hours

Excretion: Urine (~38%; parent drug 6%); feces <1%

Dosing

Adult

Anaplastic astrocytoma (refractory): Oral, I.V.: Initial dose: 150 mg/m²/day for 5 days; repeat every 28 days. Subsequent doses of 100-200 mg/m²/day for 5 days per treatment cycle; based upon hematologic tolerance.

Dosage modification for toxicity:

ANC <1000/mm³ or platelets <50,000/mm³ on day 22 or day 29 (day 1 of next cycle): Postpone therapy until ANC >1500/mm³ and platelets >100,000/mm³; reduce dose by 50 mg/m²/day for subsequent cycle

ANC 1000-1500/mm³ or platelets 50,000-100,000/mm³ on day 22 or day 29 (day 1 of next cycle): Postpone therapy until ANC >1500/mm³ and platelets >100,000/mm³; maintain initial dose

ANC ≥1500/mm³ and platelets ≥100,000/mm³ on day 22 or day 29 (day 1 of next cycle): Increase dose to or maintain dose at 200 mg/m²/day for 5 days for subsequent cycle

Glioblastoma multiforme (newly diagnosed, high-grade glioma): Oral, I.V.:

Concomitant phase: 75 mg/m²/day for 42 days with focal radiotherapy (60 Gy administered in 30 fractions). **Note:** PCP prophylaxis is required during concomitant phase and should continue in patients who develop lymphocytopenia until lymphocyte recovery to ≤grade 1. Obtain weekly CBC.

Continue at 75 mg/m²/day throughout the 42-day concomitant phase (up to 49 days) as long as ANC ≥1500/mm³, platelet count ≥100,000/mm³, and nonhematologic toxicity ≤grade 1 (excludes alopecia, nausea/vomiting)

Dosage modification for toxicity:

ANC ≥500/mm³ but <1500/mm³ **or** platelet count ≥10,000/mm³ but <100,000/mm³ **or** grade 2 nonhematologic toxicity (excludes alopecia, nausea/vomiting): Interrupt therapy

ANC <500/mm³ **or** platelet count <10,000/mm³ **or** grade 3/4 nonhematologic toxicity (excludes alopecia, nausea/vomiting): Discontinue therapy

Maintenance phase (consists of 6 treatment cycles): Begin 4 weeks after concomitant phase completion. **Note:** Each subsequent cycle is 28 days (consisting of 5 days of drug treatment followed by 23 days without treatment). Draw CBC within 48 hours of day 22; hold next cycle and do weekly CBC until ANC >1500/mm³ and platelet count >100,000/mm³; dosing modification should be based on lowest blood counts and worst nonhematologic toxicity during the previous cycle.

Cycle 1: 150 mg/m²/day for 5 days; repeat every 28 days

Cycles 2-6: May increase to 200 mg/m^2/day for 5 days every 28 days (if ANC ≥1500/mm^3, platelets ≥100,000/mm^3 and nonhematologic toxicities for cycle 1 are ≤grade 2 [excludes alopecia, nausea/vomiting]); **Note:** If dose was not escalated at the onset of cycle 2, do not increase for cycles 3-6)

Dosage modification (during maintenance phase) for toxicity:

ANC <1000/mm^3, platelet count <50,000/mm^3, or grade 3 nonhematologic toxicity (excludes for alopecia, nausea/vomiting) during previous cycle: Decrease dose by 1 dose level (by 50 mg/m^2/day for 5 days), unless dose has already been lowered to 100 mg/m^2/day, then discontinue therapy.

If dose reduction <100 mg/m^2/day is required or grade 4 nonhematologic toxicity (excludes for alopecia, nausea/vomiting), or if the same grade 3 nonhematologic toxicity occurs after dose reduction: Discontinue therapy

Glioblastoma multiforme (recurrent glioma): *Canadian labeling (unlabeled use in the U.S.):* 200 mg/m^2/day for 5 days every 28 days; if previously treated with chemotherapy, initiate at 150 mg/m^2/day for 5 days every 28 days and increase to 200 mg/m^2/day for 5 days every 28 days with cycle 2 if no hematologic toxicity (Brada, 2001; Yung, 2000)

Ewing's sarcoma, recurrent or progressive (unlabeled use): Oral: 100 mg/m^2/dose days 1-5 every 21 days (in combination with irinotecan) (Casey, 2009)

Melanoma, advanced or metastatic (unlabeled use): Oral: 200 mg/m^2/day for 5 days every 28 days (for up to 12 cycles). For subsequent cycles reduce dose to 75% of the original dose for grade 3/4 hematologic toxicity and reduce the dose to 50% of the original dose for grade 3/4 nonhematologic toxicity (Middleton, 2000).

Neuroendocrine tumors, advanced (unlabeled use): Oral: 150 mg/m^2/day for 7 days every 14 days in combination with thalidomide (Kulke, 2006)

Primary CNS lymphoma, refractory (unlabeled use): Oral: 150 mg/m^2/day for 5 days every 28 days, initially in combination with rituximab, followed by temozolomide monotherapy: 150 mg/m^2/day for 5 days every 28 days (Wong, 2004) **or** 150 mg/m^2/day for 7 days every 14 days, initially in combination with rituximab, followed by temozolomide monotherapy: 150 mg/m^2/day for 5 days every 28 days (Enting, 2004)

Soft tissue sarcoma (unlabeled use): Oral: 75 mg/m^2/day for 6 weeks (Garcia del Muro, 2005)

Geriatric Refer to adult dosing. **Note:** Patients ≥70 years of age in the anaplastic astrocytoma study had a higher incidence of grade 4 neutropenia and thrombocytopenia in the first cycle of therapy than patients <70 years of age.

Pediatric

Ewing's sarcoma, recurrent or progressive (unlabeled use): Oral: Refer to adult dosing.

Neuroblastoma, relapsed or refractory (unlabeled use): Oral: 100 mg/m^2/dose days 1-5 days every 21 days (in combination with irinotecan) for up to 6 cycles (Bagatell, 2011)

Renal Impairment Oral:

Cl_{cr} ≥36 mL/minute/m^2: No effect on temozolomide clearance was demonstrated.

Severe renal impairment (Cl_{cr} <36 mL/minute/m^2): Use with caution.

Dialysis patients: Use has not been studied.

Hepatic Impairment Severe hepatic impairment: Use with caution.

Combination Regimens

Primary CNS Lymphoma: Temozolomide-Rituximab (CNS Lymphoma) on page 1754

Sarcoma: Irinotecan-Temozolomide (Ewing's Sarcoma) on page 1697

Administration Standard antiemetics may be administered if needed.

Oral: Swallow capsules whole with a glass of water. Absorption is affected by food. Administer consistently either with food or without food (was administered in studies under fasting and nonfasting conditions). May administer on an empty stomach or at bedtime to reduce nausea and vomiting. Do not repeat if vomiting occurs after dose is administered; wait until the next scheduled dose. Do not open or chew capsules; avoid contact with skin if capsules are accidentally opened or damaged.

I.V.: Infuse over 90 minutes. Flush line before and after administration. May be administered through the same I.V. line as sodium chloride 0.9%; do not administer other medications through the same I.V. line.

Emetic Potential Moderate (30% to 90%)

Extemporaneous Preparations Hazardous agent: Use appropriate precautions for handling and disposal.

A 10 mg/mL temozolomide oral suspension may be compounded in a vertical flow hood. Mix the contents of ten 100 mg capsules and 500 mg of povidone K-30 powder in a glass mortar; add 25 mg anhydrous citric acid dissolved in 1.5 mL purified water and mix to a uniform paste; mix while adding 50 mL Ora-Plus® in incremental proportions. Transfer to an amber plastic bottle, rinse mortar 4 times with small portions of either Ora-Sweet® or Ora-Sweet® SF, and add quantity of Ora-Sweet® or Ora-Sweet® SF sufficient to make 100 mL. Store in plastic amber prescription bottles; label "shake well" and "refrigerate"; include the beyond-use date. Stable for 7 days at room temperature or 60 days refrigerated (preferred).

Trissel LA, Yanping Z, and Koontz SE, "Temozolomide Stability in Extemporaneously Compounded Oral Suspension," *Int J Pharm Compound*, 2006, 10(5):396-9.

Monitoring Parameters CBC with differential and platelets (prior to each cycle; weekly during glioma concomitant phase treatment; at or within 48 hours of day 22 and weekly until ANC >1500/mm^3 for glioma maintenance and astrocytoma treatment)

Dietary Considerations The incidence of nausea/vomiting is decreased when taken on an empty stomach. Take capsules consistently either with food or without food (absorption is affected by food).

Dosage Forms Excipient information presented when available (limited, particularly for generics); consult specific product labeling.

Capsule, oral:

Temodar®: 5 mg, 20 mg, 100 mg, 140 mg, 180 mg, 250 mg

Injection, powder for reconstitution:

Temodar®: 100 mg [contains polysorbate 80]

References

Bagatell R, London WB, Wagner LM, et al, "Phase II Study of Irinotecan and Temozolomide in Children With Relapsed or Refractory Neuroblastoma: A Children's Oncology Group Study," *J Clin Oncol*, 2011, 29(2):208-13.

Brada M, Hoang-Xuan K, Rampling R, et al, "Multicenter Phase II Trial of Temozolomide in Patients With Glioblastoma Multiforme at First Relapse," *Ann Oncol*, 2001, 12(2):259-66.

Casey DA, Wexler LH, Merchant MS, et al, "Irinotecan and Temozolomide for Ewing Sarcoma: The Memorial Sloan-Kettering Experience," *Pediatr Blood Cancer*, 2009, 53(6):1029-34.

Enting RH, Demopoulos A, DeAngelis LM, et al, "Salvage Therapy for Primary CNS Lymphoma With a Combination of Rituximab and Temozolomide," *Neurology*, 2004, 63(5):901-3.

Gan HK, Rosenthal MA, Dowling A, et al, "A Phase II Trial of Primary Temozolomide in Patients With Grade III Oligodendroglial Brain Tumors," *Neuro Oncol*, 2010, 12(5):500-7.

Garcia del Muro X, Lopez-Pousa A, Martin J, et al, "A Phase II Trial of Temozolomide as a 6-Week, Continuous, Oral Schedule in Patients With Advanced Soft Tissue Sarcoma: A Study by the Spanish Group for Research on Sarcomas," *Cancer*, 2005, 104(8):1706-12.

Hegi ME, Diserens AC, Gorlia T, et al, "MGMT Gene Silencing and Benefit From Temozolomide in Glioblastoma," *N Engl J Med*, 2005, 352(10):997-1003.

Hegi ME, Liu L, Herman JG, et al, "Correlation of O6-Methylguanine Methyltransferase (MGMT) Promoter Methylation With Clinical Outcomes in Glioblastoma and Clinical Strategies to Modulate MGMT Activity," *J Clin Oncol*, 2008, 26(25):4189-99.

Kulke MH, Stuart K, Enzinger PC, et al, "Phase II Study of Temozolomide and Thalidomide in Patients With Metastatic Neuroendocrine Tumors," *J Clin Oncol*, 2006, 24(3):401-6.

Middleton MR, Grob JJ, Aaronson N, et al, "Randomized Phase III Study of Temozolomide Versus Dacarbazine in the Treatment of Patients With Advanced Metastatic Malignant Melanoma," *J Clin Oncol*, 2000, 18(1):158-66.

Mikkelsen T, Doyle T, Anderson J, et al, "Temozolomide Single-Agent Chemotherapy for Newly Diagnosed Anaplastic Oligodendroglioma," *J Neurooncol*, 2009, 92(1):57-63.

Perry JR, Bélanger K, Mason WP, et al, "Phase II Trial of Continuous Dose-Intense Temozolomide in Recurrent Malignant Glioma: RESCUE Study," *J Clin Oncol*, 2010, 28(12):2051-7.

Stupp R, Dietrich PY, Ostermann Kraljevic S, et al, "Promising Survival for Patients With Newly Diagnosed Glioblastoma Multiforme Treated With Concomitant Radiation Plus Temozolomide Followed by Adjuvant Temozolomide," *J Clin Oncol*, 2002, 20(5):1375-82.

Stupp R, Gander M, Leyvraz S, et al, "Current and Future Developments in the Use of Temozolomide for the Treatment of Brain Tumours," *Lancet Oncol*, 2001, 2(9):552-60.

Stupp R, Hegi ME, Mason WP, et al, "Effects of Radiotherapy With Concomitant and Adjuvant Temozolomide Versus Radiotherapy Alone on Survival in Glioblastoma in a Randomised Phase III Study: 5-year Analysis of the EORTC-NCIC Trial," *Lancet Oncol*, 2009, 10(5):459-66.

Stupp R, Mason WP, van den Bent MJ, et al, "Radiotherapy Plus Concomitant and Adjuvant Temozolomide for Glioblastoma," *N Engl J Med*, 2005, 352(10):987-96.

Tani M, Fina M, Alinari L, et al, "Phase II Trial of Temozolomide in Patients With Pretreated Cutaneous T Cell Lymphoma," *Haematologica*, 2005, 90(9):1283-4.

Wong ET, Tishler R, Barron L, et al, "Immunochemotherapy With Rituximab and Temozolomide for Central Nervous System Lymphomas," *Cancer*, 2004, 101(1):139-45.

Yung WK, Albright RE, Olson J, et al, "A Phase II Study of Temozolomide vs Procarbazine in Patients With Glioblastoma Multiforme at First Relapse," *Br J Cancer*, 2000, 83(5):588-93.

Yung WK, Prados MD, Yaya-Tur R, et al, "Multicenter Phase II Trial of Temozolomide in Patients With Anaplastic Astrocytoma or Anaplastic Oligoastrocytoma at First Relapse," *J Clin Oncol*, 1999, 17(9):2762-71.

Temsirolimus (tem sir OH li mus)

Related Information

Management of Chemotherapy-Induced Nausea and Vomiting *on page 1780*

Principles of Anticancer Therapy *on page 1878*

Safe Handling of Hazardous Drugs *on page 1904*

Brand Names: U.S. Torisel®

Brand Names: Canada Torisel®

Index Terms CCI-779

Generic Availability (U.S.) No

Pharmacologic Category Antineoplastic Agent, mTOR Kinase Inhibitor

Use Treatment of advanced renal cell cancer (RCC)

Labeled Contraindications Bilirubin >1.5 times the upper limit of normal (ULN)

Canadian labeling: Additional contraindications (not in U.S. labeling): History of anaphylaxis after exposure to temsirolimus, sirolimus, or any component of the formulation

Pregnancy Risk Factor D

Lactation Excretion in breast milk unknown/not recommended

Warnings/Precautions Hazardous agent - use appropriate precautions for handling and disposal.

Hypersensitivity/infusion reactions (eg, anaphylaxis, apnea, dyspnea, flushing, loss of consciousness, hypotension, and/or chest pain) have been reported. Infusion reaction may occur during the initial infusion (early in infusion) or with subsequent infusions. Premedicate with an antihistamine (H_1 antagonist) prior to infusion; monitor throughout infusion (appropriate supportive care should be available); interrupt infusion for hypersensitivity reaction and observe patient for 30-60 minutes. With discretion, treatment may be resumed at a slower infusion rate; administer an H_1 antagonist (if not given as premedication) and/or an I.V. H_2 antagonist ~30 minutes prior to resuming infusion. For severe infusion reactions, asses risk versus benefit of continued treatment. Use with caution in patients with hypersensitivity temsirolimus, sirolimus (a metabolite), or polysorbate 80. Angioneurotic edema has been reported; concurrent use with other drugs known to cause angioedema (eg, ACE inhibitors) may increase risk.

Temsirolimus is predominantly cleared by the liver; use with caution and reduce dose in patients with mild hepatic impairment (bilirubin >1-1.5 x ULN or AST >ULN with bilirubin ≤ULN). Toxicities were increased in patients with baseline bilirubin >1.5 x ULN. Use is contraindicated in patients with moderate-to-severe hepatic impairment (bilirubin >1.5 x ULN).

Avoid concomitant use with strong CYP3A4 inhibitors and strong CYP3A4 inducers (see Drug Interactions); consider alternative agents that avoid or lessen the potential for CYP-mediated interactions. Patients should not be immunized with live, viral vaccines during or shortly after treatment and should avoid close contact with recently vaccinated (live vaccine) individuals. Patients who are receiving anticoagulant therapy or those with CNS tumors/metastases may be at increased risk for developing intracerebral bleeding. Combination therapy with temsirolimus and sunitinib has resulted in dose-limiting toxicities, including grade 3 or 4 rash, gout, and/or cellulitis.

Increases in serum glucose commonly occur during treatment; initiation or alteration of insulin and/or oral hypoglycemic therapy may be required; monitor serum glucose before and during treatment; use with caution in patients with diabetes. Use with caution in patients with hyperlipidemia; may increase serum lipids (cholesterol and triglycerides); initiation or dosage adjustment of of antihyperlipidemic agents may be required; monitor cholesterol/triglyceride panel. Treatment may result in immunosuppression, may increase risk of opportunistic infections and/or sepsis. Interstitial lung disease (ILD), sometimes fatal, has been reported; symptoms include dyspnea, cough, hypoxia, and/or fever, although asymptomatic or mild cases may present; promptly evaluate worsening respiratory symptoms; may require corticosteroids, antibiotic therapy, and/or treatment discontinuation; baseline chest radiographic assessment (CT scan or xray) is recommended. Cases of bowel perforation (fatal) have occurred (usually presenting with abdominal pain, bloody stools, diarrhea, fever, or metabolic acidosis); promptly evaluate any new or worsening abdominal pain or bloody stools. Temsirolimus may be associated with impaired wound healing; use caution in the perioperative period. Cases of acute renal failure with rapid progression have been reported (unrelated to disease progression), including cases unresponsive to dialysis. An increased incidence of rash, infection and dose interruptions have been reported in patients with renal insufficiency (Cl_{cr} ≤60 mL/minute) who received mTOR inhibitors for the treatment of renal cell cancer (Gupta, 2011).

Adverse Reactions

>10%:

Cardiovascular: Edema (35%), peripheral edema (27%), chest pain (16%)

Central nervous system: Pain (28%), fever (24%), headache (15%), insomnia (12%)

Dermatologic: Rash (47%), pruritus (19%), nail disorder/thinning (14%), dry skin (11%)

Endocrine & metabolic: Hyperglycemia (26% to 89%, grades 3/4: 16%), hypercholesterolemia (24% to 87%; grades 3/4: 2%), hypertriglyceridemia (83%; grades 3/4: 44%), hypophosphatemia (49%; grades 3/4: 18%), hyperlipidemia (27%), hypokalemia (21%; grades 3/4: 5%)

Gastrointestinal: Mucositis (41%), nausea (37%), anorexia (32%), diarrhea (27%), abdominal pain (21%), constipation (20%), stomatitis (20%), taste disturbance (20%), vomiting (19%), weight loss (19%)

Genitourinary: Urinary tract infection (15%)

Hematologic: Anemia (45% to 94%; grades 3/4: 20%), lymphopenia (53%; grades 3/4: 16%), thrombocytopenia (14% to 40%; grades 3/4: 1%; dose-limiting toxicity), leukopenia (6% to 32%; grades 3/4: 1%), neutropenia (7% to 19%; grades 3/4: 3% to 5%)

Hepatic: Alkaline phosphatase increased (68%; grades 3/4: 3%), AST increased (8% to 38%; grades 3/4: 1% to 2%)

Neuromuscular & skeletal: Weakness (51%), back pain (20%), arthralgia (18%)

Renal: Creatinine increased (14% to 57%; grades 3/4: 3%)

Respiratory: Dyspnea (28%), cough (26%), epistaxis (12%), pharyngitis (12%)

Miscellaneous: Infection (20% to 27%; includes abscess, bronchitis, cellulitis, herpes simplex, herpes zoster)

1% to 10%:

Cardiovascular: Hypertension, thrombophlebitis, venous thromboembolism (includes DVT and PE)

Central nervous system: Chills, depression

Dermatologic: Acne, wound healing impaired

Gastrointestinal: Bowel perforation

Hepatic: Hyperbilirubinemia

Neuromuscular & skeletal: Myalgia

Ocular: Conjunctivitis

Respiratory: Interstitial lung disease (ILD), pneumonia, rhinitis, upper respiratory tract infection

Miscellaneous: Allergic/hypersensitivity/infusion reaction (includes anaphylaxis, apnea, chest pain, dyspnea, flushing, hypotension, loss of consciousness)

<1%, postmarketing, and/or case reports: Acute renal failure, angioneurotic edema, glucose intolerance, infusion site extravasation (with pain, swelling, warmth, erythema), pericardial effusion, pleural effusion, pneumonitis, reflex sympathetic dystrophy, rhabdomyolysis, seizure, Stevens-Johnson syndrome

Drug Interactions

Metabolism/Transport Effects Substrate of CYP3A4 (major), P-glycoprotein; **Note:** Assignment of Major/Minor substrate status based on clinically relevant drug interaction potential; **Inhibits** CYP2D6 (weak), CYP3A4 (weak)

Avoid Concomitant Use

Avoid concomitant use of Temsirolimus with any of the following: BCG; CloZAPine; Conivaptan; Natalizumab; Pimecrolimus; Pimozide; SUNItinib; Tacrolimus (Systemic); Tacrolimus (Topical); Vaccines (Live)

Increased Effect/Toxicity

Temsirolimus may increase the levels/effects of: ACE Inhibitors; ARIPiprazole; CloZAPine; CycloSPORINE (Systemic); Leflunomide; Natalizumab; Pimozide; SUNItinib; Tacrolimus (Systemic); Tacrolimus (Topical); Vaccines (Live)

The levels/effects of Temsirolimus may be increased by: Conivaptan; CYP3A4 Inhibitors (Moderate); CYP3A4 Inhibitors (Strong); Dasatinib; Denosumab; Fluconazole; Itraconazole; Ivacaftor; Ketoconazole (Systemic); Macrolide Antibiotics; Mifepristone; P-glycoprotein/ABCB1 Inhibitors; Pimecrolimus; Posaconazole; Protease Inhibitors; Roflumilast; Tacrolimus (Systemic); Tacrolimus (Topical); Trastuzumab

Decreased Effect

Temsirolimus may decrease the levels/effects of: BCG; Coccidioidin Skin Test; Sipuleucel-T; Tacrolimus (Systemic); Vaccines (Inactivated); Vaccines (Live)

The levels/effects of Temsirolimus may be decreased by: CarBAMazepine; CYP3A4 Inducers (Strong); Deferasirox; Echinacea; Fosphenytoin; Herbs (CYP3A4 Inducers); P-glycoprotein/ABCB1 Inducers; Phenytoin; Rifamycin Derivatives; Tocilizumab

Ethanol/Nutrition/Herb Interactions

Food: Grapefruit and grapefruit juice may increase the levels/effects of sirolimus. Management: Avoid grapefruit and grapefruit juice.

Herb/Nutraceutical: Herbs with hypoglycemic properties may increase the risk of temsirolimus-induced hypoglycemia. St John's wort may decrease sirolimus (the active metabolite of temsirolimus) levels. Management: Avoid concurrent use of St John's wort. Avoid alfalfa, aloe, bilberry, bitter melon, burdock, celery, damiana, fenugreek, garcinia, garlic, ginger, ginseng (American), gymnema, marshmallow, and stinging nettle.

Storage/Stability Store intact vials refrigerated at 2°C to 8°C (36°F to 46°F). Diluted solution in the vial (10 mg/mL) is stable for 24 hours at room temperature. Solutions diluted for infusion (in NS) must be infused within 6 hours of preparation. Protect from light during storage, preparation, and handling.

Reconstitution Use appropriate precautions for handling and disposal. Preparation requires a two-step dilution process (do not add undiluted temsirolimus to aqueous solution; addition to aqueous solution prior to step 1 will result in precipitation). *Step 1:* Total amount in undiluted vial is 30 mg/1.2 mL (25 mg/mL concentration); contains overfill. Vials should initially be diluted with 1.8 mL of provided diluent to a concentration of 10 mg/mL. Once diluted with provided diluent, mix by inverting vial. *Step 2:* After allowing air bubbles to subside, the intended dose should be withdrawn from the 10 mg/mL diluted vial (ie, 2.5 mL for a 25 mg dose) and further diluted in 250 mL of NS in a non-DEHP/non-PVC container (glass, polyolefin, or polypropylene). Mix by inverting bottle or bag; avoid excessive shaking (may result in foaming).

Mechanism of Action Temsirolimus and its active metabolite, sirolimus, are targeted inhibitors of mTOR (mammalian target of rapamycin) kinase activity. Temsirolimus (and sirolimus) bind to FKBP-12, an intracellular protein, to form a complex which inhibits mTOR signaling, halting the cell cycle at the G1 phase in tumor cells. In renal cell carcinoma, mTOR inhibition also exhibits anti-angiogenesis activity by reducing levels of HIF-1 and HIF-2 alpha (hypoxia inducible factors) and vascular endothelial growth factor (VEGF).

Pharmacodynamics/Kinetics

Distribution: V_{dss}: 172 L

Metabolism: Hepatic; via CYP3A4 to sirolimus (primary active metabolite) and 4 minor metabolites

Half-life elimination: Temsirolimus: ~17 hours; Sirolimus: ~55 hours

Time to peak, plasma: Temsirolimus: At end of infusion; Sirolimus: 0.5-2 hours after temsirolimus infusion

Excretion: Feces (78%); urine (<5%)

Dosing

Adult & Geriatric Note: For infusion reaction prophylaxis, premedicate with an H_1 antagonist (eg, diphenhydramine 25-50 mg I.V.) 30 minutes prior to infusion.

Renal cell cancer (RCC), advanced: I.V.: 25 mg once weekly; continue until disease progression or unacceptable toxicity

Dosage adjustment for concomitant CYP3A4 inhibitors/inducers:

CYP3A4 inhibitors: Avoid concomitant administration with strong CYP3A4 inhibitors (eg, clarithromycin, itraconazole, ketoconazole, nefazodone, protease inhibitors, telithromycin, voriconazole); if concomitant administration with a strong CYP3A4 inhibitor cannot be avoided, consider a dose reduction to 12.5 mg/week. When a strong CYP3A4 inhibitor is discontinued; allow ~1 week to elapse prior to adjusting the temsirolimus upward to the dose used prior to initiation of the CYP3A4 inhibitor.

CYP3A4 inducers: Avoid concomitant administration with strong CYP3A4 inducers (eg, carbamazepine, dexamethasone, phenobarbital, phenytoin, rifampin, St John's wort); if concomitant administration with a strong CYP3A4 inducer cannot be avoided, consider adjusting temsirolimus dose up to 50 mg/week. If the strong CYP3A4 enzyme inducer is discontinued, reduce the temsirolimus to the dose used prior to initiation of the CYP3A4 inducer.

Renal Impairment No adjustment necessary (renal impairment is not expected to significantly impact exposure). Has not been studied in hemodialysis patients.

Hepatic Impairment

Mild hepatic impairment (bilirubin >1-1.5 x ULN or AST >ULN with bilirubin ≤ULN): Reduce dose to 15 mg once weekly.

Moderate-to-severe hepatic impairment (bilirubin >1.5 x ULN): Use is contraindicated.

Adjustment for Toxicity

Hematologic toxicity: ANC <1000/mm^3 or platelets <75,000/mm^3: Withhold treatment until resolves and reinitiate treatment with the dose reduced by 5 mg/week; minimum dose: 15 mg/week if adjustment for toxicity is needed.

Nonhematologic toxicity: Any toxicity ≥grade 3: Withhold treatment until resolves to ≤grade 2; reinitiate treatment with the dose reduced by 5 mg/week; minimum dose: 15 mg/week if adjustment for toxicity is needed.

Infusion/hypersensitivity reaction: Interrupt infusion and observe for 30-60 minutes; treatment may be resumed with discretion at a slower infusion rate (up to 60 minutes); administer an H1 antagonist (if not given as premedication) and/or an I.V. H_2 antagonist 30 minutes prior to resuming infusion.

Interstitial lung disease: Consider withholding treatment for clinically significant respiratory symptoms until after recovery of symptoms or radiographic improvement.

Combination Regimens

Renal cell cancer: Temsirolimus (RCC Regimen) *on page* 1754

Administration Infuse over 30-60 minutes via an infusion pump (preferred). Use polyethylene-lined non-DEHP administration tubing. Administer through an inline polyethersulfone filter ≤5 micron; if set does not contain an inline filter, a polyethersulfone end filter (0.2-5 micron) should be added (do not use both an inline and an end filter). Premedicate with an H_1 antagonist (eg, diphenhydramine 25-50 mg I.V.) ~30 minutes prior to infusion. Monitor during infusion; interrupt infusion for hypersensitivity/infusion reaction; monitor for 30-60 minutes; may reinitiate at a reduced infusion rate (over 60 minutes) with discretion, 30 minutes after administration of a histamine H_1 antagonist and/or a histamine H_2 antagonist (eg, famotidine or ranitidine). Administration should be completed within 6 hours of admixture.

Emetic Potential Low (10% to 30%)

Monitoring Parameters CBC with differential and platelets (weekly), serum chemistries including glucose (baseline and every other week), serum cholesterol and triglycerides (baseline and periodic), liver function (baseline and periodic), renal function tests (baseline and periodic)

Monitor for infusion reactions; infection; symptoms of ILD (or radiographic changes), symptoms of hyperglycemia (excessive thirst, polyuria)

Dietary Considerations Avoid grapefruit juice (may increase the levels of the major metabolite, sirolimus).

Dosage Forms Excipient information presented when available (limited, particularly for generics); consult specific product labeling.

Injection, solution [concentrate]:

Torisel®: 25 mg/mL (1.2 mL) [contains dehydrated ethanol, dehydrated ethanol (in diluent), polyethylene glycol 400, polysorbate 80 (in diluent), propylene glycol; supplied with diluent]

References

Bellmunt J, Szczylik C, Feingold J, et al, "Temsirolimus Safety Profile and Management of Toxic Effects in Patients With Advanced Renal Cell Carcinoma and Poor Prognostic Features," *Ann Oncol*, 2008, 19(8):1387-92.

Dutcher JP, de Souza P, McDermott D, et al, "Effect of Temsirolimus Versus Interferon-Alpha on Outcome of Patients With Advanced Renal Cell Carcinoma of Different Tumor Histologies," *Med Oncol*, 2009, 26(2):202-9.

Gupta S, Parsa VB, Heilbrun LK, et al, "Safety and Efficacy of Molecularly Targeted Agents in Patients With Metastatic Kidney Cancer With Renal Dysfunction," *Anticancer Drugs*, 2011, 22 (8):794-800.

Hudes G, Carducci M, Tomczak P, et al, "Temsirolimus, Interferon Alfa, or Both for Advanced Renal-Cell Carcinoma," *N Engl J Med*, 2007, 356(22):2271-81.

Teniposide (ten i POE side)

Related Information

Management of Drug Extravasations *on page 1800*

Safe Handling of Hazardous Drugs *on page 1904*

Brand Names: U.S. Vumon®

Brand Names: Canada Vumon®

Index Terms EPT; PTG; VM-26

Generic Availability (U.S.) No

Pharmacologic Category Antineoplastic Agent, Podophyllotoxin Derivative

Use Treatment of refractory childhood acute lymphoblastic leukemia (ALL) in combination with other chemotherapy

Unlabeled Use Treatment of refractory acute lymphoblastic leukemia (ALL) in adults

Labeled Contraindications Hypersensitivity to teniposide, polyoxyethylated castor oil (Cremophor® EL), or any component of the formulation

Pregnancy Risk Factor D

Lactation Excretion in breast milk unknown/not recommended

Warnings/Precautions Hazardous agent - use appropriate precautions for handling and disposal.

[U.S. Boxed Warning]: Severe myelosuppression resulting in infection or bleeding may occur; may be dose-limiting; monitor blood counts. Patients with Down syndrome and leukemia may be more sensitive to the myelosuppressive effects; reduced initial doses are recommended. **[U.S. Boxed Warning]: Hypersensitivity reactions, including anaphylaxis-like reactions, have been reported;** hypersensitivity reactions may include bronchospasm, dyspnea, hypertension, hypotension, tachycardia, flushing, chills, fever, or urticaria. Monitor closely during infusion (observe continuously for first 60 minutes, frequently thereafter). Stop infusion for signs of anaphylaxis; immediate treatment for anaphylactic reaction should be available during administration (may require treatment with epinephrine, corticosteroids, antihistamines, pressors, or volume expanders). Patients experiencing prior hypersensitivity are at risk for recurrence; retreat only if the potential benefit outweighs the risk of hypersensitivity; premedication (with corticosteroids and antihistamines) is recommended for retreatment. Hypotension may occur with rapid infusion; infuse slowly over at least 30-60 minutes; discontinue for clinically significant hypotension; if infusion is restarted after being withheld for hypotension, reinitiate at a slower infusion rate.

Use with caution in patients with renal or hepatic impairment; may require dosage reduction in patients with significant impairment. For I.V. use only; monitor infusion site; may cause local tissue necrosis or thrombophlebitis if extravasation occurs. Since teniposide is highly bound to plasma proteins, carefully monitor patients with hypoalbuminemia. Product contains benzyl alcohol which has been associated with "gasping syndrome" in neonates. Product contains about 43% alcohol. Acute CNS depression, hypotension and metabolic acidosis have been reported; these events occurred in patients who received high-dose teniposide (investigation protocol) and were premedicated with antiemetics, which along with the alcohol content of teniposide, may have contributed to the depression. Neurotoxicity and severe neuropathy have been reported when teniposide is used in combination with vincristine. **[U.S. Boxed Warning]: Should be administered under the supervision of an experienced cancer chemotherapy physician**

Adverse Reactions

>10%:

- Gastrointestinal: Mucositis (76%), diarrhea (33%), nausea/vomiting (29%; mild to moderate)
- Hematologic: Neutropenia (95%), leukopenia (89%), anemia (88%), thrombocytopenia (85%), myelosuppression (75%)
- Miscellaneous: Infection (12%)

1% to 10%:

- Cardiovascular: Hypotension (2%; associated with rapid [<30 minutes] infusions)
- Central nervous system: Fever (3%)
- Dermatologic: Alopecia (9%; usually reversible), rash (3%)
- Hematologic: Bleeding (5%)

Miscellaneous: Hypersensitivity reactions (5%; includes bronchospasm, chills, dyspnea, fever, flushing, hyper-/hypotension, tachycardia, or urticaria)

1% (Limited to important or life-threatening): Arrhythmia, CNS depression, confusion, headache, hepatic dysfunction, intractable hypotension, metabolic abnormality, metabolic acidosis, neuropathy (severe), neurotoxicity, renal dysfunction, thrombophlebitis, tissue necrosis (upon extravasation), weakness

Drug Interactions

Metabolism/Transport Effects Substrate of CYP3A4 (major), P-glycoprotein; **Note:** Assignment of Major/Minor substrate status based on clinically relevant drug interaction potential; **Inhibits** CYP2C9 (weak), CYP3A4 (weak)

Avoid Concomitant Use

Avoid concomitant use of Teniposide with any of the following: BCG; CloZAPine; Conivaptan; Natalizumab; Pimecrolimus; Pimozide; Tacrolimus (Topical); Vaccines (Live)

Increased Effect/Toxicity

Teniposide may increase the levels/effects of: ARIPiprazole; CloZAPine; Leflunomide; Natalizumab; Pimozide; Vaccines (Live); VinCRIStine; VinCRIStine (Liposomal)

The levels/effects of Teniposide may be increased by: Conivaptan; CYP3A4 Inhibitors (Moderate); CYP3A4 Inhibitors (Strong); Dasatinib; Denosumab; Ivacaftor; Mifepristone; P-glycoprotein/ABCB1 Inhibitors; Pimecrolimus; Roflumilast; Tacrolimus (Topical); Trastuzumab

Decreased Effect

Teniposide may decrease the levels/effects of: BCG; Coccidioidin Skin Test; Sipuleucel-T; Vaccines (Inactivated); Vaccines (Live)

The levels/effects of Teniposide may be decreased by: Barbiturates; CYP3A4 Inducers (Strong); Deferasirox; Echinacea; Fosphenytoin; Herbs (CYP3A4 Inducers); P-glycoprotein/ABCB1 Inducers; Phenytoin; Tocilizumab

Ethanol/Nutrition/Herb Interactions Herb/Nutraceutical: St John's wort may decrease teniposide levels.

Storage/Stability Store ampuls in refrigerator at 2°C to 8°C (36°F to 46°F). Protect from light. Solutions diluted for infusion to a concentration of 0.1, 0.2, or 0.4 mg/mL are stable at room temperature for up to 24 hours after preparation; solutions diluted to 1 mg/mL should be used within 4 hours of preparation. Because precipitation may occur at any concentration, the manufacturer recommends administrating as soon as possible after preparation. Use appropriate precautions for handling and disposal. Do not refrigerate solutions prepared for infusion.

Reconstitution Use appropriate precautions for handling and disposal. Precipitation may occur at any concentration. Teniposide must be diluted with either D_5W or 0.9% sodium chloride solutions to a final concentration of 0.1, 0.2, 0.4, or 1 mg/mL. **Solutions should be prepared in non-DEHP-containing containers such as glass or polyolefin containers.** The use of polyvinyl chloride (PVC) containers is not recommended. Because precipitation may occur at any concentration, the manufacturer recommends administrating as soon as possible after preparation. Use appropriate precautions for handling and disposal.

Mechanism of Action Teniposide does not inhibit microtubular assembly; it has been shown to delay transit of cells through the S phase and arrest cells in late S or early G_2 phase, preventing cells from entering mitosis. Teniposide is a topoisomerase II inhibitor, and appears to cause DNA strand breaks by inhibition of strand-passing and DNA ligase action.

Pharmacodynamics/Kinetics

Distribution: V_{dss}: Adults: 8-44 L/m^2; Children: 3-11 L/m^2; crosses blood-brain barrier to a limited extent

Protein binding: 99.4%

Metabolism: Extensively hepatic

Half-life elimination: Children: 5 hours

Excretion: Urine (44%, 4% to 12% as unchanged drug); feces (≤10%)

Dosing

Adult Note: Patients with Down syndrome and leukemia may be more sensitive to the myelosuppressive effects; administer the first course at half the usual dose and adjust dose in subsequent cycles upward based on degree of toxicities (myelosuppression and mucositis) in the previous course(s).

Acute lymphoblastic leukemia (ALL) consolidation treatment (unlabeled use; combination chemotherapy): I.V.: 165 mg/m^2/dose days 1, 4, 8, and 11 of alternating consolidation cycles (Linker, 1991)

Pediatric Note: Patients with Down syndrome and leukemia may be more sensitive to the myelosuppressive effects; administer the first course at half the usual dose and adjust dose in subsequent cycles upward based on degree of toxicities (myelosuppression and mucositis) in the previous course(s).

Acute lymphoblastic leukemia (ALL; combination chemotherapy): I.V.: 165 mg/m^2 twice weekly for 8-9 doses **or** 250 mg/m^2 weekly for 4-8 weeks **or** (unlabeled dosing) 165 mg/m^2/dose days 1 and 2 of weeks 3, 13, and 23 (Lauer, 2001)

Renal Impairment Data is insufficient, but dose adjustments may be necessary in patient with significant renal impairment.

Hepatic Impairment Data is insufficient, but dose adjustments may be necessary in patient with significant hepatic impairment.

Combination Regimens

Leukemia, acute lymphocytic: Linker Protocol (ALL) on page 1703

Administration I.V.; must be administered slowly (over at least 30-60 minutes); do not administer by rapid I.V. injection. Administer through non-DEHP-containing administration sets. Incompatible with heparin; flush infusion line with D_5W or NS before and after infusion. Precipitation may occur at any concentration; administer as soon as possible after preparation; inspect solution prior to administration. Observe patient continuously for at least the first 60 minutes of infusion, observe frequently thereafter. Stop infusion for signs of anaphylaxis (may require treatment with epinephrine, corticosteroids, antihistamines, pressors, or volume expanders); discontinue for clinically significant hypotension during infusion; if infusion is restarted after being withheld for hypotension, reinitiate at a slower infusion rate.

Vesicant/Extravasation Risk May be an irritant

Monitoring Parameters CBC, platelet count, renal and hepatic function tests; blood pressure; monitor for hypersensitivity reaction (observe continuously for first 60 minutes of infusion, frequently thereafter)

Dosage Forms Excipient information presented when available (limited, particularly for generics); consult specific product labeling.

Injection, solution:
Vumon®: 10 mg/mL (5 mL) [contains benzyl alcohol, dehydrated ethanol 42.7%, polyoxyethylated castor oil]

References

Lauer SJ, Shuster JJ, Mahoney DH Jr, et al, "A Comparison of Early Intensive Methotrexate/Mercaptopurine With Early Intensive Alternating Combination Chemotherapy for High-Risk B-Precursor Acute Lymphoblastic Leukemia: A Pediatric Oncology Group Phase III Randomized Trial," *Leukemia*, 2001, 15(7):1038-45.
Linker CA, Levitt LJ, O'Donnell M, et al, "Treatment of Adult Acute Lymphoblastic Leukemia With Intensive Cyclical Chemotherapy: A Follow-up Report," *Blood*, 1991 78(11):2814-22.
Salzer WL, Devidas M, Carroll WL, et al, "Long-Term Results of the Pediatric Oncology Group Studies for Childhood Acute Lymphoblastic Leukemia 1984-200: A Report From the Children's Oncology Group," *Leukemia*, 2010, 24(2):355-70.

◆ **TESPA** *see* Thiotepa *on page 1357*
◆ **Tetrahydrocannabinol** *see* Dronabinol *on page 484*
◆ **Teva-Acyclovir (Can)** *see* Acyclovir (Systemic) *on page 30*
◆ **Teva-Anastrozole (Can)** *see* Anastrozole *on page 96*
◆ **Teva-Chlorpromazine (Can)** *see* ChlorproMAZINE *on page 274*
◆ **Teva-Flutamide (Can)** *see* Flutamide *on page 635*
◆ **Teva-Hydromorphone (Can)** *see* HYDROmorphone *on page 724*
◆ **Teva-Medroxyprogesterone (Can)** *see* MedroxyPROGESTERone *on page 916*
◆ **Teva-Morphine SR (Can)** *see* Morphine (Systemic) *on page 1004*
◆ **Teva-Nabilone (Can)** *see* Nabilone *on page 1023*
◆ **Teva-Olanzapine (Can)** *see* OLANZapine *on page 1056*
◆ **Teva-Olanzapine OD (Can)** *see* OLANZapine *on page 1056*
◆ **Teva-Ondansetron (Can)** *see* Ondansetron *on page 1068*
◆ **Teva-Raloxifene (Can)** *see* Raloxifene *on page 1222*
◆ **Teva-Tamoxifen (Can)** *see* Tamoxifen *on page 1324*
◆ **Texacort™** *see* Hydrocortisone (Topical) *on page 719*
◆ **TG** *see* Thioguanine *on page 1354*
◆ **6-TG (error-prone abbreviation)** *see* Thioguanine *on page 1354*

Thalidomide (tha LI doe mide)

Related Information

Chemotherapy and Cancer Treatment During Pregnancy *on page 1829*
Hematopoietic Stem Cell Transplantation *on page 1887*
Management of Chemotherapy-Induced Nausea and Vomiting *on page 1786*
Principles of Anticancer Therapy *on page 1878*
Safe Handling of Hazardous Drugs *on page 1904*

Brand Names: U.S. Thalomid®

Brand Names: Canada Thalomid®

Generic Availability (U.S.) No

Pharmacologic Category Angiogenesis Inhibitor; Immunomodulator, Systemic; Tumor Necrosis Factor (TNF) Blocking Agent

Use Treatment of newly-diagnosed multiple myeloma; treatment and maintenance of cutaneous manifestations of erythema nodosum leprosum (ENL)

Unlabeled Use Treatment of refractory Crohn's disease; treatment of chronic graft-versus-host disease (GVHD) in hematopoietic stem cell transplantation;

AIDS-related aphthous stomatitis; Waldenström's macroglobulinemia; maintenance therapy of multiple myeloma (following autologous stem cell transplant)

Labeled Contraindications Hypersensitivity to thalidomide or any component of the formulation; patient unable to comply with STEPS® program (including males); women of childbearing potential unless alternative therapies are inappropriate and adequate precautions are taken to avoid pregnancy; pregnancy

Canadian labeling: Additional contraindications (not in U.S. labeling): Hypersensitivity to lenalidomide; breast-feeding

Pregnancy Risk Factor X

Lactation Excretion in breast milk unknown/not recommended

Warnings/Precautions Hazardous agent - use appropriate precautions for handling and disposal. **[U.S. Boxed Warning]: Thalidomide should only be prescribed to patients (male and female) who can understand and comply with the conditions of the S.T.E.P.S.® program. Distribution is restricted; physicians, pharmacists, and patients must be registered with the S.T.E.P.S.® program. [U.S. Boxed Warning]: Thalidomide is a known teratogen; effective contraception must be used for at least 4 weeks before initiating therapy, during therapy, and for 4 weeks following discontinuation of thalidomide for women of childbearing potential.** Use caution with drugs which may decrease the efficacy of hormonal contraceptives.

[U.S. Boxed Warning]: Thrombotic events have been reported, generally in patients with other risk factors for thrombosis (neoplastic disease, inflammatory disease, or concurrent therapy with combination chemotherapy. Use in combination with dexamethasone is associated with increased risk for deep vein thrombosis (DVT) and pulmonary embolism (PE), monitor for signs and symptoms of thromboembolism; patients at risk may benefit from prophylactic anticoagulation or aspirin. The NCCN multiple myeloma guidelines (v.1.2011) recommend anticoagulant prophylaxis with thalidomide-based therapy. Anticoagulant prophylaxis should be individualized and selected based on the venous thromboembolism risk of the combination treatment regimen, using the safest and easiest to administer (Palumbo, 2008). The Canadian labeling recommends anticoagulant prophylaxis for at least the first 5 months of thalidomide-based therapy.

May cause sedation; patients must be warned to use caution when performing tasks which require alertness. Use caution in patients with neurological disorders or constipation. Thalidomide has been associated with the development of peripheral neuropathy, which may be irreversible; generally occurs following chronic use (over months), but may occur with short-term use; use caution with other medications which may cause peripheral neuropathy. Consider immediate discontinuation (if clinically appropriate) in patients who develop neuropathy. May cause seizures; use caution in patients with a history of seizures, concurrent therapy with drugs which alter seizure threshold, or conditions which predispose to seizures. May cause neutropenia; discontinue therapy if absolute neutrophil count decreases to <750/mm^3. Use caution in patients with HIV infection; has been associated with increased viral loads. May cause orthostasis and/or bradycardia; use with caution in patients with cardiovascular disease or in patients who would not tolerate transient hypotensive episodes. Hypersensitivity, Stevens-Johnson syndrome (SJS) and toxic epidermal necrolysis (TEN) have been reported; withhold therapy and evaluate with skin rashes; permanently discontinue if rash is exfoliative, purpuric, bullous or if SJS or TEN is suspected.

Adverse Reactions

>10%:

Cardiovascular: Edema (57%), thrombosis/embolism (23%; grade 3: 13%, grade 4: 9%), hypotension (16%)

Central nervous system: Fatigue (79%; grade 3: 14%, grade 4: 3%), somnolence (36% to 38%), dizziness (4% to 20%), sensory neuropathy (54%), confusion (28%), anxiety/agitation (9% to 26%), fever (19% to 23%), motor neuropathy (22%), headache (13% to 19%)

Dermatologic: Rash/desquamation (21% to 30%; grade 3: 4%), dry skin (21%), maculopapular rash (4% to 19%), acne (3% to 11%)

Endocrine & metabolic: Hypocalcemia (72%)

Gastrointestinal: Constipation (3% to 55%), nausea (4% to 28%), anorexia (3% to 28%), weight loss (23%), weight gain (22%), diarrhea (4% to 19%), oral moniliasis (4% to 11%)

Hematologic: Leukopenia (17% to 35%), neutropenia (31%), anemia (6% to 13%), lymphadenopathy (6% to 13%)

Hepatic: AST increased (3% to 25%), bilirubin increased (14%)

Neuromuscular & skeletal: Muscle weakness (40%), tremor (4% to 26%), weakness (6% to 22%), myalgia (17%), paresthesia (6% to 16%), arthralgia (13%)

Renal: Hematuria (11%)

Respiratory: Dyspnea (42%)

Miscellaneous: Diaphoresis (13%)

1% to 10%:

Cardiovascular: Peripheral edema (3% to 8%), facial edema (4%)

Central nervous system: Insomnia (9%), nervousness (3% to 9%), malaise (8%), vertigo (8%), pain (3% to 8%)

Dermatologic: Dermatitis (fungal 4% to 9%), pruritus (3% to 8%), nail disorder (3% to 4%)

Endocrine & metabolic: Hyperlipemia (6% to 9%)

Gastrointestinal: Xerostomia (8% to 9%), flatulence (8%), tooth pain (4%)

Genitourinary: Impotence (3% to 8%)

Hepatic: LFTs abnormal (9%)

Neuromuscular & skeletal: Neuropathy (8%), back pain (4% to 6%), neck pain (4%), neck rigidity (4%)

Renal: Albuminuria (3% to 8%)

Respiratory: Pharyngitis (4% to 8%), rhinitis (4%), sinusitis (3% to 8%)

Miscellaneous: Infection (6% to 8%)

Postmarketing and/or case reports (limited to important or life-threatening): Acute renal failure, alkaline phosphatase increased, ALT increased, amenorrhea, aphthous stomatitis, arrhythmia, atrial fibrillation, bile duct obstruction, bradycardia, BUN increased, CML, creatinine clearance decreased, creatinine increased, deafness, depression, diplopia, dysesthesia, ECG abnormalities, enuresis, eosinophilia, epistaxis, erythema multiforme, erythema nodosum, erythroleukemia, exfoliative dermatitis, febrile neutropenia, foot drop, galactorrhea, granulocytopenia, gynecomastia, hepatomegaly, Hodgkin's disease, hypercalcemia, hyper-/hypokalemia, hypersensitivity, hypertension, hyper-/hypothyroidism, hyperuricemia, hypomagnesemia, hyponatremia, hypoproteinemia, intestinal obstruction, intestinal perforation, interstitial pneumonitis, LDH increased, lethargy, leukocytosis, lymphedema, lymphopenia, mental status changes, metrorrhagia, myxedema, nystagmus, oliguria, orthostatic hypotension, pancytopenia, paresthesia, petechiae, peripheral neuritis, photosensitivity, pleural effusion, prothrombin time changes, psychosis, pulmonary embolus, pulmonary hypertension, purpura, Raynaud's syndrome, seizure, status epilepticus, Stevens-Johnson syndrome, stomach ulcer, stupor, suicide attempt, syncope, tachycardia, thrombocytopenia, toxic epidermal necrolysis, tumor lysis syndrome

Drug Interactions

Metabolism/Transport Effects None known.

Avoid Concomitant Use

Avoid concomitant use of Thalidomide with any of the following: Abatacept; Anakinra; Azelastine (Nasal); BCG; Canakinumab; Certolizumab Pegol; CloZAPine; Methadone; Mirtazapine; Natalizumab; Paraldehyde; Pimecrolimus; Rilonacept; Tacrolimus (Topical); Vaccines (Live)

Increased Effect/Toxicity

Thalidomide may increase the levels/effects of: Abatacept; Alcohol (Ethyl); Anakinra; Azelastine (Nasal); Buprenorphine; Canakinumab; Certolizumab Pegol; CloZAPine; CNS Depressants; Leflunomide; Methadone; Methotrimeprazine; Metyrosine; Mirtazapine; Natalizumab; Pamidronate; Paraldehyde; Pramipexole; Rilonacept; ROPINIRole; Rotigotine; Selective Serotonin Reuptake Inhibitors; Vaccines (Live); Zoledronic Acid; Zolpidem

The levels/effects of Thalidomide may be increased by: Denosumab; Dexamethasone (Systemic); Droperidol; HydrOXYzine; Methotrimeprazine; Perampanel; Pimecrolimus; Roflumilast; Tacrolimus (Topical); Trastuzumab

Decreased Effect

Thalidomide may decrease the levels/effects of: BCG; Coccidioidin Skin Test; Sipuleucel-T; Vaccines (Inactivated); Vaccines (Live)

The levels/effects of Thalidomide may be decreased by: Echinacea

Ethanol/Nutrition/Herb Interactions

Ethanol: May increase CNS depression; monitor for increased effects with coadministration. Caution patients about effects.

Herb/Nutraceutical: Avoid cat's claw and echinacea (have immunostimulant properties; consider therapy modifications).

Storage/Stability Store at 25°C (77°F); excursions permitted to 15°C to 30°C (59°F to 86°F). Protect from light. Keep in original package.

Mechanism of Action Immunomodulatory and antiangiogenic characteristics; immunologic effects may vary based on conditions; may suppress excessive tumor necrosis factor-alpha production in patients with ENL, yet may increase plasma tumor necrosis factor-alpha levels in HIV-positive patients. In multiple myeloma, thalidomide is associated with an increase in natural killer cells and increased levels of interleukin-2 and interferon gamma. Other proposed mechanisms of action include suppression of angiogenesis, prevention of free-radical-mediated DNA damage, increased cell mediated cytotoxic effects, and altered expression of cellular adhesion molecules.

Pharmacodynamics/Kinetics

Protein binding: 55% to 66%

Metabolism: Nonenzymatic hydrolysis in plasma; forms multiple metabolites

Bioavailability: Capsule: 90%

Half-life elimination: 5-7 hours

Time to peak, plasma: 3-6 hours

Excretion: Urine (<1% as unchanged drug)

Dosing

Adult & Geriatric

Cutaneous ENL: Oral: Initial: 100-300 mg once daily

Adjustments to initial dose:

Patients weighing <50 kg: Initiate at lower end of the dosing range

Severe cutaneous reaction or patients previously requiring high dose may be initiated at 400 mg/day; doses may be divided, but taken 1 hour after meals

Duration and tapering/maintenance:

Maintenance: Dosing should continue until active reaction subsides (usually at least 2 weeks), then tapered in 50 mg decrements every 2-4 weeks

Patients who flare during tapering or with a history of requiring prolonged maintenance should be maintained on the minimum dosage necessary to control the reaction. Efforts to taper should be repeated every 3-6 months, in decrements of 50 mg every 2-4 weeks.

Multiple myeloma: Oral: **Note:** Details concerning dosing for multiple myeloma with combination regimens should also be consulted.

200 mg once daily at bedtime (in combination with dexamethasone 40 mg daily on days 1-4, 9-12, and 17-20 of a 28-day treatment cycle)

In combination with melphalan and prednisone (unlabeled combination in U.S.): 200-400 mg once daily (Facon, 2007) **or** 100 mg once daily (Palumbo, 2008)

Canadian labeling: Adults ≥65 years: 200 mg once daily (in combination with melphalan and prednisone)

AIDS-related aphthous stomatitis (unlabeled use): Oral: 200 mg once daily at bedtime for up to 8 weeks, if no response, then 200 mg twice daily for 4 weeks (Jacobson, 1997)

Chronic graft-versus-host disease (refractory), treatment (unlabeled second-line use; optimum dose not determined): Oral: Initial: 100 mg at bedtime, with dose escalation up to 400 mg/day in 3-4 divided doses (Wolff, 2010) **or** Initial: 50-100 mg 3 times/day; maximum dose: 600-1200 mg/day (Kulkarni, 2003) **or** 200 mg 4 times/day (dose adjusted to goal thalidomide concentration of ≥5 mcg/mL 2 hours postdose) (Vogelsang, 1992) **or** 100-300 mg 4 times/day (Parker, 1995)

Crohn's disease, refractory (unlabeled use): Oral: 50-100 mg/day at bedtime (Vasiliauskas, 1999) **or** 200-300 mg/day at bedtime (Ehrenpreis, 1999)

Multiple myeloma, maintenance (following autologous stem cell transplant; unlabeled use): Oral: 200 mg/day starting 3-6 months after transplant; continue until disease progression or unacceptable toxicity (Brinker, 2006) **or** 100 mg/day starting 42-60 days following transplant; increase to 200 mg/day after 2 weeks if tolerated; continue for up to 12 months (in combination with prednisolone) (Spencer, 2009)

Waldenström's macroglobulinemia (unlabeled use): Oral: 200 mg/day for up to 52 weeks (in combination with rituximab) (Treon, 2008)

Pediatric Cutaneous ENL: Children ≥12 years: Oral: Refer to adult dosing.

Chronic graft-versus-host disease (refractory), treatment (unlabeled second-line use; limited data): Children ≥3 years: Oral: 3 mg/kg 4 times/day (dose adjusted to goal thalidomide concentration of ≥5 mcg/mL 2 hours postdose) (Vogelsang, 1992) **or** Initial: 3-6 mg/kg/day in 2-4 divided doses; target dose 12 mg/kg/day; Maximum daily dose: 800 mg (Rovelli, 1998)

Renal Impairment No adjustment is required for patients with renal impairment and on dialysis (per manufacturer). In a study of 6 patients with end-stage renal disease on dialysis, although clearance was increased by dialysis, a supplemental dose was not needed (Eriksson, 2003).

Multiple myeloma: An evaluation of 29 newly-diagnosed myeloma patients with renal failure (serum creatinine ≥2 mg/dL) treated with thalidomide and dexamethasone (some also received cyclophosphamide) found that toxicities and efficacy were similar to patients with normal renal function (Seol, 2010). A study evaluating induction therapy with thalidomide and dexamethasone in 31 newly-diagnosed myeloma patients with renal failure (Cl_{cr} <50 mL/minute), including 16 patients with severe renal impairment (Cl_{cr} <30 mL/minute) and 7 patients on chronic hemodialysis found that toxicities were similar to patients without renal impairment and that thalidomide and dexamethasone could be administered safely (Tosi, 2009).

Hepatic Impairment Thalidomide does not appear to undergo significant hepatic metabolism; the pharmacokinetics of thalidomide have not been studied in patients with liver dysfunction (per manufacturer).

Adjustment for Toxicity

ANC ≤750/mm^3: Withhold treatment if clinically appropriate

Multiple myeloma:

U.S. labeling: Constipation, oversedation, peripheral neuropathy: Temporarily withhold or continue with a reduced dose

Canadian labeling:

ANC <1500/mm^3: Withhold melphalan and prednisone for 1 week; resume melphalan and prednisone after 1 week if ANC >1500/mm^3 **or** if ANC 1000-1500/mm^3 reduce melphalan dose by 50% **or** if ANC <1000/mm^3 adjust chemotherapy dose based on clinical status of patient.

Constipation, oversedation: Temporarily withhold thalidomide treatment or continue with a reduced dose

Peripheral neuropathy, Grade 1 (paresthesia, weakness and/or loss of reflexes) without loss of function): Evaluate patient and consider dose reduction with worsening of symptoms; symptom improvement may not follow dose reduction, however.

Peripheral neuropathy, Grade 2 (interferes with function but not with daily activities), Grade 3 (interferes with daily activities), or Grade 4 (disabling neuropathy): Discontinue thalidomide treatment

Thromboembolic events: Withhold therapy and initiate standard anticoagulant treatment; may resume thalidomide therapy at original dose following stabilization of patient and resolution of thromboembolic event; maintain anticoagulant treatment for duration of thalidomide therapy

Combination Regimens

Multiple myeloma:

Bortezomib-Melphalan-Prednisone-Thalidomide on page 1537

DTPACE on page 1620

Melphalan-Prednisone-Thalidomide (Multiple Myeloma) on page 1710

Thalidomide-Dexamethasone (MM) on page 1754

Administration Administer orally with water, preferably at bedtime once daily on an empty stomach, at least 1 hour after the evening meal. Doses >400 mg/day may be given in 2-3 divided doses. For missed doses, if <12 hours patient may receive dose; if >12 hours wait till next dose due.

Avoid extensive handling of capsules; capsules should remain in blister pack until ingestion. If exposed to the powder content from broken capsules or body fluids from patients receiving thalidomide, the exposed area should be washed with soap and water.

Emetic Potential Low (10% to 30%)

Extemporaneous Preparations Hazardous agent: Use appropriate precautions for handling and disposal.

A 20 mg/mL oral suspension may be prepared with capsules and a 1:1 mixture of Ora-Sweet® and Ora-Plus®. Empty the contents of twelve 100 mg capsules into a glass mortar. Add small portions of the vehicle and mix to a uniform paste; mix while adding the vehicle in incremental proportions to almost 60 mL; transfer to an amber calibrated bottle, rinse mortar with vehicle, and add quantity of vehicle sufficient to make 60 mL. Label "shake well," "protect from light," and "refrigerate". Stable for 35 days refrigerated.

Kraft S, Johnson CE, and Tyler RP, "Stability of an Extemporaneously Prepared Thalidomide Suspension," *Am J Health Syst Pharm*, 2011, 69(1):56-8.

Monitoring Parameters CBC with differential, platelets; signs of neuropathy monthly for the first 3 months, then periodically during treatment; consider monitoring of sensory nerve application potential amplitudes (at baseline and every 6 months) to detect asymptomatic neuropathy. Monitor for signs and symptoms of thromboembolism (shortness of breath, chest pain, arm/leg swelling). In HIV-seropositive patients: viral load after 1 and 3 months, then every 3 months. Pregnancy testing (sensitivity of at least 50 mIU/mL) is required within 24 hours prior to initiation of therapy, weekly during the first 4 weeks, then every 4 weeks in women with regular menstrual cycles or every 2 weeks in women with irregular menstrual cycles.

Dietary Considerations Should be taken at least 1 hour after the evening meal.

Prescribing and Access Restrictions U.S.: As a requirement of the REMS program, access to this medication is restricted. Thalidomide is approved for marketing only under a special distribution program. This program, called the "System for Thalidomide Education and Prescribing Safety" (STEPS® 1-888-423-5436), has been approved by the FDA. Prescribers and pharmacists must be registered with the program. No more than a 4-week supply should be dispensed. Blister packs should be dispensed intact (do not repackage capsules). Prescriptions must be filled within 7 days. Subsequent prescriptions may be filled only if fewer than 7 days of therapy remain on the previous prescription. A new prescription is required for further dispensing (a telephone prescription may not be accepted.) Pregnancy testing is required for females of childbearing potential.

Canada: Access to thalidomide is restricted through a controlled distribution program called RevAid®. Only physicians and pharmacists enrolled in this program are authorized to prescribe or dispense thalidomide. Patients must be enrolled in the program by their physicians. Further information is available by calling 1-888-738-2431.

Medication Guide Available Yes

Dosage Forms Excipient information presented when available (limited, particularly for generics); consult specific product labeling.

Capsule, oral:

Thalomid®: 50 mg, 100 mg, 150 mg, 200 mg

References

Brinker BT, Walker EK, Leong T, et al, "Maintenance Therapy With Thalidomide Improves Overall Survival After Autologous Hematopoietic Progenitor Cell Transplantation for Multiple Myeloma," *Cancer*, 2006, 106(10):2171-80.

Cavo M, Tacchetti P, Patriarca F, et al, "Bortezomib With Thalidomide Plus Dexamethasone Compared With Thalidomide Plus Dexamethasone as Induction Therapy Before, and Consolidation Therapy After, Double Autologous Stem-Cell Transplantation in Newly Diagnosed Multiple Myeloma: A Randomised Phase 3 Study," *Lancet*, 2010, 376(9758):2075-85.

Ehrenpreis ED, Kane SV, Cohen LB, et al, "Thalidomide Therapy for Patients With Refractory Crohn's Disease: An Open-Label Trial," *Gastroenterology*, 1999, 117(6):1271-7.

Eriksson T, Höglund P, Turesson I, et al, "Pharmacokinetics of Thalidomide in Patients With Impaired Renal Function and While On and Off Dialysis," *J Pharm Pharmacol*, 2003, 55 (12):1701-6.

Facon T, Mary JY, Hulin C, et al, "Melphalan and Prednisone Plus Thalidomide Versus Melphalan and Prednisone Alone or Reduced-Intensity Autologous Stem Cell Transplantation in Elderly Patients With Multiple Myeloma (IFM 99-06): A Randomised Trial," *Lancet*, 2007, 370 (9594):1209-18.

Hamuryudan V, Mat C, Saip S, et al, "Thalidomide in the Treatment of the Mucocutaneous Lesions of the Behçet Syndrome. A Randomized, Double-Blind, Placebo-Controlled Trial," *Ann Intern Med*, 1998, 128(6):443-50.

Hulin C, Facon T, Rodon P, et al, "Efficacy of Melphalan and Prednisone Plus Thalidomide in Patients Older Than 75 Years With Newly Diagnosed Multiple Myeloma: IFM 01/01 Trial," *J Clin Oncol*, 2009, 27(22):3664-70.

Jacobson JM, Greenspan JS, Spritzler J, et al, "Thalidomide for the Treatment of Oral Aphthous Ulcers in Patients With Human Immunodeficiency Virus Infection. National Institute of Allergy and Infectious Diseases AIDS Clinical Trials Group," *N Engl J Med*, 1997, 336(21):1487-93.

Kulkarni S, Powles R, Sirohi B, et al, "Thalidomide After Allogeneic Haematopoietic Stem Cell Transplantation: Activity in Chronic But Not in Acute Graft-Versus-Host Disease," *Bone Marrow Transplant*, 2003, 32(2):165-70.

Lokhorst HM, van der Holt B, Zweegman S, et al, "A Randomized Phase 3 Study on the Effect of Thalidomide Combined With Adriamycin, Dexamethasone, and High-Dose Melphalan, Followed by Thalidomide Maintenance in Patients With Multiple Myeloma," *Blood*, 2010, 115(6):1113-20.

National Comprehensive Cancer Network® (NCCN), "Clinical Practice Guidelines In Oncology™: Multiple Myeloma," Version 1.2011. Available at http://www.nccn.org/professionals/physician_gls/PDF/myeloma.pdf

Palumbo A, Bringhen S, Liberati AM, et al, "Oral Melphalan, Prednisone, and Thalidomide in Elderly Patients With Multiple Myeloma: Updated Results of a Randomized Controlled Trial," *Blood*, 2008, 112(8):3107-14.

Palumbo A, Bringhen S, Rossi D, et al, "Bortezomib-Melphalan-Prednisone-Thalidomide Followed by Maintenance With Bortezomib-Thalidomide Compared With Bortezomib-Melphalan-Prednisone for Initial Treatment of Multiple Myeloma: a Randomized Controlled Trial," *J Clin Oncol*, 2010, 28(34):5101-9.

Palumbo A, Rajkumar SV, Dimopoulos MA, et al, "Prevention of Thalidomide- and Lenalidomide-Associated Thrombosis in Myeloma," *Leukemia*, 2008, 22(2): 414-23.

Parker PM, Chao N, Nademanee A, et al, " Thalidomide as Salvage Therapy for Chronic Graft-Versus Host Disease," *Blood*, 1995, 86(9):3604-9.

Rajkumar SV, Blood E, Vesole D, et al, "Phase III Clinical Trial of Thalidomide Plus Dexamethasone Compared With Dexamethasone Alone in Newly Diagnosed Multiple Myeloma: A Clinical Trial Coordinated by the Eastern Cooperative Oncology Group," *J Clin Oncol*, 2006, 24(3):431-6.

Rovelli A, Arrigo C, Nesi F, et al, "The Role of Thalidomide in the Treatment of Refractory Chronic Graft-Versus-Host Disease Following Bone Marrow Transplantation in Children," *Bone Marrow Transplant*, 1998, 21(6):577-81.

Seol Y, Chung J, Kwon R, et al, "Treatment for Patients With Multiple Myeloma Complicated by Renal Failure by Thalidomide-Based Regimens," *J Clin Oncol*, 2010, 28(suppl):e13093 [abstract e13093 from 2010 ASCO Annual Meeting].

Spencer A, Prince HM, Roberts AW, et al, "Consolidation Therapy With Low-Dose Thalidomide and Prednisolone Prolongs the Survival of Multiple Myeloma Patients Undergoing a Single Autologous Stem-Cell Transplantation Procedure," *J Clin Oncol*, 2009, 27(11):1788-93.

Tosi P, Zamagni E, Tacchetti P, et al, "Thalidomide-Dexamethasone as Induction Therapy Prior to Autologous Stem-Cell Transplantation in Patients With Newly Diagnosed Multiple Myeloma and Renal Failure," *Blood*, 2009, 114(22):4934 [abstract 4934 from 2009 ASH Annual Meeting].

Treon SP, Soumerai JD, Branagan AR, et al, "Thalidomide and Rituximab in Waldenstrom Macroglobulinemia," *Blood*, 2008, 112(12):4552-7.

Vasiliauskas EA, Kam LY, Abreu-Martin MT, et al, "An Open-Label Pilot Study of Low-Dose Thalidomide in Chronically Active, Steroid-Dependent Crohn's Disease," *Gastroenterology*, 1999, 117(6):1278-87.

Vogelsang GB, Farmer ER, Hess AD, et al, "Thalidomide for the Treatment of Chronic Graft-Versus-Host Disease," *N Engl J Med*, 1992, 326(16):1055-8.

Wijermans P, Schaafsma M, Termorshuizen F, et al, "Phase III Study of the Value of Thalidomide Added to Melphalan Plus Prednisone in Elderly Patients With Newly Diagnosed Multiple Myeloma: the HOVON 49 Study," *J Clin Oncol*, 2010, 28(19):3160-6.
Wolff D, Schleuning M, von Harsdorf S, et al, "Consensus Conference on Clinical Practice in Chronic GVHD: Second-Line Treatment of Chronic Graft-versus-Host Disease," *Biol Blood Marrow Transplant*, 2010, 17(1):1-17.

◆ **Thalomid®** *see* Thalidomide *on page 1346*

◆ **THC** *see* Dronabinol *on page 484*

◆ **TheraCys®** *see* BCG *on page 153*

Thioguanine (thye oh GWAH neen)

Related Information

Chemotherapy and Cancer Treatment During Pregnancy *on page 1829*
Management of Chemotherapy-Induced Nausea and Vomiting *on page 1786*
Safe Handling of Hazardous Drugs *on page 1904*

Brand Names: U.S. Tabloid®

Brand Names: Canada Lanvis®

Index Terms 2-Amino-6-Mercaptopurine; 6-TG (error-prone abbreviation); 6-Thioguanine (error-prone abbreviation); TG; Tioguanine

Generic Availability (U.S.) No

Pharmacologic Category Antineoplastic Agent, Antimetabolite (Purine Analog)

Use Treatment of acute myelogenous (nonlymphocytic) leukemia (AML)

Unlabeled Use Treatment of pediatric acute lymphoblastic leukemia (ALL)

Labeled Contraindications Prior resistance to thioguanine (or mercaptopurine)

Canadian labeling: Additional contraindications (not in US labeling): Hypersensitivity to thioguanine or any component of the formulation

Pregnancy Risk Factor D

Lactation Excretion in breast milk unknown/not recommended

Warnings/Precautions Hazardous agent - use appropriate precautions for handling and disposal.

Not recommended for maintenance therapy or long-term continuous treatment; long-term continuous therapy or maintenance treatment is associated with a high risk for hepatotoxicity, hepatic sinusoidal obstruction syndrome (SOS; formerly called veno-occlusive disease), or portal hypertension; monitor liver function carefully for liver toxicity and discontinue in patients with evidence of hepatic SOS (eg, hyperbilirubinemia, hepatomegaly [tender], and weight gain due to ascites and fluid retention) or portal hypertension (eg, splenomegaly, thrombocytopenia, esophageal varices); hepatotoxicity with or without transaminase elevations may occur; pathologic findings of hepatotoxicity include hepatoportal sclerosis, nodular regenerative hyperplasia, peliosis hepatitis, and periportal fibrosis.

Myelosuppression (anemia, leukopenia, and/or thrombocytopenia) is a common dose-related toxicity (may be delayed); monitor for infection (due to leukopenia) or bleeding(due to thrombocytopenia); withhold treatment with abnormally significant drop in blood counts. Patients with genetic enzyme deficiency of thiopurine methyltransferase (TPMT) or who are receiving drugs which inhibit this enzyme (mesalazine, olsalazine, sulfasalazine) may be highly sensitive to myelosuppressive effects and may require substantial dose reductions.

Hyperuricemia occurs commonly with treatment; institute adequate hydration and prophylactic allopurinol. Thioguanine is potentially carcinogenic. Cross resistance with mercaptopurine generally occurs. Avoid vaccination with live vaccines during treatment.

Adverse Reactions Frequency not defined.

Endocrine & metabolic: Fluid retention, hyperuricemia (common)

Gastrointestinal: Anorexia, intestinal necrosis, intestinal perforation, nausea, splenomegaly, stomatitis, vomiting, weight gain

Hematologic: Anemia (may be delayed), bleeding, granulocytopenia, leukopenia (common; may be delayed), marrow hypoplasia, pancytopenia, thrombocytopenia (common; may be delayed)

Hepatic: Ascites, esophageal varices, hepatic necrosis (centrilobular), hepatic sinusoidal obstruction syndrome (SOS; veno-occlusive disease), hepatitis, hepatomegaly [tender], hepatoportal sclerosis, hepatotoxicity, hyperbilirubinemia, jaundice, LFTs increased, nodular regenerative hyperplasia, peliosis hepatitis, periportal fibrosis, portal hypertension

Miscellaneous: Infection

Drug Interactions

Metabolism/Transport Effects None known.

Avoid Concomitant Use

Avoid concomitant use of Thioguanine with any of the following: BCG; CloZAPine; Natalizumab; Pimecrolimus; Tacrolimus (Topical); Vaccines (Live)

Increased Effect/Toxicity

Thioguanine may increase the levels/effects of: CloZAPine; Leflunomide; Natalizumab; Vaccines (Live)

The levels/effects of Thioguanine may be increased by: 5-ASA Derivatives; Denosumab; Pimecrolimus; Roflumilast; Tacrolimus (Topical); Trastuzumab

Decreased Effect

Thioguanine may decrease the levels/effects of: BCG; Coccidioidin Skin Test; Sipuleucel-T; Vaccines (Inactivated); Vaccines (Live)

The levels/effects of Thioguanine may be decreased by: Echinacea

Ethanol/Nutrition/Herb Interactions Ethanol: Avoid; may increase the risk for hepatotoxicity.

Storage/Stability Store tablet at room temperature at 15°C to 25°C (59°F to 77°F). Protect from moisture.

Mechanism of Action Purine analog that is incorporated into DNA and RNA resulting in the blockage of synthesis and metabolism of purine nucleotides

Pharmacodynamics/Kinetics

Absorption: ~30% (range: 14% to 46%; highly variable)

Distribution: Does not reach therapeutic concentrations in the CSF

Metabolism: Hepatic; rapidly and extensively via thiopurine methyltransferase (TPMT) to 2-amino-6-methylthioguanine (MTG; active) and inactive compounds

Half-life elimination: Terminal: 5-9 hours

Time to peak, serum: Within 8 hours; predominantly metabolite(s)

Dosing

Pediatric Pediatric ALL (unlabeled use; combination therapy): Oral: Delayed intensification treatment phase: 60 mg/m^2/day for 14 days (Lange, 2002; Nachman, 1998)

Renal Impairment Children: No adjustment required (Aronoff, 2007).

Hepatic Impairment Deterioration in transaminases, alkaline phosphatase or bilirubin, toxic hepatitis, biliary stasis, clinical jaundice, evidence of hepatic sinusoidal obstruction syndrome (veno-occlusive disease), or evidence of portal hypertension: Discontinue treatment.

Combination Regimens

Leukemia, acute lymphocytic: Larson Regimen (ALL) on page 1699

Administration Administer orally; total daily dose can be given at one time.

Emetic Potential Very low (<10%)

Extemporaneous Preparations Hazardous agent: Use appropriate precautions for handling and disposal.

A 20 mg/mL oral suspension may be made with tablets, methylcellulose 1%, and simple syrup NF. Crush fifteen 40 mg tablets in a mortar and reduce to a fine powder. Add 10 mL methylcellulose 1% in incremental proportions and mix to a uniform paste. Transfer to a graduated cylinder, rinse mortar with simple syrup, and add quantity of simple syrup sufficient to make 30 mL. Label "shake well" and "refrigerate". Stable for 84 days refrigerated (preferred) or at room temperature.

Dressman JB and Poust RI, "Stability of Allopurinol and Five Antineoplastics in Suspension," *Am J Hosp Pharm*, 1983, 40(4):616-8.

Nahata MC, Pai VB, and Hipple TF, *Pediatric Drug Formulations*, 5th ed, Cincinnati, OH: Harvey Whitney Books Co, 2004.

Monitoring Parameters CBC with differential and platelet count; liver function tests (weekly when beginning therapy then monthly, more frequently in patients with liver disease or concurrent hepatotoxic drugs); serum uric acid; some laboratories offer testing for TPMT deficiency

Hepatotoxicity may present with signs of portal hypertension (splenomegaly, esophageal varices, thrombocytopenia) or sinusoidal obstruction syndrome (veno-occlusive disease; fluid retention, ascites, hepatomegaly with tenderness, or hyperbilirubinemia)

Dosage Forms Excipient information presented when available (limited, particularly for generics); consult specific product labeling.

Tablet, oral:

Tabloid®: 40 mg [scored]

References

Aronoff GR, Bennett WM, Berns JS, et al, *Drug Prescribing in Renal Failure: Dosing Guidelines for Adults and Children*, 5th ed. Philadelphia, PA: American College of Physicians; 2007, p 173.

Estlin EJ, "Continuing Therapy for Childhood Acute Lymphoblastic Leukaemia: Clinical and Cellular Pharmacology of Methotrexate, 6-Mercaptopurine and 6-Thioguanine," *Cancer Treat Rev*, 2001, 27(6):351-63.

Lange BJ, Bostrom BC, Cherlow JM, et al, "Double-Delayed Intensification Improves Event-Free Survival for Children With Intermediate-Risk Acute Lymphoblastic Leukemia: A Report From the Children's Cancer Group," *Blood*, 2002, 99(3):825-33.

Nachman JB, Sather HN, Sensel MG, et al, "Augmented Post-Induction Therapy for Children With High-Risk Acute Lymphoblastic Leukemia and a Slow Response to Initial Therapy," *N Engl J Med*, 1998, 338(23):1663-71.

Vora A, Mitchell CD, Lennard L, et al, "Toxicity and Efficacy of 6-Thioguanine Versus 6-Mercaptopurine in Childhood Lymphoblastic Leukaemia: A Randomised Trial," *Lancet*, 2006, 368(9544):1339-48.

◆ **6-Thioguanine (error-prone abbreviation)** *see* Thioguanine *on page 1354*

◆ **Thiophosphoramide** *see* Thiotepa *on page 1357*

◆ **Thioplex** *see* Thiotepa *on page 1357*

◆ **Thiosulfuric Acid Disodium Salt** *see* Sodium Thiosulfate *on page 1289*

Thiotepa (thye oh TEP a)

Related Information

Chemotherapy and Obesity *on page 1834*
Management of Chemotherapy-Induced Nausea and Vomiting *on page 1786*
Management of Drug Extravasations *on page 1800*
Safe Handling of Hazardous Drugs *on page 1904*

Index Terms TESPA; Thiophosphoramide; Thioplex; Triethylenethiophosphoramide; TSPA

Generic Availability (U.S.) Yes

Pharmacologic Category Antineoplastic Agent, Alkylating Agent

Use Treatment of superficial papillary bladder cancer; palliative treatment of adenocarcinoma of breast or ovary; controlling intracavitary effusions caused by metastatic tumors

Unlabeled Use Intrathecal treatment of leptomeningeal metastases

Labeled Contraindications Hypersensitivity to thiotepa or any component of the formulation

Note: May be contraindicated in certain circumstances of hepatic, renal, and/or bone marrow failure; evaluate on an individual basis as lower dose treatment (with close monitoring) may still be appropriate if the potential benefit outweighs the risks

Pregnancy Risk Factor D

Lactation Excretion in breast milk unknown/not recommended

Warnings/Precautions Hazardous agent - use appropriate precautions for handling and disposal. Myelosuppression is common; monitor for infection or bleeding. Myelosuppression has also been reported with intravesicular administration (due to systemic absorption). Potentially teratogenic, mutagenic, and carcinogenic; myelodysplastic syndrome and acute myeloid leukemia (AML) have been reported. Reduce dosage and use extreme caution in patients with hepatic, renal, or bone marrow damage. Use may be contraindicated with impairment/damage and should be limited to cases where benefit outweighs risk.

When used for intrathecal administration, should not be prepared during the preparation of any other agents; after preparation, keep intrathecal medications in an isolated location or container clearly marked with a label identifying as "intrathecal" use only; delivery of intrathecal medications to the patient should only be with other medications intended for administration into the central nervous system (Jacobson, 2009).

Adverse Reactions

Frequency not defined:

- Central nervous system: Chills, dizziness, fatigue, fever, headache
- Dermatologic: Alopecia, contact dermatitis, depigmentation (with topical treatment), dermatitis, rash, urticaria
- Endocrine & metabolic: Amenorrhea, spermatogenesis inhibition
- Gastrointestinal: Abdominal pain, anorexia, nausea, vomiting
- Genitourinary: Dysuria, urinary retention
- Hematologic: Anemia, bleeding, leukopenia, thrombocytopenia
- Local: Injection site pain
- Neuromuscular & skeletal: Weakness
- Ocular: Blurred vision, conjunctivitis
- Renal: Hematuria

Respiratory: Asthma, epistaxis, laryngeal edema, wheezing
Miscellaneous: Allergic reaction, anaphylactic shock, infection

Infrequent, postmarketing, and/or case reports: Acute myeloid leukemia (AML), chemical cystitis (bladder instillation), hemorrhagic cystitis (bladder instillation), myelodysplastic syndrome

Drug Interactions

Metabolism/Transport Effects Inhibits CYP2B6 (strong)

Avoid Concomitant Use

Avoid concomitant use of Thiotepa with any of the following: BCG; CloZAPine; Natalizumab; Pimecrolimus; Tacrolimus (Topical); Vaccines (Live)

Increased Effect/Toxicity

Thiotepa may increase the levels/effects of: CloZAPine; CYP2B6 Substrates; Leflunomide; Natalizumab; Vaccines (Live)

The levels/effects of Thiotepa may be increased by: Denosumab; Pimecrolimus; Roflumilast; Tacrolimus (Topical); Trastuzumab

Decreased Effect

Thiotepa may decrease the levels/effects of: BCG; Coccidioidin Skin Test; Sipuleucel-T; Vaccines (Inactivated); Vaccines (Live)

The levels/effects of Thiotepa may be decreased by: Echinacea

Ethanol/Nutrition/Herb Interactions

Ethanol: Avoid ethanol (due to GI irritation).

Herb/Nutraceutical: Avoid black cohosh, dong quai in estrogen-dependent tumors.

Storage/Stability Store intact vials under refrigeration (2°C to 8°C). Protect from light. Reconstituted solutions (10 mg/mL) are stable for up to 28 days under refrigeration (4°C to 8°C) or 7 days at room temperature (25°C), although the manufacturer recommends use within 8 hours when reconstituted solutions are stored under refrigeration. Solutions further diluted (for I.V. use) in NS to 1 mg/mL are stable for 24 hours and to 3 mg/mL are stable for 48 hours at room temperature, although the manufacturer recommends immediate use. After preparation, keep intrathecal medications in an isolated location or container clearly marked with a label identifying as "intrathecal" use only.

Reconstitution Hazardous agent; use appropriate precautions for handling and disposal. Reconstitute each 15 mg vial with 1.5 mL SWFI to a concentration of 10 mg/mL. Solutions for I.V. use should be further diluted in 0.9% sodium chloride injection prior to infusion. Filter through a 0.22 micron filter (polysulfone membrane [eg, Sterile Aerodisc®] or triton-free cellulose mixed ester [eg, Millex®-GS]) prior to administration; do not use solutions which precipitate or remain opaque after filtering. Solutions for intravesicular administration should be diluted in 30-60 mL NS. Solutions for intrathecal administration should be diluted to a concentration of 1-5 mg/mL in preservative-free NS. Intrathecal medications should not be prepared during the preparation of any other agents.

Mechanism of Action Alkylating agent that reacts with DNA phosphate groups to produce cross-linking of DNA strands leading to inhibition of DNA, RNA, and protein synthesis; mechanism of action has not been explored as thoroughly as the other alkylating agents, it is presumed that the aziridine rings open and react as nitrogen mustard; reactivity is enhanced at a lower pH

Pharmacodynamics/Kinetics

Absorption: Intracavitary instillation: Unreliable (10% to 100%) through bladder mucosa

Metabolism: Extensively hepatic; major metabolite (active): TEPA

Half-life elimination: Terminal (dose-dependent clearance): ~2 hours
Excretion: Urine (as metabolites and unchanged drug)

Dosing

Adult & Geriatric

Bladder cancer: Intravesical: 60 mg in 30-60 mL NS retained for 2 hours once weekly for 4 weeks

Ovarian, breast cancer: I.V.: 0.3-0.4 mg/kg by rapid I.V. administration every 1-4 weeks

Effusions: Intracavitary: 0.6-0.8 mg/kg

Leptomeningeal metastases (unlabeled use): Intrathecal: 10 mg twice a week for 4 weeks, then (if CSF cytology is negative) weekly for 4 weeks, then monthly for 4 doses (NCCN CNS cancer guidelines v.1.2010)

HSCT for CNS malignancy (unlabeled use; combination chemotherapy): I.V.: 250 mg/m^2/day for 3 days beginning 9 days prior to transplant (Soussain, 2008) **or** 150 mg/m^2/dose every 12 hours for 6 doses, followed by stem cell reinfusion 96 hours after completion of thiotepa (Abrey, 2006)

Pediatric HSCT for CNS malignancy (unlabeled use; combination chemotherapy): 300 mg/m^2/day for 3 days beginning 8 days prior to transplant (Gilheeney, 2010) **or** 300 mg/m^2/day for 3 days beginning 5 days prior to transplant (Dunkel, 2010; Grodman, 2009)

Renal Impairment Use with extreme caution, reduced dose may be warranted. Use may be contraindicated with existing renal impairment and should be limited to cases where benefit outweighs risk.

Hepatic Impairment Use with extreme caution, reduced dose may be warranted. Use may be contraindicated with existing hepatic impairment and should be limited to cases where benefit outweighs risk.

Adjustment for Toxicity I.V.: **Note:** Use may be contraindicated with preexisting marrow damage and should be limited to cases where benefit outweighs risk.

WBC ≤3000/mm^3: Discontinue treatment
Platelets ≤150,000/mm^3: Discontinue treatment

Administration

I.V.: Administer as a rapid injection. Infusion times may be longer for high-dose (unlabeled use) treatment; refer to specific protocols

Intravesical instillation: Instill directly into the bladder and retain for 2 hours; patient should be repositioned every 15-30 minutes for maximal exposure

Emetic Potential Low (10% to 30%)

Vesicant/Extravasation Risk May be an irritant

Monitoring Parameters CBC with differential and platelet count (monitor weekly during treatment and for at least 3 weeks after treatment), renal and liver function tests; uric acid, urinalysis

Dosage Forms Excipient information presented when available (limited, particularly for generics); consult specific product labeling.

Injection, powder for reconstitution: 15 mg

References

Abrey LE, Childs BH, Paleologos N, et al, "High-Dose chemotherapy With Stem Cell Rescue as Initial Therapy for anaplastic Oligodendroglioma: Long-Term Follow-Up," *J Neurooncol*, 2008, 89 (2):187-93.

DeAngelis LM and Butros D, "Leptomeningeal Metastasis," *Cancer Invest*, 2005, 23(2):145-54.

de Lemos ML, Monfared S, Denyssevych T, et al, "Evaluation of Osmolality and pH of Various Concentrations of Methotrexate, Cytarabine, and Thiotepa Prepared in Normal Saline, Sterile Water for Injection, and Lactated Ringer's Solution for Intrathecal Administration," *J Oncol Pharm Pract*, 2009, 15(1):45-52.

Dunkel IJ, Gardner SL, Garvin JH Jr, et al, "High-Dose Carboplatin, Thiotepa, and Etoposide With Autologous Stem Cell Rescue for Patients With Previously Irradiated Recurrent Medulloblastoma," *Neuro Oncol*, 2010, 12(3):297-303.

Gilheeney SW, Khakoo Y, Souweidane M, et al, "Thiotepa/Topotecan/Carboplatin With Autologous Stem Cell Rescue in Recurrent/Refractory/Poor Prognosis Pediatric Malignancies of the Central Nervous System," *Pediatr Blood Cancer*, 2010, 54(4):591-5.

Grodman H, Wolfe L, and Kretschmar C, "Outcome of Patients With Recurrent Medulloblastoma or Central Nervous System Germinoma Treated With Low Dose Continuous Intravenous Etoposide Along With Dose-Intensive Chemotherapy Followed by Autologous Hematopoietic Stem Cell Rescue," *Pediatr Blood Cancer*, 2009, 53(1):33-6.

Jacobson JO, Polovich M, McNiff KK, et al, "American Society of Clinical Oncology/Oncology Nursing Society Chemotherapy Administration Safety Standards," *J Clin Oncol*, 2009, 27 (32):5469-75.

National Comprehensive Cancer Network® (NCCN), "Clinical Practice Guidelines in Oncology™: Central Nervous System Cancers," Version 1.2010. Available at http://www.nccn.org/professionals/physician_gls/PDF/cns.pdf

Soussain C, Hoang-Xuan K, Taillandier L, et al, "Intensive Chemotherapy Followed by Hematopoietic Stem-Cell Rescue for Refractory and Recurrent Primary CNS and Intraocular Lymphoma: Société Française de Greffe de Moëlle Osseuse-Thérapie Cellulaire," *J Clin Oncol*, 2008, 26(15):2512-8.

◆ **Thorazine** *see* ChlorproMAZINE *on page 274*

◆ **Thrombate III®** *see* Antithrombin *on page 107*

◆ **Thymocyte Stimulating Factor** *see* Aldesleukin *on page 37*

◆ **Thymoglobulin®** *see* Antithymocyte Globulin (Rabbit) *on page 115*

◆ **Thyrogen®** *see* Thyrotropin Alfa *on page 1360*

Thyrotropin Alfa (thye roe TROH pin AL fa)

Brand Names: U.S. Thyrogen®

Brand Names: Canada Thyrogen®

Index Terms Human Thyroid Stimulating Hormone; Recombinant Human Thyrotropin; Rh-TSH; Thyrotropin Alpha; TSH

Generic Availability (U.S.) No

Pharmacologic Category Diagnostic Agent

Use An adjunctive diagnostic tool for serum thyroglobulin (Tg) testing (with or without radioiodine imaging) in patients with well-differentiated thyroid cancer; adjunctive treatment for radioiodine ablation of thyroid tissue remnants after total or near-total thyroidectomy in patients with well-differentiated thyroid cancer without evidence of metastatic disease

Potential clinical uses include: Patients with an undetectable Tg on thyroid hormone suppressive therapy to exclude the diagnosis of residual or recurrent thyroid cancer, patients requiring serum Tg testing and radioiodine imaging who are unwilling to undergo thyroid hormone withdrawal testing and whose treating physician believes that use of a less sensitive test is justified, patients who are either unable to mount an adequate endogenous TSH response to thyroid hormone withdrawal or in whom withdrawal is medically contraindicated, and patients without evidence of metastatic disease to ablate thyroid remnants (in combination with radioiodine [I^{131}]) following near-total thyroidectomy.

Labeled Contraindications There are no contraindications listed within the manufacturer's labeling.

Pregnancy Risk Factor C

Lactation Excretion in breast milk unknown/use caution

Warnings/Precautions For I.M. use only (NOT for I.V. administration). Caution should be exercised when administered to patients who have been previously treated with bovine TSH and, in particular, to those patients who have experienced hypersensitivity reactions to bovine TSH. In patients with significant residual thyroid tissue, thyrotropin will cause significant increases in thyroid hormone levels; use caution in patients with known history of heart disease or serious underlying illness; may lead to serious complications. Deaths within 24 hours of thyrotropin administration have been reported. Thyrotropin-induced hyperthyroidism may result in serious complications in patients with certain risk factors (heart disease, extensive metastatic disease or with underlying serious illness); consider hospitalization for administration and subsequent observation. Acute hemiplegia or hemiparesis have been reported in patients with CNS metastases; may be associated with sudden/rapid tumor growth. Postmarketing reports of stroke or unilateral weakness within3 days of administration have been reported in women (without known CNS metastases). Patients should be advised to seek immediate care for any neurologic symptoms following thyrotropin alfa administration. Sudden, rapid, and painful locally recurring papillary carcinoma growth has been reported within 12-48 hours of administration; may be associated with dyspnea, stridor, or dysphonia. Prompt improvement has occurred with glucocorticoids. Consider glucocorticoid premedication in patients where local tumor enlargement may compromise vital structures (trachea, CNS, or extensive macroscopic lung metastases).

Thyrotropin elimination is significantly reduced in dialysis-dependent end-stage renal impairment, leading to prolonged elevation of TSH levels. Thyrotropin use in elderly (with functioning thyroid tumors) may result in palpitations or cardiac rhythm disorders; arrhythmia has been reported in elderly patients with pre-existing cardiac disease; carefully evaluate risk versus benefit.

Considerations in the use of thyrotropin alfa.

1. There remains a meaningful risk of missing the diagnosis of thyroid cancer or of underestimating the extent of disease when thyrotropin-stimulated Tg testing is performed even in combination with radioiodine imaging. Thyroid hormone withdrawal Tg testing with radioiodine imaging is the standard diagnostic to assess presence, location and extent of thyroid cancer.
2. Thyrotropin Tg levels are generally lower than, and do not correlate with, Tg levels after thyroid hormone withdrawal.
3. Newly detectable Tg level or a Tg level rising over time after thyrotropin or a high index of suspicion of metastatic disease, even in the setting of a negative or low-stage thyrotropin radioiodine scan, should prompt further evaluation such as thyroid hormone withdrawal to definitively establish the location and extent of thyroid cancer.
4. Decision to perform a thyrotropin radioiodine scan in conjunction with a thyrotropin serum Tg test and whether or when to withdraw a patient from thyroid hormones are complex. Pertinent factors in this decision include the sensitivity of the Tg assay used, the thyrotropin Tg level obtained, and the index of suspicion of recurrent or persistent local or metastatic disease.
5. The signs and symptoms of hypothyroidism which accompany thyroid hormone withdrawal are avoided with thyrotropin use.
6. Clinical experience in thyroid remnant ablation with thyrotropin is limited; long-term outcome data have not been established compared to withholding thyroid hormone.
7. Thyrotropin studies for thyroid remnant ablation used I^{131} activity of 100 mCi ± 10%; activity of I^{131} used in clinical practice may vary; lower radioiodine doses may not be as effective.

Adverse Reactions

>10%: Gastrointestinal: Nausea (3% to 12%)

1% to 10%:

Central nervous system: Headache (1% to 7%), dizziness (≤3%), fatigue (1% to 3%), insomnia (≤2%)

Endocrine & metabolic: Hypercholesterolemia (≤3%), cholesterol abnormal (≤1%)

Gastrointestinal: Vomiting (1% to 3%), diarrhea (≤1%)

Neuromuscular & skeletal: Paresthesia (≤2%), weakness (≤2%)

Respiratory: Nasopharyngitis (≤1%)

Adverse reactions which may be related to local edema or hemorrhage at metastatic sites: Acute visual loss; enlargement of locally-recurring papillary carcinoma (accompanied by dyspnea, stridor, or dysphonia); hemiplegia, hemiparesis, laryngeal edema with respiratory distress, pain

<1%, postmarketing, and/or case reports: Atrial arrhythmia; flu-like syndrome (arthralgia, chills, fever, myalgia, shivering); hypersensitivity reactions (eg, flushing, pruritus, rash, respiratory difficulty, urticaria); hyperthyroidism, MI, pain, stroke, taste loss, thyrotropin alfa antibody formation, unilateral weakness

Drug Interactions

Metabolism/Transport Effects None known.

Avoid Concomitant Use There are no known interactions where it is recommended to avoid concomitant use.

Increased Effect/Toxicity There are no known significant interactions involving an increase in effect.

Decreased Effect There are no known significant interactions involving a decrease in effect.

Storage/Stability Store intact vials at 2°C to 8°C (36°F to 46°F). If necessary, the reconstituted solution can be stored for up to 24 hours at 2°C to 8°C (36°F to 46°F). Protect from light.

Reconstitution Reconstitute each vial with 1.2 mL of sterile water for injection to a final concentration of 0.9 mg/mL. Each vial should be reconstituted immediately prior to use.

Mechanism of Action Thyrotropin alfa, derived from a recombinant DNA source, has the identical amino acid sequence as endogenous human thyroid stimulating hormone (TSH). As a diagnostic tool in conjunction with serum thyroglobulin (Tg) testing, thyrotropin alfa stimulates the secretion of Tg from any remaining thyroid tissues (remnants). Under conditions of successful thyroidectomy and complete ablation, very little serum Tg should be detected under TSH stimulatory conditions; conversely, elevated Tg levels suggest the presence of remnant thyroid tissues. Since the source of TSH is exogenous, stimulation of Tg synthesis can be achieved in euthyroid patients, avoiding the need for thyroid hormone withdrawal.

As an adjunctive agent for radioiodine ablation treatment of thyroid cancer tissue remnants, thyrotropin alfa binds to TSH receptors on these tissues, stimulating the uptake and organification of iodine, including radiolabeled iodine (I^{131}). Cancerous tissue is destroyed via gamma emission from the radioiodine concentrated in these tissues.

Pharmacodynamics/Kinetics

Half-life elimination: 25 ± 10 hours

Time to peak: Median: 10 hours (range: 3-24 hours)

Dosing

Adult & Geriatric Radioiodine imaging or ablation: I.M.: 0.9 mg, followed 24 hours later by a second 0.9 mg dose

For radioiodine imaging or remnant ablation, radioiodine administration should be given 24 hours following the second thyrotropin injection. Diagnostic scanning should be performed 48 hours after radioiodine administration (72 hours after the second thyrotropin injection). Post-therapy scanning may be delayed (additional days) to allow decline of background activity.

For serum Tg testing, serum Tg should be obtained 72 hours after final injection of thyrotropin.

Pediatric Diagnostic aid: Children >16 years: Refer to adult dosing.

Renal Impairment Although thyrotropin alfa elimination is significantly reduced in dialysis-dependent end-stage renal impairment, no dosage adjustment provided in the manufacturer's labeling.

Administration Administer I.M. into the buttock.

Monitoring Parameters Neurologic adverse events (hemiplegia, hemiparesis, stroke, weakness); dyspnea, dysphonia, stridor or other symptoms of local tumor growth

Test Interactions Thyroglobulin assay may be confounded by thyroglobulin antibodies, possibly leading to misinterpreted or difficult to interpret thyroglobulin levels.

Dosage Forms Excipient information presented when available (limited, particularly for generics); consult specific product labeling. [DSC] = Discontinued product

Injection, powder for reconstitution:

Thyrogen®: 1.1 mg [DSC] [derived from or manufactured using Chinese hamster ovary cells]

Thyrogen®: 1.1 mg [derived from or manufactured using Chinese hamster ovary cells; supplied with diluent]

References

Mallick U, Harmer C, Yap B, et al, "Ablation With Low-Dose Radioiodine and Thyrotropin Alfa in Thyroid Cancer," *N Engl J Med*, 2012, 366(18):1674-85.

Pacini F, Ladenson PW, Schlumberger M, et al, "Radioiodine Ablation of Thyroid Remnants After Preparation With Recombinant Human Thyrotropin in Differentiated Thyroid Carcinoma: Results of an International, Randomized, Controlled Study," *J Clin Endocrinol Metab*, 2006, 91(3):926-32.

Schlumberger M, Catargi B, Borget I, et a, "Strategies of Radioiodine Ablation In Patients With Low-Risk Thyroid Cancer," *N Engl J Med*, 2012, 366(18):1663-73.

Schroeder PR, Haugen BR, Pacini F, et al, "A Comparison of Short-Term Changes in Health-Related Quality of Life in Thyroid Carcinoma Patients Undergoing Diagnostic Evaluation With Recombinant Human Thyrotropin Compared With Thyroid Hormone Withdrawal," *J Clin Endocrinol Metab*, 2006, 91(3):878-84.

◆ **Thyrotropin Alpha** *see* Thyrotropin Alfa *on page 1360*

Ticarcillin and Clavulanate Potassium

(tye kar SIL in & klav yoo LAN ate poe TASS ee um)

Brand Names: U.S. Timentin®

Brand Names: Canada Timentin®

Index Terms Ticarcillin and Clavulanic Acid

Generic Availability (U.S.) No

Pharmacologic Category Antibiotic, Penicillin

Use Treatment of lower respiratory tract, urinary tract, skin and skin structures, bone and joint, gynecologic (endometritis) and intra-abdominal (peritonitis) infections, and septicemia caused by susceptible organisms. Clavulanate expands activity of ticarcillin to include beta-lactamase producing strains of *S. aureus*, *H. influenzae*, *Bacteroides* species, and some other gram-negative bacilli

Labeled Contraindications Hypersensitivity to ticarcillin, clavulanate, any penicillin, or any component of the formulation

Pregnancy Risk Factor B

Lactation Enters breast milk/use caution

Warnings/Precautions Use with caution and modify dosage in patients with renal impairment; serious and occasionally severe or fatal hypersensitivity (anaphylactoid) reactions have been reported in patients on penicillin therapy (especially with a history of beta-lactam hypersensitivity and/or a history of sensitivity to multiple allergens); use with caution in patients with seizures and in patients with HF due to high sodium load. Particularly in patients with renal impairment, bleeding disorders have been observed; discontinue if thrombocytopenia or bleeding occurs. Prolonged use may result in fungal or bacterial superinfection, including *C. difficile*-associated diarrhea (CDAD) and pseudomembranous colitis; CDAD has been observed >2 months postantibiotic treatment.

Storage/Stability

Vials: Store intact vials at <24°C (<75°F). Reconstituted solution is stable for 6 hours at room temperature and 72 hours when refrigerated. I.V. infusion in NS or LR is stable for 24 hours at room temperature, 7 days when refrigerated, or 30 days when frozen. I.V. infusion in D_5W solution is stable for 24 hours at room temperature, 3 days when refrigerated, or 7 days when frozen. After freezing, thawed solution is stable for 8 hours at room temperature. Darkening of drug indicates loss of potency of clavulanate potassium.

Premixed solution: Store frozen at ≤-20°C (-4°F). Thawed solution is stable for 24 hours at room temperature or 7 days under refrigeration; do not refreeze.

Mechanism of Action Inhibits bacterial cell wall synthesis by binding to one or more of the penicillin-binding proteins (PBPs); which in turn inhibits the final transpeptidation step of peptidoglycan synthesis in bacterial cell walls, thus inhibiting cell wall biosynthesis. Bacteria eventually lyse due to ongoing activity of cell wall autolytic enzymes (autolysins and murein hydrolases) while cell wall assembly is arrested.

Pharmacodynamics/Kinetics

Absorption: Ticarcillin: Not absorbed orally

Protein binding: Ticarcillin: ~45%; Clavulanic acid: ~25%

Metabolism: Clavulanic acid: Hepatic

Half-life elimination: Ticarcillin: 1.1 hours; Clavulanic acid: 1.1 hours

Excretion: Ticarcillin: Urine (60% to 70%); Clavulanic acid: Urine (35% to 45% as unchanged drug)

Clearance: Clavulanic acid does not affect clearance of ticarcillin

Dosing

Adult Note: Timentin® (ticarcillin/clavulanate) is a combination product; each 3.1 g dosage form contains 3 g ticarcillin disodium and 0.1 g clavulanic acid.

Systemic infections: I.V.: 3.1 g (ticarcillin 3 g plus clavulanic acid 0.1 g) every 4-6 hours (maximum: 24 g of ticarcillin component/day)

Amnionitis, cholangitis, diverticulitis, endometritis, epididymo-orchitis, mastoiditis, orbital cellulitis, peritonitis, pneumonia (aspiration): I.V.: 3.1 g every 6 hours

Intra-abdominal infection, complicated, community-acquired, mild-to-moderate: I.V.: 3.1 g every 6 hours for 4-7 days (provided source controlled)

Liver abscess, parafascial space infections, septic thrombophlebitis: I.V.: 3.1 g every 4 hours

***Pseudomonas* infections:** I.V.: 3.1 g every 4 hours

Urinary tract infections: I.V.: 3.1 g every 6-8 hours

Geriatric I.V.: 3.1 g every 4-6 hours; adjust for renal function.

Pediatric Note: Timentin® (ticarcillin/clavulanate) is a combination product; each 3.1 g dosage form contains 3 g ticarcillin disodium and 0.1 g clavulanic acid.

Systemic infections:

Children <60 kg: 200-300 mg of ticarcillin component/kg/day in divided doses every 4-6 hours

Children ≥60 kg: 3.1 g (ticarcillin 3 g plus clavulanic acid 0.1 g) every 4-6 hours; maximum: 24 g of ticarcillin component/day

Bite wounds (animal): 200 mg of ticarcillin component/kg/day in divided doses

Neutropenic fever: 75 mg of ticarcillin component/kg every 6 hours (maximum: 3.1 g/dose)

Pneumonia (nosocomial): 300 mg of ticarcillin component/kg/day in 4 divided doses (maximum: 18-24 g of ticarcillin component/day)

Renal Impairment

Loading dose: I.V.: 3.1 g one dose, followed by maintenance dose based on creatinine clearance:

Cl_{cr} 30-60 mL/minute: Administer 2 g of ticarcillin component every 4 hours or 3.1 g every 8 hours

Cl_{cr} 10-30 mL/minute: Administer 2 g of ticarcillin component every 8 hours or 3.1 g every 12 hours

Cl_{cr} <10 mL/minute: Administer 2 g of ticarcillin component every 12 hours

Cl_{cr} <10 mL/minute with concomitant hepatic dysfunction: 2 g of ticarcillin component every 24 hours

Intermittent hemodialysis (IHD) (administer after hemodialysis on dialysis days): Dialyzable (20% to 50%): 2 g of ticarcillin component every 12 hours; supplemented with 3.1 g (ticarcillin/clavulanate) after each dialysis session. Alternatively, administer 2 g every 8 hours without a supplemental dose for deep-seated infections (Heintz, 2009). **Note:** Dosing dependent on the assumption of 3 times/week, complete IHD sessions.

Peritoneal dialysis (PD): 3.1 g every 12 hours

Continuous renal replacement therapy (CRRT) (Heintz, 2009; Trotman, 2005): Drug clearance is highly dependent on the method of renal replacement, filter type, and flow rate. Appropriate dosing requires close monitoring of pharmacologic response, signs of adverse reactions due to drug accumulation, as well as drug concentrations in relation to target trough (if appropriate). The following are general recommendations only (based on dialysate flow/ultrafiltration rates of 1-2 L/hour and minimal residual renal function) and should not supersede clinical judgment:

CVVH: Loading dose of 3.1g followed by 2 g every 6-8 hours

CVVHD: Loading dose of 3.1 g followed by 3.1 g every 6-8 hours

CVVHDF: Loading dose of 3.1 g followed by 3.1 g every 6 hours

Note: Do not administer in intervals exceeding every 8 hours. Clavulanate component is hepatically eliminated; extending the dosing interval beyond 8 hours may result in loss of beta-lactamase inhibition.

Hepatic Impairment With concomitant renal dysfunction (Cl_{cr} <10 mL/minute): 2 g of ticarcillin component every 24 hours.

Administration Infuse over 30 minutes.

Some penicillins (eg, carbenicillin, ticarcillin, and piperacillin) have been shown to inactivate aminoglycosides *in vitro*. This has been observed to a greater extent with tobramycin and gentamicin, while amikacin has shown greater stability against inactivation. Concurrent use of these agents may pose a risk of reduced antibacterial efficacy *in vivo*, particularly in the setting of profound renal impairment. However, definitive clinical evidence is lacking. If combination penicillin/aminoglycoside therapy is desired in a patient with renal dysfunction, separation of doses (if feasible), and routine monitoring of aminoglycoside levels, CBC, and clinical response should be considered.

Test Interactions Positive Coombs' test, false-positive urinary proteins

Some penicillin derivatives may accelerate the degradation of aminoglycosides *in vitro*, leading to a potential underestimation of aminoglycoside serum concentration.

Dosage Forms Excipient information presented when available (limited, particularly for generics); consult specific product labeling.

Infusion [premixed, frozen]: Ticarcillin 3 g and clavulanic acid 0.1 g (100 mL) [contains sodium 4.51 mEq and potassium 0.15 mEq per g]

Injection, powder for reconstitution: Ticarcillin 3 g and clavulanic acid 0.1 g (3.1 g, 31 g) [contains sodium 4.51 mEq and potassium 0.15 mEq per g]

- **Ticarcillin and Clavulanic Acid** *see* Ticarcillin and Clavulanate Potassium *on page 1363*
- **TICE® BCG** *see* BCG *on page 153*
- **Tigan®** *see* Trimethobenzamide *on page 1411*
- **Timentin®** *see* Ticarcillin and Clavulanate Potassium *on page 1363*
- **Tioguanine** *see* Thioguanine *on page 1354*
- **TMP-SMX** *see* Sulfamethoxazole and Trimethoprim *on page 1302*
- **TMP-SMZ** *see* Sulfamethoxazole and Trimethoprim *on page 1302*
- **TMZ** *see* Temozolomide *on page 1331*
- **TOBI®** *see* Tobramycin (Systemic, Oral Inhalation) *on page 1366*
- **TOBI® Podhaler® (Can)** *see* Tobramycin (Systemic, Oral Inhalation) *on page 1366*

Tobramycin (Systemic, Oral Inhalation) (toe bra MYE sin)

Brand Names: U.S. TOBI®

Brand Names: Canada TOBI®; TOBI® Podhaler®; Tobramycin Injection, USP

Index Terms Bethkis®; Tobramycin Sulfate

Generic Availability (U.S.) Yes: Excludes solution for nebulization

Pharmacologic Category Antibiotic, Aminoglycoside

Use Treatment of documented or suspected infections caused by susceptible gram-negative bacilli, including *Pseudomonas aeruginosa*. Tobramycin solution for inhalation and powder for inhalation (Canadian availability; not available in the U.S.) are indicated for the management of cystic fibrosis patients (>6 years of age) with *Pseudomonas aeruginosa*.

Labeled Contraindications Hypersensitivity to tobramycin, other aminoglycosides, or any component of the formulation; pregnancy

Pregnancy Risk Factor D

Lactation Enters breast milk/not recommended

Warnings/Precautions [U.S. Boxed Warning]: Aminoglycosides may cause neurotoxicity and/or nephrotoxicity; usual risk factors include pre-existing renal impairment, concomitant neuro-/nephrotoxic medications, advanced age, and dehydration. Ototoxicity may be directly proportional to the amount of drug given and the duration of treatment; tinnitus or vertigo are indications of vestibular injury and impending hearing loss; renal damage is usually reversible. May cause neuromuscular blockade and respiratory paralysis, especially when given soon after anesthesia or muscle relaxants.

Not intended for long-term therapy due to toxic hazards associated with extended administration; use caution in pre-existing renal insufficiency, vestibular or cochlear impairment, myasthenia gravis, hypocalcemia, and conditions which depress neuromuscular transmission. Dosage modification required in patients with impaired renal function. Prolonged use may result in fungal or bacterial superinfection, including *C. difficile*-associated diarrhea (CDAD) and pseudomembranous colitis; CDAD has been observed >2 months postantibiotic treatment. Solution may contain sodium metabisulfate; use caution in patients with sulfite allergy.

Storage/Stability

Injection: Stable at room temperature both as the clear, colorless solution and as the dry powder. Reconstituted solutions remain stable for 24 hours at room temperature and 96 hours when refrigerated.

Powder, for inhalation (TOBI® Podhaler®) [Canadian availability; not available in the U.S.]): Store in original package at 15°C to 30°C (59°F to 86°F). Protect from moisture.

Solution, for inhalation (TOBI®): Store under refrigeration at 2°C to 8°C (36°F to 46°F). May be stored in foil pouch at room temperature of 25°C (77°F) for up to 28 days. Avoid intense light. Solution may darken over time; however, do not use if cloudy or contains particles.

Reconstitution Dilute in 50-100 mL NS, D_5W for I.V. infusion.

Mechanism of Action Interferes with bacterial protein synthesis by binding to 30S and 50S ribosomal subunits, resulting in a defective bacterial cell membrane

Pharmacodynamics/Kinetics

Absorption:
- Oral: Poorly absorbed
- I.M.: Rapid and complete
- Inhalation: Peak serum concentrations:
  - Solution for inhalation: ~1 mcg/mL following a 300 mg dose
  - Powder for inhalation: ~1 mcg/mL (range: 0.49-1.55 mcg/mL) following a 112 mg dose

Distribution: V_d: 0.2-0.3 L/kg; Pediatrics: 0.2-0.7 L/kg; to extracellular fluid, including serum, abscesses, ascitic, pericardial, pleural, synovial, lymphatic, and peritoneal fluids; poor penetration into CSF, eye, bone, prostate
- Inhalation: Tobramycin remains concentrated primarily in the airways

Protein binding: <30%

Half-life elimination:
- Neonates: ≤1200 g: 11 hours; >1200 g: 2-9 hours
- Adults: 2-3 hours; directly dependent upon glomerular filtration rate
- Adults with impaired renal function: 5-70 hours

Time to peak, serum: I.M.: 30-60 minutes; I.V.: ~30 minutes

Excretion: Normal renal function: Urine (~90% to 95%) within 24 hours

Dosing

Adult Note: Individualization is **critical** because of the low therapeutic index.

Use of ideal body weight (IBW) for determining the mg/kg/dose appears to be more accurate than dosing on the basis of total body weight (TBW). In morbid obesity, dosage requirement may best be estimated using a dosing weight of IBW + 0.4 (TBW - IBW).

Initial and periodic plasma drug levels (eg, peak and trough with conventional dosing) should be determined, particularly in critically-ill patients with serious infections or in disease states known to significantly alter aminoglycoside pharmacokinetics (eg, cystic fibrosis, burns, or major surgery).

Severe life-threatening infections: I.M., I.V.:

Conventional: 1-2.5 mg/kg/dose every 8-12 hours; to ensure adequate peak concentrations early in therapy, higher initial dosage may be considered in selected patients when extracellular water is increased (edema, septic shock, postsurgical, and/or trauma)

Once-daily: 4-7 mg/kg/dose once daily; some clinicians recommend this approach for all patients with normal renal function; this dose is at least as efficacious with similar, if not less, toxicity than conventional dosing.

Brucellosis: I.M., I.V.: 240 mg (I.M.) daily or 5 mg/kg (I.V.) daily for 7 days; either regimen recommended in combination with doxycycline

Cholangitis: I.M., I.V.: 4-6 mg/kg once daily with ampicillin

CNS shunt infection: Intrathecal (unlabeled route): 5-20 mg/day (Tunkel, 2004)

Cystic fibrosis: Inhalation:

TOBI®: 300 mg every 12 hours (do not administer doses <6 hours apart); administer in repeated cycles of 28 days on drug followed by 28 days off drug.

TOBI® Podhaler® (Canadian availability; not available in the U.S.): 112 mg (4 x 28 mg capsules) every 12 hours (do not administer doses <6 hours apart); administer in repeated cycles of 28 days on drug followed by 28 days off drug.

Diverticulitis, complicated: I.M., I.V.: 1.5-2 mg/kg every 8 hours (with ampicillin and metronidazole)

Infective endocarditis or synergy (for gram-positive infections): I.M., I.V.: 1 mg/kg every 8 hours (with ampicillin)

Meningitis *(Enterococcus or Pseudomonas aeruginosa)*: I.V.: 5 mg/kg/day in divided doses every 8 hours (administered with another bacteriocidal drug)

Pelvic inflammatory disease: I.M., I.V.: Loading dose: 2 mg/kg, then 1.5 mg/kg every 8 hours **or** 4.5 mg/kg once daily

Plague *(Yersinia pestis)*: I.M., I.V.: Treatment: 5 mg/kg/day, followed by postexposure prophylaxis with doxycycline

Pneumonia, hospital- or ventilator-associated: I.M., I.V.: 7 mg/kg/day (with antipseudomonal beta-lactam or carbapenem)

Prophylaxis against endocarditis (dental, oral, upper respiratory procedures, GI/GU procedures): I.M., I.V.: 1.5 mg/kg with ampicillin (50 mg/kg) 30 minutes prior to procedure. **Note:** AHA guidelines now recommend prophylaxis only in patients undergoing invasive procedures and in whom underlying cardiac conditions may predispose to a higher risk of adverse outcomes should infection occur. As of April 2007, routine prophylaxis no longer recommended by the AHA.

Tularemia: I.M., I.V.: 5 mg/kg/day divided every 8 hours for 1-2 weeks
Urinary tract infection: I.M., I.V.: 1.5 mg/kg/dose every 8 hours

Geriatric Dosage should be based on an estimate of ideal body weight.
I.M., I.V.: 1.5-5 mg/kg/day in 1-2 divided doses
I.V.: Once daily or extended interval: 5-7 mg/kg/dose given every 24, 36, or 48 hours based on creatinine clearance

Pediatric Individualization is **critical** because of the low therapeutic index
Use of ideal body weight (IBW) for determining the mg/kg/dose appears to be more accurate than dosing on the basis of total body weight (TBW). In morbid obesity, dosage requirement may best be estimated using a dosing weight of IBW + 0.4 (TBW - IBW).

Usual dosage range: I.M., I.V.:
Infants and Children <5 years: 2.5 mg/kg/dose every 8 hours
Children >5 years: 2-2.5 mg/kg/dose every 8 hours
CNS shunt infection: Intrathecal (unlabeled route): Refer to adult dosing.
Cystic fibrosis:
I.M., I.V.: 2.5-3.3 mg/kg every 6-8 hours. **Note:** Some patients may require larger or more frequent doses if serum levels document the need (eg, cystic fibrosis or febrile granulocytopenic patients).
Inhalation: TOBI® or TOBI® Podhaler® (Canadian availability; not available in the U.S.): Children ≥6 years: Refer to adult dosing.

Renal Impairment I.M., I.V.:
Conventional dosing:
Cl_{cr} ≥60 mL/minute: Administer every 8 hours.
Cl_{cr} 40-60 mL/minute: Administer every 12 hours.
Cl_{cr} 20-40 mL/minute: Administer every 24 hours.
Cl_{cr} 10-20 mL/minute: Administer every 48 hours.
Cl_{cr} <10 mL/minute: Administer every 72 hours.
High-dose therapy: Interval may be extended (eg, every 48 hours) in patients with moderate renal impairment (Cl_{cr} 30-59 mL/minute) and/or adjusted based on serum level determinations.
Intermittent hemodialysis (IHD) (administer after hemodialysis on dialysis days) (Heintz, 2009): Dialyzable (25% to 70%; variable; dependent on filter, duration, and type of HD): I.V.:
Loading dose of 2-3 mg/kg, followed by:
Mild UTI or synergy: I.V.: 1 mg/kg every 48-72 hours; consider redosing for pre-HD or post-HD concentrations <1mg/L
Moderate-to-severe UTI: I.V.: 1-1.5 mg/kg every 48-72 hours; consider redosing for pre-HD concentrations <1.5-2 mg/L or post-HD concentrations <1 mg/l
Systemic gram-negative infection: I.V.: 1.5-2 mg/kg every 48-72 hours; consider redosing for pre-HD concentrations <3-5 mg/L or post-HD concentrations <2 mg/L
Note: Dosing dependent on the assumption of 3 times/week, complete IHD sessions.
Peritoneal dialysis (PD):
Administration via peritoneal dialysis (PD) fluid:
Gram-negative infection: 4-8 mg/L (4-8 mcg/mL) of PD fluid
Gram-positive infection (ie, synergy): 3-4 mg/L (3-4 mcg/mL) of PD fluid
Administration IVPB/I.M.: Dose as for Cl_{cr} <10 mL/minute and follow levels

Continuous renal replacement therapy (CRRT) (Heintz, 2009; Trotman, 2005): Drug clearance is highly dependent on the method of renal replacement, filter type, and flow rate. Appropriate dosing requires close monitoring of pharmacologic response, signs of adverse reactions due to drug accumulation, as well as drug concentrations in relation to target trough (if appropriate). The following are general recommendations only (based on dialysate flow/ultrafiltration rates of 1-2 L/hour and minimal residual renal function) and should not supersede clinical judgment:

CVVH/CVVHD/CVVHDF: I.V.: Loading dose of 2-3 mg/kg, followed by:

Mild UTI or synergy: I.V. 1 mg/kg every 24-36 hours (redose when concentration <1 mg/L)

Moderate-severe UTI: I.V.: 1-1.5 mg/kg every 24-36 hours (redose when concentration <1.5-2 mg/L)

Systemic gram-negative infection: I.V.: 1.5-2.5 mg/kg every 24-48 hours (redose when concentration <3-5 mg/L)

Hepatic Impairment No dosage adjustment necessary in hepatic impairment; monitor plasma concentrations as appropriate.

Administration

I.V.: Infuse over 30-60 minutes. Flush with saline before and after administration.

Inhalation:

TOBI®: To be inhaled over ~15 minutes using a handheld nebulizer (PARI-LC PLUS™). If multiple different nebulizer treatments are required, administer bronchodilator first, followed by chest physiotherapy, any other nebulized medications, and then TOBI® last. Do not mix with other nebulizer medications.

TOBI® Podhaler® (Canadian availability; not available in the U.S.): Capsules should be administered by oral inhalation via Podhaler® device following manufacturer recommendations for use and handling. Capsules should not be swallowed. Patients requiring bronchodilator therapy should administer the bronchodilator 15-90 minutes prior to TOBI® Podhaler®. The sequence of chest physiotherapy and additional inhaled therapies is at the discretion of the healthcare provider however TOBI® Podhaler® should always be administered last.

Some penicillins (eg, carbenicillin, ticarcillin, and piperacillin) have been shown to inactivate aminoglycosides *in vitro*. This has been observed to a greater extent with tobramycin and gentamicin, while amikacin has shown greater stability against inactivation. Concurrent use of these agents may pose a risk of reduced antibacterial efficacy *in vivo*, particularly in the setting of profound renal impairment. However, definitive clinical evidence is lacking. If combination penicillin/aminoglycoside therapy is desired in a patient with renal dysfunction, separation of doses (if feasible), and routine monitoring of aminoglycoside levels, CBC, and clinical response should be considered.

Test Interactions Some penicillin derivatives may accelerate the degradation of aminoglycosides *in vitro*, leading to a potential underestimation of aminoglycoside serum concentration.

Dosage Forms Excipient information presented when available (limited, particularly for generics); consult specific product labeling.

Infusion, premixed in NS: 80 mg (100 mL)

Injection, powder for reconstitution: 1.2 g

Injection, solution: 10 mg/mL (2 mL); 40 mg/mL (2 mL, 30 mL, 50 mL)

Solution, for nebulization [preservative free]:

TOBI®: 300 mg/5 mL (56s)

Dosage Forms: Canada Excipient information presented when available (limited, particularly for generics); consult specific product labeling.
Powder, for oral inhalation [capsule]:
TOBI® Podhaler®: 28 mg/capsule (224s)

- ◆ **Tobramycin Injection, USP (Can)** *see* Tobramycin (Systemic, Oral Inhalation) *on page* 1366
- ◆ **Tobramycin Sulfate** *see* Tobramycin (Systemic, Oral Inhalation) *on page* 1366
- ◆ **Tomudex® (Can)** *see* Raltitrexed *on page* 1226
- ◆ **Toposar®** *see* Etoposide *on page* 538

Topotecan (toe poe TEE kan)

Related Information

Chemotherapy and Obesity *on page* 1834
Management of Chemotherapy-Induced Nausea and Vomiting *on page* 1786
Management of Drug Extravasations *on page* 1800
Safe Handling of Hazardous Drugs *on page* 1904

Brand Names: U.S. Hycamtin®

Brand Names: Canada Hycamtin®; Topotecan For Injection; Topotecan Hydrochloride For Injection

Index Terms Hycamptamine; SKF 104864; SKF 104864-A; Topotecan Hydrochloride

Generic Availability (U.S.) Yes: Injection

Pharmacologic Category Antineoplastic Agent, Camptothecin; Antineoplastic Agent, Natural Source (Plant) Derivative; Antineoplastic Agent, Topoisomerase I Inhibitor

Use Treatment of metastatic ovarian cancer, relapsed or refractory small cell lung cancer, recurrent or resistant (stage IVB) cervical cancer (in combination with cisplatin)

Unlabeled Use Treatment of central nervous system lesions (metastatic from lung cancer), central nervous system lymphoma (primary), Ewing's sarcoma, merkel cell cancer, osteosarcoma, rhabdomyosarcoma (pediatrics), neuroblastoma (pediatrics)

Labeled Contraindications Hypersensitivity to topotecan or any component of the formulation; severe bone marrow depression

Canadian labeling: Additional contraindications (not in U.S. labeling): Severe renal impairment (Cl_{cr} <20 mL/minute); pregnancy, breast-feeding

Pregnancy Risk Factor D

Lactation Excretion in breast milk unknown/not recommended

Warnings/Precautions Hazardous agent - use appropriate precautions for handling and disposal. **[U.S. Boxed Warning]: May cause neutropenia, which may be severe or lead to infection or fatalities. Monitor blood counts frequently. Do NOT administer to patients with baseline neutrophils <1500/mm^3 and platelets <100,000/mm^3.** The dose-limiting toxicity is bone marrow suppression (primarily neutropenia); may also cause thrombocytopenia and anemia. Neutropenia is not cumulative overtime. In a clinical study comparing I.V. to oral topotecan, G-CSF support was administered in a higher percentage of patients receiving oral topotecan (Eckerd, 2007). Topotecan-induced neutropenia may lead to neutropenic colitis (including fatalities); should be considered in patients presenting with neutropenia, fever and abdominal pain.

Diarrhea has been reported with oral topotecan; may be severe (requiring hospitalization); incidence may be higher in the elderly; educate patients on early recognition and proper management, including diet changes, increase in fluid intake, antidiarrheals, and antibiotics. Interstitial lung disease (ILD) (with fatalities) has been reported; discontinue use in patients with confirmed ILD; risk factors for ILD include a history of ILD, pulmonary fibrosis, lung cancer, thoracic radiation, and the use of colony-stimulating factors or medication with pulmonary toxicity; monitor pulmonary symptoms (cough, fever, dyspnea, and/or hypoxia) and discontinue if ILD is diagnosed. Use caution in renal impairment; may require dose adjustment (use in severe renal impairment is contraindicated in the Canadian labeling). Topotecan exposure is increased when oral topotecan is used concurrently with P-glycoprotein inhibitors; avoid concurrent use.

Adverse Reactions

>10%:

Central nervous system: Fatigue (6% to 29%), fever (5% to 28%), pain (5% to 23%), headache (18%)

Dermatologic: Alopecia (10% to 49%), rash (16%)

Gastrointestinal: Nausea (8% to 64%), vomiting (10% to 45%), diarrhea (6% to 32%; Oral: grade 3: 4%; grade 4: ≤1%; onset: 9 days), constipation (5% to 29%), abdominal pain (5% to 22%), anorexia (7% to 19%), stomatitis (18%)

Hematologic: Anemia (89% to 98%; grade 4: 7% to 37%; nadir: 15 days), neutropenia (83% to 97%; grade 4: 32% to 80%; nadir 12-15 days; duration: 7 days), leukopenia (86% to 97%; grade 4: 15% to 32%), thrombocytopenia (69% to 81%; grade 4: 6% to 27%; nadir: 15 days; duration: 3-5 days), neutropenic fever/sepsis (2% to 43%)

Neuromuscular & skeletal: Weakness (3% to 25%)

Respiratory: Dyspnea (6% to 22%), cough (15%)

Miscellaneous: Infection (≤17%)

1% to 10%:

Gastrointestinal: Obstruction (5%)

Hepatic: Liver enzymes increased (transient; 8%; grades 3/4: 4%), bilirubin increased (grades 3/4: <2%)

Neuromuscular & skeletal: Paresthesia (7%)

Respiratory: Pneumonia (8%)

Miscellaneous: Sepsis (grades 3/4: 5%)

<1%, postmarketing, and/or case reports: Allergic reactions, anaphylactoid reactions, angioedema, bleeding (severe, associated with thrombocytopenia), dermatitis (severe), extravasation (inadvertent), interstitial lung disease (ILD), neutropenic colitis, pancytopenia, pruritus (severe)

Drug Interactions

Metabolism/Transport Effects None known.

Avoid Concomitant Use

Avoid concomitant use of Topotecan with any of the following: BCG; CloZAPine; Natalizumab; P-glycoprotein/ABCB1 Inhibitors; Pimecrolimus; Tacrolimus (Topical); Vaccines (Live)

Increased Effect/Toxicity

Topotecan may increase the levels/effects of: CloZAPine; Leflunomide; Natalizumab; Vaccines (Live)

The levels/effects of Topotecan may be increased by: BCRP/ABCG2 Inhibitors; Denosumab; Filgrastim; P-glycoprotein/ABCB1 Inhibitors; Pimecrolimus; Platinum Derivatives; Roflumilast; Tacrolimus (Topical); Trastuzumab

Decreased Effect

Topotecan may decrease the levels/effects of: BCG; Coccidioidin Skin Test; Sipuleucel-T; Vaccines (Inactivated); Vaccines (Live)

The levels/effects of Topotecan may be decreased by: Echinacea

Ethanol/Nutrition/Herb Interactions Ethanol: Avoid ethanol (due to GI irritation).

Storage/Stability

I.V.:

Solution for injection: Store intact vials at 2°C to 8°C (36°F to 45°F). Protect from light. Single-use vials should be discarded after initial vial entry; solutions for infusion are stable for 24 hours at room temperature after diluted.

Lyophilized powder: Store intact vials at room temperature of 20°C to 25°C (68°F to 77°F). Protect from light. Reconstituted solution is stable for up to 28 days at room temperature of 20°C to 25°C (68°F to 77°F), although the manufacturer recommends use immediately after reconstitution. Further dilute in 50-100 mL D_5W or NS. This solution is stable for 24 hours at room temperature (manufacturer recommendation) or up to 7 days under refrigeration (Craig, 1997).

Oral: Store at 2°C to 8°C (36°F to 46°F). Protect from light.

Reconstitution Reconstitute lyophilized powder with 4 mL SWFI. Further dilute in 50-100 mL D_5W or NS for infusion.

Mechanism of Action Binds to topoisomerase I and stabilizes the cleavable complex so that religation of the cleaved DNA strand cannot occur. This results in the accumulation of cleavable complexes and single-strand DNA breaks. Topotecan acts in S phase of the cell cycle.

Pharmacodynamics/Kinetics

Absorption: Oral: Rapid

Distribution: V_{dss} of the lactone is high (mean: 87.3 L/mm^2; range: 25.6-186 L/mm^2), suggesting wide distribution and/or tissue sequestering

Protein binding: ~35%

Metabolism: Undergoes a rapid, pH-dependent hydrolysis of the lactone ring to yield a relatively inactive hydroxy acid in plasma; metabolized in the liver to N-demethylated metabolite

Bioavailability: Oral: ~40%

Half-life elimination: I.V.: 2-3 hours; renal impairment: 5 hours; Oral: 3-6 hours

Time to peak, plasma: Oral: 1-2 hours; delayed with high-fat meal (3-4 hours)

Excretion:

I.V.: Urine (51%; 3% as N-desmethyl topotecan); feces (18%; 2% as N-desmethyl topotecan)

Oral: Urine (20%; 2% as N-desmethyl topotecan); feces (33%; <2% as N-desmethyl topotecan)

Dosing

Adult & Geriatric Details concerning dosing in combination regimens should also be consulted: **Note:** Baseline neutrophil count should be ≥1500/mm^3 and platelets should be ≥100,000/mm^3 prior to treatment; for retreatment, neutrophil count should be >1000/mm^3; platelets >100,000/mm^3 and hemoglobin ≥9 g/dL:

Small cell lung cancer:

IVPB: 1.5 mg/m^2/day for 5 days; repeated every 21 days, minimum of 4 cycles recommended in the absence of tumor progression

Oral: 2.3 mg/m^2/day for 5 days; repeated every 21 days (round dose to the nearest 0.25 mg); if patient vomits after dose is administered, do not give a replacement dose.

Metastatic ovarian cancer: IVPB: 1.5 mg/m^2/day for 5 days; repeated every 21 days, minimum of 4 cycles recommended in the absence of tumor progression

Cervical cancer: IVPB: 0.75 mg/m^2/day for 3 days (followed by cisplatin 50 mg/m^2 on day 1 only, [with hydration]); repeated every 21 days

Renal Impairment

Manufacturer's labeling recommends the following dosage adjustment:

I.V.:

Cl_{cr} ≥40 mL/minute: No dosage adjustment required

Cl_{cr} 20-39 mL/minute: Reduce to 0.75 mg/m^2/dose

Cl_{cr} <20 mL/minute: Insufficient data available for dosing recommendation (contraindicated in the Canadian labeling)

Note: For topotecan in combination with cisplatin for cervical cancer, do not initiate treatment in patients with serum creatinine >1.5 mg/dL; consider discontinuing treatment in patients with serum creatinine >1.5 mg/dL in subsequent cycles.

Oral:

Cl_{cr} ≥50 mL/minute: No dosage adjustment required

Cl_{cr} 30-49 mL/minute: Reduce dose to 1.8 mg/m^2/day

Cl_{cr} <30 mL/minute: Insufficient data available for dosing recommendation

The following guidelines have been used by some clinicians:

Aronoff, 2007: *I.V.:*

Children:

Cl_{cr} 30-50 mL/minute: Administer 75% of dose

Cl_{cr} 10-29 mL/minute: Administer 50% of dose or reduce by 0.75 mg/m^2/dose

Cl_{cr} <10 mL/minute: Administer 25% of dose

Hemodialysis: 0.75 mg/m^2

Continuous renal replacement therapy (CRRT): Administer 50% of dose or reduce by 0.75 mg/m^2/dose

Adults:

Cl_{cr} >50 mL/minute: Administer 75% of dose

Cl_{cr} 10-50 mL/minute: Administer 50% of dose

Cl_{cr} <10 mL/minute: Administer 25% of dose

Hemodialysis: Avoid use

Continuous ambulatory peritoneal dialysis (CAPD): Avoid use

Continuous renal replacement therapy (CRRT): 0.75 mg/m^2

Kintzel, 1995: *I.V.:*

Cl_{cr} 46-60 mL/minute: Administer 80% of dose

Cl_{cr} 31-45 mL/minute: Administer 75% of dose

Cl_{cr} <30 mL/minute: Administer 70% of dose

Hepatic Impairment Manufacturer's labeling recommends the following:

I.V.: Bilirubin 1.7-15 mg/dL (U.S. labeling) or >1.5-<10 mg/dL (Canadian labeling): No adjustment necessary (the half-life is increased slightly; usual doses are generally tolerated).

Oral: Bilirubin >1.5 mg/dL: No adjustment necessary.

Adjustment for Toxicity

I.V.:

Ovarian and small cell lung cancer: Dosage adjustment for hematological effects: Severe neutropenia (<500/mm^3) or platelet count <25,000/mm^3: Reduce dose to 1.25 mg/m^2/day for subsequent cycles (may consider G-CSF support [beginning on day 6] prior to instituting dose reduction for severe neutropenia). **Note:** The Canadian labeling states that the dose may be further reduced to 1 mg/m^2/day if necessary.

Cervical cancer (cisplatin may also require dosage adjustment): Severe febrile neutropenia (<500/mm^3 with temperature of 38°C) or platelet count <25,000/mm^3: Reduce topotecan to 0.6 mg/m^2/day for subsequent cycles (may consider G-CSF support [beginning on day 4] prior to instituting dose reduction for neutropenic fever.

For neutropenic fever despite G-CSF use, reduce dose to 0.45 mg/m^2/day for subsequent cycles.

Oral:

Small cell lung cancer: Severe neutropenia (neutrophils <500/mm^3 associated with fever or infection or lasting >7 days) or prolonged neutropenia (neutrophils ≥500/mm^3 to ≤1000/mm^3 lasting beyond day 21) or platelets <25,000/mm^3 or grades 3/4 diarrhea: Reduce dose by 0.4 mg/m^2/day for subsequent cycles (may consider same dosage reduction for grade 2 diarrhea if clinically indicated).

Combination Regimens

Cervical cancer: Cisplatin-Topotecan (Cervical Cancer) on page 1583

Lung cancer, small cell:

Topotecan Intravenous (Small Cell Lung Cancer Regimen) on page 1756

Topotecan Oral (Small Cell Lung Cancer Regimen) on page 1757

Ovarian cancer: Topotecan Oral Regimen (Ovarian Cancer) on page 1757

Sarcoma: Topotecan-Cyclophosphamide (Ewing's Sarcoma) on page 1756

Administration

I.V.: Administer IVPB over 30 minutes. For combination chemotherapy with cisplatin, administer pretreatment hydration.

Oral: Administer without regard to meals. Swallow whole; do not crush, chew, or divide capsule. If vomiting occurs after dose, do not take replacement dose.

Emetic Potential Moderate (30% to 90%)

Vesicant/Extravasation Risk Inadvertent extravasation, generally mild (although severe cases have been reported).

Monitoring Parameters CBC with differential and platelet count, renal function tests, bilirubin; monitor for symptoms of interstitial lung disease

Test Interactions None known

Dietary Considerations May be taken without regard to meals.

Dosage Forms Excipient information presented when available (limited, particularly for generics); consult specific product labeling.

Capsule, oral:

Hycamtin®: 0.25 mg, 1 mg

Injection, powder for reconstitution: 4 mg
Hycamtin®: 4 mg
Injection, solution [concentrate]: 1 mg/mL (4 mL)

References

Aronoff GR, Bennett WM, Berns JS, et al, *Drug Prescribing in Renal Failure: Dosing Guidelines for Adults and Children*, 5th ed. Philadelphia, PA: American College of Physicians; 2007, p 102, 174.

Eckardt JR, von Pawel J, Pujol JL, et al, "Phase III Study of Oral Compared With Intravenous Topotecan as Second-Line Therapy in Small-Cell Lung Cancer," *J Clin Oncol*, 2007, 25 (15):2086-92.

Gronlund B, Hansen HH, Hogdall C, et al, "Efficacy of Low-Dose Topotecan in Second-Line Treatment for Patients With Epithelial Ovarian Carcinoma," *Cancer*, 2002, 95(8):1656-62.

Hoskins P, Vergote I, Cervantes A, et al, "Advanced Ovarian Cancer: Phase III Randomized Study of Sequential Cisplatin-Topotecan and Carboplatin-Paclitaxel vs Carboplatin-Paclitaxel," *J Natl Cancer Inst*, 2010, 102(20):1547-56.

Hunold A, Weddeling N, Paulussen M, et al, "Topotecan and Cyclophosphamide in Patients With Refractory or Relapsed Ewing Tumors," *Pediatr Blood Cancer*, 2006, 47(6):795-800.

Kintzel PE and Dorr RT, "Anticancer Drug Renal Toxicity and Elimination: Dosing Guidelines for Altered Renal Function," *Cancer Treat Rev*, 1995, 21(1):33-64.

Korfel A, Oehm C, von Pawel J, et al, "Response to Topotecan of Symptomatic Brain Metastases of Small-Cell Lung Cancer Also After Whole-Brain Irradiation. a Multicentre Phase II Study," *Eur J Cancer*, 2002, 38(13):1724-9.

Kruijtzer CMF, Beijnen JH, Rosing H, et al, "Increased Oral Bioavailability of Topotecan in Combination With the Breast Cancer Resistance Protein and P-Glycoprotein Inhibitor GF120918," *J Clin Oncol*, 2002, 20(13):2943-50.

Levy T, Inbar M, Menczer J, et al, "Phase II Study of Weekly Topotecan in Patients With Recurrent or Persistent Epithelial Ovarian Cancer," *Gynecol Oncol*, 2004, 95(3):686-90.

London WB, Frantz CN, Campbell LA, et al, "Phase II Randomized Comparison of Topotecan Plus Cyclophosphamide Versus Topotecan Alone in Children With Recurrent or Refractory Neuroblastoma: A Children's Oncology Group Study," *J Clin Oncol*, 2010, 28(24):3808-15.

Long HJ 3rd, Bundy BN, Grendys EC Jr, et al, "Randomized Phase III Trial of Cisplatin With or Without Topotecan in Carcinoma of the Uterine Cervix: A Gynecologic Oncology Group Study," *J Clin Oncol*, 2005, 23(21):4626-33.

Monk BJ, Sill MW, McMeekin DS, et al, "Phase III Trial of Four Cisplatin-Containing Doublet Combinations in Stage IVB, Recurrent, or Persistent Cervical Carcinoma: A Gynecologic Oncology Group Study," *J Clin Oncol*, 2009, 27(28):4649-55.

Muderspach LI, Blessing JA, Levenback C, et al, "A Phase II Study of Topotecan in Patients with Squamous Cell Carcinoma of the Cervix: A Gynecologic Oncology Group Study," *Gyn Oncol*, 2001, 81(2):213-5.

O'Brien ME, Ciuleanu TE, Tsekov H, et al, "Phase III Trial Comparing Supportive Care Alone With Supportive Care With Oral Topotecan in Patients With Relapsed Small-Cell Lung Cancer," *J Clin Oncol*, 2006, 24(34):5441-7.

Saylors RL 3rd, Stine KC, Sullivan J, et al, "Cyclophosphamide Plus Topotecan in Children With Recurrent or Refractory Solid Tumors: A Pediatric Oncology Group Phase II Study," *J Clin Oncol*, 2001, 19(15):3463-9.

Voloschin AD, Betensky R, Wen PY, et al, "Topotecan as Salvage Therapy for Relapsed or Refractory Primary Central Nervous System Lymphoma," *J Neurooncol*, 2008, 86(2):211-5.

◆ **Topotecan For Injection (Can)** *see* Topotecan *on page* *1371*

◆ **Topotecan Hydrochloride** *see* Topotecan *on page* *1371*

◆ **Topotecan Hydrochloride For Injection (Can)** *see* Topotecan *on page* *1371*

Toremifene (tore EM i feen)

Related Information

Safe Handling of Hazardous Drugs *on page* *1904*

Brand Names: U.S. Fareston®

Brand Names: Canada Fareston®

Index Terms FC1157a; Toremifene Citrate

Generic Availability (U.S.) No

Pharmacologic Category Antineoplastic Agent, Estrogen Receptor Antagonist; Selective Estrogen Receptor Modulator (SERM)

Use Treatment of metastatic breast cancer in postmenopausal women with estrogen receptor positive or estrogen receptor status unknown

Unlabeled Use Treatment of soft tissue sarcoma (desmoid tumors)

Labeled Contraindications Hypersensitivity to toremifene or any component of the formulation; long QT syndrome (congenital or acquired QT prolongation), uncorrected hypokalemia, uncorrected hypomagnesemia

Pregnancy Risk Factor D

Lactation Excretion in breast milk unknown/not recommended

Warnings/Precautions Hazardous agent - use appropriate precautions for handling and disposal.

[U.S. Boxed Warning]: May prolong the QT interval; QT_c prolongation is dose-dependent and concentration dependent. Torsade de pointes, syncope, seizure and/or sudden death may occur. Use is contraindicated in patients with congenital or acquired long QT syndrome, uncorrected hypokalemia, or uncorrected hypomagnesemia. Avoid use with other medications known to prolong the QT interval and with strong CYP3A4 inhibitors. Use with caution in patients with heart failure, hepatic impairment, or electrolyte abnormalities. Monitor electrolytes; correct hypokalemia and hypomagnesemia prior to treatment. Obtain ECG at baseline and as clinically indicated in patients at risk for QT prolongation

Hypercalcemia and tumor flare have been reported during the first weeks of treatment in some breast cancer patients with bone metastases; monitor closely for hypocalcemia. Institute appropriate measures if hypercalcemia occurs, and if severe, discontinue treatment. Tumor flare consists of diffuse musculoskeletal pain and erythema with initial increased size of tumor lesions that later regress; is often accompanied by hypercalcemia. Tumor flare does not imply treatment failure or represent tumor progression. Drugs that decrease renal calcium excretion (eg, thiazide diuretics) may increase the risk of hypercalcemia in patients receiving toremifene. Leukopenia and thrombocytopenia have been reported rarely; monitor leukocyte and platelet counts. Endometrial hyperplasia has been reported; some patients have developed endometrial cancer, although a role of toremifene in endometrial cancer development has not been established. Avoid long-term use in patients with pre-existing endometrial hyperplasia. Use with caution in patients with hepatic failure. Avoid use in patients with a history of thromboembolic disease.

Adverse Reactions

>10%:

- Endocrine & metabolic: Hot flashes (35%)
- Gastrointestinal: Nausea (14%)
- Genitourinary: Vaginal discharge (13%)
- Hepatic: Alkaline phosphatase increased (8% to 19%), AST increased (5% to 19%)
- Miscellaneous: Diaphoresis (20%)

1% to 10%:

- Cardiovascular: Edema (5%), arrhythmia (≤2%), CVA/TIA (≤2%), thrombosis (≤2%), cardiac failure (≤1%), MI (≤1%)
- Central nervous system: Dizziness (9%)
- Endocrine & metabolic: Hypercalcemia (≤3%)
- Gastrointestinal: Vomiting (4%)
- Genitourinary: Vaginal bleeding (2%)
- Hepatic: Bilirubin increased (1% to 2%)
- Local: Thrombophlebitis (≤2%)

Ocular: Cataracts (≤10%), xerophthalmia (≤9%), visual field abnormal (≤4%), corneal keratopathy (≤2%), glaucoma (≤2%), vision abnormal/diplopia (≤2%)

Respiratory: Pulmonary embolism (≤2%)

<1%, postmarketing, and/or case reports: Alopecia, angina, anorexia, arthritis, ataxia, blurred vision, constipation, corneal opacity (reversible), corneal verticulata, depression, dermatitis, dyspnea, endometrial cancer, endometrial hyperplasia, fatigue, hepatitis (toxic), incoordination, ischemic attack, jaundice, lethargy, leukopenia, paresis, pruritus, QT prolongation, rigors, skin discoloration, thrombocytopenia, tremor, tumor flare, vertigo, weakness

Drug Interactions

Metabolism/Transport Effects Substrate of CYP1A2 (minor), CYP3A4 (major); **Note:** Assignment of Major/Minor substrate status based on clinically relevant drug interaction potential

Avoid Concomitant Use

Avoid concomitant use of Toremifene with any of the following: CYP3A4 Inducers (Strong); CYP3A4 Inhibitors (Strong); Highest Risk QTc-Prolonging Agents; Mifepristone; Moderate Risk QTc-Prolonging Agents

Increased Effect/Toxicity

Toremifene may increase the levels/effects of: Highest Risk QTc-Prolonging Agents; Vitamin K Antagonists

The levels/effects of Toremifene may be increased by: CYP3A4 Inhibitors (Strong); Mifepristone; Moderate Risk QTc-Prolonging Agents; QTc-Prolonging Agents (Indeterminate Risk and Risk Modifying); Thiazide Diuretics

Decreased Effect

The levels/effects of Toremifene may be decreased by: CYP3A4 Inducers (Strong); Deferasirox; Herbs (CYP3A4 Inducers); Tocilizumab

Ethanol/Nutrition/Herb Interactions

Food: Grapefruit juice may increase toremifene levels. Management: Avoid grapefruit juice.

Herb/Nutraceutical: St John's wort may decrease toremifene levels. Management: Avoid St John's wort.

Storage/Stability Store at 25°C (77°F); excursions permitted to 15°C to 30°C (59°F to 86°F); protect from heat. Protect from light.

Mechanism of Action Nonsteroidal, triphenylethylene derivative with potent antiestrogenic properties (also has estrogenic effects). Competitively binds to estrogen receptors on tumors and other tissue targets, producing a nuclear complex that decreases DNA synthesis and inhibits estrogen effects. Competes with estrogen for binding sites in breast and other tissues; cells accumulate in the G_0 and G_1 phases; therefore, toremifene is cytostatic rather than cytocidal.

Pharmacodynamics/Kinetics

Absorption: Well absorbed

Distribution: V_d: 580 L (range: 457-958 L)

Protein binding, plasma: >99.5%, primarily to albumin

Metabolism: Extensively hepatic, principally by CYP3A4 to N-demethyltoremifene (a weak antiestrogen)

Bioavailability: Not affected by food

Half-life elimination: Toremifene: ~5 days; N-demethyltoremifene: 6 days

Time to peak, serum: ≤3 hours

Excretion: Primarily feces; urine (10%) during a 1-week period

Dosing

Adult & Geriatric Metastatic breast cancer (postmenopausal): Oral: 60 mg once daily, continue until disease progression

Administration Administer orally, as a single daily dose, with or without food.

Monitoring Parameters CBC with differential, electrolytes (calcium, magnesium, and potassium), hepatic function. Obtain ECG in patients at risk for QT prolongation. In patients with bone metastases, monitor closely for hypercalcemia during the first few weeks of treatment.

Dietary Considerations May be taken with or without food. Avoid grapefruit juice.

Dosage Forms Excipient information presented when available (limited, particularly for generics); consult specific product labeling.

Tablet, oral:

Fareston®: 60 mg

References

Gianni L, Panzini I, Li, S, et al, "Ocular Toxicity During Adjuvant Chemoendocrine Therapy for Early Breast Cancer," *Cancer*, 2006, 106(3):505-13.

National Comprehensive Cancer Network® (NCCN), "Clinical Practice Guidelines in Oncology™: Breast Cancer, Version 2.2011," Available at http://www.nccn.org/professionals/physician_gls/PDF/breast.pdf

National Comprehensive Cancer Network® (NCCN), "Clinical Practice Guidelines in Oncology™: Soft Tissue Sarcoma," Version 1.2011. Available at http://www.nccn.org/professionals/physician_gls/PDF/sarcoma.pdf

Pagani O, Gelber S, Price K, et al, "Toremifene and Tamoxifen are Equally Effective for Early-Stage Breast Cancer: First Results of International Breast Cancer Study Group Trials 12-93 and 14-93," *Ann Oncol*, 2004, 15(12):1749-59.

◆ **Toremifene Citrate** *see* Toremifene *on page 1376*

◆ **Torisel®** *see* Temsirolimus *on page 1337*

◆ **Tositumomab I-131** *see* Tositumomab and Iodine I 131 Tositumomab *on page 1379*

Tositumomab and Iodine I 131 Tositumomab

(toe si TYOO mo mab & EYE oh dyne eye one THUR tee one toe si TYOO mo mab)

Related Information

Safe Handling of Hazardous Drugs *on page 1904*

Brand Names: U.S. Bexxar®

Index Terms 131 I Anti-B1 Antibody; 131 I-Anti-B1 Monoclonal Antibody; Anti-CD20-Murine Monoclonal Antibody I 131; Iodine I 131 Tositumomab and Tositumomab; Tositumomab I-131

Generic Availability (U.S.) No

Pharmacologic Category Antineoplastic Agent, Monoclonal Antibody; Radiopharmaceutical

Use Treatment of relapsed or refractory CD20 positive, low-grade, follicular, or transformed non-Hodgkin's lymphoma (NHL), with progression during or after rituximab treatment

Labeled Contraindications There are no contraindications listed in the manufacturer's labeling.

Pregnancy Risk Factor D

Lactation Enters breast milk/not recommended

Warnings/Precautions Radiopharmaceutical - use appropriate precautions for handling and disposal. **[U.S. Boxed Warning]: Serious hypersensitivity reactions (including anaphylaxis) have been reported; permanently discontinue for severe reaction; medications for the treatment of reactions**

should be readily available in the event of severe reactions. Signs and symptoms of severe allergic reactions include fever, rigors/chills, sweating, hypotension, dyspnea, bronchospasm, or nausea; may occur during or within 48 hours of infusion. Patients should be premedicated to prevent infusion-related reactions. Premedicate with acetaminophen and diphenhydramine prior to both the dosimetric and therapeutic doses. **[U.S. Boxed Warning]: Severe and prolonged cytopenias, including neutropenia and thrombocytopenia are common; do not administer in patients with >25% lymphoma marrow involvement, platelet count <100,000/mm^3 or neutrophil count <1500/mm^3.** Hematologic toxicity is reported to be the most common adverse effect with 27% patients requiring supportive care; cytopenias may be prolonged and severe. The duration of severe hematologic toxicity may be prolonged in the elderly.

[U.S. Boxed Warning]: Treatment involves radioactive isotopes and should only be administered by or under supervision of physicians enrolled in the Bexxar® therapeutic regimen certification program; appropriate precautions for handling and administration must be followed. Patients must be instructed in measures to minimize exposure of others. Women of childbearing potential should be advised of potential fetal risk; effective contraceptive measures should be used during and for 12 months following treatment (males and females). Treatment may lead to hypothyroidism; patients should receive thyroid-blocking medications beginning at least 24 hours prior to the dosimetric dose and continued for 2 weeks after the therapeutic dose; evaluate TSH and for signs and symptoms of hypothyroidism at baseline and annually thereafter. Secondary malignancies (eg, myelodysplastic syndrome, acute leukemia, skin cancer and solid tumors) have been reported.

Safety has not been established in patients with renal impairment; excretion is primarily renal; impaired renal function may increase exposure. The safety and efficacy of live vaccines in patients who have received therapy with tositumomab have not been established; avoid live vaccine administration in patients recently treated with tositumomab.

Adverse Reactions

>10%:

Central nervous system: Fever (37%), pain (19%), chills (18%), headache (16%)

Dermatologic: Rash (17%; grades 3/4: <1%)

Endocrine & metabolic: Hypothyroidism (7% to 19%)

Gastrointestinal: Nausea (36%), abdominal pain (15%), vomiting (15%), anorexia (14%), diarrhea (12%)

Hematologic: Myelosuppression (grades 3/4: 71%; nadir: 4-7 weeks; duration: ~30 days), neutropenia (grades 3/4: 63%; median duration: 31 days; grade 4: 25%), thrombocytopenia (grades 3/4: 53%; median duration: 32 days; grade 4: 21%), lymphocytopenia (recovery: ~12 weeks after treatment), anemia (grades 3/4: 29%; median duration: 23 days; grade 4: 5%), secondary leukemia/myelodysplastic syndrome (overall: 3% to 10%; 2-year follow-up: 2% to 5%; 5-year follow-up: 6% to 15%), hemorrhage (12%)

Neuromuscular & skeletal: Weakness (46%), myalgia (13%)

Respiratory: Cough (21%), pharyngitis (12%), dyspnea (11%)

Miscellaneous: Infusion-related reactions (29%, occurred within 14 days of infusion, included bronchospasm, chills, dyspnea, fever, hypotension, nausea, rigors, diaphoresis); infection (21% to 45%, serious: 9%); HAMA-positive seroconversion (10% to 11%)

1% to 10%:

Cardiovascular: Hypotension (7%), peripheral edema (9%), chest pain (7%), vasodilation (5%)

Central nervous system: Dizziness (5%), somnolence (5%)

Dermatologic: Pruritus (10%)

Gastrointestinal: Constipation (6%), dyspepsia (6%), weight loss (6%)

Local: Injection site hypersensitivity

Neuromuscular & skeletal: Arthralgia (10%), back pain (8%), neck pain (6%)

Respiratory: Rhinitis (10%), pneumonia (6%)

Miscellaneous: Diaphoresis (8%), hypersensitivity/allergic reaction (6%), secondary malignancies (nonhematologic: 5%)

<1%, postmarketing, and/or case reports: Anaphylactic reaction, angioedema, bacteremia, bronchitis, dehydration, flu-like syndrome, herpes virus infection, laryngismus, neuropathy (axonal), pleural effusion, septicemia, serum sickness, skin infections

Drug Interactions

Metabolism/Transport Effects None known.

Avoid Concomitant Use

Avoid concomitant use of Tositumomab and Iodine I 131 Tositumomab with any of the following: BCG; CloZAPine; Natalizumab; Pimecrolimus; Tacrolimus (Topical); Vaccines (Live)

Increased Effect/Toxicity

Tositumomab and Iodine I 131 Tositumomab may increase the levels/effects of: CloZAPine; Leflunomide; Natalizumab; Vaccines (Live); Vitamin K Antagonists

The levels/effects of Tositumomab and Iodine I 131 Tositumomab may be increased by: Anticoagulants; Antiplatelet Agents; Denosumab; Pimecrolimus; Roflumilast; Tacrolimus (Topical); Trastuzumab

Decreased Effect

Tositumomab and Iodine I 131 Tositumomab may decrease the levels/effects of: BCG; Cardiac Glycosides; Coccidioidin Skin Test; Sipuleucel-T; Vaccines (Inactivated); Vaccines (Live); Vitamin K Antagonists

The levels/effects of Tositumomab and Iodine I 131 Tositumomab may be decreased by: Echinacea

Storage/Stability

Tositumomab: Store under refrigeration at 2°C to 8°C (36°F to 46°F); do not freeze. Protect from strong light. Following dilution, tositumomab is stable for 24 hour when refrigerated or 8 hours at room temperature.

Iodine I 131 tositumomab: Store frozen at less than or equal to -20°C in the original lead pots. Allow ~60 minutes for thawing at ambient temperature. Thawed doses are stable for up to 8 hours at 2°C to 8°C (36°F to 46°F) or room temperature. Solutions diluted for infusion should be refrigerated prior to administration; do not freeze.

Reconstitution

Tositumomab: Withdraw and discard 32 mL of saline from a 50 mL bag of NS. Add contents of both 225 mg vials of tositumomab (total 32 mL) to remaining NS to make a final volume of 50 mL. Gently mix by inverting bag; do not shake.

Iodine I 131 tositumomab: Calculate volume required for an iodine I 131 tositumomab activity of 5 mCi (specification sheet provided with product). If the amount of tositumomab contained in the iodine I 131 tositumomab solution contains <35 mg of tositumomab, use the 35 mg vial of tositumomab to prepare a final concentration of tositumomab 35 mg. Using NS, the final volume should equal 30 mL. Gently mix by inverting or rotating; do not shake.

Mechanism of Action Tositumomab is a murine IgG_{2a} lambda monoclonal antibody which binds to the CD20 antigen, expressed on B-lymphocytes and on >90% of B-cell non-Hodgkin's lymphomas. Iodine I 131 tositumomab is a radio-iodinated derivative of tositumomab covalently linked to iodine 131. The possible actions of the regimen include apoptosis, complement-dependent cytotoxicity, antibody-dependent cellular cytotoxicity, and radiation-induced cell death. Administration results in depletion of CD20 positive cells.

Pharmacodynamics/Kinetics

Onset: CD20-positive cell depletion: ≤7 weeks

Duration: CD20-positive cell recovery begins at ~12 weeks

Distribution: Tositumomab: V_d increased with high tumor burden, splenomegaly, or bone marrow involvement

Half-life elimination: Tositumomab: 67 hours (range: 28-115 hours); decreased with high tumor burden, splenomegaly, or bone marrow involvement

Excretion: Iodine-131 elimination occurs by decay and urinary excretion; after 5 days total body clearance is 67% of a dose (98% in urine)

Dosing

Adult & Geriatric Non-Hodgkin's lymphoma (NHL), relapsed or refractory: I.V.: Dosing consists of four components administered in 2 steps. Refer to manufacturer's labeling for additional details. Indicated for a single treatment course. Thyroid protective agents (SSKI, Lugol's solution or potassium iodide) should be administered beginning at least 24 hours prior to step 1 (Refer to Additional Information). Premedicate with acetaminophen 650 mg and diphenhydramine 50 mg orally 30 minutes prior to step 1 and step 2.

Step 1: Dosimetric step (Day 0):

Tositumomab 450 mg administered over 60 minutes

Iodine I 131 tositumomab (containing I-131 5 mCi and tositumomab 35 mg) administered over 20 minutes

Note: Whole body dosimetry and biodistribution should be determined on Day 0; days 2, 3, or 4; and day 6 or 7 prior to administration of Step 2. If biodistribution is not acceptable, do not administer the therapeutic step. On day 6 or 7, calculate the patient specific activity of iodine I 131 tositumomab to deliver 75 cGy total body dose (TBD) or 65 cGy TBD (in mCi).

Step 2: Therapeutic step (one dose administered 7-14 days after step 1):

Tositumomab 450 mg administered over 60 minutes

Iodine I 131 tositumomab:

Platelets ≥150,000/mm^3: Iodine I 131 calculated to deliver 75 cGy total body irradiation and tositumomab 35 mg over 20 minutes

Platelets ≥100,000/mm^3 and <150,000/mm^3: Iodine I 131 calculated to deliver 65 cGy total body irradiation and tositumomab 35 mg over 20 minutes

Adjustment for Toxicity

Infusion-related toxicity (with tositumomab or iodine I-131 tositumomab):

Mild-to-moderate: Reduce infusion rate by 50%

Severe: Interrupt infusion; after complete resolution, resume with previous infusion rate reduced by 50%

Serious allergic reaction: Discontinue infusion.

Administration I.V.: Refer to manufacturer's labeling for additional details.

Tositumomab: Infuse over 60 minutes

Iodine I 131 tositumomab: Infuse over 20 minutes

Administer via an I.V. tubing set with an in-line 0.22 micron filter; do not change primary infusion set or filter at any time during the dosimetric or therapeutic step; changing the filter may result in up to a 7% loss of the iodine I 131 tositumomab dose (use the same infusion set and filter for tositumomab and iodine I 131 tositumomab). Flush with NS after iodine I 131 tositumomab infusion.

Prior to infusion, patients should be premedicated (with acetaminophen and an antihistamine) and a thyroid-protective agent should be started. Reduce the rate of tositumomab or iodine 131 tositumomab infusion by 50% for mild-to-moderate infusion-related toxicities; interrupt for severe infusion reaction (once severe infusion reaction has resolved, infusion may be restarted at half the previous rate). Discontinue for serious allergic reaction.

Monitoring Parameters CBC with differential (baseline and weekly for up to 12 weeks, or longer for persistent severe cytopenia); signs and symptoms of hypothyroidism and TSH (prior to therapy and yearly); renal function; signs/symptoms of infusion or allergic reaction

Following infusion of the iodine I 131 tositumomab dosimetric dose, the total body gamma camera counts and whole body images should be taken within 1 hour of the infusion and prior to urination, and 2-4 days after the infusion and following urination, and 6-7 days after the infusion and following urination.

Additional Information Thyroid protective agent: One of the following agents should be used starting at least 24 hours prior to the dosimetric dose and continued for 2 weeks after the therapeutic dose. Therapy should not begin without using one of the following agents 24 hours prior to Step 1:

SSKI: Oral: 4 drops 3 times/day

Lugol's solution: Oral: 20 drops 3 times/day

Potassium iodide: Oral: 130 mg once daily

Dosage Forms Excipient information presented when available (limited, particularly for generics); consult specific product labeling.

Note: Not all components are shipped from the same facility. When ordering, ensure that all will arrive on the same day.

Kit [dosimetric package]: Tositumomab 225 mg/16.1 mL [2 vials], tositumomab 35 mg/2.5 mL [1 vial], and iodine I 131 tositumomab 0.1 mg/mL and 0.61mCi/mL (20 mL) [1 vial]

Kit [therapeutic package]: Tositumomab 225 mg/16.1 mL [2 vials], tositumomab 35 mg/2.5 mL [1 vial], and iodine I 131 tositumomab 1.1 mg/mL and 5.6 mCi/mL (20 mL) [1 or 2 vials]

References

Kaminski MS, Radford JA, Gregory S, et al, "Re-Treatment With I-131 Tositumomab in Patients With Non-Hodgkin's Lymphoma Who Had Previously Responded to I-131 Tositumomab," *J Clin Oncol*, 2005, 23(31):7985-93.

Kaminski MS, Tuck M, Estes J, et al, "131I-Tositumomab Therapy as Initial Treatment for Follicular Lymphoma," *N Engl J Med*, 2005, 352(5):441-9.

Kaminski MS, Zelenetz AD, Press OW, et al, "Pivotal Study of Iodine I 131 Tositumomab for Chemotherapy-Refractory Low-Grade or Transformed Low-Grade B-Cell Non-Hodgkin's Lymphomas," *J Clin Oncol*, 2001, 19(19):3918-28.

Press OW, Unger JM, Braziel RM, et al, "Phase II Trial of CHOP Chemotherapy Followed by Tositumomab/Iodine I-131 Tositumomab for Previously Untreated Follicular Non-Hodgkin's Lymphoma: Five-Year Follow-up of Southwest Oncology Group Protocol S9911," *J Clin Oncol*, 2006, 24(25):4143-9.

Press OW, Unger JM, LeBlanc ML, et al, "A Phase III Randomized Intergroup Trial (S0016) Comparing CHOP Plus Rituximab With CHOP Plus Iodine-131-Tositumomab for Front-Line Treatment of Follicular Lymphoma: Results of Subset Analyses and a Comparison of Prognostic Models," *J Clin Oncol*, 2012, 30(15s):8001 [abstract 8001 from 2012 ASCO Annual Meeting].

- **Totect®** *see* Dexrazoxane *on page 448*
- **tPA** *see* Alteplase *on page 55*
- **tRA** *see* Tretinoin (Systemic) *on page 1405*

Trabectedin (tra BEK te din)

Related Information

Management of Drug Extravasations *on page 1800*

Brand Names: Canada Yondelis™

Index Terms Ecteinascidin; Ecteinascidin 743; ET-743

Pharmacologic Category Antineoplastic Agent, Miscellaneous

Use Canadian labeling: Treatment of relapsed ovarian cancer (in combination with doxorubicin liposomal)

Unlabeled Use Treatment of refractory soft tissue sarcoma

Labeled Contraindications Hypersensitivity to trabectedin or any component of the formulation; concurrent serious or uncontrolled infection; breastfeeding

Lactation Excretion in breast milk unknown/contraindicated

Warnings/Precautions Hazardous agent - use appropriate precautions for handling and disposal. Use is not recommended in patients with elevated bilirubin above the upper limit of normal (ULN), alkaline phosphatase, ALT and AST >2.5 times ULN, albumin <25 g/L, or in patients with clinically relevant liver disease (eg, active chronic hepatitis). Acute (reversible) increases in ALT and AST have been reported when used in combination with doxorubicin liposomal; transaminase elevations are not cumulative and the incidence and magnitude generally diminish from cycle to cycle; premedication with dexamethasone appears to reduce the frequency and severity of transaminase elevations. The median onset for grades 3 and 4 transaminase elevations is 8 days and return to below grade 3 within 8 days. Monitor bilirubin, ALT, AST, and alkaline phosphatase. Systemic exposure and the risk for hepatotoxicity is increased in patients with hepatic impairment. Use in combination with other medications associated with hepatotoxicity may increase the risk for hepatotoxicity. Avoid concomitant use with alcohol.

Neutropenia and thrombocytopenia are common; may be severe and/or dose-limiting. Neutropenic fever, infection, and sepsis may occur due to neutropenia; bleeding due to thrombocytopenia may occur. Do not administer if baseline neutrophils <1500/mm^3 or platelets <100,000/mm^3. Dose reduction recommended for severe neutropenia (ANC <500/mm^3) lasting >5 days or associated with fever or infection.

Rhabdomyolysis has been reported with use rarely, usually in association with myelosuppression, severe liver impairment, or renal failure (not recommended for use if CPK >2.5 times ULN). Monitor CPK closely, especially if muscle weakness/pain or symptoms of renal failure develop. If rhabdomyolysis occurs, institute supportive care and discontinue trabectedin until recovery. Combination therapy with doxorubicin liposomal is not recommended in patients with Cl_{cr} <60 mL/minute; monitor renal function.

Adverse cardiovascular events have been observed with use in combination with doxorubicin liposomal. Heart failure, including left ventricular dysfunction, cardiac failure, congestive heart failure and ventricular dysfunction have been observed. Obtain baseline MUGA scan or (2-D) echocardiogram prior to treatment; do not treat if left ventricular ejection fraction is below the normal limit. QT_c prolongation has been reported (single case report). Cases of pulmonary embolism have been reported with doxorubicin liposomal combination therapy.

HMG-CoA reductase inhibitors may increase the risk for rhabdomyolysis when used in combination with trabectedin. Concurrent use of trabectedin with antiemetic regimens containing dexamethasone have been reported to increase the trabectedin AUC; concurrent use is recommended however, due to the hepatoprotective and antiemetic effect of dexamethasone. Nausea and vomiting are common; corticosteroid premedication is recommended; other antiemetics may be needed. Patients should not be immunized with live viral vaccines during or shortly after treatment. Administer through a central line; peripheral administration may cause severe injection site reactions. Extravasation of trabectedin with subsequent tissue necrosis requiring debridement has been reported (case reports).

Adverse Reactions Note: Adverse reactions as reported for combination therapy with doxorubicin liposomal unless otherwise noted.

>10%:

- Central nervous system: Fatigue (46%), fever (20%), headache (16%)
- Dermatologic: Hand-foot syndrome (24%), alopecia (12%), rash (11%)
- Endocrine & metabolic: Hypokalemia (11% to 42%), hypophosphatemia (monotherapy: 34%)
- Gastrointestinal: Nausea (74%, grade 3: 10%), vomiting (56%; grade 3: 12%; grade 4: <1%), anorexia (32%), constipation (32%), diarrhea (26%), abdominal pain (20%), stomatitis (20%), weight gain (monotherapy: 20%), dyspepsia (13%), mucosal inflammation (12%)
- Hematologic: Anemia (48% to 95%; grade 3: 10% to 13%; grade 4: 3% to 6%), leukopenia (48% to 95%; grade 3: 25% to 45%; grade 4: 8% to 18%), neutropenia (77% to 92%; grade 3: 29% to 30%; grade 4: 34% to 42%), thrombocytopenia (36% to 64%; grade 3: 10% to 12%, grade 4: 8% to 11%)
- Hepatic: ALT increased (96%; grade 3: 46%; grade 4: 5%), AST increased (89%, grade 3: 12%; grade 4: 2%), alkaline phosphatase increased (61%; grade 3: 2%), hyperbilirubinemia (16% to 25%; grade 3:<1%)
- Local: Phlebitis (monotherapy: 15%), injection/catheter site reactions (14%)
- Neuromuscular & skeletal: CPK increased (2% to 22%; grade 3: 1%, grade 4: 1%), weakness (17%), arthralgia (monotherapy: 12%), paresthesia (monotherapy: 11%)
- Renal: Creatinine increased (28%: grade 3: <1%; grade 4: <1%)
- Respiratory: Dyspnea (15%), cough (12%)

1% to 10%:

- Cardiovascular: Peripheral edema (9%), palpitation (4%), edema (3%), heart failure events (2%), syncope (2%), left ventricular dysfunction (1%; grade 3: <1%)
- Central nervous system: Insomnia (10%)
- Dermatologic: Hyperpigmentation (6%)
- Endocrine & metabolic: Dehydration (5%)
- Gastrointestinal: Taste disorder (5%)
- Hematologic: Neutropenic fever (8%, grade 3: 6%, grade 4: 2%), bone marrow failure (2%), granulocytopenia (2%). pancytopenia (2%)

Hepatic: Hepatotoxicity (2%; grade 3: 1%)
Local: Catheter site pain (3%), catheter site inflammation (2%), catheter site erythema (2%)
Neuromuscular & skeletal: Myalgia (5%), peripheral neuropathy (5%), musculoskeletal pain (4%)
Renal: Renal failure (2%; grade 3: 1%; grade 4: <1%)
Respiratory: Pulmonary embolism (5%), pulmonary edema (1%)
Miscellaneous: Neutropenic infection (1%; grade 3: 1%), neutropenic sepsis (1%; grade 3: <1%; grade 4: <1%)

<1%, postmarketing, and/or case reports: Extravasation (with tissue necrosis, requiring debridement), QT_c prolongation, rhabdomyolysis

Drug Interactions

Metabolism/Transport Effects Substrate of CYP3A4 (major), P-glycoprotein; **Note:** Assignment of Major/Minor substrate status based on clinically relevant drug interaction potential

Avoid Concomitant Use

Avoid concomitant use of Trabectedin with any of the following: Alcohol (Ethyl); BCG; CloZAPine; Conivaptan; Natalizumab; Pimecrolimus; Tacrolimus (Topical); Vaccines (Live)

Increased Effect/Toxicity

Trabectedin may increase the levels/effects of: CloZAPine; Leflunomide; Natalizumab; Vaccines (Live); Vitamin K Antagonists

The levels/effects of Trabectedin may be increased by: Alcohol (Ethyl); Conivaptan; CYP3A4 Inhibitors (Moderate); CYP3A4 Inhibitors (Strong); Dasatinib; Denosumab; HMG-CoA Reductase Inhibitors; Ivacaftor; Mifepristone; P-glycoprotein/ABCB1 Inhibitors; Pimecrolimus; Roflumilast; Tacrolimus (Topical); Trastuzumab

Decreased Effect

Trabectedin may decrease the levels/effects of: BCG; Cardiac Glycosides; Coccidioidin Skin Test; Sipuleucel-T; Vaccines (Inactivated); Vaccines (Live); Vitamin K Antagonists

The levels/effects of Trabectedin may be decreased by: CYP3A4 Inducers (Strong); Deferasirox; Echinacea; Herbs (CYP3A4 Inducers); P-glycoprotein/ABCB1 Inducers; Tocilizumab

Ethanol/Nutrition/Herb Interactions Herb/Nutraceutical: Avoid St John's wort (may increase the clearance of trabectedin).

Storage/Stability Store intact vials under refrigeration at 2°C to 8°C (36°F to 46°F). Reconstituted solutions are stable for up to 24 hours at room temperature, although the manufacturer recommends use immediately. Solutions diluted for infusion may be stored at room temperature and should be used within 30 hours of initial reconstitution.

Reconstitution Reconstitute the 1 mg vial with 20 mL sterile water for injection (SWFI) and the 0.25 mg vial with 5 mL SWFI, resulting in a reconstituted concentration of 0.05 mg/mL. Shake until completely dissolved. Further dilute for infusion in 500 mL sodium chloride 0.9% or D_5W. Use appropriate precautions for handling and disposal.

Mechanism of Action A marine-derived compound which blocks the cell cycle at the G_2/M phase by covalently binding to the minor DNA groove, bending the helix toward the major groove and altering DNA transcription. Also alters DNA repair mechanism.

Pharmacodynamics/Kinetics

Distribution: V_d: >5000 L; distributes extensively into peripheral tissues
Protein binding: >97%; to plasma proteins
Metabolism: Extensively hepatic; oxidized via CYP3A4
Excretion: Feces (predominantly); urine (minor)

Dosing

Adult & Geriatric Note: Prior to each treatment cycle, ANC should be ≥1500/mm³, platelets ≥100,000/mm³, hemoglobin ≥9 g/dL, bilirubin ≤ULN; alkaline phosphatase (nonosseous origin), ALT, and AST ≤2.5 times ULN; albumin ≥25 g/L; serum creatinine ≤1.5 mg/dL or creatinine clearance ≥60 mL/minute; and CPK ≤2.5 times ULN. Premedication with dexamethasone I.V. 20 mg 30 minutes before infusion is recommended for hepatoprotective and antiemetic effects; additional antiemetics may be administered.

Ovarian cancer, relapsed (Canadian labeling; not approved for use in the U.S.): 1.1 mg/m² every 3 weeks (in combination with doxorubicin liposomal)

Soft tissue sarcoma, refractory (unlabeled/investigational use): I.V.: 1.5 mg/m² every 3 weeks (Yovine, 2004)

Renal Impairment Cl_{cr} <60 mL/minute: Combination therapy with doxorubicin liposomal is not recommended.

Hepatic Impairment Bilirubin >ULN, clinically relevant liver disease (eg, active chronic hepatitis): Use is not recommended.

Adjustment for Toxicity

Delay the next treatment cycle for up to 3 weeks if ANC <1500/mm³, platelets <100,000/mm³, hemoglobin <9 g/dL, bilirubin >ULN; alkaline phosphatase (nonosseous origin), ALT, and AST >2.5 times ULN; albumin <25 g/L, or serum creatinine >1.5 mg/dL or creatinine clearance <60 mL/minute; if persists beyond 3 weeks, consider discontinuing treatment.

Reduce dose if the following occur in between cycles: ANC <500/mm³, platelets <25,000/mm³, bilirubin >ULN, alkaline phosphatase (nonosseous origin) >2.5 times ULN, ALT or AST >5 times ULN which has not recovered by day 21, or any other grade 3 or 4 adverse reaction (eg, nausea, vomiting, fatigue):

- First occurrence: Reduce trabectedin dose to 0.9 mg/m² (reduce doxorubicin liposomal dose to 25 mg/m²)
- Second occurrence: Reduce trabectedin dose to 0.75 mg/m² (reduce doxorubicin liposomal dose to 20 mg/m²)
- Third occurrence: Consider treatment discontinuation

CPK >2.5 times ULN: Discontinue trabectedin treatment until full recovery

In the treatment of refractory soft tissue sarcoma (unlabeled use), the following dosage adjustments for toxicity were used in clinical trials (Garcia Carbonero, 2005; Yovine, 2004).

- Febrile neutropenia, infection, grade 4 neutropenia lasting ≥5 days or grade 4 thrombocytopenia: Reduce dose to 1.2 mg/m² over 24 hours every 3 weeks
- Cardiac or neurologic toxicity grade 2, or other nonhematologic toxicity ≥ grade 3 lasting >21 days: Reduce dose to 1.2 mg/m² over 24 hours every 3 weeks
- Recurrent severe toxicity: Further reduce dose to 1 mg/m² over 24 hours every 3 weeks
- Cardiac or neurologic toxicity ≥ grade 3 lasting >35 days: Discontinue treatment

Combination Regimens

Ovarian cancer: Trabectedin-Doxorubicin (Liposomal) (Ovarian Cancer) on page 1757

Administration Infuse through a central line. Premedicate with a corticosteroid (eg, dexamethasone 20 mg I.V.) prior to treatment; additional antiemetics may be needed.

Combination therapy with doxorubicin liposomal: Administer doxorubicin first, flush line with D_5W, then follow with trabectedin infusion over 3 hours.

Monotherapy (for soft tissue sarcoma; unlabeled use): Infuse as a continuous infusion over 24 hours; antiemetic prophylaxis was utilized in clinical trials (Yovine, 2004).

Vesicant/Extravasation Risk Vesicant

Monitoring Parameters CBC with differential (baseline, weekly for first 2 cycles, then once between cycles), bilirubin, alkaline phosphatase (consider hepatic isoenzymes 5 nucleotidase or GGT to differentiate from elevations of non-osseous origin), ALT, AST (baseline, weekly for first 2 cycles, then once between cycles), renal function (baseline and during treatment), CPK (weekly for first 2 cycles, then between subsequent cycles)

Product Availability Not commercially available in the U.S. (investigational agent)

Prescribing and Access Restrictions Not approved for use in the U.S. (investigational agent)

Dosage Forms: Canada Excipient information presented when available (limited, particularly for generics); consult specific product labeling.

Injection, powder for reconstitution:

Yondelis™: 0.25 mg, 1 mg [contains sucrose]

References

Garcia-Carbonero R, Supko JG, Maki RG, et al, "Ecteinascidin-743 (ET-743) for Chemotherapy-Naive Patients With Advanced Soft Tissue Sarcomas: Multicenter Phase II and Pharmacokinetic Study," *J Clin Oncol*, 2005, 23(24):5484-92.

Le Cesne A, Blay JY, Judson I, et al, "Phase II Study of ET-743 in Advanced Soft Tissue Sarcomas: A European Organisation for the Research and Treatment of Cancer (EORTC) Soft Tissue and Bone Sarcoma Group Trial," *J Clin Oncol*, 2005, 23(3):576-84.

Monk BJ, Herzog TJ, Kaye SB, et al, "Trabectedin Plus Pegylated Liposomal Doxorubicin in Recurrent Ovarian Cancer," *J Clin Oncol*, 2010, 28(19):3107-14.

Yovine A, Riofrio M, Blay JY, et al, "Phase II Study of Ecteinascidin-743 in Advanced Pretreated Soft Tissue Sarcoma Patients," *J Clin Oncol*, 2004, 22(5):890-9.

TraMADol (TRA ma dole)

Brand Names: U.S. ConZip™; Rybix™ ODT; Ryzolt™; Ultram®; Ultram® ER

Brand Names: Canada Durela™; Ralivia™; Tridural™; Ultram®; Zytram® XL

Index Terms Tramadol Hydrochloride

Generic Availability (U.S.) Yes: Excludes tablet (orally disintegrating)

Pharmacologic Category Analgesic, Opioid

Use Relief of moderate to moderately-severe pain

Extended release formulations are indicated for patients requiring around-the-clock management of moderate to moderately-severe pain for an extended period of time

Labeled Contraindications Hypersensitivity to tramadol, opioids, or any component of the formulation

Additional contraindications for Ultram®, Rybix™ ODT, and Ultram® ER: Any situation where opioids are contraindicated, including acute intoxication with alcohol, hypnotics, centrally-acting analgesics, opioids, or psychotropic drugs

Additional contraindications for ConZip™, Ryzolt™: Severe/acute bronchial asthma, hypercapnia, or significant respiratory depression in the absence of appropriately monitored setting and/or resuscitative equipment

Canadian product labeling:

Tramadol is contraindicated during or within 14 days following MAO inhibitor therapy

Extended release formulations: Additional contraindications:

Ralivia™, Tridural™: Severe (Cl_{cr} <30 mL/minute) renal dysfunction, severe (Child-Pugh class C) hepatic dysfunction

Durela™ and Zytram® XL: Severe (Cl_{cr} <30 mL/minute) renal dysfunction, severe (Child-Pugh class C) hepatic dysfunction; known or suspected mechanical GI obstruction or any disease/condition that affects bowel transit; mild, intermittent or short-duration pain that can be managed with other pain medication; management of peri-operative pain; obstructive airway, acute respiratory depression, cor pulmonale, delirium tremens, seizure disorder, severe CNS depression, increased cerebrospinal or intracranial pressure, head injury, breast-feeding, pregnancy; use during labor and delivery

Pregnancy Risk Factor C

Lactation Enters breast milk/not recommended

Warnings/Precautions Rare but serious anaphylactoid reactions (including fatalities) often following initial dosing have been reported. Pruritus, hives, bronchospasm, angioedema, toxic epidermal necrolysis (TEN) and Stevens-Johnson syndrome also have been reported with use. Previous anaphylactoid reactions to opioids may increase risks for similar reactions to tramadol. Caution patients to swallow extended release tablets whole. Rapid release and absorption of tramadol from extended release tablets that are broken, crushed, or chewed may lead to a potentially lethal overdose. May cause CNS depression, which may impair physical or mental abilities; patients must be cautioned about performing tasks which require mental alertness (eg, operating machinery or driving). May cause CNS depression and/or respiratory depression, particularly when combined with other CNS depressants. Use with caution and reduce dosage when administered to patients receiving other CNS depressants. An increased risk of seizures may occur in patients receiving serotonin reuptake inhibitors (SSRIs or anorectics), tricyclic antidepressants or other cyclic compounds (including cyclobenzaprine, promethazine), neuroleptics, drugs which may lower seizure threshold, or drugs which impair metabolism of tramadol (ie, CYP2D6 and 3A4 inhibitors). Patients with a history of seizures, or with a risk of seizures (head trauma, metabolic disorders, CNS infection, or malignancy, or during ethanol/drug withdrawal) are also at increased risk. Avoid use, if possible, with serotonergic agents such as TCAs, MAO inhibitors (use with extreme caution; contraindicated in Canadian product labeling), triptans, venlafaxine, trazodone, lithium, sibutramine, meperidine, dextromethorphan, St John's wort, SNRIs, and SSRIs; use caution with drugs which impair metabolism of tramadol (ie, CYP2D6 and 3A4 inhibitors); concomitant may increase the risk of serotonin syndrome.

Elderly (particularly >75 years of age), debilitated patients and patients with chronic respiratory disorders may be at greater risk of adverse events. Use with caution in patients with increased intracranial pressure or head injury. Avoid use in patients who are suicidal or addiction prone; use with caution in patients taking tranquilizers and/or antidepressants, or those with an emotional disturbance including depression. Healthcare provider should be alert to problems of abuse, misuse, and diversion. Use caution in heavy alcohol users. Use caution in treatment of acute abdominal conditions; may mask pain. Use tramadol with caution and reduce dosage in patients with liver disease or renal dysfunction. Avoid using extended release tablets in severe hepatic impairment. Do not use Ryzolt™ in any degree of hepatic impairment. Tolerance or drug dependence may result from extended use (withdrawal symptoms have been reported); abrupt discontinuation should be avoided. Tapering of dose at the time of discontinuation limits the risk of withdrawal symptoms. Some products may contain phenylalanine.

Ethanol/Nutrition/Herb Interactions

Ethanol: May increase CNS depression; monitor for increased effects with coadministration. Caution patients about effects.

Food:

Immediate release tablet: Rate and extent of absorption were not significantly affected.

Extended release:

ConZip™: Rate and extent of absorption were unaffected.

Ryzolt™: Increased C_{max}; no effect on AUC.

Ultram® ER: High-fat meal reduced C_{max} and AUC, and increased T_{max} by 3 hours.

Orally disintegrating tablet: Food delays the time to peak serum concentration by 30 minutes; extent of absorption was not significantly affected.

Herb/Nutraceutical: Avoid valerian, St John's wort, kava kava, gotu kola (may increase CNS depression).

Storage/Stability Store at 25°C (77°F); excursions permitted to 15°C to 30°C (59°F to 86°F).

Mechanism of Action Tramadol and its active metabolite (M1) binds to μ-opiate receptors in the CNS causing inhibition of ascending pain pathways, altering the perception of and response to pain; also inhibits the reuptake of norepinephrine and serotonin, which also modifies the ascending pain pathway

Pharmacodynamics/Kinetics

Onset of action: Immediate release: ~1 hour

Duration: 9 hours

Absorption: Immediate release formulation: Rapid and complete; Extended release formulation: Delayed

Distribution: V_d: 2.5-3 L/kg

Protein binding, plasma: ~20%

Metabolism: Extensively hepatic via demethylation (mediated by CYP3A4 and CYP2B6), glucuronidation, and sulfation; has pharmacologically active metabolite formed by CYP2D6 (M1; O-desmethyl tramadol)

Bioavailability: Immediate release: 75%; Extended release: Ultram® ER: 85% to 90% (as compared to immediate release), Zytram® XL, Tridural™: 70%, Ryzolt™: ~95% (as compared to immediate release)

Half-life elimination: Tramadol: ~6-8 hours; Active metabolite: 7-9 hours; prolonged in elderly, hepatic or renal impairment; Zytram® XL: Apparent half-life: ~16 hours; Durela™, Ralivia™, Ryzolt™, Tridural™: ~5-9 hours

Time to peak: Immediate release: ~2 hours; Extended release: ConZip™: ~10-12 hours, Ryzolt™, Tridural™: ~4 hours; Durela™, Ultram® ER: ~12 hours

Excretion: Urine (30% as unchanged drug; 60% as metabolites)

Dosing

Adult Moderate-to-severe pain: Oral:

Immediate release: 50-100 mg every 4-6 hours (not to exceed 400 mg/day). For patients not requiring rapid onset of effect, tolerability may be improved by starting dose at 25 mg/day and titrating dose by 25 mg every 3 days, until reaching 25 mg 4 times/day. The total daily dose may then be increased by 50 mg every 3 days as tolerated, to reach dose of 50 mg 4 times/day. After titration, 50-100 mg may be given every 4-6 hours as needed up to a maximum 400 mg/day.

Orally-disintegrating tablet (Rybix™ ODT): 50-100 mg every 4-6 hours (not to exceed 400 mg/day); for patients not requiring rapid onset of effect, tolerability may be improved by starting dose at 50 mg/day and titrating dose by 50 mg every 3 days, until reaching 50 mg 4 times/day. After titration, 50-100 mg may be given every 4-6 hours as needed up to a maximum 400 mg/day.

Extended release:

U.S. labeling: ConZip™, Ryzolt™, Ultram® ER:

Patients not currently on immediate-release tramadol: 100 mg once daily; titrate every 5 days (ConZip™, Ultram® ER) or every 2-3 days (Ryzolt™); maximum dose: 300 mg daily

Patients currently on immediate-release tramadol: Calculate 24-hour immediate release total dose and initiate total extended release daily dose (round dose to the next lowest 100 mg increment); titrate as tolerated to desired effect (maximum: 300 mg daily)

Canadian labeling: **Note:** Patients currently on immediate-release tramadol: When switching to extended release, initiate at the same or lowest nearest total daily tramadol dose. Not to exceed recommended maximum daily dosing.

Durela™, Ralivia™, Tridural™: Patients not currently on immediate-release tramadol or opioids: Initial: 100 mg once daily; titrate every 5 days (Durela™, Ralivia™) or every 2 days (Tridural™) as needed based on clinical response and severity of pain (maximum: 300 mg daily)

Zytram® XL: Patients not currently on immediate-release tramadol or opioids: 150 mg once daily; if pain relief is not achieved may titrate by increasing dosage incrementally, with sufficient time to evaluate effect of increased dosage; generally not more often than every 7 days (maximum: 400 mg daily)

Geriatric Elderly >65 years: Oral: Use caution and initiate at the lower end of the dosing range. Refer to adult dosing.

Elderly >75 years:

Immediate release: Do not exceed 300 mg/day; see dosing adjustments for renal and hepatic impairment.

Extended release: Use with great caution; see dosing for adults, renal, and hepatic impairment.

Pediatric Moderate-to-severe pain: Oral: Children ≥17 years: Refer to adult dosing.

Renal Impairment

Immediate release: Cl_{cr} <30 mL/minute: Administer 50-100 mg dose every 12 hours (maximum: 200 mg/day).

Extended release: Should not be used in patients with Cl_{cr} <30 mL/minute.

Hepatic Impairment

Immediate release: Cirrhosis: Recommended dose: 50 mg every 12 hours.

Extended release: Should not be used in patients with severe (Child-Pugh class C) hepatic dysfunction; Ryzolt™ should not be used in any degree of hepatic impairment

Administration

Immediate release: Administer without regard to meals.

Extended release: Swallow whole; do not crush, chew, or split. **Note:** Durela™, Ralivia™, and Tridural™: Canadian availability; products not available in U.S.:

ConZip™, Zytram® XL, Durela™: May administer without regard to meals.

Ultram® ER, Ralivia™, Tridural™: May administer without regard to meals, but administer in a consistent manner of either with or without meals.

Orally-disintegrating tablet: Remove from foil blister by peeling back (do not push tablet through the foil). Place tablet on tongue and allow to dissolve (may take ~1 minute); water is not needed, but may be administered with water. Do not chew, break, or split tablet.

Test Interactions May interfere with urine detection of PCP (false-positive).

Dosage Forms Excipient information presented when available (limited, particularly for generics); consult specific product labeling.

Capsule, variable release, oral, as hydrochloride: 150 mg [37.5 mg (immediate release) and 112.5 mg (extended release)]

ConZip™: 100 mg [25 mg (immediate release) and 75 mg (extended release)]

ConZip™: 200 mg [50 mg (immediate release) and 150 mg (extended release)]

ConZip™: 300 mg [50 mg (immediate release) and 250 mg (extended release)]

Tablet, oral, as hydrochloride: 50 mg

Ultram®: 50 mg [scored]

Tablet, extended release, oral, as hydrochloride: 100 mg, 200 mg, 300 mg

Ryzolt™: 100 mg, 200 mg, 300 mg

Ultram® ER: 100 mg, 200 mg, 300 mg

Tablet, orally disintegrating, oral, as hydrochloride:

Rybix™ ODT: 50 mg [contains aspartame; mint flavor]

Dosage Forms: Canada Excipient information presented when available (limited, particularly for generics); consult specific product labeling.

Tablet, extended release, as hydrochloride

Durela™: 100 mg, 200 mg, 300 mg

Ralivia™: 100 mg, 200 mg, 300 mg

Tridural™: 100 mg, 200 mg, 300 mg

Zytram® XL: 75 mg, 150 mg, 200 mg, 300 mg, 400 mg

◆ **Tramadol Hydrochloride** *see* TraMADol *on page 1388*

Tranexamic Acid (tran eks AM ik AS id)

Brand Names: U.S. Cyklokapron®; Lysteda™

Brand Names: Canada Cyklokapron®; Tranexamic Acid Injection BP

Generic Availability (U.S.) Yes: Injection

Pharmacologic Category Antifibrinolytic Agent; Antihemophilic Agent; Hemostatic Agent; Lysine Analog

Use

Solution for injection: Short-term use (2-8 days) in hemophilia patients to reduce or prevent hemorrhage and reduce need for replacement therapy during and following tooth extraction

Tablet: Treatment of cyclic heavy menstrual bleeding

Unlabeled Use Trauma-associated hemorrhage; treatment of traumatic hyphema; topical treatment (mouth rinse) of bleeding associated with dental procedures in patients on oral anticoagulant therapy; prevention of perioperative bleeding associated with cardiac surgery; prevention of bleeding associated with craniosynostosis surgery, extracorporeal membrane oxygenation (ECMO), orthognathic surgery, spinal surgery (eg, spinal fusion), total knee replacement surgery, or transurethral prostatectomy; reduction of blood loss associated with cesarean delivery; hereditary angioedema (long-term prophylaxis)

Labeled Contraindications

Solution for injection: Hypersensitivity to tranexamic acid or any component of the formulation; acquired defective color vision; active intravascular clotting; subarachnoid hemorrhage

Tablet: Hypersensitivity to tranexamic acid or any component of the formulation; active thromboembolic disease (eg, cerebral thrombosis, DVT, or PE); history of thrombosis or thromboembolism, including retinal vein or retinal artery occlusion; intrinsic risk of thrombosis or thromboembolism (eg, hypercoagulopathy, thrombogenic cardiac rhythm disease, thrombogenic valvular disease)

Pregnancy Risk Factor B

Lactation Enters breast milk/not recommended

Warnings/Precautions Venous and arterial thrombosis or thromboembolism, including central retinal artery/vein obstruction, has been reported. Use the injection with caution in patients with thromboembolic disease; oral formulation is contraindicated. Use the injection with caution in patients with upper urinary tract bleeding, ureteral obstruction due to clot formation has been reported. Use with extreme caution in patients with DIC requiring antifibrinolytic therapy; patients should be under strict supervision of a physician experienced in treating this disorder. Use with caution in patients with uncorrected cardiovascular or cerebrovascular disease due to complications of thrombosis. Patients taking hormonal contraceptives were excluded from clinical trials for heavy menstrual bleeding. Risk vs benefit should be weighed before using hormonal contraceptives concurrently with oral tranexamic acid; risk of thromboembolism (eg, MI, stroke) may be further increased, particularly in patients who are obese or >35 years of age and smoke. Avoid use of oral formulation in patients taking higher than approved doses of hormonal contraceptives. Use oral tranexamic acid with caution in patients taking tretinoin; concurrent use may exacerbate procoagulant effects.

Visual defects (eg, color vision change, visual loss) and retinal venous and arterial occlusions have been reported; discontinue treatment if changes in vision occur; prompt ophthalmic examination should be performed by an ophthalmologist. Use of the injection is contraindicated in patients with acquired defective color vision since this would prohibit monitoring one endpoint as a measure of ophthalmic toxicity. Seizures have been reported with use; most often with intraoperative use (eg, open chamber cardiac surgery) and in older patients. Ligneous conjunctivitis has been reported with the oral formulation, but usually resolved upon discontinuation of therapy. Use with caution in patients with renal impairment; dosage modification may be required.

Adverse Reactions

Injection: Frequency not defined:

Cardiovascular: Hypotension (with rapid I.V. injection)
Central nervous system: Giddiness
Dermatologic: Allergic dermatitis
Endocrine & metabolic: Unusual menstrual discomfort
Gastrointestinal: Diarrhea, nausea, vomiting
Ocular: Blurred vision

Oral:

>10%:

Central nervous system: Headache (50%)
Gastrointestinal: Abdominal pain (20%)
Neuromuscular & skeletal: Back pain (21%), muscle pain (11%)
Respiratory: Nasal/sinus symptoms (25%)

1% to 10%:

Central nervous system: Fatigue (5%)
Hematologic: Anemia (6%)
Neuromuscular & skeletal: Arthralgia (7%), muscle cramps/spasms (7%)

All formulations: <1%, postmarketing, and/or case reports: Allergic skin reaction, anaphylactic shock, anaphylactoid reactions, cerebral thrombosis, deep vein thrombosis (DVT), diarrhea, dizziness, nausea, pulmonary embolism, renal cortical necrosis, retinal artery/vein obstruction, seizure, ureteral obstruction, visual disturbances (including impaired color vision and loss), vomiting

Drug Interactions

Metabolism/Transport Effects None known.

Avoid Concomitant Use

Avoid concomitant use of Tranexamic Acid with any of the following: Anti-inhibitor Coagulant Complex

Increased Effect/Toxicity

Tranexamic Acid may increase the levels/effects of: Anti-inhibitor Coagulant Complex; Fibrinogen Concentrate (Human)

The levels/effects of Tranexamic Acid may be increased by: Contraceptives (Estrogens); Contraceptives (Progestins); Fibrinogen Concentrate (Human); Tretinoin (Systemic)

Decreased Effect There are no known significant interactions involving a decrease in effect.

Storage/Stability Store at 25°C (77°F); excursions permitted to 15°C to 30°C (59°F to 86°F).

Reconstitution For intravenous infusion, tranexamic acid may be further diluted with dextrose, saline, or other compatible solutions. The mixture should be used on the same day as prepared.

Mechanism of Action Forms a reversible complex that displaces plasminogen from fibrin resulting in inhibition of fibrinolysis; it also inhibits the proteolytic activity of plasmin

With reduction in plasmin activity, tranexamic acid also reduces activation of complement and consumption of C1 esterase inhibitor (C1-INH), thereby decreasing inflammation associated with hereditary angioedema.

Pharmacodynamics/Kinetics

Distribution: V_d: 9-27 L
Protein binding: ~3%, primarily to plasminogen
Bioavailability: Oral: ~45%
Half-life elimination: ~2-11 hours
Time to peak: Oral: ~3 hours
Excretion: Urine (>95% as unchanged drug)

Dosing

Adult & Geriatric

Elective cesarean section, blood loss reduction (unlabeled use): I.V.: 1000 mg over 5 minutes at least 10 minutes prior to skin incision (Gungorduk, 2011)

Hereditary angioedema (HAE) (unlabeled use):

Long-term prophylaxis: Oral: 1000-1500 mg 2-3 times daily; reduce to 500 mg/dose once or twice daily when frequency of attacks reduces (Gompels, 2005; Levy, 2010) **or** 25 mg/kg/dose administered 2-3 times daily (Bowen, 2004)

Short-term prophylaxis (eg, for dental work): Oral: 75 mg/kg/day divided 2-3 times daily for 5 days before and 2 days after the event (Bowen, 2004) **or** 1000 mg 4 times/day for 48 hours before and after procedure (Gompels, 2005)

Treatment of acute HAE attack: Oral, I.V.: 25 mg/kg/dose (maximum single dose: 1000 mg) every 3-4 hours (maximum: 75 mg/kg/day) (Bowen, 2004) **or** 1000 mg 4 times/day for 48 hours (Gompels, 2005)

Menorrhagia: Oral: 1300 mg 3 times/day (3900 mg/day) for up to 5 days during monthly menstruation

Orthognathic surgery, blood loss reduction (unlabeled use): I.V.: 20 mg/kg over 15 minutes prior to incision (Choi, 2009)

Prevention of dental procedure bleeding in patients on oral anticoagulant therapy (unlabeled use): Oral rinse: 4.8% solution: Hold 10 mL in mouth and rinse for 2 minutes then spit out. Repeat 4 times/day for 2 days after procedure. **Note:** Patient should not eat or drink for 1 hour after using oral rinse (Carter, 2003).

Prevention of perioperative bleeding associated with cardiac surgery (unlabeled use): I.V.: Loading dose of 30 mg/kg over 30 minutes (total loading dose includes a test dose administered over the first 10 minutes followed by the remainder of dose) prior to incision, followed by 16 mg/kg/hour until sternal closure; add an additional 2 mg/kg to cardiopulmonary bypass circuit (Fergusson, 2008)

or

Loading dose of 10 mg/kg over 20 minutes prior to incision followed by 2 mg/kg/hour continued for 2 hours after transfer to ICU; add a prime dose of 50 mg for a 2.5 L cardiopulmonary bypass circuit; maintenance infusion adjusted for renal insufficiency (Nuttall, 2008)

or

Loading dose of 10-15 mg/kg over 10-15 minutes, followed by 1-1.5 mg/kg/hour. The authors suggest adding 2–2.5 mg/kg to cardiopulmonary bypass circuit; however, amounts have varied widely in clinical trials (Gravlee, 2008).

Prevention of perioperative bleeding associated with spinal surgery (eg, spinal fusion) (unlabeled use): I.V.: 2000 mg over 20 minutes prior to incision followed by 100 mg/hour during surgery and for 5 hours postoperatively (Elwatidy, 2008) **or** 10 mg/kg prior to incision followed by

1 mg/kg/hour for the remainder of the surgery; discontinue at time of wound closure (Wong, 2008)

Total knee replacement surgery, blood loss reduction (unlabeled use): I.V.: 10 mg/kg over 30 minutes before inflation of tourniquet and 3 hours after first dose (Camarasa, 2006)

or

10 mg/kg over 10 minutes before inflation of tourniquet with a second dose (10 mg/kg) administered immediately after tourniquet release (Lozano, 2008)

or

10 mg/kg administered 30 minutes before deflation of tourniquet followed by 1 mg/kg/hour beginning at the end of the operation and continuing for 6 hours postoperatively (Alvarez, 2008)

Tooth extraction in patients with hemophilia (in combination with appropriate factor replacement therapy): I.V.: 10 mg/kg immediately before surgery, then 10 mg/kg/dose 3-4 times/day; may be used for 2-8 days

Transurethral prostatectomy, blood loss reduction (unlabeled use): Oral: 2000 mg 3 times/day on the operative and first postoperative day (Rannikko, 2004)

Trauma-associated hemorrhage (unlabeled use): I.V.: Loading dose: 1000 mg over 10 minutes, followed by 1000 mg over the next 8 hours. **Note:** Clinical trial included patients with significant hemorrhage (SBP <90 mm Hg, heart rate >110 bpm, or both) or those at risk of significant hemorrhage. Treatment began within 8 hours of injury (CRASH-2 Trial Collaborators, 2010).

Traumatic hyphema (unlabeled use): Oral: 25 mg/kg administered 3 times/day for 5-7 days (Rahmani, 1999; Vangsted, 1983; Varnek, 1980). **Note:** This same regimen may also be used for secondary hemorrhage after an initial traumatic hyphema event.

Pediatric

Hereditary angioedema (HAE) (unlabeled use): Oral:

Long-term prophylaxis: 20-40 mg/kg/day in 2-3 divided doses (maximum dose: 3000 mg/day) (Farkas, 2007) **or** 50 mg/kg/day (or 1000-2000 mg/day; depending on age and size of patient); may consider alternate-day regimen or twice-weekly regimen when frequency of attacks reduces; diarrhea may be a dose-limiting side effect (Gompels, 2005)

Short-term prophylaxis: 20-40 mg/kg/day in 2-3 divided doses (maximum dose: 3000 mg/day) (Farkas, 2007) **or** 500 mg 4 times/day (Gompels, 2005). **Note:** For short-term prophylaxis (eg, dental work), initiate 2-5 days before and continue for 2 days after the procedure (Bowen, 2004; Gompels, 2005).

Prevention of perioperative bleeding associated with cardiac surgery (unlabeled use): I.V.: 10 mg/kg given over 30 minutes prior to incision, 10 mg/kg while on cardiopulmonary bypass, and 10 mg/kg administered after protamine reversal (Chauhan, 2004; Chauhan, 2004)

or

Loading dose of 100 mg/kg over 15 minutes prior to incision, followed by 10 mg/kg/hour infusion (continued until ICU transport); add 100 mg/kg to pump reservoir when cardiopulmonary bypass initiated (Reid, 1997)

Prevention of perioperative bleeding associated with craniosynostosis surgery (unlabeled use): I.V.: Loading dose of 50 mg/kg over 15 minutes prior to incision, followed by 5 mg/kg/hour (Goobie, 2011) **or** 15 mg/kg over

15 minutes prior to incision, followed by 10 mg/kg/hour until skin closure (Dadure, 2011)

Prevention of perioperative bleeding associated with spinal surgery (eg, spinal fusion) (unlabeled use): Children and Adolescents: I.V.: 10 mg/kg given over 15 minutes prior to incision followed by 1 mg/kg/hour for the remainder of the surgery; discontinue at time of wound closure (Neilipovitz, 2001; Verma, 2010)

or

100 mg/kg over 15 minutes prior to incision followed by 10 mg/kg/hour until skin closure (Sethna, 2005)

or

30 mg/kg over 20 minutes prior to incision followed by 1 mg/kg/hour during surgery and for 5 hours postoperatively (Elwatidy, 2008)

Tooth extraction in patients with hemophilia (in combination with appropriate factor replacement therapy): Children and Adolescents: I.V.: Refer to adult dosing.

Traumatic hyphema (unlabeled use): Oral: Refer to adult dosing.

Renal Impairment

I.V. formulation:

Tooth extraction in patients with hemophilia:

Serum creatinine 1.36-2.83 mg/dL: Maintenance dose of 10 mg/kg/dose twice daily

Serum creatinine 2.83-5.66 mg/dL: Maintenance dose of 10 mg/kg/dose once daily

Serum creatinine >5.66 mg/dL: Maintenance dose of 10 mg/kg/dose every 48 hours **or** 5 mg/kg/dose once daily

Cardiac surgery (the following dose adjustments have been recommended [Nuttall, 2008]):

Serum creatinine 1.6-3.3 mg/dL: Reduce maintenance infusion to 1.5 mg/kg/hour (based on a 25% reduction from 2 mg/kg/hour)

Serum creatinine 3.3-6.6 mg/dL: Reduce maintenance infusion to 1 mg/kg/hour (based on a 50% reduction from 2 mg/kg/hour)

Serum creatinine >6.6 mg/dL: Reduce maintenance infusion to 0.5 mg/kg/hour (based on a 75% reduction from 2 mg/kg/hour)

Oral formulation: *Heavy menstrual bleeding:*

Serum creatinine >1.4-2.8 mg/dL: 1300 mg twice daily (2600 mg/day) for up to 5 days

Serum creatinine 2.9-5.7 mg/dL: 1300 mg once daily for up to 5 days

Serum creatinine >5.7 mg/dL: 650 mg once daily for up to 5 days

Administration

Injection: May be administered by direct I.V. injection at a maximum rate of 100 mg/minute; use plastic syringe only for I.V. push

In general, tranexamic acid loading doses are diluted in 50-250 mL and are administered over 5-30 minutes.

Tablet: Administer without regard to meals. Should be swallowed whole; do not break, chew, or crush.

Extemporaneous Preparations A 5% (50 mg/mL) oral solution may be prepared by diluting 5 mL of 10% (100 mg/mL) tranexamic acid injection with 5 mL sterile water. Label "refrigerate". Stable for 5 days refrigerated.

A 25 mg/mL oral suspension may be prepared with tablets. Place one 500 mg tablet (strength not available in U.S.) into 20 mL water and let stand ~2-5 minutes. Begin stirring and continue until the tablet is completely disintegrated, forming a fine particulate suspension (dispersion time for each 500 mg tablet is ~2-5 minutes). Administer immediately after preparation.

Lam MS, "Extemporaneous Compounding of Oral Liquid Dosage Formulations and Alternative Drug Delivery Methods for Anticancer Drugs," *Pharmacotherapy*, 2011, 31(2):164-92.

Monitoring Parameters Injection: Ophthalmic examination (visual acuity, color vision, eye-ground, and visual fields) at baseline and regular intervals during the course of therapy in patients being treated for longer than several days

Dietary Considerations Take tablet without regard to meals.

Additional Information Tranexamic acid is 6-10 times more potent in plasminogen/plasmin binding compared to epsilon-aminocaproic acid.

Dosage Forms Excipient information presented when available (limited, particularly for generics); consult specific product labeling.

Injection, solution: 100 mg/mL (10 mL)

Cyklokapron®: 100 mg/mL (10 mL)

Tablet, oral:

Lysteda™: 650 mg

References

Alvarez JC, Santiveri FX, Ramos I, et al, "Tranexamic Acid Reduces Blood Transfusion in Total Knee Arthroplasty Even When a Blood Conservation Program is Applied," *Transfusion*, 2008, 48 (3):519-25.

Bowen T, Cicardi M, Farkas H, et al, "Canadian 2003 International Consensus Algorithm for the Diagnosis, Therapy, and Management of Hereditary Angioedema," *J Allergy Clin Immunol*, 2004, 114(3):629-37.

Camarasa MA, Ollé G, Serra-Prat M, et al, "Efficacy of Aminocaproic, Tranexamic Acids in the Control of Bleeding During Total Knee Replacement: A Randomized Clinical Trial," *Br J Anaesth*, 2006, 96(5):576-82.

Carter G and Goss A. "Tranexamic Acid Mouthwash – A Prospective Randomized Study of a 2-Day Regimen vs 5-Day Regimen to Prevent Postoperative Bleeding in Anticoagulated Patients Requiring Dental Extractions," *Int J Oral Maxillofac Surg*, 2003, 32(5):504-7.

Chauhan S, Bisoi A, Kumar N, et al, "Dose Comparison of Tranexamic Acid in Pediatric Cardiac Surgery," *Asian Cardiovasc Thorac Ann*, 2004, 12(2):121-4.

Chauhan S, Das SN, Bisoi A, et al, "Comparison of Epsilon Aminocaproic Acid and Tranexamic Acid in Pediatric Cardiac Surgery," *J Cardiothorac Vasc Anesth*, 2004, 18(2):141-3.

CRASH-2 Trial Collaborators, "Effects of Tranexamic Acid on Death, Vascular Occlusive Events, and Blood Transfusion in Trauma Patients With Significant Haemorrhage (CRASH-2): A Randomized, Placebo-Controlled Trial," *Lancet*, 2010, 376(9734):23-32.

Choi WS, Irwin MG, and Samman N, "The Effect of Tranexamic Acid on Blood Loss During Orthognathic Surgery: A Randomized Controlled Trial," *J Oral Maxillofac Surg*, 2009, 67 (1):125-33.

Dadure C, Sauter M, Bringuier S, et al, "Intraoperative Tranexamic Acid Reduces Blood Transfusion in Children Undergoing Craniosynostosis Surgery: A Randomized Double-Blind Study," *Anesthesiology*, 2011, 114(4):856-61.

Elwatidy S, Jamjoom Z, Elgamal E, et al, "Efficacy and Safety of Prophylactic Large Dose of Tranexamic Acid in Spine Surgery: A Prospective, Randomized, Double-Blind, Placebo-Controlled Study," *Spine*, 2008, 33(24):2577-80.

Fergusson DA, Hébert PC, Mazer CD, et al, "A Comparison of Aprotinin and Lysine Analogues in High-Risk Cardiac Surgery," *N Engl J Med*, 2008, 358(22):2319-31.

Gompels MM, Lock RJ, Abinun M, et al, "C1 Inhibitor Deficiency: Consensus Document," *Clin Exp Immunol*, 2005, 139(3):379-94.

Gravlee GP and Spiess B, "Pharmacologic Prophylaxis for Post-Cardiopulmonary Bypass Bleeding," *Cardiopulmonary Bypass: Principles and Practice*, 3rd ed, Philadelphia, PA: Lippincott Williams & Wilkins, 2008, 522-42.

Gungorduk K, Yildirim G, Asıcıoğlu O, et al, "Efficacy of Intravenous Tranexamic Acid In Reducing Blood Loss After Elective Cesarean Section: A Prospective, Randomized, Double-Blind, Placebo-Controlled Study," *Am J Perinatol*, 2011, 28(3):233-40.

Lozano M, Basora M, Peidro L, et al, "Effectiveness and Safety of Tranexamic Acid Administration During Total Knee Arhthroplasty," *Vox San*, 2008, 95(1):39-44.

Nuttall GA, Gutierrez MC, Dewey JD, et al, "A Preliminary Study of a New Tranexamic Acid Dosing Schedule for Cardiac Surgery," *J Cardiothorac Vasc Anesth*, 2008, 22(2):230-5.

Rahmani B and Jahadi HR, "Comparison of Tranexamic Acid and Prednisolone in the Treatment of Traumatic Hyphema," *Ophthalmology*, 1999, 106(2):375-9.

Rannikko A, Pétas A, and Taari K, "Tranexamic Acid in Control of Primary Hemorrhage During Transurethral Prostatectomy," *Urology*, 2004, 64(5):955-8.

Sethna NF, Zurakowski D, Brustowicz RM, et al, "Tranexamic Acid Reduces Intraoperative Blood Loss in Pediatric Patients Undergoing Scoliosis Surgery," *Anesthesiology*, 2005, 102(4):727-32.

Seto AH and Dunlap DS, "Tranexamic Acid in Oncology," *Ann Pharmacother*, 1996, 30 (7-8):868-70.

van der Staak FH, de Haan AF, Geven WB, et al, "Surgical Repair of Congenital Diaphragmatic Hernia During Extracorporeal Membrane Oxygenation: Hemorrhagic Complications and the Effect of Tranexamic Acid," *J Ped Surg*, 1997, 32(4):594-9.

Vangsted P and Nielsen PJ, "Tranexamic Acid and Traumatic Hyphaema, A Prospective Study," *Acta Ophthalmol (Copenh)*, 1983, 61(3):447-53.

Varnek L, Dalsgaard C, Hansen A, et al, "The Effect of Tranexamic Acid on Secondary Haemorrhage after Traumatic Hyphaema," *Acta Ophthalmol (Copenh)*, 1980, 58(5):787-793.

Wong J, El Beheiry H, Rampersaud YR, et al, "Tranexamic Acid Reduces Perioperative Blood Loss in Adult Patients Having Spinal Fusion Surgery," *Anesth Analg*, 2008, 107(5):1479-86.

◆ **Tranexamic Acid Injection BP (Can)** *see* Tranexamic Acid *on page 1392*

◆ **Transderm-V® (Can)** *see* Scopolamine (Systemic) *on page 1274*

◆ **Transderm Scōp®** *see* Scopolamine (Systemic) *on page 1274*

◆ ***trans*-Retinoic Acid** *see* Tretinoin (Systemic) *on page 1405*

◆ ***trans* Vitamin A Acid** *see* Tretinoin (Systemic) *on page 1405*

Trastuzumab (tras TU zoo mab)

Related Information

Management of Chemotherapy-Induced Nausea and Vomiting *on page 1786*

Principles of Anticancer Therapy *on page 1878*

Safe Handling of Hazardous Drugs *on page 1904*

Brand Names: U.S. Herceptin®

Brand Names: Canada Herceptin®

Index Terms anti-c-erB-2; anti-ERB-2; MOAB HER2; rhuMAb HER2

Generic Availability (U.S.) No

Pharmacologic Category Antineoplastic Agent, Anti-HER2; Antineoplastic Agent, Monoclonal Antibody; Monoclonal Antibody

Use Treatment (adjuvant) of HER2 overexpressing breast cancer as part of a combination regimen with doxorubicin, cyclophosphamide, and either paclitaxel or docetaxel; in combination with docetaxel and carboplatin; as a single agent following anthracycline-based combination treatment; treatment of HER2 overexpressing metastatic breast cancer in combination with paclitaxel as first-line treatment or as a single agent in patients who have received prior chemotherapy regimens for treatment of metastatic disease; treatment of HER2 overexpressing metastatic gastric or gastroesophageal junction adenocarcinoma in combination with cisplatin and either capecitabine or fluorouracil in patients who have not received prior treatment for metastatic disease

Unlabeled Use Treatment of HER2-positive metastatic breast cancer (in combination with pertuzumab and docetaxel) in patients who have not received prior anti-HER2 therapy or chemotherapy to treat metastatic disease; treatment of HER2 overexpressing metastatic breast cancer (in combination with lapatinib) which had progressed on prior trastuzumab containing therapy

Labeled Contraindications There are no contraindications listed within the manufacturer's labeling.

Canadian labeling: Hypersensitivity to trastuzumab, Chinese hamster ovary (CHO) cell proteins, or any component of the formulation

Pregnancy Risk Factor D

Lactation Excretion in breast milk unknown/not recommended

Warnings/Precautions Hazardous agent - use appropriate precautions for handling and disposal. **[U.S. Boxed Warning]: Trastuzumab is associated with symptomatic and asymptomatic reductions in left ventricular ejection fraction (LVEF) and heart failure (HF); the incidence is highest in patients receiving trastuzumab with an anthracycline-containing chemotherapy regimen. Evaluate LVEF in all patients prior to and during treatment; discontinue for cardiomyopathy.** Extreme caution should be used in patients with pre-existing cardiac disease or dysfunction. Prior or concurrent exposure to anthracyclines or radiation therapy significantly increases the risk of cardiomyopathy; other potential risk factors include advanced age, high or low body mass index, smoking, diabetes, and hyper/hypothyroidism. Discontinuation should be strongly considered in patients who develop a clinically significant reduction in LVEF during therapy; treatment with HF medications (eg, ACE inhibitors, beta-blockers) should be initiated. Withhold treatment for ≥16% decrease from pretreatment levels or LVEF below normal limits and ≥10% decrease from baseline (see Dosage Adjustment for Cardiotoxicity). Cardiomyopathy due to trastuzumab is generally reversible over a period of 1-3 months after discontinuation. Trastuzumab is also associated with arrhythmias, hypertension, mural thrombus formation, stroke, and even cardiac death.

[U.S. Boxed Warning]: Serious adverse events, including hypersensitivity reaction (anaphylaxis), infusion reactions (including fatalities), and pulmonary events (including acute respiratory distress syndrome [ARDS]) have been associated with trastuzumab. Discontinue for anaphylaxis, angioedema, ARDS or interstitial pneumonitis. Most of these events occur with the first infusion; pulmonary events may occur during or within 24 hours of the first infusion; delayed reactions have occurred. Interrupt infusion for dyspnea or significant hypotension; monitor until symptoms resolve. Infusion reactions may consist of fever and chills, and may also include nausea, vomiting, pain, headache dizziness, dyspnea, hypotension, rash and weakness. Retreatment of patients who experienced severe hypersensitivity reactions has been attempted (with premedication). Some patients tolerated retreatment, while others experienced a second severe reaction. When used in combination with myelosuppressive chemotherapy, trastuzumab may increase the incidence of neutropenia (moderate-to-severe) and febrile neutropenia; the incidence of anemia may be higher when trastuzumab is added to chemotherapy. Rare cases of nephrotic syndrome with evidence of glomerulopathy have been reported, with an onset of 4-18 months from trastuzumab initiation; complications may include volume overload and HF. The incidence of renal impairment was increased in metastatic gastric cancer patients when trastuzumab is added to chemotherapy.

May cause serious pulmonary toxicity (dyspnea, hypoxia, interstitial pneumonitis, pulmonary infiltrates, pleural effusion, noncardiogenic pulmonary edema, pulmonary insufficiency, acute respiratory distress syndrome, and/or pulmonary fibrosis); use caution in patients with pre-existing pulmonary disease or patients with extensive pulmonary tumor involvement. Establish HER2 status prior to treatment; has only been studied in patients with evidence of HER2 protein overexpression, either by validated immunohistochemistry (IHC) assay or fluorescence in situ hybridization (FISH) assay. Tests appropriate for the specific tumor type (breast or gastric) should be used to assess HER2 status. **[U.S. Boxed Warning]: Trastuzumab exposure during pregnancy may**

result in oligohydramnios and oligohydramnios sequence (pulmonary hypoplasia, skeletal malformations and neonatal death). Effective contraception is recommended during and for 6 months after treatment for women of childbearing potential.

Adverse Reactions Note: Percentages reported with single-agent therapy.

>10%:

- Cardiovascular: LVEF decreased (4% to 22%)
- Central nervous system: Pain (47%), fever (6% to 36%), chills (5% to 32%), headache (10% to 26%), insomnia (14%), dizziness (4% to 13%)
- Dermatologic: Rash (4% to 18%)
- Gastrointestinal: Nausea (6% to 33%), diarrhea (7% to 25%), vomiting (4% to 23%), abdominal pain (2% to 22%), anorexia (14%)
- Neuromuscular & skeletal: Weakness (4% to 42%), back pain (5% to 22%)
- Respiratory: Cough (5% to 26%), dyspnea (3% to 22%), rhinitis (2% to 14%), pharyngitis (12%)
- Miscellaneous: Infusion reaction (21% to 40%, chills and fever most common; severe: 1%), infection (20%)

1% to 10%:

- Cardiovascular: Peripheral edema (5% to 10%), edema (8%), HF (2% to 7%; severe: <1%), tachycardia (5%), hypertension (4%), arrhythmia (3%), palpitation (3%)
- Central nervous system: Depression (6%)
- Dermatologic: Acne (2%), nail disorder (2%), pruritus (2%)
- Gastrointestinal: Constipation (2%), dyspepsia (2%)
- Genitourinary: Urinary tract infection (3% to 5%)
- Hematologic: Anemia (4%), leukopenia (3%)
- Neuromuscular & skeletal: Paresthesia (2% to 9%), bone pain (3% to 7%), arthralgia (6% to 8%), myalgia (4%), muscle spasm (3%), peripheral neuritis (2%), neuropathy (1%)
- Respiratory: Sinusitis (2% to 9%), nasopharyngitis (8%), upper respiratory infection (3%), epistaxis (2%), pharyngolaryngeal pain (2%)
- Miscellaneous: Flu-like syndrome (2% to 10%), accidental injury (6%), influenza (4%), allergic reaction (3%), herpes simplex (2%)

<1%, postmarketing, and/or case reports (as a single-agent or with combination chemotherapy): Acute respiratory distress syndrome (ARDS), amblyopia, anaphylaxis, anaphylactoid reaction, angioedema, apnea, ascites, asthma, ataxia, bone necrosis, bronchospasm, cardiac arrest, cardiomyopathy, cellulitis, coagulopathy, colitis, confusion, deafness, esophageal ulcer, gastroenteritis, glomerulonephritis (membranous, focal and fibrillary), glomerulopathy, glomerulosclerosis, hematemesis, hemorrhage, hemorrhagic cystitis, hepatic failure, hepatitis, herpes zoster, hydrocephalus, hydronephrosis, hypercalcemia, hypersensitivity, hypotension, hypothyroidism, hypoxia, ileus, intestinal obstruction, interstitial pneumonitis, laryngitis, leukemia (acute), lymphangitis, mania, mural thrombosis, myopathy, nephrotic syndrome, neutropenia, oligohydramnios, pancreatitis, pancytopenia, paroxysmal nocturnal dyspnea, pathological fracture, pericardial effusion, pleural effusion, pneumonitis, pneumothorax, pulmonary edema (noncardiogenic), pulmonary fibrosis, pulmonary hypertension, pulmonary infiltrate, pyelonephritis, radiation injury, renal failure, respiratory distress, respiratory failure, seizure, sepsis, shock, skin ulcers, stroke, syncope, stomatitis, thyroiditis (autoimmune), vascular thrombosis, ventricular dysfunction, volume overload

Drug Interactions

Metabolism/Transport Effects None known.

Avoid Concomitant Use

Avoid concomitant use of Trastuzumab with any of the following: Belimumab

Increased Effect/Toxicity

Trastuzumab may increase the levels/effects of: Antineoplastic Agents (Anthracycline, Systemic); Belimumab; Immunosuppressants

The levels/effects of Trastuzumab may be increased by: Abciximab; PACLitaxel

Decreased Effect

Trastuzumab may decrease the levels/effects of: PACLitaxel

Storage/Stability Prior to reconstitution, store intact vials under refrigeration at 2°C to 8°C (36°F to 46°F). Following reconstitution with bacteriostatic SWFI, the solution in the vial is stable refrigerated for 28 days from the date of reconstitution; do not freeze. Solutions reconstituted with sterile water for injection without preservatives must be used immediately. The solution diluted in 250 mL NS for infusion is stable for 24 hours refrigerated; do not freeze.

Reconstitution Reconstitute each vial with 20 mL of bacteriostatic sterile water for injection to a concentration of 21 mg/mL. Swirl gently; do not shake. Allow vial to rest for ~5 minutes. If the patient has a known hypersensitivity to benzyl alcohol, trastuzumab may be reconstituted with sterile water for injection without preservatives, which must be used immediately. Further dilute the appropriate volume for the trastuzumab dose in 250 mL NS prior to administration. Gently invert bag to mix.

Mechanism of Action Trastuzumab is a monoclonal antibody which binds to the extracellular domain of the human epidermal growth factor receptor 2 protein (HER-2); it mediates antibody-dependent cellular cytotoxicity by inhibiting proliferation of cells which overexpress HER-2 protein.

Pharmacodynamics/Kinetics

Distribution: V_d: 44 mL/kg; not likely to cross the (intact) blood-brain barrier (due to the large molecule size)

Half-life elimination: Weekly dosing: Mean: 6 days (range: 1-32 days); every 3 week regimen: Mean: 16 days (range: 11-23 days)

Dosing

Adult & Geriatric Details concerning dosing in combination regimens should also be consulted.

Note: Missed dose recommendation (Canadian labeling, 2010): If a dose is missed by ≤1 week, the usual maintenance dose (based on patient's schedule) should be administered as soon as possible (do not wait until the next planned cycle); if a dose is missed by >1 week, then a loading dose (4 mg/kg if patient receives trastuzumab weekly; 8 mg/kg if on an every-3-week schedule) should be administered, followed by the usual maintenance dose and schedule.

Breast cancer, adjuvant treatment, HER2+: I.V. infusion:

With concurrent paclitaxel or docetaxel:

Initial loading dose: 4 mg/kg infused over 90 minutes, followed by

Maintenance dose: 2 mg/kg infused over 30 minutes weekly for total of 12 weeks, followed 1 week later (when concurrent chemotherapy completed) by 6 mg/kg infused over 30-90 minutes every 3 weeks for total therapy duration of 52 weeks

With concurrent docetaxel/carboplatin:

Initial loading dose: 4 mg/kg infused over 90 minutes, followed by

Maintenance dose: 2 mg/kg infused over 30 minutes weekly for total of 18 weeks, followed 1 week later (when concurrent chemotherapy completed) by 6 mg/kg infused over 30-90 minutes every 3 weeks for total therapy duration of 52 weeks

Following completion of anthracycline-based chemotherapy:

Initial loading dose: 8 mg/kg infused over 90 minutes, followed by

Maintenance dose: 6 mg/kg infused over 30-90 minutes every 3 weeks for total therapy duration of 52 weeks

Breast cancer, metastatic, HER2+ (either as a single agent or in combination with paclitaxel): I.V. infusion:

Initial loading dose: 4 mg/kg infused over 90 minutes, followed by

Maintenance dose: 2 mg/kg infused over 30 minutes weekly until disease progression

Gastric cancer, metastatic, HER2+ (in combination with cisplatin and either capecitabine or fluorouracil for 6 cycles followed by trastuzumab monotherapy; Bang, 2010; Van Cutsem, 2009): I.V. infusion:

Initial loading dose: 8 mg/kg infused over 90 minutes, followed by

Maintenance dose: 6 mg/kg infused over 30-90 minutes every 3 weeks until disease progression

Breast cancer, metastatic, HER2+ (unlabeled combinations):

Trastuzumab, pertuzumab, and docetaxel (in patients with no prior anti-HER2 therapy or chemotherapy to treat metastatic disease): Initial: 8 mg/kg followed by a maintenance dose of 6 mg/kg every 3 weeks until disease progression or unacceptable toxicity (Baselga, 2012)

Trastuzumab and lapatinib (in patients with progression on prior trastuzumab containing therapy): Initial: 4 mg/kg followed by a maintenance dose of 2 mg/kg every week (Blackwell, 2010; Blackwell, 2012)

Renal Impairment No dosage adjustment provided in manufacturer's labeling, although data suggest that the disposition of trastuzumab is not altered based on serum creatinine (up to 2 mg/dL)

Hepatic Impairment

No dosage adjustment provided in manufacturer's labeling.

Adjustment for Toxicity

Cardiotoxicity: LVEF ≥16% decrease from baseline or LVEF below normal limits and ≥10% decrease from baseline: Withhold treatment for at least 4 weeks and repeat LVEF every 4 weeks. May resume trastuzumab treatment if LVEF returns to normal limits within 4-8 weeks and remains at ≤15% decrease from baseline value. Discontinue permanently for persistent (>8 weeks) LVEF decline or for >3 incidents of treatment interruptions for cardiomyopathy.

Infusion-related events:

Mild-moderate infusion reactions: Decrease infusion rate.

Dyspnea, clinically significant hypotension: Interrupt infusion.

Severe or life-threatening infusion reactions: Discontinue.

Combination Regimens

Breast cancer:

AC-Paclitaxel-Trastuzumab on page 1518
Capecitabine-Trastuzumab on page 1541
Docetaxel-Pertuzumab-Trastuzumab (Breast) on page 1614
Docetaxel-Trastuzumab on page 1615
Docetaxel-Trastuzumab-Carboplatin on page 1615
Docetaxel-Trastuzumab-Cisplatin on page 1616
Docetaxel-Trastuzumab-FEC on page 1616

Docetaxel (Weekly)-Trastuzumab on page 1617
Lapatinib-Trastuzumab (Breast Cancer) on page 1698
Trastuzumab-Paclitaxel on page 1759
Trastuzumab-Paclitaxel-Carboplatin on page 1760
Trastuzumab-Paclitaxel (Weekly) on page 1760
Vinorelbine-Trastuzumab on page 1775
Vinorelbine-Trastuzumab-FEC on page 1775

Gastric cancer:

Trastuzumab-Cisplatin-Capecitabine (Gastric Cancer) on page 1757
Trastuzumab-Cisplatin-Fluorouracil (Gastric Cancer) on page 1758

Administration Administered by I.V. infusion; loading doses are infused over 90 minutes; maintenance doses may be infused over 30 minutes if tolerated. Do not administer with D_5W. **Do not administer I.V. push or by rapid bolus.**

Observe patients closely during the infusion for fever, chills, or other infusion-related symptoms. Treatment with acetaminophen, diphenhydramine, and/or meperidine is usually effective for managing infusion-related events.

Emetic Potential Low (10% to 30%)

Monitoring Parameters Assessment for HER2 overexpression and HER2 gene amplification by validated immunohistochemistry (IHC) or fluorescence *in situ* hybridization (FISH) methodology (pretherapy); test should be specific for cancer type (breast vs gastric cancer). Pregnancy test (prior to treatment). Monitor vital signs during infusion; signs and symptoms of cardiac dysfunction; LVEF (baseline, every 3 months during treatment, upon therapy completion and if component of adjuvant therapy, every 6 months for at least 2 years; if treatment is withheld for significant LVEF dysfunction, monitor LVEF at 4-week intervals); signs and symptoms of infusion reaction; if pregnancy inadvertently occurs during treatment, monitor amniotic fluid volume

Dosage Forms Excipient information presented when available (limited, particularly for generics); consult specific product labeling.

Injection, powder for reconstitution:

Herceptin®: 440 mg [contains benzyl alcohol (in diluent)]

References

Bader AA, Schlembach D, Tamussino KF, et al, "Anhydramnios Associated With Administration of Trastuzumab and Paclitaxel for Metastatic Breast Cancer During Pregnancy," *Lancet Oncol*, 2007, 8(1):79-81.

Bang YJ, Van Cutsem E, Feyereislova A, et al, "Trastuzumab in Combination With Chemotherapy Versus Chemotherapy Alone for Treatment of HER2-Positive Advanced Gastric or Gastro-Oesophageal Junction Cancer (ToGA): A Phase 3, Open-Label, Randomised Controlled Trial," *Lancet*, 2010, 376(9742):687-97.

Baselga J, Carbonell X, Castaneda-Soto NJ, et al, "Phase II Study of Efficacy, Safety, and Pharmacokinetics of Trastuzumab Monotherapy Administered on a 3-Weekly Schedule," *J Clin Oncol*, 2005, 23(10):2162-71.

Baselga J, Cortés J, Kim SB, et al, "Pertuzumab Plus Trastuzumab Plus Docetaxel for Metastatic Breast Cancer," *N Engl J Med*, 2012, 366(2):109-19.

Blackwell KL, Burstein HJ, Storniolo AM, et al, "Overall Survival Benefit With Lapatinib in Combination With Trastuzumab for Patients With Human Epidermal Growth Factor Receptor 2-Positive Metastatic Breast Cancer: Final Results From the EGF104900 Study," *J Clin Oncol*, 2012, 30(21):2585-92.

Blackwell KL, Burstein HJ, Storniolo AM, et al, "Randomized Study of Lapatinib Alone or in Combination With Trastuzumab in Women With ErbB2-Positive, Trastuzumab-Refractory Metastatic Breast Cancer," *J Clin Oncol*, 2010, 28(7):1124-30.

Floyd JD, Nguyen DT, Lobins RL, et al, "Cardiotoxicity of Cancer Therapy," *J Clin Oncol*, 2005, 23 (30):7685-96.

Leyland-Jones B, Gelmon K, Ayoub JP, et al, "Pharmacokinetics, Safety, and Efficacy of Trastuzumab Administered Every Three Weeks in Combination With Paclitaxel," *J Clin Oncol*, 2003, 21(21):3965-71.

National Comprehensive Cancer Network® (NCCN), "Clinical Practice Guidelines in Oncology™: Breast Cancer," Version 3.2010. Available at http://www.nccn.org/professionals/physician_gls/PDF/breast.pdf

Procter M, Suter TM, de Azambuja E, et al, "Longer-Term Assessment of Trastuzumab-Related Cardiac Adverse Events in the Herceptin Adjuvant (HERA) Trial," *J Clin Oncol*, 2010, 28 (21):3422-8.

Romond EH, Perez EA, Bryant J, et al, "Trastuzumab Plus Adjuvant Chemotherapy for Operable HER2-Positive Breast Cancer,"*N Engl J Med*, 2005, 353(16):1673-84.

Van Cutsem E, Kang Y, Chung H, et al, "Efficacy Results From the ToGA Trial: A Phase III Study of Trastuzumab Added to Standard Chemotherapy (CT) in First-Line Human Epidermal Growth Factor Receptor 2 (HER2) Positive Advanced Gastric Cancer (GC)," *J Clin Oncol*, 2009, 27(18s): LBA4509 [abstract LBA4509 from 2009 ASCO Annual Meeting].

◆ **Treanda®** *see* Bendamustine *on page* 158

◆ **Trelstar®** *see* Triptorelin *on page* 1413

Tretinoin (Systemic) (TRET i noyn)

Related Information

Chemotherapy and Cancer Treatment During Pregnancy *on page* 1829
Management of Chemotherapy-Induced Nausea and Vomiting *on page* 1786
Principles of Anticancer Therapy *on page* 1878
Safe Handling of Hazardous Drugs *on page* 1904

Brand Names: Canada Vesanoid®

Index Terms *trans* Vitamin A Acid; *trans*-Retinoic Acid; All-*trans* Retinoic Acid; All-*trans* Vitamin A Acid; ATRA; Ro 5488; tRA; Tretinoinum; Vesanoid

Generic Availability (U.S.) Yes

Pharmacologic Category Antineoplastic Agent, Miscellaneous; Retinoic Acid Derivative

Use Induction of remission in patients with acute promyelocytic leukemia (APL), French American British (FAB) classification M3 (including the M3 variant) characterized by t(15;17) translocation and/or PML/RARα gene presence

Unlabeled Use Post consolidation and maintenance therapy in APL; combination therapy (with arsenic trioxide) for remission induction in APL

Labeled Contraindications Hypersensitivity to tretinoin, other retinoids, parabens, or any component of the formulation

Pregnancy Risk Factor D

Lactation Excretion in breast milk unknown/not recommended

Warnings/Precautions Hazardous agent - use appropriate precautions for handling and disposal.

[U.S. Boxed Warning]: About 25% of patients with APL treated with tretinoin have experienced APL differentiation syndrome (formerly called retinoic acid-APL [RA-APL] syndrome), which is characterized by fever, dyspnea, acute respiratory distress, weight gain, radiographic pulmonary infiltrates and pleural or pericardial effusions, edema, and hepatic, renal, and/or multiorgan failure. DS usually occurs during the first month of treatment, with some cases reported following the first dose. DS has been observed with or without concomitant leukocytosis and has occasionally been accompanied by impaired myocardial contractility and episodic hypotension; endotracheal intubation and mechanical ventilation have been required in some cases due to progressive hypoxemia, and several patients have expired with multiorgan failure. About one-half of DS cases are severe, which is associated with increased mortality. Management has not been defined, although high-dose steroids given at the first suspicion appear to reduce morbidity and mortality. Regardless of the leukocyte count, at the first signs suggestive of DS, immediately initiate steroid therapy with dexamethasone 10 mg I.V. every 12 hours for 3-5 days; taper off over 2 weeks. Most patients do not require termination of tretinoin therapy during treatment of DS.

[U.S. Boxed Warning]: During treatment, ~40% of patients will develop rapidly evolving leukocytosis. A high WBC at diagnosis increases the risk for further leukocytosis and may be associated with a higher risk of life-threatening complications. If signs and symptoms of the APL-DS syndrome are present together with leukocytosis, initiate treatment with high-dose steroids immediately. Consider adding full-dose chemotherapy (including an anthracycline, if not contraindicated) to the tretinoin therapy on day 1 or 2 for patients presenting with a WBC count of >5 x 10^9/L. Consider adding chemotherapy immediately in patients who presented with a WBC count of <5 x 10^9/L, yet the WBC count reaches ≥6 x 10^9/L by day 5, or ≥10 x 10^9/L by day 10, or ≥15 x 10^9/L by day 28.

[U.S. Boxed Warning]: High risk of teratogenicity; if treatment with tretinoin is required in women of childbearing potential, two reliable forms of contraception should be used during and for 1 month after treatment. Repeat pregnancy testing and contraception counseling monthly throughout the period of treatment. If possible, initiation of treatment with tretinoin should be delayed until negative pregnancy test result is confirmed.

Retinoids have been associated with pseudotumor cerebri (benign intracranial hypertension), especially in children. Concurrent use of other drugs associated with this effect (eg, tetracyclines) may increase risk. Early signs and symptoms include papilledema, headache, nausea, vomiting, visual disturbances, intracranial noises, or pulsate tinnitus.

Up to 60% of patients experienced hypercholesterolemia or hypertriglyceridemia, which were reversible upon completion of treatment. Venous thrombosis and MI have been reported in patient without risk factors for thrombosis or MI; the risk for thrombosis (arterial and venous) is increased during the first month of treatment. Use with caution with antifibrinolytic agents; thrombotic complications have been reported (rarely) with concomitant use. Elevated liver function test results occur in 50% to 60% of patients during treatment. Carefully monitor liver function test results during treatment and give consideration to a temporary withdrawal of tretinoin if test results reach >5 times the upper limit of normal. Most liver function test abnormalities will resolve without interruption of treatment or after therapy completion. May cause headache, malaise, and/or dizziness; caution patients about performing tasks which require mental alertness (eg, operating machinery or driving). Patients with APL are at high risk and can have severe adverse reactions to tretinoin. **[U.S. Boxed Warning]: Should be administered under the supervision of an experienced cancer chemotherapy physician.** Tretinoin treatment for APL should be initiated early, discontinue if pending cytogenetic analysis does not confirm APL by t (15;17) translocation or the presence of the PML/RARα fusion protein (caused by translocation of the promyelocytic [PML] gene on chromosome 15 and retinoic acid receptor [RAR] alpha gene on chromosome 17).

Adverse Reactions Most patients will experience drug-related toxicity, especially headache, fever, weakness and fatigue. These are seldom permanent or irreversible and do not typically require therapy interruption.

>10%:

- Cardiovascular: Peripheral edema (52%), chest discomfort (32%), edema (29%), arrhythmias (23%), flushing (23%), hypotension (14%), hypertension (11%)
- Central nervous system: Headache (86%), fever (83%), malaise (66%), pain (37%), dizziness (20%), anxiety (17%), depression (14%), insomnia (14%), confusion (11%)
- Dermatologic: Skin/mucous membrane dryness (77%), rash (54%), pruritus (20%), alopecia (14%), skin changes (14%)
- Endocrine & metabolic: Hypercholesterolemia and/or hypertriglyceridemia (≤60%)
- Gastrointestinal: Nausea/vomiting (57%), GI hemorrhage (34%), abdominal pain (31%), mucositis (26%), diarrhea (23%), weight gain (23%), anorexia (17%), constipation (17%), weight loss (17%), dyspepsia (14%), abdominal distention (11%)
- Hematologic: Hemorrhage (60%), leukocytosis (40%), disseminated intravascular coagulation (DIC) (26%)
- Hepatic: Liver function tests increased (50% to 60%)
- Local: Phlebitis (11%)
- Neuromuscular & skeletal: Bone pain (77%), paresthesia (17%), myalgia (14%)
- Ocular: Ocular disorder (17%), visual disturbances (17%)
- Otic: Earache/ear fullness (23%)
- Renal: Renal insufficiency (11%)
- Respiratory: Upper respiratory tract disorders (63%), dyspnea (60%), respiratory insufficiency (26%), pleural effusion (20%), expiratory wheezing (14%), pneumonia (14%), rales (14%)
- Miscellaneous: Shivering (63%), infections (58%), retinoic acid-acute promyelocytic leukemia syndrome differentiation syndrome (≤25%), diaphoresis (20%)

1% to 10%:

- Cardiovascular: Cerebral hemorrhage (9%), cardiac failure (6%), facial edema (6%), pallor (6%), cardiac arrest (3%), cardiomyopathy (3%), heart enlarged (3%), heart murmur (3%), ischemia (3%), MI (3%), myocarditis (3%), pericarditis (3%), stroke (3%)
- Central nervous system: Agitation (9%), intracranial hypertension (9%), hallucination (6%), aphasia (3%), cerebellar edema (3%), CNS depression (3%), coma (3%), dementia (3%), encephalopathy (3%), facial paralysis (3%), forgetfulness (3%), hypotaxia (3%), hypothermia (3%), light reflex absent (3%), seizure (3%), slow speech (3%), somnolence (3%), spinal cord disorder (3%), unconsciousness (3%)
- Dermatologic: Cellulitis (8%)
- Endocrine & metabolic: Fluid imbalance (6%), acidosis (3%)
- Gastrointestinal: Hepatosplenomegaly (9%), ulcer (3%)
- Genitourinary: Dysuria (9%), micturition frequency (3%), prostate enlarged (3%)
- Hepatic: Ascites (3%), hepatitis (3%)
- Neuromuscular & skeletal: Flank pain (9%), abnormal gait (3%), asterixis (3%), bone inflammation (3%), dysarthria (3%), hemiplegia (3%), hyporeflexia (3%), leg weakness (3%), tremor (3%)
- Ocular: Visual acuity change (6%), agnosia (3%), visual field deficit (3%)
- Otic: Hearing loss (6%)
- Renal: Acute renal failure (3%), renal tubular necrosis (3%)

Respiratory: Lower respiratory tract disorders (9%), pulmonary infiltration (6%), bronchial asthma (3%), larynx edema (3%), pulmonary hypertension (3%)

Miscellaneous: Lymph disorder (6%)

<1%, postmarketing, and/or case reports: Arterial thrombosis, basophilia, erythema nodosum, genital ulceration, hypercalcemia, hyperhistaminemia, irreversible hearing loss, myositis, organomegaly, pancreatitis, pseudotumor cerebri, renal infarct, Sweet's syndrome, thrombocytosis, vasculitis (skin), venous thrombosis

Drug Interactions

Metabolism/Transport Effects Substrate of CYP2A6 (minor), CYP2B6 (minor), CYP2C8 (major), CYP2C9 (minor); **Note:** Assignment of Major/Minor substrate status based on clinically relevant drug interaction potential; **Inhibits** CYP2C9 (weak); **Induces** CYP2E1 (weak/moderate)

Avoid Concomitant Use

Avoid concomitant use of Tretinoin (Systemic) with any of the following: BCG; Multivitamins/Minerals (with ADEK, Folate, Iron); Natalizumab; Pimecrolimus; Tacrolimus (Topical); Tetracycline Derivatives; Vaccines (Live); Vitamin A

Increased Effect/Toxicity

Tretinoin (Systemic) may increase the levels/effects of: Antifibrinolytic Agents; Leflunomide; Natalizumab; Porfimer; Vaccines (Live); Vitamin A

The levels/effects of Tretinoin (Systemic) may be increased by: CYP2C8 Inhibitors (Moderate); CYP2C8 Inhibitors (Strong); Deferasirox; Denosumab; Mifepristone; Multivitamins/Minerals (with ADEK, Folate, Iron); Pimecrolimus; Roflumilast; Tacrolimus (Topical); Tetracycline Derivatives; Trastuzumab

Decreased Effect

Tretinoin (Systemic) may decrease the levels/effects of: BCG; Coccidioidin Skin Test; Contraceptives (Estrogens); Contraceptives (Progestins); Sipuleucel-T; Vaccines (Inactivated); Vaccines (Live)

The levels/effects of Tretinoin (Systemic) may be decreased by: CYP2C8 Inducers (Strong); Echinacea

Ethanol/Nutrition/Herb Interactions

Ethanol: Avoid ethanol (may increase CNS depression).

Food: Absorption of retinoids has been shown to be enhanced when taken with food.

Herb/Nutraceutical: St John's wort may decrease tretinoin levels. Avoid dong quai, St John's wort (may also cause photosensitization). Avoid additional vitamin A supplementation; may lead to vitamin A toxicity.

Storage/Stability Store capsule at 15°C to 30°C (59°F to 86°F). Protect from light.

Mechanism of Action Tretinoin appears to bind one or more nuclear receptors and decreases proliferation and induces differentiation of APL cells; initially produces maturation of primitive promyelocytes and repopulates the marrow and peripheral blood with normal hematopoietic cells to achieve complete remission

Pharmacodynamics/Kinetics

Absorption: Well absorbed

Protein binding: >95%, predominantly to albumin

Metabolism: Hepatic via CYP; primary metabolite: 4-oxo-all-*trans*-retinoic acid; displays autometabolism

Half-life elimination: Terminal: Parent drug: 0.5-2 hours

Time to peak, serum: 1-2 hours
Excretion: Urine (63%); feces (30%)

Dosing

Adult & Geriatric Details concerning dosing in combination regimens should also be consulted. **Note:** Induction treatment of APL with tretinoin should be initiated early; discontinue if pending cytogenetic analysis does not confirm t (15;17) translocation or the presence of the PML/RARα fusion protein.

Acute promyelocytic leukemia (APL): Oral:

Remission induction: 45 mg/m^2/day in 2 equally divided doses until documentation of complete remission (CR); discontinue 30 days after CR or after 90 days of treatment, whichever occurs first

Remission induction (in combination with an anthracycline; unlabeled use): 45 mg/m^2/day in 2 equally divided doses until complete remission or 90 days (Sanz, 2004; Sanz, 2008)

Consolidation therapy, intermediate- and high-risk patients (unlabeled use): 45 mg/m^2/day in 2 equally divided doses for 15 days each month for 3 months (Sanz, 2004)

Maintenance therapy, intermediate- and high-risk patients (unlabeled use): 45 mg/m^2/day in 2 equally divided doses for 15 days every 3 months for 2 years (Sanz, 2004)

Pediatric Details concerning dosing in combination regimens should also be consulted. **Note:** Induction treatment of APL with tretinoin should be initiated early; discontinue if pending cytogenetic analysis does not confirm t(15;17) translocation or the presence of the PML/RARα fusion protein.

Acute promyelocytic leukemia (APL): Oral:

Remission induction: 45 mg/m^2/day in 2 equally divided doses until documentation of complete remission (CR); discontinue 30 days after CR or after 90 days of treatment, whichever occurs first

Remission induction (in combination with an anthracycline; unlabeled use): 25 mg/m^2/day in 2 equally divided doses until complete remission or 90 days (Ortega, 2005)

Consolidation therapy, intermediate- and high-risk patients (unlabeled use): 25 mg/m^2/day in 2 equally divided doses for 15 days each month for 3 months (Ortega, 2005)

Maintenance therapy, intermediate- and high-risk patients (unlabeled use): 25 mg/m^2/day in 2 equally divided doses for 15 days every 3 months for 2 years (Ortega, 2005)

Adjustment for Toxicity

APL differentiation syndrome: Initiate dexamethasone 10 mg I.V. every 12 hours for 3-5 days; consider interrupting tretinoin until resolution of hypoxia

Liver function tests >5 times the upper limit of normal: Consider temporarily withholding treatment

Combination Regimens

Leukemia, acute promyelocytic:

Tretinoin-Arsenic Trioxide (APL) on page 1761
Tretinoin-Daunorubicin (APL) on page 1762
Tretinoin-Daunorubicin-Cytarabine (APL) on page 1762
Tretinoin-Idarubicin (APL) on page 1764

Administration Administer orally with a meal; do not crush capsules.

Although the manufacturer does not recommend the use of the capsule contents to extemporaneously prepare tretinoin suspension, there are limited case reports of use in patients who are unable to swallow the capsules whole. In a patient with a nasogastric (NG) tube, tretinoin capsules were cut open, with partial aspiration of the contents into a glass syringe, the residual capsule contents were mixed with soy bean oil and aspirated into the same syringe and administered (Shaw, 1995). Tretinoin capsules have also been mixed with sterile water (~20 mL) and heated in a water bath (37°C) to melt the capsules and create an oily suspension for NG tube administration (Bargetzi, 1996). Tretinoin has also been administered sublingually by squeezing the capsule contents beneath the tongue (Kueh, 1999). Low plasma concentrations have been reported when tretinoin has been administered through a feeding tube, although patient-specific impaired absorption or a lack of excipient (eg, soybean oil) may have been a contributing factor (Takitani, 2004).

Emetic Potential Low (10% to 30%)

Extemporaneous Preparations Hazardous agent: Use appropriate precautions for handling and disposal.

Although the manufacturer does not recommend the use of the capsule contents to extemporaneously prepare a suspension of tretinoin (due to reports of low plasma levels) (Vesanoid® data on file), there are limited case reports of use in patients who are unable to swallow the capsules whole. In a patient with a nasogastric (NG) tube, tretinoin capsules were cut open, with partial aspiration of the contents aspirated into a glass syringe. The residual capsule contents were mixed with soybean oil, aspirated into the syringe, and administered (Shaw, 1995). Tretinoin capsules have also been mixed with sterile water (~20 mL) and heated in a water bath to melt the capsules and create an oily suspension for NG tube administration (Bargetzi, 1996). Tretinoin has also been administered sublingually by squeezing the capsule contents beneath the tongue (Kueh, 1999).

Bargetzi MJ, Tichelli A, Gratwohl A, et al, "Oral All-Transretinoic Acid Administration in Intubated Patients With Acute Promyelocytic Leukemia," *Schweiz Med Wochenschr*, 1996, 126 (45):1944-5.

Kueh YK, Liew PP, Ho PC, et al, "Sublingual Administration of All-*Trans*-Retinoic Acid to a Comatose Patient With Acute Promyelocytic Leukemia," *Ann Pharmacother*, 1999, 33(4):503-5.

Shaw PJ, Atkins MC, Nath CE, et al, "ATRA Administration in the Critically Ill Patient," *Leukemia*, 1995, 9(7):1288.

Vesanoid® data on file, Roche Pharmaceuticals

Monitoring Parameters Bone marrow cytology to confirm t(15;17) translocation or the presence of the PML/RARα fusion protein (do not withhold treatment initiation for results); monitor CBC with differential, coagulation profile, liver function test results, and triglyceride and cholesterol levels frequently; monitor closely for signs of APL differentiation syndrome (eg, monitor volume status, pulmonary status, temperature, respiration)

Dietary Considerations The absorption of retinoids (as a class) is enhanced when taken with food. Capsule contains soybean oil.

Dosage Forms Excipient information presented when available (limited, particularly for generics); consult specific product labeling.

Capsule, oral: 10 mg

References

Bargetzi MJ, Tichelli A, Gratwohl A, et al, "Oral All-Transretinoic Acid Administration in Intubated Patients With Acute Promyelocytic Leukemia," *Schweiz Med Wochenschr*, 1996, 126 (45):1944-5.

Gregory J, Kim H, Alonzo T, et al, "Treatment of Children With Acute Promyelocytic Leukemia: Results of the First North American Intergroup Trial INT0129," *Pediatr Blood Cancer*, 2009, 53 (6):1005-10.

Kueh YK, Liew PP, Ho PC, et al, "Sublingual Administration of All-*Trans*-Retinoic Acid to a Comatose Patient With Acute Promyelocytic Leukemia," *Ann Pharmacother*, 1999, 33(4):503-5.

Montesinos P, Bergua JM, Vellenga E, et al, "Differentiation Syndrome in Patients With Acute Promyelocytic Leukemia Treated with All-*Trans* Retinoic Acid and Anthracycline Chemotherapy: Characteristics, Outcomes, and Prognostic Factors," *Blood*, 2009, 113(4):775-83.

Ortega JJ, Madero L, Martin G, et al, "Treatment With All-*Trans* Retinoic Acid and Anthracycline Monochemotherapy for Children With Acute Promyelocytic Leukemia: A Multicenter Study by the PETHEMA Group," *J Clin Oncol*, 2005, 23(30):7632-40.

Sanz MA, Grimwade D, Tallman MS, et al, "Management of Acute Promyelocytic Leukemia: Recommendations From an Expert Panel on Behalf of the European LeukemiaNet," *Blood*, 2009, 113(9):1875-91.

Sanz MA, Martin G, Gonzalez M, et al, "Risk-Adapted Treatment of Acute Promyelocytic Leukemia With All-*Trans*-Retinoic Acid and Anthracycline Monochemotherapy: A Multicenter Study by the PETHEMA Group," *Blood*, 2004, 103(4):1237-43.

Sanz MA, Montesinos P, Vellenga E, et al, "Risk-Adapted Treatment of Acute Promyelocytic Leukemia With All-*Trans*-Retinoic Acid and Anthracycline Monochemotherapy: Long-Term Outcome of the LPA 99 Multicenter Study by the PETHEMA Group," *Blood*, 2008, 112(8):3130-4.

Shaw PJ, Atkins MC, Nath CE, et al, "ATRA Administration in the Critically Ill Patient," *Leukemia*, 1995, 9(7):1288.

Smith MA, Adamson PC, Balis FM, et al, "Phase I and Pharmacokinetic Evaluation of All-*trans*-Retinoic Acid in Pediatric Patients With Cancer," *J Clin Oncol*, 1992, 10(11):1666-73.

Takitani K, Nakao Y, Kosada Y, et al, "Low Plasma Levels of All-*Trans* Retinoic Acid After Feeding Tube Administration for Acute Promyelocytic Leukemia," *Am J Hematol*, 2004, 76(1):97-8.

◆ **Tretinoinum** *see* Tretinoin (Systemic) *on page 1405*

◆ **Trexall™** *see* Methotrexate *on page 949*

◆ **Triacetyluridine** *see* Uridine Triacetate *on page 1419*

◆ **Tridural™ (Can)** *see* TraMADol *on page 1388*

◆ **Triethylenethiophosphoramide** *see* Thiotepa *on page 1357*

Trimethobenzamide (trye meth oh BEN za mide)

Related Information

Management of Chemotherapy-Induced Nausea and Vomiting *on page 1786*

Brand Names: U.S. Tigan®

Brand Names: Canada Tigan®

Index Terms Trimethobenzamide Hydrochloride

Generic Availability (U.S.) Yes

Pharmacologic Category Antiemetic

Use Treatment of postoperative nausea and vomiting; treatment of nausea associated with gastroenteritis

Labeled Contraindications Hypersensitivity to trimethobenzamide or any component of the formulation; injection contraindicated in children

Lactation Excretion in breast milk unknown

Warnings/Precautions May mask emesis due to Reye's syndrome or mimic CNS effects of Reye's syndrome in patients with emesis of other etiologies. Antiemetic effects may mask toxicity of other drugs or conditions (eg, intestinal obstruction). May cause drowsiness; patient should avoid tasks requiring alertness (eg, driving, operating machinery). May cause extrapyramidal symptoms (EPS) which may be confused with CNS symptoms of primary disease responsible for emesis. Avoid use in the elderly due to the risk of EPS adverse effects combined with lower efficacy, as compared to other antiemetics (Beers Criteria). Risk of CNS adverse effects (eg, coma, EPS, seizure) may be increased in patients with acute febrile illness, dehydration, electrolyte imbalance, encephalitis, or gastroenteritis; use caution. Allergic-type skin reactions have been reported with use; discontinue with signs of sensitization. Trimethobenzamide clearance is predominantly renal; dosage reductions may be recommended in patient with renal impairment. Use capsule formulation with caution in children; antiemetics are not recommended for uncomplicated vomiting in children, limit antiemetic use to prolonged vomiting of known etiology. Use of injection is contraindicated in children.

Adverse Reactions Frequency not defined.

Cardiovascular: Hypotension (I.V. administration)

Central nervous system: Coma, depression, disorientation, dizziness, drowsiness, EPS, headache, Parkinson-like symptoms, seizure

Dermatologic: Allergic-type skin reactions

Gastrointestinal: Diarrhea

Hematologic: Blood dyscrasias

Hepatic: Jaundice

Local: Injection site burning, pain, redness, stinging, or swelling

Neuromuscular & skeletal: Muscle cramps, opisthotonos

Ocular: Blurred vision

Miscellaneous: Hypersensitivity reactions

Drug Interactions

Metabolism/Transport Effects None known.

Avoid Concomitant Use

Avoid concomitant use of Trimethobenzamide with any of the following: Aclidinium; Ipratropium (Oral Inhalation); Tiotropium

Increased Effect/Toxicity

Trimethobenzamide may increase the levels/effects of: AbobotulinumtoxinA; Anticholinergics; Cannabinoids; Mirabegron; OnabotulinumtoxinA; Potassium Chloride; RimabotulinumtoxinB; Tiotropium; Topiramate

The levels/effects of Trimethobenzamide may be increased by: Aclidinium; Ipratropium (Oral Inhalation); Pramlintide

Decreased Effect

Trimethobenzamide may decrease the levels/effects of: Acetylcholinesterase Inhibitors (Central); Secretin

The levels/effects of Trimethobenzamide may be decreased by: Acetylcholinesterase Inhibitors (Central)

Ethanol/Nutrition/Herb Interactions Ethanol: Concomitant use should be avoided (sedative effects may be additive).

Storage/Stability Store capsules and injection solution at room temperature of 25°C (77°F); excursions permitted to 15°C to 30°C (59°F to 86°F).

Mechanism of Action Acts centrally to inhibit the medullary chemoreceptor trigger zone by blocking emetic impulses to the vomiting center

Pharmacodynamics/Kinetics

Onset of action: Antiemetic: Oral: 10-40 minutes; I.M.: 15-35 minutes

Duration: 3-4 hours

Metabolism: Via oxidation, forms metabolite trimethobenzamide N-oxide

Bioavailability: Oral: 60% to 100%

Half-life elimination: 7-9 hours

Time to peak: Oral: ~45 minutes; I.M.: ~30 minutes

Excretion: Urine (30% to 50%, as unchanged drug)

Dosing

Adult

Nausea, vomiting:

Oral: 300 mg 3-4 times/day

I.M.: 200 mg 3-4 times/day

Postoperative nausea and vomiting (PONV): I.M.: 200 mg, followed 1 hour later by a second 200 mg dose

Geriatric Refer to adult dosing. Consider dosage reduction or increasing dosing interval in elderly patients with renal impairment (specific adjustment guidelines are not provided in the manufacturer's labeling).

Pediatric Nausea, vomiting: Children >40 kg: Oral: Refer to adult dosing. (Injection is contraindicated in children.)

Renal Impairment Cl_{cr} ≤70 mL/minute: Consider dosage reduction or increasing dosing interval (specific adjustment guidelines are not provided in the manufacturer's labeling)

Administration

Injection: Administer I.M. only; not for I.V. administration. Inject deep into upper outer quadrant of gluteal muscle.

Capsule: Administer capsule orally without regard to meals.

Monitoring Parameters Renal function (at baseline)

Dosage Forms Excipient information presented when available (limited, particularly for generics); consult specific product labeling.

Capsule, oral, as hydrochloride: 300 mg
Tigan®: 300 mg

Injection, solution, as hydrochloride: 100 mg/mL (20 mL)
Tigan®: 100 mg/mL (20 mL)

Injection, solution, as hydrochloride [preservative free]: 100 mg/mL (2 mL)
Tigan®: 100 mg/mL (2 mL)

References

ACOG (American College of Obstetricians and Gynecologists) Practice Bulletin: "Nausea and Vomiting of Pregnancy," *Obstet Gynecol*, 2004, 103(4):803-14.

American Geriatrics Society 2012 Beers Criteria Update Expert Panel, "American Geriatrics Society Updated Beers Criteria for Potentially Inappropriate Medication Use in Older Adults," *J Am Geriatr Soc*, 2012, 60(4):616-31.

Ginsburg CM and Clahsen J, "Evaluation of Trimethobenzamide Hydrochloride (Tigan®) Suppositories for Treatment of Nausea and Vomiting in Children," *J Pediatr*, 1980, 96(4):767-9.

◆ **Trimethobenzamide Hydrochloride** *see* Trimethobenzamide *on page 1411*

◆ **Trimethoprim and Sulfamethoxazole** *see* Sulfamethoxazole and Trimethoprim *on page 1302*

Triptorelin (trip toe REL in)

Related Information

Safe Handling of Hazardous Drugs *on page 1904*

Brand Names: U.S. Trelstar®

Brand Names: Canada Decapeptyl®; Trelstar®

Index Terms AY-25650; CL-118,532; D-Trp(6)-LHRH; Detryptoreline; Triptorelin Pamoate; Tryptoreline

Generic Availability (U.S.) No

Pharmacologic Category Gonadotropin Releasing Hormone Agonist

Use Palliative treatment of advanced prostate cancer

Decapeptyl® (Canadian labeling; not available in U.S.): Adjunctive therapy in women undergoing controlled ovarian hyperstimulation for assisted reproductive technologies (ART)

Unlabeled Use Treatment of endometriosis, *in vitro* fertilization, precocious puberty, uterine sarcoma; treatment of paraphilia/hypersexuality

Labeled Contraindications Hypersensitivity to triptorelin or any component of the formulation, other GnRH agonists or GnRH; pregnancy

Canadian labeling: Additional contraindications (not in U.S. labeling): Breast-feeding women

Pregnancy Risk Factor X

Lactation Excretion in breast milk unknown/contraindicated

Warnings/Precautions Hazardous agent - use appropriate precautions for handling and disposal. Transient increases in testosterone can lead to worsening symptoms (bone pain, hematuria, bladder outlet obstruction, neuropathy, spinal cord compression) of prostate cancer during the first few weeks of therapy. Androgen-deprivation therapy may increase the risk for cardiovascular disease (Levine, 2010) and for decreased bone mineral density. Hyperglycemia has been reported with androgen deprivation therapy (in prostate cancer) and may manifest as diabetes or worsening of pre-existing diabetes; monitor blood glucose and/or Hb A_{1c}. Cases of spinal cord compression have been reported with GnRH agonists. Closely observe (during the first 2 weeks of treatment) patients with metastatic vertebral lesions or urinary tract obstruction. Hypersensitivity reactions including angioedema, anaphylaxis and anaphylactic shock have rarely occurred; discontinue if severe reaction occurs. Patients with preexisting depression should be monitored closely during therapy; mood changes including depression have been reported with use. Rare cases of pituitary apoplexy (frequently secondary to pituitary adenoma) have been observed with GnRH agonist administration (onset from 1 hour to usually <2 weeks); may present as sudden headache, vomiting, visual or mental status changes, and infrequently cardiovascular collapse; immediate medical attention required.

Decapeptyl® (Canadian availability; not available in U.S.) may increase the risk of ovarian hyperstimulation syndrome (OHSS) and ovarian cysts. OHSS is characterized by severe ovarian enlargement, abdominal pain/distention, nausea, vomiting, diarrhea, dyspnea, and oliguria, and may be accompanied by ascites, pleural effusion, hypovolemia, electrolyte imbalance, hemoperitoneum, and thromboembolic events. If severe hyperstimulation occurs, stop treatment and hospitalize patient. This syndrome develops rapidly with 24 hours to several days and generally occurs during the 7-10 days immediately following treatment.

Adverse Reactions **Prostate cancer:** As reported with all strengths; frequency of effect may vary by strength:

>10%:

- Endocrine & metabolic: Hot flashes (59% to 73%), glucose increased, testosterone levels increased (peak: days 2-4; decline to low levels by weeks 3-4)
- Hematologic: Hemoglobin decreased, RBC count decreased
- Hepatic: Alkaline phosphatase increased (2% to >10%), ALT increased, AST increased
- Neuromuscular & skeletal: Skeletal pain (12% to 13%)
- Renal: BUN increased

1% to 10%:

- Cardiovascular: Leg edema (6%), hypertension (1% to 4%), chest pain (2%), edema (2%), peripheral edema (≤1%)
- Central nervous system: Headache (2% to 7%), pain (2% to 3%), dizziness (1% to 3%), fatigue (2%), insomnia (1% to 2%), emotional lability (1%)
- Dermatologic: Rash (2%), pruritus (1%)
- Endocrine & metabolic: Breast pain (2%), gynecomastia (2%), libido decreased (2%)
- Gastrointestinal: Nausea (3%), anorexia (2%), constipation (2%), dyspepsia (2%), vomiting (2%), abdominal pain (1%), diarrhea (1%)

Genitourinary: Erectile dysfunction (10%), testicular atrophy (8%), impotence (2% to 7%), dysuria (5%), urinary retention (≤1%), urinary tract infection (≤1%)
Hematologic: Anemia (1%)
Local: Injection site pain (4%)
Neuromuscular & skeletal: Leg pain (2% to 5%), back pain (1% to 3%), leg cramps (2%), arthralgia (1% to 2%), extremity pain (1%), myalgia (1%), weakness (1%)
Ocular: Conjunctivitis (1%), eye pain (1%)
Respiratory: Cough (2%), dyspnea (1%), pharyngitis (1%) **Reproductive studies:**

>10%:
Central nervous system: Headache (4% to 27%)
Gastrointestinal: Abdominal pain (9% to 15%)
Genitourinary: Vaginal hemorrhage (2% to 24%)
Local: Injection site inflammation (10% to 12%)

1% to 10%:
Cardiovascular: Flushing (4%)
Central nervous system: Dizziness (4% to 5%), fatigue (3% to 4%), malaise (2%)
Endocrine & metabolic: Spontaneous abortion (7%), dysmenorrhea (2% to 6%), OHSS (3%), hot flashes (2%), ovarian cyst (1%)
Gastrointestinal: Nausea (3% to 10%), vomiting (3%), abdominal distension (2%), diarrhea (2%)
Genitourinary: Pelvic pain (8%), adnexa uteri pain (2%), leukorrhea (2%)
Local: Injection site pain (4% to 7%), injection site bruising (3%), injection site reaction (2% to 3%)
Neuromuscular & skeletal: Postprocedural pain (4%), back pain (3%), post-operative pain (3%)
Respiratory: Upper respiratory tract infection (4%), pharyngitis (3%), dyspnea (2%), rhinitis (2%)
Miscellaneous: Influenza-like symptoms (3%)

Postmarketing and/or case reports: Allergic reaction, anaphylaxis, angioedema, bladder outlet obstruction, hematuria, hypersensitivity reactions, circulatory collapse, hematuria, hypersensitivity reactions, injection site necrosis, neuropathy, pituitary apoplexy, renal dysfunction, spinal cord compression; thromboembolic events (cerebrovascular events, DVT, MI, pulmonary emboli, thrombophlebitis, TIA); tumor flare, urethral obstruction

Drug Interactions

Metabolism/Transport Effects None known.

Avoid Concomitant Use There are no known interactions where it is recommended to avoid concomitant use.

Increased Effect/Toxicity There are no known significant interactions involving an increase in effect.

Decreased Effect

Triptorelin may decrease the levels/effects of: Antidiabetic Agents

Storage/Stability Trelstar®:

U.S. labeling: Store at 20°C to 25°C (68°F to 77°F). Do not freeze MIXJECT® system. Reconstitute with 2 mL sterile water for injection. Shake well to obtain a uniform suspension. Solution will appear milky. Administer immediately after reconstitution.

MIXJECT® System: Follow manufacturer's instructions for mixing prior to use.

Canadian labeling:

Trelstar® with MIXJECT system: Store at 20°C to 25°C (68°F to 77°F). Protect from light. Do not freeze MIXJECT® system. Reconstitute with 2 mL sterile water for injection. Shake well to obtain a uniform suspension. Solution will appear milky. Administer immediately after reconstitution.

Trelstar® vials without MIXJECT system: Store at 4°C to 25 °C (39°F to 77°F); do not freeze. Protect from light.

Decapeptyl® (Canadian availability; not available in U.S.): Store at 2°C to 8°C (36°F to 46°F); do not freeze. Protect from light.

Reconstitution Trelstar®: Reconstitute with 2 mL sterile water for injection. Shake well to obtain a uniform suspension. Solution will appear milky. Administer immediately after reconstitution. When using MIXJECT® system, follow manufacturer's instructions for mixing prior to use.

Mechanism of Action Causes suppression of ovarian and testicular steroidogenesis due to decreased levels of LH and FSH with subsequent decrease in testosterone (male) and estrogen (female) levels. After chronic and continuous administration, usually 2-4 weeks after initiation, a sustained decrease in LH and FSH secretion occurs. When used for ART, prevents premature LH surge in women undergoing controlled ovarian hyperstimulation.

Pharmacodynamics/Kinetics

Distribution: V_d: 30-33 L

Protein binding: None

Metabolism: Unknown; unlikely to involve CYP; no known metabolites

Half-life elimination: 2.8 ± 1.2 hours

Moderate-to-severe renal impairment: 6.5-7.7 hours

Hepatic impairment: 7.6 hours

Time to peak: 1-3 hours

Excretion: Urine (42% as intact peptide); hepatic

Dosing

Adult & Geriatric

Advanced prostate carcinoma: I.M.:

3.75 mg once every 4 weeks **or**

11.25 mg once every 12 weeks **or**

22.5 mg once every 24 weeks

Controlled ovarian hyperstimulation for assisted reproductive technologies (ART) (adjunctive therapy): *Canadian labeling (Decapeptyl®; not available in U.S.):* Females: SubQ: Usual dose: 0.1 mg once daily initiated on day 2 or 3 or days 21-23 of cycle (or 5-7 days prior to expected onset of menses). Dose may be adjusted according to ovarian response as measured by ovarian ultrasound with or without serum estradiol levels. Treatment is continued until follicles achieve suitable size (typically 4-7 weeks).

Treatment of paraphilia/hypersexuality (unlabeled use; Guay, 2009; Thibaut, 1993): Males:

Note: May cause an initial increase in androgen concentrations which may be treated with an antiandrogen (eg, flutamide, cyproterone) for 1-2 months (Guay, 2009). Avoid use in patients with osteoporosis or active pituitary pathology.

SubQ: Test dose: 1 mg (observe for hypersensitivity)

I.M.: 3.75 mg monthly

Renal Impairment No dosage adjustment provided in manufacturer's labeling; however, compared to healthy subjects, triptorelin exposure was increased in moderate to severe renal impairment; the significance of these findings has not been determined.

Hepatic Impairment No dosage adjustment provided in manufacturer's labeling; however, compared to healthy subjects, triptorelin exposure was increased in hepatic impairment (degree not specified); the significance of these findings has not been determined.

Administration

Administer by I.M. injection into the buttock; alternate injection sites. Administer immediately after reconstitution.

Decapeptyl® (Canadian availability; not available in U.S.) is administered by subcutaneous injection into the lower abdomen. If a dose is missed, it can be administered on the same day; however, do not double doses.

Monitoring Parameters Serum testosterone levels, prostate-specific antigen, glucose and Hb A_{1c} (periodically)

Decapeptyl® (Canadian availability; not available in U.S.): Negative pregnancy test prior to initiation of therapy; signs/symptoms of allergic reaction for 30 minutes after administration; ultrasound and/or estradiol levels to assess follicle development; ultrasound to assess number and size of follicles

Treatment of paraphilia/hypersexuality (unlabeled use): The following monitoring has been recommended for other GnRH agonists: CBC (baseline, monthly for 4 months then every 6 months); serum testosterone (baseline, monthly for 4 months then every 6 months); serum LH (baseline and every 6 months), FSH (baseline), serum BUN and creatinine (baseline and every 6 months); bone density (baseline and yearly); ECG (baseline) (Reilly, 2000)

Test Interactions Pituitary-gonadal function may be suppressed with chronic administration and for up to 8 weeks after triptorelin therapy has been discontinued.

Dosage Forms Excipient information presented when available (limited, particularly for generics); consult specific product labeling.

Injection, powder for reconstitution:

Trelstar®: 3.75 mg, 11.25 mg, 22.5 mg [contains polylactide-co-glycolide, polysorbate 80]

Dosage Forms: Canada Excipient information presented when available (limited, particularly for generics); consult specific product labeling.

Injection, solution, as acetate [preservative free]:

Decapeptyl®: 100 mcg/mL (equivalent to 95.6 mcg triptorelin free base) (1 mL) [prefilled syringe]

References

Guay DR, "Drug Treatment of Paraphilic and Nonparaphilic Sexual Disorders," *Clin Ther*, 2009, 31(1):1-31.

Levine GN, D'Amico AV, Berger P, et al, "Androgen-Deprivation Therapy in Prostate Cancer and Cardiovascular Risk. A Science Advisory From the American Heart Association, American Cancer Society, and American Urological Association," *Circulation*, 2010, 121:833-40.

Reilly DR, Delva NJ, and Hudson RW, "Protocols for the Use of Cyproterone, Medroxyprogesterone, and Leuprolide in the Treatment of Paraphilia," *Can J Psychiatry*, 2000, 45(6):559-63.

Thibaut F, Cordier B, and Kuhn JM, "Effect of a Long-Lasting Gonadotrophin Hormone-Releasing Hormone Agonist in Six Cases of Severe Male Paraphilia," *Acta Psychiatr Scand*, 1993, 87(6):445-50.

Thibaut F, De La Barra F, Gordon H, et al, "The World Federation of Societies of Biological Psychiatry (WFSBP) Guidelines for the Biological Treatment of Paraphilias," *World J Biol Psychiatry*, 2010, 11(4):604-55.

◆ **Triptorelin Pamoate** *see* Triptorelin *on page* 1413

◆ **Trisenox®** *see* Arsenic Trioxide *on page* 122

◆ **Tryptoreline** *see* Triptorelin *on page* 1413

◆ **TSH** *see* Thyrotropin Alfa *on page* 1360

◆ **TSPA** *see* Thiotepa *on page 1357*
◆ **Tykerb®** *see* Lapatinib *on page 854*
◆ **506U78** *see* Nelarabine *on page 1028*
◆ **U-Cort®** *see* Hydrocortisone (Topical) *on page 719*

UFT

Related Information

Management of Chemotherapy-Induced Nausea and Vomiting *on page 1786*

Brand Names: U.S. Orzel® [DSC]

Index Terms Uracil and Ftorafur; Uracil and Tegafur; Uracil and Tetrahydrofuranyl-5-Fluorouracil

Generic Availability (U.S.) No

Pharmacologic Category Antineoplastic Agent, Antimetabolite (Pyrimidine Antagonist)

Unlabeled Use Treatment of unresectable or metastatic colorectal cancer

Warnings/Precautions Hazardous agent - use appropriate precautions for handling and disposal.

Adverse Reactions Frequency not defined.

Central nervous system: Fatigue, cerebellar toxicity (rare)
Dermatologic: Rash, skin pigmentation, photosensitivity, hand-foot syndrome (rare)
Gastrointestinal: Nausea, vomiting, anorexia, diarrhea (may be dose limiting)
Hematologic: Neutropenia (may be dose limiting)
Neuromuscular & skeletal: Neurotoxicity (peripheral neuropathy)
Ocular: Lacrimation

Mechanism of Action Tegafur is a prodrug of fluorouracil. It is converted *in vivo* to fluorouracil through hepatic microsomal cytochrome P450, and also via thymidine phosphorylase and spontaneous anabolic conversion. Uracil is a competitive inhibitor of dihydropyrimidine dehydrogenase (DPD), the enzyme responsible for catabolism of approximately 85% of fluorouracil to fluoro-β alanine.

Pharmacodynamics/Kinetics

Plasma levels: Tegafur > uracil > fluorouracil
Time to C_{pmax}: Tegafur: 0.6-2.1 hours; uracil: 0.6-4.1 hours; fluorouracil: 0.7-2.0 hours; the relationship between UFT dose and fluorouracil C_{pmax} is not linear

Dosing

Adult & Geriatric Refer to individual protocols.

Oral: 300 mg/m^2/day (expressed as tegafur) in combination with oral leucovorin calcium

Emetic Potential Moderate (30% to 90%)

Dosage Forms Excipient information presented when available (limited, particularly for generics); consult specific product labeling. [DSC] = Discontinued product

Capsule:
Orzel® [DSC]: Tegafur 100 mg and uracil 224 mg

References

Ho DH, Covington WP, Pazdur R, et al, "Clinical Pharmacology of Combined Oral Uracil and Ftorafur," *Drug Metab Disp*, 1992, 20(6):936-40.
Sun W and Haller D, "UFT in the Treatment of Colorectal and Breast Cancer," *Oncology (Huntingt)*, 2001, 15(1 Suppl 2):49-56.

- **UK109496** *see* Voriconazole *on page 1473*
- **Ultram®** *see* TraMADol *on page 1388*
- **Ultram® ER** *see* TraMADol *on page 1388*
- **Unipen® (Can)** *see* Nafcillin *on page 1026*
- **Uracil and Ftorafur** *see* UFT *on page 1418*
- **Uracil and Tegafur** *see* UFT *on page 1418*
- **Uracil and Tetrahydrofuranyl-5-Fluorouracil** *see* UFT *on page 1418*
- **Urate Oxidase** *see* Rasburicase *on page 1229*

Uridine Triacetate (URE i deen trye AS e tate)

Index Terms PN401; Triacetyluridine; Vistonuridine

Pharmacologic Category Antidote

Unlabeled Use Antidote for fluorouracil overdose or overexposure

Drug Interactions

Metabolism/Transport Effects None known.

Avoid Concomitant Use There are no known interactions where it is recommended to avoid concomitant use.

Increased Effect/Toxicity There are no known significant interactions involving an increase in effect.

Decreased Effect There are no known significant interactions involving a decrease in effect.

Mechanism of Action Uridine triacetate (formerly called vistonuridine), a prodrug of uridine, is converted to uridine triphosphate (UTP) which competes with FUTP for incorporation into RNA, thereby preventing cell death and dose-limiting fluorouracil toxicity.

Pharmacodynamics/Kinetics Metabolism: Deacetylated (by esterases) to uridine

Dosing

Adult & Geriatric Fluorouracil overdose (unlabeled use): Oral: 10 g every 6 hours for 20 doses beginning as soon as possible (8 hours to 4 days) after fluorouracil overdose (von Borstel, 2009)

Administration Administer orally (tablets); begin as soon as possible following of fluorouracil overdose (within 8-96 hours).

Monitoring Parameters CBC with differential; gastrointestinal toxicity

Additional Information Oncology Comment: Uridine triacetate has been studied in a limited number of cases of fluorouracil overdose. Of 17 patients receiving uridine triacetate beginning within 8-96 hours after fluorouracil overdose, all patients fully recovered (von Borstel, 2009). Updated data has described a total of 28 patients treated with uridine triacetate for fluorouracil overdose (including overdoses related to continuous infusions delivering fluorouracil at rates faster than prescribed), all of which recovered fully (Bamat, 2010).

Prescribing and Access Restrictions Uridine triacetate (formerly called vistonuridine) is supplied for emergency use under a single-patient Investigational New Drug (IND) provision. Procurement information is available from Wellstat Therapeutics at 1-443-831-5626.

References

Bamat MK, Tremmel R, O'Neil JD, et al, "Uridine Triacetate: An Orally Administered Life-Saving Antidote for 5-FU Overdose," *J Clin Oncol*, 28(15s):9084 [abstract 9084 from 2010 ASCO Annual Meeting].

von Borstel R, O'Neil J, and Bamat M, "Vistonuridine: An Orally Administered, Life-Saving Antidote for 5-Fluorouracil (5FU) Overdose," *J Clin Oncol*, 2009, 27(15S):9616 [abstract 9616 from 2009 ASCO Annual Meeting].

von Borstel R, O'Neil JD, Saydoff JA, et al, "Uridine Triacetate for Lethal 5-FU Toxicity Due to Dihydropyrimidine Dehydrogenase (DPD) Deficiency," *J Clin Oncol*, 2010, 28(15s):e13505 [abstract e13505 from 2010 ASCO Annual Meeting].

◆ **Uromitexan (Can)** *see* Mesna *on page 940*

Valacyclovir (val ay SYE kloe veer)

Brand Names: U.S. Valtrex®

Brand Names: Canada Apo-Valacyclovir®; CO Valacyclovir; DOM-Valacyclovir; Mylan-Valacyclovir; PHL-Valacyclovir; PMS-Valacyclovir; PRO-Valacyclovir; Riva-Valacyclovir; Valtrex®

Index Terms Valacyclovir Hydrochloride

Generic Availability (U.S.) Yes

Pharmacologic Category Antiviral Agent; Antiviral Agent, Oral

Use Treatment of herpes zoster (shingles) in immunocompetent patients; treatment of first-episode and recurrent genital herpes; suppression of recurrent genital herpes and reduction of transmission of genital herpes in immunocompetent patients; suppression of genital herpes in HIV-infected individuals; treatment of herpes labialis (cold sores); chickenpox in immunocompetent children

Unlabeled Use Prophylaxis of cancer-related HSV, VZV, and CMV infections; treatment of cancer-related HSV, VZV infection

Labeled Contraindications Hypersensitivity to valacyclovir, acyclovir, or any component of the formulation

Pregnancy Risk Factor B

Lactation Enters breast milk/use caution

Warnings/Precautions Thrombotic thrombocytopenic purpura/hemolytic uremic syndrome has occurred in immunocompromised patients (at doses of 8 g/day). Safety and efficacy have not been established for treatment/suppression of recurrent genital herpes or disseminated herpes in patients with profound immunosuppression (eg, advanced HIV with CD4 <100 cells/mm^3). CNS adverse effects (including agitation, hallucinations, confusion, delirium, seizures, and encephalopathy) have been reported. Use caution in patients with renal impairment, the elderly, and/or those receiving nephrotoxic agents. Acute renal failure has been observed in patients with renal dysfunction; dose adjustment may be required. Decreased precipitation in renal tubules may occur leading to urinary precipitation; adequately hydrate patient. For cold sores, treatment should begin at with earliest symptom (tingling, itching, burning). For genital herpes, treatment should begin as soon as possible after the first signs and symptoms (within 72 hours of onset of first diagnosis or within 24 hours of onset of recurrent episodes). For herpes zoster, treatment should begin within 72 hours of onset of rash. For chickenpox, treatment should begin with earliest sign or symptom. Use with caution in the elderly; CNS effects have been reported. Safety and efficacy have not been established in patients <2 years of age.

Storage/Stability Store at 15°C to 25°C (59°F to 77°F).

Mechanism of Action Valacyclovir is rapidly and nearly completely converted to acyclovir by intestinal and hepatic metabolism. Acyclovir is converted to acyclovir monophosphate by virus-specific thymidine kinase then further converted to acyclovir triphosphate by other cellular enzymes. Acyclovir triphosphate inhibits DNA synthesis and viral replication by competing with deoxyguanosine triphosphate for viral DNA polymerase and being incorporated into viral DNA.

Pharmacodynamics/Kinetics

Absorption: Rapid

Distribution: Acyclovir is widely distributed throughout the body including brain, kidney, lungs, liver, spleen, muscle, uterus, vagina, and CSF

Protein binding: ~14% to 18%

Metabolism: Hepatic; valacyclovir is rapidly and nearly completely converted to acyclovir and L-valine by first-pass effect; acyclovir is hepatically metabolized to a very small extent by aldehyde oxidase and by alcohol and aldehyde dehydrogenase (inactive metabolites)

Bioavailability: ~55% once converted to acyclovir

Half-life elimination: Normal renal function: Adults: Acyclovir: 2.5-3.3 hours, Valacyclovir: ~30 minutes; End-stage renal disease: Acyclovir: 14-20 hours; During hemodialysis: 4 hours

Excretion: Urine, primarily as acyclovir (89%); **Note:** Following oral administration of radiolabeled valacyclovir, 46% of the label is eliminated in the feces (corresponding to nonabsorbed drug), while 47% of the radiolabel is eliminated in the urine.

Dosing

Adult & Geriatric

CMV prophylaxis in allogeneic HSCT recipients (unlabeled use): 2 g 4 times daily

Herpes labialis (cold sores): Oral: 2 g twice daily for 1 day (separate doses by ~12 hours)

Herpes zoster (shingles): Oral: 1 g 3 times daily for 7 days

HSV, VZV in cancer patients (unlabeled use):

Prophylaxis: 500 mg 2-3 times daily

Treatment: 1 g 3 times daily

Genital herpes: Oral:

Initial episode: 1 g twice daily for 10 days

Recurrent episode: 500 mg twice daily for 3 days

Reduction of transmission: 500 mg once daily (source partner)

Suppressive therapy:

Immunocompetent patients: 1 g once daily (500 mg once daily in patients with <9 recurrences per year)

HIV-infected patients (CD4 ≥100 cells/mm^3): 500 mg twice daily

Pediatric

Chickenpox: Children 2 to <18 years: 20 mg/kg/dose 3 times daily for 5 days (maximum: 1 g 3 times daily)

Herpes labialis (cold sores): Children ≥12 years: Refer to adult dosing.

Renal Impairment

Herpes zoster: Adults:

U.S. labeling:

Cl_{cr} 30-49 mL/minute: 1 g every 12 hours

Cl_{cr} 10-29 mL/minute: 1 g every 24 hours

Cl_{cr} <10 mL/minute: 500 mg every 24 hours

Canadian labeling:
Cl_{cr} >30 mL/minute: No dosage adjustment required
Cl_{cr} 15-30 mL/minute: 1 g every 12 hours
Cl_{cr} <15 mL/minute: 1 g every 24 hours

Genital herpes: Adults:
U.S. labeling:
Initial episode:
Cl_{cr} 10-29 mL/minute: 1 g every 24 hours
Cl_{cr} <10 mL/minute: 500 mg every 24 hours
Recurrent episode: Cl_{cr} <29 mL/minute: 500 mg every 24 hours
Suppressive therapy: Cl_{cr} <29 mL/minute:
For usual dose of 1 g every 24 hours, decrease dose to 500 mg every 24 hours
For usual dose of 500 mg every 24 hours, decrease dose to 500 mg every 48 hours
HIV-infected patients: 500 mg every 24 hours
Canadian labeling:
Initial episode:
Cl_{cr} 15-30 mL/minute: 1 g every 24 hours
Cl_{cr} <15 mL/minute: 500 mg every 24 hours
Recurrent episode:
Cl_{cr} 15-30 mL/minute: 500 mg every 12 hours
Cl_{cr} <15 mL/minute: 500 mg every 24 hours
Suppressive therapy:
Cl_{cr} 15-30 mL/minute: 500 mg every 24 hours
Cl_{cr} <15 mL/minute:
Immunocompetent or HIV-infected patients: 500 mg every 24 hours
Immunocompetent patients and ≤9 recurrences/year: 500 mg every 48 hours

Herpes labialis: Adolescents and Adults *(U.S. labeling)* or Adults *(Canadian labeling)*:
Cl_{cr} 30-49 mL/minute: 1 g every 12 hours for 2 doses
Cl_{cr} 10-29 mL/minute: 500 mg every 12 hours for 2 doses
Cl_{cr} <10 mL/minute: 500 mg as a single dose

Hemodialysis: Dialyzable (~33% removed during 4-hour session); administer dose postdialysis

Chronic ambulatory peritoneal dialysis/continuous arteriovenous hemofiltration dialysis: Pharmacokinetic parameters are similar to those in patients with ESRD; supplemental dose not needed following dialysis

Hepatic Impairment No adjustment required.

Administration If GI upset occurs, administer with meals.

Dosage Forms Excipient information presented when available (limited, particularly for generics); consult specific product labeling.
Caplet, oral: 500 mg, 1 g
Valtrex®: 500 mg
Valtrex®: 1 g [scored]
Tablet, oral: 500 mg, 1 g

◆ **Valacyclovir Hydrochloride** *see* Valacyclovir *on page 1420*

◆ **Valcyte®** *see* ValGANciclovir *on page 1423*

ValGANciclovir (val gan SYE kloh veer)

Brand Names: U.S. Valcyte®

Brand Names: Canada Valcyte®

Index Terms Valganciclovir Hydrochloride

Generic Availability (U.S.) No

Pharmacologic Category Antiviral Agent

Use Treatment of cytomegalovirus (CMV) retinitis in patients with acquired immunodeficiency syndrome (AIDS), prevention of CMV disease in high-risk patients (donor CMV positive/recipient CMV negative) undergoing kidney, heart, or kidney/pancreas transplantation

Labeled Contraindications Hypersensitivity to valganciclovir, ganciclovir, or any component of the formulation

Pregnancy Risk Factor C

Lactation Excretion in breast milk unknown/not recommended

Warnings/Precautions Hazardous agent - use appropriate precautions for handling and disposal. **[U.S. Boxed Warning]: May cause dose- or therapy-limiting granulocytopenia, anemia, and/or thrombocytopenia;** do not use in patients with an absolute neutrophil count <500/mm^3, platelet count <25,000/mm^3, or hemoglobin <8 g/dL. Use with caution in patients with impaired renal function (dose adjustment required). Acute renal failure (ARF) may occur; ensure adequate hydration and use with caution in patients receiving concomitant nephrotoxic agents. Elderly patients with or without pre-existing renal impairment may develop ARF; use with caution and adjust dose as needed. **[U.S. Boxed Warning]: Ganciclovir may be teratogenic, carcinogenic, and cause aspermatogenesis.** Due to its teratogenic potential, contraceptive precautions for female and male patients need to be followed during and for at least 90 days after therapy with the drug. Fertility may be temporarily or permanently impaired in males and females. Due to differences in bioavailability, valganciclovir tablets cannot be substituted for ganciclovir capsules on a one-to-one basis. The preferred dosage form for pediatric patients is the oral solution; however, valganciclovir tablets may used so long as the calculated dose is within 10% of the available tablet strength (450 mg). Not indicated for use in liver transplant patients (higher incidence of tissue-invasive CMV relative to oral ganciclovir was observed in trials). Use of valganciclovir for the treatment of congenital CMV disease has not been evaluated.

Ethanol/Nutrition/Herb Interactions Food: Coadministration with a high-fat meal increased AUC by 30%. Management: Valganciclovir should be taken with meals.

Storage/Stability

Oral solution: Store dry powder at 25°C (77°F); excursions permitted to 15°C to 30°C (59°F to 86°F). Store oral solution under refrigeration at 2°C to 8°C (36°F to 46°F); do not freeze. Discard any unused medication after 49 days.

Tablet: Store at 25°C (77°F); excursions permitted to 15°C to 30°C (59°F to 86°F).

Reconstitution Oral solution: Prior to dispensing, prepare the oral solution by adding 91 mL of purified water to the bottle; shake well. Discard any unused medication after 49 days. A reconstituted 100 mL bottle will only provide 88 mL of solution for administration.

Mechanism of Action Valganciclovir is rapidly converted to ganciclovir in the body. The bioavailability of ganciclovir from valganciclovir is increased 10-fold compared to oral ganciclovir. A dose of 900 mg achieved systemic exposure of ganciclovir comparable to that achieved with the recommended doses of intravenous ganciclovir of 5 mg/kg. Ganciclovir is phosphorylated to a substrate which competitively inhibits the binding of deoxyguanosine triphosphate to DNA polymerase resulting in inhibition of viral DNA synthesis.

Pharmacodynamics/Kinetics

Absorption: Well absorbed; high-fat meal increases AUC by 30%

Distribution: V_{dss}: Ganciclovir: 0.7 L/kg; widely to all tissue including CSF and ocular tissue

Protein binding: Ganciclovir: 1% to 2%

Metabolism: Converted to ganciclovir by intestinal mucosal cells and hepatocytes

Bioavailability: With food: 60%

Half-life elimination: Ganciclovir: 4.08 hours; prolonged with renal impairment; Severe renal impairment: Up to 68 hours

Time to peak: Ganciclovir: 1-3 hours

Excretion: Urine (primarily as ganciclovir)

Dosing

Adult & Geriatric

CMV retinitis: Oral:

Induction (active retinitis): 900 mg twice daily for 21 days

Maintenance: Following induction treatment, or for patients with inactive CMV retinitis who require maintenance therapy: 900 mg once daily

Prevention of CMV disease following transplantation: 900 mg once daily beginning within 10 days of transplantation; continue therapy until 100 days (heart or kidney-pancreas transplant) or 200 days (kidney transplant) post-transplantation

Pediatric

Prevention of CMV disease following kidney or heart transplantation: Oral:

Children 4 months to 16 years: Dose (mg) = 7 x body surface area x creatinine clearance* once daily beginning within 10 days of transplantation; continue therapy until 100 days post-transplantation. Doses should be rounded to the nearest 25 mg increment; maximum dose: 900 mg/day

*Cl_{cr} (mL/minute/1.73 m^2) = [k x Height (cm)] divided by serum creatinine (mg/dL)

Note: If the calculated Cl_{cr} is >150 mL/minute/1.73 m^2, then a maximum value of 150 mL/minute/1.73 m^2 should be used to calculate the dose.

Note: Calculated using *modified* Schwartz formula where k is as follows:

Patients <2 years: k = 0.45

Girls 2-16 years: k = 0.55

Boys 2 to <13 years: k = 0.55

Boys 13-16 years: k = 0.7

Children >16 years: Refer to adult dosing.

Renal Impairment

Children 4 months to 16 years: No additional dosage adjustments required; calculation for all patients adjusts for renal function.

Children >16 years and Adults:

Induction dose:

Cl_{cr} 40-59 mL/minute: 450 mg twice daily

Cl_{cr} 25-39 mL/minute: 450 mg once daily

Cl_{cr} 10-24 mL/minute: 450 mg every 2 days

Maintenance dose:

Cl_{cr} 40-59 mL/minute: 450 mg once daily

Cl_{cr} 25-39 mL/minute: 450 mg every 2 days

Cl_{cr} 10-24 mL/minute: 450 mg twice weekly

Note: Valganciclovir is not recommended in patients receiving hemodialysis. For patients on hemodialysis (Cl_{cr} <10 mL/minute), it is recommended that ganciclovir be used (dose adjusted as specified for ganciclovir).

Hepatic Impairment Use has not been studied.

Administration Valganciclovir should be taken with meals. The preferred dosage form for pediatric patients is the oral solution; however, valganciclovir tablets may used so long as the calculated dose is within 10% of the available tablet strength (450 mg).

Due to the carcinogenic and mutagenic potential, avoid direct contact with broken or crushed tablets, powder for oral solution, and oral solution. Consideration should be given to handling and disposal according to guidelines issued for antineoplastic drugs. However, there is no consensus on the need for these precautions.

Dosage Forms Excipient information presented when available (limited, particularly for generics); consult specific product labeling.

Powder for solution, oral:

Valcyte®: 50 mg/mL (100 mL) [contains sodium benzoate; tutti frutti flavor]

Tablet, oral [strength expressed as base]:

Valcyte®: 450 mg

◆ **Valganciclovir Hydrochloride** *see* ValGANciclovir *on page* 1423

Valrubicin (val ROO bi sin)

Related Information

Management of Chemotherapy-Induced Nausea and Vomiting *on page* 1786

Safe Handling of Hazardous Drugs *on page* 1904

Brand Names: U.S. Valstar®

Brand Names: Canada Valtaxin®

Index Terms *N*-trifluoroacetyladriamycin-14-valerate; AD32

Generic Availability (U.S.) No

Pharmacologic Category Antineoplastic Agent, Anthracycline

Use Intravesical treatment of BCG-refractory bladder carcinoma *in situ*

Labeled Contraindications Hypersensitivity to anthracyclines, polyoxyl castor oil (Cremophor® EL), or any component of the formulation; concurrent urinary tract infection; small bladder capacity (unable to tolerate a 75 mL instillation)

Pregnancy Risk Factor C

Lactation Excretion in breast milk unknown/not recommended

Warnings/Precautions Hazardous agent - use appropriate precautions for handling and disposal. Delay valrubicin therapy for at least 2 weeks after transurethral resection and/or fulguration. Evaluate bladder status prior to instillation; do not administer if mucosal integrity of bladder has been compromised or bladder perforation is present (delay treatment until restoration of bladder integrity). Use aseptic technique to prevent urinary tract infection or traumatizing urinary mucosa. Although clamping of the urinary catheter after administration is not recommended, use caution and appropriate medical supervision if performed. Irritable bladder symptoms may occur during instillation and retention, and for a brief time after voiding. Use caution in patients with severe irritable bladder symptoms. Red-tinged urine is typical for the first 24 hours after instillation. Prolonged symptoms or discoloration should prompt contact with the physician.

Contains polyoxyl castor oil (Cremophor® EL) which is associated with hypersensitivity reactions; use is contraindicated in patients with hypersensitivity to polyoxyl castor oil. Delaying cystectomy during treatment may lead to metastatic bladder cancer; reconsider cystectomy if complete response to treatment does not occur within 3 months.

Adverse Reactions Note: In general, local adverse reactions occur during or shortly after instillation and resolve within 1-7 days.

>10%: Genitourinary: Bladder irritation (88%), urinary frequency (61%), urinary urgency (57%), dysuria (56%), bladder spasm (31%), hematuria (29%; gross: 1%), bladder pain (28%), urinary incontinence (22%), cystitis (15%), urinary tract infection (15%), urine red-tinged

1% to 10%:

Cardiovascular: Chest pain (3%), vasodilation (2%), peripheral edema (1%)

Central nervous system: Headache (4%), malaise (4%), dizziness (3%), fever (2%)

Dermatologic: Rash (3%)

Endocrine & metabolic: Hyperglycemia (1%)

Gastrointestinal: Abdominal pain (5%), nausea (5%), diarrhea (3%), vomiting (2%), flatulence (1%)

Genitourinary: Nocturia (7%), burning symptoms (5%), urinary retention (4%), urethral pain (3%), pelvic pain (1%), hematuria (microscopic) (3%)

Hematologic: Anemia (2%)

Neuromuscular & skeletal: Weakness (4%), back pain (3%), myalgia (1%)

Respiratory: Pneumonia (1%)

<1%, postmarketing, and/or case reports: Hematologic toxicity (following instillation into perforated bladder), nonprotein nitrogen increased, pruritus, skin irritation (local), taste loss, tenesmus, urine flow decreased, urethritis

Drug Interactions

Metabolism/Transport Effects None known.

Avoid Concomitant Use There are no known interactions where it is recommended to avoid concomitant use.

Increased Effect/Toxicity There are no known significant interactions involving an increase in effect.

Decreased Effect There are no known significant interactions involving a decrease in effect.

Storage/Stability Store unopened vials refrigerated at 2°C to 8°C (36°F to 48°F). Stable for 12 hours at room temperature when diluted in 0.9% sodium chloride.

Reconstitution Allow vials to slowly warm to room temperature (without heating) prior to use. A waxy precipitate (due to polyoxyl castor oil) may form at temperatures <4°C, warm vial in the hand until solution is clear (do not use vial if particulate still present). Use appropriate precautions for handling and disposal. Dilute 800 mg (20 mL) with 55 mL NS (total volume of 75 mL). Use non-PVC containers (glass, polyolefin, or polypropylene) and administration sets to avoid leaching of DEHP plasticizers. Stable for 12 hours at room temperature when diluted in 0.9% sodium chloride. Do not mix with other drugs.

Mechanism of Action Blocks function of DNA topoisomerase II; inhibits DNA synthesis, causes extensive chromosomal damage, and arrests cell development (G_2 phase); unlike other anthracyclines, does not appear to intercalate DNA; readily penetrates cells.

Pharmacodynamics/Kinetics

Absorption: Intravesical: Penetrates into bladder wall; negligible systemic absorption (dependent on bladder wall condition; trauma to mucosa may increase absorption, bladder wall perforation may significantly increase absorption and systemic myelotoxicity).

Metabolism: Negligible after intravesical instillation and 2-hour retention

Excretion: Urine (post 2-hour retention): 98.6% as intact drug; 0.4% as *N*-trifluoroacetyladriamycin)

Dosing

Adult & Geriatric Bladder cancer: Intravesical: 800 mg once weekly (retain for 2 hours) for 6 weeks

Adjustment for Toxicity In clinical trials (Steinberg, 2000), treatment was delayed for 1 week for the following adverse events: Grade 3 dysuria (not controlled with phenazopyridine), frequency/urgency lasting >24 hours, grade 2 gross hematuria (without clots) lasting >48 hours, grade 3 hematuria (with clots) lasting >48 hours. For local toxicities <grade 4 (eg, dysuria [not controlled with phenazopyridine] or severe bladder spasm), anticholinergic therapy (systemic or topical) or topical anesthesia was administered prior to subsequent instillations.

Administration Intravesicular bladder instillation: Insert urinary catheter, empty bladder prior to instillation, slowly by gravity flow, instill 800 mg/75 mL (in 0.9% sodium chloride injection), remove catheter. Retain in the bladder for 2 hours, then void. Administer through non-PVC tubing due to the polyoxyl castor oil (Cremophor® EL) diluent. Maintain adequate hydration following treatment. Use appropriate protective gown, goggles, and gloves during administration.

Monitoring Parameters Cystoscopy, biopsy, and urine cytology every 3 months for recurrence or progression

Dosage Forms Excipient information presented when available (limited, particularly for generics); consult specific product labeling.

Injection, solution [preservative free]:

Valstar®: 40 mg/mL (5 mL) [contains dehydrated ethanol 50%, polyoxyl castor oil]

References

Newling DW, Hetherington J, Sundaram SK, et al, "The Use of Valrubicin for the Chemoresection of Superficial Bladder Cancer – A Marker Lesion Study," *Eur Urol*, 2001, 39(6):643-7.

Steinberg G, Bahnson R, Brosman S, et al, "Efficacy and Safety of Valrubicin for the Treatment of Bacillus Calmette Guerin Refractory Carcinoma *in situ* of the Bladder: The Valrubicin Study Group," *J Urol*, 2000, 163(3):761-7.

- **Valstar®** *see* Valrubicin *on page* 1425
- **Valtaxin® (Can)** *see* Valrubicin *on page* 1425
- **Valtrex®** *see* Valacyclovir *on page* 1420
- **Val-Vancomycin (Can)** *see* Vancomycin *on page* 1428
- **Vancocin®** *see* Vancomycin *on page* 1428

Vancomycin (van koe MYE sin)

Brand Names: U.S. Vancocin®

Brand Names: Canada PMS-Vancomycin; Sterile Vancomycin Hydrochloride, USP; Val-Vancomycin; Vancocin®; Vancomycin Hydrochloride for Injection, USP

Index Terms Vancomycin Hydrochloride

Generic Availability (U.S.) Yes

Pharmacologic Category Glycopeptide

Use

I.V.: Treatment of patients with infections caused by staphylococcal species and streptococcal species

Oral: Treatment of *C. difficile*-associated diarrhea and treatment of enterocolitis caused by *Staphylococcus aureus* (including methicillin-resistant strains)

Unlabeled Use Bacterial endophthalmitis; treatment of infections caused by gram-positive organisms in patients who have serious allergies to beta-lactam agents; treatment of beta-lactam resistant gram-positive infections; surgical prophylaxis

Labeled Contraindications Hypersensitivity to vancomycin or any component of the formulation

Pregnancy Risk Factor B (oral); C (injection)

Lactation Enters breast milk/not recommended

Warnings/Precautions May cause nephrotoxicity although limited data suggest direct causal relationship; usual risk factors include pre-existing renal impairment, concomitant nephrotoxic medications, advanced age, and dehydration (nephrotoxicity has also been reported following treatment with oral vancomycin, typically in patients >65 years of age). If multiple sequential (≥2) serum creatinine concentrations demonstrate an increase of 0.5 mg/dL or ≥50% increase from baseline (whichever is greater) in the absence of an alternative explanation, the patient should be identified as having vancomycin-induced nephrotoxicity (Rybak, 2009). Discontinue treatment if signs of nephrotoxicity occur; renal damage is usually reversible.

May cause neurotoxicity; usual risk factors include pre-existing renal impairment, concomitant neuro-/nephrotoxic medications, advanced age, and dehydration. Ototoxicity, although rarely associated with monotherapy, is proportional to the amount of drug given and the duration of treatment. Tinnitus or vertigo may be indications of vestibular injury and impending bilateral irreversible damage. Discontinue treatment if signs of ototoxicity occur. Prolonged therapy (>1 week) or total doses exceeding 25 g may increase the risk of neutropenia; prompt reversal of neutropenia is expected after discontinuation of therapy. Prolonged use may result in fungal or bacterial superinfection, including *C. difficile*-associated diarrhea (CDAD) and pseudomembranous colitis; CDAD has been observed >2 months postantibiotic treatment. Use with caution in patients with renal impairment or those receiving other nephrotoxic or ototoxic drugs; dosage modification required in patients with impaired renal function (especially elderly). Accumulation may occur after multiple oral doses of vancomycin in patients with renal impairment; consider monitoring trough concentrations in this circumstance.

Rapid I.V. administration may result in hypotension, flushing, erythema, urticaria, and/or pruritus. Oral vancomycin is only indicated for the treatment of pseudomembranous colitis due to *C. difficile* and enterocolitis due to *S. aureus* and is not effective for systemic infections; parenteral vancomycin is not effective for the treatment of colitis due to *C. difficile* and enterocolitis due to *S. aureus*. Clinically significant serum concentrations have been reported in patients with inflammatory disorders of the intestinal mucosa who have taken oral vancomycin (multiple doses) for the treatment of *C. difficile*-associated diarrhea. Although use may be warranted, the risk for adverse reactions may be higher in this situation; consider monitoring serum trough concentrations, especially with renal insufficiency, severe colitis, concurrent rectal vancomycin administration, and/or concomitant I.V. aminoglycosides. The IDSA suggests that it is appropriate to obtain trough concentrations when a patient is receiving long courses of ≥2 g/day (Cohen, 2010). **Note:** The Infectious Disease Society of America (IDSA) recommends the use of oral metronidazole for initial treatment of mild-to-moderate *C. difficile* infection and the use of oral vancomycin for initial treatment of severe *C. difficile* infection (Cohen, 2010).

Storage/Stability

Capsules: Store at controlled room temperature of 15°C to 30°C (59°F to 86°F).

Injection: Reconstituted 500 mg and 1 g vials are stable for at either room temperature or under refrigeration for 14 days. **Note:** Vials contain no bacteriostatic agent. Solutions diluted for administration in either D_5W or NS are stable under refrigeration for 14 days or at room temperature for 7 days.

Reconstitution Injection: Reconstitute vials with 20 mL of SWFI for each 1 g of vancomycin (10 mL/500 mg vial; 20 mL/1 g vial; 100 mL/5 g vial; 200 mL/10 g vial). The reconstituted solution must be further diluted with at least 100 mL of a compatible diluent per 500 mg of vancomycin prior to parenteral administration.

Intrathecal (unlabeled route): Vancomycin is available as a powder for injection and may be diluted to 1-5 mg/mL concentration in preservative free 0.9% sodium chloride for administration into the CSF.

Mechanism of Action Inhibits bacterial cell wall synthesis by blocking glycopeptide polymerization through binding tightly to D-alanyl-D-alanine portion of cell wall precursor

Pharmacodynamics/Kinetics

Absorption: Oral: Poor; may be enhanced with bowel inflammation; I.M.: Erratic; Intraperitoneal: ~38%

Distribution: V_d: 0.4-1 L/kg; Distributes widely in body tissue and fluids, except for CSF

Relative diffusion from blood into CSF: Good only with inflammation (exceeds usual MICs)

Uninflamed meninges: 0-4 mcg/mL; serum concentration dependent

Inflamed meninges: 6-11 mcg/mL; serum concentration dependent

CSF:blood level ratio: Normal meninges: Nil; Inflamed meninges: 20% to 30%

Protein binding: ~50%

Half-life elimination: Biphasic: Terminal:

Newborns: 6-10 hours

Infants and Children 3 months to 4 years: 4 hours

Children >3 years: 2.2-3 hours

Adults: 5-11 hours; significantly prolonged with renal impairment

End-stage renal disease: 200-250 hours

Time to peak, serum: I.V.: Immediately after completion of infusion

Excretion: I.V.: Urine (80% to 90% as unchanged drug); Oral: Primarily feces

Dosing

Adult & Geriatric

Usual dosage range: Initial intravenous dosing should be based on actual body weight; subsequent dosing adjusted based on serum trough vancomycin concentrations.

I.V.: 2000-3000 mg/day (or 30-60 mg/kg/day) in divided doses every 8-12 hours (Rybak, 2009); **Note:** Dose requires adjustment in renal impairment

Oral: 500-2000 mg/day in divided doses every 6 hours

Indication-specific dosing:

Catheter-related infections: Antibiotic lock technique (Mermel, 2009): 2 mg/mL ± 10 units heparin/mL **or** 2.5 mg/mL ± 2500 **or** 5000 units heparin/mL **or** 5 mg/mL ± 5000 units heparin/mL (preferred regimen); instill into catheter port with a volume sufficient to fill the catheter (2-5 mL). **Note:** May use SWFI/NS or D_5W as diluents. Do not mix with any other solutions. Dwell times generally should not exceed 48 hours before renewal of lock solution. Remove lock solution prior to catheter use, then replace.

C. difficile **-associated diarrhea (CDAD):**

Oral:

Manufacturer recommendations: 125 mg 4 times/day for 10 days

IDSA guideline recommendations: Severe infection: 125 mg every 6 hours for 10-14 days; Severe, complicated infection: 500 mg every 6 hours with or without concurrent I.V. metronidazole. May consider vancomycin retention enema (in patients with complete ileus) (Cohen, 2010).

Rectal (unlabeled route): Retention enema (in patients with complete ileus): SHEA/IDSA guideline recommendations: Severe, complicated infection in patients with ileus: 500 mg every 6 hours (in 100 mL 0.9% sodium chloride) with oral vancomycin with or without concurrent I.V. metronidazole (Cohen, 2010)

Complicated infections in seriously-ill patients: I.V.: Loading dose: 25-30 mg/kg (based on actual body weight) may be used to rapidly achieve target concentration; then 15-20 mg/kg/dose every 8-12 hours (Rybak, 2009)

Enterocolitis *(S. aureus)*: Oral: 500-2000 mg/day in 3-4 divided doses for 7-10 days (usual dose: 125-500 mg every 6 hours)

Meningitis:

I.V.: 30-60 mg/kg/day in divided doses every 8-12 hours (Rybak, 2009) **or** 500-750 mg every 6 hours (with third-generation cephalosporin for PCN-resistant *Streptococcus pneumoniae*)

Alternate regimen: *S. aureus* (methicillin-resistant) (unlabeled use; Liu, 2011): 15-20 mg/kg/dose every 8-12 hours for 2 weeks (some experts combine with rifampin

Intrathecal, intraventricular (unlabeled route): 5-20 mg/day

Pneumonia: I.V.:

Community-acquired pneumonia (CAP): S. aureus (methicillin-resistant): 45-60 mg/kg/day divided every 8-12 hours (maximum: 2000 mg/dose) for 7-21 days depending on severity (Liu, 2011)

Healthcare-associated pneumonia (HAP): S. aureus (methicillin-resistant): 45-60 mg/kg/day divided every 8-12 hours (maximum: 2000 mg/dose) for 7-21 days depending on severity (American Thoracic Society [ATS], 2005; Liu, 2011; Rybak 2009)

Prophylaxis against infective endocarditis: I.V.:

Dental, oral, or upper respiratory tract surgery: 1000 mg 1 hour before surgery. **Note:** AHA guidelines now recommend prophylaxis only in patients undergoing invasive procedures and in whom underlying cardiac conditions may predispose to a higher risk of adverse outcomes should infection occur

GI/GU procedure: 1000 mg plus 1.5 mg/kg gentamicin 1 hour prior to surgery. **Note:** As of April 2007, routine prophylaxis no longer recommended by the AHA.

Susceptible (MIC ≤1 mcg/mL) gram-positive infections: I.V.: 15-20 mg/kg/dose (usual: 750-1500 mg) every 8-12 hours (Rybak, 2009). **Note:** If MIC >2 mcg/mL, alternative therapies are recommended.

Bacteremia (*S. aureus* [methicillin-resistant]) (unlabeled use; Liu, 2011): I.V.: 15-20 mg/kg/dose every 8-12 hours for 2-6 weeks depending on severity

Brain abscess, subdural empyema, spinal epidural abscess (*S. aureus* [methicillin-resistant]) (unlabeled use; Liu, 2011): I.V.: 15-20 mg/kg/dose every 8-12 hours for 4-6 weeks (some experts combine with rifampin)

Endocarditis:

Native valve (*Enterococcus*, vancomycin MIC ≤4 mg/L) (unlabeled use; Gould, 2012): I.V.: 1000 mg every 12 hours for 4-6 weeks (combine with gentamicin for 4-6 weeks)

Native valve (*S. aureus* [methicillin-resistant]) (unlabeled use; Liu, 2011): I.V.: 15-20 mg/kg/dose every 8-12 hours for 6 weeks (European guidelines support the entire duration of therapy to be 4 weeks and in combination with rifampin [Gould, 2012])

Native or prosthetic valve (streptococcal [penicillin MIC >0.5 mg/L or patient intolerant to penicillin]) (unlabeled use; Gould, 2012): I.V.: 1000 mg every 12 hours for 4-6 weeks (combine with gentamicin for at least the first 2 weeks); **Note:** The longer duration of treatment (ie, 6 weeks) should be used for patients with prosthetic valve endocarditis.

Prosthetic valve (*Enterococcus*, vancomycin MIC ≤4 mg/L) (unlabeled use; Gould, 2012): I.V.: 1000 mg every 12 hours for 6 weeks (combine with gentamicin for 4-6 weeks)

Prosthetic valve (*S. aureus* [methicillin-resistant]) (unlabeled use; Liu, 2011): I.V.: 15-20 mg/kg/dose every 8-12 hours for at least 6 weeks (combine with rifampin for the entire duration of therapy and gentamicin for the first 2 weeks)

Endophthalmitis (unlabeled use): Intravitreal: Usual dose: 1 mg/0.1 mL NS instilled into vitreum; may repeat administration if necessary in 3-4 days, usually in combination with ceftazidime or an aminoglycoside. **Note:** Some clinicians have recommended using a lower dose of 0.2 mg/0.1 mL, based on concerns for retinotoxicity.

Osteomyelitis (*S. aureus* [methicillin-resistant]) (unlabeled use; Liu, 2011): I.V.: 15-20 mg/kg/dose every 8-12 hours for a minimum of 8 weeks (some experts combine with rifampin)

Septic arthritis (*S. aureus* [methicillin-resistant]) (unlabeled use; Liu, 2011): I.V.: 15-20 mg/kg/dose every 8-12 hours for 3-4 weeks

Septic thrombosis of cavernous or dural venous sinus (*S. aureus* [methicillin-resistant]) (unlabeled use; Liu, 2011): I.V.: 15-20 mg/kg/dose every 8-12 hours for 4-6 weeks (some experts combine with rifampin)

Skin and skin structure infections, complicated (*S. aureus* [methicillin-resistant]) (unlabeled use; Liu, 2011): I.V.: 15-20 mg/kg/dose every 8-12 hours for 7-14 days

Surgical prophylaxis (unlabeled use): I.V.: 1000 mg or 10-15 mg/kg over 60 minutes (longer infusion time if dose >1000 mg) (Bratzler, 2004)

The Society of Thoracic Surgeons recommends 1000-1500 mg or 15 mg/kg over 60 minutes with completion within 1 hour of skin incision. Although not well established, a second dose of 7.5 mg/kg may be considered during cardiopulmonary bypass (Engelman, 2007).

Pediatric

Usual dosage range: Infants >1 month and Children: I.V.: 10-15 mg/kg every 6 hours

Indication-specific dosing:

***C. difficile*-associated diarrhea (CDAD):** Infants >1 month and Children: Oral: 40 mg/kg/day in 3-4 divided doses for 7-10 days (maximum: 2000 mg/day)

Enterocolitis *(S. aureus)*: Infants >1 months and Children: Oral: 40 mg/kg/day in 3-4 divided doses for 7-10 days (maximum: 2000 mg/day)

Meningitis: Infants >1 month and Children:

I.V.: 15 mg/kg every 6 hours (Tunkel, 2004)

Alternate regimen: *S. aureus* (methicillin-resistant) (unlabeled use; Liu, 2011): 15-20 mg/kg/dose every 8-12 hours for 2 weeks (some experts combine with rifampin)

Intrathecal, intraventricular (unlabeled route): 5-20 mg/day (Tunkel, 2004)

Pneumonia:

Community-acquired pneumonia (CAP) (IDSA/PIDS, 2011): Infants >3 months and Children: I.V.: **Note:** In children ≥5 years, a macrolide antibiotic should be added if atypical pneumonia cannot be ruled out. Also consider if community-acquired MRSA suspected.

Group A *Streptococcus* (alternative to ampicillin or penicillin in beta-lactam allergic patients): 40-60 mg/kg/day divided every 6-8 hours

Presumed bacterial (in addition to recommended antibiotic therapy), *S. pneumoniae*, moderate-to-severe infection (MICs to penicillin ≤2.0 mcg/mL) (alternative to ampicillin or penicillin): 40-60 mg/kg/day divided every 6-8 hours

S. aureus (methicillin-susceptible) (alternative to cefazolin/oxacillin): 40-60 mg/kg/day divided every 6-8 hours

S. aureus, moderate-to-severe infection (methicillin-resistant +/- clindamycin susceptible) (preferred): 40-60 mg/kg/day divided every 6-8 hours **or** dosing to achieve AUC/MIC >400

Alternate regimen: 60 mg/kg/day divided every 6 hours for 7-21 days, depending on severity (Liu, 2011)

S. pneumoniae, moderate-to-severe infection (MICs to penicillin ≥4.0 mcg/mL) (alternative to ceftriaxone in beta-lactam allergic patients): 40-60 mg/kg/day divided every 6-8 hours

Healthcare-associated pneumonia (HAP), S. aureus (methicillin-resistant): I.V.: Infants and Children: 60 mg/kg/day divided every 6 hours for 7-21 days depending on severity (Liu, 2011)

Prophylaxis against infective endocarditis: Children: I.V.:

Dental, oral, or upper respiratory tract surgery: 20 mg/kg/dose administered 1 hour prior to the procedure. **Note:** American Heart Association (AHA) guidelines recommend prophylaxis only in patients undergoing invasive procedures and in whom underlying cardiac conditions may predispose to a higher risk of adverse outcomes should infection occur.

GI/GU procedure: 20 mg/kg (plus gentamicin 1.5 mg/kg) administered 1 hour prior to surgery. **Note:** Routine prophylaxis no longer recommended by the AHA.

Susceptible gram-positive infections (MIC ≤1 mcg/mL; Rybak, 2009): I.V.: Infants >1 month and Children: 10 mg/kg/dose every 6 hours (manufacturer recommendations) **or** 15 mg/kg/dose (maximum: 2000 mg/dose) every 6 hours (Liu, 2011). **Note:** If MIC ≥2 mcg/mL, alternative therapies are recommended.

Bacteremia (*S. aureus* [methicillin-resistant]) (unlabeled use; Liu, 2011): Children: I.V.: 15 mg/kg/dose every 6 hours for 2-6 weeks depending on severity

Brain abscess, subdural empyema, spinal epidural abscess (*S. aureus* [methicillin-resistant]) (unlabeled use; Liu, 2011): Children: I.V.: 15 mg/kg/dose every 6 hours for 4-6 weeks (some experts combine with rifampin)

Endocarditis, native valve (*S. aureus* [methicillin-resistant]) (unlabeled use; Liu, 2011): Children: I.V.: 15 mg/kg/dose every 6 hours for 6 weeks

Endocarditis, prosthetic valve (*S. aureus* [methicillin-resistant]) (unlabeled use; Liu, 2011): Children: I.V.:15 mg/kg/dose every 6 hours for at least 6 weeks

Osteomyelitis (*S. aureus* [methicillin-resistant]) (unlabeled use; Liu, 2011): Children: I.V.: 15 mg/kg/dose every 6 hours for 4-6 weeks

Septic arthritis (*S. aureus* [methicillin-resistant]) (unlabeled use; Liu, 2011): Children: I.V.: 15 mg/kg/dose every 6 hours for minimum of 3-4 weeks

Septic thrombosis of cavernous or dural venous sinus (*S. aureus* [methicillin-resistant]) (unlabeled use; Liu, 2011): Children: I.V.: 15 mg/kg/dose every 6 hours for 4-6 weeks (some experts combine with rifampin)

Skin and skin structure infections, complicated (*S. aureus* [methicillin-resistant]) (unlabeled use; Liu, 2011): Children: I.V.: 15 mg/kg/dose every 6 hours for 7-14 days

Renal Impairment Vancomycin levels should be monitored in patients with any renal impairment: I.V.:

Cl_{cr} >50 mL/minute: Start with 15-20 mg/kg/dose (usual: 750-1500 mg) every 8-12 hours

Cl_{cr} 20-49 mL/minute: Start with 15-20 mg/kg/dose (usual: 750-1500 mg) every 24 hours

Cl_{cr} <20 mL/minute: Will need longer intervals; determine by serum concentration monitoring

Note: In the critically-ill patient with renal insufficiency, the initial loading dose (25-30 mg/kg) should not be reduced. However, subsequent dosage adjustments should be made based on renal function and trough serum concentrations.

Poorly dialyzable by intermittent hemodialysis (0% to 5%); however, use of high-flux membranes and continuous renal replacement therapy (CRRT) increases vancomycin clearance, and generally requires replacement dosing.

Intermittent hemodialysis (IHD) (administer after hemodialysis on dialysis days): Following loading dose of 15-25 mg/kg, give either 500-1000 mg **or** 5-10 mg/kg after each dialysis session. (Heintz, 2009). **Note:** Dosing dependent on the assumption of 3 times/week, complete IHD sessions.

Redosing based on pre-HD concentrations:

<10 mg/L: Administer 1000 mg after HD

10-25 mg/L: Administer 500-750 mg after HD

>25 mg/L: Hold vancomycin

Redosing based on post-HD concentrations: <10-15 mg/L: Administer 500-1000 mg

Peritoneal dialysis (PD):

Administration via PD fluid: 15-30 mg/L (15-30 mcg/mL) of PD fluid

Systemic: Loading dose of 1000 mg, followed by 500-1000 mg every 48-72 hours with close monitoring of levels

Continuous renal replacement therapy (CRRT) (Heintz, 2009; Trotman, 2005): Drug clearance is highly dependent on the method of renal replacement, filter type, and flow rate. Appropriate dosing requires close monitoring of pharmacologic response, signs of adverse reactions due to drug accumulation, as well as drug concentrations in relation to target trough (if appropriate). The following are general recommendations only (based on dialysate flow/ultrafiltration rates of 1-2 L/hour and minimal residual renal function) and should not supersede clinical judgment:

CVVH: Loading dose of 15-25 mg/kg, followed by either 1000 mg every 48 hours **or** 10-15 mg/kg every 24-48 hours

CVVHD: Loading dose of 15-25 mg/kg, followed by either 1000 mg every 24 hours **or** 10-15 mg/kg every 24 hours

CVVHDF: Loading dose of 15-25 mg/kg, followed by either 1000 mg every 24 hours **or** 7.5-10 mg/kg every 12 hours

Note: Consider redosing patients receiving CRRT for vancomycin concentrations <10-15 mg/L.

Hepatic Impairment Degrees of hepatic dysfunction do not affect the pharmacokinetics of vancomycin (Marti, 1996).

Oral: No adjustment provided in the manufacturer's labeling.

Administration

Intravenous: Administer vancomycin with a final concentration not to exceed 5 mg/mL by I.V. intermittent infusion over at least 60 minutes (recommended infusion period of ≥30 minutes for every 500 mg administered).

If a maculopapular rash appears on the face, neck, trunk, and/or upper extremities (red man syndrome), slow the infusion rate to over 1½ to 2 hours and increase the dilution volume. Hypotension, shock, and cardiac arrest (rare) have also been reported with too rapid of infusion. Reactions are often treated with antihistamines and steroids.

Intrathecal (unlabeled route): Vancomycin is available as a powder for injection and may be diluted to 1-5 mg/mL concentration in preservative free 0.9% sodium chloride for intrathecal administration.

Intravitreal: May be administered by intravitreal injection (unlabeled use).

Oral: Vancomycin powder for injection may be reconstituted and used for oral administration (Cohen, 2010). Reconstituted powder for injection (not premixed solution) may be administered orally by diluting the reconstituted solution in 30 mL of water; common flavoring syrups may be added to improve taste. The unflavored, diluted solution may also be administered via nasogastric tube.

Rectal (unlabeled route): May be administered as a retention enema per rectum (Cohen, 2010)

Not for I.M. administration.

Extravasation treatment: Monitor I.V. site closely; extravasation will cause serious injury with possible necrosis and tissue sloughing. Rotate infusion site frequently.

Dosage Forms Excipient information presented when available (limited, particularly for generics); consult specific product labeling.

Capsule, oral: 125 mg, 250 mg

Vancocin®: 125 mg, 250 mg

Infusion, premixed iso-osmotic dextrose solution: 500 mg (100 mL); 750 mg (150 mL); 1 g (200 mL)

Injection, powder for reconstitution: 500 mg, 750 mg, 1 g, 5 g, 10 g

- **Vancomycin Hydrochloride** *see* Vancomycin *on page 1428*
- **Vancomycin Hydrochloride for Injection, USP (Can)** *see* Vancomycin *on page 1428*

Vandetanib (van DET a nib)

Related Information

Management of Chemotherapy-Induced Nausea and Vomiting *on page 1786*

Principles of Anticancer Therapy *on page 1878*

Brand Names: U.S. Caprelsa®

Brand Names: Canada Caprelsa®

Index Terms AZD6474; Zactima; ZD6474; Zictifa

Generic Availability (U.S.) No

Pharmacologic Category Antineoplastic Agent, Tyrosine Kinase Inhibitor; Epidermal Growth Factor Receptor (EGFR) Inhibitor; Vascular Endothelial Growth Factor (VEGF) Inhibitor

Use Treatment of metastatic or unresectable locally advanced medullary thyroid cancer (symptomatic or progressive)

Labeled Contraindications Congenital long QT syndrome

Canadian labeling: Additional contraindications (not in U.S. labeling): Hypersensitivity to vandetanib or any component of the formulation; persistent Fridericia-corrected QT interval (QTcF) ≥500 ms; uncorrected hypokalemia, hypomagnesemia, or hypocalcemia; uncontrolled hypertension

Pregnancy Risk Factor D

Lactation Excretion in breast milk unknown/not recommended

Warnings/Precautions Hazardous agent – use appropriate precautions for handling and disposal. **[U.S. Boxed Warning]: May prolong the QT interval; torsade de pointes and sudden death have been reported. Do not use in patients with hypocalcemia, hypokalemia, hypomagnesemia, or long QT syndrome. Correct electrolyte imbalance prior to initiating therapy. Monitor electrolytes and ECG (to monitor QT interval) at baseline, at 2-4 weeks, at 8-12 weeks, and every 3 months thereafter; monitoring (at the same frequency) is required following dose reductions for QT prolongation or with dose interruptions >2 weeks. Avoid the use of QT-prolonging agents; if concomitant use with QT prolonging agents cannot be avoided, monitor ECG more frequently. Vandetanib has a long half-life (19 days), therefore, adverse reactions (including QT prolongation) may resolve slowly; monitor appropriately.** Ventricular tachycardia has also been reported. The potential for QT prolongation is dose-dependent. Do not initiate treatment unless QT interval, Fridericia-corrected QT interval (QTcF) is <450 msec. During treatment, if QTcF >500 msec, withhold vandetanib and resume at a reduced dose when QTcF is <450 msec. Avoid use in patients with a history of torsade de pointes, congenital long QT syndrome, bradyarrhythmias or uncompensated heart failure. Patients with ventricular arrhythmias or recent MI were excluded from clinical trials. To reduce the risk of QT prolongation, maintain serum calcium and magnesium within normal limits and maintain serum potassium ≥4 mEq/L. Heart failure (HF) has been reported; monitor for signs and symptoms of HF; may require discontinuation (HF may not be reversible upon discontinuation). Hypertension and hypertensive crisis have been observed with vandetanib; monitor blood pressure and initiate or adjust antihypertensive therapy as needed; may require vandetanib dosage adjustment or treatment interruption; discontinue vandetanib (permanently) if blood pressure cannot be adequately controlled. Canadian labeling contraindicates use in uncontrolled hypertension.

Diarrhea has been reported with use; may cause electrolyte imbalance (closely monitor electrolytes); routine antidiarrheals are recommended; withhold vandetanib treatment until resolution for severe diarrhea; dose reduction is recommended when treatment is resumed. Stevens-Johnson syndrome and other serious skin reactions (including fatal) have been reported. Mild-to-moderate skin reactions, including acne, dermatitis, dry skin, palmar-plantar erythrodysesthesia syndrome, pruritus, and rash have also been reported. Withhold treatment for dermatologic toxicity of grade 3 or higher; consider a reduced dose or permanent discontinuation upon improvement in symptoms. Severe dermatologic toxicity has been managed with corticosteroids (systemic) and treatment discontinuation; mild-to-moderate toxicity has responded to corticosteroids (systemic or topical), oral antihistamines, and antibiotics (topical or systemic). Increased risk of photosensitivity is associated with use; effective sunscreen and protective clothing are recommended during and for at least 4 months after treatment discontinuation.

Reversible posterior leukoencephalopathy syndrome (RPLS) been observed with vandetanib; symptoms of RPLS include altered mental function, confusion, headache, seizure, or visual disturbances; generally associated with hypertension; consider discontinuing treatment if RPLS occurs. Serious and sometimes fatal hemorrhagic events have been reported with use; discontinue in patients with severe hemorrhage; do not administer in patients with a recent history of hemoptysis with ≥2.5 mL of red blood. Ischemic cerebrovascular events (some fatal) have been observed with vandetanib; discontinue treatment in patients with severe ischemic events (the safety of resuming treatment after an ischemic event has not been studied). Interstitial lung disease (ILD) or pneumonitis (including fatalities) has been reported with vandetanib. Patients should be advised to report any new or worsening respiratory symptoms; ILD should be suspected with nonspecific respiratory symptoms such as hypoxia, pleural effusion, cough or dyspnea. If asymptomatic (or minimal symptoms) although with radiologic evidence of ILD, may continue treatment with close monitoring; consider interrupting treatment for moderate symptoms (may require corticosteroids or antibiotics). Discontinue treatment for severe symptoms; may require corticosteroids and antibiotics, and permanent discontinuation.

Increased doses of thyroid replacement therapy have been required in patients with prior thyroidectomy; obtain TSH at baseline, at 2-4 weeks, 8-12 weeks, and every 3 months after vandetanib initiation; if signs and symptoms of hypothyroidism occur during treatment, evaluate thyroid hormone levels and adjust replacement therapy if needed. Dosage reduction is recommended in patients with moderate-to-severe renal impairment. Exposure is increased in patients with impaired renal function; closely monitor QT interval; has not been studied in patients with end stage renal disease requiring dialysis. Not recommended for use in patients with moderate-to-severe hepatic impairment.

Avoid concurrent use with strong CYP3A4 inducers, including St John's wort and with QT-prolonging agents. Due to the risk for serious treatment-related adverse events, use in patients whose disease is not progressive or symptomatic should be only be undertaken after careful consideration. **[U.S. Boxed Warning]: Vandetanib is only available through a restricted access program; prescribers and pharmacies must be certified with the restricted distribution program to prescribe and dispense vandetanib.**

Adverse Reactions

>10%:

Cardiovascular: Hypertension (33%; grades 3/4: 9%), QT prolongation (14%; grades 3/4: 8%)

Central nervous system: Headache (26%), fatigue (24%), insomnia (13%)

Dermatologic: Rash (53%; grades 3/4: 5%), dermatitis acneiform/acne (35%; grades 3/4: 1%), dry skin (15%), photosensitivity (13%), pruritus (11%)

Endocrine & metabolic: Hypocalcemia (11% to 57%), hypoglycemia (24%)

Gastrointestinal: Diarrhea/colitis (57%; grades 3/4: 11%), nausea (33%), abdominal pain (21%), appetite decreased (21%), vomiting (15%), dyspepsia (11%)

Hematologic: Leukopenia (19%), anemia (13%; grades 3/4: <1%), hemorrhage (13% to 14%)

Hepatic: ALT increased (51%), bilirubin increased (13%)

Neuromuscular & skeletal: Weakness (15%)

Ocular: Corneal abnormalities (corneal edema, corneal opacity, corneal dystrophy, corneal pigmentation, keratopathy, arcus lipoides, corneal deposits, acquired corneal dystrophy: 13%)

Renal: Creatinine increased (16%)

Respiratory: Upper respiratory tract infection (23%), cough (11%), nasopharyngitis (11%)

1% to 10%:

Cardiovascular: Cardiac failure (2%)

Central nervous system: Depression (10%)

Dermatologic: Nail disorder (inflammation, tenderness, paronychia: 9%), alopecia (8%)

Endocrine & metabolic: Hypercalcemia (7%), hypomagnesemia (7%), hyperkalemia (6%), hypokalemia (6%), hyperglycemia (5%), hypermagnesemia (3%)

Gastrointestinal: Weight loss (10%), xerostomia (9%), abnormal taste (8%)

Hematologic: Neutropenia (10%; grades 3/4: <1%), thrombocytopenia (9%)

Neuromuscular & skeletal: Muscle spasms (6%)

Ocular: Blurred vision (9%)

Renal: Proteinuria (10%)

Respiratory: Aspiration pneumonia (2%), respiratory arrest (2%), respiratory failure (2%)

Miscellaneous: Sepsis (2%)

<1%, postmarketing, and/or case reports: Arthralgia, cardiopulmonary arrest, fever, heart failure, interstitial lung disease, ischemic cerebrovascular events, palmar-plantar erythrodysesthesia syndrome, pancreatitis, pneumonitis, reversible posterior leukoencephalopathy syndrome (RPLS), Stevens-Johnson syndrome, torsade de pointes, ventricular tachycardia

Drug Interactions

Metabolism/Transport Effects Substrate of CYP3A4 (major); **Note:** Assignment of Major/Minor substrate status based on clinically relevant drug interaction potential; **Inhibits** BCRP, P-glycoprotein

Avoid Concomitant Use

Avoid concomitant use of Vandetanib with any of the following: Bosutinib; CYP3A4 Inducers (Strong); Highest Risk QTc-Prolonging Agents; Mifepristone; Moderate Risk QTc-Prolonging Agents; Silodosin; St Johns Wort; VinCRIStine (Liposomal)

Increased Effect/Toxicity

Vandetanib may increase the levels/effects of: Bosutinib; Colchicine; Dabigatran Etexilate; Everolimus; Highest Risk QTc-Prolonging Agents; P-glycoprotein/ABCB1 Substrates; Prucalopride; Rivaroxaban; Silodosin; Topotecan; VinCRIStine (Liposomal); Vitamin K Antagonists

The levels/effects of Vandetanib may be increased by: Mifepristone; Moderate Risk QTc-Prolonging Agents; QTc-Prolonging Agents (Indeterminate Risk and Risk Modifying)

Decreased Effect

Vandetanib may decrease the levels/effects of: Cardiac Glycosides; Vitamin K Antagonists

The levels/effects of Vandetanib may be decreased by: CYP3A4 Inducers (Strong); Deferasirox; St Johns Wort; Tocilizumab

Ethanol/Nutrition/Herb Interactions Herb/Nutraceutical: Avoid St John's wort (may decrease vandetanib exposure).

Storage/Stability Store at 25°C (77°F); excursions permitted to 15°C to 30°C (59°F to 86°F).

Mechanism of Action Multikinase inhibitor; inhibits tyrosine kinases including epidermal growth factor reception (EGFR), vascular endothelial growth factor (VEGF), rearranged during transfection (RET), protein tyrosine kinase 6 (BRK), TIE2, EPH kinase receptors and SRC kinase receptors, selectively blocking intracellular signaling, angiogenesis and cellular proliferation

Pharmacodynamics/Kinetics

Absorption: Slow

Protein binding: ~90%; to albumin and alpha 1-acid-glycoprotein

Distribution: V_d: ~7450 L

Metabolism: Hepatic, via CYP3A4 to N-desmethyl vandetanib and via flavin-containing monooxygenase enzymes to vandetanib-N-oxide

Bioavailability: Not affected by food

Half life, elimination: 19 days

Time to peak: 6 hours (range: 4-10 hours)

Excretion: Feces (~44%); urine (~25%)

Dosing

Adult & Geriatric Note: Do not initiate treatment unless QTcF <450 msec. Avoid concomitant use of QT-prolonging agents and strong CYP3A4 inducers. To reduce the risk of QT prolongation, maintain serum calcium and magnesium within normal limits and maintain serum potassium ≥4 mEq/L.

Medullary thyroid cancer, locally advanced or metastatic: Oral: 300 mg once daily, continue treatment until no longer clinically benefiting or until unacceptable toxicity

Renal Impairment

Cl_{cr} ≥50 mL/minute: No dosage adjustment necessary.

Cl_{cr} <50 mL/minute: Reduce initial dose to 200 mg once daily; closely monitor QT interval.

Hepatic Impairment

Mild impairment: No dosage adjustment provided in manufacturer's labeling.

Moderate and severe impairment (Child-Pugh class B or C): Use is not recommended.

Adjustment for Toxicity

QTcF >500 msec: Withhold dose until QTcF returns to <450 msec, then resume at a reduced dose

Toxicity ≥grade 3: Interrupt dose until resolves or improves to grade 1, then resume at a reduced dose

Dosage reduction: Reduce from 300 mg once daily to 200 mg once daily, further reduce if needed to 100 mg once daily

Management of specific toxicities:

Diarrhea (severe): Withhold treatment until resolution. Dose reduction is recommended when treatment is resumed. Routine antidiarrheals are recommended. Closely monitor electrolytes.

Heart failure: May require discontinuation.

Hemorrhage (severe): Discontinue.

Hypertension: Initiate or adjust antihypertensive therapy as needed; may require vandetanib dosage adjustment or treatment interruption; discontinue permanently if blood pressure cannot be adequately controlled.

Interstitial lung disease (ILD)/pneumonitis: If asymptomatic (or minimal symptoms) with radiologic evidence of ILD, may continue treatment with close monitoring. Consider interrupting treatment for moderate symptoms (may require corticosteroids or antibiotics). Discontinue treatment for severe symptoms; may require corticosteroids and antibiotics, and even permanent discontinuation.

Ischemic cerebrovascular events (severe): Discontinue treatment (safety of resuming treatment after an ischemic event has not been studied).

Reversible posterior leukoencephalopathy syndrome (RPLS): Consider discontinuing treatment.

Skin reactions: Withhold treatment for dermatologic toxicity of grade 3 or higher. Consider a reduced dose or permanent discontinuation upon improvement in symptoms. Severe dermatologic toxicity has been managed with corticosteroids (systemic) and treatment discontinuation; mild-to-moderate toxicity has responded to corticosteroids (systemic or topical), oral antihistamines, and antibiotics (topical or systemic).

Administration May be administered with or without food. Missed doses should be omitted if within 12 hours of the next scheduled dose. Do not crush tablet. If unable to swallow tablet whole or if nasogastric or gastrostomy tube administration is necessary, disperse one tablet in 2 ounces of water (noncarbonated only) and stir for 10 minutes to disperse (will not dissolve completely) and administer immediately. Rinse residue in glass with additional 4 ounces of water (noncarbonated only) and administer. Use appropriate handling precautions (hazardous agent).

Emetic Potential Low (10% to 30%)

Extemporaneous Preparations Hazardous agent: Use appropriate precautions for handling and disposal.

An oral solution may be prepared using the tablet. Disperse one tablet in 2 ounces of water (noncarbonated only) and stir for 10 minutes to disperse (will not dissolve completely) and administer immediately. Rinse residue in glass with additional 4 ounces of water (noncarbonated only) and administer.

Monitoring Parameters Monitor electrolytes (calcium, magnesium, potassium), TSH, and ECG (QT interval) at baseline, at 2-4 weeks, at 8-12 weeks, and every 3 months thereafter; also monitor QT interval at same frequency for dose reduction due to QT interval or treatment delays >2 weeks (monitor electrolytes and ECG more frequently if diarrhea). Monitor renal function, hepatic function, blood pressure; monitor for signs and symptoms of heart failure and pulmonary toxicities.

Dietary Considerations May be taken with or without food.

Prescribing and Access Restrictions As a requirement of the REMS program, access to vandetanib is restricted. Vandetanib is approved for marketing under a Food and Drug Administration (FDA) approved, risk management program, and through a restricted distribution program, the Vandetanib REMS Program (1-800-236-9933). Prescribers and pharmacies must be certified with the program to prescribe or dispense vandetanib.

In Canada, vandetanib is available only through the CAPRELSA Restricted Distribution Program. Prescribers and pharmacies must be certified with the program to prescribe or dispense vandetanib. Further information may be obtained at 1-800-668-6000.

Medication Guide Available Yes

Dosage Forms Excipient information presented when available (limited, particularly for generics); consult specific product labeling.

Tablet, oral: 100 mg, 300 mg

Caprelsa®: 100 mg, 300 mg

References

Robinson BG, Paz-Ares L, Krebs A, et al, "Vandetanib (100 mg) in Patients With Locally Advanced or Metastatic Hereditary Medullary Thyroid Cancer," *J Clin Endocrinol Metab*, 2010, 95 (6):2664-71.

Wells SA Jr, Gosnell JE, Gagel RF, et al, "Vandetanib for the Treatment of Patients With Locally Advanced or Metastatic Hereditary Medullary Thyroid Cancer," *J Clin Oncol*, 2010, 28(5):767-72.

Wells SA, Robinson BG, Gagel RF, et al, "Vandetanib (VAN) in Locally Advanced or Metastatic Medullary Thyroid Cancer (MTC): A Randomized, Double-Blind Phase III Trial (ZETA)," *J Clin Oncol*, 2010, 28(15s):5503 [abstract 5503 from 2010 ASCO Annual Meeting].

◆ **Vantas®** *see* Histrelin *on page 707*

◆ **Vascular Endothelial Growth Factor Trap** *see* Ziv-Aflibercept (Systemic) *on page 1484*

◆ **Vectibix®** *see* Panitumumab *on page 1115*

◆ **Vectical®** *see* Calcitriol *on page 215*

◆ **VEGF Trap** *see* Ziv-Aflibercept (Systemic) *on page 1484*

◆ **VEGF Trap R1R2** *see* Ziv-Aflibercept (Systemic) *on page 1484*

◆ **Velban** *see* VinBLAStine *on page 1445*

◆ **Velcade®** *see* Bortezomib *on page 187*

Vemurafenib (vem ue RAF e nib)

Related Information

Principles of Anticancer Therapy *on page 1878*

Brand Names: U.S. Zelboraf™

Brand Names: Canada Zelboraf™

Index Terms BRAF(V600E) Kinase Inhibitor RO5185426; PLX4032; RG7204; RO5185426

Generic Availability (U.S.) No

Pharmacologic Category Antineoplastic Agent, BRAF Kinase Inhibitor

Use Treatment of unresectable or metastatic melanoma in patients with a $BRAF^{V600E}$ mutation (as detected by an FDA-approved test)

Note: Not recommended in patients with wild-type BRAF melanoma

Labeled Contraindications There are no contraindications listed within the manufacturer's labeling.

Canadian labeling: Hypersensitivity to vemurafenib or any component of the formulation.

Pregnancy Risk Factor D

Lactation Excretion in breast milk unknown/not recommended

Warnings/Precautions Only patients with a $BRAF^{V600}$ mutation-positive melanoma (including $BRAF^{V600E}$) will benefit from treatment; mutation must be detected and confirmed by an FDA-approved test prior to treatment. The cobas® 4800 BRAF V600 Mutation Test was used in clinical trials and is FDA-approved to detect $BRAF^{V600E}$ mutation.

Cases of skin and keratoacanthomas cutaneous squamous cell carcinoma (cuSCC) have been reported; generally occurring early the treatment course (median onset 7-8 weeks) and is managed with excision. Potential risk factors for cuSCC include age ≥65 years, history of skin cancer or chronic sun exposure. Monitor for skin lesions (with dermatology evaluation) at baseline and every 2 months during treatment; consider continued monitoring for 6 months after treatment. New primary melanoma lesions were observed during treatment and were managed with excision while continuing treatment (at the same dose); continue to monitor for skin lesions.

Dermatologic reactions have been observed, including case reports of Stevens-Johnson syndrome and toxic epidermal necrolysis; discontinue (permanently) for severe dermatologic toxicity. Photosensitivity ranging from mild to severe has been reported. Advise patients to avoid sun exposure and wear protective clothing and use effective UVA/UVB sunscreen and lip balm (SPF ≥30) when outdoors. Dosage modification are recommended for intolerable photosensitivity consisting of erythema ≥10% to 30% of body surface area. Uveitis cases have been reported; monitor for signs and symptoms; may be managed with corticosteroid and mydriatic eye drops. Cases of blurred vision, iritis, photophobia, and a single case of retinal vein occlusion have been reported in clinical trials.

QT prolongation (dose-dependent) has been observed; may lead to increased risk for ventricular arrhythmia, including torsade de pointes. Monitor electrolytes (calcium, magnesium and potassium) at baseline and with dosage adjustments. Monitor ECG at baseline, 15 days after initiation, then monthly for 3 months, then every 3 months thereafter (more frequently if clinically appropriate); also monitor with dosage adjustments. Do not initiate treatment if baseline QT_c >500 msec. During treatment, if QT_c >500 msec, temporarily interrupt treatment; correct electrolytes and control other risk factors for QT prolongation. May reinitiate once with a dose reduction once QT_c falls to <500 msec. Discontinue (permanently), if after correction of risk factors, both the QT_c continues to increase >500 msec and there is >60 msec change above baseline. Use is not recommended in patients with electrolyte abnormalities which are not correctable, long QT syndrome, or taking concomitant medication known to prolong the QT interval.

Increases in liver function tests have been reported. Monitor transaminases, alkaline phosphatase and bilirubin. Severe hypersensitivity, including anaphylaxis, rash (generalized), erythema, or hypotension were reported with use and following reinitiation of treatment. Discontinue (permanently) with severe hypersensitivity reaction. Elderly patients may be at increased risk for adverse effects; in clinical trials, there was an increased incidence of cuSCC and keratoacanthoma, atrial fibrillation, peripheral edema, and nausea/decreased appetite in patients ≥65 years of age.

Adverse Reactions

>10%:

Cardiovascular: Peripheral edema (17% to 23%)

Central nervous system: Fatigue (38% to 54%), headache (23% to 27%), fever (17% to 19%)

Dermatologic: Rash (37% to 52%; grade 3: 7% to 8%), photosensitivity (33% to 49%; grade 3: 3%), alopecia (36% to 45%), pruritus (23% to 30%), skin papilloma (21% to 30%), hyperkeratosis (24% to 28%), cutaneous squamous cell carcinoma (24%; grade 3: 22% to 24%), maculopapular rash (9% to 21%), dry skin (16% to 19%), actinic keratosis (8% to 17%), seborrheic keratosis (10% to 14%), sunburn (10% to 14%), erythema (8% to 14%), papular rash (5% to 13%)

Gastrointestinal: Nausea (35% to 37%; grade 3: 2%), diarrhea (28% to 29%; grade 3: <1%), vomiting (18% to 26%; grade 3: 1% to 2%), appetite decreased (18% to 21%), constipation (12% to 16%), taste alteration (11% to 14%)

Hepatic: GGT increased (5% to 15%)

Neuromuscular & skeletal: Arthralgia (53% to 67%), myalgia (13% to 24%), limb pain (9% to 18%), back pain (8% to 11%), musculoskeletal pain (8% to 11%), weakness (2% to 11%)

Respiratory: Cough (8% to 12%)

≤10% and/or case reports:

Cardiovascular: Atrial fibrillation, hypotension, QT prolongation, vasculitis

Central nervous system: Dizziness, nerve paralysis (VII)

Dermatologic: Basal cell carcinoma, erythema nodosum, folliculitis, keratosis pilaris, melanoma (new primary), palmar-plantar erythrodysesthesia, Stevens-Johnson syndrome, toxic epidermal necrolysis

Gastrointestinal: Weight loss

Hepatic: Alkaline phosphatase increased, ALT increase, AST increased, bilirubin increased

Neuromuscular & skeletal: Arthritis, peripheral neuropathy

Ocular: Blurred vision, iritis, photophobia, retinal vein occlusion, uveitis

Renal: Creatinine increased

Miscellaneous: Anaphylaxis, hypersensitivity

Drug Interactions

Metabolism/Transport Effects Substrate of CYP3A4 (minor), P-glycoprotein; **Note:** Assignment of Major/Minor substrate status based on clinically relevant drug interaction potential; **Inhibits** CYP1A2 (moderate), CYP2D6 (weak), P-glycoprotein; **Induces** CYP3A4 (weak/moderate)

Avoid Concomitant Use

Avoid concomitant use of Vemurafenib with any of the following: Axitinib; Bosutinib; Highest Risk QTc-Prolonging Agents; Mifepristone; Moderate Risk QTc-Prolonging Agents; Silodosin; Topotecan; VinCRIStine (Liposomal)

Increased Effect/Toxicity

Vemurafenib may increase the levels/effects of: ARIPiprazole; Bosutinib; Colchicine; CYP1A2 Substrates; Dabigatran Etexilate; Everolimus; Highest Risk QTc-Prolonging Agents; P-glycoprotein/ABCB1 Substrates; Prucalopride; Rivaroxaban; Silodosin; Topotecan; VinCRIStine (Liposomal); Vitamin K Antagonists

The levels/effects of Vemurafenib may be increased by: CYP3A4 Inhibitors (Strong); Mifepristone; Moderate Risk QTc-Prolonging Agents; P-glycoprotein/ABCB1 Inhibitors; QTc-Prolonging Agents (Indeterminate Risk and Risk Modifying)

Decreased Effect

Vemurafenib may decrease the levels/effects of: ARIPiprazole; Axitinib; Cardiac Glycosides; Saxagliptin; Vitamin K Antagonists

The levels/effects of Vemurafenib may be decreased by: CYP3A4 Inducers (Strong); P-glycoprotein/ABCB1 Inducers; Tocilizumab

Storage/Stability Store at room temperature of 20°C to 25°C (68°F to 77°F); excursions permitted to 15°C and 30°C (59°F and 86°F).

Mechanism of Action BRAF kinase inhibitor (potent) which inhibits tumor growth in melanomas by inhibiting kinase activity of certain mutated forms of BRAF, including BRAF with V600E mutation, thereby blocking cellular proliferation in melanoma cells with the mutation. Does not have activity against cells with wild-type BRAF. $BRAF^{V600E}$ activating mutations present in ~50% of melanomas; V600E mutation involves the substitution of glutamic acid for valine at amino acid 600. The cobas® 4800 BRAF V600 mutation test is approved to detect $BRAF^{V600E}$ mutation.

Pharmacodynamics/Kinetics

Distribution: V_d: ~106 L

Protein binding: >99%, to albumin and α_1-acid glycoprotein

Half-life, elimination: 57 hours (range: 30-120 hours)

Time to peak: ~3 hours

Excretion: Feces (~94%); urine (~1%)

Dosing

Adult & Geriatric Melanoma, metastatic or unresectable (with $BRAF^{V600E}$ mutation): Oral: 960 mg twice daily; continue until disease progression or unacceptable toxicity

Renal Impairment

Mild-to-moderate impairment (pre-existing): No adjustments recommended.

Severe impairment (pre-existing): Data is insufficient to determine if dosage adjustment necessary; use with caution

Hepatic Impairment

Mild-to-moderate impairment (pre-existing): No adjustments recommended

Severe impairment (pre-existing): Data is insufficient to determine if dosage adjustment necessary; use with caution.

Adjustment for Toxicity Note: Dose reductions resulting in a dose below 480 mg twice daily are not recommended

Grade 1 or grade 2 (tolerable) toxicity: No adjustment recommended.

Grade 2 (intolerable) or grade 3 toxicity:

First incident: Interrupt treatment until toxicity returns to grade 0 or 1, then resume at 720 mg twice daily

Second incident: Interrupt treatment until toxicity returns to grade 0 or 1, then resume at 480 mg twice daily

Third incident: Discontinue permanently.

Grade 4 toxicity:

First incident: Interrupt treatment until toxicity returns to grade 0 or 1, then resume at 480 mg twice daily **or** discontinue permanently

Second incident: Discontinue permanently.

Specific toxicities:

Severe hypersensitivity or severe dermatologic toxicity: Discontinue permanently.

QT_c >500 msec: Temporarily withhold treatment, correct electrolytes and control risk factors for QT prolongation; may reinitiate with a dose reduction once QT_c <500 msec.

QT_c persistently >500 msec and >60 msec above baseline: Discontinue permanently.

Combination Regimens

Melanoma: Vemurafenib (Melanoma Regimen) on page 1770

Administration Doses should be administered orally in the morning and evening, ~12 hours apart. Swallow whole with a glass of water; do not crush or chew. May be taken with or without a meal. If a dose is missed, may be taken up to 4 hours prior to the next scheduled dose to maintain a twice daily schedule; both doses should **not** be taken at the same time.

Monitoring Parameters Liver transaminases, alkaline phosphatase and bilirubin at baseline and monthly during treatment (or as clinically appropriate). Electrolytes (calcium, magnesium and potassium) at baseline and after dosage modification. ECG at baseline, 15 days after initiation, then monthly for 3 months, then every 3 months thereafter (more frequently if clinically appropriate) and with dosage adjustments. Dermatology evaluation (for new skin lesions) at baseline and every 2 months during treatment; also consider continued monitoring for 6 months after completion of treatment.

Dietary Considerations May be taken with or without food.

Prescribing and Access Restrictions Available through specialty pharmacies. Further information may be obtained from the manufacturer, Genentech, at 1-888-249-4918, or at http://www.zelboraf.com.

Medication Guide Available Yes

Dosage Forms Excipient information presented when available (limited, particularly for generics); consult specific product labeling.

Tablet, oral:

Zelboraf™: 240 mg

References

Bloom KJ, Anderson SM, Schilling RC, et al, "Molecular Testing for BRAF V600 Mutations in the BRIM-2 Trial of the BRAF Inhibitor Vemurafenib in Metastatic Melanoma," *J Clin Oncol*, 2011, 29 (15s):10523 [abstract 10523 from ASCO 2011 Annual Meeting].

Bollag G, Hirth P, Tsai J, et al, "Clinical Efficacy of a RAF Inhibitor Needs Broad Target Blockade in BRAF-Mutant Melanoma," *Nature*, 2010, 467(7315):596-9.

Chapman PB, Hauschild A, Robert C, et al, "Improved Survival With Vemurafenib in Melanoma With BRAF V600E Mutation," *N Engl J Med*, 2011, 364(26):2507-16.

Flaherty KT, Puzanov I, Kim KB, et al, "Inhibition of Mutated, Activated BRAF in Metastatic Melanoma," *N Engl J Med*, 2010, 363(9):809-19.

Ribas A, Kim KB, Schuchter LM, et al, "BRIM-2: An Open-Label, Multicenter Phase II Study of Vemurafenib in Previously Treated Patients With BRAF V600E Mutation-Positive Metastatic Melanoma," *J Clin Oncol*, 2011, 29(15s):8509 [abstract 8509 from ASCO 2011 Annual Meeting].

Su F, Yang H, Higgins B, et al, "Molecular Mechanisms Underlying Disease Relapse on Treatment With Selective BRAF Inhibitor Vemurafenib (PLX4032)," *J Clin Oncol*, 2011, 29(15s):8517 [abstract 8517 from ASCO 2011 Annual Meeting].

◆ **Venofer®** *see* Iron Sucrose *on page 827*

◆ **VePesid** *see* Etoposide *on page 538*

◆ **Vepesid™ (Can)** *see* Etoposide *on page 538*
◆ **Veripred™ 20** *see* PrednisoLONE (Systemic) *on page 1193*
◆ **Vesanoid** *see* Tretinoin (Systemic) *on page 1405*
◆ **Vesanoid® (Can)** *see* Tretinoin (Systemic) *on page 1405*
◆ **VFEND®** *see* Voriconazole *on page 1473*
◆ **Vidaza®** *see* AzaCITIDine *on page 140*

VinBLAStine (vin BLAS teen)

Related Information

Management of Chemotherapy-Induced Nausea and Vomiting *on page 1786*
Management of Drug Extravasations *on page 1800*
Safe Handling of Hazardous Drugs *on page 1904*

Index Terms Velban; Vinblastine Sulfate; Vincaleukoblastine; VLB

Generic Availability (U.S.) Yes

Pharmacologic Category Antineoplastic Agent, Natural Source (Plant) Derivative; Antineoplastic Agent, Vinca Alkaloid

Use Treatment of Hodgkin's and non-Hodgkin's lymphoma; testicular cancer; breast cancer; mycosis fungoides; Kaposi's sarcoma; histiocytosis (Letterer-Siwe disease); choriocarcinoma

Unlabeled Use Treatment of bladder cancer, melanoma, nonsmall cell lung cancer (NSCLC), ovarian cancer, soft tissue sarcoma (desmoid tumors)

Labeled Contraindications Significant granulocytopenia; presence of bacterial infection; I.T. administration is contraindicated (may result in death)

Pregnancy Risk Factor D

Lactation Excretion in breast milk unknown/not recommended

Warnings/Precautions Hazardous agent - use appropriate precautions for handling and disposal. **[U.S. Boxed Warning]: For I.V. use only. Intrathecal administration may result in death.** Must be dispensed in overwrap which bears the statement **"Do not remove covering until the moment of injection. Fatal if given intrathecally. For I.V. use only." [U.S. Boxed Warning]: Vinblastine is a moderate vesicant; avoid extravasation. Individuals administering should be experienced in vinblastine administration;** assure proper needle or catheter placement prior to administration. Leukopenia is common; granulocytopenia may be severe with higher doses. Leukopenia may be more pronounced in cachectic patients and patients with skin ulceration. Thrombocytopenia and anemia may occur rarely.

Use with caution in patients with hepatic impairment; toxicity may be increased; may require dosage modification. Neurotoxicity is rare at clinical doses; may occur with high doses (symptoms are similar to vincristine toxicity, including peripheral neuropathy, loss of deep tendon reflexes, headache, weakness, urinary retention, and GI symptoms). May rarely cause disabling neurotoxicity (usually reversible). Itraconazole may decrease the metabolism of vinblastine via CYP3A4 inhibition and may increase the effects of vinblastine via P-glycoprotein effects; severe myelosuppression and neurotoxicity may occur. Acute shortness of breath and severe bronchospasm have been reported, most often in association with concurrent administration of mitomycin; may occur within minutes to several hours following vinblastine administration or up to 14 days following mitomycin administration; use caution in patients with pre-existing pulmonary disease. Use with caution in patients with ischemic heart disease. **[U.S. Boxed Warning]: Should be administered under the supervision of an experienced cancer chemotherapy**

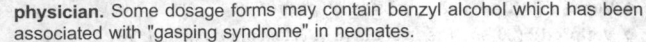

physician. Some dosage forms may contain benzyl alcohol which has been associated with "gasping syndrome" in neonates.

Adverse Reactions Frequency not defined.

Common:

Cardiovascular: Hypertension

Central nervous system: Malaise

Dermatologic: Alopecia

Gastrointestinal: Constipation

Hematologic: Myelosuppression, leukopenia/granulocytopenia (nadir: 5-10 days; recovery: 7-14 days; dose-limiting toxicity)

Neuromuscular & skeletal: Bone pain, jaw pain, tumor pain

Less common:

Cardiovascular: Angina, cerebrovascular accident, coronary ischemia, ECG abnormalities, limb ischemia, MI, myocardial ischemia, Raynaud's phenomenon

Central nervous system: Depression, dizziness, headache, neurotoxicity (duration: >24 hours), seizure, vertigo

Dermatologic: Dermatitis, photosensitivity (rare), rash, skin blistering

Endocrine & metabolic: Aspermia, hyperuricemia, SIADH

Gastrointestinal: Abdominal pain, anorexia, diarrhea, gastrointestinal bleeding, hemorrhagic enterocolitis, ileus, metallic taste, nausea (mild), paralytic ileus, rectal bleeding, stomatitis, toxic megacolon, vomiting (mild)

Genitourinary: Urinary retention

Hematologic: Anemia, thrombocytopenia (recovery within a few days), thrombotic thrombocytopenic purpura

Local: Cellulitis (with extravasation), irritation, phlebitis (with extravasation), radiation recall

Neuromuscular & skeletal: Deep tendon reflex loss, myalgia, paresthesia, peripheral neuritis, weakness

Ocular: Nystagmus

Otic: Auditory damage, deafness, vestibular damage

Renal: Hemolytic uremic syndrome

Respiratory: Bronchospasm, dyspnea, pharyngitis

Drug Interactions

Metabolism/Transport Effects Substrate of CYP2D6 (minor), CYP3A4 (major), P-glycoprotein; **Note:** Assignment of Major/Minor substrate status based on clinically relevant drug interaction potential; **Inhibits** CYP2D6 (weak), CYP3A4 (weak); **Induces** P-glycoprotein

Avoid Concomitant Use

Avoid concomitant use of VinBLAStine with any of the following: BCG; CloZAPine; Conivaptan; Dabigatran Etexilate; Natalizumab; Pimecrolimus; Pimozide; Tacrolimus (Topical); Vaccines (Live); VinCRIStine (Liposomal)

Increased Effect/Toxicity

VinBLAStine may increase the levels/effects of: ARIPiprazole; CloZAPine; Leflunomide; MitoMYcin (Systemic); Natalizumab; Pimozide; Tolterodine; Vaccines (Live)

The levels/effects of VinBLAStine may be increased by: Conivaptan; CYP3A4 Inhibitors (Moderate); CYP3A4 Inhibitors (Strong); Dasatinib; Denosumab; Itraconazole; Ivacaftor; Lopinavir; Macrolide Antibiotics; MAO Inhibitors; Mifepristone; P-glycoprotein/ABCB1 Inhibitors; Pimecrolimus; Posaconazole; Ritonavir; Roflumilast; Tacrolimus (Topical); Trastuzumab; Voriconazole

Decreased Effect

VinBLAStine may decrease the levels/effects of: BCG; Coccidioidin Skin Test; Dabigatran Etexilate; Linagliptin; P-glycoprotein/ABCB1 Substrates; Sipuleucel-T; Vaccines (Inactivated); Vaccines (Live); VinCRIStine (Liposomal)

The levels/effects of VinBLAStine may be decreased by: CYP3A4 Inducers (Strong); Deferasirox; Echinacea; Herbs (CYP3A4 Inducers); Peginterferon Alfa-2b; P-glycoprotein/ABCB1 Inducers; Tocilizumab

Ethanol/Nutrition/Herb Interactions Herb/Nutraceutical: Avoid St John's wort (may decrease vinblastine levels). Avoid black cohosh, dong quai in estrogen-dependent tumors.

Storage/Stability Note: Must be dispensed in overwrap which bears the statement "Do not remove covering until the moment of injection. Fatal if given intrathecally. For I.V. use only." Syringes should be labeled: "Fatal if given intrathecally. For I.V. use only."

Store intact vials under refrigeration at 2°C to 8°C (36°F to 46°F). Protect from light. Solutions reconstituted in bacteriostatic NS are stable for 28 days under refrigeration.

Reconstitution Reconstitute lyophilized powder to a concentration of 1 mg/mL with NS or bacteriostatic NS. For infusion, may dilute in 50 mL NS or D_5W; dilution in larger volumes (≥100 mL) of I.V. fluids is not recommended. Use appropriate precautions for handling and disposal.

Mechanism of Action Vinblastine binds to tubulin and inhibits microtubule formation, therefore, arresting the cell at metaphase by disrupting the formation of the mitotic spindle; it is specific for the M and S phases. Vinblastine may also interfere with nucleic acid and protein synthesis by blocking glutamic acid utilization.

Pharmacodynamics/Kinetics

Distribution: V_d: 27.3 L/kg; binds extensively to tissues; does not penetrate CNS or other fatty tissues; distributes to liver

Protein binding: 99%

Metabolism: Hepatic to active metabolite

Half-life elimination: Biphasic: Initial: 4 minutes; Terminal: 25 hours

Excretion: Feces (95%); urine (<1% as unchanged drug)

Dosing

Adult & Geriatric Details concerning dosing in combination regimens should also be consulted. **Note:** Frequency and duration of therapy may vary by indication, concomitant combination chemotherapy and hematologic response. **For I.V. use only.**

Antineoplastic (typical dosages): I.V.: Initial: 3.7 mg/m²; adjust dose every 7 days (based on white blood cell response) up to 5.5 mg/m² (second dose); 7.4 mg/m² (third dose); 9.25 mg/m² (fourth dose); and 11.1 mg/m² (fifth dose); do not administer more frequently than every 7 days.

Usual range: 5.5-7.4 mg/m² every 7 days; Maximum dose: 18.5 mg/m²; dosage adjustment goal is to reduce white blood cell count to ~3000/mm³

Indication-specific dosing:

Hodgkin's disease: Usual dose: 6 mg/m² every 2 weeks (as part of a combination chemotherapy regimen) (Bartlett, 1995; Horning, 2002)

Testicular cancer: Usual dose: 0.11 mg/kg daily for 2 days every 3 weeks (as part of a combination chemotherapy regimen) (Loehrer, 1998) **or** 6 mg/m²/day for 2 days every 3-4 weeks (as part of a combination chemotherapy regimen) (Clemm, 1986)

Bladder cancer (unlabeled use): Usual dose: 3 mg/m^2 every 7 days for 3 out of 4 weeks (as part of combination chemotherapy) (Sternberg, 2001) **or** 3 mg/m^2 days 2, 15, and 22 of a 28-day treatment cycle (as part of a combination chemotherapy regimen) (von der Maase, 2000)

Melanoma (unlabeled used): 2 mg/m^2 days 1-4 and 22-25 of a 6-week treatment cycle (as part of a combination chemotherapy regimen) (Eton, 2002)

Nonsmall cell lung cancer (unlabeled use): 4 mg/m^2 days 1, 8, 15, 22, and 29, then every 2 weeks (as part of combination chemotherapy) (Arriagada, 2004)

Ovarian cancer (unlabeled use): 0.11 mg/kg daily for 2 days every 3 weeks (as part of a combination chemotherapy regimen) (Loehrer, 1998)

Pediatric Details concerning dosing in combination regimens should also be consulted. **Note:** Frequency and duration of therapy may vary by indication, concomitant combination chemotherapy and hematologic response. **For I.V. use only.**

Hodgkin's disease: I.V.: Initial dose: 6 mg/m^2; do not administer more frequently than every 7 days

Letterer-Siwe disease: I.V.: Initial dose: 6.5 mg/m^2; do not administer more frequently than every 7 days

Testicular cancer: I.V.: Initial dose: 3 mg/m^2; do not administer more frequently than every 7 days

Renal Impairment According to FDA-approved labeling, no adjustment is necessary in patients with renal impairment.

Hepatic Impairment

The FDA-approved labeling recommends the following guidelines: Serum bilirubin >3 mg/dL: Administer 50% of dose

The following guidelines have been used by some clinicians:

Serum bilirubin >3.1 or transaminases >3 times ULN: Avoid use (Floyd, 2006) **or**

Serum bilirubin 1.5-3 mg/dL or AST 60-180 units: Administer 50% of dose

Serum bilirubin 3-5 mg/dL: Administer 25% of dose

Serum bilirubin >5 mg/dL or AST >180 units: Avoid use

Combination Regimens

Bladder cancer:

CMV on page 1589

M-VAC (Bladder Cancer) on page 1718

Lung cancer (nonsmall cell): Cisplatin-Vinblastine (NSCLC) on page 1585

Lymphoma, Hodgkin:

ABVD Early Stage (Hodgkin) on page 1516

ABVD (Hodgkin) on page 1516

ChlVPP (Hodgkin) on page 1562

C-MOPP/ABV Hybrid (Hodgkin) on page 1588

MOPP/ABVD (Hodgkin) on page 1714

MOPP/ABV Hybrid (Hodgkin) on page 1715

Stanford V (Hodgkin) on page 1752

VAMP (Hodgkin) on page 1769

Vinblastine (Hodgkin Regimen) on page 1771

Melanoma:

Cisplatin-Vinblastine-Dacarbazine (Melanoma) on page 1584

CVD-Interleukin-Interferon (Melanoma) on page 1597

Prostate cancer:

Doxorubicin + Ketoconazole/Estramustine + Vinblastine on page 1619

Estramustine-Vinblastine on page 1638

Soft tissue sarcoma (Desmoid tumor): Methotrexate-Vinblastine (Desmoid tumor) on page 1710

Testicular cancer:

PVB on page 1744

VBP on page 1770

VIP (Vinblastine) (Testicular Cancer) on page 1777

Administration **FATAL IF GIVEN INTRATHECALLY**. For I.V. administration only, usually as a slow (2-3 minutes) push, or a bolus (5-15 minutes) infusion; the manufacturer recommends an undiluted 1-minute infusion to prevent venous irritation/extravasation. Prolonged administration times and/or increased administration volumes may the risk of vein irritation and extravasation. Assure proper needle or catheter placement prior to administration.

Emetic Potential Very low (<10%)

Vesicant/Extravasation Risk Vesicant; see Management of Drug Extravasations on page 1800.

Monitoring Parameters CBC with differential and platelet count, serum uric acid, hepatic function tests

Dosage Forms Excipient information presented when available (limited, particularly for generics); consult specific product labeling.

Injection, powder for reconstitution, as sulfate: 10 mg

Injection, solution, as sulfate: 1 mg/mL (10 mL)

References

Arriagada R, Bergman B, Dunant A, et al, "Cisplatin-Based Adjuvant Chemotherapy in Patients With Completely Resected Non-Small-Cell Lung Cancer," *N Engl J Med*, 2004, 350(4):351-60.

Bartlett NL, Rosenberg SA, Hoppe RT, et al, "Brief Chemotherapy, Stanford V, and Adjuvant Radiotherapy for Bulky or Advanced-Stage Hodgkin's Disease: A Preliminary Report," *J Clin Oncol*, 1995, 13(5):1080-8.

Clemm C, Hartenstein R, Willich N, et al, "Vinblastine-Ifosfamide-Cisplatin Treatment of Bulky Seminoma," *Cancer*, 1986, 58(10):2203-7.

Eton O, Legha SS, Bedikian AY, et al, "Sequential Biochemotherapy Versus Chemotherapy for Metastatic Melanoma: Results From a Phase III Randomized Trial," *J Clin Oncol*, 2002, 20(8):2045-52.

Floyd J, Mirza I, Sachs B, et al, "Hepatotoxicity of Chemotherapy," *Semin Oncol*, 2006, 33(1):50-67.

Horning SJ, Hoppe RT, Breslin S, et al, "Stanford V and Radiotherapy for Locally Extensive and Advanced Hodgkin's Disease: Mature Results of a Prospective Clinical Trial," *J Clin Oncol*, 2002, 20(3):630-7.

Loehrer PJ Sr, Gonin R, Nichols CR, et al, "Vinblastine Plus Ifosfamide Plus Cisplatin as Initial Salvage Therapy in Recurrent Germ Cell Tumor," *J Clin Oncol*, 1998, 16(7):2500-4.

Morgan C, Tillett T, Braybrooke J, et al, "Management of Uncommon Chemotherapy Induced Emergencies," *Lancet Oncol*, 2011, 12(8):806-14.

Sternberg CN, de Mulder PH, Schornagel JH, et al, "Randomized Phase III Trial of High-Dose-Intensity Methotrexate, Vinblastine, Doxorubicin, and Cisplatin (M-VAC) Chemotherapy and Recombinant Human Granulocyte Colony-Stimulating Factor Versus Classic M-VAC in Advanced Urothelial Tract Tumors: European Organization for Research and Treatment of Cancer Protocol No. 30924," *J Clin Oncol*, 2001, 19(10):2638-46.

van der Maase H, Hansen SW, Roberts JT, et al, "Gemcitabine and Cisplatin Versus Methotrexate, Vinblastine, Doxorubicin, and Cisplatin in Advanced or Metastatic Bladder Cancer: Results of a Large, Randomized, Multinational, Multicenter, Phase III Study," *J Clin Oncol*, 2000, 18(17):3068-77.

- **Vinblastine Sulfate** *see* VinBLAStine *on page 1445*
- **Vincaleukoblastine** *see* VinBLAStine *on page 1445*
- **Vincasar PFS®** *see* VinCRIStine *on page 1450*

VinCRIStine (vin KRIS teen)

Related Information

Chemotherapy and Cancer Treatment During Pregnancy *on page 1829*
Chemotherapy and Obesity *on page 1834*
Chronic Pain Management (Cancer) *on page 1840*
Management of Chemotherapy-Induced Nausea and Vomiting *on page 1786*
Management of Drug Extravasations *on page 1800*
Safe Handling of Hazardous Drugs *on page 1904*

Brand Names: U.S. Vincasar PFS®

Brand Names: Canada Vincristine Sulfate Injection

Index Terms Conventional Vincristine; Leurocristine Sulfate; Oncovin; Vincristine (Conventional); Vincristine Sulfate

Generic Availability (U.S.) Yes

Pharmacologic Category Antineoplastic Agent, Natural Source (Plant) Derivative; Antineoplastic Agent, Vinca Alkaloid

Use Treatment of acute lymphocytic leukemia (ALL), Hodgkin lymphoma, non-Hodgkin lymphomas, Wilms' tumor, neuroblastoma, rhabdomyosarcoma

Unlabeled Use Treatment of central nervous system tumors, chronic lymphocytic leukemia (CLL), Ewing's sarcoma, gestational trophoblastic tumors (high-risk), multiple myeloma, ovarian germ cell tumors, retinoblastoma, small cell lung cancer (SCLC)

Labeled Contraindications Patients with the demyelinating form of Charcot-Marie-Tooth syndrome

Pregnancy Risk Factor D

Lactation Excretion in breast milk unknown/not recommended

Warnings/Precautions Hazardous agent - use appropriate precautions for handling and disposal; avoid eye contamination.

[U.S. Boxed Warning]: For I.V. administration only; inadvertent intrathecal administration usually results in death. To prevent administration errors, the World Health Organization recommends dispensing vincristine diluted in a minibag (WHO, 2007), **if not dispensed in a minibag, affix an auxiliary label stating "For intravenous use only - fatal if given by other routes" and also place in an overwrap labeled "Do not remove covering until moment of injection."** Vincristine should **NOT** be prepared during the preparation of any intrathecal medications. After preparation, keep vincristine in a location **away** from the separate storage location recommended for intrathecal medications. Vincristine should **NOT** be delivered to the patient at the same time with any medications intended for central nervous system administration.

[U.S. Boxed Warning]: Vincristine is a vesicant; avoid extravasation. Ensure proper catheter or needle position prior to (and during) infusion, individuals administering should be experienced in vincristine administration. Discontinue administration immediately if extravasation occurs and initiate appropriate extravasation management, including local injection of hyaluronidase and moderate heat application to the affected area. Use a separate vein to complete administration.

Neurotoxicity, including alterations in mental status such as depression, confusion, or insomnia may occur; neurologic effects are dose-limiting (may require dosage reduction) and may be additive with those of other neurotoxic agents and spinal cord irradiation. Use with caution in patients with pre-existing neuromuscular disease and/or with concomitant neurotoxic agents. Constipation, paralytic ileus, intestinal necrosis and/or perforation may occur; constipation may present as upper colon impaction with an empty rectum (may require flat film of abdomen for diagnosis); generally responds to high enemas and laxatives. All patients should be on a prophylactic bowel management regimen.

Use with caution in patients receiving concurrent therapy which alters CYP3A4 activity, may require therapy alterations. Acute shortness of breath and severe bronchospasm have been reported with vinca alkaloids, usually when used in combination with mitomycin. Onset may be several minutes to hours after vincristine administration and up to 2 weeks after mitomycin. Progressive dyspnea may occur. Permanently discontinue vincristine if pulmonary dysfunction occurs.

Use with caution in patients with hepatic impairment; dosage modification required. May be associated with hepatic sinusoidal obstruction syndrome (SOS; formerly called veno-occlusive disease), increased risk in children <3 years of age; use with caution in hepatobillary dysfunction. Monitor for signs or symptoms of hepatic SOS, including bilirubin >1.4 mg/dL, unexplained weight gain, ascites, hepatomegaly, or unexplained right upper quadrant pain (Arndt, 2004). Acute uric acid nephropathy has been reported with vincristine. Use with caution in the elderly; may cause or exacerbate syndrome of inappropriate antidiuretic hormone secretion or hyponatremia; monitor sodium closely with initiation or dosage adjustments in older adults (Beers Criteria).

Adverse Reactions Frequency not defined.

Cardiovascular: Edema, hyper-/hypotension, MI, myocardial ischemia

Central nervous system: Ataxia, coma, cranial nerve dysfunction (auditory damage, extraocular muscle impairment, laryngeal muscle impairment, paralysis, paresis, vestibular damage, vocal cord paralysis), dizziness, fever, headache, neurotoxicity (dose-related), neuropathic pain (common), seizure, vertigo

Dermatologic toxicity: Alopecia (common), rash

Endocrine & metabolic: Hyperuricemia, parotid pain, SIADH (rare)

Gastrointestinal: Abdominal cramps, abdominal pain, anorexia, constipation (common), diarrhea, intestinal necrosis, intestinal perforation, nausea, oral ulcers, paralytic ileus, vomiting, weight loss

Genitourinary: Bladder atony, dysuria, polyuria, urinary retention

Hematologic: Anemia (mild), leukopenia (mild), thrombocytopenia (mild), thrombotic thrombocytopenic purpura

Hepatic: Hepatic sinusoidal obstruction syndrome (SOS, veno-occlusive liver disease)

Local: Phlebitis, tissue irritation/necrosis (if infiltrated)

Neuromuscular & skeletal: Back pain, bone pain, deep tendon reflex loss, difficulty walking, foot drop, gait changes, jaw pain, limb pain, motor difficulties, muscle wasting, myalgia, paralysis, paresthesia, peripheral neuropathy (common), sensorimotor dysfunction, sensory loss

Ocular: Cortical blindness (transient), nystagmus, optic atrophy with blindness

Otic: Deafness

Renal: Acute uric acid nephropathy, hemolytic uremic syndrome

Respiratory: Bronchospasm, dyspnea, pharyngeal pain

Miscellaneous: Allergic reactions (rare), anaphylaxis (rare), hypersensitivity (rare)

Drug Interactions

Metabolism/Transport Effects Substrate of CYP3A4 (major), P-glycoprotein; **Note:** Assignment of Major/Minor substrate status based on clinically relevant drug interaction potential; **Inhibits** CYP3A4 (weak)

Avoid Concomitant Use

Avoid concomitant use of VinCRIStine with any of the following: BCG; Conivaptan; Natalizumab; Pimecrolimus; Pimozide; Tacrolimus (Topical); Vaccines (Live)

Increased Effect/Toxicity

VinCRIStine may increase the levels/effects of: ARIPiprazole; Leflunomide; MitoMYcin (Systemic); Natalizumab; Pimozide; Vaccines (Live); Vitamin K Antagonists

The levels/effects of VinCRIStine may be increased by: Conivaptan; CYP3A4 Inhibitors (Moderate); CYP3A4 Inhibitors (Strong); Dasatinib; Denosumab; Itraconazole; Ivacaftor; Lopinavir; Macrolide Antibiotics; MAO Inhibitors; Mifepristone; NIFEdipine; P-glycoprotein/ABCB1 Inhibitors; Pimecrolimus; Posaconazole; Ritonavir; Roflumilast; Tacrolimus (Topical); Teniposide; Trastuzumab; Voriconazole

Decreased Effect

VinCRIStine may decrease the levels/effects of: BCG; Cardiac Glycosides; Coccidioidin Skin Test; Fosphenytoin; Phenytoin; Sipuleucel-T; Vaccines (Inactivated); Vaccines (Live); Vitamin K Antagonists

The levels/effects of VinCRIStine may be decreased by: CYP3A4 Inducers (Strong); Deferasirox; Echinacea; Fosphenytoin; Herbs (CYP3A4 Inducers); P-glycoprotein/ABCB1 Inducers; Phenytoin; Tocilizumab

Ethanol/Nutrition/Herb Interactions Herb/Nutraceutical: St John's wort may decrease vincristine levels.

Storage/Stability Store intact vials under refrigeration. Protect from light.

I.V. solution: Diluted in 25-50 mL NS or D_5W, stable for 7 days under refrigeration, or 2 days at room temperature. In ambulatory pumps, solution is stable for 7 days at room temperature. After preparation, keep vincristine in a location away from the separate storage location recommended for intrathecal medications.

Reconstitution Use appropriate precautions for handling and disposal. Solutions for I.V. infusion may be mixed in NS or D_5W. **Note:** In order to prevent inadvertent intrathecal administration the World Health Organization (WHO) and the Institute for Safe Medical Practices (ISMP) recommend dispensing vincristine in a minibag (rather than a syringe). Vincristine should **NOT** be prepared during the preparation of any intrathecal medications. If dispensing vincristine in a syringe, affix an auxiliary label stating **"For intravenous use only - fatal if given by other routes"** to the syringe, and the syringe must also be packaged in the manufacturer-provided overwrap which bears the statement **"Do not remove covering until the moment of injection. For intravenous use only. Fatal if given intrathecally."**

Mechanism of Action Binds to tubulin and inhibits microtubule formation, therefore, arresting the cell at metaphase by disrupting the formation of the mitotic spindle; it is specific for the M and S phases. Vincristine may also interfere with nucleic acid and protein synthesis by blocking glutamic acid utilization.

Pharmacodynamics/Kinetics

Distribution: Rapidly removed from bloodstream and tightly bound to tissues; penetrates blood-brain barrier poorly

Metabolism: Extensively hepatic, via CYP3A4

Half-life elimination: Terminal: 85 hours (range: 19-155 hours)

Excretion: Feces (~80%); urine (10% to 20%; <1% as unchanged drug)

Dosing

Adult & Geriatric Note: Doses may be capped at a maximum of 2 mg/dose. Dosing and frequency may vary by protocol and/or treatment phase; refer to specific protocol.

Doses in the manufacturer's U.S. labeling: I.V.: 1.4 mg/m^2/dose; frequency may vary based on protocol

Additional dosing in combination therapy; indication-specific and/or unlabeled dosing:

Acute lymphocytic leukemia (ALL): I.V.:

Hyper-CVAD regimen: 2 mg/dose days 4 and 11 during odd-numbered cycles (cycles 1, 3, 5, 7) of an 8-cycle phase, followed by maintenance treatment (if needed) of 2 mg monthly for 2 years (Kantarjian, 2004)

Larson (CALBG 8811) regimen: Induction phase: 2 mg/dose days 1, 8, 15, and 22 (4-week treatment cycle); Early intensification phase: 2 mg/dose days 15, and 22 (4-week treatment cycle, repeat once); Late intensification phase: 2 mg/dose days 1, 8, 15 (8-week treatment cycle); Maintenance phase: 2 mg/dose day 1 every 4 weeks until 24 months from diagnosis (Larson, 1995)

Central nervous system tumors: I.V.: PCV regimen: 1.4 mg/m^2/dose (maximum dose: 2 mg) on days 8 and 29 of a 6-week treatment cycle for a total of 6 cycles (van de Bent, 2006) **or** 1.4 mg/m^2/dose (no maximum dose) on days 8 and 29 of a 6-week treatment cycle for up to 4 cycles (Cairncross, 2006)

Hodgkin lymphoma: I.V.:

BEACOPP regimen: 1.4 mg/m^2/dose (maximum dose: 2 mg) on day 8 of a 21-day treatment cycle (Diehl, 2003)

Stanford-V regimen: 1.4 mg/m^2/dose (maximum dose: 2 mg) in weeks 2, 4, 6, 8, 10, and 12 (Horning, 2000; Horning, 2002)

Non-Hodgkin lymphoma: I.V.:

CHOP regimen: 1.4 mg/m^2/dose (maximum dose: 2 mg) on day 1 of a 21-day treatment cycle for 8 cycles (Coiffier, 2002)

CVP regimen: 1.4 mg/m^2/dose (maximum dose: 2 mg) on day 1 of a 21-day treatment cycle for 8 cycles (Marcus, 2005)

EPOCH regimen: 0.4 mg/m^2/day continuous infusion for 4 days (over 96 hours) (total 1.6 mg/m^2/cycle; dose not usually capped) of a 21-day treatment cycle (Wilson, 2002)

Ewing's sarcoma (unlabeled use): I.V.: VAC/IE regimen: VAC: 2 mg/m^2 (maximum dose: 2 mg) on day 1 of a 21-day treatment cycle (in combination with doxorubicin and cyclophosphamide), alternates with IE (ifosfamide and etoposide) for a total of 17 cycles (Grier, 2003)

Gestational trophoblastic tumors, high-risk (unlabeled use): I.V.: EMA/CO regimen: 1 mg/m^2 on day 8 of 2-week treatment cycle (in combination with etoposide methotrexate, dactinomycin, and cyclophosphamide), continue for at least 2 treatment cycles after a normal hCG level (Escobar, 2003)

Multiple myeloma (unlabeled use): I.V.:

DVD regimen: 1.4 mg/m^2/dose (maximum dose: 2 mg) on day 1 of a 28-day treatment cycle (Rifkin, 2006)

VAD regimen: 0.4 mg/day continuous infusion for 4 days (over 96 hours) (total 1.6 mg/cycle) of a 28-day treatment cycle (Rifkin, 2006)

Ovarian cancer (unlabeled use): I.V.: VAC regimen: 1.5 mg/m^2/dose (maximum dose: 2 mg) weekly for 8-12 weeks (Slayton, 1985)

Small cell lung cancer (unlabeled use): I.V.: CAV regimen: 1.4 mg/m^2/dose day 1 of a 21-day treatment cycle (Hong, 1989) **or** 2 mg/dose on day 1 of a 21-day treatment cycle (von Pawel, 1999)

Dosing adjustment in obesity: Dose should be capped at a maximum of 2 mg due to neurotoxicity concerns (Griggs, 2012)

Pediatric Note: Doses may be capped at a maximum of 2 mg/dose. Dosing and frequency may vary by protocol and/or treatment phase; refer to specific protocol.

Doses in the manufacturer's U.S. labeling: I.V.:

Children ≤10 kg: 0.05 mg/kg/dose once weekly

Children >10 kg: 1.5-2 mg/m^2/dose; frequency may vary based on protocol

Additional dosing in combination therapy; indication-specific and/or unlabeled dosing:

Acute lymphocytic lymphoma (ALL): I.V.: Induction phase: 1.5 mg/m^2/dose days 0, 7, 14, and 21; Consolidation phase: 1.5 mg/m^2/dose days 0, 28, and 56; Delayed intensification phase: 1.5 mg/m^2/dose days 0, 7, and 14; Maintenance phase: 1.5 mg/m^2/dose days 0, 28, and 56 (Bostrom, 2003) **or** Induction phase: 1.5 mg/m^2/dose days 0, 7, 14, and 21; Consolidation phase: 1.5 mg/m^2/dose days 0, 28, and 56; Interim maintenance phases: 1.5 mg/m^2/dose days 0 and 28; Delayed intensification phase: 1.5 mg/m^2/dose days 0, 7, and 14; Maintenance phase: 1.5 mg/m^2/dose every 4 weeks (Avramis, 2002)

Ewing's sarcoma (unlabeled use): I.V.: 2 mg/m^2/dose (maximum dose: 2 mg) on day 1 of a 21-day cycle, administer either every cycle or during odd-numbered cycles (Grier, 2003) **or** 0.67 mg/m^2/day continuous infusion days 1, 2, and 3 (total 2 mg/m^2/cycle; maximum dose/cycle: 2 mg) during cycles 1, 2, 3, and 6 (Kolb, 2003)

Hodgkin lymphoma: I.V.: BEACOPP regimen: 2 mg/m^2/dose (maximum dose: 2 mg) on day 7 of a 21-day treatment cycle (Kelly, 2002)

Neuroblastoma: I.V.:

CE-CAdO regimen: 1.5 mg/m^2 (maximum dose: 2 mg) days 1 and 5 every 21 days for 2 cycles (Rubie, 1998) **or** 0.05 mg/kg days 1 and 5 for 2 cycles (Rubie, 2001)

CAV-P/VP regimen (unlabeled dosing): 0.033 mg/kg/day continuous infusion days 1, 2, and 3, then 1.5 mg/m^2 bolus day 9 of courses 1, 2, 4, and 6 (Kushner, 1994)

Retinoblastoma (unlabeled use): I.V.:

Children: 0.05 mg/kg on day 1 every 21 days (in combination with carboplatin) for 8 cycles (Rodriguez-Galindo, 2003)\

or

Children ≤36 months: 0.05 mg/kg on day 0 every 28 days (in combination with carboplatin and etoposide) for 6 cycles (Freidman, 2000)

or

Children >36 months: 1.5 mg/m^2 (maximum dose: 2 mg) on day 0 every 28 days (in combination with carboplatin and etoposide) for 6 cycles (Friedman, 2000)

Rhabdomyosarcoma: I.V.:

VA regimen: 1.5 mg/m^2/dose (maximum dose: 2 mg) weeks 1-8, weeks 13-20, and weeks 25-32 (Crist, 2001)

VAC regimen: 1.5 mg/m²/dose (maximum dose: 2 mg) weeks 0-12, week 16, weeks 20-25; Continuation therapy: Weeks 29-34, and weeks 38-43 (Crist, 2001)

Wilms' tumor: I.V.:

Children <1 year: 0.75 mg/m²/dose weekly for 10-11 weeks, then every 3 weeks for 15 additional weeks (total 25-26 weeks) (Pritchard, 1995)

Children ≥1 year: 1.5 mg/m²/dose weekly for 10-11 weeks, then every 3 weeks for 15 additional weeks (total 25-26 weeks) (Pritchard, 1995)

or

Children ≤30 kg: 0.05 mg/kg/dose (maximum dose: 2 mg) weeks 1, 2, 4, 5, 6, 7, 8, 10, and 11, followed by 0.067 mg/kg/dose (maximum dose: 2 mg) weeks 12, 13, 18, and 24 (Green, 2007)

Children >30 kg: 1.5 mg/m²/dose (maximum dose: 2 mg) weeks 1, 2, 4, 5, 6, 7, 8, 10, and 11, followed by 2 mg/m²/dose (maximum dose: 2 mg) weeks 12, 13, 18, and 24 (Green, 2007)

Renal Impairment No dosage adjustment necessary (Kintzel, 1995).

Hepatic Impairment The manufacturer's labeling recommends the following adjustment: Serum bilirubin >3 mg/dL: Administer 50% of normal dose.

The following adjustments have also been recommended:

Floyd, 2006: Serum bilirubin 1.5-3 mg/dL or transaminases 2-3 times ULN or alkaline phosphatase increased: Administer 50% of dose.

Superfin, 2007:

Serum bilirubin 1.5-3 mg/dL: Administer 50% of dose.

Serum bilirubin >3 mg/dL: Avoid use.

Combination Regimens

Brain tumors:
COPE on page 1596
MOPP (Medulloblastoma) on page 1717
PCV (Brain Tumor Regimen) on page 1736
POC on page 1740
Gestational trophoblastic tumor: EMA/CO on page 1622
Leukemia, acute lymphocytic:
DVP on page 1621
Hyper-CVAD + Imatinib on page 1680
Hyper-CVAD (Leukemia, Acute Lymphocytic) on page 1681
Larson Regimen (ALL) on page 1699
Linker Protocol (ALL) on page 1703
MTX/6-MP/VP (Maintenance) on page 1717
POMP on page 1741
PVA (POG 8602) on page 1742
PVDA on page 1745
VAD/CVAD on page 1768
Leukemia, chronic lymphocytic: CVP (Leukemia) on page 1598
Lung cancer (small cell): CAV (Small Cell Lung Cancer) on page 1554
Lymphoma, Hodgkin:
BEACOPP-14 (Hodgkin) on page 1522
BEACOPP Escalated (Hodgkin) on page 1522
BEACOPP Escalated Plus Standard (Hodgkin) on page 1523
BEACOPP Standard (Hodgkin) on page 1525
C-MOPP/ABV Hybrid (Hodgkin) on page 1588
MOPP/ABVD (Hodgkin) on page 1714
MOPP/ABV Hybrid (Hodgkin) on page 1715

MOPP (Hodgkin) on page 1716
Stanford V (Hodgkin) on page 1752
Lymphoma, non-Hodgkin's:
CHOP (NHL) on page 1564
CNOP on page 1589
CODOX-M on page 1590
COMLA on page 1595
COP-BLAM on page 1595
COPP on page 1596
CVP (Lymphoma, non-Hodgkin's) on page 1598
EPOCH Dose-Adjusted (AIDS-Related Lymphoma) on page 1628
EPOCH Dose-Adjusted (NHL) on page 1628
EPOCH (Dose-Adjusted)-Rituximab (NHL) on page 1629
EPOCH (NHL) on page 1630
EPOCH-Rituximab (NHL) on page 1631
Hyper-CVAD (Lymphoma, non-Hodgkin's) on page 1687
MACOP-B on page 1704
m-BACOD on page 1706
Pro-MACE-CytaBOM on page 1741
R-CVP on page 1745
Rituximab-CHOP (NHL) on page 1748
Lymphoma, non-Hodgkin's (Burkitt): CODOX-M/IVAC on page 1591
Lymphoma, non-Hodgkin's (Mantle cell): Hyper-CVAD + Rituximab on page 1688
Multiple myeloma:
Doxorubicin (Liposomal)-Vincristine-Dexamethasone on page 1620
Hyper-CVAD (Multiple Myeloma) on page 1687
VAD on page 1767
VBMCP (Multiple Myeloma) on page 1769
VCAP on page 1770
Neuroblastoma:
CAV-P/VP (Neuroblastoma) on page 1554
CE-CAdO (Neuroblastoma) on page 1555
Ovarian cancer: Vincristine-Dactinomycin-Cyclophosphamide (Ovarian Cancer) on page 1771
Retinoblastoma:
Carboplatin-Etoposide-Vincristine (Retinoblastoma) on page 1546
Carboplatin-Vincristine (Retinoblastoma) on page 1552
Rhabdomyosarcoma:
CEV on page 1562
VAC Pulse on page 1767
VAC (Rhabdomyosarcoma) on page 1767
Sarcoma:
CYVADIC on page 1605
VAC Alternating With IE (Ewing's Sarcoma) on page 1766
Wilms' tumor:
EE-4A (Wilms' Tumor) on page 1621
DD-4A (Wilms' Tumor) on page 1606
Regimen I (Wilms' Tumor) on page 1745
VAD (Wilms' Tumor) on page 1768

Administration For I.V. administration only. FATAL IF GIVEN INTRATHECALLY.

Vincristine should **NOT** be delivered to the patient at the same time with any medications intended for central nervous system administration.

I.V.: Usually administered as short 5-10 minute infusion (preferred); may also be administered as a slow (1 minute) push or by a 24-hour continuous infusion (depending on the protocol).

Vincristine is a vesicant; ensure proper needle or catheter placement prior to and during infusion; avoid extravasation. If extravasation occurs, stop infusion immediately and initiate appropriate extravasation management, including moderate heat application for 15-20 minutes at least 4 times a day for 1-2 days and local injection of hyaluronidase to the area of infiltration (Polovich, 2009). Remaining portion of the dose should be infused through a separate vein.

Emetic Potential Very low (<10%)

Vesicant/Extravasation Risk Vesicant; see Management of Drug Extravasations on page 1800.

Monitoring Parameters Serum electrolytes (sodium), hepatic function tests, CBC with differential, serum uric acid; monitor infusion site; neurologic examination, monitor for constipation and for signs/symptoms of peripheral neuropathy

Dosage Forms Excipient information presented when available (limited, particularly for generics); consult specific product labeling.

Injection, solution, as sulfate [preservative free]: 1 mg/mL (1 mL, 2 mL)

Vincasar PFS®: 1 mg/mL (1 mL, 2 mL)

References

Arndt C, Hawkins, D, Anderson JR, et al, "Age is a Risk Factor for Chemotherapy-Induced Hepatopathy With Vincristine, Dactinomycin and Cyclophosphamide," *J Clin Oncol*, 2004, 22 (10):1894-901.

Aronoff GR, Bennett WM, Berns JS, et al, *Drug Prescribing in Renal Failure: Dosing Guidelines for Adults and Children*, 5th ed. Philadelphia, PA: American College of Physicians; 2007, p 102, 174.

Avramis VI, Sencer S, Periclou AP, et al, "A Randomized Comparison of Native *Escherichia coli* Asparaginase and Polyethylene Glycol Conjugated Asparaginase for Treatment of Children With Newly Diagnosed Standard-Risk Acute Lymphoblastic Leukemia: A Children's Cancer Group Study," *Blood*, 2002, 99(6):1986-94.

Bostrom BC, Sensel MR, Sather HN, et al, "Dexamethasone Versus Prednisone and Daily Oral Versus Weekly Intravenous Mercaptopurine for Patients With Standard-Risk Acute Lymphoblastic Leukemia: A Report from the Children's Cancer Group," *Blood*, 2003, 101(10):3809-17.

Cairncross G, Berkey B, Shaew, et al, "Phase III Trial of Chemotherapy Plus Radiotherapy Compared With Radiotherapy Alone for Pure and Mixed Anaplastic Oligodendroglioma: Intergroup Radiation Therapy Oncology Group Trial 9402," *J Clin Oncol*, 2006, 24(18):2707-14.

Coiffier B, Lepage E, Briere J, et al, "CHOP Chemotherapy Plus Rituximab Compared With CHOP Alone in Elderly Patients With Diffuse Large-B-Cell Lymphoma," *N Engl J Med*, 2002, 346 (4):235-42.

Crist WM, Anderson JR, Meza JL, et al, "Intergroup Rhabdomyosarcoma Study-IV. Results for Patients With Nonmetastatic Disease," *J Clin Oncol*, 2001, 19(12):3091-102.

Diehl V, Franklin J, Pfreundschuh M, et al, "Standard and Increased-Dose BEACOPP Chemotherapy Compared With COPP-ABVD for Advanced Hodgkin's Disease," *N Engl J Med*, 2003, 348(24):2386-95.

Escobar PF, Lurain JR, Singh DK, et al, "Treatment of High-Risk Gestational Trophoblastic Neoplasia With Etoposide, Methotrexate, Actinomycin D, Cyclophosphamide, and Vincristine Chemotherapy," *Gynecol Oncol*, 2003, 91(3):552-7.

Floyd J, Mirza I, Sachs B, et al, "Hepatotoxicity of Chemotherapy," *Semin Oncol*, 2006, 33 (1):50-67.

Friedman DL, Himelstein B, Shields CL, et al, "Chemoreduction and Local Ophthalmic Therapy for Intraocular Retinoblastoma," *J Clin Oncol*, 2000, 18(1):12-7.

Green DM, Cotton CA, Malogolowkin M, et al, "Treatment of Wilms Tumor Relapsing After Initial Treatment With Vincristine and Actinomycin D: A Report From the National Wilms Tumor Study Group," *Pediatr Blood Cancer*, 2007, 48(5):493-9.

Grier HE, Krailo MD, Tarbell NJ, et al, "Addition of Ifosfamide and Etoposide to Standard Chemotherapy for Ewing's Sarcoma and Primitive Neuroectodermal Tumor of Bone," *N Engl J Med*, 2003, 348(8):694-701.

Hong WK, Nicaise C, Larson R, et al, "Etoposide Combined With Cyclophosphamide Plus Vincristine Compared With Doxorubicin Plus Cyclophosphamide Plus Vincristine and With High-Dose Cyclophosphamide Plus Vincristine in the Treatment of Small-Cell Carcinoma of the Lung: A Randomized Trial of the Bristol Lung Cancer Study Group," *J Clin Oncol*, 1989, 7 (4):450-6.

Horning SJ, Hoppe RT, Breslin S, et al, "Stanford V and Radiotherapy for Locally Extensive and Advanced Hodgkin's Disease: Mature Results of a Prospective Clinical Trial," *J Clin Oncol*, 2002, 20(3):630-7.

Horning SJ, Williams J, Bartlett NL, et al, "Assessment of the Stanford V Regimen and Consolidative Radiotherapy for Bulky and Advanced Hodgkin's Disease: Eastern Cooperative Oncology Group Pilot Study E1492," *J Clin Oncol*, 2000, 18(5):972-80.

Jacobson JO, Polovich M, McNiff KK, et al, "American Society of Clinical Oncology/ Oncology Nursing Society Chemotherapy Administration Safety Standards," *J Clin Oncol*, 2009, 27 (32):5469-75.

Kantarjian H, Thomas D, O'Brien S, et al, "Long-Term Follow-Up Results of Hyperfractionated Cyclophosphamide, Vincristine, Doxorubicin, and Dexamethasone (Hyper-CVAD), A Dose-Intensive Regimen, in Adult Acute Lymphocytic Leukemia," *Cancer*, 2004, 101(12):2788-801.

Kelly KM, Hutchinson RJ, Sposto R, et al, "Feasibility of Upfront Dose-Intensive Chemotherapy in Children With Advanced-Stage Hodgkin's Lymphoma: Preliminary Results From the Children's Cancer Group Study CCG-59704," *Ann Oncol*, 2002, 13(Suppl 1):107-11.

Kintzel PE and Dorr RT, "Anticancer Drug Renal Toxicity and Elimination: Dosing Guidelines for Altered Renal Function," *Cancer Treat Rev*, 1995, 21(1):33-64.

Kolb EA, Kushner BH, Gorlick R, et al, "Long-Term Event-Free Survival After Intensive Chemotherapy for Ewing's Family of Tumors in Children and Young Adults," *J Clin Oncol*, 2003, 21 (18):3423-30.

Kushner BH, LaQuaglia MP, Bonilla MA, et al, "Highly Effective Induction Therapy for Stage 4 Neuroblastoma in Children Over 1 Year of Age," *J Clin Oncol*, 1994, 12(12):2607-13.

Larson RA, Dodge RK, Burns CP, et al, "A Five-Drug Remission Induction Regimen With Intensive Consolidation for Adults With Acute Lymphoblastic Leukemia: Cancer and Leukemia Group B Study 8811," *Blood*, 1995, 85(8):2025-37.

Legha SS, "Vincristine Neurotoxicity. Pathophysiology and Management," *Med Toxicol*, 1986, 1 (6):421-7.

Marcus R, Imrie K, Belch A, et al, "CVP Chemotherapy Plus Rituximab Compared With CVP as First-Line Treatment for Advanced Follicular Lymphoma," *Blood*, 2005, 105(4):1417-23.

Morgan C, Tillett T, Braybrooke J, et al, "Management of Uncommon Chemotherapy-Induced Emergencies," *Lancet Oncol*, 2011, 12(8):806-14.

Pritchard J, Imeson J, Barnes J, et al, "Results of the United Kingdom Children's Cancer Study Group first Wilms' Tumor Study," *J Clin Oncol*, 1995, 13(1):124-33.

Rifkin RM, Gregory SA, Mohrbacher A, et al, "Pegylated Liposomal Doxorubicin, Vincristine, and Dexamethasone Provide Significant Reduction in Toxicity Compared With Doxorubicin, Vincristine, and Dexamethasone in Patients With Newly Diagnosed Multiple Myeloma: A Phase III Multicenter Randomized Trial," *Cancer*, 2006, 106(4):848-58.

Rodriguez-Galindo C, Wilson MW, Haik BG, et al, "Treatment of Intraocular Retinoblastoma With Vincristine and Carboplatin," *J Clin Oncol*, 2003, 21(10):2019-25.

Rubie H, Plantaz D, Coze C, et al, "Localised and Unresectable Neuroblastoma in Infants: Excellent Outcome With Primary Chemotherapy. Neuroblastoma Study Group, Société Française d'Oncologie Pédiatrique," *Med Pediatr Oncol*, 2001, 36(1):247-50.

Slayton RE, Park RC, Silverberg SG, et al, "Vincristine, Dactinomycin, and Cyclophosphamide in the Treatment of Malignant Germ Cell Tumors of the Ovary. A Gynecologic Oncology Group Study (A Final Report)," *Cancer*, 1985, 56(2):243-8.

Stefanou A and Dooley M, "Simple Method to Eliminate the Risk of Inadvertent Intrathecal Vincristine Administration," *J Clin Oncol*, 2006, 21(10):2044.

Superfin D, Iannucci AA, and Davies AM, "Commentary: Oncologic drugs in Patients With Organ Dysfunction: A Summary," *Oncologist*, 2007, 12(9):1070-83.

van den Bent MJ, Carpentier AF, Brandes AA, et al, "Adjuvant Procarbazine, Lomustine, and Vincristine Improves Progression-Free Survival But Not Overall Survival in Newly Diagnosed Anaplastic Oligodendrogliomas and Oligoastrocytomas: A Randomized European Organisation for Research and Treatment of Cancer Phase III Trial," *J Clin Oncol*, 2006, 24(18):2715-22.

von Pawel J, Schiller JH, Shepherd FA, et al, "Topotecan Versus Cyclophosphamide, Doxorubicin, and Vincristine for the Treatment of Recurrent Small-Cell Lung Cancer," *J Clin Oncol*, 1999, 17 (2):658-67.

Wilson WH, Grossbard ML, Pittaluga S, et al, "Dose-Adjusted EPOCH Chemotherapy for Untreated Large B-Cell Lymphomas: A Pharmacodynamic Approach With High Efficacy," *Blood*, 2002, 99(8):2685-93.

VinCRIStine (Liposomal) (vin KRIS teen lye po SO mal)

Index Terms Liposomal Vincristine; Liposome Vincristine; Marqibo®; Vincristine Liposome; Vincristine Sulfate Liposome; VSLI

Generic Availability (U.S.) No

Pharmacologic Category Antineoplastic Agent, Natural Source (Plant) Derivative; Antineoplastic Agent, Vinca Alkaloid

Use Treatment of relapsed Philadelphia chromosome-negative (Ph-) acute lymphoblastic leukemia (ALL) in adult patients whose disease has progressed after two or more antileukemic therapies

Labeled Contraindications

Hypersensitivity to vincristine, liposomal vincristine, or any component of the formulation; patients with Charcot-Marie-Tooth syndrome or other demyelinating conditions; administration via the intrathecal route

Pregnancy Risk Factor D

Lactation Excretion in breast milk unknown/not recommended

Warnings/Precautions Hazardous agent - use appropriate precautions for handling and disposal. **[U.S. Boxed Warning]: For I.V. administration only. Intrathecal administration is contraindicated; inadvertent intrathecal administration has resulted in death.** Liposomal vincristine should **NOT** be prepared during the preparation of any intrathecal medications. After preparation, keep liposomal vincristine in a location **away** from the separate storage location recommended for intrathecal medications. Liposomal vincristine should **NOT** be delivered to the patient at the same time with any medications intended for central nervous system administration.

[U.S. Boxed Warning]: Vincristine LIPOSOME and conventional vincristine are NOT interchangeable. Dosing differs between formulations; verify intended product and dose prior to preparation and administration to avoid overdoses. All vincristine formulations are vesicants; avoid extravasation. Only individuals experienced with vesicant administration should administer liposomal vincristine. Check for proper needle placement; if extravasation occurs, discontinue liposomal vincristine infusion immediately and institute appropriate extravasation management procedures.

Grade 3 and greater neutropenia, anemia, and thrombocytopenia were observed in clinical trials. Monitor blood counts closely and adjust dose or withhold therapy if necessary. Constipation, ileus, bowel obstruction, and colonic pseudo-obstruction have occurred with liposomal vincristine. Patients should be initiated on a prophylactic bowel regimen including a stool softener, dietary fiber, and hydration; laxative treatments may be considered. Severe fatigue was noted in clinical trials; treatment delay, dosage adjustment, or discontinuation may be necessary.

Neuropathies (sensory and motor) are common and cumulative. Neuropathy symptoms may include paresthesia, hyper-/hypoesthesia, hyporeflexia or areflexia, neuralgia, jaw pain, cranial neuropathy, ileus, arthralgia, myalgia, muscle spasm, and/or weakness. Evaluate neurologic status of patients closely prior to liposomal vincristine administration; neurologic toxicity risk is greater when given to patients with preexisting neuromuscular conditions or when used concomitantly with other neurotoxic agents. Treatment delay, dosage adjustment, and/or discontinuation may be necessary. Tumor lysis syndrome may occur as a consequence of therapy; monitor closely for signs and symptoms and manage accordingly.

Hepatotoxicity (including fatal cases) and increased AST have been reported. Monitor hepatic function tests; reduce dose or interrupt therapy if necessary. Use caution in patients with hepatic impairment; liposomal vincristine has not been studied in patients with severe hepatic impairment. In a study in a limited number of melanoma patients with moderate (Child-Pugh class B) hepatic impairment secondary to liver metastases, C_{max} and AUC were comparable to those in patients with normal hepatic function; patients with hepatic impairment received a dose of 1 mg/m^2 every 2 weeks versus 2 mg/m^2 in subjects with normal hepatic function (Bedikian, 2011). Avoid concomitant therapy with strong CYP3A4 or P-glycoprotein (P-gp) inducers or inhibitors. Use with caution in the elderly patient population; conventional vincristine may cause or exacerbate hyponatremia or syndrome of inappropriate antidiuretic hormone secretion; monitor sodium closely with therapy initiation or dosage adjustments (Beers Criteria).

Adverse Reactions

>10%:

Central nervous system: Fever (43%), fatigue (41%), insomnia (32%)

Gastrointestinal: Constipation (57%), nausea (52%), diarrhea (37%), appetite decreased (33%)

Hematologic: Neutropenic fever (38%; grades 3/4: 31%), anemia (34%; grades 3/4: 17%), neutropenia (grades 3/4: 18%), thrombocytopenia (grades 3/4: 17%)

Hepatic: AST increased (grades 3/4: 6% to 11%)

Neuromuscular & skeletal: Peripheral neuropathy (39%; grades 3/4: 17%)

1% to 10%:

Cardiovascular: Cardiac arrest (grades 3/4: 6%), hypotension (grades 3/4: 6%)

Central nervous system: Pain (grades 3/4: 8%), mental status changes (grades 3/4: 4%)

Gastrointestinal: Abdominal pain (grades 3/4: 8%), ileus (grades 3/4: 6%)

Neuromuscular & skeletal: Weakness (grades 3/4: 5%), muscle weakness (grades 3/4: 1%)

Respiratory: Pneumonia (grades 3/4: 8%), respiratory distress (grades 3/4: 6%), respiratory failure (grades 3/4: 5%)

Miscellaneous: Septic shock (grades 3/4: 6%), staphylococcal bacteremia (grades 3/4: 6%)

Drug Interactions

Metabolism/Transport Effects Substrate of CYP3A4 (major), P-glycoprotein; **Note:** Assignment of Major/Minor substrate status based on clinically relevant drug interaction potential; **Inhibits** CYP3A4 (weak)

Avoid Concomitant Use

Avoid concomitant use of VinCRIStine (Liposomal) with any of the following: BCG; CloZAPine; CYP3A4 Inducers (Strong); CYP3A4 Inhibitors (Strong); Natalizumab; P-glycoprotein/ABCB1 Inducers; P-glycoprotein/ABCB1 Inhibitors; Pimecrolimus; Pimozide; St Johns Wort; Tacrolimus (Topical); Vaccines (Live)

Increased Effect/Toxicity

VinCRIStine (Liposomal) may increase the levels/effects of: ARIPiprazole; CloZAPine; Leflunomide; MitoMYcin (Systemic); Natalizumab; Pimozide; Vaccines (Live); Vitamin K Antagonists

The levels/effects of VinCRIStine (Liposomal) may be increased by: CYP3A4 Inhibitors (Moderate); CYP3A4 Inhibitors (Strong); Dasatinib; Denosumab; Itraconazole; Ivacaftor; Lopinavir; Macrolide Antibiotics; MAO Inhibitors; Mifepristone; NIFEdipine; P-glycoprotein/ABCB1 Inhibitors; Pimecrolimus; Posaconazole; Ritonavir; Roflumilast; Tacrolimus (Topical); Teniposide; Trastuzumab; Voriconazole

Decreased Effect

VinCRIStine (Liposomal) may decrease the levels/effects of: BCG; Cardiac Glycosides; Coccidioidin Skin Test; Sipuleucel-T; Vaccines (Inactivated); Vaccines (Live); Vitamin K Antagonists

The levels/effects of VinCRIStine (Liposomal) may be decreased by: CYP3A4 Inducers (Strong); Deferasirox; Echinacea; P-glycoprotein/ABCB1 Inducers; St Johns Wort; Tocilizumab

Storage/Stability Store intact kit (containing vincristine vial, sphingomyelin/cholesterol liposome vial, and sodium phosphate vial) refrigerated at 2°C to 8°C (36°F to 46°F); do not freeze. Use appropriate precautions for handling and disposal. Once prepared, liposomal vincristine is stable for no more than 12 hours at room temperature. After preparation, keep liposomal vincristine in a location away from the separate storage location recommended for intrathecal medications.

Reconstitution Vincristine liposome preparation requires 60-90 minutes of dedicated time utilizing the manufacturer supplied kit. Do not reuse kit components with future doses. Use appropriate precautions for handling and disposal.

1). Outside the sterile area, fill a water bath to a depth of at least 8 cm (3.2 inches); water should be heated to and maintained at **63°C to 67°C** (145.4°F to 152.6°F) for the entire procedure (use calibrated thermometer to monitor temperature). Maintain water depth of at least 8 cm (3.2 inches) throughout process. Water bath must remain outside the sterile area.

2). In a biological safety cabinet, vent the sodium phosphate vial with a sterile venting needle (with a 0.2 micron filter or other suitable venting device). Venting needle should always be kept above liquid level. Remove 1 mL of sphingomyelin/cholesterol liposome injection and inject into the sodium phosphate vial. Withdraw 5 mL of vincristine sulfate injection and inject into the sodium phosphate vial. Remove the venting needle and gently invert the sodium phosphate vial 5 times to mix (do **not** shake). Place flotation ring on the sodium phosphate vial.

3). Confirm the water bath is maintained between **63°C to 67°C** (145.4°F to 152.6°F). Outside the sterile area, place constituted sodium phosphate vial in the water bath for 10 minutes. Record constitution start and stop time, as well as starting and ending water temperature. After 10 minutes, remove the vial (with tongs), remove flotation ring, then dry the vial, affix vial overlabel, and gently invert 5 times to mix (do **not** shake). Allow the vial to equilibrate for at least 30 minutes at room temperature of 15°C to 30°C (59°F to 86°F), but for no longer than 12 hours. Once prepared, vincristine sulfate liposome concentration is 5 mg/31 mL (0.16 mg/mL).

4). Return vial to biologic safety cabinet. Calculate patient's vincristine liposome dose (based on actual BSA); remove corresponding volume from 100 mL NS or D_5W infusion bag. Inject vincristine liposome dose into the infusion bag (final volume of 100 mL). Do not use if a precipitate or other foreign matter is present in the vial or infusion bag. The amount contained in each vial may exceed the prescribed dose; use care with dosage and volume calculations. Discard unused portion of the vial. After preparation, keep liposomal vincristine in a location away from the separate storage location recommended for intrathecal medications.

Mechanism of Action Vincristine is a cell cycle specific agent which binds to tubulin, leading to microtubule depolymerization and cellular apoptosis. The liposomal formulation increases the half-life, allowing for enhanced cytotoxic activity in tumor cells.

Pharmacodynamics/Kinetics

Distribution: V_{dss}: 2.7 L (Bedikian, 2006)

Metabolism: Primarily hepatic

Half-life elimination: 45 hours (urinary half-life); dependent on rate of vincristine release from sphingosome (Bedikian, 2006)

Excretion: Feces (69%); urine (<8%)

Dosing

Adult & Geriatric Note: Vincristine liposomal and conventional vincristine are **NOT** interchangeable. Dosing differs between formulations; verify intended product and dose prior to preparation and administration. The liposomal vincristine dose is based on actual body surface area (BSA) and was not capped in studies (O'Brien, 2009; Rodriguez, 2009; Silverman, 2010).

Acute lymphoblastic leukemia (ALL; Philadelphia chromosome-negative), relapsed: I.V.: 2.25 mg/m^2 once every 7 days

Renal Impairment No dosage adjustment provided in manufacturer's labeling (has not been studied); however, liposomal vincristine is minimally excreted by the kidney and like the conventional formulation, likely does not require dosage adjustment in renal impairment.

Hepatic Impairment

Moderate impairment (Child-Pugh class B): In a study in a limited number of melanoma patients with moderate (Child-Pugh class B) hepatic impairment secondary to liver metastases, C_{max} and AUC were comparable to those in patients with normal hepatic function; patients with hepatic impairment received a dose of 1 mg/m^2 every 2 weeks versus 2 mg/m^2 in subjects with normal hepatic function (Bedikian, 2011).

Severe impairment (Child-Pugh class C): No dosage adjustment provided in manufacturer's labeling (has not been studied).

Hepatotoxicity during treatment: Reduce dose or interrupt treatment.

Adjustment for Toxicity

Fatigue, severe: Consider dose delay, reduction, or therapy discontinuation.

Hematologic toxicity: Grade 3 or 4 neutropenia, thrombocytopenia, or anemia: Consider dose reduction or modification.

Hepatic toxicity: Reduce dose or interrupt treatment.

Peripheral neuropathy:

Grade 3 or persistent grade 2 toxicity: Interrupt therapy until recovery to grade 1 or 2, then reduce dose to 2 mg/m^2. If grade 3 toxicity persists or if grade 4 toxicity occurs, discontinue liposomal vincristine.

Persistent grade 2 toxicity after first dose reduction to 2 mg/m^2: Interrupt therapy for up to 7 days until recovery to grade 1, then reduce dose to 1.825 mg/m^2. If neuropathy increases to grade 3 or 4, discontinue liposomal vincristine.

Persistent grade 2 toxicity after second dose reduction to 1.825 mg/m^2: Interrupt therapy for up to 7 days until recovery to grade 1, then reduce dose to 1.5 mg/m^2. If neuropathy increases to grade 3 or 4, discontinue liposomal vincristine.

Pre-existing neuropathy, severe: Assess treatment benefit versus risk.

Administration Vesicant; avoid extravasation. **For I.V. administration only. FATAL IF GIVEN INTRATHECALLY.** Liposomal vincristine should **NOT** be delivered to the patient at the same time as any medications intended for central nervous system administration.

I.V.: Infuse over 1 hour. Do not administer I.V. push or bolus; do not use with in-line filters. Infusion must be completed within 12 hours of preparation.

Monitoring Parameters CBC with differential and platelets; hepatic function; signs/symptoms of peripheral neuropathy or other neurologic toxicities; sodium (in elderly patients; conventional vincristine may cause or exacerbate hyponatremia or syndrome of inappropriate antidiuretic hormone secretion); signs/symptoms of tumor lysis syndrome; symptoms of constipation; monitor infusion site for extravasation

Additional Information The liposomal formulation of vincristine consists of vincristine encapsulated in sphingosomes, which are composed of sphingomyelin and cholesterol (Bedikian, 2006).

Product Availability Marqibo®: FDA approved August 9, 2012; availability is currently undetermined. Consult prescribing information for additional information.

References

American Geriatrics Society 2012 Beers Criteria Update Expert Panel, "American Geriatrics Society Updated Beers Criteria for Potentially Inappropriate Medication Use in Older Adults," *J Am Geriatr Soc*, 2012, 60(4):616-31.

Bedikian AY, Silverman JA, Papadopoulos NE, et al, "Pharmacokinetics and Safety of Marqibo (Vincristine Sulfate Liposomes Injection) in Cancer Patients With Impaired Liver Function," *J Clin Pharmacol*, 2011, 51(8):1205-12.

Bedikian AY, Vardeleon A, Smith T, et al, "Pharmacokinetics and Urinary Excretion of Vincristine Sulfate Liposomes Injection in Metastatic Melanoma Patients," *J Clin Pharmacol*, 2006, 46 (7):727-37.

Heffner L, "A New Formulation of Vincristine for Acute Lymphoblastic Leukemia," *Clin Adv Hematol Oncol*, 2011, 9(4):314-6.

O'brien S, Schiller G, Damon LF, et al, "Pivotal Phase 2 Study of Weekly Vincristine Sulfate Liposomes Injection (VSLI, Marqibo®) in Adults With Philadelphia Chromosome-Negative Acute Lymphoblastic Leukemia (ALL) in Second Relapse or Progressing Following Two Anti-Leukemia Treatment Lines," *Blood*, 2009, 114(22):3088 [abstract 3088 from 2009 ASH Annual Meeting].

O'brien S, Thomas DA, Heffner LT, et al, "Marqibo® (Vincristine Sulfate Liposomes Injection; VSLI) in the Treatment of Adult Patients With Advanced, Relapsed/Refractory Acute Lymphoblastic Leukemia (ALL): A Combined Analysis of the VSLI-06 and RALLY Studies," *Blood*, 2010, 116 (21):2143 [abstract 2143 from 2010 ASH Annual Meeting].

Schiller GJ, Lister J, Heffner LT, et al, "Vincristine Sulfate Liposomes Injection (Marqibo®) Facilitates Durable Remissions and Potentially Curative Hematopoietic Stem Cell Transplantation in Adults With Advanced, Relapsed and/or Refractory Acute Lymphoblastic Leukemia," *Blood*, 2011, 118(21):4235 [abstract 4235 from 2011 ASH Annual Meeting].

Silverman JA, Aulitzky WE, Lister J, et al, "Marqibo® (Vincristine Sulfate Liposomes Injection; VSLI) Optimizes the Dosing, Delivery, and Pharmacokinetic (PK) Profile of Vincristine Sulfate (VCR) in Adults With Relapsed or Refractory Acute Lymphoblastic Leukemia (ALL)," *Blood*, 2010, 116(21):2142 [abstract 2142 from 2010 ASH Annual Meeting].

◆ **Vincristine (Conventional)** *see* VinCRIStine *on page* *1450*

◆ **Vincristine Liposome** *see* VinCRIStine (Liposomal) *on page* *1459*

◆ **Vincristine Sulfate** *see* VinCRIStine *on page* *1450*

◆ **Vincristine Sulfate Injection. (Can)** *see* VinCRIStine *on page* *1450*

◆ **Vincristine Sulfate Liposome** *see* VinCRIStine (Liposomal) *on page* *1459*

Vindesine (VIN de seen)

Related Information

Management of Drug Extravasations *on page 1800*

Safe Handling of Hazardous Drugs *on page 1904*

Index Terms DAVA; Deacetyl Vinblastine Carboxamide; Desacetyl Vinblastine Amide Sulfate; DVA; Eldisine Lilly 99094; Lilly CT-3231; Vindesine Sulfate

Generic Availability (U.S.) No

Pharmacologic Category Antineoplastic Agent, Vinca Alkaloid

Unlabeled Use Management of acute lymphocytic leukemia, chronic myelogenous leukemia; advanced breast cancer; malignant melanoma; lymphomas (Hodgkin and non-Hodgkin's)

Labeled Contraindications Hypersensitivity to vindesine, vinca alkaloids, or any component of the formulation; intrathecal administration (fatal); demyelinating form of Charcot-Marie-Tooth syndrome; severe granulocytopenia ($<1500/mm^3$) or severe thrombocytopenia; bacterial infection

Lactation Excretion in breast milk unknown/not recommended

Warnings/Precautions Hazardous agent - use appropriate precautions for handling and disposal. Vindesine should be used cautiously, if at all, in patients with impaired hepatic function or neurologic problems. **Intrathecal administration may be fatal**. Vindesine has been reported to be cross-resistance with vincristine. Vinca alkaloids are vesicants; avoid extravasation.

Adverse Reactions

>10%:

- Central nervous system: Pyrexia, malaise (up to 60%)
- Dermatologic: Alopecia (6% to 92%)
- Gastrointestinal: Mild nausea and vomiting (7% to 27%), constipation (10% to 17%) - related to the neurotoxicity
- Hematologic: Leukopenia (50%) and thrombocytopenia (14% to 26%), may be dose limiting; thrombocytosis (20% to 28%)
  - Nadir: 6-12 days
  - Recovery: Days 14-18
- Neuromuscular & skeletal: Paresthesia (40% to 70%); loss of deep tendon reflexes (35% to 60%, may be dose limiting); myalgia (up to 60%)

1% to 10%:

- Dermatologic: Rashes
- Gastrointestinal: Loss of taste
- Hematologic: Anemia
- Local: Phlebitis
- Neuromuscular & skeletal: Facial paralysis

<1%: Acute chest pain, ECG changes, paralytic ileus, jaw pain, photophobia

Storage/Stability Reconstituted solutions are stable for 30 days under refrigeration (2°C to 8°C/36°F to 46°F). Solutions diluted in dextrose or saline for I.V. infusion are stable for 24 hours at room temperature (15°C to 30°C/59°F to 86°F). **The drug will precipitate at pH >6.**

Reconstitution Use appropriate precautions for handling and disposal. The powder is reconstituted to a concentration of 1 mg/mL.

Mechanism of Action Vindesine is a semisynthetic vinca alkaloid, having a mechanism of action similar to the other vinca derivatives. It arrests cell division in metaphase through inhibition of microtubular formation of the mitotic spindle. The drug is cell-cycle specific for the S phase.

Pharmacodynamics/Kinetics

Distribution: V_d: 8 L/kg; minimal distribution to adipose tissue or CNS

Metabolism: Hepatic

Half-life elimination:

Triphasic; Alpha: 2 minutes; Beta: 1 hour

Terminal: 24 hours

Excretion: Feces; urine (~3% to 25% of dose as unchanged drug)

Dosing

Adult & Geriatric Refer to individual protocols. I.V.:

3-4 mg/m^2 /week **or**

1-2 mg/m^2 days 1 and 2 every 2 weeks **or**

1-2 mg/m^2 days 1-5 (continuous infusion) every 2-4 weeks **or**

1-2 mg/m^2 days 1-5 every 3-4 weeks

Dosage adjustment in hepatic impairment: Dosage reductions of 50% to 75% have been suggested for "severe" hepatic dysfunction; however, specific guidelines have not been published.

Hepatic Impairment Dosage reductions of 50% to 75% have been suggested for "severe" hepatic dysfunction; however, specific guidelines have not been published.

Administration Usually administered as a rapid I.V. push (2-3 minutes) or short (15-20 minutes) infusion; 24-hour continuous infusions are occasionally used. Avoid extravasation.

Vesicant/Extravasation Risk Vesicant; see Management of Drug Extravasations on page 1800

Prescribing and Access Restrictions Investigational agent in the U.S.

Dosage Forms Excipient information presented when available (limited, particularly for generics); consult specific product labeling.

Injection, powder for reconstitution: 5 mg

References

Dancey J and Steward WP, "The Role of Vindesine in Oncology - Recommendations After 10 Years' Experience," *Anticancer Drugs*, 1995, 6(6):625-36.

Rhomberg W, Eiter H, Soltesz E, et al, "Long-Term Application of Vindesine: Toxicity and Tolerance," *J Cancer Res Clin Oncol*, 1990, 116(6):651-3.

Sorenson JB and Hansen HH, "Is There a Role for Vindesine in the Treatment of Nonsmall Cell Lung Cancer?" *Invest New Drugs*, 1993, 11(2-3):103-33.

◆ **Vindesine Sulfate** *see* Vindesine *on page 1464*

Vinorelbine (vi NOR el been)

Related Information

Management of Chemotherapy-Induced Nausea and Vomiting *on page 1786*

Management of Drug Extravasations *on page 1800*

Safe Handling of Hazardous Drugs *on page 1904*

Brand Names: U.S. Navelbine®

Brand Names: Canada Navelbine®; Vinorelbine Injection, USP; Vinorelbine Tartrate for Injection

Index Terms Dihydroxydeoxynorvinkaleukoblastine; Vinorelbine Tartrate

Generic Availability (U.S.) Yes

Pharmacologic Category Antineoplastic Agent, Natural Source (Plant) Derivative; Antineoplastic Agent, Vinca Alkaloid

Use Treatment of nonsmall cell lung cancer (NSCLC)

Unlabeled Use Treatment of breast cancer (metastatic), cervical cancer, ovarian cancer, malignant pleural mesothelioma, and soft tissue sarcoma

Labeled Contraindications Pretreatment granulocyte counts <1000/mm^3

Pregnancy Risk Factor D

Lactation Excretion in breast milk unknown/not recommended

Warnings/Precautions Hazardous agent - use appropriate precautions for handling and disposal. **[U.S. Boxed Warning]: For I.V. use only; do not administer intrathecally;** intrathecal administration may result in death. **[U.S. Boxed Warning]: Avoid extravasation;** infiltration may cause irritation, thrombophlebitis and/or local tissue necrosis. **[U.S. Boxed Warning]: Severe granulocytopenia may occur with treatment;** granulocytopenia is a dose-limiting toxicity; granulocyte counts should be ≥1000/mm^3 prior to treatment initiation; monitor closely for infections and/or fever; may require dosage adjustment. The incidence of granulocytopenia is significantly higher when given in combination with cisplatin when compared to single-agent vinorelbine. Use with caution in patients with compromised marrow reserve due to prior chemotherapy therapy or prior radiation therapy.

Fatal cases of interstitial pulmonary changes and ARDS have been reported (with single-agent therapy); promptly evaluate changes in baseline pulmonary symptoms or any new onset pulmonary symptoms. Acute shortness of breath and severe bronchospasm have been reported rarely; usually associated with the concurrent administration of mitomycin.

Vinorelbine should **NOT** be prepared during the preparation of any intrathecal medications. After preparation, store vinorelbine in a location **away** from the separate storage location recommended for intrathecal medications. Dosage modification required in patients with impaired hepatic function and neurotoxicity; use with caution. May cause new onset or worsening of pre-existing neuropathy; use with caution in patients with neuropathy. May cause severe constipation (grade 3-4), paralytic ileus, intestinal obstruction, necrosis, and/or perforation. May have radiosensitizing effects with prior or concurrent radiation therapy; radiation recall reactions may occur in patients who have received prior radiation therapy. Avoid eye contamination (exposure may cause severe irritation). **[U.S. Boxed Warning]: Should be administered under the supervision of an experienced cancer chemotherapy physician.**

Adverse Reactions Note: Reported with single-agent therapy.

>10%:

Central nervous system: Fatigue (27%)

Dermatologic: Alopecia (12% to 30%)

Gastrointestinal: Nausea (31% to 44%; grade 3: 1% to 2%), constipation (35%; grade 3: 3%), vomiting (20% to 31%; grade 3: 1% to 2%), diarrhea (12% to 17%)

Hematologic: Leukopenia (83% to 92%; grade 4: 6% to 15%), granulocytopenia (90%; grade 4: 36%; nadir: 7-10 days; recovery 14-21 days; dose-limiting), neutropenia (85%; grade 4: 28%), anemia (83%; grades 3/4: 9%)

Hepatic: AST increased (67%; grade 3: 5%; grade 4: 1%), total bilirubin increased (5% to 13%; grade 3: 4%; grade 4: 3%)

Local: Injection site reaction (22% to 28%; includes erythema, vein discoloration), injection site pain (16%)

Neuromuscular & skeletal: Weakness (36%), peripheral neuropathy (25%; grade 3: 1%; grade 4: <1%)

Renal: Creatinine increased (13%)

1% to 10%:

- Cardiovascular: Chest pain (5%)
- Dermatologic: Rash (<5%)
- Gastrointestinal: Paralytic ileus (1%)
- Hematologic: Neutropenic fever/sepsis (8%; grade 4: 4%), thrombocytopenia (3% to 5%; grades 3/4: 1%)
- Local: Phlebitis (7% to 10%)
- Neuromuscular & skeletal: Loss of deep tendon reflexes (<5%), myalgia (<5%), arthralgia (<5%), jaw pain (<5%)
- Otic: Ototoxicity (≤1%)
- Respiratory: Dyspnea (7%)

<1%, postmarketing, and/or case reports: Abdominal pain, allergic reactions, anaphylaxis, angioedema, back pain, DVT, dysphagia, esophagitis, flushing, gait instability, headache, hemolytic uremic syndrome, hemorrhagic cystitis, hyper-/hypotension, hyponatremia, intestinal necrosis, intestinal obstruction, intestinal perforation, interstitial pulmonary changes, local rash, local urticaria, MI (rare), mucositis, muscle weakness, myocardial ischemia, pancreatitis, paralytic ileus, pneumonia, pruritus, pulmonary edema, pulmonary embolus, radiation recall (dermatitis, esophagitis), skin blistering, syndrome of inappropriate ADH secretion, tachycardia, thromboembolic events, thrombotic thrombocytopenic purpura, tumor pain, urticaria, vasodilation

Drug Interactions

Metabolism/Transport Effects Substrate of CYP2D6 (minor), CYP3A4 (major); **Note:** Assignment of Major/Minor substrate status based on clinically relevant drug interaction potential; **Inhibits** CYP2D6 (weak), CYP3A4 (weak)

Avoid Concomitant Use

Avoid concomitant use of Vinorelbine with any of the following: BCG; CloZAPine; Conivaptan; Natalizumab; Pimecrolimus; Pimozide; Tacrolimus (Topical); Vaccines (Live)

Increased Effect/Toxicity

Vinorelbine may increase the levels/effects of: ARIPiprazole; CloZAPine; Leflunomide; MitoMYcin (Systemic); Natalizumab; Pimozide; Vaccines (Live)

The levels/effects of Vinorelbine may be increased by: CISplatin; Conivaptan; CYP3A4 Inhibitors (Moderate); CYP3A4 Inhibitors (Strong); Dasatinib; Denosumab; Gefitinib; Itraconazole; Ivacaftor; Macrolide Antibiotics; Mifepristone; PACLitaxel; PACLitaxel (Protein Bound); Pimecrolimus; Posaconazole; Roflumilast; Tacrolimus (Topical); Trastuzumab; Voriconazole

Decreased Effect

Vinorelbine may decrease the levels/effects of: BCG; Coccidioidin Skin Test; Sipuleucel-T; Vaccines (Inactivated); Vaccines (Live)

The levels/effects of Vinorelbine may be decreased by: CYP3A4 Inducers (Strong); Deferasirox; Echinacea; Herbs (CYP3A4 Inducers); Peginterferon Alfa-2b; Tocilizumab

Ethanol/Nutrition/Herb Interactions Herb/Nutraceutical: Avoid St John's wort (may decrease vinorelbine levels).

Storage/Stability Store intact vials under refrigeration at 2°C to 8°C (36°F to 46°F); do not freeze. Protect from light. Intact vials are stable at room temperature of 25°C (77°F) for up to 72 hours. Dilutions in D_5W or NS are stable for 24 hours at room temperature. After preparation, store vinorelbine in a location **away** from the separate storage location recommended for intrathecal medications.

Reconstitution Dilute in D_5W or NS to a final concentration of 1.5-3 mg/mL (for syringe) or 0.5-2 mg/mL (for I.V. bag). Vinorelbine should **NOT** be prepared during the preparation of any intrathecal medications.

Mechanism of Action Semisynthetic vinca alkaloid which binds to tubulin and inhibits microtubule formation, therefore, arresting the cell at metaphase by disrupting the formation of the mitotic spindle; it is specific for the M and S phases. Vinorelbine may also interfere with nucleic acid and protein synthesis by blocking glutamic acid utilization.

Pharmacodynamics/Kinetics

Absorption: Unreliable; must be given I.V.

Distribution: V_d: 25-40 L/kg; binds extensively to human platelets and lymphocytes (80% to 91%)

Protein binding: 80% to 91%

Metabolism: Extensively hepatic, via CYP3A4, to two metabolites, deacetylvinorelbine (active) and vinorelbine N-oxide

Bioavailability: Oral (not approved in the U. S.): 26% to 45%

Half-life elimination: Triphasic: Terminal: 28-44 hours

Excretion: Feces (46%); urine (18%, 10% to 12% as unchanged drug)

Clearance: Plasma: Mean: 0.97-1.26 L/hour/kg

Dosing

Adult & Geriatric Details concerning dosing in combination regimens should also be consulted.

Nonsmall cell lung cancer: I.V.:

Single-agent therapy: 30 mg/m²/dose every 7 days

Combination therapy with cisplatin: 25-30 mg/m²/dose every 7 days (in combination with cisplatin)

Breast cancer (unlabeled use): I.V.: 25 mg/m²/dose every 7 days (Zelek, 2001)

Cervical cancer (unlabeled use): I.V.: 30 mg/m²/dose days 1 and 8 of a 21-day treatment cycle (Muggia, 2004; Muggia, 2005)

Malignant pleural mesothelioma (unlabeled use): I.V.: 30 mg/m²/dose (maximum dose: 60 mg) every 7 days for 6 weeks (Stebbing, 2009) **or** 30 mg/m²/dose (maximum dose: 60 mg) every 7 days for 6 weeks, off 2 weeks, then repeat cycle (Muers, 2008)

Ovarian cancer (unlabeled use): I.V.: 25 mg/m²/dose every 7 days (Bajetta, 1996) **or** 30 mg/m²/dose days 1 and 8 of a 21-day treatment cycle (Rothenberg, 2004)

Soft tissue sarcoma (unlabeled use; in combination with gemcitabine): I.V.: 25 mg/m²/dose days 1 and 8 of a 21-day treatment cycle (Dileo, 2007)

Renal Impairment No adjustment is necessary.

Hepatic Impairment

Note: In patients with concurrent hematologic toxicity and hepatic impairment, administer the lower of the doses determined from the adjustment recommendations.

The FDA-approved labeling guidelines are as follows: Vinorelbine should be administered with caution in patients with hepatic insufficiency. In patients who develop hyperbilirubinemia during treatment with vinorelbine, the dose should be adjusted for total bilirubin as follows:

Serum bilirubin ≤2 mg/dL: Administer 100% of dose

Serum bilirubin 2.1-3 mg/dL: Administer 50% of dose

Serum bilirubin >3 mg/dL: Administer 25% of dose

Adjustment for Toxicity

Note: In patients with concurrent hematologic toxicity and hepatic impairment, administer the lower of the doses determined from the adjustment recommendations.

Dosage adjustment in hematological toxicity (based on granulocyte counts):

Granulocytes ≥1500 cells/mm³ on day of treatment: Administer 100% of starting dose.

Granulocytes 1000-1499 cells/mm³ on day of treatment: Administer 50% of starting dose.

Granulocytes <1000 cells/mm³ on day of treatment: Do not administer. Repeat granulocyte count in 1 week. If 3 consecutive doses are held because granulocyte count is <1000 cells/mm³, discontinue vinorelbine.

Adjustment: For patients who, during treatment, have experienced fever or sepsis while granulocytopenic or had 2 consecutive weekly doses held due to granulocytopenia, subsequent doses of vinorelbine should be:

75% of starting dose for granulocytes ≥1500 cells/mm³

37.5% of starting dose for granulocytes 1000-1499 cells/mm³

Dosage adjustment for neurotoxicity: Neurotoxicity ≥grade 2: Discontinue treatment

Combination Regimens

Breast cancer:

Paclitaxel-Vinorelbine on page 1732
Vinorelbine-FEC on page 1773
Vinorelbine-Trastuzumab on page 1775
Vinorelbine-Trastuzumab-FEC on page 1775

Cervical cancer: Cisplatin-Vinorelbine (Cervical Cancer) on page 1585

Lung cancer (nonsmall cell):

Cetuximab-Cisplatin-Vinorelbine (NSCLC) on page 1558
Gemcitabine-Vinorelbine (NSCLC) on page 1677
Vinorelbine-Cisplatin on page 1772

Lung cancer (small cell): Vinorelbine (Small Cell Lung Cancer Regimen) on page 1774

Lymphoma, Hodgkin:

GVD (Hodgkin) on page 1679
IGEV (Hodgkin) on page 1690
Vinorelbine (Hodgkin Regimen) on page 1774

Malignant pleural mesothelioma: Vinorelbine (Mesothelioma Regimen) on page 1774

Ovarian cancer: Vinorelbine (Ovarian Regimen) on page 1774

Prostate cancer: Estramustine + Vinorelbine on page 1638

Soft tissue sarcoma: Gemcitabine-Vinorelbine (Sarcoma) on page 1677

Administration FATAL IF GIVEN INTRATHECALLY. Administer as a direct intravenous push or rapid bolus, over 6-10 minutes (up to 30 minutes). Longer infusions may increase the risk of pain and phlebitis. Intravenous doses should be followed by at least 75-125 mL of saline or D_5W to reduce the incidence of phlebitis and inflammation. Assure proper needle or catheter position prior to administration.

Emetic Potential
Oral: Moderate (30% to 90%)
I.V.: Very low (<10%)

Vesicant/Extravasation Risk Vesicant; see Management of Drug Extravasations on page 1800.

Monitoring Parameters CBC with differential and platelet count, hepatic function tests; monitor for new-onset pulmonary symptoms (or worsening from baseline); monitor for neuropathy

Dosage Forms Excipient information presented when available (limited, particularly for generics); consult specific product labeling. [DSC] = Discontinued product
Injection, solution: 10 mg/mL (1 mL [DSC], 5 mL [DSC])
Injection, solution [preservative free]: 10 mg/mL (1 mL, 5 mL)
Navelbine®: 10 mg/mL (1 mL, 5 mL)

References

Dileo P, Morgan JA, Zahrieh D, et al, "Gemcitabine and Vinorelbine Combination Chemotherapy for Patients With Advanced Soft Tissue Sarcomas," *Cancer*, 2007, 109(9):1863-9.

Jacobson JO, Polovich M, McNiff KK, et al, "American Society of Clinical Oncology/ Oncology Nursing Society Chemotherapy Administration Safety Standards," *J Clin Oncol*, 2009, 27 (32):5469-75.

Morgan C, Tillett T, Braybrooke J, et al, "Management of Uncommon Chemotherapy-Induced Emergencies," *Lancet Oncol*, 2011, 12(8):806-14.

Muers MF, Stephens RJ, Fisher P, et al, "Active Symptom Control With or Without Chemotherapy in the Treatment of Patients With Malignant Pleural Mesothelioma (MS01): A Multicentre Randomised Trial," *Lancet*, 2008, 371(9625):1685-94.

Muggia FM, Blessing JA, Method M, et al, "Evaluation of Vinorelbine in Persistent or Recurrent Squamous Cell Carcinoma of the Cervix: A Gynecologic Oncology Group Study," *Gynecol Oncol*, 2004, 92(2):639-43.

Muggia FM, Blessing JA, Waggoner S, et al, "Evaluation of Vinorelbine in Persistent or Recurrent Nonsquamous Carcinoma of the Cervix: A Gynecologic Oncology Group Study," *Gynecol Oncol*, 2005, 96(1):108-11.

Rothenberg ML, Liu PY, Wilczynski s, et al, "Phase II Trial of Vinorelbine for Relapsed Ovarian Cancer: A Southwest Oncology Group Study," *Gynecol Oncol*, 2004, 95(3):506-12.

Stebbing J Powles T, McPherson K, et al, "The Efficacy and Safety of Weekly Vinorelbine on Relapsed Malignant Pleural Mesothelioma," *Lung Cancer*, 2009, 63(1):94-7.

Zelek L, Barthier S, Riofrio M, et al, "Weekly Vinorelbine is an Effective Palliative Regimen After Failure With Anthracyclines and Taxanes in Metastatic Breast Carcinoma," *Cancer*, 2001, 92 (9):2267-72.

◆ **Vinorelbine Injection, USP (Can)** *see* Vinorelbine *on page 1465*

◆ **Vinorelbine Tartrate** *see* Vinorelbine *on page 1465*

◆ **Vinorelbine Tartrate for Injection (Can)** *see* Vinorelbine *on page 1465*

Vismodegib (vis moe DEG ib)

Brand Names: U.S. Erivedge™

Index Terms GDC-0449; Hedgehog Antagonist GDC-0449

Generic Availability (U.S.) No

Pharmacologic Category Antineoplastic Agent, Hedgehog Pathway Inhibitor

Use Treatment of metastatic basal cell carcinoma, or locally-advanced basal cell carcinoma that has recurred following surgery or in patients who are not candidates for surgery, and not candidates for radiation therapy

Labeled Contraindications There are no contraindications listed within the manufacturer's labeling.

Pregnancy Risk Factor D

Lactation Excretion in breast milk unknown/not recommended

Warnings/Precautions [U.S. Boxed Warnings]: May result in severe birth defects or embryo-fetal death. Teratogenic effects (severe midline defects, missing digits, and other irreversible malformations), embryotoxic, and fetotoxic events were observed in animal reproduction studies. Verify pregnancy status prior to initiating treatment and advise patients (female and male) of the risk of birth defects, the need for contraception and risk of exposure through semen. Amenorrhea was observed in women of reproductive potential; it is unknown if this is reversible.

Advise patients not to donate blood or blood products during vismodegib treatment and for at least 7 months after the last vismodegib dose.

Adverse Reactions

>10%:

Central nervous system: Fatigue (40%)

Dermatologic: Alopecia (64%)

Endocrine & metabolic: Amenorrhea (30%)

Gastrointestinal: Abnormal taste (55%), weight loss (45%), nausea (30%), diarrhea (29%), appetite decreased (25%), constipation (21%), vomiting (14%), loss of taste perception (11%)

Neuromuscular & skeletal: Muscle spasm (72%), arthralgia (16%)

1% to 10%:

Endocrine & metabolic: Hyponatremia (grade 3: 4%), hypokalemia (grade 3: 1%)

Renal: Azotemia (grade 3: 2%)

<1%, postmarketing, and/or case reports: Abdominal pain, alkaline phosphatase increased, aspiration, atrial fibrillation, back pain, corneal abrasion, dehydration, dyspnea, hyperkalemia, hypocalcemia, keratitis, lymphopenia, pneumonia, urinary tract infection

Drug Interactions

Metabolism/Transport Effects Substrate of CYP2C9 (minor), CYP3A4 (minor), P-glycoprotein; **Note:** Assignment of Major/Minor substrate status based on clinically relevant drug interaction potential; **Inhibits** BCRP, CYP2C19 (weak), CYP2C8 (weak), CYP2C9 (weak)

Avoid Concomitant Use There are no known interactions where it is recommended to avoid concomitant use.

Increased Effect/Toxicity

The levels/effects of Vismodegib may be increased by: P-glycoprotein/ABCB1 Inhibitors

Decreased Effect

The levels/effects of Vismodegib may be decreased by: Antacids; H2-Antagonists; P-glycoprotein/ABCB1 Inducers; Proton Pump Inhibitors; Tocilizumab

Storage/Stability Store at 20°C to 25°C (68°F to 77°F); excursions permitted to 15°C to 30°C (59°F to 86°F).

Mechanism of Action

Basal cell cancer is associated with mutations in Hedgehog pathway components. Hedgehog regulates cell growth and differentiation in embryogenesis; while generally not active in adult tissue, Hedgehog mutations associated with basal cell cancer can activate the pathway resulting in unrestricted proliferation of skin basal cells. Vismodegib is a selective Hedgehog pathway inhibitor which binds to and inhibits Smoothened homologue (SMO), the transmembrane protein involved in Hedgehog signal transduction.

Pharmacodynamics/Kinetics

Distribution: V_d: 16.4-26.6 L

Protein binding: >99%; primarily to serum albumin and alpha$_1$ acid glycoprotein (AAG)

Metabolism: Metabolized by oxidation, glucuronidation, and pyridine ring cleavage, although >98% of circulating components are as the parent drug

Bioavailability: ~32%

Half-life, elimination: Continuous daily dosing: ~4 days; Single dose: ~12 days

Time to peak: ~2.4 days (Graham, 2011)

Excretion: Feces (82%); urine (4%)

Dosing

Adult Basal cell cancer, metastatic or locally advanced: Oral: 150 mg once daily until disease progression or unacceptable toxicity.

Renal Impairment No dosage adjustment provided in the manufacturer's labeling (has not been studied).

Hepatic Impairment No dosage adjustment provided in the manufacturer's labeling (has not been studied).

Combination Regimens

Basal cell carcinoma: Vismodegib (Basal Cell Regimen) on page 1778

Administration Oral: May be taken with or without food. Swallow capsules whole; do not open or crush. If a dose is missed, do not make up; resume dosing with the next scheduled dose.

Monitoring Parameters Pregnancy test within 1 week prior to treatment initiation.

Dietary Considerations May be taken without regard to food.

Additional Information In a study of vismodegib in patients with basal cell nevus syndrome (not an approved use), with discontinuation of vismodegib treatment, taste alteration and muscle cramps abated within 1 month, and scalp and body hair began to regrow within 3 months (Tang, 2012).

Prescribing and Access Restrictions Available at specialty pharmacies through the Erivedge Access Solutions program. Further information may be obtained from the manufacturer, Genentech, at 1-888-249-4918, or at www.-ErivedgeAccessSolutions.com

Medication Guide Available Yes

Dosage Forms Excipient information presented when available (limited, particularly for generics); consult specific product labeling.

Capsule, oral:

Erivedge™: 150 mg

References

Graham RA, Lum BL, Cheeti S, et al, "Pharmacokinetics of Hedgehog Pathway Inhibitor Vismodegib (GDC-0449) in Patients With Locally Advanced or Metastatic Solid Tumors: The Role of Alpha-1-Acid Glycoprotein Binding," *Clin Cancer Res*, 2011, 17(8):2512-20.

Sekulik A, Migden M, Oro AE, et al, "Efficacy and Safety of Vismodegib in Advanced Basal-Cell Carcinoma," *New Engl J Med*, 2012, 366(23):2171-9.

Tang JY, Mackay-Wiggan JM, Aszterbaum M, et al, "Inhibiting the Hedgehog Pathway in Patients With the Basal-Cell Nevus Syndrome," *New Engl J Med*, 2012, 366(23):2180-8.

Von Hoff DD, LoRusso PM, Rudin CM, et al, "Inhibition of the Hedgehog Pathway in Advanced Basal-Cell Carcinoma," *N Engl J Med*, 2009, 361(12):1164-72.

◆ **Vistaril®** *see* HydrOXYzine *on page 736*

◆ **Vistonuridine** *see* Uridine Triacetate *on page 1419*

◆ **Vitamin K** *see* Phytonadione *on page 1169*

◆ **Vitamin K$_1$** *see* Phytonadione *on page 1169*

- **Vitrase®** *see* Hyaluronidase *on page 711*
- **VLB** *see* VinBLAStine *on page 1445*
- **VM-26** *see* Teniposide *on page 1342*
- **Voraxaze** *see* Glucarpidase *on page 680*
- **Voraxaze®** *see* Glucarpidase *on page 680*

Voriconazole (vor i KOE na zole)

Brand Names: U.S. VFEND®

Brand Names: Canada VFEND®

Index Terms UK109496

Generic Availability (U.S.) Yes: Excludes powder for suspension

Pharmacologic Category Antifungal Agent, Oral; Antifungal Agent, Parenteral

Use Treatment of invasive aspergillosis; treatment of esophageal candidiasis; treatment of candidemia (in non-neutropenic patients); treatment of disseminated *Candida* infections of the skin and viscera; treatment of serious fungal infections caused by *Scedosporium apiospermum* and *Fusarium* spp (including *Fusarium solani*) in patients intolerant of, or refractory to, other therapy

Unlabeled Use Fungal infection prophylaxis in intermediate or high risk neutropenic cancer patients with myelodysplastic syndrome (MDS) or acute myelogenous leukemia (AML), neutropenic allogeneic hematopoietic stem cell recipients, and patients with significant graft versus-host disease; empiric antifungal therapy (second-line) for persistent neutropenic fever; empiric treatment of fungal meningitis or osteoarticular infections

Labeled Contraindications Hypersensitivity to voriconazole or any component of the formulation (cross-reaction with other azole antifungal agents may occur but has not been established, use caution); coadministration of CYP3A4 substrates which may lead to QT_c prolongation (cisapride, pimozide, or quinidine); coadministration with barbiturates (long acting), carbamazepine, efavirenz (with standard [eg, not adjusted] voriconazole and efavirenz doses), ergot derivatives, rifampin, rifabutin, ritonavir (≥800 mg/day), sirolimus, St John's wort

Pregnancy Risk Factor D

Lactation Excretion in breast milk unknown/not recommended

Warnings/Precautions Visual changes, including blurred vision, changes in visual acuity, color perception, and photophobia, are commonly associated with treatment; postmarketing cases of optic neuritis and papilledema (lasting >1 month) have also been reported. Patients should be warned to avoid tasks which depend on vision, including operating machinery or driving. Changes are reversible on discontinuation following brief exposure/treatment regimens (≤28 days).

Serious hepatic reactions (including hepatitis, cholestasis, and fulminant hepatic failure) have occurred during treatment, primarily in patients with serious concomitant medical conditions. However, hepatotoxicity has occurred in patients with no identifiable risk factors. Use caution in patients with pre-existing hepatic impairment (dose adjustment or discontinuation may be required).

Voriconazole tablets contain lactose; avoid administration in hereditary galactose intolerance, Lapp lactase deficiency, or glucose-galactose malabsorption. Suspension contains sucrose; use caution with fructose intolerance, sucrase-isomaltase deficiency, or glucose-galactose malabsorption. Avoid/limit use of intravenous formulation in patients with renal impairment; intravenous formulation contains excipient cyclodextrin (sulfobutyl ether beta-cyclodextrin), which may accumulate in renal insufficiency. Acute renal failure has been observed in severely ill patients; use with caution in patients receiving concomitant nephrotoxic medications. Anaphylactoid-type infusion-related reactions may occur with intravenous dosing. Consider discontinuation of infusion if reaction is severe.

Use caution in patients taking strong cytochrome P450 inducers, CYP2C9 inhibitors, and major 3A4 substrates; consider alternative agents that avoid or lessen the potential for CYP-mediated interactions. QT interval prolongation has been associated with voriconazole use; rare cases of arrhythmia (including torsade de pointes), cardiac arrest, and sudden death have been reported, usually in seriously ill patients with comorbidities and/or risk factors (eg, prior cardiotoxic chemotherapy, cardiomyopathy, electrolyte imbalance, or concomitant QT_c-prolonging drugs). Use with caution in these patient populations; correct electrolyte abnormalities (eg, hypokalemia, hypomagnesemia, hypocalcemia) prior to initiating therapy. Do not infuse concomitantly with blood products or short-term concentrated electrolyte solutions, even if the two infusions are running in separate intravenous lines (or cannulas).

Rare cases of malignancy (melanoma, squamous cell carcinoma) have been reported in patients (mostly immunocompromised) with prior onset of severe photosensitivity reactions and exposure to long-term voriconazole therapy. Other serious exfoliative cutaneous reactions, including Stevens-Johnson syndrome, have also been reported. Patient should avoid strong, direct exposure to sunlight; may cause photosensitivity, especially with long-term use. Discontinue use in patients who develop an exfoliative cutaneous reaction or a skin lesion consistent with squamous cell carcinoma or melanoma. Periodic total body skin examinations should be performed, particularly with prolonged use.

Monitor pancreatic function in patients (children and adults) at risk for acute pancreatitis (eg, recent chemotherapy or hematopoietic stem cell transplantation); there have been postmarketing reports of pancreatitis in children.

Ethanol/Nutrition/Herb Interactions

Food: Food may decrease voriconazole absorption. Grapefruit juice may decrease voriconazole levels. Management: Oral voriconazole should be taken 1 hour before or 1 hour after a meal. Avoid grapefruit juice. Maintain adequate hydration unless instructed to restrict fluid intake.

Herb/Nutraceutical: St John's wort may decrease voriconazole levels. Management: Concurrent use of St John's wort with voriconazole is contraindicated.

Storage/Stability

Powder for injection: Store at 15°C to 30°C (59°F to 86°F). Reconstituted solutions are stable for up to 24 hours under refrigeration at 2°C to 8°C (36°F to 46°F).

Powder for oral suspension: Store at 2°C to 8°C (36°F to 46°F). Reconstituted oral suspension may be stored at 15°C to 30°C (59°F to 86°F).

Tablets: Store at 15°C to 30°C (59°F to 86°F).

Reconstitution

Powder for injection: Reconstitute 200 mg vial with 19 mL of sterile water for injection (use of automated syringe is not recommended). Resultant solution (20 mL) has a concentration of 10 mg/mL. Prior to infusion, must dilute to 0.5-5 mg/mL with NS, LR, D_5WLR, D_5W½NS, D_5W, D_5W with KCl 20 mEq, ½NS, or D_5WNS. Do not dilute with 4.2% sodium bicarbonate infusion.

Powder for oral suspension: Add 46 mL of water to the bottle to make 40 mg/mL suspension. Discard unused portion after 14 days.

Mechanism of Action Interferes with fungal cytochrome P450 activity (selectively inhibits 14-alpha-lanosterol demethylation), decreasing ergosterol synthesis (principal sterol in fungal cell membrane) and inhibiting fungal cell membrane formation.

Pharmacodynamics/Kinetics

Absorption: Well absorbed after oral administration; administration of crushed tablets is considered bioequivalent to whole tablets

Distribution: V_d: 4.6 L/kg

Protein binding: 58%

Metabolism: Hepatic, via CYP2C19 (major pathway) and CYP2C9 and CYP3A4 (less significant); saturable (may demonstrate nonlinearity)

Bioavailability: 96%

Half-life elimination: Variable, dose-dependent

Time to peak: Oral: 1-2 hours; 0.5 hours (crushed tablet)

Excretion: Urine (as inactive metabolites; <2% as unchanged drug)

Dosing

Adult & Geriatric

Aspergillosis, invasive, including disseminated and extrapulmonary infection: Duration of therapy should be a minimum of 6-12 weeks or throughout period of immunosuppression (Walsh, 2008):

I.V.: Initial: Loading dose: 6 mg/kg every 12 hours for 2 doses; followed by maintenance dose of 4 mg/kg every 12 hours

Oral: Maintenance dose:

Manufacturer's recommendations:

Patients <40 kg: 100 mg every 12 hours; maximum: 300 mg/day

Patients ≥40 kg: 200 mg every 12 hours; maximum: 600 mg/day

IDSA recommendations (Walsh, 2008): May consider oral therapy in place of I.V. with dosing of 4 mg/kg (rounded up to convenient tablet dosage form) every 12 hours; however, I.V. administration is preferred in serious infections since comparative efficacy with the oral formulation has not been established.

Scedosporiosis, fusariosis:

I.V.: Initial: Loading dose: 6 mg/kg every 12 hours for 2 doses; followed by maintenance dose of 4 mg/kg every 12 hours

Oral: Maintenance dose:

Patients <40 kg: 100 mg every 12 hours; maximum 300 mg/day

Patients ≥40 kg: 200 mg every 12 hours; maximum: 600 mg/day

Candidemia and other deep tissue *Candida* infections: Treatment should continue for a minimum of 14 days following resolution of symptoms or following last positive culture, whichever is longer.

I.V.: Initial: Loading dose 6 mg/kg every 12 hours for 2 doses; followed by maintenance dose of 3-4 mg/kg every 12 hours

Oral:

Manufacturer's recommendations: Maintenance dose:

Patients <40 kg: 100 mg every 12 hours; maximum: 300 mg/day

Patients ≥40 kg: 200 mg every 12 hours; maximum: 600 mg/day

IDSA recommendations (Pappas, 2009): Initial: Loading dose: 400 mg every 12 hours for 2 doses; followed by 200 mg every 12 hours

Endophthalmitis, fungal (unlabeled use; Pappas, 2009): I.V.: 6 mg/kg every 12 hours for 2 doses, then 3-4 mg/kg every 12 hours

Esophageal candidiasis: Oral: Treatment should continue for a minimum of 14 days, and for at least 7 days following resolution of symptoms:

Patients <40 kg: 100 mg every 12 hours; maximum: 300 mg/day

Patients ≥40 kg: 200 mg every 12 hours; maximum: 600 mg/day

Meningitis (secondary to contaminated [eg, *Exserohilum rostratum*] steroid products) (unlabeled use) (CDC [parameningeal], 2012; Kauffman, 2012): Note: Consult an infectious disease specialist and current CDC guidelines for specific treatment recommendations. Therapy duration is ≥3 months; trough serum concentrations must be maintained between 2-5 mcg/mL.

I.V.: 6 mg/kg every 12 hours. If patient does not improve or has severe disease, consider adding amphotericin B (liposomal)

Oral (only in mild disease in adherent patients whose trough concentrations/ response to therapy can be closely monitored): 6 mg/kg every 12 hours (CDC [parameningeal], 2012)

Osteoarticular infection involving the spine, discitis, epidural abscess or vertebral osteomyelitis (secondary to contaminated [eg, *Exserohilum rostratum*] steroid products) (unlabeled use) (CDC [osteoarticular], 2012; Kauffmann, 2012): I.V.: 6 mg/kg every 12 hours for ≥3 months. **Note:** Consult an infectious disease specialist and current CDC guidelines for specific treatment recommendations. Trough serum concentrations must be maintained between 2-5 mcg/mL. If patient has severe disease, consider adding amphotericin B (liposomal). Patients may be switched to oral therapy if condition has improved or stabilized.

Osteoarticular infection not involving the spine (secondary to contaminated [eg, *Exserohilum rostratum*] steroid products) (unlabeled use) (CDC [osteoarticular], 2012; Kauffman, 2012): Note: Consult an infectious disease specialist and current CDC guidelines for specific treatment recommendations. Therapy duration is ≥3 months. Trough serum concentrations must be maintained between 2-5 mcg/mL.

I.V.: 6 mg/kg every 12 hours for 2 doses, then 4 mg/kg every 12 hours. If patient has severe disease, consider adding amphotericin B (liposomal)

Oral (only in mild disease in adherent patients whose trough concentrations/ response to therapy can be closely monitored): 6 mg/kg every 12 hours for 2 doses, then 4 mg/kg every 12 hours

Dosage adjustment in patients unable to tolerate treatment:

I.V.: Dose may be reduced to 3-4 mg/kg every 12 hours, depending upon condition

Oral: Dose may be reduced in 50 mg decrements to a minimum dosage of 200 mg every 12 hours in patients weighing ≥40 kg (100 mg every 12 hours in patients <40 kg)

Dosage adjustment in patients receiving concomitant CYP450 enzyme inducers or substrates:

Efavirenz: Oral: Increase maintenance dose of voriconazole to 400 mg every 12 hours and reduce efavirenz dose to 300 mg once daily; upon discontinuation of voriconazole, return to the initial dose of efavirenz

Phenytoin:

I.V.: Increase voriconazole maintenance dosage to 5 mg/kg every 12 hours

Oral: Increase voriconazole dose to 400 mg every 12 hours in patients ≥40 kg (200 mg every 12 hours in patients <40 kg)

Pediatric

Aspergillosis, invasive including disseminated and extrapulmonary infection in HIV-exposed/-positive patients: (unlabeled; CDC, 2009): Children >2 to <12 years:

Oral: Loading dose: 8 mg/kg/dose (maximum: 400 mg/dose) every 12 hours for 2 doses on day 1, followed by maintenance dose of 7 mg/kg/dose (maximum: 200 mg/dose) every 12 hours for ≥12 weeks

I.V.: Loading dose: 6-8 mg/kg/dose (maximum: 400 mg/dose) every 12 hours for 2 doses on day 1, followed by maintenance dose of 7 mg/kg/dose (maximum: 200 mg/dose) every 12 hours for ≥12 weeks

Children ≥12 years: Refer to adult dosing.

Renal Impairment In patients with Cl_{cr} <50 mL/minute, accumulation of the intravenous vehicle (cyclodextrin) occurs. After initial I.V. loading dose, oral voriconazole should be administered to these patients, unless an assessment of the benefit:risk to the patient justifies the use of I.V. voriconazole. Monitor serum creatinine and change to oral voriconazole therapy when possible.

Oral: Poorly dialyzed; no supplemental dose or dosage adjustment necessary, including patients on intermittent hemodialysis, peritoneal dialysis, or continuous renal replacement therapy (eg, CVVHD)

Note: I.V. dosing **NOT** recommended since cyclodextrin vehicle is cleared at half the rate of voriconazole and may accumulate.

Hepatic Impairment

Mild-to-moderate hepatic dysfunction (Child-Pugh class A or B): Following standard loading dose, reduce maintenance dosage by 50%

Severe hepatic impairment: Should only be used if benefit outweighs risk; monitor closely for toxicity

Administration

Oral: Administer 1 hour before or 1 hour after a meal.

I.V.: Infuse over 1-2 hours (rate not to exceed 3 mg/kg/hour). Do not infuse concomitantly into same line or cannula with other drug infusions, including TPN.

Dosage Forms Excipient information presented when available (limited, particularly for generics); consult specific product labeling.

Injection, powder for reconstitution: 200 mg

VFEND®: 200 mg [contains cyclodextrin]

Powder for suspension, oral:

VFEND®: 40 mg/mL (70 mL) [contains sodium benzoate, sucrose; orange flavor]

Tablet, oral: 50 mg, 200 mg

VFEND®: 50 mg, 200 mg [contains lactose]

Vorinostat (vor IN oh stat)

Related Information

Management of Chemotherapy-Induced Nausea and Vomiting *on page 1786*
Principles of Anticancer Therapy *on page 1878*
Safe Handling of Hazardous Drugs *on page 1904*

Brand Names: U.S. Zolinza®

Brand Names: Canada Zolinza®

Index Terms SAHA; Suberoylanilide Hydroxamic Acid

Generic Availability (U.S.) No

Pharmacologic Category Antineoplastic Agent, Histone Deacetylase Inhibitor

Use Treatment of progressive, persistent, or recurrent cutaneous T-cell lymphoma (CTCL)

Labeled Contraindications Severe hepatic impairment.

Canadian labeling: Hypersensitivity to vorinostat or any component of the formulation; severe hepatic impairment (total bilirubin ≥3 times ULN)

Pregnancy Risk Factor D

Lactation Excretion in breast milk unknown/not recommended

Warnings/Precautions Hazardous agent - use appropriate precautions for handling and disposal. Pulmonary embolism and deep vein thrombosis (DVT) have been reported; monitor. Use caution in patients with a history of thrombotic events. Dose-related thrombocytopenia and/or anemia may occur; may require dosage adjustments or discontinuation. QT_c prolongation has been observed; baseline and periodic ECGs were done in clinical trials (Duvic, 2007; Olsen, 2007). Correct electrolyte abnormalities prior to treatment and monitor and correct potassium, calcium, and magnesium levels during therapy. Use caution in patients with a history of QT_c prolongation or with medications known to prolong the QT interval. May cause hyperglycemia; monitor and use with caution in diabetics; may require diet and/or therapy modifications. Nausea, vomiting, and diarrhea may occur; antiemetics and antidiarrheals may be required; control pre-existing nausea and vomiting prior to treatment initiation; replace fluids and electrolytes to avoid dehydration. May cause dizziness or fatigue; caution patients about performing tasks which require mental alertness (eg, operating machinery or driving). Use with caution in patients with mild-to-moderate hepatic impairment (elimination is predominantly hepatic); contraindicated in severe hepatic impairment. In the Canadian labeling, use is also not recommended in patients with moderate hepatic impairment (total bilirubin 1.5-3 times ULN).

Adverse Reactions

>10%:

Cardiovascular: Peripheral edema (13%)

Central nervous system: Fatigue (52%), chills (16%), dizziness (15%), headache (12%), fever (11%)

Dermatologic: Alopecia (19%), pruritus (12%)

Endocrine & metabolic: Hyperglycemia (8% to 69%; grade 3: 5%), dehydration (1% to 16%)

Gastrointestinal: Diarrhea (52%), nausea (41%), taste alteration (28%), anorexia (24%), weight loss (21%), xerostomia (16%), constipation (15%), vomiting (15%), appetite decreased (14%)

Hematologic: Thrombocytopenia (26%; grades 3/4: 6%), anemia (14%; grades 3/4: 2%)

Neuromuscular & skeletal: Muscle spasm (20%)
Renal: Proteinuria (51%), creatinine increased (16% to 47%)
Respiratory: Cough (11%), upper respiratory infection (11%)

1% to 10%:

Cardiovascular: QT_c prolongation (3% to 4%)
Dermatologic: Squamous cell carcinoma (4%)
Respiratory: Pulmonary embolism (5%)

<1%, postmarketing, and/or case reports: Abdominal pain, angioneurotic edema, blurred vision, chest pain, cholecystitis, deafness, diverticulitis, dysphagia, DVT, enterococcal infection, exfoliative dermatitis, gastrointestinal bleeding, gastrointestinal hemorrhage, Guillain-Barré syndrome, hemoptysis, hypertension, hypokalemia, hyponatremia, infection, lethargy, leukopenia, MI, neutropenia, pneumonia, renal failure, sepsis, spinal cord injury, streptococcal bacteremia, stroke (ischemic), syncope, T-cell lymphoma, tumor hemorrhage, ureteric obstruction, ureteropelvic junction obstruction, urinary retention, vasculitis, weakness

Drug Interactions

Metabolism/Transport Effects None known

Avoid Concomitant Use

Avoid concomitant use of Vorinostat with any of the following: CloZAPine

Increased Effect/Toxicity

Vorinostat may increase the levels/effects of: CloZAPine; Highest Risk QTc-Prolonging Agents; Moderate Risk QTc-Prolonging Agents; Vitamin K Antagonists

The levels/effects of Vorinostat may be increased by: Divalproex; Mifepristone; Valproic Acid

Decreased Effect There are no known significant interactions involving a decrease in effect.

Storage/Stability Store at 20°C to 25°C (68°F to 77°F); excursions permitted to 15°C to 30°C (59°F to 86°F).

Mechanism of Action Inhibition of histone deacetylase enzymes, HDAC1, HDAC2, HDAC3, and HDAC6, which catalyze acetyl group removal from protein lysine residues (including histones and transcription factors). Inhibition of histone deacetylase results in accumulation of acetyl groups, leading to alterations in chromatin structure and transcription factor activation causing termination of cell growth leading to cell death.

Pharmacodynamics/Kinetics

Protein binding: ~71%
Metabolism: Glucuronidated and hydrolyzed (followed by beta-oxidation) to inactive metabolites
Bioavailability: Fasting: ~43%
Half-life elimination: ~2 hours
Time to peak, plasma: With high-fat meal: ~4 hours (range: 2-10 hours)
Excretion: Urine: 52% (<1% as unchanged drug, ~52% as inactive metabolites)

Dosing

Adult & Geriatric Cutaneous T-cell lymphoma: Oral: 400 mg once daily until disease progression or unacceptable toxicity

Renal Impairment No dosage adjustment provided in manufacturer's labeling (not studied); however, based on the minimal renal elimination, adjustment not expected.

Hepatic Impairment

U.S. labeling:

Mild-to-moderate impairment: No dosage adjustment provided in manufacturer's labeling; use with caution (based on predominant hepatic metabolism).

Severe impairment: Use is contraindicated

Canadian labeling:

Moderate impairment (total bilirubin 1.5-3 times ULN): Use is not recommended

Severe impairment (total bilirubin >3 times ULN): Use is contraindicated

Adjustment for Toxicity

Intolerance: Reduce dose to 300 mg once daily; may further reduce to 300 mg daily for 5 consecutive days per week

In clinical trials, **dose reductions** were instituted for the following adverse events: Increased serum creatinine, decreased appetite, hypokalemia, leukopenia, nausea, neutropenia, thrombocytopenia, and vomiting. Vorinostat was **discontinued** for the following adverse events: Anemia, angioneurotic edema, weakness, chest pain, exfoliative dermatitis, DVT, ischemic stroke, lethargy, pulmonary embolism, and spinal cord injury.

Treatment was withheld in clinical trials for grade 4 anemia or thrombocytopenia or other grade 3 or 4 drug related toxicity, until resolved to ≤grade 1. Therapy was reinitiated with dose modification (Olsen, 2007).

Administration Administer with food. Do not open, crush, or chew capsules. Maintain adequate hydration (≥2 L/day fluids) during treatment.

Emetic Potential Low (10% to 30%)

Extemporaneous Preparations Hazardous agent: Use appropriate precautions for handling and disposal.

Although not recommended by the manufacturer, a 50 mg/mL oral suspension may be prepared with capsules. Add 20 mL Ora-Plus® into a glass bottle (≥4 oz). Add the contents of twenty 100 mg capsules and shake thoroughly to disperse (may take up to 3 minutes). Add 20 mL Ora-Sweet® and shake to disperse. Label "shake well". Stable for 14 days at room temperature.

Fouladi M, Park JR, Stewart CF, et al, "Pediatric Phase I Trial and Pharmacokinetic Study of Vorinostat: A Children's Oncology Group Phase I Consortium Report," *J Clin Oncol*, 2010, 28 (22):3623-9.

Monitoring Parameters CBC with differential and serum chemistries, including calcium, magnesium, potassium, glucose and creatinine (baseline, then every 2 weeks for 2 months, then monthly), fluid status. Baseline and periodic ECGs were done in clinical trials.

Dietary Considerations Take with food.

Dosage Forms Excipient information presented when available (limited, particularly for generics); consult specific product labeling.

Capsule, oral:

Zolinza®: 100 mg

References

Duvic M, Talpur R, Ni X, et al, "Phase II Trial of Oral Vorinostat (Suberoylanilide Hydroxamic Acid, SAHA) for Refractory Cutaneous T-Cell Lymphoma (CTCL)," *Blood*, 2007, 109(1):31-9.

Olsen EA, Kim YH, Kuzel TM, et al, "Phase IIb Multicenter Trial of Vorinostat in Patients With Persistent, Progressive, or Treatment Refractory Cutaneous T-Cell Lymphoma," *J Clin Oncol*, 2007, 25(21):3109-15.

◆ **Votrient™** *see* Pazopanib *on page* 1129

◆ **VP-16** *see* Etoposide *on page* 538

◆ **VP-16-213** *see* Etoposide *on page* 538

- ◆ **VSLI** *see* VinCRIStine (Liposomal) *on page 1459*
- ◆ **Vumon®** *see* Teniposide *on page 1342*
- ◆ **Westcort®** *see* Hydrocortisone (Topical) *on page 719*
- ◆ **Winpred™ (Can)** *see* PredniSONE *on page 1199*
- ◆ **WinRho® SDF** *see* Rh_o(D) Immune Globulin *on page 1237*
- ◆ **WR-2721** *see* Amifostine *on page 65*
- ◆ **WR-135675** *see* Gallium Nitrate *on page 654*
- ◆ **WR-139007** *see* Dacarbazine *on page 367*
- ◆ **WR-139013** *see* Chlorambucil *on page 270*
- ◆ **WR-139021** *see* Carmustine *on page 243*
- ◆ **Xalkori®** *see* Crizotinib *on page 317*
- ◆ **Xalkori™ (Can)** *see* Crizotinib *on page 317*
- ◆ **Xeloda®** *see* Capecitabine *on page 223*
- ◆ **Xgeva®** *see* Denosumab *on page 428*
- ◆ **XRP6258** *see* Cabazitaxel *on page 210*
- ◆ **Xtandi®** *see* Enzalutamide *on page 506*
- ◆ **Xyntha®** *see* Antihemophilic Factor (Recombinant) *on page 103*
- ◆ **Xyntha® Solofuse™** *see* Antihemophilic Factor (Recombinant) *on page 103*
- ◆ **Y-90 Ibritumomab** *see* Ibritumomab *on page 744*
- ◆ **Y-90 Zevalin** *see* Ibritumomab *on page 744*
- ◆ **Yervoy™** *see* Ipilimumab *on page 809*
- ◆ **YM-00310** *see* Amifostine *on page 65*
- ◆ **Yondelis™ (Can)** *see* Trabectedin *on page 1384*
- ◆ **Z4942** *see* Ifosfamide *on page 752*
- ◆ **Zactima** *see* Vandetanib *on page 1435*
- ◆ **Zaltrap®** *see* Ziv-Aflibercept (Systemic) *on page 1484*
- ◆ **Zanosar®** *see* Streptozocin *on page 1298*
- ◆ **ZD1033** *see* Anastrozole *on page 96*
- ◆ **ZD1694** *see* Raltitrexed *on page 1226*
- ◆ **ZD1839** *see* Gefitinib *on page 659*
- ◆ **ZD6474** *see* Vandetanib *on page 1435*
- ◆ **ZD9238** *see* Fulvestrant *on page 651*
- ◆ **ZDX** *see* Goserelin *on page 683*
- ◆ **Zelboraf™** *see* Vemurafenib *on page 1440*
- ◆ **Zevalin®** *see* Ibritumomab *on page 744*

Ziconotide (zi KOE no tide)

Brand Names: U.S. Prialt®

Generic Availability (U.S.) No

Pharmacologic Category Analgesic, Nonopioid; Calcium Channel Blocker, N-Type

Use Management of severe chronic pain in patients requiring intrathecal (I.T.) therapy and who are intolerant or refractory to other therapies

Labeled Contraindications Hypersensitivity to ziconotide or any component of the formulation; history of psychosis; I.V. administration

I.T. administration is contraindicated in patients with infection at the injection site, uncontrolled bleeding, or spinal canal obstruction that impairs CSF circulation

Pregnancy Risk Factor C

Lactation Excretion in breast milk unknown/not recommended

Warnings/Precautions **[U.S Boxed Warning]: Severe psychiatric symptoms and neurological impairment have been reported;** interrupt or discontinue therapy if cognitive impairment, hallucinations, mood changes, or changes in consciousness occur. May cause or worsen depression and/or risk of suicide. Cognitive impairment may appear gradually during treatment and is generally reversible after discontinuation (may take up to 2 weeks for cognitive effects to reverse). Use caution in the elderly; may experience a higher incidence of confusion. Patients should be instructed to use caution in performing tasks which require alertness (eg, operating machinery or driving). May have additive effects with opiates or other CNS-depressant medications; may potentiate opioid-induced decreased GI motility; does not interact with opioid receptors or potentiate opiate-induced respiratory depression. Will not prevent or relieve symptoms associated with opiate withdrawal and opiates should not be abruptly discontinued. Unlike opioids, ziconotide therapy can be interrupted abruptly or discontinued without evidence of withdrawal.

Meningitis may occur with use of I.T. pumps; monitor for signs and symptoms of meningitis; treatment of meningitis may require removal of system and discontinuation of intrathecal therapy. Elevated serum creatine kinase can occur, particularly during the first 2 months of therapy; consider dose reduction or discontinuing if combined with new neuromuscular symptoms (myalgias, myasthenia, muscle cramps, weakness) or reduction in physical activity. Safety and efficacy have not been established with renal or hepatic dysfunction, or in pediatric patients. Should not be used in combination with intrathecal opiates.

Ethanol/Nutrition/Herb Interactions Ethanol: May increase CNS depression; monitor for increased effects with coadministration. Caution patients about effects.

Storage/Stability Prior to use, store vials at 2°C to 8°C (36°F to 46°F). Once diluted, may be stored at 2°C to 8°C (36°F to 46°F) for 24 hours; refrigerate during transit. Do not freeze. Protect from light.

When using the Medtronic SynchroMed® EL or SynchroMed® II Infusion System, solutions expire as follows:

25 mcg/mL: Undiluted:

- Initial fill: Use within 14 days.
- Refill: Use within 84 days.

100 mcg/mL:

- Undiluted: Refill: Use within 84 days.
- Diluted: Refill: Use within 40 days.

Reconstitution Preservative free NS should be used when dilution is needed.

CADD-Micro® ambulatory infusion pump: Initial fill: Dilute to final concentration of 5 mcg/mL.

Medtronic SynchroMed® EL or SynchroMed® II infusion system: Prior to initial fill, rinse internal pump surfaces with 2 mL ziconotide (25 mcg/mL), repeat twice. Only the 25 mcg/mL concentration (undiluted) should be used for initial pump fill.

Mechanism of Action Ziconotide selectively binds to N-type voltage-sensitive calcium channels located on the nociceptive afferent nerves of the dorsal horn in the spinal cord. This binding is thought to block N-type calcium channels, leading to a blockade of excitatory neurotransmitter release and reducing sensitivity to painful stimuli.

Pharmacodynamics/Kinetics

Distribution: I.T.: V_d: ~140 mL

Protein binding: ~50%

Metabolism: Metabolized via endopeptidases and exopeptidases present on multiple organs including kidney, liver, lung; degraded to peptide fragments and free amino acids

Half-life elimination: I.V.: 1-1.6 hours (plasma); I.T.: 2.9-6.5 hours (CSF)

Excretion: I.V.: Urine (<1%)

Dosing

Adult Chronic pain: I.T.: Initial dose: ≤2.4 mcg/day (0.1 mcg/hour)

Dose may be titrated by ≤2.4 mcg/day (0.1 mcg/hour) at intervals ≤2-3 times/week to a maximum dose of 19.2 mcg/day (0.8 mcg/hour) by day 21; average dose at day 21: 6.9 mcg/day (0.29 mcg/hour). A faster titration should be used only if the urgent need for analgesia outweighs the possible risk to patient safety.

Geriatric Refer to adult dosing. Use with caution.

Adjustment for Toxicity

Cognitive impairment: Reduce dose or discontinue. Effects are generally reversible within 3-15 days of discontinuation.

Reduced level of consciousness: Discontinue until event resolves.

CK elevation with neuromuscular symptoms: Consider dose reduction or discontinuation.

Administration **Not for I.V. administration. For I.T. administration only** using Medtronic SynchroMed® EL, SynchroMed® II Infusion System, or CADD-Micro® ambulatory infusion pump.

Medtronic SynchroMed® EL or SynchroMed® II Infusion Systems:

Naive pump priming (first time use with ziconotide): Use 2 mL of undiluted ziconotide 25 mcg/mL solution to rinse the internal surfaces of the pump; repeat twice for a total of 3 rinses

Initial pump fill: Use only undiluted 25 mcg/mL solution and fill pump after priming. Following the initial fill only, adsorption on internal device surfaces will occur, requiring the use of the undiluted solution and refill within 14 days.

Pump refills: Contents should be emptied prior to refill. Subsequent pump refills should occur at least every 40 days if using diluted solution or at least every 84 days if using undiluted solution.

CADD-Micro® ambulatory infusion pump: Refer to manufacturers' manual for initial fill and refill instructions

Dosage Forms Excipient information presented when available (limited, particularly for generics); consult specific product labeling.

Infusion, intrathecal, as acetate [preservative free]:

Prialt®: 25 mcg/mL (20 mL); 100 mcg/mL (1 mL, 5 mL)

- **Zictifa** *see* Vandetanib *on page 1435*
- **Zinecard®** *see* Dexrazoxane *on page 448*

Ziv-Aflibercept (Systemic) (ziv a FLIB er sept)

Brand Names: U.S. Zaltrap®

Index Terms Aflibercept I.V.; Vascular Endothelial Growth Factor Trap; VEGF Trap; VEGF Trap R1R2

Generic Availability (U.S.) No

Pharmacologic Category Antineoplastic Agent; Vascular Endothelial Growth Factor (VEGF) Inhibitor

Use Treatment of metastatic colorectal cancer (in combination with fluorouracil, leucovorin, and irinotecan [FOLFIRI]) in patients who are resistant to or have progressed on an oxaliplatin-based regimen

Labeled Contraindications There are no contraindications listed in the manufacturer's labeling.

Pregnancy Risk Factor C

Lactation Excretion in breast milk unknown/not recommended

Warnings/Precautions The risk for hemorrhage is increased with ziv-aflibercept. **[U.S. Boxed Warning]: Severe and occasionally fatal hemorrhage, including gastrointestinal (GI) bleeding, has been reported with ziv-aflibercept/FOLFIRI. Monitor for signs and symptoms of GI and other severe bleeding events; do not administer to patients with severe hemorrhage;** discontinue if severe hemorrhage develops. Hemorrhagic events have also included hematuria, postprocedure hemorrhage, intracranial hemorrhage, and pulmonary hemorrhage/hemoptysis.

[U.S. Boxed Warning]: Severe or fatal GI perforation is a possibility; discontinue ziv-aflibercept if GI perforation occurs; monitor for signs/symptoms of GI perforation. The risk for GI and non-GI fistulas is increased with ziv-aflibercept; fistula sites have included anal, enterovesical, enterocutaneous, colovaginal and intestinal; discontinue in patients who develop fistula. Severe diarrhea and dehydration have been reported; the incidence of diarrhea is increased in patients ≥65 years of age; monitor elderly patients closely for diarrhea.

Proteinuria, nephrotic syndrome, and thrombotic microangiopathy (TMA) have been associated with ziv-aflibercept. Evaluate for proteinuria during treatment with urine dipstick and urinary protein creatinine ratio (UPCR); if UPCR >1, obtain 24-hour urine collection. Withhold ziv-aflibercept for proteinuria ≥2 g/day; for recurrent proteinuria, withhold treatment until <2 g/day and then resume with permanent dose reduction. Discontinue treatment for nephrotic syndrome or TMA.

The risk for grades 3/4 hypertension is increased; onset is generally within the first 2 treatment cycles. Monitor blood pressure every 2 weeks (more frequently if clinically indicated); treat with appropriate antihypertensive therapy (may require adjustment of existing antihypertensives); temporarily withhold treatment with uncontrolled hypertension; may reinitiate with permanent dose reduction when controlled. Discontinue for hypertensive crisis or encephalopathy. Patients with NYHA class III or IV heart failure were excluded from clinical trials.

[U.S. Boxed Warning]: Severely compromised wound healing may occur with ziv-aflibercept/FOLFIRI. Discontinue ziv-aflibercept with compromised wound healing. Withhold ziv-aflibercept at least 4 weeks prior to elective surgery. Do not resume treatment until at least 4 weeks after major surgery AND until the surgical wound is completely healed. For minor surgeries (eg, central venous access port placement, biopsy, or tooth extraction), ziv-aflibercept may be resumed or initiated as soon as the surgical wound is fully healed.

A higher incidence of neutropenia and complications due to neutropenia (neutropenic fever and infection) occurred in patients receiving ziv-aflibercept; leukopenia and thrombocytopenia were also observed in clinical trials; monitor blood counts (baseline and prior to each cycle); delay treatment until ANC is ≥1500/mm^3. Cases of reversible posterior leukoencephalopathy syndrome (RPLS) have been reported; confirm diagnosis with MRI; discontinue ziv-aflibercept if verified; symptoms generally resolve or improve within days, although persistent neurologic symptoms and death have been reported. Arterial thrombotic events (ATE), including transient ischemic attack, cerebrovascular accidents, and angina have occurred. Discontinue ziv-aflibercept in patients who experience ATEs. Certain adverse events, such as diarrhea and dehydration, occurred at a higher incidence in elderly compared to younger adults; monitor closely during treatment.

Adverse Reactions **Note:** Reactions reported in combination therapy with fluorouracil, leucovorin, and irinotecan (FOLFIRI).

>10%:

Cardiovascular: Hypertension (41%; grades 3/4: 19%)

Central nervous system: Fatigue (48%), dysphonia (25%), headache (22%)

Dermatologic: Palmar-plantar erythrodysesthesia (11%)

Gastrointestinal: Diarrhea (69%), stomatitis (50%), appetite decreased (32%), weight loss (32%), abdominal pain (27%), upper abdominal pain (11%)

Hematologic: Leukopenia (78%; grades 3/4: 16%), neutropenia (67%; grades 3/4: 37%), thrombocytopenia (48%; grades 3/4: 3%), bleeding (38%; grades 3/4: 3%)

Hepatic: AST increased (62%), ALT increased (50%)

Neuromuscular & skeletal: Weakness (18%)

Renal: Proteinuria (62%, grades 3/4: 8%), creatinine increased (23%)

Respiratory: Epistaxis (28%), dyspnea (12%)

Miscellaneous: Infection (46%)

1% to 10%:

Cardiovascular: Venous thromboembolic events (9%), arterial thromboembolic events (3%; grades 3/4: 2%)

Central nervous system: Reversible posterior encephalopathy syndrome (RPLS) (1%)

Dermatologic: Hyperpigmentation (8%)

Endocrine & metabolic: Dehydration (9%)

Gastrointestinal: Hemorrhoids (6%), proctalgia (5%), rectal hemorrhage (5%), gastrointestinal perforation (1%)

Genitourinary: Urinary tract infection (9%)

Hematologic: Neutropenic fever (grades 3/4: 4%), neutropenic infection/ sepsis (grades 3/4: 2%)

Renal: Nephrotic syndrome (1%)

Respiratory: Oropharyngeal pain (8%), rhinorrhea (6%), pulmonary embolism (5%)

Miscellaneous: Antibody formation (3%), fistula formation (2%; grades 3/4: <1%)

<1%: Hypersensitivity reactions, thrombotic microangiopathy, wound healing impaired

Drug Interactions

Metabolism/Transport Effects None known.

Avoid Concomitant Use

Avoid concomitant use of Ziv-Aflibercept (Systemic) with any of the following: CloZAPine

Increased Effect/Toxicity

Ziv-Aflibercept (Systemic) may increase the levels/effects of: CloZAPine

Decreased Effect There are no known significant interactions involving a decrease in effect.

Storage/Stability Store intact vials refrigerated at 2°C to 8°C (36°F to 46°F). Protect from light (store in original outer carton). Stable for up to 4 hours refrigerated after diluted for infusion.

Reconstitution Prior to infusion, dilute in D_5W or NS to a final concentration of 0.6-8 mg/mL. Use polyvinyl chloride (PVC) bags containing DEHP or polyolefin bags. After initial vial puncture, do not re-enter; discard unused portion of the vial. Do not mix with other medications.

Mechanism of Action Also known as VEGF-trap, ziv-aflibercept is a recombinant fusion protein which is comprised of portions of binding domains for vascular endothelial growth factor (VEGF) receptors 1 and 2, attached to the Fc portion of human IgG1. Ziv-aflibercept acts as a decoy receptor for VEGF-A, VEGF-B, and placental growth factor (PIGF) which prevent VEGF receptor binding/activation to their receptors (an action critical to angiogenesis), thus leading to antiangiogenesis and tumor regression.

Pharmacodynamics/Kinetics Half-life elimination: ~6 days (range: 4-7 days)

Dosing

Adult & Geriatric Colorectal cancer, metastatic: I.V.: 4 mg/kg every 2 weeks (in combination with fluorouracil, leucovorin, and irinotecan [FOLFIRI]), continue until disease progression or unacceptable toxicity

Renal Impairment No dosage adjustment provided in manufacturer's labeling; however, need for adjustment is not likely because exposure in patients with mild, moderate, and severe impairment was similar to that of patients with normal renal function.

Hepatic Impairment

Mild (total bilirubin >1-1.5 times ULN) to moderate (total bilirubin >1.5-3 times ULN) impairment: No dosage adjustment provided in manufacturer's labeling; however, need for adjustment is not likely because exposure was similar to that of patients with normal hepatic function.

Severe impairment (total bilirubin >3 times ULN): No dosage adjustment provided in the manufacturer's labeling (no data available).

Adjustment for Toxicity

Arterial thrombotic events: Discontinue treatment.

Fistula formation: Discontinue treatment.

Gastrointestinal perforation: Discontinue treatment.

Hemorrhage, severe: Discontinue treatment.

Hypertension:

Recurrent or severe hypertension: Temporarily withhold treatment until controlled and then resume with a permanent dose reduction to 2 mg/kg every 2 weeks.

Hypertensive crisis or hypertensive encephalopathy: Discontinue treatment.

Neutropenia: Temporarily withhold treatment until ANC is $\geq 1500/mm^3$.

Renal effects:

Proteinuria (≥2 g/24 hours): Temporarily withhold treatment until proteinuria <2 g/24 hours and then resume at previous dose.

Recurrent proteinuria: Temporarily withhold treatment until proteinuria <2 g/24 hours and then resume with a permanent dose reduction to 2 mg/kg every 2 weeks.

Nephrotic syndrome or thrombotic microangiopathy: Discontinue treatment

Reversible posterior leukoencephalopathy syndrome (RPLS): Discontinue treatment.

Surgery/ wound healing impairment:

Elective surgery: Temporarily withhold treatment for at least 4 weeks prior to elective surgery; do not resume until at least 4 weeks after major surgery AND until wound is fully healed; for minor surgery (eg, biopsy, central venous port placement, tooth extraction), may be resumed after wound is fully healed.

Wound healing impaired: Discontinue treatment.

Note: For toxicities related to FOLFIRI, refer to individual Fluorouracil or Irinotecan monographs.

Combination Regimens

Colorectal cancer: Ziv-Aflibercept + FOLFIRI (Colorectal) on page 1779

Administration I.V.: Infuse over 1 hour. Do not administer I.V. push or bolus. Administer prior to any FOLFIRI component. Do not administer other medications through the same intravenous line.

Infuse via a 0.2 micron polyethersulfone filter; do not use filters made of polyvinylidene fluoride (PVDF) or nylon. Administer with one of the following types of infusion sets: Polyvinyl chloride (PVC) containing DEHP, DEHP-free PVC containing trioctyl-trimellitate (TOTM), polypropylene, polyethylene lined PVC, or polyurethane.

Monitoring Parameters CBC with differential (baseline and prior to each cycle); urine protein (dipstick analysis and urinary protein creatinine ratio [UPCR], obtain 24-hour urine collection if UPCR >1); blood pressure (every 2 weeks; more frequently if clinically indicated); monitor for signs/symptoms of hemorrhage or GI perforation; monitor elderly patients closely for diarrhea and/or dehydration. Monitor wounds for healing impairment

Dosage Forms Excipient information presented when available (limited, particularly for generics); consult specific product labeling.

Injection, solution [preservative free]:

Zaltrap®: 25 mg/mL (4 mL, 8 mL) [contains sucrose 20%; derived from or manufactured using Chinese hamster ovary cells]

References

Allegra CJ, Lakomy R, Tabernero J, et al, "Effects of Prior Bevacizumab (B) Use on Outcomes From the VELOUR Study: A Phase III Study of Aflibercept (Afl) and FOLFIRI in Patients (Pts) With Metastatic Colorectal Cancer (Mcrc) After Failure of an Oxaliplatin Regimen," *J Clin Oncol*, 2012, 30(15s):3505 [abstract 3505 from ASCO 2012 Annual Meeting].

Isambert N, Freyer G, Zanetta S, et al, "Phase I Dose-Escalation Study of Intravenous Aflibercept in Combination With Docetaxel in Patients With Advanced Solid Tumors," *Clin Cancer Res*, 2012, 18(6):1743-50.

Joulian F, Van Cutsem E, Iqbal SU, et al, "Aflibercept versus Placebo in Combination With FOLFIRI in Previously Treated Metastatic Colorectal Cancer (Mcrc): Mean Overall Survival (OS) Estimation From a Phase III Trial (VELOUR)," *J Clin Oncol*, 2012, 30(15s):3602 [abstract 3602 from ASCO 2012 Annual Meeting].

Lockhart AC, Rothenberg ML, Dupont J, et al, "Phase I Study of Intravenous Vascular Endothelial Growth Factor Trap, Aflibercept, in Patients With Advanced Solid Tumors," *J Clin Oncol*, 2010, 28 (2):207-14.

Van Cutsem E, Tabernero J, Lakomy R, et al, "Addition of Aflibercept to Fluorouracil, Leucovorin, and Irinotecan Improves Survival in a Phase III Randomized Trial in Patients With Metastatic Colorectal Cancer Previously Treated With an Oxaliplatin-Based Regimen," *J Clin Oncol*, 2012, 30(28):3499-506.

- **Zofran®** *see* Ondansetron *on page 1068*
- **Zofran® ODT** *see* Ondansetron *on page 1068*
- **Zol 446** *see* Zoledronic Acid *on page 1488*
- **Zoladex®** *see* Goserelin *on page 683*
- **Zoladex® LA (Can)** *see* Goserelin *on page 683*
- **Zoledronate** *see* Zoledronic Acid *on page 1488*

Zoledronic Acid (zoe le DRON ik AS id)

Related Information

Chronic Pain Management (Cancer) *on page 1840*

Hypercalcemia of Malignancy *on page 1860*

Safe Handling of Hazardous Drugs *on page 1904*

Brand Names: U.S. Reclast®; Zometa®

Brand Names: Canada Aclasta®; Zometa®

Index Terms CGP-42446; Zol 446; Zoledronate

Generic Availability (U.S.) No

Pharmacologic Category Antidote; Bisphosphonate Derivative

Use

Oncology-related uses: Treatment of hypercalcemia of malignancy (albumin-corrected serum calcium >12 mg/dL); treatment of multiple myeloma; treatment of bone metastases of solid tumors

Nononcology uses: Treatment of Paget's disease of bone; treatment of osteoporosis in postmenopausal women (to reduce the incidence of fractures or to reduce the incidence of new clinical fractures in patients with low-trauma hip fracture); prevention of osteoporosis in postmenopausal women, treatment of osteoporosis in men (to increase bone mass); treatment and prevention of glucocorticoid-induced osteoporosis (in patients initiating or continuing prednisone ≥7.5 mg/day [or equivalent] and expected to remain on glucocorticoids for at least 12 months)

Unlabeled Use Prevention of bone loss associated with aromatase inhibitor therapy in postmenopausal women with breast cancer; prevention of bone loss associated with androgen deprivation therapy in prostate cancer

Labeled Contraindications

U.S. labeling:

All indications: Hypersensitivity to zoledronic acid or any component of the formulatio

Nononcology uses: Additional contraindications: Hypocalcemia; use in patients with creatinine clearance (Cl_{cr}) <35 mL/minute and use in patients with evidence of acute renal impairment due to an increased risk of renal failure

Canadian labeling:

All indications: Hypersensitivity to zoledronic acid or other bisphosphonates, or any component of the formulation; pregnancy, breast-feeding

Nononcology uses: Additional contraindications: Uncorrected hypocalcemia at the time of infusion, use in patients with Cl_{cr} <35 mL/minute and use in patients with evidence of acute renal impairment due to an increased risk of renal failure

Pregnancy Risk Factor D

Lactation Excretion in breast milk unknown/not recommended

Warnings/Precautions Hazardous agent - use appropriate precautions for handling and disposal. Osteonecrosis of the jaw (ONJ) has been reported in patients receiving bisphosphonates. Risk factors include invasive dental procedures (eg, tooth extraction, dental implants, boney surgery); a diagnosis of cancer, with concomitant chemotherapy, radiotherapy, or corticosteroids; poor oral hygiene, ill-fitting dentures; and comorbid disorders (anemia, coagulopathy, infection, pre-existing dental disease). Most reported cases occurred after I.V. bisphosphonate therapy; however, cases have been reported following oral therapy. A dental exam and preventative dentistry should be performed prior to placing patients with risk factors on chronic bisphosphonate therapy. The manufacturer's labeling states that there are no data to suggest whether discontinuing bisphosphonates in patients requiring invasive dental procedures reduces the risk of ONJ. However, other experts suggest that there is no evidence that discontinuing therapy reduces the risk of developing ONJ (Assael, 2009). The benefit/risk must be assessed by the treating physician and/or dentist/surgeon prior to any invasive dental procedure. Patients developing ONJ while on bisphosphonates should receive care by an oral surgeon.

Atypical, low energy, or low trauma femur fractures have been reported in patients receiving bisphosphonates for treatment/prevention of osteoporosis. The fractures include subtrochanteric femur (bone just below the hip joint) and diaphyseal femur (long segment of the thigh bone). Some patients experience prodromal pain weeks or months before the fracture occurs. It is unclear if bisphosphonate therapy is the cause for these fractures; atypical femur fractures have also been reported in patients not taking bisphosphonates, and in patients receiving glucocorticoids. Patients receiving long-term (>3-5 years) bisphosphonate therapy may be at an increased risk. Patients presenting with thigh or groin pain with a history of receiving bisphosphonates should be evaluated for femur fracture. Consider interrupting bisphosphonate therapy in patients who develop a femoral shaft fracture; assess for fracture in the contralateral limb.

Infrequently, severe (and occasionally debilitating) musculoskeletal (bone, joint, and/or muscle) pain have been reported during bisphosphonate treatment. The onset of pain ranged from a single day to several months. Consider discontinuing therapy in patients who experience severe symptoms; symptoms usually resolve upon discontinuation. Some patients experienced recurrence when rechallenged with same drug or another bisphosphonate; avoid use in patients with a history of these symptoms in association with bisphosphonate therapy.

May cause a significant risk of hypocalcemia in patients with Paget's disease, in whom the pretreatment rate of bone turnover may be greatly elevated. Hypocalcemia must be corrected before initiation of therapy in patients with Paget's disease and osteoporosis. Ensure adequate calcium and vitamin D intake during therapy. Use caution in patients with disturbances of calcium and mineral metabolism (eg, hypoparathyroidism, thyroid/parathyroid, surgery, malabsorption syndromes, excision of small intestine).

Nononcology indications: Use is contraindicated in patients with Cl_{cr} <35 mL/minute and in patients with evidence of acute renal impairment due to an increased risk of renal failure. Re-evaluate the need for continued therapy for the treatment of osteoporosis periodically; the optimal duration of treatment has not yet been determined.

Oncology indications: Use caution in mild-to-moderate renal dysfunction; dosage adjustment required. In cancer patients, renal toxicity has been reported with doses >4 mg or infusions administered over 15 minutes. Risk factors for renal deterioration include pre-existing renal insufficiency and repeated doses of zoledronic acid and other bisphosphonates. Dehydration and the use of other nephrotoxic drugs which may contribute to renal deterioration should be identified and managed. Use is not recommended in patients with severe renal impairment (serum creatinine >3 mg/dL or Cl_{cr} <30 mL/minute) and bone metastases (limited data); use in patients with hypercalcemia of malignancy and severe renal impairment (serum creatinine >4.5 mg/dL for hypercalcemia of malignancy) should only be done if the benefits outweigh the risks. Diuretics should not be used before correcting hypovolemia. Renal deterioration, resulting in renal failure and dialysis has occurred in patients treated with zoledronic acid after single and multiple infusions at recommended doses of 4 mg over 15 minutes. Assess renal function prior to treatment and withhold for renal deterioration [increase in serum creatinine of 0.5 mg/dL (if baseline level normal) or increase of 1 mg/dL (if baseline level abnormal)]; treatment should be withheld until renal function returns to within 10% of baseline.

According to the American Society of Clinical Oncology (ASCO) guidelines for bisphosphonates in multiple myeloma, treatment with zoledronic acid is not recommended for asymptomatic (smoldering) or indolent myeloma or with solitary plasmacytoma (Kyle, 2007). The National Comprehensive Cancer Network® (NCCN) multiple myeloma guidelines (v.1.2013) also do not recommend the use of bisphosphonates in stage 1 or smoldering disease, unless part of a clinical trial.

Adequate hydration is required during treatment (urine output ~2 L/day); avoid overhydration, especially in patients with heart failure. Pre-existing renal compromise, severe dehydration, and concurrent use with diuretics or other nephrotoxic drugs may increase the risk for renal impairment. Single and multiple infusions in patients with both normal and impaired renal function have been associated with renal deterioration, resulting in renal failure and dialysis or death (rare). Patients with underlying moderate-to-severe renal impairment, increased age, concurrent use of nephrotoxic or diuretic medications, or severe dehydration prior to or after zoledronic acid administration may have an increased risk of acute renal impairment or renal failure. Others with increased risk include patients with renal impairment or dehydration secondary to fever, sepsis, gastrointestinal losses, or diuretic use. If history or physical exam suggests dehydration, treatment should not be given until the patient is normovolemic. Creatinine clearance (using actual body weight) should be calculated with the Cockcroft-Gault formula prior to each administration. Transient increases in serum creatinine may be more pronounced in patients with impaired renal function; consider monitoring creatinine clearance in at-risk patients taking other renally-eliminated drugs.

Use caution in patients with aspirin-sensitive asthma (may cause bronchoconstriction) and the elderly. Rare cases of urticaria and angioedema and very rare cases of anaphylactic reactions/shock have been reported. Women of childbearing age should be advised against becoming pregnant. Not approved for use in children. Do not administer Zometa® and Reclast® to the same patient for different indications.

Adverse Reactions Note: An acute reaction (eg, arthralgia, fever, flu-like symptoms, myalgia) may occur within the first 3 days following infusion in up to 44% of patients; usually resolves within 3-4 days of onset, although may take up to 14 days to resolve. The incidence may be decreased with acetaminophen (prior to infusion and for 72 hours postinfusion).

Oncology indications:

>10%:

Cardiovascular: Leg edema (5% to 21%), hypotension (11%)

Central nervous system: Fatigue (39%), fever (32% to 44%), headache (5% to 19%), dizziness (18%), insomnia (15% to 16%), anxiety (11% to 14%), depression (14%), agitation (13%), confusion (7% to 13%), hypoesthesia (12%)

Dermatologic: Alopecia (12%), dermatitis (11%)

Endocrine & metabolic: Dehydration (5% to 14%), hypophosphatemia (13%), hypokalemia (12%), hypomagnesemia (11%)

Gastrointestinal: Nausea (29% to 46%), vomiting (14% to 32%), constipation (27% to 31%), diarrhea (17% to 24%), anorexia (9% to 22%), abdominal pain (14% to 16%), weight loss (16%), appetite decreased (13%)

Genitourinary: Urinary tract infection (12% to 14%)

Hematologic: Anemia (22% to 33%), neutropenia (12%)

Neuromuscular & skeletal: Bone pain (55%), weakness (5% to 24%), myalgia (23%), arthralgia (5% to 21%), back pain (15%), paresthesia (15%), limb pain (14%), skeletal pain (12%), rigors (11%)

Renal: Renal deterioration (8% to 17%; up to 40% in patients with abnormal baseline creatinine)

Respiratory: Dyspnea (22% to 27%), cough (12% to 22%)

Miscellaneous: Cancer progression (16% to 20%), moniliasis (12%)

1% to 10%:

Cardiovascular: Chest pain (5% to 10%)

Central nervous system: Somnolence (5% to 10%)

Endocrine & metabolic: Hypocalcemia (5% to 10%; grades 3/4: ≤1%), hypermagnesemia (grade 3: 2%)

Gastrointestinal: Dyspepsia (10%), dysphagia (5% to 10%), mucositis (5% to 10%), stomatitis (8%), sore throat (8%)

Hematologic: Granulocytopenia (5% to 10%), pancytopenia (5% to 10%), thrombocytopenia (5% to 10%)

Renal: Serum creatinine increased (grades 3/4: ≤2%)

Respiratory: Upper respiratory tract infection (10%)

Miscellaneous: Infection (nonspecific; 5% to 10%)

Nononcology indications:

>10%:

Cardiovascular: Hypertension (5% to 13%)

Central nervous system: Pain (2% to 24%), fever (9% to 22%), headache (4% to 20%), chills (2% to 18%), fatigue (2% to 18%)

Endocrine & metabolic: Hypocalcemia (≤3%; Paget's disease 21%)

Gastrointestinal: Nausea (5% to 18%)

Neuromuscular & skeletal: Arthralgia (9% to 27%), myalgia (5% to 23%), back pain (4% to 18%), limb pain (3% to 16%), musculoskeletal pain (≤12%)

Miscellaneous: Acute phase reaction (4% to 25%), flu-like syndrome (1% to 11%)

1% to 10%:

Cardiovascular: Chest pain (1% to 8%), peripheral edema (3% to 6%), atrial fibrillation (1% to 3%), palpitation (≤3%)

Central nervous system: Dizziness (2% to 9%), malaise (1% to 7%), hypoesthesia (≤6%), lethargy (3% to 5%), vertigo (1% to 4%), hyperthermia (≤2%)

Dermatologic: Rash (2% to 3%), hyperhidrosis (≤3%)

Gastrointestinal: Abdominal pain (1% to 9%), diarrhea (5% to 8%), vomiting (2% to 8%), constipation (6% to 7%), dyspepsia (2% to 7%), abdominal discomfort/distension (1% to 2%), anorexia (1% to 2%)

Neuromuscular & skeletal: Bone pain (3% to 9%), arthritis (2% to 9%), rigors (8%), shoulder pain (≤7%), neck pain (1% to 7%), weakness (2% to 6%), muscle spasm (2% to 6%), stiffness (1% to 5%), jaw pain (2% to 4%), joint swelling (≤3%), paresthesia (2%)

Ocular: Eye pain (≤2%)

Renal: Serum creatinine increased (2%)

Respiratory: Dyspnea (5% to 7%)

Miscellaneous: C-reactive protein increased (≤5%)

All indications: <1%, postmarketing, and/or case reports: Acute renal failure (requiring hospitalization/dialysis), allergic reaction, anaphylactic reaction/shock, angioedema, blurred vision, bradycardia, bronchoconstriction, conjunctivitis, diaphoresis, episcleritis, femur fracture (diaphyseal or subtrochanteric), hematuria, hyperesthesia, hyperkalemia, hypernatremia, hyperparathyroidism, hypersensitivity, hypertension, injection site reaction (eg, itching, pain, redness), iridocyclitis, iritis, joint and/or muscle pain (sometimes severe and/or incapacitating), muscle cramps, orbital edema, orbital inflammation, osteonecrosis (primarily of the jaws), proteinuria, pruritus, rash, renal impairment, scleritis, taste perversion, toxic acute renal tubular necrosis, tremor, urticaria, uveitis, weight gain, xerostomia

Drug Interactions

Metabolism/Transport Effects None known.

Avoid Concomitant Use There are no known interactions where it is recommended to avoid concomitant use.

Increased Effect/Toxicity

Zoledronic Acid may increase the levels/effects of: Deferasirox; Phosphate Supplements; SUNItinib

The levels/effects of Zoledronic Acid may be increased by: Aminoglycosides; Nonsteroidal Anti-Inflammatory Agents; Thalidomide

Decreased Effect

The levels/effects of Zoledronic Acid may be decreased by: Proton Pump Inhibitors

Storage/Stability

Aclasta® (Canadian availability): Store at room temperature of 15°C to 30°C (59°F to 86°F).

Reclast®: Store at room temperature of 25°C (77°F); excursions permitted to 15°C to 30°C (59°F to 86°F). After opening, stable for 24 hours at 2°C to 8°C (36°F to 46°F).

Zometa®: Store concentrate vials and ready-to-use bottles at 25°C (77°F); excursions permitted to 15°C to 30°C (59°F to 86°F). Diluted solutions for infusion which are not used immediately after preparation should be refrigerated at 2°C to 8°C (36°F to 46°F). Infusion of solution must be completed within 24 hours of preparation. The ready-to-use bottles are for single use only; if any preparation is necessary (preparing reduced dosage for patients with renal impairment), the prepared, diluted solution may be refrigerated at 2°C to 8°C (36°F to 46°F) if not used immediately. Infusion of solution must be completed within 24 hours of preparation. The previously withdrawn volume from the ready-to-use solution should be discarded; do not store or reuse.

Reconstitution Use appropriate precautions for handling and disposal.

Zometa® concentrate vials: Further dilute in 100 mL NS or D_5W prior to administration.

Zometa® ready-to use bottles: No further preparation necessary. If reduced doses are necessary for patients with renal impairment, withdraw the appropriate volume of solution and replace with an equal amount of NS or D_5W.

Mechanism of Action A bisphosphonate which inhibits bone resorption via actions on osteoclasts or on osteoclast precursors; inhibits osteoclastic activity and skeletal calcium release induced by tumors. Decreases serum calcium and phosphorus, and increases their elimination. In osteoporosis, zoledronic acid inhibits osteoclast-mediated resorption, therefore reducing bone turnover.

Pharmacodynamics/Kinetics

Distribution: Binds to bone

Protein binding: 28% to 53%

Half-life elimination: Triphasic; Terminal: 146 hours

Excretion: Urine (39% ± 16% as unchanged drug) within 24 hours; feces (<3%)

Dosing

Adult Note: Acetaminophen administration after the infusion may reduce symptoms of acute phase reactions. Patients treated for multiple myeloma, osteoporosis, and Paget's disease should receive a daily calcium supplement and multivitamin containing vitamin D (if dietary intake is inadequate).

Hypercalcemia of malignancy (albumin-corrected serum calcium ≥12 mg/dL) (Zometa®): I.V.: 4 mg (maximum) given as a single dose. Wait at least 7 days before considering retreatment.

Multiple myeloma or metastatic bone lesions from solid tumors (Zometa®): I.V.: 4 mg every 3-4 weeks

Osteoporosis, glucocorticoid-induced, treatment and prevention (Reclast®, Aclasta® [Canadian availability]): I.V.: 5 mg once a year

Osteoporosis, prevention: I.V.:

Reclast®: 5 mg once every 2 years

Aclasta® (Canadian availability): 5 mg as a single (one-time) dose

Osteoporosis, treatment (Reclast®, Aclasta® [Canadian availability]): I.V.: 5 mg once a year

Paget's disease: I.V.:

Reclast®: 5 mg as a single dose. **Note:** Data concerning retreatment is not available; retreatment may be considered for relapse (increase in alkaline phosphatase) if appropriate, for inadequate response, or in patients who are symptomatic.

Aclasta® (Canadian availability): 5 mg as a single (one-time) dose

Prevention of aromatase inhibitor-induced bone loss in breast cancer (unlabeled use): I.V.: 4 mg every 6 months for 5 years (Brufsky, 2012)

Prevention of androgen deprivation-induced bone loss in nonmetastatic prostate cancer (unlabeled use): I.V.: 4 mg every 3 months for 1 year (Smith, 2003) or 4 mg every 12 months (Michaelson, 2007)

Geriatric Refer to adult dosing. **Note:** Acetaminophen administration after infusion may reduce symptoms of acute-phase reactions. Patients treated for multiple myeloma, osteoporosis, and Paget's disease should receive a daily calcium supplement with vitamin D.

Renal Impairment

Nononcology uses:

Cl_{cr} ≥35 mL/minute: No dosage adjustment required.

Cl_{cr} <35 mL/minute: Use is contraindicated.

Oncology uses:

Multiple myeloma and bone metastases:

Cl_{cr} >60 mL/minute: 4 mg (no dosage adjustment necessary)

Cl_{cr} 50-60 mL/minute: Reduce dose to 3.5 mg

Cl_{cr} 40-49 mL/minute: Reduce dose to 3.3 mg

Cl_{cr} 30-39 mL/minute: Reduce dose to 3 mg

Cl_{cr} <30 mL/minute: Use is not recommended.

Hypercalcemia of malignancy:

Mild-to-moderate impairment: No dosage adjustment necessary.

Severe impairment (serum creatinine >4.5 mg/dL):

U.S. labeling: Evaluate risk versus benefit

Canadian labeling: Use is not recommended.

Dosage adjustment for renal toxicity (during treatment):

Hypercalcemia of malignancy: Evidence of renal deterioration: Evaluate risk versus benefit.

Multiple myeloma and bone metastases: Evidence of renal deterioration: Withhold dose until renal function returns to within 10% of baseline; renal deterioration defined as follows:

Normal baseline creatinine: Increase of 0.5 mg/dL

Abnormal baseline creatinine: Increase of 1 mg/dL

Reinitiate therapy at the same dose administered prior to treatment interruption.

Multiple myeloma: Albuminuria >500 mg/24 hours (unexplained): Withhold dose until return to baseline, then re-evaluate every 3-4 weeks; consider reinitiating with a longer infusion time of at least 30 minutes (Kyle, 2007).

Hepatic Impairment No dosage adjustment provided in the manufacturer's labeling (has not been studied).

Administration Infuse over at least 15 minutes. Flush I.V. line with 10 mL NS flush following infusion. Infuse in a line separate from other medications. Patients should be appropriately hydrated prior to treatment. Acetaminophen after administration may reduce the incidence of acute reaction (eg, arthralgia, fever, flu-like symptoms, myalgia).

Monitoring Parameters Prior to initiation of therapy, dental exam and preventative dentistry for patients at risk for osteonecrosis, including all cancer patients

Nononcology uses: Serum creatinine prior to each dose, especially in patients with risk factors, calculate creatinine clearance before each treatment (consider interim monitoring in patients at risk for acute renal failure), evaluate fluid status and adequately hydrate patients prior to and following administration.

Osteoporosis: Bone mineral density as measured by central dual-energy x-ray absorptiometry (DXA) of the hip or spine (prior to initiation of therapy and at least every 2 years; after 6-12 months of combined glucocorticoid and zoledronic acid treatment); annual measurements of height and weight, assessment of chronic back pain; serum calcium and 25(OH)D; phosphorus and magnesium; may consider monitoring biochemical markers of bone turnover

Paget's disease: Alkaline phosphatase; pain; serum calcium and 25(OH)D; phosphorus and magnesium

Oncology uses: Serum creatinine prior to each dose; serum electrolytes, phosphate, magnesium, and hemoglobin/hematocrit should be evaluated regularly. Monitor serum calcium to assess response and avoid overtreatment. In patients with multiple myeloma, monitor urine every 3-6 months for albuminuria.

Test Interactions Bisphosphonates may interfere with diagnostic imaging agents such as technetium-99m-diphosphonate in bone scans.

Dietary Considerations

Multiple myeloma or metastatic bone lesions from solid tumors: Take daily calcium supplement (500 mg) and daily multivitamin (with 400 units vitamin D).

Osteoporosis: Ensure adequate calcium and vitamin D supplementation; general requirements are calcium 1200 mg/day and vitamin D 800-1000 units/day.

Paget's disease: Take elemental calcium 1500 mg/day (750 mg twice daily or 500 mg 3 times/day) and vitamin D 800 units/day, particularly during the first 2 weeks after administration.

Additional Information Oncology Comment:

Metastatic breast cancer: The American Society of Clinical Oncology (ASCO) guidelines on the role of bone-modifying agents (BMAs) in the prevention and treatment of skeletal-related events for metastatic breast cancer patients were updated (Van Poznak, 2011). The guidelines recommend initiating a BMA (denosumab, pamidronate, zoledronic acid) in patients with a diagnosis of metastatic breast cancer to the bone. There is currently no literature indicating the superiority of one particular BMA over another. The optimal duration has yet to be defined; however, the guidelines recommend continuing therapy until substantial decline in patient's performance status. In patients with normal creatinine clearance (>60 mL/minute), no dosage/interval/infusion rate changes for pamidronate or zoledronic acid are necessary. For patients with Cl_{cr} <30 mL/minute, pamidronate and zoledronic acid are not recommended. While no renal dose adjustments are recommended for denosumab, close monitoring is advised for risk of hypocalcemia in patients with Cl_{cr} <30 mL/minute or on dialysis. The ASCO guidelines are in alignment with package insert guidelines for dosing, renal dose adjustments, infusion times, prevention and management of osteonecrosis of the jaw, and monitoring of laboratory parameter recommendations. BMAs are not the first-line therapy for pain. BMAs are to be used as adjunctive therapy for cancer-related bone pain associated with bone metastasis, demonstrating a modest pain control benefit. BMAs should be used in conjunction with agents such as NSAIDS, opioid and nonopioid analgesics, corticosteroids, radiation/surgery, interventional procedures.

Multiple myeloma: The American Society of Clinical Oncology (ASCO) also has guidelines published on the use of bisphosphonates for prevention and treatment of bone disease in multiple myeloma (Kyle, 2007). Pamidronate or zoledronic acid use is recommended in multiple myeloma patients with lytic bone destruction or compression spine fracture from osteopenia. Clodronate (not available in the U.S.; available in Canada), administered orally or I.V., is an alternative treatment. The use of the bisphosphonates pamidronate and zoledronic acid may be considered in patients with pain secondary to osteolytic disease, adjunct therapy to stabilize fractures or impending fractures, and I.V. bisphosphonates for multiple myeloma patients with osteopenia but no radiographic evidence of lytic bone disease. Bisphosphonates are not recommended in patients with solitary plasmacytoma, smoldering (asymptomatic) or indolent myeloma, or monoclonal gammopathy of undetermined significance. The guidelines recommend monthly treatment for a period of 2 years. At that time, physicians need to consider discontinuing in responsive and stable patients, and reinitiate if new-onset skeletal-related event occurs. The ASCO guidelines are in alignment with package insert guidelines for dosing, renal dose adjustments, infusion times, prevention and management of osteonecrosis of the jaw, and monitoring of laboratory parameter recommendations. The guidelines also state in patients with a serum creatinine >3 mg/dL or Cl_{cr} <30 mL/minute or extensive bone disease, pamidronate at a dose of 90 mg over 4-6 hours is recommended (unless pre-existing renal disease at which a reduced dose should be considered). The ASCO committee also recommends monitoring for the presence of albuminuria every 3-6 months. In patients with albuminuria >500 mg/24 hours, withhold the dose until level returns to baseline, then recheck every 3-4 weeks. Pamidronate may be reinitiated at a dose not to exceed 90 mg every 4 weeks with a longer infusion time of at least 4 hours. The committee also recommends considering increasing the infusion time of zoledronic acid to at least 30 minutes. However, one study has demonstrated that extending the infusion to 30 minutes did not change the safety profile (Berenson, 2011).

Medication Guide Available Yes

Dosage Forms Excipient information presented when available (limited, particularly for generics); consult specific product labeling.

Infusion, premixed:

Reclast®: 5 mg (100 mL)

Zometa®: 4 mg (100 mL)

Injection, solution [concentrate]:

Zometa®: 4 mg/5 mL (5 mL)

Dosage Forms: Canada Excipient information presented when available (limited, particularly for generics); consult specific product labeling.

Infusion, solution [premixed]:

Aclasta®: 5 mg (100 mL)

References

Assael LA, "Oral Bisphosphonates as a Cause of Bisphosphonate-Related Osteonecrosis of the Jaws: Clinical Findings, Assessment of Risks, and Preventive Strategies," *J Oral Maxillofac Surg*, 2009, 67(5 Suppl):35-43.

Berenson JR, Boccia R, Lopez T, et al, "Results of a Multicenter Open-Label Randomized Trial Evaluating Infusion Duration of Zoledronic Acid in Multiple Myeloma Patients (the ZMAX Trial), *J Support Oncol*, 2011, 9(1):32-40.

Black DM, Delmas PD, Eastell R, et al, "Once-Yearly Zoledronic Acid for Treatment of Postmenopausal Osteoporosis," *New Engl J Med*, 2007, 356(18):1809-22.

Boonen S, Sellmeyer DE, Lippuner K, et al, "Renal Safety of Annual Zoledronic Acid Infusions in Osteoporotic Postmenopausal Women," *Kidney Int*, 2008, 74(5):641-8.

Brufsky A, Harker WG, Beck JT, et al, "Zoledronic Acid Inhibits Adjuvant Letrozole-Induced Bone Loss in Postmenopausal Women With Early Breast Cancer," *J Clin Oncol* 2007, 25(7):829-36.

Brufsky AM, Harker WG, Beck JT, et al, "Final 5-year results of Z-FAST Trial: Adjuvant Zoledronic Acid Maintains Bone Mass in Postmenopausal Breast Cancer Patients Receiving Letrozole," *Cancer*, 2012, 118(5):1192-201.

Durie BG, Katz M, and Crowley J, "Osteonecrosis of the Jaw and Bisphosphonates," *N Engl J Med*, 2005, 353(1):99-102.

Gnant M, Mlineritsch B, Schippinger W, et al, "Endocrine Therapy Plus Zoledronic Acid in Premenopausal Breast Cancer," *N Engl J Med*, 2009, 360(7):679-91.

Hadji P, Aapro MS, Body JJ, et al, "Management of Aromatase Inhibitor-Associated Bone Loss in Postmenopausal Women With Breast Cancer: Practical Guidance for Prevention and Treatment," *Ann Oncol*, 2011 [epub ahead of print].

Hillner BE, Ingle JN, Chlebowski RT, et al, "American Society of Clinical Oncology 2003 Update on the Role of Bisphosphonates and Bone Health Issues in Women With Breast Cancer," *J Clin Oncol*, 2003, 21(21):4042-57.

Kyle RA, Yee GC, Somerfield MR, et al, "American Society of Clinical Oncology 2007 Clinical Practice Guideline Update on the Role of Bisphosphonates in Multiple Myeloma," *J Clin Oncol*, 2007, 25(17):2464-72.

Lyles KW, Colon-Emeric CS, Magaziner JS, et al, "Zoledronic Acid and Clinical Fractures and Mortality After Hip Fracture," *N Engl J Med*, 2005, 357(18):1799-809.

"Management of Osteoporosis in Postmenopausal Women: 2010 Position Statement of The North American Menopause Society," *Menopause*, 2010, 17(1):25-54.

McClung M, Miller P, Recknor C, et al, "Zoledronic Acid for the Prevention of Bone Loss in Postmenopausal Women With Low Bone Mass: A Randomized Controlled Trial," *Obstet Gynecol*, 2009, 114(5):999-1007.

Michaelson MD, Kaufman DS, Lee H, et al, "Randomized Controlled Trial of Annual Zoledronic Acid to Prevent Gonadotropin-Releasing Hormone Agonist-Induced Bone Loss in Men With Prostate Cancer," *J Clin Oncol*, 2007, 25(9):1038-42.

National Comprehensive Cancer Network® (NCCN), "Clinical Practice Guidelines in Oncology™: Multiple Myeloma," Version 1.2013. Available at http://www.nccn.org/professionals/physician_gls/PDF/myeloma.pdf

National Osteoporosis Foundation, "Clinician's Guide to Prevention and Treatment of Osteoporosis," Washington, DC, 2010. Available at http://www.nof.org

Reid DM, Devogelaer JP, Saag K, et al, "Zoledronic Acid and Risedronate in the Prevention and Treatment of Glucocorticoid-Induced Osteoporosis (HORIZON): A Multicentre, Double-Blind, Double-Dummy, Randomised Controlled Trial," *Lancet*, 2009, 373(9671):1253-63.

Ruggiero SL, Dodson TB, Assael LA, et al, "American Association of Oral and Maxillofacial Surgeons Position Paper on Bisphosphonate-Related Osteonecrosis of the Jaws-2009 Update," *J Oral Maxillofac Surg*, 2009, 67(5 Suppl):2-12.

Sellmeyer DE, "Atypical Fractures as a Potential Complication of Long-term Bisphosphonate Therapy," *JAMA*, 2010, 304(13):1480-4.

Smith MR, Eastham J, Gleason DM, et al, "Randomized Controlled Trial of Zoledronic Acid to Prevent Bone Loss in Men Receiving Androgen Deprivation Therapy for Nonmetastatic Prostate Cancer," *J Urol*, 2003, 169(6):2008-12.

Van Poznak CH, Temin S, Yee GC, et al, "American Society of Clinical Oncology Executive Summary of the Clinical Practice Guideline Update on the Role of Bone-Modifying Agents in Metastatic Breast Cancer," *J Clin Oncol*, 2011, 29(9):1221-7.

◆ **Zolinza®** *see* Vorinostat *on page 1170*

◆ **Zometa®** *see* Zoledronic Acid *on page 1488*

◆ **Zortress®** *see* Everolimus *on page 552*

◆ **Zosyn®** *see* Piperacillin and Tazobactam *on page 1175*

◆ **Zovirax®** *see* Acyclovir (Systemic) *on page 30*

◆ **Zovirax®** *see* Acyclovir (Topical) *on page 35*

◆ **Zuplenz®** *see* Ondansetron *on page 1068*

◆ **Zuplenz®** *see* Ondansetron *on page 1068*

◆ **Zyloprim®** *see* Allopurinol *on page 51*

◆ **ZYM-Fluconazole (Can)** *see* Fluconazole *on page 612*

◆ **ZYM-Ondansetron (Can)** *see* Ondansetron *on page 1068*

◆ **ZyPREXA®** *see* OLANZapine *on page 1056*

◆ **Zyprexa® (Can)** *see* OLANZapine *on page 1056*

◆ **ZyPREXA® IntraMuscular** *see* OLANZapine *on page 1056*

◆ **Zyprexa® Intramuscular (Can)** *see* OLANZapine *on page 1056*

◆ **ZyPREXA® Relprevv™** *see* OLANZapine *on page 1056*

◆ **Zyprexa Zydis** *see* OLANZapine *on page 1056*

- **ZyPREXA® Zydis®** *see* OLANZapine *on page 1056*
- **Zyprexa® Zydis® (Can)** *see* OLANZapine *on page 1056*
- **Zytiga™** *see* Abiraterone Acetate *on page 26*
- **Zytram® XL (Can)** *see* TraMADol *on page 1388*
- **Zyvox®** *see* Linezolid *on page 898*
- **Zyvoxam® (Can)** *see* Linezolid *on page 898*

CHEMOTHERAPY REGIMEN INDEX

CHEMOTHERAPY REGIMEN INDEX

AMYLOIDOSIS

Bortezomib-Dexamethasone (Amyloidosis) on page 1534

BRAIN TUMORS

Bevacizumab-Irinotecan (Glioblastoma) on page 1531
CDDP/VP-16 on page 1555
COPE on page 1596
MOPP (Medulloblastoma) on page 1717
PCV (Brain Tumor Regimen) on page 1736
POC on page 1740

Neuroblastoma

A3 (Neuroblastoma) on page 1515
CAV-P/VP (Neuroblastoma) on page 1554
CE-CAdO (Neuroblastoma) on page 1555
Cisplatin-Doxorubicin-Etoposide-Cyclophosphamide (Neuroblastoma) on page 1568
New A1 (Neuroblastoma) on page 1721

Primary CNS Lymphoma

Temozolomide-Rituximab (CNS Lymphoma) on page 1754

BREAST CANCER

AC on page 1517
AC/Paclitaxel (Sequential) on page 1517
AC-Paclitaxel-Trastuzumab on page 1518
Bevacizumab-Capecitabine (Breast Cancer) on page 1528
CAF on page 1538
Capecitabine + Docetaxel (Breast Cancer) on page 1539
Capecitabine + Lapatinib (Breast Cancer) on page 1541
Capecitabine-Trastuzumab on page 1541
CEF on page 1556
CMF on page 1588
CMF-IV on page 1588
Docetaxel-Bevacizumab on page 1608
Docetaxel-Cyclophosphamide (TC) on page 1611
Docetaxel-Doxorubicin (Breast Cancer) on page 1611
Docetaxel-FEC on page 1611
Docetaxel-Pertuzumab-Trastuzumab (Breast) on page 1614
Docetaxel-Trastuzumab on page 1615
Docetaxel-Trastuzumab-Carboplatin on page 1615
Docetaxel-Trastuzumab-Cisplatin on page 1616
Docetaxel-Trastuzumab-FEC on page 1616
Docetaxel (Weekly)-Trastuzumab on page 1617
Dox-CMF (Sequential) on page 1617
Doxorubicin (Liposomal)-Docetaxel (Breast Cancer) on page 1619
Everolimus-Exemestane (Breast) on page 1640
FAC on page 1641
FEC on page 1642
Gemcitabine-Paclitaxel (Breast Cancer) on page 1675
Ixabepilone-Capecitabine on page 1698

Lapatinib-Letrozole (Breast Cancer) on page 1698
Lapatinib-Trastuzumab (Breast Cancer) on page 1698
Paclitaxel-Bevacizumab on page 1725
Paclitaxel-Vinorelbine on page 1732
TAC on page 1753
Trastuzumab-Paclitaxel on page 1759
Trastuzumab-Paclitaxel Carboplatin on page 1760
Trastuzumab-Paclitaxel (Weekly) on page 1760
Vinorelbine-FEC on page 1773
Vinorelbine-Trastuzumab on page 1775
Vinorelbine-Trastuzumab-FEC on page 1775

GASTROINTESTINAL

Anal Cancer

Fluorouracil-Mitomycin (Anal Cancer) on page 1659

Biliary Adenocarcinoma

CAPOX (Biliary Cancer) on page 1542
Gemcitabine-Capecitabine (Biliary Cancer) on page 1668
Gemcitabine-Cisplatin (Biliary Cancer) on page 1669
GEMOX (Biliary Cancer) on page 1678

Colorectal Cancer

Bevacizumab-Fluorouracil-Leucovorin on page 1530
Bevacizumab + FOLFIRI (Colorectal) on page 1530
Bevacizumab-Oxaliplatin-Fluorouracil-Leucovorin on page 1531
Bevacizumab + XELOX (Colorectal) on page 1532
Cetuximab Biweekly (Colorectal Regimen) on page 1556
Cetuximab (Biweekly)-Irinotecan on page 1557
Cetuximab (Colorectal Regimen) on page 1559
Cetuximab + FOLFIRI (Colorectal) on page 1559
Cetuximab-FOLFOX4 on page 1560
Cetuximab-Irinotecan (Colorectal) on page 1561
FLOX (Colorectal) on page 1645
Fluorouracil-Leucovorin on page 1653
Fluorouracil-Leucovorin-Irinotecan (Saltz Regimen) on page 1656
FOLFIRI (Colorectal Cancer) on page 1659
FOLFOX1 (Colorectal) on page 1662
FOLFOX2 (Colorectal) on page 1662
FOLFOX3 (Colorectal) on page 1662
FOLFOX4 (Colorectal) on page 1663
FOLFOX6 and mFOLFOX6 (Colorectal) on page 1663
FOLFOX7 (Colorectal) on page 1664
FOLFOXIRI (Colorectal) on page 1665
FU-LV-CPT-11 on page 1666
Irinotecan (Colorectal Regimen) on page 1695
Panitumumab (Colorectal Regimen) on page 1733
Panitumumab + FOLFIRI (Colorectal) on page 1733
Panitumumab + FOLFOX4 (Colorectal) on page 1733
Regorafenib (Colorectal Regimen) on page 1747
XELOX (Colorectal) on page 1778
Ziv-Aflibercept + FOLFIRI (Colorectal) on page 1779

Esophageal Cancer

Cisplatin-Capecitabine (Esophageal Cancer) on page 1566
Cisplatin-Fluorouracil (Esophageal Cancer) on page 1572
Docetaxel-Cisplatin-Fluorouracil (Gastric/Esophageal Cancer) on page 1609
Docetaxel-Oxaliplatin-Fluorouracil (Esophageal Cancer) on page 1613
Docetaxel-Oxaliplatin-Leucovorin-Fluorouracil (Esophageal Cancer) on page 1613
Epirubicin-Cisplatin-Capecitabine (Esophageal Cancer) on page 1626
Epirubicin-Cisplatin-Fluorouracil (Gastric/Esophageal Cancer) on page 1626
Epirubicin-Oxaliplatin-Capecitabine on page 1627
Epirubicin-Oxaliplatin-Fluorouracil (Esophageal Cancer) on page 1627
Fluorouracil-Leucovorin-Oxaliplatin (Esophageal Cancer) on page 1656
Irinotecan-Capecitabine (Esophageal Cancer) on page 1693
Irinotecan-Cisplatin (Esophageal Cancer) on page 1694
Irinotecan-Fluorouracil-Leucovorin (Esophageal Cancer) on page 1696
Oxaliplatin-Fluorouracil (Esophageal Cancer) on page 1724
Paclitaxel-Carboplatin (Esophageal Cancer) on page 1726
Paclitaxel-Cisplatin (Esophageal Cancer) on page 1727
Paclitaxel-Cisplatin-Fluorouracil (Esophageal Cancer) on page 1728
Paclitaxel-Fluorouracil (Esophageal Cancer) on page 1729

Gastric Cancer

Capecitabine-Docetaxel (Gastric Cancer) on page 1539
Cisplatin-Capecitabine (Gastric Cancer) on page 1566
Cisplatin-Fluorouracil (Gastric Cancer) on page 1574
Docetaxel-Cisplatin-Fluorouracil (Gastric/Esophageal Cancer) on page 1609
Epirubicin-Cisplatin-Fluorouracil (Gastric/Esophageal Cancer) on page 1626
Epirubicin-Oxaliplatin-Capecitabine on page 1627
Fluorouracil-Leucovorin-Oxaliplatin (Gastric Cancer) on page 1657
Irinotecan-Capecitabine (Gastric Cancer) on page 1693
Irinotecan-Cisplatin (Gastric Cancer) on page 1695
Irinotecan-Leucovorin-Fluorouracil (Gastric Cancer) on page 1697
Trastuzumab-Cisplatin-Capecitabine (Gastric Cancer) on page 1757
Trastuzumab-Cisplatin-Fluorouracil (Gastric Cancer) on page 1758

Hepatoblastoma

IPA on page 1692
PA-CI on page 1725

Pancreatic Cancer

Capecitabine-Gemcitabine (Pancreatic) on page 1540
CAPOX (Pancreatic) on page 1543
Cisplatin-Gemcitabine (Pancreatic) on page 1579
Erlotinib-Gemcitabine (Pancreatic Cancer) on page 1632
Fluorouracil-Leucovorin (Pancreatic) on page 1658
FOLFIRINOX (Pancreatic) on page 1661
FOLFOX (Pancreatic) on page 1665
Gemcitabine Fixed Dose Rate (Pancreatic Regimen) on page 1672
Gemcitabine-Oxaliplatin (Pancreatic) on page 1674
Gemcitabine-Paclitaxel (Protein Bound) (Pancreatic) on page 1675
Gemcitabine Standard Infusion (Pancreatic Regimen) on page 1676

GENITOURINARY

Bladder Cancer

Cisplatin-Fluorouracil (Bladder Cancer) on page 1571
CMV on page 1589
Gemcitabine-Carboplatin (Bladder Cancer) on page 1668
Gemcitabine-Cisplatin (Bladder Cancer) on page 1669
M-VAC (Bladder Cancer) on page 1718
Paclitaxel-Carboplatin (Bladder Cancer) on page 1726
Paclitaxel-Carboplatin-Gemcitabine on page 1726
Paclitaxel-Gemcitabine on page 1729
Pemetrexed (Bladder Cancer Regimen) on page 1737

Prostate Cancer

Abiraterone-Prednisone (Prostate Cancer) on page 1516
Bicalutamide-Goserelin on page 1533
Bicalutamide-Leuprolide on page 1533
Cabazitaxel-Prednisone (Prostate Cancer) on page 1538
Docetaxel-Prednisone on page 1614
Docetaxel (Weekly Regimen) on page 1617
Doxorubicin + Ketoconazole on page 1619
Doxorubicin + Ketoconazole/Estramustine + Vinblastine on page 1619
Enzalutamide (Prostate Regimen) on page 1625
Estramustine + Docetaxel on page 1634
Estramustine + Docetaxel + Calcitriol on page 1635
Estramustine + Docetaxel + Carboplatin on page 1636
Estramustine + Docetaxel + Hydrocortisone on page 1636
Estramustine + Docetaxel + Prednisone on page 1636
Estramustine + Etoposide on page 1636
Estramustine-Paclitaxel on page 1637
Estramustine-Vinblastine on page 1638
Estramustine + Vinorelbine on page 1638
FL on page 1642
FZ on page 1667
Mitoxantrone + Hydrocortisone on page 1713
Mitoxantrone-Prednisone (Prostate Cancer) on page 1713
Paclitaxel + Estramustine + Carboplatin on page 1728
Paclitaxel + Estramustine + Etoposide on page 1729

Renal Cell Cancer

Bevacizumab-Interferon Alfa (RCC) on page 1530
Bevacizumab (RCC Regimen) on page 1532
Everolimus (RCC Regimen) on page 1640
Gemcitabine-Capecitabine (RCC) on page 1668
Gemcitabine-Fluorouracil (RCC) on page 1672
Interleukin 2-Interferon Alfa-2 (RCC) on page 1692
Pazopanib (RCC Regimen) on page 1734
Sorafenib (RCC Regimen) on page 1751
Sunitinib (RCC Regimen) on page 1753
Temsirolimus (RCC Regimen) on page 1754

Testicular Cancer

BEP (Ovarian Cancer, Testicular Cancer) on page 1526
BEP (Testicular Cancer) on page 1527
Carboplatin (Testicular Regimen) on page 1552

EP (Testicular Cancer) on page 1631
Gemcitabine-Oxaliplatin-Paclitaxel (Testicular) on page 1674
Gemcitabine-Paclitaxel (Testicular) on page 1675
GEMOX (Testicular) on page 1678
Paclitaxel-Ifosfamide-Cisplatin on page 1730
PVB on page 1744
VBP on page 1770
VIP (Etoposide) (Testicular Cancer) on page 1776
VIP (Vinblastine) (Testicular Cancer) on page 1777

Wilms' Tumor
EE-4A (Wilms' Tumor) on page 1621
DD-4A (Wilms' Tumor) on page 1606
Regimen I (Wilms' Tumor) on page 1745
VAD (Wilms' Tumor) on page 1768

GYNECOLOGIC

Cervical Cancer
Carboplatin-Paclitaxel (Cervical Cancer) on page 1549
Cisplatin-Fluorouracil (Cervical Cancer) on page 1571
Cisplatin-Gemcitabine (Cervical Cancer) on page 1578
Cisplatin-Paclitaxel (Cervical Cancer) on page 1581
Cisplatin-Topotecan (Cervical Cancer) on page 1583
Cisplatin-Vinorelbine (Cervical Cancer) on page 1585

Endometrial Cancer
AP on page 1520

Gestational Trophoblastic Tumor
EMA/CO on page 1622
EP/EMA on page 1625

Ovarian Cancer
BEP (Ovarian Cancer) on page 1526
BEP (Ovarian Cancer, Testicular Cancer) on page 1526
Carboplatin-Docetaxel (Ovarian) on page 1543
Carboplatin-Doxorubicin (Liposomal) (Ovarian) on page 1544
Carboplatin-Gemcitabine (Ovarian) on page 1548
Carboplatin-Paclitaxel (Ovarian) on page 1550
Cisplatin-Paclitaxel Intraperitoneal (Ovarian) on page 1582
Cisplatin-Paclitaxel (Ovarian) on page 1582
Docetaxel (Ovarian Regimen) on page 1612
Docetaxel-Oxaliplatin (Ovarian Cancer) on page 1613
Doxorubicin (Liposomal) (Ovarian Regimen) on page 1618
Etoposide-Carboplatin (Ovarian Cancer) on page 1639
Etoposide (Ovarian Regimen) on page 1639
Gemcitabine (Ovarian Regimen) on page 1673
Gemcitabine-Paclitaxel (Ovarian Cancer) on page 1675
PAC (CAP) on page 1725
Paclitaxel Maintenance (Ovarian Cancer) on page 1730
Paclitaxel (Ovarian Regimen) on page 1730
Pemetrexed (Ovarian Regimen) on page 1739
Topotecan Oral Regimen (Ovarian Cancer) on page 1757
Trabectedin-Doxorubicin (Liposomal) (Ovarian Cancer) on page 1757

Vincristine-Dactinomycin-Cyclophosphamide (Ovarian Cancer) on page 1771
Vinorelbine (Ovarian Regimen) on page 1774

HEAD AND NECK CANCER

Carboplatin-Cetuximab (Head and Neck Cancer) on page 1543
Cetuximab-Carboplatin-Fluorouracil (Head and Neck Cancer) on page 1557
Cetuximab-Cisplatin-Fluorouracil (Head and Neck Cancer) on page 1558
Cisplatin-Cetuximab (Head and Neck Cancer) on page 1566
Cisplatin-Fluorouracil (Head and Neck Cancer) on page 1575
Cisplatin-Paclitaxel (Head and Neck Cancer) on page 1581
Docetaxel-Cisplatin-Fluorouracil (Head and Neck Cancer) on page 1610
Fluorouracil-Carboplatin (Head and Neck Cancer) on page 1652
Fluorouracil-Hydroxyurea (Head and Neck Cancer) on page 1653
Paclitaxel-Cetuximab on page 1727

HEMATOLOGIC/LEUKEMIA

Leukemia, Acute Lymphocytic

DVP on page 1621
Hyper-CVAD + Imatinib on page 1680
Hyper-CVAD (Leukemia, Acute Lymphocytic) on page 1681
Larson Regimen (ALL) on page 1699
Linker Protocol (ALL) on page 1703
MTX/6-MP/VP (Maintenance) on page 1717
POMP on page 1741
PVA (POG 8602) on page 1742
PVDA on page 1745
VAD/CVAD on page 1768

Leukemia, Acute Myeloid

5 + 2 (Cytarabine-Daunorubicin) (AML Induction) on page 1512
5 + 2 (Cytarabine-Daunorubicin) (AML Postremission) on page 1512
5 + 2 (Cytarabine-Idarubicin) (AML Consolidation) on page 1512
5 + 2 (Cytarabine-Mitoxantrone) (AML Consolidation) on page 1512
5 + 2 + 5 (Cytarabine-Daunorubicin-Etoposide) (AML Consolidation) on page 1513
7 + 3 (Cytarabine-Daunorubicin) (AML Induction) on page 1513
7 + 3 (Cytarabine-Idarubicin) (AML Induction) on page 1514
7 + 3 (Cytarabine-Mitoxantrone) (AML Induction) on page 1514
7 + 3 + 7 (Cytarabine-Daunorubicin-Etoposide) (AML Induction) on page 1515
Azacitidine (AML Regimen) on page 1521
CLAG (AML Induction) on page 1586
CLAG-M (AML Induction) on page 1586
Clofarabine (AML Consolidation) on page 1587
Clofarabine (AML Induction) on page 1587
Clofarabine-Cytarabine (AML Consolidation) on page 1587
Clofarabine-Cytarabine (AML Induction) on page 1587
Cytarabine (High Dose)-Daunorubicin (AML Induction) on page 1602
Cytarabine (High Dose)-Daunorubicin-Etoposide (AML Induction) on page 1602
Cytarabine (High-Dose Single-Agent AML Induction Regimen) on page 1603
Cytarabine (Single-Agent AML Consolidation Regimen) on page 1603
Cytarabine (SubQ Single-Agent AML Induction Regimen) on page 1604
Decitabine (AML Regimen) on page 1606
FLAG (AML Induction) on page 1643
FLAG-IDA on page 1644

Hydroxyurea (AML Regimen) on page 1680
MEC (AML Induction) on page 1706
MEC-G (AML Induction) on page 1707
Mitoxantrone-Etoposide (AML Induction) on page 1713

Leukemia, Acute Promyelocytic
Tretinoin-Arsenic Trioxide (APL) on page 1761
Tretinoin-Daunorubicin (APL) on page 1762
Tretinoin-Daunorubicin-Cytarabine (APL) on page 1762
Tretinoin-Idarubicin (APL) on page 1764

Leukemia, Chronic Lymphocytic
Chlorambucil (CLL Regimen) on page 1563
Chlorambucil-Prednisone (CLL) on page 1563
CVP (Leukemia) on page 1598
Cyclophosphamide-Fludarabine-Alemtuzumab-Rituximab (CLL) on page 1601
Fludarabine-Alemtuzumab (CLL) on page 1645
Fludarabine-Cyclophosphamide (CLL) on page 1646
Fludarabine-Cyclophosphamide-Rituximab (CLL) on page 1648
Fludarabine-Rituximab (CLL) on page 1651
OFAR (CLL) on page 1722
PCR on page 1735
Pentostatin-Cyclophosphamide on page 1739

Leukemia, Chronic Myelogenous
Bosutinib (CML Regimen) on page 1538
Dasatinib (CML Regimen) on page 1605
Imatinib (CML Regimen) on page 1690
Nilotinib (CML Regimen) on page 1722

LUNG CANCER

Nonsmall Cell Lung Cancer
Bevacizumab-Carboplatin-Paclitaxel (NSCLC) on page 1528
Bevacizumab-Carboplatin-Pemetrexed (NSCLC) on page 1529
Bevacizumab-Cisplatin-Gemcitabine (NSCLC) on page 1529
Carboplatin-Gemcitabine (NSCLC) on page 1547
Carboplatin-Pemetrexed (NSCLC) on page 1551
Carbo-Tax (NSCLC) on page 1552
CaT (NSCLC) on page 1553
Cetuximab-Cisplatin-Vinorelbine (NSCLC) on page 1558
Cisplatin-Etoposide (NSCLC) on page 1568
Cisplatin-Irinotecan (NSCLC) on page 1580
Cisplatin-Pemetrexed (NSCLC) on page 1583
Cisplatin-Vinblastine (NSCLC) on page 1585
Crizotinib (NSCLC Regimen) on page 1596
Docetaxel-Cisplatin on page 1609
Docetaxel (NSCLC Regimen) on page 1612
EC (NSCLC) on page 1621
EP (NSCLC) on page 1628
EP/PE on page 1631
Erlotinib (NSCLC Regimen) on page 1632
Gemcitabine-Cisplatin (NSCLC) on page 1670
Gemcitabine-Vinorelbine (NSCLC) on page 1677
Paclitaxel (Protein Bound) (NSCLC Regimen) on page 1731

PC (NSCLC) on page 1734
Pemetrexed (NSCLC Regimen) on page 1738
Vinorelbine-Cisplatin on page 1772

Small Cell Lung Cancer

Carboplatin-Etoposide (Small Cell Lung Cancer) on page 1546
Carboplatin-Irinotecan (Small Cell Lung Cancer) on page 1548
CAV (Small Cell Lung Cancer) on page 1554
Cisplatin-Etoposide (Small Cell Lung Cancer) on page 1569
Cisplatin-Irinotecan (Small Cell Lung Cancer) on page 1580
Docetaxel (Small Cell Lung Cancer Regimen) on page 1614
Etoposide Oral (Small Cell Lung Cancer Regimen) on page 1640
Gemcitabine (Small Cell Lung Cancer Regimen) on page 1676
Irinotecan (Small Cell Lung Cancer Regimen) on page 1697
Paclitaxel (Small Cell Lung Cancer Regimen) on page 1732
Topotecan Intravenous (Small Cell Lung Cancer Regimen) on page 1756
Topotecan Oral (Small Cell Lung Cancer Regimen) on page 1757
Vinorelbine (Small Cell Lung Cancer Regimen) on page 1774

LYMPHOID TISSUE (LYMPHOMA)

Lymphoma, Hodgkin

ABVD Early Stage (Hodgkin) on page 1516
ABVD (Hodgkin) on page 1516
BEACOPP-14 (Hodgkin) on page 1522
BEACOPP Escalated (Hodgkin) on page 1522
BEACOPP Escalated Plus Standard (Hodgkin) on page 1523
BEACOPP Standard (Hodgkin) on page 1525
ChlVPP (Hodgkin) on page 1562
C-MOPP/ABV Hybrid (Hodgkin) on page 1588
Dexa-BEAM (Hodgkin) on page 1607
DHAP (Hodgkin) on page 1608
ESHAP (Hodgkin) on page 1634
GDP (Hodgkin) on page 1667
Gemcitabine (Hodgkin Regimen) on page 1672
GVD (Hodgkin) on page 1679
ICE (Hodgkin) on page 1688
IGEV (Hodgkin) on page 1690
MINE-ESHAP (Hodgkin) on page 1711
mini-BEAM (Hodgkin) on page 1712
MOPP/ABVD (Hodgkin) on page 1714
MOPP/ABV Hybrid (Hodgkin) on page 1715
MOPP (Hodgkin) on page 1716
Stanford V (Hodgkin) on page 1752
VAMP (Hodgkin) on page 1769
VIM-D (Hodgkin) on page 1770
Vinblastine (Hodgkin Regimen) on page 1771
Vinorelbine (Hodgkin Regimen) on page 1774

Lymphoma, Non-Hodgkin's

Bendamustine-Rituximab on page 1525
CEPP(B) on page 1556
CHOP (NHL) on page 1564
Cisplatin-Cytarabine-Dexamethasone (NHL Regimen) on page 1567
CNOP on page 1589

CODOX-M on page 1590
COMLA on page 1595
COP-BLAM on page 1595
COPP on page 1596
CVP (Lymphoma, non-Hodgkin's) on page 1598
EPOCH Dose-Adjusted (AIDS-Related Lymphoma) on page 1628
EPOCH Dose-Adjusted (NHL) on page 1628
EPOCH (Dose-Adjusted)-Rituximab (NHL) on page 1629
EPOCH (NHL) on page 1630
EPOCH-Rituximab (NHL) on page 1631
ESHAP on page 1633
Fludarabine-Cyclophosphamide-Mitoxantrone-Rituximab on page 1647
Fludarabine-Cyclophosphamide-Rituximab (NHL-Follicular) on page 1649
Fludarabine-Mitoxantrone on page 1649
Fludarabine-Mitoxantrone-Dexamethasone (NHL) on page 1650
Fludarabine-Mitoxantrone-Dexamethasone-Rituximab on page 1650
Fludarabine-Mitoxantrone-Rituximab on page 1651
Fludarabine-Rituximab (NHL-Follicular) on page 1651
Gemcitabine-Oxaliplatin-Rituximab (NHL) on page 1674
Hyper-CVAD (Lymphoma, non-Hodgkin's) on page 1687
ICE (Lymphoma, non-Hodgkin's) on page 1689
IMVP-16 on page 1691
MACOP-B on page 1704
m-BACOD on page 1706
MINE on page 1711
MINE-ESHAP (NHL) on page 1712
Oxaliplatin-Cytarabine-Dexamethasone (NHL Regimen) on page 1723
Pro-MACE-CytaBOM on page 1741
R-CVP on page 1745
RICE on page 1747
Rituximab-CHOP (NHL) on page 1748

Lymphoma, Non-Hodgkin's (Burkitt)
CODOX-M/IVAC on page 1591

Lymphoma, Non-Hodgkin's (Mantle cell)
Bendamustine-Rituximab on page 1525
Fludarabine-Cyclophosphamide (NHL-Mantle Cell) on page 1648
Hyper-CVAD + Rituximab on page 1688

MALIGNANT PLEURAL MESOTHELIOMA

Carboplatin-Pemetrexed (Mesothelioma) on page 1551
Cisplatin-Gemcitabine (Mesothelioma) on page 1578
Cisplatin-Pemetrexed (Mesothelioma) on page 1582
Cisplatin-Raltitrexed (Mesothelioma) on page 1583
Gemcitabine (Mesothelioma Regimen) on page 1673
Pemetrexed (Mesothelioma Regimen) on page 1738
Vinorelbine (Mesothelioma Regimen) on page 1774

MULTIPLE MYELOMA

Bortezomib-Dexamethasone (Multiple Myeloma) on page 1534
Bortezomib-Doxorubicin-Dexamethasone on page 1535
Bortezomib-Doxorubicin (Liposomal) on page 1536
Bortezomib-Doxorubicin (Liposomal)-Dexamethasone on page 1536
Bortezomib-Melphalan-Prednisone-Thalidomide on page 1537

Carfilzomib (Multiple Myeloma Regimen) on page 1553
Cyclophosphamide-Bortezomib-Dexamethasone (Multiple Myeloma) on page 1599
Doxorubicin (Liposomal)-Vincristine-Dexamethasone on page 1620
DTPACE on page 1620
Hyper-CVAD (Multiple Myeloma) on page 1687
Lenalidomide-Bortezomib-Dexamethasone (Multiple Myeloma) on page 1702
Lenalidomide-Dexamethasone on page 1702
Lenalidomide-Dexamethasone (Low Dose) on page 1703
Melphalan-Prednisone-Bortezomib (Multiple Myeloma) on page 1708
Melphalan-Prednisone (Multiple Myeloma) on page 1709
Melphalan-Prednisone-Thalidomide (Multiple Myeloma) on page 1710
Thalidomide-Dexamethasone (MM) on page 1754
VAD on page 1767
VBMCP (Multiple Myeloma) on page 1769
VCAP on page 1770

MYELODYSPLASTIC SYNDROME

Azacitidine (MDS Regimen) on page 1521
Decitabine (MDS Regimen) on page 1607

RETINOBLASTOMA

Carboplatin-Etoposide (Retinoblastoma) on page 1545
Carboplatin-Etoposide-Vincristine (Retinoblastoma) on page 1546
Carboplatin-Vincristine (Retinoblastoma) on page 1552

SARCOMA

CYVADIC on page 1605
Irinotecan-Temozolomide (Ewing's Sarcoma) on page 1697
MAID (Sarcoma) on page 1704
Topotecan-Cyclophosphamide (Ewing's Sarcoma) on page 1756
VAC Alternating With IE (Ewing's Sarcoma) on page 1768

Osteosarcoma

Gemcitabine-Docetaxel (Sarcoma) on page 1671
HDMTX on page 1679
ICE (Sarcoma) on page 1689
MTX-CDDPAdr on page 1717
POG-8651 on page 1740

Rhabdomyosarcoma

CEV on page 1562
VAC Pulse on page 1767
VAC (Rhabdomyosarcoma) on page 1767

Soft Tissue Sarcoma

AD (Soft Tissue Sarcoma) on page 1519
AI on page 1520
Gemcitabine-Docetaxel (Sarcoma) on page 1671
Gemcitabine-Vinorelbine (Sarcoma) on page 1677
ICE (Sarcoma) on page 1689
IE on page 1690
Methotrexate-Vinblastine (Desmoid Tumor) on page 1710
Pazopanib (Soft Tissue Sarcoma Regimen) on page 1734

SKIN CANCER, MELANOMA

Cisplatin-Vinblastine-Dacarbazine (Melanoma) on page 1584
CVD-Interleukin-Interferon (Melanoma) on page 1597
Ipilimumab (Melanoma Regimen) on page 1692
Vemurafenib (Melanoma Regimen) on page 1770

SKIN CANCER, NON-MELANOMA

Basal Cell Carcinoma

Vismodegib (Basal Cell Regimen) on page 1778

THYROID CANCER

Pazopanib (Thyroid Cancer Regimen) on page 1734

UNKNOWN PRIMARY (ADENOCARCINOMA)

Carboplatin-Docetaxel (Unknown Primary) on page 1544
Carboplatin-Etoposide-Paclitaxel (Unknown Primary) on page 1545
Carboplatin-Gemcitabine-Paclitaxel (Unknown Primary) on page 1548
Carboplatin-Paclitaxel (Unknown Primary) on page 1551
Cisplatin-Docetaxel (Unknown Primary) on page 1568
Cisplatin-Gemcitabine (Unknown Primary) on page 1580
Docetaxel-Gemcitabine (Unknown Primary) on page 1611

UNKNOWN PRIMARY (SQUAMOUS CELL)

Cisplatin-Docetaxel-Fluorouracil (Unknown Primary) on page 1568
Cisplatin-Fluorouracil-Paclitaxel (Unknown Primary) on page 1577

WALDENSTROM'S MACROGLOBULINEMIA

Bortezomib-Dexamethasone-Rituximab (Waldenstrom's Macroglobulinemia) on page 1535
Bortezomib-Rituximab (Waldenstrom's Macroglobulinemia) on page 1537
Bortezomib (Waldenstrom's Macroglobulinemia) on page 1537

ALPHABETICAL LISTING OF CHEMOTHERAPY REGIMENS

5 + 2 (Cytarabine-Daunorubicin) (AML Induction)

Index Terms Cytarabine-Daunorubicin (5 + 2) (AML); Daunorubicin-Cytarabine (5 + 2) (AML)

Use Leukemia, acute myeloid

Regimen

Cytarabine: I.V.: 100 mg/m^2/day continuous infusion days 1 to 5
[total dose/cycle = 500 mg/m^2]

Daunorubicin: I.V.: 45 mg/m^2/day I.V. bolus days 1 and 2
[total dose/cycle = 90 mg/m^2]

May administer a second induction cycle if needed

References

Rai KR, Holland JF, Glidewell OJ, et al, "Treatment of Acute Myelocytic Leukemia: A Study by Cancer and Leukemia Group B," *Blood*, 1981, 58(6):1203-12.

5 + 2 (Cytarabine-Daunorubicin) (AML Postremission)

Index Terms Cytarabine-Daunorubicin (5 + 2) (AML); Daunorubicin-Cytarabine (5 + 2) (AML)

Use Leukemia, acute myeloid

Regimen

Cytarabine: I.V.: 100 mg/m^2/day continuous infusion days 1 to 5
[total dose/cycle = 500 mg/m^2]

Daunorubicin: I.V.: 45 mg/m^2/day I.V. bolus days 1 and 2
[total dose/cycle = 90 mg/m^2]

Administer 2 courses

References

Wiernik PH, Banks P, Case Jr DC, et al, "Cytarabine Plus Idarubicin or Daunorubicin as Induction and Consolidation Therapy for Previously Untreated Adult Patients With Acute Myeloid Leukemia," *Blood*, 1992, 79(2):313-9.

5 + 2 (Cytarabine-Idarubicin) (AML Consolidation)

Index Terms Cytarabine-Idarubicin (5 + 2) (AML Consolidation); Idarubicin-Cytarabine (5 + 2) (AML Consolidation)

Use Leukemia, acute myeloid

Regimen

Cytarabine: I.V.: 100 mg/m^2/day continuous infusion days 1 to 5
[total dose/cycle = 500 mg/m^2]

Idarubicin: I.V.: 13 mg/m^2/day I.V. bolus days 1 and 2
[total dose/cycle = 26 mg/m^2]

Administer 2 courses

References

Wiernik PH, Banks P, Case Jr DC, et al, "Cytarabine Plus Idarubicin or Daunorubicin as Induction and Consolidation Therapy for Previously Untreated Adult Patients With Acute Myeloid Leukemia," *Blood*, 1992, 79(2):313-9.

5 + 2 (Cytarabine-Mitoxantrone) (AML Consolidation)

Index Terms Cytarabine-Mitoxantrone (5 + 2) (AML Consolidation)

Use Leukemia, acute myeloid

Regimen

Cytarabine: I.V.: 100 mg/m^2/day continuous infusion days 1 to 5
[total dose/cycle = 500 mg/m^2]

Mitoxantrone: I.V.: 12 mg/m^2/day days 1 and 2
[total dose/cycle = 24 mg/m^2]

Administered every 28 days for a total of 2 cycles

References

Arlin Z, Case DC Jr, Moore J, et al, "Randomized Multicenter Trial of Cytosine Arabinoside With Mitoxantrone or Daunorubicin in Previously Untreated Adult Patients With Acute Nonlymphocytic Leukemia (ANLL). Lederle Cooperative Group," *Leukemia*, 1990, 4(3):177-83.

5 + 2 + 5 (Cytarabine-Daunorubicin-Etoposide) (AML Consolidation)

Index Terms Cytarabine-Daunorubicin-Etoposide (5 + 2 + 5) (AML Consolidation)

Use Leukemia, acute myeloid

Regimen

Cytarabine: I.V.: 100 mg/m^2/day continuous infusion days 1 to 5
[total dose/cycle = 500 mg/m^2]

Daunorubicin: I.V.: 50 mg/m^2/day I.V. bolus days 1 and 2
[total dose/cycle = 100 mg/m^2]

Etoposide: I.V.: 75 mg/m^2/day over 1 hour days 1 to 5
[total dose/cycle = 375 mg/m^2]

Administer 2 courses

References

Bishop JF, Lowenthal RM, Joshua D, et al, "Etoposide in Acute Nonlymphocytic Leukemia, Australian Leukemia Study Group," *Blood*, 1990, 75(1):27-32.

Bishop JF, Matthews JP, Young GA, et al, "A Randomized Study of High-Dose Cytarabine in Induction in Acute Myeloid Leukemia," *Blood*, 1996, 87(5):1710-7.

7 + 3 (Cytarabine-Daunorubicin) (AML Induction)

Index Terms Cytarabine-Daunorubicin (7 + 3) (AML Induction)

Use Leukemia, acute myeloid

Regimen NOTE: Multiple variations are listed.

Variation 1:

Cytarabine: I.V.: 100 mg/m^2/day continuous infusion days 1 to 7
[total dose/cycle = 700 mg/m^2]

Daunorubicin: I.V.: 45 mg/m^2/day I.V. bolus days 1, 2, and 3
[total dose/cycle = 135 mg/m^2]

May administer a second induction cycle if needed

Variation 2 (≥60 years of age):

Cytarabine: I.V.: 100 mg/m^2/day continuous infusion days 1 to 7
[total dose/cycle = 700 mg/m^2]

Daunorubicin: I.V.: 30 mg/m^2/day days 1, 2, and 3
[total dose/cycle = 90 mg/m^2]

May administer a second induction cycle if needed (at a reduced dose of daunorubicin [45 mg/m^2])

Variation 3 (between 17 and 60 years of age):

Cytarabine: I.V.: 100 mg/m^2/day continuous infusion days 1 to 7
[total dose/cycle = 700 mg/m^2]

Daunorubicin: I.V.: 90 mg/m^2/day I.V. bolus days 1, 2, and 3
[total dose/cycle = 270 mg/m^2]

May administer a second induction cycle if needed

Variation 4 (<60 years of age):

Cytarabine: I.V.: 200 mg/m^2/day continuous infusion days 1 to 7
[total dose/cycle = 1400 mg/m^2]

Daunorubicin: I.V.: 45 mg/m^2/day I.V. bolus days 1, 2, and 3
[total dose/cycle = 135 mg/m^2]

May administer a second induction cycle if needed

References

Variation 1:

Dillman RO, Davis RB, Green MR, et al, "A Comparative Study of Two Different Doses of Cytarabine for Acute Myeloid Leukemia: A Phase III Trial of Cancer and Leukemia Group B," *Blood*, 1991, 78(10):2520-6.

Rai KR, Holland JF, Glidewell OJ, et al, "Treatment of Acute Myelocytic Leukemia: A Study by Cancer and Leukemia Group B," *Blood*, 1981, 58(6):1203-12.

Yates J, Glidewell O, Wiernik P, et al, "Cytosine Arabinoside With Daunorubicin or Adriamycin® for Therapy of Acute Myelocytic Leukemia: A CALGB Study," *Blood*, 1982, 60(2):454-62.

Variation 2:

Dillman RO, Davis RB, Green MR, et al, "A Comparative Study of Two Different Doses of Cytarabine for Acute Myeloid Leukemia: A Phase III Trial of Cancer and Leukemia Group B," *Blood*, 1991, 78(10):2520-6.

Variation 3:

Fernandez HF, Sun Z, Yao X, et al, "Anthracycline Dose Intensification in Acute Myeloid Leukemia," *N Engl J Med*, 2009, 361(13):1249-59.

Variation 4:

Dilman RO, Davis RB, Green MR, et al, "A Comparative Study of Two Different Doses of Cytarabine for Acute Myeloid Leukemia: A Phase III Trial of Cancer and Leukemia Group B," *Blood*, 1991, 78(10):2520-6.

7 + 3 (Cytarabine-Idarubicin) (AML Induction)

Index Terms Cytarabine-Idarubicin (7 + 3) (AML Induction)

Use Leukemia, acute myeloid

Regimen NOTE: Multiple variations are listed.

Variation 1:

Cytarabine: I.V.: 100 mg/m^2/day continuous infusion days 1 to 7 [total dose/cycle = 700 mg/m^2]

Idarubicin: I.V.: 12 mg/m^2/day slow I.V. infusion days 1, 2, and 3 [total dose/cycle = 36 mg/m^2]

May administer a second induction cycle if needed

Variation 2:

Cytarabine: I.V.: 100 mg/m^2/day continuous infusion days 1 to 7 [total dose/cycle = 700 mg/m^2]

Idarubicin: I.V.: 13 mg/m^2/day slow I.V. infusion days 1, 2, and 3 [total dose/cycle = 39 mg/m^2]

May administer a second induction cycle if needed

References

Variation 1:

Vogler WR, Velez-Garcia E, Weiner RS, et al, "A Phase III Trial Comparing Idarubicin and Daunorubicin in Combination With Cytarabine in Acute Myelogenous Leukemia: A Southeastern Cancer Study Group Study," *J Clin Oncol*, 1992, 10(7):1103-11.

Variation 2:

Wiernik PH, Banks P, Case Jr DC, et al, "Cytarabine Plus Idarubicin or Daunorubicin as Induction and Consolidation Therapy for Previously Untreated Adult Patients With Acute Myeloid Leukemia," *Blood*, 1992, 79(2):313-9.

7 + 3 (Cytarabine-Mitoxantrone) (AML Induction)

Index Terms Cytarabine-Mitoxantrone (7 + 3) (AML Induction)

Use Leukemia, acute myeloid

Regimen

Induction:

Cytarabine: I.V.: 100 mg/m^2/day continuous infusion days 1 to 7 [total dose/cycle = 700 mg/m^2]

Mitoxantrone: I.V.: 12 mg/m^2/day days 1, 2, and 3 [total dose/cycle = 36 mg/m^2]

Reinduction if needed:
Cytarabine: I.V.: 100 mg/m^2/day continuous infusion days 1 to 5
[total dose/cycle = 500 mg/m^2]
Mitoxantrone: I.V.: 12 mg/m^2/day days 1 and 2
[total dose/cycle = 24 mg/m^2]

References

Arlin Z, Case DC Jr, Moore J, et al, "Randomized Multicenter Trial of Cytosine Arabinoside With Mitoxantrone or Daunorubicin in Previously Untreated Adult Patients With Acute Nonlymphocytic Leukemia (ANLL). Lederle Cooperative Group," *Leukemia*, 1990, 4(3):177-83.

7 + 3 + 7 (Cytarabine-Daunorubicin-Etoposide) (AML Induction)

Index Terms Cytarabine-Daunorubicin-Etoposide (7 + 3 + 7) (AML Induction)
Use Leukemia, acute myeloid
Regimen
Cytarabine: I.V.: 100 mg/m^2/day continuous infusion days 1 to 7
[total dose/cycle = 700 mg/m^2]
Daunorubicin: I.V.: 50 mg/m^2/day days 1, 2, and 3
[total dose/cycle = 150 mg/m^2]
Etoposide: I.V.: 75 mg/m^2/day over 1 hour days 1 to 7
[total dose/cycle = 525 mg/m^2]
Up to 3 induction cycles may be given based on individual response

References

Bishop JF, Lowenthal RM, Joshua D, et al, "Etoposide in Acute Nonlymphocytic Leukemia, Australian Leukemia Study Group," *Blood*, 1990, 75(1):27-32.
Bishop JF, Matthews JP, Young GA, et al, "A Randomized Study of High Dose Cytarabine in Induction in Acute Myeloid Leukemia," *Blood*, 1996, 87(5):1710-7.
Bishop JF, Matthews JP, Young GA, et al, "Intensified Induction Chemotherapy With High Dose Cytarabine and Etoposide for Acute Myeloid Leukemia: A Review and Updated Results of the Australian Leukemia Study Group," *Leuk Lymphoma*, 1998, 28(3-4):315-27.

◆ **A1 (NEW) (Neuroblastoma)** *see* New A1 (Neuroblastoma) *on page 1721*

A3 (Neuroblastoma)

Index Terms Cyclophosphamide, Doxorubicin, Etoposide, Cisplatin (Neuroblastoma); Regimen A3 (Neuroblastoma)
Use Neuroblastoma
Regimen
Cycle 1 (New A1):
Cyclophosphamide: I.V.: 1200 mg/m^2 over 6 hours day 1
[total dose/cycle = 1200 mg/m^2]
Doxorubicin: I.V.: 40 mg/m^2 day 3
[total dose/cycle = 40 mg/m^2]
Etoposide: I.V.: 100 mg/m^2/day days 1 to 5
[total dose/cycle = 500 mg/m^2]
Cisplatin: I.V.: 90 mg/m^2 day 5
[total dose/cycle = 90 mg/m^2]
Treatment cycle is 28 days
Cycles 2-5 (A3):
Cyclophosphamide: I.V.: 1200 mg/m^2/day over 6 hours days 1 and 2
[total dose/cycle = 2400 mg/m^2]
Doxorubicin: I.V.: 40 mg/m^2 day 3
[total dose/cycle = 40 mg/m^2]
Etoposide: I.V.: 100 mg/m^2/day days 1 to 5
[total dose/cycle = 500 mg/m^2]

Cisplatin: I.V.: 25 mg/m²/day continuous infusion days 1 to 5 [total dose/cycle = 125 mg/m²]

Repeat cycle every 28 days for 5 cycles (total of 6 cycles, cycle 1 administer New A1, cycles 2 to 5 administer A3)

References

Kaneko M, Nishihira H, Mugishima H, et al, "Stratification of Treatment of Stage 4 Neuroblastoma Patients Based on N-myc Amplification Status. Study Group of Japan for Treatment of Advanced Neuroblastoma, Tokyo, Japan," *Med Pediatr Oncol*, 1998, 31(1):1-7.

Kaneko M, Tsuchida Y, Mugishima H, et al, "Intensified Chemotherapy Increases the Survival Rates in Patients With Stage 4 Neuroblastoma With MYCN Amplification," *J Pediatr Hematol Oncol*, 2002, 24(8):613-21.

Abiraterone-Prednisone (Prostate Cancer)

Use Prostate cancer

Regimen

Abiraterone acetate: Oral: 1000 mg once a day

Prednisone: Oral: 5 mg twice a day

References

Danila DC, Morris MJ, de Bono JS, et al, "Phase II Multicenter Study of Abiraterone Acetate Plus Prednisone Therapy in Patients With Docetaxel-Treated Castration-Resistant Prostate Cancer," *J Clin Oncol*, 2010, 28(9):1496-501.

de Bono JS, Logothetis CJ, Fizazi K, et al, "Aberitarone Acetate (AA) Plus Low Dose Prednisone (P) Improves Overall Survival in Patients (PTS) With Metastatic Castration-Resistant Prostate Cancer (MCRPC) Who Have Progressed After Docetaxel-Based Chemotherapy (CHEMO): Results of COU-AA-301, a Randomized Double-Blind Placebo-Controlled Phase III Study," *Ann Oncol*, 2010, 21(8s):LBA5 [abstract LBA5 from 2010 ESMO Annual Meeting].

de Bono JS, Logothetis CJ, Molina A, et al, "Abiraterone and Increased Survival in Metastatic Prostate Cancer," *New Engl J Med*, 2011, 364(21):1995-2005.

ABVD Early Stage (Hodgkin)

Index Terms Doxorubicin, Bleomycin, Vinblastine, Dacarbazine (Hodgkin)

Use Lymphoma, Hodgkin

Regimen

Doxorubicin: I.V.: 25 mg/m²/day days 1 and 14 [total dose/cycle = 50 mg/m²]

Bleomycin: I.V.: 10 units/m²/day days 1 and 14 [total dose/cycle = 20 units/m²]

Vinblastine: I.V.: 6 mg/m²/day days 1 and 14 [total dose/cycle = 12 mg/m²]

Dacarbazine: I.V.: 375 mg/m²/day days 1 and 14 [total dose/cycle = 750 mg/m²]

Repeat cycle every 28 days for a total of 2 cycles

References

Engert A, Franklin J, Eich HT, et al, "Two Cycles of Doxorubicin, Bleomycin, Vinblastine, and Dacarbazine Plus Extended-Field Radiotherapy Is Superior to Radiotherapy Alone in Early Favorable Hodgkin's Lymphoma: Final Results of the GHSG HD7 Trial," *J Clin Oncol*, 2007, 25(23):3495-502.

ABVD (Hodgkin)

Index Terms Doxorubicin-Bleomycin-Vinblastine-Dacarbazine (Hodgkin)

Use Lymphoma, Hodgkin

Regimen

Doxorubicin: I.V.: 25 mg/m²/day days 1 and 15 [total dose/cycle = 50 mg/m²]

Bleomycin: I.V.: 10 units/m²/day days 1 and 15 [total dose/cycle = 20 units/m²]

Vinblastine: I.V.: 6 mg/m²/day days 1 and 15
[total dose/cycle = 12 mg/m²]
Dacarbazine: I.V.: 375 mg/m²/day days 1 and 15
[total dose/cycle = 750 mg/m²]
Repeat cycle every 28 days for 6-8 cycles

References

Bonadonna G and Santoro A, "ABVD Chemotherapy in the Treatment of Hodgkin's Disease," *Cancer Treat Rev*, 1982, 9(1):21-35.

Canellos GP, Anderson JR, Propert KJ, et al, "Chemotherapy of Advanced Hodgkin's Disease With MOPP, ABVD, or MOPP Alternating With ABVD," *N Engl J Med*, 1992, 327(21):1478-84.

Viviani S, Zinzani PL, Rambaldi A, et al, "ABVD Versus BEACOPP for Hodgkin's Lymphoma When High-Dose Salvage Is Planned," *N Engl J Med*, 2011, 365(3):203-12.

AC

Use Breast cancer

Regimen NOTE: Multiple variations are listed.

Variation 1: AC (conventional):
Doxorubicin: I.V.: 60 mg/m² day 1
[total dose/cycle = 60 mg/m²]
Cyclophosphamide: I.V.: 600 mg/m² day 1
[total dose/cycle = 600 mg/m²]
Repeat cycle every 21 days

Variation 2:
Cyclophosphamide: Oral: 200 mg/m²/day days 3 to 6
[total dose/cycle = 800 mg/m²]
Doxorubicin: I.V.: 40 mg/m² day 1
[total dose/cycle = 40 mg/m²]
Repeat cycle every 3 weeks for 3 cycles, then every 4 weeks

References

Variation 1:

Fisher B, Brown AM, Dimitrov NV, et al, "Two Months of Doxorubicin-Cyclophosphamide With and Without Interval Reinduction Therapy Compared With 6 Months of Cyclophosphamide, Methotrexate, and Fluorouracil in Positive-Node Breast Cancer Patients With Tamoxifen-Nonresponsive Tumors: Results From the National Surgical Adjuvant Breast and Bowel Project B-15," *J Clin Oncol*, 1990, 8(9):1483-96.

Variation 2:

Jones SE, Durie BG, and Salmon SE, "Combination Chemotherapy With Adriamycin and Cyclophosphamide for Advanced Breast Cancer," *Cancer*, 1975, 36(1):90-7.

AC/Paclitaxel (Sequential)

Use Breast cancer

Regimen

Variation 1: AC + Paclitaxel (conventional):
Doxorubicin: I.V.: 60 mg/m² day 1
[total dose/cycle = 60 mg/m²]
Cyclophosphamide: I.V.: 600 mg/m² day 1
[total dose/cycle = 600 mg/m²]
Repeat cycle every 21 days for 4 cycles
followed by
Paclitaxel: I.V.: 175 mg/m² day 1
[total dose/cycle = 175 mg/m²]
Repeat cycle every 21 days for 4 cycles

Variation 2: AC + Paclitaxel (dose dense):
Doxorubicin: I.V.: 60 mg/m² day 1
[total dose/cycle = 60 mg/m²]

Cyclophosphamide: I.V.: 600 mg/m^2 day 1
[total dose/cycle = 600 mg/m^2]
Filgrastim: SubQ: 5 mcg/kg/day days 3 to 10
[total dose/cycle = 40 mcg/kg]
Repeat cycle every 14 days for 4 cycles
followed by
Paclitaxel: I.V.: 175 mg/m^2 day 1
[total dose/cycle = 175 mg/m^2]
Filgrastim: SubQ: 5 mcg/kg/day days 3 to 10
[total dose/cycle = 40 mcg/kg]
Repeat cycle every 14 days for 4 cycles

References

Variation 1:
Henderson IC, Berry DA, Demetri GD, et al, "Improved Outcomes From Adding Sequential Paclitaxel but Not From Escalating Doxorubicin Dose in an Adjuvant Chemotherapy Regimen for Patients With Node-Positive Primary Breast Cancer," *J Clin Oncol*, 2003, 21(6):976-83.
Variation 2:
Citron ML, Berry DA, Cirrincione C, et al, "Randomized Trial of Dose-Dense Versus Conventionally Scheduled and Sequential Versus Concurrent Combination Chemotherapy as Postoperative Adjuvant Treatment of Node-Positive Primary Breast Cancer: First Report of Intergroup Trial C9741/Cancer Leukemia Group B Trial 9741," *J Clin Oncol*, 2003, 21(8):1431-9.

AC-Paclitaxel-Trastuzumab

Use Breast cancer
Regimen NOTE: Multiple variations are listed.
Variation 1:
Doxorubicin: I.V.: 60 mg/m^2 day 1
[total dose/cycle = 60 mg/m^2]
Cyclophosphamide: I.V.: 600 mg/m^2 day 1
[total dose/cycle = 600 mg/m^2]
Repeat cycle every 21 days for 4 cycles
followed by
Paclitaxel: I.V.: 175 mg/m^2 day 1
[total dose/cycle = 175 mg/m^2]
Trastuzumab: I.V.: 4 mg/kg (loading dose) day 1 (cycle 1 only)
[total dose/cycle = 4 mg/kg]
followed by I.V.: 2 mg/kg/day days 8 and 15 (cycle 1)
[total dose/cycle = 4 mg/kg]
then I.V.: 2 mg/kg/day days 1, 8, and 15 (cycles 2, 3, and 4)
[total dose/cycle = 6 mg/kg]
Repeat cycle every 21 days for 4 cycles
followed by
Trastuzumab: I.V.: 2 mg/kg weekly for 40 weeks
Variation 2:
Doxorubicin: I.V.: 60 mg/m^2 day 1
[total dose/cycle = 60 mg/m^2]
Cyclophosphamide: I.V.: 600 mg/m^2 day 1
[total dose/cycle = 600 mg/m^2]
Repeat cycle every 21 days for 4 cycles
followed by
Paclitaxel: I.V.: 80 mg/m^{2}day 1 week 13
[total dose/cycle = 80 mg/m^2]

Trastuzumab: I.V.: 4 mg/kg (loading dose) day 1 week 13 only
[total dose/cycle = 4 mg/kg]
followed by
Paclitaxel: I.V.: 80 mg/m^2 weekly
[total dose/cycle = 80 mg/m^2]
Trastuzumab: I.V.: 2 mg/kg /weekly
[total dose/cycle = 2 mg/kg]
Repeat cycle every week for 11 cycles
followed by
Trastuzumab: I.V.: 2 mg/kg/weekly for 40 weeks

References

Romond EH, Perez EA, Bryant J, et al, "Trastuzumab Plus Adjuvant Chemotherapy for Operable HER2-Positive Breast Cancer," *N Engl J Med*, 2005, 353(16):1673-84.

AD (Soft Tissue Sarcoma)

Index Terms Doxorubicin-Dacarbazine (Soft Tissue Sarcoma)

Use Soft tissue sarcoma

Regimen

NOTE: Multiple variations are listed.

Variation 1 (metastatic):
Doxorubicin: I.V.: 15 mg/m^2/day continuous infusion days 1 to 4
[total dose/cycle = 60 mg/m^2]
Dacarbazine: I.V.: 187.5 mg/m^2/day continuous infusion days 1 to 4
[total dose/cycle = 750 mg/m^2]
Repeat cycle every 21 days; maximum lifetime doxorubicin dose of 450 mg/m^2

Variation 2 (metastatic):
Doxorubicin: I.V.: 60 mg/m^2 I.V. bolus day 1
[total dose/cycle = 60 mg/m^2]
Dacarbazine: I.V.: 750 mg/m^2/day I.V. bolus day 1
[total dose/cycle = 750 mg/m^2]
Repeat cycle every 21 days; maximum lifetime doxorubicin dose of 450 mg/m^2

Variation 3 (metastatic):
Doxorubicin: I.V.: 15 mg/m^2/day continuous infusion days 1 to 4
[total dose/cycle = 60 mg/m^2]
Dacarbazine: I.V.: 250 mg/m^2/day continuous infusion days 1 to 4
[total dose/cycle = 1000 mg/m^2]
Repeat cycle every 21 days

Variation 4 (metastatic):
Doxorubicin: I.V.: 60 mg/m^2 day 1
[total dose/cycle = 60 mg/m^2]
Dacarbazine: I.V.: 250 mg/m^2/day days 1 to 5
[total dose/cycle = 1250 mg/m^2]
Repeat cycle every 21 days until disease progression; when maximum lifetime doxorubicin dose received, continue with single agent dacarbazine

References

Variations 1 and 2:
Zalupski M, Metch B, Fletcher WS, et al, "Phase III Comparison of Doxorubicin and Dacarbazine Given by Bolus Versus Infusion in Patients With Soft-Tissue Sarcomas: A Southwest Oncology Group Study," *J Natl Cancer Inst*, 1991, 83(13):926-32.
Variation 3:
Antman K, Crowley J, Balcerzak SP, et al, "An Intergroup Phase III Randomized Study of Doxorubicin and Dacarbazine With or Without Ifosfamide and Mesna in Advanced Soft Tissue and Bone Sarcomas," *J Clin Oncol*, 1993, 11(7):1276-85.

Variation 4:
Borden EC, Amato DA, Rosenbaum C, et al, "Randomized Comparison of Three Adriamycin Regimens for Metastatic Soft Tissue Sarcomas," *J Clin Oncol*, 1987, 5(6):840-50.

AI

Use Soft tissue sarcoma

Regimen NOTE: Multiple variations are listed.

Variation 1:

Doxorubicin: I.V.: 25 mg/m²/day continuous infusion days 1, 2, and 3
[total dose/cycle = 75 mg/m²]

Ifosfamide: I.V.: 2 g/m²/day days 1 to 5
[total dose/cycle = 10 g/m²]

Mesna: I.V.: 400 mg/m² day 1
followed by I.V.: 1200 mg/m²/day continuous infusion days 1 to 5
[total dose/cycle = 6400 mg/m²]

Repeat cycle every 3 weeks

Variation 2:

Doxorubicin: I.V.: 30 mg/m²/day continuous infusion days 1, 2, and 3
[total dose/cycle = 90 mg/m²]

Ifosfamide: I.V.: 2.5 g/m²/day days 1 to 4
[total dose/cycle = 10 g/m²]

Mesna: I.V.: 500 mg/m² day 1
followed by I.V.: 1500 mg/m²/day continuous infusion days 1 to 4
[total dose/cycle = 6500 mg/m²]

Filgrastim: SubQ: 5 mcg/kg/day days 5 through ANC recovery

Repeat cycle every 3 weeks

References

Patel SR, Vadhan-Raj S, Burgess MA, et al, "Results of Two Consecutive Trials of Dose-Intensive Chemotherapy With Doxorubicin and Ifosfamide in Patients With Sarcomas," *Am J Clin Oncol*, 1998, 21(3):317-21.

◆ **Aldesleukin-Interferon Alfa-2 (RCC)** *see* Interleukin 2-Interferon Alfa-2 (RCC) *on page 1692*

◆ **Alemtuzumab-Fludarabine (CLL)** *see* Fludarabine-Alemtuzumab (CLL) *on page 1645*

◆ **AlinC 14** *see* PVA (POG 8602) *on page 1742*

AP

Use Endometrial cancer

Regimen

Doxorubicin: I.V.: 60 mg/m² day 1
[total dose/cycle = 60 mg/m²]

Cisplatin: I.V.: 60 mg/m² day 1
[total dose/cycle = 60 mg/m²]

Repeat cycle every 21-28 days

References

Barrett RJ, Blessing JA, Homesley HD, et al, "Circadian-Timed Combination Doxorubicin-Cisplatin Chemotherapy for Advanced Endometrial Carcinoma. A Phase II Study of the Gynecologic Oncology Group," *Am J Clin Oncol*, 1993, 16(6):494-6.

◆ **Arsenic Trioxide-ATRA (APL)** *see* Tretinoin-Arsenic Trioxide (APL) *on page 1761*

◆ **AT (Breast Cancer)** *see* Docetaxel-Doxorubicin (Breast Cancer) *on page 1611*

- **ATC** *see* TAC *on page 1753*
- **ATRA-Arsenic Trixoide (APL)** *see* Tretinoin-Arsenic Trioxide (APL) *on page 1761*
- **ATRA-Daunorubicin (APL)** *see* Tretinoin-Daunorubicin (APL) *on page 1762*
- **ATRA-Daunorubicin-Cytarabine (APL)** *see* Tretinoin-Daunorubicin-Cytarabine (APL) *on page 1762*
- **ATRA-Idarubicin (APL)** *see* Tretinoin-Idarubicin (APL) *on page 1764*

Azacitidine (AML Regimen)

Use Leukemia, acute myeloid

Regimen

Azacitidine: SubQ: 75 mg/m²/day days 1 to 7
[total dose/cycle = 525 mg/m²]

Repeat cycle every 28 days (for a minimum of 6 cycles [Fenaux, 2010]) as long as tolerated and maintaining response

References

Fenaux P, Mufti GJ, Hellstrom-Lindberg E, et al, "Azacitidine Prolongs Overall Survival Compared With Conventional Care Regimens in Elderly Patients With Low Bone Marrow Blast Count Acute Myeloid Leukemia," *J Clin Oncol*, 2010, 28(4):562-9.

Sudan N, Rossetti JM, Shadduck RK, et al, "Treatment of Acute Myelogenous Leukemia With Outpatient Azacitidine," *Cancer*, 2006, 107(8):1839-43.

Azacitidine (MDS Regimen)

Use Myelodysplastic syndrome

Regimen NOTE: Multiple variations are listed.

Variation 1:

Azacitidine: SubQ: 75 mg/m²/day days 1 to 7
[total dose/cycle = 525 mg/m²]

Repeat cycle every 28 days

Variation 2:

Azacitidine: I.V.: 75 mg/m²/day days 1 to 7
[total dose/cycle = 525 mg/m²]

Repeat cycle every 28 days

Variation 3:

Azacitidine: SubQ: 75 mg/m²/day days 1 to 5 (Mon-Fri), 2 days of rest (Sat, Sun), then 75 mg/m²/day days 1 and 2 (Mon, Tues)
[total dose/cycle = 525 mg/m²]

Repeat cycle every 28 days for a total of 6 cycles

Variation 4:

Azacitidine: SubQ: 50 mg/m²/day days 1 to 5 (Mon-Fri), 2 days of rest (Sat, Sun), then 50 mg/m²/day days 1 to 5 (Mon-Fri)
[total dose/cycle = 500 mg/m²]

Repeat cycle every 28 days for a total of 6 cycles

Variation 5:

Azacitidine: SubQ: 75 mg/m²/day days 1 to 5 (Mon-Fri)
[total dose/cycle = 375 mg/m²]

Repeat cycle every 28 days for a total of 6 cycles

References

Variation 1:

Fenaux P, Mufti GJ, Hellstrom-Lindberg E, et al, "Efficacy of Azacitidine Compared With That of Conventional Care Regimens in the Treatment of Higher-Risk Myelodysplastic Syndromes: A Randomised, Open-Label, Phase III Study," *Lancet Oncol*, 2009, 10(3):223-32.

Variation 2:

Marcucci G, Silverman L, Eller M, et al, "Bioavailability of Azacitidine Subcutaneous Versus Intravenous in Patients With the Myelodysplastic Syndromes," *J Clin Pharmacol*, 2005, 45 (5):597-602.

Sekeres MA, Maciejewski JP, Donley DW, et al, "A Study Comparing Dosing Regimens and Efficacy of Subcutaneous to Intravenous Azacitidine (ASA) for the Treatment of Myelodysplastic Syndromes (MDS), *Blood*, 2009, 114(22) [abstract 3797 from 2009 ASH Annual Meeting].

Variations 3, 4, and 5:

Lyons RM, Cosgriff TM, Modi SS, et al, "Hematologic Response to Three Alternative Dosing Schedules of Azacitidine in Patients With Myelodysplastic Syndrome," *J Clin Oncol*, 2009, 27 (11):1850-6.

- **Baby Brain I** *see* COPE *on page* 1596
- **BDR (Waldenstrom's Macroglobulinemia)** *see* Bortezomib-Dexamethasone-Rituximab (Waldenstrom's Macroglobulinemia) *on page* 1535

BEACOPP-14 (Hodgkin)

Index Terms Bleomycin, Etoposide, Doxorubicin, Cyclophosphamide, Vincristine, Procarbazine, Prednisone (Hodgkin)

Use Lymphoma, Hodgkin

Regimen

Bleomycin: I.V.: 10 units/m^2 day 8
[total dose/cycle = 10 units/m^2]

Etoposide: I.V.: 100 mg/m^2/day days 1, 2, and 3
[total dose/cycle = 300 mg/m^2]

Doxorubicin: I.V.: 25 mg/m^2 day 1
[total dose/cycle = 25 mg/m^2]

Cyclophosphamide: I.V.: 650 mg/m^2 day 1
[total dose/cycle = 650 mg/m^2]

Vincristine: I.V.: 1.4 mg/m^2 (maximum dose: 2 mg) day 8
[total dose/cycle = 1.4 mg/m^2; maximum: 2 mg]

Procarbazine: Oral: 100 mg/m^2/day days 1 to 7
[total dose/cycle = 700 mg/m^2]

Prednisone: Oral: 80 mg/m^2/day days 1 to 7
[total dose/cycle = 560 mg/m^2]

Filgrastim: SubQ: 300 mcg/day (patients <75 kg) or 480 mcg/day (patients ≥75 kg) days 8 to13

Repeat cycle every 14 days for a total of 8 cycles

References

Sieber M, Bredenfeld H, Josting A, et al, "14-Day Variant of the Bleomycin, Etoposide, Doxorubicin, Cyclophosphamide, Vincristine, Procarbazine, and Prednisone Regimen in Advanced-Stage Hodgkin's Lymphoma: Results of a Pilot Study of the German Hodgkin's Lymphoma Study Group," *J Clin Oncol*, 2003, 21(9):1734-9.

- **BEACOPP Baseline (Hodgkin)** *see* BEACOPP Standard (Hodgkin) *on page* 1525

BEACOPP Escalated (Hodgkin)

Index Terms Bleomycin, Etoposide, Doxorubicin, Cyclophosphamide, Vincristine, Procarbazine, Prednisone (Hodgkin)

Use Lymphoma, Hodgkin

Regimen

Bleomycin: I.V.: 10 units/m^2 day 8
[total dose/cycle = 10 units/m^2]

Etoposide: I.V.: 200 mg/m^2/day days 1, 2, and 3
[total dose/cycle = 600 mg/m^2]

Doxorubicin: I.V.: 35 mg/m^2 day 1
[total dose/cycle = 35 mg/m^2]
Cyclophosphamide: I.V.: 1200 mg/m^2 day 1
[total dose/cycle = 1200 mg/m^2]
Vincristine: I.V.: 1.4 mg/m^2 (maximum dose: 2 mg) day 8
[total dose/cycle = 1.4 mg/m^2: maximum: 2 mg]
Procarbazine: Oral: 100 mg/m^2/day days 1 to 7
[total dose/cycle = 700 mg/m^2]
Prednisone: Oral: 40 mg/m^2/day days 1 to 14
[total dose/cycle = 560 mg/m^2]
Filgrastim: SubQ: 300 or 480 mcg/day (depending on weight of 75 kg) day 8 until leukocyte recovery (3 days at >1000/mm^3)
Repeat cycle every 21 days for a total of 8 cycles

References

Diehl V, Franklin J, Hasenclever D, et al, "BEACOPP, A New Dose-Escalated and Accelerated Regimen, Is at Least as Effective as COPP/ABVD in Patients With Advanced-Stage Hodgkin's Lymphoma: Interim Report From a Trial of the German Hodgkin's Lymphoma Study Group," *J Clin Oncol*, 1998, 16(12):3810-21.

Diehl V, Franklin J, Pfreundschuh M, et al, "Standard and Increased-Dose BEACOPP Chemotherapy Compared With COPP-ABVD for Advanced Hodgkin's disease," *N Engl J Med*, 2003, 348(24):2386-95.

Engert A, Diehl V, Franklin J, et al, "Escalated-Dose BEACOPP in the Treatment of Patients With Advanced-Stage Hodgkin's Lymphoma: 10 Years of Follow-Up of the GHSG HD9 Study," *J Clin Oncol*, 2009, 27(27):4548-54.

BEACOPP Escalated Plus Standard (Hodgkin)

Index Terms Bleomycin, Etoposide, Doxorubicin, Cyclophosphamide, Vincristine, Procarbazine, Prednisone (Hodgkin)

Use Lymphoma, Hodgkin

Regimen NOTE: Multiple variations are listed.

Variation 1: BEACOPP Escalated for 4 cycles **followed by** 2 cycles of BEACOPP Standard

BEACOPP Escalated for 4 cycles:
Bleomycin: I.V.: 10 units/m^2 day 8
[total dose/cycle = 10 units/m^2]
Etoposide: I.V.: 200 mg/m^2/day days 1, 2, and 3
[total dose/cycle = 600 mg/m^2]
Doxorubicin: I.V.: 35 mg/m^2 day 1
[total dose/cycle = 35 mg/m^2]
Cyclophosphamide: I.V.: 1250 mg/m^2 day 1
[total dose/cycle = 1250 mg/m^2]
Vincristine: I.V.: 1.4 mg/m^2 (maximum dose: 2 mg) day 8
[total dose/cycle = 1.4 mg/m^2: maximum: 2 mg]
Procarbazine: Oral: 100 mg/m^2/day days 1 to 7
[total dose/cycle = 700 mg/m^2]
Prednisone: Oral: 40 mg/m^2/day days 1 to 14
[total dose/cycle = 560 mg/m^2]
Filgrastim: SubQ: 300 mcg/day day 8 until neutrophil recovery (>500/mm^3)
Repeat cycle every 21 days for a total of 4 cycles

Followed by BEACOPP Standard for 2 cycles:
Bleomycin: I.V.: 10 units/m^2 day 8
[total dose/cycle = 10 units/m^2]
Etoposide: I.V.: 100 mg/m^2/day days 1, 2, and 3
[total dose/cycle = 300 mg/m^2]

Doxorubicin: I.V.: 25 mg/m^2 day 1
[total dose/cycle = 25 mg/m^2]
Cyclophosphamide: I.V.: 650 mg/m^2 day 1
[total dose/cycle = 650 mg/m^2]
Vincristine: I.V.: 1.4 mg/m^2 (maximum dose: 2 mg) day 8
[total dose/cycle = 1.4 mg/m^2: maximum: 2 mg]
Procarbazine: Oral: 100 mg/m^2/day days 1 to 7
[total dose/cycle = 700 mg/m^2]
Prednisone: Oral: 40 mg/m^2/day days 1 to 14
[total dose/cycle = 560 mg/m^2]
Filgrastim: SubQ: 300 mcg/day day 8 until neutrophil recovery (>500/mm^3)
Repeat cycle every 21 days for a total of 2 cycles

Variation 2: BEACOPP Escalated for 4 cycles **followed by** 4 cycles of BEACOPP Standard

BEACOPP Escalated for 4 cycles:
Bleomycin: I.V.: 10 units/m^2 day 8
[total dose/cycle = 10 units/m^2]
Etoposide: I.V.: 200 mg/m^2/day days 1, 2, and 3
[total dose/cycle = 600 mg/m^2]
Doxorubicin: I.V.: 35 mg/m^2 day 1
[total dose/cycle = 35 mg/m^2]
Cyclophosphamide: I.V.: 1250 mg/m^2 day 1
[total dose/cycle = 1250 mg/m^2]
Vincristine: I.V.: 1.4 mg/m^2 (maximum dose: 2 mg) day 8
[total dose/cycle = 1.4 mg/m^2: maximum: 2 mg]
Procarbazine: Oral: 100 mg/m^2/day days 1 to 7
[total dose/cycle = 700 mg/m^2]
Prednisone: Oral: 40 mg/m^2/day days 1 to 14
[total dose/cycle = 560 mg/m^2]
Filgrastim: SubQ: 300 mcg/day day 8 until neutrophil count >1000/mm^3 for 3 consecutive days)
Repeat cycle every 21 days for a total of 4 cycles

Followed by BEACOPP Standard for 4 cycles:
Bleomycin: I.V.: 10 units/m^2 day 8
[total dose/cycle = 10 units/m^2]
Etoposide: I.V.: 100 mg/m^2/day days 1, 2, and 3
[total dose/cycle = 300 mg/m^2]
Doxorubicin: I.V.: 25 mg/m^2 day 1
[total dose/cycle = 25 mg/m^2]
Cyclophosphamide: I.V.: 650 mg/m^2 day 1
[total dose/cycle = 650 mg/m^2]
Vincristine: I.V.: 1.4 mg/m^2 (maximum dose: 2 mg) day 8
[total dose/cycle = 1.4 mg/m^2: maximum: 2 mg]
Procarbazine: Oral: 100 mg/m^2/day days 1 to 7
[total dose/cycle = 700 mg/m^2]
Prednisone: Oral: 40 mg/m^2/day days 1 to 14
[total dose/cycle = 560 mg/m^2]
Filgrastim: SubQ: 300 mcg/day day 8 until neutrophil count >1000/mm^3 for 3 consecutive days)
Repeat cycle every 21 days for a total of 4 cycles

References

Variation 1:

Federico M, Luminari S, Iannitto E, et al, "ABVD Compared With BEACOPP Compared With CEC for the Initial Treatment of Patients With Advanced Hodgkin's Lymphoma: Results From the HD2000 Gruppo Italiano per lo Studio dei Linfomi Trial," *J Clin Oncol*, 2009, 27(5):805-11.

Variation 2:

Viviani S, Zinzani PL, Rambaldi A, et al, "ABVD Versus BEACOPP for Hodgkin's Lymphoma When High-Dose Salvage Is Planned," *N Engl J Med*, 2011, 365(3):203-12.

BEACOPP Standard (Hodgkin)

Index Terms BEACOPP Baseline (Hodgkin); Bleomycin, Etoposide, Doxorubicin, Cyclophosphamide, Vincristine, Procarbazine, Prednisone (Hodgkin)

Use Lymphoma, Hodgkin

Regimen

Bleomycin: I.V.: 10 units/m^2 day 8
[total dose/cycle = 10 units/m^2]

Etoposide: I.V.: 100 mg/m^2/day days 1, 2, and 3
[total dose/cycle = 300 mg/m^2]

Doxorubicin: I.V.: 25 mg/m^2 day 1
[total dose/cycle = 25 mg/m^2]

Cyclophosphamide: I.V.: 650 mg/m^2 day 1
[total dose/cycle = 650 mg/m^2]

Vincristine: I.V.: 1.4 mg/m^2 (maximum dose: 2 mg) day 8
[total dose/cycle = 1.4 mg/m^2; maximum: 2 mg]

Procarbazine: Oral: 100 mg/m^2/day days 1 to 7
[total dose/cycle = 700 mg/m^2]

Prednisone: Oral: 40 mg/m^2/day days 1 to 14
[total dose/cycle = 560 mg/m^2]

Repeat cycle every 21 days for a total of 8 cycles

References

Diehl V, Franklin J, Hasenclever D, et al, "BEACOPP, a New Dose-Escalated and Accelerated Regimen, Is at Least as Effective as COPP/ABVD in Patients With Advanced-Stage Hodgkin's Lymphoma: Interim Report From a Trial of the German Hodgkin's Lymphoma Study Group," *J Clin Oncol*, 1998, 16(12):3810-21.

Diehl V, Sieber M, Rüffer U, et al, "BEACOPP: An Intensified Chemotherapy Regimen in Advanced Hodgkin's Disease. The German Hodgkin's Lymphoma Study Group," *Ann Oncol*, 1997, 8 (2):143-8.

Bendamustine-Rituximab

Index Terms Rituximab-Bendamustine

Use Lymphoma, non-Hodgkin's (Mantle cell or low-grade NHL)

Regimen NOTE: Multiple variations are listed.

Variation 1:

Pretreatment:

Rituximab: I.V.: 375 mg/m^2 1 week before the start of cycle 1
[total dose/pretreatment = 375 mg/m^2]

Cycles:

Rituximab: I.V.: 375 mg/m^2 day 1
[total dose/cycle = 375 mg/m^2]

Bendamustine: I.V.: 90 mg/m^2 days 2 and 3
[total dose/cycle = 180 mg/m^2]

Repeat cycle every 4 weeks for up to 4 cycles

Post-Treatment:

Rituximab: I.V.: 375 mg/m^2 4 weeks after the last cycle
[total dose/post-treatment = 375 mg/m^2]

Variation 2:
Pretreatment:
Rituximab: I.V.: 375 mg/m² 1 week before the start of cycle 1
[total dose/pretreatment = 375 mg/m²]
Cycles:
Rituximab: I.V.: 375 mg/m² day 1
[total dose/cycle = 375 mg/m²]
Bendamustine: I.V.: 90 mg/m² days 2 and 3
[total dose/cycle = 180 mg/m²]
Repeat cycle every 4 weeks for 4-6 cycles
Post-Treatment:
Rituximab: I.V.: 375 mg/m² 4 weeks after the last cycle
[total dose/post-treatment = 375 mg/m²]

References

Variation 1:
Rummel MJ, Al-Batran SE, Kim SZ, et al, "Bendamustine Plus Rituximab Is Effective and Has a Favorable Toxicity Profile in the Treatment of Mantle Cell and Low-Grade Non-Hodgkin's Lymphoma," *J Clin Oncol*, 2005, 23(15):3383-9.
Variation 2:
Robinson KS, Williams ME, van der Jagt RH, et al, "Phase II Multicenter Study of Bendamustine Plus Rituximab in Patients With Relapsed Indolent B-Cell and Mantle Cell Non-Hodgkin's Lymphoma," *J Clin Oncol*, 2008, 26(27):4473-9.

BEP (Ovarian Cancer)

Use Ovarian cancer

Regimen

Bleomycin: I.V.: 20 units/m² (maximum dose: 30 units) day 1
[total dose/cycle = 20 units/m²]
Etoposide: I.V.: 75 mg/m²/day days 1 to 5
[total dose/cycle = 375 mg/m²]
or I.V.: 75 mg/m²/day days 1 to 4 (if received prior radiation therapy)
[total dose/cycle = 300 mg/m²]
Cisplatin: I.V.: 20 mg/m²/day days 1 to 5
[total dose/cycle = 100 mg/m²]
Repeat cycle every 3 weeks for 4 cycles

References

Homesley HD, Bundy BN, Hurteau JA, et al, "Bleomycin, Etoposide, and Cisplatin Combination Therapy of Ovarian Granulosa Cell Tumors and Other Stromal Malignancies: A Gynecologic Oncology Group Study," *Gynecol Oncol*, 1999, 72(2):131-7.

BEP (Ovarian Cancer, Testicular Cancer)

Use Ovarian cancer; Testicular cancer

Regimen

Bleomycin: I.V.: 30 units/day days 2, 9, and 16
[total dose/cycle = 90 units]
Etoposide: I.V.: 100 mg/m²/day days 1 to 5
[total dose/cycle = 500 mg/m²]
or I.V.: 120 mg/m²/day days 1, 2, and 3
[total dose/cycle = 360 mg/m²]
Cisplatin: I.V.: 20 mg/m²/day days 1 to 5
[total dose/cycle = 100 mg/m²]
Repeat cycle every 21 days

References

Horwich A, Sleijfer DT, Fossa SD, et al, "Randomized Trial of Bleomycin, Etoposide, and Cisplatin Compared With Bleomycin, Etoposide, and Carboplatin in Good-Prognosis Metastatic Nonseminomatous Germ Cell Cancer: A Multiinstitutional Medical Research Council/European Organization for Research and Treatment of Cancer Trial," *J Clin Oncol*, 1997, 15(5):1844-52.

Nichols CR, Catalano PJ, Crawford ED, et al, "Randomized Comparison of Cisplatin and Etoposide and Either Bleomycin or Ifosfamide in Treatment of Advanced Disseminated Germ Cell Tumors: An Eastern Cooperative Oncology Group, Southwest Oncology Group, and Cancer and Leukemia Group B Study," *J Clin Oncol*, 1998, 16(4):1287-93.

Williams S, Blessing JA, Liao SY, et al, "Adjuvant Therapy of Ovarian Germ Cell Tumors With Cisplatin, Etoposide, and Bleomycin: A Trial of the Gynecologic Oncology Group," *J Clin Oncol*, 1994, 12(4):701-6.

BEP (Testicular Cancer)

Index Terms Bleomycin–Etoposide–Cisplatin (Testicular Cancer)

Use Testicular cancer

Regimen NOTE: Multiple variations are listed.

Variation 1:

Bleomycin: I.V.: 30 units/day days 1, 8, and 15
[total dose/cycle = 90 units]

Etoposide: I.V.: 100 mg/m²/day days 1 to 5
[total dose/cycle = 500 mg/m²]

Cisplatin: I.V.: 20 mg/m²/day days 1 to 5
[total dose/cycle = 100 mg/m²]

Repeat cycle every 21 days for 3-4 cycles

Variation 2:

Bleomycin: I.V.: 30 units/day days 2, 9, and 16
[total dose/cycle = 90 units]

Etoposide: I.V.: 100 mg/m²/day days 1 to 5
[total dose/cycle = 500 mg/m²]

Cisplatin: I.V.: 20 mg/m²/day days 1 to 5
[total dose/cycle = 100 mg/m²]

Repeat cycle every 21 days

Variation 3:

Bleomycin: I.V.: 30 units once weekly
[total dose/cycle = 90 units]

Etoposide: I.V.: 120 mg/m²/day days 1, 3, and 5
[total dose/cycle = 360 mg/m²]

Cisplatin: I.V.: 20 mg/m²/day days 1 to 5
[total dose/cycle = 100 mg/m²]

Repeat cycle every 21 days

Variation 4:

Bleomycin: I.V.: 30 units/day days 1, 8, and 15
[total dose/cycle = 90 units]

Etoposide: I.V.: 165 mg/m²/day days 1, 2, and 3
[total dose/cycle = 495 mg/m²]

Cisplatin: I.V.: 50 mg/m²/day days 1 and 2
[total dose/cycle = 100 mg/m²]

Repeat cycle every 21 days

References

Variation 1:

Saxman SB, Finch D, Gonin R, et al, "Long-Term Follow-Up of a Phase III Study of Three Versus Four Cycles of Bleomycin, Etoposide, and Cisplatin in Favorable-Prognosis Germ-Cell Tumors: The Indian University Experience," *J Clin Oncol*, 1998, 16(2):702-6.

Variation 2:
Williams SD, Birch R, Einhorn LH, et al, "Treatment of Disseminated Germ-Cell Tumors With Cisplatin, Bleomycin, and Either Vinblastine or Etoposide," *N Engl J Med*, 1987, 316 (23):1435-40.
Variation 3:
de Wit R, Stoter G, Sleijfer DT, et al, "Four Cycles of BEP Vs Four Cycles of VIP in Patients With Intermediate-Prognosis Metastatic Testicular Nonseminoma: A Randomized Study of the EORTC Genitourinary Tract Cancer Cooperative Group. European Organization for Research and Treatment of Cancer," *Br J Cancer*, 1998, 78(6):828-32.
Variation 4:
de Wit R, Roberts JT, Wilkinson PM, et al, "Equivalence of Three or Four Cycles of Bleomycin, Etoposide, and Cisplatin Chemotherapy and of a 3- or 5-Day Schedule in Good-Prognosis Germ Cell Cancer: A Randomized Study of the European Organization for Research and Treatment of Cancer Genitourinary Tract Cancer Cooperative Group and the Medical Research Council," *J Clin Oncol*, 2001, 19(6):1629-40.

Bevacizumab-Capecitabine (Breast Cancer)

Index Terms Capecitabine-Bevacizumab (Breast Cancer)

Use Breast cancer

Regimen NOTE: Multiple variations are listed.

Variation 1:

Capecitabine: Oral: 1250 mg/m^2 twice daily days 1 to 14
[total dose/cycle = 35,000 mg/m^2]

Bevacizumab: I.V.: 15 mg/kg day 1
[total dose/cycle = 15 mg/kg]

Repeat cycle every 21 days for up to 35 cycles

Variation 2:

Capecitabine: Oral: 2000 mg/m^2/day days 1 to 14
[total dose/cycle = 28,000 mg/m^2]

Bevacizumab: I.V.: 15 mg/kg day 1
[total dose/cycle = 15 mg/kg]

Repeat cycle every 21 days

References

Variation 1:
Miller KD, Chap LI, Holmes FA, et al, "Randomized Phase III Trial of Capecitabine Compared With Bevacizumab Plus Capecitabine in Patients With Previously Treated Metastatic Breast Cancer," *J Clin Oncol*, 2005, 23(4):792-9.
Variation 2:
Robert NJ, Dieras V, Glaspy J, et al, "RIBBON-1: Randomized, Double-Blind, Placebo-Controlled, Phase III Trial of Chemotherapy With or Without Bevacizumab (B) for First-Line Treatment of HER2-Negative Locally Recurrent or Metastatic Breast Cancer (MBC)," *J Clin Oncol*, 2009, 27 (15s):1005 [abstract from 2009 ASCO Annual Meeting].

Bevacizumab-Carboplatin-Paclitaxel (NSCLC)

Index Terms Bevacizumab-Paclitaxel-Carboplatin (NSCLC); Carboplatin-Paclitaxel-Bevacizumab (NSCLC)

Use Lung cancer, nonsmall cell (nonsquamous cell histology)

Regimen

Paclitaxel: I.V.: 200 mg/m^2 day 1
[total dose/cycle = 200 mg/m^2]

Carboplatin: I.V.: AUC 6 day 1
[total dose/cycle = AUC = 6]

Bevacizumab: I.V.: 15 mg/kg day 1
[total dose/cycle = 15 mg/kg]

Repeat cycle every 21 days for 6 cycles

followed by

Bevacizumab: I.V.: 15 mg/kg day 1
[total dose/cycle = 15 mg/kg]

Repeat cycle every 21 days until disease progression or unacceptable toxicity

References

Sandler A, Gray R, Perry MC, et al, "Paclitaxel-Carboplatin Alone or With Bevacizumab for Nonsmall-Cell Lung Cancer," *N Engl J Med*, 2006, 355(24):2542-50.

Bevacizumab-Carboplatin-Pemetrexed (NSCLC)

Index Terms Carboplatin-Pemetrexed-Bevacizumab (NSCLC); Pemetrexed-Carboplatin-Bevacizumab (NSCLC)

Use Lung cancer, nonsmall cell

Regimen

Pemetrexed: I.V.: 500 mg/m^2 over 10 minutes day 1
[total dose/cycle = 500 mg/m^2]

Carboplatin: I.V.: AUC 6 day 1
[total dose/cycle = AUC = 6]

Bevacizumab: I.V.: 15 mg/kg day 1
[total dose/cycle = 15 mg/kg]

Repeat cycle every 21 days for 6 cycles

followed by

Pemetrexed: I.V.: 500 mg/m^2 over 10 minutes day 1
[total dose/cycle = 500 mg/m^2]

Bevacizumab: I.V.: 15 mg/kg day 1
[total dose/cycle = 15 mg/kg]

Repeat cycle every 21 days until disease progression or unacceptable toxicity

References

Patel JD, Hensing TA, Rademaker A, et al, "Phase II Study of Pemetrexed and Carboplatin Plus Bevacizumab With Maintenance Pemetrexed and Bevacizumab as First-Line Therapy for Nonsquamous Non-Small-Cell Lung Cancer," *J Clin Oncol*, 2009, 27(20):3284-9.

Bevacizumab-Cisplatin-Gemcitabine (NSCLC)

Index Terms Cisplatin-Gemcitabine-Bevacizumab (NSCLC)

Use Lung cancer, nonsmall cell

Regimen

Cisplatin: I.V.: 80 mg/m^2 day 1
[total dose/cycle = 80 mg/m^2]

Gemcitabine: I.V.: 1250 mg/m^2/day days 1 and 8
[total dose/cycle = 2500 mg/m^2]

Bevacizumab: I.V.: 7.5 or 15 mg/kg day 1
[total dose/cycle = 7.5 or 15 mg/kg]

Repeat cycle every 21 days for up to 6 cycles

followed by

Bevacizumab: I.V.: 7.5 or 15 mg/kg day 1
[total dose/cycle = 7.5 or 15 mg/kg]

Repeat cycle every 21 days until disease progression or unacceptable toxicity

References

Reck M, von Pawel J, Zatloukal P, et al, "Overall Survival With Cisplatin-Gemcitabine and Bevacizumab or Placebo as First-Line Therapy for Nonsquamous Non-Small-Cell Lung Cancer: Results From a Randomised Phase III Trial AVAiL," *Ann Oncol*, 2010, 21(9):1804-9.

Reck M, von Pawel J, Zatloukal P, et al, "Phase III Trial of Cisplatin Plus Gemcitabine With Either Placebo or Bevacizumab as First-Line Therapy for Nonsquamous Non-Small-Cell Lung Cancer: AVAiL," *J Clin Oncol*, 2009, 27(8):1227-34.

◆ **Bevacizumab-Docetaxel** *see* Docetaxel-Bevacizumab *on page* *1608*

Bevacizumab-Fluorouracil-Leucovorin

Index Terms Fluorouracil-Leucovorin-Bevacizumab

Use Colorectal cancer

Regimen

Bevacizumab: I.V.: 5 mg/kg/day days 1, 15, 29, and 43
[total dose/cycle = 20 mg/kg]

Leucovorin: I.V.: 500 mg/m^2/day days 1, 8, 15, 22, 29, and 36
[total dose/cycle = 3000 mg/m^2]

Fluorouracil: I.V.: 500 mg/m^2/day days 1, 8, 15, 22, 29, and 36
[total dose/cycle = 3000 mg/m^2]

Repeat cycle every 56 days

References

Kabbinavar FF, Schulz J, McCleod M, et al, "Addition of Bevacizumab to Bolus Fluorouracil and Leucovorin in First-Line Metastatic Colorectal Cancer: Results of a Randomized Phase II Trial," *J Clin Oncol*, 2005, 23(16):3697-705.

Bevacizumab + FOLFIRI (Colorectal)

Index Terms Bevacizumab, Irinotecan, Leucovorin, Fluorouracil (Colorectal)

Use Colorectal cancer

Regimen

Bevacizumab: I.V.: 5 mg/kg day 1
[total dose/cycle = 5 mg/kg]

Irinotecan: I.V.: 180 mg/m^2 over 90 minutes day 1
[total dose/cycle = 180 mg/m^2]

Leucovorin: I.V.: 400 mg/m^2 over 2 hours day 1
[total dose/cycle = 400 mg/m^2]

Fluorouracil: I.V. bolus: 400 mg/m^2 day 1
followed by I.V.: 2400 mg/m^2 continuous infusion (CI) over 46 hours beginning day 1
[total fluorouracil dose/cycle (bolus and CI) = 2800 mg/m^2]

Repeat cycle every 14 days until disease progression or unacceptable toxicity

References

Fuchs CS, Marshall J, Mitchell E, et al, "Randomized, Controlled Trial of Irinotecan Plus Infusional, Bolus, or Oral Fluoropyrimidines in First-Line Treatment of Metastatic Colorectal Cancer: Results From the BICC-C Study," *J Clin Oncol*, 2007, 25(30):4779-86.

◆ **Bevacizumab-Interferon Alfa 2b (RCC)** *see* Bevacizumab-Interferon Alfa (RCC) *on page* 1530

Bevacizumab-Interferon Alfa (RCC)

Index Terms Bevacizumab-Interferon Alfa 2b (RCC); Interferon Alfa 2b-Bevacizumab (RCC); Interferon Alfa-Bevacizumab (RCC)

Use Renal cell cancer

Regimen

Interferon Alfa-2b: SubQ: 9 million units on 3 nonconsecutive days per week
[total dose/cycle = 108 million units]

Bevacizumab: I.V.: 10 mg/kg days 1 and 15
[total dose/cycle = 20 mg/kg]

Repeat cycle every 28 days until disease progression or unacceptable toxicity

References

Rini BI, Halabi S, Rosenberg JE, et al, "Bevacizumab Plus Interferon Alfa Compared With Interferon Alfa Monotherapy in Patients With Metastatic Renal Cell Carcinoma: CALGB 90206," *J Clin Oncol*, 2008, 26(33):5422-8.

Rini BI, Halabi S, Rosenberg JE, et al, "Phase III Trial of Bevacizumab Plus Interferon Alfa Versus Interferon Alfa Monotherapy in Patients With Metastatic Renal Cell Carcinoma: Final Results of CALGB 90206," *J Clin Oncol*, 2010, 28(13):2137-43.

Bevacizumab-Irinotecan (Glioblastoma)

Index Terms Irinotecan-Bevacizumab (Glioblastoma)

Use Brain tumors

Regimen NOTE: Patients receiving concurrent antiepileptic enzyme-inducing drugs received an increased dose of irinotecan (340 mg/m^2/dose).

Bevacizumab: I.V.: 10 mg/kg day 1
[total dose/cycle = 10 mg/kg]

Irinotecan: I.V.: 125 mg/m^2 day 1
[total dose/cycle = 125 mg/m^2]

Repeat cycle every 14 days

References

Vredenburgh JJ, Desjardins A, Herndon JE 2nd, et al, "Bevacizumab Plus Irinotecan in Recurrent Glioblastoma Multiforme," *J Clin Oncol*, 2007, 25(30):4722-9.

◆ **Bevacizumab, Irinotecan, Leucovorin, Fluorouracil (Colorectal)** *see* Bevacizumab + FOLFIRI (Colorectal) *on page 1530*

Bevacizumab-Oxaliplatin-Fluorouracil-Leucovorin

Index Terms Bevacizumab-Oxaliplatin-Leucovorin-Fluorouracil; Oxaliplatin-Fluorouracil-Leucovorin-Bevacizumab

Use Colorectal cancer

Regimen

Bevacizumab: I.V.: 10 mg/kg day 1
[total dose/cycle = 10 mg/kg]

Oxaliplatin: I.V.: 85 mg/m^2 day 1
[total dose/cycle = 85 mg/m^2]

Leucovorin: I.V.: 200 mg/m^2/day days 1 and 2
[total dose/cycle = 400 mg/m^2]

Fluorouracil: I.V. bolus: 400 mg/m^2/day days 1 and 2
followed by I.V.: 600 mg/m^2 continuous infusion over 22 hours days 1 and 2
[total dose/cycle = 2000 mg/m^2]

Repeat cycle every 14 days

References

Giantonio BJ, Catalano PJ, Meropol NJ, et al, "Bevacizumab in Combination With Oxaliplatin, Fluorouracil, and Leucovorin (FOLFOX4) for Previously Treated Metastatic Colorectal Cancer: Results From the Eastern Cooperative Oncology Group Study E3200," *J Clin Oncol*, 2007, 25 (12):1539-44.

◆ **Bevacizumab-Oxaliplatin-Leucovorin-Fluorouracil** *see* Bevacizumab-Oxaliplatin-Fluorouracil-Leucovorin *on page 1531*

◆ **Bevacizumab-Paclitaxel** *see* Paclitaxel-Bevacizumab *on page 1725*

◆ **Bevacizumab-Paclitaxel-Carboplatin (NSCLC)** *see* Bevacizumab-Carboplatin-Paclitaxel (NSCLC) *on page 1528*

Bevacizumab (RCC Regimen)

Use Renal cell cancer

Regimen

Bevacizumab: I.V.: 10 mg/kg day 1
[total dose/cycle = 10 mg/kg]
Repeat cycle every 14 days until disease progression or unacceptable toxicity

References

Yang JC, Haworth L, Sherry RM, et al, "A Randomized Trial of Bevacizumab, an Anti-Vascular Endothelial Growth Factor Antibody, for Metastatic Renal Cancer," *N Engl J Med*, 2003, 349 (5):427-34.

Bevacizumab + XELOX (Colorectal)

Index Terms Bevacizumb-Capecitabine-Oxaliplatin (Colorectal Cancer); Bevacizumb-CapeOx (Colorectal Cancer); Bevacizumb-CAPOX (Colorectal Cancer); Bevacizumb-Oxaliplatin-Capecitabine (Colorectal Cancer)

Use Colorectal cancer

Regimen NOTE: Multiple variations are listed.

Variation 1:
Bevacizumab: I.V.: 7.5 mg/kg day 1
[total dose/cycle = 7.5 mg/kg]
Oxaliplatin: I.V.: 130 mg/m^2 day 1
[total dose/cycle = 130 mg/m^2]
Capecitabine: Oral: 850 mg/m^2 twice daily days 1 (beginning with evening dose) to 15 (ending with morning dose)
[total dose/cycle = 23,800 mg/m^2]
Repeat cycle every 21 days

Variation 2:
Bevacizumab: I.V.: 7.5 mg/kg over 30-90 minutes day 1
[total dose/cycle = 7.5 mg/kg]
Oxaliplatin: I.V.: 130 mg/m^2 over 2 hours day 1
[total dose/cycle = 130 mg/m^2]
Capecitabine: Oral: 1000 mg/m^2 twice daily days 1 to 14
[total dose/cycle = 28,000 mg/m^2]
Repeat cycle every 21 days

References

Variation 1:
Hochster HS, Hart LL, Ramanathan RK, et al, "Safety and Efficacy of Oxaliplatin and Fluoropyrimidine Regimens With or Without Bevacizumab as First-Line Treatment of Metastatic Colorectal Cancer: Results of the TREE Study," *J Clin Oncol*, 2008, 26(21):3523-9.
Variation 2:
Saltz LB, Clarke S, Díaz-Rubio E, et al, "Bevacizumab in Combination With Oxaliplatin-Based Chemotherapy as First-Line Therapy in Metastatic Colorectal Cancer: A Randomized Phase III Study," *J Clin Oncol*, 2008, 26(12):2013-9.

◆ **Bevacizumb-Capecitabine-Oxaliplatin (Colorectal Cancer)** *see* Bevacizumab + XELOX (Colorectal) *on page 1532*

◆ **Bevacizumb-CapeOx (Colorectal Cancer)** *see* Bevacizumab + XELOX (Colorectal) *on page 1532*

◆ **Bevacizumb-CAPOX (Colorectal Cancer)** *see* Bevacizumab + XELOX (Colorectal) *on page 1532*

◆ **Bevacizumb-Oxaliplatin-Capecitabine (Colorectal Cancer)** *see* Bevacizumab + XELOX (Colorectal) *on page 1532*

Bicalutamide-Goserelin

Index Terms Goserelin-Bicalutamide

Use Prostate cancer

Regimen

Bicalutamide: Oral: 50 mg/day
[total dose/cycle = 1400 mg]

Goserelin acetate: SubQ: 3.6 mg day 1
[total dose/cycle = 3.6 mg]

Repeat cycle every 28 days

References

Schellhammer PF, Scharifi R, Block NL, et al, "A Controlled Trial of Bicalutamide Versus Flutamide, Each in Combination With Luteinizing Hormone-Releasing Hormone Analogue Therapy, in Patients With Advanced Prostate Cancer. Casodex Combination Study Group," *Urology*, 1995, 45(5):745-52.

Schellhammer PF, Sharifi R, Block NL, et al, "Clinical Benefits of Bicalutamide Compared With Flutamide in Combined Androgen Blockade for Patients With Advanced Prostatic Carcinoma: Final Report of a Double-Blind, Randomized, Multicenter Trial. Casodex Combination Study Group," *Urology*, 1997, 50(3):330-6.

Bicalutamide-Leuprolide

Index Terms Leuprolide-Bicalutamide

Use Prostate cancer

Regimen

Bicalutamide: Oral: 50 mg/day
[total dose/cycle = 1400 mg]

Leuprolide depot: I.M.: 7.5 mg day 1
[total dose/cycle = 7.5 mg]

Repeat cycle every 28 days

References

Schellhammer PF, Scharifi R, Block NL, et al, "A Controlled Trial of Bicalutamide Versus Flutamide, Each in Combination With Luteinizing Hormone-Releasing Hormone Analogue Therapy, in Patients With Advanced Prostate Cancer. Casodex Combination Study Group," *Urology*, 1995, 45(5):745-52.

Schellhammer PF, Sharifi R, Block NL, et al, "Clinical Benefits of Bicalutamide Compared With Flutamide in Combined Androgen Blockade for Patients With Advanced Prostatic Carcinoma: Final Report of a Double-Blind, Randomized, Multicenter Trial. Casodex Combination Study Group," *Urology*, 1997, 50(3):330-6.

◆ **Biweekly Cetuximab (Colorectal Regimen)** *see* Cetuximab Biweekly (Colorectal Regimen) *on page* 1556

◆ **Bleomycin, Etoposide, Doxorubicin, Cyclophosphamide, Vincristine, Procarbazine, Prednisone (Hodgkin)** *see* BEACOPP-14 (Hodgkin) *on page* 1522

◆ **Bleomycin, Etoposide, Doxorubicin, Cyclophosphamide, Vincristine, Procarbazine, Prednisone (Hodgkin)** *see* BEACOPP Escalated (Hodgkin) *on page* 1522

◆ **Bleomycin, Etoposide, Doxorubicin, Cyclophosphamide, Vincristine, Procarbazine, Prednisone (Hodgkin)** *see* BEACOPP Escalated Plus Standard (Hodgkin) *on page* 1523

◆ **Bleomycin, Etoposide, Doxorubicin, Cyclophosphamide, Vincristine, Procarbazine, Prednisone (Hodgkin)** *see* BEACOPP Standard (Hodgkin) *on page* 1525

◆ **Bleomycin–Etoposide–Cisplatin (Testicular Cancer)** *see* BEP (Testicular Cancer) *on page* 1527

Bortezomib-Dexamethasone (Amyloidosis)

Index Terms Dexamethasone-Bortezomib (Amyloidosis)

Use Systemic light chain amyloidosis

Regimen

Bortezomib: I.V.: 1.3 mg/m^2/dose days 1, 4, 8, and 11 [total dose/cycle = 5.2 mg/m^2]

Dexamethasone: Oral: 40 mg/day days 1 to 4 [total dose/cycle = 160 mg]

Repeat cycle every 21 days

References

Kastritis E, Wechalekar AD, Dimopoulos MA, et al, "Bortezomib With or Without Dexamethasone in Primary Systemic (Light Chain) Amyloidosis," *J Clin Oncol*, 2010, 28(6):1031-7.

Bortezomib-Dexamethasone (Multiple Myeloma)

Index Terms Dexamethasone-Bortezomib (Multiple myeloma)

Use Multiple myeloma

Regimen NOTE: Multiple variations are listed.

Variation 1:

Cycles 1 and 2:

Bortezomib: I.V.: 1.3 mg/m^2/day days 1, 4, 8, and 11 [total dose/cycle = 5.2 mg/m^2]

Dexamethasone: Oral: 40 mg/day days 1 to 4 and days 9 to 12 [total dose/cycle = 320 mg]

Treatment cycle is 21 days

Cycles 3 and 4:

Bortezomib: I.V.: 1.3 mg/m^2/day days 1, 4, 8, and 11 [total dose/cycle = 5.2 mg/m^2]

Dexamethasone: Oral: 40 mg/day days 1 to 4 [total dose/cycle = 160 mg]

Treatment cycle is 21 days

Variation 2:

Cycles 1 and 2:

Bortezomib: I.V.: 1.3 mg/m^2/day days 1, 4, 8, and 11 [total dose/cycle = 5.2 mg/m^2]

Treatment cycle is 21 days

Cycles 3 through 6 (begin dexamethasone after cycle 2 if partial response not achieved or after cycle 4 if complete response not achieved):

Bortezomib: I.V.: 1.3 mg/m^2/day days 1, 4, 8, and 11 [total dose/cycle = 5.2 mg/m^2]

Dexamethasone: Oral: 40 mg/day days 1 and 2 [total dose/cycle = 80 mg]

Treatment cycle is 21 days (for up to a total of 6 cycles)

References

Variation 1:

Harousseau JL, Attal M, Leleu X, et al, "Bortezomib Plus Dexamethasone as Induction Treatment Prior to Autologous Stem Cell Transplantation in Patients With Newly Diagnosed Multiple Myeloma: Results of an IFM Phase II Study," *Haematologica*, 2006, 91(11):1498-505.

Harousseau JL, Mathiot C, Attal M, et al, "VELCADE/Dexamethasone (Vel/D) Versus VAD as Induction Treatment Prior to Autologous Stem Cell Transplantation (ASCT) in Newly Diagnosed Multiple Myeloma (MM): Updated Results of the IFM 2005/01 Trial," *Blood*, 2007, 110(11): 450, ASH 2007 Annual Meeting Abstract 450.

Variation 2:

Jagannath S, Durie BG, Wolf J, et al, "Bortezomib Therapy Alone and in Combination With Dexamethasone for Previously Untreated Symptomatic Multiple Myeloma," *Br J Haematol*, 2005, 129(6):776-83.

Bortezomib-Dexamethasone-Rituximab (Waldenstrom's Macroglobulinemia)

Index Terms BDR (Waldenstrom's Macroglobulinemia)

Use Waldenstrom's Macroglobulinemia

Regimen

Bortezomib: I.V.: 1.3 mg/m^2 days 1, 4, 8, and 11
[total dose/cycle = 5.2 mg/m^2]

Dexamethasone: I.V.: 40 mg days 1, 4, 8, and 11
[total dose/cycle = 160 mg]

Rituximab: I.V.: 375 mg/m^2 day 11
[total dose/cycle = 375 mg/m^2]

Repeat cycle every 21 days for 4 cycles, followed by a 12 week interruption, then repeat cycle every 12 weeks for 4 cycles

References

Treon SP, Ioakimidis L, Soumerai JD, et al, "Primary Treatment of Waldenstrom Macroglobulinemia With Bortezomib, Dexamethasone, and Rituximab: WMCTG Clinical Trial 05-180," *J Clin Oncol*, 2009, 27(23):3830-5.

Bortezomib-Doxorubicin-Dexamethasone

Index Terms Dexamethasone-Bortezomib-Doxorubicin; Doxorubicin-Dexamethasone-Bortezomib; PAD

Use Multiple myeloma

Regimen NOTE: Multiple variations are listed.

Variation 1:

Cycle 1:

Bortezomib: I.V.: 1.3 mg/m^2/day days 1, 4, 8, and 11
[total dose/cycle = 5.2 mg/m^2]

Dexamethasone: Oral: 40 mg/day days 1 to 4, 8 to 11, and 15 to 18
[total dose/cycle = 480 mg]

Doxorubicin: I.V.: 4.5 or 9 mg/m^2/day days 1 to 4
[total dose/cycle = 18 or 36 mg/m^2]

Treatment cycle is 21 days

Cycles 2-4:

Bortezomib: I.V.: 1.3 mg/m^2/day days 1, 4, 8, and 11
[total dose/cycle = 5.2 mg/m^2]

Dexamethasone: Oral: 40 mg/day days 1 to 4
[total dose/cycle = 160 mg]

Doxorubicin: I.V.: 4.5 or 9 mg/m^2/day days 1 to 4
[total dose/cycle = 18 or 36 mg/m^2]

Treatment cycle is 21 days

Variation 2:

Cycle 1:

Bortezomib: I.V.: 1 mg/m^2/day days 1, 4, 8, and 11
[total dose/cycle = 4 mg/m^2]

Dexamethasone: Oral: 40 mg/day days 1 to 4, 8 to 11, and 15 to 18
[total dose/cycle = 480 mg]

Doxorubicin: I.V.: 9 mg/m^2/day days 1 to 4
[total dose/cycle = 36 mg/m^2]

Treatment cycle is 21 days

Cycles 2-4:

Bortezomib: I.V.: 1 mg/m^2/day days 1, 4, 8, and 11
[total dose/cycle = 4 mg/m^2]

Dexamethasone: Oral: 40 mg/day days 1 to 4
[total dose/cycle = 160 mg]
Doxorubicin: I.V.: 9 mg/m^2/day days 1 to 4
[total dose/cycle = 36 mg/m^2]
Treatment cycle is 21 days

Variation 3:
Bortezomib: I.V.: 1.3 mg/m^2/day days 1, 4, 8, and 11
[total dose/cycle = 5.2 mg/m^2]
Dexamethasone: Oral: 40 mg/day days 1 to 4
[total dose/cycle = 160 mg]
Doxorubicin: I.V.: 20 mg/m^2/day days 1 and 4
[total dose/cycle = 40 mg/m^2]
Repeat cycle every 28 days for up to 6 cycles

References

Variation 1:

Oakervee HE, Popat R, Curry N, et al, "PAD Combination Therapy (PS-341/Bortezomib, Doxorubicin and Dexamethasone) for Previously Untreated Patients With Multiple Myeloma," *Br J Haematol*, 2005, 129(6):755-62.

Popat R, Oakervee HE, Hallam S, et al, "Bortezomib, Doxorubicin and Dexamethasone (PAD) Front-Line Treatment of Multiple Myeloma: Updated Results After Long-Term Follow-Up," *Br J Haematol*, 2008, 41(4):512-6.

Variation 2:

Popat R, Oakervee HE, Hallam S, et al, "Bortezomib, Doxorubicin and Dexamethasone (PAD) Front-Line Treatment of Multiple Myeloma: Updated Results After Long-Term Follow-Up," *Br J Haematol*, 2008, 41(4):512-6.

Variation 3:

Palumbo A, Gay F, Bringhen S, et al, "Bortezomib, Doxorubicin and Dexamethasone in Advanced Multiple Myeloma," *Ann Oncol*, 2008, 19(6):1160-5.

Bortezomib-Doxorubicin (Liposomal)

Index Terms Doxorubicin (Liposomal)-Bortezomib

Use Multiple myeloma

Regimen

Bortezomib: I.V.: 1.3 mg/m^2/day days 1, 4, 8, and 11
[total dose/cycle = 5.2 mg/m^2]
Doxorubicin (liposomal): I.V.: 30 mg/m^2 day 4
[total dose/cycle = 30 mg/m^2]
Repeat cycle every 21 days for up to 8 cycles

References

Biehn SE, Moore DT, Voorhees PM, et al, "Extended Follow-Up of Outcome Measures in Multiple Myeloma Patients Treated on a Phase I Study With Bortezomib and Pegylated Liposomal Doxorubicin," *Ann Hematol*, 2007, 86(3):211-6.

Orlowski RZ, Nagler A, Sonneveld P, et al, "Randomized Phase III Study of Pegylated Liposomal Doxorubicin Plus Bortezomib Compared With Bortezomib Alone in Relapsed or Refractory Multiple Myeloma: Combination Therapy Improves Time to Progression," *J Clin Oncol*, 2007, 25(25):3892-901.

Orlowski RZ, Voorhees PM, Garcia RA, et al, "Phase 1 Trial of the Proteasome Inhibitor Bortezomib and Pegylated Liposomal Doxorubicin in Patients With Advanced Hematologic Malignancies," *Blood*, 2005, 105(8):3058-65.

Bortezomib-Doxorubicin (Liposomal)-Dexamethasone

Index Terms Dexamethasone-Bortezomib-Doxorubicin (Liposomal); Doxorubicin (Liposomal)-Dexamethasone-Bortezomib

Use Multiple myeloma

Regimen

Bortezomib: I.V.: 1.3 mg/m^2/day days 1, 4, 8, and 11
[total dose/cycle = 5.2 mg/m^2]

Doxorubicin (Liposomal): I.V.: 30 mg/m^2 day 1
[total dose/cycle = 30 mg/m^2]
Dexamethasone: Oral: 40 mg/day days 1 to 4
[total dose/cycle = 160 mg]
Repeat cycle every 28 days for up to 6 cycles

References

Palumbo A, Gay F, Bringhen S, et al, "Bortezomib, Doxorubicin and Dexamethasone in Advanced Multiple Myeloma," *Ann Oncol*, 2008, 19(6):1160-5.

◆ **Bortezomib-Melphalan-Prednisone (Multiple Myeloma)** *see* Melphalan-Prednisone-Bortezomib (Multiple Myeloma) *on page 1708*

Bortezomib-Melphalan-Prednisone-Thalidomide

Index Terms Melphalan-Prednisone-Bortezomib-Thalidomide; VMPT

Use Multiple myeloma

Regimen

Bortezomib: I.V.: 1-1.3 mg/m^2/day days 1, 4, 15, and 22
[total dose/cycle = 4-5.2 mg/m^2]
Melphalan: Oral: 6 mg/m^2/day days 1 to 5
[total dose/cycle = 30 mg/m^2]
Prednisone: Oral: 60 mg/m^2/day days 1 to 5
[total dose/cycle = 300 mg/m^2]
Thalidomide: Oral: 50 mg/day days 1 to 35
[total dose/cycle = 1750 mg]
Repeat cycle every 35 days for 6 cycles

References

Palumbo A, Ambrosini MT, Benevolo G, et al, "Bortezomib, Melphalan, Prednisone, and Thalidomide for Relapsed Multiple Myeloma," *Blood*, 2007, 109(7):2767-72.

Bortezomib-Rituximab (Waldenstrom's Macroglobulinemia)

Index Terms Rituximab-Bortezomib (Waldenstrom's Macroglobulinemia)

Use Waldenstrom's Macroglobulinemia

Regimen

Bortezomib: I.V.: 1.6 mg/m^2/day days 1, 8, and 15 (cycles 1 to 6)
[total dose/cycle = 4.8 mg/m^2]
Rituximab: I.V.: 375 mg/m^2/day days 1, 8, 15, and 22 (cycles 1 and 4 only)
[total dose/cycle (cycles 1 and 4 only) = 1500 mg/m^2]
Repeat cycle every 28 days for a total of 6 cycles; bortezomib administered for all 6 cycles and rituximab administered cycles 1 and 4 only

References

Ghobrial IM, Hong F, Padmanabhan S, et al, "Phase II Trial of Weekly Bortezomib in Combination With Rituximab in Relapsed or Refractory and Refractory Waldenstrom Macroglobulinemia," *J Clin Oncol*, 2010, 28(8):1422-8.

Bortezomib (Waldenstrom's Macroglobulinemia)

Use Waldenstrom's Macroglobulinemia

Regimen

Bortezomib: I.V.: 1.3 mg/m^2/day days 1, 4, 8, and 11
[total dose/cycle = 5.2 mg/m^2]
Repeat cycle every 21 days until disease progression or until 2 cycles after a complete response

References

Chen CI, Kouroukis CT, White D, et al, "Bortezomib is Active in Patients With Untreated or Relapsed Waldenstrom's Macroglobulinemia: A Phase II Study of the National Cancer Institute of Canada Clinical Trials Group," *J Clin Oncol*, 2007, 25(12):1570-5.

Bosutinib (CML Regimen)

Use Leukemia, chronic myelogenous

Regimen

Bosutinib: Oral: 500 mg once daily
[total dose/cycle = 14,000 mg]

Repeat cycle every 28 days until disease progression or unacceptable toxicity

References

Cortes JE, Kim, DW, Kantarjian HM, et al, "Bosutinib Versus Imatinib in Newly Diagnosed Chronic-Phase Chronic Myeloid Leukemia: Results From the BELA Trial," *J Clin Oncol*, 2012, 30 (28):3486-92.

Khoury HJ, Cortes JE, Kantarjian HM, et al, "Bosutinib Is Active in Chronic Phase Chronic Myeloid Leukemia After Imatinib and Dasatinib and/or Nilotinib Therapy Failure," *Blood*, 2012, 199 (5):3403-12.

Cabazitaxel-Prednisone (Prostate Cancer)

Use Prostate cancer

Regimen

Cabazitaxel: I.V.: 25 mg/m^2/dose day 1
[total dose/cycle = 25 mg/m^2]

Prednisone: Oral: 10 mg once daily
[total dose/cycle = 210 mg]

Repeat cycle every 21 days

References

De Bono JS, Oudard S, Ozguroglu M, et al, "Cabazitaxel or Mitoxantrone With Prednisone in Patients With Metastatic Castration-Resistant Prostate Cancer (mCRPC) Previously Treated With Docetaxel: Final Results of a Multinational Phase III Trial (TROPIC)," *J Clin Oncol*, 2010, 28 (15s):4508 [abstract 4508 from 2010 ASCO Annual Meeting].

Sartor AO, Oudard S, Ozguroglu M, et al, "Cabazitaxel or Mitoxantrone With Prednisone in Patients With Metastatic Castration-Resistant Prostate Cancer (mCRPC) Previously Treated With Docetaxel: Final Results of a Multinational Phase III Trial (TROPIC)," 2010 [abstract 9 from 2010 ASCO Genitourinary Cancers Symposium].

CAF

Use Breast cancer

Regimen NOTE: Multiple variations are listed.

Variation 1:

Cyclophosphamide: Oral: 100 mg/m^2/day days 1 to 14
[total dose/cycle = 1400 mg/m^2]

Doxorubicin: I.V.: 30 mg/m^2/day days 1 and 8
[total dose/cycle = 60 mg/m^2]

Fluorouracil: I.V.: 500 mg/m^2/day days 1 and 8
[total dose/cycle = 1000 mg/m^2]

Repeat cycle every 28 days

Variation 2:

Cyclophosphamide: Oral: 100 mg/m^2/day days 1 to 14
[total dose/cycle = 1400 mg/m^2]

Doxorubicin: I.V.: 25 mg/m^2/day days 1 and 8
[total dose/cycle = 50 mg/m^2]

Fluorouracil: I.V.: 500 mg/m^2/day days 1 and 8
[total dose/cycle = 1000 mg/m^2]

Repeat cycle every 28 days

References

Variation 1:

Bull JM, Tormey DC, Li SH, et al, "A Randomized Comparative Trial of Adriamycin® Versus Methotrexate in Combination Drug Therapy," *Cancer*, 1978, 41(5):1649-57.

Variation 2:

Aisner J, Weinberg V, Perloff M, et al, "Chemotherapy Versus Chemoimmunotherapy (CAF v CAFVP v CMF each +/- MER) for Metastatic Carcinoma of the Breast," *J Clin Oncol*, 1987, 5 (10):1523-33.

- **CAF-IV** *see* FAC *on page 1641*
- **CALGB 8811 ALL Regimen** *see* Larson Regimen (ALL) *on page 1699*
- **Capecitabine-Bevacizumab (Breast Cancer)** *see* Bevacizumab-Capecitabine (Breast Cancer) *on page 1528*
- **Capecitabine-Cisplatin (Esophageal Cancer)** *see* Cisplatin-Capecitabine (Esophageal Cancer) *on page 1566*
- **Capecitabine-Cisplatin (Gastric Cancer)** *see* Cisplatin-Capecitabine (Gastric Cancer) *on page 1566*
- **Capecitabine-Cisplatin-Trastuzumab (Gastric Cancer)** *see* Trastuzumab-Cisplatin-Capecitabine (Gastric Cancer) *on page 1757*

Capecitabine + Docetaxel (Breast Cancer)

Use Breast cancer

Regimen NOTE: Multiple variations are listed.

Variation 1:

Capecitabine: Oral: 1250 mg/m^2 twice daily days 1 to 14
[total dose/cycle = 35,000 mg/m^2]

Docetaxel: I.V.: 75 mg/m^2 day 1
[total dose/cycle = 75 mg/m^2]

Repeat cycle every 3 weeks

Variation 2:

Capecitabine: Oral: 1000 mg/m^2 twice daily days 2 to 15
[total dose/cycle = 28,000 mg/m^2]

Docetaxel: I.V.: 75 mg/m^2 day 1
[total dose/cycle = 75 mg/m^2]

Repeat cycle every 3 weeks

Variation 3:

Capecitabine: Oral: 937.5 mg/m^2 twice daily days 2 to 15
[total dose/cycle = 26,250 mg/m^2]

Docetaxel: I.V.: 60 mg/m^2 day 1
[total dose/cycle = 60 mg/m^2]

Repeat cycle every 3 weeks

References

Variation 1:

O'Shaughnessy J, Miles D, Vukelja S, et al, "Superior Survival With Capecitabine Plus Docetaxel Combination Therapy in Anthracycline-Pretreated Patients With Advanced Breast Cancer: Phase III Trial Results," *J Clin Oncol*, 2002, 20(12):2812-23.

Variations 2 and 3:

Lebowitz PF, Eng-Wong J, Swain SM, et al, "A Phase II Trial of Neoadjuvant Docetaxel and Capecitabine for Locally Advanced Breast Cancer," *Clin Cancer Res*, 2004, 10(20):6764-9.

Capecitabine-Docetaxel (Gastric Cancer)

Index Terms Docetaxel-Capecitabine (Gastric Cancer)

Use Gastric cancer

Regimen NOTE: Multiple variations are listed.

Variation 1:
Capecitabine: Oral: 1000 mg/m^2 twice daily days 1 to 14
[total dose/cycle = 28,000 mg/m^2]
Docetaxel: I.V.: 75 mg/m^2 day 1
[total dose/cycle = 75 mg/m^2]
Repeat cycle every 3 weeks for up to 9 cycles or until disease progression or unacceptable toxicity

Variation 2:
Capecitabine: Oral: 1000 mg/m^2 twice daily days 1 to 14
[total dose/cycle = 28,000 mg/m^2]
Docetaxel: I.V.: 36 mg/m^2 days 1 and 8
[total dose/cycle = 72 mg/m^2]
Repeat cycle every 3 weeks until disease progression or unacceptable toxicity

Variation 3:
Capecitabine: Oral: 825 mg/m^2 twice daily days 1 to 14
[total dose/cycle = 23,100 mg/m^2]
Docetaxel: I.V.: 75 mg/m^2 day 1
[total dose/cycle = 75 mg/m^2]
Repeat cycle every 3 weeks until disease progression

Variation 4:
Capecitabine: Oral: 1250 mg/m^2 twice daily days 1 to 14
[total dose/cycle = 35,000 mg/m^2]
Docetaxel: I.V.: 75 mg/m^2 day 1
[total dose/cycle = 75 mg/m^2]
Repeat cycle every 3 weeks until disease progression for up to a maximum of 6 cycles

References

Variation 1:
Kim JG, Sohn SK, Kim DH, et al, "Phase II Study of Docetaxel and Capecitabine in Patients With Metastatic or Recurrent Gastric Cancer," *Oncology*, 2005, 68(2-3):190-5.
Variation 2:
Chun JH, Kim HK, Lee JS, et al, "Weekly Docetaxel in Combination With Capecitabine in Patients With Metastatic Gastric Cancer," *Am J Clin Oncol*, 2005, 28(2):188-94.
Variation 3:
Giordano KF, Jatoi A, Stella PJ, et al, "Docetaxel and Capecitabine in Patients With Metastatic Adenocarcinoma of the Stomach and Gastroesophageal Junction: A Phase II Study From the North Central Cancer Treatment Group," *Ann Oncol*, 2006, 17(4):652-6.
Variation 4:
Park YH, Ryoo BY, Choi SJ, et al, "A Phase II Study of Capecitabine and Docetaxel Combination Chemotherapy in Patients With Advanced Gastric Cancer," *Br J Cancer*, 2004, 90(7):1329-33.

◆ **Capecitabine-Gemcitabine (Biliary Cancer)** *see* Gemcitabine-Capecitabine (Biliary Cancer) *on page 1668*

Capecitabine-Gemcitabine (Pancreatic)

Index Terms GEM-CAP (Pancreatic); Gemcitabine-Capecitabine (Pancreatic)

Use Pancreatic cancer

Regimen NOTE: Multiple variations are listed.

Variation 1:
Gemcitabine: I.V.: 1000 mg/m^2/day over 30 minutes days 1 and 8
[total dose/cycle = 2000 mg/m^2]
Capecitabine: Oral: 650 mg/m^2/dose twice daily days 1 to 14
[total dose/cycle = 18,200 mg/m^2]
Repeat cycle every 21 days until disease progression (maximum duration: 24 weeks)

Variation 2:

Gemcitabine: I.V.: 1000 mg/m²/day over 30 minutes days 1, 8, and 15 [total dose/cycle = 3000 mg/m²]

Capecitabine: Oral: 830 mg/m²/dose twice daily days 1 to 21 [total dose/cycle = 34,860 mg/m²]

Repeat cycle every 28 days until disease progression or unacceptable toxicity

References

Variation 1:

Herrmann R, Bodoky G, Ruhstaller T, et al, "Gemcitabine Plus Capecitabine Compared With Gemcitabine Alone in Advanced Pancreatic Cancer: A Randomized, Multicenter, Phase III Trial of the Swiss Group for Clinical Cancer Research and the Central European Cooperative Oncology Group," *J Clin Oncol*, 2007, 25(16):2212-7.

Variation 2:

Cunningham D, Chau I, Stocken DD, et al, "Phase III Randomized Comparison of Gemcitabine Versus Gemcitabine Plus Capecitabine in Patients With Advanced Pancreatic Cancer," *J Clin Oncol*, 2009, 27(33):5513-8.

- **Capecitabine-Gemcitabine (RCC)** *see* Gemcitabine-Capecitabine (RCC) *on page 1668*
- **Capecitabine-Irinotecan (Esophageal Cancer)** *see* Irinotecan-Capecitabine (Esophageal Cancer) *on page 1693*
- **Capecitabine-Irinotecan (Gastric Cancer)** *see* Irinotecan-Capecitabine (Gastric Cancer) *on page 1693*
- **Capecitabine-Ixabepilone** *see* Ixabepilone-Capecitabine *on page 1698*

Capecitabine + Lapatinib (Breast Cancer)

Index Terms Lapatinib-Capecitabine (Breast Cancer)

Use Breast cancer

Regimen

Capecitabine: Oral: 1000 mg/m² twice daily days 1 to 14 [total dose/cycle = 28,000 mg/m²]

Lapatinib: Oral: 1250 mg/day days 1 to 21 [total dose/cycle = 26,250 mg]

Repeat cycle every 3 weeks

References

Geyer CE, Forster J, Lindquist D, et al, "Lapatinib Plus Capecitabine for HER2-Positive Advanced Breast Cancer," *N Engl J Med*, 2006, 355(26):2733-43.

- **Capecitabine-Oxaliplatin (Biliary Cancer)** *see* CAPOX (Biliary Cancer) *on page 1542*
- **Capecitabine-Oxaliplatin (Colorectal)** *see* XELOX (Colorectal) *on page 1778*
- **Capecitabine-Oxaliplatin-Epirubicin** *see* Epirubicin-Oxaliplatin-Capecitabine *on page 1627*
- **Capecitabine-Oxaliplatin (Pancreatic)** *see* CAPOX (Pancreatic) *on page 1543*

Capecitabine-Trastuzumab

Index Terms Trastuzumab-Capecitabine

Use Breast cancer

Regimen NOTE: Multiple variations are listed.

Variation 1:

Cycle 1:

Capecitabine: Oral: 1250 mg/m^2 twice daily days 1 to 14 [total dose/cycle 1 = 35,000 mg/m^2]

Trastuzumab: I.V.: 4 mg/kg (loading dose) day 1 cycle 1 **followed by** I.V.: 2 mg/kg/day days 8 and 15 cycle 1 [total dose/cycle 1 = 8 mg/kg]

Treatment cycle is 21 days

Subsequent cycles:

Capecitabine: Oral: 1250 mg/m^2 twice daily days 1 to 14 [total dose/cycle = 35,000 mg/m^2]

Trastuzumab: I.V.: 2 mg/kg/day days 1, 8, and 15 [total dose/cycle = 6 mg/kg]

Repeat cycle every 21 days

Variation 2:

Cycle 1:

Capecitabine: Oral: 1250 mg/m^2 twice daily days 1 to 14 [total dose/cycle 1 = 35,000 mg/m^2]

Trastuzumab: I.V.: 8 mg/kg (loading dose) day 1 cycle 1 [total dose/cycle 1 = 8 mg/kg]

Treatment cycle is 21 days

Subsequent cycles:

Capecitabine: Oral: 1250 mg/m^2 twice daily days 1 to 14 [total dose/cycle = 35,000 mg/m^2]

Trastuzumab: I.V.: 6 mg/kg day 1 [total dose/cycle = 6 mg/kg]

Repeat cycle every 21 days

References

Variation 1:

Schaller G, Fuchs I, Gonsch T, et al, "Phase II Study of Capecitabine Plus Trastuzumab in Human Epidermal Growth Factor Receptor 2 Overexpressing Metastatic Breast Cancer Pretreated With Anthracyclines or Taxanes," *J Clin Oncol*, 2007, 25(22):3246-50.

Variation 2:

Bartsch R, Wenzel C, Altorjai G, et al, "Capecitabine and Trastuzumab in Heavily Pretreated Metastatic Breast Cancer," *J Clin Oncol*, 2007, 25(25):3853-8.

◆ **CapeOx (Colorectal)** *see* XELOX (Colorectal) *on page 1778*

CAPOX (Biliary Cancer)

Index Terms Capecitabine-Oxaliplatin (Biliary Cancer); Oxaliplatin-Capecitabine (Biliary Cancer)

Use Biliary adenocarcinoma

Regimen

Capecitabine: Oral: 1000 mg/m^2/dose twice daily days 1 to 14 [total dose/cycle = 28,000 mg/m^2]

Oxaliplatin: I.V.: 130 mg/m^2 over 2 hours day 1 [total dose/cycle = 130 mg/m^2]

Repeat cycle every 3 weeks

References

Nehls O, Oettle H, Hartmann JT, et al, "Capecitabine Plus Oxaliplatin as First-Line Treatment in Patients With Advanced Biliary System Adenocarcinoma: A Prospective Multicentre Phase II Trial," *Br J Cancer*, 2008, 98(2):309-15.

◆ **CAPOX (Colorectal)** *see* XELOX (Colorectal) *on page 1778*

CAPOX (Pancreatic)

Index Terms Capecitabine-Oxaliplatin (Pancreatic); Oxaliplatin-Capecitabine (Pancreatic); XELOX (Pancreatic)

Use Pancreatic cancer

Regimen NOTE: Multiple variations are listed.

Variation 1 (patients <65 years of age and ECOG PS <2):

Capecitabine: Oral: 1000 mg/m² twice daily days 1 to 14
[total dose/cycle = 28,000 mg/m²]

Oxaliplatin: I.V.: 130 mg/m² over 2 hours day 1
[total dose/cycle = 130 mg/m²]

Repeat cycle every 21 days until disease progression or unacceptable toxicity

Variation 2 (patients >65 years of age, ECOG PS of 2, or significant comorbidities):

Capecitabine: Oral: 750 mg/m² twice daily days 1 to 14
[total dose/cycle = 21,000 mg/m²]

Oxaliplatin: I.V.: 110 mg/m² over 2 hours day 1
[total dose/cycle = 110 mg/m²]

Repeat cycle every 21 days until disease progression or unacceptable toxicity

References

Variations 1 and 2:

Xiong HQ, Varadhachary GR, Blais JC, et al, "Phase 2 Trial of Oxaliplatin Plus Capecitabine (XELOX) as Second-Line Therapy for Patients With Advanced Pancreatic Cancer," *Cancer*, 2008, 113(8):2046-52.

Carboplatin-Cetuximab (Head and Neck Cancer)

Index Terms Cetuximab-Carboplatin (Head and Neck Cancer)

Use Head and neck cancer

Regimen

Cycle 1:

Cetuximab: I.V.: 400 mg/m² (loading dose) day 1 (week 1, cycle 1 only)
[total loading dose = 400 mg/m²]

followed by I.V.: 250 mg/m²/day days 8 and 15
[total dose/cycle 1 = 900 mg/m²]

Carboplatin: I.V.: AUC 5 day 1
[total dose/cycle = AUC = 5]

Treatment cycle is 3 weeks

Subsequent cycles:

Cetuximab: I.V.: 250 mg/m²/day days 1, 8, and 15
[total dose/cycle = 750 mg/m²]

Carboplatin: I.V.: AUC 5 day 1
[total dose/cycle = AUC = 5]

Repeat cycle every 3 weeks until disease progression or unacceptable toxicity for up to a maximum of 8 cycles

References

Chan AT, Hsu MM, Goh BC, et al, "Multicenter, Phase II Study of Cetuximab in Combination With Carboplatin in Patients With Recurrent or Metastatic Nasopharyngeal Carcinoma," *J Clin Oncol*, 2005, 23(15):3568-76.

Carboplatin-Docetaxel (Ovarian)

Index Terms Docetaxel-Carboplatin (Ovarian)

Use Ovarian cancer

Regimen NOTE: Multiple variations are listed.

Variation 1:
Docetaxel: I.V.: 60 mg/m^2 over 60 minutes day 1
[total dose/cycle = 60 mg/m^2]
Carboplatin: I.V.: AUC 6 over 30 minutes day 1
[total dose/cycle = AUC = 6]
Repeat cycle every 21 days for 6 cycles
Variation 2:
Docetaxel: I.V.: 75 mg/m^2 over 60 minutes day 1
[total dose/cycle = 75 mg/m^2]
Carboplatin: I.V.: AUC 5 over 30-60 minutes day 1
[total dose/cycle = AUC = 5]
Repeat cycle every 21 days for 6 cycles
Variation 3:
Docetaxel: I.V.: 35 mg/m^2 over 60 minutes days 1, 8, and 15
[total dose/cycle = 105 mg/m^2]
Carboplatin: I.V.: AUC 2 over 30 minutes days 1, 8, and 15
[total dose/cycle = AUC = 6]
Repeat cycle every 28 days until disease progression or unacceptable toxicity or 2 cycles post complete response

References

Variation 1:
Markman M, Kennedy A, Webster K, et al, "Combination Chemotherapy With Carboplatin and Docetaxel in the Treatment of Cancers of the Ovary and Fallopian Tube and Primary Carcinoma of the Peritoneum," *J Clin Oncol*, 2001, 19(7):1901-5.
Variation 2:
Strauss HG, Henze A, Teichmann A, et al, "Phase II Trial of Docetaxel and Carboplatin in Recurrent Platinum-Sensitive Ovarian, Peritoneal, and Tubal Cancer," *Gynecol Oncol*, 2007, 104(3):612-6.
Vasey PA, Jayson GC, Gordon A, et al, "Phase III Randomized Trial of Docetaxel-Carboplatin Versus Paclitaxel-Carboplatin as First-line Chemotherapy for Ovarian Carcinoma," *J Natl Cancer Inst*, 2004, 96(22):1682-91.
Variation 3:
Kushner DM, Connor JP, Sanchez F, et al, "Weekly Docetaxel and Carboplatin for Recurrent Ovarian and Peritoneal Cancer," *Gynecol Oncol*, 2007, 105(2):358-64.

Carboplatin-Docetaxel (Unknown Primary)

Index Terms Docetaxel-Carboplatin (Unknown Primary)

Use Unknown primary (adenocarcinoma)

Regimen

Docetaxel: I.V.: 65 mg/m^2 over 1 hour day 1
[total dose/cycle = 65 mg/m^2]
Carboplatin: I.V.: AUC 6 over 20 minutes day 1
[total dose/cycle = AUC = 6]
Repeat cycle every 21 days for up to a total of 8 cycles

References

Greco FA, Erland JB, Morrissey LH, et al, "Carcinoma of Unknown Primary Site: Phase II Trials With Docetaxel Plus Cisplatin or Carboplatin," *Ann Oncol*, 2000, 11(2):211-5.

Carboplatin-Doxorubicin (Liposomal) (Ovarian)

Index Terms Doxorubicin (Liposomal)-Carboplatin (Ovarian)

Use Ovarian cancer

Regimen NOTE: Multiple variations are listed.

Variation 1:
Doxorubicin (liposomal): I.V.: 30 mg/m^2 day 1
[total dose/cycle = 30 mg/m^2]

Carboplatin: I.V.: AUC 5 day 1
[total dose/cycle = AUC = 5]
Repeat cycle every 28 days until disease progression or unacceptable toxicity
Variation 2:
Doxorubicin (liposomal): I.V.: 30 mg/m^2 over 60 minutes day 1
[total dose/cycle = 30 mg/m^2]
Carboplatin: I.V.: AUC 5 over 30 minutes day 1
[total dose/cycle = AUC = 5]
Repeat cycle every 21 days for 6 cycles

References

Variation 1:
Pujade-Lauraine E, Wagner U, Aavall-Lundqvist E, et al, "Pegylated Liposomal Doxorubicin and Carboplatin Compared With Paclitaxel and Carboplatin for Patients With Platinum-Sensitive Ovarian Cancer in Late Relapse," *J Clin Oncol*, 2010, 28(20):3323-9.
Variation 2:
Pignata S, Scambia G, Ferrandina G, et al, "Carboplatin Plus Paclitaxel Versus Carboplatin Plus Pegylated Liposomal Doxorubicin as First-Line Treatment for Patients With Ovarian Cancer: The MITO-2 Randomized Phase III Trial," *J Clin Oncol*, 2011, 29(27):3628-35.

◆ **Carboplatin, Etoposide, Cyclophosphamide, Doxorubicin, Vincristine (Neuroblastoma)** *see* CE-CAdO (Neuroblastoma) *on page 1555*

Carboplatin-Etoposide-Paclitaxel (Unknown Primary)

Index Terms Paclitaxel-Carboplatin-Etoposide (Unknown Primary)
Use Unknown primary, adenocarcinoma
Regimen
Paclitaxel: I.V.: 200 mg/m^2 over 1 hour day 1
[total dose/cycle = 200 mg/m^2]
Carboplatin: I.V.: AUC 6 over 20-30 minutes day 1
[total dose/cycle = AUC = 6]
Etoposide: Oral: 50 mg/day days 1, 3, 5, 7, and 9
and Oral: 100 mg/day days 2, 4, 6, 8, and 10
[total dose/cycle = 750 mg]
Repeat cycle every 21 days for a total of 4-8 cycles

References

Greco FA, Burris HA 3rd, Erland JB, et al, "Carcinoma of Unknown Primary Site," *Cancer*, 2000, 89 (12):2655-60.

Carboplatin-Etoposide (Retinoblastoma)

Index Terms Etoposide-Carboplatin (Retinoblastoma)
Use Retinoblastoma
Regimen
Etoposide: I.V.: 100 mg/m^2/day over 1 hour days 1 to 5
[total dose/cycle = 500 mg/m^2]
Carboplatin: I.V.: 160 mg/m^2/day over 1 hour days 1 to 5
[total dose/cycle = 800 mg/m^2]
Repeat cycle in 21 to 28 days for a total of 2 cycles

References

Doz F, Neuenschwander S, Plantaz D, et al, "Etoposide and Carboplatin in Extraocular Retinoblastoma: A Study by the Societe Francaise d'Oncologie Pediatrique," *J Clin Oncol*, 1995, 13 (4):902-9.

Carboplatin-Etoposide (Small Cell Lung Cancer)

Index Terms EC (Small Cell Lung Cancer); Etoposide-Carboplatin (Small Cell Lung Cancer)

Use Lung cancer, small cell

Regimen NOTE: Multiple variations are listed.

Variation 1 (limited stage with thoracic radiotherapy):

Carboplatin: I.V.: AUC 6 over 1 hour day 1
[total dose/cycle = AUC = 6]

Etoposide: I.V.: 100 mg/m^2/day over 2 hours days 1, 2, and 3
[total dose/cycle = 300 mg/m^2]

Repeat cycle every 21 days for 6 cycles

Variation 2 (extensive):

Carboplatin: I.V.: AUC 5 day 1
[total dose/cycle = AUC = 5]

Etoposide: I.V.: 100 mg/m^2/day days 1, 2, and 3
[total dose/cycle = 300 mg/m^2]

Repeat cycle every 21 days for 6 cycles

Variation 3 (elderly, limited, and extensive):

Carboplatin: I.V.: AUC 5 over 1 hour day 1
[total dose/cycle = AUC = 5]

Etoposide: I.V.: 100 mg/m^2/day over 1 hour days 1, 2, and 3
[total dose/cycle = 300 mg/m^2]

Repeat cycle every 28 days for 4 cycles

References

Variation 1:

Skarlos DV, Samantas E, Briassoulis E, et al, "Randomized Comparison of Early Versus Late Hyperfractionated Thoracic Irradiation Concurrently With Chemotherapy in Limited Disease Small-Cell Lung Cancer: A Randomized Phase II Study of the Hellenic Cooperative Oncology Group (HeCOG)," *Ann Oncol*, 2001, 12(9):1231-8.

Variation 2:

Socinski MA, Smit EF, Lorigan P, et al, "Phase III Study of Pemetrexed Plus Carboplatin Compared With Etoposide Plus Carboplatin in Chemotherapy-Naïve Patients With Extensive-Stage Small Cell-Cell Lung Cancer," *J Clin Oncol*, 2009, 27(28):4787-92.

Variation 3:

Okamoto H, Watanabe K, Nishiwaki Y, et al, "Phase II Study of Area Under the Plasma-Concentration-Versus-Time Curve-Based Carboplatin Plus Standard-Dose Intravenous Etoposide in Elderly Patients With Small-Cell Lung Cancer," *J Clin Oncol*, 1999, 17(11):3540-5.

Carboplatin-Etoposide-Vincristine (Retinoblastoma)

Index Terms Etoposide-Carboplatin-Vincristine (Retinoblastoma); Vincristine-Carboplatin-Etoposide (Retinoblastoma)

Use Retinoblastoma

Regimen NOTE: Multiple variations are listed.

Variation 1 (<1 year of age):

Carboplatin: I.V.: 20 mg/kg day 1
[total dose/cycle = 20 mg/kg]

Etoposide Phosphate: I.V.: 5 mg/kg day 1
[total dose/cycle = 5 mg/kg]

Vincristine: I.V.: 0.05 mg/kg day 1
[total dose/cycle = 0.05 mg/kg]

Variation 2 (age >1 year):

Carboplatin: I.V.: 550-600 mg/m^2 day 1
[total dose/cycle = 550-600 mg/m^2]

Etoposide Phosphate: I.V.: 150 mg/m^2 day 1
[total dose/cycle = 150 mg/m^2]

Vincristine: I.V.: 1.5-2 mg/m^2 day 1
[total dose/cycle = 1.5-2 mg/m^2]

Variation 3 (≤36 months of age):

Carboplatin: I.V.: 18.6 mg/kg day 1
[total dose/cycle = 18.6 mg/kg]

Etoposide: I.V.: 5 mg/kg days 1 and 2
[total dose/cycle = 10 mg/kg]

Vincristine: I.V.: 0.05 mg/kg day 1 (maximum dose: 2 mg)
[total dose/cycle = 0.05 mg/kg; maximum dose: 2 mg]

Repeat cycle every 28 days for a total of 6 cycles

Variation 4 (>36 months of age):

Carboplatin: I.V.: 560 mg/m^2 day 1
[total dose/cycle = 560 mg/m^2]

Etoposide: I.V.: 150 mg/m^2 days 1 and 2
[total dose/cycle = 300 mg/m^2]

Vincristine: I.V.: 1.5 mg/m^2 day 1 (maximum dose: 2 mg)
[total dose/cycle = 1.5 mg/m^2; maximum dose: 2 mg]

Repeat cycle every 28 days for a total of 6 cycles

References

Variations 1 and 2:

Sussman DA, Escalona-Benz E, Benz MS, et al, "Comparison of Retinoblastoma Reduction for Chemotherapy vs External Beam Radiotherapy," *Arch Ophthalmol*, 2003, 121(7):979-84.

Variations 3 and 4:

Friedman DL, Himelstein B, Shields CL, et al, "Chemoreduction and Local Ophthalmic Therapy for Intraocular Retinoblastoma," *J Clin Oncol*, 2000, 18(1):12-7.

Shields CL, Honavar SG, Meadows AT, et al, "Chemoreduction for Unilateral Retinoblastoma," *Arch Ophthalmol*, 2002, 120(12):1653-8.

◆ **Carboplatin-Fluorouracil-Cetuximab (Head and Neck Cancer)** *see* Cetuximab-Carboplatin-Fluorouracil (Head and Neck Cancer) *on page 1557*

◆ **Carboplatin-Fluorouracil (Head and Neck Cancer)** *see* Fluorouracil-Carboplatin (Head and Neck Cancer) *on page 1652*

Carboplatin-Gemcitabine (NSCLC)

Index Terms GC (NSCLC); Gemcitabine-Carboplatin (NSCLC)

Use Lung cancer, nonsmall cell

Regimen NOTE: Multiple variations are listed.

Variation 1:

Gemcitabine: I.V.: 1000 mg/m^2/day over 30 minutes days 1, 8, and 15
[total dose/cycle = 3000 mg/m^2]

Carboplatin: I.V.: AUC 5 day 1
[total dose/cycle = AUC = 5]

Repeat cycle every 28 days for up to 4 cycles

Variation 2:

Gemcitabine: I.V.: 1000 mg/m^2/day days 1 and 8
[total dose/cycle = 2000 mg/m^2]

Carboplatin: I.V.: AUC 5 day 1
[total dose/cycle = AUC = 5]

Repeat cycle every 21 days for up to 4 cycles

References

Variation 1:

Danson S, Middleton MR, O'Byrne KJ, et al, "Phase III Trial of Gemcitabine and Carboplatin Versus Mitomycin, Ifosfamide, and Cisplatin or Mitomycin, Vinblastine, and Cisplatin in Patients With Advanced Nonsmall Cell Lung Carcinoma," *Cancer*, 2003, 98(3):542-53.

Variation 2:

Grønberg BH, Bremnes RM, Fløtten O, et al, "Phase III Study by the Norwegian Lung Cancer Study Group: Pemetrexed Plus Carboplatin Compared With Gemcitabine Plus Carboplatin as First-Line Chemotherapy in Advanced Non-Small-Cell Lung Cancer," *J Clin Oncol*, 2009, 27 (19):3217-24

Carboplatin-Gemcitabine (Ovarian)

Index Terms Gemcitabine-Carboplatin (Ovarian)

Use Ovarian cancer

Regimen

Gemcitabine: I.V.: 1000 mg/m^2/day days 1 and 8
[total dose/cycle = 2000 mg/m^2]

Carboplatin: I.V.: AUC 4 day 1
[total dose/cycle = AUC = 4]

Repeat cycle every 21 days for 6-10 cycles

References

Pfisterer J, Plante M, Vergote I, et al, "Gemcitabine Plus Carboplatin Compared With Carboplatin in Patients With Platinum-Sensitive Recurrent Ovarian Cancer: An Intergroup Trial of the AGO-OVAR, the NCIC CTG, and the EORTC GCG," *J Clin Oncol*, 2006, 24(29):4699-707.

Carboplatin-Gemcitabine-Paclitaxel (Unknown Primary)

Index Terms Gemcitabine-Carboplatin-Paclitaxel (Unknown Primary); Paclitaxel-Carboplatin-Gemcitabine (Unknown Primary)

Use Unknown primary (adenocarcinoma)

Regimen

Paclitaxel: I.V.: 200 mg/m^2 over 1 hour day 1
[total dose/cycle = 200 mg/m^2]

Carboplatin: I.V.: AUC 5 over 20-30 minutes day 1
[total dose/cycle = AUC = 5]

Gemcitabine: I.V.: 1000 mg/m^2/day days 1 and 8
[total dose/cycle = 2000 mg/m^2]

Repeat cycle every 21 days for a total of 4 cycles

Followed by:

Paclitaxel: I.V.: 70 mg/m^2 days 1, 8, 15, 22, 29, 36
[total dose/cycle = 420 mg/m^2]

Repeat cycle every 56 days for a total of 3 cycles

References

Greco FA, Burris HA 3rd, Litchy S, et al, "Gemcitabine, Carboplatin, and Paclitaxel for Patients With Carcinoma of Unknown Primary Site: A Minnie Pearl Cancer Research Network Study," *J Clin Oncol*, 2002, 20(6):1651-6.

Carboplatin-Irinotecan (Small Cell Lung Cancer)

Index Terms IC (Small Cell Lung Cancer); IP (Small Cell Lung Cancer); Irinotecan-Carboplatin (Small Cell Lung Cancer)

Use Lung cancer, small cell

Regimen NOTE: Multiple variations are listed.

Variation 1:

Carboplatin: I.V.: AUC 5 (Calvert formula) day 1
[total dose/cycle = AUC = 5]

Irinotecan: I.V.: 175 mg/m^2 day 1
[total dose/cycle = 175 mg/m^2]

Repeat cycle every 21 days for a total of 4 cycles

Variation 2:

Carboplatin: I.V.: AUC 5 (Calvert formula) over 1 hour day 1
[total dose/cycle = AUC = 5]

Irinotecan: I.V.: 50 mg/m^2/day over 30 minutes days 1, 8, and 15
[total dose/cycle = 150 mg/m^2]

Repeat cycle every 28 days

References

Variation 1:

Hermes A, Bergman B, Bremnes R, et al, "Irinotecan Plus Carboplatin Versus Oral Etoposide Plus Carboplatin in Extensive Small-Cell Lung Cancer: A Randomized Phase III Trial," *J Clin Oncol*, 2008, 26(26):4261-7.

Variation 2:

Schmittel A, Fischer von Weikersthal L, Sebastian M, et al, "A Randomized Phase II Trial of Irinotecan Plus Carboplatin Versus Etoposide Plus Carboplatin Treatment in Patients With Extended Disease Small-Cell Lung Cancer," *Ann Oncol*, 2006, 17(4):663-7.

Schmittel A, Sebastian M, Fischer von Weikersthal L, et al, "A German Multicenter, Randomized Phase III Trial Comparing Irinotecan-Carboplatin With Etoposide-Carboplatin as First-Line Therapy for Extensive-Disease Small-Cell Lung Cancer," *Ann Oncol*, 2011, 22(8):1798-804.

◆ **Carboplatin-Paclitaxel-Bevacizumab (NSCLC)** *see* Bevacizumab-Carboplatin-Paclitaxel (NSCLC) *on page 1528*

◆ **Carboplatin-Paclitaxel (Bladder Cancer)** *see* Paclitaxel-Carboplatin (Bladder Cancer) *on page 1726*

Carboplatin-Paclitaxel (Cervical Cancer)

Index Terms Paclitaxel-Carboplatin (Cervical Cancer)

Use Cervical cancer

Regimen NOTE: Multiple variations are listed.

Variation 1:

Paclitaxel: I.V.: 175 mg/m^2 over 3 hours day 1 (reduce to 155 mg/m^2 over 3 hours day 1 if prior pelvic irradiation)
[total dose/cycle = 175 (or 155) mg/m^2]

Carboplatin: I.V.: AUC 5 or 6 day 1
[total dose/cycle = AUC = 5 or 6]

Repeat cycle every 28 days for up to a total of 6-9 cycles

Variation 2:

Paclitaxel: I.V.: 175 mg/m^2 over 3 hours day 1
[total dose/cycle = 175 mg/m^2]

Carboplatin: I.V.: AUC 5 day 1
[total dose/cycle = AUC = 5]

Repeat cycle every 21 days for 6-9 cycles

References

Variation 1:

Tinker AV, Bhagat K, Swenerton KD, et al, "Carboplatin and Paclitaxel for Advanced and Recurrent Cervical Carcinoma: The British Columbia Cancer Agency Experience," *Gynecol Oncol*, 2005, 98 (1):54-8.

Variation 2:

Pectasides D, Fountzilas G, Papaxoinis G, et al, "Carboplatin and Paclitaxel in Metastatic or Recurrent Cervical Cancer," *Int J Gynecol Cancer*, 2009, 19(4):777-81.

◆ **Carboplatin-Paclitaxel (Esophageal Cancer)** *see* Paclitaxel-Carboplatin (Esophageal Cancer) *on page 1726*

Carboplatin-Paclitaxel (Ovarian)

Index Terms Paclitaxel-Carboplatin (Ovarian)

Use Ovarian cancer

Regimen NOTE: Multiple variations are listed.

Variation 1:

Paclitaxel: I.V.: 175 mg/m^2 over 3 hours day 1
[total dose/cycle = 175 mg/m^2]

Carboplatin: I.V.: AUC 7.5 day 1
[total dose/cycle = AUC = 7.5]

Repeat cycle every 21 days for a total of 6 cycles

Variation 2:

Paclitaxel: I.V.: 175-185 mg/m^2 over 3 hours day 1
[total dose/cycle = 175-185 mg/m^2]

Carboplatin: I.V.: AUC 5-6 day 1
[total dose/cycle = AUC = 5-6]

Repeat cycle every 21 days

Variation 3:

Paclitaxel: I.V.: 175 mg/m^2 over 3 hours day 1
[total dose/cycle = 175 mg/m^2]

Carboplatin: I.V.: AUC 5 day 1
[total dose/cycle = AUC = 5]

Repeat cycle every 21 days

Variation 4:

Paclitaxel: I.V.: 175 mg/m^2 over 3 hours day 1
[total dose/cycle = 175 mg/m^2]

Carboplatin: I.V.: AUC 7.5 over 30 minutes day 1
[total dose/cycle = AUC = 7.5]

Repeat cycle every 21 days for 3-6 cycles

Variation 5:

Paclitaxel: I.V.: 80 mg/m^2 over 1 hour days 1, 8, and 15
[total dose/cycle = 240 mg/m^2]

Carboplatin: I.V.: AUC 6 over 1 hour day 1
[total dose/cycle = AUC = 6]

Repeat cycle every 21 days for a total of 6 cycles

References

Variation 1:

Ozols RF, Bundy BN, Greer BE, et al, "Phase III Trial of Carboplatin and Paclitaxel Compared With Cisplatin and Paclitaxel in Patients With Optimally Resected Stage III Ovarian Cancer: A Gynecologic Oncology Group Study," *J Clin Oncol*, 2003, 21(17):3194-200.

Variation 2:

Parmar MK, Ledermann JA, Colombo N, et al, "Paclitaxel Plus Platinum-Based Chemotherapy Versus Conventional Platinum-Based Chemotherapy in Women With Relapsed Ovarian Cancer: The ICON4/AGO-OVAR-2.2 Trial," *Lancet*, 2003, 361(9375):2099-106.

Variation 3:

Neijt JP, Engelholm SA, Tuxen MK, et al, "Exploratory Phase III Study of Paclitaxel and Cisplatin Versus Paclitaxel and Carboplatin in Advanced Ovarian Cancer," *J Clin Oncol*, 2000, 18 (17):3084-92.

Vasey PA, Jayson GC, Gordon A, et al, "Phase III Randomized Trial of Docetaxel-Carboplatin Versus Paclitaxel-Carboplatin as First-Line Chemotherapy for Ovarian Carcinoma," *J Natl Cancer Inst*, 2004, 96(22):1682-91.

Variation 4:

Bell J, Brady MF, Young RC, et al, "Randomized Phase III Trial of Three Versus Six Cycles of Adjuvant Carboplatin and Paclitaxel in Early Stage Epithelial Ovarian Carcinoma: A Gynecologic Oncology Group Study," *Gynecol Oncol*, 2006, 102(3):432-9.

Variation 5:
Katsumata N, Yasuda M, Takahashi F, et al, "Dose-Dense Paclitaxel Once a Week in Combination With Carboplatin Every 3 Weeks for Advanced Ovarian Cancer: A Phase III, Open-Label, Randomised Trial," *Lancet*, 2009, 374(9698):1331-8.

Carboplatin-Paclitaxel (Unknown Primary)

Index Terms Carbo-Tax (Unknown Primary); Paclitaxel-Carboplatin (Unknown Primary)

Use Unknown primary (adenocarcinoma)

Regimen

Carboplatin: I.V.: Target AUC 6 day 1
[total dose/cycle = AUC = 6]

followed by

Paclitaxel: I.V.: 200 mg/m^2 infused over 3 hours day 1
[total dose/cycle = 200 mg/m^2]

Filgrastim: SubQ: 300 mcg/day days 5 to 12
[total dose/cycle = 2400 mcg]

Repeat cycle every 21 days for a total of 6 or 8 cycles

References

Briasoulis E, Kalofonos H, Bafaloukos D, et al, "Carboplatin Plus Paclitaxel in Unknown Primary Carcinoma: A Phase II Hellenic Cooperative Oncology Group Study," *J Clin Oncol*, 2000, 18 (17):3101-7.

◆ **Carboplatin-Pemetrexed-Bevacizumab (NSCLC)** *see* Bevacizumab-Carboplatin-Pemetrexed (NSCLC) *on page* 1529

Carboplatin-Pemetrexed (Mesothelioma)

Index Terms Pemetrexed-Carboplatin (Mesothelioma)

Use Malignant pleural mesothelioma

Regimen

Pemetrexed: I.V.: 500 mg/m^2 over 10 minutes day 1
[total dose/cycle = 500 mg/m^2]

Carboplatin: I.V.: AUC 5 over 30 minutes day 1 (start 30 minutes after pemetrexed)
[total dose/cycle = AUC = 5]

Repeat cycle every 21 days

References

Ceresoli GL, Zucali PA, Favaretto AG, et al, "Phase II Study of Pemetrexed Plus Carboplatin in Malignant Pleural Mesothelioma," *J Clin Oncol*, 2006, 24(9):1443-8.
Santoro A, O'Brien ME, Stahel RA, et al, "Pemetrexed Plus Cisplatin or Pemetrexed Plus Carboplatin for Chemonaïve Patients With Malignant Pleural Mesothelioma: Results of the International Expanded Access Program," *J Thorac Oncol*, 2008, 3(7):756-63.

Carboplatin-Pemetrexed (NSCLC)

Index Terms Pemetrexed-Carboplatin (NSCLC)

Use Lung cancer, nonsmall cell

Regimen

Pemetrexed: I.V.: 500 mg/m^2 day 1
[total dose/cycle = 500 mg/m^2]

Carboplatin: I.V.: AUC 5 day 1
[total dose/cycle = AUC = 5]

Repeat cycle every 21 days for a maximum of 4 cycles

References

Gronberg BH, Bremnes RM, Flotten O, et al, "Phase III Study by the Norwegian Lung Cancer Study Group: Pemetrexed Plus Carboplatin Compared With Gemcitabine Plus Carboplatin as First-Line Chemotherapy in Advanced Non-Small-Cell Lung Cancer," *J Clin Oncol*, 2009, 27(19):3217-24.

Carboplatin (Testicular Regimen)

Use Testicular cancer

Regimen NOTE: Multiple variations are listed.

Variation 1:

Carboplatin: I.V.: AUC 7 day 1

[total dose/cycle = AUC = 7]

This is administered as a one-time infusion

Variation 2:

Carboplatin: I.V.: AUC 7 day 1

[total dose/cycle = AUC = 7]

Repeat cycle every 21 days for a total of 2 cycles

References

Variation 1:

Oliver RT, Mason MD, Mead GM, et al, "Radiotherapy Versus Single-Dose Carboplatin in Adjuvant Treatment of Stage I Seminoma: A Randomised Trial," *Lancet*, 2005, 366(9482):293-300.

Oliver RT, Mead GM, Rustin G, et al, "Randomized Trial of Carboplatin Versus Radiotherapy for Stage I Seminoma: Mature Results on Relapse and Contralateral Testis Cancer Rates in MRC TE19/EORTC 30982 Study (ISRCTN27163214)," *J Clin Oncol*, 2011, 29(8):957-62.

Variation 2:

Aparicio J, Germa JR, Garcia del Muro X, et al, "Risk-Adapted Management for Patients With Clinical Stage I Seminoma: The Second Spanish Germ Cell Cancer Cooperative Group Study," *J Clin Oncol*, 2005, 23(34):8717-23.

Carboplatin-Vincristine (Retinoblastoma)

Index Terms Vincristine-Carboplatin (Retinoblastoma)

Use Retinoblastoma

Regimen NOTE: Multiple variations are listed.

Variation 1 (GFR >50 mL/minute/m^2):

Carboplatin: I.V.: 560 mg/m^2 day 1

[total dose/cycle = 560 mg/m^2]

Vincristine: I.V.: 0.05 mg/kg day 1

[total dose/cycle = 0.05 mg/kg]

Repeat for up to a total of 8 cycles

Variation 2 (GFR <50 mL/minute/m^2):

Carboplatin: I.V.: AUC 6.5 day 1

[total dose/cycle = AUC 6.5]

Vincristine: I.V.: 0.05 mg/kg day 1

[total dose/cycle = 0.05 mg/kg]

Repeat for up to a total of 8 cycles

References

Rodriguez-Galindo C, Wilson MW, Haik BG, et al, "Treatment of Intraocular Retinoblastoma With Vincristine and Carboplatin," *J Clin Oncol*, 2003, 21(10):2019-25.

◆ **Carboplatin–Etoposide (Ovarian Cancer)** *see* Etoposide-Carboplatin (Ovarian Cancer) *on page* 1639

Carbo-Tax (NSCLC)

Index Terms Paclitaxel-Carboplatin (Nonsmall Cell Lung Cancer)

Use Lung cancer, nonsmall cell

Regimen

Paclitaxel: I.V.: 135-215 mg/m^2 infused over 24 hours day 1

[total dose/cycle = 135-215 mg/m^2]

or I.V.: 175 mg/m^2 infused over 3 hours day 1

[total dose/cycle = 175 mg/m^2]

followed by

Carboplatin: I.V.: Target AUC 7.5

[total dose/cycle = AUC = 7.5]

Repeat cycle every 21 days

References

Langer CJ, Leighton JC, Comis RL, et al, "Paclitaxel By 24- or 1-Hour Infusion in Combination With Carboplatin in Advanced Nonsmall-Cell Lung Cancer: The Fox Chase Cancer Center Experience," *Semin Oncol*, 1995, 22(4 Suppl 9):18-29.

◆ **Carbo-Tax (Unknown Primary)** *see* Carboplatin-Paclitaxel (Unknown Primary) *on page* 1551

Carfilzomib (Multiple Myeloma Regimen)

Use Multiple myeloma

Regimen

Cycle 1:

Carfilzomib: I.V.: 20 mg/m^2/day over 2-10 minutes days 1, 2, 8, 9, 15, and 16

[total dose/cycle = 120 mg/m^2]

Treatment cycle is 28 days

Cycles 2-12:

Carfilzomib: I.V.: 27 mg/m^2/day over 2-10 minutes days 1, 2, 8, 9, 15, and 16

[total dose/cycle = 162 mg/m^2]

Repeat cycle every 28 days

References

Siegel DS, Martin T, Wang M, et al, "A Phase 2 Study of Single-Agent Carfilzomib (PX-171-003-A01) in Patients With Relapsed and Refractory Multiple Myeloma," *Blood*, 2012, 120:2817-25.

Vij R, Wang M, Kaufman JL, et al, "An Open-Label, Single-Arm, Phase 2 (PX-171-004) Study of Single-Agent Carfilzomib in Bortezomib-Naïve Patients With Relapsed and/or Refractory Multiple Myeloma," *Blood*, 2012, 119:5661-70.

◆ **Carmustine-Etoposide-Cytarabine-Melphalan (Hodgkin)** *see* mini-BEAM (Hodgkin) *on page* 1712

CaT (NSCLC)

Use Lung cancer, nonsmall cell

Regimen NOTE: Multiple variations are listed.

Variation 1:

Paclitaxel: I.V.: 175 mg/m^2 day 1

[total dose/cycle = 175 mg/m^2]

or I.V.: 135 mg/m^2 continuous infusion day 1

[total dose/cycle = 135 mg/m^2]

Carboplatin: I.V.: AUC 7.5 day 1 or 2

[total dose/cycle = AUC = 7.5]

Repeat cycle every 21 days

Variation 2:

Paclitaxel: I.V.: 225 mg/m^2 day 1

[total dose/cycle = 225 mg/m^2]

Carboplatin: I.V.: AUC 6 day 1

[total dose/cycle = AUC = 6]

Repeat cycle every 21 days

References

Variation 1:

Langer CJ, Leighton JC, Comis RL, et al, "Paclitaxel by 24- or 1-Hour Infusion in Combination With Carboplatin in Advanced Nonsmall-Cell Lung Cancer: The Fox Chase Cancer Center Experience," *Semin Oncol*, 1995, 22(4 Suppl 9):18-29.

Variation 2:

Schiller JH, Harrington D, Belani CP, et al, "Comparison of Four Chemotherapy Regimens for Advanced Nonsmall-Cell Lung Cancer," *N Engl J Med*, 2002, 346(2):92-8.

CAV-P/VP (Neuroblastoma)

Index Terms Cyclophosphamide, Doxorubicin, Vincristine, Etoposide, Cisplatin (Neuroblastoma); N6 Protocol (Neuroblastoma)

Use Neuroblastoma

Regimen

Note: The interval between courses is not fixed; the next course to begin upon hematologic recovery (ANC ≥500/mm^3 and platelets ≥100,000/mm^3)

Course 1, 2, 4, and 6 (CAV):

Cyclophosphamide: I.V.: 70 mg/kg/day over 6 hours days 1 and 2
[total dose/cycle = 140 mg/kg]

Doxorubicin: I.V.: 25 mg/m^2/day continuous infusion days 1, 2, and 3
[total dose/cycle = 75 mg/m^2]

Vincristine: I.V.: 0.033 mg/kg/day continuous infusion days 1, 2, and 3
[total dose/cycle = 0.099 mg/kg]

Vincristine: I.V.: 1.5 mg/m^2 bolus day 9
[total dose/cycle = 1.5 mg/m^2]

Course 3, 5, and 7 (P/VP):

Etoposide: I.V.: 200 mg/m^2/day over 2 hours days 1, 2, and 3
[total dose/cycle = 600 mg/m^2]

Cisplatin: I.V.: 50 mg/m^2/day over 1 hour days 1 to 4
[total dose/cycle = 200 mg/m^2]

References

Kushner BH, LaQuaglia MP, Bonilla MA, et al, "Highly Effective Induction Therapy for Stage 4 Neuroblastoma in Children Over 1 Year of Age," *J Clin Oncol*, 1994, 12(12):2607-13.

CAV (Small Cell Lung Cancer)

Index Terms Cyclophosphamide, Doxorubicin, Vincristine (Small Cell Lung Cancer)

Use Lung cancer, small cell

Regimen

Cyclophosphamide: I.V.: 1000 mg/m^2 day 1
[total dose/cycle = 1000 mg/m^2; maximum: 2000 mg]

Doxorubicin: I.V.: 45 mg/m^2 day 1
[total dose/cycle = 45 mg/m^2; maximum: 100 mg]

Vincristine: I.V.: 2 mg day 1
[total dose/cycle = 2 mg]

Repeat cycle every 21 days

References

von Pawel J, Schiller JH, Shephard FA, et al, "Topotecan Versus Cyclophosphamide, Doxorubicin, and Vincristine for the Treatment of Recurrent Small-Cell Lung Cancer," *J Clin Oncol*, 1999, 17 (2):658-67.

CDDP/VP-16

Use Brain tumors

Regimen

Cisplatin: I.V.: 90 mg/m^2 day 1
[total dose/cycle = 90 mg/m^2]

Etoposide: I.V.: 150 mg/m^2/day days 3 and 4
[total dose/cycle = 300 mg/m^2]

Repeat cycle every 21 days

References

Kovnar EH, Kellie SJ, Horowitz ME, et al, "Preirradiation Cisplatin and Etoposide in the Treatment of High-Risk Medulloblastoma and Other Malignant Embryonal Tumors of the Central Nervous System: A Phase II Study," *J Clin Oncol*, 1990, 8(2):330-6.

CE-CAdO (Neuroblastoma)

Index Terms Carboplatin, Etoposide, Cyclophosphamide, Doxorubicin, Vincristine (Neuroblastoma)

Use Neuroblastoma

Regimen

Variation 1:

Cycles 1 and 2 (CE):

Carboplatin: I.V.: 200 mg/m^2/day days 1, 2, and 3
[total dose/cycle = 600 mg/m^2]

Etoposide: I.V.: 150 mg/m^2/day days 1, 2, and 3
[total dose/cycle = 450 mg/m^2]

Repeat CE cycle once at 21 days, then follow with

Cycles 3 and 4 (CAdO):

Cyclophosphamide: I.V.: 300 mg/m^2/day days 1 to 5
[total dose/cycle = 1500 mg/m^2]

Doxorubicin: I.V.: 60 mg/m^2 day 5
[total dose/cycle = 60 mg/m^2]

Vincristine: I.V.: 1.5 mg/m^2 (maximum dose: 2 mg) days 1 and 5
[total dose/cycle = 3 mg/m^2 (maximum: 2 mg/dose)]

Repeat CAdO cycle once at 21 days

Variation 2:

Cycles 1 and 2 (CE):

Carboplatin: I.V.: 6.6 mg/kg/day days 1, 2, and 3
[total dose/cycle = 19.8 mg/kg]

Etoposide: I.V.: 5 mg/kg/day days 1, 2, and 3
[total dose/cycle = 15 mg/kg]

Repeat CE cycle once, then follow with

Cycles 3 and 4 (CAdO):

Cyclophosphamide: I.V.: 10 mg/kg/day days 1 to 5
[total dose/cycle = 50 mg/kg]

Doxorubicin: I.V.: 2 mg/kg day 5
[total dose/cycle = 2 mg/kg]

Vincristine: I.V.: 0.05 mg/kg days 1 and 5
[total dose/cycle = 0.1 mg/kg]

Repeat CAdO cycle once

References

Variation 1:

Rubie H, Michon J, Plantaz D, et al, "Unresectable Localized Neuroblastoma: Improved Survival After Primary Chemotherapy Including Carboplatin-Etoposide. Neuroblastoma Study Group of the Societe Francaise d'Oncologie Pediatrique (SFOP)," *Br J Cancer*, 1998, 77(12):2310-7.

Variation 2:

Rubie H, Plantaz D, Coze C, et al, "Localised and Unresectable Neuroblastoma in Infants: Excellent Outcome With Primary Chemotherapy. Neuroblastoma Study Group, Société Française d'Oncologie Pédiatrique," *Med Pediatr Oncol*, 2001, 36(1):247-50.

CEF

Use Breast cancer

Regimen

Cyclophosphamide: Oral: 75 mg/m^2/day days 1 to 14
[total dose/cycle = 1050 mg/m^2]

Epirubicin: I.V.: 60 mg/m^2/day days 1 and 8
[total dose/cycle = 120 mg/m^2]

Fluorouracil: I.V.: 500 mg/m^2/day days 1 and 8
[total dose/cycle = 1000 mg/m^2]

Repeat cycle every 28 days

References

Levine MN, Bramwell VH, Pritchard KI, et al, "Randomized Trial of Intensive Cyclophosphamide, Epirubicin, and Fluorouracil Chemotherapy Compared With Cyclophosphamide, Methotrexate, and Fluorouracil in Premenopausal Women With Node-Positive Breast Cancer, National Cancer Institute of Canada Clinical Trials Group," *J Clin Oncol*, 1998, 16(8):2651-8.

CEPP(B)

Use Lymphoma, non-Hodgkin's

Regimen

Cyclophosphamide: I.V.: 600-650 mg/m^2/day days 1 and 8
[total dose/cycle = 1200-1300 mg/m^2]

Etoposide: I.V.: 70-85 mg/m^2/day days 1, 2, and 3
[total dose/cycle = 210-255 mg/m^2]

Procarbazine: Oral: 60 mg/m^2/day days 1 to 10
[total dose/cycle = 600 mg/m^2]

Prednisone: Oral: 60 mg/m^2/day days 1 to 10
[total dose/cycle = 600 mg/m^2]

Bleomycin: I.V.: 15 units/m^2/day days 1 and 15 (Bleomycin is sometimes omitted)
[total dose/cycle = 30 units/m^2]

Repeat cycle every 28 days

References

Chao NJ, Rosenberg SA, and Horning SJ, "CEPP(B): An Effective and Well-Tolerated Regimen in Poor-Risk, Aggressive Non-Hodgkin's Lymphoma," *Blood*, 1990, 76(7):1293-8.

Cetuximab Biweekly (Colorectal Regimen)

Index Terms Biweekly Cetuximab (Colorectal Regimen); Every 2 Weeks Cetuximab (Colorectal Regimen)

Use Colorectal cancer

Regimen

Cetuximab: I.V.: 500 mg/m^2 day 1; over 120 minutes for the first infusion, and over 60 minutes for subsequent infusions

[total dose/cycle = 500 mg/m^2]

Repeat cycle every 14 days until disease progression or unacceptable toxicity

References

Bouchahda M, Marcarulla T, Liedo G, et al, "Feasibility of Cetuximab Given With a Simplified Schedule of Every 2 Weeks in Advanced Colorectal Cancer: A Multicenter, Retrospective Analysis," *Med Oncol*, 2011, 28(Suppl 1):S253-8.

Tabernero J, Pfeiffer P, and Cervantes A, "Administration of Cetuximab Every 2 Weeks in the Treatment of Metastatic Colorectal Cancer: An Effective, More Convenient, Alternative to Weekly Administration," *Oncologist*, 2008, 13(2):113-9.

Cetuximab (Biweekly)-Irinotecan

Index Terms Irinotecan-Biweekly Cetuximab

Use Colorectal cancer

Regimen

Cycle 1:

Cetuximab: I.V.: 500 mg/m^2 over 120 minutes day 1 (cycle 1 only)

[total dose/cycle = 500 mg/m^2]

Irinotecan: I.V.: 180 mg/m^2 day 1

[total dose/cycle = 180 mg/m^2]

Subsequent cycles:

Cetuximab: I.V.: 500 mg/m^{2}over 60 minutes day 1

[total dose/cycle = 500 mg/m^2]

Irinotecan: I.V.: 180 mg/m^2 day 1

[total dose/cycle = 180 mg/m^2]

Repeat cycle every 14 days

References

Pfeiffer P, Nielsen D, Bjerregaard J, et al, "Biweekly Cetuximab and Irinotecan as Third-Line Therapy in Patients With Advanced Colorectal Cancer After Failure to Irinotecan, Oxaliplatin and 5-Fluorouracil," *Ann Oncol*, 2008, 19(6):1141-5.

Cetuximab-Carboplatin-Fluorouracil (Head and Neck Cancer)

Index Terms Carboplatin-Fluorouracil-Cetuximab (Head and Neck Cancer)

Use Head and neck cancer

Regimen

Cycle 1:

Cetuximab: I.V.: 400 mg/m^2 (loading dose) day 1 (week 1, cycle 1 only)

[total loading dose = 400 mg/m^2]

followed by I.V.: 250 mg/m^2/day days 8 and 15

[total dose/cycle 1 = 900 mg/m^2]

Carboplatin: I.V.: AUC 5 day 1

[total dose/cycle = AUC = 5]

Fluorouracil: I.V.: 1000 mg/m^2/day continuous infusion days 1 to 4

[total dose/cycle = 4000 mg/m^2]

Treatment cycle is 3 weeks

Subsequent cycles:

Cetuximab: I.V.: 250 mg/m^2/day days 1, 8, and 15

[total dose/cycle = 750 mg/m^2]

Carboplatin: I.V.: AUC 5 day 1

[total dose/cycle = AUC = 5]

Fluorouracil: I.V.: 1000 mg/m^2/day continuous infusion days 1 to 4
[total dose/cycle = 4000 mg/m^2]
Repeat cycle every 3 weeks for a total of up to 6 cycles (cetuximab monotherapy may be continued thereafter until disease progression or unacceptable toxicity)

References

Vermorken JB, Mesia R, Rivera F, et al, "Platinum-Based Chemotherapy Plus Cetuximab in Head and Neck Cancer," *N Engl J Med*, 2008, 359(11):1116-27.

◆ **Cetuximab-Carboplatin (Head and Neck Cancer)** *see* Carboplatin-Cetuximab (Head and Neck Cancer) *on page 1543*

Cetuximab-Cisplatin-Fluorouracil (Head and Neck Cancer)

Index Terms Cisplatin-Fluorouracil-Cetuximab (Head and Neck Cancer)

Use Head and neck cancer

Regimen

Cycle 1:
Cetuximab: I.V.: 400 mg/m^2 (loading dose) day 1 (week 1, cycle 1 only)
[total loading dose = 400 mg/m^2]
followed by I.V.: 250 mg/m^2/day days 8 and 15
[total dose/cycle 1 = 900 mg/m^2]
Cisplatin: I.V.: 100 mg/m^2 day 1
[total dose/cycle = 100 mg/m^2]
Fluorouracil: I.V.: 1000 mg/m^2/day continuous infusion days 1 to 4
[total dose/cycle = 4000 mg/m^2]
Treatment cycle is 3 weeks
Subsequent cycles:
Cetuximab: I.V.: 250 mg/m^2/day days 1, 8, and 15
[total dose/cycle = 750 mg/m^2]
Cisplatin: I.V.: 100 mg/m^2 day 1
[total dose/cycle = 100 mg/m^2]
Fluorouracil: I.V.: 1000 mg/m^2/day continuous infusion days 1 to 4
[total dose/cycle = 4000 mg/m^2]
Repeat cycle every 3 weeks for a total of up to 6 cycles (cetuximab monotherapy may be continued thereafter until disease progression or unacceptable toxicity)

References

Vermorken JB, Mesia R, Rivera F, et al, "Platinum-Based Chemotherapy Plus Cetuximab in Head and Neck Cancer," *N Engl J Med*, 2008, 359(11):1116-27.

◆ **Cetuximab-Cisplatin (Head and Neck Cancer)** *see* Cisplatin-Cetuximab (Head and Neck Cancer) *on page 1566*

Cetuximab-Cisplatin-Vinorelbine (NSCLC)

Index Terms Cisplatin-Vinorelbine-Cetuximab (NSCLC)

Use Lung cancer, nonsmall cell

Regimen

Cycle 1:
Cetuximab: I.V.: 400 mg/m^2 (loading dose) over 2 hours day 1 (week 1, cycle 1 only)
[total loading dose = 400 mg/m^2]
followed by I.V.: 250 mg/m^2/day over 1 hour days 8 and 15
[total dose/cycle 1 = 900 mg/m^2]

Cisplatin: I.V.: 80 mg/m^2 day 1
[total dose/cycle = 80 mg/m^2]
Vinorelbine: I.V.: 25 mg/m^2/day days 1 and 8
[total dose/cycle = 50 mg/m^2]
Treatment cycle is 21 days
Cycles 2-6:
Cetuximab: I.V.: 250 mg/m^2/day over 1 hour days 1, 8, and 15
[total dose/cycle = 750 mg/m^2]
Cisplatin: I.V.: 80 mg/m^2 day 1
[total dose/cycle = 80 mg/m^2]
Vinorelbine: I.V.: 25 mg/m^2/day days 1 and 8
[total dose/cycle = 50 mg/m^2]
Repeat cycle every 21 days
followed by
Cetuximab: I.V.: 250 mg/m^2/day over 1 hour days 1, 8, and 15
[total dose/cycle = 750 mg/m^2]
Repeat cycle every 21 days until disease progression or unacceptable toxicity

References

Pirker R, Pereira JR, Szczesna A, et al, "Cetuximab Plus Chemotherapy in Patients With Advanced Non-Small-Cell Lung Cancer (FLEX): An Open-Label Randomised Phase III Trial," Lancet, 2009, 373(9674):1525-31.

Cetuximab (Colorectal Regimen)

Use Colorectal cancer

Regimen

Cycle 1:
Cetuximab: I.V.: 400 mg/m^2 (loading dose) over 120 minutes day 1 (week 1, cycle 1 only)
followed by I.V.: 250 mg/m^2/day over 60 minutes days 8, 15, and 22 (cycle 1)
[total dose/cycle 1 = 1150 mg/m^2]
Treatment cycle is 28 days
Subsequent cycles:
Cetuximab: I.V.: 250 mg/m^2/day over 60 minutes days 1, 8, 15, and 22
[total dose/cycle = 1000 mg/m^2]
Repeat cycle every 28 days until disease progression or unacceptable toxicity

References

Cunningham D, Humblet Y, Siena S, et al, "Cetuximab Monotherapy and Cetuximab Plus Irinotecan in Irinotecan-Refractory Metastatic Colorectal Cancer," *N Engl J Med*, 2004, 351 (4):337-45.

Jonker DJ, O'Callaghan CJ, Karapetis CS, "Cetuximab for the Treatment of Colorectal Cancer," *N Engl J Med*, 2007, 357(20):2040-8.

Karapetis CS, Khambata-Ford S, Jonker DJ, et al, "K-ras Mutations and Benefit From Cetuximab in Advanced Colorectal Cancer," *N Engl J Med*, 2008, 359(17):1757-65.

Cetuximab + FOLFIRI (Colorectal)

Index Terms Cetuximab, Irinotecan, Leucovorin, Fluorouracil (Colorectal)

Use Colorectal cancer

Regimen

Cycle 1:

Cetuximab: I.V.: 400 mg/m^2 (loading dose) over 120 minutes day 1 (week 1, cycle 1 only)

followed by I.V.: 250 mg/m^2/day over 60 minutes day 8

[total dose/cycle 1 = 650 mg/m^2]

Irinotecan: I.V.: 180 mg/m^2 over 30-90 minutes day 1

[total dose/cycle = 180 mg/m^2]

Leucovorin (racemic): I.V.: 400 mg/m^2 over 120 minutes day 1

[total dose/cycle = 400 mg/m^2]

Fluorouracil: I.V. bolus: 400 mg/m^2 day 1

followed by I.V.: 2400 mg/m^2 continuous infusion (CI) over 46 hours beginning day 1

[total fluorouracil dose/cycle (bolus and CI) = 2800 mg/m^2]

Treatment cycle is 14 days

Subsequent cycles:

Cetuximab: I.V.: 250 mg/m^2/day over 60 minutes days 1 and 8

[total dose/cycle = 500 mg/m^2]

Irinotecan: I.V.: 180 mg/m^2 over 30-90 minutes day 1

[total dose/cycle = 180 mg/m^2]

Leucovorin (racemic): I.V.: 400 mg/m^2 over 120 minutes day 1

[total dose/cycle = 400 mg/m^2]

Fluorouracil: I.V. bolus: 400 mg/m^2 day 1

followed by I.V.: 2400 mg/m^2 CI over 46 hours beginning day 1

[total fluorouracil dose/cycle (bolus and CI) = 2800 mg/m^2]

Repeat cycle every 14 days until disease progression or unacceptable toxicity

References

Van Custem E, Köhne CH, Hitre E, et al, "Cetuximab and Chemotherapy as Initial Treatment for Metastatic Colorectal Cancer," *N Engl J Med*, 2009, 360(14):1408-17.

Van Custem E, Köhne CH, Láng I, et al, "Cetuximab Plus Irinotecan, Fluorouracil, and Leucovorin as First-Line Treatment for Metastatic Colorectal Cancer: Updated Analysis of Overall Survival According to Tumor KRAS and BRAF Mutation Status," *J Clin Oncol*, 2011, 29(15):2011-9.

Cetuximab-FOLFOX4

Index Terms FOLFOX4-Cetuximab

Use Colorectal cancer

Regimen

Cycle 1:

Cetuximab: I.V.: 400 mg/m^2 (loading dose) day 1 (week 1, cycle 1 only)

followed by I.V.: 250 mg/m^2/day day 8

[total dose/cycle 1 = 650 mg/m^2]

Oxaliplatin: I.V.: 85 mg/m^2 (over 2 hours) day 1

[total dose/cycle = 85 mg/m^2]

Leucovorin: I.V.: 200 mg/m^2/day (over 2 hours) days 1 and 2

[total dose/cycle = 400 mg/m^2]

Fluorouracil: I.V. bolus: 400 mg/m^2/day days 1 and 2

followed by I.V.: 600 mg/m^2 continuous infusion (over 22 hours) days 1 and 2

[total dose/cycle = 2000 mg/m^2]

Note: Bolus fluorouracil and continuous infusion are both given on each day.

Treatment cycle is 14 days

Subsequent cycles:
Cetuximab: I.V.: 250 mg/m²/day days 1 and 8
[total dose/cycle = 500 mg/m²]
Oxaliplatin: I.V.: 85 mg/m² day 1
[total dose/cycle = 85 mg/m²]
Leucovorin: I.V.: 200 mg/m²/day (over 2 hours) days 1 and 2
[total dose/cycle = 400 mg/m²]
Fluorouracil: I.V. bolus: 400 mg/m²/day days 1 and 2
followed by I.V.: 600 mg/m² continuous infusion (over 22 hours) days 1 and 2
[total dose/cycle = 2000 mg/m²]
Note: Bolus fluorouracil and continuous infusion are both given on each day.
Repeat cycle every 14 days

References

Tabernero J, Van Cutsem E, Díaz-Rubio E, et al, "Phase II Trial of Cetuximab in Combination With Fluorouracil, Leucovorin, and Oxaliplatin in the First-Line Treatment of Metastatic Colorectal Cancer," *J Clin Oncol*, 2007, 25(33):5225-32.

Cetuximab-Irinotecan (Colorectal)

Index Terms Irinotecan-Cetuximab

Use Colorectal cancer

Regimen NOTE: Multiple variations are listed.

Variation 1:
Cycle 1:
Cetuximab: I.V.: 400 mg/m² (loading dose) day 1 (week 1, cycle 1 only)
followed by I.V.: 250 mg/m²/day days 8, 15, 22, 29, and 36
[total dose/cycle 1 = 1650 mg/m²]
Irinotecan: I.V.: 125 mg/m²/day days 1, 8, 15, and 22
[total dose/cycle = 500 mg/m²]
Treatment cycle is 42 days (6 weeks)
Subsequent cycles:
Cetuximab: I.V.: 250 mg/m²/day days 1, 8, 15, 22, 29, and 36
[total dose/cycle = 1500 mg/m²]
Irinotecan: I.V.: 125 mg/m²/day days 1, 8, 15, and 22
[total dose/cycle = 500 mg/m²]
Repeat cycle every 42 days (6 weeks) until disease progression or unacceptable toxicity

Variation 2:
Cycle 1:
Cetuximab: I.V.: 400 mg/m² (loading dose) day 1 (week 1, cycle 1 only)
followed by I.V.: 250 mg/m²/day days 8 and 15
[total dose/cycle 1 = 900 mg/m²]
Irinotecan: I.V.: 350 mg/m² day 1
[total dose/cycle = 350 mg/m²]
Treatment cycle is 21 days
Subsequent cycles:
Cetuximab: I.V.: 250 mg/m²/day days 1, 8, and 15
[total dose/cycle = 750 mg/m²]
Irinotecan: I.V.: 350 mg/m² day 1
[total dose/cycle = 350 mg/m²]
Repeat cycle every 21 days until disease progression or unacceptable toxicity

References

Variation 1 and 2:

Cunningham D, Humblet Y, Siena S, et al, "Cetuximab Monotherapy and Cetuximab Plus Irinotecan in Irinotecan-Refractory Metastatic Colorectal Cancer," *N Engl J Med*, 2004, 351 (4):337-45.

Variation 2:

Sobrero AF, Maurel J, Fehrenbacher L, et al, "EPIC: Phase III Trial of Cetuximab Plus Irinotecan After Fluoropyrimidine and Oxaliplatin Failure in Patients With Metastatic Colorectal Cancer," *J Clin Oncol*, 2008, 26(14):2311-9.

◆ **Cetuximab, Irinotecan, Leucovorin, Fluorouracil (Colorectal)** *see* Cetuximab + FOLFIRI (Colorectal) *on page 1559*

◆ **Cetuximab-Paclitaxel** *see* Paclitaxel-Cetuximab *on page 1727*

CEV

Use Rhabdomyosarcoma

Regimen

Carboplatin: I.V.: 500 mg/m^2 day 1
[total dose/cycle = 500 mg/m^2]

Epirubicin: I.V.: 150 mg/m^2 day 1
[total dose/cycle = 150 mg/m^2]

Vincristine: I.V.: 1.5 mg/m^2/day days 1 and 7
[total dose/cycle = 3 mg/m^2]

Repeat cycle every 21 days

References

Frascella E, Pritchard-Jones K, Modak S, et al, "Response of Previously Untreated Metastatic Rhabdomyosarcoma to Combination Chemotherapy With Carboplatin, Epirubicin and Vincristine," *Eur J Cancer*, 1996, 32A(5):821-5.

◆ **CFAR (CLL)** *see* Cyclophosphamide-Fludarabine-Alemtuzumab-Rituximab (CLL) *on page 1601*

◆ **CF (Esophageal Cancer)** *see* Cisplatin-Fluorouracil (Esophageal Cancer) *on page 1572*

◆ **CF (Gastric Cancer)** *see* Cisplatin-Fluorouracil (Gastric Cancer) *on page 1574*

◆ **CF (Head and Neck Cancer)** *see* Cisplatin-Fluorouracil (Head and Neck Cancer) *on page 1575*

◆ **CF (NHL-Mantle Cell)** *see* Fludarabine-Cyclophosphamide (NHL-Mantle Cell) *on page 1648*

ChlVPP (Hodgkin)

Index Terms Chlorambucil, Vinblastine, Procarbazine, Prednisolone (Hodgkin); Chlorambucil, Vinblastine, Procarbazine, Prednisone (Hodgkin); CHLVPP (Hodgkin)

Use Lymphoma, Hodgkin

Regimen NOTE: Multiple variations are listed.

Variation 1:

Chlorambucil: Oral: 6 mg/m^2/day (maximum dose: 10 mg/day) days 1 to 14
[total dose/cycle = 84 mg/m^2; maximum: 140 mg/cycle]

Vinblastine: I.V.: 6 mg/m^2/day (maximum dose: 10 mg/dose) days 1 and 8
[total dose/cycle = 12 mg/m^2; maximum: 20 mg/cycle]

Procarbazine: Oral: 100 mg/m^2/day (maximum dose: 150 mg/day) days 1 to 14
[total dose/cycle = 1400 mg/m^2; maximum: 2100 mg/cycle]

Prednisone or Prednisolone: Oral: 40 mg/day days 1 to 14
[total dose/cycle = 560 mg]
Repeat cycle every 28 days to complete remission plus 2 cycles; minimum of 6 cycles, maximum of 8 cycles

Variation 2:

Chlorambucil: Oral: 6 mg/m²/day days 1 to 14
[total dose/cycle = 84 mg/m²]
Vinblastine: I.V.: 6 mg/m²/day days 1 and 8
[total dose/cycle = 12 mg/m²]
Procarbazine: Oral: 100 mg/m²/day days 1 to 14
[total dose/cycle = 1400 mg/m²]
Prednisone: Oral: 40 mg/day days 1 to 14
[total dose/cycle = 560 mg]
Repeat cycle every 28 days for 6 cycles

References

Variation 1:

The International ChlVPP Treatment Group, "ChlVPP Therapy for Hodgkin's Disease: Experience of 960 Patients," *Ann Oncol*, 1995, 6(2):167-72.

Selby P, Patel P, Milan S, et al, "ChlVPP Combination Chemotherapy for Hodgkin's Disease: Long Term Results," *Br J Cancer*, 1990, 62(2):279-85.

Variation 2:

Vose JM, Bierman PJ, Anderson JR, et al, "CHLVPP Chemotherapy With Involved-Field Irradiation for Hodgkin's Disease: Favorable Results With Acceptable Toxicity," *J Clin Oncol*, 1991, 9 (8):1421-5.

Chlorambucil (CLL Regimen)

Use Leukemia, chronic lymphocytic

Regimen NOTE: Multiple variations are listed.

Variation 1:

Chlorambucil: Oral: 0.4 mg/kg day 1 (may increase by 0.1 mg/kg with each treatment course to a maximum dose of 0.8 mg/kg)
[total dose/cycle = 0.4-0.8 mg/kg]
Repeat cycle every 14 days for a maximum of 24 cycles

Variation 2:

Chlorambucil: Oral: 40 mg/m² day 1
[total dose/cycle = 40 mg/m²]
Repeat cycle every 28 days for a maximum of 12 cycles

References

Variation 1:

Eichhorst BF, Busch R, Stilgenbauer S, et al, "First Line Therapy With Fludarabine Compared With Chlorambucil Does Not Result in a Major Benefit for Elderly Patients With Advanced Chronic Lymphocytic Leukemia," *Blood*, 2009, 114(16):3382-91.

Variation 2:

Rai KR, Peterson BL, Appelbaum FR, et al, "Fludarabine Compared With Chlorambucil as Primary Therapy for Chronic Lymphocytic Leukemia," *N Engl J Med*, 2000, 343(24):1750-7.

Chlorambucil-Prednisone (CLL)

Index Terms Prednisone–Chlorambucil (CLL)

Use Leukemia, chronic lymphocytic

Regimen

Chlorambucil: Oral: 30 mg/m² day 1
[total dose/cycle = 30 mg/m²]
Prednisone: Oral: 80 mg/day days 1 to 5
[total dose/cycle = 400 mg]

Repeat cycle every 14 days until disease progression for a maximum duration of 9 months (if no response at 9 months), 15 months (if complete response at 9 months), or 18 months (if partial response at 9 months)

References

Raphael B, Anderson JW, Silber R, et al, "Comparison of Chlorambucil and Prednisone Versus Cyclophosphamide, Vincristine, and Prednisone as Initial Treatment for Chronic Lymphocytic Leukemia: Long-Term Follow-up of an Eastern Cooperative Oncology Group Randomized Clinical Trial," *J Clin Oncol*, 1991, 9(5):770-6.

◆ **Chlorambucil, Vinblastine, Procarbazine, Prednisolone (Hodgkin)** *see* ChlVPP (Hodgkin) *on page 1562*

◆ **Chlorambucil, Vinblastine, Procarbazine, Prednisone (Hodgkin)** *see* ChlVPP (Hodgkin) *on page 1562*

◆ **CHLVPP (Hodgkin)** *see* ChlVPP (Hodgkin) *on page 1562*

CHOP (NHL)

Use Lymphoma, non-Hodgkin's

Regimen NOTE: Multiple variations are listed.

Variation 1:

Cyclophosphamide: I.V.: 750 mg/m^2 day 1
[total dose/cycle = 750 mg/m^2]
Doxorubicin: I.V.: 50 mg/m^2 day 1
[total dose/cycle = 50 mg/m^2]
Vincristine: I.V.: 1.4 mg/m^2 (maximum dose: 2 mg) day 1
[total dose/cycle = 1.4 mg/m^2; maximum: 2 mg]
Prednisone: Oral: 100 mg/day days 1 to 5
[total dose/cycle = 500 mg]
Repeat cycle every 21 days for 6 to 8 cycles

Variation 2 (dose intensity/dose-dense):

Cyclophosphamide: I.V.: 1600 mg/m^2 day 1
[total dose/cycle = 1600 mg/m^2]
Doxorubicin: I.V.: 65 mg/m^2 day 1
[total dose/cycle = 65 mg/m^2]
Vincristine: I.V.: 1.4 mg/m^2 day 1
[total dose/cycle = 1.4 mg/m^2]
Prednisone: Oral: 100 mg/day days 1 to 5
[total dose/cycle = 500 mg]
Filgrastim: SubQ: 5 mcg/kg days 2 to 11 or until ANC >10,000/mm^3
Repeat cycle every 14 days for 6 cycles

Variation 3 (dose-dense):

Cyclophosphamide: I.V.: 750 mg/m^2 day 1
[total dose/cycle = 750 mg/m^2]
Doxorubicin: I.V.: 50 mg/m^2 day 1
[total dose/cycle = 50 mg/m^2]
Vincristine: I.V.: 2 mg day 1
[total dose/cycle = 2 mg]
Prednisone: Oral: 100 mg/day days 1 to 5
[total dose/cycle = 500 mg]
Filgrastim: SubQ: 300 mcg/day (<75 kg patient) or 480 mcg/day (≥75 kg patient) days 4 to 13
Repeat cycle every 14 days for 6 cycles

Variation 4 (localized disease; chemotherapy plus radiotherapy):
 Cyclophosphamide: I.V.: 750 mg/m^2 day 1
  [total dose/cycle = 750 mg/m^2]
 Doxorubicin: I.V.: 50 mg/m^2 day 1
  [total dose/cycle = 50 mg/m^2]
 Vincristine: I.V.: 1.4 mg/m^2 (maximum dose: 2 mg) day 1
  [total dose/cycle = 1.4 mg/m^2; maximum: 2 mg]
 Prednisone: Oral: 100 mg/day days 1 to 5
  [total dose/cycle = 500 mg]
 Repeat cycle every 21 days for 3 cycles followed by radiation therapy

Variation 5 (HIV-associated NHL):
 Cyclophosphamide: I.V.: 750 mg/m^2 day 1
  [total dose/cycle = 750 mg/m^2]
 Doxorubicin: I.V.: 50 mg/m^2 day 1
  [total dose/cycle = 50 mg/m^2]
 Vincristine: I.V.: 1.4 mg/m^2 (maximum dose: 2 mg) day 1
  [total dose/cycle = 1.4 mg/m^2; maximum: 2 mg]
 Prednisone: Oral: 100 mg/day days 1 to 5
  [total dose/cycle = 500 mg]
 Filgrastim: SubQ: 300 mcg/day (<70 kg patient) or 480 mcg/day (>70 kg patient) days 4 to 13
 Repeat cycle every 21 days; minimum of 4 cycles or 2 cycles beyond complete remission

References

Variation 1:

Fisher RI, Gaynor ER, Dahlberg S, et al, "Comparison of a Standard Regimen (CHOP) With Three Intensive Chemotherapy Regimens for Advanced Non-Hodgkin's Lymphoma," *N Engl J Med*, 1993,328(14):1002-6.

McKelvey EM, Gottlieb JA, Wilson HE, et al, "Hydroxyldaunomycin (Adriamycin®) Combination Chemotherapy in Malignant Lymphoma," *Cancer*, 1976, 38(4):1484-93.

van Oers MH, Klasa R, Marcus RE, et al, "Rituximab Maintenance Improves Clinical Outcome of Relapsed/Resistant Follicular Non-Hodgkin Lymphoma in Patients Both With and Without Rituximab During Induction: Results of a Prospective Randomized Phase 3 Intergroup Trial," *Blood*, 2006, 108(10):3295-301.

Variation 2:

Blayney DW, LeBlanc ML, Grogan T, et al, "Dose-Intense Chemotherapy Every 2 Weeks With Dose-Intense Cyclophosphamide, Doxorubicin, Vincristine, and Prednisone May Improve Survival in Intermediate- and High-Grade Lymphoma: A Phase II Study of the Southwest Oncology Group (SWOG 9349)," *J Clin Oncol*, 2003, 21(13): 2466-73.

Variation 3:

Pfreundschuh M, Trumper L, Kloess M, et al, "Two-Weekly or 3-Weekly CHOP Chemotherapy With or Without Etoposide for the Treatment of Elderly Patients With Aggressive Lymphomas: Results of the NHL-B2 Trial of the DSHNHL," *Blood*, 2004, 104(3):634-41.

Variation 4:

Miller TP, Dahlberg S, Cassady JR, et al, "Chemotherapy Alone Compared With Chemotherapy Plus Radiotherapy for Localized Intermediate- and High-Grade Non-Hodgkin's Lymphoma," *N Engl J Med*, 1998, 339(1):21-6.

Variation 5:

Ratner L, Lee J, Tang S, et al, "Chemotherapy for Human Immunodeficiency Virus-Associated Non-Hodgkin's Lymphoma in Combination With Highly Active Antiretroviral Therapy," *J Clin Oncol*, 2001, 19(8):2171-8.

◆ **CHOP-Rituximab (NHL)** *see* Rituximab-CHOP (NHL) *on page 1748*

◆ **Cisplatin-5FU (Cervical Cancer)** *see* Cisplatin-Fluorouracil (Cervical Cancer) *on page 1571*

Cisplatin-Capecitabine (Esophageal Cancer)

Index Terms Capecitabine-Cisplatin (Esophageal Cancer)

Use Esophageal cancer

Regimen

Cisplatin: I.V.: 80 mg/m^2 over 2 hours day 1
[total dose/cycle = 80 mg/m^2]

Capecitabine: Oral: 1000 mg/m^2/dose twice daily, days 1 to 14
[total dose/cycle = 28,000 mg/m^2]

Repeat cycle every 3 weeks until disease progression or unacceptable toxicity

References

Kang YK, Kang WK, Shin DB, et al, "Capecitabine/Cisplatin Versus 5-Fluorouracil/Cisplatin as First-Line Therapy in Patients With Advanced Gastric Cancer: A Randomised Phase III Non-inferiority Trial," *Ann Oncol*, 2009, 20(4):666-73.

Cisplatin-Capecitabine (Gastric Cancer)

Index Terms Capecitabine-Cisplatin (Gastric Cancer)

Use Gastric cancer

Regimen

Cisplatin: I.V.: 80 mg/m^2 over 2 hours day 1
[total dose/cycle = 80 mg/m^2]

Capecitabine: Oral: 1000 mg/m^2/dose twice daily, days 1 to 14
[total dose/cycle = 28,000 mg/m^2]

Repeat cycle every 3 weeks until disease progression or unacceptable toxicity

References

Kang YK, Kang WK, Shin DB, et al, "Capecitabine/Cisplatin Versus 5-Fluorouracil/Cisplatin as First-Line Therapy in Patients With Advanced Gastric Cancer: A Randomised Phase III Non-inferiority Trial," *Ann Oncol*, 2009, 20(4):666-73.

◆ **Cisplatin-Capecitabine-Trastuzumab (Gastric Cancer)** *see* Trastuzumab-Cisplatin-Capecitabine (Gastric Cancer) *on page* 1757

Cisplatin-Cetuximab (Head and Neck Cancer)

Index Terms Cetuximab-Cisplatin (Head and Neck Cancer)

Use Head and neck cancer

Regimen NOTE: Multiple variations are listed.

Variation 1:

Cycle 1:

Cetuximab: I.V.: 400 mg/m^2 (loading dose) day 1 (week 1, cycle 1 only)
[total loading dose = 400 mg/m^2]

followed by I.V.: 250 mg/m^2/day days 8, 15, and 22
[total dose/cycle 1 = 1150 mg/m^2]

Cisplatin: I.V.: 100 mg/m^2 day 1
[total dose/cycle = 100 mg/m^2]

Treatment cycle is 4 weeks

Subsequent cycles:

Cetuximab: I.V.: 250 mg/m^2/day days 1, 8, 15, and 22
[total dose/cycle = 1000 mg/m^2]

Cisplatin: I.V.: 100 mg/m^2 day 1
[total dose/cycle = 100 mg/m^2]

Repeat cycle every 4 weeks

Variation 2:
Cycle 1:
Cetuximab: I.V.: 400 mg/m^2 (loading dose) day 1 (week 1, cycle 1 only)
[total loading dose = 400 mg/m^2]
followed by I.V.: 250 mg/m^2/day days 8 and 15
[total dose/cycle 1 = 900 mg/m^2]
Cisplatin: I.V.: 75-100 mg/m^2 day 1
[total dose/cycle = 75-100 mg/m^2]
Treatment cycle is 3 weeks
Subsequent cycles:
Cetuximab: I.V.: 250 mg/m^2/day days 1, 8, and 15
[total dose/cycle = 750 mg/m^2]
Cisplatin: I.V.: 75-100 mg/m^2 day 1
[total dose/cycle = 75-100 mg/m^2]
Repeat cycle every 3 weeks

References

Variation 1:
Burtness B, Goldwasser MA, Flood W, et al, "Phase III Randomized Trial of Cisplatin Plus Placebo Compared With Cisplatin Plus Cetuximab in Metastatic/Recurrent Head and Neck Cancer: An Eastern Cooperative Oncology Group Study," *J Clin Oncol*, 2005, 23(34):8646-54.
Variation 2:
Herbst RS, Arquette M, Shin DM, et al, "Phase II Multicenter Study of the Epidermal Growth Factor Receptor Antibody Cetuximab and Cisplatin for Recurrent and Refractory Aquamous Cell Carcinoma of the Head and Neck," *J Clin Oncol*, 2005, 23(24):5578-87.

Cisplatin-Cytarabine-Dexamethasone (NHL Regimen)

Index Terms DHAP (NHL Regimen)
Use Lymphoma, non-Hodgkin's
Regimen NOTE: Multiple variations are listed.
Variation 1:
Dexamethasone: I.V. or Oral: 40 mg/day days 1 to 4
[total dose/cycle = 160 mg]
Cisplatin: I.V.: 100 mg/m^2 over 24 hours day 1
[total dose/cycle = 100 mg/m^2]
Cytarabine: I.V.: 2000 mg/m^2 every 12 hours for 2 doses day 2 (begins at the end of the cisplatin infusion)
[total dose/cycle = 4000 mg/m^2]
Repeat cycle every 3-4 weeks for 6-10 cycles
Variation 2 (patients >70 years of age):
Dexamethasone: I.V. or Oral: 40 mg/day days 1 to 4
[total dose/cycle = 160 mg]
Cisplatin: I.V.: 100 mg/m^2 over 24 hours day 1
[total dose/cycle = 100 mg/m^2]
Cytarabine: I.V.: 1000 mg/m^2 every 12 hours for 2 doses day 2 (begins at the end of the cisplatin infusion)
[total dose/cycle = 2000 mg/m^2]
Repeat cycle every 3-4 weeks for 6-10 cycles

References

Variation 1 and 2:
Velasquez WS, Cabanillas F, Salvador P, et al, "Effective Salvage Therapy for Lymphoma With Cisplatin in Combination With High-Dose Ara-C and Dexamethasone (DHAP)," *Blood*, 1988, 71 (1):117-22.

Cisplatin-Docetaxel-Fluorouracil (Unknown Primary)

Index Terms Fluorouracil-Cisplatin-Docetaxel (Unknown Primary); TPF (Unknown Primary)

Use Unknown primary (squamous cell)

Regimen

Docetaxel: I.V.: 75 mg/m^2 day 1
[total dose/cycle = 75 mg/m^2]

Cisplatin: I.V.: 75 mg/m^2 day 1
[total dose/cycle = 75 mg/m^2]

Fluorouracil: I.V.: 750 mg/m^2/day continuous infusion days 1 to 5
[total dose/cycle = 3750 mg/m^2]

Repeat cycle every 21 days for a total of 3 cycles

References

Pointreau Y, Garaud P, Chapet S, et al, "Randomized Trial of Induction Chemotherapy With Cisplatin and 5-Fluorouracil With or Without Docetaxel for Larynx Preservation," *J Natl Cancer Inst*, 2009, 101(7):498-506.

Cisplatin-Docetaxel (Unknown Primary)

Index Terms Docetaxel-Cisplatin (Unknown Primary)

Use Unknown primary (adenocarcinoma)

Regimen

Docetaxel: I.V.: 75 mg/m^2 over 1 hour day 1
[total dose/cycle = 75 mg/m^2]

Cisplatin: I.V.: 75 mg/m^2 over 1 hour day 1
[total dose/cycle = 75 mg/m^2]

Repeat cycle every 21 days for up to a total of 8 cycles

References

Greco FA, Erland JB, Morrissey LH, et al, "Carcinoma of Unknown Primary Site: Phase II Trials With Docetaxel Plus Cisplatin or Carboplatin," *Ann Oncol*, 2000, 11(2):211-5.

Cisplatin-Doxorubicin-Etoposide-Cyclophosphamide (Neuroblastoma)

Use Neuroblastoma

Regimen

Cisplatin: I.V.: 60 mg/m^2 over 6 hours day 0
[total dose/cycle = 60 mg/m^2]

Doxorubicin: I.V.: 30 mg/m^2 day 2
[total dose/cycle = 30 mg/m^2]

Etoposide: I.V.: 100 mg/m^2/day days 2 and 5
[total dose/cycle = 200 mg/m^2]

Cyclophosphamide: I.V.: 1000 mg/m^2/day days 3 and 4
[total dose/cycle = 2000 mg/m^2]

Repeat cycle every 28 days for a total of 5 cycles

References

Matthay KK, Villablanca JG, Seeger RC, et al, "Treatment of High-Risk Neuroblastoma With Intensive Chemotherapy, Radiotherapy, Autologous Bone Marrow Transplantation, and 13-*cis*-Retinoic Acid. Children's Cancer Group," *N Engl J Med*, 1999, 341(16):1165-73.

Cisplatin-Etoposide (NSCLC)

Index Terms Etoposide-Cisplatin

Use Lung cancer, nonsmall cell

Regimen NOTE: Multiple variations are listed.

Variation 1:
Cisplatin: I.V.: 80 mg/m^2 day 1
[total dose/cycle = 80 mg/m^2]
Etoposide: I.V.: 100 mg/m^2/day days 1, 2, and 3
[total dose/cycle = 300 mg/m^2]
Repeat cycle every 21 days for a total of 4 cycles
Variation 2:
Cisplatin: I.V.: 100 mg/m^2 day 1
[total dose/cycle = 100 mg/m^2]
Etoposide: I.V.: 100 mg/m^2/day days 1, 2, and 3
[total dose/cycle = 300 mg/m^2]
Repeat cycle every 28 days for a total of 3 cycles
Variation 3:
Cisplatin: I.V.: 100 mg/m^2 day 1
[total dose/cycle = 100 mg/m^2]
Etoposide: I.V.: 100 mg/m^2/day days 1, 2, and 3
[total dose/cycle = 300 mg/m^2]
Repeat cycle every 28 days for a total of 4 cycles
Variation 4:
Cisplatin: I.V.: 120 mg/m^2/day days 1, 29, and 71
[total dose/treatment = 360 mg/m^2]
Etoposide: I.V.: 100 mg/m^2/day days 1, 2, 3, 29, 30, 31, 71, 72, and 73
[total dose/treatment = 900 mg/m^2]
Variation 5:
Cisplatin: I.V.: 75 mg/m^2 day 1
[total dose/cycle = 75 mg/m^2]
Etoposide: I.V.: 100 mg/m^2/day days 1, 2, and 3
[total dose/cycle = 300 mg/m^2]
Repeat cycle every 21 days for up to 10 cycles

References

Variations 1-4:
Arriagada R, Bergman B, Dunant A, et al, "Cisplatin-Based Adjuvant Chemotherapy in Patients With Completely Resected Non-Small-Cell Lung Cancer," *N Engl J Med*, 2004, 350(4):351-60.
Variation 5:
Belani CP, Lee JS, Socinski MA, et al, "Randomized Phase III Trial Comparing Cisplatin-Etoposide to Carboplatin-Paclitaxel in Advanced or Metastatic Non-Small Cell Lung Cancer," *Ann Oncol*, 2005, 16(7):1069-75.

Cisplatin–Etoposide (Small Cell Lung Cancer)

Index Terms EP (Small Cell Lung Cancer); Etoposide-Cisplatin (Small Cell Lung Cancer); PE (Small Cell Lung Cancer)

Use Lung cancer, small cell

Regimen NOTE: Multiple variations are listed.

Variation 1: (limited stage with concurrent thoracic radiotherapy)
Etoposide: I.V.: 120 mg/m^2/day days 1, 2, and 3
[total dose/cycle = 360 mg/m^2]
Cisplatin: I.V.: 60 mg/m^2 day 1
[total dose/cycle = 60 mg/m^2]
Repeat cycle every 21 days for 4 cycles
Variation 2: (limited stage with concurrent thoracic radiotherapy)
Etoposide: I.V.: 100 mg/m^2/day days 1, 2, and 3
[total dose/cycle = 300 mg/m^2]

Cisplatin: I.V.: 80 mg/m^2 day 1
[total dose/cycle = 80 mg/m^2]
Repeat cycle every 28 days for 4 cycles

Variation 3: (extensive stage)
Etoposide: I.V.: 100 mg/m^2/day days 1, 2, and 3
[total dose/cycle = 300 mg/m^2]
Cisplatin: I.V.: 80 mg/m^2 day 1
[total dose/cycle = 80 mg/m^2]
Repeat cycle every 21 days for 4 cycles

Variation 4: (extensive stage)
Etoposide: I.V.: 100 mg/m^2 day 1
[total I.V. dose/cycle = 100 mg/m^2]
followed by: Etoposide: Oral: 200 mg/m^2/day days 2, 3, and 4
[total oral dose/cycle = 600 mg/m^2]
Cisplatin: I.V.: 75 mg/m^2 day 1
[total dose/cycle = 75 mg/m^2]
Repeat cycle every 21 days for a maximum of 5 cycles

Variation 5: (extensive stage)
Etoposide: I.V.: 80 mg/m^2/day days 1, 2, and 3
[total dose/cycle = 240 mg/m^2]
Cisplatin: I.V.: 80 mg/m^2 day 1
[total dose/cycle = 80 mg/m^2]
Repeat cycle every 21 days for maximum of 8 cycles

Variation 6: (extensive stage)
Etoposide: I.V.: 100 mg/m^2/day days 1, 2, and 3
[total dose/cycle = 300 mg/m^2]
Cisplatin: I.V.: 25 mg/m^2/day days 1, 2, and 3
[total dose/cycle = 75 mg/m^2]
Repeat cycle every 21 to 28 days for 6 cycles

Variation 7: (extensive stage)
Etoposide: I.V.: 80 mg/m^2/day days 1 to 5
[total dose/cycle = 400 mg/m^2]
Cisplatin: I.V.: 20 mg/m^2/day days 1 to 5
[total dose/cycle = 100 mg/m^2]
Repeat cycle every 21 days for 4 cycles

References

Variation 1:

Turrisi AT, Kyungmann K, Blum R, et al, "Twice-Daily Compared With Once-Daily Thoracic Radiotherapy in Limited Small-Cell Lung Cancer Treated Concurrently With Cisplatin and Etoposide," *N Engl J Med*, 1999, 340(4):265-71.

Variation 2:

Takada M, Fukuoka M, Kawahara M, et al, "Phase III Study of Concurrent Verses Sequential Thoracic Radiotherapy in Combination With Cisplatin and Etoposide for Limited-Stage Small-Cell Lung Cancer: Results of the Japan Clinical Oncology Group Study 9104," *J Clin Oncol*, 2002, 20 (14):3054-60.

Variation 3:

Lara Jr PN, Natale R, Crowley J, et al, "Phase III Trial of Irinotecan/Cisplatin Compared With Etoposide/Cisplatin in Extensive-Stage Small-Cell Lung Cancer: Clinical and Pharmacogenomic Results From SWOG S0124," *J Clin Oncol*, 2009, 27(15):2530-5.

Variation 4:

Sundstrom S, Bremnes RM, Kaasa S, et al, "Cisplatin and Etoposide Regimen Is Superior to Cyclophosphamide, Epirubicin, and Vincristine Regimen in Small-Cell Lung Cancer: Results From a Randomized Phase III Trial With 5 Years' Follow-Up," *J Clin Oncol*, 2002, 20(24):4665-72.

Variation 5:

Ihde DC, Mulshine JL, Kramer BS, et al, "Prospective Randomized Comparison of High-Dose and Standard-Dose Etoposide and Cisplatin Chemotherapy in Patients With Extensive-Stage Small-Cell Lung Cancer," *J Clin Oncol*, 1994, 12(10):2022-34.

Variation 6:

Evans WK, Shepherd FA, Feld R, et al, "VP-16 and Cisplatin as First-Line Therapy for Small-Cell Lung Cancer," *J Clin Oncol*, 1985, 3(11):1471-7.

Variation 7:

Roth BJ, Johnson DH, Einhorn LH, et al, "Randomized Study of Cyclophosphamide, Doxorubicin, and Vincristine Versus Etoposide and Cisplatin Versus Alternation of These Two Regimens in Extensive Small-Cell Lung Cancer: A Phase III Trial of the Southeastern Cancer Study Group," *J Clin Oncol*, 1992, 10(2):281-91.

Cisplatin-Fluorouracil (Bladder Cancer)

Index Terms Fluorouracil-Cisplatin (Bladder Cancer)

Use Bladder cancer

Regimen In combination with radiation therapy

Note: Begin infusion(s) 2 hours before radiation therapy on days 1, 3, 15, and 17:

Cisplatin: I.V.: 15 mg/m^2/day over 2 hours days 1, 2, 3, 15, 16, and 17
[total dose/cycle = 90 mg/m^2]

Fluorouracil: I.V.: 400 mg/m^2/day over 2 hours days 1, 2, 3, 15, 16, and 17
[total dose/cycle = 2400 mg/m^2]

References

Housset M, Maulard C, Chretien Y, et al, "Combined Radiation and Chemotherapy for Invasive Transitional-Cell Carcinoma of the Bladder: A Prospective Study," *J Clin Oncol*, 1993, 11 (11):2150-7.

Cisplatin-Fluorouracil (Cervical Cancer)

Index Terms 5FU-Cisplatin (Cervical Cancer); Cisplatin-5FU (Cervical Cancer); Fluorouracil-Cisplatin (Cervical Cancer)

Use Cervical cancer

Regimen NOTE: Multiple variations are listed.

Variation 1 (with concurrent radiation therapy):

Cisplatin: I.V.: 75 mg/m^2 day 1
[total dose/cycle = 75 mg/m^2]

Fluorouracil: I.V.: 1000 mg/m^2/day continuous infusion days 1 to 4 (96 hours)
[total dose/cycle = 4000 mg/m^2]

Repeat cycle every 21 days for a total 3 cycles

Variation 2 (with concurrent radiation therapy):

Cisplatin: I.V.: 50 mg/m^2 day 1 starting 4 hours before radiotherapy
[total dose/cycle = 50 mg/m^2]

Fluorouracil: I.V.: 1000 mg/m^2/day continuous infusion days 2 to 5 (96 hours)
[total dose/cycle = 4000 mg/m^2]

Repeat cycle every 28 days for a total of 2 cycles

Variation 3 (cycles 1 and 2 are with concurrent radiation therapy):

Cisplatin: I.V.: 70 mg/m^2 day 1
[total dose/cycle = 70 mg/m^2]

Fluorouracil: I.V.: 1000 mg/m^2/day continuous infusion days 1 to 4 (96 hours)
[total dose/cycle = 4000 mg/m^2]

Repeat cycle every 21 days for a total of 4 cycles

References

Variation 1:

Morris M, Eifel PJ, Lu J, et al, "Pelvic Radiation With Concurrent Chemotherapy Compared With Pelvic and Para-aortic Radiation for High-Risk Cervical Cancer," *N Engl J Med*, 1999, 340 (15):1137-43.

Variation 2:

Whitney CW, Sause W, Bundy BN, et al, "Randomized Comparison of Fluorouracil Plus Cisplatin Versus Hydroxyurea as an Adjunct to Radiation Therapy in Stage IIB-IVA Carcinoma of the Cervix With Negative Para-aortic Lymph Nodes: A Gynecologic Oncology Group and Southwest Oncology Group Study," *J Clin Oncol*, 1999, 17(5):1339-48.

Variation 3:
Peters WA 3rd, Liu PY, Barrett RJ 2nd, et al, "Concurrent Chemotherapy and Pelvic Radiation Therapy Compared With Pelvic Radiation Therapy Alone as Adjuvant Therapy After Radical Surgery in High-Risk Early-Stage Cancer of the Cervix," *J Clin Oncol*, 2000, 18(8):1606-13.

◆ **Cisplatin-Fluorouracil-Cetuximab (Head and Neck Cancer)** *see* Cetuximab-Cisplatin-Fluorouracil (Head and Neck Cancer) *on page 1558*

Cisplatin-Fluorouracil (Esophageal Cancer)

Index Terms CF (Esophageal Cancer); Fluorouracil-Cisplatin (Esophageal Cancer)

Use Esophageal cancer

Regimen NOTE: Multiple variations are listed.

Variation 1:
Cisplatin: I.V.: 100 mg/m^2/dose day 1
[total dose/cycle = 100 mg/m^2]
Fluorouracil: I.V.: 1000 mg/m^2/day continuous infusion days 1 to 5
[total dose/cycle = 5000 mg/m^2]
Repeat cycle every 28 days until disease progression or unacceptable toxicity.

Variation 2:
Cycles 1 to 3 (prior to surgery):
Cisplatin: I.V.: 100 mg/m^2/dose day 1
[total dose/cycle = 100 mg/m^2]
Fluorouracil: I.V.: 1000 mg/m^2/day continuous infusion days 1 to 5
[total dose/cycle = 5000 mg/m^2]
Treatment cycles 1-3 are 28 days each
Cycles 4 and 5 (postoperative):
Cisplatin: I.V.: 75 mg/m^2/dose day 1
[total dose/cycle = 75 mg/m^2]
Fluorouracil: I.V.: 1000 mg/m^2/day continuous infusion days 1 to 5
[total dose/cycle = 5000 mg/m^2]
Treatment cycles 4 and 5 are 28 days each

Variation 3 (in combination with radiation therapy):
Cycle 1:
Cisplatin: I.V.: 75 mg/m^2/dose day 1
[total dose/cycle = 75 mg/m^2]
Fluorouracil: I.V.: 1000 mg/m^2/day continuous infusion days 1 to 4
[total dose/cycle = 4000 mg/m^2]
Treatment cycle is 28 days
Cycles 2 to 4:
Cisplatin: I.V.: 75 mg/m^2/dose day 1
[total dose/cycle = 75 mg/m^2]
Fluorouracil: I.V.: 1000 mg/m^2/day continuous infusion days 1 to 4
[total dose/cycle = 4000 mg/m^2]
Repeat cycle every 21 days for 3 more cycles (total of 4 cycles)

Variation 4 (in combination with radiation therapy):
Cisplatin: I.V.: 100 mg/m^2/dose day 1
[total dose/cycle = 100 mg/m^2]
Fluorouracil: I.V.: 1000 mg/m^2/day continuous infusion days 1 to 4
[total dose/cycle = 4000 mg/m^2]
Repeat cycle every 28 days for total of 2 cycles

Variation 5 (in combination with radiation therapy):
Cisplatin: I.V.: 75 mg/m^2/dose day 1
[total dose/cycle = 75 mg/m^2]
Fluorouracil: I.V.: 1000 mg/m^2/day continuous infusion days 1 to 4
[total dose/cycle = 4000 mg/m^2]
Repeat cycle every 28 days for 4 cycles

Variation 6 (in combination with radiation therapy):
Cycles 1 and 2:
Cisplatin: I.V.: 75 mg/m^2/dose day 1
[total dose/cycle = 75 mg/m^2]
Fluorouracil: I.V.: 1000 mg/m^2/day continuous infusion days 1 to 4
[total dose/cycle = 4000 mg/m^2]
Treatment cycles 1 and 2 are 28 days each; cycle 2 is followed by a 2-week rest
Cycles 3 and 4 (begin cycle 3 at week 11):
Cisplatin: I.V.: 75 mg/m^2/dose day 1
[total dose/cycle = 75 mg/m^2]
Fluorouracil: I.V.: 1000 mg/m^2/day continuous infusion days 1 to 4
[total dose/cycle = 4000 mg/m^2]
Treatment cycles 3 and 4 are 28 days each

Variation 7 (in combination with radiation therapy):
Cycles 1 to 4:
Cisplatin: I.V.: 15 mg/m^2/day days 1 to 5
[total dose/cycle = 75 mg/m^2]
Fluorouracil: I.V.: 800 mg/m^2/day continuous infusion days 1 to 5
[total dose/cycle = 4000 mg/m^2]
Repeat cycles 1-4 every 21 days; cycle 4 is followed by a 1-week rest
Cycles 5 (begin cycle 5 at week 14):
Cisplatin: I.V.: 15 mg/m^2/day days 1 to 5
[total dose/cycle = 75 mg/m^2]
Fluorouracil: I.V.: 800 mg/m^2/day continuous infusion days 1 to 5
[total dose/cycle = 4000 mg/m^2]

Variation 8:
Cisplatin: I.V.: 80 mg/m^2/dose day 1
[total dose/cycle = 80 mg/m^2]
Fluorouracil: I.V.: 800 mg/m^2/day continuous infusion days 1 to 5
[total dose/cycle = 4000 mg/m^2]
Repeat cycle every 21 days until disease progression or unacceptable toxicity.

References

Variation 1:

Ajani JA, Moiseyenko VM, Tjulandin S, et al, "Quality of Life With Docetaxel Plus Cisplatin and Fluorouracil Compared With Cisplatin and Fluorouracil From a Phase III Trial for Advanced Gastric or Gastroesophageal Adenocarcinoma: The V-325 Study Group," *J Clin Oncol*, 2007, 25 (22):3210-6.

Dank M, Zaluski J, Barone C, et al, "Randomized Phase III Study Comparing Irinotecan Combined With 5-Fluorouracil and Folinic Acid to Cisplatin Combined With 5-Fluorouracil in Chemotherapy Naive Patients With Advanced Adenocarcinoma of the Stomach or Esophagogastric Junction," *Ann Oncol*, 2008, 19(8):1450-7.

Van Cutsem E, Moiseyenko VM, Tjulandin S, et al, "Phase III Study of Docetaxel and Cisplatin Plus Fluorouracil Compared With Cisplatin and Fluorouracil As First-Line Therapy for Advanced Gastric Cancer: A Report of the V325 Study Group," *J Clin Oncol*, 2006, 24(31):4991-7.

Variation 2:

Kelsen DP, Ginsberg R, Pajak TF, et al, "Chemotherapy Followed by Surgery Compared With Surgery Alone for Localized Esophageal Cancer," *N Engl J Med*, 1998, 339(27):1979-84.

Variation 3:
Cooper JS, Guo MD, Herskovic A, et al, "Chemoradiotherapy of Locally Advanced Esophageal Cancer: Long-Term Follow-Up of a Prospective Randomized Trial (RTOG 85-01). Radiation Therapy Oncology Group," *JAMA*, 1999, 281(17):1623-7.
Variation 4:
Tepper J, Krasna MJ, Niedzwiecki D, et al, "Phase III Trial of Trimodality Therapy With Cisplatin, Fluorouracil, Radiotherapy, and Surgery Compared With Surgery Alone for Esophageal Cancer: CALGB 9781," *J Clin Oncol*, 2008, 26(7):1086-92.
Variation 5 and 6:
Minsky BD, Pajak TF, Ginsberg RJ, et al, "INT 0123 (Radiation Therapy Oncology Group 94-05) Phase III Trial of Combined-Modality Therapy for Esophageal Cancer: High-Dose Versus Standard-Dose Radiation Therapy," *J Clin Oncol*, 2002, 20(5):1167-74.
Variation 7:
Bedenne L, Michel P, Bouché O, et al, "Chemoradiation Followed by Surgery Compared With Chemoradiation Alone in Squamous Cancer of the Esophagus: FFCD 9102," *J Clin Oncol*, 2007, 25(10):1160-8.
Variation 8:
Kang YK, Kang WK, Shin DB, et al, "Capecitabine/Cisplatin Versus 5-Fluorouracil/Cisplatin as First-Line Therapy in Patients With Advanced Gastric Cancer: A Randomised Phase III Non-inferiority Trial," *Ann Oncol*, 2009, 20(4):666-73.

Cisplatin-Fluorouracil (Gastric Cancer)

Index Terms CF (Gastric Cancer); Fluorouracil-Cisplatin (Gastric Cancer)

Use Gastric cancer

Regimen NOTE: Multiple variations are listed.

Variation 1:
Cisplatin: I.V.: 100 mg/m^2 day 1
[total dose/cycle = 100 mg/m^2]
Fluorouracil: I.V.: 1000 mg/m^2/day continuous infusion days 1 to 5
[total dose/cycle = 5000 mg/m^2]
Repeat cycle every 4 weeks until disease progression or unacceptable toxicity

Variation 2:
Cisplatin: I.V.: 80 mg/m^2 over 2 hours day 1
[total dose/cycle = 80 mg/m^2]
Fluorouracil: I.V.: 800 mg/m^2/day continuous infusion days 1 to 5
[total dose/cycle = 4000 mg/m^2]
Repeat cycle every 21 days until disease progression or unacceptable toxicity

Variation 3:
Fluorouracil: I.V.: 1000 mg/m^2/day continuous infusion days 1 to 5
[total dose/cycle = 5000 mg/m^2]
Cisplatin: I.V.: 100 mg/m^2 day 2
[total dose/cycle = 100 mg/m^2]
Repeat cycle every 4 weeks

References

Variation 1:
Ajani JA, Moiseyenko VM, Tjulandin S, et al, "Clinical Benefit With Docetaxel Plus Fluorouracil and Cisplatin Compared With Cisplatin and Fluorouracil in a Phase III Trial of Advanced Gastric or Gastroesophageal Cancer Adenocarcinoma: The V-325 Study Group," *J Clin Oncol*, 2007, 25 (22):3205-9.
Dank M, Zaluski J, Barone C, et al, "Randomized Phase III Study Comparing Irinotecan Combined With 5-Fluorouracil and Folinic Acid to Cisplatin Combined With 5-Fluorouracil in Chemotherapy Naive Patients With Advanced Adenocarcinoma of the Stomach or Esophagogastric Junction," *Ann Oncol*, 2008, 19(8):1450-7.
Van Cutsem E, Moiseyenko VM, Tjulandin S, "Phase III Study of Docetaxel and Cisplatin Plus Fluorouracil Compared With Cisplatin and Fluorouracil as First-Line Therapy for Advanced Gastric Cancer: A Report of the V325 Study Group," *J Clin Oncol*, 2006, 24(31):4991-7.

Variation 2:
Kang YK, Kang WK, Shin DB, "Capecitabine/Cisplatin Versus 5-Fluorouracil/Cisplatin as First-Line Therapy in Patients With Advanced Gastric Cancer: A Randomised Phase III Noninferiority Trial," *Ann Oncol*, 2009, 20(4):666-73.
Variation 3:
Vanhoefer U, Rougier P, Wilke H, et al, "Final Results of a Randomized Phase III Trial of Sequential High-Dose Methotrexate, Fluorouracil, and Doxorubicin Versus Etoposide, Leucovorin, and Fluorouracil Versus Infusional Fluorouracil and Cisplatin in Advanced Gastric Cancer: A Trial of the European Organization for Research and Treatment of Cancer Gastrointestinal Tract Cancer Cooperative Group," *J Clin Oncol*, 2000, 18(14):2648-57.

Cisplatin-Fluorouracil (Head and Neck Cancer)

Index Terms CF (Head and Neck Cancer); Fluorouracil-Cisplatin (Head and Neck Cancer)

Use Head and neck cancer

Regimen NOTE: Multiple variations are listed.

Variation 1:
Cisplatin: I.V.: 100 mg/m^2 day 1
[total dose/cycle = 100 mg/m^2]
Fluorouracil: I.V.: 1000 mg/m^2/day continuous infusion days 1 to 4
[total dose/cycle = 4000 mg/m^2]
Repeat cycle every 3 weeks

Variation 2:
Cisplatin: I.V.: 100 mg/m^2 day 1
[total dose/cycle = 100 mg/m^2]
Fluorouracil: I.V.: 1000 mg/m^2/day continuous infusion days 1 to 4
[total dose/cycle = 4000 mg/m^2]
Repeat cycle every 3 or 4 weeks

Variation 3:
Cisplatin: I.V.: 100 mg/m^2 day 1
[total dose/cycle = 100 mg/m^2]
Fluorouracil: I.V.: 1000 mg/m^2/day continuous infusion days 1 to 5
[total dose/cycle = 5000 mg/m^2]
Repeat cycle every 3 or 4 weeks

Variation 4:
Cisplatin: I.V.: 60 mg/m^2 day 1
[total dose/cycle = 60 mg/m^2]
Fluorouracil: I.V.: 800 mg/m^2/day continuous infusion days 1 to 5
[total dose/cycle = 4000 mg/m^2]
Repeat cycle every 14 days

Variation 5:
Cisplatin: I.V.: 20 mg/m^2/day days 1 to 5
[total dose/cycle = 100 mg/m^2]
Fluorouracil: I.V.: 200 mg/m^2/day days 1 to 5
[total dose/cycle = 1000 mg/m^2]
Repeat cycle every 3 weeks

Variation 6:
Cisplatin: I.V.: 80 mg/m^2 continuous infusion day 1
[total dose/cycle = 80 mg/m^2]
Fluorouracil: I.V.: 800 mg/m^2/day continuous infusion days 2 to 6
[total dose/cycle = 4000 mg/m^2]
Repeat cycle every 3 weeks

Variation 7:
Cisplatin: I.V.: 75 mg/m^2 day 1
[total dose/cycle = 75 mg/m^2]
Fluorouracil: I.V.: 1000 mg/m^2/day continuous infusion days 1 to 4
[total dose/cycle = 4000 mg/m^2]
Repeat cycle every 4 weeks
Variation 8:
Cisplatin: I.V.: 120 mg/m^2 day 1
[total dose/cycle = 120 mg/m^2]
Fluorouracil: I.V.: 1000 mg/m^2/day continuous infusion days 1 to 5
[total dose/cycle = 5000 mg/m^2]
Repeat cycle every 3 weeks
Variation 9:
Cisplatin: I.V.: 25 mg/m^2/day continuous infusion days 1 to 4
[total dose/cycle = 100 mg/m^2]
Fluorouracil: I.V.: 1000 mg/m^2/day days 1 to 4
[total dose/cycle = 4000 mg/m^2]
Repeat cycle every 3 weeks
Variation 10:
Fluorouracil: I.V.: 350 mg/m^2/day continuous infusion days 1 to 5
[total dose/cycle = 1750 mg/m^2]
Cisplatin: I.V.: 50 mg/m^2 day 6
[total dose/cycle = 50 mg/m^2]
Repeat cycle every 3 weeks
Variation 11:
Cisplatin: I.V.: 5 mg/m^2/day continuous infusion days 1 to 14
[total dose/cycle = 70 mg/m^2]
Fluorouracil: I.V.: 200 mg/m^2/day continuous infusion days 1 to 14
[total dose/cycle = 2800 mg/m^2]
With concurrent radiation therapy, cycle does not repeat
Variation 12 (administer during the final 2 weeks of radiation therapy; weeks 6 and 7):
Cisplatin: I.V.: 10 mg/m^2/day days 1 to 5 beginning week 6
[total dose/week = 50 mg/m^2]
Fluorouracil: I.V.: 400 mg/m^2/day continuous infusion days 1 to 5 beginning week 6
[total dose/week = 2000 mg/m^2]
Repeat cycle one time in week 7
Variation 13:
Cisplatin: I.V.: 100 mg/m^2/day day 1 (concurrent with radiation therapy)
[total dose/cycle = 100 mg/m^2]
Repeat cycle every 3 weeks for a total of 3 cycles
Followed by (postradiation chemotherapy; begin 4 weeks after radiotherapy or the last cisplatin dose):
Cisplatin: I.V.: 80 mg/m^2 day 1
[total dose/cycle = 80 mg/m^2]
Fluorouracil: I.V.: 1000 mg/m^2/day continuous infusion days 1 to 4
[total dose/cycle = 4000 mg/m^2]
Repeat cycle every 4 weeks for a total of 3 cycles

References

Variation 1:
Forastiere AA, Metch B, Schuller DE, et al, "Randomized Comparison of Cisplatin Plus Fluorouracil and Carboplatin Plus Fluorouracil Versus Methotrexate in Advanced Squamous-Cell Carcinoma of the Head and Neck: A Southwest Oncology Group Study," *J Clin Oncol*, 1992, 10(8):1245-51.

Gibson MK, Li Y, Murphy B, et al, "Randomized Phase III Evaluation of Cisplatin Plus Fluorouracil Versus Cisplatin Plus Paclitaxel in Advanced Head and Neck Cancer (E1395): An Intergroup Trial of the Eastern Cooperative Oncology Group," *J Clin Oncol*, 2005, 23(15):3562-7.

Variation 2:

Kish J, Drelichman A, Jacobs J, et al, "Clinical Trial of Cisplatin and 5-FU Infusion as Initial Treatment for Advanced Squamous Cell Carcinoma of the Head and Neck," *Cancer Treat Rep*, 1982, 66(3):471-4.

Mercier RJ, Neal GD, Mattox DE, et al, "Cisplatin and 5-Fluorouracil Chemotherapy in Advanced or Recurrent Squamous Cell Carcinoma of the Head and Neck," *Cancer*, 1987, 60(11):2609-12.

Variation 3:

Dasmahapatra KS, Citrin P, Hill GJ, et al, "A Prospective Evaluation of 5-Fluorouracil Plus Cisplatin in Advanced Squamous-Cell Cancer of the Head and Neck," *J Clin Oncol*, 1985, 3(11):1486-9.

Rooney M, Kish J, Jacobs J, et al, "Improved Complete Response Rate and Survival in Advanced Head and Neck Cancer After Three-Course Induction Therapy With 120-Hour 5-FU Infusion and Cisplatin," *Cancer*, 1985, 55(5):1123-8.

Variation 4:

Taylor SG 4th, Murthy AK, Showel JL, et al, "Improved Control in Advanced Head and Neck Cancer With Simultaneous Radiation and Cisplatin/5-FU Chemotherapy," *Cancer Treat Rep*, 1985, 69 (9):933-9.

Variation 5:

Merlano M, Tatarek R, Grimaldi A, et al, "Phase I-II Trial With Cisplatin and 5-FU in Recurrent Head and Neck Cancer: An Effective Outpatient Schedule," *Cancer Treat Rep*, 1985, 69(9):961-4.

Variation 6:

Amrein PC and Weitzman SA, "Treatment of Squamous-Cell Carcinoma of the Head and Neck With Cisplatin and 5-Fluorouracil," *J Clin Oncol*, 1985, 3(12):1632-9.

Variation 7:

Adelstein DJ, Li Y, Adams GL, et al, "An Intergroup Phase III Comparison of Standard Radiation and Two Schedules of Concurrent Chemoradiotherapy in Patients With Unresectable Squamous Cell Head and Neck Cancer," *J Clin Oncol*, 2003, 21(1):92-8.

Adelstein DJ, Sharan VM, Earle AS, et al, "Chemoradiotherapy as Initial Management in Patients With Squamous Cell Carcinoma of the Head and Neck," *Cancer Treat Rep*, 1986, 70(6):761-7.

Variation 8:

Paredes J, Hong WK, Felder TB, et al, "Prospective Randomized Trial of High-Dose Cisplatin and Fluorouracil Infusion With or Without Sodium Diethyldithiocarbamate in Recurrent and/or Metastatic Squamous Cell Carcinoma of the Head and Neck," *J Clin Oncol*, 1988, 6(6):955-62.

Variation 9:

Bernal AG, Cruz JJ, Sanchez P, et al, "Four-Day Continuous Infusion of Cisplatin and 5-Fluorouracil in Head and Neck Cancer," *Cancer*, 1989, 63(10):1927-30.

Variation 10:

Denham JW and Abbott RL, "Concurrent Cisplatin, Infusional Fluorouracil, and Conventionally Fractionated Radiation Therapy in Head and Neck Cancer: Dose-Limiting Mucosal Toxicity," *J Clin Oncol*, 1991, 9(3):458-63.

Variation 11:

Arcangeli G, Saracino B, Danesi DT, et al, "Accelerated Hyperfractionated Radiotherapy and Concurrent Protracted Venous Infusion Chemotherapy in Locally-Advanced Head and Neck Cancer," *Am J Clin Oncol*, 2002, 25(5):431-7.

Variation 12:

Garden AS, Harris J, Vokes EE, et al, "Preliminary Results of Radiation Therapy Oncology Group 97-03: A Randomized Phase II Trial of Concurrent Radiation and Chemotherapy for Advanced Squamous Cell Carcinomas of the Head and Neck," *J Clin Oncol*, 2004, 22(14):2856-64.

Variation 13:

Al-Sarraf M, LeBlanc M, Giri PG, et al, "Chemoradiotherapy Versus Radiotherapy in Patients With Advanced Nasopharyngeal Cancer: Phase III Randomized Intergroup Study 0099," *J Clin Oncol*, 1998, 16(4):1310-7.

Cisplatin-Fluorouracil-Paclitaxel (Unknown Primary)

Index Terms Cisplatin-Paclitaxel-Fluorouracil (Unknown Primary); PCF (Unknown Primary)

Use Unknown primary (squamous cell)

Regimen

Paclitaxel: I.V.: 175 mg/m^2 over 3 hours day 1
[total dose/cycle = 175 mg/m^2]

Cisplatin: I.V.: 100 mg/m^2 day 2
[total dose/cycle = 100 mg/m^2]
Fluorouracil: I.V.: 500 mg/m^2/day continuous infusion days 2 to 6
[total dose/cycle = 2500 mg/m^2]
Repeat cycle every 21 days for a total of 3 cycles

References

Hitt R, López-Pousa A, Martínez-Trufero J, et al, "Phase III Study Comparing Cisplatin Plus Fluorouracil to Paclitaxel, Cisplatin, and Fluorouracil Induction Chemotherapy Followed by Chemoradiotherapy in Locally Advanced Head and Neck Cancer," *J Clin Oncol*, 2005, 23 (34):8636-45.

- **Cisplatin-Fluorouracil-Trastuzumab (Gastric Cancer)** *see* Trastuzumab-Cisplatin-Fluorouracil (Gastric Cancer) *on page 1758*
- **Cisplatin-Gemcitabine-Bevacizumab (NSCLC)** *see* Bevacizumab-Cisplatin-Gemcitabine (NSCLC) *on page 1529*
- **Cisplatin-Gemcitabine (Biliary Cancer)** *see* Gemcitabine-Cisplatin (Biliary Cancer) *on page 1669*

Cisplatin-Gemcitabine (Cervical Cancer)

Index Terms Gemcitabine-Cisplatin (Cervical Cancer)

Use Cervical cancer

Regimen NOTE: Multiple variations are listed.

Variation 1:
Gemcitabine: I.V.: 1250 mg/m^2/day days 1 and 8
[total dose/cycle = 2500 mg/m^2]
Cisplatin: I.V.: 50 mg/m^2 day 1
[total dose/cycle = 50 mg/m^2]
Repeat cycle every 21 days for up to a total of 6 cycles

Variation 2:
Gemcitabine: I.V.: 1000 mg/m^2/day days 1 and 8
[total dose/cycle = 2000 mg/m^2]
Cisplatin: I.V.: 50 mg/m^2 day 1
[total dose/cycle = 50 mg/m^2]
Repeat cycle every 21 days for up to a total of 6 cycles; responders may continue beyond 6 cycles

References

Variation 1:
Burnett AF, Roman LD, Garcia AA, "A Phase II Study of Gemcitabine and Cisplatin in Patients With Advanced, Persistent, or Recurrent Squamous Cell Carcinoma of the Cervix," *Gynecol Oncol*, 2000, 76(1):63-6.
Variation 2:
Monk BJ, Sill MW, McMeekin DS, et al, "Phase III Trial of Four Cisplatin-Containing Doublet Combinations in Stage IVB, Recurrent, or Persistent Cervical Carcinoma: A Gynecologic Oncology Group Study," *J Clin Oncol*, 2009, 27(28):4649-55.

Cisplatin-Gemcitabine (Mesothelioma)

Index Terms Gemcitabine-Cisplatin (Mesothelioma)

Use Malignant pleural mesothelioma

Regimen NOTE: Multiple variations are listed.

Variation 1:
Cisplatin: I.V.: 100 mg/m^2 over 1 hour day 1
[total dose/cycle = 100 mg/m^2]
Gemcitabine: I.V.: 1000 mg/m^2/day over 30 minutes days 1, 8, and 15
[total dose/cycle = 3000 mg/m^2]
Repeat cycle every 28 days for up to a total of 6 cycles

Variation 2:

Gemcitabine: I.V.: 1250 mg/m^2/day over 30 minutes days 1 and 8
[total dose/cycle = 2500 mg/m^2]

Cisplatin: I.V.: 80 mg/m^2 over 3 hours day 1
[total dose/cycle = 80 mg/m^2]

Repeat cycle every 21 days for up to a total of 6 cycles

Variation 3:

Gemcitabine: I.V.: 1000 mg/m^2/day over 30 minutes days 1, 8, and 15
[total dose/cycle = 3000 mg/m^2]

Cisplatin: I.V.: 30 mg/m^2/day over 30 minutes days 1, 8, and 15
[total dose/cycle = 90 mg/m^2]

Repeat cycle every 28 days

References

Variation 1:

Nowak AK, Byrne MJ, Williamson R, et al, "A Multicentre Phase II Study of Cisplatin and Gemcitabine for Malignant Mesothelioma," *Br J Cancer*, 2002, 87(5):491-6.

Variation 2:

van Haarst JM, Baas P, Manegold Ch, et al, "Multicentre Phase II Study of Gemcitabine and Cisplatin in Malignant Pleural Mesothelioma," *Br J Cancer*, 2002, 86(3):342-5.

Variation 3:

Kalmadi SR, Rankin C, Kraut MJ, et al, "Gemcitabine and Cisplatin in Unresectable Malignant Mesothelioma of the Pleura: A Phase II Study of the Southwest Oncology Group (SWOG 9810)," *Lung Cancer*, 2008, 60:259-63.

◆ **Cisplatin-Gemcitabine (NSCLC)** *see* Gemcitabine-Cisplatin (NSCLC) *on page 1670*

Cisplatin-Gemcitabine (Pancreatic)

Index Terms GemCis (Pancreatic); Gemcitabine-Cisplatin (Pancreatic)

Use Pancreatic cancer

Regimen NOTE: Multiple variations are listed.

Variation 1:

Cisplatin: I.V.: 50 mg/m^2/day over 1 hour days 1 and 15
[total dose/cycle = 100 mg/m^2]

Gemcitabine: I.V.: 1000 mg/m^2/day over 30 minutes days 1 and 15
[total dose/cycle = 2000 mg/m^2]

Repeat cycle every 28 days

Variation 2:

Cycle 1:

Cisplatin: I.V.: 25 mg/m^2/day days 1, 8, 15, 29, 36, and 43 (cycle 1 only)
[total dose/cycle 1 = 150 mg/m^2]

Gemcitabine: I.V.: 1000 mg/m^2/day over 30 minutes days 1, 8, 15, 22, 29, 36, and 43 (cycle 1 only), 1 hour after cisplatin
[total dose/cycle 1 = 7000 mg/m^2]

Treatment cycle is 56 days

Subsequent cycles:

Cisplatin: I.V.: 25 mg/m^2/day days 1, 8, and 15
[total dose/cycle = 75 mg/m^2]

Gemcitabine: I.V.: 1000 mg/m^2/day over 30 minutes days 1, 8, and 15, 1 hour after cisplatin
[total dose/cycle = 3000 mg/m^2]

Repeat cycle every 28 days until disease progression or unacceptable toxicity

References

Variation 1:

Heinemann V, Quietzsch D, Gieseler F, et al, "Randomized Phase III Trial of Gemcitabine Plus Cisplatin Compared With Gemcitabine Alone in Advanced Pancreatic Cancer," *J Clin Oncol*, 2006, 24(24):3946-52.

Variation 2:

Colucci G, Labianca R, Di Costanzo F, et al, "Randomized Phase III Trial of Gemcitabine Plus Cisplatin Compared With Single-Agent Gemcitabine As First-Line Treatment of Patients With Advanced Pancreatic Cancer: The GIP-1 Study," *J Clin Oncol*, 2010, 28(10):1645-51.

Cisplatin-Gemcitabine (Unknown Primary)

Index Terms Gemcitabine-Cisplatin (Unknown Primary)

Use Unknown primary (adenocarcinoma)

Regimen

Gemcitabine: I.V.: 1250 mg/m^2/day days 1 and 8
[total dose/cycle = 2500 mg/m^2]

Cisplatin: I.V.: 100 mg/m^2 day 1
[total dose/cycle = 100 mg/m^2]

Repeat cycle every 21 days

References

Culine S, Lortholary A, Voigt JJ, et al, "Cisplatin in Combination With Either Gemcitabine or Irinotecan in Carcinomas of Unknown Primary Site: Results of a Randomized Phase II Study - Trial for the French Study Group on Carcinomas of Unknown Primary (GEFCAPI 01)," *J Clin Oncol*, 2003, 21(18):3479-82.

◆ **Cisplatin-Ifosfamide-Paclitaxel** *see* Paclitaxel-Ifosfamide-Cisplatin *on page 1730*

◆ **Cisplatin-Irinotecan (Esophageal Cancer)** *see* Irinotecan-Cisplatin (Esophageal Cancer) *on page 1694*

◆ **Cisplatin-Irinotecan (Gastric Cancer)** *see* Irinotecan-Cisplatin (Gastric Cancer) *on page 1695*

Cisplatin-Irinotecan (NSCLC)

Index Terms Irinotecan-Cisplatin (NSCLC)

Use Lung cancer, nonsmall cell

Regimen

Cisplatin: I.V.: 80 mg/m^2 day 1
[total dose/cycle = 80 mg/m^2]

Irinotecan: I.V.: 60 mg/m^2/dose days 1, 8, and 15
[total dose/cycle = 180 mg/m^2]

Repeat cycle every 28 days for at least 3 more cycles or until disease progression or unacceptable toxicity

References

Ohe Y, Ohashi Y, Kubota K, et al, "Randomized Phase III Study of Cisplatin Plus Irinotecan Versus Carboplatin Plus Paclitaxel, Cisplatin Plus Gemcitabine, and Cisplatin Plus Vinorelbine for Advanced Non-Small-Cell Lung Cancer: Four-Arm Cooperative Study in Japan," *Ann Oncol*, 2007, 18(2):317-23.

Cisplatin-Irinotecan (Small Cell Lung Cancer)

Index Terms IP (Small Cell Lung Cancer); Irinotecan-Cisplatin (Small Cell Lung Cancer)

Use Lung cancer, small cell

Regimen NOTE: Multiple variations are listed.

Variation 1:
Cisplatin: I.V.: 60 mg/m^2 day 1
[total dose/cycle = 60 mg/m^2]
Irinotecan: I.V.: 60 mg/m^2/day days 1, 8, and 15
[total dose/cycle = 180 mg/m^2]
Repeat cycle every 28 days for 4 cycles
Variation 2:
Cisplatin: I.V.: 30 mg/m^2/day days 1 and 8
[total dose/cycle = 60 mg/m^2]
Irinotecan: I.V.: 65 mg/m^2/day days 1 and 8
[total dose/cycle = 130 mg/m^2]
Repeat cycle every 21 days for at least 4 cycles

References

Variation 1:

Lara PN Jr, Natale R, Crowley J, et al, "Phase III Trial of Irinotecan/Cisplatin Compared With Etoposide/Cisplatin in Extensive-Stage Small-Cell Lung Cancer: Clinical and Pharmacogenomic Results from SWOG S0124," *J Clin Oncol*, 2009, 27(15):2530-5.

Noda K, Nishiwaki Y, Kawahara M, et al, "Irinotecan Plus Cisplatin Compared With Etoposide Plus Cisplatin for Extensive Small-Cell Lung Cancer," *N Engl J Med*, 2002, 346(2):85-91.

Variation 2:

Hanna N, Bunn PA Jr, Langer C, et al, "Randomized Phase III Trial Comparing Irinotecan/Cisplatin With Etoposide/Cisplatin in Patients With Previously Untreated Extensive-Stage Disease Small-Cell Lung Cancer," *J Clin Oncol*, 2006, 24(13):2038-43.

Cisplatin-Paclitaxel (Cervical Cancer)

Index Terms Paclitaxel-Cisplatin (Cervical Cancer)

Use Cervical cancer

Regimen

Paclitaxel: I.V.: 135 mg/m^2 continuous infusion over 24 hours day 1
[total dose/cycle = 135 mg/m^2]
Cisplatin: I.V.: 50 mg/m^2 day 2
[total dose/cycle = 50 mg/m^2]
Repeat cycle every 21 days for up to a total of 6 cycles; responders may continue beyond 6 cycles

References

Monk BJ, Sill MW, McMeekin DS, et al, "Phase III Trial of Four Cisplatin-Containing Doublet Combinations in Stage IVB, Recurrent, or Persistent Cervical Carcinoma: A Gynecologic Oncology Group Study," *J Clin Oncol*, 2009, 27(28):4649-55.

Moore DH, Blessing JA, McQuellon RP, et al, "Phase III Study of Cisplatin With or Without Paclitaxel in Stage IVB, Recurrent, or Persistent Squamous Cell Carcinoma of the Cervix: A Gynecologic Oncology Group Study," *J Clin Oncol*, 2004, 22(15):3113-9.

♦ **Cisplatin-Paclitaxel (Esophageal Cancer)** *see* Paclitaxel-Cisplatin (Esophageal Cancer) *on page 1727*

♦ **Cisplatin-Paclitaxel-Fluorouracil (Unknown Primary)** *see* Cisplatin-Fluorouracil-Paclitaxel (Unknown Primary) *on page 1577*

Cisplatin-Paclitaxel (Head and Neck Cancer)

Index Terms Paclitaxel-Cisplatin (Head and Neck Cancer)

Use Head and neck cancer

Regimen NOTE: Multiple variations are listed.

Variation 1 (with concurrent radiation therapy):
Paclitaxel: I.V.: 30 mg/m^2 day 1
[total dose/week = 30 mg/m^2]

Cisplatin: I.V.: 20 mg/m² day 2
[total dose/week = 20 mg/m²]
Repeat every week for a total of 7 weeks

Variation 2:

Paclitaxel: I.V.: 175 mg/m² dose over 3 hours day 1
[total dose/cycle = 175 mg/m²]
Cisplatin: I.V.: 75 mg/m²/dose day 1
[total dose/cycle = 75 mg/m²]
Repeat cycle every 3 weeks

References

Variation 1:

Garden AS, Harris J, Vokes EE, et al, "Preliminary Results of Radiation Therapy Oncology Group 97-03: A Randomized Phase II Trial of Concurrent Radiation and Chemotherapy for Advanced Squamous Cell Carcinomas of the Head and Neck," *J Clin Oncol*, 2004, 22(14):2856-64.

Variation 2:

Gibson MK, Li Y, Murphy B, et al, "Randomized Phase III Evaluation of Cisplatin Plus Fluorouracil Versus Cisplatin Plus Paclitaxel in Advanced Head and Neck Cancer (E1395): An Intergroup Trial of the Eastern Cooperative Oncology Group," *J Clin Oncol*, 2005, 23(15):3562-7.

Cisplatin-Paclitaxel Intraperitoneal (Ovarian)

Index Terms Paclitaxel-Cisplatin Intraperitoneal (Ovarian)

Use Ovarian cancer

Regimen Note: I.P. therapies administered in 2 liters warmed saline

Paclitaxel: I.V.: 135 mg/m² continuous infusion over 24 hours day 1
[total I.V. dose/cycle = 135 mg/m²]
Cisplatin: I.P.: 100 mg/m² day 2
[total I.P. dose/cycle = 100 mg/m²]
Paclitaxel: I.P.: 60 mg/m² day 8
[total I.P. dose/cycle = 60 mg/m²]
Repeat cycle every 21 days for 6 cycles

References

Armstrong DK, Bundy B, Wenzel L, et al, "Intraperitoneal Cisplatin and Paclitaxel in Ovarian Cancer," *N Engl J Med*, 2006, 354(1):34-43.

Cisplatin-Paclitaxel (Ovarian)

Index Terms Paclitaxel-Cisplatin (Ovarian)

Use Ovarian cancer

Regimen

Paclitaxel: I.V.: 135 mg/m² continuous infusion over 24 hours day 1
[total dose/cycle = 135 mg/m²]
Cisplatin: I.V.: 75 mg/m² day 2
[total dose/cycle = 75 mg/m²]
Repeat cycle every 21 days for a total of 6 cycles

References

McGuire WP, Hoskins WJ, Brady MF, et al, "Cyclophosphamide and Cisplatin Compared With Paclitaxel and Cisplatin in Patients With Stage III and Stage IV Ovarian Cancer," *N Engl J Med*, 1996, 334(1):1-6.

Muggia FM, Braly PS, Brady MF, et al, "Phase III Randomized Study of Cisplatin Versus Paclitaxel Versus Cisplatin and Paclitaxel in Patients With Suboptimal Stage III or IV Ovarian Cancer: A Gynecologic Oncology Group Study," *J Clin Oncol*, 2000, 18(1):106-15.

Cisplatin-Pemetrexed (Mesothelioma)

Index Terms Pemetrexed-Cisplatin (Mesothelioma)

Use Malignant pleural mesothelioma

Regimen

Pemetrexed: I.V.: 500 mg/m^2 over 10 minutes day 1
[total dose/cycle = 500 mg/m^2]

Cisplatin: I.V.: 75 mg/m^2 over 2 hours day 1 (start 30 minutes after pemetrexed)
[total dose/cycle = 75 mg/m^2]

Repeat cycle every 21 days

References

Santoro A, O'Brien ME, Stahel RA, et al, "Pemetrexed Plus Cisplatin or Pemetrexed Plus Carboplatin for Chemonaïve Patients With Malignant Pleural Mesothelioma: Results of the International Expanded Access Program," *J Thorac Oncol*, 2008, 3(7):756-63.

Vogelzang NJ, Rusthoven JJ, Symanowski J, et al, "Phase III Study of Pemetrexed in Combination With Cisplatin Versus Cisplatin Alone in Patients With Malignant Pleural Mesothelioma," *J Clin Oncol*, 2003, 21(14):2636-44.

Cisplatin-Pemetrexed (NSCLC)

Index Terms Pemetrexed-Cisplatin (NSCLC)

Use Lung cancer, nonsmall cell

Regimen

Pemetrexed: I.V.: 500 mg/m^2 day 1
[total dose/cycle = 500 mg/m^2]

Cisplatin: I.V.: 75 mg/m^2 day 1
[total dose/cycle = 75 mg/m^2]

Repeat cycle every 21 days for up to 6 cycles

References

Scagliotti GV, Parikh P, von Pawel J, et al, "Phase III Study Comparing Cisplatin Plus Gemcitabine With Cisplatin Plus Pemetrexed in Chemotherapy-Naive Patients With Advanced-Stage Non-Small-Cell Lung Cancer," *J Clin Oncol*, 2008, 26(21):3543-51.

Cisplatin-Raltitrexed (Mesothelioma)

Index Terms Raltitrexed-Cisplatin (Mesothelioma)

Use Malignant pleural mesothelioma

Regimen

Raltitrexed: I.V.: 3 mg/m^2 over 15 minutes day 1
[total dose/cycle = 3 mg/m^2]

Cisplatin: I.V.: 80 mg/m^2 over 1-2 hours day 1
[total dose/cycle = 80 mg/m^2]

Repeat cycle every 21 days until disease progression or unacceptable toxicity.

References

Bottomley A, Coens C, Efficace F, et al, "Symptoms and Patient-Reported Well-Being: Do They Predict Survival in Malignant Pleural Mesothelioma? A Prognostic Factor Analysis of EORTC-NCIC 08983: Randomized Phase III Study of Cisplatin With or Without Raltitrexed in Patients With Malignant Pleural Mesothelioma," *J Clin Oncol*, 2007, 25(36):5770-6.

van Meerbeeck JP, Gaafar R, Manegold C, et al, "Randomized Phase III Study of Cisplatin With or Without Raltitrexed in Patients With Malignant Pleural Mesothelioma: An Intergroup Study of the European Organisation for Research and Treatment of Cancer Lung Cancer Group and the National Cancer Institute of Canada," *J Clin Oncol*, 2005, 23(28):6881-9.

Cisplatin-Topotecan (Cervical Cancer)

Index Terms Topotecan-Cisplatin (Cervical Cancer)

Use Cervical cancer

Regimen NOTE: Multiple variations are listed.

Variation 1 (Body surface area capped at 2 m^2 maximum):

Topotecan: I.V.: 0.75 mg/m^2/day days 1, 2, and 3
[total dose/cycle = 2.25 mg/m^2]

Cisplatin: I.V.: 50 mg/m^2 day 1 only
[total dose/cycle = 50 mg/m^2]
Repeat cycle every 21 days for up to a total of 6 cycles; responders may continue beyond 6 cycles

Variation 2:
Topotecan: I.V.: 0.75 mg/m^2/day days 1, 2, and 3
[total dose/cycle = 2.25 mg/m^2]
Cisplatin: I.V.: 50 mg/m^2 day 1 only
[total dose/cycle = 50 mg/m^2]
Repeat cycle every 21 days for up to a total of 6 cycles; responders may continue beyond 6 cycles

References

Variation 1:

Long HJ 3rd, Bundy BN, Grendys EC Jr, et al, "Randomized Phase III Trial of Cisplatin With or Without Topotecan in Carcinoma of the Uterine Cervix: A Gynecologic Oncology Group Study," *J Clin Oncol*, 2005, 23(21):4626-33.

Variation 2:

Monk BJ, Sill MW, McMeekin DS, et al, "Phase III Trial of Four Cisplatin-Containing Doublet Combinations in Stage IVB, Recurrent, or Persistent Cervical Carcinoma: A Gynecologic Oncology Group Study," *J Clin Oncol*, 2009, 27(28):4649-55.

◆ **Cisplatin-Vinblastine-Dacarbazine-Interleukin-Interferon (Melanoma)** *see* CVD-Interleukin-Interferon (Melanoma) *on page 1597*

Cisplatin-Vinblastine-Dacarbazine (Melanoma)

Index Terms CVD; Dacarbazine-Cisplatin-Vinblastine; Vinblastine-Cisplatin-Dacarbazine

Use Melanoma

Regimen NOTE: Multiple variations are listed.

Variation 1:
Cisplatin: I.V.: 20 mg/m^2/day days 2 to 5
[total dose/cycle = 80 mg/m^2]
Vinblastine: I.V.: 1.6 mg/m^2/day days 1 to 5
[total dose/cycle = 8 mg/m^2]
Dacarbazine: I.V.: 800 mg/m^2 day 1
[total dose/cycle = 800 mg/m^2]
Repeat cycle every 21 days

Variation 2:
Cisplatin: I.V.: 20 mg/m^2/day days 1 to 4
[total dose/cycle = 80 mg/m^2]
Vinblastine: I.V.: 2 mg/m^2/day days 1 to 4
[total dose/cycle = 8 mg/m^2]
Dacarbazine: I.V.: 800 mg/m^2 day 1
[total dose/cycle = 800 mg/m^2]
Repeat cycle every 21 days

References

Variation 1:

Legha SS, Ring S, Papadopoulos N, et al, "A Prospective Evaluation of a Triple-Drug Regimen Containing Cisplatin, Vinblastine, and Dacarbazine (CVD) for Metastatic Melanoma," *Cancer*, 1989, 64(10):2024-9.

Variation 2:

Eton O, Legha SS, Bedikian AY, et al, "Sequential Biochemotherapy Versus Chemotherapy for Metastatic Melanoma: Results From a Phase III Randomized Trial," *J Clin Oncol*, 2002, 20 (8):2045-52.

Cisplatin-Vinblastine (NSCLC)

Index Terms Vinblastine-Cisplatin

Use Lung cancer, nonsmall cell

Regimen NOTE: Multiple variations are listed.

Variation 1:

Cisplatin: I.V.: 80 mg/m^2/day days 1, 22, 43, and 64
[total dose/treatment = 320 mg/m^2]

Vinblastine: I.V.: 4 mg/m^2/day days 1, 8, 15, 22, 29, 43, and 57
[total dose/treatment = 28 mg/m^2]

Variation 2:

Cisplatin: I.V.: 100 mg/m^2/day days 1, 29, and 57
[total dose/treatment = 300 mg/m^2]

Vinblastine: I.V.: 4 mg/m^2/day days 1, 8, 15, 22, 29, 43, and 57
[total dose/treatment = 28 mg/m^2]

Variation 3:

Cisplatin: I.V.: 100 mg/m^2/day days 1, 29, 57, and 85
[total dose/treatment = 400 mg/m^2]

Vinblastine: I.V.: 4 mg/m^2/day days 1, 8, 15, 22, 29, 43, 57, 71, and 85
[total dose/treatment = 36 mg/m^2]

Variation 4:

Cisplatin: I.V.: 120 mg/m^2/day days 1, 29, and 71
[total dose/treatment = 360 mg/m^2]

Vinblastine: I.V.: 4 mg/m^2/day days 1, 8, 15, 22, 29, 43, 57, and 71
[total dose/treatment = 32 mg/m^2]

References

Arriagada R, Bergman B, Dunant A, et al, "Cisplatin-Based Adjuvant Chemotherapy in Patients With Completely Resected Non-Small-Cell Lung Cancer," *N Engl J Med*, 2004, 350(4):351-60.

◆ **Cisplatin-Vinorelbine** *see* Vinorelbine-Cisplatin *on page* 1772

Cisplatin-Vinorelbine (Cervical Cancer)

Index Terms Vinorelbine-Cisplatin (Cervical Cancer)

Use Cervical cancer

Regimen NOTE: Multiple variations are listed.

Variation 1:

Cisplatin: I.V.: 50 mg/m^2 day 1
[total dose/cycle = 50 mg/m^2]

Vinorelbine: I.V.: 30 mg/m^2/day days 1 and 8
[total dose/cycle = 60 mg/m^2]

Repeat cycle every 21 days for up to a total of 6 cycles; responders may continue beyond 6 cycles

Variation 2:

Cisplatin: I.V.: 80 mg/m^2 day 1
[total dose/cycle = 80 mg/m^2]

Vinorelbine: I.V.: 25 mg/m^2/day days 1 and 8
[total dose/cycle = 50 mg/m^2]

Repeat cycle every 21 days for a total of 3-6 cycles

References

Variation 1:

Monk BJ, Sill MW, McMeekin DS, et al, "Phase III Trial of Four Cisplatin-Containing Doublet Combinations in Stage IVB, Recurrent, or Persistent Cervical Carcinoma: A Gynecologic Oncology Group Study," *J Clin Oncol*, 2009, 27(28):4649-55.

Variation 2:
Gebbia V, Caruso M, Testa A, et al, "Vinorelbine and Cisplatin for the Treatment of Recurrent and/or Metastatic Carcinoma of the Uterine Cervix," *Oncology*, 2002, 63(1):31-7.
Pignata S, Silvestro G, Ferrari E, et al, "Phase II Study of Cisplatin and Vinorelbine as First-Line Chemotherapy in Patients With Carcinoma of the Uterine Cervix," *J Clin Oncol*, 1999, 17 (3):756-60.

- **Cisplatin-Vinorelbine-Cetuximab (NSCLC)** *see* Cetuximab-Cisplatin-Vinorelbine (NSCLC) *on page 1558*
- **Cladribine-Cytarabine-G-CSF** *see* CLAG (AML Induction) *on page 1586*
- **Cladribine-Cytarabine-Mitoxantrone-G-CS** *see* CLAG-M (AML Induction) *on page 1586*

CLAG (AML Induction)

Index Terms Cladribine-Cytarabine-G-CSF

Use Leukemia, acute myeloid

Regimen

Cladribine: I.V.: 5 mg/m²/day over 2 hours days 1 to 5
[total dose/cycle = 25 mg/m²]

Cytarabine: I.V.: 2 g/m²/day over 4 hours days 1 to 5 (begin 2 hours after cladribine)
[total dose/cycle = 10 g/m²]

Filgrastim: SubQ: 300 mcg daily days 0 to 5 (start 24 hours prior to chemotherapy; for a total of 6 days)
[total dose/cycle = 1800 mcg]

May administer a second induction cycle if needed

References

Robak T, Wrzesień-Kuś A, Lech-Marańda E, et al, "Combination Regimen of Cladribine (2-Chlorodeoxyadenosine), Cytarabine and G-CSF (CLAG) as Induction Therapy for Patients With Relapsed or Refractory Acute Myeloid Leukemia," *Leuk Lymphoma*, 2000, 39(1-2):121-9.
Wrzesień-Kuś A, Robak T, Lech-Marańda E, et al, "A Multicenter, Open, Non-Comparative Phase II Study of the Combination of Cladribine (2-Chlorodeoxyadenosine), Cytarabine, and G-CSF as Induction Therapy in Refractory Acute Myeloid Leukemia – A Report of the Polish Adult Leukemia Group (PALG)," *Eur J Haematol*, 2003;71(3):155–62.

CLAG-M (AML Induction)

Index Terms Cladribine-Cytarabine-Mitoxantrone-G-CS

Use Leukemia, acute myeloid

Regimen

Cladribine: I.V.: 5 mg/m²/day over 2 hour days 1 to 5
[total dose/cycle = 25 mg/m²]

Cytarabine: I.V.: 2 g/m²/day over 4 hours days 1 to 5 (begin 2 hours after cladribine)
[total dose/cycle = 10 g/m²]

Mitoxantrone: I.V.: 10 mg/m²/day days 1 to 3
[total dose/cycle = 30 mg/m²]

Filgrastim: SubQ: 300 mcg daily days 0 to 5 (start 24 hours prior to chemotherapy; for a total of 6 days)
[total dose/cycle = 1800 mcg]

May administer a second induction cycle if needed

References

Wierzbowska A, Robak T, Pluta A, et al, "Cladribine Combined With High Doses of Arabinoside Cytosine, Mitoxantrone, and G-CSF (CLAG-M) is a Highly Effective Salvage Regimen in Patients With Refractory and Relapsed Acute Myeloid Leukemia of the Poor Risk: A Final Report of the Polish Adult Leukemia Group," *Eur J Haematol* 2008; 80(2):115-26.

Clofarabine (AML Consolidation)

Use Leukemia, acute myeloid

Regimen

Clofarabine: I.V.: 20 mg/m^2/day over 1 hour days 1 to 5
[total dose/cycle = 100 mg/m^2]

Up to a maximum total of 6 cycles (including induction/reinduction) may be administered

References

Kantarjian HM, Erba HP, Claxton D, et al, "Phase II Study of Clofarabine Monotherapy in Previously Untreated Older Adults With Acute Myeloid Leukemia and Unfavorable Prognostic Factors," *J Clin Oncol*, 2010, 28(4):549-55.

Clofarabine (AML Induction)

Use Leukemia, acute myeloid

Regimen

Induction:

Clofarabine: I.V.: 30 mg/m^2/day over 1 hour days 1 to 5
[total dose/cycle = 150 mg/m^2]

Reinduction (if needed) after day 28 of induction:

Clofarabine: I.V.: 20 mg/m^2/day over 1 hour days 1 to 5
[total dose/cycle = 100 mg/m^2]

References

Kantarjian HM, Erba HP, Claxton D, et al, "Phase II Study of Clofarabine Monotherapy in Previously Untreated Older Adults With Acute Myeloid Leukemia and Unfavorable Prognostic Factors," *J Clin Oncol*, 2010, 28(4):549-55.

Clofarabine-Cytarabine (AML Consolidation)

Use Leukemia, acute myeloid

Regimen

Clofarabine: I.V.: 30 mg/m^2/day infusion over 1 hour on days 1, 2, and 3
[total dose/cycle = 90 mg/m^2]

Cytarabine: SubQ: 20 mg/m^2/day days 1 to 7 (4 hours after clofarabine on days 1, 2, and 3)
[total dose/cycle = 140 mg/m^2]

Repeat cycle every 4 to 7 weeks; up to a total of 12 consolidation cycles may be administered

References

Faderl S, Ravandi F, Huang X, et al, "A Randomized Study of Clofarabine Versus Clofarabine Plus Low-Dose Cytarabine as Front-Line Therapy for Patients Aged 60 Years and Older With Acute Myeloid Leukemia and High-Risk Myelodysplastic Syndrome," *Blood*, 2008, 112(5):1638-45.

Clofarabine-Cytarabine (AML Induction)

Use Leukemia, acute myeloid

Regimen

Clofarabine: I.V.: 30 mg/m^2/day infusion over 1 hour on days 1 to 5
[total dose/cycle = 150 mg/m^2]

Cytarabine: SubQ: 20 mg/m^2/day days 1 to 14 (4 hours after clofarabine on days 1 to 5)
[total dose/cycle = 280 mg/m^2]

A second induction cycle may be administered if needed

References

Faderl S, Ravandi F, Huang X, et al, "A Randomized Study of Clofarabine Versus Clofarabine Plus Low-Dose Cytarabine as Front-Line Therapy for Patients Aged 60 Years and Older With Acute Myeloid Leukemia and High-Risk Myelodysplastic Syndrome," *Blood*, 2008, 112(5):1638-45.

CMF

Use Breast cancer

Regimen NOTE: Multiple variations are listed.

Variation 1:

Methotrexate: I.V.: 40 mg/m^2/day days 1 and 8
[total dose/cycle = 80 mg/m^2]

Fluorouracil: I.V.: 600 mg/m^2/day days 1 and 8
[total dose/cycle = 1200 mg/m^2]

Cyclophosphamide: Oral: 100 mg/m^2/day days 1 to 14
[total dose/cycle = 1400 mg/m^2]

Repeat cycle every 28 days

Variation 2 (>60 years of age):

Methotrexate: I.V.: 30 mg/m^2/day days 1 and 8
[total dose/cycle = 60 mg/m^2]

Fluorouracil: I.V.: 400 mg/m^2/day days 1 and 8
[total dose/cycle = 800 mg/m^2]

Cyclophosphamide: Oral: 100 mg/m^2/day days 1 to 14
[total dose/cycle = 1400 mg/m^2]

Repeat cycle every 28 days

References

Variations 1 and 2:

Bonadonna G, Brusamolino E, Valagussa P, et al, "Combination Chemotherapy as an Adjuvant Treatment in Operable Breast Cancer," *N Engl J Med*, 1976, 294(8):405-10.

Canellos GP, Pocock SJ, Taylor SG III, et al, "Combination Chemotherapy for Metastatic Breast Carcinoma, Prospective Comparison of Multiple Drug Therapy With L-Phenylalanine Mustard," *Cancer*, 1976, 38(5):1882-6.

CMF-IV

Use Breast cancer

Regimen

Cyclophosphamide: I.V.: 600 mg/m^2 day 1
[total dose/cycle = 600 mg/m^2]

Methotrexate: I.V.: 40 mg/m^2 day 1
[total dose/cycle = 40 mg/m^2]

Fluorouracil: I.V.: 600 mg/m^2 day 1
[total dose/cycle = 600 mg/m^2]

Repeat cycle every 21 or 28 days

References

Bonadonna G, Veronesi U, Brambilla C, et al, "Primary Chemotherapy to Avoid Mastectomy in Tumors With Diameters of Three Centimeters or More," *J Natl Cancer Inst*, 1990, 82(19):1539-45.

Tannock IF, Boyd NF, DeBoer G, et al, "A Randomized Trial of Two Dose Levels of Cyclophosphamide, Methotrexate, and Fluorouracil Chemotherapy for Patients With Metastatic Breast Cancer," *J Clin Oncol*, 1988, 6(9):1377-87.

◆ **C MOPP** *see* COPP *on page* *1596*

C-MOPP/ABV Hybrid (Hodgkin)

Index Terms Cyclophosphamide-Vincristine-Procarbazine-Prednisone-Doxorubicin-Bleomycin-Vinblastine (Hodgkin)

Use Lymphoma, Hodgkin

Regimen

Cyclophosphamide: I.V.: 650 mg/m²/day day 1
[total dose/cycle = 650 mg/m²]
Vincristine: I.V.: 1.4 mg/m²/day (maximum dose: 3 mg) day 1
[total dose/cycle = 1.4 mg/m²; maximum dose/cycle: 3 mg]
Procarbazine: Oral: 100 mg/m²/day days 1 to 7
[total dose/cycle = 700 mg/m²]
Prednisone: Oral: 40 mg/m²/day days 1 to 14
[total dose/cycle = 560 mg/m²]
Doxorubicin: I.V.: 35 mg/m²/day day 8
[total dose/cycle = 35 mg/m²]
Bleomycin: I.V.: 10 units/m²/day day 8
[total dose/cycle = 10 units/m²]
Vinblastine: I.V.: 6 mg/m²/day day 8
[total dose/cycle = 6 mg/m²]
Repeat cycles every 28 days for a total of 8 cycles

References

Montoto S, Camós M, López-Guillermo A, et al, "Hybrid Chemotherapy Consisting of Cyclophosphamide, Vincristine, Procarbazine, Prednisone, Doxorubicin, Bleomycin, and Vinblastine (C-MOPP/ABV) as First-Line Treatment for Patients With Advanced Hodgkin Disease," *Cancer*, 2000;88(9):2142-8.

CMV

Use Bladder cancer

Regimen

Cisplatin: I.V.: 100 mg/m² infused over 4 hours (start at least 12 hours after methotrexate) day 2
[total dose = 100 mg/m²]
Methotrexate: I.V.: 30 mg/m²/day days 1 and 8
[total dose = 60 mg/m²]
Vinblastine: I.V.: 4 mg/m²/day days 1 and 8
[total dose = 8 mg/m²]
Repeat cycle every 21 days

References

Harker WG, Meyers FJ, Freiha FS, et al, "Cisplatin, Methotrexate, and Vinblastine (CMV): An Effective Chemotherapy Regimen for Metastatic Transitional Cell Carcinoma of the Urinary Tract. A Northern California Oncology Group Study," *J Clin Oncol*, 1985, 3(11):1463-70.

CNOP

Use Lymphoma, non-Hodgkin's

Regimen

Cyclophosphamide: I.V.: 750 mg/m² day 1
[total dose/cycle = 750 mg/m²]
Mitoxantrone: I.V.: 10 mg/m² day 1
[total dose/cycle = 10 mg/m²]
Vincristine: I.V.: 1.4 mg/m² day 1
[total dose/cycle = 1.4 mg/m²]
Prednisone: Oral: 50 mg/m²/day days 1 to 5
[total dose/cycle = 250 mg/m²]
Repeat cycle every 21 days

References

Pavlovsky S, Santarelli MT, Erazo A, et al, "Results of a Randomized Study of Previously Untreated Intermediate and High Grade Lymphoma Using CHOP Versus CNOP," *Ann Oncol*, 1992, 3(3):205-9.

CODOX-M

Use Lymphoma, non-Hodgkin's

Regimen NOTE: Multiple variations are listed.

Variation 1:

Cyclophosphamide: I.V.: 800 mg/m^2 day 1
followed by I.V.: 200 mg/m^2/day days 2 to 5
[total dose/cycle = 1600 mg/m^2]

Vincristine: I.V.: 1.5 mg/m^2/dose (no maximum dose) days 1 and 8
[total dose/cycle = 3 mg/m^2]

Doxorubicin: I.V.: 40 mg/m^2/dose day 1
[total dose/cycle = 40 mg/m^2]

Methotrexate: I.V.: 1200 mg/m^2 (loading dose) over 1 hour
followed by I.V.: 240 mg/m^2/hour for 23 hours day 10
[total dose/cycle = 6720 mg/m^2]

Leucovorin: I.V.: 192 mg/m^2/dose day 11 (begin 36 hours after the start of methotrexate infusion)
followed by I.V.: 12 mg/m^2/dose every 6 hours until methotrexate level <5 x 10^{-8}M

Cytarabine: I.T.: 70 mg/dose (adjust to age-appropriate dose if <3 years of age) day 1
[total dose/cycle = 70 mg]

Methotrexate: I.T.: 12 mg/dose (adjust to age-appropriate dose if <3 years of age) day 3
[total dose/cycle = 12 mg]

Repeat cycle when ANC >1000/m^3 for a total of three cycles

Variation 2:

Cyclophosphamide: I.V.: 800 mg/m^2/dose day 1
followed by I.V.: 200 mg/m^2/dose days 2 to 5
[total dose/cycle = 1600 mg/m^2]

Vincristine: I.V.: 1.5 mg/m^2/dose (maximum dose: 2 mg) days 1 and 8
[total dose/cycle = 3 mg/m^2; maximum: 4 mg/cycle]

Doxorubicin: I.V.: 40 mg/m^2/dose day 1
[total dose/cycle = 40 mg/m^2]

Methotrexate: I.V.: 1200 mg/m^2 (loading dose) over 1 hour
followed by I.V.: 240 mg/m^2/hour for 23 hours day 10
[total dose/cycle = 6720 mg/m^2]

Leucovorin: I.V.: 192 mg/m^2/dose day 11 (begin 36 hours after the start of methotrexate infusion)
followed by I.V.: 12 mg/m^2/dose every 6 hours until methotrexate level <5 x 10^{-8}M

Cytarabine: I.T.: 70 mg/dose days 1 and 3
[total dose/cycle = 140 mg]

Methotrexate: I.T.: 12 mg/dose day 15
[total dose/cycle = 12 mg]

Leucovorin: Oral: 15 mg/dose day 16 (24 hours after I.T. methotrexate)

Filgrastim: 5 mcg/kg/day beginning day 13, continue until ANC >1000/mm^3

Repeat cycle when ANC >1000/mm^3 for a total of three cycles

Variation 3:

Cyclophosphamide: I.V.: 800 mg/m^2/dose days 1 and 2
[total dose/cycle = 1600 mg/m^2]

Vincristine: I.V.: 1.4 mg/m^2/dose (maximum dose: 2 mg) days 1 and 10
[total dose/cycle = 2.8 mg/m^2; maximum: 4 mg/cycle]

Doxorubicin: I.V.: 50 mg/m^2/dose day 1
[total dose/cycle = 50 mg/m^2]
Methotrexate: I.V.: 3 g/m^2 day 10
[total dose/cycle = 3 g/m^2]
Leucovorin: I.V.: 200 mg/m^2/dose day 11
followed by Oral, I.V.: 15 mg/m^2/dose every 6 hours until methotrexate level <0.1 Mmol/L
Cytarabine: I.T.: 50 mg/dose day 1
[total dose/cycle = 50 mg]
Hydrocortisone: I.T.: 50 mg/dose day 1
[total dose/cycle = 50 mg]
Methotrexate: I.T.: 12 mg/dose day 1
[total dose/cycle = 12 mg]
Filgrastim: SubQ: Dose not specified; days 3 to 8 and day 12 until ANC >1000/mm^3
Repeat cycle when ANC >1000/mm^3 for a total of three cycles

References

Variation 1:

Magrath I, Adde M, Shad A, et al, "Adults and Children With Small Non-Cleaved-Cell Lymphoma Have a Similar Excellent Outcome When Treated With the Same Chemotherapy Regimen," *J Clin Oncol*, 1996, 14(3):925-34.

Variation 2:

Mead GM, Sydes MR, Walewski J, et al, "An International Evaluation of CODOX-M and CODOX-M Alternating With IVAC in Adult Burkitt's Lymphoma: Results of United Kingdom Lymphoma Group LY06 Study," *Ann Oncol*, 2002, 13(8):1264-74.

Variation 3:

Lacasce A, Howard O, Lib S, et al, "Modified Magrath Regimens for Adults With Burkitt and Burkitt Like Lymphomas: Preserved Efficacy With Decreased Toxicity," *Leuk Lymphoma*, 2004, 45 (4):761-7.

CODOX-M/IVAC

Use Lymphoma, non-Hodgkin's (Burkitt)

Regimen NOTE: Multiple variations are listed.

Variation 1:

CODOX-M (Cycles 1 and 3; cycles begin when ANC >1000/mm^3)

Cyclophosphamide: I.V.: 800 mg/m^2/dose day 1
followed by I.V.: 200 mg/m^2/dose days 2 to 5
[total dose/cycle = 1600 mg/m^2]
Vincristine: I.V.: 1.5 mg/m^2/dose (no maximum dose) days 1 and 8 (cycle 1) and days 1, 8, and 15 (cycle 3)
[total dose/cycle = 3-4.5 mg/m^2]
Doxorubicin: I.V.: 40 mg/m^2/dose day 1
[total dose/cycle = 40 mg/m^2]
Methotrexate: I.V.: 1200 mg/m^2 (loading dose) over 1 hour
followed by I.V.: 240 mg/m^2/hour for 23 hours day 10
[total dose/cycle = 6720 mg/m^2]
Leucovorin: I.V.: 192 mg/m^2/dose day 11 (begin 36 hours after the start of methotrexate infusion)
followed by I.V.: 12 mg/m^2/dose every 6 hours until methotrexate level <5 x 10^{-8}M
Cytarabine: I.T.: 70 mg/dose (adjust to age-appropriate dose if <3 years of age) days 1 and 3
[total dose/cycle = 140 mg]

Methotrexate: I.T.: 12 mg/dose (adjust to age-appropriate dose if <3 years of age) day 15
[total dose/cycle = 12 mg]
Sargramostim: SubQ: 7.5 mcg/kg/day beginning day 13, continue until ANC >1000/mm^3
Note: If CNS disease present, administer additional I.T. treatment in cycle 1: Cytarabine 70 mg/dose (adjust to age-appropriate dose if <3 years of age) on day 5 and methotrexate 12 mg/dose (adjust to age-appropriate dose if <3 years of age) on day 17

IVAC (Cycles 2 and 4; cycles begin when ANC >1000/mm^3)
Ifosfamide: I.V.: 1500 mg/m^2/dose days 1 to 5
[total dose/cycle = 7500 mg/m^2]
Mesna: I.V.: 360 mg/m^2/dose every 3 hours days 1 to 5
Etoposide: I.V.: 60 mg/m^2/dose days 1 to 5
[total dose/cycle = 300 mg/m^2]
Cytarabine: I.V.: 2 g/m^2/dose every 12 hours, for 4 doses, days 1 and 2
[total dose/cycle = 8 g/m^2]
Methotrexate: I.T.: 12 mg/dose day 5
[total dose/cycle = 12 mg]
Sargramostim: SubQ: 7.5 mcg/kg/day beginning day 7, continue until ANC >1000/mm^3
Note: If CNS disease present, administer additional I.T. treatment in cycle 2: Cytarabine 70 mg/dose (adjust to age-appropriate dose if <3 years of age) on days 7 and 9

Variation 2:

CODOX-M (Cycles 1 and 3; cycles begin when ANC >1000/mm^3)
Cyclophosphamide: I.V.: 800 mg/m^2/dose day 1
followed by I.V.: 200 mg/m^2/dose days 2 to 5
[total dose/cycle = 1600 mg/m^2]
Vincristine: I.V.: 1.5 mg/m^2/dose (maximum dose: 2 mg) days 1 and 8
[total dose/cycle = 3 mg/m^2; maximum: 4 mg/cycle]
Doxorubicin: I.V.: 40 mg/m^2/dose day 1
[total dose/cycle = 40 mg/m^2]
Methotrexate: I.V.: 300 mg/m^2 (100 mg/m^2 if >65 years of age) (loading dose) over 1 hour
followed by I.V.: 2700 mg/m^2 (900 mg/m^2 if >65 years of age) over 23 hours day 10
[total dose/cycle = 3000 mg/m^2 (1000 mg/m^2 if >65 years of age)]
Leucovorin: I.V.: 15 mg/m^2/dose every 3 hours beginning day 11 (begin 36 hours after the start of methotrexate infusion) for 5 doses
followed by I.V.: 15 mg/m^2/dose every 6 hours until methotrexate level $<5 \times 10^{-8}$M
Cytarabine: I.T.: 70 mg/dose days 1 and 3
[total dose/cycle = 140 mg]
Methotrexate: I.T.: 12 mg/dose day 15
[total dose/cycle = 12 mg]
Leucovorin: Oral: 15 mg/dose day 16 (24 hours after I.T. methotrexate)
Filgrastim: SubQ: 5 mcg/kg/day beginning day 13, continue until ANC >1000/mm^3
Note: If CNS disease present, administer additional I.T. treatment: Cytarabine 70 mg/dose on day 5 and methotrexate 12 mg/dose (with leucovorin rescue) on day 17

IVAC (Cycles 2 and 4; cycles begin when ANC >1000/mm^3)
Ifosfamide: I.V.: 1500 mg/m^2/dose (1000 mg/m^2/dose if >65 years of age) days 1 to 5
[total dose/cycle = 7500 mg/m^2 (5000 mg/m^2 if >65 years of age)]
Mesna: I.V.: 300 mg/m^2/dose (200 mg/m^2/dose if >65 years of age) mixed with each ifosfamide dose
followed by I.V.: 300 mg/m^2/dose (200 mg/m^2/dose if >65 years of age) every 4 hours for 2 doses/day days 1 to 5
[total dose/cycle = 4500 mg/m^2 (3000 mg/m^2/dose if >65 years of age)]
Etoposide: I.V.: 60 mg/m^2/dose days 1 to 5
[total dose/cycle = 300 mg/m^2]
Cytarabine: I.V.: 2 g/m^2/dose (1 g/m^2/dose if >65 years of age) every 12 hours, for 4 doses, days 1 and 2
[total dose/cycle = 8 g/m^2 (4 g/m^2 if >65 years of age)]
Methotrexate: I.T.: 12 mg day 5
[total dose/cycle = 12 mg]
Leucovorin: Oral: 15 mg/dose day 6 (24 hours after I.T. methotrexate)
Filgrastim: SubQ: 5 mcg/kg/day beginning day 7, continue until ANC >1000/mm^3
Note: If CNS disease present, administer additional I.T. treatment: Cytarabine 70 mg/dose on days 7 and 9

Variation 3:

CODOX-M (Cycles 1 and 3; cycles begin when ANC >1000/mm^3)
Cyclophosphamide: I.V.: 800 mg/m^2/dose day 1
followed by I.V.: 200 mg/m^2/dose days 2 to 5
[total dose/cycle = 1600 mg/m^2]
Vincristine: I.V.: 1.5 mg/m^2/dose (maximum dose: 2 mg) days 1 and 8
[total dose/cycle = 3 mg/m^2; maximum: 4 mg/cycle]
Doxorubicin: I.V.: 40 mg/m^2/dose day 1
[total dose/cycle = 40 mg/m^2]
Methotrexate: I.V.: 1200 mg/m^2 (loading dose) over 1 hour
followed by I.V.: 240 mg/m^2/hour for 23 hours day 10
[total dose/cycle = 6720 mg/m^2]
Leucovorin: I.V.: 192 mg/m^2/dose day 11 (begin 36 hours after the start of methotrexate infusion)
followed by I.V.: 12 mg/m^2/dose every 6 hours until methotrexate level <5 x 10^{-8}M
Cytarabine: I.T.: 70 mg/dose days 1 and 3
[total dose/cycle = 140 mg]
Methotrexate: I.T.: 12 mg/dose day 15
[total dose/cycle = 12 mg]
Leucovorin: Oral: 15 mg/dose day 16 (24 hours after I.T. methotrexate)
Filgrastim: SubQ: 5 mcg/kg/day beginning day 13, continue until ANC >1000/mm^3
Note: If CNS disease present, administer additional I.T. treatment in cycle 1: Cytarabine 70 mg/dose (15 mg if via Ommaya reservoir) on day 5 and methotrexate 12.5 mg/dose (2 mg if via Ommaya reservoir) on day 17

IVAC (Cycles 2 and 4; cycles begin when ANC >1000/mm^3)
Ifosfamide: I.V.: 1500 mg/m^2/dose days 1 to 5
[total dose/cycle = 7500 mg/m^2]
Mesna: I.V.: 360 mg/m^2/dose mixed with each ifosfamide dose
followed by I.V.: 360 mg/m^2/dose every 3 hours for 7 doses/day days 1 to 5
[total dose/cycle = 14,400 mg/m^2]

Etoposide: I.V.: 60 mg/m^2/dose days 1 to 5
[total dose/cycle = 300 mg/m^2]
Cytarabine: I.V.: 2 g/m^2/dose every 12 hours, for 4 doses, days 1 and 2
[total dose/cycle = 8 g/m^2]
Methotrexate: I.T.: 12 mg/dose day 5
[total dose/cycle = 12 mg]
Leucovorin: Oral: 15 mg/dose day 6 (24 hours after I.T. methotrexate)
Filgrastim: SubQ: 5 mcg/kg/day beginning day 7, continue until ANC >1000/mm^3
Note: If CNS disease present, administer additional I.T. treatment in cycle 2:
Cytarabine 70 mg/dose (15 mg if via Ommaya reservoir) on days 7 and 9

Variation 4:

CODOX-M (Cycles 1 and 3; cycles begin when ANC >1000/mm^3)
Cyclophosphamide: I.V.: 800 mg/m^2/dose days 1 and 2
[total dose/cycle = 1600 mg/m^2]
Vincristine: I.V.: 1.4 mg/m^2/dose (maximum dose: 2 mg) days 1 and 10
[total dose/cycle = 2.8 mg/m^2; maximum: 4 mg/cycle]
Doxorubicin: I.V.: 50 mg/m^2/dose day 1
[total dose/cycle = 50 mg/m^2]
Methotrexate: I.V.: 3 g/m^2 day 10
[total dose/cycle = 3 g/m^2]
Leucovorin: I.V.: 200 mg/m^2/dose day 11
followed by Oral, I.V.: 15 mg/m^2/dose every 6 hours until methotrexate level <0.1 Mmol/L
Cytarabine: I.T.: 50 mg/dose days 1 and 3
[total dose/cycle = 100 mg]
Hydrocortisone: I.T.: 50 mg/dose days 1 and 3
[total dose/cycle = 100 mg]
Methotrexate: I.T.: 12 mg/dose day 1
[total dose/cycle = 12 mg]
Filgrastim: SubQ: Dose not specified, days 3 to 8 and day 12 until ANC >1000 mm^3
Note: If CNS disease present, administer additional I.T. treatment in cycle 1:
Cytarabine 50 mg/dose on day 5 and methotrexate 12 mg/dose on day 10

IVAC (Cycles 2 and 4; cycles begin when ANC >1000/mm^3)
Ifosfamide: I.V.: 1500 mg/m^2/dose days 1 to 5
[total dose/cycle = 7500 mg/m^2]
Mesna: I.V.: 1500 mg/m^2/day (in divided doses) days 1 to 5
[total dose/cycle = 7500 mg/m^2]
Etoposide: I.V.: 60 mg/m^2/dose days 1 to 5
[total dose/cycle = 300 mg/m^2]
Cytarabine: I.V.: 2 g/m^2/dose every 12 hours, for 4 doses, days 1 and 2
[total dose/cycle = 8 g/m^2]
Methotrexate: I.T.: 12 mg/dose day 5
[total dose/cycle = 12 mg]
Hydrocortisone: I.T.: 50 mg/dose day 5
[total dose/cycle = 50 mg]
Filgrastim: SubQ: Dose not specified, daily beginning day 6 until ANC >1000 mm^3
Note: If CNS disease present, administer additional I.T. treatment in cycle 2:
Cytarabine 50 mg/dose on days 3 and 5

References

Variation 1:

Magrath I, Adde M, Shad A, et al, "Adults and Children With Small Non-Cleaved-Cell Lymphoma Have a Similar Excellent Outcome When Treated With the Same Chemotherapy Regimen," *J Clin Oncol*, 1996, 14(3):925-34.

Variation 2:

Mead GM, Barrans SL, Qian W, et al, "A Prospective Clinicopathologic Study of Dose-Modified CODOX-M/IVAC in Patients With Sporadic Burkitt Lymphoma Defined Using Cytogenetic and Immunophenotypic Criteria (MRC/NCRI LY10 Trial)," *Blood*, 2008, 112(6):2248-60.

Variation 3:

Mead GM, Sydes MR, Walewski J, et al, "An International Evaluation of CODOX-M and CODOX-M Alternating With IVAC in Adult Burkitt's Lymphoma: Results of United Kingdom Lymphoma Group LY06 Study," *Ann Oncol*, 2002, 13(8):1264-74.

Variation 4:

Lacasce A, Howard O, Lib S, et al, "Modified Magrath Regimens for Adults With Burkitt and Burkitt-Like Lymphomas: Preserved Efficacy With Decreased Toxicity," *Leuk Lymphoma*, 2004, 45 (4):761-7.

COMLA

Use Lymphoma, non-Hodgkin's

Regimen

Cyclophosphamide: I.V.: 1500 mg/m^2 day 1
[total dose/cycle = 1500 mg/m^2]

Vincristine: I.V.: 1.4 mg/m^2/day (maximum dose: 2 mg) days 1, 8, and 15
[total dose/cycle = 4.2 mg/m^2]

Methotrexate: I.V.: 120 mg/m^2/day days 22, 29, 36, 43, 50, 57, 64, and 71
[total dose/cycle = 960 mg/m^2]

Leucovorin: Oral: 25 mg/m^2 every 6 hours for 4 doses (beginning 24 hours after each methotrexate dose)
[total dose/cycle = 800 mg/m^2]

Cytarabine: I.V.: 300 mg/m^2/day days 22, 29, 36, 43, 50, 57, 64, and 71
[total dose/cycle = 2400 mg/m^2]

Repeat cycle every 85 days

References

Sweet DL, Golomb HM, Ultmann JE, et al, "Cyclophosphamide, Vincristine, Methotrexate With Leucovorin Rescue, and Cytarabine (COMLA) Combination Sequential Chemotherapy for Advanced Diffuse Histiocytic Lymphoma," *Ann Intern Med*, 1980, 92(6):785-90.

COP-BLAM

Use Lymphoma, non-Hodgkin's

Regimen

Cyclophosphamide: I.V.: 400 mg/m^2 day 1
[total dose/cycle = 400 mg/m^2]

Vincristine: I.V.: 1 mg/m^2 day 1
[total dose/cycle = 1 mg/m^2]

Prednisone: Oral: 40 mg/m^2/day days 1 to 10
[total dose/cycle = 400 mg/m^2]

Bleomycin: I.V.: 15 mg day 14
[total dose/cycle = 15 mg]

Doxorubicin: I.V.: 40 mg/m^2 day 1
[total dose/cycle = 40 mg/m^2]

Procarbazine: Oral: 100 mg/m^2/day days 1 to 10
[total dose/cycle = 1000 mg/m^2]

References

Salles G, Shipp MA, and Coiffier B, "Chemotherapy of Non-Hodgkin's Aggressive Lymphomas," *Semin Hematol*, 1994, 31(1):46-69.

Urba WJ, Duffey PL, and Longo DL, "Treatment of Patients With Aggressive Lymphomas: An Overview," *J Natl Cancer Inst Monogr*, 1990, (10):29-37.

COPE

Index Terms Baby Brain I

Use Brain tumors

Regimen

Cycle A:

Vincristine: I.V.: 0.065 mg/kg/day (maximum dose: 1.5 mg) days 1 and 8
[total dose/cycle = 0.13 mg/kg]

Cyclophosphamide: I.V.: 65 mg/kg day 1
[total dose/cycle = 65 mg/kg]

Cycle B:

Cisplatin: I.V.: 4 mg/kg day 1
[total dose/cycle = 4 mg/kg]

Etoposide: I.V.: 6.5 mg/kg/day days 3 and 4
[total dose/cycle = 13 mg/kg]

Repeat cycle every 28 days in the following sequence: AABAAB

References

Duffner PK, Horowitz ME, Krischer JP, et al "Postoperative Chemotherapy and Delayed Radiation in Children Less Than Three Years of Age With Malignant Brain Tumors," *N Engl J Med*, 1993, 328(24):1725-31.

COPP

Index Terms C MOPP

Use Lymphoma, non-Hodgkin's

Regimen

Cyclophosphamide: I.V.: 450-650 mg/m^2/day days 1 and 8
[total dose/cycle = 900-1300 mg/m^2]

Vincristine: I.V.: 1.4-2 mg/m^2/day (maximum dose: 2 mg) days 1 and 8
[total dose/cycle = 2.8-4 mg/m^2]

Procarbazine: Oral: 100 mg/m^2/day days 1 to 14
[total dose/cycle = 1400 mg/m^2]

Prednisone: Oral: 40 mg/m^2/day days 1 to 14
[total dose/cycle = 560 mg/m^2]

Repeat cycle every 3-4 weeks

References

Brereton HD, Young RC, Longo DL, et al, "A Comparison Between Combination Chemotherapy and Total Body Irradiation Plus Combination Chemotherapy in Non-Hodgkin's Lymphoma," *Cancer*, 1979, 43(6):2227-31.

Crizotinib (NSCLC Regimen)

Use Lung cancer, nonsmall cell

Regimen

Crizotinib: Oral: 250 mg twice daily days 1 to 28
[total dose/cycle = 14,000 mg]

Repeat cycle every 28 days until disease progression or unacceptable toxicity

References

Kwak EL, Bang YJ, Camidge R, et al, "Anaplastic Lymphoma Kinase Inhibition in Non-Small-Cell Lung Cancer," *N Engl J Med*, 2010, 363(18):1693-703.

◆ **CVD** *see* Cisplatin-Vinblastine-Dacarbazine (Melanoma) *on page 1584*

◆ **CVD-IL-2-IFN (Melanoma)** *see* CVD-Interleukin-Interferon (Melanoma) *on page 1597*

CVD-Interleukin-Interferon (Melanoma)

Index Terms Cisplatin-Vinblastine-Dacarbazine-Interleukin-Interferon (Melanoma); CVD-IL-2-IFN (Melanoma)

Use Melanoma

Regimen NOTE: Multiple variations are listed.

Variation 1:

Cisplatin: I.V.: 20 mg/m^2/day days 1 to 4 and 22 to 25
[total dose/cycle = 160 mg/m^2]

Vinblastine: I.V.: 1.5 mg/m^2/day days 1 to 4 and 22 to 25
[total dose/cycle = 12 mg/m^2]

Dacarbazine: I.V.: 800 mg/m^2/day days 1 and 22
[total dose/cycle = 1600 mg/m^2]

Aldesleukin: I.V.: 9 million units/m^2/day continuous infusion days 5 to 8, 17 to 20, and 26 to 29
[total dose/cycle = 108 million units/m^2]

Interferon alfa-2b: SubQ: 5 million units/m^2/day days 5 to 9, 17 to 21, and 26 to 30
[total dose/cycle = 75 million units/m^2]

Repeat every 42 days (maximum of five 21-day cycles for cytokine [interleukin and interferon] component)

Variation 2:

Cisplatin: I.V.: 20 mg/m^2/day days 1 to 4
[total dose/cycle = 80 mg/m^2]

Vinblastine: I.V.: 1.6 mg/m^2/day days 1 to 4
[total dose/cycle = 6.4 mg/m^2]

Dacarbazine: I.V.: 800 mg/m^2 day 1
[total dose/cycle = 800 mg/m^2]

Aldesleukin: I.V.: 9 million units/m^2/day continuous infusion days 1 to 4
[total dose/cycle = 36 million units/m^2]

Interferon alfa-2a: SubQ: 5 million units/m^2/day days 1 to 5, 7, 9, 11, and 13
[total dose/cycle = 45 million units/m^2]

Repeat cycle every 21 days for a total of 6 cycles

Variation 3:

Cisplatin: I.V.: 20 mg/m^2/day days 1 to 4
[total dose/cycle = 80 mg/m^2]

Vinblastine: I.V.: 1.2 mg/m^2/day days 1 to 4
[total dose/cycle = 4.8 mg/m^2]

Dacarbazine: I.V.: 800 mg/m^2 day 1
[total dose/cycle = 800 mg/m^2]

Aldesleukin: I.V.: 9 million units/m^2/day continuous infusion days 1 to 4
[total dose/cycle = 36 million units/m^2]

Interferon alfa-2b: SubQ: 5 million units/m^2/day days 1 to 5, 8, 10, and 12
[total dose/cycle = 40 million units/m^2]

Repeat cycle every 21 days (maximum: 4 cycles)

References

Variation 1:

Eton O, Legha SS, Bedikian AY, et al, "Sequential Biochemotherapy Versus Chemotherapy for Metastatic Melanoma: Results From a Phase III Randomized Trial," *J Clin Oncol*, 2002, 20 (8):2045-52.

Variation 2:
Legha SS, Ring S, Eton O, et al, "Development of a Biochemotherapy Regimen With Concurrent Administration of Cisplatin, Vinblastine, Dacarbazine, Interferon Alfa, and Interleukin-2 for Patients With Metastatic Melanoma," *J Clin Oncol*, 1998, 16(5):1752-9.
Variation 3:
McDermott DF, Mier JW, Lawrence DP, et al, "A Phase II Pilot Trial of Concurrent Biochemotherapy With Cisplatin, Vinblastine, Dacarbazine, Interleukin 2, and Interferon Alpha-2B in Patients With Metastatic Melanoma," *Clin Cancer Res*, 2000, 6(6):2201-8.

CVP (Leukemia)

Use Leukemia, chronic lymphocytic

Regimen NOTE: Multiple variations are listed.

Variation 1:
Cyclophosphamide: Oral: 300 or 400 mg/m^2/day days 1 to 5
[total dose/cycle = 1500 or 2000 mg/m^2]
Vincristine: I.V.: 1.4 mg/m^2 (maximum dose: 2 mg) day 1
[total dose/cycle = 1.4 mg/m^2]
Prednisone: Oral: 100 mg/m^2/day days 1 to 5
[total dose/cycle = 500 mg/m^2]
Repeat cycle every 21 days

Variation 2:
Cyclophosphamide: I.V.: 800 mg/m^2 day 1
[total dose/cycle = 800 mg/m^2]
Vincristine: I.V.: 1.4 mg/m^2 (maximum dose: 2 mg) day 1
[total dose/cycle = 1.4 mg/m^2]
Prednisone: Oral: 100 mg/m^2/day days 1 to 5
[total dose/cycle = 500 mg/m^2]
Repeat cycle every 21 days

References

Variation 1:
Bagley CM, DeVita VT, Berard CW, et al, "Advanced Lymphosarcoma: Intensive Cyclical Combination Chemotherapy With Cyclophosphamide, Vincristine, and Prednisone," *Ann Int Med*, 1972, 76(2):227-34.
Raphael B, Anderson JW, Silber R, et al, "Comparison of Chlorambucil and Prednisone Versus Cyclophosphamide, Vincristine, and Prednisone as Initial Treatment for Chronic Lymphocytic Leukemia: Long-Term Follow-up of an Eastern Cooperative Oncology Group Randomized Clinical Trial," *J Clin Oncol*, 1991, 9(5):770-6.
Variation 2:
Oken MM and Kaplan ME, "Combination Chemotherapy With Cyclophosphamide, Vincristine, and Prednisone in the Treatment of Refractory Chronic Lymphocytic Leukemia," *Cancer Treat Rep*, 1979, 63(3):441-7.

CVP (Lymphoma, non-Hodgkin's)

Index Terms Cyclophosphamide-Vincristine-Prednisone (NHL)

Use Lymphoma, non-Hodgkin's

Regimen NOTE: Multiple variations are listed.

Variation 1:
Cyclophosphamide: I.V.: 750 mg/m^2 day 1
[total dose/cycle = 750 mg/m^2]
Vincristine: I.V.: 1.2 mg/m^2 day 1
[total dose/cycle = 1.2 mg/m^2]
Prednisone: Oral: 40 mg/m^2/day days 1 to 5
[total dose/cycle = 200 mg/m^2]
Repeat cycle every 21 days for up to 10 cycles

Variation 2:
Cyclophosphamide: I.V.: 750 mg/m^2 day 1
[total dose/cycle = 750 mg/m^2]

Vincristine: I.V.: 1.2 mg/m^2 day 1 (maximum dose: 2 mg)
[total dose/cycle = 1.2 mg/m^2 (maximum: 2 mg)]
Prednisone: Oral: 40 mg/m^2/day days 1 to 5
[total dose/cycle = 200 mg/m^2]
Repeat cycle every 28 days for up to 8 cycles

Variation 3:
Cyclophosphamide: I.V.: 750 mg/m^2 day 1
[total dose/cycle = 750 mg/m^2]
Vincristine: I.V.: 1.4 mg/m^2 day 1 (maximum dose: 2 mg)
[total dose/cycle = 1.4 mg/m^2 (maximum: 2 mg)]
Prednisone: Oral: 40 mg/m^2/day days 1 to 5
[total dose/cycle = 200 mg/m^2]
Repeat cycle every 21 days for up to 8 cycles

Variation 4:
Cyclophosphamide: Oral: 400 mg/m^2/day days 1 to 5
[total dose/cycle = 2000 mg/m^2]
Vincristine: I.V.: 1.4 mg/m^2 day 1 (maximum dose: 2 mg)
[total dose/cycle = 1.4 mg/m^2 (maximum: 2 mg)]
Prednisone: Oral: 100 mg/m^2/day days 1 to 5
[total dose/cycle = 500 mg/m^2]
Repeat cycle every 21 days

References

Variation 1:
Klasa RJ, Meyer RM, Shustik C, et al, "Randomized Phase III Study of Fludarabine Phosphate Versus Cyclophosphamide, Vincristine, and Prednisone in Patients With Recurrent Low-Grade Non-Hodgkin's Lymphoma Previously Treated With an Alkylating Agent or Alkylator-Containing Regimen," *J Clin Oncol*, 2002, 20(24):4649-54.
Variation 2:
Hagenbeek A, Eghbali H, Monfardini S, et al, "Phase III Intergroup Study of Fludarabine Phosphate Compared With Cyclophosphamide, Vincristine, and Prednisone Chemotherapy in Newly Diagnosed Patients With Stage III and IV Low-Grade Malignant Non-Hodgkin's Lymphoma," *J Clin Oncol*, 2006, 24(10):1590-6.
Variation 3:
Marcus R, Imrie K, Belch A, et al, "CVP Chemotherapy Plus Rituximab Compared With CVP as First-Line Treatment for Advanced Follicular Lymphoma," *Blood*, 2005, 105(4):1417-23.
Variation 4:
Bagley CM Jr, Devita VT Jr, Berard CW, et al, "Advanced Lymphosarcoma: Intensive Cyclical Combination Chemotherapy With Cyclophosphamide, Vincristine, and Prednisone," *Ann Intern Med*, 1972, 76(2):227-34.
Portlock CS, Rosenberg SA, Glatstein E, et al, "Treatment of Advanced Non-Hodgkin's Lymphomas With Favorable Histologies: Preliminary Results of a Prospective Trial," *Blood*, 1976, 47(5):747-56.

◆ **CVP-R** *see* R-CVP *on page* 1745

◆ **CyBorD (Multiple Myeloma)** *see* Cyclophosphamide-Bortezomib-Dexamethasone (Multiple Myeloma) *on page* 1599

Cyclophosphamide-Bortezomib-Dexamethasone (Multiple Myeloma)

Index Terms CyBorD (Multiple Myeloma)

Use Multiple myeloma

Regimen NOTE: Multiple variations are listed.

Variation 1:
Cycles 1 through 4:
Cyclophosphamide: P.O.: 300 mg/m^2/day on days 1, 8, 15, and 22
[total dose/cycle = 1200 mg/m^2]

Bortezomib: I.V. or SubQ: 1.3 mg/m^2/day on days 1, 4, 8, and 11 [total dose/cycle = 5.2 mg/m^2]
Dexamethasone: P.O.: 40 mg/day on days 1-4, 9-12, and 17-20 [total dose/cycle = 480 mg]
Treatment cycle is 28 days

Variation 2:

Cycles 1 and 2:
Cyclophosphamide: P.O.: 300 mg/m^2/day on days 1, 8, 15, and 22 [total dose/cycle = 1200 mg/m^2]
Bortezomib: I.V. or SubQ: 1.5 mg/m^2/day on days 1, 8, 15, and 22 [total dose/cycle = 6 mg/m^2]
Dexamethasone: P.O.: 40 mg/day on days 1-4, 9-12, and 17-20 [total dose/cycle = 480 mg]
Treatment cycle is 28 days

Cycles 3 and 4:
Cyclophosphamide: P.O.: 300 mg/m^2/day on days 1, 8, 15, and 22 [total dose/cycle = 1200 mg/m^2]
Bortezomib: I.V. or SubQ: 1.5 mg/m^2/day on days 1, 8, 15, and 22 [total dose/cycle = 6 mg/m^2]
Dexamethasone: P.O.: 40 mg/day on days 1, 8, 15, and 22 [total dose/cycle = 160 mg]
Treatment cycle is 28 days

Variation 3:
Cyclophosphamide: P.O.: 500 mg/m^2/day on days 1, 8, and 15 [total dose/cycle = 1500 mg/m^2]
Bortezomib: I.V. or SubQ: 1.3 mg/m^2/day on days 1, 4, 8, and 11 [total dose/cycle = 5.2 mg/m^2]
Dexamethasone: P.O.: 40 mg/day on days 1, 8, and 15 [total dose/cycle = 120 mg]
Repeat cycle every 21 days for up to 8 cycles

Variation 4:
Cyclophosphamide: P.O.: 500 mg/m^2/day on days 1 and 8 [total dose/cycle = 1000 mg/m^2]
Bortezomib: I.V. or SubQ: 1.3 mg/m^2/day on days 1, 4, 8, and 11 [total dose/cycle = 5.2 mg/m^2]
Dexamethasone: P.O.: 40 mg/day on days 1, 8, and 15 [total dose/cycle = 120 mg]
Repeat cycle every 21 days for up to 8 cycles

References

Variations 1 and 2:

Reeder CB, Reece DE, Kukrati V, et al, "Cyclophosphamide, Bortezomib and Dexamethasone Induction for Newly Diagnosed Multiple Myeloma: High Response Rates in a Phase II Clinical Trial," *Leukemia*, 2009, 23(7):1887-41.

Reeder CB, Reece DE, Kukreti V, et al, "Once- Versus Twice-Weekly Bortezomib Induction Therapy With CyBorD in Newly Diagnosed Multiple Myeloma," *Blood*, 2010, 115(16):3416-7.

Variations 3 and 4:

Kumar S, Flinn IW, Richardson PG, et al, "Novel Three- and Four-Drug Combination Regimens of Bortezomib, Dexamethasone, Cyclophosphamide, and Lenalidomide, for Previously Untreated Multiple Myeloma: Results From the Multi-Center, Randomized, Phase 2 EVOLUTION Study," *Blood*, 2010, 116:621 [abstract 621 from ASH 2010 Annual Meeting].

◆ **Cyclophosphamide, Doxorubicin, Etoposide, Cisplatin (Neuroblastoma)**
see A3 (Neuroblastoma) *on page 1515*

◆ **Cyclophosphamide, Doxorubicin, Etoposide, Cisplatin (Neuroblastoma)**
see New A1 (Neuroblastoma) *on page 1721*

- **Cyclophosphamide, Doxorubicin, Vincristine, Etoposide, Cisplatin (Neuroblastoma)** *see* CAV-P/VP (Neuroblastoma) *on page 1554*
- **Cyclophosphamide, Doxorubicin, Vincristine (Small Cell Lung Cancer)** *see* CAV (Small Cell Lung Cancer) *on page 1554*
- **Cyclophosphamide-Fludarabine (CLL)** *see* Fludarabine-Cyclophosphamide (CLL) *on page 1646*

Cyclophosphamide-Fludarabine-Alemtuzumab-Rituximab (CLL)

Index Terms CFAR (CLL); Fludarabine-Cyclophosphamide-Alemtuzumab-Rituximab (CLL)

Use Leukemia, chronic lymphocytic

Regimen

Variation 1:

Cyclophosphamide: I.V.: 200 mg/m²/day days 3, 4, and 5 [total dose/cycle = 600 mg/m²]

Fludarabine: I.V.: 20 mg/m²/day days 3, 4, and 5 [total dose/cycle = 60 mg/m²]

Rituximab: I.V.: 375-500 mg/m²/dose day 2 [total dose/cycle = 375-500 mg/m²]

Alemtuzumab: I.V.: 30 mg/dose days 1, 3, and 5 [total dose/cycle = 90 mg]

Repeat cycle every 28 days for up to a total of 6 cycles

Variation 2:

Cyclophosphamide: I.V.: 200 mg/m²/day days 3, 4, and 5 [total dose/cycle = 600 mg/m²]

Fludarabine: I.V.: 20 mg/m²/day days 3, 4, and 5 [total dose/cycle = 60 mg/m²]

Rituximab: I.V.: 375-500 mg/m²/dose day 2 [total dose/cycle = 375-500 mg/m²]

Alemtuzumab: I.V.: 30 mg/dose days 1, 3, and 5 [total dose/cycle = 90 mg]

Pegfilgrastim: SubQ: 6 mg with each cycle

Repeat cycle every 28 days for a total of 6 cycles

Variation 3:

Cyclophosphamide: I.V.: 250 mg/m²/day days 3, 4, and 5 [total dose/cycle = 750 mg/m²]

Fludarabine: I.V.: 25 mg/m²/day days 3, 4, and 5 [total dose/cycle = 75 mg/m²]

Rituximab: I.V.: 375-500 mg/m²/dose day 2 [total dose/cycle = 375-500 mg/m²]

Alemtuzumab: I.V.: 30 mg/dose days 1, 3, and 5 [total dose/cycle = 90 mg]

Repeat cycle every 28 days for a total of 6 cycles

References

Variation 1:

Wierda WG, O'Brien SM, Faderl SH, et al, "CFAR, An Active Frontline Regimen for High-Risk Patients With CLL, Including Those With Del 17p," *Blood*, 2008, 112(11):2095 [abstract 2095 from 2008 Annual ASH meeting].

Variation 2:

Parikh SA, Keating M, O'Brien S, et al, "Frontline Combined Chemoimmunotherapy With Fludarabine, Cyclophosphamide, Alemtuzumab and Rituximab (CFAR) in High-Risk Chronic Lymphocytic Leukemia," *Blood*, 2009, 114(22):208 [abstract 208 from 2009 Annual ASH meeting].

Variation 3:

Badoux XC, Keating M, O'Brien S, et al, "Chemoimmunotherapy With Cyclophosphamide, Fludarabine, Alemtuzumab and Rituximab (CFAR) Is Effective in Relapsed Patients With Chronic Lymphocytic Leukemia (CLL)," *Blood*, 2009, 114(22):3141 [abstract 3141 from 2009 Annual ASH meeting].

◆ **Cyclophosphamide-Fludarabine (NHL-Mantle Cell)** *see* Fludarabine-Cyclophosphamide (NHL-Mantle Cell) *on page 1648*

◆ **Cyclophosphamide-Topotecan (Ewing's Sarcoma)** *see* Topotecan-Cyclophosphamide (Ewing's Sarcoma) *on page 1756*

◆ **Cyclophosphamide-Vincristine-Prednisone (NHL)** *see* CVP (Lymphoma, non-Hodgkin's) *on page 1598*

◆ **Cyclophosphamide-Vincristine-Procarbazine-Prednisone-Doxorubicin-Bleomycin-Vinblastine (Hodgkin)** *see* C-MOPP/ABV Hybrid (Hodgkin) *on page 1588*

◆ **Cytarabine-Daunorubicin (5 + 2) (AML)** *see* 5 + 2 (Cytarabine-Daunorubicin) (AML Induction) *on page 1512*

◆ **Cytarabine-Daunorubicin (5 + 2) (AML)** *see* 5 + 2 (Cytarabine-Daunorubicin) (AML Postremission) *on page 1512*

◆ **Cytarabine-Daunorubicin (7 + 3) (AML Induction)** *see* 7 + 3 (Cytarabine-Daunorubicin) (AML Induction) *on page 1513*

◆ **Cytarabine-Daunorubicin-Etoposide (5 + 2 + 5) (AML Consolidation)** *see* 5 + 2 + 5 (Cytarabine-Daunorubicin-Etoposide) (AML Consolidation) *on page 1513*

◆ **Cytarabine-Daunorubicin-Etoposide (7 + 3 + 7) (AML Induction)** *see* 7 + 3 + 7 (Cytarabine-Daunorubicin-Etoposide) (AML Induction) *on page 1515*

◆ **Cytarabine-Etoposide-Mitoxantrone-CSF (AML Induction)** *see* MEC-G (AML Induction) *on page 1707*

Cytarabine (High Dose)-Daunorubicin (AML Induction)

Index Terms HDAC-Daunorubicin (AML Induction); HIDAC-Daunorubicin (AML Induction)

Use Leukemia, acute myeloid

Regimen

Cytarabine: I.V.: 2 g/m^2/day over 1 hour every 12 hours days 1 to 6 (12 total doses)
[total dose/cycle = 24 g/m^2]

Daunorubicin: I.V.: 45 mg/m^2/day I.V. bolus days 7 to 9
[total dose/cycle = 135 mg/m^2]

References

Weick JK, Kopecky KJ, Appelbaum FR, et al, "A Randomized Investigation of High-Dose Versus Standard-Dose Cytosine Arabinoside With Daunorubicin in Patients With Previously Untreated Acute Myeloid Leukemia: A Southwest Oncology Group Study," *Blood*, 1996, 88(8):2841-51.

Cytarabine (High Dose)-Daunorubicin-Etoposide (AML Induction)

Index Terms HIDAC-3-7 (AML Induction)

Use Leukemia, acute myeloid

Regimen

Daunorubicin: I.V.: 50 mg/m^2/day days 1, 2, and 3
[total dose/cycle = 150 mg/m^2]

Cytarabine: I.V.: 3 g/m^2/dose over 3 hours every 12 hours days 1, 3, 5, and 7 (8 total doses)
[total dose/cycle = 24 g/m^2]
Etoposide: I.V.: 75 mg/m^2/day days 1 to 7
[total dose/cycle = 525 mg/m^2]
Up to 3 induction cycles may be given based on individual response

References

Bishop JF, Matthews JP, Young GA, et al, "A Randomized Study of High-Dose Cytarabine in Induction in Acute Myeloid Leukemia," *Blood*, 1996, 87(5):1710-7.

Cytarabine (High-Dose Single-Agent AML Induction Regimen)

Index Terms HD Cytarabine (Single Agent AML Induction); HIDAC (Single Agent AML Induction)

Use Leukemia, acute myeloid

Regimen NOTE: Multiple variations are listed.

Variation 1 (ages 14 to 50 years):
Cytarabine: I.V.: 3 g/m^2 over 2 hours every 12 hours days 1 to 6 (total of 12 doses)
[total dose/cycle = 36 g/m^2]
May administer a second induction cycle if needed

Variation 2 (ages >50 years):
Cytarabine: I.V.: 2 g/m^2 over 2 hours every 12 hours days 1 to 6 (total of 12 doses)
[total dose/cycle = 24 g/m^2]
May administer a second induction cycle if needed

References

Karanes C, Kopecky KJ, Head DR, et al "A Phase III Comparison of High Dose ARA-C (HIDAC) Versus HIDAC Plus Mitoxantrone in the Treatment of First Relapsed or Refractory Acute Myeloid Leukemia - Southwest Oncology Group Study," *Leuk Res*, 1990, 20(9):787-94.

◆ **Cytarabine-Idarubicin (5 + 2) (AML Consolidation)** *see* 5 + 2 (Cytarabine-Idarubicin) (AML Consolidation) *on page* *1512*

◆ **Cytarabine-Idarubicin (7 + 3) (AML Induction)** *see* 7 + 3 (Cytarabine-Idarubicin) (AML Induction) *on page* *1514*

◆ **Cytarabine-Mitoxantrone (5 + 2) (AML Consolidation)** *see* 5 + 2 (Cytarabine-Mitoxantrone) (AML Consolidation) *on page* *1512*

◆ **Cytarabine-Mitoxantrone (7 + 3) (AML Induction)** *see* 7 + 3 (Cytarabine-Mitoxantrone) (AML Induction) *on page* *1514*

Cytarabine (Single-Agent AML Consolidation Regimen)

Use Leukemia, acute myeloid

Regimen NOTE: Multiple variations are listed.

Variation 1:
Cytarabine: I.V.: 3 g/m^2 over 3 hours every 12 hours on days 1, 3, and 5 (total of 6 doses)
[total dose/cycle = 18 g/m^2]
Repeat cycle every 4 to 5 weeks (depending on marrow recovery) for a total of 4 postremission cycles

Variation 2:
Cytarabine: I.V.: 400 mg/m^2/day continuous infusion on days 1 to 5 [total dose/cycle = 2000 mg/m^2]
Repeat cycle every 4 to 5 weeks (depending on marrow recovery) for a total of 4 postremission cycles
Variation 3:
Cytarabine: I.V.: 100 mg/m^2/day continuous infusion on days 1 to 5 [total dose/cycle = 500 mg/m^2]
Repeat cycle every 4 to 5 weeks (depending on marrow recovery) for a total of 4 postremission cycles
Variation 4 (≥60 years of age):
Cytarabine: I.V.: 100 mg/m^2/day continuous infusion on days 1 to 5 [total dose/cycle = 500 mg/m^2]
Repeat cycle every 28 days for a total of 4 consolidation cycles
Variation 5 (≤50 years of age):
Cytarabine: I.V.: 3 g/m^2 every 12 hours on days 1 to 3 (total of 6 doses) [total dose/cycle = 18 g/m^2]
Administer a total of 3 consolidation cycles
Variation 6 (>50 years of age)
Cytarabine: I.V.: 2 g/m^2 every 12 hours on days 1 to 3 (total of 6 doses) [total dose/cycle = 12 g/m^2]
Administer a total of 3 consolidation cycles
Variation 7(>65 years of age):
Cytarabine: SubQ: 10 mg/m^2/dose every 12 hours days 1 to 14 [total dose/cycle = 280 mg/m^2]
Repeat cycle every 6 weeks for 18 months

References

Variations 1, 2, and 3:
Mayer RJ, Davis RB, Schiffer CA, et al, "Intensive Postremission Chemotherapy in Adults With Acute Myeloid Leukemia, Cancer and Leukemia Group B," *N Engl J Med*, 1994, 331 (14):896-903.
Variation 4:
Stone RM, Berg DT, George SL, et al, "Postremission Therapy in Older Patients With *de novo* Acute Myeloid Leukemia: A Randomized Trial Comparing Mitoxantrone and Intermediate-Dose Cytarabine With Standard-Dose Cytarabine," *Blood*, 2001, 98(3):548-53.
Variations 5 and 6:
Karanes C, Kopecky K.J, Head DR, et al "A Phase III Comparison of High Dose ARA-C (HIDAC) Versus HIDAC Plus Mitoxantrone in the Treatment of First Relapsed or Refractory Acute Myeloid Leukemia - Southwest Oncology Group Study," *Leuk Res*, 1999, 23(9): 787-94.
Variation 7:
Tilly H, Castaigne S, Bordessoule D, et al, "Low-Dose Cytarabine Versus Intensive Chemotherapy in the Treatment of Acute Nonlymphocytic Leukemia in the Elderly," *J Clin Oncol*, 1990, 8 (2):272-9.

Cytarabine (SubQ Single-Agent AML Induction Regimen)

Use Leukemia, acute myeloid

Regimen NOTE: Multiple variations are listed.
Variation 1 (>50 years of age):
Cytarabine: SubQ: 20 mg/m^2/day days 1 to 14 [total dose/cycle = 280 mg/m^2]
Repeat cycle every 28 days for at least 4 cycles
Variation 2 (>65 years of age):
Cytarabine: SubQ: 10 mg/m^2/day every 12 hours days 1 to 21 [total dose/cycle = 420 mg/m^2]
After 15 days, a second induction course may be administered if needed

References

Variation 1:

Fenaux P, Mufti GJ, Hellstrom-Lindberg E, et al, "Azacitidine Prolongs Overall Survival Compared With Conventional Care Regimens in Elderly Patients With Low Bone Marrow Blast Count Acute Myeloid Leukemia, *J Clin Oncol*, 2010, 28(4):562-9.

Variation 2:

Tilly H, Castaigne S, Bordessoule D, et al, "Low-Dose Cytarabine Versus Intensive Chemotherapy in the Treatment of Acute Nonlymphocytic Leukemia in the Elderly," *J Clin Oncol*, 1990, 8 (2):272-9.

CYVADIC

Use Sarcoma

Regimen

Cyclophosphamide: I.V.: 500 mg/m^2 day 1
[total dose/cycle = 500 mg/m^2]

Vincristine: I.V.: 1.4 mg/m^2/day days 1 and 5
[total dose/cycle = 2.8 mg/m^2]

Doxorubicin: I.V.: 50 mg/m^2 day 1
[total dose/cycle = 50 mg/m^2]

Dacarbazine: I.V.: 250 mg/m^2/day days 1 to 5
[total dose/cycle = 1250 mg/m^2]

Repeat cycle every 21 days

References

Pinedo HM, Bramwell VH, Mouridsen HT, et al, "Cyvadic in Advanced Soft Tissue Sarcoma: A Randomized Study Comparing Two Schedules. A Study of the EORTC Soft Tissue and Bone Sarcoma Group," *Cancer*, 1984, 53(9):1825-32.

◆ **Dacarbazine-Cisplatin-Vinblastine** *see* Cisplatin-Vinblastine-Dacarbazine (Melanoma) *on page 1584*

◆ **Dactinomycin-Vincristine (Wilms' Tumor)** *see* EE-4A (Wilms' Tumor) *on page 1621*

◆ **Dactinomycin–Doxorubicin–Vincristine (Wilms' Tumor)** *see* DD-4A (Wilms' Tumor) *on page 1606*

Dasatinib (CML Regimen)

Use Leukemia, chronic myelogenous

Regimen NOTE: Multiple variations are listed.

Variation 1 (chronic phase):

Dasatinib: Oral: 100 mg once daily
[total dose/cycle = 2800 mg]

Repeat cycle every 28 days until disease progression or unacceptable toxicity

Variation 2 (accelerated and blast phase resistant or intolerant to imatinib):

Dasatinib: Oral: 140 mg once daily
[total dose/cycle = 3920 mg]

Repeat cycle every 28 days until disease progression or unacceptable toxicity

References

Variation 1:

Kantarjian H, Shah NP, Hochhaus A, et al, "Dasatinib Versus Imatinib in Newly Diagnosed Chronic-Phase Chronic Myeloid Leukemia," *N Engl J Med*, 2010, 362(24):2260-70.

Shah NP, Kantarjian HM, Kim DW, et al, "Intermittent Target Inhibition With Dasatinib 100 mg Once Daily Preserves Efficacy and Improves Tolerability in Imatinib-Resistant and -Intolerant Chronic-Phase Chronic Myeloid Leukemia," *J Clin Oncol*, 2008, 26(19):3204-12.

Variation 2:
Kantarjian H, Cortes J, Kim DW, et al, "Phase 3 Study of Dasatinib 140 mg Once Daily Versus 70 mg Twice Daily in Patients With Chronic Myeloid Leukemia in Accelerated Phase Resistant or Intolerant to Imatinib: 15-Month Median Follow-up," *Blood*, 2009, 113(25):6322-9.
Saglio G, Hochhaus A, Goh YT, et al, "Dasatinib in Imatinib-Resistant or Imatinib-Intolerant Chronic Myeloid Leukemia in Blast Phase After 2 Years of Follow-up in a Phase 3 Study: Efficacy and Tolerability of 140 Milligrams Once Daily and 70 Milligrams Twice Daily," *Cancer*, 2010, 116 (16):3852-61.

◆ **Daunorubicin-ATRA (APL)** *see* Tretinoin-Daunorubicin (APL) *on page 1762*
◆ **Daunorubicin-Cytarabine (5 + 2) (AML)** *see* 5 + 2 (Cytarabine-Daunorubicin) (AML Induction) *on page 1512*
◆ **Daunorubicin-Cytarabine (5 + 2) (AML)** *see* 5 + 2 (Cytarabine-Daunorubicin) (AML Postremission) *on page 1512*
◆ **Daunorubicin-Tretinoin (APL)** *see* Tretinoin-Daunorubicin (APL) *on page 1762*
◆ **DCF (Gastric/Esophageal Cancer)** *see* Docetaxel-Cisplatin-Fluorouracil (Gastric/Esophageal Cancer) *on page 1609*
◆ **DD4A (Wilms' Tumor)** *see* DD-4A (Wilms' Tumor) *on page 1606*

DD-4A (Wilms' Tumor)

Index Terms Dactinomycin–Doxorubicin–Vincristine (Wilms' Tumor); DD4A (Wilms' Tumor); Regimen DD-4A (Wilms' Tumor)

Use Wilms' tumor

Regimen

Dactinomycin: I.V.: 45 mcg/kg day 1 of weeks 0, 6, 12, 18, 24, 30, 36, 42, 48, and 54
[total dose = 450 mcg/kg]
Doxorubicin: I.V.: 45 mg/m^2 days 1 of weeks 3 and 9
Followed by
Doxorubicin: I.V.: 30 mg/m^2 days 1 of weeks 15, 21, 27, 33, 39, 45, and 51
[total dose = 300 mg/m^2]
Vincristine: I.V.: 1.5 mg/m^2 day 1 of weeks 1 to 10
Followed by
Vincristine: I.V.: 2 mg/m^2 day 1 of weeks 12, 15, 18, 21, 24, 27, 30, 33, 36, 39, 42, 45, 48, 51, and 54
[total dose = 45 mg/m^2]
Treatment course duration is week 0 through week 54

References

Green DM, Breslow NE, Beckwith JB, et al, "Effect of Duration of Treatment on Treatment Outcome and Cost of Treatment for Wilms' Tumor: A Report From the National Wilms' Tumor Study Group," *J Clin Oncol*, 1998, 16(12):3744-51.

Decitabine (AML Regimen)

Use Leukemia, acute myeloid

Regimen

Decitabine: I.V.: 20 mg/m^2/day over 1 hour days 1 to 5
[total dose/cycle = 100 mg/m^2]
Repeat cycle every 28 days

References

Cashen AF, Schiller GJ, O'Donnell MR, et al, "Multicenter Phase II Study of Decitabine for the First-Line Treatment of Older Patients With Acute Myeloid Leukemia," *J Clin Oncol*, 2010, 28 (4):556-61.

Decitabine (MDS Regimen)

Use Myelodysplastic syndrome

Regimen NOTE: Multiple variations are listed.

Variation 1:

Decitabine: I.V.: 20 mg/m²/day over 1 hour days 1 to 5 [total dose/cycle = 100 mg/m²]

Repeat cycle every 28 days

Variation 2:

Decitabine: I.V.: 15 mg/m²/dose over 3 hours every 8 hours days 1 to 3 (total of 45 mg/m²/day) [total dose/cycle = 135 mg/m²]

Repeat cycle every 6 weeks

References

Variation 1:

Kantarjian H, Oki Y, Garcia-Manero G, et al, "Results of a Randomized Study of 3 Schedules of Low-Dose Decitabine in Higher-Risk Myelodysplastic Syndrome and Chronic Myelomonocytic Leukemia," *Blood*, 2007, 109(1):52-7.

Steensma DP, Baer MR, Slack JL, et al, "Multicenter Study of Decitabine Administered Daily for 5 Days Every 4 Weeks to Adults With Myelodysplastic Syndromes: The Alternative Dosing for Outpatient Treatment (ADOPT) Trial," *J Clin Oncol*, 2009, 27(23):3842-8.

Variation 2:

Kantarjian H, Issa JP, Rosenfeld CS, et al, "Decitabine Improves Patient Outcomes in Myelodysplastic Syndromes," *Cancer*, 2006, 106(8):1794-803.

Dexa-BEAM (Hodgkin)

Index Terms Dexamethasone, Carmustine, Etoposide, Cytarabine, Melphalan (Hodgkin)

Use Lymphoma, Hodgkin

Regimen

Dexamethasone: Oral: 8 mg every 8 hours days 1 to 10 [total dose/cycle = 240 mg]

Carmustine: I.V.: 60 mg/m² day 2 [total dose/cycle = 60 mg/m²]

Etoposide: I.V.: 75 mg/m²/day days 4 to 7 [total dose/cycle = 300 mg/m²]

Cytarabine: I.V.: 100 mg/m²/dose every 12 hours days 4 to 7 (total of 8 doses) [total dose/cycle = 800 mg/m²]

Melphalan: I.V.: 20 mg/m² day 3 [total dose/cycle = 20 mg/m²]

Repeat cycle every 28 days; consider stem cell transplantation after 2 cycles in responding patients and a maximum of 4 cycles (total) in nontransplant candidates

References

Pfreundschuh MG, Rueffer U, Lathan B, et al, "Dexa-BEAM in Patients With Hodgkin's Disease Refractory to Multidrug Chemotherapy Regimens: A Trial of the German Hodgkin's Disease Study Group," *J Clin Oncol*, 1994, 12(3):580-6.

◆ **Dexamethasone-Bortezomib (Amyloidosis)** *see* Bortezomib-Dexamethasone (Amyloidosis) *on page 1534*

◆ **Dexamethasone-Bortezomib-Doxorubicin** *see* Bortezomib-Doxorubicin-Dexamethasone *on page 1535*

◆ **Dexamethasone-Bortezomib-Doxorubicin (Liposomal)** *see* Bortezomib-Doxorubicin (Liposomal)-Dexamethasone *on page 1536*

◆ **Dexamethasone-Bortezomib (Multiple myeloma)** *see* Bortezomib-Dexamethasone (Multiple Myeloma) *on page 1534*

◆ **Dexamethasone, Carmustine, Etoposide, Cytarabine, Melphalan (Hodgkin)** *see* Dexa-BEAM (Hodgkin) *on page 1607*

◆ **Dexamethasone-Cisplatin-Cytarabine (Hodgkin)** *see* DHAP (Hodgkin) *on page 1608*

◆ **Dexamethasone-Lenalidomide** *see* Lenalidomide-Dexamethasone *on page 1702*

◆ **Dexamethasone (Low Dose)-Lenalidomide** *see* Lenalidomide-Dexamethasone (Low Dose) *on page 1703*

◆ **Dexamethasone-Thalidomide (MM)** *see* Thalidomide-Dexamethasone (MM) *on page 1754*

DHAP (Hodgkin)

Index Terms Dexamethasone-Cisplatin-Cytarabine (Hodgkin)

Use Lymphoma, Hodgkin

Regimen

Salvage treatment:

Dexamethasone: I.V.: 40 mg/day days 1 to 4
[total dose/cycle = 160 mg]

Cisplatin: I.V.: 100 mg/m^2 continuous infusion for 24 hours day 1
[total dose/cycle = 100 mg/m^2]

Cytarabine: I.V.: 2000 mg/m^2 over 3 hours every 12 hours day 2 (total of 2 doses)
[total dose/cycle = 4000 mg/m^2]

Filgrastim: SubQ: 5 mcg/kg/day beginning 24 hours after last dose of cytarabine, continue until leukocytes ≥2500/mm^3 for 3 days

Administer 2 cycles

References

Josting A, Rudolph C, Reiser M, et al, "Time-Intensified Dexamethasone/Cisplatin/Cytarabine: An Effective Salvage Therapy With Low Toxicity in Patients With Relapsed and Refractory Hodgkin's Disease," *Ann Oncol*, 2002, 13(10):1628-35.

◆ **DHAP (NHL Regimen)** *see* Cisplatin-Cytarabine-Dexamethasone (NHL Regimen) *on page 1567*

◆ **DHAX (NHL Regimen)** *see* Oxaliplatin-Cytarabine-Dexamethasone (NHL Regimen) *on page 1723*

Docetaxel-Bevacizumab

Index Terms Bevacizumab-Docetaxel

Use Breast cancer

Regimen NOTE: Multiple variations are listed.

Variation 1:

Docetaxel: I.V.: 100 mg/m^2 day 1
[total dose/cycle = 100 mg/m^2]

Bevacizumab: I.V.: 7.5 mg/kg day 1
[total dose/cycle = 7.5 mg/kg]

Repeat cycle every 21 days (administer docetaxel for up to 9 cycles, bevacizumab until disease progression or unacceptable toxicity)

Variation 2:

Docetaxel: I.V.: 100 mg/m^2 day 1
[total dose/cycle = 100 mg/m^2]

Bevacizumab: I.V.: 15 mg/kg day 1
[total dose/cycle = 15 mg/kg]
Repeat cycle every 21 days (administer docetaxel for up to 9 cycles, bevacizumab until disease progression or unacceptable toxicity)

References

Miles D, Chan A, Romieu G, et al, "Randomized, Double-Blind, Placebo-Controlled, Phase III Study of Bevacizumab With Docetaxel or Docetaxel With Placebo as First-Line Therapy for Patients With Locally Recurrent or Metastatic Breast Cancer (mBC): AVADO," [LBA1011abstract from 2008 ASCO Annual Meeting].

◆ **Docetaxel-Capecitabine (Gastric Cancer)** *see* Capecitabine-Docetaxel (Gastric Cancer) *on page 1539*

◆ **Docetaxel-Carboplatin (Ovarian)** *see* Carboplatin-Docetaxel (Ovarian) *on page 1543*

◆ **Docetaxel-Carboplatin (Unknown Primary)** *see* Carboplatin-Docetaxel (Unknown Primary) *on page 1544*

Docetaxel-Cisplatin

Use Lung cancer, nonsmall cell

Regimen

Docetaxel: I.V.: 75 mg/m^2 day 1
[total dose/cycle = 75 mg/m^2]
Cisplatin: I.V.: 75 mg/m^2 day 1
[total dose/cycle = 75 mg/m^2]
Repeat cycle every 21 days

References

Zalcberg J, Millward M, Bishop J, et al, "Phase II Study of Docetaxel and Cisplatin in Advanced Nonsmall-Cell Lung Cancer," *J Clin Oncol*, 1998, 16(5):1948-53.

Docetaxel-Cisplatin-Fluorouracil (Gastric/Esophageal Cancer)

Index Terms DCF (Gastric/Esophageal Cancer); TCF (Gastric/Esophageal Cancer)

Use Esophageal cancer; Gastric cancer

Regimen NOTE: Multiple variations are listed.

Variation 1:
Docetaxel: I.V.: 75 mg/m^2 day 1
[total dose/cycle = 75 mg/m^2]
Cisplatin: I.V.: 75 mg/m^2 day 1
[total dose/cycle = 75 mg/m^2]
Fluorouracil: I.V.: 750 mg/m^2/day continuous infusion days 1 to 5
[total dose/cycle = 3750 mg/m^2]
Repeat cycle every 21 days until disease progression or unacceptable toxicity

Variation 2:
Docetaxel: I.V.: 75 mg/m^2 day 1
[total dose/cycle = 75 mg/m^2]
Cisplatin: I.V.: 75 mg/m^2 over 4 hours day 1
[total dose/cycle = 75 mg/m^2]
Fluorouracil: I.V.: 300 mg/m^2/day continuous infusion days 1 to 14
[total dose/cycle = 4200 mg/m^2]
Repeat cycle every 21 days until disease progression or unacceptable toxicity for up to a maximum of 8 cycles

References

Variation 1:

Ajani JA, Fodor MB, Tjulandin SA, et al, "Phase II Multi-Institutional Randomized Trial of Docetaxel Plus Cisplatin With or Without Fluorouracil in Patients With Untreated, Advanced Gastric, or Gastroesophageal Adenocarcinoma," *J Clin Oncol*, 2005, 23(24):5660-7.

Ajani JA, Moiseyenko VM, Tjulandin S, et al, "Quality of Life With Docetaxel Plus Cisplatin and Fluorouracil Compared With Cisplatin and Fluorouracil From a Phase III Trial for Advanced Gastric or Gastroesophageal Adenocarcinoma: The V-325 Study Group," *J Clin Oncol*, 2007, 25 (22):3210-6.

Van Cutsem E, Moiseyenko VM, Tjulandin S, et al, "Phase III Study of Docetaxel and Cisplatin Plus Fluorouracil Compared With Cisplatin and Fluorouracil as First-Line Therapy for Advanced Gastric Cancer: A Report of the V325 Study Group," *J Clin Oncol*, 2006, 24(31):4991-7.

Variation 2:

Roth AD, Fazio N, Stupp R, et al, "Docetaxel, Cisplatin, and Fluorouracil; Docetaxel and Cisplatin; and Epirubicin, Cisplatin, and Fluorouracil as Systemic Treatment for Advanced Gastric Carcinoma: A Randomized Phase II Trial of the Swiss Group for Clinical Cancer Research," *J Clin Oncol*, 2007, 25(22):3217-23.

Docetaxel-Cisplatin-Fluorouracil (Head and Neck Cancer)

Index Terms TPF

Use Head and neck cancer

Regimen NOTE: Multiple variations are listed.

Variation 1:

Docetaxel: I.V.: 75 mg/m^2 day 1
[total dose/cycle = 75 mg/m^2]

Cisplatin: I.V.: 75 mg/m^2 day 1
[total dose/cycle = 75 mg/m^2]

Fluorouracil: I.V.: 750 mg/m^2/day continuous infusion days 1 to 5
[total dose/cycle = 3750 mg/m^2]

Repeat cycle every 21 days for 4 cycles

Variation 2:

Docetaxel: I.V.: 75 mg/m^2 day 1
[total dose/cycle = 75 mg/m^2]

Cisplatin: I.V.: 75-100 mg/m^2 day 1
[total dose/cycle = 75-100 mg/m^2]

Fluorouracil: I.V.: 1000 mg/m^2/day continuous infusion days 1 to 4
[total dose/cycle = 4000 mg/m^2]

Repeat cycle every 21 days for total of 3 cycles

References

Variation 1:

Schrijvers D, van Herpen C, Kerger J, et al, "Docetaxel, Cisplatin and 5-Fluorouracil in Patients With Locally Advanced Unresectable Head and Neck Cancer: A Phase I-II Feasibility Study," *Ann Oncol*, 2004, 15(4):638-45.

Vermorken JB, Remenar E, van Herpen C, et al, "Cisplatin, Fluorouracil, and Docetaxel in Unresectable Head and Neck Cancer," *N Engl J Med*, 2007, 357(17):1695-1704.

Variation 2:

Posner MR, Glisson B, Frenette G, et al, "Multicenter Phase I-II Trial of Docetaxel, Cisplatin, and Fluorouracil Induction Chemotherapy for Patients With Locally Advanced Squamous Cell Cancer of the Head and Neck," *J Clin Oncol*, 2001, 19(4):1096-104.

Posner MR, Hershock DM, Blajman CR, et al, "Cisplatin and Fluorouracil Alone or With Docetaxel in Head and Neck Cancer," *N Engl J Med*, 2007, 357(17):1705-15.

◆ **Docetaxel-Cisplatin (Unknown Primary)** *see* Cisplatin-Docetaxel (Unknown Primary) *on page* 1568

Docetaxel-Cyclophosphamide (TC)

Index Terms TC

Use Breast cancer

Regimen

Docetaxel: I.V.: 75 mg/m^2 day 1
[total dose/cycle = 75 mg/m^2]
Cyclophosphamide: I.V.: 600 mg/m^2 day 1
[total dose/cycle = 600 mg/m^2]
Repeat cycle every 21 days for 4 cycles

References

Jones SE, Savin MA, Holmes FA, et al, "Phase III Trial Comparing Doxorubicin Plus Cyclophosphamide With Docetaxel Plus Cyclophosphamide as Adjuvant Therapy for Operable Breast Cancer," *J Clin Oncol*, 2006, 24(34):5381-7.

Docetaxel-Doxorubicin (Breast Cancer)

Index Terms AT (Breast Cancer); Doxorubicin-Docetaxel (Breast Cancer)

Use Breast cancer

Regimen

Doxorubicin: I.V.: 50 mg/m^2 day 1
[total dose/cycle = 50 mg/m^2]
Docetaxel: I.V.: 75 mg/m^2 day 1
[total dose/cycle = 75 mg/m^2]
Repeat cycle every 3 weeks for up to 8 cycles

References

Nabholtz JM, Falkson C, Campos D, et al, "Docetaxel and Doxorubicin Compared With Doxorubicin and Cyclophosphamide as First-Line Chemotherapy for Metastatic Breast Cancer: Results of a Randomized, Multicenter, Phase III Trial," *J Clin Oncol*, 2003, 21(6):968-75.

◆ **Docetaxel-Doxorubicin Liposomal (Breast Cancer)** *see* Doxorubicin (Liposomal)-Docetaxel (Breast Cancer) *on page 1619*

Docetaxel-FEC

Index Terms FEC-Docetaxel

Use Breast cancer

Regimen

Cycles 1, 2, and 3:
Docetaxel: I.V.: 80-100 mg/m^2 day 1
[total dose/cycle = 80-100 mg/m^2]
Repeat cycle every 21 days for 3 cycles
Cycles 4, 5, and 6 (FEC):
Fluorouracil: I.V.: 600 mg/m^2 day 1
[total dose/cycle = 600 mg/m^2]
Epirubicin: I.V.: 60 mg/m^2 day 1
[total dose/cycle = 60 mg/m^2]
Cyclophosphamide: I.V.: 600 mg/m^2 day 1
[total dose/cycle = 600 mg/m^2]
Repeat FEC cycle every 21 days for total of 3 cycles

References

Joensuu H, Kellokumpu-Lehtinen PL, Bono P, et al, "Adjuvant Docetaxel or Vinorelbine With or Without Trastuzumab for Breast Cancer," *N Engl J Med*, 2006, 354(8):809-20.

Docetaxel-Gemcitabine (Unknown Primary)

Index Terms Gemcitabine-Docetaxel (Unknown Primary)

Use Unknown primary (adenocarcinoma)

Regimen

Gemcitabine: I.V.: 1000 mg/m^2/day over 30 minutes days 1 and 8
[total dose/cycle = 2000 mg/m^2]

Docetaxel: I.V.: 75 mg/m^2 over 1 hour day 8
[total dose/cycle = 75 mg/m^2]

Repeat cycle every 21 days for up to a total of 6 cycles

References

Pouessel D, Culine S, Becht C, et al, "Gemcitabine and Docetaxel as Front-Line Chemotherapy in Patients With Carcinoma of an Unknown Primary Site," *Cancer*, 2004, 100(6):1257-61.

Docetaxel (NSCLC Regimen)

Use Lung cancer, nonsmall cell

Regimen NOTE: Multiple variations are listed.

Variation 1:

Docetaxel: I.V.: 75 mg/m^2 over 1 hour day 1
[total dose/cycle = 75 mg/m^2]

Repeat cycle every 21 days

Variation 2:

Docetaxel: I.V.: 35 mg/m^2 days 1, 8, and 15
[total dose/cycle = 105 mg/m^2]

Repeat cycle every 28 days for a maximum of 8 cycles

Variation 3:

Docetaxel: I.V.: 36 mg/m^2/day over 1 hour days 1, 8, 15, 22, 29, and 36
[total dose/cycle = 216 mg/m^2]

Repeat cycle every 56 days for up to 4 cycles

Variation 4 (maintenance therapy):

Docetaxel: I.V.: 75 mg/m^2 over 1 hour day 1
[total dose/cycle = 75 mg/m^2]

Repeat cycle every 21 days for a maximum of 6 cycles

References

Variation1:

Fossella FV, DeVore R, Kerr RN, et al, "Randomized Phase III Trial of Docetaxel Versus Vinorelbine or Ifosfamide in Patients With Advanced Non-Small-Cell Lung Cancer Previously Treated With Platinum-Containing Chemotherapy Regimens," *J Clin Oncol*, 2000, 18 (12):2354-62.

Variation 2:

Schuette W, Nagel S, Blankenburg T, et al, "Phase III Study of Second-Line Chemotherapy for Advanced Non-Small-Cell Lung Cancer With Weekly Compared With 3-Weekly Docetaxel," *J Clin Oncol*, 2005, 23(33):8389-95.

Variation 3:

Hainsworth JD, Burris HA, Litchy S, et al, "Weekly Docetaxel in the Treatment of Elderly Patients With Advanced Nonsmall Cell Lung Cancer: A Minnie Pearl Cancer Research Network Phase II Trial," *Cancer*, 2000, 89(2):328-33.

Variation 4:

Fidias PM, Dakhill SR, Lyss AP, et al, "Phase III Study of Immediate Compared With Delayed Docetaxel After Front-Line Therapy With Gemcitabine Plus Carboplatin in Advanced Non-Small-Cell Lung Cancer," *J Clin Oncol*, 2009, 27(4):591-8.

Docetaxel (Ovarian Regimen)

Use Ovarian cancer

Regimen

Docetaxel: I.V.: 100 mg/m^2 over 1 hour day 1
[total dose/cycle = 100 mg/m^2]

Repeat cycle every 21 days

References

Rose PG, Blessing JA, Ball HG, et al, "A Phase II Study of Docetaxel in Paclitaxel-Resistant Ovarian and Peritoneal Carcinoma: A Gynecologic Oncology Group Study," *Gynecol Oncol*, 2003, 88(2):130-5.

Docetaxel-Oxaliplatin-Fluorouracil (Esophageal Cancer)

Index Terms Oxaliplatin-Docetaxel-Fluorouracil (Esophageal Cancer)

Use Esophageal cancer

Regimen

Docetaxel: I.V.: 50 mg/m^2 day 1
[total dose/cycle = 50 mg/m^2]

Oxaliplatin: I.V.: 85 mg/m^2 day 1
[total dose/cycle = 85 mg/m^2]

Fluorouracil: I.V.: 2400 mg/m^2 continuous infusion over 46 hours starting day 1
[total dose/cycle = 2400 mg/m^2]

Repeat cycle every 14 days.

References

Shankaran V, Mulcahy MF, Hochster HS, et al, "Docetaxel, Oxaliplatin and 5-Fluorouracil for the Treatment of Metastatic or Unresectable Gastric or Gastroesophageal Junction (GEJ) Adenocarcinomas: Preliminary Results of a Phase II Study," *Gastrointestinal Symposium*, 2009:47 [abstract 47 from 2009 ASCO Gastrointestinal Cancers Symposium].

Docetaxel-Oxaliplatin-Leucovorin-Fluorouracil (Esophageal Cancer)

Index Terms FLOT (Esophageal Cancer); Oxaliplatin-Docetaxel-Leucovorin-Fluorouracil (Esophageal Cancer)

Use Esophageal cancer

Regimen

Docetaxel: I.V.: 50 mg/m^2 day 1
[total dose/cycle = 50 mg/m^2]

Oxaliplatin: I.V.: 85 mg/m^2 day 1
[total dose/cycle = 85 mg/m^2]

Leucovorin: I.V.: 200 mg/m^2 day 1
[total dose/cycle = 200 mg/m^2]

Fluorouracil: I.V.: 2600 mg/m^2/day continuous infusion over 24 hours day 1
[total dose/cycle = 2600 mg/m^2]

Repeat cycle every 14 days until disease progression or unacceptable toxicity for up to a total of 8 cycles.

References

Al-Batran SE, Hartmann JT, Hofheinz R, et al, "Biweekly Fluorouracil, Leucovorin, Oxaliplatin, and Docetaxel (FLOT) for Patients With Metastatic Adenocarcinoma of the Stomach or Esophagogastric Junction: A Phase II Trial of the Arbeitsgemeinschaft Internistische Onkologie," *Ann Oncol*, 2008, 19(11):1882-7.

Docetaxel-Oxaliplatin (Ovarian Cancer)

Index Terms Oxaliplatin-Docetaxel (Ovarian Cancer)

Use Ovarian cancer

Regimen

Docetaxel: I.V.: 75 mg/m^2/dose over 60 minutes day 1
[total dose/cycle = 75 mg/m^2]

Oxaliplatin: I.V.: 100 mg/m^2/dose over 2 hours day 1
[total dose/cycle = 100 mg/m^2]

Repeat cycle every 21 days

References

Ferrandina G, Ludovisi M, De Vincenzo R, et al, "Docetaxel and Oxaliplatin in the Second-Line Treatment of Platinum-Sensitive Recurrent Ovarian Cancer: A Phase II Study," *Ann Oncol*, 2007, 18(8):1348-53.

Docetaxel-Pertuzumab-Trastuzumab (Breast)

Index Terms Pertuzumab-Trastuzumab-Docetaxel (Breast); Trastuzumab-Pertuzumab-Docetaxel (Breast)

Use Breast cancer, metastatic HER2+

Regimen

Cycle 1:

Trastuzumab: I.V.: 8 mg/kg (loading dose) day 1 cycle 1
[total dose/cycle 1 = 8 mg/kg]

Docetaxel: I.V.: 75 mg/m^2 day 1
[total dose/cycle 1 = 75 mg/m^2]

Pertuzumab: I.V.: 840 mg (loading dose) day 1 cycle 1
[total dose/cycle 1 = 840 mg]

Treatment cycle is 21 days

Subsequent cycles:

Trastuzumab: I.V.: 6 mg/kg day 1
[total dose/cycle = 6 mg/kg]

Docetaxel: I.V.: 75 mg/m^2 day 1
[total dose/cycle = 75 mg/m^2]

Pertuzumab: I.V.: 420 mg day 1
[total dose/cycle = 420 mg]

Repeat cycle every 21 days until disease progression or unacceptable toxicity (minimum of 6 cycles of docetaxel)

References

Baselga J, Cortés J, Kim SB, et al, "Pertuzumab Plus Trastuzumab Plus Docetaxel for Metastatic Breast Cancer," *N Engl J Med*, 2012, 366(2):109-19.

Docetaxel-Prednisone

Use Prostate cancer

Regimen

Docetaxel: I.V.: 75 mg/m^2 day 1
[total dose/cycle = 75 mg/m^2]

Prednisone: Oral: 5 mg twice daily
[total dose/cycle = 210 mg]

Repeat cycle every 21 days for up to 10 cycles

References

Dagher R, Li N, Abraham S, et al, "Approval Summary: Docetaxel in Combination With Prednisone for the Treatment of Androgen-Independent Hormone-Refractory Prostate Cancer," *Clin Cancer Res*, 2004, 10(24):8147-51.

Tannock IF, de Wit R, Berry WR, et al, "Docetaxel Plus Prednisone or Mitoxantrone Plus Prednisone for Advanced Prostate Cancer," *N Engl J Med*, 2004, 351(15):1502-12

Docetaxel (Small Cell Lung Cancer Regimen)

Use Lung cancer, small cell

Regimen

Docetaxel: I.V.: 100 mg/m^2 over 1 hour day 1
[total dose/cycle = 100 mg/m^2]

Repeat cycle every 21 days

References

Smyth JF, Smith IE, Sessa C, et al, "Activity of Docetaxel (Taxotere) in Small Cell Lung Cancer," *Eur J Cancer*, 1994, 30A(8):1058-60.

Docetaxel-Trastuzumab

Index Terms Trastuzumab-Docetaxel

Use Breast cancer

Regimen

Cycle 1:

Docetaxel: I.V.: 100 mg/m^2 day 1
[total dose/cycle 1 = 100 mg/m^2]

Trastuzumab: I.V.: 4 mg/kg (loading dose) day 1 cycle 1
followed by I.V.: 2 mg/kg/day days 8 and 15 cycle 1
[total dose/cycle 1 = 8 mg/kg]

Treatment cycle is 21 days

Subsequent cycles:

Docetaxel: I.V.: 100 mg/m^2 day 1
[total dose/cycle = 100 mg/m^2]

Trastuzumab: I.V.: 2 mg/kg/day days 1, 8, and 15
[total dose/cycle = 6 mg/kg]

Repeat cycle every 21 days for a total of at least 6 cycles (continue weekly trastuzumab until disease progression)

References

Marty M, Cognetti F, Maraninchi D, et al, "Randomized Phase II Trial of the Efficacy and Safety of Trastuzumab Combined With Docetaxel in Patients With Human Epidermal Growth Factor Receptor 2-Positive Metastatic Breast Cancer Administered as First-Line Treatment: The M77001 Study Group," *J Clin Oncol*, 2005, 23(19):4265-74.

Docetaxel-Trastuzumab-Carboplatin

Index Terms Trastuzumab-Docetaxel-Carboplatin

Use Breast cancer

Regimen

Cycle 1:

Trastuzumab: I.V.: 4 mg/kg (loading dose) day 1 cycle 1
followed by I.V.: 2 mg/kg/day days 8 and 15 cycle 1
[total dose/cycle 1 = 8 mg/kg]

Docetaxel: I.V.: 75 mg/m^2 day 2
[total dose/cycle 1 = 75 mg/m^2]

Carboplatin: I.V.: AUC 6 day 2
[total dose/cycle 1 = AUC = 6]

Treatment cycle is 21 days

Subsequent cycles:

Trastuzumab: I.V.: 2 mg/kg/day days 1, 8, and 15
[total dose/cycle = 6 mg/kg]

Docetaxel: I.V.: 75 mg/m^2 day 1
[total dose/cycle = 75 mg/m^2]

Carboplatin: I.V.: AUC 6 day 1
[total dose/cycle = AUC = 6]

Repeat cycle every 21 days for a total of ~6 cycles (continue weekly trastuzumab for 1 year after chemotherapy, or until disease progression or unacceptable toxicity)

References

Pegram MD, Pienkowski T, Northfelt DW, et al, "Results of Two Open-Label, Multicenter Phase II Studies of Docetaxel, Platinum Salts, and Trastuzumab in HER2-Positive Advanced Breast Cancer," *J Natl Cancer Inst*, 2004, 96(10):759-69.

Docetaxel-Trastuzumab-Cisplatin

Index Terms Trastuzumab-Docetaxel-Cisplatin

Use Breast cancer

Regimen

Cycle 1:

Trastuzumab: I.V.: 4 mg/kg (loading dose) day 1 cycle 1
followed by I.V.: 2 mg/kg/day days 8 and 15 cycle 1
[total dose/cycle 1 = 8 mg/kg]

Docetaxel: I.V.: 75 mg/m^2 day 2
[total dose/cycle 1 = 75 mg/m^2]

Cisplatin: I.V.: 75 mg/m^2 day 2
[total dose/cycle 1 = 75 mg/m^2]

Treatment cycle is 21 days

Subsequent cycles:

Trastuzumab: I.V.: 2 mg/kg/day days 1, 8, and 15
[total dose/cycle = 6 mg/kg]

Docetaxel: I.V.: 75 mg/m^2 day 1
[total dose/cycle = 75 mg/m^2]

Cisplatin: I.V.: 75 mg/m^2 day 1
[total dose/cycle = 75 mg/m^2]

Repeat cycle every 21 days for a total of ~6 cycles (continue weekly trastuzumab for 1 year after chemotherapy, or until disease progression or unacceptable toxicity)

References

Pegram MD, Pienkowski T, Northfelt DW, et al, "Results of Two Open-Label, Multicenter Phase II Studies of Docetaxel, Platinum Salts, and Trastuzumab in HER2-Positive Advanced Breast Cancer," *J Natl Cancer Inst*, 2004, 96(10):759-69.

Docetaxel-Trastuzumab-FEC

Index Terms Trastuzumab-Docetaxel-FEC

Use Breast cancer

Regimen

Cycle 1:

Trastuzumab: I.V.: 4 mg/kg (loading dose) day 1 cycle 1
followed by I.V.: 2 mg/kg/day days 8 and 15 cycle 1
[total dose/cycle 1 = 8 mg/kg]

Docetaxel: I.V.: 80-100 mg/m^2 day 1
[total dose/cycle 1 = 80-100 mg/m^2]

Treatment cycle is 21 days

Cycles 2 and 3:

Trastuzumab: I.V.: 2 mg/kg/day days 1, 8, and 15
[total dose/cycle = 6 mg/kg]

Docetaxel: I.V.: 80-100 mg/m^2 day 1
[total dose/cycle = 80-100 mg/m^2]

Treatment cycle is 21 days

Cycles 4, 5, and 6 (FEC):

Fluorouracil: I.V.: 600 mg/m^2 day 1
[total dose/cycle = 600 mg/m^2]

Epirubicin: I.V.: 60 mg/m^2 day 1
[total dose/cycle = 60 mg/m^2]

Cyclophosphamide: I.V.: 600 mg/m^2 day 1
[total dose/cycle = 600 mg/m^2]

Repeat FEC cycle every 21 days for total of 3 cycles

References

Joensuu H, Kellokumpu-Lehtinen PL, Bono P, et al, "Adjuvant Docetaxel or Vinorelbine With or Without Trastuzumab for Breast Cancer," *N Engl J Med*, 2006, 354(8):809-20.

Docetaxel (Weekly Regimen)

Use Prostate cancer

Regimen

Docetaxel: I.V.: 40 mg/m^2 days 1, 8, and 15
[total dose/cycle = 120 mg/m^2]

Repeat cycle every 4 weeks

References

Joshua AM, Nordman I, Venkataswaran R, et al, "Weekly Docetaxel as Second Line Treatment After Mitozantrone for Androgen-Independent Prostate Cancer," *Intern Med J*, 2005, 35 (8):468-72.

Docetaxel (Weekly)-Trastuzumab

Index Terms Trastuzumab-Docetaxel (Weekly)

Use Breast cancer

Regimen

Cycle 1:

Docetaxel: I.V.: 35 mg/m^2/day days 1, 8, and 15
[total dose/cycle 1 = 105 mg/m^2]

Trastuzumab: I.V.: 4 mg/kg (loading dose) day 0 cycle 1
followed by I.V.: 2 mg/kg/day days 8 and 15 cycle 1
[total dose/cycle 1 = 8 mg/kg]

Treatment cycle is 28 days

Subsequent cycles:

Docetaxel: I.V.: 35 mg/m^2/day days 1, 8, and 15
[total dose/cycle = 105 mg/m^2]

Trastuzumab: I.V.: 2 mg/kg/day days 1, 8, and 15
[total dose/cycle = 6 mg/kg]

Repeat cycle every 28 days

References

Esteva FJ, Valero V, Booser D, et al, "Phase II Study of Weekly Docetaxel and Trastuzumab for Patients With HER-2-Overexpressing Metastatic Breast Cancer," *J Clin Oncol*, 2002, 20 (7):1800-8.

◆ **Dose-Adjusted EPOCH (AIDS-Related Lymphoma)** *see* EPOCH Dose-Adjusted (AIDS-Related Lymphoma) *on page 1628*

◆ **Dose-Adjusted EPOCH (NHL)** *see* EPOCH Dose-Adjusted (NHL) *on page 1628*

◆ **Dose-Adjusted Etoposide-Vincristine-Doxorubicin-Cyclophosphamide-Prednisone (NHL)** *see* EPOCH Dose-Adjusted (NHL) *on page 1628*

Dox-CMF (Sequential)

Use Breast cancer

Regimen

Doxorubicin: I.V.: 75 mg/m^2 day 1
[total dose/cycle = 75 mg/m^2]

Repeat cycle every 21 days for 4 cycles

followed by (after completing Cycle 4)

Cyclophosphamide: I.V.: 600 mg/m^2 day 1
[total dose/cycle = 600 mg/m^2]

Methotrexate: I.V.: 40 mg/m^2 day 1
[total dose/cycle = 40 mg/m^2]
Fluorouracil: I.V.: 600 mg/m^2 day 1
[total dose/cycle = 600 mg/m^2]
Repeat cycle every 21 days for 8 cycles

References

Bonadonna G, Zambetti M, Velagussa P, "Sequential or Alternating Doxorubicin and CMF Regimens in Breast Cancer With More Than Three Positive Nodes. Ten-Year Results," *JAMA*, 1995, 273(7):542-7.

Doxorubicin (Liposomal) (Ovarian Regimen)

Use Ovarian cancer

Regimen NOTE: Multiple variations are listed.

Variation 1:
Doxorubicin (liposomal): I.V.: 50 mg/m^2 over 60 minutes day 1
[total dose/cycle = 50 mg/m^2]
Repeat cycle every 28 days until disease progression or unacceptable toxicity

Variation 2:
Doxorubicin (liposomal): I.V.: 40 mg/m^2 over 60 minutes day 1
[total dose/cycle = 40 mg/m^2]
Repeat cycle every 28 days until disease progression or unacceptable toxicity

References

Variation 1:

Gordon AN, Tonda M, Sun S, et al, "Long-Term Survival Advantage for Women Treated With Pegylated Liposomal Doxorubicin Compared With Topotecan in a Phase III Randomized Study of Recurrent and Refractory Epithelial Ovarian Cancer," *Gynecol Onc*, 2004, 95(1):1-8.

Mutch DG, Orlando M, Goss T, et al, "Randomized Phase III Trial of Gemcitabine Compared With Pegylated Liposomal Doxorubicin in Patients With Platinum-Resistant Ovarian Cancer," *J Clin Oncol*, 2007, 25(19):2811-8.

Variation 2:

Ferrandina G, Ludovisi M, Lorusso D, et al, "Phase III Trial of Gemcitabine Compared With Pegylated Liposomal Doxorubicin in Progressive or Recurrent Ovarian Cancer," *J Clin Oncol*, 2008, 26(6):890-6.

Rose PG, Maxson JH, Fusco N, et al, "Liposomal Doxorubicin in Ovarian, Peritoneal, and Tubal Carcinoma: A Retrospective Comparative Study of Single-Agent Dosages," *Gynecol Oncol*, 2001, 82(2):323-8.

◆ **Doxorubicin, Bleomycin, Vinblastine, Dacarbazine (Hodgkin)** *see* ABVD Early Stage (Hodgkin) *on page 1516*

◆ **Doxorubicin-Bleomycin-Vinblastine-Dacarbazine (Hodgkin)** *see* ABVD (Hodgkin) *on page 1516*

◆ **Doxorubicin-Dacarbazine-Ifosfamide-Mesna (Sarcoma)** *see* MAID (Sarcoma) *on page 1704*

◆ **Doxorubicin-Dacarbazine (Soft Tissue Sarcoma)** *see* AD (Soft Tissue Sarcoma) *on page 1519*

◆ **Doxorubicin-Dexamethasone-Bortezomib** *see* Bortezomib-Doxorubicin-Dexamethasone *on page 1535*

◆ **Doxorubicin-Docetaxel (Breast Cancer)** *see* Docetaxel-Doxorubicin (Breast Cancer) *on page 1611*

Doxorubicin + Ketoconazole

Use Prostate cancer

Regimen

Doxorubicin: I.V.: 20 mg/m^2 continuous infusion day 1
[total dose/cycle = 20 mg/m^2]
Ketoconazole: Oral: 400 mg 3 times/day days 1 to 7
[total dose/cycle = 8400 mg]
Repeat cycle every 7 days

References

Sella A, Kilbourn R, Amato R, et al, "Phase II Study of Ketoconazole Combined With Weekly Doxorubicin in Patients With Androgen-Independent Prostate Cancer," *J Clin Oncol*, 1994, 12 (4):683-8.

Doxorubicin + Ketoconazole/Estramustine + Vinblastine

Use Prostate cancer

Regimen

Doxorubicin: I.V.: 20 mg/m^2/day days 1, 15, and 29
[total dose/cycle = 60 mg/m^2]
Ketoconazole: Oral: 400 mg 3 times/day days 1 to 7, 15 to 21, and 29 to 35
[total dose/cycle = 25,200 mg]
Estramustine: Oral: 140 mg 3 times/day days 8 to 14, 22 to 28, and 36 to 42
[total dose/cycle = 8820 mg]
Vinblastine: I.V.: 5 mg/m^2/day days 8, 22, and 36
[total dose/cycle = 15 mg/m^2]
Repeat cycle every 8 weeks

References

Ellerhorst JA, Tu SM, Amato RJ, et al, "Phase II Trial of Alternating Weekly Chemohormonal Therapy for Patients With Androgen-Independent Prostate Cancer," *Clin Cancer Res*, 1997, 3(12 Pt 1):2371-6.

◆ **Doxorubicin (Liposomal)-Bortezomib** *see* Bortezomib-Doxorubicin (Liposomal) *on page 1536*

◆ **Doxorubicin (Liposomal)-Carboplatin (Ovarian)** *see* Carboplatin-Doxorubicin (Liposomal) (Ovarian) *on page 1544*

◆ **Doxorubicin (Liposomal)-Dexamethasone-Bortezomib** *see* Bortezomib-Doxorubicin (Liposomal)-Dexamethasone *on page 1536*

Doxorubicin (Liposomal)-Docetaxel (Breast Cancer)

Index Terms Docetaxel-Doxorubicin Liposomal (Breast Cancer)

Use Breast cancer

Regimen

Doxorubicin (liposomal): I.V.: 30 mg/m^2 over 1 hour day 1
[total dose/cycle = 30 mg/m^2]
Docetaxel: I.V.: 60 mg/m^2 over 1 hour day 1
[total dose/cycle = 60 mg/m^2]
Repeat cycle every 3 weeks until disease progression or unacceptable toxicity

References

Sparano JA, Makhson AN, Semiglazov VF, et al, "Pegylated Liposomal Doxorubicin Plus Docetaxel Significantly Improves Time to Progression Without Additive Cardiotoxicity Compared With Docetaxel Monotherapy in Patients With Advanced Breast Cancer Previously Treated With Neoadjuvant-Adjuvant Anthracycline Therapy: Results From a Randomized Phase III Study," *J Clin Oncol*, 2009, 27(27):4522-9.

◆ **Doxorubicin Liposomal-Trabectedin (Ovarian Cancer)** *see* Trabectedin-Doxorubicin (Liposomal) (Ovarian Cancer) *on page 1757*

Doxorubicin (Liposomal)-Vincristine-Dexamethasone

Index Terms DVd; DVD

Use Multiple myeloma

Regimen NOTE: Multiple variations are listed.

Variation 1:

Doxorubicin, liposomal: I.V.: 40 mg/m^2 day 1
[total dose/cycle = 40 mg/m^2]

Vincristine: I.V.: 2 mg day 1
[total dose/cycle = 2 mg]

Dexamethasone: Oral or I.V.: 40 mg/day days 1 to 4
[total dose/cycle = 160 mg]

Repeat cycle every 4 weeks

Variation 2:

Doxorubicin, liposomal: I.V.: 40 mg/m^2 day 1
[total dose/cycle = 40 mg/m^2]

Vincristine: I.V.: 1.4 mg/m^2 (maximum dose: 2 mg) day 1
[total dose/cycle = 1.4 mg/m^2; maximum: 2 mg]

Dexamethasone: Oral: 40 mg/day days 1 to 4
[total dose/cycle = 160 mg]

Repeat cycle every 4 weeks

References

Variation 1:

Hussein MA, Wood L, Hsi E, et al, "A Phase II Trial of Pegylated Liposomal Doxorubicin, Vincristine, and Reduced-Dose Dexamethasone Combination Therapy in Newly Diagnosed Multiple Myeloma Patients," *Cancer*, 2002, 95(10):2160-8.

Variation 2:

Rifkin RM, Gregory SA, Mohrbacher A, et al, "Pegylated Liposomal Doxorubicin, Vincristine, and Dexamethasone Provide Significant Reduction in Toxicity Compared With Doxorubicin, Vincristine, and Dexamethasone in Patients With Newly Diagnosed Multiple Myeloma: A Phase III Multicenter Randomized Trial," *Cancer*, 2006, 106(4):848-58.

DTPACE

Use Multiple myeloma

Regimen

Dexamethasone: Oral: 40 mg/day days 1 to 4
[total dose/cycle = 160 mg]

Thalidomide: Oral: 400 mg/day
[total dose/cycle = 11,200 - 16,800 mg]

Cisplatin: I.V.: 10 mg/m^2/day continuous infusion days 1 to 4
[total dose/cycle = 40 mg/m^2]

Doxorubicin: I.V.: 10 mg/m^2/day continuous infusion days 1 to 4
[total dose/cycle = 40 mg/m^2]

Cyclophosphamide: I.V.: 400 mg/m^2 continuous infusion days 1 to 4
[total dose/cycle = 1600 mg/m^2]

Etoposide: I.V.: 40 mg/m^2 continuous infusion days 1 to 4
[total dose/cycle = 160 mg/m^2]

Repeat cycle every 4-6 weeks

References

Lee CK, Barlogie B, Munshi N, et al, "DTPACE: An Effective, Novel Combination Chemotherapy With Thalidomide for Previously Treated Patients With Myeloma," *J Clin Oncol*, 2003, 21 (14):2732-9.

◆ **DVd** *see* Doxorubicin (Liposomal)-Vincristine-Dexamethasone *on page 1620*

DVP

Use Leukemia, acute lymphocytic

Regimen Induction:

Daunorubicin: I.V.: 25 mg/m²/day days 1, 8, and 15
[total dose/cycle = 75 mg/m²]

Vincristine: I.V.: 1.5 mg/m²/day (maximum dose: 2 mg) days 1, 8, 15, and 22
[total dose/cycle = 6 mg/m²]

Prednisone: Oral: 60 mg/m²/day days 1 to 28 then taper over next 14 days
[total dose/cycle = 1680 mg/m² + taper over next 14 days]

Administer single cycle; used in conjunction with intrathecal chemotherapy

References

Belasco JB, Luery N, and Scher C, "Multiagent Chemotherapy in Relapsed Acute Lymphoblastic Leukemia in Children," *Cancer*, 1990, 66(12):2492-7.

◆ **ECF (Gastric/Esophageal Cancer)** *see* Epirubicin-Cisplatin-Fluorouracil (Gastric/Esophageal Cancer) *on page 1626*

EC (NSCLC)

Use Lung cancer, nonsmall cell

Regimen

Etoposide: I.V.: 120 mg/m²/day days 1, 2, and 3
[total dose/cycle = 360 mg/m²]

Carboplatin: I.V.: AUC 6 day 1
[total dose/cycle = AUC = 6]

Repeat cycle every 21-28 days

References

Birch R, Weaver CH, Hainsworth JD, et al, "A Randomized Study of Etoposide and Carboplatin With or Without Paclitaxel in the Treatment of Small Cell Lung Cancer," *Semin Oncol*, 1997, 24(4 Suppl 12):S12-135, 137.

◆ **EC (Small Cell Lung Cancer)** *see* Carboplatin-Etoposide (Small Cell Lung Cancer) *on page 1546*

◆ **ECX (Esophageal Cancer)** *see* Epirubicin-Cisplatin-Capecitabine (Esophageal Cancer) *on page 1626*

◆ **EE4A (Wilms' Tumor)** *see* EE-4A (Wilms' Tumor) *on page 1621*

EE-4A (Wilms' Tumor)

Index Terms Dactinomycin-Vincristine (Wilms' Tumor); EE4A (Wilms' Tumor); Regimen EE-4A (Wilms' Tumor); Vincristine-Dactinomycin (Wilms' Tumor)

Use Wilms' tumor

Regimen

Dactinomycin: I.V.: 45 mcg/kg day 1 of weeks 0, 3, 6, 9, 12, 15, and 18
[total dose = 315 mcg/kg]

Vincristine: I.V.: 1.5 mg/m² day 1 of weeks 1 to 10

Followed by

Vincristine: I.V.: 2 mg/m² day 1 of weeks 12, 15, and 18
[total dose = 21 mg/m²]

Treatment course duration is week 0 through week 18

References

Green DM, Breslow NE, Beckwith JB, et al, "Effect of Duration of Treatment on Treatment Outcome and Cost of Treatment for Wilms' Tumor: A Report From the National Wilms' Tumor Study Group," *J Clin Oncol*, 1998, 16(12):3744-51.

◆ **EMA 86 (AML Induction)** *see* MEC (AML Induction) *on page 1706*

EMA/CO

Use Gestational trophoblastic tumor

Regimen NOTE: Multiple variations are listed.

Variation 1:

Etoposide: I.V.: 100 mg/m^2/day days 1 and 2
[total dose/cycle = 200 mg/m^2]

Methotrexate: I.V.: 300 mg/m^2 continuous infusion over 12 hours day 1
[total dose/cycle = 300 mg/m^2]

Dactinomycin: I.V. push: 0.5 mg/day days 1 and 2
[total dose/cycle = 1 mg]

Leucovorin: Oral, I.M.: 15 mg twice daily for 2 days (start 24 hours after the start of methotrexate) days 2 and 3
[total dose/cycle = 60 mg]

Alternate weekly with:

Cyclophosphamide: I.V.: 600 mg/m^2 day 1
[total dose/cycle = 600 mg/m^2]

Vincristine: I.V. push: 0.8 mg/m^2 (maximum dose: 2 mg) day 1
[total dose/cycle = 0.8 mg/m^2]

Repeat cycle every 2 weeks

Variation 2:

Dactinomycin: I.V.: 0.5 mg/day days 1 and 2
[total dose/cycle = 1 mg]

Etoposide: I.V.: 100 mg/m^2/day days 1 and 2
[total dose/cycle = 200 mg/m^2]

Methotrexate: I.V. bolus: 100 mg/m^2 then 200 mg/m^2 continuous infusion over 12 hours day 1
[total dose/cycle = 300 mg/m^2]

Leucovorin: Oral, I.M.: 15 mg every 12 hours for 4 doses (start 24 hours after methotrexate) days 2 and 3
[total dose/cycle = 60 mg]

Vincristine: I.V.: 1 mg/m^2 day 8
[total dose/cycle = 1 mg/m^2]

Cyclophosphamide: I.V.: 600 mg/m^2 day 8
[total dose/cycle = 600 mg/m^2]

Repeat cycle every 2 weeks

Variation 3:

Dactinomycin: I.V.: 0.5 mg/day days 1 and 2
[total dose/cycle = 1 mg]

Etoposide: I.V.: 100 mg/m^2/day days 1 and 2
[total dose/cycle = 200 mg/m^2]

Methotrexate: I.V.: 300 mg/m^2 continuous infusion over 12 hours day 1
[total dose/cycle = 300 mg/m^2]

Leucovorin: Oral, I.M.: 15 mg every 12 hours for 4 doses (start 24 hours after start of methotrexate) days 2 and 3
[total dose/cycle = 60 mg]

Vincristine: I.V.: 1 mg/m^2 day 8
[total dose/cycle = 1 mg/m^2]

Cyclophosphamide: I.V.: 600 mg/m^2 day 8
[total dose/cycle = 600 mg/m^2]

Repeat cycle every 2 weeks

Variation 4:
Dactinomycin: I.V.: 0.35 mg/m^2/day days 1 and 2
[total dose/cycle = 0.7 mg/m^2]
Etoposide: I.V.: 100 mg/m^2/day days 1 and 2
[total dose/cycle = 200 mg/m^2]
Methotrexate: I.V. bolus: 100 mg/m^2 then 200 mg/m^2 continuous infusion over 12 hours day 1
[total dose/cycle = 300 mg/m^2]
Leucovorin: Oral, I.M.: 15 mg every 12 hours for 4 doses (start 24 hours after start of methotrexate) days 2 and 3
[total dose/cycle = 60 mg]
Vincristine: I.V.: 1 mg/m^2 day 8
[total dose/cycle = 1 mg/m^2]
Cyclophosphamide: I.V.: 600 mg/m^2 day 8
[total dose/cycle = 600 mg/m^2]
Repeat cycle every 2 weeks

Variation 5 (patients with brain metastases):
Dactinomycin: I.V.: 0.5 mg/day days 1 and 2
[total dose/cycle = 1 mg]
Etoposide:I.V.: 100 mg/m^2/day days 1 and 2
[total dose/cycle = 200 mg/m^2]
Methotrexate: I.V.: 1 g/m^2 continuous infusion over 12 hours day 1
[total dose/cycle = 1 g/m^2]
Leucovorin: I.M.: 20 mg/m^2 every 6 hours for 12 doses (start 24 hours after start of methotrexate) days 2, 3, and 4
[total dose/cycle = 240 mg/m^2]
Vincristine: I.V.: 1 mg/m^2 day 8
[total dose/cycle = 1 mg/m^2]
Cyclophosphamide: I.V.: 600 mg/m^2 day 8
[total dose/cycle = 600 mg/m^2]
Repeat cycle every 2 weeks

Variation 6 (patients with brain metastases):
Dactinomycin: I.V.: 0.5 mg/day days 1 and 2
[total dose/cycle = 1 mg]
Etoposide: I.V.: 100 mg/m^2/day days 1 and 2
[total dose/cycle = 200 mg/m^2]
Methotrexate: I.V.: 1 g/m^2 continuous infusion over 12 hours day 1
[total dose/cycle = 1 g/m^2]
Leucovorin: Oral, I.M.: 30 mg/m^2 every 12 hours for 6 doses (start 32 hours after start of methotrexate) days 2, 3, and 4
[total dose/cycle = 180 mg/m^2]
Vincristine: I.V.: 1 mg/m^2 day 8
[total dose/cycle = 1 mg/m^2]
Cyclophosphamide: I.V.: 600 mg/m^2 day 8
[total dose/cycle = 600 mg/m^2]
Repeat cycle every 2 weeks

Variation 7:
Dactinomycin: I.V.: 0.5 mg/day days 1 and 2
[total dose/cycle = 1 mg]
Etoposide: I.V.: 100 mg/m^2/day days 1 and 2
[total dose/cycle = 200 mg/m^2]
Methotrexate: I.V.: 1 g/m^2 continuous infusion over 24 hours day 1
[total dose/cycle = 1 g/m^2]

Leucovorin: Oral, I.M.: 15 mg every 8 hours for 9 doses (start 32 hours after start of methotrexate) days 2, 3, and 4
[total dose/cycle = 135 mg/m^2]
Vincristine: I.V.: 1 mg/m^2 day 8
[total dose/cycle = 1 mg/m^2]
Cyclophosphamide: I.V.: 600 mg/m^2 day 8
[total dose/cycle = 600 mg/m^2]
Repeat cycle every 2 weeks

Variation 8 (patients with lung metastases):
Dactinomycin: I.V.: 0.5 mg/day days 1 and 2
[total dose/cycle = 1 mg]
Etoposide: I.V.: 100 mg/m^2/day days 1 and 2
[total dose/cycle = 200 mg/m^2]
Methotrexate: I.V. bolus: 100 mg/m^2 then 200 mg/m^2 continuous infusion over 12 hours day 1
[total dose/cycle = 300 mg/m^2]
Leucovorin: Oral, I.M.: 15 mg every 12 hours for 4 doses (start 24 hours after start of methotrexate) days 2 and 3
[total dose/cycle = 60 mg]
Vincristine: I.V.: 1 mg/m^2 day 8
[total dose/cycle = 1 mg/m^2]
Cyclophosphamide: I.V.: 600 mg/m^2 day 8
[total dose/cycle = 600 mg/m^2]
Methotrexate: I.T.: 10 mg day 1 (every other cycle)
[total dose/cycle = 10 mg, every other cycle]
Repeat cycle every 2 weeks

Variation 9 (patients with lung metastases):
Dactinomycin: I.V.: 0.5 mg/day days 1 and 2
[total dose/cycle = 1 mg]
Etoposide: I.V.: 100 mg/m^2/day days 1 and 2
[total dose/cycle = 200 mg/m^2]
Methotrexate: I.V. bolus: 100 mg/m^2 then 200 mg/m^2 continuous infusion over 12 hours day 1
[total dose/cycle = 300 mg/m^2]
Leucovorin: Oral, I.M.: 15 mg every 12 hours for 4 doses (start 24 hours after start of methotrexate) days 2 and 3
[total dose/cycle = 60 mg]
Vincristine: I.V.: 1 mg/m^2 day 8
[total dose/cycle = 1 mg/m^2]
Cyclophosphamide: I.V.: 600 mg/m^2 day 8
[total dose/cycle = 600 mg/m^2]
Methotrexate: I.T.: 12.5 mg day 8
[total dose/cycle = 12.5 mg]
Repeat cycle every 2 weeks

References

Variation 1:

Bagshawe KD, "High-Risk Metastatic Trophoblastic Disease," *Obstet Gynecol Clin North Am*, 1988, 15(3):531-43.

Variation 2:

Newlands ES, Bagshawe KD, Begent RH, et al, "Developments in Chemotherapy for Medium- and High-Risk Patients With Gestational Trophoblastic Tumours (1979-1984)," *Br J Obstet Gynaecol*, 1986, 93(1):63-9.

Variation 3:
Newlands ES, Bagshawe KD, Begent RH, et al, "Results With the EMA/CO (Etoposide, Methotrexate, Actinomycin D, Cyclophosphamide, Vincristine) Regimen in High-Risk Gestational Trophoblastic Tumours, 1979 to 1989," *J Obstet Gynaecol*, 1991, 98(6):550-7.
Variation 4:
Soper JT, Evans AC, Clarke-Pearson DL, et al, "Alternating Weekly Chemotherapy With Etoposide-Methotrexate-Dactinomycin/Cyclophosphamide-Vincristine for High-Risk Gestational Trophoblastic Disease," *Obstet Gynecol*, 1994, 83(1):113-7.
Variation 5:
Bolis G, Bonazzi C, Landoni F, et al, "EMA/CO Regimen in High-Risk Gestational Trophoblastic Tumor (GTT)," *Gynecol Oncol*, 1988, 31(3):439-44.
Variation 6:
Schink JC, Singh Dk, Rademaker AW, et al, "Etoposide, Methotrexate, Actinomycin-D, Cyclophosphamide, and Vincristine for the Treatment of Metastatic, High-Risk Gestational Trophoblastic Disease," *Obstet Gynecol*, 1992, 80(5):817-20.
Variation 7:
Newlands ES, Bagshawe KD, Begent RH, et al, "Results With the EMA/CO (Etoposide, Methotrexate, Actinomycin D, Cyclophosphamide, Vincristine) Regimen in High-Risk Gestational Trophoblastic Tumours, 1979 to 1989," *Br J Obstet Gynaecol*, 1991, 98(6):550-7.
Variation 8:
Bolis G, Bonazzi C, Landoni F, et al, "EMA/CO Regimen in High-Risk Gestational Trophoblastic Tumor (GTT)," *Gynecol Oncol*, 1988, 31(3):439-44.
Variation 9:
Newlands ES, Bagshawe KD, Begent RH, et al, "Developments in Chemotherapy for Medium- and High-Risk Patients With Gestational Trophoblastic Tumours (1979-1984)," *Br J Obstet Gynaecol*, 1986, 93(1):63-9.

◆ **EMA/EP** *see* EP/EMA *on page 1625*

◆ **EMA-G (AML Induction)** *see* MEC-G (AML Induction) *on page 1707*

Enzalutamide (Prostate Regimen)

Use Prostate cancer

Regimen

Enzalutamide: Oral: 160 mg once daily
[total dose/cycle = 4480 mg]

Repeat cycle every 28 days until disease progression or unacceptable toxicity

References

Scher HI, Fizazi K, Saad F, et al, "Increased Survival With Enzalutamide in Prostate Cancer After Chemotherapy," *N Engl J Med*, 2012, 367(13):1187-97.

◆ **EOF (Esophageal Cancer)** *see* Epirubicin-Oxaliplatin-Fluorouracil (Esophageal Cancer) *on page 1627*

◆ **EOX** *see* Epirubicin-Oxaliplatin-Capecitabine *on page 1627*

EP/EMA

Index Terms EMA/EP

Use Gestational trophoblastic tumor

Regimen NOTE: Multiple variations are listed.

Variation 1:

Etoposide: I.V.: 150 mg/m^2 day 1
[total dose/cycle = 150 mg/m^2]

Cisplatin: I.V.: 25 mg/m^2 infused over 4 hours for 3 consecutive doses, day 1
[total dose/cycle = 75 mg/m^2]

Alternate weekly with:

Etoposide: I.V.: 100 mg/m^2 day 1
[total dose/cycle = 100 mg/m^2]

Methotrexate: I.V.: 300 mg/m^2 infused over 12 hours day 1
[total dose/cycle = 300 mg/m^2]

Dactinomycin: I.V. push: 0.5 mg day 1
[total dose/cycle = 0.5 mg]
Leucovorin: Oral, I.M.: 15 mg twice daily for 2 days (start 24 hours after the start of methotrexate) days 2 and 3
[total dose/cycle = 60 mg]
Variation 2:
Dactinomycin: I.V.: 0.5 mg/day days 1 and 2
[total dose/cycle = 1 mg]
Etoposide: I.V.: 100 mg/m^2/day days 1 and 2
[total dose/cycle = 200 mg/m^2]
Methotrexate: I.V.: 300 mg/m^2 continuous infusion over 12 hours day 1
[total dose/cycle = 300 mg/m^2]
Leucovorin: Oral, I.M.: 15 mg every 12 hours for 4 doses (start 24 hours after start of methotrexate) days 2 and 3
[total dose/cycle = 60 mg]
Etoposide: I.V.: 150 mg/m^2 day 8
[total dose/cycle = 150 mg/m^2]
Cisplatin: I.V.: 75 mg/m^2 day 8
[total dose/cycle = 75 mg/m^2]
Repeat cycle every 2 weeks

References

Variation 1:
Newlands ES, Bower M, Holden L, et al, "Management of Resistant Gestational Trophoblastic Tumors," *J Reprod Med*, 1998, 43(2):111-8.
Variation 2:
Newlands ES, Bagshawe KD, Begent RH, et al, "Results With the EMA/CO (Etoposide, Methotrexate, Actinomycin D, Cyclophosphamide, Vincristine) Regimen in High Risk Gestational Trophoblastic Tumours, 1979 to 1989," *J Obstet Gynaecol*, 1991, 98(6):550-7.

Epirubicin-Cisplatin-Capecitabine (Esophageal Cancer)

Index Terms ECX (Esophageal Cancer)
Use Esophageal cancer
Regimen
Epirubicin: I.V.: 50 mg/m^2 day 1
[total dose/cycle = 50 mg/m^2]
Cisplatin: I.V.: 60 mg/m^2 day 1
[total dose/cycle = 60 mg/m^2]
Capecitabine: Oral: 625 mg/m^2 twice daily days 1 to 21
[total dose/cycle = 26,250 mg/m^2]
Repeat cycle every 21 days for up to 8 cycles

References

Cunningham D, Starling N, Rao S, et al, "Capecitabine and Oxaliplatin for Advanced Esophagogastric Cancer," *N Engl J Med*, 2008, 358(1):36-46.

Epirubicin-Cisplatin-Fluorouracil (Gastric/Esophageal Cancer)

Index Terms ECF (Gastric/Esophageal Cancer)
Use Esophageal cancer; Gastric cancer
Regimen NOTE: Multiple variations are listed.
Variation 1:
Epirubicin: I.V.: 50 mg/m^2 day 1
[total dose/cycle = 50 mg/m^2]

Cisplatin: I.V.: 60 mg/m^2 day 1
[total dose/cycle = 60 mg/m^2]
Fluorouracil: I.V.: 200 mg/m^2/day continuous infusion days 1 to 21
[total dose/cycle = 4200 mg/m^2]
Repeat cycle every 3 weeks for up to a maximum of 8 cycles

Variation 2:
Epirubicin: I.V.: 50 mg/m^2 day 1
[total dose/cycle = 50 mg/m^2]
Cisplatin: I.V.: 60 mg/m^2 day 1
[total dose/cycle = 60 mg/m^2]
Fluorouracil: I.V.: 200 mg/m^2/day continuous infusion days 1 to 21
[total dose/cycle = 4200 mg/m^2]
Repeat cycle every 3 weeks for up to 6 cycles (3 cycles before surgery and 3 cycles postoperatively)

References

Variation 1:
Cunningham D, Starling N, Rao S, et al, "Capecitabine and Oxaliplatin for Advanced Esophagogastric Cancer," *N Engl J Med*, 2008, 358(1):36-46.
Ross P, Nicolson M, Cunningham D, et al, "Prospective Randomized Trial Comparing Mitomycin, Cisplatin, and Protracted Venous-Infusion Fluorouracil (PVI 5-FU) With Epirubicin, Cisplatin, and PVI 5-FU in Advanced Esophagogastric Cancer," *J Clin Oncol*, 2002, 20(8):1996-2004.
Roth AD, Fazio N, Stupp R, et al, "Docetaxel, Cisplatin, and Fluorouracil; Docetaxel and Cisplatin; and Epirubicin, Cisplatin, and Fluorouracil as Systemic Treatment for Advanced Gastric Carcinoma: A Randomized Phase II Trial of the Swiss Group for Clinical Cancer Research," *J Clin Oncol*, 2007, 25(22):3217-23.
Webb A, Cunningham D, Scarffe JH, et al, "Randomized Trial Comparing Epirubicin, Cisplatin, and Fluorouracil Versus Fluorouracil, Doxorubicin, and Methotrexate in Advanced Esophagogastric Cancer," *J Clin Oncol*, 1997, 15(1):261-7.
Variation 2:
Cunningham D, Allum WH, Stenning SP, et al, "Perioperative Chemotherapy Versus Surgery Alone for Resectable Gastroesophageal Cancer," *N Engl J Med*, 2006, 355(1):11-20.

Epirubicin-Oxaliplatin-Capecitabine

Index Terms Capecitabine-Oxaliplatin-Epirubicin; EOX; Oxaliplatin-Capecitabine-Epirubicin

Use Esophageal cancer; Gastric cancer

Regimen

Epirubicin: I.V.: 50 mg/m^2 day 1
[total dose/cycle = 50 mg/m^2]
Oxaliplatin: I.V.: 130 mg/m^2 day 1
[total dose/cycle = 130 mg/m^2]
Capecitabine: Oral: 625 mg/m^2 twice daily days 1 to 21
[total dose/cycle = 26,250 mg/m^2]
Repeat cycle every 21 days for up to 8 cycles

References

Cunningham D, Starling N, Rao S, et al, "Capecitabine and Oxaliplatin for Advanced Esophagogastric Cancer," *N Engl J Med*, 2008, 358(1):36-46.

Epirubicin-Oxaliplatin-Fluorouracil (Esophageal Cancer)

Index Terms EOF (Esophageal Cancer)

Use Esophageal cancer

Regimen

Epirubicin: I.V.: 50 mg/m^2 day 1
[total dose/cycle = 50 mg/m^2]

Oxaliplatin: I.V.: 130 mg/m^2 day 1
[total dose/cycle = 130 mg/m^2]
Fluorouracil: I.V.: 200 mg/m^2/day continuous infusion days 1 to 21
[total dose/cycle = 4200 mg/m^2]
Repeat cycle every 21 days for up to 8 cycles

References

Cunningham D, Starling N, Rao S, et al, "Capecitabine and Oxaliplatin for Advanced Esophagogastric Cancer," *N Engl J Med*, 2008, 358(1):36-46.

EP (NSCLC)

Use Lung cancer, nonsmall cell

Regimen

Etoposide: I.V.: 80-120 mg/m^2/day days 1, 2, and 3
[total dose/cycle = 240-360 mg/m^2]
Cisplatin: I.V.: 80-100 mg/m^2 day 1
[total dose/cycle = 80-100 mg/m^2]
Repeat cycle every 21-28 days

References

Goldhirsch A, Joss RA, Cavalli F, et al, "Cis-Dichlorodiammineplatinum (II) and VP 16-213 Combination Chemotherapy for Nonsmall-Cell Lung Cancer," *Med Pediatr Oncol*, 1981, 9 (3):205-8.

EPOCH Dose-Adjusted (AIDS-Related Lymphoma)

Index Terms Dose-Adjusted EPOCH (AIDS-Related Lymphoma)

Use Lymphoma, AIDS-related

Regimen

Etoposide: I.V.: 50 mg/m^2/day continuous infusion days 1 to 4
[total dose/cycle = 200 mg/m^2]
Vincristine: I.V.: 0.4 mg/m^2/day continuous infusion days 1 to 4
[total dose/cycle = 1.6 mg/m^2]
Doxorubicin: I.V.: 10 mg/m^2/day continuous infusion days 1 to 4
[total dose/cycle = 40 mg/m^2]
Cyclophosphamide: I.V.: 375 mg/m^2 day 5 for CD4+ cells ≥100/mm^3 **or** 187 mg/m^2 day 5 for CD4+ cells <100/mm^3
[total dose/cycle = 187-375 mg/m^2]
Prednisone: Oral: 60 mg/m^2/day days 1 to 5
[total dose/cycle = 300 mg/m^2]
Filgrastim: SubQ: 5 mcg/kg/day beginning day 6; continue until ANC >5000/mm^3 (past nadir)
Repeat cycle every 21 days for 6 cycles with cyclophosphamide dose adjusted based on previous cycle nadir according to the following schedule:
Nadir ANC >500/mm^3: Increase cyclophosphamide dose by 187 mg/m^2 above previous cycle dose (maximum dose: 750 mg/m^2)
Nadir ANC <500/mm^3 or platelet <25,000/mm^3: Decrease cyclophosphamide dose by 187 mg/m^2 below previous cycle dose

References

Little RF, Pittaluga S, Grant N, et al, "Highly Effective Treatment of Acquired Immunodeficiency Syndrome-Related Lymphoma With Dose-Adjusted EPOCH: Impact of Antiretroviral Therapy Suspension and Tumor Biology," *Blood*, 2003, 101(12):4653-9.

EPOCH Dose-Adjusted (NHL)

Index Terms Dose-Adjusted EPOCH (NHL); Dose-Adjusted Etoposide-Vincristine-Doxorubicin-Cyclophosphamide-Prednisone (NHL)

Use Lymphoma, non-Hodgkin's

Regimen

Etoposide: I.V.: 50 mg/m²/day continuous infusion days 1 to 4
[total dose/cycle = 200 mg/m²]

Vincristine: I.V.: 0.4 mg/m²/day continuous infusion days 1 to 4
[total dose/cycle = 1.6 mg/m²]

Doxorubicin: I.V.: 10 mg/m²/day continuous infusion days 1 to 4
[total dose/cycle = 40 mg/m²]

Cyclophosphamide: I.V.: 750 mg/m² day 5
[total dose/cycle = 750 mg/m²]

Prednisone: Oral: 60 mg/m²/day (given once daily or in 2 divided doses) days 1 to 5 or days 1 to 6
[total dose/cycle = 300-360 mg/m²]

Filgrastim: SubQ: 5 mcg/kg/day beginning day 6 or 8; continue until ANC recovery

Repeat cycle every 21 days with etoposide, doxorubicin, and cyclophosphamide dose adjustments (based on CBC 2 times/week) according to the following schedule:

Nadir ANC ≥500/mm³: 20% to 25% increase (above previous cycle) for etoposide, doxorubicin, and cyclophosphamide

Nadir ANC <500/mm³ (on 1 or 2 measurements): Same doses as previous cycle

Nadir ANC <500/mm³ (on ≥3 measurements) or nadir platelet <25,000/mm³ (on 1 measurement): 20% to 25% decrease below previous cycle for etoposide, doxorubicin, and cyclophosphamide (dosing adjustments below starting dose levels only apply to cyclophosphamide)

References

Gutierrez M, Chabner BA, Pearson D, et al, "Role of a Doxorubicin-Containing Regimen in Relapsed and Resistant Lymphomas: An 8-Year Follow-Up Study of EPOCH," *J Clin Oncol*, 2000, 18(21):3633-42.

Wilson WH, Bryant G, Bates S, et al, "EPOCH Chemotherapy: Toxicity and Efficacy in Relapsed and Refractory Non-Hodgkin's Lymphoma," *J Clin Oncol*, 1993, 11(8):1573-82.

Wilson WH, Grossbard ML, Pittaluga S, et al, "Dose-Adjusted EPOCH Chemotherapy for Untreated Large B-Cell Lymphomas: A Pharmacodynamic Approach With High Efficacy," *Blood*, 2002, 99(8):2685-93.

EPOCH (Dose-Adjusted)-Rituximab (NHL)

Index Terms EPOCH (Dose-Adjusted)-R (NHL); R-EPOCH Dose Adjusted (NHL); Rituxan-Etoposide-Prednisone-Vincristine-Cyclophosphamide-Doxorubicin (Dose-Adjusted) (NHL); Rituximab-EPOCH Dose Adjusted (NHL)

Use Lymphoma, non-Hodgkin's

Regimen

Rituximab: I.V.: 375 mg/m² day 1
[total dose/cycle = 375 mg/m²]

Etoposide: I.V.: 50 mg/m²/day continuous infusion days 1 to 4
[total dose/cycle = 200 mg/m²]

Vincristine: I.V.: 0.4 mg/m²/day continuous infusion days 1 to 4
[total dose/cycle = 1.6 mg/m²]

Doxorubicin: I.V.: 10 mg/m²/day continuous infusion days 1 to 4
[total dose/cycle = 40 mg/m²]

Cyclophosphamide: I.V.: 750 mg/m² day 5
[total dose/cycle = 750 mg/m²]

Prednisone: Oral: 60 mg/m²/day (given once daily or in 2 divided doses) days 1 to 5
[total dose/cycle = 300 mg/m²]

Filgrastim: SubQ: 5 mcg/kg/day beginning day 6; continue until ANC recovery

Repeat cycle every 21 days (for at least 2 cycles beyond best response; minimum of 6 cycles and maximum of 8 cycles) with etoposide, doxorubicin, and cyclophosphamide dose adjustments (based on CBC 2 times/week) according to the following schedule:

Nadir ANC ≥500/mm^3: 20% increase (above previous cycle) for etoposide, doxorubicin, and cyclophosphamide

Nadir ANC <500/mm^3 (on 1 or 2 measurements): Same doses as previous cycle

Nadir ANC <500/mm^3 (on ≥3 measurements): 20% decrease below previous cycle for etoposide, doxorubicin, and cyclophosphamide (dosing adjustments below starting dose levels only apply to cyclophosphamide)

References

García-Suárez J, Bañas H, Arribas I, et al, "Dose-Adjusted EPOCH Plus Rituximab Is an Effective Regimen in Patients With Poor-Prognostic Untreated Diffuse Large B-Cell Lymphoma: Results From a Prospective Observational Study," *Br J Haematol*, 2007, 136(2):276-85.

Wilson WH, Gutierrez M, O'Connor P, et al, "The Role of Rituximab and Chemotherapy in Aggressive B-Cell Lymphoma: A Preliminary Report of Dose-Adjusted EPOCH-R," *Semin Oncol*, 2002, 29(1 Suppl 2):41-7.

◆ **EPOCH (Dose-Adjusted)-R (NHL)** *see* EPOCH (Dose-Adjusted)-Rituximab (NHL) *on page 1629*

EPOCH (NHL)

Use Lymphoma, non-Hodgkin's

Regimen NOTE: Multiple variations are listed.

Variation 1:

Etoposide: I.V.: 50 mg/m^2/day continuous infusion days 1 to 4 [total dose/cycle = 200 mg/m^2]

Vincristine: I.V.: 0.4 mg/m^2/day continuous infusion days 1 to 4 [total dose/cycle = 1.6 mg/m^2]

Doxorubicin: I.V.: 10 mg/m^2/day continuous infusion days 1 to 4 [total dose/cycle = 40 mg/m^2]

Cyclophosphamide: I.V.: 750 mg/m^2 day 5 [total dose/cycle = 750 mg/m^2]

Prednisone: Oral: 60 mg/m^2/day days 1 to 5 [total dose/cycle = 300 mg/m^2]

Repeat cycle (with cyclophosphamide dose adjustments if needed based on ANC) every 21 days (best response seen in a median of 4 cycles)

Variation 2:

Etoposide: I.V.: 50 mg/m^2/day continuous infusion days 1 to 4 [total dose/cycle = 200 mg/m^2]

Vincristine: I.V.: 0.4 mg/m^2/day continuous infusion days 1 to 4 [total dose/cycle = 1.6 mg/m^2]

Doxorubicin: I.V.: 10 mg/m^2/day continuous infusion days 1 to 4 [total dose/cycle = 40 mg/m^2]

Cyclophosphamide: I.V.: 750 mg/m^2 day 6 [total dose/cycle = 750 mg/m^2]

Prednisone: Oral: 60 mg/m^2/day days 1 to 6 [total dose/cycle = 360 mg/m^2]

Repeat cycle (with cyclophosphamide dose adjustments if needed based on ANC) every 21 days (best response seen in a median of 4 cycles)

References

Variation 1:

Gutierrez M, Chabner BA, Pearson D, et al, "Role of a Doxorubicin-Containing Regimen in Relapsed and Resistant Lymphomas: An 8-Year Follow-Up Study of EPOCH," *J Clin Oncol*, 2000, 18(21):3633-42.

Variation 2:

Wilson WH, Bryant G, Bates S, et al, "EPOCH Chemotherapy: Toxicity and Efficacy in Relapsed and Refractory Non-Hodgkin's Lymphoma," *J Clin Oncol*, 1993, 11(8):1573-82.

EPOCH-Rituximab (NHL)

Index Terms EPOCH-R (NHL); R-EPOCH (NHL); Rituximab-EPOCH (NHL)

Use Lymphoma, non-Hodgkin's

Regimen

Rituximab: I.V.: 375 mg/m^2 day 1
[total dose/cycle = 375 mg/m^2]

Etoposide: I.V.: 65 mg/m^2/day continuous infusion days 2, 3, and 4
[total dose/cycle = 195 mg/m^2]

Vincristine: I.V.: 0.5 mg/m^2/day continuous infusion days 2, 3, and 4
[total dose/cycle = 1.5 mg/m^2]

Doxorubicin: I.V.: 15 mg/m^2/day continuous infusion days 2, 3, and 4
[total dose/cycle = 45 mg/m^2]

Cyclophosphamide: I.V.: 750 mg/m^2 day 5
[total dose/cycle = 750 mg/m^2]

Prednisone: Oral: 60 mg/m^2/day days 1 to 14
[total dose/cycle = 840 mg/m^2]

Repeat cycle every 21 days for 4-6 cycles

References

Jermann M, Jost LM, Taverna Ch, et al, "Rituximab-EPOCH, An Effective Salvage Therapy for Relapsed, Refractory or Transformed B-Cell Lymphomas: Results of a Phase II Study," *Ann Oncol*, 2004, 15(3):511-6.

◆ **EPOCH-R (NHL)** *see* EPOCH-Rituximab (NHL) *on page* 1631

EP/PE

Use Lung cancer, nonsmall cell

Regimen

Etoposide: I.V.: 120 mg/m^2/day days 1, 2, and 3
[total dose/cycle = 360 mg/m^2]

Cisplatin: I.V.: 60-120 mg/m^2 day 1
[total dose/cycle = 60-120 mg/m^2]

Repeat cycle every 21-28 days

References

Weick JK, Crowley J, Natale RB, et al, "A Randomized Trial of Five Cisplatin-Containing Treatments in Patients With Metastatic Nonsmall-Cell Lung Cancer: A Southwest Oncology Group Study," *J Clin Oncol*, 1991, 9(7):1157-62.

◆ **EP (Small Cell Lung Cancer)** *see* Cisplatin–Etoposide (Small Cell Lung Cancer) *on page* 1569

EP (Testicular Cancer)

Use Testicular cancer

Regimen NOTE: Multiple variations are listed.

Variation 1:

Etoposide: I.V.: 100 mg/m^2/day days 1 to 5
[total dose/cycle = 500 mg/m^2]

Cisplatin: I.V.: 20 mg/m^2/day days 1 to 5
[total dose/cycle = 100 mg/m^2]
Repeat cycle every 21 days
Variation 2:
Etoposide: I.V.: 120 mg/m^2/day days 1, 2, and 3
[total dose/cycle = 360 mg/m^2]
Cisplatin: I.V.: 20 mg/m^2/day days 1 to 5
[total dose/cycle = 100 mg/m^2]
Repeat cycle every 3 or 4 weeks
Variation 3:
Etoposide: I.V.: 120 mg/m^2/day days 1, 3, and 5
[total dose/cycle = 360 mg/m^2]
Cisplatin: I.V.: 20 mg/m^2/day days 1 to 5
[total dose/cycle = 100 mg/m^2]
Repeat cycle every 3 weeks

References

Variation 1:
Hainsworth JD, Williams SD, Einhorn LH, et al, "Successful Treatment of Resistant Germinal Neoplasms With VP-16 and Cisplatin: Results of a Southeastern Cancer Study Group Trial," *J Clin Oncol*, 1985, 3(5):666-71.
Variation 2:
Peckham MJ, Horwich A, Blackmore C, et al, "Etoposide and Cisplatin With or Without Bleomycin as First-Line Chemotherapy for Patients With Small-Volume Metastases of Testicular Non-seminoma," *Cancer Treat Rep*, 1985, 69(5):483-8.
Variation 3:
de Wit R, Stoter G, Kaye SB, et al, "Importance of Bleomycin in Combination Chemotherapy for Good-Prognosis Testicular Nonseminoma: A Randomized Study of the European Organization for Research and Treatment of Cancer Genitourinary Tract Cancer Cooperative Group," *J Clin Oncol*, 1997, 15(5):1837-43.

Erlotinib-Gemcitabine (Pancreatic)

Index Terms Gemcitabine-Erlotinib (Pancreatic)
Use Pancreatic cancer
Regimen
Cycle 1:
Gemcitabine: I.V.: 1000 mg/m^2/day over 30 minutes days 1, 8, 15, 22, 29, 36, and 43 (cycle 1 only)
[total dose/cycle 1 = 7000 mg/m^2]
Erlotinib: Oral: 100 mg once daily days 1 to 56
[total dose/cycle 1 = 5600 mg]
Treatment cycle is 56 days
Subsequent cycles:
Gemcitabine: I.V.: 1000 mg/m^2/day over 30 minutes days 1, 8, and 15
[total dose/cycle = 3000 mg/m^2]
Erlotinib: Oral: 100 mg once daily days 1 to 28
[total dose/cycle = 2800 mg]
Repeat cycle every 28 days

References

Moore MJ, Goldstein D, Hamm J, et al, "Erlotinib Plus Gemcitabine Compared With Gemcitabine Alone in Patients With Advanced Pancreatic Cancer: A Phase III Trial of the National Cancer Institute of Canada Clinical Trials Group," *J Clin Oncol*, 2007, 25(15):1960-6.

Erlotinib (NSCLC Regimen)

Use Lung cancer, nonsmall cell
Regimen NOTE: Multiple variations are listed.

Variation 1 (refractory):
Erlotinib: Oral: 150 mg once daily days 1 to 28
[total dose/cycle = 4200 mg]
Repeat cycle every 28 days
Variation 2 (maintenance):
Erlotinib: Oral: 150 mg once daily days 1 to 28
[total dose/cycle = 4200 mg]
Repeat cycle every 28 days until disease progression or unacceptable toxicity
Variation 3 (first-line):
Erlotinib: Oral: 150 mg once daily days 1 to 28
[total dose/cycle = 4200 mg]
Repeat cycle every 28 days until disease progression or unacceptable toxicity

References

Variation 1:

Ciuleanu T, Stelmakh L, Cicenas S, et al, "Efficacy and Safety of Erlotinib Versus Chemotherapy in Second-Line Treatment of Patients With Advanced, Non-Small-Cell Lung Cancer With Poor Prognosis (TITAN): A Randomised Multicentre, Open-Label, Phase 3 Study," *Lancet Oncol*, 2012, 13(3):300-8.

Sheppherd FA, Pereira JR, Ciuleanu T, et al, "Erlotinib in Previously Treated Non-Small-Cell Lung Cancer," *N Engl J Med*, 2005, 353(2):123-32.

Variation 2:

Cappuzzo F, Ciuleanu T, Stelmakh L, et al, "Erlotinib as Maintenance Treatment in Advanced Non-Small-Cell Lung Cancer: A Multicentre, Randomised, Placebo-Controlled Phase 3 Study," *Lancet Oncol*, 2010, 11(6):521-9.

Variation 3:

Rosell R, Carcereny E, Gervais R, et al, "Erlotinib Versus Standard Chemotherapy as First-Line Treatment for European Patients With Advanced EGFR Mutation-Positive Non-Small-Cell Lung Cancer (EURTAC): A Multicentre, Open-Label, Randomised, Phase 3 Trial," *Lancet Oncol*, 2012, 13(3):239-46.

Zhou C, Wu YL, Chen G, et al, "Erlotinib Versus Chemotherapy as First-Line Treatment for Patients With Advanced EGFR Mutation-Positive Non-Small-Cell Lung Cancer (OPTIMAL, CTONG-0802): A Multicentre, Open-Label, Randomised, Phase 3 Study," *Lancet Oncol*, 2011, 12 (8):735-42.

ESHAP

Use Lymphoma, non-Hodgkin's

Regimen NOTE: Multiple variations are listed.

Variation 1:
Etoposide: I.V.: 40 mg/m^2/day days 1 to 4
[total dose/cycle = 160 mg/m^2]
Methylprednisolone: I.V.: 250-500 mg/day days 1 to 5
[total dose/cycle = 1250-2500 mg]
Cytarabine: I.V.: 2000 mg/m^2 day 5
[total dose/cycle = 2000 mg/m^2]
Cisplatin: I.V.: 25 mg/m^2/day continuous infusion days 1 to 4
[total dose/cycle = 100 mg/m^2]
Repeat cycle every 21-28 days
Variation 2:
Etoposide: I.V.: 40 mg/m^2/day days 1 to 4
[total dose/cycle = 160 mg/m^2]
Methylprednisolone: I.V.: 500 mg/day days 1 to 5
[total dose/cycle = 2500 mg]
Cytarabine: I.V.: 2000 mg/m^2 day 5
[total dose/cycle = 2000 mg/m^2]

Cisplatin: I.V.: 25 mg/m^2/day continuous infusion days 1 to 4
[total dose/cycle = 100 mg/m^2]
Repeat cycle every 21-28 days

Variation 3:

Etoposide: I.V.: 60 mg/m^2/day days 1 to 4
[total dose/cycle = 240 mg/m^2]
Methylprednisolone: I.V.: 500 mg/day days 1 to 4
[total dose/cycle = 2000 mg]
Cytarabine: I.V.: 2000 mg/m^2 day 5
[total dose/cycle = 2000 mg/m^2]
Cisplatin: I.V.: 25 mg/m^2/day continuous infusion days 1 to 4
[total dose/cycle = 100 mg/m^2]
Repeat cycle every 21 days

References

Variation 1:
Velasquez WF, McLaughlin P, Tucker S, et al, "ESHAP - An Effective Chemotherapy Regimen in Refractory and Relapsing Lymphoma: A 4-Year Follow-up Study," *J Clin Oncol*, 1994, 12 (6):1169-76.
Variation 2:
Wang WS, Chiou TJ, Liu JH, et al, "ESHAP as Salvage Therapy for Refractory Non-Hodgkin's Lymphoma: Taiwan Experience," *Jpn J Clin Oncol*, 1999, 29(1):33-7.
Variation 3:
Rodriguez MA, Cabanillas FC, Velasquez W, et al, "Results of a Salvage Treatment Program for Relapsing Lymphoma: MINE Consolidated With ESHAP," *J Clin Oncol*, 1995, 13(7):1734-41.

ESHAP (Hodgkin)

Index Terms Etoposide-Methylprednisolone-Cytarabine-Cisplatin (Hodgkin)

Use Lymphoma, Hodgkin

Regimen

Etoposide: I.V.: 40 mg/m^2 /day days 1 to 4
[total dose/cycle = 160 mg/m^2]
Methylprednisolone: I.V.: 500 mg/day days 1 to 4
[total dose/cycle = 2000 mg]
Cisplatin: I.V.: 25 mg/m^2/day days 1 to 4
[total dose/cycle = 100 mg/m^2]
Cytarabine: I.V.: 2000 mg/m^2 day 5
[total dose/cycle = 2000 mg/m^2]
Filgrastim: SubQ: 5 mcg/kg/day days 6 to 18
Repeat cycle every 21 to 28 days for 3 cycles (if transplant candidate) or 6 cycles (nontransplant candidate)

References

Aparicio J, Segura A, Garcerá S, et al, "ESHAP is an Active Regimen for Relapsing Hodgkin's Disease," *Ann Oncol*, 1999, 10(5):593-5.

Estramustine + Docetaxel

Use Prostate cancer

Regimen NOTE: Multiple variations are listed.

Variation 1:

Docetaxel: I.V.: 20-80 mg/m^2 day 2
[total dose/cycle = 20-80 mg/m^2]
Estramustine: Oral: 280 mg 3 times/day days 1 to 5
[total dose/cycle = 4200 mg]
Repeat cycle every 21 days

Variation 2:
Docetaxel: I.V.: 20-80 mg/m^2 day 2
[total dose/cycle = 20-80 mg/m^2]
Estramustine: Oral: 14 mg/kg/day days 1 to 21
[total dose/cycle = 294 mg/kg]
Repeat cycle every 21 days
Variation 3:
Docetaxel: I.V.: 35 mg/m^2/day days 2 and 9
[total dose/cycle = 70 mg/m^2]
Estramustine: Oral: 420 mg 3 times/day for 4 doses, then 280 mg 3 times/day for 5 doses days 1, 2, 3, 8, 9, and 10
[total dose/cycle = 6160 mg]
Repeat cycle every 21 days
Variation 4:
Docetaxel: I.V.: 60 mg/m^2 day 2 cycle 1
[total dose/cycle = 60 mg/m^2]
followed by I.V.: 60-70 mg/m^2 day 2 (subsequent cycles)
[total dose/cycle = 60-70 mg/m^2]
Estramustine: Oral: 280 mg 3 times/day days 1 to 5
[total dose/cycle = 4200 mg]
Repeat cycle every 21 days for up to 12 cycles

References

Variation 1:
Petrylak DP, Macarthur RB, O'Connor J, et al, "Phase I Trial of Docetaxel With Estramustine in Androgen-Independent Prostate Cancer," *J Clin Oncol*, 1999, 17(3):958-67.
Variation 2:
Kreis W, Budman DR, Fetten J, et al, "Phase I Trial of The Combination of Daily Estramustine Phosphate and Intermittent Docetaxel in Patients With Metastatic Hormone Refractory Prostate Carcinoma," *Ann Oncol*, 1999, 10(1):33-8.
Variation 3:
Sitka Copur M, Ledakis P, Lynch J, et al, "Weekly Docetaxel and Estramustine in Patients With Hormone-Refractory Prostate Cancer," *Semin Oncol*, 2001, 28(4 Suppl 15):16-21.
Variation 4:
Petrylak DP, Tangen CM, Hussain MH, et al, "Docetaxel and Estramustine Compared With Mitoxantrone and Prednisone for Advanced Refractory Prostate Cancer," *N Engl J Med*, 2004, 351(15):1513-20.

Estramustine + Docetaxel + Calcitriol

Use Prostate cancer

Regimen

Cycle 1:
Calcitriol: Oral: 60 mcg (in divided doses) day 1
[total dose/cycle = 60 mcg]
Estramustine: Oral: 280 mg 3 times/day days 1 to 5
[total dose/cycle = 4200 mg]
Docetaxel: I.V.: 60 mg/m^2 day 2
[total dose/cycle = 60 mg/m^2]
Treatment cycle is 21 days
Subsequent cycles:
Calcitriol: Oral: 60 mcg (in divided doses) day 1
[total dose/cycle = 60 mcg]
Estramustine: Oral: 280 mg 3 times/day days 1 to 5
[total dose/cycle = 4200 mg]
Docetaxel: I.V.: 70 mg/m^2 day 2
[total dose/cycle = 70 mg/m^2]
Repeat cycle every 21 days for up to 12 cycles

References

Tiffany NM, Ryan CW, Garzotto M, et al, "High Dose Pulse Calcitriol, Docetaxel and Estramustine for Androgen Independent Prostate Cancer: A Phase I/II Study," *J Urol*, 2005, 174(3):888-92.

Estramustine + Docetaxel + Carboplatin

Use Prostate cancer

Regimen

Docetaxel: I.V.: 70 mg/m^2 day 2
[total dose/cycle = 70 mg/m^2]
Estramustine: Oral: 280 mg 3 times/day days 1 to 5
[total dose/cycle = 4200 mg]
Carboplatin: I.V.: Target AUC 5 day 2
[total dose/cycle = AUC = 5]
Repeat cycle every 3 weeks

References

Oh WK, Halabi S, Kelly WK, et al, "A Phase II Study of Estramustine, Docetaxel, and Carboplatin (EDC) with G-CSF Support in Men With Hormone Refractory Prostate Cancer: CALGB 99813," *Proc Am Soc Clin Oncol*, 2002, 21:195a.

Oh WK, Halabi S, Kelly WK, et al, "A Phase II Study of Estramustine, Docetaxel, and Carboplatin With Granulocyte-Colony-Stimulating Factor Support in Patients With Hormone-Refractory Prostate Carcinoma: Cancer and Leukemia Group B 99813," *Cancer*, 2003, 98(12):2592-8.

Estramustine + Docetaxel + Hydrocortisone

Use Prostate cancer

Regimen

Docetaxel: I.V.: 70 mg/m^2 day 2
[total dose/cycle = 70 mg/m^2]
Estramustine: Oral: 10 mg/kg/day days 1 to 5
[total dose/cycle = 50 mg/kg]
Hydrocortisone: Oral: 40 mg daily
[total dose/cycle = 840 mg]
Repeat cycle every 3 weeks

References

Savarese DM, Halabi S, Hars V, et al, "Phase II Study of Docetaxel, Estramustine, and Low-Dose Hydrocortisone in Men With Hormone-Refractory Prostate Cancer: A Final Report of CALGB 9780. Cancer and Leukemia Group B," *J Clin Oncol*, 2001, 19(9):2509-16.

Estramustine + Docetaxel + Prednisone

Use Prostate cancer

Regimen

Estramustine: Oral: 280 mg 3 times/day days 1 to 5 and days 7 to 11
[total dose/cycle = 8400 mg]
Docetaxel: I.V.: 70 mg/m^2 day 2
[total dose/cycle = 70 mg/m^2]
Prednisone: Oral: 10 mg daily
[total dose/cycle = 210 mg]
Repeat cycle every 21 days for up to 6 cycles

References

Boehmer A, Anastasiadis AG, Feyerabend S, et al, "Docetaxel, Estramustine and Prednisone for Hormone-Refractory Prostate Cancer: A Single-Center Experience," *Anticancer Res*, 2005, 25 (6C):4481-6.

Estramustine + Etoposide

Use Prostate cancer

Regimen NOTE: Multiple variations are listed.

Variation 1:
Estramustine: Oral: 15 mg/kg/day days 1 to 21
[total dose/cycle = 315 mg/kg]
Etoposide: Oral: 50 mg/m^2/day days 1 to 21
[total dose/cycle = 1050 mg/m^2]
Repeat cycle every 4 weeks
Variation 2:
Estramustine: Oral: 10 mg/kg/day days 1 to 21
[total dose/cycle = 210 mg/kg]
Etoposide: Oral: 50 mg/m^2/day days 1 to 21
[total dose/cycle = 1050 mg/m^2]
Repeat cycle every 4 weeks
Variation 3:
Estramustine: Oral: 140 mg 3 times/day days 1 to 21
[total dose/cycle = 8820 mg]
Etoposide: Oral: 50 mg/m^2/day days 1 to 21
[total dose/cycle = 1050 mg/m^2]
Repeat cycle every 4 weeks

References

Variation 1:
Pienta KJ, Redman B, Hussain M, et al, "Phase II Evaluation of Oral Estramustine and Oral Etoposide in Hormone-Refractory Adenocarcinoma of the Prostate," *J Clin Oncol*, 1994, 12 (10).2005-12.
Variation 2:
Pienta KJ, Redman BG, Bandekar R, et al, "A Phase II Trial of Oral Estramustine and Oral Etoposide in Hormone Refractory Prostate Cancer," *Urology*, 1997, 50(3):401-6; discussion 406-7.
Variation 3.
Dimopoulos MA, Panopoulos C, Bamia C, et al, "Oral Estramustine and Oral Etoposide for Hormone-Refractory Prostate Cancer," *Urology*, 1997, 50(5):754-8.

Estramustine-Paclitaxel

Index Terms Paclitaxel-Estramustine; PE (Prostate Cancer)
Use Prostate cancer
Regimen NOTE: Multiple variations are listed.
Variation 1:
Paclitaxel: I.V.: 30-35 mg/m^2/day continuous infusion (given in 2-3 divided doses daily) either days 1 to 4 or days 2 to 5
[total dose/cycle = 120-140 mg/m^2]
Estramustine: Oral: 600 mg/m^2/day days 1 to 21
[total dose/cycle = 12,600 mg/m^2]
Repeat cycle every 21 days
Variation 2:
Paclitaxel: I.V. 60-107 mg/m^2 infused over 3 hours weekly for 6 weeks
[total dose/cycle = 360-642 mg/m^2]
Estramustine: Oral: 280 mg twice daily 3 days/week for 6 weeks
[total dose/cycle = 3360 mg]
Repeat cycle every 8 weeks
Variation 3:
Paclitaxel: I.V. 150 mg/m^2/day days 2, 9, and 16
[total dose/cycle = 450 mg/m^2]
Estramustine: Oral: 280 mg 3 times/day days 1, 2, 3, 8, 9, 10, 15, 16, and 17
[total dose/week = 7560 mg/m^2]
Repeat cycle every 4 weeks

Variation 4:
Paclitaxel: I.V.: 100 mg/m^2/day days 2, 9, and 16
[total dose/cycle = 300 mg/m^2]
Estramustine: Oral: 280 mg 3 times/day days 1, 2, 3, 8, 9, 10, 15, 16, and 17
[total dose/cycle = 7560 mg]
Repeat cycle every 4 weeks

References

Variation 1:
Hudes GR, Nathan FE, Khater C, et al, "Paclitaxel Plus Estramustine in Metastatic Hormone-Refractory Prostate Cancer," *Semin Oncol*, 1995, 22(5 Suppl 12):41-5.
Hudes GR, Nathan F, Khater C, et al, "Phase II Trial of 96-Hour Paclitaxel Plus Oral Estramustine Phosphate in Metastatic Hormone-Refractory Prostate Cancer," *J Clin Oncol*, 1997, 15 (9):3156-63.
Variation 2:
Haas N, Roth B, Garay C, et al, "Phase I Trial of Weekly Paclitaxel Plus Oral Estramustine Phosphate in Patients With Hormone-Refractory Prostate Cancer," *Urology*, 2001, 58(1):59-64
Variation 3:
Vaishampayan U, Fontana J, Du W, et al, "An Active Regimen of Weekly Paclitaxel and Estramustine in Metastatic Androgen-Independent Prostate Cancer," *Urology*, 2002, 60 (6):1050-4.
Variation 4:
Berry W, Gregurich M, Dakhil S, et al, "Phase II Randomized Trial of Weekly Paclitaxel With or Without Estramustine Phosphate in Patients With Symptomatic, Hormone-Refractory Metastatic Carcinoma of the Prostate." *Proc Am Soc Clin Oncol*, 2001, 20:175a.

Estramustine-Vinblastine

Index Terms EV

Use Prostate cancer

Regimen NOTE: Multiple variations are listed.

Variation 1:
Estramustine: Oral: 10 mg/kg/day days 1 to 42
[total dose/cycle = 420 mg/kg]
Vinblastine: I.V.: 4 mg/m^2/day days 1, 8, 15, 22, 29, and 36
[total dose/cycle = 24 mg/m^2]
Repeat cycle every 8 weeks

Variation 2:
Estramustine: Oral: 600 mg/m^2/day days 1 to 42
[total dose/cycle = 25,200 mg/m^2]
Vinblastine: I.V.: 4 mg/m^2/day days 1, 8, 15, 22, 29, and 36
[total dose/cycle = 24 mg/m^2]
Repeat cycle every 8 weeks

References

Variation 1:
Seidman AD, Scher HI, Petrylak D, et al, "Estramustine and Vinblastine: Use of Prostate Specific Antigen as a Clinical Trial Endpoint for Hormone Refractory Prostatic Cancer," *J Urol*, 1992, 147 (3 Pt 2):931-4.
Variation 2:
Hudes GR, Greenberg R, Krigel RL, et al, "Phase II Study of Estramustine and Vinblastine, Two Microtubule Inhibitors, in Hormone-Refractory Prostate Cancer," *J Clin Oncol*, 1992, 10 (11):1754-61.

Estramustine + Vinorelbine

Use Prostate cancer

Regimen NOTE: Multiple variations are listed.

Variation 1:
Estramustine: Oral: 140 mg 3 times/day days 1 to 14
[total dose/cycle = 5880 mg]

Vinorelbine: I.V.: 25 mg/m²/day days 1 and 8
[total dose/cycle = 50 mg/m²]
Repeat cycle every 21 days
Variation 2:
Estramustine: Oral: 280 mg 3 times/day days 1, 2, and 3
[total dose/cycle = 2520 mg/m²]
Vinorelbine: I.V.: 15 or 20 mg/m² day 2
[total dose/cycle = 15 or 20 mg/m²]
Repeat cycle weekly for 8 weeks, then every other week

References

Variation 1:
Smith MR, Kaufman D, Oh W, et al, "Vinorelbine and Estramustine in Androgen-Independent Metastatic Prostate Cancer: A Phase II Study," *Cancer*, 2000, 89(8):1824-8.
Variation 2:
Sweeney CJ, Monaco FJ, Jung SH, et al, "A Phase II Hoosier Oncology Group Study of Vinorelbine and Estramustine Phosphate in Hormone-Refractory Prostate Cancer," *Ann Oncol*, 2002, 13(3):435-40.

Etoposide (Ovarian Regimen)

Use Ovarian cancer

Regimen NOTE: Multiple variations are listed.
Variaition 1: (no prior radiation therapy)
Etoposide: Oral: 50 mg/m²/day days 1 to 21
[total dose/cycle = 1050 mg/m²]
Repeat cycle every 28 days
Variation 2: (prior radiation therapy)
Etoposide: Oral: 30 mg/m²/day days 1 to 21
[total dose/cycle = 630 mg/m²]
Repeat cycle every 28 days

References

Variations 1 and 2:
Rose PG, Blessing JA, Mayer AR, et al, "Prolonged Oral Etoposide as Second-Line Therapy for Platinum-Resistant and Platinum-Sensitive Ovarian Carcinoma: A Gynecologic Oncology Group Study," *J Clin Oncol*, 1998, 16(2):405-10.

Etoposide-Carboplatin (Ovarian Cancer)

Index Terms Carboplatin–Etoposide (Ovarian Cancer)

Use Ovarian cancer

Regimen
Etoposide: I.V.: 120 mg/m²/day days 1, 2, and 3
[total dose/cycle = 360 mg/m²]
Carboplatin: I.V.: 400 mg/m² day 1
[total dose/cycle = 400 mg/m²]
Repeat cycle every 28 days for a total of 3 cycles

References

Williams SD, Kauderer J, Burnett AF, et al, "Adjuvant Therapy of Completely Resected Dysgerminoma With Carboplatin and Etoposide: A Trial of the Gynecologic Oncology Group," *Gynecol Oncol*, 2004, 95(3):496-9.

◆ **Etoposide-Carboplatin (Retinoblastoma)** *see* Carboplatin-Etoposide (Retinoblastoma) *on page* 1545

◆ **Etoposide-Carboplatin (Small Cell Lung Cancer)** *see* Carboplatin-Etoposide (Small Cell Lung Cancer) *on page* 1546

◆ **Etoposide-Carboplatin-Vincristine (Retinoblastoma)** *see* Carboplatin-Etoposide-Vincristine (Retinoblastoma) *on page* 1546

◆ **Etoposide-Cisplatin** *see* Cisplatin-Etoposide (NSCLC) *on page 1568*

◆ **Etoposide-Cisplatin (Small Cell Lung Cancer)** *see* Cisplatin–Etoposide (Small Cell Lung Cancer) *on page 1569*

◆ **Etoposide-Ifosfamide-Mitoxantrone-Dexamethasone (Hodgkin)** *see* VIM-D (Hodgkin) *on page 1770*

◆ **Etoposide-Methylprednisolone-Cytarabine-Cisplatin (Hodgkin)** *see* ESHAP (Hodgkin) *on page 1634*

Etoposide Oral (Small Cell Lung Cancer Regimen)

Use Lung cancer, small cell

Regimen

Etoposide: Oral: 50 mg/m^2/day in the morning for 21 days
[total oral dose/cycle = 1050 mg/m^2]

Repeat cycle every 21 days

References

Einhorn LH, Pennington K, and McClean J, "Phase II Trial of Daily Oral VP-16 in Refractory Small Cell Lung Cancer: A Hoosier Oncology Group Study," *Semin Oncol*, 1990, 17(1 Suppl 2):32-5.

Johnson DH, Greco FA, Strupp J, et al, "Prolonged Administration of Oral Etoposide in Patients With Relapsed or Refractory Small-Cell Lung Cancer: A Phase II Trial," *J Clin Oncol*, 1990, 8 (10):1613-7.

◆ **EV** *see* Estramustine-Vinblastine *on page 1638*

Everolimus-Exemestane (Breast)

Index Terms Exemestane-Everolimus (Breast)

Use Breast cancer

Regimen

Everolimus: Oral: 10 mg once daily

Exemestane: Oral: 25 mg once daily

Continue until disease progression or unacceptable toxicity

References

Baselga J, Campone M, Piccart M, et al, "Everolimus in Postmenopausal Hormone-Receptor-Positive Advanced Breast Cancer," *N Engl J Med*, 2012, 366(6):520-9.

Everolimus (RCC Regimen)

Use Renal cell cancer

Regimen

Everolimus: Oral: 10 mg once daily
[total dose/cycle = 280 mg]

Repeat cycle every 28 days until disease progression or unacceptable toxicity

References

Motzer RJ, Escudier B, Oudard S, et al, "Efficacy of Everolimus in Advanced Renal Cell Carcinoma: A Double-Blind, Randomised, Placebo-Controlled Phase III Trial," *Lancet*, 2008, 372(9637):449-56.

Motzer RJ, Escudier B, Oudard S, et al, "Phase 3 Trial of Everolimus for Metastatic Renal Cell Carcinoma: Final Results and Analysis of Prognostic Factors," *Cancer*, 2010, 116(18):4256-65.

◆ **Every 2 Weeks Cetuximab (Colorectal Regimen)** *see* Cetuximab Biweekly (Colorectal Regimen) *on page 1556*

◆ **Exemestane-Everolimus (Breast)** *see* Everolimus-Exemestane (Breast) *on page 1640*

◆ **F-CL** *see* Fluorouracil-Leucovorin *on page 1653*

FAC

Index Terms CAF-IV; IVCAF

Use Breast cancer

Regimen NOTE: Multiple variations are listed.

Variation 1:

Fluorouracil: I.V.: 500 mg/m²/day days 1 and 8
[total dose/cycle = 1000 mg/m²]
or 500 mg/m² day 1
[total dose/cycle = 500 mg/m²]

Doxorubicin: I.V.: 50 mg/m² day 1
[total dose/cycle = 50 mg/m²]

Cyclophosphamide: I.V.: 500 mg/m² day 1
[total dose/cycle = 500 mg/m²]

Repeat cycle every 21-28 days

Variation 2:

Fluorouracil: I.V.: 200 mg/m²/day days 1, 2, and 3
[total dose/cycle = 600 mg/m²]

Doxorubicin: I.V.: 40 mg/m² day 1
[total dose/cycle = 40 mg/m²]

Cyclophosphamide: I.V.: 400 mg/m² day 1
[total dose/cycle = 400 mg/m²]

Repeat cycle every 28 days

Variation 3:

Fluorouracil: I.V.: 400 mg/m²/day days 1 and 8
[total dose/cycle = 800 mg/m²]

Doxorubicin: I.V.: 40 mg/m² day 1
[total dose/cycle = 40 mg/m²]

Cyclophosphamide: I.V.: 400 mg/m² day 1
[total dose/cycle = 400 mg/m²]

Repeat cycle every 28 days

Variation 4:

Fluorouracil: I.V.: 600 mg/m²/day days 1 and 8
[total dose/cycle = 1200 mg/m²]

Doxorubicin: I.V.: 60 mg/m² day 1
[total dose/cycle = 60 mg/m²]

Cyclophosphamide: I.V.: 600 mg/m² day 1
[total dose/cycle = 600 mg/m²]

Repeat cycle every 28 days

Variation 5:

Fluorouracil: I.V.: 300 mg/m²/day days 1 and 8
[total dose/cycle = 600 mg/m²]

Doxorubicin: I.V.: 30 mg/m² day 1
[total dose/cycle = 30 mg/m²]

Cyclophosphamide: I.V.: 300 mg/m² day 1
[total dose/cycle = 300 mg/m²]

Repeat cycle every 28 days

References

Variation 1:

Smalley RV, Carpenter J, Bartolucci A, et al, "A Comparison of Cyclophosphamide, Adriamycin®, 5-Fluorouracil (CAF), and Cyclophosphamide, Methotrexate, 5-Fluorouracil, Vincristine, Prednisone (CMFVP) in Patients With Metastatic Breast Cancer: A Southeastern Cancer Study Group Project," *Cancer*, 1977, 40(2):625-32.

Swenerton KD, Legha SS, Smith T, et al, "Prognostic Factors in Metastatic Breast Cancer Treated With Combination Chemotherapy," *Cancer Res*, 1979, 39(5):1552-62.

Variation 2:
Nemoto T, Horton J, Simon R, et al, "Comparison of Four-Combination Chemotherapy Programs in Metastatic Breast Cancer: Comparison of Multiple Drug Therapy With Cytoxan, 5-FU, and Prednisone, Versus Cytoxan and Adriamycin, Versus Cytoxan, 5-FU, and Adriamycin, Versus Cytoxan, 5-FU, and Prednisone Alternation With Cytoxan and Adriamycin," *Cancer*, 1982, 49 (10):1988-93.
Variation 3-5:
Wood WC, Budman DR, Korzun AH, et al, "Dose and Dose Intensity of Adjuvant Chemotherapy for State II, Node-Positive Breast Carcinoma," *N Engl J Med*, 1994, 330(18):1253-9.

◆ **FC (CLL)** *see* Fludarabine-Cyclophosphamide (CLL) *on page 1646*

◆ **FCMR (NHL)** *see* Fludarabine-Cyclophosphamide-Mitoxantrone-Rituximab *on page 1647*

◆ **FC (NHL-Mantle Cell)** *see* Fludarabine-Cyclophosphamide (NHL-Mantle Cell) *on page 1648*

◆ **FCR (CLL)** *see* Fludarabine-Cyclophosphamide-Rituximab (CLL) *on page 1648*

◆ **FCR (NHL-Follicular)** *see* Fludarabine-Cyclophosphamide-Rituximab (NHL-Follicular) *on page 1649*

FEC

Use Breast cancer

Regimen

Fluorouracil: I.V.: 500 mg/m^2 day 1
[total dose/cycle = 500 mg/m^2]
Cyclophosphamide: I.V.: 500 mg/m^2 day 1
[total dose/cycle = 500 mg/m^2]
Epirubicin: I.V.: 100 mg/m^2 day 1
[total dose/cycle = 100 mg/m^2]
Repeat cycle every 21 days

References

Bonneterre J, Roché H, Bremond A, et al, "Results of a Randomized Trial of Adjuvant Chemotherapy With FEC 50 vs FEC 100 in High Risk Node-Positive Breast Cancer Patients," *Proc Am Soc Clin Oncol*, 1998, 17:124a (abstract 473).

◆ **FEC-Docetaxel** *see* Docetaxel-FEC *on page 1611*

◆ **FEC-Vinorelbine** *see* Vinorelbine-FEC *on page 1773*

FL

Index Terms Flutamide + Leuprolide

Use Prostate cancer

Regimen NOTE: Multiple variations are listed.

Variation 1:
Flutamide: Oral: 250 mg every 8 hours
[total dose/cycle = 21,000 mg]
Leuprolide acetate: SubQ: 1 mg/day
[total dose/cycle = 28 mg]
Repeat cycle every 28 days

Variation 2:
Flutamide: Oral: 250 mg every 8 hours
[total dose/cycle = 67,500 mg]
Leuprolide acetate depot: I.M.: 22.5 mg day 1
[total dose/cycle = 22.5 mg]
Repeat cycle every 3 months

References

Variation 1:

Crawford ED, Eisenberger MA, McLeod DG, et al, "A Controlled Trial of Leuprolide With and Without Flutamide in Prostatic Carcinoma," *N Engl J Med*, 1989, 17:321(7):419-24.

Variation 2:

McLeod DG, Schellhammer PF, Vogelzang NJ, et al, "Exploratory Analysis on the Effect of Race on Clinical Outcome in Patients With Advanced Prostate Cancer Receiving Bicalutamide or Flutamide, Each in Combination With LHRH Analogues. The Casodex Combination Study Group." *Prostate*, 1999, 1:40(4):218-24.

FLAG (AML Induction)

Index Terms Fludarabine-ARAC-GCSF (AML Induction); Fludarabine-Cytarabine-Filgrastim (AML Induction)

Use Leukemia, acute myeloid

Regimen NOTE: Multiple variations are listed.

Variation 1:

Fludarabine: I.V.: 30 mg/m^2/day over 30 minutes days 1 to 5
[total dose/cycle = 150 mg/m^2]

Cytarabine: I.V.: 2 g/m^2/day over 4 hours days 1 to 5 (begin 4 hours after fludarabine infusion)
[total dose/cycle = 10 g/m^2]

Filgrastim: SubQ: 300 mcg 12 hours prior to start of fludarabine then 300 mcg/day days 2 through 5
[total dose/cycle = 1500 mcg]

followed by Filgrastim: SubQ: 300 mcg/day beginning one week after the end of treatment and continuing until complete neutrophil recovery

Variation 2:

Fludarabine: I.V.: 30 mg/m^2/day over 30 minutes days 1 to 5
[total dose/cycle = 150 mg/m^2]

Cytarabine: I.V.: 2 g/m^2/day over 4 hours days 1 to 5 (begin 3.5 hours after end of fludarabine infusion)
[total dose/cycle = 10 g/m^2]

Filgrastim: SubQ: 5 mcg/kg/day beginning 24 hours prior to start of fludarabine and continuing until ANC >500 mm^3

May repeat cycle one time for partial remission

Variation 3:

Fludarabine: I.V.: 30 mg/m^2/day over 30 minutes days 1 to 5
[total dose/cycle = 150 mg/m^2]

Cytarabine: I.V.: 2 g/m^2/day over 2 hours days 1 to 5 (begin 4 hours after the start of fludarabine infusion)
[total dose/cycle = 10 g/m^2]

Filgrastim: SubQ or I.V.: 300 mcg/day beginning the day prior to start of chemotherapy and continuing during chemotherapy and until ANC >1000 mm^3

May receive a second cycle

Variation 4:

Fludarabine: I.V.: 25 mg/m^2/day over 30 minutes days 1 to 5
[total dose/cycle = 125 mg/m^2]

Cytarabine: I.V.: 2 g/m^2/day over 4 hours days 1 to 5 (begin 4 hours after start of fludarabine infusion)
[total dose/cycle = 10 g/m^2]

Filgrastim: SubQ: 5 mcg/kg/day beginning 24 hours prior to start of cytarabine and continuing until ANC >500 mm^3

May repeat cycle in patients with complete remission and partial remission

References

Variation 1:
Clavio M, Carrara P, Miglino M, et al, "High Efficacy of Fludarabine-Containing Therapy (FLAG-FLANG) in Poor Risk Acute Myeloid Leukemia," *Haematologica*, 1996, 81(6):513-20.
Variation 2:
Montillo M, Mirto S, Petti MC, et al, "Fludarabine, Cytarabine, and G-CSF (FLAG) for the Treatment of Poor Risk Acute Myeloid Leukemia," *Am J Hematol*, 1998, 58(2):105-9.
Variation 3:
Virchis A, Koh M, Rankin P, et al, "Fludarabine, Cytosine Arabinoside, Granulocyte-Colony Stimulating Factor With or Without Idarubicin in the Treatment of High Risk Acute Leukaemia or Myelodysplastic Syndromes," *Br J Haematol*, 2004, 124(1):26-32.
Variation 4:
Ossenkoppele GJ, Graveland WJ, Sonneveld P, et al, "The Value of Fludarabine in Addition to ARA-C and G-CSF in the Treatment of Patients With High-Risk Myelodysplastic Syndromes and AML in Elderly Patients," *Blood*, 2004, 103(8):2908-13.

FLAG-IDA (AML Induction)

Use Leukemia, acute myeloid

Regimen NOTE: Multiple variations are listed.

Variation 1:

Fludarabine: I.V.: 30 mg/m²/day over 30 minutes days 1 to 5
[total dose/cycle = 150 mg/m²]

Cytarabine: I.V.: 2 g/m²/day over 4 hours days 1 to 5 (begin 4 hours after the start of fludarabine)
[total dose/cycle = 10 g/m²]

Idarubicin: I.V.: 10 mg/m²/day days 1, 2, and 3
[total dose/cycle = 30 mg/m²]

Filgrastim: SubQ: 5 mcg/kg from day 6 until ANC >500/mm³

Variation 2:

Fludarabine: I.V.: 30 mg/m²/day over 30 minutes days 1 to 5
[total dose/cycle = 150 mg/m²]

Cytarabine: I.V.: 2 g/m²/day over 2 hours days 1 to 5 (begin 4 hours after the start of fludarabine infusion)
[total dose/cycle = 10 g/m²]

Idarubicin: I.V.: 8 mg/m²/day over 30 minutes days 1, 2, and 3
[total dose/cycle = 24 mg/m²]

Filgrastim: SubQ or I.V.: 300 mcg/day beginning the day prior to start of chemotherapy and continuing during chemotherapy and until ANC >1000/mm³

May receive up to 2 cycles

Variation 3:

Fludarabine: I.V.: 30 mg/m²/day over 30 minutes days 1 to 4
[total dose/cycle = 120 mg/m²]

Cytarabine: I.V.: 2 g/m²/day over 4 hours days 1 to 4 (begin 4 hours after fludarabine treatment)
[total dose/cycle = 8 g/m²]

Idarubicin: I.V.: 10 mg/m²/day days 1, 2, and 3
[total dose/cycle = 30 mg/m²]

Filgrastim: Sub Q: see article for dose and frequency

References

Variation 1:
Pastore D, Specchia G, Carluccio P, et al, "FLAG-IDA in the Treatment of Refractory/Relapsed Acute Myeloid Leukemia: Single-Center Experience," *Ann Hematol*, 2003, 82(4):231-5.
Variation 2:
Virchis A, Koh M, Rankin P, et al, "Fludarabine, Cytosine Arabinoside, Granulocyte-Colony Stimulating Factor With or Without Idarubicin in the Treatment of High Risk Acute Leukaemia or Myelodysplastic Syndromes," *Br J Haematol*, 2004, 124(1):26-32.

Variation 3:
De la Rubia J, Regadera AI, Martin G, et al, "FLAG-IDA Regimen in the Treatment of Patients With High-Risk Myeloid Malignancies," *Leuk Res*, 2002, 26(8):725-30.

- **FLO (Esophageal Cancer)** *see* Fluorouracil-Leucovorin-Oxaliplatin (Esophageal Cancer) *on page 1656*
- **FLO (Gastric Cancer)** *see* Fluorouracil-Leucovorin-Oxaliplatin (Gastric Cancer) *on page 1657*
- **FLOT (Esophageal Cancer)** *see* Docetaxel-Oxaliplatin-Leucovorin-Fluorouracil (Esophageal Cancer) *on page 1613*

FLOX (Colorectal)

Index Terms Oxaliplatin-Leucovorin-Fluorouracil (Colorectal)

Use Colorectal cancer

Regimen

Oxaliplatin: I.V.: 85 mg/m^2 over 2 hours days 1, 15, and 29
[total dose/cycle = 255 mg/m^2]

Leucovorin: I.V.: 500 mg/m^2/day over 2 hours weekly for 6 weeks on days 1, 8, 15, 22, 29, and 36
[total dose/cycle = 3000 mg/m^2]

Fluorouracil: I.V.: 500 mg/m^2/day bolus (1 hour after beginning the leucovorin infusion) weekly for 6 weeks on days 1, 8, 15, 22, 29, and 36
[total dose/cycle = 3000 mg/m^2]

Repeat cycle every 8 weeks for a total of 3 cycles

References

Kuebler JP, Wieand HS, O'Connell MJ, et al, "Oxaliplatin Combined With Weekly Bolus Fluorouracil and Leucovorin as Surgical Adjuvant Chemotherapy for Stage II and III Colon Cancer: Results From NSABP C-07," *J Clin Oncol*, 2007, 25(16):2198-204.

- **FluCam (CLL)** *see* Fludarabine-Alemtuzumab (CLL) *on page 1645*

Fludarabine-Alemtuzumab (CLL)

Index Terms Alemtuzumab-Fludarabine (CLL); FluCam (CLL)

Use Leukemia, chronic lymphocytic

Regimen

Prior to Cycle 1 (days -14 to -1):

Alemtuzumab dose escalation (on consecutive days): I.V.: 3 mg/dose/day (repeat until tolerated); when tolerated, increase to 10 mg/dose/day (repeat until tolerated); when tolerated, increase to 30 mg/dose

Cycle 1 (begin when alemtuzumab successfully escalated to 30 mg, but no more than 14 days from dose escalation protocol):

Alemtuzumab: I.V.: 30 mg/dose over 2 hours days 1, 2, and 3
[total dose/cycle = 90 mg]

Fludarabine: I.V.: 30 mg/m^2/day over 15-30 minutes days 1, 2, and 3 (begin with alemtuzumab at full dose)
[total dose/cycle = 90 mg/m^2]

Repeat cycle in 28 days

Cycles 2-4:

Alemtuzumab: I.V.: 30 mg/dose (over 4 hours day 1; over 2 hours days 2 and 3) days 1, 2, and 3
[total dose/cycle = 90 mg]

Fludarabine: I.V.: 30 mg/m^2/day over 15-30 minutes days 1, 2, and 3
[total dose/cycle = 90 mg/m^2]

Repeat cycle every 28 days; may administer an additional 2 cycles (cycles 5 and 6) if respond (and tolerate)

References

Elter T, Borchmann P, Schulz H, et al, "Fludarabine in Combination With Alemtuzumab Is Effective and Feasible in Patients With Relapsed or Refractory B-Cell Chronic Lymphocytic Leukemia: Results of a Phase II Trial," *J Clin Oncol*, 2005, 23(28):7024-31.

- **Fludarabine-ARAC-GCSF (AML Induction)** *see* FLAG (AML Induction) *on page 1643*
- **Fludarabine-Cyclophosphamide-Alemtuzumab-Rituximab (CLL)** *see* Cyclophosphamide-Fludarabine-Alemtuzumab-Rituximab (CLL) *on page 1601*

Fludarabine-Cyclophosphamide (CLL)

Index Terms Cyclophosphamide-Fludarabine (CLL); FC (CLL)

Use Leukemia, chronic lymphocytic

Regimen NOTE: Multiple variations are listed.

Variation 1:

Fludarabine: I.V.: 25 mg/m^2/day days 1, 2, and 3
[total dose/cycle = 75 mg/m^2]

Cyclophosphamide: I.V.: 250 mg/m^2/day days 1, 2, and 3
[total dose/cycle = 750 mg/m^2]

Repeat cycle every 4 weeks for up to 6 cycles

Variation 2:

Fludarabine: I.V.: 30 mg/m^2/day days 1, 2, and 3
[total dose/cycle = 90 mg/m^2]

Cyclophosphamide: I.V.: 250 mg/m^2/day days 1, 2, and 3
[total dose/cycle = 750 mg/m^2]

Repeat cycle every 4 weeks for up to 6 cycles

Variation 3:

Cyclophosphamide: I.V.: 600 mg/m^2 day 1
[total dose/cycle = 600 mg/m^2]

Fludarabine: I.V.: 20 mg/m^2/day days 1 to 5
[total dose/cycle = 100 mg/m^2]

Repeat cycle every 4 weeks for up to 6 cycles

Variation 4:

Fludarabine: I.V.: 30 mg/m^2/day days 1, 2, and 3
[total dose/cycle = 90 mg/m^2]

Cyclophosphamide: I.V.: 300 mg/m^2/day days 1, 2, and 3
[total dose/cycle = 900 mg/m^2]

Repeat cycle every 4 weeks for up to 6 cycles

Variation 5:

Fludarabine: I.V.: 30 mg/m^2/day days 1, 2, and 3
[total dose/cycle = 90 mg/m^2]

Cyclophosphamide: I.V.: 300 mg/m^2/day days 1, 2, and 3
[total dose/cycle = 900 mg/m^2]

Repeat cycle every 4-6 weeks for up to 6 cycles

References

Variation 1:

Catovsky D, Richards S, Matutes E, et al, "Assessment of Fludarabine Plus Cyclophosphamide for Patients With Chronic Lymphocytic Leukaemia (The LRF CLL4 Trial): A Randomised Controlled Trial," *Lancet*, 2007, 370(9583):230-9.

O'Brien S, Moore JO, Boyd TE, et al, "Randomized Phase III Trial of Fludarabine Plus Cyclophosphamide With or Without Oblimersen Sodium (Bcl-2 Antisense) in Patients With Relapsed or Refractory Chronic Lymphocytic Leukemia," *J Clin Oncol*, 2007, 25(9):1114-20.

Variation 2:

Eichhorst BF, Busch R, Obwandner T, et al, "Health-Related Quality of Life in Younger Patients With Chronic Lymphocytic Leukemia Treated With Fludarabine Plus Cyclophosphamide or Fludarabine Alone for First-Line Therapy: A Study by the German CLL Study Group," *J Clin Oncol*, 2007, 25(13):1722-31.

Variation 3:

Flinn IW, Neuberg DS, Grever MR, et al, "Phase III Trial of Fludarabine Plus Cyclophosphamide Compared With Fludarabine for Patients With Previously Untreated Chronic Lymphocytic Leukemia: US Intergroup Trial E2997," *J Clin Oncol*, 2007, 25(7):793-8.

Variation 4:

Wierda W, O'Brien S, Faderl S, et al, "A Retrospective Comparison of Three Sequential Groups of Patients With Recurrent/Refractory Chronic Lymphocytic Leukemia Treated With Fludarabine-Based Regimens," *Cancer*, 2006, 106(2):337-45.

Variation 5:

O'Brien SM, Kantarjian HM, Cortes J, et al, "Results of the Fludarabine and Cyclophosphamide Combination Regimen in Chronic Lymphocytic Leukemia," *J Clin Oncol*, 2001, 19(5):1414-20.

Fludarabine-Cyclophosphamide-Mitoxantrone-Rituximab

Index Terms FCMR (NHL); R-FCM (NHL); Rituximab-Fludarabine-Cyclophosphamide-Mitoxantrone

Use Lymphoma, non-Hodgkin's

Regimen NOTE: Multiple variations are listed.

Consider pretherapy cytoreduction with cyclophosphamide 200 mg/m²/day for 3-5 days for patients with high tumor burden and/or lymphocytes >20,000/mm³

Variation 1:

Rituximab: I.V.: 375 mg/m²/dose day 1
[total dose/cycle = 375 mg/m²]

Fludarabine: I.V.: 25 mg/m²/day days 2, 3, and 4
[total dose/cycle = 75 mg/m²]

Cyclophosphamide: I.V.: 200 mg/m²/day days 2, 3, and 4
[total dose/cycle = 600 mg/m²]

Mitoxantrone: I.V.: 8 mg/m²/dose day 2
[total dose/cycle = 8 mg/m²]

Repeat cycle every 28 days for total of 4 cycles

Variation 2 (with maintenance rituximab):

Rituximab: I.V.: 375 mg/m²/dose day 1
[total dose/cycle = 375 mg/m²]

Fludarabine: I.V.: 25 mg/m²/day days 2, 3, and 4
[total dose/cycle = 75 mg/m²]

Cyclophosphamide: I.V.: 200 mg/m²/day days 2, 3, and 4
[total dose/cycle = 600 mg/m²]

Mitoxantrone: I.V.: 8 mg/m²/dose day 2
[total dose/cycle = 8 mg/m²]

Repeat cycle every 28 days for total of 4 cycles

followed by:

Maintenance rituximab (begin 3 months after completion of cycle 4):

Rituximab: I.V.: 375 mg/m²/dose day 1, 8, 15, and 22
[total dose/cycle = 1500 mg/m²]

Repeat maintenance cycle (once) in 6 months

References

Variation 1:

Forstpointner R, Dreyling M, Repp R, et al, "The Addition of Rituximab to a Combination of Fludarabine, Cyclophosphamide, Mitoxantrone (FCM) Significantly Increases the Response Rate and Prolongs Survival as Compared With FCM Alone in Patients With Relapsed and Refractory Follicular and Mantle Cell Lymphomas: Results of a Prospective Randomized Study of the German Low-Grade Lymphoma Study Group," *Blood*, 2004, 104(10):3064-71.

Variation 2:

Forstpointner R, Unterhalt M, Dreyling M, et al, "Maintenance Therapy With Rituximab Leads to a Significant Prolongation of Response Duration After Salvage Therapy With a Combination of Rituximab, Fludarabine, Cyclophosphamide, and Mitoxantrone (R-FCM) in Patients With Recurring and Refractory Follicular and Mantle Cell Lymphomas: Results of a Prospective Randomized Study of the German Low Grade Lymphoma Study Group (GLSG)," *Blood*, 2006, 108 (13):4003-8.

Fludarabine-Cyclophosphamide (NHL-Mantle Cell)

Index Terms CF (NHL-Mantle Cell); Cyclophosphamide-Fludarabine (NHL-Mantle Cell); FC (NHL-Mantle Cell)

Use Lymphoma, non-Hodgkin's (Mantle cell)

Regimen NOTE: Multiple variations are listed.

Variation 1:

Fludarabine: I.V.: 20 mg/m^2/day days 1 to 5
[total dose/cycle = 100 mg/m^2]

Cyclophosphamide: I.V.: 800 mg/m^2/dose day 1
[total dose/cycle = 800 mg/m^2]

Repeat cycle every 3-4 weeks for up to a total of 5 cycles

Variation 2:

Fludarabine: I.V.: 20 mg/m^2/day days 1 to 5
[total dose/cycle = 100 mg/m^2]

Cyclophosphamide: I.V.: 1000 mg/m^2/dose day 1
[total dose/cycle = 1000 mg/m^2]

Repeat cycle every 3-4 weeks for up to a total of 5 cycles

Variation 3:

Fludarabine: I.V.: 25 mg/m^2/day days 1 to 4
[total dose/cycle = 100 mg/m^2]

Cyclophosphamide: I.V.: 1000 mg/m^2/dose day 1
[total dose/cycle = 1000 mg/m^2]

Repeat cycle every 3-4 weeks for up to a total of 5 cycles

References

Variations 1-3:

Cohen BJ, Moskowitz C, Straus D, et al, "Cyclophosphamide/Fludarabine (CF) Is Active in the Treatment of Mantle Cell Lymphoma," *Leuk Lymphoma*, 2001, 42(5):1015-22.

Fludarabine-Cyclophosphamide-Rituximab (CLL)

Index Terms FCR (CLL); Rituximab-Fludarabine-Cyclophosphamide (CLL)

Use Leukemia, chronic lymphocytic

Regimen

Cycle 1:

Rituximab: I.V.: 375 mg/m^2 day 1
[total dose/cycle = 375 mg/m^2]

Fludarabine: I.V.: 25 mg/m^2/day days 2, 3, and 4
[total dose/cycle = 75 mg/m^2]

Cyclophosphamide: I.V.: 250 mg/m^2/day days 2, 3, and 4
[total dose/cycle = 750 mg/m^2]

Treatment cycle is 4 weeks

Cycles 2-6:
Rituximab: I.V.: 500 mg/m^2 day 1
[total dose/cycle = 500 mg/m^2]
Fludarabine: I.V.: 25 mg/m^2/day days 1, 2, and 3
[total dose/cycle = 75 mg/m^2]
Cyclophosphamide: I.V.: 250 mg/m^2/day days 1, 2, and 3
[total dose/cycle = 750 mg/m^2]
Repeat cycle every 4 weeks

References

Keating MJ, O'Brien S, Albitar M, et al, "Early Results of a Chemoimmunotherapy Regimen of Fludarabine, Cyclophosphamide, and Rituximab as Initial Therapy for Chronic Lymphocytic Leukemia," *J Clin Oncol*, 2005, 23(18):4079-88.

Wierda W, O'Brien S, Wen S, et al, "Chemoimmunotherapy With Fludarabine, Cyclophosphamide, and Rituximab for Relapsed and Refractory Chronic Lymphocytic Leukemia," *J Clin Oncol*, 2005, 23(18):4070-8.

Fludarabine-Cyclophosphamide-Rituximab (NHL-Follicular)

Index Terms FCR (NHL-Follicular); Rituximab-Fludarabine-Cyclophosphamide (NHL-Follicular)

Use Lymphoma, non-Hodgkin's (Follicular lymphoma)

Regimen

Cycle 1:
Rituximab: I.V.: 375 mg/m^2 day 15
[total dose/cycle = 375 mg/m^2]
Fludarabine: I.V.: 25 mg/m^2/day days 1, 2, and 3
[total dose/cycle = 75 mg/m^2]
Cyclophosphamide: I.V.: 300 mg/m^2/day days 1, 2, and 3
[total dose/cycle = 900 mg/m^2]
Treatment cycle is 3 weeks
Cycles 2-4:
Rituximab: I.V.: 375 mg/m^2 day 1
[total dose/cycle = 375 mg/m^2]
Fludarabine: I.V.: 25 mg/m^2/day days 1, 2, and 3
[total dose/cycle = 75 mg/m^2]
Cyclophosphamide: I.V.: 300 mg/m^2/day days 1, 2, and 3
[total dose/cycle = 900 mg/m^2]
Each treatment cycle is 3 weeks

References

Sacchi S, Pozzi S, Marcheselli R, et al, "Rituximab in Combination With Fludarabine and Cyclophosphamide in the Treatment of Patients With Recurrent Follicular Lymphoma," *Cancer*, 2007, 110(1):121-8.

♦ **Fludarabine-Cytarabine-Filgrastim (AML Induction)** see FLAG (AML Induction) *on page 1643*

Fludarabine-Mitoxantrone

Index Terms FM (NHL)

Use Lymphoma, non-Hodgkin's

Regimen

Fludarabine: I.V.: 25 mg/m^2/day days 1, 2, and 3
[total dose/cycle = 75 mg/m^2]
Mitoxantrone: I.V.: 10 mg/m^2/dose day 1
[total dose/cycle = 10 mg/m^2]
Repeat cycle every 21 days for total of 6 cycles

References

Zinzani PL, Pulsoni A, Perrotti A, et al, "Fludarabine Plus Mitoxantrone With and Without Rituximab Versus CHOP With and Without Rituximab as Front-Line Treatment for Patients With Follicular Lymphoma," *J Clin Oncol*, 2004, 22(13):2654-61.

Fludarabine-Mitoxantrone-Dexamethasone (NHL)

Index Terms FND (NHL)

Use Lymphoma, non-Hodgkin's

Regimen

Fludarabine: I.V.: 25 mg/m^2/day days 1, 2, and 3
[total dose/cycle = 75 mg/m^2]

Mitoxantrone: I.V.: 10 mg/m^2/dose day 1
[total dose/cycle = 10 mg/m^2]

Dexamethasone: I.V. or Oral: 20 mg/day days 1 to 5
[total dose/cycle = 100 mg]

Repeat cycle every 28 days for up to a total of 8 cycles

References

McLaughlin P, Hagemeister FB, Romaguera JE, et al, "Fludarabine, Mitoxantrone, and Dexamethasone: An Effective New Regimen for Indolent Lymphoma," *J Clin Oncol*, 1996, 14(4):1262-8.

Tsimberidou AM, McLaughlin P, Younes A, et al, "Fludarabine, Mitoxantrone, Dexamethasone (FND) Compared With an Alternating Triple Therapy (ATT) Regimen in Patients With Stage IV Indolent Lymphoma," *Blood*, 2002, 100(13):4351-7.

Fludarabine-Mitoxantrone-Dexamethasone-Rituximab

Index Terms FNDR (NHL); Rituximab-Fludarabine-Mitoxantrone-Dexamethasone

Use Lymphoma, non-Hodgkin's

Regimen

Cycle 1:

Rituximab: I.V.: 375 mg/m^2/day days 1 and 8
[total dose/cycle = 750 mg/m^2]

Fludarabine: I.V.: 25 mg/m^2/day days 1, 2, and 3
[total dose/cycle = 75 mg/m^2]

Mitoxantrone: I.V.: 10 mg/m^2/dose day 1
[total dose/cycle = 10 mg/m^2]

Dexamethasone: I.V. or Oral: 20 mg/m^2/day days 1 to 5
[total dose/cycle = 100 mg/m^2]

Treatment cycle is 28 days

Cycles 2-5:

Rituximab: I.V.: 375 mg/m^2 day 1
[total dose/cycle = 375 mg/m^2]

Fludarabine: I.V.: 25 mg/m^2/day days 2, 3, and 4
[total dose/cycle = 75 mg/m^2]

Mitoxantrone: I.V.: 10 mg/m^2/dose day 2
[total dose/cycle = 10 mg/m^2]

Dexamethasone: I.V. or Oral: 20 mg/m^2/day days 1 to 5
[total dose/cycle = 100 mg/m^2]

Repeat cycle every 28 days

Cycles 6-8:

Fludarabine: I.V.: 25 mg/m^2/day days 1, 2, and 3
[total dose/cycle = 75 mg/m^2]

Mitoxantrone: I.V.: 10 mg/m^2/dose day 1
[total dose/cycle = 10 mg/m^2]

Dexamethasone: I.V. or Oral: 20 mg/m^2/day days 1 to 5
[total dose/cycle = 100 mg/m^2]
Repeat cycle every 28 days
followed by:
Interferon maintenance:
Interferon alfa-2b: SubQ: 3 million units/m^2 days 1 to 14
[total dose/cycle = 42 million units/m^2]
Dexamethasone: Oral: 8 mg/day days 1, 2, and 3
[total dose/cycle = 24 mg]
Repeat cycle every month for 1 year

References

McLaughlin P, Hagemeister FB, Rodriguez MA, et al, "Safety of Fludarabine, Mitoxantrone, and Dexamethasone Combined With Rituximab in the Treatment of Stage IV Indolent Lymphoma," *Semin Oncol*, 2000, 27(6 Suppl 12):37-41.

Fludarabine-Mitoxantrone-Rituximab

Index Terms FMR (NHL); RFM (NHL); Rituximab-Fludarabine-Mitoxantrone

Use Lymphoma, non-Hodgkin's

Regimen

Fludarabine: I.V.: 25 mg/m^2/day days 1, 2, and 3
[total dose/cycle = 75 mg/m^2]
Mitoxantrone: I.V.: 10 mg/m^2/dose day 1
[total dose/cycle = 10 mg/m^2]
Repeat cycle every 21 days for total of 6 cycles
followed by:
Sequential rituximab (after completion of cycle 6):
Rituximab: I.V.: 375 mg/m^2/dose weekly for 4 doses
[total dose/4 weeks = 1500 mg/m^2]

References

Zinzani PL, Pulsoni A, Perrotti A, et al, "Fludarabine Plus Mitoxantrone With and Without Rituximab Versus CHOP With and Without Rituximab as Front-Line Treatment for Patients With Follicular Lymphoma," *J Clin Oncol*, 2004, 22(13):2654-61.

Fludarabine-Rituximab (CLL)

Use Leukemia, chronic lymphocytic

Regimen

Rituximab: I.V.: 375 mg/m^2/day days 1 and 4 (cycle 1); day 1 (cycles 2 to 6)
Fludarabine: I.V.: 25 mg/m^2/day days 1 to 5
Repeat cycle every 4 weeks

References

Byrd JC, Peterson BL, Morrison VA, et al, "Randomized Phase 2 Study of Fludarabine With Concurrent vs Sequential Treatment With Rituximab in Symptomatic, Untreated Patients With B-Cell Chronic Lymphocytic Leukemia: Results From Cancer and Leukemia Group B 9712 (CALGB 9712)," *Blood*, 2003, 101(1):6-14.

Fludarabine-Rituximab (NHL-Follicular)

Index Terms Rituximab-Fludarabine (NHL-Follicular)

Use Lymphoma, non-Hodgkin's (Follicular lymphoma)

Regimen

Week 1:
Rituximab: I.V.: 375 mg/m^2/dose for 2 doses 4 days apart
[total dose/week = 750 mg/m^2]

Week 2:
Fludarabine: I.V.: 25 mg/m²/day days 1 to 5
[total dose/week = 125 mg/m²]
Week 5:
Rituximab: I.V.: 375 mg/m²/dose day 5
[total dose/week = 375 mg/m²]
Week 6:
Fludarabine: I.V.: 25 mg/m²/day days 1 to 5
[total dose/week = 125 mg/m²]
Week 10:
Fludarabine: I.V.: 25 mg/m²/day days 1 to 5
[total dose/week = 125 mg/m²]
Week 13:
Rituximab: I.V.: 375 mg/m²/dose day 5
[total dose/week = 375 mg/m²]
Week 14:
Fludarabine: I.V.: 25 mg/m²/day days 1 to 5
[total dose/week = 125 mg/m²]
Week 18:
Fludarabine: I.V.: 25 mg/m²/day days 1 to 5
[total dose/week = 125 mg/m²]
Week 21:
Rituximab: I.V.: 375 mg/m²/dose day 5
[total dose/week = 375 mg/m²]
Week 22:
Fludarabine: I.V.: 25 mg/m²/day days 1 to 5
[total dose/week = 125 mg/m²]
Week 26:
Rituximab: I.V.: 375 mg/m²/dose for 2 doses 4 days apart
[total dose/week = 750 mg/m²]

References

Czuczman MS, Koryzna A, Mohr A, et al, "Rituximab in Combination With Fludarabine Chemotherapy in Low-Grade or Follicular Lymphoma," *J Clin Oncol*, 2005, 23(4):694-704.

Fluorouracil-Carboplatin (Head and Neck Cancer)

Index Terms Carboplatin-Fluorouracil (Head and Neck Cancer)

Use Head and neck cancer

Regimen NOTE: Multiple variations are listed.

Variation 1:
Fluorouracil: I.V.: 600 mg/m²/day continuous infusion days 1 to 4
[total dose/cycle = 2400 mg/m²]
Carboplatin: I.V.: 70 mg/m²/day days 1 to 4
[total dose/cycle = 280 mg/m²]
Repeat cycle every 3 weeks for 3 cycles

Variation 2:
Fluorouracil: I.V.: 1000 mg/m²/day continuous infusion days 1 to 4
[total dose/cycle = 4000 mg/m²]
Carboplatin: I.V.: 300 mg/m²/dose day 1 (may escalate to 360 mg/m²/dose in future cycles for grade 0 or 1 hematologic toxicity)
[total dose/cycle = 300-360 mg/m²]
Repeat cycle every 28 weeks

Variation 3:
Carboplatin: I.V.: 400 mg/m² day 1
[total dose/cycle = 400 mg/m²]

Fluorouracil: I.V.: 1000 mg/m²/day continuous infusion days 1 to 4 [total dose/cycle = 4000 mg/m²]

Repeat cycle every 28 days for a total of 2 or 3 cycles

References

Variation 1:

Denis F, Garaud P, Bardet E, et al, "Final Results of the 94-01 French Head and Neck Oncology and Radiotherapy Group Randomized Trial Comparing Radiotherapy Alone With Concomitant Radiochemotherapy in Advanced-Stage Oropharynx Carcinoma," *J Clin Oncol*, 2004, 22 (1):69-76.

Variation 2:

Forastiere AA, Metch B, Schuller DE, et al, "Randomized Comparison of Cisplatin Plus Fluorouracil and Carboplatin Plus Fluorouracil Versus Methotrexate in Advanced Squamous-Cell Carcinoma of the Head and Neck: A Southwest Oncology Group Study," *J Clin Oncol*, 1992, 10(8):1245-51.

Gregoire V, Beauduin M, Humblet Y, et al, "A Phase I-II Trial of Induction Chemotherapy With Carboplatin and Fluorouracil in Locally Advanced Head and Neck Squamous Cell Carcinoma: A Report From the UCL-Oncology Group, Belgium," *J Clin Oncol*, 1991, 9(8):1385-92.

- **Fluorouracil-Cisplatin (Bladder Cancer)** *see* Cisplatin-Fluorouracil (Bladder Cancer) *on page 1571*
- **Fluorouracil-Cisplatin (Cervical Cancer)** *see* Cisplatin-Fluorouracil (Cervical Cancer) *on page 1571*
- **Fluorouracil-Cisplatin-Docetaxel (Unknown Primary)** *see* Cisplatin-Docetaxel-Fluorouracil (Unknown Primary) *on page 1568*
- **Fluorouracil-Cisplatin (Esophageal Cancer)** *see* Cisplatin-Fluorouracil (Esophageal Cancer) *on page 1572*
- **Fluorouracil-Cisplatin (Gastric Cancer)** *see* Cisplatin-Fluorouracil (Gastric Cancer) *on page 1574*
- **Fluorouracil-Cisplatin (Head and Neck Cancer)** *see* Cisplatin-Fluorouracil (Head and Neck Cancer) *on page 1575*
- **Fluorouracil-Cisplatin-Trastuzumab (Gastric Cancer)** *see* Trastuzumab-Cisplatin-Fluorouracil (Gastric Cancer) *on page 1758*
- **Fluorouracil-Gemcitabine (RCC)** *see* Gemcitabine-Fluorouracil (RCC) *on page 1672*

Fluorouracil-Hydroxyurea (Head and Neck Cancer)

Index Terms Hydroxyurea-Fluorouracil (Head and Neck Cancer)

Use Head and neck cancer

Regimen NOTE: Administered with concurrent radiation therapy

Fluorouracil: I.V.: 800 mg/m²/day continuous infusion days 1 to 5 [total dose/cycle = 4000 mg/m²]

Hydroxyurea: Oral: 1000 mg/dose every 12 hours for 11 doses beginning day 1 [total dose/cycle = 11,000 mg]

Repeat cycle every other week for a total therapy duration of 13 weeks

References

Garden AS, Harris J, Vokes EE, et al, "Preliminary Results of Radiation Therapy Oncology Group 97-03: A Randomized Phase II Trial of Concurrent Radiation and Chemotherapy for Advanced Squamous Cell Carcinomas of the Head and Neck," *J Clin Oncol*, 2004, 22(14):2856-64.

Fluorouracil-Leucovorin

Index Terms F-CL; FU-LV; FU/Leucovorin

Use Colorectal cancer

Regimen NOTE: Multiple variations are listed.

Variation 1 (Mayo Regimen):
Fluorouracil: I.V.: 370-425 mg/m^2/day days 1 to 5
[total dose/cycle = 1850-2125 mg/m^2]
Leucovorin: I.V.: 20 mg/m^2/day days 1 to 5
[total dose/cycle = 100 mg/m^2]
Repeat cycle at 4 weeks, 8 weeks, and every 5 weeks thereafter

Variation 2:
Fluorouracil: I.V.: 400 mg/m^2/day days 1 to 5
[total dose/cycle = 2000 mg/m^2]
Leucovorin: I.V.: 20 mg/m^2/day days 1 to 5
[total dose/cycle = 100 mg/m^2]
Repeat cycle every 28 days

Variation 3:
Fluorouracil: I.V.: 500 mg/m^2 day 1
[total dose/cycle = 500 mg/m^2]
Leucovorin: I.V.: 20 mg/m^2 (2-hour infusion) day 1
[total dose/cycle = 20 mg/m^2]
Repeat cycle weekly

Variation 4:
Fluorouracil: I.V.: 600 mg/m^2 weekly for 6 weeks
[total dose/cycle = 3600 mg/m^2]
Leucovorin: I.V.: 500 mg/m^2 (3-hour infusion) weekly for 6 weeks
[total dose/cycle = 3000 mg/m^2]
Repeat cycle every 8 weeks

Variation 5:
Fluorouracil: I.V.: 600 mg/m^2 weekly for 6 weeks
[total dose/cycle = 3600 mg/m^2]
Leucovorin: I.V.: 500 mg/m^2 (2-hour infusion) weekly for 6 weeks
[total dose/cycle = 3000 mg/m^2]
Repeat cycle every 8 weeks

Variation 6:
Fluorouracil: I.V.: 600 mg/m^2 weekly
[total dose/cycle = 600 mg/m^2]
Leucovorin: I.V.: 500 mg/m^2 (2-hour infusion) weekly
[total dose/cycle = 500 mg/m^2]
Repeat cycle weekly

Variation 7:
Fluorouracil: I.V.: 2600 mg/m^2 continuous infusion over 24 hours day 1
[total dose/cycle = 2600 mg/m^2]
Leucovorin: I.V.: 500 mg/m^2 continuous infusion over 24 hours day 1
[total dose/cycle = 500 mg/m^2]
Repeat cycle weekly

Variation 8:
Fluorouracil: I.V.: 2600 mg/m^2 continuous infusion over 24 hours day 1
[total dose/cycle = 2600 mg/m^2]
Leucovorin: I.V.: 300 mg/m^2 (maximum dose: 500 mg) continuous infusion over 24 hours day 1
[total dose/cycle = 300 mg/m^2; maximum: 500 mg]
Repeat cycle weekly

Variation 9:
Fluorouracil: I.V.: 2600 mg/m^2 continuous infusion over 24 hours once weekly for 6 weeks
[total dose/cycle = 15,600 mg/m^2]

Leucovorin: I.V.: 500 mg/m^2 over 2 hours once weekly for 6 weeks
[total dose/cycle = 3000 mg/m^2]
Repeat cycle every 8 weeks

Variation 10:
Fluorouracil: I.V.: 2300 mg/m^2 continuous infusion over 24 hours day 1
[total dose/cycle = 2300 mg/m^2]
Leucovorin: I.V.: 50 mg/m^2 continuous infusion over 24 hours day 1
[total dose/cycle = 50 mg/m^2]
Repeat cycle weekly

Variation 11:
Fluorouracil: I.V.: 200 mg/m^2/day continuous infusion days 1 to 14
[total dose/cycle = 2800 mg/m^2]
Leucovorin: I.V.: 5 mg/m^2/day continuous infusion days 1 to 14
[total dose/cycle = 70 mg/m^2]
Repeat cycle every 28 days

Variation 12:
Cycle 1:
Fluorouracil: I.V.: 200 mg/m^2/day continuous infusion for 4 weeks
[total dose/cycle = 5600 mg/m^2]
Leucovorin: I.V.: 20 mg/m^2/day days 1, 8, 15, 22
[total dose/cycle = 80 mg/m^2]
Treatment cycle is 6 weeks
Subsequent cycles (starting week 7):
Fluorouracil: 200 mg/m^2 continuous infusion days 1 to 21
[total dose/cycle = 4200 mg/m^2]
Leucovorin: I.V.: 20 mg/m^2/day days 1, 8, and 15
[total dose/cycle = 60 mg/m^2]
Repeat cycle every 4 weeks

References

Variation 1:

Poon MA, O'Connell MJ, Moertel CG, et al, "Biochemical Modulation of Fluorouracil: Evidence of Significant Improvement of Survival and Quality of Life in Patients With Advanced Colorectal Carcinoma," *J Clin Oncol*, 1989, 7(10):1407-18.

Variation 2:

Borner MM, Castiglione M, Bacchi M, et al "The Impact of Adding Low-Dose Leucovorin to Monthly 5-Fluorouracil in Advanced Colorectal Carcinoma: Results of a Phase III Trial. Swiss Group for Clinical Cancer Research (SAKK)," *Ann Oncol*, 1998, 9(5):535-41.

Variation 3:

Jager E, Heike M, Bernhard H, et al, "Weekly High-Dose Leucovorin Versus Low-Dose Leucovorin Combined With Fluorouracil in Advanced Colorectal Cancer: Results of a Randomized Multicenter Trial. Study Group for Palliative Treatment of Metastatic Colorectal Cancer Study Protocol 1," *J Clin Oncol*, 1996, 14(8):2274-9.

Variation 4:

Leichman CG, Fleming TR, Muggia FM, et al, "Phase II Study of Fluorouracil and Its Modulation in Advanced Colorectal Cancer: A Southwest Oncology Group Study," *J Clin Oncol*, 1995, 13 (6):1303-11.

Variation 5:

Buroker TR, O'Connell MJ, Wieand HS, et al, "Randomized Comparison of Two Schedules of Fluorouracil and Leucovorin in the Treatment of Advanced Colorectal Cancer," *J Clin Oncol*, 1994, 12(1):14-20.

Variation 6:

Nobile MT, Rosso R, Sertoli MR, et al, "Randomised Comparison of Weekly Bolus 5-Fluorouracil With or Without Leucovorin in Metastatic Colorectal Carcinoma," *Eur J Cancer*, 1992, 28A (11):1823-7.

Variation 7:

Ardalan B, Chua L, Tian EM, et al, "A Phase II Study of Weekly 24-Hour Infusion With High-Dose Fluorouracil With Leucovorin in Colorectal Carcinoma," *J Clin Oncol*, 1991, 9(4):625-30.

Variation 8:
Yeh KH, Cheng AL, Lin MT, et al, "A Phase II Study of Weekly 24-Hour Infusion of High-Dose 5-Fluorouracil and Leucovorin (HDFL) in the Treatment of Recurrent or Metastatic Colorectal Cancers," *Anticancer Res*, 1997, 17(5B):3867-72.
Variation 9:
Kohne CH, Schoffski P, Wilke H, et al, "Effective Biomodulation by Leucovorin of High-Dose Infusion Fluorouracil Given as a Weekly 24-Hour Infusion: Results of a Randomized Trial in Patients With Advanced Colorectal Cancer," *J Clin Oncol*, 1998, 16(2):418-26.
Variation 10:
Haas NB, Schilder RJ, Nash S, et al, "A Phase II Trial of Weekly Infusional 5-Fluorouracil in Combination With Low-Dose Leucovorin in Patients With Advanced Colorectal Cancer," *Invest New Drugs*, 1995, 13(3):229-33.
Variation 11:
Falcone A, Allegrini G, Lencioni M, et al, "Protracted Continuous Infusion of 5-Fluorouracil and Low-Dose Leucovorin in Patients With Metastatic Colorectal Cancer Resistant to 5-Fluorouracil Bolus-Based Chemotherapy: A Phase II Study," *Cancer Chemother Pharmacol*, 1999, 44 (2):159-63.
Variation 12:
Leichman CG, Leichman L, Spears CP, et al, "Prolonged Continuous Infusion of Fluorouracil With Weekly Bolus Leucovorin: A Phase II Study in Patients With Disseminated Colorectal Cancer," *J Natl Cancer Inst*, 1993, 85(1):41-4.

◆ **Fluorouracil-Leucovorin-Bevacizumab** *see* Bevacizumab-Fluorouracil-Leucovorin *on page 1530*

◆ **Fluorouracil-Leucovorin-Irinotecan** *see* FU-LV-CPT-11 *on page 1666*

◆ **Fluorouracil-Leucovorin-Irinotecan (Esophageal Cancer)** *see* Irinotecan-Fluorouracil-Leucovorin (Esophageal Cancer) *on page 1696*

◆ **Fluorouracil-Leucovorin-Irinotecan (Gastric Cancer)** *see* Irinotecan-Leucovorin-Fluorouracil (Gastric Cancer) *on page 1697*

Fluorouracil-Leucovorin-Irinotecan (Saltz Regimen)

Index Terms FU-LV-CPT-11 (Saltz Regimen); Irinotecan-Fluorouracil-Leucovorin (Saltz Regimen); Saltz Regimen

Use Colorectal cancer

Regimen

Fluorouracil: I.V.: 500 mg/m^2/day days 1, 8, 15, and 22
[total dose/cycle = 2000 mg/m^2]

Leucovorin: I.V.: 20 mg/m^2/day days 1, 8, 15, and 22
[total dose/cycle = 80 mg/m^2]

Irinotecan: I.V.: 125 mg/m^2/day days 1, 8, 15, and 22
[total dose/cycle = 500 mg/m^2]

Repeat cycle every 42 days

References

Saltz LB, Cox JV, Blanke C, et al, "Irinotecan Plus Fluorouracil and Leucovorin for Metastatic Colorectal Cancer, Irinotecan Study Group," *N Engl J Med*, 2000, 343(13):905-14.

◆ **Fluorouracil, Leucovorin, Oxaliplatin (Colorectal)** *see* FOLFOX4 (Colorectal) *on page 1663*

◆ **Fluorouracil-Leucovorin-Oxaliplatin (Colorectal)** *see* FOLFOX6 and mFOLFOX6 (Colorectal) *on page 1663*

Fluorouracil-Leucovorin-Oxaliplatin (Esophageal Cancer)

Index Terms FLO (Esophageal Cancer); Oxaliplatin-Fluorouracil-Leucovorin (Esophageal Cancer); Oxaliplatin-Leucovorin-Fluorouracil (Esophageal Cancer)

Use Esophageal Cancer

Regimen NOTE: Multiple variations are listed.

Variation 1:

Oxaliplatin: I.V.: 85 mg/m^2/dose over 2 hours day 1
[total dose/cycle = 85 mg/m^2]

Leucovorin: I.V.: 200 mg/m^2/dose over 2 hours day 1
[total dose/cycle = 200 mg/m^2]

Fluorouracil: I.V.: 2600 mg/m^2/dose continuous infusion over 24 hours day 1
[total dose/cycle = 2600 mg/m^2]

Repeat cycle every 2 weeks until disease progression or unacceptable toxicity.

Variation 2:

Oxaliplatin: I.V.: 85 mg/m^2/dose over 2 hours day 1
[total dose/cycle = 85 mg/m^2]

Leucovorin: I.V.: 500 mg/m^2/day over 2 hours days 1 and 2
[total dose/cycle = 1000 mg/m^2]

Fluorouracil: I.V. bolus: 400 mg/m^2/day days 1 and 2
followed by I.V.: 600 mg/m^2/day continuous infusion over 22 hours days 1 and 2
[total dose/cycle = 2000 mg/m^2]

Repeat cycle every 2 weeks for 4 cycles (if achieve stable disease or response, continue until disease progression or unacceptable toxicity).

Variation 3:

Oxaliplatin: I.V.: 85 mg/m^2/dose day 1
[total dose/cycle = 85 mg/m^2]

Leucovorin: I.V.: 200 mg/m^2/day over 2 hours days 1 and 2
[total dose/cycle = 400 mg/m^2]

Fluorouracil: I.V. bolus: 400 mg/m^2/day days 1 and 2
followed by I.V.: 600 mg/m^2/day continuous infusion over 22 hours days 1 and 2
[total dose/cycle = 2000 mg/m^2]

Repeat cycle every 2 weeks for 6 cycles (3 cycles with radiation therapy and 3 cycles after completion of radiation therapy).

References

Variation 1:

Al-Batran SE, Hartmann JT, Probst S, et al, "Phase III Trial in Metastatic Gastroesophageal Adenocarcinoma With Fluorouracil, Leucovorin Plus Either Oxaliplatin or Cisplatin: A Study of the Arbeitsgemeinschaft Internistische Onkologie," *J Clin Oncol*, 2008, 26(9):1435-42.

Variation 2:

Mauer AM, Kraut EH, Krauss SA, et al, "Phase II Trial of Oxaliplatin, Leucovorin and Fluorouracil in Patients With Advanced Carcinoma of the Esophagus," *Ann Oncol*, 2005, 16(8):1320-5.

Variation 3:

Conroy T, Yataghène Y, Etienne PL, et al, "Phase II Randomised Trial of Chemoradiotherapy With FOLFOX4 or Cisplatin Plus Fluorouracil in Oesophageal Cancer," *Br J Cancer*, 2010, 103(9):1049-56.

Fluorouracil-Leucovorin-Oxaliplatin (Gastric Cancer)

Index Terms FLO (Gastric Cancer); Oxaliplatin–Leucovorin–Fluorouracil (Gastric Cancer)

Use Gastric cancer

Regimen NOTE: Multiple variations are listed.

Variation 1:

Oxaliplatin: I.V.: 85 mg/m^2/dose over 2 hours day 1
[total dose/cycle = 85 mg/m^2]

Leucovorin: I.V.: 200 mg/m^2/dose over 2 hours day 1
[total dose/cycle = 200 mg/m^2]

Fluorouracil: I.V.: 2600 mg/m²/dose continuous infusion over 24 hours day 1
[total dose/cycle = 2600 mg/m²]
Repeat cycle every 2 weeks until disease progression or unacceptable toxicity

Variation 2:
Oxaliplatin: I.V.: 100 mg/m²/dose over 2 hours day 1
[total dose/cycle = 100 mg/m²]
Leucovorin: I.V.: 400 mg/m²/dose over 2 hours day 1
[total dose/cycle = 400 mg/m²]
Fluorouracil: I.V. bolus: 400 mg/m²/dose over 10 minutes day 1
followed by I.V.: 3000 mg/m² continuous infusion over 46 hours beginning day 1
[total dose/cycle = 3400 mg/m²]
Repeat cycle every 2 weeks until disease progression or unacceptable toxicity for at least 6 cycles

Variation 3:
Oxaliplatin: I.V.: 85 mg/m²/dose over 2 hours day 1
[total dose/cycle = 85 mg/m²]
Leucovorin: I.V.: 500 mg/m²/dose over 2 hours day 1
[total dose/cycle = 500 mg/m²]
Fluorouracil: I.V.: 2600 mg/m²/dose continuous infusion over 24 hours day 1
[total dose/cycle = 2600 mg/m²]
Repeat cycle every 2 weeks until disease progression or unacceptable toxicity

References

Variation 1:
Al-Batran SE, Hartmann JT, Probst S, et al, "Phase III Trial in Metastatic Gastroesophageal Adenocarcinoma With Fluorouracil, Leucovorin Plus Either Oxaliplatin or Cisplatin: A Study of the Arbeitsgemeinschaft Internistische Onkologie," *J Clin Oncol*, 2008, 26(9):1435-42.
Variation 2:
Louvet C, André T, Tigaud JM, et al, "Phase II Study of Oxaliplatin, Fluorouracil, and Folinic Acid in Locally Advanced or Metastatic Gastric Cancer Patients," *J Clin Oncol*, 2002, 20(23):4543-8.
Variation 3:
Al-Batran SE, Atmaca A, Hegewisch-Becker S, et al, "Phase II Trial of Biweekly Infusional Fluorouracil, Folinic Acid, and Oxaliplatin in Patients With Advanced Gastric Cancer," *J Clin Oncol*, 2004, 22(4):658-63.

◆ **Fluorouracil, Leucovorin, Oxaliplatin (Pancreatic)** *see* FOLFOX (Pancreatic) *on page 1665*

Fluorouracil-Leucovorin (Pancreatic)

Index Terms 5FU-Folinic Acid (Pancreatic); 5FU-Leucovorin (Pancreatic); 5FU-LV (Pancreatic)

Use 5FU-Folinic Acid (Pancreatic)

Regimen

Leucovorin: I.V.: 20 mg/m²/day bolus days 1 to 5
[total dose/cycle = 100 mg/m²]
Fluorouracil: I.V.: 425 mg/m²/day bolus days 1 to 5
[total dose/cycle = 2125 mg/m²]
Repeat cycle every 28 days for 6 cycles

References

Neoptolemos JP, Stocken DD, Bassi C, et al, "Adjuvant Chemotherapy With Fluorouracil Plus Folinic Acid Vs Gemcitabine Following Pancreatic Cancer Resection: A Randomized Controlled Trial," *JAMA*, 2010, 304(10):1073-81.

Neoptolemos JP, Stocken DD, Friess H, et al, "A Randomized Trial of Chemoradiotherapy and Chemotherapy After Resection of Pancreatic Cancer," *N Engl J Med*, 2004, 350(12):1200-10.
Neoptolemos JP, Stocken DD, Smith CT, et al, "Adjuvant 5-Fluorouracil and Folinic Acid Vs Observation for Pancreatic Cancer: Composite Data From the ESPAC-1 and -3 (v1) Trials," *Br J Cancer*, 2009, 100(2):246-50.

Fluorouracil-Mitomycin (Anal Cancer)

Index Terms Mitomycin–Fluorouracil (Anal Cancer)

Use Anal cancer

Regimen NOTE: Multiple variations are listed.

Variation 1 (in combination with radiotherapy):

Fluorouracil: I.V.: 1000 mg/m^2/day continuous infusion days 1 to 4 and days 29 to 32
[total dose/cycle = 8000 mg/m^2]

Mitomycin: I.V.: 10 mg/m^2/day (maximum dose: 20 mg) days 1 and 29
[total dose/cycle = 20 mg/m^2; maximum: 40 mg]

Variation 2 (in combination with radiotherapy):

Fluorouracil: I.V.: 1000 mg/m^2/day continuous infusion days 1 to 4
[total dose/cycle = 4000 mg/m^2]

Mitomycin: I.V.: 10 mg/m^2/dose (maximum dose: 20 mg) day 1
[total dose/cycle = 10 mg/m^2; maximum: 20 mg]

Repeat cycle in 28 days (total of 2 cycles)

References

Variation 1:
Ajani JA, Winter KA, Gunderson LL, et al, "Fluorouracil, Mitomycin, and Radiotherapy vs Fluorouracil, Cisplatin, and Radiotherapy for Carcinoma of the Anal Canal: A Randomized Controlled Trial," *JAMA*, 2008, 299(16):1914-21.
Variation 2:
Flam M, John M, Pajak TF, et al, "Role of Mitomycin in Combination With Fluorouracil and Radiotherapy, and of Salvage Chemoradiation in the Definitive Nonsurgical Treatment of Epidermoid Carcinoma of the Anal Canal: Results of a Phase III Randomized Intergroup Study," *J Clin Oncol*, 1996, 14(9):2527-39.

- **Fluorouracil-Oxaliplatin (Esophageal Cancer)** *see* Oxaliplatin-Fluorouracil (Esophageal Cancer) *on page 1724*
- **Fluorouracil-Paclitaxel (Esophageal Cancer)** *see* Paclitaxel-Fluorouracil (Esophageal Cancer) *on page 1729*
- **Flutamide + Goserelin** *see* FZ *on page 1667*
- **Flutamide + Leuprolide** *see* FL *on page 1642*
- **FM (NHL)** *see* Fludarabine-Mitoxantrone *on page 1649*
- **FMR (NHL)** *see* Fludarabine-Mitoxantrone-Rituximab *on page 1651*
- **FND (NHL)** *see* Fludarabine-Mitoxantrone-Dexamethasone (NHL) *on page 1650*
- **FNDR (NHL)** *see* Fludarabine-Mitoxantrone-Dexamethasone-Rituximab *on page 1650*

FOLFIRI (Colorectal Cancer)

Use Colorectal cancer

Regimen NOTE: Multiple variations are listed.

Variation 1:

Cycles 1 and 2:

Irinotecan: I.V.: 180 mg/m^2 over 90 minutes day 1
[total dose/cycle = 180 mg/m^2]

Leucovorin: I.V.: 400 mg/m^2 over 2 hours day 1
[total dose/cycle = 400 mg/m^2]
Fluorouracil: I.V. bolus: 400 mg/m^2 day 1
followed by I.V.: 2400 mg/m^2 continuous infusion (over 46 hours) beginning day 1
[total fluorouracil dose/cycle = 2800 mg/m^2]
Repeat cycle in 14 days

Subsequent cycles:
Irinotecan: I.V.: 180 mg/m^2 over 90 minutes day 1
[total dose/cycle = 180 mg/m^2]
Leucovorin: I.V.: 400 mg/m^2 over 2 hours day 1
[total dose/cycle = 400 mg/m^2]
Fluorouracil: I.V. bolus: 400 mg/m^2 day 1
followed by I.V.: 3000 mg/m^2 continuous infusion (over 46 hours) beginning day 1
[total fluorouracil dose/cycle = 3400 mg/m^2]
Repeat cycle every 14 days until disease progression or unacceptable toxicity

Variation 2:
Irinotecan: I.V.: 180 mg/m^2 over 90 minutes day 1
[total dose/cycle = 180 mg/m^2]
Leucovorin: I.V.: 200 mg/m^2/day over 2 hours days 1 and 2
[total dose/cycle = 400 mg/m^2]
Fluorouracil: I.V. bolus: 400 mg/m^2/day days 1 and 2
followed by I.V.: 600 mg/m^2/day continuous infusion (over 22 hours each day) on days 1 and 2
[total fluorouracil dose/cycle = 2000 mg/m^2]
Repeat cycle every 14 days until disease progression or unacceptable toxicity

Variation 3:
Irinotecan: I.V.: 180 mg/m^2 over 1 hour day 1
[total dose/cycle = 180 mg/m^2]
Leucovorin: I.V.: 100 mg/m^2/day over 2 hours days 1 and 2
[total dose/cycle = 200 mg/m^2]
Fluorouracil: I.V. bolus: 400 mg/m^2/day days 1 and 2
followed by I.V.: 600 mg/m^2/day continuous infusion (over 22 hours each day) on days 1 and 2
[total fluorouracil dose/cycle = 2000 mg/m^2]
Repeat cycle every 14 days for up to 12 cycles or until disease progression or unacceptable toxicity

Variation 4:
Irinotecan: I.V.: 180 mg/m^2 over 90 minutes day 1
[total dose/cycle = 180 mg/m^2]
Leucovorin: I.V.: 400 mg/m^2 over 2 hours day 1
[total dose/cycle = 400 mg/m^2]
Fluorouracil: I.V. bolus: 400 mg/m^2 day 1
followed by I.V.: 2400 mg/m^2 continuous infusion (over 46 hours) beginning day 1
[total fluorouracil dose/cycle = 2800 mg/m^2]
Repeat cycle every 14 days until disease progression or unacceptable toxicity

References

Variation 1:

André T, Louvet C, Maindrault-Goebel F, et al, "CPT-11 (Irinotecan) Addition to Bimonthly, High-Dose Leucovorin and Bolus and Continuous-Infusion 5-Fluorouracil (FOLFIRI) for Pretreated Metastatic Colorectal Cancer. GERCOR," *Eur J Cancer*, 1999, 35(9):1343-7.

Tournigand C, André T, Achille E, "FOLFIRI Followed by FOLFOX6 or the Reverse Sequence in Advanced Colorectal Cancer: A Randomized GERCOR Study," *J Clin Oncol*, 2004, 22(2):229-37.

Variation 2:

Aranda E, Valladares M, Martinez-Villacampa M, et al, "Randomized Study of Weekly Irinotecan Plus High-Dose 5-Fluorouracil (FUIRI) Versus Biweekly Irinotecan Plus 5-Fluorouracil/Leucovorin (FOLFIRI) as First-Line Chemotherapy for Patients With Metastatic Colorectal Cancer: A Spanish Cooperative Group for the Treatment of Digestive Tumors Study," *Ann Oncol*, 2009, 20 (2):251-7.

Douillard JY, Cunningham D, Roth AD, et al, "Irinotecan Combined With Fluorouracil Compared With Fluorouracil Alone as First-Line Treatment for Metastatic Colorectal Cancer: A Multicentre Randomised Trial," *Lancet*, 2000, 355(9209):1041-7.

Variation 3:

Falcone A, Ricci S, Brunetti I, et al, "Phase III Trial of Infusional Fluorouracil, Leucovorin, Oxaliplatin, and Irinotecan (FOLFOXIRI) Compared With Infusional Fluorouracil, Leucovorin, and Irinotecan (FOLFIRI) as First-Line Treatment for Metastatic Colorectal Cancer: The Gruppo Oncologico Nord Ovest," *J Clin Oncol*, 2007, 25(13):1670-6.

Variation 4:

Fuchs CS, Marshall J, Mitchell E, et al, "Randomized, Controlled Trial of Irinotecan Plus Infusional, Bolus, or Oral Fluoropyrimidines in First-Line Treatment of Metastatic Colorectal Cancer: Results From the BICC-C Study," *J Clin Oncol*, 2007, 25(30):4779-86.

FOLFIRINOX (Pancreatic)

Index Terms Irinotecan-Oxaliplatin-Fluorouracil-Leucovorin (Pancreatic); Oxaliplatin-Irinotecan-Fluorouracil-Leucovorin (Pancreatic)

Use Pancreatic cancer

Regimen

Oxaliplatin: I.V.: 85 mg/m² over 2 hours day 1
[total dose/cycle = 85 mg/m²]

Leucovorin: I.V.: 400 mg/m² over 2 hours day 1
[total dose/cycle = 400 mg/m²]

Irinotecan: I.V.: 180 mg/m² over 90 minutes day 1
[total dose/cycle = 180 mg/m²]

Fluorouracil: I.V. bolus: 400 mg/m² day 1
followed by I.V.: 2400 mg/m² continuous infusion (CI) over 46 hours beginning day 1
[total fluorouracil dose/cycle (bolus and CI) = 2800 mg/m²]

Note: Bolus and CI fluorouracil are both given on day 1

Repeat cycle every 14 days until disease progression or unacceptable toxicity, 12 cycles recommended

References

Conroy T, Desseigne F, Ychou M, et al, "FOLFIRINOX Versus Gemcitabine for Metastatic Pancreatic Cancer," *N Engl J Med*, 2011, 364(19):1817-25.

Conroy T, Paillot B, François E, et al, "Irinotecan Plus Oxaliplatin and Leucovorin-Modulated Fluorouracil in Advanced Pancreatic Cancer–A Groupe Tumeurs Digestives of the Federation Nationale des Centres de Lutte Contre le Cancer Study," *J Clin Oncol*, 2005, 23(6):1228-36.

◆ **FOLFOX4-Cetuximab** *see* Cetuximab-FOLFOX4 *on page 1560*

◆ **FOLFOX 6 (Pancreatic)** *see* FOLFOX (Pancreatic) *on page 1665*

FOLFOX1 (Colorectal)

Index Terms Oxaliplatin-Leucovorin-Fluorouracil (Colorectal)

Use Colorectal cancer

Regimen

Oxaliplatin: I.V.: 130 mg/m^2 over 2 hours day 1 (every other cycle)
[total dose/cycle = 130 mg/m^2]

Leucovorin: I.V.: 500 mg/m^2/day over 2 hours days 1 and 2
[total dose/cycle = 1000 mg/m^2]

Fluorouracil: I.V.: 1500-2000 mg/m^2/day continuous infusion over 22 hours days 1 and 2
[total dose/cycle = 3000-4000 mg/m^2]

Repeat cycle every 14 days until disease progression or unacceptable toxicity

References

de Gramont A, Tournigand C, Louvet C, et al, "Oxaliplatin, Folinic Acid, and 5-Fluorouracil (FOLFOX) in Pretreated Patients With Metastatic Advanced Cancer, The GERCOD," *Rev Med Interne*, 1997, 18(10):769-75.

FOLFOX2 (Colorectal)

Index Terms Oxaliplatin-Leucovorin-Fluorouracil (Colorectal)

Use Colorectal cancer

Regimen

Oxaliplatin: I.V.: 100 mg/m^2 over 2 hours day 1
[total dose/cycle = 100 mg/m^2]

Leucovorin: I.V.: 500 mg/m^2/day over 2 hours days 1 and 2
[total dose/cycle = 1000 mg/m^2]

Fluorouracil: I.V.: 1500-2000 mg/m^2/day continuous infusion over 22 hours days 1 and 2
[total dose/cycle = 3000-4000 mg/m^2]

Repeat cycle every 14 days until disease progression or unacceptable toxicity

References

de Gramont A, Tournigand C, Louvet C, et al, "Oxaliplatin, Folinic Acid and 5-Fluorouracil (Folfox) in Pretreated Patients With Metastatic Advanced Cancer. The GERCOD," *Rev Med Interne*, 1997, 18(10):769-75

de Gramont A, Vignoud J, Tournigand C, et al, "Oxaliplatin With High-Dose Leucovorin and 5-Fluorouracil 48-Hour Continuous Infusion in Pretreated Metastatic Colorectal Cancer," *Eur J Cancer*, 1997, 33(2):214-9.

FOLFOX3 (Colorectal)

Index Terms Oxaliplatin-Leucovorin-Fluorouracil (Colorectal)

Use Colorectal cancer

Regimen

Oxaliplatin: I.V.: 85 mg/m^2 over 2 hours day 1
[total dose/cycle = 85 mg/m^2]

Leucovorin: I.V.: 500 mg/m^2/day over 2 hours days 1 and 2
[total dose/cycle = 1000 mg/m^2]

Fluorouracil: I.V.: 1500-2000 mg/m^2/day continuous infusion over 22 hours days 1 and 2
[total dose/cycle = 3000-4000 mg/m^2]

Repeat cycle every 14 days until disease progression or unacceptable toxicity

References

de Gramont A, Tournigand C, Louvet C, et al, "Oxaliplatin, Folinic Acid, and 5-Fluorouracil (FOLFOX) in Pretreated Patients With Metastatic Advanced Cancer, The GERCOD," *Rev Med Interne*, 1997, 18(10):769-75.

FOLFOX4 (Colorectal)

Index Terms Fluorouracil, Leucovorin, Oxaliplatin (Colorectal); Oxaliplatin, Leucovorin, Fluorouracil (Colorectal)

Use Colorectal cancer

Regimen NOTE: Multiple variations are listed.

Variation 1:

Oxaliplatin: I.V.: 85 mg/m² over 2 hours day 1
[total dose/cycle = 85 mg/m²]

Leucovorin: I.V.: 200 mg/m²/day over 2 hours days 1 and 2
[total dose/cycle = 400 mg/m²]

Fluorouracil: I.V. bolus: 400 mg/m²/day days 1 and 2
followed by I.V.: 600 mg/m²/day continuous infusion (CI) over 22 hours days 1 and 2
[total dose/cycle (bolus and CI) = 2000 mg/m²]

Repeat cycle every 14 days for a total of 12 cycles in the adjuvant setting; and until disease progression or unacceptable toxicity in the metastatic setting.

Variation 2:

Oxaliplatin: I.V.: 85 mg/m² over 2 hours day 1
[total dose/cycle = 85 mg/m²]

Leucovorin (L-isomer): I.V.: 100 mg/m²/day over 2 hours days 1 and 2
[total dose/cycle = 200 mg/m²]

Fluorouracil: I.V. bolus: 400 mg/m²/day days 1 and 2
followed by I.V.: 600 mg/m²/day continuous infusion (CI) over 22 hours days 1 and 2
[total dose/cycle (bolus and CI) = 2000 mg/m²]

Repeat cycle every 14 days

References

Variation 1:

Andre T, Boni C, Mounedji-Boudiaf L, et al, "Oxaliplatin, Fluorouracil, and Leucovorin as Adjuvant Treatment for Colon Cancer," *N Engl J Med*, 2004, 350(23):2343-51.

Andre T, Boni C, Navarro M, et al, "Improved Overall Survival With Oxaliplatin, Fluorouracil, and Leucovorin as Adjuvant Treatment in Stage II or III Colon Cancer In the MOSAIC Trial," *J Clin Oncol*, 2009, 27(19):3109-16.

de Gramont A, Figer A, Seymour M, et al, "Leucovorin and Fluorouracil With or Without Oxaliplatin as First-Line Treatment in Advanced Colorectal Cancer," *J Clin Oncol*, 2000, 18(16):2938-47.

Variation 2:

Colucci G, Gebbia V, Paoletti G, et al, "Phase III Randomized Trial of FOLFIRI Versus FOLFOX4 in the Treatment of Advanced Colorectal Cancer: A Multicenter Study Gruppo Oncologico Dell'Italia Meridionale," *J Clin Oncol*, 2005, 23(22):4866-75.

FOLFOX6 and mFOLFOX6 (Colorectal)

Index Terms Fluorouracil-Leucovorin-Oxaliplatin (Colorectal), mFOLFOX6 and FOLFOX6 (Colorectal), Modified Fluorouracil-Leucovorin-Oxaliplatin (Colorectal); Modified FOLFOX6 (Colorectal); Oxaliplatin-Leucovorin-Fluorouracil (Colorectal)

Use Colorectal cancer

Regimen NOTE: Multiple variations are listed.

Variation 1:

Cycles 1 and 2:

Oxaliplatin: I.V.: 100 mg/m² over 2 hours day 1
[total dose/cycle = 100 mg/m²]

Leucovorin: I.V.: 400 mg/m² over 2 hours day 1
[total dose/cycle = 400 mg/m²]

Fluorouracil: I.V. bolus: 400 mg/m^2 day 1
followed by I.V.: 2400 mg/m^2 continuous infusion (CI) over 46 hours beginning day 1
[total fluorouracil dose/cycle (bolus and CI) = 2800 mg/m^2]
Repeat cycle every 14 days for 2 cycles
Subsequent Cycles:
Oxaliplatin: I.V.: 100 mg/m^2 over 2 hours day 1
[total dose/cycle = 100 mg/m^2]
Leucovorin: I.V.: 400 mg/m^2 over 2 hours day 1
[total dose/cycle = 400 mg/m^2]
Fluorouracil: I.V. bolus: 400 mg/m^2 day 1
followed by I.V.: 3000 mg/m^2 continuous infusion (CI) over 46 hours beginning day 1
[total fluorouracil dose/cycle (bolus and CI) = 3400 mg/m^2]
Repeat cycle every 14 days until disease progression or unacceptable toxicity
Variation 2:
Oxaliplatin: I.V.: 85 mg/m^2 over 2 hours day 1
[total dose/cycle = 85 mg/m^2]
Leucovorin: I.V.: 350 mg over 2 hours day 1
[total dose/cycle = 350 mg]
Fluorouracil: I.V. bolus: 400 mg/m^2 day 1
followed by I.V.: 2400 mg/m^2 continuous infusion (CI) over 46 hours beginning day 1
[total fluorouracil dose/cycle (bolus and CI) = 2800 mg/m^2]
Repeat cycle every 14 days until disease progression or unacceptable toxicity

References

Variation 1:
Maindrault-Goebel F, Louvet C, Andre T, et al, "Oxaliplatin Added to the Simplified Bimonthly Leucovorin and 5-Fluorouracil Regimen as Second-Line Therapy for Metastatic Colorectal Cancer (FOLFOX6), GERCOR," *Eur J Cancer*, 1999, 35(9):1338-42.
Tournigand C, André T, Achille E, et al, "FOLFIRI Followed by FOLFOX6 or the Reverse Sequence in Advanced Colorectal Cancer: A Randomized GERCOR Study," *J Clin Oncol*, 2004, 22 (2):229-37.
Variation 2:
Cheesman SL, Joel SP, Chester JD, et al, "A 'Modified de Gramont' Regimen of Fluorouracil, Alone and With Oxaliplatin, for Advanced Colorectal Cancer," *Br J Cancer*, 2002, 87(4): 393-9.
Hochster HS, Hart LL, Ramanathan RK, et al, "Safety and Efficacy of Oxaliplatin and Fluoropyrimidine Regimens With or Without Bevacizumab as First-Line Treatment of Metastatic Colorectal Cancer: Results of the TREE Study," *J Clin Oncol*, 2008, 26(21):3523-9.

FOLFOX7 (Colorectal)

Use Colorectal cancer

Regimen

Oxaliplatin: I.V.: 130 mg/m^2 over 2 hours day 1
[total dose/cycle = 130 mg/m^2]
Leucovorin: I.V.: 400 mg/m^2 over 2 hours day 1
[total dose/cycle = 400 mg/m^2]
Fluorouracil: I.V. bolus: 400 mg/m^2 day 1
followed by I.V.: 2400 mg/m^2 continuous infusion (CI) over 46 hours beginning on day 1
total fluorouracil dose/cycle (bolus and CI) = 2800 mg/m^2
Repeat cycle every 14 days for a total of 8 cycles; evaluate every 2 months; may resume if disease progression

References

Maindrault-Goebel F, de Gramont A, Louvet C, et al, "High-Dose Intensity Oxaliplatin Added to the Simplified Bimonthly Leucovorin and 5-Fluorouracil Regimen as Second-Line Therapy for Metastatic Colorectal Cancer (FOLFOX 7)," *Eur J Cancer*, 2001, 37(8):1000-5.

FOLFOXIRI (Colorectal)

Index Terms Irinotecan, Oxaliplatin, Leucovorin, Fluorouracil (Colorectal)

Use Colorectal cancer

Regimen

Irinotecan: I.V.: 165 mg/m^2 over 1 hour day 1
[total dose/cycle = 165 mg/m^2]

Oxaliplatin: I.V.: 85 mg/m^2 over 2 hours day 1
[total dose/cycle = 85 mg/m^2]

Leucovorin: I.V.: 200 mg/m^2 over 2 hours day 1
[total dose/cycle = 200 mg/m^2]

Fluorouracil: I.V.: 3200 mg/m^2 continuous infusion over 48 hours beginning day 1
[total dose/cycle = 3200 mg/m^2]

Repeat cycle every 14 days for a maximum of 12 cycles

References

Falcone A, Ricci S, Brunetti I, et al, "Phase III Trial of Infusional Fluorouracil, Leucovorin, Oxaliplatin, and Irinotecan (FOLFOXIRI) Compared With Infusional Fluorouracil, Leucovorin, and Irinotecan (FOLFIRI) as First-Line Treatment for Metastatic Colorectal Cancer: The Gruppo Oncologico Nord Ovest," *J Clin Oncol*, 2007, 25(13):1670-6.

FOLFOX (Pancreatic)

Index Terms Fluorouracil, Leucovorin, Oxaliplatin (Pancreatic); FOLFOX 6 (Pancreatic); Oxaliplatin, Fluorouracil, Leucovorin (Pancreatic)

Use Pancreatic cancer

Regimen

Oxaliplatin: I.V.: 100 mg/m^2 day 1
[total dose/cycle = 100 mg/m^2]

Leucovorin: I.V.: 400 mg/m^2 day 1
[total dose/cycle = 400 mg/m^2]

Fluorouracil: I.V. bolus: 400 mg/m^2 day 1
followed by I.V.: 3000 mg/m^2 continuous infusion (CI) over 46 hours beginning day 1
[total fluorouracil dose/cycle (bolus and CI) = 3400 mg/m^2]

Repeat cycle every 14 days until disease progression or unacceptable toxicity

References

Ghosn M, Farhat F, Kattan J, et al, "FOLFOX-6 Combination as the First-Line Treatment of Locally Advanced and/or Metastatic Pancreatic Cancer," *Am J Clin Oncol*, 2007, 30(1):15-20.

- **FU-LV** *see* Fluorouracil-Leucovorin *on page 1653*
- **FU-LV-CPT-11 (Saltz Regimen)** *see* Fluorouracil-Leucovorin-Irinotecan (Saltz Regimen) *on page 1656*
- **5FU-LV (Pancreatic)** *see* Fluorouracil-Leucovorin (Pancreatic) *on page 1658*
- **5FU-Cisplatin (Cervical Cancer)** *see* Cisplatin-Fluorouracil (Cervical Cancer) *on page 1571*
- **5FU-Folinic Acid (Pancreatic)** *see* Fluorouracil-Leucovorin (Pancreatic) *on page 1658*
- **FU/Leucovorin** *see* Fluorouracil-Leucovorin *on page 1653*

◆ **5FU-Leucovorin (Pancreatic)** *see* Fluorouracil-Leucovorin (Pancreatic) *on page 1658*

FU-LV-CPT-11

Index Terms Fluorouracil-Leucovorin-Irinotecan; Irinotecan-Fluorouracil-Leucovorin

Use Colorectal cancer

Regimen NOTE: Multiple variations are listed.

Variation 1:

Irinotecan: I.V.: 350 mg/m^2 day 1
[total dose/cycle = 350 mg/m^2]
Leucovorin: I.V.: 20 mg/m^2/day days 22 to 26
[total dose/cycle = 100 mg/m^2]
Fluorouracil: I.V.: 425 mg/m^2/day days 22 to 26
[total dose/cycle = 2125 mg/m^2]
Repeat cycle every 6 weeks

Variation 2:

Irinotecan: I.V.: 80 mg/m^2 day 1
[total dose/cycle = 80 mg/m^2]
Fluorouracil: I.V.: 2300 mg/m^2 continuous infusion day 1
[total dose/cycle = 2300 mg/m^2]
Leucovorin: I.V.: 500 mg/m^2 day 1
[total dose/cycle = 500 mg/m^2]
Repeat cycle weekly

or

Irinotecan: I.V.: 180 mg/m^2 day 1
[total dose/cycle = 180 mg/m^2]
Leucovorin: I.V.: 200 mg/m^2/day days 1 and 2
[total dose/cycle = 400 mg/m^2]
Fluorouracil: I.V.: 400 mg/m^2/day days 1 and 2
[total dose/cycle = 800 mg/m^2]
followed by I.V.: 600 mg/m^2/day continuous infusion days 1 and 2
[total dose/cycle = 1200 mg/m^2]
Repeat cycle every 2 weeks

Variation 3:

Irinotecan: I.V.: 175 mg/m^2 day 1
[total dose/cycle = 175 mg/m^2]
Leucovorin: I.V.: 250 mg/m^2 day 2
[total dose/cycle = 250 mg/m^2]
Fluorouracil: I.V.: 950 mg/m^2 day 2
[total dose/cycle = 950 mg/m^2]

or

Irinotecan: I.V.: 200 mg/m^2 day 1
[total dose/cycle = 200 mg/m^2]
Leucovorin: I.V.: 250 mg/m^2 day 2
[total dose/cycle = 250 mg/m^2]
Fluorouracil: I.V.: 850 mg/m^2 day 2
[total dose/cycle = 850 mg/m^2]
Repeat cycle every other week

References

Variation 1:

Van Cutsem E, Pozzo C, Starkhammar H, et al, "A Phase II Study of Irinotecan Alternated With Five Days Bolus of 5-Fluorouracil and Leucovorin in First-Line Chemotherapy of Metastatic Colorectal Cancer," *Ann Oncol*, 1998, 9(11):1199-204.

Variation 2:

Douillard JY, Cunningham D, Roth AD, et al, "Irinotecan Combined With Fluorouracil Compared With Fluorouracil Alone as First-Line Treatment for Metastatic Colorectal Cancer: A Multicentre Randomised Trial," *Lancet*, 2000, 355(9209):1041-7.

Variation 3:

Comella P, Casaretti F, De Vita F, et al, "Concurrent Irinotecan and 5-Fluorouracil Plus Levo-Folinic Acid Given Every Other Week in the First-Line Management of Advanced Colorectal Carcinoma: A Phase I Study of the Southern Italy Cooperative Oncology Group," *Ann Oncol*, 1999, 10 (8):915-21.

FZ

Index Terms Flutamide + Goserelin

Use Prostate cancer

Regimen NOTE: Multiple variations are listed.

Variation 1:

Flutamide: Oral: 250 mg every 8 hours
[total dose/cycle = 21,000 mg]

Goserelin acetate: SubQ: 3.6 mg day 1
[total dose/cycle = 3.6 mg]

Repeat cycle every 28 days

Variation 2:

Flutamide: Oral: 250 mg every 8 hours
[total dose/cycle = 67,500 mg]

Goserelin acetate: SubQ: 10.8 mg day 1
[total dose/cycle = 10.8 mg]

Repeat cycle every 3 months

References

McLeod DG, Schellhammer PF, Vogelzang NJ, et al, "Exploratory Analysis on the Effect of Race on Clinical Outcome in Patients With Advanced Prostate Cancer Receiving Bicalutamide or Flutamide, Each in Combination With LHRH Analogues. The Casodex Combination Study Group," *Prostate*, 1999, 40(4):218-24.

◆ **GC (NSCLC)** *see* Carboplatin-Gemcitabine (NSCLC) *on page 1547*

GDP (Hodgkin)

Index Terms Gemcitabine-Dexamethasone-Cisplatin (Hodgkin)

Use Lymphoma, Hodgkin

Regimen

Gemcitabine: I.V.: 1000 mg/m^2 over 30 minutes days 1 and 8
[total dose/cycle = 2000 mg/m^2]

Dexamethasone: Oral: 40 mg/day (divided doses) days 1 to 4
[total dose/cycle = 160 mg]

Cisplatin: I.V.: 75 mg/m^2 over 1 hour day 1, administer after gemcitabine
[total dose/cycle = 75 mg/m^2]

Repeat cycle every 21 days; consider stem cell transplantation after 2 cycles in responding patients; and a maximum of 6 cycles in nontransplant candidates

References

Baetz T, Belch A, Couban S, et al, "Gemcitabine, Dexamethasone and Cisplatin is an Active and Non-Toxic Chemotherapy Regimen in Relapsed or Refractory Hodgkin's Disease: A Phase II Study by the National Cancer Institute of Canada Clinical Trials," *Ann Oncol*, 2003, 14 (12):1762-7.

◆ **GEM-CAP (Pancreatic)** *see* Capecitabine-Gemcitabine (Pancreatic) *on page 1540*

◆ **GemCis (Pancreatic)** *see* Cisplatin-Gemcitabine (Pancreatic) *on page 1579*

Gemcitabine-Capecitabine (Biliary Cancer)

Index Terms Capecitabine-Gemcitabine (Biliary Cancer)

Use Biliary adenocarcinoma

Regimen

Gemcitabine: I.V.: 1000 mg/m^2/day over 30 minutes days 1 and 8
[total dose/cycle = 2000 mg/m^2]

Capecitabine: Oral: 650 mg/m^2 twice daily days 1 to 14
[total dose/cycle = 18,200 mg/m^2]

Repeat cycle every 21 days until disease progression or unacceptable toxicity

References

Knox JJ, Hedley D, Oza A, et al, "Combining Gemcitabine and Capecitabine in Patients With Advanced Biliary Cancer: A Phase II Trial," *J Clin Oncol*, 2005, 23(10):2332-8.

◆ **Gemcitabine-Capecitabine (Pancreatic)** *see* Capecitabine-Gemcitabine (Pancreatic) *on page 1540*

Gemcitabine-Capecitabine (RCC)

Index Terms Capecitabine-Gemcitabine (RCC)

Use Renal cell cancer

Regimen NOTE: Multiple variations are listed.

Variation 1:

Gemcitabine: I.V.: 1000 mg/m^2/day days 1, 8, and 15
[total dose/cycle = 3000 mg/m^2]

Capecitabine: Oral: 830 mg/m^2/dose twice daily on days 1 to 21
[total dose/cycle = 34,860 mg/m^2]

Repeat cycle every 28 days

Variation 2 (for patients with Cl_{cr} 30-50 mL/minute):

Gemcitabine: I.V.: 1000 mg/m^2/day days 1, 8, and 15
[total dose/cycle = 3000 mg/m^2]

Capecitabine: Oral: 622 mg/m^2/dose twice daily on days 1 to 21
[total dose/cycle = 26,124 mg/m^2]

Repeat cycle every 28 days

Variation 3:

Gemcitabine: I.V.: 1200 mg/m^2/day days 1 and 8
[total dose/cycle = 2400 mg/m^2]

Capecitabine: Oral: 1300 mg/m^2/dose twice daily on days 1 to 14
[total dose/cycle = 36,400 mg/m^2]

Repeat cycle every 21 days for up to 6 cycles

References

Variations 1 and 2:

Tannir NM, Thall PF, Ng CS, et al, "A Phase II Trial of Gemcitabine Plus Capecitabine for Metastatic Renal Cell Cancer Previously Treated With Immunotherapy and Targeted Agents," *J Urol*, 2008, 180(3):867-72.

Variation 3:

Waters JS, Moss C, Pyle L, et al, "Phase II Clinical Trial of Capecitabine and Gemcitabine Chemotherapy in Patients With Metastatic Renal Carcinoma," *Br J Cancer*, 2004, 91(10):1763-8.

Gemcitabine-Carboplatin (Bladder Cancer)

Use Bladder cancer

Regimen

Gemcitabine: I.V.: 1000 mg/m^2/day days 1 and 8
[total dose/cycle = 2000 mg/m^2]

Carboplatin: I.V.: AUC 5 day 1
[total dose/cycle = AUC = 5]
Repeat cycle every 21 days for up to 6 cycles

References

Bamias A, Moulopoulos LA, Koutras A, et al, "The Combination of Gemcitabine and Carboplatin as First-Line Treatment in Patients With Advanced Urothelial Carcinoma. A Phase II Study of the Hellenic Cooperative Oncology Group," *Cancer*, 2006, 106(2):297-303.

◆ **Gemcitabine-Carboplatin (NSCLC)** *see* Carboplatin-Gemcitabine (NSCLC) *on page 1547*

◆ **Gemcitabine-Carboplatin (Ovarian)** *see* Carboplatin-Gemcitabine (Ovarian) *on page 1548*

◆ **Gemcitabine-Carboplatin-Paclitaxel (Unknown Primary)** *see* Carboplatin-Gemcitabine-Paclitaxel (Unknown Primary) *on page 1548*

Gemcitabine-Cisplatin (Biliary Cancer)

Index Terms Cisplatin-Gemcitabine (Biliary Cancer)

Use Biliary adenocarcinoma

Regimen NOTE: Multiple variations are listed.

Variation 1:
Gemcitabine: I.V.: 1250 mg/m^2/dose days 1 and 8
[total dose/cycle = 2500 mg/m^2]
Cisplatin: I.V.: 75 mg/m^2/dose day 1
[total dose/cycle = 75 mg/m^2]
Repeat cycle every 3 weeks

Variation 2:
Gemcitabine: I.V.: 1000 mg/m^2/dose days 1 and 8
[total dose/cycle = 2000 mg/m^2]
Cisplatin: I.V.: 70 mg/m^2/dose day 1
[total dose/cycle = 70 mg/m^2]
Repeat cycle every 3 weeks (maximum: 6 cycles)

References

Variation 1:
Thongprasert S, Napapan S, Charoentum C, et al, "Phase II Study of Gemcitabine and Cisplatin as First-Line Chemotherapy in Inoperable Biliary Tract Carcinoma," *Ann Oncol*, 2005, 16(2):279-81.
Variation 2:
Doval DC, Sekhon JS, Gupta SK, et al, "A Phase II Study of Gemcitabine and Cisplatin in Chemotherapy-Naive, Unresectable Gall Bladder Cancer," *Br J Cancer*, 2004, 90(8):1516-20.

Gemcitabine-Cisplatin (Bladder Cancer)

Use Bladder cancer

Regimen

Gemcitabine: I.V.: 1000 mg/m^2/day days 1, 8, and 15
[total dose/cycle = 3000 mg/m^2]
Cisplatin: I.V.: 70 mg/m^2 day 2
[total dose/cycle = 70 mg/m^2]
Repeat cycle every 28 days for 6 cycles

References

von der Maase H, Hansen SW, Roberts JT, et al, "Gemcitabine and Cisplatin Versus Methotrexate, Vinblastine, Doxorubicin, and Cisplatin in Advanced or Metastatic Bladder Cancer: Results of a Large, Randomized, Multinational, Multicenter, Phase III Study," *J Clin Oncol*, 2000, 18 (17):3068-77.

◆ **Gemcitabine-Cisplatin (Cervical Cancer)** *see* Cisplatin-Gemcitabine (Cervical Cancer) *on page 1578*

◆ **Gemcitabine-Cisplatin (Mesothelioma)** *see* Cisplatin-Gemcitabine (Mesothelioma) *on page 1578*

Gemcitabine-Cisplatin (NSCLC)

Index Terms Cisplatin-Gemcitabine (NSCLC)

Use Lung cancer, nonsmall cell

Regimen NOTE: Multiple variations are listed.

Variation 1:

Gemcitabine: I.V.: 1000 mg/m^2/day days 1, 8, and 15
[total dose/cycle = 3000 mg/m^2]

Cisplatin: I.V.: 100 mg/m^2 day 1
[total dose/cycle = 100 mg/m^2]

Repeat cycle every 28 days

Variation 2:

Gemcitabine: I.V.: 1250 mg/m^2/day days 1 and 8
[total dose/cycle = 2500 mg/m^2]

Cisplatin: I.V.: 100 mg/m^2 day 1
[total dose/cycle = 100 mg/m^2]

Repeat cycle every 21 days

Variation 3:

Gemcitabine: I.V.: 1000 mg/m^2/day days 1 and 8
[total dose/cycle = 2000 mg/m^2]

Cisplatin: I.V.: 80 mg/m^2 day 1
[total dose/cycle = 80 mg/m^2]

Repeat cycle every 21 days

Variation 4:

Gemcitabine: I.V.: 1250 mg/m^2/day days 1 and 8
[total dose/cycle = 2500 mg/m^2]

Cisplatin: I.V.: 75 mg/m^2 day 1
[total dose/cycle = 75 mg/m^2]

Repeat cycle every 21 days for up to 6 cycles

Variation 5:

Gemcitabine: I.V.: 1000 mg/m^2/day days 1, 8, and 15
[total dose/cycle = 3000 mg/m^2]

Cisplatin: I.V.: 100 mg/m^2 day 15
[total dose/cycle = 100 mg/m^2]

Repeat cycle every 28 days

Variation 6:

Gemcitabine: I.V.: 1000 mg/m^2/day days 1, 8, and 15
[total dose/cycle = 3000 mg/m^2]

Cisplatin: I.V.: 100 mg/m^2 day 2
[total dose/cycle = 100 mg/m^2]

Repeat cycle every 28 days for 5 cycles

Variation 7:

Gemcitabine: I.V.: 1200 mg/m^2/day days 1, 8, and 15
[total dose/cycle = 3600 mg/m^2]

Cisplatin: I.V.: 100 mg/m^2 day 15
[total dose/cycle = 100 mg/m^2]

Repeat cycle every 28 days for up to 6 cycles

Variation 8 (patients ≥70 years of age):

Gemcitabine: I.V.: 1000 mg/m^2/day days 1 and 8
[total dose/cycle = 2000 mg/m^2]

Cisplatin: I.V.: 60 mg/m^2 day 1
[total dose/cycle = 60 mg/m^2]
Repeat cycle every 21 days for up to 6 cycles

References

Variation 1:
Comella P, Frasci G, Panza N, et al, "Randomized Trial Comparing Cisplatin, Gemcitabine, and Vinorelbine With Either Cisplatin and Gemcitabine or Cisplatin and Vinorelbine in Advanced Non-Small-Cell Lung Cancer: Interim Analysis of a Phase III Trial of the Southern Italy Cooperative Oncology Group," *J Clin Oncol*, 2000, 18(7):1451-7.
Sandler AB, Nemunaitis J, Denham C, et al, "Phase III Trial of Gemcitabine Plus Cisplatin Versus Cisplatin Alone in Patients With Locally Advanced or Metastatic Nonsmall-Cell Lung Cancer," *J Clin Oncol*, 2000, 18(1):122-30.
Schiller JH, Harrington D, Belani CP, et al, "Comparison of Four Chemotherapy Regimens for Advanced Non-Small-Cell Lung Cancer," *N Engl J Med*, 2002, 346(2):92-8.
Variation 2:
Cardenal F, López-Cabrerizo MP, Antón A, et al, "Randomized Phase III Study of Gemcitabine-Cisplatin Versus Etoposide-Cisplatin in the Treatment of Locally Advanced or Metastatic Non-Small-Cell Lung Cancer," *J Clin Oncol*, 1999, 17(1):12-8.
Variation 3:
Ohe Y, Ohashi Y, Kubota K, et al, "Randomized Phase III Study of Cisplatin Plus Irinotecan Versus Carboplatin Plus Paclitaxel, Cisplatin Plus Gemcitabine, and Cisplatin Plus Vinorelbine for Advanced Non-Small-Cell Lung Cancer: Four-Arm Cooperative Study in Japan," *Ann Oncol*, 2007, 18(2):317-23.
Variation 4:
Scagliotti GV, Parikh P, von Pawel J, et al, "Phase III Study Comparing Cisplatin Plus Gemcitabine With Cisplatin Plus Pemetrexed in Chemotherapy-Naive Patients With Advanced-Stage Non-Small-Cell Lung Cancer," *J Clin Oncol*, 2008, 26(21):3543-51.
Variation 5:
Abratt RP, Bezwoda WR, Goedhals L, et al, "Weekly Gemcitabine With Monthly Cisplatin: Effective Chemotherapy for Advanced Nonsmall-Cell Lung Cancer," *J Clin Oncol*, 1997, 15(2):744-9.
Variation 6:
Crino L, Scagliotti G, Marangolo M, et al, "Cisplatin-Gemcitabine Combination in Advanced Nonsmall-Cell Lung Cancer: A Phase II Study," *J Clin Oncol*, 1997, 15(1):297-303
Variation 7:
Anton A, Diaz-Fernandez N, Gonzalez Larriba JL, et al, "Phase II Trial Assessing the Combination of Gemcitabine and Cisplatin in Advanced Non-Small Cell Lung Cancer (NSCLC)," *Lung Cancer*, 1998, 22(2):139-48.
Variation 8:
Gridelli C, Maione P, Illiano A, et al, "Cisplatin Plus Gemcitabine or Vinorelbine for Elderly Patients With Advanced Non Small-Cell Lung Cancer: The MILES-2P Studies," *J Clin Oncol*, 2007, 25 (29):4663-9.

◆ **Gemcitabine-Cisplatin (Pancreatic)** *see* Cisplatin-Gemcitabine (Pancreatic) *on page 1579*

◆ **Gemcitabine-Cisplatin (Unknown Primary)** *see* Cisplatin-Gemcitabine (Unknown Primary) *on page 1580*

◆ **Gemcitabine-Dexamethasone-Cisplatin (Hodgkin)** *see* GDP (Hodgkin) *on page 1667*

Gemcitabine-Docetaxel (Sarcoma)

Use Osteosarcoma; Soft tissue sarcoma

Regimen

Gemcitabine: I.V.: 675 mg/m^2/day days 1 and 8
[total dose/cycle = 1350 mg/m^2]
Docetaxel: I.V.: 100 mg/m^2 day 8
[total dose/cycle = 100 mg/m^2]
Repeat cycle every 21 days

References

Leu KM, Ostruszka LJ, Shewach D, et al, "Laboratory and Clinical Evidence of Synergistic Cytotoxicity of Sequential Treatment With Gemcitabine Followed by Docetaxel in the Treatment of Sarcoma," *J Clin Oncol*, 2004, 22(9):1706-12.

- **Gemcitabine-Docetaxel (Unknown Primary)** *see* Docetaxel-Gemcitabine (Unknown Primary) *on page 1611*
- **Gemcitabine-Erlotinib (Pancreatic)** *see* Erlotinib-Gemcitabine (Pancreatic) *on page 1632*

Gemcitabine Fixed Dose Rate (Pancreatic Regimen)

Use Pancreatic cancer

Regimen

Gemcitabine: I.V.: 1500 mg/m^2/day over 150 minutes (10 mg/m^2/minute) days 1, 8, and 15
[total dose/cycle = 4500 mg/m^2]

Repeat cycle every 28 days until disease progression or unacceptable toxicity

References

Tempero M, Plunkett W, Ruiz van Haperen VW, et al, "Randomized Phase II Comparison of Dose-Intense Gemcitabine: Thirty-Minute Infusion and Fixed Dose Rate Infusion in Patients With Pancreatic Adenocarcinoma," *J Clin Oncol*, 2003, 21(18):3402-8.

Poplin E, Feng Y, Berlin J, et al, "Phase III, Randomized Study of Gemcitabine and Oxaliplatin Versus Gemcitabine (Fixed-Dose Rate Infusion) Compared With Gemcitabine (30-Minute Infusion) in Patients With Pancreatic Carcinoma E6201: A Trial of the Eastern Cooperative Oncology Group," *J Clin Oncol*, 2009, 27(23):3778-85.

Gemcitabine-Fluorouracil (RCC)

Index Terms Fluorouracil-Gemcitabine (RCC)

Use Renal cell cancer

Regimen

Gemcitabine: I.V.: 600 mg/m^2/day days 1, 8, and 15
[total dose/cycle = 1800 mg/m^2]

Fluorouracil: I.V.: 150 mg/m^2/day continuous infusion days 1 to 21
[total dose/cycle = 3150 mg/m^2]

Repeat cycle every 28 days for at least 2 cycles

References

Rini BI, Vogelzang NJ, Dumas MC, et al, "Phase II Trial of Weekly Intravenous Gemcitabine With Continuous Infusion Fluorouracil in Patients With Metastatic Renal Cell Cancer," *J Clin Oncol*, 2000, 18(12):2419-26.

Gemcitabine (Hodgkin Regimen)

Use Lymphoma, Hodgkin

Regimen NOTE: Multiple variations are listed.

Variation 1:

Gemcitabine: I.V.: 1250 mg/m^2/day over 30 minutes days 1, 8, and 15
[total dose/cycle = 3750 mg/m^2]

Repeat cycles every 28 days

Variation 2:

Gemcitabine: I.V.: 1200 mg/m^2/day over 30 minutes days 1, 8, and 15
[total dose/cycle = 3600 mg/m^2]

Repeat cycles every 28 days for a total of 6 cycles

Variation 3:

Cycle 1:

Gemcitabine: I.V.: 1000 mg/m^2/day over 30 minutes weekly for 7 weeks, followed by one week rest
[total dose/cycle = 7000 mg/m^2]

Treatment cycle is 8 weeks

Subsequent Cycles:

Gemcitabine: I.V.: 1000 mg/m^2/day over 30 minutes days 1, 8, and 15
[total dose/cycle = 3000 mg/m^2]

Repeat cycle every 28 days until disease progression or drug intolerance

References

Variation 1:

Santoro A, Bredenfeld H, Devizzi L, et al, "Gemcitabine in the Treatment of Refractory Hodgkin's Disease: Results of a Multicenter Phase II Study," *J Clin Oncol*, 2000, 18(13):2615-9.

Variation 2:

Zinzani PL, Bendandi M, Stefoni V, et al, "Value of Gemcitabine Treatment in Heavily Pretreated Hodgkin's Disease Patients," *Haematologica*, 2000, 85(9):926-9.

Variation 3:

Savage DG, Rule SA, Tighe M, et al, "Gemcitabine for Relapsed or Resistant Lymphoma," *Ann of Oncol*, 2000, 11(5):595-7.

Gemcitabine (Mesothelioma Regimen)

Use Malignant pleural mesothelioma

Regimen

Gemcitabine: I.V.: 1250 mg/m^2/day over 30 minutes days 1, 8, and 15
[total dose/cycle = 3750 mg/m^2]

Repeat cycle every 28 days for up to a total of 10 cycles

References

van Meerbeeck JP, Baas P, Debruyne C, et al, "A Phase II Study of Gemcitabine in Patients With Malignant Pleural Mesothelioma," *Cancer*, 1999, 85(12):2577-82.

◆ **Gemcitabine-nab Paclitaxel (Pancreatic)** *see* Gemcitabine-Paclitaxel (Protein Bound) (Pancreatic) *on page* 1675

Gemcitabine (Ovarian Regimen)

Use Ovarian cancer

Regimen NOTE: Multiple variations are listed.

Variation 1:

Gemcitabine: I.V.: 1000 mg/m^2/dose over 30-60 minutes days 1 and 8
[total dose/cycle = 2000 mg/m^2]

Repeat cycle every 21 days until disease progression or unacceptable toxicity

Variation 2:

Gemcitabine: I.V.: 1000 mg/m^2/dose over 30 minutes days 1, 8, and 15
[total dose/cycle = 3000 mg/m^2]

Repeat cycle every 28 days until disease progression or unacceptable toxicity

References

Variation 1:

Mutch DG, Orlando M, Goss T, et al, "Randomized Phase III Trial of Gemcitabine Compared With Pegylated Liposomal Doxorubicin in Patients With Platinum-Resistant Ovarian Cancer," *J Clin Oncol*, 2007, 25(19):2811-8.

Variation 2:

Ferrandina G, Ludovisi M, Lorusso D, et al, "Phase III Trial of Gemcitabine Compared With Pegylated Liposomal Doxorubicin in Progressive or Recurrent Ovarian Cancer," *J Clin Oncol*, 2008, 26(6):890-6.

Gemcitabine-Oxaliplatin-Paclitaxel (Testicular)

Index Terms GOP (Testicular); Oxaliplatin-Gemcitabine-Paclitaxel (Testicular); Paclitaxel-Gemcitabine-Oxaliplatin (Testicular)

Use Testicular cancer

Regimen

Gemcitabine: I.V.: 800 mg/m^2/day over 30 minutes days 1 and 8
[total dose/cycle = 1600 mg/m^2]

Paclitaxel: I.V.: 80 mg/m^2/day over 1 hour days 1 and 8
[total dose/cycle = 160 mg/m^2]

Oxaliplatin: I.V.: 130 mg/m^2 over 2 hours day 1
[total dose/cycle = 130 mg/m^2]

Repeat cycle every 21 days for 2 cycles beyond best response, maximum of 8 cycles

References

Bokemeyer C, Oechsle K, Honecker F, et al, "Combination Chemotherapy With Gemcitabine, Oxaliplatin, and Paclitaxel in Patients With Cisplatin-Refractory or Multiply Relapsed Germ-Cell Tumors: A Study of the German Testicular Cancer Study Group," *Ann Oncol*, 2008, 19(3):448-53.

Gemcitabine-Oxaliplatin (Pancreatic)

Index Terms GEMOX (Pancreatic); Oxaliplatin-Gemcitabine (Pancreatic)

Use Pancreatic cancer

Regimen

Gemcitabine: I.V.: 1000 mg/m^2 over 100 minutes (10 mg/m^2/minute) day 1
[total dose/cycle = 1000 mg/m^2]

Oxaliplatin: I.V.: 100 mg/m^2 over 2 hours day 2
[total dose/cycle = 100 mg/m^2]

Repeat cycle every 14 days until disease progression or unacceptable toxicity

References

Demols A, Peeters M, Polus M, et al, "Gemcitabine and Oxaliplatin (GEMOX) in Gemcitabine Refractory Advanced Pancreatic Adenocarcinoma: A Phase II Study," *Br J Cancer*, 2006, 94 (4):481-5.

Louvet C, Labianca R, Hammel P, et al, "Gemcitabine in Combination With Oxaliplatin Compared With Gemcitabine Alone in Locally Advanced or Metastatic Pancreatic Cancer: Results of a GERCOR and GISCAD Phase III Trial," *J Clin Oncol*, 2005, 23(15):3509-16.

Poplin E, Feng Y, Berlin J, et al, "Phase III, Randomized Study of Gemcitabine and Oxaliplatin Versus Gemcitabine (Fixed-Dose Rate Infusion) Compared With Gemcitabine (30-Minute Infusion) in Patients With Pancreatic Carcinoma E6201: A Trial of the Eastern Cooperative Oncology Group," *J Clin Oncol*, 2009, 27(23):3778-85.

Gemcitabine-Oxaliplatin-Rituximab (NHL)

Index Terms GEMOX-R (NHL); Oxaliplatin-Gemcitabine-Rituximab (NHL)

Use Lymphoma, non-Hodgkin's

Regimen

Oxaliplatin: I.V.: 100 mg/m^2/dose day 1
[total dose/cycle = 100 mg/m^2]

Gemcitabine: I.V.: 1000 mg/m^2/dose day 1
[total dose/cycle = 1000 mg/m^2]

Rituximab: I.V.: 375 mg/m^2/dose day 1
[total dose/cycle = 375 mg/m^2]

Repeat cycle every 3 weeks (for a total of 6-8 cycles)

References

López A, Gutiérrez A, Palacios A, et al, "GEMOX-R Regimen is a Highly Effective Salvage Regimen in Patients With Refractory/Relapsing Diffuse Large-Cell Lymphoma: A Phase II Study," *Eur J Haematol*, 2008, 80(2):127-32.

Rodríguez J, Gutierrez A, Palacios A, et al, "Rituximab, Gemcitabine and Oxaliplatin: An Effective Regimen in Patients With Refractory and Relapsing Mantle Cell Lymphoma," *Leuk Lymphoma*, 2007, 48(11):2172-8.

- **Gemcitabine-Oxaliplatin (Testicular)** *see* GEMOX (Testicular) *on page 1678*
- **Gemcitabine-Paclitaxel** *see* Paclitaxel-Gemcitabine *on page 1729*

Gemcitabine-Paclitaxel (Breast Cancer)

Index Terms Paclitaxel-Gemcitabine (Breast Cancer)

Use Breast cancer

Regimen

Paclitaxel: I.V.: 175 mg/m^2 (infused over 3 hours) day 1
[total dose/cycle = 175 mg/m^2]

Gemcitabine: I.V.: 1250 mg/m^2/day days 1 and 8
[total dose/cycle = 2500 mg/m^2]

Repeat cycle every 21 days until disease progression or unacceptable toxicity

References

Albain KS, Nag SM, Calderillo-Ruiz G, et al, "Gemcitabine Plus Paclitaxel Versus Paclitaxel Monotherapy in Patients With Metastatic Breast Cancer and Prior Anthracycline Treatment," *J Clin Oncol*, 2008, 26(24):3950-7.

Gemcitabine-Paclitaxel (Ovarian Cancer)

Index Terms Paclitaxel-Gemcitabine (Ovarian Cancer)

Use Ovarian cancer

Regimen

Paclitaxel: I.V.: 110 mg/m^2/dose over 1 hour days 1, 8, and 15
[total dose/cycle = 330 mg/m^2]

Gemcitabine: I.V.: 1000 mg/m^2/dose days 1, 8, and 15
[total dose/cycle = 3000 mg/m^2]

Repeat cycle every 4 weeks for a maximum of 6 cycles

References

Hinton S, Catalano P, Einhorn LH, et al, "Phase II Study of Paclitaxel Plus Gemcitabine in Refractory Germ Cell Tumors (E9897): A Trial of the Eastern Cooperative Oncology Group," *J Clin Oncol*, 2002, 20(7):1859-63.

Gemcitabine-Paclitaxel (Protein Bound) (Pancreatic)

Index Terms Gemcitabine-nab Paclitaxel (Pancreatic); Paclitaxel (Protein Bound)-Gemcitabine (Pancreatic)

Use Pancreatic cancer

Regimen

Gemcitabine: I.V.: 1000 mg/m^2/day days 1, 8, and 15
[total dose/cycle = 3000 mg/m^2]

Paclitaxel (Protein Bound): I.V.: 125 mg/m^2/day days 1, 8, and 15
[total dose/cycle = 375 mg/m^2]

Repeat cycle every 28 days until disease progression or unacceptable toxicity

References

Von Hoff DD, Ramanathan RK, Borad MJ, et al, "Gemcitabine Plus Nab-Paclitaxel Is an Active Regimen in Patients With Advanced Pancreatic Cancer: A Phase I/II Trial," *J Clin Oncol*, 2011, 29 (34):4548-54.

Gemcitabine-Paclitaxel (Testicular)

Index Terms Paclitaxel-Gemcitabine (Testicular)

Use Testicular cancer

Regimen

Paclitaxel: I.V.: 100 mg/m^2/day over 1 hour days 1, 8, and 15 [total dose/cycle = 300 mg/m^2]

Gemcitabine: I.V.: 1000 mg/m^2/day over 30 minutes days 1, 8, and 15 [total dose/cycle = 3000 mg/m^2]

Repeat cycle every 28 days for a maximum of 6 cycles

References

Einhorn LH, Brames MJ, Juliar B, et al, "Phase II Study of Paclitaxel Plus Gemcitabine Salvage Chemotherapy for Germ Cell Tumors After Progression Following High-Dose Chemotherapy With Tandem Transplant," *J Clin Oncol*, 2007, 25(5):513-6.

Mulherin BP, Brames MJ, Einhorn LH, at el, "Long-Term Survival With Paclitaxel and Gemcitabine for Germ Cell Tumors After Progression Following High-Dose Chemotherapy With Tandem Transplants," *J Clin Oncol*, 2011, 29:4562 [abstract 4562 from 2011 ASCO Annual Meeting].

Gemcitabine (Small Cell Lung Cancer Regimen)

Use Lung cancer, small cell

Regimen NOTE: Multiple variations are listed.

Variation 1:

Gemcitabine: I.V.: 1000 mg/m^2/day over 30 minutes days 1, 8, and 15 [total dose/cycle = 3000 mg/m^2]

Repeat cycle every 28 days

Variation 2:

Gemcitabine: I.V.: 1250 mg/m^2/day over 30 minutes days 1 and 8 [total dose/cycle = 2500 mg/m^2]

Repeat cycle every 21 days

References

Variation1:

Masters GA, Declerck L, Blanke C, et al, "Phase II Trial of Gemcitabine in Refractory or Relapsed Small-Cell Lung Cancer: Eastern Cooperative Oncology Group Trial 1597," *J Clin Oncol*, 2003, 21(8):1550-5.

van der Lee I, Smit EF, van Putten JWG, et al, "Single-Agent Gemcitabine in Patients With Resistant Small-Cell Lung Cancer," *Ann Oncol*, 2001, 12(4):557-61.

Variation 2:

Hoang T, Kim K, Jaslowski A, et al, "Phase II Study of Second-Line Gemcitabine in Sensitive or Refractory Small Cell Lung Cancer," *Lung Cancer*, 2003, 42(1):97-102.

Gemcitabine Standard Infusion (Pancreatic Regimen)

Use Pancreatic cancer

Regimen NOTE: Multiple variations are listed.

Variation 1: (advanced)

Cycle 1:

Gemcitabine: I.V.: 1000 mg/m^2/day over 30 minutes days 1, 8, 15, 22, 29, 36, and 43 (cycle 1 only) [total dose/cycle 1 = 7000 mg/m^2]

Treatment cycle is 56 days

Subsequent cycles:

Gemcitabine: I.V.: 1000 mg/m^2/day over 30 minutes days 1, 8, and 15 [total dose/cycle = 3000 mg/m^2]

Repeat cycle every 28 days until disease progression or unacceptable toxicity

Variation 2: (adjuvant)

Gemcitabine: I.V.: 1000 mg/m^2/day over 30 minutes days 1, 8, and 15 [total dose/cycle = 3000 mg/m^2]

Repeat cycle every 28 days until for 6 cycles

References

Variation 1:

Burris HA 3rd, Moore MJ, Andersen J, et al, "Improvements in Survival and Clinical Benefit With Gemcitabine as First-Line Therapy for Patients With Advanced Pancreas Cancer: A Randomized Trial," *J Clin Oncol*, 1997, 15(6):2403-13.

Variation 2:

Neoptolemos JP, Stocken DD, Bassi C, et al, "Adjuvant Chemotherapy With Fluorouracil Plus Folinic Acid Vs Gemcitabine Following Pancreatic Cancer Resection: A Randomized Controlled Trial," *JAMA*, 2010, 304(10):1073-81.

Oettle H, Post S, Neuhaus P, et al, "Adjuvant Chemotherapy With Gemcitabine Vs Observation in Patients Undergoing Curative-Intent Resection of Pancreatic Cancer: A Randomized Controlled Trial," *JAMA*, 2007, 297(3):267-77.

◆ **Gemcitabine-Vinorelbine-Doxorubicin (Liposomal) (Hodgkin)** *see* GVD (Hodgkin) *on page 1679*

Gemcitabine-Vinorelbine (NSCLC)

Index Terms Vinorelbine-Gemcitabine (NSCLC)

Use Lung cancer, nonsmall cell

Regimen NOTE: Multiple variations are listed.

Variation 1:

Gemcitabine: I.V.: 1200 mg/m^2/day days 1 and 8 [total dose/cycle = 2400 mg/m^2]

Vinorelbine: I.V.: 30 mg/m^2/day days 1 and 8 [total dose/cycle = 60 mg/m^2]

Repeat cycle every 21 days for 6 cycles

Variation 2:

Gemcitabine: I.V.: 1000 mg/m^2/day days 1, 8, and 15 [total dose/cycle = 3000 mg/m^2]

Vinorelbine: I.V.: 20 mg/m^2/day days 1, 8, and 15 [total dose/cycle = 60 mg/m^2]

Repeat cycle every 28 days for a maximum of 6 cycles

Variation 3:

Gemcitabine: I.V.: 800 mg/m^2/day days 1, 8, and 15 [total dose/cycle = 2400 mg/m^2]

Vinorelbine: I.V.: 20 mg/m^2/day days 1, 8, and 15 [total dose/cycle = 60 mg/m^2]

Repeat cycle every 28 days for up to 6 cycles

References

Variation 1:

Frasci G, Lorusso V, Panza N, et al, "Gemcitabine Plus Vinorelbine Versus Vinorelbine Alone in Elderly Patients With Advanced Non-Small-Cell Lung Cancer," *J Clin Oncol*, 2000, 18 (13):2529-36.

Variation 2:

Hainsworth JD, Burris HA 3rd, Litchy S, et al, "Gemcitabine and Vinorelbine in the Second-Line Treatment of Nonsmall Cell Lung Carcinoma Patients: A Minnie Pearl Cancer Research Network Phase II Trial," *Cancer*, 2000, 88(6):1353-8.

Variation 3:

Chen YM, Perng RP, Yang KY, et al, "A Multicenter Phase II Trial of Vinorelbine Plus Gemcitabine in Previously Untreated Inoperable (Stage IIIB/IV) Non-Small-Cell Lung Cancer," *Chest*, 2000, 117(6):1583-9.

Gemcitabine-Vinorelbine (Sarcoma)

Index Terms Vinorelbine-Gemcitabine (Sarcoma)

Use Soft tissue sarcoma

Regimen NOTE: Multiple variations are listed.

Variation 1:
Vinorelbine: I.V.: 25 mg/m^2/dose over 10 minutes days 1 and 8 [total dose/cycle = 50 mg/m^2]
Gemcitabine: I.V.: 800 mg/m^2/dose over 90 minutes days 1 and 8 [total dose/cycle = 1600 mg/m^2]
Repeat cycle every 21 days until disease progression or unacceptable toxicity
Variation 2 (modification for toxicity):
Vinorelbine: I.V.: 25 mg/m^2/dose over 10 minutes days 1 and 15 [total dose/cycle = 50 mg/m^2]
Gemcitabine: I.V.: 800 mg/m^2/dose over 90 minutes days 1 and 15 [total dose/cycle = 1600 mg/m^2]
Repeat cycle every 28 days until disease progression or unacceptable toxicity

References

Variations 1 and 2:
Dileo P, Morgan JA, Zahrieh D, et al, "Gemcitabine and Vinorelbine Combination Chemotherapy for Patients With Advanced Soft Tissue Sarcomas: Results of a Phase II Trial," *Cancer*, 2007, 109 (9):1863-9.

GEMOX (Biliary Cancer)

Use Biliary adenocarcinoma

Regimen

Gemcitabine: I.V.: 1000 mg/m^2 day 1 [total dose/cycle = 1000 mg/m^2]
Oxaliplatin: I.V.: 100 mg/m^2 day 2 [total dose/cycle = 100 mg/m^2]
Repeat cycle every 2 weeks

References

Andre T, Tournigand C, Rosmorduc O, et al, "Gemcitabine Combined With Oxaliplatin (GEMOX) in Advanced Biliary Tract Adenocarcinoma: A GERCOR Study," *Ann Oncol*, 2004, 15(9):1339-43.

◆ **GEMOX (Pancreatic)** *see* Gemcitabine-Oxaliplatin (Pancreatic) *on page 1674*

◆ **GEMOX-R (NHL)** *see* Gemcitabine-Oxaliplatin-Rituximab (NHL) *on page 1674*

GEMOX (Testicular)

Index Terms Gemcitabine-Oxaliplatin (Testicular); Oxaliplatin-Gemcitabine (Testicular)

Use Testicular cancer

Regimen NOTE: Multiple variations are listed.

Variation 1:
Gemcitabine: I.V.: 1000 mg/m^2/day over 30 minutes days 1 and 8 [total dose/cycle = 2000 mg/m^2]
Oxaliplatin: I.V.: 130 mg/m^2 over 2 hours day 1 [total dose/cycle = 130 mg/m^2]
Repeat cycle every 21 days for a total of at least 2 cycles (maximum: 6 cycles)
Variation 2:
Gemcitabine: I.V.: 1250 mg/m^2/day over 30 minutes days 1 and 8 [total dose/cycle = 2500 mg/m^2]

Oxaliplatin: I.V.: 130 mg/m² over 2 hours day 1
[total dose/cycle = 130 mg/m²]
Repeat cycle every 21 days for a maximum of 6 cycles

References

Variation 1:
Kollmannsberger C, Beyer J, Liersch R, et al, "Combination Chemotherapy With Gemcitabine Plus Oxaliplatin in Patients With Intensively Pretreated or Refractory Germ Cell Cancer: A Study of the German Testicular Cancer Study Group," *J Clin Oncol*, 2004, 22(1):108-14.
Pectasides D, Pectasides M, Farmakis D, et al, "Gemcitabine and Oxaliplatin (GEMOX) in Patients With Cisplatin-Refractory Germ Cell Tumors: A Phase II Study," *Ann Oncol*, 2004, 15(3):493-7.
Variation 2:
De Giorgi U, Rosti G, Aieta M, et al, "Phase II Study of Oxaliplatin and Gemcitabine Salvage Chemotherapy in Patients With Cisplatin-Refractory Nonseminomatous Germ Cell Tumor," *Eur Urol*, 2006, 50(5):1032-8.

◆ **GOP (Testicular)** *see* Gemcitabine-Oxaliplatin-Paclitaxel (Testicular) *on page 1674*

◆ **Goserelin-Bicalutamide** *see* Bicalutamide-Goserelin *on page 1533*

GVD (Hodgkin)

Index Terms Gemcitabine-Vinorelbine-Doxorubicin (Liposomal) (Hodgkin)
Use Lymphoma, Hodgkin
Regimen NOTE: Multiple variations are listed.

Variation 1 (for transplant-naive patients):
Vinorelbine: I.V.: 20 mg/m²/day over 6-10 minutes days 1 and 8
[total dose/cycle = 40 mg/m²]
Gemcitabine: I.V.: 1000 mg/m²/day over 30 minutes days 1 and 8
[total dose/cycle = 2000 mg/m²]
Doxorubicin liposomal: I.V.: 15 mg/m²/day over 30-60 minutes days 1 and 8
[total dose/cycle = 30 mg/m²]
Repeat cycle every 21 days for a total of 2 to 6 cycles

Variation 2 (for patients with prior transplant):
Vinorelbine: I.V.: 15 mg/m²/day over 6-10 minutes days 1 and 8
[total dose/cycle = 30 mg/m²]
Gemcitabine: I.V.: 800 mg/m²/day over 30 minutes days 1 and 8
[total dose/cycle = 1600 mg/m²]
Doxorubicin liposomal: I.V.: 10 mg/m²/day over 30-60 minutes days 1 and 8
[total dose/cycle = 20 mg/m²]
Repeat cycle every 21 days for a total of 2 to 6 cycles

References

Variations 1 and 2:
Bartlett NL, Niedzwiecki D, Johnson JL, et al, "Gemcitabine, Vinorelbine, and Pegylated Liposomal Doxorubicin (GVD), A Salvage Regimen in Relapsed Hodgkin's Lymphoma: CALGB 59804," *Ann Oncol*, 2007, 18(6):1071-9.

◆ **HDAC-Daunorubicin (AML Induction)** *see* Cytarabine (High Dose)-Daunorubicin (AML Induction) *on page 1602*

◆ **HD Cytarabine (Single Agent AML Induction)** *see* Cytarabine (High-Dose Single-Agent AML Induction Regimen) *on page 1603*

HDMTX

Use Osteosarcoma
Regimen

Methotrexate: I.V.: 12 g/m²/week for 2-12 weeks
[total dose/cycle = 24-144 g/m²]

Leucovorin calcium rescue: Oral, I.V.: 15 mg/m^2 every 6 hours (beginning 30 hours after the beginning of the 4-hour methotrexate infusion) for 10 doses; **serum methotrexate levels must be monitored**
[total dose/cycle = 150 mg/m^2]

References

Camitta BM and Holcenberg JS, "Safety of Delayed Leucovorin 'Rescue' Following High-Dose Methotrexate in Children," *Med Pediatr Oncol*, 1978, 5(1):55-9.

◆ **HIDAC-3-7 (AML Induction)** *see* Cytarabine (High Dose)-Daunorubicin-Etoposide (AML Induction) *on page 1602*

◆ **HIDAC-Daunorubicin (AML Induction)** *see* Cytarabine (High Dose)-Daunorubicin (AML Induction) *on page 1602*

◆ **HIDAC (Single Agent AML Induction)** *see* Cytarabine (High-Dose Single-Agent AML Induction Regimen) *on page 1603*

Hydroxyurea (AML Regimen)

Use Leukemia, acute myeloid

Regimen

Hydroxyurea: Oral: 25 mg/kg/dose 4 times/day for a maximum of 30 days
[total maximum dose/cycle = 3000 mg/kg]

Administer treatment until achievement of bone marrow aplasia, for a maximum of 30 days

References

Petti MC, Tafuri A, Latagliata R, et al, "High-Dose Hydroxyurea in the Treatment of Poor-Risk Myeloid Leukemias," *Ann Hematol*, 2003, 82(8):476-80.

◆ **Hydroxyurea-Fluorouracil (Head and Neck Cancer)** *see* Fluorouracil-Hydroxyurea (Head and Neck Cancer) *on page 1653*

Hyper-CVAD + Imatinib

Use Leukemia, acute lymphocytic

Regimen

Cycle A: (Cycles 1, 3, 5, and 7)

Imatinib: Oral: 400 mg/day days 1 to 14
[total dose/cycle = 5600 mg]

Cyclophosphamide: I.V.: 300 mg/m^2 every 12 hours, for 6 doses, days 1, 2, and 3
[total dose/cycle = 1800 mg/m^2]

Mesna: I.V. 600 mg/m^2/day continuous infusion days 1, 2, and 3
[total dose/cycle = 1800 mg/m^2]

Vincristine: I.V.: 2 mg/day days 4 and 11
[total dose/cycle = 4 mg]

Doxorubicin: I.V.: 50 mg/m^2/day continuous infusion day 4
[total dose/cycle = 50 mg/m^2]

Dexamethasone: Oral, I.V.: 40 mg/day days 1 to 4 and 11 to 14
[total dose/cycle = 320 mg]

Cycle B: (Cycles 2, 4, 6, and 8)

Imatinib: Oral: 400 mg/day days 1 to 14
[total dose/cycle = 5600 mg]

Methotrexate: I.V.: 1 g/m^2/day continuous infusion day 1
[total dose/cycle = 1 g/m^2]

Leucovorin: I.V.: 50 mg then 15 mg every 6 hours, for 8 doses (start 12 hours after the end of the methotrexate infusion)
[total dose/cycle = 170 mg]

Cytarabine: I.V.: 3 g/m^2 every 12 hours for 4 doses, days 2 and 3
[total dose/cycle = 12 g/m^2]
Repeat every 6 weeks in the following sequence: ABABABAB
CNS Prophylaxis
Methotrexate: I.T.: 12 mg/day day 2
[total dose/cycle = 12 mg/day]
or 6 mg into Ommaya day 2
[total dose/cycle = 6 mg/day]
Cytarabine: I.T.: 100 mg/day day 7 or 8
[total dose/cycle = 100 mg/day]
Repeat cycle every 3 weeks for 3 or 4 cycles
Maintenance (POMP)
Imatinib: Oral: 600 mg/day
[total dose/cycle = 18,000 mg]
Vincristine: I.V.: 2 mg/day day 1
[total dose/cycle = 2 mg]
Prednisone: Oral: 200 mg/day days 1 to 5
[total dose/cycle = 1000 mg/m^2]
Repeat cycle every month (except months 6 and 13) for 13 months
Intensification
Imatinib: Oral: 400 mg/day days 1 to 14
[total dose/cycle = 5600 mg]
Cyclophosphamide: I.V.: 300 mg/m^2 every 12 hours, for 6 doses, days 1, 2, and 3
[total dose/cycle = 1800 mg/m^2]
Mesna: I.V.: 600 mg/m^2/day continuous infusion days 1, 2, and 3
[total dose/cycle = 1800 mg/m^2]
Vincristine: I.V.: 2 mg/day days 4 and 11
[total dose/cycle = 4 mg]
Doxorubicin: 50 mg/m^2/day continuous infusion day 4
[total dose/cycle = 50 mg/m^2]
Dexamethasone: I.V. or Oral: 40 mg/day days 1 to 4 and 11 to 14
[total dose/cycle = 320 mg]
Cycle is given in months 6 and 13 during maintenance

References

Thomas DA, Faderl S, Cortes J, et al, "Treatment of Philadelphia Chromosome-Positive Acute Lymphocytic Leukemia With Hyper-CVAD and Imatinib Mesylate," *Blood*, 2004, 103 (12):4396-407.

Hyper-CVAD (Leukemia, Acute Lymphocytic)

Use Leukemia, acute lymphocytic
Regimen NOTE: Multiple variations are listed.
Variation 1:
Cycle A: (Cycles 1, 3, 5, and 7)
Cyclophosphamide: I.V.: 300 mg/m^2 every 12 hours, for 6 doses, days 1, 2, and 3
[total dose/cycle = 1800 mg/m^2]
Mesna: I.V.: 1200 mg/m^2/day continuous infusion days 1, 2, and 3
[total dose/cycle = 3600 mg/m^2]
Vincristine: I.V.: 2 mg/day days 4 and 11
[total dose/cycle = 4 mg]
Doxorubicin: I.V.: 50 mg/m^2 day 4
[total dose/cycle = 50 mg/m^2]

Dexamethasone: (route not specified): 40 mg/day days 1 to 4 and 11 to 14
[total dose/cycle = 320 mg]
Cycle B: (Cycles 2, 4, 6, and 8)
Methotrexate: I.V.: 1 g/m^2 continuous infusion day 1
[total dose/cycle = 1g/m^2]
Leucovorin: (route not specified): 15 mg every 6 hours, for 8 doses (start 12 hours after end of methotrexate infusion)
[total dose/cycle = 120 mg]
Cytarabine: I.V.: 3 g/m^2 every 12 hours, for 4 doses, days 2 and 3
[total dose/cycle = 12 g/m^2]
Methylprednisolone: I.V.: 50 mg twice daily, for 6 doses, days 1, 2, and 3
[total dose/cycle = 300 mg/m^2]
Repeat every 6 weeks in the following sequence: ABABABAB

CNS Prophylaxis

Methotrexate: I.T.: 12 mg/day day 2
[total dose/cycle = 12 mg]
or 6 mg/day into Ommaya day 2
[total dose/cycle = 6 mg]
Cytarabine: I.T: 100 mg day 8
[total dose/cycle = 100 mg]
Repeat cycle every 3 weeks

Maintenance (POMP)

Mercaptopurine: Oral: 50 mg 3 times/day
[total dose/cycle = 4200-4650 mg]
Vincristine: I.V.: 2 mg day 1
[total dose/cycle = 2 mg]
Methotrexate: Oral: 20 mg/m^2/day days 1, 8, 15, and 22
[total dose/cycle = 80 mg/m^2]
Prednisone: Oral: 200 mg/day days 1 to 5
[total dose/cycle = 1000 mg/m^2]
or
Mercaptopurine: I.V.: 1 g/m^2/day days 1 to 5
[total dose/cycle = 5 g/m^2]
Vincristine: I.V.: 2 mg day 1
[total dose/cycle = 2 mg]
Methotrexate: I.V.: 10 mg/m^2/day days 1 to 5
[total dose/cycle = 50 mg/m^2]
Prednisone: Oral: 200 mg/day days 1 to 5
[total dose/cycle = 1000 mg/m^2]
Repeat cycles every month for 2 years

Variation 2:
Cycle A: (Cycles 1, 3, 5, and 7)
Cyclophosphamide: I.V.: 300 mg/m^2 every 12 hours, for 6 doses, days 1, 2, and 3
[total dose/cycle = 1800 mg/m^2]
Mesna: I.V.: 600 mg/m^2/day continuous infusion days 1, 2, and 3
[total dose/cycle = 1800 mg/m^2]
Vincristine: I.V.: 2 mg/day days 4 and 11
[total dose/cycle = 4 mg]
Doxorubicin: I.V.: 50 mg/m^2 day 4
[total dose/cycle = 50 mg/m^2]
Dexamethasone: Oral, I.V.: 40 mg/day days 1 to 4 and 11 to 14
[total dose/cycle = 320 mg]

Cycle B: (Cycles 2, 4, 6, and 8)
Methotrexate: I.V.: 1 g/m^2 continuous infusion day 1
[total dose/cycle = 1 g/m^2]
Leucovorin: I.V.: 50 mg (start 12 hours after end of methotrexate infusion)
followed by I.V.: 15 mg every 6 hours, for 8 doses
[total dose/cycle = 170 mg]
Cytarabine: I.V.: 3 g/m^2 every 12 hours, for 4 doses, days 2 and 3
[total dose/cycle = 12 g/m^2]
Repeat every 6 weeks in the following sequence: ABABABAB

CNS Prophylaxis
Methotrexate: I.T.: 12 mg day 2
[total dose/cycle = 12 mg]
or 6 mg into Ommaya day 2
[total dose/cycle = 6 mg]
Cytarabine: I.T.: 100 mg day 7
[total dose/cycle = 100 mg]
Repeat cycle every 3 weeks

Variation 3:
Cycle A: (Cycles 1, 3, 5, and 7)
Cyclophosphamide: I.V.: 300 mg/m^2 every 12 hours, for 6 doses, days 1, 2, and 3
[total dose/cycle = 1800 mg/m^2]
Mesna: I.V.: 600 mg/m^2/day continuous infusion days 1, 2, and 3
[total dose/cycle = 1800 mg/m^2]
Vincristine: I.V.: 2 mg/day days 4 and 11
[total dose/cycle = 4 mg]
Doxorubicin: I.V.: 50 mg/m^2 continuous infusion day 4
[total dose/cycle = 50 mg/m^2]
Dexamethasone: Oral, I.V.: 40 mg/day days 1 to 4 and 11 to 14
[total dose/cycle = 320 mg]
Cycle B: (Cycles 2, 4, 6, and 8)
Methotrexate: I.V.: 200 mg/m^2 day 1
followed by I.V.: 800 mg/m^2 continuous infusion day 1
[total dose/cycle = 1 g/m^2]
Leucovorin: I.V.: 50 mg (start 12 hours after end of methotrexate infusion)
followed by I.V.: 15 mg every 6 hours, for 8 doses
[total dose/cycle = 170 mg/m^2]
Cytarabine: I.V.: 3 g/m^2 every 12 hours, for 4 doses, days 2 and 3
[total dose/cycle = 12 g/m^2]
Repeat every 6 weeks in the following sequence: ABABABAB

CNS Prophylaxis
Methotrexate: I.T.: 12 mg day 2
[total dose/cycle = 12 mg]
or 6 mg into Ommaya day 2
[total dose/cycle = 6 mg]
Cytarabine: I.T.: 100 mg day 7 **or** 8
[total dose/cycle = 100 mg]
Repeat cycles every 3 weeks for 6 or 8 cycles

Maintenance (POMP)
Mercaptopurine: Oral: 50 mg 3 times/day
[total dose/cycle = 4200-4650 mg]
Vincristine: I.V.: 2 mg day 1
[total dose/cycle = 2 mg]

Methotrexate: Oral, I V: 20 mg/m^2/ day days 1, 8, 15, and 22
[total dose/cycle = 80 mg/m^2]
Prednisone: Oral: 200 mg/day days 1 to 5
[total dose/cycle = 1000 mg/m^2]
or
Mercaptopurine: I.V.: 1 g/m^2/day days 1 to 5
[total dose/cycle = 5 g/m^2]
Vincristine: I.V.: 2 mg day 1
[total dose/cycle = 2 mg]
Methotrexate: I.V.: 10 mg/m^2/day days 1 to 5
[total dose/cycle = 50 mg/m^2]
Prednisone: Oral: 200 mg/day days 1 to 5
[total dose/cycle = 1000 mg]
Repeat cycles every month (except months 7 and 11 or 9 and 12) for 2 years

Intensification
Etoposide: I.V.: 100 mg/m^2/day days 1 to 5
[total dose/cycle = 500 mg/m^2]
Pegaspargase: I.V.: 2500 units/m^2 day 1
[total dose/cycle = 2500 units/m^2]
Given during months 9 and 12 of maintenance
or
Methotrexate: I.V.: 100 mg/m^2/day days 1, 8, 15, and 22
[total dose/cycle = 400 mg/m^2]
Asparaginase: I.V.: 20,000 units/day days 2, 9, 16, and 23
[total dose/cycle = 80,000 units]
Given during months 7 and 11 of maintenance

Variation 4:
Cycle A: (Cycles 1, 3, 5, and 7)
Cyclophosphamide: I.V.: 300 mg/m^2 every 12 hours, for 6 doses, days 1, 2, and 3
[total dose/cycle = 1800 mg/m^2]
Mesna: I.V.: 600 mg/m^2/day continuous infusion days 1, 2, and 3
[total dose/cycle = 1800 mg/m^2]
Vincristine: I.V.: 2 mg/day days 4 and 11
[total dose/cycle = 4 mg]
Doxorubicin: I.V.: 50 mg/m^{2}day 4
[total dose/cycle = 50 mg/m^2]
Dexamethasone: (route not specified): 40 mg/day days 1 to 4 and 11 to 14
[total dose/cycle = 320 mg]
Cycle B: (Cycles 2, 4, 6, and 8)
Methotrexate: I.V.: 200 mg/m^2 day 1
followed by I.V.: 800 mg/m^2 continuous infusion day 1
[total dose/cycle = 1 g/m^2]
Leucovorin: (route not specified): 15 mg every 6 hours, for 8 doses (start 24 hours after end of methotrexate infusion)
[total dose/cycle = 120 mg]
Cytarabine: I.V.: 3 g/m^2 every 12 hours, for 4 doses, days 2 and 3
[total dose/cycle = 12 g/m^2]
Repeat every 6 weeks in the following sequence: ABABABAB

CNS Prophylaxis
Methotrexate: I.T.: 12 mg day 2
[total dose/cycle = 12 mg]

Cytarabine: I.T.: 100 mg day 8
[total dose/cycle = 100 mg]
Repeat cycle every 3 weeks for 4 or 8 cycles

Maintenance (POMP)

Mercaptopurine: Oral: 50 mg 3 times/day
[total dose/cycle = 4200-4650 mg]
Vincristine: I.V.: 2 mg day 1
[total dose/cycle = 2 mg]
Methotrexate: Oral: 20 mg/m^2/day days 1, 8, 15, and 22
[total dose/cycle = 80 mg/m^2]
Prednisone: Oral: 200 mg/day days 1 to 5
[total dose/cycle = 1000 mg/m^2]

or

Mercaptopurine: I.V.: 1 g/m^2/day days 1 to 5
[total dose/cycle = 5 g/m^2]
Vincristine: I.V.: 2 mg day 1
[total dose/cycle = 2 mg]
Methotrexate: I.V.: 10 mg/m^2/day days 1 to 5
[total dose/cycle = 50 mg/m^2]
Prednisone: Oral: 200 mg/day days 1 to 5
[total dose/cycle = 1000 mg/m^2]

or

Interferon alfa: SubQ: 5 million units/m^2 daily
[total dose/cycle = 140-155 million units/m^2]
Cytarabine: SubQ: 10 mg daily
[total dose/cycle = 280-310 mg]
Repeat cycles every month for 2 years

Variation 5:

Cycle A: (Cycles 1, 4, 6, and 8)

Cyclophosphamide: I.V.: 300 mg/m^2 every 12 hours, for 6 doses, days 1, 2, and 3
[total dose/cycle = 1800 mg/m^2]
Mesna: I.V.: 600 mg/m^2/day continuous infusion days 1, 2, and 3
[total dose/cycle = 1800 mg/m^2]
Vincristine: I.V.: 2 mg/day days 4 and 11
[total dose/cycle = 4 mg]
Doxorubicin: I.V.: 50 mg/m^2 continuous infusion day 4
[total dose/cycle = 50 mg/m^2]
Dexamethasone: Oral, I.V.: 40 mg/day days 1 to 4 and 11 to 14
[total dose/cycle = 320 mg]

Cycle B: (Cycles 3, 5, 7, and 9)

Methotrexate: I.V.: 200 mg/m^2 day 1
followed by I.V.: 800 mg/m^2 continuous infusion day 1
[total dose/cycle = 1 g/m^2]
Leucovorin: I.V.: 50 mg (start 12 hours after end of methotrexate infusion)
followed by I.V.: 15 mg every 6 hours, for 8 doses
[total dose/cycle = 170 mg]
Cytarabine: I.V.: 3 g/m^2 every 12 hours, for 4 doses, days 2 and 3
[total dose/cycle = 12 g/m^2]

Cycle C: Liposomal Daunorubicin/Cytarabine (Cycle 2):

Daunorubicin, liposomal: I.V.: 150 mg/m^2/day days 1 and 2
[total dose/cycle = 300 mg/m^2]

Cytarabine: I.V.: 1.5 g/m^2/day continuous infusion days 1 and 2
[total dose/cycle = 3 g/m^2]
Prednisone: Oral: 200 mg/day days 1 to 5
[total dose/cycle = 1000 mg]
Administer in the following sequence: ACBABABA (Cycle C does not repeat)

CNS Prophylaxis

Methotrexate: I.T.: 12 mg day 2
[total dose/cycle = 12 mg]
or 6 mg into Ommaya day 2
[total dose/cycle = 6 mg]
Cytarabine: I.T.: 100 mg day 7 **or** 8
[total dose/cycle = 100 mg]
Repeat cycle every 3 weeks for 6 or 8 cycles

Maintenance (POMP)

Mercaptopurine: I.V.: 1 g/m^2/day days 1 to 5
[total dose/cycle = 5 g/m^2]
Vincristine: I.V.: 2 mg day 1
[total dose/cycle = 2 mg]
Methotrexate: I.V.: 10 mg/m^2/day days 1 to 5
[total dose/cycle = 50 mg/m^2]
Prednisone: Oral: 200 mg/day days 1 to 5
[total dose/cycle = 1000 mg]
Repeat cycles monthly, except months 6, 7, 18, and 19 for 3 years

Intensification

Methotrexate: I.V.: 100 mg/m^2/day days 1, 8, 15, and 22
[total dose/cycle = 400 mg/m^2]
Asparaginase: I.V.: 20,000 units/day days 2, 9, 16, and 23
[total dose/cycle = 80,000 units]
Given during months 6 and 18 of maintenance
Cyclophosphamide: I.V.: 300 mg/m^2 every 12 hours, for 6 doses, days 1, 2, and 3
[total dose/cycle = 1800 mg/m^2]
Mesna: I.V.: 600 mg/m^2/day continuous infusion days 1, 2, and 3
[total dose/cycle = 1800 mg/m^2]
Vincristine: I.V.: 2 mg/day days 4 and 11
[total dose/cycle = 4 mg]
Doxorubicin: I.V.: 50 mg/m^2/day continuous infusion day 4
[total dose/cycle = 50 mg/m^2]
Dexamethasone: Oral, I.V.: 40 mg/day days 1 to 4 and 11 to 14
[total dose/cycle = 320 mg]
Given during months 7 and 19 of maintenance

References

Variation 1:
Kantarjian H, Thomas D, O'Brien S, et al, "Long-Term Follow-Up Results of Hyperfractionated Cyclophosphamide, Vincristine, Doxorubicin, and Dexamethasone (Hyper-CVAD), A Dose-Intensive Regimen, in Adult Acute Lymphocytic Leukemia," *Cancer*, 2004, 101(12):2788-2801.
Variation 2:
Thomas DA, Cortes J, O'Brien S, et al, "Hyper-CVAD Program in Burkitt's-Type Adult Acute Lymphoblastic Leukemia," *J Clin Oncol*, 1999, 17(8):2461-70.
Variation 3:
Thomas DA, O'Brien S, Cortes J, et al, "Outcome With the Hyper-CVAD Regimens in Lymphoblastic Lymphoma," *Blood*, 2004, 104(6):1624-30.
Variation 4:
Kantarjian HM, O'Brien S, Smith TL, et al, "Results of Treatment With Hyper-CVAD, A Dose-Intensive Regimen, in Adult Acute Lymphocytic Leukemia," *J Clin Oncol*, 2000, 18(3): 547-61.

Variation 5:
Thomas DA, O'Brien S, Cortes J, et al, "Outcome With the Hyper-CVAD Regimens in Lymphoblastic Lymphoma," *Blood*, 2004, 104(6):1624-30.

Hyper-CVAD (Lymphoma, non-Hodgkin's)

Use Lymphoma, non-Hodgkin's

Regimen

Cycle A: (Cycles 1, 3, 5, and 7)

Cyclophosphamide: I.V.: 300 mg/m² every 12 hours, for 6 doses, days 1, 2, and 3
[total dose/cycle = 1800 mg/m²]

Vincristine: I.V.: 2 mg/day days 4 and 11
[total dose/cycle = 4 mg]

Doxorubicin: I.V.: 25 mg/m²/day continuous infusion days 4 and 5
[total dose/cycle = 50 mg/m²]

Dexamethasone: Oral, I.V.: 40 mg/day days 1 to 4 and 11 to 14
[total dose/cycle = 320 mg]

Cycle B: (Cycles 2, 4, 6, and 8)

Methotrexate: I.V.: 200 mg/m² day 1
followed by I.V.: 800 mg/m² continuous infusion day 1
[total dose/cycle = 1 g/m²]

Leucovorin: Oral: 50 mg
followed by Oral: 15 mg every 6 hours, for 8 doses (start 24 hours after end of methotrexate infusion)
[total dose/cycle = 170 mg]

Cytarabine: I.V.: 3 g/m² every 12 hours, for 4 doses, days 2 and 3
[total dose/cycle = 12 g/m²]

Repeat every 6 weeks in the following sequence: ABABABAB

References

Khouri IF, Romaguera J, Kantarjian H, et al, "Hyper-CVAD and High-Dose Methotrexate/Cytarabine Followed by Stem-Cell Transplantation: An Active Regimen for Aggressive Mantle-Cell Lymphoma," *J Clin Oncol*, 1998, 16(12):3803-9.

Hyper-CVAD (Multiple Myeloma)

Use Multiple myeloma

Regimen

Cyclophosphamide: I.V.: 300 mg/m² every 12 hours, for 6 doses, days 1, 2, and 3
[total dose/cycle = 1800 mg/m²]

Mesna: I.V.: 600 mg/m²/day continuous infusion days 1, 2, and 3
[total dose/cycle = 1800 mg/m²]

Doxorubicin: I.V.: 25 mg/m²/day continuous infusion days 4 and 5
[total dose/cycle = 50 mg/m²]

Vincristine: I.V.: 1 mg/day continuous infusion days 4 and 5
followed by I.V.: 2 mg day 11
[total dose/cycle = 4 mg]

Dexamethasone: Oral, I.V.: 20 mg/m²/day days 1 to 5 and 11 to 14
[total dose/cycle = 180 mg/m²]

Repeat cycle once if ≥50% reduction in myeloma protein

Maintenance

Cyclophosphamide: Oral: 125 mg/m² every 12 hours, for 10 doses, days 1 to 5
[total dose/cycle = 1250 mg/m²]

Dexamethasone: Oral: 20 mg/m^2/day days 1 to 5
[total dose/cycle = 100 mg/m^2]
Repeat maintenance cycle every 5 weeks

References

Dimopoulos MA, Weber D, Kantarjian H, et al, "HyperCVAD for VAD-Resistant Multiple Myeloma," *Am J Hematol*, 1996, 52(2):77-81.

Hyper-CVAD + Rituximab

Use Lymphona, non-Hodgkin's (Mantle cell)

Regimen

Cycle A: (Cycles 1, 3, 5 [and 7, if needed])
Rituximab: I.V.: 375 mg/m^2 day 1
[total dose/cycle = 375 mg/m^2]
Cyclophosphamide: I.V.: 300 mg/m^2 every 12 hours, for 6 doses, days 2, 3, and 4
[total dose/cycle = 1800 mg/m^2]
Mesna: I.V.: 600 mg/m^2 continuous infusion days 2, 3, and 4
[total dose/cycle = 1800 mg/m^2]
Vincristine: I.V.: 1.4 mg/m^2 (maximum dose: 2 mg) days 5 and 12
[total dose/cycle = 2.8 mg/m^2; maximum: 4 mg]
Doxorubicin: I.V.: 16.7 mg/m^2 continuous infusion days 5, 6, and 7
[total dose/cycle = 50.1 mg/m^2]
Dexamethasone: Oral, I.V.: 40 mg/day days 2 to 5 and 12 to 15
[total dose/cycle = 320 mg]
Cycle B: (Cycles 2, 4, 6 [and 8, if needed])
Rituximab: I.V.: 375 mg/m^2 day 1
[total dose/cycle = 375 mg/m^2]
Methotrexate: I.V.: 200 mg/m^2 day 2
followed by I.V.: 800 mg/m^2 continuous infusion day 2
[total dose/cycle = 1000 mg/m^2]
Leucovorin: Oral: 50 mg (start 12 hours after the end of the methotrexate infusion)
followed by Oral: 15 mg every 6 hours, for 8 doses
[total dose/cycle = 170 mg]
Cytarabine: I.V.: 3 g/m^2 every 12 hours, for 4 doses, day 3 and 4
[total dose/cycle = 12 g/m^2]
Repeat every 6 weeks in the following sequence: ABABABAB

References

Romaguera JE, Fayad L, Rodriguez MA, et al, "High Rate of Durable Remissions After Treatment of Newly Diagnosed Aggressive Mantle-Cell Lymphoma With Rituximab Plus Hyper-CVAD Alternating With Rituximab Plus High-Dose Methotrexate and Cytarabine," *J Clin Oncol*, 2005, 23(28):7013-23.

ICE (Hodgkin)

Index Terms Ifosfamide-Carboplatin-Etoposide (Hodgkin)

Use Lymphoma, Hodgkin

Regimen

Etoposide: I.V.: 100 mg/m^2/day days 1 to 3
[total dose/cycle = 300 mg/m^2]
Carboplatin: I.V.: AUC 5 day 2 (maximum dose: 800 mg)
[total dose/cycle = AUC 5, maximum dose/cycle: 800 mg]
Ifosfamide: I.V.: 5 g/m^2/day continuous infusion for 24 hours day 2
[total dose/cycle = 5 g/m^2]

Mesna: I.V.: 5 g/m^2/day continuous infusion for 24 hours day 2
[total dose/cycle = 5 g/m^2]
Filgrastim: 5 mcg/kg/day days 5 to 12 (except during PBPC mobilization)
Repeat cycle every 14 days for 2 cycles

References

Moskowitz CH, Nimer SD, Zelenetz AD, et al, "A 2-Step Comprehensive High-Dose Chemoradiotherapy Second-Line Program for Relapsed and Refractory Hodgkin Disease: Analysis by Intent to Treat and Development of a Prognostic Model," *Blood*, 2001, 97(3):616-23.

ICE (Lymphoma, non-Hodgkin's)

Use Lymphoma, non-Hodgkin's

Regimen

Etoposide: I.V.: 100 mg/m^2/day days 1, 2, and 3
[total dose/cycle = 300 mg/m^2]
Carboplatin: I.V.: AUC 5 (maximum dose: 800 mg) day 2
[total dose/cycle = AUC = 5]
Ifosfamide: I.V.: 5000 mg/m^2 continuous infusion day 2
[total dose/cycle = 5000 mg/m^2]
Mesna: I.V.: 5000 mg/m^2 continuous infusion day 2
[total dose/cycle = 5000 mg/m^2]
Filgrastim: SubQ: 5 mcg/kg/day days 5-12 (cycles 1 and 2 only)
[total dose/cycle = 40 mcg/kg]
followed by SubQ: 10 mcg/kg/day day 5 through completion of leukapheresis (cycle 3 only)
Repeat cycle every 2 weeks for 3 cycles

References

Moskowitz CH, Bertino JR, Glassman JR, et al, "Ifosfamide, Carboplatin, and Etoposide: A Highly Effective Cytoreduction and Peripheral-Blood Progenitor-Cell Mobilization Regimen for Transplant-Eligible Patients With Non-Hodgkin's Lymphoma," *J Clin Oncol*, 1999, 17(12):3776-85.

ICE (Sarcoma)

Use Osteosarcoma; Soft tissue sarcoma

Regimen

Ifosfamide: I.V.: 1500 mg/m^2/day days 1, 2, and 3
[total dose/cycle = 4500 mg/m^2]
Carboplatin: I.V.: 300-635 mg/m^2 day 3
[total dose/cycle = 300-635 mg/m^2]
Etoposide: I.V.: 100 mg/m^2/day days 1, 2, and 3
[total dose/cycle = 300 mg/m^2]
Mesna: I.V.: 500 mg/m^2 prior to each ifosfamide, and every 3 hours for 2 more doses/day days 1, 2, and 3
[total dose/cycle = 4500 mg/m^2]
Repeat cycle every 21-28 days

References

Kung FH, Desai SJ, Dickerman JD, et al, "Ifosfamide/Carboplatin/Etoposide (ICE) for Recurrent Malignant Solid Tumors of Childhood: A Pediatric Oncology Group Phase I/II Study," *J Pediatr Hematol Oncol*, 1995, 17(3):265-9.

◆ **IC (Small Cell Lung Cancer)** *see* Carboplatin-Irinotecan (Small Cell Lung Cancer) *on page 1548*

◆ **Idarubicin-ATRA (APL)** *see* Tretinoin-Idarubicin (APL) *on page 1764*

◆ **Idarubicin-Cytarabine (5 + 2) (AML Consolidation)** *see* 5 + 2 (Cytarabine-Idarubicin) (AML Consolidation) *on page 1512*

◆ **Idarubicin-Tretinoin (APL)** *see* Tretinoin-Idarubicin (APL) *on page 1764*

IE

Use Soft tissue sarcoma

Regimen

Etoposide: I.V.: 100 mg/m²/day days 1, 2, and 3
[total dose/cycle = 300 mg/m²]

Ifosfamide: I.V.: 2500 mg/m²/day days 1, 2, and 3
[total dose/cycle = 7500 mg/m²]

Mesna: I.V.: 500 mg/m² prior to ifosfamide, after ifosfamide, and every 4 hours for 3 more doses (total of 5 doses/day) days 1, 2, and 3
[total dose/cycle = 7500 mg/m²]

Repeat cycle every 28 days

References

Edmonson JH, Buckner JC, Long HJ, et al, "Phase II Study of Ifosfamide-Etoposide-Mesna in Adults With Advanced Nonosseous Sarcomas," *J Natl Cancer Inst*, 1989, 81(11):863-6.

- **Ifosfamide-Carboplatin-Etoposide (Hodgkin)** *see* ICE (Hodgkin) *on page 1688*
- **Ifosfamide, Gemcitabine, Vinorelbine, Prednisolone (Hodgkin)** *see* IGEV (Hodgkin) *on page 1690*

IGEV (Hodgkin)

Index Terms Ifosfamide, Gemcitabine, Vinorelbine, Prednisolone (Hodgkin)

Use Lymphoma, Hodgkin

Regimen

Ifosfamide: I.V.: 2000 mg/m²/day over 2 hours days 1 to 4
[total dose/cycle = 8000 mg/m²]

Mesna: I.V.: 2600 mg/m²/day days 1 to 4
[total dose/cycle = 10,400 mg/m²]

Gemcitabine: I.V.: 800 mg/m² days 1 and 4
[total dose/cycle = 1600 mg/m²]

Vinorelbine: I.V.: 20 mg/m² day 1
[total dose/cycle = 20 mg/m²]

Prednisolone: I.V.: 100 mg days 1 to 4
[total dose/cycle = 400 mg/m²]

Filgrastim: Days 7 to 12 of each course or up to apheresis in the course of mobilization

Repeat cycle every 21 days for a total of 4 cycles

References

Santoro A, Magagnoli M, Spina M, et al, "Ifosfamide, Gemcitabine, and Vinorelbine: A New Induction Regimen for Refractory and Relapsed Hodgkin's Lymphoma," *Haematologica*, 2007, 92(1):35-41.

- **IL-2-Interferon Alfa 2 (RCC)** *see* Interleukin 2-Interferon Alfa-2 (RCC) *on page 1692*

Imatinib (CML Regimen)

Use Leukemia, chronic myelogenous

Regimen NOTE: Multiple variations are listed.

Variation 1 (chronic phase):

Imatinib: Oral: 400 mg once daily
[total dose/cycle = 11,200 mg]

Repeat cycle every 28 days until disease progression or unacceptable toxicity

Variation 2 (accelerated phase and blast crisis):
  Imatinib: Oral: 600 mg once daily
    [total dose/cycle = 16,800 mg]
  Repeat cycle every 28 days until disease progression or unacceptable toxicity
Variation 3 (chronic phase high dose):
  Imatinib: Oral: 400 mg twice daily
    [total dose/cycle = 22,400 mg]
  Repeat cycle every 28 days until disease progression or unacceptable toxicity

References

Variation 1:

Deininger M, O'Brien SG, Guilhot F, et al, "International Randomized Study of Interferon Vs STI571 (IRIS) 8-Year Follow Up: Sustained Survival and Low Risk for Progression or Events in Patients With Newly Diagnosed Chronic Myeloid Leukemia in Chronic Phase (CML-CP) Treated With Imatinib," *Blood*, 2009, 114:abstract 1126.

Druker BJ, Guilhot F, O'Brien SG, et al, "Five-Year Follow-Up of Patients Receiving Imatinib for Chronic Myeloid Leukemia," *N Engl J Med*, 2006, 355(23):2408-17.

O'Brien SG, Guilhot F, Larson RA, et al, "Imatinib Compared With Interferon and Low-Dose Cytarabine for Newly Diagnosed Chronic-Phase Chronic Myeloid Leukemia," *N Engl J Med*, 2003, 348(11):994-1004.

Variation 2:

Sawyers CL, Hochhaus A, Feldman E, et al, "Imatinib Induces Hematologic and Cytogenetic Responses in Patients With Chronic Myelogenous Leukemia in Myeloid Blast Crisis: Results of a Phase II Study," *Blood*, 2002, 99(10):3530-9.

Talpaz M, Silver RT, Druker BJ, et al, "Imatinib Induces Durable Hematologic and Cytogenetic Responses in Patients With Accelerated Phase Chronic Myeloid Leukemia: Results of a Phase 2 Study," *Blood*, 2002, 99(6):1928-37.

Variation 3:

Cortes JE, Baccarani M, Guilhot F, et al, "Phase III, Randomized, Open-Label Study of Daily Imatinib Mesylate 400 mg Versus 800 mg in Patients With Newly Diagnosed, Previously Untreated Chronic Myeloid Leukemia in Chronic Phase Using Molecular End Points: Tyrosine Kinase Inhibitor Optimization and Selectivity Study," *J Clin Oncol*, 2010, 28(3):424-30.

IMVP-16

Use Lymphoma, non-Hodgkin's

Regimen

Ifosfamide: I.V.: 4 g/m^2 continuous infusion over 24 hours day 1
  [total dose/cycle = 4 g/m^2]
Mesna: I.V.: 800 mg/m^2 bolus prior to ifosfamide, then 4 g/m^2 continuous infusion over 12 hours concurrent with ifosfamide, then 2.4 g/m^2 continuous infusion over 12 hours after ifosfamide infusion day 1
  [total dose/cycle = 7.2 g/m^2]
Methotrexate: I.V.: 30 mg/m^2/day days 3 and 10
  [total dose/cycle = 60 mg/m^2]
Etoposide: I.V.: 100 mg/m^2/day days 1, 2, and 3
  [total dose/cycle = 300 mg/m^2]
Repeat cycle every 21-28 days

References

Cabanillas F, Hagemeister FB, Bodey GP, et al, "IMVP-16: An Effective Regimen for Patients With Lymphoma Who Have Relapsed After Initial Combination Chemotherapy," *Blood*, 1982, 60 (3):693-7.

◆ **Interferon Alfa 2b-Bevacizumab (RCC)** *see* Bevacizumab-Interferon Alfa (RCC) *on page 1530*

◆ **Interferon Alfa 2-Interleukin (RCC)** *see* Interleukin 2-Interferon Alfa-2 (RCC) *on page 1692*

◆ **Interferon Alfa-Bevacizumab (RCC)** *see* Bevacizumab-Interferon Alfa (RCC) *on page 1530*

Interleukin 2-Interferon Alfa-2 (RCC)

Index Terms Aldesleukin-Interferon Alfa-2 (RCC); IL-2-Interferon Alfa 2 (RCC); Interferon Alfa 2-Interleukin (RCC)

Use Renal cell cancer

Regimen

Induction (2 cycles):

Aldesleukin: I.V.: 18 million units/m^2/day continuous infusion days 1 to 5 and days 12 to 16

[total dose/cycle = 180 million units/m^2]

Repeat aldesleukin induction cycle one time (total of 2 cycles) after a 3-week rest between cycles

Interferon Alfa-2: SubQ: 6 million units/dose 3 times weekly continuously (no rest break) during induction cycles

[total dose/week = 18 million units/week]

Maintenance (begin after a 3-week aldesleukin rest):

Aldesleukin: I.V.: 18 million units/m^2/day continuous infusion days 1 to 5

[total dose/cycle = 90 million units/m^2]

Repeat aldesleukin maintenance cycle 3 times (total of 4 maintenance cycles) after 3-week rest between cycles

Interferon Alfa-2: SubQ: 6 million units/dose 3 times weekly continuously (no rest break) during maintenance cycles

[total dose/week = 18 million units/week]

References

Negrier S, Escudier B, Lasset C, et al, "Recombinant Human Interleukin-2, Recombinant Human Interferon Alfa-2a, or Both in Metastatic Renal-Cell Carcinoma. Groupe Français d'Immunothérapie," *N Engl J Med*, 1998, 338(18):1272-8.

IPA

Use Hepatoblastoma

Regimen

Ifosfamide: I.V.: 500 mg/m^2 day 1

[total dose/cycle = 500 mg/m^2]

followed by I.V.: 1000 mg/m^2/day continuous infusion days 1 to 3

[total dose/cycle = 3000 mg/m^2]

Cisplatin: I.V.: 20 mg/m^2/day days 4 to 8

[total dose/cycle = 100 mg/m^2]

Doxorubicin: I.V.: 30 mg/m^2/day continuous infusion days 9 and 10

[total dose/cycle = 60 mg/m^2]

Repeat cycle every 21 days

References

von Schweinitz D, Byrd DJ, Hecker H, et al, "Efficiency and Toxicity of Ifosfamide, Cisplatin, and Doxorubicin in the Treatment of Childhood Hepatoblastoma. Study Committee of the Cooperative Paediatric Liver Tumour Study HB89 of the German Society for Paediatric Oncology and Haematology," *Eur J Cancer*, 1997, 33(8):1243-9.

Ipilimumab (Melanoma Regimen)

Use Melanoma

Regimen

Ipilimumab: I.V.: 3 mg/kg day 1

[total dose/cycle = 3 mg/kg]

Repeat cycle every 21 days for 4 cycles

References

Hodi FS, O'Day SJ, McDermott DF, et al, "Improved Survival With Ipilimumab in Patients With Metastatic Melanoma," *N Engl J Med*, 2010, 363(8):711-23.

- **IP (Small Cell Lung Cancer)** *see* Carboplatin-Irinotecan (Small Cell Lung Cancer) *on page 1548*
- **IP (Small Cell Lung Cancer)** *see* Cisplatin-Irinotecan (Small Cell Lung Cancer) *on page 1580*
- **Irinotecan-Bevacizumab (Glioblastoma)** *see* Bevacizumab-Irinotecan (Glioblastoma) *on page 1531*
- **Irinotecan-Biweekly Cetuximab** *see* Cetuximab (Biweekly)-Irinotecan *on page 1557*

Irinotecan-Capecitabine (Esophageal Cancer)

Index Terms Capecitabine-Irinotecan (Esophageal Cancer)

Use Esophageal cancer

Regimen NOTE: Multiple variations are listed.

Variation 1:

Irinotecan: I.V.: 250 mg/m^2/dose day 1
[total dose/cycle = 250 mg/m^2]

Capecitabine: Oral: 1000 mg/m^2/dose twice daily days 1 to 14
[total dose/cycle = 28000 mg/m^2]

Repeat cycle every 21 days until disease progression or unacceptable toxicity

Variation 2:

Irinotecan: I.V.: 250 mg/m^2/dose day 1
[total dose/cycle = 250 mg/m^2]

Capecitabine: Oral: 1000 mg/m^2/dose twice daily days 1 to 14
[total dose/cycle = 28000 mg/m^2]

Repeat cycle every 21 days for up to 24 weeks

References

Variation 1:

Moehler M, Kanzler S, Geissler M, et al, "A Randomized Multicenter Phase II Study Comparing Capecitabine With Irinotecan or Cisplatin in Metastatic Adenocarcinoma of the Stomach or Esophagogastric Junction," *Ann Oncol*, 2010, 21(1):71-7.

Variation 2:

Leary A, Assersohn L, Cunningham D, et al, "A Phase II Trial Evaluating Capecitabine and Irinotecan as Second Line Treatment in Patients With Oesophago-Gastric Cancer Who Have Progressed on, or Within 3 Months of Platinum-Based Chemotherapy," *Cancer Chemother Pharmacol*, 2009, 64(3):455-62.

Irinotecan-Capecitabine (Gastric Cancer)

Index Terms Capecitabine-Irinotecan (Gastric Cancer)

Use Gastric cancer

Regimen NOTE: Multiple variations are listed.

Variation 1:

Irinotecan: I.V.: 250 mg/m^2/dose day 1
[total dose/cycle = 250 mg/m^2]

Capecitabine: Oral: 1000 mg/m^2/dose twice daily days 1 to 14
[total dose/cycle = 28000 mg/m^2]

Repeat cycle every 21 days until disease progression or unacceptable toxicity

Variation 2:
Irinotecan: I.V.: 250 mg/m^2/dose day 1
[total dose/cycle = 250 mg/m^2]
Capecitabine: Oral: 1000 mg/m^2/dose twice daily days 1 to 14
[total dose/cycle = 28000 mg/m^2]
Repeat cycle every 21 days for up to 24 weeks

References

Variation 1:
Moehler M, Kanzler S, Geissler M, et al, "A Randomized Multicenter Phase II Study Comparing Capecitabine With Irinotecan or Cisplatin in Metastatic Adenocarcinoma of the Stomach or Esophagogastric Junction," *Ann Oncol*, 2010, 21(1):71-7.
Variation 2:
Leary A, Assersohn L, Cunningham D, et al, "A Phase II Trial Evaluating Capecitabine and Irinotecan as Second Line Treatment in Patients With Oesophago-Gastric Cancer Who Have Progressed on, or Within 3 Months of Platinum-Based Chemotherapy," *Cancer Chemother Pharmacol*, 2009, 64(3):455-62.

◆ **Irinotecan-Carboplatin (Small Cell Lung Cancer)** *see* Carboplatin-Irinotecan (Small Cell Lung Cancer) *on page 1548*

◆ **Irinotecan-Cetuximab** *see* Cetuximab-Irinotecan (Colorectal) *on page 1561*

Irinotecan-Cisplatin (Esophageal Cancer)

Index Terms Cisplatin-Irinotecan (Esophageal Cancer)

Use Esophageal cancer

Regimen NOTE: Multiple variations are listed.

Variation 1:
Cisplatin: I.V.: 30 mg/m^2/dose days 1, 8, 15, and 22
[total dose/cycle = 120 mg/m^2]
Irinotecan: I.V.: 65 mg/m^2/dose days 1, 8, 15, and 22
[total dose/cycle = 260 mg/m^2]
Repeat cycle every 6 weeks until disease progression.

Variation 2 (with concurrent radiation therapy):
Cisplatin: I.V.: 30 mg/m^2/dose on day 1 and 8
[total dose/cycle = 60 mg/m^2]
Irinotecan: I.V.: 65 mg/m^2/dose day 1 and 8
[total dose/cycle = 130 mg/m^2]
Treatment cycle is 21 days; cycle is not repeated.

Variation 3:
Cisplatin: I.V.: 30 mg/m^2/dose on days 1, 8, 22, and 29
[total dose/cycle = 120 mg/m^2]
Irinotecan: I.V.: 50 mg/m^2/dose on days 1, 8, 22, and 29
[total dose/cycle = 200 mg/m^2]
Administered (with concurrent radiation therapy) over one 5-week treatment cycle.
Followed by: Postoperative therapy:
Cisplatin: I.V.: 30 mg/m^2/dose on days 1 and 8
[total dose/cycle = 60 mg/m^2]
Irinotecan: I.V.: 65 mg/m^2/dose on days 1 and 8
[total dose/cycle = 130 mg/m^2]
Repeat postop cycle every 21 days for a total of 3 cycles.

Variation 4:
Cisplatin: I.V.: 30 mg/m^2/dose on day 1 and 8
[total dose/cycle = 60 mg/m^2]

Irinotecan: I.V.: 65 mg/m²/dose day 1 and 8
[total dose/cycle = 130 mg/m²]
Repeat cycle every 21 days.

References

Variation 1:
Ilson DH, Saltz L, Enzinger P, et al, "Phase II Trial of Weekly Irinotecan Plus Cisplatin in Advanced Esophageal Cancer," *J Clin Oncol*, 1999, 17(10):3270-5.
Variation 2:
Sharma R, Yang GY, Nava HR, et al, "A Single Institution Experience With Neoadjuvant Chemoradiation (CRT) With Irinotecan (I) and Cisplatin (C) in Locally Advanced Esophageal Carcinoma (LAEC)," *J Clin Oncol*, 2009, 27(15S):e15619 [abstract e15619 from 2009 annual ASCO meeting].
Variation 3:
Kleinberg L, Powell ME, Forastiere AA, et al, "Survival Outcome of E1201: An Eastern Cooperative Oncology Group (ECOG) Randomized Phase II Trial of Neoadjuvant Preoperative Paclitaxel/Cisplatin/Radiotherapy (RT) or Irinotecan/Cisplatin/RT in Endoscopy With Ultrasound (EUS) Staged Esophageal Adenocarcinoma," *J Clin Oncol*, 2008, 26(15S):4532 [abstract 4532 from 2008 annual ASCO meeting].
Variation 4:
Ilson DH, "Phase II Trial of Weekly Irinotecan/Cisplatin in Advanced Esophageal Cancer," *Oncology (Williston Park)*, 2004, 18(14 Supp14):22-5.

Irinotecan-Cisplatin (Gastric Cancer)

Index Terms Cisplatin-Irinotecan (Gastric Cancer)

Use Gastric cancer

Regimen

Irinotecan: I.V.: 65 mg/m²/dose over 90 minutes days 1, 8, 15, and 22
[total dose/cycle = 260 mg/m²]
Cisplatin: I.V.: 30 mg/m²/dose over 1 hour days 1, 8, 15, and 22
[total dose/cycle = 120 mg/m²]
Repeat cycle every 6 weeks until disease progression or unacceptable toxicity

References

Ajani JA, Baker J, Pisters PW, et al, "CPT-11 Plus Cisplatin in Patients With Advanced, Untreated Gastric or Gastroesophageal Junction Carcinoma: Results of a Phase II Study," *Cancer*, 2002, 94 (3):641-6.

◆ **Irinotecan-Cisplatin (NSCLC)** *see* Cisplatin-Irinotecan (NSCLC) *on page 1580*

◆ **Irinotecan-Cisplatin (Small Cell Lung Cancer)** *see* Cisplatin-Irinotecan (Small Cell Lung Cancer) *on page 1580*

Irinotecan (Colorectal Regimen)

Use Colorectal cancer

Regimen NOTE: Multiple variations are listed.

Variation 1:
Irinotecan: I.V.: 125 mg/m²/week over 90 minutes weekly for 4 weeks on days 1, 8, 15, and 22
[total dose/cycle = 500 mg/m²]
Repeat cycle every 6 weeks until disease progression or unacceptable toxicity

Variation 2:
Irinotecan: I.V.: 350 mg/m² over 90 minutes day 1
[total dose/cycle = 350 mg/m²]
Repeat cycle every 21 days until disease progression or unacceptable toxicity

Variation 3 (patients ≥70 years, ECOG PS 2, previous pelvic irradiation):
Irinotecan: I.V.: 300 mg/m^2 over 90 minutes day 1
[total dose/cycle = 300 mg/m^2]
Repeat cycle every 21 days until disease progression or unacceptable toxicity

References

Variation 1, 2, 3:
Fuchs CS, Moore MR, Harker G, et al, "Phase III Comparison of Two Irinotecan Dosing Regimens in Second-Line Therapy of Metastatic Colorectal Cancer," *J Clin Oncol*, 2003, 21(5):807-14.

◆ **Irinotecan-Fluorouracil-Leucovorin** *see* FU-LV-CPT-11 *on page 1666*

Irinotecan-Fluorouracil-Leucovorin (Esophageal Cancer)

Index Terms Fluorouracil-Leucovorin-Irinotecan (Esophageal Cancer); Irinotecan-Leucovorin-Fluorouracil (Esophageal cancer)

Use Esophageal cancer

Regimen NOTE: Multiple variations are listed.

Variation 1:
Irinotecan: I.V.: 80 mg/m^2/dose days 1, 8, 15, 22, 29, and 36
[total dose/week = 480 mg/m^2]
Fluorouracil: I.V.: 2000 mg/m^2/dose continuous infusion over 24 hours days 1, 8, 15, 22, 29, and 36
[total dose/cycle = 12,000 mg/m^2]
Leucovorin: I.V.: 500 mg/m^2/dose continuous infusion over 24 hours days 1, 8, 15, 22, 29, and 36
[total dose/week = 3000 mg/m^2]
Repeat cycle every 8 weeks until disease progression or unacceptable toxicity.

Variation 2:
Irinotecan: I.V.: 80 mg/m^2/dose day 1
[total dose/cycle = 80 mg/m^2]
Leucovorin: I.V.: 500 mg/m^2/dose over 2 hours day 1
[total dose/cycle = 500 mg/m^2]
Fluorouracil: I.V.: 2000 mg/m^2/dose continuous infusion over 22 hours day 1 (begin immediately after leucovorin)
[total dose/cycle = 2000 mg/m^2]
Repeat every week for 6 weeks followed by a 1-week rest, continue until disease progression or unacceptable toxicity.

References

Variation 1:
Wolff K, Wein A, Reulbach U, et al, "Weekly High-Dose 5-Fluorouracil as a 24-h Infusion and Sodium Folinic Acid (AIO Regimen) Plus Irinotecan in Patients With Locally Advanced Non-resectable and Metastatic Adenocarcinoma or Squamous Cell Carcinoma of the Oesophagus: A Phase II Trial," *Anticancer Drugs*, 2009, 20(3):165-73.
Variation 2:
Dank M, Zaluski J, Barone C, et al, "Randomized Phase III Study Comparing Irinotecan Combined With 5-Fluorouracil and Folinic Acid to Cisplatin Combined With 5-Fluorouracil in Chemotherapy Naive Patients With Advanced Adenocarcinoma of the Stomach or Esophagogastric Junction," *Ann Oncol*, 2008, 19(8):1450-7.

◆ **Irinotecan-Fluorouracil-Leucovorin (Saltz Regimen)** *see* Fluorouracil-Leucovorin-Irinotecan (Saltz Regimen) *on page 1656*

◆ **Irinotecan-Leucovorin-Fluorouracil (Esophageal cancer)** *see* Irinotecan-Fluorouracil-Leucovorin (Esophageal Cancer) *on page 1696*

Irinotecan-Leucovorin-Fluorouracil (Gastric Cancer)

Index Terms Fluorouracil-Leucovorin-Irinotecan (Gastric Cancer)

Use Gastric cancer

Regimen NOTE: Multiple variations are listed.

Variation 1:

Irinotecan: I.V.: 80 mg/m^2/dose day 1
[total dose/week = 80 mg/m^2]

Leucovorin: I.V.: 500 mg/m^2/dose over 2 hours day 1
[total dose/week = 500 mg/m^2]

Fluorouracil: I.V.: 2000 mg/m^2/dose continuous infusion over 22 hours day 1
[total dose/week = 2000 mg/m^2]

Repeat cycle weekly for 6 weeks followed by a 1-week rest; repeat until disease progression or unacceptable toxicity

Variation 2:

Irinotecan: I.V.: 180 mg/m^2/dose day 1
[total dose/cycle = 180 mg/m^2]

Leucovorin: I.V.: 200 mg/m^2/dose over 2 hours days 1 and 2
[total dose/cycle = 400 mg/m^2]

Fluorouracil: I.V. bolus: 400 mg/m^2 days 1 and 2
followed by I.V.: 600 mg/m^2/dose continuous infusion over 22 hours days 1 and 2
[total dose/cycle = 2000 mg/m^2]

Repeat cycle every 14 days for at least 4 cycles or until disease progression or unacceptable toxicity

References

Variation 1:

Dank M, Zaluski J, Barone C, et al, "Randomized Phase III Study Comparing Irinotecan Combined With 5-Fluorouracil and Folinic Acid to Cisplatin Combined With 5-Fluorouracil in Chemotherapy Naive Patients With Advanced Adenocarcinoma of the Stomach or Esophagogastric Junction," *Ann Oncol*, 2008, 19(8):1450-7.

Variation 2:

Bouché O, Raoul JL, Bonnetain F, et al, "Randomized Multicenter Phase II Trial of a Biweekly Regimen of Fluorouracil and Leucovorin (LV5FU2), LV5FU2 Plus Cisplatin, or LV5FU2 Plus Irinotecan in Patients With Previously Untreated Metastatic Gastric Cancer: A Federation Francophone de Cancerologie Digestive Group Study–FFCD 9803," *J Clin Oncol*, 2004, 22 (21):4319-28.

◆ **Irinotecan-Oxaliplatin-Fluorouracil-Leucovorin (Pancreatic)** *see* FOLFIRINOX (Pancreatic) *on page* 1661

◆ **Irinotecan, Oxaliplatin, Leucovorin, Fluorouracil (Colorectal)** *see* FOLFOXIRI (Colorectal) *on page* 1665

Irinotecan (Small Cell Lung Cancer Regimen)

Use Lung cancer, small cell

Regimen

Irinotecan: I.V.: 100 mg/m^2/day over 90 minutes days 1, 8, 15, and 22
[total dose/cycle = 400 mg/m^2]

Repeat cycle every 28 days

References

Masuda N, Fukuoka M, Kusunoki Y, et al, "CPT-11: A New Derivative of Camptothecin for the Treatment of Refractory or Relapsed Small-Cell Lung Cancer," *J Clin Oncol*, 1992, 10(8):1225-9.

Irinotecan-Temozolomide (Ewing's Sarcoma)

Index Terms Temozolomide-Irinotecan (Ewing's Sarcoma)

Use Ewing's sarcoma

Regimen

Irinotecan: I.V.: 20 mg/m²/dose days 1 to 5 and days 8 to 12
[total dose/cycle = 200 mg/m²]

Temozolomide: Oral: 100 mg/m²/dose days 1 to 5
[total dose/cycle = 500 mg/m²]

Repeat cycle every 21 days

References

Casey DA, Wexler LH, Merchant MS, et al, "Irinotecan and Temozolomide for Ewing Sarcoma: The Memorial Sloan-Kettering Experience," *Pediatr Blood Cancer*, 2009, 53(6):1029-34.

◆ **IVCAF** *see* FAC *on page* 1641

Ixabepilone-Capecitabine

Index Terms Capecitabine-Ixabepilone

Use Breast cancer

Regimen

Capecitabine: Oral: 1000 mg/m² twice daily days 1 to 14
[total dose/cycle = 28,000 mg/m²]

Ixabepilone: I.V.: 40 mg/m² day 1
[total dose/cycle = 40 mg/m²]

Repeat cycle every 3 weeks

References

Thomas ES, Gomez HL, Li RK, et al, "Ixabepilone Plus Capecitabine for Metastatic Breast Cancer Progressing After Anthracycline and Taxane Treatment," *J Clin Oncol*, 2007, 25(33):5210-7.

Vahdat LT, Thomas E, Li R, et al, "Phase III Trial of Ixabepilone Plus Capecitabine Compared to Capecitabine Alone in Patients With Metastatic Breast Cancer (MBC) Previously Treated or Resistant to an Anthracycline and Resistant to Taxanes," *J Clin Onc*, 2007, 25(18S):1006 [abstract from 2007 Proceedings of ASCO Annual Meeting].

◆ **Lapatinib-Capecitabine (Breast Cancer)** *see* Capecitabine + Lapatinib (Breast Cancer) *on page* 1541

Lapatinib-Letrozole (Breast Cancer)

Index Terms Letrozole-Lapatinib (Breast Cancer)

Use Breast cancer

Regimen

Lapatinib: Oral: 1500 mg/day days 1 to 28
[total dose/cycle = 42,000 mg]

Letrozole: Oral: 2.5 mg/day days 1 to 28
[total dose/cycle = 70 mg]

Repeat cycle every 28 days until disease progression

References

Johnston S, Pippen J Jr, Pivot X, et al, "Lapatinib Combined With Letrozole Versus Letrozole and Placebo as First-Line Therapy for Postmenopausal Hormone Receptor-Positive Metastatic Breast Cancer," *J Clin Oncol*, 2009, 27(33):5538-46.

Lapatinib-Trastuzumab (Breast Cancer)

Index Terms Trastuzumab-Lapatinib (Breast Cancer)

Use Breast cancer

Regimen

Week 1:

Trastuzumab: I.V.: 4 mg/kg (loading dose) day 1
[total dose/week 1 = 4 mg/kg]

Lapatinib: Oral: 1000 mg/day days 1 to 7
[total dose/week = 7000 mg]

Subsequent weeks:

Trastuzumab: I.V.: 2 mg/kg day 1
[total dose/week = 2 mg/kg]

Lapatinib: Oral: 1000 mg/day days 1 to 7
[total dose/week = 7000 mg]

Repeat weekly

References

O'Shaughnessy J, Blackwell KL, Burstein H, et al, "A Randomized Study of Lapatinib Alone or in Combination With Trastuzumab in Heavily Pretreated HER2+ Metastatic Breast Cancer Progressing on Trastuzumab Therapy," *J Clin Oncol*, 2008, 26(15s):1015 [abstract 1015 from 2008 ASCO Annual Meeting].

Storniolo AM, Pegram MD, Overmoyer B, et al, "Phase I Dose Escalation and Pharmacokinetic Study of Lapatinib in Combination With Trastuzumab in Patients With Advanced ErbB2-Positive Breast Cancer," *J Clin Oncol*, 2008, 26(20):3317-23.

◆ **Larson ALL Regimen** *see* Larson Regimen (ALL) *on page 1699*

Larson Regimen (ALL)

Index Terms CALGB 8811 ALL Regimen; Larson ALL Regimen

Use Leukemia, acute lymphocytic

Regimen NOTE: Multiple variations are listed.

Variation 1 (CALGB 8811):

Induction, patients <60 years of age (4-week cycle):

Cyclophosphamide: I.V.: 1200 mg/m^2 day 1
[total dose/cycle = 1200 mg/m^2]

Daunorubicin: I.V.: 45 mg/m^2/dose days 1, 2, and 3
[total dose/cycle = 135 mg/m^2]

Vincristine: I.V.: 2 mg/dose days 1, 8, 15, and 22
[total dose/cycle = 8 mg]

Prednisone: Oral: 60 mg/m^2/dose days 1 to 21
[total dose/cycle = 1260 mg/m^2]

Asparaginase: SubQ: 6000 units/m^2/dose days 5, 8, 11, 15, 18, and 22
[total dose/cycle = 36,000 units/m^2]

Induction, patients ≥60 years of age (4-week cycle):

Cyclophosphamide: I.V.: 800 mg/m^2 day 1
[total dose/cycle = 800 mg/m^2]

Daunorubicin: I.V.: 30 mg/m^2/dose days 1, 2, and 3
[total dose/cycle = 90 mg/m^2]

Vincristine: I.V.: 2 mg/dose days 1, 8, 15, and 22
[total dose/cycle = 8 mg]

Prednisone: Oral: 60 mg/m^2/dose days 1 to 7
[total dose/cycle = 420 mg/m^2]

Asparaginase: SubQ: 6000 units/m^2/dose days 5, 8, 11, 15, 18, and 22
[total dose/cycle = 36,000 units/m^2]

Early intensification (4-week cycle; repeat cycle once):

Methotrexate: I.T.: 15 mg/dose day 1
[total dose/cycle = 15 mg]

Cyclophosphamide: I.V.: 1000 mg/m^2 day 1
[total dose/cycle = 1000 mg/m^2]

Mercaptopurine: Oral: 60 mg/m^2/dose days 1 to 14
[total dose/cycle = 840 mg/m^2]

Cytarabine: SubQ: 75 mg/m^2/dose days 1 to 4 and 8 to 11
[total dose/cycle = 600 mg/m^2]

Vincristine: I.V.: 2 mg/dose days 15 and 22
[total dose/cycle = 4 mg]

Asparaginase: SubQ: 6000 units/m^2/dose days 15, 18, 22, and 25 [total dose/cycle = 24,000 units/m^2]

CNS prophylaxis/interim maintenance (12 week duration; with cranial irradiation days 1 to 12):

Methotrexate: I.T.: 15 mg/dose days 1, 8, 15, 22, and 29 [total dose/cycle = 75 mg]

Mercaptopurine: Oral: 60 mg/m^2/dose days 1 to 70 [total dose/cycle = 4200 mg/m^2]

Methotrexate: Oral: 20 mg/m^2/dose days 36, 43, 50, 57, and 64 [total dose/cycle = 100 mg/m^2]

Late intensification (8-week cycle):

Doxorubicin: I.V.: 30 mg/m^2/dose days 1, 8, and 15 [total dose/cycle = 90 mg/m^2]

Vincristine: I.V.: 2 mg/dose days 1, 8, and 15 [total dose/cycle = 6 mg]

Dexamethasone: Oral: 10 mg/m^2/dose days 1 to 14 [total dose/cycle = 140 mg/m^2]

Cyclophosphamide: I.V.: 1000 mg/m^2 day 29 [total dose/cycle = 1000 mg/m^2]

Thioguanine: Oral: 60 mg/m^2/dose days 29 to 42 [total dose/cycle = 840 mg/m^2]

Cytarabine: SubQ: 75 mg/m^2/dose days 29 to 32 and 36 to 39 [total dose/cycle = 600 mg/m^2]

Maintenance (continue until 24 months from diagnosis):

Vincristine: I.V. 2 mg/dose day 1 every 4 weeks [total dose/4 weeks = 2 mg]

Prednisone: Oral: 60 mg/m^2/dose days 1 to 5 every 4 weeks [total dose/4 weeks = 300 mg/m^2]

Methotrexate: Oral: 20 mg/m^2/dose days 1, 8, 15, and 22 [total dose/phase = 80 mg/m^2]

Mercaptopurine: Oral: 60 mg/m^2/dose days 1 to 28 [total dose/phase = 1680 mg/m^2]

Variation 2 (with G-CSF; CALGB 9111):

Induction, patients <60 years of age (4-week cycle):

Cyclophosphamide: I.V.: 1200 mg/m^2 day 1 [total dose/cycle = 1200 mg/m^2]

Daunorubicin: I.V.: 45 mg/m^2/dose days 1, 2, and 3 [total dose/cycle = 135 mg/m^2]

Vincristine: I.V.: 2 mg/dose days 1, 8, 15, and 22 [total dose/cycle = 8 mg]

Prednisone: Oral: 60 mg/m^2/dose days 1 to 21 [total dose/cycle = 1260 mg/m^2]

Asparaginase: SubQ, I.M.: 6000 units/m^2/dose days 5, 8, 11, 15, 18, and 22 [total dose/cycle = 36,000 units/m^2]

Filgrastim: SubQ: 5 mcg/kg/day starting day 4; continue for at least 7 days and until ANC ≥1000/mm^3 on two draws, 24 hours apart

Induction, patients ≥60 years of age (4-week cycle):

Cyclophosphamide: I.V.: 800 mg/m^2 day 1 [total dose/cycle = 800 mg/m^2]

Daunorubicin: I.V.: 30 mg/m^2/dose days 1, 2, and 3 [total dose/cycle = 90 mg/m^2]

Vincristine: I.V.: 2 mg/dose days 1, 8, 15, and 22 [total dose/cycle = 8 mg]

Prednisone: Oral: 60 mg/m²/dose days 1 to 7
[total dose/cycle = 420 mg/m²]
Asparaginase: SubQ, I.M.: 6000 units/m²/dose days 5, 8, 11, 15, 18, and 22
[total dose/cycle = 36,000 units/m²]
Filgrastim: SubQ: 5 mcg/kg/day starting day 4; continue for at least 7 days and until ANC ≥1000/mm³ on two draws, 24 hours apart

Early intensification (4-week cycle; repeat cycle once):
Methotrexate: I.T.: 15 mg/dose day 1
[total dose/cycle = 15 mg]
Cyclophosphamide: I.V.: 1000 mg/m² day 1
[total dose/cycle = 1000 mg/m²]
Mercaptopurine: Oral: 60 mg/m²/dose days 1 to 14
[total dose/cycle = 840 mg/m²]
Cytarabine: SubQ: 75 mg/m²/dose days 1 to 4 and 8 to 11
[total dose/cycle = 600 mg/m²]
Vincristine: I.V.: 2 mg/dose days 15 and 22
[total dose/cycle = 4 mg]
Asparaginase: SubQ, I.M.: 6000 units/m²/dose days 15, 18, 22, and 25
[total dose/cycle = 24,000 units/m²]
Filgrastim: SubQ: 5 mcg/kg/day starting day 2; continue at least 14 days and until ANC ≥5000/mm³ on two draws, 24 hours apart

CNS prophylaxis/interim maintenance (12-week duration; with cranial irradiation days 1 to 12):
Methotrexate: I.T.: 15 mg/dose days 1, 8, 15, 22, and 29
[total dose/cycle = 75 mg]
Mercaptopurine: Oral: 60 mg/m²/dose days 1 to 70
[total dose/cycle = 4200 mg/m²]
Methotrexate: Oral: 20 mg/m²/dose days 36, 43, 50, 57, and 64
[total dose/cycle = 100 mg/m²]

Late intensification (8-week cycle):
Doxorubicin: I.V.: 30 mg/m²/dose days 1, 8, and 15
[total dose/cycle = 90 mg/m²]
Vincristine: I.V.: 2 mg/dose days 1, 8, and 15
[total dose/cycle = 6 mg]
Dexamethasone: Oral: 10 mg/m²/dose days 1 to 14
[total dose/cycle = 140 mg/m²]
Cyclophosphamide: I.V.: 1000 mg/m² day 29
[total dose/cycle = 1000 mg/m²]
Thioguanine: Oral: 60 mg/m²/dose days 29 to 42
[total dose/cycle = 840 mg/m²]
Cytarabine: SubQ: 75 mg/m²/dose days 29 to 32 and 36 to 39
[total dose/cycle = 600 mg/m²]

Maintenance (continue until 24 months from diagnosis):
Vincristine: I.V.: 2 mg/dose day 1 every 4 weeks
[total dose/4 weeks = 2 mg]
Prednisone: Oral: 60 mg/m²/dose days 1 to 5 every 4 weeks
[total dose/4 weeks = 300 mg/m²]
Methotrexate: Oral: 20 mg/m²/dose days 1, 8, 15, and 22
[total dose/phase = 80 mg/m²]
Mercaptopurine: Oral: 60 mg/m²/dose days 1 to 28
[total dose/phase = 1680 mg/m²]

References

Variation 1:

Larson RA, Dodge RK, Burns CP, et al, "A Five-Drug Remission Induction Regimen With Intensive Consolidation for Adults With Acute Lymphoblastic Leukemia: Cancer and Leukemia Group B Study 8811," *Blood*, 1995, 85(8):2025-37.

Variation 2:

Larson RA, Dodge RK, Linker CA, et al, "A Randomized Controlled Trial of Filgrastim During Remission Induction and Consolidation Chemotherapy for Adults With Acute Lymphoblastic Leukemia: CALGB Study 9111," *Blood*, 1998, 92(5):1556-64.

Lenalidomide-Bortezomib-Dexamethasone (Multiple Myeloma)

Index Terms RVD (Multiple Myeloma)

Use Multiple myeloma

Regimen NOTE: Multiple variations are listed.

Variation 1:

Lenalidomide: P.O.: 25 mg daily on days 1-14
[total dose/cycle = 350 mg]

Bortezomib: I.V. or SubQ: 1.3 mg/m^2/day on days 1, 4, 8, and 11
[total dose/cycle = 5.2 mg/m^2]

Dexamethasone: P.O.: 20 mg/day on days 1, 2, 4, 5, 8, 9, 11, and 12
[total dose/cycle = 160 mg]

Repeat cycle every 21 days for up to 8 cycles

Variation 2:

Lenalidomide: P.O.: 25 mg daily on days 1-14
[total dose/cycle = 350 mg]

Bortezomib: I.V. or SubQ: 1.3 mg/m^2/day on days 1, 4, 8, and 11
[total dose/cycle = 5.2 mg/m^2]

Dexamethasone: P.O.: 40 mg/day on days 1, 8, and 15
[total dose/cycle = 120 mg]

Repeat cycle every 21 days for up to 8 cycles

References

Variation 1:

Richardson PG, Weller E, Lonial S, et al, "Lenalidomide, Bortezomib, and Dexamethasone Combination Therapy in Patients With Newly Diagnosed Multiple Myeloma," *Blood*, 2010, 116 (5):679-86.

Variation 2:

Kumar S, Flinn IW, Richardson PG, et al, "Novel Three- and Four-Drug Combination Regimens of Bortezomib, Dexamethasone, Cyclophosphamide, and Lenalidomide, for Previously Untreated Multiple Myeloma: Results From the Multi-Center, Randomized, Phase 2 EVOLUTION Study," *Blood*, 2010, 116:621 [abstract 621 from ASH 2010 Annual Meeting].

Lenalidomide-Dexamethasone

Index Terms Dexamethasone-Lenalidomide

Use Multiple myeloma

Regimen

Lenalidomide: Oral: 25 mg/day days 1 to 21
[total dose/cycle = 525 mg]

Dexamethasone: Oral: 40 mg/day days 1 to 4, 9 to 12, and 17 to 20 (cycles 1 to 4)
[total dose/cycle = 480 mg]

Dexamethasone: Oral 40 mg/day days 1 to 4 (cycle 5 and beyond)
[total dose/cycle = 160 mg]

Repeat cycle every 28 days

References

Dimopoulos M, Spencer A, Attal M, et al, "Lenalidomide Plus Dexamethasone for Relapsed or Refractory Multiple Myeloma," *N Engl J Med*, 2007, 357(21):2123 32.
Rajkumar SV, Hayman SR, Lacy MQ, et al, "Combination Therapy With Lenalidomide Plus Dexamethasone (Rev/Dex) for Newly Diagnosed Myeloma," *Blood*, 2005, 106(13):4050-3.
Weber DM, Chen C, Niesvizky R, et al, "Lenalidomide Plus Dexamethasone for Relapsed Multiple Myeloma in North America," *N Engl J Med*, 2007, 357(21):2133-42.

Lenalidomide-Dexamethasone (Low Dose)

Index Terms Dexamethasone (Low Dose)-Lenalidomide

Use Multiple myeloma

Regimen

Lenalidomide: Oral: 25 mg/day days 1 to 21
[total dose/cycle = 525 mg]
Dexamethasone: Oral: 40 mg/day days 1, 8, 15, and 22
[total dose/cycle = 160 mg]
Repeat cycle every 28 days

References

Rajkumar SV, Jacobus S, Callander N, et al, "A Randomized Phase III Trial of Lenalidomide Plus High-Dose Dexamethasone Versus Lenalidomide Plus Low-Dose Dexamethasone in Newly Diagnosed Multiple Myeloma (E4A03): A Trial Coordinated by the Eastern Cooperative Oncology Group," *Blood*, 2006, 108(11), ASH Abstract 799.
Rajkumar SV, Jacobus S, Callander N, et al, "Phase III Trial of Lenalidomide Plus High-Dose Dexamethasone Versus Lenalidomide Plus Low-Dose Dexamethasone in Newly Diagnosed Multiple Myeloma (E4A03): A Trial Coordinated by the Eastern Cooperative Oncology Group, *J Clin Onc*, 2007, 25(18S), ASCO Abstract LBA8025.

◆ **Letrozole-Lapatinib (Breast Cancer)** *see* Lapatinib-Letrozole (Breast Cancer) *on page 1698*

◆ **Leuprolide-Bicalutamide** *see* Bicalutamide-Leuprolide *on page 1533*

Linker Protocol (ALL)

Use Leukemia, acute lymphocytic

Regimen

Remission induction:

Daunorubicin: I.V.: 50 mg/m^2/day days 1, 2, and 3
[total dose/cycle = 150 mg/m^2]
Vincristine: I.V.: 2 mg/day days 1, 8, 15, and 22
[total dose/cycle = 8 mg]
Prednisone: Oral: 60 mg/m^2/day days 1 to 28
[total dose/cycle = 1680 mg/m^2]
Asparaginase: I.M.: 6000 units/m^2/day days 17 to 28
[total dose/cycle = 72,000 units/m^2]

If residual leukemia in bone marrow on day 14:

Daunorubicin: I.V.: 50 mg/m^2 day 15
[total dose/cycle = 50 mg/m^2]

If residual leukemia in bone marrow on day 28:

Daunorubicin: I.V.: 50 mg/m^2/day days 29 and 30
[total dose/cycle = 100 mg/m^2]
Vincristine: I.V.: 2 mg/day days 29 and 36
[total dose/cycle = 4 mg]
Prednisone: Oral: 60 mg/m^2/day days 29 to 42
[total dose/cycle = 840 mg/m^2]
Asparaginase: I.M.: 6000 units/m^2/day days 29 to 35
[total dose/cycle = 42,000 units/m^2]

Consolidation therapy:

Treatment A (cycles 1, 3, 5, and 7)

Daunorubicin: I.V.: 50 mg/m^2/day days 1 and 2
[total dose/cycle = 100 mg/m^2]

Vincristine: I.V.: 2 mg/day days 1 and 8
[total dose/cycle = 4 mg]

Prednisone: Oral: 60 mg/m^2/day days 1 to 14
[total dose/cycle = 840 mg/m^2]

Asparaginase: I.M.: 12,000 units/m^2/day days 2, 4, 7, 9, 11, and 14
[total dose/cycle = 72,000 units/m^2]

Treatment B (cycles 2, 4, 6, and 8)

Teniposide: I.V.: 165 mg/m^2/day days 1, 4, 8, and 11
[total dose/cycle = 660 mg/m^2]

Cytarabine: I.V.: 300 mg/m^2/day days 1, 4, 8, and 11
[total dose/cycle = 1200 mg/m^2]

Treatment C (cycle 9)

Methotrexate: I.V.: 690 mg/m^2 continuous infusion over 42 hours day 1
[total dose/cycle = 690 mg/m^2]

Leucovorin: I.V.: 15 mg/m^2 every 6 hours for 12 doses (start at end of methotrexate infusion)
[total dose/cycle = 180 mg/m^2]

Administer remission induction regimen for one cycle only. Repeat consolidation cycle every 28 days.

References

Linker CA, Levitt LJ, O'Donnell M, et al, "Treatment of Adult Acute Lymphoblastic Leukemia With Intensive Cyclical Chemotherapy: A Follow-up Report," *Blood*, 1991 78(11):2814-22.

MACOP-B

Use Lymphoma, non-Hodgkin's

Regimen

Methotrexate: I.V. bolus: 100 mg/m^2 weeks 2, 6, 10
followed by I.V.: 300 mg/m^2 over 4 hours weeks 2, 6, and 10
[total dose/cycle = 1200 mg/m^2]

Doxorubicin: I.V.: 50 mg/m^2 weeks 1, 3, 5, 7, 9, and 11
[total dose/cycle = 300 mg/m^2]

Cyclophosphamide: I.V.: 350 mg/m^2 weeks 1, 3, 5, 7, 9, and 11
[total dose/cycle = 2100 mg/m^2]

Vincristine: I.V.: 1.4 mg/m^2 (maximum dose: 2 mg) weeks 2, 4, 6, 8, 10, and 12
[total dose/cycle = 8.4 mg/m^2; maximum: 12 mg]

Bleomycin: I.V.: 10 units/m^2 weeks 4, 8, and 12
[total dose/cycle = 30 units/m^2]

Prednisone: Oral: 75 mg/day for 12 weeks, then taper over 2 weeks

Leucovorin calcium: Oral: 15 mg/m^2 every 6 hours, for 6 doses (beginning 24 hours after methotrexate) weeks 2, 6, and 10
[total dose/cycle = 270 mg/m^2]

Administer one cycle

References

Klimo P and Conors JM, "MACOP-B Chemotherapy for the Treatment of Diffuse Large-Cell Lymphoma," *Ann Intern Med*, 1985, 102(5):596-602.

MAID (Sarcoma)

Index Terms Doxorubicin-Dacarbazine-Ifosfamide-Mesna (Sarcoma); Mesna-Doxorubicin-Ifosfamide-Dacarbazine (Sarcoma)

Use Sarcoma

Regimen NOTE: Multiple variations are listed.

Variation 1:

Mesna: I.V.: 2000 mg/m^2/day continuous infusion days 1 to 4 [total dose/cycle = 8000 mg/m^2]

Doxorubicin: I.V.: 15 mg/m^2/day continuous infusion days 1 to 4 [total dose/cycle = 60 mg/m^2]

Ifosfamide: I.V.: 2000 mg/m^2/day continuous infusion days 1, 2, and 3 [total dose/cycle = 6000 mg/m^2]

Dacarbazine: I.V.: 250 mg/m^2/day continuous infusion days 1 to 4 [total dose/cycle = 1000 mg/m^2]

Repeat cycle every 21 days until disease progression or until maximum lifetime cumulative doxorubicin dose of 450 mg/m^2

Variation 2:

Mesna: I.V.: 2500 mg/m^2/day continuous infusion days 1 to 4 [total dose/cycle = 10,000 mg/m^2]

Doxorubicin: I.V.: 20 mg/m^2/day continuous infusion days 1, 2, and 3 [total dose/cycle = 60 mg/m^2]

Ifosfamide: I.V.: 2500 mg/m^2/day continuous infusion days 1, 2, and 3 [total dose/cycle = 7500 mg/m^2]

Dacarbazine: I.V.: 300 mg/m^2/day continuous infusion days 1, 2, and 3 [total dose/cycle = 900 mg/m^2]

Repeat cycle every 21 days (delay 1 week for leukopenia or thrombocytopenia)

Variation 3 (if prior pelvic irradiation):

Mesna: I.V.: 2500 mg/m^2/day continuous infusion days 1 to 4 [total dose/cycle = 10,000 mg/m^2]

Doxorubicin: I.V.: 20 mg/m^2/day continuous infusion days 1, 2, and 3 [total dose/cycle = 60 mg/m^2]

Ifosfamide: I.V.: 1500 mg/m^2/day continuous infusion days 1, 2, and 3 [total dose/cycle = 4500 mg/m^2]

Dacarbazine: I.V.: 300 mg/m^2/day continuous infusion days 1, 2, and 3 [total dose/cycle = 900 mg/m^2]

Repeat cycle every 21 days (delay 1 week for leukopenia or thrombocytopenia)

Variation 4:

Mesna: I.V.: 2500 mg/m^2/day continuous infusion days 1 to 4 [total dose/cycle = 10,000 mg/m^2]

Doxorubicin: I.V.: 15 mg/m^2/day continuous infusion days 1 to 4 [total dose/cycle = 60 mg/m^2]

Ifosfamide: I.V.: 2000 mg/m^2/day continuous infusion days 1, 2, and 3 [total dose/cycle = 6000 mg/m^2]

Dacarbazine: I.V.: 250 mg/m^2/day continuous infusion days 1 to 4 [total dose/cycle = 1000 mg/m^2]

Repeat cycle every 21 days (or when adequate hematologic recovery)

References

Variation 1:

Antman K, Crowley J, Balcerzak SP, et al, "A Southwest Oncology Group and Cancer and Leukemia Group B Phase II Study of Doxorubicin, Dacarbazine, Ifosfamide, and Mesna in Adults With Advanced Osteosarcoma, Ewing's Sarcoma, and Rhabdomyosarcoma," *Cancer*, 1998, 82 (7):1288-95.

Variations 2 and 3:

Elias A, Ryan L, Sulkes A, et al, "Response to Mesna, Doxorubicin, Ifosfamide, and Dacarbazine in 108 Patients With Metastatic or Unresectable Sarcoma and No Prior Chemotherapy," *J Clin Oncol*, 1989, 7(9):1208-16.

Variation 4:

Antman K, Crowley J, Balcerzak SP, et al, "An Intergroup Phase III Randomized Study of Doxorubicin and Dacarbazine With or Without Ifosfamide and Mesna in Advanced Soft Tissue and Bone Sarcomas," *J Clin Oncol*, 1993, 11(7):1276-85.

m-BACOD

Use Lymphoma, non-Hodgkin's

Regimen

Methotrexate: I.V.: 200 mg/m²/day days 8 and 15
[total dose/cycle = 400 mg/m²]

Leucovorin calcium: Oral: 10 mg/m² every 6 hours for 8 doses (beginning 24 hours after each methotrexate dose) days 9 and 16
[total dose/cycle = 160 mg/m²]

Bleomycin: I.V.: 4 units/m² day 1
[total dose/cycle = 4 units/m²]

Doxorubicin: I.V.: 45 mg/m² day 1
[total dose/cycle = 45 mg/m²]

Cyclophosphamide: I.V.: 600 mg/m² day 1
[total dose/cycle = 600 mg/m²]

Vincristine: I.V.: 1 mg/m² day 1
[total dose/cycle = 1 mg/m²]

Dexamethasone: Oral: 6 mg/m²/day days 1 to 5
[total dose/cycle = 30 mg/m²]

Repeat cycle every 21 days

References

Salles G, Shipp MA, and Coiffier B, "Chemotherapy of Non-Hodgkin's Aggressive Lymphomas," *Semin Hematol*, 1994, 31(1):46-69.

Urba WJ, Duffey PL, and Longo DL, "Treatment of Patients With Aggressive Lymphomas: An Overview," *J Natl Cancer Inst Monogr*, 1990, (10):29-37.

MEC (AML Induction)

Index Terms EMA 86 (AML Induction); Mitoxantrone-Etoposide-Cytarabine (AML Induction)

Use Leukemia, acute myeloid

Regimen

Variation 1:

Mitoxantrone: I.V.: 12 mg/m²/day over 30 minutes days 1, 2, and 3
[total dose/cycle = 36 mg/m²]

Cytarabine: I.V.: 500 mg/m²/day continuous infusion days 1, 2, and 3 and days 8, 9, and 10
[total dose/cycle = 3000 mg/m²]

Etoposide: I.V.: 200 mg/m²/day continuous infusion days 8, 9, and 10
[total dose/cycle = 600 mg/m²]

May administer a second induction cycle if needed

Variation 2:

Etoposide: I.V.: 80 mg/m²/day over 1 hour days 1 to 6
[total dose/cycle = 480 mg/m²]

Cytarabine: I.V.: 1 g/m²/day over 6 hours days 1 to 6
[total dose/cycle = 6 g/m²]

Mitoxantrone: I.V.: 6 mg/m²/day I.V. bolus days 1 to 6 (3 hours after the end of the cytarabine infusion)
[total dose/cycle = 36 mg/m²]

References

Variation 1:

Archimbaud E, Leblond V, Michallet M, et al ""Intensive Sequential Chemotherapy With Mitoxantrone and Continuous Infusion Etoposide and Cytarabine for Previously Treated Acute Myelogenous Leukemia," *Blood*, 1991, 77(9):1894-900.

Archimbaud E, Thomas X, Leblond V, et al, "Timed Sequential Chemotherapy for Previously Treated Patients With Acute Myeloid Leukemia: Long-Term Follow-Up of the Etoposide, Mitoxantrone, and Cytarabine-86 Trial," *J Clin Oncol*, 1995, 13(1):11-8.

Variation 2:

Amadori S, Arcese W, Isacchi G, et al, "Mitoxantrone, Etoposide, and Intermediate-Dose Cytarabine: An Effective and Tolerable Regimen for the Treatment of Refractory Acute Myeloid Leukemia," *J Clin Oncol*, 1991, 9(7):1210-4.

MEC-G (AML Induction)

Index Terms Cytarabine-Etoposide-Mitoxantrone-CSF (AML Induction); EMA-G (AML Induction)

Use Leukemia, acute myeloid

Regimen

Variation 1:

Mitoxantrone: I.V.: 12 mg/m²/day days 1, 2, and 3
[total dose/cycle = 36 mg/m²]

Cytarabine: I.V.: 500 mg/m²/day continuous infusion days 1, 2, and 3 and days 8, 9, and 10
[total dose/cycle = 3000 mg/m²]

Etoposide: I.V.: 200 mg/m²/day continuous infusion days 8, 9, and 10
[total dose/cycle = 600 mg/m²]

Sargramostim: I.V.: 5 mcg/kg/day over 6 hours days 4 to 8

Variation 2:

Mitoxantrone: I.V.: 12 mg/m²/day I.V. bolus days 1, 2, and 3
[total dose/cycle = 36 mg/m²]

Cytarabine: I.V.: 500 mg/m²/day continuous infusion days 1, 2, and 3 and days 8, 9, and 10
[total dose/cycle = 3000 mg/m²]

Etoposide: I.V.: 200 mg/m²/day continuous infusion days 8, 9, and 10
[total dose/cycle = 600 mg/m²]

Filgrastim: SubQ: 5 mcg/kg/day starting on day 4 til ANC >500/mm³ for 2 consecutive days

Administer one cycle only

References

Variation 1:

Archimbaud E, Fenaux P, Reiffers J, et al, "Granulocyte Macrophage Colony-Stimulating Factor in Association to Timed-Sequential Chemotherapy With Mitoxantrone, Etoposide, and Cytarabine for Refractory Acute Myelogenous Leukemia," *Leukemia*, 1993, 7(3):372-7.

Variation 2:

He XY, Elson P, Pohlman B, et al, "Timed Sequential Chemotherapy With Concomitant Granulocyte Colony Stimulating Factor for High-Risk Acute Myelogenous Leukemia: A Single Arm Clinical Trial," *BMC Cancer*, 2002, 2:12.

He XY, Pohlman B, Lichtin A, et al, "Timed-Sequential Chemotherapy With Concomitant Granulocyte Colony-Stimulating Factor for Newly Diagnosed De Novo Acute Myelogenous Leukemia," *Leukemia*, 2003, 17(6):1078-84.

◆ **Mechlorethamine, Doxorubicin, Vinblastine, Vincristine, Bleomycin, Etoposide, Prednisone (Hodgkin)** *see* Stanford V (Hodgkin) *on page 1752*

◆ **Mechlorethamine, Vincristine, Procarbazine, Prednisone, Doxorubicin, Bleomycin, Vinblastine, Dacarbazine (Hodgkin)** *see* MOPP/ABVD (Hodgkin) *on page 1714*

◆ **Mechlorethamine, Vincristine, Procarbazine, Prednisone, Doxorubicin, Bleomycin, Vinblastine (Hodgkin)** *see* MOPP/ABV Hybrid (Hodgkin) *on page 1715*

◆ **Mechlorethamine, Vincristine, Procarbazine, Prednisone (Hodgkin)** *see* MOPP (Hodgkin) *on page 1716*

Melphalan-Prednisone-Bortezomib (Multiple Myeloma)

Index Terms Bortezomib-Melphalan-Prednisone (Multiple Myeloma); VMP (Multiple Myeloma)

Use Multiple myeloma

Regimen NOTE: Multiple variations are listed.

Variation 1:

Bortezomib: I.V.: 1.3 mg/m^2/day days 1, 4, 8, 11, 22, 25, 29, and 32
[total dose/cycle = 10.4 mg/m^2]

Melphalan: Oral: 9 mg/m^2/day days 1 to 4
[total dose/cycle = 36 mg/m^2]

Prednisone: Oral: 60 mg/m^2/day days 1 to 4
[total dose/cycle = 240 mg/m^2]

Repeat cycle every 42 days for 4 cycles

followed by

Bortezomib: I.V.: 1.3 mg/m^2/day days 1, 8, 22, and 29
[total dose/cycle = 5.2 mg/m^2]

Melphalan: Oral: 9 mg/m^2/day days 1 to 4
[total dose/cycle = 36 mg/m^2]

Prednisone: Oral: 60 mg/m^2/day days 1 to 4
[total dose/cycle = 240 mg/m^2]

Repeat cycle every 42 days for 5 cycles

Variation 2:

Bortezomib: I.V.: 1-1.3 mg/m^2/day days 1, 4, 8, 11, 22, 25, 29, and 32
[total dose/cycle = 8-10.4 mg/m^2]

Melphalan: Oral: 9 mg/m^2/day days 1 to 4
[total dose/cycle = 36 mg/m^2]

Prednisone: Oral: 60 mg/m^2/day days 1 to 4
[total dose/cycle = 240 mg/m^2]

Repeat cycle every 42 days for 4 cycles

followed by

Bortezomib: I.V.: 1-1.3 mg/m^2/day days 1, 8, 15, and 22
[total dose/cycle = 4-5.2 mg/m^2]

Melphalan: Oral: 9 mg/m^2/day days 1 to 4
[total dose/cycle = 36 mg/m^2]

Prednisone: Oral: 60 mg/m^2/day days 1 to 4
[total dose/cycle = 240 mg/m^2]

Repeat cycle every 35 days for 5 cycles

References

Variation 1:

Dimopoulos MA, Richardson PG, Schlag R, et al, "VMP (Bortezomib, Melphalan, and Prednisone) Is Active and Well Tolerated in Newly Diagnosed Patients With Multiple Myeloma With Moderately Impaired Renal Function, and Results in Reversal of Renal Impairment: Cohort Analysis of the Phase III VISTA Study," *J Clin Oncol*, 2009, 27(36):6086-93.

San Miguel JF, Schlag R, Khuageva NK, et al, "Bortezomib Plus Melphalan and Prednisone for Initial Treatment of Multiple Myeloma," *N Engl J Med*, 2008, 359(9):906-17.

Variation 2:

Mateos MV, Hernández JM, Hernández MT, et al, "Bortezomib Plus Melphalan and Prednisone in Elderly Untreated Patients With Multiple Myeloma: Results of a Multicenter Phase 1/2 Study," *Blood*, 2006, 108(7):2165-72.

Mateos MV, Hernández JM, Hernández MT, et al, "Bortezomib Plus Melphalan and Prednisone in Elderly Untreated Patients With Multiple Myeloma: Updated Time-to-Events Results and Prognostic Factors for Time to Progression," *Haematologica*, 2008, 93(4):560-5.

◆ **Melphalan-Prednisone-Bortezomib-Thalidomide** *see* Bortezomib-Melphalan-Prednisone-Thalidomide *on page* 1537

Melphalan-Prednisone (Multiple Myeloma)

Index Terms MP (Multiple Myeloma)

Use Multiple myeloma

Regimen NOTE: Multiple variations are listed.

Variation 1:

Melphalan: Oral: 0.25 mg/kg/dose days 1 to 4
[total dose/cycle = 1 mg/kg]

Prednisone: Oral: 2 mg/kg/dose days 1 to 4
[total dose/cycle = 8 mg/kg]

Repeat cycle every 6 weeks for a total of 12 cycles

Variation 2:

Melphalan: Oral: 4 mg/m^2/dose days 1 to 7
[total dose/cycle = 28 mg/m^2]

Prednisone: Oral: 40 mg/m^2/dose days 1 to 7
[total dose/cycle = 280 mg/m^2]

Repeat cycle every 4 weeks for a total of 6 cycles

Variation 3:

Melphalan: Oral: 9 mg/m^2/dose days 1 to 4
[total dose/cycle = 36 mg/m^2]

Prednisone: Oral: 60 mg/m^2/dose days 1 to 4
[total dose/cycle = 240 mg/m^2]

Repeat cycle every 6 weeks for a total of 9 cycles

Variation 4:

Melphalan: Oral: 6 mg/m^2/dose days 1 to 7
[total dose/cycle = 42 mg/m^2]

Prednisone: Oral: 60 mg/m^2/dose days 1 to 7
[total dose/cycle = 420 mg/m^2]

Repeat cycle every 4 weeks for a total of 6 cycles

Followed by (in responders):

Interferon alfa: SubQ: 3 million units/dose 3 times/week until relapse

Dexamethasone: Oral: 40 mg/dose days 1 to 4 every 2 months until relapse

References

Variation 1:

Facon T, Mary JY, Hulin C, et al, "Melphalan and Prednisone Plus Thalidomide Versus Melphalan and Prednisone Alone or Reduced-Intensity Autologous Stem Cell Transplantation in Elderly Patients With Multiple Myeloma (IFM 99 06): A Randomised Trial," *Lancet*, 2007, 370 (9594):1209-18.

Facon T, Mary JY, Pégourie B, et al, "Dexamethasone-Based Regimens Versus Melphalan-Prednisone for Elderly Multiple Myeloma Patients Ineligible for High-Dose Therapy," *Blood*, 2006, 107(4):1292-8.

Variation 2:

Palumbo A, Bringhen S, Caravita T, et al, "Oral Melphalan and Prednisone Chemotherapy Plus Thalidomide Compared With Melphalan and Prednisone Alone in Elderly Patients With Multiple Myeloma: Randomised Controlled Trial," *Lancet*, 2006, 367(9513):825-31.

Palumbo A, Bringhen S, Liberati AM, et al, "Oral Melphalan, Prednisone, and Thalidomide in Elderly Patients With Multiple Myeloma: Updated Results of a Randomized Controlled Trial," *Blood*, 2008, 112(8):3107-14.

Variation 3:

San Miguel JF, Schlag R, Khuageva NK, et al, "Bortezomib Plus Melphalan and Prednisone for Initial Treatment of Multiple Myeloma," *N Engl J Med*, 2008, 359(9):906-17.

Variation 4:
Palumbo A, Bringhen S, Petrucci MT, et al, "Intermediate-Dose Melphalan Improves Survival of Myeloma Patients Aged 50 to 70: Results of a Randomized Controlled Trial," *Blood*, 2004, 104 (10):3052-7.

Melphalan-Prednisone-Thalidomide (Multiple Myeloma)

Index Terms MPT (Multiple Myeloma)

Use Multiple myeloma

Regimen NOTE: Multiple variations are listed.

Variation 1:

Melphalan: Oral: 4 mg/m^2/day days 1 to 7
[total dose/cycle = 28 mg/m^2]

Prednisone: Oral: 40 mg/m^2/day days 1 to 7
[total dose/cycle = 280 mg/m^2]

Thalidomide: Oral: 100 mg/day days 1 to 28
[total dose/cycle = 2800 mg]

Repeat cycle every 28 days for 6 cycles

followed by

Thalidomide: Oral: 100 mg daily (as maintenance)

Variation 2:

Melphalan: Oral: 0.25 mg/kg/dose days 1 to 4
[total dose/cycle = 1 mg/kg]

Prednisone: Oral: 2 mg/kg/dose days 1 to 4
[total dose/cycle = 8 mg/kg]

Thalidomide: Oral: 100-400 mg/day days 1 to 42
[total dose/cycle = 4200-16,800 mg]

Repeat cycle every 6 weeks for a total of 12 cycles (discontinue thalidomide on day 4 of the last cycle)

References

Variation 1:
Palumbo A, Bertola A, Musto P, et al, "Oral Melphalan, Prednisone, and Thalidomide for Newly Diagnosed Patients With Myeloma," *Cancer*, 2005, 104(7):1428-33.
Palumbo A, Bringhen S, Caravita T, et al, "Oral Melphalan and Prednisone Chemotherapy Plus Thalidomide Compared With Melphalan and Prednisone Alone in Elderly Patients With Multiple Myeloma: Randomised Controlled Trial," *Lancet*, 2006, 367(9513):825-31.
Palumbo A, Bringhen S, Liberati AM, et al, "Oral Melphalan, Prednisone, and Thalidomide in Elderly Patients With Multiple Myeloma: Updated Results of a Randomized Controlled Trial," *Blood*, 2008, 112(8):3107-14.
Variation 2:
Facon T, Mary JY, Hulin C, et al, "Melphalan and Prednisone Plus Thalidomide Versus Melphalan and Prednisone Alone or Reduced-Intensity Autologous Stem Cell Transplantation in Elderly Patients With Multiple Myeloma (IFM 99-06): A Randomised Trial," *Lancet*, 2007, 370 (9594):1209-18.

◆ **Mesna-Doxorubicin-Ifosfamide-Dacarbazine (Sarcoma)** *see* MAID (Sarcoma) *on page 1704*

◆ **Mesna-Ifosfamide-Mitoxantrone-Etoposide and Etoposide-Methylprednisolone-Cytarabine-Cisplatin (Hodgkin)** *see* MINE-ESHAP (Hodgkin) *on page 1711*

◆ **Mesna-Ifosfamide-Mitoxantrone-Etoposide and Etoposide-Methylprednisolone-Cytarabine-Cisplatin(NHL)** *see* MINE-ESHAP (NHL) *on page 1712*

Methotrexate-Vinblastine (Desmoid Tumor)

Index Terms Vinblastine-Methotrexate (Desmoid Tumor)

Use Soft tissue sarcoma (Desmoid tumor)

Regimen

Methotrexate: I.V.: 30 mg/m^2 every 7-10 days
[total dose/treatment = 30 mg/m^2]
Vinblastine: I.V.: 6 mg/m^2 every 7-10 days
[total dose/treatment = 6 mg/m^2]
Continue treatment for 1 year (52 treatments)

References

Azzarelli A, Gronchi A, Bertulli R, et al, "Low-Dose Chemotherapy With Methotrexate and Vinblastine for Patients With Advanced Aggressive Fibromatosis," *Cancer*, 2001, 92(5):1259-64.

◆ **mFOLFOX6 and FOLFOX6 (Colorectal)** *see* FOLFOX6 and mFOLFOX6 (Colorectal) *on page* 1663

MINE

Use Lymphoma, non-Hodgkin's

Regimen

Mesna: I.V.: 1.33 g/m^2/day concurrent with ifosfamide dose, then 500 mg orally (4 hours after each ifosfamide infusion) days 1, 2, and 3
[total dose/cycle = 3.99 g/m^2/1500 mg]
Ifosfamide: I.V.: 1.33 g/m^2/day days 1, 2, and 3
[total dose/cycle = 3.99 g/m^2]
Mitoxantrone: I.V.: 8 mg/m^2 day 1
[total dose/cycle = 8 mg/m^2]
Etoposide: I.V.: 65 mg/m^2/day days 1, 2, and 3
[total dose/cycle = 195 mg/m^2]
Repeat cycle every 28 days

References

Rodriguez-Monge EJ and Cabanillas F, "Long-Term Follow-up of Platinum-Based Lymphoma Salvage Regimens. The M.D. Anderson Cancer Center Experience," *Hematol Oncol Clin North Am*, 1997, 11(5):937-47.

MINE-ESHAP (Hodgkin)

Index Terms Mesna-Ifosfamide-Mitoxantrone-Etoposide and Etoposide-Methylprednisolone-Cytarabine-Cisplatin (Hodgkin)

Use Lymphoma, Hodgkin

Regimen

Refractory disease (alternate MINE regimen with ESHAP regimen for a total of 2 MINE cycles and 2 ESHAP cycles):

MINE Regimen:
Mesna: I.V.: 2250 mg/m^2/day days 1, 2, and 3
[total dose/cycle = 6750 mg/m^2]
Ifosfamide: I.V.: 1500 mg/m^2/day days 1, 2, and 3
[total dose/cycle = 4500 mg/m^2]
Mitoxantrone: I.V.: 10 mg/m^2 day 1
[total dose/cycle = 10 mg/m^2]
Etoposide: I.V.: 80 mg/m^2/day days 1, 2, and 3
[total dose/cycle = 240 mg/m^2]
Treatment cycle is 28 days

ESHAP Regimen:
Etoposide: I.V.: 40 mg/m^2/day days 1 to 4
[total dose/cycle = 160 mg/m^2]
Methylprednisolone: I.V.: 250 mg/day days 1 to 4
[total dose/cycle = 1000 mg]

Cisplatin: I.V.: 25 mg/m^2/day continuous infusion over 21 hours days 1 to 4
[total dose/cycle = 100 mg/m^2]
Cytarabine: I.V.: 2000 mg/m^2 day 5
[total dose/cycle = 2000 mg/m^2]
Treatment cycle is 28 days

References

Fernandex de Larrea C, Martinez C, Gaya A, et al, "Salvage Chemotherapy With Alternating MINE-ESHAP Regimen in Relapsed or Refractory Hodgkin's Lymphoma Followed By Autologous Stem-Cell Transplantation," *Ann Oncol*, 2010, 21(6):1211-6.

MINE-ESHAP (NHL)

Index Terms Mesna-Ifosfamide-Mitoxantrone-Etoposide and Etoposide-Methylprednisolone-Cytarabine-Cisplatin(NHL)

Use Lymphoma, non-Hodgkin's

Regimen

Relapsed NHL (In patients achieving a complete remission, administer 6 cycles of MINE regimen, followed by 3 cycles of ESHAP regimen):

MINE regimen:

Mesna: I.V.: 1330 mg/m^2/day over 1 hour days 1, 2, and 3
[total I.V. dose/cycle = 4000 mg/m^2]
Followed by Mesna: Oral: 500 mg (4 hours after ifosfamide) days 1, 2, and 3
[total oral dose/cycle = 1500 mg]
Ifosfamide: I.V.: 1330 mg/m^2/day over 1 hour days 1, 2, and 3
[total dose/cycle = 4000 mg/m^2]
Mitoxantrone: I.V.: 8 mg/m^2 day 1
[total dose/cycle = 8 mg/m^2]
Etoposide: I.V.: 65 mg/m^2/day over 1 hour days 1, 2, and 3
[total dose/cycle = 195 mg/m^2]
Repeat MINE cycle every 21 days for 6 cycles, followed by 3 cycles of ESHAP

ESHAP Regimen:

Etoposide: I.V.: 60 mg/m^2/day over 1 hour days 1 to 4
[total dose/cycle = 240 mg/m^2]
Methylprednisolone: I.V.: 500 mg/day days 1 to 4
[total dose/cycle = 2000 mg]
Cisplatin: I.V.: 25 mg/m^2/day continuous infusion days 1 to 4
[total dose/cycle = 100 mg/m^2]
Cytarabine: I.V.: 2000 mg/m^2 over 2 hours day 5
[total dose/cycle = 2000 mg/m^2]
Repeat ESHAP cycle every 21 days for 3 cycles

References

Rodriguez MA, Cabanillas FC, Velasquez W, et al, "Results of a Salvage Treatment Program for Relapsing Lymphoma: MINE Consolidated With ESHAP," *J Clin Oncol*, 1995, 13(7):1734-41.

mini-BEAM (Hodgkin)

Index Terms Carmustine-Etoposide-Cytarabine-Melphalan (Hodgkin)

Use Lymphoma, Hodgkin

Regimen

Carmustine: I.V.: 60 mg/m^2 over 30 minutes day 1
[total dose/cycle = 60 mg/m^2]
Etoposide: I.V.: 75 mg/m^2/day over 30 minutes days 2 to 5
[total dose/cycle = 300 mg/m^2]

Cytarabine: I.V.: 100 mg/m^2 every 12 hours days 2 to 5 (total of 8 doses) [total dose/cycle = 800 mg/m^2]
Melphalan: I.V.: 30 mg/m^2 over 15 minutes day 6 [total dose/cycle = 30 mg/m^2]
Repeat cycle every 4 to 6 weeks

References

Colwill R, Crump M, Couture F, et al, "Mini-BEAM as Salvage Therapy for Relapsed or Refractory Hodgkin's Disease Before Intensive Therapy and Autologous Bone Marrow Transplantation," *J Clin Oncol*, 1995, 13(2):396-402.

Martín A, Fernández-Jiménez MC, Caballero MD, et al, "Long-Term Follow-Up in Patients Treated With Mini-BEAM as Salvage Therapy for Relapsed or Refractory Hodgkin's Disease," *Br J Haematol*, 2001, 113(1):161-71.

◆ **Mitomycin–Fluorouracil (Anal Cancer)** *see* Fluorouracil-Mitomycin (Anal Cancer) *on page 1659*

Mitoxantrone-Etoposide (AML Induction)

Index Terms MV (AML Induction)

Use Leukemia, acute myeloid

Regimen

Mitoxantrone: I.V.: 10 mg/m^2/day over ≤15 minutes days 1 to 5 [total dose/cycle = 50 mg/m^2]
Etoposide: I.V.: 100 mg/m^2/day over 30 minutes days 1 to 5 [total dose/cycle = 500 mg/m^2]
May administer a second induction cycle if needed

References

Ho AD, Lipp T, Ehninger G, et al, "Combination of Mitoxantrone and Etoposide in Refractory Acute Myelogenous Leukemia an Active and Well-Tolerated Regimen," *J Clin Oncol*, 1988, 6(2):213-17.

◆ **Mitoxantrone-Etoposide-Cytarabine (AML Induction)** *see* MEC (AML Induction) *on page 1706*

Mitoxantrone + Hydrocortisone

Use Prostate cancer

Regimen

Mitoxantrone: I.V.: 14 mg/m^2 day 1 [total dose/cycle = 14 mg/m^2]
Hydrocortisone: Oral: 40 mg daily [total dose/cycle = 840 mg]
Repeat cycle every 3 weeks

References

Kantoff PW, Halabi S, Conaway M, et al, "Hydrocortisone With or Without Mitoxantrone in Men With Hormone-Refractory Prostate Cancer: Results of the Cancer and Leukemia Group B 9182 Study," *J Clin Oncol*, 1999, 17(8):2506-13.

Mitoxantrone-Prednisone (Prostate Cancer)

Index Terms MP (Prostate Cancer); Prednisone-Mitoxantrone (Prostate Cancer)

Use Prostate cancer

Regimen NOTE: Multiple variations are listed.

Variation 1:

Mitoxantrone: I.V.: 12 mg/m^2 day 1 [total dose/cycle = 12 mg/m^2]

Prednisone: Oral: 5 mg twice daily
[total dose/cycle = 210 mg]
Repeat cycle every 21 days for up to a total of 10 cycles
Variation 2:
Cycle 1:
Mitoxantrone: I.V.: 12 mg/m^2 day 1
[total dose/cycle = 12 mg/m^2]
Prednisone: Oral: 5 mg twice daily
[total dose/cycle = 210 mg]
Treatment cycle is 21 days
Cycle 2 and beyond:
Mitoxantrone: I.V.: 12-14 mg/m^2 day 1 (increase to 14 mg/m^2 if no grade 3/4 adverse events)
[total dose/cycle = 12-14 mg/m^2]
Prednisone: Oral: 5 mg twice daily
[total dose/cycle = 210 mg]
Repeat cycle every 21 days for up to a maximum cumulative mitoxantrone dose of 144 mg/m^2
Variation 3:
Cycle 1:
Mitoxantrone: I.V.: 12 mg/m^2 day 1
[total dose/cycle = 12 mg/m^2]
Prednisone: Oral: 5 mg twice daily
[total dose/cycle = 210 mg]
Treatment cycle is 21 days
Cycles 2-8:
Mitoxantrone: I.V.: 12-14 mg/m^2 day 1 (increase to 14 mg/m^2 if granulocyte nadir is >1000/mm^3 and platelet nadir >50,000/mm^3)
[total dose/cycle = 12-14 mg/m^2]
Prednisone: Oral: 5 mg twice daily
[total dose/cycle = 210 mg]
Treatment cycle is 21 days for up to a total of 8 cycles

References

Variation 1:
Tannock IF, de Wit R, Berry WR, et al, "Docetaxel Plus Prednisone or Mitoxantrone Plus Prednisone for Advanced Prostate Cancer," *N Engl J Med*, 2004, 351(15):1502-12.
Variation 2:
Petrylak DP, Tangen CM, Hussain MH, et al, "Docetaxel and Estramustine Compared With Mitoxantrone and Prednisone for Advanced Refractory Prostate Cancer," *N Engl J Med*, 2004, 351(15):1513-20.
Variation 3:
Moore MJ, Osoba D, Murphy K, et al, "Use of Palliative Endpoints to Evaluate the Effects of Mitoxantrone and Low-Dose Prednisone in Patients With Hormonally Resistant Prostate Cancer," *J Clin Oncol*, 1994, 12(4):689-94.

◆ **Modified Fluorouracil-Leucovorin-Oxaliplatin (Colorectal)** *see* FOLFOX6 and mFOLFOX6 (Colorectal) *on page 1663*

◆ **Modified FOLFOX6 (Colorectal)** *see* FOLFOX6 and mFOLFOX6 (Colorectal) *on page 1663*

MOPP/ABVD (Hodgkin)

Index Terms Mechlorethamine, Vincristine, Procarbazine, Prednisone, Doxorubicin, Bleomycin, Vinblastine, Dacarbazine (Hodgkin)

Use Lymphoma, Hodgkin

Regimen NOTE: Multiple variations are listed.

Variation 1:

Mechlorethamine: I.V.: 6 mg/m²/day days 1 and 8
[total dose/cycle = 12 mg/m²]

Vincristine: I.V.: 1.4 mg/m²/day days 1 and 8
[total dose/cycle = 2.8 mg/m²]

Procarbazine: Oral: 100 mg/m²/day days 1 to 14
[total dose/cycle = 1400 mg/m²]

Prednisone: Oral: 40 mg/m²/day days 1 to 14 (during cycles 1, 4, 7, and 10 **only**)
[total dose/cycle = 560 mg/m²]

Doxorubicin: I.V.: 25 mg/m²/day days 29 and 43
[total dose/cycle = 50 mg/m²]

Bleomycin: I.V.: 10 units/m²/day days 29 and 43
[total dose/cycle = 20 units/m²]

Vinblastine: I.V.: 6 mg/m²/day days 29 and 43
[total dose/cycle = 12 mg/m²]

Dacarbazine: I.V.: 375 mg/m²/day days 29 and 43
[total dose/cycle = 750 mg/m²]

Repeat cycle every 56 days for a total of 6 cycles.

Variation 2:

Mechlorethamine: I.V.: 6 mg/m²/day days 1 and 8
[total dose/cycle = 12 mg/m²]

Vincristine: I.V.: 1.4 mg/m²/day (maximum dose: 2 mg) days 1 and 8
[total dose/cycle = 2.8 mg/m²; maximum dose/cycle: 4 mg]

Procarbazine: Oral: 100 mg/m²/day days 1 to 14
[total dose/cycle = 1400 mg/m²]

Prednisone: Oral: 40 mg/m²/day days 1 to 14 (during cycles 1 and 7 **only**)
[total dose/cycle = 560 mg/m²]

Doxorubicin: I.V.: 25 mg/m²/day days 29 and 43
[total dose/cycle = 50 mg/m²]

Bleomycin: I.V.: 10 units/m²/day days 29 and 43
[total dose/cycle = 20 units/m²]

Vinblastine: I.V.: 6 mg/m²/day days 29 and 43
[total dose/cycle = 12 mg/m²]

Dacarbazine: I.V.: 375 mg/m²/day days 29 and 43
[total dose/cycle = 750 mg/m²]

Repeat cycle every 56 days for a total of 6 cycles.

References

Variation 1:

Bonadonna G, Valagussa P, and Santoro A, "Alternating Noncross-Resistant Combination Chemotherapy or MOPP in State IV Hodgkin's Disease. A Report of 8-Year Results," *Ann Int Med*, 1986, 104(6):739-46.

Variation 2:

Canellos, GP, Anderson JR, Propert KJ, et al, "Chemotherapy of Advanced Hodgkin's Disease With MOPP, ABVD, or MOPP Alternating With ABVD," *N Engl J Med*, 1992, 327(21):1478-84.

MOPP/ABV Hybrid (Hodgkin)

Index Terms Mechlorethamine, Vincristine, Procarbazine, Prednisone, Doxorubicin, Bleomycin, Vinblastine (Hodgkin)

Use Lymphoma, Hodgkin

Regimen

Mechlorethamine: I.V.: 6 mg/m² day 1
[total dose/cycle = 6 mg/m²]

Vincristine: I.V.: 1.4 mg/m^2 (maximum dose: 2 mg) day 1
[total dose/cycle = 1.4 mg/m^2; maximum: 2 mg/cycle]
Procarbazine: Oral: 100 mg/m^2/day days 1 to 7
[total dose/cycle = 700 mg/m^2]
Prednisone: Oral: 40 mg/m^2/day days 1 to 14
[total dose/cycle = 560 mg/m^2]
Doxorubicin: I.V.: 35 mg/m^2 day 8
[total dose/cycle = 35 mg/m^2]
Bleomycin: I.V.: 10 units/m^2 day 8
[total dose/cycle = 10 units/m^2]
Vinblastine: I.V.: 6 mg/m^2 day 8
[total dose/cycle = 6 mg/m^2]
Repeat cycle every 28 days for a maximum of 8 cycles

References

Conners JM, Klimo P, Adams G, et al, "Treatment of Advanced Hodgkin's Disease With Chemotherapy – Comparison of MOPP/ABV Hybrid Regimen With Alternating Courses of MOPP and ABVD: A Report From the National Cancer Institute of Canada Clinical Trials," *J Clin Oncol*, 1997, 15(4):1638-45.

Klimo P and Connors JM, "MOPP/ABV Hybrid Program: Combination Chemotherapy Based on Early Introduction of Seven Effective Drugs for Advanced Hodgkin's Disease," *J Clin Oncol*, 1985, 3(9):1174-82.

MOPP (Hodgkin)

Index Terms Mechlorethamine, Vincristine, Procarbazine, Prednisone (Hodgkin)

Use Lymphoma, Hodgkin

Regimen NOTE: Multiple variations are listed.

Variation 1:
Mechlorethamine: I.V.: 6 mg/m^2/day days 1 and 8
[total dose/cycle = 12 mg/m^2]
Vincristine: I.V.: 1.4 mg/m^2/day days 1 and 8
[total dose/cycle = 2.8 mg/m^2]
Procarbazine: Oral: 100 mg/m^2/day days 1 to 14
[total dose/cycle = 1400 mg/m^2]
Prednisone: Oral: 40 mg/m^2/day days 1 to 14 (cycles 1 and 4)
[total dose/cycle = 560 mg/m^2]
Repeat cycle every 28 days for 6 cycles

Variation 2:
Mechlorethamine: I.V.: 6 mg/m^2/day days 1 and 8
[total dose/cycle = 12 mg/m^2]
Vincristine: I.V.: 1.4 mg/m^2/day (maximum dose: 2 mg) days 1 and 8
[total dose/cycle = 2.8 mg/m^2; maximum dose/cycle: 4 mg]
Procarbazine: Oral: 100 mg/m^2/day days 1 to 14
[total dose/cycle = 1400 mg/m^2]
Prednisone: Oral: 40 mg/m^2/day days 1 to 14 (cycles 1 and 4)
[total dose/cycle = 560 mg/m^2]
Repeat cycle every 28 days for 6-8 cycles

References

Variation 1:
Devita VT Jr, Serpick AA, and Carbone PP, "Combination Chemotherapy in the Treatment of Advanced Hodgkin's Disease," *Ann Intern Med*, 1970, 73(6):881-95.
Variation 2:
Canellos GP, Anderson JR, Propert KJ, et al, "Chemotherapy of Advanced Hodgkin's Disease With MOPP, ABVD, or MOPP Alternating With ABVD," *N Engl J Med*, 1992, 327(21):1478-84.

MOPP (Medulloblastoma)

Use Brain tumors

Regimen

Mechlorethamine: I.V.: 3 mg/m²/day days 1 and 8
[total dose/cycle = 6 mg/m²]
Vincristine: I.V.: 1.4 mg/m²/day (maximum dose: 2 mg) days 1 and 8
[total dose/cycle = 2.8 mg/m²]
Prednisone: Oral: 40 mg/m²/day days 1 to 10
[total dose/cycle = 400 mg/m²]
Procarbazine: Oral: 50 mg day 1
[total dose/cycle = 50 mg]
followed by Oral: 100 mg day 2
[total dose/cycle = 100 mg]
followed by Oral: 100 mg/m²/day days 3 to 10
[total dose/cycle = 800 mg/m²]
Repeat cycle every 28 days

References

Krischer JP, Ragab AH, Kun L, et al, "Nitrogen Mustard, Vincristine, Procarbazine, and Prednisone as Adjuvant Chemotherapy in the Treatment of Medulloblastoma. A Pediatric Oncology Group Study," *J Neurosurg*, 1991, 74(6):905-9.

◆ **MP (Multiple Myeloma)** *see* Melphalan-Prednisone (Multiple Myeloma) *on page 1709*

◆ **MP (Prostate Cancer)** *see* Mitoxantrone-Prednisone (Prostate Cancer) *on page 1713*

◆ **MPT (Multiple Myeloma)** *see* Melphalan-Prednisone-Thalidomide (Multiple Myeloma) *on page 1710*

MTX/6-MP/VP (Maintenance)

Use Leukemia, acute lymphocytic

Regimen

Methotrexate: Oral: 20 mg/m² weekly
[total dose/cycle = 80 mg/m²]
Mercaptopurine: Oral: 75 mg/m²/day
[total dose/cycle = 2250 mg/m²]
Vincristine: I.V.: 1.5 mg/m² day 1
[total dose/cycle = 1.5 mg/m²]
Prednisone: Oral: 40 mg/m²/day days 1 to 5
[total dose/cycle = 200 mg/m²]
Repeat monthly for 2-3 years

References

Bleyer WA, Sather HN, Nickerson HJ, et al, "Monthly Pulses of Vincristine and Prednisone Prevent Bone Marrow and Testicular Relapse in Low-Risk Childhood Acute Lymphoblastic Leukemia: A Report of the CCG 101 Study by the Childrens Cancer Study Group," *J Clin Oncol*, 1991, 9 (6):1012-21.

MTX-CDDPAdr

Use Osteosarcoma

Regimen

Cisplatin: I.V.: 75 mg/m² day 1 of cycles 1-7, then 120 mg/m² for cycles 8, 9, and 10
Doxorubicin: I.V.: 25 mg/m²/day days 1, 2, and 3 of cycles 1 to 7
Methotrexate: I.V.: 12 g/m²/day days 21 and 28

Leucovorin calcium rescue: I.V.: 20 mg/m^2 every 3 hours (beginning 16 hours after completion of methotrexate) for 8 doses, then orally every 6 hours for 8 doses

References

Meyers PA, Heller G, Healey J, et al, "Chemotherapy for Nonmetastatic Osteogenic Sarcoma: The Memorial Sloan-Kettering Experience," *J Clin Oncol*, 1992, 10(1):5-15.

M-VAC (Bladder Cancer)

Use Bladder cancer

Regimen NOTE: Multiple variations are listed.

Variation 1:
- Methotrexate: I.V.: 30 mg/m^2/day days 1, 15, and 22
  [total dose/cycle = 90 mg/m^2]
- Vinblastine: I.V.: 3 mg/m^2/day days 2, 15, and 22
  [total dose/cycle = 9 mg/m^2]
- Doxorubicin: I.V.: 30 mg/m^2 day 2
  [total dose/cycle = 30 mg/m^2]
- Cisplatin: I.V.: 70 mg/m^2 day 2
  [total dose/cycle = 70 mg/m^2]
- Repeat cycle every 4 weeks

Variation 2:
- Methotrexate: I.V.: 40 or 50 mg/m^2/day days 1, 15, and 22
  [total dose/cycle = 120 or 150 mg/m^2]
- Vinblastine: I.V.: 4 or 5 mg/m^2/day days 2, 15, and 22
  [total dose/cycle = 12 or 15 mg/m^2]
- Doxorubicin: I.V.: 40 or 50 mg/m^2 day 2
  [total dose/cycle = 40 or 50 mg/m^2]
- Cisplatin: I.V.: 100 mg/m^2 day 2
  [total dose/cycle = 100 mg/m^2]
- Repeat cycle every 4 weeks

Variation 3:
- Methotrexate: I.V.: 30 mg/m^2/day days 1, 15, and 22
  [total dose/cycle = 90 mg/m^2]
- Vinblastine: I.V.: 3 mg/m^2 day 2
  [total dose/cycle = 3 mg/m^2]
- Doxorubicin: I.V.: 30 mg/m^2 day 2
  [total dose/cycle = 30 mg/m^2]
- Cisplatin: I.V.: 70 mg/m^2 day 2
  [total dose/cycle = 70 mg/m^2]
- Repeat cycle every 4 weeks

Variation 4:
- Methotrexate: I.V.: 60 mg/m^2 day 1
  [total dose/cycle = 60 mg/m^2]
  followed by I.V.: 30 mg/m^2 day 16
  [total dose/cycle = 30 mg/m^2]
- Vinblastine: I.V.: 4 mg/m^2/day days 2 and 16
  [total dose/cycle = 8 mg/m^2]
- Doxorubicin: I.V.: 60 mg/m^2 day 2
  [total dose/cycle = 60 mg/m^2]
- Cisplatin: I.V.: 100 mg/m^2 day 2
  [total dose/cycle = 100 mg/m^2]
- Repeat cycle every 23 days

Variation 5:
- Methotrexate: I.V.: 30 mg/m^2/day days 1, 16, and 23 [total dose/cycle = 90 mg/m^2]
- Vinblastine: I.V.: 4 mg/m^2/day days 1, 16, and 23 [total dose/cycle = 12 mg/m^2]
- Doxorubicin: I.V.: 60 mg/m^2 day 2 [total dose/cycle = 60 mg/m^2]
- Cisplatin: I.V.: 100 mg/m^2 day 2 [total dose/cycle = 100 mg/m^2]
- Repeat cycle every 23 days

Variation 6:
- Methotrexate: I.V.: 30 or 35 mg/m^2 day 1 [total dose/cycle = 30 or 35 mg/m^2]
- Vinblastine: I.V.: 3 or 3.5 mg/m^2 day 2 [total dose/cycle = 3 or 3.5 mg/m^2]
- Doxorubicin: I.V.: 30 or 35 mg/m^2 day 2 [total dose/cycle = 30 or 35 mg/m^2]
- Cisplatin: I.V.: 70 or 80 mg/m^2 day 2 [total dose/cycle = 70 or 80 mg/m^2]
- Repeat cycle every 2 weeks

Variation 7:
- Methotrexate: I.V.: 30 mg/m^2 day 1 [total dose/cycle = 30 mg/m^2]
- Vinblastine: I.V.: 3 mg/m^2 day 2 [total dose/cycle = 3 mg/m^2]
- Doxorubicin: I.V.: 30 mg/m^2 day 2 [total dose/cycle = 30 mg/m^2]
- Cisplatin: I.V.: 70 mg/m^2 day 2 [total dose/cycle = 70 mg/m^2]
- Repeat cycle every 14 days

Variation 8:
- Methotrexate: I.V.: 30 mg/m^2/day days 1, 15, and 22 [total dose/cycle = 90 mg/m^2]
- Vinblastine: I.V.: 3 mg/m^2/day days 1, 15, and 22 [total dose/cycle = 9 mg/m^2]
- Doxorubicin: I.V.: 45 mg/m^2 day 2 [total dose/cycle = 45 mg/m^2]
- Cisplatin: I.V.: 70 mg/m^2 day 2 [total dose/cycle = 70 mg/m^2]
- Repeat cycle every 4 weeks

Variation 9:
- Methotrexate: I.V.: 40 mg/m^2/day days 1 and 16 [total dose/cycle = 80 mg/m^2]
- Vinblastine: I.V.: 4 mg/m^2/day days 1, 16, and 23 [total dose/cycle = 12 mg/m^2]
- Doxorubicin: I.V.: 60 mg/m^2 day 2 [total dose/cycle = 60 mg/m^2]
- Cisplatin: I.V.: 100 mg/m^2 day 2 [total dose/cycle = 100 mg/m^2]
- Repeat cycle every 23 days

Variation 10:
- Methotrexate: I.V.: 30 mg/m^2/day days 1, 15, and 22 [total dose/cycle = 90 mg/m^2]

Vinblastine: I.V.: 3 mg/m²/day days 1, 16, and 22
[total dose/cycle = 9 mg/m²]
Doxorubicin: I.V.: 30 mg/m² day 1
[total dose/cycle = 30 mg/m²]
Cisplatin: I.V.: 70 mg/m² day 1
[total dose/cycle = 70 mg/m²]
Repeat cycle every 4 weeks

Variation 11:
Methotrexate: I.V.: 30 mg/m²/day days 1, 15, and 22
[total dose/cycle = 90 mg/m²]
Vinblastine: I.V.: 3 mg/m²/day days 2, 15, and 22
[total dose/cycle = 9 mg/m²]
Doxorubicin: I.V.: 30 mg/m² day 2
[total dose/cycle = 30 mg/m²]
Cisplatin: I.V.: 70 mg/m² day 2
[total dose/cycle = 70 mg/m²]
Leucovorin: Oral: 15 mg every 6 hours for 4 doses days 2, 16, and 23
[total dose/cycle = 180 mg]
Repeat cycle every 4 weeks

Variation 12:
Methotrexate: I.V.: 30 mg/m²/day days 1 and 15
[total dose/cycle = 60 mg/m²]
Vinblastine: I.V.: 3 mg/m²/day days 2 and 15
[total dose/cycle = 6 mg/m²]
Doxorubicin: I.V.: 30 or 40 mg/m² day 3
[total dose/cycle = 30 or 40 mg/m²]
Cisplatin: I.V.: 70 mg/m² day 2
[total dose/cycle = 70 mg/m²]
Repeat cycle every 4 weeks

Variation 13:
Methotrexate: I.V.: 30 mg/m²/day days 1 and 15
[total dose/cycle = 60 mg/m²]
Vinblastine: I.V.: 3 mg/m²/day days 2 and 15
[total dose/cycle = 6 mg/m²]
Doxorubicin: I.V.: 30 or 40 mg/m² day 2
[total dose/cycle = 30 or 40 mg/m²]
Cisplatin: I.V.: 70 mg/m² day 2
[total dose/cycle = 70 mg/m²]
Repeat cycle every 4 weeks

References

Variation 1:

Sternberg CN, de Mulder PH, Schornagel JH, et al, "Randomized Phase III Trial of High-Dose-Intensity Methotrexate, Vinblastine, Doxorubicin, and Cisplatin (MVAC) Chemotherapy and Recombinant Human Granulocyte Colony-Stimulating Factor Versus Classic MVAC in Advanced Urothelial Tract Tumors: European Organization for Research and Treatment of Cancer Protocol No. 30924," *J Clin Oncol*, 2001, 19(10):2638-46.

Sternberg CN, Yagoda A, Scher HI, et al, "Preliminary Results of M-VAC (Methotrexate, Vinblastine, Doxorubicin, and Cisplatin) for Transitional Cell Carcinoma of the Urothelium," *J Urol*, 1985, 133(3):403-7.

Variation 2:

Loehrer PJ Sr, Elson P, Dreicer R, et al, "Escalated Dosages of Methotrexate, Vinblastine, Doxorubicin, and Cisplatin Plus Recombinant Human Granulocyte Colony-Stimulating Factor in Advanced Urothelial Carcinoma: An Eastern Cooperative Oncology Group Trial," *J Clin Oncol*, 1994, 12(3):483-8.

Variation 3:

Loehrer PJ Sr, Einhorn LH, Elson PJ, et al, "A Randomized Comparison of Cisplatin Alone or in Combination With Methotrexate, Vinblastine, and Doxorubicin in Patients With Metastatic Urothelial Carcinoma: A Cooperative Group Study," *J Clin Oncol*, 1992, 10(7):1066-73.

Variation 4:

Logothetis CJ, Finn LD, Smith T, et al, "Escalated MVAC With or Without Recombinant Human Granulocyte-Macrophage Colony-Stimulating Factor for the Initial Treatment of Advanced Malignant Urothelial Tumors: Results of a Randomized Trial," *J Clin Oncol*, 1995, 13(9):2272-7.

Variation 5:

Logothetis CJ, Dexeus FH, Sella A, et al, "Escalated Therapy for Refractory Urothelial Tumors: Methotrexate-Vinblastine-Doxorubicin-Cisplatin Plus Unglycosylated Recombinant Human Granulocyte-Macrophage Colony-Stimulating Factor," *J Natl Cancer Inst*, 1990, 82(8):667-72.

Variation 6:

Sternberg CN, de Mulder PH, van Oosterom AT, et al, "Escalated M-VAC Chemotherapy and Recombinant Human Granulocyte-Macrophage Colony Stimulating Factor (rhGM-CSF) in Patients With Advanced Urothelial Tract Tumors," *Ann Oncol*, 1993, 4(5):403-7.

Variation 7:

Sternberg CN, de Mulder PH, Schornagel JH, et al, "Randomized Phase III Trial of High-Dose-Intensity Methotrexate, Vinblastine, Doxorubicin, and Cisplatin (M-VAC) Chemotherapy and Recombinant Human Granulocyte Colony-Stimulating Factor Versus Classic M-VAC in Advanced Urothelial Tract Tumors: European Organization for Research and Treatment of Cancer Protocol No. 30924," *J Clin Oncol*, 2001, 19(10):2638-46.

Variation 8 and 9:

Seidman AD, Scher HI, Gabrilove JL, et al, "Dose-Intensification of MVAC With Recombinant Granulocyte Colony-Stimulating Factor as Initial Therapy in Advanced Urothelial Cancer," *J Clin Oncol*, 1993, 11(3):408-14.

Variation 10:

Bamias A, Aravantinos G, Deliveliotis C, et al, "Docetaxel and Cisplatin With Granulocyte Colony-Stimulating Factor (G-CSF) Versus M-VAC With G-CSF in Advanced Urothelial Carcinoma: A Multicenter, Randomized, Phase III Study From the Hellenic Cooperative Oncology Group," *J Clin Oncol*, 2004, 22(2):220-8.

Variation 11:

Simon SD and Srougi M, "Neoadjuvant M-VAC Chemotherapy and Partial Cystectomy for Treatment of Locally Invasive Transitional Cell Carcinoma of the Bladder," *Prog Clin Biol Res*, 1990, 353:169-74.

Variation 12:

Farah R, Chodak GW, Vogelzang NJ, et al, "Curative Radiotherapy Following Chemotherapy for Invasive Bladder Carcinoma (A Preliminary Report)," *Int J Radiat Oncol Biol Phys*, 1991, 20 (3):413-7.

Variation 13:

Vogelzang NJ, Moormeier JA, Awan AM, et al, "Methotrexate, Vinblastine, Doxorubicin, and Cisplatin Followed by Radiotherapy or Surgery for Muscle Invasive Bladder Cancer: The University of Chicago Experience," *J Urol*, 1993, 149(4):753-7.

◆ **MV (AML Induction)** *see* Mitoxantrone-Etoposide (AML Induction) *on page 1713*

◆ **N6 Protocol (Neuroblastoma)** *see* CAV-P/VP (Neuroblastoma) *on page 1554*

◆ **nab Paclitaxel (NSCLC Regimen)** *see* Paclitaxel (Protein Bound) (NSCLC Regimen) *on page 1731*

◆ **NEW A1 (Neuroblastoma)** *see* New A1 (Neuroblastoma) *on page 1721*

New A1 (Neuroblastoma)

Index Terms A1 (NEW) (Neuroblastoma); Cyclophosphamide, Doxorubicin, Etoposide, Cisplatin (Neuroblastoma); NEW A1 (Neuroblastoma); Regimen new A1 (Neuroblastoma)

Use Neuroblastoma

Regimen

Cyclophosphamide: I.V.: 1200 mg/m^2 over 6 hours day 1
[total dose/cycle = 1200 mg/m^2]

Doxorubicin: I.V.: 40 mg/m^2 day 3
[total dose/cycle = 40 mg/m^2]
Etoposide: I.V.: 100 mg/m^2/day days 1 to 5
[total dose/cycle = 500 mg/m^2]
Cisplatin: I.V.: 90 mg/m^2 day 5
[total dose/cycle = 90 mg/m^2]
Repeat cycle every 28 days for up to a total of 6 cycles

References

Kaneko M, Nishihira H, Mugishima H, et al, "Stratification of Treatment of Stage 4 Neuroblastoma Patients Based on N-myc Amplification Status. Study Group of Japan for Treatment of Advanced Neuroblastoma, Tokyo, Japan," *Med Pediatr Oncol*, 1998, 31(1):1-7.

Kaneko M, Tsuchida Y, Mugishima H, et al, "Intensified Chemotherapy Increases the Survival Rates in Patients With Stage 4 Neuroblastoma With MYCN Amplification," *J Pediatr Hematol Oncol*, 2002, 24(8):613-21.

Nilotinib (CML Regimen)

Use Leukemia, chronic myelogenous

Regimen NOTE: Multiple variations are listed.

Variation 1 (newly diagnosed chronic phase):
Nilotinib: Oral: 300 mg twice daily
[total dose/cycle = 16,800 mg]
Repeat cycle every 28 days until disease progression or unacceptable toxicity

Variation 2 (chronic or accelerated phase resistant or intolerant to imatinib):
Nilotinib: Oral: 400 mg twice daily
[total dose/cycle = 22,400 mg]
Repeat cycle every 28 days until disease progression or unacceptable toxicity

References

Variation 1:

Larson RA, Kim D, Rosti G, et al, "Comparison of Nilotinib and Imatinib in Patients (Pts) With Newly Diagnosed Chronic Myeloid Leukemia in Chronic Phase (CML-CP): ENESTnd 24-Month Follow-Up," *J Clin Oncol*, 2011, 29(Suppl 15):6511 [abstract].

Saglio G, Kim DW, Issaragrisil S, et al, "Nilotinib Versus Imatinib for Newly Diagnosed Chronic Myeloid Leukemia," *N Engl J Med*, 2010, 362(24):2251-9.

Variation 2:

Kantarjian HM, Giles F, Gattermann N, et al, "Nilotinib (Formerly AMN107), a Highly Selective BCR-ABL Tyrosine Kinase Inhibitor, Is Effective in Patients With Philadelphia Chromosome-Positive Chronic Myelogenous Leukemia in Chronic Phase Following Imatinib Resistance and Intolerance," *Blood*, 2007, 110(10):3540-6.

Kantarjian HM, Giles FJ, Bhalla KN, et al, "Nilotinib Is Effective in Patients With Chronic Myeloid Leukemia in Chronic Phase After Imatinib Resistance or Intolerance: 24-Month Follow-up Results," *Blood*, 2011, 117(4):1141-5.

le Coutre P, Ottmann OG, Giles F, et al, "Nilotinib (Formerly AMN107), a Highly Selective BCR-ABL Tyrosine Kinase Inhibitor, Is Active in Patients With Imatinib-Resistant or -Intolerant Accelerated-Phase Chronic Myelogenous Leukemia," *Blood*, 2008, 111(4):1834-9.

OFAR (CLL)

Index Terms Oxaliplatin-Fludarabine-Cytarabine-Rituximab (CLL)

Use Leukemia, chronic lymphocytic

Regimen

Cycle 1:
Oxaliplatin: I.V.: 25 mg/m^2/dose day 1 to 4
[total dose/cycle = 100 mg/m^2]
Fludarabine: I.V.: 30 mg/m^2/dose days 2 and 3
[total dose/cycle = 60 mg/m^2]

Cytarabine: I.V.: 1000 mg/m²/dose over 2 hours days 2 and 3
[total dose/cycle = 2000 mg/m²]
Rituximab: I.V.: 375 mg/m² day 3
[total dose/cycle = 375 mg/m²]
Treatment cycle is 4 weeks
Cycles 2-6:
Oxaliplatin: I.V.: 25 mg/m²/dose day 1 to 4
[total dose/cycle = 100 mg/m²]
Fludarabine: I.V.: 30 mg/m²/dose days 2 and 3
[total dose/cycle = 60 mg/m²]
Cytarabine: I.V.: 1000 mg/m²/dose over 2 hours days 2 and 3
[total dose/cycle = 2000 mg/m²]
Rituximab: I.V.: 375 mg/m² day 1
[total dose/cycle = 375 mg/m²]
Repeat cycle every 4 weeks (maximum: 6 cycles)

References

Tsimberidou AM, Wierda WG, Plunkett W, et al, "Phase I-II Study of Oxaliplatin, Fludarabine, Cytarabine, and Rituximab Combination Therapy in Patients With Richter's Syndrome or Fludarabine-Refractory Chronic Lymphocytic Leukemia," *J Clin Oncol*, 2008, 26(2):196-203.

◆ **Oxaliplatin-Capecitabine (Biliary Cancer)** *see* CAPOX (Biliary Cancer) *on page 1542*

◆ **Oxaliplatin-Capecitabine (Colorectal)** *see* XELOX (Colorectal) *on page 1778*

◆ **Oxaliplatin-Capecitabine-Epirubicin** *see* Epirubicin-Oxaliplatin-Capecitabine *on page 1627*

◆ **Oxaliplatin-Capecitabine (Pancreatic)** *see* CAPOX (Pancreatic) *on page 1543*

Oxaliplatin-Cytarabine-Dexamethasone (NHL Regimen)

Index Terms DHAX (NHL Regimen)

Use Lymphoma, non-Hodgkin's

Regimen

Dexamethasone: I.V. or Oral: 40 mg/day days 1 to 4
[total dose/cycle = 160 mg]
Oxaliplatin: I.V.: 130 mg/m² over 2 hours day 1
[total dose/cycle = 130 mg/m²]
Cytarabine: I.V.: 2000 mg/m² over 3 hours every 12 hours for 2 doses day 2
[total dose/cycle = 4000 mg/m²]
Repeat cycle every 3 weeks

References

Chau I, Webb A, Cunningham D, et al, "An Oxaliplatin-Based Chemotherapy in Patients With Relapsed or Refractory Intermediate and High-Grade Non-Hodgkin's Lymphoma," *Br J Haematol*, 2001, 115(4):786-92.

◆ **Oxaliplatin-Docetaxel-Fluorouracil (Esophageal Cancer)** *see* Docetaxel-Oxaliplatin-Fluorouracil (Esophageal Cancer) *on page 1613*

◆ **Oxaliplatin-Docetaxel-Leucovorin-Fluorouracil (Esophageal Cancer)** *see* Docetaxel-Oxaliplatin-Leucovorin-Fluorouracil (Esophageal Cancer) *on page 1613*

◆ **Oxaliplatin-Docetaxel (Ovarian Cancer)** *see* Docetaxel-Oxaliplatin (Ovarian Cancer) *on page 1613*

◆ **Oxaliplatin-Fludarabine-Cytarabine-Rituximab (CLL)** *see* OFAR (CLL) *on page 1722*

Oxaliplatin-Fluorouracil (Esophageal Cancer)

Index Terms Fluorouracil-Oxaliplatin (Esophageal Cancer)

Use Esophageal cancer

Regimen In combination with radiation therapy:

Oxaliplatin: I.V.: 85 mg/m²/day over 2 hours days 1, 15, and 29 [total dose/cycle = 255 mg/m²]

Fluorouracil: I.V.: 180 mg/m²/day continuous infusion days 8 to 42 [total dose/cycle = 6300 mg/m²]

References

Khushalani NI, Leichman CG, Proulx G, et al, "Oxaliplatin in Combination With Protracted-Infusion Fluorouracil and Radiation: Report of a Clinical Trial for Patients With Esophageal Cancer," *J Clin Oncol*, 2002, 20(12):2844-50.

◆ **Oxaliplatin-Fluorouracil-Leucovorin-Bevacizumab** *see* Bevacizumab-Oxaliplatin-Fluorouracil-Leucovorin *on page 1531*

◆ **Oxaliplatin-Fluorouracil-Leucovorin (Esophageal Cancer)** *see* Fluorouracil-Leucovorin-Oxaliplatin (Esophageal Cancer) *on page 1656*

◆ **Oxaliplatin, Fluorouracil, Leucovorin (Pancreatic)** *see* FOLFOX (Pancreatic) *on page 1665*

◆ **Oxaliplatin-Gemcitabine-Paclitaxel (Testicular)** *see* Gemcitabine-Oxaliplatin-Paclitaxel (Testicular) *on page 1674*

◆ **Oxaliplatin-Gemcitabine (Pancreatic)** *see* Gemcitabine-Oxaliplatin (Pancreatic) *on page 1674*

◆ **Oxaliplatin-Gemcitabine-Rituximab (NHL)** *see* Gemcitabine-Oxaliplatin-Rituximab (NHL) *on page 1674*

◆ **Oxaliplatin-Gemcitabine (Testicular)** *see* GEMOX (Testicular) *on page 1678*

◆ **Oxaliplatin-Irinotecan-Fluorouracil-Leucovorin (Pancreatic)** *see* FOLFIRINOX (Pancreatic) *on page 1661*

◆ **Oxaliplatin-Leucovorin-Fluorouracil (Colorectal)** *see* FLOX (Colorectal) *on page 1645*

◆ **Oxaliplatin-Leucovorin-Fluorouracil (Colorectal)** *see* FOLFOX1 (Colorectal) *on page 1662*

◆ **Oxaliplatin-Leucovorin-Fluorouracil (Colorectal)** *see* FOLFOX2 (Colorectal) *on page 1662*

◆ **Oxaliplatin-Leucovorin-Fluorouracil (Colorectal)** *see* FOLFOX3 (Colorectal) *on page 1662*

◆ **Oxaliplatin, Leucovorin, Fluorouracil (Colorectal)** *see* FOLFOX4 (Colorectal) *on page 1663*

◆ **Oxaliplatin-Leucovorin-Fluorouracil (Colorectal)** *see* FOLFOX6 and mFOLFOX6 (Colorectal) *on page 1663*

◆ **Oxaliplatin-Leucovorin-Fluorouracil (Esophageal Cancer)** *see* Fluorouracil-Leucovorin-Oxaliplatin (Esophageal Cancer) *on page 1656*

◆ **Oxaliplatin–Leucovorin–Fluorouracil (Gastric Cancer)** *see* Fluorouracil-Leucovorin-Oxaliplatin (Gastric Cancer) *on page 1657*

PAC (CAP)

Use Ovarian cancer

Regimen

Cisplatin: I.V.: 50 mg/m^2 day 1
[total dose/cycle = 50 mg/m^2]

Doxorubicin: I.V.: 50 mg/m^2 day 1
[total dose/cycle = 50 mg/m^2]

Cyclophosphamide: I.V.: 1000 mg/m^2 day 1
[total dose/cycle = 1000 mg/m^2]

Repeat cycle every 21 days for 8 cycles

References

Omura GA, Bundy BN, Berek JS, et al, "Randomized Trial of Cyclophosphamide Plus Cisplatin With or Without Doxorubicin in Ovarian Carcinoma: A Gynecologic Oncology Group Study," *J Clin Oncol*, 1989, 7(4):457-65.

PA-CI

Use Hepatoblastoma

Regimen NOTE: Multiple variations are listed.

Variation 1:

Cisplatin: I.V.: 90 mg/m^2 day 1
[total dose/cycle = 90 mg/m^2]

Doxorubicin: I.V.: 20 mg/m^2/day continuous infusion days 2 to 5
[total dose/cycle = 80 mg/m^2]

Repeat cycle every 21 days

Variation 2:

Cisplatin: I.V.: 20 mg/m^2/day days 1 to 4
[total dose/cycle = 80 mg/m^2]

Doxorubicin: I.V.: 100 mg/m^2 continuous infusion day 1
[total dose/cycle = 100 mg/m^2]

Repeat cycle every 21-28 days

References

Variation 1:

Ortega JA, Douglass EC, Feusner JH, et al, "Randomized Comparison of Cisplatin/Vincristine/Fluorouracil and Cisplatin/Continuous Infusion Doxorubicin for Treatment of Pediatric Hepatoblastoma: A Report From the Children's Cancer Group and the Pediatric Oncology Group," *J Clin Oncol*, 2000, 18(14):2665-75.

Variation 2:

Ortega JA, Krailo MD, Haas JE, et al, "Effective Treatment of Unresectable or Metastatic Hepatoblastoma With Cisplatin and Continuous Infusion Doxorubicin Chemotherapy: A Report From the Childrens Cancer Study Group," *J Clin Oncol*, 1991, 9(12):2167-76.

Paclitaxel-Bevacizumab

Index Terms Bevacizumab Paclitaxel

Use Breast cancer

Regimen

Paclitaxel: I.V.: 90 mg/m^2/day days 1, 8, and 15
[total dose/cycle = 270 mg/m^2]

Bevacizumab: I.V.: 10 mg/kg/day days 1 and 15
[total dose/cycle = 20 mg/kg]

Repeat cycle every 28 days

References

Miller KD, "E2100: A Phase III Trial of Paclitaxel Versus Paclitaxel/Bevacizumab for Metastatic Breast Cancer," *Clin Breast Cancer*, 2003, 3(6):421-2.

Miller K, Wang M, Gralow J, et al, "Paclitaxel Plus Bevacizumab Versus Paclitaxel Alone for Metastatic Breast Cancer," *N Engl J Med*, 2007, 357(26):2666-76.

Paclitaxel-Carboplatin (Bladder Cancer)

Index Terms Carboplatin-Paclitaxel (Bladder Cancer); PC (Bladder Cancer)

Use Bladder cancer

Regimen

Paclitaxel: I.V.: 200 mg/m^2 or 225 mg/m^2 day 1
[total dose/cycle = 200 or 225 mg/m^2]

Carboplatin: I.V.: AUC 5-6 day 1
[total dose/cycle = AUC = 5-6]

Repeat cycle every 21 days

References

Vaughn DJ, Malkowicz SB, Zoltick B, et al, "Paclitaxel Plus Carboplatin in Advanced Carcinoma of the Urothelium: An Active and Tolerable Outpatient Regimen," *J Clin Oncol*, 1998, 16(1):255-60.

◆ **Paclitaxel-Carboplatin (Cervical Cancer)** *see* Carboplatin-Paclitaxel (Cervical Cancer) *on page 1549*

Paclitaxel-Carboplatin (Esophageal Cancer)

Index Terms Carboplatin-Paclitaxel (Esophageal Cancer)

Use Esophageal cancer

Regimen

Paclitaxel: I.V.: 50 mg/m^2/dose over 1 hour days 1, 8, 15, 22, and 29
[total dose/cycle = 250 mg/m^2]

Carboplatin: I.V.: AUC = 2 days 1, 8, 15, 22, and 29
[total dose/cycle = AUC = 10]

Administer with concurrent radiation therapy; cycle does not repeat.

References

van Meerten E, Muller K, Tilanus HW, et al ""Neoadjuvant Concurrent Chemoradiation With Weekly Paclitaxel and Carboplatin for Patients With Oesophageal Cancer: A Phase II Study," *Br J Cancer*, 2006, 94(10):1389-94.

◆ **Paclitaxel-Carboplatin-Etoposide (Unknown Primary)** *see* Carboplatin-Etoposide-Paclitaxel (Unknown Primary) *on page 1545*

Paclitaxel-Carboplatin-Gemcitabine

Use Bladder cancer

Regimen

Paclitaxel: I.V.: 200 mg/m^2 day 1
[total dose/cycle = 200 mg/m^2]

Gemcitabine: I.V.: 1000 mg/m^2/day days 1 and 8
[total dose/cycle = 2000 mg/m^2]

Carboplatin: I.V.: AUC 5 day 1
[total dose/cycle = AUC = 5]

Repeat cycle every 21 days

References

Hainsworth JD, Meluch AA, Litchy S, et al, "Paclitaxel, Carboplatin, and Gemcitabine in the Treatment of Patients With Advanced Transitional Cell Carcinoma of the Urothelium," *Cancer*, 2005, 103(11):2298-303

◆ **Paclitaxel-Carboplatin-Gemcitabine (Unknown Primary)** *see* Carboplatin-Gemcitabine-Paclitaxel (Unknown Primary) *on page 1548*

◆ **Paclitaxel-Carboplatin (Nonsmall Cell Lung Cancer)** *see* Carbo-Tax (NSCLC) *on page 1552*

◆ **Paclitaxel-Carboplatin (Ovarian)** *see* Carboplatin-Paclitaxel (Ovarian) *on page 1550*

- **Paclitaxel-Carboplatin-Trastuzumab** *see* Trastuzumab-Paclitaxel-Carboplatin *on page 1760*
- **Paclitaxel-Carboplatin (Unknown Primary)** *see* Carboplatin-Paclitaxel (Unknown Primary) *on page 1551*

Paclitaxel-Cetuximab

Index Terms Cetuximab-Paclitaxel

Use Head and neck cancer

Regimen

Week 1:

Paclitaxel: I.V.: 80 mg/m^2 day 1
[total dose/week 1 = 80 mg/m^2]

Cetuximab: I.V.: 400 mg/m^2 (loading dose) day 1 (week 1 only)
[total loading dose (week 1) = 400 mg/m^2]

Subsequent weeks:

Paclitaxel: I.V.: 80 mg/m^2 day 1
[total dose/week = 80 mg/m^2]

Cetuximab: I.V.: 250 mg/m^2 day 1
[total dose/week = 250 mg/m^2]

References

Hitt R, Irigoyen H, Nunez J, et al, "Phase II Study of Combination Cetuximab and Weekly Paclitaxel in Patients With Metastatic/Recurrent Squamous Cell Carcinama of Head and Neck (SCCHN): Spanish Head and Neck Cancer Group (TTCC)," *J Clin Oncol*, 2007, 25(18S) [abstract 6012 from 2007 ASCO Annual Meeting].

- **Paclitaxel-Cisplatin (Cervical Cancer)** *see* Cisplatin-Paclitaxel (Cervical Cancer) *on page 1581*

Paclitaxel-Cisplatin (Esophageal Cancer)

Index Terms Cisplatin-Paclitaxel (Esophageal Cancer)

Use Esophageal cancer

Regimen NOTE: Multiple variations are listed.

Variation 1:

Paclitaxel: I.V.: 50 mg/m^2/dose over 1 hour days 1, 8, 15, 22, and 29
[total dose/cycle = 250 mg/m^2]

Cisplatin: I.V.: 30 mg/m^2/dose days 1, 8, 15, 22, and 29
[total dose/cycle = 150 mg/m^2]

Administered (with concurrent radiation therapy) over one 5 week treatment cycle.

Followed by: Postoperative therapy:

Paclitaxel: I.V.: 175 mg/m^2/dose day 1
[total dose/cycle = 175 mg/m^2]

Cisplatin: I.V.: 75 mg/m^2/dose day 1
[total dose/cycle = 75 mg/m^2]

Repeat postop cycle every 21 days for a total of 3 cycles.

Variation 2:

Paclitaxel: I.V.: 60 mg/m^2/dose over 3 hours days 1, 8, 15, and 22
[total dose/cycle = 240 mg/m^2]

Cisplatin: I.V.: 75 mg/m^2/dose over 2 hours day 1
[total dose/cycle = 75 mg/m^2]

Filgrastim: SubQ: 5 mcg/kg/day starting day 23; continue until ANC >10,000/mm^3

Administer with concurrent radiation therapy; cycle does not repeat.

Variation 3:

Paclitaxel: I.V.: 90 mg/m²/dose over 3 hours day 1
[total dose/cycle = 90 mg/m²]

Cisplatin: I.V.: 50 mg/m²/dose over 1 hour day 1
[total dose/cycle = 50 mg/m²]

Repeat cycle every 14 days until disease progression or unacceptable toxicity.

References

Variation 1:

Kleinberg L, Powell ME, Forastiere AA, et al, "Survival Outcome of E1201: An Eastern Cooperative Oncology Group (ECOG) Randomized Phase II Trial of Neoadjuvant Preoperative Paclitaxel/Cisplatin/Radiotherapy (RT) or Irinotecan/Cisplatin/RT in Endoscopy With Ultrasound (EUS) Staged Esophageal Adenocarcinoma," *J Clin Oncol*, 2008, 26(15S):4532 [abstract 4532 from 2008 annual ASCO meeting].

Variation 2:

Urba SG, Orringer MB, Ianettonni M, et al, "Concurrent Cisplatin, Paclitaxel, and Radiotherapy as Preoperative Treatment for Patients With Locoregional Esophageal Carcinoma," *Cancer*, 2003, 98(10):2177-83.

Variation 3:

Petrasch S, Welt A, Reinacher A, et al, "Chemotherapy With Cisplatin and Paclitaxel in Patients With Locally Advanced, Recurrent or Metastatic Oesophageal Cancer," *Br J Cancer*, 1998, 78 (4):511-4.

Paclitaxel-Cisplatin-Fluorouracil (Esophageal Cancer)

Index Terms Paclitaxel-Fluorouracil-Cisplatin (Esophageal Cancer); TCF (Esophageal Cancer)

Use Esophageal cancer

Regimen

Paclitaxel: I.V.: 175 mg/m² over 3 hours day 1
[total dose/cycle = 175 mg/m²]

Cisplatin: I.V.: 20 mg/m²/day days 1 to 5 for cycles 1, 2, and 3
[total dose/cycle = 100 mg/m²]
then 15 mg/m²/day days 1 to 5
[total dose/cycle = 75 mg/m²]

Fluorouracil: I.V.: 750 mg/m²/day continuous infusion days 1 to 5
[total dose/cycle = 3750 mg/m²]

Repeat cycle every 28 days

References

Ilson DH, Ajani J, Bhalla K, et al, "Phase II Trial of Paclitaxel, Fluorouracil, and Cisplatin in Patients With Advanced Carcinoma of the Esophagus," *J Clin Oncol*, 1998, 16(5):1826-34.

◆ **Paclitaxel-Cisplatin (Head and Neck Cancer)** *see* Cisplatin-Paclitaxel (Head and Neck Cancer) *on page 1581*

◆ **Paclitaxel-Cisplatin Intraperitoneal (Ovarian)** *see* Cisplatin-Paclitaxel Intraperitoneal (Ovarian) *on page 1582*

◆ **Paclitaxel-Cisplatin (Ovarian)** *see* Cisplatin-Paclitaxel (Ovarian) *on page 1582*

◆ **Paclitaxel-Estramustine** *see* Estramustine-Paclitaxel *on page 1637*

Paclitaxel + Estramustine + Carboplatin

Use Prostate cancer

Regimen

Paclitaxel: I.V.: 100 mg/m² day 3 each week
[total dose/cycle = 400 mg/m²]

Estramustine: Oral: 10 mg/kg/day days 1 to 5 each week
[total dose/cycle = 200 mg/kg]
Carboplatin: I.V.: Target AUC 6 day 3
[total dose/cycle = AUC = 6]
Repeat cycle every 28 days

References

Kelly WK, Curley T, Slovin S, et al, "Paclitaxel, Estramustine Phosphate, and Carboplatin in Patients With Advanced Prostate Cancer," *J Clin Oncol*, 2001, 19(1):44-53.

Paclitaxel + Estramustine + Etoposide

Use Prostate cancer

Regimen

Paclitaxel: I.V.: 135 mg/m^2 day 2
[total dose/cycle = 135 mg/m^2]
Estramustine: Oral: 280 mg 3 times/day days 1 to 14
[total dose/cycle = 11,760 mg]
Etoposide: Oral: 100 mg/day days 1 to 14
[total dose/cycle = 1400 mg]
Repeat cycle every 21 days

References

Smith DC, Esper P, Strawderman M, et al, "Phase II Trial of Oral Estramustine, Oral Etoposide, and Intravenous Paclitaxel in Hormone-Refractory Prostate Cancer," *J Clin Oncol*, 1999, 17 (6):1664-71.

◆ **Paclitaxel-Fluorouracil-Cisplatin (Esophageal Cancer)** *see* Paclitaxel-Cisplatin-Fluorouracil (Esophageal Cancer) *on page 1728*

Paclitaxel-Fluorouracil (Esophageal Cancer)

Index Terms Fluorouracil-Paclitaxel (Esophageal Cancer)

Use Esophageal cancer

Regimen

Paclitaxel: I.V.: 45 mg/m^2/dose over 3 hours day 1
[total dose/cycle = 45 mg/m^2]
Fluorouracil: I.V.: 300 mg/m^2/day continuous infusion days 1 to 5
[total dose/cycle = 1500 mg/m^2]
Repeat cycle weekly for 5 weeks; administer concurrent with radiation therapy; cycle does not repeat.

References

Schnirer II, Komaki R, Yao JC, et al, "Pilot Study of Concurrent 5-Fluorouracil/Paclitaxel Plus Radiotherapy in Patients With Carcinoma of the Esophagus and Gastroesophageal Junction," *Am J Clin Oncol*, 2001, 24(1):91-5.

Paclitaxel-Gemcitabine

Index Terms Gemcitabine-Paclitaxel

Use Bladder cancer

Regimen

Paclitaxel: I.V.: 200 mg/m^2 day 1
[total dose/cycle = 200 mg/m^2]
Gemcitabine: I.V.: 1000 mg/m^2/day days 1, 8, and 15
[total dose/cycle = 3000 mg/m^2]
Repeat cycle every 21 days for a maximum of 6 cycles

References

Meluch AA, Greco FA, Burris HA 3rd, et al, "Paclitaxel and Gemcitabine Chemotherapy for Advanced Transitional-Cell Carcinoma of the Urothelial Tract: A Phase II Trial of the Minnie Pearl Cancer Research Network," *J Clin Oncol*, 2001, 19(12):3018-24.

- **Paclitaxel-Gemcitabine (Breast Cancer)** *see* Gemcitabine-Paclitaxel (Breast Cancer) *on page 1675*
- **Paclitaxel-Gemcitabine (Ovarian Cancer)** *see* Gemcitabine-Paclitaxel (Ovarian Cancer) *on page 1675*
- **Paclitaxel-Gemcitabine-Oxaliplatin (Testicular)** *see* Gemcitabine-Oxaliplatin-Paclitaxel (Testicular) *on page 1674*
- **Paclitaxel-Gemcitabine (Testicular)** *see* Gemcitabine-Paclitaxel (Testicular) *on page 1675*

Paclitaxel-Ifosfamide-Cisplatin

Index Terms Cisplatin-Ifosfamide-Paclitaxel

Use Testicular cancer

Regimen

Paclitaxel: I.V.: 250 mg/m^2 continuous infusion day 1
[total dose/cycle = 250 mg/m^2]

Ifosfamide: I.V.: 1500 mg/m^2/day days 2 to 5
[total dose/cycle = 6000 mg/m^2]

Cisplatin: I.V.: 25 mg/m^2/day days 2 to 5
[total dose/cycle = 100 mg/m^2]

Mesna: I.V.: 500 mg/m^2 prior to ifosfamide and every 4 hours for 2 doses, days 2 to 5
[total dose/cycle = 6000 mg/m^2]

Repeat cycle every 21 days for 4 cycles

References

Kondagunta GV, Bacik J, Donadio A, et al, "Combination of Paclitaxel, Ifosfamide, and Cisplatin is an Effective Second-Line Therapy for Patients With Relapsed Testicular Germ Cell Tumors," *J Clin Oncol*, 2005, 23(27):6549-55.

Paclitaxel Maintenance (Ovarian Cancer)

Use Ovarian cancer

Regimen

Paclitaxel: I.V.: 175 mg/m^2 over 3 hours day 1
[total dose/cycle = 175 mg/m^2]

Repeat cycle every 28 days for 12 cycles

References

Markman M, Liu PY, Wilczynsi S, et al, "Phase III Randomized Trial of 12 Versus 3 Months of Maintenance Paclitaxel in Patients With Advanced Ovarian Cancer After Complete Response to Platinum and Paclitaxel-Based Chemotherapy: A Southwest Oncology Group and Gynecologic Oncology Group Trial," *J Clin Oncol*, 2003, 21(13):2460-5.

Paclitaxel (Ovarian Regimen)

Use Ovarian cancer

Regimen NOTE: Multiple variations are listed.

Variation 1:

Paclitaxel: I.V.: 80 mg/m^2/day days 1, 8, and 15
[total dose/cycle = 240 mg/m^2]

Repeat cycle every 28 days for 6-9 cycles or until disease progression or unacceptable toxicity

Variation 2:

Paclitaxel: I.V.: 80 mg/m^2/day over 1 hour days 1, 8, 15, and 21
[total dose/cycle = 320 mg/m^2]

Repeat cycle every 28 days for 3 cycles

Followed by:

Paclitaxel: I.V.: 80 mg/m^2/day days 1, 8, and 15
[total dose/cycle = 240 mg/m^2]

Repeat cycle every 28 days until disease progression or unacceptable toxicity

Variation 3:

Paclitaxel: I.V.: 175 mg/m^2 over 3 hours day 1
[total dose/cycle = 175 mg/m^2]

Repeat cycle every 21 days for 6-10 cycles

Variation 4 (heavily pretreated or poor performance status patients):

Paclitaxel: I.V.: 135 mg/m^2 over 3 hours day 1
[total dose/cycle = 135 mg/m^2]

Repeat cycle every 21 days for 6-10 cycles

References

Variation 1:

Lortholary A, Largiller R, Weber B, et al, "Weekly Paclitaxel as a Single Agent or in Combination With Carboplatin or Weekly Topotecan in Patients With Resistant Ovarian Cancer: The CARTAXHY Randomized Phase II Trial From Groupe d'Investigateurs Nationaux pour l'Etude des Cancers Ovarianens (GINECO)," *Ann Oncol*, 2012, 23(2):346-52.

Variation 2:

Markman M, Blessing J, Rubin SC, et al, "Phase II Trial of Weekly Paclitaxel (80mg/m^2) in Platinum and Paclitaxel-Resistant Ovarian and Primary Peritoneal Cancers: A Gynecologic Group Study," *Gynecol Oncol*, 2006, 101(3):436-40.

Variation 3 and 4:

Bruzzone M, Catsafados E, Miglietta L, et al, "Salvage Chemotherapy With Paclitaxel in Platinum-Resistant Advanced Ovarian Cancer Patients," *Oncology*, 1996, 53(5):349-53.

◆ **Paclitaxel (Protein Bound)-Gemcitabine (Pancreatic)** *see* Gemcitabine-Paclitaxel (Protein Bound) (Pancreatic) *on page 1675*

Paclitaxel (Protein Bound) (NSCLC Regimen)

Index Terms nab Paclitaxel (NSCLC Regimen)

Use Lung cancer, nonsmall cell

Regimen NOTE: Multiple variations are listed:

Variation 1:

Paclitaxel (Protein Bound): I.V.: 260 mg/m^2 over 30 minutes day 1
[total dose/cycle = 260 mg/m^2]

Repeat cycle every 21 days until disease progression or unacceptable toxicity

Variation 2:

Paclitaxel (Protein Bound): I.V.: 125 mg/m^2/day over 30 minutes days 1, 8, and 15
[total dose/cycle = 375 mg/m^2]

Repeat cycle every 28 days until disease progression or unacceptable toxicity

References

Variation 1:

Green MR, Manikhas GM, Orlov S, et al, "Abraxane®, a Novel Cremophor®-Free, Albumin-Bound Particle Form of Paclitaxel for the Treatment of Advanced Non-Small-Cell Lung Cancer," *Ann Oncol*, 2006, 17(8):1263-8.

Variation 2:

Rizvi NA, Riely GJ, Azzoli CG, et al, "Phase I/II Trial of Weekly Intravenous 130-nm Albumin-Bound Paclitaxel As Initial Chemotherapy in Patients With Stage IV Non-Small-Cell Lung Cancer," *J Clin Oncol*, 2008, 26(4):639-43.

Paclitaxel (Small Cell Lung Cancer Regimen)

Use Lung cancer, small cell

Regimen NOTE: Multiple variations are listed.

Variation 1:

Paclitaxel: I.V.: 175 mg/m^2 over 3 hours day 1
[total dose/cycle = 175 mg/m^2]

Repeat cycle every 21 days

Variation 2:

Paclitaxel: I.V.: 80 mg/m^2/day over 1 hour days 1, 8, 15, 22, 29, and 36
[total dose/cycle = 480 mg/m^2]

Repeat cycle every 56 days

References

Variation 1:
Smit EF, Fokkema E, Biesma B, et al, "A Phase II Study of Paclitaxel in Heavily Pretreated Patients With Small-Cell Lung Cancer," *Br J Cancer*, 1998, 77(2):347-51.
Variation 2:
Yamamoto N, Tsurutani J, Yoshimura N, et al, "Phase II Study of Weekly Paclitaxel for Relapsed and Refractory Small Cell Lung Cancer," *Anticancer Res*, 2006, 26(1B):777-82.

◆ **Paclitaxel-Trastuzumab** *see* Trastuzumab-Paclitaxel *on page* *1759*

Paclitaxel-Vinorelbine

Use Breast cancer

Regimen NOTE: Multiple variations are listed.

Variation 1:

Paclitaxel: I.V.: 135 mg/m^2 day 1
[total dose/cycle = 135 mg/m^2]

Vinorelbine: I.V.: 30 mg/m^2 day 1
[total dose/cycle = 30 mg/m^2]

Repeat cycle every 21 days

Variation 2:

Paclitaxel: I.V.: 150 mg/m^2 day 1
[total dose/cycle = 150 mg/m^2]

Vinorelbine: I.V.: 25 mg/m^2 day 1
[total dose/cycle = 25 mg/m^2]

Repeat cycle every 21 days

Variation 3:

Paclitaxel: I.V.: 135 mg/m^2 day 1
[total dose/cycle = 135 mg/m^2]

Vinorelbine: I.V.: 30 mg/m^2/day days 1 and 8
[total dose/cycle = 60 mg/m^2]

Repeat cycle every 28 days

References

Variation 1:
Martin M, Lluch A, Casado A, et al, "Paclitaxel Plus Vinorelbine: An Active Regimen in Metastatic Breast Cancer Patients With Prior Anthracycline Exposure," *Ann Oncol*, 2000, 11(1):85-9.
Variation 2:
Vici P, Amodio A, Di Lauro L, et al, "First-Line Chemotherapy With Vinorelbine and Paclitaxel As Simultaneous Infusion in Advanced Breast Cancer," *Oncology*, 2000, 58(1):3-7.
Variation 3:
Romero Acuna LR, Langhi M, Perez J, et al, "Vinorelbine and Paclitaxel as First-Line Chemotherapy in Metastatic Breast Cancer," *J Clin Oncol*, 1999, 17(1):74-81.

◆ **Paclitaxel (Weekly)-Trastuzumab** *see* Trastuzumab-Paclitaxel (Weekly) *on page* *1760*

◆ **PAD** *see* Bortezomib-Doxorubicin-Dexamethasone *on page* *1535*

Panitumumab (Colorectal Regimen)

Use Colorectal cancer

Regimen

Panitumumab: I.V.: 6 mg/kg over 60 minutes day 1
[total dose/cycle = 6 mg/kg]

Repeat cycle every 14 days until disease progression or unacceptable toxicity

References

Amado RG, Wolf M, Peeters M, et al, "Wild-Type *KRAS* Is Required for Panitumumab Efficacy in Patients With Metastatic Colorectal Cancer," *J Clin Oncol*, 2008, 26(10):1626-34.

Van Cutsem E, Peeters M, Siena S, et al, "Open-Label Phase III Trial of Panitumumab Plus Best Supportive Care Compared With Best Supportive Care Alone in Patients With Chemotherapy-Refractory Metastatic Colorectal Cancer," *J Clin Oncol*, 2007, 25(13):1658-64.

Panitumumab + FOLFIRI (Colorectal)

Use Colorectal cancer

Regimen

Panitumumab: I.V.: 6 mg/kg over 30-60 minutes day 1
[total dose/cycle = 6 mg/kg]

Irinotecan: I.V.: 180 mg/m^2 day 1
[total dose/cycle = 180 mg/m^2]

Leucovorin (racemic): I.V.: 400 mg/m^2 day 1
[total dose/cycle = 400 mg/m^2]

Fluorouracil: I.V. bolus: 400 mg/m^2 day 1
followed by I.V.: 2400 mg/m^2 continuous infusion (CI) over 46 hours beginning day 1
[total fluorouracil dose/cycle (bolus and CI) = 2800 mg/m^2]

Repeat cycle every 14 days until disease progression or unacceptable toxicity

References

Peeters M, Price TJ, Cervantes A, et al, "Randomized Phase III Study of Panitumumab With Fluorouracil, Leucovorin, and Irinotecan (FOLFIRI) Compared With FOLFIRI Alone as Second-Line Treatment in Patients With Metastatic Colorectal Cancer," *J Clin Oncol*, 2010, 28 (31):4706-13.

Panitumumab + FOLFOX4 (Colorectal)

Use Colorectal cancer

Regimen

Panitumumab: I.V.: 6 mg/kg over 30-60 minutes day 1
[total dose/cycle = 6 mg/kg]

Oxaliplatin: I.V.: 85 mg/m^2 day 1
[total dose/cycle = 85 mg/m^2]

Leucovorin: I.V.: 200 mg/m^2/day days 1 and 2
[total dose/cycle = 400 mg/m^2]

Fluorouracil: I.V. bolus: 400 mg/m^2/day days 1 and 2
followed by I.V.: 600 mg/m^2 continuous infusion (CI) over 22 hours days 1 and 2
[total fluorouracil dose/cycle (bolus and CI) = 2000 mg/m^2]

Note: Bolus fluorouracil and continuous infusion fluorouracil are both given on each day

Repeat cycle every 14 days until disease progression or unacceptable toxicity

References

Douillard JY, Siena S, Cassidy J, et al, "Randomized, Phase III Trial of Panitumumab With Infusional Fluorouracil, Leucovorin, and Oxaliplatin (FOLFOX4) Versus FOLFOX4 Alone as First-Line Treatment in Patients With Previously Untreated Metastatic Colorectal Cancer: The PRIME Study," *J Clin Oncol*, 2010, 28(31):4697-705.

Pazopanib (RCC Regimen)

Use Renal cell cancer

Regimen

Pazopanib: Oral: 800 mg once daily
[total dose/cycle = 22,400 mg]

Repeat cycle every 28 days until disease progression or unacceptable toxicity

References

Sternberg CN, Davis ID, Mardiak J, et al, "Pazopanib in Locally Advanced or Metastatic Renal Cell Carcinoma: Results of a Randomized Phase III Trial," *J Clin Oncol*, 2010, 28(6): 1061-8.

Pazopanib (Soft Tissue Sarcoma Regimen)

Use Soft tissue sarcoma

Regimen

Pazopanib: Oral: 800 mg once daily
[total dose/cycle = 22,400 mg]

Repeat cycle every 28 days until disease progression or unacceptable toxicity

References

Van Der Graaf WT, Blay J, Chawla SP, et al, "PALETTE: A Randomized, Double-Blind, Phase III Trial of Pazopanib Versus Placebo in Patients (PTS) With Soft-Tissue Sarcoma (STS) Whose Disease has Progressed During or Following Prior Chemotherapy – An EORTC STBSG Global Network Study (EORTC 62072)," *J Clin Oncol*, 29 (Suppl 18):LBA10002 [abstract LBA10002 from 2011 ASCO Annual Meeting].

Pazopanib (Thyroid Cancer Regimen)

Use Thyroid cancer

Regimen

Pazopanib: Oral: 800 mg once daily
[total dose/cycle = 22,400 mg]

Repeat cycle every 28 days until disease progression or unacceptable toxicity

References

Bible KC, Suman VJ, Molina JR, et al, "Efficacy of Pazopanib in Progressive, Radioiodine-Refractory, Metastatic Differentiated Thyroid Cancers: Results of a Phase 2 Consortium Study," *Lancet Oncol*, 2010, 11(10): 962-72.

◆ **PC (Bladder Cancer)** *see* Paclitaxel-Carboplatin (Bladder Cancer) *on page 1726*

◆ **PCF (Unknown Primary)** *see* Cisplatin-Fluorouracil-Paclitaxel (Unknown Primary) *on page 1577*

PC (NSCLC)

Use Lung cancer, nonsmall cell

Regimen NOTE: Multiple variations are listed.

Variation 1:

Paclitaxel: I.V.: 175-225 mg/m^2 day 1
[total dose/cycle = 175-225 mg/m^2]

Carboplatin: I.V.: Target AUC 5-7 day 1
[total dose/cycle = AUC = 5-7]

Repeat cycle every 21 days for 2-8 cycles

Variation 2:

Paclitaxel: I.V.: 175 mg/m^2 day 1
[total dose/cycle = 175 mg/m^2]

Cisplatin: I.V.: 80 mg/m^2 day 1
[total dose/cycle = 80 mg/m^2]

Repeat cycle every 21 days

Variation 3:

Paclitaxel: I.V.: 135 mg/m^2 continuous infusion day 1
[total dose/cycle = 135 mg/m^2]

Carboplatin: I.V.: AUC 7.5 day 2
[total dose/cycle = AUC = 7.5]

Repeat cycle every 21 days

Variation 4:

Paclitaxel: I.V.: 135 mg/m^2 continuous infusion day 1
[total dose/cycle = 135 mg/m^2]

Cisplatin: I.V.: 75 mg/m^2 day 2
[total dose/cycle = 75 mg/m^2]

Repeat cycle every 21 days

References

Variation 1:

Hainsworth JD, Urba WJ, Hon JK, et al, "One-Hour Paclitaxel Plus Carboplatin in the Treatment of Advanced Nonsmall-Cell Lung Cancer: Results of a Multicentre, Phase II Trial," *Eur J Cancer*, 1998, 34(5):654-8.

Helsing M, Thaning L, Sederholm C, et al, "Treatment With Paclitaxel 1-H Infusion and Carboplatin of Patients With Advanced Nonsmall-Cell Lung Cancer: A Phase II Multicentre Trial. Joint Lung Cancer Study Group," *Lung Cancer*, 1999, 24(2):107-13.

Kosmidis PA, Mylonakis N, Fountzilas G, et al, "Paclitaxel and Carboplatin in Inoperable Nonsmall-Cell Lung Cancer: A Phase II Study," *Ann Oncol*, 1997, 8(7):697-9.

Laohavinij S, Maoleekoonpairoj S, Cheirsilpa A, et al, "Phase II Study of Paclitaxel and Carboplatin for Advanced Nonsmall-Cell Lung Cancer," *Lung Cancer*, 1999, 26(3):175-85.

Variation 2:

Giaccone G, Splinter TA, Debruyne C, et al, "Randomized Study of Paclitaxel-Cisplatin Versus Cisplatin-Teniposide in Patients With Advanced Nonsmall-Cell Lung Cancer. The European Organization for Research and Treatment of Cancer Lung Cancer Cooperative Group," *J Clin Oncol*, 1998, 16(6):2133-41.

Variation 3:

Langer CJ, Leighton JC, Comis RL, et al, "Paclitaxel by 24- or 1-Hour Infusion in Combination With Carboplatin in Advanced Nonsmall Cell Lung Cancer: The Fox Chase Cancer Center Experience," *Semin Oncol*, 1995, 22(4 Suppl 9):18-29.

Variation 4:

Schiller JH, Harrington D, Belani CP, et al, "Comparison of Four Chemotherapy Regimens for Advanced Nonsmall-Cell Lung Cancer," *N Engl J Med*, 2002, 346(2):92-8.

PCR

Index Terms Pentostatin-Cyclophosphamide-Rituximab

Use Leukemia, chronic lymphocytic

Regimen NOTE: Multiple variations are listed.

Variation 1:

Cycle 1:

Cyclophosphamide: I.V.: 600 mg/m^2 day 1
[total dose/cycle = 600 mg/m^2]

Pentostatin: I.V.: 4 mg/m^2 day 1
[total dose/cycle = 4 mg/m^2]

Treatment cycle is 3 weeks

Cycles 2-6:

Cyclophosphamide: I.V.: 600 mg/m^2 day 1
[total dose/cycle = 600 mg/m^2]

Pentostatin: I.V.: 4 mg/m^2 day 1
[total dose/cycle = 4 mg/m^2]

Rituximab: I.V.: 375 mg/m^2 day 1
[total dose/cycle = 375 mg/m^2]

Repeat cycle every 3 weeks

Variation 2:
Cycle 1:
Pentostatin: I.V.: 2 mg/m^2 day 1
[total dose/cycle = 2 mg/m^2]
Cyclophosphamide: I.V.: 600 mg/m^2 day 1
[total dose/cycle = 600 mg/m^2]
Rituximab: I.V.: 100 mg/m^2 day 1 only
followed by I.V.: 375 mg/m^2/day days 3 and 5 only
[total dose/cycle 1 = 850 mg/m^2]
Treatment cycle is 3 weeks
Cycles 2-6:
Pentostatin: I.V.: 2 mg/m^2 day 1
[total dose/cycle = 2 mg/m^2]
Cyclophosphamide: I.V.: 600 mg/m^2 day 1
[total dose/cycle = 600 mg/m^2]
Rituximab: I.V.: 375 mg/m^2 day 1
[total dose/cycle = 375 mg/m^2]
Repeat cycle every 3 weeks

References

Variation 1:
Lamanna N, Kalaycio M, Maslak P, et al, "Pentostatin, Cyclophosphamide, and Rituximab Is an Active, Well-Tolerated Regimen for Patients With Previously Treated Chronic Lymphocytic Leukemia," *J Clin Oncol*, 2006, 24(10):1575-81.
Variation 2:
Kay NE, Geyer SM, Call TG, et al, "Combination Chemoimmunotherapy With Pentostatin, Cyclophosphamide, and Rituximab Shows Significant Clinical Activity With Low Accompanying Toxicity in Previously Untreated B Chronic Lymphocytic Leukemia," *Blood*, 2007, 109(2):405-11.

PCV (Brain Tumor Regimen)

Index Terms Procarbazine-CCNU-Vincristine; Procarbazine-Lomustine-Vincristine

Use Brain tumors

Regimen NOTE: Multiple variations are listed.
Variation 1:
Lomustine: Oral: 110 mg/m^2 day 1
[total dose/cycle = 110 mg/m^2]
Procarbazine: Oral: 60 mg/m^2/day days 8 to 21
[total dose/cycle = 840 mg/m^2]
Vincristine: I.V.: 1.4 mg/m^2/day (maximum dose: 2 mg) days 8 and 29
[total dose/cycle = 2.8 mg/m^2; maximum: 4 mg]
Repeat cycle every 6 weeks for a total of 6 cycles
Variation 2:
Lomustine: Oral: 110 mg/m^2 day 1
[total dose/cycle = 110 mg/m^2]
Procarbazine: Oral: 60 mg/m^2/day days 8 to 21
[total dose/cycle = 840 mg/m^2]
Vincristine: I.V.: 1.4 mg/m^2/day (maximum dose: 2 mg) days 8 and 29
[total dose/cycle = 2.8 mg/m^2; maximum: 4 mg]
Repeat cycle every 6 weeks for a total of 7 cycles
Variation 3:
Procarbazine: Oral: 75 mg/m^2/day days 8 to 21
[total dose/cycle = 1050 mg/m^2]
Lomustine: Oral: 130 mg/m^2 day 1
[total dose/cycle = 130 mg/m^2]

Vincristine: I.V.: 1.4 mg/m^2/day (no maximum) days 8 and 29
[total dose/cycle = 2.8 mg/m^2; no maximum]
Repeat cycle every 6 weeks for a total of 6 cycles
Variation 4:
Procarbazine: Oral: 75 mg/m^2/day days 8 to 21
[total dose/cycle = 1050 mg/m^2]
Lomustine: Oral: 130 mg/m^2 day 1
[total dose/cycle = 130 mg/m^2]
Vincristine: I.V.: 1.4 mg/m^2/day (no maximum) days 8 and 29
[total dose/cycle = 2.8 mg/m^2; no maximum]
Repeat cycle every 6 weeks for up to a total of 4 cycles
Variation 5:
Lomustine: Oral: 110 mg/m^2 day 1
[total dose/cycle = 110 mg/m^2]
Procarbazine: Oral: 60 mg/m^2/day days 8 to 21
[total dose/cycle = 840 mg/m^2]
Vincristine: I.V.: 1.4 mg/m^2/day days 8 and 29
[total dose/cycle = 2.8 mg/m^2]
Repeat cycle every 6-8 weeks for 1 year

References

Variation 1:
van den Bent MJ, Carpentier AF, Brandes AA, et al, "Adjuvant Procarbazine, Lomustine, and Vincristine Improves Progression-Free Survival But Not Overall Survival in Newly Diagnosed Anaplastic Oligodendrogliomas and Oligoastrocytomas: A Randomized European Organisation for Research and Treatment of Cancer Phase III Trial," *J Clin Oncol*, 2006, 24(18):2715-22.
Variation 2:
Levin VA, Uhm JH, Jaeckle KA, et al, "Phase III Randomized Study of Postradiotherapy Chemotherapy With Alpha Difluoromethylornithine-Procarbazine, N-(2-Chloroethyl)-N'-Cyclohexyl-N-Nitrosurea, Vincristine (DFMO-PCV) Versus PCV for Glioblastoma Multiforme," *Clin Cancer Res*, 2000, 6(10):3878-84.
Variation 3:
Cairncross G, Macdonald D, Ludwin S, et al, "Chemotherapy for Anaplastic Oligodendroglioma, National Cancer Institute of Canada Clinical Trials Group," *J Clin Oncol*, 1994, 12(10):2013-21.
Variation 4:
Intergroup Radiation Therapy Oncology Group Trial 9402, Cairncross G, Berkey B, et al, "Phase III Trial of Chemotherapy Plus Radiotherapy Compared With Radiotherapy Alone for Pure and Mixed Anaplastic Oligodendroglioma: Intergroup Radiation Therapy Oncology Group Trial 9402," *J Clin Oncol*, 2006, 24(18):2707-14.
Variation 5:
Levin VA, Silver P, Hannigan J, et al, "Superiority of Post-Radiotherapy Adjuvant Chemotherapy With CCNU, Procarbazine, and Vincristine (PCV) Over BCNU for Anaplastic Gliomas: NCOG 6G61 Final Report," *Int J Radiat Oncol Biol Phys*, 1990, 18(2):321-4.

Pemetrexed (Bladder Cancer Regimen)

Use Bladder cancer

Regimen

Pemetrexed: I.V.: 500 mg/m^2 infused over 10 minutes day 1
[total dose/cycle = 500 mg/m^2]
Repeat cycle every 21 days

References

Sweeney CJ, Roth BJ, Kabbinavar FF, et al, "Phase II Study of Pemetrexed for Second-Line Treatment of Transitional Cell Cancer of the Urothelium," *J Clin Oncol*, 2006, 24(21):3451-7.

- **Pemetrexed-Carboplatin-Bevacizumab (NSCLC)** *see* Bevacizumab-Carboplatin-Pemetrexed (NSCLC) *on page 1529*
- **Pemetrexed-Carboplatin (Mesothelioma)** *see* Carboplatin-Pemetrexed (Mesothelioma) *on page 1551*

- ◆ **Pemetrexed-Carboplatin (NSCLC)** *see* Carboplatin-Pemetrexed (NSCLC) *on page 1551*
- ◆ **Pemetrexed-Cisplatin (Mesothelioma)** *see* Cisplatin-Pemetrexed (Mesothelioma) *on page 1582*
- ◆ **Pemetrexed-Cisplatin (NSCLC)** *see* Cisplatin-Pemetrexed (NSCLC) *on page 1583*

Pemetrexed (Mesothelioma Regimen)

Use Malignant pleural mesothelioma

Regimen

Pemetrexed: I.V.: 500 mg/m^2 over 10 minutes day 1
[total dose/cycle = 500 mg/m^2]

Repeat cycle every 21 days

References

Jassem J, Ramlau R, Santoro A, et al, "Phase III Trial of Pemetrexed Plus Best Supportive Care Compared With Best Supportive Care in Previously Treated Patients With Advanced Malignant Pleural Mesothelioma," *J Clin Oncol*, 2008, 26(10):1698-1704.

Taylor P, Castagneto B, Dark G, et al, "Single-Agent Pemetrexed for Chemonaïve and Pretreated Patients With Malignant Pleural Mesothelioma: Results of an International Expanded Access Program," *J Thorac Oncol*, 2008, 3(7):764-71.

Pemetrexed (NSCLC Regimen)

Use Lung cancer, nonsmall cell

Regimen NOTE: Multiple variations are listed.

Variation 1 (second-line):

Pemetrexed: I.V.: 500 mg/m^2 over 10 minutes day 1
[total dose/cycle = 500 mg/m^2]

Repeat cycle every 21 days until disease progression or unacceptable toxicity

Variation 2 (maintenance therapy):

Pemetrexed: I.V.: 500 mg/m^2 day 1
[total dose/cycle = 500 mg/m^2]

Repeat cycle every 21 days until disease progression or unacceptable toxicity

References

Variation 1:

Hanna N, Shephard FA, Fossella FV, et al, "Randomized Phase III Trial of Pemetrexed Versus Docetaxel in Patients With Non-Small-Cell Lung Cancer Previously Treated With Chemotherapy," *J Clin Oncol*, 2004, 22(9):1589-97.

Variation 2:

Ciuleanu T, Brodowicz T, Zielinski C, et al, "Maintenance Pemetrexed Plus Best Supportive Care Versus Palcebo Plus Best Supportive Care For Non-Small-Cell Lung Cancer: A Randomised, Double-Blind, Phase 3 Study," *Lancet*, 2009, 374(9699):1432-40.

Pemetrexed (Ovarian Regimen)

Use Ovarian cancer

Regimen NOTE: Multiple variations are listed.

Variation 1:

Pemetrexed: I.V.: 500 mg/m^2 day 1
[total dose/cycle = 500 mg/m^2]

Repeat cycle every 21 days

Variation 2 (no prior radiation):

Pemetrexed: I.V.: 900 mg/m^2 over 10 minutes day 1
[total dose/cycle = 900 mg/m^2]

Repeat cycle every 21 days until disease progression or unacceptable toxicity

Variation 3 (prior radiation):

Pemetrexed: I.V.: 700 mg/m^2 over 10 minutes day 1
[total dose/cycle = 700 mg/m^2]

Repeat cycle every 21 days until disease progression or unacceptable toxicity

References

Variation 1:

Vergote I, Calvert H, Kania M, et al, "A Randomised, Double-Blind, Phase II Study of Two Doses of Pemetrexed in the Treatment of Platinum-Resistant, Epithelial Ovarian or Primary Peritoneal Cancer," *Eur J Cancer*, 2009, 45(8):1415-23.

Variation 2 and 3:

Miller DS, Blessing JA, Krasner CN, et al, "Phase II Evaluation of Pemetrexed in the Treatment of Recurrent or Persistent Platinum-Resistant Ovarian or Primary Peritoneal Carcinoma: A Study of the Gynecologic Oncology Group," *J Clin Oncol*, 2009, 27(16):2686-91.

Pemetrexed (Ovarian Regimen)

Use Ovarian cancer

Regimen NOTE: Multiple variations are listed.

Variation 1:

Pemetrexed: I.V.: 500 mg/m^2 day 1
[total dose/cycle = 500 mg/m^2]

Repeat cycle every 21 days

Variation 2 (no prior radiation):

Pemetrexed: I.V.: 900 mg/m^2 over 10 minutes day 1
[total dose/cycle = 900 mg/m^2]

Repeat cycle every 21 days until disease progression or unacceptable toxicity

Variation 3 (prior radiation):

Pemetrexed: I.V.: 700 mg/m^2 over 10 minutes day 1
[total dose/cycle = 700 mg/m^2]

Repeat cycle every 21 days until disease progression or unacceptable toxicity

References

Variation 1:

Vergote I, Calvert H, Kania M, et al, "A Randomised, Double-Blind, Phase II Study of Two Doses of Pemetrexed in the Treatment of Platinum-Resistant, Epithelial Ovarian or Primary Peritoneal Cancer," *Eur J Cancer*, 2009, 45(8):1415-23.

Variation 2 and 3:

Miller DS, Blessing JA, Krasner CN, et al, "Phase II Evaluation of Pemetrexed in the Treatment of Recurrent or Persistent Platinum-Resistant Ovarian or Primary Peritoneal Carcinoma: A Study of the Gynecologic Oncology Group," *J Clin Oncol*, 2009, 27(16):2686-91

Pentostatin-Cyclophosphamide

Use Leukemia, chronic lymphocytic

Regimen

Cyclophosphamide: I.V.: 600 mg/m^2 day 1
[total dose/cycle = 600 mg/m^2]

Pentostatin: I.V.: 4 mg/m^2 day 1
[total dose/cycle = 4 mg/m^2]

Repeat cycle every 3 weeks for up to 6 cycles

References

Weiss MA, Maslak PG, Jurcic JG, et al, "Pentostatin and Cyclophosphamide: An Effective New Regimen in Previously Treated Patients With Chronic Lymphocytic Leukemia," *J Clin Oncol*, 2003, 21(7):1278-84.

- **Pentostatin-Cyclophosphamide-Rituximab** *see* PCR *on page 1735*
- **PE (Prostate Cancer)** *see* Estramustine-Paclitaxel *on page 1637*
- **Pertuzumab-Trastuzumab-Docetaxel (Breast)** *see* Docetaxel-Pertuzumab-Trastuzumab (Breast) *on page 1614*
- **PE (Small Cell Lung Cancer)** *see* Cisplatin–Etoposide (Small Cell Lung Cancer) *on page 1569*

POC

Use Brain tumors

Regimen

Prednisone: Oral: 40 mg/m^2/day days 1 to 14
[total dose/cycle = 560 mg/m^2]

Vincristine: I.V.: 1.5 mg/m^2/day (maximum dose: 2 mg) days 1, 8, and 15
[total dose/cycle = 4.5 mg/m^2]

Lomustine: Oral: 100 mg/m^2 day 1
[total dose/cycle = 100 mg/m^2]

Repeat cycle every 6 weeks

References

Finlay JL, Boyett JM, Yates AJ, et al, "Randomized Phase III Trial in Childhood High-Grade Astrocytoma Comparing Vincristine, Lomustine, and Prednisone With the Eight-Drugs-In-1-Day Regimen. Childrens Cancer Group," *J Clin Oncol*, 1995, 13(1):112-23.

POG-8651

Use Osteosarcoma

Regimen

(Surgery at week 10)

Methotrexate: I.V.: 12 g/m^2 weeks 0, 1, 5, 6, 13, 14, 18, 19, 23, 24, 37, and 38
[total dose/cycle = 144 g/m^2]

Leucovorin: (route not specified): 15 mg every 6 hours for 10 doses, weeks 0, 1, 5, 6, 13, 14, 18, 19, 23, 24, 37, and 38
[total dose/cycle = 1800 mg]

Doxorubicin: I.V.: 37.5 mg/m^2/dose days 1 and 2 of weeks 2, 7, 25, and 28
followed by I.V.: 30 mg/m^2/dose days 1, 2, and 3 of week 20
[total dose/cycle = 390 mg/m^2]

Cisplatin: I.V.: 60 mg/m^2/day days 1 and 2, weeks 2, 7, 25, and 28
[total dose/cycle = 480 mg/m^2]

Cyclophosphamide: I.V.: 600 mg/m^2/day days 1, 2, and 3, weeks 15, 31, 34, 39, and 42
[total dose/cycle = 9000 mg/m^2]

Bleomycin: I.V.: 15 units/m^2/day days 1, 2, and 3, weeks 15, 31, 34, 39, and 42
[total dose/cycle = 225 units/m^2]

Dactinomycin: I.V.: 0.6 mg/m^2/day days 1, 2, and 3, weeks 15, 31, 34, 39, and 42
[total dose/cycle = 9 mg/m^2]

or

(Surgery at week 0)

Methotrexate: 12 g/m^2 weeks 3, 4, 8, 9, 13, 14, 18, 19, 23, 24, 37, and 38
[total dose/cycle = 144 g/m^2]

Leucovorin: (route not specified): 15 mg every 6 hours for 10 doses, weeks 3, 4, 8, 9, 13, 14, 18, 19, 23, 24, 37, and 38
[total dose/cycle = 1800 mg]

Doxorubicin: I.V.: 37.5 mg/m^2/day days 1 and 2, weeks 5, 10, 25, and 28 and 30 mg/m^2 days 1, 2, and 3, week 20
[total dose/cycle = 390 mg/m^2]
Cisplatin: I.V.: 60 mg/m^2/day days 1 and 2, weeks 5, 10, 25, and 28
[total dose/cycle = 480 mg/m^2]
Cyclophosphamide: I.V.: 600 mg/m^2/day days 1, 2, and 3, weeks 15, 31, 34, 39, and 42
[total dose/cycle = 9000 mg/m^2]
Bleomycin: I.V.: 15 units/m^2/day days 1, 2, and 3, weeks 15, 31, 34, 39, and 42
[total dose/cycle = 225 units/m^2]
Dactinomycin: I.V.: 0.6 mg/m^2/day days 1, 2, and 3, weeks 15, 31, 34, 39, and 42
[total dose/cycle = 9 mg/m^2]

References

Goorin AM, Schwartzentruber DJ, Devidas M, et al, "Presurgical Chemotherapy Compared With Immediate Surgery and Adjuvant Chemotherapy for Nonmetastatic Osteosarcoma: Pediatric Oncology Group Study POG-8651," *J Clin Oncol*, 2003, 21(8):1574-80.

POMP

Use Leukemia, acute lymphocytic

Regimen Maintenance:

Mercaptopurine: Oral: 50 mg 3 times/day
[total dose/cycle = 4200-4650 mg]
Methotrexate: Oral: 20 mg/m^2 once weekly
[total dose/cycle = 80 mg/m^2]
Vincristine: I.V.: 2 mg day 1
[total dose/cycle = 2 mg]
Prednisone: Oral: 200 mg/day days 1 to 5
[total dose/cycle = 1000 mg]
Repeat cycle monthly for 2 years

References

Kantarjian HM, O'Brien S, Smith TL, et al, "Results of Treatment With Hyper-CVAD, a Dose-Intensive Regimen, in Adult Acute Lymphocytic Leukemia," *J Clin Oncol*, 2000, 18(3):547-61.

- **Prednisone-Mitoxantrone (Prostate Cancer)** *see* Mitoxantrone-Prednisone (Prostate Cancer) *on page 1713*
- **Prednisone-Chlorambucil (CLL)** *see* Chlorambucil-Prednisone (CLL) *on page 1563*
- **Procarbazine-CCNU-Vincristine** *see* PCV (Brain Tumor Regimen) *on page 1736*
- **Procarbazine-Lomustine-Vincristine** *see* PCV (Brain Tumor Regimen) *on page 1736*

Pro-MACE-CytaBOM

Use Lymphoma, non-Hodgkin's

Regimen

Prednisone: Oral: 60 mg/m^2/day days 1 to 14
[total dose/cycle = 840 mg/m^2]
Doxorubicin: I.V.: 25 mg/m^2 day 1
[total dose/cycle = 25 mg/m^2]
Cyclophosphamide: I.V.: 650 mg/m^2 day 1
[total dose/cycle = 650 mg/m^2]
Etoposide: I.V.: 120 mg/m^2 day 1
[total dose/cycle = 120 mg/m^2]

Cytarabine: I.V.: 300 mg/m^2 day 8
[total dose/cycle = 300 mg/m^2]
Bleomycin: I.V.: 5 units/m^2 day 8
[total dose/cycle = 5 units/m^2]
Vincristine: I.V.: 1.4 mg/m^2 (maximum dose: 2 mg) day 8
[total dose/cycle = 1.4 mg/m^2]
Methotrexate: I.V.: 120 mg/m^2 day 8
[total dose/cycle = 120 mg/m^2]
Leucovorin: Oral: 25 mg/m^2 every 6 hours for 4 doses (start 24 hours after methotrexate dose) day 9
[total dose/cycle = 100 mg/m^2]
Repeat cycle every 21 days

References

Longo DL, DeVita VT Jr, Duffey PL, et al, "Superiority of ProMACE-CytaBOM Over ProMACE-MOPP in the Treatment of Advanced Diffuse Aggressive Lymphoma: Results of a Prospective Randomized Trial," *J Clin Oncol*, 1991, 9(1):25-38.

PVA (POG 8602)

Index Terms AlinC 14

Use Leukemia, acute lymphocytic

Regimen

Induction:

Prednisone: Oral: 40 mg/m^2/day (maximum dose: 60 mg) given in 3 divided doses days 0 to 28
[total dose/cycle = 1160 mg/m^2]
Vincristine: I.V.: 1.5 mg/m^2/day (maximum dose: 2 mg) days 0, 7, 14, and 21
[total dose/cycle = 6 mg/m^2; maximum: 8 mg]
Asparaginase: I.M.: 6000 units/m^2 3 times per week for 2 weeks
[total dose/cycle = 36,000 units/m^2]
Intrathecal therapy (triple): Days 0 and 22
Leucovorin: Route and dose not specified: Single dose 24 hours after every intrathecal treatment days 1 and 23
Administer one cycle only

CNS consolidation:

Mercaptopurine: Oral: 75 mg/m^2/day days 29 to 43
[total dose/cycle = 1125 mg/m^2]
Intrathecal therapy (triple): Days 29 and 36
Leucovorin: Route and dose not specified: Single dose 24 hours after every intrathecal treatment days 30 and 37
Administer one cycle only

Intensification:

Regimen A:

Methotrexate: I.V.: 1000 mg/m^2 continuous infusion over 24 hours day 1
[total dose/cycle = 1000 mg/m^2]
Cytarabine: I.V.: 1000 mg/m^2 continuous infusion over 24 hours day 1 (start 12 hours after start of methotrexate)
[total dose/cycle = 1000 mg/m^2]
Leucovorin: I.M., I.V., or Oral: 30 mg/m^2 at 24 and 36 hours after the start of methotrexate
[total dose/cycle = 60 mg/m^2]
followed by I.M., I.V., or Oral: 3 mg/m^2 at 48, 60, and 72 hours after the start of methotrexate
[total dose/cycle = 9 mg/m^2]

Repeat cycle every 3 weeks for 6 cycles (administered weeks 7, 10, 13, 16, 19, and 22)
Intrathecal therapy (triple): Weeks 9, 12, 15, and 18
Leucovorin: Route and dose not specified: Single dose 24 hours after every intrathecal treatment weeks 9, 12, 15, and 18
or
Regimen B:
Methotrexate: I.V.: 1000 mg/m^2 continuous infusion over 24 hours day 1 [total dose/cycle = 1000 mg/m^2]
Cytarabine: I.V.: 1000 mg/m^2 continuous infusion over 24 hours day 1 (start 12 hours after methotrexate)
[total dose/cycle = 1000 mg/m^2]
Leucovorin: I.M., I.V., or Oral: 30 mg/m^2 at 24 and 36 hours after the start of methotrexate
[total dose/cycle = 60 mg/m^2]
followed by I.M., I.V., or Oral: 3 mg/m^2 at 48, 60, and 72 hours after the start of methotrexate
[total dose/cycle = 9 mg/m^2]
Repeat cycle every 12 weeks for 6 cycles (administer weeks 7, 19, 31, 43, 55, and 67)
Intrathecal therapy (triple): Weeks 9, 12, 15, and 18
Leucovorin: Route and dose not specified: Single dose 24 hours after every intrathecal treatment weeks 9, 12, 15, and 18

Maintenance:
Regimen A:
Methotrexate: I.M.: 20 mg/m^2 weekly, weeks 25 to 156
[total dose/cycle = 2640 mg/m^2]
Mercaptopurine: Oral: 75 mg/m^2 daily, weeks 25 to 156
[total dose/cycle = 69,300 mg/m^2]
Intrathecal therapy (triple): Every 8 weeks, weeks 26 through 105
Leucovorin: Route and dose not specified: Single dose 24 hours after every intrathecal treatment weeks 26 through 105
Prednisone: Oral: 40 mg/m^2/day (maximum dose: 60 mg) days 1 to 7 (given in 3 divided doses), weeks 8, 17, 25, 41, 57, 73, 89, and 105
[total dose/cycle = 2240 mg/m^2; maximum: 3360 mg]
Vincristine: I.V.: 1.5 mg/m^2/day (maximum dose: 2 mg) day 1, weeks 8, 9, 17, 18, 25, 26, 41, 42, 57, 58, 73, 74, 89, 90, 105, and 106
[total dose/cycle = 24 mg/m^2; maximum: 32 mg]
or
Regimen B:
Methotrexate: I.M.: 20 mg/m^2 weekly, weeks 22-28, 34-40, 46-52, and 58-64
[total dose/cycle = 560 mg/m^2]
Mercaptopurine: Oral: 75 mg/m^2 daily for 7 weeks, weeks 22-28, 34-40, 46-52, and 58-64
[total dose/cycle = 14700 mg/m^2]
followed by
Methotrexate: I.M.: 20 mg/m^2 weekly, weeks 70 to 156
[total dose/cycle = 1720 mg/m^2]
Mercaptopurine: Oral: 75 mg/m^2 daily, weeks 70 to 156
[total dose/cycle = 45,150 mg/m^2]

Intrathecal therapy (triple): Every 8 weeks, weeks 26 through 105
Leucovorin: Route and dose not specified: Single dose 24 hours after every intrathecal treatment weeks 26 through 105
Prednisone: Oral: 40 mg/m²/day (maximum dose: 60 mg) days 1 to 7 (given in 3 divided doses), weeks 8, 17, 25, 41, 57, 73, 89, and 105 [total dose/cycle = 2240 mg/m²]
Vincristine: I.V.: 1.5 mg/m²/day (maximum dose: 2 mg) day 1, weeks 8, 9, 17, 18, 25, 26, 41, 42, 57, 58, 73, 74, 89, 90, 105, and 106 [total dose/cycle = 24 mg/m²; maximum dose: 32 mg]

References

Land VJ, Shuster JJ, Crist WM, et al, "Comparison of Two Schedules of Intermediate-Dose Methotrexate and Cytarabine Consolidation Therapy for Childhood B-Precursor Cell Acute Lymphoblastic Leukemia: A Pediatric Oncology Group Study," *J Clin Oncol*, 1994, 12(9):1939-45.

PVB

Use Testicular cancer

Regimen NOTE: Multiple variations are listed.

Variation 1:
Cisplatin: I.V.: 20 mg/m²/day days 1 to 5 [total dose/cycle = 100 mg/m²]
Vinblastine: I.V.: 0.2 mg/kg/day days 1 and 2 [total dose/cycle = 0.4 mg/kg]
Bleomycin: I.V.: 30 units/day days 2, 9, and 16 [total dose/cycle = 90 units]
Repeat cycle every 3 weeks

Variation 2:
Cisplatin: I.V.: 20 mg/m²/day days 1 to 5 [total dose/cycle = 100 mg/m²]
Vinblastine: I.V.: 0.15 mg/kg/day days 1 and 2 [total dose/cycle = 0.3 mg/kg]
Bleomycin: I.V.: 30 units/day days 2, 9, and 16 [total dose/cycle = 90 units]
Repeat cycle every 3 weeks

Variation 3:
Cisplatin: I.V.: 20 mg/m²/day days 1 to 5 [total dose/cycle = 100 mg/m²]
Vinblastine: I.V.: 6 mg/m²/day days 1 and 2 [total dose/cycle = 12 mg/m²]
Bleomycin: I.M.: 30 units/day days 2, 9, and 16 [total dose/cycle = 90 units]
Repeat cycle every 3 weeks

References

Variation 1:
Einhorn LH and Donohue J, "Cis-Diamminedichloroplatinum, Vinblastine, and Bleomycin Combination Chemotherapy in Disseminated Testicular Cancer," *Ann Intern Med*, 1977, 87(3):293-8.
Variation 2:
Williams SD, Birch R, Einhorn LH, et al, "Treatment of Disseminated Germ-Cell Tumors With Cisplatin, Bleomycin, and Either Vinblastine or Etoposide," *N Engl J Med*, 1987, 316 (23):1435-40.
Variation 3:
Bodrogi I, Baki M, Horti J, et al, "Vinblastine, Cisplatin, and Bleomycin Treatment of Advanced Nonseminomatous Testicular Tumors," *Neoplasma*, 1990, 37(4):445-50.

◆ **PVB** *see* VBP *on page 1770*

PVDA

Use Leukemia, acute lymphocytic

Regimen Induction:

Prednisone: Oral: 60 mg/m^2/day days 1 to 28
[total dose/cycle = 1680 mg/m^2]

Vincristine: I.V.: 1.5 mg/m^2/day days 1, 8, 15, and 22
[total dose/cycle = 6 mg/m^2]

Daunorubicin: I.V.: 25 mg/m^2/day days 1, 8, 15, and 22
[total dose/cycle = 100 mg/m^2]

Asparaginase: I.M., SubQ, or I.V.: 5000 units/m^2/day days 1 to 14
[total dose/cycle = 70,000 units/m^2]

Administer one cycle only; used in conjunction with intrathecal chemotherapy

References

Hoelzer D, Thiel E, Loffler H, et al, "Intensified Therapy in Acute Lymphoblastic and Acute Undifferentiated Leukemia in Adults," *Blood*, 1984, 64(1):38-47.

◆ **Raltitrexed-Cisplatin (Mesothelioma)** *see* Cisplatin-Raltitrexed (Mesothelioma) *on page 1583*

◆ **R-CHOP (NHL)** *see* Rituximab-CHOP (NHL) *on page 1748*

R-CVP

Index Terms CVP-R; Rituximab-CVP; Rituximab-Cyclophosphamide-Vincristine-Prednisone

Use Lymphoma, non-Hodgkin's

Regimen

Rituximab: I.V.: 375 mg/m^2 day 1
[total dose/cycle = 375 mg/m^2]

Cyclophosphamide: I.V.: 750 mg/m^2 day 1
[total dose/cycle = 750 mg/m^2]

Vincristine: I.V.: 1.4 mg/m^2 day 1
[total dose/cycle = 1.4 mg/m^2]

Prednisone: Oral: 40 mg/m^2/day days 1 to 5
[total dose/cycle = 200 mg/m^2]

Repeat cycle every 21 days

References

Marcus R, Imrie K, Belch A, et al, "CVP Chemotherapy Plus Rituximab Compared With CVP as First-Line Treatment for Advanced Follicular Lymphoma," *Blood*, 2005, 105(4):1417-23.

◆ **Regimen DD-4A (Wilms' Tumor)** *see* DD-4A (Wilms' Tumor) *on page 1606*

◆ **Regimen A3 (Neuroblastoma)** *see* A3 (Neuroblastoma) *on page 1516*

◆ **Regimen EE-4A (Wilms' Tumor)** *see* EE-4A (Wilms' Tumor) *on page 1621*

Regimen I (Wilms' Tumor)

Index Terms Vincristine, Doxorubicin, Cyclophosphamide, Mesna, Etoposide

Use Wilms' tumor

Regimen NOTE: Multiple variations are listed.

Variation 1 (patients ≤30 kg):

Vincristine: I.V.: 0.05 mg/kg (maximum dose: 2 mg) I.V. push day 1 of weeks 1, 2, 4 to 8, 10 and 11

Followed by

Vincristine 0.067 mg/kg (maximum dose: 2 mg) I.V. push day 1 of weeks 12, 13, 18, and 24
[total dose = 0.718 mg/kg; maximum: 26 mg]

Doxorubicin: I.V.: 1.5 mg/kg I.V. push day 1 of weeks 0, 6, 12, 18, and 24
[total dose = 7.5 mg/kg]
Cyclophosphamide: I.V.: 14.7 mg/kg/day days 1 to 5 of weeks 3, 9, 15, and 21
[total dose = 294 mg/kg]
Mesna: I.V.: 3 mg/kg/dose 4 doses/day (after cyclophosphamide) days 1 to 5 of weeks 3, 9, 15, and 21
[total dose = 240 mg/kg]
Cyclophosphamide: I.V.: 14.7 mg/kg/day days 1 to 3 of weeks 6, 12, 18, and 24
[total dose = 176.4 mg/kg]
Mesna: I.V.: 3 mg/kg/dose 4 doses/day (after cyclophosphamide) days 1 to 3 of weeks 6, 12, 18, and 24
[total dose = 144 mg/kg]
Etoposide: I.V.: 3.3 mg/kg/day days 1 to 5 of weeks 3, 9, 15, and 21
[total dose = 66 mg/kg]
Filgrastim: SubQ: 5 mcg/kg/day beginning 24 hours after last dose of chemotherapy and continued until ANC ≥10,000/mm^3 or for a minimum of 1 week
Treatment course duration is week 0 through week 24

Variation 2 (patients >30 kg):
Vincristine: I.V.: 1.5 mg/m^2 (maximum dose: 2 mg) I.V. push day 1 of weeks 1, 2, 4 to 8, 10 and 11
Followed by
Vincristine 2 mg/m^2 (maximum dose: 2 mg) I.V. push days 1 of weeks 12, 13, 18, and 24
[total dose = 21.5 mg/m^2; maximum: 26 mg]
Doxorubicin: I.V.: 45 mg/m^2 I.V. push day 1 of weeks 0, 6, 12, 18, and 24
[total dose = 225 mg/m^2]
Cyclophosphamide: I.V.: 440 mg/m^2/day days 1 to 5 of weeks 3, 9, 15, and 21
[total dose = 8800 mg/m^2]
Mesna: I.V.: 90 mg/m^2/dose 4 doses/day (after cyclophosphamide) days 1 to 5 of weeks 3, 9, 15, and 21
[total dose = 7200 mg/m^2]
Cyclophosphamide: I.V.: 440 mg/m^2/day days 1 to 3 of weeks 6, 12, 18, and 24
[total dose = 5280 mg/m^2]
Mesna: I.V.: 90 mg/m^2/dose 4 doses/day (after cyclophosphamide) days 1 to 3 of weeks 6, 12, 18, and 24
[total dose = 4320 mg/m^2]
Etoposide: I.V.: 100 mg/m^2/day days 1 to 5 of weeks 3, 9, 15, and 21
[total dose = 2000 mg/m^2]
Filgrastim: SubQ: 5 mcg/kg/day beginning 24 hours after last dose of chemotherapy and continued until ANC ≥10,000/mm^3 or for a minimum of 1 week
Treatment course duration is week 0 through week 24

References

Variations 1 and 2:
Green DM, Cotton CA, Malogolowkin M, et al, "Treatment of Wilms Tumor Relapsing After Initial Treatment With Vincristine and Actinomycin D: A Report From the National Wilms Tumor Study Group," *Pediatr Blood Cancer*, 2007, 48(5):493-9.

◆ **Regimen new A1 (Neuroblastoma)** *see* New A1 (Neuroblastoma) *on page 1721*

Regorafenib (Colorectal Regimen)

Use Colorectal cancer

Regimen

Regorafenib: Oral: 160 mg once daily for 21 days
[total dose/cycle = 3360 mg]

Repeat cycle every 28 days, continue until disease progression or unacceptable toxicity

References

Grothey A, Sobrero AF, Siena S, et al, "Results of a Phase III Randomized, Double-Blind, Placebo-Controlled, Multicenter Trial (CORRECT) of Regorafenib Plus Best Supportive Care (BSC) Versus Placebo Plus BSC in Patients (Pts) With Metastatic Colorectal Cancer (mCRC) Who Have Progressed After Standard Therapies," *J Clin Oncol*, 2012, 30(suppl 4):LBA385 [abstract LBA385 from 2012 ASCO Gastrointestinal Cancers Symposium].

◆ **R-EPOCH Dose Adjusted (NHL)** *see* EPOCH (Dose-Adjusted)-Rituximab (NHL) *on page 1629*

◆ **R-EPOCH (NHL)** *see* EPOCH-Rituximab (NHL) *on page 1631*

◆ **R-FCM (NHL)** *see* Fludarabine-Cyclophosphamide-Mitoxantrone-Rituximab *on page 1647*

◆ **RFM (NHL)** *see* Fludarabine-Mitoxantrone-Rituximab *on page 1651*

RICE

Index Terms R-ICE; Rituximab-ICE

Use Lymphoma, non-Hodgkin's

Regimen

Rituximab: I.V.: 375 mg/m^2/day days 2 and 1 (cycle 1)
[total dose/cycle = 750 mg/m^2]

Rituximab: I.V.: 375 mg/m^2 day 1 (cycles 2 and 3)
[total dose/cycle = 375 mg/m^2]

Etoposide: I.V.: 100 mg/m^2/day days 3, 4, and 5
[total dose/cycle = 300 mg/m^2]

Carboplatin: I.V.: AUC = 5 (maximum dose: 800 mg) day 4
[total dose/cycle = AUC = 5]

Ifosfamide: I.V.: 5000 mg/m^2 continuous infusion day 4
[total dose/cycle = 5000 mg/m^2]

Mesna: I.V.: 5000 mg/m^2 continuous infusion day 4
[total dose/cycle = 5000 mg/m^2]

Filgrastim: SubQ: 5 mcg/kg/day days 7 to 14 (cycles 1 and 2)
[total dose/cycle = 40 mcg/kg]

Filgrastim: SubQ: 10 mcg/kg/day days 7 to 14 (cycle 3)
[total dose/cycle = 80 mcg/kg]

Repeat cycle every 2 weeks

References

Kewalramani T, Zelenetz AD, Nimer SD, et al, "Rituximab and ICE as Second-Line Therapy before Autologous Stem Cell Transplantation for Relapsed or Primary Refractory Diffuse Large B-Cell Lymphoma," *Blood*, 2004, 103(10):3684-8.

◆ **R-ICE** *see* RICE *on page 1747*

◆ **Rituxan-Etoposide-Prednisone-Vincristine-Cyclophosphamide-Doxorubicin (Dose-Adjusted) (NHL)** *see* EPOCH (Dose-Adjusted)-Rituximab (NHL) *on page 1629*

◆ **Rituximab-Bendamustine** *see* Bendamustine-Rituximab *on page 1525*

◆ **Rituximab-Bortezomib (Waldenstrom's Macroglobulinemia)** *see* Bortezomib-Rituximab (Waldenstrom's Macroglobulinemia) *on page 1537*

Rituximab-CHOP (NHL)

Index Terms CHOP-Rituximab (NHL); R-CHOP (NHL); RCHOP (NHL)

Use Lymphoma, non-Hodgkin's

Regimen NOTE: Multiple variations are listed.

Variation 1 (diffuse large B-cell lymphoma):

Rituximab: I.V.: 375 mg/m^2 day 1
[total dose/cycle = 375 mg/m^2]
Cyclophosphamide: I.V.: 750 mg/m^2 day 1
[total dose/cycle = 750 mg/m^2]
Doxorubicin: I.V.: 50 mg/m^2 day 1
[total dose/cycle = 50 mg/m^2]
Vincristine: I.V.: 1.4 mg/m^2 (maximum dose: 2 mg) day 1
[total dose/cycle = 1.4 mg/m^2; maximum: 2 mg]
Prednisone: Oral: 40 mg/m^2/day days 1 to 5
[total dose/cycle = 200 mg/m^2]
Repeat cycle every 21 days for a total of 8 cycles

Variation 2 (low-grade or follicular lymphoma):

Rituximab: I.V.: 375 mg/m^2 administer 7 and 2 days prior to the start of cycle 1 of CHOP, 2 days prior to the start of cycles 3 and 5 of CHOP, and after the 6th cycle of CHOP on days 134 and 141 (total of 6 doses of rituximab)
CHOP:
Cyclophosphamide: I.V.: 750 mg/m^2 day 1
[total dose/cycle = 750 mg/m^2]
Doxorubicin: I.V.: 50 mg/m^2 day 1
[total dose/cycle = 50 mg/m^2]
Vincristine: I.V.: 1.4 mg/m^2 (maximum dose: 2 mg) day 1
[total dose/cycle = 1.4 mg/m^2; maximum: 2 mg]
Prednisone: Oral: 100 mg/m^2/day days 1 to 5
[total dose/cycle = 500 mg/m^2]
Repeat each CHOP cycle every 21 days for a total of 6 CHOP cycles

Variation 3 (dose-dense R-CHOP in aggressive CD20-expressing B-cell lymphomas):

Pre-treatment (to improve performance status and diminish adverse effects to cycle 1):
Vincristine: I.V.: 1 mg 1 week before cycle 1
Prednisone: Oral: 100 mg/day for 7 days 1 week before cycle 1
Rituximab: I.V.: 375 mg/m^2 day 1
[total dose/cycle = 375 mg/m^2]
Cyclophosphamide: I.V.: 750 mg/m^2 day 1
[total dose/cycle = 750 mg/m^2]
Doxorubicin: I.V.: 50 mg/m^2 day 1
[total dose/cycle = 50 mg/m^2]
Vincristine: I.V.: 2 mg day 1
[total dose/cycle = 2 mg]
Prednisone: Oral: 100 mg/day days 1 to 5
[total dose/cycle = 500 mg]
Filgrastim (dose and route not specified): Daily beginning day 4 until leukocyte recovery
Repeat cycle every 14 days for a total of 6 cycles

Variation 4 (diffuse large B-cell lymphoma):
- Rituximab: I.V.: 375 mg/m^2 days -7, 1, 22, and 43
  [total dose/cycle = 1400 mg/m^2]
- Cyclophosphamide: I.V.: 750 mg/m^2 days 3, 24, and 45
  [total dose/cycle = 2250 mg/m^2]
- Doxorubicin: I.V.: 50 mg/m^2 days 3, 24, and 45
  [total dose/cycle = 150 mg/m^2]
- Vincristine: I.V.: 1.4 mg/m^2 (maximum dose: 2 mg) days 3, 24, and 45
  [total dose/cycle = 4.2 mg/m^2; maximum: 6 mg/cycle]
- Prednisone: Oral: 100 mg/day for 5 days starting on days 3, 24, and 45
  [total dose/cycle = 1500 mg]
- Cycle does not repeat; followed by radiation therapy beginning on day 66

Variation 5 (diffuse large B-cell lymphoma):
- Rituximab: I.V.: 375 mg/m^2 administer 7 and 3 days prior to the start of cycle 1 of CHOP, 2 days prior to the start of cycles 3 and 5 of CHOP, and 2 days before cycle 7 (if administered)
- CHOP:
- Cyclophosphamide: I.V.: 750 mg/m^2 day 1
  [total dose/cycle = 750 mg/m^2]
- Doxorubicin: I.V.: 50 mg/m^2 day 1
  [total dose/cycle = 50 mg/m^2]
- Vincristine: I.V.: 1.4 mg/m^2 (maximum dose: 2 mg) day 1
  [total dose/cycle = 1.4 mg/m^2, maximum: 2 mg]
- Prednisone: Oral: 100 mg/m^2/day days 1 to 5
  [total dose/cycle = 500 mg/m^2]
- Repeat each CHOP cycle every 21 days for a total of 6 CHOP cycles

Variation 6 (mantle cell lymphoma):
- Rituximab: I.V.: 375 mg/m^2 day 0 (administer the day before CHOP)
  [total dose/cycle = 375 mg/m^2]
- Cyclophosphamide: I.V.: 750 mg/m^2 day 1
  [total dose/cycle = 750 mg/m^2]
- Doxorubicin: I.V.: 50 mg/m^2 day 1
  [total dose/cycle = 50 mg/m^2]
- Vincristine: I.V.: 1.4 mg/m^2 (maximum dose: 2 mg) day 1
  [total dose/cycle = 1.4 mg/m^2; maximum: 2 mg]
- Prednisone: Oral: 100 mg/m^2/day days 1 to 5
  [total dose/cycle = 500 mg/m^2]
- Repeat cycle every 21 days for a total of 6 cycles

Variation 7 (follicular lymphoma):
- Rituximab: I.V.: 375 mg/m^2 day 0 (administer the day before CHOP)
  [total dose/cycle = 375 mg/m^2]
- Cyclophosphamide: I.V.: 750 mg/m^2 day 1
  [total dose/cycle = 750 mg/m^2]
- Doxorubicin: I.V.: 50 mg/m^2 day 1
  [total dose/cycle = 50 mg/m^2]
- Vincristine: I.V.: 1.4 mg/m^2 (maximum dose: 2 mg) day 1
  [total dose/cycle = 1.4 mg/m^2; maximum: 2 mg]
- Prednisone: Oral: 100 mg/m^2/day days 1 to 5
  [total dose/cycle = 500 mg/m^2]
- Repeat cycle every 21 days for a total of 6-8 cycles

Variation 8 (follicular lymphoma):
- Rituximab: I.V.: 375 mg/m^2 day 1
  [total dose/cycle = 375 mg/m^2]

Cyclophosphamide: I.V.: 750 mg/m^2 day 1
[total dose/cycle = 750 mg/m^2]
Doxorubicin: I.V.: 50 mg/m^2 day 1
[total dose/cycle = 50 mg/m^2]
Vincristine: I.V.: 1.4 mg/m^2 (maximum dose: 2 mg) day 1
[total dose/cycle = 1.4 mg/m^2; maximum: 2 mg]
Prednisone: Oral: 100 mg/day days 1 to 5
[total dose/cycle = 500 mg]
Repeat cycle every 21 days for a total of 6 cycles
followed by (maintenance rituximab):
Rituximab: I.V.: 375 mg/m^2 day 1
[total dose/cycle = 375 mg/m^2]
Repeat every 3 months until relapse or for a maximum of 2 years

References

Variation 1:

Coiffier B, Lepage E, Briere J, et al, "CHOP Chemotherapy Plus Rituximab Compared With CHOP Alone in Elderly Patients With Diffuse Large-B-Cell Lymphoma," *N Engl J Med*, 2002, 346 (4):235-42.

Coiffier B, Thieblemont C, Van Den Neste E, et al, "Long-Term Outcome of Patients in the LNH-98.5 Trial, the First Randomized Study Comparing Rituximab-CHOP to Standard CHOP Chemotherapy in DLBCL Patients: A Study by the Groupe d'Etudes des Lymphomes de l'Adulte," *Blood*, 2010, 116(12):2040-5.

Feugier P, Van Hoof A, Sebban C, et al, "Long-Term Results of the R-CHOP Study in the Treatment of Elderly Patients With Diffuse Large B-Cell Lymphoma: A Study by the Groupe d'Etude des Lymphomes de l'Adulte," *J Clin Oncol*, 2005, 23(18):4117-26.

Variation 2:

Czuczman MS, Grillo-López AJ, White CA, et al, "Treatment of Patients With Low-Grade B-Cell Lymphoma With the Combination of Chimeric Anti-CD20 Monoclonal Antibody and CHOP Chemotherapy," *J Clin Oncol*, 1999, 17(1):268-76.

Czuczman MS, Weaver R, Alkuzweny B, et al, "Prolonged Clinical and Molecular Remission in Patients With Low-Grade or Follicular Non-Hodgkin's Lymphoma Treated With Rituximab Plus CHOP Chemotherapy: 9-Year Follow-Up," *J Clin Oncol*, 2004, 22(23):4711-6.

Variation 3:

Pfreundschuh M, Schubert J, Ziepert M, et al, "Six Versus Eight Cycles of Bi-Weekly CHOP-14 With or Without Rituximab in Elderly Patients With Aggressive CD20+ B-cell Lymphomas: A Randomised Controlled Trial (RICOVER-60)," *Lancet Oncol*, 2008, 9(2):105-16.

Variation 4:

Persky DO, Unger JM, Spier CM, et al, "Phase II Study of Rituximab Plus Three Cycles of CHOP and Involved-Field Radiotherapy for Patients With Limited-Stage Aggressive B-Cell Lymphoma: Southwest Oncology Group Study 0014," *J Clin Oncol*, 2008, 26(14):2258-63.

Variation 5:

Habermann TM, Weller EA, Morrison VA, et al, "Rituximab-CHOP Versus CHOP Alone or With Maintenance Rituximab in Older Patients With Diffuse Large B-cell Lymphoma," *J Clin Oncol*, 2006, 24(19):3121-7.

Variation 6:

Lenz G, Dreyling M, Hoster E, et al, "Immunochemotherapy With Rituximab and Cyclophosphamide, Doxorubicin, Vincristine, and Prednisone Significantly Improves Response and Time to Treatment Failure, but Not Long-Term Outcome in Patients With Previously Untreated Mantle Cell Lymphoma: Results of a Prospective Randomized Trial of the German Low Grade Lymphoma Study Group (GLSG)," *J Clin Oncol*, 2005, 23(9):1984-92

Variation 7:

Hiddemann W, Kneba M, Dreyling M, et al, "Frontline Therapy With Rituximab Added to the Combination of Cyclophosphamide, Doxorubicin, Vincristine, and Prednisone (CHOP) Significantly Improves the Outcome for Patients With Advanced-Stage Follicular Lymphoma Compared With Therapy With CHOP Alone: Results of a Prospective Randomized Study of the German Low-Grade Lymphoma Study Group," *Blood*, 2005, 106(12):3725-32.

Variation 8:

van Oers MH, Klasa R, Marcus RE, et al, "Rituximab Maintenance Improves Clinical Outcome of Relapsed/Resistant Follicular Non-Hodgkin Lymphoma in Patients Both With and Without Rituximab During Induction: Results of a Prospective Randomized Phase 3 Intergroup Trial," *Blood*, 2006, 108(10):3295-301.

van Oers MH, Van Glabbeke M, Giurgea L, et al, "Rituximab Maintenance Treatment of Relapsed/Resistant Follicular Non-Hodgkin's Lymphoma: Long-Term Outcome of the EORTC 20981 Phase III Randomized Intergroup Study," *J Clin Oncol*, 2010, 28(17):2853-8.

◆ **Rituximab-CVP** *see* R-CVP *on page 1745*

◆ **Rituximab-Cyclophosphamide-Vincristine-Prednisone** *see* R-CVP *on page 1745*

◆ **Rituximab-EPOCH Dose Adjusted (NHL)** *see* EPOCH (Dose-Adjusted)-Rituximab (NHL) *on page 1629*

◆ **Rituximab-EPOCH (NHL)** *see* EPOCH-Rituximab (NHL) *on page 1631*

◆ **Rituximab-Fludarabine-Cyclophosphamide (CLL)** *see* Fludarabine-Cyclophosphamide-Rituximab (CLL) *on page 1648*

◆ **Rituximab-Fludarabine-Cyclophosphamide-Mitoxantrone** *see* Fludarabine-Cyclophosphamide-Mitoxantrone-Rituximab *on page 1647*

◆ **Rituximab-Fludarabine-Cyclophosphamide (NHL-Follicular)** *see* Fludarabine-Cyclophosphamide-Rituximab (NHL-Follicular) *on page 1649*

◆ **Rituximab-Fludarabine-Mitoxantrone** *see* Fludarabine-Mitoxantrone-Rituximab *on page 1651*

◆ **Rituximab-Fludarabine-Mitoxantrone-Dexamethasone** *see* Fludarabine-Mitoxantrone-Dexamethasone-Rituximab *on page 1650*

◆ **Rituximab-Fludarabine (NHL-Follicular)** *see* Fludarabine-Rituximab (NHL-Follicular) *on page 1651*

◆ **Rituximab-ICE** *see* RICE *on page 1747*

◆ **Rituximab-Temozolomide (CNS Lymphoma)** *see* Temozolomide-Rituximab (CNS Lymphoma) *on page 1754*

◆ **RVD (Multiple Myeloma)** *see* Lenalidomide-Bortezomib-Dexamethasone (Multiple Myeloma) *on page 1702*

◆ **Saltz Regimen** *see* Fluorouracil-Leucovorin-Irinotecan (Saltz Regimen) *on page 1656*

Sorafenib (RCC Regimen)

Use Renal cell cancer

Regimen NOTE: Multiple variations are listed.

Variation 1 (refractory):

Sorafenib: Oral: 400 mg twice daily

Continue until disease progression or unacceptable toxicity.

Variation 2 (first-line):

Sorafenib: Oral: 400 mg twice daily; if disease progression, may escalate to 600 mg twice daily

Continue until disease progression or unacceptable toxicity.

References

Variation 1:

Escudier B, Eisen T, Stadler WM, et al, "Sorafenib for Treatment of Renal Cell Carcinoma: Final Efficacy and Safety Results of the Phase III Treatment Approaches in Renal Cancer Global Evaluation Trial," *J Clin Oncol*, 2009, 27(20):3312-8.

Escudier B, Eisen T, Stadler WM, et al, "Sorafenib in Advanced Clear-Cell Renal-Cell Carcinoma," *N Engl J Med*, 2007, 356(2):125-34.

Variation 2:

Escudier B, Szczylik C, Hutson TE, et al, "Randomized Phase II Trial of First-Line Treatment With Sorafenib Versus Interferon Alfa-2a in Patients With Metastatic Renal Cell Carcinoma," *J Clin Oncol*, 2009, 27(8):1280-9.

Stanford V (Hodgkin)

Index Terms Mechlorethamine, Doxorubicin, Vinblastine, Vincristine, Bleomycin, Etoposide, Prednisone (Hodgkin)

Use Lymphoma, Hodgkin

Regimen NOTE: Multiple variations are listed.

Variation 1:

Mechlorethamine: I.V.: 6 mg/m^2/dose weeks 1, 5, and 9
[total dose/cycle = 18 mg/m^2]

Doxorubicin: I.V.: 25 mg/m^2/dose weeks 1, 3, 5, 7, 9, and 11
[total dose/cycle = 150 mg/m^2]

Vinblastine: I.V.: 6 mg/m^2/dose weeks 1, 3, 5, 7, 9, and 11
[total dose/cycle = 36 mg/m^2]

Vincristine: I.V.: 1.4 mg/m^2/dose (maximum dose: 2 mg) weeks 2, 4, 6, 8, 10, and 12
[total dose/cycle = 8.4 mg/m^2; maximum: 12 mg]

Bleomycin: I.V.: 5 units/m^2/dose weeks 2, 4, 6, 8, 10, and 12
[total dose/cycle = 30 units/m^2]

Etoposide: I.V.: 60 mg/m^2/day for 2 consecutive days, weeks 3, 7, and 11
[total dose/cycle = 360 mg/m^2]

Prednisone: Oral: 40 mg/m^2 every other day for 10 weeks
[total dose prior to taper = 1400 mg/m^2]
followed by tapering of prednisone dose during weeks 11 and 12

Treatment cycle is 12 weeks

Variation 2:

Mechlorethamine: I.V.: 6 mg/m^2/dose weeks 1 and 5
[total dose/cycle = 12 mg/m^2]

Doxorubicin: I.V.: 25 mg/m^2/dose weeks 1, 3, 5, and 7
[total dose/cycle = 100 mg/m^2]

Vinblastine: I.V.: 6 mg/m^2/dose weeks 1, 3, 5, and 7
[total dose/cycle = 24 mg/m^2]

Vincristine: I.V.: 1.4 mg/m^2/dose (maximum dose: 2 mg) weeks 2, 4, 6, and 8
[total dose/cycle = 5.6 mg/m^2; maximum: 8 mg]

Bleomycin: I.V.: 5 units/m^2/dose weeks 2, 4, 6, and 8
[total dose/cycle = 20 units/m^2]

Etoposide: I.V.: 60 mg/m^2/day days 15 and 16 and 43 and 44
[total dose/cycle = 240 mg/m^2]

Prednisone: Oral: 40 mg/m^2 days 1 to 36
[total dose prior to taper = 1440 mg/m^2]
followed by tapering of prednisone dose during weeks 7 and 8

Treatment cycle is 8 weeks

References

Variation 1:

Horning SJ, Hoppe RT, Breslin S, et al, "Stanford V and Radiotherapy for Locally Extensive and Advanced Hodgkin's Disease: Mature Results of a Prospective Clinical Trial," *J Clin Oncol*, 2002, 20(3):630-7.

Gordon LI, Hong F, Fisher RI, et al, "A Randomized Comparison of the Stanford V Regimen and ABVD in the Treatment of Advanced Hodgkin's Lymphoma: An Intergroup Study Coordinated by the Eastern Cooperative Oncology Group (E2496)," *Blood*, 2010, 116:415 [abstract 415 from ASH 2010 Annual Meeting].

Variation 2:

Horning SJ, Hoppe RT, Advan R, et al, "Efficacy and Late Effects of Stanford V Chemotherapy and Radiotherapy in Untreated Hodgkin's Disease: Mature Data in Early and Advanced Stage Patients" *Blood*, 2004, 104:308a [abstract 308a from ASH 2004 Annual Meeting].

Sunitinib (RCC Regimen)

Use Renal cell cancer

Regimen

Sunitinib: Oral: 50 mg once daily for 4 weeks, followed by 2 weeks of rest [total dose/cycle = 1400 mg]

Repeat cycle every 6 weeks until disease progression or unacceptable toxicity

References

Motzer RJ, Hutson TE, Tomczak P, et al, "Overall Survival and Updated Results for Sunitinib Compared With Interferon Alfa in Patients With Metastatic Renal Cell Carcinoma," *J Clin Oncol*, 2009, 27(22):3584-90.

Motzer RJ, Hutson TE, Tomczak P, et al, "Sunitinib Versus Interferon Alfa in Metastatic Renal-Cell Carcinoma," *N Engl J Med*, 2007, 356(2):115-24.

TAC

Index Terms ATC

Use Breast cancer

Regimen NOTE: Multiple variations are listed.

Variation 1:

Docetaxel: I.V.: 75 mg/m^2 day 1
[total dose/cycle = 75 mg/m^2]

Doxorubicin: I.V.: 50 mg/m^2 day 1
[total dose/cycle = 50 mg/m^2]

Cyclophosphamide: I.V.: 500 mg/m^2 day 1
[total dose/cycle = 500 mg/m^2]

Repeat cycle every 3 weeks

Variation 2:

Docetaxel: I.V.: 60 mg/m^2 day 1
[total dose/cycle = 60 mg/m^2]

Doxorubicin: I.V.: 60 mg/m^2 day 1
[total dose/cycle = 60 mg/m^2]

Cyclophosphamide: I.V.: 600 mg/m^2 day 1
[total dose/cycle = 600 mg/m^2]

Repeat cycle every 3 weeks

References

Variation 1:

Martin M, Pienkowski T, Mackey J, et al, "Adjuvant Docetaxel for Node-Positive Breast Cancer," *N Engl J Med*, 2005, 352(22):2302-13.

Nabholtz JM, Smylie M, Mackey JR, et al, "Docetaxel/Doxorubicin/Cyclophosphamide in the Treatment of Metastatic Breast Cancer," *Oncology (Williston Park)*, 1997, 11(6 Suppl 6):25-7.

Variation 2:

Smith RE, Anderson SJ, Brown A, et al,"Phase II Trial of Doxorubicin/Docetaxel/Cyclophosphamide for Locally Advanced and Metastatic Breast Cancer: Results From NSABP Trial BP-58," *Clin Breast Cancer*, 2002, 3(5):333-40.

◆ **TC** *see* Docetaxel-Cyclophosphamide (TC) *on page 1611*

◆ **TCF (Esophageal Cancer)** *see* Paclitaxel-Cisplatin-Fluorouracil (Esophageal Cancer) *on page 1728*

◆ **TCF (Gastric/Esophageal Cancer)** *see* Docetaxel-Cisplatin-Fluorouracil (Gastric/Esophageal Cancer) *on page 1609*

◆ **Temozolomide-Irinotecan (Ewing's Sarcoma)** *see* Irinotecan-Temozolomide (Ewing's Sarcoma) *on page 1697*

Temozolomide-Rituximab (CNS Lymphoma)

Index Terms Rituximab-Temozolomide (CNS Lymphoma)

Use Primary CNS lymphoma

Regimen NOTE: Multiple variations are listed.

Variation 1:

Combination therapy (cycles 1-4):

Rituximab: I.V.: 375 mg/m^2/dose day 1
[total dose/cycle = 375 mg/m^2]

Temozolomide: Oral: 150 mg/m^2/day days 1 to 5
[total dose/cycle = 750 mg/m^2]

Repeat cycle every 28 days for a total of 4 cycles

followed by

Maintenance therapy:

Temozolomide: Oral: 150 mg/m^2/day days 1 to 5
[total dose/cycle = 750 mg/m^2]

Repeat cycle every 28 days for a total of 8 cycles

Variation 2:

Combination therapy (cycles 1 and 2):

Rituximab: I.V.: 750 mg/m^2/dose days 1, 8, 15, and 22
[total dose/cycle = 3000 mg/m^2]

Temozolomide: Oral: 150 mg/m^2/day days 1 to 7
[total dose/cycle = 1050 mg/m^2]

Repeat cycle every 28 days for a total of 2 cycles

followed by

Maintenance therapy:

Temozolomide: Oral: 150 mg/m^2/day days 1 to 5
[total dose/cycle = 750 mg/m^2]

Repeat cycle every 28 days

References

Variation 1:

Wong ET, Tishler R, Barron L, et al, "Immunochemotherapy With Rituximab and Temozolomide for Central Nervous System Lymphomas," *Cancer*, 2004, 101(1):139-45.

Variation 2:

Enting RH, Demopoulos A, DeAngelis LM, et al, "Salvage Therapy for Primary CNS Lymphoma With a Combination of Rituximab and Temozolomide," *Neurology*, 2004, 63(5):901-3.

Temsirolimus (RCC Regimen)

Use Renal cell cancer

Regimen

Temsirolimus: I.V.: 25 mg over 30 minutes day 1
[total dose/cycle = 25 mg]

Repeat cycle every week until disease progression or unacceptable toxicity

References

Hudes G, Carducci M, Tomczak P, et al, "Temsirolimus, Interferon Alfa, or Both for Advanced Renal-Cell Carcinoma," *N Engl J Med*, 2007, 356(22):2271-81.

Thalidomide-Dexamethasone (MM)

Index Terms Dexamethasone-Thalidomide (MM)

Use Multiple myeloma

Regimen NOTE: Multiple variations are listed.

Variation 1 (refractory):

Thalidomide: Oral: 100 mg/day days 1 to 28
[total dose/cycle = 2800 mg]

Dexamethasone: Oral: 40 mg/day days 1 to 4
[total dose/cycle = 160 mg]
Repeat cycle every 28 days
Variation 2 (refractory):
Thalidomide: Oral: 200 mg/day days 1 to 14 (cycle 1)
followed by Oral: 400 mg/day days 15 to 28 (cycle 1)
[total dose/cycle = 8400 mg]
Thalidomide: Oral: 400 mg/day days 1 to 28 (subsequent cycles)
[total dose/cycle = 11,200 mg]
Dexamethasone: Oral: 20 mg/m^2/day days 1 to 4, 9 to 12, and 17 to 20 (cycle 1)
[total dose/cycle = 240 mg/m^2]
followed by Oral: 20 mg/m^2/day days 1 to 4 (subsequent cycles)
[total dose/cycle = 80 mg/m^2]
Repeat cycle every 28 days
Variation 3 (newly diagnosed):
Thalidomide: Oral: 200 mg/day days 1 to 28
[total dose/cycle = 5600 mg]
Dexamethasone: Oral: 40 mg/day days 1 to 4, 9 to 12, and 17 to 20
[total dose/cycle = 480 mg]
Repeat cycle every 28 days
Variation 4 (newly diagnosed):
Thalidomide: Oral: 50 mg/day days 1 to 14
followed by Oral: 100 mg/day days 15 to 28 (cycle 1)
[total dose/cycle 1 = 2100 mg]
followed by Oral: 200 mg/day days 1 to 28 (starting with cycle 2 and subsequent cycles)
[total dose/cycle = 5600 mg]
Dexamethasone: Oral: 40 mg/day days 1 to 4, 9 to 12, and 17 to 20 (cycles 1 to 4)
[total dose/cycle 1 to 4 = 480 mg]
followed by Oral: 40 mg/day days 1 to 4 (starting with cycle 5 and subsequent cycles)
[total dose/cycle = 160 mg]
Repeat cycle every 28 days until disease progression or unacceptable toxicity
Variation 5 (newly diagnosed):
Thalidomide: Oral: 100 mg/day days 1 to 14
followed by Oral: 200 mg/day days 15 to 28 (cycle 1)
[total dose/cycle = 4200 mg]
followed by Oral: 200 mg/day days 1 to 28 (starting with cycle 2 and subsequent cycles)
[total dose/cycle = 5600 mg]
Dexamethasone: Oral: 40 mg/day days 1 to 4, 9 to 12, and 17 to 20 (odd cycles)
[total dose/cycle = 480 mg]
Dexamethasone: Oral: 40 mg/day days 1 to 4 (even cycles)
[total dose/cycle = 160 mg]
Repeat cycle every 28 days for a total of 4 cycles
Variation 6 (newly diagnosed induction):
Thalidomide: Oral: 50 mg/day; may escalate by 50 mg per week to a maximum dose of 400 mg/day
[total dose/cycle = up to 14,000 mg]

Dexamethasone: Oral: 40 mg/day days 1 to 4, 9 to 12, and 17 to 20 [total dose/cycle = 480 mg]

Repeat cycle every 35 days for a total of 3 cycles

References

Variation 1:

Palumbo A, Giaccone L, Bertola A, et al, "Low-Dose Thalidomide Plus Dexamethasone Is an Effective Salvage Therapy for Advanced Myeloma," *Haematologica*, 2001, 86(4):399-403.

Variation 2:

Dimopoulos MA, Zervas K, Kouvatseas G, et al, "Thalidomide and Dexamethasone Combination for Refractory Multiple Myeloma," *Ann Oncol*, 2001, 12(7):991-5.

Variation 3:

Rajkumar SV, Blood E, Vesole D, et al, "Phase III Clinical Trial of Thalidomide Plus Dexamethasone Compared With Dexamethasone Alone in Newly Diagnosed Multiple Myeloma: A Clinical Trial Coordinated by the Eastern Cooperative Oncology Group," *J Clin Oncol*, 2006, 24(3):431-6.

Variation 4:

Rajkumar SV, Rosiñol L, Hussein M, et al, "Multicenter, Randomized, Double-Blind, Placebo-Controlled Study of Thalidomide Plus Dexamethasone Compared With Dexamethasone as Initial Therapy for Newly Diagnosed Multiple Myeloma," *J Clin Oncol*, 2008, 26(13):2171-7.

Variation 5:

Cavo M, Zamagni E, Tosi P, et al, "Superiority of Thalidomide and Dexamethasone Over Vincristine-Doxorubicin-Dexamethasone (VAD) as Primary Therapy in Preparation for Autologous Transplantation for Multiple Myeloma," *Blood*, 2005, 106(1):35-9.

Variation 6:

Hussein MA, Bolejack V, Zonder JA, et al, "Phase II Study of Thalidomide Plus Dexamethasone Induction Followed by Tandem Melphalan-Based Autotransplantation and Thalidomide-Plus-Prednisone Maintenance for Untreated Multiple Myeloma: A Southwest Oncology Group Trial (S0204)," *J Clin Oncol*, 2009, 27(21):3510-7.

◆ **Topotecan-Cisplatin (Cervical Cancer)** *see* Cisplatin-Topotecan (Cervical Cancer) *on page 1583*

Topotecan-Cyclophosphamide (Ewing's Sarcoma)

Index Terms Cyclophosphamide-Topotecan (Ewing's Sarcoma)

Use Ewing's sarcoma

Regimen

Cyclophosphamide: I.V.: 250 mg/m^2/dose days 1 to 5 [total dose/cycle = 1250 mg/m^2]

Topotecan: I.V.: 0.75 mg/m^2/dose days 1 to 5 [total dose/cycle = 3.75 mg/m^2]

Repeat cycle every 21 days

References

Hunold A, Weddeling N, Paulussen M, et al, "Topotecan and Cyclophosphamide in Patients With Refractory or Relapsed Ewing Tumors," *Pediatr Blood Cancer*, 2006, 47(6):795-800.

Topotecan Intravenous (Small Cell Lung Cancer Regimen)

Use Lung cancer, small cell

Regimen

Topotecan: I.V.: 1.5 mg/m^2/day over 30 minutes days 1 to 5 [total dose/cycle = 7.5 mg/m^2]

Repeat cycle every 21 days

References

Eckardt JR, von Pawel J, Pujol JL, et al, "Phase III Study of Oral Compared With Intravenous Topotecan as Second-Line Therapy in Small-Cell Lung Cancer," *J Clin Oncol*, 2007, 25 (15):2086-92.

van Pawel J, Gatzemeier U, Pujol JL, et al, "Phase II Comparator Study of Oral Versus Intravenous Topotecan in Patients With Chemosensitive Small-Cell Lung Cancer," *J Clin Oncol*, 2001, 19 (6):1743-9.

von Pawel J, Schiller JH, Shephard FA, et al, "Topotecan Versus Cyclophosphamide, Doxorubicin, and Vincristine for the Treatment of Recurrent Small-Cell Lung Cancer," *J Clin Oncol*, 1999, 17 (2):658-67.

Topotecan Oral Regimen (Ovarian Cancer)

Use Ovarian cancer

Regimen

Topotecan: Oral: 2.3 mg/m^2/day days 1 to 5
[total dose/cycle = 11.5 mg/m^2]

Repeat cycle every 21 days until disease progression or for at least 4 cycles after achieve stable disease

References

Clarke-Pearson DL, Van Le L, Iveson T, et al, "Oral Topotecan as Single-Agent Second-Line Chemotherapy in Patients With Advanced Ovarian Cancer," *J Clin Oncol*, 2001, 19(19):3967-75.

Topotecan Oral (Small Cell Lung Cancer Regimen)

Use Lung cancer, small cell

Regimen

Topotecan: Oral: 2.3 mg/m^2/day days 1 to 5
[total dose/cycle = 11.5 mg/m^2]

Repeat cycle every 21 days

References

Eckardt JR, von Pawel J, Pujol JL, et al, "Phase III Study of Oral Compared With Intravenous Topotecan as Second-Line Therapy in Small-Cell Lung Cancer," *J Clin Oncol*, 2007, 25 (15):2086-92.

O'Brien ME, Ciuleanu TE, Tsekov H, et al, "Phase III Trial Comparing Supportive Care Alone With Supportive Care With Oral Topotecan in Patients With Relapsed Small-Cell Lung Cancer," *J Clin Oncol*, 2006, 24(34):5441-7.

◆ **TPF** *see* Docetaxel-Cisplatin-Fluorouracil (Head and Neck Cancer) *on page 1610*

◆ **TPF (Unknown Primary)** *see* Cisplatin-Docetaxel-Fluorouracil (Unknown Primary) *on page 1568*

Trabectedin-Doxorubicin (Liposomal) (Ovarian Cancer)

Index Terms Doxorubicin Liposomal-Trabectedin (Ovarian Cancer)

Use Ovarian cancer

Regimen

Doxorubicin (liposomal): I.V.: 30 mg/m^2 over 90 minutes day 1
[total dose/cycle = 30 mg/m^2]

Trabectedin: I.V.: 1.1 mg/m^2 over 3 hours (via central line) day 1
[total dose/cycle = 1.1 mg/m^2]

Repeat cycle every 3 weeks until disease progression or for 2 cycles beyond confirmed complete response.

References

Monk BJ, Herzog TJ, Kaye SB, et al, "Trabectedin Plus Pegylated Liposomal Doxorubicin in Recurrent Ovarian Cancer," *J Clin Oncol*, 2010, 28(19):3107-14.

◆ **Trastuzumab-Capecitabine** *see* Capecitabine-Trastuzumab *on page 1541*

Trastuzumab-Cisplatin-Capecitabine (Gastric Cancer)

Index Terms Capecitabine-Cisplatin-Trastuzumab (Gastric Cancer); Cisplatin-Capecitabine-Trastuzumab (Gastric Cancer)

Use Gastric cancer

Regimen

Cycle 1:

Capecitabine: Oral: 1000 mg/m²/dose twice daily days 1 to 14 [total dose/cycle = 28,000 mg/m²]

Cisplatin: I.V.: 80 mg/m²/dose day 1 [total dose/cycle = 80 mg/m²]

Trastuzumab: I.V.: 8 mg/kg/dose (loading dose) day 1 [total dose/cycle 1 = 8 mg/kg]

Treatment cycle is 21 days

Cycles 2-6:

Capecitabine: Oral: 1000 mg/m²/dose twice daily days 1 to 14 [total dose/cycle = 28,000 mg/m²]

Cisplatin: I.V.: 80 mg/m²/dose day 1 [total dose/cycle = 80 mg/m²]

Trastuzumab: I.V.: 6 mg/kg/dose day 1 [total dose/cycle = 6 mg/kg]

Treatment cycle is 21 days

Subsequent cycles:

Trastuzumab: I.V.: 6 mg/kg/dose day 1 [total dose/cycle = 6 mg/kg]

Repeat cycle every 3 weeks until disease progression or unacceptable toxicity

References

Bang YJ, Van Cutsem E, Feyereislova A, et al, "Trastuzumab in Combination With Chemotherapy Versus Chemotherapy Alone for Treatment of HER2-Positive Advanced Gastric or Gastro-Oesophageal Junction Cancer (ToGA): A Phase 3, Open-Label, Randomised Controlled Trial," *Lancet*, 2010, 376(9742):687-97.

Trastuzumab-Cisplatin-Fluorouracil (Gastric Cancer)

Index Terms Cisplatin-Fluorouracil-Trastuzumab (Gastric Cancer); Fluorouracil-Cisplatin-Trastuzumab (Gastric Cancer)

Use Gastric cancer

Regimen

Cycle 1:

Fluorouracil: I.V.: 800 mg/m²/day continuous infusion days 1 to 5 [total dose/cycle = 4000 mg/m²]

Cisplatin: I.V.: 80 mg/m²/dose day 1 [total dose/cycle = 80 mg/m²]

Trastuzumab: I.V.: 8 mg/kg/dose (loading dose) day 1 [total dose/cycle 1 = 8 mg/kg]

Treatment cycle is 21 days

Cycles 2-6:

Fluorouracil: I.V.: 800 mg/m²/day continuous infusion days 1 to 5 [total dose/cycle = 4000 mg/m²]

Cisplatin: I.V.: 80 mg/m²/dose day 1 [total dose/cycle = 80 mg/m²]

Trastuzumab: I.V.: 6 mg/kg/dose day 1 [total dose/cycle = 6 mg/kg]

Treatment cycle is 21 days

Subsequent cycles:

Trastuzumab: I.V.: 6 mg/kg/dose day 1 [total dose/cycle = 6 mg/kg]

Repeat cycle every 3 weeks until disease progression or unacceptable toxicity

References

Bang YJ, Van Cutsem E, Feyereislova A, et al, "Trastuzumab in Combination With Chemotherapy Versus Chemotherapy Alone for Treatment of HER2-Positive Advanced Gastric or Gastro-Oesophageal Junction Cancer (ToGA): A Phase 3, Open-Label, Randomised Controlled Trial," *Lancet*, 2010, 376(9742):687-97.

◆ **Trastuzumab-Docetaxel** *see* Docetaxel-Trastuzumab *on page 1615*

◆ **Trastuzumab-Docetaxel-Carboplatin** *see* Docetaxel-Trastuzumab-Carboplatin *on page 1615*

◆ **Trastuzumab-Docetaxel-Cisplatin** *see* Docetaxel-Trastuzumab-Cisplatin *on page 1616*

◆ **Trastuzumab-Docetaxel-FEC** *see* Docetaxel-Trastuzumab-FEC *on page 1616*

◆ **Trastuzumab-Docetaxel (Weekly)** *see* Docetaxel (Weekly)-Trastuzumab *on page 1617*

◆ **Trastuzumab-Lapatinib (Breast Cancer)** *see* Lapatinib-Trastuzumab (Breast Cancer) *on page 1698*

Trastuzumab-Paclitaxel

Index Terms Paclitaxel-Trastuzumab

Use Breast cancer

Regimen NOTE: Multiple variations are listed.

Variation 1:

Cycle 1:

Paclitaxel: I.V.: 175 mg/m^2 day 1
[total dose/cycle = 175 mg/m^2]

Trastuzumab: I.V.: 4 mg/kg (loading dose) day 1
followed by I.V.: 2 mg/kg/day days 8 and 15
[total dose/cycle 1 = 8 mg/kg]

Treatment cycle is 21 days

Subsequent cycles:

Paclitaxel: I.V.: 175 mg/m^2 day 1
[total dose/cycle = 175 mg/m^2]

Trastuzumab: I.V.: 2 mg/kg/day days 1, 8, and 15
[total dose/cycle = 6 mg/kg]

Repeat cycle every 21 days for a total of at least 6 cycles

Variation 2:

Cycle 1:

Trastuzumab: I.V.: 4 mg/kg (loading dose) day 1
followed by I.V.: 2 mg/kg/day days 8 and 15
[total dose/cycle 1 = 8 mg/kg]

Paclitaxel: I.V.: 175 mg/m^2 day 2
[total dose/cycle = 175 mg/m^2]

Treatment cycle is 21 days

Subsequent cycles:

Trastuzumab: I.V.: 2 mg/kg/day days 1, 8, and 15
[total dose/cycle = 6 mg/kg]

Paclitaxel: I.V.: 175 mg/m^2 day 2
[total dose/cycle = 175 mg/m^2]

Repeat cycle every 21 days for a total of at least 6 cycles (continue weekly trastuzumab after chemotherapy until disease progression or unacceptable toxicity)

References

Variation 1:

Slamon DJ, Leyland-Jones B, Shak S, et al, "Use of Chemotherapy Plus a Monoclonal Antibody Against HER2 for Metastatic Breast Cancer That Overexpresses HER2," *N Engl J Med*, 2001, 344(11):783-92.

Variation 2:

Robert N, Leyland-Jones B, Asmar L, et al, "Randomized Phase III Study of Trastuzumab, Paclitaxel, and Carboplatin Compared With Trastuzumab and Paclitaxel in Women With HER-2-Overexpressing Metastatic Breast Cancer," *J Clin Oncol*, 2006, 24(18):2786-92.

Trastuzumab-Paclitaxel-Carboplatin

Index Terms Paclitaxel-Carboplatin-Trastuzumab

Use Breast cancer

Regimen

Cycle 1:

Trastuzumab: I.V.: 4 mg/kg (loading dose) day 1

followed by I.V.: 2 mg/kg/day days 8 and 15

[total dose/cycle 1 = 8 mg/kg]

Paclitaxel: I.V.: 175 mg/m^2 day 2

[total dose/cycle = 175 mg/m^2]

Carboplatin: I.V.: AUC 6 day 2

[total dose/cycle = AUC = 6]

Treatment cycle is 21 days

Subsequent cycles:

Trastuzumab: I.V.: 2 mg/kg/day days 1, 8, and 15

[total dose/cycle = 6 mg/kg]

Paclitaxel: I.V.: 175 mg/m^2 day 2

[total dose/cycle = 175 mg/m^2]

Carboplatin: I.V.: AUC 6 day 2

[total dose/cycle = AUC = 6]

Repeat cycle every 21 days for a total of at least 6 cycles (continue weekly trastuzumab after chemotherapy until disease progression or unacceptable toxicity)

References

Robert N, Leyland-Jones B, Asmar L, et al, "Randomized Phase III Study of Trastuzumab, Paclitaxel, and Carboplatin Compared With Trastuzumab and Paclitaxel in Women With HER-2-Overexpressing Metastatic Breast Cancer," *J Clin Oncol*, 2006, 24(18):2786-92.

Trastuzumab-Paclitaxel (Weekly)

Index Terms Paclitaxel (Weekly)-Trastuzumab

Use Breast cancer

Regimen NOTE: Multiple variations are listed.

Variation 1:

Week 1:

Trastuzumab: I.V.: 4 mg/kg (loading dose) day 1

[total dose/week 1 = 4 mg/kg]

Paclitaxel: I.V.: 90 mg/m^2 day 2

[total dose/week 1 = 90 mg/m^2]

Subsequent weeks:

Paclitaxel: I.V.: 90 mg/m^2 day 1

[total dose/week = 90 mg/m^2]

Trastuzumab: I.V.: 2 mg/kg day 1

[total dose/week = 2 mg/kg]

Repeat weekly

Variation 2:
Week 1:
Trastuzumab: I.V.: 4 mg/kg (loading dose) day 1
[total dose/week 1 = 4 mg/kg]
Paclitaxel: I.V.: 80 mg/m^2 day 1
[total dose/week 1 = 80 mg/m^2]
Subsequent weeks:
Trastuzumab: I.V.: 2 mg/kg day 1
[total dose/week = 2 mg/kg]
Paclitaxel: I.V.: 80 mg/m^2 day 1
[total dose/week = 80 mg/m^2]
Repeat weekly

References

Variation 1:
Seidman AD, Fornier MN, Esteva FJ, et al, "Weekly Trastuzumab and Paclitaxel Therapy for Metastatic Breast Cancer With Analysis of Efficacy by HER2 Immunophenotype and Gene Amplification," *J Clin Oncol*, 2001, 19(10):2587-95.
Variation 2:
Seidman AD, Berry D, Cirrincione C, et al, "Randomized Phase III Trial of Weekly Compared With Every-3-Weeks Paclitaxel for Metastatic Breast Cancer, With Trastuzumab for all HER-2 Over-expressors and Random Assignment to Trastuzumab or Not in HER-2 Nonoverexpressors: Final Results of Cancer and Leukemia Group B Protocol 9840," *J Clin Oncol*, 2008, 26(10):1642-9.

◆ **Trastuzumab-Pertuzumab-Docetaxel (Breast)** *see* Docetaxel-Pertuzumab-Trastuzumab (Breast) *on page* 1614

◆ **Trastuzumab-Vinorelbine** *see* Vinorelbine-Trastuzumab *on page* 1775

Tretinoin-Arsenic Trioxide (APL)

Index Terms Arsenic Trioxide-ATRA (APL); ATRA-Arsenic Trixoide (APL)
Use Leukemia, acute promyelocytic
Regimen
Induction (continue until <5% blasts in marrow and no abnormal promyelocytes):
Tretinoin: Oral: 45 mg/m^2/day (in 2 divided doses) day 1 up to day 85
[total induction dose = up to 3825 mg/m^2]
Arsenic Trioxide: I.V.: 0.15 mg/kg/day over 1 hour beginning day 10 up to day 85
[total induction dose = up to 11.25 mg/kg]
Postremission therapy (beginning with complete remission):
Tretinoin: Oral: 45 mg/m^2/day weeks 1, 2, 5, 6, 9, 10, 13, 14, 17, 18, 21, 22, 25, 26
[total postremission dose = 4410 mg/m^2]
Arsenic Trioxide: I.V.: 0.15 mg/kg/day Monday through Friday weeks 1 to 4, 9 to 12, 17 to 20, and 25 to 28
[total postremission dose = 12 mg/kg]

References

Estey E, Garcia-Manero G, Ferrajoli A, et al, "Use of All-*Trans* Retinoic Acid Plus Arsenic Trioxide as an Alternative to Chemotherapy in Untreated Acute Promyelocytic Leukemia," *Blood*, 2006, 107(9):3469-73.
Ravandi F, Estey E, Jones D, et al, "Effective Treatment of Acute Promyelocytic Leukemia With All-*Trans*-Retinoic Acid, Arsenic Trioxide, and Gemtuzumab Ozogamicin," *J Clin Oncol*, 2009, 27 (4):504-10.

Tretinoin-Daunorubicin (APL)

Index Terms ATRA-Daunorubicin (APL); Daunorubicin-ATRA (APL); Daunorubicin-Tretinoin (APL)

Use Leukemia, acute promyelocytic

Regimen

Induction:

Tretinoin: Oral: 45 mg/m^2/day (in 2 divided doses) day 1 until hematologic complete remission

Daunorubicin: I.V.: 60 mg/m^2/day days 1, 2, and 3
[total dose/cycle = 180 mg/m^2]

Consolidation:

Course 1:

Daunorubicin: I.V.: 60 mg/m^2/day days 1, 2, and 3
[total dose/cycle = 180 mg/m^2]

Course 2:

Daunorubicin: I.V.: 45 mg/m^2/day days 1, 2, and 3
[total dose/cycle = 135 mg/m^2]

Maintenance:

Mercaptopurine: Oral: 90 mg/m^2 daily
[total dose/cycle = 8100 mg/m^2 (90 days)]

Methotrexate: Oral: 15 mg/m^2 weekly
[total dose/cycle = 180 mg/m^2]

Tretinoin: Oral: 45 mg/m^2/day (in 2 divided doses) days 1 to 15
[total dose/cycle = 675 mg/m^2]

Repeat cycle every 3 months for 2 years

References

Adès L, Chevret S, Raffoux E, et al, "Is Cytarabine Useful in the Treatment of Acute Promyelocytic Leukemia? Results of a Randomized Trial From the European Acute Promyelocytic Leukemia Group," *J Clin Oncol*, 2006, 24(36):5703-10.

Tretinoin-Daunorubicin-Cytarabine (APL)

Index Terms ATRA-Daunorubicin-Cytarabine (APL)

Use Leukemia, acute promyelocytic

Regimen NOTE: Multiple variations are listed.

Variation 1 (patients ≤60 years of age and WBC <10,000/mm^3):

Induction:

Tretinoin: Oral: 45 mg/m^2/day (in 2 divided doses) day 1 until hematologic complete remission

Daunorubicin: I.V.: 60 mg/m^2/day days 1, 2, and 3
[total dose/cycle = 180 mg/m^2]

Cytarabine: I.V.: 200 mg/m^2/day days 3 to 10
[total dose/cycle = 1400 mg/m^2]

Consolidation:

Course 1:

Daunorubicin: I.V.: 60 mg/m^2/day days 1, 2, and 3
[total dose/cycle = 180 mg/m^2]

Cytarabine: I.V.: 200 mg/m^2/day days 1 to 7
[total dose/cycle = 1400 mg/m^2]

Course 2:

Daunorubicin: I.V.: 45 mg/m^2/day days 1, 2, and 3
[total dose/cycle = 135 mg/m^2]

Cytarabine: I.V.: 1000 mg/m^2/dose every 12 hours for 8 doses
[total dose/cycle = 8000 mg/m^2]

Maintenance:

Mercaptopurine: Oral: 90 mg/m^2 daily
[total dose/cycle = 8100 mg/m^2 (90 days)]

Methotrexate: Oral: 15 mg/m^2 weekly
[total dose/cycle = 180 mg/m^2]

Tretinoin: Oral: 45 mg/m^2/day (in 2 divided doses) days 1 to 15
[total dose/cycle = 675 mg/m^2]

Repeat cycle every 3 months for 2 years

Variation 2 (patients ≤60 years of age and WBC ≥10,000/mm^3):

Induction:

Tretinoin: Oral: 45 mg/m^2/day (in 2 divided doses) day 1 until hematologic complete remission

Daunorubicin: I.V.: 60 mg/m^2/day days 1, 2, and 3
[total dose/cycle = 180 mg/m^2]

Cytarabine: I.V.: 200 mg/m^2/day days 3 to 10
[total dose/cycle = 1400 mg/m^2]

Consolidation:

Course 1:

Daunorubicin: I.V.: 60 mg/m^2/day days 1, 2, and 3
[total dose/cycle = 180 mg/m^2]

Cytarabine: I.V.: 200 mg/m^2/day days 1 to 7
[total dose/cycle = 1400 mg/m^2]

Course 2:

Daunorubicin: I.V.: 45 mg/m^2/day days 1, 2, and 3
[total dose/cycle = 135 mg/m^2]

Cytarabine: I.V.: 2000 mg/m^2/dose every 12 hours for 10 doses
[total dose/cycle = 20,000 mg/m^2]

Intrathecal prophylaxis: Five intrathecal injections. First dose in between induction and consolidation and 2 doses during each consolidation phase:

Methotrexate (preservative free): I.T.: 15 mg

Cytarabine (preservative free): I.T.: 50 mg

Corticosteroids (preservative free): I.T.: Dose unspecified

Maintenance:

Mercaptopurine: Oral: 90 mg/m^2 daily
[total dose/cycle = 8100 mg/m^2 (90 days)]

Methotrexate: Oral: 15 mg/m^2 weekly
[total dose/cycle = 180 mg/m^2]

Tretinoin: Oral: 45 mg/m^2/day (in 2 divided doses) days 1 to 15
[total dose/cycle = 675 mg/m^2]

Repeat cycle every 3 months for 2 years

Variation 3 (patients >60 years of age and WBC >10,000/mm^3):

Induction:

Tretinoin: Oral: 45 mg/m^2/day (in 2 divided doses) day 1 until hematologic complete remission

Daunorubicin: I.V.: 60 mg/m^2/day days 1, 2, and 3
[total dose/cycle = 180 mg/m^2]

Cytarabine: I.V.: 200 mg/m^2/day days 3 to 10
[total dose/cycle = 1400 mg/m^2]

Consolidation:

Course 1:

Daunorubicin: I.V.: 60 mg/m^2/day days 1, 2, and 3
[total dose/cycle = 180 mg/m^2]

Cytarabine: I.V.: 200 mg/m^2/day days 1 to 7
[total dose/cycle = 1400 mg/m^2]

Course 2:
Daunorubicin: I.V.: 45 mg/m^2/day days 1, 2, and 3
[total dose/cycle = 135 mg/m^2]
Cytarabine: I.V.: 1000 mg/m^2/dose every 12 hours for 8 doses
[total dose/cycle = 8,000 mg/m^2]

Intrathecal prophylaxis: Five intrathecal injections: First dose in between induction and consolidation and 2 doses during each consolidation phase:
Methotrexate (preservative free): I.T.: 15 mg
Cytarabine (preservative free): I.T.: 50 mg
Corticosteroids (preservative free): I.T.: Dose unspecified

Maintenance:
Mercaptopurine: Oral: 90 mg/m^2 daily
[total dose/cycle = 8100 mg/m^2 (90 days)]
Methotrexate: Oral: 15 mg/m^2 weekly
[total dose/cycle = 180 mg/m^2]
Tretinoin: Oral: 45 mg/m^2/day (in 2 divided doses) days 1 to 15
[total dose/cycle = 675 mg/m^2]
Repeat cycle every 3 months for 2 years

References

Variations 1, 2, and 3:
Adès L, Chevret S, Raffoux E, et al, "Is Cytarabine Useful in the Treatment of Acute Promyelocytic Leukemia? Results of a Randomized Trial From the European Acute Promyelocytic Leukemia Group," *J Clin Oncol*, 2006, 24(36):5703-10.

Tretinoin-Idarubicin (APL)

Index Terms ATRA-Idarubicin (APL); Idarubicin-ATRA (APL); Idarubicin-Tretinoin (APL)

Use Leukemia, acute promyelocytic

Regimen NOTE: Multiple variations are listed.

Variation 1:

Induction:
Tretinoin: Oral: 45 mg/m^2/day (in 2 divided doses) day 1 up to 90 days
[total dose/cycle = up to 4050 mg/m^2]
≤20 years: Oral: 25 mg/m^2/day (in 2 divided doses) day 1 up to 90 days
[total dose/cycle = up to 2250 mg/m^2]
Idarubicin: I.V.: 12 mg/m^2/day days 2, 4, 6, and 8 (omit day 8 for patients >70 years of age)
[total dose/cycle = 36-48 mg/m^2]

Consolidation (administer courses sequentially at 1-month intervals for 3 months):

Course 1:
Idarubicin: I.V.: 5 mg/m^2/day days 1 to 4
[total dose/cycle = 20 mg/m^2]
or
Idarubicin: I.V.: 7 mg/m^2/day days 1 to 4
[total dose/cycle = 28 mg/m^2]
Tretinoin: Oral: 45 mg/m^2/day (in 2 divided doses) days 1 to 15
[total dose/cycle = 675 mg/m^2]

Course 2:
Mitoxantrone: I.V.: 10 mg/m^2/day days 1 to 5
[total dose/cycle = 50 mg/m^2]
or
Mitoxantrone: I.V.: 10 mg/m^2/day days 1 to 5
[total dose/cycle = 50 mg/m^2]

Tretinoin: Oral: 45 mg/m²/day (in 2 divided doses) days 1 to 15
[total dose/cycle = 675 mg/m²]

Course 3:

Idarubicin: I.V.: 12 mg/m² day 1
[total dose/cycle = 12 mg/m²]

or

Idarubicin: I.V.: 12 mg/m²/day days 1 and 2
[total dose/cycle = 24 mg/m²]

Tretinoin: Oral: 45 mg/m²/day (in 2 divided doses) days 1 to 15
[total dose/cycle = 675 mg/m²]

Maintenance:

Mercaptopurine: Oral: 50 mg/m² daily
[total dose/cycle = 4500 mg/m² (90 days)]

Methotrexate: I.M.: 15 mg/m² weekly
[total dose/cycle = 180 mg/m²]

Tretinoin: Oral: 45 mg/m²/day (in 2 divided doses) days 1 to 15
[total dose/cycle = 675 mg/m²]

Repeat cycle every 3 months for 2 years

Variation 2:

Induction:

Tretinoin: Oral: 45 mg/m²/day (in 2 divided doses) day 1 up to 90 days
[total dose/cycle = up to 4050 mg/m²]

<15 years: Oral: 25 mg/m²/day (in 2 divided doses) day 1 up to 90 days
[total dose/cycle = up to 2250 mg/m²]

Idarubicin: I.V.: 12 mg/m²/day days 2, 4, 6, and 8
[total dose/cycle = 48 mg/m²]

Consolidation (administer courses sequentially at 1-month intervals for 3 months):

Course 1:

Idarubicin: I.V.: 5 mg/m²/day days 1 to 4
[total dose/cycle = 20 mg/m²]

Course 2:

Mitoxantrone: I.V.: 10 mg/m²/day days 1 to 5
[total dose/cycle = 50 mg/m²]

Course 3:

Idarubicin: I.V.: 12 mg/m² day 1
[total dose/cycle = 12 mg/m²]

Maintenance:

Mercaptopurine: Oral: 90 mg/m² daily
[total dose/cycle = 8100 mg/m²(90 days)]

Methotrexate: I.M.: 15 mg/m² weekly
[total dose/cycle = 180 mg/m²]

Tretinoin: Oral: 45 mg/m²/day (in 2 divided doses) days 1 to 15
[total dose/cycle = 675 mg/m²]

Repeat cycle every 3 months for 2 years

Variation 3 (patients ≥60 years of age):

Induction:

Tretinoin: Oral: 45 mg/m²/day (in 2 divided doses) day 1 up to 90 days
[total dose/cycle = up to 4050 mg/m²]

Idarubicin: I.V.: 12 mg/m²/day days 2, 4, 6, and 8 (omit day 8 for patients ≥70 years of age)
[total dose/cycle = 36-48 mg/m²]

Consolidation (administer courses sequentially at 1-month intervals for 3 months):

Course 1:

Idarubicin: I.V.: 5 mg/m^2/day days 1 to 4
[total dose/cycle = 20 mg/m^2]

Tretinoin: Oral: 45 mg/m^2/day (in 2 divided doses) days 1 to 15 (if intermediate or high risk)
[total dose/cycle = 675 mg/m^2]

Course 2:

Mitoxantrone: I.V.: 10 mg/m^2/day days 1 to 5
[total dose/cycle = 50 mg/m^2]

Tretinoin: Oral: 45 mg/m^2/day (in 2 divided doses) days 1 to 15 (if intermediate or high risk)
[total dose/cycle = 675 mg/m^2]

Course 3:

Idarubicin: I.V.: 12 mg/m^2 day 1
[total dose/cycle = 12 mg/m^2]

Tretinoin: Oral: 45 mg/m^2/day (in 2 divided doses) days 1 to 15 (if intermediate or high risk)
[total dose/cycle = 675 mg/m^2]

Maintenance:

Mercaptopurine: Oral: 50 mg/m^2 daily
[total dose/cycle = 4500 mg/m^2 (90 days)]

Methotrexate: I.M.: 15 mg/m^2 weekly
[total dose/cycle = 180 mg/m^2]

Tretinoin: Oral: 45 mg/m^2/day (in 2 divided doses) days 1 to 15
[total dose/cycle = 675 mg/m^2]

Repeat cycle every 3 months for 2 years

References

Variation 1:

Sanz MA, Martin G, Gonzalez M, et al, "Risk-Adapted Treatment of Acute Promyelocytic Leukemia With All-*Trans*-Retinoic Acid and Anthracycline Monochemotherapy: A Multicenter Study by the PETHEMA Group," *Blood*, 2004, 103(4):1237-43.

Variation 2:

Sanz MA, Martin G, Rayon C, et al, "A Modified AIDA Protocol With Anthracycline-Based Consolidation Results in High Antileukemic Efficacy and Reduced Toxicity in Newly Diagnosed PML/RARalpha-Positive Acute Promyelocytic Leukemia," *Blood*, 1999, 94(9):3015-21.

Variation 3:

Sanz MA, Vellenga E, Rayón C, et al, "All-*Trans* Retinoic Acid and Anthracycline Monochemotherapy for the Treatment of Elderly Patients With Acute Promyelocytic Leukemia," *Blood*, 2004, 104(12):3490-3.

VAC Alternating With IE (Ewing's Sarcoma)

Use Ewing's sarcoma

Regimen

Cycle A: (Odd numbered cycles)

Cyclophosphamide: I.V.: 1200 mg/m^2 day 1 (followed by mesna; dose not specified)
[total dose/cycle = 1200 mg/m^2]

Vincristine: I.V.: 2 mg/m^2 (maximum dose: 2 mg) day 1
[total dose/cycle = 2 mg/m^2; maximum: 2 mg]

Doxorubicin: I.V.: 75 mg/m^2 day 1, for 5 cycles (maximum cumulative dose: 375 mg/m^2)
[total dose/cycle = 75 mg/m^2; maximum cumulative dose: 375 mg/m^2]

Dactinomycin: I.V.: 1.25 mg/m^2 day 1, begin cycle 11 (after reaching maximum cumulative doxorubicin dose)
[total dose/cycle = 1.25 mg/m^2]
Cycle B: (Even numbered cycles)
Ifosfamide: I.V.: 1800 mg/m^2/day days 1 to 5 (given with mesna)
[total dose/cycle = 9000 mg/m^2]
Etoposide: I.V.: 100 mg/m^2/day days 1 to 5
[total dose/cycle = 500 mg/m^2]
Alternate Cycles A and B, administering a cycle every 3 weeks (alternating in the following sequence: ABABAB) for 17 cycles

References

Grier HE, Krailo MD, Tarbell NJ, et al, "Addition of Ifosfamide and Etoposide to Standard Chemotherapy for Ewing's Sarcoma and Primitive Neuroectodermal Tumor of Bone," *N Engl J Med*, 2003, 348(8):694-701.

◆ **VAC (Ovarian Cancer)** *see* Vincristine-Dactinomycin-Cyclophosphamide (Ovarian Cancer) *on page 1771*

VAC Pulse

Use Rhabdomyosarcoma

Regimen

Vincristine: I.V.: 2 mg/m^2/dose (maximum dose: 2 mg/dose) every 7 days, for 12 weeks
Dactinomycin: I.V.: 0.015 mg/kg/day (maximum dose: 0.5 mg/day) days 1 to 5, every 3 months for 5 courses
Cyclophosphamide: Oral, I.V.: 10 mg/kg/day for 7 days, repeat every 6 weeks

References

Wilbur JR, Sutow WW, Sullivan MP, et al, "Chemotherapy of Sarcomas," *Cancer*, 1975, 36 (2):765-9.

VAC (Rhabdomyosarcoma)

Use Rhabdomyosarcoma

Regimen

Induction (weeks 1 to 17):
Vincristine: I.V. push: 1.5 mg/m^2 (maximum dose: 2 mg) day 1 of weeks 1 to 13, then one dose at week 17
Dactinomycin: I.V. push: 0.015 mg/kg/day (maximum dose: 0.5 mg) days 1 to 5 of weeks 1, 4, 7, and 17
Cyclophosphamide: I.V.: 2.2 g/m^2 day 1 of weeks 1, 4, 7, 10, 13, and 17
Continuation (weeks 21 to 44):
Vincristine: I.V. push: 1.5 mg/m^2 (maximum dose: 2 mg) day 1 of weeks 21 to 26, 30 to 35, and 39 to 44
Dactinomycin: I.V. push: 0.015 mg/kg/day (maximum dose: 0.5 mg) days 1 to 5 of weeks 21, 24, 30, 33, 39, and 42
Cyclophosphamide: I.V.: 2.2 g/m^2 day 1 of weeks 21, 24, 30, 33, 39, and 42

References

Baker KS, Anderson JR, Link MP, et al, "Benefit of Intensified Therapy for Patients With Local or Regional Embryonal Rhabdomyosarcoma: Results From the Intergroup Rhabdomyosarcoma Study IV," *J Clin Oncol*, 2000, 18(12):2427-34.

VAD

Use Multiple myeloma

Regimen

Vincristine: I.V.: 0.4 mg/day continuous infusion days 1 to 4
[total dose/cycle = 1.6 mg]

Doxorubicin: I.V.: 9 mg/m^2/day continuous infusion days 1 to 4
[total dose/cycle = 36 mg/m^2]
Dexamethasone: Oral: 40 mg/day days 1 to 4, 9 to 12, and 17 to 20
[total dose/cycle = 480 mg]
Repeat cycle every 28-35 days

References

Barlogie B, Smith L, and Alexanian R, "Effective Treatment of Advanced Multiple Myeloma Refractory to Alkylating Agents," *N Engl J Med*, 1984, 310(21):1353-6.

VAD/CVAD

Use Leukemia, acute lymphocytic

Regimen Induction cycle:

Vincristine: I.V.: 0.4 mg/day continuous infusion days 1 to 4 and 24 to 27
[total dose/cycle = 3.2 mg]
Doxorubicin: I.V.: 12 mg/m^2/day continuous infusion days 1 to 4 and 24 to 27
[total dose/cycle = 96 mg/m^2]
Dexamethasone: Oral: 40 mg/day days 1 to 4, 9 to 12, 17 to 20, 24 to 27, 32 to 35, and 40 to 43
[total dose/cycle = 960 mg]
Cyclophosphamide: I.V.: 1 g/m^2 day 24
[total dose/cycle = 1 g/m^2]
Administer one cycle only

References

Kantarjian H, Walters RS, Keating MJ, et al, "Results of the Vincristine, Doxorubicin, and Dexamethasone Regimen in Adults With Standard and High-Risk Acute Lymphocytic Leukemia," *J Clin Oncol*, 1990, 8(6):994-1004.

VAD (Wilms' Tumor)

Index Terms Vincristine, Dactinomycin, Doxorubicin (Wilms' Tumor)

Use Wilms' tumor

Regimen NOTE: Multiple variations are listed.

Variation 1 (Stage III favorable disease; children ≥1 year):
Vincristine: I.V.: 1.5 mg/m^2 weekly for 10 to 11 weeks
Followed by:
Vincristine: I.V.: 1.5 mg/m^2 every 3 weeks
Dactinomycin: I.V.: 1.5 mg/m^2 every 6 weeks
Doxorubicin: I.V.: 40 mg/m^2 every 6 weeks
NOTE: Alternate dactinomycin and doxorubicin; administer dactinomycin at 3 weeks and doxorubicin in 3 weeks
Treatment continued for 1 year

Variation 2 (Stage III favorable disease; children <1 year):
Vincristine: I.V.: 0.75 mg/m^2 weekly for 10 to 11 weeks
Followed by:
Vincristine: I.V.: 0.75 mg/m^2 every 3 weeks
Dactinomycin: I.V.: 0.75 mg/m^2 every 6 weeks
Doxorubicin: I.V.: 20 mg/m^2 every 6 weeks
NOTE: Alternate dactinomycin and doxorubicin; administer dactinomycin at 3 weeks and doxorubicin in 3 weeks
Treatment continued for 1 year

References

Variations 1 and 2:
Pritchard J, Imeson J, Barnes J, et al, "Results of the United Kingdom Children's Cancer Study Group First Wilms' Tumor Study," *J Clin Oncol*, 1995, 13(1):124-33.

VAMP (Hodgkin)

Index Terms Vinblastine, Doxorubicin, Methotrexate, Prednisone (Hodgkin)

Use Lymphoma, Hodgkin

Regimen NOTE: Patients < 21 years old

Vinblastine: I.V.: 6 mg/m^2/day days 1 and 15
[total dose/cycle = 12 mg/m^2]

Doxorubicin: I.V.: 25 mg/m^2/day days 1 and 15
[total dose/cycle = 50 mg/m^2]

Methotrexate: I.V.: 20 mg/m^2/day days 1 and 15
[total dose/cycle = 40 mg/m^2]

Prednisone: Oral: 40 mg/m^2/day days 1 to 14 (omit after mediastinal radiation)
[total dose/cycle = 560 mg/m^2]

Repeat cycle every 28 days for a total of 4 cycles

References

Donaldson SS, Link MP, Weinstein HJ, et al, "Final Results of a Prospective Clinical Trial With VAMP and Low-Dose Involved Radiation for Children With Low-Risk Hodgkin's Disease," *J Clin Oncol*, 2007, 25(3):332-7.

VBMCP (Multiple Myeloma)

Use Multiple myeloma

Regimen NOTE: Multiple variations are listed.

Variation 1:

Vincristine: I.V.: 1.2 mg/m^2 day 1
[total dose/cycle = 1.2 mg/m^2]

Carmustine: I.V.: 20 mg/m^2 day 1
[total dose/cycle = 20 mg/m^2]

Melphalan: Oral: 8 mg/m^2/day days 1 to 4
[total dose/cycle = 32 mg/m^2]

Cyclophosphamide: I.V.: 400 mg/m^2 day 1
[total dose/cycle = 400 mg/m^2]

Prednisone: Oral: 40 mg/m^2/day days 1 to 7
[total dose/cycle = 280 mg/m^2]

Repeat cycle every 35 days for up to 2 years or until disease progression

Variation 2:

Vincristine: I.V.: 1.2 mg/m^2 (maximum dose: 2 mg) day 1
[total dose/cycle = 1.2 mg/m^2; maximum: 2 mg]

Carmustine: I.V.: 20 mg/m^2 day 1
[total dose/cycle = 20 mg/m^2]

Melphalan: Oral: 8 mg/m^2/day days 1 to 4
[total dose/cycle = 32 mg/m^2]

Cyclophosphamide: I.V.: 400 mg/m^2 day 1
[total dose/cycle = 400 mg/m^2]

Prednisone: Oral: 40 mg/m^2/day days 1 to 7 (all cycles)
[total dose/cycle = 280 mg/m^2]

followed by Oral: 20 mg/m^2/day days 8 to 14 (first 3 cycles only)
[total dose/cycle = 140 mg/m^2]

Repeat cycle every 35 days

References

Variation 1:

Kyle RA, Leong T, Li S, et al, "Complete Response in Multiple Myeloma: Clinical Trial E9486, an Eastern Cooperative Oncology Group Study Not Involving Stem Cell Transplantation," *Cancer*, 2006, 106(9):1958-66.

Variation 2:
Oken MM, Harrington DP, Abramson N, et al, "Comparison of Melphalan and Prednisone With Vincristine, Carmustine, Melphalan, Cyclophosphamide, and Prednisone in the Treatment of Multiple Myeloma: Results of Eastern Cooperative Oncology Group Study E2479," *Cancer*, 1997, 79(8):1561-7.

VBP

Index Terms PVB

Use Testicular cancer

Regimen

Vinblastine: I.V.: 0.15 mg/kg/day days 1 and 2
[total dose/cycle = 0.3 mg/kg]

Bleomycin: I.V.: 30 units/day days 2, 9, and 16
[total dose/cycle = 90 units]

Cisplatin: I.V.: 20 mg/m^2/day days 1 to 5
[total dose/cycle = 100 mg/m^2]

Repeat cycle every 21 days for 4 cycles

References

Williams SD, Birch R, Einhorn LH, et al, "Treatment of Disseminated Germ-Cell Tumors With Cisplatin, Bleomycin, and Either Vinblastine or Etoposide," *N Engl J Med*, 1987, 316 (23):1435-40.

◆ **VC** *see* Vinorelbine-Cisplatin *on page 1772*

VCAP

Use Multiple myeloma

Regimen

Vincristine: I.V.: 1 mg/m^2 (maximum dose: 1.5 mg) day 1
[total dose/cycle = 1 mg/m^2]

Cyclophosphamide: Oral: 125 mg/m^2/day days 1 to 4
[total dose/cycle = 500 mg/m^2]

Doxorubicin: I.V.: 30 mg/m^2 day 1
[total dose/cycle = 30 mg/m^2]

Prednisone: Oral: 60 mg/m^2/day days 1 to 4
[total dose/cycle = 240 mg/m^2]

Repeat cycle every 21 days for 6-12 months

References

Salmon SE, Haut A, Bonnet JD, et al, "Alternating Combination Chemotherapy and Levamisole Improves Survival in Multiple Myeloma: A Southwest Oncology Group Study," *J Clin Oncol*, 1983, 1(8):453-61.

Vemurafenib (Melanoma Regimen)

Use Melanoma

Regimen

Vemurafenib: Oral: 960 mg twice daily

Continue until disease progression or unacceptable toxicity

References

Chapman PB, Hauschild A, Robert C, et al, "Improved Survival With Vemurafenib in Melanoma With BRAF V600E Mutation," *N Engl J Med*, 2011, 364(26):2507-16.
Sosman JA, Kim KB, Schuchter L, et al, "Survival in BRAF V600-Mutant Advanced Melanoma Treated With Vemurafenib," *N Engl J Med*, 2012, 366(8):707-14.

VIM-D (Hodgkin)

Index Terms Etoposide-Ifosfamide-Mitoxantrone-Dexamethasone (Hodgkin)

Use Lymphoma, Hodgkin

Regimen

Etoposide: I.V.: 100 mg/m^2 over 30 minutes day 1
[total dose/cycle = 100 mg/m^2]
Ifosfamide: I.V.: 4 g/m^2 continuous infusion over 24 hours day 1
[total dose/cycle = 4 g/m^2]
Mesna: I.V.: 1 g/m^2 I.V. bolus day 1
followed by: Mesna: I.V.: 6 g/m^2 continuous infusion over 36 hours
[total dose/cycle = 7 g/m^2]
Mitoxantrone: I.V.: 10 mg/m^2 I.V. bolus day 1
[total dose/cycle = 10 mg/m^2]
Dexamethasone: Oral: 40 mg/day days 1 to 5
[total dose/cycle = 200 mg]
Repeat cycle every 28 days; treat 3 cycles post remission

References

Phillips JK, Spearing RL, Davies JM, et al, "VIM-D Salvage Chemotherapy in Hodgkin's Disease," *Cancer Chemother Pharmacol*, 1990, 27(2):161-3.

- **Vinblastine-Cisplatin** *see* Cisplatin-Vinblastine (NSCLC) *on page 1585*
- **Vinblastine-Cisplatin-Dacarbazine** *see* Cisplatin-Vinblastine-Dacarbazine (Melanoma) *on page 1584*
- **Vinblastine, Doxorubicin, Methotrexate, Prednisone (Hodgkin)** *see* VAMP (Hodgkin) *on page 1769*

Vinblastine (Hodgkin Regimen)

Use Lymphoma, Hodgkin

Regimen

Vinblastine: I.V.: 4-6 mg/m^2/day I.V. bolus day 1
[total dose/cycle = 4-6 mg/m^2]
Repeat cycle every 1 to 2 weeks until disease progression

References

Little R, Wittes RE, Longo DL, et al, "Vinblastine for Recurrent Hodgkin's Disease Following Autologous Bone Marrow Transplant," *J Clin Oncol*, 1998, 16(2):584-8.

- **Vinblastine-Methotrexate (Desmoid Tumor)** *see* Methotrexate-Vinblastine (Desmoid Tumor) *on page 1710*

Vincristine-Dactinomycin-Cyclophosphamide (Ovarian Cancer)

Index Terms VAC (Ovarian Cancer)

Use Ovarian cancer (germ cell tumor)

Regimen NOTE: Multiple variations are listed.

Variation 1:
Vincristine: I.V.: 1.5 mg/m^2 (maximum dose: 2 mg) days 1, 8, 15, and 22 for 2-3 cycles
[total dose/cycle = 6 mg/m^2 (maximum: 8 mg)] for 2-3 cycles
Dactinomycin: I.V.: 300 mcg/m^2/day days 1 to 5
[total dose/cycle = 1500 mcg/m^2]
Cyclophosphamide: I.V.: 150 mg/m^2/day days 1 to 5
[total dose/cycle = 750 mg/m^2]
Repeat cycle every 4 weeks for at least 10 cycles; vincristine is only administered for 8-12 weeks

Variation 2:
Vincristine: I.V.: 1-1.5 mg/m^2 day 1
[total dose/cycle = 1-1.5 mg/m^2]
Dactinomycin: I.V.: 500 mcg/day days 1 to 5
[total dose/cycle = 2500 mcg]
Cyclophosphamide: I.V.: 5-7 mg/kg/day days 1 to 5
[total dose/cycle = 25-35 mg/kg]
Repeat cycle every 4 weeks for up to 12 cycles

References

Variation 1:
Slayton RE, Park RC, Silverberg SG, et al, "Vincristine, Dactinomycin, and Cyclophosphamide in the Treatment of Malignant Germ Cell Tumors of the Ovary. A Gynecologic Oncology Group Study (A Final Report)," *Cancer*, 1985, 56(2):243-8.
Variation 2:
Gershenson DM, Copeland LJ, Kavanagh JJ, et al, "Treatment of Malignant Nondysgerminomatous Germ Cell Tumors of the Ovary With Vincristine, Dactinomycin, and Cyclophosphamide," *Cancer*, 1985, 56(12):2756-61.

◆ **Vincristine-Carboplatin-Etoposide (Retinoblastoma)** *see* Carboplatin-Etoposide-Vincristine (Retinoblastoma) *on page 1546*

◆ **Vincristine-Carboplatin (Retinoblastoma)** *see* Carboplatin-Vincristine (Retinoblastoma) *on page 1552*

◆ **Vincristine, Dactinomycin, Doxorubicin (Wilms' Tumor)** *see* VAD (Wilms' Tumor) *on page 1768*

◆ **Vincristine-Dactinomycin (Wilms' Tumor)** *see* EE-4A (Wilms' Tumor) *on page 1621*

◆ **Vincristine, Doxorubicin, Cyclophosphamide, Mesna, Etoposide** *see* Regimen I (Wilms' Tumor) *on page 1745*

Vinorelbine-Cisplatin

Index Terms Cisplatin-Vinorelbine; VC

Use Lung cancer, nonsmall cell

Regimen NOTE: Multiple variations are listed.

Variation 1:
Cisplatin: I.V.: 50 mg/m^2/day days 1 and 8
[total dose/cycle = 100 mg/m^2]
Vinorelbine: I.V.: 25 mg/m^2/day days 1, 8, 15, and 22
[total dose/cycle = 100 mg/m^2]
Repeat cycle every 28 days for total of 4 cycles

Variation 2:
Vinorelbine: I.V.: 25 mg/m^2/day days 1, 8, 15, and 22
[total dose/cycle = 100 mg/m^2]
Cisplatin: I.V.: 100 mg/m^2 day 1
[total dose/cycle = 100 mg/m^2]
Repeat cycle every 28 days

Variation 3:
Vinorelbine: I.V.: 30 mg/m^2 weekly
Cisplatin: I.V.: 120 mg/m^2/day days 1 and 29, then once every 6 weeks

Variation 4:
Vinorelbine: I.V.: 30 mg/m^2/day days 1, 8, and 15
[total dose/cycle = 90 mg/m^2]
Cisplatin: I.V.: 80 mg/m^2 day 1
[total dose/cycle = 80 mg/m^2]
Repeat cycle every 21 days for total of 4 cycles

Note: Vinorelbine treatment is discontinued after day 1 of cycle 4

Variation 5:

Vinorelbine: I.V.: 30 mg/m²/day days 1, 8, 15, and 22
[total dose/cycle = 120 mg/m²]

Cisplatin: I.V.: 100 mg/m² day 1
[total dose/cycle = 100 mg/m²]

Repeat cycle every 28 days for total of 3 or 4 cycles

Note: Vinorelbine treatment is discontinued after day 1 of last treatment cycle

References

Variation 1:

Winton T, Livingston R, Johnson D, et al, "Vinorelbine Plus Cisplatin Vs. Observation in Resected Non-Small-Cell Lung Cancer," *N Engl J Med*, 2005, 352(25):2589-97.

Variation 2:

Kelly K, Crowley J, Bunn PA Jr, et al, "Randomized Phase III Trial of Paclitaxel Plus Carboplatin Versus Vinorelbine Plus Cisplatin in the Treatment of Patients With Advanced Nonsmall-Cell Lung Cancer: A Southwest Oncology Group Trial," *J Clin Oncol*, 2001, 19(13):3210-8.

Wozniak AJ, Crowley JJ, Balcerzak SP, et al, "Randomized Trial Comparing Cisplatin With Cisplatin Plus Vinorelbine in the Treatment of Advanced Nonsmall-Cell Lung Cancer: A Southwest Oncology Group Study," *J Clin Oncol*, 1998, 16(7):2459-65.

Variation 3:

Le Chevalier T, Brisgand D, Douillard JY, et al, "Randomized Study of Vinorelbine and Cisplatin Versus Vindesine and Cisplatin Versus Vinorelbine Alone in Advanced Nonsmall-Cell Lung Cancer: Results of a European Multicenter Trial Including 612 Patients," *J Clin Oncol*, 1994, 12(2):360-7.

Le Chevalier T, Pujol JL, Douillard JY, et al, "A Three-Arm Trial of Vinorelbine (Navelbine) Plus Cisplatin, Vindesine Plus Cisplatin, and Single-Agent Vinorelbine in the Treatment of Nonsmall Cell Lung Cancer: An Expanded Analysis," *Semin Oncol*, 1994, 21(5 Suppl 10):28-33; discussion 33-4.

Variations 4 and 5:

Arriagada R, Bergman B, Dunant A, et al, "Cisplatin-Based Adjuvant Chemotherapy in Patients With Completely Resected Non-Small-Cell Lung Cancer," *N Engl J Med*, 2004, 350(4):351-60.

◆ **Vinorelbine-Cisplatin (Cervical Cancer)** *see* Cisplatin-Vinorelbine (Cervical Cancer) *on page* 1585

Vinorelbine-FEC

Index Terms FEC-Vinorelbine

Use Breast cancer

Regimen

Cycles 1 and 2:

Vinorelbine: I.V.: 25 mg/m²/day days 1, 8, and 15
[total dose/cycle = 75 mg/m²]

Treatment cycle is 21 days

Cycle 3:

Vinorelbine: I.V.: 25 mg/m²/day days 1 and 8
[total dose/cycle 3 = 50 mg/m²]

Treatment cycle is 21 days

Cycles 4, 5, and 6 (FEC):

Fluorouracil: I.V.: 600 mg/m² day 1
[total dose/cycle = 600 mg/m²]

Epirubicin: I.V.: 60 mg/m² day 1
[total dose/cycle = 60 mg/m²]

Cyclophosphamide: I.V.: 600 mg/m² day 1
[total dose/cycle = 600 mg/m²]

Repeat FEC cycle every 21 days for total of 3 cycles

References

Joensuu H, Kellokumpu-Lehtinen PL, Bono P, et al, "Adjuvant Docetaxel or Vinorelbine With or Without Trastuzumab for Breast Cancer," *N Engl J Med*, 2006, 354(8):809-20.

◆ **Vinorelbine-Gemcitabine (NSCLC)** *see* Gemcitabine-Vinorelbine (NSCLC) *on page 1677*

◆ **Vinorelbine-Gemcitabine (Sarcoma)** *see* Gemcitabine-Vinorelbine (Sarcoma) *on page 1677*

Vinorelbine (Hodgkin Regimen)

Use Lymphoma, Hodgkin

Regimen

Vinorelbine: I.V.: 30 mg/m^2/day day 1
[total dose/cycle = 30 mg/m^2]

Repeat cycle every 7 days, maximum of 24 doses

References

Devizzi L, Santoro A, Bonfante V, et al, "Vinorelbine: An Active Drug for the Management of Patients With Heavily Pretreated Hodgkin's Disease," *Ann Oncol*, 1994, 5(9):817-20.

Vinorelbine (Mesothelioma Regimen)

Use Malignant pleural mesothelioma

Regimen

Vinorelbine: I.V.: 30 mg/m^2 (maximum dose: 60 mg) over 5 minutes weekly on days 1, 8, 15, 22, 29, and 36
[total dose/cycle = 180 mg/m^2]

Repeat cycle every 42 days

References

Stebbing J, Powles T, McPherson K, et al, "The Efficacy and Safety of Weekly Vinorelbine in Relapsed Malignant Pleual Mesothelioma," *Lung Cancer*, 2009, 63(1):94-7.

Steele JP, Shamash J, Evans T, et al, "Phase II Study of Vinorelbine in Patients With Malignant Pleural Mesothelioma," *J Clin Oncol*, 2000, 18(23):3912-7.

Vinorelbine (Ovarian Regimen)

Use Ovarian cancer

Regimen

Vinorelbine: I.V.: 30 mg/m^2/day days 1 and 8
[total dose/cycle = 60 mg/m^2]

Repeat cycle every 21 days

References

Rothenberg ML, Liu PY, Wilczynski S, et al, "Phase II Trial of Vinorelbine for Relapsed Ovarian Cancer: A Southwest Oncology Group Study," *Gynecol Oncol*, 2004, 95(3):506-12.

Sorensen P, Høyer M, Jakobsen A, et al, "Phase II Study of Vinorelbine in the Treatment of Platinum-Resistant Ovarian Carcinoma," *Gynecol Oncol*, 2001, 81(1):58-62.

Vinorelbine (Small Cell Lung Cancer Regimen)

Use Lung cancer, small cell

Regimen NOTE: Multiple variations are listed:

Variation 1:

Vinorelbine: I.V.: 30 mg/m^2 day 1
[total dose/cycle = 30 mg/m^2]

Repeat cycle every 7 days until disease progression or unacceptable toxicity

Variation 2:

Vinorelbine: I.V.: 25 mg/m^2 day 1
[total dose/cycle = 25 mg/m^2]

Repeat cycle every 7 days until disease progression, no response after 4 cycles, or unacceptable toxicity

References

Variation 1:

Jassem J, Karnicka-Mlodkowska H, van Pottelsberghe C, et al, "Phase II Study of Vinorelbine (Navelbine) in Previously Treated Small Cell Lung Cancer Patients. EORTC Lung Cancer Cooperative Group," *Eur J Cancer*, 1993, 29(12):1720-2.

Variation 2:

Furuse K, Kubota K, Kawahara M, et al, "Phase II Study of Vinorelbine in Heavily Previously Treated Small Cell Lung Cancer. Japan Lung Cancer Vinorelbine Study Group," *Oncology*, 1996, 53(2):169-172.

Vinorelbine-Trastuzumab

Index Terms Trastuzumab-Vinorelbine

Use Breast cancer

Regimen

Week 1:

Trastuzumab: I.V.: 4 mg/kg (loading dose) day 1 week 1
[total dose/week 1 = 4 mg/kg]

Vinorelbine: I.V.: 25 mg/m^2 day 1
[total dose/week 1 = 25 mg/m^2]

Subsequent weeks:

Trastuzumab: I.V.: 2 mg/kg (loading dose) day 1
[total dose/week = 2 mg/kg]

Vinorelbine: I.V.: 25 mg/m^2 day 1
[total dose/week = 25 mg/m^2]

Repeat weekly

References

Burstein HJ, Kuter I, Campos SM, et al, "Clinical Activity of Trastuzumab and Vinorelbine in Women With HER2-Overexpressing Metastatic Breast Cancer," *J Clin Oncol*, 2001, 19(10):2722-30.

Vinorelbine-Trastuzumab-FEC

Index Terms Vinorelbine-Trastuzumab-FEC

Use Breast cancer

Regimen

Cycle 1:

Trastuzumab: I.V.: 4 mg/kg (loading dose) day 1 cycle 1
followed by I.V.: 2 mg/kg/day days 8 and 15 cycle 1
[total dose/cycle 1 = 8 mg/kg]

Vinorelbine: I.V.: 25 mg/m^2/day days 1, 8, and 15
[total dose/cycle 1 = 75 mg/m^2]

Treatment cycle is 21 days

Cycle 2:

Trastuzumab: I.V.: 2 mg/kg/day days 1, 8, and 15
[total dose/cycle = 6 mg/kg]

Vinorelbine: I.V.: 25 mg/m^2/day days 1, 8, and 15
[total dose/cycle 2 = 75 mg/m^2]

Treatment cycle is 21 days

Cycle 3:

Trastuzumab: I.V.: 2 mg/kg/day days 1, 8, and 15
[total dose/cycle = 6 mg/kg]

Vinorelbine: I.V.: 25 mg/m^2/day days 1 and 8
[total dose/cycle 3 = 50 mg/m^2]

Treatment cycle is 21 days

Cycles 4, 5, and 6 (FEC):

Fluorouracil: I.V.: 600 mg/m^2 day 1
[total dose/cycle = 600 mg/m^2]

Epirubicin: I.V.: 60 mg/m^2 day 1
[total dose/cycle = 60 mg/m^2]
Cyclophosphamide: I.V.: 600 mg/m^2 day 1
[total dose/cycle = 600 mg/m^2]
Repeat FEC cycle every 21 days for total of 3 cycles

References

Joensuu H, Kellokumpu-Lehtinen PL, Bono P, et al, "Adjuvant Docetaxel or Vinorelbine With or Without Trastuzumab for Breast Cancer," *N Engl J Med*, 2006, 354(8):809-20.

◆ **Vinorelbine-Trastuzumab-FEC** *see* Vinorelbine-Trastuzumab-FEC *on page 1775*

VIP (Etoposide) (Testicular Cancer)

Use Testicular cancer

Regimen NOTE: Multiple variations are listed.

Variation 1:
Etoposide: I.V.: 75 mg/m^2/day days 1 to 5
[total dose/cycle = 375 mg/m^2]
Ifosfamide: I.V.: 1200 mg/m^2/day days 1 to 5
[total dose/cycle = 6000 mg/m^2]
Cisplatin: I.V.: 20 mg/m^2/day days 1 to 5
[total dose/cycle = 100 mg/m^2]
Mesna: I.V.: 400 mg/m^2 day 1 only
followed by I.V.: 1200 mg/m^2/day continuous infusion days 1 to 5
[total dose/cycle = 6400 mg/m^2]
Repeat cycle every 21 days for 4 cycles

Variation 2:
Etoposide: I.V.: 100 mg/m^2/day days 1 to 5
[total dose/cycle = 500 mg/m^2]
Ifosfamide: I.V.: 1200 mg/m^2/day days 1 to 5
[total dose/cycle = 6000 mg/m^2]
Cisplatin: I.V.: 20 mg/m^2/day days 1 to 5
[total dose/cycle = 100 mg/m^2]
Mesna: I.V.: 200 mg/m^2 every 4 hours, for 3 doses each day, days 1, 2, and 3
[total dose/cycle = 1800 mg/m^2]
Repeat cycle every 21 days

Variation 3:
Ifosfamide: I.V.: 2500 mg/m^2/day days 1 and 2
[total dose/cycle = 5000 mg/m^2]
Mesna: I.V.: 2400 mg/m^2/day days 1 and 2
[total dose/cycle = 4800 mg/m^2]
Etoposide: I.V.: 100 mg/m^2/day days 3, 4, and 5
[total dose/cycle = 300 mg/m^2]
Cisplatin: I.V.: 40 mg/m^2/day days 3, 4, and 5
[total dose/cycle = 120 mg/m^2]
Repeat cycle every 21 days

Variation 4:
Etoposide: I.V.: 75 mg/m^2/day days 1 to 5
[total dose/cycle = 375 mg/m^2]
Ifosfamide: I.V.: 1200 mg/m^2/day days 1 to 5
[total dose/cycle = 6000 mg/m^2]
Cisplatin: I.V.: 20 mg/m^2/day days 1 to 5
[total dose/cycle = 100 mg/m^2]

Mesna: I.V.: 120 mg/m^2 day 1 only
followed by I.V.: 1200 mg/m^2/day continuous infusion days 1 to 5
[total dose/cycle = 6120 mg/m^2]
Repeat cycle every 21 days for 4 cycles

References

Variation 1:

Loehrer PJ Sr, Lauer R, Roth BJ, et al, "Salvage Therapy in Recurrent Germ Cell Cancer: Ifosfamide and Cisplatin Plus Either Vinblastine or Etoposide," *Ann Intern Med*, 1988, 109 (7):540-6.

"Correction: Incomplete Dosage Information in Article on Germ Cell Cancer," *Ann Intern Med*, 1988, 109(10):846.

Variation 2:

Harstrick A, Schmoll HJ, Wilke H, et al, "Cisplatin, Etoposide, and Ifosfamide Salvage Therapy for Refractory or Relapsing Germ Cell Carcinoma," *J Clin Oncol*, 1991, 9(9):1549-55.

Variation 3:

Pizzocaro G, Salvioni R, Piva L, et al, "Modified Cisplatin, Etoposide (or Vinblastine) and Ifosfamide Salvage Therapy for Male Germ-Cell Tumors. Long-Term Results," *Ann Oncol*, 1992, 3(3):211-6.

Variation 4:

Nichols CR, Catalano PJ, Crawford ED, et al, "Randomized Comparison of Cisplatin and Etoposide and Either Bleomycin or Ifosfamide in Treatment of Advanced Disseminated Germ Cell Tumors: An Eastern Cooperative Oncology Group, Southwest Oncology Group, and Cancer and Leukemia Group B Study," *J Clin Oncol*, 1998, 16(4):1287-93.

VIP (Vinblastine) (Testicular Cancer)

Use Testicular cancer

Regimen NOTE: Multiple variations are listed.

Variation 1:
Vinblastine: I.V.: 0.11 mg/kg/day days 1 and 2
[total dose/cycle = 0.22 mg/kg]
Ifosfamide: I.V.: 1200 mg/m^2/day days 1 to 5
[total dose/cycle = 6000 mg/m^2]
Cisplatin: I.V.: 20 mg/m^2/day days 1 to 5
[total dose/cycle = 100 mg/m^2]
Mesna: I.V.: 400 mg/m^2 day 1
followed by I.V.: 1200 mg/m^2/day continuous infusion days 1 to 5
[total dose/cycle = 6400 mg/m^2]
Repeat cycle every 21 days for 4 cycles

Variation 2:
Vinblastine: I.V.: 6 mg/m^2/day days 1 and 2
[total dose/cycle = 12 mg/m^2]
Ifosfamide: I.V.: 1500 mg/m^2/day days 1 to 5
[total dose/cycle = 7500 mg/m^2]
Cisplatin: I.V.: 20 mg/m^2/day days 1 to 5
[total dose/cycle = 100 mg/m^2]
Mesna: I.V.: 300 mg/m^2 3 times/day days 1 to 5
[total dose/cycle = 4500 mg/m^2]
Repeat cycle every 21 days for 4 cycles

References

Variation 1:

Loehrer PJ Sr, Lauer R, Roth BJ, et al, "Salvage Therapy in Recurrent Germ Cell Cancer: Ifosfamide and Cisplatin Plus Either Vinblastine or Etoposide," *Ann Intern Med*, 1988, 109 (7):540-6.

"Correction: Incomplete Dosage Information in Article on Germ Cell Cancer," *Ann Intern Med*, 1988, 109(10):846.

Variation 2:

Clemm C, Hartenstein R, Willich N, et al, "Vinblastine-Ifosfamide-Cisplatin Treatment of Bulky Seminoma," *Cancer*, 1986, 58(10):2203-7.

Vismodegib (Basal Cell Regimen)

Use Basal cell carcinoma

Regimen

Vismodegib: Oral: 150 mg once daily
[total dose/cycle = 4200 mg]

Repeat cycle every 28 days until disease progression or unacceptable toxicity

References

Sekulic A, Migden MR, Oro AE, et al, "Efficacy and Safety of Vismodegib in Advanced Basal-Cell Carcinoma," *N Engl J Med*, 2012, 366(23):2171-9.

◆ **VMP (Multiple Myeloma)** *see* Melphalan-Prednisone-Bortezomib (Multiple Myeloma) *on page* 1708

◆ **VMPT** *see* Bortezomib-Melphalan-Prednisone-Thalidomide *on page* 1537

XELOX (Colorectal)

Index Terms Capecitabine-Oxaliplatin (Colorectal); CapeOx (Colorectal); CAPOX (Colorectal); Oxaliplatin-Capecitabine (Colorectal)

Use Colorectal cancer

Regimen NOTE: Multiple variations are listed.

Variation 1 (adjuvant):

Oxaliplatin: I.V.: 130 mg/m^2 over 2 hours day 1
[total dose/cycle = 130 mg/m^2]

Capecitabine: Oral: 1000 mg/m^2 twice daily days 1 to 14
[total dose/cycle = 28,000 mg/m^2]

Repeat cycle every 21 days for 8 cycles

Variation 2 (metastatic):

Oxaliplatin: I.V.: 130 mg/m^2 over 2 hours day 1
[total dose/cycle = 130 mg/m^2]

Capecitabine: Oral: 1000 mg/m^2 twice daily days 1 (beginning with evening dose) to 15 (ending with morning dose)
[total dose/cycle = 28,000 mg/m^2]

Repeat cycle every 21 days

Variation 3 (metastatic):

Oxaliplatin: I.V.: 130 mg/m^2 day 1
[total dose/cycle = 130 mg/m^2]

Capecitabine: Oral: 850 mg/m^2 twice daily days 1 (beginning with evening dose) to 15 (ending with morning dose)
[total dose/cycle = 23,800 mg/m^2]

Repeat cycle every 21 days

References

Variation 1:

Haller DG, Tabernero J, Maroun J, et al, "Capecitabine Plus Oxaliplatin Compared With Fluorouracil and Folinic Acid as Adjuvant Therapy for Stage III Colon Cancer," *J Clin Oncol*, 2011, 29 (11):1465-71.

Variation 2:

Cassidy J, Clarke S, Díaz-Rubio E, et al, "Randomized Phase III Study of Capecitabine Plus Oxaliplatin Compared With Fluorouracil/Folinic Acid Plus Oxaliplatin as First-Line Therapy for Metastatic Colorectal Cancer," *J Clin Oncol*, 2008, 26(12):2006-12.

Cassidy J, Tabernero J, Twelves C, et al, "XELOX (Capecitabine Plus Oxaliplatin): Active First-Line Therapy for Patients With Metastatic Colorectal Cancer," *J Clin Oncol*, 2004, 22(11):2084-91.

Variation 3:

Hochster HS, Hart LL, Ramanathan RK, et al, "Safety and Efficacy of Oxaliplatin and Fluoropyrimidine Regimens With or Without Bevacizumab as First-Line Treatment of Metastatic Colorectal Cancer: Results of the TREE Study," *J Clin Oncol*, 2008, 26(21):3523-9.

◆ **XELOX (Pancreatic)** *see* CAPOX (Pancreatic) *on page* 1543

Ziv-Aflibercept + FOLFIRI (Colorectal)

Index Terms Ziv-Aflibercept, Irinotecan, Leucovorin, Fluorouracil (Colorectal)

Use Colorectal cancer

Regimen

Ziv-Aflibercept: I.V.: 4 mg/kg over 1 hour day 1
[total dose/cycle = 4 mg/kg]

Irinotecan: I.V.: 180 mg/m^2 over 90 minutes day 1
[total dose/cycle = 180 mg/m^2]

Leucovorin: I.V.: 400 mg/m^2 over 2 hours day 1
[total dose/cycle = 400 mg/m^2]

Fluorouracil: I.V. bolus: 400 mg/m^2 day 1
followed by I.V.: 2400 mg/m^2 continuous infusion (CI) over 46 hours beginning day 1
[total fluorouracil dose/cycle (bolus and CI) = 2800 mg/m^2]

Repeat cycle every 14 days until disease progression or unacceptable toxicity

References

Van Cutsem E, Tabernero J, Lakomy R, et al, "Addition of Aflibercept to Fluorouracil, Leucovorin, and Irinotecan Improves Survival in a Phase III Randomized Trial in Patients With Metastatic Colorectal Cancer Previously Treated With an Oxaliplatin-Based Regimen," *J Clin Oncol*, 2012 [epub ahead of print].

◆ **Ziv-Aflibercept, Irinotecan, Leucovorin, Fluorouracil (Colorectal)** *see* Ziv-Aflibercept + FOLFIRI (Colorectal) *on page 1779*

[illegible]

SPECIAL TOPICS

Cancer Treatment-Related Complications
Fertility and Cancer Therapy ... 1782
Management of Chemotherapy-Induced Nausea and Vomiting ... 1786
Management of Drug Extravasations ... 1800
Management of Infections ... 1809
Oral Mucositis/Stomatitis ... 1814
Tumor Lysis Syndrome ... 1822

Cancer-Related Topics
Chemotherapy and Cancer Treatment During Pregnancy ... 1829
Chemotherapy and Obesity ... 1834
Chronic Pain Management (Cancer) ... 1840
Common Toxicity Criteria ... 1848
Hospice (End of Life) Care ... 1857
Hypercalcemia of Malignancy ... 1860
Malignant Pleural Effusions ... 1865
Palliative Care Medicine (Cancer) ... 1871
Principles of Anticancer Therapy ... 1878
Venous Thromboembolism in the Cancer Patient ... 1883

Stem Cell Transplantation
Hematopoietic Stem Cell Transplantation ... 1887

Drug Development, Approval, and Distribution
Drug Development Process ... 1898
Investigational Drug Service ... 1901

Hazardous Drugs
Safe Handling of Hazardous Drugs ... 1904

FERTILITY AND CANCER THERAPY

Antineoplastic therapy (chemotherapy, radiation, surgery) or cancer itself can affect fertility and/or sexual function in both men and women. Temporary or permanent sequelae that impact pregnancy outcomes, neonatal development, pubertal development, and gonadal function are possible in cancer survivors. Factors influencing fertility and reproduction in cancer survivors include the type and intensity of therapy, duration of therapy, age, and gender.

Primary Antineoplastic Agents Associated With Sterility

Women	Men
Busulfan	Busulfan
Chlorambucil	Chlorambucil
Cyclophosphamide	Cyclophosphamide
Mechlorethamine	Mechlorethamine
Melphalan	Nitrosoureas
Procarbazine	Procarbazine
Other alkylating agents	Other alkylating agents
	Cisplatin

FEMALES

Antineoplastic drugs can stop the development of follicles (vesicles within ovarian that contain oocytes) or damage oocytes (female egg cells). Prepubertal gonads may be more resistant than postpubertal gonads, possibly due to a larger number of follicles as compared to ovaries in older patients. Gonadal destruction causes clinical findings associated with estrogen deficiency such as amenorrhea, endometrial hypoplasia, vaginal atrophy and dryness, and hot flashes. Follicle stimulating hormone (FSH) levels become elevated and estrogen levels decrease with impaired ovarian function. The onset and duration of symptoms is dose- and age-related. Younger patients are able to tolerate higher doses of chemotherapy before symptoms develop and have a higher likelihood of the return of menses when therapy is stopped.

The effect of radiation on fertility depends on the age of the patient, the number of remaining oocytes at the time of radiation, and the exposure dose and field. Childhood cancer survivors who have received a hypothalamic/pituitary radiation dose of 30 gray (Gy) (RR = 0.61) or more or an ovarian uterine radiation dose exceeding 5 Gy (RR = 0.56) are less likely to ever become pregnant than their female siblings.

In vitro fertilization with embryo cryopreservation is an option for circumventing the gonadotoxic effect of antineoplastic therapy. Ovarian stimulation for oocyte collection generally involves estrogenic therapy and may be risky in women with hormonally-responsive cancers. In addition, this method can only be used when the consequent delay in chemotherapy administration is not deleterious to the expected outcome of anticancer therapy. Some women may choose to make use of a gestational surrogate to carry their child through pregnancy. Investigational procedures for fertility preservation may be considered when *in vitro* fertilization is not advisable for medical reasons or impractical for women without a partner to provide sperm. Pertinent investigational techniques include oocyte cryopreservation, ovarian follicle cryopreservation, ovarian tissue cryopreservation, and *in vitro* follicle maturation. It should be noted that potential risks to the patient and prospective offspring from investigational fertility preservation are still being identified and delineated. Inadvertent reimplantation of cancer cells is possible with autotransplantation of cryopreserved ovarian tissue. Genetic and *in vivo* analysis of frozen ovarian tissue from patients with acute lymphoblastic leukemia and chronic myeloid leukemia have demonstrated the presence of viable malignant cells in the cryopreserved specimens.

Gonadotropin releasing hormone (GnRH) agonists are under investigation as a tool to preserve female fertility throughout chemotherapy administration. GnRH agonists cause medical castration which may provide a gonadoprotective effect by decreasing the number of follicles entering the differentiation phase, the stage most sensitive to chemotherapy. In addition, decreased serum estrogen concentrations reduce ovarian perfusion, thereby reducing ovarian exposure to systemic chemotherapy. Additional proposed mechanisms of GnRh agonist gonadoprotection during chemotherapy administration include a direct effect of the GnRH on the ovary, indirect antiapoptotic effects, and protection of germ line cells. Women older than 36 years of age may not have an adequate follicular reserve to benefit from gonadoprotection from GnRh therapy during chemotherapy administration. One comparative trial evaluated return of spontaneous menstruation and ovulation in 80 women with breast cancer undergoing treatment with chemotherapy with or without goserelin. All women were younger than 40 years of age and received treatment with FAC (fluorouracil-doxorubicin-cyclophosphamide). Following completion of treatment, menses returned within 3-8 months for 90% of women in the cohort treated with chemotherapy and goserelin and 33% of women receiving chemotherapy alone. Ovulation returned for 69% of women in the goserelin cohort and 26% the control patients. This trial suggests a positive effect of GnRH agonist therapy for protection of female fertility during chemotherapy; however, continued research is required to substantiate these findings in a broader patient population and with longer follow-up. At present, most clinical evidence supporting use of a GnRh agonist to protect female fertility during chemotherapy is based on noncomparative phase II trials, case series, and case reports.

MALES

Antineoplastic drugs and radiation destroy epithelial germ cells in a dose-dependent fashion. This damage results in increased FSH levels, decreased testosterone levels, oligospermia, or azoospermia. Spermatogenesis is more susceptible than testosterone production; and postpubertal testes are more susceptible to damage than prepubertal testes. Azoospermia may or may not be reversible. When it does recover, return of spermatogenesis may take up to 49 months.

Effects of radiation therapy on the testes are dependent on the dose, stage of germ cell development, and pubertal stage of the patient. Spermatogonia (precursor cell for spermatocyte) are the most sensitive to radiation damage, followed in decreasing sensitivity by spermatocytes (produce spermatid by meiosis) and spermatids (precursor for spermatozoa that fertilize ovum). Prepubertal boys may have oligo- or azoospermia once they reach sexual maturation. They may also have delayed sexual maturation due to destruction of Leydig cells and thus decreased testosterone production. Prolonged azoospermia generally occurs following a cumulative radiation dose of 2.5 Gy to the testis.

Surgery can affect male sexuality and fertility. Surgery for testicular cancer includes orchiectomy (surgical castration) and retroperitoneal lymph node resection which can result in decreased semen volume, erectile dysfunction, and low sexual desire. Prostate cancer surgery can also produce erectile dysfunction and changes in semen volume or ejaculatory problems.

Impaired spermatogenesis is present at the time of diagnosis for 60% to 70% men with testicular cancer. Elevated serum levels of β-human chorionic gonadotropin (β-hCG), which is a finding in many cases of testicular cancer, is associated with inferior spermatogenesis relative to cases with normal β-hCG levels.

In men, cryopreservation of sperm is a viable alternative and should be offered. The clinical pregnancy success rate of cryopreserved sperm is 36% by intrauterine insemination and 50% with *in vitro* fertilization and intracytoplasmic sperm injection. During *in vitro* fertilization sperm fertilize ovum in a liquid medium. Intracytoplasmic sperm injection is a more advanced process that injects one sperm into one oocyte for fertilization.

OUTCOMES OF PREGNANCY

Improved survival for cancer patients introduces the concern of long term treatment- and disease-related sequelae, including pregnancy outcome. The Childhood Cancer Survivor Study is a collaborative effort involving 25 health care institutions in the United States and Canada to facilitate research pertaining to the long term health outcomes of childhood cancer survivors. Over 14,000 subjects surviving 5 years or more following the diagnosis of childhood cancer are participating in this project.

Analysis of data from the Childhood Cancer Survivor Study demonstrated that offspring of female cancer survivors were more likely to be born preterm (OR, 1.9; $P<0.001$) than offspring from their female siblings. Moreover, previous treatment with a cumulative radiation dose exceeding 0.5 Gy to the uterus was associated with preterm birth (OR, 3.5; $P=0.003$), low birth weight (<2.5 g) (OR, 6.8; $P=0.001$), and small for gestational age (OR, 4; $P=0.003$). Data from the Childhood Cancer Survivor Study was also evaluated to assess pregnancy outcome for the female partners of male cancer survivors. Pregnant partners of male cancer survivors were less likely to yield a live born infant (RR, 0.77) than the control group ($P=0.007$). This was particularly evident when anticancer treatment included radiation with the treatment field affecting the testicles with or without shielding. The offspring of male cancer survivors treated with nonalkylating chemotherapy were more likely to have low birth weight than offspring from the survivor's male siblings (RR, 3.03; $P=0.025$). Otherwise, there was no difference in birth weight between offspring of the male cancer survivors in comparison to the control group. The male:female ratio of offspring fathered by male cancer survivors was 1:1.03; whereas, the male:female ratio of offspring from the survivor's male siblings was 1.24:1.0 ($P=0.016$).

A British survey of 10,483 childhood cancer survivors examined pregnancy outcome and reported that women treated with radiation to the abdomen or brain produced markedly fewer offspring than expected. Women treated with abdominal radiation were threefold and twofold more likely to have preterm or low birth weight babies. In addition, the risk of miscarriage was slightly increased in this group.

The impact of malignant disease and antineoplastic treatment on pregnancy outcome is not fully defined. However, patients with cancer should be informed of the known risks and potential options for fertility and reproduction.

SELECTED READINGS

Badawy A, Elnashar A, El-Ashry M, et al, "Gonadotropin-Releasing Hormone Agonists For Prevention of Chemotherapy-Induced Ovarian Damage: Prospective Randomized Study," *Fertil Steril*, 2009, 91(3):694-7.

Blumenfeld Z, "How to Preserve Fertility In Young Women Exposed to Chemotherapy? The Role of GnRH Agonist Cotreatment In Addition to Cryopreservation of Embrya, Oocytes, or Ovaries," *Oncologist*, 2007, 12(9):1044-54.

de Bruin D, de Jong IJ, Arts EG, et al, "Semen Quality in Men With Disseminated Testicular Cancer: Relation With Human Chorionic Gonadotropin Beta-Subunit and Pituitary Gonadal Hormones," *Fertil Steril*, 2009, 91(6):2481-6.

Dolmans MM, Marinescu C, Saussoy P, et al, "Reimplantation of Cryopreserved Ovarian Tissue From Patients With Acute Lymphoblastic Leukemia is Potentially Unsafe," *Blood*, 2010, Jul 1. [Epub ahead of print]

Green DM, Kawashima T, Stovall M, et al, "Fertility of Female Survivors of Childhood Cancer: A Report From the Childhood Cancer Survivor Study," *J Clin Oncol*, 2009, 27(16):2677-85.

Green DM, Whitton JA, Stovall M, et al, "Pregnancy Outcome of Partners of Male Survivors of Childhood Cancer: A Report From the Childhood Cancer Survivor Study," *J Clin Oncol*, 2003, 21 (4):716-21.

Krychman ML and King T, "Pregnancy After Breast Cancer: A Case Study Resolving the Reproductive Challenge With a Gestational Surrogate," *Breast J*, 2006, 12(4):363-5.

Neal MS, Nagel K, Duckworth J, et al, "Effectiveness of Sperm Banking In Adolescents and Young Adults With Cancer: A Regional Experience," *Cancer*, 2007, 110(5):1125-9.

Lee SJ, Schover LR, Partridge AH, et al, "American Society of Clinical Oncology Recommendations on Fertility Preservation in Cancer Patients," *J Clin Oncol*, 2006, 24(18):2917-31.

Pentheroudakis G, Pavlidis N, and Castiglione M, "Cancer, Fertility and Pregnancy: ESMO Clinical Recommendations For Diagnosis, Treatment and Follow-Up," *Ann Oncol*, 2009, 20 (Suppl 4):178-81.

Reulen RC, Zeegers MP, Wallace WH, et al,"Pregnancy Outcomes Among Adult Survivors of Childhood Cancer In the British Childhood Cancer Survivor Study," *Cancer Epidemiol Biomarkers Prev*, 2009, 18(8):2239-47.

Robison LL, Mertens AC, Boice JD, et al, "Study Design and Cohort Characteristics of the Childhood Cancer Survivor Study: A Multi-Institutional Collaborative Project," *Med Pediatr Oncol*, 2002, 38(4):229-39.

Signorello LB, Cohen SS, Bosetti C, et al, "Female Survivors of Childhood Cancer: Preterm Birth and Low Birth Weight Among Their Children," *J Natl Cancer Inst*, 2006, 98(20):1453-61.

MANAGEMENT OF CHEMOTHERAPY-INDUCED NAUSEA AND VOMITING

Nausea: The feeling or sensation of an imminent desire to vomit.

Vomiting: The forceful upward expulsion of gastric contents.

Retching: Rhythmic, labored, spasmodic respiratory movements involving the diaphragm, chest wall, and abdominal muscles.

Nausea and vomiting are common side effects of many antineoplastic agents. Studies, both prior to the advent of serotonin antagonists and after their introduction, have been conducted asking chemotherapy patients to rank the five most distressing symptoms in order from most to least severe. Nausea and vomiting remained among the top three most distressing symptoms, despite the use of serotonin antagonists for prevention or management of acute chemotherapy-induced nausea and vomiting. Uncontrolled nausea and vomiting can have a significant impact on a patient's overall attitude, quality of life, compliance, and response to treatment. Uncontrolled nausea and vomiting can result in dehydration, electrolyte imbalances, weight loss, and malnutrition. Prolonged vomiting and retching can cause esophageal and/or gastric ruptures (Mallory-Weiss tears, Boerhaave's syndrome) and bleeding. Even in the absence of actual emesis, patients may experience varying degrees of nausea, often accompanied by anorexia.

Table 1. Other Causes of Nausea or Vomiting

Abdominal Emergencies
- Appendicitis
- Cholecystitis
- GI obstruction
- Peritonitis

Acute Systemic Infections
- Bacterial
- Parasitic
- Viral

Cardiovascular Disorders
- Congestive heart failure
- Hypotension
- Myocardial infarction
- Syncope

Neurologic
- Increased intracranial pressure
- Mènière's disease
- Otitis interna
- Severe or chronic pain
- Anticipatory nausea and vomiting
- Vestibular dysfunction

Drugs
- Anesthetics
- Antibiotics
- Antineoplastics
- Aspirin
- Cardiac glycosides
- Ethanol
- Levodopa
- Nonsteroidal anti-inflammatory agents
- Opiates
- Quinidine
- Steroids
- Theophylline

Endocrine Disorders
- Adrenal insufficiency
- Diabetes mellitus

Gastrointestinal Disorders
- Dyspepsia
- Gastric outlet obstruction
- Gastroparesis
- Heartburn
- Partial or complete bowel obstruction
- Constipation
- Hepatic metastases

Metabolic
- Hypercalcemia
- Hyperglycemia
- Hyponatremia
- Uremia

Pregnancy

Psychogenic Stimuli

Therapy-Related
- Postsurgical
- Radiation Therapy

Patterns of Drug-Induced Nausea / Vomiting

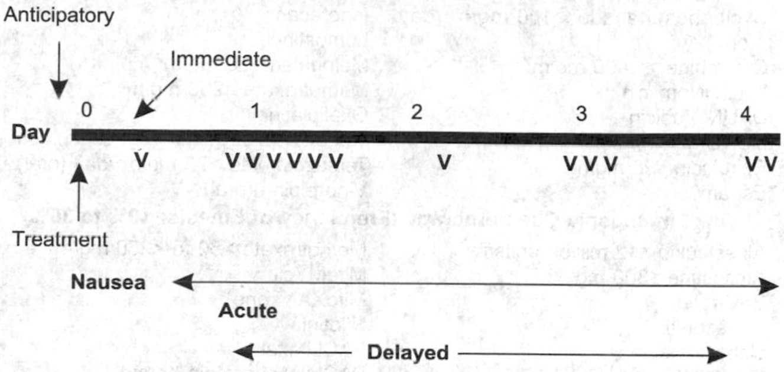

Table 2 describes the emetogenic potential of many of the antineoplastic agents. This table has been developed based on various guidelines and publications including: American Society of Clinical Oncology (ASCO), Multinational Association of Supportive Care in Cancer (MASCC), and National Comprehensive Cancer Network (NCCN). Several factors affect the emetic potential of these agents. For some drugs, such as cyclophosphamide or methotrexate, the dose administered has a significant effect on the drug's emetogenicity. Higher doses of these agents are much more emetogenic than low doses. The method of administration can also affect the incidence of nausea. Cytarabine, when given as a continuous infusion, is generally moderately emetogenic; however, higher cytarabine doses with short infusion times can produce a much higher incidence and severity of nausea and vomiting. Patient-related risk factors for nausea and vomiting include: Age, gender, prior experiences with chemotherapy, psychosocial factors (anxiety, depression), history of morning sickness with pregnancies, and history of motion sickness.

Table 2. Emetogenic Potential of Antineoplastic Agents

Highly Emetogenic Chemotherapy (Frequency of Emesis: >90%)

AC (either doxorubicin or epirubicin in combination with cyclophosphamide)	DOXOrubicin >60 mg/m^2
Carmustine >250 mg/m^2	Epirubicin >90 mg/m^2
CISplatin ≥50 mg/m^2	Ifosfamide ≥10 g/m^2
Cyclophosphamide >1,500 mg/m^2	Mechlorethamine
Dacarbazine	Procarbazine (oral)
	Streptozocin

Moderately Emetogenic Chemotherapy (Frequency of Emesis: 30% to 90%)

Aldesleukin >12-15 million units/m^2	AzaCITIDine
Alemtuzumab	Bendamustine
Altretamine	Busulfan (I.V.) or ≥4 mg/day (oral)
Amifostine >300 mg/m^2	CARBOplatin
Arsenic trioxide	Carmustine ≤250 mg/m^2

CISplatin <50 mg/m^2
Clofarabine
Cyclophosphamide ≤1,500 mg/m^2 (I.V.)
Cyclophosphamide ≥100 mg/m^2/day (oral)
Cytarabine >1,000 mg/m^2
DACTINomycin
DAUNOrubicin
DOXOrubicin ≤60 mg/m^2
Epirubicin ≤90 mg/m^2
Estramustine
IDArubicin
Ifosfamide <10 g/m^2
Imatinib
Interferon alfa ≥10 million units/m^2
Irinotecan
Lomustine
Melphalan >50 mg/m^2
Methotrexate ≥250 mg/m^2
Oxaliplatin
Temozolomide (I.V.)
Temozolomide >75 mg/m^2/day (oral)
Vinorelbine (oral)

Low Emetogenic Chemotherapy (Frequency of Emesis: 10% to 30%)

Aldesleukin ≤12 million units/m^2
Amifostine ≤300 mg
Bexarotene
Bortezomib
Cabazitaxel
Capecitabine
Cytarabine 100-200 mg/m^2
DOCEtaxel
DOXOrubicin (liposomal)
Eribulin
Etoposide (I.V.)
Etoposide (oral)
Everolimus
Fludarabine (oral)
Fluorouracil
Gemcitabine
Interferon alfa >5 million to <10 million units/m^2
Ixabepilone
Lapatinib
Lenalidomide
Methotrexate >50 to <250 mg/m^2
MitoMYcin
MitoXANtrone
Nilotinib
PACLitaxel
PACLitaxel protein bound
Panitumumab
PEMEtrexed
Pentostatin
PRALAtrexate
RomiDEPsin
SUNItinib
Temsirolimus
Thalidomide
Thiotepa
Topotecan
Trastuzumab
Tretinoin
UFT (oral)
Vandetanib
Vorinostat

Minimal Emetogenic Chemotherapy (Frequency of Emesis: <10%)

Asparaginase
Bevacizumab
Bleomycin
Busulfan <4 mg/day
Cetuximab
Chlorambucil
Cladribine
Cyclophosphamide <100 mg/m^2/day (oral)
Cytarabine <100 mg/m^2
Dasatinib
Decitabine
Denileukin diftitox
Dexrazoxane
Erlotinib
Fludarabine (I.V.)
Gefitinib
Gemtuzumab ozogamicin
Hydroxyurea
Interferon alfa <5 million units/m^2
Ipilimumab
Melphalan (oral, low dose)
Mercaptopurine
Methotrexate ≤50 mg/m^2
Methotrexate (oral)
Nelarabine
Ofatumumab
Pazopanib
Pegaspargase
Peginterferons
RiTUXimab
SORAfenib
Temozolomide ≤75 mg/m^2/day (oral)
Thioguanine (oral)
Valrubicin
VinBLAStine
VinCRIStine
Vinorelbine (I.V.)

Nausea and vomiting caused by cytotoxic therapy generally falls into one of five categories: Acute, delayed, anticipatory, breakthrough, or refractory.

Acute nausea or vomiting is seen within the first 18-24 hours of drug administration, with the peak incidence seen at 4-6 hours. Acute nausea and vomiting tends to be responsive to drug therapy. Guidelines support the use of a neurokinin-1 receptor antagonist, serotonin antagonist, and dexamethasone combination for the prevention of acute nausea and vomiting in a patient receiving a highly emetogenic regimen. Patients receiving regimens classified as moderately emetogenic are recommended to be given a serotonin antagonist and dexamethasone. For multi-day chemotherapy regimens, antiemetics should be administered for each day of chemotherapy and for 2 days after (Basch, 2011).

Delayed nausea or vomiting usually begins after the first 18-24 hours of drug administration but may occur up to 5 days after chemotherapy, with the peak incidence in 2-3 days. The classic causative agent for delayed nausea and vomiting is cisplatin; however the phenomenon has also been described with cyclophosphamide, doxorubicin, carboplatin, and ifosfamide administration. The exact cause of this side effect is not clear; however, it is believed to have a separate mechanism from acute nausea or vomiting. Gastritis, tissue destruction, electrolyte fluctuations, or effects on the central or peripheral nervous system have all been postulated as possible mechanisms for delayed nausea and vomiting.

Delayed nausea and vomiting is not as responsive to drug therapy when compared to acute nausea and vomiting. The ASCO and MASCC guidelines recommend the use of dexamethasone and aprepitant for the prevention of delayed emesis associated with high emetic risk chemotherapy. For prevention of delayed emesis associated with moderate emetic risk chemotherapy, the ASCO guidelines recommend aprepitant as a single agent for cyclophosphamide and doxorubicin (AC) and single agent dexamethasone or a serotonin antagonist. The NCCN guidelines (v.1.2012) suggest that palonosetron is of use in preventing delayed emesis.

While not drug-induced *per se*, anticipatory nausea and vomiting is also a relatively common complication of antineoplastic therapy. Anticipatory nausea and vomiting occurs due to inadequate control of nausea and vomiting in the past. Sights, smells, or sounds can also trigger anticipatory nausea and vomiting. This type of nausea and vomiting occurs before the administration of chemotherapy and has a variable response to drug therapy. The most active antiemetic regimen appropriate for the chemotherapy treatment is recommended, these antiemetics should be administered with the initial chemotherapy, as opposed to retrospective assessment of response with a less active antiemetic regimen (Basch, 2011).

Breakthrough nausea and vomiting is defined as nausea and/or vomiting despite adequate prophylaxis therapy and requires rescue therapy. Refractory nausea and vomiting on the other hand occurs during subsequent cycles of chemotherapy when antiemetic prophylaxis or rescue therapy (or both) has failed in earlier cycles.

Before changing a patient's antiemetic regimen, it is important to determine when the patient experienced the nausea and vomiting. Basing the decision on the timing of the episode(s) will help guide the change(s) in the regimen. If the patient experienced nausea and vomiting within the first 24 hours, it would be appropriate to change the patient's acute regimen. If the patient had no episodes until day 2, it would be more appropriate to change the delayed regimen for the patient.

A number of possible alternatives exist when changing a patient's acute regimen, including switching to another serotonin antagonist, adding a neurokinin receptor antagonist (eg, aprepitant, fosaprepitant) to the previous serotonin antagonist/steroid regimen, switching to a nonserotonin modulating antiemetic, or adding an benzodiazepine prophylactically. When changing the delayed regimen, there are numerous possibilities including: Adding a neurokinin receptor antagonist, dopamine antagonists, benzodiazepines, or cannabinoids, depending on the specific patient situation. Olanzapine is a thienobenzodiazepine antipsychotic that blocks multiple receptors associated with nausea or vomiting, including dopamine, histamine, muscarinic, and serotonin receptors. A few small trials have reported olanzapine effective (in combination with a steroid and serotonin antagonist) for prevention of delayed nausea and vomiting.

Table 3. Classification of Antiemetic Agents

Antihistamines	DiphenhydrAMINE, hydroxyzine, promethazine
Anticholinergics	Scopolamine
Benzodiazepines	Diazepam, LORazepam
Butyrophenones	Droperidol, haloperidol
Cannabinoids	Dronabinol, nabilone
Corticosteroids	Dexamethasone, methylprednisolone
Neurokinin antagonists	Aprepitant, fosaprepitant
Phenothiazines	Chlorpromazine, perphenazine, prochlorperazine, thiethylperazine,[1] triflupromazine, (promethazine)
Serotonin antagonists	Dolasetron, granisetron, ondansetron, palonosetron, tropisetron[1]
Substituted benzamides	Metoclopramide, trimethobenzamide
Thienobenzodiazepines	OLANZapine

[1]Not commercially available in the United States

Table 4. Site of Action of Antiemetic Agents

Emetic center	Antihistamines, anticholinergics, serotonin antagonists, thienobenzodiazepines(?)
Chemoreceptor trigger zone (CTZ)	Benzamides, butyrophenones, phenothiazines, thienobenzodiazepines(?)
Cerebral cortex	Antihistamines, benzodiazepines, cannabinoids, (corticosteroids), neurokinin antagonists(?), thienobenzodiazepines(?)
Peripheral	Metoclopramide, neurokinin antagonists, serotonin antagonists, thienobenzodiazepines(?)
Unknown	Corticosteroids

Table 5. Equitherapeutic Serotonin Antagonist Doses

Drug	Oral	I.V.	Transdermal
Dolasetron	100-200 mg	(contraindicated)	
Granisetron	2 mg	10 mcg/kg or 1 mg	3.1 mg/24 h
Ondansetron	8-24 mg	8-10 mg	
Palonosetron		0.25 mg	

Receptors for a large number of different neurotransmitters, including dopamine, serotonin, substance P, endocannabinoids, acetylcholine, histamine, opiates, and benzodiazepines, are involved in the vomiting reflex. Blockade of one or more of these receptors is the basic mechanism of action of most antiemetic agents.

Anticholinergics. Alkaloids (eg, atropine and scopolamine) exhibit some antiemetic activity, primarily postoperative nausea and vomiting, and motion sickness. The apparent mechanism of action is blockage of central muscarinic receptors. Toxicities, such as sedation, restlessness, blurred vision, and dry mouth, limit the systemic use of these agents. Transdermal application of scopolamine is is most useful in patients whose nausea is positional or due to motion. Scopolamine is also helpful as an adjunct in chemotherapy-induced delayed nausea or in treating prolonged mild nausea.

Antihistamines. The antihistamines block H_1 receptors both centrally and in the middle ear. A number of drugs in this class are effective against motion sickness and labyrinth disorders, but only diphenhydramine, hydroxyzine, and promethazine seem to have any activity against chemotherapy-induced nausea or vomiting. The major toxicities seen with these drugs are drowsiness, sedation, and dry mouth. These agents are most commonly used to enhance the efficacy of combination antiemetic regimens, although hydroxyzine or promethazine are occasionally used to treat mild-to-moderate nausea in patients who cannot tolerate, or are refractory to, other antiemetics. Diphenhydramine can be used in combination with dopamine antagonists to prevent extrapyramidal reactions seen with these agents at high doses.

Benzodiazepines. The exact antiemetic mechanism or location of action of the benzodiazepines is unclear. An inhibitory effect on the vomiting center, anxiolytic activity, and general CNS depression have all been postulated. Possible sites of action include the limbic system, vomiting center, cerebrum, and brain stem. The most common side effects include sedation, drowsiness, disinhibition, motor incoordination, and amnesia. In this setting, the anterograde amnesia induced by the benzodiazepine is usually considered a desired therapeutic effect rather than an adverse reaction. Benzodiazepines are commonly used as adjuncts to conventional antiemetics in the prophylaxis and treatment of chemotherapy-induced acute, breakthrough, and refractory nausea and vomiting. The benzodiazepines are also highly effective in the prevention of anticipatory nausea and vomiting. As single agents, the benzodiazepines have only mild antiemetic activity. Lorazepam is the most commonly used benzodiazepine for chemotherapy induced nausea and vomiting, but midazolam and diazepam have also been used.

Butyrophenones. A group of dopamine antagonists that can be effective in treating chemotherapy-induced nausea and vomiting are the butyrophenones. Both haloperidol and droperidol have been reported to have antiemetic activity against highly, moderately, and mild emetogenic chemotherapy, although their use may be reserved for use in chemotherapy with low emetic potential. Droperidol has been associated with cardiovascular toxicities, particularly QT prolongation and torsade de points. These toxicities, some fatal, occurred in patients receiving recommended doses or lower and also in patients with no known risk factors, which has ultimately limited the use of this agent. However, one trial comparing ondansetron and droperidol found no difference in the incidence or severity of QT_c interval changes between the two drugs. As with most other antiemetics, the optimum response to the butyrophenones is seen in multidrug regimens. Like other dopamine blockers, extrapyramidal reactions, restlessness, sedation, and hypotension are relatively common side effects.

Cannabinoids. Proper evaluation of the antiemetic activity of cannabinoid derivatives has been hindered by social and political stigmas associated with marijuana use. Tetrahydrocannabinol, levonantradol, and nabilone are all reported to be effective in treating chemotherapy-induced nausea and vomiting. The specific site and mechanism of activity is unclear. Inhibition of endorphins in the emetic center, suppression of prostaglandin synthesis, and inhibition of medullary activity through an unspecified cortical action have all been postulated. Cannabinoids can inhibit buildup of cyclic adenosine monophosphate and cannabinoid receptors have been identified in the hippocampus, hypothalamus, and cortex. Cannabinoids used by the oral route seem to be most effective against mild-to-moderately emetogenic chemotherapy. Blurred vision, hypotension, and tachycardia, and a number of CNS complications, including euphoria, dysphoria, hallucinations, and sedation can be seen with cannabinoid therapy. Cannabinoids offer an alternative in patients unable to tolerate, or who are refractory to, other antiemetic agents.

Corticosteroids. The mechanism of antiemetic activity for the steroids is unknown, although alterations of cell permeability and inhibition of prostaglandin activity have been postulated. In spite of this uncertainty, corticosteroids, particularly dexamethasone, are frequent components of combination antiemetic regimens for high-to-moderately emetogenic chemotherapy. Studies have demonstrated a synergistic activity with metoclopramide and serotonin antagonists resulting in a 20% increase in effectiveness. For delayed nausea and vomiting, monotherapy dexamethasone appears to be more effective than, serotonin antagonists for delayed nausea and vomiting. Side effects from single or short term dosing of dexamethasone are infrequent, but may include euphoria, anxiety, insomnia, increased appetite, and hyperglycemia. For patients in whom a corticosteroid is not clearly contraindicated, these agents are an important component of antiemetic therapy.

Neurokinin-1 (NK_1) Receptor Antagonists. Neurokinin, or substance P, antagonists are the latest class of antiemetics. Substance P is a tachykinin (neurokinin) located in neurons of the central and peripheral nervous system. It is associated with a variety of functions, including emesis, depression, inflammatory pain and inflammatory/immune responses in asthma, and other diseases. Substance P's activity is mediated by the NK_1 receptor, a G-protein receptor coupled to the inositol phosphate signal pathway. Blocking this receptor is a mechanism to treat conditions mediated at least in part by substance P. Several neurokinin receptor antagonists, including aprepitant (MK-869, L-754030), its prodrug L-758298, ezlopitant (CJ-11974), fosaprepitant, vofopitant (GR-205171), and CP-122721 have been studied; aprepitant and fosaprepitant are approved for marketing.

NK_1 antagonists are effective in preventing cisplatin-induced nausea and vomiting, when used in conjunction with a serotonin antagonist and steroid. Addition of a neurokinin antagonist to a serotonin antagonist and steroid combination increases control of acute nausea by 10% to 15%, and control of delayed nausea by 20% to 30%. Most studies indicate the neurokinin receptors are less effective then serotonin antagonists, particularly for prevention of acute nausea within the first 8-12 hours. However, the neurokinin antagonists appear to be more effective than serotonin antagonists in preventing delayed nausea (days 2-5). Aprepitant has a very complex metabolism. Aprepitant is a substrate of 3A4 and when administered for 3 days is an inhibitor of 3A4, and an inducer of 3A4 and 2C9 if administered for more than 14 days. Caution should be used when administering with oral contraceptives, warfarin, dexamethasone, midazolam, and 3A4 inhibitors and inducers. Side effects, although similar to placebo, may include asthenia/fatigue, dizziness, hiccups, gastritis/heartburn, diarrhea, and mild and transient increase in LFTs. Current guidelines recommend aprepitant or fosaprepitant as initial therapy for highly emetogenic regimens (including high dose cisplatin) or moderately emetogenic regimens that contain both doxorubicin and cyclophosphamide.

Phenothiazines. Phenothiazines were the first class of drugs accepted as antiemetic therapy for antineoplastic chemotherapy. Blockade of dopamine (D_2) receptors in the area postrema (chemoreceptor trigger zone and vomiting center) appears to be their primary mechanism of action. A number of different drugs, including chlorpromazine, perphenazine, prochlorperazine, promethazine, and thiethylperazine (no longer marketed in the United States), have antiemetic activity. Common toxicities such as extrapyramidal reactions, restlessness, sedation, and hypotension limit the use of these drugs. Phenothiazines are most effective against mild-to-moderate nausea or vomiting, but have little impact on emesis from highly emetogenic agents such as dacarbazine or cisplatin. Higher doses of these agents may have increased activity, but the increased incidence and severity of side effects prohibits their use. Since the serotonin antagonists became available, use of the phenothiazines generally has been limited to prevention of nausea from mildly emetogenic chemotherapy, treatment of breakthrough nausea or vomiting in patients refractory to a serotonin blocker, or in association with dexamethasone to treat delayed nausea.

Serotonin ($5\text{-}HT_3$) Antagonists. A major advance in antiemetic therapy was the introduction of the serotonin ($5\text{-}HT_3$) antagonists. These agents have been shown to block serotonin in two ways: Peripheral antagonism by blocking release from enterochromaffin cells in the GI tract and central antagonism of receptors in the medulla. The high efficacy rate of these agents in preventing acute nausea and vomiting for highly and moderately emetogenic agents, coupled with their low incidence of side effects, has made them the standard of care in these settings.

Studies comparing serotonin antagonist plus dexamethasone with dexamethasone monotherapy or serotonin antagonist monotherapy have demonstrated that the combination regimen is significantly better than either agent alone. The addition of corticosteroids is synergistic and results in an increase in response of approximately 20%. Conversely, serotonin antagonists are not as efficacious as corticosteroids for delayed nausea and vomiting.

A transdermal patch formulation of the serotonin antagonist granisetron is available. The patch contains 34.3 mg of granisetron and releases 3.1 mg/day. The patch was approved based on a noninferiority study compared to oral granisetron in the setting of highly and moderately emetogenic chemotherapy. The patch is recommended to be applied 24-48 hours prior to chemotherapy.

The currently-available serotonin antagonists have relatively flat dose/response curves. Dose response studies have demonstrated that granisetron's efficacy seems to reach a plateau at 10 mcg/kg. There appears to be no difference in efficacy between granisetron doses of 10 mcg/kg and 40 mcg/kg. A few small studies suggest higher doses of granisetron (3 mg I.V. or 40-240 mcg/kg) may be effective in treating breakthrough nausea; however, none of these reports found the improvement to be statistically significant. A similar limitation exists for dolasetron, ondansetron, and palonosetron. A number of reports suggest that ondansetron doses between 20-32 mg have comparable efficacy in preventing nausea induced by a variety of antineoplastic drugs. Daily doses >32 mg seem to provide no increase in response. Data are also lacking on the value of using a different serotonin antagonist to treat nausea or vomiting resulting from the failure of the initial serotonin antagonist regimen.

Toxicities with these agents, including headache, constipation or diarrhea, and elevated transaminases, have been minimal. QT_c prolongation and/or ECG abnormalities have been observed with dolasetron, granisetron, ondansetron, and palonosetron. Due to the risk for torsades de points, the use of the I.V. formulation of dolesetron is contraindicated in the prevention of chemotherapy-induced nausea and vomiting and the maximum recommended single I.V. ondansetron dose is 16 mg.

Substituted Benzamides. Metoclopramide is the most commonly used antiemetic drug in this category. Prior to introduction of the serotonin antagonists, high-dose (1-3 mg/kg) metoclopramide was the preferred drug for prevention of nausea or vomiting from highly emetogenic chemotherapy. Metoclopramide's ability to block central and peripheral dopamine receptors was believed to be the mechanism of its antiemetic activity. Recognition that high doses also blocked peripheral serotonin receptors in the intestines led to the identification of the role serotonin inhibition has in preventing nausea or vomiting, and, ultimately, to development of the serotonin antagonists. Like the phenothiazines, use of metoclopramide is complicated by extrapyramidal reactions, restlessness, sedation, and hypotension. Diarrhea is also a significant side effect, especially with the high doses used for antiemetic therapy. Also like the phenothiazines, the current use of metoclopramide is generally limited to prevention of nausea from mild-to-moderately emetogenic chemotherapy and treatment of breakthrough nausea or vomiting.

Olanzapine is a thienobenzodiazepine antipsychotic that blocks multiple receptors associated with nausea or vomiting, including dopamine, histamine, muscarinic, and serotonin receptors. A few small trials have reported olanzapine effective (in combination with a steroid and 5-HT_3-antagonist) for prevention of delayed nausea and vomiting.

REPRESENTATIVE ANTIEMETIC REGIMENS

HIGHLY EMETOGENIC CHEMOTHERAPY

Aprepitant 125 mg orally or fosaprepitant 115 mg I.V. day 1, followed by aprepitant 80 mg orally days 2 and 3 or fosaprepitant 150 mg I.V. on day 1 only **plus**

Dexamethasone 12 mg orally or I.V. day 1, followed by 8 mg once daily days 2-4 (with aprepitant) or dexamethasone 12 mg day 1, followed by 8 mg orally day 2, followed by 8 mg twice daily days 3 and 4 (with fosaprepitant 150 mg) or dexamethasone 20 mg day 1, followed by 8 mg twice daily for 3-4 days (if no aprepitant or fosaprepitant) **plus**

Serotonin antagonist as follows:

- Dolasetron 100 mg orally day 1 **or**
- Granisetron 1-2 mg/day orally or 0.01 mg/kg (maximum: 1 mg) I.V. day 1 or 34.3 mg transdermal patch (3.1 mg/24 hours; maximum duration: 7 days) applied 24-48 hours prior to first chemotherapy dose **or**
- Ondansetron 16-24 mg orally or 8-16 mg I.V. or 0.15 mg/kg (maximum dose: 16 mg) I.V. day 1 **or**
- Palonosetron 0.25 mg I.V. day 1

± LORazepam 0.5-2 mg orally, I.V., or sublingual every 4-6 hours days 1-4, if needed

± H_2-blocker or proton pump inhibitor (PPI)

MODERATELY EMETOGENIC CHEMOTHERAPY

Palonosetron 0.25 mg I.V. day 1 (may substitute granisetron or ondansetron if palonosetron not available), **plus** dexamethasone days 1-3, ± aprepitant **or**:

Day 1:

Aprepitant 125 mg orally or fosaprepitant 115 mg I.V. (in selected patients; eg, with AC) **plus**

Dexamethasone 8-12 mg orally or I.V. or 8 mg orally (if aprepitant/fosaprepitant not included) **plus**

Serotonin antagonist as follows:

- Dolasetron 100 mg orally **or**
- Granisetron 1-2 mg/day orally or 0.01 mg/kg (maximum: 1 mg) I.V. or 34.3 mg transdermal patch (3.1 mg/24 hours; maximum duration: 7 days) applied 24-48 hours prior to first chemotherapy dose **or**
- Ondansetron 16-24 mg orally or 8-12 mg I.V. or 0.15 mg/kg (maximum dose: 16 mg) I.V. **or**
- Palonosetron 0.25 mg I.V.

± LORazepam 0.5-2 mg orally, I.V., or sublingual every 4-6 hours days 1-4, if needed

± H_2 blocker or PPI

Day 2 (and beyond):

Aprepitant 80 mg orally days 2 and 3 (if aprepitant/fosaprepitant included day 1) **or**

± Dexamethasone 8-12 mg/day orally or I.V. for 2 days or 8 mg/day for 2-3 days **or**

Serotonin antagonist as follows:

- Dolasetron 100 mg orally **or**
- Granisetron 1-2 mg/day orally or 0.01 mg/kg (maximum: 1 mg) I.V. **or**
- Ondansetron 16 mg/day orally or 8 mg I.V. or 0.15 mg/kg (maximum dose: 16 mg) I.V.

± LORazepam 0.5-2 mg orally, I.V., or sublingual every 4-6 hours days 1-4, if needed

± H_2 blocker or PPI

LOW EMETOGENIC CHEMOTHERAPY

Dexamethasone 12 mg orally or I.V. daily or 4-8 mg orally daily prior to chemotherapy **or**

Metoclopramide 10-40 mg orally or I.V. prior to chemotherapy and then every 4-6 hours if needed **or**

Prochlorperazine 10 mg orally or I.V. prior to chemotherapy and then every 4-6 hours if needed

± LORazepam 0.5-2 mg orally, I.V., or sublingual every 4-6 hours days 1-4 if needed

± H_2 blocker or PPI

ORAL CHEMOTHERAPY

High-to-moderate emetogenic risk:

Serotonin Antagonists (oral): Granisetron 2 mg/day or ondansetron 16-24 mg daily

± LORazepam 0.5-2 mg orally or sublingual every 4-6 hours days 1-4, if needed

± H_2 blocker or PPI

Low-to-minimal emetogenic risk:

Metoclopramide 10-40 mg orally prior to chemotherapy and then every 4-6 hours **or**

Prochlorperazine 10 mg orally prior to chemotherapy and then every 4-6 hours

± LORazepam 0.5-2 mg orally every 4-6 hours days 1-4, if needed

± H_2 blocker or PPI

BREAKTHROUGH TREATMENT OPTIONS

Prochlorperazine 25 mg rectally every 12 hours or 10 mg orally or I.V. every 4-6 hours **or**

Metoclopramide 10-40 mg orally or I.V. every 4-6 hours **or**

Promethazine 12.5-25 mg orally or I.V. every 4 hours **or**

Haloperidol 1-2 mg orally every 4-6 hours as needed **or**

LORazepam 0.5-2 mg orally every 4-6 hours **or**

Dolasetron 100 mg orally **or**

Granisetron 1-2 mg/day orally or 0.01 mg/kg (maximum: 1 mg) I.V. or 34.3 mg transdermal patch (3.1 mg/24 hours; maximum duration: 7 days) **or**

Ondansetron 16 mg/day orally or I.V. **or**

Dronabinol 5-10 mg orally every 3-6 hours **or**

Nabilone 1-2 mg orally twice a day **or**

Dexamethasone 12 mg orally or I.V. daily **or**

OLANZapine 2.5-5 mg twice daily **or**

Scopolamine one patch every 72 hours

GENERAL PRINCIPLES FOR MANAGING NAUSEA AND VOMITING

Key to prevention is aggressively prescribing the most effective antiemetic regimen during initial therapy.

A. **Prevention**

a. **Antiemetics are most effective when given prophylactically.**

b. Depending on the antiemetic agent(s) and route(s) of administration, pretreatment may range from 1 hour to 5 minutes prior to administration of the antineoplastic agent(s).

c. **Emetogenic potential is additive and may be different on different days of the regimen.**

d. **Provide patient with delayed nausea regimen for 2-3 days and PRN antiemetics while at home.**

e. In most cases, **combination antiemetics are required for optimum control of nausea.** Two or more agents, from *different pharmacologic categories*, may be required to achieve optimal results.

f. **Avoid duplication of agents from the same pharmacologic category.**

g. **Doses and intervals of the antiemetic regimen need to be individualized for each patient.** "PRN" regimens should not be used. A fixed schedule of drug administration is preferable.

h. **If a patient has had no nausea for 24 hours** while on their scheduled antiemetic regimen, **it is usually possible to switch to a "PRN" regimen.** The patient should be advised to resume the fixed schedule ***at the FIRST sign of recurrent nausea***, and continue it until they have had at least 24 hours without nausea.

i. **Titrate antiemetic dose to patient tolerance.**

j. **Anticipatory nausea and vomiting can often be minimized if the patient receives effective prophylaxis against nausea from the first cycle of therapy.**

k. **If anticipatory nausea does develop, an anxiolytic agent is usually the drug of choice.**

l. **"If it's not broken – DON'T fix it!"** Regardless of your own preferences, if the patient's current antiemetic regimen is working, don't change it.

B. **Antiemetics**

a. **The serotonin antagonists have a "ceiling" dose**, above which there is little or no added antiemetic effect.

b. **Serotonin antagonists are most effective within the first 24 hours.** Most studies of multiple day dosing show a sharp decline in the efficacy of the serotonin antagonists after the second or third day.

c. **Neurokinin antagonists are not very effective as single agents**, and should only be used in combination with a serotonin antagonist and steroid.

d. **Serotonin and neurokinin blockers are most effective in scheduled prophylactic regimens;** rather than in "PRN" regimens to chase existing vomiting.

e. **Serotonin and neurokinin antagonists have limited efficacy in stopping nausea or vomiting once it has begun.** A dopamine blocker may be more effective.

f. **Other antiemetics, such as cannabinoids, antihistamines, or anticholinergics, have limited use as initial therapy.** They are best used in combination with more effective agents (steroids, dopamine, or serotonin blockers); or, as second- or third-line therapy.

SELECTED READINGS

Aapro M, "5-HT_3-Receptor Antagonists in the Management of Nausea and Vomiting in Cancer and Cancer Treatment," *Oncology*, 2005, 69(2):97-109.

Basch E, Prestrud AA, Hesketh PJ, et al, "Antiemetics: American Society of Clinical Oncology Clinical Practice Guideline Update," *J Clin Oncol*, 2011, 29(31):4189-98.

Geling O and Eichler HG, "Should 5-Hydroxytryptamine-3 Receptor Antagonists Be Administered Beyond 24 Hours After Chemotherapy to Prevent Delayed Emesis? Systematic Re-evaluation of Clinical Evidence and Drug Cost Implications," *J Clin Oncol*, 2005, 23(6):1289-94.

Graves T, "Emesis as a Complication of Cancer Chemotherapy: Pathophysiology, Importance, and Treatment," *Pharmacotherapy*, 1992, 12(4):337-45.

Grunberg SM and Hesketh PJ, "Control of Chemotherapy-Induced Emesis," *N Engl J Med*, 1993, 329(24):1790-6.

Grunberg SM, Warr D, Gralla RJ, et al, "Evaluation of New Antiemetic Agents and Definition of Antineoplastic Agent Emetogenicity – State of the Art," *Support Care Cancer*, 2011, 19(Suppl 1): S43-7.

Hesketh PJ, "Chemotherapy-Induced Nausea and Vomiting," *N Engl J Med*, 2008, 358 (23):2482-94.

Hesketh PJ, Kris MG, Grunberg SM, et al, "Proposal for Classifying the Acute Emetogenicity of Cancer Chemotherapy," *J Clin Oncol*, 1997, 15(1):103-9.

Hesketh PJ, Van Belle S, Aapro M, et al, "Differential Involvement of Neurotransmitters Through the Time Course of Cisplatin-Induced Emesis as Revealed by Therapy With Specific Receptor Antagonists," *Eur J Cancer*, 2003, 39(8):1074-80.

Holdsworth MT, "Ethical Issues Regarding Study Designs Used in Serotonin-Antagonist Drug Development," *Ann Pharmacother*, 1996, 30(10):1182-4.

Horiot JC, "Antiemetic Therapy in Cancer: An Update," *Expert Opin Pharmacother*, 2005, 6 (10):1713-23.

Jordan K, Schmoll HJ, and Aapro MS, "Comparative Activity of Antiemetic Drugs," *Crit Rev Oncol Hematol*, 2007, 61(2):162-75.

Kris MG, Hesketh PJ, Somerfield MR, et al, "American Society of Clinical Oncology Guideline for Antiemetics in Oncology: Update 2006," *J Clin Oncol*, 2006, 24(18)2932-47.

Multinational Association of Supportive Care in Cancer, "MASCC/ESMO Antiemetic Guideline 2011." Updated April 2011. Available at http://data.memberclicks.com/site/mascc/MASCC_Guidelines_English_2011.pdf

National Comprehensive Cancer Network® (NCCN), "NCCN Clinical Practice Guidelines in Oncology™: Antiemesis," V.1.2012. Available at http://www.nccn.org/professionals/physician_gls/PDF/antiemesis.pdf

Navari RM, "Prevention of Emesis From Multiple-Day and High-Dose Chemotherapy Regimens," *J Natl Compr Canc Netw*, 2007, 5(1):51-9.

Oo TH and Hesketh PJ, "Drug Insight: New Antiemetics in the Management of Chemotherapy-Induced Nausea and Vomiting," *Nat Clin Pract Oncol*, 2005, 2(4):196-201.

Roila F, Herrstedt J, Aapro M, et al, "Guideline Update for MASCC and ESMO in the Prevention of Chemotherapy- and Radiotherapy-Induced Nausea and Vomiting: Results of the Perugia Consensus Conference," *Ann Oncol*, 2010, 21(Suppl 5):v232-43.

MANAGEMENT OF DRUG EXTRAVASATIONS

Vesicant: An agent that has the potential to cause blistering, severe tissue injury, or tissue necrosis when extravasated.

Irritant: An agent that causes aching, tightness, and phlebitis with or without inflammation, but does not typically cause tissue necrosis. Irritants can cause necrosis if the extravasation is severe or left untreated.

Extravasation: Unintentional leakage (or instillation) of fluid out of a blood vessel into surrounding tissue.

Flare: Local, nonpainful, possibly allergic reaction often accompanied by reddening along the vein.

A potential complication of drug therapy is extravasation caused by leakage of the drug solution or instillation out of the vein. A variety of symptoms, including erythema, ulceration, pain, tissue sloughing, and necrosis, is possible. This problem is not unique to antineoplastic therapy; a variety of drugs have been reported to cause tissue damage if extravasated. See table.

Vesicant Agents

Antineoplastic Agents	Nonantineoplastic Agents
Amsacrine[1]	Acyclovir (>7 mg/mL)
CISplatin (≥0.5 mg/mL)	Aminophylline
DACTINomycin	Calcium chloride (>10%)
DAUNOrubicin	Calcium gluconate
DOXOrubicin	Calcium gluceptate[1]
Epirubicin	ChlordiazePOXIDE
IDArubicin	Contrast media
Mechlorethamine	Crystalline amino acids (4.25%)
MitoMYcin	Dantrolene
MitoXANtrone	Dextrose (>10%)
Oxaliplatin	Diazepam
Streptozocin	Digoxin
Trabectedin[1]	DOPamine
VinBLAStine	EPINEPHrine
VinCRIStine	Esmolol
Vindesine[1]	HydrOXYzine
Vinorelbine	Mannitol (>5%)
	Nafcillin
	Nitroglycerin
	Norepinephrine
	Phenylephrine
	Phenytoin
	Potassium acetate (>0.1 mEq/mL)
	Potassium chloride (>0.1 mEq/mL)
	Promethazine
	Propylene glycol
	Sodium bicarbonate (≥8.4%)
	Sodium chloride (>1%)
	Sodium thiopental
	Tromethamine
	Vasopressin

[1]Not commercially available in the U.S.

Antineoplastic Agents Associated With Irritation or Occasional Extravasation Reactions

- Arsenic Trioxide
- Bendamustine
- Bleomycin
- Bortezomib
- Busulfan
- CARBOplatin
- Carmustine
- CISplatin (<0.5 mg/mL)
- Cladribine
- Cyclophosphamide
- Dacarbazine
- DAUNOrubicin Citrate (Liposomal)
- DOCEtaxel
- DOXOrubicin (Liposomal)
- Etoposide
- Floxuridine
- Fluorouracil
- Gemcitabine
- Ibritumomab
- Ifosfamide
- Irinotecan
- Melphalan
- PACLitaxel
- PACLitaxel (Protein Bound)
- Teniposide
- Thiotepa
- Topotecan

The actual incidence of drug extravasations is unknown. Some of the uncertainty stems from varying definitions of incidence. Incidence rates have been reported based on total number of drug doses administered, number of vesicant doses administered, number of treatments, number of patients treated with vesicants, and total number of patients treated. Most estimates place the incidence of extravasations with cytotoxic agents to be in the range of 1% to 7%.

The best management for extravasation is prevention, education, and close monitoring. Although it is not possible to prevent all accidents, a few simple precautions can minimize the risk to the patient. The vein used should be a large, intact vessel with good blood flow. Veins in the forearm (ie, basilic, cephalic, and median antebrachial) are usually good options for peripheral infusions. To minimize the risk of dislodging the catheter, veins in the hands, dorsum of the foot, and any joint space (eg, antecubital) should be avoided. It is also important to remember to not administer chemotherapy distal to a recent venipuncture.

A frequently recommended precaution against drug extravasation is the use of a central venous catheter. Use of a central line has several advantages, including high patient satisfaction, reliable venous access, high flow rates, and rapid dilution of the drug. Many institutions encourage or require use of a vascular access device for administration of vesicant agents. Despite their benefit, central lines are not an absolute solution. Vascular access devices are subject to a number of complications. Misplacement/migration of the catheter or improper placement of the needle in accessing injection ports, and cuts, punctures, infections, or rupture of the catheter itself have all been reported.

Education of both the patient and practitioner is imperative. Educate the patient to immediately report any signs of pain, itching, tingling, burning, redness, or discomfort, all of which could be signs of extravasation. Ensure the healthcare team is informed of the risks and management strategies for both prevention and treatment of extravasations.

The nurse administering the chemotherapy agents needs to monitor the patient and I.V. site frequently. Prior to drug administration, the patency of the I.V. line should be verified. The line should be flushed with 5-10 mL of a saline or dextrose solution (depending on compatibility) and the drug(s) infused through the side of a free-flowing I.V. line over 2-5 minutes. If an extravasation occurs, it is important to monitor the site closely at 24 hours, 1 week, 2 weeks, and as necessary for any signs and symptoms of extravasation.

When a drug extravasation does occur, a number of immediate actions are recommended.

1. **Stop the infusion.** At the first suspicion of extravasation, the drug infusion and I.V. fluids should be stopped.
2. **Do NOT remove the catheter/needle.** The I.V. tubing should be disconnected, but the catheter/needle should not be removed. It should be left in place to facilitate aspiration of fluid from the extravasation site and, if appropriate, administration of an antidote.
3. **Aspirate fluid.** To the extent possible, the extravasated drug solution should be removed from the subcutaneous tissues. It is important to avoid any friction or pressure to the area.
4. **Do NOT flush the line.** Flooding the infiltration site with saline or dextrose in an attempt to dilute the drug solution is not recommended.
5. **Remove the catheter/needle.** If an antidote is not going to be injected into the extravasation site, the catheter/needle should be removed. If an antidote is to be injected into the area, it should be injected through the catheter to ensure delivery of the antidote to the extravasation site. When this has been accomplished, the catheter should then be removed.
6. In addition, the affected extremity should be elevated, marked, and photographed if possible. Documentation of the event and follow-up is also highly recommended.

Two issues for which there is less consensus are the application of heat or cold and the use of various antidotes. A variety of recommendations exists for each of these concerns; however, there is no consensus concerning the proper approach.

Cold: Intermittent cooling of the area of extravasation results in vasoconstriction, potentially restricting the spread of the drug and decreasing the pain and inflammation in the area. Application of cold is usually recommended as immediate treatment for most drug extravasations, except the vinca alkaloids and epipodophyllotoxins (eg, etoposide).

Heat: Application of heat results in a localized vasodilation and increased blood flow. Increased circulation is believed to facilitate removal of the drug from the area of extravasation. Heat is generally recommended for treatment for vinca alkaloid and epipodophyllotoxin extravasations. Most data are from animal studies with relatively few human case reports. Animal models indicate application of heat exacerbates the damage from anthracycline extravasations.

For some agents, such as cisplatin, epipodophyllotoxins, mechlorethamine, and paclitaxel, there are conflicting recommendations. Some reports recommend application of cold; others recommend heat. At least one report suggests neither cold nor heat is effective for paclitaxel extravasations.

EXTRAVASATION-SPECIFIC ANTIDOTES

A very wide variety of agents have been reported as possible antidotes for extravasated drugs, with no consensus on their proper use. For a number of reasons, evaluation of the various reports is difficult.

Agents Used as Antidotes

Dexrazoxane	Sodium thiosulfate
Hyaluronidase	Dimethyl sulfoxide

Dexrazoxane: Dexrazoxane, a derivative of EDTA, is an intracellular chelating agent used as a cardioprotective agent in patients receiving anthracycline therapy. It is believed that the cardioprotective effect of dexrazoxane is a result of chelating iron following intracellular hydrolysis. Dexrazoxane is not an effective chelator itself but is hydrolyzed intracellularly to an open-ring chelator form, which complexes with iron, other heavy metals, and doxorubicin complexes to inhibit the generation of free radicals. It has been postulated that dexrazoxane's chelating effect and its ability to stabilize topoisomerase II may be useful in preventing tissue damage from anthracycline extravasations.

Dexrazoxane was FDA-approved in 2007 for the treatment of anthracycline-induced extravasations. Approval was based on two clinical trials, including a total of 80 patients with anthracycline extravasations. Dexrazoxane was administered as 3 I.V. infusions over 1-2 hours through a different venous access location: 1000 mg/m^2 within 6 hours, 1000 mg/m^2 after 24 hours, and 500 mg/m^2 after 48 hours of the actual extravasation up to a maximum total dose of 2000 mg on days 1 and 2 and 1000 mg on day 3, respectively. Although localized cooling was permitted (except within 15 minutes of dexrazoxane infusion) in the trials, the number of patients in which this was used was not reported. Fifty-four of the 80 patients were evaluable. The primary endpoint was rate of surgical resection and necrosis. One patient (2%) required surgery and two patients (4%) developed tissue necrosis. Seventy-one percent of the patients were able to maintain chemotherapy appointments on schedule. Treatment has been associated with neutropenia, leukopenia, and thrombocytopenia. Hematological and liver function tests should be monitored. Other common yet reversible adverse events include nausea and vomiting, diarrhea, stomatitis, and infusion site burning. The proportion of toxicities that were attributable to dexrazoxane or as a result of primary antineoplastic therapy was not clear. Prior to administering dexrazoxane, discontinue DMSO as studies suggest the single agent is more effective than when used in combinations with DMSO.

Hyaluronidase: Hyaluronidase is an enzyme that destroys hyaluronic acid, an essential component of connective tissue. This results in increased permeability of the tissue, facilitating diffusion and absorption of fluids. It is postulated that increasing the diffusion of extravasated fluids results in more rapid absorption, thereby limiting tissue damage. In individual case reports, hyaluronidase has been reported effective in preventing tissue damage from a wide variety of agents, including vinca alkaloids, epipodophyllotoxins, and taxanes. The recommended total dose is 1 mL (150 units) administered as 5 separate 0.2 mL SubQ injections via a 24-gauge or smaller needle. It is recommended to use a new syringe for each injection site.

Sodium thiosulfate: Sodium thiosulfate (1/6 molar) has been recommended for treatment of mechlorethamine, dacarbazine, and cisplatin extravasations. Sodium thiosulfate provides a substrate for alkylation by mechlorethamine, preventing the alkylation and subsequent destruction in subcutaneous tissue. The use of sodium thiosulfate to treat mechlorethamine extravasations is based almost exclusively on *in vitro* and animal data. A single case report of successful sodium thiosulfate treatment of an accidental intramuscular mechlorethamine injection has been published. Thus far, no reports of sodium thiosulfate treatment of mechlorethamine infiltrations have been published.

Preparation of a 1/6 molar solution of sodium thiosulfate:

- Dilute 4 mL of a sodium thiosulfate 10% solution into a syringe with 6 mL of sterile water for injection, resulting in 10 mL of 1/6 molar solution

  or

- Dilute 1.6 mL of a sodium thiosulfate 25% solution with 8.4 mL of sterile water for injection, resulting in 10 mL of 1/6 molar solution

Inject 1-5 mL of the 1/6 molar sodium thiosulfate solution subcutaneously around the edge of the extravasation site using a tuberculin syringe. The dose of sodium thiosulfate depends on the amount of drug extravasated. For mechlorethamine, administer 2 mL of sodium thiosulfate 1/6 molar for every estimated 1 mg of mechlorethamine extravasated. For a cisplatin extravasation, it is recommended to inject 2 mL of sodium thiosulfate for each estimated 100 mg of cisplatin extravasated. It is recommended to use a new syringe for each injection site.

Dimethyl sulfoxide (DMSO): A number of case reports and small clinical trials have suggested that the application of DMSO is an effective treatment for chemotherapy extravasations. It is believed DMSO's protective effect is due to its ability to act as a free radical scavenger. DMSO may be considered as a treatment option for extravasations due to anthracyclines, mitomycin C, and actinomycin D. The optimal dose and duration is unknown. Common doses are to apply 1.5 mL of 50% DMSO topically with a saturated gauze pad every 6 hours for 7-14 days. Gently paint DMSO solution onto an area twice the size of the extravasation. Allow the site to dry. Do not cover with a dressing, as severe blistering may result. During application, DMSO may cause mild local burning, blistering, erythema, and itching.

There are a number of limitations for the use of DMSO. Results in animal models have been equivocal, with some reports indicating DMSO is beneficial and some showing little or no effect. Clinical reports of its use are extremely difficult to interpret due to variations in DMSO concentration (50% to 99%), number of applications/day, duration of therapy, inclusion of nonvesicants in studies, and concomitant treatments. A number of different treatments, including cold, steroids, vitamin E, and sodium bicarbonate, have been used in conjunction with DMSO. Also, most reports that suggest DMSO is effective in preventing tissue damage used DMSO concentrations >90%, which is not available for clinical use in the United States. The product is only commercially available in the United States at a concentration 50% (vol/vol) solution in water; however, higher concentrations may be purchased at health food stores. And lastly, the only FDA-approved indication is symptomatic relief interstitial cystitis (intravesicular administration). Based on these limitations, many institutions, ONS, and the prescribing information do not include DMSO as a treatment option for anthracycline extravasations.

Accepted Treatment Regimens for Specific Drug Extravasations

Medication Extravasated	Treatment	Dose	Route	Duration	Preparation	Administration	Concomitant Therapy
Anthracycline (DAUNOrubicin, DOXOrubicin, epirubicin, IDArubicin)	Children <18 years: Dimethyl sulfoxide[1]	90% to 99% every 6-8 hours	Topical	7-14 days	N/A	Topical; apply to area twice the size of the extravasation; do not cover with dressing	Cold[2]
	Adults: Dexrazoxane	1000 mg/m² 500 mg/m²	I.V.	Days 1 and 2 Day 3	1000 mL NS	I.V. (in a large vein remote from extravasation) over 1-2 hours	Cold[2,4] **Note:** Withhold cooling for 15 min before dexrazoxane infusion; may reinstitute cooling 15 minutes after infusion complete
MitoMYcin	Dimethyl sulfoxide[1]	90% to 99% every 6-8 hours	Topical	7-14 days	N/A	Topical	Cold[2]
Aminophylline, calcium salts, nafcillin, phenytoin, potassium	Hyaluronidase	150-900 units (total)	I.V., SubQ	One time	Reconstitute with 1 mL NS[6]	1-6 mL into I.V. line of extravasated solution (if still accessed) or SubQ; typical dose of 1 mL per each mL extravasated or 5 injections (0.2 mL) SubQ into area of extravasation in a clockwise manner	Use of either heat or cold therapy has not been determined
Epipodophyllotoxins (eg, etoposide, teniposide)[5], Vinca alkaloids (eg, vinBLAStine, vinCRIStine, vinorelbine)	Hyaluronidase	150-900 units (total)	I.V., SubQ	One time	Reconstitute with 1 mL NS[6]	1-6 mL into I.V. line of extravasated solution (if still accessed) or SubQ; typical dose of 1 mL per each mL extravasated or 5 injections (0.2 mL) SubQ into area of extravasation in a clockwise manner	Heat[3]

Accepted Treatment Regimens for Specific Drug Extravasations *continued*

Medication Extravasated	Treatment	Dose	Route	Duration	Preparation	Administration	Concomitant Therapy
Amino acid solutions, contrast media[4], dextrose, mannitol	Hyaluronidase	150-900 units (total)	I.V., SubQ	One time	Reconstitute with 1 mL NS[6]	1-6 mL into I.V. line of extravasated solution (if still accessed) or SubQ; typical dose of 1 mL per each mL extravasated or 5 injections (0.2 mL) SubQ into area of extravasation in a clockwise manner	Cold[2]
Docetaxel, paclitaxel							Cold[2]
Mechlorethamine, CISplatin	Sodium thiosulfate	1/6M	I.V., SubQ	One time	Mix 4 mL of 10% sodium thiosulfate with 6 mL sterile water	Mechlorethamine: Inject 2 mL for each 1 mg of mechlorethamine; Cisplatin: Inject locally 2 mL for each 100 mL of cisplatin infiltrated (cisplatin >20 mL and >0.5 mg/mL)	Cold[2]

Accepted Treatment Regimens for Specific Drug Extravasations *continued*

Medication Extravasated	Treatment	Dose	Route	Duration	Preparation	Administration	Concomitant Therapy
Vasopressors (DOPamine, EPINEPHrine, norepinephrine, phenylephrine)	Phentolamine	5 mg	SubQ	1 day	Mix 5 mg with 9 mL NS	Inject small amount(s) of solution into area of extravasation. Blanching should reverse immediately; if blanching should recur, additional injections may be needed.	None
				or			
	Terbutaline **Note:** Phentolamine is the preferred antidote for these extravasations; terbutaline has been used during phentolamine shortage	1 mg	SubQ	One time	Larger extravasations: Mix 1 mg in 10 mL NS Smaller extravasations (eg, accidental epinephrine autoinjection into digit): Mix 1 mg in 1 mL NS	Inject small amount(s) of solution into area of extravasation. Blanching should reverse immediately; if blanching should recur, additional injections may be needed.	None

N/A = not applicable, I.V. = intravenous SubQ = subcutaneous, I.D. = intradermal

[1]DMSO concentration >50% are not available for human use in the U.S.

[2] **Cold therapy:** Mechlorethamine: Apply ice for 6-12 hours (after sodium thiosulfate); for most other antineoplastic agents (when cold is recommended): Apply cold pack for 15 minutes at least 4 times/day for 24 hours. For all other (nonantineoplastic) agents: Apply cold pack for 15 minutes 4 times/day for 3-4 days.

[3] **Heat therapy:** For vinca alkaloids and epipodophyllotoxins: Apply warm pack for 15-20 minutes at least 4 times/day for 1-2 days.

[4]Large extravasations only

[5]In some instances (eg, small extravasations or diluted solution), the use of hyaluronidase for epipodophyllotoxin extravasation may not be necessary.

[6] **Hyaluronidase:** Some institutions utilize a 1:10 dilution in infants and children; prepare by mixing 0.1 mL of 150 units/mL solution with 0.9 mL NS in 1 mL syringe to make final concentration = 15 units/mL

SELECTED READINGS

Bellin MF, Jakobsen JA, Tomassin I, et al, "Contrast Medium Extravasation Injury: Guidelines for Prevention and Management," *Eur Radiol*, 2002, 12(11):2807-12.

Bertelli G, "Prevention and Management of Extravasation of Cytotoxic Drugs," *Drug Saf*, 1995, 12 (4):245-55.

Boyle DM and Engelking C, "Vesicant Extravasation: Myths and Realities," *Oncol Nurs Forum*, 1995, 22(1):57-67.

Doellman D, Hadaway L, Bowe-Geddes LA, et al, "Infiltration and Extravasation: Update on Prevention and Management," *J Infus Nurs*, 2009, 32(4):203-11.

Dorr RT, "Antidotes to Vesicant Chemotherapy Extravasations," *Blood Rev*, 1990, 4(1):41-60.

Dorr RT, Soble M, and Alberts DS, "Efficacy of Sodium Thiosulfate as a Local Antidote to Mechlorethamine Skin Toxicity in the Mouse," *Cancer Chemother Pharmacol*, 1988, 22 (4):299-302.

Ener RA, Meglathery SB, and Styler M, "Extravasation of Systemic Hemato-Oncological Therapies," *Ann Oncol*, 2004, 15(6):858-62.

Hadaway L, "Infiltration and Extravasation," *Am J Nurs*, 2007, 107(8):64-72.

Kurul S, Saip P, and Aydin T, "Totally Implantable Venous-Access Ports: Local Problems and Extravasation Injury," *Lancet Oncol*, 2002, 3(11):684-92.

Larson DL, "Alterations in Wound Healing Secondary to Infusion Injury," *Clin Plast Surg*, 1990, 17 (3):509-17.

Larson DL, "Treatment of Tissue Extravasation by Antitumor Agents," *Cancer*, 1982, 49(9):1796-9.

Larson DL, "What Is the Appropriate Management of Tissue Extravasation by Antitumor Agents?" *Plast Reconstr Surg*, 1985, 75(3):397-405.

MacCara ME, "Extravasation: A Hazard of Intravenous Therapy," *Drug Intell Clin Pharm*, 1983, 17 (10):713-7.

Mouridsen HT, Langer SW, Buter J, et al, "Treatment of Anthracycline Extravasation With Savene (Dexrazoxane): Results From Two Prospective Clinical Multicentre Studies," *Ann Oncol*, 2007, 18 (3):546-50.

Perry MC, "Extravasation," *The Chemotherapy Source Book*, 4th ed, Philadelphia, PA, 2008.

Polovich M, Whitford JN and Olsen M, *Chemotherapy and Biotherapy Guidelines and Reccomendations for Practice*, 3rd ed, Pittsburgh, PA: Oncology Nursing Society, 2009.

Schrijvers DL, "Extravasation: A Dreaded Complication of Chemotherapy," *Ann Oncol*, 2003, 14 Suppl 3:iii26-30.

Schulmeister L and Camp-Sorrell D, "Chemotherapy Extravasation From Implanted Ports," *Oncol Nurs Forum*, 2000, 27(3):531-8.

Schulmeister L, "Preventing and Managing Vesicant Chemotherapy Extravasations," *J Support Oncol*, 2010, 8(5):212-5.

Stier PA, Bogner MP, Webster K, et al, "Use of Subcutaneous Terbutaline to Reverse Peripheral Ischemia," *Am J Emerg Med*, 1999, 17(1):91-4.

Wang CL, Cohan RH, Ellis JH, et al, "Frequency, Management, and Outcome of Extravasation of Nonionic Iodinated Contrast Medium in 69,657 Intravenous Injections," *Radiology*, 2007, 243 (1):80-7.

MANAGEMENT OF INFECTIONS

Certain oncology patients are at increased risk of morbidity and mortality from infectious complications secondary to disease- or treatment-related loss of immunity (see table). Impaired immunity is generally associated with malignancies that arise from hematologic cells and lymphoid tissues. The most common iatrogenic reasons for impaired immunity are related to repeated courses of chemotherapy or radiation that are toxic to normal cells of the immune system or from a loss of innate barrier, such as mucositis, and central venous access device placement. Patients undergoing allogeneic hematopoietic stem cell (bone marrow) transplantation are at great risk for infectious complications because they generally have a hematologic malignancy, receive intensive chemotherapy prior to the bone marrow transplant, and require chronic immunosuppression to prevent graft-versus-host disease.

Disease-Related Risks for Infections

Cancer	Corresponding Normal Cell	Infectious Risk
Hodgkin lymphoma	Reed Sternberg cell (lymphocyte)	Encapsulated bacteria; *Pneumocystis jirovecii*; herpes simplex virus and varicella zoster virus; extensive chemotherapy/ radiation
Non-Hodgkin lymphoma	B cells (90%) T cells (10%)	*Pneumocystis jirovecii*; herpes simplex virus and varicella zoster virus; extensive chemotherapy/radiation
Acute lymphoblastic leukemia	B cells (90%) T cells (10%)	Extensive chemotherapy/radiation
Acute myeloid leukemia	Myeloid blood cell	Extensive chemotherapy/radiation
Chronic lymphocytic leukemia	B cells (90%) T cells (10%)	Atypical infections secondary to chronic immune impairment with protracted indolent course of disease

Neutropenia increases the risk of developing infection. The likelihood of morbidity or mortality from infection increases as the depth, rate of decline, and duration of neutropenia increase. The underlying cause of neutropenia is often anticancer treatment; however, it can also be secondary to the patient's malignant disease. It is important to distinguish the neutrophil count from the white blood cell count. The white blood cell count represents the sum of different types of white blood cells, including neutrophils, monocytes, lymphocytes, basophils, and mast cells. Patients with leukemias can present with a normal or markedly elevated white blood cell count, and at the same time, can be profoundly neutropenic because the vast majority of their circulating blood cells are blasts (malignant hematologic cells). An absolute neutrophil count (ANC) <500 cells/mm^3 blood increases the risk of infectious complications. In fact, patients are considered "high-risk" neutropenics when the ANC is ≤100 cells/mm^3 blood for ≥7 days. Additional clinical criteria for identification of patients at high risk for infection-related morbidity include unstable vital signs, pneumonia, new onset abdominal pain, and neurologic changes. The ANC is calculated as follows:

ANC = WBC x [(% segmented neutrophils + % band neutrophils) / 100]

Most anticancer treatments reduce immunity by causing neutropenia and mucositis. However, some products also impair the adaptive arm of immunity, which includes cell mediated immunity and antibody production. Monoclonal antibodies that impair adaptive immunity include alemtuzumab, denileukin diftitox, and rituximab. Bortezomib and the cytotoxic purine nucleotides (eg, clofarabine, fludarabine, nelarabine) inhibit adaptive immunity. In addition, corticosteroids, such as dexamethasone and methylprednisolone, are used in the treatment of some lymphoid malignancies.

The most frequent source of opportunistic pathogens is the patient or close human contacts. Common causes of gram-positive bacterial infections include *Staphylococcus aureus*, *Staphylococcus epidermidis*, *Streptococcus pneumoniae*, *Streptococcus pyogenes*, *Streptococcus viridans*, *Enterococcus faecalis*, *Enterococcus faecium*, and *Corynebacterium* spp. Common causes of gram-negative bacterial infections include *Escherichia coli*, *Klebsiella pneumoniae*, and *Pseudomonas* spp. *Candida albicans* generally colonizes mucous membranes of the gastrointestinal and urogenital tract. Environmental sources of opportunistic pathogens include the surface of fresh fruits and vegetables (bacteria), dried foliage, tobacco, marijuana leaves (*Aspergillus* spp); recent construction or renovation (*Aspergillus* spp); and tap water (*Legionella* spp). Rarely, viruses can be transmitted by blood products (packed red blood cells, platelets, stem cells) or plasma-derived products (intravenous immune globulin).

Thorough and frequent handwashing reduces the risk of transmitting opportunistic pathogens to neutropenic patients. In addition, limitation of the number of visitations and personal contacts also reduces opportunity for transmission of opportunistic pathogens. Additional preventive measures which are generally implemented to reduce the risk of infection in patients at greatest risk (eg, allogeneic bone marrow transplant patients) include hospital room-specific instrumentation, HEPA filtration of patient rooms or nursing units, total room clean following discharge, low microbial diets, and diligent mouth care. HEPA filtration involves circulation of room air through a filter 8-12 times/hour to remove small airborne particles. Low microbial diets prohibit ingestion of fresh fruits and vegetables, or undercooked meat. Diligent mouth care requires swishing and expectoration of mouthwash 4-6 times daily. Mouthwashes may be 0.9% NaCl or dilute bicarbonate solution (sodium bicarbonate 50 mEq/L in sterile water), because the greatest utility of mouth care is to remove oral debris and thereby prohibit microbial growth. Chlorhexidine 0.12% may also be used as a mouthwash; however, this product contains alcohol which can have a drying and irritating effect on damaged mucous membranes.

Selective gut decontamination using sulfamethoxazole-trimethoprim or a fluoroquinolone is used to reduce gram-negative colonization in patient undergoing intensive chemotherapy. Selective gut decontamination allows continued colonization of the lower gastrointestinal tract with anaerobic bacteria, which reduces the possibility of fungal overgrowth. High-risk patients undergoing treatment with intensive chemotherapy, such as allogeneic hematopoietic stem cell transplant recipients, or patients with acute myeloid leukemia undergoing induction chemotherapy, may also receive prophylactic acyclovir (or an equivalent antiviral) and fluconazole. Allogeneic bone marrow transplant recipients at risk for cytomegalovirus infection may receive prophylactic ganciclovir following engraftment. Sulfamethoxazole-trimethoprim is administered chronically to prevent *Pneumocystis jirovecii* pneumonia in some patients undergoing repeated chemotherapy treatments or alemtuzumab therapy for lymphoid malignancies.

The management of infections in cancer patients is directed by the nature and degree of immune compromise and the identified or suspected pathogen(s). Cancer patients without disease-related or treatment-related immune suppression are managed as appropriate for the type and severity of infection. A comprehensive discussion on all potential infections in cancer patients is outside of the scope of this chapter. For information on specific infections, such as pneumonia or cellulitis occurring in the cancer patient, the reader is referred to the National Comprehensive Cancer Network Clinical Practice Guidelines in Oncology™ "Prevention and Treatment of Cancer-Related Infections" (available at http://www.nccn.org)

Fever is frequently the only sign of infection in the neutropenic patient. Febrile neutropenic patients are empirically managed for presumed infection. Fever is defined as single oral temperature exceeding 38.3°C (101°F), or oral temperature 38°C (100.4°F) for at least 60 minutes. Evaluation of the febrile neutropenic patient should include history and physical examination, chest radiograph, blood cultures drawn from the central venous line (all ports), blood cultures drawn by peripheral venipuncture, specimens of urine and diarrheal stool, plus additional specimens as indicated by history and physical examination. Blood cultures must be drawn prior to initiation of antibiotics to increase the likelihood of acquiring a positive culture; although, blood cultures generally remain negative due to the small inoculum of microbes needed to cause infection in the neutropenic host and due to the early initiation of broad spectrum antibacterials. Empiric treatment with aggressive intravenous doses of broad spectrum, bactericidal antibiotics should be initiated as soon as possible after blood cultures have been collected. Choice of therapy greatly depends on the clinical status of the patient (ie, high vs. low risk), as well as the presumed origin of infection based on clinical presentation. Antibiotics should be infused through alternating central venous line ports.

Vancomycin is not recommended as a routine component of initial empiric therapy in the neutropenic patient due to concerns of emerging resistant organisms. Vancomycin should only be considered for patients considered high-risk for serious gram-positive infections. Criteria for use of vancomycin in the febrile neutropenia patient are listed in the table below. Vancomycin should be used in combination with a bactericidal agent that has activity against gram-negative organisms, including *Pseudomonas* spp (eg, cefepime, a carbapenem, or piperacillin/tazobactam). Aztreonam is a bactericidal alternative for the treatment of gram-negative microbes in patients who are allergic to penicillins, cephalosporins, or carbapenems. To minimize the development of resistant organisms, treatment with vancomycin should be discontinued in 2-3 days if resistant gram-positive organisms have not been identified. If history or cultures suggest vancomycin-resistant organisms (eg, enterococci), treatment options include daptomycin or linezolid. Monitor serum creatine kinase (CPK) levels at baseline and at least once weekly for patients receiving treatment with daptomycin. Myelosuppression is a reported side effect of linezolid. Use of this product in patients undergoing treatment with chemotherapy is reported in the medical literature; however, linezolid should be used with caution in any patients with additional risk factors for leukopenia, thrombocytopenia, or anemia.

Criteria for Use of Vancomycin in Febrile Neutropenia

- Clinically apparent, serious, catheter-related infection
- Positive blood cultures for gram positive bacterial prior to final identification and susceptibility testing

- Colonization with penicillin/cephalosporin-resistant pneumococci or methicillin resistant *Staphylococcus aureus*
- Clinically unstable (eg, hypotension, shock) without an identified pathogen
- Soft tissue infection
- Risk factors for viridans group streptococcal infections, such as prophylaxis with sulfamethoxazole/trimethoprim or fluoroquinolones antimicrobials, severe mucositis

When criteria for use of vancomycin is not met, the patient may receive monotherapy (eg, cefepime or carbapenem), or dual therapy (aminoglycoside or ciprofloxacin plus an antipseudomonal penicillin) should be initiated. The antipseudomonal beta lactam can be replaced with aztreonam for penicillin allergic patients. The choice for monotherapy versus dual therapy is determined by the patient's history and physical examination. The effect of antimicrobial therapy should be assessed in 72 hours or as indicated by the patient's clinical status.

The low-risk febrile neutropenic patient who defervesces within 72 hours following appropriate antibiotic therapy and is free of signs and symptoms of infection, may be converted to oral antibiotics (second generation cephalosporin or fluoroquinolone). Criteria for considering a patient high risk and continuing intravenous antibiotics include signs and symptoms of sepsis at presentation, additional signs of infection such as pneumonia or endocarditis, moderate-to-severe mucositis, dermal or mucosal loss of integrity, impending invasive procedure(s), or impending immunosuppressive therapy. If the patient remains febrile despite 72 hours of broad spectrum antibiotic coverage, the selection of antibiotics can be changed or additional antibiotics can be started. Vancomycin can be discontinued in patients who are clinically stable. Additional antibiotics should be added to patients who appear acutely ill from infection or are at high risk for infectious complications. The choice of antibiotic, which is dependent on current antimicrobial therapy in addition to the patient's history and physical examination, may include vancomycin, second gram-negative agent, antifungal with activity against invasive mold infections (voriconazole, caspofungin, an amphotericin product), or antianaerobic agent. Treatment with an antifungal should be started for patients with persistent fevers despite 5-7 days of appropriate empiric antibiotic therapy. Atypical pathogens, including *Legionella pneumoniae*, invasive molds (*Aspergillus* spp, *Fusarium* spp, mucormycoses), and viruses (cytomegalovirus [CMV], adenovirus, herpes simplex), should be considered in the chronically immunosuppressed patient. Appropriate empiric treatment for suspected viral infection would include acyclovir, but valacyclovir or famciclovir are reasonable alternatives. Treatment with ganciclovir, valganciclovir, or foscarnet is recommended if there is concern for CMV. Ganciclovir plus intravenous immune globulin are administered for CMV pneumonitis. Positive cultures and antibiotic sensitivity reports may streamline therapy in the stable patient. However, the high-risk patient may continue receiving broad spectrum antibacterials because the finding of a specific pathogen does not exclude the possibility of additional infecting organisms in the neutropenic patient. Caspofungin or fluconazole are used for the treatment of mucocutaneous candidiasis in the neutropenic patient. Prolonged and persistent neutropenia is a risk factor for invasive aspergillosis. Initial antifungal therapy for presumed or microbiologically documented aspergillosis is voriconazole, or an amphotericin product, or caspofungin. Itraconazole has activity against antiaspergillus; however, characteristics of the formulation(s) make it a less attractive option. Central venous line removal is done judiciously due to the ongoing need for intravenous fluids, drugs, and blood products in the neutropenic and thrombocytopenic patient, and the risk of infection or bleeding with insertion of a new central venous line. Empiric antibiotics should be continued until the patient is afebrile and clinically stable. Empiric antibiotics can be discontinued after 7 days in the low-risk neutropenic patient. One may consider discontinuation of empiric antibiotics in the high-risk neutropenic patient following 5-7 days without fever. Although, antibiotics should be continued until the ANC is at least 500 cells/mm^3 and severe mucositis, or signs and symptoms of sepsis have resolved. Four to 5 days following resolution of neutropenia, discontinuation of antibiotics may be considered in the low-risk, neutropenic, clinically stable patient with persistent fevers. With close observation and follow-up, antibiotics may be discontinued after 2 weeks of therapy in the clinically stable patient with persistent fever and persistent neutropenia.

Colony stimulating factors, which reduce the duration of neutropenia, are helpful in reducing hospital admission for neutropenic fevers in patients with a history of febrile neutropenia or prolonged neutropenia following outpatient chemotherapy.

Patients with chronic lymphocytic leukemia do not produce antibodies effectively and may require periodic administration of intravenous immune globulin to maintain normal serum immunoglobulin levels.

SELECTED READINGS

Freifeld AG, Bow EJ, Sepkowitz KA, et al, "Clinical Practice Guideline for the Use of Antimicrobial Agents in Neutropenic Patients With Cancer: 2010 Update by the Infectious Diseases Society of America," *Clin Infect Dis*, 2011, 52(4):427-31.

Maki DG, Alvarado CJ, Hassemer CA, et al, "Relation of the Inanimate Hospital Environment to Endemic Nosocomial Infection," *N Engl J Med*, 1982, 307(25):1562-6.

National Comprehensive Cancer Network® (NCCN), "NCCN Clinical Practice Guidelines in Oncology™ – Prevention and Treatment of Cancer-Related Infections," V 2.2011. Available at http://www.nccn.org/professionals/physician_gls/PDF/infections.pdf

ORAL MUCOSITIS/STOMATITIS

Also known as mucosal barrier injury, mucositis and stomatitis are general terms for the erythema, edema, desquamation, and ulceration of the gastrointestinal tract caused by many antineoplastic drugs and external beam radiation therapy (radiotherapy). Stomatitis refers to the finding of mucositis in the mouth or oropharynx. Gastrointestinal complications of mucositis include pain, xerostomia, bloating, diarrhea, malabsorption, and dysmotility. Airway compromise can develop from severe tissue damage and inflammation. Mucositis is defined as severe (grade 3-4) when the pain and anatomic damage prevent adequate oral hydration and oral nutrition, or airway compromise is evident (Table 1). Severe mucositis increases the risk of infectious complications. Moreover, some opportunistic infections, such as herpesvirus, cause and exacerbate mucositis. In addition, severe and prolonged mucositis contributes to anticancer treatment dosage reductions and delays, and increases the cost of therapy.

Table 1. National Cancer Institute (NCI) Common Toxicity Criteria Grading for Mucositis

Grade 0	Grade 1	Grade 2	Grade 3	Grade 4
No signs or symptoms	Painless ulcers, erythema, or mild soreness in the absence of lesions	Painful erythema, edema, or ulcers, but can eat or swallow	Painful erythema, edema, or ulcers requiring I.V. hydration	Severe ulceration or requires parenteral or enteral nutritional support or prophylactic intubation

The severity of chemotherapy-associated mucositis is related to drug selection, increased dose, combination versus single agent chemotherapy, extended infusion of cell cycle-specific chemotherapy drugs, concurrent radiotherapy, and female gender. The frequency of severe mucositis for patients undergoing standard dose therapy and high dose therapy is 5% to 40% and 60% to 100%, respectively. Major organ impairment that prolongs the clearance of anticancer treatments can increase the likelihood and severity of mucositis. Patients with Down syndrome or carriers of the methylenetetrahydrofolate reductase *677 TT* genotype have an increased risk of severe mucositis following methotrexate administration. The severity of mucositis secondary to radiotherapy is related to the anatomic site of radiation exposure, radiation dose, and dosage fractionation. Grade 3-4 mucositis occurs in more than 50% of patients undergoing radiotherapy to the head and neck, abdomen, or pelvis. Table 2 lists various anticancer treatments associated with severe mucositis. The duration and severity of regimen-related mucositis can be increased by concurrent infections from opportunistic bacterial or viral pathogens affecting the gastrointestinal tract. Moreover, graft-versus-host disease can worsen regimen-related mucositis following allogeneic hematopoietic stem cell transplantation.

Table 2. Standard Dose Regimens Associated With Grade 3-4 Mucositis

Occurring in ≥30% of Patients	Occurring in ≥10% of Patients
Anthracycline + DOCEtaxel + fluorouracil	Anthracycline + cyclophosphamide
Taxane + radiotherapy	Anthracycline + taxane
DOCEtaxel + fluorouracil	Anthracycline + cyclophosphamide + DOCEtaxel
PACLitaxel + fluorouracil + radiotherapy	Anthracycline + cyclophosphamide + PACLitaxel
Taxane + platinum + radiotherapy	Anthracycline + DOCEtaxel + platinum
Taxane + platinum + fluorouracil	Capecitabine + DOCEtaxel
Oxaliplatin + radiotherapy	DOCEtaxel
Platinum + taxane + radiotherapy	Platinum + radiotherapy
Fluorouracil CIV[1] + platinum + radiotherapy	Platinum + gemcitabine + taxane
Fluorouracil + leucovorin + taxane	Platinum + taxane + irinotecan
Irinotecan	Platinum + methotrexate + leucovorin
Irinotecan + fluorouracil + radiotherapy	Fluorouracil CIV[1]
Irinotecan + fluorouracil + leucovorin	Fluorouracil CIV[1] + radiotherapy
Irinotecan + fluorouracil + leucovorin + platinum	Fluorouracil CIV[1] + platinum
	Fluorouracil + leucovorin
	Fluorouracil + leucovorin + mitoMYcin
	Irinotecan + taxane

[1]CIV, continuous intravenous infusion; adapted from Sonis ST, Elting LS, Keefe D, et al, "Perspectives on Cancer Therapy-Induced Mucosal Injury: Pathogenesis, Measurement, Epidemiology, and Consequences for Patients," *Cancer*, 2004, 100(9 Suppl):1995-2025.

MUCOSITIS PREVENTION AND TREATMENT

Good oral hygiene is an essential constituent of routine supportive care for stomatitis and mucositis. Regular, gentle brushing with a soft toothbrush or cotton swab several times a day is helpful in removing dental plaque. Rinsing the mouth with a saline/bicarbonate solution helps remove debris and increases the pH, slowing the growth of oral flora. Use of mouthwashes containing alcohol may be painful or may dry the oral mucosa; phenol may promote mucosal ulceration.

Palifermin is a recombinant human keratinocyte growth factor that works in a receptor-mediated manner to reduce the duration and severity of mucositis by promoting epithelial cell proliferation, differentiation, and migration. Palifermin is indicated to decrease the incidence and duration of severe oral mucositis in patients with hematologic malignancies receiving myelotoxic therapy requiring hematopoietic stem cell support. The 2008 American Society of Clinical Oncology (ASCO) guidelines for the use of chemotherapy and radiotherapy protectants recommend palifermin to decrease the incidence of severe mucositis in patients undergoing autologous stem-cell transplantation with a total body irradiation (TBI) conditioning regimen. Additionally, palifermin may be considered in patients undergoing myeloablative allogeneic stem-cell transplantation with a TBI conditioning regimen. Data are insufficient however, for autologous and allogeneic transplant, to recommend palifermin when the conditioning regimen is chemotherapy only (Hensley, 2009). The labeled dose for palifermin is 60 mcg/kg/day I.V. for 3 doses prior to myelotoxic therapy, with the 3rd dose given at least 24 hours before the chemotherapy and then 60 mcg/kg/day for 3 doses after myelotoxic therapy beginning on the same day as hematopoietic stem cell infusion.

Weekly administration of palifermin for reduction of mucositis secondary to chemoradiotherapy for head and neck cancer was tested in two randomized, double-blind, placebo-controlled clinical trials (Henke, 2011; Le, 2011). In both studies, palifermin administration reduced the incidence, time to onset, and duration of severe mucositis. However, in both studies, patient reported mouth soreness scores and interruptions in therapy were similar for palifermin- and placebo-treated cohorts. Overall survival and disease response were similar for the palifermin- and placebo-treated patients. Single-dose palifermin prior to doxorubicin-based chemotherapy for the treatment of soft tissue sarcoma reduced patient-reported symptoms of oral mucositis (Vandhan-Raj, 2010).

Administration of palifermin concurrently with chemotherapy can cause increased severity of mucositis because epithelial cells are stimulated to proliferate when exposed to the systemic cytotoxic therapy. Precautions from the manufacturer include the lack of safety and efficacy data in patients with solid tumors. The effect of palifermin on tumor growth in patients has not been established; however, palifermin promotes *in vitro* and *in vivo* epithelial tumor growth in experimental models.

Amifostine has been studied for reduction of chemotherapy-associated mucositis; however, the findings are equivocal. Due to insufficient data, the ASCO guidelines for the use of chemotherapy and radiotherapy protectants do not recommend amifostine to reduce the incidence of radiation therapy-induced mucositis associated with head and neck cancer or to prevent esophagitis due to concurrent chemoradiotherapy in patients with nonsmall cell lung cancer. Amifostine use to prevent xerostomia in patients with head and neck cancer receiving concurrent platinum-based chemotherapy is not supported; however, the guidelines suggest that the use of amifostine may be considered to reduce the incidence of xerostomia in patients with head and neck cancer undergoing radiation therapy alone (Hensley, 2009).

Supplementation with oral glutamine throughout chemotherapy administration may reduce the rate of clinically significant or severe mucositis. Regular gum chewing by pediatric patients to promote salivation as a means for preventing chemotherapy-induced mucositis did not reduce the rate of severe stomatitis following administration of intensive treatment regimens. However, the frequency of grades 1-4 stomatitis was significantly reduced with gum chewing five times daily with lower intensity chemotherapy regimens. In the multivariate analysis, the risk of oral mucositis was related only to the type of chemotherapy regimen used. Additional pharmaceutical agents and interventions that have been employed to reduce the duration and severity of mucositis, but lack sufficient evidence to support routine use, include allopurinol-cryotherapy, celecoxib, chlorhexidine, doxepin rinse, histamine gel, pilocarpine, sargramostim, vitamin E, and zinc sulfate.

Cryotherapy reduces oral mucositis associated with intravenous bolus administration of fluorouracil, methotrexate, and high-dose melphalan. Cryotherapy requires that the patient hold ice in their mouth for 30-60 minutes before and following chemotherapy administration. Cryotherapy purportedly reduces local oromucosal blood flow and consequently reduces chemotherapy exposure to the effected area. Patient tolerance limits the duration of cryotherapy treatments and reduces the utility of cryotherapy for chemotherapy with prolonged systemic clearance or drugs administered by protracted continuous infusion.

Therapy of stomatitis consists primarily of symptomatic support.

Pain control is a crucial part of stomatitis therapy. In addition to making the patient more comfortable, adequate pain control allows the patient to communicate and eat normally, thereby improving quality of life and reducing nutritional complications. Narcotic analgesia is frequently required for management of moderate-to-severe pain from mucositis. Gabapentin may be useful as an adjunct to opioid therapy when additional analgesia is warranted (Bar, 2010). Topical application of local anesthetics is the most common approach to management of mild-to-moderate pain from stomatitis. Local application of cold sometimes provides adequate relief. Diphenhydramine has been used, but may cause drying of local tissues and sedation. Most products also contain significant amounts of alcohol which can exacerbate symptomatology. Local anesthetics (eg, benzocaine, lidocaine, tetracaine) are more potent than diphenhydramine, and are not associated with significant drying of local tissues. However, the numbing effect of these agents can impair swallowing. In addition, most of these products are unpalatable, and some are relatively expensive. The following table lists some of the commonly used agents.

Table 3. Various Mouth Care Products

Product	Concentration(s)	Dosage
Anesthetics		
Benzocaine	5% to 20%	1-5 mL; swish and expectorate q4-6h
DiphenhydrAMINE	12.5 mg/5 mL	5 mL; swish and expectorate (or swallow) q4-6h
Lidocaine	1%	5 mL; swish and expectorate (or swallow) q2-3h
Antimicrobials		
Amphotericin B	100 mg/mL	1 mL qid; swish in mouth as long as possible; swallow or expectorate
Chlorhexidine gluconate	0.12%	15 mL q4-6h; swish and expectorate
Clotrimazole	10 mg	1 troche tid (prophylaxis) One 5 times/day for 14 days (treatment)
Nystatin	100,000 units/mL	5 mL; swish and expectorate (or swallow) q4-6h
	100,000 units (vaginal tablet)	1 q4-6h (dissolve in mouth)
Mouth Rinses		
Sodium bicarbonate (8.4 g/50 mEq/0.9% NaCl [1000 mL] mixture)	0.5 mEq/10 mL	5-15 mL q3-4h
Sodium chloride	0.9%	5-15 mL q3-4h

Many institutions and prescribers use locally compounded anesthetic formulations for treatment of stomatitis pain. Although the exact formulae may vary tremendously, the general rubric includes a local anesthetic to which one or more of the following are added: A second anesthetic, aluminum hydroxide/magnesium hydroxide suspension, diphenhydramine, hydrocortisone, kaolin/pectin suspension, sucralfate suspension, nystatin, tetracycline, and/or water. Controlled trials comparing various formulations with each other, or with the various individual ingredients are not available. However, these products often form the mainstay of symptomatic treatment for stomatitis. Examples of recipes for a few such formulations are found in Table 4.

Sucralfate is basic aluminum sucrose sulfate, a sulfate disaccharide, used primarily as an antiulcer agent. The activity of sucralfate appears to be local, rather than systemic. The drug forms a viscous material that adheres to the surface of gastric and duodenal ulcers, forming a protective barrier over the ulcer. Protected from the activity of gastric enzymes and acid, ulcers are able to heal naturally. This local activity stimulated investigation of sucralfate as a treatment for oral ulcers. A number of groups have studied sucralfate as a therapy for various oral ulcerative conditions with equivocal results. Although the results published to date do not demonstrate a real advantage to sucralfate therapy, some patients may benefit from its use. Sucralfate is commercially available as a tablet (1 g) or suspension (1 g/10 mL). When placed into water, the tablet readily absorbs the fluid and forms a gelatinous suspension.

Table 4. Examples of Extemporaneously Compounded Oral Stomatitis Products

Anesthetics

Diphenhydramine syrup 5 mL + lidocaine 2% 5-10 mL + aluminum/magnesium hydroxide suspension 5-15 mL (Maalox®/Mylanta®) (may also be referred to as "BMX"). **Note:** Avoid diphenhydramine products containing alcohol.

Lidocaine 2% 45 mL + diphenhydramine elixir 30 mL + sodium bicarbonate 8.4 g + 0.9% sodium chloride qs 1000 mL

Intubation: Nondepolarizing neuromuscular blockade should be used for the patient with severe mucositis requiring intubation to support the airway. One case report describes succinylcholine-induced hyperkalemia in a patient with severe mucositis following treatment chemotherapy.

Xerostomia

Xerostomia often accompanies stomatitis, particularly in patients who have received radiation to the neck and lower jaw. The condition can result in severe pain, dysphagia, malnutrition, and secondary infections. Subcutaneous or intravenous push administration of amifostine 200 mg/m^2 15-30 minutes prior to radiotherapy of the head and neck reduces acute and chronic xerostomia. The dose of amifostine for reduction of radiation-associated xerostomia and mucositis can be standardized to 500 mg in 0.9% sodium chloride 2.5 mL. Benzydamine oral rinse (not available in the United States), which has local anesthetic and anti-inflammatory properties, may be used for the prevention of radiation-induced mucositis in head and neck cancer patients. Artificial saliva substitutes can provide symptomatic relief from dry mouth and throat discomfort following chemotherapy and radiotherapy. Saliva substitutes, which generally contain a mixture of electrolytes, sugars(s), and carboxymethylcellulose, are available without a prescription.

Infections

In spite of good oral hygiene, some patients develop oral infections. This is particularly common in the patient with additional sources of immunosuppression, such as severe neutropenia, treatment with exogenous immunosuppressions, or disease-related immune impairment. One organism most commonly seen in such infections is *Candida albicans*. Topical treatment with nystatin or clotrimazole is usually sufficient to control these infections. Such treatments are usually well tolerated and produce minimal systemic effects. Nystatin 400,000-600,000 units (4-6 mL) four times a day, swished in the mouth for at least 2 minutes, then swallowed is recommended. Alternatively, nystatin vaginal tablets can be used orally. Clotrimazole 10 mg five times a day is another effective treatment for these infections. Troches are placed under the tongue or in a buccal cavity and allowed to dissolve. In some patients, clotrimazole used three times a day is an effective prophylaxis against oral *Candida* infections. Patients with significant xerostomia may have trouble dissolving the nystatin or clotrimazole tablets, and may require an artificial saliva product to moisten the mouth. Oral or intravenous administration of fluconazole 100-200 mg daily may be necessary for treatment of microbiologically documented or presumed oromucosal candidiasis in the patient with moderate-to-severe mucositis extending proximally beyond the mouth or the patient with additional sources of immune suppression. Fluconazole should be continued for at least 2 weeks, and until microbiologic and clinical evidence of infectious disease have resolved and the patient's immune recovery is considered adequate. Alternative systemic antifungal agents that can be considered for treatment of oromucosal and esophageal candidiasis include caspofungin, itraconazole, posaconazole, voriconazole, and amphotericin B products.

Herpes simplex virus is another common pathogen causing oral and other gastrointestinal infections in the patient with moderate-to-severe mucositis. The risk for oral Herpes simplex infection is greatest in patients with an additional source of immune compromise. Systemic treatment with acyclovir, famciclovir, or valacyclovir is required for oromucosal or gastrointestinal Herpes simplex infection. Alternative systemic antiviral agents for treatment of resistant Herpes simplex infections include ganciclovir, valganciclovir, and foscarnet.

SELECTED READINGS

Aisa Y, Mori T, Kudo M, et al, "Oral Cryotherapy for the Prevention of High-Dose Melphalan-Induced Stomatitis in Allogeneic Hematopoietic Stem Cell Transplant Recipients," *Support Care Cancer*, 2005, 13(4):266-9.

Al-Khafaji AH, Dewhirst WE, Cornell CJ Jr, et al, "Succinylcholine-Induced Hyperkalemia in a Patient With Mucositis Secondary to Chemotherapy," *Crit Care Med*, 2001, 29(6):1274-6.

Alterio D, Jereczek-Fossa BA, Zuccotti GF, et al, "Tetracaine Oral Gel in Patients Treated With Radiotherapy for Head-and-Neck Cancer: Final Results of a Phase II Study," *Int J Radiat Oncol Biol Phys*, 2006, 64(2):392-5.

Aquino VM, Harvey AR, Garvin JH, et al, "A Double-Blind Randomized Placebo-Controlled Study of Oral Glutamine in the Prevention of Mucositis in Children Undergoing Hematopoietic Stem Cell Transplantation: A Pediatric Blood and Marrow Transplant Consortium Study," *Bone Marrow Transplant*, 2005, 36(7):611-6.

Awidi A, Homsi U, Kakail RI, et al, "Double-Blind, Placebo-Controlled Cross-Over Study of Oral Pilocarpine for the Prevention of Chemotherapy-Induced Oral Mucositis in Adult Patients With Cancer," *Eur J Cancer*, 2001, 37(16):2010-4.

Bar Ad V, Weinstein G, Dutta PR, et al, "Gabapentin for the Treatment of Pain Related to Radiation-Induced Mucositis in Patients With Head and Neck Tumors Treated With Intensity-Modulated Radiation Therapy," *Head Neck*, 2010, 32(2):173-7.

Berger A, Henderson M, Nadoolman W, et al, "Oral Capsaicin Provides Temporary Relief for Oral Mucositis Pain Secondary to Chemotherapy/Radiation Therapy," *J Pain Symptom Manage*, 1995, 10(3):243-8.

Cerchietti LC, Navigante AH, Lutteral MA, et al, "Double-Blinded, Placebo-Controlled Trial on Intravenous L-Alanyl-L-Glutamine in the Incidence of Oral Mucositis Following Chemoradiotherapy in Patients With Head-and-Neck Cancer," *Int J Radiat Oncol Biol Phys*, 2006, 65(5):1330-7.

Chan A and Ignoffo RJ, "Survey of Topical Oral Solutions for the Treatment of Chemo-Induced Oral Mucositis," *J Oncol Pharm Pract*, 2005, 11(4):139-43.

Chiara S, Nobile MT, Vincenti M, et al, "Sucralfate in the Treatment of Chemotherapy-Induced Stomatitis: A Double-Blind, Placebo-Controlled Pilot Study," *Anticancer Res*, 2001, 21 (5):3707-10.

Choi K, Lee SS, Oh SJ, et al, "The Effect of Oral Glutamine on 5-Fluorouracil/Leucovorin-Induced Mucositis/Stomatitis Assessed by Intestinal Permeability Test," *Clin Nutr*, 2007, 26(1):57-62.

Dodd MJ, Miaskowski C, Greenspan D, et al, "Radiation-Induced Mucositis: A Randomized Clinical Trial of Micronized Sucralfate Versus Salt & Soda Mouthwashes," *Cancer Invest*, 2003, 21 (1):21-33.

Elad S, Ackerstein A, Bitan M, et al, "A Prospective, Double-Blind Phase II Study Evaluating the Safety and Efficacy of a Topical Histamine Gel for the Prophylaxis of Oral Mucositis in Patients Post Hematopoietic Stem Cell Transplantation," *Bone Marrow Transplant*, 2006, 37(8):757-62.

El-Housseiny AA, Saleh SM, El-Masry AA, et al, "The Effectiveness of Vitamin "E" in the Treatment of Oral Mucositis in Children Receiving Chemotherapy," *J Clin Pediatr Dent*, 2007, 31(3):167-70.

Epstein JB, Epstein JD, Epstein MS, et al, "Oral Doxepin Rinse: The Analgesic Effect and Duration of Pain Reduction in Patients With Oral Mucositis Due to Cancer Therapy," *Anesth Analg*, 2006, 103(2):465-70.

Epstein JB, Silverman S Jr, Paggiarino DA, et al, "Benzydamine HCl for Prophylaxis of Radiation-Induced Oral Mucositis: Results From a Multicenter, Randomized, Double-Blind, Placebo-Controlled Clinical Trial," *Cancer*, 2001, 92(4):875-85.

Ertekin MV, Koc M, Karslioglu I, et al, "Zinc Sulfate in the Prevention of Radiation-Induced Oropharyngeal Mucositis: A Prospective, Placebo-Controlled, Randomized Study," *Int J Radiat Oncol Biol Phys*, 2004, 58(1):167-74.

Franzen L, Henriksson R, Littbrand B, et al, "Effects of Sucralfate on Mucositis During and Following Radiotherapy of Malignancies in the Head and Neck Region, A Double-Blind Placebo-Controlled Study," *Acta Oncol*, 1995, 34(2):219-23.

Gandemer V, Le Deley MC, Dollfus C, et al, "Multicenter Randomized Trial of Chewing Gum for Preventing Oral Mucositis in Children Receiving Chemotherapy," *J Pediatr Hematol Oncol*, 2007, 29(2):86-94.

Garre ML, Relling MV, Kalwinsky D, et al, "Pharmacokinetics and Toxicity of Methotrexate in Children With Down Syndrome and Acute Lymphocytic Leukemia," *J Pediatr*, 1987, 111 (4):606-12.

Gori E, Arpinati M, Bonifazi F, et al, "Cryotherapy in the Prevention of Oral Mucositis in Patients Receiving Low-Dose Methotrexate Following Myeloablative Allogeneic Stem Cell Transplantation: A Prospective Randomized Study of the Gruppo Italiano Trapianto Di Midollo Osseo Nurses Group," *Bone Marrow Transplant*, 2007, 39(6):347-52.

Henke M, Alfonsi M, Foa P, et al, "Palifermin Decreases Severe Oral Mucositis of Patients Undergoing Postoperative Radiochemotherapy for Head and Neck Cancer: A Randomized, Placebo-Controlled Trial," *J Clin Oncol*, 2011, 29(20):2815-20.

Hensley ML, Hagerty KL, Kewalramani T, et al, "American Society of Clinical Oncology 2008 Clinical Practice Guideline Update: Use of Chemotherapy and Radiotherapy Protectants," *J Clin Oncol*, 2009, 27(1): 127-45.

Huang EY, Leung SW, Wang CJ, et al, "Oral Glutamine to Alleviate Radiation-Induced Oral Mucositis: A Pilot Randomized Trial," *Int J Radiat Oncol Biol Phys*, 2000, 46(3):535-9.

Javle MM, Cao S, Durrani FA, et al, "Celecoxib and Mucosal Protection: Translation From an Animal Model to a Phase I Clinical Trial of Celecoxib, Irinotecan, and 5-Fluorouracil," *Clin Cancer Res*, 2007, 13(3):965-71.

Keefe DM, Schubert MM, Elting LS, et al, "Updated Clinical Practice Guidelines for the Prevention and Treatment of Mucositis," *Cancer*, 2007, 109(5):820-31.

Le QT, Kim HE, Schneider CJ, et al, "Palifermin Reduces Severe Mucositis in Definitive Chemoradiotherapy of Locally Advanced Head and Neck Cancer: A Randomized, Placebo-Controlled Study," *J Clin Oncol*, 2011, 29(20):2808-14.

Lilleby K, Garcia P, Gooley T, et al, "A Prospective, Randomized Study of Cryotherapy During Administration of High-Dose Melphalan to Decrease the Severity and Duration of Oral Mucositis in Patients With Multiple Myeloma Undergoing Autologous Peripheral Blood Stem Cell Transplantation," *Bone Marrow Transplant*, 2006, 37(11):1031-5.

Lin LC, Que J, Lin LK, et al, "Zinc Supplementation to Improve Mucositis and Dermatitis in Patients After Radiotherapy for Head-and-Neck Cancers: A Double-Blind, Randomized Study," *Int J Radiat Oncol Biol Phys*, 2006, 65(3):745-50.

Makkonen TA, Bostrom P, Vilja P, et al, "Sucralfate Mouth Washing in the Prevention of Radiation-Induced Mucositis: A Placebo-Controlled Double-Blind Randomized Study," *Int J Radiat Oncol Biol Phys*, 1994, 30:177-82.

McAleese JJ, Bishop KM, A'Hern R, et al, "Randomized Phase II Study of GM-CSF to Reduce Mucositis Caused by Accelerated Radiotherapy of Laryngeal Cancer," *Br J Radiol*, 2006, 79 (943):608-13.

Mori T, Yamazaki R, Aisa Y, et al, "Brief Oral Cryotherapy for the Prevention of High-Dose Melphalan-Induced Stomatitis in Allogeneic Hematopoietic Stem Cell Transplant Recipients," *Support Care Cancer*, 2006, 14(4):392-5.

"National Cancer Institute Common Terminology Criteria for Adverse Events (CTCAE) Version 3." Available at http://ctep.cancer.gov/protocolDevelopment/electronic_applications/docs/ctcaev3.pdf. Last accessed August 9, 2007.

Okuno SH, Woodhouse CO, Loprinzi CL, et al, "Phase III Controlled Evaluation of Glutamine for Decreasing Stomatitis in Patients Receiving Fluorouracil (5-FU)-Based Chemotherapy," *Am J Clin Oncol*, 1999, 22(3):258-61.

Peterson DE, Jones JB, and Petit RG 2nd, "Randomized, Placebo-Controlled Trial of Saforis for Prevention and Treatment of Oral Mucositis in Breast Cancer Patients Receiving Anthracycline-Based Chemotherapy," *Cancer*, 2007, 109(2):322-31.

Pfeiffer P, Madsen EL, Hansen O, et al, "Effect of Prophylactic Sucralfate Suspension on Stomatitis Induced by Cancer Chemotherapy: A Randomized, Double-Blind Cross-Over Study," *Acta Oncol*, 1990, 29(2):171-3.

Pitten FA, Kiefer T, Buth C, et al, "Do Cancer Patients With Chemotherapy-Induced Leukopenia Benefit From an Antiseptic Chlorhexidine Based Oral Rinse? A Double-Blind, Block-Randomized, Controlled Study," *J Hosp Infect*, 2003, 53(4):283-91.

Potting CM, Uitterhoeve R, Op Reimer WS, et al, "The Effectiveness of Commonly Used Mouthwashes for the Prevention of Chemotherapy-Induced Oral Mucositis: A Systematic Review," *Eur J Cancer Care (Engl)*, 2006, 15(5):431-9.

Quintiliani R, Owens NJ, Quercia RA, et al, "Treatment and Prevention of Oropharyngeal Candidiasis," *Am J Med*, 1984, 77(4D):44-8.

Rattan J, Schneider M, Arber N, et al, "Sucralfate Suspension as a Treatment of Recurrent Aphthous Stomatitis," *J Intern Med*, 1994, 236(3):341-3.

Rossi A, Rosati G, Colarusso D, et al, "Subcutaneous Granulocyte-Macrophage Colony-Stimulating Factor in Mucositis Induced by an Adjuvant 5-Fluorouracil Plus Leucovorin Regimen. A Phase II Study and Review of the Literature," *Oncology*, 2003, 64(4):353-60.

Ryu JK, Swann S, LeVeque F, et al, "The Impact of Concurrent Granulocyte Macrophage-Colony Stimulating Factor on Radiation-Induced Mucositis in Head and Neck Cancer Patients: A Double-Blind Placebo-Controlled Prospective Phase III Study by Radiation Therapy Oncology Group 9901," *Int J Radiat Oncol Biol Phys*, 2007, 67(3):643-50.

Saarilahti K, Kajanti M, Joensuu T, et al, "Comparison of Granulocyte-Macrophage Colony-Stimulating Factor and Sucralfate Mouthwashes in the Prevention of Radiation-Induced Mucositis: A Double-Blind Prospective Randomized Phase III Study," *Int J Radiat Oncol Biol Phys*, 2002, 54(2):479-85.

Scarantino C, LeVeque F, Swann RS, et al, "Effect of Pilocarpine During Radiation Therapy: Results of RTOG 97-09, a Phase III Randomized Study in Head and Neck Cancer Patients," *J Support Oncol*, 2006, 4(5):252-8.

Sonis ST, Elting LS, Keefe D, et al, "Perspectives on Cancer Therapy-Induced Mucosal Injury: Pathogenesis, Measurement, Epidemiology, and Consequences for Patients," *Cancer*, 2004, 100 (9 Suppl):1995-2025.

Stokman MA, Wachters FM, Koopmans P, et al, "Outcome of Local Application of Amifostine (WR-1065) on Epirubicin-Induced Oral Mucositis. A Phase II Study," *Anticancer Res*, 2004, 24 (5B):3263-7.

Sung L, Tomlinson GA, Greenberg ML, et al, "Serial Controlled N-of-1 Trials of Topical Vitamin E as Prophylaxis for Chemotherapy-Induced Oral Mucositis in Paediatric Patients," *Eur J Cancer*, 2007, 43(8):1269-75.

Ulrich CM, Yasui Y, Storb R, et al, "Pharmacogenetics of Methotrexate: Toxicity Among Marrow Transplantation Patients Varies With the Methylenetetrahydrofolate Reductase C677T Polymorphism," *Blood*, 2001, 98(1):231-4.

Vadhan-Raj S, Trent J, Patel S, et al, "Single-Dose Palifermin Prevents Severe Oral Mucositis During Multicycle Chemotherapy in Patients With Cancer: A Randomized Trial," *Ann Intern Med*, 2010, 153(6):358-67.

Vokurka S, Bystricka E, Koza V, et al, "Higher Incidence of Chemotherapy Induced Oral Mucositis in Females: A Supplement of Multivariate Analysis to a Randomized Multicentre Study," *Support Care Cancer*, 2006, 14(9):974-6.

Yokomizo H, Yoshimatsu K, Hashimoto M, et al, "Prophylactic Efficacy of Allopurinol Ice Ball for Leucovorin/5-Fluorouracil Therapy-Induced Stomatitis," *Anticancer Res*, 2004, 24(2C):1131-4.

TUMOR LYSIS SYNDROME

INTRODUCTION

Tumor lysis syndrome (TLS) is a potentially life-threatening disorder that is characterized as an acute metabolic disturbance resulting from the rapid destruction of tumor cells. Cellular destruction releases intracellular constituents (nucleic acids, anions, cations, peptides) that overwhelm the body's normal mechanisms for their utilization, excretion, and elimination. Signs and symptoms of TLS often develop within 72 hours of beginning cytotoxic chemotherapy in patients with newly diagnosed acute leukemias (acute lymphoblastic leukemia [ALL] and acute myeloid leukemia [AML]) or lymphoproliferative malignancies (Burkitt's and non-Burkitt's lymphomas). Moreover, TLS can occur spontaneously in malignant diseases with vigorous cell turnover. Although most commonly reported in patients with hematologic and lymphoid malignancies, TLS has also been reported with solid tumors such as breast cancer, colon cancer, melanoma, ovarian cancer, prostate cancer, small cell lung cancer, and testicular cancer. Acute TLS attributed to administration of a corticosteroid, imatinib, rituximab, sorafenib, and zoledronic acid in patients with treatment-sensitive tumors have been reported in the medical literature. Additional treatment and diagnostic procedures attributed with causing tumor lysis syndrome include total body irradiation, splenic irradiation, staging laparotomy, laparoscopic splenectomy preceded by splenic artery embolization, and radiofrequency interstitial thermal ablation of metastatic hepatic lesions. Metabolic abnormalities associated with acute TLS include hyperphosphatemia, hyperkalemia, hyperuricemia, azotemia, hypocalcemia, and metabolic acidosis. Cardiac arrhythmias, seizures, and major organ failure can occur in severe cases of TLS. Hyperkalemia, hyperuricemia, and hypocalcemia can produce cardiac arrhythmias, tetany, and sudden death. Acute renal failure can occur due to precipitation of uric acid and calcium phosphate in the renal tubules.

PREDISPOSING FACTORS

1. Bulky disease (>10 cm); leukemia with high white blood cell count (>25,000/mm^3) or rapidly increasing peripheral blast count
2. Acute myeloid leukemia with history of chronic myelomonocytic leukemia
3. Marked sensitivity of the tumor to a particular treatment modality
4. Renal impairment, including pre-existing volume depletion
5. Elevated pretreatment lactic dehydrogenase serum concentrations (>2 times ULN)
6. Elevated pretreatment uric acid serum concentrations (>7.5 mg/dL) independent of renal impairment

CLINICAL FEATURES AND TREATMENT

Classification and Risk Stratification

TLS can be described as either laboratory (LTLS) or clinical (CTLS) type. LTLS is the presence of 2 or more abnormal lab values or a 25% change in lab values within 3 days before or 7 days after chemotherapy. Laboratory values to monitor include uric acid, potassium, phosphorus, and calcium. CTLS is defined as LTLS with at least one clinical manifestation such as renal insufficiency, seizures, cardiac arrhythmias, or sudden death.

Certain patients have greater risk for developing LTLS and/or CTLS and should be treated more aggressively to prevent its occurrence. Risk stratification guides what type of prophylaxis and management therapies should be used for which patients. Patients classified as high risk should have aggressive prophylactic treatment with hydration and rasburicase while being monitored closely in an ICU or similarly monitored setting. Intermediate risk patients should receive prophylactic treatment with hydration and allopurinol; if hyperuricemia does develop in these patients, consider rasburicase. Initial management of pediatric patients at intermediate risk may include rasburicase. Patients at low risk for developing TLS require no prophylactic therapy but should be monitored closely and treated as necessary.

Risk Stratification

Type of Cancer	High Risk	Intermediate Risk	Low Risk
Non-Hodgkin's lymphoma (NHL)	Burkitt's, Burkitt's-ALL (B-ALL), lymphoblastic lymphoma	Diffuse large B-cell lymphoma (DLBCL)	Indolent NHL
Acute lymphoblastic leukemia (ALL)	WBC ≥100,000 cells/mm^3	WBC 50,000-100,000 cells/mm^3	WBC ≤50,000 cells/mm^3
Acute myeloid leukemia (AML)	WBC ≥50,000 cells/mm^3; monoblastic; rapidly increasing peripheral blast count	WBC 10,000-50,000 cells/mm^3	WBC ≤10,000 cells/mm^3
Chronic lymphocytic leukemia (CLL)		WBC 10,000-100,000 cells/mm^3; treatment with fludarabine	WBC ≤10,000 cells/mm^3
Other hematologic malignancies (chronic myeloid leukemia [CML], multiple myeloma) and solid tumors		Rapid proliferation with expected rapid response to therapy	Remainder of patients

Monitoring

High risk patients should have laboratory and clinical parameters (serum uric acid, phosphate, calcium, creatinine, LDH, and fluid input and output) monitored 4-6 hours after initiating chemotherapy. For all patients treated with rasburicase, monitor serum uric acid 4 hours after administration, then every 6-8 hours thereafter until resolution of TLS occurs. Frequent assessment of serum chemistries and fluid balance is necessary to avert pathophysiologic adverse events and guide the duration of rasburicase therapy. Electrolyte and fluid abnormalities must be addressed at the time that they are identified. However, rasburicase is administered no more frequently than once daily to achieve uric acid control for a duration of 5-7 doses (has also been administered as a single dose schedule with repeat doses, if needed, based on serum uric acid level).

Intermediate risk patients should be monitored throughout and for at least 24 hours after completion of chemotherapy. If rasburicase is not used, laboratory parameters should be monitored 8 hours after initiation of chemotherapy and regularly thereafter according to the patient's clinical condition and institutional practice.

Low risk patients should be monitored as determined by the institution and patient factors. If TLS has not occurred within 2 days, development is very unlikely.

General Principles

Prevention and early management of TLS are aimed at decreasing the risk of morbidity and mortality from cardiac arrhythmias, seizures, and organ failure. In patients with high or intermediate risk, vigorous hydration is the cornerstone of the initial management for acute or potential TLS. Patients should be hydrated with 2-3 L/m^2/day (200 mL/kg/day if ≤10 kg) intravenous fluid (Children: $D_5W^1/_4NS$; Adults: Not specified) to maintain urine output of 80-100 mL/m^2/hour (4-6 mL/kg/hour if ≤10 kg), with diuretic use if necessary (avoid or minimize diuretic use in patients with hypovolemia or obstructive uropathy). Due to the tendency for calcium phosphate nephrocalcinosis and the potential for metabolic alkalosis, urinary alkalinization with sodium bicarbonate is no longer universally recommended for the treatment and prevention of TLS (Coiffier, 2008).

Allopurinol should be administered to intermediate risk patients to decrease endogenous uric acid production and reduce associated urinary obstruction; dose reductions may be required for renal dysfunction (Coiffier, 2008). In adult or pediatric patients, give 150-300 mg/m^2/day (or 10 mg/kg/day in pediatric patients) divided every 8 hours (maximum: 800 mg/day) orally or 200-400 mg/m^2/day I.V. (in 1-3 divided doses; maximum: 600 mg/day). The time to maximum effect of allopurinol is 27 hours. While allopurinol decreases uric acid production, it is ineffective in reducing markedly elevated uric acid concentrations which may allow renotubular crystal formation and obstruction despite its administration. In addition, allopurinol impedes the clearance of purine analogues such as mercaptopurine and azathioprine.

Rasburicase is administered to rapidly reduce uric acid concentrations; significant reduction in plasma uric acid concentrations is measurable four hours following drug administration. Rasburicase, which is a recombinant form of urate oxidase produced in *Saccharomyces cerevisiae*, catalyzes the degradation of uric acid to allantoin which is more soluble and readily excreted by the kidneys. Rasburicase is reserved for patients at high risk for TLS (or considered in intermediate risk pediatric patients), patients with elevated uric acid concentrations, or patients with signs of moderate-to-severe renal impairment or other major organ dysfunction. The major risks associated with administration of rasburicase include anaphylaxis, hypersensitivity reactions, methemoglobinemia, and hemolysis. Rasburicase is contraindicated in patients with glucose-6-phosphate dehydrogenase deficiency due to an increased risk of hemolysis. An additional concern with rasburicase administration is the development of neutralizing antibodies. This phenomenon was observed in 64% of 28 normal, healthy volunteers studied; the effect of neutralizing antibodies on the efficacy of this product with repeated usage is unknown. Rasburicase appears to be less immunogenic in patients with hematologic or lymphoid malignancies receiving chemotherapy. One study reported detection of neutralizing antibodies in 2% of 184 patients with hematologic or lymphoid malignancies treated with rasburicase before and throughout chemotherapy (Cortes, 2010).

Rasburicase is approved for use in pediatric and adult patients, with the labeled dose of 0.2 mg/kg/dose daily for up to five days. Due to the costs and risks of therapy plus the immediate and measurable effects of rasburicase, some centers administer a single dose which is repeated daily as warranted by plasma uric acid concentrations. The following doses (based on risk for TLS) and duration of treatment based on plasma uric acid concentrations have been recommended for children: 0.2 mg/kg once daily (duration based on plasma uric acid concentrations) for high risk patients, 0.15 mg/kg once daily (duration based on plasma uric acid concentrations) for intermediate risk, and 0.05-0.1 mg/kg once daily (duration based on clinical judgment) if used for low-risk patients (Coiffier, 2008). Weight- and risk-based dosing as detailed above has been reported in adults. Fixed-dose rasburicase, ranging from 3-7.5 mg as a single dose (Hutcherson, 2006; McDonnell, 2006; Reeves, 2008; Trifilio, 2006) with doses (1.5-6 mg) repeated if needed (based on serum uric acid concentrations) has also been reported in adults. The optimal timing of rasburicase administration (with respect to chemotherapy administration) is not specified in the manufacter's labeling. In some studies, chemotherapy was administered 4-24 hours after the first rasburicase dose (Cortes, 2010; Kikuchi, 2009; Vadhan-Raj, 2012); however, rasburicase generally may be administered irrespective of chemotherapy timing.

Upon rasburicase administration, serum uric acid levels generally decrease within 4 hours. In order to allow for appropriate therapeutic effect and to accurately assess the need for a repeat dose, repeat uric acid levels should be drawn no earlier than 4 hours post-rasburicase dose. Rasburicase will degrade uric acid *in vitro* when the blood sample is stored at room temperature. Consequently, to prevent artifactually depressed uric acid concentrations, plasma samples must be collected in prechilled tubes, then immediately placed in an ice water bath until centrifuged at 4°C. Plasma must be analyzed within four hours of collection.

Clinical features and treatment for specific metabolic disorders are discussed in the following sections.

Hyperuricemia

Cytolysis during TLS releases purine and pyrimidine nucleotides into the bloodstream and extracellular tissues. Oxidation of the purines hypoxanthine and xanthine yields uric acid, which can precipitate in the renal tubules and cause oliguric renal failure. A high concentration of uric acid and an acidic urine pH promote uric acid crystallization and renotubular precipitation. Maintenance of urine flow is utilized to reduce purine precipitation and preserve renal function. Allopurinol blocks the endogenous production of uric acid by inhibiting the enzyme xanthine oxidase, which oxidizes hypoxanthine and xanthine to uric acid. Allopurinol is used prophylactically during the early management of TLS in intermediate risk patients. Rasburicase decreases existing uric acid concentrations by conversion of this molecule to the inactive and soluble metabolite allantoin, which is readily excreted by the kidneys. Rasburicase should be used prophylactically in high risk patients or in patients with pre-existing hyperuricemia or acute renal impairment.

Hyperkalemia

Potassium is primarily an intracellular ion that is released during massive cellular breakdown. Increasing concentrations of serum potassium can be dangerous, leading to cardiac arrhythmias or sudden death, especially in the presence of hypocalcemia (see following discussion). Standard treatments to remove potassium from the blood stream and extracellular fluids should be initiated as warranted by the patient's serum potassium concentration and electrocardiographic abnormalities. Other sources of potassium intake (including nutritional sources, medications, and intravenous solutions) should be eliminated in patients at risk for or with TLS. Pharmaceutical measures routinely used to manage hyperkalemia in patients with TLS include volume expansion with forced diuresis, administration of insulin with glucose, and the cation exchange product sodium polystyrene sulfonate. Sodium bicarbonate can be administered I.V. push to induce influx of potassium into cells. Textbook algorithms for management of hyperkalemia include instructions for administration of calcium as a cardioprotective measure; however, this is **not** a standard intervention in the setting of TLS. Calcium gluconate administration must be done judiciously in the patient with TLS as it can precipitate as calcium phosphate in highly perfused tissues. Monitor patient ECG and cardiac rhythm closely for arrhythmias.

Hyperphosphatemia

The release of intracellular inorganic phosphate following massive cellular breakdown sets into motion several important clinical features. Serum phosphate concentrations will quickly exceed the threshold for normal renal excretion, with phosphate excretion becoming limited by the glomerular filtration rate. Any azotemia that develops during therapy will hinder phosphate excretion. Treatment includes the use of phosphate binders such as aluminum hydroxide, sevelamer, calcium carbonate (avoid use in patients with hypercalcemia and limit use to pediatric patients), or lanthanum carbonate (avoid use in pediatric patients). In severe cases of hyperphosphatemia, hemodialysis or hemofiltration may be necessary.

Hypocalcemia

High phosphate concentrations will also cause reciprocal hypocalcemia. Although generally asymptomatic, hypocalcemia may cause neuromuscular irritation, tetany, and cardiac dysrhythmias. Symptomatic patients may receive calcium gluconate intravenously (slowly, with ECG monitoring) to increase serum calcium concentrations. Unfortunately, despite hypocalcemia, the solubility product of calcium and phosphate may be exceeded in acute TLS due to high concentrations of phosphate, resulting in tissue calcification and organ failure. For this reason, calcium gluconate should be administered cautiously and only if necessary.

Hemodialysis/Hemofiltration

Due to the unpredictability of TLS, renal replacement therapy may be needed and can be lifesaving. Hemodialysis or hemofiltration may be used to control and maintain fluid volume and/or to remove uric acid, phosphate, and potassium from serum. Intermittent hemodialysis, continuous arteriovenous hemodialysis, or continuous veno-venous hemodiafiltration should be considered as warranted by the severity of serum chemistry abnormalities, major organ dysfunction, and the patient's response to pharmaceutical treatments.

Leukoreduction/Plasmapheresis

Leukoreduction, which utilizes plasmapheresis and hydroxyurea to rapidly decrease the peripheral white blood cell count, is performed in some cases of acute myeloid leukemia. The primary goal of leukoreduction is to reduce the risk of complications from serum hyperviscosity syndrome consequent to a very high white blood cell count. However, leukoreduction can indirectly reduce the risk of TLS as removal of circulating blasts diminishes the primary source of cells undergoing lysis in patients with acute myeloid leukemia. Plasmapheresis is used infrequently and very cautiously in patients with acute promyelocytic leukemia due to the inherent disease-related risks of coagulopathy, hemorrhage, and hypotension in this population. Plasmapheresis is rarely used for leukoreduction in patients with lymphocytic or lymphoblastic leukemias as these patients are at lower risk for hyperviscosity syndrome despite a high white blood cell count. This is because lymphocytes do not have the same 'sticky' quality as myeloid cells. Hydroxyurea can be used without plasmapheresis to achieve leukoreduction.

REFERENCES

Abu-Alfa AK and Younes A, "Tumor Lysis Syndrome and Acute Kidney Injury: Evaluation, Prevention, and Management," *Am J Kidney Dis*, 2010, 55(5 Suppl 3):S1-13.

Al-Kali A, Farooq S, and Tfayli A, "Tumor Lysis Syndrome After Starting Treatment With Gleevec in a Patient With Chronic Myelogenous Leukemia," *J Clin Pharm Ther*, 2009, 34(5):607-10.

Arnold TM, Reuter JP, Delman BS, et al, "Use of Single-Dose Rasburicase in an Obese Female," *Ann Pharmacother*, 2004, 38(9):1428-31.

Barry BD, Kell MR, and Redmond HP, "Tumor Lysis Syndrome Following Endoscopic Radio-frequency Interstitial Thermal Ablation of Colorectal Liver Metastases," *Surg Endosc*, 2002, 16 (7):1109.

Cairo MS and Bishop M, "Tumour Lysis Syndrome: New Therapeutic Strategies and Classification," *Br J Haematol*, 2004, 127(1):3-11.

Cairo MS, Coiffier B, Reiter A, et al, "Recommendations for the Evaluation of Risk and Prophylaxis of Tumour Lysis Syndrome (TLS) in Adults and Children With Malignant Diseases: An Expert TLS Panel Consensus," *Br J Haematol*, 2010, 149(4):578-86.

Chen SW, Hwang WS, Tsao CJ, et al, "Hydroxyurea and Splenic Irradiation-Induced Tumour Lysis Syndrome: A Case Report and Review of the Literature," *J Clin Pharm Ther*, 2005, 30(6):623-5.

Coiffier B, Altman A, Pui CH, et al, "Guidelines for the Management of Pediatric and Adult Tumor Lysis Syndrome: An Evidence-Based Review," *J Clin Oncol*, 2008, 26(16):2767-78.

Coiffier B, Mounier N, Bologna S, et al, "Efficacy and Safety of Rasburicase (Recombinant Urate Oxidase) for the Prevention and Treatment of Hyperuricemia During Induction Chemotherapy of Aggressive Non-Hodgkin's Lymphoma: Results of the GRAAL1 (Groupe d'Etude Des Lymphomes De l'Adulte Trial on Rasburicase Activity in Adult Lymphoma) Study," *J Clin Oncol*, 2003, 21(23):4402-6.

Cortes J, Moore JO, Maziarz RT, et al, "Control of Plasma Uric Acid in Adults at Risk for Tumor Lysis Syndrome: Efficacy and Safety of Rasburicase Alone and Rasburicase Followed by Allopurinol Compared With Allopurinol Alone – Results of a Multicenter Phase III Study," *J Clin Oncol*, 2010, 28(27):4207-13.

Duzova A, Cetin M, Gümrük F, et al, "Acute Tumour Lysis Syndrome Following a Single-Dose Corticosteroid in Children With Acute Lymphoblastic Leukaemia," *Eur J Haematol*, 2001, 66 (6):404-7.

Gemici C, "Tumour Lysis Syndrome in Solid Tumours," *Clin Oncol (R Coll Radiol)*, 2006, 18 (10):773-80.

Habib GS and Saliba WR, "Tumor Lysis Syndrome After Hydrocortisone Treatment in Metastatic Melanoma: A Case Report and Review of the Literature," *Am J Med Sci*, 2002, 323(3):155-7.

Huang WS and Yang CH, "Sorafenib Induced Tumor Lysis Syndrome in an Advanced Hepatocellular Carcinoma Patient," *World J Gastroenterol*, 2009, 15(35):4464-6.

Hutcherson DA, Gammon DC, Bhatt MS, et al, "Reduced-Dose Rasburicase in the Treatment of Adults With Hyperuricemia Associated With Malignancy," *Pharmacotherapy*, 2006, 26(2):242-7.

Jabr FI, "Acute Tumor Lysis Syndrome Induced by Rituximab in Diffuse Large B-Cell Lymphoma," *Int J Hematol*, 2005, 82(4):312-4.

Kikuchi A, Kigasawa H, Tsurusawa M, et al, "A Study of Rasburicase for the Management of Hyperuricemia in Pediatric Patients With Newly Diagnosed Hematologic Malignancies at High Risk for Tumor Lysis Syndrome," *Int J Hematol*, 2009, 90(4):492-500.

Kurt M, Onal IK, Elkiran T, et al, "Acute Tumor Lysis Syndrome Triggered by Zoledronic Acid in a Patient With Metastatic Lung Adenocarcinoma," *Med Oncol*, 2005, 22(2):203-6.

Lee MH, Cheng KI, Jang RC, et al, "Tumour Lysis Syndrome Developing During an Operation," *Anaesthesia*, 2007, 62(1):85-7.

Lee AC, Li CH, So KT, et al, "Treatment of Impending Tumor Lysis With Single-Dose Rasburicase," *Ann Pharmacother*, 2003, 37(11):1614-7.

Leibowitz AB, Adamsky C, Gabrilove J, et al, "Intraoperative Acute Tumor Lysis Syndrome During Laparoscopic Splenectomy Preceded by Splenic Artery Embolization," *Surg Laparosc Endosc Percutan Tech*, 2007, 17(3):210-1.

Lerza R, Botta M, Barsotti B, et al, "Dexamethazone-Induced Acute Tumor Lysis Syndrome in a T-Cell Malignant Lymphoma," *Leuk Lymphoma*, 2002, 43(5):1129-32.

Linck D, Basara N, Tran V, et al, "Peracute Onset of Severe Tumor Lysis Syndrome Immediately After 4 Gy Fractionated TBI as Part of Reduced Intensity Preparative Regimen in a Patient With T-ALL With High Tumor Burden," *Bone Marrow Transplant*, 2003, 31(10):935-7.

Liu CY, Sims-McCallum RP, and Schiffer CA, "A Single Dose of Rasburicase is Sufficient for the Treatment of Hyperuricemia in Patients Receiving Chemotherapy," *Leuk Res*, 2005, 29(4):463-5.

Mato AR, Riccio BE, Qin L, et al, "A Predictive Model for the Detection of Tumor Lysis Syndrome During AML Induction Therapy," *Leuk Lymphoma*, 2006, 47(5):877-83.

McDonnell AM, Lenz KL, Frei-Lahr DA, et al, "Single-Dose Rasburicase 6 Mg in the Management of Tumor Lysis Syndrome in Adults," *Pharmacotherapy*, 2006, 26(6):806-12.

National Comprehensive Cancer Network® (NCCN), "Practice Guidelines in Oncology: Acute Myeloid Leukemia, Version 1.2011." Available at http://www.nccn.org/professionals/physician_gls/PDF/aml.pdf

Oztop I, Demirkan B, Yaren A, et al, "Rapid Tumor Lysis Syndrome in a Patient With Metastatic Colon Cancer as a Complication of Treatment With 5-Fluorouracil/Leucoverin and Irinotecan," *Tumori*, 2004, 90(5):514-6.

Reeves DJ and Bestul DJ, "Evaluation of a Single Fixed Dose of Rasburicase 7.5 mg for the Treatment of Hyperuricemia in Adults With Cancer," *Pharmacother*, 2008; 28(6):685–90.

Riccio B, Mato A, Olson EM, et al, "Spontaneous Tumor Lysis Syndrome in Acute Myeloid Leukemia: Two Cases and a Review of the Literature," *Cancer Biol Ther*, 2006, 5(12):1614-7.

Rostom AY, El-Hussainy G, Kandil A, et al, "Tumor Lysis Syndrome Following Hemi-Body Irradiation for Metastatic Breast Cancer," *Ann Oncol*, 2000, 11(10):1349-51.

Sorscher SM, "Tumor Lysis Syndrome Following Docetaxel Therapy for Extensive Metastatic Prostate Cancer," *Cancer Chemother Pharmacol*, 2004, 54(2):191-2.

Theodorou D, Lagoudianakis E, Pattas M, et al, "Pretreatment Tumor Lysis Syndrome Associated With Bulky Retroperitoneal Tumors. Recognition is the Mainstay of Therapy," *Tumori*, 2006, 92 (6):540-1.

Trifilio S, Gordon L, Singhal S, et al, "Reduced-Dose Rasburicase (Recombinant Xanthine Oxidase) in Adult Cancer Patients With Hyperuricemia," *Bone Marrow Transplant*, 2006, 37 (11):997-1001.

Vadhan-Raj S, Fayad LE, Fanale MA, et al, "A Randomized Trial of a Single-Dose Rasburicase Versus Five-Daily Doses in Patients at Risk for Tumor Lysis Syndrome," *Ann Oncol*, 2012, 23 (6):1640-5.

Yahata T, Nishikawa N, Aoki Y, et al, "Tumor Lysis Syndrome Associated With Weekly Paclitaxel Treatment in a Case With Ovarian Cancer," *Gynecol Oncol*, 2006, 103(2):752-4.

Zigrossi P, Brustia M, Bobbio F, et al, "Flare and Tumor Lysis Syndrome With Atypical Features After Letrozole Therapy in Advanced Breast Cancer. A Case Report," *Ann Ital Med Int*, 2001, 16 (2):112-7.

CHEMOTHERAPY AND CANCER TREATMENT DURING PREGNANCY

Cancer is the second leading cause of death in women between the ages of 20-39 years and it complicates up to 1 in 1000 pregnancies. The most common malignancies occurring during pregnancy are the same as those diagnosed in comparative nonpregnant females: Breast cancer, cervical cancer, lymphoma, and melanoma. Medical management of the pregnant patient with cancer must consider both maternal and fetal outcomes. Disease prognosis, natural history, and symptomatology are important considerations with respect to maternal outcome because these determine the urgency of treatment initiation. In addition, hematologic and major organ toxicity from anticancer treatment greatly increase the risk of maternal complications from pregnancy and delivery. Anticancer therapy can be delayed until after delivery when this is not deleterious to the patient's prognosis or does not unacceptably exacerbate cancer-related morbidity (Pereg, 2008). Unfortunately, in some cases, the risks of anticancer treatments to fetal or maternal health are considered unacceptable; in such cases, therapeutic abortion is generally recommended (Pereg, 2008).

One retrospective analysis of data from an international registry evaluated pregnancy outcome in 215 women from Belgium (68%), Netherlands (26%), and Czech Republic (6%) diagnosed with cancer while pregnant (Van Calsteren, 2010). The leading diagnosis was breast cancer, affecting 46% of the women, followed by hematologic malignancy (18%), dermatologic cancer (10%), and cervical cancer (9%). The mean maternal age at cancer diagnosis was 33 years ± 5 years. The diagnosis of cancer was made in the first, second, and third trimesters in 24%, 43%, and 33% of cases, respectively. Fifty-eight women (27%) were able to delay treatment until after delivery. For 122 patients (57%), anticancer treatment (single agent or combination therapy) was initiated at mean gestational age 20 weeks ± 9 weeks. Spontaneous miscarriage occurred prior to initiation of anticancer therapy in five women (2%) at mean gestational age of 11 weeks ± 5 weeks. Pregnancy was terminated at mean gestational age of 11 weeks ± 7 weeks for 30 cases (14%). Treatment included chemotherapy, non-cytotoxic anticancer therapy, and/or radiation therapy for 73 women (60% of treated patients). Surgery was the only treatment for 49 women (40% of treated patients). A gestational complication occurred in 27 (15%) of the 180 pregnancies that progressed to delivery. The rate of preterm labor was increased for women treated with chemotherapy or radiation therapy relative to the general population (p=0.012). The incidence of preterm premature rupture of membranes was similar to that of the general population (p=0.000). Delivery occurred at gestational age of <32 weeks, 32-37 weeks, and at term for 8%, 46%, and 46% of children, respectively. More babies exposed *in utero* to anticancer treatment were small for their gestational age (p=0.012) in comparison to infants not exposed to anticancer treatment *in utero*. Low birth weight was noted in 24% of babies born following *in utero* exposure to chemotherapy or radiation treatment. The frequency of major and minor congenital physical abnormalities for babies born to treated and untreated mothers were similar to that expected of the general population. Two infants born following 2 weeks of maternal chemotherapy treatment for acute leukemia required white blood cell colony stimulating factor support for neutropenia. Neonatal intensive care unit admission was required by 75 babies for prematurity.

Gestational age is an important consideration with respect to fetal outcome. Gestation refers to the period of time that the fetus is developing in the uterus, which is normally a period of about 38 weeks. Pertinent phases of fetal development include implantation, organogenesis, and growth. Implantation, which begins with conception and lasts for about 2 weeks, often ends in spontaneous abortion subsequent to toxic drug or radiation exposure. Organogenesis begins shortly after implantation and continues throughout the first trimester. During this period, toxic drug or radiation exposure can yield organ dysgenesis (malformation) and fetal death. The fetal liver can metabolize medications as early as gestational weeks 7-8; however, the degree to which this contributes to drug detoxification is unknown. The fetal growth phase occurs from the second trimester to term. Toxic exposures during this period of fetal development can lead to growth retardation with low birth weight and complications, including abnormal brain development with learning disabilities (Pereg, 2008).

There is a great degree of interpatient variability for systemic exposure to most pharmaceutical anticancer treatments (Baker, 2002). Physiologic changes that occur normally in pregnancy can enhance pharmacokinetic variability by influencing the systemic exposure to anticancer treatments. Pregnancy increases plasma volume and alters plasma protein expression. In addition, systemic medication elimination is increased due to enhanced mixed function oxidase activity and increased glomerular filtration rate. The intestinal absorption of medications is reduced in pregnant patients due to delayed gastric emptying and reduced gut motility. Enterohepatic circulation is increased with pregnancy, which increases the absorption of certain medications.

Systemic anticancer treatments are generally mutagenic, teratogenic, or fetotoxic in preclinical models. Most chemotherapy drugs are assigned a Pregnancy Teratogenic Risk Category designation of D or X (see Table). However, the true risk of chemotherapy administration during pregnancy is not well-delineated because relevant clinical information is based primarily on case series and anecdotal reports. Controlled clinical trials evaluating the risks of chemotherapy administration throughout pregnancy are not feasible because of the relatively infrequent and sporadic occurrence of cancer diagnosis during pregnancy and the ethical concerns related to chemotherapy administration during certain gestational periods. The overall risk of major fetal malformations attributed to chemotherapy administration during the first trimester of pregnancy is 10% to 20% (Pereg, 2008). Successful pregnancy despite systemic anticancer therapy during pregnancy is reported; however, it is imperative to recognize that due to the lack of stringently evaluated scientific data, these cases **do not verify** the safety of systemic anticancer therapy during pregnancy. In fact, one report describes *in utero* exposure of fraternal twins to cyclophosphamide and prednisone throughout the first 33 weeks of gestation with divergent outcomes for the male and female offspring. The male twin was affected with multiple congenital anomalies affecting the right arm, esophagus, inferior vena cava, and renal collecting system (Zemlickis, 1993). In addition, the male twin was diagnosed with papillary thyroid cancer at 11 years of age and neuroblastoma at 14 years of age. In contrast, the female twin was born without congenital anomalies and demonstrated normal growth and development until her last follow-up at 22 years of age. The greatest risk for spontaneous abortion occurs with systemic anticancer therapy or radiation administered during the first 2-3 weeks of pregnancy (Azim, 2010). The greatest risk of congenital abnormalities occurs with anticancer treatment during organogenesis and the first trimester of pregnancy. Following organogenesis, the central nervous system, eyes, hematopoietic system, and genitalia remain sensitive to the toxic effects of systemic anticancer therapy and radiation exposure (Pereg, 2008). Anticancer treatments given after the first trimester should be scheduled in such a manner as to reduce the risk of complications at the time of delivery.

Pregnancy Category Indicating Teratogenic Risk

Category	Criteria
A	Adequate and well-controlled studies in pregnant women have not shown that the drug increases the risk of fetal abnormalities.
B	Animal reproduction studies show no evidence of impaired fertility or harm to the fetus; however, no adequate and well-controlled studies have been conducted in pregnant women. **or** Animal reproduction studies have shown adverse events; however, studies in pregnant women have not shown that the drug increases the risk of abnormalities.
C	Animal reproduction studies have shown an adverse effect on the fetus. There are no adequate and well-controlled studies in humans and the benefits from the use of the drug in pregnant women may be acceptable, despite its potential risks. **or** Animal reproduction studies have not been conducted.
D	Based on human data, the drug can cause fetal harm when administered to pregnant women, but the potential benefits from the use of the drug may be acceptable, despite its potential risks.
X	Studies in animals or humans have demonstrated fetal abnormalities (or there is positive evidence of fetal risk based on reports and/or marketing experience) and the risk of using the drug in pregnant women clearly outweighs any possible benefit (for example, safer drugs or other forms of therapy are available).

The most common abnormality attributed to *in utero* exposure to anticancer therapy is low birth weight for gestational age (Briggs, 2011). *In utero* exposure to cytotoxic chemotherapy during the second and third trimesters can yield growth retardation and premature delivery. Numerous congenital anomalies affecting bone and cartilage, major organs, gastrointestinal tract, vascular system, and limbs have been identified after *in utero* exposure to anticancer therapy during the first trimester. Congenital anomalies have occurred following first trimester exposure to cyclophosphamide, cytarabine, doxorubicin, fluorouracil, imatinib, methotrexate, procarbazine, tamoxifen, thalidomide, thioguanine, and vincristine (Briggs, 2011; Paskulin, 2005; Vaux, 2003). Medication-specific congenital abnormalities are implicated with *in utero* exposure to methotrexate, imatinib, and tretinoin (Briggs, 2011; Pye, 2008). Methotrexate is an abortifacient, fetotoxic, and teratogenic compound. The fetal aminopterin/methotrexate syndrome is characterized by fetal growth deficiency, severe lack of ossification of the calvarium (portion of the skull), prominent eyes due to defective supraorbital ridge formation, small low-set ears, micronagthia (undersized jaw), and limb abnormalities (Del Campo, 1999). Mispositioned heart, anomalous ribs, and digit malformations are also reported following *in utero* methotrexate exposure (Briggs, 2011). Mental retardation, motor impediment, and postnatal growth delay can occur from prenatal exposure to methotrexate. Tretinoin is a retinoid, so it carries the class risk of retinoic acid embryopathy characterized by growth delays, skull and facial malformations, central nervous system abnormalities, and cardiac anomalies (Briggs, 2011). Microphthalmos (small eye diameter), polyhydramnios (increased amniotic fluid volume), and oligohydramnios (reduced amniotic fluid volume) are reported after *in utero* exposure to cisplatin (Mir, 2008). Doxorubicin and daunorubicin concentrations have been detected in amniotic fluid, placental tissue, and fetal tissues (Germann, 2004). Albeit for many anticancer treatments, including the aforementioned products, congenital anomalies do not conform to a medication-specific array of abnormalities (Briggs, 2011).

Molecularly targeted therapy and endocrine therapy also present a risk to the mother and fetus. Pregnancy and fetal outcome in 125 women treated with imatinib included normal delivery (50%), elective pregnancy termination (28%), spontaneous abortion (14%), live birth with congenital anomaly (6%), and stillborn with fetal abnormalities (1%) (Pye, 2008). Six of eight live births with congenital anomalies and the single case of stillbirth occurred following *in utero* exposure to imatinib during the first trimester of pregnancy. Birth defects demonstrated by more than one child were exomphalos (umbilical protrusion), right renal dysgenesis, and scoliosis or vertebral anomalies. Oligohydramnios has been reported with *in utero* exposure to erlotinib, lapatinib, and trastuzumab (Robinson, 2007). Craniofacial abnormalities are attributed to *in utero* exposure to tamoxifen and retinoids, such as tretinoin (Berger, 2008). Thalidomide is a known teratogen. Absent or short limbs, bone defects, external ear abnormalities, eye defects, and congenital heart defects are attributed to *in utero* exposure to thalidomide exposure (Briggs, 2011). Due to similar pharmacology and preclinical teratogenicity, lenalidomide is presumed to carry the same risks.

One retrospective series describes fetal outcome following maternal treatment with chemotherapy for breast cancer during (one patient) and after the first trimester (27 patients) (Ring, 2005). Chemotherapy regimens used were cyclophosphamide/methotrexate/fluorouracil (CMF), doxorubicin/cyclophosphamide (AC), and epirubicin/cyclophosphamide (EC) for 43%, 39%, and 18% of cases, respectively. The median gestational age at birth was 37 weeks (range: 30-40 weeks); no fetal anomalies were identified for the 28 births, none of the infants had a birth weight lower than the 10th percentile for their gestational age, and five newborns required neonatal intensive care unit support. Another case report describes congenital anomalies in a child born at 38 weeks gestational age following *in utero* exposure (during the first 16 weeks of pregnancy) to cyclophosphamide/doxorubicin/fluorouracil (CAF) for treatment of maternal breast cancer; the abnormalities included high-arched palate, small head circumference, a flat nasal bridge, bilateral syndactyly (skin webbing between fingers), and finger nail dystrophy (Paskulin, 2005). This child had a low birth weight and retarded postnatal development. The use of trastuzumab during pregnancy is associated with reports with oligohydroamnios (Pant, 2008; Sekar, 2007).

Chemotherapy administration during the second and third trimester of pregnancy can cause treatment-related toxicity to the fetus due to drug distribution through the placental barrier (Briggs, 2011). Transient renal impairment with resolution on postpartum day 8 was noted following *in utero* exposure to cisplatin (Mir, 2008). Cases of cardiotoxicity are reported following second and third trimester *in utero* exposure to anthracyclines (Germann, 2004). Fetal myelosuppression can occur secondary to maternal chemotherapy treatments during the second and third trimesters. Hematologic abnormalities are reported in some babies born to women receiving rituximab for the treatment of non-Hodgkin lymphoma and management of nonmalignant disorders (Chakravarty, 2011). Neonatal lymphopenia, B cell lymphopenia or depletion, leukopenia, thrombocytopenia, and anemia have been reported in babies born following *in utero* exposure to rituximab. In addition, perinatal infectious complications, including cytomegalovirus infection (vertical transmission), bronchiolitis, acute chorioamnionitis (diagnosed in placental pathology), and fever (presumably from viral infection), have been reported following *in utero* exposure to rituximab. Detectable levels of cisplatin have been measured in neonatal blood (Mir, 2008).

The threshold dose of radiation for inducing congenital abnormalities during fetal organogenesis is 0.1-0.2 Gy; a decrease in intelligence quotient can result from fetal central nervous system exposure to radiation 0.1 Gy during gestational weeks 8-25 and there is a 40% risk of severe mental retardation if the fetus is exposed to radiation 1 Gy during gestation weeks 8-25 (Pereg, 2008). Fetal exposure to radiation therapy increases the risk of developing malignant disease during the first ten years of life. Therapeutic radiation should be delayed until the postpartum period whenever possible. Radiation to the flank area for the treatment of pediatric unilateral Wilms tumor can yield pathophysiologic changes affecting pregnancies that occur decades following treatment. These cancer survivors are more likely to have hypertension complicating pregnancy, fetal malposition, and premature labor and their babies are more likely to be born prematurely and have a low birth weight for their gestational age (Green, 2010).

REFERENCES

Amant F, Loibl S, Neven P, et al, "Breast Cancer in Pregnancy," *Lancet*, 2012, 379(9815):570-9.

Azim HA Jr, Peccatori FA, and Pavlidis N, "Treatment of the Pregnant Mother With Cancer: A Systematic Review on the Use of Cytotoxic, Endocrine, Targeted Agents and Immunotherapy During Pregnancy. Part I: Solid Tumors," *Cancer Treat Rev*, 2010, 36(2):101-9.

Baker SD, Verweij J, Rowinsky EK, et al, "Role of Body Surface Area in Dosing of Investigational Anticancer Agents in Adults, 1991-2001," *J Natl Cancer Inst*, 2002, 94(24):1883-8.

Berger JC and Clericuzio CL, "Pierre Robin Sequence Associated With First Trimester Fetal Tamoxifen Exposure," *Am J Med Genet A*, 2008, 146A(16):2141-4.

Briggs GG, Freeman RK, and Yaffe SJ, "Drugs in Pregnancy and Lactation," 9th ed, Philadelphia: Lipincott Williams & Wilkins, 2011.

Chakravarty EF, Murray ER, Kelman A, et al, "Pregnancy Outcomes After Maternal Exposure to Rituximab," *Blood*, 2011, 117(5):1499-506.

Del Campo M, Kosaki K, Bennett FC, et al, "Developmental Delay in Fetal Aminopterin/Methotrexate Syndrome," *Teratology*, 1999, 60(1):10-2.

Germann N, Goffinet F, and Goldwasser F, "Anthracyclines During Pregnancy: Embryo-Fetal Outcome in 160 Patients," *Ann Oncol*, 2004, 15(1):146-50.

Green DM, Lange JM, Peabody EM, et al, "Pregnancy Outcome After Treatment for Wilms Tumor: A Report From the National Wilms Tumor Long-Term Follow-Up Study," *J Clin Oncol*, 2010, 28 (17):2824-30.

Mir O, Berveiller P, Ropert S, et al, "Use of Platinum Derivatives During Pregnancy," *Cancer*, 2008, 113(11):3069-74.

Pant S, Landon MB, Blumenfeld M, et al, "Treatment of Breast Cancer With Trastuzumab During Pregnancy," *J Clin Oncol*, 2008, 26(9):1567-9.

Paskulin GA, Gazzola Zen PR, de Camargo Pinto LL, et al, "Combined Chemotherapy and Teratogenicity," *Birth Defects Res A Clin Mol Teratol*, 2005, 73(9):634-7.

Pereg D, Koren G, and Lishner M, "Cancer in Pregnancy: Gaps, Challenges and Solutions," *Cancer Treat Rev*, 2008, 34(4):302-12.

Pye SM, Cortes J, Ault P, et al, "The Effects of Imatinib on Pregnancy Outcome," *Blood*, 2008, 111 (12):5505-8.

Reynoso EE, Shepherd FA, Messner HA, et al, "Acute Leukemia During Pregnancy: The Toronto Leukemia Study Group Experience With Long-Term Follow-Up of Children Exposed *in utero* to Chemotherapeutic Agents," *J Clin Oncol*, 1987, 5(7):1098-106.

Ring AE, Smith IE, Jones A, et al, "Chemotherapy for Breast Cancer During Pregnancy: An 18-Year Experience From Five London Teaching Hospitals," *J Clin Oncol*, 2005, 23(18):4192-7.

Robinson AA, Watson WJ, and Leslie KK, "Targeted Treatment Using Monoclonal Antibodies and Tyrosine-Kinase Inhibitors in Pregnancy," *Lancet Oncol*, 2007, 8(8):738-43.

Sekar R and Stone PR, "Trastuzumab Use for Metastatic Breast Cancer in Pregnancy," *Obstet Gynecol*, 2007, 110(2 Pt 2):507-10.

Van Calsteren K, Heyns L, De Smet F, et al, "Cancer During Pregnancy: An Analysis of 215 Patients Emphasizing the Obstetrical and the Neonatal Outcomes," *J Clin Oncol*, 2010, 28 (4):683-9.

Vaux KK, Kahole NC, and Jones KL, "Cyclophosphamide, Methotrexate, and Cytarabine Embropathy: Is Apoptosis the Common Pathway?" *Birth Defects Res A Clin Mol Teratol*, 2003, 67 (6):403-8.

Zemlickis D, Lishner M, Erlich R, et al, "Teratogenicity and Carcinogenicity in a Twin Exposed *in utero* to Cyclophosphamide," *Teratog Carcinog Mutagen*, 1993, 13(3):139-43.

CHEMOTHERAPY AND OBESITY

Obesity increases the risk for development of certain cancers and is associated with poorer outcome. The World Health Organization defines obesity in terms of body mass index (BMI): Underweight, <18.5 kg/m^2; normal weight, 18.5-24.9 kg/m^2; overweight, 25-29.9 kg/m^2; moderately obese, 30-34.9 kg/m^2; severely obese, 35-39.9 kg/m^2; morbidly obese, >40 kg/m^2. For the purpose of this text, the term obese refers to any BMI >30 kg/m^2 unless specified otherwise.

Obesity confounds optimal dosing of chemotherapy. Chemotherapy has a narrow therapeutic index and it is generally administered at a dosage that is one level below the amount associated with unacceptable toxicity. Presumably, the safety and efficacy of treatment correlate with systemic drug exposure. Much of the data defining systemic exposure to chemotherapy and other medications is based on pharmacokinetic studies performed in nonobese patients. Obesity can alter chemotherapy pharmacokinetics due to increased vasculature with excess adipose tissue and blood flow redistribution with respect to major organs, such as the liver, kidneys, and heart (Navarro, 2003). Volume of distribution is often altered in obesity due to increased vascular space and possibly due to altered plasma protein content (Jain, 2011). Obese patients may have increased or decreased alpha$_1$-acid glycoprotein concentrations which may impact the distribution of basic drugs. The findings of altered alpha$_1$-acid glycoprotein levels in obesity are confounded by comorbidities commonly affecting this population that increase the expression of this plasma protein; there is inconsistent data in the primary literature regarding this matter (Jain, 2011). Hepatic fatty infiltration can yield liver damage in morbidly obese patients; obesity may affect enzymatic drug metabolism (Jain, 2011). The activity of CYP2E1, which metabolizes fatty acid, ketones, and ethanol, increases proportionally with obesity; the effect of obesity on other CYP isoforms is confounded by inconsistent data in the primary literature (Jain, 2011). According to one study, glomerular filtration rate (GFR) determined by inulin clearance is increased in obese patients, although the difference abates when normalized for lean body mass (Janmahasatian, 2008). Obesity can prolong the systemic absorption of subcutaneously administered medications (Jain, 2011).

The relationship between body size and the pharmacokinetics of chemotherapy is variable and not fully delineated. Lean body mass correlates well with drug clearance for many medications (Jain, 2011). However, several chemotherapy drugs may have increased or decreased clearance depending on the drug and the patient's body size (Sparreboom, 2007). Most chemotherapy doses are calculated using body surface area (BSA). BSA is advantageous to use because the value of this parameter increases disproportionately less than weight with increasing obesity. For a patient whose actual body weight is double that of their ideal body weight, the BSA increases approximately 1.4-fold instead of 2-fold.

The American Society of Clinical Oncology (ASCO) Clinical Practice Guidelines provide evidence-based recommendations for dosing chemotherapy to treat cancer in obese patients (Griggs, 2012). The ASCO Clinical Practice Guidelines are based on the clinical evidence that the use of actual body weight for chemotherapy dose calculation does not increase acute or chronic regimen-related toxicity. Interestingly, when chemotherapy doses are calculated using actual body weight, the subsequent myelosuppression is similar or reduced in obese patients relative to their nonobese counterparts. In addition, the premise that the use of actual body weight to calculate chemotherapy doses for obese patients improves the efficacy of treatment is inherent to the ASCO guidelines.

Key Points of the ASCO Clinical Practice Guidelines for Dosing Chemotherapy in Obesity

- Calculate chemotherapy doses using the actual body weight; this is especially important for curative therapy.
- Manage regimen-related toxicities in obese patients in the same manner as for nonobese patients.
- If chemotherapy dose reduction is utilized in response to toxicity, resumption of full actual body weight-based dosing should be considered as possible by the patient's clinical status and major organ function. There is no evidence to support greater dose reductions for obese patients compared to nonobese patients.
- Use of fixed-dose cytotoxic chemotherapy is rarely justified, except for a few agents. Stated exceptions:
  - Carboplatin dose calculated using Calvert formula and maximum creatinine clearance of 150 mL/minute
  - Vincristine dose cap for neurotoxicity
  - Bleomycin set dose (due to pulmonary toxicity)

Well-intentioned empiric adjustment of chemotherapy dosage in obese patients carries the risk of lessening therapeutic efficacy without improving safety. Ultimately, the decision of whether to adjust chemotherapy dosages empirically for obesity must take into consideration the same factors that are considered for the nonobese cancer patient; the goal of treatment (curative versus palliative), the patient's ability to tolerate treatment, and the nature of regimen-related toxicity (transient versus potentially debilitating).

Use of actual body weight for body surface area-based chemotherapy dose calculations did not yield greater toxicity in 408 obese patients (BMI ≥27.3 kg/m^2) receiving FAC (fluorouracil-doxorubicin-cyclophoshamide) as adjuvant therapy for breast cancer relative to their 818 nonobese counterparts in the clinical trial (CALBG 8541) (Rosner, 1996); severe hematologic and nonhematologic adverse events were similar with the first treatment cycle and throughout the entire course of therapy for all patients. Administration of adjuvant chemotherapy for breast cancer using actual body weight in the dose calculations for obese women is reported. One retrospective analysis included 662 women with breast cancer receiving adjuvant FEC (fluorouracil-epirubicin-cyclophosphamide). The population consisted of underweight (1%), normal weight (44%), overweight (37%), obese (16%), and morbidly obese (2%) patients (Jenkins, 2007). The relative dose intensity (RDI) for FEC was ≥92.8% for all patients. In this report, patients with BMI >25 kg/m^2 were less likely to experience cycle delays due to prolonged myelosuppression ($p < 0.001$), particularly toward the end of the treatment course.

Empiric dosage reduction of chemotherapy used for the adjuvant treatment of breast cancer is reported. One analysis of socioeconomic status and BMI in 764 women found that RDI of ordered treatment versus standard therapy was <0.85 for 10%, 14%, 18%, and 27% of normal or underweight, overweight, obese, and morbidly obese patients, respectively (Griggs, 2007). A retrospective analysis of 9672 breast cancer patients receiving adjuvant therapy with AC (doxorubicin-cyclophosphamide) demonstrated reduced RDI for obese patients; empiric first cycle dose reductions to <0.9-times the standard dose were done for 9%, 11%, 20%, and 37% of healthy weight, overweight, obese, and very obese women, respectively. Reduced RDI is also suggested by fewer admissions for febrile neutropenia in the very obese patients (Griggs, 2005).

The rate of breast cancer recurrence and mortality were similar for 3385 women who received adjuvant therapy with tamoxifen for breast cancer on clinical trial NSABP B-14; approximately 50% of the women enrolled in this study were overweight or obese (Dignam, 2003). In NSABP B-14, breast cancer recurrence was not significantly increased for obese women [HR = 0.98, 95% confidence interval (CI) = 0.80 to 1.18]; breast cancer mortality was not significantly increased for obese women (HR = 1.20, 95% CI = 0.97 to 1.49); however, the obese women in this study did fare worse with respect to development of contralateral breast cancer (HR = 1.58, 95% CI = 1.1 to 2.25), risk of other primary cancers (HR = 1.62, 95% CI = 1.16-2.24), all cause mortality (HR = 1.31, 95% CI = 1.12-1.54), and risk of mortality unrelated to breast cancer (HR = 1.49, 95% CI = 1.15-1.92) (Dignam, 2003).

Obesity may influence the pharmacodynamics of aromatase inhibitor therapy. The augmented amount of peripheral adipose tissue in obese patients increases aromatase activity for peripheral estradiol production. The clinical significance of this effect is not fully established. A disparity of breast cancer recurrence rate relative to BMI was identified in the ATAC (Arimidex, Tamoxifen Alone or in Combination) trial, which prospectively compared anastrozole 1 mg daily (n=2469) vs tamoxifen 20 mg daily (n=2470) vs the combination of these products as adjuvant therapy for postmenopausal breast cancer in a prospective, randomized, and double-blind manner; the combination arm was terminated early and omitted from the final analysis (Baum, 2003). An analysis of outcome relative to body size reported that disease recurrence occurred more often in women with BMI >35 kg/m^2 vs women with BMI <23 kg/m^2 (adjusted hazard ratio [HR], 1.39; 95% CI: 1.06-1.82; $P_{heterogeneity}$ = 0.03) (Sestak, 2010). The analysis reported similar efficacy for tamoxifen across all BMI values when compared to the lowest quintile ($P_{heterogeneity}$ = 0.54). However, the efficacy of anastrozole was superior for women with BMI <28 kg/m^2 than for women with BMI >30 kg/m^2 ($P_{heterogeneity}$ = 0.01) (Sestak, 2010). A retrospective analysis of results from the Austrian Breast and Colorectal Cancer Study Group (ABCSG)-12 trial reported divergent outcome data for obese vs nonobese women (Pfeiler, 2011). The ABCSG-12 trial compared anastrozole 1 mg daily vs tamoxifen 20 mg daily as adjuvant therapy for premenopausal women with breast cancer receiving ovarian ablation (goserelin 3.6 mg monthly) with or without zoledronic acid 4 mg monthly. For patients receiving anastrozole, women with BMI >25 kg/m^2 had an increased risk of disease recurrence (HR, 1.60; 95% CI: 1.06-2.41; P=0.02) or death (HR, 2.14; 95% CI: 1.17-3.92; P=0.01) compared to their nonobese counterparts. Overweight or obese patients treated with anastrozole had an increased risk of disease recurrence (HR, 1.49; 95% CI: 0.93-2.38; P=0.08) or death (HR, 3.03; 95% CI: 1.35-6.82; P=0.004) compared to all women treated with tamoxifen (Pfeiler, 2011). One small study compared estradiol suppression in 44 postmenopausal women who received therapy with anastrozole 1 mg daily and letrozole 2.5 mg daily for 3-month intervals in a treatment crossover manner. Both treatments reduced endogenous estradiol concentrations, although mean estradiol levels were greater for five women with BMI >35 kg/m^2 in comparison to their leaner counterparts. Estradiol suppression was more pronounced with letrozole treatment for all body sizes (Folkerd, 2012).

The pharmacokinetics of carboplatin, cisplatin, docetaxel, doxorubicin, irinotecan, paclitaxel, topotecan, and troxcitabine in obese patients (n=162) relative to nonobese patients (n=1044) were analyzed with respect to BSA calculations. The body size descriptors actual body weight, body mass index, ideal body weight, adjusted ideal body weight, lean body mass, and predicted normal weight were used (Sparreboom, 2007). This study identified significantly increased absolute clearance for cisplatin (p=0.007), paclitaxel (p=0.023), and troxcitabine (p=0.016) for obese patients by a factor of 13%, 20%, and 19%, respectively. However, statistical significance was not sustained when drug clearance for the aforementioned products was normalized to body surface area using the actual body weight for calculation. The relative systemic exposure was increased 1.33-fold for docetaxel and 1.25-fold for doxorubicin in obese patients. Interestingly, the relative doxorubicin clearance for obese patients relative to nonobese patients was 0.69 for women and 1.11 for men. The study did not identify an advantage to using parameters other than actual body weight for irinotecan, carboplatin, or topotecan dosage calculation. In addition, the findings of this study suggest the risk of notable underdosing with use of parameters other than actual body weight for calculation of cisplatin, paclitaxel, and troxcitabine doses.

Clinical studies and reports indicate that body size impacts the accuracy of pharmacokinetically based carboplatin dose calculations. Carboplatin with dosage calculation using the Calvert method to achieve an area under the plasma concentration-time curve (AUC) of 7.5 in combination with paclitaxel was administered to 358 women enrolled in the GOG 158 clinical trial (Wright, 2008). The Calvert method of dosing carboplatin calculates a patient's dose according to a target AUC and the GFR. In clinical practice, the patient's GFR is generally estimated by the calculated creatinine clearance. For women treated in GOG 158, the Jelliffe formula [creatinine clearance = {98 - [0.8 × (age - 20)]} / (creatinine) × 0.9 was used as a GFR estimate. Notably, the Jelliffe formula does not include a factor for body size. Subsequently, for a given GFR calculation, overweight and obese patients received a lower surface area-based carboplatin dose than the normal weight patients. The women in this cohort were normal weight (50%), overweight (32%), and obese (18%). Patient tolerance suggests that the obese women received a less intensive systemic exposure than their normal weight counterparts. The proportional reduction in platelet count was less for obese (25% reduction) than normal weight (61% decrease) patients (p=0.01). Treatment-related reduction in hemoglobin (p=0.006) and hematocrit were also less for the obese patients (p=0.002). Chemotherapy dose reductions due to adverse events were less in obese (21%) than normal weight (34%) patients (p=0.004). The obese women were less likely to experience moderate-to-severe thrombocytopenia, leukopenia, and neutropenia during the entire treatment course than the normal weight subjects. Treatment schedule delays and dose reductions were more common in the normal weight women.

The Cockcroft-Gault formula is another GFR estimation tool used in the Calvert method for carboplatin dose calculation. The Cockcroft-Gault formula utilizes weight, age, gender, and serum creatinine as variable factors for calculation of creatinine clearance. The utility of various body weight descriptors for use in the Cockcroft-Gault equation to estimate GFR was tested with pharmacokinetic data from 240 patients and 380 carboplatin administrations (Ekhart, 2009). For normal body weight and underweight individuals, lean body weight provided the best fit dose calculation for target AUC; for obese and very obese patients (with normal renal function), adjusted ideal body weight provided the best fit dose calculation for target AUC. Interestingly, the study demonstrated that the best fit for all patients was the use of actual body weight with a maximum creatinine clearance value of 140 mL/minute (Ekhart, 2009). This finding is aligned with the Food and Drug Administration recommendation to cap the creatinine clearance value at 125 mL/minute when used for pharmacokinetically-derived carboplatin doses. A case illustrating the inaccuracy of using actual body weight for calculation of creatinine clearance with the Cockcroft-Gault formula for AUC-based carboplatin dosing is presented in the arena of high-dose chemotherapy (De Jonge, 2002). The measured carboplatin AUC was 1.7-fold greater than the targeted AUC for a 167 cm, 130 kg patient receiving CTC (cyclophosphamide-thiotepa-carboplatin) prior to autologous hematopoietic stem cell transplantation. Her calculated BSA and BMI were 2.34 m^2 and 47 kg/m^2. This patient's actual body weight was used for the calculation of creatinine clearance using the Cockcroft-Gault equation. Another study evaluating patient gender, weight, creatinine, and age as variables predicting carboplatin clearance demonstrated that average body weight was the most accurate weight variable for use in overweight and obese patients; this study analyzed carboplatin pharmacokinetics in 25 subjects who were 1.2- to 1.7-times their ideal body weight (Bénézet, 1997).

REFERENCES

Baum M, Buzdar A, Cuzick J, et al, "Anastrozole Alone or in Combination With Tamoxifen Versus Tamoxifen Alone for Adjuvant Treatment of Postmenopausal Women With Early-Stage Breast Cancer: Results of the ATAC (Arimidex, Tamoxifen Alone or in Combination) Trial Efficacy and Safety Update Analyses," *Cancer*, 2003, 98(9):1802-10.

Bénézet S, Guimbaud R, Chatelut E, et al, "How to Predict Carboplatin Clearance From Standard Morphological and Biological Characteristics in Obese Patients," *Ann Oncol*, 1997, 8(6):607-9.

Centers for Disease Control and Prevention, "About BMI for Adults." Available at http://www.cdc.gov/healthyweight/assessing/bmi/adult_bmi/index.html. Accessed October 10, 2011.

De Jonge ME, Mathôt RA, Van Dam SM, et al, "Extremely High Exposures in an Obese Patient Receiving High-Dose Cyclophosphamide, Thiotepa and Carboplatin," *Cancer Chemother Pharmacol*, 2002, 50(3):251-5.

Dignam JJ, Wieand K, Johnson KA, et al, "Obesity, Tamoxifen Use, and Outcomes in Women With Estrogen Receptor-Positive Early-Stage Breast Cancer," *J Natl Cancer Inst*, 2003, 95 (19):1467-76.

Efstathiou JA, Bae K, Shipley WU, et al, "Obesity and Mortality in Men With Locally Advanced Prostate Cancer: Analysis of RTOG 85-31," *Cancer*, 2007, 110(12):2691-9.

Ekhart C, Rodenhuis S, Schellens JH, et al, "Carboplatin Dosing in Overweight and Obese Patients With Normal Renal Function, Does Weight Matter?" *Cancer Chemother Pharmacol*, 2009, 64 (1):115-22.

Ewertz M, Jensen MB, Gunnarsdóttir KÁ, et al, "Effect of Obesity on Prognosis After Early-Stage Breast Cancer," *J Clin Oncol*, 2011, 29(1):25-31.

Folkerd EJ, Dixon JM, Renshaw L, et al, "Suppression of Plasma Estrogen Levels by Letrozole and Anastrozole Is Related to Body Mass Index in Patients With Breast Cancer," *J Clin Oncol*, 2012, 30(24):2977-80.

Geyer SM, Morton LM, Habermann TM, et al, "Smoking, Alcohol Use, Obesity, and Overall Survival From Non-Hodgkin Lymphoma: A Population-Based Study," *Cancer*, 2010, 116(12):2993-3000.

Gong Z, Agalliu I, Lin DW, et al, "Obesity Is Associated With Increased Risks of Prostate Cancer Metastasis and Death After Initial Cancer Diagnosis in Middle-Aged Men," *Cancer*, 2007, 109 (6):1192-202.

Griggs JJ, Culakova E, Sorbero ME, et al, "Effect of Patient Socioeconomic Status and Body Mass Index on the Quality of Breast Cancer Adjuvant Chemotherapy," *J Clin Oncol*, 2007, 25 (3):277-84.

Griggs JJ, Mangu PB, Anderson H, et al, "Appropriate Chemotherapy Dosing for Obese Adult Patients With Cancer: American Society of Clinical Oncology Clinical Practice Guideline," *J Clin Oncol*, 2012, 30(13):1553-61.

Griggs JJ, Sorbero ME, and Lyman GH, "Undertreatment of Obese Women Receiving Breast Cancer Chemotherapy," *Arch Intern Med*, 2005, 165(11):1267-73.

Jain R, Chung SM, Jain L, et al, "Implications of Obesity for Drug Therapy: Limitations and Challenges," *Clin Pharmacol Ther*, 2011, 90(1):77-89.

Janmahasatian S, Duffull SB, Chagnac A, et al, "Lean Body Mass Normalizes the Effect of Obesity on Renal Function," *Br J Clin Pharmacol*, 2008, 65(6):964-5.

Jenkins P, Elyan S, and Freeman S, "Obesity Is Not Associated With Increased Myelosuppression in Patients Receiving Chemotherapy for Breast Cancer," *Eur J Cancer*, 2007, 43(3):544-8.

Key TJ, Appleby PN, Reeves GK, et al, "Body Mass Index, Serum Sex Hormones, and Breast Cancer Risk in Postmenopausal Women," *J Natl Cancer Inst*, 2003, 95(16):1218-26.

Litton JK, Gonzalez-Angulo AM, Warneke CL, et al, "Relationship Between Obesity and Pathologic Response to Neoadjuvant Chemotherapy Among Women With Operable Breast Cancer," *J Clin Oncol*, 2008, 26(25):4072-7.

McWilliams RR, Matsumoto ME, Burch PA, et al, "Obesity Adversely Affects Survival in Pancreatic Cancer Patients," *Cancer*, 2010, 116(21):5054-62.

Meloni G, Proia A, Capria S, et al, "Obesity and Autologous Stem Cell Transplantation in Acute Myeloid Leukemia," *Bone Marrow Transplant*, 2001, 28(4):365-7.

Navarro WH, "Impact of Obesity in the Setting of High-Dose Chemotherapy," *Bone Marrow Transplant*, 2003, 31(11):961-6.

Park SM, Lim MK, Shin SA, et al, "Impact of Prediagnosis Smoking, Alcohol, Obesity, and Insulin Resistance on Survival in Male Cancer Patients: National Health Insurance Corporation Study," *J Clin Oncol*, 2006, 24(31):5017-24.

Pavelka JC, Brown RS, Karlan BY, et al, "Effect of Obesity on Survival in Epithelial Ovarian Cancer," *Cancer*, 2006, 107(7):1520-4.

Pfeiler G, Königsberg R, Fesl C, et al, "Impact of Body Mass Index on the Efficacy of Endocrine Therapy in Premenopausal Patients With Breast Cancer: An Analysis of the Prospective ABCSG-12 Trial," *J Clin Oncol*, 2011, 29(19):2653-9.

Rosner GL, Hargis JB, Hollis DR, et al, "Relationship Between Toxicity and Obesity in Women Receiving Adjuvant Chemotherapy for Breast Cancer: Results From Cancer and Leukemia Group B Study 8541," *J Clin Oncol*, 1996, 14(11):3000-8.

Sestak I, Distler W, Forbes JF, et al, "Effect of Body Mass Index on Recurrences in Tamoxifen and Anastrozole Treated Women: An Exploratory Analysis From the ATAC Trial," *J Clin Oncol*, 2010, 28(21):3411-5.

Sparreboom A, Wolff AC, Mathijssen RH, et al, "Evaluation of Alternate Size Descriptors for Dose Calculation of Anticancer Drugs in the Obese," *J Clin Oncol*, 2007, 25(30):4707-13.

Wright JD, Tian C, Mutch DG, et al, "Carboplatin Dosing in Obese Women With Ovarian Cancer: A Gynecologic Oncology Group Study," *Gynecol Oncol*, 2008, 109(3):353-8.

CHRONIC PAIN MANAGEMENT (CANCER)

DEFINITION AND INCIDENCE

Pain is defined by the International Society for the Study of Pain as "an unpleasant sensory and emotional experience associated with actual or potential tissue damage, or described in terms of such damage". The reported incidence of pain in cancer patients varies with the method used to determine the presence of pain, and the type and stage of cancer. It is estimated that 51% of patients with various stages of cancer experience pain, and patients with advanced disease are more likely to have severe pain. Pain in cancer patients may be due to the disease itself (eg, metastatic bone disease, visceral involvement); it may be secondary to some treatments (eg, painful neuropathy from vincristine or paclitaxel, or postoperative pain); it may result from complications associated with cancer (eg, postherpetic neuralgia); or it may have been present prior to the diagnosis of cancer and be unrelated to cancer (eg, arthritis). Most often, treatment guidelines and discussions focus on the management of chronic pain associated with progressive disease.

NONOPIOID ANALGESICS

The World Health Organization recommends a stepwise approach to the management of cancer pain (see figure).

WHO Three-Step Analgesic Ladder

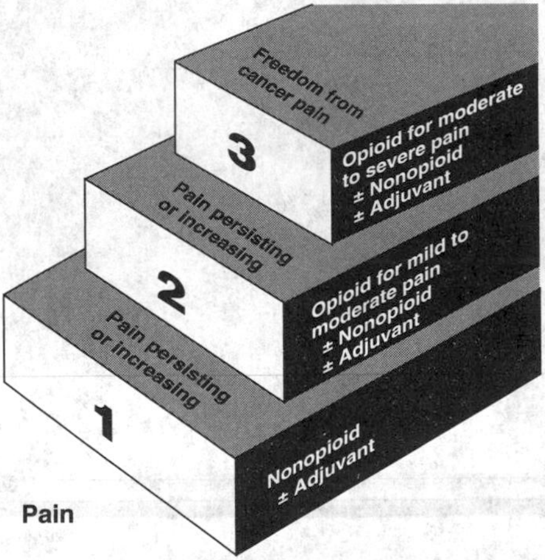

This approach recommends that the choice of therapy match the severity of pain (ie, strong opioids for moderate to severe pain). Nonopioids for (mild) cancer pain include acetaminophen, nonsteroidal anti-inflammatory drugs (NSAIDs), and aspirin. All of these have a ceiling above which increasing the dose will not enhance pain relief and will increase the likelihood of side effects. Although nonopioid analgesics are traditionally WHO step 1 products, they do have a role in the management of moderate-to-severe cancer pain. One blinded, placebo-controlled study reports that acetaminophen added to a strong opioid regimen in cancer patients improves pain control and well being.

Acetaminophen is commonly used for the management of mild-to-moderate pain. Use (including amounts contained in combination products) should be limited to a maximum daily dose of acetaminophen 4000 mg per 24 hours (acute use) or 3000 mg per 24 hours (chronic use) to reduce the risk of hepatotoxicity. Concerns regarding the use of NSAIDs in chronic cancer pain include the reversible inhibition of platelet aggregation, and the potential for gastropathy and nephrotoxicity. Aspirin is frequently avoided because of the potential for gastropathy and inhibition of platelet aggregation. Platelets exposed to aspirin become acetylated and permanently impaired. Celecoxib and nonacetylated salicylates, such as choline salicylate and magnesium salicylate, do not inhibit platelet aggregation.

OPIOID ANALGESICS

Opioid analgesic therapy should be initiated when adequate doses of nonopioid analgesics provide inadequate pain control or they are poorly tolerated.

Opioid analgesics for severe, persistent pain should be given "around-the-clock", not on an "as needed" or "PRN" basis. It is easier to prevent pain from recurring than to treat it once it has recurred. Titration of opioids to pain relief is easiest and safest using short-acting drugs (average duration of pain relief of 4 hours) or a continuous parenteral infusion. Once adequate pain relief is achieved, the 24-hour opioid dose can be given as a long-acting preparation (eg, sustained release morphine or oxycodone, transdermal fentanyl). In fact, opioid requirements can be increased in a similar manner for patients with worsening chronic pain daily. Short-acting medication for breakthrough pain, which is a transient worsening of otherwise stable pain in a patient taking an opioid, should always be available. Doses for breakthrough pain (ie, rescue doses) are commonly 5% to 15% of the 24-hour opioid dose, and may be administered every 1-2 hours as needed.

The oral route of administration for opioid analgesics is preferred whenever possible. All opioids undergo a high first-pass effect, which must be considered when converting from one route of administration to another. The parenteral to oral ratios for effectiveness of the different opioids vary from 1:2 to 1:6. The parenteral to oral dose ratio for morphine is 1:3 and 1:6 for the treatment of chronic pain and acute pain, respectively. Opioid equianalgesic doses are listed in the table that follows. Dose titration of opioid analgesics is based on pain control and patient tolerance; there is no maximum dosage for administration of opioid analgesics. Tolerance develops to most of the medication-related adverse effects except constipation and myoclonus.

Table 1. Opioid Analgesics

Drug	Route of Administration	Approx Equianalgesic Dose (mg)	Approx Duration[1] (h)
Codeine	I.M., I.V.	100-130	4-6
	Oral	200	
FentaNYL[2]	I.V.	0.1	0.5-2
HYDROcodone	Oral	30-45	4-6
HYDROmorphone	I.M., I.V., SubQ	1.5	2-5
	Oral, rectal	7.5	
Meperidine	I.M., I.V., SubQ	75	2-4
	Oral	300	
Methadone	I.M., I.V., SubQ	Variable	6-12
	Oral	See Guidelines for Conversion to Oral Methadone in Adults	
Morphine	I.M., I.V., SubQ	10	3-4[3]
	Oral, rectal	30	
OxyCODONE	Oral	20	4-6[3]
Oxymorphone	Oral	10	3-6[3]

Guidelines for Conversion to Oral Methadone in Adults[4]

Oral Morphine Dose or Equivalent (mg/day)	Oral Morphine:Oral Methadone (Conversion Ratio)
<90	4:1
90-300	8:1
>300	12:1

[1]Parenteral or immediate-release products

[2]Transdermal fentanyl conversion presented in separate table that follows

[3]Duration for sustained release dosage forms is 8-12 hours (MS Contin®, Oramorph SR®), 24 hours (Kadian®), 12 hours (OxyCONTIN®), unknown (Opana® ER)

[4]Conversion of higher doses may be guided by the following (consult a pain or palliative care specialist if unfamiliar with methadone prescribing): As the total daily chronic dose of morphine increases, the equianalgesic dose ratio (morphine:methadone) changes (American Pain Society, 2008). Total daily dose should be divided by 3; delivered every 8 hours. Methadone is significantly more potent with repetitive dosing (due to its active metabolite). Begin methadone at lower doses and gradually titrate. Applicability to pediatric patients is unknown.

Meperidine is not recommended for chronic use. This is because of the potential for accumulation of a neurotoxic metabolite, normeperidine (see following information). Meperidine administration is best reserved for incident pain (ie, before a painful manipulation or procedure).

Tolerance is characterized by the requirement for a higher dose of opioid in order to produce the same effect previously seen with a lower dose. Tolerance develops to many side effects of opioids: respiratory depression, sedation, nausea, and vomiting. Tolerance does not usually develop to constipation or myoclonus. When a given dose of opioid is not effective, for whatever reason, and if side effects are tolerable, the dose can be increased. Physical dependence occurs with regular use of opioids, but is only of clinical importance if the opioid is abruptly discontinued or an opioid antagonist (eg, naloxone) is administered, in which cases a withdrawal syndrome can be seen. Opioids should be tapered in patients whose pain improves. Signs and symptoms of withdrawal can be reduced by maintaining at least 25% of the previous day's opioid dose. The opioid can be discontinued when the total daily dose is the equivalent of 10-15 mg of intramuscular morphine. Psychological dependence is defined as a "pattern of compulsive drug use characterized by a continued craving for an opioid and the need to use the opioid for effects other than pain relief." Unlike tolerance and physical dependence, psychological dependence is a characteristic of the patient, and is a function of environmental, social, economic, and personality factors. Psychological dependence or addiction, can develop in patients requiring management of chronic pain; however, this is **not** a valid reason to undertreat pain.

The most troublesome side effect associated with chronic opioid use is constipation, and, as noted above, tolerance to constipation does not occur. Regular use of stimulant laxatives is often required.

Tolerance does develop to opioid-induced respiratory depression, allowing safe dose escalation. In the event of an acute overdose, or in the case of respiratory depression not responding to supportive measures, naloxone can be used. Naloxone administration is reserved for serious situations because it precipitates withdrawal symptoms and the prompt return of pain in patients physically dependent on opioids. Other side effects of naloxone administration include nausea, vomiting, sedation, sweating, itching, dry mouth, and tremulousness. Initiate naloxone therapy with low doses (0.1-0.2 mg) repeated and increased as warranted by respiratory rate and patient comfort. Naltrexone is only available as an oral formulation, which limits its utility for acute reversal of opioid toxicity. Tolerance develops to nausea and vomiting, and these effects are more likely to occur when opioid therapy is initiated. Phenothiazines can be used to treat nausea and vomiting. Dimenhydrinate or meclizine can also be used to treat this side effect. Tolerance usually develops to sedation. For those patients in whom persistent or profound sedation limits opioid dose escalation and therefore pain relief, the use of stimulants (eg, dextroamphetamine, methylphenidate) should be considered. Sweating and itching are thought to be due to histamine release. Morphine and meperidine are notable for causing histamine release. Switching to another opioid should be considered for patients with intolerable sweating or itching. Seizures associated with opioids are generally attributed to accumulation of neurotoxic metabolites or large overdoses that presumably cause hypoxia. Normeperidine, a metabolite of meperidine that can accumulate with frequent repeated doses or in patients with renal insufficiency, is the most well known of these neurotoxic metabolites. Distinct from seizures, myoclonic jerks may be seen with the use of high doses of opioids. Occasional reports indicate that they may also be seen with relatively lower doses. Benzodiazepines have been suggested to control this side effect as tolerance does not typically develop to this adverse event.

Opioid-induced hyperalgesia (OIH) should be suspected when analgesic efficacy is inexplicably lost or when generalized or worsening pain develops during aggressive opioid titration. OIH is a rare consequence of opioid therapy in cancer patients, and most often seen with aggressive morphine titration. The underlying mechanism is thought to be related to inhibition of glycinergic activity at the level of the spinal cord by phenanthrene-type opioids that promotes a strychnine-like excitatory effect. Additional biochemical mechanisms implicated in OIH include upregulation of intracellular phosphokinase C which activates the NMDA receptor system, and intraspinal dynorphin-mediated substance P and glutamate release.

In the scenario of OIH, continued dose escalation aggravates pain which then improves with dose reduction. Management of OIH includes dose reduction or interruption of treatment with the offending agent. Replacing a phenanthrene derivative to a piperidine-type opioid, such as fentanyl or methadone, is recommended.

As previously noted, the oral route of administration for opioids is generally preferred. When oral administration is not possible, several other routes are available (see Table 1). Morphine and hydromorphone are also available in rectal suppositories. The recommended rectal dose is the same as the oral dose. Continuous subcutaneous or intravenous infusions administered with an infusion control device are useful when oral administration is impossible. Continuous parenteral infusion of opioids provides more consistent pain relief and patient tolerance compared to intermittent injections which result in peaks and valleys of pain relief or side effects. Continuous infusions also allow for quick titration of opioid in patients with uncontrolled pain. Patient-controlled analgesia provides a continuous infusion of opioid with a capacity for patient-administered bolus injections for breakthrough pain. This is not unlike the concept of regularly scheduled sustained release oral opioid with immediate release tablets for breakthrough, as previously discussed. Assessment of the use of breakthrough doses, whether oral or parenteral, provides a basis for adjusting the dose/rate of the underlying opioid. Transdermal fentanyl is another alternative, long-acting, analgesic for patients unable to take oral opioids. Transdermal fentanyl should be avoided when initiating chronic analgesia in opioid-naive patients to reduce the risk of profound respiratory depression. As is the case with sustained release oral opioids, it is preferable to titrate to pain relief using short-acting drugs, and then switch to transdermal fentanyl. The manufacturer recommends equianalgesic conversion to the fentanyl patch as presented in Table 2. This schema represents a conservative conversion from an oral or parenteral opioid to the fentanyl transdermal system, so the tabulated information should **not** be used to convert from fentanyl transdermal to an oral or parenteral opioid analgesic.

Table 2. Dosing Guidelines for Conversion to FentaNYL Transdermal Systems

Current Analgesic	Daily Dosage (mg/day)			
Morphine (oral)	60-134	135-224	225-314	315-404
Morphine (parenteral)	10-22	23-37	38-52	53-67
HYDROmorphone (oral)	8-17	17.1-28	28.1-39	39.1-51
HYDROmorphone (parenteral)	1.5-3.4	3.5-5.6	5.7-7.9	8-10
OxyCODONE (oral)	30-67	67.5-112	112.5-157	157.5-202
Meperidine (parenteral)	75-165	166-278	279-390	391-503
FentaNYL transdermal recommended dose[1]	**25 mcg/h**	**50 mcg/h**	**75 mcg/h**	**100 mcg/h**

[1]Recommendations are based on U.S. product labeling and differ from Canadian transdermal product labeling; see current Canadian product label.

One method for switching transdermal fentanyl and oral methadone is described by using the transdermal fentanyl:oral methadone conversion factor of 1:20 (daily dose:daily dose) to change patients (N=31) with inadequate pain control from one product to another (Mercandante, 2005). Oral methadone was administered in divided doses every eight hours. Fentanyl patches were removed when the first dose of methadone was administered. Conversely, for patients transitioning to transdermal fentanyl, the patch was applied with administration of the last methadone dose. This method was used successfully in 24 of 31 patients (78%) with improved pain control reported within 24 hours of product conversion and acceptable patient tolerance. Inadequate symptom control (6 patients) and adverse effects (1 patient) were the reasons for unsuccessful switching in seven patients. Using this conversion ratio, treatment with transdermal fentanyl 200 mcg/hour is switched to oral methadone 96 mg daily administered in divided doses as 30 mg every eight hours.

A similar method has been described which calculates the appropriate methadone dose using two steps (Benitez-Rosario, 2004). First, the patient's daily transdermal fentanyl dose is converted to the equivalent oral morphine dose using a ratio of fentanyl:oral morphine of 1:100. The resultant value is converted to the equivalent daily dose of oral methadone using the ratio of oral morphine: oral methadone ratio of 5:1 or 10:1. The calculated methadone dose is divided for administration every 8-12 hours beginning 8-24 hours following removal of the transdermal fentanyl system. Using this method, a patient with adequate pain control from transdermal fentanyl 100 mcg/hour would be receiving a daily dose of fentanyl 2.4 mg every 24 hours, which converts to oral morphine 240 mg per 24-hour, which converts to oral methadone 24-48 mg per 24 hours. So, 8-24 hours after removing the fentanyl patch, a dosage of oral methadone 15 mg administered every 8 or 12 hours can be started.

Intraspinal administration of opioids should be reserved for patients in whom systemic administration of opioids results in unacceptable or unmanageable toxicity. Epidural morphine is 5-10 times more potent than parenteral morphine, and intrathecal morphine is 10 times more potent than epidural morphine. Bupivacaine, clonidine, and ketamine have been added to epidural morphine infusions to enhance effectiveness.

Partial opioid agonists (eg, buprenorphine) or agonist-antagonists (eg, pentazocine, butorphanol, dezocine, nalbuphine) are generally not recommended for use in chronic cancer pain management. They have a ceiling for analgesic effectiveness, above which side effects are much more likely to increase, and they may precipitate withdrawal in patients receiving opioid agonists (eg, morphine). Naloxone may not be effective in reversing respiratory depression caused by buprenorphine.

Tramadol is a synthetic opioid that inhibits the neuronal reuptake of norepinephrine and serotonin. This product is indicated for the management of moderate pain and it has been tested in the management of mild-to-moderate cancer pain. Its use is limited by the risk of seizures which have occurred in patients taking the usual and recommended dosage. One comparative study reported that the rate of vomiting, dizziness, anorexia, and weakness was greater with tramadol than codeine or hydrocodone when used for cancer pain (Rodriguez, 2007). Abrupt discontinuation of tramadol can precipitate withdrawal symptoms, such as tremors, sweating, diarrhea, upper respiratory symptoms, and rarely, hallucinations. The dosage of tramadol must be adjusted for impaired renal function.

ADJUVANT ANALGESICS

Adjuvant analgesics are frequently used in addition to, rather than instead of, opioid analgesics. Adjuvants are often drugs that have primary indications other than pain, but may provide pain relief in certain situations. NSAIDs are commonly used for pain due to bone metastases (see individual NSAID monographs).

Gabapentin and pregabalin are commonly used as adjunctive therapy for neuropathic pain. Additional drugs that have been used for this purpose include tricyclic antidepressants (eg, amitriptyline, nortriptyline), anticonvulsants (eg, carbamazepine), corticosteroids, and antiarrhythmics (eg, topical lidocaine). Methadone and ketamine are thought to improve neuropathic pain through blockade of the N-methyl-D-aspartate (NMDA) receptor. Neuropathic pain, often characterized by sharp, shooting, lancinating sensations, may result from nerve compression, infiltration, or destruction by tumor or from other associated conditions (eg, postherpetic neuralgia). Pain relief is usually not complete and, as is the case with NSAIDs in bone pain, these drugs are generally used in addition to opioids. Baclofen has also been used as an adjuvant analgesic for various types of neuropathic pain. Strontium-89 is a radiopharmaceutical that is reported to decrease the need for analgesics in patients with osteoblastic bone metastases. Prostate cancer is the most frequent malignancy associated with painful osteoblastic lesions. The bisphosphonates pamidronate and zoledronic acid are used to decrease pain and adverse skeletal events in patients with multiple myeloma and breast cancer. Capsaicin is a topically applied adjuvant analgesic that depletes substance P, a "painful" neurotransmitter. Capsaicin is recommended for use in postherpetic neuralgia and other painful neuropathies.

REFERENCES

Axelrod DJ and Reville B, "Using Methadone to Treat Opioid-Induced Hyperalgesia and Refractory Pain," *J Opioid Manag*, 2007, 3(2):113-4.

Benítez-Rosario MA, Feria M, Salinas-Martín A, et al, "Opioid Switching From Transdermal Fentanyl to Oral Methadone in Patients With Cancer Pain," *Cancer*, 2004, 101(12):2866-73.

Benrath J, Scharbert G, Gustorff B, et al, "Long-Term Intrathecal S(+)-Ketamine in a Patient With Cancer-Related Neuropathic Pain," *Br J Anaesth*, 2005, 95(2):247-9.

Berenson JR, Lichtenstein A, Porter L, et al, "Efficacy of Pamidronate in Reducing Skeletal Events in Patients With Advanced Multiple Myeloma. Myeloma Aredia Study Group," *N Engl J Med*, 1996, 334(8):488-93.

Cordell GA and Araujo OE, "Capsaicin: Identification, Nomenclature, and Pharmacotherapy," *Ann Pharmacother*, 1993, 27(3):330-6.

Davis MP, Shaiova LA, and Angst MS, "When Opioids Cause Pain," *J Clin Oncol*, 2007, 25 (28):4497-8.

Elsner F, Radbruch L, Loick G, et al, "Intravenous Versus Subcutaneous Morphine Titration in Patients With Persisting Exacerbation of Cancer Pain," *J Palliat Med*, 2005, 8(4):743-50.

Fromm GH, "Baclofen as an Adjuvant Analgesic," *J Pain Symptom Manage*, 1994, 9(8):500-9.

Højsted J and Sjøgren P, "Addiction to Opioids in Chronic Pain Patients: A Literature Review," *Eur J Pain*, 2007, 11(5):490-518.

Holdsworth MT, Adams VR, Chavez CM, et al, "Continuous Midazolam Infusion for the Management of Morphine-Induced Myoclonus," *Ann Pharmacother*, 1995, 29(1):25-9.

Jackson KC 2nd, "Pharmacotherapy for Neuropathic Pain," *Pain Pract*, 2006, 6(1):27-33.

Jacox A, Carr DB, Payne R, et al, "Management of Cancer Pain," *Clinical Practice Guideline No. 9, AHCPR Publication No. 94-0592*, Rockville, MD: Agency for Health Care Policy and Research, U.S. Department of Health and Human Services, Public Health Service, March 1994.

Laizure SC, "Considerations in Morphine Therapy," *Am J Hosp Pharm*, 1994, 51(16):2042-3.

Levy MH, Chwistek M, and Mehta RS, "Management of Chronic Pain in Cancer Survivors," *Cancer J*, 2008, 14(6):401-9.

Levy MH, "Pharmacologic Treatment of Cancer Pain," *N Engl J Med*, 1996, 335(15):1124-32.

Lossignol DA, Obiols-Portis M, and Body JJ, "Successful Use of Ketamine for Intractable Cancer Pain," *Support Care Cancer*, 2005, 13(3):188-93.

Mercadante SL, Berchovich M, Casuccio A, et al, "A Prospective Randomized Study of Corticosteroids as Adjuvant Drugs to Opioids in Advanced Cancer Patients," *Am J Hosp Palliat Care*, 2007, 24(1):13-9.

Mercadante S, Ferrera P, Villari P, et al, "Rapid Switching Between Transdermal Fentanyl and Methadone in Cancer Patients," *J Clin Oncol*, 2005, 23(22):5229-34.

Potter JM, Reid DB, Shaw RJ, et al, "Myoclonus Associated With Treatment With High Doses of Morphine: The Role of Supplemental Drugs," *BMJ*, 1989, 299(6692):150-3.

"Principles of Analgesic Use in the Treatment of Acute Pain and Cancer Pain," 6th ed, Glenview, IL: American Cancer Pain Society, 2008.

Robinson RG, Preston DF, Baxter KG, et al, "Clinical Experience With Strontium-89 in Prostatic and Breast Cancer Patients," *Semin Oncol*, 1993, 20(3 Suppl 2):44-8.

Rodriguez RF, Bravo LE, Castro F, et al, "Incidence of Weak Opioids Adverse Events in the Management of Cancer Pain: A Double-Blind Comparative Trial," *J Palliat Med*, 2007, 10 (1):56-60.

Rodriguez RF, Castillo JM, Del Pilar Castillo M, et al, "Codeine/Acetaminophen and Hydrocodone/Acetaminophen Combination Tablets for the Management of Chronic Cancer Pain in Adults: A 23-Day, Prospective, Double-Blind, Randomized, Parallel-Group Study," *Clin Ther*, 2007, 29 (4):581-7.

Stearns L, Boortz-Marx R, Du Pen S, et al, "Intrathecal Drug Delivery for the Management of Cancer Pain: A Multidisciplinary Consensus of Best Clinical Practices," *J Support Oncol*, 2005, 3 (6):399-408.

Stockler M, Vardy J, Pillai A, et al, "Acetaminophen (Paracetamol) Improves Pain and Well-Being in People With Advanced Cancer Already Receiving a Strong Opioid Regimen: A Randomized, Double-Blind, Placebo-Controlled Cross-Over Trial," *J Clin Oncol*, 2004, 22(16):3389-94.

Svendsen KB, Andersen S, Arnason S, et al, "Breakthrough Pain in Malignant and Non-Malignant Diseases: A Review of Prevalence, Characteristics and Mechanisms," *Eur J Pain*, 2005, 9 (2):195-206.

Szeto HH, Inturrisi CE, Houde R, et al, "Accumulation of Normeperidine, an Active Metabolite of Meperidine in Patients With Renal Failure of Cancer," *Ann Intern Med*, 1977, 86(6):738-41.

Tsavaris N, Kopterides P, Kosmas C, et al, "Analgesic Activity of High-Dose Intravenous Calcitonin in Cancer Patients With Bone Metastases," *Oncol Rep*, 2006, 16(4):871-5.

Vranken JH, van der Vegt MH, Kal JE, et al, "Treatment of Neuropathic Cancer Pain With Continuous Intrathecal Administration of S +-Ketamine," *Acta Anaesthesiol Scand*, 2004, 48 (2):249-52.

Wellington K and Goa KL, "Zoledronic Acid: A Review of Its Use in the Management of Bone Metastases and Hypercalcaemia of Malignancy," *Drugs*, 2003, 63(4):417-37.

Yucel A, Ozyalcin S, Koknel Talu G, et al, "The Effect of Venlafaxine on Ongoing and Experimentally Induced Pain In Neuropathic Pain Patients: A Double Blind, Placebo Controlled Study," *Eur J Pain*, 2005, 9(4):407-16.

COMMON TOXICITY CRITERIA

Selected Common Toxicity Criteria[1]

Toxicity	Grade 0	Grade 1	Grade 2	Grade 3	Grade 4
Hematologic					
Leukocytes (WBC)	WNL	3000/mm^3 to <LLN	2000 to <3000/mm^3	1000 to <2000/mm^3	<1000/mm^3
Neutrophils (ANC)	WNL	1500/mm^3 to <LLN	1000 to <1500/mm^3	500 to <1000/mm^3	≤500/mm^3
Lymphocytes	WNL	800/mm^3 to <LLN	500 to <800/mm^3	200 to <500/mm^3	<200/mm^3
Anemia (Hgb)	WNL	10 g/dL to <LLN	8 to <10 g/dL	v3: 6.5 to <8 g/dL v4: <8 g/dL	v3: <6.5 g/dL v4: Life-threatening
Platelets	WNL	75,000/mm^3 to <LLN	50,000 to <75,000/mm^3	25,000 to <50,000/mm^3	<25,000/mm^3
Hemorrhage	None	Mild, no intervention indicated	Intervention indicated (symptomatic or medical)	Transfusion (and/or other intervention) indicated	Life-threatening; major intervention indicated
Cardiovascular					
Hypotension	None	v3: Changes v4: Asymptomatic; no treatment required	v3: Brief (<24 hours) treatment (eg, fluid replacement or other therapy) required v4: Nonurgent medical intervention indicated	v3: Sustained (>24 hours) treatment required; resolves without persisting physiologic consequences v4: Medical intervention indicated	v3: Shock v4: Life-threatening; urgent intervention indicated
Hypertension	None	v3: Increase of DBP >20 mm Hg or to >150/100; treatment not required v4: Prehypertension (SBP 120-139 mm Hg or DBP 80-89 mm Hg)	v3: Recurrent or persistent grade 1 level; may require monotherapy treatment v4: Stage 1 (SBP 140-159 mm Hg or DBP 90-99 mm Hg); medical intervention indicated; recurrent or persistent (≥24 hours); symptomatic increase of >20 mm Hg (DBP) or to >140/90; monotherapy indicated	v3: More intensive treatment or >1 drug required v4: Stage 2 (SBP ≥16- mm Hg or DBP ≥100 mm Hg); medical intervention indicated; >1 drug or more intensive therapy indicated	v3: Life-threatening (eg, hypertensive crisis) v4: Life-threatening (eg, malignant hypertension, hypertensive crisis); urgent intervention indicated

Selected Common Toxicity Criteria[1] *continued*

Toxicity	Grade 0	Grade 1	Grade 2	Grade 3	Grade 4
Pericardial effusion	None	v3: Asymptomatic effusion	v4: Small- to moderate-sized asymptomatic effusion	Physiologic consequences	Life-threatening consequences; urgent nervention indicated
QT_c prolongation	WNL	v3: QT_c >450-470 msec v4: QT_c >450-480 msec	v3: QT_c >470-500 msec; ≥60 msec increase from baseline v4: QT_c 481-500 msec	v3: QT_c >500 msec v4: QT_c ≥501 msec (on 2 separate ECGs)	v3: QT_c >500 msec with life-threatening signs or symptoms (eg, arrhythmia, CHF, hypotension, shock, syncope); Torsades de pointes v4: QT_c ≥501 msec or >60 msec change from baseline and Torsades de pointes or polymorphic ventricular tachycardia or signs/ symptoms or serious arrhythmia
Syncope	Absent			v3: Present v4: Fainting; orthostatic collapse	Life-threatening consequences
Thrombosis/ embolism	None	v4: Superficial	v3: DVT or cardiac thrombosis; intervention not indicated v4: Venous thrombosis (uncomplicated DVT); medical intervention indicated	v3: DVT or cardiac thrombosis; intervention indicated v4: Thrombosis (eg, uncomplicated pulmonary embolism, nonembolic cardiac mural thrombus); medical intervention indicated	v3: Pulmonary embolism/life threatening thrombus v4: Life-threatening (eg, pulmonary embolism, cerebrovascular event, arterial insufficiency); hemodynamic or neurologic instability; urgent intervention indicated

Selected Common Toxicity Criteria[1] *continued*

Toxicity	Grade 0	Grade 1	Grade 2	Grade 3	Grade 4
Dermatologic					
Rash (acne/ acneiform)	None	v3: Intervention not indicated v4: Papules and/or pustules covering <10% of BSA	v3: Intervention indicated v4: Papules and/or pustules covering 10% to 30% of BSA; limits ADL	v3: Pain, disfigurement, ulceration, desquamation v4: Papules and/or pustules covering >30% of BSA; limits self-care ADL; local superinfection requiring oral antibiotics	v4: Papules or pustules associated with extensive superinfection with I.V. antibiotics indicated; life-threatening consequences
Rash	None	v3: Macular or papular eruption v4: Macules or papules covering <10% of BSA	v3: Macular or papular eruption or erythema w/ pruritus affecting <50% of BSA v4: Macules or papules covering 10% to 30% of BSA; limits ADL	v3: Severe erythema/ desquamation/macular, papular, or vesicular eruption covering ≥50% of BSA v4: Macules or papules covering >30% of BSA; limits self-care ADL	v3: Generalized exfoliative, ulcerative, or bullous dermatitis
Rash (erythema multiforme)	None	v4: Lesions covering <10% of BSA	v3: Scattered eruption v4: Lesions covering 10% to 30% of BSA, associated with skin tenderness	v3: Severe eruption; I.V. fluids, tube feeding, or TPN indicated v4: Lesions covering >30% of BSA, associated with oral or genital erosions	v3: Life-threatening eruption; disabling v4: Lesions covering >30% of BSA, associated with fluid or electrolyte abnormality; ICU or burn unit indicated
Hand-foot syndrome	None	Minimal skin changes or dermatitis without pain	v3: Skin changes or pain not interfering with ADL v4: Skin changes with pain; limits ADL	v3: Ulcerative dermatitis or skin changes with pain; interferes with ADL v4: Severe skin changes (peeling, blisters, bleeding, edema, hyperkeratosis) with pain; limits self-care ADL	

Selected Common Toxicity Criteria[1] *continued*

Toxicity	Grade 0	Grade 1	Grade 2	Grade 3	Grade 4
Alopecia	None	v3: Thinning or patchy v4: Hair loss <50% (of normal)	v3: Complete v4: Hair loss ≥50% (of normal)		
Gastrointestinal					
Nausea	None	Loss of appetite/able to eat	v3: Oral intake decreased, no significant weight loss, dehydration, or malnutrition; I.V. fluids indicated <24 hours v4: Oral intake decreased, no significant weight loss, dehydration, or malnutrition	v3: Inadequate oral caloric or fluid intake/I.V. fluids required ≥24 hours v4: Inadequate oral caloric or fluid intake; tube fueeding, TPN, or hospitalization indicated	Life-threatening consequences
Vomiting	None	v3: 1 episode/24 hours v4: 1-2 episodes/24 hours	v3: 2-5 episodes/24 hours; I.V. fluids indicated <24 hours v4: 3-5 episodes/24 hours	v3: ≥6 episodes/24 hours, I.V. fluids, or TPN required ≥24 hours v4: ≥6 episodes/24 hours, I.V. fluids, tube feeding, or TPN required	Life-threatening consequences
Diarrhea	None	<4 stools/day increase over baseline	v3: 4-6 stools/day increase over baseline; I.V. fluids indicated <24 hours; does not limit ADL v4: 4-6 stools/day increase over baseline	v3: ≥7 stools/day increase over baseline; I.V. fluids required ≥24 hours; hospitalization; interferes with ADL v4: ≥7 stools/day increase over baseline; incontinence; hospitalization; limits self-care ADL	v3: Life-threatening consequences v4: Life-threatening consequences; urgent intervention indicated

Selected Common Toxicity Criteria[1] *continued*

Toxicity	Grade 0	Grade 1	Grade 2	Grade 3	Grade 4
Mucositis/stomatitis	None	v3: Mucosal erythema v4: Asymptomatic or mild	v3: Patchy ulcerations v4: Moderate pain; does not interfere with oral intake; modified diet needed	v3: Confluent ulceration, bleeding with minor trauma v4: Severe pain, interferes with oral intake	v3: Tissue necrosis/ bleeding; life-threatening v4: Life-threatening; urgent intervention indicated
GI bleeding	None	Mild; intervention not indicated	Symptomatic; mild intervention indicated	Transfusion required; intervention indicated	Life-threatening consequences; urgent intervention indicated
Amylase elevation	None	>ULN to 1.5 x ULN	>1.5 to 2 x ULN	>2 to 5 x ULN	>5 x ULN
Lipase elevation	None	>ULN to 1.5 x ULN	>1.5 to 2 x ULN	>2 to 5 x ULN	>5 x ULN
Ascites	None	Asymptomatic	Symptomatic; intervention indicated	Symptomatic; invasive intervention indicated	v3: Life-threatening consequences v4: Life-threatening consequences; urgent operative intervention indicated
Hepatic					
Alkaline phosphatase elevation	WNL	>ULN to 2.5 x ULN	>2.5 to 5 x ULN	>5 to 20 x ULN	>20 x ULN
AST elevation	WNL	v3: >ULN to 2.5 x ULN v4: >ULN to 3 x ULN	v3: >2.5 to 5 x ULN v4: >3 to 5 x ULN	>5 to 20 x ULN	>20 x ULN
ALT elevation	WNL	v3: >ULN to 2.5 x ULN v4: >ULN to 3 x ULN	v3: >2.5 to 5 x ULN v4: >3 to 5 x ULN	>5 to 20 x ULN	>20 x ULN
Hyperbilirubinemia	WNL	>ULN to 1.5 x ULN	>1.5 to 3 x ULN	>3 to 10 x ULN	>10 x ULN

Selected Common Toxicity Criteria[1] *continued*

Toxicity	Grade 0	Grade 1	Grade 2	Grade 3	Grade 4
Metabolic					
Hypoalbuminemia	WNL	3 g/dL to <LLN	2 to <3 g/dL	<2 g/dL	v4: Life-threatening; urgent intervention indicated
Hypercholesteremia	None	>ULN to 300 mg/dL	>300 to 400 mg/dL	>400 to 500 mg/dL	>500 mg/dL
Hyperglycemia	WNL	>ULN to 160 mg/dL	>160 to 250 mg/dL	>250 to 500 mg/dL	>500 mg/dL
Hypertriglyceridemia	None	v3: >ULN to 2.5 x ULN v4: 150 to 300 mg/dL	v3: >2.5 to 5 x ULN v4: >300 to 500 mg/dL	v3: >5 to 10 x ULN v4: >500 to 1000 mg/dL	v3: >10 x ULN v4: >1000 mg/dL; life-threatening
Hypoglycemia	WNL	55 mg/dL to <LLN	40 to <55 mg/dL	30 to <40 mg/dL	<30 mg/dL
Hypocalcemia	WNL	Corrected calcium: 8 mg/dL to <LLN	Corrected calcium: 7 to <8 mg/dL	v3: Corrected calcium: 6 to <7 mg/dL v4: Corrected calcium: 6 to <7 mg/dL; hospitalization indicated	v3: Corrected calcium: <6 mg/dL v4: Corrected calcium: <6 mg/dL; life-threatening
Hypokalemia	WNL	3 mmol/L to <LLN	v3: 3 mmol/L to <LLN v4: 3 mmol/L to <LNN; symptomatic; intervention indicated	v3: 2.5 to <3 mmol/L v4: 2.5 to <3 mmol/L; hospitalization indicated	v3: <2.5 mmol/L v4: <2.5 mmol/L; life-threatening
Hypomagnesemia	WNL	1.2 mg/dL to <LLN	0.9 to <1.2 mg/dL	0.7 to <0.9 mg/dL	v3: <0.7 mg/dL v4: <0.7 mg/dL; life-threatening
Hypophosphatemia	WNL	2.5 mg/dL to <LLN	2 to <2.5 mg/dL	1 to <2 mg/dL	v3: <1 mg/dL v4: <1 mg/dL; life-threatening

Selected Common Toxicity Criteria[1] *continued*

Toxicity	Grade 0	Grade 1	Grade 2	Grade 3	Grade 4
			Renal/Genitourinary		
Hematuria	None	v3: Minimal or microscopic; intervention not indicated v4: Asymptomatic; intervention not indicated	v3: Gross bleeding; intervention or irrigation required v4: Symptomatic; catheter or irrigation indicated; limits ADL	v3: Transfusion or intervention indicated v4: Gross hematuria, transfusion, I.V. medications, or hospitalization indicated; limits self-care ADL	Life-threatening consequences; urgent intervention indicated
Serum creatinine elevation	WNL	v3: >ULN to 1.5 x ULN v4: Increase of >0.3 mg/dL; 1.5 to 2 x baseline	v3: >1.5 to 3 x ULN v4: >2 to 3 x baseline	v3: >3 to 6 x ULN v4: >3 x baseline or >4 mg/dL; hospitalization indicated	v3: >6 x ULN v4: Life-threatening; dialysis indicated
			Respiratory		
Dyspnea	None	v3: Dyspnea on exertion (can walk 1 flight of stairs without stopping) v4: Dyspnea with moderate exertion	v3: Dyspnea on exertion (cannot walk 1 flight of stairs or 1 city block without stopping) v4: Dyspnea with minimal exertion; limits ADL	v3: Dyspnea with ADL v4: Dyspnea at rest; limits self-care ADL	v3: Dyspnea at rest; intubation/ventilator support indicated v4: Life-threatening; urgent intervention indicated
Epistaxis	None	Mild; no intervention indicated	Symptomatic; intervention indicated	Transfusion required; intervention indicated	Life-threatening consequences; urgent intervention indicated
Pleural effusion	None	Asymptomatic	v3: Symptomatic; intervention required (diuretics or up to 2 thoracenteses) v4: Symptomatic; intervention required (thoracentesis or tube drainage)	v3: Symptomatic, oxygen, thoracentesis, tube drainage, or pleurodesis required v4: Severe symptoms; intervention indicated	Life-threatening; intubation or urgent intervention required

Selected Common Toxicity Criteria[1] *continued*

Toxicity	Grade 0	Grade 1	Grade 2	Grade 3	Grade 4
Pneumonitis/ pulmonary infiltrates	None	Asymptomatic; radiographic findings only	Symptomatic but does not interfere with ADL	Symptomatic; interferes with ADL; oxygen indicated	Life-threatening; ventilator support indicated
CNS/Neurologic					
Fatigue/weakness	None	v3: Mild fatigue over baseline v4: Fatigue relieved by rest	v3: Moderate; some difficulty with ADL v4: Fatigue not relieved by rest; limits ADL	v3: Severe; interferes with ADL v4: Fatigue not relieved by rest; limits self-care ADL	Disabling
Neuropathy, motor	Normal	Asymptomatic; weakness on exam	Symptomatic weakness; mild difficulty with function	Weakness; interferes with ADL	Life-threatening/ disabling
Neuropathy, sensory	Normal	Asymptomatic; paresthesia/deep tendon reflex loss	v3: Paresthesia/sensory loss; interferes with function but not ADL v4: Moderate symptoms; limits ADL	v3: Sensory loss/ paresthesia; interferes w/ ADL v4: Severe symptoms; limits self-care ADL	v3: Disabling v4: Life-threatening/ disabling
Miscellaneous					
Allergic reaction	None	Transient flushing or rash, drug fever <38°C	v3: Rash, flushing, urticaria, dyspnea, drug fever ≥38°C v4: Intervention or interruption of infusion indicated	v3: Symptomatic bronchospasm; parenteral medications indicated v4: Prolonged recurrence of symptoms after initial improvement	Life-threatening; urgent intervention indicated
Anaphylaxis	None			Symptomatic bronchospasm; parenteral treatment required; allergy-related edema, angioedema, hypotension	Life-threatening; urgent intervention indicated

Selected Common Toxicity Criteria[1] *continued*

Toxicity	Grade 0	Grade 1	Grade 2	Grade 3	Grade 4
Infusion-related reaction	None	Mild, transient; infusion interruption or intervention not indicated	Interruption indicated; responds promptly to symptomatic treatment; prophylactic medications indicated ≤24 hours	Prolonged reaction (not initially responding to symptomatic treatment); symptoms recur following initial improvement; hospitalization indicated	Life-threatening; urgent intervention indicated
Fever	None	38°C to 39°C (100.4°F to 102.2°F)	>39°C to 40°C (102.3°F to 104°F)	>40°C (104°F) for ≤24 h	>40°C (104°F) for >24 h
Neutropenic fever	None			v3: ANC <1000/mm^3 with temperature ≥38.3°C (101.3°F) v4: ANC <1000/mm^3 with single temperature >38.3°C (101.3°F) or sustained temperature ≥38°C (100.4°F) for >1 hour	Life-threatening; urgent intervention indicated

DBP = diastolic blood pressure, SBP = systolic blood pressure, BSA = body surface area, ADL = activities of daily living, WNL = within normal limits, LLN = lower limits of normal, ULN = upper limits of normal

[1]The National Cancer Institute (NCI) Cancer Therapy Evaluation Program (CTEP) has developed version 4.0 of the Common Terminology Criteria for Adverse Events (CTCAE). While version 4 is transitioning into practice, protocols and/or dosage reduction recommendations may be based on version 3. When version 4 differs from version 3, the differences are noted.

Adapted from the NCI Common Terminology Criteria for Adverse Events (CTCAE) versions 3.0 and 4.0. Available at http://ctep.cancer.gov/protocolDevelopment/electronic_applications/ctc.htm#ctc_40_conversion. Last accessed October 2012.

HOSPICE (END OF LIFE) CARE

Hospice care is provided to maintain comfort and control symptoms in the dying patient. Most patients receiving hospice care have a life expectancy of less than a few months. The pharmaceutical component of hospice care is one aspect pertaining to the quality of dying and death. The quality of dying and death entails the physical experience, psychological experience, social and cultural comprehension, spiritual or existential understanding, life closure and death preparation, and the circumstances of death. For cancer patients the type and stage of malignant disease and their health care experience impact the quality of dying and death.

Important communications between the patient and loved one or the patient and health care professional is best conducted early during hospice care rather than later. Many people are unable to effectively communicate within hours to days before death occurs. The percentage of patients who are awake, drowsy, or comatose one week prior to death is 56%, 44%, and zero, respectively. In comparison, 24 hours before death 26% of patients are awake, 62% of patients are drowsy, and 12% are comatose. And within 6 hours of death 8% of patients are awake, 42% of patients are drowsy, and 50% are comatose.

It is difficult to predict the expected time of impending death. Some patients become progressively less responsive until they die; whereas, other experience symptomatology portending death. Noisy respirations (also known as death rattle) occur when patients are obtunded or too weak to expectorate secretions. The noise is generated by secretions that accumulate in the hypopharynx and bronchial tree and oscillate with the movement of air during inspiration and exhalation. Noisy respirations generally develop within 2-3 days of death. Respiration with involuntary mandibular movement, cyanosis of the extremities, and loss of radial pulse occur approximately eight hours, five hours, and three hours, respectively, prior to death. Interestingly, the time from respiration with mandibular movement or cyanosis to death is markedly prolonged in patients with primary lung cancer or metastatic malignant disease affecting the lungs. Additional adverse events associated with dying include agitation or restlessness, delirium, dyspnea, incontinence of urine or stool, irregular breathing including gasping or 20-30 second interruptions in respiration, nausea, and swelling of the extremities.

It is important to provide safe and appropriate therapy relative to the expected outcome of therapy. Medications utilized in hospice care are often for off-label uses and are administered outside of the usual dosage range. In addition, many medications used for symptom control are prone to diversion for recreational use. In order to effectively deliver pharmacologic medication therapy for hospice care, it is important for institutions to develop policies and procedures governing the management and use of drugs for end of life care.

Noisy respirations are generally managed by placement of the patient in a semiprone position, reduction of parenteral hydration, explanation of the situation to family members and visitors, gentle nasopharyngeal or tracheal suctioning, and administration of anticholinergic medications. Transdermal scopolamine and parenteral glycopyrrolate are used in the management of noisy respirations. The commercially available patch delivers scopolamine 1 mg over 72 hours. A single patch may be sufficient for reduction of noisy respirations; however, additional patches can be applied without exceeding the daily dose of subcutaneous scopolamine administered to European hospice patients. Administration of scopolamine 1.2 mg per 24 hours by continuous subcutaneous infusion for reduction of noisy respirations is reported in the medical literature. Application of four patches is expected to deliver scopolamine 1.3 mg per 24 hours. Parenteral scopolamine is not licensed for use in the United States. Glycopyrrolate 0.2 mg can be administered by subcutaneous or intravenous bolus. Administration of glycopyrrolate 0.6 mg per 24 hours by continuous subcutaneous infusion for management of noisy respirations is reported in the medical literature. Administration of parenteral medications can be difficult for patients who are dying at home or outside of a hospital. In such circumstances, ipratropium bromide 0.03% nasal solution may provide an alternative to glycopyrrolate. Sublingual administration of ipratropium bromide 0.03% nasal solution two sprays 1-3 times daily is reportedly effective for reduction of drug induced sialorrhea. One drawback to sublingual administration may be erratic absorption for patients with excess secretions in the oral cavity. Atropine 1% ophthalmic drops are a suboptimal selection because each drop of solution delivers 0.5 mg of atropine, which is a pharmacologic dose that can modulate heart rate.

Opioid therapy is the cornerstone of treatment for pain and dyspnea in hospice care. Opioid requirements tend to increase in the dying patient. The proportion of dying patients requiring opioids expands from 42% one week before death to 78% during the final 48 hours of life. In addition, the daily opioid dose increases 2-3 fold during the same time frame. Increased opioid requirements are thought to be due to progression of the patient's underlying pathophysiologic problems instead of the development of tolerance. (Refer to Chronic Pain Management (Cancer) on page 1840 and Palliative Care Medicine (Cancer) on page 1871.)

Pharmacologic sedation is often required for end of life delirium restlessness and agitation. Normally the goal of sedation is to manage symptoms without appreciably reducing the patient's level of consciousness. End of life sedation has not been shown to shorten survival. Sedation during hospice care can include proportional palliative sedation (PPS) or, less commonly, palliative sedation to achieve unconsciousness (PSU). The goal of PPS is to provide an adequate amount of sedation for symptom control and maintain consciousness, as much as possible. Gradual titration of a benzodiazepine is commonly used for PPS. Two of the most commonly studied benzodiazepines for end of life sedation are midazolam and lorazepam. Additional drugs that have been utilized for end of life sedation are propofol and phenobarbital. Respiratory depression caused by phenobarbital should be considered when this product is administered. Limited information describes use of chlorpromazine and haloperidol for end of life restlessness and agitation. Chlorpromazine is suboptimal because it lowers the seizure threshold. Haloperidol should be reserved for use in patients with concurrent delirium. The potential for QT_c interval prolongation with haloperidol should be considered with use of this product. The goal of PSU is to induce unconsciousness. This is reserved for refractory cases with unbearable symptoms. PSU is generally accomplished by rapid titration of a benzodiazepine to the state of unconsciousness, with continuation of adequate doses to maintain unconsciousness.

SELECTED READINGS

Back IN, Jenkins K, Blower A, et al, "A Study Comparing Hyoscine Hydrobromide and Glycopyrrolate in the Treatment of Death Rattle," *Palliat Med*, 2001, 15(4):329-36.

Hales S, Zimmermann C, and Rodin G, "The Quality of Dying and Death," *Arch Intern Med*, 2008, 168(9):912-8.

Hugel H, Ellershaw J, and Gambles M, "Respiratory Tract Secretions in the Dying Patient: A Comparison Between Glycopyrronium snd Hyoscine Hydrobromide," *J Palliat Med*, 2006, 9 (2):279-84.

Kåss RM and Ellershaw J, "Respiratory Tract Secretions in the Dying Patient: A Retrospective Study," *J Pain Symptom Manage*, 2003, 26(4):897-902.

Kehl KA, "Treatment of Terminal Restlessness: A Review of the Evidence," *J Pain Palliat Care Pharmacother*, 2004, 18(1):5-30.

Kintzel PE, Chase SL, Thomas W, et al, "Anticholinergic Medications for Managing Noisy Respirations in Adult Hospice Patients," *Am J Health Syst Pharm*, 2009, 66(5):458-64.

Maltoni M, Scarpi E, Rosati M, et al, "Palliative Sedation in End-of-Life Care and Survival: A Systematic Review," *J Clin Oncol*, 2012, 30(12):1378-83.

Morita T, Ichiki T, Tsunoda J, et al, "A Prospective Study on the Dying Process in Terminally Ill Cancer Patients," *Am J Hosp Palliat Care*, 1998, 15(4):217-22.

Pantilat SZ and Isaac M, "End-of-Life Care for the Hospitalized Patient," *Med Clin North Am*, 2008, 92(2):349-70.

Quill TE, Lo B, Brock DW, et al, "Last-Resort Options for Palliative Sedation," *Ann Intern Med*, 2009, 151(6):421-4.

HYPERCALCEMIA OF MALIGNANCY

INTRODUCTION

Hypercalcemia of malignancy (HCM) affects 20% to 30% of patients with advanced cancer. It is the most frequently occurring life-threatening metabolic disorder in this patient population. The highest incidence is seen in patients with lung, breast, and renal cell cancers. In addition to these solid tumors, HCM is also commonly observed in patients with the hematologic malignancies multiple myeloma and human T-cell lymphotropic virus type I (HTLV-1)-associated T-cell lymphoma. Even with appropriate treatment, 30-day mortality rates following the HCM diagnosis approach 50% (Stewart, 2005). Poor prognostic indicators include corrected serum calcium exceeding 11.3 mg/dL (hazard ratio [HR]: 2.21), serum albumin <3.6 g/dL (HR: 2.41), squamous cell carcinoma (HR: 2.64), and metastatic disease affecting the bone (HR: 1.44) or liver (HR: 2.22) (Penel, 2008).

PATHOPHYSIOLOGY

The primary cause of HCM is increased bone resorption secondary to osteoclast activation which is mediated by proteins and cytokines released by tumor cells or their microenvironment. HCM can be classified into 4 types (local humoral, osteolytic, calcitriol secreting lymphomas, and ectopic hyperparathyroidism). Parathyroid-hormone-related protein (PTHrP)-mediated hypercalcemia (or humoral HCM) is the most common cause in solid tumors without bone metastasis. PTHrP released by the tumor initially stimulates osteoblasts to secrete receptor activator of nuclear factor-kappa ligand (RANKL). RANKL activates osteoclasts, resulting in increased bone resorption. PTHrP also promotes calcium renal tubular reabsorption. In patients with bone metastasis, local osteoclastic bone resorption is increased in the areas surrounding the tumor within the marrow space. Some lymphomas produce calcitriol ($1,25(OH)_2D3$), leading to hypercalcemia due to increased osteoclastic bone resorption and enhanced intestinal absorption of calcium. Lastly, a very rare cause of HCM is ectopic secretion of parathyroid hormone (PTH).

SYMPTOMS AND DIAGNOSIS

One early sign of hypercalcemia is polyuria, which develops as the body tries to eliminate excess ionized calcium from the serum. Polyuria causes intravascular volume depletion and dehydration, which signals the body to retain sodium. The ensuing renotubular reabsorption of sodium promotes concurrent reabsorption of calcium which fuels the hypercalcemia. Acute renal impairment may occur due to intravascular volume depletion and calcium-phosphate precipitation in the renal tubules. Neurologic adverse effects are generally the most serious sequelae of hypercalcemia. Confusion is common and patients can progress to somnolence and coma. Malaise and muscle weakness occur. Gastrointestinal adverse effects include anorexia, constipation, ileus, nausea, and vomiting. Cardiac effects include bradycardia and other dysrhythmias. Symptom severity is related to the degree of hypercalcemia and the rate at which the serum calcium increased.

Diagnosis of HCM is confirmed with laboratory measurement of serum calcium levels. As total calcium levels are associated with patients' albumin stores, it is important to calculate the serum ionized calcium level using the equation [corrected Ca++ (mg/dL) = measured serum Ca++ (mg/dL) + 0.8 x (4 - measured serum albumin in g/dL)]. However, this equation may not always accurately reflect true ionized calcium levels; in such cases, directly measuring serum ionized calcium is prudent. PTH and PTHrP may be measured in the occasional cases in which the cause of hypercalcemia is not clear. Likewise, 1,25$(OH)_2$D3 levels may be assessed if sarcoidosis or other granulomatous conditions, or the 1,25 $(OH)_2$D3 lymphoma syndrome, is in the differential diagnosis.

Body System	Symptoms
General	Dehydration, weight loss, pruritis, polydipsia
Neuromuscular	Fatigue, lethargy, muscle weakness, hyporeflexia, confusion, psychosis, seizure, obtundation, coma
Gastrointestinal	Anorexia, nausea, vomiting, constipation, ileus
Renal	Polyuria, renal insufficiency
Cardiac	Bradycardia, prolonged PR, shortened QT, wide T wave, arrhythmias

MANAGEMENT

The first treatment priority of HCM is reversal of dehydration to reduce the serum calcium concentration and preserve renal function. Once normovolemia is restored, furosemide is often added; however, the primary role of a loop diuretic in this situation is to prevent volume overload. First-line therapies to reduce bone resorption include bisphosphonates and calcitonin. Second-line therapies include corticosteroids for multiple myeloma and lymphoid malignancies, and gallium nitrate. Hemodialysis may be necessary in severe cases of hypercalcemia. Treatment of the underlying malignancy is also an option for reducing HCM for some patients. However, the metabolic benefits of effective anticancer treatment may not be clinically evident for a period of weeks to months. Unfortunately, many patients with HCM have cancer that has progressed despite the standard anticancer therapies.

Treatment is based on symptomatology and the serum calcium level. The criteria for initiation of treatment are generally hypercalcemia with signs of toxicity (polyuria, mental status changes, renal dysfunction, cardiac dysrhythmias) attributed to hypercalcemia. A total calcium level exceeding 13 mg/dL is cited as criteria for initiation of therapy; although, it is unusual for HCM to present without related symptomatology.

0.9% Sodium Chloride

The intravenous fluid used for rehydration is 0.9% sodium chloride because it effectively improves intravascular volume and promotes renal excretion of calcium. The rate of administration of sodium chloride depends on the degree of dehydration, the severity of hypercalcemia, and the cardiopulmonary status of the patient. Ideally, patients should receive 0.9% sodium chloride at a rate of 2-3 L/m^2 per 24 hours; however, this often must be attenuated relative to what the patient's cardiopulmonary status can accommodate. Hydration rates as high as 5 L/m^2 per 24 hours have been used in severe cases. Following rehydration, proximal tubular reabsorption of sodium, and therefore calcium, will decrease. Further, other treatments for hypercalcemia require prior volume replacement in order to minimize toxicities. Sodium chloride can lower serum calcium by approximately 2 mg/dL. Saline hydration has an immediate but transient effect. Even if normocalcemia is achieved, serum calcium will increase again unless additional treatments aimed at reducing bone resorption or treating the underlying malignancy are administered.

Furosemide

The major use of furosemide in the management of cancer-associated hypercalcemia is to prevent and manage fluid overload in order to facilitate the administration of sodium chloride for volume replacement. A usual starting dose of furosemide is 10-20 mg by intravenous push every 6-12 hours around the clock or as needed to maintain an acceptable rate of urine output. Loop diuretics are not effective agents for enhancing renal excretion of calcium. Loop diuretics should be used with caution to avoid intravascular volume depletion with exacerbation of hypercalcemia and renal impairment.

Bisphosphonates

Bisphosphonates bind to hydroxyapatite in bone and inhibit osteoclastic bone resorption. Pamidronate and zoledronic acid are the most commonly used bisphosphonates for management of HCM. Intravenous ibandronate is also a treatment option for this condition. The dose of intravenous ibandronate used for HCM in clinical trials is 2 mg or 4 mg. In a randomized, double-blind comparison with 275 of 287 subjects evaluable for efficacy zoledronic acid was superior to pamidronate for normalization of serum calcium by day 4 (50% versus 33% of patients) and day 10 (88% versus 70% of patients) of therapy. The median duration of normocalcemia was 32 days for zoledronic acid 4 mg and 18 days for pamidronate 90 mg. However, the frequency of renal impairment was greater in the zoledronic acid treatment arm.

Bisphosphonates should be used with caution in patients with severe renal impairment because these products are eliminated by the kidneys and can cause nephrotoxicity. Pamidronate has not been studied in patients with serum creatinine exceeding 3 mg/dL or creatinine clearance less than 30 mL/minute. Renal dosage adjustment of zoledronic acid administered for the treatment of HCM is not warranted when the serum creatinine is less than 4.5 mg/dL. The manufacturer of intravenous ibandronate recommends against use of this product for serum creatinine exceeding 2.3 mg/dL or creatinine clearance less than 30 mL/min.

Common side effects of bisphosphonates are mild and include fever and infusion site reactions, such as phlebitis. Avascular osteonecrosis of the jaw (ONJ) is an infrequent but serious adverse effect of bisphosphonate therapy. ONJ can be an extremely painful condition. Most reported cases of ONJ involve cancer patients receiving intravenous bisphosphonate therapy while undergoing dental procedures. Risk factors for ONJ during bisphosphonate therapy include cancer, chemotherapy, radiotherapy, corticosteroids, poor oral hygiene, pre-existing dental disease or infection, anemia, and coagulopathy. Patients should maintain good oral hygiene and have a dental examination with preventive dentistry prior to treatment with bisphosphonates. Another adverse effect identified in women receiving bisphosphonate therapy for postmenopausal osteoporosis is severe musculoskeletal pain that develops within days, weeks or months of beginning treatment. This condition may become debilitating and necessitate discontinuation of bisphosphonate therapy.

Calcitonin

Calcitonin works in a receptor-mediated manner to inhibit bone resorption and enhance urinary excretion of calcium. It is the fastest acting of the agents used to treat hypercalcemia and may be given safely before rehydration is complete. The usual starting dose of calcitonin is 4 units/kg by subcutaneous injection every 12 hours. Side effects are mild and infrequent and include nausea, abdominal cramps, and flushing. Calcitonin lowers serum calcium by approximately 2 mg/dL. Resistance to the pharmacologic effects of calcitonin generally develops with a few days of therapy. In fact, this can become apparent clinically as rebound hypercalcemia.

Corticosteroids

Corticosteroid administration is added to therapy when the underlying malignancy is a steroid-responsive disease, such as multiple myeloma, and lymphoma.

Gallium Nitrate

Gallium nitrate decreases serum calcium by adsorbing to hydroxyapatite and inhibiting bone resorption. It is given as a continuous intravenous infusion at a dose of 200 mg/m^2/day for 5 days. Most patients respond to gallium nitrate; however, its use is limited by the risk of nephrotoxicity and the cumbersome administration schedule. Gallium nitrate reduces serum calcium approximately 3 mg/dL after a complete 5-day course of therapy. Gallium nitrate was initially tested as an anticancer drug at higher daily doses than those used for hypercalcemia administered intravenously over 15-30 minutes. Dose limiting adverse effects were nephrotoxicity, neurotoxicity, and hypocalcemia. Nephrotoxicity attributed to gallium nitrate administration has been reported in patients treated for hypercalcemia. Nephrotoxicity may be potentiated by other nephrotoxic drugs. Gallium should not be used in patients with serum creatinine >2.5 mg/dL. Because of the potential for nephrotoxicity and the inconvenient dosing schedule relative to other agents, gallium should not be considered a first-line treatment for hypercalcemia.

Other

Bortezomib has a dual anticancer and bone stabilizing effect. This medication, which is used in the treatment of multiple myeloma and mantle cell lymphoma, stimulates osteoblast differentiation, and inhibits osteoclast formation and bone resorption independently of its anticancer effect. The human monoclonal antibody denosumab targets the mediator of bone resorption RANKL. Denosumab is effective in reducing the incidence of skeletal-related events in patients with bone metastases due to solid tumors, such as lung, breast, and prostate. While not indicated for treatment of HCM, denosumab has been used in a patient (case report) who was unable to receive bisphosphonate therapy (Bech, 2012). Hypocalcemia has been reported with denosumab use; monitor serum calcium levels accordingly.

Drug	Usual Dose	Onset of Effect (h)	Duration of Effect
Bisphosphonates			
Pamidronate	60 or 90 mg	24-48	Median 10 days (1-30)
Zoledronic acid	4 mg	24-48	Median 10 days (1-30)
Calcitonin	4 units/kg q12h	4	Median 2 day (1-6)
Gallium nitrate	200 mg/m^2/24 h x 5 d	24-48	Median 6 days
0.9% sodium chloride	2-3 L/m^2/24-hr	12-48	Transient

Treatments are listed in alphabetical order. See text for guidance on priority and order of use.

REFERENCES

Bech A and de Boer H, "Denosumab for Tumor-Induced Hypercalcemia Complicated by Renal Failure," *Ann Intern Med*, 2012, 156(12):906-7.

LeGrand SB, Leskuski D, and Zama I, "Narrative Review: Furosemide for Hypercalcemia: An Unproven Yet Common Practice," *Ann Intern Med*, 2008, 149(4):259-63.

Lumachi F, Brunello A, Roma A, et al, "Cancer-Induced Hypercalcemia," *Anticancer Res*, 2009, 29 (5):1551-5.

Major P, Lortholary A, Hon J, et al, "Zoledronic Acid Is Superior to Pamidronate in the Treatment of Hypercalcemia of Malignancy: A Pooled Analysis of Two Randomized, Controlled Clinical Trials," *J Clin Oncol*, 2001, 19(2):558-67.

Nussbaum SR, Younger J, Vandepol CJ, et al, "Single-Dose Intravenous Therapy With Pamidronate for the Treatment of Hypercalcemia of Malignancy: Comparison of 30-, 60-, and 90-mg Dosages," *Am J Med*, 1993, 95(3):297-304.

Penel N, Dewas S, Doutrelant P, et al, "Cancer-Associated Hypercalcemia Treated With Intravenous Diphosphonates: A Survival and Prognostic Factor Analysis," *Support Care Cancer*, 2008, 16(4):387-92.

Perlia CP, Gubisch NJ, Wolter J, et al, "Mithramycin Treatment of Hypercalcemia," *Cancer*, 1970, 25:389-94.

Shemerdiak WP, Kukreja SC, Lad TE, et al, "Evaluation of Routine Ionized Calcium Determination in Cancer Patients," *Clin Chem*, 1981, 27:1621-2.

Stewart AF, "Clinical Practice. Hypercalcemia Associated With Cancer," *N Engl J Med*, 2005, 352 (4):373-9.

Warrell RP Jr, Israel R, Frisone M, et al, "Gallium Nitrate for Acute Treatment of Cancer-Related Hypercalcemia. A Randomized, Double-Blind Comparison to Calcitonin," *Ann Intern Med*, 1988, 108(5):699-74.

MALIGNANT PLEURAL EFFUSIONS

Malignant pleural effusion is an accumulation of fluid in the pleural space separating the lung and chest wall. It may be attributed to primary tumor growth, direct extension of tumor from an adjacent anatomic structure, or metastatic dissemination to the affected area. By definition, malignant pleural effusion must contain cancer cells. Breast, lung, and lymphoid malignancies account for two-thirds of malignant pleural effusions, but they are also found with gastric cancer, ovarian carcinomas, and mesothelioma. Case reports describe malignant pleural effusions with juvenile granulose cell tumor, pulmonary leiomyosarcoma, pleural liposarcoma, malignant melanoma, primitive neuroendocrine tumor, renal medullary carcinoma, and salivary gland cancer. A malignant pleural effusion may be the presenting sign of cancer, but most often it is a complication of a previously diagnosed malignancy. The median duration of survival following the diagnosis of malignant pleural effusion is 4 months; however, prolonged survival is possible in some cases. Predictors of less favorable outcome include high-risk tumors, poor performance status, lower pleural fluid glucose levels, leukocytosis, hypoxemia, and hypoalbuminemia.

PATHOPHYSIOLOGY

The pleura is a thin membrane that covers the lungs and chest wall. It is composed of the visceral pleura (covering the surface of the lungs) and the parietal pleura (covering the thoracic cavity). The interface between the two surfaces is the pleural space. Normally, pleural fluid production is <100 mL/day. Movement of fluid within the pleural space is governed by hydrostatic and oncotic pressures that follow Starling's law of transcapillary exchange. Hydrostatic pressure in the parietal capillaries is higher, causing a net movement into the pleural space. Reabsorption of the fluid occurs primarily through lymphatics on the parietal surface and less prominently via lymphatics on the visceral surface. Changes in pleural fluid production, reabsorption, or both produce a pleural effusion.

Malignancies can cause a fluid imbalance within the pleural space in several ways. Malignant cells in the pleural space can cause an inflammatory response that increases both capillary permeability and the net filtration of fluid, proteins, and cells into the pleural space. In addition, malignant obstruction of lymphatic channels and changes in pleural fluid protein content can impair reabsorption and drainage of fluid from the pleural space. The resulting fluid accumulation is exudative and is characterized by an increased concentration of protein and cells, decreased glucose levels compared to the serum, and an absence of eosinophils.

CLINICAL SYMPTOMS AND DIAGNOSIS

The most common symptom is dyspnea, often in conjunction with cough, chest pain, tachypnea, and reduced exercise tolerance. Symptoms are often related not to the amount of pleural fluid present, but to the rate of fluid accumulation. Patients with pleural effusions may be asymptomatic. A diagnosis often begins with a chest x-ray, which will demonstrate fluid accumulation on the posteroanterior (PA) and lateral decubitus film. Physical findings include dullness to percussion, decreased breath sounds, decreased diaphragmatic excursion, and possible contralateral tracheal deviation. In asymptomatic patients, malignant pleural effusion is generally diagnosed incidentally from radiographic imaging performed for other reasons.

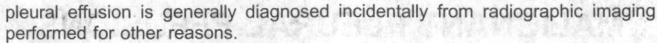

TREATMENT PRINCIPLES

The goal of treatment is to effectively provide symptomatic relief with the least amount of risk and discomfort to the patient. Mainstays of therapy include fluid drainage (thoracentesis) with prevention of fluid reaccumulation by way of pleurodesis or an implanted pleural catheter. Successful palliation of dyspnea is possible with either pleurodesis or chronic drainage. Not all patients benefit from treatment. Some patients with effusions are asymptomatic and may not require treatment until symptoms develop. Individuals with a life expectancy of <1 month might only require oxygen, opioids, and possibly thoracentesis.

SYSTEMIC AND RADIATION THERAPY

Malignant pleural effusions arising from treatment-sensitive cancers are managed with systemic or radiation therapy intended to reduce the effusion by treating the underlying malignant cause. Improvement of malignant pleural effusions with systemic or radiation therapy is most likely to occur when the underlying cause is lymphoma, small cell lung cancer, germ cell tumor, breast cancer, ovarian cancer, prostate cancer, or thyroid cancer. Systemic therapy may be administered in addition to local therapy (effusion drainage) and pleurodesis (local instillation of treatment).

LOCAL THERAPY

Thoracentesis is the process of removing fluid from the pleural space using a specialized catheter and syringe under local anesthetic. This procedure can be done at the bedside and is utilized frequently for symptomatic patients. Thoracentesis is ineffective for long-term control of the malignant pleural effusion. Recurrence is frequent and repeated procedures carry a risk of increased complications, such as pneumothorax; ultrasound-guided thoracentesis can be performed to reduce this risk.

Tube thoracostomy (chest tube) is effective in controlling a malignant pleural effusion for a short period of time. Its 30-day success rate is approximately 70%. However, it is ineffective in the long-term control of effusions. Tubal thoracostomy is most useful in draining the fluid from the pleural space prior to instilling a sclerosing agent.

Indwelling pleural catheters with small bore tubing can be placed subcutaneously to provide long-term drainage of malignant pleural effusions. Patients can be educated to drain the catheters on a routine basis or as needed for symptom relief. The most common complication is pain or other symptoms due to intrapleural loculations, which occur in approximately 8% of cases. Additional complications reported in <5% of cases include unsuccessful insertion, asymptomatic loculations, cellulitis, empyema, and pneumothorax. Pleuroperitoneal shunts represent another tool that can be used for management of malignant pleural effusion.

PLEURODESIS

Pleurodesis, or sclerosis, should be considered in patients who experience symptomatic relief from thoracentesis with complete lung re-expansion and who have a life expectancy of at least weeks to months. The primary goals of pleurodesis are prevention of effusion reaccumulation and reduced hospitalizations for thoracentesis. Sclerosing agents act by promoting an inflammatory response in the pleura that causes fibrin adhesions of the visceral and parietal pleura. This results in fixed obliteration of the pleural space, which is prohibitive to recurrent effusion accumulation. Sclerosing agents are administered via a thoracostomy tube following demonstration of adequate effusate drainage (<200 mL/day).

The efficacy of pleurodesis is categorized as complete success, partial success, or failure. Criteria for complete success are long-term symptom relief and absence of fluid reaccumulation. Criteria for partial success are improved symptomatology with <50% of fluid reaccumulation without additional thoracentesis. Any less of a response is categorized as pleurodesis failure.

Successful use of a sclerosing agent depends on its uniform distribution in the pleural space and the dose of selected drug. The presence of loculations within the pleural space can interfere with distribution of the sclerosing agent. Immediate and complete lung expansion is desirable for pleurodesis. However, the clinical outcome for patients experiencing partial lung expansion is similar with respect to quality of life, procedure-related complications, extent of effusion drainage, hospital stay duration, and overall survival. Effective lung expansion and durable prevention of effusion reaccumulation may be related to tumor type. Patients with lung cancer and mesothelioma tend to have a less favorable response to pleurodesis in comparison to patients with breast or other cancers. Another factor that influences the efficacy of pleurodesis is the extent of tumor involving the pleural space. Preclinical data suggests that inhibition of vascular endothelial growth factor is deleterious to successful pleurodesis due to impeded adhesion formation (Teixeira, 2011).

SCLEROSING AGENTS

Talc is one of the oldest and most effective sclerosing agents for treatment of malignant pleural effusions. Successful talc pleurodesis is achieved in 70% to 96% of patients. Meta-analysis infers that talc is a more effective sclerosing agent than bleomycin or tetracycline and tetracycline analogues. Pharmaceutical grade sterile asbestos-free talc is commercially available for use as a sclerosing agent. Talc powder is prepared as a sterile slurry for bedside administration through a chest tube. The usual dose of talc slurry is 5 g in 50-100 mL of 0.9% sodium chloride. Powdered talc is also available in a pressurized spray canister for administration under video-assisted thoracic surgery (VATS, thoracoscopy) or open thoracotomy. Aerosolized talc is available in single use 4 g canisters; the usual dose is 4-8 g. Pain and fever are the most common acute side effects of pleurodesis. Rare serious adverse effects of talc pleurodesis include adult respiratory distress syndrome (ARDS), pneumonia, empyema, hemoptysis, bronchopleural fistula, tachycardia, hypotension, and infection. Cases of ARDS have occurred in patients receiving instillations of talc slurry 10 g.

The TIME2 study compared symptom control with talc pleurodesis vs an indwelling pleural catheter in 106 cases of previously untreated malignant pleural effusion. A 100 mm visual analogue scale (VAS) was used to measure dyspnea; a score of 0 mm indicated no dyspnea and a score of 100 mm indicated maximal dyspnea. Dyspnea was similarly improved in both groups for the initial 6 weeks of therapy (p=0.96). Assessment at 6 months identified a mean VAS score difference of 14 mm favoring symptom palliation in the group with implanted pleural catheters. This finding was statistically significant (p=0.01); however, it did not translate into a difference in quality of life between the two groups (p=0.14). More patients treated with talc pleurodesis (22%) required additional pleural procedures for symptom control compared to those with implanted pleural catheters (6%) (p=0.03). In addition, pleurodesis required hospitalization for a median 4 days (interquartile range, 2-6 days); whereas, catheter implantation was generally an entirely outpatient procedure (initial hospitalization for median 0 days [interquartile range: 0-1 days]). Treatment-related adverse events were more common in patients with implanted pleural catheters (40%) than in patients treated with pleurodesis (13%) (p=0.002) (Davies, 2012).

Bleomycin 1 mg/kg (1 unit/kg) in 100 mL of 0.9% sodium chloride is an effective agent for controlling malignant pleural effusions. The range of intrapleural bleomycin doses reported in the literature is 24-240 mg. However, due to a lack of increased efficacy at doses >60 mg, some authors have recommended limiting the dose to 60 mg or 1 mg/kg body weight. Bleomycin has not demonstrated an efficacy advantage over talc and the acquisition cost of bleomycin is substantially greater than that of talc (Haddad, 2004). Common toxicities associated with intrapleural bleomycin include pain, fever, and gastrointestinal adverse effects (nausea, vomiting, diarrhea). Serious adverse effects are more common in patients with elderly age or reduced renal function.

Parenteral tetracycline was one of the most widely used sclerosing agents prior to its removal from the market in the mid-1990s. Doxycycline 500 mg injection mixed in 50-100 mL of 0.9% sodium chloride effectively treats pleural effusions in 50% to 75% of patients; however, repeated instillations are generally required to achieve results similar to tetracycline. Intrapleural minocycline following VATS for spontaneous pneumothorax reduced prolonged postoperative air leaks, chest drainage, and hospital days for 313 patients relative to 51 consecutive historical controls (Chen, 2004). The author reported administration of minocycline 300-400 mg injection in 20 mL of 0.9% sodium chloride through a chest tube. Due to a lack of stability information, this dose of minocycline should be prepared immediately before use. Chest pain was a common complaint after pleurodesis with minocycline.

Additional products that have been used as sclerosing agents for pleurodesis are povidone iodine, silver nitrate, distilled water, quinacrine, *Corynebacterium parvum*, interferon-α, and interferon-β.

OTHER

Intrapleural administration of cytotoxic chemotherapy is reported. Its use is based on the premise that cytotoxic chemotherapy can exert anticancer and proinflammatory actions. In addition, intrapleural administration of chemotherapy may yield a regional advantage with intrapleural drug levels greatly exceeding drug levels in the plasma (Heffner, 2008; Lombardi, 2010). The reader is cautioned that the safety and efficacy of intrapleural administration of cytotoxic chemotherapy is not extensively tested.

A phase II study tested intrapleural administration of paclitaxel 120 mg/m^2 for the treatment of malignant pleural effusion in 18 patients with ovarian cancer (11 patients) or breast cancer (7 patients). Paclitaxel was infused after thoracentesis. The catheter used for paclitaxel administration was clamped for a period of 24 hours, after which it remained in place until drainage was <200 mL over 24 hours. Objective response (complete plus partial success rate) at 1 month and 2 months following treatment was reported in 78% and 89% of patients, respectively. Common side effects included chest pain, fever, and dyspnea. Pleural fluid paclitaxel concentrations were approximately 10,000-fold greater than those measured in the plasma. The half-life of intrapleural paclitaxel was approximately

68 hours (Lombardi, 2012). A phase I study with pharmacokinetic analysis of intrapleural docetaxel 50-125 mg/m^2 reported a 1000-fold difference in concurrent drug concentrations measured in the pleural fluid relative to those in the plasma. This relative AUC from 0-36 hours for docetaxel in pleural fluid was 2000-7000 times greater than the corresponding plasma AUC (Jones, 2010).

GENERAL PLEURODESIS PROCEDURE

Effusate is drained via a chest tube until the fluid production is <200 mL/day. The patient is premedicated with systemic analgesia (usually a parenteral opioid), sedation, and intrapleural administration of a topical anesthetic (typically lidocaine 1%). The sclerosing agent is instilled through the chest tube and the tube is clamped for 30 minutes to 2 hours. Some procedures include frequent repositioning of the patient during the time that the chest tube is clamped to facilitate uniform distribution of the sclerosing agent, although the efficacy of repositioning is untested and its use is controversial. The tube is then unclamped, reconnected to water-seal suction until production is <100-200 mL/day, and the chest tube is removed.

COMPLICATIONS

Management of malignant pleural effusions is associated with several complications. Pain from insertion of the chest tube or instillation of the sclerosing agent should be pretreated with parenteral opioids. Traction pneumothorax results from repeated attempts to re-expand the lung. Cough is caused by lung re-expansion and is self-limiting. Fluid loculation is associated with drainage and pleurodesis. Lysis of adhesions may be necessary prior to pleurodesis. Empyema (purulent fluid) formation from contamination or bronchopulmonary communication should be treated with appropriate antibiotics.

REFERENCES

Antonangelo L, Rosa AG, Corá AP, et al, "Uncommon Pleural Effusion: Pleuropulmonary Metastasis From Primitive Neuroectodermal Tumor," *J Bras Pneumol*, 2009, 35(6):606-9.

Bielsa S, Hernández P, Rodriguez-Panadero F, et al, "Tumor Type Influences the Effectiveness of Pleurodesis in Malignant Effusions," *Lung*, 2011, 189(2):151-5.

Chen JS, Hsu HH, Kuo SW, et al, "Effects of Additional Minocycline Pleurodesis After Thoracoscopic Procedures For Primary Spontaneous Pneumothorax," *Chest*, 2004, 125(1):50-5.

Dagli AF, Pehlivan S, Ozercan MR, et al, "Pleural Liposarcoma Mimicking Carcinoma in Pleural Effusion Cytology: A Case Report," *Acta Cytol*, 2010, 54(4):601-4.

Davies HE, Mishra EK, Kahan BC, et al, "Effect of an Indwelling Pleural Catheter Vs Chest Tube and Talc Pleurodesis for Relieving Dyspnea in Patients With Malignant Pleural Effusion: The TIME2 Randomized Controlled Trial," *JAMA*, 2012, 307(22):2383-9.

Ellis CL, Burroughs F, Michael CW, et al, "Cytology of Metastatic Renal Medullary Carcinoma in Pleural Effusion: A Study of Two Cases," *Diagn Cytopathol*, 2009, 37(11):843-8.

Haddad FJ, Younes RN, Gross JL, et al, "Pleurodesis in Patients With Malignant Pleural Effusions: Talc Slurry or Bleomycin? Results of a Prospective Randomized Trial," *World J Surg*, 2004, 28(8):749-53.

Heffner JE and Klein JS, "Recent Advances in the Diagnosis and Management of Malignant Pleural Effusions," *Mayo Clin Proc*, 2008, 83(2):235-50.

Hirata T, Yonemori K, Hirakawa A, et al, "Efficacy of Pleurodesis for Malignant Pleural Effusions in Breast Cancer Patients," *Eur Respir J*, 2011, 38(6):1425-30.

Jones DR, Taylor MD, Petroni GR, et al, "Phase I Trial of Intrapleural Docetaxel Administered Through an Implantable Catheter in Subjects With a Malignant Pleural Effusion," *J Thorac Oncol*, 2010, 5(1):75-81.

Kaifi JT, Toth JW, Gusani NJ, et al, "Multidisciplinary Management of Malignant Pleural Effusion," *J Surg Oncol*, 2012, 105(7):731-8.

Kaur H, Bagga R, Saha SC, et al, "Juvenile Granulosa Cell Tumor of the Ovary Presenting With Pleural Effusion and Ascites," *Int J Clin Oncol*, 2009, 14(1):78-81.

Kriegel I, Daniel C, Falcou MC, et al, "Use of a Subcutaneous Implantable Pleural Port in the Management of Recurrent Malignant Pleurisy: Five-Year Experience Based on 168 Subcutaneous Implantable Pleural Ports," *J Palliat Med*, 2011, 14(7):829-34

Kubo A, Koh Y, Kawaguchi T, et al, "Malignant Pleural Effusion From Lung Adenocarcinoma Treated by Gefitinib," *Intern Med*, 2011, 50(7):745-8.

Lombardi G, Nicoletto MO, Gusella M, et al, "Intrapleural Paclitaxel for Malignant Pleural Effusion From Ovarian and Breast Cancer: A Phase II Study With Pharmacokinetic Analysis," *Cancer Chemother Pharmacol*, 2012, 69(3):781-7.

Lombardi G, Zustovich F, Nicoletto MO, et al, "Diagnosis and Treatment of Malignant Pleural Effusion: A Systematic Literature Review and New Approaches," *Am J Clin Oncol*, 2010, 33 (4):420-3.

Mitra S, Kundu S, Pattari SK, et al, "Metastatic Pleural Effusion: A Rare Presentation of Salivary Gland Adenoid Cystic Carcinoma," *Indian J Chest Dis Allied Sci*, 2011, 53(2):107-10.

Ozyurtkan MO, Balci AE, and Cakmak M, "Predictors of Mortality Within Three Months in the Patients With Malignant Pleural Effusion," *Eur J Intern Med*, 2010, 21(1):30-4.

Passamonte PM and Luger AM, "Primary Pulmonary Leiomyosarcoma With Digital Clubbing and Pleural Effusion. Case Report," *Mo Med*, 1984, 81(10):667-8.

Pilling JE, Dusmet ME, Ladas G, et al, "Prognostic Factors for Survival After Surgical Palliation of Malignant Pleural Effusion," *J Thorac Oncol*, 2010, 5(10):1544-50.

Rodriguez-Panadero F and Montes-Worboys A, "Mechanisms of Pleurodesis," *Respiration*, 2012, 83(2):91-8.

Shameem M, Akhtar J, Baneen U, et al, "Malignant Melanoma Presenting as an Isolated Pleural Effusion," *Monaldi Arch Chest Dis*, 2011, 75(2):138-40.

Shaw P and Agarwal R, "Pleurodesis For Malignant Pleural Effusions," *Cochrane Database Syst Rev*, 2004, (1):CD002916.

Suzuki K, Servais EL, Rizk NP, et al, "Palliation and Pleurodesis in Malignant Pleural Effusion: The Role for Tunneled Pleural Catheters," *J Thorac Oncol*, 2011, 6(4):762-7.

Teixeira LR, Vargas FS, Acencio MM, et al, "Blockage of Vascular Endothelial Growth Factor (VEGF) Reduces Experimental Pleurodesis," *Lung Cancer*, 2011, 74(3):392-5.

Terra RM, Junqueira JJ, Teixeira LR, et al, "Is Full Postpleurodesis Lung Expansion a Determinant of a Successful Outcome After Talc Pleurodesis?" *Chest*, 2009, 136(2):361-8.

PALLIATIVE CARE MEDICINE (CANCER)

SCOPE OF PALLIATIVE CARE MEDICINE

The National Consensus Project for Quality Palliative Care (2009) states "The goal of palliative care is to prevent and relieve suffering and to support the best possible quality of life for patients and their families, regardless of the stage of the disease or the need for other therapies. Palliative care is both a philosophy of care and an organized, highly structured system for delivering care. Palliative care expands traditional disease-model medical treatments to include the goals of enhancing quality of life for patient and family, optimizing function, helping with decision-making, and providing opportunities for personal growth. As such, it can be delivered concurrently with life-prolonging care or as the main focus of care." Palliative care is appropriate at any stage of a disease process as the primary approach to symptom management or in combination with standard therapy. Palliative care addresses symptoms arising from serious, life-threatening diseases and intractable symptoms from benign conditions that depreciate quality of life. Palliative care is often used in the management of patients with life expectancies extending months, years, or decades; however, it can also be an essential part of end-of-life (hospice) care.

The American Society of Clinical Oncology (ASCO) published a provisional clinical opinion stating that palliative care should be offered in addition to standard anticancer therapy at the time of initial diagnosis of metastatic nonsmall cell lung cancer (NSCLC) (Smith, 2012). Demonstration of improved patient and caregiver outcomes with addition of palliative care to standard therapy in randomized controlled clinical trials provided the impetus for this statement. Advantages conferred with palliative care in the management of metastatic NSCLC include improvement in symptom control, mood, patient satisfaction, and reduced caregiver burden (Pirl, 2012; Smith, 2012). In addition, appropriate utilization of hospice services and reduced futile intensive terminal care were substantiated with early initiation of palliative care. Longer median survival (P=0.02), despite less aggressive end-of-life care, was reported for 77 patients with metastatic NSCLC randomized to receive palliative care (in addition to standard anticancer therapy) at the time of initial diagnosis vs a cohort of 74 patients randomized to receive standard anticancer therapy without formalized palliative care services (Temel, 2010). Palliative care achieves these benefits without causing harm to the patient or caregiver, and without increasing the overall cost of care (Smith, 2012). The ASCO provisional clinical opinion acknowledges that stringently performed palliative care research is in its infancy and recommends the following investigative priorities: Optimal timing and venue (inpatient, outpatient/community) for palliative care, reimbursement models, interventions providing greatest benefit, benefit in diseases other than lung cancer, and impact of palliative care across the continuum of care (especially during the delivery of anticancer therapy).

Palliative care is provided most effectively by an interdisciplinary team specializing in this area of medicine. Clinical and regulatory challenges related to delivery of pharmaceutical products for palliative care impact the pharmacy department. One aspect of palliative care is symptom control for intractable situations following an adequate trial of the therapeutic standard of care. Subsequently, medications may be prescribed for off-label indications at doses outside of the norm and for administration by atypical routes. Moreover, since palliative care medicine is an evolving field, medical literature supporting the safety and efficacy of certain interventions may be scant. Some medications used for symptom control are controlled substances or prone to diversion, so stringent methods of drug accountability must be adhered to. Pharmacy departments should formalize policies and procedures to support the delivery of palliative pharmaceutical care.

SYMPTOM MANAGEMENT

Pain

The management of pain should be optimized as per standard clinical practice. Refer to Chronic Pain Management (Cancer) on page 1840. Opioid and non-opioid analgesic therapy should be optimized. Nonsteroidal anti-inflammatory drugs, bisphosphonates, and radiotherapy should be used as appropriate for bone pain. External beam radiation may be helpful for tumor size reduction with pain relief in some cases. Nonsteroidal anti-inflammatory drugs or corticosteroids should be used as warranted for inflammatory pain. Gabapentin, pregabalin, and antidepressants may improve neuropathic pain.

High doses of opioid analgesia may be required for intractable pain. The oral route of administration is preferred whenever possible. Opioid administration by continuous subcutaneous or intravenous infusion with or without patient-controlled PRN boluses is an option. Subcutaneous infusion of methadone should be avoided due to local irritation. Patients may require intraspinal opioid administration to achieve and tolerate adequate pain control.

Methadone can be administered by continuous intravenous infusion and patient-controlled analgesia. However, this intervention is often reserved for select patients as a bridge to intraspinal therapy because methadone prolongs the QT_c interval and there is discordance between the pharmacokinetics and pharmacodynamics of this drug. The risk of torsade de pointes is increased when the QT_c interval exceeds 500 milliseconds. Consensus guidelines (Shaiova, 2008) pertaining to intravenous administration of methadone recommend assessment of the QT_c interval at baseline, 24 hours and 4 days after initiation of methadone, and following any significant dose increase or at the discretion of the practitioner. More frequent monitoring of the QT_c interval should be considered for patients with a QT_c interval exceeding 450 milliseconds. Patients should be advised of the risk of dysrhythmias with methadone, so that they may make an informed decision about their therapy. Since the half-life of methadone exceeds the duration of analgesia, the consensus guidelines state that the initial rate titration must be done at least 12 hours after initiation of the infusion to allow evolution of side effects. Subsequent rate titrations should be done once daily. Liberal use of PRN boluses are recommended by the consensus guidelines before and between rate titration for methadone by continuous intravenous infusion. Due to incomplete cross-tolerance between methadone and high-dose morphine, the consensus guidelines recommend the following conversion factors (Shaiova, 2008). In addition, a 25% to 50% reduction in the calculated methadone dose at infusion initiation is recommended for patients requiring more than 50 mg/hour of morphine.

Opioid	Basal Rate (mg/h)	Methadone	
		Basal Rate (mg/h)	PRN Bolus Available Every 15 Minutes
Morphine	10	1	1
HYDROmorphone	1.5	0.3	0.3
FentaNYL	0.25	1.25	1.25

Intravenous lidocaine is used for severe intractable neuropathic pain. The efficacy of lidocaine is greater in the treatment of peripheral sensory neuropathy vs symptoms caused by a central pain syndrome. Small studies report administration of intravenous lidocaine 1-5 mg/kg over a period of 30 minutes to 6 hours. Some centers use a set dose of 100-150 mg infused intravenously over a period of 30-60 minutes. Analgesia superior to placebo is reported in crossover design trials. The reported time to maximum analgesia is 1-6 hours, with the reported duration of analgesia ranging from hours to days to weeks. Common adverse effects include lightheadedness, vertical nystagmus, feeling drunk, and sedation. The rapid metabolism of lidocaine probably allows administration of 1-5 mg/kg over a period of 30 minutes to 6 hours without cardiac or central nervous system toxicity. Caution should be exercised when using intravenous lidocaine in patients who are elderly, debilitated, or have poor hepatic function. One case series of three patients with neuropathic cancer pain describes chronic administration of lidocaine 100-160 mg/hour by continuous subcutaneous infusion. Periodic assessment of serum lidocaine levels should be considered with administration by continuous infusion.

Ketamine is used as an adjunct to opioid therapy for intractable cancer pain and neuropathic pain. Ketamine can be administered orally, intravenously, and subcutaneously. Ketamine can be administered intramuscularly; however, this route is rarely used for repeated administration. The dose of oral ketamine is 20-60 mg 3-4 times daily plus PRN administration of ketamine 20 mg every 3 hours. Tapering the dose at a rate of 25% per 24 hours may reduce the likelihood of dysphoria when ketamine is being discontinued. Ketamine is commercially available as a parenteral formulation. The oral dose can be mixed in cola immediately prior to ingestion. To reduce the risk of drug diversion or inadvertent ingestion by a family member, some institutions have the nurse squirt the dose of ketamine from an oral syringe into the patient's mouth with cola or another beverage to follow. Intravenous ketamine is generally given as a continuous infusion starting at 1-2 mg/hour. Administration of intravenous ketamine 0.1-0.4 mg/kg as an intravenous bolus is reported in the literature. Ketamine may cause hallucinations, drowsiness, and confusion. At anesthetic doses (1-4.5 mg/kg intravenous bolus), ketamine causes hypertension and tachycardia.

Dyspnea

Opioid (usually morphine) administration is the cornerstone of medication therapy for reducing the sensation of chronic dyspnea in advanced cancer patients. The sensation of dyspnea is a complex disorder that is influenced by many pathophysiologic changes within and outside of the cardiopulmonary system. Morphine (or an equivalent opioid) can be administered to cancer patients with mild-to-severe dyspnea for symptom control without having a deleterious effect on SaO_2, $PaCO_2$, or heart rate. These findings are consistent when evaluated relative to whether the patient was hypoxic (SaO_2 <90%) at baseline or opioid-naïve. Opioid medications should always be used cautiously. However, medical literature supports the safety and efficacy of opioid administration for management of chronic dyspnea in patients with advanced cancer. For opioid-naïve patients, morphine doses in the range of 1-3 mg by intravenous push or 5-10 mg orally every 4 hours as needed may be sufficient to improve dyspnea. Opioid-tolerant patients will need higher doses to relieve dyspnea. There is no advantage to administration of morphine by nebulization vs use of the subcutaneous, intravenous, or oral routes.

Treatment of anxiety using lorazepam or another suitable product may improve the sensation of dyspnea. Addition of furosemide to therapy should be considered when heart failure may be contributing to the sensation of dyspnea. Long acting β-agonists improve dyspnea for patients with chronic obstructive pulmonary disease. The use of oxygen therapy is controversial due to conflicting information about its efficacy in the medical literature. Patients with chronic obstructive pulmonary disease are most likely to benefit from oxygen therapy.

Cough/Hiccups

Initial symptomatic treatment of persistent cough due to chronic disease affecting the lungs includes guaifenesin, dextromethorphan, and benzonatate. For intractable cough despite usual therapies, nebulized lidocaine may provide relief. Symptomatic relief occurs rapidly for responding patients. Common adverse effects include oropharyngeal numbness and an unpleasant taste. It is important to note that nebulized lidocaine causes a transient loss of gag reflex. Nebulized lidocaine for intractable cough is often administered as follows:

Nebulized Lidocaine for Intractable Cough Administration

Lidocaine 4% preservative-free 2.5 mL
Administer by nebulization every 4 hours as needed.
Note: Patient should have nothing by mouth for 30 minutes before and 2 hours after each dose.

Intractable hiccups, which are generally defined as hiccups lasting more than 1 month, impair the quality and activities of daily life. Hiccups are caused by repeated involuntary spasmodic contractions of the diaphragm followed by a sudden closure of the glottis which blocks the incoming air to produce the characteristic sounds. Hiccups can be secondary to gastric extension and diaphragmatic irritation. Drugs credited with causing intractable hiccups include aprepitant, dexamethasone, doxycycline, etoposide, megestrol acetate, and perphenazine. Interruption of therapy should be tried when hiccups are thought to be medication-related. Nonpharmacologic methods for hiccup cessation should be attempted prior to drug therapy. Examples of nonpharmacologic therapy include holding one's breath, breathing inside of a paper (nonplastic) grocery bag, gasping with sudden fright, the Valsalva maneuver, hyperventilation, slowly drinking water, and drinking water from the "wrong side" of a glass.

Medications used for intractable hiccups include chlorpromazine, metoclopramide, baclofen, and gabapentin. Chlorpromazine 25-50 mg administered orally or intravenously 3-4 times daily as needed or around the clock may be used for control of hiccups. Chlorpromazine may also be administered intramuscularly; however, this route is seldom utilized for repeated administration. Metoclopramide 10 mg is generally administered 4 times daily for management of hiccups. Metoclopramide may be administered orally or intravenously. The dosage of baclofen for intractable hiccups is 5-10 mg by mouth 3-4 times daily. Gabapentin

300-400 mg 3 times daily by mouth for control of hiccups is reported in the medical literature. Gabapentin has a wide margin of safety and doses up to 3600 mg/day are well-tolerated in patients with adequate renal function. Metoclopramide, baclofen, and gabapentin are administered on a scheduled basis around the clock (instead of PRN) for the management of intractable hiccups. Combination therapy using drugs with different pharmacologic mechanisms of action and nonoverlapping toxicity may be tried for patients not responding to single-agent therapy.

Hiccups that continue despite an adequate trial of chlorpromazine, metoclopramide, and baclofen may respond to nebulized lidocaine. The dosage, time to effect, and safety of nebulized lidocaine is described in the preceding section pertaining to management of intractable cough.

Fatigue

Pharmacologic therapy may be added to physical and behavioral therapy for the management of moderate-to-severe fatigue in cancer patients. Prior to adding pharmacologic management, it is essential to identify and address any underlying contributing factors arising from medical conditions or medication adverse effects. Stimulant medications used to manage fatigue in cancer patients are dexmethylphenidate, methylphenidate, and modafinil (Campos, 2011). A randomized, double-blind study compared dexmethylphenidate 5 mg twice daily (n=75 patients) to placebo (n=77 patients) for the management of chemotherapy-related fatigue and cognitive impairment in breast cancer (78% of patients), ovarian cancer (13% of patients), or other cancer (9% of patients) (Lower, 2009). Patients receiving dexmethylphenidate demonstrated improved fatigue scores according to the Functional Assessment of Chronic Illness Therapy-Fatigue Subscale (p=0.02) and Clinical Global Impression-Severity Scores (p=0.02). Cognitive function was not significantly improved in either cohort during the 8-week follow-up period. Adverse effects attributed to medication therapy occurred more commonly in patients treated with active drug (63% vs 28%) and discontinuation of medication therapy due to regimen-related adverse effects occurred more frequently in the active treatment group (11% vs 1.3%). Headache was a common side effect in both treatment groups, nausea and xerostomia were more common in the dexmethylphenidate cohort, and diarrhea and insomnia occurred more commonly in the placebo cohort.

A study in cancer patients enrolled in hospice care randomized patients to methylphenidate (15 patients) or placebo (15 patients). The initial dose of methylphenidate was 10 mg daily, which was divided for administration as 5 mg at 0800 and 5 mg at 1300 daily, with the daily dose increased in increments of 10 mg every 3 days (per patient tolerance and response) to a maximum daily dose of 40 mg. At day 14 of follow-up, the mean effective daily dose of methylphenidate was 20 mg (Kerr, 2012). Fatigue scores (Piper Fatigue Score) for the group receiving methylphenidate improved significantly (compared to baseline) throughout a 14-day monitoring period (p<0.05). In addition, indicators of depression improved in the methylphenidate group as assessed using the Center for Epidemiologic Studies-Depression Scale (p=0.002), Beck Depression Inventory-II score (p=0.028), and Edmonton Symptom Assessment Scale (p=0.05) depression scores. Fatigue and depression scores did not improve in the patients receiving placebo. The author reported that no significant adverse effects occurred (Kerr, 2012). In small, open-label studies, methylphenidate is credited with improving mood, appetite, nausea, pain, drowsiness, cognition, and functional ability in cancer patients according to the reports of noncomparative studies (Campos, 2011).

A multicenter, randomized, double-blind, placebo-controlled trial evaluated modafinil 200 mg daily (315 patients) with placebo (316 patients) for the treatment of cancer-related fatigue. Patient condition was evaluated using the following scales: Brief Fatigue Inventory, Epworth Sleepiness Scale, and Center for Epidemiological Study-Depression, Profile of Mood States-Depression/Dejection. Patients with severe baseline fatigue benefited from modafinil ($p=0.017$); patients with mild or moderate baseline fatigue did not experience significant improvement in their fatigue scores with modafinil. Modafinil did not positively impact depression scores ($p>0.05$). The frequency and severity of adverse effects was similar between the two treatment groups (Jean-Pierre, 2010). Small, open-label studies also suggest benefit of modafinil for the treatment of fatigue in cancer patients (Campos, 2011).

The use of corticosteroids, progestational steroids, antidepressants, and vitamins as management of cancer-related fatigue has been reported (Campos, 2011).

Anemia is a common condition affecting cancer patients which may cause fatigue. Patients with anemia should be evaluated for underlying contributing factors, such as iron deficiency, vitamin B_{12} or folate deficiency, hemolysis, blood loss, renal dysfunction, and treatment with myelosuppressive therapy. Blood transfusions or erythropoietin-stimulating agents (ESAs) may benefit patients with anemia that persists despite correction of treatable causes. The ESAs epoetin and darbepoetin are considered to be therapeutically equivalent for the management of anemia in cancer patients. Blood transfusions are advantageous to ESAs when rapid improvement in hemoglobin is warranted. Risks specific to blood transfusion for anemia include blood-borne infection(s) and immune-mediated adverse effects. The use of ESAs can reduce the need for blood transfusions. However, ESA use in cancer patients confers an increased risk of thromboembolic disorders and shortened survival. ESA therapy is guided by a Food and Drug Administration-mandated Risk-Evaluation-Mitigation-Strategy (REMS) program that was implemented to support informed decision-making by healthcare professionals and patients with regard to medication-related risks. The ESA APPRISE Oncology Program is a piece of the REMS program implemented in order to reduce the risk of decreased survival or worse tumor outcomes in cancer patients. Guidelines for the use of ESAs in cancer patients are jointly published by the American Society of Clinical Oncology and the American Society of Hematology (Rizzo, 2010). Benefit from ESAs is greatest for cases in which the baseline hemoglobin is ≤10 g/dL. ESAs should be administered at the lowest possible dose to achieve a hemoglobin value greater than 10 g/dL. An adequate trial of ESA use is considered to be 6-8 weeks. Patients without an adequate response to ESAs administered according to the product labeling should not continue to receive treatment with these agents beyond a period of 6-8 weeks. The ASCO ASH guidelines support the use of ESAs for cancer patients undergoing treatment with myelosuppressive therapy who have baseline hemoglobin <10 g/dL. The guidelines also support the use of ESAs for patients with low-risk myelodysplastic syndromes who are not undergoing treatment with chemotherapy.

REFERENCES

Attal N, Rouaud J, Brasseur L, et al, "Systemic Lidocaine in Pain Due to Peripheral Nerve Injury and Predictors of Response," *Neurology*, 2004, 62(2):218-25.

Brose WG and Cousins MJ, "Subcutaneous Lidocaine for Treatment of Neuropathic Cancer Pain," *Pain*, 1991, 45(2):145-8.

Campos MP, Hassan BJ, Riechelmann R, et al, "Cancer-Related Fatigue: A Practical Review," *Ann Oncol*, 2011, 22(6):1273-9.

Clemens KE, Quednau I, and Klaschik E, "Use of Oxygen and Opioids in the Palliation of Dyspnoea in Hypoxic and Nonhypoxic Palliative Care Patients: A Prospective Study," *Support Care Cancer*, 2009, 17(4):367-77.

Clinical Practice Guidelines for Quality Palliative Care, 2nd ed, Pittsburgh, PA: National Consensus Project for Quality Palliative Care, 2009. Available at:http://www.nationalconsensusproject.org/guideline.pdf.

Dy SM, Lorenz KA, Naeem A, et al, "Evidence-Based Recommendations for Cancer Fatigue, Anorexia, Depression, and Dyspnea," *J Clin Oncol*, 2008, 26(23):3886-95.

Enarson MC, Haye H, and Woodroffe MA, "Clinical Experience With Oral Ketamine," *J Pain Symptom Manage*, 1999, 17(5):384-6.

Jean-Pierre P, Morrow GR, Roscoe JA, et al, "A Phase 3 Randomized, Placebo-Controlled, Double-Blind, Clinical Trial of the Effect of Modafinil on Cancer-Related Fatigue Among 631 Patients Receiving Chemotherapy: A University of Rochester Cancer Center Community Clinical Oncology Program Research Base Study," *Cancer*, 2010, 116(14):3513-20.

Kannan TR, Saxena A, Bhatnagar S, et al, "Oral Ketamine as an Adjuvant to Oral Morphine for Neuropathic Pain in Cancer Patients," *J Pain Symptom Manage*, 2002, 23(1):60-5.

Kerr CW, Drake J, Milch RA, et al, "Effects of Methylphenidate on Fatigue and Depression: A Randomized, Double-Blind, Placebo-Controlled Trial," *J Pain Symptom Manage*, 2012, 43 (1):68-77.

Lower EE, Fleishman S, Cooper A, et al, "Efficacy of Dexmethylphenidate for the Treatment of Fatigue After Cancer Chemotherapy: A Randomized Clinical Trial," *J Pain Symptom Manage*, 2009, 38(5):650-62.

Midgren B, Hansson L, Karlsson JA, et al, "Capsaicin-Induced Cough in Humans," *Am Rev Respir Dis*, 1992, 146(2):347-51.

Neeno TA and Rosenow EC 3rd, "Intractable Hiccups. Consider Nebulized Lidocaine," *Chest*, 1996, 110(4):1129-30.

Pirl WF, Greer JA, Traeger L, et al, "Depression and Survival in Metastatic Non-Small-Cell Lung Cancer: Effects of Early Palliative Care," *J Clin Oncol*, 2012, 30(12):1310-5.

Qaseem A, Snow V, Shekelle P, et al, "Evidence-Based Interventions to Improve the Palliative Care of Pain, Dyspnea, and Depression at the End of Life: A Clinical Practice Guideline From the American College of Physicians," *Ann Intern Med*, 2008, 148(2):141-6.

Rizzo JD, Brouwers M, Hurley P, et al, "American Society of Clinical Oncology/American Society of Hematology Clinical Practice Guideline Update on the Use of Epoetin and Darbepoetin in Adult Patients With Cancer," *J Clin Oncol*, 2010, 28(33):4996-5010.

Shaiova L, Berger A, Blinderman CD, et al, "Consensus Guideline on Parenteral Methadone Use in Pain and Palliative Care," *Palliat Support Care*, 2008, 6(2):165-76.

Smith TJ, Temin S, Alesi ER, et al, "American Society of Clinical Oncology Provisional Clinical Opinion: The Integration of Palliative Care Into Standard Oncology Care," *J Clin Oncol*, 2012, 30 (8):880-7.

Temel JS, Greer JA, Muzikansky A, et al, "Early Palliative Care for Patients With Metastatic Non-Small-Cell Lung Cancer," *N Engl J Med*, 2010, 363(8):733-42.

Tremont-Lukats IW, Hutson PR, and Backonja MM, "A Randomized, Double-Masked, Placebo Controlled Pilot Trial of Extended I.V. Lidocaine Infusion for Relief of Ongoing Neuropathic Pain," *Clin J Pain*, 2006, 22(3):266-71.

PRINCIPLES OF ANTICANCER THERAPY

Treatment options for cancer include systemic therapy, radiation therapy, and surgical procedures. The wide array of treatment options is warranted by the great complexity of treating cancer. The diagnosis of cancer actually encompasses a multitude of malignant diseases with differing symptomatology and prognosis relative to the tumor's site of origin, natural history, and biologic characteristics. In addition, the intent of therapy can be curative, palliative, or supportive, or it may be investigational. Curative therapy is expected to eradicate cancer from the body, whereas palliative therapy is intended to reduce the body's tumor burden to improve disease-related adverse events. A greater degree of transient and supportable treatment-related toxicity is considered acceptable with curative therapy than with palliative therapy. Best supportive care, which is provided when curative therapy and palliative therapy are not established for a particular cancer, manages disease-related symptomatology without impacting the progression of malignant disease. Investigational therapy adds to the body of knowledge directing the standard of care for cancer patients.

Selection of specific anticancer treatment options is based on disease-related and patient-specific factors. Resource availability is also a consideration. Primary disease-related factors that determine selection of anticancer therapy are the cancer type, stage, and biologic characteristics. The type of cancer (breast cancer, lymphoma, sarcoma) is defined by the cell of origin and is determined by pathologic analysis of tissue or hematology specimens. The stage of disease refers to the body's tumor burden and how advanced the disease process has become. Early stage cancer tends to be localized in the area of initial growth, whereas advanced cancer has often spread to distant sites within the body. Biologic characteristics of cancer can vary, even within a particular tumor type. As an example, breast cancer specimens are tested to determine the amount of estrogen receptor, progesterone receptor, and Her-2 expression. These characteristics vary between patients and influence the selection of treatment options.

The patient's ability to withstand anticancer treatments is an important consideration. Comorbidities that impair major organ function increase the likelihood of serious treatment-related adverse events because the body is more sensitive to drug toxicity and may be less able to effectively eliminate systemic therapies. Life expectancy guides selection of anticancer therapy. As an example, androgen deprivation therapy for localized prostate cancer is generally deferred for patients with a life expectancy of less than 10 years because the chronic cardiovascular and endocrine side effects of therapy outweigh its benefits. Patient and family wishes also factor into treatment-related decisions for cancer patients.

Resource availability that affects selection of anticancer therapy includes reimbursement and accessible level of care. The product acquisition cost of anticancer therapy spans a sizable range from economical to very expensive. Optimal treatment of malignant disease is provided by trained oncologists and an interdisciplinary team. Some treatments, such as hematopoietic stem cell transplantation and major surgeries, are performed only at regional treatment centers.

Systemic therapy is used for the treatment of localized and metastatic sites of disease. The most extensively used type of systemic therapy is cytotoxic chemotherapy. Cytotoxic chemotherapy has a narrow therapeutic index and the overall efficacy of therapy is often based on a balance of tumor sensitivity and patient tolerance. In order to optimize anticancer treatment, cytotoxic chemotherapy is generally administered as combination therapy. Combination of specific chemotherapy drugs (see Table 1) is based on principles intended to provide the greatest anticancer effect with acceptable regimen-related toxicity. Proven efficacy against the tumor type being treated is essential to justify inclusion of a particular agent in combination therapy. Combination of chemotherapy drugs with different pharmacologic mechanisms of action yields increased sites of pharmacologic damage to the cancer. In addition, an increased number of pharmacologic mechanisms of action provides stronger overall anticancer efficacy when the malignant cells comprising a patient's tumor vary with respect to drug target sensitivity. Administration of chemotherapy drugs susceptible to different mechanisms of anticancer drug resistance improves treatment efficacy because a specific mechanism of cellular resistance will only impede a proportion of the regimen's overall anticancer activity. Selection of anticancer drugs with nonoverlapping serious toxicities for use in combination therapy is important in order to maintain acceptable toxicity with respect to anticipated outcome and to allow administration of the maximum dose for each drug in the regimen. The anticancer activity of most chemotherapy drugs correlates with the dose administered, so use of the maximum tolerated dose of each drug within a regimen is warranted for optimal efficacy. The maximum tolerated dose of chemotherapy drugs is often lower when administered in combination vs single agent therapy. In addition, combination chemotherapy must be scheduled such that cycles are repeated with the shortest possible time interval between administrations. The time interval should be adequate to allow recovery of nonmalignant tissues, such as gastrointestinal mucosa and bone marrow, and otherwise as short as possible to impede malignant cellular repair and tumor progression.

Table 1: Principles of Combination Chemotherapy

- Proven efficacy against the tumor type being treated
- Different pharmacologic mechanisms of action
- Different spectrum of drug resistance
- Nonoverlapping serious toxicities
- Maximum tolerated dose
- Shortest possible interval between cyclic administrations

Additional models used for evaluating and optimizing the delivery of efficacious anticancer therapy include dose intensity, alternating or sequential noncross-resistant chemotherapy, and dose density. Dose intensity is mathematically defined by the equation mg/m^2/week of chemotherapy. Increased dose intensity was initially investigated for its correlation with disease response and relapse-free survival in the treatment of localized and metastatic breast cancer and has since been examined in other tumor types. Initial findings supported a correlation of increased dose intensity with improved disease response and relapse-free survival in breast cancer patients. Several aspects of the initial work evaluating dose intensity have been criticized, including its retrospective evaluation of protocol-directed vs actual drug administration and failure to consider the impact of different administration routes. However, dose intensity provides a useful tool for assessing the efficacy and safety of chemotherapy administration. Relative dose intensity is used to evaluate the efficacy and safety of varying the interval between administrations of a particular chemotherapy regimen (see Table 2). In addition, the relative dose intensity of planned vs actual drug administration provides a measure of patient tolerance relative to treatment efficacy. Alternating or sequential noncross-resistant chemotherapy delivers alternating or sequentially repeated cycles of chemotherapy with known activity against a particular tumor type at the full doses tested to demonstrate anticancer efficacy. This approach utilizes the efficacy advantage of combination chemotherapy without the need to reduce chemotherapy doses for patient tolerance. An example of sequential chemotherapy is AC → T which administers four cycles of cyclophosphamide 600 mg/m^2/dose and doxorubicin 60 mg/m^2/dose every 21 days, followed by four cycles of paclitaxel 175 mg/m^2/dose administered every 21 days for the treatment of breast cancer. Dose density refers to the practice of shortening the interval between chemotherapy administration to reduce the time allowed for malignant cellular repair and tumor progression. Patient tolerance is maintained throughout administration of dose-dense chemotherapy by the use of white blood cell colony-stimulating factors. An example of dose-dense chemotherapy is AC → T with chemotherapy cycles shortened to 14-day intervals and white blood cell colony-stimulating factor support.

Table 2: Relative Dose Intensity of AC Regimen Administered at 21-Day or 28-Day Intervals

Dose intensity of AC with 21-day administration schedule: Cyclophosphamide 600 mg/m^2/dose every 21 days x 4 cycles = 200 mg/m^2/week Doxorubicin 60 mg/m^2/dose every 21 days x 4 cycles = 20 mg/m^2/week
Dose intensity of AC with 28-day administration schedule: Cyclophosphamide 600 mg/m^2/dose every 28 days x 4 cycles = 150 mg/m^2/week Doxorubicin 60 mg/m^2/dose every 28 days x 4 cycles = 15 mg/m^2/week
Relative dose intensity of cyclophosphamide: 200 mg/m^2/week *divided by* 150 mg/m^2/week = 1.33
Relative dose intensity of doxorubicin: 20 mg/m^2/week *divided by* 15 mg/m^2/week = 1.33

Endocrine therapy is effective in cancers that utilize a hormone-dependent pathway for growth and survival. The greatest utility of endocrine therapy is in the treatment of breast cancer and prostate cancer. A major advantage to endocrine therapy is patient tolerance of these products relative to the side effect profile of cytotoxic chemotherapy. Antiestrogenic therapy is part of curative therapy for most cases of estrogen-receptor positive localized breast cancer and it is utilized as primary therapy for many estrogen-receptor positive advanced and metastatic cases of breast cancer. Medical castration using LHRH agonist, LHRH antagonist, and androgen-receptor blocking therapy is the initial systemic therapy for prostate cancer that is advancing or metastatic. Most side effects from endocrine therapy are transient and manageable, consisting of hot flashes, fatigue, fluid retention, vaginal discharge, and mood changes. However, for some patients, the immediate side effects can be dose-limiting and major organ sequelae can occur with chronic administration. A troublesome and sometimes dose-limiting side effect of aromatase inhibitor therapy is arthralgias. Chronic administration of aromatase inhibitors is associated with loss of bone mineral density. Chronic administration of tamoxifen is associated with endometrial cancer, thromboembolic disorders, and cataract formation. Chronic androgen deprivation is associated with the development of metabolic syndrome and increased cardiovascular morbidity.

Targeted anticancer therapy is designed to inactivate or disrupt a molecular process or biochemical pathway that is unique to malignant cell growth and viability. The efficacy of molecularly targeted anticancer agents is related to their ability to interfere with an essential malignant process. The utility of targeted therapy may be limited by redundancies occurring in some cellular processes that circumvent the damage done by these agents. Small molecule tyrosine kinase inhibitors and multikinase inhibitors represent the largest number of targeted products that are commercially available (see Table 3). Additional molecules and pathways targeted by commercially available anticancer therapy include angiogenesis, histone deacetylase, and proteasome activity (see Table 3). Many types of biologic therapy have a targeted mechanism of action. Targeted therapy is less toxic than cytotoxic chemotherapy because it does not predictably exert the classic severe dose-related effects of bone marrow suppression, mucositis, and emesis. However, side effects associated with targeted therapy that are mild-to-moderate in severity can be dose-limiting due to the negative impact on quality of life with the chronic nature of drug administration. Examples include diarrhea and skin problems from tyrosine kinase inhibitor therapy. In addition, targeted therapy with antiVEGF activity can cause or exacerbate adverse effects deleterious to cardiovascular and renal function, which can limit the use of these products.

Table 3: Molecularly Targeted Anticancer Therapy

Drug	Product Type	Molecular Target-Mechanism
Abiraterone	Small molecule	CYP17 inhibitor
Aldesleukin	Recombinant cytokine	Interleukin-2 receptor agonist
Alemtuzumab	Monoclonal antibody	CD52 ligand
Bevacizumab	Monoclonal antibody	Vascular endothelial growth factor (VEGF) inhibitor
Bortezomib	Small molecule	Proteosome inhibitor
Brentuximab vedotin	Conjugated monoclonal antibody	CD30, tubulin
Cetuximab	Monoclonal antibody	Epidermal growth factor receptor (EGFR) tyrosine kinase inhibitor (TKI)
Dasatinib	Small molecule	BCR-ABL TKI
Denileukin diftitox	Fusion protein	CD25 ligand
Erlotinib	Small molecule	EGFR TKI
Everolimus	Small molecule	m-TOR inhibitor
Imatinib	Small molecule	BCR-ABL TKI
Ipilimumab	Monoclonal antibody	CTLA-4 ligand
Lapatinib	Small molecule	EGFR TKI, HER-2 TKI
Lenalidomide	Small molecule	Multiple mechanisms
Nilotinib	Small molecule	BCR-ABL TKI
Ofatumumab	Monoclonal antibody	CD20 ligand
Panitumumab	Monoclonal antibody	EGFR ligand
Pazopanib	Small molecule	Multityrosine kinase inhibitor (MTKI)
Rituximab	Monoclonal antibody	CD20 ligand

Table 3: Molecularly Targeted Anticancer Therapy *(continued)*

Drug	Product Type	Molecular Target-Mechanism
Romidepsin	Small molecule	Histone deactylase inhibitor
Sorafenib	Small molecule	MTKI
Sunitinib	Small molecule	MTKI
Temsirolimus	Small molecule	m-TOR inhibitor
Thalidomide	Small molecule	Multiple mechanisms
Trastuzumab	Monoclonal antibody	HER-2 ligand
Tretinoin	Small molecule	Nuclear retinoic acid receptor isotypes α, β, γ
Vandetanib	Small molecule	MTKI
Vemurafenib	Monoclonal antibody	$BRAF^{V600E}$ TKI
Vorinostat	Small molecule	Histone deactylase inhibitor

REFERENCES

Citron ML, Berry DA, Cirrincione C, et al, "Randomized Trial of Dose-Dense Versus Conventionally Scheduled and Sequential Versus Concurrent Combination Chemotherapy as Postoperative Adjuvant Treatment of Node-Positive Primary Breast Cancer: First Report of Intergroup Trial C9741/Cancer and Leukemia Group B Trial 9741," *J Clin Oncol*, 2003, 21(8):1431-9.

DeVita VT Jr, Young RC, and Canellos GP, "Combination Versus Single Agent Chemotherapy: A Review of the Basis for Selection of Drug Treatment of Cancer," *Cancer*, 1975, 35(1):98-110.

Felson DT and Cummings SR, "Aromatase Inhibitors and the Syndrome of Arthralgias With Estrogen Deprivation," *Arthritis Rheum*, 2005, 52(9):2594-8.

Hryniuk W and Bush H, "The Importance of Dose Intensity in Chemotherapy of Metastatic Breast Cancer," *J Clin Oncol*, 1984, 2(11):1281-8.

Hryniuk W and Levine MN, "Analysis of Dose Intensity for Adjuvant Chemotherapy Trials in Stage II Breast Cancer," *J Clin Oncol*, 1986, 4(8):1162-70.

Kintzel PE, Chase SL, Schultz LM, et al, "Increased Risk of Metabolic Syndrome, Diabetes Mellitus, and Cardiovascular Disease in Men Receiving Androgen Deprivation Therapy for Prostate Cancer," *Pharmacotherapy*, 2008, 28(12):1511-22.

Marill J, Idres N, Capron CC, et al, "Retinoic Acid Metabolism and Mechanism of Action: A Review," *Curr Drug Metab*, 2003, 4(1):1-10.

VENOUS THROMBOEMBOLISM IN THE CANCER PATIENT

INTRODUCTION

Venous thromboembolism (VTE) is a common and life-threatening complication in cancer patients. Overall, approximately 500,000 new cases of VTE are diagnosed annually, 1 in 5 of which are diagnosed in cancer patients. Patients with active cancer have at least a 6- to 7-fold increased risk of VTE. Diagnosis of VTE or superficial venous thrombosis in a young or middle-aged person without an identifiable cause is suspicious for underlying malignancy. VTE is generally diagnosed in cancer patients within the first few months of malignant disease and may be related to a number of intrinsic (eg, aggressiveness) or extrinsic (eg, surgery, radiation) factors. Development of VTE is a major source of mortality in this population; it may increase the likelihood of death by up to 47-fold in certain patients (Khorana, 2007). Pathophysiologic causes for VTE in cancer patients include hypercoagulability, vessel wall damage, and vessel stasis from direct compression by tumors. Given the significant morbidity and mortality caused by VTE, it is important for the clinician to recognize patients at risk for VTE and to offer appropriate prophylactic and treatment strategies.

VTE RISK ASSESSMENT

VTE risk factors for the cancer patient can be separated into three categories: Patient-related (ie, intrinsic and extrinsic factors), cancer-related, and treatment-related. Patient-related factors include an active cancer diagnosis, previous VTE, hypercoagulable state (eg, factor V Leiden, lupus anticoagulant, anticardiolipin antibodies), >70 years of age, obesity (BMI ≥30 kg/m^2), hospitalization, and bed rest/immobility (for at least 3 days). Increased comorbid burden defined by coexisting conditions, such as pulmonary disease, kidney disease, and infections, is associated with a greater risk of VTE.

Cancer type also influences VTE risk. A diagnosis of metastatic cancer arising from the pancreas, stomach, bladder, uterus, kidney, and lung confers a greater risk for VTE, as do diagnoses of acute leukemia, multiple myeloma, and non-Hodgkin lymphoma. Lower risk for VTE is associated with breast cancer, prostate cancer, and head and neck cancers. In addition, histologic subtype also plays a role in VTE prevalence, with adenocarcinomas having a higher risk vs squamous cell cancers. Advanced stage of disease, poor patient performance status, and the finding of leukocytosis or thrombocytosis (platelet count >350,000/microliter) at presentation all may put patients at risk for thrombosis. Lastly, VTE risk factors specific to multiple myeloma include M-spike >1.6 g/dL, progressive disease, and hyperviscosity syndrome.

Treatment-related and iatrogenic factors, such as surgery, the presence of a central venous access device (CVAD), and chemotherapy and/or radiotherapy administration place cancer patients in jeopardy for developing VTE. The reported incidence of ultrasound-detected upper extremity deep venous thrombosis (DVT) is variable (2% to 67%) (Rooden, 2005); the incidence of PE on autopsy reports was up to 50% (Verso, 2003) in cancer patients with CVADs. The 3 main classes of cancer drugs which may lead to VTE include cytotoxic chemotherapy, hormonal therapy with estrogenic properties, and anti-angiogenic medications. Administration of cytotoxic chemotherapy is associated with a 2- to 6-fold increased risk of VTE. Selective estrogen receptor modulator (tamoxifen) administration is associated with 2- to 5-fold increased risk of VTE among women with breast cancer (Kahn, 2012). The immune modulating products lenalidomide and thalidomide are thrombogenic, especially when administered in combination with a corticosteroid or cytotoxic chemotherapy. Treatment of multiple myeloma and lymphoid malignancies often includes chronic or episodic corticosteroid administration which further increases the risk of VTE. The findings of one meta-analysis indicate that the incidence of VTE is 12% with bevacizumab administration. Ancillary therapies used to prevent and manage disease and treatment-related adverse events can also increase the likelihood of VTE. Two such examples are erythopoietin-stimulating agents (ESA) administered for anemia and corticosteroids which may be administered for antiemesis and many other medical purposes.

VTE PROPHYLAXIS

Most hospitalized patients with cancer meet conditions for prophylactic anticoagulation based on the standard risk assessment criteria discussed above. In such cases, prophylactic anticoagulation using a low molecular weight heparin (LMWH) or unfractionated heparin should be administered according to standard guidelines, such as the American College of Chest Physicians (ACCP) or the National Cancer Center Network (NCCN). In patients for whom anticoagulation is absolutely or relatively contraindicated (eg, recent central nervous system bleeding, major active bleeding, recent lumbar puncture, low platelet count), intermittent pneumatic venous compression devices (IPCs) may be considered for VTE prophylaxis.

Criteria for VTE prophylaxis in the outpatient cancer setting are not clearly delineated. However, some surgical and medical oncology patients are at high risk for VTE and may benefit from outpatient prophylaxis. For surgical oncology patients (particularly those undergoing abdominal or pelvic surgery), the NCCN Guidelines support continued administration of VTE prophylaxis after hospital discharge for a period of up to 4 weeks following major surgery. Multiple myeloma patients receiving thrombotic anticancer therapy (lenalidomide or thalidomide in combination with dexamethasone >480 mg monthly or doxorubicin or multiagent chemotherapy) also may require outpatient VTE prophylaxis. The NCCN Guidelines discuss continuation of VTE prophylaxis following hospital discharge for patients with 2 or more VTE risk factors. LMWHs, unfractionated heparin, and warfarin are the primary agents used for VTE prophylaxis in cancer patients. Aspirin can be considered for VTE prophylaxis in patients with multiple myeloma at relatively low-risk for VTE (no more than one VTE risk factor). Risk stratification criteria based on tumor site, prechemotherapy platelet count, prechemotherapy leukocyte count, anemia and ESA administration, and body size have been proposed (Dutia, 2012). However, primary pharmacologic prophylaxis administered to prevent a first VTE in ambulatory cancer patients remains controversial because it increases the risk of bleeding with indeterminate efficacy for prevention of VTE.

VTE TREATMENT

Initial treatment of VTE in cancer patients is similar to that of noncancer patients, with unfractionated heparin, LMWHs, and warfarin (or vitamin K antagonist [VKA]) providing the cornerstone of anticoagulant therapy. Initial assessment and management of VTE in cancer patients is handled according to clinical practice guidelines provided by ACCP, NCCN, and institutional policy. The minimum duration of anticoagulant therapy is 3-6 months for DVT and 6-12 months for pulmonary embolism (PE). The ACCP suggests the use of LMWH over a VKA in cancer patients who develop DVT of the leg or PE. According to the NCCN Guidelines, anticoagulation with LMWH for a 6-month duration is recommended for proximal DVT, PE, and recurrent VTE in patients with advanced or metastatic cancer. For patients with active cancer or continuing VTE risk factors, anticoagulation should be continued indefinitely. The duration of anticoagulant therapy for catheter-related DVT is at least 3 months and for such time as long as the catheter remains in place.

Special situations related to cancer and its treatments may complicate delivery of safe and effective therapeutic anticoagulation. Low platelet counts due to hematologic malignancies or cytotoxic treatments may be present in cancer patients requiring anticoagulation. Unfortunately, limited options exist for patients with an active clotting process, despite a low platelet count. Inferior vena cava (IVC) filter placement is one method for reducing the risk of PE in patients with DVT. Drawbacks to IVC filter placement include lack of systemic anticoagulant effect and increased risk of recurrent DVT. Management of therapeutic anticoagulation in the setting of thrombocytopenia must be handled judiciously on a case-by-case basis. Cancer patients requiring anticoagulation may also need intrathecal administration of chemotherapy. Anticoagulation must be interrupted for spinal injection and intrathecal medication administration. The American Society of Regional Anesthesia and Pain Medicine (ASRA) recommends withholding LMWH administration for at least 24 hours and unfractionated heparin for at least 1 hour before spinal injection for delivery of analgesia. Warfarin should be held for 4-5 days prior to spinal injection.

ANTICOAGULANT SELECTION

Anticoagulant selection may be influenced by cancer and its treatments. The anticoagulant activity of warfarin is readily affected by diet, drug interactions, liver function, and certain physiologic stressors. Food intake in the cancer patient can vary relative to disease- and treatment-related factors that alter taste sensation, reduce appetite, and cause adverse gastrointestinal events. Numerous therapeutic and ancillary medications used in the management of cancer interact with the anticoagulant intensity of warfarin. Due to the extensive and expanding list of medications that interact with warfarin, the reader should refer to specific drug monographs for detailed information about particular medications. Hepatic function can be impaired due to primary or metastatic tumor growth in the liver. Any physiologic stressor, such as infection, can alter the anticoagulant effect of warfarin in the cancer patient.

LMWHs are not prone to altered anticoagulant intensity by the myriad of dietary, drug, and physiologic factors affecting warfarin therapy. However, all commercially available LMWHs are excreted renally and may require dosage adjustments in patients with renal dysfunction; anti-Xa monitoring may facilitate appropriate administration in this clinical scenario. Unfractionated heparin should be considered as an alternative to LMWH for use in patients with severely impaired renal function.

Anticoagulant Comparison Table

Name	Use	DVT and PE Dose (SubQ unless otherwise noted)	Adjust Dose for Renal Impairment?
Low Molecular Weight Heparins			
Dalteparin	Prophylaxis	2500-5000 units/day	Yes
	Treatment	Month 1: 200 units/kg once daily Months 2-6: 150 units/kg once daily	
Enoxaparin	Prophylaxis	30 mg q12h or 40 mg once daily	Yes
	Treatment	1 mg/kg q12h	
Heparin			
Heparin	Prophylaxis	5000 units q8-12h	No
	Treatment	80 units/kg IVP, then 18 units/kg/hour	
Selective Anti-Xa Inhibitor			
Fondaparinux	Prophylaxis	≥50 kg: 2.5 mg once daily (prophylactic use is contraindicated in patients <50 kg)	Yes
	Treatment	≤50 kg: 5 mg once daily 50-100 kg: 7.5 mg once daily ≥100 kg: 10 mg once daily	
Coumarin Derivatives			
Warfarin	Prophylaxis	Variable	No
	Treatment	Variable	

REFERENCES

Battinelli EM, Murphy DL, and Connors JM, "Venous Thromboembolism Overview," *Hematol Oncol Clin North Am*, 2012, 26(2):345-67.

Dutia M, White RH, and Wun T, "Risk Assessment Models for Cancer-Associated Venous Thromboembolism," *Cancer*, 2012, 118(14):3468-76.

Horlocker TT, Wedel DJ, Rowlingson JC, et al, "Regional Anesthesia in the Patient Receiving Antithrombotic or Thrombolytic Therapy: American Society of Regional Anesthesia and Pain Medicine Evidence-Based Guidelines (Third Edition)," *Reg Anesth Pain Med*, 2010, 35 (1):64-101.

Kahn SR, Lim W, Dunn AS, et al, "Prevention of VTE in Nonsurgical Patients: Antithrombotic Therapy and Prevention of Thrombosis, 9th ed: American College of Chest Physicians Evidence-Based Clinical Practice Guidelines," *Chest*, 2012, 141(2 Suppl):e195S-226S.

Kearon C, Akl EA, Comerota AJ, et al, "Antithrombotic Therapy for VTE Disease: Antithrombotic Therapy and Prevention of Thrombosis, 9th ed: American College of Chest Physicians Evidence-Based Clinical Practice Guidelines," *Chest*, 2012, 141(2 Suppl):e419S-94S.

Khorana AA, Francis CW, Culakova E, et al, "Thromboembolism Is a Leading Cause of Death in Cancer Patients Receiving Outpatient Chemotherapy," *J Thromb Haemost*, 2007, 5(3):632-4.

National Comprehensive Cancer Network® (NCCN), "Clinical Practice Guidelines in Oncology™: Venous Thromboembolic Disease," Version 1.2012. Available at http://www.nccn.org/professionals/physician_gls/pdf/vte.pdf

Palumbo A, Cavo M, Bringhen S, et al, "Aspirin, Warfarin, or Enoxaparin Thromboprophylaxis in Patients With Multiple Myeloma Treated With Thalidomide: A Phase III, Open-Label, Randomized Trial," *J Clin Oncol*, 2011, 29(8):986-93.

Rooden CJ, Tesselaar ME, Osanto S, et al, "Deep Vein Thrombosis Associated With Central Venous Catheters − a Review," *J Thromb Haemost*, 2005, 3(11):2409-19.

Sørensen HT, Sværke C, Farkas DK, et al, "Superficial and Deep Venous Thrombosis, Pulmonary Embolism and Subsequent Risk of Cancer," *Eur J Cancer*, 2012, 48(4):586-93.

Verso M and Agnelli G, "Venous Thromboembolism Associated With Long-Term Use of Central Venous Catheters in Cancer Patients," *J Clin Oncol*, 2003, 21(19):3665-75.

HEMATOPOIETIC STEM CELL TRANSPLANTATION

INTRODUCTION

Hematopoietic stem cell transplantation (HSCT) involves the infusion of hematopoietic stem and progenitor cells into a patient in order to treat malignant disease and nonmalignant hematologic, lymphopoietic, congenital, and other disorders. Hematopoietic stem cells are immature cells that mature and differentiate into the various functional myeloid (eg, neutrophils, monocytes, macrophages, megakaryocytes, erythrocytes) and lymphoid cells (eg, T lymphocytes, B lymphocytes, natural killer cells) of the hematopoietic system. Hematopoietic stem cells are transplanted in order to replace diseased hematopoietic cells, reduce the duration of pancytopenia following administration of high dose chemotherapy, or to generate antitumor immunity in cancer patients. Allogeneic stem cell transplants require donation of stem cells from a healthy donor; whereas, autologous transplantation uses stem cells previously collected from the patient undergoing treatment. Allogeneic stem cell transplants are further classified as related transplants (donor and recipient are siblings), unrelated transplants (donor and recipient are not related by pedigree), or syngeneic transplants (donor and recipient are identical twins). Immunologic likeness of the donor and recipient is determined by comparison of the genotype of donor and recipient class I and class II major histocompatibility (MHC) antigens. MHC Class I antigens (HLA-A, HLA-B, HLA-C) are present on all nucleated cells in the body and provide a means for the immune system to differentiate self vs nonself. MHC Class II proteins (HLA-D) are present on antigen presenting cells, such as macrophages, dendritic cells, B lymphocytes, and activated endothelial cells, and are critical in initiation and maintenance of long-lasting immunity and tolerance.

Stem cell transplants are classified according to the intensity of the pretransplant preparative regimen. Myeloablative chemotherapy regimens administer the highest possible dose of chemotherapy, with the doses limited by regimen-related nonhematologic toxicity. The goal of the myeloablative regimen is to achieve the maximum anticancer effect and complete immunosuppression through the effects of the high dose cytotoxic agents. The goal of the nonmyeloablative preparative regimen is to inhibit the recipient immune system adequately to allow engraftment of the donated hematopoietic cells. Complete donor engraftment following nonmyeloablative transplantation typically occurs after a period of mixed chimerism (coexistence of donor and recipient hematologic cells) and is associated with antitumor effect mediated by donor immune cells.

Terms that are synonymous with hematopoietic stem cell transplantation include bone marrow transplantation, peripheral blood cell transplantation, and peripheral blood cell rescue. The following table lists clinical uses for allogeneic and autologous myeloablative hematopoietic stem cell transplantation.

Condition	Allogeneic	Autologous
Acute lymphocytic leukemia (ALL)	+	+
Acute myelogenous leukemia (AML)	+	+
Myelodysplastic syndrome	+	-
Chronic lymphocytic leukemia (CLL)	+	-
Chronic myelogenous leukemia (CML)	+	-
Non-Hodgkin's lymphoma (NHL)	+	+
Hodgkin's lymphoma	+	+
Multiple myeloma (MM)	+	+
Severe aplastic anemia (SAA)	+	-
Sickle cell disease (SCD)	+	-
Congenital immunodeficiency syndromes	+	-
Adult autoimmune disorders (eg, scleroderma, multiple sclerosis, rheumatoid arthritis)	-	+
Germ cell/testicular cancer	-	+
Neuroblastoma	-	+
Congenital hematopoietic disorders	+	-
Inborn errors of metabolism	+	-
Paroxysmal nocturnal hemoglobinuria	+	-
Thalassemia major	+	-
Wiskott-Aldrich syndrome	+	-

SOURCES, COLLECTION, AND PROCESSING OF HEMATOPOIETIC PROGENITOR CELLS

The hematopoietic progenitor cells for transplantation are generally gathered from the peripheral blood. The hematopoietic stem and progenitor cells are removed via leukapheresis, which is routinely done in an ambulatory setting. Cells collected for autologous transplantation are processed and cryopreserved for future use. Cells collected for allogeneic transplantation are processed and infused immediately (within 24 hours). Leukapheresis involves the processing of approximately 10 L of peripheral blood over a 2- to 6-hour period. The usual goal is a product containing at least 2 x 10^6/kg and ideally 5 x 10^6/kg of recipient weight of $CD34^+$ cells, which closely correlate with the content of stem and progenitor cells collected. This may be accomplished by 1 or several leukaphereses. Donors may require calcium supplementation during leukapheresis due to the citrate anticoagulant used during the procedure. Common medical risks to the allogeneic donor of peripheral hematopoietic stem cells include adverse effects from treatment with a colony-stimulating factor (bone pain) and adverse events associated with leukapheresis (acute hypocalcemia, catheter-related discomfort). Although no long-term toxicity has been reported in donors treated with colony-stimulating factors, rare serious toxicity such as splenic rupture can occur and the donor must be screened carefully prior to donation.

The peripheral blood concentration of hematopoietic stem cells and progenitor cells must be increased to facilitate successful collection. This process is known as peripheral progenitor cell mobilization. After administration of chemotherapy, colony-stimulating factors, or a combination of the two agents, the numbers of circulating early and late progenitor cells greatly magnifies. A colony-stimulating factor, such as filgrastim or sargramostim, is used for this purpose in the healthy allogeneic donor. For the autologous donor, a colony-stimulating factor is administered alone or prescribed following chemotherapy. Mobilization of hematopoietic progenitor cells can be more difficult in patients with hematologic malignancies, or a history of extensive treatment with chemotherapy and radiation. The following table provides the dosage and schedule for some of the more commonly used mobilization regimens. Selection of the chemotherapy for mobilization in the autologous donor is primarily based on the type of cancer being treated.

Mobilization Agent	Dosage and Duration
Filgrastim (G-CSF)	10 mcg/kg/day SubQ for 5-7 days or until target WBC; dose escalation to 16-32 mcg/kg/day has been used to improve inadequate mobilization
Sargramostim (GM-CSF)	250 mg/m^2/day SubQ for 5-7 days or until target WBC
Etoposide (VP-16)	2 g/m^2 I.V. over 2 hours followed in 24 hours by G-CSF or GM-CSF until target WBC
Cyclophosphamide	4 g/m^2 (range of 1.5-7 g/m^2) I.V. over 2 hours followed at 24 hours by G-CSF 5-10 mcg/kg/day until target WBC; higher doses are also used (7 g/m^2)
Cytarabine plus etoposide	2 g/m^2 I.V. q12h x 8 doses + 40 mg/kg VP-16 over 4 days then G-CSF 10 mcg/kg/day from day 14 until cells collected
Plerixafor (in combination with filgrastim)	0.24 mg/kg SubQ once daily for up to 4 consecutive days beginning ~11 hours prior to apheresis; maximum dose: 40 mg/day

Historically, the bone marrow was the primary source of hematopoietic stem cells for transplantation and it still represents an equivalent, if not better, stem cell source in the setting of allogeneic transplantation. The bone marrow contains populations of hematopoietic cells ranging from the pluripotent stem cell, early progenitor cells, and later, more differentiated progenitor cells that all exist within and are supported by the bone marrow stroma (matrix composed of connective tissue, reticuloendothelial cells, adipose cells). Compared to blood, the concentration of T lymphocytes is significantly lower in the marrow. Bone marrow can be harvested by removing an adequate volume of marrow (approximately 10 mL/kg) from the posterior iliac crests of the donor or patient. This is generally done in an operating room and requires general or local anesthesia. Common medical risks to the donor of bone marrow include the risks of undergoing anesthesia, and transient moderate pain in the area of cell harvesting. Severe anemia can also develop. The frequency of life-threatening complications, which have included thromboembolic disorders, aspiration pneumonia, and cardiac dysrhythmias, is ≤0.3%. Hematopoietic engraftment (normalization of the peripheral white blood cell count) occurs earlier following peripheral stem cell transplantation than following bone marrow transplantation. However, chronic graft-versus-host disease (GVHD) risk is lower with the bone marrow source.

Umbilical cord blood (UCB) is another source of hematopoietic progenitor cells. The product, which is harvested from the placenta and umbilical cord immediately after birth, can be processed and transplanted or frozen for future use. The product obtained from UCB contains a high proportion of pluripotent stem cells and natural killer cells, and a low proportion of mature lymphocytes. The time to engraftment is generally longer following UCB transplantation than following peripheral blood or bone marrow hematopoietic stem cell transplantation.

Moreover, UCB transplantation is generally reserved for children and small adults because the number of stem cells that can be collected from cord blood may be inadequate to support timely engraftment for larger patients. The risk for severe GVHD is lower with UCB even when HLA matching is not perfect. The process of harvesting UCB does not present a medical risk to the donor, because the actual collection of cells is done after the placenta is extruded as part of the birthing process.

The hematopoietic progenitor cells may be treated prior to transplantation to eradicate tumor cell contamination in the product following autologous donation or reduce the number of T lymphocytes that may promote graft-versus-host disease in an allogeneic recipient. The term purging refers to the removal of tumor cells by various techniques such as binding to specific monoclonal antibodies or incubation with cytotoxic drugs, such as 4-hydroperoxycyclophosphamide, that spare the immature stem cells. *Ex vivo* T lymphocyte reduction, also known as T cell depletion, is generally achieved using monoclonal antibodies directed against surface proteins expressed on T lymphocytes. Engraftment is generally delayed following transplantation of hematopoietic progenitor cells that have undergone *ex vivo* purging or T cell depletion.

AUTOLOGOUS MYELOABLATIVE TRANSPLANTATION

Chemotherapy and dosage selection for autologous myeloablative HSCT is based on three important principles:

1. Certain drugs such as alkylating agents and etoposide exhibit steep dose-response curves when used to treat susceptible malignancies. Therefore, when the dose-limiting adverse effect of these drugs is myelosuppression, high doses can be administered with hematopoietic stem cell rescue to achieve high response rates.
2. High doses of chemotherapy with nonoverlapping nonhematologic major organ toxicity can be combined without compromising dose.
3. Cryopreserved bone marrow and/or blood progenitor cells can rescue the patient from the myeloablative effects of the high-dose chemotherapy.

Administration of filgrastim or sargramostim following reinfusion of the autologous hematopoietic progenitor cells significantly shortens the duration of neutropenia associated with myeloablative chemotherapy (refer to filgrastim or sargramostim monographs for dosing, etc). The hematopoietic recovery period following HSCT is generally 1-2 weeks, which is shorter than that for bone marrow or UCB transplants which require 2-4 weeks. The monocytes and neutrophils engraft first followed by the platelets about a week later. The most common complications associated with autologous HSCT are febrile neutropenia, serum electrolyte abnormalities, infection, bleeding, gastrointestinal toxicities (mucositis, nausea, vomiting, and diarrhea), and less commonly, other organ toxicities that are related to the specific chemotherapy administered. Palifermin is approved for use to decrease the incidence and duration of severe oral mucositis in patients with hematologic malignancies undergoing HSCT. The following table lists commonly used chemotherapy agents with their dose-limiting toxicities in SCT.

Chemotherapy	Standard Dose[1]	Maximum SCT Dose as Single Agent[2]	Maximum SCT Dose in Combination[2]	Dose-Limiting Toxicity
Busulfan (oral)	4 mg/d	16 mg/kg	16 mg/kg	GI, liver (SOS), CNS (seizure), pulmonary
Busulfan (I.V.)		12 mg/kg	12 mg/kg	GI, liver (SOS), CNS (seizure), pulmonary
CARBOplatin	400 mg/m^2	2000 mg/m^2	1300 mg/m^2	Liver, renal
Carmustine	200 mg/m^2	800 mg/m^2	600 mg/m^2	Liver, pulmonary
CISplatin	50-100 mg/m^2	180-200 mg/m^2	165-200 (in BEP) mg/m^2	Renal, neuropathy
Cyclophosphamide	600-1875 mg/m^2	200 mg/kg or 7.5 g/m^2	200 mg/kg or 7.5 g/m^2	Cardiac, hemorrhagic cystitis, liver (SOS)
Etoposide	100 mg/m^2/dose x 1-5 days	2400 mg/m^2	2400 mg/m^2	GI, hypotension
Melphalan	40 mg/m^2	220 mg/m^2	140-180 mg/m^2	GI
MitoXANtrone	12 mg/m^2/d x 3	90 mg/m^2	60-80 mg/m^2	GI, cardiac

[1]Usual dose for therapy that does not include HSCT.

[2]Maximum dose is divided for administration over 2 or more days.

ALLOGENEIC MYELOABLATIVE TRANSPLANTATION

The principle behind allogeneic myeloablative hematopoietic stem cell transplantation is that hematological disease can be cured by complete marrow ablation with profound immunosuppression so that the donor cells can engraft and successfully replace the patient's diseased hematopoietic system. Post-transplant immunosuppressive therapy is essential for successful engraftment of donor cells and prevention of graft-versus-host disease (GVHD). Preparative regimens for allogeneic transplantation are based on the need for both marrow ablation and immunosuppression. Commonly used regimens are listed below.

Acronym	Chemotherapy Drugs (Total Dose)	Dosages and Scheduling
BuCy	Busulfan (12-16 mg/kg)	0.875-1 mg/kg/dose P.O. q6h x 16 doses; or 1 mg/kg/dose P.O. q6h x 12 doses; or 0.8 mg/kg I.V. q6h x 16 doses
	Cyclophosphamide (120 mg/kg)	60 mg/kg/dose I.V. q24h x 2 doses
FTBI/Cy, or CyTBI	Fractionated total body irradiation	1200-1500 cGy divided bid over 3-5 days
	Cyclophosphamide (120-200 mg/kg)	50 mg/kg/dose I.V. q24h x 4 doses or 60 mg/kg/dose I.V. q24h x 2 doses
TBI-VP16-Cy	Fractionated total body irradiation	1200-1400 cGy divided bid over 3-5 days
	Etoposide (30 mg/kg)	30 mg/kg/dose I.V. x 1 dose
	Cyclophosphamide (120 mg/kg)	60 mg/kg/dose I.V. q24h x 2 doses
Bu/Mel	Busulfan (16 mg/kg)	1 mg/kg/dose P.O. q6h x 16 doses
	Melphalan (135-140 mg/m^2)	45 mg/m^2/dose I.V. q24h x 3, or 140 mg/m^2 once
FTBI/Mel	Fractionated total body irradiation	1200-1500 cGy divided bid over 3-5 days
	Melphalan (135-140 mg/m^2)	45 mg/m^2/dose I.V. q24h x 2, or 70 mg/m^2/dose I.V. q24h x 2; or 140 mg/m^2 once
CyATG	Cyclophosphamide (200 mg/kg)	50 mg/kg/dose I.V. q24h x 4
	Lymphocyte immune globulin (90-160 mg/kg)	30-40 mg/kg/dose I.V. q24-48h x 3-4 doses

Lymphocyte immune globulin or antithymocyte globulin is included in the preparative regimen for patients with severe aplastic anemia. Lymphocyte immune globulin or antithymocyte globulin is often added to the preparative regimen for allogeneic transplants when the donor and recipient are immunologically mismatched or unrelated, and for umbilical cord blood transplants. This added immunosuppression improves engraftment and may decrease acute GVHD.

Hematopoietic growth factors (filgrastim or sargramostim) are usually administered after infusion of allogeneic donor blood cells. The doses range from 5-10 mcg/kg/day and administration is begun either on day 0 or +1 or may be delayed up to 6 days post-cell infusion. The colony stimulating factors are discontinued when the absolute neutrophil count reaches a designated target, which is often in the range of 5000-10,000/mm^3.

Allogeneic HSCT recipients are at risk for all of the common complications associated with administration of high-dose chemotherapy, including febrile neutropenia, serum electrolyte abnormalities, infection, bleeding, gastrointestinal toxicities (mucositis, nausea, vomiting, and diarrhea), and less commonly, other organ toxicities that are related to the specific chemotherapy administered.

NONMYELOABLATIVE TRANSPLANTS

Nonmyeloablative or reduced intensity conditioning (RIC) HSCT is achieved by administration of immunosuppressive conditioning regimens that are less directly cytotoxic to bone marrow and nonhematopoietic tissue(s). Nonmyeloablative transplantation utilizes the graft-versus-leukemia effect as part of the overall treatment. The safety impetus for use of RIC is to allow allogeneic HSCT in patients unable to tolerate the myeloablative preparative regimens, such as the elderly, or patients with an extensive history of chemotherapy treatment, impaired major organ function, or comorbid conditions. Clinical trials and case series describe use of nonmyeloablative hematopoietic stem cell transplantation for the following diseases: Congenital immunodeficiency syndromes, acute myelogenous leukemia, myelodysplastic syndrome, acute lymphocytic leukemia, multiple myeloma, non-Hodgkin's lymphoma, Hodgkin's disease, sickle cell disease, renal cell carcinoma, and various advanced solid tumors. Most of the published studies and case series report use of this procedure in patients with relapsed or refractory disease, elderly patients, or those unable to tolerate myeloablative preparative regimens.

The premise supporting nonmyeloablative transplantation is that nonmyeloablative, but sufficiently immunosuppressive conditioning regimens, yield a state of mixed chimerism in the recipient, which gradually converts to full donor chimerism. The chimeric engraftment supports a graft-versus-malignancy effect. Complete donor engraftment, also known as 100% donor chimerism, occurs when all of the detectable hematopoietic cells are of donor origin. Complete donor chimerism occurring within 30-90 days following transplantation is generally associated with disease response. Because antitumor effects of nonmyeloablative allogeneic transplants appear somewhat late (2-3 months after the procedure), patients with active or poorly controlled malignancies do not appear to be optimal candidates for this type of transplantation.

Examples of reduced-intensity preparative regimens are listed in the following table.

Acronym	Chemotherapy Drugs (Total Dose)	Dosages and Scheduling
Flu/ATG	Lymphocyte immune globulin 40 mg/kg (Atgam®)	10 mg/kg/day I.V. on 4 consecutive days
	Antithymoglobulin 10 mg/kg (Thymoglobulin®)	2.5 mg/kg/day I.V. on 4 consecutive days
	Fludarabine 125 mg/m^2	25 mg/m^2/day I.V. on 5 consecutive days
FC-ATG	Fludarabine 125 mg/m^2	25 mg/m^2/day I.V. on days -6 to -2
	Cyclophosphamide 120 mg/kg	60 mg/kg/day I.V. on days -3 and -2
	Lymphocyte immune globulin 60 mg/kg (Atgam®)	20 mg/kg/day I.V. on 3 consecutive days
TBI/Flu	Total body irradiation 4 Gy	2 Gy/day on days -8 and -7
	Fludarabine 125 mg/m^2	25 mg/m^2/day I.V. on days -6 to -2

(continued)

Acronym	Chemotherapy Drugs (Total Dose)	Dosages and Scheduling
Flu/Mel/ATG	Fludarabine 125 mg/m^2	25 mg/m^2/day I.V. on days -6 to -2
	Melphalan 140-180 mg/m^2	70-90 mg/m^2/day I.V. on days -3 and -2
	Lymphocyte immune globulin 120 mg/kg (Atgam®)	30 mg/kg/day I.V. on days -4 to -1
Bu/Flu/ATG	Busulfan 8 mg/kg	1 mg/kg/dose P.O. q6h X8 doses on days -6 and -5
	Fludarabine 125 mg/m^2	25 mg/m^2/day I.V. on days -6 to -2
	Antithymocyte globulin (Fresnius) 10 mg/kg	2.5 mg/kg/day I.V. on 4 consecutive days
Cy/Flu/TBI	Cyclophosphamide 50 mg/kg	50 mg/kg I.V. on day -6
	Fludarabine 200 mg/m^2	40 mg/m^2/day I.V. on days -6 to -2
	TBI 200 cGy	TBI 200 cGy on day -1

GVHD prophylaxis generally includes cyclosporine or tacrolimus plus mycophenolate mofetil. Treatment of moderate-to-severe GVHD is similar to the approach taken for treatment of GVHD following myeloablative allogeneic hematopoietic stem cell transplantation (see Postransplant Complications). Most complications following nonmyeloablative hematopoietic stem cell transplantation are related to GVHD and the immunosuppression required for treatment of GVHD. Infectious complications from cytomegalovirus, herpes virus, candidiasis, aspergillosis, and other opportunistic microbes are common.

Less regimen-related toxicity occurs with RIC, so it is considered as an alternative therapeutic modality for patients unable to tolerate the adverse effects inherent to myeloablative therapy. However, patients undergoing nonmyeloablative transplantation must have adequate organ function and physiologic reserve for chronic administration of immunosuppressive therapy and management of opportunistic infections that may arise.

POSTTRANSPLANT COMPLICATIONS

Graft-Versus-Host Disease

GVHD is an immune-mediated reaction initiated by donor T-cell recognition of recipient tissues as nonself. GVHD which occurs before 100 days post-transplant is classified as acute GVHD, and after 100 days, it is classified as chronic GVHD. Acute GVHD primarily affects the skin, gastrointestinal tract, and liver. It is graded based on extent of organ involvement from grade I (mild) to grade IV (life-threatening). Chronic GVHD affects the skin, gastrointestinal tract, liver, and other organs and tissues, including the lungs, lacrimal glands, and connective tissue. Chronic GVHD is generally graded as limited or extensive disease. Mortality ranges from 10% to 30%. There is a strong positive correlation between development of acute or chronic GVHD and decreased risk of malignancy recurrence due to associated graft vs malignancy effect.

Given the high morbidity and mortality associated with severe GVHD, posttransplant care is directed to prevent this complication. A combination of 2-3 immunosuppressants is used to prevent GVHD. The selection of prophylactic immunosuppressants used is based on the degree of risk for GVHD and the risk of malignant relapse. In general, as the depth and duration of immunosuppression increase, so does the risk of malignant relapse, and infectious disease. Commonly used prophylactic immunosuppressants include cyclosporine or tacrolimus plus methotrexate, with addition of a methylprednisolone for patients at high risk for GVHD.

GVHD Prophylactic Agents	Usual Dose and Schedule
CycloSPORINE	2.5-4 mg/kg/day I.V. continuous infusion or divided q12h over 2-6 hours. Adjust dose according to toxicity and blood concentrations. Convert to oral dose when appropriate.
Tacrolimus	0.03 mg/kg/day I.V. continuous infusion. Adjust dose according to toxicity and blood concentrations. Transition (using appropriate conversion) to oral dose when appropriate.
Methotrexate	15 mg/m^2/dose on day + 1, 10 mg/m^2/dose on days +3, +6, and +11; give I.V. push.
MethylPREDNISolone	Variable; 0.5-1 mg/kg/day divided q6-12h then taper. May start day +1 up to +7; increase dose for acute GVHD reactions.
Mycophenolate mofetil	1 g/dose I.V. or P.O. q12h; or 15 mg/kg/dose I.V. or P.O. q12h

Initial treatment of GVHD includes addition of a corticosteroid or a dosage increase of ongoing corticosteroid treatment. Other agents used for the treatment of steroid-refractory acute GVHD include lymphocyte immune globulin or antithymocyte globulin, interleukin-2 receptor antagonists (basiliximab), tumor necrosis factor antagonists (etanercept, infliximab), sirolimus, and pentostatin. Thalidomide, pentostatin, PUVA (8-methoxypsoralen plus UV-A radiation), and rituximab also have been utilized in the setting of steroid-refractory GVHD.

Infection

Allogeneic stem cell transplantation is associated with a wide range of infectious complications that occur during identifiable time periods after the transplant. The early period of neutropenia is most commonly associated with bacterial infections, fungal infections (*Candida* species), and herpes simplex virus (HSV) reactivation. *Pneumocystis jirovecii pneumoniae* (PCP) risk increases with duration of immunosuppressive therapy. Other life-threatening opportunistic infections typically occurring 2-3 months post-transplant include aspergillosis and CMV (disseminated or pneumonitis). Other serious atypical viral and fungal infections can also be seen at this later time. Infections with rhinovirus and coronavirus are common during the first 100 days following allogeneic HSCT and tend to present as symptoms of rhinorrhea, congestion, postnasal drip, sputum production, and cough. Lower respiratory tract infections attributed to rhinovirus or coronavirus occur in approximately 2% of infected patients.

Prophylaxis for certain infections is routine while others are treated when they are diagnosed. Trimethoprim-sulfamethoxazole or a fluoroquinolone is given during the preparative regimen for selective gut decontamination. Trimethoprim-sulfamethoxazole is also administered after hematopoietic recovery on a 2-3 times weekly schedule as PCP prophylaxis. The major concern with trimethoprim-sulfamethoxazole is the myelosuppressive effect. Alternative antimicrobials for patients allergic to sulfonamide antimicrobials include inhaled pentamidine or oral dapsone. Fungal prophylaxis is routinely given as well. This generally consists of fluconazole, voriconazole, or an amphotericin B product. Inhalational amphotericin B can also be used to decrease risk of pulmonary aspergillosis. Acyclovir is routinely used to prevent HSV reinfection. The role of acyclovir for prevention of

CMV infection is controversial. Some centers routinely prescribe acyclovir immediately following the transplant for prevention of CMV or HSV infection. After cellular recovery, the patient may be switched to ganciclovir or valganciclovir therapy. The hematologic toxicity of ganciclovir and valganciclovir precludes its routine use at an earlier point in the transplant; however, CMV therapy is started preemptively before engraftment with the finding of CMV DNA by polymerase chain reaction in the peripheral white blood cells. The role of antibacterial prophylaxis or continued gut decontamination varies with transplant centers but is often used in some form. Prophylactic antimicrobials are generally administered throughout the duration of exogenous immunosuppression following allogeneic hematopoietic stem cell transplantation.

Sinusoidal Obstruction Syndrome

Hepatic sinusoidal obstruction syndrome (SOS), formerly known as hepatic veno-occlusive disease (VOD), can occur as a result of the pretransplant conditioning regimen. Risk factors for hepatic SOS include pre-existing liver disease, malignant involvement of the liver, serum ferritin level exceeding 1000 ng/mL, malnutrition, prior extensive chemotherapy treatment, and previous treatment with busulfan, imatinib, or gemtuzumab ozogamicin. SOS, which usually presents within the first 3 weeks after transplant, results from obstruction of blood flow in the small hepatic veins. Signs and symptoms include right upper quadrant pain or tenderness, hepatomegaly, weight gain, ascites, hyperbilirubinemia, and thrombocytopenia. Treatment options include supportive care, alteplase (has a high incidence of bleeding complications), and antithrombin. Defibrotide is an investigational agent with antithrombotic, thrombolytic, and anti-ischemic properties which has been used in the prevention and treatment of SOS. Low-dose heparin or ursodiol have also been used for SOS prophylaxis.

FUTURE DIRECTIONS

Proteasome Inhibition and GVHD

Trials of the proteasome inhibitor bortezomib for GVHD prophylaxis and for treatment of steroid-refractory GVHD are ongoing (Reddy, 2012). Bortezomib inhibits nuclear factor-κB (NF-κB), induces apoptosis, reduces interleukin-6-mediated cell growth, and possibly has antiangiogenic properties. Through such mechanisms, bortezomib appears to reduce cytokine production and immunostimulatory activity, which are important in the pathogenesis of GVHD. In addition to depleting T-lymphocytes, bortezomib may also enhance the graft vs tumor effect by downregulating major histocompatibility complex I expression on tumor cell surfaces and promoting their NK-mediated destruction (Reddy, 2012).

Histone Deacetylase Inhibition and GVHD

Histone deacetylase inhibitors (HDACis), such as vorinostat, inhibit histone deacetylase (HDAC) enzymes. Such inhibition causes alterations in chromatin structure and increased gene transcription, ultimately resulting in cell death. Through preclinical studies, histone deacetylase inhibitors have been found to have potent anti-inflammatory and immunoregulatory effects (Reddy, 2012). Phase II clinical trials of vorinostat, in combination with standard GVHD prophylaxis, are underway to determine if histone deacetylase inhibition further reduces the incidence of acute GVHD in patients receiving reduced-intensity conditioning regimens (Reddy, 2012).

REFERENCES

Bacigalupo A, "Second EBMT Workshop on Reduced Intensity Allogeneic Hemopoietic Stem Cell Transplants (RI-HSCT)," *Bone Marrow Transplant*, 2002, 29:191-5.

Barker JN, Weisdorf DJ, DeFor TE, et al, "Rapid and Complete Donor Chimerism in Adult Recipients of Unrelated Donor Umbilical Cord Blood Transplantation After Reduced-Intensity Conditioning," *Blood*, 2003, 102(5):1915-9.

Cairo MS and Wagner JE, "Placental and/or Umbilical Cord Blood: An Alternative Source of Hematopoietic Stem Cells for Transplantation," *Blood*, 1997, 90:4665-78.

Champlin R, Khouri I, Anderlini P, et al, "Nonmyeloablative Preparative Regimens for Allogeneic Hematopoietic Transplantation," *Bone Marrow Transplant*, 2001, 27 Suppl 2:S13-22.

Chopra R, Eaton JD, Grassi A, et al, "Defibrotide for the Treatment of Hepatic Veno-Occlusive Disease: Results of the European Compassionate-Use Study," *Br J Haematol*, 2000, 111 (4):1122-9.

Copelan EA, "Hematopoietic Stem-Cell Transplantation," *N Engl J Med*, 2006, 354(17):1813-26.

Gyurkocza B, Storb R, Storer BE, et al, "Nonmyeloablative Allogeneic Hematopoietic Cell Transplantation in Patients With Acute Myeloid Leukemia," *J Clin Oncol*, 2010, 28(17):2859-67.

Ho VT and Soiffer RJ, "The History and Future of T-Cell Depletion as Graft-Versus-Host Disease Prophylaxis for Allogeneic Hematopoietic Stem Cell Transplantation," *Blood*, 2001, 98:3192-204.

Klingebiel T and Schlegel PG, "GVHD: Overview on Pathophysiology, Incidence, Clinical and Biological Features," *Bone Marrow Transplant*, 1998, 21 (Suppl 2):S45-9.

Kumar S, DeLeve LD, Kamath PS, et al, "Hepatic Veno-Occlusive Disease (Sinusoidal Obstruction Syndrome) After Hematopoietic Stem Cell Transplantation," *Mayo Clin Proc*, 2003, (78):589-98.

Maradei SC, Maiolino A, de Azevedo AM, et al, "Serum Ferritin as Risk Factor for Sinusoidal Obstruction Syndrome of the Liver in Patients Undergoing Hematopoietic Stem Cell Transplantation," *Blood*, 2009, 114(6):1270-5.

McClune BL, Weisdorf DJ, Pedersen TL, et al, "Effect of Age on Outcome of Reduced-Intensity Hematopoietic Cell Transplantation for Older Patients With Acute Myeloid Leukemia in First Complete Remission or With Myelodysplastic Syndrome," *J Clin Oncol*, 2010, 28(11):1878-87.

Milano F, Campbell AP, Guthrie KA, et al, "Human Rhinovirus and Coronavirus Detection Among Allogeneic Hematopoietic Stem Cell Transplantation Recipients," *Blood*, 2010, 115(10):2088-94.

Mogul MJ, "Unrelated Cord Blood Transplantation Vs Matched Unrelated Donor Bone Marrow Transplantation: The Risks and Benefits of Each Choice," *Bone Marrow Transplant*, 2000, 25 (Suppl 2):S58-60.

Pegram AA and Kennedy LD, "Prevention and Treatment of Veno-Occlusive Disease," *Ann Pharmacother*, 2001, 35(7-8):935-42.

Reddy P, de Lima M, and Koreth J, "Emerging Therapies in Hematopoietic Stem Cell Transplantation," *Biol Blood Marrow Transplant*, 2012, 18(1 Suppl):S125-31.

Richardson PG, Soiffer RJ, Antin JH, et al, "Defibrotide for the Treatment of Severe Hepatic Veno-Occlusive Disease and Multiorgan Failure After Stem Cell Transplantation: A Multicenter, Randomized, Dose-Finding Trial," *Biol Blood Marrow Transplant*, 2010, 16(7):1005-17.

Ringdén O, Labopin M, Ehninger G, et al, "Reduced Intensity Conditioning Compared With Myeloablative Conditioning Using Unrelated Donor Transplants in Patients With Acute Myeloid Leukemia," *J Clin Oncol*, 2009, 27(27):4570-7.

Rowe JM, Ciobanu N, Ascensao J, et al, "Recommended Guidelines for the Management of Autologous and Allogeneic Bone Marrow Transplantation. A Report From the Eastern Cooperative Oncology Group (ECOG)," *Ann Intern Med*, 1994, 120:143-58.

Stiff P, "Mucositis Associated With Stem Cell Transplantation: Current Status and Innovative Approaches to Management," *Bone Marrow Transplant* , 2001, 27 (Suppl 2):S3-S11.

Storb R, Deeg HJ, Whitehead J, et al, "Methotrexate and Cyclosporine Compared With Cyclosporine Alone for Prophylaxis of Acute Graft Versus Host Disease After Marrow Transplantation for Leukemia," *N Engl J Med*, 1986, 314:729-35.

Vogelsang GB and Arai S, "Mycophenolate Mofetil for the Prevention and Treatment of Graft-Versus-Host Disease Following Stem Cell Transplantation: Preliminary Findings," *Bone Marrow Transplant*, 2001, 27:1255-62.

DRUG DEVELOPMENT PROCESS

Drug development describes the process required to bring a drug from its original identity to becoming a commercially available product for use in human beings. The drug development process involves scientific, clinical, and regulatory activities. Bringing a new molecular entity or new active substance through the drug development process takes years of time and hundreds of millions to billions of dollars.

SCIENTIFIC CONTRIBUTION

The major scientific contribution is drug discovery and drug design. Candidates for drug development arise from biotechnologic or chemical synthesis and natural product extraction. Selection of drug candidates is often based on their ability *in vitro* to bind a molecular target or exert a biologic effect. This is an inefficient low-yield process despite the use of automated high throughput screening methods that can test thousands of drug candidates daily. A challenge of drug discovery is the myriad of factors that can abrogate the utility or efficacy of drug candidates as they proceed through preclinical and clinical testing.

Preclinical testing is done in several species of animals to evaluate toxicity, pharmacodynamics, and pharmacokinetics. Acute toxicity, chronic toxicity, fetotoxicity, teratogenicity, and carcinogenicity are tested in animals to identify common sites of toxicity and potentially use-limiting toxicity, such as neurologic adverse effects or carcinogenicity. Drug pharmacodynamics and pharmacokinetics are evaluated in animals to extrapolate a first in human (FIH) dose when the drug advances to clinical trials.

Additional scientific contributions to drug development include chemical characterization and pharmaceutical development of drug candidates.

REGULATORY PROCESS

In the United States, clinical trials administering drugs to human beings are regulated by the Food and Drug Administration (FDA). Regulation is directed and implemented through an application process required for various levels of clinical drug development. The Investigational New Drug (IND) application is required prior to testing a drug in human subjects or distributing it across state lines. The IND (Form 1571) contains preclinical data, proposed clinical protocol, investigator's brochure (if available), and manufacturing information. An Exploratory IND allows administration of subtherapeutic doses to a small number of subjects to assess whether the preclinically tested drug-target interaction occurs in humans. An Emergency IND allows distribution of an investigational drug on a patient-specific basis for management of a serious condition. Investigational drugs must have demonstrated a certain degree of efficacy and safety for an Emergency IND application to be granted. The New Drug Application (NDA) is reviewed by the FDA to determine whether drug testing is sufficient for product approval and consumer use. The NDA is a comprehensive document containing data supporting all of the chemical, pharmacologic, pharmaceutical, preclinical, therapeutic, safety, and pharmacokinetic information and claims required for product approval. Approval of generic equivalents can be achieved with an Abbreviated New Drug Application (ANDA). Generic drugs are reviewed using the ANDA because the efficacy and safety of these products was previously established by the original brand (innovator drug). Approval of a generic drug is based on scientific data demonstrating that the generic product is bioequivalent to the innovator product. Biologic products, such as monoclonal antibodies and vaccines, are approved for commercial use using a Biologic License Application (BLA). An abbreviated licensure pathway for biological products that are "bio-similar" to or "interchangeable" with an FDA-licensed biological product is in development.

The conduct of clinical trials is approved, monitored, and reviewed by an institutional review board (IRB), also known as human subjects committee, independent ethics committee, ethical review board, etc. The IRB is responsible for overseeing the conduct of biomedical and behavioral research involving human subjects. The IRB ensures that biomedical and behavioral research is ethical, informed consent is sufficient, and appropriate safeguards are established. The FDA Department of Health and Human Services Office for Human Research Protection empowers IRBs to approve, require modifications, or disapprove research conducted under their domain. Most IRBs are based at academic institutions or health care systems. However, independent commercial for profit IRBs exist that adhere to the same federal regulations as local committees.

CLINICAL TRIALS

Clinical trials include Phase 0, Phase I, Phase II, and Phase III analysis of a drug in humans. Phase 0 studies evaluate clinical drug-target interaction(s). Phase I testing is done to assess drug safety and pharmacokinetics. Phase 0 and Phase I clinical trials are FIH drug studies that are unlikely to provide any therapeutic benefit to the participating subjects. Phase II clinical trials test the efficacy of a drug in the management of a specific disease or pathophysiologic process. The purpose of Phase III clinical trials is to compare the investigational treatment to the standard of care. Phase IV testing (postmarketing surveillance) generally involves pharmacovigilance or additional pharmacokinetic or drug interaction characterization in FDA-approved medications. Phase IV testing is often done independently by academic investigators or it may be a requirement imposed by the FDA.

Oncology Agents

Phase 0 clinical trials are an attempt to reduce the consumption of valuable time and resources that occur when promising preclinical candidates fail in Phase II clinical trials. Specifically, small doses of drug are administered to 15 or fewer subjects for a short period of time to evaluate whether the therapeutic drug-target interaction occurs in human beings. Drugs tested in Phase 0 clinical trials must have a wide margin of safety and a validated method for testing drug-target interaction(s).

Phase I clinical trials for anticancer treatments are used to identify safety. For cytotoxic products, phase I studies determine the maximum tolerated dose (MTD). The FIH dose of cytotoxic chemotherapy is generally a small fraction (1/10th) of the preclinical dose that produced lethality in 10% of the most sensitive animal model. The dose is increased in a stepwise fashion until the dose-limiting toxicity (DLT) is reached in >33% of a patient cohort. The dose at which <33% of patients have DLT is utilized in Phase II studies. Dose calculation based on body surface area or weight is used as a tool to extrapolate clinical doses from those administered to animals in preclinical testing. Unlike Phase I clinical trials for nononcology medications conducted in normal human subjects, only patients with advanced cancer refractory to treatment and with normal organ function, are utilized for Phase I oncology studies. The dose of targeted anticancer treatments, such as monoclonal antibodies and tyrosine kinase inhibitors, that is designated for Phase II testing is generally based on receptor saturation or another surrogate marker of efficacy instead of MTD. Phase I methodology should be used when anticancer treatments with an established dose for single agent therapy or administered as combination therapy.

Phase II trials evaluate drug safety and efficacy in a group of patients with a disease the drug is intended to treat. Data is collected on adverse effects and response to the therapy. Phase II clinical trials may report efficacy based on tumor response (tumor shrinkage), which is a much less stringent measure of efficacy than survival.

Phase III studies involve a larger number of patients with a particular tumor. Patients are randomized to the new treatment or the current standard of care. A placebo arm is used for Phase III analysis of novel treatments for which there is no comparable standard of care; use of placebo can be controversial when studying treatments for life-threatening diseases. Primary endpoints for Phase III clinical trials evaluating anticancer treatments generally include disease response, duration of disease-free survival, duration of overall survival, and safety. As was the case with gemcitabine in pancreatic cancer, a clinical benefit response may be an endpoint that is measured.

COST(S)

Investigational new drugs are generally provided free of charge to the patient. However, there are cases when the manufacturer can seek FDA authorization to charge for use of an investigational new drug to recover costs necessary to continue drug development.

SELECTED READINGS

Daugherty CK, Ratain MJ, Emanuel EJ, et al, "Ethical, Scientific, and Regulatory Perspectives Regarding the Use of Placebos in Cancer Clinical Trials," *J Clin Oncol*, 2008, 26(8):1371-8.

"Drug Development and Approval Process." Available at http://www.fda.gov/Drugs/DevelopmentApprovalProcess/default.htm. Last accessed August 2012.

Egorin MJ, "Horseshoes, Hand Grenades, and Body-Surface Area-Based Dosing: Aiming For a Target," *J Clin Oncol*, 2003, 21(2):182-3.

Fojo T and Grady C, "How Much Is Life Worth: Cetuximab, Non-Small Cell Lung Cancer, and the $440 Billion Question," *J Natl Cancer Inst*, 2009, 101(15):1044-8.

Hamberg P and Verweij J, "Phase I Drug Combination Trial Design: Walking the Tightrope," *J Clin Oncol*, 2009 [epub ahead of print].

"Health and Human Services, Office for Human Research Protections (OHRP)." Available at http://www.hhs.gov/ohrp

Mordenti J, Thomsen K, Licko V, et al, "Efficacy and Concentration-Response of Murine Anti-VEGF Monoclonal Antibody In Tumor-Bearing Mice and Extrapolation to Humans," *Toxicol Pathol*, 1999, 27(1):14-21.

Rowan K, "Oncology's First Phase 0 Trial," *J Natl Cancer Inst*, 2009, 101(14):978-9.

INVESTIGATIONAL DRUG SERVICE

An Investigational Drug Service (IDS) is an organized pharmacy-based service that controls the inventory, preparation, and dispensing of investigational drugs. Investigational drugs are administered only to patients who have, in an informed manner, signed a consent form to participate in the particular study using these investigational drugs. A patient formally enrolled to participate in a clinical study is known as a "subject". Investigational drugs used in this manner are frequently new drugs undergoing First in Human, Phase I, Phase II, or Phase III evaluation prior to FDA approval for a medical purpose. In addition, investigational drugs can be commercially available drugs used under the direction of a protocol for a nonlabeled indication or as a supportive measure for a new drug. An IDS should be under the direction of an appropriately trained pharmacist with technical support as warranted by the workload.

A study protocol is the document describing the scientific background providing the basis for doing the study, specific study objectives and endpoints, treatments and tests done as part of the study, study drug information, statistical methodology, means for assurance of patient confidentiality, and the subject consent form. Some studies provide an Investigator's Drug Brochure, which presents very detailed and comprehensive study drug information. Each study is assigned a unique identifier (eg, SWOG S0927) that generally includes an abbreviation for the research consortium (Southwest Oncology Group), a truncation of the year of study development (2009), and its position within a series of studies (27). Study protocols and Investigator's Drug Brochures are confidential, and frequently proprietary documents. Prior to study activation at an institution, the planned research must be approved by the institutional Investigational review board. All departments needed to provide personnel or resources for study implementation should review the protocol prior to study implementation to ensure that study activities can reasonably be supported with available resources. The IDS pharmacist should scrutinize each study protocol prior to study activation to determine the impact of study implementation on pharmacy department personnel and resources.

Investigational drug inventory must be stored at the appropriate conditions and separate from commercial drug inventory. An ongoing drug-specific inventory must be maintained for all investigational drugs housed within a pharmacy. Some studies will require lot number-specific, or subject-specific inventory for study drugs. Minimal inventory documentation should include study identification number, study drug dosage form and lot number, study drug expiration date or date of preparation, transaction date, transaction type (receipt, dispensing, return, waste), and current number of dosage forms available. Although it may be kept separately from individual study drug inventories, the pharmacy must maintain an ongoing refrigerator, freezer, and ambient temperature log for study drug storage facilities. All inventory records should be kept in a secure, yet accessible, location by the pharmacy, even after study closure. In addition, study drug should be shipped directly to the Pharmacy Department rather than the Principal Investigator's office. This will ensure that the Pharmacy Department has shipping receipts and shipment invoices to verify receipt of the packaged contents. This will also reduce the possibility of prolonged study drug storage at inappropriate conditions, such as the institutional loading dock.

Study drug preparation should be described in the protocol or Investigator's Drug Brochure. Unfortunately, extensive admixture stability and compatibility information is not available for many injectable study drugs. Subsequently, these may have to be prepared on a dose-by-dose basis. Departmental inservices to acquaint professional and technical personnel with each new study are helpful tools for increasing staff familiarity with new studies and study drug preparation. Pharmacy department personnel should have 24-hour access to information about study drug preparation. Ideally, this is in the form of an easy-to-read and readily accessible fast facts sheet. Study protocols and Investigator's Drug Brochures should also be available to Pharmacy Department personnel around the clock for questions that arise outside of standard business hours. The Investigational Drug Service must develop a plan such that study drug doses are labeled in the manner directed by the study, are consistent with institutional policies and procedures, and are in accordance with state and federal regulations.

Study drug doses prepared for administration within a hospital or clinic should be dispensed directly to the study or institutional nurse for delivery to the patient's bedside for administration or placed directly into the subject's secured medication bin on the nursing unit. Generally, study drug doses should not be intermixed with standard medication doses transported via the routine intra-institutional delivery system. Although the risk of inadvertent misplacement of a study drug dose may be low, the consequences can have ethical and legal implications. As an example, a study drug dose inadvertently transported to the wrong nursing unit may be mistakenly administered to a patient with a name similar to that of the actual study subject. Consequently, the study drug dose could be administered to a person who did not consent to receive an investigational drug.

Pharmacy support of blinded studies can involve additional responsibilities and challenges. Pharmacy-related activities may include randomization (treatment assignment) of subjects when the Principal Investigator and other study personnel are blinded to the study treatment. Randomization for treatment assignment can be done for some studies by simply following a list of treatment assignments sequentially for consecutive subjects. However, randomization for large multicenter studies may require contacting a central randomization center with provision of patient-specific information. When pharmacy activities include randomization, it is important for the Investigational Drug Service to ensure that a workable plan is in place prior to study activation. Moreover, labeling of blinded study drug doses can be challenging since the traditional role of pharmacy labeling is to provide a completely clear description of the dosage form. In contrast, to maintain a study blind, the specific contents of a study dosage form must be omitted from the pharmacy label. Several approaches have been taken to balance study methods with institutional and legislative requirements. As an example, for a blinded fictitious study, protocol #1211, evaluating the efficacy of newazole 200 mg versus placebo (0.9% NaCl 100 mL), the following labeling techniques can be utilized to identify the dosage form: newazole 200 mg or placebo; newazole study drug; protocol #1211 study drug. Nursing personnel should be consulted regarding the proposed labeling of blinded study drug to ensure that the labeling used is compatible with medication administration records maintained by nursing staff.

Investigational drugs are generally supplied free-of-charge by the study sponsor for use according to a predefined protocol. However, there are limited circumstances whereby a study sponsor can charge for use of an investigational drug. In select predetermined situations, the Food and Drug Administration (FDA) will allow a manufacturer to charge for direct drug costs when it would be otherwise impossible for drug development to proceed. In addition, a drug manufacturer can charge for costs related to expanded access (compassionate use) of investigational products. The Investigational Drug Service determines fair charges for Pharmacy Department personnel time and resources utilized in the support of study activities. As a rule, routine pharmacy charges to the patient's bill cannot be generated for investigational new drugs, or study drugs provided free-of-charge by the study sponsor. The Investigation Drug Service must charge the study funds. Thls ls generally achieved at the institutional level by generating charges to the local Principal Investigator or Clinical Trials Office.

Additional information about handling investigational drugs is available from the National Cancer Institute Pharmaceutical Management Branch. Available at http://ctep.cancer.gov/branches/pmb/idh_slideshow.htm. Accessed August 4, 2012.

Information from the FDA regarding access to investigational drugs is available at http://www.fda.gov/ForConsumers/ConsumerUpdates/ucm176845.htm.

SAFE HANDLING OF HAZARDOUS DRUGS

Early concerns regarding the identification and exposure risk of hazardous drugs in healthcare setting were primarily focused on antineoplastic medications, but now have expanded to numerous other agents (eg, antivirals, hormones, bioengineered medications). The criteria for a hazardous drug include one or more of the following characteristics:

- Carcinogenic
- Teratogenic (or other developmental toxicity)
- Causing reproductive toxicity
- Organotoxic at low doses
- Genotoxic
- New agents with structural or toxicity profiles similar to existing hazardous agents

Agencies have developed definitions, created lists, and generated guidelines to minimize risk of exposure to products considered hazardous.

Hazardous drugs must be stored, transported, prepared, administered, and disposed of under conditions that protect the healthcare worker from either acute or chronic/low level exposure. Institutional policies or guidelines to minimize occupational exposure to hazardous drugs should include a focus on the following areas:

- Development and maintenance of a facility-specific hazardous drugs list
  - Working definition/criteria of a hazardous drug
  - Volumes, formulations, and frequency of hazardous drugs handled: Injection, oral (liquid, solid), topical
  - Oral dosage forms and administration (coated tablets or capsules administered intact may not pose a risk; however, uncoated tablets or alteration of forms by crushing or preparation of oral solutions will likely result in exposure)

Each institution or facility must create its own policy or guideline, including a facility-specific list of drugs deemed hazardous. According to the Joint Commission standards, organizations should minimize risks associated with handling hazardous medications. The Environmental Protection Agency (EPA), National Institute for Occupational Safety and Health (NIOSH), and American Society of Health-System Pharmacists (ASHP) have created definitions of hazardous agents (Table 1) which may be useful. Based on their definitions, these agencies developed lists of agents which are identified as hazardous drugs (Table 2). NIOSH updated its list of antineoplastic and hazardous drugs in 2012. Table 3 provides a list of the FDA-assigned pregnancy categories D and X drugs in which studies in humans have demonstrated positive evidence of fetal risk. Until proven otherwise, most institutions consider investigational drugs to be hazardous and to be handled accordingly, particularly if the mechanism of action suggests a potential for concern. Hazardous drug procedures must include all possible routes of administration.

Additional information regarding development and implementation of an institutional policy/guideline, areas at risk, personnel at risk, risk management, spill management, personnel training, and surveillance may be found at:

ASHP Guidelines on Handling Hazardous Drugs:
http://www.ashp.org/DocLibrary/BestPractices/PrepGdlHazDrugs.aspx

Environmental Protection Agency Recommendations:
http://hercenter.org/hazmat/hazdeterm.cfm
http://hercenter.org/hazmat/pharma.cfm

NIOSH List of Antineoplastic and Other Hazardous Drugs in Healthcare settings:
http://www.cdc.gov/niosh/docs/2012-150/pdfs/2012-150.pdf

U.S. Nuclear Regulatory Commission (radiopharmaceuticals, such as ibritumomab or tositumomab):
http://www.nrc.gov/materials/miau/med-use.html

- Identification of personnel and locations in the facility at risk for occupational exposure to hazardous drugs
  - Pharmacy
    - Receiving storage and inventory
    - Dose preparation and dispensing
    - Drug waste disposal
  - Nursing Unit
    - Drug administration
    - Drug waste disposal
    - Patient waste disposal
  - Other areas
    - Laboratory
    - Operating/procedure rooms
    - Veterinary department
    - Facility shipping/receiving
    - Environmental/laundry services

While the greatest risk of occupational exposure to hazardous drugs occurs during preparation and administration of these agents, it is important to recognize that a risk to exposure can occur throughout the facility from the moment of delivery through the disposal of product and contaminated human waste. Drug preparation and administration may occur in nontraditional areas of the institution including the operating room and in veterinary facilities. Procedures should address the importance of proper labeling and packaging and separation of hazardous vs nonhazardous inventories throughout the facility. Drug containers should be examined upon their arrival at the pharmacy. Containers that show signs of damage should be handled carefully and may require quarantine and decontamination before being placed in stock. Give consideration to routinely quarantining and decontaminating all hazardous drug containers as part of the inspection process before placing in stock.

- Mechanisms/routes of occupational exposure
  - Inhalation of dust or aerosolized droplets
  - Absorption through skin
  - Ingestion from contaminated food/drink
  - Accidental injection during preparation/administration/disposal
- Risk management
  - Use and maintenance of equipment designed to minimize exposure during handling
    - Buffer/Ante transition area
    - Biological safety cabinets, isolators
    - Closed system drug-transfer devices
    - Personal protective equipment
    - Deactivation, decontamination, and cleaning procedures

Barrier protection through the use of ventilation controls and personal protective equipment is the current standard to minimize exposure when handling hazardous drugs. NIOSH and ASHP recommend the use of Class II biological safety cabinets (type B2 preferred), but other options include the totally enclosed Class III biological safety cabinets and appropriate isolators. Self-contained or closed system devices have been recommended to minimize workplace contamination by preventing escape of drug or vapor out of the device. Devices available include PhaSeal®, ONGARD™, TEVADAPTOR™, Equashield™, and CLAVE® systems; other systems may also be commercially available. Gloves, gowns, hair and shoe covers, and eye protection represent the core of personal protective equipment. Guidelines for choice of gowns and gloving, and the circumstances to employ this protection are published by ASHP, NIOSH, and in USP 797.

  - Hazardous drug spill management
    - Size and location
    - Spill kit use
    - Worker contamination

Procedures for handling spills throughout a facility are well described by ASHP and NIOSH. Institutional procedures should focus on location and size of the spill, how to handle a spill when a spill kit is not available, and how to respond to a worker contamination (emergent treatment, follow-up care).

  - Personnel training in the handling of hazardous drugs
    - Prior to handling hazardous drugs
    - Periodic and ongoing testing

Personnel throughout a facility must have training in the handling of hazardous drugs that are relevant to their job description. Pharmacy personnel who compound and dispense hazardous drugs must be fully trained in the storing, preparation, dispensing, and disposal of these agents. Such training should include didactic, as well as demonstrating hands-on technique, and such validation should be repeated on a regular schedule. Special training may be necessary for hazardous drugs administered by routes outside of traditional administration routes and when administered in settings outside of traditional settings (eg, at home).

– Environmental and medical surveillance
  - Components of a comprehensive medical surveillance program
  - Potential use of environmental sampling techniques
  - Use of common marker hazardous drugs for assay purposes

There is no current standard for environmental or medical surveillance of personnel handling hazardous drugs. It is recommended that some type of medical surveillance be employed by the facility, and may include the basic observation of employee symptom complaints or monitoring for changes in health status as part of routine checkups. Some programs follow the employee more closely, and procedures may include periodic blood counts, and a more detailed medical history and exposure history. Environmental sampling to look for surface contamination in hazardous drug preparation and administration areas may be considered, particularly in institutions with high volumes. Certain hazardous drugs serve as markers which allow for assay for measurable contamination, and can alert the facility for proper follow-up.

– Work practices regarding reproductive risks to health care workers
  - Alternative duty options

Since hazardous drugs are associated with reproductive risks, policies and guidelines should address healthcare workers whom are pregnant, attempting to conceive or father a child, and whom are breast-feeding. Workers of reproductive capability should acknowledge in writing that they understand the risk of handling hazardous drugs, and be given the opportunity for reassignment or alternate work duty.

Table 1. Criteria for Defining Hazardous Agents

EPA	NIOSH	ASHP
Meets one of the following criteria: Ignitability: Create fire (under certain conditions) or are spontaneously combustible and have a flash point <60°C (140°F) Corrosivity: Acids or bases (pH ≤2 or ≥12.5) capable of corroding metal containers Reactivity: Unstable under "normal" conditions; may cause explosions, toxic fumes, gases, or vapors if heated, compressed, or mixed with water Toxicity: Harmful or fatal if ingested or absorbed; may leach from the waste and pollute ground water when disposed of on land **OR**	Carcinogenic Teratogenic or other developmental toxicity Causing reproductive toxicity Organotoxic at low doses Genotoxic New drugs with structural and toxicity profiles similar to existing hazardous agents	Genotoxic Carcinogenic Teratogenic or impairs fertility Causes serious organ or other toxic manifestation at low doses
Appears on one of the following lists: F: Wastes (nonspecific) from common or industrial manufacturing processes from nonspecific sources K: Specific (source) wastes from specific industries (eg, petroleum or pesticides) P (acutely toxic) or U (toxic): Wastes (unused form) from certain discarded commercial chemical products		

Table 2. Drugs Listed as Hazardous

EPA:

Arsenic trioxide (P-listed)
Chloral hydrate (U-listed)
Chlorambucil (U-listed)
Cyclophosphamide (U-listed)
DAUNOrubicin, including liposomal formulation (U-listed)
Dichlorodifluoromethane (U-listed)
Diethylstilbestrol (U-listed)
EPINEPHrine (does not include epinephrine salts) (P-listed)
Formaldehyde (U-listed)
Hexachlorophene (U-listed)
Lindane (U-listed)
Melphalan (U-listed)
Mercury (U-listed)
MitoMYcin (U-listed)
Nicotine (P-listed)
Nitroglycerin (doses in "finished form" are excluded) (P-listed)
Paraldehyde (U-listed)
Phenacetin (U-listed)
Phenol (U-listed)
Physostigmine (P-listed)
Reserpine (U-listed)
Resorcinol (U-listed)
Saccharin (U-listed)
Selenium sulfide (U-listed)
Streptozocin (U-listed)
Trichloromonofluoromethane (U-listed)
Uracil mustard (U-listed)
Warfarin (<0.3% U-listed; >0.3%, P-listed)

Healthcare Environmental Resource Center (HERC), "Pharmaceutical Wastes in Healthcare Facilities." Available at http://www.hercenter.org/hazmat/pharma.cfm#listed. Last accessed Sept. 15, 2010.

Healthcare Environmental Resource Center (HERC), "Hazardous Waste Determination." Available at http://www.hercenter.org/hazmat/hazdeterm.cfm. Last accessed Sept. 15, 2010.

NIOSH:

Acitretin
Aldesleukin
Alefacept
Alitretinoin
Altretamine
Amsacrine
Ambrisentan
Anastrozole
Arsenic trioxide
Asparaginase
AzaCITIDine
AzaTHIOprine
BCG vaccine
Bendamustine
Bexarotene
Bicalutamide
Bleomycin
Bortezomib
Bosentan
Busulfan
Cabergoline
Capecitabine
CarBAMazepine
CARBOplatin
Carmustine
Cetrorelix
Chlorambucil
Chloramphenicol
Choriogonadotropin alfa
Cidofovir
CISplatin
Cladribine
Clofarabine
ClonazePAM
Colchicine
Cyclophosphamide
CycloSPORINE
Cytarabine
Dacarbazine
DACTINomycin
Dasatinib
DAUNOrubicin HCl
Decitabine
Degarelix
Denileukin
Diethylstilbestrol
Dinoprostone
Divalproex
DOCEtaxel
DOXOrubicin
Dronedarone
Dutasteride
Entecavir
EPIrubicin
Ergonovine/methylergonovine
Estradiol
Estramustine
Estrogen-progestin combinations
Estrogens, conjugated
Estrogens, esterified
Estrone
Estropipate
Etoposide
Everolimus
Exemestane
Finasteride
Floxuridine
Fludarabine
Fluorouracil
Fluoxymesterone
Flutamide
Fulvestrant
Ganciclovir
Ganirelix
Gemcitabine
Gemtuzumab ozogamicin
Gonadotropin, chorionic
Goserelin
Hydroxyurea
IDArubicin
Ifosfamide
Imatinib
Irinotecan
Ixabepilone
Leflunomide
Lenalidomide
Letrozole
Leuprolide
Lomustine
Mechlorethamine
MedroxyPROGESTERone
Megestrol
Melphalan
Menotropins
Mercaptopurine
Methotrexate
MethylTESTOSTERone
Mifepristone
MitoMYcin
Mitotane
MitoXANtrone
Mycophenolate
Nafarelin
Nelarabine

Nilotinib
Nilutamide
Oxaliplatin
OXcarbazepine
Oxytocin
PACLitaxel
Palifermin
PARoxetine
Pazopanib
Pegaspargase
PEMEtrexed
Pentamidine
Pentetate calcium trisodium
Pentostatin
Phenoxybenzamine
Pipobroman
Plerixafor
Podofilox
Podophyllum resin
PRALAtrexate
Procarbazine
Progesterone
Progestins
Raloxifene
Rasagiline
Ribavirin
RisperiDONE
RomiDEPsin
Sirolimus
SORAfenib
Streptozocin
SUNItinib
Tacrolimus
Tamoxifen
Telavancin
Temozolomide
Temsirolimus
Teniposide
Testolactone
Testosterone
Tetracycline
Thalidomide
Thioguanine
Thiotepa
Topotecan
Toremifene
Tretinoin
Trifluridine
Triptorelin
Uracil mustard
ValGANciclovir
Valproic Acid
Valrubicin
Vidarabine
Vigabatrin
VinBLAStine
VinCRIStine
Vinorelbine
Vorinostat
Zidovudine
Ziprasidone
Zoledronic Acid
Zonisamide

National Institute for Occupational Safety and Health (NIOSH), "NIOSH List of Antineoplastic and Other Hazardous Drugs in Health Care Settings, 2012." Available at http://www.cdc.gov/niosh/docs/2012-150/pdfs/2012-150.pdf. Last Accessed July 10, 2012.

Product Labeling (not on EPA or NIOSH lists): Anticancer medications

Bosutinib
Brentuximab vedotin
Cabazitaxel
Cytarabine liposomal
Dexrazoxane
DOXOrubicin liposomal
Omacetaxine
PACLitaxel protein bound
Porfimer
Raltitrexed
Vandetanib
VinCRIStine (Liposomal)
Vindesine

Table 3. Sample Listing of Teratogenic Agents

Pregnancy Risk Factor X: Anticancer medications

Abiraterone
Anastrozole
Bexarotene
Bicalutamide
Degarelix
Enzalutamide
Exemestane
Fluorouracil (topical)
Goserelin
Lenalidomide
Letrozole
Leuprolide
Methotrexate
Sodium iodide I^{131}
Thalidomide

Pregnancy Risk Factor X: Nonantineoplastic

Acetohydroxamic acid
Acitretin
Alprostadil
Ambrisentan
Amlodipine & atorvastatin
AtorvaSTATin
Benzphetamine
Bosentan
Cetrorelix
Chenodiol
Chorionic gonadotropin
ClomiPHENE
Danazol
Denosumab (Prolia®)
Diclofenac & misoprostol
Dihydroergotamine
Dronedarone
Dutasteride
Dutasteride & tamsulosin
Ergotamine
Ergotamine & caffeine
Estazolam
Estradiol
Estrogens
Ezetimibe & simvastatin
Finasteride
Fluoxymesterone
Fluvastatin
Follitropins
Ganirelix
Histrelin
ISOtretinoin
Leflunomide
Lovastatin
Lutropin alfa
MedroxyPROGESTERone
Megestrol
Menotropins
Methylene blue
MethylTESTOSTERone
Mifepristone
Miglustat
Misoprostol
MitoMYcin (ophthalmic)
Nafarelin
Norethindrone
Norgestrel
Orlistat
Oxandrolone
Oxymetholone
Phentermine
Pitavastatin
Pravastatin
Quazepam
Raloxifene
Ribavirin
Rosuvastatin
Simvastatin
Tazarotene
Temazepam
Tesamorelin
Testosterone
Triazolam
Triptorelin
Ulipristal
Urofollitropin
Vitamin A
Warfarin (D for women with mechanical heart valves)

Pregnancy Risk Factor D: Anticancer medications

Alitretinoin
Altretamine
Arsenic trioxide
AzaCITIDine
Axitinib
Bendamustine
Bleomycin
Bortezomib
Bosutinib
Brentuximab vedotin
Busulfan
Cabazitaxel
Capecitabine
CARBOplatin
Carfilzomib
Carmustine
Chlorambucil
CISplatin
Cladribine
Clofarabine
Crizotinib
Cyclophosphamide
Cytarabine (conventional)
Cytarabine (liposomal)
DACTINomycin
Dasatinib
DAUNOrubicin (conventional)
DAUNOrubicin (liposomal)

Decitabine
Dexrazoxane
DOCEtaxel
DOXOrubicin
DOXOrubicin (liposomal)
EPIrubicin
EriBULin
Erlotinib
Etoposide
Etoposide phosphate
Everolimus (Afinitor®)
Floxuridine
Fludarabine
Fluorouracil
Flutamide
Fulvestrant
Gefitinib
Gemcitabine
Goserelin
Hydroxyurea
Ibritumomab
IDArubicin
Ifosfamide
Imatinib
Irinotecan
Ixabepilone
Lapatinib
Lomustine
Mechlorethamine
Melphalan
Mercaptopurine
MitoXANtrone
Nelarabine
Nilotinib
Omacetaxine
Oxaliplatin
PACLitaxel
PACLitaxel (protein bound)
Pazopanib
PEMEtrexed
Pentostatin
Pertuzumab
Plerixafor
PRALAtrexate
Procarbazine
Regorafenib
RomiDEPsin
Samarium Sm 153 lexidronam
SORAfenib
Streptozocin
SUNItinib
Tamoxifen
Temozolomide
Temsirolimus
Teniposide
Thioguanine
Thiotepa
Topotecan
Toremifene
Tositumomab
Trastuzumab
Tretinoin
Vandetanib
Vemurafenib
VinBLAStine
VinCRIStine
VinCRIStine (Liposomal)
Vinorelbine
Vismodegib
Vorinostat

Pregnancy Risk Factor D: Nonantineoplastic

ACE inhibitors and combination products
Acetaminophen, aspirin, & caffeine
Aliskiren (2nd and 3rd trimesters)
Aliskiren combination products
ALPRAZolam
Amikacin
Amiodarone
Amitriptyline & chlordiazepoxide
Amobarbital
Angiotensin receptor blockers and combination products
Anthrax vaccine
Aspirin & dipyridamole
Atenolol
Atenolol & chlorthalidone
AzaTHIOprine
Bismuth, metronidazole, & tetracycline
Butabarbital
CarBAMazepine
Celecoxib (≥30 weeks)
Clidinium & chlordiazepoxide
ClonazePAM
Deferiprone
Demeclocycline
Denosumab (Xgeva®)
Diazepam
Diclofenac (≥30 weeks)
Divalproex
Doxycycline
Efavirenz
Efavirenz, emtricitabine, & tenofovir
Ethotoin
Fluconazole (chronic high doses)

Fosphenytoin
Gentamicin
Ibuprofen (≥30 weeks)
Kanamycin
Ketorolac nasal spray (≥30 weeks)
Lithium
LORazepam
Meloxicam (≥30 weeks)
Methimazole
Methoxsalen (systemic) (Uvadex®)
Minocycline
Mycophenolate
Neomycin
Pamidronate
Paroxetine
PenicillAMINE
PENTobarbital
Phenytoin
PrednisoLONE (systemic) (Flo-Pred™)
Propylthiouracil
Secobarbital
Smallpox vaccine
Streptomycin
Strontium-89
Tetracycline
Tigecycline
Tobramycin
Topiramate
Triamcinolone (ophthalmic)
Valproic acid
Voriconazole
Zoledronic acid

SELECTED READINGS

American Society of Hospital Pharmacists, "ASHP Guidelines on Handling Hazardous Drugs," 2006, 63(12):1172-93.

Baker ES and Connor TH, "Monitoring Occupational Exposure to Cancer Chemotherapy Drugs," *Am J Health Syst Pharm*, 1996, 53(22):2713-23.

Bos RP and Sessink PJ, "Biomonitoring of Occupational Exposures to Cytostatic Anticancer Drugs," *Rev Environ Health*, 1997, 12(1):43-58.

Connor TH, "Permeability of Nitrile Rubber, Latex, Polyurethane, and Neoprene Gloves to 18 Antineoplastic Drugs," *Am J Health Syst Pharm*, 1999, 56(23):2450-3.

Connor TH, Anderson RW, Sessink PJ, et al, "Surface Contamination With Antineoplastic Agents in Six Cancer Treatment Centers in Canada and the United States," *Am J Health Syst Pharm*, 1999, 56(14):1427-32.

Connor TH and McDiarmid MA, "Preventing Occupational Exposures to Antineoplastic Drugs in Health Care Settings," *CA Cancer J Clin*, 2006, 56(6):354-65.

Connor TH, Sessink PJ, Harrison BR, et al, "Surface Contamination of Chemotherapy Drug Vials and Evaluation of New Vial-Cleaning Techniques: Results of Three Studies," *Am J Health Syst Pharm*, 2005, 62(5):475-84.

Healthcare Environmental Resource Center (HERC), "Hazardous Waste Determination." Available at http://www.hercenter.org/hazmat/hazdeterm.cfm. Last accessed Sept. 15, 2010.

Healthcare Environmental Resource Center (HERC), "Pharmaceutical Wastes in Healthcare Facilities." Available at http://www.hercenter.org/hazmat/pharma.cfm#listed. Last accessed Sept. 15, 2010.

National Institute for Occupational Safety and Health (NIOSH), "NIOSH List of Antineoplastic and Other Hazardous Drugs in Health Care Settings, 2010." Available at http://www.cdc.gov/niosh/docs/2010-167/pdfs/2010-167.pdf. Last accessed Sept. 15, 2010.

National Institute for Occupational Safety and Health (NIOSH), "NIOSH List of Antineoplastic and Other Hazardous Drugs in Healthcare Settings 2012." Available at http://www.cdc.gov/niosh/docs/2012-150/pdfs/2012-150.pdf. Accessed July 11, 2012.

National Institute for Occupational Safety and Health (NIOSH), "Preventing Occupational Exposure to Antineoplastic and Other Hazardous Drugs in Health Care Settings." Available at http://www.cdc.gov/niosh/docs/2004-165/2004-165d.html#o. Last accessed Oct. 1, 2007.

Polovich M, *Safe Handling of Hazardous Drugs*, 2nd ed, Pittsburgh, PA: Oncology Nursing Society, 2011.

Sessink PJ, Anzion RB, Van den Broek PH, et al, "Detection of Contamination With Antineoplastic Agents in a Hospital Pharmacy Department," *Pharm Weekbl Sci*, 1992, 14(1):16-22.

Sessink PJ, Boer KA, Scheefhals AP, et al, "Occupational Exposure to Antineoplastic Agents at Several Departments in a Hospital. Environmental Contamination and Excretion of Cyclophosphamide and Ifosfamide in Urine of Exposed Workers," *Int Arch Occup Environ Health*, 1992, 64(2):105-12.

Sessink PJ and Bos RP, "Drugs Hazardous to Healthcare Workers. Evaluation of Methods for Monitoring Occupational Exposure to Cytostatic Drugs," *Drug Saf*, 1999, 20(4):347-59.

Sorsa M and Anderson D, "Monitoring of Occupational Exposure to Cytostatic Anticancer Agents," *Mutat Res*, 1996, 355(1-2):253-61.

APPENDIX TABLE OF CONTENTS

Abbreviations and Measurements
Milliequivalent and Millimole Calculations and Conversions 1916
Acid-Base Assessment 1919
Selected Clinical Equations 1921
Body Surface Area 1923
Assessment of Renal Function
Renal Function Estimation in Adult Patients 1924
Renal Function Estimation in Pediatric Patients 1928
Renal Function Tests 1931
Comparative Drug Charts
Immune Globulin Product Comparison 1934
Oral Anticoagulant Comparison Chart 1936
Oral Antiplatelet Comparison Chart 1938
Laboratory Values
Reference Values for Adults 1940

MILLIEQUIVALENT AND MILLIMOLE CALCULATIONS AND CONVERSIONS

DEFINITIONS AND CALCULATIONS

Definitions

mole	=	gram molecular weight of a substance (aka molar weight)
millimole (mM)	=	milligram molecular weight of a substance (a millimole is 1/1000 of a mole)
equivalent weight	=	gram weight of a substance which will combine with or replace 1 gram (1 mole) of hydrogen; an equivalent weight can be determined by dividing the molar weight of a substance by its ionic valence
milliequivalent (mEq)	=	milligram weight of a substance which will combine with or replace 1 milligram (1 millimole) of hydrogen (a milliequivalent is 1/1000 of an equivalent)

Calculations

$$\text{moles} = \frac{\text{weight of a substance (grams)}}{\text{molecular weight of that substance (grams)}}$$

$$\text{millimoles} = \frac{\text{weight of a substance (milligrams)}}{\text{molecular weight of that substance (milligrams)}}$$

$$\text{equivalents} = \text{moles} \times \text{valence of ion}$$

$$\text{milliequivalents} = \text{millimoles} \times \text{valence of ion}$$

$$\text{moles} = \frac{\text{equivalents}}{\text{valence of ion}}$$

$$\text{millimoles} = \frac{\text{milliequivalents}}{\text{valence of ion}}$$

$$\text{millimoles} = \text{moles} \times 1000$$

$$\text{milliequivalents} = \text{equivalents} \times 1000$$

Note: Use of equivalents and milliequivalents is valid only for those substances which have fixed ionic valences (eg, sodium, potassium, calcium, chlorine, magnesium, bromine, etc). For substances with variable ionic valences (eg, phosphorous), a reliable equivalent value cannot be determined. In these instances, one should calculate millimoles (which are fixed and reliable) rather than milliequivalents.

MILLIEQUIVALENT CONVERSIONS

To convert mg/100 mL to mEq/L the following formula may be used:

$$\frac{(\text{mg/100 mL}) \times 10 \times \text{valence}}{\text{atomic weight}} = \text{mEq/L}$$

To convert mEq/L to mg/100 mL the following formula may be used:

$$\frac{(\text{mEq/L}) \times \text{atomic weight}}{10 \times \text{valence}} = \text{mg/100 mL}$$

To convert mEq/L to volume of percent of a gas the following formula may be used:

$$\frac{(\text{mEq/L}) \times 22.4}{10} = \text{volume percent}$$

Valences and Atomic Weights of Selected Ions

Substance	Electrolyte	Valence	Molecular Wt
Calcium	Ca^{++}	2	40
Chloride	Cl^-	1	35.5
Magnesium	Mg^{++}	2	24
Phosphate	HPO_4 (80%)	1.8	96[1]
pH = 7.4	$H_2PO_4^-$ (20%)	1.8	96[1]
Potassium	K^+	1	39
Sodium	Na^+	1	23
Sulfate	SO_4^{--}	2	96[1]

[1]The molecular weight of phosphorus only is 31, and sulfur only is 32.

Approximate Milliequivalents — Weights of Selected Ions

Salt	mEq/g Salt	mg Salt/mEq
Calcium carbonate [$CaCO_3$]	20	50
Calcium chloride [$CaCl_2 \cdot 2H_2O$]	14	74
Calcium gluceptate [$Ca(C_7H_{13}O_8)_2$]	4	245
Calcium gluconate [$Ca(C_6H_{11}O_7)_2 \cdot H_2O$]	5	224
Calcium lactate [$Ca(C_3H_5O_3)_2 \cdot 5H_2O$]	7	154
Magnesium gluconate [$Mg(C_6H_{11}O_7)_2 \cdot H_2O$]	5	216
Magnesium oxide [MgO]	50	20
Magnesium sulfate [$MgSO_4$]	17	60
Magnesium sulfate [$MgSO_4 \cdot 7H_2O$]	8	123
Potassium acetate [$K(C_2H_3O_2)$]	10	98
Potassium chloride [KCl]	13	75

Approximate Milliequivalents — Weights of Selected Ions *(continued)*

Salt	mEq/g Salt	mg Salt/mEq
Potassium citrate [$K_3(C_6H_5O_7) \cdot H_2O$]	9	108
Potassium iodide [KI]	6	166
Sodium acetate [$Na(C_2H_3O_2)$]	12	82
Sodium acetate [$Na(C_2H_3O_2) \cdot 3H_2O$]	7	136
Sodium bicarbonate [$NaHCO_3$]	12	84
Sodium chloride [NaCl]	17	58
Sodium citrate [$Na_3(C_6H_5O_7) \cdot 2H_2O$]	10	98
Sodium iodine [NaI]	7	150
Sodium lactate [$Na(C_3H_5O_3)$]	9	112
Zinc sulfate [$ZnSO_4 \cdot 7H_2O$]	7	144

ACID-BASE ASSESSMENT

Henderson-Hasselbalch Equation

$pH = 6.1 + \log ([HCO_3^-] / (0.03) [PaCO_2])$

Normal arterial blood pH: 7.4 (normal range: 7.35 - 7.45)

Where:

$[HCO_3^-]$ = Serum bicarbonate concentration

$PaCO_2$ = Arterial carbon dioxide partial pressure

Alveolar Gas Equation

P_iO_2 = F_iO_2 x (total atmospheric pressure – vapor pressure of H_2O at 37°C)

= F_iO_2 x (760 mm Hg – 47 mm Hg)

PAO_2 = $P_iO_2 - (PaCO_2 / R)$

Alveolar-arterial oxygen (A-a) gradient = $PAO_2 - PaO_2$

or

A-a gradient = $[(F_iO_2 \times 713) - (PaCO_2/0.8)] - PaO_2$

A-a gradient normal ranges:

Children	15-20 mm Hg
Adults	20-25 mm Hg

where:

P_iO_2 = Oxygen partial pressure of inspired gas (mm Hg) (150 mm Hg in room air at sea level)

F_iO_2 = Fractional pressure of oxygen in inspired gas (0.21 in room air)

PAO_2 = Alveolar oxygen partial pressure

PaO_2 = Arterial oxygen partial pressure

$PaCO_2$ = Arterial carbon dioxide partial pressure

R = Respiratory exchange quotient (typically 0.8, increases with high carbohydrate diet, decreases with high fat diet)

Acid-Base Disorders

Acute metabolic acidosis:

$PaCO_2$ expected = 1.5 ($[HCO_3^-]$) + 8 ± 2 **or**

Expected decrease in $PaCO_2$ = 1.3 (1-1.5) x decrease in $[HCO_3^-]$

Acute metabolic alkalosis:

Expected increase in $PaCO_2$ = 0.6 (0.5-1) x increase in $[HCO_3^-]$

Acute respiratory acidosis (<6 h duration):

For every $PaCO_2$ increase of 10 mm Hg, $[HCO_3^-]$ increases by 1 mEq/L

Chronic respiratory acidosis (>6 h duration):
For every $PaCO_2$ increase of 10 mm Hg, $[HCO_3^-]$ increases by 4 mEq/L

Acute respiratory alkalosis (<6 h duration):
For every $PaCO_2$ decrease of 10 mm Hg, $[HCO_3^-]$ decreases by 2 mEq/L

Chronic respiratory alkalosis (>6 h duration):
For every $PaCO_2$ decrease of 10 mm Hg, $[HCO_3^-]$ increases by 5 mEq/L

SELECTED CLINICAL EQUATIONS

CORRECTED SODIUM

Corrected Na^+ = measured Na^+ + [1.5 x (glucose – 150 divided by 100)]

Note: Do not correct for glucose <150.

WATER DEFICIT

Water deficit = 0.6 x body weight [1 – (140 divided by Na^+)]

Note: Body weight is estimated weight in kg when fully hydrated; **Na^+** is serum or plasma sodium. Use corrected Na^+ if necessary. Consult medical references for recommendations for replacement of deficit.

TOTAL SERUM CALCIUM CORRECTED FOR ALBUMIN LEVEL

[(Normal albumin – patient's albumin) x 0.8] + patient's measured total calcium

OSMOLALITY

Definition: The summed concentrations of all osmotically active solute particles.

Predicted serum osmolality =

$$\text{mOsm/L} = (2 \times \text{serum } Na^{++}) + \frac{\text{serum glucose}}{18} + \frac{\text{BUN}}{2.8}$$

The normal range of serum osmolality is 285-295 mOsm/L.

Calculated Osm

Note: Osm is a term used to reconcile osmolality and osmolarity

Osmol gap = measured Osm – calculated Osm

0 to +10: Normal
>10: Abnormal
<0: Probable lab or calculation error

Drugs Causing Osmolar Gap
(by freezing-point depression, gap is >10 mOsm)
Ethanol
Ethylene glycol
Glycerol
Iodine (questionable)
Isopropanol (acetone)
Mannitol
Methanol
Sorbitol

BICARBONATE DEFICIT

HCO_3^- deficit = (0.4 x wt in kg) x (HCO_3^- desired – HCO_3^- measured)

Note: In clinical practice, the calculated quantity may differ markedly from the actual amount of bicarbonate needed or that which may be safely administered.

ANION GAP

Definition: The difference in concentration between unmeasured cation and anion equivalents in serum.

Anion gap = $Na^+ - (Cl^- + HCO_3^-)$
(The normal anion gap is 10-14 mEq/L)

Differential Diagnosis of Increased Anion Gap Acidosis

Organic anions
- Lactate (sepsis, hypovolemia, seizures, large tumor burden)
- Pyruvate
- Uremia
- Ketoacidosis (β-hydroxybutyrate and acetoacetate)
- Amino acids and their metabolites
- Other organic acids

Inorganic anions
- Hyperphosphatemia
- Sulfates
- Nitrates

Differential Diagnosis of Decreased Anion Gap

Organic cations
- Hypergammaglobulinemia

Inorganic cations
- Hyperkalemia
- Hypercalcemia
- Hypermagnesemia

Medications and toxins
- Lithium

Hypoalbuminemia

RETICULOCYTE INDEX

(% retic divided by 2) x (patient's Hct divided by normal Hct) **or**
(% retic divided by 2) x (patient's Hgb divided by normal Hgb)

Normal index: 1.0
Good marrow response: 2.0-6.0

CORRECTED QT INTERVAL EQUATIONS

Bazett (B) Formula:

QT_cB: $QT_c = QT/(R - R \text{ interval}^{0.5})$

or

QT_cB: QT_c = QT/Square root of (R - R interval)

Frederica (F) Formula:

QT_cF: $QT_c = QT/(R - R \text{ interval}^{0.33})$

BODY SURFACE AREA

Body Surface Area (BSA) – Adults and Pediatric

$$\text{BSA (m}^2\text{)} = \frac{\text{kg}^{0.425} \times \text{cm}^{0.725} \times 71.84}{10{,}000}$$

or

$$\log \text{BSA (m}^2\text{)} = \frac{(\log \text{kg} \times 0.425) + (\log \text{cm} \times 0.725) + 1.8564}{10{,}000}$$

DuBois D and DuBois EF, "A Formula to Estimate the Approximate Surface Area if Height and Weight Be Known," *Arch Intern Med*, 1916, 17:863-71.

$$\text{BSA (m}^2\text{)} = \sqrt{\frac{\text{ht (in)} \times \text{wt (lb)}}{3131}} \quad \textit{or} \quad \text{BSA (m}^2\text{)} = \sqrt{\frac{\text{ht (cm)} \times \text{wt (kg)}}{3600}}$$

Lam TK and Leung DT, "More on Simplified Calculation of Body-Surface Area," *N Engl J Med*, 1988, 318(17):1130 (letter).

Mosteller RD, "Simplified Calculation of Body Surface Area," *N Engl J Med*, 1987, 317:1098 (letter).

Ideal Body Weight

Men: 50 kg + 2.3 kg/inch >5 ft

Women: 45 kg + 2.3 kg/in >5 ft

Devine BJ, "Gentamicin Therapy," *Drug Intelligence and Clinical Pharmacy*, 1974, 8:650-5.

or

Men: 51.65 kg + 1.85 kg/in >5 ft

Women: 48.67 kg + 1.7 kg/in >5 ft

Robinson JD, Lupkiewicz SM, Palenik L, et al, "Determination of Ideal Body Weight for Drug Dosage Calculations," *Am J Hosp Pharm*, 1983, 40(6): 1016-9.

Adjusted Body Weight

Adjusted wt (kg) = ideal body weight (kg) + 0.4 [actual wt (kg) – ideal body weight (kg)]

Area Under the Curve (AUC) for Carboplatin Dosing

Carboplatin (mg) = desired AUC x (25 + GFR)

GFR = creatinine clearance (measured or estimated)

Calvert AH, Newell DR, Gumbrell LA, et al, "Carboplatin Dosage: Prospective Evaluation of a Simple Formula Based on Renal Function," *J Clin Oncol*, 1989, 7(11):1748-56.

RENAL FUNCTION ESTIMATION IN ADULT PATIENTS

Evaluation of a patient's renal function often includes the use of equations to estimate glomerular filtration rate (GFR) (eg, estimated GFR [eGFR] creatinine clearance [Cl_{Cr}]) using an endogenous filtration marker (eg, serum creatinine) and other patient variables. For example, the Cockcroft-Gault equation estimates renal function by calculating Cl_{Cr} and is typically used to steer medication dosing. Equations which calculate eGFR are primarily used to categorize chronic kidney disease (CKD) staging. The rate of creatinine clearance does not always accurately represent GFR; creatinine may be cleared by other renal mechanisms in addition to glomerular filtration and serum creatinine concentrations may be affected by non-renal factors (eg, age, gender, race, body habitus, illness, diet). In addition, these equations were developed based on studies in limited populations and may either over- or underestimate the renal function of a specific patient.

Nevertheless, most clinicians estimate renal function using Cl_{Cr} as an indicator of actual renal function for the purpose of adjusting medication doses. For medications that require dose adjustment for renal impairment, utilization of eGFR (ie, Modification of Diet in Renal Disease [MDRD]) may overestimate renal function by up to 40% which may result in supratherapeutic medication doses (Hermsen, 2009). These equations should only be used in the clinical context of patient-specific factors noted during the physical exam/work-up. Decisions regarding drug therapy and doses must be based on clinical judgment.

RENAL FUNCTION ESTIMATION EQUATIONS

Commonly used equations include the Cockcroft-Gault, Jelliffe, four-variable Modification of Diet in Renal Disease (MDRD), and six-variable MDRD (aka, MDRD extended). All of these equations were originally developed using a serum creatinine assay measured by the alkaline picrate-based (Jaffe) method. Many substances, including proteins, can interfere with the accuracy of this assay and overestimate serum creatinine concentration. The National Kidney Foundation and The National Kidney Disease Education Program (NDKEP) advocate for a universal creatinine assay, in order to ensure an accurate estimate of renal function in patients. As a result, a more specific enzymatic assay with an isotope dilution mass spectrometry (IDMS)-traceable international standard has been developed. Compared to the older methods, IDMS-traceable assays may report lower serum creatinine values and may, therefore, overestimate renal function when used in the original equations (eg, Cockcroft-Gault, Jelliffe, original MDRD). Updated four-variable MDRD and six-variable MDRD equations based on serum creatinine measured by the IDMS-traceable method has been proposed for adults (Levey, 2006); the Cockcroft-Gault and Jelliffe equations have not been re-expressed and may overestimate renal function when used with a serum creatinine measured by the IDMS-traceable method. Clinicians should be aware of the serum creatinine assay used by their institution and the ramifications the assay may have on the equations used for renal function estimation.

Regardless of the serum creatinine assay used, the following factors may contribute to an inaccurate estimation of renal function (Stevens, 2006):

- Increased creatinine generation (may underestimate renal function):
  - Black or African American patients
  - Muscular body habitus
  - Ingestion of cooked meats
- Decreased creatinine generation (may overestimate renal function):
  - Increased age
  - Female patients
  - Hispanic patients
  - Asian patients
  - Amputees
  - Malnutrition, inflammation, or deconditioning (eg, cancer, severe cardiovascular disease, hospitalized patients)
  - Neuromuscular disease
  - Vegetarian diet
- Rapidly changing serum creatinine (either up or down): In patients with rapidly rising serum creatinines (ie, increasing by >0.5-0.7 mg/dL/day), it is best to assume that the patient's renal function is severely impaired

Use extreme caution when estimating renal function in the following patient populations:

- Low body weight (actual body weight < ideal body weight)
- Liver transplant
- Elderly (>90 years of age)
- Dehydration
- Recent kidney transplantation (serum creatinine values may decrease rapidly and can lead to renal function underestimation; conversely, delayed graft function may be present)

Note: In most situations, the use of the patient's ideal body weight (IBW) is recommended for estimating renal function, except when the patient's actual body weight (ABW) is less than ideal. Use of actual body weight (ABW) in obese patients (and possibly patients with ascites) may significantly overestimate renal function. Some clinicians prefer to use an adjusted body weight in such cases [eg, IBW + 0.4 (ABW - IBW)]; the adjustment factor may vary based on practitioner and/or institutional preference.

Alkaline picrate-based (Jaffe) methods

Note: These equations have not been updated for use with serum creatinine methods traceable to IDMS. Use with IDMS-traceable serum creatinine methods may overestimate renal function; use with caution.

Method 1: MDRD equation:

$eGFR = 186 \times (Creatinine)^{-1.154} \times (Age)^{-0.203} \times (Gender) \times (Race)$

where:

eGFR = estimated GFR; calculated in mL/minute/1.73 m^2

Creatinine is input in mg/dL

Age is input in years

Gender: Females: Gender = 0.742; Males: Gender = 1

Race: Black: Race = 1.212; White or other: Race = 1

Method 2: MDRD Extended equation:

$eGFR = 170 \times (Creatinine)^{-0.999} \times (Age)^{-0.176} \times (SUN)^{-0.170} \times (Albumin)^{0.318} \times (Gender) \times (Race)$

where:

eGFR = estimated GFR; calculated in mL/minute/1.73 m^2

Creatinine is input in mg/dL

Age is input in years

SUN = Serum Urea Nitrogen; input in mg/dL

Albumin = Serum Albumin; input in g/dL

Gender: Females: Gender = 0.762; Males: Gender = 1

Race: Black: Race = 1.18; White or other: Race = 1

Method 3: Cockroft-Gault equation[1]

Males: $Cl_{Cr} = [(140 - Age) \times Weight] / (72 \times Creatinine)$

Females: $Cl_{Cr} = \{[(140 - Age) \times Weight] / (72 \times Creatinine)\} \times 0.85$

where:

Cl_{Cr} = creatinine clearance; calculated in mL/minute

Age is input in years

Weight is input in kg

Creatinine is input in mg/dL

Method 4: Jelliffe equation

Males: $Cl_{Cr} = \{98 - [0.8 \times (Age - 20)]\} / (Creatinine)$

Females: Cl_{Cr} = Use above equation, then multiply result by 0.9

where:

Cl_{Cr} = creatinine clearance; calculated in mL/minute/1.73m^2

Age is input in years

Creatinine is input in mg/dL

IDMS-traceable methods

Method 1: MDRD equation[2]:

$eGFR = 175 \times (Creatinine)^{-1.154} \times (Age)^{-0.203} \times (Gender) \times (Race)$

where:

eGFR = estimated GFR; calculated in mL/minute/1.73 m^2

Creatinine is input in mg/dL

Age is input in years

Gender: Females: Gender = 0.742; Males: Gender = 1

Race: Black: Race = 1.212; White or other: Race = 1

Method 2: MDRD Extended equation:

$$eGFR = 161.5 \times (Creatinine)^{-0.999} \times (Age)^{-0.176} \times (SUN)^{-0.170} \times (Albumin)^{0.318} \times (Gender) \times (Race)$$

where:

eGFR = estimated GFR; calculated in mL/minute/1.73 m^2

Creatinine is input in mg/dL

Age is input in years

SUN = Serum Urea Nitrogen; input in mg/dL

Albumin = Serum Albumin; input in g/dL

Gender: Females: Gender = 0.762; Males: Gender = 1

Race: Black: Race = 1.18; White or other: Race = 1

FOOTNOTES

[1]Equation typically used for adjusting medication doses

[2]Preferred equation for CKD staging National Kidney Disease Education Program

REFERENCES

Cockcroft DW and Gault MH, "Prediction of Creatinine Clearance From Serum Creatinine," *Nephron*, 1976, 16(1):31-41.

Dowling TC, Matzke GR, Murphy JE, et al, "Evaluation of Renal Drug Dosing: Prescribing Information and Clinical Pharmacist Approaches," *Pharmacotherapy*, 2010, 30(8):776-86.

Hermsen ED, Maiefski M, Florescu MC, et al, "Comparison of the Modification of Diet in Renal Disease and Cockcroft-Gault Equations for Dosing Antimicrobials," *Pharmacotherapy*, 2009, 29 (6):649-55.

Jelliffe RW, "Letter: Creatinine Clearance: Bedside Estimate," *Ann Intern Med*, 1973, 79(4):604-5.

Levey AS, Bosch JP, Lewis JB, et al, "A More Accurate Method to Estimate Glomerular Filtration Rate From Serum Creatinine. A New Prediction Equation. Modification of Diet in Renal Disease Study Group," *Ann Intern Med*, 1999, 16;130(6):461–70.

Levey AS, Coresh J, Greene T, et al, "Using Standardized Serum Creatinine Values in the Modification of Diet in Renal Disease Study Equation for Estimating Glomerular Filtration Rate," *Ann Intern Med*, 2006, 145(4):247-54.

National Kidney Disease Education Program, "GFR Calculators." Available at http://www.nkdep.nih.gov/professionals/gfr_calculators. Last accessed January 20, 2011.

Stevens LA, Coresh J, Greene T, et al, "Assessing Kidney Function - Measured and Estimated Glomerular Filtration Rate," *N Engl J Med*, 2006, 354(23):2473-83.

RENAL FUNCTION ESTIMATION IN PEDIATRIC PATIENTS

Evaluation of a patient's renal function often includes the use of equations to estimate glomerular filtration rate (GFR) (eg, estimated GFR [eGFR] creatinine clearance [Cl_{Cr}]) using an endogenous filtration marker (eg, serum creatinine) and other patient variables. For example, the Schwartz equation estimates renal function by calculating eGFR and is typically used to steer medication dosing or categorize chronic kidney disease (CKD) staging. The rate of creatinine clearance does not always accurately represent GFR; creatinine may be cleared by other renal mechanisms in addition to glomerular filtration and serum creatinine concentrations may be affected by non-renal factors (eg, age, gender, race, body habitus, illness, diet). In addition, these equations were developed based on studies in limited populations and may either over- or underestimate the renal function of a specific patient.

Nevertheless, most clinicians use an eGFR or Cl_{Cr} as an indicator of renal function in pediatric patients for the purposes of adjusting medication doses. These equations should be used in the clinical context of patient-specific factors noted during the physical exam/work-up. **Decisions regarding drug therapy and doses must be made on clinical judgment.**

RENAL FUNCTION ESTIMATION EQUATIONS

Commonly used equations include the Schwartz and Traub-Johnson equations. Both equations were originally developed using a serum creatinine assay measured by the alkaline picrate-based (Jaffe) method. Many substances, including proteins, can interfere with the accuracy of this assay and overestimate serum creatinine concentration. The National Kidney Foundation and The National Kidney Disease Education Program advocate for a universal creatinine assay, in order to ensure an accurate estimate of GFR in patients. As a result, a more specific enzymatic assay with an isotope dilution mass spectrometry (IDMS)-traceable international standard has been developed. Compared to the older methods, IDMS-traceable assays may report lower serum creatinine values and may, therefore, overestimate renal function when used in the original equations. An updated Schwartz equation (eg, Bedside Schwartz) based on serum creatinine measured by the IDMS-traceable method has been proposed for pediatrics (Schwartz, 2009); the Traub-Johnson equation has not been re-expressed. The original Schwartz and Traub-Johnson equations may overestimate renal function when used with a serum creatinine measured by the IDMS-traceable method. Clinicians should be aware of the serum creatinine assay used by their institution and the ramifications the assay may have on the equations used for renal function estimation.

Regardless of the serum creatinine assay used, the following factors may contribute to an inaccurate estimation of renal function (Stevens, 2006):

- Increased creatinine generation (may underestimate renal function):
  - Black or African American patients
  - Muscular body habitus
  - Ingestion of cooked meats

- Decreased creatinine generation (may overestimate renal function):
  - Increased age
  - Female patients
  - Asian patients
  - Amputees
  - Malnutrition, inflammation, or deconditioning (eg, cancer, severe cardiovascular disease, hospitalized patients)
  - Neuromuscular disease
  - Vegetarian diet
- Rapidly changing serum creatinine (either up or down):
  - In patients with rapidly rising serum creatinines (ie, increasing by >0.5-0.7 mg/dL/day), it is best to assume that the patient's renal function is severely impaired

Use extreme caution when estimating renal function in the following patient populations:

- Low body weight (actual body weight < ideal body weight)
- Liver transplant
- Prematurity (especially very low birth weight)
- Dehydration
- Recent kidney transplantation (serum creatinine values may decrease rapidly and can lead to renal function underestimation; conversely, delayed graft function may be present)

Alkaline picrate-based (Jaffe) methods

Note: These equations have not been updated for use with serum creatinine methods traceable to IDMS. Use with IDMS-traceable serum creatinine methods may overestimate renal function; use with caution.

Method 1: Schwartz equation

Note: This equation may not provide an accurate estimation of creatinine clearance for infants <6 months of age or for patients with severe starvation or muscle wasting.

eGFR = (k X Height) / Creatinine

where:

eGFR = estimated GFR; calculated in mL/minute/1.73 m^2

Height (length) is input in cm

k = constant of proportionality that is age-specific

<1 year preterm: 0.33

<1 year full-term: 0.45

1-12 years: 0.55

>12 years female: 0.55

>12 years male: 0.7

Creatinine is input in mg/dL

Method 2: Traub-Johnson equation

Note: This equation is for use in ages 1-18 years.
Cl_{Cr} = (0.48 X Height) / Creatinine
where:
Cl_{Cr} = estimated creatinine clearance; calculated in mL/minute/1.73 m^2
Height (length) is input in cm
Creatinine = Sr_{Cr} input in mg/dL

IDMS-traceable method: Bedside Schwartz[1]

Note: This equation is for use in ages 1-16 years.
eGFR = (0.413 X Height) / Creatinine
where:
eGFR = estimated GFR; calculated in mL/minute/1.73 m^2
Height (length) is input in cm
Creatinine = Sr_{Cr} input in mg/dL

FOOTNOTES

[1]National Kidney Disease Education Program preferred equation

REFERENCES

Dowling TC, Matzke GR, Murphy JE, et al, "Evaluation of Renal Drug Dosing: Prescribing Information and Clinical Pharmacist Approaches," *Pharmacotherapy*, 2010, 30(8):776-86.

Myers GL, Miller WG, Coresh J, et al, "Recommendations for Improving Serum Creatinine Measurement: A Report From the Laboratory Working Group of the National Kidney Disease Education Program," *Clin Chem*, 2006, 52(1):5-18.

National Kidney Disease Education Program, "GFR Calculators." Available at http://www.nkdep.nih.gov/professionals/gfr_calculators. Last accessed January 20, 2011.

Pottel H, Mottaghy FM, Zaman Z, et al, "On the Relationship Between Glomerular Filtration Rate and Serum Creatinine in Children," *Pediatr Nephrol*, 2010, 25(5):927-34.

Schwartz GJ, Brion LP, and Spitzer A, "The Use of Plasma Creatinine Concentration for Estimating Glomerular Filtration Rate in Infants, Children, and Adolescents," *Pediatr Clin North Am*, 1987, 34 (3):571-90.

Schwartz GJ, Haycock GB, Edelmann CM Jr, et al, "A Simple Estimate of Glomerular Filtration Rate in Children Derived From Body Length and Plasma Creatinine," *Pediatrics*, 1976, 58 (2):259-63.

Schwartz GJ, Muñoz A, Schneider MF, et al, "New Equations to Estimate GFR in Children With CKD," *J Am Soc Nephrol*, 2009, 20(3):629-37.

Staples A, LeBlond R, Watkins S, et al, "Validation of the Revised Schwartz Estimating Equation in a Predominantly Non-CKD Population," *Pediatr Nephrol*, 2010, 25(11):2321-6.

Stevens LA, Coresh J, Greene T, et al, "Assessing Kidney Function - Measured and Estimated Glomerular Filtration Rate," *N Engl J Med*, 2006, 354(23):2473-83.

Traub SL and Johnson CE, "Comparison of Methods of Estimating Creatinine Clearance in Children," *Am J Hosp Pharm*, 1980, 37(2):195-201.

RENAL FUNCTION TESTS

Endogenous Creatinine Clearance vs Age (timed collection)

Creatinine clearance (mL/min/1.73 m^2) = (Cr_uV/Cr_sT) (1.73/A)

where:

Cr_u = urine creatinine concentration (mg/dL)
V = total urine collected during sampling period (mL)
Cr_s = serum creatinine concentration (mg/dL)
T = duration of sampling period (min) (24 h = 1440 min)
A = body surface area (m^2)

Age-specific normal values

5-7 d	50.6 ± 5.8 mL/min/1.73 m^2
1-2 mo	64.6 ± 5.8 mL/min/1.73 m^2
5-8 mo	87.7 ± 11.9 mL/min/1.73 m^2
9-12 mo	86.9 ± 8.4 mL/min/1.73 m^2
≥18 mo	
male	124 ± 26 mL/min/1.73 m^2
female	109 ± 13.5 mL/min/1.73 m^2
Adults	
male	105 ± 14 mL/min/1.73 m^2
female	95 ± 18 mL/min/1.73 m^2

Note: In patients with renal failure (creatinine clearance <25 mL/min), creatinine clearance may be elevated over GFR because of tubular secretion of creatinine.

Calculation of Creatinine Clearance From a 24-Hour Urine Collection

Equation 1:

$$Cl_{cr} = \frac{U \times V}{P}$$

where:

Cl_{cr} = creatinine clearance
U = urine concentration of creatinine
V = total urine volume in the collection
P = plasma creatinine concentration

Equation 2:

$$Cl_{cr} = \frac{\text{(total urine volume [mL]) x (urine Cr concentration [mg/dL])}}{\text{(serum creatinine [mg/dL]) x (time of urine collection [minutes])}}$$

Occasionally, a patient will have a 12- or 24-hour urine collection done for direct calculation of creatinine clearance. Although a urine collection for 24 hours is best, it is difficult to do since many urine collections occur for a much shorter period. A 24-hour urine collection is the desired duration of urine collection because the urine excretion of creatinine is diurnal and thus the measured creatinine clearance will vary throughout the day as the creatinine in the urine varies. When the urine collection is less than 24 hours, the total excreted creatinine will be affected by the time of the day during which the collection is performed. A 24-hour urine collection is sufficient to be able to accurately average the diurnal creatinine excretion variations. If a patient has 24 hours of urine collected for creatinine clearance, equation 1 can be used for calculating the creatinine clearance. To use equation 1 to calculate the creatinine clearance, it will be necessary to know the duration of urine collection, the urine collection volume, the urine creatinine concentration, and the serum creatinine value that reflects the urine collection period. In most cases, a serum creatinine concentration is drawn anytime during the day, but it is best to have the value drawn halfway through the collection period.

Amylase:Creatinine Clearance Ratio

$$\frac{\text{Amylase}_u \times \text{creatinine}_p}{\text{Amylase}_p \times \text{creatinine}_u} \times 100$$

u = urine; p = plasma

Serum BUN:Serum Creatinine Ratio

Serum BUN (mg/dL:serum creatinine (mg/dL))

Normal BUN:creatinine ratio is 10-15

BUN:creatinine ratio >20 suggests prerenal azotemia (also seen with high urea-generation states such as GI bleeding)

BUN:creatinine ratio <5 may be seen with disorders affecting urea biosynthesis such as urea cycle enzyme deficiencies and with hepatitis.

Fractional Sodium Excretion

Fractional sodium secretion (FENa) = $Na_uCr_s/Na_sCr_u \times 100\%$

where:

Na_u = urine sodium (mEq/L)
Na_s = serum sodium (mEq/L)
Cr_u = urine creatinine (mg/dL)
Cr_s = serum creatinine (mg/dL)

FENa <1% suggests prerenal failure
FENa >2% suggest intrinsic renal failure (for newborns, normal FENa is approximately 2.5%)

Note: Disease states associated with a falsely elevated FENa include severe volume depletion (>10%), early acute tubular necrosis, and volume depletion in chronic renal disease. Disorders associated with a lowered FENa include acute glomerulonephritis, hemoglobinuric or myoglobinuric renal failure, nonoliguric acute tubular necrosis, and acute urinary tract obstruction. In addition, FENa may be <1% in patients with acute renal failure **and** a second condition predisposing to sodium retention (eg, burns, congestive heart failure, nephrotic syndrome).

Urine Calcium:Urine Creatinine Ratio (spot sample)

Urine calcium (mg/dL): urine creatinine (mg/dL)

Normal values <0.21 (mean values 0.08 males, 0.06 females)

Premature infants show wide variability of calcium:creatinine ratio, and tend to have lower thresholds for calcium loss than older children. Prematures without nephrolithiasis had mean Ca:Cr ratio of 0.75 ± 0.76. Infants with nephrolithiasis had mean Ca:Cr ratio of 1.32 ± 1.03 (Jacinto JS, Modanlou HD, Crade M, et al, "Renal Calcification Incidence in Very Low Birth Weight Infants," *Pediatrics*, 1988, 81:31.)

Urine Protein:Urine Creatinine Ratio (spot sample)

P_u / Cr_u	Total Protein Excretion (mg/m²/d)
0.1	80
1	800
10	8000

where:

P_u = urine protein concentration (mg/dL)
Cr_u = urine creatinine concentration (mg/dL)

IMMUNE GLOBULIN PRODUCT COMPARISON

Brand Name	Concentration	pH	Initial Rate		Max Rate		IgA Content (mcg/mL)	Osmolarity/ Osmolality (mOsmol/ kg)	Comments
			I.V.	SubQ	I.V.[1]	SubQ			
Carimune® NF[2]	3%	6.4-6.8	1 mL/kg/h	–	6 mL/kg/h	–	Trace[3]	192-498[4]	Contains sucrose
	12%		0.24 mL/kg/h		1.5 mL/kg/h			768-1074[4]	
Flebogamma® DIF	5%	5-6	0.6 mL/kg/h	–	6 mL/kg/h	–	<50	240-370	
	10%		0.6 mL/kg/h		4.8 mL/kg/h		<100		
GamaSTAN™ S/D		6.4-7.2	–	–	–	–	Not available	Not available	For I.M. use
Gammagard S/D®	5%	6.4-7.2	0.5 mL/kg/h	–	4 mL/kg/h	–	≤2.2[5]	636	Contains polysorbate 80
	10%		0.5 mL/kg/h		8 mL/kg/h		≤4.4[5]	1250	
Gammagard® Liquid	10%	4.6-5.1	0.5 mL/kg/h	<40 kg: 15 mL/h/ site with a maximum of 8 sites ≥40 kg: 20 mL/h/ site with a maximum of 8 sites	5 mL/kg/h	<40 kg: 20 mL/h/ site with a maximum of 8 sites; maximum **total** rate: 160 mL/h ≥40 kg: 30 mL/h/ site with a maximum of 8 sites; maximum **total** rate: 240 mL/h	37	240-300	
Gammaked™	10%	4-4.5	0.6 mL/kg/h 1.2 mL/kg/h (CIDP only)	20 mL/h/site with a maximum of 8 sites	4.8 mL/kg/h	Not determined	46	258	
Gammaplex®	5%	4.8-5	0.6 mL/kg/h	–	4.8 mL/kg/h	–	<10	420-500	Contains polysorbate 80
Gamunex® C	10%	4-4.5	0.6 mL/kg/h 1.2 mL/kg/h (CIDP only)	20 mL/h/site with a maximum of 8 sites	4.8 mL/kg/h	Not determined	46	258	

continued

Brand Name	Concen-tration	pH	Initial Rate		Max Rate		IgA Content (mcg/mL)	Osmolarity/ Osmolality (mOsmol/ kg)	Comments
			I.V.	SubQ	I.V.[1]	SubQ			
Hizentra®	20%	4.6-5.2	–	–	–	Initial infusion: 15 mL/h/site with a maximum of 4 sites; maximum **total** rate: 50 mL/h Subsequent infusions: 25 mL/h/ site with a maximum of 4 sites; maximum **total** rate: 50 mL/h	≤50	380	Contains L-proline and polysorbate 80
Octagam®	5%	5.1-6	0.6 mL/kg/h	–	4.2 mL/kg/h	–	≤200	310-380	Contains maltose
Privigen®	10%	4.6-5	0.3 mL/kg/h	–	2.4 mL/kg/h (ITP only) 4.8 mL/kg/h	–	≤25	240-440	Contains L-proline

[1]Lower infusion rates should be used in patients at risk for renal dysfunction or thrombotic complications; see specific product information for details.

[2]Other concentrations may be prepared; see product information for additional details.

[3]Per product information; other sources list IgA content as 1000-2000 mcg/mL for 6% solution (Siegel J, "Immune Globulins: Therapeutic, Pharmaceutical, Cost, and Administration Considerations," *Pharm Prac News*, 2011).

[4]Osmolarity depends on concentration and diluent used; see product information for details.

[5]Data presented is the maximum concentration; additional Gammagard S/D® formulations with a lower IgA content are available; see specific product information for details.

ORAL ANTICOAGULANT COMPARISON CHART

Medication	Mechanism of Action	Metabolism	Monitoring Parameters	Pharmacotherapy Pearls	Reversal Strategies[1]	Preoperative/ Preprocedure Management (General Guide)
Warfarin	Inhibits formation of vitamin K-dependent clotting factors II, VII, IX, X, and proteins C and S	• CYP2C9 • CYP1A2 • CYP3A4 • CYP2C19	• PT/INR (individualized; depends on INR stability)	• CYP1A2, 3A4, 2C9, and 2C19 drug interactions and vitamin K-containing food interactions • Full therapeutic effect usually seen within 5-7 days • Average half-life is 40 hours	• Vitamin K (route and dose will depend on clinical situation and INR) • For major bleeding (at any INR): Consider prothrombin complex concentrate (PCC) with vitamin K ± FFP	• Hold at least 5 days before surgery; depending on urgency of surgery/ procedure, may administer low-dose I.V. or oral vitamin K
Dabigatran (Pradaxa®)	Directly inhibits thrombin	• Hepatic glucuronidation • P-glycoprotein (P-gp) substrate	• Routine lab monitoring not required; aPTT, ECT (if available)[2], TT (most sensitive) may be used to detect presence of dabigatran • Renal function	• Compliance issues (BID dosing) • Specific conversions to/ from warfarin, I.V. anticoagulants • Dose reduction or avoidance required if used with dronedarone, ketoconazole, P-gp inhibitors • P-gp drug interactions • Renal adjustment required • Use with caution in patients ≥80 years of age	• No specific antidote; for major bleeding, may consider activated PCC (eg, Feiba NF), FFP, recombinant factor VIIa[3], or concentrates of factors II, IX, or X[4] • Use of 4-factor PCC is **not** effective • Dabigatran is ~60% dialyzable	• Cl_{Cr} ≥50 mL/minute: Hold 1-2 days before surgery • Cl_{Cr} <50 mL/minute: Hold 3-5 days before surgery • May consider holding for >5 days in patients undergoing major surgery, spinal puncture, or insertion of a spinal or epidural catheter or port

continued

Medication	Mechanism of Action	Metabolism	Monitoring Parameters	Pharmacotherapy Pearls	Reversal Strategies[1]	Preoperative/ Preprocedure Management (General Guide)
Rivaroxaban (Xarelto®)	Directly inhibits factor Xa	• CYP3A4 • CYP3A5 • CYP2J2	• Routine lab monitoring not required; may use PT to detect presence of rivaroxaban • Renal and hepatic function	• Administer doses ≥15 mg/day with food • Renal and hepatic adjustments required • Dosing frequency depends on indication • CYP3A4 drug interactions	• No specific antidote; for major bleeding, may consider PCC, activated PCC (Feiba NF), or recominant factor VIIa[4]	• Hold at least 24 hours before surgery; longer duration of treatment cessation may be necessary based on individual patient situation and physician clinical judgment
Apixaban (Eliquis®; currently not available in U.S.)	Directly inhibits factor Xa	• CYP3A4 • P-gp substrate	• Routine lab monitoring not required; PT, INR, and aPTT may be used to detect presence of apixaban	• Compliance issues (BID dosing) • Not recommended in patients with Cl_{cr} <15 mL/ minute, ESRD, or severe liver impairment • Contraindicated in patients with hepatic disease associated with coagulopathy • CYP3A4 and P-gp drug interactions	• No specific antidote; for major bleeding, may consider FFP or recombinant factor VIIa for life-threatening bleeding[4]	• No information provided; half-life is ~12 hours; allow at least 24 hours after last dose before removing epidural catheters

[1]Management of anticoagulant-associated bleeding requires careful consideration of the indication for anticoagulant therapy and bleeding extent (eg, epistaxis vs intracranial hemorrhage); minor bleeding may only require local hemostasis.

[2]Ecarin clotting time

[3]The use of rFVIIa in healthy subjects treated with another direct thrombin inhibitor, melagatran (not FDA-approved), did not reverse the anticoagulant effects of melagatran.

[4]The evidence in support of these reversal strategies is limited; an exception to this may be the use of 4-factor PCC for rivaroxaban reversal; however, only 3-factor PCCs are available in the U.S. (Bebulin® VH and Profilnine® SD).

Levi M, Eerenberg E, and Kamphuisen PW, "Bleeding Risk and Reversal Strategies for Old and New Anticoagulants and Antiplatelet Agents," *J Thromb Haemost* 2011, 9(9):1705-12.

Wolzt M, Levi M, Sarich TC, et al, "Effect of Recombinant Factor VIIa on Melagatran-Induced Inhibition of Thrombin Generation and Platelet Activation in Healthy Volunteers," *Thromb Haemost* 2004, 91(6):1090-6.

ORAL ANTIPLATELET COMPARISON CHART

Medication	Mechanism of Action	Reversible Platelet Inhibition	Prodrug	Metabolism	Pharmacotherapy Pearls	Reversal Strategies[1]	Preoperative/ Preprocedure Management (General Guide)
Aspirin	Inhibits cyclooxygenase-1 and 2	No	No	• CYP2C9	• Chronic NSAID use can compromise antiplatelet effects • Monitor for GI ulceration	• No specific antidote • Consider platelet transfusion ± DDAVP • Normal platelet function returns within 7-10 days after discontinuation	• Hold 7-10 days before surgery • May be continued through surgery for CABG or noncardiac surgery in patients with high cardiac risk
Cilostazol (Pletal®)	Inhibits platelet phosphodiesterase III	Yes	No	• CYP3A4 • CYP2C19 • CYP1A2 • CYP2D6	• Administer before or 2 hours after meals • Contraindicated in patients with heart failure of any severity • CYP3A4 and 2C19 drug interactions	• No specific antidote • Normal platelet function returns within 4 days after discontinuation	• Hold 2-3 days before surgery
Clopidogrel (Plavix®)	Inhibits $P2Y_{12}$ component of ADP receptors	No	Yes	• CYP2C19 • CYP3A4	• CYP2C19 inhibitors may reduce concentrations of active metabolite • CYP2C19 polymorphisms may affect clopidogrel efficacy	• No specific antidote • Consider platelet transfusion ± DDAVP • Normal platelet function returns within 7-10 days after discontinuation	• Hold 5-10 days before surgery[2]
Ticlopidine	Inhibits $P2Y_{12}$ component of ADP receptors	No	Yes	• CYP3A4	• Black Box warning on hematologic toxicities (aplastic anemia, TTP) • Frequent CBC monitoring required •BID dosing	• No specific antidote • Consider platelet transfusion ± DDAVP • Normal platelet function returns within 5-10 days after discontinuation	• Hold 10-14 days before surgery

continued

Medication	Mechanism of Action	Reversible Platelet Inhibition	Prodrug	Metabolism	Pharmacotherapy Pearls	Reversal Strategies[1]	Preoperative/ Preprocedure Management (General Guide)
Prasugrel (Effient®)	Inhibits $P2Y_{12}$ component of ADP receptors	No	Yes	• CYP3A4 • CYP2B6	• Reduce maintenance dose to 5 mg in patients <60 kg • Contraindicated in patients with history of stroke, TIA • Not recommended in patients ≥75 years of age	• No specific antidote • Consider platelet transfusion ± DDAVP • Normal platelet function returns within 5-9 days after discontinuation	• Hold 5-7 days before surgery[2]
Ticagrelor (Brilinta®)	Inhibits $P2Y_{12}$ component of ADP receptors	Yes	No	• CYP3A4 • CYP3A5	• Used in combination with aspirin; daily maintenance aspirin dose should not exceed 81 mg • CYP3A4 drug interactions • BID dosing • Monitor closely for dyspnea, bradyarrhythmia (including ventricular pauses)	• No specific antidote • Consider aminocaproic acid, tranexamic acid, recombinant factor VIIa • Normal platelet function returns within 3-5 days after discontinuation	• Hold at least 5 days before surgery[2]

[1]Management of antiplatelet-associated bleeding requires careful consideration of the indication for antiplatelet therapy and bleeding extent (eg, epistaxis vs intracranial hemorrhage); minor bleeding may only require local hemostasis.

[2]When urgent CABG is necessary, the ACCF/AHA CABG guidelines recommend discontinuation for at least 24 hours prior to surgery (Hillis, 2011).

Hillis LD, Smith PK, Anderson JL, et al, "2011 ACCF/AHA Guideline for Coronary Artery Bypass Graft Surgery: Executive Summary: A Report of the American College of Cardiology Foundation/American Heart Association Task Force on Practice Guidelines," *Circulation*, 2011, 124(23):2610-42.

Levi M, Eerenberg E, and Kamphuisen PW, "Bleeding Risk and Reversal Strategies for Old and New Anticoagulants and Antiplatelet Agents," *J Thromb Haemost*, 2011, 9(9):1705-12.

Patrono C, Andreotti F, Arnesen H, et al, "Antiplatelet Agents for the Treatment and Prevention of Atherothrombosis," *Eur Heart J*, 2011, 32(23):2922-32.

REFERENCE VALUES FOR ADULTS

CHEMISTRY

Test	Values	Remarks
Serum/Plasma		
Acetone	Negative	
Albumin	3.2-5 g/dL	
Alcohol, ethyl	Negative	
Aldolase	1.2-7.6 IU/L	
Ammonia	20-70 mcg/dL	Specimen to be placed on ice as soon as collected.
Amylase	30-110 units/L	
Bilirubin, direct	0-0.3 mg/dL	
Bilirubin, total	0.1-1.2 mg/dL	
Calcium	8.6-10.3 mg/dL	
Calcium, ionized	2.24-2.46 mEq/L	
Chloride	95-108 mEq/L	
Cholesterol, total	≤200 mg/dL	Fasted blood required – normal value affected by dietary habits. This reference range is for a general adult population.
HDL cholesterol	40-60 mg/dL	Fasted blood required – normal value affected by dietary habits.
LDL cholesterol	<160 mg/dL	If triglyceride is >400 mg/dL, LDL cannot be calculated accurately (Friedewald equation). Target LDL-C depends on patient's risk factors.
CO_2	23-30 mEq/L	
Creatine kinase (CK) isoenzymes		
CK-BB	0%	
CK-MB (cardiac)	0% to 3.9%	
CK-MM (muscle)	96% to 100%	
CK-MB levels must be both ≥4% and 10 IU/L to meet diagnostic criteria for CK-MB positive result consistent with myocardial injury.		
Creatine phosphokinase (CPK)	8-150 IU/L	
Creatinine	0.5-1.4 mg/dL	
Ferritin	13-300 ng/mL	
Folate	3.6-20 ng/dL	

CHEMISTRY *(continued)*

Test	Values	Remarks
GGT (gamma-glutamyltranspeptidase)		
male	11-63 IU/L	
female	8-35 IU/L	
GLDH	To be determined	
Glucose (preprandial)	<115 mg/dL	Goals different for diabetics.
Glucose, fasting	60-110 mg/dL	Goals different for diabetics.
Glucose, nonfasting (2-h postprandial)	<120 mg/dL	Goals different for diabetics.
Hemoglobin A_{1c}	<8	
Hemoglobin, plasma free	<2.5 mg/100 mL	
Hemoglobin, total glycosolated (Hb A_1)	4% to 8%	
Iron	65-150 mcg/dL	
Iron binding capacity, total (TIBC)	250-420 mcg/dL	
Lactic acid	0.7-2.1 mEq/L	Specimen to be kept on ice and sent to lab as soon as possible.
Lactate dehydrogenase (LDH)	50-194 IU/L	
Lactate dehydrogenase (LDH) isoenzymes		
LD_1	20% to 34%	
LD_2	29% to 41%	
LD_3	15% to 25%	
LD_4	1% to 12%	
LD_5	1% to 15%	
Flipped LD_1/LD_2 ratios (>1 may be consistent with myocardial injury) particularly when considered in combination with a recent CK-MB positive result.		
Lipase	23-208 units/L	
Magnesium	1.6-2.5 mg/dL	Increased by slight hemolysis.
Osmolality	289-308 mOsm/kg	
Phosphatase, alkaline		
adults 25-60 y	33-131 IU/L	
adults ≥61 y	51-153 IU/L	
infancy-adolescence	Values range up to 3-5 times higher than adults	
Phosphate, inorganic	2.8-4.2 mg/dL	
Potassium	3.5-5.2 mEq/L	Increased by slight hemolysis.
Prealbumin	>15 mg/dL	
Protein, total	6.5-7.9 g/dL	
AST	<35 IU/L (20-48)	

CHEMISTRY *(continued)*

Test	Values	Remarks
ALT (10-35)	<35 IU/L	
Sodium	134-149 mEq/L	
Thyroid stimulating hormone (TSH)		
adults ≤20 y	0.7-6.4 mIU/L	
21-54 y	0.4-4.2 mIU/L	
55-87 y	0.5-8.9 mIU/L	
Transferrin	>200 mg/dL	
Triglycerides	45-155 mg/dL	Fasted blood required.
Troponin I	<1.5 ng/mL	
Urea nitrogen (BUN)	7-20 mg/dL	
Uric acid		
male	2-8 mg/dL	
female	2-7.5 mg/dL	
Cerebrospinal Fluid		
Glucose	50-70 mg/dL	
Protein	15-45 mg/dL	CSF obtained by lumbar puncture.

Note: Bloody specimen gives erroneously high value due to contamination with blood proteins

Urine
(24-hour specimen is required for all these tests unless specified)

Test	Values	Remarks
Amylase	32-641 units/L	The value is in units/L and **not** calculated for total volume.
Amylase, fluid (random samples)		Interpretation of value left for physician, depends on the nature of fluid.
Calcium	Depends upon dietary intake	
Creatine		
male	150 mg/24 h	Higher value on children and during pregnancy.
female	250 mg/24 h	
Creatinine	1000-2000 mg/24 h	
Creatinine clearance (endogenous)		
male	85-125 mL/min	A blood sample must accompany urine specimen.
female	75-115 mL/min	
Glucose	1 g/24 h	
5-hydroxyindoleacetic acid	2-8 mg/24 h	
Iron	0.15 mg/24 h	Acid washed container required.
Magnesium	146-209 mg/24 h	
Osmolality	500-800 mOsm/kg	With normal fluid intake.
Oxalate	10-40 mg/24 h	

CHEMISTRY *(continued)*

Test	Values	Remarks
Phosphate	400-1300 mg/24 h	
Potassium	25-120 mEq/24 h	Varies with diet; the interpretation of urine electrolytes and osmolality should be left for the physician.
Sodium	40-220 mEq/24 h	
Porphobilinogen, qualitative	Negative	
Porphyrins, qualitative	Negative	
Proteins	0.05-0.1 g/24 h	
Salicylate	Negative	
Urea clearance	60-95 mL/min	A blood sample must accompany specimen.
Urea N	10-40 g/24 h	Dependent on protein intake.
Uric acid	250-750 mg/24 h	Dependent on diet and therapy.
Urobilinogen	0.5-3.5 mg/24 h	For qualitative determination on random urine, send sample to urinalysis section in Hematology Lab.
Xylose absorption test		
children	16% to 33% of ingested xylose	
Feces		
Fat, 3-day collection	<5 g/d	Value depends on fat intake of 100 g/d for 3 days preceding and during collection.
Gastric Acidity		
Acidity, total, 12 h	10-60 mEq/L	Titrated at pH 7

Blood Gases

	Arterial	Capillary	Venous
pH	7.35-7.45	7.35-7.45	7.32-7.42
pCO_2 (mm Hg)	35-45	35-45	38-52
pO_2 (mm Hg)	70-100	60-80	24-48
HCO_3 (mEq/L)	19-25	19-25	19-25
TCO_2 (mEq/L)	19-29	19-29	23-33
O_2 saturation (%)	90-95	90-95	40-70
Base excess (mEq/L)	-5 to +5	-5 to +5	-5 to +5

HEMATOLOGY

Complete Blood Count

Age	Hgb (g/dL)	Hct (%)	RBC (mill/mm^3)	RDW
0-3 d	15.0-20.0	45-61	4.0-5.9	<18
1-2 wk	12.5-18.5	39-57	3.6-5.5	<17
1-6 mo	10.0-13.0	29-42	3.1-4.3	<16.5
7 mo to 2 y	10.5-13.0	33-38	3.7-4.9	<16
2-5 y	11.5-13.0	34-39	3.9-5.0	<15
5-8 y	11.5-14.5	35-42	4.0-4.9	<15
13-18 y	12.0-15.2	36-47	4.5-5.1	<14.5
Adult male	13.5-16.5	41-50	4.5-5.5	<14.5
Adult female	12.0-15.0	36-44	4.0-4.9	<14.5

Age	MCV (fL)	MCH (pg)	MCHC (%)	Plts (x 10^3/mm^3)
0-3 d	95-115	31-37	29-37	250-450
1-2 wk	86-110	28-36	28-38	250-450
1-6 mo	74-96	25-35	30-36	300-700
7 mo to 2 y	70-84	23-30	31-37	250-600
2-5 y	75-87	24-30	31-37	250-550
5-8 y	77-95	25-33	31-37	250-550
13-18 y	78-96	25-35	31-37	150-450
Adult male	80-100	26-34	31-37	150-450
Adult female	80-100	26-34	31-37	150-450

WBC and Differential

Age	WBC (x 10^3/mm^3)	Segs	Bands	Lymphs	Monos
0-3 d	9.0-35.0	32-62	<18	19-29	5-7
1-2 wk	5.0-20.0	14-34	<14	36-45	6-10
1-6 mo	6.0-17.5	13-33	<12	41-71	4-7
7 mo to 2 y	6.0-17.0	15-35	<11	45-76	3-6
2-5 y	5.5-15.5	23-45	<11	35-65	3-6
5-8 y	5.0-14.5	32-54	<11	28-48	3-6
13-18 y	4.5-13.0	34-64	<11	25-45	3-6
Adults	4.5-11.0	35-66	<11	24-44	3-6

Age	Eosinophils	Basophils	Atypical Lymphs	No. of NRBCs
0-3 d	0-2	0-1	0-8	0-2
1-2 wk	0-2	0-1	0-8	0
1-6 mo	0-3	0-1	0-8	0
7 mo to 2 y	0-3	0-1	0-8	0
2-5 y	0-3	0-1	0-8	0
5-8 y	0-3	0-1	0-8	0
13-18 y	0-3	0-1	0-8	0
Adults	0-3	0-1	0-8	0

Segs = segmented neutrophils.
Bands = band neutrophils.
Lymphs = lymphocytes.
Monos = monocytes.

Erythrocyte Sedimentation Rates and Reticulocyte Counts

Sedimentation rate, Westergren	Children	0-20 mm/h
	Adult male	0-15 mm/h
	Adult female	0-20 mm/h
Sedimentation rate, Wintrobe	Children	0-13 mm/h
	Adult male	0-10 mm/h
	Adult female	0-15 mm/h
Reticulocyte count	Newborns	2% to 6%
	1-6 mo	0% to 2.8%
	Adults	0.5% to 1.5%

PHARMACOLOGIC CATEGORY INDEX

Abortifacient
Mifepristone ... 983

Acne Products
ISOtretinoin ... 832

Adjuvant, Chemoprotective Agent (Cytoprotective)
Amifostine ... 65

Amebicide
MetroNIDAZOLE (Systemic) ... 978

Analgesic, Nonopioid
Ziconotide ... 1481

Analgesic, Opioid
Codeine ... 311
FentaNYL ... 583
HYDROmorphone ... 724
Levorphanol ... 892
Meperidine ... 932
Methadone ... 944
Morphine (Liposomal) ... 1011
Morphine (Systemic) ... 1004
OxyCODONE ... 1084
Oxymorphone ... 1088
TraMADol ... 1388

Androgen
Fluoxymesterone ... 634

Angiogenesis Inhibitor
Lenalidomide ... 859
Thalidomide ... 1346

Anilidopiperidine Opioid
FentaNYL ... 583

Antiandrogen
Abiraterone Acetate ... 26
Cyproterone ... 344
Enzalutamide ... 506
Nilutamide ... 1037

Antibiotic, Aminoglycoside
Amikacin ... 69
Gentamicin (Systemic) ... 677
Tobramycin (Systemic, Oral Inhalation) ... 1366

Antibiotic, Carbapenem
Imipenem and Cilastatin ... 773

Antibiotic, Cephalosporin (Third Generation)
CefTAZidime ... 254
CefTRIAXone ... 258

Antibiotic, Cephalosporin (Fourth Generation)
Cefepime ... 251

Antibiotic, Miscellaneous
Aztreonam ... 145
MetroNIDAZOLE (Systemic) ... 978
Sulfamethoxazole and Trimethoprim ... 1302

Antibiotic, Oxazolidinone
Linezolid ... 898

Antibiotic, Penicillin
Nafcillin ... 1026
Piperacillin and Tazobactam ... 1175
Ticarcillin and Clavulanate Potassium ... 1363

Antibiotic, Quinolone
Ciprofloxacin (Systemic) ... 283
Levofloxacin (Systemic) ... 883
Ofloxacin (Systemic) ... 1053

Antibiotic, Sulfonamide Derivative
Sulfamethoxazole and Trimethoprim ... 1302

Anticholinergic Agent
Scopolamine (Systemic) ... 1274

Anticoagulant
Antithrombin ... 107
Heparin ... 697

Antidiarrheal
Octreotide ... 1043

Antidote
Amifostine ... 65
Calcitonin ... 214
Deferoxamine ... 414
Dexrazoxane ... 448
Glucarpidase ... 680
Leucovorin Calcium ... 870
LEVOleucovorin ... 888
Mesna ... 940
Methylene Blue ... 962
Octreotide ... 1043
Pamidronate ... 1109
Sodium Thiosulfate ... 1289
Uridine Triacetate ... 1419
Zoledronic Acid ... 1488

Antiemetic
Aprepitant ... 118

Dexamethasone
(Systemic) 440
Dolasetron 462
Dronabinol 484
Droperidol 486
Fosaprepitant 643
Granisetron 687
HydrOXYzine 736
Metoclopramide 974
Nabilone 1023
Ondansetron 1068
Palonosetron 1106
Prochlorperazine 1212
Promethazine 1218
Trimethobenzamide 1411

Antifibrinolytic Agent
Aminocaproic Acid 72
Tranexamic Acid 1392

Antifungal Agent
Pentamidine 1156

Antifungal Agent, Oral
Fluconazole 612
Flucytosine 618
Itraconazole 838
Ketoconazole (Systemic) 840
Posaconazole 1187
Voriconazole 1473

Antifungal Agent, Oral Nonabsorbed
Clotrimazole (Oral) 311
Nystatin (Oral) 1041

Antifungal Agent, Parenteral
Amphotericin B Cholesteryl Sulfate
Complex 78
Amphotericin B
(Conventional) 79
Amphotericin B (Lipid
Complex) 84
Amphotericin B (Liposomal) 87
Anidulafungin 99
Caspofungin 210
Fluconazole 612
Micafungin 981
Voriconazole 1473

Antifungal Agent, Topical
Nystatin (Topical) 1042

Antifungal Agent, Vaginal
Nystatin (Topical) 1042

Antigout Agent
Allopurinol 51

Antihemophilic Agent
Aminocaproic Acid 72
Antihemophilic Factor
(Human) 101
Antihemophilic Factor
(Recombinant) 103
Desmopressin 434
Factor IX 571
Factor IX Complex
(Human) 575
Factor VIIa (Recombinant) 568
Tranexamic Acid 1392

Anti-inflammatory Agent
Dexamethasone
(Systemic) 440

Antimanic Agent
ChlorproMAZINE 274
OLANZapine 1056

Antineoplastic Agent
Amsacrine 90
Bendamustine 158
Bortezomib 187
Carfilzomib 239
Carmustine 243
Lenalidomide 859
Lomustine 904
Ziv Aflibercept
(Systemic) 1484

Antineoplastic Agent, Alkylating Agent
Bendamustine 158
Busulfan 203
CARBOplatin 229
Carmustine 243
Chlorambucil 270
CISplatin 290
Cyclophosphamide 321
Estramustine 535
Ifosfamide 752
Lomustine 904
Melphalan 925
Oxaliplatin 1077
Procarbazine 1208
Streptozocin 1298
Thiotepa 1357

Antineoplastic Agent, Alkylating Agent (Nitrogen Mustard)
Bendamustine 158
Ifosfamide 752
Mechlorethamine 913

Antineoplastic Agent, Alkylating Agent (Nitrosourea)
Carmustine 243
Lomustine 904

Antineoplastic Agent, Alkylating Agent (Triazene)
Dacarbazine 367
Temozolomide 1331

Antineoplastic Agent, Anaplastic Lymphoma Kinase Inhibitor
Crizotinib 317

Antineoplastic Agent, Anthracenedione
MitoXANtrone 996

Antineoplastic Agent, Anthracycline
DAUNOrubicin (Conventional) 396
DAUNOrubicin (Liposomal) 400
DOXOrubicin 467
DOXOrubicin (Liposomal) 473
Epirubicin 510
IDArubicin 749
Valrubicin 1425

Antineoplastic Agent, Antiandrogen
Abiraterone Acetate 26
Bicalutamide 178
Enzalutamide 506
Flutamide 635
Nilutamide 1037

Antineoplastic Agent, Antibiotic
Bleomycin 181
DACTINomycin 371
IDArubicin 749
MitoMYcin (Systemic) 990
Pentostatin 1161

Antineoplastic Agent, Anti-HER2
Lapatinib 854
Pertuzumab 1165
Trastuzumab 1399

Antineoplastic Agent, Antimetabolite
Capecitabine 223
Cladribine 298
Cytarabine (Conventional) 348
Hydroxyurea 731
Mercaptopurine 934
Nelarabine 1028
PEMEtrexed 1151
Raltitrexed 1226

Antineoplastic Agent, Antimetabolite (Antifolate)
Methotrexate 949
PEMEtrexed 1151
PRALAtrexate 1190

Antineoplastic Agent, Antimetabolite (Purine Analog)
Cladribine 298
Clofarabine 306
Fludarabine 619
Mercaptopurine 934
Nelarabine 1028
Pentostatin 1161
Thioguanine 1354

Antineoplastic Agent, Antimetabolite (Pyrimidine Analog)
Capecitabine 223
Cytarabine (Conventional) 348
Floxuridine 610
Fluorouracil (Systemic) 627
Fluorouracil (Topical) 632
Gemcitabine 663

Antineoplastic Agent, Antimetabolite (Pyrimidine Antagonist)
Cytarabine (Liposomal) 361
UFT 1418

Antineoplastic Agent, Antimicrotubular
Cabazitaxel 210
DOCEtaxel 453
Eribulin 524
Ixabepilone 842
PACLitaxel 1092
PACLitaxel (Protein Bound) 1098

Antineoplastic Agent, Aromatase Inactivator
Exemestane 564

Antineoplastic Agent, Aromatase Inhibitor
Anastrozole 96
Letrozole 867

Antineoplastic Agent, BRAF Kinase Inhibitor
Vemurafenib 1440

Antineoplastic Agent, Camptothecin
Irinotecan 813
Topotecan 1371

Antineoplastic Agent, Cephalotaxine
Omacetaxine 1064

Antineoplastic Agent, DNA Methylation Inhibitor
AzaCITIDine 140
Decitabine 403

Antineoplastic Agent, Epothilone B Analog
Ixabepilone 842

Antineoplastic Agent, Estrogen Receptor Antagonist
Fulvestrant 651
Tamoxifen 1324
Toremifene 1376

Antineoplastic Agent, Gonadotropin-Releasing Hormone Agonist
Goserelin 683
Leuprolide 876

Antineoplastic Agent, Gonadotropin-Releasing Hormone Antagonist
Degarelix 422

Antineoplastic Agent, Hedgehog Pathway Inhibitor
Vismodegib 1470

Antineoplastic Agent, Histone Deacetylase Inhibitor
RomiDEPsin 1254
Vorinostat 1478

Antineoplastic Agent, Hormone
Estramustine 535
Megestrol 922

Antineoplastic Agent, Hormone Antagonist
Mifepristone 983

Antineoplastic Agent, Hormone (Estrogen/Nitrogen Mustard)
Estramustine 535

Antineoplastic Agent, Janus Associated Kinase Inhibitor
Ruxolitinib 1261

Antineoplastic Agent, Miscellaneous
Aldesleukin 37
Alitretinoin 50
Altretamine 63
Arsenic Trioxide 122
Asparaginase (E. coli) 130
Asparaginase (Erwinia) 126
Bexarotene (Systemic) 173
Bexarotene (Topical) 176
Denileukin Diftitox 425
ISOtretinoin 832
Mitotane 994
Pegaspargase 1135
Porfimer 1183
Trabectedin 1384
Tretinoin (Systemic) 1405

Antineoplastic Agent, Monoclonal Antibody
Alemtuzumab 43
Bevacizumab 165
Brentuximab Vedotin 199
Cetuximab 264
Gemtuzumab Ozogamicin 673
Ibritumomab 744
Ipilimumab 809
Ofatumumab 1050
Panitumumab 1115
Pertuzumab 1165
RiTUXimab 1244
Tositumomab and Iodine I 131 Tositumomab 1379
Trastuzumab 1399

Antineoplastic Agent, mTOR Kinase Inhibitor
Everolimus 552
Temsirolimus 1337

Antineoplastic Agent, Natural Source (Plant) Derivative
DOCEtaxel 450
Irinotecan 813
PACLitaxel 1092
PACLitaxel (Protein Bound) 1098
Topotecan 1371
VinBLAStine 1445
VinCRIStine 1450
VinCRIStine (Liposomal) 1459
Vinorelbine 1465

Antineoplastic Agent, Platinum Analog
CARBOplatin 229
CISplatin 290
Oxaliplatin 1077

Antineoplastic Agent, Podophyllotoxin Derivative
Etoposide 538
Etoposide Phosphate 548
Teniposide 1342

Antineoplastic Agent, Protein Synthesis Inhibitor
Omacetaxine 1064

Antineoplastic Agent, Taxane Derivative
Cabazitaxel 210
DOCEtaxel 453
PACLitaxel 1092
PACLitaxel (Protein Bound) 1098

Antineoplastic Agent, Topoisomerase I Inhibitor
Irinotecan 813
Topotecan 1371

Antineoplastic Agent, Topoisomerase II Inhibitor
Etoposide 538
Etoposide Phosphate 548

Antineoplastic Agent, Tyrosine Kinase Inhibitor
Axitinib 135
Bosutinib 195
Crizotinib 317
Dasatinib 390
Erlotinib 528
Gefitinib 659
Imatinib 762
Lapatinib 854
Nilotinib 1031
Pazopanib 1129
Regorafenib 1233
Ruxolitinib 1261
SORAfenib 1292
SUNItinib 1308
Vandetanib 1435

Antineoplastic Agent, Vinca Alkaloid
VinBLAStine 1445
VinCRIStine 1450
VinCRIStine (Liposomal) 1459
Vindesine 1464
Vinorelbine 1465

Antiplatelet Agent
Defibrotide 420

Antiprogestin
Mifepristone 983

Antiprotozoal
Pentamidine 1156

Antiprotozoal, Nitroimidazole
MetroNIDAZOLE (Systemic) 978

Antipsychotic Agent, Atypical
OLANZapine 1056

Antipsychotic Agent, Typical
Droperidol 486
Haloperidol 691

Antipsychotic Agent, Typical, Phenothiazine
ChlorproMAZINE 274
Prochlorperazine 1212

Antirheumatic, Disease Modifying
InFLIXimab 789
Methotrexate 949

Antirheumatic Miscellaneous
Cyclophosphamide 321
RiTUXimab 1244

Antitussive
Codeine 311

Antiviral Agent
Acyclovir (Systemic) 30
Famciclovir 580
Foscarnet 646
Ganciclovir (Systemic) 656
Valacyclovir 1420
Valganciclovir 1423

Antiviral Agent, Oral
Valacyclovir 1420

Antiviral Agent, Topical
Acyclovir (Topical) 35

Appetite Stimulant
Dronabinol 484
Megestrol 922

Benzodiazepine
LORazepam 907

Biological Response Modulator
Aldesleukin 37
BCG 153
Oprelvekin 1074

Bisphosphonate Derivative
Clodronate 303
Ibandronate 739
Pamidronate 1109
Zoledronic Acid 1488

Blood Product Derivative
Antihemophilic Factor (Human) 101
Antithrombin 107
Cytomegalovirus Immune Globulin (Intravenous-Human) 365
Factor IX 571
Factor IX Complex (Human) 575
Fibrinogen Concentrate (Human) 602
Immune Globulin 777
$Rh_o(D)$ Immune Globulin 1237

Bone-Modifying Agent
Denosumab 428

Calcimimetic
Cinacalcet 280

Calcineurin Inhibitor
CycloSPORINE (Systemic) 333
Tacrolimus (Systemic) 1315

Calcium Channel Blocker, N-Type
Ziconotide 1481

Calcium-Lowering Agent
Gallium Nitrate 654

Cardioprotectant
Dexrazoxane 448

Cellular Immunotherapy, Autologous
Sipuleucel-T 1279

Chelating Agent
Deferasirox 407
Deferiprone 412
Deferoxamine 414

Chemotherapy Modulating Agent
Leucovorin Calcium 870
LEVOleucovorin 888

Cholinergic Agonist
Pilocarpine (Systemic) 1173

Colony Stimulating Factor
Darbepoetin Alfa 382
Eltrombopag 494
Epoetin Alfa 516
Filgrastim 604
Pegfilgrastim 1138
RomiPLOStim 1257
Sargramostim 1270

Contraceptive
MedroxyPROGESTERone 916

Contrast Agent
Hexaminolevulinate 705
Isosulfan Blue 831

Corticosteroid, Ophthalmic
PrednisoLONE (Ophthalmic) 1198

Corticosteroid, Rectal
Hydrocortisone (Topical) 719

Corticosteroid, Systemic
Dexamethasone (Systemic) 440
Hydrocortisone (Systemic) 713
MethylPREDNISolone 967
PrednisoLONE (Systemic) 1193
PredniSONE 1199

Corticosteroid, Topical
Hydrocortisone (Topical) 719

Cortisol Receptor Blocker
Mifepristone 983

Diagnostic Agent
Thyrotropin Alfa 1360

Echinocandin
Anidulafungin 99
Caspofungin 249
Micafungin 981

Enzyme
Asparaginase (E. coli) 130
Asparaginase (Erwinia) 126
Glucarpidase 680
Hyaluronidase 711
Pegaspargase 1135
Rasburicase 1229

Enzyme, Urate-Oxidase (Recombinant)
Rasburicase 1229

Epidermal Growth Factor Receptor (EGFR) Inhibitor
Cetuximab 264
Erlotinib 528
Lapatinib 854
Panitumumab 1115
Vandetanib 1435

Erythropoiesis-Stimulating Agent (ESA)
Darbepoetin Alfa 382
Epoetin Alfa 516

Factor Xa Inhibitor
Fondaparinux 638

Gastrointestinal Agent, Miscellaneous
InFLIXimab 789
Methylnaltrexone 964
Mucosal Barrier Gel, Oral 1014
Saliva Substitute 1266

Gastrointestinal Agent, Prokinetic
Metoclopramide 974

General Anesthetic
FentaNYL 583

Glycopeptide
Vancomycin 1428

Gonadotropin Releasing Hormone Agonist
Goserelin 683
Histrelin 707
Leuprolide 876
Triptorelin 1413

Gonadotropin Releasing Hormone Antagonist
Degarelix 422

Growth Factor
Darbepoetin Alfa 382
Epoetin Alfa 516

Hematopoietic Stem Cell Mobilizer
Plerixafor 1180

Hemostatic Agent
Aminocaproic Acid 72
Desmopressin 434
Tranexamic Acid 1392

Histamine H_1 Antagonist
Cyproheptadine 342
HydrOXYzine 736
Promethazine 1218

Histamine H_1 Antagonist, First Generation
Cyproheptadine 342
HydrOXYzine 736
Promethazine 1218

Hormone
Calcitonin 214

Human Growth Factor
Oprelvekin 1074

Immune Globulin
Antithymocyte Globulin (Equine) 111
Antithymocyte Globulin (Rabbit) 115
Cytomegalovirus Immune Globulin (Intravenous-Human) 365
Immune Globulin 777
Rh_o(D) Immune Globulin 1237

Immunomodulator, Systemic
Lenalidomide 859
Thalidomide 1346

Immunosuppressant Agent
Antithymocyte Globulin (Equine) 111
Antithymocyte Globulin (Rabbit) 115
Basiliximab 149
Cyclophosphamide 321
CycloSPORINE (Systemic) 333
Everolimus 552
InFLIXimab 789
Mercaptopurine 934
Methotrexate 949
Mycophenolate 1015
RiTUXimab 1244
Sirolimus 1282
Tacrolimus (Systemic) 1315

Interferon
Interferon Alfa-2b 798
Peginterferon Alfa-2b 1140

Iron Salt
Ferric Gluconate 597
Ferumoxytol 600

Iron Dextran Complex 824
Iron Sucrose 827

Janus Associated Kinase Inhibitor
Ruxolitinib 1261

Keratinocyte Growth Factor
Palifermin 1104

Local Anesthetic
Lidocaine and Prilocaine 894

Local Anesthetic, Oral
Benzydamine 164

Low Molecular Weight Heparin
Dalteparin 376
Enoxaparin 499

Lysine Analog
Aminocaproic Acid 72
Tranexamic Acid 1392

Monoclonal Antibody
Alemtuzumab 43
Basiliximab 149
Denosumab 428
Eculizumab 490
InFLIXimab 789
Ipilimumab 809
Ofatumumab 1050
RiTUXimab 1244
Trastuzumab 1399

Monoclonal Antibody, Complement Inhibitor
Eculizumab 490

mTOR Kinase Inhibitor
Everolimus 552
Sirolimus 1282

Opioid Antagonist, Peripherally-Acting
Methylnaltrexone 964

Phenothiazine Derivative
Promethazine 1218

Phosphodiesterase-3 Enzyme Inhibitor
Anagrelide 93

Phospholipase A_2 Inhibitor
Anagrelide 93

Photosensitizing Agent, Topical
Aminolevulinic Acid 75

Piperazine Derivative
HydrOXYzine 736

Piperidine Derivative
Cyproheptadine 342

Polyclonal Antibody
Antithymocyte Globulin
(Equine) 111
Antithymocyte Globulin
(Rabbit) 115

Progestin
MedroxyPROGESTERone 916
Megestrol 922

Proteasome Inhibitor
Bortezomib 187
Carfilzomib 239

Prothrombin Complex Concentrate (PCC)
Factor IX Complex
(Human) 575

Radiopharmaceutical
Chromic Phosphate P 32 279
Gallium Citrate Ga-67 653
Ibritumomab 744
Indium In-111 Pentetreotide 788
Iobenguane I 123 800
Samarium Sm 153
Lexidronam 1268
Strontium-89 1300
Tositumomab and Iodine I 131
Tositumomab 1379

Recombinant Human Erythropoietin
Darbepoetin Alfa 382
Epoetin Alfa 516

Rescue Agent (Chemotherapy)
Leucovorin Calcium 870
LEVOleucovorin 888

Respiratory Fluoroquinolone
Levofloxacin (Systemic) 883

Retinoic Acid Derivative
Alitretinoin 50
ISOtretinoin 832
Tretinoin (Systemic) 1405

Sclerosing Agent
Talc (Sterile) 1323

Selective 5-HT$_3$ Receptor Antagonist
- Dolasetron 462
- Granisetron 687
- Ondansetron 1068
- Palonosetron 1106

Selective Estrogen Receptor Modulator (SERM)
- Raloxifene 1222
- Tamoxifen 1324
- Toremifene 1376

Somatostatin Analog
- Lanreotide 851
- Octreotide 1043

Substance P/Neurokinin 1 Receptor Antagonist
- Aprepitant 118
- Fosaprepitant 643

Thrombolytic Agent
- Alteplase 55
- Defibrotide 420

Thrombopoietic Agent
- Eltrombopag 494
- RomiPLOStim 1257

Topical Skin Product
- Aminolevulinic Acid 75
- Fluorouracil (Topical) 632
- Ingenol Mebutate 796

Tumor Necrosis Factor (TNF) Blocking Agent
- InFLIXimab 789
- Thalidomide 1346

Uroprotectant
- Mesna 940

Vaccine, Inactivated (Viral)
- Papillomavirus (Types 6, 11, 16, 18) Vaccine (Human, Recombinant) 1120
- Papillomavirus (Types 16, 18) Vaccine (Human, Recombinant) 1124

Vaccine, Live (Bacterial)
- BCG 153

Vascular Endothelial Growth Factor (VEGF) Inhibitor
- Axitinib 135
- Bevacizumab 165
- Pazopanib 1129
- Regorafenib 1233
- SORAfenib 1292
- SUNItinib 1308
- Vandetanib 1435
- Ziv-Aflibercept (Systemic) 1484

Vasopressin Analog, Synthetic
- Desmopressin 434

Vitamin D Analog
- Calcitriol 215

Vitamin, Fat Soluble
- Phytonadione 1169

Vitamin, Water Soluble
- Leucovorin Calcium 870

Xanthine Oxidase Inhibitor
- Allopurinol 51

Notes

Notes

Notes

Notes

Notes

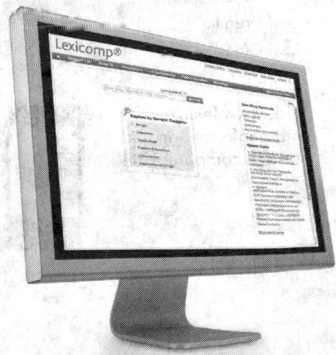

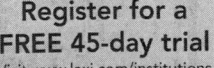